Stockley's Drug Interactions

Stockley's Drug Interactions

A source book of interactions, their mechanisms, clinical importance and management

Sixth Edition

Editor-in-Chief

Ivan H Stockley

BPharm, PhD (Nott), FRPharmS (Lond),
CBiol, MIBiol

University of Nottingham Medical School
Nottingham, UK

Sixth edition 2002

© 1981, 1983, 1991, 1994, 1999, 2002 Pharmaceutical Press

Printed in Great Britain by TJ International, Padstow, Cornwall

ISBN 0 85369 504 0

All rights reserved. No part of this publication may be reproduced, stored in a retrieval system, or transmitted in any form or by any means, without the prior written permission of the copyright holder.

The publisher makes no representation, express or implied, with regard to the accuracy of the information contained in this book and cannot accept any legal responsibility or liability for any errors or omissions that may be made.

A catalogue record for this book is available from the British Library.

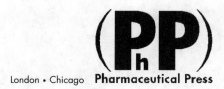

London • Chicago Pharmaceutical Press

Published by the Pharmaceutical Press
Publications division of the Royal Pharmaceutical Society of Great Britain

1 Lambeth High Street, London SE1 7JN, UK
100 South Atkinson Road, Suite 206, Grayslake, IL 60030-7820, USA

First edition 1981
Fifth edition 1999
Reprinted 2000 (twice), 2001
Sixth edition 2002

© 1981, 1991, 1994, 1996, 1999, 2002 Pharmaceutical Press

Printed in Great Britain by The Bath Press, Bath

ISBN 0 85369 504 0

O LORD, you have searched me
and you know me.
You know when I sit and when I rise;
you perceive my thoughts from afar.
You discern my going out and my lying down;
you are familiar with all my ways.
Before a word is on my tongue
you know it completely, O LORD.

You hem me in-behind and before;
you have laid your hand upon me.
Such knowledge is too wonderful for me,
too lofty for me to attain.

Where can I go from you Spirit?
Where can I flee from you presence?
If I go up to the heavens, you are there;
if I make my bed in the depths, you are there.
If I rise on the wings of the dawn,
if I settle on the far side of the sea,
even there your hand will guide me,
your right hand will hold me fast.

If I say, "Surely the darkness will hide me
and the light become night around me,"
even the darkness will not be dark to you;
the night will shine like the day,
for darkness is as light to you.

For you created my inmost being;
you knit me together in my mother's womb.
I praise you because I am fearfully and wonderfully made;
your works are wonderful.
I know that full well.
My frame was not hidden from you
when I was made in the secret place.
When I was woven together in the depths of the earth,
your eyes saw my unformed body.
All the days ordained for me
were written in your book
before one of them came to be.

How precious to me are your thoughts, O God!
How vast is the sum of them!
Were I to count them,
they would outnumber the grains of sand.
When I awake,
I am still with you.

Search me, O God, and know my heart;
test me and know my anxious thoughts.
See if there is any offensive way in me,
and lead me in the way everlasting.

Psalm 139, 1–18, 23, 24. (NIV)

STOCKLEY STAFF

Contents

Contents

Preface

This sixth edition continues the pattern of previous editions. Inevitably it has grown to accommodate the flood of new information about old and new drugs, and of course herbal remedies. Most of the old monographs have been reviewed, updated and revalidated, and literally scores of new ones (about 10%) have been added since the last edition making a total well in excess of two-and-half thousand.

I believe that no other book in the world provides such a wide and detailed coverage of drug–drug, drug–drink, drug–herb and drug–food interactions, and with the creation of an electronic version of this book (*e-Stockley*) it is now possible to provide a regular updating service.

The aim in this, as in previous editions, is to inform busy doctors, pharmacists, surgeons, nurses and other busy healthcare professionals, of the facts about interactions, without their having to do the time-consuming literature searches for themselves. These therefore are the practical questions which this book attempts to answer:

- Are the drugs in question known to interact or is the interaction only theoretical and speculative?
- If they do interact, how serious is it?
- Has it been described many times or only once?
- Are all patients affected or only a few?
- Is it best to avoid these two drugs altogether or can the interaction be accommodated in some way?
- And what alternative and safer drugs can be used instead?

To précis the mass of literature into a concise and easy-to-read form, the text has been organised into a series of individual drug–drug monographs, all with a common format and assembled into 23 chapters. There is a brief outline of the most common mechanisms of interaction in Chapter 1 so that the details of the mechanisms do not have to be endlessly repeated in individual monographs. If you need some insight into the general philosophy underlying the way all this information is handled in this book, you should have a look at the section, 'Before using this book. . .'.

The major difference about this edition is that it is no longer single authored by me. The *Pharmaceutical Press*, which is the publishing arm of the *Royal Pharmaceutical Society of Great Britain* has taken over *Stockley's Drug Interactions*, and I am delighted to have been joined by a team of highly skilled and experienced writers from the larger editorial team which produces *Martindale*, with all the resources and expertise which that implies. I would like to acknowledge here all the work put in over the last 18 months by Sean Sweetman, the editor of *Martindale*, and by Karen Baxter the now executive editor of *Stockley*, in co-ordinating the conversion of this book from a single-authored publication into a collaborative effort. Thanks are also due to Prakash Gotecha, Marian Quinn, Claire Ryan, Emma Williamson and John Wilson who have handled various aspects of the production of this book, and I am particularly grateful to Charles Fry, the Director of Publications, who has had the total oversight of the whole project. It is so good that the future of *Stockley* is now assured and in such good hands.

Inevitably this book has a national, British, flavour because all authors have a nationality and have to live and publish somewhere in the world, nevertheless this is not just a UK or European book. It is international. It has been written to be used worldwide, across national, international and continental boundaries. To facilitate this a whole range of drug synonyms have been used in the text and in the index - International drug names (rINNs), US names (USANs) as well as British Approved names (BANs) – so that it can be used anywhere where English is understood.

I continue to be grateful to so many people who, in small and large ways, have helped me. Suzanne Armour has done the basic literature searches for me, and kept my filing system and database in such excellent order. Medicines information pharmacists and others in the UK and the US pharmaceutical industries have patiently let me pick their brains and supplied me with data on company files which is not available anywhere else. They, and others in hospital Medicines Information departments, have also made constructive suggestions and helpful criticisms, and drawn my attention to reports I might otherwise have missed. And, too infrequently, but always very welcome, are the helpful letters I have had from users of the book, telling me what they like or dislike about it, and their suggestions for improvements. To all of you, thank you very much. We have a dedicated e-mail address: *stockley@rpsgb.org.uk*

I collaborate each year with Boehringer Ingelheim International in the production of the *Drug Interaction Alert* ready-reference chart which complements this book. Once again I acknowledge here their very generous support over many years. The book is written as a stand-alone, but it also complements the electronic *Stockley Interaction Alert* module which is used by *NDC Health Information Services* in the UK and by other companies in Australia and Israel. Users of all of these systems will find that this book gives the details of the interactions which their own facilities can only provide in a more concise form.

Ivan Stockley
University of Nottingham Medical School
Nottingham
England

Abbreviations

ACE—angiotensin-converting enzyme
AIDS—acquired immunodeficiency syndrome
ALL—acute lymphoblastic leukaemia
ALT—alanine aminotransferase
am—*ante meridiem* (before noon)
AML—acute myeloid leukaemia
aPPT—activated partial thromboplastin time
AST—aspartate aminotransferase
AUC—area under the time–concentration curve
$AUC_{0-12 h}$—area under the time–concentration curve measured over 0 to 12 hours
AV—atrioventricular
BNF—British National Formulary
BP—blood pressure
BP—British Pharmacopoeia
BPC—British Pharmaceutical Codex
bpm—beats per minute
BUN—blood urea nitrogen
CDC—Centers for Disease Control (USA)
Cmax—maximum serum concentration
CNS—central nervous system
COPD—chronic obstructive pulmonary disease
CPR—cardiopulmonary resuscitation
CSF—cerebrospinal fluid
CSM—Committee on Safety of Medicines (UK)
ECG—electrocardiogram
ECT—electroconvulsive therapy
EEG—electroencephalogram
e.g.—*exempli gratia* (for example)
FDA—Food and Drug Administration (USA)
FEF_{25-75}—maximum expiratory flow over the middle 50% of the vital capacity
FEV_1—forced expiratory volume in one second
ft—foot (feet)
FVC—forced vital capacity
GGT—gamma glutamyl transpeptidase
g—gram(s)

h—hour(s)
HAART—highly active antiretroviral therapy
HCV—hepatitis C virus
HIV+—human immunodeficiency virus positive
HRT—hormone replacement therapy
i.e.—*id est* (that is)
im—intramuscular
INR—international normalised ratio
ITU—intensive therapy unit
IU—International Units
iv—intravenous
IUD—intra-uterine device
kg—kilogram(s)
l—litre
lbs—pound(s) avoirdupois
μg—microgram(s)
m—metre(s)
MAOI—monoamine oxidase inhibitor
MAOI-A—monoamine oxidase inhibitor, type A
MAOI-B—monoamine oxidase inhibitor, type B
MCA—Medicines Control Agency
MIC—minimum inhibitory concentration
mEq—milliequivalent(s)
meq—milliequivalent(s)
mg—milligram(s)
min—minute(s)
ml—millilitre(s)
mmHg—millimetre(s) of mercury
μmol—micromole
mmol—millimole
mol—mole
MRSA—methicillin-resistant *Staphylococcus aureus*
ms—millisecond(s)
msec—millisecond(s)
ng—nanogram(s)
nM—nanomole

nmol—nanomole

NNRTI—non-nucleoside reverse transcriptase inhibitor

NRTI—nucleoside reverse transcriptase inhibitor

NSAID—non-steroidal anti-inflammatory drug

OTC—over-the-counter (i.e. obtainable without a prescription)

PABA—para-amino benzoic acid

PCP—*Pneumocystis carinii* pneumonia

pH—the negative logarithm of the hydrogen ion concentration

pm—*post meridiem* (after noon)

pO_2—plasma partial pressure (concentration) of oxygen

PPI—proton pump inhibitor

PTT—partial thromboplastin time

PUD—peptic ulcer disease

s—second(s)

sbp—systolic blood pressure

SSRI—selective serotonin reuptake inhibitor

STD—sexually transmitted disease

UK—United Kingdom

US and USA—United States of America

USP—The United States Pharmacopeia

UTI—urinary tract infection

Vd—volume of distribution

Vmax—maximum velocity

Before using this book . . .

. . . you should read this short explanatory section so that you know how the drug interaction data have been set out here, and why – as well as the basic philosophy that has been followed in presenting it.

The monographs

The book has over 2500 monographs with a common format which are subdivided into sections like these:

- An abstract or summary for quick reading.

- **Clinical evidence**, detailing one, two or more illustrative examples of the interaction, followed by most or all of other supportive clinical evidence currently available.

- **Mechanism**, in brief.

- **Importance and management**, a short discussion designed to aid rapid clinical decision making. For example:
  - Is the interaction established or not?
  - What is its incidence?
  - How important is it?
  - How can it be managed?
  - And what, if any, are the non-interacting alternatives?

- **References**, a list of all of the relevant references. The length of the references list gives a very fair indication of the extent of the documentation. A long list indicates a well documented interaction, whereas a short list indicates poor documentation.

Some of the monographs have been compressed into fewer subsections instead of the more usual five, simply to save space where information is limited or where there is little need to be more expansive.

The monographs do not carry my drug interaction Hazard/ Severity ratings as used in the electronic *Stockley Interactions Alerts* because of the difficulties of applying them to monographs that cover multiple pairs of drug–drug interactions, but what is written in each monograph should speaks for itself.

Quality of information on interactions

The data on interactions are of widely varying quality and reliability. The best come from clinical studies carried out on large numbers of patients under scrupulously controlled conditions. The worst are anecdotal, uncontrolled, or based solely on *animal* studies. Sometimes they are no more than speculative and theoretical scaremongering guesswork, hallowed by repeated quotation until they become virtually set in stone.

My aim has been to filter out as much useless noise as possible, so wherever possible I have avoided 'secondary' references, using instead 'primary' references which are available in good medical and scientific libraries – although sometimes I have used unpublished, good quality, in-house reports on drug company files which I have been allowed to see. I have also increasingly used drug company datasheets or product information booklets (rather than the research reports which lie behind them) because often they are initially the only source of published information about new drugs.

The quality of drug company literature is very variable. Some of it is excellent, helpful and very reliable, but regrettably a growing proportion contains a welter of speculative and self-protective statements, probably driven more by the company's medico-legal policy than anything else, and the nervousness of drug regulatory authorities. It is almost unbelievable (but true all the same) that drug companies which are scrupulous in the way they do their research, come out with statements about possible interactions which are little more than guesswork. I have done my best to separate out this kind of chaff from the real wheat.

When drawing your own conclusions

The human population is a total mixture, unlike selected batches of laboratory animals (same age, weight, sex, and strain etc.). For this reason human beings do not respond uniformly to one or more drugs. Our genetic make up, ethnic background, sex, renal and hepatic functions, diseases and nutritional states, ages and other factors (the route of administration, for example) all contribute towards the heterogeneity of our responses. This means that the outcome of giving one or more drugs to any individual for the first time is never totally predictable because it is a new and unique 'experiment'. Even so, some idea of the probable outcome of using a drug or a pair of drugs can be based on what has been seen in other patients: the more extensive the data, the firmer the predictions.

The most difficult decisions concern isolated cases of interaction, many of which only achieved prominence because they were serious. Do you ignore them as 'idiosyncratic' or do you, from that moment onwards, contraindicate the use of the two drugs totally?

There is no simple 'yes' or 'no' answer to these questions, but one simple rule-of-thumb is that isolated cases of interaction with old and very well-tried pairs of drugs are unlikely to be of general importance, whereas those with new drugs may possibly be the tip of an emerging iceberg and should therefore initially be taken much more seriously until more is known. The delicate balance between these two has then to be set against the actual severity of the reaction reported and weighed up against how essential it is to use the drug combination in question.

When deciding the possible first-time use of any two drugs in any particular patient, you need to put what is currently known about these drugs against the particular profile of your patient. Read the monograph. Consider the facts and my conclusions, and then set the whole against the backdrop of your patients unique condition (age, disease, general condition, and so forth) so that what you eventually decide to do is well thought out and soundly based. We do not usually have the luxury of knowing absolutely all the facts, so that an initial conservative approach is often the safest.

1

General considerations and an outline survey of some basic interaction mechanisms

1. What is a drug interaction?

An interaction is said to occur when the effects of one drug are changed by the presence of another drug, food, drink or by some environmental chemical agent. Much more colourful and informal definitions by patients are that it is ". . . when medicines fight each other. . .", or ". . . when medicines fizz together in the stomach . . .", or (from my then 98-year-old aunt) ". . .what happens when one medicine falls out with another. . ."

The outcome can be harmful if the interaction causes an increase in the toxicity of the drug. For example, patients on warfarin may begin to bleed if they are given azapropazone or phenylbutazone without reducing the warfarin dosage. Patients taking monoamine oxidase inhibitor antidepressants (MAOIs) may experience an acute and potentially life-threatening hypertensive crisis if they eat tyramine-rich foods such as cheese.

A reduction in efficacy due to an interaction can sometimes be just as harmful as an increase: patients on warfarin given rifampicin need more warfarin to maintain adequate and protective anticoagulation, while patients taking tetracycline or quinolone antibacterials need to avoid antacids and milky foods (or separate their ingestion) because the effects of these antibacterials can be reduced or even abolished if admixture occurs in the gut.

These unwanted and unsought-for interactions are adverse and undesirable drug reactions, but there are other interactions which can be beneficial and valuable, such as the deliberate co-prescription of antihypertensive drugs and diuretics in order to achieve antihypertensive effects possibly not obtainable with either drug alone. The mechanisms of both types of interaction, whether adverse or beneficial, are often very similar, but the adverse interactions are the focus of this book.

I have not stuck rigidly in this book to these definitions of a drug interaction because the subject inevitably overlaps into other areas of adverse reactions with drugs. So you will find in these pages some 'interactions' where one drug does not actually affect another at all, but the adverse outcome is the simple additive effects of two drugs with similar effects (for example the combined effects of two or more CNS depressants, or two drugs which affect the QT interval). I have also included a few drug-disease interactions as well (e.g. beta-blockers in patients needing medication for asthma) because many, probably most, users of this book would expect to find 'interactions' of this kind described here.

Sometimes the term 'drug interaction' is used for the physico-chemical reactions that go on if drugs are mixed in intra-venous fluids, causing precipitation or inactivation. It is also often used for the interference that drugs may have on biochemical and other assays carried out on body fluids that can upset the results. I think that the long-established and less ambiguous term for the former is 'pharmaceutical incompatibilities', but there is no brief and widely accepted term for the drug-biochemical test interactions. For my part I would reserve the simple term 'drug interactions' just for those reactions which go on within, rather than outside, the body.

2. What is the incidence of drug interactions?

The more drugs a patient takes the greater the likelihood that an adverse reaction will occur. One hospital study found that the rate was 7% in those taking 6 to 10 drugs but 40% in those taking 16 to 20 drugs which represents a disproportionate increase.[1] A possible explanation is that the drugs were interacting.

Some of the early studies on the frequency of interactions uncritically compared the drugs which had been prescribed with lists of possible drug interactions, without appreciating that many interactions may be clinically trivial or simply theoretical. As a result an unrealistically high incidence was suggested. Most of the later studies have avoided this error by looking at only potentially clinically important interactions and incidences of 4.7%,[2] 6.3%[3] and 8.8%[4] have been found. Even so, not all of these studies took into account the distinction which must be made between the incidence of potential interactions and the incidence of those where clinical problems actually arise. The simple fact is that some patients experience quite serious reactions while taking interacting drugs, while others appear not to be affected at all.

A screening of 2422 patients over a total of 25,005 days revealed that 113 (4.7%) were taking combinations of drugs that could interact, but evidence of interactions was observed in only seven patients, representing only 0.3%.[2] In another hospital study of 44 patients over a 5-day period taking 10 to 17 drugs, 77 potential drug interactions were identified, but only one probable and four possible adverse reactions (6.4%) were detected.[5] A further study among patients taking anticonvulsant drugs found that 6% of the cases of toxicity were due to drug interactions.[6] These figures are low compared with those of a hospital survey which monitored 927 patients who had received 1004 potentially interacting drug combinations. Changes in drug dosage were made in 44% of these cases.[7] A review of these and other studies found that the reported incidence rates ranged from 70.3 to 2.2%, and the percentage of patients actually experiencing problems was less than 11.1%. Another review found a 37% incidence among 639 elderly patients.[8] Yet another review of 236 geriatric patients found an 88% incidence of clinically significant interactions, and a 22% incidence of potentially serious and life-threatening interactions.[9] A 4.1% incidence of drug interactions on prescriptions presented to community pharmacists in the USA was found in a further survey,[10] whereas the incidence was only 1.9% in a Swedish study.[11] Another USA study found a 2.9% incidence.[12] An Australian study found that about 10% of hospital admissions were drug-related, of which 4.4% were due to drug interactions.[13] A very high incidence (47 to 50%) of potential drug interactions was found in a study carried out in an Emergency Department in the US.[14] One French study found that 16% of the prescriptions for a group of patients taking antihypertensive drugs were contraindicated or unsuitable,[15] whereas another study on a group of geriatrics found only a 1% incidence.[16] The incidence of problems would be expected to be higher in the elderly because ageing affects the functioning of the kidneys and liver so that many drugs are lost from the body much more slowly.[17,18]

These discordant figures need to be put into the context of the under-reporting of adverse reactions of any kind by doctors, for reasons that include pressure of work, indifference, indolence or the fear of litigation. Both doctors and patients may not recognise adverse reactions and interactions, and many outpatients simply stop taking their drugs without saying why. None of these studies gives a clear answer to the question of how frequently drug interactions occur, but even if the incidence is as low as some of the studies suggest, it still represents a very considerable number of patients who appear to be at risk when one thinks of the large numbers of drugs prescribed and handled every day by doctors and pharmacists.

3. How seriously should interactions be regarded and handled?

It would be very easy to conclude after leafing through this book that it is extremely risky to treat patients with more than one drug at a time, but this would be an over-reaction. The figures quoted in the previous section illustrate that many drugs that are known in some patients to interact, simply fail to do so in others. This partially explains why some quite important drug interactions remained virtually unnoticed for many years, a good example of this being the effect which quinidine has on serum digoxin levels (see Fig. 1.1).

Examples of this kind suggest that patients apparently tolerate adverse interactions remarkably well and that many experienced physicians accommodate the effects (such as rises or falls in serum drug levels) without consciously recognising that what they are seeing is the result of an interaction.

One of the reasons it is often difficult to detect an interaction is that, as already mentioned, patient variability is very considerable. We now know many of the predisposing and protective factors which determine whether an interaction occurs or not, but in practice it is still very difficult to predict what will happen when an individual patient is given two potentially interacting drugs. An easy solution to this practical problem is to choose a non-interacting alternative, but if none is available, it is frequently possible to give interacting drugs to-

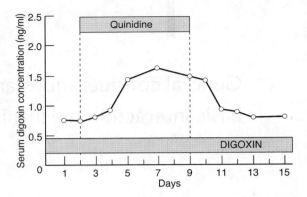

Fig. 1.1 A multiple-mechanism interaction. The effect of quinidine (1 mg daily) on the serum digoxin levels of five subjects taking constant doses of digoxin (after Doering W, N Engl J Med (1979) 301, 400, with permission). The mechanisms involved include changes in renal and non-renal (biliary) clearance, and possibly absorption and tissue binding.

gether if appropriate precautions are taken. If the effects are well monitored the effects of the interaction can often be allowed for simply by adjusting the dosages. Many interactions are dose-related so that if the dosage of the causative drug is reduced, the effects on the other drug will be reduced accordingly. For example, isoniazid causes the levels of phenytoin to rise, particularly in those individuals who are slow acetylators of isoniazid, and levels may climb into the toxic range. If the serum phenytoin levels are monitored and its dosage reduced appropriately, the concentrations can be kept within the therapeutic range. The dosage of the interacting drug may also be critical. Thus a small dosage of cimetidine may fail to inhibit the metabolism of warfarin, whereas a larger dose may have profound clinical effects.

Some interactions can be accommodated by using another member of the same group of drugs. For example, the serum levels of doxycycline can fall to subtherapeutic concentrations if phenytoin, barbiturates or carbamazepine are given, but other tetracyclines do not seem to be affected. Cimetidine causes serum warfarin levels to rise because it inhibits its metabolism, but not those of phenprocoumon because these two anticoagulants are metabolised in different ways. It is therefore clearly important not to extrapolate uncritically the interactions seen with one drug to all members of the same group.

It is interesting to note in this context that a study in two hospitals in Maryland, USA, found that when interacting drugs were given with warfarin (but not theophylline) the length of hospital stay increased by a little over 3 days, with a rise in general costs because of the need to do more tests to get the balance right.[19] So it may be easier, quicker and cheaper to use a non-interacting alternative drug (always provided that its price is not markedly greater).

The variability in patient response has lead to some extreme responses among prescribers. Some clinicians have become over-anxious about interactions so that their patients are denied useful drugs which they might reasonably be given if appropriate precautions are taken. This attitude is exacerbated by some of the more alarmist lists and charts of interactions, which fail to make a distinction between interactions that are very well documented and well established, and those that have only been encountered in a single patient and which in the final analysis are probably totally idiosyncratic. 'One swallow does not make a summer', nor does a serious reaction in a single patient mean that the drugs in question should never again be administered to anyone else. At the other extreme there are some clinicians who have personally encountered few interactions and who therefore virtually disregard their existence so that some of their patients are potentially put at risk. The responsible position lies between these two extremes because a very substantial number of interacting drugs can be given together safely if the appropriate precautions are taken, whereas there are relatively few pairs of drugs that should always be avoided.

4. Mechanisms of drug interaction

Some drugs interact together in totally unique ways, but as the many examples in this book amply illustrate, there are certain mechanisms of interaction which are encountered time and time again. Some of these common mechanisms are discussed here in greater detail than space will allow in the individual monographs so that only the briefest reference need be made there.

Mechanisms that are unusual or peculiar to particular pairs of drugs are detailed within the monographs. Very many drugs that interact do so, not by a single mechanism, but often by two or more mechanisms acting in concert, although for clarity most of the mechanisms are dealt with here as though they occur in isolation. For convenience the mechanisms of interactions can be subdivided into those which involve the pharmacokinetics of a drug and those which are pharmacodynamic.

4.1 Pharmacokinetic interactions

Pharmacokinetic interactions are those which can affect the processes by which drugs are absorbed, distributed, metabolised and excreted (the so-called ADME interactions).

4.1.1 Drug absorption interactions

Most drugs are given orally for absorption through the mucous membranes of the gastrointestinal tract, and most of the interactions that go on within the gut result in reduced rather than increased absorption. A clear distinction must be made between those that decrease the *rate* of absorption and those that alter the *total amount* absorbed. For drugs that are given chronically on a multiple dose regimen (e.g. the oral anticoagulants) the rate of absorption is usually unimportant, provided the total amount of drug absorbed is not markedly altered. On the other hand for drugs which are given as single doses intended to be absorbed rapidly (e.g. hypnotics or analgesics) where a rapidly achieved high concentration is needed, a reduction in the rate of absorption may result in failure to achieve an adequate effect. Table 1.1 lists some of the drug interactions that result from changes in absorption.

4.1.1.1 Effects of changes in gastrointestinal pH. The passage of drugs through mucous membranes by simple passive diffusion depends upon the extent to which they exist in the non-ionised lipid-soluble form. Absorption is therefore governed by the pKa of the drug, its lipid-solubility, the pH of the con-

Table 1.1 Some drug absorption interactions

Drug affected	Interacting drugs	Effect of interaction
Digoxin	Metoclopramide	Reduced digoxin absorption
	Propantheline	Increased digoxin absorption (due to changes in gut motility)
Digoxin Levothyroxine Warfarin	Colestyramine	Reduced absorption due to binding/ complexation with colestyramine
Ketoconazole	Antacids H_2-blockers	Reduced ketoconazole absorption due to reduced dissolution
Penicillamine	Antacids containing Al^{3+}, Mg^{2+}, iron preparations, food	Formation of less soluble penicillamine chelates resulting in reduced absorption of penicillamine
Penicillin	Neomycin	Neomycin-induced malabsorption state
Quinolone antibiotics	Antacids containing Al^{3+}, Mg^{2+}, milk, Zn^{2+}(?), Fe^{2+}	Formation of poorly absorbed complexes
Tetracyclines	Antacids containing Al^{3+}, Ca^{2+}, Mg^{2+}, Bi^{2+}, milk, Zn^{2+}, Fe^{2+}	Formation of poorly soluble chelates resulting in reduced antibiotic absorption (see Fig. 1.2)

tents of gut and various other parameters relating to the pharmaceutical formulation of the drug. Thus the absorption of salicylic acid by the stomach is much greater at low pH than at high. On theoretical grounds it might be expected therefore that alterations in gastric pH caused by drugs such as H_2-blockers would have a marked effect on absorption, but in practice the outcome is often uncertain because a number of other mechanisms may also come into play such as chelation, adsorption and changes in gut motility, which can considerably affect what actually happens. Rises in pH due to H_2-blockers and antacids that affect dissolution can however markedly reduce the absorption of ketoconazole, and also possibly enoxacin.

4.1.1.2 Adsorption, chelation and other complexing mechanisms. Activated charcoal is intended to act as an adsorbing agent within the gut for the treatment of drug overdosage or to remove other toxic materials, but inevitably it can affect the absorption of drugs given in therapeutic doses. Antacids can also adsorb a very considerable number of drugs, but often other mechanisms of interaction are also involved. For example the tetracycline antibacterials can chelate with a number of divalent and trivalent metallic ions such as calcium, aluminium, bismuth and iron to form complexes, which not only

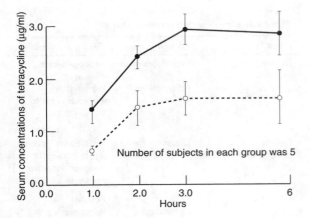

Fig. 1.2 A drug chelation interaction. Tetracycline forms a less-soluble chelate with iron if the two drugs are allowed to mix within the gut. This reduces the absorption and depresses the serum levels and the antibacterial effects (after Neuvonen PJ, *BMJ* (1970) 4, 532, with permission). The same interaction can occur with other ions such as Al^{3+}, Ca^{2+}, Mg^{2+}, Bi^{2+} and Zn^{2+}.

are poorly absorbed, but have reduced antibacterial effects (see Figure 1.2).

These metallic ions are found in dairy products and antacids. Separating the dosages by 2 to 3 h goes some way towards reducing the effects of this type of interaction. The marked reduction in the bioavailability of penicillamine by some antacids seems also to be due to chelation, although adsorption may have some part to play. Colestyramine, an anionic exchange resin intended to bind bile acids and cholesterol metabolites in the gut, binds to a considerable number of drugs if co-administered (e.g. digoxin, warfarin, levothyroxine) thereby reducing their absorption. Table 1.1 lists the drugs that chelate, complex or adsorb other drugs thereby reducing their absorption.

4.1.1.3 Changes in gastrointestinal motility. Since most drugs are largely absorbed in the upper part of the small intestine, drugs that alter the rate at which the stomach empties its contents can affect absorption. Propantheline, for example, delays gastric emptying and reduces paracetamol (acetaminophen) absorption whereas metoclopramide has the opposite effect, however the total amount of drug absorbed remains unaltered. These two drugs have quite the opposite effect on the absorption of hydrochlorothiazide. Anticholinergic drugs decrease the motility of the gut, thus the tricyclic antidepressants can increase the absorption of dicoumarol, probably because they increase the time available for dissolution and absorption, but in the case of levodopa they reduce the absorption, possibly because the exposure time to intestinal mucosal metabolism is increased. The same reduced levodopa absorption has also been seen with homatropine. On the other hand trihexyphenidyl (benzhexol) (another anticholinergic) reduces the absorption of chlorpromazine. Other examples of changes in motility that affect absorption include the reduced absorption caused by pethidine (meperidine) and diamorphine. These

examples illustrate that what actually happens is sometimes very unpredictable because the final outcome may be the result of several different mechanisms.

4.1.1.4 Malabsorption caused by drugs. Neomycin causes a malabsorption syndrome which is similar to that seen with non-tropical sprue. The effect is to impair the absorption of a number of drugs including digoxin and phenoxymethylpenicillin (penicillin V).

4.1.2 Drug displacement (protein-binding) interactions

Following absorption drugs are rapidly distributed around the body by the circulation. Some drugs are totally dissolved in the plasma water, but many others are transported with some proportion of their molecules in solution and the rest bound to plasma proteins, particularly the albumins. The extent of this binding varies enormously but some drugs are extremely highly bound. For example, dicoumarol has only four out of every 1000 molecules remaining unbound at serum concentrations of 0.5 mg%. Drugs can also become bound to albumin in the interstitial fluid, and some such as digoxin can bind to the heart muscle tissue.

The binding of drugs to the plasma proteins is reversible, an equilibrium being established between those molecules that are bound and those that are not. Only the unbound molecules remain free and pharmacologically active, while those that are bound form a circulating but pharmacologically inactive reservoir which, in the case of 'restrictive' drugs, is temporarily protected from metabolism and excretion. As the free molecules become metabolised, some of the bound molecules become unbound and pass into solution to exert their normal pharmacological actions, before they, in their turn are metabolised and excreted.

Depending on the concentrations and their relative affinities for the binding sites, one drug may successfully compete with another and displace it from the sites it is already occupying. The displaced (and now active) drug molecules pass into plasma water where their concentration rises. So for example, a drug which reduces the binding from (say) 99 to 95% would thereby increase the unbound concentration of free and active drug from 1 to 4% (a fourfold increase). This displacement is only likely to raise the number of free and active molecules significantly if the majority of the drug is within the plasma rather than the tissues, so that only drugs with a low apparent volume of distribution (V_d) will be affected. Such drugs include the sulphonylureas such as tolbutamide (96% bound, V_d 10 l), oral anticoagulants such as warfarin (99% bound, V_d 9 l) and phenytoin (90% bound, V_d 35 l). Other highly bound drugs include diazoxide, etacrynic acid, methotrexate, nalidixic acid, phenylbutazone and the sulphonamides.

Displacement of this kind happens when patients stabilised on warfarin are given chloral hydrate because its major metabolite, trichloroacetic acid, is a highly bound compound which successfully displaces warfarin, thereby increasing its anticoagulant effects. This effect is only very short-lived because the now free and active warfarin molecules become exposed to metabolism as the blood flows through the liver and the total amount of drug rapidly falls. A small but transient increase in the anticoagulant effects can be seen and the warfarin requirements fall briefly by about a third, but within about 5 days a new equilibrium becomes established with the same concentration of unbound warfarin, even though the free fraction has increased. Normally no change in the warfarin dosage is needed.[20]

In vitro many commonly used drugs are capable of being displaced by others, but in the body the effects seem almost always to be buffered so effectively that the outcome is normally clinically unimportant. It would therefore seem that the importance of this interaction mechanism has been grossly over-emphasised,[21] despite statements made to the contrary in numerous papers, reviews and drug data sheets.[22] It is difficult to find an example of a clinically important interaction due to this mechanism alone. One possible example is the marked diuresis that was seen in patients with nephrotic syndrome when they were given clofibrate.[23] Usually this mechanism has a minor part to play compared with other mechanisms that are going on at the same time. However it may need to be taken into account in some circumstances.

Suppose, for example, an epileptic patient has a total serum phenytoin concentration of 50 micromol/l of which 45 micromol/l is bound and 5 micromol/l free (i.e. 10% free). If another drug is given, which displaces a further 10%, more of the phenytoin thereby becomes exposed to metabolism and excretion, so that the total serum phenytoin concentration is halved (to 25 micromol/l) with a free concentration of 20%, but which still remains at 5 micromol/l. From the patient's point of view the effective amount of phenytoin stays the same, even though the total amount of phenytoin in circulation has halved. Under these circumstances there would be no need to change the phenytoin dosage, and to do so in order to accommodate the change in total levels might lead to overdosage.

Basic drugs as well as acidic drugs can be highly protein bound, but clinically important displacement interactions do not seem to have been described. The reasons seem to be that the binding sites within the plasma are different from those occupied by acidic drugs (alpha-1-acid glycoprotein rather than albumin) and, in addition, basic drugs have a large V_d with only a small proportion of the total amount of drug being within the plasma.

4.1.3 Drug metabolism (biotransformation) interactions

Although a few drugs are lost from the body simply by being excreted unchanged in the urine, most are chemically altered within the body to less lipid-soluble compounds which are more easily excreted by the kidneys. If this were not so, many drugs would persist in the body and continue to exert their effects for a long time. This chemical change is called 'metabolism', 'biotransformation', 'biochemical degradation' or sometimes 'detoxification'. Some drug metabolism goes on in the serum, the kidneys, the skin and the intestines, but by far the greatest proportion is carried out by enzymes that are found in the membranes of the endoplasmic reticulum of the liver cells. If liver is homogenised and then centrifuged, the reticulum breaks up into small sacs called microsomes which carry the enzymes, and it is for this reason that the metabolising enzymes of the liver are frequently referred to as the 'liver microsomal enzymes'. We metabolise drugs by two major types of reaction. The first, so-called Phase I reactions (involving oxidation, reduction or hydrolysis), turn drugs into more polar compounds, while Phase II reactions involve cou-

pling drugs with some other substance (e.g. glucuronic acid) to make usually inactive compounds.

4.1.3.1 Enzyme induction. A phenomenon familiar to prescribers is the 'tolerance' that develops to some drugs. For example, when barbiturates were widely used as hypnotics it was found necessary to keep on increasing the dosage as time went by to achieve the same hypnotic effect, the reason being that the barbiturates increase the activity of the microsomal enzymes so that pace of metabolism and excretion increases. This phenomenon of enzyme stimulation or 'induction' not only accounts for the tolerance, but if another drug is present as well, which is metabolised by the same range of enzymes (an oral anticoagulant for example), its enzymic metabolism is similarly increased and larger doses are needed to maintain the same therapeutic effect. Figure 1.3 shows the effects of an enzyme inducing agent, dichloralphenazone, on the metabolism and anticoagulant effects of warfarin. Figures 1.4 and 1.5 show the effects of another enzyme inducing agent, rifampicin (rifampin) on the serum levels of ketoconazole and ciclosporin. Table 1.2 lists some of the interactions due to enzyme induction and Table 1.3 contains some of the potent enzyme-inducing drugs.

A metabolic pathway that is commonly affected is Phase I oxidation, this term covering a number of metabolic biotransformations, all of which require the presence of NADPH and the haem-containing protein cytochrome P450. When enzyme induction occurs the amount of endoplasmic reticulum within the liver cells increases and the amount of cytochrome P450 also rises. The extent of the enzyme induction depends

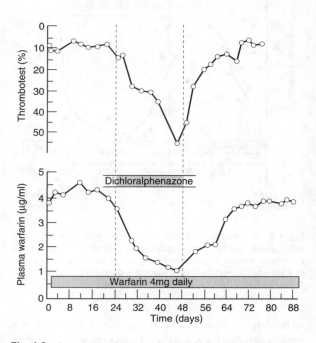

Fig. 1.3 An enzyme induction interaction. In this patient the hypnotic dichloralphenazone (Welldorm) increased the metabolism of the warfarin, thereby reducing its serum levels and its effects (thrombotest percentages) (after Breckenridge A et al., Clin Sci (1971) 40, 351, with permission).

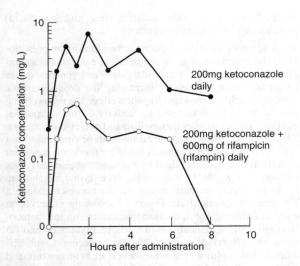

Fig. 1.4 An enzyme induction interaction. Rifampicin (600 mg daily plus isoniazid) increased the metabolism of the ketoconazole in this patient, thereby reducing the serum levels (after Brass C, Antimicrob Agents Chemother (1982) 21, 151, with permission).

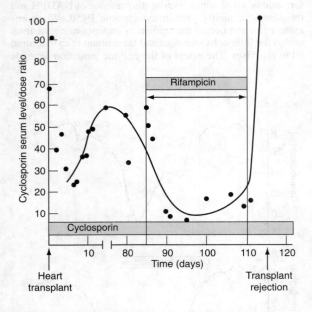

Fig. 1.5 An enzyme induction interaction. Rifampicin (rifampin) (600 mg daily) increased the metabolism of cyclosporin (ciclosporin) in this patient, thereby reducing the trough serum levels. He subsequently died because his heart transplant was rejected (after Van Buren D et al., Transplant Proc (1984) 16, 1642, with permission).

Table 1.2 Interactions due to enzyme induction

Drug affected	Inducing agent(s)	Effect of interaction
Anticoagulants (oral)	Aminoglutethimide Barbiturates Carbamazepine Dichloralphenazone Glutethimide Phenazone Rifampicin (rifampin)	Anticoagulant effects reduced (see Fig. 1.3)
Contraceptives (oral)	Barbiturates Carbamazepine Phenytoin Primidone Rifampicin (rifampin)	Contraceptive effects reduced. Break-through bleeding, contraceptive failures
Corticosteroids	Aminoglutethimide Barbiturates Carbamazepine Phenytoin Primidone Rifampicin (rifampin)	Corticosteroid effects reduced
Haloperidol	Tobacco smoke	Haloperidol effects reduced
Pentazocine	Tobacco smoke	Pentazocine effects reduced
Phenytoin	Rifampicin (rifampin)	Phenytoin effects reduced. Seizure-risk increased
Theophylline	Barbiturates Rifampicin (rifampin) Tobacco smoke	Theophylline effects reduced

Table 1.3 Enzyme-inducing drugs

Aminoglutethimide
Barbiturates
Carbamazepine
Dichloralphenazone
Glutethimide
Phenazone (antipyrine)
Phenytoin
Primidone
Rifampicin (rifampin)
Tobacco smoke

on the drug and its dosage, but it may take days or even 2 to 3 weeks to develop fully, and persist for a similar length of time when the inducing agent is stopped. This means that enzyme induction interactions are delayed in both starting and stopping. Enzyme induction is an extremely common mechanism of interaction and is not confined to drugs; it is also caused by

the chlorinated hydrocarbon insecticides such as dicophane and lindane, and after smoking tobacco.

If one drug reduces the effects of another by enzyme induction, it is possible to accommodate the interaction simply by raising the dosage of the drug affected, but this requires good monitoring, and there are obvious hazards if the inducing

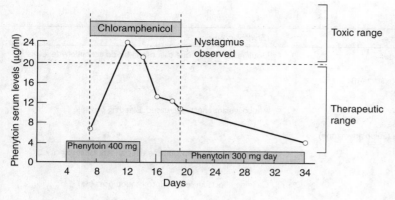

Fig. 1.6 An enzyme inhibition interaction. The chloramphenicol inhibited the metabolism of the phenytoin in this patient so that the serum levels climbed into the toxic range and intoxication developed (indicated by nystagmus). The problem was solved by stopping the phenytoin and later re-starting at a lower dosage (after Ballek RE et al., Lancet (1973) i, 150, with permission).

drug is eventually stopped without remembering to reduce the dosage again. The raised drug dosage will be an overdose when the drug metabolism has returned to normal.

4.1.3.2 Enzyme inhibition. Just as some drugs can stimulate the activity of the microsomal enzymes, so there are others, which have the opposite effect, and act as inhibitors. The normal pace of drug metabolism is slackened so that the metabolism of other drugs given concurrently is also reduced and they begin to accumulate within the body, the effect being essentially the same as when the dosage is increased. Unlike enzyme induction, which may take several days or even weeks to develop fully, enzyme inhibition can occur within 2 to 3 days resulting in the rapid development of toxicity. Figure 1.6 shows what happened when an epileptic patient on phenytoin was given chloramphenicol. The accumulating phenytoin was not detected until it reached levels at which the patient began to manifest toxicity.

Figure 1.7 illustrates the sharp and potentially hazardous rise in blood pressure which can occur if the normally protective monoamine oxidase within the gut wall and liver is inhibited by the presence of an MAO-inhibitory drug (tranylcypromine). Other mechanisms of interaction are also involved. Table 1.4 lists some other interactions due to the inhibition of microsomal and other enzymes, and Tables 1.5 and 1.8 list some enzyme-inhibiting drugs. Numerous other examples are to be found throughout this book.

The clinical significance of many enzyme inhibition interactions depends on the extent to which the serum levels of the drug rise. If the serum levels remain within the therapeutic range the interaction may be advantageous. If not, the interaction becomes adverse as the serum levels climb into the toxic range.

4.1.3.3 Cytochrome P450 isoenzymes and predicting drug interactions. Cytochrome P450 mentioned above is not a single entity but is in fact a very large family of related isoenzymes, about 30 of which have been found in human liver tissue. However in practice only a few specific subfamilies seem to be responsible for most (about 90%) of the metabolism of the commonly used drugs. These isoenzymes are called CYP1A2, CYP2C9 CYP2C19, CYP2D6 CYP3A3 and CYP3A4. There are others of lesser importance.

The isoenzyme CYP2D6 shows what is called 'genetic polymorphism' which simply means that most people possess this isoenzyme but a small proportion of the human population have little or none (about 5 to 10% in white caucasians, 0 to 2% in Asians and black people). Which group any particular individual falls into is genetically determined. The latter, smaller group, cannot metabolise drugs which normally use this isoenzyme and are therefore called 'slow metabolisers' while the majority who possess the isoenzyme are called 'fast' metabolisers. You can find out which group any particular individual falls into by looking at the way a single dose of a test or 'probe' drug is metabolised. This ability (or lack of ability) to metabolise certain drugs explains why some patients develop toxicity when given an interacting drug while others remain symptom free. CYP2C19 also shows polymorphism but other isoenzymes, such as CYP3A4, do not, although there is still some broad variation in the population without there being two clear and distinct groups.

It is interesting to know which particular isoenzyme is responsible for the metabolism of drugs, because by doing *in vitro* tests with human liver enzymes it is often possible to explain why and how some drugs interact. For example,

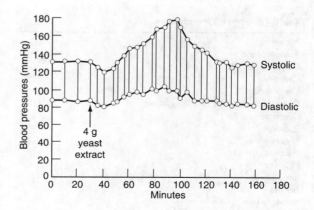

Fig. 1.7 An enzyme inhibition interaction. The effect of 4 g *Marmite* (a tyramine-rich yeast extract) on the diastolic and systolic blood pressures of a patient taking a monoamine oxidase inhibitor (tranylcypromine) (after Blackwell B, Br J Psychiatry (1967) 113, 349, with permission).

Table 1.4 Interactions due to enzyme inhibition

Drug affected	Inducing agent(s)	Clinical outcome
Alcohol	Chlorpropamide Disulfiram Latamoxef (Moxalactam) Metronidazole	Disulfiram-reaction due to a rise in blood acetaldehyde levels
Anticoagulants (oral)	Metronidazole Phenylbutazone Sulfinpyrazone (Sulphinpyrazone)	Anticoagulant effects increased. Bleeding possible
Azathioprine Mercaptopurine	Allopurinol	Azathioprine/mercaptopurine effects increased; toxicity
Caffeine	Enoxacin Idrocilamide	Caffeine effects increased. Intoxication possible
Corticosteroids	Erythromycin Troleandomycin (Triacetyloleandomycin)	Corticosteroid effects increased. Toxicity possible
Phenytoin	Chloramphenicol Isoniazid	Phenytoin effects increased. Intoxication possible (see Fig. 1.6)
Suxamethonium	Ecothiopate (Ecothiophate)	Neuromuscular blockade increased. Prolonged apnoea possible
Tolbutamide	Azapropazone Chloramphenicol Phenylbutazone	Tolbutamide effects increased. Hypoglycaemia possible
Tyramine-containing food-stuffs	Monoamine oxidase inhibitors (MAOI)	Tyramine-induced hypertensive crisis (other mechanisms also involved; see Fig. 1.7)

ciclosporin is metabolised by CYP3A4 and we know that rifampicin (rifampin) is a potent inducer of this cytochrome, whereas ketoconazole inhibits its activity, so that it comes as no surprise that the former reduces the effects of ciclosporin and the latter increases it.

What is very much more important than retrospectively finding out why two drugs interact, is the knowledge such

Table 1.5 Some enzyme inhibitors

Allopurinol
Azapropazone
Chloramphenicol
Cimetidine
Ciprofloxacin
Dextropropoxyphene (Propoxyphene)
Disulfiram
Enoxacin
Erythromycin
Fluconazole
Fluoxetine
Idrocilamide
Isoniazid
Ketoconazole
Metronidazole
Phenylbutazone
Sulphinpyrazone
Troleandomycin (Triacetyloleandomycin)
Verapamil

in vitro tests can provide about forecasting which other drugs may possibly also interact, which may reduce the numbers of expensive clinical trials in subjects and patients.[24] Such forecasting is, like weather forecasting, still a somewhat hit-and-miss business because we do not know all of the factors that may modify or interfere with metabolism. It is far too simplistic to think that we have all the answers just because we know which liver isoenzymes are concerned with the metabolism of a particular drug, but it is a very good start.

Tables 1.6, 1.7 and 1.8 are lists of which drugs are metabolised by which cytochrome isoenzymes, and which drugs are significant inducers and inhibitors of these isoenzymes. It needs to be stressed that these tables should only be used as very a broad general guide, and if you use them to try to predict which drug pairs are likely to interact, you must be prepared to get it wrong some of the time. What may happen *in vitro* may not necessarily work in clinical practice because all of the many variables which can come into play are not known (such as how much of the enzyme is available, the concentration of the drug at the site of metabolism and the affinity of the drug for the enzyme). Remember too that some drugs can be metabolised by more than one cytochrome isoenzyme; some drugs (and their metabolites) can both inhibit a particular cytochrome and be metabolised by it; and some drugs (or their metabolites) can inhibit a particular cytochrome but not be metabolised by it. With so many factors possibly impinging on the outcome of giving two or more drugs together, it is very easy to lose sight of one of the factors (or not even know about it) so that the sum of 2 + 2 may not turn out to be the 4 that you have predicted.

4.1.3.4 Changes in blood flow through the liver. After absorption in the intestine, the portal circulation takes drugs directly to the liver before they are distributed by the blood flow around the rest of the body. A number of highly lipid-soluble drugs undergo substantial biotransformation during this 'first pass' through the gut wall and liver and there is evidence that some concurrently administered drugs can have a marked effect on the extent of first pass metabolism by altering the blood flow through the liver. Cimetidine (but not ranitidine) decreases hepatic blood flow and thereby increases the bioavailability of propranolol. Propranolol also reduces both its own clearance and that of other drugs such as lidocaine (lignocaine) whereas a number of other drugs have the opposite effect and increase the flow of blood through the liver so that their metabolism is increased.

Table 1.6 Drugs metabolised by these cytochrome P450 isoenzymes

Cytochrome P450 isoenzyme	Drugs metabolised
CYP1A2	Caffeine, Clozapine, Imipramine, Maprotiline, Phenacetin, Propranolol, R-warfarin, Ropinirole, Theophylline
CYP2D6	Amitriptyline, Amfetamine (Amphetamine), Captopril, Clomipramine, Codeine, Desipramine, Dextromethorphan, Dihydrocodeine, Diphenhydramine, Flecainide, Fluoxetine, Haloperidol, Hydrocodone, Imipramine, Labetalol, Maprotiline, Metoprolol, Mexiletine, Nortriptyline, Ondensatron, Oxycodone, Papaverine, Paroxetine, Penbutolol, Perphenazine, Propafenone, Propranolol, Thioridazine, Timolol, Trimipramine, Venalfaxine, Yohimbine
CYP2C9	Diclofenac, Dofetilide, Fluvastatin, Ibuprofen, Mefenamic acid, Naproxen, Phenytoin, Piroxicam, S-warfarin, Tolbutamide
CYP2C19	Clomipramine, Diazepam, Hexobarbital (Hexobarbitone), Imipramine, Mephobarbital, Omeprazole, Phenytoin, Propranolol, Proguanil, S-mephenytoin
CYP3A4	Amiodarone, Amitriptyline, Alprazolam, Astemizole, Carbamazepine, Ciclosporin (Cyclosporin), Cisapride, Clindamycin, Clomipramine, Clonazepam, Dapsone, Dexamethasone, Dextromethorphan, Diazepam, Diltiazem, Erythromycin, Ethyl estradiol, Felodipine, Hydrocortisone (Cortisol), Imipramine, Indinavir, Lidocaine (Lignocaine), Lovastatin, Midazolam, Nefazodone, Nelfinavir, Nevirapine, Nifedipine, Nimodipine, Nisoldipine, Propafenone, Quinidine, R-warfarin, Ritonavir, Saquinavir, Sertraline, Simvastatin, Tamoxifen, Terfenadine, Testosterone, Triazolam, Venlafaxine, Verapamil, Zolpidem

This list is not exhaustive and is derived from several sources.

Table 1.7 Drugs that induce these cytochrome P450 isoenzymes

Cytochrome P450 isoenzyme	Inducing drugs
CYP1A2	Barbiturates, Omeprazole, Phenytoin, Tobacco smoke
CYP2D6	?
CYP2C9	Barbiturates, Rifampicin (Rifampin)
CYP2C19	?
CYP3A4	Barbiturates, Carbamazepine, Dexamethasone, Phenytoin, Rifabutin, Rifampicin (Rifampin)

This list is not exhaustive and is derived from several sources.

Table 1.8 Drugs that inhibit these cytochrome P450 isoenzymes

Cytochrome P450 isoenzyme	Inhibiting drugs
CYP1A2	Enoxacin, Cimetidine, Ciprofloxacin, Fluvoxamine, Furafylline, Grapefruit juice, Grepafloxacin
CYP2D6	Fluoxetine, Haloperidol, Paroxetine, Quinidine, Ritonavir, Sertraline, Thioridazine
CYP2C9	Fluconazole, Fluoxetine, Fluvoxamine, Ritonavir
CYP2C19	Fluoxetine, Fluvoxamine, Omeprazole
CYP3A4	Cimetidine, Clarithromycin, Erythromycin, Fluvoxamine, Grapefruit juice, Itraconazole, Ketoconazole, Miconazole, Nefazodone, Nelfinavir, Remacemide, Ritonavir

This list is not exhaustive and is derived from several sources.

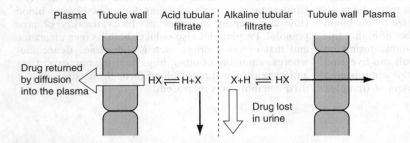

Plasma   Tubule wall   Acid tubular   Alkaline tubular   Tubule wall   Plasma
                       filtrate   filtrate

Drug returned
by diffusion
into the plasma   HX ⇌ H+X   X+H ⇌ HX

                                  Drug lost
                                  in urine

Fig. 1.8 An excretion interaction. If the tubular filtrate is acidified, most of the molecules of weakly acid drugs (HX) exist in an un-ionised lipid-soluble form and are able to return through the lipid membranes of the tubule cells by simple diffusion. Thus they are retained. In alkaline urine most of the drug molecules exist in an ionised non-lipid soluble form (X). In this form the molecules are unable to diffuse freely through these membranes and are therefore lost in the urine.

4.1.4 Interactions due to changes in excretion

With the exception of the inhalation anaesthetics, most drugs are excreted either in the bile or in the urine. Blood entering the kidneys along the renal arteries is, first of all, delivered to the glomeruli of the tubules where molecules small enough to pass through the pores of the glomerular membrane (e.g. water, salts, some drugs) are filtered through into the lumen of the tubules. Larger molecules, such as plasma proteins, and blood cells are retained. The blood flow then passes to the remaining parts of the kidney tubules where active energy-using transport systems are able to remove drugs and their metabolites from the blood and secrete them into the tubular filtrate. The tubule cells additionally possess active and passive transport systems for the reabsorption of drugs. Interference by drugs with kidney tubule fluid pH, with active transport systems and with blood flow to the kidney can alter the excretion of other drugs.

4.1.4.1 Changes in urinary pH. As with drug absorption in the gut, passive reabsorption of drugs depends upon the extent to which the drug exists in the non-ionised lipid-soluble form which in its turn depends on its pKa and the pH of the urine. Only the non-ionised form is lipid-soluble and able to diffuse back through the lipid membranes of the tubule cells. Thus at high pH values (alkaline), weakly acid drugs (pKa 3.0 to 7.5) largely exist as ionised lipid-insoluble molecules which are unable to diffuse into the tubule cells and will therefore be lost in the urine. The converse will be true for weak organic bases with pKa values of 7.5 to 10.5. Thus pH changes that increase the amount in the ionised form (alkaline urine for acidic drugs, acid for bases) increase the loss of the drug, whereas moving the pH in the opposite directions will increase their retention. Figure 1.8 illustrates the situation with a weakly acidic drug.

The clinical significance of this interaction mechanism is small, because although a very large number of drugs are either weak acids or bases, almost all are largely metabolised by the liver to inactive compounds and few are excreted in the urine unchanged. In practice therefore only a handful of drugs seem to be affected by changes in urinary pH (the exceptions include changes in the excretion of quinidine and salicylate due to alterations in urinary pH caused by antacids). In cases of overdose, deliberate urinary pH changes have been used to increase the loss of drugs such as phenobarbital and salicylates.

4.1.4.2 Changes in active kidney tubule excretion. Drugs that use the same active transport systems in the kidney tubules can compete with one another for excretion. For example, probenecid reduces the excretion of penicillin and other drugs by successfully competing for an excretory mechanism, thus the 'loser' (penicillin) is retained. But even the 'winner' (probenecid) is also later retained because it is passively reabsorbed further along the kidney tubule. See Figure 1.9. Some examples of drugs which interact in this way are given in Table 1.9.

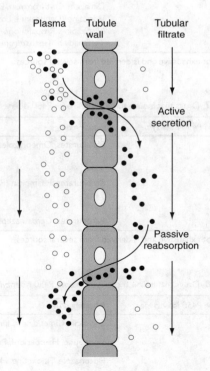

Plasma   Tubule   Tubular
          wall   filtrate

                     Active
                     secretion

                     Passive
                     reabsorption

Fig. 1.9 Competitive interaction between drugs for active tubular secretion. Probenecid (●) is able successfully to compete with some of the other drugs (○) for active secretory mechanisms in the kidney tubules which reduces their loss in the urine and raises serum levels. The probenecid is later passively reabsorbed.

Table 1.9 Interactions due to changes in renal transport

Drug affected	Interacting drugs	Results of interaction

Cephalosporins
Dapsone
Indometacin
  (Indomethacin)
Nalidixic acid
Penicillin
PAS (aminosalicylic
  acid)
	Probenecid	Serum levels of drug affected raised; possibility of toxicity with some drugs. See Fig. 1.9

Methotrexate	Salicylates and some other NSAIDs	Methotrexate serum levels raised. Serious methotrexate toxicity possible
Acetohexamide Glibenclamide Tolbutamide	Phenylbutazone	Hypoglycaemic effects increased and prolonged due to reduced renal excretion

Table 1.10 Additive, synergistic or summation interactions

Drugs	Results of interaction
Anticholinergics + anticholinergics (anti-parkinsonian agents, butyrophenones, phenothiazines, tricyclic antidepressants, etc.)	Increased anticholinergic effects; heat stroke in hot and humid conditions; adynamic ileus; toxic psychoses
Antihypertensives + drugs causing hypotension (anti-anginals, vasodilators, phenothiazines)	Increased antihypertensive effects; orthostasis
CNS depressants + CNS depressants (alcohol, anti-emetics, antihistamines, hypnosedatives, etc.)	Impaired psychomotor skills, reduced alertness, drowsiness, stupor, respiratory depression, coma, death
QT prolonging drugs + other QT prolonging drugs (Amiodarone + Disopyramide)	Additive prolongation of QT interval, increased risk of torsade de pointes
Methotrexate + co-trimoxazole	Bone marrow megaloblastosis due to folic acid antagonism
Nephrotoxic drugs + nephrotoxic drugs (gentamicin or tobramycin with cefalotin (cephalothin)	Increased nephrotoxicity
Neuromuscular blockers + drugs with neuromuscular blocking effects (e.g. aminoglycoside antibacterials)	Increased neuromuscular blockade; delayed recovery, prolonged apnoea
Potassium supplements + potassium-sparing diuretics (triamterene)	Marked hyperkalaemia

4.1.4.3 Changes in kidney blood flow. The flow of blood through the kidney is partially controlled by the production of renal vasodilatory prostaglandins. If the synthesis of these prostaglandins is inhibited (e.g. by indometacin), the renal excretion of lithium is reduced and its serum levels rise as a result.

4.1.4.4 Biliary excretion and the entero-hepatic shunt. A number of drugs are excreted in the bile, either unchanged or conjugated (e.g. as the glucuronide) to make them more water soluble. Some of the conjugates are metabolised to the parent compound by the gut flora which are then reabsorbed. This recycling process prolongs the stay of the drug within the body, but if activity of the gut flora is decimated by the presence of an antibacterial, the drug is not recycled and is lost more quickly. This may possibly explain the rare failure of the oral contraceptives that can be brought about by the concurrent use of penicillins or tetracyclines.

4.1.5 P-glycoprotein interactions. More and more evidence is accumulating to show that some drug interactions occur because of interference by drugs with the activity of P-glycoprotein. This is a 'pump' found in the membranes of certain cells, which can push metabolites and drugs out of the cells and have a considerable impact on the extent of drug absorption (via the intestine) or elimination (in the urine and bile). So, for example, the P-glycoprotein in the cells of the gut lining can eject some already-absorbed drug molecules back into the intestine so that the total amount of drug absorbed is reduced. In this way the P-glycoprotein acts as a barrier to absorption. The activity of p-glycoprotein in the endothelial cells of the blood-brain barrier can also block the entry of certain drugs into the brain.

The pumping actions of P-glycoprotein can be induced or inhibited by some drugs. So for example, the induction (or stimulation) of the activity of P-glycoprotein by rifampicin (rifampin) within the lining cells of the gut causes digoxin to be ejected into the gut more vigorously. This results in a fall in the levels of digoxin in the plasma. In contrast, ciclosporin appears to inhibit the activity of P-glycoprotein within the

kidney tubule cells so that the amount of digoxin pushed out into the urine is reduced, thereby causing a rise in plasma digoxin levels.

Thus the induction or inhibition of P-glycoprotein can have a major impact on the pharmacokinetics of some drugs.

4.2 Pharmacodynamic interactions

Pharmacodynamic interactions are those where the effects of one drug are changed by the presence of another drug at its site of action. Sometimes the drugs directly compete for particular receptors (e.g. beta-2 agonists such as salbutamol and beta-blockers such as propranolol) but often the reaction is more indirect and involves the interference with physiological mechanisms. These interactions are much less easy to classify neatly than those which are pharmacokinetic.

4.2.1 Additive or synergistic interactions and combined toxicity

If two drugs, which have the same pharmacological effect are given together, the effects can be additive. For example, alcohol depresses the CNS and, if taken in moderate amounts with

Table 1.11 Opposing or antagonistic interactions

Drug affected	Interacting drugs	Results of interaction
Anticoagulants	Vitamin K	Anticoagulant effects opposed
Carbenoxolone	Spironolactone	Ulcer-healing effects opposed
Hypoglycaemic agents	Glucocorticoids	Hypoglycaemic effects opposed
Hypnotic drugs	Caffeine	Hypnosis opposed
Levodopa	Antipsychotics (those with Parkinsonian side effects)	Antiparkinsonian effects opposed

normal therapeutic doses of any of a large number of drugs (e.g. sedatives, tranquillisers, etc.), may cause excessive drowsiness. Strictly speaking (as pointed out earlier) these are not interactions within the definition given at the beginning of this chapter, nevertheless it is convenient to consider them within the broad context of the clinical outcome of giving two drugs together. Additive effects can occur with both the main effects of the drugs as well as their side-effects, thus an additive 'interaction' can occur with anticholinergic antiparkinson drugs (main effect) or butyrophenones (side effect) that can result in serious anticholinergic toxicity. Sometimes the additive effects are solely toxic (e.g. additive ototoxicity, nephrotoxicity, bone marrow depression, QT interval prolongation). Examples of these reactions are listed in Table 1.10. It is common to use the terms 'additive', 'summation', 'synergy' or 'potentiation' to describe what happens if two or more drugs behave like this. These words have precise pharmacological definitions but they are often used rather loosely as synonyms because in practice in man it is often very difficult to know the extent of the increased activity, that is to say whether the effects are greater or smaller than the sum of the individual effects.

4.2.1.1 The Serotonin syndrome. In the 1950s a serious and life-threatening toxic reaction was reported in patients on iproniazid (an MAOI) when they were treated with pethidine (meperidine). The reasons were then not understood and even now we do not have the full picture. What happened is thought to have been due to over-stimulation of the 5-HT_{1A} and 5-HT_{2A} receptors and possibly other serotonin receptors in the central nervous system (in the brain stem and spinal cord in particular) due to the combined effects of these two drugs. It can occur exceptionally after taking only one drug, which causes over-stimulation of these 5-HT receptors, but much more usually it develops when two or more drugs (so-called serotonergic or serotomimetic drugs) act in concert. The characteristic symptoms (now known as the 'serotonin syndrome') fall into three main areas, namely altered mental status (agitation, confusion, mania), autonomic dysfunction (diaphoresis, diarrhoea, fever, shivering) and neuromuscular abnormalities (hyperreflexia, incoordination, myoclonus, tremor). These are the 'Sternbach diagnostic criteria' named after Dr Harvey Sternbach who drew up this list of clinical features and who suggested that at least three of them need to be seen before classifying this toxic reaction as the 'serotonin syndrome' rather than the 'neuroleptic malignant syndrome'.[25]

The syndrome can develop shortly after one serotonergic drug is added to another, or even if one is replaced by another without allowing a long enough washout period in between, and the problem usually resolves fairly rapidly within about 24 hours if both drugs are withdrawn and supportive measures given. Non-specific serotonin antagonists (cyproheptadine, chlorpromazine, methysergide) have also been used. Most patients recover uneventfully, but there have been a few fatalities.

Following the first report of this syndrome, many other cases have been described involving L-tryptophan and MAOIs, the tricyclic antidepressants and MAOIs, and more recently the SSRIs, but other serotonergic drugs have also been involved and the list is lengthening every year.

It is still not at all clear why many patients can take two, possibly even more, serotonergic drugs together without problems while a very small number develop this serious toxic reaction, but it certainly suggests that there are as yet other factors involved which remain to be identified. The full story is likely to be much more complex than just the simple additive effects of two drugs.

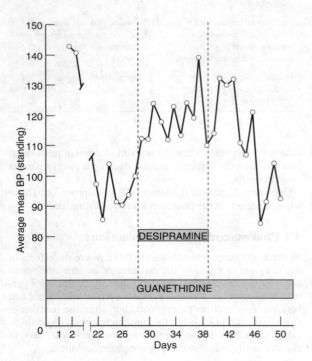

Fig. 1.10 A pharmacodynamic interaction. The desipramine (75–100 mg daily) inhibited the uptake of guanethidine (150 mg daily) into adrenergic neurones of the sympathetic nervous system thereby stopping its antihypertensive effects. As a result the blood pressure in this patient rose once again (after Oates JA et al., Ann NY Acad Sci (1971) 179, 302, with permission).

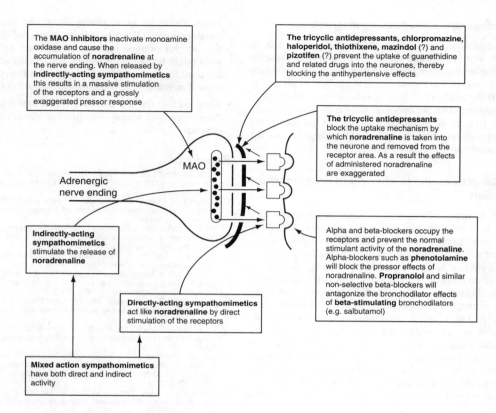

The **MAO inhibitors** inactivate monoamine oxidase and cause the accumulation of **noradrenaline** at the nerve ending. When released by **indirectly-acting sympathomimetics** this results in a massive stimulation of the receptors and a grossly exaggerated pressor response

The **tricyclic antidepressants, chlorpromazine, haloperidol, thiothixene, mazindol** (?) and **pizotifen** (?) prevent the uptake of guanethidine and related drugs into the neurones, thereby blocking the antihypertensive effects

The **tricyclic antidepressants** block the uptake mechanism by which **noradrenaline** is taken into the neurone and removed from the receptor area. As a result the effects of administered noradrenaline are exaggerated

MAO

Adrenergic nerve ending

Indirectly-acting sympathomimetics stimulate the release of **noradrenaline**

Alpha and beta-blockers occupy the receptors and prevent the normal stimulant activity of the **noradrenaline**. Alpha-blockers such as **phenotolamine** will block the pressor effects of noradrenaline. **Propranolol** and similar non-selective beta-blockers will antagonize the bronchodilator effects of **beta-stimulating** bronchodilators (e.g. salbutamol)

Directly-acting sympathomimetics act like **noradrenaline** by direct stimulation of the receptors

Mixed action sympathomimetics have both direct and indirect activity

Fig. 1.11 Interactions at adrenergic neurones. A highly simplified composite diagram of an adrenergic neurone (molecules of norepinephrine (noradrenaline) indicated as (●) contained in a single vesicle at the nerve-ending) to illustrate in outline some of the different sites where drugs can interact. More details of these interactions are to be found in individual synopses.

Table 1.12 Interactions due to changes in drug transport mechanisms

Drug affected	Interacting drugs	Results of interaction
Clonidine	Tricyclic antidepressants	Antihypertensive effects opposed, possibly due to interference in CNS with clonidine uptake
Guanethidine-like antihypertensives (debrisoquine, guanoclor, etc.)	Tricyclic antidepressants Chlorpromazine Haloperidol Tiotixene (Thiothixene) Indirectly-acting sympathomimetics	Antihypertensive effects opposed, due to inhibition of uptake into adrenergic neurones. See Fig. 1.11
Noradrenaline (norepinephrine)	Tricyclic antidepressants	Pressor effects increased due to inhibition of noradrenaline uptake into adrenergic neurones

Table 1.13 Interactions due to disturbances in fluid and electrolyte balance

Drug affected	Interacting drugs	Results of interaction
Digitalis	Potassium-depleting diuretics	Digitalis toxicity related to changes in ionic balance at the myocardium
Lithium chloride	Dietary salt restriction	Increased serum lithium levels; intoxication possible
	Increased salt intake	Reduced serum lithium levels
Lithium chloride	Thiazide and related diuretics	Increased serum lithium levels; intoxication possible
Guanethidine Chlorothiazide	Kebuzone Phenylbutazone	Antihypertensive effects opposed due to salt and water retention

4.2.2 Antagonistic or opposing interactions

In contrast to additive interactions, there are some pairs of drugs with activities which are opposed to one another. For example the oral anticoagulants can prolong the blood clotting time by competitively inhibiting the effects of dietary vitamin K. If the intake of vitamin K is increased, the effects of the oral anticoagulant are opposed and the prothrombin time can return to normal, thereby cancelling out the therapeutic benefits of anticoagulant treatment. Other examples of this type of interaction are listed in Table 1.11.

4.2.3 Interactions due to changes in drug transport mechanisms

A number of drugs whose actions occur at adrenergic neurones can be prevented from reaching those sites of action by the presence of other drugs. Thus the uptake of guanethidine and related drugs (guanoclor, betanidine (bethanidine), debrisoquine, etc.) is blocked by chlorpromazine, haloperidol, tiotixene (thiothixene), a number of indirectly-acting sympathomimetic amines and the tricyclic antidepressants so that the antihypertensive effect is prevented. This is illustrated in Figure 1.10. The tricyclic antidepressants also prevent the re-uptake of noradrenaline into peripheral adrenergic neurones so that its pressor effects are increased. The antihypertensive effects of clonidine are also prevented by the tricyclic antidepressants, one possible reason being that the uptake of clonidine within the CNS is blocked. Some of these interactions at adrenergic neurones are illustrated in Figure 1.11. See also Table 1.12.

4.2.4 Interactions due to disturbances in fluid and electrolyte balance

An increase in the sensitivity of the myocardium to the digitalis glycosides, and resultant toxicity, can result from a fall in plasma potassium concentrations brought about by potassium-depleting diuretics such as furosemide (frusemide). Plasma lithium levels can rise if thiazide diuretics are used because the clearance of the lithium by the kidney is changed, probably as a result of the changes in sodium excretion that can accompany the use of these diuretics. Table 1.13 lists some examples.

5. Conclusions

It is now quite impossible to remember all the known clinically important interactions and how they occur, which is why this reference publication has been produced, but there are some broad general principles which need little memorising:

- Be on the alert with any drugs which have a narrow therapeutic window or where it is necessary to keep serum levels at or above a suitable level (e.g. anticoagulants, anticonvulsants, antihypertensives, anti-infectives, cytotoxics, digitalis glycosides, hypoglycaemic agents, immunosuppressants, etc.).

- Remember those drugs which are enzyme inducing agents (e.g. phenytoin, barbiturates, rifampicin, etc) or enzyme inhibiting agents (e.g. cimetidine).

- Think about the basic pharmacology of the drugs under consideration so that obvious problems (additive CNS depression for example) are not overlooked, and try to think what might happen if drugs which affect the same receptors are used together. And don't forget that many drugs affect more than one type of receptor which results in side-effects.

- Keep in mind that the elderly are most at risk because of reduced liver and kidney function on which drug clearance depends.

References

1. Smith JW, Seidl LG, Cluff LE. Studies on the epidemiology of adverse drug reactions. V. Clinical factors influencing susceptibility. *Ann Intern Med* (1969) 65, 629.
2. Puckett WH, Visconti JA. An epidemiological study of the clinical significance of drug-drug interaction in a private community hospital. *Am J Hosp Pharm* (1971) 28, 247.
3. Shinn AF, Shrewsbury RP, Anderson KW. Development of a computerized drug interaction database (Medicom) for use in a patient specific environment. *Drug Inf J* (1983) 17, 205.
4. Ishikura C, Ishizuka H. Evaluation of a computerized drug interaction checking system. *Int J Biomed Comput* (1983) 14, 311.
5. Schuster BG, Fleckenstein L, Wilson JP, Peck CC. Low incidence of adverse reactions due to drug-drug interaction in a potentially high risk population of medical inpatients. *Clin Res* (1982) 30, 258A.
6. Manon-Espaillat R, Burnstine TH, Remler B, Reed RC, Osorio I. Antiepileptic drug intoxication: factors and their significance. *Epilepsia* (1991) 32, 96–100.
7. Haumschild MJ, Ward ES, Bishop JM, Haumschild MS. Pharmacy-based computer system for monitoring and reporting drug interactions. *Am J Hosp Pharm* (1987) 44, 345.
8. Manchon ND, Bercoff E, Lamarchand P, Chassagne P, Senant J, Bourreille J. Fréquence et gravité des interaction médicamenteuses dans une population âgée: étude prospective concernant 639 malades. *Rev Med Interne* (1989) 10, 521–5.
9. Lipton JL, Bero LA, Bird JA, McPhee SJ. The impact of clinical pharmacist' consultations on physicians' geriatric drug prescribing. *Medical Care* (1992) 30, 646–58.
10. Rupp MT, De Young M, Schondelmeyer SW. Prescribing problems and pharmacist interventions in community practice. *Medical Care* (1992) 30, 926–40.
11. Linnarsson R. Drug interactions in primary health care. A retrospective database study and its implications for the design of a computerized decision support system. *Scand J Prim Health Care* (1993) 11, 181–6.
12. Rotman BL, Sullivan AN, McDonald T, DeSmedt P, Goodnature D, Higgins M, Suermond HJ, Young CY, Owens DK. A randomized evaluation of a computer-based physician's workstation; design considerations and baseline results. *Proc Ann Symp Comput Appl Med Care* (1995) 693–7.
13. Stanton LA, Peterson GM, Rumble RH, Cooper GM, Polack AE. Drug-related admissions to an Australian hospital. *J Clin Pharm Ther* (1994) 19, 341–7.
14. Goldberg RM, Mabee J, Chan L, Wong S. Drug-drug and drug-disease interactions in the ED; analysis of a high-risk population. *Am J Emerg Med* (1996) 14, 447–50.
15. Paille R, Pissochet P. L'ordonnance et les interactions medicamenteuses: etude prospective chez 896 patients traites pour hypertension arterielle en medicine generale. *Therapie* (1995) 50, 253–8.
16. Di Castri A, Jacquot JM, Hemmi P, Moati L, Rouy JM, Compan B, Nachar H, Bossy-Vassal A. Interactions medicamenteuses: etude de 409 ordonnances etablies a l'issue d'une hospitalisation geriatrique. *Therapie* (1995) 50, 259–64.
17. Cadieux RJ. Drug interactions in the elderly. *Postgrad Med* (1989) 86, 179–86.
18. Tinawi M, Alguire P. The prevalence of drug interactions in hospitalized patients. *Clin Res* (1992) 40, 773A.
19. Jankel CA, McMillan JA, Martin BC. Effect of drug interactions on outcomes of patient receiving warfarin or theophylline. *Am J Hosp Pharm* (1994) 51, 661–6.
20. Boston Collaborative Drug Surveillance Program. Interaction between chloral hydrate and warfarin. *N Engl J Med* (1972) 286, 53–5.
21. Benet LZ, Hoener B-A. Changes in plasma protein binding have little clinical relevance. *Clin Pharmacol Ther* (2002) 71, 115–121.
22. MacKichan JJ. Protein binding drug displacement interactions. Fact or fiction? *Clin Pharmacokinet* (1989) 16, 65–73.
23. Bridgeman JF, Rosem SM, Thorp JM. Complications during clofibrate treatment of nephrotic syndrome hyperlipoproteinaemia. *Lancet* (1972) ii, 506.
24. Tucker GT. The rational selection of drug interaction studies: implications of recent advances in drug metabolism. *Int J Clin Pharmacol Ther Toxicol* (1992) 30, 550–3.
25. Sternbach H. The serotonin syndrome. *Am J Psychiatry* (1991) 148, 705–13.

2

Alcohol interactions

For social and historical reasons alcohol is usually bought from a store or in a bar or restaurant, rather than from a pharmacy, because it is considered to be a drink and not a drug, but pharmacologically speaking it has much in common with medicinal drugs which depress the central nervous system. Objective tests show that as blood-alcohol levels rise, the ability to perform a number of skills gradually deteriorates as the brain becomes progressively disorganised. The myth that alcohol is a stimulant has arisen because at parties and social occasions it helps people to lose some of their inhibitions and it allows them to relax and unwind. Professor JH Gaddum put it amusingly and succinctly when, describing the early effects of moderate amounts of alcohol, he wrote that "logical thought is difficult but after dinner speeches easy." The

Table 2.1 Reactions to different concentrations of alcohol in the blood

Amounts of alcohol drunk			
Man 11 stones (70 kg)	Woman 9 stones (55 kg)	Blood-alcohol levels mg% (mg per 100 ml)	Reactions to different % of alcohol in the blood
2 units	1 unit	25–30	Sense of well-being enhanced. Reaction times reduced
4 units	2 units	50–60	Mild loss of inhibition, judgement impaired, increased risk of accidents at home, at work and on the road; no overt signs of drunkenness
5 units	3 units	75–80	Physical co-ordination reduced, more marked loss of inhibition; noticeably under the influence; at the legal limit for driving in the UK
7 units	4 units	100+	Clumsiness, loss of physical control, tendency to extreme responses; definite intoxication
10 units	6 units	150	Slurred speech, possible loss of memory the following day, probably drunk and disorderly
24 units	14 units	360	Dead drunk, sleepiness, possible loss of consciousness
33 units	20 units	500	Coma and possibly death
1 unit	= half pint (300 ml medium strength beer)	= glass wine (100 ml)	= single sherry or martini (a third of a gill (50 ml))	= single spirit one-sixth gill (25 ml)

| 3–4% alcohol | 11% alcohol | 17–20% alcohol | 37–40% alcohol |

After *Which?* October 1984, page 447 and others.

expansiveness and locquaciousness which are socially acceptable, lead on, with increasing amounts of alcohol, to unrestrained behaviour in normally well-controlled individuals, through drunkenness, unconsciousness and finally death from respiratory failure. These effects are all a reflection of the progressive and deepening depression of the CNS.

Table 2.1 gives an indication in very broad terms of the reactions of men and women to different amounts and concentrations of alcohol.

On the whole women are smaller than men, they have a higher proportion of fat in which alcohol is not very soluble, their body fluids represent a smaller proportion of their total body mass and their first-pass metabolism of alcohol is less than men because they have less alcohol dehydrogenase in their stomach walls. Consequently if a man and woman of the same weight matched each other, drink for drink, the woman would finish up with a blood alcohol level about 50% higher than the man. The values shown assume that the drinkers regularly drink, have had a meal and weigh between 9 and 11 stones (55–70 kg). Higher blood alcohol levels would occur if drunk on an empty stomach and lower values in much heavier individuals. The liver metabolises about one unit per hour so that the values will fall with time.

Since alcohol impairs the skills needed to drive safely, almost all national and state authorities have imposed maximum legal blood alcohol limits. In the UK and a number of other countries this is currently set at 80 mg/100 ml (35 micrograms per 100 ml in the breath) but impairment is clearly detectable at lower concentrations, for which reason some countries have imposed much lower legal limits. Since many countries express their statutory blood-alcohol limits for driving in mg/ml or g, and breath-alcohol limits in mg/l, all of the values in Table 2.2 have been expressed in the same units for easy comparison.

Probably the most common drug interaction of all occurs if alcohol is drunk while taking other drugs which have CNS depressant activity, the result being even further CNS depression. Blood alcohol levels well within the legal driving limit may, in the presence of other CNS depressants, be equivalent to blood alcohol levels at or above the legal limit (in terms of worsened driving and other skills). This can occur with some antihistamines, analgesics, antidepressants, cough, cold and influenza remedies, hypno-sedatives, psychotropics, tranquillisers, travel-sickness remedies and others (see 'Alcohol + CNS depressants', p.26). This chapter contains a number of monographs that describe the results of formal studies of

Table 2.2 Maximum legally allowable blood alcohol limits when driving in various countries

100 mg%	Eire, Puerto Rico, Some of the States in the USA
90 mg%	Cyprus, Peru (0.99 ml%)
80 mg%	Austria, Belgium, Brazil, Canada, Denmark, Germany, Iceland, Italy, Ivory Coast, Luxembourg, Mauritius, New Zealand, Northern Ireland, Singapore, South Africa, Spain, Switzerland, Thailand, United Kingdom, Some of the States in the USA
54 mg%	Netherlands
50 mg%	Australia, Chile, Finland, France, Greece, Iceland, Japan, Norway, Portugal, Turkey, Yugoslavia
20 mg%	Poland, Sweden
0 mg%	Albania, Bahrain, Brunei, Bulgaria, Czech Republic, Egypt, Hungary, Iran, Jordan, Pakistan, Romania, Saudi Arabia, Slovak Republic

Note: For easy comparison the legally allowable blood alcohol limits have all been expressed as mg%. Thus blood alcohol levels of 80 mg% = 80 mg of alcohol in 100 ml blood = 0.8 g/L. The breath level limit equivalent to 80 mg% can vary slightly: thus UK and Eire (35 µg/L), South Africa (38 µg/L).

Some of the Australian states have different rules for certain drivers (learners, bus drivers etc), and other countries have a two-tier system with different penalties. Some of the former members of the Soviet Republic do not have blood alcohol levels specifically stated but it is an offence to drive while intoxicated. Muslim countries forbid alcohol entirely. Some of the legal limits are under review and likely to be reduced shortly to the next level (Austria, Eire, other countries of the EC, and some States in the USA). The values quoted above were assembled in 1996.

alcohol combined with a number of recognised CNS depressants, but there are still many other drugs which await study of this kind and which undoubtedly represent a real hazard.

A less common interaction which can occur between alcohol and some drugs, chemical agents and fungi is the flushing (Antabuse) reaction. This is exploited in the case of disulfiram (Antabuse) as a drink deterrent, but it can occur unexpectedly with some other drugs and be both unpleasant and possibly frightening, but it is not usually dangerous.

Alcohol + Amphetamines

Dexamfetamine (dexamphetamine) can reduce to some extent the deleterious effects of alcohol on driving skills, but some impairment still occurs and it may be unsafe to drive.

Clinical evidence

Alcohol (0.85 g/kg–2 g/kg 100 proof vodka in orange juice) worsened the performance of a SEDI task (Simulator Evaluation of Drug Impairment) in 12 normal subjects.[1] This task is believed to parallel the skills needed to drive safely and involves tests of attention, memory, recognition, decision making and reaction times. When the subjects were additionally given 0.09 or 0.18 mg/kg **dexamfetamine (dexamphetamine)**, the performance of the SEDI task was improved (dosage related) but the subjective assessment of intoxication was unchanged. Blood alcohol levels reached a maximum of about 100 g/dl (*sic*) at an hour. The bioavailability of the alcohol was slightly increased.[1]

Earlier reports using different testing methods found that in some tests **dexamfetamine** modified the effects of alcohol, but the total picture was complex.[2-5] Another study found that **dexamfetamine** failed to improve attentive motor performance made worse by alcohol if the task was long and boring.[6] A later study found that alcohol and **methylamphetamine** together actually made the subjects feel more intoxicated.[7]

Mechanism

Not understood. Although alcohol is a CNS depressant and the amphetamines are CNS stimulants, there is no simple antagonism between the two.[5]

Importance and management

This interaction has been well studied, but the conclusions to be drawn from the results are not clear cut. Although there is some evidence that the effects of alcohol are modified or reduced, none of these reports should be used to support the uncritical use of the amphetamines to sober up drinkers because their driving skills may still remain impaired to some extent, particularly after a while when boredom or fatigue is likely to have set in.

1. Perez-Reyes M, White WR, McDonald SA, Hicks RE. Interaction between ethanol and dextroamphetamines: effects on psychomotor performance. *Alcohol Clin Exp Res* (1992) 16, 75–81.
2. Kaplan HL, Forney RB, Richards AB, Hughes FW. Dextro-amphetamine, alcohol, and dextro-amphetamine-alcohol combination and mental performance. In Harger RN (Ed). Alcohol and traffic safety. Proc 4th Int Conf Alc Traffic Safety, Bloomington, Indiana. Indiana Univ Press (1966) 211–14.
3. Hughes FW, Forney RB. Dextro-amphetamine, ethanol and dextro-amphetamine-ethanol combinations on performance of human subjects stressed with delayed auditory feedback (DAF). *Psychopharmacologia* (1964) 6, 234–8.
4. Newman HW, Newman EJ. Failure of dexedrine and caffeine as practical antagonists of the depressant effect of ethyl alcohol in man. *Quart J Stud Alcohol* (1956) 17, 406–10.
5. Wilson L, Taylor JD, Nash CW, Cameron DF. The combined effects of ethanol and amphetamine sulfate on performance of human subjects. *Can Med Assoc J* (1966) 94, 478–84.
6. Brown DJ, Hughes FW, Forney RB, Richards AB. Effect of d-amphetamine and alcohol on attentive motor performance in human subjects. In Harger RN (Ed). Alcohol and traffic safety. Proc 4th Int Conf Alc Traffic Safety, Bloomington, Indiana. Indiana Univ Press (1966) 215–19.
7. Mendelson J, Jones RT, Upton R, Jacob III P. Methamphetamine and ethanol interactions in humans. *Clin Pharmacol Ther* (1995) 57, 559–68.

Alcohol + Anticholinergics

Propantheline and atropine appear not to affect blood alcohol levels but marked impairment of attention can occur if alcohol is taken in the presence of atropine or glycopyrrolate (glycopyrronium), probably making driving more hazardous. No adverse interaction appears to occur with transdermal hyoscine (scopolamine) and alcohol.

Clinical evidence, mechanism, importance and management

Neither chronic oral **propantheline** (45–120 mg daily) nor single 3-mg doses of **atropine** 2 h before alcohol appear to affect blood alcohol levels.[1] However a study in healthy subjects of the effects of 0.5 mg **atropine** or 1.0 mg **glycopyrrolate (glycopyrronium)** in combination with alcohol (0.5 g/kg) showed that while reaction times and co-ordination were unaffected or even improved, there was a marked impairment of attention which was large enough to make driving more hazardous.[2] Patients should be warned.

A double-blind crossover study in 12 normal subjects showed that a transdermal **hyoscine** (scopolamine) preparation (*Scopoderm-TTS*) did not alter the effects of alcohol on the performance of the psychometric tests used (Critical Flicker Fusion Frequency, Choice Reaction Tasks), nor was the loss of alcohol or of **hyoscine** from the body changed. Blood alcohol levels up to 80 and 130 mg% were studied.[3] No special precautions seem necessary.

1. Gibbons DO, Lant AF. Effects of intravenous and oral propantheline and metoclopramide on ethanol absorption. *Clin Pharmacol Ther* (1975) 17, 578–84.
2. Linnoila M. Drug effects on psychomotor skills related to driving: interaction of atropine, glycopyrrhonium and alcohol. *Eur J Clin Pharmacol* (1973) 6, 107–12.
3. Gleiter CH, Antonin K-H, Schoenleber W, Bieck PR. Interaction of alcohol and transdermally administered scopolamine. *J Clin Pharmacol* (1988) 28, 1123–7.

Alcohol + Antihistamines

Some antihistamines cause drowsiness which can be increased by alcohol. The detrimental effects of alcohol on driving skills are considerably increased by the use of the older more sedative antihistamines (promethazine, chlorphenamine (chlorpheniramine), diphenhydramine, etc.), but are much less marked with the less sedative antihistamines (clemastine, clemizole, cyclizine, cyproheptadine, mebhydrolin, pheniramine, tripelennamine, triprolidine, etc.) and appear to be minimal or absent with the newer ones (acrivastine, astemizole, cetirizine, desloratadine, ebastine, fexofenadine, levocabastine, loratadine, mizolastine, terfenadine). Some of the more sedative antihistamines occur in cough, cold and influenza remedies.

Clinical evidence

The antihistamines can be broadly subdivided into (a) the most sedative, (b) those which are less sedative, and (c) those which cause little or no sedation.

(a) Alcohol + the most sedative antihistamines (chlorphenamine (chlorpheniramine), dexchlorpheniramine, diphenhydramine, promethazine)

Significant impairment of psychomotor performance was seen in subjects given 12 mg **chlorphenamine (chlorpheniramine)** with alcohol (0.5 g/kg body weight).[1] Alcohol (0.75 g/kg) and **dexchlorpheniramine** (4 mg/70 kg) given to 13 subjects significantly impaired their performance of a number of tests (standing steadiness, reaction time, manual dexterity, perception, etc.).[2] Other studies also describe this interaction.[3] **Diphenhydramine** in doses of 25 or 50 mg was shown to increase the detrimental effects of alcohol on the performance of choice reaction and co-ordination tests by subjects who had taken 0.5–0.68 mg/kg alcohol; its interaction in doses of 50, 75 or 100 mg has been confirmed in other reports.[4-9] A marked interaction can also occur with **promethazine**.[10] A very marked deterioration in driving skills was clearly demonstrated in a test of car drivers given 20 ml *Beechams Night Nurse* (promethazine + dextromethorphan), 10 ml *Benylin* (diphenhydramine + dextromethorphan), or 30 ml *Lemsip Night time flu medicine* (**chlorphenamine + dextromethorphan**). Very poor scores were seen when they were additionally given a double **Scotch whisky** about 1.5 h later.[11]

(b) Alcohol + less sedative antihistamines (clemastine, clemizole, cyclizine, cyproheptadine, mebhydrolin, pheniramine, tripelennamine, triprolidine)

The effects of alcohol (blood levels about 50 mg%) and antihistamines, alone or together, on the performance of tests designed to assess mental and motor performance were examined in 16 subjects. **Clemizole** (40 mg) or **tripelennamine** (50 mg), did not significantly affect the performance under the stress of delayed auditory feedback. **Clemastine** in 3-mg doses also affected co-ordination, whereas 1.5 mg and 1 mg did not.[12,13] A study[14] on five subjects showed that the detrimental effects of 100 ml **whiskey** on the performance of driving tests on a racing car simulator (blood alcohol estimated as less than 80 mg%) were not increased by 50 mg **cyclizine**. However three of the subjects experienced drowsiness after **cyclizine**, and other studies[15] have shown that **cyclizine** alone causes drowsiness in the majority. A study in 20 subjects of the effects of alcohol and **mebhydrolin** (0.71 mg/kg) found that the performance of a number of tests on perceptual, cognitive and motor functions was impaired to some extent.[16] No interaction was detected in one study of the combined effects of 4 mg **pheniramine** or 4 mg **cyproheptadine** and alcohol (0.7 g/kg),[17] however **triprolidine** (10 mg) worsens the deterioration in driving caused by alcohol.[18,19] A marked deterioration in driving skills has been demonstrated with 10 ml *Actifed Syrup* (**triprolidine + pseudoephedrine**) alone and with a double **whiskey**.[11]

(c) Alcohol + least sedative antihistamines (acrivastine, astemizole, cetirizine, desloratadine, ebastine, fexofenadine, levocabastine, loratadine, mizolastine, terfenadine)

Acrivastine (4 and 8 mg) with and without alcohol was found in a study to behave like **terfenadine** (which interacts minimally or not at all).[20] A double blind study found that **terfenadine** alone (60 to 240 mg) did not affect psychomotor skills, nor did it affect the adverse effects of alcohol,[6] however a later study found that 240 mg slowed braking reaction times in the laboratory both alone and with alcohol.[21] Other studies have shown that **astemizole** (10 to 30 mg daily),[1,22,23] **desloratadine**,[24] **ebastine** (20 mg),[25,26] **fexofenadine** (120 to 240 mg)[5] **levocabastine** (2 nasal puffs of 0.5 mg/ml),[27] **terfenadine** (60 mg), **loratadine** (10 to 20 mg)[18,19] and **mizolastine** (10 mg)[28,29] do not interact with alcohol. **Cetirizine** 10 mg also appeared not interact with alcohol in two studies[28-30] but some slight additive effects were detected in another.[31]

Mechanism

When an interaction occurs it appears to be due to the combined or additive central nervous depressant effects of both the alcohol and the antihistamine.

Importance and management

An adverse interaction between alcohol and the **most sedative antihistamines** (diphenhydramine, chlorphenamine (chlorpheniramine), promethazine) is well established and clinically important. Marked drowsiness can occur with these antihistamines taken alone which makes driving or handling other potentially dangerous machinery much more hazardous. This can be further worsened by alcohol. Remember that some of these antihistamines appear 'in disguise' as antiemetics, sedatives and as components of cough/cold and influenza remedies (e.g. *Benylin*, *Lemsip*, *Night Nurse*) which can be bought over the counter. Patients should be strongly warned.

The situation with some of the **less sedative antihistamines** (clemastine, clemizole, cyclizine, cyproheptadine, mebhydrolin, pheniramine, tripelennamine and triprolidine) is less clear cut, and tests with some of them failed to detect an interaction with normal doses and moderate amounts of alcohol, however it has been clearly seen with *Actifed Syrup* (containing triprolidine). It would therefore be prudent to issue some cautionary warning, particularly if the patient is likely to drive.

The **newest non-sedating antihistamines** (acrivastine, astemizole, cetirizine, ebastine, fexofenadine, levocabastine, loratadine, mizolas-

tine, terfenadine) seem to cause little or no drowsiness in most patients and the risks if taken alone or with alcohol appear to be minimal or absent.

The possible interactions of alcohol with other antihistamines not cited here do not seem to have been formally studied, but increased drowsiness and increased driving risks would be expected with any which caused some sedation. Patients should be warned. The risks with non-sedating antihistamines (e.g. **azelastine, epinastine, noberastine, setastine, tazifylline, temelastine**) are probably minimal, but this needs confirmation.

1. Hindmarch I, Bhatti JZ. Psychomotor effects of astemizole and chlorpheniramine, alone and in combination with alcohol. *Int Clin Psychopharmacol* (1987) 2, 117–19.
2. Franks HM, Hensley VR, Hensley WJ, Starmer GA, Teo RKC. The interaction between ethanol and antihistamines. 1: Dexchlorpheniramine. *Med J Aust* (1978) 1, 449–52.
3. Smith RB, Rossie GV, Orzechowski RF. Interactions of chlorpheniramine-ethanol combinations: acute toxicity and antihistamine activity. *Toxicol Appl Pharmacol* (1974) 28, 240.
4. Hughes FW, Forney RB. Comparative effect of three antihistaminic and ethanol on mental and motor performance. *Clin Pharmacol Ther* (1964) 5, 414–21.
5. Vermeeren A, O'Hanlon JF. Fexofenadine's effects, alone and with alcohol, on actual driving and psychomotor performance. *J Allergy Clin Immunol* (1998) 101, 306–11.
6. Moser L, Hüther KJ, Koch-Weser J, Lundt PV. Effects of terfenadine and diphenhydramine alone or in combination with diazepam or alcohol on psychomotor performance and subjective feelings. *Eur J Clin Pharmacol* (1978) 14, 417–23.
7. Baugh R, Calvert RT. The effects of diphenhydramine alone and in combination with ethanol on histamine skin response and mental performance. *Eur J Clin Pharmacol* (1977) 12, 201–4.
8. Burns M, Moskowitz H. Effects of diphenhydramine and alcohol on skills performance. *Eur J Clin Pharmacol* (1980) 17, 259–66.
9. Burns M. Alcohol and antihistamine in combination: effects on performance. *Alcohol Clin Exp Res* (1989) 13, 341.
10. Hedges A, Hills M, Maclay WP, Newman-Taylor AJ, Turner P. Some central and peripheral effects of meclastine, a new antihistaminic drug, in man. *J Clin Pharmacol* (1971) 11, 112–19.
11. Carter N. Cold cures drug alert. *Auto Express* (1992) November Issue 218, 15–16.
12. Linnoila M. Effects of drugs on psychomotor skills related to driving: antihistamines, chlormezanone and alcohol. *Eur J Clin Pharmacol* (1973) 5, 87.
13. Franks HM, Hensley VR, Hensley WJ, Starmer GA, Teo RKC. The interaction between ethanol and antihistamines. 2. Clemastine. *Med J Aust* (1979) 1, 185.
14. Hughes DTD, Cramer F, Knight GJ. Use of a racing car simulator for medical research. The effects of marzine and alcohol on driving performances. *Med Sci Law* (1967) 7, 200–4.
15. Brand JJ, Colquhoun WP, Gould AH, Perry WLM. (–)-Hyoscine and cyclizine as motion sickness remedies. *Br J Pharmacol Chemother* (1967) 30, 463–9.
16. Franks HM, Lawrie M, Schabinsky VV, Starmer GA, Teo RKC. The interaction between ethanol and antihistamines. 3. Mebhydrolin. *Med J Aust* (1981) 2, 447–9.
17. Landauer AA, Milner G. Antihistamines, alone and together with alcohol, in relation to driving safety. *J Forensic Med* (1971) 18, 127–39.
18. Riedel WJ, Schoenmakers EAJM, O'Hanlon JF. The effects of loratadine alone and in combination with alcohol on actual driving performance. Institute for Drugs, Safety and Behavior, University of Limburg, Maastricht, The Netherlands, August 1987.
19. O'Hanlon JF. Antihistamines and driving performance: The Netherlands. *J Respir Dis* (1988) (Suppl), S12–S17.
20. Cohen AF, Hamilton MJ, Peck AW. The effects of acrivastine (BW825C), diphenhydramine and terfenadine in combination with alcohol on human CNS performance. *Eur J Clin Pharmacol* (1987) 32, 279–88.
21. Bhatti JZ, Hindmarch I. The effects of terfenadine with and without alcohol on an aspect of car driving performance. *Clin Exp Allergy* (1989) 19, 609–11.
22. Bateman DN, Chapman PH, Rawlins MD. Lack of effect of astemizole on ethanol dynamics or kinetics. *Eur J Clin Pharmacol* (1983) 25, 567–8.
23. Moser L, Plum H, Bruckmann M. Interaktionen eines neuen Antihistaminikums mit Diazepam und Alkohol. *Med Welt* (1984) 35, 296–9.
24. Rikken G, Scharf M, Danzig M, Staudinger H. Desloratadine and alcohol coadministration: no increase in impairment of performance over that induced by alcohol alone. Poster at EAACI (European Academy of Allergy and Clinical Immunology) Conference, Lisbon, Portugal. 2-4 July 2000.
25. Mattila MJ, Kuitunen T. Ebastine, a non-sedative H1-antihistamine without alcohol interaction. *Eur J Pharmacol* (1990) 183, 1653–4.
26. Mattila MJ, Kuitunen T, Plétan Y. Lack of pharmacodynamic and pharmacokinetic interactions of the antihistamine ebastine with ethanol in healthy subjects. *Eur J Clin Pharmacol* (1992) 43, 179–84.
27. Nicholls A, Janssens M, James R. The effects of levocabastine and ethanol on psychomotor performance in healthy volunteers. *Allergy* (1993) 48 (Suppl 16), 34.
28. Stubbs D, Blondin P, Patat A, Bergougnan L, Irving A, Clough W. Lack of interaction between a new antihistamine, mizolastine, and ethanol on psychomotor and driving performance in healthy volunteers. *Br J Clin Pharmacol* (1995) 39, 570P.
29. Patat A, Stubbs D, Dunmore C, Ulliac N, Sexton B, Zieleniuk I, Irving A, Jones W. Lack of interaction between two antihistamines, mizolastine and cetirizine, and ethanol in psychomotor and driving performance in healthy subjects. *Eur J Clin Pharmacol* (1995) 48, 143–50.
30. Doms M, Vanhulle G, Baelde Y, Coulie P, Dupont P, Rihoux J-P. Lack of potentiation by cetirizine of alcohol-induced psychomotor disturbances. *Eur J Clin Pharmacol* (1988) 34, 619–23.
31. Ramaekers JG, Uiterwijk MMC, O'Hanlon JF. Effects of loratadine and cetirizine on actual driving and psychometric test performance, and EEG during driving. *Eur J Clin Pharmacol* (1992) 42, 363–9.

Alcohol + Aspirin and Salicylates

A small increase in the gastrointestinal blood loss caused by aspirin occurs in patients if they drink, but any increased damage to the lining of the stomach is small and appears usually to be of minimal importance in most normal individuals. Buffered aspirin, paracetamol (acetaminophen) and diflunisal do not interact in this way. Some limited information suggests that aspirin can raise or lower blood alcohol levels.

Clinical evidence

(a) Alcohol + unbuffered aspirin: effect on blood loss

The mean daily blood loss from the gut of 13 men was 0.4 ml while taking no medication, 3.2 ml while taking 2100 mg of soluble unbuffered aspirin (*Disprin*) and 5.3 ml while also taking 180 ml Australian whiskey (31.8% w/v ethanol). Alcohol alone did not cause gastrointestinal bleeding.[1]

A not dissimilar study showed that the daily blood loss increased from 2.15 to 5.32 ml when, in addition to 2400 mg aspirin daily, the subjects drank 140 ml vodka (40% alcohol) and 200 ml table wine.[2] An epidemiological study of patients admitted to hospital with gastrointestinal haemorrhage showed a statistical association between bleeding and the ingestion of aspirin with or without alcohol.[3] Endoscopic examination reveals that aspirin and alcohol have additive damaging effects on the gastric mucosa (not on the duodenum) but the extent is small.[4]

(b) Alcohol + buffered aspirin: effect on blood loss

No increased gastrointestinal bleeding occurred in 22 normal subjects given three double whiskeys (equivalent to 142 ml 40% ethanol) and 728 g sodium acetylsalicylate.[5]

(c) Alcohol + aspirin: effect on blood alcohol levels

(i) Alcohol levels increased. Five normal subjects were given a standard breakfast with and without 1 g aspirin, and an hour later they were given 0.3 g/kg alcohol. The aspirin increased the peak blood alcohol levels by 39% (from 5.44 to 7.56 mmol/l) and the AUC by 26% (from 8.83 to 11.11 mmol/l.h).[6] 28 normal subjects were given a midday meal (two sandwiches and a cup of tea or coffee), followed an hour later by 600 mg aspirin or a placebo, and then half-an-hour later by two standard drinks (35.5 ml of 37.5% vodka (21.6 g alcohol) plus 60 ml orange juice which were drunk within 15 min. The blood alcohol levels of the men were raised 31% after 1 h (from 24.29 to 31.85 mg%) and by 18% (from 20.82 to 24.57 mg%) after 2 h. The blood alcohol levels of the women subjects were raised 31% (from 37.39 to 49.23) after 1 h and by 21% (from 37.56 to 45.54 mg%) after 2 h.[7]

(ii) Alcohol levels largely unchanged. A later study (effectively a repeat of a study[6] above) in 12 subjects failed to find any effect on blood alcohol levels, but peak aspirin levels were reduced 25%.[8] A crossover trial in 10 normal male subjects found that after taking 75 mg aspirin daily for a week, their mean blood alcohol AUC following a 0.3 g/kg dose was smaller, but not statistically significant. Individual maximum blood levels varied. One subject showed a rise, two were unchanged, and five were lowered.[9]

Mechanisms

(a) & (b). Aspirin and alcohol can damage the mucosal lining of the stomach, one measure of the injury being a fall in the gastric potential difference. An additive fall has been seen with unbuffered aspirin and alcohol, whereas an increase occurs with buffered aspirin.[10] Once the protective mucosal barrier is breached, exfoliation of the cells occurs and damage to the capillaries follows. Aspirin causes a marked prolongation in bleeding times, and this can be increased by alcohol.[11] The total picture is complex.

(c). The increased blood alcohol levels in the presence of food and aspirin may possibly occur because the aspirin reduces the enzymic oxidation of the alcohol by the gastric mucosa (by alcohol dehydrogenase), so that more remains available for absorption.[6] Any decreases with low dose aspirin may possibly be due to delayed gastric emptying.[9]

Importance and management

The combined effect of aspirin and alcohol on the stomach wall is established. 3 g aspirin daily for a period of 3–5 days induces an average blood loss of about 5 ml or so. Some increased loss undoubtedly occurs with alcohol, but it seems to be quite small and unlikely to be of much importance in most normal individuals using moderate doses. In one study it was found that alcohol was a mild damaging agent or a mild potentiating agent for other damaging drugs.[4] Buffered aspirin, paracetamol (acetaminophen) or diflunisal[2] are preferable because they do not interact with alcohol.[4] On the other hand it should be remembered that chronic and/or gross overuse of salicylates and alcohol may result in gastric ulceration.

Information about the increase in blood alcohol levels caused by aspirin after food is very limited and contradictory, and of uncertain practical importance. However no practically relevant interaction has been seen with other drugs (e.g. the H₂-blockers) which have been very extensively studied and which appear to interact by the same mechanism. The pattern for these drugs is that the increases in blood alcohol levels are appreciable with small doses of alcohol, but usually they become proportionately too small to matter with larger doses of alcohol (i.e. those which give blood and breath levels at or around the legal driving limit in the UK). More study of this interaction is needed.

1. Goulston K, Cooke AR. Alcohol, Aspirin and gastrointestinal bleeding. *BMJ* (1968) 4, 644.
2. DeSchepper PJ, Tjandramaga TB, De Roo M, Verhaest L, Daurio C, Steelman SL, Tempero KF. Gastrointestinal blood loss after diflunisal and after aspirin: effect of ethanol. *Clin Pharmacol Ther* (1978) 23, 669–76.
3. Needham CD, Kyle J, Jones PF, Johnstone SJ, Kerridge DF. Aspirin and alcohol in gastrointestinal haemorrhage. *Gut* (1971) 12, 819.
4. Lanza FL, Royer GL, Nelson RS, Rack MF, Seckman CC. Ethanol, aspirin, ibuprofen, and the gastroduodenal mucosa: an endoscopic assessment. *Gastroenterology* (1985) 80, 767–9.
5. Bouchier JAD, Williams HS. Determination of faecal blood-loss after combined alcohol and sodium acetylsalicylate intake. *Lancet* (1969) i, 178.
6. Roine R, Gentry T, Hernández-Munõz R, Baraona E, Lieber CS. Aspirin increases blood alcohol concentrations in humans after ingestion of ethanol. *JAMA* (1990) 264, 2406–8.
7. Sharma SC, Feeley J. The influence of aspirin and paracetamol on blood concentrations of alcohol in young adults. *Br J Clin Pharmacol* (1996) 41, 467P.
8. Melander O, Lidén A, Melander A. Pharmacokinetic interactions of alcohol and acetylsalicylic acid. *Eur J Clin Pharmacol* (1995) 48, 151–3.
9. Kechagias S, Jönsson K-Å, Norlander B, Carlsson B, Jones AW. Low-dose aspirin decreases blood alcohol concentrations by delaying gastric emptying. *Eur J Clin Pharmacol* (1997) 53, 241–6.
10. Murray HS, Strottman MP, Cooke AR. Effect of several drugs on gastric potential differences in man. *BMJ* (1974) 1, 19.
11. Rosove MH, Harwig SSL. Confirmation that ethanol potentiates aspirin-induced prolongation of the bleeding time. *Thromb Res* (1983) 31, 525–7.

Alcohol + Barbiturates

Alcohol and the barbiturates are CNS depressants which together can have additive (possibly more than additive) effects. Activities requiring alertness and good co-ordination, such as driving a car or handling other potentially dangerous machinery, will be made more difficult and more hazardous. Alcohol may also continue to interact next day if the barbiturate has hangover effects.

Clinical evidence

A study in man of the effects of alcohol (0.5 g/kg), taken in the morning after using 100 mg amobarbital (amylobarbitone) as a hypnotic the night before, showed that the performance of co-ordination skills was much more impaired than with either drug alone.[1]

This increased CNS depression due to combined use has been described in a number of other clinical studies,[2-4] and has featured very many times in coroners' reports of fatal accidents and suicides.[5] A study of the fatalities due to this interaction indicated that with some barbiturates the CNS depressant effects are more than additive.[6]

There is also some evidence that blood alcohol levels may be reduced in the presence of a barbiturate.[3,7,8]

Mechanisms

Both alcohol and the barbiturates are CNS depressants, and simple additive CNS depression provides part of the explanation. The Ferguson principle may account for the more than additive effects.[9] Acute alcohol ingestion may inhibit the liver enzymes concerned with the metabolism of the barbiturates.[4,10]

Importance and management

Few formal studies in normal clinical situations have been made of the alcohol/barbiturate interactions but the effects (particularly those which are fatal) are very well established, serious and of clinical importance. The most obvious hazards are increased drowsiness, lack of alertness and impaired co-ordination which make the handling of potentially dangerous machinery (e.g. car driving) more difficult and dangerous. But it has also been rightly pointed out[11] that other risks are increased: ". . . many old people may have a whiskey nightcap with their barbiturate sleeping pill. They then have to get out of bed in the middle of the night to empty their bladder; they are unsteady, they fall, they are found in the morning with a fractured femur or in a hypothermic state. No figures are available to give a reliable idea of the scale of this problem . . ." Only amobarbital (amylobarbitone) is specifically referenced here but this interaction would be expected with all of the barbiturates (e.g. **phenobarbital (phenobarbitone), methylphenobarbital (methylphenobarbitone), butobarbital (butobarbitone), secobarbital (quinalbarbitone)**, etc). Some barbiturate hangover effects may be present next morning and may therefore continue to interact significantly with alcohol. Patients should be warned.

1. Saario I, Linnoila M. Effect of subacute treatment with hypnotics alone or in combination with alcohol, on psychomotor skills relating to driving. *Acta Pharmacol Toxicol* (1976) 38, 382–92.
2. Kielholz P, Goldberg L, Obersteg JI, Pöldinger W, Ramseyer A, Schmid P. Fahrversuche zur frage der beeinträchtigung der Verkehrstüchtigkeit durch alkohol, tranquilizer und hypnotika. *Dtsch Med Wochenschr* (1969) 94, 301–6.
3. Morselli PL, Veneroni E, Zaccala M, Bizzi A. Further observations on the interaction between ethanol and psychotropic drugs. *Arzneimittelforschung* (1971) 21, 20–3.
4. Wegener VH, Kötter L. Analgetica und verkehrstüchtigkeit: wirkung einer kombination von 5-allyl-5-isobutylsäure, dimethylaminophenazon und coffeine nach einmaliger und wiederholter applikation. *Arzneimittelforschung* (1971) 21, 47–51.
5. Gupta RC, Kofoed J. Toxicological statistics for barbiturates, other sedatives, and tranquillizers in Ontario. *Can Med Assoc J* (1966) 94, 863–5.
6. Stead AH, Moffat AC. Quantification of the interaction between barbiturates and alcohol and interpretation of fatal blood concentrations. *Hum Toxicol* (1983) 2, 5–14.
7. Mould GP, Curry SH, Binns TB. Interaction of glutethimide and phenobarbitone with ethanol in man. *J Pharm Pharmacol* (1972) 24, 894–9.
8. Mezey E, Robles EA. Effects of phenobarbital administration on rates of ethanol clearance and on ethanol-oxidising enzymes in man. *Gastroenterology* (1974) 66, 248.
9. King LA. Thermodynamic interpretation of synergism in barbiturate/ethanol poisoning. *Hum Toxicol* (1985) 4, 633–5.
10. Rubin E, Lieber CS. Inhibition of drug metabolism by acute ethanol intoxication. A hepatic microsomal mechanism. *Am J Med* (1970) 49, 801.
11. Wilkes E. Are you still prescribing those outdated drugs? *MIMS Magazine* (1976) 27, 84.

Alcohol + Benzodiazepines and related drugs

Benzodiazepine and related tranquillisers increase the CNS depressant effects of alcohol to some extent, but usually less than other more obviously sedative drugs. The risks of car driving and handling other potentially dangerous machinery are increased. The risk is heightened because the patient may be unaware of being affected. Some hypnotic benzodiazepines used at night are still present in appreciable amounts next day and therefore may continue to interact if the patient carries on drinking.

Clinical evidence

It is very difficult to assess and compare the results of the very many studies of this interaction because of the differences between the tests, their duration, the dosages of the benzodiazepines and alcohol, whether given chronically or acutely, and a number of other varia-

bles. However the overall picture seems to be that **diazepam**[1-13] has a more marked effect than **chlordiazepoxide**,[1,14-19] **medazepam**,[20] or **oxazepam**,[8] but possibly the same as **triazolam**.[21,22] The effects of **lormetazepam** may be greater than **diazepam**.[23] The potencies of **adinazolam**,[24] **alpidem**,[25] **alprazolam**,[26-28] **bromazepam**,[29] **clobazam**,[30] **lorazepam**,[12,25,31,32] **oxazolam**,[33] **metaclazepam**,[34] **potassium clorazepate**[35] and **zopiclone**[36,37] are unclear, but **brotizolam** seems to have a small effect.[38] Those on **lorazepam** and **triazolam** may be unaware of the extent of the impairment which occurs[21,31] and the anxiolytic effects of **lorazepam** may be opposed by alcohol.[32] **Alprazolam** and alcohol together may possibly increase behavioural aggression.[39]

The hypnotic benzodiazepines **flurazepam**,[40-42] **nitrazepam**,[4,43] **temazepam**[41] and **flunitrazepam**[36,44] when taken the night before can interact with alcohol the next morning, but **midazolam**[45,46] **triazolam**[37] and **zopiclone**[37] appear not to do so. **Loprazolam** may mitigate the effects of alcohol and may possibly have less of a hangover effect.[47] Alcohol appears to have minimal effects on the pharmacokinetics of **zopiclone**.[48]

Mechanism

The CNS depressant actions of the benzodiazepines and alcohol are additive. Alcohol also increases the absorption and raises the serum levels of some benzodiazepines.[30,49,50]

Importance and management

Extensively studied, well established and clinically important interactions. The overall picture is that these drugs worsen the detrimental effects of alcohol.[51] Up to a 20–30% increase has been suggested.[21] The deterioration in skills will depend on the particular drug in question (see 'Clinical evidence' above), its dosage and the amounts of alcohol taken. With modest amounts of alcohol the effects may be quite small in most patients (although a few may be more markedly affected[13]), but anyone taking any of these drugs should be warned that their usual response to alcohol may be greater than expected, and their ability to drive a car, or carry out any other tasks requiring alertness, may be impaired. They may be quite unaware of the deterioration. Benzodiazepines and alcohol are frequently found in the blood of car drivers involved in traffic accidents which suggests that the risks are real.[26,51,52] The warnings apply not only to the tranquillising benzodiazepines but also to some of the hypnotic benzodiazepines as well (flunitrazepam, flurazepam, nitrazepam, temazepam) because the body may still contain enough the next morning to continue to interact with alcohol.

1. Dundee JW, Isaac M. Interaction of alcohol with sedatives and tranquillizers (a study of blood levels at loss of consciousness following rapid infusion). *Med Sci Law* (1970) 10, 220.
2. Morselli PL, Veneroni E, Zaccala M, Bizzi A. Further observations on the interaction between ethanol and psychotropic drugs. *Arzneimittelforschung* (1971) 21, 20.
3. Linnoila M, Häkkinen S. Effects of diazepam and codeine, alone and in combination with alcohol, on simulated driving. *Clin Pharmacol Ther* (1974) 15, 368–73.
4. Linnoila M. Drug interaction on psychomotor skills related to driving: hypnotics and alcohol. *Ann Med Exp Biol Fenn* (1973) 51, 118–24.
5. Missen AW, Cleary W, Eng L, McMillan S. Diazepam, alcohol and drivers. *N Z Med J* (1978) 87, 275–7.
6. Laisu U, Linnoil M, Seppälä T, Himberg JJ, Mattila MJ. Pharmacokinetic and pharmacodynamic interactions of diazepam with different alcoholic beverages. *Eur J Clin Pharmacol* (1979) 16, 263.
7. Palva ES, Linnoila M, Saario I, Mattila MJ. Acute and subacute effects of diazepam on psychomotor skills: interaction with alcohol. *Acta Pharmacol Toxicol* (1979) 45, 257–64.
8. Molander L, Duvhök C. Acute effects of oxazepam, diazepam and methylperone, alone and in combination with alcohol on sedation, coordination and mood. *Acta Pharmacol Toxicol* (1976) 38, 145–60.
9. Curry SH, Smith CM. Diazepam-ethanol interaction in humans: addition or potentiation? *Commun Psychopharmacol* (1979) 3, 101–13.
10. Smiley A, Moskowitz H. Effects of long-term administration of buspirone and diazepam on driver steering control. *Am J Med* (1986) 80 (Suppl 3B), 22–9.
11. Erwin CW, Linnoila M, Hartwell J, Erwin A and Guthrie S. Effects of buspirone and diazepam, alone and in combination with alcohol, on skilled performance and evoked potentials. *J Clin Psychopharmacol* (1986) 6, 199–209.
12. Aranko K, Seppälä T, Pellinen J, Mattila MJ. Interaction of diazepam or lorazepam with alcohol. Psychomotor effects and bioassayed serum levels after single and repeated doses. *Eur J Clin Pharmacol* (1985) 28, 559–65.
13. van Steveninck AL, Gieschke R, Schoemaker HC, Pieters MSM, Kroon JM, Breimer DD, Cohen AF. Pharmacokinetic interactions of diazepam and intravenous alcohol at pseudo steady state. *Psychopharmacology (Berl)* (1993) 110, 471–8.
14. Reggiani G, Hurlimann A, Theiss E. Some aspects of the experimental and clinical toxicology of chlordiazepoxide. *Acta Pharmacol Toxicol* (1979) 45, 256.

15. Hughes FW, Forney RB, Richards AB. Comparative effect in human subjects of chlordiazepoxide, diazepam, and placebo on mental and physical performance. *Clin Pharmacol Ther* (1965) 6, 139–45.
16. Linnoila M. Effects of diazepam, chlordiazepoxide, thioridazine, haloperidol, flupenthixol and alcohol on psychomotor skills related to driving. *Ann Med Exp Biol Fenn* (1973) 51, 125–32.
17. Linnoila M, Saario I, Olkoniemi J, Liljequist R, Himberg JJ, Mäki M. Effect of two weeks' treatment with chlordiazepoxide or flupenthixol, alone or in combination with alcohol, on psychomotor skills related to driving. *Arzneimittelforschung* (1975) 25, 1088–92.
18. Hoffer A. Lack of potentiation by chlordiazepoxide (Librium) of depression or excitation due to alcohol. *Can Med Assoc J* (1962) 87, 920–1.
19. Kielholz P, Goldberg L, Obersteg JI, Pöldinger W, Ramseyer A, Schmid P. Fahrversuche zur frage der beeinträchtigung der Verkehrstüchtigkeit durch alkohol, tranquilizer und hypnotika. *Dtsch Med Wochenschr* (1969) 94, 301–6.
20. Landauer AA, Pocock DA, Prott FW. The effect of medazepam on cognitive and motor skills used in car driving. *Psychopharmacologia* (1974) 37, 159–68.
21. Dorian P, Sellers EM, Kaplan HL, Hamilton C, Greenblatt DJ, Abernethy D. Triazolam and ethanol interaction: kinetic and dynamic consequences. *Clin Pharmacol Ther* (1985) 37, 558–62.
22. Ochs HR, Greenblatt DJ, Arendt RM, Hubbel W, Shader RI. Pharmacokinetic noninteraction of triazolam and ethanol. *J Clin Psychopharmacol* (1984) 4,106–7.
23. Willumeit H-P, Ott H, Neubert W, Hemmerling K-G, Schratzer M, Fichte K. Alcohol interaction of lormetazepam, mepindolol sulphate and diazepam measured by performance on the driving simulator. *Pharmacopsychiatry* (1984) 17, 36–43.
24. Linnoila M, Stapleton JM, Moss H, Lane E, Granger A, Greenblatt DJ, Eckardt MJ. Effects of adinazolam and diazepam, alone and in combination with ethanol, on psychomotor and cognitive performance and on autonomic nervous system reactivity in healthy volunteers. *Eur J Clin Pharmacol* (1990) 38, 371–7.
25. Allen D, Baylav A, Lader M. A comparative study of the interaction of alcohol with alpidem, lorazepam and placebo in normal studies. *Int Clin Psychopharmacol* (1988) 3, 327–41.
26. Chan AWK. Effects of combined alcohol and benzodiazepine: a review. *Drug Alcohol Depend* (1984) 13, 315–41.
27. Linnoila M, Stapleton JM, Lister R, Moss H, Lane E, Granger A, Eckardt MJ. Effects of single doses of alprazolam and diazepam, alone and in combination with ethanol, on psychomotor and cognitive performance and on autonomic nervous system reactivity in healthy volunteers. *Eur J Clin Pharmacol* (1990) 39, 21–8.
28. Rush CR, Griffiths RR. Acute participant-rated and behavioral effects of alprazolam and buspirone, alone and in combination with ethanol, in normal volunteers. *Exp Clin Psychopharmacol* (1997) 5, 28–38.
29. Seppälä T, Saario I, Mattila MJ. Two weeks' treatment with chlorpromazine, thioridazine, sulpiride, or bromazepam: actions and interactions with alcohol on psychomotor skills relating to driving. *Mod Probl Pharmacopsychiatry* (1976) 11, 85–90.
30. Tauber K, Badian M, Brettell HF, Royen Th, Rupp K, Sitting W, Uihlein M. Kinetic and dynamic interaction of clobazam and alcohol. *Br J Clin Pharmacol* (1979) 7, 91S.
31. Seppälä T, Aranko K, Mattila MJ, Shrotriya RC. Effects of alcohol on buspirone and lorazepam actions. *Clin Pharmacol Ther* (1982) 32, 201–7.
32. Lister RG, File SE. Performance impairment and increased anxiety resulting from the combination of alcohol and lorazepam. *J Clin Psychopharmacol* (1983) 3, 66–71.
33. Hopes VH, Debus G. Untersuchungen zu kombinationseffekten von oxazolam und alkohol auf leistung und befinden bei gesunden probanden. *Arzneimittelforschung* (1984) 34, 921–6.
34. Schmidt VV. Experimentelle untersuchunger zur wechselwirkung zwischen alkohol und metaclazepam. *Beitr Gerichtl Med* (1983) 41, 413–7.
35. Staak M, Raff G, Nusser W. Pharmacopsychological investigations concerning the combined effects of dipotassium clorazepate and ethanol. *Int J Clin Pharmacol Biopharm* (1979) 17, 205–12.
36. Seppälä T, Nuotto E, Dreyfus JF. Drug–alcohol interactions on psychomotor skills: zopiclone and flunitrazepam. *Pharmacology* (1983) 27, (Suppl 2), 127–35.
37. Kuitunen T, Mattila MJ, Seppälä T. Actions and interactions of hypnotics on human performance: single doses of zopiclone, triazolam and alcohol. *Int Clin Psychopharmacol* (1990) 5 (Suppl 2), 115–30.
38. Scavone JM, Greenblatt DJ, Harmatz JS, Shader RI. Kinetic and dynamic interaction of brotizolam and ethanol. *Br J Clin Pharmacol* (1986) 21, 197–204.
39. Bond AJ, Silveira JC. Behavioural aggression following the combination of alprazolam and alcohol. *J Psychopharmacol* (1990) 4, 315.
40. Saario I, Mattila M. Effect of subacute treatment with hypnotics alone or in combination with alcohol on psychomotor skills related to driving. *Acta Pharmacol Toxicol* (1976) 38, 382.
41. Betts TA, Birtle J. Effect of two hypnotic drugs on actual driving performance next morning. *BMJ* (1982) 285, 852.
42. Hindmarch I, Gudgeon AC. Loprazolam (HR158) and flurazepam with ethanol compared on tests of psychomotor ability. *Eur J Clin Pharmacol* (1982) 23, 509–12.
43. Saario I, Linnoila M, Maki M. Interaction of drugs with alcohol on human psychomotor skills related to driving: effect of sleep deprivation or two weeks' treatment with hypnotics. *J Clin Pharmacol* (1975) 15, 52–9.
44. Linnoila M, Erwin CW, Brendle A, Logue P. Effects of alcohol and flunitrazepam on mood and performance in healthy young men. *J Clin Pharmacol* (1981) 21, 430–5.
45. Hindmarch I, Subhan Z. The effects of midazolam in conjunction with alcohol on sleep, psychomotor performance and car driving ability. *Int J Clin Pharmacol Res* (1983) III, 323–9.
46. Lichtor JL, Zacny J, Korttila K, Apfelbaum JL, Lane BS, Rupani G, Thisted RA, Dohrn C. Alcohol after midazolam sedation: does it really matter? *Anesth Analg* (1991) 72, 661–6.
47. McManus IC, Ankier SI, Norfolk J, Phillips M, Priest RG. Effects of psychological performance of the benzodiazepine loprazolam alone and with alcohol. *Br J Clin Pharmacol* (1983) 16, 291–300.
48. Larivière L, Caillé G, Elie R. The effects of low and moderate doses of alcohol on the pharmacokinetic parameters of zopiclone. *Biopharm Drug Dispos* (1986) 7, 207–10.
49. MacLeod SM, Giles HG, Patzalek G, Thiessen JJ, Sellers EM. Diazepam actions and plasma concentrations following ethanol ingestion. *Eur J Clin Pharmacol* (1977) 11, 345–9.
50. Laisi U, Linnoila M, Seppälä T, Himberg J-J, Mattila MJ. Pharmacokinetic and pharmacodynamic interactions of diazepam with different alcoholic beverages. *Eur J Clin Pharmacol* (1979) 16, 263–70.
51. Schuster R, Bodem M. Evaluation of ethanol-benzodiazepine-interactions using blood sampling protocol data. *Blutalkohol* (1997) 34, 54–65.
52. Staub C, Lacalle H, Fryc O. Présence de psychotropes dans le sang de conducteurs responsable d'accidents de la route ayant consommé en même temps de l'alcool. *Soz Praeventivmed* (1994) 39, 143–9.

Alcohol + Bretazenil

A normal dose of bretazenil plus a moderate amount of alcohol can have marked sedative effects.

Clinical evidence, mechanism, importance and management

A comparative study in 12 normal subjects given single oral doses of 0.5 mg **bretazenil** or 10 mg diazepam and an intravenous infusion of alcohol to achieve a steady-state of 50 mg/100 ml found that no pharmacokinetic interactions occurred, and no clear synergistic or supra-additive pharmacodynamic interactions (as measured by various tests) were seen, but very obvious additive sedative effects occurred. With **bretazenil** or diazepam plus alcohol the subjects were highly sedated, often unable to carry out the tests adequately and tended to fall asleep.[1] In practical terms this means that combined use should be avoided by patients who need to carry out tasks requiring attention and alertness (e.g. handling machinery or driving), but it may be advantageous for those who want to sleep. A blood alcohol level of 50 mg/100 ml is achievable by a man after drinking 4 units of alcohol or by a woman after 2 units (that is to say with only moderate social amounts).

1. Van Steveninck AL, Gieschke R, Schoemaker RC, Roncari G, Tuk B, Pieters MSM, Breimer DD, Cohen AF. Pharmacokinetic and pharmacodynamic interactions of bretazenil and diazepam with alcohol. *Br J Clin Pharmacol* (1996) 41, 565–73.

Alcohol + Bromisoval or Ethinamate

The detrimental effects of alcohol on the skills related to driving are made worse by bromisoval, but the interaction with ethinamate is mild. Both show hangover effects and can interact with alcohol next morning.

Clinical evidence, mechanism, importance and management

A study on a very large number of subjects given 1 g **ethinamate** or 0.6 g **bromisoval**, either alone or with 0.5 g/kg alcohol, showed that the performance of a number of psychomotor skills related to driving was slightly impaired by **ethinamate**, but strongly impaired by **bromisoval**. There was sufficient hangover for both drugs to interact with alcohol next morning after being used as hypnotics the night before.[1] The CNS depressant effects of these hypnotics and alcohol would seem to be additive. Patients should be warned.

1. Linnoila M. Drug interaction on psychomotor skills related to driving: hypnotics and alcohol. *Ann Med Exp Biol Fenn* (1973) 51, 118–24.

Alcohol + Butyraldoxime

A disulfiram-like reaction can occur in those exposed to *N*-butyraldoxime if they drink alcohol.

Clinical evidence, mechanism, importance and management

Workers in a printing company complained of flushing of the face, shortness of breath, tachycardia and drowsiness very shortly after drinking quite small quantities of alcohol (1.5 oz of **whiskey**), and were found to have increased levels of acetaldehyde in their blood. The reason appeared to be that the printing ink they were using contained *N*-butyraldoxime, an antioxidant which, like disulfiram, can inhibit the metabolism of alcohol so that acetaldehyde accumulates (see 'Alcohol + Disulfiram', p.27).[1] This reaction would seem to be more unpleasant and socially disagreeable than serious. No treatment normally seems necessary.

1. Lewis W, Schwartz L. An occupational agent (N-butyraldoxime) causing reaction to alcohol. *Med Ann DC* (1956) 25, 485–90.

Alcohol + Caffeine

Despite popular belief, objective tests show that caffeine does not counteract the effects of alcohol. It does not sober up those who have drunk too much and may even make them more accident-prone.

Clinical evidence, mechanism, importance and management

A study on a large number of subjects given 300 mg **caffeine**, either alone or with alcohol (0.75 g/kg), found that **caffeine** did not antagonise the deleterious effect of alcohol on the performance of psychomotor skill tests. Only reaction times were reversed.[1] Two other tests also failed to find that **caffeine** antagonised the effects of alcohol.[2,3] Yet another test carried out on 8 subjects found that, contrary to expectations, **caffeine** increased the frequency of errors in the performance of a serial reaction task.[4] A further study found no evidence that **caffeine** opposed the actions of alcohol, instead it appeared to increase its detrimental effects.[5] The reasons are not understood.

As long ago as 1894 Walsh[6] claimed that ". . . those who may desire to rescue a drunkard from his bane will find no better substitute for strong, fresh-made coffee [which] must be administered without the addition of either milk or sugar . . ." Even so, despite this long standing and time-hallowed belief in the value of strong black **coffee** to sober up those who have drunk too much, it now seems that it is not effective, except possibly that the time taken to drink the coffee gives the liver just a little more time to metabolise some of the alcohol. **Coffee** and other sources of **caffeine** do not make it safe to drive or handle dangerous machinery, and it may even make drivers more accident-prone.

1. Franks HM, Hagedorn H, Hensley VR, Hensley WJ, Starmer GA. The effect of caffeine on human performance, alone and in combination with alcohol. *Psychopharmacologia* (1975) 45, 177–81.
2. Nuotto E, Mattila MJ, Seppälä T, Konno K. Coffee and caffeine and alcohol effects on psychomotor function. *Clin Pharmacol Ther* (1982) 31, 68–76.
3. Newman HW, Newman EJ. Failure of dexedrine and caffeine as practical antagonists of the depressant effect of ethyl alcohol in man. *Quart J Stud Alc* (1956) 17, 406–10.
4. Lee DJ, Lowe G. Interaction of alcohol and caffeine in a perceptual-motor task. *IRCS Med Sci* (1980) 8, 420.
5. Osborne DJ, Rogers Y. Interactions of alcohol and caffeine on human reaction time. *Aviat Space Environ Med* (1983) 54, 528–34.
6. Walsh JM. Coffee; its History, Classification and Description. Philadelphia; Winston; 1894.

Alcohol + Calcium carbimide or Nitrefazole

Alcohol causes a disulfiram-like reaction in patients taking calcium carbimide or nitrefazole. Both are used as alcohol deterrents.

Clinical evidence, mechanism, importance and management

Calcium carbimide (**calcium cyanamide**) and **nitrefazole** interact with alcohol in a similar way to disulfiram and by a similar mechanism (see 'Alcohol + Disulfiram', p.27). Both of them bind to aldehyde dehydrogenase but are said to have fewer side-effects because they do not bind to dopamine beta hydroxylase. Like disulfiram they are used to deter alcoholics from continuing to drink.[1-3]

1. Peachey JE *et al.* A comparative review of the pharmacological and toxicological properties of disulfiram and calcium carbimide. *J Clin Psychopharmacol* (1981) 1, 21–6.
2. Monteiro MG. Pharmacological treatment of alcoholism. *Aust N Z J Med* (1992) 22, 220–3.
3. Stockwell T, Sutherland G, Edwards G. The impact of a new alcohol sensitizing agent (nitrefazole) on craving in severely dependent alcoholics. *Br J Addict* (1984) 79, 403–9.

Alcohol + Calcium channel blockers

Blood alcohol levels can be raised by verapamil and may remain elevated for a much longer period of time. Alcohol may also increase the bioavailability of felodipine and nifedipine but amlodipine appears not to interact.

Clinical evidence

(a) Alcohol serum levels and effects increased

Ten normal subjects given 80 mg **verapamil** three times daily for 6 days were additionally given 0.8 g/kg alcohol on day 6. Peak serum alcohol levels were found to be raised by 16.7% (from 106.45 to 124.24 mg/dl) and the $AUC_{0-12 h}$ was raised by almost 30% (from 366 to 475 mg.h/dl). The time that serum alcohol levels exceeded 100 mg/dl was prolonged from 0.2 to 1.3 h and the subjects said they felt more intoxicated.[1] Another study carried out to find out if **verapamil** (80 or 160 mg) antagonises the effects of alcohol found no evidence that it does so.[2]

(b) Alcohol pharmacokinetics unchanged

A study in 30 normal subjects found that single and multiple doses of 10 mg **amlodipine** (with or without lisinopril and simvastatin) for 15 days had no effect on the pharmacokinetics of alcohol (0.8 g/kg) nor on subjective psychological performance.[3]

(c) Felodipine and Nifedipine effects increased

A study in 8 normal subjects given enough alcohol to maintain their blood levels at 0.8–1.2% found that their blood **felodipine** levels (following a single 10 mg oral dose) were approximately doubled (AUC + 77%, maximum serum levels + 98%). Diuresis was about doubled and heart rates were increased.[4] 0.8 g/kg alcohol (75 ml 94% alcohol + 75 ml orange juice) given to ten normal subjects increased the AUC of single 20 mg doses of **nifedipine** by 54%, but no significant changes in heart rate or blood pressure were seen.[5] Another study carried out to find out if **nifedipine** (10 or 20 mg) antagonises the effects of alcohol found no evidence that it does so.[2]

Mechanism

Not understood. It seems possible that the verapamil inhibits the metabolism of the alcohol by the liver, thereby reducing its loss from the body. Alcohol also appears to inhibit the metabolism of nifedipine.

Importance and management

Information seems to be limited to these reports and they need confirmation. An alcohol concentration rise of almost 17% by verapamil is quite small but it could be enough to lift legal blood levels to illegal levels if driving. Moreover the intoxicant effects of alcohol may persist for a much longer period of time (by a factor of five in this instance).[1] The clinical significance of the nifedipine/alcohol interaction is uncertain. Amlodipine appears not to interact.

1. Bauer LA, Schumock G, Horn J, Opheim K. Verapamil inhibits ethanol elimination and prolongs the perception of intoxication. *Clin Pharmacol Ther* (1992) 52, 6–10.
2. Perez-Reyes M, White WR, Hicks RE. Interaction between ethanol and calcium channel blockers in humans. *Alcohol Clin Exp Res* (1992) 16, 769–75.
3. Vincent J, Colangelo P, Baris B, Willavize S. Single and multiple doses of amlodipine do not alter the pharmacokinetics of alcohol in man. *Therapie* (1995) (Suppl) 50, 509.
4. Pentikainen PJ, Virolainen T, Tenhunen R, Aberg J. Acute alcohol intake increases the bioavailability of felodipine. *Clin Pharmacol Ther* (1994) 55, 148.
5. Qureshi S, Laganiere S, Caille G, Gossard D, Lacasse Y, McGilveray I. Effect of an acute dose of alcohol on the pharmacokinetics of oral nifedipine in humans. *Pharm Res* (1992) 9, 683–6.

Alcohol + Cannabis

Smoking cannabis (marijuana) alters the bioavailability of alcohol. The peak blood levels are reduced and delayed. The effects of drinking alcohol and smoking cannabis appear to be additive.

Clinical evidence, mechanism, importance and management

Fifteen normal subjects given 0.7 g/kg alcohol developed peak blood alcohol levels of 78.25 mg/dl at 50 min, but if they smoked a **cannabis cigarette** 30 min after the drink, their peak blood alcohol levels were only 54.8 mg/dl and they occurred at 105 min.[1] Combined use reduces the performance of psychomotor tests and those who use both drugs should expect the deleterious effects to be additive.[2]

1. Lukas SE, Benedikt R, Mendelson JH, Kouri E, Sholar M, Amass L. Marihuana attenuates the rise in plasma ethanol levels in human subjects. *Neuropsychopharmacology* (1992) 7, 77–81.
2. Bird K, Boleyn T, Chesher GB, Jackson DM, Starmer GA, Teo RK. Intercannabiol and cannabinoid-ethanol interactions and their effects on human performance. *Psychopharmacology (Berl)* (1980) 71, 181–8.

Alcohol + Cephalosporins

Disulfiram-like reactions can occur in those taking cefamandole (cephamandole), cefoperazone, cefmenoxime, cefotetan, latamoxef (moxalactam) and possibly cefonicid after drinking alcohol or following an injection of alcohol. This is not a general reaction of the commonly used cephalosporins but is confined to those with particular chemical structures.

Clinical evidence

A young man with cystic fibrosis was given 2 g **latamoxef (moxalactam)** intravenously every 8 h for pneumonia. After 3 days' treatment he drank, as was his custom, a can of **beer** with lunch. He rapidly became flushed with a florid macular eruption over his face and chest. This faded over the next 30 min but he complained of severe nausea and headache. A woman patient also on **latamoxef** became flushed, diaphoretic and nauseated after drinking a cocktail of **vodka** and tomato juice.[1]

This reaction has been described in at least 5 other subjects who drank alcohol while receiving **latamoxef**.[2-4] The symptoms experienced have included flushing of the face, arms and neck, shortness of breath, headache, tachycardia, dizziness, hyper- and hypotension, and vomiting. Similar reactions have been described in patients on **cefamandole (cephamandole)**,[5,6] **cefoperazone**,[7-13] **cefmenoxime**,[14] **cefonicid**[15] and **cefotetan**[16] after drinking **wine**, **beer**, or other alcoholic drinks,[17-19] and after the ingestion of an 8% alcoholic elixir.[10] It has also been seen following the injection of alcohol into the para-aortic space for celiac plexus block.[11]

Mechanism

These reactions appear to have the same pharmacological basis as the disulfiram/alcohol reaction (see 'Alcohol + Disulfiram', p.27). Three of these cephalosporins (latamoxef, cefamandole and cefoperazone) can raise blood acetaldehyde levels in *rats* when alcohol is given, but to a lesser extent than disulfiram.[2,18] It appears that it normally only occurs with cephalosporins which possess a methyltetrazolethiol group in the 3-position on the cephalosporin molecule,[20] but it has also been seen with cefonicid which possesses a methylsulphonthiotetrazole group instead.[15]

Importance and management

Established but unpredictable interactions of varying incidence. One out of 30 on **latamoxef** reacted according to one study[1] and in another

2 out of 10 did so.[4] Five out of 8 on **cefotetan** reacted.[16] The reaction appears normally to be more embarrassing or unpleasant and frightening than serious, with the symptoms subsiding spontaneously after a few hours. There is evidence that the severity varies (**cefoperazone > latamoxef > cefmetazole**.[21]). Treatment is not usually needed but there are two reports[3,5] of 2 elderly patients who needed treatment for hypotension which was life-threatening in one case;[3] plasma expanders and dopamine have been used as treatment.[3,5]

Because the reaction is unpredictable, warn all patients taking these potentially interacting cephalosporins that it can occur during and up to three days after the course of treatment is over. Advise them to avoid alcohol. Those with kidney or liver disease in whom the drug clearance is prolonged should wait a week. It should not be forgotten that some foods and pharmaceuticals contain substantial amounts of alcohol, and a reaction with some topically applied products cannot be excluded (see 'Alcohol + Disulfiram', p.27).

This disulfiram-like reaction is not a general reaction of all the cephalosporins. There are no reports of reactions in those taking **cefpirome**,[22] **cefalotin (cephalothin)**, **cefradine (cephradine)**, **cefoxitin**, **cefazolin (cephazolin)**, or **cefsulodin**.[23] Ceftizoxime is reported not interact with alcohol in man.[24] No interaction was seen with **cefonicid** in one placebo-controlled study,[25] nevertheless a case report describes a disulfiram-reaction in one patient.[15]

A number of others cephalosporins are possible candidates for this reaction because they possess the methyltetrazolethiol group in the 3-position. These include **cefminox**, **ceforanide**, **cefotiam**, **cefpiramide**, and **ceftriaxone**.[10,20]

1. Neu HC, Prince AS. Interaction between moxalactam and alcohol. *Lancet* (1980), i, 1422.
2. Buening MK, Wold JS, Isreal KS, Kammer RB. Disulfiram-like reaction to β-lactams. *JAMA* (1981) 245, 2027–8.
3. Brown KR, Guglielmo BJ, Pons VG, Jacobs RA. Theophylline elixir, moxalactam, and a disulfiram-like reaction. *Ann Intern Med* (1982) 97, 621–2.
4. Elenbaas RM, Ryan JL, Robinson WA. Singsank MJ, Harvey MJ, Klaasen CD. Investigation of the disulfiram-like activity of moxalactam. *Clin Pharmacol Ther* (1982) 32, 347–55.
5. Portier H, Chalopin JM, Freysz M, Tanter Y. Interaction between cephalosporins and alcohol. *Lancet* (1980), ii, 263.
6. Drummer S, Hauser WE, Remington JS. Antabuse-like effect of β-lactam antibiotics. *N Engl J Med* (1980) 303, 1417–18.
7. Foster TS, Raehl CL, Wilson HD. Disulfiram-like reaction associated with parenteral cephalosporin. *Am J Hosp Pharm* (1980) 37, 858–9.
8. Allaz AF, Dayer P, Fabre J, Rudhardt M, Balant L. Pharmacocinetique d'une novelle cephalosporine, la cefoperazone. *Schweiz Med Wochenschr* (1979), 109, 1999–2005.
9. Kemmerich B, Lode H. Cefoperazone — another cephalosporin associated with a disulfiram type alcohol incompatibility. *Infection* (1981) 9, 110.
10. Uri JV, Parks DB. Disulfiram-like reaction to certain cephalosporins. *Ther Drug Monit* (1983) 5, 219–24.
11. Umeda S, Arai T. Disulfiram-like reaction to moxalactam after celiac plexus alcohol block. *Anesth Analg* (1985) 64, 377–82.
12. Bailey RR, Peddie B, Blake E, Bishop V, Reddy J. Cefoperazone in the treatment of severe or complicated infections. *Drugs* (1981) 22 (Suppl 1), 76–86.
13. Ellis-Pegler RB, Lang SDR. Cefoperazone in Klebsiella Meningitis: A case report. *Drugs* (1981) 22 (Suppl 1), 69–71.
14. Kannangara DW, Gallagher K, Lefrock JL. Disulfiram-like reactions with newer cephalosporins: cefmenoxime. *Am J Med Sci* (1984) 287, 45–7.
15. Marcon G, Spolaor A, Scevola M, Zolli M, Carlassara GB. Effetto disulfiram-simile da cefonicid: prima segnalazione. *Recenti Prog Med* (1990) 81, 47–8.
16. Kline SS, Mauro VF, Forney RB, Freimer EH, Somani P. Cefotetan-induced disulfiram-type reactions and hypoprothrombinemia. *Antimicrob Agents Chemother* (1987) 31, 1328–31.
17. Reeves DS, Davies AJ. Antabuse effect with cephalosporins. *Lancet* (1980) ii, 540.
18. Yanagihara M, Okada K, Nozaki M, Tsurumi K, Fujimura H. Cephem antibiotics and alcohol metabolism. Disulfiram-like reaction resulting from intravenous administration of cephem antibiotics. *Fol Pharmacol Japon* (1982) 79, 55–60.
19. McMahon FG. Disulfiram-like reaction to a cephalosporin. *JAMA* (1980), 243, 2397.
20. Norrby SR. Adverse reactions and interactions with newer cephalosporin and cephamycin antibiotics. *Med Toxicol* (1987) 2, 32–46.
21. Nakamura K, Nakagawa A, Tanaka M. Effects of cephem antibiotics on ethanol metabolism. *Fol Pharmacol Japon* (1984) 83, 183–91.
22. Lassman HB, Hubbard JW, Chen B-L, Puri SK. Lack of interaction between cefpirome and alcohol. *J Antimicrob Chemother* (1992) 29 (Suppl A), 47–50.
23. McMahon FG. Quoted in 15 as personal communication.
24. McMahon FG, Noveck RJ. Lack of disulfiram-like reactions with ceftizoxime. *J Antimicrob Chemother* (1982) 10 (Suppl C), 129–33.
25. McMahon FG, Ryan JR, Jain AK, LaCorte W, Ginzler F. Absence of disulfiram-type reactions to single and multiple doses of cefonicid: a placebo-controlled study. *J Antimicrob Chemother* (1987) 20, 913–8.

Alcohol + Chloral hydrate

Both alcohol and chloral are CNS depressants and their effects may be additive, possibly even more than additive. Some patients may experience a disulfiram-like flushing reaction if they drink after taking chloral for several days.

Clinical evidence

Studies in 5 subjects given **chloral** (15 mg/kg) and alcohol (0.5 g/kg) found that both drugs given alone impaired their ability to carry out complex motor tasks. When taken together, the effects were additive, and possibly even more than additive. After taking **chloral** for 7 days, one of the subjects experienced a disulfiram-like reaction (bright red-purple flushing of the face, tachycardia, hypotension, anxiety and persistent headache) after drinking alcohol.[1,2]

The disulfiram-like reaction has been described in other reports.[3,4] One of these was published more than a century ago in 1872 and describes 2 patients on **chloral** who experienced this reaction after drinking only half a bottle of **beer**.[3]

Mechanism

Alcohol, chloral and trichloroethanol (to which chloral is metabolised) are all CNS depressants. During concurrent use, the metabolic pathways used for their elimination are mutually inhibited: blood-alcohol levels rise because the trichloroethanol competitively depresses the oxidation of alcohol to acetaldehyde, while trichloroethanol levels also rise because its production from chloral is increased and its further conversion and clearance as the glucuronide is inhibited. As a result the rises in the blood levels of alcohol and trichloroethanol are exaggerated, and their effects are accordingly greater.[1,2,5,6] Blood levels of acetaldehyde are raised by only 50% during the use of chloral, so that the flushing reaction, despite its resemblance to the disulfiram reaction, may possibly have a partially different basis.[2]

Importance and management

A well-documented and established interaction. Only a few references are given here. A comprehensive bibliography is to found in references 1 and 2. Patients given chloral should be warned about the extensive CNS depression which can occur if they drink, and of the disulfiram-like reaction which may occur after taking chloral for a period of time. Its incidence is uncertain. The legendary Mickey Finn which is concocted of chloral and alcohol is reputed to be so potent that deep sleep can be induced in an unsuspecting victim within minutes of ingestion, but the evidence seems largely to be anecdotal. Very large doses of both would be likely to cause serious and potentially life-threatening CNS depression.

It seems likely that **chloral betaine**, **triclofos** and other compounds closely related to chloral hydrate will interact with alcohol in a similar manner, but this requires confirmation.

1. Sellers EM, Carr G, Bernstein JG, Sellers S, Koch-Weser J. Interaction of chloral hydrate and ethanol in man. II. Hemodynamic and performance. *Clin Pharmacol Ther* (1972) 13, 50–8.
2. Sellers EM, Lang M, Koch-Weser J, LeBlanc E, Kalant H. Interaction of chloral hydrate and ethanol in man. I. Metabolism. *Clin Pharmacol Ther* (1972) 13, 37–49.
3. Bjorstrom F. On the effect of alcoholic beverages and simultaneous use of chloral. *Uppsala Lakareforenings Forhandlingar* (1872) 8, 114.
4. Bardodej Z. Intolerance alkohlu po chloralhydratu. *Cesk Farm* (1965) 14, 478.
5. Owens AH, Marshall EK, Brown GO. A comparative evaluation of the hypnotic potency of chloral hydrate and trichloroethanol. *Bull Johns Hopkins Hosp* (1955) 96, 71.
6. Wong LK, Biemann K. A study of drug interaction by gas chromatography–mass spectrometry—synergism of chloral hydrate and ethanol. *Biochem Pharmacol* (1978) 27, 1019–22.

Alcohol + Cimetidine, Famotidine, Nizatidine or Ranitidine

Although some studies have found that blood alcohol levels can be raised to some extent in those taking some H_2-blockers (cimetidine, ranitidine, nizatidine) and possibly remain elevated for longer than usual, others report that no significant interaction occurs. This interaction is not established. Drinking may worsen the gastrointestinal disease for which these H_2-blockers are being given.

Clinical evidence

(a) Evidence of an interaction

A double-blind study on 6 volunteers showed that after taking 1200 mg **cimetidine** daily for 7 days, their peak blood alcohol levels following the ingestion of 0.8 g/kg alcohol were raised about 12% (from 146 to 163 mg%). The AUC was increased about 7% (from 717 to 771 mg/100 ml/h). The subjects assessed themselves as being more intoxicated while taking **cimetidine** and alcohol than with alcohol alone.[1]

An essentially similar study[2,3] found that the blood alcohol levels were raised 17% (from 73 to 86 mg%) by **cimetidine** but not by **ranitidine**. A later study in 6 normal subjects found that 800 mg **cimetidine** daily for a week approximately doubled the AUC (from 0.89 to 1.64 mM.h) following a single 0.15 g/kg oral dose of alcohol and raised peak levels about 33%. No changes were seen when the alcohol was given intravenously.[4] Two- to threefold rises in blood alcohol concentrations are described in another study using **cimetidine** or **ranitidine**.[5] Another study in subjects given **cimetidine** or **ranitidine** for only two days showed that peak blood alcohol levels were raised by 17 and 27% respectively, and the time for which blood levels remained above the 80 mg% mark (the legal driving limit in the UK and some other countries) was prolonged by about one-third.[6] **Nizatidine** was said to inhibit the metabolism of alcohol in man, but little detail was given in the report.[7] A further study in subjects given 0.75 g/kg alcohol found that single 800 mg doses of **cimetidine**, 300 mg **nizatidine** or 300 mg **ranitidine** raised blood alcohol levels at 45 min by 26% (from 75.5 to 95.2 mg%), 17.5% (from 75.5 to 88.7 mg%) and 3.2% (75.5 to 78.0 mg%) respectively, and the AUCs at 120 min were increased by 25%, 20% and 9.8% respectively. Each of the subjects said they felt more inebriated after taking **cimetidine** or **nizatidine**.[8,9] Another study found that **cimetidine** almost doubled peak alcohol serum levels, whereas **ranitidine** raised the levels about 50%.[10]

(b) Evidence of no interaction

The makers of cimetidine (SKF) have on file three unpublished studies which failed to find any evidence that **cimetidine** or **ranitidine** significantly increased the blood levels of alcohol. One study was on 6 normal subjects given single 400 mg doses of **cimetidine**, another on 6 normal subjects given 1 g **cimetidine** daily for 14 days, and the last on 10 normal subjects given either 1 g **cimetidine** daily or 300 mg **ranitidine** daily.[11] A number of other studies also failed to demonstrate significant interactions involving either **cimetidine**, **ranitidine** or **famotidine** and a number of different alcoholic drinks.[12-20] Three other studies found that **famotidine** had no significant effect on blood alcohol levels.[8-10]

Mechanism

It would appear that the interacting H_2-blockers inhibit the activity of alcohol dehydrogenase (ADH) in the gastric mucosa so that more alcohol passes unmetabolised into the circulation, thereby raising the levels.[5,21-23]

Importance and management

The contrasting and apparently contradictory results cited here clearly show that this interaction is by no means established. An extensive review of the data concluded that the interaction is clinically insignificant.[24] Until the situation is fully resolved, it might be prudent to tell patients who are starting H_2-blockers to be alert for any increase in their response to alcohol. In any case they should restrict their drinking because alcohol may worsen peptic ulcer and other diseases.

1. Feely J, Wood AJJ. Effects of cimetidine on the elimination and actions of alcohol. *JAMA* (1982) 247, 2819–21.

2. Seitz HK, Bösche J, Czygan P, Veith S, Simon B, Kommerell B. Increased blood ethanol levels following cimetidine but not ranitidine. *Lancet* (1983) i, 760.
3. Seitz HK, Veith S, Czygan P, Bösche J, Simon B, Gugler R, Kommerell B. In vivo interactions between H₂-receptor antagonists and ethanol metabolism in man and in rats. *Hepatology* (1984) 4, 1231–4.
4. Caballeria J, Baraona E, Rodamilans M, Lieber CS. Effects of cimetidine on gastric alcohol dehydrogenase activity and blood alcohol levels. *Gastroenterology* (1989) 96, 388–92.
5. Roine R, DiPadova C, Frezza M, Hernández-Muñoz R, Baraona E, Lieber CS. Effects of omeprazole, cimetidine and ranitidine on blood ethanol concentrations. *Gastroenterology* (1990) 98, A114.
6. Webster LK, Jones DB, Smallwood RA. Influence of cimetidine and ranitidine on ethanol pharmacokinetics. *Aust N Z J Med* (1985) 15, 359–60.
7. Palmer RH. Cimetidine and alcohol absorption. *Gastroenterology* (1989) 97, 1066–8.
8. Guram M, Holt S. Are ethanol-H₂ receptor antagonist interactions "relevant"? *Gastroenterology* (1991) 100, 5 part 2, A749.
9. Holt S, Guram M, Howden CW. Evidence for an interaction between alcohol and certain H₂ receptor antagonists. *Gut* (1991) 32, A1220.
10. DiPadova C, Roine R, Frezza M, Gentry T, Baraona E, Lieber CS. Effects of ranitidine on blood alcohol levels after ethanol ingestion: comparison with other H₂-receptor antagonists. *JAMA* (1992) 267, 83–6.
11. Robson AS (Smith Kline and French). Personal communication (1989).
12. Dobrilla G, de Pretis G, Piazzi L, Chilovi F, Comberlato M, Valentini M, Pastorino A, Vallaperta P. Is ethanol metabolism affected by oral administration of cimetidine and ranitidine at therapeutic doses. *Hepatogastroenterology* (1984) 31, 35–7.
13. Johnston KI, Fenzl E, Hein B. Einfluss von Cimetidine auf den Abbau und die Wirkung des Alkohols. *Arzneimittelforschung* (1984) 34, 734–6.
14. Tanaka E, Nakamura K. Effects of H₂-receptor antagonists on ethanol metabolism in Japanese volunteers. *Br J Clin Pharmacol* (1988) 26, 96–9.
15. Tan OT, Stafford TJ, Sarkany I, Gaylarde PM, Tilsey C, Payne JP. Suppression of alcohol-induced flushing by a combination of H₁ and H₂ histamine antagonists. *Br J Dermatol* (1982) 107, 647–52.
16. Holtmann G, Singer MV. Histamine H₂ receptor antagonists and blood alcohol levels. *Dig Dis Sci* (1988) 33, 767–8.
17. Holtmann G, Singer MV, Knop D, Becker S, Goebell H. Effect of histamine-H₂-receptor antagonists on blood alcohol levels. *Gastroenterology* (1988) 94, A190.
18. Fraser AG, Prewett EJ, Hudson M, Sawyerr AM, Rosalki S, Pounder RE. Ranitidine, cimetidine and famotidine have no effect on alcohol absorption in healthy volunteers. *Gastroenterology* (1991) 100, A66.
19. Fraser AG, Prewett EJ, Hudson M, Sawyerr AM, Rosalki SB, Pounder RE. The effect of ranitidine, cimetidine or famotidine on low-dose post-prandial alcohol absorption. *Aliment Pharmacol Ther* (1991) 5, 263–72.
20. Jönsson K-Å, Jones AW, Boström H, Andersson T. No influence of omeprazole on the pharmacokinetics of ethanol in healthy men. World Congr Gastroenterology, Sydney, August 1990. Abstracts II, PD201.
21. Caballería J. Interactions between alcohol and gastric metabolizing enzymes: practical implications. *Clin Ther* (1991) 13, 511–20.
22. Fiatarone JR, Bennett MK, Kelly P, James OFW. Ranitidine but not gastritis or female sex reduces the first pass metabolism of ethanol. *Gut* (1991) 32, A594.
23. Caballería J, Baraona E, Deulofeu R, Hernández-Muñoz R, Rodés J, Lieber CS. Effects of H₂-receptor antagonists on gastric alcohol dehydrogenase activity. *Dig Dis Sci* (1991) 36, 1673–9.
24. Levitt MD. Review article: lack of clinical significance of the interaction between H₂-receptor antagonists and ethanol. *Aliment Pharmacol Ther* (1993) 7, 131–8.

Alcohol + Ciprofloxacin

Ciprofloxacin does not interact with alcohol.

Clinical evidence, mechanism, importance and management

A 3-day course of 500 mg **ciprofloxacin** twice daily had no significant effect on the pharmacokinetics of a single oral dose of **alcohol** (30 g/75 ml **vodka**) in 12 normal subjects, nor was the performance of a number of psychomotor tests affected.[1,2] There would seem to be no reason to avoid alcohol while taking **ciprofloxacin.**

1. Kamali F. Influence of ciprofloxacin on ethanol pharmacokinetics and pharmacodynamics. *Br J Clin Pharmacol* (1994) 37, 490P.
2. Kamali F. No influence of ciprofloxacin on ethanol disposition: a pharmacokinetic-pharmacodynamic interaction study. *Eur J Clin Pharmacol* (1994) 47, 71–4.

Alcohol + Cisapride

Cisapride increases blood alcohol levels to some extent but the clinical importance of this is uncertain. It is probably small.

Clinical evidence, mechanism, importance and management

A preliminary study in 16 normal subjects given 0.7 g/kg alcohol in orange juice found that 10 mg **cisapride** did not affect blood alcohol levels, but it was absorbed more quickly. The performance of a number of psychomotor tests was unaffected.[1] However a later study[2] in 5 normal subjects given 10 mg **cisapride**, followed 1 h later by a **standard meal**, and then by 0.3 g/kg alcohol diluted in orange juice, found a 34% rise in maximum blood alcohol levels (from 5.2 to 7.0 mM) and a 24% increase in the AUC over 4 h. Another study in 8 normal men found that when fasting and given 150 micrograms/kg **cisapride** 7 h and 20 min before drinking 0.5 g/kg alcohol, the peak serum alcohol levels rose 14% (from 15.6 to 17.8 mmol/l).[3] The reason appears to be that the **cisapride** speeds up the emptying of the stomach.

The extent to which these modestly increased blood alcohol levels would affect the ability to drive or handle other dangerous machinery is uncertain but it seems unlikely that the effects will be marked. The makers suggest in their datasheet that the sedative effects of alcohol will be accelerated.

1. Idzikowski C, Welburn P. An evaluation of possible interactions between ethanol and cisapride. Unpublished report N 49087 on file, Janssen Pharmaceuticals (1986).
2. Roine R, Heikkonen E, Salaspuro M. Cisapride enhances alcohol absorption and leads to high blood alcohol levels. *Gastroenterology* (1992) 102 (4 pt 2) A507.
3. Dziekan G, Contesse J, Werth B, Schwarzer G, Reinhardt WH. Cisapride increases peak plasma and saliva ethanol levels under fasting conditions. *J Intern Med* (1997) 242, 479–82.

Alcohol + Clomethiazole (Chlormethiazole)

Alcohol with clomethiazole (chlormethiazole) can cause serious, even potentially fatal, CNS depression due to additive CNS depressant effects, associated with increased clomethiazole bioavailability.

Clinical evidence, mechanism, importance and management

The following is a taken from an editorial in the British Medical Journal which was entitled 'Chlormethiazole and alcohol: a lethal cocktail':[1]

Clomethiazole (chlormethiazole) is commonly used to treat withdrawal from alcohol because of its hypnotic, anxiolytic and anticonvulsant effects. It is very effective if a rapidly reducing dosage regimen is followed over six days, but if it is used long term and drinking continues it carries several serious risks.

Alcoholics readily transfer dependency to **clomethiazole** and may visit several practitioners and hospitals to get their supplies. Tolerance develops so that very large amounts may be taken (up to 25 g daily). Often alcohol abuse continues and the combination of large amounts of alcohol and **clomethiazole** can result in coma and even fatal respiratory depression, due mainly to simple additive CNS depression. Other factors are that alcohol increases the bioavailability of **clomethiazole** (probably by impairing first pass metabolism),[2] and in the case of those with alcoholic cirrhosis, the systemic bioavailability may be increased tenfold because of venous shunting.[3]

It is suggested that **clomethiazole** should not be given long term. If General Practitioners choose to manage detoxification at home, it should be done under very close supervision, issuing prescriptions for only one day's supply to ensure daily contact and to minimise the risk of abuse. And if the patient shows evidence of tolerance or **clomethiazole** dependency or of continuing to drink, the only safe policy is rapid admission for inpatient care.[1]

Nobody appears to have checked on the combined effects of **clomethiazole** and alcohol on driving and related skills, but concurrent use would be expected to increase the risks.

1. McInnes GT. Chlormethiazole and alcohol: a lethal cocktail. *BMJ* (1987) 294, 592.
2. Neuvonen PJ, Pentikäinen PJ, Jostell KG, Syvälahti E. The pharmacokinetics of chlormethiazole in healthy subjects as affected by ethanol. *Clin Pharmacol Ther* (1981) 29, 268–9.
3. Pentikäinen PJ, Neuvonen PJ, Tarpila S, Syvälahti E. Effect of cirrhosis of the liver on the pharmacokinetics of chlormethiazole. *BMJ* (1978) ii, 861–3.

Alcohol + Clovoxamine, Femoxetine, Fluoxetine or Fluvoxamine

Clovoxamine, fluoxetine and femoxetine in therapeutic doses do not appear to interact with alcohol, but some modest interaction possibly occurs with fluvoxamine.

Clinical evidence, mechanism, importance and management

(a) Clovoxamine, Femoxetine, Fluoxetine

No sedation was seen in a study with 150 mg **clovoxamine** daily.[1] Another study in 12 subjects found no evidence that single doses of 50, 100 or 150 mg **clovoxamine** increased the effects of alcohol (0.8 g/kg) as measured by a number of psychomotor tests.[2] No significant interaction was seen in another study with **femoxetine** (200 to 600 mg) and alcohol (1 g/kg).[3] Neither **fluoxetine** (30 to 60 mg) nor alcohol (4 oz **whiskey**) affected the pharmacokinetics of the other in normal subjects, and no changes in psychomotor activity were seen (stability of stance, motor performance, manual co-ordination).[4] Blood alcohol levels of 80 mg% (80 mg/dl) impaired the performance of a number of psychomotor tests in 12 subjects but the addition of 40 mg **fluoxetine** daily taken for six days had little further effect.[5] Another study also found no change in the performance of a number of psychophysiological tests when **fluoxetine** was combined with alcohol.[6] No problems were found in a study of 76 patients on 60 mg **fluoxetine** daily when they drank alcohol.[7]

No special precautions would seem necessary with alcohol and any of these drugs.

(b) Fluvoxamine

One study found that 150 mg **fluvoxamine** daily with alcohol (0.5%) impaired alertness and attention more than alcohol alone,[8] whereas another study in subjects given 40 g alcohol (blood alcohol levels up to 70 mg/dl) failed to find evidence that the addition of 50 mg **fluvoxamine** twice daily worsened the performance of the psychomotor tests used, and even appeared to reverse some of the effects.[9,10] Another study similarly failed to find a significant interaction.[11] The pharmacokinetics of alcohol are hardly affected by **fluvoxamine**,[12] but the steady-state maximum serum levels of the **fluvoxamine** were increased by 20%.[10] The situation with **fluvoxamine** is therefore less clear than with the related drugs listed in (a) above, but it would seem prudent to give patients some warning that the effects of alcohol may possibly be modestly increased.

1. Ochs HR, Greenblatt DJ, Verburg-Ochs B, Labedski L. Chronic treatment with fluvoxamine, clovoxamine and placebo: interaction with digoxin and effects on sleep and alertness. *J Clin Pharmacol* (1989) 29, 91–5.
2. Strömberg C, Mattila MJ. Acute comparison of clovoxamine and mianserin, alone and in combination with ethanol, on human psychomotor performance. *Pharmacol Toxicol* (1987) 60, 374–9.
3. Strömberg C, Mattila MJ. Acute and subacute effects on psychomotor performance of femoxetine alone and with alcohol. *Eur J Clin Pharmacol* (1985) 28, 641–7.
4. Lemberger L, Rowe H, Bergstrom RF, Farid KZ, Enas GG. Effect of fluoxetine on psychomotor performance, physiologic response, and kinetics of ethanol. *Clin Pharmacol Ther* (1985) 37, 658–64.
5. Allen D, Lader M, Curran HV. A comparative study of the interactions of alcohol with amitriptyline, fluoxetine and placebo in normal subjects. *Prog Neuropsychopharmacol Biol Psychiatry* (1988) 12, 63–80.
6. Schaffler K. Study on performance and alcohol interaction with the antidepressant fluoxetine. *Int Clin Psychopharmacol* (1989) 4 (Suppl 1). 15–20.
7. Florkowski A, Gruszczyński W. Alcohol problems and treating patients with fluoxetine. *Pol J Pharmacol* (1995) 47, 547.
8. Herberg K-W, Menke H. Study of the effects of the antidepressant fluvoxamine on driving skills and its interaction with alcohol. Duphar Laboratories. Data on file 1981.
9. van Harten J, Wesnes K, Raghoebar M. Negligible kinetic and dynamic interaction between fluvoxamine and alcohol. *Clin Pharmacol Ther* (1991) 49, 178.
10. van Harten J, Stevens LA, Raghoebar M, Holland RL, Wesnes K, Cournot A. Fluvoxamine does not interact with alcohol or potentiate alcohol-related impairment of cognitive function. *Clin Pharmacol Ther* (1992) 52, 427–35.
11. Linnoila M, Stapleton JM, George DT, Lane E, Eckardt MJ. Effects of fluvoxamine, alone and in combination with ethanol, on psychomotor and cognitive performance and on autonomic nervous system reactivity in healthy volunteers. *J Clin Psychopharmacol* (1993) 13, 175–80.
12. van Harten J, Stevens LA, Raghoebar M. The influence of single-dose and multiple-dose administration of fluvoxamine on the pharmacokinetics of ethanol in man. *Eur J Pharmacol* (1990) 183, 2386–7.

Alcohol + CNS depressants

The concurrent use of small or moderate amounts of alcohol and therapeutic doses of drugs which are CNS depressants can increase drowsiness and reduce alertness. These drugs include analgesics, anticonvulsants, antidepressants, antihistamines, antipsychotics, antinauseants, appetite suppressants, hypno-sedatives, narcotics, neuroleptics, opioid analgesics, tranquillisers, and others. This increases the risk of accident when driving or handling other potentially dangerous machinery, and may make the performance of everyday tasks more difficult and hazardous.

Clinical evidence, mechanism, importance and management

Alcohol is a CNS depressant (see the introduction to this chapter). With only small or moderate amounts of alcohol and with blood-alcohol levels well within legal driving limits, it may be quite unsafe to drive if another CNS depressant is being taken concurrently. The details of most of the drugs which have been tested are set out in the monographs in this chapter (see the Index), but there are others which nobody seems to have tested formally. The summary above contains a list of some of those which commonly cause drowsiness. Quite apart from driving, almost everyone meets potentially dangerous situations every day at home, in the garden, in the street and at work. Crossing a busy street or even walking downstairs can become much more risky under the influence of CNS depressant drugs and drink. A cause for concern is that the patient may be partially or totally unaware of the extent of the deterioration in his skills. Patients should be warned.

Alcohol + Codeine

Codeine in 50-mg doses, both alone and with alcohol, impairs the ability to drive safely but no interaction of importance would be expected with the relatively small amounts of codeine in most compound analgesic preparations.

Clinical evidence, mechanism, importance and management

Double blind studies on a very large number of professional army drivers found that 50-mg of **codeine** and alcohol (0.5 g/kg), both alone and together, impaired their ability to drive safely on a static driving simulator. The number of 'collisions', neglected instructions and the times they 'drove off the road' were increased.[1,2] **Codeine** dosages of this order are given in the form of **Codeine Phosphate Syrup** (BPC 1973) in **Tablets of Codeine Phosphate BP** so that these preparations, particularly with alcohol, could make drivers more accident-prone, but the increased hazard is difficult to quantify. **Codeine phosphate** in doses of 15, 25 or 30 mg occurs in some elixirs and linctuses, but only relatively small amounts (5–8 mg) are found in most proprietary compound analgesic tablets. Alcohol appears not to affect the pharmacokinetics of **codeine**.[3]

1. Linnoila M, Häkkinen S. Effects of diazepam and codeine, alone and in combination with alcohol, on simulated driving. *Clin Pharmacol Ther* (1974) 15, 368–73.
2. Linnoila M, Mattila MJ. Interaction of alcohol and drugs on psychomotor skills as demonstrated by a driving simulator. *Br J Pharmacol* (1973) 47, 671P–672P.
3. Bodd E, Beylich KM. Christopherson AS, Morland J. Oral administration of codeine in the presence of ethanol: a pharmacokinetic study in man. *Pharmacol Toxicol* (1987) 61, 297–300.

Alcohol + Co-dergocrine mesilate (Ergoloid mesylates)

Co-dergocrine mesilate (ergoloid mesylates) causes a very small reduction in blood alcohol levels.

Clinical evidence, mechanism, importance and management

Thirteen subjects were given 0.5 g/kg 25% alcohol in orange juice after breakfast, before and after taking 4.5 mg **co-dergocrine mesilate** (ergoloid mesylates, *Hydergine*) every 8 h for nine doses. The **co-dergocrine** caused a small reduction in blood alcohol levels (maximum serum levels reduced from 59 to 55.7 mg/100 ml, clearance reduced from 0.11 to 0.10 g/kg/h).[1] The reason is not understood. This interaction is almost certainly not of clinical importance.

1. Savage IT, James IM. The effect of Hydergine on ethanol pharmacokinetics in man. *J Pharm Pharmacol* (1993) 45 (Suppl 2), 1119.

Alcohol + Dextropropoxyphene (Propoxyphene)

The central nervous system depressant effects of alcohol are only modestly increased by normal therapeutic doses of dextropropoxyphene. In deliberate suicidal overdosage the CNS depressant effects appear to be additive and can be fatal.

Clinical evidence

Alcohol alone (blood levels of 50 mg%) impaired the performance of various psychomotor tests (motor co-ordination, mental performance and stability of stance) in eight volunteers more than 65 mg **dextropropoxyphene** (**propoxyphene**) alone. When given together there was some evidence that the effects were greater than with either alone, but in some instances the impairment was no greater than with just alcohol. The effect of alcohol clearly predominated.[1]

Another study found that the effects of 95 mg alcohol on the performance of two psychomotor tests were not altered in subjects who had also been given two tablets of *Distalgesic* (**dextropropoxyphene** 32.5 mg + **paracetamol** (**acetaminophen**) 325 mg in each tablet).[2] A further study found no change in the psychomotor effects of alcohol (0.5 g/kg) following the addition of 130 mg **dextropropoxyphene** but the bioavailability of the **dextropropoxyphene** was raised by 25%.[3] Yet another found a 31% increase in bioavailability with blood alcohol levels of about 800–1000 mg/l.[4]

Mechanism

Not understood. Both drugs are CNS depressants and in overdosage the fatal dose of dextropropoxyphene is reduced by the presence of alcohol. Their effects seem to be additive.[5,6]

Importance and management

Numerous reports describe the severe and sometimes fatal respiratory depression which can follow alcohol/dextropropoxyphene overdosage, but information about moderate social drinking and therapeutic doses of dextropropoxyphene is limited. The objective evidence is that the interaction with moderate doses of both is quite small. Even so it would seem prudent (at the risk of being overcautious) to warn patients that dextropropoxyphene can cause drowsiness and this may be exaggerated to some extent by alcohol. They should be warned that driving or handling potentially hazardous machinery may be more risky, but total abstinence from alcohol does not seem to be necessary.

1. Kiplinger GF, Sokol G, Rodda BE. Effects of combined alcohol and propoxyphene on human performance. *Arch Int Pharmacodyn Ther* (1974) 212, 175–80.
2. Edwards C, Gard PR, Handley SL, Hunter M, Whittington RM. Distalgesic and ethanol-impaired function. *Lancet* (1982) ii, 384.
3. Girre C, Hirschhorn M, Bertaux L, Palombo S, Dellatolas F, Ngo R, Moreno M, Fournier PE. Enhancement of propoxyphene bioavailability by ethanol: relation to psychomotor and cognitive function in healthy volunteers. *Eur J Clin Pharmacol* (1991) 41, 147–52.
4. Sellers EM, Hamilton CA, Kaplan HL, Degani NC, Foltz RL. Pharmacokinetic interaction of propoxyphene with ethanol. *Br J Clin Pharmacol* (1985) 19, 398–401.
5. Carson DJL, Carson ED. Fatal dextropropoxyphene poisoning in Northern Ireland: review of 30 cases. *Lancet* (1977) i, 894–7.
6. Whittington RM, Barclay AD. The epidemiology of dextropropoxyphene (Distalgesic) overdose fatalities in Birmingham and the West Midlands. *J Clin Hosp Pharm* (1981) 6, 251–7.

Alcohol + Dimethylformamide (DMF)

A disulfiram-like reaction can occur in about 20% of those who drink alcohol after being exposed to dimethylformamide (DMF) vapour.

Clinical evidence

A three-year study in a chemical plant where **dimethylformamide** (**DMF**) was used found that about 20% (19 out of 102 men) exposed to the vapour experienced flushing of the face, and often of the neck, arms, hands and chest, after drinking alcohol. Sometimes dizziness, nausea and tightness of the chest also occurred. A single glass of **beer** was enough to induce a flush lasting 2 h. The majority of the men experienced the reaction within 24 h of exposure to **DMF**, but it could occur even after 4 days.[1]

Three further cases of this interaction are described in other reports.[2,3]

Mechanism

Men exposed to DMF vapour develop substantial amounts of DMF and its metabolite (*N*-methylformamide) in their blood and urine.[1] This latter compound in particular has been shown in *rats* given alcohol to raise their blood acetaldehyde levels by a factor of five, so it would seem probable that the *N*-methylformamide is similarly responsible for this disulfiram-like reaction in man (see 'Alcohol + Disulfiram', p.27).[4]

Importance and management

An established interaction, the incidence being about 20%.[1] Those who come into contact with DMF, even in very low concentrations, should be warned of this possible interaction with alcohol. It would appear to be more unpleasant than serious in most instances, and normally requires no treatment.

1. Lyle WH, Spence TWM, McKinneley WM, Duckers K. Dimethylformamide and alcohol intolerance. *Br J Ind Med* (1979) 36, 63–6.
2. Chivers CP. Disulfiram effect from inhalation of dimethylformamide. *Lancet* (1978) i, 331.
3. Reinl W, Urban HJ. Erkrankungen durch dimethylformamid. *Int Arch Arbeitsmed* (1965) 21, 333–46.
4. Hanasono GK, Fuller RW, Broddle WD, Gibson WR. Studies on the effects of N,N-dimethylformamide on ethanol disposition and monoamine oxidase activity in rats. *Toxicol Appl Pharmacol* (1977) 39, 461.

Alcohol + Disulfiram

The ingestion of alcohol while taking disulfiram will result in flushing and fullness of the face and neck, tachycardia, breathlessness, giddiness and hypotension, nausea and vomiting. This is called the Disulfiram or Antabuse reaction. It is used to deter alcoholic patients from drinking. A mild flushing reaction of the skin may possibly occur in particularly sensitive individuals if alcohol is applied to the skin or if the vapour is inhaled.

Clinical evidence

This toxic interaction was first observed in 1937 by Dr EE Williams[1] amongst workers in the rubber industry who were handling **tetramethylthiuram disulphide**:

"Beer will cause a flushing of the face and hands, with rapid pulse, and some of the men describe palpitations and a terrible fullness of the face, eyes and head. After a glass of beer (six ounces) the blood pressure falls about 10 points, the pulse is slightly accelerated and the skin becomes flushed in the face and wrists. In 15 min the blood pressure falls another 10 points, the heart is more rapid, and the patient complains of fullness in the head."

The later observation[2] by Hald and his colleagues of the same reaction with the *ethyl* congener (**disulfiram**) led to its introduction as a drink deterrent. Patients experience throbbing in head and neck, giddiness, sweating, nausea, vomiting, thirst, chest pain, difficulty in breathing and headache. The severity of the reaction can depend upon the amount of alcohol ingested but some individuals are extremely sensitive. Respiratory depression, cardiovascular collapse, cardiac arrhythmias, unconsciousness and convulsions may occur. There have been fatalities[3,4] (12 according to one reviewer[5]). An unusual and isolated report describes painful, intermittent and transient myoclonic jerking of the arms and legs as the only manifestation of the **disulfiram** reaction in one patient.[6]

A mild **disulfiram** reaction is said to occur in some patients who apply alcohol to the skin but it is probably largely due to inhalation of the vapour. It has been reported after using **after-shave lotion**,[7] **tar gel** (33% alcohol)[8] and a **beer-containing shampoo** (3% alcohol).[9] A **contact lens wetting solution** (containing **polyvinyl alcohol**) used to irrigate the eye has also been implicated in a reaction.[10,11] It has also been described in a patient who inhaled vapour from paint in a poorly ventilated area and from the inhalation of '**mineral spirits**'.[12] Another man experienced a reaction after using alcohol for cleaning trays in a print shop.[5] A woman on **disulfiram** reported vaginal stinging and soreness during sexual intercourse, and similar discomfort to her husband's penis which seemed to be related to the **disulfiram** dosage and how intoxicated her husband was.[13]

Mechanism

Partially understood. Alcohol is normally rapidly metabolised within the liver, firstly to acetaldehyde (by acetaldehyde dehydrogenase) and then by a series of biochemical steps to water and carbon dioxide. Disulfiram inhibits this first enzyme so that the acetaldehyde accumulates. Prostaglandin release may also be involved.[14] Not all of the symptoms of the reaction can be reproduced by injecting acetaldehyde so that some other biochemical mechanism(s) must also be involved. For example, it is thought that the inhibition of dopamine-beta-hydroxylase may have some part to play. It has been suggested that the mild skin flush which can occur if alcohol is applied to the skin is not a true disulfiram reaction.[15]

Importance and management

An extremely well-documented and important interaction exploited therapeutically to deter alcoholics from drinking. Initial treatment should be closely supervised because an extremely intense and potentially serious reaction occurs in a few individuals with even quite small doses of alcohol. Apart from the usual warnings about drinking, patients should also be warned about the unwitting ingestion of alcohol in some **pharmaceutical preparations**. The alcohol-content of nearly 500 American products has been published which is too extensive to be reproduced here.[16] The risk of a reaction is real. It has been seen following a single dose of an alcohol-containing **cough mixture**,[17] whereas the ingestion of small amounts of **communion wine** and the absorption of alcohol from a **bronchial nebuliser spray** are said not to result in any reaction.[18]

Treatment

The disulfiram reaction can be treated, if necessary, with ascorbic acid. 1 g given orally is reported to be effective in mild cases (heart rate <100 bpm and general condition good). It works within 30–45 min. Moderately severe cases (heart rate 100–150 bpm, blood pressure 150/100 mmHg) can be treated with 1 g intravenous ascorbic acid and is effective within 2–5 min. Critically ill patients may need other standard supportive emergency measures.[5]

1. Williams EE. Effects of alcohol on workers with carbon disulfide. *JAMA* (1937) 109, 1472.
2. Hald J, Jacobsen E, Larsen V. The sensitizing effects of tetraethylthiuramdisulphide (Antabuse) to ethylalcohol. *Acta Pharmacol* (1948) 4, 285–96.
3. Garber RS, Bennett RE. Unusual reaction to antabuse: report of three cases. *J Med Soc NJ* (1950) 47, 168.
4. Kwentus J, Major LF. Disulfiram in the treatment of alcoholism: a review. *J Stud Alcohol* (1979) 40, 428–46.
5. McNichol RW. Disulfiram, a strategic weapon in the battle for sobriety. In McNichol RW, Ewing JA, Fairman MD (Eds) Disulfiram (Antabuse), a unique medical aid to sobriety. History, pharmacology, research, clinical use. Springfield Il: Charles C Thomas (1987) 47–90.
6. Syed J, Moarefi G. An unusual presentation of a disulfiram-alcohol reaction. *Del Med J* (1995) 67, 183.
7. Mercurio F. Antabuse®-alcohol reaction following the use of after-shave lotion. *JAMA* (1952) 149, 82.
8. Ellis CN, Mitchell AJ, Beardsley GR. Tar gel interaction with disulfiram. *Arch Dermatol* (1979) 115, 1367–8.
9. Stoll D, King LE. Disulfiram-alcohol skin reaction to beer-containing shampoo. *JAMA* (1980) 244, 2045.
10. Newsom SR, Harper BS. Disulfiram-alcohol reaction caused by contact lens wetting solution. *Contact and Intraocular Lens Med J* (1980) 6, 407–8.
11. Refojo MF. Letter to Editor. *Contact and Intraocular Lens Med J* (1981) 7, 172.
12. Scott GE, Little FW. Disulfiram reaction to organic solvents other than ethanol. *N Engl J Med* (1982) 312, 790.
13. Chick JD. Disulfiram reaction during sexual intercourse. *Br J Psychiatry* (1988) 152, 438.
14. Truitt EB, Gaynor CR, Mehl DL. Aspirin attenuation of alcohol-induced flushing and intoxication in oriental and occidental subjects. *Alcohol Alcohol* (1987) 22 (Suppl 1), 595–9.
15. Haddock NF, Wilkin JK. Cutaneous reactions to lower aliphatic alcohols before and during disulfiram therapy. *Arch Dermatol* (1982) 118, 157–9.
16. Parker WA. Alcohol-containing pharmaceuticals. *Am J Drug Alcohol Abuse* (1982–3) 9, 195–209.
17. Koff RS, Papadimas I, Honig EG. Alcohol in cough medicines: hazards to the disulfiram user. *JAMA* (1971) 215, 1988–9.
18. Rothstein E. Use of disulfiram (Antabuse) in alcoholism. *N Engl J Med* (1970) 283, 936.

Alcohol-containing ritonavir oral solution (Norvir) + Disulfiram or Metronidazole

The makers suggest the possibility of a disulfiram-reaction with disulfiram or metronidazole and an alcohol-containing preparation of Norvir (ritonavir).

Clinical evidence, mechanism, importance and management

The makers of the **oral solution of ritonavir** (*Norvir*) say that since it contains 43% alcohol the preparation should not be taken with **disulfiram** or other drugs such as **metronidazole** because a disulfiram reaction is possible,[1] (for details of this reaction see, 'Alcohol + Disulfiram', p.27). However in practice the risk is probably fairly small because the recommended dose of **ritonavir** in this form is only 7.5 ml. No interaction will occur with ritonavir capsules because they do not contain alcohol.

1. Norvir (Ritonavir). Abbott Laboratories Ltd. Summary of product characteristics, January 2001.

Alcohol + Edible fungi

A disulfiram-like reaction can occur if alcohol is taken after eating the smooth ink(y) caps fungus (*Coprinus atramentarius*) or certain other edible fungi.

Clinical evidence

A man who drank 3 pints of **beer** 2 h after eating a meal of freshly picked and fried **inky caps** (*Coprinus atramentarius*) developed facial flushing and a blotchy red rash over the upper half of his body. His face and hands swelled and he became breathless, sweated profusely, and vomited during the 3 h when the reaction was most severe. On admission to hospital he had tachycardia and some cardiac arrhythmia. The man's wife who ate the same meal but without an alcoholic drink did not show the reaction.[1]

This reaction has been described on many occasions in medical and pharmacological reports[2-4] and in books devoted to descriptions of edible and poisonous fungi.[5] Only a few are listed here. Mild hypotension and ". . .alarming orthostatic features. . ."[6,7] are said to be common symptoms but the arrhythmia seen in the case cited here[1] appears to be rare. Recovery is usually spontaneous and uncomplicated. A similar reaction has been described after eating *Boletus luridus*,[8] and other fungi including *Coprinus micaceus*, *Clitocybe claviceps* and certain *morels*.[8] An African relative of *Coprinus atramentarius* which also causes this reaction is called by the Nigerian Yoruba people the **Ajeimutin** fungus (*Coprinus africanus*). The literal translation of this name is the 'eat-without-drinking-alcohol' mushroom.[9]

Mechanism

An early and attractive idea was that the reaction with *Coprinus atramentarius* was due to the presence of disulfiram (one group of workers actually claimed to have isolated it from the fungus[10]), but this was not confirmed by later work[11,12] and it now appears that the active ingredient is coprine (*N*-5-(1-hydroxycyclopropyl)-glutamine).[13,14] This is metabolised in the body to 1-aminocyclopropanol which appears, like disulfiram, to inhibit aldehyde dehydrogenase (see 'Alcohol + Disulfiram', p.27). The active ingredients in the other fungi are unknown.

Importance and management

An established and well documented interaction. It is said to occur up to 24 h after eating the fungus. The intensity depends upon the quantity of fungus and alcohol consumed, and the time interval between them.[1,6] Despite the widespread consumption of edible fungi and alcohol, reports of this reaction in the medical literature are few and far between, suggesting that even though it can be very unpleasant and frightening, the outcome is usually uncomplicated. Treatment appears normally not to be necessary.

The related fungus *Coprinus comatus* (the 'shaggy ink cap' or 'Lawyers wig') is said not to interact with alcohol,[7,15] nor is there anything to suggest that it ever occurs with the **common field mushroom** (*Agaricus campestris*) or the cultivated variety (*Agaricus bisporis*).[15]

1. Caley MJ, Clarke RA. Cardiac arrhythmias after mushroom ingestion. *BMJ* (1977) 2, 1633.
2. Reynolds WA, Lowe FH. Mushrooms and a toxic reaction to alcohol: report of four cases. *N Engl J Med* (1965) 272, 630–1.
3. Wildervanck LS. Alcohol en de kale inktzwam. *Ned Tijdschr Geneeskd* (1978) 122, 913–14.
4. Tottmar O, Marchner H and Lindberg P. in 'Alcohol and Aldehyde Metabolising Systems', ed Thuram RG, Williamson JR, Drott HR and Chance B. vol 2. Academic Press, NY (1977) pp. 20–12.
5. Ramsbottom J. Mushrooms and Toadstools. Collins, London (1953) p 55.
6. Buck RW. Mushroom toxins; brief review of literature. *N Engl J Med* (1961) 265, 681.
7. Broadhurst-Zingrich L. Ink caps and alcohol. *BMJ* (1978) 1, 511.
8. Budmiger H, Kocher F. Hexenröhrling (Boletus luridus) mit alkohol: ein kasuistischer beitrag. *Schweiz Med Wochenschr* (1982) 112, 1179–81.
9. Oso BA. Mushrooms and the Yoruba people of Nigeria. *Mycologia* (1975) 67, 311–19.
10. Simandl J, Franc J. Isolation of tetraethylthiuram disulfide from Coprinus atramentarius. *Chem Listy* (1956) 50, 1862.
11. Vanhaelen M, Vanhaelen-Fastré R, Hoyois J, Mardens Y. Reinvestigation of disulfiram-like activity of *Coprinus atramentarius* (Bull. *ex* Fr.) Fr. extracts. *J Pharm Sci* (1976) 65, 1774–6.
12. Wier JK, Tyler VE. An investigation of *Coprinus atramentarius* for the presence of disulfiram. *J Am Pharm Assoc* (1960) 49, 427–9.
13. Hatfield GM, Schaumberg JP. Isolation and structural studies of coprine, the disulfiram-like constituent of Coprinus atramentarius. *Lloydia* (1975) 38, 489.
14. Lindberg P, Bergman R, Wickberg B. Isolation and structure of coprine, a novel physiologically active cyclopropane derivative from Coprinus atramentarius and its synthesis via 1-amino-cyclo-propanol. *J Chem Soc Chem Commun* (1975) 946.
15. Radford AP. Ink caps and mushrooms. *BMJ* (1981) 1, 112.

Alcohol + Fentanyl-midazolam

The residual effects of fentanyl-midazolam appear not to interact adversely with alcoholic drinks taken several hours later.

Clinical evidence, mechanism, importance and management

A study with 12 normal subjects concluded that the residual effects of **fentanyl** (2 micrograms/kg) with **midazolam** (0.1 mg/kg) given intravenously for surgery were unlikely to interact significantly in outpatients if they drank when they arrived home about 4 h later. The

subjects were given enough alcohol to achieve blood levels of about 60 mg% (equivalent to 1.4 L of **beer** or 950 ml **wine** or 180 ml **spirits**).[1]

1. Lichtor JL, Zacny J, Apfelbaum JL, Lane BS, Rupani G, Thisted RA, Dohrn C, Korttila K. Alcohol after sedation with i.v. midazolam–fentanyl: effects on psychomotor functioning. *Br J Anaesth* (1991) 67, 579–84.

Alcohol + Furazolidone

A disulfiram-like reaction may occur in patients taking furazolidone if they drink alcohol.

Clinical evidence

A patient taking 200 mg **furazolidone** four times daily complained of facial flushing, lachrymation, conjunctivitis, weakness and light-headedness within 10 min of drinking **beer**. It occurred on several occasions and lasted 30–45 min.[1]

A man prescribed 100 mg **furazolidone** four times daily and who had taken only three doses, developed intense facial flushing, wheezing and dyspnoea of an hour's duration within an hour of drinking 2 oz of **brandy**. The same thing happened again the next day after drinking a **martini cocktail**. No treatment was given.[2] A report originating from the makers of **furazolidone** stated that by 1976, 43 cases of a disulfiram-like reaction had been reported, of which 14 were produced experimentally using above-normal doses of **furazolidone**.[3] A later study in 1986 described nine out of 47 patients (19%) who complained of a disulfiram-like reaction after drinking alcohol while taking 100 mg **furazolidone** four times daily for five days.[4] The report does not say whether all of them drank.[4]

Mechanism

Uncertain. It seems possible that furazolidone acts like disulfiram by inhibiting the activity of acetaldehyde dehydrogenase (see 'Alcohol + Disulfiram', p.27).

Importance and management

An established and clinically important interaction of uncertain incidence. One report suggests that possibly about 1 in 5 may be affected.[4] Reactions of this kind appear to be more unpleasant and possibly frightening than serious, and normally need no treatment, however patients should be warned about what may happen if they drink.

1. Calesnick B. Antihypertensive action of the antimicrobial agent furazolidone. *Am J Med Sci* (1958) 236, 736–46.
2. Kolodny AL. Side-effects produced by alcohol in a patient receiving furazolidone. *Md State Med J* (1962) 11, 248.
3. Chamberlain RE. (Eaton Laboratories, Norwich Pharmacal Co.) Chemotherapeutic properties of prominent nitrofurans. *J Antimicrob Chemother* (1976) 2, 325–336.
4. DuPont HL, Ericsson CD, Reves RR, Galindo E. Antimicrobial therapy for travelers' diarrhea. *Rev Infect Dis* (1986) 8, (Suppl 2), S217–S222.

Alcohol + Ginseng

Ginseng increases the clearance of alcohol from the body and lowers blood alcohol levels.

Clinical importance, mechanism, importance and management

Fourteen normal subjects, each acting as their own control, were given oral alcohol (72 g/kg body weight as a 25% solution) with and without a **ginseng** extract (3 g/kg body weight) mixed in with it. They drank the alcohol or the alcohol/**ginseng** mixture over a 45-min period in 7 portions, the first four at 5-min intervals and the next three at 10-min intervals. Measurements taken 40 min later showed that the presence of the **ginseng** lowered blood alcohol levels by an average of 35.2% (0.11% w/v compared with 0.18%). The levels of 10 subjects were lowered 32–51% by the **ginseng**, 3 showed reductions of 14–18% and one showed no changes at all.[1]

The reasons for this interaction are uncertain, but it is suggested that some of the action of the **ginseng** is possibly to increase the activity of the enzymes (alcohol and aldehyde dehydrogenase)[2] which are concerned with the metabolism of the alcohol, thereby increasing the clearance of the alcohol from the body. What this means in practical terms is not clear but the authors of the report suggest the possibility of using **ginseng** to treat alcoholic patients and those with acute alcohol intoxication.[1]

1. Lee FC, Ko JH, Park KJ, Lee JS. Effect of *Panax ginseng* on blood alcohol clearance in man. *Clin Exp Pharmacol Physiol* (1987) 14, 543–6.
2. Choi CW, Lee SI, Huh K. Effect of ginseng on the hepatic alcohol metabolizing enzyme system activity in chronic alcohol-treated mice. *Kor J Pharmacol* (1984) 20, 13–21.

Alcohol + Glutethimide

The sedative effects of glutethimide are increased by alcohol and the performance of psychomotor skills is impaired. Driving or handling other potentially dangerous machinery is made more hazardous.

Clinical evidence, mechanism, importance and management

A double-blind study on normal subjects given 250 mg **glutethimide**, either alone or with alcohol (0.5 g/kg), found that concurrent use both subjectively and objectively impaired the performance of a number of psychomotor skill tests related to driving (choice reaction, coordination, divided attention).[1] Both are CNS depressants and their effects would appear to be additive. It has also been reported that blood alcohol levels can be raised 11–30% by **glutethimide** and blood **glutethimide** levels are reduced,[2] but a later study was unable to confirm this.[1] It has also even been claimed that effects of alcohol and **glutethimide** are antagonistic rather than additive.[2]

The information is limited and somewhat contradictory, nevertheless patients should be warned about the probable results of taking **glutethimide** and alcohol together. Driving, handling dangerous machinery or undertaking any task needing alertness and full coordination is likely to be made more difficult and hazardous. There is no evidence of a hangover effect which could result in an interaction with alcohol the next day.[1]

1. Saario I, Linnoila M. Effect of subacute treatment with hypnotics, alone or in combination with alcohol, on psychomotor skills related to driving. *Acta Pharmacol Toxicol* (1976) 38, 382–92.
2. Mould GP, Curry SH, Binns TB. Interactions of glutethimide and phenobarbitone with ethanol in man. *J Pharm Pharmacol* (1972) 24, 894–9.

Alcohol + Glyceryl trinitrate

Patients who take glyceryl trinitrate (nitroglycerin) while drinking may feel faint and dizzy.

Clinical evidence, mechanism, importance and management

The results of studies[1,2] on the combined haemodynamic effects of alcohol and **glyceryl trinitrate** give support to claims made in 1965 and 1980 that concurrent use increases the risk of exaggerated hypotension and fainting.[3,4] Their vasodilatory effects[5] would appear to be additive. The greatest effect was seen when the **glyceryl trinitrate** was taken 1 h after starting to drink.[1] It is suggested that this increased susceptibility to postural hypotension should not be allowed to stop patients from using **glyceryl trinitrate** if they want to drink, but they should be warned and told what to do if they feel faint and dizzy (sit or lie down).[1]

1. Kupari M, Heikkilä J, Ylikahri R. Does alcohol intensify the hemodynamic effects of nitroglycerin? *Clin Cardiol* (1984) 7, 382–6.
2. Abrams J, Schroeder K, Raizada V, Gibbs D. Potentially adverse effects of sublingual nitroglycerin during consumption of alcohol. *J Am Coll Cardiol* (1990) 15, 226A.
3. Shafer N. Hypotension due to nitroglycerin combined with alcohol. *N Engl J Med* (1965) 272, 1169.
4. Opie. LH. Drugs and the heart. Nitrates. *Lancet* (1980) i, 750–2.
5. Allison RD, Kraner JC, Roth GM. Effects of alcohol and nitroglycerin on vascular responses in man. *Angiology* (1971) 22, 211–222.

Alcohol + Griseofulvin

An isolated case report describes a very severe disulfiram-like reaction in man on griseofulvin after drinking a can of beer. Two others developed flushing and tachycardia. A handful of others have shown increased alcohol effects.

Clinical evidence

(a) Disulfiram-like reaction

A man took 500 mg **griseofulvin** daily for about 2 weeks without problems. He drank a can of *beer*, took his usual dose of **griseofulvin** about an hour later, and within 30–60 min developed a severe disulfiram-like reaction (flushing, severe nausea, vomiting, diarrhoea, hypotension and paraesthesias of all extremities). He was successfully treated with intravenous normal saline, potassium and dopamine, and intramuscular promethazine.[1]

Two other cases of flushing and tachycardia attributed to concurrent use have also been described.[2,3]

(b) Increased alcohol effects

The descriptions of this response are very brief. One of them describes[4] a man who had "... decreased tolerance to alcohol and emotional instability manifested by crying and nervousness so severe that the drug was stopped." Another[2] states that "... a possible potentiation of the effects of alcohol has been noted in a very small number of patients."

Mechanism

Not understood. The reaction (a) described above possibly has the same pharmacological basis as the disulfiram/alcohol reaction (see 'Alcohol + Disulfiram', p.27).

Importance and management

The documentation is extremely sparse which would seem to suggest that adverse interactions between alcohol and griseofulvin are uncommon. Concurrent use need not be avoided but patients should be warned. The disulfiram-like reaction described was unusually severe.

1. Fett DL, Vukov LF. An unusual case of severe griseofulvin-alcohol interaction. *Ann Emerg Med* (1994) 24, 95–7.
2. Simon HJ, Randz LA. Reactions to antimicrobial agents. *Ann Rev Med* (1961) 12, 119.
3. Robinson MM. Griseofulvin therapy of superficial mycoses. *Antibiotics Annual* (1959–60) 7, 680–6.
4. Drowns BV, Fuhrman DL, Dennie CC. Use, abuse and limitations of griseofulvin. *Mo Med* (1960) 57, 1473.

Alcohol + Hydromorphone

A single case report describes a fatality due to the combined CNS depressant effects of hydromorphone and alcohol.

Clinical evidence, mechanism, importance and management

A young man died from the combined cardiovascular and respiratory depressant effects of **hydromorphone** (*Dilaudid*) and alcohol.[1] He fell into a sleep, the serious nature of which was not recognised by those around him. Post-mortem analysis revealed alcohol and **hydro-morphone** concentrations of 900 mg/l and 0.1 mg/l, neither of which is particularly excessive. This case emphasises the importance of warning patients about the potentially hazardous consequences of drinking while taking potent CNS depressants of this kind.

1. Levine B, Saady J, Fierro M, Valentour J. A hydromorphone and ethanol fatality. *J Forensic Sci* (1984) 29, 655–9.

Alcohol + Indometacin (Indomethacin) or Phenylbutazone

The skills related to driving are impaired by indometacin (indomethacin) and phenylbutazone. Further impairment occurs if patients drink while taking phenylbutazone, but this does not appear to occur with indometacin.

Clinical evidence, mechanism, importance and management

A study on a large number of normal subjects showed that the performance of various psychomotor skills related to driving (choice reaction, coordination, divided attention tests) were impaired by 50 mg **indometacin (indomethacin)** or 200 mg **phenylbutazone**. The concurrent ingestion of alcohol (0.5 g/kg) made things worse in those taking **phenylbutazone**, but the performance of those taking **indometacin** was improved to some extent.[1] The reasons are not understood. The study showed that the subjects were subjectively unaware of the adverse effects of **phenylbutazone**. Information is very limited, but patients should be warned if they intend to drive.

1. Linnoila M, Seppälä T, Mattila MJ. Acute effect of antipyretic analgesics, alone or in combination with alcohol, on human psychomotor skills related to driving. *Br J Clin Pharmacol* (1974) 1, 477–84.

Alcohol + Isoniazid

Isoniazid increases the hazards of driving after drinking alcohol. Isoniazid-induced hepatitis may also possibly be increased by alcohol, and the effects of isoniazid are possibly reduced.

Clinical evidence, mechanism, importance and management

The effects of 750 mg **isoniazid** with 0.5 g/kg alcohol were examined in 100 volunteers given various psychomotor tests and using a driving simulator. No major interaction was seen in the psychomotor tests, but the number of drivers who 'drove off the road' on the simulator was increased.[1,2] There would therefore appear to be some extra risks for patients on **isoniazid** who drink and drive, but the effect does not appear to be large. Patients should nevertheless be warned. The incidence of severe progressive liver damage due to **isoniazid** is said to be higher in those who drink regularly,[3,4] and the clinical effects of **isoniazid** are also said to be reduced by heavy drinking in some patients.[3]

1. Linnoila M, Mattila MJ. Effects of isoniazid on psychomotor skills related to driving. *J Clin Pharmacol* (1973) 13, 343–50.

2. Linnoila M, Mattila MJ. Interaction of alcohol and drugs on psychomotor skills as demonstrated by a driving simulator. *Br J Pharmacol* (1973) 47, 671P–672P.

3. Anonymous. Interactions of drugs with alcohol. *Med Lett Drugs Ther* (1981) 23, 33–4.

4. Kopanoff DE, Snider DE, Caras GJ. Isoniazid-related hepatitis. *Am Rev Respir Dis* (1978) 117, 991–1001.

Alcohol + Jian Bu Wan

Jian Bu Wan appears not to relieve or cure a hangover.

Clinical evidence, mechanism, importance and management

Jian Bu Wan is a Chinese traditional herbal medicine containing a bark which has anticholinergic, antibacterial, diuretic and choleretic properties. It is used to alleviate 'weakness', that is to say the cardiovascular and gastrointestinal symptoms after severe infections and acute alcohol intake. A controlled double-blind crossover study of 8 normal subjects who, the evening before, had drunk **champagne** and **vodka** (averaging 0.6 g/kg body weight), found no evidence that **Jian Bu Wan** was more effective than a placebo when given to treat a hangover the next morning. The subjects were given psychomotor function tests, a subjective evaluation of their symptoms, blood alcohol concentration tests, and their blood pressures and heart rates were measured.[1]

1. Frisk-Holmberg M, Kerth P, van der Kleyn E, Synavae P. Effects of Jian Bu Wan – a traditional Chinese medication on behavioural and cardiovascular parameters after acute alcohol intake in normal subjects. *Fundam Clin Pharmacol* (1990) 4, 11–15.

Alcohol + Kava

There is some evidence that kava may worsen the deleterious effects of alcohol.

Clinical evidence, mechanism, importance and management

Forty healthy subjects underwent a number of cognitive tests (digital symbol coding, Mackworth clock, divided attention, tracking and visual search, and a symmetry identification test) and visuomotor tests after taking alcohol alone, **kava** alone, or both together. The subjects took 0.75 g/kg alcohol (enough to give blood alcohol levels above 50 mg%) and the **kava** dose was 1 g/kg. The **kava** drink was made by mixing middle grade **Fijian kava** with water and straining it to produce about 350 ml **kava liquid**. It was found that **kava** alone had no effect on the tests, but alcohol alone reduced performance in some of the tests, and **kava** with alcohol reduced it even more. **Kava** (or **Kava-Kava**) is the pepper plant *Piper methysticum*, parts of which (usually the root) are used to make a ceremonial and recreational drink in several Pacific islands such as Fiji, Samoa, Tonga, Vanuatu and New Caledonia. It is also by some aborigines in the Northern Territory of Australia.[1]

No very strong conclusions can be drawn from the results of this study, but they do suggest that car driving and handling other machinery may possibly be more hazardous if **kava** and alcohol are taken together. The outcome of taking different doses of alcohol and **kava** seems not to have been studied.

1. Foo H, Lemon J. Acute effects of kava, alone or in combination with alcohol, on subjective measures of impairment and intoxication and on cognitive performance. *Drug Alcohol Rev* (1997) 16, 147–55.

Alcohol + Ketoconazole

Disulfiram-like reactions have been seen in a few patients taking ketoconazole after drinking alcohol.

Clinical evidence, mechanism, importance and management

One patient out of group of 12 taking 200 mg **ketoconazole** daily experienced a disulfiram-like reaction (nausea, vomiting, facial flushing) after drinking.[1] No further details are given and the report does not say whether any of the others drank alcohol. A woman on 200 mg

ketoconazole daily developed a disulfiram-like reaction when she drank.[2] Another report describes a transient 'sunburn-like' rash or flush on the face, upper chest and back of a patient taking 200 mg **ketoconazole** daily when she drank modest quantities of **wine** or **beer**.[3] One other case has been briefly reported.[4] The reasons for the reactions are not known but it seems possible that **ketoconazole** may act like disulfiram and inhibit the activity of acetaldehyde dehydrogenase (see 'Alcohol + Disulfiram', p.27). The incidence of this reaction appears to be low (these appear to be the only reports) and its importance is probably small, but patients should be warned. Reactions of this kind are usually more unpleasant than serious, the disulfiram/alcohol reaction being the possible exception.

1. Fazio RA, Wickremesinghe PC, Arsura EL. Ketoconazole therapy of candida esophagitis—a prospective study of 12 cases. *Am J Gastroenterol* (1983) 78, 261–4.
2. Meyboom RHB, Pater BW. Overgevoeligheid voor alcoholische dranken tijdens behandeling met ketoconazol. *Ned Tijdschr Geneeskd* (1989) 133, 1463–4.
3. Magnasco AJ, Magnasco LD. Interaction of ketoconazole and ethanol. *Clin Pharm* (1986) 5, 522–3.
4. Graybill JR. Quoted as personnal communication by Clissold SP. Safety in clinical practice, in 'Ketoconazole today. A review of clinical experience Manchester.' Adis Press (1987), pp 77–91.

Alcohol + Lithium carbonate

Some limited evidence suggests that lithium carbonate alone or combined with alcohol may make car driving more hazardous.

Clinical evidence, mechanism, importance and management

0.5 g/kg of alcohol raised the serum levels of **lithium carbonate** in 9 out of 10 normal subjects by 16% after taking a single 600 mg dose of **lithium**, and 4 subjects had at least a 25% increase, however this rise were not considered to be clinically important.[1] However a study on 20 normal subjects given **lithium carbonate** to achieve blood levels of 0.75 mEq/l and 0.5 g/kg alcohol, and who were subjected to various psychomotor tests (choice reaction, coordination, attention) to assess any impairment of skills related to driving, indicated that **lithium carbonate** both alone and with alcohol may increase the risk of accident.[2] Information is very limited but patients should be warned.

1. Anton RF, Paladino JA, Morton A, Thomas RW. Effect of acute alcohol consumption on lithium kinetics. *Clin Pharmacol Ther* (1985) 38, 52–5.
2. Linnoila M, Saario I, Maki M. Effects of treatment with diazepam or lithium and alcohol on psychomotor skills related to driving. *Eur J Clin Pharmacol* (1974) 7, 337–42.

Alcohol + Liv. 52

Liv. 52, an Ayurvedic herbal remedy, appears to reduce the hangover symptoms after drinking, reducing both urine and blood alcohol and acetaldehyde levels at 12 h. However it also raises the blood alcohol levels of moderate drinkers for the first few hours after drinking.

Clinical evidence

Nine volunteers who normally drank socially (40–100 g weekly) took six tablets of *Liv. 52* 2 h before drinking alcohol (four 60 ml doses of **whiskey**, equivalent to 90 g alcohol). Their blood alcohol levels at 1 h were increased 15% (from 75.0 to 86.2 mg%). After taking three tablets of *Liv. 52* daily for two weeks, their 1 h blood alcohol levels were raised 27% (from 75% to 95.3 mg%).[1] The blood alcohol levels of eight other moderate drinkers were found to be raised over the first 2 h by about 27–30% after taking three tablets of *Liv. 52* daily for two weeks, and by 16% and 14% respectively over the following 2 h.[2] Only a minor increase in the blood alcohol levels of occasional drinkers occurred.[2] Acetaldehyde levels in the blood and urine were markedly lowered at 12 h, and hangover seemed to be reduced.[1]

Mechanism

Not understood. *Liv. 52* contains the active principles from *Capparis spinosa, Cichorium intybus, Solanum nigrum, Cassia occidentalis, Terminalia arjuna, Achillea millefolium, Tamarix gallica* and *Phyllanthus amarus.*[1] These appear to increase the absorption of alcohol, or reduce its metabolism by the liver, thereby raising the blood-alcohol levels. It is suggested that the reduced hangover effects may possibly occur because it prevents the binding of acetaldehyde to cell proteins causing a more rapid elimination.[1]

Importance and management

Direct experimental evidence seems to be limited to these two studies.[1,2] *Liv. 52* appears to reduce the hangover effects after drinking, but at the same time it can significantly increase the blood alcohol levels of moderate drinkers for the first few hours after drinking. Increases of up to 30% may be enough to raise the blood alcohol from legal to illegal levels when driving. Moderate drinkers should be warned. Occasional drinkers appear to develop higher blood alcohol levels than moderate drinkers but *Liv. 52* seems not to increase them significantly.[1]

1. Chauhan BL, Kulkarni RD. Alcohol hangover and Liv.52. *Eur J Clin Pharmacol* (1991) 40, 187–8.
2. Chauhan BL, Kulkarni RD. Effect of Liv.52, a herbal preparation, on absorption and metabolism of ethanol in humans. *Eur J Clin Pharmacol* (1991) 40, 189–91.

Alcohol + Maprotiline

The sedative effects of maprotiline and alcohol combined can possibly make car driving or handling dangerous machinery more hazardous.

Clinical evidence, mechanism, importance and management

A double blind crossover trial in 12 normal subjects found that single 75-mg oral doses of **maprotiline** subjectively caused drowsiness which was increased by alcohol (1 g/kg) and worsened the performance of a number of tests.[1] However the same group later failed to find that 50 mg **maprotiline** twice daily increased the detrimental effects of alcohol. Nevertheless it would seem prudent (at the risk of being overcautious) to warn patients of the possible increased risk if they drive or handle potentially dangerous machinery.[2]

1. Strömberg C, Seppälä T, Mattila MJ. Acute effects of maprotiline, doxepin and zimeldine with alcohol in healthy volunteers. *Arch Int Pharmacodyn Ther* (1988) 291, 217–228.
2. Strömberg C, Suokas A, Seppälä T. Interaction of alcohol with maprotiline or nomifensine: echocardiographic and psychometric effects. *Eur J Clin Pharmacol* (1988) 35, 593–99.

Alcohol + Meprobamate

The intoxicant effects of alcohol can be considerably increased by the presence of normal daily doses of meprobamate. Driving or handling other potentially dangerous machinery is made much more hazardous.

Clinical evidence

A study on 24 subjects, given 2.4 mg **meprobamate** daily for a week, showed that with blood alcohol levels of 50 mg% their performance of a number of coordination and judgement tests was much more impaired than with either drug alone.[1] Some of the subjects were quite obviously drunk while taking both and showed ". . . marked muscular incoordination and little or no concern for the social proprieties . . . . Two could not walk without assistance . . . Nothing approaching this was seen with alcohol alone."

Other studies confirm this interaction, although the effects appeared to be less pronounced.[2-7]

Mechanism

Both meprobamate and alcohol are CNS depressants which appear to have additive effects. There is also evidence that alcohol may inhibit or increase meprobamate metabolism, depending on whether it is taken acutely or chronically, but the contribution of this to the enhanced CNS depression is uncertain.[8,9]

Importance and management

A well-documented and potentially serious interaction. Normal daily dosages of meprobamate in association with relatively moderate blood-alcohol concentrations, well within the UK legal limit for driving, can result in obviously hazardous intoxication. Patients should be warned.

1. Zirkle GA, McAtee OB, King PD, Van Dyke R. Meprobamate and small amounts of alcohol: effects on human ability, coordination, and judgement. *JAMA* (1960) 173, 1823–5.
2. Reisby N, Theilgaard A. The interaction of alcohol and meprobamate in man. *Acta Psychiatr Scand* (1969) (Suppl 208), 191–4.
3. Forney RB, Hughes FW. Meprobamate, ethanol or meprobamate-ethanol combinations on performance of human subjects under delayed audiofeedback (DAF). *J Psychol* (1964) 57, 431–6.
4. Goldberg L. Behavioural and physiological effects of alcohol on man. *Psychosom Med* (1966) 28, 570.
5. Ashford JR, Cobby JM. Drug interactions. The effects of alcohol and meprobamate applied singly and jointly in human subjects. IV. *J Stud Alcohol* (1975) (Suppl 7), 140.
6. Cobby JM, Ashford JR. Drug interactions. The effects of alcohol and meprobamate applied singly and jointly in human subjects. V. *J Stud Alcohol* (1975) (Suppl 7), 162.
7. Ashford JR, Carpenter JA. Drug interactions. The effects of alcohol and meprobamate applied singly and jointly in human subjects. V. Summary and conclusions. *J Stud Alcohol* (1975) (Suppl 7), 177–87.
8. Misra PS, Lefevre A, Ishi H, Rubin E, Lieber CS. Increase of ethanol, meprobamate and pentobarbital metabolism after chronic ethanol administration in man and in rats. *Am J Med* (1971) 51, 346.
9. Rubin E, Gang H, Misra PS, Lieber CS. Inhibition of drug metabolism by acute ethanol intoxication: a hepatic microsomal mechanism. *Am J Med* (1970) 49, 801–6.

Alcohol + Methaqualone or Mandrax (methaqualone + diphenhydramine)

The CNS depressant effects of alcohol and its detrimental effects on the skills relating to driving or handling other potentially dangerous machinery are increased by the concurrent use of methaqualone or Mandrax.

Clinical evidence

(a) Methaqualone

A retrospective study of drivers arrested for driving under the influence of drugs and/or drink showed that, generally speaking, those with blood-**methaqualone** levels of 1.0 mg/l or less showed no symptoms of sedation, whereas those above 2.0 mg/l demonstrated serious deterioration (staggering gait, drowsiness, incoherence and slurred speech). These effects were increased if the drivers had also been drinking. The authors write that ". . . the levels (of **methaqualone**) necessary for driving impairment are considerably lowered (by alcohol) . . .", but no precise measure of this is presented in the paper. A similar effect was seen in drivers taking **methaqualone** and diazepam.[1]

(b) Mandrax (methaqualone 250 mg + diphenhydramine 25 mg)

A double-blind study on 12 subjects given two *Mandrax* tablets showed that sedation and a reduction in cognitive skills were enhanced by alcohol (0.5 g/kg). Residual amounts of *Mandrax* continued to interact as long as 72 h after a single dose. **Methaqualone** blood levels are also raised by regular moderate amounts of alcohol.[2] Enhanced effects were also seen in another study.[3]

Mechanism

Alcohol, methaqualone and diphenhydramine are all CNS depressants, the effects of which are additive. The diphenhydramine/alcohol interaction is discussed under 'Alcohol + Antihistamines', p.17. A hangover can occur because the elimination half-life of methaqualone is long (10–40 h).

Importance and management

An established interaction of importance. Those taking either methaqualone or *Mandrax* should be warned that handling machinery, driving a car, or any other task requiring alertness and full coordination, will be made more difficult and hazardous if they drink. Doses of alcohol below the legal driving limit with normal amounts of methaqualone may cause considerable intoxication. Patients should also be told that a significant interaction may possibly occur the following day because methaqualone taken on the previous day can have a hangover effect.

1. McCurdy HH, Solomons ET, Holbrook JM. Incidence of methaqualone in driving-under-the-influence (DUI) cases in the State of Georgia. *J Anal Toxicol* (1981) 5, 270–4.
2. Roden S, Harvey P, Mitchard M. The effect of ethanol on residual plasma methaqualone concentrations and behaviour in volunteers who have taken Mandrax. *Br J Clin Pharmacol* (1977) 4, 245–7.
3. Saario I, Linnoila M. Effect of subacute treatment with hypnotics, alone or in combination with alcohol, on psychomotor skills related to driving. *Acta Pharmacol Toxicol* (1976) 38, 382–92.

Alcohol + Metoclopramide

There is some evidence that metoclopramide can increase the rate of absorption of alcohol, raise maximum blood alcohol levels and possibly increase sedation.

Clinical evidence, mechanism, importance and management

A study in 7 subjects found that 20 mg intravenous **metoclopramide** increased the rate of alcohol absorption, while the peak blood levels were raised from 55 to 86 mg/100 ml. Similar results were seen in 2 subjects given **metoclopramide** orally.[1] Another study in 7 normal subjects found that 10 mg intravenous **metoclopramide** accelerated the rate of absorption of alcohol (70 mg/kg) given orally and increased its peak levels but not to a statistically significant extent. Blood alcohol levels remained below 12 mg%. More importantly the sedative effects of the alcohol were found to be increased.[2] The reasons are not fully understood but it appears to be related to an increase in gastric emptying. These two studies were done to find out more about intestinal absorption mechanisms rather than to identify daily practicalities so that the importance of these findings is uncertain, but it seems possible that the effects of alcohol will be increased. More study is needed.

1. Gibbons DO, Lanet AF. Effects of intravenous and oral propantheline and metoclopramide on ethanol absorption. *Clin Pharmacol Ther* (1975) 17, 578–84.
2. Bateman D, Kahn C, Mashiter K and Davies DS. Pharmacokinetic and concentration-effect studies with IV metoclopramide. *Br J Clin Pharmacol* (1978) 6, 401–5.

Alcohol + Metronidazole

A disulfiram-like reaction can develop in patients on oral metronidazole who drink alcohol. There is one report of its occurrence when applied as a vaginal insert and another when metronidazole was given intravenously. The existence of this interaction is disputed in some reports.

Clinical evidence

A man who had been in a drunken stupor for three days was given two **metronidazole** tablets (total of 500 mg) 1 h apart by his wife in the belief that they might sober him up. Twenty min after the first tablet he was awake and complaining that he had been given disulfiram (which he had had some months before). Immediately after the second tablet he took another drink and developed a classic disulfiram-like reaction with flushing of the face and neck, nausea and epigastric discomfort.[1]

All 10 alcoholic patients in a test of the value of **metronidazole** (250 mg twice daily) as a possible drink-deterrent experienced some disulfiram-like reactions of varying intensity (facial flushing, head-aches, sensation of heat, fall in blood pressure, vomiting).[2] All of 60 other patients, given 250–750 mg **metronidazole** daily, developed mild to moderate disulfiram-like reactions.[3] The incidence in other reports is said to be lower: 24%,[4] 10%[5] and 2%.[6] Other individual cases have been reported.[7]

The reaction has been seen in a patient treated with **intravenous metronidazole** and a trimethoprim-sulfamethoxazole (sulphameth-oxazole) preparation containing 10% alcohol as a diluent,[8] and also reported in association with metabolic acidosis in an intoxicated man 4 h after being given **intravenous metronidazole** as prophylaxis fol-lowing injury.[9] Another report describes a reaction with a **metroni-dazole vaginal insert**.[10] A fatality occurred in a 31-year old woman attributed to cardiac dysrhythmia caused by acetaldehyde toxicity re-sulting from the alcohol/**metronidazole** interaction, linked to auto-nomic distress caused by a physical assault.[11] Alcohol is also said to taste badly[1,2] or is less pleasurable[6] while taking **metronidazole**. Some drug abusers apparently exploit the reaction for 'kicks'.[12] In contrast, there are other reports which claim that **metronidazole** has no disulfiram-like effects whatsoever.[13,14]

Mechanism

Not fully understood. Metronidazole, like disulfiram, can inhibit the activity of acetaldehyde dehydrogenase, xanthine oxidase and alde-hyde dehydrogenase.[15] The accumulation of acetaldehyde appears to be responsible for most of the symptoms (see 'Alcohol + Disulfiram', p.27).

Importance and management

An extensively studied interaction but it remains a slightly controver-sial issue, the incidence being variously reported as between 0 and 100%. Nevertheless because of its unpredictability all patients given metronidazole by mouth should be warned what may happen if they drink. The reaction, when it occurs, normally seems to be more un-pleasant and possibly frightening than serious, and usually requires no treatment, although one report describes a serious reaction when intravenous metronidazole was given to an intoxicated man,[9] and one fatality has been reported.[11] The risk of a reaction with metronidazole used intravaginally seems to be small because the absorption is low (about 20% compared with about 100% orally) but evidently it can happen, even if rarely.[10] Patients should be warned.

1. Taylor JAT. Metronidazole—a new agent for combined somatic and psychic therapy for alcoholism: a case study and preliminary report. *Bull Los Angeles Neurol Soc* (1964) 29, 158–62.
2. Ban TA, Lehmann HE, Roy P. Rapport préliminaire sur l'effect thérapeutidue du Flagyl dans l'alcoolisme. *Union Med Can* (1966) 95, 147–9.
3. Sansoy OM, Vegas L. Evaluation of metronidazole in the treatment of alcoholism. *J Indian Med Assoc* (1970) 55, 29.
4. de Mattos H. Relationship between alcoholism and the digestive system. *Hospital* (1968) 74, 281.
5. Channabasavanna SM, Kaliaperumal VG, Mathew G. Metronidazole in the treatment of alcoholism: a controlled trial. *Ind J Psychiatry* (1979) 21, 90–3.
6. Penick SB, Carrier RN, Sheldon JB. Metronidazole in the treatment of alcoholism. *Am J Psychiatry* (1969) 125, 1063–6.
7. Alexander J. 'Alcohol—Antabuse' syndrome in patients receiving metronidazole during gynaecological treatment. *Br J Clin Pract* (1985) 39, 292–3.
8. Edwards DL, Fink PC, Van Dyke PO. Disulfiram-like reaction associated with intrave-nous trimethoprim–sulphamethoxazole and metronidazole. *Clin Pharm* (1986) 5, 999–1000.
9. Harries DP, Teale KFH, Sunderland G. Metronidazole and alcohol: potential problems. *Scott Med J* (1990) 35, 179–180.
10. Plosker GL. Possible interaction between ethanol and vaginally administered metronida-zole. *Clin Pharm* (1987) 6, 189 and 192–3.
11. Cina SJ, Russell RA, Conradi SE. Sudden death due to metronidazole/ethanol interac-tion. *Am J Forensic Med Pathol* (1996) 17, 343–6.
12. Giannini AJ, DeFrance DT. Metronidazole and alcohol—potential for combinative abuse. *J Toxicol Clin Toxicol* (1983) 20, 509–15.
13. Goodwin DW. Metronidazole in the treatment of alcoholism. *Am J Psychiatry* (1968) 123, 1276–8.
14. Gelder MG, Edwards G. Metronidazole in the treatment of alcohol addiction: a control-led trial. *Br J Psychiatry* (1968) 114, 473–5.
15. Fried R, Fried LW. The effect of Flagyl on xanthine oxidase and alcohol dehydrogenase. *Biochem Pharmacol* (1966) 15, 1890.

Alcohol + Milk

Blood levels of alcohol and its intoxicant effects are reduced if milk has been drunk.

Clinical evidence, mechanism, importance and management

Ten subjects were given 25 ml alcohol (equivalent to a double **whis-key**) after drinking a pint and a half of water or **milk** during the pre-vious 90 min. Blood alcohol levels 90 min later were reduced about 40% by the presence of the **milk**, and about 25% half an hour later. The intoxicant effects of the alcohol were also clearly reduced.[1] The reasons are not understood, but a possible explanation is that the ab-sorption of the alcohol by the gut is reduced by the **milk**. These find-ings appear to confirm a long and widely held belief among drinkers, but whether this interaction can be regarded as advantageous or un-desirable is a moot point.

1. Miller DS, Stirling JL, Yudkin J. Effect of ingestion of milk on concentrations of blood alcohol. *Nature* (1966) 212, 1051.

Alcohol + Miscellaneous Anxiolytics

Buspirone with alcohol may cause drowsiness and weakness which may make driving more hazardous. Suriclone increas-es the CNS depressant effects of alcohol to some extent, but usually less than other more obviously sedative drugs.

Clinical evidence, mechanism, importance and management

Studies in 12 normal subjects showed that 10 or 20 mg **buspirone** did not appear to interact with alcohol (i.e. worsen the performance of certain psychomotor tests) but it did make them feel drowsy and weak. The tentative conclusion was drawn that patients might there-fore be more aware of feeling 'under par' than with some other drugs (e.g. the benzodiazepines) and less likely to take risks.[1,2] However an-other study in 13 normal subjects suggested that the effects of com-bining **buspirone** (15 and 30 mg/70 kg) and alcohol were broadly similar to those seen with alprazolam plus alcohol,[3] so that it would seem prudent to warn patients of the potential hazards of driving or handling other potentially dangerous machinery.

Normal subjects on 0.2 or 0.4 mg **suriclone** three times a day showed modest changes in the performance of a number of tests when also taking alcohol (blood levels of 64–67 mg/dl), similar in many re-spects to those seen with diazepam, but the differences included in-creased irritability and antagonism, and some stomach troubles (indigestion, nausea, loss of appetite).[4] As with diazepam, you should warn patients of the possible increased risks of driving or handling other potentially dangerous machinery.

1. Mattila MJ, Aranko K, Seppälä T. Acute effects of buspirone and alcohol on psychomotor skills. *J Clin Psychiatry* (1982) 43, 56–60.
2. Seppälä T, Aranko K, Mattila MJ, Shrotriya RC. Effects of alcohol on buspirone and lo-razepam actions. *Clin Pharmacol Ther* (1982) 32, 201–7.
3. Rush CR, Griffiths RR. Acute participant-rated and behavioral effects of alprazolam and buspirone, alone and in combination with ethanol, in normal volunteers. *Exp Clin Psy-chopharmacol* (1997) 5, 28–38.
4. Allen D, Lader M. The interactions of ethanol with single and repeated doses of suriclone and diazepam on physiological and psychomotor functions in normal subjects. *Eur J Clin Pharmacol* (1992) 42, 499–505.

Alcohol + Nitrofurantoin

There appears to be no good clinical evidence for an alleged nitrofurantoin/alcohol interaction.

Clinical evidence, mechanism, importance and management

Despite claims in some books and reviews, an extensive literature survey failed to find any experimental or clinical evidence for an alleged disulfiram-like reaction between alcohol and **nitrofurantoin**.[1] A study in normal subjects failed to demonstrate any such interaction[2] and a survey of the reports in the maker's database also failed to find good evidence for alcohol intolerance.[3] It is concluded that this 'interaction' is erroneous.[1]

1. Rowles B, Worthen DB. Clinical drug information: a case of misinformation. *N Engl J Med* (1982) 306, 113–4.
2. Miura K, Reckendorf HK. The nitrofurans. In Ellis GP, West GB (eds). Progress in Medicinal Chemistry. New York, Plenum Press (1967) 5, 320–81.
3. D'Arcy PF. Nitrofurantoin. *Drug Intell Clin Pharm* (1985) 19, 540–7.

Alcohol + Nitroimidazoles

It is alleged that benznidazole, nimorazole, ornidazole and tinidazole can cause a disulfiram-like reaction with alcohol.

Clinical evidence, mechanism, importance and management

It has been alleged that all of the nitroimidazoles (**benznidazole, metronidazole, nimorazole, ornidazole, tinidazole**) can cause a disulfiram-like reaction with alcohol (flushing of the face and neck, palpitations, dizziness, nausea, etc.)[1,2] but there does not appear to be any direct evidence to confirm that this actually occurs, except with **metronidazole** (see 'Alcohol + Metronidazole', p.33). Roche, the makers of **benznidazole**, also say they have no record of this interaction on their drug database.[3] So, the alleged interactions of alcohol with these other nitroimidazoles may simply be an extrapolation of the known interaction with **metronidazole**. Even if a disulfiram-like reaction were to occur it is usually more unpleasant and frightening than serious, and normally requires little or no treatment.

1. Bodino JAJ, Lopez EL. Schistosomiasis drugs. In Koren G, Prober CG, Gold R (eds), Antimicrobial therapy in infants and children, Marcel Dekker, NY (1988) pp 687–727.
2. Ralph ED. Nitroimidazoles. In Koren G, Prober CG, Gold R (eds), Antimicrobial therapy in infants and children, Marcel Dekker, NY (1988) pp 729–745.
3. Roche UK. Personal communication (1989).

Alcohol + Paraldehyde

Both alcohol and paraldehyde have CNS depressant effects which can be additive. Their concurrent use in the treatment of acute intoxication has had a fatal outcome.

Clinical evidence, mechanism, importance and management

A report describes 8 patients who died suddenly and unexpectedly after treatment for acute intoxication with 30–60 ml **paraldehyde** (normal dose range 3–30 ml; fatal dose 120 ml or more).[1] Both are CNS depressants and may therefore be expected to have additive effects at any dosage, although an *animal* study suggested that it may be less than additive.[2]

1. Kaye S, Haag HB. Study of death due to combined action of alcohol and paraldehyde in man. *Toxicol Appl Pharmacol* (1964) 6, 316–20.
2. Gessner PK, Shakarjian MP. Interactions of paraldehyde with ethanol and chloral hydrate. *J Pharmacol Exp Ther* (1985) 235, 32–6.

Alcohol + Phenothiazines, Butyrophenones and other psychotropic drugs

The detrimental effects of alcohol on the skills related to driving are made worse by chlorpromazine, flupenthixol (possibly prochlorperazine?) and to a lesser extent by thioridazine. Any interaction with amisulpride, haloperidol, sulpiride or tiapride seems to be mild or relatively unimportant. There is evidence that drinking can precipitate the emergence of extrapyramidal side-effects in patients taking neuroleptics.

Clinical evidence

(a) Effect on driving and other skills

No significant pharmacokinetic interactions were seen in 18 normal subjects given 50 and 200 mg doses of **amisulpride** with 0.8 g/kg alcohol, nor were the detrimental effects of alcohol on performance increased by the **amisulpride**.[1] 21 subjects showed a marked deterioration in the performance of a number of skills related to driving when given 200 mg **chlorpromazine** daily and alcohol (blood levels 42 mg%). Many complained of feeling sleepy, lethargic, dull, groggy and poorly coordinated and most considered themselves more unsafe to drive than with alcohol alone.[2] A later study confirmed these findings with 1 mg/kg **chlorpromazine** and blood alcohol levels of 80 mg%.[3] Increased sedation was clearly seen in another study.[4] A double-blind study in subjects given 0.5 mg **flupenthixol**, three times a day for 2 weeks found that combined with 0.5 g/kg alcohol their performance of a number of tests (choice reaction, coordination, attention) was impaired to such an extent that driving or handling other potentially dangerous machinery could be hazardous.[5,6] No interaction of any importance was seen with single 0.5 mg doses of **haloperidol**.[5,6] A study in 12 normal subjects found that 5 mg **prochlorperazine** three times daily (no alcohol) for 3 days caused carelessness and slowing of a weaving test while driving a car, with little subjective appreciation of the deterioration. No changes could be detected in the performance of kinetic visual acuity or simple reaction time tests.[7] Alcohol would be expected to increase this impairment but nobody seems to have checked on this yet, nevertheless patients should be warned. In the same study 72 mg **betahistine** daily for 3 days was found to have no detectable effect on driving performance.[7] Subjects given 150 mg **sulpiride** daily for 2 weeks demonstrated only a mild interaction with alcohol, whereas when given 30–60 mg **thioridazine** daily for 2 weeks some additive effects with alcohol were seen, with a moderately deleterious effect on attention.[6,8] Another study found that **thioridazine** and alcohol affected skills related to driving, but not as much as the effects seen with **chlorpromazine**.[3] Another study found no difference between the effects of **thioridazine** and a placebo.[9] A study in 9 alcoholics given 400 to 600 mg **tiapride** daily showed that wakefulness was not impaired when combined with alcohol (0.5 g/kg) and in fact appeared to be improved, but the effect on driving skills was not studied.[10]

(b) Precipitation of extrapyramidal side-effects

A report[11] describes in detail 7 patients who developed acute extrapyramidal side-effects (akathisia, dystonia) while taking **trifluoperazine, fluphenazine** and **chlorpromazine** when they drank alcohol. The author stated that these were examples of numerous such alcohol-induced neuroleptic toxicity reactions observed by him over an 18-year period involving phenothiazines and butyrophenones. Elsewhere he describes the emergence of drug-induced parkinsonism in a woman taking **perphenazine** and **amitriptyline** when she began to drink.[12] Eighteen cases of **haloperidol**-induced extrapyramidal reactions among young drug abusers, in most instances associated with the ingestion of alcohol, have also been described.[13]

(c) Reduced fluphenazine levels

A study in 7 schizophrenics found that when given 40 g alcohol to drink at about the same time as their regular injection of **fluphenazine decanoate** (25–125 mg every 2 weeks), their serum **fluphenazine** levels were depressed by 30% at 2 h and by 16% at 12 h.[14]

Mechanisms

Uncertain. (a) Additive CNS depressant effects are one explanation of this interaction. (b) One suggestion to account for the emergence of the drug side-effects is that alcohol lowers the threshold of resistance to the neurotoxicity of these drugs. In addition it seems possible that alcohol impairs the activity of tyrosine hydroxylase so that the dopamine/acetylcholine balance within the corpus striatum is upset.[12]

Importance and management

The documentation is limited. (a) Warn patients that if they drink while on chlorpromazine, thioridazine or flupenthixol (probably other related drugs as well) they may become very drowsy, and should not drive or handle other potentially dangerous machinery. Some risk is possible with prochlorperazine as well, but the effects of alcohol with amisulpride, haloperidol, sulpiride and tiapride appear to be minimal. (b) The author of the reports describing the emergence of serious neuroleptic side-effects in those who drink, considers that patients should routinely be advised to abstain from alcohol during neuroleptic treatment. (c) The clinical importance of reduced fluphenazine levels is uncertain. This needs more study.

1. Mattila MJ, Patat A, Seppälä T, Kalska H, Lalava M-L, Vanakoski J, Lavanant C. Single oral doses of amisulpride do not enhance the effects of alcohol on the performance and memory of healthy subjects. *Eur J Clin Pharmacol* (1996) 51, 161–6.
2. Zirkle GA, King PD, McAtee OB. Van Dyke R. Effects of chlorpromazine and alcohol on coordination and judgment. *JAMA* (1959) 171, 1496–9.
3. Milner G, Landauer AA. Alcohol, thioridazine and chlorpromazine effects on skills related to driving behaviour. *Br J Psychiatry* (1971) 118, 351–2.
4. Sutherland VC, Burbridge TN, Adams JE, Simon A. Cerebral metabolism in problem drinkers under the influence of alcohol and chlorpromazine hydrochloride. *J Appl Physiol* (1960) 15, 189–96.
5. Linnoila M. Effects of diazepam, chlordiazepoxide, thioridazine, haloperidol, flupenthixol and alcohol on psychomotor skills related to driving. *Ann Med Exp Biol Fenn* (1973) 51, 125–32.
6. Linnoila M, Saario I, Olkonieme J, Liljequist R, Himberg JJ, Maki M. Effect of two weeks treatment with chlordiazepoxide or flupenthixol, alone or in combination with alcohol, on psychomotor skills related to driving. *Arzneimittelforschung* (1975) 25, 1088.
7. Betts T, Harris D, Gadd E. The effects of two anti-vertigo drugs (betahistine and prochlorperazine) on driving skills. *Br J Clin Pharmacol* (1991) 32, 455–8.
8. Seppälä T, Saario I, Mattila MJ. Two weeks' treatment with chlorpromazine, thioridazine, sulpiride, or bromazepam: actions and interactions with alcohol on psychomotor skills related to driving. *Mod Probl Pharmacopsychiatry* (1976) 11, 85–90.
9. Saario I. Psychomotor skills during subacute treatment with thioridazine and bromazepam, and their combined effects with alcohol. *Ann Clin Res* (1976) 8, 117–23.
10. Vandel B, Bonin B, Vandel S, Blum D, Rey E, Volmat R. Étude de l'interaction entre le tiapride et l'alcool chez l'homme. *Sem Hop Paris* (1984) 60, 175–7.
11. Lutz EG. Neuroleptic-induced akathisia and dystonia triggered by alcohol. *JAMA* (1976) 236, 2422–3.
12. Lutz EG. Neuroleptic-induced parkinsonism facilitated by alcohol. *J Med Soc NJ* (1978) 75, 473–4.
13. Kenyon-David D. Haloperidol intoxication. *N Z Med J* (1981) 93, 165.
14. Soni SD, Bamrah JS, Krska J. Effects of alcohol on serum fluphenazine levels in stable chronic schizophrenics. *Hum Psychopharmacol* (1991) 6, 301–6.

Alcohol + Procarbazine

A flushing reaction has been seen in patients on procarbazine after drinking alcohol.

Clinical evidence

One report describes 5 patients taking **procarbazine** whose faces became very red and hot for a short time after drinking **wine**.[1] Another says that flushing occurred in 3 patients on **procarbazine** after drinking **beer**.[2] Two out of 40 patients in a third study complained of facial flushing after taking a small alcoholic drink, and one patient thought that the effects of alcohol were markedly increased.[3] Yet another describes a 'flush syndrome' in 3 out of 50 patients after drinking alcohol.[4]

Mechanism

Not established, but it seems possible that in man, as in *rats*,[5] the procarbazine inhibits acetaldehyde dehydrogenase in the liver causing a disulfiram-like reaction (see 'Alcohol + Disulfiram', p.27).

Importance and management

An established interaction but of uncertain incidence. It seems to be more embarrassing, possibly frightening, than serious and if it occurs it is unlikely to require treatment, however patients should be warned.

1. Mathé G, Berumen L, Schweisguth O, Brule G, Schneider M, Cattan A, Amiel JL, Schwarzenberg L. Methyl-hydrazine in the treatment of Hodgkin's disease and various forms of haematosarcoma and leukaemia. *Lancet* (1963) ii, 1077–80.
2. Dawson WB. Ibenzmethyzin in the management of late Hodgkin's disease. In 'Natulan, Ibenzmethyzin'. Report of the proceedings of a symposium, Downing College, Cambridge, June 1965. Jelliffe AM and Marks J (Eds). John Wright, Bristol (1965) p 31–4.
3. Todd IDH. Natulan in the management of late Hodgkin's disease, other lymphoreticular neoplasms, and malignant melanoma. *BMJ* (1965) 1, 326–7.
4. Brulé G, Schlumberger JR, Griscelli C. N-isopropyl-α-(2-methylhydrazino)-p-toluamide, hydrochloride (NSC-77213) in treatment of solid tumors. *Cancer Chemother Rep* (1965) 44, 31–8.
5. Vasiliou V, Malamas M, Marselos M. The mechanism of alcohol intolerance produced by various therapeutic agents. *Acta Pharmacol Toxicol* (1986) 58, 305–10.

Alcohol + Sodium cromoglicate (cromoglycate)

No adverse interaction occurs between sodium cromoglicate (cromoglycate) and alcohol.

Clinical evidence, mechanism, importance and management

A double-blind crossover trial on 17 subjects found that 40 mg **sodium cromoglicate (cromoglycate)** had little or no effect on the performance of a number of tests on human perceptual, cognitive and motor skills, whether taken alone or with alcohol (0.75 g/kg). Nor did it affect blood alcohol levels.[1] This is in line with the common experience of patients, and no special precautions seem to be necessary.

1. Crawford WA, Franks HM, Hensley VR, Hensley WJ, Starmer GA, Teo RKC. The effect of disodium cromoglycate on human performance, alone and in combination with ethanol. *Med J Aust* (1976) 1, 997–9.

Alcohol + Sulfiram (Monosulfiram)

Disulfiram-like reactions have been seen in at least 3 patients who drank alcohol after using a solution of sulfiram (monosulfiram) on the skin for the treatment of scabies.

Clinical evidence

A man who used undiluted **Tetmosol** (a solution of **sulfiram (monosulfiram)**) for 3 days on the skin all over his body developed a disulfiram-like reaction (flushing, sweating, skin swelling, severe tachycardia and nausea) on the third day after drinking three double whiskeys. The same thing happened on two subsequent evenings after drinking.[1] Similar reactions have been described in 2 other patients after drinking while using **Tetmosol** or **Ascabiol** (also containing **sulfiram**).[2,3]

Mechanism

Sulfiram (tetraethylthiuram monosulphide) is closely related to disulfiram (tetraethylthiuram disulphide) and can apparently undergo photochemical conversion to disulfiram when exposed to light. The longer it is stored, the higher the concentration.[4,5] The reaction with alcohol (inhibition of aldehyde dehydrogenase) appears therefore to be largely due to the presence of disulfiram (see 'Alcohol + Disulfiram', p.27).[6]

Importance and management

An established interaction. The makers of sulfiram (monosulfiram) preparations and others advise abstention from alcohol before, and for at least 48 h after application, but this may not always be necessary. The writer of a letter,[7] commenting on the first case cited,[1] wrote that he had never encountered this reaction when using a diluted solution of *Tetmosol* on patients at the Dreadnought Seamen's Hospital in London who ". . . are not necessarily abstemious." This would suggest that the reaction is normally uncommon and unlikely to occur if the solution is correctly diluted (usually with 2–3 parts of water) thereby reducing the amount absorbed through the skin. However one unusually sensitive patient is said to have had a reaction (flushing, sweating, tachycardia) after using diluted *Tetmosol*, but without drinking alcohol. It was suggested that she reacted to the alcohol base of the formulation passing through her skin.[8] Patients should be warned.

1. Gold S. A skinful of alcohol. *Lancet* (1966) ii, 1417.
2. Dantas W. Monosulfiram como causa de síndrome do acetaldeído. *Arq Cat Med* (1980) 9, 29–30.
3. Blanc D, Deprez Ph. Unusual adverse reaction to an acaricide. *Lancet* (1990) 335, 1291.
4. Lipsky JJ, Mays DC, Naylor S. Monosulfiram, disulfiram, and light. *Lancet* (1994) 343, 304.
5. Mays DC, Nelson AN, Benson LM, Johnson KL, Naylor S, Lipsky JJ. Photolysis of monosulfiram: a mechanism for its disulfiram-like reaction. *Clin Pharmacol Ther* (1994) 55, 191.
6. Lipsky JJ, Nelson AN, Dockter EC. Inhibition of aldehyde dehydrogenase by sulfiram. *Clin Pharmacol Ther* (1992) 51, 184.
7. Erskine D. A skinful of alcohol. *Lancet* (1967) i, 54.
8. Burgess I. Adverse reactions to monosulfiram. *Lancet* (1990) 336, 873.

Alcohol + Tetracyclic antidepressants

Mianserin can cause drowsiness and impair the ability to drive or handle other dangerous machinery, particularly during the first few days of treatment. This impairment is increased by alcohol. Pirlindole appears not to interact with alcohol.

Clinical evidence

(a) Mianserin

A double-blind crossover study in 13 normal subjects given 20 to 60 mg **mianserin** daily for eight days, with and without alcohol (1 g/kg), showed that their performance of a number of psychomotor tests (choice reaction, coordination, critical flicker frequency) were impaired by concurrent use. The subjects were aware of feeling drowsy and muzzy, and less able to carry out the tests.[1]

These results confirm the findings of other studies.[2-4]

(b) Pirlindole

A study in subjects given **pirlindole** indicated that it did not affect the performance of a number of psychomotor tests, with or without alcohol.[5]

Mechanism

The CNS depressant effects of mianserin appear to be additive with those of alcohol.

Importance and management

Drowsiness is a frequently reported side-effect of mianserin, particularly during the first few days of treatment. Patients should be warned that driving or handling dangerous machinery will be made more hazardous if they drink. Pirlindole appears not to interact.

1. Seppälä T, Strömberg C, Bergman I. Effect of zimeldine, mianserin and amitriptyline on psychomotor skills and their interaction with alcohol: a placebo controlled cross-over study. *Eur J Clin Pharmacol* (1984) 27, 181–9.
2. Mattila MJ, Liljequist R, Seppälä T. Effects of amitriptyline and mianserin on psychomotor skills and memory in man. *Br J Clin Pharmacol* (1978) 5, 53S.
3. Seppälä T. Psychomotor skills during acute and two-week treatment with mianserin (Org GB 94) and amitriptyline, and their combined effects with alcohol. *Ann Clin Res* (1977) 9, 66–72.
4. Strömberg C, Mattila MJ. Acute comparison of clovoxamine and mianserin, alone and in combination with ethanol, on human psychomotor performance. *Pharmacol Toxicol* (1987) 60, 374–9.
5. Ehlers T, Ritter M. Effects of the tetracyclic antidepressant pirlindole on sensorimotor performance and subjective condition in comparison to imipramine and during interaction of ethanol. *Neuropsychobiology* (1984) 12, 48–54.

Alcohol + Tolazoline

A disulfiram-like reaction may occur in patients on tolazoline if they drink.

Clinical evidence, mechanism, importance and management

Seven normal subjects were given 500 mg **tolazoline** daily for 4 days. Within 15 and 90 min of drinking 90 ml **port wine** (18.2% **alcohol**) 6 of the 7 experienced tingling over the head, and 4 developed warmth and fullness of the head.[1] The reasons are not understood, but this reaction is not unlike a mild disulfiram reaction and may possibly have a similar mechanism (see 'Alcohol + Disulfiram', p.27). Patients given **tolazoline** should be warned about this reaction if they drink and advised to limit their consumption. Reactions of this kind with drugs other than disulfiram are usually more unpleasant or frightening than serious, and treatment is rarely needed.

1. Boyd EM. A search for drugs with disulfiram-like activity. *Q J Stud Alcohol* (1960) 21, 23–5.

Alcohol + Trazodone

Trazodone makes driving or handling other dangerous machinery more hazardous, and further impairment may occur with alcohol.

Clinical evidence

A study in 6 normal subjects comparing the effects of **amitriptyline** (50 mg) and **trazodone** (100 mg) found that both drugs impaired the performance of a number of psychomotor tests, causing drowsiness and reducing 'clearheadedness' to approximately the same extent. Only manual dexterity was further impaired when the subjects on **trazodone** were given sufficient alcohol to give blood levels of about 40 mg%.[1]

Another study similarly found that the impairment of psychomotor performance by **trazodone** was increased by alcohol.[2]

Mechanism

Uncertain. Simple additive depression of the CNS seems a likely explanation.

Importance and management

An established interaction, and of practical importance. Patients should be warned that their ability to drive, handle dangerous machinery or to do other tasks needing complex psychomotor skills may be impaired by trazodone, and further worsened by alcohol.

1. Warrington SJ, Ankier SI, Turner P. Evaluation of possible interactions between ethanol and trazodone or amitriptyline. *Neuropsychobiology* (1986) 15 (Suppl 1), 31–7.
2. Tiller JWG. Antidepressants, alcohol and psychomotor performance. *Acta Psychiatr Scand* (1990) (Suppl 360), 13–17.

Alcohol + Trichloroethylene

A flushing skin reaction similar to a mild disulfiram reaction can occur in those exposed to trichloroethylene when they drink alcohol.

Clinical evidence

An engineer from a factory where **trichloroethylene** was being used as a degreasing agent, developed facial flushing, a sensation of increased pressure in the head, lachrymation, tachypnoea and blurred vision within 12 min of drinking 3 oz **bourbon whiskey**. The reaction did not develop when he was no longer exposed to the **trichlo-**

roethylene. Other workers in the same plant reported the same experience.[1]

Vivid red blotches in a symmetrical pattern on the face, neck, shoulders and back were seen in other workers exposed for a few hours each day to 20–220 ppm **trichloroethylene** when they drank only half-a-pint (300 ml) of **beer**,[2] and it has also been reported elsewhere.[3] It has been described as the 'degreasers flush'.[2] There is also some evidence that long-term exposure may possibly reduce mental capacity.[4]

Mechanism

Uncertain. One suggested mechanism is a disulfiram-like inhibition of acetaldehyde metabolism by trichloroethylene (see 'Alcohol + Disulfiram', p.27).

Importance and management

An established interaction. It would seem to be more unpleasant and socially disagreeable than serious, and normally requires no treatment. The whole question of whether long-term exposure to trichloroethylene is desirable does not seem to have been answered.

1. Pardys S, Brotman M. Trichloroethylene and alcohol: a straight flush. *JAMA* (1974) 229, 521–2.
2. Stewart RD, Hake CL, Peterson JE. "Degreasers' Flush": dermal response to trichloroethylene and ethanol. *Arch Environ Health* (1974) 29, 1–5.
3. Smith GF. Trichloroethylene: a review. *Br J Ind Med* (1966) 23, 249.
4. Windemuller FJB, Ettema JH. Effects of combined exposure to trichloroethylene and alcohol on mental capacity. *Int Arch Occup Environ Health* (1978) 41, 77–85.

Alcohol + Tricyclic antidepressants

The ability to drive, to handle dangerous machinery or to do other tasks requiring complex psychomotor skills may be impaired by amitriptyline and to a lesser extent by doxepin, particularly during the first few days of treatment. This impairment is increased by alcohol. Amoxapine, clomipramine, desipramine, imipramine and nortriptyline appear to interact with alcohol only minimally. Information about other tricyclics appears to be lacking. There is also evidence that alcoholics may need larger doses of desipramine and imipramine to control depression.

Clinical evidence

(a) Amitriptyline

Blood alcohol levels of about 80 mg% impaired the performance by 21 normal subjects of three motor skills tests related to driving. When additionally given 0.8 mg/kg **amitriptyline** the performance was even further impaired.[1]

Similar results have been very clearly demonstrated in considerable numbers of subjects using a variety of psychomotor skill tests,[1-7] the interaction being most marked during the first few days of treatment, but tending to wane as treatment continued.[5] There is also some limited evidence from *animal* studies that **amitriptyline** may possibly enhance the fatty changes induced in the liver by alcohol,[8] but this still needs confirmation from human studies. Unexplained blackouts lasting a few hours have also been described in 3 women after drinking only modest amounts;[9] they had been taking **amitriptyline** or **imipramine** for only a month.

(b) Doxepin

A double-blind crossover trial on 21 subjects given various combinations of alcohol and either **doxepin** or a placebo showed that with blood alcohol levels of 40–50 mg% their choice reaction test times were prolonged and the number of mistakes increased. Coordination was obviously impaired after 7 days' treatment with **doxepin**, but not after 14 days.[3] In an earlier study **doxepin** appeared to cancel out the deleterious effects of alcohol on the performance of a simulated driving test.[10]

(c) Amoxapine, Clomipramine, Desipramine, Imipramine, Nortriptyline

Studies in subjects with blood alcohol levels of 40–60 mg% showed that **clomipramine** and **nortriptyline** had only slight or no effects on various choice reaction, coordination, memory and learning tests.[3,11-13] The **amoxapine**/alcohol interaction was found to be slight[14] but two patients have been described who experienced reversible extrapyramidal symptoms (parkinsonism, akathisia) while taking **amoxapine**, apparently caused by drinking.[15] Tests in subjects given 100 mg **desipramine** indicated that no significant interaction occurs with alcohol,[16] but 150 mg **imipramine** daily tends to increase the sedative-hypnotic effects of alcohol.[17]

A comparative study in recently detoxified alcoholic men showed that the half-lives of **imipramine** and **desipramine** were about halved in recently detoxified alcoholics (8.7 and 10.9 h respectively) compared with normal subjects (19.9 and 19.6 h), and the total body clearances were about doubled.[18]

Mechanisms

Part of the explanation for the increased CNS depression is that both alcohol and some of the tricyclics, particularly amitriptyline, cause drowsiness and other CNS depressant effects which can be additive with the effects of alcohol.[6] The sedative effects are said in one review to be amitriptyline > doxepin > imipramine > nortriptyline > desipramine > protriptyline.[19] In addition alcohol causes marked increases (100–200%) in the plasma concentrations of amitriptyline, probably by inhibiting its metabolism during its first pass through the liver.[4] The reduced serum levels of imipramine and desipramine seen in abstinent alcoholics is attributable to induction by alcohol of the cytochrome P450 enzymes.[18]

Importance and management

The increased CNS depression resulting from the amitriptyline/alcohol interaction is well documented and clinically important. Warn patients that driving or handling dangerous machinery may be made more hazardous if they drink, particularly during the first few days, but the effects of the interaction diminish during continued treatment. The alcohol/doxepin interaction is less well documented and the information is conflicting, but to be on the safe side a similar warning should be given. Amoxapine, clomipramine, desipramine, imipramine and nortriptyline appear to interact only minimally with alcohol. Direct information about other tricyclics seems to be lacking, but there appear to be no particular reasons for avoiding concurrent use, however prescribers may feel it appropriate to offer some precautionary advice because during the first 1–2 weeks of treatment many tricyclics (without alcohol) may temporarily impair the skills related to driving.[14]

Also be aware that alcoholic patients may need higher doses of imipramine and desipramine (possibly doubled) to control depression, and if abstinence is achieved the dosages may then eventually need to be reduced. Information about other tricyclics seems to be lacking.

1. Landauer AA, Milner G, Patman J. Alcohol and amitriptyline effects on skills related to driving behavior. *Science* (1969) 163, 1467–8.
2. Seppälä T. Psychomotor skills during acute and two-week treatment with mianserin (ORG GB 94) and amitriptyline, and their combined effects with alcohol. *Ann Clin Res* (1977) 9, 66–72.
3. Seppälä T, Linnoila M, Elonen E, Mattila MJ, Mäki M. Effect of tricyclic antidepressants and alcohol on psychomotor skills related to driving. *Clin Pharmacol Ther* (1975) 17, 515–22.
4. Dorian P, Sellers EM, Reed KL, Warsh JJ, Hamilton C, Kaplan HL, Fan T. Amitriptyline and ethanol: pharmacokinetic and pharmacodynamic interaction. *Eur J Clin Pharmacol* (1983) 25, 325–31.
5. Seppälä T, Strömberg C, Bergman I. Effects of zimeldine, mianserin and amitriptyline on psychomotor skills and their interaction with ethanol: a placebo controlled cross-over study. *Eur J Clin Pharmacol* (1984) 27, 181–9.
6. Scott DB, Fagan D, Tiplady B. Effects of amitriptyline and zimelidine in combination with alcohol. *Psychopharmacology (Berl)* (1982) 76, 209–11.
7. Mattila M, Liljequist R, Seppälä T. Effects of amitriptyline and mianserin on psychomotor skills and memory in man. *Br J Clin Pharmacol* (1978) 5, 53S.
8. Milner G, Kakulas BA. The potentiation by amitriptyline of liver changes induced by ethanol in mice. *Pathology* (1969) 1, 113–18.
9. Hudson CJ. Tricyclic antidepressants and alcoholic blackouts. *J Nerv Ment Dis* (1981) 169, 381–2.
10. Milner G, Landauer AA. The effects of doxepin, alone and together with alcohol in relation to driving safety. *Med J Aust* (1973) 1, 837–8.
11. Hughes FW, Forney RB. Delayed audiofeedback (DAF) for induction of anxiety: effect of nortriptyline, ethanol, or nortriptyline-ethanol combinations on performance with DAF. *JAMA* (1963) 185, 556–8.

12. Liljequist R, Linnoila M, Mattila M. Effect of two weeks' treatment with chlorimipramine and nortriptyline, alone or in combination with alcohol on learning and memory. *Psychopharmacology (Berl)* (1974) 39, 181–6.
13. Berlin I, Cournot A, Zimmer R, Pedarriosse A-M, Manfredi R, Molinier P, Puech AJ. Evaluation and comparison of the interaction between alcohol and moclobemide or clomipramine in healthy subjects. *Psychopharmacology (Berl)* (1990) 100, 40–5.
14. Linnoila M, Seppälä T. Antidepressants and driving. *Accid Anal Prev* (1985) 17, 297–301.
15. Shen WW. Alcohol, amoxapine, and akathisia. *Biol Psychiatry* (1984) 19, 929–30.
16. Linnoila M, Johnson J, Dubyoski K, Buchsbaum MS, Schneinin M, Kilts C. Effects of antidepressants on skilled performance. *Br J Clin Pharmacol* (1984) 18, 109S–120S.
17. Frewer LJ, Lader M. The effects of nefazodone, imipramine and placebo, alone and combined with alcohol, in normal subjects. *Int Clin Psychopharmacol* (1993) 8, 13–20.
18. Ciraulo DA, Barnhill JG, Jaffe JJ. Clinical pharmacokinetics of imipramine and desipramine in alcoholics and normal volunteers. *Clin Pharmacol Ther* (1988) 43, 509–18.
19. Marco LA, Randels RM. Drug interactions in alcoholic patients. *Hillside J Clin Psychiatry* (1981) 3, 27–44.

Alcohol + Viqualine

No adverse interaction occurs if alcohol and viqualine are taken together.

Clinical evidence, mechanism, importance and management

Alcohol (serum levels 17–22 mmol/l) had no effect on the steady-state serum levels of **viqualine** (75 mg twice daily for three days) in 16 normal subjects, nor was there any evidence of a disulfiram-like reaction. The deleterious effects of alcohol on a number of skills (word recall, manual tracking, body sway) and self-ratings of intoxication, sedation and performance were also not altered by the **viqualine**.[1] On the basis of this study there would seem to be no good reason for those taking **viqualine** to avoid alcoholic drinks.

1. Sullivan JT, Naranjo CA, Shaw CA, Kaplan HL, Kadlec KE, Sellers EM. Kinetic and dynamic interactions of oral viqualine and ethanol in man. *Eur J Clin Pharmacol* (1989) 36, 93–6.

Alcohol + Xylene

Some individuals exposed to xylene vapour who subsequently drink alcohol may experience dizziness and nausea. A flushing skin reaction has also been seen.

Clinical evidence, mechanism, importance and management

Studies[1] in volunteers exposed to *m*-xylene vapour at concentrations of 140 or 250 ppm for 4 h who were then given alcohol to drink (0.8 g/kg) showed that about 10% experienced dizziness and nausea. One subject exposed to 300 ppm developed a conspicuous dermal flush on his face, neck, chest and back. He also showed some erythema on alcohol alone. The reasons for these reactions are not understood.

1. Riihimäki V, Laine A, Savolainen K, Sippel H. Acute solvent-ethanol interactions with special reference to xylene. *Scand J Work Environ Health* (1982) 8, 77–9.

3

Analgesic and non-steroidal anti-inflammatory drug (NSAID) interactions

The drugs dealt with in this chapter are listed in Table 3.1 with their proprietary names. In addition the list also contains other analgesic and non-steroidal anti-inflammatory drugs (NSAIDs) that act as interacting agents and are dealt with in other chapters. The Index should be consulted for the full listing. The NSAIDs are also briefly classified in Chapter 24 in Table 24.1 ('Antiasthmatic drugs + NSAIDs', p.863).

Table 3.1 Analgesics and non-steroidal anti-inflammatory drugs (NSAIDs)

Generic names	Proprietary names
Analgesics (non-narcotic)	
Alclofenac	
Azapropazone	Prolixan, Rheumox, Tolyprin
Bromfenac	
Clometacin	
Dexketoprofen	Desketo, Enantyum, Keral, Ketesse, Quiralam, Sympal
Diclofenac	3-A, Abitren, Acoflam, Agofenac, Algefit, Allvoran, Almiral, Alsidexten, Ana-Flex, Analpan, Anfenax, Apo-Diclo, Arclonac, Arthotec, Arthrex, Arthrotec, Artotec, Artren, Artrenac, Artrotec, Athrofen, Athru-Derm, Bel-Gel, Benevran, Benfofen, Betaren, Biclopan, Biofenac, Cataflam, Catalgem, Catanac, Cataren, Cinaflan, Clo-Far, Clofec, Clofen, Clofenac, Clofenak, Clofon, Clonodifen, Dealgic, Dedolor, Deflamat, Deflamm, Deflox, Delphinac, Deltaflogin, Deltaren, Demac, Di Retard, Dicfafena, Diclac, Diclax, Diclaxol, Diclo, Diclobene, Diclocular, Diclodoc, Diclodol, Diclofam, Diclofan, Diclofen, Diclofenax, Diclofenbeta, Dicloflex, Dicloftil, Diclogel, Diclogrun, Diclohexal, Diclolan, Diclomax, Diclomel, Diclomelan, Diclometin, Diclomex, Diclomol, Diclon, Diclophlogont, Dicloplast, Dicloran, Diclorengel, Dicloreum, Diclosian, Diclosifar, Diclostad, Diclosyl, Diclotard, Diclotec, Diclovol, Diclowal, Diclozip, Difelene, Difena, Difenac, Difene, Difenet, Difeno, Difnal, Dinac, Dinefec, Dioxaflex, Dirret, Dofen, Dolaren, Dolaut, Dolflam, Dolo Nervobion, Dolo-Voltaren, Dolotren, Dolpasse, Dorcalor, Dorgen, Doriflan, Dosanac, duravolten, Ecofenac, Econac, Effekton, Evadol, Fenac, Fenadol, Fenaflan, Fenaren, Fenburil, Fenil-V, Flamatak, Flameril, Flamrase, Flanaren, Flankol, Flector, Flexagen, Flexamina, Flexotard, Flogan, Flogesic, Flogiren, Flogofenac, Flogoken, Flotac, Forgenac, Fortenac, Fortfen, Fustaren, Galedol, Grofenac, Inac, Infla-Ban, Infladoren, Inflamac, Inflamax, Inflanac, Inflaren, Isclofen, Jenafenac, Lexobene, Liberalgium, Lifenac, Liroken, Lodyfen, Lofenac, Lofensaid, Luase, Luparen, Mafena, Magluphen, Masaren, Medaren, Merxil, Misofenac, Modifenac, Molfenac, Monoflam, Motifene, Myogit, Myonac, Naclof, Neo-Pyrazon, Novapirina, Novo-Difenac, Nu-Diclo, Olfen, Ortoflan, Ostaren, Painex, Panamor, Pennsaid, Posnac, Practiser, Primofenac, Putaren, Remafen, Remethan, Reutaren, Rewodina, Rhemofenax, Rheufenac, Rheumatac, Rhewlin, Rhumalgan, Rhumanol, Ribex Flu, Rumatab, Selectofen, Sigafenac, Silflam, Slofenac, Solaraze, Still, Taks, Tarjen, Tarjena, Toryxil, Trabona, Tratul, Uniren, Veenac, Veltex, Vendrex, Vicmafen, Vifenac, Vofenal, Voldal, Volfenac, Volnac, Vologen, Volraman, Volsaid, Voltaflan, Voltaflex, Voltanac, Voltaren, Voltarene, Voltarol, Voltfast, Voltrix, Volverac, Voren, Vostar, Votamed, Xenid, Zolterol, Zymamed
Diflunisal	Aflogos, Artrodol, Biartac, Difludol, Diflusal, Dolobid, Dolobis, Dolocid, Donobid, Fluniget, Unisal
Etodolac	Acudor, Articulan, Dualgan, Elderin, Etonox, Etopan, Flancox, Hypen, Lodine, Metazin, Todolac, Ultradol
Fenoprofen	Fenopron, Fepron, Nalfon, Nalgesic, Trandor
Feprazone	Brotazona, Zepelin
Floctafenine	Idalon, Idarac
Flufenamic acid	Dignodolin, Rheuma Lindofluid
Flurbiprofen	Ansaid, Antadys, Benactiv, Cebutid, Edolfene, Fenomel, Flurofen, Flurozin, Froben, Neo Artrol, Novo-Flurprofen, Ocufen, Ocuflur, Reupax, Strefen, Strepfen, Targus, Transact, Transact Lat, Tulip
Glafenine	Adalgur

Table 3.1 Analgesics and non-steroidal anti-inflammatory drugs (NSAIDs) *(Continued)*

Generic names	Proprietary names
Ibuprofen	*ACT-3, Aciril, Actimidol, Actiprofen, Adex, Advil, Aktren, Algiasdin, Algifor, Algofen, Alindrin, Altior, Ampifen, Anadin Ultra, Anadvil, Anafen, Anco, Antalgil, Antalisin, Antarene, Antiflam, Apain, Aprofen, Arfen, Arthrofen, Artofen, Artril, Avallone, Belep, Benfast, Benflogin, Benotrin, Bestafen, Betagesic, Betaprofen, Bifen, Brufen, Brufort, Brugesic, Brumed, Bruprin, Brusil, Bufigen, Bumed, Burana, Calmine, Cefen, Cibalgina Due Fast, Citalgan, Contraneural, Cunil, Cuprofen, Dalsy, Days, Decontractyl New, Dibufen, Diprodol, Dismenol N, Dismenol Neu, Doctril, Dolgit, Dolibu, Dolo-Dismenol, Dolo-Puren, Dolo-Spedifen, Dolocyl, Dolodoc, Dolofort, Dolormin, Dolprin, Dolprofen, Dolval, Dolver, Doretrim Dorival, Duafen, Duran, Dynofen, Ebufac, Ecoprofen, Edenil, Ergix, Espidifen, Esprenit, Exneural, Expanfen, Faspic, Febratic, Femaprin, Femidol, Feminalin, Fenbid, Fibraflex, Flexafen, G-Fen, Galprofen, Gelufene, Genpril, Gineflor, Ginenorm, Greatofen, Grefen, Gyno-Neuralgin, Gynofug, Haltran, Hemagene Tailleur, Ibenon, Ibrofen, Ibrufhalal, Ibu, Ibualgic, Ibubeta, Ibudolor, Ibufac, Ibufem, Ibufen, Ibuflam, Ibuflex, Ibufug, Ibugan, Ibugel, Ibuhexal, Ibulan, Ibular, Ibuleve, Ibuloid, Ibumax, Ibumed, Ibumerck, Ibumetin, Ibumousse, Ibupax, Ibuphlogont, Ibuprof, Ibupron, Iburem, Iburen, Ibureumin, Ibusal, Ibuscent, Ibusifar, Ibuslow, Ibuspray, Ibutad, Ibutop, Ibux, Ibuxin, Ilvico grippal, Imbun, Inoven, Intralgis, Inza, Ipren, Iproben, Iprogel, Irfen, Isdol, Isisfen, Jenaprofen, Junifen, Kalma, Kontagripp Mono, Kratalgin, Leonal, Librofem, Lidifen, Mafen, Malafene, Manorfen, Medifen, Melfen, Menadol, Mensoton, Migrafen, Moment, Motrin, Neobrufen, Nodolfen, Norflam T, Novaprin, Novartril, Novo-Profen, Novogent, Nuprin, Nureflex, Nurofen, Nurofen Advance, Obifen, Offeno, Optalidon, Optifen, Opturem, Oralfene, Orbifen, Ostofen, Ozonol, P-Fen, Pacifene, Panafen, Panax N, Parartrin, Parsal, Perofen, Perviam, Pfeil, Phor Pain, Phorpain, Pippen, Pocyl, Proartinal, Probufen, Profena, Profinal, Proflex, Quadrax, Rafen, Ranfen, ratioDolor, Realdrax, Relcofen, Rheumanox, Rimafen, Rolab-Antiflam, Rumasian, Rumatifen, Rupan, Sadefen, Saetil, Saleto-200, Sanafen, Schmerz-Dolgit, Schufen, Serviprofen, Siprofen, Skelan IB, Solfen, Solpaflex, Solufen, Solufena, Solvium, Spedifen, Spidifen, Spidufen, Syntofene, Tabalon, Tabcin, Tempil, Tispol Ibu-DD, Tofen, Togal N, Trauma-Dolgit, Tri-Profen, Trifene, Trofen, Upfen, Urem, Zafen, etc*
Indobufen	*Ibustrin*
Indometacin (Indomethacin)	*Aflamin, Agilisin, Aliviosin, Amuno, Antalgin, Arthrexin, Articulen, Artracin, Artrinovo, Autritis, Betacin, Bonidon, Bucin, Chibro-Amuno 3, Chrono-Indocid, Cidomel, Confortid, Dolovin, Elmetacin, Famethacin, Flamaret, Flexidin, Flexin Continus, Flogoter, Grindocin, Helvecin, Idc, Imbrilon, Imet, Inacid, Indo, Indo Framan, Indo Top, Indo-Mepha, Indo-Phlogont, Indo-paed, Indobene, Indocaf, Indocarsil, Indocid, Indocin, Indocollirio, Indocollyre, Indocontin, Indoflam, Indoftol, Indohexal, Indolar SR, Indolgina, Indom Collirio, Indoman, Indomax, Indomed, Indomee, Indomelan, Indomet, Indometacinum-mp, Indometin, Indomisal, Indomod, Indonilo, Indophtal, Indoptic, Indoptol, Indospray, Indostad, Indotard, Indotec, Indotrin, Indovis, Indoxen, Inflam, Inflamate, Infree, Inthacine, Italon, Liometacen, Luiflex, Malival, Maximet SR, Mederreumol, Mediflex, Metacen, Methacin, Methocaps, Metindo, Mobilat, Neo Decabutin, Nisaid, Novo-Methacin, Nu-Indo, Pardelprin, Putatone, Ralicid, Restameth-SR, Reumo, Reusin, Rheubalmin Indo, Rheumacin, Rhodacine, Rimacid, Rothacin, Servindomet, Sigadoc, Slo-Indo, etc*
Isoxicam	
Kebuzone	*Ketazon*
Ketoprofen	*Actron, Actroneffix, Alket, Apo-Keto, Arcental, Artrinid, Artrofene, Artrosil, Artrosilene, Bi-Profenid, Deflogix, Efiken, Extraplus, Fastum, Flexen, Gabrilen, Jomethid, K-Profen, Keduril, Kefen, Kefentech, Kenhancer, Keprodol, Ketalgesic, Ketartrium, Ketil, Keto, Ketocid, Ketodol, Ketofene, Ketoflam, Ketolist, Ketomex, Ketonal, Ketop, Ketoplus, Ketorin, Ketosolan, Ketotard, Ketotop, Ketozip, Ketum, Larafen, Meprofen, Myproflam, Novo-Keto, Oki, Orafen, Orofen, Orucote, Orudis, Orugesic, Oruject, Oruvail, Oscorel, Powergel, Prodon, Profenid, Prontoket, Provail, Reuprofen, Rhodis, Rhovail, Rofenid, Rofepain, Siduro, Spondylon, Topfena, Toprec, Toprek, Zepelindue, Zon, etc*
Ketorolac	*Acular, Aculare, Acularen, Algikey, Alidol, Celfax, Dolac, Dolotor, Droal, Estopein, Findol, Glicima, Lixidol, Onemer, Supradol, Taradyl, Toloran, Tonum, Topadol, Tora-Dol, Toradol, Toral, Tromedal*
Lornoxicam	*Acabel, Artok, Bosporon, Lornox, Telos, Xefo*
Meclofenamic acid	*Lenidolor, Movens*
Mefenamic acid	*Artriden, Conamic, Coslan, Dysman, Dyspen, Fenamic, Fenamin, Gandin, Lysalgo, Manic, Medicap, Mednil, Mefac, Mefacap, Mefalgic, mefe-basan, Mefenacide, Mefenan, Mefenix, Mefic, Meflam, Melur, Mephadolor, Namic, Namifen, Napan, Opustan, Painnox, Parkemed, Pinalgesic, Ponac, Ponalar, Ponalgic, Ponmel, Ponnac, Ponnesia, Ponstan, Ponstel, Ponstyl, Pontalon, Pontyl, Prostan, Pynamic, Sefnic, Spiralgin*
Meloxicam	*Aflamid, Diatec, Dormelox, Exel, Flamatec, Flexican, Inicox, Latonid, Leutrol, Loxam, Loxibest, Loxiflan, Masflex, Melosteral, Meloxil, Mevamox, Mobec, Mobic, Mobicox, Movalis, Movatec, Movicox, Movoxicam, Parocin, Uticox, Zilutrol*
Metamizole sodium (Dipyrone)	*Acodon, Alnex, Anador, Analgex, Analgin, Anaprol, Apixol, Avafontan, Avaldrian, Ayoral Simple, Baralgin, Berlosin, Bioscina, Cefaldina, Conmel, Dalsin, Dipydol, Dofisan, Dolgan, Dolofur, Domenal, Dornal, Exalgin, Exodalina, Fandall, Fardolpin, Fimdor, Genergin, Inalgon Neu, Indigon, Invoigin, Macodin, Magnil, Magnol, Magsons, Maxiliv, Mecoten, Medalgin, Mermid, Metapirona, Metilon, Midelin, Minalgin, Minoral, Mizoltec, Neo Melubrina, Neomelin, Neo-Melubrina, Nivagin, Nominfone, Novalgin, Novalgina, Novalgine, Novaminsulfon, Olan-Gin, Optalgin, Paleodina, Phanalgin, Piramagno, Pirandall, Pirinovag, Piromebrina, Poloren, Prodolina, Pyranol, Spasmo Inalgon Neu, Sulpyrin, Suprim, Termonil, Trisalgina, Utidol, V-Talgin*

Table 3.1 Analgesics and non-steroidal anti-inflammatory drugs (NSAIDs) *(Continued)*

Generic names	Proprietary names
Mofebutazone	Diadin M, Mofesal
Nabumetone	Artaxan, Balmox, Dolsinal, Listran, Mebutan, Nabone, Nabucox, Nabuser, Nametone, Relafen, Relif, Relifen, Relifex, Relisan, Relitone
Naproxen	Actiquim, Akudol, Aleve, Aliviomas, Alpoxen, Anaprox, Anapsyl, Anax, Annoxen, Antalgin, Aperdan, Ap-Napro-Na, Aponacin, Apo-Napro-Na, Apra-Gel, Apranax, Artagen, Arthrosin, Arthroxen, Artron, AS/85, Axer, Bioxan, Bipronyl, Bonyl, Crysanal, Dafloxen, Daprox, Deflamox, Denaxpren, Diferbest, D/N PR, Dolxen, Dysmenalgit, Femex, Fibroxyn, Flanax, Flexen, Flexin, Flogen, Floginax, Floxalin, Fuxen, Genalgen, Genoxen, Gerinap, Gesiprox, Gibinap, Gibixen, Gynestrel, Inza, Iqfasol, Laraflex, Laser, Ledox, Leniartril, Lorexen, Lundiran, Malexin, Miranax, Momendol, Nafasol, Naflapen, Napflam, Napmel, Napratec, Naprel, Naprelan, Napren, Naprex, Naprius, Naprobene, Naprocet, Naprocoat, Naprodil, Naprodol, Napro-Dorsch, Naprogesic, Naprokes, Naprometin, Napromex, Naprorex, Naproscript, Naprosian, Naproso, Naprosyn, Naprosyne, Naproval, Naprovite, Naproxi, Napxen, Narocin, Narzen, Naxen, Naxopren, Naxyn, Neo Eblimon, Neonaxil, Nitens, Nixal, Noflam, Novaxen, Novo-Naprox, Numidan, Nu-Naprox, Nycopren, Pactens, Piproxen, Point, Polyxen, Prexan, Pronat, Pronaxen, Pronaxil, Pronoxen, Proxalin, Proxen, Reuxen, Rhodiaprox, Rimoxyn, Roxen, Sertrixen, Serviproxan, Soden, Sodixen, Soproxen, Soren, Sunprox, Synalgo, Synflex, Synogin, Tacron, Tandax, Tanizona, Ticoflex, Timpron, Traumox, U-Proxyn, Velsay, Vinsen, Xenar, Zynal, etc
Nefopam	Acupan, Ajan, Nefam, Oxadol, Silentan
Nimesulide	Algimesil, Algolider, Antalgo, Antiflogil, Antifloxil, Areuma, Aulin, Biosal, Deflogen, Degorflan, Deltaflan, Domes, Donulide, Edemax, Efridol, Eskaflam, Eudolene, Fansidol, Fenisal, Flamide, Flolid, Guaxan, Isodol, Jabasulide, Laidor, Ledoren, Lidaflan, Lusemin, Maxsulid, Mesulid, Neosulida, Nerelid, Nexen, Nide, Nidol, Nimalgex, Nimed, Nimedex, Nimeflan, Nimesil, Nimesilam, Nimesulene, Nimesulin, Nimexan, Nims, Nisalgen, Nisulid, Noalgos, Nodor, Noxalide, Optaflan, Redaflam, Remov, Resulin, Scaflam, Scalid, Severin, Sintalgin, Solving, Sulidamor, Sulide, Sulimed, Teonim
Oxametacin	
Oxaprozin	Daypro, Deflam, Prozina
Oxyphenbutazone	Diflamil, Edefen, Redolet, Tanderil, Tandrex
Paracetamol (Acetaminophen)	
Penicillamine	Adalken, Artamin, Atamir, Cuprimine, Cupripen, Depen, Distamine, D-Penamine, Kelatin, Kelatine, Mercaptyl, Metalcaptase, Pemine, Sufortan, Sufortanon, Trisorcin, Trolovol
Phenazone (Antipyrine)	Aequiton-P, Aurone, Erasol, Migrane-Kranit mono, Oto-Phen, Tropex
Phenylbutazone	Ambene, Basireuma, Bloken, Bresal, Buta, Butacote, Butadion, Butalen, Butazolidin, Butazolidina, Butazolidine, Butazona, Butazone, Butazonil, Delbulasa, Demoplas, exrheudon OPT, Fezona, Inflazone, Kadol, Lorfenil, Peralgin
Piroxicam	Anartrit, Androxicam, Antiflog, Artinor, Artragil, Artroxicam, Artyflam, Baxo, Bicam, Bioximil, Brexecam, Brexicam, Brexidol, Brexin, Brexine, Brexinil, Brexivel, Brexodin, Bruxicam, Candyl, Cicladol, Ciclafast, Citoken T, Clevian, Cycladol, Dekamega, Dexicam, Dixonal, Doblexan, Dolzycam, durapirox, Euroxi, Exipan, Facicam, Fasax, Felcam, Felden, Feldexican, Feldox, Felnan, Felrox, Fexicam, Finfo, Flamadene, Flamarene, Flamatrol, Flamic, Flamostat, Flexar, Flexase, Flexirox, Flodol, Flogene, Flogobene, Flogocan, Flogoxen, Geldene, Geroxicam, Glandicin, Hotemin, Ifemed, Improntal, Inflaced, Inflamene, Inflanan, Inflanox, Inflax, Jenapirox, Lampoflex, Larapam, Lisedema, Maswin, Mobilis, Neogel, Neotica, Novo-Pirocam, Nu-Pirox, Olcam, Osteral, Oxicam, Oxicanol, Pericam, Piram, Pirax, Pirkam, Piro, Pirobeta, Pirocal, Pirocam, Pirodax, Piroflam, Piroftal, Pirohexal-D, Pirom, Piro-Phlogont, Piro-Puren, Pirorheum, PirorheumA, Pirosol, Pirox, Piroxal, Piroxam, Piroxan, pirox-basan, Piroxcin, Piroxen, Piroxene, Piroxifen, Piroxiflam, Piroxil, Piroxiplus, Piroxistad, Piroxityrol, Piroxsil, Pirox-Spondyril, Piroxy, Pirozip, Pixicam, Polipirox, Polyxicam, Posedene, Pra-Brexidol, Proxalyoc, Pyrocaps, Pyroxy, ratioMobil, Reucam, Reudene, Reumagil, Reumoxican, Reutricam, Rheugesic, Rheumitin, Riacen, Roccaxin, Rosiden, Rosig, Roxazin, Roxene, Roxenil, Roxicam, Roxiden, Roxifen, Roxycam, R-Tyflam, Rumadene, Salcacam, Salvacam, Sasulen, Sinartrol, Solicam, Sotilen, Synoxicam, Tetram, Tonimed, Vitaxicam, Xicam, Xycam, Zelis, Zofora, etc
Salicylates	
Aspirin	
Aloxiprin	
Benorilate	Benoral, Duvium, Salipran
Choline salicylate	Applicaine, Arthropan, Audax, Dinnefords Teejel, Herron Baby Teething Gel, Ora-Sed, Ora-Sed Jel, Teejel
Sodium salicylate	Dodds, Jackson's Febrifuge
Sulindac	Aclin, Apo-Sulin, Arthrocine, Artribid, Bio-Dac, Cenlidac, Citireuma, Clinoril, Copal, Daclin, Kenalin, Lyndak, Novo-Sundac, Saldac, Sulartrene, Sulen, Sulindal
Tenidap	
Tiaprofenic acid	Albert Tiafen, Anafen, Artiflam, Artroreuma, Fengam, Flamirex, Flanid, Gasam, Suralgan, Surgam, Surgamic, Surgamyl, Tiaprofen
Tenoxicam	Alganex, Artriunic, Bioreucam, Dolmen, Doxican, Legil, Menzotil, Mobiflex, Nadamen, Reutenox, Rexalgan, Seftil, Sinoral, Teconam, Tenax, Tenocam, Tenocan, Tenotec, Tenox, Tenoxen, Tenoxil, Tilatil, Tilcotil, Tiloxican, Tobitil

Table 3.1 Analgesics and non-steroidal anti-inflammatory drugs (NSAIDs) *(Continued)*

Generic names	Proprietary names
Tolfenamic acid	*Bifenac, Clotam, Clotan, Fenamic, Migea, Rociclyn*
Tolmetin	*Artrocaptin, Tolectin*

Analgesics (narcotic and related)

Alfentanil	*Alfenta, Fanaxal, Fentalim, Limifen, Rapifen*
Buprenorphine	*Anorfin, Buprenex, Buprex, Buprine, Nopan, Prefin, Subutex, Temgesic, Transtec*
Butorphanol	*Stadol*
Codeine	
(Dextro)propoxyphene	*642, Abalgin, Algifene, Darvon, Deprancol, Depronal, Develin, Dexofen, Doloxene, Doxypol, Liberen*
Dextromoramide	*Palfium*
Diamorphine (Heroin)	*Diagesil, Diamorf*
Dihydrocodeine	*Codicontin, Codidol, Contugesic, DF 118, DHC, Dicodin, Didor, Hydol, Hydrocodeinon, Paracodin, Paracodina, Paracodine, Remedacen, Rikodeine, Tiamon Mono, Tosidrin*
Fentanyl	*Actiq, Duragesic, Durogesic, Fenodid, Fentanest, Haldid, Leptanal, Sintenyl, Sublimaze, Tanyl*
Hydrocodone	*Biocodone, Dicodid, Hycodan, Robidone*
Hydromorphone	*Dilaudid, Hydal, Hydromorph, Opidol, Palladon, Palladone, Sophidone*
Methadone	*Adolan, Biodone, Dolmed, Dolophine, Eptadone, Heptadon, Ketalgine, Metasedin, Methaddict, Methadose, Methex, Pallidone, Phymet DTF, Physeptone, Pinadone DTF, Symoron, Synastone*
Morphine	*Actiskenan, Analfin, Anamorph, Astramorph, Avinza, Capros, Compensan, Contalgin, Depolan, Dimorf , Dolcontin, Doltard, Duralgin, Duralmor, Duramorph, Filnarine, Graten, Infumorph, Kadian, Kapabloc, Kapanol, LA Morph, M-beta, MCR, M-Dolor, M-Eslon, MIR, M-long, Mogetic, Morapid, Morcap, Morphitec, Morstel, MOS, Moscontin, MS Contin, MS Direct, MS Mono, MSI, MSIR, MS-Long, MSP, MSR, MST, MST Continus, M-Stada, Mundidol, MXL, Noceptin, Oglos, Onkomorphin, Oramorph, Ordine, RA Morph, RMS, Roxanol, Sevredol, Sevre-Long , Skenan, Slo-Morph, SRM-Rhotard, Statex, Stellorphinad, Stellorphine, Substitol, Uni Mist, Vendal, Zomorph etc*
Oxycodone	*Endocodone, Endone, Eubine, Oxanest, Oxycod, Oxycontin, Oxyfast, Oxygesic, OxyIR, Oxynorm, Percolone, Proladone, Roxicodone, Supeudol*
Oxymorphone	*Numorphan*
Papaveretum	*Omnopon*
Pentazocine	*Fortal, Fortalgesic, Fortral, Fortralin, Fortwin, Ospronim, Pangon, Peltazon, Pentagin, Rafazocine, Sosegon, Sosenol, Talwin*
Pethidine (Meperidine)	*Alodan, Demerol, Dolantin, Dolantina, Dolantine, Dolestine, Dolosal*
Phenoperidine	
Sufentanil	*Fastfen, Fentatienil, Sufenta*
Tramadol	*Adamon, Adolonta, Amadol, Anadol, Biodalgic, Contramal, Dolol, Dolzam, Dorless, Dromadol, Ecodolor, Fortradol, Fraxidol, Lanalget, Mabron, Madol, Madola, Mandolgin, Nobligan, Nycodol, Paxilfar, Pengesic, Predalgic, Prontalgin, Prontofort, Sefmal, Sensitram, Sylador, Theradol, Tioner, Tiparol, Topalgic, Trabar, Tradol, Tradolan, Tradonal, Tralgiol, Tralic, Trama, Tramabene, Tramabeta, Tramadex, Tramadin, Tramadolor, Trama-Dorsch, Tramadura, Tramagetic, Tramagit, Tramake, Tramal, Tramalan, Tramamed, Tramamerck, Tramastad, Tramatyrol, Trambo, Tramex, Tramo, Tramoda, Tramundal, Tramundin, Trasedal, Travex, Trexol, Trosic, Ultram, Veldrol, Volcidol-S, Zamadol, Zamudol, Zumalgic, Zydol*

Alfentanil or Sufentanil + Erythromycin, Fluconazole or Troleandomycin

Some patients may experience prolonged and increased alfentanil effects if they are treated with erythromycin, fluconazole or troleandomycin. Sufentanil appears not to interact with erythromycin.

Clinical evidence

(a) Alfentanil + Erythromycin

A 32-year old man undergoing exploratory laparotomy was given 1 g **erythromycin** and 1 g neomycin three times daily on the day before surgery. He was given pancuronium, **alfentanil** and thiopental for induction, followed by suxamethonium (succinylcholine) and N_2O/O_2. Anaesthesia was maintained with **alfentanil**. Altogether he received 20.9 mg of **alfentanil**. An hour after recovery he was found to be unrousable and with only 5 breaths per minute. He was successfully treated with naloxone.[1]

Erythromycin 500 mg twice daily for 7 days increased the mean half-life of **alfentanil** in 6 subjects by 56% (from 84 to 131 min) and decreased the clearance from 3.9 to 2.9 ml/kg/min. Some of the subjects were much more sensitive than others: 2 showed marked changes; 2 showed little changes, and the other 2 showed intermediate effects. The 2 most sensitive subjects demonstrated considerable changes with only one day of **erythromycin** treatment.[2] Another patient given **alfentanil** and **erythromycin** is said to have developed respiratory arrest during recovery.[3]

(b) Alfentanil + Troleandomycin

A study in nine healthy subjects found that when given 20 micrograms/kg **alfentanil** intravenously after taking 500 mg **troleandomycin** orally, its clearance was reduced almost 70% (to 1.5 compared with 4.9 ml/kg/min for the controls given a placebo).[4]

(c) Alfentanil + Fluconazole

A double-dummy randomised crossover study in 9 healthy subjects given intravenous **alfentanil** 20 micrograms/kg after receiving 400 mg **fluconazole** orally or by infusion found that the **fluconazole** reduced the **alfentanil** clearance by about 60%. Both the alfentanil-induced ventilatory depression and its subjective effects were increased.[5,6]

(d) Sufentanil + Erythromycin

Seven days' treatment with 500 mg **erythromycin** twice daily in 6 healthy subjects was found not to affect the pharmacokinetics of intravenous **sufentanil** (3 micrograms/kg) in the 9 hours following administration.[7] Two of the subjects were the same as those who had shown an alfentanil/erythromycin interaction cited above.

Mechanism

There is good evidence that erythromycin, fluconazole and troleandomycin[4] inhibit cytochrome P450 isoenzyme CYP3A3/4 in the liver which is concerned with the metabolism of alfentanil. Sufentanil on the other hand is a high extraction drug and therefore less likely to be affected by changes in liver metabolism.[8]

Importance and management

The interactions of alfentanil with erythromycin, fluconazole and troleandomycin appear to be established and clinically important. Ketoconazole may interact in a similar way.[9] Alfentanil should be only given in reduced amounts or avoided in those who have recently had any of these three drugs.[2] Be alert for evidence of prolonged alfentanil effects and respiratory depression. It appears not to affect all patients given erythromycin, but it is not clear whether this also occurs with fluconazole and troleandomycin. Alternatively, sufentanil can be used instead, using doses of 3 micrograms/kg or less, but much larger doses of sufentanil should only be given with caution.[7]

1. Bartkowski RR, McDonnell TE. Prolonged alfentanil effect following erythromycin administration. *Anesthesiology* (1990) 73, 566–8.
2. Bartkowski RR, Goldberg ME, Larijani GE and Boerner T. Inhibition of alfentanil metabolism by erythromycin. *Clin Pharmacol Ther* (1989) 46, 99–102.
3. Yate PM, Thomas D, Short TSM, Sebel PS, Morton J. Comparison of infusions of alfentanil or pethidine for sedation of ventilated patients on ITU. *Br J Anaesth* (1986) 58, 1091–9.
4. Kharasch ED, Russell M, Mautz D, Thummel KE, Kunze KL, Bowdle A, Cox K. The role of cytochrome P450 3A4 in alfentanil clearance. *Anesthesiology* (1997) 87, 36–50.
5. Olkkola KT, Palkama VJ, Isohanni MH, Neuvonen PJ. Effect of fluconazole on the pharmacokinetics and pharmacodynamics of iv alfentanil. *Anesthesiology* (1997) 87, A373.
6. Palkama VJ, Isohanni MH, Neuvonen PJ, Olkkola KT. The effect of intravenous and oral fluconazole on the pharmacokinetics and pharmacodynamics of intravenous alfentanil. *Anesth Analg* (1998) 87, 190–4.
7. Bartkowski RR, Goldberg ME, Huffnagle S, Epstein RH. Sufentanil disposition. Is it affected by erythromycin administration? *Anesthesiology* (1993) 78, 260–5.
8. Kharasch ED, Thummel KE. Human alfentanil metabolism by cytochrome P450 3A3/4. An explanation for the interindividual variability in alfentanil clearance? *Anesth Analg* (1993) 76, 1033–9.
9. Labroo RB, Thummel KE, Kunze KL, Podoll T, Trager WF, Kharasch ED. Catalytic role of cytochrome P4503A4 in multiple pathways of alfentanil metabolism. *Drug Metab Dispos* (1995) 23, 490–6.

Alfentanil + H$_2$-blockers

Cimetidine, but not ranitidine, increases the plasma levels of alfentanil.

Clinical evidence, mechanism, importance and management

A pharmacokinetic study[1] in 19 intensive care patients found that 1200 mg intravenous **cimetidine** daily for 2 days increased the half-life of alfentanil (single 125 micrograms/kg intravenous doses) by 75 or 62%, and reduced the clearance by 64 or 54% when compared with an oral antacid and **ranitidine** (300 mg intravenously, daily) respectively. The alfentanil plasma levels were significantly raised by the **cimetidine**, probably because the **cimetidine** inhibits the metabolism of the alfentanil, thereby reducing its loss. Whether the alfentanil effects are increased to a clinically important extent awaits assessment, however, be alert for increased alfentanil effects because pharmacokinetic changes of this size are known to be clinically important in some patients. See 'Alfentanil or Sufentanil + Erythromycin, Fluconazole or Troleandomycin', p.44. **Ranitidine** apparently does not interact significantly with alfentanil.

1. Kienlen J, Levron J-C, Aubas S, Roustan J-P, du Cailar J. Pharmacokinetics of alfentanil in patients treated with either cimetidine or ranitidine. *Drug Invest* (1993) 6, 257–62.

Alfentanil + Ondansetron

Ondansetron appears not to interact adversely with alfentanil.

Clinical evidence, mechanism, importance and management

Single doses of **ondansetron** 8 or 16 mg in healthy subjects was found to have no effect on the sedation or ventilatory depression due to alfentanil (a continuous infusion of 0.25 to 0.75 micrograms/kg following a 5 microgram/kg bolus dose) and no effect on the rate of recovery.[1] On theoretical grounds **ondansetron** (a 5-HT3 receptor antagonist) might be expected to decrease the effects of anti-nociceptive drugs (because 5-HT is thought to cause anti-nociception via presynaptic 5-HT3 receptors on primary afferent nociceptive neurones in the spinal dorsal horn), but a study found that 8 mg intravenous **ondansetron** had no effect on the reaction of 8 healthy subjects to pressure, cold or electrical stimulation, nor did it oppose the analgesic effect of 30 microgram/kg intramuscular alfentanil.[2] No special precautions would seem to be necessary during concurrent use.

1. Dershwitz M, Di Biase PM, Rosow CE, Wilson RS, Sanderson PE, Joslyn AF. Ondansetron does not affect alfentanil-induced ventilatory depression or sedation. *Anesthesiology* (1992) 77, 447–52.
2. Petersen-Felix S, Arendt-Nielsen L, Bjerring P, Bak P. Svensson P, Breivik H, Zbinden AM. Ondansetron does not inhibit the analgesic potency of alfentanil. *Acta Anaesthesiol Scand* (1993) 37 (Suppl 10), 222.

Alfentanil + Reserpine

An isolated report describes ventricular dysrhythmias in a patient on reserpine when given alfentanil during anaesthesia.

Clinical evidence, mechanism, importance and management

A hypertensive woman on 0.25 mg **reserpine** daily was given 800 micrograms alfentanil intravenously over 5 minutes before anaesthesia with thiopental (thiopentone) and suxamethonium (succinylcholine), followed during the surgery by 900 micrograms alfentanil in 9 doses and 70% N_2O/O_2. Bradycardia developed and frequent unifocal premature ventricular contractions occurred throughout the surgery, but they disappeared 3 to 4 h afterwards. The reasons are not understood.[1]

1. Jahr JS, Weber S. Ventricular dysrhythmias following an alfentanil anesthetic in a patient on reserpine for hypertension. *Acta Anaesthesiol Scand* (1991) 35, 788–9.

Alfentanil + Rifampicin (Rifampin)

There is good evidence that the effects of alfentanil are reduced by rifampicin.

Clinical evidence, mechanism, importance and management

A study in nine healthy subjects found that when given 20 micrograms/kg alfentanil intravenously after taking 600 mg **rifampicin** orally for 5 days, its clearance was increased almost threefold (13.2 compared with 4.9 ml/kg/min for the controls).[1] The reason appears to be that the **rifampicin** increases the activity of cytochrome P450 isoenzyme CYP3A4 in the liver which is concerned with the metabolism of alfentanil so that its loss from the body is increased. This study was primarily designed to investigate the role of CYP3A4 in the metabolism of alfentanil, but it also provides good evidence that alfentanil will be much less effective in patients treated with **rifampicin**. A much larger dose will almost certainly be needed.

1. Kharasch ED, Russell M, Mautz D, Thummel KE, Kunze KL, Bowdle A, Cox K. The role of cytochrome P450 3A4 in alfentanil clearance. *Anesthesiology* (1997) 36–50.

Antirheumatic agents + Mazindol

Mazindol is reported not to interact adversely with indometacin (indomethacin), salicylates and other analgesics and anti-inflammatory drugs.

Clinical evidence, mechanism, importance and management

A double-blind study of **mazindol** and a placebo was carried out on 26 obese arthritics, 15 of whom were on **salicylates**, 11 on **indometacin** (**indomethacin**) and one on **dextropropoxyphene** (**propoxyphene**) with **paracetamol** (**acetaminophen**). Additional drugs used were **ibuprofen** (4 patients), **phenylbutazone** (one patient), **dextropropoxyphene** (7 patients), **paracetamol** (3 patients) and **prednisone** (9 patients). No adverse interactions were seen.[1]

1. Thorpe PC, Isaac PF, Rodgers J. A controlled trial of mazindol (Sanjorex, Teronac) in the management of obese rheumatic patients. *Curr Ther Res* (1975) 17, 149–55.

Aspirin or Salicylates + Antacids or Urinary alkalinizers

The serum salicylate concentrations of patients taking large doses of aspirin as an anti-inflammatory agent can be reduced to subtherapeutic levels by the concurrent use of some antacids.

Clinical evidence

A child with rheumatic fever taking 0.6 g **aspirin** five times daily had a serum salicylate concentration of between 8.2 and 11.8 mg/100 ml while taking 30 ml *Maalox* (**aluminium and magnesium hydroxide suspension**). When the *Maalox* was withdrawn, the urinary pH fell from a range of 7 to 8 down to a range of 5.0 to 6.4, whereupon the serum salicylate level rose to about 38 mg/100 ml, calling for a reduction in dosage.[1] An associated study in 13 healthy subjects taking 4 g **aspirin** daily for a week showed that the concurrent use of 4 g **sodium bicarbonate** daily reduced serum salicylate levels from 27 to 15 mg/100 ml. This reflected a rise in the urinary pH from a range of 5.6 to 6.1 up to around 6.2 to 6.9.[1,2]

Similar changes have been reported in other studies.[3-7]

Mechanism

Aspirin and other salicylates are acidic compounds which are excreted by the kidney tubules and are ionised in solution. In alkaline solution, much of the drug exists in the ionised form, which is not readily reabsorbed and therefore is lost in the urine. If the urine is made more acidic, much more of the drug exists in the un-ionised form which is readily reabsorbed so that less is lost in the urine and the drug is retained in the body.[6,7] Magnesium oxide also strongly adsorbs aspirin and sodium salicylate.[8]

Importance and management

A well-established and clinically important interaction for those on chronic treatment with large doses of salicylates because the serum salicylate may be reduced to subtherapeutic levels. This interaction can occur with both 'systemic' antacids (e.g. sodium bicarbonate) as well as some 'non-systemic' antacids (e.g. magnesium-aluminium hydroxides), although some evidence suggests that some aluminium-containing antacids (*Amphojel* – aluminium hydroxide, and *Robalate* – aluminium aminoacetate) may have minimal effects on urinary pH.[1,9] Care should be taken to monitor serum salicylate levels if any antacid is started or stopped in patients where the control of salicylate levels is critical.

No important adverse interaction would be expected in those taking occasional doses of aspirin for analgesia. Some aspirin formulations actually include sodium bicarbonate to take advantage of the increased absorption rates and higher peak serum levels, which give more rapid analgesia.

1. Levy G. Interactions of salicylates with antacids. Clinical implications with respect to gastrointestinal bleeding and antiinflammatory activity. Frontiers of Internal Medicine 1974, 12th Int Congr Intern Med, Tel Aviv, 1974, p 404–8, Karger, Basel (1975).
2. Levy G, Leonards JR. Urine pH and salicylate therapy. *JAMA* (1971) 217, 81.
3. Levy G, Lampman T, Kamath BL, Garrettson LK. Decreased serum salicylate concentration in children with rheumatic fever treated with antacid. *N Engl J Med* (1975) 293, 323–5.
4. Hansten PD, Hayton WL. Effect of antacid and ascorbic acid on serum salicylate concentration. *J Clin Pharmacol* (1980) 20, 326–31.
5. Shastri RA. Effect of antacids on salicylate kinetics. *Int J Clin Pharmacol Ther Toxicol* (1985) 23, 480–4.
6. Macpherson CR, Milne MD, Evans BM. The excretion of salicylate. *Br J Pharmacol* (1955) 10, 484–9.
7. Hoffman WS, Nobe C. The influence of urinary pH on the renal excretion of salicyl derivatives during aspirin therapy. *J Lab Clin Med* (1950) 35, 237–48.
8. Naggar VF, Khalil SA, Daabis NA. The in-vitro adsorption of some antirheumatics on antacids. *Pharmazie* (1976) 31, 461–5.
9. Muirden KD, Barraclough DRE. Drug interaction in the management of rheumatoid arthritis. *Aust N Z J Med* (1976) 6 (Suppl 1), 14–21.

Aspirin or Salicylates + Caffeine

Caffeine increases the bioavailability, the rate of absorption and the plasma levels of aspirin.

Clinical evidence, mechanism, importance and management

Caffeine 120 mg increased the AUC of a single 650 mg dose of **aspirin** in healthy subjects by 36%, and increased the maximum plasma levels by 15%.[1] This confirms the results of a previous study.[2] Both of these studies suggest that there may be merit in combining these two drugs if more rapid and effective analgesia is required. There would appear to be no reason for avoiding concurrent use.

1. Thithapandha A. Effect of caffeine on the bioavailability and pharmacokinetics of aspirin. *J Med Assoc Thai* (1989) 72, 562–6.
2. Yoovathaworn KC, Sriwatanakul K, Thithapandha A. Influence of caffeine on aspirin pharmacokinetics. *Eur J Drug Metab Pharmacokinet* (1986) 11, 71–6.

Aspirin or Salicylates + Carbonic anhydrase inhibitors

A severe and even life-threatening toxic reaction can occur in those on high dose salicylate treatment if concurrently treated with carbonic anhydrase inhibitors (acetazolamide, diclofenamide (dichlorphenamide)).

Clinical evidence

A boy of 8 with chronic juvenile arthritis, well controlled on prednisolone, indometacin (indomethacin) and **aloxiprin**, was admitted to hospital with drowsiness, vomiting and hyperventilation (diagnosed as metabolic acidosis) within a month of increasing the **aloxiprin** dosage from 3 to 3.6 g daily and adding **diclofenamide (dichlorphenamide) 25 mg three times** daily for glaucoma.[1]

Other cases of toxicity (metabolic acidosis) occurred in a 22-year-old woman on **salsalate** when additionally given **acetazolamide** 250 mg four times daily,[1] and in 2 elderly women on large doses of **aspirin** when they were given **acetazolamide** or **diclofenamide**.[2] Poisoning developed in a man on **diclofenamide** within 10 days of starting to take 3.9 g **aspirin** daily.[3] Coma developed in an 85-year-old taking 3.9 g **aspirin** daily when the dosage of **acetazolamide** was increased from 0.5 to 1 g,[4] and toxicity was seen in another very old man given both drugs.[5] Levels of unbound **acetazolamide** were found to be unusually high.[5] An elderly man became confused, lethargic, incontinent and anorexic when treated with **acetazolamide** and **salsalate**. He needed intravenous hydration.[6] A 50-year-old woman treated with acetazolamide for glaucoma was admitted to hospital with confusion and cerebellar ataxia associated with hyperchloraemic acidosis 14 days after additionally taking aspirin for acute pericarditis.[7]

Mechanism

Not fully established. One idea is that these carbonic anhydrase inhibitors (acetazolamide, diclofenamide) affect the plasma pH so that more of the salicylate exists in the non-ionised (lipid-soluble) form which can enter the CNS and other tissues more easily, leading to salicylate intoxication.[2] *Animal* studies confirm that carbonic anhydrase inhibitors increase the lethality of aspirin.[3] An alternative suggestion is that because salicylate inhibits the plasma protein binding of acetazolamide and its excretion by the kidney, acetazolamide toxicity may occur which mimics salicylate toxicity.[5] It is not clear whether the increased salicylate clearance caused by the acetazolamide has any part to play.[8]

Importance and management

There are few clinical cases on record, but the interaction is established, well confirmed by *animal* studies, and potentially serious. Carbonic anhydrase inhibitors should probably be avoided in those on high dose salicylate treatment (a recommendation in one study[5]). If they are used, the patient should be well monitored for any evidence of toxicity (confusion, lethargy, hyperventilation, tinnitus) because the interaction may develop slowly and insidiously.[2] In this context other non-steroidal anti-inflammatory drugs may be safer. **Naproxen** proved to be a satisfactory substitute in one case.[1] The authors of one study suggest that **methazolamide** may possibly be a safer alternative to acetazolamide because it is minimally bound to plasma proteins. They also suggest **paracetamol (acetaminophen)** as an alternative to salicylate in patients taking acetazolamide.[5] The reports cited here concern carbonic anhydrase inhibitors given orally, not as eye drops. It is not known whether the latter interact similarly, but there appear to be no reports.

1. Cowan RA, Hartnell GG, Lowdell CP, McLean Baird I, Leak AM. Metabolic acidosis induced by carbonic anhydrase inhibitors and salicylates in patients with normal renal function. *BMJ* (1984) 289, 347–8.
2. Anderson CJ, Kaufman PL, Sturm RJ. Toxicity of combined therapy with carbonic anhydrase inhibitors and aspirin. *Am J Ophthalmol* (1978) 86, 516–19.
3. Hurwitz GA, Wingfield W, Cowart TD, Jollow DJ. Toxic interaction between salicylates and a carbonic anhydrase inhibitor: the role of cerebral edema. *Vet Hum Toxicol* (1980) 22 (Suppl), 42–4.
4. Chapron DJ, Brandt JL, Sweeny KR, Olesen-Zammett L. Interaction between acetazolamide and aspirin — a possible unrecognized cause of drug-induced coma. *J Am Geriatr Soc* (1984) 32, S18.
5. Sweeney KR, Chapron DJ, Brandt JL, Gomolin IH, Feig PU, Kramer PA. Toxic interaction between acetazolamide and salicylate: case reports and a pharmacokinetic explanation. *Clin Pharmacol Ther* (1986) 40, 518–24.
6. Rousseau P, Fuentevilla-Clifton A. Acetazolamide and salicylate interaction in the elderly: a case report. *J Am Geriatr Soc* (1993) 41, 868–9.
7. Hazouard E, Grimbert M, Jonville-Berra A-P, De Toffol M-C, Legras A. Salicylisme et glaucome: augmentation réciproque de la toxicité de l'acétazolamide et de l'acide acétyl salicylique. *J Fr Ophtalmol* (1999) 22, 73–5.
8. Macpherson CR, Milne MD, Evans BM. The excretion of salicylate. *Br J Pharmacol* (1955) 10, 484–9.

Aspirin or Salicylates + Colestyramine

Colestyramine does not have a clinically important effect on the absorption of aspirin.

Clinical evidence, mechanism, importance and management

A study in 3 healthy subjects and 3 patients, and a later study in 7 healthy subjects, found that 4 g **colestyramine** delayed the absorption of a single 500-mg dose of **aspirin** (peak levels extended from 30 to 60 min) but the total amount absorbed was only reduced by 5 to 6%. Some of the subjects had slightly higher serum **aspirin** levels while taking **colestyramine**.[1] There would seem to be little reason for avoiding concurrent use unless rapid analgesia is needed.

1. Hahn K-J, Eiden W, Schettle M, Hahn M, Walter E, Weber E. Effect of cholestyramine on the gastrointestinal absorption of phenprocoumon and acetylosalicylic acid in man. *Eur J Clin Pharmacol* (1972) 4, 142–5.

Aspirin or Salicylates + Corticosteroids or Corticotropin (Corticotrophin, ACTH)

Concurrent use is very common but the incidence of gastrointestinal bleeding and ulceration may be increased. Serum salicylate levels are reduced by corticosteroids and therefore they may rise, possibly to toxic concentrations, if the corticosteroid is withdrawn without first reducing the salicylate dosage. See also 'Corticosteroids + NSAIDs', p.637.

Clinical evidence

A 4-year-old boy chronically treated with at least 20 mg **prednisone** daily was additionally given 3.6 g **choline salicylate** daily, the prednisone gradually being tapered off to 2 mg daily over a 3-month period. Severe salicylate intoxication developed, and in a retrospective investigation of the cause, using frozen serum samples drawn for other purposes, it was found that the serum salicylate levels had climbed from about 10 mg% to 90 mg% during the withdrawal of the prednisone.[1] Later studies in 3 other patients on choline salicylate or aspirin and either prednisone or another unnamed corticosteroid, demonstrated similar but less spectacular rises (about threefold) during corticosteroid withdrawal.[1] Hydrocortisone was also found to increase the clearance of sodium salicylate in four other patients.[1]

A serum salicylate rise of similar proportions has been described in a patient on aloxiprin when prednisolone was withdrawn.[2] Other studies in considerable numbers of both adults and children show that prednisone, methylprednisolone, betamethasone and corticotropin (corticotrophin, ACTH) reduce serum salicylate levels.[3-5] Two studies also found that intra-articular doses of steroids (dexamethasone, methylprednisolone, triamcinolone) transiently reduced serum salicylate levels in patients given enteric-coated aspirin.[6,7] However one study in patients failed to show that 12 to 60 mg prednisone daily had any effect on the clearance of single doses of sodium salicylate.[8]

Mechanism

Uncertain. One idea is that the presence of the corticosteroid increases the glomerular filtration rate so that clearance of the salicylate is also increased. When the corticosteroid is withdrawn, the clearance returns to normal and the salicylate accumulates. Another suggestion is that the corticosteroids increase the metabolism of the salicylate.[3]

Importance and management

Well-established interactions. Concurrent use is very common but patients should be monitored to ensure that salicylate levels remain adequate when corticosteroids are added[4] and do not become excessive if they are withdrawn. It should also be remembered that concurrent use may increase the incidence of gastrointestinal bleeding[9] and ulceration. See also 'Corticosteroids + NSAIDs', p.637.

1. Klinenberg JR, Miller F. Effect of corticosteroids on blood salicylate concentration. JAMA (1965) 194, 601–4.
2. Muirden KD, Barraclough DRE. Drug interactions in the management of rheumatoid arthritis. Aust N Z J Med (1976) 6 (Suppl 1), 14–17.
3. Graham GG, Champion GD, Day RO, Paull PD. Patterns of plasma concentrations and urinary excretion of salicylate in rheumatoid arthritis. Clin Pharmacol Ther (1977) 22, 410–20.
4. Bardare M, Cislaghi GU, Mandelli M, Sereni F. Value of monitoring plasma salicylate levels in treating juvenile rheumatoid arthritis. Arch Dis Child (1978) 53, 381–5.
5. Koren G, Roifman C, Gelfand E, Lavi S, Suria D, Stein L. Corticosteroids-salicylate interaction in a case of juvenile rheumatoid arthritis. Ther Drug Monit (1987) 9, 177–9.
6. Edelman J, Potter JM, Hackett LP. The effect of intra-articular steroids on plasma salicylate concentrations. Br J Clin Pharmacol (1986) 21, 301–7.
7. Baer PA, Shore A, Ikeman RL. Transient fall in serum salicylate levels following intraarticular injection of steroid in patients with rheumatoid arthritis. Arthritis Rheum (1987) 30, 345–7.
8. Day RO, Harris G, Brown M, Graham GG, Champion GD. Interaction of salicylate and corticosteroids in man. Br J Clin Pharmacol (1988) 26, 334–7.
9. Carson JL, Strom BL, Schinnar R, Sim E, Maislin G, Morse ML. Do corticosteroids really cause upper GI bleeding? Clin Res (1987) 35, 340A.

Aspirin or Salicylates + Food

Avoid food if rapid analgesia is needed because it delays the absorption of aspirin.

Clinical evidence, mechanism, importance and management

A study in 25 subjects given 650 mg aspirin in five different aspirin preparations showed that food roughly halved their serum salicylate levels when measured 10 and 20 min later, compared with those seen when the same dose was taken while fasting.[1] Similar results were found in another study in subjects given 1500 mg calcium aspirin.[2] In yet another study on 8 subjects who were given 900 mg effervescent aspirin, their serum salicylate levels were roughly halved by food at 15 min, but were almost the same after an hour.[3] A possible

reason for the reduced absorption is that the aspirin becomes adsorbed onto the food. Food also delays gastric emptying. Thus if rapid analgesia is needed, aspirin should be taken without food, but if aspirin is needed long-term its administration with food can help to protect the gastric mucosa.

1. Wood JH. Effect of food on aspirin absorption. Lancet (1967) ii, 212.
2. Spiers ASD and Malone HF. Effect of food on aspirin absorption. Lancet (1967) i, 440.
3. Volans GN. Effects of food and exercise on the absorption of effervescent aspirin. Br J Clin Pharmacol (1974) 1, 137–41.

Aspirin or Salicylates + Griseofulvin

An isolated report describes a marked fall in serum salicylate levels in a child concurrently treated with aspirin and griseofulvin.

Clinical evidence, mechanism, importance and management

A boy of 8 with rheumatic fever on 110 mg/kg/day aspirin and also taking several other drugs (furosemide (frusemide), digoxin, captopril, potassium, aluminium/magnesium hydroxide and iron) showed a very marked fall in serum salicylate levels (from a range of 18.3 to 30.6 mg/dl to less than 0.2 mg/dl) within 2 days of starting 10 mg/kg griseofulvin daily. Two days after the griseofulvin was stopped, the salicylate levels were back to their former levels. The reasons are not known, but some interference with the salicylate absorption is suggested.[1] This appears to be the first and only report of this interaction so that its general importance is uncertain, but it would be prudent to monitor the effects in any patient if substantial doses of salicylates are given with griseofulvin.

1. Phillips KR, Wideman SD, Cochran EB, Becker JA. Griseofulvin significantly decreases serum salicylate concentrations. Pediatr Infect Dis J (1993) 12, 350–2.

Aspirin or Salicylates + Kaolin-pectin

Kaolin-pectin causes a small but clinically unimportant reduction in the absorption of aspirin.

Clinical evidence, mechanism, importance and management

The absorption of 975 mg aspirin in 10 healthy subjects was reduced by 5 to 10% by the concurrent use of 30 or 60 ml kaolin-pectin.[1] A likely explanation is that the aspirin becomes adsorbed by the kaolin so that the amount available for absorption through the gut wall is reduced. This small reduction in absorption is unlikely to be of clinical importance.

1. Juhl RP. Comparison of kaolin-pectin and activated charcoal for inhibition of aspirin absorption. Am J Hosp Pharm (1979) 36, 1097–8.

Aspirin or Salicylates + Levamisole

A rise in salicylate levels in a patient on aspirin when given levamisole was not confirmed in a subsequent controlled study.

Clinical evidence, mechanism, importance and management

A preliminary report of a patient who showed an increase in salicylate levels when levamisole was given with aspirin[1] prompted a study of this possible interaction. Nine healthy subjects were given 3.9 g of sustained-release aspirin daily in two divided doses over a period of 3 weeks. During this period they were also given 50 mg levamisole three times a day for a week, each subject acting as his own control. No significant changes in plasma salicylate levels were found.[2]

1. Laidlaw D'A. Rheumatoid arthritis improved by treatment with levamisole and L-histidine. *Med J Aust* (1976) 2, 382–5.
2. Rumble RH, Brooks PM, Roberts MS. Interaction between levamisole and aspirin in man. *Br J Clin Pharmacol* (1979) 7, 631–3.

Aspirin or Salicylates + Omeprazole

The antiplatelet activity and the pharmacokinetics of aspirin are not affected by omeprazole.

Clinical evidence, mechanism, importance and management

A study in 14 healthy subjects given **omeprazole** 20 mg daily for 4 days with a final dose 1 h before a single dose of **aspirin** 125 mg found that **omeprazole** did not significantly affect the plasma levels of either **aspirin** or **salicylic acid**. **Omeprazole** also did not affect the anti-platelet effects of **aspirin**.[1] No special precautions would seem to be needed, but further studies are required to confirm whether the effects of lower doses of aspirin on platelets will be similarly unaffected by omeprazole.

1. Iñarrea P, Esteva F, Corudella, Lanas A. Omeprazole does not interfere with the antiplatelet effect of low-dose aspirin in man. *Scand J Gastroenterol* (2000) 35, 242–6.

Aspirin or Salicylates + Pentazocine

Renal papillary necrosis occurred in man chronically taking large doses of aspirin when pentazocine was added.

Clinical evidence, mechanism, importance and management

An isolated report describes renal papillary necrosis in a man, regularly taking 1.8 to 2.4 g **aspirin** daily, within 6 months of additionally starting to take 800 to 850 mg **pentazocine** daily. He developed abdominal pain, nausea and vomiting, and passed tissue via his urethra. Before starting the **pentazocine** and when it was stopped, no necrosis was apparent. The postulated reason for this reaction is that the pentazocine-induced reduction in blood flow through the kidney potentiated the adverse effects of the chronic **aspirin** use.[1] The general importance of this case is uncertain, but it emphasises the risks of long-term use (possibly abuse) of **aspirin** with **pentazocine**. More study is needed.

1. Muhalwas KK, Shah GM, Winer RL. Renal papillary necrosis caused by long-term ingestion of pentazocine and aspirin. *JAMA* (1981) 246, 867–8.

Aspirin or Salicylates + Phenylbutazone

Phenylbutazone reduces the uricosuric effects of aspirin.

Clinical evidence

The observation that several patients given both drugs developed elevated serum urate levels, prompted a study in 4 patients without gout. This showed that 2 g **aspirin** daily had little effect on the excretion of uric acid in the urine, but marked uricosuria occurred with 5 g daily. When **phenylbutazone** was additionally given (200, 400 and then 600 mg daily over 3 days) the uricosuria was abolished. Serum uric acid levels rose from an average of 4 to 6 mg%. The interaction was confirmed in a patient with tophaceous gout. The retention of uric acid also occurs if the **phenylbutazone** is given first.[1]

Mechanism

Not understood. It seems almost certain that some interference occurs within the kidney tubules.

Importance and management

An established but sparsely documented interaction. If serum urate measurements are taken for diagnostic purposes, full account should be taken of this interaction. The potential problems arising from this interaction should also be recognised in any patient given both drugs.

1. Oyer JH, Wagner SL, Schmid FR. Suppression of salicylate-induced uricosuria by phenylbutazone. *Am J Med Sci* (1966) 225, 40–5.

Aspirin or Salicylates + Probenecid

The uricosuric effects of aspirin or other salicylates and probenecid are not additive as might be expected but are mutually antagonistic. Low dose, enteric-coated aspirin appears not to interact.

Clinical evidence

(a) Uricosuric effects reduced

A study showed that the urinary uric acid excretion in mg/average 24 h was found to be 673 mg with a single 3 g daily dose of **probenecid**, 909 mg with a 6 g daily dose of **sodium salicylate**, but only 114 mg when both drugs were used concurrently.[1] Similar antagonism has been seen in other studies in patients given 2.6 to 5.2 g **aspirin** daily.[2-4] No antagonism is seen until serum salicylate levels of 5 to 10 mg/100 ml are reached.[4]

(b) Uricosuric effects unchanged

A crossover study in 11 patients with gouty arthritis, stabilised on **probenecid**, found that the addition of daily doses of 325 mg **enteric-coated aspirin** taken either with the **probenecid** or 6 h later had no effect on serum urate levels or on the 24 hour urate excretion.[5]

Mechanism

Not understood. The interference probably occurs at the site of renal tubular secretion, but it also seems that both drugs can occupy the same site on plasma albumins.

Importance and management

A well established and clinically important interaction. Regular dosing with substantial amounts of salicylates should be avoided if this antagonism is to be avoided, but small very occasional analgesic doses probably do not matter. Serum salicylate levels of 5 to 10 mg/100 ml are necessary before this interaction occurs.

1. Seegmiller JE, Grayzel AI. Use of the newer uricosuric agents in the management of gout. *JAMA* (1960) 173, 1076–80.
2. Pascale LR, Dubin A, Hoffman WS. Therapeutic value of probenecid (Benemid®) in gout. *JAMA* (1952) 149, 1188–94.
3. Gutman AB, Yü TF. Benemid (p-di-n-propylsulfamyl-benzoic acid) as uricosuric agent in chronic gouty arthritis. *Trans Assoc Am Physicians* (1951) 64, 279–88.
4. Pascale LR, Dubin A, Bronsky D, Hoffman WS. Inhibition of the uricosuric action of Benemid by salicylate. *J Lab Clin Med* (1955) 45, 771–7.
5. Harris M, Bryant LR, Danaher P, Alloway J. Effect of low dose aspirin on serum urate levels and urinary excretion in patients receiving probenecid for gouty arthritis. *J Rheumatol* (2000) 27, 2873–6.

Aspirin or Salicylates + Sulfinpyrazone

The uricosuric effects of the salicylates and sulfinpyrazone are not additive, as might be expected, but are mutually antagonistic.

Clinical evidence

Sodium salicylate 6 g with **sulfinpyrazone 600 mg** daily caused a urinary uric acid excretion in a patient of only 30 mg/average 24 h, whereas when each drug was used alone in the same doses the excretion was 281 and 527 mg/average 24 h respectively.[1] A later study on five gouty men infused with **sulfinpyrazone** for about an hour

(300 mg to prime followed by 10 mg/min) showed that the additional infusion with **sodium salicylate** (3 g to prime followed by 10 to 20 mg/min) virtually abolished the uricosuria. When the drugs were given in the reverse order to three other patients the same result was seen.[2]

The uricosuria caused by 400 mg **sulfinpyrazone** daily was shown in another study to be completely abolished by 3.5 g **aspirin**.[3]

Mechanism

Not fully understood. Sulfinpyrazone competes successfully with salicylate for secretion by the kidney tubules so that salicylate excretion is reduced, but the salicylate blocks the inhibitory effect of sulfinpyrazone on the tubular reabsorption of uric acid so that the uric acid accumulates within the body.[2]

Importance and management

An established and clinically important interaction. Concurrent use for uricosuria should be avoided. Doses of aspirin as low as 700 mg can cause an appreciable fall in uric acid excretion[3] but the effects of an occasional small dose are probably of little practical importance.

1. Seegmiller JE, Grayzel AI. Use of the newer uricosuric agents in the management of gout. *JAMA* (1960) 173, 1076–80.
2. Yu TF, Dayton PG, Gutman AB. Mutual suppression of the uricosuric effects of sulfinpyrazone and salicylate: a study in interactions between drugs. *J Clin Invest* (1963) 42, 1330–9.
3. Kersley GD, Cook ER, Tovey DCJ. Value of uricosuric agents and in particular of G.28 315 in gout. *Ann Rheum Dis* (1958) 17, 326–33.

Aspirin or Salicylates + *Tamarindus indica* fruit extract

Tamarindus indica **fruit extract markedly increases the absorption and serum levels of aspirin.**

Clinical evidence, mechanism, importance and management

A study in 6 healthy subjects found that the bioavailability of a single 600-mg dose of **aspirin** was increased when taken with a meal containing *Tamarindus indica* **fruit extract**. The **aspirin** AUC rose sixfold (from 14.03 to 86.51 mg/ml.h), the maximum serum levels rose almost threefold (from 10.04 to 28.62 mg/ml) and the half-life increased moderately (from 1.04 to 1.50 h).[1] The reasons are not known, nor has the clinical importance of these large increases been evaluated, but this interaction should be borne in mind if high doses of **aspirin** are taken with this fruit extract. There would seem to be the possible risk of **aspirin** toxicity.

1. Mustapha A, Yakasai IA, Aguye IA. Effect of *Tamarindus indica L.* on the bioavailability of aspirin in health human volunteers. *Eur J Drug Metab Pharmacokinet* (1996) 21, 223–6.

Azapropazone + Miscellaneous drugs

The plasma levels of azapropazone are not significantly changed by the concurrent use of chloroquine, dihydroxy-aluminium sodium carbonate, magnesium aluminium silicate, bisacodyl or anthraquinone laxatives.

Clinical evidence, mechanism, importance and management

A study in 12 subjects given 300 mg azapropazone three times daily found that the plasma levels of azapropazone, measured at 4 h, were not affected by the concurrent use of **chloroquine**, 250 mg daily for 7 days.[1] Another study in 15 patients taking the same dosage of azapropazone found that the concurrent use of **dihydroxy-aluminium sodium carbonate, magnesium aluminium silicate, bisacodyl** or **anthraquinone laxatives** only caused a minor (5 to 7%) reduction in azapropazone plasma levels.[2] No special precautions would seem to be needed if these drugs are given together.

1. Faust-Tinnefeldt G, Geissler HE. Azapropazon und rheumatologische Basistherapie mit Chloroquin unter dem Aspekt der Arzneimittelinteraktion. *Arzneimittelforschung* (1977) 27, 2170–4.
2. Faust-Tinnefeldt G, Geissler HE, Mutschler E. Azapropazon-Plasmaspiegel unter Begleitmedikation mit einem Antacidum oder Laxans. *Arzneimittelforschung* (1977) 27, 2411–12.

Buprenorphine or Oxycodone + Amitriptyline or Ketorolac

No marked increase in the CNS and respiratory depressant effects of buprenorphine occurs if amitriptyline is given concurrently. Oxycodone similarly appears not to interact adversely with amitriptyline. A single case report describes marked respiratory depression in a man on buprenorphine when ketorolac was added.

Clinical evidence, mechanism, importance and management

(a) Buprenorphine, Oxycodone + Amitriptyline

A study in 12 healthy subjects found that both 400 micrograms **buprenorphine** given sublingually and 50 mg **amitriptyline** given orally impaired the performance of a number of psychomotor tests (digit symbol substitution, flicker fusion, Maddox wing, hand-to-eye coordination, reactive skills) and the subjects felt drowsy, feeble, mentally slow and muzzy. When given together the effects were only moderately increased and the increase in the respiratory depressant effects of the **buprenorphine** was only mild.[1] A not dissimilar study using 0.28 mg/kg **oxycodone** and 25 mg **amitriptyline** found no major pharmacodynamic interactions.[2] There seem to be no strong reasons for avoiding concurrent use but patients should be warned.

(b) Buprenorphine + Ketorolac

A man underwent thoracotomy for carcinoma of the middle third of his oesophagus. An hour after transfer to the recovery ward he complained of severe pain at the operative site and was given 150 micrograms (3 micrograms/kg) epidural **buprenorphine**, and 2 hours later 30 mg **ketorolac** intramuscularly because of continued pain. During the next hour he became more drowsy, stopped obeying commands and developed bradypnoea (6 breaths per min). He recovered after 6 h of mechanical ventilation. The authors of this report suggest that it may be necessary to use less **buprenorphine** in the presence of **ketorolac** to avoid the development of these respiratory depressant effects.[3] More study is needed of this apparent interaction.

1. Saarialho-Kere U, Mattila MJ, Paloheimo M, Seppälä T. Psychomotor, respiratory and neuroendocrinological effects of buprenorphine and amitriptyline in healthy volunteers. *Eur J Clin Pharmacol* (1987) 33, 139–46.
2. Pöyhiä R, Kalso E, Seppälä T. Pharmacodynamic interactions of oxycodone and amitriptyline in healthy volunteers. *Curr Ther Res* (1992) 51, 739–49.
3. Jain PN, Shah SC. Respiratory depression following combination of epidural buprenorphine and intramuscular ketorolac. *Anaesthesia* (1993) 48, 898–9.

Butorphanol + Cimetidine

Butorphanol and cimetidine appear not to interact.

Clinical evidence, mechanism, importance and management

The pharmacokinetics of transnasal **butorphanol** (1 mg six-hourly) and **cimetidine** (300 mg six-hourly) for 4 days were not significantly altered by concurrent use in 16 healthy subjects.[1] There would seem to be no reason for avoiding combined use.

1. Shyu WC, Barbhaiya RH. Lack of pharmacokinetic interaction between butorphanol nasal spray and cimetidine. *Br J Clin Pharmacol* (1996) 42, 513–17.

Codeine + Carbamazepine

Carbamazepine appears to increase the production of a more potent metabolite of codeine.

Clinical evidence, mechanism, importance and management

An experimental study in 7 epileptics to find out if **carbamazepine** induces the enzymes concerned with the metabolism of codeine found that it increased the production of the metabolite normorphine almost threefold. The epileptics were taking 400 to 600 mg **carbamazepine** daily and were given a single 25-mg dose of codeine.[1] Normorphine is similar to, or possibly more potent, than morphine, so that those taking both codeine and carbamazepine may possibly experience a stronger analgesic effect. This would seem to be an advantageous interaction. There would seem to be no reason for avoiding concurrent use.

1. Yue Q-Y, Tomson T, Säwe J. Carbamazepine and cigarette smoking induce differentially the metabolism of codeine in man. *Pharmacogenetics* (1994) 4, 193–8.

Codeine, Dihydrocodeine, Hydrocodone or Tramadol + Quinidine

The analgesic effects of codeine, dihydrocodeine and hydrocodone are reduced or abolished by quinidine in most patients but tramadol appears not to interact.

Clinical evidence

(a) Codeine

Sixteen extensive metabolisers were given 100 mg **codeine** with and without single 200-mg doses of **quinidine**. The **quinidine** reduced the peak morphine levels by about 80% (from a mean of 18 to less than 4 nanomol/l). **Codeine** alone increased the pain threshold (pin-prick pain test using an argon laser) but no significant analgesic effects were detectable when the **quinidine** was also present.[1]

These studies confirm those of a previous study with 100 mg **codeine** and 50-mg doses of **quinidine**.[2] The **quinidine** reduced the peak morphine plasma levels by more than 90% (by 92% in 7 extensive metabolisers, and by 97% in one poor metaboliser) and similarly abolished the analgesic effects.[2]

(b) Dihydrocodeine

A study in which 4 extensive metabolisers were given 40 or 60 mg **dihydrocodeine** found that when pretreated with 200 mg **quinidine** almost none of the morphinoid metabolites of **dihydrocodeine** normally present in the serum after taking **dihydrocodeine** could be detected.[3] The same authors found essentially the same results in a later study in 10 extensive metabolisers given 60 mg **dihydrocodeine** and 50 mg **quinidine**.[4]

(c) Hydrocodone

In a comparative study, 5 extensive metabolisers and 6 poor metabolisers were given **hydrocodone**, and 4 extensive metabolisers were given **hydrocodone** after pre-treatment with **quinidine**. The metabolism of the **hydrocodone** to its active metabolite (hydromorphone) was found to be high in the extensive metabolisers who described 'good opiate effects' but poor in the poor metabolisers and the extensive metabolisers pre-treated with **quinidine** who described 'poor opiate effects'.[5]

(d) Tramadol

A double-blind placebo controlled study in 12 healthy subjects (11 extensive metabolisers and 1 poor metaboliser) carried out to investigate the mode of action of **tramadol**, found that when given 100 mg **tramadol** with and without 50 mg **quinidine**, the **quinidine** had virtually no effect on the tramadol's analgesic effects but it weakly inhibited its effect on pupil size. The **quinidine** inhibited the production of *o*-desmethyltramadol which affects opioid receptors, but tramadol's analgesia appears to be largely due to some other mechanism.[6]

Mechanism

The evidence available shows that the conversion of codeine, dihydrocodeine and hydrocodone to their active analgesic metabolites in the body (morphine, morphinoid metabolites and hydromorphone respectively) depends upon the activity of cytochrome P450 isoenzyme CYP2D6 in the liver. If this isoenzyme is inhibited by quinidine, these conversions largely fail to occur and the analgesic effects are reduced or lost. This interaction is only likely to occur in extensive metabolisers who possess CYP2D6, but not in poor metabolisers who lack the gene for the production of CYP2D6 and who are therefore normally unlikely to find these analgesics effective.[7] Tramadol's analgesia appears to be mediated by two mechanisms: a very weak opioid mechanism and a separate and more potent effect on non-opioid receptors. Thus even marked inhibition by quinidine of the production of *o*-desmethyltramadol which affects opioid receptors is unimportant.

Importance and management

The codeine/quinidine interaction is well established and clinically important. Codeine will be virtually ineffective as an analgesic in extensive metabolisers taking quinidine. An alternative analgesic should be used. No interaction would be expected in poor metabolisers. Whether the antitussive effects of codeine are similarly affected is not established, but it seems likely.

The interactions of dihydrocodeine and hydrocodone are less well established, but the biochemical evidence suggests that their analgesic effects will similarly be reduced or lost if quinidine is used concurrently by extensive metabolisers. No interaction would be expected in poor metabolisers.

The metabolic status of a patient (i.e. whether 'extensive' or 'poor') is genetically determined so that you will not know whether these interactions are likely to occur, or whether these analgesics will normally be effective, unless the patient's status has already been identified.

The evidence available suggests that the analgesic effects of tramadol are little affected by the presence of quinidine.

1. Sindrup SH, Arendt-Nielsen L, Brøsen K, Bjerring P, Angelo HR, Eriksen B, Gram LF. The effect of quinidine on the analgesic effect of codeine. *Eur J Clin Pharmacol* (1992) 42, 587–92.

2. Desmeules J, Dayer P, Gascon M-P, Magistris M. Impact of genetic and environmental factors on codeine analgesia. *Clin Pharmacol Ther* (1989) 45, 122.

3. Hufschmid E, Theurillat R, Martin U, Thormann W. Exploration of the metabolism of dihydrocodeine via determination of its metabolites in human urine using micellar electokinetic capillary chromatography. *J Chromatogr B: Biomed Appl* (1995) 668, 159–70.

4. Hufschmid E, Theurillat R, Wilder-Smith CH, Thormann W. Characterization of the genetic polymorphism of dihydrocodeine O-demethylation in man via analysis of urinary dihydrocodeine and dihydromorphine by micellar electrokinetic capillary chromatography. *J Chromatogr B: Biomed Appl* (1996) 678, 45–51.

5. Otton SV, Schadel M, Cheung SW, Kaplan, Busto UE, Sellers EM. CYP2D6 phenotype determines the metabolic conversion of hydrocodone to hydromorphone. *Clin Pharmacol Ther* (1993) 54, 463–72.

6. Collart L, Luthy C, Dayer P. Multimodel analgesic effect of tramadol. *Clin Pharmacol Ther* (1993) 53, 223.

7. Caraco Y, Sheller J, Wood AJ. Pharmacogenetic determination of the effects of codeine and prediction of drug interactions. *J Pharmacol Exp Ther* (1996) 278, 1165–74.

Codeine + Rifampicin (Rifampin)

Some preliminary evidence suggests that rifampicin may reduce the analgesic effects of codeine.

Clinical evidence, mechanism, importance and management

A study in 9 extensive metabolisers and 6 poor metabolisers found that after taking 600 mg **rifampicin** daily for 3 weeks, the metabolism of a single 120 mg oral dose of codeine phosphate was markedly increased in the extensive metabolisers due to the increased activity of cytochrome P450 isoenzyme CYP2D6. Only small changes were seen in the poor metabolisers. The pharmacokinetic effects of the interaction were measured by looking at the reductions in the respiratory, psychomotor and pupillary effects of the codeine, but the clinically more relevant question of whether, and to what extent, the analgesic effects of the codeine were reduced by this interaction was not addressed by this study.[1] But since **rifampicin** reduces the serum levels of the morphine produced from codeine (by which codeine exerts its analgesic effects), some reduction would be expected. If therefore these drugs are used concurrently, be alert for the need to raise the codeine dosage. More study is needed.

1. Caraco Y, Sheller J, Wood AJJ. Pharmacogenetic determinants of codeine induction by rifampin: the impact on codeine's respiratory, psychomotor and miotic effects. *J Pharmacol Exp Ther* (1997) 281, 330–6.

Dextromoramide + Troleandomycin

An isolated report describes a marked increase in the effects of dextromoramide, and coma in a man when he was treated with troleandomycin.

Clinical evidence, mechanism, importance and management

A man on dextromoramide developed signs of overdosage (a morphine-like coma, mydriasis and depressed respiration) 3 days after starting treatment with **troleandomycin** for a dental infection. He recovered when treated with naloxone. A possible explanation is that the **troleandomycin** reduced the metabolism of the dextromoramide, thereby reducing its loss from the body and increasing its serum levels and effects.[1] The general importance of this interaction is uncertain but concurrent use should be well monitored. It is not clear whether other macrolide antibacterials can interact similarly.

1. Carry PV, Ducluzeau R, Jourdan C, Bourrat Ch, Vigneau C, Descotes J. De nouvelles interactions avec les macrolides? *Lyon Med* (1982) 248, 189–90.

Dextropropoxyphene (Propoxyphene) + Food

Food can delay the absorption of dextropropoxyphene, but the total amount absorbed may be slightly increased.

Clinical evidence, mechanism, importance and management

A study in healthy subjects showed that while fasting, peak plasma dextropropoxyphene levels were reached after about 2 h. **High fat** and **high carbohydrate meals** delayed peak serum levels to about 3 h, and **high protein** to about 4 h. Both the **protein and carbohydrate meals** caused a small increase in the total amount of dextropropoxyphene absorbed.[1] Likely reasons for the delay in absorption are that **food** delays gastric emptying and possibly also physically prevents the dextropropoxyphene from coming into contact with the absorbing surface of the gut. Avoid **food** if rapid analgesic effects are needed.

1. Musa MN and Lyons LL. Effect of food and liquid on the pharmacokinetics of propoxyphene. *Curr Ther Res* (1976) 19, 669–74.

Dextropropoxyphene (Propoxyphene) + Orphenadrine

An alleged adverse interaction between dextropropoxyphene and orphenadrine which is said to cause mental confusion, anxiety, and tremors seems to be very rare, if indeed it ever occurs.

Clinical evidence, mechanism, importance and management

The makers of **orphenadrine**, used to state in their package insert that mental confusion, anxiety and tremors have been reported in patients receiving **orphenadrine** and dextropropoxyphene (propoxyphene) concurrently. The makers of propoxyphene, issued a similar warning. However in correspondence with both manufacturers, two investigators[1] of this interaction were told that the basis of these statements consisted of either anecdotal reports from clinicians or cases where patients had received twice the recommended dose of **orphenadrine**, in all a total of 13 cases. In every case the adverse reactions seen were similar to those reported with either drug alone. A brief study on 5 patients given both drugs to investigate this alleged interaction failed to reveal an adverse interaction.[2]

The documentation is therefore sparse (to say the least) and no case of interaction has been firmly established. The investigators calculated that the two drugs were probably being used together on 300 000 prescriptions a year, and at that time (1970) a maximum of 13 doubtful cases had been reported.[1] There seems therefore little reason for avoiding concurrent use, although prescribers should know that the advisability of using the two drugs together has been the subject of some debate.

1. Pearson RE, Salter FJ. Drug interaction? — Orphenadrine with propoxyphene. *N Engl J Med* (1970) 282, 1215.
2. Puckett WH, Visconti JA. Orphenadrine and propoxyphene (cont.). *N Engl J Med* (1970) 283, 544.

Dextropropoxyphene (Propoxyphene) + Tobacco smoking

Dextropropoxyphene is less effective as an analgesic in smokers than in non-smokers.

Clinical evidence

A study on 835 patients who were given dextropropoxyphene (propoxyphene) hydrochloride for mild or moderate pain or headache showed that its efficacy as an analgesic was decreased by **smoking**. The drug was rated as ineffective in 10.1% of 335 non-smokers, 15% of 347 patients who **smoked** up to 20 cigarettes daily, and 20.3% of 153 patients who **smoked** more than 20 cigarettes daily.[1]

Mechanism

It is thought that tobacco smoke contains compounds which increase the activity of the liver enzymes concerned with the metabolism of dextropropoxyphene, thereby increasing its loss from the body and diminishing its effectiveness as an analgesic.[1]

Importance and management

The interaction appears to be well established. Prescribers should be aware that dextropropoxyphene is twice as likely to be ineffective in those who smoke more than 20 cigarettes a day (1 in 5) as in those who do not smoke (1 in 10).

1. Boston Collaborative Drug Surveillance Program. Decreased clinical efficacy of propoxyphene in cigarette smokers. *Clin Pharmacol Ther* (1973) 14, 259–63.

Diamorphine + Pyrithyldione

A single case report describes a fatality due to the combined CNS depressant effects of diamorphine (heroin) and pyrithyldione.

Clinical evidence, mechanism, importance and management

A heroin (diamorphine) addict was found dead after taking **pyrithyldione** (a sedative and hypnotic) and diamorphine. His blood **pyrithyldione** and brain morphine levels were found to be 590 nanograms/ml and 0.06 nanograms/g respectively, suggesting that he had taken only a therapeutic dose of the **pyrithyldione** and a moderate dose of diamorphine. The presumed cause of death was the combined CNS depressant effects of both drugs. The authors of the report draw the conclusion that the **pyrithyldione** potentiated the effects of the diamorphine.[1]

1. Jorens PG, Coucke V, Selala MI, Schepens PJC. Fatal intoxication due to the combined use of heroin and pyrithyldione. *Hum Exp Toxicol* (1992) 11, 296–7.

Diclofenac + Colestyramine or Colestipol

The absorption of diclofenac from the gut is reduced by colestyramine, and to a lesser extent by colestipol.

Clinical evidence

A three-phase crossover study in 6 healthy subjects found that 8 g **colestyramine** reduced the AUC of a single 100 mg oral dose of enteric coated diclofenac by 62% and reduced its maximum plasma levels by 75%. **Colestipol** 10 g reduced the diclofenac AUC by 33% and its maximum plasma levels by 58%.[1]

Mechanism

Colestyramine and colestipol are anion exchange resins which are intended to bind with bile acids, but which can also bind with drugs which are present in the gut so that their absorption is reduced. *In vitro* studies show that the binding capacity of colestipol is less than that of colestyramine.[1]

Importance and management

Established interactions but their clinical importance still needs assessment in patients. It seems likely that the effectiveness of diclofenac will be decreased by both resins, and particularly by colestyramine. Separating the administration of the diclofenac from the resins may not be a totally successful way of avoiding this interaction because as much as a third of the diclofenac may be secreted in the bile. Giving the drugs separately, possibly 2 h apart, may be of some help, but you may still have to raise the diclofenac dosage. More study is needed.

1. Al-Balla SR, El-Sayed YM, Al-Meshal MA, Gouda MW. The effects of cholestyramine and colestipol on the absorption of diclofenac in man. *Int J Clin Pharmacol Ther* (1994) 32, 441–5.

Diclofenac + Floctafenine

No adverse interaction appears to occur between diclofenac and floctafenine.

Clinical evidence, mechanism, importance and management

No pharmacokinetic nor any other clinically relevant interaction was seen when 6 healthy subjects were given 400 mg **floctafenine** with 75 mg diclofenac daily for a week.[1] No special precautions would seem to be necessary.

1. Sioufi A, Stierlin H, Schweizer A, Botta L, Degen PH, Theobald W, Brechbühler S. Recent findings concerning clinically relevant pharmacokinetics of diclofenac sodium. In: Voltarol — New Findings, ed Kass E. Proc Int Symp Voltarol, Paris June 22nd, 1981. 15th Int Congress of Rheumatology. p 19–30.

Diclofenac + Miscellaneous antibacterials

Doxycycline and cefadroxil do not interact with diclofenac. The biliary excretion of ceftriaxone is increased by diclofenac.

Clinical evidence, mechanism, importance and management

Neither 2 g **cefadroxil** (8 patients) nor 100 mg **doxycycline** (7 patients) when taken daily for a week had any effect on the pharmacokinetics of 100 mg diclofenac daily.[1] No special precautions are needed while taking either of these drugs and diclofenac. A pharmacokinetic study in 8 patients who had undergone cholecystectomy and who had a T drain in the common bile duct, found that while taking diclofenac (50 mg 12-hourly) the excretion of **ceftriaxone** (2 g intravenously) in the bile was increased fourfold while the urinary excretion was approximately halved.[2] The clinical importance of this is uncertain, but probably small.

1. Schumacher A, Geissler HE, Mutschler E, Osterburg M. Untersuchungen potentieller Interaktionen von Diclofenac-Natrium (Voltaren) mit Antibiotika. *Z Rheumatol* (1983) 42, 25–7.
2. Merle-Melet M, Bresler L, Lokiec F, Dopff C, Boissel P, Dureux JB. Effects of diclofenac on ceftriaxone pharmacokinetics in humans. *Antimicrob Agents Chemother* (1992) 36, 2331–3.

Diclofenac (topical) + Miscellaneous drugs

Topical diclofenac intended for use on the skin is very unlikely to interact adversely with any of the drugs which are known to interact with the diclofenac given orally

Clinical evidence, mechanism, importance and management

The makers of *Pennsaid* (a 1.5% topical solution of diclofenac in 45% (w/w) dimethylsulphoxide) say that when the maximum dosage of 1 ml is used on the skin, the maximum serum levels of diclofenac achieved are less than 10 nanograms/ml.[1] This is 50 times lower than the maximum serum levels achieved with the oral administration of 25 mg diclofenac. Despite these very low concentrations, the UK summary of product characteristics lists a whole range of potentially interacting drugs (**aspirin, digoxin, lithium, oral hypoglycaemic agents, diuretics, NSAIDs, methotrexate, ciclosporin, quinolone antibacterials and antihypertensives**).[1] This list seems to have been borrowed directly from the literature used for oral diclofenac, and it would seem to be inappropriately alarmist to apply it to the topical form of the drug. None of the drugs listed has ever been reported to interact with the topical form, and it seems unlikely that any of them ever will.

1. Pennsaid (Diclofenac). Provalis Healthcare. Summary of product characteristics, November 2001.

Diclofenac + Omeprazole or Food

Omeprazole appears not to interact to a clinically relevant extent with diclofenac, but food possibly delays the absorption of diclofenac.

Clinical evidence, mechanism, importance and management

Thirteen healthy subjects were given single doses of potassium diclofenac suspension (*Flogan*, 105 mg in 7 ml while fasting, after gastric acid secretion blockade with **omeprazole**, and after **food**. The pharmacokinetics of the diclofenac were not changed to a clinically relevant extent by either **omeprazole** or **food**, except that the **food** delayed the absorption which might possibly be important if rapid analgesia was needed.[1]

1. Poli A, Moreno RA, Ribiero W, Dias HB, Moreno H, Muscara MN, De Nucci G. Influence of gastric acid secretion blockade and food intake on the bioavailability of a potassium diclofenac suspension in healthy male volunteers. *Int J Clin Pharmacol Ther* (1996) 34, 76–9.

Diclofenac + Pentazocine

An isolated report describes grand mal seizures in a patient treated with diclofenac and pentazocine.

Clinical evidence, mechanism, importance and management

A man with Buerger's disease had a grand mal seizure while watching television 2 h after being given a single 50 mg suppository of diclofenac. He was also taking 50 mg **pentazocine** three times daily. He may possibly have had a previous seizure some months before after taking a single 100-mg slow-release diclofenac tablet.[1] The reasons for this reaction are not known, but on rare occasions diclofenac alone has been associated with seizures (said[1] to be 1 in 100 000) and seizures have also been seen with **pentazocine** alone. It is not clear what part the disease itself, or watching television, had a part to play in the development of this adverse reaction.[1]

No interaction between diclofenac and **pentazocine** is established, but be aware of this case if concurrent use is being considered, particularly in patients who are known to be seizure-prone.

1. Heim M, Nadvorna H, Azaria M. With comments by Straughan J and Hoehler HW. Grand mal seizures following treatment with diclofenac and pentazocine. *S Afr Med J* (1990) 78, 700–1.

Diclofenac + Rifampicin (Rifampin)

Preliminary data suggest that the serum levels of diclofenac are reduced by rifampicin.

Clinical evidence, mechanism, importance and management

A study in 6 healthy subjects found that after taking 450 mg **rifampicin** daily for 6 days, the maximum serum levels of diclofenac measured 8 h after a single 100-mg dose (enteric coated tablets) was reduced to 57% and the AUC to 33%. The reason is uncertain.[1] This preliminary data therefore suggests that patients on **rifampicin** will need an increase in the dosage of diclofenac. More study is needed.

1. Kumar JS, Mamidi NVSR, Chakrapani T, Krishna DR. Rifampicin pretreatment reduces bioavailability of diclofenac sodium. *Ind J Pharmacol* (1995) 27, 183–5.

Diflunisal + Antacids

Antacids containing aluminium and magnesium can reduce the absorption of diflunisal by up to 40%, but no important interaction occurs if food is taken at the same time.

Clinical evidence, mechanism, importance and management

A study on 4 healthy subjects found that when given three 15-ml doses of *Aludrox* (**aluminium hydroxide**), 2 h before, together with and 2 h after a single 500-mg oral dose of diflunisal, its absorption was reduced about 40%.[1] Another study[2] showed that the absorption of a single 500-mg dose of diflunisal was reduced 13% when given with 30 ml *Maalox* (**aluminium-magnesium hydroxides**), 21% when given 1 h later, and 32% when the antacid was given on a four-times-a-day schedule. Yet another study demonstrated a 26% reduction in absorption by 15 ml **aluminium hydroxide** gel.[3] However the bioavailability of diflunisal was not significantly altered in those taking **aluminium-magnesium hydroxides** if also taken with food.[4] Just how these antacids cause a reduced absorption is not clear but adsorption has been suggested.[4] The clinical importance of this interaction is uncertain.

1. Verbeeck R, Tjandramaga TB, Mullie A, Verbesselt R, De Schepper PJ. Effect of aluminium hydroxide on diflunisal absorption. *Br J Clin Pharmacol* (1979) 7, 519–22.
2. Holmes GI, Irvin JD, Schrogie JJ, Davies RO, Breault GO, Rogers JL, Huber PB, Zinny MA. Effects of Maalox on the bioavailability of diflunisal. *Clin Pharmacol Ther* (1979) 25, 229.
3. Tobert JA, DeSchepper P, Tjandramaga TB, Mullie A, Meisinger MAP, Buntinx AP, Huber PB, Yeh KC. The effect of antacids on the bioavailability of diflunisal. *Clin Pharmacol Ther* (1979) 25, 251.
4. Tobert JA, DeSchepper P, Tjandramaga TB, Mullie A, Buntinx AP, Meisinger MAP, Huber PB, Hall TLP, Yeh KC. Effect of antacids on the bioavailability of diflunisal in the fasting and postprandial states. *Clin Pharmacol Ther* (1981) 30, 385–9.

Diflunisal or Oxaprozin + Miscellaneous drugs

The loss of diflunisal from the body is faster in men than women, and is increased by smoking and oral contraceptives.[1] The pharmacokinetics of oxaprozin are only changed to a minor degree by conjugated oestrogens (*Premarin*).[2,3] None of the changes appeared to be large enough to be of clinical importance.

1. Macdonald JI, Herman RJ, Verbeeck RK. Sex-difference and the effects of smoking and oral contraceptive steroids on the kinetics of diflunisal. *Eur J Clin Pharmacol* (1990) 38, 175–9.
2. Scavone JM, Ochs HR, Greenblatt DJ, Matlis R. Pharmacokinetics of oxaprozin in women receiving conjugated estrogen. *Eur J Clin Pharmacol* (1988) 35, 105–8.
3. Scavone JM, Greenblatt DJ. Oxaprozin kinetics in women receiving conjugated estrogens. *J Clin Pharmacol* (1987) 27, 725.

Diflunisal + NSAIDs or Analgesics

Aspirin can reduce serum diflunisal levels. Diflunisal raises serum indometacin (indomethacin) levels two to threefold and concurrent use should be avoided. Paracetamol (acetaminophen) levels are increased by diflunisal but not those of naproxen.

Clinical evidence, mechanism, importance and management

(a) Diflunisal + Aspirin

The concurrent use of **aspirin** 600 mg four times daily has been shown to cause a 15% fall in plasma diflunisal levels after 250 mg twice daily over 3 three days.[1,2] This is probably clinically unimportant.

(b) Indometacin (Indomethacin)

A study in 16 healthy subjects showed that diflunisal 500 mg twice daily raised the steady-state plasma levels and the AUC of **indometacin** (50 mg twice daily) two to threefold.[3] Another study confirmed that plasma **indometacin** levels are approximately doubled and the CNS side-effects are increased (dizziness, nausea, tiredness, unsteadiness, light-headedness).[4] In yet another study[5] it was found that diflunisal 250 mg twice daily with **indometacin** 25 mg three times daily increased plasma indometacin levels by 30 to 35%. The reason appears to be that the diflunisal inhibits the glucuronidation of the indometacin so that it is retained in the body longer.[3,4] The diflunisal appears to have no clear effect on the blood loss in the faeces.[3] Despite evidence that diflunisal protects the human gastric mucosa against the damaging effects of **indometacin**,[6] fatal gastrointestinal haemorrhage has occurred in one patient concurrently treated with diflunisal and **indometacin**,[7] and the manufacturers advise avoidance.

(c) Paracetamol (Acetaminophen), Naproxen

Diflunisal significantly raises serum **paracetamol** levels but the total bioavailability is unchanged.[8] Diflunisal 250 mg twice daily has been found to have no effect on plasma levels of co-administered **naproxen** (250 mg twice daily).[9] Neither of these interactions has been shown to be clinically important.

1. Tempero KF, Cirillo VJ, Steelman SL. Diflunisal: a review of pharmacokinetic and pharmacodynamic properties, drug interactions and special tolerability studies in humans. *Br J Clin Pharmacol* (1977) 4, 31S–36S.
2. Perrier CV. Unpublished observations quoted in ref.1.
3. Van Hecken A, Verbesselt R, Tjandra-Maga TB, De Schepper PJ. Pharmacokinetic interaction between indomethacin and diflunisal. *Eur J Clin Pharmacol* (1989) 36, 507–12.
4. Eriksson L-O, Wåhlin-Boll E, Liedholm H, Seideman P, Melander A. Influence of chronic diflunisal treatment on the plasma levels, metabolism and excretion of indomethacin. *Eur J Clin Pharmacol* (1989) 37, 7–15.
5. De Schepper P. Unpublished observations quoted in ref.1.
6. Cohen MM. Diflunisal protects human gastric mucosa against damage by indomethacin. *Dig Dis Sci* (1983) 28, 1070–77.
7. Edwards IR. Medicines Adverse Reactions Committee: eighteenth annual report, 1983. *N Z Med J* (1984) 97, 729–32.
8. Diggins JB, (Merck Sharp Dohme). *Personal communication* (1988).
9. Dresse A, Gerard MA, Quinaux N, Fischer P, Gerardy J. Effect of diflunisal on human plasma levels and on the urinary excretion of naproxen. *Arch Int Pharmacodyn Ther* (1978) 236, 276–84.

Etodolac + Miscellaneous drugs

Etodolac appears not to interact with glibenclamide (glyburide) nor phenytoin. Food delays the absorption of etodolac, but does not significantly reduce the amount absorbed. An un-named antacid has been found not to interact.

Clinical evidence, mechanism, importance and management

A three-way crossover study in 16 healthy subjects found that 200 mg etodolac 12-hourly for 3 days had no effect on the pharmacokinetics or the pharmacological effects of either **glibenclamide (glyburide)** 3.5 mg daily or **phenytoin** (100 mg twice daily for 2 days, 100 mg on day three).[1] There would seem to be no reason for avoiding the concurrent use of either of these drugs but as clinical experience is still limited it would be prudent to monitor the outcome well. Information about other hypoglycaemic agents and anticonvulsants seems to be lacking.

A study in 18 healthy subjects found that when given 400 mg etodolac after a **high fat meal**, peak concentrations were approximately halved (from 31 to 14 micrograms/ml) and delayed (from 1.4 to 3.8 h), but the total amount absorbed was not markedly changed (from 152 to 133 micrograms.h/ml). Thus food slows the rate but not the extent of absorption. When taken with an **antacid** (not named) neither the rate nor the extent of absorption were altered.[2]

1. Zvaifler N. A review of the antiarthritic efficacy and safety of etodolac. *Clin Rheumatol* (1989) 8 (Suppl 1), 43–53.
2. Troy S, Sanda M, Dressler D, Chiang S, Latts J. The effect of food and antacid on etodolac bioavailability. *Clin Pharmacol Ther* (1990) 47, 192.

Etoricoxib + Miscellaneous drugs

Etoricoxib increases the maximum serum levels of digoxin, raises ethinylestradiol and levels and causes a small increase in INR when taken with warfarin. Ketoconazole moderately raises etoricoxib serum levels but all of these interactions seem to be of minor clinical relevance. The makers say avoid other NSAIDs and aspirin in doses above those used for antiplatelet action because of increased gastrointestinal toxicity, and they infer that some increase in the dosage of etoricoxib may be needed if rifampicin (rifampin) is taken concurrently. Suggestions have also been made about the possibility of increased toxicity risks if etoricoxib is given with ACE inhibitors, oral corticosteroids, ciclosporin, lithium, methotrexate or tacrolimus.

Clinical evidence, mechanism, importance and management

(a) Anticoagulants

Studies in healthy subjects on **warfarin** found that 120 mg etoricoxib daily caused an approximately 13% increase in INR which is unlikely to be clinically relevant. Even so the makers[1] cautiously say that ". . . patients receiving **warfarin** or similar agents should be closely monitored for their prothrombin time INR, particularly in the first few days when therapy with etoricoxib is initiated or the dose of etoricoxib is changed." Some monitoring may be appropriate because all NSAIDS can irritate the gastrointestinal tract and cause bleeding.

(b) Antihypertensives and diuretics

The makers say that **NSAIDs** in general can reduce the effects of **antihypertensives** and **diuretics**, and they point out that the concurrent use of **ACE inhibitors** and drugs which inhibit cyclo-oxygenase (which includes etoricoxib) may cause further deterioration of patients with already compromised kidney function. So far there seem to be no reports about this with etoricoxib.[1]

(c) Contraceptives, oral

A study in women taking a **combined oral contraceptive (ethinylestradiol** 35 micrograms + 0.5 to 1.0 mg **norethindrone)** for 21 days found that the addition of 120 mg etoricoxib increased the 24 hr steady-state levels of **ethinylestradiol** by 50 to 60% but the **norethindrone** levels were not raised to a clinically relevant extent. The etoricoxib was given either at the same time as the contraceptive or 12 h later. There would therefore appear to be no reason for avoiding concurrent use but the makers suggest that this increase in **ethinylestradiol** levels should be considered when choosing the oral contraceptive.[1]

(d) Corticosteroids

The makers say that in drug interaction studies etoricoxib was found not to have a clinically important effect on the pharmacokinetics of **prednisone/prednisolone**. However it should be borne in mind that the concurrent use of most **NSAIDs** and **oral corticosteroids** increase the incidences of gastrointestinal irritation and possible bleeding, so that it would be prudent to monitor the oral use of these and other **corticosteroids** with etoricoxib.[2]

(e) Digoxin

A study in healthy subjects on **digoxin** found that the addition of 120 mg etoricoxib daily for 10 days did not alter the steady-state 24-h AUC of **digoxin** or its renal elimination, but the maximum serum **digoxin** levels were increased by about 33%.[1] This change is unlikely to be clinically relevant in most patients but it might possibly affect a very small number whose **digoxin** levels are already high.

(f) Immunosuppressants

The makers say that the concurrent use of **ciclosporin** or **tacrolimus** and etoricoxib has not been studied, but based on the increased nephrotoxicity seen with some **NSAIDs** they say that kidney function should be monitored if etoricoxib is used with either drug.[1]

(g) Ketoconazole

A study in healthy subjects found that 400 mg **ketoconazole** daily for 11 days increased the AUC of a single 60-mg dose of etoricoxib by 43%, the reason being that **ketoconazole** inhibits the activity of cytochrome P450 isoenzyme CYP3A4, which is responsible for 60% of the metabolism of etoricoxib. As a result, its clearance from the body is reduced and its serum levels rise. This moderate rise in serum levels is not regarded as being clinically relevant.

(h) Lithium

The makers[1] cautiously say that "the plasma concentration of **lithium** could be increased by NSAIDs." While this is certainly true for some NSAIDs there appears to be no evidence as yet that etoricoxib itself actually affects serum **lithium** levels.

(i) Methotrexate

A study in patients taking 7.5 to 20 mg **methotrexate** weekly for rheumatoid arthritis found that the addition of 60, 90 or 120 mg etoricoxib daily had no effect on the **methotrexate** AUC or on its renal clearance. However another similar study found that 120 mg etoricoxib daily increased the **methotrexate** AUC by 28% and reduced its clearance by 13%. For this reason the makers of etoricoxib say that concurrent use should be monitored for any evidence of **methotrexate** toxicity.[1]

(j) NSAIDs

The makers say that at steady-state the concurrent use of 120 mg etoricoxib daily did not affect the antiplatelet activity of 81 mg daily doses of **aspirin** so that low-dose prophylactic cardiovascular use of **aspirin** is acceptable. But they also point out that this still carries an increased risk of gastrointestinal ulceration[1] so that good monitoring is needed. The patient should be advised to report any excessive stomach discomfort or pain. However, the makers also say that larger doses of **aspirin** or other **NSAIDs** with etoricoxib should be avoided.[1] The CSM in the UK has also issued a general warning about not using more than one **NSAID**.[2] The risk of gastrointestinal perforation/obstruction, ulceration or bleeding is more than doubled when **aspirin** is given with **other NSAIDs**.[2]

(k) Rifampicin (Rifampin)

Rifampicin has been found to reduce the serum levels of etoricoxib by 65%. The reason is that **rifampicin** is a potent inducer of cytochrome P450 isoenzyme CYP3A4 which is responsible for 60% of the metabolism of etoricoxib, as a result of which its clearance from the body is increased and its serum levels fall. The clinical relevance of this reduction has not be assessed, but the makers infer in their product literature is that it may possibly be necessary to raise the dosage of etoricoxib. Be alert for any evidence of reduced etoricoxib efficacy if both drugs are used, and raise the dosage if necessary.

1. Arcoxia (Etoricoxib). Merck Sharp & Dohme Limited. Summary of product characteristics, February 2002.
2. Committee on the Safety of Medicines/Medicines Control Agency. Non-steroidal anti-inflammatory drugs (NSAIDs) and gastrointestinal (GI) safety. Current Problems in Pharmacovigilance (2002) 28, 5.

Fenoprofen + Phenobarbital

Phenobarbital increases the loss of fenoprofen from the body.

Clinical evidence, mechanism, importance and management

Pretreatment with 15 or 60 mg **phenobarbital** 6-hourly for 10 days reduced the AUC of a single 200-mg dose of fenoprofen sodium in 6 healthy subjects by 23% and 37% respectively.[1] The clinical importance of this awaits further study.

1. Helleberg L, Rubin A, Wolen RL, Rodda BE, Ridolfo AS, Gruber CM. A pharmacokinetic interaction in man between phenobarbitone and fenoprofen, a new anti-inflammatory agent. Br J Clin Pharmacol (1974) 1, 371–4.

Fentanyl + Anticonvulsants

Patients on anticonvulsants appear to need more fentanyl than those not on anticonvulsants.

Clinical evidence, mechanism, importance and management

Twenty-eight patients, undergoing craniotomy for seizure focus excision and on long term treatment with **anticonvulsants** in various combinations, needed 48 to 144% more fentanyl during anaesthesia than a control group of 22 patients who were not on anticonvulsants. The fentanyl maintenance requirements in micrograms/kg/h were 2.7 (control group), 4 (patients on **carbamazepine**), 4.7 (patients on **carbamazepine** and **phenytoin** or **sodium valproate**), and 6.3 (patients on **carbamazepine**, **sodium valproate** and either **phenytoin** or **primidone**).[1] Similar results are reported by the same authors in a study involving 61 patients.[2]

The suggested reason is that these anticonvulsants are potent enzyme inducing agents (with the exception of **sodium valproate**) which increase the metabolism of fentanyl by the liver so that it is cleared from the body more quickly.[1] Changes in the state of opiate receptors induced by chronic anticonvulsant exposure may also be involved.[2] A marked increase in the fentanyl requirements should therefore be anticipated in any patient on long-term treatment with these interacting anticonvulsants, but not **sodium valproate**.

1. Tempelhoff R, Modica P, Spitznagel E. Increased fentanyl requirement in patients receiving long-term anticonvulsant therapy. Anesthesiology (1988) 69, A594.
2. Tempelhoff R, Modica PA, Spitznagel EL. Anticonvulsant therapy increases fentanyl requirements during anaesthesia for craniotomy. Can J Anaesth (1990) 37, 327–32.

Fentanyl + Baclofen

Fentanyl effects are increased by baclofen.

Clinical evidence, mechanism, importance and management

A study in three groups of 10 patients showed that pretreatment with 0.6 mg/kg **baclofen** intramuscularly in four doses for 5 days, or 0.6 mg/kg intravenously in 5% glucose in 100 ml 45 min before surgery, prolonged the duration of fentanyl anaesthesia from 18 to 30 min (fentanyl plus nitrous oxide in oxygen). The **baclofen** reduced the amounts of fentanyl needed by 30 to 40%.[1] The reasons are not known but a suggestion is that what happens is connected in some way with the action of baclofen on GABA receptors.[1] In practical terms this interaction means that **baclofen** can used to reduce the amount of fentanyl used for analgesia. It appears not to be an adverse interaction.

1. Panerai AE, Massei R, De Silva E, Sacerdote P, Monza G, Mantegazza P. Baclofen prolongs the analgesic effect of fentanyl in man. Br J Anaesth (1985) 57, 954–5.

Fentanyl + Benzodiazepines

Respiratory depression and hypotension can occur in adults if fentanyl is used in conjunction with diazepam or midazolam. This can occur in neonates if fentanyl is used with midazolam.

Clinical evidence

(a) Hypotension and respiratory depression in neonates

Hypotension occurred in 6 neonates with respiratory distress who were given **midazolam** (a bolus of 200 microgram/kg and/or 60 microgram/kg/h infusion) for sedation during the first 12 to 36 h of life. Five of them were also given fentanyl either as an infusion (1 to 2 microgram/kg/h) or a bolus (1.5 to 2.5 microgram/kg), or both.

Table 3.2 These figures represent the percentage of antirheumatic drug adsorbed per gram of adsorbent. The figures in brackets are the percentage eluted using either 0.01 N HCl (first figure) or 0.014 N NaHCO$_3$ (second figure)

	Magnesium trisilicate	Magnesium oxide	Aluminium hydroxide	Bismuth subcarbonate	Calcium carbonate	Kaolin
Flufenamic acid	0	90 (26.–)	10	79	37	44
Mefenamic acid	0	95 (40.–)	69	26	2	90
Oxyphenbutazone	0	24 (100.–)	27	0	0	0
Phenylbutazone	0	12 (100.100)	0	0	0	0

Blood pressures fell to values in the range 38/28 to 31/19 mmHg in 5 of them, and to less than 20 mmHg in one.[1] Another report describes respiratory arrest in a child of 14 months when given both drugs.[2]

(b) Hypotension and respiratory depression in adults

Midazolam alone (0.05 mg/kg) caused no episodes of apnoea or hypoxaemia in 12 healthy subjects, whereas fentanyl alone (2 microgram/kg) caused hypoxaemia in half (6/12) but no apnoea. When used together half (6/12) showed apnoea and most (11/12) showed hypoxaemia.[3]

Fentanyl plus **diazepam** caused more respiratory depression in 12 healthy subjects than either drug alone.[4] Hypotension has also been seen in adult patients given fentanyl with **midazolam**[5] or **diazepam**.[6]

Mechanism

Uncertain. The concomitant use of other CNS depressants may produce additive depressant effects.

Importance and management

Established interactions in neonates and adults. Significant cardiovascular and respiratory depression can occur in adults given either of these benzodiazepines with fentanyl or in neonates given midazolam with fentanyl. Concurrent use need not be totally avoided but be aware of what can happen.

1. Burtin P, Daoud P, Jacqz-Aigrain E, Mussat E, Moriette G. Hypotension with midazolam and fentanyl in the newborn. *Lancet* (1991) 337, 1545–6.
2. Yaster M, Nichols DG, Deshpande JK, Wetzel RC. Midazolam-fentanyl intravenous sedation in children: case report of respiratory arrest. *Pediatrics* (1991) 86, 463–6.
3. Bailey PL, Moll JWB, Pace NL, East KA, Stanley TH. Respiratory effects of midazolam and fentanyl: potent interaction producing hypoxemia and apnea. *Anesthesiology* (1988) 69, 3A, A813.
4. Bailey PL, Andriano KP, Pace NL, Westenskow DR, Stanley TH. Small doses of fentanyl potentiate and prolong diazepam induced respiratory depression. *Anesth Analg* (1984) 63, 183.
5. Heikkilä J, Jalonen J, Arola M, Kanto J, Laaksonen V. Midazolam as adjunct to high-dose fentanyl anaesthesia for coronary artery bypass grafting operation. *Acta Anaesthesiol Scand* (1984) 28, 683–89.
6. Tomicheck RC, Rosow CE, Philbin DM, Moss J, Teplick RS, Schneider RC. Diazepam-fentanyl interaction — hemodynamic and hormonal effects in coronary artery surgery. *Anesth Analg* (1983) 62, 881–4.

Fentanyl + Cimetidine

Some preliminary observations suggest that the effects of fentanyl may be increased by cimetidine.

Clinical evidence, mechanism, importance and management

The terminal half-life of fentanyl (100 microgram/kg) is reported to be more than doubled (from 155 to 340 min) by pretreatment with **cimetidine** (10 mg/kg the night before and 5 mg/kg 90 min before). The possible reason is that the **cimetidine** inhibits the metabolism of the fentanyl by the liver, thereby delaying its clearance from the body.[1] The clinical importance of this interaction has not been

assessed, but if both drugs are used concurrently, be alert for increased and prolonged fentanyl effects.

1. Unpublished data quoted by Maurer PM, Barkowski RR. Drug interactions of clinical significance with opioid analgesics. *Drug Safety* (1993) 8, 30–48.

Flufenamic, Mefenamic and Tolfenamic acids, Oxyphenbutazone or Phenylbutazone + Antacids

The absorption of the fenamates is markedly accelerated by magnesium hydroxide but retarded by aluminium hydroxide. Sodium bicarbonate appears not to interact, and *in vitro* studies suggest that oxyphenbutazone and phenylbutazone are little affected. See also 'Ibuprofen or Flurbiprofen + Antacids', p.57 and 'Indometacin (Indomethacin) + Antacids', p.58.

Clinical evidence

Studies in 6 healthy subjects given single 500-mg doses of **mefenamic acid** or 400 mg **tolfenamic acid** showed that **magnesium hydroxide** accelerated the absorption of both drugs (the **mefenamic acid** AUC after 1 h was increased threefold and of **tolfenamic acid** sevenfold) but the total bioavailability was only slightly increased. **Sodium bicarbonate** had no significant effect, but **aluminium hydroxide** markedly retarded the rate of absorption but no marked change in the total amount absorbed occurred.[1]

Table 3.2 summarises some *in vitro* adsorption and elution studies undertaken with a number of **antacids**, designed to mimic the conditions which occur as drugs are moved through the intestinal tract.[2]

Mechanisms

Partial or totally reversible adsorption can occur with some of these antacids. It is not understood why the absorption of both mefenamic and tolfenamic acids is increased by magnesium hydroxide.

Importance and management

Information is very limited but it would appear that if rapid analgesia is needed with either mefenamic or tolfenamic acid, magnesium hydroxide can be given concurrently but aluminium hydroxide should be avoided. Aluminium hydroxide markedly retards the speed of absorption but only reduces the total absorption by about 20%. Sodium bicarbonate does not interact. The data in the table suggest that flufenamic acid is possibly similarly affected but whether the other antacids listed interact significantly is not known. There appears to be little problem with oxyphenbutazone or phenylbutazone, however the full significance of the data in the table needs to be evaluated clinically. See also 'Ibuprofen or Flurbiprofen + Antacids', p.57 and 'Indometacin (Indomethacin) + Antacids', p.58.

1. Neuvonen PJ, Kivistö KT. Effect of magnesium hydroxide on the absorption of tolfenamic and mefenamic acids. *Eur J Clin Pharmacol* (1988) 35, 495–501.
2. Naggar VF, Khalil SA, Daabis NA. The in-vitro adsorption of some antirheumatics on antacids. *Pharmazie* (1976) 31, 461–5.

Flufenamic or Mefenamic acid + Colestyramine

The absorption of both flufenamic and mefenamic acid is markedly reduced in *animals* by the concurrent use of colestyramine, but the importance of this interaction in man is uncertain.

Clinical evidence, mechanism, importance and management

In vitro studies with physiological concentrations of bile salt anions have shown that **colestyramine** binds to both **flufenamic** and **mefenamic acid**, while reductions of 60 to 70% in the gastrointestinal absorption of both acids have been seen in the presence of **colestyramine** in *rats*.[1] The same interaction seems a possibility in man, but so far nobody appears to have carried out a clinical study.

1. Rosenberg HA, Bates TR. Inhibitory effect of cholestyramine on the absorption of flufenamic and mefenamic acids in rats. *Proc Soc Exp Biol Med* (1974) 145, 93–8.

Ibuprofen + Alcohol

Ibuprofen does not affect blood alcohol levels and aspirin appears only to have a very small damaging effect on the stomach wall when combined with alcohol. An isolated report describes acute renal failure in a young woman taking normal doses of ibuprofen when she drank a relatively large amount of rum.

Clinical evidence, mechanism, importance and management

Ibuprofen had no significant effect on blood **alcohol** levels of 19 and 12 healthy subjects,[1,2] and in a comparative study with aspirin, it was found to have only a small damaging effect on the stomach wall when combined with **alcohol**.[3] There would normally seem to be little reason for avoiding concurrent use.

After taking 400 mg ibuprofen the evening before, 400 mg the following morning, and then 375 ml of **rum** later in the day, followed by two further 400-mg tablets of ibuprofen, a normal healthy young woman with no history of renal disease developed acute renal failure.[4] The reason is not understood. One suggestion is that the **alcohol** may have made her normal kidneys susceptible to the effects of ibuprofen which, like other NSAIDs, can block the synthesis of the vasodilatory prostaglandins by the kidneys. As a result her kidneys became starved of their normal blood flow.[4] This is an isolated case and not of general importance.

1. Barron SE, Perry JR, Ferslew KE. The effect of ibuprofen on ethanol concentration and elimination rate. *J Forensic Sci* (1992) 37, 432–5.
2. Melander O, Lidén A, Melander A. Pharmacokinetic interactions of alcohol and acetylsalicylic acid. *Eur J Clin Pharmacol* (1995) 48, 151–3.
3. Lanza FL, Royer GL, Nelson RS, Rack MF, Seckman CC. Ethanol, aspirin, ibuprofen, and the gastroduodenal mucosa: an endoscopic assessment. *Am J Gastroenterol* (1985) 80, 767–9.
4. Elsasser GN, Lopez L, Evans E, Barone EJ. Reversible acute renal failure associated with ibuprofen ingestion and binge drinking. *J Fam Pract* (1988) 27, 221–2.

Ibuprofen or Flurbiprofen + Antacids

Magnesium hydroxide increases the initial absorption of ibuprofen and flurbiprofen, but not if aluminium hydroxide is also present. See also 'Flufenamic, Mefenamic and Tolfenamic acids, Oxyphenbutazone or Phenylbutazone + Antacids', p.56 and 'Indometacin (Indomethacin) + Antacids', p.58.

Clinical evidence, mechanism, importance and management

An antacid containing **aluminium and magnesium hydroxides**, given before, with and after a single 400-mg dose of **ibuprofen**, did not alter the **ibuprofen** pharmacokinetics in eight healthy subjects.[1] The absorption of **ibuprofen** formulated with **aluminium** is delayed and reduced compared to that with **ibuprofen** without aluminium.[2] Another study in 6 normal subjects found that 850 mg **magnesium hydroxide** increased the $AUC_{0-1 h}$ of a single 400-mg dose of **ibuprofen** by 65% and the peak concentration by 31%. The time to the peak was shortened by about half-an-hour. The total bioavailability was unchanged.[3]

30 ml *Maalox* (**aluminium and magnesium hydroxides**) taken 30 min before 100 mg **flurbiprofen** was found not to affect either the rate or extent of **flurbiprofen** absorption in a group of healthy subjects.[4] Another study found that **magnesium hydroxide** increased the $AUC_{0-2 h}$ by 61%, but over the $AUC_{0-8 h}$ was not changed.[5]

It would appear therefore that the initial absorption of both **ibuprofen** and **flurbiprofen** is increased by **magnesium hydroxide**, but not if **aluminium hydroxide** is present as well. Thus if rapid analgesia is needed, an antacid containing **magnesium hydroxide** but without **aluminium hydroxide** could be used. See also 'Flufenamic, Mefenamic and Tolfenamic acids, Oxyphenbutazone or Phenylbutazone + Antacids', p.56 and 'Indometacin (Indomethacin) + Antacids', p.58.

1. Gontarz N, Small RE, Comstock TJ, Stalker DJ, Johnson SM, Willis HE. Effect of antacid suspension on the pharmacokinetics of ibuprofen. *Clin Pharm* (1987) 6, 413–16.
2. Laska EM, Sunshine A, Marrero I, Olson N, Siegel C, McCormick N. The correlation between blood levels of ibuprofen and clinical analgesic response. *Clin Pharmacol Ther* (1986) 40, 1–7.
3. Neuvonen PJ. The effect of magnesium hydroxide on the oral absorption of ibuprofen, ketoprofen and diclofenac. *Br J Clin Pharmacol* (1991) 31, 263–6.
4. Caillé G, du Souich P, Vézina M, Pollock SR, Stalker DJ. Pharmacokinetic interaction between flurbiprofen and antacids in healthy volunteers. *Biopharm Drug Dispos* (1989) 10, 607–15.
5. Rao TRK, Ravisekhar K, Shobha JC, Sekhar EC, Naidu MUR, Krishna DR. Influence of magnesium hydroxide on the oral absorption of flurbiprofen. *Drug Invest* (1992) 4, 473–6.

Ibuprofen + Colestyramine or Colestipol

The absorption of ibuprofen from the gut is moderately reduced by colestyramine, but not by colestipol.

Clinical evidence

A three-phase crossover study in 6 healthy subjects found that 8 g **colestyramine** reduced the AUC of a single 400 mg oral dose of ibuprofen by 26% and reduced its maximum serum levels by 34%. The rate of absorption was also reduced. 10 g **colestipol** had no significant effect on the pharmacokinetics of ibuprofen.[1]

Mechanism

Colestyramine is an anion exchange resin which is intended to bind with bile acids, but which can also bind with drugs such as ibuprofen which are present in the gut so that its absorption is reduced.

Importance and management

The ibuprofen/colestyramine interaction is established, but its clinical importance is uncertain, but probably small. The reductions seen are only very moderate. A simple way to reduce this interaction would be to give the drugs separately, to minimise their admixture in the gut. More study is needed.

1. Al-Meshal MA, El-Sayed YM, Al-Balla SR, Gouda MW. The effect of colestipol and cholestyramine on ibuprofen bioavailability in man. *Biopharm Drug Dispos* (1994) 15, 463–71.

Indometacin (Indomethacin) + Allopurinol

Allopurinol does not affect serum indometacin levels.

Clinical evidence, mechanism, importance and management

Eight patients were treated for 5 days with 300 mg **allopurinol** each morning and 50 mg indometacin (indomethacin) eight-hourly. The **allopurinol** had no significant effect on the AUC of indometacin and the amounts of indometacin excreted in the urine were not significantly altered.[1,2] There seems to be no reason for avoiding concurrent use.

1. Pullar T, Myall O, Dixon JS, Haigh JRM, Lowe JR, Bird HA. Allopurinol has no effect on steady-state concentrations of indometacin. *Br J Clin Pharmacol* (1988) 25, 672P.

2. Pullar T, Myall O, Haigh JRM, Lowe JR, Dixon JS, Bird HA. The effect of allopurinol on the steady-state pharmacokinetics of indometacin. *Br J Clin Pharmacol* (1988) 25, 755–7.

Indometacin (Indomethacin) + Antacids

The irritation of the gut caused by indometacin can be relieved by the concurrent use of antacids, but serum indometacin levels may be reduced to some extent as a result. This appears not to be clinically important. See also 'Flufenamic, Mefenamic and Tolfenamic acids, Oxyphenbutazone or Phenylbutazone + Antacids', p.56 and 'Ibuprofen or Flurbiprofen + Antacids', p.57

Clinical evidence

The absorption of a single 50-mg dose of indometacin (indomethacin) in 12 healthy subjects was reduced by 35% when taken with 80% *Mergel* (an antacid formulation of **aluminium hydroxide, magnesium carbonate and hydroxide**).[1]

In another study in normal subjects 700 mg **aluminium hydroxide** suspension caused a marked fall in peak indometacin serum levels,[2] whereas in yet another study 30 ml **magnesium-aluminium hydroxide** caused only slight changes in the absorption of a 50-mg dose of indometacin.[3]

Mechanism

In vitro studies have shown that indometacin can be adsorbed by various antacids (magnesium trisilicate, magnesium oxide, magnesium hydroxide, bismuth oxycarbonate, calcium carbonate).[4] This may explain some of the reduction in gastrointestinal absorption, but other mechanisms may also be involved.

Importance and management

Adequately but not extensively documented. Some reduction in serum levels is possible. Despite this the makers of indometacin recommend that it is taken with food, milk or an antacid to minimise gastrointestinal disturbances. Check that the indometacin remains effective.

See also 'Flufenamic, Mefenamic and Tolfenamic acids, Oxyphenbutazone or Phenylbutazone + Antacids', p.56 and 'Ibuprofen or Flurbiprofen + Antacids', p.57

1. Galeazzi RL. The effect of an antacid on the bioavailability of indometacin. *Eur J Clin Pharmacol* (1977) 12, 65–8.

2. Garnham JC, Kaspi T, Kaye CM and Oh VMS. The different effects of sodium bicarbonate and aluminium hydroxide on the absorption of indometacin in man. *Postgrad Med J* (1977) 53, 126–9.

3. Emori HW, Paulus H, Bluestone R, Champion GD, Pearson C. Indomethacin serum concentrations in man. Effects of dosage, food and antacid. *Ann Rheum Dis* (1976) 35, 333–8.

4. Naggar VF, Khalil SA, Daabis NA. The in-vitro adsorption of some antirheumatics on antacids. *Pharmazie* (1976) 31, 461–5.

Indometacin (Indomethacin) + Cimetidine or Ranitidine

Cimetidine can cause a small reduction in the plasma levels of indometacin but its anti-inflammatory effects do not seem to be significantly altered.

Clinical evidence, mechanism, importance and management

Ten patients with rheumatoid arthritis on 100 to 200 mg indometacin (indomethacin) daily for over a year were additionally given 1 g **cimetidine** daily for a 2 weeks. Their plasma indometacin levels fell by an average of 18% (from 1.64 to 1.34 nanograms/ml) but there was no significant change in the clinical effectiveness of the anti-inflammatory treatment (as measured by articular index, pain, grip strength and ESR). The fall in indometacin levels is thought to be due to some alteration in the absorption from the gut.[1] Another study found no changes in the pharmacokinetics of indometacin in healthy subjects given **ranitidine**.[2] No marked changes in the bioavailability of either **cimetidine** or **ranitidine** with indometacin was seen in a single dose study of both drugs in healthy subjects.[3]

No special precautions would therefore seem to be necessary during concurrent use of indometacin and either of these H2-blockers.

1. Howes CA, Pullar T, Sourindhrin I, Mistra PC, Capel H, Lawson DH, Tilstone WJ. Reduced steady-state plasma concentrations of chlorpromazine and indometacin in patients receiving cimetidine. *Eur J Clin Pharmacol* (1983) 24, 99–102.

2. Kendall MJ, Gibson R, Walt RP. Co-administration of misoprostol or ranitidine with indomethacin: effects on pharmacokinetics, abdominal symptoms and bowel habit. *Aliment Pharmacol Ther* (1992) 6, 437–46.

3. Delhotal-Landes B, Flouvat B, Liote F, Abel L, Meyer P, Vinceneux P, Carbon C. Pharmacokinetic interactions between NSAIDs (indomethacin or sulindac) and H2-receptor antagonists (cimetidine or ranitidine) in human volunteers. *Clin Pharmacol Ther* (1988) 44, 442–52.

Indometacin (Indomethacin) + Cocaine

An isolated report describes marked oedema, anuria and haematemesis in a premature child attributed to an interaction between the cocaine and indometacin taken earlier by the mother before the birth.

Clinical evidence, mechanism, importance and management

A woman in premature labour was unsuccessfully treated with terbutaline and magnesium sulphate. Indometacin proved to be more effective, but after being given 400 mg over 2 days she gave birth to a boy estimated at 34 to 35 weeks. Before birth the child was noted to be anuric and at birth showed marked oedema, and later haematemesis. The suggested reasons are that the anuria and oedema were due to renal vascular constriction of the foetus caused by the **cocaine** (the mother had been abusing cocaine), combined with some interference by the indometacin with ADH-mediated water reabsorption. Both drugs can cause gastrointestinal bleeding which would account for the haematemesis. The authors of this report point out that one of the side-effects of **cocaine** is premature labour, and that the likelihood is high that indometacin may be used to control it. They advise screening likely addicts in premature labour for evidence of **cocaine** usage before indometacin is given.[1]

1. Carlan SJ, Stromquist C, Angel JL, Harris M, O'Brien WF. Cocaine and indomethacin: fetal anuria, neonatal edema and gastrointestinal bleeding. *Obstet Gynecol* (1991) 78, 501–3.

Indometacin (Indomethacin) + Probenecid

Serum indometacin levels can be doubled by the concurrent use of probenecid. This can result in clinical improvement in patients with arthritic diseases, but indometacin toxicity may also occur, particularly in those whose kidney function is impaired. The uricosuric effects of probenecid are not affected.

Clinical evidence

A study on 28 patients with osteoarthritis, taking 50 to 150 mg indometacin (indomethacin) daily by mouth or rectally, showed that 0.5 to 1 g **probenecid** daily roughly doubled their indometacin plasma levels and this paralleled the increased effectiveness (relief of morning stiffness, joint tenderness and raised grip strength indices). But 4 patients demonstrated indometacin toxicity.[1]

Other studies have also demonstrated the marked rise in plasma indometacin levels caused by **probenecid**.[2-4] Clear signs of indometacin toxicity (nausea, headache, tinnitus, confusion and a rise in blood urea) occurred in a woman with stable mild renal impairment when given **probenecid**.[5] The uricosuric effects of **probenecid** are not altered.[2]

Mechanism

Uncertain. It seems possible that the indometacin and probenecid compete for the same kidney tubule secretory mechanisms, which leads to a decrease in the loss of the indometacin.[2] There may also be some reduction in biliary excretion of indometacin as well.[6]

Importance and management

An established and adequately documented interaction. Concurrent use should be well monitored because, while clinical improvement can undoubtedly occur, some patients may develop indometacin toxicity (headache, dizziness, light-headedness, nausea, etc.). This is particularly likely in those with some impaired kidney function. Reduce the indometacin dosage as necessary.

1. Brooks PM, Bell MA, Sturrock RD, Famaey JP, Dick WC. The clinical significance of indomethacin-probenecid interaction. *Br J Clin Pharmacol* (1974) 1, 287–90.
2. Skeith MD, Simkin PA, Healey LA. The renal excretion of indomethacin and its inhibition by probenecid. *Clin Pharmacol Ther* (1968) 9, 89–93.
3. Emori W, Paulus HE, Bluestone R, Pearson CM. The pharmacokinetics of indomethacin in serum. *Clin Pharmacol Ther* (1973) 14, 134.
4. Baber N, Halliday L, Littler T, Orme ML'E, Sibeon R. Clinical studies of the interaction between indomethacin and probenecid. *Br J Clin Pharmacol* (1978) 5, 364P.
5. Sinclair H, Gibson T. Interaction between probenecid and indomethacin. *Br J Rheumatol* (1986) 25, 316–17.
6. Duggan DE, Hooke KF, White SD, Noll RM, Stevenson CR. The effects of probenecid upon the individual components of indomethacin elimination. *J Pharmacol Exp Ther* (1977) 201, 463.

Indometacin (Indomethacin) + Vaccines

Some very limited evidence suggests that the response of the body to immunisation with live vaccines may be more severe than usual in the presence of indometacin.

Clinical evidence

A man with ankylosing spondylitis on 25 mg indometacin (indomethacin) three times a day had a strong primary type reaction 12 days after **smallpox vaccination**. He experienced 3 days of severe malaise, headache and nausea, as well as enlarged lymph nodes. The scab that formed was unusually large (3 cm diameter) but he suffered no long term ill-effects.[1]

Mechanism

Uncertain. The suggestion is that the indometacin alters the response of the body to viral infections, whether originating from vaccines or not.[1] For example, a child taking indometacin who developed haem-

orrhagic chickenpox during a ward outbreak of the disease suffered severe scarring.[2] The makers of indometacin state that indometacin may mask the signs and symptoms of infection.

Importance and management

Information is very sparse and the interaction is not adequately established, but be aware that a more severe reaction may possibly occur if live vaccines (e.g. rubella, measles, etc.) are used in patients using indometacin.

1. Maddocks AC. Indomethacin and vaccination. *Lancet* (1973) ii, 210–11.
2. Rodriguez RS, Barbabosa E. Hemorrhagic chickenpox after indomethacin. *N Engl J Med* (1971) 285, 690.

Isoxicam + Miscellaneous drugs

Aspirin may possibly cause changes in the plasma levels of isoxicam but the importance of this is uncertain. Blood loss is increased. Isoxicam is reported not to be affected by phenytoin.

Clinical evidence, mechanism, importance and management

Isoxicam 200 to 300 mg once daily and **aspirin** 600 mg three times daily for 14 days in healthy subjects was found to cause small rises in the plasma levels of both drugs. Gastrointestinal blood loss was significantly increased.[1] In contrast another study found that **aspirin** 1.95 g twice daily approximately halved the plasma levels of isoxicam 200 mg daily.[2] Reduced plasma **isoxicam** levels were seen in another study.[3] Whether any of these changes has any important effect on the clinical efficacy of isoxicam is uncertain but the possible increase in gastrointestinal blood loss should not be overlooked.

Another study found that **phenytoin** does not change the pharmacokinetics of isoxicam.[4]

1. Farnham DJ. Studies of isoxicam in combination with aspirin, warfarin sodium and cimetidine. *Sem Arthritis Rheum* (1982) 12 (Suppl 2), 179–183.
2. Grace EM, Mewa AAM, Sweeney GD, Rosenfeld JM, Darke AC, Buchanan WW. Lowering of plasma isoxicam concentrations with acetylsalicylic acid. *J Rheumatol* (1986) 13, 1119–21.
3. Esquivel M, Cussenot F, Ogilvie RI, East DS, Shaw DH. Interaction of isoxicam with acetylsalicylic acid. *Br J Clin Pharmacol* (1984) 18, 567–71.
4. Caille A. The effect of administration of phenytoin on the pharmacokinetics of isoxicam. In preparation. Quoted by Downie WW, Gluckman MI, Ziehmer BA, Boyle JA. *Clin Rheum Dis* (1984) 10, 385–99.

Ketoprofen + Metoclopramide

Metoclopramide reduces the bioavailability of ketoprofen.

Clinical evidence, mechanism, importance and management

Four healthy subjects given 50 mg ketoprofen in capsule form (*Profenid*) showed reductions in their AUCs when concurrently given 10 mg **metoclopramide**. The AUC was reduced by about 28%. The maximum plasma levels were almost halved and the time to reach this maximum was prolonged by 30%.[1] The probable reason is that the **metoclopramide** speeds up the gastric emptying so that the relatively poorly soluble ketoprofen spends less time in the stomach where it dissolves. As a result less is available for absorption in the small intestine.

The clinical importance of this interaction awaits assessment but the authors of this study recommend that ketoprofen (and possibly other NSAIDs which are poorly soluble) should be taken 1 to 2 h before the **metoclopramide**.

1. Etman MA, Ismail FA, Nada AH. Effect of metoclopramide on ketoprofen pharmacokinetics in man. *Int J Pharmaceutics* (1992) 88, 433–5.

Ketorolac + Miscellaneous drugs

Ketorolac is contraindicated with anti-asthmatic and anti-ulcer drugs, NSAIDs and pentoxifylline (oxpentifylline). An isolated report describes temporary acute kidney failure and gastrointestinal bleeding following ketorolac and vancomycin.

Clinical evidence, mechanism, importance and management

The makers and the CSM in the UK say that ketorolac is contraindicated in patients with a history of peptic ulcer or gastrointestinal bleeding because of the risk of serious gastrointestinal bleeding, and also in patients with a history of asthma because of the risk of bronchospasm. This means that ketorolac should not normally be given to patients on **anti-ulcer drugs** or **anti-asthmatics**. The makers also say that ketorolac is contraindicated with other **NSAIDs** because of the risk of serious bleeding and additive side-effects (see Index for other NSAID + NSAID interactions). An increased risk of bleeding is also said to exist with **pentoxifylline (oxpentifylline)** so that this drug combination should be also be avoided.[1-3]

A previously healthy middle-aged man developed complete kidney shut down and subsequent gastrointestinal bleeding following uncomplicated surgery when treated with ketorolac trometamol and **vancomycin**. The reason for the temporary kidney failure is not known, but the authors of the report suggest that the ketorolac inhibited the normal production of the vasodilatory renal prostaglandins so that renal blood flow was reduced. This would seem to have been additive with nephrotoxic effects of the **vancomycin**.[4] Ketorolac alone can cause dose-related and transient renal dysfunction.[4] It has also been suggested that the trometamol component may be associated with hyperkalaemia.[5] The gastrointestinal bleeding appeared to be due to the direct irritant effects of the ketorolac, possibly made worse by the previous use of **piroxicam**.[4] The general importance of this interaction is uncertain.

1. *Committee on Safety of Medicines. Current Problems in Pharmacovigilance* (1993) 19, 5–6.
2. Toradol (Ketorolac trometamol) Roche Products Limited. Summary of Product Characteristics, October 2000.
3. Syntex Pharmaceuticals Limited. Personal communication, January 1995.
4. Murray RP, Watson RC. Acute renal failure and gastrointestinal bleed associated with postoperative Toradol and vancomycin. *Orthopedics* (1993) 16, 1361–3.
5. Waters JH. Ketorolac-induced hyperkalaemia. *Am J Kidney Dis* (1995) 26, 266.

Leflunomide + Miscellaneous drugs

The serum levels of the active metabolite of leflunomide are reduced by activated charcoal or colestyramine. The makers advise the avoidance of the concurrent use of alcohol, other DMARDs, or live vaccines, and they also advise caution with phenytoin, tolbutamide and warfarin (a single case of raised INR has been seen). No clinically relevant interaction occurs with cimetidine, corticosteroids, NSAIDs, oral contraceptives or rifampicin.

(a) Alcohol

The makers say that because of the potential for additive hepatotoxic effects, it is recommended that **alcohol** should be avoided while taking leflunomide.[1]

(b) Cimetidine

A crossover trial in 12 healthy subjects found that the serum levels of the active metabolite of leflunomide (A771726) were similar, with or without pretreatment with 300 mg **cimetidine** four times daily for 6 days.[1,2] No special precautions would therefore seem to be needed if both drugs are used.

(c) Colestyramine, Activated charcoal,

Studies in healthy subjects found that 8 g **colestyramine** three times daily reduced the serum levels of the active metabolite of leflunomide (A771726) by 48% after 24 h and by 49–65% after 48 h. Treatment with 50 mg **activated charcoal** 6-hourly for 24 h, either orally or by nasogastric tube, reduced A771726 levels by 37% after 24 h and by 48% after 48 h. The reason is believed to be that these drugs bind with the A771726 in the gut, thereby interrupting the enterohepatic cycle or possibly its gastrointestinal dialysis.[1,3] Patients should therefore not be given either **colestyramine** or **activated charcoal** and leflunomide concurrently, unless the intention is to remove the leflunomide, for example following overdosage or when there is any other good reason to clear leflunomide from the body more quickly.[1,3]

(d) Contraceptives, oral

Leflunomide 100 mg daily was given to 32 premenopausal women on a **triphasic oral contraceptive** containing 30 micrograms **ethinylestradiol** (*Triphasil*) on days 1 to 3 of the cycle and then leflunomide 20 mg daily was given for the next 17 days were additionally given. During the trial which extended over about 12 weeks it was found that the leflunomide had no effect on the pharmacokinetics or the activity of the **oral contraceptive** and the pharmacokinetics of the active metabolite of leflunomide (A771726) were not changed to a clinically relevant extent.[1,2] No special precautions would therefore appear to be needed.

(e) DMARDs (Disease modifying antirheumatic drugs) other than methotrexate

The makers say that the concurrent use of leflunomide and other DMARDs (they list **azathioprine, chloroquine, hydroxychloroquine**, intramuscular or oral **gold** and **penicillamine**) has not yet been studied but they say that combined use is currently not advisable.[1]

(f) Methotrexate

No pharmacokinetic interaction was seen in patients while taking **methotrexate** (mean dose 17.2 mg per week) to which was added leflunomide 100 mg daily for 2 days as a loading dose followed by 10 to 20 mg daily.[4] However elevated liver enzyme levels have been seen following concurrent use. Because of the possible risks of additive or supra-additive liver toxicity or haematotoxicity, particularly when used long-term, the makers say that the concurrent use of **methotrexate** is not advisable.[1] They recommend close liver enzyme monitoring if switching between these drugs.[1]

(g) Non-steroidal anti-inflammatory drugs (NSAIDs), Corticosteroids

Leflunomide inhibits the activity of cytochrome P450 isoenzyme CYP3A4 *in vitro* and might therefore be expected to increase the serum levels of **NSAIDs** which are metabolised by this isoenzyme (e.g. **diclofenac, ibuprofen**) but the makers say that no safety problems were seem in clinical trials with leflunomide and **NSAIDs**. No special precautions would seem to be needed if any of these or any other **NSAID** drugs are given concurrently.[1] The makers also say that **corticosteroids** may continue to be used if leflunomide is given.[1]

(h) Phenytoin, Tolbutamide, Warfarin

The makers advise caution if leflunomide is given together with **phenytoin, tolbutamide** or **warfarin**.[1] The reason is that the active metabolite of leflunomide (A771726) has been shown by *in vitro* studies to be an inhibitor of cytochrome P450 isoenzyme CYP2C9 which is concerned with the metabolism of these three drugs. If this inhibition were to occur *in vivo* it could possibly lead to a decrease in their metabolism and an increase in their toxicity.

So far there has only been a single case report involving a woman whose INR more than doubled within a few days of adding leflunomide to **warfarin**.[5] To be on the safe side it would therefore now be prudent to be alert for evidence of unexplained bruising or bleeding (or raised INR) if added to **warfarin**, increased side-effects if added to **phenytoin**, or of hypoglycaemia if added to **tolbutamide**.

(i) Rifampicin

A crossover study in normal subjects found that after taking 600 mg **rifampicin** daily for 8 days the serum levels of the active metabolite of leflunomide (A771726) were increased by 40% (from 8.2 to

11.4 mg/l) but the AUC was unchanged.[1,2] The reasons are not understood. There would seem to be no reason for avoiding concurrent use.

(j) Vaccines

The makers say that there is no clinical data about the safety of vaccination with **live attenuated vaccines**, but it is not recommended.[1]

1. Arava (Leflunomide), Aventis Pharma Ltd. Summary of product characteristics, March 2002.
2. Hoechst Marion Roussel (Kansas City). Arava – Drug Interactions. Data on file, 1998.
3. Hoechst Marion Roussel (Kansas City). Arava-washout with cholestyramine and activated charcoal. Data on file, 1998.
4. Weinblatt ME, Kremer JM, Coblyn JS, Maier AL, Helfgott SM, Morrell M, Byrne VM, Kaymakcian MV, Strand V. Pharmacokinetics, safety, and efficacy of combination treatment with methotrexate and leflunomide in patients with active rheumatoid arthritis. *Arthritis Rheum* (1999) 42, 1322–8.
5. Mason JP. Warfarin and leflunomide. *Pharm J* (2000) 265, 267.

Levacetylmethadol + Miscellaneous drugs

Direct interaction studies with levacetylmethadol appear to be lacking, but for theoretical reasons the makers contraindicate the concurrent use of MAOIs or drugs which prolong the QT interval. They warn about the possible effects of inducers or inhibitors of cytochrome P450 isoenzyme CYP3A4 which may increase or reduce its activity, the additive effects of alcohol or other CNS depressants, and the possible risk of oral contraceptive failure. They also advise the avoidance of pethidine (meperidine), dextropropoxyphene (propoxyphene) or naloxone (except when used for overdosage).

Clinical evidence, mechanisms and management

No interaction studies in man appear to have been carried out with levacetylmethadol, but on the basis of *in vitro* and other studies and for theoretical reasons the makers have issued a number of interaction warnings in their product literature as follows:

(a) Alcohol or other CNS depressants

The makers point out that levacetylmethadol can cause drowsiness so that there is the risk of marked drowsiness if taken with **alcohol** or other **CNS depressants**. They warn that since the peak activity of levacetylmethadol is not immediate there is a risk of fatal overdosage if combined with other CNS depressants, especially with the first few doses.[1]

(b) Drugs which prolong the QT interval

The makers have on record 5 cases of torsade de pointes (causing syncope and 3 cases of cardiac arrest) due to levacetylmethadol from an estimated 10,000 patient exposures.[2] There is also another case on record of a patient also taking fluoxetine and intravenous cocaine who developed torsade de pointes.[2] For this reason the makers contraindicate the concurrent use of a whole range of drugs which similarly cause QT prolongation because of the risk that these adverse effects may be additive. The drug groups they name are as follows: **Class I** or **Class III antiarrhythmic agents**. This would therefore include **quinidine, procainamide, disopyramide, tiracizine, mexiletine, tocainide, diprafenone, encainide, flecainide** and **propafenone** in Class I, and **amiodarone, bretylium, dofetilide, ibutilide** and **sotalol** in Class III. The makers also name the following: antihistamines (**astemizole** and **terfenadine**), antimalarials (**chloroquine, halofantrine, quinine**), some calcium channel blockers (**bepridil, lidoflazine, prenylamine, terodiline**), antipsychotics (**chlorpromazine, haloperidol, pimozide, sertindole, sultopride, thioridazine**), antidepressants (**amitriptyline, doxepin, imipramine, maprotiline**) and other medicinal products (**cisapride,** intravenous **erythromycin, ketanserin,** intravenous **pentamidine, sparfloxacin, spiramycin**). The makers similarly contraindicate drugs known to induce hypokalaemia or hypomagnesaemia which may prolong the QT interval and they list **diuretics** and **laxatives** (none named) and the supraphysiological use of mineralocorticoids such as systemic **fludrocortisone**.[1] All of these drugs should therefore be avoided for reasons of safety.

(c) Enzyme inducing and inhibiting drugs

Levacetylmethadol acts like a pro-drug which needs to be metabolised within the body to its long-acting and active metabolites. The primary enzyme invloved in the conversion (to nor- and dinor-acetylmethadol) is cytochrome P450 isoenzyme CYP3A4, which is found in the gut and liver.[3] Thus the first-pass metabolism of levacetylmethadol does not decrease its effectiveness, unlike most first-pass effects, but increases it. Therefore drugs which increase the activity of CYP3A4 (i.e. enzyme inducers) would be expected to produce increased amounts of metabolites thereby increasing their activity and/or shortening their duration of action. Typical inducers of CYP3A4 activity which are named by the makers are **rifampicin, phenobarbital, phenytoin** and **carbamazepine**. On the other hand enzyme inhibitors are predicted to slow the onset, lower the activity and/or increase the duration of action. Typical inhibitors of CYP3A4 are **erythromycin, cimetidine, ketoconazole, itraconazole, ritonavir, indinavir** and **ciclosporin**.[1] Studies with human liver microsomes confirm that **ketoconazole** can interact with levacetylmethadol *in vitro*.[3] It needs however to be emphasised that although the makers list these as potentially interacting drugs in their product literature, they point out that the outcome of concurrent use is unpredictable.[1] At the moment there is no clinical confirmation that any clinically relevant interactions actually occur with these drugs, but for safety you should monitor the concurrent use of any of them (or any others which are potent CYP3A4 inducers or inhibitors), being alert for the need to adjust the levacetylmethadol dosage if necessary.

(d) Monoamine Oxidase inhibitors (MAOIs)

The makers contraindicate levacetylmethadol with **MAOIs**[1] but there appears to be no direct evidence as yet that any interaction actually occurs. This appears to be a 'blanket' warning which many drug manufacturers issue in the absence of any direct information, simply to be on the safe side.

(e) Opioid agonists or agonists/antagonists

The makers say that ". . . agonists such as **meperidine** (**pethidine**) and **dextropropoxyphene** (**propoxyphene**) which are *N*-demethylated to long-acting excitatory metabolites should not be used with levacetylmethadol because they would be ineffective unless given in such high doses that the risk of toxic effects of the metabolites would become unacceptable." They also say that the concurrent use of **naloxone** is contraindicated except for the treatment of overdosage.[1]

(f) Oral contraceptives

The makers say that the effectiveness of **oral contraceptives** during levacetylmethadol treatment has not been established, but they recommend that an alternative method of contraception – e.g. a barrier method – should be also be used.[1] It is not clear why this recommendation is made because there appear to be no reports of contraceptive failures nor obvious theoretical reasons for thinking that failure might occur.

1. OrLAAM (Levacetylmethadol), Prescribing Information, Britannia Pharmaceuticals UK, January 2000.
2. Deamer RL, Wilson DR, Clark DS, Prichard JG. Torsades de pointes associated with high dose levomethadyl acetate (ORLAAM). *J Addict Dis* (2001) 20, 7–15.
3. Moody DE, Alburges ME, Parker RJ, Collins JM, Strong JM. The involvement of cytochrome P450 3A4 in the *N*-demethylation of l-α-acetylmethadol (LAAM), norLaam and methadone. *Drug Metab Dispos* (1997) 25, 1347–53.

Lornoxicam + Antacids

Lornoxicam (chlortenoxicam) does not interact adversely with tripotassium dicitratobismuthate, Maalox or Solugastril.

Clinical evidence, mechanism, importance and management

Neither 10 ml *Maalox* (**aluminium and magnesium hydroxides**) nor 10 g *Solugastril* (**aluminium hydroxide and calcium carbonate**) had any effect on the pharmacokinetic profile of lornoxicam in

18 healthy subjects when given as a 4 mg film-coated tablet.[1] A later study similarly found no changes in the absorption or pharmacokinetics of the same lornoxicam formulation when given with 120 mg **bismuth chelate** twice daily.[2] There would seem to be no reason for avoiding concurrent use.

1. Dittrich P, Radhofer-Welte S, Magometschnigg D, Kukovetz WR, Mayerhofer S, Ferber HP. The effect of concomitantly administered antacids on the bioavailability of lornoxicam, a novel highly potent NSAID. *Drugs Exp Clin Res* (1990) 16, 57–62.
2. Ravic M, Johnston A, Turner P, Foley K, Rosenow D. Does bismuth chelate influence lornoxicam absorption? *Hum Exp Toxicol* (1992) 11, 59–60.

Lornoxicam + H$_2$-blockers

Cimetidine, but not usually ranitidine, causes a small rise in serum lornoxicam (chlortenoxicam) levels. However, a marked increase in serum lornoxicam levels has been seen in one patient taking ranitidine.

Clinical evidence, mechanism, importance and management

Cimetidine 400 mg twice daily increased the maximum serum levels of lornoxicam (8 mg twice daily) and its AUC by 28% and 9% respectively in 12 healthy subjects. The reason is thought to be that the **cimetidine** inhibits the metabolism (hydroxylation) of the lornoxicam by the liver, thereby allowing it to accumulate. **Ranitidine** 150 mg twice daily had no significant effect on the lornoxicam pharmacokinetics, except that one subject showed a very marked increase in serum lornoxicam levels while taking both drugs. It is not clear what part, if any, the **ranitidine** had to play. He dropped out of the trial after 6 days because of severe gastric irritation.[1]

The increases caused by **cimetidine** are small and unlikely to be of clinical importance, and no interaction normally occurs with **ranitidine**. However the marked changes seen in one of the subjects highlights the importance of checking the response in anyone when first given lornoxicam with or without either of these H$_2$-blockers.

1. Ravic M, Salas-Herrera I, Johnston A, Turner P, Foley K, Rosenow DE. A pharmacokinetic interaction between cimetidine or ranitidine and lornoxicam. *Postgrad Med J* (1993) 69, 865–66.

Lornoxicam + Miscellaneous drugs

Lornoxicam (chlortenoxicam) causes a small increase in the effects of glibenclamide (glyburide) and in the serum levels of digoxin but neither is probably clinically important.

Clinical evidence, mechanism, importance and management

(a) Digoxin

The concurrent use of 4 mg lornoxicam twice daily (taken for 14 days) and 0.25 mg **digoxin** daily (taken for 24 days) in 12 healthy subjects had only a small effect on the pharmacokinetics of each drug. The apparent clearance of the **digoxin** was decreased by 14% while the maximum serum level of the lornoxicam was decreased by 21% and its elimination half-life increased by 36%.[1] None of these changes is probably clinically important, but until more is known it would seem prudent to monitor the effects if these two drugs are given to patients.

(b) Glibenclamide (glyburide)

Lornoxicam 4 mg twice daily for 6 days had no effect on the pharmacokinetics of a single 5-mg dose of **glibenclamide (glyburide)** in 15 healthy subjects. The pharmacokinetics of lornoxicam also remained unchanged. However concurrent use significantly increased plasma insulin levels (AUC 47%) and lowered serum glucose levels (8%), the suggested reason being that the lornoxicam displaces the **glibenclamide (glyburide)** from its plasma protein binding sites so that its unbound (and active) levels rise, thereby increasing the secretion of

insulin. However the changes seen are believed to be too small to be clinically relevant.[1] This needs confirmation in diabetic patients.

1. Warrington SJ, Debbas NMG, Turner P, Ravic M. Chlortenoxicam and glibenclamide in normal subjects: interaction study. Charterhouse Clinical Research Unit. Internal study (1989). Unpublished data. Quoted by Ravic M, Johnston A, Turner P. Clinical pharmacological studies of some possible interactions of lornoxicam with other drugs. *Postgrad Med J* (1990) 66 (Suppl 4), S30–S34.

Meclofenamic acid + Miscellaneous drugs

Aspirin can cause a small and probably clinically unimportant reduction in plasma meclofenamate levels, but intestinal bleeding is increased. Dextropropoxyphene (propoxyphene) and meclofenamate do not interact.

Clinical evidence, mechanism, importance and management

Twenty healthy subjects given 600 mg **aspirin** and 100 mg sodium meclofenamate both three times daily for 14 days showed no significant reductions in plasma salicylate levels, but plasma meclofenamate levels were depressed to some extent. The clinical significance of this is uncertain, but it is probably limited. The gastrointestinal blood loss was approximately doubled compared with either drug alone.[1] The concurrent use of 260 mg **dextropropoxyphene (propoxyphene)** daily and 400 mg sodium meclofenamate daily was found to have no effect on the plasma levels of either drug.[1]

1. Baragar FD, Smith TC. Drug interaction studies with sodium meclofenamate (Meclomen®). *Curr Ther Res* (1978) 23 (April Suppl), S51–S59.

Meloxicam + Miscellaneous drugs

Meloxicam does not interact with cimetidine or *Maalox*, and only a small clinically irrelevant interaction appears to occur with aspirin.

Clinical evidence, mechanism, importance and management

In an open, randomised, crossover study a group of 9 healthy subjects was given 30 mg meloxicam alone, or with 1 g **aspirin** three times daily for 4 days, or with 200 mg **cimetidine** four times daily for 5 days. Another group was similarly given 30 mg meloxicam alone or with *Maalox* suspension (600 mg **magnesium hydroxide**, 900 mg **aluminium hydroxide**) four times daily for 4 days. The **aspirin** increased the maximum plasma levels of the meloxicam by 25% and its AUC by 10%, but neither **cimetidine** nor *Maalox* had a significant effect on the pharmacokinetics of the meloxicam. The small interaction with aspirin was not considered by the authors of the study to be clinically relevant, and they concluded that no adjustments of the dosage of meloxicam are needed if given with **aspirin**, **cimetidine** or *Maalox*.[1]

1. Busch U, Heinzel G, Narjes H, Nehmiz G. Interaction of meloxicam with cimetidine, Maalox or aspirin. *J Clin Pharmacol* (1996) 36, 79–84.

Metamizole sodium (Dipyrone) + Miscellaneous drugs

Metamizole sodium (dipyrone) appears not to interact with alcohol, aluminium hydroxide-magnesium hydroxide gel or

glibenclamide (glyburide), but the pharmacokinetics of rifampicin (rifampin) are changed to some extent.

Clinical evidence, mechanism, importance and management

Metamizole sodium (dipyrone) is often considered an unsafe drug because, like the related aminophenazone (amidopyrine), it can cause potentially fatal agranulocytosis. For this reason it is banned in several countries and it has been stated that it should be considered unsuitable for use.[1] However an international comparative study of the risks of agranulocytosis with various NSAIDs found the following, expressed in cases of agranulocytosis per million users in one treatment week: metamizole sodium (1.1), butazones (0.2), salicylates (0.06), indometacin (0.4).[2]

The following interaction studies have been carried out:

(a) Alcohol

The pharmacokinetics of **alcohol** (1 g/kg) and the results of performance tests were found to be similar in subjects given 1 g metamizole sodium (dipyrone) or a placebo.[3] No special precautions seem to be necessary.

(b) Antacids

The concurrent use of 20 ml *Maaloxan* (**aluminium hydroxide/magnesium hydroxide** gel) is reported to have had no effect on the pharmacokinetics of metabolites of metamizole sodium (dipyrone).[4] No special precautions seem to be necessary.

(c) Glibenclamide (glyburide)

Six non-insulin dependent diabetics taking **glibenclamide (glyburide)** showed no changes in their blood glucose profiles while taking 1 g metamizole sodium (dipyrone) daily for 2 days.[5] No special precautions seem to be necessary. There seems to be no information about other oral hypoglycaemic agents.

(d) Rifampicin (Rifampin)

A study in untreated patients with leprosy showed that the pharmacokinetics of a single 600-mg dose of **rifampicin** were not markedly changed by 1 g metamizole sodium (dipyrone), but peak serum **rifampicin** levels occurred sooner (at 3 instead of 4 h) and were about 50% higher.[6] The clinical importance of this is uncertain.

1. Sweetman SC, editor. Martindale: The complete drug reference. 33rd ed. London: Pharmaceutical Press; 2002 p.13.
2. Kaufman DW, Kelly JP, Levy M et al. The drug etiology of agranulocytosis and aplastic anemia. Oxford: Oxford University Press (1991).
3. Badian LM, Rosenkrantz B. Quoted as personal communication by Levy M, Zylber-Katz E, Rosenkranz B. Clinical pharmacokinetics of dipyrone and its metabolites. *Clin Pharmacokinet* (1995) 28, 216–34.
4. Scholz W, Rosenkrantz B. Quoted as personal communication by Levy M, Zylber-Katz E, Rosenkranz B. Clinical pharmacokinetics of dipyrone and its metabolites. *Clin Pharmacokinet* (1995) 28, 216–34.
5. Haupt E, Hoppe FU, Bamberg E. Zur frage der Wecheslwirkugen von Analgetika und oralen Antidiabetika — Metamizol-Glibenclamid. *Med Welt* (1989) 40, 681–3.
6. Krishna DR, Appa Rao AVN, Ramanakar TV, Reddy KSC, Prabhakar MC. Pharmacokinetics of rifampin in the presence of dipyrone in leprosy patients. *Drug Dev Ind Pharm* (1984) 10, 101–110.

Methadone + Anticonvulsants

Methadone levels can be reduced by the concurrent use of carbamazepine, phenobarbital or phenytoin. An increase in the methadone dosage may be needed. Sodium valproate appears not to interact.

Clinical evidence

(a) Carbamazepine

A study in 37 patients on methadone maintenance found that only those on enzyme-inducing drugs (10 patients) had low trough methadone levels (less than 100 nanograms/ml). One was taking **carbamazepine** and he complained of daily withdrawal symptoms and had signs of opioid abstinence.[1] The other 9 were taking **phenobar-**

bital or **phenytoin**, see below.[1] Withdrawal symptoms were also seen in another patient given **carbamazepine**.[2]

(b) Phenobarbital

In the study cited above, 5 patients on methadone maintenance who were on **phenobarbital** had low trough serum methadone levels.[1] Another former heroin addict controlled with methadone complained of withdrawal symptoms when he started to take **phenobarbital.** His methadone plasma levels were found to be depressed.[3]

(c) Phenytoin

Methadone withdrawal symptoms developed in five patients within 3 to 4 days of starting to take 300 to 500 mg **phenytoin** daily. Methadone plasma levels were depressed about 60%. The symptoms disappeared within 2 to 3 days of stopping the **phenytoin** and the plasma methadone levels rapidly climbed to their former values.[4] Reduced serum methadone levels and withdrawal symptoms have been described in other patients taking **phenytoin**.[1,2,5,6] See also (a) and (d).

(d) Sodium valproate

Two patients who had had methadone withdrawal symptoms while on 300 to 400 mg **phenytoin** daily, and one of them later when on 600 mg **carbamazepine** daily, became free from withdrawal symptoms when given **sodium valproate** instead. It was also found possible to virtually halve their daily methadone dosage.[2]

Mechanism

Not fully established, but all of these anticonvulsants (except sodium valproate which does not interact) are recognised enzyme-inducing agents which can increase the metabolism of other drugs by the liver, thereby hastening their loss from the body. In one study it was found that while taking phenytoin the excretion into the urine of the main metabolite of methadone was increased.[4]

Importance and management

Information is limited but the interaction between methadone and these anticonvulsants appears to be established and of clinical importance. Anticipate the need to increase the methadone dosage in patients taking carbamazepine, phenytoin or phenobarbital. It may be necessary to give the methadone twice daily to prevent withdrawal symptoms appearing towards the end of the day. It seems probable that **primidone** will interact similarly because it is metabolised to phenobarbital. Also be aware of the need to reduce the methadone dose if any enzyme inducing anticonvulsant is stopped. Sodium valproate appears to be a possible non-interacting alternative.

1. Bell J, Seres V, Bowron P, Lewis J, Batey R. The use of serum methadone levels in patients receiving methadone maintenance. *Clin Pharmacol Ther* (1988) 43, 623–9.
2. Saxon AJ, Whittaker S, Hawker CS. Valproic acid, unlike other anticonvulsants, has no effect on methadone metabolism: two cases. *J Clin Psychiatry* (1989) 50, 228–9.
3. Liu S-J, Wang RIH. Case report of barbiturate-induced enhancement of methadone metabolism and withdrawal syndrome. *Am J Psychiatry* (1984) 141, 1287–8.
4. Tong TG, Pond SM, Kreek MJ, Jaffery NF, Benowitz NL. Phenytoin-induced methadone withdrawal. *Ann Intern Med* (1981) 94, 349–51.
5. Finelli PF. Phenytoin and methadone tolerance. *N Engl J Med* (1976) 294, 227.
6. Knoll B, Haefeli WE, Ladewig D, Stohler R. Early recurrence of withdrawal symptoms under phenytoin and chronic alcohol use. *Pharmacopsychiatry* (1997) 30, 72–3.

Methadone + Cimetidine

Two isolated reports describe two elderly patients on methadone who developed apnoea when additionally treated with cimetidine.

Clinical evidence, mechanism, importance and management

An elderly patient on 25 mg methadone daily developed apnoea 2 days after starting 1200 mg **cimetidine** daily.[1] Another elderly patient on methadone and morphine also developed apnoea (two breaths per minute) after taking 1200 mg **cimetidine** daily for 6 days.[2] This was controlled with naloxone.

The reasons for this marked increase in the effects of methadone are not known, but **cimetidine** inhibits the activity of the liver enzymes concerned with the *N*-demethylation of methadone (demonstrated with *rat*-liver microsomes[1]) so that it could accumulate in the body, thereby exaggerating its respiratory depressant effects. Liver impairment might possibly have contributed towards, or even been largely responsible for, the development of this interaction because both patients were elderly.

It seems doubtful if this interaction is of any general importance when the two isolated reports cited here are viewed against the background of the wide-spread use of both of these two drugs for a good number of years and the lack of other published adverse reports.

1. Dawson GW, Vestal RE. Cimetidine inhibits the *in vitro* N-demethylation of methadone. *Res Commun Chem Pathol Pharmacol* (1984) 46, 301–4.
2. Sorkin EM, Ogawa GS. Cimetidine potentiation of narcotic action. *Drug Intell Clin Pharm* (1983) 17, 60–1.

Methadone + Ciprofloxacin

A case is reported of sedation, confusion and respiratory depression attributed to the inhibition of methadone metabolism by ciprofloxacin.

Clinical evidence

A woman stabilised on methadone 140 mg daily for 6 years to manage pain due to chronic intestinal pseudo-obstruction was admitted to hospital because of a urinary tract infection and started on **ciprofloxacin** 750 mg twice daily. Two days later she became sedated and confused. **Ciprofloxacin** was replaced with co-trimoxazole and the patient recovered within 48 h. She was treated with **ciprofloxacin** for recurrent urinary-tract infections a further three times and each occasion the patient became sedated and normal alertness was regained on discontinuing **ciprofloxacin**. On the last occasion, when venlafaxine which she had also been taking was replaced by fluoxetine, she also developed respiratory depression, which was reversed with naloxone.[1]

Mechanism

The cytochrome P450 isoenzymes, CYP1A2, CYP2D6 and CYP3A4 are involved in the metabolism of methadone. Ciprofloxacin is a potent inhibitor of CYP1A2 and possibly CYP3A4. It is therefore probable that the confusion and sedation seen in the patient were due to the inhibition of methadone metabolism. The use of fluoxetine and the fact that the patient was a smoker may also have contributed. See also 'Methadone + Selective serotonin re-uptake inhibitors', p.66.

Importance and management

This seems to be the only report of this interaction but it would appear to be of clinical importance. Care should be exercised if the two are given concurrently, especially if there are other factors such as smoking or the use of other enzyme inhibitors, which may also contribute to the interaction. Be alert for the need to change methadone dosage.

1. Herrlin K, Segerdahl M, Gustafsson LL, Kalso E. Methadone, ciprofloxacin, and adverse drug reactions. *Lancet* (2000) 356, 2069–70.

Methadone + Disulfiram

No adverse interaction was seen in patients treated concurrently with methadone and disulfiram.

Clinical evidence, mechanism, importance and management

Seven opiate addicts, without chronic alcoholism or liver disease, and who were on methadone maintenance treatment (45 to 65 mg daily) showed an increase in the urinary excretion of the major pyrrolidine metabolite of methadone (an indicator of increased *N*-demethylation)

when given 500 mg **disulfiram** daily for 7 days, but there was no effect on the degree of opiate intoxication, nor were withdrawal symptoms experienced.[1] No special precautions would seem to be necessary.

1. Tong TG, Benowitz NL, Kreek MJ. Methadone-disulfiram interaction during methadone maintenance. *J Clin Pharmacol* (1980) 20, 506–13.

Methadone + Efavirenz

Methadone plasma levels can be markedly reduced by efavirenz. Increasing the methadone dosage may prevent the development of withdrawal symptoms.

Clinical evidence

A woman with HIV who had been on methadone for over a year began to complain of discomfort within 4 weeks of having nelfinavir replaced by 600 mg **efavirenz** daily, and by 8 weeks typical methadone withdrawal symptoms were occurring late in the afternoon. It was found that the levels of (*R*)-methadone (the active enantiomer) had fallen from 168 to 90 nanograms/ml, and those of (*S*)-methadone from 100 to 28 nanograms/ml. The methadone dosage had to be increased from 100 mg daily to 180 mg daily before the symptoms disappeared.[1] A further case is reported in which a man on methadone maintenance (30 mg daily) stopped taking co-administered **efavirenz** 600 mg daily because of the occurrence of withdrawal symptoms in spite of increased methadone dosage.[2]

Eleven patients on methadone (35 to 100 mg daily) were additionally started on **efavirenz** plus dual nucleoside analogues. Nine of the patients developed methadone withdrawal symptoms and needed dose increases of 15 to 30 mg. A pharmacokinetic study of these patients showed that 3 weeks after starting the efavirenz their mean methadone AUCs were reduced to 43% and their maximum plasma levels to 52%.[3,4] In another retrospective study, 6 out of 7 patients needed methadone dosage increases within 2 weeks to 8 months of additionally taking **efavirenz**.[5]

Mechanism

It is believed that **efavirenz** induces the activity of cytochrome P450 isoenzyme CYP3A4 which is concerned with the metabolism of methadone, the effect of which would be to increase its loss from the body, thereby reducing its effects.

Importance and management

An established interaction of clinical importance. If efavirenz is added to established treatment with methadone, be alert for the need to raise the methadone dosage, although as the case above illustrates, this may not always satisfactorily prevent withdrawal symptoms.[2] Some patients may need a doubled dose. The interaction can apparently develop within 2 to 3 weeks in some patients but may take much longer in others.

1. Marzolini C, Troillet N, Telenti A, Baumann P, Decosterd LA, Eap CB. Efavirenz decreases methadone blood concentrations. *AIDS* (2000) 14, 1291–2.
2. Pinzani V, Faucherre V, Peyriere H, Blayac J-P. Methadone withdrawal symptoms with nevirapine and efavirenz. *Ann Pharmacother* (2000) 34, 405–7.
3. Clarke S, Mulcahy F, Barry M, Gibbons S, Tjia J, Reynolds H, Back DJ. The pharmacokinetics and tolerability of methadone and efavirenz in injecting drug users with HIV infection. Poster presented at 7th Eur Conf Clinical Aspects and Treatment of HIV-infection, Lisbon, Portugal, October 23-7, 1999 (Poster 1210).
4. Clarke SM, Mulcahy FM, Tjia J, Reynolds HE, Gibbons SE, Barry MG, Back DJ. The pharmacokinetics of methadone in HIV-positive patients receiving the non-nucleoside reverse transcriptase inhibitor efavirenz. *Br J Clin Pharmacol* (2001) 51, 213–7.
5. Tashima K, Bose T, Gormley J, Sousa H, Flanigan TP. The potential impact of efavirenz on methadone maintenance. Poster presented at 9th European Conference on Clinical Microbiology and Infectious Diseases, Berlin, March 23rd 1999 (Poster PO552).

Methadone + Fluconazole

Fluconazole causes a moderate increase in the serum levels of methadone, but no reduction in the dosage of methadone is needed.

Clinical evidence, mechanism, importance and management

A randomised, double-blind, placebo-controlled study in 25 methadone-maintained patients found that 200 mg **fluconazole** daily for 2 weeks increased the steady-state serum methadone levels and the AUC by about 30%, but no signs of methadone overdosage were seen and no changes in the methadone dosage were needed.[1,2] The reasons for this interaction are not understood, but a likely explanation is that the **fluconazole** inhibits the metabolism of the methadone to some extent. The authors of the report concluded that although a statistically significant pharmacokinetic interaction occurs, it is of no clinical importance.[1,2] Information appears to be limited to this report, but no special precautions would appear to be necessary if these drugs are used concurrently.

1. Cobb M, Desai J, Brown LS, Zannikos P, Trapnell C, Rainey P. The effect of fluconazole on the clinical pharmacokinetics of methadone. 11th Int Conf AIDS (1996), Vancouver, vol 1, 88 (Mo.B/1196)
2. Cobb MN, Desai J, Brown LS, Zannikos PN, Rainey PM. The effect of fluconazole on the clinical pharmacokinetics of methadone. *Clin Pharmacol Ther* (1998) 63, 655–62.

Methadone + Fusidic acid or Zidovudine

One report says that fusidic acid and zidovudine can reduce the effects of methadone. Others say that methadone is not affected by zidovudine but that the zidovudine serum levels can rise.

Clinical evidence

(a) Methadone effects reduced or unaffected

Two drug abusers with AIDS needed an increase in their methadone dosages, one from 40 to 60 mg daily, and the other from 60 to 80 mg daily, the first within a month of beginning treatment with 1 g **zidovudine** daily and the other within 6 months of starting to take 1500 mg **fusidic acid** daily.[1]

In contrast, two related studies found no evidence of any change in the pharmacokinetics of methadone in HIV+ patients treated with **zidovudine**. No methadone withdrawal symptoms occurred.[2,3] A third study in 16 HIV+ patients found that a fixed combination of **zidovudine** 300 mg + 150 mg **lamivudine** *(Combivir)* had no statistical or clinically relevant effects on the pharmacokinetics of methadone, and there was no evidence of withdrawal or toxicity.[4]

(b) Zidovudine effects increased

In the study already cited above[2] and the earlier related study by the same workers,[3] the AUC of the **zidovudine** was increased on average by 43% by the methadone, and in 4 of the 9 patients it was doubled.[2] Five HIV+ patients showed a 52% increase in **zidovudine** AUC when given orally and a 30% increase when given intravenously.[5] Increased **zidovudine** plasma levels are described in another report.[6]

Mechanisms

(a). Both patients showed evidence of liver enzyme induction (using antipyrine as a marker of induction), from which it was concluded that these two drugs increase the metabolism and loss of methadone from the body.[1]

(b). Methadone apparently reduces the glucuronidation of the zidovudine by the liver, resulting in an increase in its serum levels.[3,7] Methadone may also reduce renal clearance of zidovudine.[8]

Importance and management

Information appears to be limited to these somewhat inconsistent reports. Concurrent use need not be avoided but the outcome is uncertain. Be alert for any evidence of methadone underdosage and of increased zidovudine effects and possible toxicity.

1. Brockmeyer NH, Mertins L, Goos M. Pharmacokinetic interaction of antimicrobial agents with levomethadon in drug-addicted AIDS patients. *Klin Wschr* (1991) 69, 16–18.
2. Schwartz EL, Brechbühl A-B, Kahl P, Miller MA, Selwyn PA, Friedland GH. Pharmacokinetic interactions of zidovudine and methadone in intravenous drug-using patients with HIV infection. *J Acquir Immune Defic Syndr* (1992) 5, 619–26.
3. Schwartz EL, Brechbühl A-B, Kahl P, Miller MH, Selwyn PA, Friedland GH. Altered pharmacokinetics of zidovudine in former IV drug-using patients receiving methadone. 6th International Conference on AIDS, San Francisco (1990) Abstract SB432.
4. Rainey PM, Friedland G, Snidow J, McCance-Katz E, Mitchell SM, Lane B, Jatlow P. Effects of zidovudine plus lamivudine on methadone disposition. *Clin Pharmacol Ther* (2000) 67, 165.
5. Jatlow P, McCance EF, Rainey PM, Trapnell CB, Friedland G. Methadone increases zidovudine exposure in HIV-infected injection drug users. Infect Dis Soc Am Nat Inst Health, Centres IDS control Prev 3rd Conf on Retroviruses and opportunistic infections, Washington DC, (1996) Abstract 129.
6. Burger DM, Meenhorst PL, ten Napel CHH, Mulder JW, Neef C, Koks CHW, Bult A, Beijnen JH. Pharmacokinetic variability of zidovudine in HIV-infected individuals: subgroup analysis and drug interactions. *AIDS* (1994) 8, 1683–9.
7. Cretton-Scott E, de Sousa G, Nicolas F, Rahmani R, Sommadossi J-P. Methadone and its metabolite N-demethyl methadone, inhibit AZT glucuronidation in vitro. *Clin Pharmacol Ther* (1996) 59, 168.
8. McCance-Katz EF, Rainey PM, Jatlow P, Friedland G. Methadone effects on zidovudine disposition (AIDS clinical trials group 262). *J Acquir Immune Defic Syndr Hum Retrovirol* (1998) 18, 435–43.

Methadone + Protease inhibitors

Methadone serum levels can be reduced by ritonavir and nelfinavir. An increased methadone dosage may be needed in some patients to prevent opiate withdrawal. No interaction appears to occur with indinavir or possibly saquinavir

Clinical evidence

(a) Indinavir

A multiple dose, randomised, two period, crossover study in 12 patients on methadone maintenance found that the pharmacokinetics of the methadone were unchanged when 800 mg **indinavir** was given 8-hourly for 8 days. A small decrease in maximum **indinavir** levels and a small increase in trough levels occurred.[1] There are clinical reports about two patients whose methadone levels appeared to be unaltered while taking **indinavir** but who later showed reduced levels when treated with nelfinavir or ritonavir (see (b) and (c) below).[2,3] This would seem to confirm that **indinavir** does not have a clinically relevant effect on maintenance with methadone. Another study in 6 HIV+ patients on methadone and two nucleoside analogues similarly found that methadone serum levels remained unchanged when **indinavir** was added.[4,5]

(b) Nelfinavir

An HIV+ man who had been stable on 100 mg methadone daily for several years and taking 800 mg indinavir and 0.75 mg zalcitabine three times daily, developed opiate withdrawal symptoms within 6 weeks of additionally starting stavudine and 750 mg **nelfinavir** three times daily. His methadone dosage was increased to 285 mg daily before therapeutic serum levels were achieved. When his antiretroviral treatment was withdrawn, his methadone dosage was then reduced to 125 mg daily.[3] Two other patients on nucleoside analogues showed a 40 to 50% fall in serum methadone levels when **nelfinavir** was added.[4,5] However the makers of **nelfinavir** say that in a pharmacokinetic study it was found that **nelfinavir** reduced the concentrations of methadone and its metabolites by 29 to 47% but none of the subjects developed withdrawal symptoms.[6]

(c) Ritonavir

A patient taking 90 mg methadone daily and on HIV treatment with indinavir, lamivudine and zidovudine, developed withdrawal symptoms and was hospitalised within a week of stopping these HIV drugs and starting 400 mg **ritonavir**, 400 mg saquinavir and 40 mg stavudine daily. The patient was later restabilised on 130 mg methadone daily.[2] Another patient on lamivudine and zidovudine showed a marked decrease in methadone serum levels when **ritonavir** was added.[4,5]

Eleven normal subjects were given a single 20-mg dose of methadone on day 1 of a study, followed by a 2-week washout period and then **ritonavir** on days 15 to 28. On day 25 a single 5 mg dose of methadone was given. It was found that the **ritonavir** reduced the maximum serum levels of the methadone by 37.8% and the AUC by 36.3%.[7]

(d) Saquinavir

A study in an HIV+ patient on methadone and two nucleoside analogues found that methadone serum levels remained unchanged when **saquinavir** was added.[4,5] An *in vitro* study with human liver microsomes predicted that no methadone/**saquinavir** interaction is likely.[8]

Mechanism

Not fully established but the most likely explanation for the interactions with nelfinavir and ritonavir is that these drugs increase the metabolism of the methadone, probably by inducing the activity of the cytochrome P450 isoenzyme CYP3A4, resulting in an increased clearance of the methadone from the body.

Importance and management

Information is limited but the interactions with ritonavir and nelfinavir would appear to be established, however the picture seems to be that not all patients experience withdrawal symptoms if given either of these two drugs. Monitor well so that those who do need a dosage increase can be identified. Indinavir appears not to interact and very limited evidence suggests that saquinavir does not either.

1. Cantilena L, McCrea J, Blazes D, Winchell G, Carides A, Royce C, Deutsch P. Lack of a pharmacokinetic interaction between indinavir and methadone. *Clin Pharmacol Ther* (1999) 65, 135.
2. Geletko SM, Erickson AD. Decreased methadone effect after ritonavir initiation. *Pharmacotherapy* (2000) 20, 93-4.
3. McCance-Katz EF, Farber S, Selwyn PA, O'Connor A. Decrease in methadone levels with nelfinavir mesylate. *Am J Psychiatry* (2000) 157, 481.
4. Touzeau D, Beauverie P, Bouchez J, Poisson N, Edel Y, Dessalles M-C, Lherm J, Furlan V, Lagarde B. Méthadone et nouveau anti-rétroviraux. Résultats du suivi thérapeutique. *Ann Med Interne (Paris)* (1999) 150, 355-6.
5. Beauverie P, Taburet A-M, Dessalles M-C, Furlan V, Touzeau D. Therapeutic monitoring of methadone in HIV-infected patients receiving protease inhibitors. *AIDS* (1998) 12, 2510-11.
6. Viracept (Nelfinavir). Roche Products Limited. Summary of product characteristics, March 2001.
7. Hsu A, Granneman GR, Carothers L, Dennis S, Chiu Y-L, Valdes J, Sun E. Ritonavir does not increase methadone exposure in healthy volunteers. Abbott Laboratories. Personal communication 2000.
8. Guibert A, Furlan V, Martino J, Taburet AM. *In vitro* effect of HIV protease inhibitors on methadone metabolism. *Intersci Conf Antimicrob Agents Chemother* (1997) 37, 12.

Methadone + Rifampicin (Rifampin) or Rifabutin

Serum methadone levels can be markedly reduced by rifampicin. A dosage increase may be needed by many patients to prevent the development of withdrawal symptoms. Rifabutin appears to interact to a lesser extent so that fewer patients are likely to be affected. Isoniazid appears not to interact.

Clinical evidence

(a) Rifampicin

Following the observation that former heroin addicts on methadone maintenance complained of withdrawal symptoms when given **rifampicin**, a study was made on 30 patients on methadone. Twenty-one of them developed withdrawal symptoms within 1 to 33 days of starting 600 to 900 mg **rifampicin** and **isoniazid** daily. In 6 of the 7 most severely affected the symptoms developed within a week, their plasma methadone concentrations falling by 33 to 68%. None of 56 other patients on methadone and other anti-tubercular treatment (which included **isoniazid** but not **rifampicin**) showed withdrawal symptoms.[1-3]

Other cases of this interaction have been reported.[4-8] Some patients needed two to threefold increases in the methadone dosage while taking **rifampicin** to control the withdrawal symptoms.[5,6,8]

(b) Rifabutin

A study in 24 HIV+ patients on **methadone** maintenance found that after taking 300 mg **rifabutin** daily for 13 days the pharmacokinetics of the **methadone** were minimally changed, however 75% of them reported at least one mild symptom of methadone withdrawal but it was not enough for any of them to withdraw from the study. Only 3 of them asked for and received an increase in dosage. The authors offered the opinion that over-reporting of withdrawal symptoms was likely due to the warnings that the patients had received.[9,10]

Mechanism

Rifampicin is a potent enzyme-inducing agent which increases the activity of the liver enzymes concerned with the metabolism of methadone, as a result of which its clearance from the body is markedly increased. In 4 patients in the study cited the urinary excretion of the major metabolite of methadone rose by 150%.[1] Rifabutin has only a small enzyme inducing effect.

Importance and management

The methadone/rifampicin interaction is established, adequately documented and of clinical importance. The incidence is high. Two-thirds (21) of the narcotic-dependent patients in the study cited[1] developed this interaction, 14 of whom were able to continue treatment. Withdrawal symptoms may develop within 24 h. The analgesic effects of methadone would also be expected to be reduced. Concurrent use need not be avoided, but the effects should be monitored and appropriate dosage increases (as much as two to threefold) made where necessary.

Rifabutin appears to interact to a very much lesser extent so that fewer patients may need a methadone dosage increase. Isoniazid appears not to interact with methadone.

1. Kreek MJ, Garfield JW, Gutjahr CL, Giusti LM. Rifampin-induced methadone withdrawal. *N Engl J Med* (1976) 294, 1104–6.
2. Garfield JW, Kreek MJ, Giusti L. Rifampin-methadone relationship. 1. The clinical effects of rifampin-methadone interaction. *Am Rev Respir Dis* (1975) 111, 926.
3. Kreek MJ, Garfield JW, Gutjahr CL, Bowen D, Field F, Rothschild M. Rifampin-methadone relationship. 2. Rifampin effects on plasma concentration, metabolism, and excretion of methadone. *Am Rev Respir Dis* (1975) 111, 926–7.
4. Bending MR, Skacel PO. Rifampicin and methadone withdrawal. *Lancet* (1977) i, 1211.
5. Van Leeuwen DJ. Rifampicine leidt tot onthoudingsverschijnselen bij methadongebruikers. *Ned Tijdschr Geneeskd* (1986) 130, 548–50.
6. Brockmeyer NH, Mertins L, Goos M. Pharmacokinetic interaction of antimicrobial agents with levomethadon in drug-addicted AIDS patients. *Klin Wochenschr* (1991) 69, 16–18.
7. Holmes VF. Rifampin-induced methadone withdrawal in AIDS. *J Clin Psychopharmacol* (1990) 10, 443–4.
8. Raistrick D, Hay A, Wolff K. Methadone maintenance and tuberculosis treatment. *BMJ* (1996) 313, 925–6.
9. Brown LS, Sawyer RC, Li R, Cobb MN, Colborn DC, Narang PK. Lack of a pharmacologic interaction between rifabutin and methadone in HIV-infected former injecting drug users. *Drug Alcohol Depend* (1996) 43, 71–7.
10. Sawyer RC, Brown LS, Li RC, Colborn DC, Narang PK. Lack of effect of concomitant rifabutin on methadone safety and pharmacokinetics in HIV+ injecting drug users. *Intersci Conf Antimicrob Agents Chemother* (1995) 35, 7.

Methadone + Selective serotonin re-uptake inhibitors (SSRIs)

Methadone serum levels may rise if fluvoxamine is added, possibly resulting in increased side-effects. Sertraline may also increase methadone levels, but no interaction appears to occur with fluoxetine.

Clinical evidence, mechanism, importance and management

(a) Fluoxetine

Nine patients were given methadone, 30 to 100 mg daily, and 20 mg **fluoxetine** daily (two of them were also taking **fluvoxamine**). Although there were possible compliance problems with some of the patients, the methadone plasma/dose ratio of the group as a whole was not altered by the addition of the **fluoxetine**.[1] This is consistent with the results of another study which found that **fluoxetine** did not appear to alter the plasma methadone levels of 16 patients treated for cocaine dependence.[2] No special precautions would therefore seem to be necessary if **fluoxetine** is added to methadone treatment.

(b) Fluvoxamine

Five patients on maintenance treatment with methadone were additionally given **fluvoxamine**. Two of them showed an approximately 20% increase in the methadone plasma/dose ratio, while the other 3 showed 40 to 100% rises. One of them developed asthenia, marked drowsiness and nausea which disappeared when both drug dosages were reduced.[3] One patient has been described who was unable to maintain adequate methadone levels, despite a daily dosage of 200 mg, and experienced withdrawal symptoms until **fluvoxamine** was added.[4] Another patient on methadone 70 mg daily and diazepam 2 mg twice daily was admitted to hospital with an acute exacerbation of asthma and intractable cough three weeks after additionally starting **fluvoxamine** 100 mg daily. Blood gas measurements indicated severe hypoxaemia and hypercapnia. The symptoms resolved when the methadone dose was reduced to 50 mg daily and diazepam was gradually withdrawn; methadone levels fell by about 23% (from 262 to 202 nanograms/ml).[5] The reason appears to be that the **fluvoxamine** can inhibit the liver metabolism of the methadone by cytochrome P450 isoenzyme CYP3A4 (confirmed by *in vitro* studies[6]) thereby allowing it to accumulate in the body. Information is limited but it indicates that the effects of starting or stopping **fluvoxamine** should be monitored in patients on methadone, being alert for the need to adjust the methadone dosage.

(c) Sertraline

A placebo-controlled study in 31 depressed methadone-maintained patients found that **sertraline** significantly increased the methadone plasma level/dose ratio by 26% while patients on placebo showed a 16% decrease after 6 weeks treatment, but by 12 weeks ratios had shifted towards baseline values. Side effects were similar in both groups. As **sertraline** may inhibit methadone metabolism during the first few weeks of co-administration, monitoring should be considered.[7]

1. Bertschy G, Eap CB, Powell K, Baumann P. Fluoxetine addition to methadone in addicts: pharmacokinetic aspects. *Ther Drug Monit* (1996) 18, 570–2.
2. Batki SL, Manfredi LB, Jacob P, Jones RT. Fluoxetine for cocaine dependence in methadone maintenance: quantitative plasma and urine cocaine-benzoylecgonine concentrations. *J Clin Psychopharmacol* (1993) 13, 243–50.
3. Bertschy G, Baumann P, Eap CB, Baettig D. Probable metabolic interaction between methadone and fluvoxamine in addict patients. *Ther Drug Monit* (1994) 16, 42–5.
4. DeMaria PA, Serota RD. A therapeutic use of the methadone fluvoxamine drug interaction. *J Addict Dis* (1999) 18, 5–12.
5. Alderman CP, Frith PA. Fluvoxamine-methadone interaction. *Aust N Z J Psychiatry* (1999) 33, 99–101.
6. Iribarne C, Picart D, Dreano Y, Berthou F. In vitro interactions between fluoxetine or fluvoxamine and methadone or buprenorphine. *Fundam Clin Pharmacol* (1998) 12, 194–9.
7. Hamilton SP, Nunes EV, Janal M, Weber L. The effect of sertraline on methadone plasma levels in methadone-maintenance patients. *Am J Addict* (2000) 9, 63–9.

Methadone + Urinary acidifiers or alkalinizers

The loss of methadone from the body in the urine is increased if the urine is made acid and reduced if it is made alkaline.

Clinical evidence

A study in patients on methadone found that the urinary clearance in those with urinary pHs of less than 6 was greater than those with higher urinary pHs.[1] When one subject's urinary pH was lowered from 6.2 to 5.5, the loss of unchanged methadone in the urine was nearly doubled.[2]

A pharmacokinetic study in 5 healthy subjects given 10-mg doses of methadone intramuscularly found that the plasma half-life was 19.5 h when the urine was made acidic (pH 5.2) with **ammonium chloride** compared with 42.1 h when the urine was made alkaline (pH 7.8) with **sodium bicarbonate**. The body clearance of the meth-

adone fell from 134 to 91.9 ml/min when the urine was changed from acidic to alkaline.[3]

Mechanism

Methadone is eliminated from the body both by liver metabolism and excretion of unchanged methadone in the urine. Above pH 6 the urinary excretion is less important, but with urinary pH below 6 the half-life becomes dependent on both excretion (30%) and metabolism (70%).[2-4] Methadone is a weak base (pKa 8.4) so that in acid urine little of the drug is in the un-ionised form and little is reabsorbed by simple passive diffusion. On the other hand in alkaline solution most of the drug is in the un-ionised form which is readily reabsorbed by the kidney tubules and little is lost in the urine.

Importance and management

An established interaction but of uncertain importance. Be alert for any evidence of reduced methadone effects in patients whose urine becomes acidic because they are taking large doses of ammonium chloride or acetazolamide. Lowering the pH to 5 with ammonium chloride to increase the clearance can also be used to treat intoxication.

1. Bellward GD, Warren PM, Howald W, Axelson JE, Abbott FS. Methadone maintenance: effect of urinary pH on renal clearance in chronic high and low doses. *Clin Pharmacol Ther* (1977) 22, 92–9.
2. Inturrisi CE, Verebely K. Disposition of methadone in man after a single oral dose. *Clin Pharmacol Ther* (1972) 13, 923–30.
3. Nilsson M-I, Widerlöv E, Meresaar U, Änggård E. Effect of urinary pH on the disposition of methadone in man. *Eur J Clin Pharmacol* (1982) 22, 337–42.
4. Baselt RC, Casarett LJ. Urinary excretion of methadone in man. *Clin Pharmacol Ther* (1972) 13, 64–70.

Morphine + Cimetidine or Ranitidine

Clinically important interactions between morphine and these H$_2$-blockers appear to be rare. A slight and unimportant increase in respiratory depression may occur with cimetidine, and no interaction normally occurs with ranitidine. An isolated report describes an adverse reaction in one patient on morphine or papaveretum and cimetidine, and there is another isolated report involving morphine and ranitidine.

Clinical evidence

(a) Cimetidine

Cimetidine (300 mg four times daily for 4 days) given to 7 healthy subjects had no effect on the pharmacokinetics of morphine. The extent and duration of the morphine-induced pupillary miosis was unchanged.[1] In other healthy subjects it was found that 600 mg **cimetidine** 1 h before 10 mg morphine (intramuscularly) prolonged the respiratory depression due to morphine, but the extent was small and clinically insignificant.[2]

An acutely ill patient with grand mal epilepsy, gastrointestinal bleeding and an intertrochanteric fracture who was undergoing haemodialysis three times a week, was being treated with 300 mg **cimetidine** three times daily. After being given the sixth dose of morphine (15 mg four-hourly) he became apnoeic (three respirations per minute) which was controlled with naloxone. He remained confused and agitated for the next 80 h with muscular twitching and further periods of apnoea controlled with naloxone. He had nine 10-mg doses of morphine on a previous occasion in the absence of **cimetidine** without problems. About a month later he experienced the same adverse reactions when given **papaveretum** while still taking **cimetidine**.[3]

(b) Ranitidine

A man with terminal cancer on 150 mg **ranitidine** intravenously eight-hourly became confused, disorientated and agitated when given the **ranitidine** after an intravenous infusion of morphine (50 mg daily) was started. When the **ranitidine** was stopped his mental state improved but worsened when he was given **ranitidine** again 8 h and

16 h later. He improved when the **ranitidine** was stopped.[4]

Another report describes hallucinations in a patient given sustained-release morphine and **ranitidine**, but the author discounted the possibility of an interaction.[5]

Mechanism

In vitro studies have shown that the conjugation of morphine is not affected by cimetidine or ranitidine.[6] The isolated cases of interaction remain unexplained.[3,4] It would seem that unidentified factors conspired to cause these reactions.

Importance and management

The virtual absence of a generally important morphine/cimetidine interaction is adequately documented. Concurrent use normally causes only a slight and normally unimportant prolongation of the respiratory depression due to morphine but it might possibly have some importance in patients with pre-existing breathing disorders. *In vitro* evidence suggests that ranitidine is unlikely to interact with morphine,[6] however the isolated cases cited here underline the importance of monitoring the concurrent use of morphine or papaveretum and H$_2$-blockers.

1. Mojaverian P, Fedder IL, Vlasses PH, Rotmensch HH, Rocci ML, Swanson BN, Ferguson RK. Cimetidine does not alter morphine disposition in man. *Br J Clin Pharmacol* (1982) 14, 809–13.
2. Lam AM, Clement JL. Effect of cimetidine premedication on morphine-induced ventilatory depression. *Can Anaesth Soc J* (1984) 31, 36–43.
3. Fine A, Churchill DN. Potentially lethal interaction of cimetidine and morphine. *Can Med Assoc J* (1981) 124, 1434–6.
4. Martinez-Abad M, Delgado Gomis F, Ferrer JM, Morales-Olivas FJ. Ranitidine-induced confusion with concomitant morphine. *Drug Intell Clin Pharm* (1988) 22, 914–5.
5. Jellema JG. Hallucination during sustained-release morphine and methadone administration. *Lancet* (1987) ii, 392.
6. Knodell RG, Holtzman JL, Crankshaw DL, Steele NM, Stanley LN. Drug metabolism by rat and human hepatic microsomes in response to interaction with H$_2$-receptor antagonists. *Gastroenterology* (1982) 82, 84–8.

Morphine + Contraceptives, oral

The clearance of morphine is approximately doubled by the concurrent use of the oral contraceptives.

Clinical evidence, mechanism, importance and management

The clearance of intravenous morphine (1 mg) was increased by 75%, and of oral morphine (10 mg) by 120%, in 6 young women taking an **oral contraceptive**.[1] The suggested reason is that the oestrogen component of the contraceptive increases the activity of one of the liver enzymes (glucuronyl transferase) concerned with the metabolism of the morphine. This implies that the dosage of morphine would need to be virtually doubled to achieve the same degree of analgesia. Whether this is so in practice requires confirmation.

1. Watson KJR, Ghabrial H, Mashford ML, Harman PJ, Breen KJ, Desmond PV. The oral contraceptive pill increases morphine clearance but does not increase hepatic blood flow. *Gastroenterology* (1986) 90, 1779.

Morphine + Dexamfetamine (Dextroamphetamine) or Methylphenidate

Both of these drugs increase the analgesic effects of morphine and reduce some of its side-effects.

Clinical evidence, mechanism, importance and management

Dexamfetamine (dextroamphetamine) increases the analgesic effects of morphine and reduces to some extent its respiratory depressant effects.[1] **Methylphenidate** similarly increases the analgesic effects and reduces the sedation.[2] There would seem to be advantages in using these drugs in combination.

1. Bourke DL, Allen PD, Rosenberg M, Mendes RW, Karabelas AN. Dextroamphetamine with morphine: respiratory effects. *J Clin Pharmacol* (1983) 23, 65–70.
2. Bruera E, Chadwick S, Brenneis C, Hanson J, MacDonald RN. Methylphenidate associated with narcotics for the treatment of cancer pain. *Cancer Treat Rep* (1987) 71, 67–70.

Morphine + Fluoxetine

No significant pharmacokinetic interaction appears to occur between morphine and fluoxetine, but fluoxetine may increase the analgesic effects of morphine and reduce some of its side-effects.

Clinical evidence, mechanism, importance and management

A double-blind crossover study in 15 healthy subjects found that a single 60-mg dose of **fluoxetine** did not affect the pharmacokinetics of morphine sulphate in doses tailored to produce and maintain steady-state plasma levels of 15, 30 and 60 nanograms/ml for 60 min. Morphine administration was found not to affect plasma levels of **fluoxetine** or **norfluoxetine**. Analgesia was slightly improved by 3 to 8% and the subjects experienced less nausea and drowsiness. Psychomotor function and respiratory depression were not affected. There seems to be no reason to avoid concurrent use.[1]

1. Erjavec MK, Coda BA, Nguyen Q, Donaldson G, Risler L, Shen DD. Morphine-fluoxetine interactions in healthy volunteers: analgesia and side effects. *J Clin Pharmacol* (2000) 40, 1286–95.

Morphine + Food

Food increases the bioavailability of oral morphine and produces a sustained serum level.

Clinical evidence, mechanism, importance and management

Twelve patients with chronic pain were given 50 mg morphine hydrochloride by mouth in 200 ml water either while fasting or after a **high fat breakfast** (fried eggs and bacon, toast with butter, and milk). The maximum blood morphine concentrations and the time to achieve these concentrations were not significantly altered by the presence of the **food**, but the AUC was increased by 34% and blood morphine levels were maintained at higher levels over the period from 4 to 10 h after being given the morphine.[1] The reasons are not understood. The inference to be drawn is that pain relief is likely to be increased if the morphine is given with **food**. This appears to be an advantageous interaction. More confirmatory study is needed.

1. Gourlay GK, Plummer JL, Cherry DA, Foate JA, Cousins MJ. Influence of a high-fat meal on the absorption of morphine from oral solutions. *Clin Pharmacol Ther* (1989) 46, 463–8.

Morphine + Local Anaesthetics

Chloroprocaine can reduce epidural morphine analgesia when compared with lidocaine (lignocaine). Lidocaine does not appear to increase respiratory depressant effects of morphine, and may have synergistic analgesic effects with mor-

phine. Morphine given as an intravenous bolus does not alter lidocaine (lignocaine) serum levels given as a continuous intravenous infusion.

Clinical evidence, mechanism, importance and management

(a) Chloroprocaine

Two studies[1,2] have found that **chloroprocaine** decreases the duration of epidural **morphine** analgesia (16 h for **chloroprocaine** compared with 24 h for **lidocaine (lignocaine)**[1]. A third study showed that morphine requirements after caesarean section were much higher in those women who had received **chloroprocaine** for epidural anaesthesia than those receiving **lidocaine**.[3] The authors of one of the studies suggest that **chloroprocaine** should be avoided if epidural **morphine** therapy is used.[1]

(b) Lignocaine

A double-blind controlled study in 10 patients who were receiving continuous **lidocaine (lignocaine)** infusions during suspected myocardial infarction found that a 10-mg intravenous morphine sulphate bolus did not significantly alter the steady-state serum levels of lidocaine (about 2.45 micrograms/ml).[4] In another study, the coadministration of **lidocaine** with extradural morphine did not increase the risk of respiratory depression associated with morphine.[5] However, in one case, respiratory depression occurred within 5 min of giving intravenous **lidocaine** for an episode of ventricular tachycardia in a patient who had previously been given spinal opioids (fentanyl and morphine). Naloxone successfully reversed this.[6] Numerous studies[7] in *animals* have shown that **lidocaine** and morphine have synergistic analgesic effects (reference 7 is cited as an example).

1. Eisenach JC, Schlairet TJ, Dobson CE, Hood DH. Effect of prior anesthetic solution on epidural morphine analgesia. *Anesth Analg* (1991) 73, 119–23.
2. Phan CQ, Azar I, Osborn IP, Lear E. The quality of epidural morphine analgesia following epidural anesthesia with chloroprocaine or chloroprocaine mixed with epinephrine for cesarean delivery. *Anesth Analg* (1997) 41, 774–8.
3. Karambelkar DJ, Ramanathan S. 2-Chloroprocaine antagonism of epidural morphine analgesia. *Acta Anaesthesiol Scand* (1997) 41, S171.
4. Vacek JL, Wilson DB, Hurwitz A, Gollub SB, Dunn MI. The effect of morphine sulfate on serum lidocaine levels. *Clin Res* (1988) 36, 325A.
5. Saito Y, Sakura S, Kaneko M, Kosaka Y. Interaction of extradural morphine and lignocaine on ventilatory response. *Br J Anaesth* (1995) 75, 394–8.
6. Jensen E, Nader ND. Potentiation of narcosis after intravenous lidocaine in a patient given spinal opioids. *Anesth Analg* (1999) 89, 758–9.
7. Maves TJ, Gebhart GF. Antinociceptive synergy between intrathecal morphine and lidocaine during visceral and somatic nociception in the rat. *Anesthesiology* (1992) 76, 91–9.

Morphine + Metoclopramide

Metoclopramide increases the rate of absorption of oral morphine and increases its sedative effects.

Clinical evidence

Ten mg of oral **metoclopramide** markedly increased the extent and speed of sedation due to a 20 mg oral dose of modified-release morphine (*MST Continus Tablets*) over a period of 3 to 4 h in 10 patients undergoing surgery. Peak plasma morphine levels and the total absorption remained unaltered.[1]

Mechanism

Metoclopramide increases the rate of gastric emptying so that the rate of morphine absorption from the small intestine is increased. An alternative idea is that both drugs act additively on opiate receptors to increase sedation.[1]

Importance and management

An established interaction which can be usefully exploited in anaesthetic practice, but the increased sedation may also represent a problem if the morphine is being given long-term.

1. Manara AR, Shelly MP, Quinn K, Park GR. The effect of metoclopramide on the absorption of oral controlled release morphine. *Br J Clin Pharmacol* (1988) 25, 518–21.

Morphine + Miscellaneous drugs

Some supplemental drugs appear to increase the myoclonus caused by high doses of morphine. Ketoprofen may reduce morphine-associated respiratory depression. Diclofenac may not alter morphine bioavailability but levels of an active metabolite of morphine may remain high in the presence of diclofenac.

Clinical evidence, mechanism, importance and management

The incidence of myoclonus in 19 patients with malignant disease on high doses of morphine (daily doses of 500 mg or more orally or 250 mg or more parenterally) appeared to be increased by the presence of other drugs including antidepressants (**amitriptyline, doxepin**), antipsychotics (**chlorpromazine, haloperidol**), NSAIDs (**indometacin, naproxen, piroxicam, aspirin**) and an antiemetic (**thiethylperazine**).[1] The reasons are not understood. The authors conclude that the best way to treat this problem is to change the supplemental drugs. More study is needed.

Ketoprofen reduces the respiratory depression associated with morphine and it has been suggested the combination may be useful for post-operative analgesia.[2] A study in 6 patients found that **diclofenac** does not significantly affect the pharmacokinetics of morphine, also suggesting that they can be used together without any risk of morphine overdosage.[3] However, in contrast to these reports, a study in 7 patients on the first postoperative day after spinal surgery found that administration of **diclofenac** 100 mg rectally reduced patient-controlled morphine consumption by 20 % but the concentration of an active metabolite, morphine-6-glucuronide was unchanged. Respiratory rates were significantly lower after **diclofenac** administration.[4] There may be a risk of respiratory depression and other side effects due to persistently high levels of morphine-6-glucuronide. Until more information is available, the possibility that NSAIDs may increase opioid-associated toxicity should be borne in mind if such combinations are used.

1. Potter JM, Reid DB, Shaw RJ, Hackett P, Hickman PE. Myoclonus associated with treatment with high doses of morphine: the role of supplemental drugs. *BMJ* (1989) 299, 150–3.
2. Moren J, Francois T, Blanloeil Y, Pinaud M. The effects of a nonsteroidal antiinflammatory drug (ketoprofen) on morphine respiratory depression: a double-blind, randomized study in volunteers. *Anesth Analg* (1997) 85, 400–5.
3. De Conno F, Ripamonti C, Bianchi M, Ventafridda V, Panerai AE. Diclofenac does not modify morphine bioavailability in cancer patients. *Pain* (1992) 48, 401–2.
4. Tighe KE, Webb AM, Hobbs GJ. Persistently high plasma morphine-6-glucuronide levels despite decreased hourly patient-controlled analgesia morphine use after single-dose diclofenac: potential for opioid-related toxicity. *Anesth Analg* (1999) 88, 1137–42.

Morphine + Rifampicin (Rifampin)

A study found that rifampicin increases the loss of morphine from the body, abolishing its analgesic effects.

Clinical evidence, mechanism, importance and management

In a randomised, double-blind crossover study, 10 healthy subjects were given either 10 mg morphine sulphate orally or a placebo on days 1, 4, 15 and 18, and from days 5 to 18 they were additionally given 600 mg **rifampicin** daily. It was found that the **rifampicin** increased the clearance of the morphine by 49% and its analgesic effects (using a modified cold pressor test) were abolished.[1,2] The presumed reason is that the **rifampicin** (a recognised potent enzyme inducing agent) increases the metabolism of the morphine so that it is cleared from the body much more quickly and its effects are therefore lost.[1,2]

This seems to be the only direct evidence of this interaction, but it is consistent with the way rifampicin affects many other drugs, including methadone (see 'Methadone + Rifampicin', p.66). You should be alert for the need to use an increased dosage of morphine in patients treated with rifampicin. More study is needed.

1. Eckhardt K, Fromm MF, Li S, Hofmann U, Mikus G, Eichelbaum M. Induction of morphine metabolism by rifampicin leads to a loss of analgesia. *Naunyn Schmiedebergs Arch Pharmacol* (1996) 353 (4 Suppl), R145.

2. Fromm MF, Eckhardt K, Li S, Schänzle G, Hofmann U, Mikus G, Eichelbaum M. Loss of analgesic effect of morphine due to coadministration of rifampin. *Pain* (1997) 72, 261–7.

Morphine + Ritonavir

The makers of ritonavir predict that ritonavir will decrease the serum levels of morphine but the clinical relevance of this is uncertain.

Clinical evidence, mechanism, importance and management

The makers of **ritonavir** say that although pharmacokinetic data on the concurrent use of morphine and **ritonavir** is not available, they say that they have unpublished data indicating that **ritonavir** will induce the hepatic enzymes responsible for the glucuronidation of morphine (its principal route of metabolism), and their prediction is that morphine serum levels will be decreased.[1,2] However there seems to be no confirmatory clinical evidence of this interaction and no published data to show whether this interaction is important or not.

1. Norvir (Ritonavir). Abbott Laboratories Limited. Summary of product characteristics, January 2001.

2. Abbott Laboratories Ltd (UK). Personal communication, March 1998.

Morphine + Secobarbital (Quinalbarbitone)

Secobarbital (quinalbarbitone) increases the respiratory depressant effects of morphine, whereas diazepam appears not to interact in this way with pethidine (meperidine).

Clinical evidence, mechanism, importance and management

In 30 healthy subjects it was found that **secobarbital (quinalbarbitone)** and morphine depressed respiration when given alone, a much greater and more prolonged depression occurring when given together.[1] Other respiratory depressant drugs (e.g. other narcotic, opiate analgesics) can also have additive effects. See 'Pethidine (Meperidine) + Chlorpromazine or other Phenothiazines', p.84. **Diazepam** is an alternative tranquillising and sedative drug which appears neither to depress respiration nor to add to the respiratory depressant effects of **pethidine** (**meperidine**), even in patients with chronic obstructive pulmonary disease.[2,3]

1. Zsigmond EK, Flynn K. Effect of secobarbital and morphine on arterial blood gases in healthy human volunteers. *J Clin Pharmacol* (1993) 33, 453–7.

2. Zsigmond EK, Flynn K, Martinez OA. Diazepam and meperidine on arterial blood gases in healthy volunteers. *J Clin Pharmacol* (1974) 14, 377–81.

3. Zsigmond EK, Shively JG, Flynn K. Diazepam and meperidine on arterial blood gases in patients with chronic obstructive pulmonary disease. *J Clin Pharmacol* (1975) 15, 464–68.

Morphine + Tricyclic antidepressants

The bioavailability and the degree of analgesia of oral morphine is increased by the concurrent use of clomipramine, desipramine and possibly amitriptyline. In some circumstances this may be a useful interaction.

Clinical evidence, mechanism, importance and management

Clomipramine or **amitriptyline** in daily doses of 20 or 50 mg increased the AUC of oral morphine by amounts ranging from 28 to 111% in 24 patients being treated for cancer pain. The half-life of morphine was also prolonged.[1] A previous study[2] found that **desipramine** but not **amitriptyline** increased and prolonged morphine analgesia, and a later one by the same group confirmed the value of **desipramine**.[3] The reasons are not understood. The increased analgesia may be due not only to the increased serum levels of morphine, but possibly also to some alteration in the way the morphine affects its receptors. The tricyclics do not appear to possess inherent analgesic activity.

In some circumstances this may be a useful interaction, but the possibility of increased morphine toxicity should also be borne in mind. Whether other tricyclic antidepressants behave similarly is uncertain.

1. Ventafridda V, Ripamonti C, De Conno F, Bianchi M, Pazzuconi F, Panerai AE. Antidepressants increase bioavailability of morphine in cancer patients. *Lancet* (1987) i, 1204.

2. Levine JD, Gordon NC, Smith R, McBryde R. Desipramine enhances opiate postoperative analgesia. *Pain* (1986) 27, 45–9.

3. Gordon NC, Heller PH, Gear RW, Levine JD. Temporal factors in the enhancement of morphine analgesia by desipramine. *Pain* (1993) 53, 273–6.

Nabumetone + Miscellaneous drugs

Nabumetone normally does not interact with acenocoumarol (nicoumalone) or warfarin, but an isolated report describes a raised INR and haemarthrosis in one patient on warfarin attributed to an interaction with nabumetone. Nabumetone appears not to interact with antihypertensive drugs and it is not affected by aluminium hydroxide, paracetamol (acetaminophen) or aspirin, but its absorption is increased by food and milk.

Clinical evidence, mechanism, importance and management

(a) Anticoagulants

Nabumetone has been found not to affect significantly the anticoagulant effects of **warfarin** in either normal subjects[1] or patients,[2,3] moreover it also appears not to affect bleeding time, platelet aggregation or prothrombin times in the absence of an anticoagulant.[4] However an isolated and unexplained report describes an increased INR and haemarthrosis in a patient on **warfarin** a week after nabumetone was added.[5] Another clinical study in osteoarthritis patients also found that nabumetone did not affect the anticoagulant effects of **acenocoumarol** (**nicoumalone**).[6,7] However if anticoagulants are used concurrently, bear in mind that nabumetone can irritate the gut and thereby increase the risk of gastrointestinal bleeding so that good monitoring would be a prudent precaution. Information about other anticoagulants seems to be lacking.

b) Aluminium hydroxide, aspirin, antihypertensives, food, milk, phenytoin, sulphonylureas

Single-dose studies have shown that the absorption of nabumetone is not significantly altered by **aluminium hydroxide**, **aspirin** or **paracetamol** but it is increased by **food** and **milk**.[8] No significant changes in blood pressure were seen in large numbers of hypertensive patients when given nabumetone.[9] Because the active metabolite of nabumetone is highly protein bound and can displace other highly protein bound drugs, the makers of nabumetone say that the effects of hydantoin anticonvulsants (**phenytoin**) and the **sulphonylureas** may possibly be increased,[9] but the risk is theoretical rather than real and the makers say they have no reports of adverse interactions with either of these groups of drugs.[10]

1. Fitzgerald DE. Double blind study to establish whether there is any interaction between nabumetone and warfarin in healthy adult male volunteers. *Roy Soc Med Int Congr Symp* (1985) Series 69, 47–53.
2. Hilleman DE, Mohiuddin SM, Lucas BD. Nonsteroidal antiinflammatory drug use in patients receiving warfarin: emphasis on nabumetone. *Am J Med* (1993) 95 (Suppl 2A), 30S–34S.
3. Hilleman DE, Mohiuddin SM, Lucas BD. Hypoprothrombinemic effect of nabumetone in warfarin-treated patients. *Pharmacotherapy* (1993) 13, 270–1.
4. Al Balla S, Al Momen AK, Al Arfaj H, Al Sugair S, Gader AMA. Interaction between nabumetone — a new non-steroidal anti-inflammatory drug — and the haemostatic system ex vivo. *Haemostasis* (1990) 20, 270–5.
5. Dennis VC, Thomas BK, Hanlon JE. Potentiation of oral anticoagulation and hemarthrosis associated with nabumetone. *Pharmacotherapy* (2000) 20, 234–9.
6. Pardo A, García-Losa M, Fernández-Pavón A, del Castillo S, Pascual-García T, García-Méndez E, Dal-Ré R. A placebo-controlled study of interaction between nabumetone and acenocoumarol. *Br J Clin Pharmacol* (1999) 47, 441–4.
7. Pardo A, Garcia-Losa M, Fernández-Pavón, A, Del Castillo S, Pascual T, García-Méndez E, Dal-Ré R. Drug interaction with acenocoumarol: nabumetone not different from placebo. *Methods Find Exp Clin Pharmacol* (1998) 20 (Suppl A), 69.
8. Schrader HWv, Buscher G, Dierdorf D, Mügge H, Wolf D. Nabumetone — a novel anti-inflammatory drug: the influence of food, milk, antacids, and analgesics on bioavailability of single oral doses. *Int J Clin Pharmacol Ther Toxicol* (1983) 21, 311–21.
9. Relifex (Nabumetone). Summary of product characteristics, May 2002.
10. Bencard, Personal Communication, September 1993.

Naproxen + Amoxicillin

An isolated report describes acute interstitial nephritis with nephrotic syndrome associated with the use of naproxen and amoxicillin.

Clinical evidence, mechanism, importance and management

A man without any previous kidney problems developed acute interstitial nephritis with nephrotic syndrome after taking naproxen for 4 days (4 g) and **amoxicillin** for 10 days (24 g). He appeared to recover when the drugs were stopped, but 3 months later he developed kidney failure and needed haemodialysis. Some months later he had a kidney graft.[1] This is not only a rare syndrome (reported to be only 55 cases in the world literature in 1988)[1] but this is the first and case involving both of these drugs. No special precautions would normally seem to be necessary.

1. Nortier J, Depierreux M, Bourgeois V, Dupont P. Acute interstitial nephritis with nephrotic syndrome after intake of naproxen and amoxycillin. *Nephrol Dial Transplant* (1990) 5, 1055.

Naproxen + Antacids

There is evidence that the absorption of naproxen can be altered (increased or decreased) by some antacids, but the clinical importance of this is uncertain.

Clinical evidence, mechanism, importance and management

Sodium bicarbonate 700 or 1400 mg increased the rate and extent of absorption of single 300-mg doses of naproxen in 14 healthy subjects, whereas 700 mg **magnesium oxide** or **aluminium hydroxide** had the opposite effect and reduced both. On the other hand when 15 or 60 ml *Maalox* were given, the rate and extent of absorption were slightly increased.[1] The reasons are not fully understood, but naproxen becomes more soluble as the pH rises which may account for the increased absorption with **sodium bicarbonate**, whereas **magnesium** and **aluminium** may form less soluble complexes.[2] The clinical importance of these observations is uncertain because single dose, short term studies (these studies only extended over 3 h) do not reliably predict what may happen when multiple doses are taken. Concurrent use need not be avoided but the effectiveness of the naproxen should be monitored if antacids are also given.

1. Segre EJ, Sevelius H, Varady J. Effects of antacids on naproxen absorption. *N Engl J Med* (1974) 291, 582–3.
2. Segre EJ. Drug interactions with naproxen. *Eur J Rheumatol Inflamm* (1979) 2, 12–18.

Naproxen + Colestyramine

Colestyramine delays but does not reduce the absorption of naproxen.

Clinical evidence, mechanism, importance and management

The absorption of naproxen (a single 250-mg dose) was delayed but not reduced in 8 healthy subjects when given with **colestyramine** (4 g in 100 ml orange juice). The amount absorbed after 2 h was reduced from 96 to 51%, but was complete after 5 h.[1] Since naproxen is given chronically, this delay is probably not important. This needs confirmation.

1. Calvo MV, Dominguez-Gil A. Interaction of naproxen with cholestyramine. *Biopharm Drug Dispos* (1984) 5, 33–42.

Naproxen or Diclofenac + Diazepam

Diazepam may affect the pharmacokinetics of naproxen but the combination appears not to produce changes in mood or attention. Diazepam may also affect the pharmacokinetics of diclofenac.

Clinical evidence, mechanism, importance and management

A double-blind crossover study failed to find any clinically important changes in mood or attention in healthy subjects given naproxen and **diazepam**.[1] A single-dose study in 10 healthy subjects found that peak serum concentrations of naproxen 500 mg were reduced by 23%, the time to peak concentration was increased (1.36 to 2 h) and the absorption rate constant was decreased (4.07 to 2.42 h^{-1}) by co-administration of **diazepam** 10 mg. Other pharmacokinetic parameters were not affected.[2] No special precautions appear to be necessary.

In another study in 8 healthy subjects diazepam increased the peak serum levels of diclofenac by 68 and 112% and increased the AUC by 60% while the clearance was reduced by 36%.[3] The effects of **diazepam** on diclofenac appeared to depend on time of co-administration and may reflect time-dependent effects of **diazepam** on gastrointestinal function. More study is needed.

1. Stitt FW, Latour R, Frane JW. A clinical study of naproxen-diazepam drug interaction on tests of mood and attention. *Curr Ther Res* (1977) 21, 149–56.
2. Rao BR, Rambhau D. Influence of diazepam on the pharmacokinetic properties of orally administered naproxen. *Drug Invest* (1992) 4, 416–21.
3. Mahender VN, Rambhau D, Rao BR, Rao VVS, Venkateshwarlu G. Time-dependent influence of diazepam on the pharmacokinetics of orally administered diclofenac sodium in human subjects. *Clin Drug Invest* (1995) 10, 296–301.

Naproxen + Sulglycotide

Sulglycotide does not affect the absorption of naproxen.

Clinical evidence, mechanism, importance and management

Sulglycotide 200 mg had no significant effects on the pharmacokinetics of single 500-mg doses of naproxen in 12 healthy subjects.[1] **Sulglycotide** may therefore be used to protect the gastric mucosa from possible injury by naproxen without altering its absorption.

1. Berté F, Feletti F, De Bernardi di Valserra M, Nazzari M, Cenedese A, Cornelli U. Lack of influence of sulglycotide on naproxen bioavailability in healthy volunteers. *Int J Clin Pharmacol Ther Toxicol* (1988) 26, 125–8.

Narcotic analgesics + Benzodiazepines

The respiratory depressant effects of opioids such as diamorphine and phenoperidine appear to be opposed by the presence of benzodiazepines. Patients on methadone who are given diazepam may experience increased drowsiness and possibly enhanced opiate effects.

Clinical evidence, mechanism, importance and management

A 14-year-old boy with staphylococcal pneumonia secondary to influenza developed adult respiratory distress syndrome. It was decided to suppress his voluntary breathing with opiates and use assisted ventilation and he was therefore given **phenoperidine** and **diazepam** for 11 days, and later **diamorphine** with **lorazepam**. Despite very high doses (19.2 g **diamorphine** in 24 h) his respiratory drive was not suppressed. On day 17, despite serum **morphine** and **lorazepam** levels of 320 and 5.3 micrograms/ml respectively, he remained conscious and his pupils were not constricted.[1] Later *animal* studies confirmed that **lorazepam** opposed the respiratory depressant effects of **morphine**.[1] In this situation this was an unwanted interaction, but under some circumstances it might be used to advantage. The effects on analgesia were not measured.

Four addicts, maintained on **methadone** for at least 6 months, were given 0.3 mg/kg **diazepam** for 9 days. The pharmacokinetics were unaltered and the opiate effects of the **methadone** remained unchanged, but all 4 were sedated.[2] The CNS depressant effects of both drugs would seem to be additive. The lack of a pharmacokinetic interaction was confirmed by another studies.[3] However, another study[4] by the same group of authors suggested that the opiate effects of methadone may be enhanced by diazepam. It has been suggested that the absence of this in the earlier study[2] may possibly be explained by the relatively low daily doses of diazepam they used, in contrast to the higher more intermittent doses used in the later study,[4] which is the pattern of dosage reportedly used by patients.

Concurrent use involving low-to-moderate diazepam dosage need not be avoided but patients given both drugs are likely to experience increased drowsiness, and with a high diazepam dose the possibility of opiate enhancement should be borne in mind.

1. McDonald CF, Thomson SA, Scott NC, Scott W, Grant IWB, Crompton GK. Benzodiazepine-opiate antagonism — a problem in intensive-care therapy. *Intensive Care Med* (1986) 12, 39–42.
2. Pond SM, Tong TG, Benowitz NL, Jacob P, Rigod J. Lack of effect of diazepam on methadone metabolism in methadone-maintained addicts. *Clin Pharmacol Ther* (1982) 31, 139–43.
3. Preston KL, Griffiths RR, Cone EJ, Darwin WD, Gorodetzky CW. Diazepam and methadone blood levels following concurrent administration of diazepam and methadone. *Drug Alcohol Depend* (1986) 18, 195–202.
4. Preston KL, Griffiths RR, Stitzer ML, Bigelow GE, Liebson IA. Diazepam and methadone interactions in methadone maintenance. *Clin Pharmacol Ther* (1984) 36, 534–41.

Narcotic analgesics + Promethazine

Although promethazine can be used to reduce the dosage of many narcotic analgesics, it has potent sedative effects which would be expected to be additive with CNS depressant effects of the narcotics.

Clinical evidence, mechanism, importance and management

The analgesic requirements of more than 300 patients treated with a variety of narcotic analgesics (**morphine, pethidine (meperidine), oxymorphone, hydromorphone, fentanyl, pentazocine**) were reduced 28 to 44% when they were given **promethazine**, 50 mg/70 kg body weight.[1] This possible advantageous interaction would be expected to be accompanied by increased sedation since promethazine is a potent CNS depressant which would be additive with the CNS depressant effects of the narcotics. See also 'Pethidine (Meperidine) + Chlorpromazine or other Phenothiazines', p.84.

1. Keèri-Szàntò M. The mode of action of promethazine in potentiating narcotic drugs. *Br J Anaesth* (1974) 46, 918–24.

Nefopam + Miscellaneous drugs

Nefopam should not be given to patients taking anticonvulsants or the MAOIs. Be cautious with tricyclic antidepressants, anticholinergics and sympathomimetics. The intensity and incidence of side-effects are somewhat increased when nefopam is given with codeine, pentazocine or dextropropoxyphene (propoxyphene).

Clinical evidence, mechanism, importance and management

Detailed information about adverse interactions between nefopam and other drugs seems not to be available, but convulsions have been seen in a few patients and the makers say that nefopam is contraindicated in patients with **a history of convulsive disorders**. Caution should be exercised with the **tricyclic antidepressants** and other drugs with **anticholinergic side-effects** because the convulsive threshold may be lowered and the side-effects may be additive. The CSM in the UK has a number of reports of **urinary retention** caused by nefopam[1], which would be expected to be worsened by drugs with **anticholinergic activity**. Nefopam appears to have **sympathomimetic activity** and the makers say it should not be given with the **MAOIs**. A controlled trial in 45 healthy subjects divided into nine groups of five, each given 60 mg nefopam three times daily for 3 days with either 650 mg **aspirin**, 5 mg **diazepam**, 60 mg **phenobarbital**, 65 mg **dextropropoxyphene (propoxyphene)**, 60 mg **codeine**, 50 mg **pentazocine**, 25 mg **indometacin (indomethacin)** or 50 mg **hydroxyzine pamoate** (all three times daily) found that the only changes were possibly an additive increase in the intensity and incidence of side-effects with nefopam and **codeine, pentazocine** or **dextropropoxyphene**.[2] The incidence of sedation with nefopam is 20 to 30% which, depending on the circumstances, may present a problem if given with **other sedative drugs**.[3]

1. Committee on Safety of Medicines (CSM). Nefopam hydrochloride (Acupan). Current Problems No 24, January 1989.
2. Lasseter KC, Cohen A, Back EL. Nefopam HCl interaction study with eight other drugs. *J Int Med Res* (1976) 4, 195–201.
3. Heel RC, Brogden RN, Pakes GE, Speight TM, Avery GS. Nefopam: a review of its pharmacological properties and therapeutic efficacy. *Drugs* (1980) 19, 249–57.

Nimesulide + Miscellaneous drugs

Nimesulide reduces the serum levels of furosemide (frusemide) and also reduces its sodium depleting effects, but the clinical importance of this has still to be assessed. Nimesulide appears not to interact with digoxin, hypoglycaemic agents or theophylline, but good monitoring has been suggested if it is added to warfarin.

Clinical evidence, mechanism, importance and management

(a) Anticoagulants

A pilot study in 6 patients stabilised on **acenocoumarol (nicoumalone)** found that a single 100-mg dose of nimesulide did not affect the clotting mechanisms, although the platelet aggregating response to adenosine diphosphate, adrenaline (epinephrine) and collagen were reduced for 2 to 4 h.[1] Ten patients on 5 mg **warfarin** daily showed no significant changes in their prothrombin times, partial thromboplastin time or bleeding times when concurrently treated with 100 mg nimesulide twice daily for a week.[2] However since a few patients showed some increased anticoagulant effects, good monitoring has been recommended.[1]

(b) Digoxin

Nimesulide 100 mg twice daily for 7 days had little effect on the pharmacokinetics of **digoxin** in 9 patients with mild heart failure taking 250 micrograms of **digoxin** daily. No major change in their clinical condition occurred.[3] Another, possibly related, study also found no changes.[1] There would seem to be no reason for avoiding concurrent use.

(c) Furosemide (Frusemide)

Nimesulide 200 mg twice daily for 5 days reduced the AUC of **furosemide** 40 mg twice daily by about 25%. The urinary recovery was also reduced to a similar extent, suggesting that one of the interaction mechanisms is a reduction in the absorption from the gut.[4] Inhibition of renal cyclo-oxygenase is also believed to take place and a reduction in the loss of sodium by the kidney occurs.[4] The clinical importance of this interaction awaits assessment, but it is suggested that nimesulide should be used with caution if given with drugs known to have an adverse effect on the blood flow in the kidney.[1]

(d) Hypoglycaemic agents

Although a preliminary report suggested a slight increase in the effects of **glibenclamide (glyburide)** by nimesulide,[1] a later study using various (unnamed) **sulphonylureas** failed to find that it affected fasting blood sugar levels or the glucose tolerance of diabetic patients.[1] No special precautions would therefore seem necessary.

(e) Theophylline

Nimesulide 100 mg twice daily for 7 days did not affect lung function in 10 patients with chronic obstructive airways disease taking 200 mg slow-release **theophylline** twice daily, although there was a slight, clinically insignificant fall in **theophylline** levels, possibly due to enzyme induction. The pharmacokinetics of the nimesulide were unchanged.[5] No special precautions seem to be necessary.

1. Perucca E. Drug interactions with nimesulide. *Drugs* (1993) 46 (Suppl 1), 79–82.
2. Auteri A, Bruni F, Blardi P, Di Renzo M, Pasqui AL, Saletti M, Verzuri MS, Scaricabarozzi I, Vargiu G, Di Perri T. Clinical study on pharmacological interaction between nimesulide and warfarin. *Int J Clin Pharmacol Res* (1991) 11, 267–70.
3. Baggio E, Maraffi F, Montalto C, Nava ML, Torti L, Casciarri I. A clinical assessment of the potential for pharmacological interaction between nimesulide and digoxin in patients with heart failure. *Drugs* (1993) 46 (Suppl 1), 91–4.
4. Steinhäuslin F, Munafo A, Buclin T, Macciocchi A, Biollaz J. Renal effects of nimesulide in furosemide-treated subjects. *Drugs* (1993) 46 (Suppl 1), 257–62.
5. Auteri A, Blardi P, Bruni F, Domini L, Pasqui AL, Saletti M, Verzuri MS, Scaricabarozzi I, Vargiu G, Di Perri T. Pharmacokinetics and pharmacodynamics of slow-release theophylline during treatment with nimesulide. *Int J Clin Pharmacol Res* (1991) 11, 211–7.

NSAIDs + Antacids

The absorption of ketorolac, suprofen, tolmetin and zomepirac is not significantly affected by the concurrent use of magnesium-aluminium hydroxide but a small reduction can occur with ketoprofen. Diclofenac is not affected by aluminium hydroxide, neither ketoprofen nor diclofenac are affected by magnesium hydroxide and ketoprofen is not affected by dimeticone.

Clinical evidence, mechanism, importance and management

Five healthy subjects showed a 22% reduction in the absorption of 50 mg **ketoprofen** (as measured by the amount excreted in the urine) when given 1 g **aluminium hydroxide**, largely as a result of the adsorption of the **ketoprofen** by the antacid.[1] Another study in 12 healthy subjects showed that **dimeticone**, which may be used similarly to antacids to reduce the gastrointestinal effects of NSAIDs, did not significantly affect the bioavailability of a single dose of **ketoprofen** 100 mg.[2] Two teaspoonfuls of a 5.8% suspension of **aluminium hydroxide** had no effect on the bioavailability of a single 50-mg dose of **diclofenac** in 7 healthy subjects.[3] In another study 850 mg **magnesium hydroxide** was found to have no significant effect on the absorption of 50 mg **ketoprofen** or 50 mg **diclofenac**.[4] *Aluco Gel*

(**aluminium hydroxide + magnesium hydroxide**) was also found not to have a clinically important effect on the absorption of enteric-coated **diclofenac**. The AUC of **ketorolac** (10 mg orally) was found to be reduced 11% when taken with an unstated amount of *Maalox* by 12 healthy subjects.[5] Twenty-four healthy subjects were given 200 mg **suprofen** with either 8 oz water or 30 ml *Maalox* and water after an overnight fast. The bioavailability of the **suprofen** was not significantly affected by the antacid.[6] A detailed pharmacokinetic study on 24 healthy subjects similarly showed that *Maalox*, given as single 20 ml doses four times a day over a 3-day period, had no significant effect on the absorption from the gut of **tolmetin** given as single 400-mg doses.[7] Neither single dose nor longer-term administration of 20 ml doses of *Maalox* affects the absorption or the plasma elimination half-life of 100-mg doses of **zomepirac**.[8]

No particular precautions would seem to be needed if these antacids are given with **diclofenac**, **ketorolac**, **suprofen**, **tolmetin** or **zomepirac**, and it seems doubtful if the effects of **ketoprofen** will be reduced to any great extent by **aluminium hydroxide**.

1. Ismail FA, Khalafallah N, Khalil SA. Adsorption of ketoprofen and bumadizone calcium on aluminium-containing antacids and its effect on ketoprofen bioavailability in man. *Int J Pharmaceutics* (1987) 34, 189–96.
2. Presle N, Lapicque F, Gillet P, Herrmann M-A, Bannwarth B, Netter P. Effect of dimethicone (polysilane gel) on the stereoselective pharmacokinetics of ketoprofen. *Eur J Clin Pharmacol* (1998) 54, 351–4.
3. Schumacher A, Faust-Tinnefeldt G, Geissler HE, Gilfrich HJ, Mutschler E. Untersuchungen potentieller Interaktionen von Diclofenac-Natrium (Voltaren) mit einem Antazidum und mit Digitoxin. *Therapiewoche* (1983) 33, 2619–25.
4. Neuvonen PJ. The effect of magnesium hydroxide on the oral absorption of ibuprofen, ketoprofen and diclofenac. *Br J Clin Pharmacol* (1991) 31, 263–6.
5. Mroszczak EJ, Jung D, Yee J, Bynum L, Sevelius H, Massey I. Ketorolac tromethamine pharmacokinetics and metabolism after intravenous, intramuscular, and oral administration in humans and animals. *Pharmacotherapy* (1990) 10 (Suppl 6), 33S–39S.
6. Abrams LS, Marriott TB, Van Horn A. The effect of *Maalox* on the bioavailability of suprofen. *Clin Res* (1983) 31, 626A.
7. Ayres JW, Weidler DJ, MacKichan J, Sakmar E, Hallmark MR, Lemanowicz EF, Wagner JG. Pharmacokinetics of tolmetin with and without concomitant administration of antacid in man. *Eur J Clin Pharmacol* (1977) 12, 421–8.
8. Nayak RK, Ng KT, Gottlieb S. Effect of acute and chronic antacid administration on zomepirac pharmacokinetics. *Clin Pharmacol Ther* (1980) 27, 275.

NSAIDs + Aspirin or NSAIDs

Aspirin is reported to increase, decrease or have no effect on serum indometacin (indomethacin) levels. It reduces serum diclofenac, fenoprofen, flurbiprofen, ibuprofen, ketoprofen, naproxen, pirprofen, tenoxicam and tolmetin levels but not those of piroxicam or sudoxicam. Indometacin and flurbiprofen appear not to affect each other's pharmacokinetics but choline magnesium trisalicylate reduces serum naproxen levels. None of these changes has been clearly shown to improve or worsen treatment but concurrent use is believed to increase gastrointestinal damage. See the Index for other NSAID combinations.

Clinical evidence

The overall picture with **aspirin** and **indometacin** (indomethacin) is confusing and contradictory. Some studies report that **aspirin** reduces serum **indometacin** levels and/or its effects.[1-6] Others claim that no interaction occurs[7-10] and no changes in clinical effectiveness take place.[9,11] Yet other studies using **buffered aspirin** claim that it increases the rate of absorption of **indometacin** and is associated with an increase in side-effects.[12,13] **Aspirin** more than halves the serum levels of **ibuprofen**[14,15] and **tenoxicam**,[16] and reduces the AUC of **flurbiprofen** to about a third[17] but without any clear changes in clinical effectiveness.[18] The pharmacokinetics of the **aspirin** are unchanged by **flurbiprofen**.[17] **Aspirin** also virtually halves the AUC of **fenoprofen**[1] and reduces the AUCs of **ketoprofen**,[19] **diclofenac**[20] and **pirprofen**[21] by about one-third. **Piroxicam**[22] and **sudoxicam**[23] are not significantly affected by **aspirin**, and **naproxen** serum levels are only minimally depressed (AUC decreased by 10-15%).[24,25] **Salicylate** levels are unaffected by **piroxicam**.[22] No clinically significant changes in the pharmacokinetics of either **indometacin** or **flurbiprofen** occur if given concurrently.[26] **Choline magnesium trisalicylate** increases the clearance of **naproxen** by 56% and decreases its serum levels by 26%;[27] the value of concurrent naproxen and salicylate is debatable.[27,28] Plasma **tolmetin** levels are slightly reduced by **aspirin**.[29]

Mechanism

Not resolved. Changes in the rates of absorption and renal clearance have been proposed. The damaging effects of the NSAIDs on the gut appear to be additive.

Importance and management

Although extensively studied, there seems to be no clear evidence, one way or the other, that there are either marked treatment advantages or disadvantages in using any of these drugs concurrently. However it would be prudent to check on the effectiveness of concurrent use and in particular to assess the possible adverse effects of long-term use on the gastrointestinal tract since they all increase the risk of gastric and duodenal ulcers and their complications (bleeding, perforation and death).[30] The CSM in the UK suggests that the risk of adverse reactions with the oral NSAIDs can be reduced by not using more than one NSAID.[31] Some NSAIDs cause more gastrointestinal toxicity than others, a suggested broad 'rank order' of seven NSAIDs commonly used in the UK is as follows, based on epidemiological studies and the yellow card database. Highest risk (**azapropazone**); intermediate risk (**diclofenac, indometacin, ketoprofen and naproxen**, with **piroxicam** more risky than the others); lowest risk (**ibuprofen**).[31] The overall risks associated with the use of NSAIDs are by no means unimportant. One extensive hospital study of emergency admissions and deaths from upper gastrointestinal crises, linked to the use of NSAIDs, suggested that, if extrapolated to the UK population (55 million) as a whole, 62,000 emergency admissions and 4000 deaths annually would be expected.[32]

1. Rubin A, Rodda BE, Warrick P, Gruber CM, Ridolfo AS. Interactions of aspirin with nonsteroidal antiinflammatory drugs in man. *Arthritis Rheum* (1973) 16, 635–45.
2. Kaldestad E, Hansen T, Brath HK. Interaction of indomethacin and acetylsalicylic acid as shown by the serum concentrations of indomethacin and salicylate. *Eur J Clin Pharmacol* (1975) 9, 199–207.
3. Jeremy R, Towson J. Interaction between aspirin and indomethacin in the treatment of rheumatoid arthritis. *Med J Aust* (1970) 3, 127–9.
4. Lei BW, Kwan KC, Duggan DE, Breault GO, Davis RL, Besselaar GH, Czerwinski AW. The influence of aspirin on the absorption and disposition of indomethacin. *Clin Pharmacol Ther* (1976) 19, 110.
5. Kwan KC, Breault GO, Davis RL, Lei BW, Czerwinski AW, Besselaar GH, Duggan DE. Effects of concomitant aspirin administration on the pharmacokinetics of indomethacin in man. *J Pharmacokinet Biopharm* (1978) 6, 451–76.
6. Pawlotsky Y, Chales G, Grosbois B, Miane B, Bourel M. Comparative interaction of aspirin with indomethacin and sulindac in chronic rheumatic diseases. *Eur J Rheumatol Inflamm* (1978) 1, 18–20.
7. Champion D, Mongan E, Paulus H, Sarkissian E, Okun R, Pearson C. Effect of concurrent aspirin (ASA) administration on serum concentrations of indomethacin (I). *Arth Rheum* (1971) 14, 375.
8. Lindquist B, Jensen KM, Johansson H, Hansen T. Effect of concurrent administration of aspirin and indomethacin on serum concentrations. *Clin Pharmacol Ther* (1974) 15, 247–52.
9. Brooks PM, Walker JJ, Bell MA, Buchanan WW, Rhymer AR. Indomethacin—aspirin interaction: a clinical appraisal. *BMJ* (1975) 3, 69–71.
10. Barraclough DRE, Muirden KD, Laby B. Salicylate therapy and drug interaction in rheumatoid arthritis. *Aust N Z J Med* (1975) 5, 518–23.
11. The Cooperating Clinics Committee of the American Rheumatism Association. A three-month trial of indomethacin in rheumatoid arthritis, with special reference to analysis and inference. *Clin Pharmacol Ther* (1967) 8, 11–37.
12. Turner P,Garnham JC. Indomethacin-aspirin interaction. *BMJ* (1975) 2, 368.
13. Garnham JC, Raymond K, Shotton E, Turner P. The effect of buffered aspirin on plasma indomethacin. *Eur J Clin Pharmacol* (1975) 8, 107–13.
14. Albert KS, Gernaat CM. Pharmacokinetics of ibuprofen. *Am J Med* (1984) 77(1A), 40–6.
15. Grennan DM, Ferry DG, Ashworth ME, Kenny RE, Mackinnon M. The aspirin-ibuprofen interaction in rheumatoid arthritis. *Br J Clin Pharmacol* (1979) 8, 497–503.
16. Day RO, Paull PD, Lam S, Swanson BR, Williams KM, Wade DN. The effect of concurrent aspirin upon plasma concentrations of tenoxicam. *Br J Clin Pharmacol* (1988) 26, 455–62.
17. Kaiser DG, Brooks CD, Lomen PL. Pharmacokinetics of flurbiprofen. *Am J Med* (1986) 80 (Suppl 3A), 10–15.
18. Brooks PM, Khong TK. Flurbiprofen-aspirin interaction: a double-blind crossover study. *Curr Med Res Opin* (1977) 5, 53–7.
19. Williams RL, Upton RA, Buskin JN, Jones RM. Ketoprofen-aspirin interactions. *Clin Pharmacol Ther* (1981) 30, 226–31.
20. Willis JV, Kendall MJ, Jack DB. A study of the effect of aspirin on the pharmacokinetics of oral and intravenous diclofenac sodium. *Eur J Clin Pharmacol* (1980) 18, 415–8.
21. Luders RC, Bartlett MF, Maggio-Cavaliere MB, Chao DK, Gum OB, Proctor JD. Effect of aspirin on the disposition of pirprofen in man. *Curr Ther Res* (1982) 31, 413–21.
22. Hobbs DC, Twomey TM. Piroxicam pharmacokinetics in man: aspirin and antacid interaction studies. *J Clin Pharmacol* (1979) 19, 270–81.
23. Wiseman EH, Chang Y-H, Hobbs DC. Interaction of sudoxicam and aspirin in animals and man. *Clin Pharmacol Ther* (1975) 18, 441–8.
24. Segre EJ, Chaplin M, Forchielli E, Runkel R, Sevelius H. Naproxen-aspirin interactions in man. *Clin Pharmacol Ther* (1974) 15, 374–9.
25. Segre E, Sevelius H, Chaplin M, Forchielli E, Runkel R, Rooks W. Interaction of naproxen and aspirin in the rat and in man. *Scand J Rheumatol* (1973) (Suppl 2), 37–42.
26. Rudge SR, Lloyd-Jones JK, Hind ID. Interaction between flurbiprofen and indomethacin in rheumatoid arthritis. *Br J Clin Pharmacol* (1982) 13, 448–51.
27. Furst DE, Sarkissian E, Blocka K, Cassell S, Dromgoole S, Harris ER, Hirschberg JM, Josephson N, Paulus HE. Serum concentrations of salicylate and naproxen during concurrent therapy in patients with rheumatoid arthritis. *Arthritis Rheum* (1987) 30, 1157–61.
28. Willkens RF, Segre EJ. Combination therapy with naproxen and aspirin in rheumatoid arthritis. *Arthritis Rheum* (1976) 19, 677–82.
29. Cressman WA, Wortham GF, Plostnieks J. Absorption and excretion of tolmetin in man. *Clin Pharmacol Ther* (1976) 19, 224–33.
30. Levi S, Shaw-Smith C. Non-steroidal anti-inflammatory drugs: how do they damage the gut? *Br J Rheumatol* (1994) 33, 605–12.
31. Committee on the Safety of Medicines. *Current Problems in Pharmacovigilance* (1994) 20, 9–11.
32. Blower AL, Brooks A, Hill A, Fenn GC, Pearce MY, Morant S, Bardhan KD. Emergency admissions and deaths from upper gastro-intestinal crises in relation to NSAID use. *Gastroenterology* (1994) 106 (4 Suppl), A55.

NSAIDs + Food

Gastric upset caused by indometacin (indomethacin) or suprofen can be minimised by taking them with food or milk. Absorption of ketoprofen may be affected by the calorie/fat content of food. Any interaction seems to be of minimal importance.

Clinical evidence, mechanism, importance and management

Studies in patients and healthy subjects, given single or multiple oral doses of **indometacin (indomethacin)**, have shown that **food** causes marked and complex changes in the immediate serum **indometacin** levels (peak levels are delayed and altered), but fluctuations in levels are somewhat ironed out.[1] However another study comparing **indometacin** concentrations in serum and synovial fluids found that they were about the same 5 to 9 h after taking the **indometacin**,[2] so it would seem that the fluctuations and alterations which go on during the first 5 h are probably much less important than overall serum levels. **Food** also reduces the peak plasma levels of **suprofen** (to 44%) and its bioavailability (to 81%).[3] The likelihood of an undesirable interaction with either of these NSAIDs seems to be small, whereas the advantages of taking them at meal times to avoid gastric upset (a makers recommendation) are considerable. Absorption of **ketoprofen** (as a gastric-juice resistant, sustained-release formulation) was greater when given 4 h before a **low-calorie/low-fat diet** rather than a **high-calorie/high-fat diet**. The effect may be linked to differences in gastric-emptying rate but is unlikely to be of clinical importance.[4]

1. Emori HW, Paulus H, Bluestone R, Champion GD, Pearson GH. Indomethacin serum concentrations in man. Effects of dosage, food, and antacid. *Ann Rheum Dis* (1976) 35, 333–8.
2. Emori HW, Champion GD, Bluestone R, Paulus HE. Simultaneous pharmacokinetics of indomethacin in serum and synovial fluid. *Ann Rheum Dis* (1973) 32, 433–5.
3. Chaikin P, Marriott TB, Simon D, Weintraub HS. Comparative bioavailability of suprofen after coadministration with food or milk. *J Clin Pharmacol* (1988) 28, 1132–5.
4. Le Liboux A, Teule M, Frydman A, Oosterhuis B, Jonkman JHG. Effect of diet on the single- and multiple-dose pharmacokinetics of sustained-release ketoprofen. *Eur J Clin Pharmacol* (1994) 47, 361–6.

NSAIDs + Gold

Gold appears to increase the risk of aspirin-induced liver damage. Fenoprofen seems to be safer.

Clinical evidence, mechanism, importance and management

A study in rheumatoid patients given 3.9 g **aspirin** or 2.4 g **fenoprofen calcium** daily suggested that concurrent gold induction therapy (**sodium aurothiomalate**, by intramuscular injection to a total dose of 985 mg over 6 months) can increase aspirin-induced hepatotoxicity. Levels of AST, LDH and alkaline phosphatase were higher during **aspirin** than during **fenoprofen** treatment. These indicators of liver dysfunction suggest that **fenoprofen** is safer than **aspirin** in this context. Concurrent gold/NSAID treatment was more effective than the NSAIDs alone.[1] **Fenoprofen** would therefore seem to be preferable to **aspirin**.

1. Davis JD, Turner RA, Collins RL, Ruchte IR, Kaufmann JS. Fenoprofen, aspirin, and gold induction in rheumatoid arthritis. *Clin Pharmacol Ther* (1977) 21, 52–61.

NSAIDs + H$_2$-blockers

The H$_2$-blockers (cimetidine, famotidine, nizatidine, ranitidine) have no effect or cause only modest and normally clinically unimportant changes in the serum levels of aspirin, diclofenac, flurbiprofen, ibuprofen, isoxicam, ketoprofen, piroxicam, naproxen and tenoxicam. More importantly they may protect the gastric mucosa from the irritant effects of the NSAIDs.

Clinical evidence

(a) Aspirin and salicylates

Only a modest increase occurred in the serum salicylate levels of 3 out of 6 healthy subjects given 1200 mg **aspirin** 1 h after 300 mg **cimetidine**.[1] The total amount of **aspirin** absorbed was unaltered, but serum levels were slightly raised (from 161 to 180 micrograms/ml) in 13 patients with rheumatoid arthritis on **enteric-coated aspirin** after taking **cimetidine** 300 mg four times daily for 7 days.[2] Six healthy subjects showed little change in the pharmacokinetics of a single 1-g dose of **aspirin** after being given 150 mg **ranitidine** twice daily for a week.[3] **Famotidine** has been found to cause some small changes in the pharmacokinetics of **aspirin**, but this is of doubtful clinical importance.[4]

(b) Azapropazone

A randomised pharmacokinetic study in 12 healthy subjects found that after taking 300 mg **cimetidine** 6-hourly for 6 days the AUC of single 600-mg doses of **azapropazone** was increased by 25%, and of **cimetidine** by 16%. No significant changes in laboratory values (blood counts, enzyme levels) were seen, and adverse effects were small (headaches in 3 subjects).[5]

(c) Diclofenac

Famotidine 40 mg raised the peak plasma levels of **diclofenac** (100 mg in enteric-coated form) in 14 healthy subjects from 5.84 to 7.04 mg/l and they occurred more rapidly (2.0 v 2.75 h). The extent of the absorption was unchanged.[6] **Diclofenac** does not affect the pharmacokinetics of **ranitidine** nor its ability to suppress gastric pH.[7] The pharmacokinetics of **diclofenac** are unaffected by **ranitidine**.[8]

(d) Flurbiprofen

Cimetidine 300 mg three times daily for 2 weeks increased the maximal serum level of **flurbiprofen** (150 to 300 mg daily) in 30 patients with rheumatoid arthritis, but 150 mg **ranitidine** twice daily had no effect. The efficacy of the **flurbiprofen** (assessed by Ritchie score, 50 ft walking time, grip strength) was not altered.[9] Another study in healthy subjects taking single 200-mg doses of **flurbiprofen** found that **flurbiprofen** serum levels were very slightly raised by **cimetidine** 300 mg four times daily and the AUC was raised 13%, but no significant interaction occurred with **ranitidine** 150 mg twice daily.[10]

(e) Ibuprofen

Cimetidine 400 mg three times daily raised the peak serum **ibuprofen** levels (single 600-mg dose) of 13 healthy subjects by 14% (from 56 to 64 micrograms/ml) and AUCs by 6%. No changes were seen with 300 mg **ranitidine** daily.[11] Another study found larger increases (AUC for *R*-ibuprofen of 37%, for *S*-ibuprofen of 19% but these were not statistically significant).[12] However no changes were seen in 5 other studies with **ibuprofen** and **cimetidine** or **ranitidine**,[13–17] one of which also found no interaction between **ibuprofen** and **nizatidine**.[14] However analysis of the results of one study showed that peak serum **ibuprofen** levels in black subjects (USA) were 54% higher

and occurred sooner, whereas in white subjects (USA) they were 27% lower and delayed.[15,18]

(f) Isoxicam

Cimetidine 300 mg four times daily had no effect on the rate and extent of absorption of a single 200-mg dose of **isoxicam** in 11 healthy subjects.[19]

(g) Ketoprofen

Cimetidine 600 mg twice daily was found not to affect the pharmacokinetics of 100 mg enteric-coated **ketoprofen** twice daily in 12 healthy subjects.[20]

(h) Naproxen

One study found no adverse interaction between **naproxen** and **cimetidine** and no alteration in the beneficial effects of **cimetidine** on gastric acid secretion,[21] but another study found a moderate (39 to 60%) decrease in the **naproxen** half-life.[22,23] In the latter study the half-life of **naproxen** was reduced by about 40% by **ranitidine** and 50% by **famotidine**.[23] **Nizatidine** does not affect the pharmacokinetics of **naproxen**.[24]

(i) Piroxicam

Cimetidine 300 mg four times daily for 7 days slightly increased the half-life and the AUC of a single dose of **piroxicam** 20 mg (by 8 and 16% respectively) in 10 healthy subjects.[25] Another study found a 15% rise in the AUC of **piroxicam**,[26] whereas yet another in 12 healthy subjects found that the half-life and AUC of a single dose of **piroxicam** were increased by 41% and 31% respectively by **cimetidine** 200 mg three times daily, and the plasma levels were raised accordingly.[27] For example, at 4 h they were raised almost 25%.[27] **Ranitidine** does not affect the pharmacokinetics of **piroxicam**.[28] No clinically significant changes occurred in the steady-state serum levels of **piroxicam** in yet another study when either **cimetidine** or **nizatidine** were given.[29]

(j) Tenoxicam

The pharmacokinetics of a single 20 mg oral dose of **tenoxicam** was unaltered in 6 healthy subjects after taking 1 g **cimetidine** daily for 7 days.[30]

Mechanisms

Uncertain. Piroxicam serum levels are possibly increased because its metabolism is reduced by the cimetidine.[27]

Importance and management

Most of these interactions between the NSAIDs and cimetidine, famotidine, nizatidine or ranitidine appear to be of no particular clinical importance. The H$_2$-blockers as a group may protect the gastric mucosa from the irritant effects of the NSAIDs and concurrent use may therefore be advantageous.

1. Khoury W, Geraci K, Askari A, Johnson M. The effect of cimetidine on aspirin absorption. *Gastroenterology* (1979) 76, 1169.
2. Willoughby JS, Paton TW, Walker SE, Little AH. The effect of cimetidine on enteric-coated ASA disposition. *Clin Pharmacol Ther* (1983) 33, 268.
3. Corrocher R, Bambara LM, Caramaschi P, Testi R, Girelli M, Pellegatti M, Lomeo A. Effect of ranitidine on the absorption of aspirin. *Digestion* (1987) 37, 178–83.
4. Domecq C, Fuentes A, Hurtado C, Arancibia A. Effect of famotidine on the bioavailability of acetylsalicylic acid. *Med Sci Res* (1993) 21, 219–20.
5. Maggon KK, Lam GM. IV. Interaction between azapropazone and cimetidine, in 'Azapropazone: 20 years of clinical use.' Edited by Rainsford KD (1989), p. 136–45.
6. Suryakumar J, Chakrapani T, Krishna DR. Famotidine affects the pharmacokinetics of diclofenac sodium. *Drug Invest* (1992) 4, 66–8.
7. Blum RA, Alioth C, Chan KKH, Furst DE, Ziehmer BA, Schentag JJ. Diclofenac does not affect the pharmacodynamics of ranitidine. *Clin Pharmacol Ther* (1992) 51, 192.
8. Dammann HG, Simon-Schultz J, Steinhoff I, Damaschke A, Schmoldt A, Sallowsky E. Differential effects of misoprostol and ranitidine on the pharmacokinetics of diclofenac and gastrointestinal symptoms. *Br J Clin Pharmacol* (1993) 36, 345–9.
9. Kreeft JH, Bellamy N, Freeman D. Do H$_2$-antagonists alter the kinetics and effects of chronically-administered flurbiprofen in rheumatoid arthritis? *Clin Invest Med* (1987) 10 (4 Suppl B), B58.
10. Sullivan KM, Small RE, Rock WL, Cox SR, Willis HE. Effects of cimetidine or ranitidine on the pharmacokinetics of flurbiprofen. *Clin Pharm* (1986) 5, 586–9.
11. Ochs HR, Greenblatt DJ, Matlis R, Weinbrenner J. Interaction of ibuprofen with the H-2 receptor antagonists ranitidine and cimetidine. *Clin Pharmacol Ther* (1985) 38, 648–51.
12. Li G, Treiber G, Klotz U. The ibuprofen-cimetidine interaction. Stereochemical considerations. *Drug Invest* (1989) 1, 11–17.
13. Conrad KA, Mayersohn M, Bliss M. Cimetidine does not alter ibuprofen kinetics after a single dose. *Br J Clin Pharmacol* (1984) 18, 624–6.

14. Forsyth DR, Jayasinghe KSA, Roberts CJC. Do nizatidine and cimetidine interact with ibuprofen? *Eur J Clin Pharmacol* (1988) 35, 85–8.
15. Stephenson DW, Small RE, Wood JH, Willis HE, Johnson SM, Karnes HT, Rajas-ekharaiah K. Effect of ranitidine and cimetidine on ibuprofen pharmacokinetics. *Clin Pharm* (1988) 7, 317–21.
16. Evans AM, Nation RL, Sansom LN. Lack of effect of cimetidine on the pharmacokinetics of R(-)- and S(+)-ibuprofen. *Br J Clin Pharmacol* (1989) 28, 143–9.
17. Small RE, Wilmot-Pater MG, McGee BA, Willis HE. Effects of misoprostol or ranitidine on ibuprofen pharmacokinetics. *Clin Pharm* (1991) 10, 870–2.
18. Small RE, Wood JH. Influence of racial differences on effects of ranitidine and cimetidine on ibuprofen pharmacokinetics. *Clin Pharm* (1989) 8, 471–2.
19. Farnham DJ. Studies of isoxicam in combination with aspirin, warfarin sodium, and cimetidine. *Sem Arth Rheum* (1982) 12 (Suppl 2), 179–83.
20. Verbeeck RK, Corman CL, Wallace SM, Herman RJ, Ross SG, Le Morvan P. Single and multiple dose pharmacokinetics of enteric coated ketoprofen: effect of cimetidine. *Eur J Clin Pharmacol* (1988) 35, 521–7.
21. Holford NHG, Altman D, Riegelman S, Buskin JN, Upton RA. Pharmacokinetic and pharmacodynamic study of cimetidine administered with naproxen. *Clin Pharmacol Ther* (1981) 29, 251–2.
22. Vree TB, van den Biggelaar-Martea M, Verwey-van Wissen CPWGM, Vree ML, Guelen PJM. The pharmacokinetics of naproxen, its metabolite *O*-desmethylnaproxen, and their acyl glucuronides in humans. Effect of cimetidine. *Br J Clin Pharmacol* (1993) 35, 467–72.
23. Vree TB, van den Biggelaar-Martea M, Verwey-van Wissen CPWGM, Vree ML, Guelen PJM. The effects of cimetidine, ranitidine and famotidine on the single-dose pharmacokinetics of naproxen and its metabolites in humans. *Int J Clin Pharmacol Ther Toxicol* (1993) 31, 597–601.
24. Satterwhite JH, Bowsher RR, Callaghan JT, Cerimele BJ, Levine LR. Nizatidine: lack of drug interaction with naproxen. *Clin Res* (1992) 40, 706A.
25. Mailhot C, Dahl SL, Ward JR. The effect of cimetidine on serum concentrations of piroxicam. *Pharmacotherapy* (1986) 6, 112–17.
26. Freeman DJ, Danter WR, Carruthers SG. Pharmacokinetic interaction between cimetidine and piroxicam in normal subjects. *Clin Invest Med* (1988) 11, C19.
27. Said SA, Foda AM. Influence of cimetidine on the pharmacokinetics of piroxicam in rat and man. *Arzneimittlforschung* (1989) 39, 790–2.
28. Dixon JS, Lacey LF, Pickup ME, Langley SJ, Page MC. A lack of pharmacokinetic interaction between ranitidine and piroxicam. *Eur J Clin Pharmacol* (1990) 39, 583–6.
29. Milligan PA, McGill PE, Howden CW, Kelman AW, Whiting B. The consequences of H₂ receptor antagonist-piroxicam coadministration in patients with joint disorders. *Eur J Clin Pharmacol* (1993) 45, 507–12.
30. Day RO, Geisslinger G, Paull P, Williams KM. Neither cimetidine nor probenecid affect the pharmacokinetics of tenoxicam in normal volunteers. *Br J Clin Pharmacol* (1994) 37, 79–81.

NSAIDs + Probenecid

Probenecid reduces the loss of carprofen, diflunisal, ketoprofen, ketorolac, naproxen, sodium meclofenamate and tenoxicam from the body, and raises their serum levels. Some increased effects would be expected. Ketorolac and probenecid are contraindicated according to the makers. See Index for other probenecid/NSAID interactions (aspirin, sodium salicylate).

Clinical evidence

Probenecid 1 g approximately doubled the plasma levels of **carprofen** in subjects after a single 100-mg dose and modestly increased its half-life, while the uricosuric effects of the **probenecid** remained virtually unchanged.[1] **Probenecid** 500 mg twice daily increased the steady-state plasma levels of **diflunisal** (250 mg twice daily) by 65% in 8 healthy subjects, and reduced the clearances of the glucuronide metabolites.[2] **Probenecid** 500 mg six-hourly reduced the **ketoprofen** clearance in 6 healthy subjects by 67% when given 50 mg six-hourly.[3] **Probenecid** 500 mg four times daily for 4 days increased the total AUC of a single 10-mg dose of **ketorolac** in 8 subjects more than threefold, increased its half-life from 6.6 to 15.1 h, raised its maximum plasma levels by 24% and reduced its clearance by 67%.[4] **Probenecid** 500 mg twice daily increased the plasma **naproxen** levels of 12 healthy subjects by 50% while taking 250 mg twice daily.[5] Single dose studies on the pharmacokinetics of 100 mg **sodium meclofenamate** in 6 healthy subjects found that pretreatment with **probenecid** (dosage unstated) increased its AUC by an unstated amount and reduced its apparent plasma clearance to 40%, due primarily to a decrease in non-renal clearance.[6] **Probenecid** 1 g twice daily for 4 days increased the maximum serum levels of **tenoxicam** (single 20 mg oral dose) by 25% (from 2.8 to 3.5 micrograms/ml). None of the other pharmacokinetic parameters was significantly altered.[7]

Mechanism

Probenecid possibly inhibits the metabolism (conjugation) of ketoprofen, the glucuronidation of diflunisal[2] and apparently inhibits the loss of conjugates and unchanged naproxen in the urine (half-life prolonged from 14 to 37 h). It also alters its metabolism by the liver.[5] The interactions with the other NSAIDs are not understood.

Importance and management

Information is limited but these interactions appear to be established. The clinical importance of most of them is uncertain, but probably small. Reports of adverse effects seems to be lacking, however be alert for any evidence of increased side-effects. Reduce the NSAID dosage if necessary. The exception is ketorolac which its makers[8] and the British National Formulary suggest should be avoided with probenecid because of the marked changes seen.

1. Yü T-F, Perel J. Pharmacokinetic and clinical studies of carprofen in gout. *J Clin Pharmacol* (1980) 20, 347–51.
2. Macdonald JI, Wallace SM, Herman RJ, Verbeeck RK. Effect of probenecid on the formation and elimination kinetics of the sulphate and glucuronide conjugates of diflunisal. *Eur J Clin Pharmacol* (1995) 47, 519–23.
3. Upton RA, Williams RL, Buskin JN, Jones RM. Effects of probenecid on ketoprofen kinetics. *Clin Pharmacol Ther* (1982) 31, 705–12.
4. Mroszczak EJ, Combs DL, Goldblum R, Yee J, McHugh D, Tsina I, Fratis T. The effect of probenecid on ketorolac pharmacokinetics after oral dosing of ketorolac tromethamine. *Clin Pharmacol Ther* (1992) 51, 154.
5. Runkel R, Mroszczak E, Chaplin M, Sevelius H, Segre E. Naproxen-probenecid interaction. *Clin Pharmacol Ther* (1978) 24, 706–13.
6. Waller ES. The effect of probenecid on the disposition of meclofenamate sodium. *Drug Intell Clin Pharm* (1983) 17, 453–4.
7. Day RO, Geisslinger G, Paull P, Williams KM. Neither cimetidine nor probenecid affect the pharmacokinetics of tenoxicam in normal volunteers. *Br J Clin Pharmacol* (1994) 37, 79–81.
8. Toradol (Ketorolac trometamol). Roche Products Limited. Summary of product characteristics, October 2000.

NSAIDs + Prostaglandins

Isolated cases of adverse neurological side effects have been seen with naproxen or phenylbutazone given with misoprostol. Misoprostol also increases the abdominal pain and other side-effects of diclofenac and indometacin (indomethacin). NSAIDs are reported not to affect the abortive effects of misoprostol. Paracetamol (acetaminophen) intensifies pain if given with mifepristone and sulprostone used to induce abortion. No important adverse or pharmacokinetic interactions seem to occur between aspirin, ibuprofen and misoprostol, between aspirin and arbaprostil.

Clinical evidence, mechanism, importance and management

(a) Aspirin, Ibuprofen

No clinically important pharmacokinetic interactions have been found to occur between 975 mg **aspirin** and 200 micrograms **misoprostol**,[1] between **ibuprofen** and **misoprostol**,[2] or between **aspirin** and **arbaprostil**.[3] No special precautions seem necessary. The makers say that **aspirin** and other **NSAIDs** should be avoided ". . . at least until the follow-up visit 8 to 12 days after **mifepristone** administration . . ." because of a theoretical risk that these prostaglandin synthetase inhibitors might alter the efficacy of the **mifepristone**.[4,5] However a study involving 416 women given **misoprostol** to induce early abortion found that the concurrent use of **NSAIDs** did not interfere with the action of misoprostol to induce abortion.[6]

(b) Diclofenac

An increase in the incidence of abdominal pain, diarrhoea, nausea and dyspepsia occurs if **diclofenac** is combined with **misoprostol**.[7,8] One study found no significant pharmacokinetic changes[9] whereas another found a 20% decrease in the AUC of **diclofenac**.[8] The changes in serum **diclofenac** levels do not seem to be clinically relevant, but warn patients about the possibility of increased stomach pain and diarrhoea. A combined **diclofenac-misoprostol** product is available.

(c) Indometacin (indomethacin)

One study found that 200 micrograms **misoprostol** raised steady-state **indometacin** levels (50 mg three times daily) by about 30%,[10] whereas another found that 400 micrograms **misoprostol** twice daily reduced the AUC of **indometacin** 50 mg twice daily after one dose by 13% and the maximum steady-state plasma concentration by 24%. Concurrent use also resulted in an increase in frequency and severity of abdominal symptoms, frequency of bowel movements and a decrease in faecal consistency.[11] The changes in serum **indometacin** levels do not seem to be clinically important, but warn patients about the possibility of increased stomach pain and diarrhoea.

(d) Naproxen, Etodolac, Phenylbutazone

A man with rheumatoid arthritis on long-term **naproxen** developed ataxic symptoms a few hours after starting **misoprostol**. He said he felt like a drunk person, staggering all over and vomiting. He rapidly improved when he stopped the **misoprostol** but the adverse symptoms recurred on two further occasions when he restarted **misoprostol**.[12] Three patients taking 200 to 400 mg **phenylbutazone** daily developed adverse effects when also given 400 to 800 micrograms **misoprostol** daily.[13] One had headaches, dizziness and ambulatory instability which disappeared and then reappeared when the **misoprostol** was stopped and then restarted. No problems occurred when the **phenylbutazone** was replaced by 400 mg **etodolac** daily. The other 2 developed symptoms including headache, tingles, dizziness, hot flushes and transient diplopia.[13,14] No problems developed when one of them was given **naproxen** and **misoprostol**.[14] The reasons are not understood (possibly a potentiation of the neurological side-effects of **phenylbutazone**?). Although **misoprostol** appears to prevent gastric ulcers caused by the use of NSAIDs and its use is usually uneventful, these adverse reports emphasise that good monitoring may be advisable.

(e) Paracetamol

A study in 45 women undergoing abortion with mifepristone and **sulprostone** found that **paracetamol** (**acetaminophen**) given as a 600-mg suppository intensified rather than reduced their pain, and approximately doubled its duration. The reason is not understood. The women had had the mifepristone 2 days earlier and the **paracetamol** was given 30 min before the intramuscular injection of 0.5 mg **sulprostone**.[15] **Paracetamol** therefore appears not to be a satisfactory analgesic in the presence of sulprostone.

1. Karim A, Rozek LF, Leese PT. Absorption of misoprostol (Cytotec), an antiulcer prostaglandin, is not affected when given concomitantly to healthy human subjects. *Gastroenterology* (1987) 92, 1742.
2. Small RE, Wilmot-Pater MG, McGee BA, Willis HE. Effects of misoprostol or ranitidine on ibuprofen pharmacokinetics. *Clin Pharm* (1991) 10, 870–2.
3. Hsyu P-H, Cox JW, Pullen RH, Gee WL, Euler AR. Pharmacokinetic interactions between arbaprostil and aspirin in humans. *Biopharm Drug Dispos* (1989) 10, 411–22.
4. Mifegyne (Mifepristone), Exelgyn Laboratories. Summary of product characteristics, August 2001.
5. Roussel Laboratories. Personal Communication, August 1995.
6. Creinin MD, Shulman T. Effect of nonsteroidal anti-inflammatory drugs on the action of misoprostol in a regimen for early abortion. *Contraception* (1997) 56, 165–8.
7. Gagnier P. Review of the safety of diclofenac/misoprostol. *Drugs* (1993) 45 (Suppl 1), 31–5.
8. Dammann HG, Simon-Schultz J, Steinhoff I, Damaschke A, Schmoldt A, Sallowsky E. Differential effects of misoprostol and ranitidine on the pharmacokinetics of diclofenac and gastrointestinal symptoms. *Br J Clin Pharmacol* (1993) 36, 345–9.
9. Karim A. Pharmacokinetics of diclofenac and misoprostol when administered alone or as a combination product. *Drugs* (1993) 45 (Suppl 1), 7–14.
10. Rainsford KD, James C, Hunt RH, Stetsko PI, Rischke JA, Karim A, Nicholson PA, Smith M, Hantsbarger G. Effects of misoprostol on the pharmacokinetics of indometacin in human volunteers. *Clin Pharmacol Ther* (1992) 51, 415–21.
11. Kendall MJ, Gibson R, Walt RP. Co-administration of misoprostol or ranitidine with indomethacin: effects on pharmacokinetics, abdominal symptoms and bowel habit. *Aliment Pharmacol Ther* (1992) 6, 437–46.
12. Huq M. Neurological adverse effects of naproxen and misoprostol combination. *Br J Gen Pract* (1990) 40, 432.
13. Jacquemier JM, Lassoued S, Laroche M, Mazières B. Neurosensory adverse effects after phenylbutazone and misoprostol combined treatment. *Lancet* (1989) 2, 1283.
14. Chassagne Ph, Humez C, Gourmelen O, Moore N, Le Loet X, Deshayes P. Neurosensory adverse effects after combined phenylbutazone and misoprostol. *Br J Rheumatol* (1991) 30, 392.
15. Weber B, Fontan J-E. Acetaminophen as a pain enhancer during voluntary interruption of pregnancy with mifepristone and sulprostone. *Eur J Clin Pharmacol* (1990) 39, 609.

NSAIDs + Sucralfate

Sucralfate appears not to interact adversely with aspirin, choline-magnesium trisalicylate, diclofenac, ibuprofen, indometacin (indomethacin), ketoprofen, piroxicam or naproxen.

Clinical evidence, mechanism, importance and management

Eighteen healthy subjects were given 2 g **sucralfate** half-an-hour before taking single doses of either 50 mg **ketoprofen**, 50 mg **indometacin** (**indomethacin**) or 500 mg **naproxen**. Some significant changes were seen (reduced maximal serum concentrations of **ketoprofen**, **naproxen** and **indometacin**, reduced rate of absorption of **naproxen** and **indometacin**, increased time to achieve maximal serum concentrations with **indometacin**) but no alterations in bioavailability occurred.[1] A delay, but no reduction in the total absorption of **naproxen** is described in two studies.[2,3] It is unlikely that its clinical efficacy will be reduced.[2] **Sucralfate** 1 g four times daily for 2 days was found not to decrease the rate of absorption of single 400-mg doses of **ibuprofen**[4] nor of 650-mg doses of **aspirin**.[5] **Sucralfate** 5 g in divided doses did not significantly alter the absorption of single 600-mg doses of **ibuprofen**.[6] **Sucralfate** 2 g was found not to affect significantly the pharmacokinetics of either 20 mg **piroxicam** or 50 mg **diclofenac**.[7] **Sucralfate** 1 g six-hourly was found not to affect the pharmacokinetics of **choline-magnesium trisalicylate** 1.5 g every 12 h.[8]

Single dose studies do not necessarily reliably predict what will happen when patients take drugs regularly, but most of the evidence available suggests that sucralfate is unlikely to have an adverse effect on treatment with these NSAIDs.

1. Caillé G, Du Souich P, Gervais P, Besner J-G. Single dose pharmacokinetics of ketoprofen, indometacin, and naproxen taken alone or with sucralfate. *Biopharm Drug Dispos* (1987) 8, 173–83.
2. Caille G, du Souich P, Gervais P, Besner JG, Vezina M. Effects of concurrent sucralfate administration on pharmacokinetics of naproxen. *Am J Med* (1987) 83 (Suppl 3B), 67–73.
3. Lafontaine D, Mailhot C, Vermeulen M, Bissonnette B, Lambert C. Influence of chewable sucralfate or a standard meal on the bioavailability of naproxen. *Clin Pharm* (1990) 9, 773–7.
4. Anaya AL, Mayersohn M, Conrad KA, Dimmitt DC. The influence of sucralfate on ibuprofen absorption in healthy adult males. *Biopharm Drug Dispos* (1986) 7, 443–51.
5. Lau A, Chang C-W, Schlesinger P. Evaluation of a potential drug interaction between sucralfate and aspirin. *Gastroenterology* (1985) 88, 1465.
6. Pugh MC, Small RE, Garnett WR, Townsend RJ, Willis HE. Effect of sucralfate on ibuprofen absorption in normal volunteers. *Clin Pharm* (1984) 3, 630–3.
7. Ungethüm W. Study on the interaction between sucralfate and diclofenac/piroxicam in healthy volunteers. *Arzneimittelforschung* (1991) 41, 797–800.
8. Schneider DK, Gannon RH, Sweeney KR, DeFusco PA. Influence of sucralfate on trisilate bioavailability. *J Clin Pharmacol* (1991) 31, 377–9.

Oxycodone + Fluoxetine

An isolated report describes a marked reduction in the analgesic effects of oxycodone in a patient treated with fluoxetine.

Clinical evidence, mechanism, importance and management

A man with advanced multiple sclerosis found that when he began to take 20 mg **fluoxetine** daily for depression he needed to increase his analgesic dosage of oxycodone (for painful muscle spasms) about fourfold, from 13 to 15 tablets of 5 mg to about 50 to 55 daily. The reason is thought to be that the **fluoxetine** inhibits the activity of cytochrome P450 isoenzyme CYP2D6 within the liver so that the metabolism of oxycodone to an active metabolite (oxymorphone) is reduced.[1] This patient was found to be a 'poor' metaboliser (about 7% of the population) so that this interaction would not be expected to occur in the majority of patients.

1. Otton SV, Wu D, Joffe RT, Cheung SW, Sellers EM. Inhibition by fluoxetine of cytochrome P450 2D6 activity. *Clin Pharmacol Ther* (1993) 53, 401–9.

Oxyphenbutazone or Phenylbutazone + Anabolic steroids

Serum oxyphenbutazone levels are raised about 40% by the use of methandienone (methandrostenolone). Phenylbutazone appears to be unaffected.

Clinical evidence

Oxyphenbutazone levels were raised 43% (range 5 to 100%) in 6 subjects on 300 to 400 mg **oxyphenbutazone** daily for 2 to 5 weeks when given **methandienone**. Neither 5 mg **prednisone** nor 1.5 mg **dexamethasone** daily were found to affect oxyphenbutazone levels.[1]

Two other studies confirm this interaction with **oxyphenbutazone**.[2,3] One of them found no interaction with **phenylbutazone**.[2]

Mechanism

Uncertain. One idea is that the anabolic steroids alter the distribution of oxyphenbutazone between the tissues and plasma so that more remains in circulation. There may also possibly be some changes in metabolism. Phenylbutazone possibly does not interact because it displaces oxyphenbutazone (its normal metabolite) from the plasma binding sites, thereby raising the levels of unbound oxyphenbutazone and obliterating the effect of the steroid.

Importance and management

The interaction is established but its importance is uncertain. There seem to be no reports of toxicity arising from concurrent use but the possibility should be borne in mind.

1. Weiner M, Siddiqui AA, Shahani RT, Dayton PG. Effect of steroids on disposition of oxyphenbutazone in man. *Proc Soc Exp Biol Med* (1967) 124, 1170–3.
2. Hvidberg E, Dayton PG, Read JM, Wilson CH. Studies of the interaction of phenylbutazone, oxyphenbutazone and methandrostenolone in man. *Proc Soc Exp Biol Med* (1968) 129, 438–43.
3. Weiner M, Siddiqui AA, Bostanci N, Dayton PG. Drug interactions.The effect of combined administration on the half-life of coumarin and pyrazolone drugs in man. *Fedn Proc* (1965) 24, 153.

Paracetamol (Acetaminophen) + Alcohol

Severe liver damage, fatal in some instances, can occur in some alcoholics and persistent heavy drinkers who take only moderate doses of paracetamol. Occasional and moderate drinkers do not seem to be at risk.

Clinical evidence

Three chronic **alcoholic** patients developed severe liver damage after taking paracetamol (acetaminophen). They demonstrated AST levels of about 7000 to 10,000 IU. Two of them had taken only 10 g paracetamol over 24 or 48 h before admission (normal dosage is up to 4 g daily) but the third patient had taken about 50 g paracetamol over 72 h. One of them died in hepatic coma and a post mortem revealed typical paracetamol toxicity. Two of them also developed renal failure.[1]

There are other reports of liver toxicity in a total of about 30 alcoholics attributed to the concurrent use of **alcohol** and paracetamol. About one-third had been taking daily doses within the recommended daily maximum (4 g daily), and one-third had had doses within the range 4 to 8 g daily.[2-18] Fasting possibly makes things worse.[19] A survey describes a total of another 67 patients, many of whom were **alcoholics** (64%) who developed liver toxicity after taking paracetamol (60% taking daily doses not exceeding 6 g daily). Forty percent were taking less than 4 g daily. More than 90% of them developed AST levels ranging from 3000 to 48,000 IU.[20]

Paracetamol 1 g was found to have no effect on the single-dose pharmacokinetics of **alcohol** in 12 healthy subjects.[21] Another study found that blood **alcohol** levels were raised by 1 g paracetamol but this was not statistically significant.[22]

Mechanism

Only partially understood. Paracetamol (acetaminophen) is normally predominantly metabolised by the liver to non-toxic sulphate and glucuronide conjugates. Persistent heavy drinking stimulates a normally minor biochemical pathway involving cytochrome P450 CYP2E1 which allows the production of unusually large amounts of highly hepatotoxic metabolites. Unless sufficient glutathione is present to detoxify these metabolites (alcoholics often have an inadequate intake of protein), they become covalently bound to liver macromolecules and damage results. In fact alcoholics may possibly be most susceptible to toxicity during alcohol withdrawal because, while drinking, alcohol may possibly compete with the paracetamol for metabolism and even inhibit it. Acute ingestion of alcohol by non-alcoholics appears to protect them against damage because the damaging biochemical pathway is inhibited rather than stimulated.

Importance and management

The incidence of this interaction is uncertain, but possibly fairly small, bearing in mind the very wide-spread use of paracetamol and alcohol. However the damage, when it occurs, can be serious and therefore alcoholics and those who persistently drink heavily should be advised to avoid paracetamol or limit their intake considerably. The normal daily recommended 'safe' maximum of 4 g seems to be too high in some alcoholics. The risk for non-alcoholics, moderate drinkers and those who very occasionally drink a lot appears to be low.

1. McClain CJ, Kromhout JP, Peterson FJ, Holtzman JL. Potentiation of acetaminophen hepatotoxicity by alcohol. *JAMA* (1980) 244, 251–3.
2. Emby DJ, Fraser BN. Hepatotoxicity of paracetamol enhanced by ingestion of alcohol. *S Afr Med J* (1977) 51, 208–9.
3. Goldfinger R, Ahmed KS, Pitchumoni CS, Weseley SA. Concomitant alcohol and drug abuse enhancing acetaminophen toxicity. *Am J Gastroenterol* (1978) 70, 385–8.
4. Barker JD, de Carle DJ, Anuras S. Chronic excessive acetaminophen use and liver damage. *Ann Intern Med* (1977) 87, 299–301.
5. O'Dell JR, Zetterman RK, Burnett DA. Centrilobular hepatic fibrosis following acetaminophen-induced hepatic necrosis in an alcoholic. *JAMA* (1986) 255, 2636–7.
6. McJunkin B, Barwick KW, Little WC, Winfield JB. Fatal massive hepatic necrosis following acetaminophen overdosage. *JAMA* (1976) 236, 1874–5.
7. LaBrecque DR, Mitros FA. Increased hepatotoxicity of acetaminophen in the alcoholic. *Gastroenterology* (1980) 78, 1310.
8. Johnson MW, Friedman PA, Mitch WE. Alcoholism, nonprescription drugs and hepatotoxicity. The risk from unknown acetaminophen ingestion. *Am J Gastroenterol* (1981) 76, 530–3.
9. Licht H, Seeff LB, Zimmerman HJ. Apparent potentiation of acetaminophen hepatotoxicity by alcohol. *Ann Intern Med* (1980) 92, 511.
10. Black M, Cornell JF, Rabin L, Shachter N. Late presentation of acetaminophen hepatotoxicity. *Dig Dis Sci* (1982) 27, 370–4.
11. Fleckenstein JL. *Nyquil* and acute hepatic necrosis. *N Engl J Med* (1985) 313, 48.
12. Gerber MA, Kaufmann H, Klion F, Alpert LI. Acetaminophen associated hepatic injury: report of two cases showing unusual portal tract reactions. *Hum Pathol* (1980) 11, 37–42.
13. Leist MH, Gluskin LE, Payne JA. Enhanced toxicity of acetaminophen in alcoholics: report of three cases. *J Clin Gastroenterol* (1985) 7, 55–9.
14. Himmelstein DU, Woolhandler SJ, Adler RD. Elevated SGOT/SGPT ratio in alcoholic patients with acetaminophen hepatotoxicity. *Am J Gastroenterol* (1984) 79, 718–20.
15. Levinson M. Ulcer, back pain and jaundice in an alcoholic. *Hosp Pract* (1983) 18, 48N, 48S.
16. Seeff LB, Cuccherini BA, Zimmerman HJ, Adler E, Benjamin SB. Acetaminophen hepatotoxicity in alcoholics. A therapeutic misadventure. *Ann Intern Med* (1986) 104, 399–404.
17. Florén C-H, Thesleff P, Nilsson Å. Severe liver damage caused by therapeutic doses of acetaminophen. *Acta Med Scand* (1987) 222, 285–8.
18. Edwards R, Oliphant J. Paracetamol toxicity in chronic alcohol abusers – a plea for greater consumer awareness. *N Z Med J* (1992) 105, 174–5.
19. Whitcomb DC, Block GD. Association of acetaminophen hepatotoxicity with fasting and ethanol use. *JAMA* (1994) 272, 1845–50.
20. Zimmerman HJ, Maddrey WC. Acetaminophen (paracetamol) hepatotoxicity with regular intake of alcohol: analysis of instances of therapeutic misadventure. *Hepatology* (1995) 22, 767–73.
21. Melander O, Lidén A, Melander A. Pharmacokinetic interactions of alcohol and acetylsalicylic acid. *Eur J Clin Pharmacol* (1995) 48, 151–3.
22. Sharma SC, Feely J. The influence of aspirin and paracetamol on blood concentrations of alcohol in young adults. *Br J Clin Pharmacol* (1996) 41, 467P.

Paracetamol (Acetaminophen) + Anticholinergic agents

Anticholinergic drugs can delay gastric emptying so that the onset of analgesia with paracetamol may be delayed.

Clinical evidence, mechanism, importance and management

Propantheline 30 mg intravenously delayed the peak serum levels of paracetamol (acetaminoiphen) (1.5 g) in 6 convalescent patients from about 1 h to 3 h. Peak concentrations were lowered by about one-third, but the total amount of paracetamol absorbed was unchanged.[1] The reason is that **propantheline** is an anticholinergic drug which slows the rate at which the stomach empties so that the rate of absorption in the gut is reduced. The practical consequence of this is likely to be that rapid pain relief with single doses of paracetamol may be delayed and reduced by anticholinergics (e.g. some antiparkinson drugs, tricyclic antidepressants, some phenothiazines and antihistamines, etc.) but this needs clinical confirmation. Nobody seems to have studied any of these drugs except **propantheline**. If the paracetamol is being taken in repeated doses over extended periods it seems unlikely to be an important interaction because the total amount absorbed is unchanged.

1. Nimmo J, Heading RC, Tothill P, Prescott LF. Pharmacological modification of gastric emptying: effects of propantheline and metoclopramide on paracetamol absorption. *BMJ* (1973) 1, 587–9.

Paracetamol (Acetaminophen) + Anticonvulsants

The effects of paracetamol are possibly reduced in patients taking anticonvulsants (carbamazepine, phenytoin, phenobarbital, primidone). Anticonvulsant serum levels are unaffected. Two isolated reports describe hepatotoxicity in two patients on phenobarbital after taking normal doses of paracetamol. Paracetamol modestly increases the loss of lamotrigine from the body but appears not to affect phenytoin or carbamazepine.

Clinical evidence

(a) Paracetamol (acetaminophen) clearance increased

The AUC of 1 g paracetamol taken orally was found to be 40% lower in 6 epileptic subjects than in 6 healthy subjects. Five of the epileptics were taking at least two of the following drugs: **carbamazepine, phenobarbital, primidone, phenytoin**. One was taking only **phenytoin**.[1] Another study found that these anticonvulsants shortened the half-life of paracetamol.[2] Yet another found that the clearance of paracetamol was increased 46% by **phenytoin** and **carbamazepine**.[3]

(b) Anticonvulsant levels unaffected

The serum levels of **phenytoin** and **carbamazepine** in 10 epileptics were found not to be significantly affected by 1500 mg paracetamol daily for 3 days.[4]

(c) Hepatotoxicity

An epileptic on 100 mg **phenobarbital** daily developed hepatitis after taking 1 g paracetamol daily for 3 months for headaches. Within two weeks of stopping the paracetamol her serum transaminase levels had fallen within the normal range which implied that her hepatitis was due to drug-induced liver damage.[5] Another patient on **phenobarbital** developed liver and kidney toxicity after taking only 9 g paracetamol over 48 h.[6] **Phenobarbital** also appeared to have increased the toxic effects of paracetamol in an adolescent who took an overdose of both drugs, which resulted in fatal hepatic encephalopathy.[7]

(d) Lamotrigine effects reduced

A study in 8 normal healthy found that 2.7 g paracetamol daily reduced the AUC of a 300-mg dose of **lamotrigine** by 20% and reduced its half-life by 15%.[8]

Mechanisms

(a). The increased paracetamol clearance is due to the well-recognised enzyme inducing effects of the anticonvulsants which increase its metabolism (glucuronidation and oxidation) and loss from the body.

(b). The liver enzyme induction caused by the phenobarbital apparently resulted in an increase in the production of the hepatotoxic metabolites of paracetamol which exceeded the normal glutathione binding capacity, leading to liver damage.

(c). It seems possible that paracetamol increases the metabolism of the lamotrigine.

Importance and management

Information is limited. The clinical importance of none of these interactions is established and further study is needed. Paracetamol is possibly a less effective analgesic in patients taking the interacting anticonvulsants. The risk of liver damage after overdosage is possibly increased, and perhaps after prolonged consumption[3] although only one case seems to have been reported (cited above).[7] The prolonged use of paracetamol should therefore probably be avoided by patients on these anticonvulsants. It is unlikely that the lamotrigine/paracetamol interaction is of practical importance, but this needs confirmation.

1. Perucca E, Richens A. Paracetamol disposition in normal subjects and in patients treated with antiepileptic drugs. *Br J Clin Pharmacol* (1979) 7, 201–6.
2. Prescott LF, Critchley JAJH, Balali-Mood M, Pentland B. Effects of microsomal enzyme induction on paracetamol metabolism in man. *Br J Clin Pharmacol* (1981) 12, 149–53.
3. Miners JO, Attwood J, Birkett DJ. Determinants of acetaminophen metabolism: effect of inducers and inhibitors of drug metabolism on acetaminophen's metabolic pathways. *Clin Pharmacol Ther* (1984) 35, 480–6.
4. Neuvonen PJ, Lehtovaara R, Bardy A, Elomaa E. Antipyretic analgesics in patients on antiepileptic drug therapy. *Eur J Clin Pharmacol* (1979) 15, 263–8.
5. Pirotte JH. Apparent potentiation by phenobarbital of hepatotoxicity from small doses of acetaminophen. *Ann Intern Med* (1984) 101, 403.
6. Marsepoil T, Mahassani B, Roudiak N, Sebbah JL, Caillard G. Potentialisation de la toxicité hépatique et rénale du paracétamol par le phénobarbital. *JEUR* (1989) 2, 118–20.
7. Wilson JT, Kasantikul V, Harbison R, Martin D. Death in an adolescent following an overdose of acetaminophen and phenobarbital. *Am J Dis Child* (1978) 132, 466–73.
8. Depot M, Powell JR, Messenheimer JA, Cloutier G, Dalton MJ. Kinetic effects of multiple oral doses of acetaminophen on a single oral dose of lamotrigine. *Clin Pharmacol Ther* (1990) 48, 346–55.

Paracetamol (Acetaminophen) + Colestyramine

The absorption of paracetamol may possibly be reduced if colestyramine is given at the same time, but the reduction in absorption is small if given an hour later.

Clinical evidence

When 4 healthy subjects took 12 g **colestyramine** and 2 g paracetamol (acetaminophen) together, the absorption of the paracetamol was reduced by 60% (range 30 to 98%) at 2 h but the results were said not to be statistically significant. When the **colestyramine** was given 1 h after the paracetamol, the absorption was reduced by only 16%.[1]

Mechanism

Colestyramine reduces the absorption, presumably because it binds with the paracetamol in the gut. Separating the dosages minimises mixing in the gut.

Importance and management

An established interaction. The colestyramine should not be given within 1 h of the paracetamol if maximal analgesia is to be achieved.

1. Dordoni B, Willson RA, Thompson RPH, Williams R. Reduction of absorption of paracetamol by activated charcoal and cholestyramine: a possible therapeutic measure. *BMJ* (1973) 3, 86–7.

Paracetamol (Acetaminophen) + Contraceptives, oral or Conjugated oestrogens

Paracetamol is cleared from the body more quickly in women taking oral contraceptives and the analgesic effects are expected to be reduced. Conjugated oestrogens appear not to interact with paracetamol. Paracetamol also increases the absorption of ethinylestradiol from the gut by about 20%.

Clinical evidence

(a) Effect of oral contraceptives or conjugated oestrogens on paracetamol (acetaminophen)

While taking **oral contraceptives** the plasma clearance of paracetamol in seven healthy women, following a single 1.5 g dose, was increased by 64% (from 287 to 470 ml/min) and the elimination half-life decreased by 30% (from 2.40 to 1.67 h), when compared with 7 healthy women not taking **oral contraceptives**.[1]

Other studies have found increases in paracetamol clearance of 41%, 49% and 30%, and corresponding half-life decreases in women on **oral contraceptives**.[2-4]

One study found that conjugated oestrogens taken for at least 3 months did not affect the pharmacokinetics of single doses of paracetamol 650 mg intravenously.[5]

(b) Effect of paracetamol on oral contraceptives

Paracetamol 1 g increased the AUC of **ethinylestradiol** by 21.6% in 6 healthy women.[6,7]

Mechanism

The evidence suggests that the oral contraceptives increase the metabolism (both oxidation and glucuronidation) by the liver of the paracetamol so that it is cleared from the body more quickly.[3] The increased absorption of the ethinylestradiol is probably because the paracetamol reduces its metabolism by the gut wall during absorption.[6,7] It has been suggested that the differences between the effects of oral contraceptives and conjugated oestrogens on paracetamol may be attributable to the influence of progestogens on glucuronide and sulphate conjugation.[5] This needs confirmation.

Importance and management

The pharmacokinetic interaction of the oral contraceptives on paracetamol is well-established but its clinical importance has not been directly studied. It seems likely that an increase in the dosage of paracetamol (acetaminophen) may be needed to achieve optimal analgesic effects in women on the pill but nobody seems to have checked on this. The clinical importance of the increased ethinylestradiol absorption is uncertain.

1. Mitchell MC, Hanew T, Meredith CG, Schenker S. Effects of oral contraceptive steroids on acetaminophen metabolism and elimination. *Clin Pharmacol Ther* (1983) 34, 48–53.
2. Abernethy DR, Divoll M, Ochs HR, Ameer B, Greenblatt DJ. Increased metabolic clearance of acetaminophen with oral contraceptive use. *Obstet Gynecol* (1982) 60, 338–41.
3. Miners JO, Attwood J, Birkett DJ. Influence of sex and oral contraceptive steroids on paracetamol metabolism. *Br J Clin Pharmacol* (1983) 16, 503–9.
4. Mucklow JC, Fraser HS, Bulpitt CJ, Kahn C, Mould G, Dollery CT. Environmental factors affecting paracetamol metabolism in London factory and office workers. *Br J Clin Pharmacol* (1980) 10, 67–74.
5. Scavone JM, Greenblatt DJ, Blyden GT, Luna BG, Harmatz JS. Acetaminophen pharmacokinetics in women receiving conjugated estrogen. *Eur J Clin Pharmacol* (1990) 38, 97–8.
6. Rogers SM, Back DJ, Stevenson P, Grimmer SFM, Orme ML'E. Paracetamol interaction with oral contraceptive steroids. *Br J Clin Pharmacol* (1987) 23, 615P.
7. Rogers SM, Back DJ, Stevenson PJ, Grimmer SFM, Orme ML'E. Paracetamol interaction with oral contraceptive steroids: increased plasma concentration of ethinyloestradiol. *Br J Clin Pharmacol* (1987) 23, 721–5.

Paracetamol (Acetaminophen) + Disulfiram

Disulfiram does not appear to interact adversely with paracetamol.

Clinical evidence, mechanism, importance and management

After taking 200 mg **disulfiram** daily for 5 days, the clearance of paracetamol (a single 500-mg intravenous dose) was reduced by about 10% in 5 healthy subjects without liver disease and 5 others with alcoholic liver cirrhosis.[1] The reason is uncertain. Among the conclusions drawn are that **disulfiram** does not interact adversely with paracetamol, and it might even reduce the risks of paracetamol overdose.[1,2]

1. Poulson HE, Ranek L, Jørgensen L. The influence of disulfiram on acetaminophen metabolism in man. *Xenobiotica* (1991) 21, 243–9.
2. Poulson HE, Loft S, Andersen JR, Andersen M. Disulfiram therapy — adverse drug reactions and interactions. *Acta Psychiatr Scand* (1992) 86 (Suppl 369), 59–66.

Paracetamol (Acetaminophen) + Food

Low and high protein meals do not appear to significantly alter the pharmacokinetics of paracetamol.[1] Another study in South African subjects (Tswanas) found that a high fat meal reduced paracetamol absorption the most, while a high fibre meal delayed absorption the most.[2] The clinical importance of these findings is uncertain.

1. Robertson DRC, Higginson I, Macklin BS, Renwick AG, Waller DG, George CF. The influence of protein containing meals on the pharmacokinetics of levodopa in healthy volunteers. *Br J Clin Pharmacol* (1991) 31, 413–17.
2. Wessels JC, Koeleman HA, Boneschans B, Steyn HS. The influence of different types of breakfast on the absorption of paracetamol among members of an ethnic group. *Int J Clin Pharmacol Ther Toxicol* (1992) 30, 208–13.

Paracetamol (Acetaminophen) + H₂-blockers

Co-administered paracetamol and cimetidine do not interact, but administration of cimetidine one hour before paracetamol may affect paracetamol pharmacokinetics. Ranitidine does not interact with paracetamol.

Clinical evidence, mechanism, importance and management

No clinically important interaction has been seen when paracetamol (acetaminophen) and cimetidine are used concurrently.[1] However, a study in 8 healthy subjects found that although cimetidine 400 mg did not alter the salivary pharmacokinetics of co-administered paracetamol 1 g, delayed administration of paracetamol 1 h after cimetidine resulted in a significant reduction in peak salivary concentration and absorption rate constant of paracetamol, while time to peak concentration and elimination half-life were significantly increased.[2] Ranitidine does not affect the pharmacokinetics of paracetamol.[3] No special precaution would seem to be necessary with ranitidine but the efficacy of paracetamol may be affected if paracetamol is administered after rather than concurrently with cimetidine. More study is required.

1. Chen MM, Lee CS. Cimetidine-acetaminophen interaction in humans. *J Clin Pharmacol* (1985) 25, 227–9.
2. Garba M, Odunola MT, Ahmed BH. Effect of study protocol on the interactions between cimetidine and paracetamol in man. *Eur J Drug Metab Pharmacokinet* (1999) 24, 159–62.
3. Thomas M, Michael MF, Andrew P, Scully N. A study to investigate the effects of ranitidine on the metabolic disposition of paracetamol in man. *Br J Clin Pharmacol* (1988) 25, 671P.

Paracetamol (Acetaminophen) + Isoniazid

A number of reports suggest that the toxicity of paracetamol may be increased by isoniazid so that normal daily analgesic dosages (4 g) may not be safe in some individuals.

Clinical evidence

A woman of 21 who had been taking 300 mg **isoniazid** for 6 months took ten 325-mg tablets of paracetamol (paracetamol) for abdominal cramping. Within about 6 hours she developed marked evidence of liver damage (prolonged prothrombin time, elevated ammonia, transaminases, hyperbilirubinaemia).[1]

A young woman on **isoniazid** who had ingested not more than 11.5 g paracetamol in a suicide gesture, developed life-threatening hepatic and renal toxicity despite the fact that her serum paracetamol levels 13 h later were only 15 micromol/l (toxicity normally associated with levels > 26 micromol/l.)[2]

Six other possible cases of this toxic interaction have been described.[3-5] Three of them had taken only 2 to 6 g paracetamol daily and were under treatment with **isoniazid**, rifampicin and pyrazinamide.[5]

Mechanism

Not established. A possible reason is that the isoniazid induces the mixed-function oxidase enzymes (cytocrome P450 isoenzyme CYP2E1) in both liver and kidneys, resulting in a greater proportion of the paracetamol being converted into toxic metabolites than would normally occur[2] (possibly similar to the increased toxicity of paracetamol seen in chronic alcoholics). The results of an experimental study contrast with this suggestion because there was evidence that isoniazid actually reduces the formation of the toxic metabolite of paracetamol.[6] In some instances the patients were also taking rifampicin and pyrazinamide which may have exacerbated the hepatotoxicity.[5]

Importance and management

Information is limited, but it would now seem prudent to warn patients taking isoniazid to limit their use of paracetamol because it seems that some individuals risk possible paracetamol-induced liver toxicity, even with normal recommended doses. More study is needed to clarify the situation.

1. Crippin JS. Acetaminophen hepatotoxicity: potentiation by isoniazid. *Am J Gastroenterol* (1993) 88, 590–2.
2. Murphy R, Swartz R, Watkins P B. Severe acetaminophen toxicity in a patient receiving isoniazid. *Ann Intern Med* (1990) 113, 799–800.
3. Moulding TS, Redeker AG, Kanel GC. Twenty isoniazid-associated deaths in one state. *Am Rev Respir Dis* (1989) 140, 700–5.
4. Moulding TS, Redeker AG, Kanel GC. Acetaminophen, isoniazid, and hepatic toxicity. *Ann Intern Med* (1991) 114, 431.
5. Nolan CM, Sandblom RE, Thummel KE, Slattery JT, Nelson SD. Hepatotoxicity associated with acetaminophen usage in patients receiving multiple drug therapy for tuberculosis. *Chest* (1994) 105, 408–11.
6. Epstein MM, Nelson SD, Slattery JT, Kalhorn TF, Wall RA, Wright JM. Inhibition of the metabolism of paracetamol by isoniazid. *Br J Clin Pharmacol* (1991) 31, 139–42.

Paracetamol (Acetaminophen) + Kakkonto

Single-dose studies in healthy subjects found no pharmacokinetic interaction with paracetamol and kakkonto, but *animal* studies found increased paracetamol levels.

Clinical evidence, mechanism, importance and management

A study in 6 healthy subjects found that 5 g of **Kakkonto extract**, a Chinese herbal medicine containing extracts of *Puerariae, Ephedrae, Zingiberis, Cinnamomi, Glycyrrhizae, Paeoniae* and *Zizphi* spp. had no effects on the pharmacokinetics of a single 12 mg/kg dose of paracetamol (acetaminophen). A further study in 19 healthy subjects found that 1.25 g **Kakkonto** had no effect on the pharmacokinetics of paracetamol 150 mg (from a preparation also containing salicylamide, caffeine and promethazine-methylene-disalicylate). Because in *animal* studies high doses of **Kakkonto** for 7 days were found to significantly increase serum levels of paracetamol, the authors concluded that further investigations were required to assess safety and efficacy of concurrent use.[1]

1. Qi J, Toyoshima A, Honda Y, Mineshita S. Pharmacokinetic study on acetaminophen: interaction with a Chinese medicine. *J Med Dent Sci* (1997) 44, 31–5.

Paracetamol (Acetaminophen) + Metoclopramide

Metoclopramide increases the rate of absorption of paracetamol and raises its maximum plasma levels.

Clinical evidence, mechanism, importance and management

Metoclopramide 10 mg intravenously increased the peak plasma levels of paracetamol (acetaminophen) by 64% in 5 healthy subjects (slow absorbers of paracetamol) after taking a single 1.5-g dose, and increased its rate of absorption (peak levels reached in 48 instead of 120 min), but the total amount absorbed remained virtually unaltered.[1] Oral **metoclopramide** also increases the rate of paracetamol absorption,[2] probably because the rate of gastric emptying is increased. This interaction is exploited in *Paramax* (a proprietary oral preparation containing both drugs) to increase the effectiveness and onset of analgesia for the treatment of migraine. This is obviously an advantageous interaction in this situation.

1. Nimmo J, Heading RC, Tothill P, Prescott LF. Pharmacological modification of gastric emptying: effects of propantheline and metoclopramide on paracetamol absorption. *BMJ* (1973) 1, 587-9.
2. Crome P, Kimber GR, Wainscott G, Widdop B. The effect of the simultaneous administration of oral metoclopramide on the absorption of paracetamol in healthy volunteers. *Br J Clin Pharmacol* (1981) 11, 430P-431P.

Paracetamol (Acetaminophen) and other drugs + Opioid analgesics

Morphine, pethidine and diamorphine delay gastric emptying so that the rate of absorption of other drugs given orally may be reduced.

Clinical evidence, mechanism, importance and management

The absorption of a single 20-mg/kg dose of paracetamol (acetaminophen) 8 healthy subjects was markedly delayed and reduced 30 min after an intramuscular injection of either **pethidine** 150 mg or **diamorphine** 10 mg. Peak plasma paracetamol levels were reduced from 20 to 13.8 and 5.2 micrograms/ml respectively, and delayed from 22 to 114 and 142 min respectively.[1] This interaction was also observed by the same study group in women in labour who had been given opiate analgesics.[2] **Pethidine** (100 mg intramuscularly) and **morphine** (10 mg intramuscularly) similarly delay the absorption of **diazepam**. Diazepam levels were found to be lower and peak levels were not reached in the 90-min study period compared with peak levels at 60 min in the control group.[3]

The underlying mechanism of these interactions is that the opiate analgesics delay gastric emptying so that the rate of absorption of the other drugs is reduced, but the total amount absorbed is not affected. These were largely investigational studies on interaction mechanisms, and the combined use of the drugs cited seem unlikely to have serious or important clinical consequences.

1. Nimmo WS, Heading RC, Wilson J, Tothill P, Prescott LF. Inhibition of gastric emptying and drug absorption by narcotic analgesics. *Br J Clin Pharmacol* (1975) 2, 509–13.

2. Nimmo WS, Wilson J, Prescott LF. Narcotic analgesics and delayed gastric emptying during labour. *Lancet* (1975) i, 890–3.
3. Gamble JAS, Gaston JH, Nair SG, Dundee JW. Some pharmacological factors influencing the absorption of diazepam following oral administration. *Br J Anaesth* (1976) 48, 1181–5.

Paracetamol (Acetaminophen) + Probenecid

Probenecid reduces the loss of paracetamol from the body.

Clinical evidence, mechanism, importance and management

A metabolic study in 10 healthy subjects found that the clearance of paracetamol (1500 mg) was almost halved (from 6.23 to 3.42 ml/min) when taken 1 h after 1 g **probenecid**. The amount of unchanged paracetamol in the urine stayed the same, but the amount of paracetamol glucuronide fell sharply. This suggests that the reduced clearance is probably largely due to inhibition by of the paracetamol glucuronidation by the liver. Another study in 11 subjects also found that while taking 500 mg **probenecid** 6-hourly the paracetamol (650 mg intravenously) clearance was almost halved (from 5.05 to 2.72 ml/min/kg).[2] The practical consequences of this interaction are uncertain but there seem to be no adverse reports.

1. Kamali F. The effect of probenecid on paracetamol metabolism and pharmacokinetics. *Eur J Clin Pharmacol* (1993) 45, 551–3.
2. Abernethy DR, Ameer B, Greenblatt DJ. Probenecid inhibition of acetaminophen and lorazepam glucuronidation. *Clin Pharmacol Ther* (1984) 35, 224.

Paracetamol (Acetaminophen) + Rifampicin (Rifampin) or Sulfinpyrazone

Sulfinpyrazone and rifampicin (rifampin) increase the loss of paracetamol from the body.

Clinical evidence, mechanism, importance and management

Sulfinpyrazone has been found to increase the clearance of paracetamol (acetaminophne) (+ 23%) as a result of increased metabolism (glucuronidation, oxidation) by the liver. It has been suggested that, as a result, the risk of liver damage may be increased after overdosage and perhaps during prolonged consumption, but this has yet to be confirmed.[1] **Rifampicin** (600 mg daily) was also found to increase the clearance of paracetamol in two patients but no precise data were given in the report.[2] The clinical importance of these findings awaits further study, however see also 'Paracetamol (Acetaminophen) + Isoniazid', p.81.

1. Miners JO, Attwood J, Birkett DJ. Determinants of acetaminophen metabolism: effect of inducers and inhibitors of drug metabolism on acetaminophen's metabolic pathways. *Clin Pharmacol Ther* (1984) 35, 480–6.
2. Prescott LF, Critchley JAJH, Balali-Mood M, Pentland B. Effects of microsomal enzyme induction on paracetamol metabolism in man. *Br J Clin Pharmacol* (1981) 12, 149–53.

Paracetamol (Acetaminophen) + Sucralfate

No change in the bioavailability of 1 g paracetamol was found in 6 healthy subjects when given 1 g sucralfate, using salivary paracetamol levels over 4 h as a measure.[1] Concurrent use need not be avoided.

1. Kamali F, Fry JR, Smart HL, Bell GD. A double-blind placebo-controlled study to examine effects of sucralfate on paracetamol absorption. *Br J Clin Pharmacol* (1985) 19, 113–4.

Penicillamine + Antacids

The absorption of penicillamine from the gut can be reduced by 30 to 40% if antacids containing aluminium and magnesium hydroxides are taken concurrently.

Clinical evidence

Maalox-plus (**aluminium hydroxide, magnesium hydroxide, simeticone**) 30 ml reduced the absorption of a single 500-mg dose of penicillamine in six healthy subjects by a third.[1] Another study found that 30 ml *Aludrox* (**aluminium and magnesium hydroxides**) reduced the absorption by about 40%.[2]

Mechanism

The most likely explanation is that the penicillamine forms less soluble chelates with magnesium and aluminium ions in the gut which reduces its absorption.[2] Another idea is that the penicillamine is possibly less stable at the higher pH values caused by the antacid.[1]

Importance and management

An established interaction of clinical importance. If maximal absorption is needed the administration of the two drugs should be separated to avoid mixing in the gut. Two hours or so has been found enough for most other drugs which interact similarly. There seems to be nothing documented about other antacids.

1. Osman MA, Patel RB, Schuna A, Sundstrom WR, Welling PG. Reduction in oral penicillamine absorption by food, antacid and ferrous sulphate. *Clin Pharmacol Ther* (1983) 33, 465–70.
2. Ifan A, Welling PG. Pharmacokinetics of oral 500-mg penicillamine: effect of antacids on absorption. *Biopharm Drug Dispos* (1986) 7, 401–5.

Penicillamine + Food

Food can reduce the absorption of penicillamine by as much as a half.

Clinical evidence

The presence of **food** reduced the plasma penicillamine levels by about 50% (from 3.05 to 1.52 micrograms/ml) in healthy subjects given 500 mg. The total amount absorbed was reduced similarly.[1,2]

These figures are in good agreement with previous findings.[3]

Mechanism

Uncertain. One suggestion is that food delays stomach emptying so that the penicillamine is exposed to more prolonged degradation in the stomach.[2] Another idea is that the protein in food reduces penicillamine absorption.

Importance and management

An established interaction. If maximal effects are required the penicillamine should not be taken with food.

1. Schuna A, Osman MA, Patel RB, Welling PG, Sundstrom WR. Influence of food on the bioavailability of penicillamine. *J Rheumatol* (1983) 10, 95–7.
2. Osman MA, Patel RB, Schuna A, Sundstrom WR, Welling PG. Reduction in oral penicillamine absorption by food, antacid and ferrous sulphate. *Clin Pharmacol Ther* (1983) 33, 465–70.
3. Bergstrom RF, Kay DR, Harkcom TM, Wagner JG. Penicillamine kinetics in normal subjects. *Clin Pharmacol Ther* (1981) 30, 404–13.

Penicillamine + Iron preparations

The absorption of penicillamine can be reduced as much as two-thirds by the concurrent use of oral iron preparations.

Clinical evidence

Ferrous iron (as *Fersamal*) 90 mg reduced the absorption of 250 mg penicillamine in 5 healthy subjects by about two-thirds (using the cupruretic effects of penicillamine as a measure).[1]

A two-thirds reduction in absorption has been described in 6 other subjects given 500 mg penicillamine and 300 mg **ferrous sulphate**.[2] Other studies confirm this interaction.[3,4] There is also evidence that withdrawal of **iron** from patients stabilized on penicillamine without a reduction in the dosage can lead to the development of toxicity (nephropathy).[5]

Mechanism

It is believed that the iron and penicillamine form a chemical complex or chelate within the gut which is less easily absorbed.

Importance and management

An established and clinically important interaction. For maximal absorption give the iron at least 2 h after the penicillamine. This should reduce their admixture in the gut.[1] Do not withdraw iron suddenly from patients stabilized on penicillamine because the marked increase in absorption which follows may precipitate penicillamine toxicity. The toxic effects of penicillamine seem to be dependent on the size of the dose and possibly also related to the rate at which the dosage is increased.[5] Only ferrous sulphate and fumarate have been studied but other iron preparations would be expected to interact similarly.

1. Lyle WH. Penicillamine and iron. *Lancet* (1976) ii, 420.
2. Osman MA, Patel RB, Schuna A, Sundstrom WR, Welling PG. Reduction in oral penicillamine absorption by food, antacid, and ferrous sulphate. *Clin Pharmacol Ther* (1983) 33, 465–70.
3. Lyle WH, Pearcey DF, Hui M. Inhibition of penicillamine-induced cupruresis by oral iron. *Proc R Soc Med* (1977) 70 (Suppl 3), 48–9.
4. Hall ND, Blake DR, Alexander GJM, Vaisey C, Bacon PA. Serum SH reactivity: a simple assessment of D-penicillamine absorption? *Rheumatol Int* (1981) 1, 39–41.
5. Harkness JAL, Blake DR. Penicillamine nephropathy and iron. *Lancet* (1982) ii, 1368–9.

Penicillamine + Miscellaneous drugs

Penicillamine plasma levels are increased by chloroquine and to a lesser extent by indometacin (indomethacin). An increase in penicillamine toxicity is a possibility. An isolated report describes penicillamine-induced breast enlargement in a woman when given a combined oral contraceptive.

Clinical evidence, mechanism, importance and management

(a) Penicillamine + Chloroquine or Indometacin (Indomethacin)

Studies in which **chloroquine** was given to patients on penicillamine found that it was more effective, less effective, or indistinguishable from penicillamine alone, however in some instances penicillamine toxicity was reported to be increased.[1] A pharmacokinetic study in patients with rheumatoid arthritis on 250 mg penicillamine daily found that single doses of **chloroquine phosphate** (250 mg) increased the AUC by 34%, and raised the peak plasma levels by about 55%.[1] It seems possible therefore that any increased toxicity is simply a reflection of increased plasma penicillamine levels. Be alert for evidence of toxicity if both drugs are used. **Indometacin** was also found in the study cited to increase the AUC of penicillamine by 26% and the peak plasma levels by about 22%.[1]

(b) Penicillamine + Oral contraceptives, Corticosteroids, Cimetidine

A woman with Wilson's disease began to develop dark facial hair about 10 months after starting treatment with 1250 to 1500 mg penicillamine daily. When her testosterone levels were found to be slightly raised, after 20 months she was started on a combined **oral contraceptive**, but within a month her breasts began to enlarge and become more tender, and after a further 6 months the penicillamine was replaced by trientine hydrochloride.[2] The reasons are not understood, but the authors of the report suggest that the penicillamine was the prime cause of the macromastia, but it possibly needed the presence of a 'second trigger' (i.e. the **oral contraceptive**) to set things in motion.[2] There are 12 other cases of macromastia and gynaecomastia on record associated with the use of penicillamine, in some of which the second trigger may possibly have been a **corticosteroid** or **cimetidine**.[2] Macromastia appears to be an unusual side-effect of penicillamine and there would seem to be no general reason for patients taking penicillamine to avoid **oral contraceptives**.

1. Seideman P, Lindström B. Pharmacokinetic interactions of penicillamine in rheumatoid arthritis. *J Rheumatol* (1989) 16, 473–4.
2. Rose BI, LeMaire WJ, Jeffers LJ. Macromastia in a woman treated with penicillamine and oral contraceptives. *J Reprod Med* (1990) 35, 43–5.

Pentazocine + Amitriptyline

Concurrent use appears not to increase the impairment of psychomotor skills (such as those needed for driving) more than each drug given alone, but respiratory depression is increased.

Clinical evidence, mechanism, importance and management

Eleven healthy subjects found that both pentazocine and **amitriptyline** caused them to feel drowsy, muzzy and clumsy, and both reduced the performance of a number of psychomotor tests. However when they were given 30 mg pentazocine intramuscularly after taking **amitriptyline** 50 mg daily for a week, the combination of drugs appeared not to impair driving or occupational skills more than either drug given alone.[1] Even so, patients should be warned of the side-effects of each drug. Respiratory depression was increased which may be undesirable in patients with a restricted respiratory capacity.[1]

1. Saarialho-Kere U, Mattila MJ, Seppälä T. Parenteral pentazocine: effects on psychomotor skills and respiration, and interactions with amitriptyline. *Eur J Clin Pharmacol* (1988) 35, 483–9.

Pentazocine + Tobacco smoking or Environmental pollution

Those who smoke or who live in urban areas where the air is heavily polluted may need about 50% more pentazocine to achieve satisfactory analgesia than those who do not smoke or who live where the air is clean.

Clinical evidence, mechanism, importance and management

A study in which pentazocine was used to supplement nitrous oxide relaxant anaesthesia found that patients who came from an urban environment needed about 50% more pentazocine than those who lived in the country (3.6 compared with 2.4 micrograms/kg/min). Roughly the same difference was seen between those who **smoked** and those who did not (3.8 compared with 2.5 micrograms/kg/min).[1] In another study it was found that those who smoked metabolized 40% more pentazocine than non-smokers.[2]

The likely reason for these differences is that **tobacco smoke** and **polluted city air** contain chemical compounds which act as enzyme inducing agents which increase the rate at which the liver metabolises pentazocine (and probably other drugs as well). Smokers and urban

dwellers from polluted areas may need about 40 to 50% more pentazocine than country dwellers and non-smokers to achieve the equivalent amount of analgesia.

1. Keeri-Szanto M, Pomeroy JR. Atmospheric pollution and pentazocine metabolism. *Lancet* (1971) i, 947–9.
2. Vaughan DP, Beckett AH, Robbie DS. The influence of smoking on the intersubject variation in pentazocine elimination. *Br J Clin Pharmacol* (1976) 3, 279–83.

Pethidine (Meperidine) + Aciclovir

An isolated report describes pethidine toxicity associated
with the concurrent use of high dose aciclovir.

Clinical evidence, mechanism, importance and management

A man with Hodgkin's disease was treated with high dose **aciclovir**
for localised herpes zoster, and with pethidine, methadone and carbi-
dopa-levodopa for pain. On the second day he experienced nausea,
vomiting and confusion, and later dysarthria, lethargy and ataxia. Despite vigorous treatment he later died. It was concluded that some of
the adverse effects were due to pethidine toxicity arising from norpethidine accumulation, associated with renal impairment due to the
aciclovir.[1]

1. Johnson R, Douglas J, Corey L, Krasney H. Adverse effects with acyclovir and meperidine. *Ann Intern Med* (1985) 103, 962–3.

Pethidine (Meperidine) + Barbiturates

A single case report describes greatly increased sedation with
severe CNS toxicity in a woman given pethidine after receiving phenobarbital for a 2 weeks. The analgesic effects of
pethidine can be reduced by barbiturates.

Clinical evidence

(a) Increased pethidine toxicity

A woman whose pain had been satisfactorily controlled with pethidine without particular CNS depression, showed prolonged sedation
with severe CNS toxicity when later given pethidine after being treated with **phenobarbital** 30 mg four times daily for a 2 weeks as anticonvulsant therapy.[1]

(b) Pethidine effects reduced

Studies in women undergoing dilatation and curettage found that **thiopental** and **pentobarbital** increased their sensitivity to pain, and opposed the analgesic effects of pethidine.[2] This confirmed the findings
of a previous study.[3] A marked anti-analgesic effect has been seen
with large doses of **thiopental** up to 5 hours after commonly used
doses of **thiopental**.[2] This anti-analgesic effect is also said to be produced by **phenobarbital**.[2]

Mechanism

Studies in the patient cited, in 4 other patients and in 2 normal subjects revealed that phenobarbital stimulates the liver enzymes concerned with the metabolism (*N*-demethylation) of pethidine so that
the production of its more toxic metabolite (norpethidine, normeperidine) is increased. The toxicity seen appears to be the combined effects of this compound and the directly sedative effects of the
barbiturate.[1,4]

Importance and management

There is only one report of toxicity, but the metabolic changes described under 'Mechanism' were seen in other patients and subjects.
The general clinical importance is uncertain but concurrent use
should be undertaken with care. It has also been suggested that if the
pethidine is continued but the barbiturate suddenly withdrawn, the

toxic concentrations of norpethidine might lead to convulsions in the
absence of the anticonvulsant.[1] Whether other barbiturates behave
similarly is not clear, but it is possible. More study is needed to confirm these possibilities. Be aware that the barbiturates reduce analgesia. The metabolic product of pethidine is a less effective analgesic
than the parent compound.

1. Stambaugh JE, Wainer IW, Hemphill DM, Schwartz I. A potentially toxic drug interaction between pethidine (meperidine) and phenobarbitone. *Lancet* (1977) i, 398–9.
2. Dundee JW. Alterations in response to somatic pain associated with anaesthesia. II. The
   effect of thiopentone and pentobarbitone. *Br J Anaesth* (1960) 32, 407–14.
3. Clutton Brock JC. Some pain threshold studies with particular reference to thiopentone.
   Anaesthesia (1960) 15, 71.
4. Stambaugh JE, Wainer IW, Schwartz I. The effect of phenobarbital on the metabolism of
   meperidine in normal volunteers. *J Clin Pharmacol* (1978) 18, 482–90.

Pethidine (Meperidine) + Chlorpromazine or other Phenothiazines

Pethidine (meperidine) and chlorpromazine can be used together for increased analgesia and for premedication before
anaesthesia, but increased respiratory depression, sedation,
CNS toxicity and hypotension can also occur. Other phenothiazines such as levomepromazine (methotrimeprazine),
promethazine, prochlorperazine, propiomazine and thioridazine may also interact to cause some of these effects.

Clinical evidence

A study in 6 healthy subjects found that pethidine (meperidine) alone
(100 mg/70 kg body-weight) caused respiratory depression whereas
chlorpromazine alone (25 mg/70 kg body weight) had no consistent
effects. But together the respiratory depressant effects were greater
than with pethidine alone. One subject showed marked respiratory
depression, beginning about half-an-hour after receiving both drugs
and lasting 2 h.[1] No change in the pharmacokinetics of pethidine
(meperidine) when **chlorpromazine** was given was found in a single
dose study in healthy subjects, but the excretion of the metabolites of
pethidine was increased. The symptoms of light-headedness, dry
mouth and lethargy were significantly increased and 4 subjects experienced such marked debilitation that they required assistance to continue the study. Systolic and diastolic blood pressures were also
depressed.[2]

Studies with other phenothiazines have shown that **promethazine**[3]
prolongs the analgesic effects of pethidine, and **promethaz-
ine/pentobarbital**,[4] **propiomazine**[5,6] and **levomepromazine (methotrimeprazine)**[7] can all increase its respiratory depressant effects,
but the effects of **prochlorperazine**[8] on respiration were not statistically significant. A 12-year-old patient on chronic **thioridazine** treatment (50 mg twice daily) given premedication with pethidine,
diphenhydramine and glycopyrrolate was very lethargic after surgery
and stopped breathing. He responded to naloxone.[9] Increased respiratory depression has also been seen with **hydroxyzine** (not a phenothiazine) in one study,[6] but not in two others.[10,11]

Mechanism

There is evidence that chlorpromazine can increase the activity of the
liver microsomal enzymes so that the metabolism of pethidine to
normeperidine and normeperidinic acid are increased. These are toxic
and probably account for the lethargy and hypotension seen in one
study.[2] The effects of the phenothiazines on pethidine-induced respiratory depression may be related.

Importance and management

Lower doses of pethidine can be used if chlorpromazine is given,[12]
but concurrent use is clearly not without its problems. A marked increase in respiratory depression can occur in some susceptible individuals.[1] The authors of one study[2] offer the opinion that ". . . the
debilitation observed after pethidine-chlorpromazine combinations
again raises the question as to whether the clinical use of this combi-

nation is justified. The risks of increased CNS toxicity and hypotension outweigh the uncertain advantages, and the use of the combination as an analgesic should probably be discontinued."

Information about other adverse pethidine/phenothiazine interactions seems to be very limited. The pethidine/thioridazine interaction cited here seems to be the only one recorded.[9] Increased analgesia may occur but it may be accompanied by increased respiratory depression[3,5] which is undesirable in patients with existing respiratory insufficiency.

1. Lambertsen CJ, Wendel H, Longenhagen JB. The separate and combined respiratory effects of chlorpromazine and meperidine in normal men controlled at 46 mmHg alveolar pCO₂. *J Pharm Exp Ther* (1961) 131, 381–93.
2. Stambaugh JE, Wainer IW. Drug interaction: meperidine and chlorpromazine, a toxic combination. *J Clin Pharmacol* (1981) 21, 140–6.
3. Keèri-Szàntò M. The mode of action of promethazine in potentiating narcotic drugs. *Br J Anaesth* (1974) 46, 918–24.
4. Pierce JA, Garofalvo ML. Preoperative medication and its effect on blood gases. *JAMA* (1965) 194, 487.
5. Hoffman JC, Smith TC. The respiratory effects of meperidine and propiomazine in man. *Anesthesiology* (1970) 32, 325–31.
6. Reier CE, Johnstone RE. Respiratory depression: narcotic versus narcotic-tranquillizer combinations. *Anesth Analg* (1970) 49, 119–124.
7. Zsigmond EK, Flynn K. The effect of methotrimeprazine on arterial blood gases in human volunteers. *J Clin Pharmacol* (1988) 28, 1033–7.
8. Steen SN, Yates M. The effects of benzquinamide and prochlorperazine, separately and combined, on the human respiratory center. *Anesthesiology* (1972) 36, 519–20.
9. Grothe DR, Ereshefsky L, Jann MW, Fidone GS. Clinical implications of the neuroleptic-opioid interaction. *Drug Intell Clin Pharm* (1986) 20, 75–7.
10. Zsigmond EK, Flynn K, Shively JG. Effect of hydroxyzine and meperidine on arterial blood gases in healthy human volunteers. *J Clin Pharmacol* (1989) 29, 85–90.
11. Zsigmond EK, Flynn K, Shively JG. Effect of hydroxyzine and meperidine on arterial blood gases in patients with chronic obstructive pulmonary disease. *Int J Clin Pharmacol Ther Toxicol* (1993) 31, 124–9.
12. Sadove MS, Levin MJ, Rose RF, Schwartz L, Witt FW. Chlorpromazine and narcotics in the management of pain of malignant lesions. *JAMA* (1954) 155, 626–8.

Pethidine (Meperidine) + Cimetidine or Ranitidine

Cimetidine reduces the loss of pethidine from the body, but the extent to which this increases its analgesic and toxic effects is uncertain. It is probably not large. Ranitidine does not interact.

Clinical evidence

Cimetidine 600 mg twice daily for one week reduced the total body clearance of single 70 mg intravenous doses of pethidine (meperidine) in 8 healthy subjects by 22%.[1]

Mechanism

The probable reason is that the cimetidine inhibits the liver microsomal enzymes concerned with metabolism of the pethidine, because it was found that the production of the normal metabolite of pethidine, norpethidine, was reduced by 23%.[1] This is supported by other studies with both *animal* and human liver microsomes.[2]

Importance and management

Information about the pethidine/cimetidine interaction is very limited, and its clinical importance is uncertain but probably small. Since the effects of the pethidine, both analgesic and toxic, would be expected to be increased to some extent, concurrent use should be monitored. An alternative would be to use ranitidine which has been shown not to interact.[3]

1. Guay DRP, Meatherall RC, Chalmers JL, Grahame GR. Cimetidine alters pethidine disposition in man. *Br J Clin Pharmacol* (1984) 18, 907–14.
2. Knodell RG, Holtzman JL, Crankshaw DL, Steele NM, Stanley LN. Drug metabolism by rat and human hepatic microsomes in response to interaction with H₂-receptor antagonists. *Gastroenterology* (1982) 82, 84–8.
3. Guay DRP, Meatherall RC, Chalmers JL, Grahame GR, Hudson RJ. Ranitidine does not alter pethidine disposition in man. *Br J Clin Pharmacol* (1985) 20, 55–9.

Pethidine (Meperidine) + Furazolidone

On the basis of *animal* experiments it has been suggested that if pethidine and furazolidone are used concurrently in man, a serious hyperpyrexic reaction may occur similar to that seen with the antidepressant MAOIs. This has yet to be confirmed.

Clinical evidence, mechanism, importance and management

Fatal hyperpyrexia followed the injection of pethidine (meperidine) in *rabbits* given oral **furazolidone** for 4 days.[1] On the basis of this observation, linked with the known MAO-inhibitory properties of **furazolidone** in man[2] and the well-documented MAOI/pethidine interaction in man, there would seem to be the possibility of some risk if these two drugs are used together. More study is needed to find out if this is a clinically important interaction or not.

1. Eltayeb IB, and Osman OH. Furazolidoine-pethidine interactions in rabbits. *Br J Pharmacol* (1975) 55, 497–501.
2. Pettinger WA, Soyangco FG, and Oates JA. Monoamine-oxidase inhibition by furazolidone in man. *Clin Res* (1966) 14, 258.

Pethidine (Meperidine) + Phenytoin

An isolated report describes pethidine toxicity in a man taking phenytoin. Other studies confirm that phenytoin increases the production of the toxic metabolite of pethidine.

Clinical evidence

A man of 61 who was addicted to pethidine (meperidine) (5 to 10 g weekly) is reported to have developed repeated seizures and myoclonus despite, even possibly because, he was also taking **phenytoin** (see Mechanism below). The problem resolved when both drugs were stopped.[1]

Mechanism

It is known that phenytoin increases the production of normeperidine, the metabolic product of pethidine which is believed to be responsible for the neurotoxicity of pethidine (seizures, myoclonus, tremors etc). Studies[2,3] in healthy subjects found that 300 mg phenytoin daily for nine days decreased the elimination half-life of pethidine (100 mg orally and 50 mg intravenously) from 6.4 to 4.3 h, and the systemic clearance increased from 14.3 to 18.2 ml/min/kg. Phenytoin is a well recognised and potent enzyme inducing agent.

Importance and management

This seems to be the only report[1] of an adverse pethidine/phenytoin interaction so that its general importance is uncertain, however it would be prudent to monitor concurrent use in any patient. Since the studies cited[2,3] found that pethidine given orally produced more of the toxic metabolite (normeperidine) than when given intravenously, it may be preferable to give pethidine intravenously in patients taking phenytoin.

1. Hochman MS. Meperidine-associated myoclonus and seizures in long-term hemodialysis patients. *Ann Neurol* (1983) 14, 593.
2. Pond SM, Kretzschmar KM. Decreased bioavailability and increased clearance of meperidine during phenytoin administration. *Clin Pharmacol Ther* (1981) 29, 273.
3. Pond SM, Kretschmar KM. Effect of phenytoin on meperidine clearance and normeperidine formation. *Clin Pharmacol Ther* (1981) 30, 680–6.

Phenazone (Antipyrine) + Miscellaneous drugs

Changes in the half-life of phenazone (reduced by liver enzyme-inducers, prolonged by liver enzyme-inhibitors) are used to detect the possible effects of drugs on liver enzyme activity.

Clinical evidence, mechanism, importance and management

Phenazone (antipyrine) is metabolised by mixed function oxidase enzymes in the liver, for which reason it is extensively used as a model drug for studying whether other drugs stimulate (induce) or inhibit liver enzymes. For example, **barbiturates** reduce the half-life of phenazone. In one study **phenobarbital** caused about a 40% reduction thereby demonstrating that the liver enzymes were being stimulated to metabolise the phenazone more rapidly.[1] In contrast, other drugs which are enzyme inhibitors cause the half-life of phenazone to be prolonged which shows that the activity of the metabolising enzymes is reduced. Equally it may be that the drug neither stimulates nor inhibits the enzymes which metabolise phenazone (for example, **spiramycin**[2]).

Thus phenazone often features in drug interaction studies because it provides predictive information about whether a particular drug is likely or not to stimulate or inhibit the metabolism of other drugs, but phenazone itself usually has only a minor role to play as an analgesic and antipyretic.

1. Vesell ES, Page JG. Genetic control of the phenobarbital-induced shortening of plasma antipyrine half-lives in man. *J Clin Invest* (1969) 48, 2202–9.
2. Descotes J, Evreux J Cl. Drug interactions with spiramycin: lack of influence on antipyrine pharmacokinetics. *Chemioterapia* (1987) 6, 337–8.

Phenoperidine + Antacids

An antacid has been shown to increase the plasma levels of phenoperidine given intravenously.

Clinical evidence

Andursil (**aluminium and magnesium hydroxides, magnesium carbonate, simeticone**) considerably increased the plasma levels of phenoperidine in 6 healthy subjects over the 20 min period following a 15 microgram/kg intravenous dose. The peak level rose 60% (from 9.1 to 14.7 nanograms/ml) but fell after 20 min to about the same levels. The AUC over this period was increased by 47%. The secondary peaks in the plasma concentrations were also ironed out.[1]

Mechanism

Uncertain. A possible reason is that changes in gastric pH caused by the antacid may alter the secretion of phenoperidine into the stomach (this also occurs with pethidine).

Importance and management

The clinical significance of this study is uncertain, but it seems possible that in the presence of antacids there may be an increase in both the analgesic and respiratory depressant effects of phenoperidine. More study is needed.

1. Calvey TN, Milne LA, Williams NE, Chan K, Murray GR. Effect of antacids on the plasma concentration of phenoperidine. *Br J Anaesth* (1983) 55, 535–9.

Phenoperidine + Beta-blockers

An isolated report describes a patient with tetanus who showed a very marked fall in blood pressure when given phenoperidine following a dose of propranolol.

Clinical evidence, mechanism, importance and management

A patient with tetanus was treated uneventfully with 2 mg phenoperidine on five occasions over 24 h. Later 2 mg **propranolol** intrave-

nously was used to reduce the heart rate from 150 to 120 bpm, without any fall in blood pressure. When 2 mg phenoperidine was subsequently given, the systolic blood pressure fell to 30 mmHg (heart rate 100 to 120 bpm) and this persisted for 5 to 10 min until reversed by naloxone.[1] The reasons for this marked hypotensive response are not understood. The general importance of this is uncertain because this incident occurred in the context of tetanus.

1. Woods KL. Hypotensive effect of propranolol and phenoperidine in tetanus. *Br Med J* (1978) 2, 1164.

Phenylbutazone + Allopurinol

Allopurinol appears not to interact significantly with phenylbutazone.

Clinical evidence, mechanism, importance and management

Allopurinol 100 mg three times daily in 6 healthy subjects for a month had no effect on the elimination of a 200-mg daily dose of phenylbutazone, and no effect on the steady-state plasma levels of phenylbutazone in three patients taking 200 or 300 mg daily.[1] In another study on 8 patients with acute gouty arthritis it was found that 100 mg **allopurinol** 8 hourly produced small but clinically unimportant effects on the half-life of phenylbutazone (6 mg/kg).[2] No special precautions would seem necessary if both drugs are given.

1. Rawlins MD, Smith SE. Influence of allopurinol on drug metabolism in man. *Br J Pharmacol* (1973) 48, 693–8.
2. Horwitz D, Thorgeirsson SS, Mitchell JR. The influence of allopurinol and size of dose on the metabolism of phenylbutazone in patients with gout. *Eur J Clin Pharmacol* (1977) 12, 133–6.

Phenylbutazone + Barbiturates

Some reduction in the plasma levels of phenylbutazone may be expected if phenobarbital is given concurrently, but the practical importance of this is uncertain.

Clinical evidence, mechanism, importance and management

The half-life of phenylbutazone was reduced by 22 hours after pretreatment with 90 mg **phenobarbital** daily for 3 days.[1] Other studies confirm that it increases the loss of phenylbutazone from the body.[2,3] The probable reason is that the **phenobarbital** increases the metabolism of phenylbutazone by the liver, thereby hastening its clearance.

The clinical importance of this interaction is uncertain (probably small) but be alert for any evidence of reduced phenylbutazone effects if **phenobarbital** is added. Other barbiturates are likely to behave similarly because they are all potent enzyme inducing agents.

1. Levi AJ, Sherlock S, Walker D. Phenylbutazone and isoniazid metabolism in patients with liver disease in relation to previous drug therapy. *Lancet* (1968) i, 1275–9.
2. Whittaker JA, Price Evans DA. Genetic control of phenylbutazone metabolism in man. *BMJ* (1970) 4, 323–8.
3. Anderson KE, Peterson CM, Alvares AP, Kappas A. Oxidative drug metabolism and inducibility by phenobarbital in sickle cell anemia. *Clin Pharmacol Ther* (1977) 22, 580–7.

Phenylbutazone + Colestyramine

Animal **studies suggest that colestyramine may delay the absorption of phenylbutazone, but the clinical importance of this is uncertain.**

Clinical evidence, mechanism, importance and management

An *in vitro* study found that phenylbutazone becomes markedly bound (98%) to **colestyramine**.[1] In *rats* it was found that 71.5 mg/kg and 357.5 mg/kg **colestyramine** reduced phenylbutazone absorption by 32% and 49% respectively after 1 h, and by 22% and 47% after 2 h, but after 4 h the lower dose group showed a 29% increase in absorption and the higher dose group was the same as the control.[1] These results indicate that **colestyramine** reduces the rate of absorption of phenylbutazone initially, however the total amount absorbed was not measured. Nobody seems to have checked on this interaction in man, but until more is known it would seem reasonable, and easy, to separate the dosages as much as possible to prevent admixture in the gut.

1. Gallo D G, Bailey K R, Sheffner A L. The interaction between cholestyramine and drugs. *Proc Soc Exp Biol Med* (1965) 120, 60–5.

Phenylbutazone + Indometacin (Indomethacin)

An isolated report describes transient deterioration in renal function in a patient during recovery from phenylbutazone-induced renal failure when given 25 mg indometacin (indomethacin) three times a day.[1] A possible reason is that the indometacin displaced the residual phenylbutazone from its plasma protein binding sites.[2] This possible interaction does not seem to be of general importance. See the Index for other combinations.

1. Kimberly R, Brandstetter RD. Exacerbation of phenylbutazone-related renal failure by indomethacin. *Arch Intern Med* (1978) 138, 1711–12.
2. Solomon HM, Schrogie JJ, Williams D. The displacement of phenylbutazone-¹⁴C and warfarin-¹⁴C from human albumin by various drugs and fatty acids. *Biochem Pharmacol* (1968) 17, 143–51.

Phenylbutazone + Methylphenidate

Serum phenylbutazone levels are raised by methylphenidate.

Clinical evidence, mechanism, importance and management

Single dose and chronic studies in man using normal daily doses of phenylbutazone (200 to 400 mg) and **methylphenidate** showed that serum phenylbutazone levels were significantly increased in 5 out of 6 subjects, due, it is suggested to inhibition of liver metabolising enzymes.[1] The clinical importance of this is uncertain.

1. Dayton PG, Perel JM, Israili ZH, Faraj BA, Rodewig K, Black N and Goldberg LI. Studies with methylphenidate: drug interactions and metabolism. Int Symp Alc Drug Addiction. Toronto, Ontario, October 1973. (Ed Sellers, EM) Clinical Pharmacology of Psychoactive Drugs, Addiction Res Foundation. ISBN-0-88868-007-4, pages 183–202.

Phenylbutazone + Pesticides

Chronic exposure to lindane and other chlorinated pesticides can increase the rate of metabolism of phenylbutazone.

Clinical evidence, mechanism, importance and management

The plasma half-life of phenylbutazone in a group of men who regularly used **chlorinated insecticide** sprays (mainly **lindane**) as part of their work, was found to be shorter (51 h) than in a control group (64 h), due, it is believed, to the enzyme-inducing effects of the **insecticides**.[1] This is of doubtful direct clinical importance, but it illustrates

the changed metabolism which can occur in those exposed to environmental chemical agents.

1. Kolmodin-Hedman B. Decreased plasma half-life of phenylbutazone in workers exposed to chlorinated pesticides. *Eur J Clin Pharmacol* (1973) 5, 195–8.

Phenylbutazone + Tobacco smoking

The loss of phenylbutazone from the body is greater in smokers than in non-smokers.

Clinical evidence, mechanism, importance and management

The half-life of a single 6-mg/kg dose of phenylbutazone was 37 h in a group of smokers (10 or more **cigarettes** daily for 2 years) compared with 64 h in a group of non-smokers. The metabolic clearance was approximately doubled.[1] The conclusion to be drawn is that those who smoke may possibly need larger or more frequent doses of phenylbutazone to achieve the same therapeutic response, but this needs confirmation.

1. Garg SK, Kiran TNR. Effect of smoking on phenylbutazone disposition. *Int J Clin Pharmacol Ther Toxicol* (1983) 20, 289–90.

Phenylbutazone or Oxyphenbutazone + Tricyclic antidepressants

The tricyclic antidepressants can delay the absorption of phenylbutazone and oxyphenbutazone from the gut, but their antirheumatic effects are probably not affected.

Clinical evidence, mechanism, importance and management

When treated with 75 mg **desipramine** daily the absorption of **phenylbutazone** in 4 depressed women was considerably delayed, but the total amount absorbed (measured by the urinary excretion of oxyphenbutazone) remained unchanged.[1] In another 5 depressed women the half-life of **oxyphenbutazone** was found to be unaltered by 75 mg **desipramine** or **nortriptyline** daily.[2] *Animal* studies have confirmed that the absorption of **phenylbutazone** and **oxyphenbutazone** are delayed by the **tricyclic antidepressants**, probably because their anticholinergic effects reduce the motility of the gut,[3,4] but there seems to be no direct clinical evidence that the antirheumatic effects of either drug are reduced by this interaction. No particular precautions appear to be needed.

1. Consolo S, Morselli PL, Zaccala M, Garattini S. Delayed absorption of phenylbutazone caused by desmethylimipramine in humans. *Eur J Pharmacol* (1970) 10, 239–42.
2. Hammer W, Mårtens S, Sjöqvist F. A comparative study of the metabolism of desmethylimipramine, nortriptyline, and oxyphenbutazone in man. *Clin Pharmacol Ther* (1969) 10, 44–9.
3. Consolo S. An interaction between desipramine and phenylbutazone. *J Pharm Pharmacol* (1968) 20, 574–5.
4. Consolo S, Garattini S. Effect of desipramine on intestinal absorption of phenylbutazone and other drugs. *Eur J Pharmacol* (1969) 6, 322–6.

Piroxicam + Antacids

A multiple-dose study found that Mylanta and Amphojel did not significantly affect the bioavailability of piroxicam.[1] Concurrent use need not be avoided.

1. Hobbs DC, Twomey TM. Piroxicam pharmacokinetics in man: aspirin and antacid interaction studies. *J Clin Pharmacol* (1979) 19, 270–81.

Piroxicam, Meloxicam or Tenoxicam + Colestyramine

Colestyramine increases the loss of meloxicam, piroxicam, and tenoxicam from the body and their therapeutic effects would therefore be expected to be reduced accordingly.

Clinical evidence

(a) Meloxicam

A study in 12 healthy subjects found that 4 g **colestyramine** taken 2 h before a 30 mg intravenous dose of **meloxicam** increased its clearance by 49% and reduced its mean residence time in the body by 39%.[1]

(b) Piroxicam, Tenoxicam

A study on the enterohepatic recycling of **piroxicam** and **tenoxicam** in 8 healthy subjects found that when given 4 g **colestyramine** three times a day, the clearances of 20 mg oral doses of **piroxicam** and 20 mg intravenous doses of **tenoxicam** were increased by 52% and 105% respectively, and their half-lives reduced by 40 and 52% respectively. The **colestyramine** was not given until after the **piroxicam** had been absorbed.[2] Other studies have found similar results.[3,4] The elimination half-life of both analgesics was approximately doubled by 24 g **colestyramine** daily.[3]

Mechanism

Colestyramine binds with some drugs in the gut. Since the colestyramine was not given until the piroxicam had been absorbed and the meloxicam and tenoxicam were given intravenously,[2] it would seem likely that the colestyramine binds with these drugs following their excretion in the bile, thereby preventing their reabsorption and increasing their loss in the faeces.

Importance and management

Direct information appears to be limited to these studies. Unlike the situation with a number of other drugs, this interaction can be reduced but not avoided by separating the dosages. Monitor the effects of concurrent use and increase the NSAID dosages as necessary. Alternatively use other NSAIDs or hypolipidaemic drugs. Colestyramine can be used to speed the removal of piroxicam and tenoxicam following overdosage.[3]

1. Busch U, Heinzel G, Narjes H. The effect of cholestyramine on the pharmacokinetics of meloxicam, a new non-steroidal anti-inflammatory drug (NSAID), in man. *Eur J Clin Pharmacol* (1995) 48, 269–72.
2. Guentert TW, Defoin R, Mosberg H. Accelerated elimination of tenoxicam and piroxicam by cholestyramine. *Clin Pharmacol Ther* (1988) 43, 179.
3. Benveniste C, Striberni R, Dayer P. Indirect assessment of the enterohepatic recirculation of piroxicam and tenoxicam. *Eur J Clin Pharmacol* (1990) 38, 547–9.
4. Ferry DG, Gazeley LR, Busby WJ, Beasley DMG, Edwards IR, Campbell AJ. Enhanced elimination of piroxicam by administration of activated charcoal or cholestyramine. *Eur J Clin Pharmacol* (1990) 39, 599–601.

Sufentanil + Midazolam or Lorazepam

Marked and sudden hypotension has been seen in a few patients premedicated with midazolam or lorazepam when anaesthesia has been induced with sufentanil. Preliminary evidence suggests that midazolam can also reduce the efficacy of sufentanil.

Clinical evidence, mechanism, importance and management

(a) Acute hypotension

A man of 50 scheduled for a heart valve replacement and on clonidine, captopril and furosemide (frusemide) was premedicated with 5 mg **midazolam** intramuscularly, glycopyrrolate intravenously and anaesthetised with 150 micrograms sufentanil over 4 min. His blood pressure fell from 130/60 to 76/40 mmHg and his pulse fell from 90 to 55 bpm. He responded to repeated doses of 0.4 mg atropine and 10 mg ephedrine intravenously.[1] This is consistent with another report of sudden hypotension during anaesthetic induction in four patients given high-dose sufentanil who had received **lorazepam** prior to induction.[2] On the basis of this limited evidence it would now seem prudent to be alert for sudden hypotension in patients given benzodiazepines and sufentanil. More study is needed.

(b) Reduced sufentanil effects

An analysis of 43 patients who were mechanically ventilated following major trauma, and who were given infusions of sufentanil alone or sufentanil plus **midazolam**, found that **midazolam** appeared to reduce the efficacy of the sufentanil. The rate of sufentanil infusion in the group given both drugs (21 patients) was increased more than 50% above the group given sufentanil alone (22 patients). It was found possible to reduce the sufentanil infusion in 8 of patients given sufentanil alone, whereas this was possible in only one patient given both drugs.[3] More study is needed to confirm and evaluate this report.

1. West JM, Estrada S, Heerdt M. Sudden hypotension associated with midazolam and sufentanil. *Anesth Analg* (1987) 66, 693–4.
2. Spiess BD, Sathoff RH, El-Ganzouri ARS, Ivankovich AD. High-dose sufentanil: four cases of sudden hypotension on induction. *Anesth Analg* (1986) 65, 703–5.
3. Luger TJ, Morawetz RF. Clinical evidence for a midazolam-sufentanil interaction in patients with major trauma. *Clin Pharmacol Ther* (1991) 49, 133.

Sulindac + Colestyramine

Colestyramine markedly reduces the absorption of sulindac, even when their administration is separated by as much as 3 h.

Clinical evidence

Colestyramine 4 g twice daily was found to reduce the AUC of 400 mg sulindac by 78% and of its sulphide metabolite by 84% when given to 6 healthy subjects. Even when the sulindac was given 3 h before the **colestyramine**, its AUC was reduced by 44% and that of its sulphide metabolite by 55%.[1]

Mechanism

Colestyramine is a non-absorbable anion exchange resin which can bind to drugs such as sulindac in the gut, thereby reducing the amount available for absorption. Even staggering the dosages apparently only partially prevents their admixture in the gut because sulindac is recycled by the enterohepatic shunt (i.e. it is absorbed and then re-secreted in the bile).

Importance and management

Information is limited but the interaction appears to be established. Separating the dosages only goes some way towards reducing the effects of this interaction. On the basis of this study it would seem that you may need approximately to double the sulindac dosage even if the sulindac and colestyramine are separated by 3 h.

1. Malloy MJ, Ravis WR, Pennell AT, Hagan DR, Betagari S, Doshi DH. Influence of cholestyramine resin administration on single dose sulindac pharmacokinetics. *Int J Clin Pharmacol Ther* (1994) 32, 286–9.

Sulindac + Dimethyl sulfoxide (DMSO)

A single case report describes a patient on sulindac who developed a serious peripheral neuropathy when he applied DMSO to his skin.

Clinical evidence, mechanism, importance and management

A man with a long history of degenerative arthritis was treated uneventfully with 400 mg sulindac daily for 6 months until, without his doctor's knowledge, he began regularly to apply a topical preparation containing 90% **DMSO** to his upper and lower extremities. Soon afterwards he began to experience pain, weakness in all his extremities, and difficulty in standing or walking. He was found to have both segmental demyelination and axonal neuropathy. He made a partial recovery but was unable to walk without an artificial aid.[1] The reason for this reaction is not known, but studies in *rats* have shown that **DMSO** can inhibit a reductase enzyme by which sulindac is metabolised,[2] and it may be that the high concentrations of unmetabolised sulindac increased the neurotoxic activity of the **DMSO**. Although there is only this case on record, its seriousness suggests that patients should not use sulindac and **DMSO**-containing preparations concurrently.

1. Reinstein L, Mahon R, Russo GL. Peripheral neuropathy after concomitant dimethyl sulfoxide use and sulindac therapy. *Arch Phys Med Rehabil* (1982) 63, 581–4.
2. Swanson BN, Mojaverian P, Boppana VK, Dudash M. Dimethylsulfoxide (DMSO) interaction with sulindac (SO). *Pharmacologist* (1981) 23, 196.

Tenidap + Miscellaneous drugs

Tenidap increases the serum levels of lithium[1] and also causes a very small rise in blood pressure in patients on enalapril,[2] but it appears not to interact to a clinically relevant extent with cimetidine,[3] digoxin,[4] food,[5] Maalox,[5] oral contraceptives,[6] tolbutamide,[7] thiazide diuretics[8] or warfarin.[9] The serum levels of free phenytoin[10] may rise. The development of tenidap for use in arthritis has stopped because of concerns about its effect on bone mineral density and at present this drug is not available.

1. Apseloff G, Wilner KD, Von Deutsch DA, Gerber N. Tenidap sodium decreases renal clearance and increases steady-state concentrations of lithium in healthy volunteers. *Br J Clin Pharmacol* (1995) 39 (Suppl 1), 25S–28S.
2. Rapeport WG, Grimwood VC, Hosie J, Sloan PM, Korlipara K, Silvert BD, James I, Mechie GL, Anderton JL. The effect of tenidap on the anti-hypertensive efficacy of ACE inhibitors in patients treated for mild to moderate hypertension. *Br J Clin Pharmacol* (1995) 39 (Suppl 1), 57S–61S.
3. Wilner KD, Gardner MJ. Cimetidine does not alter the clearance or plasma binding of tenidap in healthy male volunteers. *Br J Clin Pharmacol* (1995) 39 (Suppl 1), 21S–24S.
4. Dewland PM, Grimwood VC, Rapeport WG, Coates PE. Effect of tenidap sodium on digoxin pharmacokinetics in healthy young men. *Br J Clin Pharmacol* (1995) 39 (Suppl 1), 43S–46S.
5. Coates PE, Mesure R. Pharmacokinetics of tenidap sodium administered with food or antacid in healthy volunteers. *Br J Clin Pharmacol* (1995) 39 (Suppl 1), 17S–19S.
6. Coates PE, Mesure R. An investigation into the effect of tenidap sodium on the pharmacokinetics of a combined oral contraceptive. *Br J Clin Pharmacol* (1995) 39 (Suppl 1), 47S–50S.
7. Wilner KD, Gardner MJ. Tenidap sodium does not alter the clearance or plasma protein binding of tolbutamide in healthy male volunteers. *Br J Clin Pharmacol* (1995) 39 (Suppl 1), 39S–42S.
8. Rapeport WG, Grimwood VC, Korlipara K, Grillage MG, James I, Anderton JL, Selfridge DI. The effect of tenidap on the anti-hypertensive efficacy of thiazide diuretics in patients treated for mild to moderate hypertension. *Br J Clin Pharmacol* (1995) 39 (Suppl 1), 51S–55S.
9. Apseloff G, Wilner KD, Gerber N. Effect of tenidap on the pharmacodynamics and plasma protein binding of warfarin in healthy volunteers. *Br J Clin Pharmacol* (1995) 39 (Suppl 1), 29S–33S.
10. Blum RA, Schentag JJ, Gardner MJ, Wilner KD. The effect of tenidap sodium on the disposition and plasma protein binding of phenytoin in healthy male volunteers. *Br J Clin Pharmacol* (1995) 39 (Suppl 1), 35S–38S.

Tenoxicam + Antacids or Food

Food and antacids appear not have a clinically important effect on the absorption of tenoxicam.

Clinical evidence, mechanism, importance and management

The bioavailability of 20 mg tenoxicam was found to be unaffected in 12 healthy subjects by **aluminium hydroxide** (*Amphojel*) or **aluminium/magnesium hydroxide** (*Mylanta*) whether taken before, at the same time, or afterwards. **Food** delayed the achievement of peak serum levels.[1] No special precautions seem necessary.

1. Day RO, Lam S, Paull P, Wade D. Effect of food and various antacids on the absorption of tenoxicam. *Br J Clin Pharmacol* (1987) 24, 323–8.

Tramadol + Miscellaneous drugs

Tramadol has been reported to increase the anticoagulant effects of warfarin and phenprocoumon in a few patients. The plasma levels and analgesic effects of tramadol are reduced by carbamazepine, but cimetidine does not interact. The CSM in the UK advises caution with tricyclic and SSRI antidepressants because of the possible risk of convulsions, and the avoidance of tramadol in epileptics. The makers suggest the theoretical possibility of adverse interactions with CNS depressants and those drugs which affect monoaminergic transmission (MAOIs, lithium). The serotonin syndrome developed in one patient on iproniazid and tramadol, and delirium in another given tramadol shortly after stopping phenelzine.

Clinical evidence, mechanism, importance and management

(a) Anticoagulants

A brief report describes 5 elderly patients (ages 71 to 84), anticoagulated with **warfarin** or **phenprocoumon** and on a range of other drugs, who showed clinically important rises in INRs (up to threefold) a few days after starting to take tramadol. One of the patients bled. In some of the cases it was possible to manage the situation by reducing the anticoagulant dosage.[1]

A 61-year old woman with a mitral valve replacement on **warfarin** developed ecchymoses about 2 weeks after starting 50-mg tramadol 6-hourly. Her prothrombin time was found to have risen to 39.6 s and her INR was 10.6. These values returned to normal when the tramadol was withdrawn and the **warfarin** temporarily stopped.[2] Another patient on **warfarin** developed a prothrombin time of 27.8 s, an INR of 7.31 and some bleeding about 5 weeks after starting 150 mg tramadol daily.[3] Two further patients on **phenprocoumon** developed raised INRs (5 and 8.5 respectively) shortly after starting 50 to 100 mg tramadol four times daily, but this report is complicated by use of 4 g paracetamol (acetaminophen) daily which can also interact with coumarin anticoagulants.[4]

In contrast, 19 patients anticoagulated with **phenprocoumon** showed unchanged mean INR values when concurrently given 50 mg tramadol three times daily for a week, but one patient showed an INR rise from 4 to 7.5, and another from a just under 5 to 6.[5,6] The reasons for this interaction, when it occurs, are not understood.

These reports clearly show that some patients on anticoagulants may develop clinically important INR rises and even bleeding when given tramadol. The incidence is not known but because the interaction is unpredictable it would now be prudent to monitor prothrombin times closely in any patient on anticoagulants when tramadol is first added, being alert for the need to reduce the anticoagulant dosage. Information about anticoagulants other than **warfarin** and **phenpro-**

coumon is lacking but the same precautions would be appropriate. More study is needed.

(b) Anticonvulsants and drugs affecting the convulsive threshold

The CSM has publicised 27 reports of convulsions and one of worsening epilepsy with tramadol, a reporting rate of 1 in 7000 patients. Some of them were given doses well in excess of those recommended and one patient was also taking **propofol** (recognised to be associated with convulsions), while some of the others were also taking **tricyclic antidepressants** (8 patients) and **SSRIs** (5 patients), both of which are known to reduce the convulsive threshold. For this reason the CSM recommend the avoidance of tramadol in patients with a history of epilepsy unless compelling reasons exist, and caution in its use with both of these two groups of drugs.[7]

An unpublished study by the makers found that the maximum plasma levels of tramadol and the elimination half-life of a single 50-mg dose were reduced by 50% after using 400 mg **carbamazepine** twice daily for 9 days.[8] On the basis of this study the makers say that the analgesic effectiveness of tramadol and its duration of action would be expected to be reduced.[8,9] However in the light of the CSM warning it would seem prudent to avoid concurrent use if the **carbamazepine** is being used to control epilepsy.

(c) Cimetidine

The makers say that only clinically insignificant changes occur in the serum concentrations of tramadol if **cimetidine** is given concurrently.[9] No special precautions would therefore seem necessary.

(d) Monoamine oxidase inhibitors

The makers of tramadol first contraindicated its use with the **MAOIs** on the grounds that it is an opioid agonist, like pethidine (meperidine).[8,9] This may mean the serotonin syndrome could develop. Later this prediction was confirmed by a report[10] of the development of the serotonin syndrome (myoclonus, tremor, sweating, hyper-reflexia, tachycardia) in a patient on **iproniazid** when tramadol was added to his drug regimen. When the tramadol was stopped the patient recovered within 48 h. Another single case report describes the development of severe delirium in a patient within 3 days of stopping long term treatment with 45 mg **phenelzine** daily and starting 100 mg intramuscular tramadol three times daily. The patient became anxious and confused, and developed visual hallucinations and persecutory ideation. The symptoms disappeared within 48 h of stopping the tramadol.[11] There are therefore sound practical and theoretical reasons for patients on MAOIs to avoid tramadol.

(e) Other drugs

The makers say that the concurrent use of other **CNS depressants** including **alcohol** may potentiate the CNS depressant effects of tramadol, although sedation does not seem to be a significant side-effect. They also suggest that an interaction could occur with **lithium** because, in common with tramadol, it might enhance monoaminergic neurotransmission, and for this reason good monitoring is appropriate. These warnings would seem to be based on theoretical considerations and so far there appear to be no reports of any serious adverse interactions arising from concurrent use.

1. Jensen K. Interaktion mellem tramadol og orale antikoagulantia. *Ugeskr Laeger* (1997) 159, 785–6.
2. Sabbe JR, Sims PJ, Sims MH. Tramadol-warfarin interaction. *Pharmacotherapy* (1998) 18, 871–3.
3. Scher ML, Huntington NH, Vitillo JA. Potential interaction between tramadol and warfarin. *Ann Pharmacother* (1997) 31, 646–7.
4. Madsen H, Rasmussen JM, Brøsen K. Interaction between tramadol and phenprocoumon. *Lancet* (1997) 350, 637.
5. Boeijinga JK, van Meegen E. Pharmacodynamic/-kinetic influence of tramadol on the anticoagulant coumarin derivative phenprocoumon in patients. Data on file, Searle 1997.
6. Boeijinga JK, van Meegen E, van den Ende R, Schook CE, Cohen AF. Is there interaction between tramadol and phenprocoumon? *Lancet* (1997) 350, 1552.
7. Committee on Safety of Medicines. *Current Problems in Pharmacovigilance* (1996) 22, 11.
8. GD Searle. Personal Communication, November 1994.
9. Zydol (Tramadol) Pharmacia. Summary of product characteristics, October 1998.
10. de Larquier A, Vial T, Bréjoux G, Descotes J. Syndrome sérotoninergique lors de l'association tramadol et iproniazide. *Therapie* (1999) 54, 767–8.
11. Calvisi V, Ansseau M. Confusion mentale liée à l'administration de tramadol chez une patiente sous IMAO. *Rev Med Liege* (1999) 54, 912–3.

4

Antiarrhythmic drug interactions

This chapter is concerned with the Class I antiarrhythmic agents that possess some local anaesthetic properties and with Class III drugs (see Table 4.2). Antiarrhythmic agents that fall into other classes are dealt with in the chapters devoted to specific groups of drugs (beta-blockers, digitalis glycosides, calcium channel blockers). Some antiarrhythmics that do not fit into this usual classification are also included in this chapter (e.g. adenosine). Interactions in which the antiarrhythmic drug is the affecting agent, rather than the drug whose activity is altered, are dealt with in other chapters. Consult the Index for a full listing.

Predicting interactions between two antiarrhythmic drugs

It is difficult to know exactly what is likely to happen if two antiarrhythmics are used together. The hope is always that a combination will work better than just one drug, and many

Table 4.1 Antiarrhythmic agents

Generic names	Proprietary names
Adenosine	Adenocard, Adenocor, Adenoscan, Adenyl, Adesinon-P, Adrekar, Ampecyclal, Atepadene, Atepodin, Bio-Regenerat S 3, Krenosin, Krenosine, Myoviton
Ajmaline	Gilurytmal
Amiodarone	Amidox, Amiobeta, Amiodacore, Amiodar, Amiodarex, Amiogamma, Amiohexal, Amirone, Ancoron, Angiodarona, Aratac, Atlansil, Braxan, Cardinorm, Cor Mio, Corbionax, Cordarex, Cordarone, Cordarone X, Diodarone, Escodarone, Forken, Hexarone, Miodaron, Miodrone, Pacerone, Procor, Rivodarone, Sedacoron, Tachydaron, Taquicord, Trangorex
Aprindine	Amidonal, Fiboran
Bretylium	Bretylate
Cibenzoline (Cifenline)	Cipralan, Exacor
Diprafenone	
Disopyramide	Dicorantil, Dicorynan, Dimodan, Dirythmin, Dirytmin, Disomet, Diso-Duriles, Durbis, Isomide, Isorythm, Norpace, Ritmodan, Ritmoforine, Rythmical, Rythmodan, Rythmodul
Dofetilide	Tikosyn
Encainide	
Flecainide	Almarytm, Apocard, Aristocor, Flecaine, Flecatab, Tambocor
Ibutilide	Corvert
Lidocaine (Lignocaine)	Basicaina, Curadent, Dentipatch, Dilocaine, Docaine, Duo-Trach Kit, Dynexan, Ecocain, ELA-Max, Esracain, Gelicain, Laryng-O-Jet, Licain, Lident Adrenalina, Lident Andrenor, Lidesthesin, Lidocation, Lidocaton, Lidodan, Lidoject, Lidonostrum, Lidosen, Lidrian, Lignospan, Lignostab-A, Lincaina, Linisol, Llorentecaina Noradrenal, Luan, Mesocaine, Neo-Lidocaton, Neo-Sinedol, Neo-Xylestesin, Nervocaine, Nurocain, Octocaine, Odontalg, Ortodermina, Peterkaien, Pisacaina, Rapidocaine, Remicaine, Rowo-629, Sagittaproct, Sedagul, Xilo-Mynol, Xilonibsa, Xilonibsa , Xylanaest, Xylesine, Xylestesin, Xylocain, Xylocaina, Xylocaine, Xylocitin, Xyloneural, Xylonor, Xylotox
Lorcainide	
Mexiletine	Mexilen, Mexitil, Ritalmex
Moracizine (Moricizine)	Ethmozine
Pirmenol	
Procainamide	Biocoryl, Procamide, Procan, Procanbid, Pronestyl
Propafenone	Arythmol, Asonacor, Cuxafenon, Homopafen, Nistaken, Norfenon, Propafen, Propamerck, Prorynorm, Rhythmocor, Ritmonorm, Rythmex, Rythmol, Rytmogenat, Rytmonorm, Rytmonorma, Rytmo-Puren
Quinidine	Biquin, Cardioquin, Cardioquine, Chinteina, Kinidin, Kinidine, Kinidine Durettes, Kiniduron, Longachin, Longacor, Naticardina, Natisedina, Quinaglute, Quini, Quinicardine, Quinidex, Quiniduran, Quinora, Ritmocor
Tocainide	Tonocard, Xylotocan

drug trials have confirmed that hope, but sometimes the combinations are unsafe. Predicting these is difficult, but there are some very broad general rules that can be applied if the general pharmacology of the drugs is understood.

If drugs with similar effects are used together, whether they act on the myocardium itself or on the conducting tissues, the total effect is likely to be increased (additive). The classification of the antiarrhythmics in Table 4.2 helps to predict what is likely to happen, but remember that the classification is not rigid so that drugs in one class can share some characteristics with others. Here are some examples:

1. Combinations of antiarrhythmics from the same class

The drugs in Class Ia can prolong the QT interval so combining drugs from this class would be expected to show an increased effect on the QT interval. This prolongation carries the risk of causing torsade de pointes arrhythmias (see the monograph, 'Drugs that prolong the QT interval + Other drugs that prolong the QT interval', p.103). It would also be expected that the negative inotropic effects of quinidine would be increased by procainamide or any of the others within Class Ia. For safety therefore it is sometimes considered best to avoid drugs that fall into the same subclass or only use them together with caution.

2. Combinations of antiarrhythmics from different classes

Class III antiarrhythmics such as amiodarone can also prolong the QT interval, so they would also be expected to inter-

Table 4.2 Modified Vaughan Williams classification of the oral antiarrhythmic drugs

Class I: Membrane stabilising drugs
(a) Quinidine, Procainamide, Disopyramide, Tiracizine
(b) Lidocaine (Lignocaine), Mexiletine, Tocainide, Phenytoin
(c) Diprafenone, Encainide, Flecainide, Propafenone
Difficult to classify – Moracizine
Class II: Beta-blockers
Propranolol, Atenolol
Class III: Inhibitors of depolarisation
Amiodarone, Bretylium, Dofetilide, Ibutilide, Sotalol
Class IV: Calcium channel blockers
Verapamil, Diltiazem

act with drugs in other classes that do the same, namely Class Ia drugs (see 'Drugs that prolong the QT interval + Other drugs that prolong the QT interval', p.103). Verapamil comes into Class IV and has negative inotropic effects, so it can interact with other drugs with similar effects, such as the beta-blockers, which fall into Class III. For safety you should always look at the whole drug profile and take care with any two drugs, from any class, that share a common pharmacological action.

Adenosine + Dipyridamole

Dipyridamole markedly reduces the bolus dose of adenosine necessary to convert supraventricular tachycardia to sinus rhythm (by about fourfold).

Clinical evidence

Adenosine by rapid intravenous bolus (10 to 200 micrograms/kg in stepwise doses) was found to restore sinus rhythm in 10 of 14 episodes of tachycardia in 7 patients with supraventricular tachycardia. The mean dose was 8.8 mg compared with only 1 mg in two patients also taking oral **dipyridamole**.[1] Another study in 6 patients found that **dipyridamole** (0.56 mg/kg intravenous bolus, followed by a continuous infusion of 5 micrograms/kg/min) reduced the minimum effective bolus dose of intravenous adenosine required to stop the supraventricular tachycardia fourfold (from 68 to 17 micrograms/kg) in 5 patients. In the other patient, dipyridamole alone stopped the supraventricular tachycardia.[2]

Other studies in normal subjects have clearly shown that **dipyridamole** reduced the dose of adenosine required to produce an equivalent cardiovascular effect by fourfold[3] or six- to sixteenfold.[4] A brief report describes a woman on **dipyridamole** (dosage not stated) with paroxysmal supraventricular tachycardia who lost ventricular activity for 18 secs when given 6 mg adenosine intravenously.[5] Another report describes 3 of 4 patients given adenosine 3 to 6 mg by central venous bolus who had heart block of 3, 9 and 21-second duration. The patient with the most profound heart block was also being treated with **dipyridamole**, which was thought to have contributed to the reaction.[6]

Mechanism

Not fully understood. Part of the explanation is that dipyridamole increases plasma levels of endogenous adenosine by inhibiting its uptake into cells.[2,4,7]

Importance and management

An established interaction. Patients will need much less adenosine to treat arrhythmias while taking dipyridamole. Initial dosage reductions of adenosine of twofold[5] or fourfold[2] have been suggested. The makers actually advise the avoidance of adenosine in patients on dipyridamole. If it must be used for supraventricular tachycardia in a patient on dipyridamole, they suggest that the initial bolus adenosine dose should be reduced about fourfold (from 3 to 0.5 to 1 mg).[8] If adenosine is considered necessary for myocardial imaging in a patient on dipyridamole, they suggest that the dipyridamole should be stopped 24 hours before, or the dose of adenosine should be greatly reduced.[6]

1. Watt AH, Bernard MS, Webster J, Passani SL, Stephens MR, Routledge PA. Intravenous adenosine in the treatment of supraventricular tachycardia: a dose-ranging study and interaction with dipyridamole. *Br J Clin Pharmacol* (1986) 21, 227–30.
2. Lerman BB, Wesley RC, Belardinelli L. Electrophysiologic effects of dipyridamole on atrioventricular nodal conduction and supraventricular tachycardia. Role of endogenous adenosine. *Circulation* (1989) 80, 1536–43.
3. Biaggioni I, Onrot J, Hollister AS, Robertson D. Cardiovascular effects of adenosine infusion in man and their modulation by dipyridamole. *Life Sci* (1986) 39, 2229–36.
4. Conradson T-BG, Dixon CMS, Clarke B, Barnes PJ. Cardiovascular effects of infused adenosine in man: potentiation by dipyridamole. *Acta Physiol Scand* (1987) 129, 387–91.
5. Mader TJ. Adenosine: adverse interactions. *Ann Emerg Med* (1992) 21, 453.
6. McCollam PL, Uber WE, Van Bakel AB. Adenosine-related ventricular asystole. *Ann Intern Med* (1993) 118, 315–16.
7. German DC, Kredich NM, Bjornsson TD. Oral dipyridamole increases plasma adenosine levels in human beings. *Clin Pharmacol Ther* (1989) 45, 80–4.
8. Adenoscan (Adenosine). Sanofi Winthrop Limited. Summary of product characteristics, February 1997.

Adenosine + Nicotine

Nicotine appears to enhance the effects of adenosine, but the clinical relevance of this is unclear.

Clinical evidence, mechanism, importance and management

Nicotine chewing gum 2 mg (approximately equal to 1 cigarette) increased the circulatory effects of 0.07 mg/kg/min adenosine infusion in 10 healthy subjects. The increase in heart rate due to nicotine (5.5 bpm) was further increased to 14.9 bpm by concomitant adenosine. The diastolic blood pressure rise due to nicotine (7 mmHg) was reduced to 1.1 mmHg by concomitant adenosine.[1] In another study, **nicotine** chewing gum 2 mg increased chest pain and the duration of AV block when given with intravenous bolus doses of adenosine in 7 healthy subjects.[2] What this means in practical terms is uncertain, but be aware that the effects of adenosine may be modified to some extent by nicotine-containing products (**tobacco smoking**, **nicotine gum**, etc.).

1. Smits P, Eijsbouts A, Thien T. Nicotine enhances the circulatory effects of adenosine in human beings. *Clin Pharmacol Ther* (1989) 46, 272–8.
2. Sylvén C, Beerman B, Kaijser L, Jonzon B. Nicotine enhances angina pectoris-like chest pain and atrioventricular blockade provoked by intravenous bolus of adenosine in healthy volunteers. *J Cardiovasc Pharmacol* (1990) 16, 962–5.

Adenosine + Xanthines

Caffeine and theophylline can inhibit the effects of adenosine infusion used in conjunction with radionuclide myocardial imaging. They should be withheld 12 to 24 hours prior to the procedure or they will interfere with test results. They have been used to terminate persistent adverse effects of the adenosine infusion.

Clinical evidence

Experimental studies in healthy subjects on the way xanthine drugs possibly interact with adenosine have shown that **caffeine** and **theophylline** (but not **enprofylline**) reduced the increased heart rate and the changes in blood pressure caused by infusions of adenosine,[1-4] and attenuated adenosine-induced vasodilation.[5,6] **Theophylline** also attenuated adenosine-induced respiratory effects and chest pain.[3,4] Similarly, adenosine infusion antagonised the haemodynamic effects of a single dose of **theophylline** in healthy subjects, but did not reduce the metabolic effects (reductions in plasma potassium and magnesium).[3]

Mechanism

The reason is that caffeine and theophylline have an antagonistic effect on adenosine receptors.[7] They appear to have opposite effects on the circulatory system: caffeine and theophylline cause vasoconstriction whereas adenosine infusion generally causes vasodilation.[1]

Importance and management

The makers of adenosine state that theophylline, aminophylline and other xanthines should be avoided for 24 h before using adenosine infusion for radionuclide myocardial imaging, and that xanthine-containing drinks (tea, coffee, chocolate, '*Coke*' etc.) should be avoided for at least 12 h before.[8] In a recent study in 70 patients, measurable caffeine serum levels were found in 74% of patients after 12 h self-reported abstention from caffeine-containing products. Patients with caffeine serum levels of at least 2.9 mg/l had significantly fewer stress symptoms (chest tightness, chest pain, headache, dyspnoea, nausea, dizziness) than those with lower serum levels. The authors suggest that 12-h abstention from **caffeine** containing products may be insufficient, and could result in false-negative results.[9] Xanthines, such as intravenous aminophylline, may be used to terminate persistent adverse effects of adenosine infusion given for myocardial imaging.[8]

The effect of caffeine and theophylline on the negative chronotropic effect of adenosine bolus injection appears not to have been studied. Whether adenosine bolus can stop theophylline-induced supraventricular tachycardia also appears not to have been studied.

1. Smits P, Schouten J, Thien T. Cardiovascular effects of two xanthines and the relation to adenosine antagonism. *Clin Pharmacol Ther* (1989) 45, 593–9.
2. Smits P, Boekema P, De Abreu R, Thien T, van 't Laar A. Evidence for an antagonism between caffeine and adenosine in the human cardiovascular system. *J Cardiovasc Pharmacol* (1987) 10, 136–43.
3. Minton NA, Henry JA. Pharmacodynamic interactions between infused adenosine and oral theophylline. *Hum Exp Toxicol* (1991) 10, 411–18.
4. Maxwell DL, Fuller RW, Conradson T-B, Dixon CMS, Aber V, Hughes JMB, Barnes PJ. Contrasting effects of two xanthines, theophylline and enprofylline, on the cardio-respiratory stimulation of infused adenosine in man. *Acta Physiol Scand* (1987) 131, 459–65.
5. Taddei S, Pedrinelli R, Salvetti A. Theophylline is an antagonist of adenosine in human forearm arterioles. *Am J Hypertens* (1991) 4, 256–9.
6. Smits P, Lenders JWM, Thien T. Caffeine and theophylline attenuate adenosine-induced vasodilation in humans. *Clin Pharmacol Ther* (1990) 48, 410–18.
7. Fredholm BB. On the mechanism of action of theophylline and caffeine. *Acta Med Scand* (1985) 217, 149–53.
8. Adenoscan (Adenosine). Sanofi Winthrop Limited. Summary of product characteristics, February 1997.
9. Majd-Ardekani J, Clowes P, Menash-Bonsu V, Nunan TO. Time for abstention from caffeine before an adenosine myocardial perfusion scan. *Nuclear Med Comm* (2000) 21, 361–4.

Ajmaline + Miscellaneous drugs

An isolated report describes cardiac failure in a patient given ajmaline and lidocaine (lignocaine) concurrently. Quinidine causes a very considerable increase in the plasma levels of ajmaline, and phenobarbital appears to cause a marked reduction.

Clinical evidence, mechanism, importance and management

A woman showed marked aggravation of cardiac failure when treated with ajmaline orally and **lidocaine (lignocaine)** intravenously for repeated ventricular tachycardias.[1]

A study[2] in 4 healthy subjects found that if a single 200-mg oral dose of **quinidine** was given with a single 50-mg oral dose of ajmaline, the AUC of ajmaline was increased 10- to 30-fold and the maximal plasma concentrations increased from 0.018 to 0.141 micrograms/ml. Another single-dose study in 5 healthy subjects found that the metabolism of ajmaline was inhibited by **quinidine**, possibly because the quinidine becomes competitively bound to the metabolising enzymes.[3]

The clearance of intravenous ajmaline was almost twice as high in 3 patients receiving **phenobarbital** when compared with 5 patients who were not, so that its clinical effects would be expected to be markedly diminished.[4]

The clinical importance of all of these interactions is uncertain but concurrent use should be well monitored.

1. Bleifeld W. Side effects of antiarrhythmics. *Naunyn Schmiedebergs Arch Pharmacol* (1971) 269, 282–97.
2. Hori R, Okumura K, Inui K-I, Yasuhara M, Yamada K, Sakurai T, Kawai C. Quinidine-induced rise in ajmaline plasma concentration. *J Pharm Pharmacol* (1984) 36, 202–4.
3. Köppel C, Tenczer J, Arndt I. Metabolic disposition of ajmaline. *Eur J Drug Metab Pharmacokinet* (1989) 14, 309–16.
4. Köppel C, Wagemann A, Martens F. Pharmacokinetics and antiarrhythmic efficacy of intravenous ajmaline in ventricular arrhythmia of acute onset. *Eur J Drug Metab Pharmacokinet* (1989) 14, 161–7.

Amiodarone + Anaesthetics

There is some evidence that the presence of amiodarone possibly increases the risk of complications (atropine-resistant bradycardia, hypotension, decreased cardiac output) during general anaesthesia.

Clinical evidence

(i) Evidence for no complications

The preliminary report of one study in 21 patients taking amiodarone (mean dose 538 mg daily) and undergoing defibrillator implantation suggested that haemodynamic changes during surgery were not significantly different from those in matched controls not taking amiodarone.[1] Similarly, another study found no difference in haemodynamic status or pacemaker dependency between patients on short-term amiodarone and a control group during valve replacement surgery with **thiopentone-fentanyl** anaesthesia. The amiodarone group received 600 mg daily for 1 week then 400 mg daily for 2 weeks prior to surgery.[2] In a double-blind trial, there was no significant difference in haemodynamic instability during **fentanyl-isoflurane** anaesthesia between patients randomised to receive short-term amiodarone (3.4 g over 5 days or 2.2 g over 24 h) or placebo before cardiac surgery. In this study, haemodynamic instability was assessed by fluid balance, use of dopamine or other vasopressor agents, and use of a phosphodiesterase inhibitor or intra-aortic balloon pump.[3]

(ii) Evidence for complications

Several case reports[4-6] and two studies[7,8] suggest that severe intra-operative complications may occur in patients receiving amiodarone (atropine-resistant bradycardia, myocardial depression, hypotension). One of these, a comparative retrospective review of patients (16 receiving amiodarone 300 to 800 mg daily and 30 controls) having operations under anaesthesia (mainly cardio-pulmonary bypass surgery), showed that the incidence of slow nodal rhythm, complete heart block or pacemaker dependency rose from 17% in controls to 66% in amiodarone-treated patients. Intra-aortic balloon pump augmentation was 7% compared with 50%, and low systemic vascular resistance/high cardiac output rose from 0 to 13% in controls and amiodarone-treated patients, respectively. Mortality was 19% in the amiodarone group and 0% in the control group. **Fentanyl** was used for all of the patients, often combined with **diazepam**, and sometimes also **isoflurane**, **enflurane** or **halothane**.[7] Another study of 37 patients receiving amiodarone (mean dose about 250 mg daily) found no problems in 8 undergoing non-cardiac surgery. Of the 29 undergoing cardiac surgery, 52% had postoperative dysrhythmic complications and 24% required a pacemaker, which was not considered exceptional for the type of surgery. However, one patient had fatal vasoplegia (a hypotensive syndrome) after cardio-pulmonary bypass, which was considered amiodarone-related. Anaesthesia in all patients was **fentanyl**-based.[8] It was suggested in one case report that serious hypotension in 2 patients on amiodarone undergoing surgery may have been further compounded by **ACE inhibitor** therapy.[6]

Mechanism

In vitro and *in vivo* studies in *animals* suggest that amiodarone has additive cardiodepressant and vasodilator effects with volatile anaesthetics such as halothane, enflurane and isoflurane.[5,9]

Importance and management

The assessment of this interaction is complicated by the problem of conducting studies in anaesthesia, most being retrospective and using matched controls. The only randomised study used short-term amiodarone to assess its safety if used for prevention of post-operative atrial fibrillation, and its findings may not be relevant to patients on long-term therapy.[3] It appears that potentially severe complications may occur in some patients taking amiodarone undergoing general anaesthesia including bradycardia unresponsive to atropine, hypotension, conduction disturbances, and decreased cardiac output. Anaesthetists should take particular care in patients on amiodarone undergoing coronary bypass surgery.[10] Amiodarone persists in the body for many weeks, which usually means it cannot be withdraw before surgery if there are risks in delaying surgery,[8] or it is being used for serious arrhythmias.[10]

1. Elliott PL, Schauble JF, Rogers MC, Reid PR. Risk of decompensation during anesthesia in presence of amiodarone. *Circulation* (1983) 68 (Suppl 3), 280.
2. Chassard D, George M, Guiraud M, Lehot JJ, Bastien O, Hercule C, Villard J, Estanove S. Relationship between preoperative amiodarone treatment and complications observed during anaesthesia for valvular cardiac surgery. *Can J Anaesth* (1990) 37, 251–4.
3. White CM, Dunn A, Tsikouris J, Waberski W, Felton K, Freeman-Bosco L, Giri S, Kluger J. An assessment of the safety of short-term amiodarone therapy in cardiac surgical patients with fentanyl-isoflurane anesthesia. *Anesth Analg* (1999) 89, 585–9.
4. Gallagher JD, Lieberman RW, Meranze J, Spielman SR, Ellison N. Amiodarone-induced complications during coronary artery surgery. *Anesthesiology* (1981) 55, 186–8.
5. MacKinnon G, Landymore R, Marble A. Should oral amiodarone be used for sustained ventricular tachycardia in patients requiring open-heart surgery? *Can J Surg* (1983) 26, 355–7.
6. Mackay JH, Walker IA, Bethune DW. Amiodarone and anaesthesia: concurrent therapy with ACE inhibitors—an additional cause for concern? *Can J Anaesth* (1991) 38, 687.
7. Liberman BA, Teasdale SJ. Anaesthesia and amiodarone. *Can Anaesth Soc J* (1985) 32, 629–38.
8. Van Dyck M, Baele P, Rennotte MT, Matta A, Dion R, Kestens-Servaye Y. Should amiodarone be discontinued before cardiac surgery? *Acta Anaesth Belg* (1988) 39, 3–10.
9. Rooney RT, Marijic J, Stommel KA, Bosnjak ZJ, Aggarwai A, Kampine JP, Stowe DF. Additive cardiac depression by volatile anesthetics in isolated hearts after chronic amiodarone treatment. *Anesth Analg* (1995) 80, 917–24.
10. Teasdale S, Downar E. Amiodarone and anaesthesia. *Can J Anaesth* (1990) 37, 151–5.

Amiodarone + Beta-blockers

Hypotension, bradycardia, ventricular fibrillation and asystole have been seen in a few patients given amiodarone with propranolol, metoprolol or sotalol (for sotalol, see also 'Drugs that prolong the QT interval + Other drugs that prolong the QT interval', p.103). However, analysis of clinical trials suggests that the combination can be beneficial.

Clinical evidence

A woman of 64 was treated for hypertrophic cardiomyopathy with amiodarone (1200 mg daily) and **atenolol** (50 mg daily). Five days later the **atenolol** was replaced by **metoprolol** (100 mg daily). Within 3 h she complained of dizziness, weakness and blurred vision. On examination she was found to be pale and sweating with a pulse rate of 20 per min. Her systolic pressure was 60 mmHg. Atropine 2 mg did not produce chronotropic or haemodynamic improvement. She responded to isoprenaline (isoproterenol).[1] Severe hypotension has been reported in another patient on **sotalol** when given intravenous amiodarone (total dose 250 mg).[2] Another report describes a cardiac arrest in one patient on amiodarone, and severe bradycardia and ventricular fibrillation (requiring defibrillation) in another, within 1.5 and 2 h of starting to take **propranolol**.[3] In contrast to the above case reports, an analysis of data from two large clinical trials of the use of amiodarone for arrhythmias post-myocardial infarction found that the combination of un-named **beta-blockers** and amiodarone was beneficial (reduced cardiac deaths, arrhythmic deaths and resuscitated cardiac arrest) compared with either drug alone, or neither drug.[4] Similarly, in the analysis of another trial in heart failure, the benefits of the beta-blocker **carvedilol** were still apparent in those patients already receiving amiodarone, and the combination was not associated with a greater incidence of adverse effects (worsened heart failure, hypotension/dizziness, bradycardia/atrioventricular block, aggravation of angina) than either drug alone.[5]

Mechanism

Not understood. The clinical picture is that of excessive beta-blockade, and additive pharmacodynamic effects are possible. The time course of the interaction makes it unlikely that amiodarone affected the hepatic metabolism of propranolol and metoprolol, although a pharmacokinetic interaction based on altered volume of distribution (due to protein binding changes) has been suggested.[1] Increased bradycardia and other ECG changes have been seen with amiodarone and practolol.[6]

Importance and management

The isolated reports of adverse reactions cited here (they seem to be the only ones so far documented) emphasise the need for caution when amiodarone is used with beta-blockers. The maker of amiodarone recommends that the combination should not be used because potentiation of negative chronotropic properties and conduction slowing effects may occur.[7] However, the concurrent use of beta-blockers and amiodarone is not uncommon and may be therapeutically useful. The authors of one of the analyses suggest that post-myocardial infarction, if possible, beta-blockers should be continued in patients for whom amiodarone is indicated.[4] See also 'Drugs that prolong the QT interval + Other drugs that prolong the QT interval', p.103, which deals with the possible risks of using amiodarone and sotalol.

1. Leor J, Levartowsky D, Sharon C, Farfel Z. Amiodarone and β-adrenergic blockers: an interaction with metoprolol but not with atenolol. *Am Heart J* (1988) 116, 206–7.
2. Warren R, Vohra J, Hunt D, Hamer A. Serious interactions of sotalol with amiodarone and flecainide. *Med J Aust* (1990) 152, 277.
3. Derrida JP, Ollagnier J, Benaim R, Haiat R, Chiche P. Amiodarone et propranolol; une association dangereuse? *Nouv Presse Med* (1979) 8, 1429.
4. Boutitie F, Boissel J-P, Connolly SJ, Camm AJ, Cairns JA, Julian DG, Gent M, Janse MJ, Dorian P, Frangin G. Amiodarone interaction with β-blockers: analysis of the merged EMIAT (European Myocardial Infarct Amiodarone Trial) and CAMIAT (Canadian Amiodarone Myocardial Infarction Trial) databases. *Circulation* (1999) 99, 2268–75.
5. Krum H, Shusterman N, MacMahon S, Sharpe N. Efficacy and safety of carvedilol in patients with chronic heart failure receiving concomitant amiodarone therapy. *J Card Fail* (1998) 4, 281–8.
6. Antonelli G, Cristallo E, Cesario S, Calabrese P. Modificazioni elettrocardiografiche indotte dalla somministrazione di amiodarone associato a practolilo. *Boll Soc Ital Cardiol* (1973) 18, 236–42.
7. Cordarone X (Amiodarone hydrochloride). Sanofi Synthelabo. Summary of product characteristics. January 2000.

Amiodarone + Calcium channel blockers

Increased cardiac depressant effects would be expected if amiodarone is used with diltiazem or verapamil. One case of sinus arrest and serious hypotension has been reported in a woman on diltiazem when given amiodarone.

Clinical evidence, mechanism, importance and management

A woman with compensated congestive heart failure, paroxysmal atrial fibrillation and ventricular arrhythmias was treated with **furosemide (frusemide)** and 90 mg **diltiazem** six-hourly. Four days after starting additional treatment with amiodarone, 600 mg 12-hourly, she developed sinus arrest and a life-threatening low cardiac output state (systolic pressure 80 mmHg) with oliguria. **Diltiazem** and amiodarone were stopped and she was treated with pressor drugs and ventricular pacing. She had previously had no problems on **diltiazem** or **verapamil** alone, and later she did well on 400 mg amiodarone daily without **diltiazem.** The reason for this reaction is thought to be the additive effects of both drugs on myocardial contractility, and on sinus and atrioventricular nodal function.[1] Before this isolated case report was published, another author predicted this interaction with **diltiazem** or **verapamil** on theoretical grounds and warned of the risks if dysfunction of the sinus node, such as bradycardia or sick sinus syndrome is suspected, or if partial AV block exists.[2] The makers state that the use of amiodarone with certain calcium channel blockers (**diltiazem**, **verapamil**) is not recommended because potentiation of negative chronotropic properties and conduction slowing effects may occur.[3] There do not appear to be any reports of adverse effects attributed to the use of amiodarone with the dihydropyridine class of calcium channel blockers (e.g. **nifedipine**), which typically have little or no negative inotropic activity at usual doses.

1. Lee TH, Friedman PL, Goldman L, Stone PH, Antman EM. Sinus arrest and hypotension with combined amiodarone-diltiazem therapy. *Am Heart J* (1985) 109, 163–4.
2. Marcus FI. Drug interactions with amiodarone. *Am Heart J* (1983) 106, 924–30.
3. Cordarone X (Amiodarone hydrochloride). Sanofi Synthelabo. Summary of product characteristics, January 2000.

Amiodarone + Cimetidine

Cimetidine possibly causes a rise in the serum levels of amiodarone in some patients.

Clinical evidence

The preliminary report of one study notes that the mean amiodarone serum levels of 12 patients on long-term treatment (200 mg twice daily) rose by an average of 38% (from 1.4 to 1.93 micrograms/ml) when given 1200 mg **cimetidine** daily for a week. The desethyl-amiodarone levels rose by 54%. However, these increases were not statistically significant, and only 8 of the 12 showed any rise.[1]

Mechanism

Not understood. Cimetidine is a well-recognised enzyme inhibitor which reduces the metabolism of many drugs (and therefore possibly amiodarone as well) so that they are cleared more slowly.

Importance and management

Information seems to be limited to this study but this interaction may be clinically important. Monitor the serum amiodarone levels if possible when cimetidine is started, anticipating a rise. Not all patients appear to be affected. Remember that amiodarone is lost from the body very slowly (half-life 25–100 days) so that the results of the one-week study cited here may possibly not adequately reflect the magnitude of this interaction. More study is needed.

1. Hogan C, Landau S, Tepper D and Somberg J. Cimetidine-amiodarone interaction. *J Clin Pharmacol* (1988) 28, 909.

Amiodarone + Colestyramine

Colestyramine appears to reduce the serum levels of amiodarone.

Clinical evidence

When four 4 g doses of **colestyramine** were given to 11 patients at 1 h intervals starting 1.5 h after a single 400-mg dose of amiodarone, the serum amiodarone levels 7.5 h later were depressed by about 50%.[1] In a further study, the amiodarone half-life was lower (23.5, 29 and 32 days) in 3 patients given **colestyramine** 4 g daily after discontinuing long-term amiodarone compared with that in 8 patients discontinuing amiodarone and not given **colestyramine** (35 to 58 days).[1]

Mechanism

The probable reason is that the colestyramine binds with the amiodarone in the gut, thereby reducing its absorption, and it may also affect the enterohepatic recirculation of amiodarone.[1] This is consistent with the way colestyramine interacts with other drugs.

Importance and management

Information is very limited but a reduced response to the amiodarone may be expected. Separating the dosages to avoid admixture in the gut would reduce or prevent any effects on absorption from the gut, but not the effects due to reduction in enterohepatic recirculation. Monitor the effects closely and raise the amiodarone dosage if necessary.

1. Nitsch J, Liideritz B. Beschleunigte Elimination von Amiodaron durch Colestyramin. *Dtsch Med Wochenschr* (1986) 111, 1241–4.

Amiodarone + Disopyramide

The risk of QT interval prolongation and torsade de pointes (also described as AVT, atypical ventricular tachycardia) seems to be increased if amiodarone is used with disopyramide.

Clinical evidence

A brief report describes 2 patients who developed torsade de pointes during the concurrent use of amiodarone and **disopyramide**. Their QT intervals became markedly prolonged (more than 0.50 sec).[1] In another study 2 patients who had been taking **disopyramide** 300 mg daily for a number of months developed prolonged QT intervals of 0.64 and 0.68 sec and torsade de pointes 2 and 5 days after starting amiodarone 800 mg daily.[2]

Mechanism

Amiodarone is a class III antiarrhythmic and can prolong the QT interval. Disopyramide is in class 1a and also prolongs the QT interval. Their additive effects can result in the development of torsade de pointes arrhythmias.

Importance and management

Established and potentially serious interaction. In general, Class Ia antiarrhythmics such as disopyramide (see Table 4.2) should be avoided or used with great caution with amiodarone because of their additive effects in delaying conduction. The makers of amiodarone contraindicate its use with class Ia antiarrhythmics.[3] However, the successful and apparently safe use of amiodarone (100–600 mg daily) with disopyramide (300–500 mg daily)[4] has also been described, although the results on long-term follow-up were not reported in all cases. See also 'Drugs that prolong the QT interval + Other drugs that prolong the QT interval', p.103, 'Procainamide + Amiodarone', p.115, and 'Quinidine + Amiodarone', p.119.

1. Tartini R, Kappenberger L, Steinbrunn W. Gefährliche Interaktionen zwischen Amiodaron und Antiarrhythmika der Klass I. *Schweiz Med Wochenschr* (1982) 112, 1585–7.
2. Keren A, Tzivoni D, Gavish D, Levi J, Gottlieb S, Benhorin J, Stern S. Etiology, warning signs and therapy of Torsade de Pointes. *Circulation* (1981) 64, 1167–74.
3. Cordarone X (Amiodarone hydrochloride). Sanofi Synthelabo. Summary of product characteristics, January 2000.
4. James MA, Papouchado M, Vann Jonec J. Combined therapy with disopyramide and amiodarone: a report of 11 cases. *Int J Cardiol* (1986) 13, 248–52.

Amiodarone + Lithium

Hypothyroidism developed very rapidly in two patients on amiodarone when lithium was added.

Clinical evidence, mechanism, importance and management

A patient on 400 mg amiodarone daily for more than a year developed acute manic depression. He was started on 600 mg **lithium** (salt unknown) daily, but within 2 weeks he developed clinical signs of hypothyroidism, which was confirmed by clinical tests. He made a complete recovery within 3 weeks of stopping the amiodarone while continuing the **lithium**.[1] Similarly, another patient on amiodarone rapidly developed hypothyroidism when additionally given **lithium** (dose and salt unknown), which resolved when the amiodarone was stopped.[1] Both **lithium** and amiodarone on their own can cause hypothyroidism, but usually only when taken chronically. In these two cases the effects appear to have been additive, and very rapid.

These two cases appear to be the first report of this interaction. Its general importance is therefore still uncertain, but it would be prudent to monitor for any signs of hypothyroidism (lethargy, weakness, depression, weight gain, hoarseness) in any patient when given both drugs. More study is needed. Lithium therapy has rarely been associated with cardiac QT prolongation, and consequently the maker of amiodarone contraindicates its combined use.[2] See also 'Drugs that prolong the QT interval + Other drugs that prolong the QT interval', p.103.

1. Ahmad S. Sudden hypothyroidism and amiodarone-lithium combination: an interaction. *Cardiovasc Drug Ther* (1995) 9, 827–8.

2. Cordarone X (Amiodarone hydrochloride). Sanofi Synthelabo. Summary of product characteristics, January 2000.

Amiodarone + Protease inhibitors

A case is reported of enhanced serum levels of amiodarone during concomitant indinavir administration. Nelfinavir, ritonavir and, possibly, saquinavir are predicted to act similarly.

Clinical evidence

A patient on amiodarone 200 mg daily was additionally given zidovudine, lamivudine, and **indinavir** for 4 weeks, as post HIV-exposure prophylaxis after a needlestick injury. Amiodarone serum levels increased, from 0.9 mg/l before antiretroviral prophylaxis, to 1.3 mg/l during therapy, and gradually decreased to 0.8 mg/l during the 77 days after stopping prophylaxis. Although the reference range for amiodarone levels is not established, these levels were not outside those usually considered to achieve good antiarrhythmic control.[1]

Mechanism

HIV protease inhibitors such as **indinavir** are metabolised by cytochrome P450 enzymes and pharmacokinetic interactions are therefore possible. It was considered that the increase in serum amiodarone in this case was due to decreased metabolism of amiodarone, although no decrease in the serum levels of desethylamiodarone were observed.[1]

Importance and management

Although in the case cited the interaction was not clinically relevant, the authors considered it could be in patients with higher initial amiodarone levels. They recommend monitoring amiodarone therapy if indinavir is coadministered.[1] Other HIV protease inhibitors are also predicted to inhibit the metabolism of amiodarone. See index.

1. Lohman JJHM, Reichert LJM, Degen LPM. Antiretroviral therapy increases serum concentrations of amiodarone. *Ann Pharmacother* (1999) 33, 645–6.

Amiodarone + Sertraline

In an isolated report, a slight to moderate rise in plasma amiodarone levels has been attributed to the concurrent use of sertraline.

Clinical evidence, mechanism, importance and management

When a depressed patient on 200 mg amiodarone twice daily had his concurrent treatment with carbamazepine (200 mg twice daily) and **sertraline** (100 mg daily) stopped, just before ECT treatment, it was noted that by day 4 his plasma amiodarone levels had fallen by nearly 20%. The authors of the report drew the conclusion that while taking all three drugs, the amiodarone levels had become slightly raised due to the enzyme inhibitory effects of the **sertraline**, despite the potential enzyme-inducing activity of the carbamazepine.[1] The patient showed no changes in his cardiac status while on the reduced amiodarone levels, suggesting that this interaction (if such it is) is of no

clinical importance. However it may be worth considering an antidepressant with low affinity for cytochrome P450 isoenzyme CYP3A4 such as paroxetine or venlafaxine if concurrent use is required with amiodarone.

1. DeVane CL, Gill HS, Markowitz JS, Carson WH. Awareness of potential drug interactions may aid avoidance. *Ther Drug Monit* (1997) 19, 366–7.

Amiodarone + Trazodone

An isolated report describes the development of torsade de pointes in a woman on amiodarone when given trazodone.

Clinical evidence, mechanism, importance and management

A 74-year-old woman with a pacemaker on nifedipine, furosemide (frusemide), aspirin and 200 mg amiodarone daily began to have dizzy spells but no loss of consciousness soon after starting **trazodone** (initially 50 mg and eventually 150 mg daily by the end of 2 weeks). Both the amiodarone and **trazodone** were stopped when she was hospitalised. She showed prolonged QT, QTc and JTc intervals on the ECG and recurrent episodes of torsade de pointes arrhythmia, which were controlled by increasing the ventricular pacing rate. The ECG intervals shortened and she was later discharged on amiodarone again without the **trazodone**, showing an ECG pattern similar to that seen 4 months before hospitalisation.[1] No general conclusions can be drawn from this apparent interaction, but prescribers should be aware of this case. The makers note that trazodone does have the potential to be arrhythmogenic.[2] See also, 'Drugs that prolong the QT interval + Other drugs that prolong the QT interval', p.103.

1. Mazur A, Strasberg B, Kusniec J, Sclarovsky S. QT prolongation and polymorphous ventricular tachycardia association with trazodone-amiodarone combination. *Int J Cardiol* (1995) 52, 27–9.

2. Molipaxin (Trazodone). Hoechst Marion Roussel Ltd. Summary of product characteristics, June 2000.

Aprindine + Amiodarone

Serum aprindine levels can be increased by the concurrent use of amiodarone. Toxicity may occur unless the dosage is reduced.

Clinical evidence, mechanism, importance and management

The serum aprindine levels of two patients rose, accompanied by signs of toxicity (nausea, ataxia, etc.), when additionally treated with **amiodarone**. One of them on 100 mg aprindine daily showed a progressive rise in trough serum levels from 2.3 to 3.5 mg/l over a 5-week period when given 1200 mg and later 600 mg **amiodarone** daily. Even when the aprindine dosage was reduced, serum levels remained higher than before beginning the **amiodarone**.[1] The authors say that those given both drugs generally need less aprindine than those on aprindine alone. This interaction has been briefly reported elsewhere.[2] Its mechanism is not understood. Monitor the effects of concurrent use and reduce the dosage of aprindine as necessary.

1. Southworth W, Friday KJ, Ruffy R. Possible amiodarone-aprindine interaction. *Am Heart J* (1982) 104, 323.

2. Zhang Z, Wang G, Wang H, Zhang J. Effect of amiodarone on the plasma concentration of aprindine. *Zhongguo Yaoxue Zazhi* (1991) 26, 156–9. *Abstract 115: 197745u in Chemical Abstracts* (1991) 115, 22.

Cibenzoline (Cifenline) + Cimetidine or Ranitidine

Cimetidine increases the plasma levels of cibenzoline, but ranitidine does not interact.

Clinical evidence, mechanism, importance and management

Cimetidine 1200 mg daily raised the maximum plasma levels of cibenzoline (single 160-mg doses) in 12 healthy subjects by 27%, increased the AUC by 44%, and prolonged its half-life by 30%. Ranitidine 300 mg daily had no effect.[1] The probable reason is that the cimetidine reduces the metabolism of the cibenzoline by the liver, whereas ranitidine does not. The clinical importance of this interaction is not known but be alert for increased cibenzoline effects. More study is needed.

1. Massarella JW, Defeo TM, Liguori J, Passe S, Aogaichi K. The effects of cimetidine and ranitidine on the pharmacokinetics of cifenline. Br J Clin Pharmacol (1991) 31, 481–3.

Disopyramide or Procainamide + Antacids or Antidiarrhoeals

There is some inconclusive evidence that some antacids may possibly cause a small reduction in the absorption of these antiarrhythmic agents. Kaolin-pectin appears to reduce the bioavailability of procainamide.

Clinical evidence, mechanism, importance and management

A single 11 g dose of an aluminium phosphate antacid had no statistically significant effect on the pharmacokinetics of a single 200 mg oral dose of disopyramide in 10 patients, but did affect the pharmacokinetics of a single 750 mg oral dose of procainamide. However the antacid appeared to reduce the absorption of both antiarrhythmic agents to a some extent in individual subjects.[1] The clinical importance of this interaction is uncertain, but probably small.

Kaolin-pectin was found to and reduce the peak saliva concentrations and AUC of a single 250-mg dose of procainamide by about 30% in 4 healthy subjects. Kaolin-pectin and a variety of antacids (Pepto-bismol, Simeco, and magnesium trisilicate) absorbed procainamide in vitro.[2] The clinical importance of this awaits further study.

1. Albin H, Vincon G, Bertolaso D, Dangoumau J. Influence du phosphate d'aluminium sur la biodisponibilité de la procaïnamide et du disopyramide. Therapie (1981) 36, 541–6.

2. Al-Shora HI, Moustafa MA, Niazy EM, Gaber M, Gouda MW. Interactions of procainamide, verapamil, guanethidine and hydralazine with adsorbent antacids and antidiarrhoeal mixtures. Int J Pharmaceutics (1988) 47, 209–13.

Disopyramide + Beta-blockers

Severe bradycardia has been described in 3 cases (1 fatal) after the use of intravenous practolol then intravenous disopyramide; in one case (fatal) after oral pindolol and oral disopyramide; and in one case when oral metoprolol was added to disopyramide. Another patient given intravenous sotalol developed asystole (see also 'Drugs that prolong the QT interval + Other drugs that prolong the QT interval', p.103).

Atenolol modestly decreased disopyramide clearance in one study. Oral propranolol and disopyramide have been combined without any increase in negative inotropic effects or pharmacokinetic changes in healthy subjects.

Clinical evidence

Two patients with supraventricular tachycardia (180 bpm) were treated, firstly with intravenous practolol (20 and 10 mg respectively) and shortly afterwards with disopyramide (150 and 80 mg respectively). The first patient rapidly developed sinus bradycardia of 25 bpm, lost consciousness and became profoundly hypotensive. He failed to respond to 600 micrograms atropine, but later his heart rate increased to 60 bpm while a temporary pacemaker was being inserted.[1] He was successfully treated with disopyramide 150 mg alone for a later episode of tachycardia. The second patient also developed severe bradycardia and asystole, despite the use of atropine. He was resuscitated with epinephrine (adrenaline) but later died.[1] Severe bradycardia has been reported in another patient, similarly treated with intravenous practolol and then disopyramide.[2] One other patient has been described who developed severe bradycardia and died when treated for supraventricular tachycardia with pindolol 5 mg and disopyramide 250 mg (both orally).[3] Another patient on oral disopyramide 250 mg twice daily developed asystole when given a total of 60 mg of intravenous sotalol.[4]

A patient with hypertrophic obstructive cardiomyopathy and paroxysmal atrial fibrillation on disopyramide 450 mg daily developed hypotension, bradycardia and cardiac conduction disturbances 5 days after starting metoprolol 50 mg daily. It was suggested that disopyramide, especially when given with metoprolol, has the potential to induce adverse effects in patients with normal cardiac conduction and ventricular function.[5]

Atenolol (100 mg daily) has been shown to increase the serum disopyramide steady-state levels from 3.46 to 4.25 micrograms/ml and reduce the clearance of disopyramide by 16% (from 1.9 to 1.59 ml/kg/min) in healthy subjects and patients with ischaemic heart disease.[6] None of the subjects developed any adverse reactions or symptoms of heart failure, apart from one of the volunteers who showed transient first degree heart block.[6]

In contrast, studies in healthy subjects have shown that the negative inotropic effect was no greater when oral propranolol and disopyramide were used concurrently,[7,8] nor were the pharmacokinetics of either drug affected.[9]

Mechanism

Not understood. Both disopyramide and the beta-blockers can depress the contractility and conductivity of the heart muscle.

Importance and management

The general clinical importance of this interaction is uncertain. A clear risk seems to exist in patients who are treated with disopyramide and practolol or sotalol given intravenously. Considerable caution should be exercised in these patients. More study is needed to find out what contributes to the development of this potentially serious interaction. The makers of disopyramide suggest that the combination of disopyramide and beta-blockers should generally be avoided.[10,11]

The makers of sotalol also warn that both sotalol and disopyramide can prolong the QT interval, which may therefore increase the risk of torsade de pointes arrhythmia if both are used together.[12] See also 'Drugs that prolong the QT interval + Other drugs that prolong the QT interval', p.103.

1. Cumming AD, Robertson C. Interaction between disopyramide and practolol. BMJ (1979) 2, 1264.
2. Gelipter D, Hazell M. Interaction between disopyramide and practolol. BMJ (1980) 1, 52.
3. Pedersen C, Josephsen P, Lindvig K. Interaktion mellem disopyramid og pindolol efter oral indgift. Ugeskr Laeger (1983) 145, 3266.
4. Bystedt T, Vitols S. Sotalol-disopyramid ledde till asystoli. Lakartidningen (1994) 91, 2241.
5. Pernat A, Pohar B, Horvat M, Heart conduction disturbances and cardiovascular collapse after disopyramide and low-dose metoprolol in a patient with hypertrophic obstructive cardiomyopathy. J Electrocardiology (1997) 30, 341–4.
6. Bonde J, Bødtker S, Angelo HR, Svendsen TL, Kampmann JP. Atenolol inhibits the elimination of disopyramide. Eur J Clin Pharmacol (1986) 28, 41–3.

7. Cathcart-Rake WF, Coker JE, Atkins FL, Huffman DH, Hassanein KM, Shen DD, Azarnoff DL. The effect of concurrent oral administration of propranolol and disopyramide on cardiac function in healthy men. *Circulation* (1980) 61, 938–45.
8. Cathcart-Rake W, Coker J, Shen D, Huffman D, Azarnoff D. The pharmacodynamics of concurrent disopyramide and propranolol. *Clin Pharmacol Ther* (1979) 25, 217.
9. Karim A, Nissen C, Azarnoff DL. Clinical pharmacokinetics of disopyramide. *J Pharmacokinet Biopharm* (1982) 10, 465–94.
10. Dirythmin (Disopyramide). AstraZeneca. Summary of product characteristics. October 1995.
11. Rythmodan (Disopyramide). Borg Medicare. Summary of product characteristics. June 1998.
12. Beta-Cardone (Sotalol). Celltech Pharmaceuticals Limited. Summary of product characteristics, April 2001.

Disopyramide + Cimetidine or Ranitidine

A single-dose study has shown that cimetidine can slightly increase the serum levels of oral disopyramide, but whether this would also occur with multiple doses is not known. Cimetidine did not affect the pharmacokinetics of intravenous disopyramide. Ranitidine appears not to interact.

Clinical evidence, mechanism, importance and management

Cimetidine 400 mg twice daily by mouth for 14 days did not alter the pharmacokinetics of a single 150 mg intravenous dose of disopyramide in 7 healthy subjects.[1] Another study in 6 normal subjects showed that a single 400-mg dose of **cimetidine** increased the AUC following a single 300 mg oral dose of disopyramide by 8.5% and increased the maximum serum levels by 18.5%, but did not significantly affect the metabolism of disopyramide. **Ranitidine** 150 mg was found not to interact significantly.[2] The reasons are not known, but the authors of the report suggest that **cimetidine** may have increased disopyramide absorption. Cimetidine is only a weak inhibitor of disopyramide metabolism *in vitro*.[3] Whether an interaction would occur in a more clinically realistic situation, using multiple oral doses of both drugs, awaits further study.

1. Bonde J, Pedersen LE, Nygaard E, Ramsing T, Angelo HR, Kampmann JP. Stereoselective pharmacokinetics of disopyramide and interaction with cimetidine. *Br J Clin Pharmacol* (1991) 31, 708–10.
2. Jou M-J, Huang S-C, Kiang F-M, Lai M-Y, Chao P-DL. Comparison of the effects of cimetidine and ranitidine on the pharmacokinetics of disopyramide in man. *J Pharm Pharmacol* (1997) 49, 1072–5.
3. Echuzen H, Kawasaki H, Chiba K, Tani M, Ishizaki T. A potent inhibitory effect of erythromycin and other macrolide antibiotics on the mono-N-dealkylation metabolism of disopyramide with human liver microsomes. *J Pharmacol Exp Ther* (1993) 264, 1425–31.

Disopyramide + Macrolide antibacterials

The serum disopyramide levels of two patients rose when given erythromycin and cardiac arrhythmias developed. One patient given both drugs developed heart block. Yet another developed ventricular fibrillation when given clarithromycin with disopyramide and two other patients developed severe hypoglycaemia. Ventricular fibrillation occurred in a patient treated with azithromycin and disopyramide. *In vitro* studies suggest that josamycin may interact similarly. See also 'Drugs that prolong the QT interval + Other drugs that prolong the QT interval', p.103.

Clinical evidence

(a) Azithromycin

A patient on disopyramide 150 mg three times daily developed ventricular tachycardia (requiring cardioversion) 11 days after starting **azithromycin** 250 mg daily.[1] Her disopyramide level was found to have risen from 2.6 to 11.1 mg/l.

(b) Clarithromycin

A woman of 74 who had been taking 200 mg disopyramide twice daily for 7 years collapsed with ventricular fibrillation 6 days after start-

ing to take 40 mg omeprazole, 800 mg metronidazole and 500 mg **clarithromycin** daily. After successful resuscitation, her QTc, which had never previously been above 440 ms, was found to have risen to 625 ms. Her disopyramide plasma level was also elevated (4.6 micrograms/ml) and the half-life was markedly prolonged (40 h). The QTc interval normalised as her plasma disopyramide levels fell.[2]

A haemodialysis patient, receiving disopyramide 50 mg daily because of paroxysmal atrial fibrillation, was hospitalised with hypoglycaemic coma after additional treatment with clarithromycin 600 mg daily. Serum disopyramide levels increased from 1.5 micrograms/ml to 8 micrograms/ml during treatment with clarithromycin. QT and QTc intervals were prolonged, but torsade de pointes did not occur.[3] Hypoglycaemic coma during concomitant disopyramide and clarithromycin treatment has also been reported in another patient.[4]

(c) Erythromycin

A woman with ventricular ectopy taking disopyramide (300 mg alternating with 150 mg six-hourly) developed new arrhythmias (ventricular asystoles and later polymorphic ventricular tachycardia – torsade de pointes) within 36 h of starting 1 g **erythromycin lactobionate** intravenously 6-hourly and cefamandole (cephamandole). Her QTc interval had increased from 0.39 to 0.6 sec and her serum disopyramide level was found to be 16 micromol/l. The problem resolved when the disopyramide was stopped and bretylium given, but it returned when the disopyramide was restarted. It resolved again when the **erythromycin** was stopped.[5] Another patient with ventricular tachycardia, well controlled over 5 years with 200 mg disopyramide four times daily, developed polymorphic ventricular tachycardia within a few days of starting 500 mg **erythromycin base** four times daily. His QTc interval had increased from 0.43 to 0.63 sec and serum disopyramide levels were found to be elevated (30 micromol/l). The problem resolved when both drugs were withdrawn and antiarrhythmics given.[5] Heart block is said to have developed in another patient treated with both drugs.[6]

Mechanism

Not fully established. An *in vitro* study using human liver microsomes indicated that erythromycin inhibits the metabolism (mono-*N*-dealkylation) of disopyramide which, *in vivo*, would be expected to reduce its loss from the body and increase its serum levels.[7] Clarithromycin and azithromycin probably do the same. The increased serum levels of disopyramide can result in adverse effects such as QT prolongation and torsade de pointes, and may result in enhanced insulin secretion and hypoglycaemia.[3,4] There are also a number of cases on record of prolongation of the QT interval and torsade de pointes associated with the use of intravenous erythromycin alone.[8] Therefore, disopyramide and intravenous erythromycin may have additive effects on the QT interval in addition to the pharmacokinetic interaction.

Importance and management

Direct information seems to be limited to these 6 cases[1-6] and the *in vitro* study cited.[7] Even so the effects of concurrent use should be well monitored if azithromycin, clarithromycin or erythromycin is added to disopyramide, being alert for the development of raised plasma disopyramide levels and prolongation of the QT interval. One of the makers of disopyramide recommends[9] avoiding the combination of disopyramide with macrolides that inhibit cytochrome P450 isoenzyme CYP3A, and this would certainly be prudent in situations where close monitoring is not possible. Direct clinical information about other macrolides is lacking but *in vitro* studies with human liver microsomes[7] indicate that **josamycin** is likely to interact similarly. More study is needed. See also 'Drugs that prolong the QT interval + Other drugs that prolong the QT interval', p.103.

1. Granowitz EV, Tabor KJ, Kirchhoffer JB. Potentially fatal interaction between azithromycin and disopyramide. *Pacing Clin Electrophysiol* (2000) 23, 1433–5.
2. Paar D, Terjung B, Sauerbruch T. Life-threatening interaction between clarithromycin and disopyramide. *Lancet* (1997) 349, 326–7.
3. Iida H, Morita T, Suzuki E, Iwasawa K, Toyo-oka T, Nakajima T. Hypoglycemia induced by interaction between clarithromycin and disopyramide. *Jpn Heart J* (1999) 40, 91–6.

4. Morlet-Barla N, Narbonne H, Vialettes B. Hypoglycémie grave et récidivante secondaire á l'interaction disopyramide-clarithromicine. *Presse Med* (2000) 29, 1351.
5. Ragosta M, Weihl AC, Rosenfeld LE. Potentially fatal interaction between erythromycin and disopyramide. *Am J Med* (1989) 86, 465–6.
6. Beeley L, Cunningham H, Carmichael A, Brennan A. Bulletin of the W. *Midlands Centre for Adverse Drug Reaction Reporting* (1992) 35, 13.
7. Echizen H, Kawasaki H, Chiba K, Tani M. Ishizaki T. A potent inhibitory effect of erythromycin and other macrolide antibiotics on the mono-N-dealkylation metabolism of disopyramide with human liver microsomes. *J Pharmacol Exp Ther* (1993) 264, 1425–31.
8. Gitler B, Berger LS, Buffa SD. Torsades de pointes induced by erythromycin. *Chest* (1994) 105, 368–72.
9. Rythmodan (Disopyramide). Borg Medicare. Summary of product characteristics. June 1998.

Disopyramide + Phenobarbital

Serum disopyramide levels are reduced by the concurrent use of phenobarbital.

Clinical evidence

After taking 100 mg **phenobarbital** daily for 21 days, the half-life and AUC of a single 200-mg dose of disopyramide were reduced by about 35%. The apparent metabolic clearance more than doubled, and the fraction recovered in urine as metabolite increased. Sixteen normal subjects took part in the study and no significant differences were seen between those who smoked and those who did not.[1]

Mechanism

It seems probable that the phenobarbital (a known enzyme inducing agent) increases the metabolism of disopyramide by the liver, and thereby increases its loss from the body.

Importance and management

This interaction appears to be established, but its clinical importance is uncertain. The extent to it would reduce the control of arrhythmias by disopyramide in patients is unknown, but monitor the effects and the serum levels of disopyramide if phenobarbital is added or withdrawn. One maker of disopyramide recommends avoiding using it in combination with inducers of cytochrome P450 isoenzyme CYP3A such as phenobarbital.[2] Other barbiturates would be expected to interact similarly.

1. Kapil RP, Axelson JE, Mansfield IL, Edwards DJ, McErlane B, Mason MA, Lalka D, Kerr CR. Disopyramide pharmacokinetics and metabolism: effect of inducers. *Br J Clin Pharmacol* (1987) 24, 781–91.
2. Rythmodan (Disopyramide). Borg Medicare. Summary of product characteristics. June 1998.

Disopyramide + Phenytoin

Serum disopyramide levels are reduced by the concurrent use of phenytoin and may fall below therapeutic concentrations. Loss of arrhythmic control may occur.

Clinical evidence

Eight patients with ventricular tachycardia treated with disopyramide (600–2000 mg daily) showed a 54% fall in their serum disopyramide levels (from a mean of 3.99 to 1.82 micrograms/ml) when concurrently treated with **phenytoin** (200–600 mg daily) for a week. Two of the patients who responded to disopyramide and underwent Holter monitoring showed a 53- and 2000-fold increase in ventricular premature beat frequency as a result of this interaction.[1]

In other reports, 3 patients who had low levels of disopyramide and high levels of its metabolite were noted to be simultaneously taking phenytoin,[2] and 1 patient receiving both drugs required an unusually high dose of disopyramide.[3] A marked fall in serum disopyramide levels (75% in one case) was seen in 2 patients after taking **phenytoin** (300–400 mg daily) for up to two weeks.[4] Pharmacokinetic studies in two[5] and ten[3] healthy subjects confirm this interaction. In addition,

one healthy epileptic taking **phenytoin** had about 50% lower disopyramide AUC and elimination half-life than control subjects.[5]

Mechanism

Phenytoin, which is a known enzyme-inducing agent, increases the metabolism of the disopyramide by the liver. The major metabolite (N-dealkyldisopyramide) also possesses antiarrhythmic activity nevertheless the net effect is a reduction in arrhythmic control.[1]

Importance and management

An established interaction of clinical importance. Some loss of arrhythmic control can occur during concurrent use. Serum disopyramide levels and the antiarrhythmic response should be well monitored. An increase in the dosage of disopyramide may be necessary. Serum disopyramide levels return to normal within two weeks of withdrawing the phenytoin.

1. Matos JA, Fisher JD, Kim SG. Disopyramide-phenytoin interaction. *Clin Res* (1981) 29, 655A.
2. Aitio M-L, Vuorenmaa T. Enhanced metabolism and diminished efficacy of disopyramide by enzyme induction? *Br J Clin Pharmacol* (1980) 9, 149–152.
3. Nightingale J, Nappi JM. Effect of phenytoin on serum disopyramide concentrations. *Clin Pharm* (1987) 6, 46–50.
4. Kessler JM, Keys PW, Stafford RW. Disopyramide and phenytoin interaction. *Clin Pharm* (1982) 1, 263–4.
5. Aitio M-L, Mansury L, Tala E, Haataja M, Aitio A. The effect of enzyme induction on the metabolism of disopyramide in man. *Br J Clin Pharmacol* (1981) 11, 279–85.

Disopyramide + Quinidine

Disopyramide serum levels may be slightly raised by quinidine. Both drugs prolong the QT interval, and this may be additive on combined use.

Clinical evidence, mechanism, importance and management

After taking **quinidine** 200 mg four times a day, the peak serum levels of disopyramide, given as single 150-mg doses to 16 normal subjects, were raised by 20% (from 2.68 to 3.23 micrograms/ml), and by 14% when given chronically as 150 mg four times a day. Serum **quinidine** levels were decreased by 26%. However, there was no change in the half-life of either drug. Both quinidine and disopyramide caused a slight lengthening of the QTc interval, and when quinidine was added to disopyramide therapy additional lengthening of the QT interval occurred. The frequency of adverse effects such as dry mouth, blurred vision, urine retention and nausea were also somewhat increased.[1] The mechanism of the effect on serum levels is not understood. The anticholinergic side-effects of disopyramide may be increased. Disopyramide and quinidine are both class Ia antiarrhythmics that prolong the QT interval, and, in general, such combinations should be avoided (see also 'Drugs that prolong the QT interval + Other drugs that prolong the QT interval', p.103).

1. Baker BJ, Gammill J, Massengill J, Schubert E, Karin A, Doherty JE. Concurrent use of quinidine and disopyramide: evaluation of serum concentrations and electrocardiographic effects. *Am Heart J* (1983) 105, 12–15.

Disopyramide + Rifampicin

The serum levels of disopyramide can be markedly reduced by the concurrent use of rifampicin.

Clinical evidence

After taking **rifampicin** for 14 days the plasma levels of disopyramide in 11 patients with tuberculosis who had taken single 200 or 300-mg doses were approximately halved.[1] The AUCs before and after were 20.3 and 8.22 micrograms ml^{-1} h, respectively, and the half-life was reduced from 5.9 to 3.25 h. A woman who had been receiving **rifampicin** for 2 weeks initially showed only subtherapeutic serum levels of disopyramide (0.9 micromol/l) when first started on 100 mg 8-hourly. The dosage of disopyramide was increased to 300 mg 8-hourly, and the rifampicin was discontinued, although its effects persisted for 5 days. Three days after discontinuing rifampicin the disopyramide level was 3.6 micromol/l and after 5 days it was 8.1 micromol/l. The patient was eventually maintained on disopyramide 250 mg 8-hourly.[2]

Mechanism

The most probable explanation is that rifampicin (a well known enzyme inducer) markedly increases the metabolism of the disopyramide by the liver so that it is cleared from the body much more quickly.

Importance and management

Information seems to be limited to these studies, but they indicate that the dosage of disopyramide will need to be increased in most patients taking rifampicin.

1. Aitio M-L, Mansury L, Tala E, Haataja M, Aitio A. The effect of enzyme induction on the metabolism of disopyramide in man. *Br J Clin Pharmacol* (1981) 11, 279–85.
2. Staum JM. Enzyme induction: rifampin-disopyramide interaction. *DICP Ann Pharmacother* (1990) 24, 701–3.

Disopyramide + Verapamil

Profound hypotension and collapse has occurred in a small number of patients on verapamil given disopyramide.

Clinical evidence, mechanism, importance and management

A group of clinicians who had given single 400 mg oral doses of disopyramide successfully and with few side-effects for reverting acute supraventricular arrhythmias, also reported five cases of profound hypotension and collapse. Three of the patients developed severe epigastric pain. All five had previous myocardial disease and/or were taking myocardial depressants — beta-blockers or **verapamil** in small quantities (not specified).[1]

On the basis of this report, on reports of studies in *animals*,[2] and from the known risks associated with the concurrent use of beta-blockers (see 'Disopyramide + Beta-blockers', p.98), the makers warn about combining disopyramide and other drugs [such as **verapamil**] that may have additive negative inotropic effects. However, they do point out that in some specific circumstances the combination may be beneficial. They note that hypotension has usually been associated with cardiomyopathy or uncompensated congestive heart failure.[3,4]

1. Manolas EG, Hunt D, Dowling JT, Luxton M, Vohra J. Collapse after oral administration of disopyramide. *Med J Aust* (1979) Jan 13.
2. Lee JT, Davy J-M, Kates RE. Evaluation of combined administration of verapamil and disopyramide in dogs. *J Cardiovasc Pharmacol* (1985) 7, 501–7.
3. Rythmodan (Disopyramide). Borg Medicare. Summary of product characteristics, June 1998.
4. Dirythmin (Disopyramide). AstraZeneca. Summary of product characteristics, October 1995.

Dofetilide + Miscellaneous drugs

Cimetidine, ketoconazole and trimethoprim markedly increase plasma dofetilide levels, and hence increase dofetilide-induced QT prolongation and the risk of torsade de pointes arrhythmias. Verapamil transiently increases dofetilide plasma levels and QTc prolongation, and has been associated with an increased risk of torsade de pointes. Their combined use with dofetilide should probably be avoided. Dofetilide appears not to interact with antacids, digoxin, omeprazole, phenytoin, ranitidine, theophylline or warfarin.

Clinical evidence

(a) Cimetidine or ranitidine

A placebo-controlled study in 24 healthy subjects indicated that the co-administration of **cimetidine** 400 mg twice daily with dofetilide 500 micrograms twice daily for 7 days significantly decreased the renal clearance of dofetilide (by 44%), and increased its AUC (by 58%) and peak blood levels (by 50%), without significantly altering the QTc interval.[1] In a further study it was found that **cimetidine** 100 or 400 mg twice daily for 4 days reduced the renal clearance of single doses of dofetilide 500 micrograms by 13 and 33% respectively. In addition, the respective cimetidine doses increased the QTc interval by 22 and 33%. **Ranitidine** 150 mg twice daily did not significantly affect the pharmacokinetics or pharmacodynamics of dofetilide

(b) Digoxin

In a placebo-controlled study in 13 subjects, 250 micrograms dofetilide twice daily for 5 days had no effect on the steady-state pharmacokinetics of **digoxin**, administered at a dose of 250 micrograms daily after a loading dose.[2-4]

(c) Ketoconazole

The maker of dofetilide notes that **ketoconazole** 400 mg daily administered concurrently with dofetilide 500 micrograms twice daily for 7 days increased the dofetilide peak levels by 53% and 97%, and AUC by 41% and 69%, in males and females, respectively.[5]

(d) Omeprazole or Antacids

A study in 12 healthy subjects found that altering gastric pH by pretreatment with either **omeprazole** 40 mg (10 or 2 h before dofetilide), or **Maalox** 30 ml (10, 2 and 0.5 h before dofetilide) did not affect the pharmacokinetics of dofetilide 500 micrograms nor the dofetilide-induced change in QTc interval.[6]

(e) Phenytoin

In one study, 24 healthy subjects were stabilised on **phenytoin** to achieve steady-state plasma levels of 8–20 micrograms/ml and then either 1 mg dofetilide daily or placebo was co-administered. No effects on **phenytoin** pharmacokinetics or cardiac effects were seen.[7] Another study by the same researchers in 24 subjects given 500 micrograms dofetilide 12-hourly found that the concurrent use of 300 mg **phenytoin** daily did not have a clinically important effect on either the pharmacokinetics of the **dofetilide** or on its pharmacodynamics (QTc, PR, QRS, RR intervals).[8]

(f) Theophylline

Studies in healthy subjects found that the concurrent use of **theophylline** 450 mg every 12 hours and dofetilide 500 micrograms every 12 hours was well tolerated and the steady-state pharmacokinetics and pharmacodynamics of both dofetilide and theophylline were not affected by the co-administration of either drug.[9,10]

(g) Trimethoprim

The maker of dofetilide notes that **trimethoprim** 160 mg (in combination with **sulfamethoxazole** 800 mg) twice daily administered concurrently with dofetilide 500 micrograms twice daily for 4 days increased dofetilide peak levels by 93% and AUC by 103%.[5]

(h) Verapamil

A study in 12 healthy subjects found that concurrent administration of **verapamil** 80 mg three times daily and dofetilide 500 micrograms daily caused an increase in peak plasma levels of dofetilide from 2.4 to 3.43 ng/ml (42%). There was a transient increase in AUC over the first 4 hours from 7.4 to 9.3 ng.h/ml, which was associated with a transient simultaneous increase in QTc from 20 ms for dofetilide alone to 26 ms in the presence of **verapamil**.[11] The maker notes that an analysis of clinical trial data for dofetilide revealed a higher occurrence of torsade de pointes when **verapamil** was used with dofetilide.[5]

(i) Warfarin

The prothrombin time response to a single 40-mg dose of **warfarin** was found to be unchanged when given on day 5 of an 8-day course of 750 micrograms dofetilide twice daily in 14 healthy subjects.[2]

Mechanism

At least 50% of a dofetilide dose is eliminated unchanged in the urine by an active renal tubular secretion mechanism.[5,12] Drugs that inhibit this mechanism, such as cimetidine, ketoconazole and trimethoprim, increase dofetilide plasma levels.[5,13] These drugs may increase the risk of dofetilide-induced torsade de pointes arrhythmias since there is a linear relationship between plasma dofetilide concentrations and prolongation of the QT interval.[5] Verapamil is postulated to interact with dofetilide by affecting hepatic blood flow.[11]

An *in vitro* study showed a lack of cytochrome P450 inhibition by dofetilide suggesting that dofetilide is unlikely to affect the metabolism of other drugs.[14] This has been confirmed for phenytoin, theophylline, and warfarin. However, dofetilide is partially metabolised by the liver, primarily by cytochrome P450 isoenzyme CYP3A4,[14] and therefore an effect of CYP3A4 inhibitors on dofetilide metabolism cannot be discounted.[5]

Importance and management

The concomitant use of verapamil with dofetilide appears to be associated with an increased risk of torsade de pointes and should be avoided. Drugs that have been shown to markedly increase dofetilide plasma concentrations such as cimetidine, ketoconazole, and trimethoprim, should probably be avoided because they are also likely to increase the risk of torsade de pointes arrhythmias. The manufacturer also suggests the avoidance of other drugs that inhibit the renal mechanism by which dofetilide is eliminated, such as **prochlorperazine** and **megestrol**,[5] although these have not been directly studied. The manufacturer suggests[5] that there is a potential for dofetilide plasma levels to be increased by other drugs undergoing active renal secretion (e.g. **amiloride, metformin** and **triamterene**), and by inhibitors of cytochrome P450 isoenzyme CYP3A4.

No special precautions appear to be necessary with antacids, digoxin, omeprazole, phenytoin, ranitidine, theophylline and warfarin.

1. Vincent J, Gardner MJ, Apseloff G, Baris B, Willavize S, Friedman HL. Cimetidine inhibits renal elimination of dofetilide without altering QTc activity on multiple dosing in healthy subjects. *Clin Pharmacol Ther* (1998) 63, 210.
2. Nichols DJ, Dalrymple I, Newgreen MW, Kleinermans D. The effect of dofetilide on pharmacodynamics of warfarin and pharmacokinetics of digoxin. *Eur Heart J* (1999) 20 (Abstr Suppl), 586.
3. Rasmussen HS, Kleinermans D, Walker D, Rapeport WG. A double-blind, placebo controlled parallel group study of the effect of UK-68,798, a novel class III antiarrhythmic agent, on the pharmacokinetics and pharmacodynamics of digoxin. *Eur Heart J* (1990) 11 (Suppl), S57.
4. Kleinermans D, Nichols DJ, Dalrymple I. Effect of dofetilide on the pharmacokinetics of digoxin. *Am J Cardiol* (2001) 87, 248–50.
5. Tikosyn (Dofetilide). Pfizer Labs. US prescribing information, December 1999.
6. Vincent J, Gardner MJ, Baris B, Willavize SA. Concurrent administration of omeprazole and antacid does not alter the pharmacokinetics and pharmacodynamic of dofetilide in healthy subjects. *Clin Pharmacol Ther* (1996) 59, 182.
7. Vincent J, Gardner M, Scavone J, Ashton H, Willavize S, Friedman HL. The effect of dofetilide on the steady-state PK and cardiac effects of phenytoin in healthy subjects. *Clin Pharmacol Ther* (1997) 61, 233.
8. Gardner MJ, Ashton HM, Willavize SA, Friedman HL, Vincent J. The effects of phenytoin on the steady-state PK and PD of dofetilide in healthy subjects. *Clin Pharmacol Ther* (1997) 61, 205.
9. Gardner MJ, Ashton HM, Willavize SA, Vincent J. The effects of concomitant dofetilide therapy on the pharmacokinetics and pharmacodynamics of theophylline. *Clin Pharmacol Ther* (1996) 59, 181.
10. Gardner MJ, Ashton HM, Willavize SA, Vincent J. The effects of orally administered theophylline on the pharmacokinetics and pharmacodynamics of dofetilide. *Clin Pharmacol Ther* (1996) 59, 182.
11. Johnson BF, Cheng SL, Venitz J. Transient kinetic and dynamic interactions between verapamil and dofetilide, a class III antiarrhythmic. *J Clin Pharmacol* (2001) 41, 1248–56.
12. Rasmussen HS, Allen MJ, Blackburn KJ, Butrous GS, Dalrymple HW. Dofetilide, a novel class III antiarrhythmic agent. *J Cardiovasc Pharmacol* (1992) 20 (Suppl 2), S96–S105.
13. Abel S, Nichols DJ, Brearly CJ, Eve MD. Effect of cimetidine and ranitidine on pharmacokinetics and pharmacodynamics of a single dose of dofetilide. *Br J Clin Pharmacol* (2000) 49, 64–71.
14. Walker DK, Alabaster CT, Congrave GS, Hargreaves MB, Hyland R, Jones BC, Reed LJ, Smith DA. Significance of metabolism in the disposition and action of the antidysrhythmic drug, dofetilide. *In vitro* studies and correlation with *in vivo* data. *Drug Metab Dispos* (1996) 24, 447–55.

Table 4.3 Drugs causing QT prolongation and torsade de pointes

Antiarrhythmics

Amiodarone (1,2)
Disopyramide (1,2)
Dofetilide (4)
Procainamide (1,2)
Quinidine (1,2)
Sotalol (1,2)

Antihistamines

Astemizole (1,2,3)
Terfenadine (1,2,3)

Anti-infectives

Artemether (3)
Chloroquine (2)
Clarithromycin (3)
Co-trimoxazole (2)
Erythromycin (2,3)
Gatifloxacin (3)
Grepafloxacin (3)
Halofantrine (1,2,3)
Ketoconazole (3)
Moxifloxacin (3)
Pentamidine (2,3)
Quinine (2,3)
Sparfloxacin (3)
Spiramycin (2,3)

Antidepressants

Fluoxetine (3)
Maprotiline (2)
Tricyclic antidepressants (2,3)

Antipsychotics

Chlorpromazine (2,3)
Droperidol (1,3)
Haloperidol (2,3)
Lithium (2)
Pimozide (1,2,3)
Sertindole (3)
Thioridazine (1,2,3)

Calcium channel blockers

Bepridil (2)
Lidoflazine (2)
Prenylamine (2)
Terodiline (2)

Miscellaneous drugs

Chloral hydrate (2)
Cisapride (2)
Ketanserin (2)
Organophosphates (2)
Probucol (2,3)
Suxamethonium (Succinylcholine) (2)
Tacrolimus (3)
Tamoxifen (3)
Vasopressin (2)

This list is not exhaustive.

Drugs that prolong the QT interval + Other drugs that prolong the QT interval

The consensus of opinion is that the concurrent use of two or more drugs that prolong the QT interval should be avoided because of the risk of additive effects, leading to the possible development of serious and potentially life-threatening torsade de pointes cardiac arrhythmia.

Clinical evidence, mechanism, importance and management

If the QT interval on the ECG becomes excessively prolonged, ventricular arrhythmias can develop, in particular a type of polymorphic tachycardia known as 'torsade de pointes'. On the ECG this arrhythmia can appear as an intermittent series of rapid spikes during which the heart fails to pump effectively, the blood pressure falls and the patient will feel dizzy and may possibly lose consciousness. Usually the condition is self-limiting but it may progress and degenerate into ventricular fibrillation which can cause sudden death.

There are a number of reasons why QT interval prolongation can occur. These include congenital conditions, cardiac disease and some metabolic disturbances (hypokalaemia, hypomagnesaemia), but probably the most important cause is the use of various drugs including some antiarrhythmics, antipsychotics, antihistamines, antimalarials and others.

It is thought that torsade de pointes arrhythmia is unlikely to develop until the corrected QT (QTc) interval exceeds 500 ms, but this is not an exact figure and the risks are uncertain and unpredictable. Because of these uncertainties, many drug manufacturers and regulatory agencies now contraindicate the concurrent use of drugs known to prolong the QT interval, and a 'blanket' warning is often issued because the QT prolonging effects of the drugs are expected to be additive. The UK CSM/MCA advise avoiding concurrent use of more than one of these drugs (the drugs specifically named by the CSM/MCA in 1996 are indicated by a (1) in Table 4.3). The extent of the drug-induced prolongation usually depends on the dosage of the drug and the particular drugs in question.

Table 4.3 is a list of drugs (derived from the sources indicated[1-4]) that are known to prolong the QT interval and cause torsade de pointes, but it needs to be made very clear that in many cases the prediction of possible additive effects is only based on a reasonable supposition. In many cases interactions have yet to been shown to occur in clinical practice, and to be of importance. Some of the drug pairs are dealt with in individual monographs. See the Index. Drugs that do not themselves prolong the QT interval, but potentiate the effect of drugs that do (e.g. by pharmacokinetic mechanisms) are not included in Table 4.3. The interactions of these drugs (e.g. azole antifungals or macrolides with cisapride) are dealt with in individual monographs. See the Index.

1. Committee on Safety of Medicines/Medicines Control Agency. Drug-induced prolongation of the QT interval. *Current Problems* (1996) 22, 2.
2. Thomas SHL. Drugs, QT interval abnormalities and ventricular arrhythmias. *Adverse Drug React Toxicol Rev* (1994) 13, 77–102.
3. De Ponti F, Poluzzi E, Montanaro N. QT-interval prolongation by non-cardiac drugs: lessons to be learned from recent experience. *Eur J Clin Pharmacol* (2000) 56, 1–18.
4. Rasmussen HS, Allen MJ, Blackburn KJ, Butrous GS, Dalrymple HW. Dofetilide, a novel class III antiarrhythmic agent. *J Cardiovasc Pharmacol* (1992) 20 (Suppl 2), S96–S105.

Flecainide + Amiodarone

Serum flecainide levels are increased by amiodarone. The flecainide dosage should be reduced by between one-third and one-half. An isolated report describes torsade de pointes in a patient on amiodarone when given flecainide.

Clinical evidence

Seven patients on oral flecainide (200–500 mg daily) were given reduced doses when **amiodarone** was added (1200 mg daily for 10 to 14 days as a loading dose, later reduced to 600 mg daily) because it was observed that the trough plasma levels of flecainide were increased by about 50%. The flecainide dosage was reduced by one-third (averaging a reduction from 325 to 225 mg daily) to keep the flecainide levels constant. Observations in two patients suggest that the interaction begins soon after the **amiodarone** is added, and it takes two weeks or more to develop fully.[1]

Other authors have reported this interaction, and suggest reducing the flecainide dosage by between one-third to one-half when amiodarone is added.[2-4] Another study found that amiodarone raised steady-state flecainide plasma levels by 37% in extensive metabolisers, and 55% in poor metabolisers, of dextromethorphan (a probe drug for cytochrome P450 isoenzyme CYP2D6 activity).[5] In a later report of this study the authors concluded that these differences were not clinically important, and that CYP2D6 phenotype does not affect the extent of the flecainide-amiodarone interaction.[6] An isolated report describes torsade de pointes in a patient on **amiodarone** when given flecainide.[7]

Mechanism

Amiodarone inhibits cytochrome P450 isoenzyme CYP2D6 activity, so that the flecainide is metabolised by the liver more slowly. Amiodarone also inhibits CYP2D6-independent mechanisms of flecainide elimination.[6]

Importance and management

An established interaction, but the documentation is limited. Reduce the flecainide dosage by between one-third to one-half if amiodarone is added.[1-4,6] The maker of flecainide recommends a 50% reduction in dose if amiodarone is given, and that plasma levels should be monitored.[8] There seems to be no need to treat extensive metabolisers differently from poor metabolisers.[6] Remember that the interaction may take two weeks or more to develop fully, and also that amiodarone is cleared from the body exceptionally slowly so that this interaction may persist for some weeks after it has been withdrawn.

1. Shea P, Lal R, Kim SS, Schechtman K, Ruffy R. Flecainide and amiodarone interaction. *J Am Coll Cardiol* (1986) 7, 1127–30.
2. Leclercq JF, Coumel P. La flécaïnide: un nouvel antiarrhythmique. *Arch Mal Coeur* (1983) 76, 1218–29.
3. Fontaine G, Frank R, Tonet JL. Association amiodarone-flécaïnide dans le traitement des troubles du rythme ventriculaires graves. *Arch Mal Coeur* (1984) 77, 1421.
4. Leclercq JF, Coumel P. Association amiodarone-flécaïnide dans le traitement des troubles du rythme ventriculaires graves. Résponse. *Arch Mal Coeur* (1984) 77, 1421–2.
5. Funck-Brentano C, Kroemer HK, Becquemont L, Bühl K, Eichelbaum M, Jaillon P. The interaction between amiodarone and flecainide is genetically determined. *Circulation* (1992) 86, (Suppl I), I–720.
6. Funck-Brentano C, Becquemont L, Kroemer HK, Bühl K, Knebel NG, Eichelbaum M, Jaillon P. Variable disposition kinetics and electrocardiographic effects of flecainide during repeated dosing in humans: contribution of genetic factors, dose-dependent clearance, and interaction with amiodarone. *Clin Pharmacol Ther* (1994) 55, 256–69.
7. Andrivet P, Beaslay V, Canh VD. Torsades de pointe with flecainide-amiodarone therapy. *Int Care Med* (1990) 16, 342–3.
8. Tambocor (Flecainide). 3M Health Care Ltd. Summary of product characteristics, July 2001.

Flecainide + Anticonvulsants

No clinically important interaction appears to occur if phenytoin or phenobarbital is given to patients on flecainide.

Clinical evidence, mechanism, importance and management

A controlled study with epileptic patients on **phenytoin** or **phenobarbital** found that the pharmacokinetics of a single 2 mg/kg intravenous dose of flecainide were not statistically different from those in a group of normal subjects. The authors[1] say that ". . .a modest reduction in flecainide half-life is possible, but may not require any adjustment in the flecainide dosage."

1. Pentikäinen PJ, Halinen MO, Hiepakorpi S, Chang SF, Conard GJ, McQuinn RL. Pharmacokinetics of flecainide in patients receiving enzyme inducers. *Acta Pharmacol Toxicol* (1986) 59 (Suppl 5), 91.

Flecainide + Cimetidine

Cimetidine can increase flecainide plasma levels.

Clinical evidence

The flecainide plasma levels of 8 healthy subjects taking 200 mg daily were raised by up to 28% and the clearance reduced by up to 27% after taking 1 g **cimetidine** daily for a week.[1-3] In another study, 1 g **cimetidine** for 5 days almost doubled the plasma flecainide levels (from 160–245 to 380–455 ng/ml) in 11 patients taking 200 mg flecainide daily.[4]

Mechanism

Uncertain, but it is thought that the cimetidine reduces both the renal clearance, and the metabolism of the flecainide by the liver.[1-4]

Importance and management

An established but as yet not extensively documented interaction. The clinical importance appears not to have been assessed, but be alert for the need to reduce the flecainide dosage if cimetidine is added. Caution is recommended in patients with impaired renal function. More study is needed to assess the clinical implications.

1. Tjandra Maga TB, Verbesselt R, Van Hecken A, Van Melle P, De Schepper PJ. Oral flecainide elimination kinetics: effects of cimetidine. *Circulation* (1983) 68 (Supp III), 416.

2. Tjandra-Maga TB, Van Hecken A, Van Melle P, Verbesselt R, De Schepper PJ. Altered pharmacokinetics of oral flecainide by cimetidine. *Br J Clin Pharmacol* (1986) 22, 108–110.

3. Verbesselt R, Tjandra Maga TB, Van Hecken A, Van Melle P, De Schepper PJ. Effects of cimetidine on the elimination of oral flecainide. *Eur Heart J* (1984) 5, 136.

4. Nitsch J, Köhler U, Neyses L, Lüderitz B. Flecainid-Plasmakonzentraionen bei Hemmung des hepatischen Metabolismus durch Cimetidin. *Klin Wochenschr* (1987) 65 (Suppl IX), 250.

Flecainide + Colestyramine

An isolated report describes reduced plasma flecainide levels in a patient given colestyramine. Studies in other subjects failed to demonstrate any interaction.

Clinical evidence, mechanism, importance and management

A patient on 100 mg flecainide twice daily had unusually low trough plasma levels (100 ng/ml) while taking **colestyramine**. When he stopped taking the **colestyramine** (4 g three times daily) his plasma flecainide levels rose. However a later study in 3 healthy subjects given 100 mg flecainide once daily and 4 g **colestyramine** three times daily, found little or no evidence of an interaction (steady-state flecainide levels of 63.1 and 59.1 ng/ml without and with **colestyramine**). *In vitro* studies also failed to demonstrate any binding between flecainide and **colestyramine** which might result in reduced absorption from the gut.[1] The authors however postulate that the citric acid contained in the **colestyramine** formulation might have altered the urinary pH which could have increased the renal clearance of the flecainide.[1]

Information seems to be limited to this report. Its general importance seems to be minor, nevertheless the outcome of concurrent use should be monitored so that any unusual cases can be identified.

1. Stein H, Hoppe U. Is there an interaction between flecainide and cholestyramine? *Naunyn Schmiedebergs Arch Pharmacol* (1989) 339 (Suppl), R114.

Flecainide + Food or Antacids

The absorption of flecainide is not significantly altered if taken with food or an aluminium hydroxide antacid in adults, but it may possibly be reduced by milk in infants.

Clinical evidence, mechanism, importance and management

Neither **food** nor 15 ml of *Aldrox* (280 mg **aluminium hydroxide** per 5 ml had any significant effect on the absorption of a single 200-mg dose of flecainide in healthy adult subjects.[1] No special precautions seem necessary if taken together.

A premature baby being treated for refractory atrio-ventricular tachycardia with high doses of flecainide (40 mg/kg daily or 25 mg six-hourly) developed flecainide toxicity (seen as ventricular tachycardia) when his **milk feed** was replaced by **5% dextrose**. His serum flecainide levels approximately doubled, the conclusion being that the **milk** had reduced the absorption.[2] **Milk**-fed infants on high doses may therefore possibly need a reduced flecainide dosage if **milk** is reduced or stopped. Monitor the effects.

1. Tjandra-Maga TB, Verbesselt R, Van Hecken A, Mullie A, De Schepper PJ. Flecainide: single and multiple oral dose kinetics, absolute bioavailability and effect of food and antacid in man. *Br J Clin Pharmacol* (1986) 22, 309–16.

2. Russell GAB, Martin RP. Flecainide toxicity. *Arch Dis Child* (1989) 64, 860–2.

Flecainide + Quinidine or Quinine

Quinidine and quinine cause a modest reduction in the loss of flecainide from the body.

Clinical evidence, mechanism, importance and management

(a) Quinidine

A single 50 mg oral dose of **quinidine** given the night before a single 150 mg intravenous dose of flecainide acetate decreased the flecainide clearance by 23% in 6 normal subjects. The flecainide half-life was increased by 22% and its AUC by 28%.[1,2] In another study, 5 patients who were extensive metabolisers of cytochrome P450 isoenzyme CYP2D6 and on chronic flecainide treatment were given 50 mg **quinidine** six-hourly for 5 days. The plasma levels and clearance of S-(+)-flecainide were unchanged, but plasma levels of R-(−)-flecainide increased approximately 15% and its clearance reduced 15%. The effects of the flecainide were slightly but not significantly increased.[3] Quinidine inhibits CYP2D6, which is concerned with the metabolism of flecainide. The clinical importance of this interaction is uncertain, but it is probably minor.

(b) Quinine

Three 500-mg doses of **quinine** administered over 24 h increased the AUC of a single 150 mg intravenous infusion (over 30 mins) of flecainide by 21% (from 196 to 237 micrograms.min/ml) and reduced the systemic clearance by 16.5% (from 9.1 to 7.6 ml/min.kg) in 10 healthy subjects. Renal clearance remained unchanged. The increases in the PR and QRS intervals caused by flecainide were slightly, but not significantly, increased by **quinine**.[4] The evidence suggests that **quinine** reduces the metabolism of flecainide.[4] The clinical importance of this interaction is uncertain but a slight increase in the serum levels of flecainide would be expected, accompanied by some, probably minor, changes in its effects.

1. Munafo A, Buclin T, Steinhäuslin F, Biollaz J. Disposition of flecainide in subjects taking quinidine. *Clin Pharmacol Ther* (1990) 47, 156.

2. Munafo A, Buclin T, Tuto D, Biollaz J. The effect of a low dose of quinidine on the disposition of flecainide in healthy volunteers. *Eur J Clin Pharmacol* (1992) 43, 441–3.

3. Birgersdotter UM, Wong W, Turgeon J, Roden DM. Stereoselective genetically-determined interaction between chronic flecainide and quinidine in patients with arrhythmias. *Br J Clin Pharmacol* (1992) 33, 275–80.

4. Munafo A, Reymond-Michel G, Biollaz J. Altered flecainide disposition in healthy volunteers taking quinine. *Eur J Clin Pharmacol* (1990) 38, 269–73.

Flecainide + Tobacco smoking

Tobacco smokers need larger doses of flecainide than non-smokers to achieve the same therapeutic effects.

Clinical evidence

Prompted by the chance observation that **smokers** appeared to have a reduced pharmacodynamic response to flecainide than **non-smokers**, a meta-analysis[1] was undertaken of the findings of 7 premarketing pharmacokinetic studies and 5 multicentre efficacy trials in which flecainide had been studied and in which the smoking habits of the subjects/patients had been also been recorded. In the pharmacokinetic studies, the clearance of flecainide was found to be approximately 50% higher in smokers than in non-smokers. In the efficacy studies, average clinically effective flecainide doses were found to be 338 mg daily for **smokers** and 288 mg daily for **non-smokers**, while trough plasma concentrations of flecainide were 1.74 and 2.18 ng/ml/mg for the **smokers** and **non-smokers**, respectively. This confirmed that **smokers** needed higher doses of flecainide to achieve the same steady-state serum levels.[1]

Mechanism

The probable reason is that some components of the tobacco smoke stimulate the cytochrome P450 enzymes in the liver concerned with the *O*-dealkylation of flecainide, so that it is cleared from the body more quickly.[1]

Importance and management

An established interaction. Anticipate the need to give smokers higher doses of flecainide than non-smokers to achieve the required therapeutic response.

1. Holtzman JL, Weeks CE, Kvam DC, Berry DA, Mottonen L, Ekholm BP, Chang SF, Conard GJ. Identification of drug interactions by meta-analysis of premarketing trials: The effect of smoking on the pharmacokinetic and dosage requirements for flecainide acetate. *Clin Pharmacol Ther* (1989) 46, 1–8.

Flecainide + Urinary acidifiers and alkalinizers

The loss of flecainide is increased if the urine is made acidic (e.g. with ammonium chloride) and reduced if the urine is made alkaline (e.g. with sodium bicarbonate). The clinical importance of these changes is not known.

Clinical evidence

Six healthy subjects were given single 300 mg oral doses of flecainide on two occasions: once after taking 1 g **ammonium chloride** orally every 3 h, and 2 g at bedtime, for a total of 21 h to make the urine acidic (pH range 4.4 to 5.4): and the second after taking 4 g **sodium bicarbonate** every 4 h for a total of 21 h (including night periods) to make the urine alkaline (pH range 7.4–8.3). Over the next 32 h, 44.7% of the unchanged flecainide appeared in the acidic urine, but only 7.4% in alkaline urine.[1] This compares to 25% found by other researchers when urinary pH was not controlled.[1] A later similar study from the same research group broadly confirmed these findings; the elimination half-life of the flecainide being found as 10.7 h in acidic urine and 17.6 h in alkaline urine.[2] Another study also confirmed the effect of urinary pH on the excretion of flecainide, and found that the fluid load and the urinary flow rate had little effect on flecainide excretion.[3]

Mechanism

In alkaline urine at pH 8, much of the flecainide exists in the kidney tubules in the non-ionised form (non-ionised fraction 0.04) which is therefore more readily reabsorbed. In acidic urine at pH 5 more exists in the ionised form (non-ionised fraction 0.0001) which is less readily reabsorbed and is therefore lost in the urine.[3]

Importance and management

Established interactions, but their clinical importance is still uncertain. The effects of these changes on the subsequent control of arrhythmias by flecainide in patients seem not to have been studied, but the outcome should be well monitored if patients are given drugs that alter urinary pH to a significant extent (such as ammonium chloride, sodium bicarbonate). Large doses of some antacids may possibly do the same, but nobody seems to have studied this.

1. Muhiddin KA, Johnston A, Turner P. The influence of urinary pH on flecainide excretion and its serum pharmacokinetics. *Br J Clin Pharmacol* (1984) 17, 447–51.
2. Johnston A, Warrington S, Turner P. Flecainide pharmacokinetics in healthy volunteers: the influence of urinary pH. *Br J Clin Pharmacol* (1985) 20, 333–8.
3. Hertrampf R, Gundert-Remy U, Beckmann J, Hoppe U, Elsäßer W, Stein H. Elimination of flecainide as a function of urinary flow rate and pH. *Eur J Clin Pharmacol* (1991) 41, 61–3.

Flecainide + Verapamil

Although flecainide and verapamil have been used together successfully, serious and potentially life-threatening cardiogenic shock and asystole have been seen in a few patients because the cardiac depressant effects of the two drugs can be additive.

Clinical evidence

A man with triple coronary vessel disease and on 200 mg flecainide daily for recurrent ventricular tachycardia, developed severe cardiogenic shock within two days of increasing the flecainide dosage to 300 mg daily and one day of starting 80 mg **verapamil** daily. His blood pressure fell to 60/40 mmHg and he had an idioventricular rhythm of 88 bpm.[1] Another patient with atrial flutter and fibrillation was treated with **digitalis** and 120 mg **verapamil** three times daily. He was additionally given 150 mg flecainide daily for 10 days, but three days after the dosage was raised to 200 mg daily he fainted, and later developed severe bradycardia (15 bpm) and asystoles of up to 14 sec. He later died.[1]

Another report describes atrioventricular block in a patient with a pacemaker when treated with **digoxin**, flecainide and **verapamil**.[2]

Two earlier studies in patients[3] and normal subjects[4] had found that the kinetics of flecainide and **verapamil** were only minimally affected by concurrent use, but the PR interval was increased by both drugs and additive depressant effects were seen on heart contractility and AV conduction. No serious adverse responses occurred.

Mechanism

Flecainide and verapamil have little or no effects on the kinetics of each other,[3,4] but they can apparently have additive depressant effects on the heart (negative inotropic and chronotropic) in both patients and normal subjects.[1,3,4] Verapamil alone[5,6] and with beta-blockers[7,8] or digoxin,[9] and flecainide alone[10,11] have been responsible for asystole and cardiogenic shock in a few patients. In the cases cited above[1-3] the depressant effects were serious because the patients already had compromised cardiac function.

Importance and management

An established interaction, but the incidence of serious adverse effects is probably not great. The additive depressant effects on heart function are probably of little importance in many patients, but may represent 'the last straw' in a few who have seriously compromised cardiac function. The authors of the reports cited[1] advise careful monitoring if both drugs are used and emphasise the potential hazards of combining Class Ic antiarrhythmics and calcium channel blockers of the verapamil type. See also 'Beta-blockers + Flecainide', p.439.

1. Buss J, Lasserre JJ, Heene DL. Asystole and cardiogenic shock due to combined treatment with verapamil and flecainide. *Lancet* (1992) 340, 546.
2. Tworek DA, Nazari J, Ezri M, Bauman JL. Interference by antiarrhythmic agents with function of electrical cardiac devices. *Clin Pharm* (1992) 11, 48–56.
3. Landau S, Hogan C, Butler B, Somberg J. The combined administration of verapamil and flecainide. *J Clin Pharmacol* (1988) 28, 909.
4. Holtzman JL, Finley D, Mottonen L, Berry DA, Ekholm BP, Kvam DC, McQuinn RL, Miller AM. The pharmacodynamic and pharmacokinetic interaction between single doses of flecainide acetate and verapamil: Effects on cardiac function and drug clearance. *Clin Pharmacol Ther* (1989) 46, 26–32.
5. Perrot B, Danchin N, De La Chaise AT. Verapamil: a cause of sudden death in a patient with hypertrophic cardiomyopathy. *Br Heart J* (1984) 51, 532–4.
6. Cohen IL, Fein A, Nabi A. Reversal of cardiogenic shock and asystole in a septic patient with hypertrophic cardiomyopathy on verapamil. *Crit Care Med* (1990) 18, 775–6.
7. Benaim ME. Asystole after verapamil. *BMJ* (1972) 2, 169–70.
8. Frierson J, Bailly D, Shultz T, Sund S, Dimas A. Refractory cardiogenic shock and complete heart block after unsuspected verapamil-SR and atenolol overdose. *Clin Cardiol* (1992) 14, 933–5.
9. Kounis NG. Asystole after verapamil and digoxin. *Br J Clin Pract* (1980) 34, 57–8.
10. Forbes WP, Hee TT, Mohiuddin SM, Hillman DE. Flecainide-induced cardiogenic shock. *Chest* (1988) 94, 1121.
11. Echt DS, Liebson PR, Mitchell LB, Peters RW, Obias-Manno D, Barker AH, Arensberg D, Baker A, Friedman L, Greene HL, Huther ML, Richardson DW, CAST investigators. Mortality and morbidity in patients receiving encainide, flecainide or placebo. *N Engl J Med* (1991) 324, 781–8.

Ibutilide + Miscellaneous drugs

No adverse interactions appear to have been reported with ibutilide, but because it can prolong the QT interval, caution has been advised about the concurrent use of other drugs that can do the same. Ibutilide is reported not to interact with beta-blockers, calcium channel blockers or digoxin.

Clinical evidence, mechanism, importance and management

No specific drug interaction studies appear to have been undertaken with ibutilide, which is a Class III antiarrhythmic, but because it can prolong the QT interval it has been recommended that other drugs that can do the same should be administered with caution, because of the potential additive effects.[1] The maker of ibutilide specifically recommends that class Ia and other class III antiarrhythmics not be given within 4 h of ibutilide infusion.[2] The concern is that a prolongation of the QT interval is associated with an increased risk of torsade de pointes arrhythmia which is potentially life-threatening. See also 'Drugs that prolong the QT interval + Other drugs that prolong the QT interval', p.103.

The concurrent use of **beta-blockers**, **calcium channel blockers** and **digoxin** during clinical trials is reported not to affect the safety or efficacy of ibutilide.[1] Ibutilide is said[1] not to affect cytochrome P450 isoenzymes CYP3A4 or CYP2D6 so that metabolic interactions with drugs affected by these enzymes would not be expected. Study is needed to confirm all of these predictions and findings.

1. Cropp JS, Antal EG, Talbert RL. Ibutilide: a new Class III antiarrhythmic agent. *Pharmacotherapy* (1997) 17, 1–9.
2. Corvert (Ibutilide fumarate). Pharmacia & Upjohn. US prescribing information. October 2000.

Lidocaine (Lignocaine) + Amiodarone

Isolated reports describe a seizure in a man on lidocaine (lignocaine) about two days after starting to take amiodarone, and sinoatrial arrest in another man with sick sinus syn- **drome when given both drugs. There is conflicting evidence as to whether or not amiodarone affects the pharmacokinetics of lidocaine.**

Clinical evidence

(a) Increased lidocaine (lignocaine) levels, seizure

An elderly man taking digoxin, enalapril, amitriptyline and temazepam was treated for monomorphic ventricular tachycardia, firstly with procainamide, later replaced by a continuous infusion of lidocaine (2 mg/min), to which was added 600 mg **amiodarone** orally twice daily. After 12 h his lidocaine level was 5.4 mg/l (therapeutic levels 1.5–5 mg/l), but 53 h later he developed a seizure and his lidocaine level was found to have risen to 12.6 mg/l. A tomography brain scan showed no abnormalities that could have caused the seizure and it was therefore attributed to the toxic lidocaine levels.[1]

(b) Sinoatrial arrest

An elderly man with long standing brady-tachycardia was successfully treated for atrial flutter firstly with a temporary pacemaker, later withdrawn, and 600 mg **amiodarone** daily. Ten days later, and 25 min after a permanent pacemaker was inserted under local anaesthesia with 15 ml 2% lidocaine (lignocaine) when the brachiocephalic vein was exposed, severe sinus bradycardia and long sinoatrial arrest developed. He was effectively treated with atropine plus isoprenaline, and cardiac massage.[2]

(c) Pharmacokinetics of concurrent use

Six patients with symptomatic cardiac arrhythmias took part in a two-phase study. Initially, lidocaine (lignocaine) hydrochloride 1 mg/kg was given intravenously over 2 min. In phase I loading doses of **amiodarone** 500 mg daily for 6 days were given, followed by the same lidocaine (lignocaine) dose. After 19 to 21 days, when the total cumulative **amiodarone** dose was 13 g, the same lidocaine dose was given again (phase II). The lidocaine (lignocaine) AUC increased by about 20% and the systemic clearance decreased by about 20%. The elimination half-life and distribution volume at steady-state were unchanged. The pharmacokinetic parameters of lidocaine (lignocaine) in phase II were the same as those in phase I, indicating that the interaction occurs early in the loading phase of amiodarone administration.[3] This is in contrast to an earlier study, in which the pharmacokinetics of a bolus dose of lidocaine (lignocaine) (1 mg/kg over 2 min) were not altered in 10 patients after taking **amiodarone** 200–400 mg daily (following an loading dose of 800 or 1200 mg) for 4–5 weeks.[4]

Mechanisms

(a). The marked increase in lidocaine (lignocaine) may have been due to inhibition of its metabolism by amiodarone.

(b). The authors of the report suggest a synergistic depression by both drugs of the sinus node.

(c). An *in vitro* study has demonstrated that amiodarone may inhibit lidocaine (lignocaine) metabolism competitively and *vice versa*. The interaction *in vivo* may be due to inhibition of cytochrome P450 isoenzyme CYP3A4 by amiodarone and/or its main metabolite desethylamiodarone.[4]

Importance and management

Evidence of a pharmacokinetic interaction between lidocaine (lignocaine) and amiodarone is conflicting. However, the two reports of adverse interactions and the study in patients with arrhythmias illustrate the importance of good monitoring if both drugs are used.

1. Siegmund JB, Wilson JH, Imhoff TE. Amiodarone interaction with lidocaine. *J Cardiovasc Pharmacol* (1993) 21, 513–5.
2. Keidar S, Grenadier E, Palant A. Sinoatrial arrest due to lidocaine injection in sick sinus syndrome during amiodarone administration. *Am Heart J* (1982) 104, 1384–5.
3. Ha HR, Candinas R, Steiger B, Meyer UA, Follath F. Interactions between amiodarone and lidocaine. *J Cardiovasc Pharmacol* (1996) 28, 533–9.
4. Nattel S, Talajic M, Beaudoin D, Matthews C, Roy D. Absence of pharmacokinetic interaction between amiodarone and lidocaine. *Am J Cardiol* (1994) 73, 92–4.

Lidocaine (Lignocaine) + Barbiturates

Plasma lidocaine (lignocaine) levels following slow intravenous injection may be lower in patients who are taking barbiturates.

Clinical evidence

A single dose of 2 mg/kg **lidocaine (lignocaine)** was administered by slow intravenous injection (rate about 100 mg over 15 mins) to 7 epileptic patients, firstly while taking their usual antiepileptic drugs and sedatives (including **phenytoin, barbiturates,** phenothiazines, benzodiazepines) and secondly after taking only 300 mg **phenobarbital** daily for 4 weeks. The same lidocaine dose was also administered to 6 control subjects who had not received any drugs. Plasma lidocaine (lignocaine) levels were 10 to 25% higher after **phenobarbital** treatment alone in the patients with epilepsy. When compared with the levels in the 6 control subjects, plasma lidocaine (lignocaine) levels were somewhat lower in the patients, and this was statistically significant at 30 and 60 minutes (18 and 29% lower).[1]

Mechanism

Not fully understood. One suggestion is that the barbiturates increase the activity of the liver microsomal enzymes, thereby increasing the rate of metabolism of the lidocaine.[1]

Importance and management

Direct information is very limited but the interaction in man appears to be established. It may be necessary to increase the dosage of lidocaine (lignocaine) to achieve the desired therapeutic response in patients on phenobarbital or other barbiturates.

1. Heinonen J, Takki S, Jarho L. Plasma lidocaine levels in patients treated with potential inducers of microsomal enzymes. *Acta Anaesth Scand* (1970) 14, 89–95.

Lidocaine (Lignocaine) + Beta-blockers

The plasma levels of lidocaine (lignocaine) can be increased by the concurrent use of propranolol. Two cases of toxicity attributed to this interaction have been reported. Nadolol possibly interacts similarly, but there is uncertainty about metoprolol. Atenolol and pindolol appear not to interact, but the need for an increased loading dosage of lidocaine in the presence of penbutolol has been suggested.

Clinical evidence

(a) Atenolol, pindolol

Studies with oral **atenolol** (50 mg daily),[1] and intravenous **pindolol** (0.023 mg/kg)[2] found that these beta-blockers did not affect the clearance of lidocaine.

(b) Metoprolol

In 6 healthy subjects, 100 mg **metoprolol** twice daily for 2 days did not affect the pharmacokinetics of a single intravenous dose of lidocaine.[3] Similarly, another study in 7 healthy subjects failed to find any changes in the pharmacokinetics of a single oral or intravenous dose of lidocaine after one week's treatment with **metoprolol** (100 mg 12-hourly).[1] In contrast, another study found that the clearance of a single intravenous dose of lidocaine was reduced 31% by one days pretreatment with **metoprolol** 50 mg six-hourly.[4]

(c) Nadolol

A study in 6 healthy subjects receiving 30 h infusions of lidocaine (2 mg/min) showed that 3 days pretreatment with 160 mg **nadolol** daily raised the steady-state plasma lidocaine levels by 28% (from 2.1

to 2.7 micrograms/ml) and reduced the plasma clearance by 17% (from 1030 to 850 ml/min).[5]

(d) Penbutolol

In 7 healthy subjects, **penbutolol** 60 mg daily significantly increased the volume of distribution of a single intravenous dose of lidocaine 100 mg, thus prolonging its elimination half-life. However, the reduction in clearance of lidocaine did not reach significance.[6]

(e) Propranolol

A study in 6 healthy subjects receiving 30 h infusions of lidocaine (2 mg/min) showed that 3 days pretreatment with **propranolol** (80 mg eight-hourly) raised the steady-state plasma lidocaine levels by 19% (from 2.1 to 2.5 micrograms/ml) and reduced the plasma clearance by 16% (1030 to 866 ml/min).[5] Other similar studies have found a 22.5 to 30% increase in steady-state serum lidocaine levels and a 14.7 to 46% fall in plasma clearance due to the concurrent use of **propranolol**.[2,4,7] Two cases of lidocaine toxicity attributed to a lidocaine-**propranolol** interaction were revealed by a search[8] of the FDA adverse drug reaction file in 1981.

(f) Un-named beta-blockers

A matched study in 51 cardiac patients on a variety of beta-blockers (including **propranolol, metoprolol, timolol, pindolol**) found no significant differences in either total or free concentrations of lidocaine, but there was a trend towards an increase in the adverse effects of lidocaine (bradycardias) with concurrent beta-blocker treatment.[9,10]

Mechanism

Not fully agreed. There is some debate about whether the increased serum lidocaine levels largely occur because of the decreased cardiac output caused by the beta-blockers which decreases the flow of blood through the liver thereby reducing the metabolism of the lidocaine,[5] or because of direct liver enzyme inhibition.[11] There may also be a pharmacodynamic interaction, with an increased risk of myocardial depression.[10]

Importance and management

The lidocaine (lignocaine)/propranolol interaction is established and of clinical importance. Monitor the effects of concurrent use and reduce the lidocaine dosage if necessary to avoid toxicity. The situation with other beta-blockers is less clear. Nadolol appears to interact like propranolol, but it is uncertain whether metoprolol interacts or not. Atenolol and pindolol are reported not to interact pharmacokinetically. It has been suggested that a higher loading dose (but not a higher maintenance dose) of lidocaine may be needed if penbutolol is used.[6] The suggestion has been made that a significant pharmacokinetic interaction is only likely to occur with non-selective beta-blockers without intrinsic sympathomimetic activity.[11] Until the situation is better defined it would be prudent to monitor the effects of concurrent use with any beta-blocker.

Local anaesthetic preparations of lidocaine often contain epinephrine (adrenaline). See the Index for 'Anaesthetics, local + Beta-blockers', p.753.

1. Miners JO, Wing LMH, Lillywhite KJ, Smith KJ. Failure of 'therapeutic' doses of β-adrenoceptor antagonists to alter the disposition of tolbutamide and lignocaine. *Br J Clin Pharmacol* (1984) 18, 853–60.
2. Svendsen TL, Tangø M, Waldorff S, Steiness E, Trap-Jensen J. Effects of propranolol and pindolol on plasma lignocaine clearance in man. *Br J Clin Pharmacol* (1982) 13, 223S–226S.
3. Jordö L, Johnsson G, Lundborg P, Regårdh C-G. Pharmacokinetics of lidocaine in healthy individuals pretreated with multiple dose of metoprolol. *Int J Clin Pharmacol Ther Toxicol* (1984) 22, 312–15.
4. Conrad KA, Byers JM, Finley PR, Burnham L. Lidocaine elimination: effects of metoprolol and of propranolol. *Clin Pharmacol Ther* (1983) 33, 133–8.
5. Schneck DW, Luderer JR, Davis D, Vary J. Effects of nadolol and propranolol on plasma lidocaine clearance. *Clin Pharmacol Ther* (1984) 36, 584–7.
6. Ochs HR, Skanderra D, Abernethy DR, Greenblatt DJ. Effect of penbutolol on lidocaine kinetics. *Arzneimittelforschung* (1983) 33, 1680–1.
7. Ochs HR, Carstens G, Greenblatt DJ. Reduction in lidocaine clearance during continuous infusion and by co administration of propranolol. *N Engl J Med* (1980) 303, 373–7.
8. Graham CF, Turner WM, Jones JK. Lidocaine-propranolol interactions. *N Engl J Med* (1981) 304, 1301.
9. Wyse DG, Kellen J, Tam Y, Rademaker AW. Increased efficacy and toxicity of lidocaine in patients on beta blockers. *Circulation* (1986) 74, II-43.

10. Wyse DG, Kellen J, Tam Y, Rademaker AW. Increased efficacy and toxicity of lidocaine in patients on beta-blockers. *Int J Cardiol* (1988) 21, 59–70.
11. Bax NDS, Tucker GT, Lennard MS, Woods HF. The impairment of lignocaine clearance by propranolol—major contribution from enzyme inhibition. *Br J Clin Pharmacol* (1985) 19, 597–603.

Lidocaine (Lignocaine) + Cimetidine or Ranitidine

Cimetidine modestly reduces the clearance of lidocaine (lignocaine) and raises serum levels in some patients. Lidocaine toxicity may occur if the dosage is not reduced. Ranitidine appears to interact minimally. See also 'Anaesthetics, local + Cimetidine or Ranitidine', p.753.

Clinical evidence

(a) Studies with cimetidine in cardiac patients

In one study, 15 patients were given a 1 mg/kg loading dose of lidocaine (lignocaine) intravenously followed by a continuous infusion of 2 or 3 mg/min over 26 h. At 6 h they were started on **cimetidine** (initial dose 300 mg intravenously, then 300 mg six-hourly by mouth). After 26 h (20 h after cimetidine) the serum levels of lidocaine were 30% higher (5.6 micrograms/ml) than in a control group of 6 patients (4.3 micrograms/ml). The most substantial rise in levels occurred in the first 6 h after cimetidine administration. Six patients developed toxic serum levels (over 5 micrograms/ml) and two (with levels of 10 and 11 micrograms/ml) experienced lethargy and confusion attributed to toxicity, which disappeared when the lidocaine was stopped.[1]

A study in patients with suspected myocardial infarction given two 300 mg oral doses of **cimetidine** 4 h apart, starting 11–20 h after a 2 mg/min infusion of lidocaine began, showed that total lidocaine serum levels had risen by 28%, and unbound levels by 18%, 24 h after the initial cimetidine dose. In three of these patients whose diagnosis was subsequently confirmed, rises in total and unbound lidocaine serum levels of 24% and 9% occurred by 24 h.[2] In contrast, a study in six patients with suspected myocardial infarction given lidocaine infusions, followed later by a **cimetidine** infusion, failed to find a significant increase in the plasma accumulation of lidocaine.[3]

(b) Studies with cimetidine in healthy subjects

A rise in peak serum lidocaine (lignocaine) levels of 50% was seen in a study in 6 healthy subjects given 300 mg **cimetidine** six-hourly for a day. Systemic clearance fell by about 25% (from 766 to 576 ml/min) and 5 of the 6 experienced toxicity (light-headedness, paraesthesia).[4] Similarly, two further studies in healthy subjects taking 1 or 1.2 g **cimetidine** daily showed a 21 and 30% fall in lidocaine clearance, respectively.[5,6] In contrast, in another study, **cimetidine** 1.2 g daily caused only an 18% fall in lidocaine clearance, which did not reach statistical significance.[7] Similarly, **cimetidine** 300 mg four times daily orally caused a 15% reduction in lidocaine clearance under both single-dose and steady-state conditions, but this was not statistically significant. In this study, the effect of intravenous **cimetidine** 300 mg four times daily was less than that of the oral **cimetidine**.[8]

(c) Studies with ranitidine in healthy subjects

A study in 10 healthy subjects given 150 mg **ranitidine** twice daily for 5 days showed that it increased the systemic clearance of lidocaine (lignocaine) by 9%, but did not alter the oral clearance.[9] Two other studies in healthy subjects given **ranitidine** 150 mg twice daily for one to 2 days found no change in the clearance of lidocaine given intravenously.[7,10]

Mechanism

Not established. It seems possible that the metabolism of the lidocaine is reduced both by a fall in blood flow to the liver and by direct inhibition of the activity of the liver microsomal enzymes. As a result its clearance is reduced and its serum levels rise.

Importance and management

The lidocaine (lignocaine)/cimetidine interaction is well studied but controversial. It is confused by the differences between the studies (healthy subjects, patients with different diseases, different modes of drug administration, etc). A fall in the clearance of lidocaine (15% or more) and a resultant rise in the serum levels should be looked for if cimetidine is used, but a clinically significant alteration may not occur in every patient. It may possibly be of less importance in patients following a myocardial infarction because of the increased amounts of alpha-1-acid glycoprotein which alter the levels of bound and free lidocaine.[2] Monitor all patients closely for evidence of toxicity and check serum lidocaine levels regularly. A reduced infusion rate may be needed. Ranitidine would appear to be a suitable alternative to cimetidine. See also 'Anaesthetics, local + Cimetidine or Ranitidine', p.753.

1. Knapp AB, Maguire W, Keren G, Karmen A, Levitt B, Miura DS, Somberg JC. The cimetidine-lidocaine interaction. *Ann Intern Med* (1983) 98, 174–7.
2. Berk SI, Gal P, Bauman JL, Douglas JB, McCue JD, Powell JR. The effect of oral cimetidine on total and unbound serum lidocaine concentrations in patients with suspected myocardial infarction. *Int J Cardiol* (1987) 14, 91–4.
3. Patterson JH, Foster J, Powell JR, Cross R, Wargin W, Clark JL. Influence of a continuous cimetidine infusion on lidocaine plasma concentrations in patients. *J Clin Pharmacol* (1985) 25, 607–9.
4. Feely J, Wilkinson GR, McAllister CB, Wood AJJ. Increased toxicity and reduced clearance of lidocaine by cimetidine. *Ann Intern Med* (1982) 96, 592–4.
5. Wing LMH, Miners JO, Birkett DJ, Foenander T, Lillywhite K, Wanwimolruk S. Lidocaine disposition—sex differences and effects of cimetidine. *Clin Pharmacol Ther* (1984) 35, 695–701.
6. Bauer LA, Edwards WAD, Randolph FP, Blouin RA. Cimetidine-induced decrease in lidocaine metabolism. *Am Heart J* (1984) 108, 413–15.
7. Jackson JE, Bentley JB, Glass SJ, Fukui T, Gandolfi AJ, Plachetka JR. Effects of histamine-2 receptor blockade on lidocaine kinetics. *Clin Pharmacol Ther* (1985) 37, 544–8.
8. Powell JR, Foster J, Patterson JH, Cross R, Wargin W. Effect of duration of lidocaine infusion and route of cimetidine administration on lidocaine pharmacokinetics. *Clin Pharm* (1986) 5, 993–8.
9. Robson RA, Wing LMH, Miners JO, Lillywhite KJ, Birkett DJ. The effect of ranitidine on the disposition of lignocaine. *Br J Clin Pharmacol* (1985) 20, 170–3.
10. Feely J, Guy E. Lack of effect of ranitidine on the disposition of lignocaine. *Br J Clin Pharmacol* (1983) 15, 378–9.

Lidocaine (Lignocaine) + Cocaine

Limited evidence suggests lidocaine (lignocaine) use in patients with cocaine-associated myocardial infarction is not associated with significant toxicity.

Clinical evidence, mechanism, importance and management

A retrospective study, covering a 6-year period in 29 hospitals, identified 29 patients (27 available for review) who received lidocaine (lignocaine) for prophylaxis or treatment of **cocaine**-associated myocardial infarction. No patient exhibited bradycardia, sustained ventricular tachycardia or ventricular fibrillation, and no patients died.[1]

Both lidocaine (lignocaine) and **cocaine** exhibit type I antiarrhythmic effects and are proconvulsants. Lidocaine (lignocaine) may potentiate the cardiac and CNS side-effects of cocaine. Therefore the use of lidocaine (lignocaine) for **cocaine**-associated myocardial infarction is controversial. The lack of adverse effects in this study may have been due to delays of more than 5 h between last exposure to **cocaine** and lidocaine (lignocaine) therapy. The authors concluded that the cautious use of lidocaine (lignocaine) does not appear to be contraindicated in patients with **cocaine**-associated myocardial infarction who require antiarrhythmic therapy. However, extra care should be taken in patients who receive lidocaine (lignocaine) shortly after cocaine.[1]

1. Shih RD, Hollander JE, Burstein JL, Nelson LS, Hoffman RS, Quick AM. Clinical safety of lidocaine in patients with cocaine-associated myocardial infarction. *Ann Emerg Med* (1995) 26, 702–6.

Lidocaine (Lignocaine) + Dextromethorphan

Lidocaine (lignocaine) does not inhibit the activity of cytochrome P450 isoenzyme CYP2D6 and is therefore unlikely to interact with drugs that are metabolised by this isoenzyme.

Clinical evidence, mechanism, importance and management

Although *in vitro* data suggested that lidocaine (lignocaine) inhibited oxidative metabolism reactions mediated by cytochrome P450 isoenzyme CYP2D6, a later *in vivo* study in 16 patients found that, while being infused with lidocaine (serum level range 3.2–55.9 micromol/l), the metabolism of a single 30-mg dose of **dextromethorphan** remained unchanged. All of the patients were of the extensive metaboliser phenotype. Since **dextromethorphan** is a well-established marker or indicator of CYP2D6 activity, it was concluded that lidocaine is unlikely to interact with drugs that are extensively metabolised by this isoenzyme.[1]

1. Bartoli A, Gatt G, Chimienti M, Corbellini D, Perrucca E. Does lidocaine affect oxidative dextromethorphan metabolism «in vivo»? *Giornale Italiano di Chimica Clinica* (1993/4) 18, 125–9.

Lidocaine (Lignocaine) + Disopyramide

Laboratory studies show that disopyramide can increase the levels of unbound lidocaine (lignocaine), but whether in practice their combined effects have a clinically important depressant effect on the heart is not known.

Clinical evidence, mechanism, importance and management

An *in vitro* study using serum taken from 9 patients receiving lidocaine (lignocaine) for severe ventricular arrhythmias showed that there was an average 20% increase in its free (unbound) fraction when **disopyramide** in a concentration of 14.7 micromol/l was added.[1] The reason would seem to be that **disopyramide** can displace lidocaine from its binding sites on plasma proteins (alpha-1-acid glycoprotein).

The importance of this possible displacement interaction in clinical practice is uncertain. The suggestion made by the authors[1] is that, although lidocaine has only a minor cardiac depressant effect, a transient 20% increase in levels of free and active lidocaine plus the negative inotropic effects of the **disopyramide** might possibly be hazardous in patients with reduced heart function. More study is needed.

1. Bonde J, Jensen NM, Burgaard P, Angelo HR, Graudal N, Kampmann JP, Pedersen LE. Displacement of lidocaine from human plasma proteins by disopyramide. *Pharmacol Toxicol* (1987) 60, 151–5.

Lidocaine (Lignocaine) + Erythromycin

Erythromycin may markedly increase plasma levels of lidocaine (lignocaine) after oral administration, but not after intravenous administration.

Clinical evidence

Nine normal subjects were given **erythromycin** 500 mg three times daily or placebo daily for 4 days, in a randomised double-blind crossover study. **Erythromycin** increased the AUC and peak plasma levels of a single 1 mg/kg oral dose of lidocaine (lignocaine) by 50 and 40% respectively. **Erythromycin** also markedly increased the AUC of the metabolite of lidocaine, monoethylglycinexylidide (MEGX) by

60%.[1] In a similar study,[2] **erythromycin** had no effect on the AUC or peak plasma level of a single 1.5 mg/kg intravenous dose of lidocaine, but still increased the AUC of MEGX by 70%.

Mechanism

Erythromycin is an inhibitor of cytochrome P450 isoenzyme CYP3A4, and appears to markedly reduce the first-pass metabolism of orally administered lidocaine (lignocaine) so that its plasma levels rise.[1] The increase in MEGX could be due to either an increase in the production of this metabolite, or the inhibition of its further metabolism.

Importance and management

Information seems limited, and since lidocaine (lignocaine) is not usually given orally the practical importance is minor. However, lidocaine is used for oro-pharyngeal topical anaesthesia, and there have been cases of toxicity after accidental ingestion. Thus, in a patient on erythromycin, the toxicity of oral lidocaine may be markedly increased. Further study is required to assess the significance of the increase in MEGX during prolonged intravenous lidocaine (lignocaine) infusions.

1. Isohanni MH, Neuvonen PJ, Olkkola KT. Effect of erythromycin and itraconazole on the pharmacokinetics of oral lignocaine. *Pharmacol Toxicol* (1999) 84, 143–6.

2. Isohanni MH, Neuvonen PJ, Palkama VJ, Olkkola KT. Effect of erythromycin and itraconazole on the pharmacokinetics of intravenous lignocaine. *Eur J Clin Pharmacol* (1998) 54, 561–5.

Lidocaine (Lignocaine) + Itraconazole

Itraconazole may markedly increase plasma levels of lidocaine (lignocaine) after oral administration, but not after intravenous administration.

Clinical evidence

Nine normal subjects were given either **itraconazole** 200 mg once daily or placebo for 4 days, in a randomised double-blind crossover study. **Itraconazole** increased the AUC and peak plasma levels (Cmax) of a single 1 mg/kg oral dose of lidocaine (lignocaine) by 75 and 55% respectively. **Itraconazole** did not affect the concentration of the lidocaine metabolite, monoethylglycinexylidide (MEGX).[1] In a similar study, **itraconazole** had no effect on the AUC and peak plasma levels of lidocaine or MEGX after a single 1.5 mg/kg intravenous dose of lidocaine.[2]

Mechanism

Itraconazole is an inhibitor of cytochrome P450 isoenzyme CYP3A4 and appears to markedly reduce the first-pass metabolism of orally administered lidocaine (lignocaine) so that its plasma levels rise.[1]

Importance and management

Information seems limited, and since lidocaine (lignocaine) is not usually given orally the practical importance is minor. However, lidocaine is used for oro-pharyngeal topical anaesthesia, and there have been cases of toxicity after accidental ingestion. In a patient on itraconazole, the toxicity of oral lidocaine may be markedly increased.

1. Isohanni MH, Neuvonen PJ, Olkkola KT. Effect of erythromycin and itraconazole on the pharmacokinetics of oral lignocaine. *Pharmacol Toxicol* (1999) 84, 143–6.

2. Isohanni MH, Neuvonen PJ, Palkama VJ, Olkkola KT. Effect of erythromycin and itraconazole on the pharmacokinetics of intravenous lignocaine. *Eur J Clin Pharmacol* (1998) 54, 561–5.

Lidocaine (Lignocaine) + Mexiletine

Mexiletine may increase the toxicity of lidocaine (lignocaine).

Clinical evidence, mechanism, importance and management

Lidocaine (lignocaine) CNS toxicity occurred within 1 hour of administration of a total of 600 mg oral lidocaine in a patient with cardiomyopathy who was receiving **mexiletine** 300 mg twice daily. Her lidocaine concentration was raised at 26.9 micrograms/ml. Although this was a high lidocaine dose, it was also considered that the concurrent use of **mexiletine** may have contributed to the raised levels since **mexiletine** is an oral lidocaine analog.[1] The combination should be used with caution.

1. Geraets DR, Scott SD, Ballew KA. Toxicity potential of oral lidocaine in a patient receiving mexiletine. *Ann Pharmacother* (1992) 26, 1380–1.

Lidocaine (Lignocaine) + Phenytoin

The incidence of central toxic side-effects may be increased following the concurrent intravenous infusion of lidocaine (lignocaine) and phenytoin. Sinoatrial arrest has been reported in one patient. In patients taking phenytoin as an anticonvulsant, serum lidocaine levels may be slightly reduced when given intravenously, but markedly reduced if given orally.

Clinical evidence

(a) Cardiac depression and increased side-effects

A study in 5 patients with suspected myocardial infarction given 0.5–3.0 mg/min lidocaine (lignocaine) intravenously for at least 24 h, followed by additional intravenous injections or infusions of **phenytoin**, showed that plasma levels of both drugs remained normal and unchanged but the incidence of side-effects (vertigo, nausea, nystagmus, diplopia, impaired hearing) were unusually high.[1]

Sinoatrial arrest occurred in a man following a suspected myocardial infarction with heart block, after receiving 1 mg/kg lidocaine infused intravenously in 1 min, followed 3 min later by 250 mg **phenytoin** over 5 min. The patient lost consciousness and his blood pressure could not be measured, but he responded to 200 micrograms isoprenaline (isoproterenol).[2]

(b) Serum lidocaine (lignocaine) levels

In the study described above,[1] intravenous **phenytoin** had no effect on plasma lidocaine levels during continuous infusion. In another study, lidocaine 2 mg/kg was administered intravenously to 7 epileptic patients while taking their usual anticonvulsants (including **phenytoin, barbiturates**, phenothiazines, benzodiazepines), and to 6 control subjects. Plasma lidocaine levels were 27 and 43% lower in the patients at 30 and 60 minutes.[3] Another study found that the clearance of intravenous lidocaine was slightly greater in patients taking **anticonvulsants** than in normal subjects (0.85 compared with 0.77 l/min) but this difference was not statistically significant.[4] Other studies in epileptic patients and normal subjects showed that when taking **phenytoin** the bioavailability of lidocaine *given orally* was halved.[4,5]

Mechanisms

(a). Phenytoin and lidocaine appear to have additive depressant actions on the heart.

(b). The reduced lidocaine serum levels is possibly due to liver enzyme induction; when given orally the marked reduction results from the stimulation of hepatic first-pass metabolism of phenytoin.[4,5] In addition, patients taking anticonvulsants including phenytoin had higher plasma concentrations of alpha-1-acid glycoprotein, which may result in a lower free fraction of lidocaine in plasma.[6]

Importance and management

Information is limited and the importance of the interactions is not well established. (a) The case of sinoatrial arrest emphasises the need to exercise caution when giving two drugs that have depressant actions on the heart. (b) The reduction in serum lidocaine (lignocaine) levels given intravenously to patients taking anticonvulsants, including phenytoin, is small and appears not to be of any clinical significance. Since lidocaine is not usually given orally, the practical importance of the marked reduction in bioavailability would also seem to be small.

1. Karlsson E, Collste P, Rawlins MD. Plasma levels of lidocaine during combined treatment with phenytoin and procainamide. *Eur J Clin Pharmacol* (1974) 7, 455–9.
2. Wood RA. Sinoatrial arrest: an interaction between phenytoin and lidocaine. *BMJ* (1971) i, 645.
3. Heinonen J, Takki S, Jarho L. Plasma lidocaine levels in patients treated with potential inducers of microsomal enzymes. *Acta Anaesth Scand* (1970) 14, 89–95.
4. Perucca E, Richens A. Reduction of oral bioavailability of lignocaine by induction of first pass metabolism in epileptic patients. *Br J Clin Pharmacol* (1979) 8, 21–31.
5. Perucca E, Hedges A, Makki KA, Richens A. A comparative study of antipyrine and lignocaine disposition in normal subjects and in patients treated with enzyme-inducing drugs. *Br J Clin Pharmacol* (1980) 10, 491–7.
6. Routledge PA, Stargel WW, Finn AL, Barchowsky A, Shand DG. Lignocaine disposition in blood in epilepsy. *Br J Clin Pharmacol* (1981) 12, 663–6.

Lidocaine (Lignocaine) + Procainamide

An isolated case of delirium has been described in a patient given lidocaine (lignocaine) and procainamide.

Clinical evidence, mechanism, importance and management

A man with paroxysmal tachycardia, under treatment with oral **procainamide** 1 g five-hourly and increasing doses of lidocaine (lignocaine) by intravenous infusion (550 mg within 3.5 h), became restless, noisy and delirious when given a further 250 mg intravenous dose of procainamide.[1] The symptoms disappeared within 20 minutes of discontinuing the lidocaine. The reason is not understood but the symptoms suggest that the neurotoxic effects of the two drugs might be additive. Other studies in patients have shown that lidocaine plasma levels are unaffected by intravenous or oral **procainamide**.[2]

1. Ilyas M, Owens D, Kvasnicka G. Delirium induced by a combination of anti-arrhythmic drugs. *Lancet* (1969) ii, 1368–9.
2. Karlsson E, Collste P, Rawlins MD. Plasma levels of lidocaine during combined treatment with phenytoin and procainamide. *Eur J Clin Pharmacol* (1974) 7, 455–9.

Lidocaine (Lignocaine) + Propafenone

Propafenone has minimal effects on the pharmacokinetics of lidocaine (lignocaine), but the severity and duration of the CNS side-effects are increased.

Clinical evidence, mechanism, importance and management

Twelve normal subjects, who had been taking 225 mg **propafenone** 8-hourly for 4 days, were given a continuous infusion of lidocaine (lignocaine) 2 mg/kg/h for 22 h. The AUC of the lidocaine was increased by 7% (from 76.3 to 81.7 micrograms.h/ml) and the clearance was reduced by 7% (from 10.27 to 9.53 ml/min/kg). One poor metaboliser of propafenone showed an increase in lidocaine clearance. The pharmacodynamic changes seen, were increases in the PR and QRS intervals of 10–20%. Combined use increased the severity and duration of adverse effects (lightheadedness, dizziness, paraesthesia, lethargy, somnolence). One subject withdrew from the study as a result.[1]

There would therefore appear to be no marked or important pharmacokinetic interaction between these two drugs, but the increased

CNS side-effects may be poorly tolerated by some individuals, and cardiac depressant effects may be additive.

1. Ujhelyi MR, O'Rangers EA, Fan C, Kluger J, Pharand C, Chow MSS. The pharmacokinetic and pharmacodynamic interaction between propafenone and lidocaine. *Clin Pharmacol Ther* (1993) 53, 38–48.

Lidocaine (Lignocaine) or Lorcainide + Rifampicin (Rifampin)

A case report describes a marked reduction in serum lorcainide concentrations and failure to control ventricular tachycardia in a man treated with rifampicin. There is also some indirect evidence that serum lidocaine (lignocaine) levels may possibly be reduced by rifampicin.

Clinical evidence, mechanism, importance and management

(a) Lidocaine (Lignocaine)

The report cited below (b) gives no indication of whether or not the patient also needed a much higher than usual dosage of **lidocaine** in the presence of the **rifampicin**, but a later *in vitro* experimental study suggests this possibility. Using cultured human hepatocytes it was found that **rifampicin** increases the metabolism of **lidocaine**, probably because the **rifampicin** induces the cytochrome P450 isoenzyme CYP3A4 which is concerned with the metabolism of **lidocaine** to its primary metabolite.[1] It seems possible therefore that this will also occur *in vivo* as well, although so far there appear to be no case reports or clinical studies of this interaction. If **rifampicin** is given with **lidocaine**, be alert for the need to use an increased **lidocaine** dosage. More study of this interaction is needed.

(b) Lorcainide

A 62-year-old on 600 mg **rifampicin** daily for tuberculosis had his treatment for ventricular tachycardia changed from lidocaine (lignocaine) to **lorcainide**. It was found necessary to give him three times the normal dosage (800–900 mg daily instead of 200–300 mg) to control his condition and to achieve satisfactory plasma levels (0.29 micrograms/ml). The likely reason is that the **rifampicin** (a known, potent enzyme inducing agent) increased the metabolism of the **lorcainide** by the liver, thereby hastening its loss from the body and reducing the plasma levels.[2] This seems to be the first and only report of this interaction, but be alert for it in any patient receiving these drugs and anticipate the need to increase the **lorcainide** dosage.

1. Li AP, Rasmussen A, Xu L, Kaminski DL. Rifampicin induction of lidocaine metabolism in cultured human hepatocytes. *J Pharmacol Exp Ther* (1995) 274, 673–7.
2. Mauro VF, Somani P, Temesy-Armos PN. Drug interaction between lorcainide and rifampicin. *Eur J Clin Pharmacol* (1987) 31, 737–8.

Lidocaine (Lignocaine) + Tobacco smoking

Smoking reduces the bioavailability of oral but not intravenous lidocaine (lignocaine).

Clinical evidence, mechanism, importance and management

A study in normal subjects found that the bioavailability of oral lidocaine (lignocaine) was markedly reduced in **smokers** (AUCs of 15.2 micrograms. ml⁻.min⁻¹ in smokers and 47.9 in non-smokers) but when given intravenously only moderate changes were seen.[1] The reason for the changes is probably due to liver enzyme induction caused by components of **tobacco** smoke. With oral lidocaine this could result in increased first-pass hepatic clearance. In the case of intravenous lidocaine, first-pass clearance is bypassed, and the enzyme induction was opposed by a decrease in hepatic flow. In practical terms this interaction is unlikely to be of much importance because lidocaine is usually titrated for the needs of the patient.

1. Huet P-M, Lelorier J. Effects of smoking and chronic hepatitis B on lidocaine and indocyanine green kinetics. *Clin Pharmacol Ther* (1980) 28, 208–15.

Lidocaine (Lignocaine) + Tocainide

A report describes a tonic-clonic seizure in a man which occurred during the period when his treatment for arrhythmia with lidocaine (lignocaine) was being changed to tocainide.

Clinical evidence, mechanism, importance and management

An elderly man treated with furosemide (frusemide) and co-trimoxazole experienced a tonic-clonic seizure while his treatment with lidocaine (lignocaine) was being changed to **tocainide**, although the serum levels of both antiarrhythmics remained within their therapeutic ranges. The patient became progressively agitated and disoriented about 2 h after taking the second of two 600 mg (six-hourly) oral doses of **tocainide** while still receiving 2 mg/min lidocaine intravenously, and about 1 h later he had the seizure. The patient subsequently tolerated each drug separately at concentrations similar to those which preceded the seizure without problems.[1] The maker notes that concomitant use of lidocaine and **tocainide** may cause an increased incidence of adverse effects, including CNS adverse reactions such as seizure, since the two drugs have similar pharmacodynamic effects.[2] Great care must therefore be exercised if tocainide is given during lidocaine (lignocaine) administration.

1. Forrence E, Covinsky JO, Mullen C. A seizure induced by concurrent lidocaine-tocainide therapy — Is it just a case of additive toxicity? *Drug Intell Clin Pharm* (1986) 20, 56–9.
2. Tonocard (Tocainide). AstraZeneca. US prescribing information, September 2000.

Mexiletine + Antacids, Atropine or Metoclopramide

The absorption of mexiletine is slowed by almasilate and atropine and hastened by metoclopramide, but the extent of the absorption is unaltered. See also 'Mexiletine + Opioids', p.112.

Clinical evidence, mechanism, importance and management

Oral administration of the antacid **almasilate** (*Gelusil*) 1 hour before a single dose of mexiletine 400 mg resulted in a slight delay in absorption (time to maximum concentration prolonged from 1.7 to 2.9 h), but had no effect on the extent of absorption.[1]

A study in 8 healthy subjects found that single 0.6-mg doses of intravenous **atropine** reduced, and 10 mg of intravenous **metoclopramide** hastened, the rate of absorption of single 400 mg oral doses of mexiletine, but the mexiletine AUC remained unaffected.

Since the achievement of steady-state levels depends on the extent of absorption, not on its rate, it seems very unlikely that these drugs will affect the antiarrhythmic effects of mexiletine during chronic dosing.[2] These drugs may however cause variations in the antiarrhythmic effects of initial oral mexiletine doses, which may be a problem if rapid control of the arrhythmia is essential. In general, no special precautions would appear necessary.

1. Herzog P, Holtermüller KH, Kasper W, Meinertz T, Trenk D, Jähnchen E. Absorption of mexiletine after treatment with gastric antacids. *Br J Clin Pharmacol* (1982) 14, 746–7.
2. Wing LMH, Meffin PJ, Grygiel JJ, Smith KJ, Birkett DJ. The effect of metoclopramide and atropine on the absorption of orally administered mexiletine. *Br J Clin Pharmacol* (1980) 9, 505–9.

Mexiletine + Cimetidine or Ranitidine

No adverse interaction occurs if mexiletine and cimetidine or ranitidine are given concurrently. Cimetidine can reduce the gastric side-effects of mexiletine.

Clinical evidence, mechanism, importance and management

The peak and trough plasma mexiletine levels of 11 patients were un-altered when given 1.2 g **cimetidine** daily for a week, and the frequency and severity of the ventricular arrhythmias for which they were receiving treatment remained unchanged. Moreover the gastric side-effects of mexiletine were reduced in half of the patients.[1] This study in patients confirms the findings of 2 other studies using **cimetidine** or **ranitidine** in healthy subjects.[2-4] There would seem to be no problems associated with giving these drugs concurrently, and some advantages.

1. Klein AL, Sami MH. Usefulness and safety of cimetidine in patients receiving mexiletine for ventricular arrhythmia. *Am Heart J* (1985) 109, 1281–6.
2. Klein A, Sami M, Selinger K. Mexiletine kinetics in healthy subjects taking cimetidine. *Clin Pharmacol Ther* (1985) 37, 669–73.
3. Brockmeyer NH, Breithaupt H, Hattingberg MV, Ohnhaus EE. Metabolism of mexiletine alone and in combination with cimetidine and ranitidine *in vivo* and *in vitro*. *Br J Clin Pharmacol* (1987) 24, 246P.
4. Brockmeyer NH, Breithaupt H, Ferdinand W, von Hattingberg M, Ohnhaus EE. Kinetics of oral and intravenous mexiletine: lack of effect of cimetidine and ranitidine. *Eur J Clin Pharmacol* (1989) 36, 375–8.

Mexiletine + Fluconazole

Fluconazole does not interact pharmacokinetically with mexiletine.

Clinical evidence, mechanism, importance and management

Six normal subjects were given single 200-mg doses of mexiletine before and after taking 200 mg **fluconazole** daily for 7 days. Two of the subjects were given 400 mg **fluconazole** daily for a further 7 days. No significant changes in the pharmacokinetics of mexiletine were seen.[1] The clinical outcome of concurrent use in patients was not examined, but there appear to be no adverse reports in the literature. No special precautions appear to be necessary if these drugs are used concurrently.

1. Ueno K, Yamaguchi R, Tanaka K, Sakaguchi M, Morishima Y, Yamauchi K, Iwai A. Lack of a kinetic interaction between fluconazole and mexiletine. *Eur J Clin Pharmacol* (1996) 50, 129–31.

Mexiletine + Omeprazole

Omeprazole does not appear to interact pharmacokinetically with mexiletine.

Clinical evidence, mechanism, importance and management

A crossover study in 9 normal Japanese men found that when given 200 mg mexiletine after taking 40 mg **omeprazole** daily for 8 days, the mexiletine serum concentrations and its AUCs remained unchanged. It was concluded that **omeprazole** does not affect the metabolism of mexiletine,[1] and no special precautions would seem to be needed if these drugs are used concurrently.

1. Kusumoto M, Ueno K, Tanaka K, Takeda K, Mashimo K, Kameda T, Fujimura Y, Shibakawa M. Lack of pharmacokinetic interaction between mexiletine and omeprazole. *Ann Pharmacother* (1998) 32, 182–4.

Mexiletine + Opioids

The absorption of mexiletine is depressed in patients following a myocardial infarction, and very markedly depressed and delayed if diamorphine or morphine is used concurrently. A higher loading dose may be needed if oral mexiletine is required as an antiarrhythmic agent during the first few hours following an infarction.

Clinical evidence

A pharmacokinetic study in patients and normal subjects showed that the plasma levels of mexiletine (400 mg orally followed by 200 mg 2 h later) in patients who had suffered a myocardial infarction and who had been given **diamorphine** (5–10 mg) or **morphine** (10 to 15 mg) were reduced as follows: at 2 h to 33%; 3 h 40%; 4 h 53%; 6 h 70% and 8 h 80%. The peak concentrations in the subjects and patients who had not received opioids occurred at about 3 h, while the peak in patients who had received opioids occurred at 6 h.[1,2]

Mechanism

The reduced absorption of mexiletine would seem to result from inhibition by the narcotics of gastric emptying. Other mechanisms probably contribute to its delayed clearance.

Importance and management

An established interaction although information is limited. The delay and reduction in the absorption would seem to limit the value of oral mexiletine during the first few hours after a myocardial infarction, particularly if these narcotic analgesics are used. The maker suggests that a higher loading dose of oral mexiletine may be preferable in this situation. Alternatively, an intravenous dose of mexiletine may be given. In addition, they note that it may be necessary to titrate the dose against therapeutic effects and side effects.[3]

1. Prescott LF, Pottage A, Clements JA. Absorption, distribution and elimination of mexiletine. *Postgrad Med J* (1977) 53 (Suppl 1), 50–5.
2. Pottage A, Campbell RWF, Achuff SC, Murray A, Julian DC, Prescott LF. The absorption of oral mexiletine in coronary care patients. *Eur J Clin Pharmacol* (1978) 13, 393–9.
3. Mexitil (Mexiletine). Boehringer Ingelheim Ltd. Summary of product characteristics, October 1999.

Mexiletine + Other Antiarrhythmic drugs

The concurrent use of mexiletine and amiodarone, beta-blockers, propafenone, or quinidine is clinically useful. It should be noted that both propafenone and quinidine raise mexiletine serum levels in extensive metabolisers of cytochrome P450 isoenzyme CYP2D6.

Clinical evidence, mechanism, importance and management

(a) Amiodarone

Torsade de pointes has been described in a patient taking amiodarone and mexiletine (a class Ib antiarrhythmic).[1] Class Ib antiarrhythmics are not associated with QT prolongation and torsade de points, and the makers of mexiletine say that this seems to be an isolated case.[2] The two drugs have been used together successfully,[3,4] and the makers of mexiletine state that it may be used concurrently with amiodarone.[5]

(b) Beta-blockers

A study in 4 patients showed that a combination of mexiletine and **propranolol** (240 mg daily) was more effective in blocking ventricular premature depolarisation (VPD) and ventricular tachycardia than mexiletine alone, and did not increase adverse effects. Plasma mexiletine concentrations were not changed significantly by **propranolol**.[6] Success in decreasing VPDs was noted in 30% of 44 patients taking mexiletine plus a **beta-blocker** compared with only 14% of 185 subjects taking mexiletine alone.[7] The makers of mexiletine state that it may be used concurrently with **beta-blockers**.[5]

(c) Propafenone

In one study in healthy subjects, **propafenone** reduced mexiletine clearance and increased plasma mexiletine concentrations in those subjects with extensive cytochrome P450 isoenzyme CYP2D6 activity, but had no effect in those of the poor metaboliser phenotype. The pharmacokinetics of mexiletine in extensive metabolisers after **propafenone** treatment became the same as those in poor metabolisers.[8,9] Mexiletine did not affect **propafenone** pharmacokinetics.[8,10] In this study, overall changes in ECG parameters were minor during concurrent administration of mexiletine and **propafenone**.[8,11] **Propafenone** is an inhibitor of CYP2D6, and inhibits the metabolism of mexiletine by this pathway.[8] Although the use of the combination was not associated with significant ECG changes, the potentiation of drug effects could predispose to proarrhythmias in patients with ischaemic heart disease. The authors suggest that slow dose-titration of the combination may decrease the risk of adverse effects.[8]

(d) Quinidine

Mexiletine and **quinidine** given concurrently were reported to be more effective than either drug alone, and the incidence of side-effects was reduced. Mexiletine limited the **quinidine**-induced increase in QT interval.[12] A study in *animals* concluded the benefit of combined use may be due to prolonged refractoriness and conduction time in the peri-infarct zone.[13] Two studies[14-16] in healthy subjects have shown that **quinidine** reduced the metabolism and excretion of mexiletine in extensive metabolisers of cytochrome P450 isoenzyme CYP2D6 (total clearance reduced by 24%[16]), but not poor metabolisers. **Quinidine** is an inhibitor of CYP2D6, and inhibits the metabolism of mexiletine by this pathway. Thus, a pharmacokinetic mechanism may also contribute to the increased efficacy of the combination.[16] The makers of mexiletine state that it may be used concurrently with **quinidine**.[5]

1. Tartini R, Kappenberger L, Steinbrunn W. Gefährliche Interaktionen zwischen Amiodaron und Antiarrhythmika der Klasse I. *Schweiz Med Wochenschr* (1982) 112, 1585–7.
2. Boehringer Ingelheim. Personal Communication, July 1995.
3. Waleffe A, Mary-Rabine L, Legrand V, Demoulin JC, Kulbertus HE. Combined mexiletine and amiodarone treatment of refractory recurrent ventricular tachycardia. *Am Heart J* (1980) 100, 788–93.
4. Hoffmann A, Follath F, Burckhardt D. Safe treatment of resistant ventricular arrhythmias with a combination of amiodarone and quinidine or mexiletine. *Lancet* (1983) i, 704–5.
5. Mexitil (Mexiletine). Boehringer Ingelheim Ltd. Summary of product characteristics, October 1999.
6. Leahey EB, Heissenbuttel RH, Giardina E-GV, Bigger JT. Combined mexiletine and propranolol treatment of refractory ventricular tachycardia. *BMJ* (1980) 281, 357–8.
7. Quoted as unpublished data by Bigger JT. The interaction of mexiletine with other cardiovascular drugs. *Am Heart J* (1984) 107, 1079–85.
8. Labbé L, O'Hara G, Lefebvre M, Lessard É, Gilbert M, Adedoyin A, Champagne J, Hamelin B, Turgeon J. Pharmacokinetic and pharmacodynamic interaction between mexiletine and propafenone in human beings. *Clin Pharmacol Ther* (2000) 68, 44–57.
9. Labbé L, Hamelin BA, Champagne J, O'Hara G, Turgeon J. Propafenone decreases mexiletine clearance in subjects with extensive CYP2D6 activity. *Clin Pharmacol Ther* (2000) 67, 117.
10. Labbé L, Hamelin BA, Champagne J, O'Hara G, Turgeon J. Pharmacokinetic and pharmacodynamic interactions between propafenone and mexiletine. *Clin Pharmacol Ther* (2000) 67, 117.
11. Labbé L, Hamelin BA, Champagne J, Gilbert M, O'Hara G, Turgeon J. QRS intervals during combined administration of mexiletine and propafenone. *Pharmacotherapy* (1998) 18, 428.
12. Duff HJ, Roden D, Primm RK, Oates JA, Woosley RL. Mexiletine in the treatment of resistant ventricular arrhythmias: enhancement of efficacy and reduction of dose-related side effects by combination with quinidine. *Circulation* (1983) 67, 1124–8.
13. Duff HJ, Rahmberg M, Sheldon RS. Role of quinidine in the mexiletine-quinidine interaction: electrophysiological correlates of enhanced antiarrhythmic efficacy. *J Cardiovasc Pharmacol* (1990) 16, 685–91.
14. Broly F, Vandamme N, Caron J, Libersa C, Lhermitte M. Single-dose quinidine treatment inhibits mexiletine oxidation in extensive metabolizers of debrisoquine. *Life Sci* (1991) 48, PL-123–128.
15. Fiset C, Giguère R, Kroemer HK, Gilbert M, Rouleau JR, Mikus G, Nguyen NN, Eichelbaum M, Bélanger PM, Turgeon J. Genetically-determined pharmacokinetic interaction between mexiletine and quinidine in man. *Clin Invest Med* (1991) 14 (4 Suppl A), A18.
16. Turgeon J, Fiset C, Giguère R, Gilbert M, Moerike K, Rouleau JR, Kroemer HK, Eichelbaum M, Grech-Bélanger O, Bélanger PM. Influence of debrisoquine phenotype and of quinidine on mexiletine disposition in man. *J Pharmacol Exp Ther* (1991) 259, 789–98.

Mexiletine + Phenytoin

Plasma mexiletine levels are reduced by the concurrent use of phenytoin. An increase in the dosage may be necessary.

Clinical evidence

The observation that 3 patients had unusually low plasma mexiletine levels while taking **phenytoin** prompted a pharmacokinetic study in 6 healthy subjects. After taking 300 mg **phenytoin** daily for a week, the mean mexiletine AUC and its half-life following single 400-mg doses were reduced by an average of about 50% (AUC reduced from 17.7 to 8.0 micrograms/ml/h; half-life reduced from 17.2 to 8.4 h).[1]

Mechanism

The most likely explanation is that phenytoin, a potent liver enzyme-inducing agent, particularly of cytochrome P450 isoenzyme CYP1A2, increases the metabolism and clearance of mexiletine from the body.

Importance and management

Information seems to be limited to this report[1] but the interaction appears to be established. It seems likely that the fall in mexiletine levels will be clinically important in some individuals. Monitor the plasma mexiletine levels and raise the dosage if necessary.

1. Begg EJ, Chinwah PM, Webb C, Day RO, Wade DN. Enhanced metabolism of mexiletine after phenytoin administration. *Br J Clin Pharmacol* (1982) 14, 219–23.

Mexiletine + Rifampicin (Rifampin)

The clearance of mexiletine from the body is increased by the concurrent use of rifampicin. An increase in the dosage of mexiletine may be necessary.

Clinical evidence, mechanism, importance and management

After taking 600 mg **rifampicin** daily for 10 days, the half-life of a single 400-mg dose of mexiletine was reduced in 8 normal subjects by 40% (from 8.5 to 5 h) and the AUC fell by 39%.[1,2] The probable reason is that the **rifampicin** (a known, potent enzyme-inducing agent) increases the metabolism and clearance of the mexiletine from the body. It seems likely that the mexiletine dosage will need to be increased during concurrent use, but by how much is uncertain (probably by up to 50%). More study using multiple doses of mexiletine is needed to confirm the extent and clinical importance of this interaction.

1. Pentikäinen PJ, Koivula IH, Hiltunen HA. Effect of enzyme induction on pharmacokinetics of mexiletine. *Clin Pharmacol Ther* (1982) 31, 260.
2. Pentikäinen PJ, Koivula IH, Hiltunen HA. Effect of rifampicin treatment on the kinetics of mexiletine. *Eur J Clin Pharmacol* (1982) 23, 261–6.

Mexiletine + Urinary acidifiers and alkalinizers

Large changes in urinary pH caused by the concurrent use of acidifying or alkalinizing drugs can have a marked effect on the plasma levels of mexiletine in some patients.

Clinical evidence

In 4 healthy subjects, a single 200 mg intravenous dose of mexiletine was given, once when the urine was acidic (pH 5) after administration of **ammonium chloride**, and once when the urine was alkaline (pH 8) after administration of **sodium bicarbonate**. The plasma elimination half-life was significantly shorter (2.8 h) when the urine was acidic compared with when it was alkaline (8.6 h). In addition, the percentage of mexiletine excreted unchanged in the urine was 57.5% when acidic and just 0.6% when alkaline.[1] Similar results were found in another study.[2] A further study in patients with uncontrolled urine pH (range 5.04 to 7.86) given mexiletine orally for 5 days found that the plasma concentration of mexiletine correlated with urine pH. In addition, it was predicted that a normal variation in pH could cause more than a 50% variation in plasma mexiletine levels.[3] A later comprehensive pharmacokinetic study in 5 healthy subjects confirmed that renal clearance of mexiletine was markedly lower in alkaline urine (pH 8) compared with acidic urine (pH 5.2) (4 versus 168 ml/min). In 2 subjects, this resulted in an increase in plasma concentrations of 61% and 96%, but in the other 3 the increase was less than 20%. Non-renal clearance (metabolic clearance) increased in the 3 subjects with little change in plasma concentrations, but did not in the 2 with marked changes.[4]

Mechanism

Mexiletine is a basic drug, and undergoes greater reabsorption by the kidneys when in the non-ionised form in alkaline urine. Mexiletine is also extensively cleared from the body by liver metabolism and only about 10% is excreted unchanged in the urine at physiological pH, although this is variable. Any effect of urine pH altering the renal clearance of mexiletine might therefore be expected to be compensated by an increase in metabolic clearance, but this does not seem to occur in all patients.[4]

Importance and management

Although changes in urinary pH can affect the amount of mexiletine lost in the urine, the effect of diet or the concurrent use of **alkalinizers** (**sodium bicarbonate**) or **acidifiers** (**acetazolamide**, **ammonium chloride** etc.) on the plasma concentrations of mexiletine does not appear to be predictable. There appear to be no reports of adverse interactions but concurrent use should be monitored. The maker of mexiletine recommends that the concomitant use of drugs that markedly acidify or alkalinize the urine should be avoided.[5]

1. Kiddie MA, Kaye CM, Turner P, Shaw TRD. The influence of urinary pH on the elimination of mexiletine. *Br J Clin Pharmacol* (1974) 1, 229–32.
2. Beckett AH, Chidomere EC. The distribution, metabolism and excretion of mexiletine in man. *Postgrad Med J* (1977) 53 (Suppl 1), 60–6.
3. Johnston A, Burgess CD, Warrington SJ, Wadsworth J, Hamer NAJ. The effect of spontaneous changes in urinary pH on mexiletine plasma concentrations and excretion during chronic administration to healthy volunteers. *Br J Clin Pharmacol* (1979) 8, 349–52.
4. Mitchell BG, Clements JA, Pottage A, Prescott LF. Mexiletine disposition: individual variation in response to urine acidification and alkalinisation. *Br J Clin Pharmacol* (1983) 16, 281–4.
5. Mexitil (Mexiletine). Boehringer Ingelheim Ltd. Summary of product characteristics, October 1999.

Moracizine + Beta-blockers

Moracizine appears not to interact adversely with propranolol.

Clinical evidence, mechanism, importance and management

The efficacy and tolerability of the combination of **propranolol** and moracizine was compared with either drug alone in patients with ventricular arrhythmias in controlled trials. The combination was well tolerated, with no evidence of any adverse interactions, nor any beneficial interactions. However, the dose of propranolol used was fairly low (120 mg/day).[1,2] Further study is needed.

1. Pratt CM, Butman SM, Young JB, Knoll M, English LD. Antiarrhythmic efficacy of ethmozine (moricizine HCl) compared with disopyramide and propranolol. *Am J Cardiol* (1987) 60, 52F–58F.
2. Butman SM, Knoll ML, Gardin JM. Comparison of ethmozine to propranolol and the combination for ventricular arrhythmias. *Am J Cardiol* (1987) 60, 603–7.

Moracizine + Cimetidine

Cimetidine increases the plasma levels of moracizine but the clinical importance of this is uncertain.

Clinical evidence, mechanism, importance and management

After taking 300 mg **cimetidine** four times daily for 7 days, the clearance of a single 500-mg dose of moracizine in 8 normal subjects was halved (from 38.2 to 19.7 ml/kg/min) and both its half-life and the AUC were increased (from 3.3 to 4.6 h and from 5.6 to 7.8 micrograms.ml/h respectively). It is believed that this is because the **cimetidine** reduces its metabolism by the liver.[1] Despite the increase in plasma moracizine levels, the PR and QRS intervals were not further prolonged. One possible explanation (so it is postulated) is that some of the metabolites of moracizine, whose production is inhibited by **cimetidine**, could also be pharmacologically active. Concurrent use should be well monitored but measuring plasma moracizine levels may be of limited value. More study is needed.

1. Biollaz J, Shaheen O, Wood AJJ. Cimetidine inhibition of ethmozine metabolism. *Clin Pharmacol Ther* (1985) 37, 665–8.

Pirmenol + Cimetidine

Cimetidine 300 mg four times daily for 8 days in 8 normal subjects had no significant effect on the pharmacokinetics of single 150 mg oral doses of pirmenol.[1] No clinically important interaction would therefore be expected in patients given both drugs.

1. Stringer KA, Lebsack ME, Cetnarowski-Cropp AB, Goldfarb AL, Radulovic LL, Bockbrader HN, Chang T, Sedman AJ. Effect of cimetidine administration on the pharmacokinetics of pirmenol. *J Clin Pharmacol* (1992) 32, 91–4.

Pirmenol + Rifampicin (Rifampin)

Rifampicin markedly increases the loss of pirmenol from the body. A reduction in its antiarrhythmic effects is likely to occur.

Clinical evidence

Treatment with 600 mg **rifampicin** daily for 14 days markedly affected the pharmacokinetics of a single 150-mg dose of pirmenol in 12 normal subjects.[1,2] The apparent plasma clearance increased sevenfold (from 12.8 to 88.3 l/h) and the AUC decreased 83% (from 13.5 to 2.3 mg.h/l).[2]

Mechanism

The probable reason is that the rifampicin (a well-recognised enzyme inducer) increases the metabolism of the pirmenol by the liver, thereby increasing its loss from the body.

Importance and management

Direct information seems to be limited to this study but what occurred is consistent with the way rifampicin interacts with many other drugs. Anticipate the need to increase the dosage of pirmenol if rifampicin is used concurrently.

1. Stringer KA, Thomas RW, Cetnarowski AB, Goldfarb AL. Effect of rifampin on the disposition of pirmenol. *J Clin Pharmacol* (1987) 27, 709.
2. Stringer KA, Cetnarowski AB, Goldfarb AB, Lebsack ME, Chang TS, Sedman AJ. Enhanced pirmenol elimination by rifampin. *J Clin Pharmacol* (1988) 28, 1094–7.

Procainamide + Amiodarone

The QT interval prolonging effects are increased when procainamide and amiodarone are used together, therefore the combination should generally be avoided. Serum procainamide levels are increased by about 60% and of N-acetylprocainamide by about 30% if amiodarone is given concurrently. If the combination is used, the dosage of procainamide will need to be reduced to avoid toxicity.

Clinical evidence

Twelve patients were stabilised on procainamide (2–6 g daily, or about 900 mg six-hourly). When concurrently treated with **amiodarone** (600 mg loading dose 12-hourly for 5–7 days, then 600 mg daily) their mean serum procainamide levels rose by 57% (from 6.8 to 10.6 micrograms/ml) and their serum N-acetylprocainamide (NAPA) levels rose by 32% (from 6.9 to 9.1 micrograms/ml). Procainamide levels increased by more than 3.0 micrograms/ml in 6 patients. The increases usually occurred within 24 h, but in other patients as late as 4 or 5 days. Toxicity was seen in two patients. Despite lowering the procainamide dosages by 20%, serum procainamide levels were still higher (at 7.7 micrograms/ml) than before the **amiodarone** was started.[1]

In another study, intravenous procainamide was administered once before (at a mean dose of 13 mg/kg), and once during (at a 30% reduced dose—mean 9.2 mg/kg), administration of **amiodarone** 1600 mg daily for 7 to 14 days. **Amiodarone** decreased the clearance of procainamide by 23% and increased its elimination half-life by 38%. Both drugs prolonged the QRS and QTc intervals, and the extent of prolongation was significantly greater with the combination that either drug alone.[2,3]

Mechanism

The mechanism behind the pharmacokinetic interaction is not understood. The QT prolonging effects of the two drugs would be expected to be additive.

Importance and management

Information appears to be limited to these studies, but the pharmacokinetic/pharmacodynamic interaction would seem to be established and clinically important. The use of amiodarone with procainamide further prolongs the QTc interval, which can increase the risk of torsade de pointes. Therefore, the combination should generally be avoided (the makers of amiodarone contraindicate its use with class Ia antiarrhythmics such as procainamide[4]). See also 'Drugs that prolong the QT interval + Other drugs that prolong the QT interval', p.103. The pharmacokinetic component has a high incidence (11 out of 12 in the report cited), and develops rapidly. Therefore, if the two drugs are considered essential, the dosage of procainamide may need to be reduced by 20–50%, and serum levels should be monitored and patients observed for side-effects.[1,3]

1. Saal AK, Werner JA, Greene HL, Sears GK, Graham EL. Effect of amiodarone on serum quinidine and procainamide levels. *Am J Cardiol* (1984) 53, 1264–7.
2. Windle JR, Prystowsky EN, Miles WM, Zipes DP, Heger JJ. Pharmacokinetic and pharmacodynamic interaction of amiodarone and procainamide. *J Am Coll Cardiol* (1985) 5, 481.
3. Windle J, Prystowsky EN, Miles WM, Heger JJ. Pharmacokinetic and electrophysiologic interactions of amiodarone and procainamide. *Clin Pharmacol Ther* (1987) 41, 603–10.
4. Cordarone X (Amiodarone hydrochloride). Sanofi Synthelabo. Summary of product characteristics, January 2000.

Procainamide + Beta-blockers

The pharmacokinetics of procainamide are little changed by either propranolol or metoprolol. Both sotalol and procainamide have QT-interval prolonging effects, which may be additive if they are used together.

Clinical evidence, mechanism, importance and management

One study in 6 normal subjects found that long-term treatment with **propranolol** (period and dosage not stated) increased the procainamide half-life from 1.71 to 2.66 h and reduced the plasma clearance by 16%.[1] However a later study in 8 normal subjects showed that the pharmacokinetics of a single 500-mg dose of procainamide hydrochloride were only slightly altered by the concurrent use of either 80 mg **propranolol** three times daily or 100 mg **metoprolol** twice daily. The procainamide half-life increased from 1.9 to 2.2 h with **propranolol** and to 2.3 h with **metoprolol**, but no significant changes in total clearance occurred. No changes in the AUC of N-acetylprocainamide were seen.[2] It seems unlikely that a clinically important adverse interaction normally occurs between these drugs.

A clinical study describes the successful use of procainamide with **sotalol**;[3] however, both **sotalol** and procainamide can prolong the QT interval, and there may be an increased the risk of torsade de pointes arrhythmia if they are used together. See also 'Drugs that prolong the QT interval + Other drugs that prolong the QT interval', p.103.

1. Weidler DJ, Garg DC, Jallad NS, McFarland MA. The effect of long-term propranolol administration on the pharmacokinetics of procainamide in humans. *Clin Pharmacol Ther* (1981) 29, 289.
2. Ochs HR, Carstens G, Roberts G-M, Greenblatt DJ. Metoprolol or propranolol does not alter the kinetics of procainamide. *J Cardiovasc Pharmacol* (1983) 5, 392–5.
3. Dorian P, Newman D, Berman N, Hardy J, Mitchell J. Sotalol and type IA drugs in combination prevent recurrence of sustained ventricular tachycardia. *J Am Coll Cardiol* (1993) 22, 106–13.

Procainamide + H$_2$-blockers

Serum procainamide levels can be increased if cimetidine is given concurrently and toxicity may develop, particularly in those who have a reduced renal clearance such as the elderly. Ranitidine and famotidine appear to interact only minimally or not at all.

Clinical evidence

(a) Cimetidine

In one study, 36 elderly patients (65–90 years old) on sustained-release oral procainamide 6-hourly showed mean steady-state serum procainamide and N-acetylprocainamide levels rises of 55 and 36% respectively after taking 300 mg **cimetidine** 6-hourly for 3 days. This was tolerated in 24 of them without side-effects (serum procainamide and N-acetylprocainamide <12 and <15 mg/l respectively) but the other 12 had some adverse effects (nausea, weakness, malaise P-R interval increases <20%) which was dealt with by stopping one or both drugs.[1] Another report describes an elderly man who developed procainamide toxicity when given 1200 mg **cimetidine** daily. His procainamide dosage was roughly halved (from 937.5 to 500 mg every 6 hours) to bring his serum procainamide and N-acetylprocainamide levels into the accepted therapeutic range.[2]

Four studies in normal subjects have found that **cimetidine** increased the procainamide AUC by 24–43%,and decreased the loss through the kidneys by 31–40%.[3-8] A steady-state procainamide serum level increase of 43% has been seen following 1200 mg **cimetidine** daily.[7,8]

(b) Famotidine

One study found that 40 mg **famotidine** daily for 5 days did not affect the pharmacokinetics or pharmacodynamics of a single 5 mg/kg intravenous dose of procainamide in normal subjects.[9,10]

(c) Ranitidine

One study found that **ranitidine** 150 mg twice daily for one day reduced the absorption of procainamide from the gut by 10% and reduced its renal excretion by 19%, increasing the procainamide and N-acetylprocainamide AUC by about 14%.[11] However, no change in the steady-state pharmacokinetics of procainamide was found with **ranitidine** 150 mg twice daily in another study, except that **ranitidine** delayed the time to maximum plasma concentration (from 1.4 to 2.7 h).[7,8]

Mechanism

Procainamide levels in the body are increased because cimetidine reduces its kidney excretion by about one-third or more, but the precise mechanism is uncertain. One suggestion is that it interferes with the active secretion of procainamide by the kidney tubules.[4,5]

Importance and management

The procainamide/cimetidine interaction is established. Concurrent use should be undertaken with care because the safety margin of procainamide is low. Reduce the procainamide dosage as necessary. This is particularly important in the elderly because they have a reduced ability to clear both drugs. Ranitidine and famotidine appear not to interact to a clinically important extent, but it should be appreciated that what is known is based on studies in normal subjects rather than patients.

1. Bauer LA, Black D, Gensler A. Procainamide-cimetidine drug interaction in elderly male patients. *J Am Geriatr Soc* (1990) 38, 467–9.
2. Higbee MD, Wood JS, Mead RA. Case report. Procainamide-cimetidine interaction. A potential toxic interaction in the elderly. *J Am Geriatr Soc* (1984) 32, 162–4.
3. Somogyi A Heinzow B. Cimetidine reduces procainamide elimination. *N Engl J Med* (1982) 307, 1080.
4. Somogyi A, McLean A, Heinzow B. Cimetidine-procainamide pharmacokinetic interaction in man: evidence of competition for tubular secretion of basic drugs. *Eur J Clin Pharmacol* (1983) 25, 339–45.
5. Christian CD, Meredith CG, Speeg KV. Cimetidine inhibits renal procainamide clearance. *Clin Pharmacol Ther* (1984) 36, 221–7.
6. Lai MY, Jiang FM, Chung CH, Chen HC, Chao PDL. Dose dependent effect of cimetidine on procainamide disposition in man. *Int J Clin Pharmacol Ther Toxicol* (1988) 26, 118–21.
7. Paloucek F, Rodvold K, Jung D, Gallestegui J. The effects of cimetidine and ranitidine on steady-state pharmacokinetics of procainamide. *J Clin Pharmacol* (1986) 26, 557.
8. Rodvold KA, Paloucek FP, Jung D, Gallestegui J. Interaction of steady-state procainamide with H₂-receptor antagonists cimetidine and ranitidine. *Ther Drug Monit* (1987) 9, 378–83.
9. Klotz U, Arvela P, Rosenkranz B. Interaction study of diazepam and procainamide with the new H₂-receptor antagonist famotidine. *Clin Pharmacol Ther* (1985) 37, 205.
10. Klotz U, Arvela P, Rosenkranz B. Famotidine, a new H₂-receptor antagonist, does not affect hepatic elimination of diazepam or tubular secretion of procainamide. *Eur J Clin Pharmacol* (1985) 28, 671–5.
11. Somogyi A, Bochner F. Dose and concentration dependent effect of ranitidine on procainamide disposition and renal clearance in man. *Br J Clin Pharmacol* (1984) 18, 175–81.

Procainamide + Para-aminobenzoic acid (PABA)

A single case report found that para-aminobenzoic acid (PABA) increased the serum levels of procainamide and reduced the production and serum levels of the procainamide metabolite *N*-acetylprocainamide. In contrast, a later pharmacokinetic study in healthy subjects found that PABA had no effect on serum procainamide and increased serum *N*-acetylprocainamide.

Clinical evidence, mechanism, importance and management

A 61-year-old man who had sustained ventricular tachycardia, which failed to respond adequately to oral procainamide, was found to be a rapid acetylator of procainamide so that the serum levels of the procainamide metabolite (*N*-acetylprocainamide) were particularly high when compared with the procainamide levels. When he was additionally given 1.5 g **PABA** six-hourly for 30 h to suppress the production of this metabolite, the serum level of procainamide increased, that of *N*-acetylprocainamide decreased, and control of his arrhythmia improved.[1] However, a later study in 10 normal subjects who were also fast acetylators found that **PABA** did not significantly affect the pharmacokinetics of procainamide. In addition, although it inhibited the production of *N*-acetylprocainamide, it also inhibited renal excretion, so that the AUC and elimination half-life were increased. This sug-

gests that **PABA** may in fact not be useful for increasing the efficacy and safety of procainamide.[2]

These contradictory findings are difficult to explain, but neither report suggests that concurrent use need be avoided. More study is needed to clarify the situation.

1. Nylen ES, Cohen AI, Wish MH, Lima JL, Finkelstein JD. Reduced acetylation of procainamide by para-aminobenzoic acid. *J Am Coll Cardiol* (1986) 7, 185–7.
2. Tisdale JE, Rudis MI, Padhi ID, Svensson CK, Webb CR, Borzak S, Ware JA, Krepostman A, Zarowitz BJ. Inhibition of N-acetylation of procainamide by para-aminobenzoic acid in humans. *J Clin Pharmacol* (1995) 35, 902–10.

Procainamide + Probenecid

Probenecid appears not to interact with procainamide. The pharmacokinetics of a single 750 mg intravenous dose of procainamide and its effects on QT intervals were not altered by prior administration of 2 g probenecid in 6 healthy subjects.[1] No special precautions appear to be necessary.

1. Lam YWF, Boyd RA, Chin SK, Chang D, Giacomini KM. Effect of probenecid on the pharmacokinetics and pharmacodynamics of procainamide. *J Clin Pharmacol* (1991) 31, 429–32.

Procainamide + Quinidine

A single case report describes a marked increase in the plasma procainamide levels of a patient when concurrently treated with quinidine. The combination prolongs the QT interval, and should generally be avoided because of the increased risk of torsade de pointes.

Clinical evidence

A man with sustained ventricular tachycardia on high dose intravenous procainamide (2 g eight-hourly) showed a 70% increase (a rise from 9.1 to 15.4 ng/ml) in his steady-state plasma procainamide levels when concurrently treated with 324 mg **quinidine gluconate** eight-hourly. The procainamide half-life increased from 3.7 to 7.2 h and its clearance fell from 27 to 16 l/h. His QTc interval increased from 648 to 678 ms.[1] In another study in patients with ventricular arrhythmias, **quinidine** was combined with procainamide. The doses were adjusted based, in part, on the QT interval. The QTc interval was longer with the combination (499 ms) than each drug alone (quinidine 470 ms; procainamide, 460 ms) despite using reduced doses in the combination (mean **quinidine** dose reduced by 28%; procainamide by 32%).[2]

Mechanism

It was suggested that the **quinidine** interferes with one or more of renal pathways by which procainamide is cleared from the body.[1]

Importance and management

Information on the possible pharmacokinetic interaction seems to be limited to this report. Both quinidine and procainamide are class Ia antiarrhythmics and prolong the QT interval, an effect that is increased with the combination. Such combinations should generally be avoided because of the increased risk of torsade de pointes. See also 'Drugs that prolong the QT interval + Other drugs that prolong the QT interval', p.103.

1. Hughes B, Dyer JE, Schwartz AB. Increased procainamide plasma concentrations caused by quinidine: a new drug interaction. *Am Heart J* (1987) 114, 908–9.
2. Kim SG, Seiden SW, Matos JA, Waspe LE, Fisher JD. Combination of procainamide and quinidine for better tolerance and additive effects for ventricular arrhythmias. *Am J Cardiol* (1985) 56, 84–8.

Procainamide + Quinolone antibacterials

Ofloxacin causes a moderate increase in the serum levels of procainamide but the ECG appears to be unaltered in studies in healthy subjects.

Clinical evidence, mechanism, importance and management

Nine normal subjects were given a single oral 1 g dose of procainamide alone then again with the fifth dose of **ofloxacin** (400 mg given twice daily for five doses). The AUC of procainamide was increased 27% by the **ofloxacin** (from 31.1 to 39.6 mg.h/l), the maximum plasma levels were increased by 21% (from 4.8 to 5.8 micrograms/l) and the total clearance was reduced by 22% (from 34.7 to 27.2 l/h),[1] whereas the pharmacokinetics of the active metabolite of procainamide (N-acetylprocainamide) were not significantly altered. The probable reason for the interaction is that the **ofloxacin** inhibits the secretion of unchanged procainamide by the kidney tubules. Despite the pharmacokinetic changes, no ECG changes were detected. These results suggest that **ofloxacin** interacts to a modest extent with procainamide, and that it might be prudent to monitor the outcome if both drugs are given together in patients. There seems to be no information about the possible effects of other quinolone antibacterials.

1. Martin DE, Shen J, Griener J, Raasch R, Patterson JH, Cascio W. Effects of ofloxacin on the pharmacokinetics and pharmacodynamics of procainamide. *J Clin Pharmacol* (1996) 36, 85–91.

Procainamide + Sucralfate

Sucralfate appears not to affect the absorption of procainamide.

Clinical evidence, mechanism, importance and management

In 4 healthy subjects, 1g **sucralfate** taken 30 min before a single 250-mg dose of procainamide reduced the mean maximum salivary level by 5.3%, but did not significantly affect either the AUC or the rate of absorption.[1] These results need confirmation in patients taking long-term procainamide, but they suggest that a clinically significant interaction is unlikely.

1. Turkistani AAA, Gaber M, Al-Meshal MA, Al-Shora HI, Gouda MW. Effect of sucralfate on procainamide absorption. *Int J Pharmaceutics* (1990) 59, R1–R3.

Procainamide + Trimethoprim

Trimethoprim causes a marked increase in the plasma levels of procainamide and its active metabolite, N-acetylprocainamide, with the risk of toxicity.

Clinical evidence

Eight normal subjects were given 500 mg procainamide six-hourly for three days. The concurrent use of 200 mg **trimethoprim** daily increased the AUC from 0 to 12 h of procainamide by 63% and of its active metabolite, N-acetylprocainamide (NAPA), by 51%. The renal clearance of procainamide decreased by 47% and that of NAPA by 13%. The QTc prolonging effects of procainamide were increased to a significant, but slight, extent by the concomitant use of trimethoprim.[1,2] Another study found that 200 mg **trimethoprim** daily reduced the renal clearance of a single 1 g dose of procainamide by 45% and of NAPA by 26%. The QTc interval was increased from 0.4 to 0.43 sec.[3]

Mechanism

Trimethoprim decreases the losses in the urine of both procainamide and its active metabolite by competing for active tubular secretion. It may also cause a small increase in the conversion of procainamide to N-acetylprocainamide.[1]

Importance and management

An established interaction but its documentation is limited. The need to reduce the procainamide dosage should be anticipated if trimethoprim is given to patients already controlled on procainamide. In practice the effects may be greater than the studies cited suggest because the elderly lose procainamide through the kidneys more slowly than normal young healthy subjects. Remember too that the daily dosage of trimethoprim in **co-trimoxazole** (trimethoprim 160 mg + sulfamethoxazole (sulphamethoxazole) 800 mg) may equal or exceed the dosages used in the study cited.

1. Kosoglou T, Rocci ML, Vlasses PH. Evaluation of trimethoprim/procainamide interaction at steadystate in normal volunteers. *Clin Pharmacol Ther* (1988) 43, 131.
2. Kosoglou T, Rocci ML, Vlasses PH. Trimethoprim alters the disposition of procainamide and N-acetylprocainamide. *Clin Pharmacol Ther* (1988) 44, 467–77.
3. Vlasses PH, Kosoglou T, Chase SL, Greenspon AJ, Lottes S, Andress E, Ferguson RK, Rocci ML. Trimethoprim inhibition of the renal clearance of procainamide and N-acetylprocainamide. *Arch Intern Med* (1989) 149, 1350–3.

Propafenone + Barbiturates

Phenobarbital (phenobarbitone) increases the loss of propafenone from the body, and reduces its serum levels.

Clinical evidence, mechanism, importance and management

In a preliminary report of a study in 7 non-smoking subjects who were fast metabolisers of propafenone, 100 mg **phenobarbital** daily for 3 weeks reduced the peak serum propafenone level (following a single 300-mg dose) by 26–87% and the AUC by 10–89%. The intrinsic clearance increased 11–84%. The results in a further 4 heavy smokers were similar.[1] The probable reason is that **phenobarbital** (a potent stimulator of liver enzymes) increases the metabolism of the propafenone and its loss from the body. The clinical importance of this awaits assessment but check that propafenone remains effective if **phenobarbital** is added, and that toxicity does not occur if it is stopped. If the suggested mechanism is correct, other barbiturates would be expected to interact similarly. Study in patients is needed.

1. Chan GL-Y, Axelson JE, Kerr CR. The effect of phenobarbital on the pharmacokinetics of propafenone in man. *Pharm Res* (1988) 5, S153.

Propafenone + Cimetidine

Cimetidine appears to interact minimally with propafenone.

Clinical evidence, mechanism, importance and management

A study in 12 normal subjects (10 extensive metabolisers and 2 poor metabolisers of propafenone) given 225 mg propafenone eight-hourly showed that the concurrent use of 400 mg **cimetidine** eight-hourly caused some changes in the pharmacokinetics and pharmacodynamics of the propafenone with wide intersubject variability. Raised mean peak and steady-state plasma levels were seen (by 24 and 22%, respectively), but these did not reach statistical significance. A slight increase in the QRS duration also occurred.[1] None of the changes were considered clinically important.

1. Pritchett ELC, Smith WM, Kirsten EB. Pharmacokinetic and pharmacodynamic interactions of propafenone and cimetidine. *J Clin Pharmacol* (1988) 28, 619–24.

Propafenone + Erythromycin

Limited evidence suggests erythromycin may inhibit the metabolism of propafenone.

Clinical evidence, mechanism, importance and management

The preliminary results of a study in 12 normal subjects given a single dose of propafenone 300 mg with or without **erythromycin** 250 mg showed that the increase in propafenone AUC with **erythromycin** was greater in those with lower cytochrome P450 isoenzyme CYP2D6 activity. It was suggested[1] that low CYP2D6 activity shifts propafenone metabolism to the CYP3A4/1A2-mediated N-depropylpropafenone pathway increasing the interaction with **erythromycin,** which is an inhibitor of CYP3A4. This appears to be the only documentation of a possible interaction with **erythromycin** and its clinical significance is not certain. More study is needed.

1. Munoz CE, Ito S, Bend JR, Tesoro A, Freeman D, Spence JD, Bailey DG. Propafenone interaction with CYP3A4 inhibitors in man. *Clin Pharmacol Ther* (1997) 61, 154.

Propafenone + Grapefruit juice

Limited evidence suggests grapefruit juice may inhibit the metabolism of propafenone.

Clinical evidence, mechanism, importance and management

Preliminary results of a study in 12 normal subjects given a single dose of propafenone 300 mg with or without 250 ml **grapefruit juice** showed that the increase in propafenone AUC with **grapefruit juice** was greater in those with lower cytochrome P450 isoenzyme CYP2D6 activity. It was suggested[1] that low CYP2D6 activity shifts propafenone metabolism to the CYP3A4/1A2-mediated N-depropylpropafenone pathway increasing the interaction with **grapefruit juice,** which is an inhibitor of CYP3A4. The clinical significance of this finding is not certain. Further study is needed

1. Munoz CE, Ito S, Bend JR, Tesoro A, Freeman D, Spence JD, Bailey DG. Propafenone interaction with CYP3A4 inhibitors in man. *Clin Pharmacol Ther* (1997) 61, 154.

Propafenone + Ketoconazole

An isolated case report describes convulsions in a man taking propafenone within two days of starting ketoconazole.

Clinical evidence

A man who had been taking captopril and hydrochlorothiazide for 6 years and 300 mg propafenone daily for 4 years, without problems and without any history of convulsive episodes, experienced a tonic-clonic seizure while watching the TV. It was later found that he had started to take two capsules of **ketoconazole** daily two days previously for the treatment of a candidal infection.[1] The preliminary results of another study in 12 healthy subjects given a single dose of propafenone 300 mg with or without ketoconazole 200 mg showed that the increase in propafenone AUC with ketoconazole was greater in those with lower cytochrome P450 isoenzyme CYP2D6 activity.[2]

Mechanism

The authors of the case report postulate that the ketoconazole may have inhibited the metabolism of the propafenone so that this patient, in effect, may have developed an overdose.[1] However convulsions with propafenone are rare.[3] **Ketoconazole** is an inhibitor of cytochrome P450 isoenzyme CYP3A4, by which propafenone is metabolised to N-depropylpropafenone. Propafenone is also extensively

metabolised by CYP2D6 to 5-hydroxypropafenone. However, it was suggested that if CYP2D6 activity is low, propafenone metabolism may be shifted to the N-depropylpropafenone pathway increasing the possibility of an interaction with ketoconazole.[2]

Importance and management

The general importance of this interaction is uncertain. As of 1996, there had been no other cases reported to the maker of propafenone.[3] The more recent data suggests that an interaction can occur, and it would seem prudent to monitor concurrent use. More study is needed. There seems to be nothing documented about the effects of other azole antifungals.

1. Duvelleroy Hommet C, Jonville-Bera AP, Autret A, Saudeau D, Autret E, Fauchier JP. Une crise convulsive chez un patient traité par propafénone et kétoconazole. *Therapie* (1995) 50, 164–5.
2. Munoz CE, Ito S, Bend JR, Tesoro A, Freeman D, Spence JD, Bailey DG. Propafenone interaction with CYP3A4 inhibitors in man. *Clin Pharmacol Ther* (1997) 61, 154.
3. Knoll Ltd. Personal communication, February 1996.

Propafenone + Quinidine

Quinidine doubles the plasma levels of propafenone and halves the levels of its active metabolite in 'extensive' metabolisers, but the antiarrhythmic effects appear to be unaffected.

Clinical evidence

Nine patients on propafenone for frequent isolated ventricular ectopic beats, firstly had their dosage reduced to 150 mg eight-hourly and then four days later the steady-state pharmacokinetics of propafenone were determined at this new dose. Then **quinidine** was added at a dose of 50 mg eight-hourly. Four days later the steady-state plasma propafenone levels in 7 patients ('extensive' metabolisers) had more than doubled (from 408 to 1100 ng/ml), and 5-hydroxypropafenone concentrations had approximately halved, but the ECG intervals and arrhythmia frequency were unaltered. The steady-state plasma propafenone levels remained unchanged in the other two patients ('poor' metabolisers).[1] The same research group conducted a similar study in healthy subjects, which confirmed that **quinidine** increased the plasma levels of propafenone in extensive, but not poor, metabolisers. In addition, it was found that quinidine increased the extent of the beta-blockade caused by the propafenone in extensive metabolisers (assessed by a decrease in heart rate at exercise and by sensitivity to isoprenaline (isoproterenol)) to approach that seen in poor metabolisers.[2,3] Another study has shown that the inhibition of propafenone metabolism by low-dose quinidine also occurs in Chinese as well as Caucasian patients.[4]

Mechanism

Quinidine inhibits the metabolism (cytochrome P450 isoenzyme CYP2D6-dependent 5-hydroxylation) of propafenone by the liver in those who are 'extensive' metabolisers so that it is cleared more slowly. Its plasma levels are doubled as a result, but the overall antiarrhythmic effects remain effectively unchanged possibly because the production of its active antiarrhythmic metabolite (5-hydroxypropafenone) is simultaneously halved.[1] Quinidine increases the beta-blocking effects of propafenone in extensive metabolisers because only the parent drug, and not the metabolites, has beta-blocking activity.[3]

Importance and management

An established interaction but of uncertain clinical importance. The patients described above had their propafenone dosage approximately halved before the study began, and although the pharmacokinetic effects of low-dose quinidine were marked, they apparently had little clinical relevance.[1] The metabolic status of patients seems in this instance not to have been important. Further study is needed, and until then, concurrent use should be well monitored.

1. Funck-Brentano C, Kroemer HK, Pavlou H, Woosley RL, Roden DM. Genetically-determined interaction between propafenone and low dose quinidine: role of active metabolites in modulating net drug effect. Br J Clin Pharmacol (1989) 27, 435–44.
2. Mörike K, Roden D. Quinidine-enhanced β-blockade during treatment with propafenone in extensive metabolizer human subjects. Circulation (1992) 86 (4 Suppl I), I–719.
3. Mörike K, Roden D. Quinidine-enhanced β-blockade during treatment with propafenone in extensive metabolizer human subjects. Clin Pharmacol Ther (1994) 55, 28–34.
4. Fan C, Tang M, Lau C-P, Chow M. The effect of quinidine on propafenone metabolism in Chinese patients. Clin Invest Med (1998) (Suppl) S12.

Propafenone + Rifampicin (Rifampin)

Propafenone serum levels and its therapeutic effects can be markedly reduced by concurrent use of rifampicin.

Clinical evidence

A man successfully treated with propafenone showed marked falls in his plasma propafenone levels (from 993 to 176 ng/ml) with levels of its two active metabolites, 5-hydroxypropafenone and N-depropyl-propafenone changing from 195 to 64 ng/ml and from 110 to 192 ng/ml respectively within 12 days of starting to take 450 mg **rifampicin** twice daily. His arrhythmias returned. Two weeks after stopping the **rifampicin** his arrhythmias had disappeared and the propafenone and its metabolites had returned to acceptable levels (1411, 78 and 158 ng/ml respectively).[1] In a study in young healthy subjects, **rifampicin** 600 mg daily for 9 days reduced the bioavailability of a single oral dose of propafenone 300 mg from 30 to 10% in extensive metabolisers, and from 81 to 48% in poor metabolisers of cytochrome P450 isoenzyme CYP2D6. QRS prolongation decreased during enzyme induction. In contrast, in this study, **rifampicin** had no substantial effect on the pharmacokinetics of propafenone when administered intravenously.[2] Similar findings were reported in a further study by the same research group in healthy elderly subjects.[3]

Mechanism

Rifampicin induced the cytochrome P450 isoenzyme CYP3A4/1A2-mediated metabolism and phase II glucuronidation of propafenone. The effect of rifampicin on gastrointestinal clearance of propafenone was greater than that of its hepatic clearance. Rifampicin had no effect on CYP2D6-mediated metabolism of propafenone (the usual main metabolic route in extensive metabolisers).[2,3]

Importance and management

An established and clinically relevant metabolic drug interaction. The dosage of oral propafenone will need increasing during concurrent use of rifampicin.[3] Alternatively, if possible, the authors of the case report[1] advise the use of another antibacterial because of the probable difficulty in adjusting the propafenone dosage.

1. Castel JM, Cappiello E, Leopaldi D, Latini R. Rifampicin lowers plasma concentrations of propafenone and its antiarrhythmic effect. Br J Clin Pharmacol (1990) 30, 155–6.
2. Dilger K, Greiner B, Fromm MF, Hofmann U, Kroemer HK, Eichelbaum M. Consequences of rifampicin treatment on propafenone disposition in extensive and poor metabolizers of CYP2D6. Pharmacogenetics (1999) 9, 551–9.
3. Dilger K, Hofmann U, Klotz U. Enzyme induction in the elderly: Effect of rifampin on the pharmacokinetics and pharmacodynamics of propafenone. Clin Pharmacol Ther (2000) 67, 512–20.

Quinidine + Amiloride

Preliminary studies have shown that the antiarrhythmic activity of quinidine can be opposed by amiloride.

Clinical evidence

A study in 10 patients with inducible sustained ventricular tachycardia was carried out to see whether a beneficial interaction occurred between quinidine and **amiloride**. Patients were given oral quinidine until their trough serum levels reached 10 micromol/l, or the maximum well-tolerated dose was reached. After electrophysiological studies had been done, oral **amiloride** was added at a dosage of 5 mg twice daily, increased up to 10 mg twice daily (if serum potassium levels remained normal) for 3 days. The electrophysiological studies were then repeated. Unexpectedly, 7 of the 10 patients demonstrated adverse responses while taking both drugs. Three developed sustained ventricular tachycardia and 3 others had somatic side-effects (hypotension, nausea, diarrhoea) which prevented further studies being carried out. One patient had 12 episodes of sustained ventricular tachycardia while taking both drugs. **Amiloride** had no effect on quinidine levels.[1]

Mechanism

Not understood. The surface QRS duration was prolonged by the addition of the amiloride, with no further prolongation of the QT interval. Parallel electrophysiological experiments in vitro found that the maximum rate of rise of phase 0 of the action potential was decreased (43 V/sec with quinidine alone, 24 V/sec with both drugs) because of a greater degree of tonic block of Vmax (3% with quinidine alone, 14% with both drugs).[1]

Importance and management

So far the evidence seems to be limited to this single study but it suggests that amiloride can reverse (oppose) the antiarrhythmic activity of quinidine. The full clinical implications of this interaction are not yet known, but it would now clearly be prudent to monitor concurrent use very closely to confirm that the quinidine continues to be effective if amiloride is present.

1. Wang L, Sheldon RS, Mitchell B, Wyse DG, Gillis AM, Chiamvimonvat N, Duff HJ. Amiloride-quinidine interaction: adverse outcomes. Clin Pharmacol Ther (1994) 56, 659–67.

Quinidine + Amiodarone

The QT interval prolonging effects are increased when quinidine and amiodarone are used together, and torsade de pointes has occurred, therefore the combination should generally be avoided. Serum quinidine levels can be increased by the concurrent use of amiodarone. Therefore, if the combination is used, reduce the quinidine dosage appropriately to avoid quinidine toxicity.

Clinical evidence

Eleven patients were stabilised on quinidine (daily doses of 1200 to 4200 mg). When concurrently treated with **amiodarone** (600 mg loading dose 12-hourly for 5–7 days, then 600 mg daily) their mean serum quinidine levels rose by an average of 32% (from 4.4 to 5.8 micrograms/ml). Three of them had a substantial increase (+2.0 micrograms/ml). Signs of toxicity (diarrhoea, nausea, vomiting, hypotension) were seen in some, and the quinidine dosage was reduced in 9 of the 11 by an average of 37%. Even so, the quinidine serum levels were still higher (at 5.2 micrograms/ml) than before the **amiodarone** was started.[1]

A test on a normal subject showed that when 600 mg **amiodarone** was added to a daily quinidine dosage of 1200 mg, the serum quinidine levels doubled within 3 days and the QT interval was prolonged from 1.0 (no drugs) to 1.2 (quinidine alone) to 1.4 (quinidine plus **amiodarone**).[2] This report also described two patients with minor heart arrhythmias who developed QT prolongation and atypical ventricular tachycardia (AVT or 'torsade de pointes') when given both drugs.[2]

Mechanism

The mechanism behind the pharmacokinetic interaction is not understood. The QT prolonging effects of the two drugs would be expected to be additive.

Importance and management

An established and clinically important pharmacokinetic/pharmaco-dynamic interaction. The use of amiodarone with quinidine further prolongs the QT interval and increases the risk of torsade de pointes. Therefore, the combination should generally be avoided (see also 'Drugs that prolong the QT interval + Other drugs that prolong the QT interval', p.103). The pharmacokinetic component appears to occur in most patients, and to develop rapidly. Therefore, if the two drugs are considered essential, the dosage of quinidine should be reduced by about 30–50% and the serum levels should be monitored. The ECG should also be monitored for evidence of a prolongation of the QT interval when combined therapy is started.[3] Successful and uneventful concurrent use has been described in a report of 4 patients on quinidine (dose not stated) and **amiodarone** (200 mg five times weekly).[4] Another describes the successful use of a short course of quinidine to convert chronic atrial fibrillation to sinus rhythm in 9 of 15 patients on long-term amiodarone therapy. Patients were hospitalised and continuously monitored: no proarrhythmias occurred and the QT interval remained within acceptable limits.[5]

1. Saal AK, Werner JA, Greene HL, Sears GK, Graham EL. Effect of amiodarone on serum quinidine and procainamide levels. Am J Cardiol (1984) 53, 1265–7.
2. Tartini R, Kappenberger L, Steinbrunn W, Meyer UA. Dangerous interaction between amiodarone and quinidine. Lancet (1982) i, 1327–9.
3. Kinidin Durules (Quinidine). AstraZeneca. Summary of product characteristics, March 1997.
4. Hoffmann A, Follath F, Burckhardt D. Safe treatment of resistant ventricular arrhythmias with a combination of amiodarone and quinidine or mexiletine. Lancet (1983) i, 704–5.
5. Kerin NZ, Ansari-Leesar M, Faitel K, Narala C, Frumin H, Cohen A. The effectiveness and safety of the simultaneous administration of quinidine and amiodarone in the conversion of chronic atrial fibrillation. Am Heart J (1993) 125, 1017–21.

Quinidine + Antacids or Urinary alkalinizers

Large rises in urinary pH due to the concurrent use of some antacids, diuretics or alkaline salts can cause the retention of quinidine which could lead to quinidine toxicity, but there seems to be only one case on record of an adverse interaction (with *Mylanta*—magnesium and aluminium hydroxide). Aluminium hydroxide appears not to interact.

Clinical evidence

The renal clearance of quinidine in 4 normal subjects taking 200 mg six-hourly by mouth was reduced by an average of 50% (from 53 to 26 ml/min) when their urine was made alkaline (i.e. changed from pH 6–7 to pH 7–8) with **sodium bicarbonate** and **acetazolamide** (0.5 g every 12 h). Below pH 6 their urine quinidine level averaged 115 mg/l, whereas when urinary pH values rose above 7.5 their average level fell to 13 mg/l. The quinidine urinary excretion rate decreased from 103 to 31 micrograms/min. In 6 other subjects the rise in serum quinidine levels was reflected in a prolongation of the QT interval. Raising the urinary pH from about 6 to 7.5 in one individual increased serum quinidine levels from about 1.6 to 2.6 micrograms/ml.[1]

A patient on quinidine who took 8 *Mylanta* tablets daily (**aluminium hydroxide** gel 200 mg, **magnesium hydroxide** 200 mg and simethicone 20 mg) for a week and a little over 1L fruit juice (orange and grapefruit) each day developed a threefold increase in serum quinidine levels (from 8 to 25 mg/l) and toxicity. In 6 healthy subjects, this dose of *Mylanta* for 3 days produced a consistently alkaline urine in 4 subjects, and in 5 subjects when combined with fruit juice.[2] In 4 healthy subjects, 30 ml **aluminium hydroxide** gel *(Amphogel)* administered with, and one hour after, a single 200-mg dose of quinidine sulphate had no effect on serum quinidine levels, AUC or excretion (urine pH ranged from 5 to 6.2).[3] Two similar single-dose studies in normal subjects found that the absorption and elimination of 400 mg quinidine sulphate[4] or 648 mg quinidine gluconate[5] was unaffected by 30 ml **aluminium hydroxide** gel, although the change in quinidine AUC did vary from −18% to +35% in one study.[5] Urinary pH was unaffected in both studies.[4,5]

Mechanism

Quinidine is lost from the body as unchanged quinidine in the urine. In acid urine much of the quinidine excreted by the kidney tubules is in the ionised (lipid-insoluble) form which is unable to diffuse freely back into the cells and so is lost in the urine. In alkaline urine more of the quinidine is in the non-ionised (lipid-soluble) form which freely diffuses back into the cells and is retained. In this way the pH of the urine determines how much quinidine is lost or retained and thereby governs the serum levels. *In vitro* data suggest changes in pH and adsorption effects within the gut due to antacids may also possibly affect the absorption of quinidine.[6,7]

Importance and management

An established interaction, but with the exception of the one isolated case cited,[2] there seem to be no reports of problems in patients given quinidine and antacids or urinary alkalinizers. Nevertheless you should monitor the effects if drugs that can markedly change urinary pH are started or stopped. Reduce the quinidine dosage as necessary.

It is difficult to predict which antacids, if any, are likely to increase the serum levels of quinidine. As noted above, *Mylanta* (**aluminium hydroxide** gel and **magnesium hydroxide**) alkalinizes urine and can interact. Similarly, *Maalox* (**magnesium and aluminium hydroxide**) can raise the urinary pH by about 0.9 and could possibly interact.[8] *Milk of magnesia* (**magnesium hydroxide**) and *Titralac* (**calcium carbonate-glycine**) in normal doses raise the urinary pH by about 0.5, so that a smaller effect is likely.[8] *Amphogel* (**aluminium hydroxide** gel) and *Robalate* (**dihydroxyaluminium glycinate**) are reported to have no effect on urinary pH,[8] and the studies above confirm **aluminium hydroxide** gel does not generally interact. More study is needed.

1. Gerhardt RE, Knouss RF, Thyrum PT, Luchi RJ, Morris JJ. Quinidine excretion in aciduria and alkaluria. Ann Intern Med (1969) 71, 927–33.
2. Zinn MB. Quinidine intoxication from alkali ingestion. Texas Med (1970) 66, 64–6.
3. Romankiewicz JA, Reidenberg M, Drayer D, Franklin JE. The noninterference of aluminium hydroxide gel with quinidine sulfate absorption: an approach to control quinidine-induced diarrhea. Am Heart J (1978) 96, 518–20.
4. Ace LN, Jaffe JM, Kunka RL. Effect of food and antacid on quinidine bioavailability. Biopharm Drug Dispos (1983) 4, 183–90.
5. Mauro VF, Mauro LS, Fraker TD, Temesy-Armos PN, Somani P. Effect of aluminium hydroxide gel on quinidine gluconate absorption. Ann Pharmacother (1990) 24, 252–4.
6. Remon JP, Van Severen R, Braeckman P. Interaction entre antiarythmiques, antiacides et antidiarrhéiques. III. Influence d'antacides et d'antidiarrhéiques sur la réabsorption in vitro de sels de quinidine. Pharm Acta Helv (1979) 54, 19–22.
7. Moustafa MA, Al-Shora HI, Gaber M, Gouda MW. Decreased bioavailability of quinidine sulphate due to interactions with adsorbent antacids and antidiarrhoeal mixtures. Int J Pharmaceutics (1987) 34, 207–11.
8. Gibaldi M, Grundhofer B, Levy G. Effect of antacids on pH of urine. Clin Pharmacol Ther (1974) 16, 520–5.

Quinidine + Anticonvulsants

Serum quinidine levels can be reduced by the concurrent use of phenytoin, phenobarbital (phenobarbitone) or primidone. Loss of arrhythmia control is possible if the quinidine dosage is not increased.

Clinical evidence

A man on long-term **primidone** 500 mg daily was started on quinidine 300 mg four-hourly, but only attained a plasma quinidine level of 0.8 micrograms/ml with an estimated half-life of 5 h. When **primidone** was discontinued, quinidine levels rose to 2.4 micrograms/ml with a half-life of 12 h. **Phenobarbital** 90 mg daily was then started, and the quinidine level fell to 1.6 micrograms/ml with a half-life of 7.6 h. In another case, a women required doses of quinidine sulphate of up to 800 mg four-hourly to achieve therapeutic levels while taking **phenytoin.** When the **phenytoin** was stopped, quinidine toxicity occurred, and the dose was eventually halved. Further study was then made in 4 normal subjects. After four weeks treatment with either **phenytoin** or **phenobarbital** (in dosages adjusted to give 10 to 20 micrograms/ml), the elimination half-life of a single 300-mg dose of quinidine sulphate was reduced by about 50% and the total AUC by about 60%.[1]

Similar results were found with **phenytoin** in another study in 3 normal subjects.[2] Other cases have also been reported with **phenytoin, primidone, pentobarbital** and **phenobarbital**.[3-6] In one case, quinidine levels fell by 44% when **phenytoin** was added to quinidine therapy in a patient with recurrent ventricular tachycardia.[3] Quinidine levels increased from a mean of 0.8 micrograms/ml to 2.2 micrograms/ml 15 days after **pentobarbital** was discontinued in another report.[4] A 3-year-old child on both **phenobarbital** and **phenytoin** required 300 mg quinidine 4-hourly to achieve therapeutic serum quinidine levels, and had an estimated quinidine half-life of only 1.4 h.[5] Difficulty in achieving adequate serum quinidine levels was also reported in a woman on **phenytoin** and **primidone**. Her quinidine half-life was 2.7 h, approximately half that usually seen in adults.[6]

Mechanism

The evidence suggests that phenytoin, primidone or phenobarbital (all known enzyme-inducing agents) increase the metabolism by the liver of the quinidine and increase its loss from the body.[2]

Importance and management

Established interactions of clinical importance although the documentation is limited. The concurrent use of phenytoin, primidone, phenobarbital (phenobarbitone) or any other barbiturate need not be avoided, but be alert for the need to increase the quinidine dosage. If the anticonvulsants are withdrawn the quinidine dosage may need to be reduced to avoid quinidine toxicity. Quinidine serum levels should be monitored.

1. Data JL, Wilkinson GR, Nies AS. Interaction of quinidine with anticonvulsant drugs. *N Engl J Med* (1976) 294, 699–702.
2. Russo ME, Russo J, Smith RA, Pershing LK. The effect of phenytoin on quinidine pharmacokinetics. *Drug Intell Clin Pharm* (1982) 16, 480.
3. Urbano AM. Phenytoin-quinidine interaction in a patient with recurrent ventricular tachyarrhythmias. *N Engl J Med* (1983) 308, 225.
4. Chapron DJ, Mumford D, Pitegoff GI. Apparent quinidine-induced digoxin toxicity after withdrawal of pentobarbital. A case of sequential drug interactions. *Arch Intern Med* (1979) 139, 363–5.
5. Rodgers GC, Blackman MS. Quinidine interaction with anticonvulsants. *Drug Intell Clin Pharm* (1983) 17, 819–20.
6. Kroboth FJ, Kroboth PD, Logan T. Phenytoin-theophylline-quinidine interaction. *N Engl J Med* (1983) 308, 725.

Quinidine + Aspirin

A patient and two normal subjects given quinidine and aspirin showed a two- to threefold increase in bleeding times. The patient developed petechiae and gastrointestinal bleeding.

Clinical evidence, mechanism, importance and management

A patient with a prolonged history of paroxysmal atrial tachycardia was given quinidine (800 mg daily) and **aspirin** (325 mg twice daily). After a week he showed generalised petechiae and blood in his faeces. His prothrombin and partial prothrombin times were normal but the template bleeding time was more than 35 min (normal 2–10 min). Further study in two normal subjects showed that quinidine alone (975 mg daily for 5 days) and **aspirin** alone (650 mg three times a day for 5 days) prolonged bleeding times by 125% and 163% respectively; given together for 5 days the bleeding times were prolonged by 288%.[1] The underlying mechanism is not totally understood but it is believed to be the outcome of the additive effects of two drugs, both of which can reduce blood platelet aggregation.

This seems to be the only study of this adverse interaction, but what is known from other studies about the effects of both drugs on platelet function when given alone supports this report. Concurrent use in other patients should be monitored to check that bleeding does not occur.

1. Lawson D, Mehta J, Mehta P, Lipman BC, Imperi GA. Cumulative effects of quinidine and aspirin on bleeding time and platelet α₂-adrenoceptors: potential mechanism of bleeding diathesis in patients receiving this combination. *J Lab Clin Med* (1986) 108, 581–6.

Quinidine + Calcium channel blockers

A few patients have shown increased serum quinidine levels when stopping nifedipine, but others have shown no interaction and one study even suggests that quinidine serum levels may be slightly raised. Nifedipine levels may be modestly raised by quinidine. In contrast, verapamil reduces the clearance of quinidine and in one patient the serum quinidine levels doubled and quinidine toxicity developed. Acute hypotension has also been seen in three patients on quinidine when given verapamil intravenously. Felodipine and nisoldipine appear not to interact, and the situation with diltiazem is unclear.

Clinical evidence

(a) Diltiazem

A study in 10 normal subjects given 600 mg quinidine twice daily and 120 mg **diltiazem** daily for 7 days showed that the pharmacokinetics of neither drug was affected by the presence of the other.[1] These findings contrast with another crossover study in 12 healthy subjects given single doses of diltiazem 60 mg or quinidine 200 mg alone then after pretreatment with 100 mg quinidine twice daily or 90 mg **diltiazem** twice daily for five doses, respectively. The pharmacokinetics of **diltiazem** were unaffected by quinidine, but the AUC of quinidine was increased 51% by diltiazem.[2,3] When quinidine was given after diltiazem pretreatment, there were significant increases in QTc and PR intervals, and a significant decrease in heart rate and diastolic blood pressure. Pretreatment with quinidine did not significantly alter the effects of diltiazem.[3]

(b) Felodipine

Felodipine 10 mg daily for 3 days was found to have no clinically significant effect on the pharmacokinetics or haemodynamic and ECG effects of a single 400-mg dose of quinidine in 12 normal subjects. Felodipine did cause a modest 22% decrease in the AUC of the quinidine metabolite 3-hydroxyquinidine.[4,5]

(c) Nifedipine

(i) Quinidine serum levels reduced, unaffected or increased. Two patients taking 300 or 400 mg quinidine sulphate six-hourly and 10 or 20 mg **nifedipine** six or eight-hourly showed a doubling of their serum quinidine levels (from 2–2.5 to 4.6 micrograms/ml and from 1.6–1.8 to 3.5 micrograms/ml respectively) when the **nifedipine** was withdrawn. The increased serum quinidine levels were reflected in a prolongation of the QT_c interval. However, the first patient had demonstrated no change in quinidine levels when nifedipine was initially added to his existing quinidine therapy. In addition, 4 other patients failed to demonstrate this interaction.[6]

Two other reports describe a similar response:[7,8] the quinidine serum level doubled in one patient when the **nifedipine** was stopped,[7] and in the other it was found difficult to achieve adequate serum quinidine levels when nifedipine was added, even when the quinidine dosage was increased threefold. When the **nifedipine** was withdrawn, the quinidine levels rose once again.[8] A study in 12 patients found no significant change in serum quinidine levels in the group as a whole when given **nifedipine**, but one patient showed a 41% decrease.[9] Two other studies in healthy subjects found that quinidine AUC was unchanged by **nifedipine**.[4,5,10]

A further study in 12 normal subjects found that the AUC of a single 200 mg oral dose of quinidine sulphate was increased 16% by 20 mg oral **nifedipine**, its clearance was reduced by 14% and the maximum serum level was raised almost 20%. These modest changes were not considered clinically relevant.[11]

(ii) Nifedipine serum levels increased. The **nifedipine** AUC of 10 normal subjects was increased 37% when also given 200 mg quinidine sulphate eight-hourly, and heart rates were significantly increased. Quinidine levels were unchanged.[10] Another study found that quinidine had a modest inhibitory effect on the metabolism of **nifedipine** (half-life prolonged 40%).[12] A further study in 12 normal subjects found

that the AUC of a single 20 mg oral dose of **nifedipine** was increased 16% by 200 mg oral quinidine and its clearance was reduced by 17%, but these modest changes were not considered clinically relevant.[11]

(d) Nisoldipine

An open crossover study in 20 normal subjects found that 20 mg **nisoldipine** had no effect on the bioavailability of 648 mg quinidine gluconate.[13]

(e) Verapamil

After taking 80 mg **verapamil** three times daily for 3 days, the clearance of a single 400-mg dose of quinidine sulphate in 6 normal subjects was decreased by 32% (from 17 to 11.69 l/h) and the half-life was increased by 35% (from 6.87 to 9.29 h).[14]

A patient given 648 mg quinidine gluconate six-hourly showed an increase in serum levels from 2.6 to 5.7 micrograms/ml when given 80 mg **verapamil** eight-hourly for a week. He became dizzy and had blurred vision and was found to have atrioventricular block (heart rate 38 bpm) and a systolic blood pressure of 50 mmHg. In a subsequent study in this patient it was found that the **verapamil** halved the quinidine clearance and almost doubled the serum half-life.[15] Three other patients given quinidine orally showed marked hypotension when given intravenous **verapamil** 2.5 or 5 mg (blood pressure fall from 130/70 to 80/50 mmHg, systolic pressure fall from 140 to 85 mmHg and a mean arterial pressure fall from 100 to 60 mmHg, in the 3 patients respectively). In two of the patients, after quinidine was discontinued the same dose of verapamil did not cause a drop in blood pressure.[16]

Mechanisms

Suggestions for how nifedipine could alter quinidine levels include changes in cardiovascular haemodynamics,[6] and effects on metabolism.[9] Quinidine probably inhibits nifedipine metabolism by cytochrome P450 isoenzyme CYP3A4.[12] The quinidine/verapamil interaction is probably due to an inhibitory effect of verapamil on the metabolism of quinidine (inhibition of cytochrome P450 isoenzyme CYP3A).[14,17] The marked hypotension observed may be related to the antagonistic effects of the two drugs on catecholamine-induced alpha-receptor induced vasoconstriction.[16]

Importance and management

The results of studies of the quinidine/nifedipine interaction are inconsistent and contradictory so that the outcome of concurrent use is uncertain. Monitor the response, being alert for the need to modify the dosage. More study of this interaction is needed. Quinidine appears to increase nifedipine levels, but the importance of this is uncertain.

What is known about the quinidine/verapamil interaction suggests that a reduction in the dosage of the quinidine may be needed to avoid toxicity. If the verapamil is given intravenously, use with caution and be alert for evidence of acute hypotension. Monitor the effects of concurrent use closely. There is actually a fixed dose drug combination marketed in Germany (*Cordichin*). No interaction apparently occurs between quinidine and felodipine or nisoldipine. The situation with diltiazem is as yet uncertain but be alert for the need to reduce the quinidine dosage.

1. Matera MG, De Santis D, Vacca C, Fici F, Romano AR, Marrazzo R, Marmo E. Quinidine-diltiazem: pharmacokinetic interaction in humans. *Curr Ther Res* (1986) 40, 653–6.
2. Laganière S, Davies RF, Carignan G, Foris K, Goernert L, McGilveray IJ. Pharmacokinetic interaction of quinidine and diltiazem given alone and in combination in volunteers. *Pharm Res* (1994) 11 (Suppl), S-341.
3. Laganière S, Davies RF, Carignan G, Foris K, Goernert L, Carrier K, Pereira C, McGilveray I. Pharmacokinetic and pharmacodynamic interactions between diltiazem and quinidine. *Clin Pharmacol Ther* (1996) 60, 255–64.
4. Bailey DG, Melendez L, Freeman DJ, Kreeft J Carruthers SG. Evaluation of the interaction between quinidine and the calcium channel antagonists, nifedipine and felodipine. *Clin Invest Med* (1991) 14, 4 (Suppl A), A19.
5. Bailey DG, Freeman DJ, Melendez LJ, Kreeft JH, Edgar B, Carruthers SG. Quinidine interaction with nifedipine and felodipine: pharmacokinetic and pharmacodynamic evaluation. *Clin Pharmacol Ther* (1993) 53, 354–9.
6. Farringer JA, Green JA, O'Rourke RA, Linn WA, Clementi WA. Nifedipine-induced alterations in serum quinidine concentrations. *Am Heart J* (1984) 108, 1570–2.
7. Van Lith RM, Appleby DH. Quinidine-nifedipine interaction. *Drug Intell Clin Pharm* (1985) 19, 829–31.
8. Green JA, Clementi WA, Porter C, Stigelman W. Nifedipine-quinidine interaction. *Clin Pharm* (1983) 2, 461–5.
9. Munger MA, Jarvis RC, Nair R, Kasmer RJ, Nara AR, Urbancic A, Green JA. Elucidation of the nifedipine-quinidine interaction. *Clin Pharmacol Ther* (1989) 45, 411–16.
10. Bowles SK, Reeves RA, Cardozo L, Edwards DJ. Evaluation of the pharmacokinetic and pharmacodynamic interaction between quinidine and nifedipine. *J Clin Pharmacol* (1993) 33, 727–31.
11. Hippius M, Henschel L, Sigusch H, Tepper J, Brendel E. Hoffmann A. Pharmacokinetic interaction of nifedipine and quinidine. *Naunyn Schmiedebergs Arch Pharmacol* (1994) 349 (Suppl), R138.
12. Schellens JHM, Ghabrial H, van der Wart HHF, Bakker EN, Wilkinson GR, Breimer DD. Differential effects of quinidine on the disposition of nifedipine, sparteine and mephenytoin in humans. *Clin Pharmacol Ther* (1991) 50, 520–8.
13. Schall R, Müller FO, Groenewoud G, Hundt HKL, Luus HG, Van Dyk M, Van Schalkwyk AMC. Investigation of a possible pharmacokinetic interaction between nisoldipine and quinidine in healthy volunteers. *Drug Invest* (1994) 8, 162–170.
14. Lavoie R, Blevins RD, Rubenfire M. The effect of verapamil on quinidine pharmacokinetics in man. *Drug Intell Clin Pharm* (1986) 20, 457.
15. Trohman RG, Estes DM, Castellanos A, Palomo AR, Myerburg RJ, Kessler KM. Increased quinidine plasma concentrations during administration of verapamil; a new quinidine-verapamil interaction. *Am J Cardiol* (1986) 57, 706–7.
16. Maisel AS, Motulsky HJ, Insel PA. Hypotension after quinidine plus verapamil. Possible additive competition at alpha-adrenergic receptors. *N Engl J Med* (1985) 312, 167–70.
17. Kroemer HK, Gautier J-C, Beaune P, Henderson C, Wolf CR, Eichelbaum M. Identification of P450 enzymes involved in metabolism of verapamil in humans. *Naunyn Schmiedebergs Arch Pharmacol* (1993) 348, 332–7.

Quinidine + Cimetidine or Ranitidine

Quinidine serum levels can rise and toxicity may develop in some patients when concurrently treated with cimetidine. An isolated case of ventricular bigeminy occurred in a patient on quinidine and ranitidine.

Clinical evidence

Cimetidine 1.2 g daily for 7 days prolonged the elimination half-life of a single dose of quinidine sulphate 400 mg by 55% (from 5.8 to 9 h) and decreased its clearance by 37% in 6 normal subjects. Peak plasma levels were raised by 21%. These changes were reflected in ECG changes (+51% and +28% respectively, in the mean areas under the QT and QT_c time curves), but these were said not to be statistically significant.[1]

A later study, prompted by the observation of two patients who developed toxic quinidine levels when given **cimetidine**, found essentially the same. The AUC and half-life of quinidine were increased by 14.5 and 22.6% respectively, and the clearance was decreased by 25% by cimetidine 1.2 g daily in healthy subjects.[2] A further study in 4 normal subjects found that 1.2 g **cimetidine** daily for 5 days prolonged the elimination half-life of quinidine by 54% and decreased the its total clearance by 36%.[3-5] **Cimetidine** prolonged the QT interval by 30% above quinidine's effect alone.[3,5] A single case report describes marked increases in both quinidine and digitoxin concentrations in a woman when given **cimetidine**.[6] Ventricular bigeminy occurred in a man on quinidine when given **ranitidine**. His serum quinidine levels remained unchanged.[7]

Mechanism

It was originally suggested that the cimetidine depresses the metabolism of the quinidine by the liver so that it is cleared more slowly.[2] However further data suggest that cimetidine successfully competes with quinidine for its excretion by the kidneys.[8]

Importance and management

The quinidine/cimetidine interaction is established and of clinical importance. The incidence is unknown. Be alert for changes in the response to quinidine if cimetidine is started or stopped. Ideally the quinidine serum levels should be monitored and the dosage reduced as necessary. Reductions of 25% (oral) and 35% (intravenous) have been suggested.[4] Those at greatest risk are likely to be patients with impaired kidney function, patients with impaired liver function elimination of the drugs such as the elderly, and those with serum quinidine levels already at the top end of the therapeutic range.[2] The situation with ranitidine is uncertain.

1. Hardy BG, Zador IT, Golden L, Lalka D, Schentag JJ. Effect of cimetidine on the pharmacokinetics and pharmacodynamics of quinidine. *Am J Cardiol* (1983) 52, 172–5.
2. Kolb KW, Garnett WR, Small RE, Vetrovec GW, Kline BJ, Fox T. Effect of cimetidine on quinidine clearance. *Ther Drug Monit* (1984) 6, 306–12.

3. Boudoulas H, MacKichan JJ, Schaal SF. Effect of cimetidine on quinidine pharmacokinetics and pharmacodynamics. *Clin Res* (1987) 35, 874A.

4. MacKichan JJ, Boudoulas H, Schaal SF. Effect of cimetidine on quinidine bioavailability. *Biopharm Drug Dispos* (1989) 10, 121–5.

5. Boudoulas H, MacKichan JJ, Schaal SF. Effect of cimetidine on the pharmacodynamics of quinidine. *Med Sci Res* (1988) 16, 713–14.

6. Polish LB, Branch RA, Fitzgerald GA. Digitoxin-quinidine interaction: potentiation during administration of cimetidine. *South Med J* (1981) 74, 633–4.

7. Iliopoulou A, Kontogiannis D, Tsoutsos D, Mouloopoulos S. Quinidine-ranitidine adverse reaction. *Eur Heart J* (1986) 7, 360.

8. Hardy BG, Schentag JJ. Lack of effect of cimetidine on the metabolism of quinidine: effect on renal clearance. *Int J Clin Pharmacol Ther Toxicol* (1988) 26, 388–91.

Quinidine + Diazepam

A single dose study suggests that diazepam does not affect the pharmacokinetics of quinidine.

Clinical evidence, mechanism, importance and management

A comparative study in 8 normal subjects showed that the pharmacokinetics of a single 250-mg dose of quinidine sulphate was unaltered by a single 10-mg dose of **diazepam**.[1] This suggests that no interaction between these drugs is likely but it needs confirmation by further studies using multiple doses of both drugs.

1. Rao BR, Rambhau D. Absence of a pharmacokinetic interaction between quinidine and diazepam. *Drug Metabol Drug Interact* (1995) 12, 45–51.

Quinidine + Diclofenac

Diclofenac inhibits the metabolism of quinidine by *N*-oxidation but does not affect other pharmacokinetic parameters.

Clinical evidence, mechanism, importance and management

In an open study, 6 healthy subjects were given a single dose of quinidine sulphate 200 mg before and on day 5 of a 6-day course of **diclofenac** 100 mg daily. Concomitant administration of **diclofenac** reduced the *N*-oxidation of quinidine by 33%, but no other pharmacokinetic changes were found.[1] **Diclofenac** is a substrate for, and therefore a possible competitive inhibitor of, cytochrome P450 isoenzyme CYP2C9. These results suggest CYP2C9 does not appear to have a major role in quinidine metabolism,[1] and so clinically relevant pharmacokinetic interactions between quinidine and **diclofenac** would seem unlikely. No special precautions appear to be necessary during concurrent use.

1. Damkier P, Hansen LL, Brøsen K. Effect of diclofenac, disulfiram, itraconazole, grapefruit juice and erythromycin on the pharmacokinetics of quinidine. *Br J Clin Pharmacol* (1999) 48, 829–38.

Quinidine + Disulfiram

Disulfiram does not affect the pharmacokinetics of quinidine.

Clinical evidence, mechanism, importance and management

In an open study, 6 healthy subjects were given a single dose of quinidine sulphate 200 mg before and on day 5 of a 6-day course of **disulfiram** 200 mg daily. There were no changes in quinidine pharmacokinetics during **disulfiram** administration.[1] **Disulfiram** is thought to be an inhibitor of cytochrome P450 isoenzyme CYP2E1, but this isoenzyme does not appear to have a major role in quinidine metabolism.[1] Clinically relevant pharmacokinetic interactions between quinidine and **disulfiram** therefore seem unlikely. Concurrent use need not be avoided.

1. Damkier P, Hansen LL, Brøsen K. Effect of diclofenac, disulfiram, itraconazole, grapefruit juice and erythromycin on the pharmacokinetics of quinidine. *Br J Clin Pharmacol* (1999) 48, 829–38.

Quinidine + Erythromycin

Erythromycin can increase quinidine levels and cause a small further increase in the QT_c interval. An isolated report describes a moderate rise in serum quinidine levels in an elderly man attributed to the concurrent use of intravenous erythromycin, and possibly a factor in an episode of torsade de pointes. Another isolated report describes the development of torsade de pointes arrhythmia in a very old man when given both drugs. See also 'Drugs that prolong the QT interval + Other drugs that prolong the QT interval', p.103.

Clinical evidence

A man of 74 with a history of cardiac disease (coronary artery disease, by-pass graft surgery, ventricular tachycardia) under treatment with quinidine sulphate 200 mg every 6 h and several other drugs (mexiletine, hydralazine, dipyridamole, aspirin and paracetamol (acetaminophen), was hospitalised with suspected implantable cardioverter defibrillator infection. Within two days of starting 500 mg **erythromycin lactobionate** six-hourly and 1 g **ceftriaxone** daily, both given intravenously, his trough serum quinidine levels had risen by about one-third (from about 2.8 to 4.2 mg/l). On day seven 500 mg **metronidazole** 8-hourly was added and the **erythromycin** dosage was doubled, and the patient experienced an episode of torsade de pointes. By day 12 his serum quinidine levels had further risen to 5.8 mg/l, whereupon the quinidine dosage was reduced by 25%. Because an interaction between quinidine and **erythromycin** had by then been suspected, the antibacterials were replaced by **doxycycline** and **ciprofloxacin**. By day 21 the quinidine serum levels had fallen to their former levels. The patient had a prolonged QTc interval on admission (504 ms), and this did not change.[1]

A man of 95 developed QT interval prolongation, torsade de pointes arrhythmia and subsequent cardiac arrest when given oral quinidine and **erythromycin**.[2]

Preliminary results of a randomised, placebo-controlled crossover study in 12 subjects found that when given a single 400-mg dose of quinidine after taking 500 mg **erythromycin** three times daily or a placebo for 5 days, the total QT_c AUC was significantly prolonged (about 6% from 10279 to 10878 ms.h) during the **erythromycin** phase.[3] In a parallel study by the same group, peak levels of quinidine were increased by 39% (from 587 to 816 ng/ml) and the AUC by 62% (from 326 to 528 mg.min/ml) by day 5 of the **erythromycin** phase. Peak levels of the main metabolite of quinidine, 3-hydroxyquinidine, were significantly reduced.[4] Another study in 6 healthy subjects found that **erythromycin** 250 mg four times daily for 6 days reduced the total clearance of a single dose of quinidine sulphate 200 mg by 34% and increased its maximum serum concentration by 39%.[5]

Mechanism

Not fully understood, but erythromycin inhibits the metabolism of the quinidine,[4] possibly by inhibition of cytochrome P450 isoenzyme CYP3A4[5] thereby reducing its clearance from the body and increasing its effects. There are also a number of cases on record of prolongation of the QT interval and torsade de pointes associated with the use of intravenous erythromycin alone.[6] Therefore, quinidine and erythromycin may have additive effects on the QT interval in addition to the pharmacokinetic interaction.

1. Damkier P, Hansen LL, Brøsen K. Effect of diclofenac, disulfiram, itraconazole, grapefruit juice and erythromycin on the pharmacokinetics of quinidine. *Br J Clin Pharmacol* (1999) 48, 829–38.

Importance and management

Information about this interaction appears to be limited to these reports, but it would appear to be established. If erythromycin is essential in a patient taking quinidine, the effects of concurrent use should be well monitored, being alert for the development of raised plasma quinidine levels and prolongation of the QT interval (see also 'Drugs that prolong the QT interval + Other drugs that prolong the QT interval', p.103). There seems to be nothing documented about any other quinidine/macrolide antibacterial interactions.

1. Spinler SA, Cheng JWM, Kindwall KE, Charland SL. Possible inhibition of hepatic metabolism of quinidine by erythromycin. *Clin Pharmacol Ther* (1995) 57, 89–94.
2. Lin JC, Quasny HA. QT prolongation and development of torsades de pointes with the concomitant administration of oral erythromycin base and quinidine. *Pharmacotherapy* (1997) 17, 626–30.
3. Stanford RH, Geraets DR, Lee H-C, Min DI. Effect of oral erythromycin on quinidine pharmacodynamics in healthy volunteers. *Pharmacotherapy* (1997) 17, 1111.
4. Stanford RH, Park JM, Geraets Dr, Min DI, Lee H-C. Effect of oral erythromycin on quinidine pharmacokinetics in healthy volunteers. *Pharmacotherapy* (1998) 18, 426–7.
5. Damkier P, Hansen LL, Brøsen K. Effect of diclofenac, disulfiram, itraconazole, grapefruit juice and erythromycin on the pharmacokinetics of quinidine. *Br J Clin Pharmacol* (1999) 48, 829–38.
6. Gitler B, Berger LS, Buffa SD. Torsades de pointes induced by erythromycin. *Chest* (1994) 105, 368–72.

Quinidine + Fluvoxamine

Fluvoxamine appears to inhibit the metabolism and clearance of quinidine.

Clinical evidence, mechanism, importance and management

Six healthy subjects were given a single dose of quinidine sulphate 250 mg before and on day 5 of a 6-day course of **fluvoxamine** 100 mg daily.[1] The total apparent oral clearance of quinidine was reduced by 29%, and *N*-oxidation and 3-hydroxylation were reduced by 33 and 44% respectively. Renal clearance and elimination half-life were unchanged. It was concluded that **fluvoxamine** inhibited the metabolism of quinidine by cytochrome P450 isoenzyme CYP3A4 although a role for CYP1A2 and CYP2C19 was not excluded. The clinical relevance of these findings is unclear. However, it would seem prudent to monitor the concurrent use of quinidine with **fluvoxamine**. More study is needed to assess the effect of multiple dosing and to establish the clinical significance of this interaction.

1. Damkier P, Hansen LL, Brøsen K. Effect of fluvoxamine on the pharmacokinetics of quinidine. *Eur J Clin Pharmacol* (1999) 55, 451–6.

Quinidine + Grapefruit juice

Grapefruit juice delays the absorption of quinidine and reduces its metabolism to some extent, but no clinically relevant adverse interaction seems to occur.

Clinical evidence, mechanism, importance and management

In one study, 12 normal subjects were given 400 mg quinidine sulphate orally on two occasions, once with 240 ml water and once with **grapefruit juice**. The pharmacokinetics of the quinidine were unchanged, except that its absorption was delayed (the time to reach maximum plasma concentrations was doubled from 1.6 to 3.3 h), for reasons that are not understood. The AUC of its metabolite (3-hydroxyquinidine) was decreased by one-third, suggesting that the **grapefruit juice** inhibits the metabolism of the quinidine by CYP3A4.[1] No important changes in the QTc interval were seen.[1] Similarly, another study in 6 normal subjects found the total clearance of a single 200-mg dose of quinidine sulphate was reduced by 15% by 250 ml **grapefruit juice**, with no change in maximum level. There

was a small reduction in metabolite formation suggesting only minor inhibition of CYP3A4.[2] These studies suggest that it is not necessary for patients on quinidine to avoid **grapefruit juice**.

1. Min DI, Ku Y-M, Geraets DR, Lee H-c. Effect of grapefruit juice on the pharmacokinetics and pharmacodynamics of quinidine in healthy volunteers. *J Clin Pharmacol* (1996) 36, 469–76.
2. Damkier P, Hansen LL, Brøsen K. Effect of diclofenac, disulfiram, itraconazole, grapefruit juice and erythromycin on the pharmacokinetics of quinidine. *Br J Clin Pharmacol* (1999) 48, 829–38.

Quinidine + Itraconazole

Itraconazole increases the plasma levels of quinidine.

Clinical evidence

In a double-blind, randomised, two-phase crossover study, 9 normal subjects were given a single 100-mg dose of quinidine sulphate on day 4 of a four-day course of either 200 mg **itraconazole** or a placebo. The **itraconazole** caused a 1.6-fold increase in the peak plasma quinidine levels, a 2.4-fold increase in its AUC and a 1.6-fold increase in its elimination half-life and a 50% decrease in its renal clearance.[1] Similarly, another study in 6 healthy subjects found that **itraconazole** 100 mg daily for 6 days reduced the total clearance of a single dose of quinidine sulphate 200 mg by 61%, increased its elimination half-life by 35%, and decreased its renal clearance by 60%.[2]

Mechanism

The most likely explanation is that the itraconazole not only inhibits the metabolism of the quinidine by cytochrome P450 isoenzyme CYP3A4 in the gut wall and liver, but possibly also inhibits the active secretion of quinidine by the kidney tubules.[1,2]

Importance and management

Direct information appears to be limited to these studies, but the evidence suggests that this interaction is clinically important. What happens is consistent with the way itraconazole interacts with other drugs. If larger doses of itraconazole were to be used and for longer periods, it seems likely that the effects would be even greater. The concurrent use of these drugs should therefore be well monitored and the dosage of quinidine reduced accordingly. More study is needed.

1. Kaukonen K-M, Olkkola KT, Neuvonen PJ. Itraconazole increases plasma concentrations of quinidine. *Clin Pharmacol Ther* (1997) 62, 510–17.
2. Damkier P, Hansen LL, Brøsen K. Effect of diclofenac, disulfiram, itraconazole, grapefruit juice and erythromycin on the pharmacokinetics of quinidine. *Br J Clin Pharmacol* (1999) 48, 829–38.

Quinidine + Kaolin-pectin

There is some evidence that kaolin-pectin can reduce the absorption of quinidine and lower its serum levels.

Clinical evidence, mechanism, importance and management

When given with 30 ml of *Kaopectate* (kaolin-pectin), the maximal salivary quinidine concentration after a single 100 mg oral dose was reduced in 4 normal subjects by 54% and the AUC by 58%, without any effect on absorption rate.[1] There is a correlation between salivary and serum concentrations after a single (but not repeated) doses of quinidine.[2] This is consistent with *in vitro* data showing quinidine is adsorbed onto **kaolin**,[3] **pectin**,[3] and **kaolin-pectin**.[1] More study is needed to confirm these two studies, but be alert for the need to increase the quinidine dosage if **kaolin-pectin** is used concurrently.

1. Moustafa MA, Al-Shora HI, Gaber M, Gouda MW. Decreased bioavailability of quinidine sulphate due to interactions with adsorbent antacids and antidiarrhoeal mixtures. *Int J Pharmaceutics* (1987) 34, 207–11.

2. Narang PK, Carliner NH, Fisher ML, Crouthamel WG. Quinidine saliva concentrations: absence of correlation with serum concentrations at steady state. *Clin Pharmacol Ther* (1983) 34, 695–702.
3. Bucci AJ, Myre SA, Tan HSI, Shenouda LS. In vitro interaction of quinidine with kaolin and pectin. *J Pharm Sci* (1981) 70, 999–1002.

Quinidine + Ketoconazole

An isolated report describes a marked increase in plasma quinidine levels in man when additionally treated with keto-conazole.

Clinical evidence, mechanism, importance and management

An elderly man with chronic atrial fibrillation, treated with 300 mg quinidine sulphate four times daily, was additionally given 200 mg **ketoconazole** daily for candidal oesophagitis. Within 7 days his plasma quinidine levels had risen from a range of 1.4–2.7 mg/l to 6.9 mg/l (normal range 2 to 5 mg/l) but he showed no evidence of toxicity. The elimination half-life of quinidine was found to be 25 h (normal values in healthy subjects 6 to 7 h). The quinidine dosage was reduced to 200 mg twice daily, but it needed to be increased to the former dose by the end of a month. The reasons for this reaction are not understood, but may be due to inhibition of metabolic enzyme activity by ketoconazole.[1] This is an isolated case so that its general importance is uncertain, but it draws attention to the need to monitor plasma quinidine levels patients taking **ketoconazole**. Further study is needed. See also 'Quinidine + Itraconazole', p.124.

1. McNulty RM, Lazor JA, Sketch M. Transient increase in plasma quinidine concentrations during ketoconazole-quinidine therapy. *Clin Pharm* (1989) 8, 222–5.

Quinidine + Laxatives

Quinidine plasma levels can be reduced by the concurrent use of the anthraquinone laxative senna.

Clinical evidence, mechanism, importance and management

A study in 7 patients with heart arrhythmias taking 500 mg quinidine bisulphate 12-hourly showed that concurrent use of the anthraquinone laxative **senna** (*Liquedepur*) reduced plasma quinidine levels, measured 12 h after the last dose of quinidine, by about 25%.[1] This might be of clinical importance in patients whose plasma levels are barely adequate to control their arrhythmia.

1. Guckenbiehl W, Gilfrich HJ, Just H. Einfluß von Laxantien und Metoclopramid auf die Chindin-Plasmakonzentration während Langzeittherapie bei Patienten mit Herzrhythmusstörugen. *Med Welt* (1976) 27, 1273–6.

Quinidine + Lidocaine (Lignocaine)

A single case report describes a man on quinidine who had sinoatrial arrest when he was given lidocaine (lignocaine).

Clinical evidence, mechanism, importance and management

A man with Parkinson's disease was given 300 mg quinidine six-hourly for the control of ventricular ectopic beats. After receiving 600 mg he was given **lidocaine (lignocaine)** as well, initially a bolus of 80 mg, followed by an infusion of 4 mg/min because persistent premature ventricular beats developed. Within 2.5 h the patient complained of dizziness and weakness, and was found to have sinus bradycardia, SA arrest and atrioventricular escape rhythm. Normal sinus rhythm resumed when the **lidocaine (lignocaine)** was stopped. Whether quinidine was a contributing factor in this reaction is uncer-

tain.[1] However, this case emphasises the need to exercise caution when giving two drugs that have depressant actions on the heart.

1. Jeresaty RM, Kahn AH, Landry AB. Sinoatrial arrest due to lidocaine in a patient receiving quinidine. *Chest* (1972) 61, 683–5.

Quinidine + *Lomotil* (Co-phenotrope; Atropine sulphate/Diphenoxylate)

Lomotil slightly reduced the rate, but not extent, of absorption of single doses of quinidine.

Clinical evidence, mechanism, importance and management

In one study,[1] 8 normal subjects were given a single 300 mg-dose of quinidine sulphate alone and after taking two tablets of *Lomotil* (0.025 mg **atropine sulphate**, 2.5 mg **diphenoxylate; co-pheno-prope**) at midnight on the evening before and another two tablets the next morning an hour before the quinidine. It was found that the maximum plasma quinidine levels were reduced 21% (from 2.10 to 1.65 micrograms/ml) by the *Lomotil*, the time to maximum level was prolonged from 0.89 to 1.21 h, and there was a slight increase in elimination half-life (5.7 to 6.8 h). While these results were statistically significant, the changes were relatively small and it seems doubtful if they are clinically relevant, particularly as the extent of absorption (AUC) was unchanged. However it needs to be emphasised that because the quinidine formulation used was an immediate-release preparation, these results may not necessarily apply to sustained-release preparations, and also may not apply if multiple doses of quinidine are used. More study is needed.

1. Ponzillo JJ, Scavone JM, Paone RP, Lewis GP, Rayment CM, Fitzsimmons WE. Effect of diphenoxylate with atropine sulfate on the bioavailability of quinidine sulfate in healthy subjects. *Clin Pharm* (1988) 7, 139–42.

Quinidine + Metoclopramide

Metoclopramide slightly reduced the absorption of quinidine from a sustained-release formulation in one study, but increased quinidine levels in another.

Clinical evidence

A study of this interaction was prompted by the case of a patient on sustained-release quinidine (*Quinidex*) whose arrhythmia failed to be controlled when **metoclopramide** was added. Nine normal subjects were given either 10 mg **metoclopramide** six-hourly for 24 h before, and 48 h after, a single oral dose of 600 mg or 900 mg quinidine sulphate or quinidine alone, then were crossed over to receive the other treatment. It was found that the **metoclopramide** caused a mean decrease in the quinidine absorption (AUC) of 10%, although two subjects had decreases of 22.5 and 28.1%. The elimination rate constant was unaffected.[1] Another study in patients taking a sustained-release formulation of 500 mg quinidine bisulphate 12-hourly found that 10 mg **metoclopramide** three times daily increased the mean plasma levels measured 3.5 h after the last dose of quinidine by almost 20% (from 1.6 to 1.9 micrograms/ml) and at 12 h by about 16% (from 2.4 to 2.8 micrograms/ml).[2]

Mechanism

Not understood. Metoclopramide alters both the gastric emptying time and gastrointestinal motility which can affect absorption.

Importance and management

Direct information seems to be limited to these studies using different quinidine preparations. Since the outcome of concurrent use is uncertain, the effects should be well monitored. More study is needed.

1. Yuen GJ, Hansten PD, Collins J. Effect of metoclopramide on the absorption of an oral sustained-release quinidine product. *Clin Pharm* (1987) 6, 722–5.
2. Guckenbiehl W, Gilfrich HJ, Just H. Einfluß von Laxantien und Metoclopramid auf die Chindin-Plasmakonzentration während Langzeittherapie bei Patienten mit Herzrhythmusstörugen. *Med Welt* (1976) 27, 1273–6.

Quinidine + Quinolone antibacterials

Ciprofloxacin normally appears not to interact with quinidine to a clinically relevant extent.

Clinical evidence, mechanism, importance and management

The pharmacokinetics of a single 400 mg oral dose of quinidine sulphate and the ECG parameters measured (QRS and QTc prolongation) were not significantly changed in 7 normal subjects after taking 750 mg **ciprofloxacin** daily for 6 days. The mean decrease in clearance was 1%, with a range from –10% to +20%, which is unlikely to be clinically relevant.[1] However an isolated case report describes a woman who was started on quinidine gluconate 324 mg eight-hourly while she was taking **ciprofloxacin** and metronidazole. Her first trough serum quinidine levels was raised a little above normal (6.3 micrograms/ml compared with the normal range of 2 to 5 micrograms/ml) without evidence of toxicity. Quinidine therapy was continued unchanged, and her next trough serum quinidine level was only 2.3 micrograms/ml, 3 days after finishing the course of antibacterials. This was tentatively attributed to the possible enzyme inhibitory effects of **ciprofloxacin** and metronidazole. This case is far from clear so that no firm conclusions can be reached.[2] There would seem to be little reason for avoiding concurrent use. There seems to be no information as yet about the effects of other quinolone antibacterials.

1. Bleske BE, Carver PL, Annesley TM, Bleske JRM, Morady F. The effect of ciprofloxacin on the pharmacokinetic and ECG parameters of quinidine. *J Clin Pharmacol* (1990) 30, 911–15.
2. Cooke CE, Sklar GE, Nappi JM. Possible pharmacokinetic interaction with quinidine: ciprofloxacin or metronidazole? *Ann Pharmacother* (1996) 30, 364–6.

Quinidine + Rifampicin (Rifampin)

The serum levels of quinidine and its therapeutic effects can be markedly reduced by the concurrent use of rifampicin.

Clinical evidence

It was noted that the control of ventricular dysrhythmia deteriorated in a patient on quinidine sulphate 800 mg daily within a week of starting to take **rifampicin** 600 mg daily. His serum quinidine level fell from 4 to 0.5 micrograms/ml, and remained low despite increasing the quinidine dose to 1600 mg daily. The rifampicin was discontinued, and quinidine levels gradually increased over a week. Some signs of quinidine toxicity then occurred, and the quinidine dose was reduced back to 800 mg daily.[1] Further study in 4 normal subjects showed that treatment with 600 mg **rifampicin** daily for 7 days reduced the mean half-life of a single 6 mg/kg oral dose of quinidine sulphate by about 62% (from 6.1 to 2.3 h) and the AUC by 83%.[2,3] Similar findings were reported in 4 other subjects receiving the same dose of quinidine intravenously.[3]

Another case report describes a patient who failed to achieve adequate serum quinidine levels despite large daily doses of quinidine (3200 mg) while taking **rifampicin**. When the **rifampicin** was stopped, ultimately, a reduced quinidine dosage of 1800 mg daily achieved a serum level of 2 micrograms/ml (reflecting a 44% decrease in dose and a 43% increase in level).[4] In a further case, a 'double interaction' was seen in a patient on quinidine and digoxin when given **rifampicin**: the quinidine levels fell, resulting in a fall in digoxin levels.[5,6]

Mechanism

Rifampicin is a potent enzyme-inducing agent which increases the metabolism of the quinidine by the liver three to fourfold, thereby increasing its loss from the body and reducing its effects. It has been suggested that two of the quinidine metabolites (3-hydroxquinidine and 2-oxoquinidinone) may be active, which might, to some extent, offset the effects of this interaction.[5,6]

Importance and management

An established and clinically important interaction, although documentation is limited. The dosage of quinidine will need to be increased if rifampicin is given concurrently. Monitor the serum levels. Doubling the dose may not be enough.[3,5] An equivalent dosage reduction will be needed if the rifampicin is stopped.

1. Ahmad D, Mathur P, Ahuja S, Henderson R, Carruthers G. Rifampicin-quinidine interaction. *Br J Dis Chest* (1979) 73, 409–11.
2. Twum-Barima Y, Carruthers SG. Evaluation of rifampin-quinidine interaction. *Clin Pharmacol Ther* (1980) 27, 290.
3. Twum-Barima Y, Carruthers SG. Quinidine-rifampin interaction. *N Engl J Med* (1981) 304, 1466–9.
4. Schwartz A, Brown JR. Quinidine-rifampin interaction. *Am Heart J* (1984) 107, 789–90.
5. Bussey HI, Merritt GJ, Hill EG. The influence of rifampin on quinidine and digoxin. *Arch Intern Med* (1984) 144, 1021–3.
6. Bussey HI, Farringer J, Merritt GJ. Influence of rifampin (R) on quinidine (Q) and digoxin (D). *Drug Intell Clin Pharm* (1983) 17, 436.

Quinidine + Sucralfate

An isolated report describes a marked reduction in serum quinidine levels in a patient attributed to the concurrent use of sucralfate.

Clinical evidence, mechanism, importance and management

An elderly woman on multiple therapy which included warfarin, digoxin and sustained-release quinidine developed subtherapeutic levels of all three while taking **sucralfate**, even when the dosages were separated from the **sucralfate** by 2 h. When the sucralfate was stopped her serum quinidine levels rapidly climbed from 0.31 to 5.55 micromol/l.[1] The suggestion is that the **sucralfate** can bind with quinidine within the gut. The general importance of this interaction is uncertain, but be alert for any evidence of reduced effects if both drugs are given.

1. Rey AM, Gums JG. Altered absorption of digoxin, sustained-release quinidine, and warfarin with sucralfate administration. *DICP Ann Pharmacother* (1991) 25, 745–6

Tocainide + Antacids or Urinary alkalinizers

Raising the pH of the urine (e.g. with concurrent use of some antacids, diuretics or alkaline salts) can modestly reduce the loss of tocainide from the body.

Clinical evidence

Preliminary findings of a study showed that when 5 normal subjects took 30 ml of an **un-named antacid** four times a day for 48 h before and 58 h after a single 600-mg dose of tocainide, the urinary pH rose (from 5.9 to 6.9), the total clearance fell by 28%, the peak serum levels fell by 19% (from 4.2 to 3.4 micrograms/ml), the AUC rose by 33% and the half-life was prolonged from 13.2 to 15.4 h.[1]

Mechanism

Tocainide is a weak base so that its loss in the urine will be affected by the pH of the urine. Alkalinization of the urine increases the number of un-ionised molecules available for passive reabsorption, thereby reducing the urinary loss and raising the serum levels.

Importance and management

An established interaction of uncertain but probably limited clinical importance. There seem to be no reports of adverse reactions in patients as a result of this interaction, but be alert for any evidence of increased tocainide effects if other drugs are given that can raise the urinary pH significantly (e.g. **sodium bicarbonate** and **acetazolamide**). Reduce the tocainide dosage if necessary. Of the antacids, *Maalox* (magnesium and aluminium hydroxide) can raise urinary pH by about 0.9 whereas *Milk of magnesia* (**magnesium hydroxide**) and *Titralac* (**calcium carbonate-glycine**) in normal doses raise the pH by about 0.5.[2] *Amphogel* (**aluminium hydroxide**) and *Robalate* (**dihydroxyaluminium glycinate**) are reported to have no effect on urinary pH.[2] More study is needed.

1. Meneilly GP, Scavone JM, Meneilly GS, Wei JY. Tocainide: pharmacokinetic alterations during antacid-induced urinary alkalinization. *Clin Pharmacol Ther* (1987) 41, 178.
2. Gibaldi M, Grundhofer B, Levy G. Effect of antacids on pH of urine. *Clin Pharmacol Ther* (1974) 16, 520–5.

Tocainide + Cimetidine or Ranitidine

There is some evidence that cimetidine can reduce the bioavailability and serum levels of tocainide but ranitidine appears not to interact.

Clinical evidence, mechanism, importance and management

In a preliminary report of a study, four days treatment with **cimetidine** (dose not stated) in 11 healthy subjects had a small effect on the pharmacokinetics of 500 mg tocainide given intravenously over 15 min (half-life increased, clearance decreased), which was not considered clinically important.[1] In another study, 1200 mg **cimetidine** daily for two days reduced the AUC of a single 400 mg oral dose of tocainide in 7 normal subjects by about one-third (from 31.6 to 23.1 micrograms.h/ml). The peak serum levels were also reduced, from 2.81 to 1.7 micrograms/ml, but no changes in the half-life or renal clearance occurred.[2,3] The reasons for this, and its clinical impor-

tance are uncertain, but be alert for evidence of a reduced response to tocainide in the presence of **cimetidine**. **Ranitidine** 150 mg twice daily was found not to interact.[2,3]

1. Price BA, Holmes GI, Antonello J, Yeh KC, Demetriades J, Irvin JD, McMahon FG. Intravenous tocainide (T) maintains safe therapeutic levels when administered concomitantly with cimetidine (C). *Clin Pharmacol Ther* (1987), 41, 237.
2. Lalonde RL, North DS, Mattern AL, Kapil RP. Tocainide pharmacokinetics after H-2 antagonists. *Clin Pharmacol Ther* (1987) 41, 241.
3. North DS, Mattern AL, Kapil RP, Lalonde RL. The effect of histamine-2 receptor antagonists on tocainide pharmacokinetics. *J Clin Pharmacol* (1988) 28, 640–3.

Tocainide + Rifampicin (Rifampin)

The loss of tocainide from the body is increased by the concurrent use of rifampicin.

Clinical evidence

The AUC of a single 600 mg oral dose of tocainide was reduced by almost 30% (from 76.8 to 55 mg.h/l) and the half-life was also reduced about 30% (from 13.2 to 9.4 h) in 8 normal subjects given 300 mg **rifampicin** twice daily for five days.[1]

Mechanism

This response is consistent with the well-recognised enzyme inducing effects of rifampicin which increase the metabolism of drugs by the liver, thereby increasing their loss from the body and reducing their serum levels.

Importance and management

Information is limited to this single dose study in normal subjects but the interaction would seem to be established and may be of clinical importance. Monitor any patients given rifampicin for evidence of reduced tocainide serum levels and reduced effects. Increase the dosage as necessary. Reduce the tocainide dosage if the rifampicin is withdrawn. More study is needed.

1. Rice TL, Patterson JH, Celestin C, Foster JR, Powell JR. Influence of rifampin on tocainide pharmacokinetics in humans. *Clin Pharm* (1989) 8, 200–205.

5

Antibacterial and anti-infective agent drug interactions

"Most physicians . . . have the vague feeling that if one antimicrobial drug is good, two should be better, and three should cure almost everybody of almost every ailment."

This 'vague feeling' has proved to be valid in a number of instances, but there is also good evidence that sometimes the very opposite is true. This situation has fuelled a keen debate about the desirability of combining antimicrobial agents, which has gone on for many years. Various schemes have been published that try to provide a logical framework for predicting the likely outcome. One of the serious difficulties is the often poor correlation between *in vitro* and *in vivo* studies, so that it is difficult to get a thoroughly reliable indication of how antimicrobial agents will behave together in clinical practice. Some of the monographs in this chapter illustrate these difficulties very clearly.

Some of the arguments in favour of combining antimicrobial agents are as follows. Where the infections are acute and undiagnosed the presence of more than one drug increases the chance that at least one effective antimicrobial is present. This may be especially important if the patient is infected by more than one organism. The possibility of the emergence of resistant organisms is decreased by the use of more than one drug, and in some cases two drugs acting at different sites may be more effective than one drug alone. It may also be that two drugs administered below their toxic thresholds may be as ef-

fective and less toxic than one drug at a higher concentration.

In contrast there are other arguments against using antimicrobials together. One serious objection is that two drugs may actually be less effective than one on its own. In theory this could arise if a bactericidal drug, which requires actively dividing cells for it to be effective, were used with a bacteriostatic drug. However in practice this seems to be less important than might be supposed and there are relatively few well-authenticated clinical examples. Another objection is that some broad-spectrum drugs may be sub-optimal for particular organisms and may inadequately control the infection. Toxic side-effects may possibly also be increased by the use of more than one drug.

An indiscriminate and 'blunderbuss' approach to the treatment of infections is no longer in favour. The general consensus of informed opinion is that the advantages of combined antimicrobial treatment are balanced by a number of clear disadvantages, and that usually one drug alone, properly chosen, is likely to be equally effective in most cases.

Some of the monographs in this chapter are concerned with the adverse effects of combining antimicrobials together but most of them deal with the interactions caused by other agents. Some other interactions with antimicrobials are dealt with in other chapters. A complete listing is to be found in the Index.

Table 5.1 Anti-infectives

Aminoglycosides	Amikacin, Dibekacin, Dihydrostreptomycin, Framycetin, Gentamicin, Kanamycin, Neomycin, Netilmicin, Paromomycin, Ribostamycin, Sisomicin, Streptomycin, Tobramycin
Anthelmintics	Albendazole, Diethylcarbamazine, Ivermectin, Levamisole, Mebendazole, Metrifonate (Metriphonate), Niclosamide, Piperazine, Praziquantel, Pyrantel, Tiabendazole (Thiabendazole), Tetrachlorethylene
Antifungals	Amphotericin B, Amorolfine, Clotrimazole, Econazole, Fenticonazole, Fluconazole, Flucytosine, Griseofulvin, Isoconazole, Itraconazole, Ketoconazole, Miconazole, Nystatin, Terbinafine, Tinidazole, Tioconazole
Antimalarials	Chloroquine, Halofantrine, Hydroxychloroquine, Mefloquine, Mepacrine, Pamaquine, Primaquine, Proguanil, Pyrimethamine, Quinine, Sulfadoxine
Antiprotozoals	Diloxanide furoate, Metronidazole, Tinidazole
Antituberculars and Antileprotics	Aminosalicylic acid (PAS), Capreomycin, Clofazimine, Cycloserine, Dapsone, Ethambutol, Ethionamide, Isoniazid, Prothionamide, Pyrazinamide, Rifabutin, Rifampicin (Rifampin), Rifapentine
Cephalosporins	Cefacetrile (Cephacetrile), Cefaclor, Cefadroxil, Cefalexin (Cephalexin), Cefaloglycin, Cefaloridine (Cephaloridine), Cefalotin (Cephalothin), Cefamandole (Cephamandole), Cefapirin, Cefazaflur, Cefazedone, Cefazolin (Cephazolin), Cefdinir, Cefditoren pivoxil, Cefepime, Cefetamet pivoxil, Cefixime, Cefmenoxime, Cefmetazole, Cefodizime, Cefonicid, Cefoperazone, Ceforanide, Cefotaxime, Cefotetan, Cefotiam, Cefoxitin, Cefpirome, Cefpodoxime, Cefpiramide, Cefprozil, Cefradine (Cephradine), Cefsulodin, Ceftazidime, Ceftibuten, Ceftizoxime, Ceftriaxone, Cefuroxime, Latamoxef (Moxalactam)
Macrolides	Azithromycin, Clarithromycin, Erythromycin, Josamycin, Midecamycin, Roxithromycin, Spiramycin, Troleandomycin (Triacetyloleandomycin)
Penicillins	Amoxicillin (Amoxycillin), Ampicillin, Azlocillin, Bacampicillin, Benzylpenicillin (Penicillin G), Carbenicillin, Ciclacillin, Cloxacillin, Dicloxacillin, Flucloxacillin, Hetacillin, Methicillin, Mezlocillin, Nafcillin, Oxacillin, Phenethicillin, Phenoxymethylpenicillin (Penicillin V), Piperacillin, Pivampicillin, Procaine benzylpenicillin (Procaine penicillin), Temocillin, Ticarcillin
Polypeptides	Bacitracin, Colistimethate sodium, Colistin, Polymyxin B, Teicoplanin, Vancomycin
Quinolones	Amifloxacin, Ciprofloxacin, Cinoxacin, Enoxacin, Fleroxacin, Grepafloxacin, Hydroxyquinoline, Levofloxacin, Lomefloxacin, Nalidixic acid, Nitroxoline, Norfloxacin, Ofloxacin, Pefloxacin, Rufloxacin, Sparfloxacin, Temafloxacin, Tilbroquinol, Tiliquinol, Tosufloxacin, Trovafloxacin
Sulphonamides	Co-trimoxazole, Sulfadiazine (Sulphadiazine), Sulfadimethoxine, Sulfadimidine (Sulphadimidine) (-methazine, -dimerazine), Sulfafurazole (Sulphafurazole, Sulfisoxazole), Sulfalene (Sulfametopyrazine), Sulfamerazine, Sulfamethizole (Sulphamethizole), Sulfamethoxazole (Sulphamethoxazole), Sulfametoxypyridazine (Sulphamethoxypyridazine), Sulfaphenazole, Sulfathiazole (Sulphathiazole), Sulfisomidine (Sulphasomidine), Sulphapyridine
Tetracyclines	Chlortetracycline, Demeclocycline, Doxycycline, Lymecycline, Methacycline, Minocycline, Oxytetracycline, Rolitetracycline, Tetracycline
Miscellaneous	Atovaquone, Aztreonam, Biapenem, Cilastatin, Chloramphenicol, Clindamycin, Clioquinol, Fosfomycin, Furazolidone, Fusidic acid, Imipenem, Mepacrine (Quinacrine), Meropenem, Methenamine (Hexamine), Mupirocin, Nitrofurantoin, Novobiocin, Pentamidine, Spectinomycin, Stibogluconate, Trimethoprim, Trimetrexate

Table 5.2 Antivirals

Anti-herpes etc.	Aciclovir, Amantadine, Famciclovir, Inosine pranobex, Penciclovir, Rimantadine, Valaciclovir
Interferons	Interferon alpha
NNRTIs	Atevirdine, Delavirdine, Efavirenz, Nevirapine
NRTIs	Didanosine, Lamivudine, Stavudine, Zalcitabine, Zidovudine
Protease inhibitors	Indinavir, Nelfinavir, Ritonavir, Saquinavir
Miscellaneous	Cidofovir, Cycloserine, Foscarnet sodium, Ganciclovir, Ribavirin (Tribavirin), Vidarabine

NNRTIs = non-nucleoside reverse transcriptase inhibitors; NRTIs = nucleoside reverse transcriptase inhibitors.

Aciclovir or Valaciclovir + Cimetidine or Probenecid

Single dose studies have found that cimetidine and probenecid increase the bioavailability of aciclovir but this is thought unlikely to be of clinical importance.

Clinical evidence

Twelve healthy subjects were given 1 g **valaciclovir** alone, with cimetidine (800 mg taken 8 h and 1 h before), **probenecid** (1 g taken 2 h before), or both. The AUCs for the prodrug **valaciclovir** (after 3 hours) were increased 83% by **cimetidine**, 22% by **probenecid** and 196% by both together. The AUCs for the active metabolite **aciclovir** (after 24 hours) were increased 27% by **cimetidine**, 46% by **probenecid**, and 73% by both together. The urinary recovery of **aciclovir** was unchanged.[1] An earlier study had found a similar (40%) increase in the AUC of **aciclovir** caused by 1 g **probenecid**.[2]

Mechanism

The authors of the main study suggest that the increase in aciclovir AUCs is entirely attributable to a reduction in its renal excretion, probably due to competition for secretion by the kidney tubules.[1] This proposal seems confirmed by a later specific study of valaciclovir/aciclovir renal clearance.[3] It seems that, in addition to glomerular filtration, three secretory pathways are involved, an anionic pathway inhibited by cimetidine, a cationic pathway inhibited by probenecid and another as yet to be identified.[3]

Importance and management

These interactions are established but, despite the increased aciclovir AUCs with both cimetidine and probenecid, the authors of the main study suggest that they are probably clinically unimportant because aciclovir has such a wide therapeutic index.[1] It seems likely that no changes in the dosages of aciclovir or valaciclovir will be needed in patients also taking either cimetidine or probenecid.

1. Rolan PE, Maillot F, On NT, Posner J. The effects of cimetidine and probenecid on the conversion of a valine ester of acyclovir, 256U, to acyclovir and acyclovir renal clearance in healthy volunteers. *Br J Clin Pharmacol* (1993) 35, 533P.

2. Laskin OL, de Miranda P, King DH, Page DA, Longstreth JA, Rocco L, Lietman PS. Effects of probenecid on the pharmacokinetics and elimination of acyclovir in humans. *Antimicrob Agents Chemother* (1982) 21, 804–7.

3. De Bony F, Bidault R, Tod M, On N, Rolan P. Interaction of cimetidine and probenecid with valaciclovir and its metabolite acyclovir. *Intersci Conf Antimicrob Agents Chemother* (1996) 36, 6.

Aciclovir + Mycophenolate Mofetil

Aciclovir and mycophenolate mofetil appear not to interact together to a clinically relevant extent.

Clinical evidence, mechanism, importance and management

Normal subjects were given single doses of 800 mg oral aciclovir or 1 g **mycophenolate mofetil** or both drugs together in a three-period crossover study. The pharmacokinetics of both drugs were either minimally altered or unchanged by concurrent use, and it was concluded that any changes were unlikely to be clinically significant.[1]

1. Shah J, Juan D, Bullingham R, Wong B, Wong R, Fu C. A single dose drug interaction study of mycophenolate mofetil and acyclovir in normal subjects. *J Clin Pharmacol* (1994) 34, 1029.

Aminoglycosides + Amphotericin B

Nephrotoxicity attributed to the concurrent use of gentamicin and amphotericin has been described in four patients.

Clinical evidence, mechanism, importance and management

Four patients given moderate doses of **gentamicin** showed renal deterioration when additionally given **amphotericin**. Both drugs in sufficiently high doses are known to be nephrotoxic and it is suggested, on the basis of what was seen, that low doses of each may have additive nephrotoxic effects.[1] The documentation seems to be limited to this report. Until more is known it would be prudent to monitor renal function carefully if these two drugs are used.

1. Churchill DN, Seely J. Nephrotoxicity associated with combined gentamicin-amphotericin B therapy. *Nephron* (1977) 19, 176–181.

Aminoglycosides + Calcium channel blockers

Verapamil appears to protect the kidney from damage caused by gentamicin.

Clinical evidence, mechanism, importance and management

A comparative study was conducted in 9 healthy subjects who were given **gentamicin** alone (2 mg/kg loading dose, followed by 8-hourly doses to achieve a peak concentration of 5.5 mg/l and a trough concentration of 0.5 mg/l), and in 6 other subjects who were given **gentamicin** with 180 mg **verapamil** SR twice daily. The gentamicin AUCs of the two groups were virtually the same but the 24-h urinary excretion of alanine aminopeptidase (AAP) was 18% less in the group given **verapamil**, the reduction in AAP excretion being particularly marked during the first 6 days.[1] The significance of urinary AAP is that this enzyme is found primarily in the brush border membranes of the proximal renal tubules, and its excretion is an early and sensitive marker of renal damage. Thus it seems that **verapamil** protects the kidneys from damage by **gentamicin**. Whether this means that **verapamil** should be used routinely to help to reduce gentamicin-induced nephrotoxicity awaits further investigation, but this study would certainly suggest that concurrent use need not be avoided. Information about other aminoglycosides and other calcium channel blockers seems to be lacking.

1. Kazierad DJ, Wojcik GJ, Nix DE, Goldfarb AL, Schentag JJ. The effect of verapamil on the nephrotoxic potential of gentamicin as measured by urinary enzyme excretion in healthy volunteers. *J Clin Pharmacol* (1995) 35, 196–201.

Aminoglycosides + Cephalosporins

The nephrotoxic effects of gentamicin and tobramycin can be increased by the concurrent use of cefalotin. This may possibly also occur with other aminoglycosides, but some cephalosporins (cited below) appear not to interact adversely.

Clinical evidence

A randomised double-blind trial in patients with sepsis showed the following incidence of definite nephrotoxicity: **gentamicin + cefalotin** 30.4% (7 of 23); **tobramycin + cefalotin** 20.8% (5 of 24); **gentamicin + methicillin** 10% (2 of 20); **tobramycin + methicillin** 4.3% (1 of 23).[1]

A very considerable number of studies and case reports confirm this increase in the incidence of nephrotoxicity when **gentamicin**[2-10] or **tobramycin**[11,12] are used with **cefalotin**. However the opposite conclusion has been reached by a few others.[13-15] Acute renal failure developed in a patient given **gentamicin** and **cefaloridine**.[16] **Cefuroxime**[17] and **cefotaxime**[18] are reported not to increase the nephrotoxic effects of **tobramycin**. No clinically important adverse interaction occurs if **ceftazidime** and **tobramycin**[19] or **cefepime** and **amikacin**[20] are used together. Hypokalaemia has also been described in patients taking **cytotoxic drugs** for leukaemia when they were given **gentamicin** and **cefalexin**.[21]

Mechanism

Uncertain. The nephrotoxic effects of gentamicin and tobramycin are well documented and it appears that these effects can be additive with cefalotin in some patients. Doses which are well tolerated separately can be nephrotoxic when given together.[9]

Importance and management

The gentamicin/cefalotin interaction is very well documented and potentially serious, but there is less information about tobramycin with cefalotin. The risk of nephrotoxicity is probably greatest if high doses are used in those with some existing renal impairment. Concurrent use is not totally contraindicated (see the report cited above[1]) but renal function should be very closely monitored and dosages kept to a minimum. One study suggests that short courses of treatment is sometimes justified.[10] The combination of gentamicin or tobramycin and cefalotin is probably best avoided in high risk patients wherever possible. Possible alternatives with a much reduced risk of nephrotoxicity are gentamicin or tobramycin with methicillin,[1] or tobramycin with cefuroxime,[17] cefotaxime[18] or ceftazidime,[19] or amikacin with cefepime.[20] Whether other aminoglycosides interact similarly is uncertain, but the possibility should be borne in mind.

1. Wade JC, Smith CR, Petty BG, Lipsky JJ, Conrad G, Ellner J, Lietman PS. Cephalothin plus an aminoglycoside is more nephrotoxic than methicillin plus an aminoglycoside. *Lancet* (1978) ii, 604–6.
2. Opitz A, Herrman I, von Harrath D, Schaefer K. Akute niereninsuffizienz nach Gentamycin-Cephalosporin-Kombinationstherapie. *Med Welt* (1971) 22, 434–8.
3. Plager JE. Association of renal injury with combined cephalothin-gentamicin therapy among patients severely ill with malignant disease. *Cancer* (1976) 37, 1937–43.
4. The EORTC International Antimicrobial Therapy Project Group. Three antibiotic regimens in the treatment of infection in febrile granulocytopenic patients with cancer. *J Infect Dis* (1978) 137, 14–29.
5. Kleinknecht D, Ganeval D, Droz D. Acute renal failure after high doses of gentamicin and cephalothin. *Lancet* (1973) i, 1129.
6. Bobrow SN, Jaffe E, Young RC. Anuria and acute tubular necrosis associated with gentamicin and cephalothin. *JAMA* (1972) 222, 1546–7.
7. Fillastre JP, Laumonier R, Humbert G, Dubois D, Metayer J, Delpech A, Leroy J, Robert M. Acute renal failure associated with combined gentamicin and cephalothin therapy. *BMJ* (1973) 2, 396–7.
8. Cabanillas F, Burgos RC, Rodríguez RC, Baldizón C. Nephrotoxicity of combined cephalothin-gentamicin regimen. *Arch Intern Med* (1975) 135, 850–52.
9. Tvedegaard E. Interaction between gentamicin and cephalothin as cause of acute renal failure. *Lancet* (1976) ii, 581.
10. Hansen MM, Kaaber K. Nephrotoxicity in combined cephalothin and gentamicin therapy. *Acta Med Scand* (1977) 201, 463–7.
11. Tobias JS, Whitehouse JM, Wrigley PFM. Severe renal dysfunction after tobramycin/cephalothin therapy. *Lancet* (1976) i, 425.
12. Klastersky J, Hensgens C, Debusscher L. Empiric therapy for cancer patients: comparative study of ticarcillin-tobramycin, ticarcillin-cephalothin, and cephalothin-tobramycin. *Antimicrob Agents Chemother* (1975) 7, 640–45.
13. Fanning WL, Gump D, Jick H. Gentamicin- and cephalothin-associated rises in blood urea nitrogen. *Antimicrob Agents Chemother* (1976) 10, 80–82.
14. Stille W, Arndt I. Argumente gegen eine Nephrotoxizität von cephalothin und gentamycin. *Med Welt* (1972) 23, 1601–1605.
15. Wellwood JM, Simpson PM, Tighe JR, Thompson AE. Evidence of gentamicin nephrotoxicity in patients with renal allografts. *BMJ* (1975) 3, 278–81.
16. Zazgornik J, Schmidt P, Lugscheider R, Kopsa H. Akutes Nierenversagen bei kombinierter Cephaloridin-Gentamicin-Therapie. *Wien Klin Wochenschr* (1973) 85, 839–41.
17. Trollfors B, Alestig K, Rödjer S, Sandberg T, Westin J. Renal function in patients treated with tobramycin-cefuroxime or tobramycin-penicillin G. *J Antimicrob Chemother* (1983) 12, 641–5.
18. Kuhlmann J, Seidel G, Richter E, Grötsch H. Tobramycin nephrotoxicity: failure of cefotaxime to potentiate injury in patient. *Naunyn Schmiedebergs Arch Pharmacol* (1981) 316 (Suppl), R80.
19. Aronoff GR, Brier RA, Sloan RS, Brier ME. Interactions of ceftazidime and tobramycin in patients with normal and impaired renal function. *Antimicrob Agents Chemother* (1990) 34, 1139–42.
20. Barbhaiya RH, Knupp CA, Pfeffer M, Pittman KA. Lack of pharmacokinetic interaction between cefepime and amikacin in humans. *Antimicrob Agents Chemother* (1992) 36, 1382–6.
21. Young GP, Sullivan J, Hurley A. Hypokalaemia due to gentamicin/cephalexin in leukaemia. *Lancet* (1973) ii, 855.

Aminoglycosides + Clindamycin or Lincomycin

Three cases of acute renal failure have been tentatively attributed to the concurrent use of gentamicin and clindamycin. Lincomycin does not affect the pharmacokinetics of gentamicin.

Clinical evidence, mechanism, importance and management

Three patients with normal renal function developed acute renal failure when they were concurrently treated with **gentamicin** (3.9 to 4.9 mg/kg/day for 13 to 18 days) and **clindamycin** (0.9 to 1.8 mg/kg/day for 13 to 18 days). They recovered within 3 to 5 days of discontinuing the antibacterials.[1] The reasons for the renal failure are not known. Until more is known it would be prudent to monitor renal function carefully if these antibacterials are used together. **Tobramycin** with **clindamycin** is reported not to be nephrotoxic.[2]

1. Butkus DE, de Torrente A, Terman DS. Renal failure following gentamicin in combination with clindamycin. Gentamicin nephrotoxicity. *Nephron* (1976) 17, 307–13.
2. Gillett P, Wise R, Melikian V, Falk R. Tobramycin/cephalothin nephrotoxicity. *Lancet* (1976) i, 547.

Aminoglycosides + Dimenhydrinate

The makers of dimenhydrinate (diphenhydramine teoclate) suggest that it may possibly undesirably mask the ototoxic effects of streptomycin and other aminoglycoside antibacterials.

Clinical evidence, mechanism, importance and management

Dimenhydrinate can block the dizziness, nausea and vomiting which can occur during treatment with **streptomycin**.[1,2] However, the makers of **dimenhydrinate**, have warned that "caution should be used when *Dramamine* (**dimenhydrinate**) is given in conjunction with certain antibacterials which may cause ototoxicity, since *Dramamine* is capable of masking ototoxic symptoms and an irreversible state may be reached."[3] There seems to be no direct clinical evidence to confirm this, but there would seem to be an obvious hazard in not taking enough notice of the warning signs of developing ototoxicity with streptomycin or any other aminoglycoside. It is not clear whether the same warning should be made with other antihistamines which can also be used for nausea and vomiting (e.g. buclizine, chlorcyclizine, cyclizine, cinnarizine, pheniramine, meclozine).

1. Titche LL and Nady A. Control of vestibular toxic effects of streptomycin by Dramamine. *Dis Chest* (1950) 18, 386.
2. Cohen AC and Glinsky GC. Hypersensitivity to streptomycin. *J Allergy* (1951) 22, 63.
3. Dramamine tablets. Searle. Product information leaflet, November 1984.

Aminoglycosides + Etacrynic acid

The concurrent use of aminoglycoside antibacterials and etacrynic acid should be avoided because their damaging actions on the ear can be additive. Intravenous administration and renal impairment are additional causative factors. Even sequential administration may not be safe.

Clinical evidence

Four patients with some renal impairment became permanently deaf after treatment with 1 to 1.5 g **kanamycin**, given intramuscularly, and 50 to 150 mg **etacrynic acid**. One patient also received streptomycin, whilst another also received oral neomycin. Deafness took between 30 mins and almost 2 weeks to develop. In some cases deafness developed despite the doses being given on separate days and in all cases it appeared irreversible.[1]

There are other reports describing temporary, partial or total permanent deafness in man as a result of giving **etacrynic acid** with **gentamicin**,[2] **kanamycin**,[1-4] **streptomycin**,[1,3,5] or **neomycin**.[1,3,6] This interaction has been very extensively demonstrated in *animals*.

Mechanism

Both the aminoglycosides and etacrynic acid given singly can damage the ear and cause deafness, the site of action of the aminoglycosides being the hair cell and that of etacrynic acid the stria vascularis. *Animal* studies have shown that neomycin can cause a fivefold increase in the concentration of etacrynate in cochlear tissues, and it is possible that the aminoglycoside has some effect on the tissues which allows the etacrynic acid to penetrate more easily.[7] Similar results have been found with gentamicin.[8]

Importance and management

A well-established and well-documented interaction. The concurrent or sequential use of etacrynic acid with gentamicin, kanamycin, neomycin or streptomycin should be avoided because permanent deafness may result. Patients with renal impairment seem to be particularly at risk, most likely because the drugs are less rapidly cleared. Most of the reports describe deafness after intravenous administration but it has also been seen when etacrynic acid is given orally. If it is deemed absolutely necessary to use both drugs, minimal doses should be used and the effects on hearing should be monitored continuously.

Not every aminoglycoside has been implicated, but their ototoxicity is clearly established and they may be expected to interact in a similar way. For this reason the same precautions should be used.

1. Johnson AH, Hamilton CH. Kanamycin ototoxicity — possible potentiation by other drugs. *South Med J* (1970) 63, 511–13.
2. Meriwether WD, Mangi RJ, Serpick AA. Deafness following standard intravenous dose of ethacrynic acid. *JAMA* (1971) 216, 795–8.
3. Mathog RH, Klein WJ. Ototoxicity of ethacrynic acid and aminoglycoside antibiotics in uremia. *N Engl J Med* (1969) 280, 1223–4.
4. Ng PSY, Conley CE, Ing TS. Deafness after ethacrynic acid. *Lancet* (1969) i, 673–4.
5. Schneider WJ, Becker EL. Acute transient hearing loss after ethacrynic acid therapy. *Arch Intern Med* (1966) 117, 715–17.
6. Matz GJ, Beal DD, Krames L. Ototoxicity of ethacrynic acid. Demonstrated in a human temporal bone. *Arch Otolaryngol* (1969) 90, 152–5.
7. Orsulakova A, Schacht J. A biochemical mechanism of the ototoxic interaction between neomycin and ethacrynic acid. *Acta Otolaryngol (Stockh)* (1982) 93, 43–8.
8. Tran Ba Huy P, Meulemans A, Manuel C, Sterkers O, Wassef M. Critical appraisal of the experimental studies on the ototoxic interaction between ethacrynic acid and aminoglycoside antibiotics. A pharmacokinetical standpoint. In 'Ototoxic side effects of diuretics' (ed by Klinke R, Lahn W, Querfurth H, Scholtholt J). *Scand Audiol* (1981) (Suppl 14), 225–32.

Aminoglycosides + Furosemide (Frusemide) or Bumetanide

Although some patients have developed nephrotoxicity and/or ototoxicity while taking both drugs, it has not been established that the damage resulted from an interaction. Nevertheless, concurrent use should be well monitored.

Clinical evidence

An analysis of 3 prospective, controlled, randomised, double blind trials showed that the concurrent use of aminoglycosides (**gentamicin, tobramycin, amikacin**) and **furosemide** did not increase either aminoglycoside-induced nephrotoxicity, or ototoxicity. Nephrotoxicity developed in 20% (10 of 50 patients) given **furosemide** and 17% (38 of 222) not given **furosemide**. Auditory toxicity developed in 22% (5 of 23) given **furosemide** and 24% (28 of 119) not given **furosemide**.[1]

A clinical study evaluating a possible interaction found that **furosemide** increased the aminoglycoside-induced renal damage,[2] whereas two other clinical studies found no interaction.[3,4] There are clinical reports claiming that concurrent use results in ototoxicity, but usually only small numbers of patients were involved and control groups were not included.[5-8] A retrospective study of neonates suggested the possibility of increased ototoxicity but no firm conclusions could be drawn.[9] A patient on **gentamicin** has been described, who rapidly developed deafness only when **furosemide** was replaced by **etacrynic acid**.[1] There seem to be no clinical reports of an **aminoglycoside/bumetanide** interaction, but it has been described in *animals*.[10,11]

Mechanism

Both the aminoglycosides and furosemide given singly are associated with ototoxicity. Studies in patients and healthy subjects have shown that furosemide reduces the renal clearance of gentamicin[12,13] and can cause a rise in both serum gentamicin[13] and tobramycin levels.[14]

Importance and management

Although there is ample evidence of an adverse interaction in *animals*,[15] the weight of evidence suggests that furosemide does not normally increase either the nephrotoxicity or ototoxicity of the aminoglycosides in man. Nevertheless as there is still some uncertainty about the safety of concurrent use it would be prudent to monitor for any evidence of changes in aminoglycoside serum levels or of kidney or ear damage. The authors of the major study cited[1] suggest that an interaction may possibly exist if high dose infusions of furosemide are used. The same precautions would seem to be appropriate with bumetanide.

1. Smith CR, Lietman PS. Effect of furosemide on aminoglycoside-induced nephrotoxicity and auditory toxicity in humans. *Antimicrob Agents Chemother* (1983) 23, 133–7.
2. Prince RA, Ling MH, Hepler CD, Rainville EC, Kealey GP, Donta ST, LeFrock JL, Kowalsky SF. Factors associated with creatinine clearance changes following gentamicin therapy. *Am J Hosp Pharm* (1980) 37, 1489–95.
3. Bygbjerg IC, Møller R. Gentamicin-induced nephropathy. *Scand J Infect Dis* (1976) 8, 203–8.
4. Smith CR, Maxwell RR, Edwards CQ, Rogers JF, Lietman PS. Nephrotoxicity induced by gentamicin and amikacin. *Johns Hopkins Med J* (1978) 142, 85–90.
5. Gallagher KL, Jones JK. Furosemide-induced ototoxicity. *Ann Intern Med* (1979) 91, 744–5.
6. Noël P, Levy V-G. Toxicité rénale de l'association gentamicine-furosémide. Une observation. *Nouv Presse Med* (1978) 7, 351–3.
7. Brown CB, Ogg CS, Cameron JS, Bewick M. High dose frusemide in acute reversible intrinsic renal failure. A preliminary communication. *Scott Med J* (1974) 19, 35–9.
8. Thomsen J, Bech P, Szpirt W. Otological symptoms in chronic renal failure. The possible role of aminoglycoside-furosemide interaction. *Arch Otorhinolaryngol* (1976) 214, 71–9.
9. Salamy A, Eldredge L, Tooley WH. Neonatal status and hearing loss in high-risk infants. *J Pediatr* (1989) 114, 847–52.
10. Ohtani I, Ohtsuki K, Omata T, Ouchi J, Saito T. Interaction of bumetanide and kanamycin. *Otorhinolaryngol* (1978) 40, 216–25.
11. Brummett RE, Bendrick T, Himes D. Comparative ototoxicity of bumetanide and furosemide when used in combination with kanamycin. *J Clin Pharmacol* (1981) 21, 628–36.
12. Lawson DH, Tilstone WJ, Semple PF. Furosemide interactions: studies in normal volunteers. *Clin Res* (1976) 24, 3.
13. Lawson DH, Tilstone WJ, Gray JMB, Srivastava PK. Effect of furosemide on the pharmacokinetics of gentamicin in patients. *J Clin Pharmacol* (1982) 22, 254–8.
14. Kaka JS, Lyman C, Kilarski DJ. Tobramycin-furosemide interaction. *Drug Intell Clin Pharm* (1984) 18, 235–8.
15. Ohtani I, Ohtsuki K, Omata T, Ouchi J, Saito T. Potentiation and its mechanism of cochlear damage resulting from furosemide and aminoglycoside antibiotics. *ORL J Otorhinolaryngol Relat Spec* (1978) 40, 53–63.

Aminoglycosides + Indometacin (Indomethacin)

Conflicting reports claim that serum gentamicin and amikacin levels are, or are not, raised in premature babies when given indometacin to treat patent ductus arteriosus.

Clinical evidence

(a) Aminoglycoside serum levels increased

A study in 20 preterm infants with gestational ages ranging from 25 to 34 weeks, showed that the use of **indometacin** (0.2 mg/kg, 8-hourly, up to 3 doses) caused a rise in the serum levels of either **gentamicin** or **amikacin** which they were being given concurrently. Trough and peak levels of **gentamicin** were raised 48 and 33% respectively, and of **amikacin** 28 and 17%.[1] Another later study confirmed that **indometacin** (0.2, 0.1, 0.1 mg/kg iv at 0, 12 and 36 h) decreased the clearance of single 3 mg/kg daily doses of **gentamicin** by 23% (from 35 to 27 ml/h) in preterm infants of less than 1250 g.[2]

(b) Aminoglycoside serum levels unchanged

Eight out of 13 infants showed no increase in serum **gentamicin** levels when given 0.2 to 0.25 mg/kg **indometacin** 12 hourly for 3 doses. Four showed slight to moderate rises and one had a substantial rise.[3] In another study in 31 preterm babies given 0.2 mg/kg parenteral **indometacin** 12 hourly for 3 doses, no significant changes in serum **gentamicin** levels were seen.[4]

Mechanism

Indometacin reduces the filtration rate of the kidney tubules. Since the aminoglycosides are lost from the body by kidney filtration, the effect of the indometacin is possibly to cause the retention of the antibacterial at this site.

Importance and management

Information seems to be limited to these conflicting studies although supporting evidence comes from the fact that indometacin also causes the retention of digoxin in premature babies. The authors of the second study[3] suggest that the different results may be because their aminoglycoside serum levels were lower before the indometacin was given, and also because they measured the new steady-state levels after 40 to 60 h instead of 24 h. Whatever the explanation, concurrent use should be very closely monitored because toxicity is associated with raised aminoglycoside serum levels. The authors of the first study[1] suggest that the aminoglycoside dosage should be reduced before giving indometacin and the serum levels and kidney function well monitored during concurrent use. Other aminoglycosides possibly behave similarly. This interaction does not seem to have been studied in adults.

1. Zarfin Y, Koren G, Maresky D, Perlman M, MacLeod S. Possible indomethacin-aminoglycoside interaction in preterm infants. *J Pediatr* (1985) 106, 511–13.
2. Dean RP, Domanico RS, Covert RF. Prophylactic indomethacin alters gentamicin pharmacokinetics in preterm infants <1250 grams. *Pediatr Res* (1994) 35, 83A.
3. Jerome M, Davis JC. The effects of indomethacin on gentamicin serum levels. *Proc West Pharmacol Soc* (1987) 30, 85–7.
4. Grylack LJ, Scanlon JW. Interaction of indomethacin (I) and gentamicin (G) in preterm newborns. *Pediatr Res* (1988) 23, 409A.

Aminoglycosides + Magnesium salts

Respiratory arrest occurred in a baby with elevated serum magnesium levels when given gentamicin.

Clinical evidence

A baby girl born to a woman whose pre-eclampsia had been treated with **magnesium sulphate** was found to have muscle weakness and a serum magnesium concentration of 4.3 mg/dl. When 12 hours old the baby was given **ampicillin**, 100 mg/kg intravenously and **gentamicin** 2.5 mg/kg intramuscularly every 12 h. Soon after the second dose of **gentamicin** she stopped breathing and needed intubation. The **gentamicin** was stopped and the baby improved.[1] Animal studies confirmed this interaction.[1]

Mechanism

Magnesium ions and the aminoglycoside antibacterials have neuromuscular blocking activity which can be additive (see also 'Neuromuscular blockers + Magnesium salts', p.766 and 'Neuromuscular blockers and/or Anaesthetics + Aminoglycosides', p.755). In the case cited here it was enough to block the actions of the respiratory muscles.

Importance and management

Direct information about this interaction is very limited, but it is well supported by the well-recognised pharmacological actions of magne-

sium and the aminoglycosides, and their interactions with conventional neuromuscular blockers. The aminoglycosides as a group should be avoided in hypermagnesaemic infants needing antimicrobial treatment. If this is not possible, the effects on respiration should be closely monitored.

1. L'Hommedieu CS, Nicholas D, Armes DA, Jones P, Nelson T, Pickering LK. Potentiation of magnesium sulfate-induced neuromuscular weakness by gentamicin, tobramycin and amikacin. *J Pediatr* (1983) 102, 629–31.

Aminoglycosides + Miconazole

A report describes a reduction in serum tobramycin levels due to miconazole.

Clinical evidence, mechanism, importance and management

Intravenous **miconazole** significantly lowered the peak serum **tobramycin** levels (from 9.1 to 6.7 micrograms/ml) of 9 patients undergoing bone marrow transplantation. Six of them needed dosage adjustments.[1] Miconazole was stopped in 4 patients, and **tobramycin** pharmacokinetic parameters returned to normal 4 to 8 days later. The reasons for this interaction are not understood. Concurrent use should be monitored. More study is needed.[1]

1. Hatfield SM, Crane LR, Duman K, Karanes C, Kiel RJ. Miconazole-induced alteration in tobramycin pharmacokinetics. *Clin Pharm* (1986) 5, 415–19.

Aminoglycosides + Penicillins or Carbapenems

A reduction in serum levels can occur if both aminoglycosides and penicillins are given to patients with severe renal impairment or those undergoing haemodialysis. Netilmicin and piperacillin appear to be the only documented non-interacting combination. No interaction of importance appears to occur with any aminoglycoside/penicillin combination in those with normal renal function. Aminoglycosides appear not to interact significantly with carbapenems, but this awaits further confirmation.

Clinical evidence

(a) Aminoglycosides + penicillins in patients with renal impairment

A study in 6 patients with renal failure requiring dialysis, who were receiving intravenous **carbenicillin** (8 to 15 g daily administered in divided doses 3 to 6 times daily), showed that the presence of the penicillin prevented the achievement of serum **gentamicin** levels above 4 micrograms/ml even though large doses (1.2 to 2.1 mg/kg/day) were given. When the **carbenicillin** was stopped, serum **gentamicin** levels rose.[1] A similar interaction was seen with **carbenicillin** and **tobramycin**.[1]

Other reports similarly describe unusually low **gentamicin** levels in patients with impaired renal function, also given **carbenicillin**,[2-5] **ticarcillin**,[3,5] **piperacillin**,[6] or **tobramycin** with **ticarcillin**.[7] A reduction in the half-life of **gentamicin** to about a half or a third has been described as well.[3,6,8] When given **piperacillin** (4g 12-hourly), the pharmacokinetics of **netilmicin** (2 mg/kg) in 3 chronic haemodialysis patients were unchanged, whereas in another 3 patients given **tobramycin** (2 mg/kg) and **piperacillin**, the clearance was more than doubled (from 3.6 to 8.3 ml/min) and the half-life reduced from 73 to 22 h.[9] A patient showed a reduction in **tobramycin** half-life from an expected 70 h to 10.5 h when also treated with **piperacillin**.[10]

(b) Aminoglycosides + penicillins in patients with normal renal function

A patient with normal renal function was given 80 mg **gentamicin** intravenously, with and without 4 g **carbenicillin**. The serum **gentamicin** concentration profiles in both cases were very similar.[2]

No interaction was seen in 10 patients with normal renal function given **tobramycin** and **piperacillin**,[11] and another 10 healthy subjects given once daily **gentamicin** and **piperacillin/tazobactam**.[12] Only minimal changes were seen in 9 healthy subjects given **tobramycin** with **piperacillin/tazobactam**[13] and 18 other patients (adults and children) with cystic fibrosis given **tobramycin** with **ticarcillin**.[14]

(c) Aminoglycosides + Imipenem/cilastatin, or Biapenem

The suspicion that low **tobramycin** serum levels seen in a patient might have been due to an interaction with **imipenem/cilastatin** (no further details given) was not confirmed in a later *in vitro* study.[15] It has also been suggested that the nephrotoxic effects of **imipenem** and the **aminoglycosides** might possibly be additive but this awaits confirmation.[16] The pharmacokinetics of neither **tobramycin** nor **biapenem** were found to be altered when given concurrently to 12 healthy subjects,[17] No inactivation occurred in an *in vitro* assessment of these two drugs in urine.[18] No dosage adjustment would seem to be necessary.

Mechanism

In vitro, these penicillins interact chemically with the aminoglycoside antibacterials to form biologically inactive amides by a reaction between the amino groups on the aminoglycosides and the beta-lactam ring on the penicillins.[19] Thus both antibacterials are inactivated. It has been suggested that this may also occur in the plasma, causing a drop in the levels of the antibacterials.[8]

Importance and management

The interaction seems to occur most frequently in patients with renal impairment. In those cases where concurrent use is thought necessary, it has been recommended that the penicillin dosage should be adjusted to renal function and the serum levels of both antibacterials closely monitored.[1] Piperacillin appears to affect tobramycin in patients on haemodialysis, but not netilmicin.

There would seem to be no reason for avoiding concurrent use in patients with normal renal function because no significant *in vivo* inactivation appears to occur. Moreover there is good clinical evidence that concurrent use is valuable, especially in the treatment of Pseudomonas infections.[2,20] Tobramycin appears not to be affected by either **imipenem/cilastatin**[15] or **biapenem**.[17,18] See also 'Aminoglycosides + Phenoxymethylpenicillin (Penicillin V)', p.134.

1. Weibert R, Keane W, Shapiro F. Carbenicillin inactivation of aminoglycosides in patients with severe renal failure. *Trans Am Soc Artif Intern Organs* (1976) 22, 439–43.
2. Eykyn S, Phillips I, Ridley M. Gentamicin plus carbenicillin. *Lancet* (1971) i, 545–6.
3. Davies M, Morgan JR, Anand C. Interactions of carbenicillin and ticarcillin with gentamicin. *Antimicrob Agents Chemother* (1975) 7, 431–4.
4. Weibert RT, Keane WF. Carbenicillin-gentamicin interaction in acute renal failure. *Am J Hosp Pharm* (1977) 34, 1137–9.
5. Kradjan WA, Burger R. In vivo inactivation of gentamicin by carbenicillin and ticarcillin. *Arch Intern Med* (1980) 140, 1668–70.
6. Thompson MIB, Russo ME, Saxon BJ, Atkin-Thor E, Matsen JM. Gentamicin inactivation by piperacillin or carbenicillin in patients with end-stage renal disease. *Antimicrob Agents Chemother* (1982) 21, 268–73.
7. Chow MSS, Quintiliani R, Nightingale CH. In vivo inactivation of tobramycin by ticarcillin. A case report. *JAMA* (1982) 247, 658–59.
8. Riff LJ, Jackson GG. Laboratory and clinical conditions for gentamicin activation by carbenicillin. *Arch Intern Med* (1972) 130, 887–91.
9. Matzke GR, Halstenson CE, Heim KL, Abraham PA, Keane WF. Netilmicin disposition is not altered by concomitant piperacillin administration. *Clin Pharmacol Ther* (1985) 41, 210.
10. Uber WE, Brundage RC, White RL, Brundage DM, Bromley HR. In vivo inactivation of tobramycin by piperacillin. *DICP Ann Pharmacother* (1991) 25, 357–9.
11. Lau A, Lee M, Flascha S, Prasad R, Sharifi R. Effect of piperacillin on tobramycin pharmacokinetics in patients with normal renal function. *Antimicrob Agents Chemother* (1983) 24, 533–7.
12. Hitt CM, Patel KB, Nicolau DP, Zhu Z, Nightingale CH. Influence of piperacillin-tazobactam on pharmacokinetics of gentamicin given once daily. *Am J Health-Syst Pharm* (1997) 54, 2704–8.
13. Lathia C, Sia L, Lanc R, Greene D, Kuye O, Batra V, Yacobi A, Faulkner R. Pharmacokinetics of piperacillin/tazobactam IV with and without tobramycin IV in healthy adult male volunteers. *Pharm Res* (1991) 8, (10 Suppl), S-303.
14. Roberts GW, Nation RL, Jarvinen AO, Martin AJ. An *in vivo* assessment of the tobramycin/ticarcillin interaction in cystic fibrosis patients. *Br J Clin Pharmacol* (1993) 36, 372–5.
15. Ariano RE, Kassum DA, Meatherall RC, Patrick WD. Lack of in vitro inactivation of tobramycin by imipenem/cilastatin. *Ann Pharmacother* (1992) 26, 1075–7.
16. Albrecht LM, Rybak MJ. Combination imipenem-aminoglycoside therapy. *Drug Intell Clin Pharm* (1986) 20, 506.
17. Muralidharan G, Buice R, Depuis E, Carver A, Friederici D, Kinchelow T, Kinzig M, Kuye O, Sorgel F, Yacobi A, Mayer P. Pharmacokinetics of biapenem with and without tobramycin in healthy volunteers. *Pharm Res* (1993) 10 (10 Suppl) S-396.
18. Muralidharan G, Carver A, Mayer P. Lack of in vitro inactivation of tobramycin by biapenem in human urine. *Pharm Res* (1994) 11 (10 Suppl) S-398.
19. Perényi T, Graber H, Arr M. Über die Wechselwirkung der Penizilline und Aminoglykosid-Antibiotika. *Int J Clin Pharmacol Ther Toxicol* (1974) 10, 50 5.
20. Kluge RM, Standiford HC, Tatem B, Young VM, Schimpff SC, Greene WH, Calia FM, Hornick RB. The carbenicillin-gentamicin combination against *Pseudomonas aeruginosa*. Correlation of effect with gentamicin sensitivity. *Ann Intern Med* (1974) 81, 584–7.

Aminoglycosides + Phenoxymethylpenicillin (Penicillin V)

The serum levels of phenoxymethylpenicillin when given orally can be halved by the concurrent use of neomycin.

Clinical evidence, mechanism, importance and management

The serum concentrations of **phenoxymethylpenicillin** (given as a 250 mg oral dose) in 5 healthy subjects, were reduced by more than 50% after taking **neomycin** 3g four times daily for 7 days. A return to normal was not achieved until 6 days after the **neomycin** was withdrawn.[1] The probable reason is that **neomycin** causes a reversible malabsorption syndrome (histologically similar to nontropical sprue) which affects the absorption of several foodstuffs and electrolytes. It seems possible that **kanamycin** and **paromomycin** might do the same, but this needs confirmation. Parenteral administration of the **penicillin** or an increase in the oral dosage would seem to be logical answers to this problem, but whether these are effective seems not to have been documented. This study appears to be the only direct evidence of this interaction. See also 'Aminoglycosides + Penicillins or Carbapenems', p.133.

1. Cheng SH, White A. Effect of orally administered neomycin on the absorption of penicillin V. *N Engl J Med* (1962) 267, 1296-7.

Aminoglycosides + Vancomycin

Most, but not all, of the evidence suggests that the nephrotoxicity of the aminoglycosides and vancomycin may be additive.

Clinical evidence, mechanism, importance and management

Although the combination of an aminoglycoside and **vancomycin** can be valuable in the treatment of staphylococcal infections, a retrospective study of 94 patients[1] found a high incidence of nephrotoxicity in patients given both drugs (35%) compared with 5 to 10% when either drug was given alone.[2] Another study in 229 patients found that incidence of nephrotoxicity (15 to 18%) was the same in patients given **vancomycin** alone, or **vancomycin** with an aminoglycoside (not named). However, when the trough serum **vancomycin** levels were 10 micrograms/ml or more, the incidence of nephrotoxicity rose to 27% in those on **vancomycin** alone and to 42% in those taking both drugs.[3] A study using changes in alanine aminopeptidase in the urine as a possible indicator of kidney toxicity found a tenfold increase (suggesting greater renal damage) in patients given **gentamicin** and **vancomycin**.[4] In another report, nephrotoxicity developed in 28 out of 105 (27%) patients given **vancomycin** and aminoglycosides (**gentamicin** or **tobramycin**). However, 22 of the 28 had other factors known to contribute to renal failure.[5] A very brief report describes renal impairment in 2 patients in whom **vancomycin** and **gentamicin** had been used concurrently.[6] Additive nephrotoxicity has been clearly demonstrated in *rats*.[7]

In contrast to these reports, another study failed to find that concurrent use with an un-named aminoglycoside significantly increased the incidence of nephrotoxicity above the 17% seen with **vancomycin** alone.[8]

The picture presented by these reports is not totally clear. What is currently known suggests that it would certainly be prudent to monitor concurrent use carefully for nephrotoxicity, particularly in those with raised trough serum antibacterial levels or other associated risk factors (age, liver disease, peritonitis, use of amphotericin B, male sex).[6]

1. Farber BF, Moellering RC. Retrospective study of the toxicity of preparations of vancomycin from 1974 to 1981. *Antimicrob Agents Chemother* (1983) 23, 138–41.

2. Hewitt W. Gentamicin: toxicity in perspective. *Postgrad Med J* (1974) 50 (Suppl 7), 55–9.

3. Cimino MA, Rotstein C, Slaughter RL, Emrich LJ. Relationship of serum antibiotic concentrations to nephrotoxicity in cancer patients receiving concurrent aminoglycoside and vancomycin therapy. *Am J Med* (1987) 83, 1091–7.

4. Rybak MJ, Frankowski JJ, Edwards DJ, Albrecht LM. Alanine aminopeptidase and β_2-microglobulin excretion in patients receiving vancomycin and gentamicin. *Antimicrob Agents Chemother* (1987) 31, 1461–4.

5. Pauly DJ, Musa DM, Lestico MR, Lindstrom MJ, Hetsko CM. Risk of nephrotoxicity with combination vancomycin-aminoglycoside antibiotic therapy. *Pharmacotherapy* (1990) 10, 378–82.

6. Beeley L, Cunningham H, Brennan A. Bulletin W Midlands Centre for Adverse Drug Reaction Reporting. (1993) 36, 17.

7. Wold JS, Turnipseed SA. Toxicology of vancomycin in laboratory animals. *Rev Infect Dis* (1981) 3 (Suppl), S224–S229.

8. Downs NJ, Neihart RE, Dolezal JM, Hodges GR. Mild nephrotoxicity associated with vancomycin use. *Arch Intern Med* (1989) 149, 1777–81.

Aminosalicylic acid (PAS) + Alcohol

Alcohol can completely nullify the blood-lipid-lowering effects of PAS.

Clinical evidence, mechanism, importance and management

A study was conducted in a group of 63 patients, on the effectiveness of PAS-C (purified PAS recrystallised in vitamin C) and diet on the treatment of hyperlipidaemia types IIa and IIb. It was noted that when 3 of the subjects drank unstated amounts of **alcohol** (**beer** or **cocktails**), the effects of the PAS-C on lowering serum cholesterol, triglyceride and LDL-cholesterol levels were completely abolished.[1] The reasons are not understood. Patients given PAS to reduce blood-lipid levels should avoid **alcohol**. There seems to be no evidence that **alcohol** affects the treatment of tuberculosis with PAS.

1. Kuo PT, Fan WC, Kostis JB, Hayase K. Combined para-aminosalicylic acid and dietary therapy in long-term control of hypercholesterolemia and hypertriglyceridemia (types II$_a$ and II$_b$ hyperlipoproteinemia). *Circulation* (1976) 53, 338–41.

Aminosalicylic acid (PAS) + Diphenhydramine

Diphenhydramine can cause a small reduction in the absorption of aminosalicylic acid from the gut.

Clinical evidence, mechanism, importance and management

A study in 9 healthy subjects[1] (and in *rats*) showed that when 50 mg **diphenhydramine** was injected intramuscularly 10 min before giving 2 g aminosalicylic acid by mouth, the mean peak serum aminosalicylic acid levels were reduced about 15%. The possible reason is that the **diphenhydramine** reduces peristalsis in the gut which in some way reduces aminosalicylic acid absorption. The extent to which **diphenhydramine** or any other anticholinergic drug diminishes the therapeutic response to long-term treatment with aminosalicylic acid is uncertain, but it is probably small.

1. Lavigne J-G, Marchand C. Inhibition of the gastrointestinal absorption of p-aminosalicylate (PAS) in rats and humans by diphenhydramine. *Clin Pharmacol Ther* (1973) 14, 404–12.

Aminosalicylic acid (PAS) + Probenecid

The serum levels of aminosalicylic acid can be raised two to fourfold by the concurrent use of probenecid.

Clinical evidence, mechanism, importance and management

When 500 mg **probenecid** was administered 6-hourly, the serum levels of aminosalicylic acid 4 g were increased by as much as fourfold.[1] Similar results are described in another report.[2] The reasons are uncertain but it seems probable that the **probenecid** successfully competes with the aminosalicylic acid for active excretion by the kidney tubules, resulting in its retention and accumulation in the body.

The documentation of this interaction is limited but it appears to be established. Such large increases in serum aminosalicylic acid levels would be expected to lead to toxicity. It also seems possible that the dosage of aminosalicylic acid could be reduced without losing the required therapeutic response. This needs confirmation. Concurrent use should be undertaken with caution.

1. Boger WP, Pitts FW. Influence of *p*-(Di-n-propylsulfamyl)-benzoic acid, 'Benemid' on para-aminosalicylic acid (PAS) plasma concentrations. *Am Rev Tuberc* (1950) 61, 862–7.

2. Carr DT, Karlson AG, Bridge EV. Concentration of PAS and tuberculostatic potency of serum after administration of PAS with and without Benemid. *Proc Staff Meet Mayo Clin* (1952) 27, 209–15.

Amoxicillin or Ampicillin + Allopurinol

The incidence of skin rashes among those taking either ampicillin or amoxicillin is increased by the concurrent use of allopurinol.

Clinical evidence

A retrospective search through the records of 1324 patients, 67 of whom were taking **allopurinol** and **ampicillin**, showed that 15 of them (22%) developed a skin rash compared with 94 (7.5%) of the rest not taking **allopurinol**.[1] The types of rash were not defined. Another study showed similar results: 35 out of 252 patients (13.9%) taking **allopurinol** and **ampicillin** developed a rash, compared with 251 out of 4434 (5.9%) taking **ampicillin** alone.[2] A parallel study revealed that 8 out of 36 patients (22%) on **amoxicillin** and **allopurinol** developed a rash, whereas only 52 out of 887 (5.9%) did so on **amoxicillin** alone.[2]

Mechanism

Not understood. One suggestion is that the allopurinol or hyperuricaemia was responsible.[1] Another is that hyperuricaemic individuals may possibly have an altered immunological reactivity.[3]

Importance and management

An established interaction of limited importance. There would seem to be no strong reason for avoiding concurrent use, but prescribers should recognise that the development of a rash is by no means unusual. Whether this also occurs with penicillins other than ampicillin or amoxicillin is uncertain, and does not seem to have been reported.

1. Boston Collaborative Drug Surveillance Programme. Excess of ampicillin rashes associated with allopurinol or hyperuricemia. *N Engl J Med* (1972) 286, 505–7.

2. Jick H, Porter JB. Potentiation of ampicillin skin reactions by allopurinol or hyperuricemia. *J Clin Pharmacol* (1981) 21, 456–8.

3. Fessel WJ. Immunological reactivity in hyperuricemia. *N Engl J Med* (1972) 286, 1218.

Amoxicillin or Ampicillin + Khat (Catha)

Chewing khat reduces the absorption of ampicillin and, to a lesser extent, amoxicillin, but the effects are minimal 2 h after khat chewing stops.

Clinical evidence, mechanism, importance and management

Khat (the leaves and stem tips of *Catha edulis*) is chewed in some African and Arabian countries for its stimulatory properties, so a study was conducted to see if **khat** affected amoxicillin absorption. Subjects chewed **khat** for 4 h and were given a 500-mg dose of amoxicillin before, after or during chewing. Chewing **khat** resulted in variable reduction in amoxicillin bioavailability which was maximal (reduced by 78%) when it was given midway during the chewing period.[1] A study in 8 healthy Yemeni male subjects found that chewing **khat** reduced the absorption of oral **ampicillin** from the gut.[2] When the **ampicillin** (500 mg with 250 ml water) was taken 2 h before **khat** chewing started, or just before, or midway through a 4 h chewing session, the amounts of unchanged **ampicillin** in the urine fell by 46, 41 and 49% respectively. Even when taken 2 h after a chewing session had stopped, the amount fell by 12%. A parallel series of studies with 500 mg **amoxicillin** found much smaller reductions. The equivalent reductions were 14, 9, 22 and 13%. The reasons for this interaction are not known, but the authors of the report suggest that what possibly happens is that tannins from the khat form insoluble and non-absorbable complexes with the antibacterials, and possibly also directly reduce the way the gut actually absorbs the antibacterials.[2] One of the studies concluded that both **ampicillin** and **amoxicillin** should be taken 2 h after **khat** chewing to ensure that maximum absorption occurs.[2]

1. Abdel Ghani YM, Etman MA, Nada AH. Effect of khat chewing on the absorption of orally administered amoxicillin. *Acta Pharm* (1999) 49, 43–50.
2. Attef OA, Abdul-Azem A, Hassan MA. Effect of Khat chewing on the bioavailabiliy of ampicillin and amoxycillin. *J Antimicrob Chemother* (1997) 39, 523–5.

Amoxicillin + Nifedipine

Nifedipine increases the absorption of amoxicillin from the gut but this is unlikely to be clinically important.

Clinical evidence, mechanism, importance and management

When 1 g amoxicillin was given half-an-hour after 20 mg **nifedipine**, the peak serum amoxicillin levels in 8 healthy subjects were raised by 33%, the bioavailability was raised 21% and the absorption rate was raised by 70%.[1] The authors speculate that the uptake of **amoxicillin** through the gut wall is increased by **nifedipine** in some way.[1] There would seem to be no good reason for avoiding concurrent use.

1. Westphal J-F, Trouvin J-H, Deslandes A, Carbon C. Nifedipine enhances amoxicillin absorption kinetics and bioavailability in humans. *J Pharmacol Exp Ther* (1990) 255, 312–17.

Amphotericin B + Azole antifungals

There is evidence that amphotericin B with either fluconazole, itraconazole, ketoconazole or miconazole may possibly be less effective than amphotericin B alone and the side-effects may be greater.

Clinical evidence, mechanism, importance and management

Studies in a few patients and *in vitro* experiments suggest that the antifungal effects of amphotericin B and **miconazole** used together may be antagonistic, and not additive as might be expected.[1,2] In another study, 4 out of 6 patients failed to respond to amphotericin B treatment while concurrently receiving **ketoconazole**, whereas it was successful in 6 others, 5 of whom had stopped taking either prophylactic **miconazole** or **ketoconazole**. The authors suggested that the numbers are too small to draw any definite conclusions, but antagonism is certainly a possibility.[3] A comparative study in patients found that those on **itraconazole** and amphotericin B had serum itraconazole levels of less than 1.0 microgram/ml, whereas those on **itraconazole** alone had serum itraconazole levels of 3.75 micrograms/ml, which suggests that the amphotericin B actually reduces the **itraconazole** levels.[4] Other *in vitro* studies suggest that amphotericin B with **fluconazole**, **itraconazole**, **miconazole**[5] or **ketoconazole**[5,6] may possibly be less effective than amphotericin B alone, whereas a further *in vitro* study indicates that sometimes (most notably with **ketoconazole** and amphotericin B) the antifungal effects may be increased.[7] The reasons for amphotericin B/imidazole combinations having *less* antifungal activity than either drug alone are not understood.

A retrospective study of **itraconazole** use found that 11 of 12 leukaemic patients given amphotericin B and **itraconazole** had raised LFTs. These abnormalities resolved in 7 patients when the amphotericin B was discontinued. **Itraconazole** alone, given to another 8 patients did not cause and LFT abnormalities, even though it was used in high doses.[8]

The whole topic is still the subject of some considerable debate[9,10] so that until more is known it might be better to avoid concurrent use, or the outcome should be very well monitored, being alert for a reduced antifungal response, or increasing LFTs.[8] A valuable review has been written on this topic.[11]

1. Schacter LP, Owellen RJ, Rathbun HK, Buchanan B. Antagonism between miconazole and amphotericin B. *Lancet* (1976) ii, 318.
2. Cosgrove RF, Beezer AE, Miles RJ. In vitro studies of amphotericin B in combination with the imidazole antifungal compounds clotrimazole and miconazole. *J Infect Dis* (1978) 138, 681–5.
3. Meunier-Carpentier F, Cruciani M, Klastersky J. Oral prophylaxis with miconazole or ketoconazole of invasive fungal disease in neutropenic cancer patients. *Eur J Cancer Clin Oncol* (1983) 19, 43–8.
4. Pennick GJ, McGough DA, Barchiesi F, Rinaldi MG. Concomitant therapy with amphotericin B and itraconazole: Does this combination affect the serum concentration of itraconazole? *Intersci Conf Antimicrob Agents Chemother* (1994) 34, 39.
5. Petrou MA, Rogers TR. Interactions *in vitro* between polyenes and imidazoles against yeasts. *J Antimicrob Chemother* (1991) 27, 491–506.
6. Sud IJ, Feingold DS. Effect of ketoconazole on the fungicidal action of amphotericin B in *Candida albicans*. *Antimicrob Agents Chemother* (1983) 23, 185–7.
7. Odds FC. Interactions among amphotericin B, 5-fluorocytosine, ketoconazole, and miconazole against pathogenic fungi in vitro. *Antimicrob Agents Chemother* (1982) 22, 763–70.
8. Persat F, Schwartzbrod PE, Troncy J, Timour Q, Maul A, Piens MA, Picot S. Abnormalities in liver enzymes during simultaneous therapy with itraconazole and amphotericin B in leukaemic patients. *J Antimicrob Chemother* (2000) 45, 928–30.
9. Pahls S, Schaffner A. *Aspergillus fumigatus* pneumonia in neutropenic patients receiving fluconazole for infection due to *Candida* species: is amphotericin B combined with fluconazole the appropriate answer? *Clin Infect Dis* (1994) 18, 484–5.
10. Meis JF, Donnelly JP, Hoogkamp-Korstanje JA, De Pauw BE. Reply. *Clin Infect Dis* (1994) 18, 485–6.
11. Sugar AM. Use of amphotericin B with azole antifungal drugs: what are we doing? *Antimicrob Agents Chemother* (1995) 39, 1907–12.

Amphotericin B + Corticosteroids

Amphotericin B and corticosteroids can cause both potassium loss and salt and water retention which can have adverse effects on cardiac function.

Clinical evidence

Four patients treated with amphotericin B and 25 to 40 mg **hydrocortisone** daily developed cardiac enlargement and congestive heart failure. The cardiac size decreased and the failure disappeared within 2 weeks of stopping the **hydrocortisone**. The amphotericin B was continued successfully with the addition of potassium supplements.[1]

Mechanism

Amphotericin B causes potassium to be lost in the urine. Hydrocortisone can cause potassium to be lost and salt and water to be retained and occasional instances of hypernatraemia with amphotericin B have also been seen. Working in concert these could account for the hypokalaemic cardiopathy and the circulatory overload that was seen.

Importance and management

Information is limited but the interaction would seem to be established. Monitor the electrolyte and fluid balance and the cardiac function during concurrent use. The elderly would seem to be particularly at risk.

1. Chung D-K, Koenig MG. Reversible cardiac enlargement during treatment with amphotericin B and hydrocortisone. Report of three cases. *Am Rev Respir Dis* (1971) 103, 831–41.

Amphotericin B + Low salt diet

The renal toxicity of amphotericin B can be associated with sodium depletion. When the sodium is replaced the renal function improves.[1,2]

1. Feeley J, Heidemann H, Gerkens J, Roberts LJ, Branch RA. Sodium depletion enhances nephrotoxicity of amphotericin B. *Lancet* (1981) i, 1422–3.
2. Heidemann HT, Gerkens JF, Spickard WA, Jackson EK, Branch RA. Amphotericin B nephrotoxicity in humans decreased by salt repletion. *Am J Med* (1983) 75, 476–81.

Amphotericin B + Pentamidine

There is evidence that acute renal failure may develop in patients on amphotericin if pentamidine is given concurrently.

Clinical evidence, mechanism, importance and management

A retrospective study between 1985 and 1988 identified 101 patients with AIDS who had been treated with amphotericin B for various systemic mycoses. The patients were given 0.6 to 0.8 mg/kg/day for 7 to 10 days, followed by thrice-weekly dosing for about 9 weeks. Nine patients were concurrently treated for *Pneumocystis carinii* pneumonia, but only the 4 who had been given **pentamidine parenterally** developed acute and rapid reversible renal failure. No renal failure was seen in 2 others given **pentamidine** by **inhalation** or 3 given intravenous **co-trimoxazole**.[1] In all 4 cases, renal function returned to normal when the drugs were withdrawn. The reason for the kidney damage appears to be the additive nephrotoxic effects of both drugs. The reason no toxicity occurred when the **pentamidine** was given by inhalation is probably because the serum levels achieved were low. The authors of the study advise caution if both drugs are used. More study is needed.

1. Antoniskis D, Larsen RA. Acute, rapidly progressive renal failure with simultaneous use of amphotericin B and pentamidine. *Antimicrob Agents Chemother* (1990) 34, 470–2.

Antibacterials + Alcohol

No adverse or undesirable interaction normally occurs between alcohol and most antibacterials, with the exception of some cephalosporins, furazolidone, metronidazole and possibly doxycycline and erythromycin succinate.

Clinical evidence, mechanism, importance and management

A long-standing and very common belief among members of the general public (presumably derived from advice given by doctors and pharmacists) is that **alcohol** should be strictly avoided while taking any 'antibiotic'. This belief was expressed in 1965 by Dr W Kitto of Chicago who, in answer to a question posed in the Journal of the American Medical Association, claimed that **alcohol** increases the degradation of **penicillin** in the gut and reduces the amount available for absorption.[1] However, a much later study in 1987 showed that the pharmacokinetics of **phenoxymethylpenicillin (penicillin V)** were unaffected by **alcoholic drinks**.[2] Another study found that **alcohol** delayed the absorption of **amoxicillin** but did not affect the total amount absorbed.[3]

It is difficult to know how this clinical folklore arose because there is little to support it for most antibacterials. The few exceptions include **latamoxef**, **cefamandole**, **cefoperazone**, **cefmenoxime**, a few **other uncommon cephalosporins**, **furazolidone** and **metronidazole**, all of which sometimes cause an unpleasant disulfiram-like reaction with alcohol. This does not happen with most of the commonly prescribed cephalosporins. It is also known that serum **doxycycline** levels may be significantly reduced by **alcohol** in alcoholics, but not in normal subjects. The absorption of **erythromycin succinate** is also reduced by **alcohol**. Details of these interactions are to be found in the appropriate monographs, but apart from these particular antibacterials, there seems to be little reason why patients taking any of the others should avoid **alcohol**.

1. Kitto W. Antibiotics and ingestion of alcohol. *JAMA* (1965) 193, 411.
2. Lindberg RLP, Huupponen RK, Viljanen S and Pihlajamäki KK. Ethanol and the absorption of oral penicillin in man. *Int J Clin Pharmacol Ther Toxicol* (1987) 25, 536–8.
3. Morasso MI, Hip A, Márquez M, González C, Arancibia A. Amoxicillin kinetics and ethanol ingestion. *Int J Clin Pharmacol Ther Toxicol* (1988) 26, 428–31.

Antibacterials + Cimetidine

Human studies show that cimetidine does not adversely affect the bioavailability of ampicillin or co-trimoxazole.[1] The bioavailability of oral benzylpenicillin may be increased in some subjects.[2] The pharmacokinetics of azithromycin were not affected by a single 800-mg dose of cimetidine.[3]

1. Rogers HJ, James CA, Morrison PJ and Bradbrook ID. Effect of cimetidine on oral absorption of ampicillin and co-trimoxazole. *J Antimicrob Chemother* (1980) 6, 297.
2. Fairfax AJ, Adam J and Pagan FS. Effect of cimetidine on absorption of oral benzylpenicillin. *BMJ* (1977) 2, 820.
3. Foulds G, Hilligoss DM, Henry EB, Gerber N. The effects of an antacid or cimetidine on the serum concentrations of azithromycin. *J Clin Pharmacol* (1991) 31, 164–7.

Antibacterials + Immunoglobulins

Animal **studies suggest that concurrent use may be much less effective than the antibacterial alone.**

Clinical evidence, mechanism, importance and management

A study[1] in newborn *rats* infected with a group B streptococcal infection found the following mortalities: 100% with **immunoglobulin** (2 g/kg) alone, 51% with **benzylpenicillin (penicillin G)** alone, 88% with **immunoglobulin + benzylpenicillin**. Not dissimilar results were found when the penicillin was replaced by **ceftriaxone**. More study is needed to find out if this unexpected adverse effect also occurs in man.

1. Kim KS. High-dose intravenous immune globulin impairs antibacterial activity of antibiotics. *J Allergy Clin Immunol* (1989) 84, 579–88.

Anti-infectives + Sucralfate

An *in vitro* study with amphotericin B, colistin sulphate and tobramycin sulphate found that all three became markedly and irreversibly bound to sucralfate at the pH values found in the gut.

Clinical evidence, mechanism, importance and management

To simulate what might happen in the gut, 3 anti-infectives (25 mg/l **amphotericin B**, 50 mg/l **colistin sulphate**, 50 mg/l **tobramycin sulphate**) were each mixed separately with 500 mg **sucralfate** in 40 ml water at pH 3.5 and allowed to stand for 90 min at 25°C. Analysis of the solutions showed that the amounts of the anti-infectives fell rapidly and progressively over the 90 min period. Concentration/time curves showed that the **amphotericin B** concentration fell to about 20%, the **colistin** to about 40%, and the **tobramycin** to about 1%. When the pH of the mixtures was then raised to 6.5–7.0 for 90 min, there was no change in the concentrations of any of the three anti-infectives, suggesting that the interaction was irreversible.[1] The reason for these changes is not known, but the suggestion is that the **sucralfate** forms insoluble chelates with these anti-infectives.[1]

It is not known how important these interactions are likely to be in practice, but if the anti-infectives were to be used for selective decontamination of the gut, there would seem to be the risk that their concentrations might become too low to inhibit some pathogenic organisms. Separating the dosages might not be effective in some postoperative patients because their gastric function may not return to normal for up to 5 days, and some **sucralfate** might still be present when the next dose of the anti-infective was given.[1] More study is needed to find out whether any or all of these interactions is clinically important, but in the meanwhile it would seem prudent to monitor concurrent use carefully, being alert for any evidence of reduced effects.

1. Feron B, Adair CG, Gorman SP, McClurg B. Interaction of sucralfate with antibiotics used for selective decontamination of the gastrointestinal tract. *Am J Hosp Pharm* (1993) 50, 2550–3.

Antimalarials + Antacids or Antidiarrhoeals

The absorption of chloroquine is moderately reduced by magnesium trisilicate and kaolin. The absorption of proguanil is more markedly reduced by magnesium trisilicate. *In vitro* studies suggest that pyrimethamine may be affected like chloroquine.

Clinical evidence

(a) Chloroquine, Pyrimethamine + Antacids, Antidiarrhoeals

Six healthy subjects were given 1 g **chloroquine phosphate** (equivalent to 620 mg of **chloroquine** base) with either 1 g **magnesium trisilicate** or 1 g **kaolin** after an overnight fast. The **magnesium trisilicate** reduced the AUC of the **chloroquine** by 18.2% and the **kaolin** reduced it by 28.6%.[1]

Related *in vitro* studies by the same authors using segments of *rat* intestine showed that the absorption of **chloroquine** and **pyrimethamine** respectively were decreased as follows: **magnesium trisilicate** (31.3 and 37.5%), **kaolin** (46.5 and 49.9%), **calcium carbonate** (52.8 and 31.5%), and **gerdiga** (36.1 and 38.0%). Gerdiga is a clay containing hydrated silicates with sodium and potassium carbonates and bicarbonates. It is used in rural areas of the Sudan as an antacid and is similar to **attapulgite**.[2]

(b) Halofantrine + Antacids

Magnesium carbonate was shown *in vitro* to adsorb more **halofantrine** than **aluminium hydroxide** or **magnesium trisilicate** antacid preparations so its *in vivo* effects on **halofantrine** pharmacokinetics were studied in 7 healthy subjects. **Magnesium carbonate** 1 g did not affect the bioavailability of **halofantrine** 500 mg. However, clinical efficacy of **halofantrine** is thought to be related to the maximum plasma concentration, which was almost halved by concurrent administration. The active metabolite of **halofantrine**, which is equally potent was similarly affected and so it would seem inadvisable to administer **halofantrine** with **magnesium carbonate**.[3]

(c) Proguanil + Antacids

The bioavailability of a 200-mg dose of **proguanil** was reduced by almost two-thirds (AUC reduction from 3256 to 1148 ng.h.ml^{-1}) in 8 normal subjects when given **magnesium trisilicate**.[4]

Mechanism

These antacid and antidiarrhoeal compounds adsorb chloroquine and proguanil[4] thereby reducing the amount available for absorption by the gut. Pyrimethamine appears to be similarly affected.[2]

Importance and management

The chloroquine/magnesium trisilicate, chloroquine/kaolin, halofantrine/magnesium carbonate and proguanil/magnesium trisilicate interactions are established, but their clinical importance does not seem to have been assessed. The antimalarial effects of proguanil would be expected to be reduced much more than those of chloroquine. One way to minimise the interaction is to separate the dosages of the antimalarials and magnesium trisilicate or kaolin as much as possible (2 to 3 h) to reduce admixture in the gut. Nobody seems to have checked to see if other antacids behave similarly. There does not seem to be any direct clinical evidence that the pyrimethamine effects are reduced by antacids but its *in vitro* absorption pattern in *animal* studies is similar to chloroquine.[2]

1. McElnay JC, Mukhtar HA, D'Arcy PF, Temple DJ, Collier PS. The effect of magnesium trisilicate and kaolin on the *in vivo* absorption of chloroquine. *J Trop Med Hyg* (1982) 85, 159–63.
2. McElnay JC, Mukhtar HA, D'Arcy PF, Temple DJ. *In vitro* experiments on chloroquine and pyrimethamine absorption in the presence of antacid constituents of kaolin. *J Trop Med Hyg* (1982) 85, 153–8.
3. Aideloje SO, Onyeji CO, Ugwu NC. Altered pharmacokinetics of halofantrine by an antacid, magnesium carbonate. *Eur J Pharm Biopharm* (1998) 46, 299–303.
4. Onyeji CO, Babalola CP. The effect of magnesium trisilicate on proguanil absorption. *Int J Pharmaceutics* (1993) 100, 249–52.

Atovaquone + Miscellaneous drugs

Preliminary evidence suggests that of the drugs examined, only metoclopramide causes any marked changes (decreases) in the atovaquone steady-state serum levels. Atovaquone appears not to interact with phenytoin.

Clinical evidence, mechanism, importance and management

An analysis of 191 patients with AIDS, given atovaquone as part of efficacy studies found that when normalised for plasma albumin, body weight, and the absence of other drugs, the expected steady-state plasma levels of atovaquone were 14.8 micrograms/ml. Steady-state atovaquone plasma levels achieved in the presence of other drugs were examined in an attempt to identify possible interactions. **Fluconazole** and **prednisone** were associated with increases of 2.5 and 2.3 micrograms/ml respectively, whereas **paracetamol (acetaminophen)**, **aciclovir**, **opioids**, **antidiarrhoeals**, **cephalosporins**, **benzodiazepines** and **laxatives** were associated with decreases of > 3.4 micrograms/ml. **Metoclopramide** was associated with a decrease of 7.2 micrograms/ml. **Zidovudine**, **U plasma binders**, **erythromycin**, **clofazimine**, **antacids**, **clotrimazole**, **NSAIDs**, **ketoconazole**, **hydroxyzine**, **megestrol**, **antiemetics**, **other systemic steroids**, and **H$_2$ antagonists** were not associated with any change in steady-state atovaquone serum levels. **Zidovudine**, **U plasma binders**, **erythromycin** and **clofazimine** were represented by fewer than 5 subjects.[1,2]

This kind of analysis provides only the very broadest indication that interactions might or might not occur between atovaquone and these drugs, but it highlights the need to be vigilant if an apparently interacting drug is used concurrently. Only the change caused by **metoclopramide** seems likely to have any potential clinical importance.

A single dose study in 12 healthy subjects found that atovaquone does not affect the pharmacokinetics of **phenytoin**, and it was concluded that a clinically important pharmacokinetic interaction is unlikely.[3]

1. Sadler BM, Blum MR. Relationship between steady-state plasma concentrations of atovaquone (C_{ss}) and the use of various concomitant medications in AIDS patients with *Pneumocystis carinii* pneumonia. IXth Int Conf AIDS & IVth STD World Congr, Berlin (1993) June 6–11, 504.
2. Wellvone (Atovaquone). GlaxoWellcome. Summary of product characteristics, May 2001.
3. Davis JD, Dixon R, Khan AZ, Toon S, Rolan PE, Posner J. Atovaquone has no effect on the pharmacokinetics of phenytoin in healthy male volunteers. *Br J Clin Pharmacol* (1996) 42, 246–8.

Atovaquone and Proguanil + Artesunate

Artesunate does not appear to interact with atovaquone/proguanil.

Clinical evidence, mechanism, importance and management

In a study to assess the effect of **artesunate** on the pharmacokinetics of atovaquone/proguanil, 1 g atovaquone/400 mg proguanil was given to 12 healthy subjects with and without 250 mg **artesunate**. No change was noted in the pharmacokinetics of either atovaquone or proguanil and no unexpected adverse events were seen.[1] Although **artesunate** does not therefore appear to interact with atovaquone/proguanil, this needs confirmation in a multiple-dose study.

1. van Vugt M, Edstein MD, Proux S, Lay K, Ooh M, Looareesuwan S, White NJ, Nosten F. Absence of an interaction between artesunate and atovaquone – proguanil. *Eur J Clin Pharmacol* (1999) 55, 469–74.

Atovaquone + Rifampicin (Rifampin) or Rifabutin

Rifampicin reduces serum atovaquone levels whereas atovaquone raises serum rifampicin levels. No clinically relevant interaction appears to occur between atovaquone and rifabutin.

Clinical evidence

A steady-state study in 13 HIV+ patients found that concurrent treatment with atovaquone 750 mg twice daily and **rifampicin** 600 mg four times daily resulted in a more than 50% reduction in the atovaquone AUC and serum levels, but a more than 30% rise in **rifampicin** AUC and serum levels.[1] A study in 24 normal subjects given 750 mg atovaquone twice daily found that the concurrent use of 300 mg **rifabutin** caused a small (34%) decrease in the AUC of the atovaquone and a small decrease in the **rifabutin** levels, but the authors of the report suggest that no dosage adjustment is needed.[2]

Mechanism

Uncertain. Evidence from 6-beta-hydroxycortisol studies suggest that rifampicin, as expected, acts as an enzyme inducer thereby increasing the metabolism of the atovaquone, but just why atovaquone increases the serum levels of rifampicin is not known.[1]

Importance and management

Information is limited but the interactions appear to be established. Their clinical importance is unknown, but be alert for the need to increase the atovaquone dosage if rifampicin is added. More study is needed.

1. Sadler BM, Caldwell P, Scott JD, Rogers M, Blum MR. Drug interaction between rifampin and atovaquone (Mepron®) in HIV+ asymptomatic volunteers. *Intersci Conf Antimicrob Agents Chemother* (1995) 35, 7.
2. Gillotin C, Grandpierre I, Sadler BM. Pharmacokinetic interaction between atovaquone (ATVQ) suspension and rifabutin (RFB). *Clin Pharmacol Ther* (1998) 63, 229.

Azithromycin + Miscellaneous drugs

Azithromycin appears not to interact with carbamazepine cimetidine, methylprednisolone, or a number of other drugs used for analgesia, anxiety, arthritis, asthma, hypnosis or sedation. Food appears to halve azithromycin absorption and antacids may reduce its peak serum levels.

Clinical evidence, mechanism, importance and management

A study in 4000 patients, which investigated the efficacy of azithromycin, did not report any interaction with **methylprednisolone**. Concurrent treatment also occurred with **bronchodilators**, **analgesics**, **hypnotics/sedatives/anxiolytics** or **anti-arthritic drugs** (none of them specifically named) in 45% of patients, with no interaction problems encountered.[1] No pharmacokinetic interactions occurred with **carbamazepine**.[1,2]

The peak serum levels, but not the total absorption, of azithromycin was reduced in 10 healthy subjects by 30 ml *Maalox* (**aluminium/magnesium hydroxide**).[3] **Food** appears to reduce the absorption of azithromycin by about half.[1] It is suggested therefore that **azithromycin** should not be given at the same time as **antacids** or food, but should be taken at least 1 h before or 2 h after either an **antacid** or a **meal**.[1,4]

It has been suggested that **ergot alkaloids** should be avoided, because clinically important interactions have been seen between these drugs and other macrolide antibacterials related to azithromycin.[1,4,5] However there seems so far to be no direct evidence of any adverse interactions between **ergot alkaloids**.

1. Hopkins S. Clinical toleration and safety of azithromycin. *Am J Med* (1991) 91 (Suppl 3A), 40S–45S.
2. Rapeport WG, Dewland PM, Muirhead DC, Forster PL. Lack of an interaction between azithromycin and carbamazepine. *Br J Clin Pharmacol* (1992) 33, 551P.
3. Foulds G, Hilligoss DM, Henry EB, Gerber N. The effects of an antacid or cimetidine on the serum concentrations of azithromycin. *J Clin Pharmacol* (1991) 31, 164–7.
4. Zithromax (Azithromycin). Pfizer Ltd. Summary of product characteristics, May 2001.
5. Lode H. The pharmacokinetics of azithromycin and their clinical significance. *Eur J Clin Microbiol Infect Dis* (1991) 10, 807–12.

Azole antifungals + Antacids, H_2-blockers or Sucralfate

The gastrointestinal absorption of ketoconazole is markedly reduced by antacids, cimetidine and ranitidine, whereas sucralfate has a smaller effect. The absorption of itraconazole is reduced (possibly halved) by H_2-blockers, but the absorption of fluconazole appears not be to significantly affected by antacids, cimetidine, ranitidine or sucralfate.

Clinical evidence

(a) Fluconazole

Maalox forte (**aluminium** and **magnesium hydroxide**) 20 ml did not affect the absorption of single 100-mg doses of fluconazole in 14 healthy subjects.[1] The AUC over 48 h of 100 mg fluconazole given to 6 healthy subjects was reduced by only 13% when a single 400-mg dose **cimetidine** was given.[2] Two other studies found that **cimetidine**[3] and **famotidine**[4] did not affect fluconazole absorption. **Sucralfate** 2 g was found to have no significant effect on the pharmacokinetics of a single 200-mg dose of fluconazole in 10 healthy subjects, confirming the results of an *in vitro* study.[5]

(b) Itraconazole

Twelve healthy subjects were given 400 mg **cimetidine** twice daily or 150 mg **ranitidine** twice daily for 3 days before and after single 200-mg doses of itraconazole. The AUC and maximum serum levels of the itraconazole were reduced, but not significantly. The largest changes were 20% reductions in the AUC and maximum serum levels due to **ranitidine**.[6] In contrast, another study in 30 healthy subjects found that 150 mg **ranitidine** twice daily for 3 days reduced the AUC of a single 200-mg dose of itraconazole by 44%, and reduced the maximum serum levels by 52%.[7] Yet another study found that **ranitidine** and **antacids** (not named) appeared to reduce serum itraconazole serum levels.[8] A study of the bioavailability of itraconazole in 12 lung transplant patients also given **ranitidine** 150 mg twice daily and **antacid** four times daily found that the serum levels of itraconazole were highly variable. However, satisfactory levels were achieved in all patients, even though some needed their doses of itraconazole increased from 200 to 400 mg daily.[9]

Famotidine 40 mg was found to reduce serum itraconazole levels by about 50% in 12 healthy subjects given a 200-mg dose.[4] **Famotidine** 20 mg twice daily was given with itraconazole 200 mg daily for 10 days, to 16 patients undergoing chemotherapy for haematological malignancies. The minimum plasma levels of itraconazole were reduced by about 39%, and 8 patients failed to achieve the levels considered necessary to protect neutropenic patients from fungal infections.[10]

(c) Ketoconazole

A haemodialysis patient failed to respond to treatment with ketoconazole 200 mg daily while on **cimetidine**, **sodium bicarbonate** 2 g daily and **aluminium oxide** 2.5 g daily. Only when the ketoconazole dosage was increased to 200 mg four times daily did her serum levels rise. A later study in 3 healthy subjects found that when 200 mg ketoconazole was taken 2 h after 400 mg **cimetidine**, the absorption was considerably reduced (AUC reduced to about 40%). When this was repeated with 0.5 g **sodium bicarbonate** as well, the absorption was reduced to about 5%. In contrast, when this was repeated once more but with the ketoconazole in an acidic solution, the absorption was increased by about 50%[11]

Another study[3] in 24 healthy subjects found intravenous **cimetidine** titrated to give a gastric pH of 6 or more reduced the absorption by 95%. A study[12,13] in 6 healthy subjects found that 150 mg **ranitidine** given 2 h before 400 mg ketoconazole reduced its AUC by about 95%. **Sucralfate** 1 g caused a smaller reduction of about 20%.[12,13] Another study found that 1 g **sucralfate** reduced the AUC and maximum serum levels of a single 100-mg dose of ketoconazole by about 25%, but no significant changes were seen when the ketoconazole was given 2 h after the **sucralfate**.[14] A study in 4 patients found that the concurrent use of *Maalox* reduced the absorption of ketoconazole but this was not statistically significant.[15] An anecdotal report suggested that giving ketoconazole 2 h before a stomatitis cocktail containing *Maalox* seemed to prevent the cocktail reducing its effectiveness.[16]

Mechanism

Ketoconazole is a poorly soluble base which must be transformed by the acid in the stomach into the soluble hydrochloride salt. Agents which reduce gastric secretion, such as H_2-blockers or antacids, raise the pH in the stomach so that the dissolution of the ketoconazole and its absorption are reduced. Conversely, anything which increases the gastric acidity increases the dissolution and the absorption.[15,17] There is also *in vitro* evidence that an electrostatic interaction occurs between ketoconazole and sucralfate to form an ion pair which cannot pass through the gut wall.[18] The absorption of itraconazole is also affected by changes in gastric pH, but fluconazole is minimally affected.

Importance and management

The interactions with ketoconazole are clinically important but not extensively documented. Advise patients to take antacids or sucralfate, not less than 2 to 3 h before or after the ketoconazole so that absorption can take place with minimal changes in the pH of the gastric contents.[11] Monitor the effects to confirm that the ketoconazole is effective. Sucralfate would be expected to interact much more moderately than the other drugs.

The situation with itraconazole is not entirely clear, but some reduction in its absorption apparently occurs and it would therefore be prudent to confirm that it remains effective in the presence of H_2-

blockers and possibly antacids. It has been suggested that the reduction in bioavailability due to H_2-blockers can be minimised by administering itraconazole and ketoconazole with an acidic drink such as *Coca-cola*.[7]

Fluconazole is an alternative antifungal that only interacts to a small and clinically irrelevant extent with H_2-blockers and is therefore a possible alternative to ketoconazole and itraconazole. It is not expected to be affected by antacids and does not interact with sucralfate.

1. Thorpe JE, Baker N, Bromet-Petit M. Effect of oral antacid administration on the pharmacokinetics of oral fluconazole. *Antimicrob Agents Chemother* (1990) 34, 2032–3.
2. Lazar JD, Wilner KD. Drug interactions with fluconazole. *Rev Infect Dis* (1990) 12 (Suppl 3), S327–S333.
3. Blum RA, D'Andrea DT, Florentino BM, Wilton JH, Hilligoss DM, Gardner MJ, Henry EB, Goldstein H, Schentag JJ. Increased gastric pH and the bioavailability of fluconazole and ketoconazole. *Ann Intern Med* (1991) 114, 755–7.
4. Lim SG, Sawyerr AM, Hudson M, Sercombe J, Pounder RE. Short report: The absorption of fluconazole and itraconazole under conditions of low intragastric acidity. *Aliment Pharmacol Ther* (1993) 7, 317–21.
5. Carver PL, Hoeschele JD, Partipilo L, Kauffman CA, Mercer BT, Pecoraro VL. Fluconazole: a model compound for in vitro and in vivo interactions with sucralfate. *Pharmacotherapy* (1994) 14, 347.
6. Stein AG, Daneshmend TK, Warnock DW, Bhaskar N, Burke J, Hawkey CJ. The effects of H_2-receptor antagonists on the pharmacokinetics of itraconazole, a new oral antifungal. *Br J Clin Pharmacol* (1989) 27, 105P–106P.
7. Hardin J, Lange D., Wu J, Klausner M. The effect of a cola beverage on the bioavailability of itraconazole in the presence of H_2 blockers. *Intersci Conf Antimicrob Agents Chemother* (1994) 34, 39.
8. Patterson TF, Peters J, McGough DA, Fothergill AW, Levine SM, Anzueto A, Bryan CL, Sako EY, Miller OL, Calhoon JC, Rinaldi MG. Serum itraconazole levels in lung transplant patients receiving concomitant antacid/H_2-blocker therapy. *Intersci Conf Antimicrob Agents Chemother* (1994) 34, 39.
9. Patterson TF, Peters J, Levine SM, Anzueto A, Bryan CL, Sako EY, LaWayne Miller O, Calhoon JH, Rinaldi MG. Systemic availability of itraconazole in lung transplantation. *Antimicrob Agents Chemother* (1996) 40, 2217–20.
10. Kanda Y, Kami M, Matsuyama T, Mitani K, Chiba S, Yazaki Y, Hirai H. Plasma concentration of itraconazole in patients receiving chemotherapy for hematological malignancies: the effect of famotidine on the absorption of itraconazole. *Hematol Oncol* (1998) 16, 33–7.
11. Van der Meer JWM, Keuning JJ, Scheijgrond HW, Heykants J, Van Cutsem J, Brugmans J. The influence of gastric acidity on the bio-availability of ketoconazole. *J Antimicrob Chemother* (1980) 6, 552–4.
12. Goss TF, Piscitelli SC, Schentag JJ. Evaluation of ketoconazole bioavailability interactions with sucralfate and ranitidine using gastric pH monitoring. *Clin Pharmacol Ther* (1991) 49, 128.
13. Piscitelli SC, Goss TF, Wilton JH, D'Andrea DT, Goldstein H, Schentag JJ. Effects of ranitidine and sucralfate on ketoconazole bioavailability. *Antimicrob Agents Chemother* (1991) 35, 1765–71.
14. Carver PL, Berardi RR, Knapp MJ, Rider JM, Kauffman CA, Bradley SF, Atassi M. In vivo interaction of ketoconazole and sucralfate in healthy volunteers. *Antimicrob Agents Chemother* (1994) 38, 326–9.
15. Brass C, Galgiani JN, Blaschke TF, Defelice R, O'Reilly RA, Stevens DA. Disposition of ketoconazole, an oral antifungal, in humans. *Antimicrob Agents Chemother* (1982) 21, 151–8.
16. Franklin MG. Nizoral and stomatitis cocktails may not mix. *Oncol Nurs Forum* (1991) 18, 1417.
17. Sutherland C, Murphy JE, Schleifer NH. The effects of two gastric acidifying agents on the pharmacokinetics of ketoconazole. 18th Annual Midyear Clinical Meeting of the American Society of Hospital Pharmacists, Atlanta, Georgia, Dec 4–8, 1983, 141.
18. Hoeschele JD, Roy AK, Pecoraro VL, Carver PL. In vitro analysis of the interaction between sucralfate and ketoconazole. *Antimicrob Agents Chemother* (1994) 38, 319–25.

Azole antifungals + Cytotoxic agents

Preliminary evidence suggests that the pharmacokinetics of fluconazole are less likely to be affected by cytotoxic drugs than itraconazole, and it may therefore be the drug of choice for treating fungal infections in patients receiving chemotherapy. Itraconazole can increase the toxicity of vincristine.

Clinical evidence, mechanism, importance and management

(a) Effect of cytotoxics on azole antifungals

A study in 10 leukaemic patients (AML and ALL) found that the pharmacokinetics of 100 mg **fluconazole** were not affected by 15 days of chemotherapy. The cytotoxic drugs used were **daunorubicin**, **cytarabine**, **vincristine**, **prednisone**, **asparaginase** and **idarubicin**, either alone or in combination. In contrast, a parallel study in another 10 leukaemic patients suggested that there may be some changes in the pharmacokinetics of **itraconazole** in individual patients. There was no consistent pattern of changes in the AUCs for these patients. The scatter was wide, and some AUCs were raised while others were lowered. The cytotoxics used were as before.[1]

On the basis of these findings the authors of the report suggest that because of the apparent risk of over- or underdosage with **itraconazole** in these patients, **fluconazole** may be the more reliable agent for the prevention and treatment of candidiasis in the presence of these cytotoxic drugs.[1] It needs to be emphasised that these results were derived from only a relatively small number of patients, taking different combinations of drugs, so that the conclusions should only be regarded as preliminary. Much more study is still needed. See also (b) for a serious reaction with **itraconazole** and **vincristine**.

(b) Effect of azole antifungals on cytotoxics

Four out of 14 patients with ALL given induction chemotherapy with weekly injections of **vincristine** (with prednisone, daunorubicin and asparaginase) and antifungal prophylaxis with 400 mg **itraconazole** daily, developed severe and early **vincristine**-induced neurotoxicity (paraesthesia and muscle weakness of the hands and feet, paralytic ileus, mild laryngeal nerve paralysis). The degree and early onset of these neurotoxic reactions were unusual, and were all reversible except for mild paraesthesia in one patient. The complications were more serious than in a previous series of 460 patients previously treated with **vincristine** but without the **itraconazole** (29% compared to 6%).[2] Five children with ALL developed severe **vincristine** toxicity attributed to concurrent treatment with **itraconazole**. They were also receiving **nifedipine** which is known to reduce the clearance of **vincristine** and which may have made things worse.[3] Other studies similarly indicate that greater **vincristine** toxicity may occur in patients given **itraconazole**.[3] The reasons for this interaction are not understood, but among the suggestions are that the **itraconazole** inhibits the metabolism of **vincristine** by cytochrome P450-dependent enzymes so that it is cleared from the body less quickly or, less likely, that **itraconazole** inhibits the P-glycoprotein efflux pump.[2] The authors of one report[2] suggest that **itraconazole** should be avoided, and the makers of **vincristine** also issue a warning about the increased risks.[4]

1. Lazo de la Vega S, Volkow P, Yeates RA, Pfaff G. Administration of the antimycotic agents fluconazole and itraconazole to leukaemia patients: a comparative pharmacokinetic study. *Drugs Exp Clin Res* (1994) 20, 69–75.
2. Böhme A, Ganser A, Hoelzer D. Aggravation of vincristine-induced neurotoxicity by itraconazole in the treatment of adult ALL. *Ann Hematol* (1995) 71, 311–12.
3. Murphy JA, Ross LM, Gibson BES. Vincristine toxicity in five children with acute lymphoblastic leukaemia. *Lancet* (1995) 346, 443.
4. Oncovin (Vincristine). Eli Lilly and Company Limited. Summary of product characteristics, October 1998.

Azole antifungals + Food

Itraconazole capsules should be taken with or after food to achieve the best results from treatment, whereas solution should be taken before food. The makers advise taking ketoconazole with food, but the background evidence supporting this is confusing and contradictory.

Clinical evidence

(a) Fluconazole

A study in 12 healthy subjects found that there was no therapeutically relevant effect of **food** on the pharmacokinetics of **fluconazole**.[1]

(b) Itraconazole

A study in 24 patients with superficial dermatophyte, *Candida albicans* and pityriasis versicolor infections given 50 or 100-mg doses of **itraconazole** daily showed that taking the drug with or after **breakfast** produced higher serum levels and gave much better treatment results than taking it before **breakfast**.[2] A later study found that the relative **itraconazole** bioavailabilities were 54% on an empty stomach, 86% after a **light meal** and 100% after a **full meal**.[1]

In contrast to these results with **itraconazole** capsules, studies with the oral solution give different results. A study in 30 healthy males given 200 mg **itraconazole** solution daily, either on an empty stomach or with a standard **breakfast**, showed that the bioavailability was 29% higher when taken in the fasted state.[3]

In another study of 20 HIV+ patients, glutamic acid (1360 mg), giv-

en to acidify the stomach, either with or without food did not enhance **itraconazole** absorption.[4]

(c) Ketoconazole

One study found that the AUC and peak serum concentrations of a single 200-mg dose of **ketoconazole** were reduced by about 40% (from 14.4 to 8.6 micrograms.h/ml and from 4.1 to 2.3 micrograms/ml respectively) when taken by 10 healthy subjects after a **standardised meal**.[5] Another study found that **high carbohydrate** and **fat** diets tended to reduce the rate, but not the overall amount of **ketoconazole** absorbed.[6] A third study found that the absorption of single 200 or 800-mg doses of **ketoconazole** in eight healthy subjects was not altered when taken after a **standardised breakfast** although the peak serum levels were delayed. The absorption of single 400 and 600 mg doses were somewhat increased by **food**.[7]

Mechanism

Not understood.

Importance and management

There appears to be no relevant food/fluconazole interaction. Itraconazole absorption from capsule formulation is best with or after food, whereas absorption form the acidic solution appears to be better before food. A confusing and conflicting picture is presented by the studies with ketoconazole. However the manufacturers of ketoconazole say that "absorption of ketoconazole is maximal when taken during a meal, as it depends on stomach acidity" and "should always be taken with meals".

1. Zimmermann T, Yeates RA, Laufen H, Pfaff G, Wildfeuer A. Influence of concomitant food intake on the oral absorption of two triazole antifungal agents, itraconazole and fluconazole. *Eur J Clin Pharmacol* (1994) 46, 147–150.
2. Wishart JM. The influence of food on the pharmacokinetics of itraconazole in patients with superficial fungal infection. *J Am Acad Dermatol* (1987) 17, 220–3.
3. Barone JA, Moskovitz BL, Guarnieri J, Hassell AE, Colaizzi JL, Bierman RH, Jessen L. Food interaction and steady-state pharmacokinetics of itraconazole oral solution in healthy volunteers. *Pharmacotherapy* (1998) 18, 295–301.
4. Carver P, Welage L, Kauffman C. The effect of food and gastric pH on the oral bioavailability of itraconazole in HIV+ patients. *Intersci Conf Antimicrob Agents Chemother* (1996) 36, 6.
5. Männistö PT, Mäntylä R, Nykänen S, Lamminsivu U, Ottoila P. Impairing effect of food on ketoconazole absorption. *Antimicrob Agents Chemother* (1982) 21, 730–33.
6. Lelawongs P, Barone JA, Colaizzi JL, Hsuan ATM, Mechlinski W, Legendre R, Guarnieri J. Effect of food and gastric acidity on absorption of orally administered ketoconazole. *Clin Pharm* (1988) 7, 228–16.
7. Daneshmend TK, Warnock DW, Ene MD, Johnson EM, Potten MR, Richardson MD, Williamson PJ. Influence of food on the pharmacokinetics of ketoconazole. *Antimicrob Agents Chemother* (1984) 25, 1–3.

Azole antifungals + Proton pump inhibitors

Omeprazole reduces the acidity of the stomach and markedly reduces the bioavailability of ketoconazole. Rabeprazole also reduces the bioavailability of ketoconazole. Other proton pump inhibitors are expected to behave similarly.

Clinical evidence

(a) Omeprazole

Itraconazole 200 mg was given to 11 healthy subjects after 14 days pre-treatment with **omeprazole** 40 mg daily. The AUC and maximum serum level of **itraconazole** were both reduced by about 65%.[1]

A three-way crossover study in 9 healthy subjects found that when 200 mg **ketoconazole** was taken with 60 mg **omeprazole**, the AUC of the ketoconazole was reduced to about 20% (a reduction from 17.9 to 3.5 mg.h/l).[2] Another study was carried out in 10 healthy subjects (both 'extensive' and 'poor' metabolisers) to find out how much cytochrome P450 isoenzyme CYP3A4 is involved in the metabolism (sulfoxidation) of **omeprazole**. This revealed that 100 to 200 mg **ketoconazole,** a known inhibitor of CYP3A4, led to a fall in the formation of the **omeprazole sulfone** in both groups, and a doubling of serum **omeprazole** levels in the poor metabolisers.[3]

(b) Rabeprazole

In a randomised placebo-controlled study 18 healthy subjects were given 400 mg **ketoconazole** before and after taking 20 mg **rabeprazole** or a placebo daily for 7 days. Significant decreases in the **ketoconazole** AUC and in the maximum serum levels were found, representing about a reduction in its bioavailability.[4] There was no evidence that the **rabeprazole** affected the **ketoconazole** metabolism.

Mechanism

Ketoconazole and itraconazole are a poorly soluble bases, which must be transformed by the acid in the stomach into the soluble hydrochloride salt. Agents which reduce gastric secretions, such as proton pump inhibitors, H_2-blockers or antacids, raise the pH in the stomach so that the dissolution and absorption of drugs such as itraconazole or ketoconazole are reduced. Conversely, anything that increases the gastric acidity increases its dissolution and absorption. The rise in omeprazole levels caused by ketoconazole is almost certainly because the metabolism of omeprazole by cytochrome CYP3A4 is inhibited.

Importance and management

The ketoconazole/omeprazole interaction appears to be established and of clinical importance. Direct evidence seems to be limited to this study but other drugs that raise the gastric pH have a similar effect (see 'Azole antifungals + Antacids, H_2-blockers or Sucralfate', p.139). Such a large reduction in the absorption of ketoconazole would be expected to result in the failure of treatment. Separating the dosages of the two drugs is unlikely to be the answer because the effect of omeprazole is so prolonged. A better solution might be to use fluconazole instead, the bioavailability of which is not affected by omeprazole.[5] The authors of the itraconazole study suggest that if the combination cannot be avoided higher doses of itraconazole should be used.[1] The rise in the serum omeprazole levels caused by the ketoconazole is of uncertain clinical importance.

The ketoconazole/rabeprazole interaction is also established but the reduction in the bioavailability is only moderate (30%) and it may be possible to accommodate this by raising the dosage, although the makers suggest that consideration should be given to stopping the rabeprazole. It seems possible that fluconazole may not interact with rabeprazole but this needs confirmation.

There appear to be no reports about ketoconazole and other proton pump inhibitors (pantoprazole, lansoprazole) but they are also expected to interact to reduce the bioavailability of the ketoconazole, but the extent is not known. These predictions all need confirmation.

1. Jararatanasirikul S, Sriwiriyajan S. Effect of omeprazole on the pharmacokinetics of itraconazole. *Eur J Clin Pharmacol* (1998) 54, 159–61.
2. Chin TWF, Leob M, Fong IW. Effects of an acidic beverage (Coca-Cola) on absorption of ketoconazole. *Antimicrob Agents Chemother* (1995) 39, 1671–5.
3. Böttiger Y, Tybring G, Götharson E, Bertilsson L. Inhibition of the sulfoxidation of omeprazole by ketoconazole in poor and extensive metabolizers of S-mephenytoin. *Clin Pharmacol Ther* (1997) 62, 384–91.
4. Humphries TJ, Nardi RV, Spera AC, Lazar JD, Laurent AL, Spanyers SA. Coadministration of rabeprazole sodium (E3810) and ketoconazole results in a predictable interaction with ketoconazole. *Gastroenterology* (1996) 110 (Suppl), A138.
5. Zimmermann T, Yeates RA, Riedel K-D, Lach P, Laufen H. The influence of gastric pH on the pharmacokinetics of fluconazole: the effect of omeprazole. *Int J Clin Pharmacol Ther* (1994) 32, 491–6.

Bacampicillin + Miscellaneous drugs

Bacampicillin appears not to be affected by food, but a reduction in its bioavailability may possibly occur if the gastric pH is increased.

Clinical evidence, mechanism, importance and management

Bacampicillin is a prodrug, without appreciable antibacterial properties of its own, which is hydrolysed in the body to active ampicillin. Although direct clinical evidence is largely lacking, it would be expected to interact like ampicillin (see the Index). One very limited study suggested that **food** decreases the bioavailability of bacampicillin about 26%, and when given with 300 mg **ranitidine** and 4 g **sodium bicarbonate**, either with or without **breakfast**, the bioavailability was also reduced, by 84% and 55% respectively.[1] However, these results have been criticised.[2] On the basis of other work which suggests that no important interaction occurs with food,[3] the makers say that bacampicillin can be given without regard to time of **food** intake. The observations regarding **ranitidine** and **sodium bicarbonate** remain unconfirmed, and their clinical significance is uncertain.

1. Sommers DK, van Wyk M, Moncrieff J, Schoeman HS. Influence of food and reduced gastric acidity on the bioavailability of bacampicillin and cefuroxime axetil. *Br J Clin Pharmacol* (1984) 18, 535–9.
2. Upjohn Limited, Personal communication, April 1993.
3. Magni L, Sjöberg B, Sjövall J, Wessman J. Clinical pharmacological studies with bacampicillin, in Chemotherapy (1976) 5, 109–114, edited by Williams JD, Geddes AM. Plenum Publishing Corp, NY.

Caspofungin + Itraconazole

Caspofungin and itraconazole appear not to interact.

Clinical evidence, mechanism, importance and management

Caspofungin 70 mg on day 1 and 50 mg for the next 13 days did not alter the pharmacokinetics of **itraconazole** 200 mg daily.[1] The pharmacokinetics of caspofungin were also unaltered by concurrent administration.

1. Stone JA, McCrea JB, Wickersham PJ, Holland SD, Deutsch PJ, Bi S, Cicero T, Greenberg H, Waldman SA. A phase I study of caspofungin evaluating the potential for drug interactions with itraconazole, the effect of gender and the use of a loading dose regimen. *Intersci Conf Antimicrob Agents Chemother* (2000) 40, 26.

Cefalotin + Colistimethate sodium

Renal failure has been attributed to the concurrent use of cefalotin and colistimethate sodium.

Clinical evidence, mechanism, importance and management

Four patients developed acute renal failure, which appeared to be reversible, during treatment with **colistimethate sodium (colistin sulphomethate sodium)**. Three were given cefalotin concurrently and the fourth had previously been treated with this antibacterial.[1] An increase in renal toxicity associated with concurrent use has been described in another report.[2] The reason for this reaction is not known. What is known suggests that renal function should be closely monitored if these antibacterials are given concurrently or sequentially.

1. Adler S, Segal DP. Nonoliguric renal failure secondary to sodium colistimethate: a report of four cases. *Am J Med Sci* (1971) 262, 109–14.
2. Koch-Weser J, Sidel VW, Federman EB, Kanarek P, Finer DC, Eaton AE. Adverse effects of sodium colistimethate. Manifestations and specific reaction rates during 317 courses of therapy. *Ann Intern Med* (1970) 72, 857–68.

Cefotaxime + Ofloxacin

Cefotaxime appears not to interact with ofloxacin.

Clinical evidence, mechanism, importance and management

In a study of 11 healthy subjects, the pharmacokinetics of cefotaxime and **ofloxacin** were similar, whether given singly or in combination, and the antimicrobial effect of the combination was additive for *S. au-*

reus, S. pneumoniae, E. cloacae and *K. pneumoniae*, but not against *P. aeruginosa*.[1] This suggests that the combination can be given safely.

1. Nix DE, Wilton JH, Hyatt J, Thomas J, Strenkoski-Nix LC, Forrest A, Schentag JJ. Pharmacodynamic modeling of the in vivo interaction between cefotaxime and ofloxacin by using serum ultrafiltrate inhibitory titers. *Antimicrob Agents Chemother* (1997) 41, 1108–14.

Cephalosporins + Antacids, H₂-blockers or Pirenzepine

No clinically significant interactions appear to occur between *Maalox* and cefalexin, cefetamet pivoxil, cefixime or cefprozil; between *Alka-Seltzer* and cefixime; between cefditoren pivoxil and either aluminium hydroxide or cimetidine; between cefetamet pivoxil or ranitidine; between cefalexin or pirenzepine, or between ceftibuten and *Mylanta* or ranitidine. Maalox and famotidine reduce the bioavailability of cefpodoxime proxetil, while ranitidine with sodium bicarbonate reduces the bioavailability of cefuroxime axetil. *Maalox* and cimetidine also cause a small reduction in the bioavailability of cefaclor AF.

Clinical evidence, mechanism, importance and management

(a) Cefaclor + Maalox

A study of **cefaclor AF** (a formulation with a slower rate of release) found that 800 mg **cimetidine** the night before reduced its maximum serum concentration by 12%, whereas *Maalox* given one hour after the **cefaclor AF** in the fed state reduced the AUC by 18%.[1] These reductions are small and unlikely to be clinically important, but this needs confirmation.

(b) Cefetamet pivoxil + Maalox or Ranitidine

Eighteen healthy subjects were given 1 g **cefetamet pivoxil** after breakfast for 3 study periods. In the first, the pharmacokinetics of **cefetamet** alone were assessed, in the second they were additionally given 80 ml *Maalox 70* the evening before and again 2 h before and after breakfast, and in the third they were additionally given 150 mg **ranitidine** twice daily for 4 days. The pharmacokinetics of the **cefetamet** were similar in all study periods.[2] No special precautions seem to be needed if given concurrently.

(c) Cefixime, Cefalexin or Cefprozil + Maalox, Pirenzepine or Alka-Seltzer

Maalox (10 doses of 10 ml), **ranitidine** (150 mg for 3 doses) or **pirenzepine** (50 mg for 4 doses) had only small and therapeutically unimportant effects on the pharmacokinetics of 1 g **cefalexin**.[3] *Maalox* and *Alka-Seltzer* do not significantly affect the absorption of **cefixime**,[4,5] and *Maalox* does not affect the bioavailability of **cefprozil**.[6] No special precautions would seem necessary if any of these drugs is used concurrently.

(d) Cefpodoxime proxetil or Cefuroxime axetil + Maalox, Famotidine, Ranitidine or Sodium bicarbonate

A study in 10 healthy subjects showed that 10 ml *Maalox* or 40 mg **famotidine** reduced the bioavailability of **cefpodoxime proxetil** by about 40%, thought to be due to reduced dissolution at increased gastric pH values.[7] This confirms the findings of a previous study.[8] It has been recommended that **cefpodoxime** is given at least 2 h after antacids or H₂-blockers which can raise the gastric pH.[7]

Ranitidine 300 mg with 4 g **sodium bicarbonate** reduced the AUC of 1 g **cefuroxime axetil** in one study by over 65% and the urinary recovery fell by over 35%.[9] It would seem reasonable to follow the same precautions with **cefuroxime** as those recommended for **cefpodoxime** (see above), although the clinical importance of neither of these two interactions seems to have been studied. Other anti-ulcer drugs (H₂-blockers, proton pump inhibitors, **antacids etc**) which can raise the pH would be expected to interact similarly.

(e) Ceftibuten + Mylanta or Ranitidine

60 ml *Mylanta II* was found not to affect the pharmacokinetics of 400 mg **ceftibuten** in 18 healthy subjects, whereas 150 mg **ranitidine** 12-hourly for 3 days raised the maximum serum levels of **ceftibuten** by 23% and the AUC by 16%. However these values lie within the normal ranges seen in healthy subjects and no dosage adjustment is thought to be needed.[10,11]

1. Satterwhite JH, Cerimele BJ, Coleman DL, Hatcher BL, Kisicki J, DeSante KA. Pharmacokinetics of cefaclor AF: effects of age, antacids and H₂-receptor antagonists. *Postgrad Med J* (1992) 68 (Suppl 3), S3–S9.

2. Blouin RA, Kneer J, Ambros RJ, Stoeckel K. Influence of antacid and ranitidine on the pharmacokinetics of oral cefetamet pivoxil. *Antimicrob Agents Chemother* (1990) 34, 1744–8.

3. Deppermann K-M, Lode H, Höffken G, Tschink G, Kalz C, Koeppe P. Influence of ranitidine, pirenzepine, and aluminum magnesium hydroxide on the bioavailability of various antibiotics, including amoxicillin, cephalexin, doxycycline and amoxicillinclavulanic acid. *Antimicrob Agents Chemother* (1989) 33, 1901–1907.

4. Petitjean O, Brion N, Tod M, Montagne A, Nicolas P. Étude de l'interaction pharmacocinétique entre le céfixime et deux antiacides. Résultats préliminaires. *Presse Med* (1989) 18, 1596–8.

5. Healy DP, Sahai JV, Sterling LP, Racht EM. Influence of an antacid containing aluminum and magnesium on the pharmacokinetics of cefixime. *Antimicrob Agents Chemother* (1989) 33, 1994–7.

6. Shyu WC, Wilber RB, Pittman KA, Barbhaiya RH. Effect of antacid on the bioavailability of cefprozil. *Antimicrob Agents Chemother* (1992) 36, 962–5.

7. Saathoff N, Lode H, Neider K, Depperman KM, Borner K, Koeppe P. Pharmacokinetics of cefpodoxime proxetil and interactions with an antacid and an H₂ receptor antagonist. *Antimicrob Agents Chemother* (1992) 36, 796–800.

8. Hughes GS, Heald DL, Barker KB, Patel RK, Spillers CR, Watts KC, Batts DH, Euler AR. The effects of gastric pH and food on the pharmacokinetics of a new oral cephalosporin, cefpodoxime proxetil. *Clin Pharmacol Ther* (1989) 46, 674–85.

9. Sommers De K, Van Wyk M, Moncrieff J, Schoeman HS. Influence of food and reduced gastric acidity on the bioavailability of bacampicillin and cefuroxime axetil. *Br J Clin Pharmacol* (1984) 18, 535–9.

10. Radwanski E, Nomeir A, Cutler D, Fettner S, Lin C, Affrime M, Batra V. Pharmacokinetics of ceftibuten administered with and without Mylanta II or ranitidine. *Pharm Res* (1993) 10 (10 Suppl), S-310.

11. Radwanski E, Nomeir A, Cutler D, Affrime M, Lin C-C. Pharmacokinetic drug interaction study: administration of ceftibuten concurrently with the antacid Mylanta double-strength liquid or with ranitidine. *Am J Ther* (1998) 5, 67–72.

Cephalosporins + Calcium channel blockers

Nifedipine increases the serum levels of cefixime but this is unlikely to be clinically important. Neither nifedipine nor diltiazem affect the pharmacokinetics of cefpodoxime proxetil.

Clinical evidence, mechanism, importance and management

The AUC of a single 200-mg dose of **cefixime** was increased by about 70% in 8 healthy subjects and the peak serum levels increased almost 50% when taken 30 min after a 20-mg dose of **nifedipine**. The rate of absorption was also increased. No adverse responses were seen. One suggested reason is that the **nifedipine** increases the absorption of the **cefixime** by affecting the carrier system across the epithelial wall of the gut.[1] It seems doubtful if this increased **cefixime** bioavailability is clinically important (the combination was well-tolerated) and no particular precautions would seem to be necessary with concurrent use.

The pharmacokinetics of single 200-mg doses of **cefpodoxime proxetil** in 12 healthy subjects were found to be unchanged by single doses of either 60 mg **diltiazem** or 20 mg **nifedipine** in another study.[2] No special precautions during concurrent use would seem necessary. Information about other cephalosporins and calcium channel blockers seems to be lacking.

1. Duverne C, Bouten A, Deslandes A, Westphal J-F, Trouvin J-H, Farinotti R, Carbon C. Modification of cefixime bioavailability by nifedipine in humans: involvement of the dipeptide carrier system. *Antimicrob Agents Chemother* (1992) 36, 2462–7.

2. Deslandes A, Camus F, Lacroix C, Carbon C, Farinotti R. Effects of nifedipine and diltiazem on pharmacokinetics of cefpodoxime following its oral administration. *Antimicrob Agents Chemother* (1996) 40, 2879–81.

Cephalosporins + Colestyramine

Colestyramine binds with cefadroxil and cefalexin in the gut, which delays their absorption. The importance of this is uncertain but probably small.

Clinical evidence

The peak serum levels of cefadroxil (after a 500 mg oral dose) were reduced and delayed in 4 subjects when the antibacterial was taken with 10 g colestyramine, but the total amount absorbed was not affected.[1] Similar results were found in a study involving cefalexin and colestyramine.[2]

Mechanism

Colestyramine is an ion-exchange resin, which binds with these two cephalosporins in the gut. This prevents the early and rapid absorption of the antibacterial, but as the colestyramine/cephalosporin complex passes along the gastro-intestinal tract, the antibacterial is progressively released and eventually virtually all of it becomes available for absorption.[1]

Importance and management

Direct information seems to be limited to the studies cited. The clinical significance is uncertain, but as the total amount of antibacterial absorbed is not reduced this interaction is probably of little importance. This needs confirmation. Information about other cephalosporins seems to be lacking.

1. Marino EL, Vicente MT and Dominguez-Gil A. Influence of cholestyramine on the pharmacokinetic parameters of cefadroxil after simultaneous administration. *Int J Pharmaceutics* (1983) 16, 23–30.
2. Parsons RL, Paddock GM. Absorption of two antibacterial drugs, cephalexin and co-trimoxazole, in malabsorption syndromes. *J Antimicrob Chemother* (1975) 1 (Suppl), 59–67.

Cephalosporins + Food or Miscellaneous drugs

The pharmacokinetics of cefprozil are minimally affected by food, propantheline and metoclopramide,[1] and the pharmacokinetics of cefpodoxime proxetil are minimally affected by food[2] and acetylcysteine.[3] None of these interactions is likely to be clinically important. However, the clearance of ceftazidime is significantly reduced by indometacin in neonates and dosage adjustments are likely to be necessary.[4]

1. Shukla UA, Pittman KA, Barbhaiya RH. Pharmacokinetic interactions of cefprozil with food, propantheline, metoclopramide, and probenecid in healthy volunteers. *J Clin Pharmacol* (1992) 32, 725–31.
2. Borin MT, Forbes KK. Effect of food on absorption of cefpodoxime proxetil oral suspension in adults. *Antimicrob Agents Chemother* (1995) 273–5.
3. Kees F, Wellenhofer M, Bröhl K, Grobecker H. Bioavailability of cefpodoxime proxetil with co-administered acetylcysteine. *Arzneimittelforschung* (1996) 46, 435–8.
4. van den Anker JN, Hop WCJ, Schoemaker RC, Van der Heijden BJ, Neijens HJ, De Groot R. Ceftazidime pharmacokinetics in preterm infants: effect of postnatal age and postnatal exposure to indometacin. *Br J Clin Pharmacol* (1995) 40, 439–43.

Cephalosporins + Furosemide (Frusemide)

The nephrotoxic effects of cefaloridine appear to be increased by the concurrent use of furosemide (frusemide) and there is some limited evidence of nephrotoxicity with cefalotin and cefacetrile. Cefradine brain levels are reduced by furosemide. No important interactions appear to occur between furosemide and either cefoxitin, ceftazidime or ceftriaxone.

Clinical evidence

(a) Nephrotoxicity

Nine out of 36 patients who developed acute renal failure while taking cefaloridine had also been treated with a diuretic, furosemide (frusemide) being used in 7 cases. Other factors such as age and dosage may also have been involved. The authors of this report related their observations to previous *animal* studies which showed that potent diuretics such as furosemide and etacrynic acid enhanced the incidence and extent of tubular necrosis.[1] Several other reports describe nephrotoxicity in patients given both cephaloridine and furosemide (frusemide).[2-4] There is a question mark hanging over cefalotin and cefacetrile because *animal* studies have demonstrated increased nephrotoxicity,[5,6] and there is a single report describing nephrotoxicity in one patient on cefalotin and furosemide.[2]

(b) Changes in serum levels and clearance

A clinical study showed that 80 mg furosemide (frusemide) increased the serum half-life of cefaloridine by 25%[7] and in another study its clearance was reduced.[8,9] Another study found that brain concentrations of cefradine are markedly reduced by furosemide.[10]

Mechanism

Cefaloridine is nephrotoxic, but why this should be increased by furosemide is not understood. It may possibly be related to the fall in its clearance[8,9] and an increase in its serum half-life.[7]

Importance and management

The cefaloridine/furosemide (frusemide) interaction is not well-established, but there is enough evidence to suggest that concurrent use should be undertaken with care. Age and/or renal impairment may possibly be predisposing factors. Renal function should be checked frequently. A pharmacokinetic study suggests that the development of this adverse interaction may possibly depend on the time relationship of drug administration, and it has been recommended that furosemide should be avoided 3 or 4 h before the cefaloridine.[11]

Although the makers of ceftazidime issue a caution about its use with other nephrotoxic drugs, they say that clinical experience has not shown this to be a problem at the recommended doses.[12] The rest of the information about other cephalosporins and furosemide is fairly sparse. Most appear not to interact adversely, with a few possible exceptions, namely cefalotin (nephrotoxicity in a single case[2] and *animal* studies[5]) and cephacetrile (nephrotoxicity in *animal* studies[6]). Care is clearly needed with these two cephalosporins. Cefoxitin seems to be relatively free of nephrotoxicity alone or with furosemide.[13] Ceftriaxone does not interfere with the diuretic effects of furosemide in man.[14]

1. Dodds MG, Foord RD. Enhancement by potent diuretics of renal tubular necrosis induced by cephaloridine. *Br J Pharmacol* (1970) 4, 227–36.
2. Simpson IJ. Nephrotoxicity and acute renal failure associated with cephalothin and cephaloridine. *N Z Med J* (1971) 74, 312–15.
3. Kleinknecht D, Jungers P, Fillastre J-P. Nephrotoxicity of cephaloridine. *Ann Intern Med* (1974) 80, 421–2.
4. Lawson DH, Macadam RF, Singh H, Gavras H, Linton AL. The nephrotoxicity of cephaloridine. *Postgrad Med J* (1970) 46 (Suppl), 36–9.
5. Lawson DH, Macadam RF, Singh H, Gavras H, Hartz S, Turnbull D, Linton AL. Effect of furosemide on antibiotic-induced renal damage in rats. *J Infect Dis* (1972) 126, 593–600.
6. Luscombe DK, Nichols PJ. Possible interaction between cephacetrile and frusemide in rabbits and rats. *J Antimicrob Chemother* (1975) 1, 67–77.
7. Norrby R, Stenqvist K, Elgefors B. Interaction between cephaloridine and furosemide in man. *Scand J Infect Dis* (1976) 8, 209–212.
8. Lawson DH, Tilstone WJ, Semple PF. Furosemide interactions: studies in normal volunteers. *Clin Res* (1976) 24, 3.
9. Tilstone WJ, Semple PF, Lawson DH, Boyle JA. Effects of furosemide on glomerular filtration rate and clearance of practolol, digoxin, cephaloridine and gentamicin. *Clin Pharmacol Ther* (1977) 22, 389–94.
10. Adam D, Jacoby W, Raff WK. Beeinflussung der Antibiotika-Konzentration im Gewebe durch ein Saluretikum. *Klin Wochenschr* (1978) 56, 247–51.
11. Kosmidis J, Polyzos A, Daikos GK. Pharmacokinetic interactions between cephalosporins and furosemide are influenced by administration time relationships. Curr Chemother Infect Dis. PISF Int Congr Chemother 11th (1979 and 1980) 673–5.
12. Fortum for injection (Ceftazidime). Glaxo Wellcome. Summary of product characteristics, December 1999.
13. Trollfors B, Norrby R, Kristianson K, Nilsson NJ. Effects on renal function of treatment with cefoxitin alone or in combination with furosemide. *Scand J Infect Dis* (1978) (Suppl), 13, 73–7.
14. Korn A, Eichler HG, Gasic S. A drug interaction study of ceftriaxone and frusemide in healthy volunteers. *Int J Clin Pharmacol Ther Toxicol* (1986) 24, 262–4.

Cephalosporins + Iron preparations

Ferrous sulphate markedly reduces the absorption of cefdinir.

Clinical evidence

When 6 healthy subjects were given **ferrous sulphate** (1050 mg *Fero-Gradumet*, sustained release, equivalent to 210 mg **elemental iron**) with 200 mg **cefdinir**, the bioavailability of the **cefdinir** was reduced by 93%, as measured by the AUC. When the **ferrous sulphate** was taken 3 h after the **cefdinir**, the absorption of the **cefdinir** remained unchanged for 3 h and then rapidly fell, the total AUC over 12 h being reduced by 36%.[1]

Mechanism

It is believed that the ferrous sulphate chelates with the cefdinir in the gut to produce a poorly absorbed complex.

Importance and management

An established interaction of clinical importance. Avoid ferrous sulphate and other iron salts while taking cefdinir. It is not yet known how far apart these drugs must be separated to avoid this interaction but 3 h improves the situation considerably even if it does not totally solve it. No other cephalosporins appear to interact in this way.

1. Ueno K, Tanaka K, Tsujimura K, Morishima Y, Iwashige H, Yamazaki K, Nakata I. Impairment of cefdinir absorption by iron ion. *Clin Pharmacol Ther* (1993) 54, 473–5.

Cephalosporins + Penicillins

Mezlocillin reduces the loss of cefotaxime from the body in the presence of normal renal function.

Clinical evidence, mechanism, importance and management

When **cefotaxime** (30 mg/kg) and **mezlocillin** (50 mg/kg) were infused together, over 30 min, in 8 healthy subjects, the pharmacokinetics of the **mezlocillin** were unchanged but the clearance of the **cefotaxime** was reduced by 40 to 42%. In 5 concurrently studied patients with end-stage renal-disease no significant decrease in **cefotaxime** clearance was seen. The clinical significance of this interaction is uncertain.[1,2]

1. Flaherty J, Barriere S, Gambertoglio J. Interaction between cefotaxime (C) and mezlocillin (M). *Clin Pharmacol Ther* (1985) 37, 196.
2. Rodondi LC, Flaherty JF, Schoenfeld P, Barriere SL, Gambertoglio JG. Influence of coadministration on the pharmacokinetics of mezlocillin and cefotaxime in healthy volunteers and in patients with renal failure. *Clin Pharmacol Ther* (1989) 45, 527–34.

Cephalosporins + Phenobarbital

A marked increase in serious skin reactions has been seen in children given cefotaxime and high-dose phenobarbital.

Clinical evidence, mechanism, importance and management

A 30-month study observed a very marked increase in drug-induced reactions in children in intensive care who were treated with high-dose **phenobarbital** and beta-lactam antibacterials, mainly **cefotaxime**. Twenty-four out of 49 children developed drug-induced reactions, which were mainly exanthematous skin reactions.[1] The

reasons are not known. More study is needed to confirm these findings.

1. Harder S, Schneider W, Bae ZU, Bock U, Zielen S. Unerwünschte Arzneimittelreaktionen bei gleichzeitiger Gabe von hochdosiertem Phenobarbital und Betalaktam-Antibiotika. *Klin Padiatr* (1990) 202, 404–7.

Cephalosporins + Probenecid

The serum levels of many cephalosporins are raised by probenecid. This may possibly increase the risk of nephrotoxicity with some cephalosporins such as cefaloridine and cefalotin.

Clinical evidence

Ten healthy subjects given single 500-mg oral doses of **cefradine** or **cefaclor** developed markedly raised serum antibacterial concentrations when given **probenecid** (500-mg doses taken 25, 13 and 2 h before the antibacterial). Peak serum levels of the antibacterial were very roughly doubled.[1] Similar results were obtained in another study in healthy subjects given **cefradine** by mouth or intramuscularly.[2]

The following cephalosporins interact with **probenecid** similarly but not identically, the overall picture being that their clearance is reduced, their serum levels are raised and sometimes their half-lives are prolonged: **cefalotin**,[3,4] **cefacetrile**,[5] **cefalexin**,[4,6] **cefamandole**,[4,7] **cefazolin**,[4,8,9] **cefadroxil**,[4] **cefazedone**,[4] **cefmenoxime**,[4] **cefmetazole**,[4,10] **cefonicid**,[4] **cefotaxime**,[4] **cefoxitin**,[4,11-13] **cefprozil**,[14] **cefradine**,[4] **cefaclor**,[4] **ceftizoxime**,[4,15] **cefuroxime**,[4,16] **cefaloglycin**[17] and **cefaloridine**.[18]

Probenecid is reported to lack a significant effect on the pharmacokinetics of **ceforanide**,[4,19] **ceftazidime**,[4] **ceftriaxone**[4] and **latamoxef**.[4]

Mechanism

Probenecid inhibits the excretion of most cephalosporins by the kidney tubules by successfully competing for the excretory mechanisms. A fuller explanation of this mechanism is set out in the introductory chapter. Thus the cephalosporin is retained in the body and its serum levels rise. The extent of the rise cannot always be fully accounted for by this mechanism alone and it is suggested that some change in tissue distribution may sometimes have a part to play.[1]

Importance and management

An extremely well-documented interaction. Only a few representative references are listed below to save space, but the details of many are well reviewed in reference 18. The serum levels of many (but not all) cephalosporins will be higher if probenecid is used concurrently, but no special precautions are normally needed. Elevated serum levels of some cephalosporins, in particular cefaloridine and cefalotin, might possibly increase the risk of nephrotoxicity.

1. Welling PG, Dean S, Selen A, Kendall MJ, Wise R. Probenecid: an unexplained effect on cephalosporin pharmacology. *Br J Clin Pharmacol* (1979) 8, 491–5.
2. Mischler TW, Sugerman AA, Willard DA, Brannick LJ, Neiss ES. Influence of probenecid and food on the bioavailability of cephradine in normal male subjects. *J Clin Pharmacol* (1974) 14, 604–11.
3. Tuano SB, Brodie JL, Kirby WMM. Cephaloridine versus cephalothin: relation of the kidney to blood level differences after parenteral administration. *Antimicrob Agents Chemother* (1966) 6, 101–6.
4. Brown GR. Cephalosporin-probenecid drug interactions. *Clin Pharmacokinet* (1993) 24, 289–300.
5. Wise R, Reeves DS. Pharmacological studies on cephacetrile in human volunteers. *Curr Med Res Opin* (1974) 2, 249–55.
6. Taylor WA, Holloway WJ. Cephalexin in the treatment of gonorrhea. *Int J Clin Pharmacol Ther Toxicol* (1972) 6, 7–9.
7. Griffith RS, Black HR, Brier GL, Wolny JD. Effect of probenecid on the blood levels and urinary excretion of cefamandole. *Antimicrob Agents Chemother* (1977) 11, 809–12.
8. Duncan WC. Treatment of gonorrhea with cefazolin plus probenecid. *J Infect Dis* (1974) 130, 398–401.
9. Brown G, Zemcov SJV, Clarke AM. Effect of probenecid on cefazolin serum concentrations. *J Antimicrob Chemother* (1993) 31, 1009–1011.
10. Ko H, Cathcart KS, Griffith DL, Peters GR, Adams WJ. Pharmacokinetics of intravenously administered cefmetazole and cefoxitin and effects of probenecid on cefmetazole elimination. *Antimicrob Agents Chemother* (1989) 33, 356–61.
11. Bint AJ, Reeves DS, Holt HA. Effect of probenecid on serum cefoxitin concentrations. *J Antimicrob Chemother* (1977) 3, 627–8.

12. Reeves DS, Bullock DW, Bywater MJ, Holt HA, White LO, Thornhill DP. The effect of probenecid on the pharmacokinetics and distribution of cefoxitin in healthy volunteers. *Br J Clin Pharmacol* (1981) 11, 353–9.

13. Vlasses PH, Holbrook AM, Schrogie JJ, Rogers JD, Ferguson RK, Abrams WB. Effect of orally administered probenecid on the pharmacokinetics of cefoxitin. *Antimicrob Agents Chemother* (1980) 17, 847–55.

14. Shukla UA, Pittman KA, Barbhaiya RH. Pharmacokinetic interactions of cefprozil with food, propantheline, metoclopramide, and probenecid in healthy volunteers. *J Clin Pharmacol* (1992) 32, 725–31.

15. LeBel M, Paone RP, Lewis GP. Effect of probenecid on the pharmacokinetics of ceftizoxime. *J Antimicrob Chemother* (1983) 12, 147–55.

16. Garton AM, Rennie RP, Gilpin J, Marrelli M, Shafran SD. Comparison of dose doubling with probenecid for sustaining serum cefuroxime levels. *J Antimicrob Chemother* (1997) 40, 903–6.

17. Applestein JM, Crosby EB, Johnson WD, Kaye D. In-vitro antimicrobial activity and human pharmacology of cephaloglycin. *Appl Microbiol* (1968) 16, 1006–10.

18. Kaplan KS, Reisberg BE, Weinstein L. Cephaloridine: antimicrobial activity and pharmacologic behaviour. *Am J Med Sci* (1967) 253, 667–74.

19. Jovanovich JF, Saravolatz LD, Burch K, Pohlod DJ. Failure of probenecid to alter the pharmacokinetics of ceforanide. *Antimicrob Agents Chemother* (1981) 20, 530–2.

Chloramphenicol + Anticonvulsants

Studies in children show that phenobarbital, and in one case phenytoin, can markedly depress serum chloramphenicol levels. There is a single report, in one adult, of markedly increased serum phenobarbital levels caused by the use of chloramphenicol.

Clinical evidence

(a) Decreased serum chloramphenicol concentrations

A study in a group of infants and children (1 month to 12 years) on chloramphenicol 25 mg/kg 6-hourly found that 6 of them also on **phenobarbital** had reduced serum chloramphenicol levels compared with 17 controls. The peak and trough levels were lowered by 34 and 44% (from 25.3 to 16.6 micrograms/ml, and from 13.4 to 7.5 micrograms/ml respectively).[1] Two children (3 and 7 months old) were treated for *H. influenzae* meningitis with 100 mg/kg/day chloramphenicol, initially intravenously, and later orally. The chloramphenicol levels halved over the first 2 days of treatment, while the children were concurrently receiving **phenobarbital** (10 mg/kg/day) to prevent convulsions. One child had serum chloramphenicol levels of only 5 micrograms/ml or less until the chloramphenicol dosage was doubled, when they rose to 7 to 11 micrograms/ml. The initial doses used were expected to give levels of 15 to 25 micrograms/ml.[2]

Another study confirmed that this interaction can occur in neonates (20 patients), but no statistically significant effect was confirmed in infants (40 patients).[3] Decreased chloramphenicol levels have been described in a single case report of a child who was also being treated with **phenytoin** and **phenobarbital**. The serum chloramphenicol levels were 35.1 micrograms/ml prior to the anticonvulsants, 19.1 micrograms/ml after 2 days of **phenytoin** and 13.2 micrograms/ml a month after the further addition of **phenobarbital**.[4]

(b) Increased serum chloramphenicol concentrations

A study in a group of infants and children (1 month to 12 years) on chloramphenicol 25 mg/kg 6-hourly found that 6 of them also on **phenytoin** had elevated serum chloramphenicol levels. Elevated serum levels associated with less significant changes in chloramphenicol pharmacokinetics were noted in 5 other patients similarly treated.[1]

(c) Increased serum phenobarbital concentrations

A man admitted to hospital on numerous occasions for pulmonary complications associated with cystic fibrosis, had average serum **phenobarbital** concentrations of 33 micrograms/ml while taking 200 mg **phenobarbital** daily and chloramphenicol. One week after the antibacterial was withdrawn, his serum **phenobarbital** levels were 24 micrograms/ml even though the **phenobarbital** dosage was increased from 200 to 300 mg daily. A prior episode of phenytoin toxicity had also coincided with chloramphenicol treatment.[5]

Mechanism

Phenobarbital is a potent liver enzyme inducing agent which can increase the metabolism and clearance of chloramphenicol (clearly demonstrated in *rats*[6]) so that its serum levels fall and its effects are reduced. Chloramphenicol has the opposite effect and inhibits the metabolism of the phenobarbital (also demonstrated in *animals*[7]) so that the effects of the barbiturate are increased. Although phenytoin also induces hepatic enzymes it also displaces chloramphenicol from protein binding sites, thus causing an elevation in levels.[1]

Importance and management

These interactions appear to be established. The documentation is very limited but what happened is consistent with the recognised enzyme inducing actions of phenobarbital and the inhibitory actions of chloramphenicol. Concurrent use should be well monitored to ensure that chloramphenicol serum levels are adequate, and that phenobarbital levels do not become too high. Make appropriate dosage adjustments as necessary. Other barbiturates also act like phenobarbital and may be expected to interact similarly. Appropriate dose reductions may also be required with the phenytoin/chloramphenicol combination, to avoid chloramphenicol toxicity. Good monitoring is advised. Sodium valproate has little or no enzyme-inducing activity and may be a suitable anticonvulsant alternative for phenobarbital or phenytoin.[8]

1. Krasinski K, Kusmiesz H, Nelson JD. Pharmacologic interactions among chloramphenicol, phenytoin and phenobarbital. *Pediatr Infect Dis* (1982) 1, 232–5.

2. Bloxham RA, Durbin GM, Johnson T, Winterborn MH. Chloramphenicol and phenobarbitone—a drug interaction. *Arch Dis Child* (1979) 54, 76–7.

3. Windorfer A, Pringsheim W. Studies on the concentrations of chloramphenicol in the serum and cerebrospinal fluid of neonates, infants, and small children. *Eur J Pediatr* (1977) 124, 129–38.

4. Powell DA, Nahata MC, Durrell DC, Glazer JP, Hilty MD. Interactions among chloramphenicol, phenytoin, and phenobarbital in a pediatric patient. *J Pediatr* (1981) 98, 1001–1003.

5. Koup JR, Gibaldi M, McNamara P, Hilligoss DM, Colburn WA, Bruck E. Interaction of chloramphenicol with phenytoin and phenobarbital. Case report. *Clin Pharmacol Ther* (1978) 24, 571–5.

6. Bella DD, Ferrari V, Marca G, Bonanomi L. Chloramphenicol metabolism in the phenobarbital-induced rat. Comparison with thiamphenicol. *Biochem Pharmacol* (1968) 17, 2381–90.

7. Adams HR. Prolonged barbiturate anesthesia by chloramphenicol in laboratory animals. *J Am Vet Med Assoc* (1970) 157, 1908–13.

8. Oxley J, Hedges A, Makki KA, Monks A, Richens A. Lack of hepatic enzyme inducing effect of sodium valproate. *Br J Clin Pharmacol* (1979) 8, 189–90.

Chloramphenicol + Cimetidine

Two isolated reports describe fatal aplastic anaemia in two patients given intravenous chloramphenicol and cimetidine

Clinical evidence, mechanism, importance and management

Pancytopenia and aplastic anaemia developed in a man on **cimetidine** 1200 mg daily, within 18 days of being given intravenous chloramphenicol 1 g 6-hourly. It proved to be fatal.[1] Another patient similarly treated developed fatal aplastic anaemia after 19 days.[2] A possible reason is that the bone marrow depressant effects of the two drugs were additive. There are at least 8 other cases of aplastic anaemia following the use of parenteral chloramphenicol in the absence of **cimetidine**.[2] The general importance of these observations is uncertain, but the authors of one of the reports suggest that these drugs should be used with caution.

1. Farber BF, Brody JP. Rapid development of aplastic anemia after intravenous chloramphenicol and cimetidine therapy. *South Med J* (1981) 74, 1257–8.

2. West BC, DeVault GA, Clement JC, Williams DM. Aplastic anemia associated with parenteral chloramphenicol: review of 10 cases, including the second case of possible increased risk with cimetidine. *Rev Infect Dis* (1988) 10, 1048–51.

Chloramphenicol + Paracetamol (Acetaminophen)

Although there is limited evidence to suggest that paracetamol may affect chloramphenicol pharmacokinetics its validity has been criticised. Evidence of a clinically relevant interaction appears lacking.

Clinical evidence, mechanism, importance and management

Two studies report alterations in the pharmacokinetics of chloramphenicol by **paracetamol**. The first was conducted in 6 adults on ITU after an observation that the half-life of chloramphenicol was prolonged by **paracetamol** in children with kwashiorkor. The addition of 100 mg intravenous **paracetamol** increased half-life of chloramphenicol in the adults from 3.25 to 15 h.[1] However, this study has been criticised because of potential errors in the method used to calculate half life,[2] the unusual doses and routes of administration used,[2,3] and because the pharmacokinetics of the chloramphenicol with and without **paracetamol** were calculated at different times after the administration of chloramphenicol.[4] The initial observation has also been questioned, as malnutrition (e.g. kwashiorkor) can increase the elimination rate and AUC of chloramphenicol, independently of **paracetamol**.[2]

The second study demonstrated a different interaction, in that the clearance of chloramphenicol was *increased* and the half-life *reduced*.[5] This study has also been criticised as it does not account for the fact that chloramphenicol clearance increases over the duration of a treatment course, suggesting that the changes in the pharmacokinetics of chloramphenicol demonstrated may be independent of the **paracetamol**.[6]

Three other studies have failed to confirm the existence of an interaction.[2-4]

The clinical significance of these reports is unclear, and clinical evidence of toxicity or treatment failure of the chloramphenicol appears to be lacking. It would seem prudent to remain aware of the potential for interaction, especially in malnourished patients, but routine monitoring would appear unnecessary without further evidence.

1. Buchanan N, Moodley GP. Interaction between chloramphenicol and paracetamol. *BMJ* (1979) 2, 307–308.
2. Kearns GL, Bocchini JA, Brown RD, Cotter DL, Wilson JT. Absence of a pharmacokinetic interaction between chloramphenicol and acetaminophen in children. *J Pediatr* (1985) 107, 134–9.
3. Rajpurohit R, Krishnaswamy K. Lack of effect of paracetamol on the pharmacokinetics of chloramphenicol in adult human subjects. *Indian J Pharmacol* (1984) 16, 124–8.
4. Stein CM, Thornhill DP, Neill P, Nyazema NZ. Lack of effect of paracetamol on the pharmacokinetics of chloramphenicol. *Br J Clin Pharmacol* (1989) 27, 262–4.
5. Spika JS, Davis DJ, Martin SR, Beharry K, Rex J, Aranda JV. Interaction between chloramphenicol and acetaminophen. *Arch Dis Child* (1986) 61, 1121–4.
6. Choonara IA. Interaction between chloramphenicol and acetaminophen. *Arch Dis Child* (1987) 62, 319.

Chloramphenicol + Penicillins, Streptomycin or Cephalosporins

Antagonism between chloramphenicol and other antibacterials has been described in a case of staphylococcal endocarditis, in bacterial meningitis in a large group of patients and in an infant. In contrast, no antagonism and even additive antibacterial effects have been described in other infections.

Clinical evidence

(a) Antibacterial antagonism

A study in 264 patients (adults, and children of more than two months) with acute bacterial meningitis showed that when given **ampicillin** 150 mg/kg daily alone, the case-fatality ratio was 4.3% compared with 10.5% on a combination of **ampicillin**, chloramphenicol (100 mg/kg daily up to 4 g) and **streptomycin** (40 mg/kg daily

up to 2 g). The neurological sequelae (hemiparesis, deafness, cranial nerve palsies) were also markedly increased by the use of the combined drugs.[1]

Antibacterial antagonism was clearly seen in an infant of two-and-a-half months with meningitis due to *Salmonella enteritidis* when treated with chloramphenicol and **ceftazidime**.[2]

(b) Lack of antagonism and increased antibacterial effects

A report claims that no antagonism was seen in 65 of 66 patients given chloramphenicol and **benzylpenicillin** for bronchitis or bronchopneumonia.[3] **Ampicillin** with chloramphenicol is more effective than chloramphenicol alone in the treatment of typhoid,[4] and in a study of 700 patients, **procaine benzylpenicillin** with chloramphenicol was shown to be more effective than chloramphenicol alone in the treatment of gonorrhoea (failure rates of 1.8% compared with 8.5%).[5] In a study on premature and full-term neonates, infants and small children, it was found that the presence of **penicillin** markedly raised the serum concentrations of concurrently administered chloramphenicol.[6]

Mechanism

By no means fully understood. Chloramphenicol inhibits bacterial protein synthesis and can change an actively growing bacterial colony into a static one. Thus the effects of a bactericide, such as penicillin, which interferes with cell wall synthesis, are blunted, and the death of the organism occurs more slowly. This would seem to explain the antagonism seen with some organisms.

Importance and management

Proven cases of antibacterial antagonism in patients seem to be few in number. Some practitioners totally avoid concurrent use, but there is certainly insufficient evidence to impose a general prohibition because, depending on the organism, they have been used together with clear advantage.[4,5]

1. Mathies AW, Leedom JM, Ivler D, Wehrle PF, Portnoy B. Antibiotic antagonism in bacterial meningitis. *Antimicrob Agents Chemother* (1967) 7, 218–24.
2. French GL, Ling TKW, Davies DP, Leung DTY. Antagonism of ceftazidime by chloramphenicol in vitro and in vivo during treatment of gram negative meningitis. *BMJ* (1985) 291, 636–7.
3. Ardalan P. Zur Frage des Antagonismus von Penicillin und Chloramphenicolus klinischer Sicht. *Prax Pneumol* (1969) 23, 772–6.
4. De Ritis R, Giammanco G, Manzillo G. Chloramphenicol combined with ampicillin in treatment of typhoid. *BMJ* (1972) 4, 17–18.
5. Gjessing HC, Ödegaard K. Oral chloramphenicol alone and with intramuscular procaine penicillin in the treatment of gonorrhoea. *Br J Vener Dis* (1967) 43, 133–6.
6. Windorfer A, Pringsheim W. Studies on the concentrations of chloramphenicol in the serum and cerebrospinal fluid of neonates, infants and small children. *Eur J Pediatr* (1977) 124, 129–38.

Chloramphenicol + Rifampicin (Rifampin)

The chloramphenicol serum levels of four children were markedly lowered when additionally treated with rifampicin.

Clinical evidence

Two children aged 2 and 5 with *Haemophilus influenzae* meningitis were given 100 mg/kg/day chloramphenicol in four divided doses by infusion over 30 min. Within 3 days of starting **rifampicin (rifampin)** (20 mg/kg/day) their peak serum chloramphenicol levels were depressed by 86 and 64% respectively, and only returned to the therapeutic range when the chloramphenicol dosage was increased to 125 mg/kg/day.[1]

Two other children, of 5 and 18 months, with *Haemophilus influenzae* infections, are also reported to have shown marked reductions (75% and 94% respectively) in serum chloramphenicol levels when given **rifampicin** (20 mg/kg daily) for 4 days, despite 20 to 25% increases in the chloramphenicol dosage.[2]

Mechanism

It is thought that rifampicin, a potent enzyme inducing agent, markedly increased the metabolism of the chloramphenicol by the liver, thereby lowering its serum levels.[1,2] An increased clearance of chloramphenicol in the presence of rifampicin has also been demonstrated in chimpanzees.[2]

Importance and management

So far only four cases have been reported. However, the evidence is sufficiently strong for this interaction to be taken seriously. There is a risk that the serum chloramphenicol will fall to subtherapeutic levels. The authors of the second report point out that raising the chloramphenicol dosage may possibly expose the patient to a greater risk of bone marrow aplasia. They suggest delaying rifampicin prophylaxis in patients with invasive *Haemophilus influenzae* infections until the end of chloramphenicol treatment. More study is needed.

1. Prober CG. Effect of rifampin on chloramphenicol levels. *N Engl J Med* (1985) 312, 788–9.
2. Kelly HW, Couch RC, Davis RL, Cushing AH, Knott R. Interaction of chloramphenicol and rifampin. *J Pediatr* (1988) 112, 817–20.

Chloroquine + Cimetidine or Ranitidine

Cimetidine reduces the metabolism and the loss of chloroquine from the body. The clinical importance of this is still uncertain. Ranitidine appears not to interact.

Clinical evidence, mechanism, importance and management

Cimetidine 400 mg daily for 4 days approximately halved (from 0.49 to 0.23 l/d/kg) the clearance of a single dose of chloroquine (600 mg base) in 10 healthy subjects. The elimination half-life was prolonged from 3.11 to 4.62 days.[1] The suggested reason is that the **cimetidine** inhibits the metabolism of the chloroquine by the liver, thereby reducing its loss from the body. The clinical importance of this interaction is uncertain, but since the main metabolite of chloroquine has pharmacological activity it would seem prudent to be alert for any signs of chloroquine toxicity during concurrent use. A similar study by the same authors found that **ranitidine** does not interact with chloroquine.[2]

1. Ette EI, Brown-Awala EA, Essien EE. Chloroquine elimination in humans: effect of low-dose cimetidine. *J Clin Pharmacol* (1987) 27, 813–16.
2. Ette EI, Brown-Awala EA, Essien EE. Effect of ranitidine on chloroquine disposition. *Drug Intell Clin Pharm* (1987) 21, 732–4.

Chloroquine + Colestyramine

Colestyramine can reduce the absorption of chloroquine, but the clinical importance of this is uncertain.

Clinical evidence, mechanism, importance and management

Colestyramine 4g reduced the absorption of chloroquine (10 mg/kg) by about 30% in 5 children aged 6 to 13. Considerable individual differences were seen.[1] This reduced absorption is consistent with the way **colestyramine** interacts with other drugs by binding to them in the gut. The clinical importance is uncertain but separating the dosages is effective in reducing the effects of this interaction with other drugs. More study is needed.

1. Gendrel D, Verdier F, Richard-Lenoble D, Nardou M. Interaction entre cholestyramine et chloroquine. *Arch Fr Pediatr* (1990) 47, 387–8.

Chloroquine + Imipramine

No pharmacokinetic interaction was seen in six healthy subjects given single doses of 300 mg chloroquine and 50 mg imipramine.[1] However see also 'Drugs that prolong the QT interval + Other drugs that prolong the QT interval', p.103.

1. Onyeji CO, Toriola TA, Ogunbona FA. Lack of pharmacokinetic interaction between chloroquine and imipramine. *Ther Drug Monit* (1993) 15, 43–6.

Cinoxacin + Miscellaneous drugs

Warnings have been published about possible interactions between cinoxacin and other drugs but, with the possible exception of probenecid, they seem to be based solely on theoretical considerations.

Clinical evidence, mechanism, importance and management

Cinoxacin is a quinolone antibacterial which might be expected to interact like other quinolones. For this reason the makers suggest in their drug datasheet that it may increase the effects of oral anticoagulants such as **warfarin** and raise **theophylline** serum levels, so they prudently advise good monitoring.[1]

However there seems to be no direct clinical evidence that cinoxacin has ever caused problems with either of these drugs, nor that its serum levels and effects are reduced by **antacids** or **iron preparations** which are known to interact significantly with some other quinolones. A literature search by the makers of cinoxacin in 1995 failed to turn up any significant interactions[2] but **probenecid** is reported to increase serum levels of cinoxacin (see 'Quinolone antibacterials + Probenecid', p.215). Any warnings would therefore seem to be based solely on the way other quinolones behave.

1. Cinobac (Cinoxacin) Eli Lilly and Company. ABPI Compendium of Datasheets and Summaries of Product Characteristics, 1999–2000, pp. 734–5.
2. Eli Lilly, Personal communication, March 1995.

Clarithromycin + Rifamycins

Both rifabutin and rifampicin markedly reduce the serum levels of clarithromycin, but it is not clear whether this results in treatment failure. Clarithromycin increases the serum levels of rifabutin. There is an increased risk of uveitis with clarithromycin combined with rifabutin.

Clinical evidence

(a) Rifabutin

(i) Clarithromycin levels reduced. Twelve HIV+ patients were started on 500 mg clarithromycin daily, to which 300 mg **rifabutin** daily was added on day 15, as a possible regimen for the prophylaxis of *Mycobacterium avium* complex (MAC) disease. By day 42 the clarithromycin AUC was found to have fallen by more than 50%.[1] A related study by the same group in 14 patients given 500 mg clarithromycin 12-hourly and 300 mg **rifabutin** daily found that after 28 days the AUC of the **rifabutin** was increased by 77%.[2] Another group of patients with lung disease due to MAC were treated with 500 mg clarithromycin twice daily. When 600 mg **rifabutin** was added the levels fell by 63% (from 5.4 to 2.0 micrograms/ml).[3]

(ii) Uveitis or arthralgias. Uveitis, and in some cases pseudojaundice, aphthous stomatitis and an arthralgia syndrome have been described in patients treated with both clarithromycin 1 to 2 g daily and **rifabutin** (300 to 600 mg daily).[4-7]

One report describes 5 HIV+ patients who developed uveitis 6 weeks to 9 months after starting treatment with 450 to 600 mg **rifab-**

utin, 1.5 to 2 g clarithromycin and 100 to 400 mg fluconazole daily. One further patient who developed uveitis was taking **rifabutin** and clarithromycin, but not fluconazole.[5] In a study of 68 HIV+ patients taking a variety of treatments for MAC, 10 developed uveitis within 27 to 370 days. All of these 10 patients had been given clarithromycin 1 to 2 g daily and **rifabutin** 300 to 600 mg daily. A further episode of uveitis occurred in a patient on **rifabutin** and **ethambutol**. Many patients were also taking fluconazole, but this showed no statistical association with the development of uveitis. Further statistical analysis showed the risk of uveitis was greater with **rifabutin** plus clarithromycin than **rifabutin** alone, or **rifabutin** with other anti-MAC treatments.[6]

(b) Rifampicin

Patients with lung disease due to MAC were treated with 500 mg clarithromycin twice daily. When 600 mg **rifampicin** daily was added, the mean serum levels of clarithromycin fell by almost 90% (from 5.4 to 0.7 micrograms/ml).[3]

Mechanism

Both rifabutin and rifampicin are known enzyme inducing agents which can increase the metabolism of other drugs by the liver, thereby reducing their serum levels. Rifampicin is recognised as being the more potent inducer. The reason for the uveitis is not known, but based on *animal* studies it has been suggested that it is associated with effective treatment of MAC and is due to release of a mycobacterial protein, rather than a toxic effect of the drugs.[8]

Importance and management

Direct information appears to be limited to these reports but the interactions would appear to be established. What happens is certainly consistent with the way these rifamycins interact with other drugs. What is not entirely clear is whether this interaction results in treatment failures because of the potentially subtherapeutic clarithromycin serum levels. This does not seem to have been assessed. If therefore you add either of these rifamycins to clarithromycin you should be alert for evidence of reduced efficacy.

Rifabutin is known to cause polyarthritis on rare occasions, but in conjunction with clarithromycin it appears to happen at much lower doses.[7] Careful monitoring is necessary. Also be aware of the increased risk of uveitis with clarithromycin and rifabutin (CSM warning[9]) and of the raised rifabutin levels. If uveitis occurs the rifabutin should be stopped and the patient should be referred to an ophthalmologist.[9] Because of the increased risk of uveitis the CSM says that consideration should be given to reducing the dosage of rifabutin to 300 mg daily. See also 'Rifabutin (Ansamycin) + Azithromycin', p.218.

1. The DATRI 001 Study group. Clarithromycin (CL) plus rifabutin (RFB) for MAC prophylaxis. Evidence for a drug interaction. Abstracts of 1st Nat Conf Human Retrovirus related infections (1993) Dec 12-16, Washington DC, p 106.
2. The DATRI 001 Study group. Coadministration of clarithromycin (CL) alters the concentration-time profile of rifabutin (RFB). *Intersci Conf Antimicrob Agents Chemother* (1994) 34, 3.
3. Wallace RJ, Brown BA, Griffith DE, Girard W, Tanaka K. Reduced serum levels of clarithromycin in patients treated with multidrug regimens including rifampin or rifabutin for *Mycobacterium avium-M. intracellulare* infection. *J Infect Dis* (1995) 171, 747–50.
4. Shafren SD, Deschênes J, Miller M, Phillips P, Toma E. Uveitis and pseudojaundice during a regimen of clarithromycin, rifabutin, and ethambutol. *N Engl J Med* (1994) 330, 438–9.
5. Becker K, Schimkat M, Jablonowski H, Häussinger D. Anterior uveitis associated with rifabutin medication in AIDS patients. *Infection* (1996) 24, 34–6.
6. Kelleher P, Helbert M, Sweeney J, Anderson J, Parkin J, Pinching A. Uveitis associated with rifabutin and macrolide therapy for *Mycobacterium avium intracellulare* infections in AIDS patients. *Genitourin Med* (1996) 72, 419–21.
7. Le Gars L, Collon T, Picard O, Kaplan G, Berenbaum F. Polyarthralgia-arthritis syndrome induced by low doses of rifabutin. *J Rheumatol* (1999) 26, 1201–2.
8. Opremcak EM, Cynamon M. Uveitogenic activity of rifabutin and clarithromycin in the *Mycobacterium avium*-infected beige mice. Am Soc Microbiol 2nd Nat Conf. Human retroviruses and related infections. Washington DC, Jan 29—Feb 2 1995, 74.
9. Committee on the Safety of Medicines. Rifabutin (Mycobutin) – uveitis. *Current Problems* (1994) 20, 4.

Clindamycin or Lincomycin + Food or Drinks

The serum levels of lincomycin are markedly depressed (by up to two-thirds) if taken in the presence of food, but clindamycin is not significantly affected. Cyclamate sweeteners can also reduce the absorption of lincomycin.

Clinical evidence

The mean peak serum levels of **lincomycin** achieved after single 500 mg oral doses in 10 normal subjects were approximately 3 micrograms/ml when taken 4 h before breakfast, 2 micrograms/ml when taken 1 h before **breakfast**, and less than 1 microgram/ml when taken after **breakfast**. The mean total amounts of **lincomycin** recovered from the urine were respectively 40.4, 23.8 and 8.9 mg. There were considerable individual variations.[1]

Depressed serum **lincomycin** levels due to the presence of **food** have been described in other reports,[2,3] but the absorption of **clindamycin** is not affected.[3,4] **Sodium cyclamate** used as an artificial sweetener in diet foods, drinks and some pharmaceuticals can also markedly reduce the absorption of **lincomycin** (reduction in AUC of about 75% using 1 Molar equivalent with 500 mg **lincomycin**).[5]

Mechanism

Not understood.

Importance and management

The food interaction with lincomycin is well established and of clinical importance. Lincomycin should not be taken with food or within several hours of eating a meal if adequate serum levels are to be achieved. An alternative is clindamycin, a synthetic derivative of lincomycin, which has the same antibacterial spectrum but the absorption of which is not affected by the presence of food.

1. McCall CE, Steigbigel NH, Finland M. Lincomycin: activity *in vitro* and absorption and excretion in normal young men. *Am J Med Sci* (1967) 254, 144–55.
2. Kaplan K, Chew WH, Weinstein L. Microbiological, pharmacological and clinical studies of lincomycin. *Am J Med Sci* (1965) 250, 137–46.
3. McGehee RF, Smith CB, Wilcox C, Finland M. Comparative studies of antibacterial activity in vitro and absorption and excretion of lincomycin and clinimycin. *Am J Med Sci* (1968) 256, 279–92.
4. Wagner JG, Novak E, Patel NC, Chidester CG, Lummis WL. Absorption, excretion and half-life of clinimycin in normal adult males. *Am J Med Sci* (1968) 256, 25–37.
5. Wagner JG. Aspects of pharmacokinetics and biopharmaceutics in relation to drug activity. *Am J Pharm Sci Support Public Health* (1969) 141, 5–20.

Clindamycin or Lincomycin + Kaolin

Kaolin-containing antidiarrhoeal preparations can markedly reduce the absorption of lincomycin by the gut. This can be avoided by giving the lincomycin two hours after the kaolin. Lincomycin-induced diarrhoea is a potential hazard. The rate but not the extent of clindamycin absorption is altered by kaolin-pectin.

Clinical evidence

About 85 ml (3 fl oz) of *Kaopectate* (**kaolin-pectin**) reduced the absorption of 500 mg **lincomycin** by about 90% in 8 normal subjects. Giving the *Kaopectate* 2 h before the antibacterial had little or no effect on its absorption, whereas when given 2 h after, the absorption was reduced about 50%. The absorption rate of **clindamycin** is markedly prolonged by **kaolin**, but the extent of its absorption remains unaffected.[1]

Mechanism

It seems probable that the lincomycin becomes adsorbed onto the kaolin, thereby reducing its bioavailability. The kaolin also coats the lining of the gut and acts as a physical barrier to absorption.[2]

Importance and management

Information seems to be limited to this study, but the lincomycin-kaolin interaction appears to be established and of clinical importance. For good absorption and a good antibacterial response separate their administration as much as possible, ideally giving the kaolin 2 h before the antibacterial. Remember that lincomycin itself can cause diarrhoea in a fairly large proportion of patients, which in some cases has lead to the development of fatal pseudomembraneous colitis. Marked diarrhoea, according to the makers, is an indication that the lincomycin should be stopped immediately. Clindamycin appears to be a suitable alternative to lincomycin.

1. Albert KS, DeSante KA, Welch RD, DiSanto AR. Pharmacokinetic evaluation of a drug interaction between kaolin-pectin and clindamycin. *J Pharm Sci* (1978) 67, 1579–82.
2. Wagner JG. Design and data analysis of biopharmaceutical studies in man. *Can J Pharm Sci* (1966) 1, 55–68.

Co-trimoxazole + Azithromycin

Azithromycin does not alter the pharmacokinetics of co-trimoxazole.

Clinical evidence, mechanism, importance and management

A study in 12 healthy subjects given **co-trimoxazole** 960 mg daily for 7 days found that a single dose of azithromycin 1200 mg given on day 7 did not alter the **co-trimoxazole** pharmacokinetics to a clinically relevant extent.[1]

1. Amsden GW, Foulds G, Thakker K. Pharmacokinetic study of azithromycin with fluconazole and cotrimoxazole (trimethoprim-sulfamethoxazole) in healthy volunteers. *Clin Drug Invest* (2000) 20, 135–42.

Co-trimoxazole + Kaolin-pectin

Kaolin-pectin can cause a small but probably clinically unimportant reduction in serum co-trimoxazole levels.

Clinical evidence, mechanism, importance and management

Co-trimoxazole suspension (160 mg trimethoprim + 800 mg sulfamethoxazole was given to 8 healthy subjects, with and without 20 ml **kaolin-pectin** suspension. The **kaolin-pectin** reduced the AUC of the trimethoprim by about 12% and the maximal serum levels were reduced by about 20%. Changes in the sulfamethoxazole pharmacokinetics were not significant.[1] The probable reason is that the drugs, particularly trimethoprim, are adsorbed onto the **kaolin-pectin** which reduces their bioavailability. The reductions are small and unlikely to be clinically relevant, but this needs confirmation.

1. Gupta KC, Desai NK, Satoskar RS, Gupta C, Goswami SN. Effect of pectin and kaolin on bioavailability of co-trimoxazole suspension. *Int J Clin Pharmacol Ther Toxicol* (1987) 25, 320–1.

Co-trimoxazole + Prilocaine/Lidocaine (Lignocaine) cream

Methaemoglobinaemia developed in a baby treated with co-trimoxazole when *Emla* (prilocaine/lidocaine) cream was applied to his skin.

Clinical evidence, mechanism, importance and management

A 12-week-old child on co-trimoxazole for 2 months for pyelitis was treated with 5 g of *Emla* cream (25 mg **prilocaine** + 25 mg **lidocaine** per gram) applied to the back of his hands and in the cubital regions.

Unfortunately his operation was delayed, and 5 h later, just before the operation began, his skin was noted to be pale and his lips had a brownish cyanotic colour. This was found to be due to the presence of 28% methaemoglobin.[1] The authors of the report suggest that the **prilocaine** together with the sulfamethoxazole (both known to be able to cause methaemoglobin formation) suppressed the activity of two enzymes (NADH-dehydrogenase and NADP-diaphorase) which normally keep blood levels of methaemoglobin to a minimum.[1] Other studies[2,3] in children confirm that *Emla* cream can increase methaemoglobin levels up to 2%. As the methaemoglobin levels remained elevated after 24 hours, daily administration may lead to accumulation, and a greater risk of toxicity.[2]

The report cited[1] appears to be unusual, but it has been suggested that there may be a special risk of methaemoglobinaemia with *Emla* in children with pre-existing anaemia, reduced renal excretion of the metabolites of prilocaine, or the concurrent use of sulphonamides.[2]

1. Jakobson B, Nilsson A. Methemoglobinemia associated with a prilocaine-lidocaine cream and trimetoprim-sulphamethoxazole. A case report. *Acta Anaesthesiol Scand* (1985) 29, 453–55.
2. Frayling IM, Addison GM, Chattergee K, Meakin G. Methaemoglobinaemia in children treated with prilocaine-lignocaine cream. *BMJ* (1990) 301, 153–4.
3. Engberg G, Danielson K, Henneberg S, Nilsson A. Plasma concentrations of prilocaine and lidocaine and methaemoglobin formation in infants after epicutaneous application of a 5% lidocaine-prilocaine cream (Emla). *Acta Anaesthesiol Scand* (1987) 31, 624–8.

Co-trimoxazole or Trimethoprim + Rifamycins

Both rifabutin (ansamycin) and rifampicin (rifampin) appear to affect the clearance of trimethoprim but neither interaction appears to be clinically important in healthy subjects, although it may be significant in HIV+ patients. Sulfamethoxazole appears to be unaffected by rifabutin.

Clinical evidence, mechanism, importance and management

(a) Rifabutin

Twelve HIV+ patients taking one **co-trimoxazole** tablet (strength not stated) twice daily for 7 days were additionally given **rifabutin** 300 mg daily for a further 14 days. The **sulfamethoxazole** component remained unaffected but the **trimethoprim** AUC was decreased by 22%. This small reduction is not expected to be clinically significant.[1]

(b) Rifampicin

No significant pharmacokinetic interaction seems to occur when healthy subjects are given **trimethoprim** 240 mg daily with **rifampicin** 900 mg daily (both in divided doses). After 4 to 5 days, less **trimethoprim** is recovered in the urine as more is metabolized prior to excretion due to the enzyme inducing activity of **rifampicin**.[2,3] This does not appear to be of clinical importance. However, a study in 10 HIV+ subjects given **rifampicin** 600 mg daily with **co-trimoxazole** 960 mg daily found that the AUCs of **trimethoprim** and **sulfamethoxazole** were reduced by 56% and 28% respectively. It is anticipated that these changes are large enough to reduce the efficacy of **co-trimoxazole** treatment.[4]

1. Lee BL, Lampiris H, Colborn DC, Lewis RC, Narang PK, Sullam P. The effect of rifabutin (RBT) on the pharmacokinetics (PK) of trimethoprim-sulfamethoxazole (TMP-SMX) in HIV-infected patients. *Intersci Conf Antimicrob Agents Chemother* (1995) 35, 7.
2. Buniva G, Palminteri R, Berti M. Kinetics of a rifampicin-trimethoprim combination. *Int J Clin Pharmacol Biopharm* (1979) 17, 256–9.
3. Emmerson AM, Grüneberg RN, Johnson ES. The pharmacokinetics in man of a combination of rifampicin and trimethoprim. *J Antimicrob Chemother* (1978) 4, 523–31.
4. Ribera E, Pou L, Fernandez-Sola A, Campos F, Lopez RM, Ocaña I, Ruiz I, Pahissa A. Rifampin reduces concentrations of trimethoprim and sulfamethoxazole in serum in human immunodeficiency virus infected patients. *Antimicrob Agents Chemother* (2001) 45, 3238–41.

Cycloserine + Miscellaneous drugs

Cycloserine is reported to increase the effects of alcohol. Its CNS side-effects are increased by isoniazid.

Clinical evidence, mechanism, importance and management

A brief report describes an enhancement of the effects of **alcohol** in 2 patients on cycloserine.[1] Patients should be warned. In a report about the concurrent use of cycloserine and **isoniazid**, both an increase and a decrease in serum cycloserine levels were seen, but the mean values were not significantly changed. Only one out of 11 patients on cycloserine alone developed CNS effects (drowsiness, dizziness, unstable gait), but when cycloserine was given in conjunction with **isoniazid**, 9 of the 11 developed these effects.[2] Cycloserine is contraindicated in epilepsy because it can cause convulsions.

1. Glaß F, Mallach HJ, Simsch A. Beobachtungen und Untersuchungen über die gemeinsame Wirkung von Alkohol und D-Cycloserin. *Arzneimittelforschung* (1965) 15, 684–8.
2. Mattila MJ, Nieminen E, Tiitinen H. Serum levels, urinary excretion, and side-effects of cycloserine in the presence of isoniazid and p-aminosalicylic acid. *Scand J Respir Dis* (1969) 50, 291–300.

Dapsone + Antacids

The absorption of dapsone is unaltered by *Mylanta II* (hydrated aluminium hydroxide, magnesium hydroxide, simethicone).

Clinical evidence, mechanism, importance and management

A study to see whether changes in gastric pH might affect the absorption of dapsone found that when a single 100-mg dose of dapsone, taken with the second of 11 hourly doses of *Mylanta II*, the absorption of the dapsone remained unchanged. The mean gastric pH rose from 2.3 before using the antacid, to 4.5 or higher while taking dapsone and antacid.[1] No special precautions would therefore seem to be needed if *Mylanta* is used, nor any other similar antacid. See also 'Nucleoside reverse transcriptase inhibitors + Dapsone', p.182.

1. Breen GA, Brocavich JM, Etzel JV, Shah V, Schaefer P, Forlenza S. Evaluation of effects of altered gastric pH on absorption of dapsone in healthy volunteers. *Antimicrob Agents Chemother* (1994) 38, 2227–9.

Dapsone + Cimetidine, Omeprazole or Ranitidine

Cimetidine raises serum dapsone levels. Cimetidine, ranitidine and omeprazole do not appear to affect the outcome of dapsone prophylaxis against *Pneumocystis carinii* pneumonia (PCP).

Clinical evidence, mechanism, importance and management

The AUC of a single 100-mg dose of dapsone was increased by 40% (from 31 to 43.3 micrograms^{-1}ml^{-1}h) in 7 healthy subjects after taking 400 mg **cimetidine** three times daily for 3 days.[1] The probable reason is that the **cimetidine** (a known enzyme inhibitor) inhibits the metabolism of the dapsone by the liver. This might be expected to increase the risk of haematological side-effects of dapsone by raising its serum levels, but the **cimetidine** also apparently markedly reduces the production of dapsone hydroxylamine (the AUC fell by more than half). Dapsone hydroxylamine appears to be responsible for the methaemoglobinaemia and haemolysis that may occur with dapsone treatment.[1] These findings were later confirmed in 8 patients on chronic dapsone therapy (50 to 100 mg daily) given 1600 mg cimetidine daily

for 3 months. Steady-state serum dapsone levels rose about 30% accompanied by a fall in serum methaemoglobin levels from 5.5 to 3.9% (normal range < 2%) by week 3. However, a sustained decrease in methaemoglobin was not seen, with levels returning to baseline at week 12, despite the continuance of the **cimetidine**.[2] Another report on a small number of patients, comparing those treated with **cimetidine**, **ranitidine** or **omeprazole** to those not, found no difference in the outcome of dapsone prophylaxis for PCP in HIV patients.[3] More study is needed to confirm these findings.

1. Coleman MD, Scott AK, Breckenridge AM, Park BK. The use of cimetidine as a selective inhibitor of dapsone *N*-hydroxylation in man. *Br J Clin Pharmacol* (1990) 30, 761–7.
2. Rhodes LE, Tingle MD, Park BK, Chu P, Verbov JL, Friedmann PS. Cimetidine improves the therapeutic/toxic ratio of dapsone in patients on chronic dapsone therapy. *Br J Dermatol* (1995) 132, 257–62.
3. Huengsberg M, Castelino S, Sherrard J, O'Farrell N, Bingham J. Does drug interaction cause failure of PCP prophylaxis with dapsone? *Lancet* (1993) 341, 48.

Dapsone + Clofazimine

Dapsone can reduce the anti-inflammatory effects of clofazimine but clofazimine does not affect the pharmacokinetics of dapsone.

Clinical evidence, mechanism, importance and management

Fourteen out of 16 patients with severe recurrent erythema nodosum leprosum (ENL) failed to respond adequately when given dapsone and **clofazimine** and needed additional therapy with corticosteroids. When the dapsone was stopped the patients responded to **clofazimine** alone, and in some instances they were controlled on smaller doses.[1] Further evidence of this interaction comes from a laboratory study which suggests that the actions of **clofazimine** may be related to its ability to inhibit neutrophil migration (resulting in decreased numbers of neutrophils in areas of inflammation), whereas dapsone can have the opposite effect.[1] Although the information is very limited, it would seem prudent to avoid concurrent use in the treatment of ENL. The authors of this report[1] are at great pains to emphasise that what they describe only relates to the effects of dapsone on the anti-inflammatory effects of **clofazimine**, and not to the beneficial effects of combined use when treating drug-resistant *Mycobacterium leprae*.

Three studies in patients on isoniazid or rifampicin as well as **clofazimine** and dapsone suggest that **clofazimine** does not affect the pharmacokinetics of dapsone.[2-4]

1. Imkamp FMJH, Anderson R, Gatner EMS. Possible incompatibility of dapsone with clofazimine in the treatment of patients with erythema nodosum leprosum. *Lepr Rev* (1982) 53, 148–9.
2. Venkatesan K, Mathur A, Girdhar BK, Bharadwaj VP. The effect of clofazimine on the pharmacokinetics of rifampicin and dapsone in leprosy. *J Antimicrob Chemother* (1986) 18, 715–18.
3. Pieters FAJM, Woonink F, Zuidema J. Influence of once-monthly rifampicin and daily clofazimine on the pharmacokinetics of dapsone in leprosy patients in Nigeria. *Eur J Clin Pharmacol* (1988) 34, 73–6.
4. Venkatesan K, Bharadwaj VP, Ramu R, Desikan KV. Study on drug interactions. *Lepr India* (1980) 52, 229–35.

Dapsone + Probenecid

The serum levels of dapsone can be markedly raised by the concurrent use of probenecid.

Clinical evidence

Twelve patients with quiescent tuberculoid leprosy were given 300 mg dapsone with 500 mg **probenecid**, and 5 h later another 300 mg dapsone. At 4 h, the dapsone serum levels were raised about 50%. The urinary excretion of dapsone and its metabolites were found to be reduced.[1]

Mechanism

Not fully examined. It seems probable that the probenecid inhibits the renal excretion of dapsone by the kidney.

Importance and management

The documentation is very limited. It is likely that the probenecid will raise the serum levels of dapsone given chronically. The importance of this is uncertain, but the extent of the rise and the evidence that the haematological toxicity of dapsone may be dose-related[2] suggests that it may well have some clinical importance. This needs confirmation.

1. Goodwin CS, Sparell G. Inhibition of dapsone excretion by probenecid. *Lancet* (1969) ii, 884–5.
2. Ellard GA, Gammon PT, Savin JA, Tan RS-H. Dapsone acetylation in dermatitis herpetiformis. *Br J Dermatol* (1974) 90, 441–4.

Dapsone + Proguanil

Dapsone and proguanil appear not to interact pharmacokinetically and they have been successfully used together for protection against malaria.

Clinical evidence, mechanism, importance and management

A comparative study in 6 healthy subjects found that 200 mg **proguanil** daily had no effect on the pharmacokinetics of 10 mg dapsone daily, nor on its principal metabolite (monoacetyldapsone). The authors of this report however are ultra-cautious because, despite this lack of a pharmacokinetic interaction at these dosages, they say that increased dapsone toxicity cannot be ruled out.[1] Combined use (dapsone 25 mg, **proguanil** 200 mg daily) was successfully used for malarial prophylaxis in the Vietnam war,[2] and the same regimen, but with dapsone dosage every third day was successful as prophylaxis against **proguanil**-resistant falciparum malaria in Papua New Guinea.[1] More recently a different dosage (dapsone 4 or 12.5 mg, **proguanil** 200 mg daily) used as prophylaxis in Thailand was found to be well tolerated over a period of 80 days.[3]

1. Edstein MD, Rieckmann KH. Lack of effect of proguanil on the pharmacokinetics of dapsone in healthy volunteers. *Chemotherapy* (1993) 39, 235–41.
2. Black RH. Malaria in the Australian army in South Vietnam. Successful use of a proguanil-dapsone combination for chemoprophylaxis of chloroquine-resistant falciparum malaria. *Med J Aust* (1973) 1, 1265–70.
3. Shanks GD, Edstein MD, Suriyamongkol V, Timsaad S, Webster HK. Malaria prophylaxis using proguanil/dapsone combinations on the Thai-Cambodian border. *Am J Trop Med Hyg* (1992) 46, 643–8.

Dapsone + Rifampicin (Rifampin) or Clarithromycin

Rifampicin increases the excretion of dapsone, lowers its serum levels and increases the risk of toxicity (methaemoglobinaemia).

Clinical evidence

A study in 7 patients with leprosy given single doses of dapsone 100 mg and **rifampicin** 600 mg, alone or together, showed that while the pharmacokinetics of **rifampicin** were not significantly changed by dapsone, the half-life of the dapsone was approximately halved and the AUC was reduced by about 20%.[1] This confirms previous studies in patients given both drugs for several days, which showed reduced dapsone serum levels and an increased urinary excretion.[2,3] Another study in 12 healthy subjects given single 100-mg doses of dapsone before and after taking 600 mg **rifampicin** daily for 10 days, found that the clearance of the dapsone was considerably increased (from 2.01 to 7.17 L/h). Of equal importance was finding that the production of the N-hydroxylation metabolite of dapsone, which appears

to be responsible for the haematological toxicity (methaemoglobinaemia), was markedly increased. The AUC_{0-24} of methaemoglobin was increased by more than 60%.[4] A parallel study found no such interaction between dapsone and **clarithromycin**.[4]

Mechanism

It appears that the rifampicin, well recognised as a potent liver-enzyme inducing agent, increases the metabolism and loss of dapsone from the body and also increases the blood levels of the toxic metabolite of dapsone.

Importance and management

The dapsone/rifampicin interaction is established but of uncertain clinical importance. Concurrent use should be well monitored to confirm that treatment is effective. It may be necessary to raise the dosage of dapsone. It has been pointed out that there is the risk of treatment failures for *Pneumocystis carinii* pneumonia as well as for leprosy.[5] Also be alert for any evidence of methaemoglobinaemia.

1. Krishna DR, Appa Rao AVN, Ramanakar TV, Prabhakar MC. Pharmacokinetic interaction between dapsone and rifampicin in leprosy patients. *Drug Dev Ind Pharm* (1986) 12, 443–59.
2. Balakrishnan S, Seshadri PS. Drug interactions – the influence of rifampicin and clofazimine on the urinary excretion of DDS. *Lepr India* (1981) 53, 17–22.
3. Peters JH, Murray JF, Gordon GR, Gelber RH, Laing ABG, Waters MFR. Effect of rifampin on the disposition of dapsone in Malaysian leprosy patients. *Fedn Proc* (1977) 36, 996.
4. Occhipinti DJ, Choi A, Deyo K, Danziger LH, Fischer JH. Influence of rifampin and clarithromycin on dapsone (D) disposition and methemoglobin concentrations. *Clin Pharmacol Ther* (1995) 57, 163.
5. Jorde UP, Horowitz HW, Wormser GP. Significance of drug interactions with rifampin in *Pneumocystis carinii* pneumonia prophylaxis. *Arch Intern Med* (1992) 152, 2348.

Dapsone + Trimethoprim

The serum levels of each drug are possibly raised by the presence of the other. Both increased efficacy and dapsone toxicity have been seen.

Clinical evidence

Eighteen patients with AIDS, under treatment for *Pneumocystis carinii* pneumonia (PCP) and taking dapsone (100 mg daily), were compared with 30 other patients taking dapsone and **trimethoprim** (20 mg/kg daily). The combined treatment group developed plasma dapsone levels which were 40% higher (a rise from 1.5 to 2.1 micrograms/ml) at 7 days (steady-state). Dapsone toxicity (methaemoglobinaemia) was also increased.

Trimethoprim plasma levels were 48.4% higher in the 30 patients taking dapsone and **trimethoprim** than in another group of 30 patients given dapsone and **co-trimoxazole**), but the incidence of toxicity was higher in the latter group.[1] However a later study by the same authors in 8 asymptomatic HIV+ patients given 100 mg dapsone daily and 200 mg **trimethoprim** 12-hourly found that the steady-state pharmacokinetics of neither drug were unaffected by the other, although the single dose pharmacokinetics showed increased serum levels.[2]

Mechanism

Not understood. Dapsone and trimethoprim appear to have mutually inhibitory effects on clearance.

Importance and management

Information is limited. The difference between the results of the two studies may be because the first was carried out on AIDS patients with PCP and the second on asymptomatic HIV+ patients whose drug metabolism may possibly be different. Concurrent use appears to be an effective form of treatment, but be alert for evidence of increased dapsone toxicity (methaemoglobinaemia).

1. Lee BL, Medina I, Benowitz NL, Jacob P, Wofsy CB, Mills J. Dapsone, trimethoprim, and sulfamethoxazole plasma levels during treatment of pneumocystis pneumonia in patients with acquired immunodeficiency syndrome (AIDS). *Ann Intern Med* (1989) 110, 606–11.
2. Lee BL, Safrin S, Makrides V, Gambertoglio JG. Zidovudine, trimethoprim, and dapsone pharmacokinetic interactions in patients with human immunodeficiency virus infection. *Antimicrob Agents Chemother* (1996) 40, 1231–6.

Diethylcarbamazine + Urinary acidifiers or alkalinizers

Urinary alkalinizers can reduce the loss of diethylcarbamazine in the urine, whereas urinary acidifiers can increase the loss. The clinical importance of this is unknown.

Clinical evidence

Two studies, one in normal subjects[1] and the other in patients with onchocerciasis,[2] found that making the urine alkaline with **sodium bicarbonate** markedly increased the retention of the diethylcarbamazine in the body. The urinary excretion of diethylcarbamazine was 62.3% of the administered dose (50 mg) when the urine was made acidic with **ammonium chloride** (pH less than 5.5), but only 5.1% when the urine was made alkaline with **sodium bicarbonate** (pH more than 7.5). The elimination half-life of the diethylcarbamazine was 9.6 h when the urine was alkaline, and 4 h when acid.[1]

Mechanism

The reason appears to be that in alkaline urine most of the diethylcarbamazine is non-ionised and is therefore easily reabsorbed in the kidney by simple diffusion through the lipid membrane. However, the conclusion was reached that in practice there is no advantage in making the urine alkaline in order to be able to use smaller doses of diethylcarbamazine because the severity of the adverse reactions (the Mazzotti reaction) is not reduced, and the microfilarial counts at the end of a month are not significantly different.[2]

Importance and management

The clinical importance of any unsought for changes in the urinary pH brought about by the use of other drugs during diethylcarbamazine treatment has not been assessed, but be aware that its pharmacokinetics and possibly the severity of its side-effects can be changed.

1. Edwards G, Breckenridge AM, Adjepon-Yamoah KK, Orme M L'E, Ward SA. The effect of variations in urinary pH on the pharmacokinetics of diethylcarbamazine. *Br J Clin Pharmacol* (1981) 12, 807–12.
2. Awadzi K, Adjepon-Yamoah KK, Edwards G, Orme M L'E, Breckenridge AM, Gilles HM. The effect of moderate urine alkalinisation on low dose diethylcarbamazine therapy in patients with onchocerciasis. *Br J Clin Pharmacol* (1986) 21, 669–76.

Erythromycin + Alcohol

Alcohol can cause a moderate reduction in the absorption of erythromycin ethylsuccinate. There is some evidence that erythromycin can raise blood alcohol levels but the extent and the practical importance of this is unknown.

Clinical evidence, mechanism, importance and management

(a) Erythromycin absorption reduced

When single 500-mg doses of erythromycin ethylsuccinate were taken by 9 healthy subjects with 150 ml of an **alcoholic drink**, followed 150 min later by another 150 ml, the erythromycin AUC was decreased by about 27% and the absorption delayed. One subject showed a paradoxical 185% increase in absorption. The alcoholic drink was **pisco sour** which contains lemon juice, sugar and **pisco** (**alcohol** obtained by distilling grape juice). Blood **alcohol** levels achieved were about 50 mg% (0.5 g/l).[1] The reason for the reduced absorption is not understood but it is suggested that the slight delay is because alcohol delays gastric emptying so that the erythromycin reaches its absorption site in the duodenum a little later.[1] The extent to which this reduced absorption might affect the control of an infection is uncertain. More study is needed to assess the clinical importance of this interaction.

(b) Alcohol effects

A study in 10 healthy subjects found that while taking 500 mg erythromycin base three times daily the pharmacokinetics of oral **alcohol** (0.8 g/kg) were unchanged and the subjects' perception of intoxication was unaltered.[2] In contrast, another study in 8 healthy subjects, primarily investigating the effects of erythromycin lactobionate (3 mg/kg iv) on gastric emptying, found that when given a liquid meal of orange juice, 0.5 g/kg **alcohol** and 10 g lactulose immediately after a solid meal, the mean peak blood **alcohol** levels were raised about 40% and the AUC over the first hour was increased 33%. After that the curve was virtually the same as that seen with a saline placebo. The reason for the increased blood **alcohol** levels is thought to be that the erythromycin causes more rapid gastric emptying so that the **alcohol** is exposed to metabolism by the gastric mucosa for a shorter time.[3] What this means in terms of an increase in the effects of alcohol (e.g. on driving) is not known, but more study of this interaction is needed using oral erythromycin.

1. Morasso MI, Chávez J, Gai MN, Arancibia A. Influence of alcohol consumption on erythromycin ethylsuccinate kinetics. *Int J Clin Pharmacol Ther Toxicol* (1990) 28, 426–9.
2. Min DI, Noormohamed SE, Flanigan MJ. Effect of erythromycin on ethanol's pharmacokinetics and perception of intoxication. *Pharmacotherapy* (1995) 15, 164–9.
3. Edelbroek MAL, Horowitz M, Wishart JM, Akkermans LMA. Effects of erythromycin on gastric emptying, alcohol absorption and small intestinal transit in normal subjects. *J Nucl Med* (1993) 34, 582–8.

Erythromycin + Antacids

Mylanta can prolong the absorption of erythromycin but the clinical importance of this is uncertain.

Clinical evidence, mechanism, importance and management

Mylanta (**aluminium hydroxide, magnesium hydroxide, dimeticone**) 30 ml given with 500 mg erythromycin stearate to 8 healthy subjects had no significant effect on the AUC, peak serum concentration, or time to peak serum concentration of the erythromycin, but the mean elimination rate constant was 0.44 compared with 0.2 h^{-1}. Thus the total amount of erythromycin absorbed remained unaltered. It was suggested that the effect on elimination may be due to a possible prolonging of absorption.[1] The reason for this is not clear nor is its clinical importance known, but it is probably minor.

1. Yamreudeewong W, Scavone JM, Paone RP, Lewis GP. Effect of antacid coadministration on the bioavailability of erythromycin stearate. *Clin Pharm* (1989) 8, 352–4.

Erythromycin + Cimetidine

Cimetidine can almost double the serum levels of erythromycin. A single case report describes reversible deafness attributed to this interaction.

Clinical evidence

A 64-year-old woman was admitted to hospital with cough, dyspnoea and pleuritic pain. Her right lung was found to be consolidated and *Streptococcus milleri* was isolated from her sputum. All her antihypertensive treatment (methyldopa, propranolol, co-amilofruse) was stopped, due to hypotension, and her treatment for duodenal ulcer was changed from ranitidine 150 mg twice daily to 400 mg **cimetidine** at night. She was then started on 500 mg amoxicillin three times daily and 1 g erythromycin stearate four times daily for atypical pneumonia. Two days later she complained of 'fuzzy hearing' and audiometry showed a bilateral hearing loss. The erythromycin was stopped and her hearing returned to normal after 5 days.[1]

A study of this possible interaction in 8 healthy subjects given 250 mg erythromycin found that 400 mg **cimetidine** twice daily increased the AUC of a single 250-mg dose of erythromycin by 73%. Maximum serum erythromycin levels were doubled.[1]

Mechanism

Cimetidine is known to inhibit the *N*-demethylation of erythromycin so that it is metabolised and cleared from the body more slowly and its serum levels rise. Deafness is known to be one of the side effects of erythromycin,[1] probably exacerbated by the increased levels in this patient and made worse by her renal impairment.

Importance and management

Clinical information seems to be limited to this case and the associated human study. The general clinical importance of this interaction is uncertain, but it would now be prudent to monitor concurrent use. The makers say that reversible hearing loss has been reported with erythromycin alone, usually in doses greater than 4 g daily and usually by the intravenous route[2] (the patient cited above was taking 4 g daily). The other side-effects of erythromycin (nausea, vomiting, diarrhoea, abdominal discomfort) would also be expected to be exaggerated by cimetidine. Famotidine, nizatidine and ranitidine are possible non-interacting alternatives because they normally do not have enzyme inhibitory effects.

1. Mogford N, Pallett A, George C. Erythromycin deafness and cimetidine treatment. *BMJ* (1994) 309, 1620.
2. Erymax Capsules (Erythromycin). Elan Pharma Ltd. Summary of product characteristics, April 2001.

Erythromycin + Other antibacterials

There is some *in vitro* evidence that antagonism may occur between erythromycin, a bacteriostatic agent, and other antibacterials (e.g. penicillins, lincomycin).[1,2] However, evidence for this in practice is apparently lacking, and the combination has been used together successfully on a number of occasions.[3] The general points for and against concurrent treatment with antibacterials are outlined in the introduction to this chapter.

1. Manten A. Synergism and antagonism between antibiotic mixtures containing erythromycin. *Antibiot Chemother* (1954) 4, 1228–33.
2. Griffin LJ, Ostrander WE, Mullins CG, Beswick DE. Drug antagonism between lincomycin and erythromycin. *Science* (1965) 147, 746–7.
3. Bach MC, Monaco AP, Finland M. Pulmonary nocardiosis therapy with minocycline and with erythromycin plus ampicillin. *JAMA* (1973) 224, 1378–81.

Erythromycin + Sucralfate

Sucralfate appears not to interact adversely with erythromycin.

Clinical evidence, mechanism, importance and management

The pharmacokinetics (elimination rate constant, half-life, AUC) of a single 400-mg dose of erythromycin ethylsuccinate were not significantly altered by 1 g **sucralfate** in 6 healthy subjects. It was conclud-

ed that the therapeutic effects of erythromycin are unlikely to be affected by concurrent use.[1]

1. Miller LG, Prichard JG, White CA, Vytla B, Feldman S, Bowman RC. Effect of concurrent sucralfate administration on the absorption of erythromycin. *J Clin Pharmacol* (1990) 30, 39–44.

Erythromycin + Urinary acidifiers or alkalinizers

In the treatment of urinary tract infections, the antibacterial activity of erythromycin is maximal in alkaline urine and minimal in acid urine.

Clinical evidence

Urine taken from 7 subjects taking 1 g erythromycin 8-hourly, was tested against 5 genera of Gram-negative bacilli (*Escherichia coli*, *Klebsiella pneumoniae*, *P. mirabilis*, *Ps. aeruginosa* and *Serratia* sp.) both before and after treatment with **acetazolamide** or **sodium bicarbonate**. A direct correlation was found between the activity of the antibacterial and the pH of the urine. Normally acid urine had little or no antibacterial activity, whereas alkalinized urine had activity.[1]

Clinical studies have confirmed the increased antibacterial effectiveness of erythromycin in the treatment of bacteriuria when the urine is made alkaline.[2,3]

Mechanism

The pH of the urine does not apparently affect the way the kidney handles the antibacterial (most of it is excreted actively rather than passively) but it does have a direct influence on the way the antibacterial affects the micro-organisms. Mechanisms suggested include effects on bacterial cell receptors, the induction of active transport mechanisms on bacterial cell walls, and changes in ionisation of the antibacterial which enables it to enter the bacterial cell more effectively.

Importance and management

An established interaction, which can be exploited. The effectiveness of the antibacterial in treating urinary tract infections can be maximised by making the urine alkaline (for example with acetazolamide or sodium bicarbonate). Treatment with urinary acidifiers will minimise the activity of the erythromycin and should be avoided.

1. Sabath LD, Gerstein DA, Loder PB, Finland M. Excretion of erythromycin and its enhanced activity in urine against gram-negative bacilli with alkalinization. *J Lab Clin Med* (1968) 72, 916–23.
2. Zinner SH, Sabath LD, Casey JI, Finland M. Erythromycin and alkalinisation of the urine in the treatment of urinary-tract infections due to gram-negative bacilli. *Lancet* (1971) i, 1267–8.
3. Zinner SH, Sabath LD, Casey JI, Finland M. Erythromycin plus alkalinization in treatment of urinary infections. *Antimicrob Agents Chemother* (1969) 9, 413–16.

Ethambutol + Antacids

Aluminium hydroxide can cause a small, and probably clinically unimportant, reduction in the absorption of ethambutol in some patients.

Clinical evidence, mechanism, importance and management

A study in 13 patients with tuberculosis, given single 50 mg/kg doses of ethambutol, showed that when they were also given 1.5 g **aluminium hydroxide gel** at the same time, and repeated 15 and 30 min later, their serum ethambutol levels were delayed and reduced. The average urinary excretion of ethambutol over a 10-h period was reduced about 15%, but there were marked variations between individual patients. Some showed no interaction, and others showed increased absorption. However, no interaction was seen in 6 healthy subjects similarly treated.[1] A further study in 14 healthy subjects found decreases in the ethambutol AUC by 10% and in the maximum serum levels by 29% when ethambutol 25 mg/kg was given with 30 ml **aluminium-magnesium hydroxide** antacid.[2] Just why this interaction occurs is not understood, but **aluminium hydroxide** can affect gastric emptying. The reduction in absorption is generally small and variable, and it seems doubtful if it will have a significant effect on the treatment of tuberculosis. However, the authors of the second study suggest avoiding giving antacid at the same time as ethambutol.[2]

1. Mattila MJ, Linnoila M, Seppälä T, Koskinen R. Effect of aluminium hydroxide and gly-copyrrhonium on the absorption of ethambutol and alcohol in man. *Br J Clin Pharmacol* (1978) 5, 161–6.
2. Peloquin CA, Bulpitt AE, Jaresko GS, Jelliffe RW, Childs JM, Nix DE. Pharmacokinetics of ethambutol under fasting conditions, with food, and with antacids. *Antimicrob Agents Chemother* (1999) 43, 568–72.

Ethambutol + Food

The pharmacokinetics of ethambutol given with a high fat breakfast were only slightly different to the pharmacokinetics when given in the fasting state.[1]

1. Peloquin CA, Bulpitt AE, Jaresko GS, Jelliffe RW, Childs JM, Nix DE. Pharmacokinetics of ethambutol under fasting conditions, with food, and with antacids. *Antimicrob Agents Chemother* (1999) 43, 568–72.

Ethambutol + Rifabutin (Ansamycin)

Ethambutol appears not to interact adversely with rifabutin.

Clinical evidence, mechanism, importance and management

Ten healthy subjects were given a single 1200-mg dose of ethambutol before and after taking 300 mg **rifabutin** daily for a week. No clinically relevant changes in the pharmacokinetics of ethambutol were seen. Five of the subjects experienced moderate to severe chills, and one had transient thrombocytopenia.[1] However, these reactions are unlikely to have been due to an interaction. No special precautions would appear to be necessary during concurrent use.

1. Benedetti MS, Breda M, Pellizzoni C, Poggesi I, Sassella D, Dolfi L, Rimoldi R. Effect of rifabutin on ethambutol pharmacokinetics in healthy volunteers. *Therapie* (1995) 50 (Suppl), 503.

Ethionamide + Miscellaneous drugs

Ethionamide has been associated in a few cases with mental depression, psychiatric disturbances, hypoglycaemia, hypothyroidism and alcohol-related psychotoxicity.

Clinical evidence, mechanism, importance and management

Ethionamide can cause depression, mental disturbances and hypoglycaemia.[1,2] Caution has been advised in patients under treatment for these **psychiatric conditions** and **diabetes mellitus**.[3] Hypothyroidism and thyroid enlargement have also been reported in a few patients treated with ethionamide and particular care may therefore be necessary in patients under treatment for **thyroid malfunction**.[4] A psychotoxic reaction has also been seen in a patient on ethionamide attributed to the heavy consumption of **alcohol**.[5] The incidence and importance of all of these reactions is uncertain, but prescribers should take them into account if ethionamide is prescribed with other drugs.

1. Narang RK. Acute psychotic reaction probably caused by ethionamide. *Tubercle* (1972) 53, 137–8.
2. Sharma GS, Gupta PK, Jain NK, Shanker A, Nanawati V. Toxic psychosis to isoniazid and ethionamide in a patient with pulmonary tuberculosis. *Tubercle* (1979) 60, 171–2.
3. Sweetman SC, editor. Martindale: The complete drug reference. 33rd ed. London: Pharmaceutical Press; 2002 p.206.
4. Moulding T, Fraser R. Hypothyroidism related to ethionamide. *Am Rev Respir Dis* (1970) 101, 90–94.
5. Lansdown FS, Beran M, Litwak T. Psychotoxic reaction during ethionamide therapy. *Am Rev Respir Dis* (1967) 95, 1053–5.

Famciclovir + Miscellaneous drugs

No clinically important interactions appear to occur if famciclovir is given with allopurinol, cimetidine, digoxin or theophylline. On theoretical grounds it has been suggested that the renal excretion of the active metabolite of famciclovir might be reduced by probenecid.

Clinical evidence, mechanism, importance and management

No clinically relevant changes in the pharmacokinetics of either **allopurinol** or famciclovir were seen in 12 healthy subjects given 500 mg famciclovir after taking 300 mg **allopurinol** daily for 5 days.[1,2] **Cimetidine** 800 mg daily for 6 days increased the AUC of 500 mg famciclovir in 12 healthy subjects by about 18%, but this small change is unlikely to be of clinical importance.[3] No clinically significant pharmacokinetic interactions were seen in healthy subjects given famciclovir with **theophylline**[4] or **digoxin**.[5,6] No special precautions would therefore seem necessary if any of these drugs is used with famciclovir.

The renal excretion of aciclovir, ganciclovir and valaciclovir is reduced by **probenecid**, and for this reason the makers suggest that a similar interaction might also occur with famciclovir, resulting in an increase in the serum levels of penciclovir (the active metabolite of famciclovir)[7,8] with the implied possibility of increased toxicity. But this is totally theoretical,[8] and as yet there is no experimental or clinical evidence to show that this interaction occurs or that it is likely to be clinically important.

1. Fowles SE, Pierce D, Laroche J, Pratt SK, Prince WT, Thomas D, Woodward A. An investigation into the potential interaction between allopurinol and oral famciclovir in non-patient volunteers. *Br J Clin Pharmacol* (1992) 34, 449P–450P.
2. Fowles SE, Pratt SK, Laroche J, Prince WT. Lack of a pharmacokinetic interaction between oral famciclovir and allopurinol in healthy volunteers. *Eur J Clin Pharmacol* (1994) 46, 355–9.
3. Pratt SK, Fowles SE, Pierce DM, Prince WT. An investigation of the potential interaction between cimetidine and famciclovir in non-patient volunteers. *Br J Clin Pharmacol* (1991) 32, 656P.
4. Fairless AJ, Pratt SK, Pue MA, Fowles SE, Wolf D, Daniels S, Prince WT. An investigation into the potential interaction between theophylline and famciclovir in healthy male volunteers. *Br J Clin Pharmacol* (1992) 34, 171P–172P.
5. Pue MA, Saporito M, Laroche J, Lua S, Bygate E, Daniels S, Broom C. An investigation of the potential interaction between digoxin and oral famciclovir in healthy male volunteers. *Br J Clin Pharmacol* (1993) 36, 177P.
6. Siederer S, Scott S, Fowles S, Haveresch L, Hust R. Lack of interaction between steady-state digoxin and famciclovir. *Intersci Conf Antimicrob Agents Chemother* (1996) 36, A33.
7. Famvir (Famciclovir). Novartis Pharmaceuticals UK Ltd. Summary of product characteristics, March 2000.
8. SmithKline Beecham, Personal Communication, November 1995.

Fenticonazole + Miscellaneous drugs

Fenticonazole in the form of pessaries is absorbed very poorly from the vagina so that the risk of an interaction with other drugs given systemically is small.

Clinical evidence, mechanism, importance and management

A study in 14 women (5 of them normal, 4 with relapsing vulvovaginal candidiasis, and 5 with cervico-carcinoma) found that the systemic absorption of fenticonazole nitrate from a single 1000 mg vaginal dose was very small indeed. The amount absorbed, based on the amount recovered from the urine and faeces over 5 days ranged from 0.58 to 1.81% of the original dose.[1] The risk of a clinically relevant interaction with other drugs which may be present in the body would therefore seem to be very small. None appears to have been reported.

1. Upjohn Limited. Personal communication, May 1995.

Fluconazole + Hydrochlorothiazide

A very brief report describes a 40% increase in fluconazole serum levels in a small group of normal subjects when given hydrochlorothiazide.[1] However it is suggested that no change in the fluconazole dosage is needed.[1]

1. Quoted as unpublished data on file, Pfizer, by Grant SM, Clissold SP. Fluconazole. A review of its pharmacodynamic and pharmacokinetic properties, and therapeutic potential in superficial and systemic mycoses. *Drugs* (1990) 39, 877–916.

Fluconazole + Rifamycins

Although rifampicin (rifampin) causes only a modest increase in the loss of fluconazole from the body, the reduction in its effects may possibly be clinically important. Rifabutin levels are increased by fluconazole which carries an increased risk of uveitis.

Clinical evidence

(a) Rifampicin

Healthy subjects taking 600 mg **rifampicin** daily for 20 days were given 200 mg fluconazole on day 14. The AUC of the fluconazole was decreased by 23% and the half-life decreased by 22%.[1] **Rifampicin** 600 mg daily for 19 days in another 16 healthy subjects reduced the fluconazole AUC by 23%.[2]

Three patients with AIDS being treated for cryptococcal meningitis with fluconazole 400 mg daily relapsed when **rifampicin** was added.[3] Another undetailed report says that one of 5 patients on fluconazole needed an increased dosage or a replacement antifungal when given **rifampicin**.[4] However, a study in 11 AIDS patients with cryptococcal meningitis found that 200 mg fluconazole twice daily for 14 days had no effect on the pharmacokinetics of 300 mg **rifampicin** daily.[5]

(b) Rifabutin (Ansamycin)

Twelve HIV+ patients were given 500 mg zidovudine daily from day 1 to 44, fluconazole 200 mg daily from days 3 to 30 and 300 mg **rifabutin** from days 17 to 44. No significant changes in the pharmacokinetics of fluconazole occurred between days 16 and 30.[6]

In a similar, related study the AUC of **rifabutin** was increased by over 70% by fluconazole in patients also taking zidovudine,[7] and in a later study the same group found an 82% increase in the **rifabutin** AUC in 12 HIV+ patients when given fluconazole.[8] The prophylactic treatment of *M. avium* complex disease need not be changed as a result of this interaction,[7] but the increased rifabutin levels also carry an increased risk of uveitis.[9] Uveitis developed in 6 HIV+ patients on **rifabutin** (450 to 600 mg daily) and fluconazole. Of these, 5 were also taking clarithromycin.[10] Uveitis has been attributed to the concurrent use of **rifabutin** and fluconazole in other reports.[11,12]

Mechanism

Rifampicin increases the metabolism of the fluconazole by the liver, thereby increasing its loss from the body.[2] However, fluconazole (unlike ketoconazole) is mainly excreted unchanged in the urine so that changes in its metabolism would not be expected to have a marked effect. Fluconazole apparently increases the rifabutin levels by inhibiting its metabolism. The increased incidence of uveitis with rifabutin and ketoconazole is not understood but it seems to be related to the increased rifabutin levels.

Importance and management

Information is limited but the rifampicin/fluconazole interaction appears to be established and of clinical importance. Although rifampicin has only a relatively small effect on fluconazole (compared with its considerable effects on ketoconazole),[1,2] the cases of relapse cited above[3] and the need for an increased dosage[4] indicate that this interaction can be clinically important. Monitor concurrent use and increase the fluconazole dosage if necessary.

The rifabutin/fluconazole interaction is established, the general picture being that concurrent use can be advantageous but because of the increased risk of uveitis, the CSM in the UK says that full consideration should be given to reducing the dosage of rifabutin to 300 mg daily. The rifabutin should be stopped if uveitis develops and the patient referred to an ophthalmologist.[13]

1. Lazar J D, Wilner KD. Drug interactions with fluconazole. *Rev Infect Dis* (1990) 12 (Suppl 3), S327–S333.
2. Apseloff G, Hilligoss M, Gardner MJ, Henry EB, Inskeep PB, Gerber N, Lazar JD. Induction of fluconazole metabolism by rifampin: *in vivo* study in humans. *J Clin Pharmacol* (1991) 31, 358–61.
3. Coker RJ, Tomlinson DR, Parkin J, Harris JRW, Pinching AJ. Interaction between fluconazole and rifampicin. *BMJ* (1990) 301, 818.
4. Tett S, Carey D, Lee H-S. Drug interactions with fluconazole. *Med J Aust* (1992) 156, 365.
5. Jaruratanasirikul S, Kleepaew A. Lack of effect of fluconazole on the pharmacokinetics of rifampicin in AIDS patients. *J Antimicrob Chemother* (1996) 38, 877–80.
6. Trapnell CB, Lavelle JP, O'Leary CR, James DS, Li R, Colburn D, Woosely RL, Narang PK. Rifabutin does not alter fluconazole pharmacokinetics. *Clin Pharmacol Ther* (1993) 53, 196.
7. Trapnell CB, Narang PK, Li R, Lewis R, Colborn D, Lavelle J. Fluconazole (FLU) increases rifabutin (RIF) absorption in HIV(+) patients on stable zidovudine (ZDV) therapy. IXth Int Conf AIDS & IVth STD World Congr, Berlin, June 6-11, 1993. Abstr PO-B31-2212.
8. Trapnell CB, Narang PK, Li R, Lavelle JP. Increased plasma rifabutin levels with concomitant fluconazole therapy in HIV-infected patients. *Ann Intern Med* (1996) 124, 573–6.
9. Narang PK, Trapnell CB, Schoenfelder JR, Lavelle JP, Bianchine JR. Fluconazole and enhanced effect of rifabutin prophylaxis. *N Engl J Med* (1994) 330, 1316–17.
10. Becker K, Schimkat M, Jablonowski H, Häussinger D. Anterior uveitis associated with rifabutin medication in AIDS patients. *Infection* (1996) 24, 34–6.
11. Fuller JD, Stanfield LED, Craven DE. Rifabutin prophylaxis and uveitis. *N Engl J Med* (1994) 330, 1315–16.
12. Kelleher P, Helbert M, Sweeney J, Anderson J, Parkin J, Pinching A. Uveitis associated with rifabutin and macrolide therapy for *Mycobacterium avium intracellulare* infections in AIDS patients. *Genitourin Med* (1996) 72, 419–21.
13. Committee on Safety of Medicines/Medicines Control Agency. Stop Press: Rifabutin (Mycobutin) — uveitis. *Current Problems* (1994) 20, 4.

Flucytosine + Cytarabine

Some very limited evidence suggests that cytarabine may oppose the activity of flucytosine.

Clinical evidence, mechanism, importance and management

A man with Hodgkin's disease treated for cryptococcal meningitis with 100 mg/kg flucytosine daily showed a fall in his serum and CSF levels from a range of 30 to 40 mg/l down to undetectable levels when given **cytarabine** intravenously. When the **cytarabine** was replaced by procarbazine in the patient, his body fluid levels of flucytosine returned to their former values. *In vitro* tests showed that 1 mg/l **cytarabine** completely abolished the activity of up to 50 mg/l flucytosine against the patient's strain of cryptococcus, whereas procarbazine did not.[1] In another study in a patient with acute myeloid leukaemia it was found that the predose and postdose flucytosine levels fell from 65 and 80 mg/l to 42 and 53 mg/l respectively while concurrently receiving **cytarabine** and **daunorubicin**. These were still within the therapeutic range.[2] The drop in levels was attributed to an improvement in renal function rather than antagonism between the two drugs.[2] No changes in the activity of flucytosine against 14 out of 16 wild isolates of cryptococcus in the presence of **cytarabine** was seen in an *in vitro* study. In the remaining two, an increase was seen in one and a decrease in the other.[2]

The evidence for this interaction is therefore very limited indeed and its general clinical importance remains uncertain, but the manufacturers warn against concurrent use. It has been suggested that if both drugs are used, the flucytosine should be given 3 h or more after the **cytarabine** when the serum levels will have fallen.[3]

1. Holt RJ. Clinical problems with 5-fluorocytosine. *Mykosen* (1978) 21, 363–9.
2. Wingfield HJ. Absence of fungistatic antagonism between flucytosine and cytarabine *in vitro* and *in vivo*. *J Antimicrob Chemother* (1987) 20, 523–7.
3. Pfizer Limited. Personal communication, February 1988.

Flucytosine + Miscellaneous drugs

The interactions of flucytosine with amphotericin B and aluminium hydroxide-magnesium hydroxide do not appear to be of clinical importance.

Clinical evidence, mechanism, importance and management

The combined use of flucytosine and **amphotericin B** is more effective than flucytosine alone in the treatment of cryptococcal meningitis, but **amphotericin B** can cause deterioration in kidney function, which may result in raised flucytosine blood levels and a possible increase in flucytosine toxicity. Nevertheless combined use is thought to be useful.[1] **Aluminium hydroxide-magnesium hydroxide** delays the absorption of flucytosine from the gut, but the total amount absorbed remains unaffected.[2]

1. Bennett JE, Dismukes WE, Duma RJ, Medoff G, Sande MA, Gallis H, Leonard J, Fields BT, Bradshaw M, Haywood H, McGee ZA, Cate TR, Cobbs CG, Warner JF, Alling DW. A comparison of amphotericin B alone and combined with flucytosine in the treatment of cryptoccal meningitis. *N Engl J Med* (1979) 301, 126–31.
2. Cutler RE, Blair AD, Kelly MR. Flucytosine kinetics in subjects with normal and impaired renal function. *Clin Pharmacol Ther* (1978) 24, 333–42.

Foscarnet + Ciprofloxacin

Two patients developed tonic-clonic seizures when treated with foscarnet and ciprofloxacin.

Clinical evidence

An HIV+ patient on multiple therapy (including **ciprofloxacin**, clarithromycin, cimetidine, fluconazole, morphine, rifampicin, vancomycin) was additionally prescribed intravenous foscarnet 60 mg/kg 8-hourly for cytomegalovirus infection. He was only given half of the first dose, but 9 hours later he developed a tonic-clonic seizure. About 45 min after the start of administration of the remainder of the foscarnet infusion he again had seizures. No further seizures occurred when the foscarnet was stopped.[1] Another HIV+ patient was given the same foscarnet regimen and dosage for 10 days without problems, until he was additionally started on **ciprofloxacin**, clofazimine, ethambutol, pyrazinamide and rifampicin for mycobacterial sepsis. Within 2 days he developed a seizure a few minutes after the start of the foscarnet infusion. This stopped when the foscarnet was stopped, and reoccurred when the foscarnet was restarted.[1] The **ciprofloxacin** dosage given to both patients was 750 mg twice daily.

Mechanism

Not understood. Both foscarnet and ciprofloxacin have the potential to cause seizures and it seems that some enhancement of this activity occurs if they are used in combination.

Importance and management

Direct information seems to be limited to these two cases. It is impossible to know for certain if the seizures were due to the combined effects of these two drugs or not, but the evidence seems to point in that direction. The general importance of this interaction is uncertain, but you should monitor very closely if these drugs are used together. Oth-

er quinolones may possibly be no safer because they also have epileptogenic activity. More study is needed.

1. Fan-Havard P, Sanchorawala V, Oh J, Moser EM, Smith SP. Concurrent use of foscarnet and ciprofloxacin may increase the propensity for seizures. *Ann Pharmacother* (1994) 28, 869–72.

Foscarnet + Miscellaneous drugs

Four patients showed marked hypocalcaemia when concurrently treated with foscarnet and pentamidine. One of them died. Foscarnet and probenecid do not appear to interact adversely.

Clinical evidence, mechanism, importance and management

(a) Pentamidine

Four patients with suspected AIDS-related cytomegaloviral infections of the chest developed signs of hypocalcaemia within 10 days of starting treatment with foscarnet and **pentamidine** (dosages not stated). All 4 had paraesthesia of the hands and feet, and 3 of them had Chvosteks's and Trousseau's signs (signs of tetany). The serum calcium levels of 3 of them fell but normalised when one of the drugs was stopped. The fourth patient died with severe hypocalcaemia (1.42 mmol/l). Both drugs have been associated with hypocalcaemia in HIV patients, and in these 4 patients their effects appear to have been additive. The authors of the report advise very close monitoring if both drugs are used.[1]

(b) Probenecid

A study in 6 HIV+ patients found that 1 g **probenecid** twice daily for 3 days had no effect on the pharmacokinetics of foscarnet 90 mg/kg given intravenously as a sustained infusion. The authors conclude that, because of the lack of interaction with **probenecid**, almost all of the renal elimination of foscarnet is by glomerular filtration, with only a minimal contribution of active tubular secretion.[2] No special precautions seem to be necessary.

1. Youle MS, Clarbour J, Gazzard B, Chanas A. Severe hypocalcaemia in AIDS patients treated with foscarnet and pentamidine. *Lancet* (1988) 1, 1455–6.
2. Noormohamed FH, Youle MS, Higgs CJ, Gazzard BG, Lant AF. Pharmacokinetics of intravenous foscarnet in AIDS patients: lack of effect of probenecid pretreatment. *Br J Clin Pharmacol* (1994) 37, 519P.

Foscarnet + Nucleoside reverse transcriptase inhibitors

No pharmacokinetic interactions occur between foscarnet and didanosine, zalcitabine or zidovudine.

Clinical evidence, mechanism, importance and management

(a) Didanosine

In 3 phases, 12 HIV+ patients were given 4 doses of foscarnet (90 mg/kg iv), 4 doses of **didanosine** (200 mg orally), and 4 doses of both drugs together. Based on the data obtained from these patients (drug clearance, volume of distribution, half-life, mean residence time), no pharmacokinetic interactions were seen to occur between these two drugs. This suggests that no dosage adjustments will be needed during concurrent use.[1]

(b) Zalcitabine

Foscarnet 90 mg/kg 12-hourly and **zalcitabine** 750 micrograms 8-hourly were given to 12 HIV+ subjects for 2 days. There were no clinically significant alterations in the pharmacokinetics of either drug.[2]

(c) Zidovudine

The antiviral effects of foscarnet and **zidovudine** appear to be additive or synergistic. However, no significant alteration in the pharmacokinetics of either drug was seen in a 14-day study in 5 AIDS patients given both drugs.[3] Foscarnet does not appear to affect **zidovudine** intracellular activation.[4] Concurrent use would seem to be valuable.

1. Aweeka FT, Mathur V, Dorsey R, Jacobson MA, Martin-Munley S, Pirrung D, Franco J, Lizak P, Johnson J, Gambertoglio J. Concomitant foscarnet and didanosine: a pharmacokinetic (PK) evaluation in patients with HIV disease. American Society of Microbiology 2nd National Conference on Human Retroviruses and Related infections, Washington DC, 1995. Abstract 492.
2. Aweeka FT, Brody SR, Jacobson M, Jacobson K, Martin-Munley S. Is there a pharmacokinetic interaction between foscarnet and zalcitabine during concomitant administration? *Clin Ther* (1998) 20, 232–43.
3. Aweeka FT, Gambertoglio JG, van der Horst C, Raasch R, Jacobson MA. Pharmacokinetics of concomitantly administered foscarnet and zidovudine for treatment of human immunodeficiency virus infection (AIDS clinical trials group protocol 053). *Antimicrob Agents Chemother* (1992) 36, 1773–8.
4. Brody SR, Aweeka FT. Pharmacokinetics of intracellular zidovudine and its phosphorylated anabolites in the absence and presence of other antiviral agents using an in vitro human PBMC model. *Clin Pharmacol Ther* (1997) 61, 149.

Fosfomycin trometamol + Cimetidine or Metoclopramide

Cimetidine does not affect the pharmacokinetics of fosfomycin trometamol. Metoclopramide reduces its bioavailability but the evidence suggests that this probably does not affect the control of urinary tract infections.

Clinical evidence, mechanism, importance and management

Nine healthy subjects were given 20 mg **metoclopramide** 30 min before fosfomycin 50 mg/kg and then a week later, **cimetidine**, 400 mg on the night before and 400 mg 30 min before fosfomycin 50 mg/kg. **Cimetidine** had almost no effect on the pharmacokinetics of fosfomycin trometamol, whereas **metoclopramide** reduced the peak serum levels by 42% and the AUC by 27%. The reason seems to be that the **metoclopramide** speeds the transit through the gut, so that less time is available for good absorption. However, despite these reductions the urinary concentrations remained above the minimum levels required for common urinary pathogens for at least 36 h after giving the antibacterial.[1] This suggests that the interaction is possibly not clinically important.

1. Bergan T, Mastropaolo G, Di Mario F, Naccarato R. Pharmacokinetics of fosfomycin and influence of cimetidine and metoclopramide on the bioavailability of fosfomycin trometamol. New Trends in Urinary Tract Infections (eds Neu and Williams) Int Symp Rome 1987, pp 157–66. Published in 1988.

Furazolidone + Sympathomimetics (directly and indirectly-acting)

After 5 to 10 days use furazolidone has MAO-inhibitory activity approximately equivalent to the antidepressant and antihypertensive MAOIs. The concurrent use of sympathomimetic amines with indirect activity (amphetamines, phenylpropanolamine, ephedrine, etc.) or tyramine-rich foods and drinks may be expected to result in a potentially serious rise in blood pressure, although direct evidence of accidental adverse reactions of this kind seem not to have been reported. The pressor effects of norepinephrine (noradrenaline) are unchanged.

Clinical evidence

After 6 days treatment with 400 mg furazolidone daily, the pressor responses to **tyramine** or **dexamfetamine (dextroamphetamine)** in 4 hypertensive patients had increased two to threefold, and after

13 days about tenfold. These responses were approximately the same as those found in two other patients on **pargyline**.[1] The MAO-inhibitory activity of furazolidone was confirmed by measurements taken on jejunal specimens. The pressor effects of **norepinephrine (noradrenaline)** were unchanged.[1]

Mechanism

The MAO-inhibitory activity of furazolidone is not immediate and may in fact be due to a metabolite of furazolidone.[2] It develops gradually so that after 5 to 10 days use, indirectly-acting sympathomimetics will interact with furazolidone in the same way as they do in the presence of other MAOIs.[3,4] More details of the mechanisms of this interaction are to be found elsewhere (see 'Monoamine oxidase inhibitors (MAOIs) + Tyramine-rich foods', p.685, 'Monoamine oxidase inhibitors (MAOIs) + Sympathomimetics (indirectly-acting)', p.680).

Importance and management

The MAO-inhibitory activity of furazolidone after 5 to 10 days use is established, but reports of hypertensive crises either with sympathomimetics or tyramine-containing foods or drinks appear to be lacking. Notwithstanding, it would seem prudent to warn patients given furazolidone not to take any of the drugs, foods or drinks which are prohibited to those on antidepressant or antihypertensive MAOIs (e.g. cough, cold and influenza remedies containing phenylpropanolamine, phenylephrine, pseudoephedrine, etc., appetite-suppressants containing sympathomimetics, or tyramine-rich foods or drinks). See the appropriate monographs for more detailed lists of these drugs, foods and drinks ('Monoamine oxidase inhibitors (MAOIs) + Tyramine-rich foods', 'Monoamine oxidase inhibitors (MAOIs) + Tyramine-rich drinks', p.684). No adverse interaction would be expected with norepinephrine (noradrenaline).

1. Pettinger WA, Oates JA. Supersensitivity to tyramine during monoamine oxidase inhibition in man. Mechanism at the level of the adrenergic neurone. *Clin Pharmacol Ther* (1968) 9, 341–4.
2. Stern IJ, Hollifield RD, Wilk S, Buzard JA. The anti-monoamine oxidase effects of furazolidone. *J Pharmacol Exp Ther* (1967) 156, 492–9.
3. Pettinger WA, Soyangco FG, Oates JA. Monoamine-oxidase inhibition by furazolidone in man. *Clin Res* (1966) 14, 258.
4. Pettinger WA, Soyangco FG, Oates JA. Inhibition of monoamine oxidase in man by furazolidone. *Clin Pharmacol Ther* (1968) 9, 442–7.

Ganciclovir + Probenecid

Probenecid reduces the renal excretion of ganciclovir and increases its serum levels, but this is of uncertain importance.

Clinical evidence, mechanism, importance and management

A pharmacokinetic study in HIV+ patients found that 500 mg **probenecid** 6-hourly increased the AUC of oral ganciclovir 1 g 8-hourly by 53.1%, and the renal clearance was reduced 12.3%. The presumed mechanism is that the two drugs compete for renal tubular secretion.[1]

The clinical importance of this interaction is uncertain, but be alert for increased ganciclovir effects and toxicity if **probenecid** is used concurrently.

1. Gaines K, Wong R, Jung D, Cimoch P, Lavelle J, Pollard R. Pharmacokinetic interactions with oral ganciclovir: zidovudine, didanosine, probenecid. Abstract book of the 10th Int Conf AIDS 1994 August 7–12, Yokohama (Japan) (1994) 1,7.

Ganciclovir + Trimethoprim

Ganciclovir and trimethoprim do not appear to interact.

Clinical evidence, mechanism, importance and management

Ganciclovir 1000 mg 8-hourly was given to 11 HIV+ subjects with **trimethoprim** 200 mg daily for 7 days. Ganciclovir clearance was decreased by 13%, and the half life increased by 18% while the **trimethoprim** minimum serum concentration was raised by 13%. The combination was well tolerated and none of these changes were considered clinically significant, so no dose alteration appears necessary on concurrent use.[1]

1. Jung D, AbdelHameed MH, Hunter J, Teitelbaum P, Dorr A, Griffy K. The pharmacokinetics and safety profile of oral ganciclovir in combination with trimethoprim in HIV- and CMV-seropositive patients. *Br J Clin Pharmacol* (1999) 47, 255–9.

Griseofulvin + Phenobarbital

The antifungal effects of griseofulvin can be reduced or even abolished by the concurrent use of phenobarbital.

Clinical evidence

Two epileptic children of 7 and 8 taking 40 mg **phenobarbital** daily failed to respond to long-term treatment for tinea capitis with griseofulvin, 125 mg three times daily, until the **barbiturate** was withdrawn.[1]

Five other patients (3 also taking **phenytoin**) have been reported who similarly failed to respond to griseofulvin while taking **phenobarbital**.[2-4] Two studies, in a total of 14 healthy subjects, found that while taking 30 mg **phenobarbital** three times daily the serum levels of griseofulvin given orally were reduced by about a third[5] and the absorption reduced from 58.1% without **phenobarbital** to 40.6% in the presence of **phenobarbital**.[6]

Mechanism

Not fully understood. Initially it was thought that the phenobarbital increased the metabolism and clearance of the griseofulvin,[7] but it has also been suggested that it reduces the absorption of griseofulvin from the gut.[6] One idea is that the phenobarbital increases peristalsis so that the opportunity for absorption is diminished.[6] Another suggestion is that the phenobarbital forms a complex with the griseofulvin which makes an already poorly soluble drug even less soluble, and therefore less readily absorbed.[8]

Importance and management

An established interaction of clinical importance, although the evidence seems to be limited to the reports cited. If the barbiturate must be given, it has been suggested that the griseofulvin should be given in divided doses three times a day to give it a better chance of being absorbed,[6] although divided doses were used when the interaction occurred in one of the studies cited.[1] The effect of increasing the dosage of griseofulvin appears not to have been studied. An alternative is to exchange the phenobarbital for a non-interacting anticonvulsant such as sodium valproate. This proved to be successful in one of the cases cited.[1]

1. Beurey J, Weber M, Vignaud J-M. Traitement des teignes microsporiques. Interférence métabolique entre phénobarbital et griséofulvine. *Ann Dermatol Venereol* (1982) 109, 567–70.
2. Lorenc E. A new factor in griseofulvin treatment failures. *Mo Med* (1967) 64, 32–3.
3. Stepanova ZV, Sheklakova AA. Liuminal kak prichina neudachi griseofulvinoterapii bol'nogo mikrospoviei. *Vestn Dermatol Venerol* (1975) 12, 63–5.
4. Hay RJ, Clayton YM, Moore MK, Midgely G. An evaluation of itraconazole in the management of onychomycosis. *Br J Dermatol* (1988) 119, 359–66.
5. Busfield D, Child KJ, Atkinson RM, Tomich EG. An effect of phenobarbitone on blood-levels of griseofulvin in man. *Lancet* (1963) ii, 1042-3.
6. Riegelman S, Rowland M, Epstein WL. Griseofulvin-phenobarbital interaction in man. *JAMA* (1970) 213, 426–31.
7. Busfield D, Child KJ, Tomich EG. An effect of phenobarbitone on griseofulvin metabolism in the rat. *Br J Pharmacol* (1964) 22, 137–42.
8. Abougela IKA, Bigford DJ, McCorquodale I, Grant DJW. Complex formation and other physico-chemical interactions between griseofulvin and phenobarbitone. *J Pharm Pharmacol* (1976) 28, 44P.

Halofantrine + Miscellaneous drugs

The CSM in the UK recommends that halofantrine should not be used with other drugs that can prolong the QT interval because of the risk of cardiac arrhythmias. Halofantrine appears not to be an enzyme inhibitor.

Clinical evidence, mechanism, importance and management

Halofantrine in recommended doses can prolong the QT interval in the majority of patients, causing ventricular arrhythmias in a very small number. The effect is increased if taken with **fatty foods** because of the markedly increased absorption. A preliminary clinical study suggests that *Fansidar* (**pyrimethamine** and **sulfadoxine**) may raise the AUC and peak plasma levels of halofantrine, which could lead to an increased incidence of arrhythmias.[1] World-wide, 14 cases of cardiac arrhythmias have been reported and 8 patients are known to have died. In order to reduce the likelihood of arrhythmias, the UK CSM now advises that halofantrine should not be taken with **meals**, or with certain other drugs that may induce arrhythmias. They list **chloroquine**, **mefloquine** and **quinine**, **tricyclic antidepressants**, **antipsychotics**, **certain antiarrhythmic agents**, **terfenadine** and **astemizole**, as well as drugs causing electrolyte disturbances.[2] A study into the enzyme inhibitory actions of concurrent **chloroquine** and halofantrine found that both drugs inhibited the cytochrome P450 isoenzyme CYP2D6, which reinforces the recommendation that they should not be used together.[3] Although not listed, it would seem prudent to avoid other drugs that prolong the QT interval. For a list, see 'Drugs that prolong the QT interval + Other drugs that prolong the QT interval', p.103. Halofantrine should also not be given to patients with an already prolonged QT interval or ventricular arrhythmia (e.g. coronary heart disease, cardiomyopathy, congenital heart disease).[2] *In vitro* and *animal* studies suggest that halofantrine is not a potent inhibitor of cytochrome P450-mediated drug metabolism.[4] However, drugs such as **ketoconazole**, **quinidine** and **quinine** have been shown *in vitro* to inhibit the metabolism of halofantrine by the cytochrome P450 isoenzyme CYP3A4, and so may increase halofantrine levels, which could reasonably be expected to increase toxicity.[5] Confirmatory studies of these potential interactions are needed in a clinical practice.

1. Hombhanje FW. Effect of a single dose of Fansidar™ on the pharmacokinetics of halofantrine in healthy volunteers: a preliminary report. *Br J Clin Pharmacol* (2000) 49, 283–4.
2. Committee on Safety of Medicines/Medicines Control Agency. Cardiac arrhythmias with halofantrine (Halfan). *Current Problems* (1994) 20, 6.
3. Simooya OO, Sijumbil G, Lennard MS, Tucker GT. Halofantrine and chloroquine inhibit CYP2D6 activity in healthy Zambians. *Br J Clin Pharmacol* (1998) 45, 315–17.
4. Karbwang J, Bangchang KN. Clinical pharmacokinetics of halofantrine. *Clin Pharmacokinet* (1994) 27, 104–119.
5. Baune B, Furlan V, Taburet AM, Farinotti R. Effect of selected antimalarial drugs and inhibitors of cytochrome P-450 3A4 on halofantrine metabolism by human liver microsomes. *Drug Metab Dispos* (1999) 27, 565–8.

Hetacillin + Miscellaneous drugs

No changes in serum antibacterial levels were seen in 12 patients concurrently treated with hetacillin and anticonvulsants (which included carbamazepine, clonazepam, di-

azepam, phenytoin, phenobarbital, primidone, valproic acid) or in 12 other patients treated with chlorpromazine.[1] No special precautions would seem to be necessary.

1. Galanopoulou P, Karageorgiou C, Dimakopoulou K. Effect of enzyme induction on bioavailability of hetacillin in patients treated with anticonvulsants and chlorpromazine. *Eur J Drug Metab Pharmacokinet* (1990) 15, 15–18.

Hydroxychloroquine + Rifampicin

The control of discoid lupus with hydroxychloroquine in a woman was rapidly lost when rifampicin was added. Control was regained when the hydroxychloroquine dosage was doubled.

Clinical evidence, mechanism, importance and management

A woman with discoid lupus, well controlled with 200 mg hydroxychloroquine daily, was additionally given **rifampicin**, isoniazid and pyrazinamide for tuberculosis. Within 1 to 2 weeks the discoid lupus flared-up again but it rapidly responded when the hydroxychloroquine dosage was doubled. The reason is not known for certain but the authors of the report suggest that the **rifampicin** (a recognised and potent cytochrome P450 microsomal enzyme inducing agent) increased the metabolism and clearance of the hydroxychloroquine so that it was no longer effective.[1] It is already known that discoid lupus flare-ups can occur within 2 weeks of stopping hydroxychloroquine,[2] which gives support to this suggested mechanism. Neither isoniazid nor pyrazinamide is likely to have been responsible for what happened.

This seems to be the first and only report of this interaction, but what happened is consistent with the way **rifampicin** interacts with many other drugs. If therefore **rifampicin** is added to hydroxychloroquine, the outcome should be well monitored. Be alert for the need to increase the hydroxychloroquine dosage.

1. Harvey CJ, Bateman NT, Lloyd ME, Hughes GRV. Influence of rifampicin on hydroxychloroquine. *Clin Exp Rheumatol* (1995) 13, 536.
2. The Canadian Hydroxychloroquine Study Group. A randomized study of the effect of withdrawing hydroxychloroquine sulfate in systemic lupus erythematosus. *N Engl J Med* (1991) 324, 150–4.

Hydroxyquinoline + Zinc oxide

The presence of zinc oxide inhibits the therapeutic effects of 8-hydroxyquinoline in ointments.

Clinical evidence

The observation that a patient had an allergic reaction to 8-hydroxyquinoline in ointments with a paraffin base, but not a zinc oxide base, prompted further study of a possible incompatibility. The subsequent study in 13 patients confirmed that **zinc oxide** reduces the eczematogenic (allergic) properties of the 8-hydroxyquinoline. However, it also inhibits its antibacterial and antimycotic effects as well, and appears to stimulate the growth of *Candida albicans*.[1]

Mechanism

It seems almost certain that the zinc ions form chelates with 8-hydroxyquinoline, which have little or no antibacterial properties.[1,2]

Importance and management

The documentation is limited but the reaction appears to be established. There is no point in using zinc oxide to reduce the allergic properties of the 8-hydroxyquinoline if, at the same time, the therapeutic effects disappear.

1. Fischer T. On 8-hydroxyquinoline-zinc oxide incompatibility. *Dermatologica* (1974) 149, 129–35.

2. Albert A, Rubbo SD, Goldacre RJ, Balfour BG. The influence of chemical constitution on antibacterial activity. Part III: A study of 8-hydroxyquinoline (oxine) and related compounds. *Br J Exp Path* (1947) 28, 69–87.

Influenza vaccine + Miscellaneous drugs

Paracetamol does not affect influenza vaccine and appears to reduce its side-effects. The pharmacokinetics of alprazolam, lorazepam and paracetamol are not affected by influenza vaccine.

Clinical evidence, mechanism, importance and management

The pharmacokinetics of single doses of 650 mg intravenous **paracetamol** (**acetaminophen**), 1 mg oral **alprazolam**, or 2 mg intravenous **lorazepam** remained unaffected in normal subjects when measured 7 and 14 days after 0.5 ml influenza vaccine given intramuscularly.[1] **Paracetamol** (**acetaminophen**) 1 g four times daily for 2 days had no effect on the production of *H. influenzae* antibodies in a group of 29 elderly patients concurrently given inactivated influenza virus vaccine, and appeared to reduce the adverse effects of the vaccine (fever, etc).[2] There would seem to be no reason for avoiding the concurrent use of these drugs and, in the case of **paracetamol**, some advantage.

1. Scavone JM, Blyden GT, LeDuc BW, Greenblatt DJ. Effect of influenza vaccine on acetaminophen, alprazolam, antipyrine and lorazepam pharmacokinetics. *J Clin Pharmacol* (1986) 26, 556.
2. Gross P, Bonelli J, Weksler M, Russo C, Munk G, Dran S, Levandowski R. Acetaminophen prevents adverse effects but does not reduce antibody responses to inactivated influenza virus vaccine in the elderly. *Intersci Conf Antimicrob Agents Chemother* (1992) 32, 179.

Interferons + ACE inhibitors

Preliminary evidence indicates that severe granulocytopenia can develop if ACE inhibitors and interferon are given concurrently.

Clinical evidence, mechanism, importance and management

Patients with cryoglobulinaemia were treated with 3 million units of recombinant **interferon alfa-2a** (35 patients) or natural **interferon beta** (3 patients), both daily or on alternate days for periods of 6 to 17 months. Severe toxicity developed in 3 patients, who were the only ones amongst the group to also be treated with ACE inhibitors. Granulocytopenia developed in 2 patients within a few days of starting **enalapril** 10 mg daily or **captopril** 50 mg daily, and subsided 1 to 2 weeks after the both drugs were stopped. Another patient, already on **enalapril** 5 mg daily, developed severe granulocytopenia when interferon was started, and again when re-challenged with both drugs. None of the other 35 patients on interferon alone developed any significant haematological problems. The reasons for this severe reaction are not understood but the authors of the report postulate that it may be an autoimmune response.[1]

A follow-up letter commenting on this report described 2 further patients with hepatitis C infection, cryoglobulinaemia and glomerulonephritis on 3 million units daily of recombinant **interferon alfa-2a** who showed granulocytopenia within 9 days of being given 75 mg **captopril** or 20 mg **enalapril** daily. Counts returned to normal with both drug dosages unchanged. Another patient with multiple myeloma given **interferon alfa-2a** (3 million units 3 times weekly) and long-term **benazepril** 10 mg daily showed a normal granulocyte count after 3 months.[2]

Whatever the explanation for these findings, the extent of this severe and potentially life-threatening response certainly suggests that if the decision is made to give ACE inhibitors and interferons concurrently, the outcome should be very closely monitored. It remains to be seen whether the interaction is confined to patients with cryoglob-ulinaemia.

1. Casato M, Pucillo LP, Leoni M, di Lullo L, Gabrielli A, Sansonno D, Dammacco F, Danieli G, Bonomo L. Granulocytopenia after combined therapy with interferon and angiotensin-converting enzyme inhibitors: evidence of synergistic hematological toxicity. Am J Med (1995) 99, 386–91.
2. Jacquot C, Caudwell V, Belenfant X. Granulocytopenia after combined therapy with interferon and angiotensin-converting enzyme inhibitors: evidence for a synergistic hematologic toxicity. Am J Med (1996) 101, 235–6.

Interferons + Miscellaneous drugs

Aspirin and paracetamol (acetaminophen) appear neither to reduce the effects of interferon nor its side-effects. Prednisone also does not reduce its side-effects but it may possibly reduce its biological activity.

Clinical evidence

A single intramuscular dose of 18 million units of recombinant human interferon α_{2a} was given alone, or after one day of an 8-day course of either **aspirin** (650 mg four-hourly), **paracetamol** (650 mg four-hourly) or **prednisone** (40 mg daily) to 8 healthy subjects. None of these additional drugs reduced the interferon side-effects of fever, chills, headache or myalgia. However the **prednisone** appeared to reduce the biological response to interferon by approximately half.[1]

Mechanism

Not understood.

Importance and management

This study would seem to suggest there is no point in using either aspirin or paracetamol to reduce the side effects of interferon, but apparently no adverse interaction occurs either. In the case of prednisone (and possibly other corticosteroids) the reduction in the biological activity of the interferon would seem to be a disadvantage but more confirmatory study of this is needed.

1. Witter FR, Woods AS, Griffin MD, Smith CR, Nadler P, Lietman PS. Effects of prednisone, aspirin and acetaminophen on an in vivo biologic response to interferon in humans. Clin Pharmacol Ther (1988) 44, 239–43.

Interferons + Ribavirin

Interferon and ribavirin appear to interact together advantageously and not adversely.

Clinical evidence, mechanism, importance and management

A meta-analysis of three trials involving 186 patients, which studied the efficacy and tolerability of combining **ribavirin** and interferon for the treatment for chronic hepatitis C, showed no serious adverse effects and the therapy was enhanced two to threefold compared to interferon therapy alone.[1] The report failed to say which form of interferon was used. Another study using interferon α-2b found similar results.[2]

1. Schalm SW, Hansen BE, Chemello L, Bellobuono A, Brouwer JT, Weiland O, Cavalletto L, Schvarcz R, Ideo G, Alberti A. Ribavirin enhances the efficacy but not the adverse effects of interferon in chronic hepatitis C. Meta-analysis of individual patient data from European centers. J Hepatol (1997) 26, 961–6.
2. Khakoo S, Glue P, Grellier L, Wells B, Bell A, Dash C, Murray-Lyon I, Lypnyj D, Flannery B, Walters K, Dusheiko GM. Ribavirin and interferon alfa-2b in chronic hepatitis C: assessment of possible pharmacokinetic and pharmacodynamic interactions. Br J Clin Pharmacol (1998) 46, 563–70.

Isoniazid + Aminosalicylic acid (PAS)

Isoniazid serum levels are raised by the concurrent use of aminosalicylic acid.

Clinical evidence, mechanism, importance and management

A study in man showed that the concurrent administration of **aminosalicylic acid** significantly increased the serum levels and half-lives of isoniazid due, it is suggested, to the inhibition of the isoniazid metabolism by the **aminosalicylic acid**. The effect was most marked among the 'fast' acetylators of isoniazid.[1] No precise figures were stated. There seem to be no reports of isoniazid toxicity arising from this interaction.

1. Boman G, Borgå O, Hanngren Å, Malmborg A-S, Sjöqvist F. Pharmacokinetic interactions between the tuberculostatics rifampicin, para-aminosalicylic acid and isoniazid. Acta Pharmacol Toxicol (1970) 28 (Suppl 1), 15.

Isoniazid + Antacids

The absorption of isoniazid from the gut is reduced by the concurrent use of aluminium hydroxide. Isoniazid should be given at least an hour before the antacid to minimise the effects of this interaction.

Clinical evidence

10 patients with tuberculosis were given 45 ml **aluminium hydroxide (Amphojel)** at 6, 7 and 8 am, followed immediately by isoniazid and any other medication they were receiving. 1 h serum isoniazid levels and the AUCs were depressed, and peak serum concentrations occurring between 1 and 2 h after ingestion were reduced about 16% (or expressed in micrograms/ml/mg of isoniazid/kg body weight to allow for different dosages, by 25%).[1] The effect of **magaldrate (hydrated magnesium aluminate)** was less,[1] and in another study **magnesium-aluminium hydroxide** had no effect.[2]

Mechanism

Aluminium hydroxide delays gastric emptying (demonstrated in man and rats[3,4]), causing retention of the isoniazid in the stomach. Since isoniazid is largely absorbed from the intestine, the decrease in serum isoniazid concentrations is explained. Aluminium hydroxide also appears to inhibit absorption as well.

Importance and management

This interaction appears to be established, although information is limited. Its clinical importance is uncertain, but because single high doses of isoniazid are more effective in arresting tuberculosis than the same amount of drug in divided doses[5,6] it would seem wise to avoid this interaction by following the recommendations made in the study cited, namely to give the isoniazid at least an hour before **aluminium hydroxide**.[1] There seems to be no information about the effects of other antacids. **Didanosine** tablets contain antacids (**magnesium/aluminium hydroxide**) in the formulation to raise the pH within the stomach, but it has been shown that there is too little to affect the bioavailability of isoniazid if given concurrently.[7]

1. Hurwitz A, Schlozman DL. Effects of antacids on gastrointestinal absorption of isoniazid in rat and man. Am Rev Respir Dis (1974) 109, 41–7.
2. Peloquin CA, Namdar S, Dodge AA, Nix DE. Pharmacokinetics of isoniazid under fasting conditions, with food, and with antacids. Int J Tuberc Lung Dis (1999) 3, 703–710.
3. Hava M, Hurwitz A. The relaxing effect of aluminium and lanthanum on rat and human gastric smooth muscle in vitro. Eur J Pharmacol (1973) 22, 156–61.
4. Vats TS, Hurwitz A, Robinson RG, Herrin W. Effects of antacids on gastric emptying in children. Pediatr Res (1973) 7, 340.
5. Fox W. General considerations in intermittent drug therapy of pulmonary tuberculosis. Postgrad Med J (1971) 47, 729–36.

6. Hudson LD, Sbarbaro JA. Twice weekly tuberculosis chemotherapy. *JAMA* (1973) 223, 139–43.
7. Gallicano K, Sahai J, Zaror-Behrens G, Pakuts A. Effect of antacids in didanosine tablet on bioavailability of isoniazid. *Antimicrob Agents Chemother* (1994) 38, 894–7.

Isoniazid + Cheese or Fish

Patients taking isoniazid who eat some foods such as cheese, and particularly fish from the scombroid family (tuna, mackerel, salmon) which are not fresh, may experience an exaggerated histamine poisoning reaction.

Clinical evidence

Three months after starting to take 300 mg isoniazid daily, a woman experienced a series of unpleasant reactions 10 to 30 min after eating **cheese**. These reactions included chills, headache (sometimes severe), itching of the face and scalp, slight diarrhoea, flushing of the face (and on one occasion the whole body), variable and mild tachycardia and a bursting sensation in the head. Blood pressure measurements showed only a modest rise (from her normal level of 95/65 to 110/80 mmHg). No physical or biochemical abnormalities were found.[1]

Headache, dizziness, blurred vision, tachycardia, flushing and itching of the skin, redness of the eyes, burning sensation of the body, difficulty in breathing, abdominal colic, diarrhoea, vomiting, sweating and wheezing have all been described in other patients on isoniazid after eating **cheese**.[2-5] Certain **tropical fish**, including **tuna** (**skipjack** or **bonito**—*Katsuwanus pelamis*),[6-10] *Sardinella (Amblygaster) sirm*,[11] *Rastrigella kanagurta*[12] and others[13] are also implicated. There are a few hundred cases of this reaction on record.

Mechanism

What occurs appears to be an exaggeration of the histamine poisoning that can occur after eating some foods such as cheese and members of the scombroid family of fish (tuna, mackerel, salmon, etc) if not fresh and adequately refrigerated. These fish have a high histidine content and under poor storage circumstances the histine is decarboxylated by bacteria to produce unusually large amounts of histamine. Normally this is inactivated by histaminase in the body, but in the presence of isoniazid, which is a potent inhibitor of this enzyme it can be absorbed largely unchanged and histamine poisoning develops.[14] Histamine survives all but very prolonged cooking. Tuna fish can contain 180 to 500 mg histamine per 100 g, other types of fish may contain as little as 0.5 to 7.5 mg.[9]

Importance and management

An established interaction of clinical importance but the incidence appears to be small. With the exception of one patient who appeared to have had a cerebrovascular accident,[8] the reactions experienced by the others were unpleasant and alarming but usually not serious nor life-threatening, and required little or no treatment, although 'scombroid poisoning' in the absence of isoniazid is sometimes more serious. Two reports say that treatment with antihistamines can be effective.[9,13] Isoniazid has been in use since 1956 and there is little need now to introduce any general dietary restrictions, but if any of these reactions is experienced, examine the patient's diet and advise the avoidance of any probable offending foodstuffs. Very mature cheese and fish of the scombroid family (tuna, mackerel, salmon and other varieties of dark meat fish) which are not fresh are to be treated with suspicion, but there is no way one can guess the likely histamine content of food without undertaking a detailed analysis.

1. Smith CK, Durack DT. Isoniazid and reaction to cheese. *Ann Intern Med* (1978) 88, 520–1.
2. Uragoda CG, Lodha SC. Histamine intoxication in a tuberculous patient after ingestion of cheese. *Tubercle* (1979) 60, 59–61.
3. Lejonc JL, Gusmini D, Brochard P. Isoniazid and reaction to cheese. *Ann Intern Med* (1979) 91, 793.
4. Hauser MJ, Baier H. Interactions of isoniazid with foods. *Drug Intell Clin Pharm* (1982) 16, 617–18.
5. Toutoungi M, Carroll R, Dick P. Isoniazide (INH) and tyramine-rich food. *Chest* (1986) 89 (Suppl 6), 540S.
6. Uragoda CG, Kottegoda SR. Adverse reactions to isoniazid on ingestion of fish with a high histamine content. *Tubercle* (1977) 58, 83–9.
7. Uragoda CG. Histamine poisoning in tuberculous patients after ingestion of tuna fish. *Am Rev Respir Dis* (1980) 121, 157–9.
8. Senanayake N, Vyravanathan S, Kanagasuriyam S. Cerebrovascular accident after a 'skipjack' reaction in a patient taking isoniazid. *BMJ* (1978) 2, 1127–8.
9. Senanayake N, Vyravanathan S. Histamine reactions due to ingestion of tuna fish (*Thunnus argentivittatus*) in patients on antituberculosis therapy. *Toxicon* (1981) 19, 184–5.
10. Morinaga S, Kawasaki A, Hirata H, Suzuki S, Mizushima Y. Histamine poisoning after ingestion of spoiled raw tuna in a patient taking isoniazid. *Intern Med* (1997) 36, 198–200.
11. Uragoda CG. Histamine poisoning in tuberculous patients on ingestion of tropical fish. *J Trop Med Hyg* (1978) 81, 243–5.
12. Uragoda CG. Histamine intoxication with isoniazid and a species of fish. *Ceylon Med J* (1978) 23, 109–10.
13. Diao Y *et al.* Histamine like reaction in tuberculosis patients taking fishes containing much of histamine under treatment with isoniazid in 277 cases. *Chin J Tubercul Resp Dis* (1986) 9, 267–9, 317–18.
14. O'Sullivan TL. Drug-food interaction with isoniazid resembling anaphylaxis. *Ann Pharmacother* (1997) 31, 928–9.

Isoniazid + Cimetidine or Ranitidine

Pharmacokinetic evidence suggests that neither cimetidine nor ranitidine interact with isoniazid.

Clinical evidence, mechanism, importance and management

400 mg **cimetidine** or 300 mg **ranitidine**, three times a day, for three days had no effect on the pharmacokinetics of single 10 mg/kg doses of isoniazid in 13 healthy subjects. Neither the absorption nor the metabolism of isoniazid were changed.[1] The absence of an interaction indicated by this study needs clinical confirmation.

1. Paulsen O, Höglund P, Nilsson L-G, Gredeby H. No interaction between H₂ blockers and isoniazid. *Eur J Respir Dis* (1986) 68, 286–90.

Isoniazid + Corticosteroids

Prednisolone can lower serum isoniazid levels, but this may not be clinically important.

Clinical evidence, mechanism, importance and management

Isoniazid 10 mg/kg daily was given to 26 patients with tuberculosis. The 13 slow inactivators of isoniazid showed a 23% fall in plasma isoniazid levels when additionally given 20 mg **prednisolone**, while the 13 rapid inactivators showed a 38% fall over 8.5 h. The reasons are not understood, but changes in the metabolism and/or the excretion of the isoniazid by the kidney are possibilities. Despite these changes, the response to treatment was excellent.[1] In another group of 49 patients, both slow and rapid inactivators, the additional use of 12 mg/kg **rifampicin** largely counteracted the isoniazid-lowering effects of the **prednisolone**.[1]

None of these interactions were of clinical importance, but the authors point out that if the dosage of isoniazid had been lower, its effects might have been reduced. Be alert for any evidence of a reduced response during concurrent use, and raise the isoniazid dosage if necessary. There seems to be no information about other corticosteroids.

1. Sarma GR, Kailasam S, Nair NGK, Narayana ASL, Tripathy SP. Effect of prednisolone and rifampin on isoniazid metabolism in slow and rapid inactivators of isoniazid. *Antimicrob Agents Chemother* (1980) 18, 661–6.

Isoniazid + Disulfiram

Most patients taking isoniazid and disulfiram have no problems, but one report describes seven patients on isoniazid who experienced difficulties in co-ordination and changes in affect and behaviour after taking disulfiram concurrently. Four others became drowsy.

Clinical evidence

Seven patients with tuberculosis who had been taking isoniazid for not less than 30 days, without problems, experienced adverse reactions within 2 to 8 days of starting to take 500 mg **disulfiram** daily. Among the symptoms were dizziness, disorientation, a staggering gait, insomnia, irritability and querulous behaviour, listlessness and lethargy. One patient showed hypomania. Most of them were also taking chlordiazepoxide and other drugs including PAS, streptomycin and phenobarbital. The adverse reactions decreased or disappeared when the **disulfiram** was either reduced to 250 to 125 mg daily, or withdrawn. These 7 patients represented less than a third of those who received both drugs. Because **disulfiram** is known to inhibit the metabolism of chlordiazepoxide,[1] another 4 patients were given only isoniazid and **disulfiram**. Although their reaction was not as severe, all 4 showed drowsiness and depression.[2]

In contrast, another report describes the concurrent use of both drugs in 200 patients without problems.[3] No interaction was also seen in one other patient taking **disulfiram** with isoniazid and **rifampicin (rifampin)**.[4]

Mechanism

Not understood. One idea is that some kind of synergy occurs between the two drugs because both can produce not dissimilar side effects if given in high doses. The authors of the report cited[2] speculate that isoniazid and disulfiram together inhibit two of three biochemical pathways concerned with the metabolism of dopamine. One of these metabolises dopamine by dopamine beta-hydroxylase to norepinephrine (noradrenaline), and then by MAO to 3,4-dihydrophenyl acetic acid. This leaves a third pathway open, catalysed by COMT, which produces a number of methylated products of dopamine. These may possibly have been responsible for the mental and physical reactions seen.

Importance and management

Information about this interaction in man appears to be limited to the report cited above.[2] Its incidence is uncertain but apparently quite small. Two-thirds of this particular group failed to show this interaction, and 200 other patients showed no interaction.[3] No interaction was seen in another patient taking both drugs and rifampicin (rifampin).[4] It would seem therefore that concurrent use need not be avoided, but the response should be monitored and, if necessary, the dosage of disulfiram should be reduced, or it should be withdrawn.

1. Antabuse (Disulfiram). Dumex Limited. Summary of product characteristics, August 1999.
2. Whittington HG, Grey L. Possible interaction between disulfiram and isoniazid. *Am J Psychiatry* (1969) 125, 1725–9.
3. McNichol RW. Disulfiram (Antabuse), a strategic weapon in the battle for sobriety. In McNichol RW, Ewing JA, Fairman MD (Eds.) Disulfiram (Antabuse), a unique medical aid to sobriety. History, pharmacology, research, clinical use. Springfield Il: Charles C Thomas (1987) 47–90.
4. Rothstein E. Rifampin with disulfiram. *JAMA* (1972) 219, 1216.

Isoniazid + Ethambutol

There is experimental evidence that ethambutol does not affect serum isoniazid levels but there is also some evidence which suggests that the optic neuropathy of ethambutol may be increased by the concurrent use of isoniazid.

Clinical evidence, mechanism, importance and management

The mean serum levels of isoniazid after taking a single 300-mg dose were not significantly changed in 10 patients with tuberculosis when they were also given a single 20 mg/kg dose of **ethambutol**.[1] The possible effects of concurrent use over a period of time were not stud-

ied. However there is some evidence that the optic neuropathy of **ethambutol** may be increased by the concurrent use of isoniazid.[2-5]

1. Singhal KC, Varshney DP, Rathi R, Kishore K, Varshney SC. Serum concentration of isoniazid administered with and without ethambutol in pulmonary tuberculosis patients. *Indian J Med Res* (1986) 83, 360–2.
2. Renard G, Morax PV. Nevrite optique au cours des traitements antituberculeux. *Ann Oculist (Paris)* (1977) 210, 53–61.
3. Karmon G, Savir H, Zevin D, Levi J. Bilateral optic neuropathy due to combined ethambutol and isoniazid treatment. *Ann Ophthalmol* (1979) 11, 1013–17.
4. Garret CR. Optic neuritis in a patient on ethambutol and isoniazid evaluated by visual evoked potentials: Case report. *Mil Med* (1985) 150, 43–6.
5. Jimenez-Lucho VE, del Busto R, Odel J. Isoniazid and ethambutol as a cause of optic neuropathy. *Eur J Respir Dis* (1987) 71, 42–5.

Isoniazid + Fluconazole

Fluconazole appears not to interact with isoniazid.

Clinical evidence, mechanism, importance and management

A double blind crossover study in 16 healthy subjects (8 "fast" and 8 "slow" acetylators of isoniazid) found that 400 mg **fluconazole** daily for a week had no clinically significant effect on the pharmacokinetics of isoniazid.[1] No special precautions would appear necessary during concurrent use.

1. Buss DC, Routledge PA, Hutchings A, Brammer KW, Thorpe JE. The effect of fluconazole on the acetylation of isoniazid. *Hum Exp Toxicol* (1991) 10, 85–6.

Isoniazid + Food

The absorption of isoniazid is reduced by food. See also 'Isoniazid + Cheese or Fish', p.162.

Clinical evidence

The mean peak serum isoniazid levels of 9 healthy subjects given 10 mg/kg were delayed and reduced to 21% when given with **breakfast** rather than when fasting. The AUC was reduced to 57%.[1] In another study in 14 healthy subjects given isoniazid with a **full fat breakfast**, the maximum serum levels were decreased by 51%, absorption was delayed, and the AUC was decreased by 12%.[2] Similar results have been found in another study.[3]

Mechanism

Uncertain. Food delays gastric emptying so that absorption further along the gut is also delayed, but the reduction in absorption is not understood.

Importance and management

Information is limited but the interaction seems to be established. Since single high doses of isoniazid are more effective in arresting tuberculosis than the same amount of drug in divided doses[3-5] it seems probable that this interaction is clinically important. For maximal absorption isoniazid should be taken without food, hence the maker's guidance to take it at least 30 mins before or 2 h after food.[6] See also 'Isoniazid + Cheese or Fish', p.162.

1. Melander A, Danielson K, Hanson A, Jansson L, Rerup C, Scherstén B, Thulin T, Wåhlin E. Reduction of isoniazid bioavailability in normal men by concomitant intake of food. *Acta Med Scand* (1976) 200, 93–7.
2. Peloquin CA, Namdar S, Dodge AA, Nix DE. Pharmacokinetics of isoniazid under fasting conditions, with food, and with antacids. *Int J Tuberc Lung Dis* (1999) 3, 703–710.
3. Männisto P, Mäntylä R, Klinge R, Nykänen S, Koponen A, Lamminsivu U. Influence of various diets on the bioavailability of isoniazid. *J Antimicrob Chemother* (1982) 10, 427–34.
4. Fox W. General considerations in intermittent drug therapy of pulmonary tuberculosis. *Postgrad Med J* (1971) 47, 729–36.
5. Hudson LD, Sbarbaro JA. Twice weekly tuberculosis chemotherapy. *JAMA* (1973) 223, 139–43.
6. Isoniazid. Celltech Manufacturing Services Limited. Summary of product characteristics, July 2001.

Isoniazid + Levodopa

An isolated case report describes hypertension, tachycardia, flushing and tremor in a patient attributed to the concurrent use of isoniazid and levodopa.

Clinical evidence, mechanism, importance and management

A patient being treated with **levodopa** developed hypertension, agitation, tachycardia, flushing and severe non-parkinsonian tremor after starting to take isoniazid. He recovered when the isoniazid was stopped.[1] The reasons are not understood. The author suggested that it might be related in some way to the MAOI/levodopa interaction, but the MAO-inhibitory properties of isoniazid are small. Some of the symptoms seen were not dissimilar to those experienced by patients on isoniazid who ate cheese or fish (see 'Isoniazid + Cheese or Fish', p.162). Concurrent use should be monitored.

1. Morgan JP. Isoniazid and levodopa. *Ann Intern Med* (1980) 92, 434.

Isoniazid + Pethidine (Meperidine)

An isolated case report describes hypotension and lethargy in a patient following the concurrent use of isoniazid and pethidine (meperidine).

Clinical evidence, mechanism, importance and management

A patient became lethargic and his blood pressure fell from 124/68 to 84/50 mmHg within 20 min of being given 75 mg **pethidine** (**meperidine**) intramuscularly. An hour before he had been given isoniazid. There was no evidence of fever or heart arrhythmias, and his serum electrolytes, glucose levels and blood gases were normal. His blood pressure returned to normal over the next 3 h. He had previously had both **pethidine** and isoniazid separately without incident. He was subsequently treated with intravenous **morphine sulphate**, 4 mg every 2 to 4 h uneventfully.[1] The authors of the report attribute this reaction to the MAO-inhibitory properties of the isoniazid and equate it with the severe and potentially fatal MAOI-**pethidine** interaction, but in reality this reaction was mild and lacked many of the characteristics of the more serious reaction. Moreover isoniazid possesses little MAO-inhibitory properties and does not normally interact to the same extent as the potent antidepressant and antihypertensive MAOIs.

There is too little evidence to forbid concurrent use, but clearly it should be undertaken with caution.

1. Gannon R, Pearsall W, Rowley R. Isoniazid, meperidine, and hypotension. *Ann Intern Med* (1983) 99, 415.

Isoniazid + Propranolol

Propranolol causes a small reduction in the clearance of isoniazid from the body. It seems unlikely to be of much practical importance.

Clinical evidence, mechanism, importance and management

The clearance of single 600 mg intravenous doses of isoniazid was found in 6 healthy subjects to have been reduced by 21% (from 16.4 to 13.0 l/h) after they had been taking 40 mg **propranolol** three times daily for 3 days.[1] A suggested reason is that the **propranolol** inhibits the acetylation of the isoniazid by liver enzymes.[1] However the increase in isoniazid levels is likely to be only modest, and this interaction is probably of little clinical importance.

1. Santoso B. Impairment of isoniazid clearance by propranolol. *Int J Clin Pharmacol Ther Toxicol* (1985) 23, 134–6.

Isoniazid + Rifabutin (Ansamycin)

Rifabutin does not alter the pharmacokinetics of isoniazid.

Clinical evidence, mechanism, importance and management

Rifabutin 300 mg daily for 7 days had no significant effect on the plasma pharmacokinetics of isoniazid (after a single 300-mg dose) or the metabolite acetylisoniazid in 6 healthy subjects. Two of the 6 were rapid acetylators of isoniazid.[1] Although both drugs have been effectively used together in the treatment of tuberculosis, it is not clear is whether concurrent use increases the incidence of hepatotoxicity, as occurs with isoniazid and **rifampicin**. Combined use should therefore be well monitored.

1. Breda M, Painezzola E, Benedetti MS, Efthymiopoulos C, Carpentieri M, Sassella D, Rimoldi R. A study of the effects of rifabutin on isoniazid pharmacokinetics and metabolism in healthy volunteers. *Drug Metabol Drug Interact* (1993) 10, 323–40.

Isoniazid + Rifampicin (Rifampin)

Although concurrent use is common and therapeutically valuable, there is evidence that the incidence of isoniazid hepatotoxicity, particularly in slow acetylators, may be increased.

Clinical evidence, mechanism, importance and management

These drugs used together have a valuable part to play in the treatment of tuberculosis. Studies in man have shown that the serum levels and half-lives of both drugs are unaffected by concurrent use.[1,2] However, there is some evidence that the incidence and severity of hepatotoxicity rises if both drugs are used concurrently.[3] Reports from India suggest that the incidence can be as high as 8 to 10% while much lower figures of 2 to 3%, are reported in the West.[4] There is certainly one case report which appears to prove that hepatotoxicity can arise rapidly from the use of both drugs. In this case the patient tolerated both drugs individually, but hepatotoxicity reappeared on concurrent use.[5] Increased isoniazid hepatotoxicity caused by **rifampicin** has been demonstrated *in vitro*.[6] The reasons for the hepatotoxicity are not fully understood but **rifampicin** or isoniazid alone can cause liver damage by their own toxic action. One suggestion is that the **rifampicin** alters the metabolism of isoniazid, resulting in the formation of hydrazine, which is a proven hepatotoxic agent.[4,5,7] Higher plasma levels of hydrazine are said to occur in slow acetylators of isoniazid,[4] but one study failed to confirm that this is so.[8] It would be prudent to be on the watch for signs of liver damage if both drugs are given, and especially in patients also exposed to other potent enzyme inducers such as **phenytoin** and the **barbiturates**. There has certainly been one fatality caused by this combination.[9] The makers of isoniazid say that hepatotoxicity can occur particularly in those with pre-existing liver disorders, the elderly, the very young and the malnourished. They suggest that liver function tests should be reviewed regularly and that treatment should be withdrawn if AST reaches three times the upper limit of normal, or if there is a rise in bilirubin levels.[10]

1. Boman G. Serum concentration and half-life of rifampicin after simultaneous oral administration of aminosalicylic acid or isoniazid. *Eur J Clin Pharmacol* (1974) 7, 217–25.
2. Sarma GR, Kailasam S, Nair NGK, Narayana ASL, Tripathy SP. Effect of prednisolone and rifampin on isoniazid metabolism in slow and rapid inactivators of isoniazid. *Antimicrob Agents Chemother* (1980) 18, 661–6.

3. Steele MA, Burk RF, DesPrez RM. Toxic hepatitis with isoniazid and rifampin. A meta-analysis. *Chest* (1991) 99, 465–71.

4. Gangadharam PRJ. Isoniazid, rifampin and hepatotoxicity. *Am Rev Respir Dis* (1986) 133, 963–5.

5. Askgaard DS, Wilcke T, Døssing M. Hepatotoxicity caused by the combined action of isoniazid and rifampicin. *Thorax* (1995) 50, 213–14.

6. Nicod L, Viollon C, Regnier A, Jacqueson A, Richert L. Rifampicin and isoniazid increase acetaminophen and isoniazid cytotoxicity in human HepG2 hepatoma cells. *Hum Exp Toxicol* (1997) 16(1), 28–34.

7. Pessayre D, Bentata M, Degott C, Nouel O, Miguet J-P, Rueff B, Benhamou J-P. Isoniazid-rifampin fulminant hepatitis. A possible consequence of the enhancement of isoniazid hepatotoxicity by enzyme induction. *Gastroenterology* (1977) 72, 284–9.

8. Jenner PJ, Ellard GA. Isoniazid-related hepatotoxicity: a study of the effect of rifampicin administration on the metabolism of acetylisoniazid in man. *Tubercle* (1989) 70, 93–101.

9. Lenders JWM, Bartelink AKM, van Herwaarden CLA, van Haelst UJGM, van Tongeren JHM. Dodelijke levercelnecrose na kort durende toediening van isoniazide en rifampicine aan een patiënt die reeds werd behandeld met anti-epileptica. *Ned Tijdschr Geneeskd* (1983) 127, 420–3.

10. Isoniazid. Celltech Manufacturing Services Limited. Summary of product characteristics, July 2001.

Isoniazid + Selective serotonin re-uptake inhibitors (SSRIs) or related antidepressants

No important interaction appears to occur between isoniazid and the SSRIs or nefazodone. However, adverse reactions have been seen during concurrent use but they are thought unlikely to have been due to an interaction.

Clinical evidence

Two HIV+ patients on 20 mg **fluoxetine** daily were additionally started on isoniazid. One of them tolerated the use of both drugs, but the other developed vomiting and diarrhoea, and after 10 days the **fluoxetine** was stopped. Another HIV+ patient on isoniazid who had previously suffered nausea and vomiting 2 days after his dosage of **moclobemide** was increased, later tolerated the use of isoniazid and **fluoxetine** without adverse effects. The authors of this report were doubtful whether any of the adverse effects seen could be attributed to an isoniazid/antidepressant reaction.[1]

A woman who had been hospitalised for serious depression was started on 300 mg **nefazodone** daily. A few days later she began to take also 300 mg isoniazid daily, and was later discharged on an increased **nefazodone** dose of 400 mg daily. She was reported to have had no problems while taking both drugs over a 5 month period.[2]

A woman identified as having tuberculosis and taking 300 mg isoniazid daily presented with depression and was additionally given 50 mg **sertraline** daily, later raised to 150 mg, without problems. She responded well and was reported to have taken both drugs together for 8 months without problems.[2]

Mechanism, importance and management

Direct information about the concurrent use of isoniazid and SSRIs seems to be limited, but the reports cited here and the absence of any other reports of adverse reactions would suggest that the combination of isoniazid and these SSRIs is normally without problems.

In theory isoniazid could interact with the SSRIs[3] because it has some weak MAO inhibitory activity. However, it does not normally behave like the MAOIs. This is because isoniazid seems to lack activity on mitochondrial MAO even though it has activity on plasma MAO. Therefore no adverse MAOI/SSRI interaction would be expected.

1. Judd FK, Mijch AM, Cockram A, Norman TR. Isoniazid and antidepressants: is there cause for concern? *Int Clin Psychopharmacol* (1994) 9, 123–5.

2. Malek-Ahmadi P, Chavez M, Contreras SA. Coadministration of isoniazid and antidepressant drugs. *J Clin Psychiatry* (1996) 57, 550.

3. Evans ME, Kortas KJ. Potential interaction between isoniazid and selective serotonin re-uptake inhibitors. *Am J Health-Syst Pharm* (1995) 52, 2135–6.

Isoniazid + Sodium valproate

An isolated report describes liver toxicity attributed to the concurrent use of isoniazid and sodium valproate.

Clinical evidence, mechanism, importance and management

A girl of 13 with epilepsy and tuberculosis was treated with 300 mg isoniazid and 750 mg primidone daily. Within 2 days of adding 600 mg **sodium valproate** daily she developed stomach ache, loss of appetite, vomiting and drowsiness. Her liver enzymes (AST, ALT, GGT) were found to have risen and her fibrinogen levels fell. The **sodium valproate** was stopped and recovery from these adverse effects occurred while taking only phenobarbital. She had previously had both isoniazid alone and **sodium valproate** alone without problems.[1] Just why concurrent use should cause liver toxicity of this kind is not understood, but both drugs are known to be hepatotoxic alone. The general importance of this reaction is uncertain but be alert for any evidence of an adverse response in any patient given both drugs.

1. Dockweiler U. Isoniazid-induced valproic-acid toxicity, or vice versa. *Lancet* (1987) ii, 152.

Itraconazole + Anticonvulsants

Phenytoin causes a very marked fall in serum itraconazole levels, thereby reducing or abolishing its antifungal effects. Phenobarbital and carbamazepine appear to interact similarly.

Clinical evidence

After taking 300 mg oral doses of **phenytoin** for 15 days, the AUC of a single 200-mg dose of itraconazole given to 13 healthy subjects was reduced more than 90%. The half-life of itraconazole fell from 22.3 to 3.8 h. A parallel study[1] in another group found that 200 mg itraconazole for 15 days increased the **phenytoin** AUC by 10.3%.

Two patients on **phenytoin** and two on **phenytoin** with **carbamazepine** failed to respond to treatment with 400 mg itraconazole daily for aspergillosis, coccidioidomycosis or cryptococcosis, or suffered a relapse. All of them had undetectable or substantially reduced serum itraconazole levels compared with other patients on itraconazole alone.[2] Two other patients also had very low serum itraconazole serum levels while taking **phenytoin** and **phenobarbital**.[3]

The serum itraconazole levels of a patient taking 200 mg daily were very low (0.01 to 0.03 mg/l, therapeutic range 0.25 to 2 mg/l) while taking **phenobarbital**. Two months after stopping the **phenobarbital** they were higher (0.15 mg/l), but still below the therapeutic range, apparently because **carbamazepine** had been recently started. However, 2 months later itraconazole serum levels were undetectable. Carbamazepine was stopped, and 3 weeks later the itraconazole serum levels were 0.36 mg/l.[4]

Mechanism

It seems almost certain that these anticonvulsants can increase the metabolism and clearance of itraconazole by the liver, thereby reducing its serum levels and its effects.

Importance and management

The phenytoin/itraconazole interaction is established, clinically important and its incidence appears to be high. Because such a marked fall in itraconazole levels occurs, it is difficult to predict by how much its dosage should be increased, for which reason the authors of one report advise using another antifungal instead.[1] The small rise in serum phenytoin levels caused by itraconazole is unlikely to be clinically important.

The interactions of itraconazole with the carbamazepine and phenobarbital are relatively poorly documented and their incidence is unknown, but if itraconazole is given to patients taking these anticonvulsants, be alert for the need to increase the itraconazole dosage. More study is needed.

1. Ducharme MP, Slaughter RL, Warbasse LH, Chandrasekar PH, Van der Velde V, Mannens G, Edwards DJ. Itraconazole and hydroxyitraconazole serum concentrations are reduced more than tenfold by phenytoin. *Clin Pharmacol Ther* (1995) 58, 617–24.
2. Tucker RM, Denning DW, Hanson LH, Rinaldi MG, Graybill JR, Sharkey PK, Pappagianis D, Stevens DA. Interaction of azoles with rifampin, phenytoin, and carbamazepine: in vitro and clinical observations. *Clin Infect Dis* (1992) 14, 165–74.
3. Hay RJ, Clayton YM, Moore MK, Midgely G. An evaluation of itraconazole in the management of onychomycosis. *Br J Dermatol* (1988) 119, 359–66.
4. Bonay M, Jonville-Bera AP, Diot P, Lemarie E, Lavandier M, Autret E. Possible interaction between phenobarbital, carbamazepine and itraconazole. *Drug Safety* (1993) 9, 309–11.

Itraconazole + Antitubercular drugs

Rifampicin very markedly reduces serum itraconazole serum levels. This can reduce or abolish the antifungal effects of the itraconazole, possibly depending on the infection being treated.

Clinical evidence

A patient on anti-tubercular treatment including 600 mg **rifampicin** and 300 mg **isoniazid** daily was additionally started on 200 mg itraconazole daily. After 2 weeks his serum itraconazole levels were negligible (0.011 mg/l). Even when the dosage was doubled the levels only reached a maximum of 0.056 mg/l. Later when the antitubercular drugs had been stopped and while taking 300 mg itraconazole daily, his serum itraconazole level was 3.23 mg/l, and on 200 mg daily it was 2.35 to 2.60 mg/l.[1]

A later study in 8 other patients confirmed that itraconazole levels were reduced by **rifampicin** but the clinical outcome depended on the mycosis being treated. Four out of 5 patients responded to treatment for a *Cryptococcus neoformans* infection, despite undetectable itraconazole levels, apparently because there is synergy between the 2 drugs. In contrast, 2 patients with coccidioidomycosis failed to respond, and 2 others with cryptococcosis suffered a relapse or persistence of seborrhoeic dermatitis (possibly due to *M. furfur*) while taking both drugs.[2] The serum itraconazole levels of an AIDS patient taking 400 to 600 mg daily were undetectable while taking **rifampicin,** and took 3 to 5 days to recover after the **rifampicin** was stopped.[3] Undetectable itraconazole levels occurred in another patient when given **rifampicin**, whilst taking itraconazole for histoplasmosis.[4] A study found that the AUC of itraconazole in 6 healthy subjects was reduced to 20% after taking 600 mg **rifampicin** for 3 days.[5] Very markedly reduced serum itraconazole levels (undetectable in some instances) were also been seen in other normal subjects and AIDS patients when given **rifampicin**.[6,7]

Mechanism

The suggested reason is that the rifampicin increases the metabolism of the itraconazole within the liver, and hastens its loss from the body. This is consistent with the way rifampicin interacts with many other drugs.

Importance and management

An established and clinically important interaction. Monitor the effects of concurrent use, being alert for the need to increase the itraconazole dosage. The effect on serum itraconazole levels can be very marked indeed. The clinical importance of this interaction can apparently depend on the mycosis being treated.

1. Blomley M, Teare EL, de Belder A, Thway Y, Weston M. Itraconazole and anti-tuberculosis drugs. *Lancet* (1990) ii, 1255.
2. Tucker RM, Denning DW, Hanson LH, Rinaldi MG, Graybill JR, Sharkey PK, Pappagianis D, Stevens DA. Interaction of azoles with rifampin, phenytoin and carbamazepine: in vitro and clinical observations. *Clin Infect Dis* (1992) 14, 165–74.
3. Drayton J, Dickinson G, Rinaldi MG. Coadministration of rifampin and itraconazole leads to undetectable levels of serum itraconazole. *Clin Infect Dis* (1994) 18, 266.

4. Hecht FM, Wheat J, Korzun AH, Hafner R, Skahan KJ, Larsen R, Limjoco MT, Simpson M, Schneider D, Keefer MC, Clark R, Lai KK, Jacobsen JM, Squires K, Bartlett JA, Powderly W. Itraconazole maintenance treatment for histoplasmosis in AIDS: a prospective, multicenter trial. *J Acquir Immune Defic Syndr Hum Retrovirol* (1997) 16, 100–107.
5. Heykants J, Michiels M, Meuldermans W, Monbaliu J, Lavrijsen K, Van Peer A, Levron JC, Woestenborghs R, Cauwenbergh G. The pharmacokinetics of itraconazole in *animals* and man: an overview. In Recent Trends in the Discovery, Development and Evaluation of Antifungal Agents. Fromtling RA (Ed), JR Prous Science Publishers, SA (1987) p 223–49.
6. Jaruratanasirikul S, Sriwiriyajan S. Effect of rifampicin on the pharmacokinetics of itraconazole in normal volunteers and AIDS patients. *Eur J Clin Pharmacol* (1997) 52 (Suppl), A133.
7. Jaruratanasirikul S, Sriwiriyajan S. Effect of rifampicin on the pharmacokinetics of itraconazole in normal volunteers and AIDS patients. *Eur J Clin Pharmacol* (1998) 54, 155–8.

Itraconazole + Clarithromycin

Clarithromycin can almost double the serum levels of itraconazole.

Clinical evidence, mechanism, importance and management

A study in 8 AIDS patients taking 200 mg itraconazole daily found that when 500 mg **clarithromycin** twice daily was added for 14 days, the maximum serum levels and the AUC of the itraconazole were increased by 90% and 92% respectively.[1] Both **clarithromycin** and itraconazole are known to compete for the hepatic cytochrome P450 isoenzyme CYP3A4 and it is therefore probable that this leads to a reduction in the clearance of itraconazole from the body. This report does not comment on the outcome of this almost twofold increase in itraconazole levels, but it would seem prudent to be alert for the need to reduce its dosage. More study is needed.

1. Hardin TC, Summers KS, Rinaldi MG, Sharkey PK. Evaluation of the pharmacokinetic interaction between itraconazole and clarithromycin following chronic oral dosing in HIV-infected patients. *Pharmacotherapy* (1997) 17, 195.

Itraconazole or Ketoconazole + Cola drinks

Some cola drinks can lower the stomach pH in patients with achlorhydria or hypochlorhydria which improves the bioavailability of itraconazole and ketoconazole. Normally a useful interaction but good monitoring is needed to ensure that the azole serum levels do not become excessive.

Clinical evidence

Eight healthy subjects were given 100 mg **itraconazole** with either 325 ml of water or *Coca-Cola* (pH 2.5). Their peak serum **itraconazole** levels were more than doubled when given with *Coca-Cola* and the AUC was increased by 80%. Two of the subjects failed to demonstrate this effect.[1,2]

Another study in 18 fasted AIDS patients who absorbed **itraconazole** poorly, found that the absorption was restored to that of fasted healthy subjects when administered with a **cola drink**.[3] Yet another study used omeprazole to raise the pH and *Coca-Cola Classic* to lower it. Absorption was greatest when **ketoconazole** was given alone, and least when given with omeprazole. However, *Coca-Cola* increased the absorption of **ketoconazole** in the presence of omeprazole.[4]

Mechanism

Itraconazole and ketoconazole are poorly soluble bases, which must be transformed by the acid in the stomach into a soluble hydrochloride salt. Therefore any clinical condition which reduces gastric secretion (or any drug which raises stomach pH) can reduce the dissolution and the absorption of these antifungals. Agents which lower the pH (such as some Cola drinks) can increase the absorption.

Importance and management

The interactions of itraconazole and ketoconazole with Cola drinks, which lower the gastric pH, are established. The interaction can be exploited to improve the absorption of these antifungals in patients with achlorhydria or hypochlorhydria, but some caution is needed to ensure that serum levels do not rise excessively which could lead to toxicity.

Coca-Cola Classic, Pepsi and *Canada Dry Ginger Ale* can be used because they can achieve stomach pH values of less than 3, but none of the other beverages examined in one study produced such a low pH. The authors suggest that these would be less effective, although they were not actually studied. They included *Diet Coca-Cola, Diet Pepsi, Diet 7-Up, Diet Canada Dry Ginger Ale, Diet Canada Dry Orange juice, 7-Up* and *Canada Dry Orange juice*.[4]

1. Jaruratanasirikul S, Kleepkaew A. Influence of an acidic beverage (Coca-Cola) on absorption of itraconazole. *Clin Pharmacol Ther* (1997) 61, 149.
2. Jaruratanasirikul S, Kleepkaew A. Influence of an acidic beverage (Coca-Cola) on absorption of itraconazole. *Eur J Clin Pharmacol* (1997) 52, 235–7.
3. Hardin J, Lange D, Heykants J, Ding C, Van de Velde V, Slusser C, Klausner M. The effect of co-administration of a cola beverage on the bioavailability of itraconazole in AIDS patients. *Intersci Conf Antimicrob Agents Chemother* (1995) 35, 6.
4. Chin TWF, Leob M, Fong IW. Effects of an acidic beverage (Coca-Cola) on absorption of ketoconazole. *Antimicrob Agents Chemother* (1995) 39, 1671–5.

Itraconazole + Grapefruit juice

Grapefruit juice impairs the absorption of itraconazole, but the clinical significance of this is unknown.

Clinical evidence, mechanism, importance and management

As **grapefruit juice** is an inhibitor of intestinal cytochrome P450 isoenzyme CYP3A4, the major enzyme involved in itraconazole metabolism, a study[1] was conducted to see if it could be used to enhance itraconazole absorption. Either 240 ml of double strength **grapefruit juice** or 240 ml water were given with, and 2 h after a single 200-mg dose of itraconazole. When given with **grapefruit juice**, the AUC of itraconazole unexpectedly decreased, on average by 43% (range −81% to +105%). The results were in line with decreased absorption, rather than altered metabolism and so the authors suggest that **grapefruit juice** may impair the absorption of itraconazole either by affecting P-glycoprotein or lowering the duodenal pH. However, another study found that **grapefruit juice** had no effect on itraconazole pharmacokinetics.[2] The clinical significance of these results is not known, but it would seem prudent to avoid concurrent administration until more information is available. More study is needed.

1. Penzak SR, Gubbins PO, Gurley BJ, Wang P-L, Saccente M. Grapefruit juice decreases the systemic availability of itraconazole capsules in healthy volunteers. *Ther Drug Monit* (1999) 21, 304–309.
2. Kawakami M, Suzuki K, Ishizuka T, Hidaka T, Matsuki Y, Nakumara H. Effect of grapefruit juice on pharmacokinetics of itraconazole in healthy subjects. *Int J Clin Pharmacol Ther* (1998) 36, 306–308.

Itraconazole + Rifabutin (Ansamycin)

Rifabutin reduces the plasma levels of itraconazole. An isolated report describes increased serum rifabutin levels associated with uveitis.

Clinical evidence

(a) Itraconazole serum levels reduced

Six HIV+ patients were given three periods of treatment: (a) 200 mg itraconazole daily for 14 days, (b) 300 mg **rifabutin** daily for 10 days, and then (c) a period of 14 days on both drugs. It was found that the **rifabutin** reduced the peak plasma levels of the itraconazole by 71% and its AUC by 74%.[1]

(b) Rifabutin serum levels raised

A 49-year-old HIV+ man on 300 mg **rifabutin** daily was started on itraconazole 600 mg daily. Because of low plasma levels the itraconazole dose was increased to 900 mg daily after 3 weeks. A week later the patient developed anterior uveitis. It was found that the itraconazole trough serum levels were normal but **rifabutin** trough serum levels were raised to 153 nanograms/ml (expected to be less than 50 nanograms/ml after 24 h). Rifabutin was stopped and the uveitis was treated. Symptoms resolved after 5 days.[2]

Mechanisms

The presumed reasons are that the rifabutin increases the metabolism of the itraconazole by the liver so that its serum levels fall, and the itraconazole inhibits the metabolism of the rifabutin so that its serum levels rise, thereby precipitating uveitis.

Importance and management

Information is very limited but be alert for both of these interactions if both drugs are used. Monitor for reduced antifungal activity, raising the itraconazole dosage as necessary, and watch for increased rifabutin levels and toxicity (in particular uveitis).

More study is needed to confirm these interactions and to assess their general importance.

1. Smith JA, Hardin TC, Patterson TF, Rinaldi MG, Graybill JR. Rifabutin (RIF) decreases itraconazole (ITRA) plasma levels in patients with HIV-infection. Am Soc Microbiol 2nd Nat Conf. Human retroviruses and related infections. Washington DC, Jan 29—Feb 2 1995, 77.
2. Lefort A, Launay O, Carbon C. Uveitis associated with rifabutin prophylaxis and itraconazole therapy. *Ann Intern Med* (1996) 125, 939–40.

Ketoconazole + Anticonvulsants

Four patients showed reduced serum ketoconazole levels and reduced antifungal effects while taking phenytoin. Two were also taking phenobarbital. Ketoconazole appears not to affect serum phenytoin levels.

Clinical evidence

A man being treated for coccidioidal meningitis with ketoconazole 400 mg daily relapsed when given 300 mg **phenytoin** daily. A pharmacokinetic study showed that his peak serum ketoconazole levels and AUC were reduced compared with the values seen before the **phenytoin** was started. Even though the ketoconazole dose was increased to 600 mg, and later 1200 mg his serum levels remained low when compared with other patients taking only 400 or 600 mg of ketoconazole.[1]

Coccidioidomycosis progressed in another patient on **phenytoin** despite the use of ketoconazole.[2] Low serum ketoconazole levels were seen in one patient[3] taking **phenytoin** and **phenobarbital**. It appears that ketoconazole does not affect the serum levels of **phenytoin**.[4]

Mechanism

Not established, but a likely explanation is that the phenytoin, a known potent enzyme-inducing agent, increases the metabolism and clearance of the ketoconazole from the body. Phenobarbital probably acts in the same way.

Importance and management

Information appears to be limited to these reports but be alert for any signs of a reduced antifungal response in any patient given either or both of these anticonvulsants. It may be necessary to increase the dosage of the ketoconazole.

1. Brass C, Galgiani JN, Blaschke TF, Defelice R, O'Reilly RA, Stevens DA. Disposition of ketoconazole, an oral antifungal, in humans. *Antimicrob Agents Chemother* (1982) 21, 151–8.

2. Tucker RM, Denning DW, Hanson LH, Rinaldi MG, Graybill JR, Sharkey PK, Pappagianis D, Stevens DA. Interaction of azoles with rifampin, phenytoin and carbamazepine: in vitro and clinical observations. *Clin Infect Dis* (1992) 14, 165–74.
3. Stockley RJ, Daneshmend TK, Bredow MT, Warnock DW, Richardson MD, Slade RR. Ketoconazole pharmacokinetics during chronic dosing in adults with haematological malignancy. *Eur J Clin Microbiol* (1986) 5, 513–17.
4. Touchette MA, Chandrasekar PH, Millad MA, Edwards DJ. Differential effects of ketoconazole and fluconazole on phenytoin and testosterone concentrations in man. *Pharmacotherapy* (1991) 11, 275.

Ketoconazole + Rifampicin (Rifampin) and/or Isoniazid

The serum levels of ketoconazole can be markedly reduced (50 to 90%) by the concurrent use of rifampicin and/or isoniazid. Serum rifampicin levels can also be halved by the concurrent use of ketoconazole, but are possibly unaffected if the drugs are given 12 h apart.

Clinical evidence

(a) Effect on serum ketoconazole levels

The serum ketoconazole levels of a patient taking 200 mg daily were approximately halved (AUC reduced from 17.33 to 9.15 micrograms.h/ml) when concurrently treated with 600 mg **rifampicin**. After 5 months of concurrent use with **rifampicin** and 300 mg **isoniazid** daily, there was a ninefold decrease in peak serum levels (AUC reduced from 17.33 to 2.02 micrograms.h/ml)[1].

A study in a 3-year-old child who had responded poorly to treatment showed that peak serum ketoconazole levels were reduced by about 65 to 80% by the concurrent use of **rifampicin** and/or **isoniazid**, and the AUCs were similarly reduced. The interaction also occurred when the dosages were separated by 12 h. When all three drugs were given together the ketoconazole serum levels were undetectable.[2] Other reports confirm these interactions can occur,[3-10] although one of them found an 80% reduction in the AUC of ketoconazole but no reduction in **rifampicin** levels.[6]

(b) Effect on serum rifampicin levels

A study in the child cited above showed that **rifampicin** serum levels were approximately halved by the concurrent use of ketoconazole, but when given 12 h after the ketoconazole, the serum levels of **rifampicin** remained unaffected.[2] Other studies also show a reduction in **rifampicin** levels caused by ketoconazole.[5,7,8,10]

Mechanisms

It seems probable that rifampicin reduces the serum levels of ketoconazole by increasing its rate of metabolism within the liver, thereby hastening its clearance from the body. Just how isoniazid interacts is uncertain. It is suggested that ketoconazole impairs the absorption of rifampicin from the gut.

Importance and management

The ketoconazole/rifampicin interactions appear to be established and of clinical importance, but there is very much less information about the ketoconazole/isoniazid interaction. The effects on rifampicin can apparently be avoided by giving the ketoconazole at a different time (12 h apart seems to be effective) but this does not solve the problem of the effects on ketoconazole. The dosage of at least one of the drugs will need to be increased to achieve both good antitubercular and antifungal responses. Concurrent use should be well monitored and dosage increases made if necessary.

1. Brass C, Galgiani JN, Blaschke TF, Defelice R, O'Reilly RA, Stevens DA. Disposition of ketoconazole, an oral antifungal, in humans. *Antimicrob Agents Chemother* (1982) 21, 151–8.
2. Engelhard D, Stutman HR, Marks MI. Interaction of ketoconazole with rifampin and isoniazid. *N Engl J Med* (1984) 311, 1681–3.
3. Drouhet E, Dupont B. Laboratory and clinical assessment of ketoconazole in deep-seated mycoses. *Am J Med* (1983) 74, 30–47.
4. Meunier-Carpentier F, Heymans C, Snoeck R, Taterman J. Interaction of rifampin (Rif) with ketoconazole (Ke) and Bayer n7133 (Bay) in normal volunteers (Vol.). *Intersci Conf Antimicrob Agents Chemother* (1983) 23, 265.
5. Doble N, Hykin P, Shaw R, Keal EE. Pulmonary mycobacterium tuberculosis in acquired immune deficiency syndrome. *BMJ* (1985) 291, 849–50.
6. Doble H, Shaw R, Rowland-Hill C, Lush M, Warnock DW, Keal EE. Pharmacokinetic study of the interaction between rifampicin and ketoconazole. *J Antimicrob Chemother* (1988) 21, 633–5.
7. Abadie-Kemmerly S, Pankey GA, Dalvisio JR. Failure of ketoconazole treatment of *Blastomyces dermatidis* due to interaction of isoniazid and rifampin. *Ann Intern Med* (1988) 109, 844–5.
8. Pilheu JA et al. Interaction of ketoconazole with isoniazid and rifampicin. *Eur Respir J* (1988) 1 (Suppl 2), 274s.
9. Tucker RM, Denning DW, Hanson LH, Rinaldi MG, Graybill JR, Sharkey PK, Pappagianis D, Stevens DA. Interaction of azoles with rifampin, phenytoin and carbamazepine: in vitro and clinical observations. *Clin Infect Dis* (1992) 14, 165–74.
10. Pilheu JA, Galati MR, Yunis AS, De Salvo MC, Negroni R, Garcia Fernandez JC, Mingolla L, Rubio MC, Masana M, Acevedo C. Interaccion farmacocinetica entre ketoconazol, isoniacida y rifampicina. *Medicina (B Aires)* (1989) 49, 43–7.

Linezolid + Miscellaneous drugs

Because of its weak MAO-inhibitory properties, the makers of linezolid contraindicate use with adrenergic bronchodilators salbutamol (albuterol), indirectly-acting sympathomimetics (phenylpropanolamine, pseudoephedrine), pethidine (meperidine) and SSRIs, although there is evidence suggesting that serious interactions are unlikely. For theoretical reasons they also contraindicate buspirone, MAOIs, dopaminergic agents and vasopressors, and warn that excessive amounts of tyramine-rich foods and drinks should be avoided. No clinically relevant interaction occurs with warfarin or phenytoin, and no pharmacokinetic interaction with aztreonam or gentamicin.

Clinical evidence, mechanism, importance and management

Linezolid is an oxazolidinone antibacterial which causes weak, reversible and non-selective inhibition of monoamine oxidase but without antidepressants effects at the doses used for antibacterial therapy. Most of the interaction contraindications and warnings issued by the makers appear to be based on what can happen with potent antidepressant MAOIs, and not on direct clinical evidence about linezolid which only has weak MAO-inhibitory activity. Indeed what is known suggests that serious problems of the kind seen with the antidepressant MAOIs are unlikely to occur.

(a) Antibacterials

The makers report that the pharmacokinetics of neither aztreonam nor gentamicin are altered by the concurrent use of linezolid.[1]

(b) Dextromethorphan

A group of 14 healthy subjects given two 20-mg doses of **dextromethorphan** 4 h apart, with and without linezolid, showed no evidence of the serotonin syndrome which has been described when **dextromethorphan** was taken by patients also taking antidepressant MAOIs. Although there were modest changes in the pharmacokinetics of **dextromethorphan** these were not considered sufficient to warrant any dosing alterations. There would therefore appear to be no reason for avoiding concurrent use.[2]

(c) Indirectly-acting sympathomimetics

In a placebo controlled study, 14 healthy patients were given two 60-mg doses of **pseudoephedrine** or two 25-mg dose of **phenylpropanolamine** 4 h apart, with and without linezolid. The mean maximum blood pressure rise was 11 mmHg with placebo, 15 mmHg with linezolid and placebo, 18 mmHg with **pseudoephedrine** and 14 mmHg with **phenylpropanolamine.** When the subjects were given linezolid plus **pseudoephedrine** the rise was 32 mmHg, which was similar to the 38 mmHg rise seen with linezolid plus **phenylpropanolamine**. However, these rises were transient, resolving in about 2 h. No effects were seen on linezolid pharmacokinetics.[2]

The reason for the increased rise in blood pressure is believed to be that linezolid acts as a weak MAO-inhibitor which allows the accumulation of some norepinephrine at adrenergic nerve endings associated with arterial blood vessels. These two indirectly-acting sympathomimetics can release these above-normal amounts of norepinephrine resulting in blood vessel constriction and a rise in blood pressure. The makers caution the use of sympathomimetics with linezolid unless there are facilities available for close observation of the patient and monitoring of blood pressure. Some sympathomimetics occur in cough and cold remedies which can be bought OTC. To keep in line with the makers caution, patients should be told to avoid these preparations. However, it should be said that the evidence available indicates that blood pressure rises are only very moderate and certainly unlikely to be of the hypertensive crisis proportions seen with the antidepressant MAOIs. Other similar sympathomimetics with indirect activity are to be found in the monograph 'Monoamine oxidase inhibitors (MAOIs) + Sympathomimetics (indirectly-acting)', p.680.

(d) Monoamine oxidase inhibitors (MAOIs)

The makers contraindicate the concurrent use of linezolid and any other drug which inhibits either monoamine oxidase A or B, or within 2 weeks of taking either drug,[3] because their MAO-inhibitory activities are predicted to be additive. **Isocarboxazid**, **moclobemide**, **phenelzine** and **selegiline** are named, although if any adverse interaction were to occur it would also be likely to occur with a number of other MAOIs. It is not entirely clear what the outcome of any additional MAO-inhibition might be.

(e) Other miscellaneous drugs

The makers of linezolid contraindicate **buspirone**, **directly-acting sympathomimetics**, **vasopressors**, **dopaminergic agents** and **tricyclic antidepressants**.[3] The reasons are that some of these drugs have interacted adversely with conventional antidepressant MAOIs so that to be on the safe side these drugs are listed as contraindicated with linezolid. There seems to be no direct clinical evidence that linezolid interacts with any of these drugs. These contraindications are therefore based solely on theoretical considerations.

(f) Pethidine (Meperidine)

11 normal subjects taking linezolid were given either a placebo or 50 mg intramuscular **pethidine** followed by 100 mg 4 h later. There was no evidence of the serotonin syndrome which sometimes occurs in patients concurrently given **pethidine** while taking antidepressant MAOIs.[1] Despite this evidence, the makers currently contraindicate **pethidine**.[3] This contraindication would therefore seem to be based on theoretical considerations, despite the direct clinical evidence which is available.

(g) Salbutamol (Albuterol)

14 normal subjects taking 600 g linezolid twice daily were additionally given a placebo, 2.5 mg oral **salbutamol** or 2.5 mg inhaled **salbutamol**. No differences in blood pressure, heart rate or respiratory rate were seen.[1] Even so, the makers of linezolid currently contraindicate adrenergic bronchodilators which would include **salbutamol**.[3] This contraindication would therefore seem to be based on theoretical considerations, despite the direct clinical evidence which is available.

(h) Selective serotonin re-uptake inhibitors (SSRIs)

18 normal subjects were given 20 mg **paroxetine** daily for a week and then 40 mg daily for a further 4 days. From day 5 to 11 of the study they were additionally given either a placebo (6 subjects) or 600 mg linezolid (12 subjects) twice daily.[1] No interaction was seen and there was no evidence of the serotonin syndrome which has sometimes been seen in patients concurrently taking SSRIs and antidepressant MAOIs. However symptomless and transient hypertension (a rise from 130/80 mmHg to 180/130 mmHg after 1.5 h) was seen in 92-year-old with multiple problems and medications (aspirin, indoramin, frusemide, salbutamol, glyceryl trinitrate and **fluoxetine**) when given linezolid. The **fluoxetine** was stopped on the day the linezolid was started.[1] It is not known whether what happened was linked to the sequential use of these two drugs.

Despite the weight of evidence which suggests that problems are unlikely to occur, the makers currently contraindicate the concurrent use of linezolid and **any SSRI**.[3] This contraindication would therefore seem to be based largely on theoretical considerations rather than on the any direct clinical evidence.

(i) Tyramine-rich foods and drinks

A phase I pharmacokinetic study in normal subjects, given 625 mg linezolid twice daily, found that 100 mg **tyramine** raised the blood pressure by 30 mmHg but no significant rise was seen with doses of less than 100 mg **tyramine**.[1] The reason for the rise is that linezolid acts as a weak MAO-inhibitor which allows the accumulation of some norepinephrine at adrenergic nerve endings associated with arterial blood vessels. **Tyramine** is an indirectly-acting sympathomimetic which can release these above-normal amounts of norepinephrine resulting in an exaggerated blood vessel constriction and a rise in blood pressure. A much more detailed explanation of this mechanism of interaction is to be found in the monograph 'Monoamine oxidase inhibitors (MAOIs) + Tyramine-rich foods', p.685.

The makers of linezolid therefore recommend that patients should avoid excessive amounts **tyramine-rich food and drinks** and should not consume more than 100 mg **tyramine** per meal.[3] A list of tyramine-containing foods is to be found in the monograph already referred to above.

The stringent dietary restrictions imposed on patients taking nonselective MAOIs are therefore unnecessary in those treated with linezolid, but the avoidance of very large amounts of **tyramine** is a prudent precaution (a maker's recommendation). A severe hypertensive reaction crisis of the proportions possible with the antidepressant MAOIs seems unlikely.

(j) Warfarin, Phenytoin and Cytochrome P450 studies

A study in which **warfarin** was added to linezolid at steady-state found that a 10% reduction in the mean maximum INR and a 5% reduction in the AUC (area under the curve) INR occurred.[1] The makers also report that linezolid does not substantially alter the pharmacokinetics of (S)-warfarin which is extensively metabolised by cytochrome P450 isoenzyme CYP2C9. Thus any INR changes are small and the makers say that **warfarin** may be given with linezolid without dosage adjustments.[1]

The makers also say that because linezolid is not detectably metabolised by cytochrome P450 enzymes and does not inhibit human cytochrome isoenzymes CYP1A2, CYP2C9, CYP2C19, CYP2D6, CYP2E1, or CYP3A4, no interactions mediated by cytochrome induction or inhibition are expected with linezolid. On the basis of these observations they say that **phenytoin**, which is a CYP2C9 substrate, may be given with linezolid without any dosage adjustments.[1]

1. Data on file, Pharmacia, Zyvox (linezolid) Clinical information Pack, 2000.
2. Hendershot PE, Antal EJ, Welshman IR, Batts DH, Hopkins NK. Linezolid: pharmacokinetic and pharmacodynamic evaluation of coadministration with pseudoephedrine HCl, phenylpropanolamine HCl, and dextromethorphan HBr. *J Clin Pharmacol* (2001) 41, 563–72.
3. Zyvox (Linezolid). Pharmacia. Summary of product characteristics, August 2001.

Loracarbef + Probenecid

Probenecid increases the half-life of loracarbef by about 50% but the clinical importance of this is unknown.[1]

1. Force RW, Nahata MC. Loracarbef: a new orally administered carbacephem antibiotic. *Ann Pharmacother* (1993) 27, 321–9.

Lumefantrine + Mefloquine

The levels of lumefantrine (as co-artemether) are reduced by mefloquine, but the changes are not thought to be clinically significant.

Clinical evidence, mechanism, importance and management

In a study 6 doses of co-artemether (artemether 80 mg/lumefantrine 480 mg each) were given over 60 h to 42 healthy subjects 12 h after a short course of **mefloquine** (3 doses totalling 1000 mg over 12 h). The pharmacokinetics of the **mefloquine** and the artemether were unaffected by concurrent use, but lumefantrine maximum plasma concentrations and the AUC were reduced by 29% and 41% respectively. However, given that the plasma levels of lumefantrine are usually highly variable these changes were not thought large enough to affect the efficacy of treatment.[1]

In another study these drugs in combination were found not to affect the QT interval, and levels were also considered adequate for treatment.[2]

1. Lefèvre G, Bindschedler M, Ezzet F, Schaeffer N, Meyer I, Thomsen MS. Pharmacokinetic interaction trial between co-artemether and mefloquine. *Eur J Pharm Sci* (2000) 10, 141–51.
2. Bindschedler M, Lefèvre G, Ezzet F, Schaeffer N, Meyer I, Thomsen MS. Cardiac effects of co-artemether (artemether/lumefantrine) and mefloquine given alone or in combination to healthy volunteers. *Eur J Clin Pharmacol* (2000) 56, 375–81.

Macrolide antibacterials + Antacids or H₂-blockers

Maalox (aluminium and magnesium hydroxide) and ranitidine are reported not to affect the pharmacokinetics of clarithromycin[1] or roxithromycin.[2,3] Cimetidine prolongs the absorption of clarithromycin, but this is unlikely to be of significance.[4] There would seem to be no reason for avoiding concurrent use.

1. Zündorf H, Wischmann L, Fassenbender M, Lode H, Borner K, Koeppe P. Pharmacokinetics of clarithromycin and possible interaction with H₂ blockers and antacids. *Intersci Conf Antimicrob Agents Chemother* (1991) 31, 185.
2. Nilsen OG. Roxithromycin. A new molecule, a new pharmacokinetic profile. *Drug Invest* (1991) 3 (Suppl 3), 28–32.
3. Boeckh M, Lode H, Höffken G, Daeschlein S, Koeppe P. Pharmacokinetics of roxithromycin and influence of H₂-blockers and antacids on gastrointestinal absorption. *Eur J Clin Microbiol Infect Dis* (1992) 11, 465–8.
4. Amsden GW, Cheng KL, Peloquin CA, Nafziger AN. Oral cimetidine prolongs clarithromycin absorption. *Antimicrob Agents Chemother* (1998) 42, 1578–80.

Macrolide antibacterials + Fluconazole

Fluconazole causes a small to moderate increase in the plasma levels of clarithromycin which is unlikely to be of clinical importance. Azithromycin does not appear to be affected.

Clinical evidence, mechanism, importance and management

(a) Azithromycin

Single doses of **fluconazole** 800 mg and **azithromycin** 1200 mg were given to 18 healthy subjects alone and together without any significant change in the pharmacokinetics of either drug.[1]

(b) Clarithromycin

Twenty healthy subjects were given 500 mg **clarithromycin** twice daily for 8 days. **Fluconazole** 400 mg daily was added on day 5, and then 200 mg daily on days 6 to 8. The **fluconazole** increased the minimum plasma levels of the **clarithromycin** by 33% and the AUC_{0-12} by 18%.[2] These relatively small changes in the pharmacokinetics of **clarithromycin** are almost certainly of little or no clinical importance.

1. Amsden GW, Foulds G, Thakker K. Pharmacokinetic study of azithromycin with fluconazole and cotrimoxazole (trimethoprim-sulfamethoxazole) in healthy volunteers. *Clin Drug Invest* (2000) 20, 135–42.
2. Gustavson LE, Shi H, Palmer RN, Siepman NC, Craft JC. Drug interaction between clarithromycin and fluconazole in healthy subjects. *Clin Pharmacol Ther* (1996) 59, 185.

Macrolide antibacterials + Proton pump inhibitors

Proton pump inhibitors do not appear to interact with macrolide antibacterials.

Clinical evidence, mechanism, importance and management

A study of roxithromycin 300 mg twice daily, alone, with **omeprazole** 20 mg twice daily or with **lansoprazole** 30 mg twice daily, for 6 days found no significant pharmacokinetic differences between any of the 3 regimens.[1] Therefore no precautions would seem necessary if these drugs are taken together.

1. Kees F, Holstege A, Ittner KP, Zimmermann M, Lock G, Schölmerich J, Grobecker H. Pharmacokinetic interaction between proton pump inhibitors and roxithromycin in volunteers. *Aliment Pharmacol Ther* (2000) 14, 407–12.

Mebendazole + Miscellaneous drugs

Cimetidine raises serum mebendazole levels and increases its effectiveness. Phenytoin and carbamazepine, but not sodium valproate, lower serum mebendazole levels.

Clinical evidence, mechanism, importance and management

(a) Anticonvulsants

The same report cited bekow found that both **phenytoin** and **carbamazepine** lowered serum mebendazole levels, presumably due to their well-recognised enzyme inducing effects which increase the metabolism and loss of mebendazole from the body.[2] **Sodium valproate** tended to increase mebendazole levels, but it is unclear whether or not this rise is significant.[2] This interaction is only likely to be important when treating organisms within the tissues, rather than when treating infections in the gut. For tissue infections it may be necessary to increase the mebendazole dosage in the presence of **phenytoin** and **carbamazepine**. Monitor the outcome of concurrent use.

(b) Cimetidine

A study[1] in 8 patients (5 with peptic ulcers and 3 with hydatid cysts) taking 1.5 g mebendazole three times daily found that **cimetidine** 400 mg three times daily for 30 days raised the maximum serum mebendazole levels by 48%. The previously unresponsive hepatic hydatid cysts resolved totally. However, previous study had suggested that the rises in serum mebendazole levels are too small to be useful.[2] It is suggested that the interaction is caused by the enzyme inhibitory actions of **cimetidine** reducing the metabolism of mebendazole.[1] There would seem to be no reason for avoiding concurrent use, but be alert for any evidence of mebendazole toxicity (allergic reactions, leucopenia, alopecia).

1. Bekhti A, Pirotte J. Cimetidine increases serum mebendazole concentrations. Implications for treatment of hepatic hydatid cysts. *Br J Clin Pharmacol* (1987) 24, 390–2.
2. Luder PJ, Siffert B, Witassek F, Meister F, Bircher J. Treatment of hydatid disease with high oral doses of mebendazole. Long-term follow-up of plasma mebendazole levels and drug interactions. *Eur J Clin Pharmacol* (1986) 31, 443–8.

Mefloquine + Alcohol

Mefloquine appears normally not to interact with alcohol. An isolated report describes two incidents of severe psychosis and depression in a man on mefloquine after drinking large quantities of alcohol.

Clinical evidence, mechanism, importance and management

Mefloquine 250 mg, or placebo was given to 2 groups of 20 healthy subjects on days 1, 2, 3, 8, 15, 22 and 29. They were tested on days 4, 23 and 30 after taking enough **alcohol** to achieve blood levels of about 35 mg%. The mefloquine did not affect blood alcohol levels, nor did it increase the effects of **alcohol** on two real highway driving tests or on psychomotor tests done in the laboratory. In fact the mefloquine group actually drove better than placebo group.[1]

A 40-year old man with no previous psychiatric history taking 250 mg mefloquine weekly for malarial prophylaxis had no problems with the first 2 doses. However, on two separate occasions when taking the third and fourth doses he concurrently drank about half a litre of **whiskey**, whereupon he developed severe paranoid delusions, hallucinations and became suicidal. When he stopped drinking he had no further problems while taking subsequent doses of mefloquine. He was used to drinking such large amounts of **alcohol** and had experienced no problems while previously taking **proguanil/chloroquine**.[2]

The broad picture is that mefloquine appears not to worsen the effects of moderate amounts of **alcohol** (blood levels of 35 mg%) and it seems unlikely that it will have a marked effect with larger doses, but this needs confirmation. Just why an unusual toxic reaction developed in one individual is not known.

1. Vuurman EFPM, Muntjewerff ND, Uiterwijk MMC, van Veggel LMA, Crevoisier C, Haglund L, Kinzig M, O'Hanlon JF. Effects of mefloquine alone and with alcohol on psychomotor and driving performance. *Eur J Clin Pharmacol* (1996) 50, 475–82.

2. Wittes RC, Saginur R. Adverse reaction to mefloquine associated with ethanol ingestion. *Can Med Assoc J* (1995) 152, 515–17.

Mefloquine + Antimalarials

Primaquine can increase both the serum levels and the side-effects of mefloquine. Mefloquine serum levels may possibly be increased by quinine. In theory there is an increased risk of convulsions if mefloquine is given with quinine or chloroquine. Artemisinin derivatives do not appear to adversely affect the pharmacokinetics of mefloquine.

Clinical evidence, mechanism, importance and management

(a) Artemisinin derivatives

In a single-dose three-way crossover study, 10 healthy subjects were given either 750 mg mefloquine, 300 mg **dihydroartemisinin** or both drugs together. The pharmacokinetics of the drugs were unchanged on concurrent use, except for the rate of absorption of mefloquine, which was increased, and the activity against *Plasmodium falciparum* was synergistic, rather than additive.[1]

(b) Primaquine

A randomised crossover study in 14 healthy subjects given 1 g mefloquine found that the addition of 15 or 30 mg **primaquine** raised the peak serum levels of mefloquine by 48% (from 1.64 to 2.42 micrograms/ml) and 29% (from 2.52 to 3.24 micrograms/ml) respectively. Those taking the larger dose of **primaquine** showed a transient increase in peak **primaquine** serum levels, and its conversion to its inactive carboxyl metabolite also increased. Significant CNS symptoms were also experienced by those taking the larger dose of **primaquine**.[2] *In vitro* studies suggest that **primaquine** is a potent inhibitor of mefloquine metabolism.[3] However, these results contrast with a single dose study in 8 healthy subjects given single oral doses of 750 mg mefloquine and 45 mg **primaquine** in which no increased side-effects attributable to concurrent use were seen.[4] The clinical significance of this interaction is uncertain, but combined used may increase the mefloquine side-effects.

(c) Quinine, Chloroquine

Mefloquine 750 mg alone, or followed 24 h later by **quinine** 600 mg, was given to 7 healthy subjects. The combination did not affect the pharmacokinetics of either drug, but the number of side effects and the period of prolongation of the QT interval was greater with the combination, although no symptomatic cardiotoxicity was seen.[5] This absence of a change in pharmacokinetics is contrary to earlier *in vitro* data and unpublished clinical observations,[3] which suggested that **quinine** may inhibit the metabolism of mefloquine, thereby raising its serum levels. The makers of mefloquine say that it should not be administered with **quinine** or **related compounds** (e.g. **quinidine, chloroquine**) since this could increase the risk of ECG abnormalities and convulsions. Patients treated initially for 2 to 3 days with **quinine** given intravenously should have the dose of mefloquine delayed until at least 12 h after the last dosing of **quinine** to largely prevent interactions leading to adverse events.[6] However, there seem to be no documented adverse reports of this interaction leading to convulsions.

1. Na-Bangchang K, Tippawangkosol P, Thanavibul A, Ubalee R, Karbwang J. Pharmacokinetic and pharmacodynamic interactions of mefloquine and dihydroartemisinin. *Int J Clin Pharmacol Res* (1999) 19, 9–17.

2. Macleod CM, Trenholme GM, Nora MV, Bartley EA, Frischer H. Interaction of primaquine with mefloquine in healthy males. *Intersci Conf Antimicrob Agents Chemother* (1990) 30, 213.

3. Bangchang KN, Karbwang J, Back DJ. Mefloquine metabolism by human liver microsomes. Effect of other antimalarial drugs. *Biochem Pharmacol* (1992) 43, 1957–61.

4. Karbwang J, Bangchang KN, Thanavibul A, Back DJ, Bunnag D. Pharmacokinetics of mefloquine in the presence of primaquine. *Eur J Clin Pharmacol* (1992) 42, 559–60.

5. Na-Bangchang K, Tan-Ariya P, Thanavibul A, Reingchainam S, Shrestha SB, Karbwang J. Pharmacokinetic and pharmacodynamic interactions of mefloquine and quinine. *Int J Clin Pharmacol Res* (1999) 19, 73–82.

6. Lariam (Mefloquine). Roche Products Limited. Summary of product characteristics, August 2000.

Mefloquine + Cardioactive drugs

Mefloquine prolongs the QT interval and an isolated report describes cardiopulmonary arrest in one patient taking propranolol. The WHO have issued a warning about the concurrent use of anti-arrhythmics, beta-blockers, calcium-channel blockers antihistamines or phenothiazines.

Clinical evidence, mechanism, importance and management

A WHO report[1] advises that "The co-administration of mefloquine with **anti-arrhythmic agents**, **beta-adrenergic blocking agents**, **calcium channel blockers**, **antihistamines** including H_1-blocking agents and **phenothiazines** might contribute to the prolongation of QT_c intervals. However, in the light of information currently available, co-administration of mefloquine with such drugs is not contraindicated." It is also suggested that "mefloquine and related drugs (e.g. **quinine** or **quinidine**) should only be given concomitantly under close medical supervision because of possible additive cardiotoxicity".[1]

The makers of mefloquine also give this warning, pointing out that the interaction is theoretical.[2]

No formal studies on the possible adverse effects of combining any of these drugs with mefloquine seem to have been done, but ECG changes have been seen in some individuals. There is a single case report of cardiopulmonary arrest in a patient on **propranolol** when given a single dose of mefloquine.[3] It remains to be confirmed whether the effects of mefloquine and these other drugs on cardiac function are normally additive, and whether the outcome is clinically important. However until more is known it would seem prudent to err on the side of caution and to follow this cautionary advice. More study is needed.

1. WHO. International travel and health: vaccination requirements and health advice. Geneva: WHO, 2001.

2. Lariam (Mefloquine). Roche Products Limited. Summary of product characteristics, August 2000.

3. Anon. Mefloquine for malaria. *Med Lett Drugs Ther* (1990) 31, 13–14.

Mefloquine + Cimetidine

The loss of mefloquine from the body is reduced by the concurrent use of cimetidine, but the clinical importance of this is uncertain.

Clinical evidence, mechanism, importance and management

A single 500-mg dose of mefloquine was given to 10 healthy subjects before and after taking 800 mg **cimetidine** daily for 28 days. The **cimetidine** had no effect on the mefloquine serum levels or on its AUC, but its half-life increased by 50% (from 9.6 to 14.4 days) and the oral clearance decreased by almost 40%.[1] The probable reason is that **cimetidine** (a recognised enzyme inhibitor) reduces the metabolism of the mefloquine by the liver so that it is lost from the body more slowly. The clinical importance of this is uncertain, but to be on the safe side prescribers should be alert for any evidence of increased mefloquine side-effects (dizziness, nausea, vomiting, abdominal pain) and toxicity during concurrent use. The CSM say that patients should be informed about the adverse effects of mefloquine and they should seek medical advice if necessary before the next dose is due.[2]

1. Sunbhanichi M, Ridtitid W, Wongnawa M, Akesiripong S, Chamnongchob P. Effect of cimetidine on an oral single-dose mefloquine pharmacokinetics in humans. *Asia Pacific J Pharmacol* (1997) 12, 51–5.
2. Committee on Safety of Medicines/Medicines Control Agency. Mefloquine (Lariam) and neuropsychiatric reactions. *Current Problems* (1996) 22, 6.

Mefloquine + Metoclopramide

Although metoclopramide increases the rate of absorption of mefloquine and increases its peak blood levels, its side-effects are possibly reduced.

Clinical evidence, mechanism, importance and management

When 10 mg **metoclopramide** was taken 15 min before a single 750-mg dose of mefloquine, the absorption half-life of the mefloquine in 7 normal subjects was reduced from 3.2 to 2.4 h and the peak blood levels were raised by 31%. However, although the rate of absorption was increased, the total amount absorbed was unchanged. A possible reason for these changes is that the **metoclopramide** increases the gastric emptying so that the mefloquine reaches the small intestine more quickly, which would increase the rate of absorption. Despite these changes, the toxicity of mefloquine (dizziness, nausea, vomiting, abdominal pain) were noted to be reduced.[1] It is not clear what the outcome of chronic use might be but it would be prudent to monitor the outcome closely. More study is needed.

1. Bangchang KN, Karbwang J, Bunnag D, Harinasuta T, Back DJ. The effect of metoclopramide on mefloquine pharmacokinetics. *Br J Clin Pharmacol* (1991) 32, 640–1.

Mefloquine + Quinolone antibacterials

Three non-epileptic patients developed convulsions when concurrently treated for fever with mefloquine and quinolone antibacterials.

Clinical evidence, mechanism, importance and management

A large scale survey in India of the adverse effects of mefloquine identified 3 cases of convulsions out of a total of 150 patients concurrently treated with **ciprofloxacin**, **ofloxacin** or **sparfloxacin**. All 3 patients were not epileptic, and had no family history of epilepsy. All were being treated for fever, which was due to *Plasmodium vivax* in one case, *P. falciparum* in the second, and was not established in the

third. None of the patients had severe or complicated malaria. The **ofloxacin** was given 2 days before the mefloquine, and the other two **quinolones** were given together with the mefloquine.[1] The reason for the seizures is not known, but seizures are among the recognised side-effects of both mefloquine and these quinolones. These adverse, apparently additive, side-effects are rare, but prescribers should be aware of the potential problems of prescribing these drugs together.

1. Mangalvedhekar SS, Gogtay NJ, Wagh VR, Waran MS, Mane D, Kshirsager NA. Convulsions in non-epileptics due to mefloquine-fluoroquinolone co-administration. *Natl Med J India* (2000) 13, 47.

Mefloquine + Rifampicin

Rifampicin significantly reduces the plasma concentrations of mefloquine.

Clinical evidence, mechanism, importance and management

Mefloquine 500 mg was given to 7 healthy subjects after 7 days pretreatment with **rifampicin** 600 mg daily. The maximum plasma level of mefloquine decreased by 19% and the AUC decreased by 68%. This is thought to be due to **rifampicin** causing enhanced metabolism of mefloquine in the liver and gut wall. Simultaneous use of rifampicin and mefloquine should be avoided to prevent treatment failure and the risk of *P. falciparum* resistance to mefloquine.[1]

1. Ridtitid W, Wongnawa M, Mahattanatrakul W, Chaipol P, Sunbhanich M. Effect of rifampicin on plasma concentrations of mefloquine in healthy volunteers. *J Pharm Pharmacol* (2000) 52, 1265–9.

Mefloquine + Tetracycline

Mefloquine serum levels are increased by tetracycline.

Clinical evidence, mechanism, importance and management

The maximum serum levels of mefloquine following a single 750-mg dose were increased by 38% (from 1160 to 1600 ng/ml) in 20 healthy Thai men after taking 250 mg **tetracycline** four times daily for a week. The AUC (0–7 days) was increased 30% and the half-life reduced from 19.3 to 14.4 days, without evidence of any increase in side-effects. The suggested reason for the increased mefloquine levels is that its enterohepatic recycling is reduced because of competition for biliary excretion.[1] The authors of the report conclude that concurrent use may be valuable for treating multi-drug resistant falciparum malaria because higher mefloquine levels are associated with a more effective response. However, more study is needed to confirm these findings. There seems to be no reason for avoiding concurrent use.

1. Karbwang J, Bangchang KN, Back DJ, Bunnag D, Rooney W. Effect of tetracycline on mefloquine pharmacokinetics in Thai males. *Eur J Clin Pharmacol* (1992) 43, 567–9.

Meropenem + Probenecid

Probenecid increases the serum levels of meropenem.

Clinical evidence, mechanism, importance and management

Probenecid (1 g orally 2 h before and 500 mg orally, 1.5 h after meropenem) increased the AUC of 500 mg meropenem by 43% (from 28.1 to 40.2 micrograms.h/ml) in 6 healthy subjects.[1] Another study found that **probenecid** (1.5 g in divided doses the day before and 500 mg 1 h before meropenem) increased the AUC of 1 g meropenem in 6 healthy subjects by up to 55% (from 61.5 to 95.4 mg.h/l) and increased its half-life 33% (from 0.98 to 1.3 h).[2] In both studies the serum levels of meropenem were increased modestly. This is possibly because meropenem and probenecid compete for active kidney tubular secretion.[3] The makers say that because the potency and duration of meropenem are adequate without **probenecid**, they do not recommend co-administration.[3]

1. Ishida Y, Matsumoto F, Sakai O, Yoshida M, Shiba K. The pharmacokinetic study of meropenem: effect of probenecid and hemodialysis. *J Chemother* (1993) 5 (Suppl 1), 124–6.
2. Bax RP, Bastain W, Featherstone A, Wilkinson DM, Hutchison M, Haworth SJ. The pharmacokinetics of meropenem in volunteers. *J Antimicrob Chemother* (1989) 24 (Suppl A), 311–20.
3. Meronem (Meropenem). AstraZeneca. Summary of product characteristics, August 2001.

Methenamine (Hexamine) compounds + Urinary acidifiers, Alkalinizers or Sulphonamides

Urinary alkalinizers (e.g. potassium or sodium citrate) and those antacids which can raise the urinary pH above 5.5 should not be used during treatment with methenamine (hexamine) compounds. If some of the older less-soluble sulphonamides are used with methenamine there is the risk of kidney damage due to crystalluria at low urinary pH values.

Clinical evidence, mechanism, importance and management

(a) Methenamine (hexamine) + urinary acidifiers or alkalinizers

Methenamine and methenamine mandelate are only effective as urinary antiseptics if the pH is about 5.5 or lower, when formaldehyde is released. This is normally achieved by giving urinary acidifiers such as **ammonium chloride**, **ascorbic acid**[1,2] or **sodium acid phosphate**. In the case of methenamine hippurate, the acidification of the urine is achieved by the presence of hippuric acid. The concurrent use of compounds which raise the urinary pH such as **acetazolamide**, **sodium bicarbonate**, **potassium** or **sodium citrate** is clearly contraindicated. **Potassium citrate mixture BPC** at normal therapeutic doses has been shown to raise the pH by more than 1 thereby making the urine sufficiently alkaline to interfere with the activation of methenamine to formaldehyde.[3] Concurrent use should therefore be avoided. Some **antacids** can also cause a very significant rise in the pH of the urine.[4]

(b) Methenamine (hexamine) + urinary acidifiers + sulphonamides

At pH values of 5.5 and below at which methenamine is effective, many of the older sulphonamides (e.g. **sulphapyridine, sulfadiazine, sulfamethizole**) are insoluble and can crystallise in the kidney tubules causing physical damage. Although this is much less likely to occur with the newer, more soluble **sulphonamides**, it would seem preferable to avoid the problem by using some other form of treatment.

1. Strom JG. Jun HW. Effect of urine pH and ascorbic acid on the rate of conversion of methenamine to formaldehyde. *Biopharm Drug Dispos* (1993) 14, 61–9.
2. Nahata MC, Cummins BA, McLeod DC, Schondelmeyer SW, Butler R. Effect of urinary acidifiers on formaldehyde concentration and efficacy with methenamine therapy. *Eur J Clin Pharmacol* (1982) 22, 281–4.
3. Lipton JH. Incompatibility between sulfamethizole and methenamine mandelate. *N Engl J Med* (1963) 268, 92.
4. Levy G. Interaction of salicylates with antacids. Clinical implications with respect to gastrointestinal bleeding and antiinflammatory activity. Frontiers of Internal Medicine 1974, 12th Int Congr Intern Med, Tel Aviv 1974. Karger, Basel (1975) p 404–8.

Metronidazole + Antacid, Kaolin-pectin or Colestyramine

The absorption of metronidazole from the gut is unaffected by kaolin-pectin, but a small reduction occurs if either an aluminium hydroxide antacid or colestyramine is given concurrently.

Clinical evidence, mechanism, importance and management

The bioavailability of single 500-mg doses of metronidazole in 5 healthy subjects was not significantly changed by 30 ml of a **kaolin-pectin antidiarrhoeal mixture**, but a 14.5% reduction occurred with 30 ml of an **aluminium hydroxide/simethicone** suspension, and a 21.3% reduction with 4 g **colestyramine**.[1] The clinical importance of these reductions is uncertain, but probably small, however clinical studies using repeated doses are needed to confirm this. Advise patients to separate the dosages to minimise admixture of the drugs within the gut.

1. Molokhia AM, Al-Rahman S. Effect of concomitant oral administration of some adsorbing drugs on the bioavailability of metronidazole. *Drug Dev Ind Pharm* (1987) 13, 1229–37.

Metronidazole + Antiulcer drugs

Cimetidine reduces the loss of metronidazole from the body to some extent, but the clinical importance of this is probably small. Omeprazole has no effect on metronidazole pharmacokinetics.

Clinical evidence, mechanism, importance and management

(a) Cimetidine

The half-life of metronidazole (400 mg intravenous dose) in 6 healthy subjects was increased from 6.2 to 7.9 h after taking **cimetidine** 400 mg twice daily for 6 days. The total plasma clearance was reduced by almost 30%.[1] It is believed that this is due to inhibition by **cimetidine** of the metabolism of the metronidazole by the liver. However in another study in 6 patients with Crohn's disease, **cimetidine** 600 mg twice daily for 7 days was found not to affect either the AUC or the half-life of metronidazole,[2,3] and no evidence of an interaction was found in a further study in 6 healthy subjects.[4]

The effect of this interaction, if and when it occurs, is not large and it seems unlikely that clinical effects will be marked. There appear to be no reports of metronidazole toxicity during concurrent use.

(b) Omeprazole

The pharmacokinetics of a single dose of metronidazole were unaffected by 5 days pre-treatment with **omeprazole** 20 mg twice daily in 14 healthy subjects.[5]

1. Gugler R, Jensen JC. Interaction between cimetidine and metronidazole. *N Engl J Med* (1983) 309, 1518–19.
2. Eradiri O, Jamali F, Thomson ABR. Interaction of metronidazole with cimetidine and phenobarbital in Crohn's disease. *Clin Pharmacol Ther* (1987) 41, 235.
3. Eradiri O, Jamali F, Thomson ABR. Interaction of metronidazole with phenobarbital, cimetidine, prednisone, and sulfasalazine in Crohn's disease. *Biopharm Drug Dispos* (1988) 9, 219–27.
4. Loft S, Døssing M, Sonne J, Dalhof K, Bjerrum K, Poulsen HE. Lack of effect of cimetidine on the pharmacokinetics and metabolism of a single oral dose of metronidazole. *Eur J Clin Pharmacol* (1988) 35, 65–8.
5. David FL, Da Silva CMF, Mendes FD, Ferraz JGP, Muscara MN, Moreno H, De Nucci G, Pedrazzoli J. *Aliment Pharmacol Ther* (1998) 12, 349–54.

Metronidazole + Barbiturates

Phenobarbital markedly increases the loss of metronidazole from the body so that larger doses are needed. Conventional doses of metronidazole in the presence of phenobarbital failed to clear up trichomoniasis in a woman, and giardiasis or amoebiasis in children.

Clinical evidence

A woman with vaginal trichomoniasis was given metronidazole on several occasions over the course of a year, but the infection flared up again as soon as it was stopped. When it was realised that she was also taking 100 mg **phenobarbital** daily, the metronidazole dosage was doubled to 500 mg three times daily, for seven days, and she was cured.[1] A pharmacokinetic study found that the metronidazole was being cleared from her body much more rapidly than usual (half-life 3.5 h compared with the normal 8 to 9 h).[1]

A retrospective study in children who had failed to respond to metronidazole for giardiasis or amoebiasis found that 80% of them had been on long-term **phenobarbital** treatment. A prospective study in 36 children the normal recommended dosage had to be increased threefold (to 60 mg/kg) to achieve a cure. The half-life of metronidazole in 15 other children on **phenobarbital** was found to be 3.5 h compared with the normal 8 to 9 h.[2] **Phenobarbital** 60 mg twice daily reduced the metronidazole AUC in 6 patients with Crohn's disease by about a third,[3] and in another 7 healthy subjects 100 mg **phenobarbital** for 7 days increased the clearance of metronidazole 1.5-fold.[4]

Mechanism

Phenobarbital is a known, potent liver enzyme-inducing agent, which increases the metabolism and loss of metronidazole from the body.

Importance and management

An established and clinically important interaction. Monitor the effects of concurrent use and anticipate the need to increase the metronidazole dosage two-three fold if phenobarbital is given concurrently. All of the barbiturates are potent liver enzyme inducing agents and would be expected to interact similarly.

1. Mead PB, Gibson M, Schentag JJ, Ziemniak JA. Possible alteration of metronidazole metabolism by phenobarbital. *N Engl J Med* (1982) 306, 1490.
2. Gupte S. Phenobarbital and metabolism of metronidazole. *N Engl J Med* (1983) 308, 529.
3. Eradiri O, Jamali F, Thomson ABR. Interaction of metronidazole with cimetidine and phenobarbital in Crohn's disease. *Clin Pharmacol Ther* (1987) 41, 235.
4. Loft S, Sonne J, Poulsen HE, Petersen KT, Jørgensen BG, Døssing M. Inhibition and induction of metronidazole and antipyrine metabolism. *Eur J Clin Pharmacol* (1987) 32, 35–41.

Metronidazole + Chloroquine

An isolated report describes acute dystonia in a patient on metronidazole when given a single dose of chloroquine.

Clinical evidence, mechanism, importance and management

A patient was given a 7-day course of metronidazole and ampicillin, following a laparoscopic investigation. She developed acute dystonic reactions (facial grimacing, coarse tremors, and an inability to maintain posture) on day 6, within 10 min of being given a single dose of **chloroquine phosphate** (equivalent to 200 mg base), plus 25 mg intramuscular promethazine. The dystonic symptoms started to subside within 15 min of being given 5 mg diazepam intravenously, and had completely resolved within 2 h. She had previously had **chloroquine** without problems, and later had metronidazole and ampicillin without problems. Although extrapyramidal reactions to **chloroquine** appear to be rare the authors of the report suggest that *Fansidar* (**pyrimethamine/sulfadoxine**) should be used for malarial prophylaxis in patients on metronidazole.[1]

1. Achumba JI, Ette EI, Thomas WOA, Essien EE. Chloroquine-induced acute dystonic reactions in the presence of metronidazole. *Drug Intell Clin Pharm* (1988) 22, 308–10.

Metronidazole + Corticosteroids

Prednisone increases the loss of metronidazole from the body. A moderate increase in the dosage of metronidazole may be needed.

Clinical evidence

When given 10 mg **prednisone** twice daily for 6 days, the AUC of metronidazole 250 mg twice daily in 6 patients with Crohn's disease was reduced by 31% (from 78.56 to 53.83 mg.h^{-1}).[1]

Mechanism

Prednisone appears to increase the metabolism of metronidazole by enzyme induction, thereby increasing its clearance from the body.[1]

Importance and management

Information appears to be limited to this report and the interaction is probably of only moderate clinical importance. Be alert for the need to increase the metronidazole dosage. Information about other corticosteroids is lacking.

1. Eradiri O, Jamali F, Thomson ABR. Interaction of metronidazole with phenobarbital, cimetidine, prednisone, and sulfasalazine in Crohn's disease. *Biopharm Drug Dispos* (1988) 9, 219–27.

Metronidazole + Disulfiram

Acute psychoses and confusion can result from the concurrent use of metronidazole and disulfiram.

Clinical evidence

In a double-blind study on 58 hospitalised chronic alcoholics being treated with **disulfiram**, half of them were additionally given 750 mg metronidazole daily for a month, followed by 250 mg daily. Six of the 29 subjects in the group receiving metronidazole developed acute psychoses or confusion. Five of the 6 had paranoid delusions and in 3 visual and auditory hallucinations were also seen. The symptoms persisted for 2 to 3 days after the drugs were withdrawn, but disappeared at the end of a fortnight and did not reappear when **disulfiram** alone was restarted.[1] Similar reactions have been described in two other reports.[2,3]

Mechanism

Not understood

Importance and management

This appears to be an established interaction. The incidence is high. Concurrent use should be avoided or very well monitored.

1. Rothstein E, Clancy DD. Toxicity of disulfiram combined with metronidazole. *N Engl J Med* (1969) 280, 1006–7.
2. Goodhue WW. Disulfiram-metronidazole (well-identified) toxicity. *N Engl J Med* (1969) 280, 1482–3.
3. Scher JM. Psychotic reaction to disulfiram. *JAMA* (1967) 201, 1051.

Metronidazole + Rifampicin (Rifampin)

Rifampicin increases the clearance of metronidazole from the body, but the clinical importance of this is uncertain.

Clinical evidence, mechanism, importance and management

Metronidazole 500 or 1000 mg intravenously was given to 10 healthy subjects before and after taking 450 mg **rifampicin** daily for 7 days. The **rifampicin** reduced the metronidazole AUC by 33% and increased its clearance by 44%. Results were the same with both doses.[1] The reason for this interaction is almost certainly because the **rifampicin** (a well-recognised and potent enzyme inducer) increases the metabolism of the metronidazole by the liver, thereby increasing its loss from the body.

The effectiveness of the metronidazole would be expected to be reduced by this interaction, but nobody seems to have checked on whether this is of real clinical importance. However in the absence of definite reports, it would now clearly be prudent to monitor the outcome of adding **rifampicin** to metronidazole. This interaction is not likely to have any relevance when metronidazole is being used for infections within the gut.

1. Djojosaputro M, Mustofa SS, Donatus IA, Santoso B. The effects of doses and pre-treatment with rifampicin on the elimination kinetics of metronidazole. *Eur J Pharmacol* (1990) 183, 1870–1.

Metronidazole + Sucralfate

Sucralfate does not appear to interact with metronidazole.

Clinical evidence, mechanism, importance and management

Because oral triple therapy using **sucralfate** instead of bismuth to eradicate *H. pylori* has yielded inconsistent results, a 5-day study was undertaken in 14 healthy subjects to investigate whether **sucralfate** interacts with metronidazole. It was found that 2 g **sucralfate** twice daily had no effect on the pharmacokinetics of a single dose of metronidazole 400 mg.[1]

1. Amaral Moraes ME, De Almeida Pierossi M, Moraes MO, Bezerra FF, Ferreira De Silva CM, Dias HB, Muscará MN, De Nucci G, Pedrazzoli J. Short-term sucralfate administration does not alter the absorption of metronidazole in healthy male volunteers. *Int J Clin Pharmacol Ther* (1996) 34, 433–7.

Minocycline + Ethinylestradiol

There is some evidence that preparations containing ethinylestradiol may accentuate the facial pigmentation which can be caused by minocycline.

Clinical evidence

Two teenage sisters taking minocycline for severe acne vulgaris (50 mg four times daily for 14 days, then reduced to twice daily), developed dark-brown pigmentation in the acne scars when also given *Dianette* (**cyproterone acetate** and **ethinylestradiol**) for about 15 months.[1] The type of pigmentation was not identified because they both declined to have a biopsy, but in other cases it has been found to consist of haemosiderin, iron, melanin and a metabolic degradation product of minocycline.[1] Two other reports describe facial pigmentation in other patients on minocycline, two of whom were taking **oral contraceptives** containing **ethinylestradiol**.[2,3] Other young women who have developed minocycline pigmentation may also have been taking **oral contraceptives** because they fall into the right age-group, but this is not specifically stated in any of the reports.

Mechanism

Not understood. It seems possible that the facial pigmentation (melasma, chloasma) which can occur with oral contraceptives may have been additive with the effects of the minocycline.[1]

Importance and management

Evidence is very limited but it has been suggested that everyone on long-term minocycline treatment should be well screened for the development of pigmentation, particularly if they are taking other drugs such as the oral contraceptives which are known to induce hyperpigmentation.[1] Remember also that very rarely contraceptive failure has been associated with the use of minocycline and other tetracyclines, see 'Oral contraceptives + Antibacterials and Anti-infectives', p.469.

1. Eedy DJ, Burrows D. Minocycline-induced pigmentation occurring in two sisters. *Clin Exp Dermatol* (1991) 16, 55–7.
2. Ridgeway HA, Sonnex TS, Kennedy CTC. et al. Hyperpigmentation associated with oral minocycline. *Br J Dermatol* (1982) 107, 95–102.
3. Prigent F, Cavelier-Balloy B, Tollenaere C, Civatte J. Pigmentation cutanée induite par la minocycline: deux cas. *Ann Dermatol Venereol* (1986) 113, 227–33.

Nalidixic acid + Nitrofurantoin

***In vitro* studies have demonstrated antagonistic antibacterial effects when the two drugs are used together.**

Clinical evidence, mechanism, importance and management

The antibacterial activity of nalidixic acid can be inhibited by sub-inhibitory concentrations of **nitrofurantoin**. In 44 out of 53 strains of *Escherichia coli*, *Salmonella* and *Proteus* antagonism was shown.[1] Another study confirmed these findings.[2] Whether this similarly occurs if both antibacterials are given to patients is uncertain, but the advice that concurrent use should be avoided when treating urinary tract infections seems sound.[1] Other quinolone antibacterials and **nitrofurantoin** are also said to be antagonistic and it is recommended that the combination is avoided.[3]

1. Stille W and Ostner KH. Antagonismus Nitrofurantoin-Nalidixinsaure. *Klin Wochenschr* (1966) 44, 155–6.
2. Piguet D. L'action inhibitrice de la nitrofurantoïne sur le pouvoir bactériostatique *in vitro* de l'acide nalidixique. *Ann Inst Pasteur (Paris)* (1969) 116, 43–8.
3. Sweetman SC, editor. Martindale: The complete drug reference. 33rd ed. London: Pharmaceutical Press; 2002 p.231.

Niclosamide + Alcohol

Alcohol may possibly increase the side-effects of niclosamide.

Clinical evidence, mechanism, importance and management

The makers of niclosamide advise the avoidance of **alcohol** while taking niclosamide. The reasoning behind this is that while niclosamide is virtually insoluble in water, it is slightly soluble in **alcohol** which might possibly increase its absorption by the gut, resulting an increase in its side-effects. There are no formal reports of this but Bayer say they have some anecdotal information which is consistent with this suggestion.[1]

1. Bayer. Personal communication, July 1992.

Nitrofurantoin + Antacids

The antibacterial effectiveness of nitrofurantoin in the treatment of urinary tract infections is possibly reduced by magnesium trisilicate but this awaits confirmation. Aluminium hydroxide is reported not to interact. Whether other antacids interact adversely is uncertain.

Clinical evidence

Magnesium trisilicate 5 g in 150 ml water reduced the absorption of single 100 g oral doses of nitrofurantoin in 6 healthy subjects by more than 50%. The time during which the concentration of nitrofurantoin in the urine was at, or above, the minimal antibacterial inhibitory concentration of 32 micrograms/ml was also reduced.[1] The amounts of nitrofurantoin adsorbed by other antacids in *in vitro* tests were as follows: **magnesium trisilicate** and **charcoal** 99%, **bismuth oxycarbonate** and **talc** 50 to 53%, **kaolin** 31%, **magnesium oxide** 27%, **aluminium hydroxide** 2.5% and **calcium carbonate** 0%.[1]

A crossover study in 6 healthy subjects confirmed that **aluminium hydroxide gel** does not affect the absorption of nitrofurantoin from the gut (as measured by its excretion into the urine).[2] Another study in 10 healthy subjects found that an antacid containing **aluminium hydroxide**, **magnesium carbonate** and **magnesium hydroxide** reduced the absorption by 22%.[3]

Mechanism

Antacids can, to a greater or lesser extent, adsorb nitrofurantoin onto their surfaces, as a result less is available for absorption by the gut and for excretion into the urine.

Importance and management

Information appears to be limited to these reports. There seems to be nothing in the literature confirming that a clinically important nitrofurantoin/antacid interaction occurs. One reviewer offers the opinion that common antacid preparations are unlikely to interact with nitrofurantoin.[4]

It is not yet known whether magnesium trisilicate significantly reduces the antibacterial effectiveness of nitrofurantoin but the response should be monitored. Be alert for the need to increase the dosage of the nitrofurantoin. While it is known that the antibacterial action of nitrofurantoin is increased by drugs which acidify the urine (so that reduced actions would be expected if the urine were made more alkaline by antacids) this again does not seem to have been confirmed. The results of the *in vitro* studies suggest that the possible effects of the other antacids are quite small, and aluminium hydroxide is reported not to interact.

1. Naggar VF, Khalil SA. Effect of magnesium trisilicate on nitrofurantoin absorption. *Clin Pharmacol Ther* (1979) 25, 857–63.
2. Jaffe JM, Hamilton B, Jeffers S. Nitrofurantoin-antacid interaction. *Drug Intell Clin Pharm* (1976) 10, 419–20.
3. Männistö P. The effect of crystal size, gastric content and emptying rate on the absorption of nitrofurantoin in healthy human volunteers. *Int J Clin Pharmacol Biopharm* (1978) 16, 223–8.
4. D'Arcy PF. Nitrofurantoin. *Drug Intell Clin Pharm* (1985) 19, 540–7.

Nitrofurantoin + Anticholinergics or Diphenoxylate

Diphenoxylate and anticholinergic drugs such as propantheline can double the absorption of nitrofurantoin in some patients, but the clinical importance of this is uncertain.

Clinical evidence, mechanism, importance and management

Propantheline 30 mg given 45 mins before nitrofurantoin approximately doubled the absorption of 100 mg nitrofurantoin (as measured by the urinary excretion) in 6 healthy subjects.[1] In another study, 2 out of 6 men similarly showed nearly doubled nitrofurantoin absorption when given 200 mg **diphenoxylate** daily for 3 days, but the other 4 showed little effect.[2] **Atropine** 500 micrograms given subcutaneously 30 mins before a single 100-mg dose of nitrofurantoin had little effect on the bioavailability of nitrofurantoin, but the absorption and excretion into the urine is delayed.[3] It was suggested that the reduced motility of the gut caused by these drugs allows the nitrofurantoin to dissolve more completely so that it is absorbed by the gut more easily. Whether this is of any clinical importance is uncertain but it would be expected to be accompanied by an increase in the therapeutic effects of nitrofurantoin and possibly in the incidence of dose-related adverse reactions. So far there appear to be no reports of any problems arising from concurrent use.

1. Jaffe JM. Effect of propantheline on nitrofurantoin absorption. *J Pharm Sci* (1975) 64, 1729–30.
2. Callahan M, Bullock FJ, Braun J, Yesair DW. Pharmacodynamics of drug interactions with diphenoxylate (Lomotil®). *Fedn Proc* (1974) 33, 513.
3. Männistö P. The effect of crystal size, gastric content and emptying rate on the absorption of nitrofurantoin in healthy human volunteers. *Int J Clin Pharmacol Biopharm* (1978) 16, 223–8.

Nitrofurantoin + Metoclopramide

Metoclopramide reduces the absorption of nitrofurantoin.

Clinical evidence, mechanism, importance and management

The urinary excretion of nitrofurantoin in 10 healthy subjects was approximately halved when they were given a 100 mg tablet of nitrofurantoin after pretreatment with 10 mg **metoclopramide** intramuscularly and 10 mg by mouth half an hour before.[1] The reason is thought to be that the **metoclopramide** increases the gastric emptying rate, thus decreasing absorption. The practical importance of this is uncertain because there seem to be no reports describing problems, but it would be prudent to check on the effectiveness of nitrofurantoin in the presence of **metoclopramide**. It may be necessary to raise the nitrofurantoin dosage.

1. Männistö P. The effect of crystal size, gastric content and emptying rate on the absorption of nitrofurantoin in healthy human volunteers. *Int J Clin Pharmacol Biopharm* (1978) 16, 223–8.

Nitrofurantoin + Probenecid or Sulfinpyrazone

On theoretical grounds the efficacy and toxicity of nitrofurantoin may possibly be increased by probenecid or sulfinpyrazone.

Clinical evidence, mechanism, importance and management

A study of the way the kidneys handle nitrofurantoin found that **sulfinpyrazone** 2.5 mg/kg given intravenously reduced the secretion of nitrofurantoin by the kidney tubules by about 50%.[1] This reduction would therefore be expected to reduce its urinary antibacterial efficacy, and the higher serum levels might lead to increased systemic toxicity, but there do not seem to be any reports confirming or denying that this represents a real problem in practice. The same situation would also seem likely with **probenecid**, but I have not been able to find any reports confirming this interaction.

The clinical importance of both of these interactions is therefore uncertain, but it would seem prudent to be alert for any evidence of reduced antibacterial efficacy and increased systemic toxicity if either of these uricosuric agents is used with nitrofurantoin.

1. Schirmeister J, Stefani F, Willmann H, Hallauer W. Renal handling of nitrofurantoin in man. *Antimicrob Agents Chemother* (1965) 5, 223–6.

Nitroxoline + Antacids

There is *in vitro* evidence that metallic ions such as magnesium and calcium can reduce the antibacterial effects of nitroxoline, but whether in practice a clinically important interaction occurs with antacids containing these ions is not known.

Clinical evidence, mechanism, importance and management

The antibacterial effects of nitroxoline have been found to be reduced by **magnesium** and **calcium** ions *in vitro* because, like other quinolones, it can form chelates with these ions.[1] What is not known is whether in clinical practice nitroxoline would interact significantly with these ions in **antacids**, and whether this would result in inadequate urine concentrations (nitroxoline is mainly used for urinary tract infections). In the absence of any direct clinical information it would however seem prudent to monitor concurrent use for any evidence that its antibacterial effects are reduced.

1. Pelletier C, Prognon P, Bourlioux P. Roles of divalent cations and pH in mechanism of action of nitroxoline against *Escherichia coli* strains. *Antimicrob Agents Chemother* (1995) 707–13.

Non-nucleoside reverse transcriptase inhibitors + Antacids

Maalox does not interact to a clinically relevant extent with oral nevirapine, but antacids approximately halve the AUCs of atevirdine and delavirdine.

Clinical evidence, mechanism, importance and management

(a) Atevirdine

Maalox TC (**aluminium/magnesium hydroxides**) 30 ml, given while fasting, approximately halved the AUC and maximum serum levels of 600 mg **atevirdine mesilate** given to 11 HIV+ subjects.[1] If antacids like *Maalox* are used with **atevirdine**, anticipate the need to increase the **atevirdine** dosage. In theory at least it might be possible to minimise the effects of this interaction by separating the dosages. More study is needed.

(b) Delavirdine

Delavirdine is poorly soluble at pH greater than 3, so the effect of giving **delavirdine** 300 mg 10 min after **antacid** (type and dose unstated) was studied in 12 healthy subjects. The AUC and maximum serum levels of **delavirdine** were reduced by 48 and 57% respectively, suggesting that **delavirdine** should not be given with **antacids**.[2]

(c) Nevirapine

In a study in 24 healthy subjects it was found that 30 ml *Maalox* (**aluminium/magnesium hydroxides**) caused some moderate changes in the pharmacokinetics of 200 mg of **nevirapine**, but none of them was considered to be clinically relevant.[3] No special precautions would seem to be necessary.

1. Borin MT, Della-Coletta AA, Batts DH. Effects of food and antacid on bioavailability of atevirdine mesylate (ATV) in HIV+ patients. *Clin Pharmacol Ther* (1994) 55, 194.
2. Cox SR, Della-Coletta AA, Turner SW, Freimuth WW. Single-dose pharmacokinetic (PK) studies with delavirdine (DLV) mesylate: dose proportionality and effects of food and antacid. *Intersci Conf Antimicrob Agents Chemother* (1994) 34, 82.
3. Lamson MJ, Cort S, Macy H, Love J, Korpalski D, Pav J, Keirns J, Effect of food or an antacid on the bioavailability of nevirapine 200 mg tablets. 11th International Conference on AIDS, Vancouver, 1996. Abstract Tu.B.2323.

Non-nucleoside reverse transcriptase inhibitors + Azole antifungals

Fluconazole causes a moderate rise in atevirdine and efavirenz steady-state levels. It is not clear whether nevirapine and ketoconazole interact to a clinically relevant extent, but the US makers advise avoidance. Delavirdine does not appear to interact with fluconazole.

Clinical evidence, mechanism, importance and management

(a) Atevirdine

A study in HIV+ subjects found that 400 mg **fluconazole** daily for 14 days reduced the clearance of **atevirdine** 600 mg 8-hourly by almost 40% and increased its steady-state levels by 30%.[1] The importance of this interaction awaits assessment. It would seem prudent to monitor the outcome of concurrent use.

(b) Delavirdine

Delavirdine mesilate 300 mg three times daily was given to 13 HIV+ subjects for 30 days. **Fluconazole** 400 mg daily was given to 8 of them on 2 study days. No differences in the pharmacokinetics of either drug were noted between the two groups.[2] On the basis of these results, it would appear that no dosage adjustments are needed if these drugs are used together.

(c) Efavirenz

Fluconazole 400 mg daily for one day, then 200 mg **fluconazole** daily for 4 days was given to 20 healthy subjects with **efavirenz** 400 mg daily. No effects on the pharmacokinetics of **fluconazole** were noted, and although the AUC of **efavirenz** was raised by 15%, no clinically significant effects are anticipated.[3]

(d) Nevirapine

The makers of **nevirapine** quote a study in which 200 mg **nevirapine** twice daily was given with 400 mg **ketoconazole** daily. The **nevirapine** plasma levels were raised 15 to 28%, while the **ketoconazole** AUC was reduced 63% and its maximum plasma levels were reduced by 40%. The US and UK makers suggest that the clinical significance of this interaction is unknown.[4,5] The UK makers suggest that **fluconazole** might possibly be substituted (because it is eliminated renally) although clinical studies confirming the lack of a **nevirapine/fluconazole** interaction have not been conducted.[4]

1. Borin MT, Driver MR, Wajszczuk CP, Anderson RD. The effect of fluconazole (FLU) on the pharmacokinetics of atevirdine mesylate (ATV) in HIV+ patients. *Clin Pharmacol Ther* (1994) 55, 193.
2. Borin MT, Cox SR, Herman BD, Carel BJ, Anderson RD. Effect of fluconazole on the steady-state pharmacokinetics of delavirdine in human immunodeficiency virus-positive patients. *Antimicrob Agents Chemother* (1997) 41 1892–7.
3. Benedek IH, Fiske WD, White SJ, Kornhauser DM. Plasma levels of fluconazole (FL) are not altered by coadministration of DMP 266 in healthy volunteers. *Intersci Conf Antimicrob Agents Chemother* (1997) 37, 1.
4. Viramune (Nevirapine). Boehringer Ingelheim Limited. Summary of product characteristics, November 2001.
5. Viramune (Nevirapine). Boehringer Ingelheim. Full prescribing information, April 2001.

Non-nucleoside reverse transcriptase inhibitors + Food

Food has no clinically relevant effect on nevirapine or delavirdine, but it can double the bioavailability of atevirdine.

Clinical evidence, mechanism, importance and management

(a) Atevirdine

A study in 11 HIV+ patients found that a **high fat breakfast** doubled the AUC of a 600-mg dose of **atevirdine** and almost doubled the maximum serum levels when compared to the fasted state.[1] The clinical importance of this awaits assessment.

(b) Delavirdine

A randomised crossover study in 13 HIV+ patients on **delavirdine** 400 mg daily found that there were no changes in the steady-state serum levels of **delavirdine** whether taken with or without **food** for periods of 2 weeks.[2] This differed from a previous single dose study which had found a 26% fall with **food**.[3] There would appear to be no need to avoid taking **delavirdine** with **food**.

(c) Nevirapine

In a study in 24 healthy subjects it was found that **high fat breakfast** caused some moderate changes in the pharmacokinetics of 200 mg oral **nevirapine**, but the AUC was not affected and none of them was considered to be clinically relevant.[4] No special precautions would seem to be necessary.

1. Borin MT, Della-Coletta AA, Batts DH. Effects of food and antacid on bioavailability of atevirdine mesylate (ATV) in HIV+ patients. *Clin Pharmacol Ther* (1994) 55, 194.
2. Morse GD, Fischl MA, Cox SR, Thompson L, Della-Coletta AA, Freimuth WW. Effect of food on the steady-state pharmacokinetics of delavirdine (DLV) in HIV+ patients. *Intersci Conf Antimicrob Agents Chemother* (1995) 35, 210.
3. Cox SR, Della-Coletta AA, Turner SW, Freimuth WW. Single-dose pharmacokinetic (PK) studies with delavirdine (DLV) mesylate: dose proportionality and effects of food and antacid. *Intersci Conf Antimicrob Agents Chemother* (1994) 34, 82.
4. Lamson MJ, Cort S, Sabo JP, MacGregor TR, Keirns JJ, Effect of food or antacid on the bioavailability of nevirapine 200 mg in 24 healthy volunteers. *Pharm Res* (1995) 12 (9 Suppl), S-101.

Non-nucleoside reverse transcriptase inhibitors + Miscellaneous drugs

Delavirdine and clarithromycin do not appear to interact, but nevirapine may interact with the macrolide antibacterials. No interaction has been demonstrated with nevirapine and oral contraceptives, but alternative contraceptive methods have been advised. The CSM in the UK advise that St John's wort may decrease blood levels of the non-nucleoside reverse transcriptase inhibitors and so combined use should be avoided.[1]

Clinical evidence, mechanism, importance and management

A. Delavirdine

(a) Clarithromycin

No clinically significant changes in the pharmacokinetics of **delavirdine** were seen in 7 HIV+ patients given **delavirdine** 300 mg three times daily with **clarithromycin** 500 mg twice daily for 15 days, when compared with 4 other HIV+ patients taking only **delavirdine**. The combination was well tolerated and no serious events occurred.[2] No special precautions would appear to be needed.

(b) Glutamic acid

When **glutamic acid** 1360 mg three times daily was given with **delavirdine** 400 mg three times daily to 8 HIV+ subjects with gastric hypoacidity the AUC of **delavirdine** was increased by 50%. However, the clinical significance of this interaction is unknown.[3]

B. Nevirapine

(a) Macrolide antibacterials

Steady-state **nevirapine** levels are reported to have risen by 24% in 18 patients given **clarithromycin** (not specifically named),[4] due (it is believed) to the enzyme inhibitory effects of these drugs on cytochrome P450 isoenzyme CYP3A4, but these increases are almost certainly too small to be of clinical importance.

(b) Oral contraceptives

Administration of a single dose of an oral contraceptive containing **ethinylestradiol** 0.035 mg and **norethisterone** 1 mg with **nevirapine** 200 mg twice daily significantly decreased the AUCs of **17α-ethinylestradiol** and **norethisterone** by 29% and 18% respectively. The makers of **nevirapine** advise the use of alternative contraceptive measures (barrier methods) because of the risk that the **contraceptive steroid** levels, and consequently their effects might be reduced.[4,5] The dose of these hormones may need to be increased for indications such as endometriosis, if used with **nevirapine**.[4]

1. Committee on Safety of Medicines. Message from Professor A Breckenridge (Chairman of CSM) and Fact Sheet for Health Care Professionals, 29th February 2000.
2. Cox SR, Borin MT, Driver MR, Levy B, Freimuth WW. Effect of clarithromycin on the steady-state pharmacokinetics of delavirdine in HIV-1 patients. American Society for Microbiology, 2nd National Conference on Human Retroviruses, 1995. Abstract 487.
3. Morse GD, Adams JM, Shelton MJ, Hewitt RG, Cox SR, Chambers JH. Gastric acidification increases delavirdine mesylate (DLV) exposure in HIV+ subjects with gastric hypoacidity (GH). Clin Pharmacol Ther (1996) 59, 141.
4. Viramune (Nevirapine). Boehringer Ingelheim Limited. Summary of product characteristics, November 2001.
5. Viramune (Nevirapine). Boehringer Ingelheim Inc, Full Prescribing Information, April 2001.

Non-nucleoside reverse transcriptase inhibitors + Nucleoside reverse transcriptase inhibitors

Atevirdine and delavirdine absorption is reduced by didanosine. Doses should be given an hour apart. Delavirdine does not interact with zidovudine, and nevirapine does not interact significantly with didanosine, zalcitabine or zidovudine.

Clinical evidence, mechanism, importance and management

(a) Atevirdine

A single dose pharmacokinetic study in 12 HIV+ patients found that 200 mg **didanosine** (as two tablets) reduced the AUC of **atevirdine mesilate** 600 mg by about 45%, and lowered its maximum serum level fourfold. The pharmacokinetics of **didanosine** were not significantly altered.[1] It appears that the **didanosine** reduces the **atevirdine** absorption because the buffers in the **didanosine** formulation raise the pH and thereby reduce the **atevirdine** solubility. The authors suggest that dosages should be separated by at least one hour, until the results of steady-state pharmacokinetic studies are available.[1]

(b) Delavirdine

A study in 34 HIV+ patients stabilised on 200 mg **zidovudine** three times daily found that 400 to 1200 mg **delavirdine mesilate** daily for 9 days had no significant effect on the **zidovudine** pharmacokinetics.[2]

In a steady-state study, 9 HIV+ patients stabilised on 200 mg **didanosine** twice times daily were also given 400 mg **delavirdine mesilate** three times daily for 14 days. Simultaneous administration caused a 37% reduction in the maximum **delavirdine** serum levels, but when the drugs were given 1 h apart no significant effect occurred.[3] A single dose study in 12 HIV+ patients found similar results.[4] The authors of one report suggest that separating the doses by about one hour is preferable, but not essential.[3]

(c) Nevirapine

The pharmacokinetics of **didanosine/zidovudine** or **didanosine/zidovudine/nevirapine** were assessed in 175 HIV+ subjects. The bioavailability of **didanosine** was not affected, but the bioavailability of **zidovudine** was decreased by about one-third in the triple combination.[5] In a steady-state study in 24 HIV+ patients, 200 mg of **nevirapine** 12-hourly was added to regimens of **didanosine** or **didanosine/zidovudine** or **zidovudine/zalcitabine** for a 4-week period. No significant changes in the pharmacokinetics of **didanosine** or **zalcitabine** were seen. However, in the **didanosine/zidovudine** group the peak **zidovudine** plasma levels and AUC were reduced by 27% and 32% respectively. The **zidovudine** pharmacokinetics in the **zidovudine/zalcitabine** group were not affected.[6] The reasons for these changes are not clear, but the clinical consequences are thought to be small, and the safety data indicate that the concurrent use of these drugs is safe and well tolerated. The makers say that no dosage adjustments are needed if **didanosine**, **zalcitabine** or **zidovudine** is taken with **nevirapine**.[7]

1. Morse GD, Fischl MA, Shelton MJ, Borin MT, Driver MR, DeRemer M, Lee K, Wajszczuk CP. Didanosine reduces atevirdine absorption in subjects with human immunodeficiency virus infections. Antimicrob Agents Chemother (1996) 40, 767–71.
2. Morse GD, Cox SR, DeRemer MF, Batts DH, Freimuth WW. Zidovudine (ZDV) pharmacokinetics (PK) during an escalating multiple-dose study of delavirdine (DLV) mesylate. Intersci Conf Antimicrob Agents Chemother (1994) 34, 132.
3. Cox SR, Cohn SE, Greisberger C, Reichman RC, Della-Coletta AA, Freimuth WW, Morse GD. Evaluation of the steady state (SS) pharmacokinetic interaction between didanosine (ddI) and delavirdine mesylate (DLV) in HIV+ patients. Intersci Conf Antimicrob Agents Chemother (1995) 35, 210.
4. Morse GD, Fischl MA, Shelton MJ, Cox SR, Driver M, DeRemer M, Freimuth WW. Single-dose pharmacokinetics of delavirdine mesylate and didanosine in patients with human immunodeficiency virus infection. Antimicrob Agents Chemother (1997) 41, 169–74.
5. Zhou XJ, Sheiner LB, D'Aquila RT, Hughes MD, Hirsch MS, Fischl MA, Johnson VA, Myers M, Sommadossi JP and the NIAID ACTG241 Investigators. Population pharmacokinetics of nevirapine, zidovudine and didanosine after combination therapy in HIV-infected individuals. Clin Pharmacol Ther (1998) 63,182.
6. MacGregor TR, Lamson MJ, Cort S, Pav JW, Saag MS, Elvin AT, Sommadossi J-P, Myers M, Keirns JJ. Steady state pharmacokinetics of nevirapine, didanosine, zalcitabine and zidovudine combination therapy in HIV-1 positive patients. Pharm Res (1995) 12 (9 Suppl), S-101.
7. Viramune (Nevirapine), Boehringer Ingelheim Limited. Summary of product characteristics, November 2001.

Non-nucleoside reverse transcriptase inhibitors + Protease inhibitors

In general the non-nucleoside reverse transcriptase inhibitors decrease the levels of protease inhibitors, however delavirdine appears to have the opposite effect. Ritonavir has been used to elevate levels of other protease inhibitors. Dosage adjustments are most commonly needed with indinavir.

Clinical evidence, mechanism, importance and management

(a) Delavirdine

A combination of **amprenavir** plus **delavirdine** plus 2 NRTIs was given to 6 HIV+ children. This resulted in a threefold increase in the **amprenavir** maximum serum levels, as compared with monotherapy. No increase in short-term toxicity was noted.[1]

Nelfinavir 750 mg three times daily was given to 12 healthy subjects for 14 days, with **delavirdine** 400 mg three times daily added from days 8 to 14. Another group of 12 subjects was given the same drugs in the reverse order. The AUC of **nelfinavir** was approximately doubled, whereas the AUC of **delavirdine** fell by 42% during concurrent use. In total, 4 subjects had to stop both drugs before completing the study because of neutropenia, which resolved over several days.[2]

A study in healthy subjects given **delavirdine** 400 mg three times daily with either **ritonavir** 300 mg twice daily or **saquinavir** 600 mg three times daily found that the steady-state levels of **delavirdine** were either unchanged or slightly increased, by about 20%. The **ritonavir** and **saquinavir** steady state levels were altered, but this was not thought to be significant.[3] When **delavirdine** 400 or 600 mg twice daily was given with a single 400 or 800-mg dose of **indinavir** the steady state levels of **delavirdine** were either unchanged or slightly increased, by about 20%. However, the AUC of **indinavir** 800 mg given alone, was very similar to the AUC of **indinavir** 400 mg given with **delavirdine**. The authors of the report therefore suggest that no dosage adjustments are needed with **ritonavir** or **saquinavir** but they suggest that the dosage of the **indinavir** may be reduced to 400 or 600 mg three times daily.[3] This suggestion is supported by other studies with **ritonavir/delavirdine**,[4] and **indinavir/delavirdine**.[5]

(b) Efavirenz

Amprenavir 1200 mg twice daily was given in combination with **efavirenz** 600 mg daily to 7 HIV+ patients. After 7 days, 3 of 6 patients showed markedly decreased **amprenavir** levels. By 14 days, 6 of the 7 patients had **amprenavir** levels that were about one-fifth or less of those expected. In 4 patients, ritonavir 100 mg twice daily was added and the **amprenavir** dose reduced to 900 mg twice daily. This resulted in a 15 to 90-fold increase in **amprenavir** levels.[6] The addition of **efavirenz** to **amprenavir** (plus 2 NRTIs) in 2 children resulted in undetectable **amprenavir** levels. These 2 children plus two others on the same drugs had **ritonavir** 8 mg/kg twice daily added to their treatment, which resulted in therapeutic **amprenavir** levels. No short-term toxicity was noted with the combination.[1] Other studies have suggested that if **amprenavir** is to be used with **efavirenz**, the dose of **amprenavir** should be increased to 1200 mg three times daily to ensure the minimum serum levels remain high enough to ensure sufficient antiretroviral activity.[7]

A study in patients given 750 mg **nelfinavir** 8-hourly with 600 mg **efavirenz** daily for a week found that the pharmacokinetics of **efavirenz** were not affected but the AUC of the **nelfinavir** was increased by about 20%.[8] This change is unlikely to be clinically significant and dosage alterations should not be needed when both drugs are used together.

(c) Nevirapine

A study in 19 HIV+ subjects given **indinavir** 800 mg 8-hourly with **nevirapine** (200 mg daily for 14 days then 200 mg twice daily thereafter) found that the **indinavir** AUC was decreased by 27.7% while the minimum serum level was decreased by about 50%. The authors concluded that no change to the **indinavir** dosage would be required, unless other parameters (e.g. the viral load) suggested it was necessary.[9] However, another study using comparing stavudine/**indinavir**/lamivudine with stavudine/**indinavir**/nevirapine suggested that the **indinavir** dose may need to be increased from 800 mg to 1000 mg three times daily in the presence of **nevirapine**.[10]

A study of 3 patients taking 750 mg **nelfinavir** 8-hourly showed an average decrease in AUC of 46% after additionally taking **nevirapine** (dose not stated).[11]

Studies in HIV+ patients given nevirapine and **ritonavir**[12] or nevirapine and **nelfinavir**[13] found no significant changes in the serum levels of either drug.

Nevirapine 200 mg twice daily reduced the maximum serum levels and the AUC of **saquinavir** 600 mg three times daily by almost 30% in 21 HIV+ patients given the combination for 7 days.[14] The importance of this is uncertain but the makers of nevirapine point out that this may possibly be significant because the serum levels of **saquinavir** achieved with hard gelatin capsules is already marginal.[12]

For all of these three protease inhibitors, the makers say that combination with **nevirapine** appears not to affect their overall safety.[12] The reductions in the serum levels of **indinavir** and **saquinavir** are small and probably of minimal clinical importance, but this needs confirmation.

(d) Talviraline

The clearance of **indinavir** 800 mg 8-hourly was increased nearly threefold when **talviraline** 500 mg 8-hourly was given concurrently. The authors suggest that the dose of **indinavir** may need adjustment if the drugs are to be used together.[15]

1. Wintergerst U, Engelhorn C, Kurowski M, Hoffmann F, Notheis G, Belohradsky BH. Pharmacokinetic interaction of amprenavir in combination with efavirenz or delavirdine in HIV-infected children. *AIDS* (2000) 14, 1866–8.
2. Cox SR, Schneck DW, Herman BD, Carel BJ, Gullotti BR, Kerr BM, Freimuth WW. Delavirdine (DLV) and nelfinavir (NFV): A pharmacokinetic (PK) drug-drug interaction study in healthy adult volunteers. 5th Conference on Retroviruses and Opportunistic Infections, Chicago, 1998. Abstract 345.
3. Cox SR, Ferry JJ, Batts DH, Carlson GF, Schneck DW, Herman BD, Della-Coletta AA, Chambers JH, Carel BJ, Stewart F, Buss N, Brown A. Delavirdine (D) and marketed protease inhibitors (PIs) pharmacokinetic (PK) interaction studies in healthy volunteers. 4th Conference on Retroviruses and Opportunistic Infections, Washington, 1997. Abstract 372.
4. Shelton MJ, Hewitt RG, Adams JM, Baldwin J, Della-Coletta A, Cox S, Batts DH, Morse GD. Delavirdine (DLV) mesylate pharmacokinetics (PK) during combination therapy with ritonavir. *Intersci Conf Antimicrob Agents Chemother* (1997) 37, 13.
5. Ferry JJ, Herman BD, Carel BJ, Carlson GF, Batts DH. Pharmacokinetic drug-drug interaction study of delavirdine and indinavir in healthy volunteers. *J Acquir Immune Defic Syndr Hum Retrovirol* (1998) 18, 252–9.
6. Duval X, Le Moing V, Longuet P, Leport C, Vildé J-L, Lamotte C, Peytavin G, Farinotti R. Efavirenz-induced decrease in plasma amprenavir levels in human immunodeficiency virus-infected patients and correction by ritonavir. *Antimicrob Agents Chemother* (2000) 44, 2593.
7. Falloon J, Piscitelli S, Vogel S, Sadler B, Mitsuya H, Kavlick MF, Yoshimura K, Rogers M, LaFon S, Manion DJ, Lane HC, Masur H. Combination therapy with amprenavir, abacavir, and efavirenz in human immunodeficiency virus (HIV)-infected patients failing a protease-inhibitor regimen: pharmacokinetic drug interactions and antiviral activity. *Clin Infect Dis* (2000) 30, 313–18.
8. Fiske WD, Benedek LH, White SJ, Pepperess KA, Joseph JL, Kornhauser DM. Pharmacokinetic interaction between efavirenz (EFV) and nelfinavir mesylate (NFV) in healthy volunteers. 5th Conference on Retroviruses and Opportunistic Infections, Chicago, 1998. Abstract 349.
9. Murphy RL, Sommadossi J-P, Lamson M, Hall DB, Myers M, Dusek A. Antiviral effect and pharmacokinetic interaction between nevirapine and indinavir in persons infected with human immunodeficiency virus type 1. *J Infect Dis* (1999) 179, 1116–23.
10. Launay O, Peytavin G, Flandre P, Gerard L, Levy C, Joly V, Aboulker JP, Yeni P. Pharmacokinetic (PK) interaction between nevirapine (NVP) and indinavir (IDV) in ANRS 081 trial. *Intersci Conf Antimicrob Agents Chemother* (2000) 40, 331.
11. Morry C, Barry MG, Mulcahy FM, Ryan M, Back DJ. The pharmacokinetics of nelfinavir alone and in combination with nevirapine. 5th Conference on Retroviruses and Opportunistic Infections, Chicago, 1998. Abstract 351.
12. Viramune (Nevirapine), Boehringer Ingelheim Limited. Summary of product characteristics, November 2001.
13. Skowron G, Leoung G, Dusek A, Anderson R, Grosso R, Lamson M, Beebe S. Stavudine (d4T), nelfinavir (NFV) and nevirapine (NVP): Preliminary safety, activity and pharmacokinetic (PK) interactions. 5th Conference on Retroviruses and Opportunistic Infections, Chicago, 1998. Abstract 350.
14. Sahai J, Cameron W, Salgo M, Stewart F, Myers M, Lamson M, Gagnier P. Drug interaction study between saquinavir (SQV) and nevirapine (NVP). 4th Conference on Retroviruses and Opportunistic Infections, Washington, 1997. Abstract 613.
15. Hayashi S, Jayesekara D, Shah A, Jayewardene A, Thevanayagam L, Aweeka F. Multiple dose pharmacokinetic (PK) study to determine the effect of HBY-097 (HBY) on the plasma concentrations of indinavir (IND) and zidovudine (ZDV). *Clin Pharmacol Ther* (1998) 63, 181.

Non-nucleoside reverse transcriptase inhibitors + Rifamycins

Rifabutin and rifampicin cause a very marked fall in delavirdine serum levels, but only a moderate fall occurs with nevirapine.

Clinical evidence, mechanism, importance and management

(a) Delavirdine

A controlled study in 7 HIV+ patients on 400 mg **delavirdine mesilate** three times daily for 30 days found that the addition of 300 mg **rifabutin** daily from days 16 to 30 caused a fivefold increase in the **delavirdine** clearance, and an 84% fall in the steady-state plasma levels.[1] This was presumably due to the enzyme inducing effects of the **rifabutin**.

A similar study using **rifampicin** in place of rifabutin found that **rifampicin** caused a 27-fold increase in clearance of **delavirdine**, and the steady-state plasma levels became almost undetectable. It has been recommended that the **delavirdine/rifampicin** combination should be considered as contraindicated because the effects of the interaction are so large.[2] The CDC recommends that neither **rifabutin** nor **rifampicin** be used with **delavirdine**.[3]

(b) Nevirapine

A clinical studies in 14 subjects showed that the serum levels of **nevirapine** were reduced by 37% in 3 patients given **rifampicin** and by 16% in 19 patients given **rifabutin**.[4] Other information suggests that the AUC of **nevirapine** is reduced by 58% by **rifampicin**.[5] These changes are likely to be due to the enzyme inducing effects of these two rifamycins on the cytochrome P450 isoenzyme CYP3A4, which is concerned with the metabolism of **nevirapine**.[5] The US makers of **nevirapine** advise good monitoring if either **rifamycin** is used concurrently with **nevirapine**.[4] The UK makers also advise monitoring with **rifabutin** and **nevirapine**, but contraindicate the use of **rifampicin** with **nevirapine**.[5] The CDC state that the **nevirapine/rifabutin** can be used, whilst the **nevirapine/rifampicin** combination may possibly be used.[3]

1. Borin MT, Chambers JH, Carel BJ, Freimuth WW, Aksentijevich S, Piergies AA. Pharmacokinetic study of the interaction between rifabutin and delavirdine mesylate in HIV-1 infected patients. *Antiviral Res* (1997) 35, 53–63.
2. Borin MT, Chambers JH, Carel BJ, Gagnon S, Freimuth WW. Pharmacokinetic study of the interaction between rifampin and delavirdine mesylate. *Clin Pharmacol Ther* (1997) 61, 544–53.
3. Anon. CDC alters recommendations on rifamycin-antiretroviral drug use. *Am J Health-Syst Pharm* (2000) 57, 735.
4. Viramune (Nevirapine). Boehringer Ingelheim. Full prescribing information, April 2001.
5. Viramune (Nevirapine). Boehringer Ingelheim Limited. Summary of product characteristics, November 2001.

Novobiocin + Rifampicin (Rifampin)

Rifampicin reduces the half-life of novobiocin but this is unlikely to be of clinical significance.

Clinical evidence, mechanism, importance and management

When 10 healthy subjects were given 1 g novobiocin daily for 13 days with 600 mg **rifampicin** daily, the novobiocin half-life was reduced from 5.85 to 2.66 h and the AUC was reduced by almost 50%. However the plasma novobiocin levels were not significantly altered and the trough serum levels remained in excess of the MIC for 90% of the strains of MRSA tested. No significant changes in the **rifampicin** pharmacokinetics were seen.[1] No special precautions would therefore seem to be necessary during concurrent use.

1. Drusano GL, Townsend RJ, Walsh TJ, Forrest A, Antal EJ, Standiford HC. Steady-state serum pharmacokinetics of novobiocin and rifampin alone and in combination. *Antimicrob Agents Chemother* (1986) 30, 42–5.

Nucleoside reverse transcriptase inhibitors + Anticonvulsants

Sodium valproate increases the bioavailability of zidovudine. Other NRTIs have not been shown to interact.

Clinical evidence

(a) No significant changes

The makers of the nucleoside reverse transcriptase inhibitors **lamivudine**, **stavudine** and **zalcitabine** do not anticipate interactions with **anticonvulsants**. These three drugs are excreted largely unchanged in the urine. The exact metabolic pathway of **didanosine** is not known, but it also is not expected to interact. The makers of **abacavir** say that **phenobarbital** and **phenytoin** may slightly decrease **abacavir** concentrations by their action on UDP-glucuronyltransferase (see Mechanism below). **Abacavir** is metabolised by the liver but does not affect the cytochrome P450 isoenzymes CYP3A4, CYP2C9 or CYP2D6.

(b) Increased blood and CSF levels

Currently the only reports of an interaction are with **zidovudine**. **Zidovudine** 100 mg 8-hourly was given to 6 HIV+ subjects. They showed an 80% increase in the **zidovudine** plasma AUC while additionally taking 250 or 500 mg **sodium valproate** 8-hourly for 4 days. The mean plasma levels were raised by 80%. No adverse reactions, changes in hepatic or renal function, or alterations in the blood picture were reported.[1] A case report describes an AIDS patient on 100 mg **zidovudine** five times daily who showed a two- to three-fold increase in trough and peak serum **zidovudine** levels, and a 74% increase in the CSF **zidovudine** levels while taking 500 mg **sodium valproate** three times daily.[2]

Mechanism

The evidence indicates that the metabolism (glucuronidation) of the zidovudine is inhibited by the sodium valproate so that its bioavailability is increased.[1,2]

Importance and management

Information seems to be limited to the papers cited. Most of the nucleoside reverse transcriptase inhibitors appear not to interact with anticonvulsants but an interaction between zidovudine and sodium valproate would appear to be established. It would therefore seem prudent to monitor for any evidence of increased zidovudine effects and possible toxicity if sodium valproate is added.

1. Lertora JJL, Rege AB, Greenspan DL, Akula S, George WJ, Hyslop NE, Agrawal KC. Pharmacokinetic interaction between zidovudine and valproic acid in patients infected with human immunodeficiency virus. *Clin Pharmacol Ther* (1994) 56, 272–8.
2. Akula SK, Rege AB, Dreisbach AW, Dejace PMJT, Lertora JJL. Valproic acid increases cerebrospinal fluid zidovudine levels in a patient with AIDS. *Am J Med Sci* (1997) 313, 244–6.

Nucleoside reverse transcriptase inhibitors + Antitubercular drugs

Didanosine, stavudine and zalcitabine are not expected to interact with rifabutin, but the picture is less clear with zidovudine. Rifampicin appears to increase the clearance of zidovudine. Pyrazinamide and ethambutol appear not to interact with zidovudine, and neither does isoniazid with either zidovudine or zalcitabine.

Clinical evidence, mechanism, importance and management

(a) Didanosine

Rifabutin 300 to 600 mg daily for 12 days did not significantly affect the pharmacokinetics of **didanosine** 167 to 375 mg twice daily in 12 patients with AIDS.[1] No special precautions would seem necessary if both drugs are given.

(b) Stavudine

A study in 10 HIV+ subjects found that the addition of **rifabutin** 300 mg daily to **stavudine** 30 or 40 mg twice daily caused no significant effects on the pharmacokinetics of the **stavudine** and the incidence of side effects did not increase.[2] No special precautions would seem necessary if both drugs are given.

(c) Zalcitabine

A study in 12 HIV+ patients found that when given 1.5 mg **zalcitabine** three times daily and 300 mg **isoniazid** daily the pharmacokinetics of the **zalcitabine** remained unchanged but the clearance of the **isoniazid** was approximately doubled.[3] You should monitor concurrent use well.

The makers say that no significant interactions may be expected between **rifabutin** and **zalcitabine**.[4]

(d) Zidovudine

The pharmacokinetics of **rifabutin** are not affected by the concurrent use of **zidovudine** in AIDS patients.[5,6] **Rifabutin** does not affect the pharmacokinetics of **zidovudine** in HIV+ patients,[7] although in one review of concurrent treatment there was a trend towards increased clearance of **zidovudine** by **rifabutin**.[8] No increase in adverse effects appears to occur with the combination of **rifabutin** and zidovudine.[6,8] In a retrospective study of healthy subjects and HIV+ individuals the clearance of **zidovudine** was increased 132% by **rifampicin** and 50% by **rifabutin** suggesting that the enzyme inducing effects of **rifabutin** are very much less than **rifampicin**, so less significant interactions would be expected.[9]

A comparative study in HIV infected patients given **zidovudine** and antitubercular treatment (**isoniazid**, **rifampicin**, **pyrazinamide**, **ethambutol** initially, then **isoniazid** and **rifampicin**) for 8 months found no evidence of an adverse interaction. However, marked anaemia occurred in those subjects given both groups of drugs, but it was not necessary to permanently stop **zidovudine** in any patient. The authors advise careful monitoring for haematological toxicity.[10] Another study in 4 HIV+ patients found that **rifampicin** lowered the AUC and increased the clearance of **zidovudine** in all patients, probably due to the enzyme inducing activity of the **rifampicin**, which increases the glucuronidation of zidovudine. When the **rifampicin** was stopped in one patient, his **zidovudine** AUC doubled.[11] A later study of the same interaction in 8 HIV+ men found that **rifampicin** significantly induced the glucuronidation of **zidovudine** and suggested that the effect wore off 14 days after stopping the **rifampicin**. The authors of this study suggest that dosage alterations may not be necessary with concurrent use,[12] but be e alert for any evidence of a reduced response to **zidovudine** if **rifampicin** is given.

1. Li RC, Narang PK, Sahai J, Cameron W, Bianchine JR. Rifabutin absorption in the gut unaltered by concomitant administration of didanosine in AIDS patients. *Antimicrob Agents Chemother* (1997) 41, 1566–70.
2. Piscitelli SC, Kelly G, Walker RE, Kovacs J, Falloon J, Davey RT, Raje S, Masur H, Polis MA. A multiple drug interaction study of stavudine with agents for opportunistic infections in human immunodeficiency virus-infected patients. *Antimicrob Agents Chemother* (1999) 43, 647–50.
3. Lee BL, Täuber MG, Chambers HF, Gambertoglio J, Delahunty T. The effect of zalcitabine on the pharmacokinetics of isoniazid in HIV-infected patients. *Intersci Conf Antimicrob Agents Chemother* (1994) 34, 3.
4. Mycobutin (Rifabutin). Pharmacia. Summary of product characteristics, July 1997.
5. Narang PK, Nightingale S, Lewis RC, Colborn D, Wynne B, Li R. Concomitant zidovudine (ZDV) dosing does not affect rifabutin (RIF) disposition in AIDS patients. 9th International Conference AIDS & 4th STD World Congress, Berlin, June 6-11, 1993. Abstract PO-B31-2216.
6. Li RC, Nightingale S, Lewis RC, Colburn DC, Narang PK. Lack of effect of concomitant zidovudine on rifabutin kinetics in patients with AIDS-related complex. *Antimicrob Agents Chemother* (1996) 40, 1397–1402.
7. Gallicano K, Sahai J, Swick L, Seguin I, Pakuts A, Cameron DW. Effect of rifabutin on the pharmacokinetics of zidovudine in patients infected with human immunodeficiency virus. *Clin Infect Dis* (1995) 21, 1008–11.
8. Narang PK, Sale M. Population based assessment of rifabutin (R) effect on zidovudine (ZDV) disposition in AIDS patients. *Clin Pharmacol Ther* (1993) 53, 219.
9. Narang PK, Gupta S, Li RC, Strolin-Benedetti M, Della Bruna C, Bianchine JR. Assessing dosing implications of enzyme inducing potential: rifabutin (RIF) vs. rifampicin (RFM). *Intersci Conf Antimicrob Agents Chemother* (1993) 33, 228.
10. Antoniskis D, Easley AC, Espina BM, Davidson PT, Barnes PF. Combined toxicity of zidovudine and antituberculosis chemotherapy. *Am Rev Respir Dis* (1992) 145, 430–4.
11. Burger DM, Meenhorst PL, Koks CHW. Beijnen JH. Pharmacokinetic interaction between rifampin and zidovudine. *Antimicrob Agents Chemother* (1993) 37, 1426–31.
12. Gallicano KD, Sahai J, Shukla VK, Seguin I, Pakuts A, Kwok D, Foster BC, Cameron DW. Induction of zidovudine glucuronidation and animation pathways by rifampicin in HIV-infected patients. *Br J Clin Pharmacol* (1999) 48, 168–79.

Nucleoside reverse transcriptase inhibitors + Azole antifungals

Fluconazole has no significant effects on the pharmacokinetics of didanosine or stavudine but it causes an increase in serum zidovudine although the clinical importance of this is uncertain. Fluconazole serum levels remain unchanged. Itraconazole appears not to affect the pharmacokinetics of zidovudine. Serum levels of itraconazole are markedly reduced by concurrent didanosine, but the interaction can be avoided if itraconazole if taken at least 2 h before didanosine. Didanosine does not interact with ketoconazole administered at least 2 h earlier. The frequency of haematologic toxicity with zidovudine was not increased by concurrent ketoconazole.

Clinical evidence

(a) Fluconazole

A group of 12 HIV+ subjects taking **didanosine** 100 to 250 mg twice daily were additionally given **fluconazole** for 7 days (two 200-mg doses on the first day, followed by 200 mg daily). The pharmacokinetics of the **didanosine** remained unchanged in the presence of the **fluconazole**, and concurrent use was well tolerated.[1]

A study in 10 HIV+ subjects on **stavudine** 40 mg twice daily, found that the addition of **fluconazole** 200 mg daily for one week had no significant effect on the pharmacokinetics of the **stavudine**.[2]

On two occasions, 12 HIV+ men were given 200 mg **zidovudine** 8-hourly with and without 400 mg **fluconazole** daily for 7 days. While taking the **fluconazole** the AUC of the **zidovudine** increased by 74%, the maximum serum levels increased by 84%, the terminal half-life was increased 128% and the clearance was reduced 43%.[3] **Zidovudine** 500 mg daily from day 1 to 44 with 200 mg **fluconazole** daily from days 3 to 30 and 300 mg rifabutin daily from days 17 to 44 were given to 12 HIV+ subjects. No significant changes in the pharmacokinetics of **fluconazole** occurred between days 16 and 30.[4] Another study in HIV+ patients found only a very small change in the pharmacokinetics of **zidovudine** due to **fluconazole**.[5]

(b) Itraconazole

A patient of 35, with AIDS was given **itraconazole** 200 mg daily, following an episode of cryptococcal meningitis. When he relapsed it was noted that he had been taking the **itraconazole** at the same time as his **didanosine** therapy. Plasma levels indicated a delay in the peak **itraconazole** plasma concentration from 2 h post-dose to 8 h post-dose.[6] A mean peak serum **itraconazole** level of 0.9 micrograms/ml was seen in 6 healthy subjects 3 h after a single 200 mg oral dose of **itraconazole**, but the levels were undetectable when 300 mg **didanosine** was given with the **itraconazole**.[7] A later study in 12 HIV+ patients found that the AUC of **itraconazole** after a single 200-mg dose was not significantly different when taken alone or with 200 mg **didanosine** 2 or 4 h later.[8]

Itraconazole 200 mg daily for 2 weeks was reported to have no effect on the pharmacokinetics of **zidovudine** in 7 patients, but the serum levels in 2 patients were reported as being higher.[9]

(c) Ketoconazole

Twelve HIV+ patients were given 375 mg **didanosine** twice daily either alone or 2 h after 200 mg **ketoconazole** daily, for 4 days. **Didanosine** levels were slightly reduced (−12%) and no significant changes in the pharmacokinetics of the **ketoconazole** were seen.[10]

A study of **zidovudine** use in 282 AIDS patients found that haematological abnormalities (anaemia, leucopenia, neutropenia) were very common, but the concurrent use of **ketoconazole** in some of these patients did not increase the haematological toxicity.[11]

Mechanism, importance and management

There is evidence of a minor interaction between zidovudine/fluconazole, but this is unlikely to be clinically significant. A study in human liver microsomes suggests that these changes are, in part, due to fluconazole inhibiting zidovudine glucuronidation.[12] The most significant interaction occurs between didanosine and itraconazole. Itraconazole depends on stomach acidity for absorption. A raised gastric pH due to the buffers in the didanosine formulation appears to reduce the itraconazole absorption. The didanosine itself appears to have no part to play in this interaction. Patients should avoid taking both drugs at the same time, but giving the itraconazole at least 2 h before the didanosine appears to solve any problem. Ketoconazole may interact similarly so until more information is available it would seem wise to follow the same precautions as with itraconazole. The outcome of concurrent use should be well monitored. More study is needed.

1. Bruzzese VL, Gillum JG, Israel DS, Johnson GL, Kaplowitz LG, Polk RE. Effect of fluconazole on pharmacokinetics of 2′,3′-dideoxyinosine in persons seropositive for human immunodeficiency virus. *Antimicrob Agents Chemother* (1995) 39, 1050–53.
2. Piscitelli SC, Kelly G, Walker RE, Kovacs J, Falloon J, Davey RT, Raje S, Masur H, Polis MA. A multiple drug interaction study of stavudine with agents for opportunistic infections in human immunodeficiency virus-infected patients. *Antimicrob Agents Chemother* (1999) 43, 647–50.
3. Sahai J, Gallicano K, Pakuts A, Cameron DW. Effect of fluconazole on zidovudine pharmacokinetics in patients infected with human deficiency virus. *J Infect Dis* (1994) 169, 1103–7.
4. Trapnell CB, Lavelle JP, O'Leary CR, James DS, Li R, Colburn D, Woosley RL, Narang PK. Rifabutin does not alter fluconazole pharmacokinetics. *Clin Pharmacol Ther* (1993) 53, 194.
5. Brockmeyer NH, Tillmann I, Mertins L, Barthel B, Goos M. Pharmacokinetic interaction of fluconazole and zidovudine in HIV-positive patients. *Eur J Med Res* (1997) 2, 377–83.
6. Moreno F, Hardin TC, Rinaldi MG, Graybill JR. Itraconazole-didanosine excipient interaction. *JAMA* (1993) 269, 1508.
7. May DB, Drew RH, Yedinak KC, Bartlett JA. Effect of simultaneous didanosine administration on itraconazole absorption in healthy volunteers. *Pharmacotherapy* (1994) 14, 509–13.
8. Hardin TC, Sharkey-Mathis PK, Rinaldi MG, Graybill JR. Evaluation of the pharmacokinetic interaction between itraconazole and didanosine in HIV-infected subjects. *Intersci Conf Antimicrob Agents Chemother* (1995) 35, 6.
9. Henrivaux P, Fairon Y, Fillet G. Pharmacokinetics of AZT among HIV infected patients treated by itraconazole. 5th Int Conf AIDS, Montreal. 1989, Abstract M.B.P.340.
10. Knupp CA, Brater DC, Relue J, Barbhaiya RH. Pharmacokinetics of didanosine and ketoconazole after coadministration to patients seropositive for the human immunodeficiency virus. *J Clin Pharmacol* (1993) 33, 912–17.
11. Richman DD, Fischl MA, Grieco MH, Gottlieb MS, Volberding PA, Laskin OL, Leedom JM, Groopman JE, Mildvan D, Hirsch MS, Jackson GG, Durack DT, Nusinoff-Lehrman S and the AZT Collaborative Working Group. The toxicity of azidothymidine (AZT) in the treatment of patients with AIDS and AIDS-related complex. A double-blind, placebo-controlled trial. *N Engl J Med* (1987) 317, 192–7.
12. Asgari M, Back DJ. Effect of azoles on the glucuronidation of zidovudine by human liver UDP-glucuronyltransferase. *J Infect Dis* (1995) 172, 1634–5.

Nucleoside reverse transcriptase inhibitors + Cytokines

Interferon alfa does not alter the pharmacokinetics of didanosine. No special precautions would seem necessary if used concurrently. Interferon alfa and beta can cause an increase in the serum levels of zidovudine. Interleukin-2 appears not to interact significantly with zidovudine.

Clinical evidence

(a) Interferon

AIDS patients who had been taking 200 mg **zidovudine** 4-hourly for 8 weeks were additionally given 45 million units daily of **recombinant beta interferon** subcutaneously. After 3 and 15 days the **zidovudine** metabolism was reduced by 75% and 97% respectively. By day 15 the **zidovudine** half-life was increased about twofold.[1] Another study in 6 children aged 3 months to 17 years found that after 5 weeks concurrent treatment the AUC of **zidovudine** was increased by 36% by **interferon alfa**, the maximum serum levels were raised by 69% and the clearance was reduced 20%.[2]

Interferon alfa 1 to 15 million units daily was given to 26 HIV+ patients concurrently taking **didanosine** (sachet formulation) 100 to 375 mg twice daily. The interferon appeared to have no clinically significant effects on the pharmacokinetics of the **didanosine**.[3]

(b) Interleukin-2

A study found that a 4 week course of **interleukin-2** (0.25 million units/m^2 daily) by continuous infusion had no clinically significant effect on the pharmacokinetics of a 100 mg intravenous

dose of **zidovudine**.[4] Another study in 8 HIV+ males given **zidovudine** orally (200 mg 4-hourly) showed similar results.[3] No special precautions would seem necessary.

Mechanism

Beta interferon appears to inhibit the metabolism (glucuronidation) of the zidovudine by the liver.

Importance and management

Information seems to be limited to these reports. The results of the first report suggest that the zidovudine dosage may need to be reduced if beta interferon is added in order to avoid increased zidovudine toxicity. A dosage reduction of two-thirds, or even more, would seem to be needed. More study is needed to confirm these observations. Interferon alfa appears to interact to a much lesser extent.

1. Nokta M, Loh JP, Douidar SM, Ahmed AE, Pollard RB. Metabolic interaction of recombinant interferon-β and zidovudine in AIDS patients. *J Interferon Res* (1991) 11, 159–64.
2. Diaz C, Yogev R, Rodriguez J, Rege A, George W, Lertora J. ACTG-153: Zidovudine pharmacokinetics when used in combination with interferon alpha. *Intersci Conf Antimicrob Agents Chemother* (1994) 34, 79.
3. Piscitelli SC, Amantea MA, Vogel S, Bechtel C, Metcalf JA, Kovacs JA. Effects of cytokines on antiviral pharmacokinetics: an alternative approach to assessment of drug interactions using bioequivalence guidelines. *Antimicrob Agents Chemother* (1996) 40, 161–5.
4. Skinner MH, Pauloin D, Schwartz D, Merigan TC, Blaschke TF. IL-2 does not alter zidovudine kinetics. *Clin Pharmacol Ther* (1989) 45, 128.

Nucleoside reverse transcriptase inhibitors + Dapsone

The prophylactic effects of dapsone in preventing *Pneumocystis carinii* pneumonia (PCP) may be reduced or abolished in the presence of oral didanosine because of an interaction due to an ingredient of the didanosine formulation. Separating their administration may possibly be effective. Dapsone has no effect on the pharmacokinetics of zalcitabine, whereas zalcitabine causes a small rise in the serum levels of dapsone, reduces its clearance and increases its half-life. Dapsone appears not to affect the pharmacokinetics of zidovudine although concurrent use may be associated with increased blood dyscrasias.

Clinical evidence

(a) Didanosine

A report describes the development of PCP in 11 out of 28 HIV+ patients taking **dapsone** prophylaxis as well as **didanosine**. Of the 11 patients where prophylaxis failed, 4 died from respiratory failure.[1] A later report describes a similar failure of prophylaxis in 6 patients and apparent success in 19 patients given the combination. The authors say that the size of their study makes meaningful comparison difficult, but that it does not seem to support the idea that a rise in gastric pH makes **dapsone** prophylaxis ineffective.[2]

(b) Zalcitabine

A pharmacokinetic study in 12 HIV+ patients who were given 1.5 mg **zalcitabine** three times daily and 100 mg **dapsone** daily, alone or together, found that **dapsone** did not significantly affect the kinetics of the **zalcitabine**. However, **zalcitabine** decreased the clearance of **dapsone** by 21%, increased its maximum serum levels by 19% and increased its half-life by 34%.[3] These changes are relatively small and seem unlikely to have much clinical relevance, but until this is confirmed it would seem prudent to monitor the concurrent use of these two drugs.

(c) Zidovudine

A 63% decrease in the clearance of **zidovudine** was seen in 5 HIV+ patients when they were additionally given **trimethoprim** (no dosage stated) and a 71% decrease when **dapsone** (no dosage stated) was added to the combination. **Dapsone** alone had no effect.[4] These findings were confirmed in a later study by the same authors.[5] In neither case was the AUC of **zidovudine** significantly affected by **dapsone**. In a further study which considered the safety of **dapsone** in combination with **zidovudine**, **dapsone** was shown to increase the risk of blood dyscrasias that occur with **zidovudine** treatment.[6] Therefore it would seem that **dapsone** and **zidovudine** can be given concurrently, but monitoring for an increase in adverse events would seem advisable.

Mechanism

Didanosine is formulated with a citrate-phosphate buffer intended to facilitate its absorption at pH 7 to 8 by minimizing acid-induced hydrolysis in the stomach. At these high pH values the dapsone becomes very insoluble and therefore fails to be absorbed sufficiently to be effective. However a later study failed to confirm that a marked rise in gastric pH affects the absorption of dapsone (see 'Dapsone + Antacids', p.151),[7] and another study similarly failed to find that the magnesium-aluminium antacids in the didanosine formulation affected dapsone bioavailability.[8]

Importance and management

The authors of the report on didanosine suggest that the administration of the two drugs should be separated by at least two hours.[1] This is effective with didanosine and ketoconazole (also dependent on a low pH for its absorption) but confirmatory study is needed. A possible alternative would be to use co-trimoxazole instead of the didanosine which in this same study[1] was 100% effective in 17 patients. However, also see 'Dapsone + Trimethoprim', p.152. On the other hand, other NRTIs do not seem to interact, and so may be a possible alternative.

1. Metroka CE, McMechan MF, Andrada R, Laubenstein LJ, Jacobus DP. Failure of prophylaxis with dapsone in patients taking dideoxyinosine. *N Engl J Med* (1992) 325, 737.
2. Huengsberg M, Castelino S, Sherrard J, O'Farrell N, Bingham J. Does drug interaction cause failure of PCP prophylaxis with dapsone? *Lancet* (1993) 341, 48.
3. Lee BL, Tauber MG, Chambers HF, Gambertoglio J, Delahunty T. Zalcitabine (DDC) and dapsone (DAP) pharmacokinetic (PK) interaction in HIV-infected patients. *Clin Pharmacol Ther* (1995) 57, 186.
4. Lee BL, Safrin S, Makrides V, Benowitz NL, Gambertoglio JG, Mills J. Trimethoprim decreases the renal clearance of zidovudine. *Clin Pharmacol Ther* (1992) 51,183.
5. Lee BL, Safrin S, Makrides V, Gambertoglio JG. Zidovudine, trimethoprim, and dapsone pharmacokinetic interactions in patients with human immunodeficiency virus infection. *Antimicrob Agents Chemother* (1996) 40, 1231–6.
6. Pinching AJ, Helbert M, Peddle B, Robinson D, Janes K, Gor D, Jeffries DJ, Stoneham C, Mitchell D, Kocsis AE, Mann J, Forster SM, Harris JRW. Clinical experience with zidovudine for patients with acquired immune deficiency syndrome and acquired immune deficiency syndrome-related complex. *J Infect* (1989) 18 (Suppl 1), 33–40.
7. Breen GA, Brocavich JM, Etzel JV, Shah V, Schaefer P, Forlenza S. Evaluation of effects of altered gastric pH on absorption of dapsone in healthy volunteers. *Antimicrob Agents Chemother* (1994) 38, 2227–9.
8. Sahai J, Garber G, Gallicano K, Oliveras L, Cameron DW. Effects of the antacids in didanosine tablets on dapsone pharmacokinetics. *Ann Intern Med* (1995) 123, 584–7.

Nucleoside reverse transcriptase inhibitors + Food

Food can reduce the bioavailability of didanosine, possibly causing a loss in efficacy. The absorption of zidovudine is markedly reduced if taken with food.

Clinical evidence, mechanism, importance and management

(a) Didanosine

Didanosine (as two 150-mg chewable tablets) were given to 10 HIV+ subjects 30 minutes before **breakfast**, 1 h before **breakfast** 1 h after **breakfast** and 2 h after **breakfast**. When the dose was given prior to **breakfast** the results were very similar to those obtained with subjects in the fasting state. When given after a **breakfast**, the **didanosine** AUC and maximum plasma concentration were both decreased by about 50%.[1] Similar results were found in another study.[2] Another study[3] using sachets containing **didanosine**, sucrose and citratephosphate buffer, found that **food** reduced the bioavailability from 29 to 17%. The reason would appear to be that **food** delays gastric emptying so that the **didanosine** is exposed to prolonged contact with gas-

tric acid which causes decomposition with a resultant fall in bioavailability.[4] To achieve maximum bioavailability the **didanosine** should be taken while fasting, although there is little difference with administration 30 mins to 1 h before **food**, which is considerably more convenient.

(b) Zidovudine

Zidovudine was given to 13 AIDS patients either with **breakfast** or when fasting. The maximum plasma level of **zidovudine** was 2.8 greater in the fasted patients, and the AUC was reduced by 22% when **zidovudine** was given with food.[5] **Zidovudine** absorption was reduced in another study by a standard **breakfast**.[6] In a study[7] of 8 patients a **high-fat meal** reduced **zidovudine** serum levels by about 50%. In all these cases inter-individual variation in **zidovudine** absorption was high.[5-7] However, when a sustained-release formulation of **zidovudine** was used, the absorption was delayed, but the bioavailability was increased by 28% by a **high-fat meal**.[8] In contrast **zidovudine** absorption was not affected by co-administration with 25 g of a **protein supplement**.[9]

The reasons are not understood. Inter-individual variation appears high and the practical consequences of these changes are uncertain. It has been suggested **zidovudine** should be taken on an empty stomach.[6,7]

1. Knupp CA, Milbrath R, Barbhaiya RH. Effect of time of food administration on the bioavailability of didanosine from a chewable tablet formulation. *J Clin Pharmacol* (1993) 33, 568–73.
2. Shyu WC, Knupp CA, Pittman KA, Dunkle L, Barbhaiya RH. Food-induced reduction in bioavailability of didanosine. *Clin Pharmacol Ther* (1991) 50, 503–7.
3. Hartman NR, Yarchoan R, Pluda JM, Thomas RV, Wyvill KM, Flora KP, Broder S, Johns DG. Pharmacokinetics of 2′,3′-dideoxyinosine in patients with severe human immunodeficiency infection. II. The effects of different formulations and the presence of other medications. *Clin Pharmacol Ther* (1991) 50, 278–85.
4. Videx (Didanosine). Bristol-Myers Squibb Pharmaceuticals Ltd. Summary of product characteristics, June 2001.
5. Lotterer E, Ruhnke M, Trautmann M, Beyer R, Bauer FE. Decreased and variable systemic availability of zidovudine in patients with AIDS if administered with a meal. *Eur J Clin Pharmacol* (1991) 40, 305–8.
6. Ruhnke M, Bauer FE, Seifert M, Trautmann M, Hille H, Koeppe P. Effects of standard breakfast on pharmacokinetics of oral zidovudine in patients with AIDS. *Antimicrob Agents Chemother* (1993) 37, 2153–8.
7. Unadkat JD, Collier AC, Crosby SS, Cummings D, Opheim KE, Corey L. Pharmacokinetics of oral zidovudine (azidothymidine) in patients with AIDS when administered with and without a high-fat meal. *AIDS* (1990) 4, 229–32.
8. Hollister AS, Frazer HA. The effects of a high fat meal on the serum pharmacokinetics of sustained-release zidovudine. *Clin Pharmacol Ther* (1994) 55, 193.
9. Sahai J, Gallicano K, Garber G, McGilveray I, Hawley-Foss N, Turgeon N, Cameron DW. The effect of a protein meal on zidovudine pharmacokinetics in HIV-infected patients. *Br J Clin Pharmacol* (1992) 33, 657–60.

Nucleoside reverse transcriptase inhibitors + Ganciclovir

The makers of lamivudine advise the avoidance of intravenous ganciclovir. A very marked increase in haematological toxicity occurs if zidovudine and ganciclovir are used concurrently, without any increase in efficacy. Didanosine serum levels seem to be raised by ganciclovir, but one report did not find an interaction. This drug combination should be avoided. Ganciclovir does not appear to interact with stavudine or zalcitabine.

Clinical evidence

(a) Didanosine

Didanosine 200 mg twice daily was given to 11 HIV+ patients with 1 g oral **ganciclovir** three times daily. The maximum **didanosine** serum levels were raised 57.7% and the AUC 71.5% by the **ganciclovir**. When the drugs were administered 2 h apart, similar results were seen.[1] Similar increases with **ganciclovir** given intravenously[2] and high dose **ganciclovir** (2 g 8-hourly) have also been reported.[3] Yet another study found that the serum levels of **didanosine** 200 mg twice daily were approximately doubled when taken with oral **ganciclovir** 1000 mg three times daily,[4] and a large audit of 994 patients (209 on **didanosine** and **ganciclovir**) also suggested that an interaction occurs.[5] However, in contrast, a further study found that the pharmacokinetics of **didanosine** were not altered by **ganciclovir**.[6]

(b) Lamivudine

The makers say that the co-administration of **lamivudine** and intravenous **ganciclovir** is not recommended until further information becomes available.[7]

(c) Stavudine

In a study of 11 HIV+ patients, **ganciclovir** 1000 mg three times daily had no significant effect on the pharmacokinetics of **stavudine** 40 mg twice daily, nor were the **ganciclovir** pharmacokinetics affected by the **stavudine**.[8] No dosage adjustments would therefore appear necessary if these drugs are used concurrently.

(d) Zalcitabine

In a study in 10 HIV+ patients no pharmacokinetic interaction was observed between **zalcitabine** and **ganciclovir** 1000 mg three times daily.[8] No dosage adjustments would therefore appear necessary if these drugs are used concurrently.

(e) Zidovudine

The efficacy of **zidovudine** 100 or 200 mg 4-hourly alone or combined with **ganciclovir** (5 mg/kg iv twice daily for 14 days, then once daily 5 days each week) was assessed in 40 patients for the treatment of cytomegalovirus (CMV). Severe haematological toxicity occurred in all of the first 10 patients given 1200 mg **zidovudine** daily and **ganciclovir**. Consequently the dose of **zidovudine** was reduced to 600 mg daily. Overall 82% of the 40 patients enrolled experienced profound and rapid toxicity (anaemia, neutropenia, leucopenia, gastrointestinal disturbances). **Zidovudine** dosage reductions to 300 mg daily were needed by many patients.[9]

Another study in 6 AIDS patients with CMV retinitis given **zidovudine** and **ganciclovir** found increased bone marrow toxicity but no improved efficacy over **ganciclovir** alone.[10] Increased toxicity (myelotoxicity and pancytopenia) has also been reported elsewhere.[11,12]

Mechanism

It has been suggested that the increased levels are because the drugs compete with one another for active secretion by the kidney tubules.[1]

The toxicity of the zidovudine/ganciclovir combination may be simply additive,[9] but *in vitro* studies with three human cell lines showed synergistic cytotoxicity when both drugs were used.[13]

Importance and management

The interactions between ganciclovir and didanosine or zidovudine would appear to be established (although there is one discordant report) but the clinical importance is uncertain. Zidovudine seems to be associated with greater toxicity than didanosine. Close and careful monitoring is required if either combination is used. Neither stavudine nor zalcitabine appear to interact with ganciclovir.

1. Trapnell CB, Cimoch P, Gaines K, Jung D, Hale M, Lavelle J. Altered didanosine pharmacokinetics with concomitant oral ganciclovir. *Clin Pharmacol Ther* (1994) 55, 193.
2. Frascino RJ, Anderson RD, Griffy KG, Jung D, Yu S. Two multiple dose crossover studies of IV ganciclovir (GCV) and didanosine (ddI) in HIV infected persons. *Intersci Conf Antimicrob Agents Chemother* (1995) 35, 6.
3. Jung D, Griffy K, Dorr A, Raschke R, Tarnowski TL, Hulse J, Kates RE. Effect of high-dose oral ganciclovir on didanosine disposition in human immunodeficiency virus (HIV)-positive patients. *J Clin Pharmacol* (1998) 38, 1057–62.
4. Griffy KG. Pharmacokinetics of oral ganciclovir capsules in HIV-infected persons. *AIDS* (1996) 10 (Suppl 4), S3–S6.
5. Brosgart C, Craig C, Hillman D, Louis TA, Alston B, Fisher E, El-Sadr W. Final results from a randomized, placebo-controlled trial of the safety and efficacy of oral ganciclovir for prophylaxis of CMV retinal and gastrointestinal mucosal disease. 11th International Conference on AIDS, Vancouver, 1996. Abstract Th.B.301.
6. Hartman NR, Yarchoan R, Pluda JM, Thomas RV, Wyvill KM, Flora KP, Broder S, Johns DG. Pharmacokinetics of 2′,3′-dideoxyinosine in patients with severe human immunodeficiency infection. II. The effects of different oral formulations and the presence of other medications. *Clin Pharmacol Ther* (1991) 50, 278–85.
7. Epivir (Lamivudine). Glaxo Wellcome. Summary of product characteristics, July 2001.
8. Jung D, AbdelHameed MH, Teitelbaum P, Dorr A, Griffy K. The pharmacokinetics and safety profile of oral ganciclovir combined with zalcitabine or stavudine in asymptomatic HIV- and CMV-seropositive patients. *J Clin Pharmacol* (1999) 39, 505–12.
9. Hochster H, Dieterich D, Bozzette S, Reichman RC, Connor JD, Liebes L, Sonke RL, Spector SA, Valentine F, Pettinelli C, Richman DD. Toxicity of combined ganciclovir and zidovudine for cytomegalovirus disease associated with AIDS. An AIDS clinical trials group study. *Ann Intern Med* (1990) 113, 111–17.
10. Millar AB, Miller RF, Patou G, Mindel A, Marsh R, Semple SJG. Treatment of cytomegalovirus retinitis with zidovudine and ganciclovir in patients with AIDS: outcome and toxicity. *Genitourin Med* (1990) 66, 156–8.
11. Jacobsen MA, de Miranda P, Gordon SM, Blum MR, Volberding P, Mills J. Prolonged pancytopenia due to combined ganciclovir and zidovudine therapy. *J Infect Dis* (1988) 158, 489–90.
12. Pinching AJ, Helbert M, Peddle B, Robinson D, Janes K, Gor D, Jeffries DJ, Stoneham C, Mitchell D, Kocsis AE, Mann J, Forster SM, Harris JRW. *J Infect* (1989) 18 (Suppl 1), 33–40.
13. Prichard MN, Prichard LE, Baguley WA, Nassiri MR, Shipman C. Three-dimensional analysis of the synergistic cytotoxicity of ganciclovir and zidovudine. *Antimicrob Agents Chemother* (1991) 35, 1060–5.

Nucleoside reverse transcriptase inhibitors + H₂-blockers

Concurrent use results in a minor increase in the serum levels of didanosine, and a minor decrease in the serum levels of ranitidine. Both changes seem to be clinically unimportant. Lamivudine does not interact with cimetidine or ranitidine. Cimetidine raises serum zalcitabine levels, but this is of uncertain importance. Cimetidine, but not ranitidine, reduces the renal secretion of zidovudine, but neither has a significant effect on zidovudine serum levels.

Clinical evidence, mechanism, importance and management

(a) Didanosine

Didanosine 375 mg was given to 12 HIV+ subjects either alone, or 2 h after a single 150-mg dose of **ranitidine**. The **didanosine** AUC was increased 14% by the **ranitidine**.[1] The reason is not known but the **ranitidine** possibly enhances the effects of the citrate-phosphate buffer with which the **didanosine** is formulated. The **ranitidine** AUC was reduced by 16% for reasons that are not understood, but it is possible that antacids (such as the citrate-phosphate buffer) reduce the absorption of **ranitidine**[1] (see 'H₂-blockers + Antacids', p.896).

These bioavailability changes appear to be too small to matter clinically, and no particular precautions would seem necessary if the drugs are taken in this way. It is not known whether other H₂-blockers or proton pump inhibitors behave similarly.

(b) Lamivudine

Lamivudine is cleared predominantly from the body by the kidneys using the organic cationic transport system, but it has been shown not to interact with **cimetidine** and **ranitidine**, which partly use this mechanism.[2]

(c) Zalcitabine

A study in 12 HIV+ patients given a single 1.5-mg dose of **zalcitabine** found that 800 mg of **cimetidine** caused a 24% reduction in the renal clearance of **zalcitabine**, assumed to be due to a reduction in renal tubular secretion, and a 36% increase in the AUC.[3]

These changes are relatively moderate and of uncertain clinical importance, but this still awaits formal assessment. You should monitor concurrent use for possible toxicity.

(d) Zidovudine

Zidovudine 600 mg daily was given to 5 HIV+ men and one man with AIDS in a randomised crossover study. The **zidovudine** was given either alone, with 300 mg **cimetidine** four times daily, or with 150 mg **ranitidine** twice daily, each for 7 days. **Cimetidine** reduced the renal elimination of the **zidovudine** by 56%, but had no effect on the metabolism of **zidovudine**. It was suggested that the reduction in clearance was due to inhibition of tubular secretion. **Ranitidine** had no effect on **zidovudine** pharmacokinetics. No clinical toxicity occurred and the immunological parameters measured (CD4 and CD8 cells) were not significantly altered. The authors concluded that no change in the dosage of **zidovudine** is needed if either of the these H₂-blockers is given concurrently.[4] Information about other H₂-blockers seems to be lacking.

1. Knupp CA, Graziano FM, Dixon RM, Barbhaiya RH. Pharmacokinetic-interaction study of didanosine and ranitidine in patients seropositive for human immunodeficiency virus. *Antimicrob Agents Chemother* (1992) 36, 2075–9.
2. Epivir (Lamivudine). GlaxoWellcome. Summary of product characteristics, November 2001.
3. Massarella JW, Holazo AA, Koss-Twardy S, Min B, Smith B, Nazareno LA. The effects of cimetidine and Maalox® on the pharmacokinetics of zalcitabine in HIV-positive patients. *Pharm Res* (1994) 11 (10 Suppl), S-415.
4. Fletcher CV, Henry WK, Noormohamed SE, Rhame FS, Balfour HH. The effect of cimetidine and ranitidine administration with zidovudine. *Pharmacotherapy* (1995) 15, 701–8.

Nucleoside reverse transcriptase inhibitors + Macrolides

Clarithromycin causes some reduction in the bioavailability of zidovudine, but this is minimised if the two drugs are given not less than 2 h apart. Clarithromycin does not appear to interact with either didanosine, stavudine or zalcitabine and azithromycin does not interact with didanosine or zidovudine.

Clinical evidence

(a) Didanosine

Azithromycin 1200 mg daily for 14 days was given concurrently with **didanosine** 200 mg twice daily to 12 HIV+ subjects without any significant change in the pharmacokinetics of either drug.[1]

Clarithromycin 1 g twice daily for 7 days was given to 4 HIV+ patients and 8 AIDS patients already taking oral **didanosine**. For the group as a whole the pharmacokinetics of the **didanosine** remained unchanged, but there were large differences in the AUC between subjects that could have hidden an interaction.[2]

(b) Stavudine

A study in 10 HIV+ subjects found that the addition of **clarithromycin** 500 mg twice daily to **stavudine** 30 or 40 mg twice daily caused no significant effects on the pharmacokinetics of the **stavudine** and the incidence of side effects did not increase.[3] No special precautions would seem necessary if both drugs are given.

(c) Zalcitabine

A 7-day course of **clarithromycin** 500 mg twice daily was given to 12 HIV+ subjects already taking **zalcitabine**. The addition of **clarithromycin** caused no change to the pharmacokinetics of **zalcitabine**.[4]

(d) Zidovudine

Azithromycin 1200 mg daily for 14 days was given concurrently with **zidovudine** 100 mg 5 times daily to 12 HIV+ subjects without any significant change in **zidovudine** pharmacokinetics.[1] Similarly, **azithromycin** 1g given weekly caused no change in the pharmacokinetics of **zidovudine** 10 mg/kg/day given to 9 HIV+ subjects. The **azithromycin** pharmacokinetics also remained unchanged.[5]

Zidovudine 100 mg 4-hourly 5 times a day and oral **clarithromycin** 500, 1000 or 2000 mg 12-hourly, both together and alone, were given to 15 HIV+ patients. The pharmacokinetics of the **clarithromycin** were not substantially changed but the serum **zidovudine** level and AUC were reduced by 24 to 46% and 12 to 27% respectively. However, these effects were not seen in all patients.[6] Another study similarly found that **clarithromycin** caused a moderate reduction in the AUC of oral **zidovudine** (by up to 27%). No changes were seen when the **zidovudine** was given 4 or more hours after the **clarithromycin**.[7] Yet another study recorded a 25% reduction in the **zidovudine** AUC when coadministered with **clarithromycin**.[8] **Zidovudine** and **clarithromycin** were given to 16 AIDS patients 2 h apart for 4 days. The maximum serum levels of the **zidovudine** rose by about 50% (from 616 to 949 ng/ml) but the minimum levels and the AUC over 8 h did not change.[9]

Mechanism

Not understood but possibly due to some changes in absorption.

Importance and management

The overall picture is slightly confusing, but it seems that some reductions in zidovudine levels are likely if the two drugs are taken at the same time, but no important changes seem to occur if the administration of the drugs is separated. The authors of one study recommend that the clarithromycin is given at least 2 h before or after the zidovudine.[7] The authors of the report on didanosine conclude that clarithromycin may safely be given with didanosine,[2] and it also seems likely that didanosine/azithromycin, zidovudine/azithromycin, stavudine/clarithromycin or zalcitabine/clarithromycin can be used safely together. More study is needed to confirm this.

1. Amsden G, Flaherty J, Luke D. Lack of an effect of azithromycin on the disposition of zidovudine and dideoxyinosine in HIV-infected patients. *J Clin Pharmacol* (2001) 41, 210–16.
2. Gillum JG, Bruzzese VL, Israel DS, Kaplowitz LG, Polk RE. Effect of clarithromycin on the pharmacokinetics of 2′,3′-dideoxyinosine in patients who are seropositive for human immunodeficiency virus. *Clin Infect Dis* (1996) 22, 716–18.
3. Piscitelli SC, Kelly G, Walker RE, Kovacs J, Falloon J, Davey RT, Raje S, Masur H, Polis MA. A multiple drug interaction study of stavudine with agents for opportunistic infections in human immunodeficiency virus-infected patients. *Antimicrob Agents Chemother* (1999) 43, 647–50.
4. Pastore A, van Cleef G, Fisher EJ, Gillum G, LeBel M, Polk RE. Dideoxycitidine (ddC) pharmacokinetics and interaction with clarithromycin in patients seropositive for HIV. 4th Conference on Retroviruses and Opportunistic Infections, Washington DC, January 22nd-26th 1997. Abstract 613.
5. Chave J-P, Munafo A, Chatton J-Y, Dayer P, Glauser MP, Biollaz J. Once-a-week azithromycin in AIDS patients: tolerability, kinetics, and effects on zidovudine disposition. *Antimicrob Agents Chemother* (1992) 36, 1013–18.
6. Gustavson LE, Chu S-Y, Mackenthun A, Gupta SD, Craft JC. Drug interaction between clarithromycin and oral zidovudine in HIV-1 infected patients. *Clin Pharmacol Ther* (1993) 53, 163.
7. Petty B, Polis M, Haneiwich S, Dellerson M, Craft JC, Chaisson R. Pharmacokinetic assessment of clarithromycin plus zidovudine in HIV patients. Intersci Conf Antimicrob Ag Chemother, Anaheim, Calif, Oct 11–14, 1992, 32, 114.
8. Polis MA, Piscitelli SC, Vogel S, Witebsky FG, Conville PS, Petty B, Kovacs JA, Davey RT, Walker RE, Falloon J, Metcalf JA, Craft C, Lane HC, Masur H. Clarithromycin lowers plasma zidovudine levels in persons with human immunodeficiency virus infection. *Antimicrob Agents Chemother* (1997) 41, 1709–14.
9. Vance E, Watson-Bitar M, Gustavson L, Kazanjian P. Pharmacokinetics of clarithromycin and zidovudine in patients with AIDS. *Antimicrob Agents Chemother* (1995) 39, 1335–60.

Nucleoside reverse transcriptase inhibitors + Miscellaneous drugs

The makers currently contraindicate lamivudine/foscarnet. There have been case reports of interactions resulting in serious toxicity with azathioprine/lamivudine, pentamidine/zalcitabine and vancomycin/zidovudine. *In vitro* evidence suggests that stavudine/doxorubicin, zidovudine/chloramphenicol and zidovudine/ethinylestradiol may interact. The significance of interactions between zalcitabine and aminoglycosides, amphotericin or foscarnet await confirmation. Loperamide and metoclopramide do not appear to interact with didanosine. Allopurinol and hydroxycarbamide raise didanosine levels, possibly advantageously. Moderate pharmacokinetic changes not requiring dose adjustments have been seen with zalcitabine and *Maalox*, naproxen or indometacin and between zidovudine and atovaquone, bleomycin, doxorubicin, epirubicin, etoposide, vinblastine, vincristine, vinorelbine, vindesine, dipyridamole or lithium.

Clinical evidence, mechanism, importance and management

A. Lamivudine

(a) Azathioprine

A single case report describes a 51-year-old woman with a kidney transplant who developed pancreatitis after starting **lamivudine**. **Azathioprine** had been discontinued only 3 days before and it is possible (although the evidence is weak) that the residual serum **azathioprine** had interacted with **lamivudine** to cause the pancreatitis.[1] Both drugs are known to cause pancreatitis. No firm conclusions can be drawn from this very slim evidence.

(b) Foscarnet

The makers say that the co-administration of **lamivudine** and **foscarnet** is not recommended until further information becomes available.[2]

B. Didanosine

(a) Allopurinol

Didanosine 400 mg was given to 14 healthy subjects with and without **allopurinol** 300 mg daily for 7 days. Concurrent administration of **allopurinol** significantly increased **didanosine** absorption, shown by a twofold increase in the AUC and a 69% rise in the maximum serum concentration.[3]

(b) Hydroxycarbamide

Didanosine 200 to 300 mg twice daily was given with **hydroxycarbamide** 500 mg twice daily for up to 24 weeks in 9 HIV+ subjects. The peak plasma concentrations of **didanosine** were well above those needed to suppress HIV and CD4+ counts rose over the duration of the treatment period. The combination was well tolerated, although there was one episode of neutropenia.[4] **Hydroxycarbamide** is thought to augment the action of **didanosine** by favouring its incorporation into cells. An *in vitro* study demonstrated that, when given in combination with **hydroxycarbamide**, less **didanosine** is required to achieve the same antiretroviral effect.[5] This interaction appears potentially favourable and more study into it is warranted.

(c) Loperamide

The pharmacokinetics of 300 mg oral **didanosine** were found to be unaffected by 4 mg **loperamide** 19, 13, 7 and 1 h before the **didanosine** in 6 men and 6 women who were HIV+. The rate but not the extent of the **didanosine** absorption was changed. On the basis of this study the authors conclude that neither the dose nor the frequency of **didanosine** administration need be altered if **loperamide** is given concurrently.[6]

(d) Metoclopramide

The pharmacokinetics of 300 mg oral **didanosine** were found to be unaffected by 10 mg intravenous **metoclopramide** in 6 men and 6 women who were HIV+. On the basis of this study the authors conclude that neither the dose nor the frequency of **didanosine** administration need be altered if **metoclopramide** is given concurrently.[6]

C. Stavudine

(a) Doxorubicin

Nucleoside reverse transcriptase inhibitors such as **stavudine** need to be phosphorylated within cells before they become effective. *In vitro* studies using mononucleated blood cells found that **doxorubicin** interfered with phosphorylation at clinically relevant concentrations.[7] The clinical importance of this interaction awaits assessment.

D. Zalcitabine

(a) Antacid

A study in 12 HIV+ patients given a single 1.5-mg dose of **zalcitabine** found that 30 ml *Maalox* caused a 25% reduction in the bioavailability of the **zalcitabine**.[8] The changes are moderate and of uncertain clinical importance, but this still awaits formal assessment. You should monitor concurrent use well.

(b) Miscellaneous

The makers of **zalcitabine** suggest that the concurrent use of **zalcitabine** and **amphotericin**, **foscarnet** and the **aminoglycoside antibacterials** should be well monitored because these drugs may possibly decrease the renal clearance of the **zalcitabine**, thereby increasing its serum levels and its toxicity. These predicted interactions still await formal assessment.[9]

(c) Pentamidine

Fatal fulminant pancreatitis occurred in a patient given **zalcitabine** and intravenous **pentamidine**.[9] The makers suggest that if **pentamidine** is to be given, treatment with **zalcitabine** should be interrupted.[9]

E. Zidovudine

(a) Aspirin or NSAIDs

A study of **zidovudine** use in 282 AIDS patients found that haematological abnormalities were not increased by the concurrent use of **aspirin** in 47 patients.[10] An *in vitro* study using human liver microsomes found that **indometacin** and **naproxen** inhibited the glucuronidation of **zidovudine** by 50% or more.[11] This suggested that these drugs might possibly increase the effects and the toxicity of **zidovudine**. However, another study found no changes in the kinetics of a single dose of **zidovudine** with **indometacin** 25 mg twice daily for 3 days[12] or **naproxen** 0.5 to 1 g daily for 3 or 4 days.[13] No special precautions would seem necessary with these drugs.

(b) Atovaquone

A study in 14 HIV+ patients given 750 mg **atovaquone** 12-hourly and 200 mg **zidovudine** 8-hourly found that under steady-state conditions the **zidovudine** had no effect on the pharmacokinetics of **atovaquone**.[14] This confirmed the findings of a previous study.[15] However, the AUC of the **zidovudine** was increased by 31%, and its clearance was reduced by 25% by concurrent use of **atovaquone**. The reason appears to be that the **atovaquone** inhibits the metabolism (glucuronidation) of the **zidovudine**.[14]

The increased **zidovudine** AUC is only moderate and, it is suggested, is unlikely to be of clinical concern except possibly in patients taking other drugs causing bone marrow toxicity (such as ganciclovir, amphotericin B, flucytosine). If bone marrow toxicity is seen it is suggested that the **zidovudine** dosage may need to be reduced by a third.[14]

(c) Chloramphenicol

An *in vitro* study using human liver microsomes found that **chloramphenicol** inhibited the glucuronidation of **zidovudine** by 50% or more, suggesting that the effects and toxicity of **zidovudine** may be increased.[11] The effects of concurrent use in patients awaits assessment.

(d) Cytotoxic agents

The interaction of chemotherapy with **zidovudine** was assessed in HIV+ patients being treated for Kaposi's sarcoma, non-Hodgkin's lymphoma or Hodgkin's disease. The cytotoxic agents used were **bleomycin**, **cyclophosphamide**, **doxorubicin**, **epirubicin**, **etoposide**, **vinblastine**, **vincristine**, **vindesine** and **vinorelbine**. The **zidovudine** metabolism was unchanged, but a 57% decrease was noted in the maximum serum levels of **zidovudine**, which was independent of the chemotherapy given. As the **zidovudine** AUC remained unchanged and maximum serum levels have not been shown to correlate with virucidal activity, the authors concluded that dose changes of **zidovudine** were not need with the cytotoxic agents used.[16]

(e) Dipyridamole

A study in 11 asymptomatic HIV+ patients showed no significant changes in the pharmacokinetics of **zidovudine** 500 mg daily when concurrently treated with 75 to 100 mg **dipyridamole** 4-hourly for 5 days, but the **dipyridamole** side-effects (headaches, nausea) when taking the higher dose were found to be intolerable.[17] No **zidovudine** dosage adjustment seems to be necessary. The long-term safety of this drug combination awaits further study.

(f) Ethinylestradiol

An *in vitro* study using human liver microsomes found that **ethinylestradiol** inhibited the glucuronidation of **zidovudine** by 50% or more, suggesting that the effects and toxicity of **zidovudine** may be increased.[11] The effects of concurrent use in patients awaits assessment.

(g) Lithium

A study in 5 patients with AIDS found that serum **lithium carbonate** levels of 0.6 to 1.2 mEq/l increased their neutrophil counts sufficiently to allow the re-introduction of **zidovudine** previously withdrawn due to neutropenia. Withdrawal of the **lithium** resulted in a rapid fall in neutrophil levels in two patients.[18] The reasons for this effect on neutrophil production are not understood.

This report suggests that no adverse reaction occurs in patients taking **zidovudine** who are given **lithium**, and that there are some advantages. More study is needed.

(h) Vancomycin

A report describes marked neutropenia in 4 HIV+ patients on **zidovudine** when given **vancomycin** (which can also, rarely, have neutropenic effects).[19] On theoretical grounds any drug causing bone marrow suppression might be additive with the effects of **zidovudine**.

1. Van Vlierberghe H, Elewaut A. Development of a necrotising pancreatitis after starting lamivudine in a kidney transplant patient with fibrosing cholestatic hepatitis: A possible role of the interaction lamivudine and azathioprine. *Gastroenterology* (1997) 112 (4 Suppl), 1407.
2. Epivir (Lamivudine). Glaxo Wellcome. Summary of product characteristics, November 2001.
3. Liang D, Breaux K, Nornoo A Phadungpojna S, Rodriguez-Barradas M, Bates TR. Pharmacokinetic interaction between didanosine (ddI) and allopurinol in healthy volunteers. *Intersci Conf Antimicrob Agents Chemother* (1999) 39, 25.
4. Luzatti R, Fendt D, Ramarli D, Parisi S, Broccali GP, Concia E. Pharmacokinetics (PK), safety and antiviral activity of hydroxyurea (HU) in combination with didanosine (ddI) in HIV-infected individuals. *Intersci Conf Antimicrob Agents Chemother* (1997) 37, 2.
5. Rana KZ, Simmons KA, Dudley MN. Hydroxyurea reduces the 50% inhibitory concentration of didanosine in HIV-infected cells. *AIDS* (1999) 13, 2186–8.
6. Knupp CA, Milbrath RL, Barbhaiya RH. Effect of metoclopramide and loperamide on the pharmacokinetics of didanosine in HIV seropositive asymptomatic male and female patients. *Eur J Clin Pharmacol* (1993) 45, 409–13.
7. Hoggard PG, Barry MG, Khoo SH, Back DJ. Drug interactions with d4T phosphorylation *in vitro*. *Br J Clin Pharmacol* (1996) 42, 278P.
8. Massarella JW, Holazo AA, Koss-Twardy S, Min B, Smith B, Nazareno LA. The effects of cimetidine and Maalox® on the pharmacokinetics of zalcitabine in HIV-positive patients. *Pharm Res* (1994) 11 (10 Suppl), S-415.
9. Hivid (Zalcitabine), Roche Products Limited. Summary of product characteristics, December 1998.
10. Richman DD, Fischl MA, Grieco MH, Gottlieb MS, Volberding PA, Laskin OL, Leedom JM, Groopman JE, Mildvan D, Hirsch MS, Jackson GG, Durack DT, Nusinoff-Lehrman S and the AZT Collaborative Working Group. The toxicity of azidothymidine (AZT) in the treatment of patients with AIDS and AIDS-related complex. A double-blind, placebo-controlled trial. *N Engl J Med* (1987) 317, 192–7.
11. Sim SM, Back DJ, Breckenridge AM. The effect of various drugs on the glucuronidation of zidovudine (azidothymidine; AZT) by human liver microsomes. *Br J Clin Pharmacol* (1991) 32, 17–21.
12. Barry M, Howe J, Back D, Breckenridge A, Brettle R, Mitchell R, Beeching N, Nye F. Effect of non-steroidal anti-inflammatory drugs on zidovudine pharmacokinetics. *Br J Clin Pharmacol* (1992) 34, 446P.
13. Sahai J, Gallicano K, Garber G, Pakuts A, Hawley-Foss N, Huang L, McGilveray I, Cameron DW. Evaluation of the in vivo effect of naproxen on zidovudine pharmacokinetics in patients infected with human immunodeficiency virus. *Clin Pharmacol Ther* (1992) 52, 464–70.
14. Lee BL, Täuber MG, Sadler B, Goldstein D, Chambers HF. Atovaquone inhibits the glucuronidation and increases the plasma concentrations of zidovudine. *Clin Pharmacol Ther* (1996) 59, 14–21.
15. Sadler BM, Blum MR. Relationship between steady-state plasma concentrations of atovaquone (C_{ss}) and the use of various concomitant medications in AIDS patients with *Pneumocystis carinii* pneumonia. 9th International Conference AIDS & 4th STD World Congress, Berlin, June 6–11 1993. Abstract PO-B31-2213.
16. Toffoli G, Errante D, Corona G, Vaccher E, Bertola A, Robieux I, Aita P, Sorio R, Tirelli U, Boiocchi M. Interactions of antineoplastic chemotherapy with zidovudine pharmacokinetics in patients with HIV-related neoplasms. *Chemotherapy* (1999) 45, 418–28.
17. Hendrix CW, Flexner C, Szebeni J, Kuwahara S, Pennypacker S, Weinstein JN, Lietman PS. Effect of dipyridamole on zidovudine pharmacokinetics and short-term tolerance in asymptomatic human immunodeficiency virus-infected subjects. *Antimicrob Agents Chemother* (1994) 38, 1036–40.
18. Roberts DE, Berman SM, Nakasato S, Wyle FA, Wishnow RM, Segal GP. Effect of lithium carbonate on zidovudine-associated neutropenia in the acquired immunodeficiency syndrome. *Am J Med* (1988) 85, 428–31.
19. Kitchen LW, Clark RA, Hanna BJ, Pollock B, Valainis GT. Vancomycin and neutropenia in AZT-treated AIDS patients with staphylococcal infections. *J Acquir Immune Defic Syndr* (1990) 3, 925–6.

Nucleoside reverse transcriptase inhibitors + Nucleoside reverse transcriptase inhibitors

Zidovudine decreases the cellular activation of stavudine and it is recommended that concurrent use be avoided. In general the other NRTIs are well tolerated in combination, with minimal pharmacokinetics changes occurring. Those changes that do result for combined use appear to be due to changes in absorption and a metabolic interaction seems unlikely. There are some reports of additive toxicity (blood dyscrasias and neuropathy), so treatment should be carefully monitored.

Clinical evidence, mechanism, importance and management

(a) Abacavir + Lamivudine

A single dose of **lamivudine** 150 mg was given with **abacavir** 600 mg to 13 HIV+ subjects. The pharmacokinetics of **abacavir** were not significantly affected but the **lamivudine** maximum serum levels and AUC were decreased by 35 and 15%. These changes were considered to be consistent with a change in absorption. The extent of the change is not thought to be clinically significant and so no dose alteration would seem necessary on concurrent use.[1]

(b) Abacavir + Zidovudine

A single dose of **zidovudine** 300 mg was given with **abacavir** 600 mg to 13 HIV+ subjects. The pharmacokinetics of **abacavir** were not significantly affected but the **zidovudine** maximum serum level decreased by 20%, but the AUC was unchanged. This change is not thought to be clinically significant and so no dose alteration would seem necessary on concurrent use.[1] These results were confirmed in a steady-state study in which 79 HIV+ subjects received 8 weeks treatment with **abacavir** 600 to 1800 mg daily, in divided doses and **zidovudine** 600 mg daily, in divided doses.[2]

(c) Didanosine + Lamivudine

Lamivudine is cleared predominantly from the body by the kidneys using the organic cationic transport system. **Didanosine** is not cleared by this mechanism and so is unlikely to interact with **lamivudine**.[3] Nucleoside reverse transcriptase inhibitors such as **lamivudine** need to be phosphorylated within cells to a triphosphate anabolite to become active. Since **didanosine** does not affect this phosphorylation *in vitro*[4] it is predicted that no interaction is likely to occur by this mechanism.

(d) Didanosine + Stavudine

Didanosine 100 mg twice daily was given to 10 HIV+ subjects with **stavudine** 40 mg twice daily for 9 doses. The **didanosine** pharmacokinetics were unchanged by concurrent use but the half-life of the **stavudine** increased by 25.6% (1.56 to 1.96 h). However, the AUC was unchanged, adverse effects were minimal, and the authors of the report concluded that no clinically significant adverse interaction is likely if both drugs are given concurrently.[5] Combination treatment with **stavudine** and **didanosine** was given to 13 HIV+ subjects for 8 weeks. Neuropathy occurred in 3 patients, with only 2 restarting treatment. Viral load decreased and CD4 counts increased by 52 cells/mm³. The combination therefore seems relatively safe and effective.[6] Confirmation of this would appear to be provided by an *in vitro* study using human blood cells, which found that **didanosine** does not interfere with the intracellular activation of **stavudine**.[7]

(e) Didanosine + Zalcitabine

A man of 29 with persistent mild neuropathy due to **zalcitabine** developed severe neuropathy when given **didanosine** 3 weeks after discontinuing **zalcitabine**. As the **didanosine** neuropathy developed so rapidly it was suggested that it was caused by additive toxicity with **zalcitabine**.[8] The advice to monitor concurrent use of drugs that share this serious side-effect seems a sensible precaution (as recommended by the makers of both drugs). More study is needed.

(f) Didanosine + Zidovudine

A study in 8 HIV+ patients found that when given 250 mg **zidovudine** and 250 mg **didanosine** together, the pharmacokinetics of the **didanosine** were unaltered but the **zidovudine** AUC were *raised* by 35%, possibly due to altered absorption.[9]

Zidovudine serum levels were *lower* in 4 out of 5 HIV+ patients when given **didanosine** and there was an average 14% reduction in the **zidovudine** AUC. The **zidovudine** clearance was increased by 29% but the **didanosine** pharmacokinetics were unchanged.[10]

A study in over 50 subjects ranging in age from 3 months to 21 years found that when compared with day 3 (start of concurrent administration), no significant changes in AUCs occurred after 4 or 12 weeks of concurrent **zidovudine** 60 to 180 mg/m² 6-hourly and **didanosine** 60 to 180 mg/m² 12-hourly.[11] Several other studies have not found a pharmacokinetic interaction or evidence of increased toxicity when didanosine and **zidovudine** are used concurrently.[12-15]

The reports are slightly contradictory, but the weight of evidence seems to be that no clinically relevant interaction occurs. Nevertheless you should monitor well if both drugs are used.

(g) Lamivudine + Zalcitabine

Lamivudine is cleared predominantly from the body by the kidneys using the organic cationic transport system. **Zalcitabine** is not cleared by this mechanism and so is unlikely to interact with lamivudine.[3]

(h) Lamivudine + Stavudine

Nucleoside reverse transcriptase inhibitors such as **lamivudine** need to be activated by phosphorylation within cells to a triphosphate anabolite. Since **stavudine** does not affect this phosphorylation *in vitro*[4] it is predicted that no interaction is likely to occur by this mechanism.

(i) Lamivudine + Zidovudine

Lamivudine 300 mg twice daily was given to 12 HIV+ patients for 2 days, and then on day 3 they were given 300 mg **lamivudine** plus 200 mg **zidovudine**. No major changes in the pharmacokinetics of the **zidovudine** occurred and it was concluded that dosage adjustments are not needed if these two drugs are given concurrently.[16] Another study showed the same results,[1] and an extensive study in over 200 patients has shown that combined use can be safe and effective.[17]

However there are case reports of blood dyscrasias occurring with concurrent use. **Zidovudine** 500 to 600 mg daily was given with **lamivudine** 300 mg daily to 8 HIV+ men. **Zidovudine** or **lamivudine** alone had previously been given to 6 of these 8 without problem. However, when the drugs were combined, blood dyscrasias occurred in all patients within 7 weeks. Anaemia, with a 50% fall in haemoglobin occurred in 7 patients, while the other patient developed leucopenia and thrombocytopenia. The drug combination was stopped, blood transfusions were given, and all patients improved or recovered over 5 weeks. **Zidovudine** or **lamivudine** alone was later started in 5 patients without further haematological problems.[18] Similar precipitous falls in haemoglobin occurred in another two patients when **lamivudine** 300 mg daily was added to their long term **zidovudine** treatment. Again both recovered when the drugs were stopped and blood was given.[19] Anaemia is a common side-effect of **zidovudine**, but these patients had no problems until the **lamivudine** was added. The available evidence indicates that concurrent use can be safe and effective, with the adverse interactions cited here being uncommon. It has been suggested that a complete baseline blood count should be done when combined treatment is started, and then every month for the first 3 months of treatment.[19]

(j) Stavudine + Zidovudine

Nucleoside reverse transcriptase inhibitors such as **stavudine** need to be phosphorylated within cells to a triphosphate anabolite before they become effective. *In vitro* studies using mononucleated blood cells found that **zidovudine** significantly inhibited this phosphorylation.[7] The makers currently do not recommend the combination.[20]

(k) Zalcitabine + Zidovudine

In a study in 56 advanced HIV+ patients taking **zidovudine** (50 to 200 mg 8-hourly) and **zalcitabine** (0.005 to 0.01 mg/kg 8-hourly), neither drug affected the pharmacokinetics of the other and toxicity was not increased.[21] No special precautions would appear to be necessary.

1. Wang LH, Chittick GE, McDowell JA. Single-dose pharmacokinetics and safety of abacavir (1592U89), zidovudine, and lamivudine administered alone and in combination in adults with human immunodeficiency virus infection. *Antimicrob Agents Chemother* (1999) 43, 1708–15.
2. McDowell JA, Lou Y, Symonds WS, Stein DS. Multiple-dose pharmacokinetics and pharmacodynamics of abacavir alone and in combination with zidovudine in human immunodeficiency virus-infected adults. *Antimicrob Agents Chemother* (2000) 44, 2061–7.
3. Epivir (Lamivudine). Glaxo Wellcome. Summary of product characteristics. November 2001.
4. Kewn S, Veal GJ, Hoggard PG, Barry MG, Back DJ. Lamivudine (3TC). Phosphorylation and drug interactions *in vitro*. *Biochem Pharmacol* (1997) 54, 589–95.
5. Seifert RD, Stewart MB, Sramek JJ, Conrad J, Kaul S, Cutler NR. Pharmacokinetics of co-administered didanosine and stavudine in HIV-seropositive male patients. *Br J Clin Pharmacol* (1994) 38, 405–10.
6. Kalathoor S, Sinclair J, Andron L, Sension MG, High K. Combination therapy with stavudine and didanosine. 4ᵗʰ Conference on Retroviruses and Opportunistic Infections, Washington DC, Jan 22-26 1997. Abstract 552.
7. Hoggard PG, Kewn S, Barry MG, Khoo SH, Back DJ. Effects of drugs on 2',3'-dideoxy-2',3'-didehydrothymidine phosphorylation in vitro. *Antimicrob Agents Chemother* (1997) 41, 1231–6.
8. LeLacheur SF, Simon GL. Exacerbation of dideoxycytidine-induced neuropathy with dideoxyinosine. *J Acquir Immune Defic Syndr* (1991) 4, 538–9.
9. Barry M, Howe JL, Ormesher S, Back DJ, Breckenridge AM, Bergin C, Mulcahy F, Beeching N, Nye F. Pharmacokinetics of zidovudine and dideoxyinosine alone and in combination in patients with acquired immunodeficiency syndrome. *Br J Clin Pharmacol* (1994) 37, 421–6.
10. Burger DM, Meenhorst PL, Kroon FP, Mulder JW, Koks CHW, Bult A, Beijnen JH. Pharmacokinetic interaction study of zidovudine and didanosine. *J Drug Dev* (1994) 6, 187–94.
11. Mueller BU, Pizzo PA, Farley M, Husson RN, Goldsmith J, Kovacs A, Woods L, Ono J, Church JA, Brouwers P, Jarosinski P, Venzon D, Balis FM. Pharmacokinetic evaluation of the combination of zidovudine and didanosine in children with human immunodeficiency virus infection. *J Pediatr* (1994) 125, 142–6.
12. Collier AC, Coombs RW, Fischl MA, Skolnik PR, Northfelt D, Boutin P, Hooper CJ, Kaplan LD, Volberding PA, Davis LG, Henrard DR, Weller S, Corey L. Combination therapy with zidovudine and didanosine compared with zidovudine alone in HIV-1 infection. *Ann Intern Med* (1993) 119, 786–93.
13. Sahai J, Gallicano K, Seguin I, Garber G, Cameron W. Interaction between zidovudine (ZDV) and didanosine (ddI). *Intersci Conf Antimicrob Agents Chemother* (1994) 34, 82.
14. Sahai J, Gallicano K, Pakuts A, Cameron W. Pharmacokinetics of simultaneously administered zidovudine and didanosine in HIV-seropositive male patients. *J Acquir Immune Defic Syndr Hum Retrovirol* (1995) 10, 54–60.
15. Gibb D, Barry M, Ormesher S, Nokes L, Seefried M, Giaquinto C, Back D. Pharmacokinetics of zidovudine and dideoxyinosine alone and in combination in children with HIV infection. *Br J Clin Pharmacol* (1995) 39, 527–30.
16. Rana KZ, Horton CM, Yuen GJ, Pivarnik PE, Mikolich DM, Fisher AE, Mydlow PK, Dudley MN. Effect of lamivudine on zidovudine pharmacokinetics in asymptomatic HIV-infected individuals. *Intersci Conf Antimicrob Agents Chemother* (1994) 34, 83.
17. Staszewski S, Loveday C, Picazo JJ, Dellamonica P, Skinhøj P, Johnson MA, Danner SA, Harrigan PR, Hill AM, Verity L, McDade H. Safety and efficacy of lamivudine-zidovudine combination therapy in zidovudine-experienced patients. *JAMA* (1996) 276, 111–17.
18. Tseng A, Fletcher D, Gold W, Conly J, Keystone D, Walmsley S. Precipitous decline in hemoglobin with combination AZT/3TC. 4ᵗʰ Conference on Retroviruses and Opportunistic Infections, Washington, Jan 22-26, 1997. Abstract 559.
19. Hester EK, Peacock JE. Profound and unanticipated anemia with lamivudine-zidovudine combination therapy in zidovudine-experienced patients with HIV infection. *AIDS* (1998) 12, 439–51.
20. Zerit (Stavudine). Bristol-Myers Squibb Pharmaceuticals Ltd. Summary of product characteristics, July 2001.
21. Meng T-C, Fischl MA, Boota AM, Spector SA. Bennett D, Bassiakos Y, Lai S, Wright B, Richman DD. Combination therapy with zidovudine and dideoxycytidine in patients with advanced human immunodeficiency virus infection. *Ann Intern Med* (1992) 116, 13–20.

Nucleoside reverse transcriptase inhibitors + Probenecid

Probenecid reduces the loss of zalcitabine and zidovudine, increasing their serum levels. The zalcitabine/probenecid combination is well tolerated, but the incidence of side-effects is reported to be very much increased with the probenecid and zidovudine combination. Patients should be monitored for any signs of toxicity.

Clinical evidence

(a) Zalcitabine

In a single-dose study, 12 HIV+ or AIDS patients were given 1.5 mg **zalcitabine** alone or with **probenecid** (500 mg given 8 and 2 h before then 4 h after). The renal clearance of the **zalcitabine** was decreased 42% by **probenecid**, the half-life increased 47% and AUC increased 54%.[1]

(b) Zidovudine

The concurrent use of **zidovudine** and 500 mg **probenecid** 8-hourly for 3 days increased the **zidovudine** AUC in 12 patients with AIDS or AIDS-related complex by an average of 80% (range 14 to 192%).[2] Other studies in patients[3-5] and healthy subjects[6] found that **probenecid** approximately doubled the AUC of **zidovudine** when given in a variety of dosing schedules,[3,4] however the effects on **zidovudine** pharmacokinetics were lost if the two drugs were given 6 h apart.[5] Another report describes a very high incidence of rashes in 6 out of 8 HIV+ men when given **zidovudine** and **probenecid** 500 mg 6-hourly. The rash and other symptoms (such as malaise, fever and myalgia) were sufficiently severe for the **probenecid** to be withdrawn in 4 of them.[7] A later study found that when using only 250 mg

probenecid 8-hourly the **zidovudine** AUC was increased 70% but the adverse effects still occurred, although the incidence was possibly somewhat lower.[8]

Mechanism

Experimental clinical evidence indicates that probenecid reduces the metabolism (glucuronidation) of the zidovudine by the liver enzymes, thereby reducing its loss from the body.[2,4,6,9,10] The interaction with zalcitabine is presumably due to inhibition of zalcitabine secretion in the renal tubules.[1]

Importance and management

Concurrent use of zidovudine and probenecid should be well monitored to ensure that zidovudine levels do not rise excessively. Reduce the zidovudine dosage as necessary. However, the apparent increase in side effects during concurrent use (cited above[7]) should be borne in mind. Concurrent use of zalcitabine and probenecid was well tolerated, and because the zalcitabine half-life is short compared to its dosing schedule significant accumulation would not be expected.

It would seem prudent to monitor for any signs of toxicity if either drug combination is used chronically. The safety of combined use needs further assessment.

1. Massarella JW, Nazareno LA, Passe S, Min B. The effect of probenecid on the pharmacokinetics of zalcitabine in HIV-positive patients. *Pharm Res* (1996) 13, 449–52.
2. Kornhauser DM, Petty BG, Hendrix CW, Woods AS, Nerhood LJ, Bartlett JG, Lietman PS. Probenecid and zidovudine metabolism. *Lancet* (1989) 2, 473–5.
3. Hedaya MA, Elmquist WF, Sawchuk RJ. Probenecid inhibits the metabolic and renal clearances of zidovudine (AZT) in human volunteers. *Pharm Res* (1990) 7, 411–17.
4. de Miranda P, Good SS, Yarchoan R, Thomas RV, Blum MR, Myers CE, Broder S. Alteration of zidovudine pharmacokinetics by probenecid in patients with AIDS or AIDS-related complex. *Clin Pharmacol Ther* (1989) 46, 494–500.
5. McDermott J, Kennedy J, Ellis-Pegler RB, Thomas MG. Pharmacokinetics of zidovudine plus probenecid. *J Infect Dis* (1992) 166, 687–8.
6. Campion JJ, Bawdon RE, Baskin LB, Barton CI. Effect of probenecid on the pharmacokinetics of zidovudine and zidovudine glucuronide. *Pharmacotherapy* (1990) 10, 235.
7. Petty BG, Kornhauser DM, Lietman PS. Zidovudine with probenecid: a warning. *Lancet* (1990) 1, 1044–5.
8. Petty BG, Barditch-Crovo PA, Nerhood L, Kornhauser DM, Kuwahara S, Lietman PS. Unexpected clinical toxicity of probenecid (P) with zidovudine (Z) in patients with HIV infection. *Intersci Conf Antimicrob Agents Chemother* (1991) 31, 323.
9. Sim SM, Back DJ, Breckenridge AM. The effect of various drugs on the glucuronidation of zidovudine (azidothymidine; AZT) by human liver microsomes. *Br J Clin Pharmacol* (1991) 32, 17–21.
10. Kamali F, Rawlins MD. Influence of probenecid and paracetamol (acetaminophen) on zidovudine glucuronidation in human liver *in vitro*. *Biopharm Drug Dispos* (1992) 13, 403–9.

Nucleoside reverse transcriptase inhibitors + Protease Inhibitors

With the exception of didanosine and indinavir, which should be administered 1 h apart, the changes in pharmacokinetics seen when giving protease inhibitors with NRTIs do not appear to be clinically significant.

Clinical evidence, mechanism, importance and management

(a) Abacavir

A phase I study in HIV+ patients given **amprenavir** 900 mg twice daily with **abacavir** 300 mg twice daily for 3 weeks found that neither drug had any significant effect on the pharmacokinetics of the other.[1]

(b) Didanosine

The makers of **indinavir** recommend that **indinavir** and **didanosine** should be given at least one hour apart because **indinavir** may require a normal acidic gastric pH for optimal absorption whereas **didanosine** is formulated with buffering agents to raise gastric pH. Any increase in pH would therefore be expected to reduce **indinavir** absorption.[2] A study investigating how the timing of administration affected this interaction found that the pharmacokinetics of 800 mg **indinavir** were unchanged when the dose was given 1 h after 400 mg **didanosine**.[3]

The pharmacokinetics of **nelfinavir** were not significantly altered after concurrent administration with **didanosine**.[4]

Didanosine 200 mg twice daily was given with **ritonavir** 600 mg twice daily to 13 HIV+ subjects. Administration of the two drugs was separated by 2.5 hours, and treatment was given for 4 days. There was little or no change in the pharmacokinetics of **ritonavir**, and the maximum serum levels and AUC of **didanosine** were reduced by 16 and 13% respectively, which was not considered to be clinically significant. It was suggested that these changes may have been due to altered absorption in the presence of **ritonavir**.[5]

(c) Lamivudine

Lamivudine is cleared predominantly from the body by the kidneys using the organic cationic transport system and does not involve liver metabolism by the cytochrome P450 isoenzyme CYP3A4. Therefore it is unlikely that it will interact with drugs such as the **protease inhibitors** which are metabolised by this system.[6]

(d) Stavudine

The AUC of **stavudine** was increased 25% when 40 mg **stavudine** twice daily was given with 800 mg **indinavir** 8-hourly for a week, which was not considered to be clinically significant. The serum levels of **indinavir** were unchanged.[7]

Although no pharmacokinetic studies were conducted, a study found that CD4 counts increased by 80 to 195 cells/mm³ when **stavudine** was given with **nelfinavir** over a period of 28 days. Therapy was well tolerated, and adverse effects were similar to those seen when **stavudine** was given alone, although the incidence of diarrhoea did increase.[8]

(e) Zidovudine

A crossover study in 18 HIV+ subjects found that the pharmacokinetics of **ritonavir** 300 mg 6-hourly were unchanged when given with **zidovudine** 200 mg 8-hourly. However, the maximum plasma levels and AUC of the **zidovudine** were both reduced by about 25%. The lack of change in the other pharmacokinetic parameters suggested that these changes were not due to altered metabolism.[9] A study found that AUC of **zidovudine** was increased by 17% and that of **indinavir** by 13% when 200 mg **zidovudine** 8-hourly and 1 g **indinavir** 8-hourly were given together for a week.[7]

1. McDowell J, Sadler BM, Millard J, Nunnally P, Mustafa N. Evaluation of potential pharmacokinetic (PK) drug interaction between 141W94 and 1592U89 in HIV+ patients. *Intersci Conf Antimicrob Agents Chemother* (1997) 37, 13.
2. Crixivan (Indinavir). Merck Sharp & Dohme Limited. Summary of product characteristics, July 2001.
3. Shelton MJ, Mei H, Hewitt RG, Defrancesco R. If taken 1 hour before indinavir (IDV), didanosine does not affect IDV exposure, despite persistent buffering effects. *Antimicrob Agents Chemother* (2001) 45, 298–300.
4. Pedneault L, Elion R, Adler M, Anderson R, Kelleher T, Knupp C, Kaul S, Kerr B, Cross A, Dunkle L. Stavudine (d4T), didanosine (ddI), and nelfinavir combination therapy in HIV-infected subjects: antiviral effect and safety in an ongoing pilot study. 4th Conference on Retroviruses and Opportunistic Infections, Washington, 1997. Abstract 241.
5. Cato A, Qian J, Hsu A, Vomvouras S, Piergies AA, Leonard J, Granneman R. Pharmacokinetic interaction between ritonavir and didanosine when administered concurrently to HIV-infected patients. *J Acquir Immune Defic Syndr Hum Retrovirol* (1998) 18, 466–72.
6. Epivir (Lamivudine). Glaxo Wellcome. Summary of product characteristics, November 2001.
7. The Indinavir (MK 639) Pharmacokinetic Study Group. Indinavir (MK 639) drug interaction studies. 11th International Conference on AIDS, Vancouver, 1996. Abstract Mo.B.174.
8. Gathe J, Burkhardt B, Hawley P, Conant M, Peterkin J, Chapman S. A randomized phase II study of Viracept™, a novel HIV protease inhibitor, used in combination with stavudine (D4T) vs. stavudine (D4T) alone. 11th International Conference on AIDS, Vancouver, 1996. Abstract Mo.B.413.
9. Cato A, Qian J, Hsu A, Levy B, Leonard J, Granneman R. Multidose pharmacokinetics of ritonavir and zidovudine in human immunodeficiency virus-infected patients. *Antimicrob Agents Chemother* (1998) 42, 1788–93.

Nucleoside reverse transcriptase inhibitors + Ribavirin

In vitro **studies suggest that ribavirin may reduce the effects of stavudine. Ribavirin appears not to interact with didanosine.**

Clinical evidence, mechanism, importance and management

(a) Didanosine

Ribavirin 600 mg daily was given to 16 HIV+ patients who had already been taking 125 to 200 mg **didanosine** twice daily for 4 weeks. Over the 8 or 20 weeks of the study, no pharmacokinetic interaction was seen and the combination was well tolerated.[1] **Ribavirin** 6 or 10 mg/kg daily was given with **didanosine** 120 mg/m² 12-hourly to 11 HIV+ children (aged 3 months to 12 years) for 24 weeks. No significant changes were found in the pharmacokinetics of **didanosine**.[2] Information seems limited to these studies, but it appears that the combination can be safely administered.

(b) Stavudine

Nucleoside reverse transcriptase inhibitors such as **stavudine** need to be phosphorylated within cells to a triphosphate anabolite before they become effective. *In vitro* studies using mononucleated blood cells found that **ribavirin** interfered with phosphorylation at clinically relevant concentrations.[3] The clinical importance of this interaction awaits assessment.

1. Japour AJ, Lertora JJ, Meehan PM, Erice A, Connor JD, Griffith BP, Clax PA, Holden-Wiltse J, Hussey S, Walesky M, Cooney E, Pollard R, Timpone J, McLaren C, Johanneson N, Wood K, Booth DK, Bassiakos Y, Crumpacker CS. A phase-1 study of the safety, pharmacokinetics, and antiviral activity of combination didanosine and ribavirin in patients with HIV-1 disease. *J Acquir Immune Defic Syndr Hum Retrovirol* (1996) 13, 235–46.
2. Lertora JJL, Harrison M, Dreisbach AW, Van Dyke R. Lack of pharmacokinetic interaction between DDI and ribavirin in HIV infected children. *J Invest Med* (1999) 47, 106A.
3. Hoggard PG, Barry MG, Khoo SH, Back DJ. Drug interactions with d4T phosphorylation *in vitro*. *Br J Clin Pharmacol* (1996) 42, 278P.

Nucleoside reverse transcriptase inhibitors + Trimethoprim +/- Sulfamethoxazole

Co-trimoxazole reduces the loss of lamivudine, zalcitabine and zidovudine in the urine, and trimethoprim alone interacts with zalcitabine and zidovudine in the same way. However, the extent appears not to be clinically important and no increased lamivudine, zalcitabine or zidovudine toxicity would be expected. No significant adverse pharmacokinetic interaction occurs if didanosine is given with sulfamethoxazole or trimethoprim either separately or together.

Clinical evidence

(a) Didanosine

A study in 10 HIV+ subjects investigated the pharmacokinetics of **didanosine** 200 mg, **trimethoprim** 200 mg and **sulfamethoxazole** 1 g in combination. Most pharmacokinetic parameters were unchanged, however, **didanosine** clearance was reduced by 35%, **trimethoprim** clearance was decreased by 32% and **sulfamethoxazole** clearance was increased by 39%, when all 3 agents were co-administered. When only 2 of the 3 drugs were given, **trimethoprim** caused a 27% decrease in the clearance of **didanosine**, and **sulphamethoxazole** caused an 82% increase in the clearance of **sulphamethoxazole**.[1] Despite these alterations in clearance, the maximum serum concentration, AUC and half-life were minimally affected.[1]

(b) Lamivudine

In a study of 14 HIV+ patients taking **co-trimoxazole** 960 mg daily for 5 days, it was found that the AUC of a single dose of 300 mg **lamivudine** given on day 4 was increased by 43% and the renal clearance decreased 35%. The pharmacokinetics of the **trimethoprim** and the **sulfamethoxazole** were unaffected.[2]

(c) Zalcitabine

In a steady-state study, 8 HIV+ patients received 1.5 mg **zalcitabine** three times daily with and without 200 mg **trimethoprim** twice daily. The **trimethoprim** increased the AUC and decreased the clearance of the **zalcitabine** by about 35%.[3]

(d) Zidovudine

A study in 9 HIV+ patients given 3 mg/kg **zidovudine** by infusion over 1 h found that neither **trimethoprim** 150 mg nor **co-trimoxazole** 960 mg affected the metabolic clearance of the **zidovudine**. However, the renal clearances were reduced by 48 and 58% respectively, and of its glucuronide by 20 and 27% respectively.[4] Another study also found no changes in **zidovudine** pharmacokinetics.[5] Another 5 HIV+ patients showed a **zidovudine** AUC rise of 30% when also given **trimethoprim** (no dosage stated).[6] **Zidovudine** renal clearance was reduced by 58% in 8 HIV+ subjects when they were also given 200 mg **trimethoprim**, but the 6 h AUC of the **zidovudine** glucuronide/ **zidovudine** ratio was unchanged, suggesting that the metabolism was unaffected.[7]

Increases in the half-lives of **trimethoprim**, **sulfamethoxazole** and *N*-acetyl sulfamethoxazole of 72%, 39% and 115% respectively were seen when **co-trimoxazole** was given to 4 patients with AIDS taking **zidovudine** 250 mg 8-hourly for 8 days.[8]

A study of **zidovudine** use in 282 AIDS patients found that haematological abnormalities (anaemia, leucopenia, neutropenia) were common. However, the frequency was not increased in the patients (number unknown) also taking **co-trimoxazole**.[9]

Mechanism

A likely reason is that the trimethoprim inhibits the secretion of both zidovudine and its glucuronide by the kidney tubules. It is not known why the half-life of co-trimoxazole is increased. The other NRTIs that interact are likely to do so by the same mechanism.

Importance and management

Since renal clearance represents only 20-30% of the total clearance of zidovudine, the authors of two of these reports[1,5] suggest that this interaction is unlikely to be clinically important unless the glucuronidation by the liver is impaired by liver disease or other drugs. Similarly with the other NRTIs (e.g. lamivudine and zalcitabine) which are renally excreted, it is unlikely that dosage alterations are necessary unless the patient has a degree of renal impairment. However, the makers of lamivudine recommend that the co-administration of lamivudine and high dose co-trimoxazole for the treatment of *Pneumocystis carinii* pneumonia and toxoplasmosis should be avoided.[10]

In general dosage alterations are not necessary in normal renal or liver function, but concurrent use should be well monitored, especially because co-trimoxazole alone has been associated with a high incidence of adverse effects in patients with AIDS.[11]

1. Srinivas NR, Knupp CA, Batteiger B, Smith RA, Barbhaiya RH. A pharmacokinetic interaction study of didanosine coadministered with trimethoprim and/or sulphamethoxazole in HIV seropositive asymptomatic male patients. *Br J Clin Pharmacol* (1996) 41, 207–15.
2. Moore KHP, Yuen GJ, Raasch RH, Eron JJ, Martin D, Mydlow PK, Hussey EK. Pharmacokinetics of lamivudine administered alone and with trimethoprim-sulphamethoxazole. *Clin Pharmacol Ther* (1996) 59, 550–8.
3. Lee BL, Täuber MG, Chambers HF, Gambertoglio J, Delahunty T. The effect of trimethoprim (TMP) on the pharmacokinetics (PK) of zalcitabine (ddC) in HIV-infected patients. *Intersci Conf Antimicrob Agents Chemother* (1995) 35, 6.
4. Chatton JY, Munafo A, Chave JP, Steinhäuslin F, Roch-Ramel F, Glauser MP, Biollaz J. Trimethoprim, alone of in combination with sulphamethoxazole, decreases the renal excretion of zidovudine and its glucuronide. *Br J Clin Pharmacol* (1992) 34, 551–4.
5. Cañas E, Pachon J, Garcia-Pesquera F, Castillo JR, Viciana P, Cisneros JM, Jimenez-Mejias M. Absence of effect of trimethoprim-sulfamethoxazole on pharmacokinetics of zidovudine in patients infected with human immunodeficiency virus. *Antimicrob Agents Chemother* (1996) 40, 230–33.
6. Lee BL, Safrin S, Makrides V, Benowitz NL, Gambertoglio JG, Mills J. Trimethoprim decreases the renal clearance of zidovudine. *Clin Pharmacol Ther* (1992) 51,183.
7. Lee BL, Safrin S, Makrides V, Gambertoglio JG. Zidovudine, trimethoprim, and dapsone pharmacokinetic interactions in patients with human immunodeficiency virus infection. *Antimicrob Agents Chemother* (1996) 40, 1231–6.
8. Berson A, Happy K, Rousseau F, Grateau G, Farinotti R, Séréni D. Effect of zidovudine (AZT) on cotrimoxazole (TMP_SMX) kinetics: preliminary results. 9th International Conference on AIDS & 5th STD World Congress, Berlin, June 6-11 1993. Abstract PO-B30-2193.
9. Richman DD, Fischl MA, Grieco MH, Gottlieb MS, Volberding PA, Laskin OL, Leedom JM, Groopman JE, Mildvan D, Hirsch MS, Jackson GG, Durack DT, Nusinoff-Lehrman S and the AZT Collaborative Working Group. The toxicity of azidothymidine (AZT) in the treatment of patients with AIDS and AIDS-related complex. A double-blind, placebo-controlled trial. *N Engl J Med* (1987) 317, 192–7.
10. Epivir (Lamivudine). GlaxoWellcome. Summary of product characteristics, November 2001.
11. Medina I, Mills J, Leoung G, Hopefull PC, Lee B, Modin G, Benowitz N, Wofsy CB. Oral therapy for *Pneumocystis carinii* pneumonia in the acquired immunodeficiency syndrome: a controlled trial of trimethoprim-sulfamethoxazole versus trimethoprim-dapsone. *N Engl J Med* (1990) 323, 776–82.

Penicillins + Amiloride

Amiloride can cause a small, probably clinically unimportant, reduction in the absorption of amoxicillin.

Clinical evidence, mechanism, importance and management

When 8 healthy subjects were given 10 mg **amiloride**, followed 2 h later by a single 1 g oral dose of **amoxicillin**, the bioavailability and maximum serum levels of the **amoxicillin** were reduced by 27% and 25% respectively, and the time to reach maximum levels was delayed from 1 h to 1.56 h. When the **amoxicillin** was given intravenously its bioavailability was unchanged by the **amiloride**.[1] It is thought that the absorption of β-lactams like **amoxicillin** depends on a dipeptide carrier system in the cells (brush border membrane) lining the intestine. This system depends on the existence of a pH gradient between the outside and inside of the cells which is maintained by a Na-H exchanger. As this exchanger is inhibited by **amiloride** the reduced absorption would seem to be explained.

This reported reduction in the absorption of the **amoxicillin** is only small and unlikely to have very much clinical relevance, but this needs confirmation. To be on the safe side you should check that **amoxicillin** remains effective in the presence of **amiloride**. There seems to be no information about other **penicillins**.

1. Westphal JF, Jehl F, Brogard JM. Reduction of oral amoxicillin (AX) bioavailability by amiloride: role of the intestinal Na-H exchange in the dipeptide ß-lactam carrier system. *Clin Pharmacol Ther* (1995) 57, 144.

Penicillins + Antacids, Anticholinergics or H₂-blockers

Aluminium-magnesium hydroxide (*Maalox*), pirenzepine and ranitidine do not significantly affect the bioavailability of amoxicillin or amoxicillin-clavulanic acid.

Clinical evidence, mechanism, importance and management

Maalox (**aluminium magnesium hydroxide**, 10 doses of 10 ml), **pirenzepine** (50 mg for 4 doses) and **ranitidine** (150 mg for 3 doses) have only small and therapeutically unimportant effects on the pharmacokinetics of 1 g **amoxicillin** or 500 mg **amoxicillin**/125 mg **clavulanic acid**.[1] There would seem to be no reason for avoiding the concurrent use of any of these drugs.

1. Deppermann K-M, Lode H, Höffken G, Tschink G, Kalz C, Koeppe P. Influence of ranitidine, pirenzepine, and aluminium magnesium hydroxide on the bioavailability of various antibacterials, including amoxicillin, cephalexin, doxycycline, and amoxicillin-clavulanic acid. *Antimicrob Agents Chemother* (1989) 33, 1901–7.

Penicillins + Chloroquine

The absorption of ampicillin is reduced by the concurrent use of chloroquine, but bacampicillin is not affected.

Clinical evidence

Chloroquine 1 g reduced the absorption of single 1 g doses of oral **ampicillin** by about a third (from 29 to 19%) in 7 healthy subjects, as measured by its excretion in the urine.[1] Another study by the same author demonstrated that the absorption of **ampicillin** from **bacampicillin** tablets was unaffected by concurrent **chloroquine** administration.[2]

Mechanism

A possible reason is that the chloroquine irritates the gut so that the ampicillin is moved through more quickly, thereby reducing the time for absorption.

Importance and management

Information appears to be limited to the studies cited, which used large doses of chloroquine (1 g) when compared with those usually used for malarial prophylaxis (300 mg base weekly) or for rheumatic diseases (150 mg daily). The reduction in the ampicillin absorption is also only moderate (about a third). The general clinical importance of this interaction is therefore uncertain. However one report suggests separating the dosing by not less than 2 h.[1] An alternative would be to use bacampicillin (an ampicillin pro-drug) the bioavailability of which is not affected by chloroquine.[2] More study is needed to confirm and evaluate the importance of this interaction.

1. Ali HM. Reduced ampicillin bioavailability following oral coadministration with chloroquine. *J Antimicrob Chemother* (1985) 15, 781–4.
2. Ali HM. The effect of Sudanese food and chloroquine on the bioavailability of ampicillin from bacampicillin tablets. *Int J Pharmaceutics* (1981) 9, 185–90.

Penicillins + Dietary fibre

Dietary fibre can cause a small reduction the absorption of amoxicillin.

Clinical evidence, mechanism, importance and management

The AUC of single 500 mg oral doses of **amoxicillin** in 10 healthy subjects was found to be 12.17 micrograms/ml/h while on a **low fibre diet** (7.8 g of insoluble fibre daily) but only 9.65 micrograms/ml/h (about a 20% reduction) while on a **high fibre diet** (36.2 g of insoluble fibre daily). Peak serum levels were the same and occurred at 3 h. The subjects used were slum-dwellers in Santiago and the two diets represented the amounts of **fibre** normally eaten during the winter and summer seasons. A possible reason for the reduced absorption is that the **amoxicillin** becomes trapped within the **fibre**. The clinical importance of this interaction is uncertain but it is probably small. However in the absence of any more information it might be prudent to be alert for any evidence of a reduced response to **amoxicillin** in those who have a **high fibre diet**.[1]

1. Lutz M, Espinoza J, Arancibia A, Araya M, Pacheco I, Brunser O. Effect of structured dietary fiber on bioavailability of amoxicillin. *Clin Pharmacol Ther* (1987) 42, 220–4.

Penicillins + Guar gum

Guar gum causes a small reduction in the absorption of phenoxymethylpenicillin (penicillin V).

Clinical evidence, mechanism, importance and management

Guar gum 5 g (*Guarem*, **95% guar gum**) reduced the absorption of a single 1980 mg dose of **phenoxymethylpenicillin (penicillin V)** in 10 healthy subjects when taken together. Peak serum **penicillin** levels were reduced by 25% and the AUC (0 to 6 h) by 28%.[1] The reasons are not understood. The clinical significance of this interaction is uncertain, but the reduction in serum levels is only small. It would clearly only be important if the reduced amount of **penicillin** absorbed was inadequate to control infection, and for this reason the makers suggest giving **penicillin** an hour before the **guar gum** if it is important to establish maximum serum levels.[2] The effect of **guar gum** on other **penicillins** seems not to have been studied.

1. Huupponen R, Seppälä P, Iisalo E. Effect of guar gum, a fibre preparation, on digoxin and penicillin absorption in man. *Eur J Clin Pharmacol* (1984) 26, 279–81.
2. Guarem granules (Guar gum). Rybar Laboratories Limited. Summary of product characteristics, March 2001.

Penicillins + Miscellaneous drugs

Aspirin, indometacin, phenylbutazone, sulfaphenazole and sulfinpyrazone prolong the half-life of benzylpenicillin (penicillin G) significantly, whereas chlorothiazide, sulfamethizole and sulfamethoxypyridazine do not. These interactions do not seem to present any problems in practice. Some sulphonamides reduce oxacillin blood levels.

Clinical evidence, mechanism, importance and management

Studies in patients given different drugs for 5 to 7 days showed the following increases in the half-life of **benzylpenicillin (penicillin G)**: **aspirin** 63%; **indometacin** 22%; **phenylbutazone** 139%; **sulfaphenazole** 44%; **sulfinpyrazone** 65%. It seems likely that competition with these drugs and **benzylpenicillin** for excretion by the kidney tubules caused these changes. Changes in the half-life with **chlorothiazide**, **sulfamethizole** and **sulfamethoxypyridazine** were not significant.[1]

In healthy subjects, 3 g **sulfamethoxypyridazine** given 8 h before 1 g oral **oxacillin** reduced the 6 h urinary recovery by 55%. **Sulfaethidole** 3.9 g given 3 h before the **oxacillin** reduced the 6 h urinary recovery by 42%.[2]

None of the interactions listed appears to be adverse and some may be exploited. No particular precautions would seem necessary during concurrent use of these drugs and the penicillins, except to ensure that the levels of the antibacterial do not become excessive. The importance of the oxacillin-sulphonamide interaction is uncertain, but it can easily be avoided by choosing alternative drugs.

1. Kampmann J, Hansen JM, Siersboek-Nielsen K, Laursen H. Effect of some drugs on penicillin half-life in blood. *Clin Pharmacol Ther* (1972) 13, 516–19.
2. Kunin CM. Clinical pharmacology of the new penicillins. II. Effect of drugs which interfere with binding to serum proteins. *Clin Pharmacol Ther* (1966) 7, 180–88.

Penicillins + Probenecid

Probenecid reduces the excretion of the penicillins.

Clinical evidence

(a) Amoxicillin

Amoxicillin 3 g twice daily plus placebo, **amoxicillin** 1 g plus **probenecid** 1 g, both twice daily and **amoxicillin** 1 g twice daily plus **probenecid** 500 mg four times daily were given to 6 patients to treat bronchiectasis. The maximum serum concentration and half-life of both high- and low-dose **amoxicillin** were similar, but in the regimens containing **probenecid** the clearance of **amoxicillin** dropped to one-third of the level of that seen with **amoxicillin** alone.[1]

(b) Nafcillin

A study in 5 healthy subjects given 500 mg intravenous **nafcillin sodium** with **probenecid** (1 g given orally the previous night and 2 h prior to the antibacterial) showed that the urinary recovery of **nafcillin** dropped from 30% to 17% and the AUC was approximately doubled.[2]

(c) Piperacillin/Tazobactam

Probenecid 1g given 1 h prior to a single infusion of **piperacillin** 3 g/**tazobactam** 0.375 g to 10 healthy volunteers caused about a 25% decrease in the clearance of both components. The half-life of **tazobactam** was also increased, by 72%.[3]

(d) Ticarcillin

Probenecid, either 500 mg twice daily or 1 g daily or 2 g daily was added to **ticarcillin** 3 g four-hourly which was being given to treat infections in adult cystic fibrosis patients. In all cases the clearance of **ticarcillin** was reduced; to 72.7% with the 500-mg dose regimen, 67.5% with the 1 g dose regimen and 57.3% with the 2 g dose regimen.[4]

Mechanism

In each case the penicillin competes with the probenecid for excretion by the kidney tubules, although with the nafcillin, non-renal clearance may also play a part.

Importance and management

In the case of amoxicillin, nafcillin and ticarcillin the effects are of clinical significance and can be exploited to enable dose reductions. However, with the older penicillins available as generics concurrent use of probenecid is no longer as cost effective as it used to be. In the case of the ticarcillin study the authors suggest that a 12-hourly dosing regimen could be used if probenecid is given concurrently, which has implications for home treatment. With piperacillin/tazobactam the changes were not thought to provide any benefit in terms of dose reduction or alteration of the dosage interval.

1. Allen MB, Fitzpatrick RW, Barratt A, Cole RB. The use of probenecid to increase the serum amoxycillin levels in patients with bronchiectasis. *Respir Med* (1990) 84, 143–6.
2. Waller ES, Sharanevych MA, Yakatan GJ. The effect of probenecid on nafcillin disposition. *J Clin Pharmacol* (1982) 22, 482–9.
3. Ganes D, Batra V, Faulkner R, Greene D, Haynes J, Kuye O, Ruffner A, Shin K, Tonelli A, Yacobi A. Effect of probenecid on the pharmacokinetics of piperacillin and tazobactam in healthy volunteers. *Pharm Res* (1991) 8 (10 Suppl), S-299.
4. Corvaia L, Li SC, Ioannides-Demos LL, Bowes G, Spicer WJ, Spelman DW, Tong N, McLean AJ. A prospective study of the effects of oral probenecid on the pharmacokinetics of intravenous ticarcillin in patients with cystic fibrosis. *J Antimicrob Chemother* (1992) 30, 875–8.

Penicillins + Tetracyclines

Tetracyclines can reduce the effectiveness of penicillins in the treatment of pneumococcal meningitis and probably scarlet fever. It is uncertain whether a similar interaction occurs with other infections. It may possibly only be important with those infections where a rapid kill is essential.

Clinical evidence

When **chlortetracycline** originally became available it was tested as a potential treatment for meningitis. In patients with pneumococcal meningitis it was shown that **penicillin** alone (one million units, intramuscularly every 2 h) was more effective than the same regimen of **penicillin**, with **chlortetracycline** (500 mg intravenously every 6 h). Out of 43 patients given **penicillin** alone, 70% recovered compared with only 20% in another group of 14 essentially similar patients who had had both antibacterials.[1]

Another report about the treatment of pneumococcal meningitis with **penicillin** and **tetracyclines** (**chlortetracycline**, **oxytetracycline**, **tetracycline**) confirmed that the mortality was much lower in those given only **penicillin**, rather than the combination of **penicillin** and a **tetracycline**.[2] In the treatment of scarlet fever (Group A beta-haemolytic streptococci), no difference was seen in the initial response to treatment with **penicillin** and **tetracycline** or **penicillin** alone, but spontaneous re-infection occurred more frequently in those who had received **penicillin** and **chlortetracycline**.[3]

Mechanism

The generally accepted explanation is that bactericides, such as penicillin which inhibits bacterial cell wall synthesis, require cells to be actively growing and dividing to be maximally effective, a situation that will not occur in the presence of bacteriostatic antibacterials such as the tetracyclines.

Importance and management

An established and important interaction when treating pneumococcal meningitis, and probably scarlet fever as well. The documentation seems to be limited to the reports cited. Concurrent use should be avoided in these infections, but the importance of this interaction with other infections is uncertain. It has not been shown to occur when treating pneumococcal pneumonia.[4] It has been suggested that antagonism, if it occurs, may only be significant when it is essential to kill bacteria rapidly,[4] i.e. in serious infections such as meningitis. The antibacterials implicated in the interaction are penicillin, tetracycline, chlortetracycline and oxytetracycline, but any penicillin and any tetracycline would be expected to behave similarly.

1. Lepper MH, Dowling HF. Treatment of pneumococcic meningitis with penicillin compared with penicillin plus aureomycin: studies including observations on an apparent antagonism between penicillin and aureomycin. *Arch Intern Med* (1951) 88, 489–94.
2. Olsson RA, Kirby JC, Romansky MJ. Pneumococcal meningitis in the adult. Clinical, therapeutic and prognostic aspects in forty-three patients. *Ann Intern Med* (1961) 55, 545–9.
3. Strom J. The question of antagonism between penicillin and chlortetracycline, illustrated by therapeutical experiments in Scarlatina. *Antibiot Med* (1955) 1,6–12.
4. Ahern JJ, Kirby WMM. Lack of interference of aureomycin in treatment of pneumoccic pneumonia. *Arch Intern Med* (1953) 91, 197–203.

Penicillins + Vancomycin

Vancomycin does not interact to a clinically relevant extent with piperacillin/tazobactam.

Clinical evidence, mechanism, importance and management

A three-way, randomised crossover study in 9 healthy subjects found that infusions of 500 mg **vancomycin** with 3 g **piperacillin**/0.375 g **tazobactam** had little or no effect on the pharmacokinetics of any of the antibacterials, except that the **piperacillin** AUC was slightly raised by about 7%. It was concluded that no dosage adjustments are needed if these drugs are given together.[1]

1. Vechlekar D, Sia L, Lanc R, Kuye O, Yacobi A, Faulkner R. Pharmacokinetics of piperacillin/tazobactam (Pip/Taz) IV with and without vancomycin IV in healthy adult male volunteers. *Pharm Res* (1992) 9 (10 Suppl), S-322.

Piperazine + Phenothiazines

An isolated case of convulsions in a child was attributed to the use of chlorpromazine following piperazine.

Clinical evidence, mechanism, importance and management

A child given piperazine for pin worms developed convulsions when treated with **chlorpromazine** several days later.[1] In a subsequent *animal* study using 4.5 or 10 mg/kg **chlorpromazine**, many of the *animals* died from respiratory arrest after severe clonic convulsions.[1] However a later study failed to confirm these findings[2] and it is by no means certain whether the adverse reaction in the child was due to an interaction or not. Given that both drugs may cause convulsions, there is probably enough evidence to warrant caution if these drugs are used concurrently.

1. Boulos BM, Davis LE. Hazard of simultaneous administration of phenothiazine and piperazine. *N Engl J Med* (1969) 280, 1245–6.
2. Armbrecht BH. Reaction between piperazine and chlorpromazine. *N Engl J Med* (1970) 282, 1490–1.

Pivampicillin + Miscellaneous drugs

On theoretical grounds the makers of pivampicillin advise the avoidance of sodium valproate because of the increased risk of carnitine deficiency. Their warning about a potential pivampicillin/antacid interaction is probably no longer needed.

Clinical evidence, mechanism, importance and management

Pivampicillin is a prodrug of ampicillin with a higher absorption than the parent drug which, following absorption, is hydrolysed to release ampicillin, pivalic acid and formaldehyde. One of the potential prob-

lems is that the pivalic acid can react with carnitine to form pivaloyl-carnitine, which is excreted in the urine, and so the body can become depleted of carnitine. Carnitine is essential for fatty acid transport through the mitochondrial membrane and is needed for energy production in skeletal and cardiac muscle which depend on fatty acid oxidation, so that carnitine deficiency is seen as muscle weakness and cardiomyopathy.

The risks of carnitine deficiency due to pivampicillin (or pivmecillinam which similarly releases pivalic acid) seem to be small in normal adults, but the makers of pivampicillin issue a warning about long-term or frequently repeated treatment.[1] They also advise the avoidance of **valproic acid** or **valproate**[1] because they too can cause an increased carnitine loss from the body (for reasons which are not well understood).[2] However, there seem to be no reports of carnitine deficiency in patients which have resulted from the additive effects of pivampicillin and **valproic acid** or **valproate**, so that the risk as yet appears to be only theoretical.

The makers drug datasheet[1] says that "**antacid** therapy with *Pondocillin* [pivampicillin] is not recommended, since it reduces absorption of the antibacterial, and may cause underdosing." This warning in fact relates to a hydrochloride salt formulation, which needs acidic conditions for optimal absorption, whereas the basic salt formulation should not be affected by any pH change.[3]

1. Pondocillin (Pivampicillin). Leo Laboratories Ltd. ABPI Compendium of Datasheets and Summaries of Product Characteristics, 1998–99, 625–6.
2. Melegh B, Kerner J, Jaszai V, Bieber LL. Differential excretion of xenobiotic acyl-esters of carnitine due to administration of pivampicillin and valproate. *Biochem Med Metab Biol* (1990) 43, 30–8.
3. Leo Laboratories Limited. Personal communication, March 1995.

Praziquantel + Albendazole or Food

Food, but not albendazole increases the bioavailability of praziquantel. Both food and praziquantel markedly increase the bioavailability of albendazole. None of these changes appears to have adverse consequences.

Clinical evidence, mechanism, importance and management

A study in 9 healthy Sudanese men, of the possible pharmacokinetic changes which might occur during the concurrent use of praziquantel, **albendazole** and **food,** found that **albendazole** did not affect the pharmacokinetics of praziquantel. However, when praziquantel was given with **food** the AUC was increased 2.6-fold.

The pharmacokinetics of the **albendazole** were most affected. The AUC of the active metabolite of **albendazole** (**albendazole sulphoxide**) increased 4.5-fold when given with praziquantel, eightfold when given with **food**, and twelvefold when given with both **food** and praziquantel. The reasons for these changes and their practical consequences are not known, but the marked increases in **albendazole sulphoxide** levels seemed not to cause any problems.[1] On the basis of this study there do not seem to be any obvious reasons why the concurrent use of these two drugs should be avoided, but good monitoring is advisable.

1. Homeida M, Leahy W, Copeland S, Ali MMM, Harron DWG. Pharmacokinetic interaction between praziquantel and albendazole in Sudanese men. *Ann Trop Med Parasitol* (1994) 88, 551–9.

Praziquantel + Anticonvulsants and/or Cimetidine

Phenytoin and carbamazepine markedly reduce the serum levels of praziquantel. Neurocysticercosis treatment failures may occur as a result. A case report suggests that the addition of cimetidine may control this interaction, and cimetidine alone can double the serum levels of praziquantel.

Clinical evidence, mechanism, importance and management

(a) Praziquantel + Carbamazepine or Phenytoin

A comparative study of patients on chronic anticonvulsant treatment with **phenytoin**, or **carbamazepine**, and healthy subjects (10 in each group) given single oral doses of 25 mg/kg praziquantel, found that **phenytoin** and **carbamazepine** reduced the AUC of the praziquantel to 26% and 9.7% of the controls, and the maximum serum levels to 24% and 7.9% of the controls respectively.[1,2]

(b) Praziquantel + Cimetidine

A randomised crossover study in 8 healthy subjects given three oral doses of 25 mg/kg praziquantel at 2-hourly intervals found that 400 mg **cimetidine** approximately doubled the praziquantel serum levels and AUC when given 1 h before each dose of praziquantel.[3,4]

(c) Praziquantel + Phenytoin/Phenobarbital + Cimetidine

A patient with neurocysticercosis taking **phenytoin** and **phenobarbital** for a seizure disorder and also on **dexamethasone**, repeatedly failed to respond to praziquantel until 1600 mg **cimetidine** daily was added. His serum praziquantel levels then more than doubled (maximum serum levels raised from 350 to 826 ng/ml) and the AUC rose from 754 to 3050 ng.h/ml, and became similar to that found in normal controls taking praziquantel alone. The patient responded to the praziquantel but only slowly.[5]

Mechanism

Not established, but the probable reason is that these anticonvulsants (potent enzyme inducers) and dexamethasone (see 'Praziquantel or Albendazole + Corticosteroids', p.194) can increase the metabolism and loss of praziquantel by the liver, thereby hastening its loss from the body. The cimetidine (a potent enzyme inhibitor) appears to oppose this effect by inhibiting the liver enzymes concerned with the metabolism of the praziquantel.

Importance and management

Direct information appears to be limited to the reports cited, but the interactions appear to be established. When treating neurocysticercosis some authors advise increasing the praziquantel dosage from 25 to 50 mg/kg, if potent enzyme inducers such as carbamazepine or phenytoin are being used, in order to reduce the risk of treatment failure.[1] An alternative might be to add cimetidine, however the authors of another study[5] were not sure whether the improvement they saw was in fact due to the cimetidine or simply "part of the natural history of this disease." However it is clear that cimetidine alone can markedly increase praziquantel levels, and the authors say that concurrent use can reduce treatment for neurocysticercosis from 2 weeks to 1 day.[3]

1. Bittencourt PRM, Gracia CM, Martins R, Fernandes AG, Diekmann HW, Jung W. Phenytoin and carbamazepine decrease oral bioavailability of praziquantel. *Neurology* (1992) 42, 492–6.
2. Bittencourt PRM, Gracia CM, Martins R, Fernandes AG. Praziquantel is almost inactivated by carbamazepine and phenytoin. *Epilepsia* (1991) 32 (Suppl 1), 104.
3. Jung H, Medina R, Castro N, Corona T, Sotelo J. Pharmacokinetic study of praziquantel administered alone and in combination with cimetidine in a single-day therapeutic regimen. *Antimicrob Agents Chemother* (1997) 41, 1256–9.
4. Castro N, Gonzàlez-Esquivel D, Medina R, Sotelo J, Jung H. The influence of cimetidine on plasma levels of praziquantel after a single day therapeutic regimen. *Proc West Pharmacol Soc* (1997) 40, 33–4.
5. Dachman WD, Adubofour KO, Bikin DS, Johnson CH, Mullin PD, Winograd M. Cimetidine-induced rise in praziquantel levels in a patient with neurocysticercosis being treated with anticonvulsants. *J Infect Dis* (1994) 169, 689–91.

Praziquantel + Chloroquine

Chloroquine reduces the bioavailability of praziquantel which would be expected to reduce its anti-schistosomal effects.

Clinical evidence, mechanism, importance and management

Single 40 mg/kg oral doses of praziquantel were given to 8 healthy subjects alone, and 2 h after 600 mg **chloroquine**. The chloroquine reduced the praziquantel AUC by 65% and the maximum serum levels by 59%. The reasons are not understood. There were large individual variations and one subject was not affected. The effect of this interaction could be that some patients will not achieve high enough serum praziquantel levels to destroy schistosomes. After taking the **chloroquine**, the praziquantel serum levels of 4 out of the 8 subjects failed to reach the threshold of about 0.3 micrograms/ml for about 6 h (which is required to effectively kill schistosomes), compared with only 2 of 8 during the control period. The authors conclude that an increased dosage of praziquantel should be considered if **chloroquine** is given (they do not suggest how much), particularly in anyone who does not respond to initial treatment with praziquantel.[1] More study of this interaction is needed.

1. Masimirembwa CM, Naik YS, Hasler JA. The effect of chloroquine on the pharmacokinetics and metabolism of praziquantel in rats and in humans. *Biopharm Drug Dispos* (1994) 15, 33–43.

Praziquantel or Albendazole + Corticosteroids

The continuous use of dexamethasone can reduce serum praziquantel levels by 50%, but it can raise those of albendazole by 50%.

Clinical evidence

Eight patients with parenchymal brain cysticercosis treated with **praziquantel** (50 mg/kg divided into three doses 8-hourly) showed a 50% reduction in steady-state serum levels (from 3.13 to 1.55 micrograms/ml) when given 8 mg **dexamethasone** 8-hourly.[1] In a further study by the same authors, an alternative cysticidal **albendazole** was given to 8 similar patients. The plasma levels of **albendazole** (15 mg/kg daily in three divided doses) were found to be increased by about 50% by the use of 8 mg **dexamethasone** 8-hourly.[2] Another study did not detect significantly increased plasma levels of the active metabolite of **albendazole** (**albendazole sulfoxide**), but it did note a decrease in its clearance.[3]

Mechanism

Not understood.

Importance and management

Information about praziquantel and albendazole seems to be limited to this study[1] but the interaction would appear to be established. Just how much it affects the outcome of treatment for cysticercosis is unknown because the optimum praziquantel and albendazole levels are still uncertain. The authors of the reports suggest that dexamethasone should not be given continuously with praziquantel but only used transiently for the treatment of inflammatory reactions to praziquantel treatment. Conversely it would appear that albendazole can be given concurrently with dexamethasone without compromising treatment. There seems to be no information about these drugs with other corticosteroids.

1. Vazquez ML, Jung H, Sotelo J. Plasma levels of praziquantel decrease when dexamethasone is given simultaneously. *Neurology* (1987) 37, 1561–2.
2. Jung H, Hurtado M, Tulio Medina M, Sanchez M, Sotelo J. Dexamethasone increases plasma levels of albendazole. *J Neurol* (1990) 237, 279–80.
3. Takayanagui OM, Lanchote VL, Marques MPC, Bonato PS. Therapy for neurocysticercosis: pharmacokinetic interaction of albendazole sulfoxide with dexamethasone. *Ther Drug Monit* (1997) 19, 51–5.

Primaquine or Pamaquine + Mepacrine (Quinacrine)

Pamaquine elevates serum levels of mepacrine. Theoretically primaquine would be expected to interact similarly, but there are do not seem to be any reports confirming or disproving this.

Clinical evidence, mechanism, importance and management

Patients given **pamaquine**, a predecessor of primaquine almost identical in structure, showed grossly elevated serum levels when concurrently treated with **mepacrine**.[1,2] The probable reason is that the **mepacrine** occupies binding sites in the body normally also used by the **pamaquine** and, as a result, the serum levels become very high. On theoretical grounds **primaquine** might be expected to interact with **mepacrine** similarly, but there seem to be no reports confirming that a clinically important interaction actually takes place.

1. Zubrod CG, Kennedy TJ, Shannon JA. Studies on the chemotherapy of the human malarias. VIII. The physiological disposition of pamaquine. *J Clin Invest* (1948) 27 (Suppl), 114–120.
2. Earle DP, Bigelow FS, Zubrod CG, Kane CA. Studies on the chemotherapy of the human malarias. IX. Effect of pamaquine on the blood cells of man. *J Clin Invest* (1948) 27, (Suppl), 121–9.

Proguanil + Cimetidine or Omeprazole

There is some evidence that omeprazole and cimetidine can moderately reduce the production of the active metabolite of proguanil, but the clinical relevance of this is unknown.

Clinical evidence

In one study, 4 patients with peptic ulcer disease (PUD) and 6 healthy subjects were given a single 200-mg dose of proguanil on the last day of a 3-day course of **cimetidine** 400 mg twice daily. In both groups the half-life and AUC of proguanil were significantly increased, but only the healthy subjects showed an increase in the maximum serum concentration (89%). In both groups these pharmacokinetic changes resulted in lower levels of the active metabolite, cycloguanil.[1] This decrease in cycloguanil supported an earlier study, which had found a 30% decrease in the urinary recovery of cycloguanil when proguanil and **cimetidine** were given concurrently.[2]

In a steady-state study in 12 healthy subjects taking 200 mg proguanil daily it was found that 20 mg **omeprazole** daily approximately halved the AUC of the active metabolite, cycloguanil.[2] Another study however failed to detect any effect of 20 mg **omeprazole** on the urinary recovery of cycloguanil (or proguanil) following a single dose of 200 mg proguanil.[3]

Mechanism

Cimetidine and omeprazole increase the gastric pH, which may lead to an increase in the absorption of proguanil. Cimetidine[1] and omeprazole[3] are also thought to inhibit the metabolism of proguanil, due to their effects on cytochrome P450.

Importance and management

The differences between the healthy subjects and patients with PUD seen in one study may have been because the PUD modulated the effects of the cimetidine in some way.[1] Patients with PUD are also likely to have an increased gastric pH, which will lead to altered proguanil absorption. The clinical relevance of all these findings is still unclear, although the implication is that decreased cycloguanil

levels may lead to inadequate malaria prophylaxis. More study is needed.

1. Kolawole JA, Mustapha A, Abdul-Aguye I, Ochekpe N, Taylor RB. Effects of cimetidine on the pharmacokinetics of proguanil in healthy subjects and in peptic ulcer patients. *J Pharm Biomed Anal* (1999) 20, 737–43.
2. Funck-Bretano C, Becquemont L, Leneveu A, Roux A, Jaillon P, Beaune P. Inhibition by omeprazole of proguanil metabolism: mechanism of the interaction *in vitro* and prediction of *in vivo* results from the *in vitro* experiments. *J Pharmacol Exp Ther* (1997) 280, 730–8.
3. Somogyi AA, Reinhard HA, Bochner F. Effects of omeprazole and cimetidine on the urinary metabolic ratio of proguanil in healthy volunteers. *Eur J Clin Pharmacol* (1996) 50, 417–19.

Proguanil + Fluvoxamine

Proguanil fails to be converted in the body to its active metabolite in 'fast metabolisers' if fluvoxamine is being taken concurrently.

Clinical evidence

Twelve healthy subjects, 6 of whom were extensive metabolisers (i.e. who had cytochrome P450 isoenzyme CYP2C19) and 6 were poor metabolisers (i.e. lacking CYP2C19 isoenzyme), were given 200 mg proguanil daily for 8 days. This was followed by a course of 100 mg **fluvoxamine** for 8 days, to which a single 200-mg dose of proguanil was added, on day 6.

In the group of extensive metabolisers it was found that the **fluvoxamine** reduced the total clearance of the proguanil by about 40%. The partial clearance of proguanil via its two metabolites was reduced, by 85% for cycloguanil and by 89% for 4-chlorophenylbiguanide. The concentrations of these two metabolites in the plasma were hardly detectable while **fluvoxamine** was being taken. No interaction occurred in the poor metabolisers.[1]

Mechanism

Proguanil, which is a prodrug, is metabolised to its active metabolite, cycloguanil, in the body by the activity of CYP2C19. This cytochrome P450 isoenzyme is inhibited by fluvoxamine in fast metabolisers so that the proguanil fails to become activated.[2]

Importance and management

Information appears to be limited to the studies cited, the purpose of which was to confirm that fluvoxamine is an inhibitor of cytochrome P450 isoenzyme CYP2C19. However, they also demonstrate that proguanil, which is prodrug, will not be effectively converted into its active form in patients who are extensive metabolisers, if fluvoxamine is being taken concurrently. There are as yet no reports of treatment failures due to this interaction, but the activity of proguanil is expected to be virtually abolished if fluvoxamine is taken concurrently. The authors recommend that the two drugs should not be taken together.[2] More study is needed.

1. Jeppesen U, Rasmussen BB, Brøsen K. The CYP2C19 catalyzed bioactivation of proguanil is abolished during fluvoxamine intake. *Eur J Clin Pharmacol* (1997) 52 (Suppl), A134.
2. Rasmussen BB, Nielsen TL, Brøsen K. Fluvoxamine inhibits the CYP2C19-catalysed metabolism of proguanil in vitro. *Eur J Clin Pharmacol* (1998) 54, 735–40.

Proguanil + Other antimalarials

Chloroquine appears to almost double the incidence of mouth ulcers among those taking proguanil prophylactically and atovaquone appears to have a non-significant effect on the pharmacokinetics of proguanil.

Clinical evidence, mechanism, importance and management

(a) Atovaquone

Atovaquone did not affect the pharmacokinetics of proguanil in a comparative study of 4 patients taking proguanil 200 mg twice daily for 3 days and 12 patients taking proguanil 200 mg twice daily plus **atovaquone** 500 mg twice daily for 3 days.[1] Similar results were seen in 18 healthy subjects given proguanil 400 mg daily with **atovaquone** 1 g daily for 3 days.[2]

(b) Chloroquine

Following the observation that mouth ulcers appeared to be common amongst those taking prophylactic antimalarials, an extensive study was undertaken in 628 servicemen in Belize. Of those on 200 mg proguanil daily, 24% developed mouth ulcers, and in those additionally taking 150 to 300 mg **chloroquine** base weekly 37% developed mouth ulcers. The incidence of diarrhoea was also increased from 63% among those who did not develop ulcers to 83% in those that did develop ulcers (any treatment). The reasons are not understood. The authors of the study suggest that these two drugs should not be given together unnecessarily for prophylaxis against *Plasmodium falciparum*.[3]

1. Edstein MD, Looareesuwan S, Viravan C, Kyle DE. Pharmacokinetics of proguanil in malaria patients treated with proguanil plus atovaquone. *Southeast Asian J Trop Med Public Health* (1996) 27, 216–20.
2. Gillotin C, Mamet JP, Veronese L. Lack of pharmacokinetic interaction between atovaquone and proguanil. *Eur J Clin Pharmacol* (1999) 55, 311–15.
3. Drysdale SF, Phillips-Howard PA, Behrens RH. Proguanil, chloroquine, and mouth ulcers. *Lancet* (1990) 1, 164.

Protease Inhibitors + Anticonvulsants

Case reports suggests that ritonavir increases carbamazepine levels, carbamazepine reduces indinavir levels, nelfinavir reduces phenytoin levels and phenytoin induces the metabolism of indinavir. Carbamazepine or phenytoin should be used with caution in combination with protease inhibitors.

Clinical evidence, mechanism, importance and management

(a) Carbamazepine

An epileptic, HIV+ man of 20 years, who had his seizures controlled with **carbamazepine** 350 mg twice daily and zonisamide 140 mg twice daily was admitted to hospital for review of his antiretrovirals. He was to be started on **ritonavir** 200 mg three times daily, but when he was given the first dose of **ritonavir** his serum **carbamazepine** levels rose from 9.8 to 17.8 micrograms/ml. This was accompanied by intractable vomiting and vertigo, so after 2 days the **ritonavir** was stopped. Symptoms resolved over the next few days. Subsequently **ritonavir** 200 mg daily was started, with the same effect, so the dose of **carbamazepine** was reduced to one third, which resulted in carbamazepine levels of 6.2 micrograms/ml. Levels of **ritonavir** were not measured.[1] Another report describes the case of a man of 48 years whose antiretroviral therapy (**indinavir** 800 mg 8-hourly, lamivudine 150 mg twice daily and zidovudine 200 mg three times daily) became ineffective after a two and a half month course of **carbamazepine** for post-herpetic neuralgia. Over this time **indinavir** levels were up to 16 times lower than those measured in the absence of **carbamazepine**. Despite a low **carbamazepine** dose of 200 mg daily, the levels reached the therapeutic range for epilepsy.[2] A further report describes an HIV+ man whose viral load became undetectable after treatment with indinavir, zidovudine and lamivudine but, when later treated with **carbamazepine** for postherpetic neuralgia, his plasma indinavir levels fell markedly and his antiretroviral therapy failed.[3] Patients given indinavir and any of these enzyme inducing drugs should therefore be closely monitored. The authors of one report suggest that amitriptyline or gabapentin would be possible alternatives for **carbamazepine** used for pain, or valproic acid or lamotrigine for carbamazepine used for seizures.[3]

In all of these cases the **carbamazepine** levels were dramatically raised by the protease inhibitor and in the second the protease inhibitor levels became subtherapeutic, probably due to altered metabolism by the cytochrome P450 isoenzyme CYP3A. It would therefore appear that the combination of these drugs should be avoided where possible, but if both must be used then extremely close monitoring is warranted. In their summaries of product characteristics the makers of **indinavir**,[4] **lopinavir**,[5] **nelfinavir**[6] and **saquinavir**[7] all predict that protease inhibitor levels will be reduced on concurrent administration, whilst the makers of **amprenavir**[8] and **ritonavir**[9] predict that the protease inhibitor will increase **carbamazepine** levels.

(b) Phenobarbital

In the Summaries of Product Characteristics the makers of **indinavir**,[4] **lopinavir**,[5] **nelfinavir**[6] and **saquinavir**[7] all predict that protease inhibitor levels will be reduced on concurrent administration of **phenobarbital**, although this awaits confirmation in clinical practice.

(c) Phenytoin

An HIV+ man taking **phenytoin** and phenobarbital for epilepsy had been on **nelfinavir** 750 mg three times daily and stavudine 30 mg twice daily for nearly 3 months when he had a tonic-clonic seizure. After starting **nelfinavir** and stavudine serum **phenytoin** levels were found to have dropped from around 10 mg/l to around 5 mg/l.[10] An HIV+ man of 39 years, already on **phenytoin** 300 mg daily was started on **indinavir** 800 mg three times daily. When the **phenytoin** dose was reduced to 200 mg daily, the viral load dropped by almost half and his CD4+ count doubled.[11] A case report describes the intentional use of **ritonavir** 600 mg twice daily in a boy of 14 who had been having seizures of 28 days, despite the use of several anticonvulsants. **Phenytoin** at 20 mg/kg daily failed to produce satisfactory plasma levels, although it did reduce the rate of seizures. After starting the **ritonavir** his seizures were controlled and the **phenytoin** level became therapeutic. However, seizures started again after the **ritonavir** was stopped.[12] Although the combination may sometimes be useful, it would therefore seem that an alternative agent, such as sodium valproate, which does not affect the cytochrome P450 isoenzyme CYP3A may be more appropriate in patients on protease inhibitors. However, if there is no option but to use **phenytoin** close monitoring is essential. In the summaries of product characteristics the makers of **indinavir**,[4] **lopinavir**,[5] **nelfinavir**[6] and **saquinavir**[7] all predict that protease inhibitor levels will be reduced on concurrent administration of **phenytoin**.

1. Kato Y, Fujii T, Mizoguchi N, Takata N, Ueda K, Feldman MD, Kayser SR. Potential interaction between ritonavir and carbamazepine. *Pharmacotherapy* (2000) 20, 851–4.
2. Hugen PWH, Burger DM, Brinkman K, ter Hofstede HJM, Schuurman R, Koopmans PP, Hekster YA. Carbamazepine-indinavir interaction causes antiretroviral therapy failure. *Ann Pharmacother* (2000) 34, 465–70.
3. Hugen PWH, Burger DM, Brinkman K, ter Hofstede HJM, Schuurman R, Koopmans PP, Hekster YA. Carbamazepine-indinavir causes anteretroviral therapy failure. *Ann Pharmacother* (2000) 34, 465–70.
4. Crixivan (Indinavir). Merck Sharp & Dohme Limited. Summary of product characteristics, July 2001.
5. Kaletra Soft Capsules (Lopinavir). Abbott Laboratories Limited. Summary of product characteristics, March 2001.
6. Viracept (Nelfinavir). Roche Product Limited. Summary of product characteristics, October 2001.
7. Fortovase (Saquinavir). Roche Products Limited. Summary of product characteristics, January 2001.
8. Agenerase (Amprenavir). Glaxo Wellcome. Summary of product characteristics, October 2001.
9. Norvir (Ritonavir). Abbott Laboratories Limited. Summary of product characteristics, January 2001.
10. Honda M, Yasuoka A, Aoki M, Oka S. A generalized seizure following initiation of nelfinavir in a patient with human immunodeficiency virus type 1 infection, suspected due to interaction between nelfinavir and phenytoin. *Intern Med* (1999) 38, 302–3.
11. Campagna KD, Torbert A, Bedsole GD, Ravis WR. Possible induction of indinavir metabolism by phenytoin. *Pharmacotherapy* (1997) 17, 182.
12. Broderick A, Webb DW, McMenamin J, Butler K. A novel use of ritonavir. *AIDS* (1998) 12 (Suppl 12), S29.

Protease Inhibitors + Antidepressants

Fluoxetine raises levels of ritonavir. Ritonavir raises desipramine levels and is predicted to also raise the levels of other tricyclic antidepressants. A lower starting dose of desipramine is suggested and monitoring is advisable. In a

single dose study venlafaxine lowers indinavir levels, which may affect treatment.

Clinical evidence, mechanism, importance and management

(a) SSRIs

Ritonavir 600 mg was given to 16 healthy subjects before and after 8 days treatment with fluoxetine 30 mg twice daily. The maximum serum levels of ritonavir were unaffected, but the AUC rose by 19%. These changes were not considered large enough to warrant changing the dose of ritonavir.[1] The study was criticised for not achieving steady state before assessing the pharmacokinetics and thus possibly underestimating the interaction.[2] However, the authors point out that fluoxetine levels were equivalent to those seen at steady state, and multiple dosing of ritonavir is likely to induce its own metabolism, so if anything, the interaction would be lessened at steady state.[3]

The makers of ritonavir predict that the levels of other SSRIs (paroxetine, sertraline) will also be elevated[4] (not investigated in the study quoted) although nothing appears to be documented about this effect in clinical practice.

(b) Tricyclic antidepressants

A single dose of desipramine 100 mg was given to 14 healthy subjects before and after 10 days of ritonavir 500 mg twice daily. The AUC and half-life of desipramine increased nearly 2.5-fold and two-fold respectively. The maximum serum levels were also increased by 22.1%. These changes are considered to be clinically significant, so the authors suggest that a lower initial dose of desipramine should be used if it is to be started in patients on ritonavir, and careful monitoring should be carried out in the first few weeks of treatment.[5] These effects are likely to be due to the strong enzyme inhibitory effects of ritonavir. Because of this, the makers of ritonavir also predict that the levels of other tricyclic antidepressants (e.g. amitriptyline, imipramine, nortriptyline) will also be raised.[4]

(c) Venlafaxine

In a study of the effects of concurrent use of indinavir and venlafaxine, 9 healthy subjects were given a single dose of indinavir before and after 10 days of venlafaxine 75 mg twice daily. Indinavir did not affect the venlafaxine, but venlafaxine reduced the AUC and maximum serum levels of indinavir by 28 and 36% respectively. This is possibly enough to reduce the efficacy of indinavir.[6] Quite why this happens is not clear. More study is needed to establish the effects of multiple doses.

1. Ouellet D, Hsu A, Quian J, Lamm JE, Cavanaugh JH, Leonard JM, Granneman GR. Effect of fluoxetine on the pharmacokinetics of ritonavir. *Antimicrob Agents Chemother* (1998) 42, 3107–12.
2. Bellibas SE. Ritonavir-fluoxetine interaction. *Antimicrob Agents Chemother* (1999) 43, 1815.
3. Ouellet D, Hsu A. Ritonavir-fluoxetine interaction. *Antimicrob Agents Chemother* (1999) 43, 1815.
4. Norvir (Ritonavir). Abbott Laboratories Limited. Summary of product characteristics, January 2001.
5. Bertz RI, Cao G, Cavanaugh JH, Hsu A, Granneman GR, Leonard JM. Effect of ritonavir on the pharmacokinetics of desipramine. 11th International Conference on AIDS, Vancouver, 1996. Abstract Mo.B.1201.
6. Levin GM, Nelson LA, Devane CL, Preston SL, Carson SW, Eisele G. Venlafaxine and indinavir: results of a pharmacokinetic interaction study. *Intersci Conf Antimicrob Agents Chemother* (1999) 39, 25.

Protease Inhibitors + Azole antifungals

Ketoconazole and itraconazole raise the AUCs of the protease inhibitors, but on the information available so far this rarely seems to warrant a dose adjustment. Fluconazole appears not to interact.

Clinical evidence

(a) Fluconazole

Fluconazole (400 mg on day one, followed by 200 mg daily for 4 days) did not affect any of the pharmacokinetic parameters of ritonavir 200 mg 6-hourly by more than 15%, when given to 8 healthy subjects.[1] Similarly the pharmacokinetics of both indinavir 1000 mg 8-hourly and fluconazole 400 mg daily were unaffected by concurrent use in 11 HIV+ patients.[2] Another study also found no significant interaction between indinavir and fluconazole.[3]

(b) Itraconazole

Three patients (one on saquinavir/ritonavir, 2 on indinavir) were noted to have reactions similar to those seen with protease inhibitors alone (eczematous eruptions, raised serum transaminases) shortly after itraconazole was added to their treatment. This was attributed to raised levels of both medications, brought about by their concurrent use.[4] The makers of indinavir say that administering indinavir 600 mg 8-hourly with itraconazole 200 mg twice daily produces an AUC similar to that achieved when indinavir 800 mg 8-hourly is given alone.[5]

(c) Ketoconazole

When saquinavir (soft gel capsule formulation) 1200 mg three times daily was given to 12 healthy subjects with and without ketoconazole 400 mg daily for 7 days, the saquinavir AUC and maximum serum levels were raised by 190 and 171%.[6] The same study in 22 HIV+ patients, using ketoconazole 200 mg daily found that the AUC and maximum serum levels were raised by 69 and 36% respectively.[6] Pharmacokinetic changes have been seen with concurrent use of ketoconazole with amprenavir[7] (AUC increased by 32%), indinavir[8] (AUC raised by 62%) or nelfinavir[9] (AUC raised by 35%). In 12 HIV+ patients, ketoconazole 200 or 400 mg increased the AUC of saquinavir and ritonavir in combination (both 400 mg twice daily) by 37 and 29% respectively. The distribution of ritonavir was also affected, with disproportionate rises seen in CSF concentrations. All these changes appeared to be unrelated to the dose of ketoconazole used.[10] The pharmacokinetics of atazanavir 400 mg daily were not affected after 7 days concurrent treatment with ketoconazole 200 mg daily.[11]

The pharmacokinetics of ketoconazole are also affected by some protease inhibitors, amprenavir caused a 44% rise in the ketoconazole AUC,[7] and the combination of saquinavir with ritonavir caused a rise in peak plasma concentrations of ketoconazole.[10] However, saquinavir alone did not affect ketoconazole pharmacokinetics.[6]

Mechanism

Ketoconazole and itraconazole are known to inhibit the cytochrome P450 isoenzyme CYP3A4, and the protease inhibitors share this pathway of metabolism.[3,6,7,10] Thus enzyme inhibition, and competition for metabolism results in raised serum levels of both drugs. It has also been suggested that ketoconazole may inhibit P-glycoprotein transport of saquinavir, causing a decrease in its clearance.[6,10] Fluconazole is not a potent enzyme inhibitor and is therefore not expected to interact.[1,2]

Importance and management

The magnitude of the changes seen with ketoconazole are unlikely to warrant dose changes of the protease inhibitors or cause significant clinical effects. The makers of lopinavir suggest that doses greater than 200 mg a day of either ketoconazole or itraconazole are not recommended,[12] although on limited evidence from the other protease inhibitors it would seem that the interaction is not dose related. The differences seen in the study of saquinavir/ketoconazole[6] were attributed to the subjects (one group were patients the other HIV+) rather than the doses used. The information with itraconazole is more limited, but it would be expected to act in a similar way to ketoconazole. The makers of indinavir advise reducing the indinavir dose to 600 mg 8-hourly if it is to be given with itraconazole.[5] The small changes seen with fluconazole and the protease inhibitors are unlikely to be of clinical significance. Some authors suggest using an alternative azole in place of ketoconazole where possible.[6] Fluconazole would seem an appropriate choice.

1. Cato A, Cao G, Hsu A, Cavanaugh J, Leonard J, Granneman R. Evaluation of the effect of fluconazole on the pharmacokinetics of ritonavir. *Drug Metab Dispos* (1997) 25, 1104–1106.

2. De Wit S, Turner D, Debier M, Desmet M, McCrea J, Matthews C, Stone J, Carides A, Clumeck N. Absence of interaction between indinavir and fluconazole; a pharmacokinetic study in HIV patients. *Intersci Conf Antimicrob Agents Chemother* (1996) 36, 5.
3. The indinavir (MK 639) pharmacokinetic study group. Indinavir (MK 639) drug interaction studies. 11th International Conference on AIDS, Vancouver, 1996. Abstract Mo.B.174.
4. MacKenzie-Wood AR, Whitfield MJ, Ray JE. Itraconazole and HIV protease inhibitors: an important interaction. *Med J Aust* (1999) 170, 46–7.
5. Crixivan (Indinavir) . Merck Sharp & Dohme Limited. Summary of product characteristics, July 2001.
6. Grub S, Bryson H, Goggin T, Lüdin E, Jorga K. The interaction of saquinavir (soft gelatin capsule) with ketoconazole, erythromycin and rifampicin: comparison of the effect in healthy volunteers and HIV-infected patients. *Eur J Clin Pharmacol* (2001) 57, 115–21.
7. Polk RE, Israel DS, Pastor A, Sadler BM, Chittick GE, Symonds WT, Crouch M, Gouldin W, Lou Y, Rawls C, Bye A. Pharmacokinetic (PK) interaction between ketoconazole (KCZ) and the HIV protease inhibitor 141W94 after single dose administration to normal volunteers. *Intersci Conf Antimicrob Agents Chemother* (1997) 37, 12.
8. McCrea J, Woolf E, Sterrett A, Matthews C, Deutsch P, Yeh KC, Waldman S, Bjornsson T. Effects of ketoconazole and other P450 inhibitors on the pharmacokinetics of indinavir. *Pharm Res* (1996) 13 (Suppl 9), S465.
9. Kerr B, Lee C, Yuen G, Anderson R, Daniels R, Grettenberger H, Liang B-H, Quart B, Sandoval T, Shetty B, Wu E, Zhang K. Overview of *in-vitro* and *in-vivo* drug interaction studies of nelfinavir mesylate (NFV), a new HIV-1 protease inhibitor. 4th Conference on Retroviruses and Opportunistic Infections, Washington DC, 1997. Session 39, Slide 373.
10. Khaliq Y, Gallicano K, Venance S, Kravcik S, Cameron DW. Effect of ketoconazole on ritonavir and saquinavir concentrations in plasma and cerebrospinal fluid from patients infected with human immunodeficiency virus. *Clin Pharmacol Ther* (2000) 68, 637–36.
11. O'Mara EM, Randall D, Mummaneni V, Uderman H, Knox L, Schuster A, Geraldes M, Raymond R. Steady-state pharmacokinetic interaction study between BMS-232632 and ketoconazole in healthy subjects. *Intersci Conf Antimicrob Agents Chemother* (2000) 40, 335.
12. Kaletra Soft Capsules (Lopinavir). Abbott Laboratories Limited. Summary of product characteristics, March 2001.

Protease Inhibitors + Co-trimoxazole

Minor pharmacokinetic changes have been seen when co-trimoxazole is given concurrently with the protease inhibitors, but these changes are not considered to be clinically significant.

Clinical evidence

A study in 12 healthy subjects given **indinavir** 400 mg 6-hourly with **co-trimoxazole** 960 mg 12-hourly showed that neither drug had any clinically important effects on the pharmacokinetics of the other.[1] The same results were found in a similar study.[2] The pharmacokinetic changes found when **ritonavir** 500 mg twice daily was given with a single dose of **co-trimoxazole** 960 mg in 15 healthy subjects were considered too small to be of clinical relevance.[3,4] The combination of **saquinavir** 600 mg three times daily and **co-trimoxazole** 960 mg three times weekly caused no significant changes in the pharmacokinetics of **saquinavir**.[5] The makers of **lopinavir** state that they do not anticipate any interaction between **lopinavir** and **co-trimoxazole**.[6] There would seem to be no reason for avoiding using **co-trimoxazole** with any of the protease inhibitors.

1. Sturgill MG, Seibold JR, Boruchoff SE, Yeh KC, Haddix H, Deutsch P. Trimethoprim/sulfamethoxazole does not affect the steady-state disposition of indinavir. *J Clin Pharmacol* (1999) 39, 1077–84.
2. The indinavir (MK 639) pharmacokinetic study group. Indinavir (MK 639) drug interaction studies. 11th International Conference on AIDS, Vancouver, 1996. Abstract Mo.B.174.
3. Bertz RJ, Cao G, Cavanaugh JH, Hsu A, Granneman GR, Leonard JM. Effect of ritonavir on the pharmacokinetics of trimethoprim/sulfamethoxazole. 11th International Conference on AIDS, Vancouver, 1996. Abstract Mo.B.1197.
4. Norvir (Ritonavir). Abbott Laboratories Limited. Summary of product characteristics, January 2001.
5. Maserati R, Villani P, Cocchi L, Regazzi MB. Co-trimoxazole administered for *Pneumocystis carinii* pneumonia prophylaxis does not interfere with saquinavir pharmacokinetics. *AIDS* (1998) 12, 815–6.
6. Kaletra Soft Capsules (Lopinavir). Abbott Laboratories Limited. Summary of product characteristics, March 2001.

Protease Inhibitors + Food or Drink

Enteral feeds do not affect the pharmacokinetics of ritonavir. Food increases the bioavailability of nelfinavir, but decreases that of indinavir. Grapefruit juice does not have any clinically significant effects on the pharmacokinetics of either indinavir or saquinavir.

Clinical evidence, mechanism, importance and management

(a) Enteral Feeds

A 600-mg dose of **ritonavir** oral solution was mixed with 240 ml of either **Advera**, **Ensure** or water 1 h prior to dosing. The pharmacokinetics of **ritonavir** in either of the feeds were almost identical to those when **ritonavir** was administered in water.[1]

(b) Food or milk

A single dose of **indinavir** 600 mg was given to 7 HIV+ subjects immediately following a variety of types of meal. The **protein**, **carbohydrate**, **fat** and **high viscosity meals** reduced the AUC of indinavir by 68, 45, 34 and 30% respectively. The **fat meal** was associated with the largest inter-subject variability in bioavailability. The effect of the **protein meal** was attributed to the fact that it raised gastric pH and therefore impaired the absorption of **indinavir** (a weak base). The impairment of **indinavir** absorption caused by the other meals, which did not alter gastric pH, may have been due to delayed gastric emptying.[2] A similar study comparing a **full breakfast** with **light breakfasts** (toast or cereal) on **indinavir** absorption found that the full breakfast reduced the absorption of **indinavir** by 78% and the maximum serum levels by 86%, whilst the light breakfasts had no significant effect.[3] The makers advise that **indinavir** is administered 1 h before or 2 h after meals, or with light meals only.[4] Food has the opposite effect on **nelfinavir** absorption. When **nelfinavir** 400 or 800 mg was given to 12 healthy subjects in the fasted state, the AUC was only 27 to 50% of that observed when **nelfinavir** was given with a meal.[5] A 600-mg dose of **ritonavir** oral solution was mixed with 240 ml of either **chocolate milk** or water 1 h prior to dosing. The pharmacokinetics of **ritonavir** in the **milk** was almost identical to those when **ritonavir** was administered in water.[1]

(c) Grapefruit juice

Grapefruit juice (8 oz, approximately 200 ml reduced the AUC of **indinavir** 400 mg by 27% in 10 healthy subjects.[6] The effects seen in a similar study in 15 HIV+ subjects were not clinically significant.[7] In a study of the effects of concurrent use of **grapefruit juice** 400 ml and **saquinavir** 600 mg, the **grapefruit juice** was found to double the AUC of **saquinavir**, possibly by affecting intestinal CYP3A4.[8] Despite this increase, the makers of **saquinavir** advise that no dosage adjustment is necessary.[9]

1. Bertz R, Shi H, Cavanaugh J, Hsu A. Effect of three vehicles, Advera®, Ensure® and chocolate milk, on the bioavailability of an oral liquid formulation of Norvir (Ritonavir). *Intersci Conf Antimicrob Agents Chemother* (1996) 36, 5.
2. Carver PL, Fleisher D, Zhou SY, Kaul D, Kazanjian P, Li C. Meal composition effects on the oral bioavailability of indinavir in HIV-infected patients. *Pharm Res* (1999) 16, 718–24.
3. Stone JA, Ju WD, Steritt A, Woolf EJ, Yeh KC, Deutsch P, Waldman S, Bjornsson TD. Effect of food on the pharmacokinetics of indinavir in man. *Pharm Res* (1996) 13 (Suppl 9), S414.
4. Crixivan (Indinavir). Merck Sharp & Dohme Limited. Summary of product characteristics, July 2001.
5. Quart BD, Chapman SK, Peterkin J, Webber S, Oliver S. Phase I safety, tolerance, pharmacokinetics and food effect studies of AG1343--a novel HIV protease inhibitor. The American Society for Microbiology in collaboration with NIH and CDC. 2nd National Conference Human Retroviruses and Related Infections, Washington DC, 1995. Abstract LB3.
6. Wynn H, Shelton MJ, Bartos L, Difrancesco R, Hewitt RG. Grapefruit juice (GJ) increases gastric pH, but does not affect indinavir (IDV) exposure, in HIV patients. *Intersci Conf Antimicrob Agents Chemother* (1999) 39, 25.
7. McCrea J, Woolf E, Sterrett A, Matthews C, Deutsch P, Yeh KC, Waldman S, Bjornsson T. Effects of ketoconazole and other P-450 inhibitors on the pharmacokinetics of indinavir. *Pharm Res* (1996) 13 (Suppl 9), S485.
8. Kupferschmidt HHT, Fattinger KE, Ha HR, Follath F, Krähenbühl S. Grapefruit juice enhances the bioavailability of the HIV protease inhibitor saquinavir in man. *Br J Clin Pharmacol* (1998) 45, 355–9.
9. Fortovase (Saquinavir). Roche Products Limited. Summary of product characteristics, January 2001.

Protease Inhibitors + Macrolide antibacterials

Nelfinavir significantly elevates the serum levels of azithromycin, but the clinical significance of this is uncertain. Amprenavir, indinavir and ritonavir do not have clinically significant effects on the pharmacokinetics of clarithromycin.

Clinical evidence

(a) Azithromycin

A single dose of **azithromycin** 1200 mg was given to 12 healthy volunteers who had taken **nelfinavir** 750 mg 8-hourly for 8 days. The pharmacokinetics of **nelfinavir** were minimally affected, but the AUC and maximum serum levels of **azithromycin** were approximately doubled.[1]

(b) Clarithromycin

In a study in 12 healthy adults, **amprenavir** 1200 mg twice daily was given with **clarithromycin** 500 mg twice daily, for 4 days. The AUC and maximum serum levels of **amprenavir** were increased by 18% and 15% respectively, whereas the pharmacokinetics of **clarithromycin** were not significantly altered. None of the changes were considered to be clinically significant.[2] Similarly, a study into the effects of concurrent use of **clarithromycin** 500 mg 8-hourly and **indinavir** 800 mg 8-hourly found no clinically significant alterations in the pharmacokinetics of either drug in 11 healthy subjects.[3] A study of **ritonavir** 200 mg 8-hourly with **clarithromycin** 500 mg 12-hourly found that the combination produced no clinically significant effects, however, the **clarithromycin** became more dependent on renal clearance and so the authors concluded that the interaction may be significant in patients with renal failure.[4] The makers of **ritonavir** and **clarithromycin** suggest that no dosage reductions should be needed in those with normal kidney function, but they recommend a 50% reduction for those with a creatinine clearance of 30 to 60 ml/min and a 75% reduction for clearances of less than 30 ml/min. They advise avoidance of **clarithromycin** dosages exceeding 1 g daily.[5,6] Concurrent administration of **saquinavir** 1200 mg three times daily and **clarithromycin** 500 mg twice daily resulted in nearly doubled AUC and maximum serum levels of **saquinavir** and **clarithromycin** AUC and maximum serum levels 40% higher than those alone. However, the makers say that for short courses no dosage adjustment is needed.[7]

Mechanism

Clarithromycin is metabolised by the cytochrome P450 isoenzyme CYP3A, as are the protease inhibitors. However, is seems unlikely that competition is the only mechanism involved in this interaction.[2] With the azithromycin interaction, cytochrome P450 inhibition is unlikely, so it has been suggested that the nelfinavir may alter the P-glycoprotein transport of azithromycin.[1]

Importance and management

The interaction of the protease inhibitors with clarithromycin does not appear to be clinically significant. The interaction between azithromycin and nelfinavir is likely to be of clinical significance,[1] and although the outcome is presumed to be positive, this has yet to be assessed in practice. If concurrent use is necessary, monitor the outcome carefully. The makers of nelfinavir suggest that an interaction with erythromycin is unlikely, although not impossible.[8] The makers of ritonavir suggest that because erythromycin levels may rise, due to inhibition of its metabolism by ritonavir, care should be taken if both drugs are prescribed concurrently.[5] Similar warnings are issued by the makers of lopinavir regarding concurrent use of erythromycin and clarithromycin,[9] and the makers of amprenavir about erythromycin.[10] However, erythromycin and other macrolides do not seem to have been formally studied and their interactions or lack of interaction await confirmation in clinical practice.

1. Amsden GW, Nafziger AN, Foulds G, Cabelus LJ. A study of the pharmacokinetics of azithromycin and nelfinavir when coadministered in healthy volunteers. *J Clin Pharmacol* (2000) 40, 1522–7.
2. Brophy DF, Israel DS, Pastor A, Gillotin C, Chittick GE, Symonds WT, Lou Y, Sadler BM, Polk RE. Pharmacokinetic interaction between amprenavir and clarithromycin in healthy male volunteers. *Antimicrob Agents Chemother* (2000) 44, 978–84.
3. Boruchoff SE, Sturgill MG, Grasing KW, Seibold JR, McCrea J, Winchell GA, Kusma SE, Deutsch PJ. The steady-state disposition of indinavir is not altered by the concomitant administration of clarithromycin. *Clin Pharmacol Ther* (2000) 67, 351–9.
4. Ouellet D, Hsu A, Granneman GR, Carlson G, Cavanaugh J, Guenther H, Leonard JM. Pharmacokinetic interaction between ritonavir and clarithromycin. *Clin Pharmacol Ther* (1998) 64, 355–62.
5. Norvir (Ritonavir). Abbott Laboratories Limited. Summary of product characteristics, January 2001.
6. Klaricid (Clarithromycin). Abbott Laboratories Limited. Summary of product characteristics, October 2000.
7. Fortovase (Saquinavir). Roche Products Limited. Summary of product characteristics, January 2001.
8. Viracept (Nelfinavir). Roche Products Limited. Summary of product characteristics, October 2001.
9. Kaletra Soft Capsules (Lopinavir). Abbott Laboratories Limited. Summary of product characteristics, March 2001.
10. Agenerase (Amprenavir). Glaxo Wellcome. Summary of product characteristics, October 2001.

Protease Inhibitors + Miscellaneous drugs

Indinavir levels are raised by interleukin-2, lowered in some cases by omeprazole, and not affected by influenza vaccine, quinidine or mefloquine. Nelfinavir does not appear to interact with mefloquine or pancreatic enzyme supplements but significantly increases levels of terfenadine. Ritonavir increases the AUC of alprazolam but does not interact with garlic supplements. The combination of ritonavir/saquinavir and fusidic acid raises plasma levels of all three drugs.

Clinical evidence, mechanism, importance and management

(A) Evidence for or against an interaction

(a) Fusidic acid

An HIV+ man of 32 years was admitted with suspected **fusidic acid** toxicity after taking **fusidic acid** 500 mg three times daily for one week, with his usual treatment of **ritonavir** 400 mg twice daily, **saquinavir** 400 mg twice daily and stavudine 40 mg twice daily. His plasma **fusidic acid** level was found to be twice the expected level, and his **ritonavir** and **saquinavir** levels were also elevated. He improved spontaneously, however 4 days later he returned with jaundice, nausea and vomiting. All medications were stopped, but after 6 days his **fusidic acid** level was still 1.3 times that expected, his **saquinavir** level was 16.3 micrograms/ml (range 1 to 4 micrograms/ml) and his **ritonavir** level was 43.4 micrograms/ml (range (4 to 12 micrograms/ml). He was later able to restart his antivirals without problem. The authors recommend avoiding this drug combination.[1]

(b) Garlic supplements

Garlic supplements (5 mg garlic extract) was given to 10 healthy volunteers with 400 mg **ritonavir** suspension. The addition of the **garlic** did not significantly affect the pharmacokinetics of **ritonavir**.[2]

(c) Influenza vaccine

Influenza whole virus vaccine was given to 9 patients on **indinavir** containing HAART. No significant changes were found in indinavir pharmacokinetics.[3]

(d) Interleukins

In pharmacokinetic study in 9 HIV+ patients, the subjects were kept on their usual antiretrovirals and additionally given a 4 week course of **indinavir** 800 mg three times daily followed by 5 days of **interleukin-2** infusions 3 to 12 million units daily. The AUC of **indinavir** increased in 8 of the 9 subjects (average increase 88%). During this time interleukin-6 was also elevated, so it was thought that the increased **indinavir** concentrations were due to the inhibitory effects of interleukin-6 on the cytochrome P450 isoenzyme CYP3A4. Increased **indinavir** trough levels were also seen in a further 8 patients not participating in the pharmacokinetic study.[4]

(e) Mefloquine

Two HIV+ patients using HAART, one on **indinavir** 800 mg three times daily, the other on **nelfinavir** 1250 mg twice daily were given **mefloquine** 250 mg weekly, before a trip to Africa. No pharmacokinetic changes in the **mefloquine** or the protease inhibitors were found with either combination.[5]

(f) Omeprazole

A study in 8 healthy subjects given 40 mg **omeprazole** daily with a single 800-mg dose of **indinavir** found that although not all subjects showed significant pharmacokinetic changes, half of them showed a clinically significant decrease in the plasma levels of **indinavir**.[6] A review by the same authors, of 9 patients taking **omeprazole** with **indinavir** found that 4 had plasma levels of **indinavir** lower than expected. In two patients increasing the **indinavir** dose from 800 to 1000 mg three times daily resulted in acceptable plasma levels. The authors suggest careful monitoring of the combination and the use of dose adjustments as necessary.[7]

(g) Pancreatic enzymes

Combined use of **pancreatic enzymes** (pancrelipase 20,000 USP units, amylase 65,000 USP units and protease 65,000 USP units) and **nelfinavir** 1250 mg twice daily in 9 HIV+ subjects for 14 days resulted in no significant changes in the pharmacokinetics of **nelfinavir**.[8]

(h) Quinidine

Quinidine sulphate 200 mg was given to 10 healthy subjects, followed 1 h later by a single 400-mg dose of **indinavir**. **Quinidine** had no clinically significant effects on the pharmacokinetics of **indinavir**.[9]

(i) Terfenadine

When a single 60-mg dose of **terfenadine** was given after 5 days of **nelfinavir** 750 mg 8-hourly, the **terfenadine** plasma levels rose from <5 ng/ml to a range of 5 to 15 ng/ml. The pharmacokinetics of **nelfinavir** were unaffected.[10]

(B) Predicted interactions

In vitro and *in vivo* studies have shown that **ritonavir** is a potent inhibitor of cytochromes P450 isoenzymes CYP3A and CYP2D6 and to a lesser extent of CYP2C9, which are concerned with the metabolism of a large number of drugs.[11] The other protease inhibitors also affect cytochrome P450 isoenzymes to varying degrees. This means that protease inhibitors might be expected to affect the serum levels of the drugs metabolised by these isoenzymes, leading in some cases to toxicity. The makers of the protease inhibitors therefore predict a number of drug interactions in their Summaries of Product Characteristics. **Grapefruit** components have been shown *in vitro* to inhibit the CYP3A4 mediated metabolism of **saquinavir**, however, the clinical relevance of this effect is not known.[12]

1. Khaliq Y, Gallicano K, Leger R, Foster B, Badley A. A drug interaction between fusidic acid and a combination of ritonavir and saquinavir. *Br J Clin Pharmacol* (2000) 50, 82–3.
2. Choudhri SH, Gallicano K, Foster B, Leclaire T. A study of pharmacokinetic interactions between garlic supplements and ritonavir in healthy volunteers. *Intersci Conf Antimicrob Agents Chemother* (2000) 40, 332.
3. Maserati R, Villani P, Barasolo G, Mongiovetti M, Regazzi MB. Influenza immunization and indinavir pharmacokinetics. *Scand J Infect Dis* (2000) 32, 449–50.
4. Piscitelli SC, Vogel S, Figg WD, Raje S, Forrest A, Metcalf JA, Baseler M, Falloon J. Alteration in indinavir clearance during interleukin-2 infusions in patients infected with the human immunodeficiency virus. *Pharmacotherapy* (1998) 18, 1212–16.
5. Schippers EF, Hugen PWH, den Hartigh J, Burger DM, Hoetelmans RMW, Visser LG, Kroon FP. No drug-drug interaction between nelfinavir or indinavir and mefloquine in HIV-1 infected patients. *AIDS* (2000) 14, 2794–5.
6. Hugen PWH, Burger DM, ter Hofstede HJM, Koopmans PP. Concomitant use of indinavir and omeprazole; risk of antiretroviral subtherapy. *AIDS* (1998) 12 (Suppl 4), S29.
7. Burger DM, Hugen PWH, Kroon FP, Groenveld P, Brinkman K, Foudraine NA, Sprenger H, Koopmans PP, Hekster YA. *AIDS* (1998) 12, 2080–2.
8. Price J, Shalit P, Carlsen J, Becker MI, Frye J, Hsyu P. Pharmacokinetic interaction between Ultrase® MT-20 and nelfinavir in HIV-infected individuals. *Intersci Conf Antimicrob Agents Chemother* (1999) 39, 20.
9. McCrea J, Woolf E, Sterrett A, Matthews C, Deutsch P, Yeh KC, Waldman S, Bjornsson T. Effects of ketoconazole and other P-450 inhibitors on the pharmacokinetics of indinavir. *Pharm Res* (1996) 13 (9 Suppl), S485.
10. Kerr B, Yuep G, Daniels R, Quart B, Kravcik S, Sahai J, Anderson R. Strategic approach to nelfinavir mesylate (NFV) drug interactions involving CYP3A metabolism. 6th European Conference on Clinical Aspects and Treatment of HIV-infection, Hamburg, October 11–15th 1997. Abstracts.
11. Norvir (Ritonavir). Abbott Laboratories Limited. Summary of product characteristics, January 2001.
12. Eagling VA, Profit L, Back DJ. Inhibition of the CYP3A4-mediated metabolism and P-glycoprotein-mediated transport of the HIV-1 protease inhibitor saquinavir by grapefruit juice components. *Br J Clin Pharmacol* (1999) 48, 543–52.

Protease inhibitors + Protease inhibitors

The protease inhibitors are metabolised through similar metabolic pathways and so they affect the metabolism of each other to varying degrees.

Clinical evidence, mechanism, importance and management

(a) Amprenavir

A study in human liver microsomes indicated that **amprenavir** metabolism is likely to be inhibited by **indinavir**, **nelfinavir** and **ritonavir**, with **ritonavir** almost completely inhibiting **amprenavir** metabolism.[1] **Saquinavir** is unlikely to have any effect.[1]

(b) Indinavir

The effects of a range of doses of **ritonavir** (200, 300, or 400 mg 12-hourly) on **indinavir** pharmacokinetics were assessed in 39 healthy subjects. The AUC of **indinavir** (400 or 600 mg) was increased two- to five-fold by concurrent **ritonavir**. It is suggested that the combination of **indinavir** 400 mg 12-hourly with **ritonavir** 400 mg 12-hourly will result in an AUC of **indinavir** roughly equivalent to that of **indinavir** 800 mg 8-hourly, without any effect on the pharmacokinetics of **ritonavir**.[2]

Indinavir is reported to inhibit the metabolism of **saquinavir** by intestinal cytochrome P450 isoenzyme CYP3A4 *in vitro* and the authors of the study have suggested that combination therapy might therefore improve the oral bioavailability of **saquinavir**.[3] However, in another *in vitro* study of antiviral activity, the combination of **saquinavir** and **indinavir** demonstrated antagonism.[4] Neither of these studies totally precludes the concurrent use of these drugs but very close monitoring is clearly needed to ensure that the outcome is advantageous.

(c) Nelfinavir

Indinavir 1000 mg 12-hourly, given with **nelfinavir** 750 mg 12-hourly to 11 HIV+ subjects produced an AUC similar to **indinavir** 800 mg 8-hourly, given alone. The combination was well tolerated over an 8-week period.[5]

A single dose of **saquinavir** 1200 mg, given after 3 days of **nelfinavir** 750 mg 8-hourly had no effect on the pharmacokinetics of nelfinavir, however, the **nelfinavir** caused a fourfold increase in the AUC of **saquinavir**.[6] Similar two- to twelve-fold increases have been found in other studies in HIV+ subjects.[7-10] A study in which 157 patients received 12 weeks of combined **saquinavir/nelfinavir** treatment (doses unstated) found that the combination was well tolerated.[11]

(d) Ritonavir

A study in 6 patients with advanced HIV disease found that while taking 600 mg **saquinavir** three times daily the addition of 300 mg **ritonavir** twice daily increased the maximum **saquinavir** serum levels 33-fold, and increased the AUC 58-fold at steady state.[12] A pilot study in HIV+ patients given both drugs together (**saquinavir** 800 mg daily, **ritonavir** 400 to 600 mg daily) found that the **ritonavir** serum levels were unaffected. However, the **saquinavir** levels were substantially higher than those achieved with **saquinavir** alone in daily doses of 3600 to 7200 mg.[13] In a single-dose study **saquinavir** serum levels following a 200-mg dose were increased more than 50-fold by 600 mg **ritonavir**.[14] A study in 57 healthy subjects, of a range of **ritonavir** and **saquinavir** doses (200 to 600 mg) found that **saquinavir** did not affect **ritonavir** pharmacokinetics, but **ritonavir** increased the AUC of **saquinavir** 50 to 132-fold. The authors say[15] that the combination, optimally 400 mg 12-hourly of both drugs, would result in "sustained and highly suppressive concentrations of **ritonavir** and **saquinavir**." The probable reason is that the **ritonavir** inhibits cytochrome P450 isoenzyme CYP3A4 in the gut wall and liver so that the absorbed **saquinavir** escapes the normal extensive metabolism.

1. Decker CJ, Laitinen LM, Bridson GW, Rayback SA, Tung RD, Chaturvedi PR. Metabolism of amprenavir in liver microsomes: role of CYP3A4 inhibition for drug interactions. *J Pharm Sci* (1998) 87, 803–7.
2. Hsu A, Granneman GR, Cao G, Carothers L, Japour A, El-Shourbagy T, Dennis S, Berg J, Erdman K, Leonard JM, Sun E. Pharmacokinetic interaction between ritonavir and indinavir in healthy volunteers. *Antimicrob Agents Chemother* (1998) 42, 2784–91.
3. Fitzsimmons ME, Collins JM. Selective biotransformation of the human immunodeficiency virus protease inhibitor saquinavir by human small-intestinal cytochrome P4503A4: Potential contribution to high first-pass metabolism. *Drug Metab Dispos* (1997) 25, 256–66.
4. Merrill DP, Manion DJ, Chou T-C, Hirsch MS. Antagonism between human immunodeficiency virus type 1 protease inhibitors indinavir and saquinavir in vitro. *J Infect Dis* (1997) 176, 265–8.

5. Havlir DV, Riddler S, Squires K, Winslow D, Kerr B, Nguyen BY, Yeh K, Hawe L, Zhong L, Deutsch P, Saah A. Co-administration of indinavir (IDV) and nelfinavir (NFV) in a twice daily regimen: Preliminary safety, pharmacokinetic and anti-viral activity results. 5th Conference on Retroviruses and Opportunistic Infections, Chicago, 1998. Abstract 393.

6. Kerr B, Yuep G, Daniels R, Quart B, Kravcik S, Sahai J, Anderson R. Strategic approach to nelfinavir mesylate (NFV) drug interactions involving CYP3A metabolism. 6th European Conference on Clinical Aspects and Treatment of HIV-infection, Hamburg, Germany, 1997. Abstract.

7. Merry C, Ryan M, Mulchay F, Halifax K, Barry M, Back D. The effect of nelfinavir on plasma saquinavir levels. 6th European Conference on Clinical Aspects and Treatment of HIV-infection, Hamburg, Germany, 1997. Abstract 455.

8. Merry C, Barry MG, Mulcahy FM, Back DJ. Saquinavir pharmacokinetics alone and in combination with nelfinavir in HIV infected patients. 5th Conference on Retroviruses and Opportunistic Infections, Chicago, 1998. Abstract 352.

9. Gallicano K, Sahai J, Kravcik S, Seguin I, Bristow N, Cameron DW. Nelfinavir (NFV) increases plasma exposure of saquinavir in hard gel capsule (SQV-HGC) in HIV+ patients. 5th Conference on Retroviruses and Opportunistic Infections, Chicago, 1998. Abstract 353.

10. Hoetelmans RMW, Reijers MHE, Wit FW, ten Kate RW, Weige HM, Frissen PHJ, Bruisten SM, Beijnen JH, Lange JMA. Saquinavir (SQV) pharmacokinetics in combination with nelfinavir (NFV) in the ADAM study. 6th European Conference on Clinical Aspects and Treatment of HIV-infection, Hamburg, Germany, 1997. Abstract 255.

11. Posniak A and the SPICE study team. Study of protease inhibitors in combination in Europe (SPICE). 6th European Conference on Clinical Aspects and Treatment of HIV-infection, Hamburg, Germany, 1997. Abstract 209.

12. Merry C, Barry MG, Mulcahy F, Ryan M, Heavey J, Tjia JF, Gibbons SE, Breckenridge AM, Back DJ. Saquinavir pharmacokinetics alone and in combination with ritonavir in HIV-infected patients. AIDS (1997) 11, F29–F33.

13. Cameron DW, Hsu A, Granneman GR, Sun E, McMahon D, Farthing C, Poretz D, Markowitz M, Cohen C, Follansbee S, Mellors J, Ho D, Xu Y, Rode R, Salgo M, Leonard J. Pharmacokinetics of ritonavir-saquinavir combination therapy. AIDS (1996) 10 (Suppl 2), S16.

14. Kempf DJ, Marsh KC, Kumar G, Rodrigues AD, Denissen JF, McDonald E, Kukulka MJ, Hsu A, Granneman GR, Baroldi PA, Sun E, Pizzuti D, Plattner JJ, Norbeck DW, Leonard JM. Pharmacokinetic enhancement of inhibitors of the human immunodeficiency virus protease by coadministration with ritonavir. Antimicrob Agents Chemother (1997) 41, 654–60.

15. Hsu A, Granneman GR, Cao G, Carothers L, El-Shourbagy T, Baroldi P, Erdman K, Brown F, Sun E, Leonard JM. Pharmacokinetic interactions between two human immunodeficiency virus protease inhibitors, ritonavir and saquinavir. Clin Pharmacol Ther (1998) 63, 453–64.

Protease Inhibitors + Rifamycins

The use of many of the protease inhibitors with rifamycins is contraindicated by their makers, although combination antiretroviral drug therapy e.g. with saquinavir and ritonavir may make concurrent use possible. Rifabutin bioavailability is increased by amprenavir, indinavir, nelfinavir and ritonavir. Rifabutin decreases the bioavailability of indinavir, nelfinavir and saquinavir. Rifampicin reduces the bioavailability of amprenavir, indinavir, nelfinavir and saquinavir.

Clinical evidence, importance and management

(a) Amprenavir

Amprenavir 1200 mg twice daily was given with rifabutin 300 mg daily or rifampicin 600 mg daily, to two groups of 11 healthy subjects for 10 and 4 days respectively. Amprenavir caused an almost threefold increase in the AUC of rifabutin, but the rifabutin did not significantly affect the pharmacokinetics of amprenavir. The combination poorly tolerated, with 5 of 11 subjects stopping treatment between days one and 9 due to adverse events.[1] The makers of amprenavir suggest that the dose of rifabutin should be at least halved if concurrent use is necessary.[2] In the rifampicin group, the effects were reversed; amprenavir did not affect the pharmacokinetics of rifampicin, but rifampicin caused the amprenavir AUC to drop by 82%. The maximum plasma levels were also significantly affected, dropping by 70% from 9.2 to 2.78 micrograms/ml when rifampicin was added.[1] For this reason concurrent use is contraindicated.[2]

(b) Indinavir

A study in 11 AIDS patients given indinavir 800 mg 8-hourly and rifampicin 600 mg daily for 14 days showed that AUC of rifampicin was increased by 73% with concurrent use.[3] In a similar study looking at the effects of the rifampicin on indinavir, the indinavir AUC and maximum serum levels were decreased by 92 and 86% respectively.[4] For this reason concurrent use of rifampicin and indinavir is contraindicated.[5] When rifabutin 300 mg was given with indinavir

800 mg 8-hourly to 10 healthy subjects for 10 days, the indinavir maximum serum levels and AUC were reduced by about a third, whereas the rifabutin maximum serum levels and AUC were increased two- to three-fold.[6,7] A 50% dose reduction of rifabutin and a dosage increase of indinavir to 1000–1200 mg every 8 hours is suggested if concurrent use is necessary.[5,6] When the combination was used in practice, there were no treatment failures in 25 patients being treated with rifabutin whilst on HAART (containing indinavir and or nelfinavir). The rifabutin was given as 300 mg every 2 weeks and the indinavir dose was increased from 800 to 1200 mg 8-hourly to achieve satisfactory levels.[8]

(c) Nelfinavir

Rifampicin 600 mg daily for 7 days decreased the AUC of 750 mg nelfinavir 8-hourly for 6 days by 82%.[9] The makers of nelfinavir therefore suggest that this combination should be avoided.[10] In an associated study in which 300 mg rifabutin daily for 8 days was given with 750 mg nelfinavir 8-hourly for 7 to 8 days, the nelfinavir AUC was reduced 32% and the rifabutin AUC increased 207%.[9] The manufacturers therefore suggest halving the rifabutin dosage when both drugs are used together.[10] Also see indinavir above.

(d) Protease inhibitor combinations

It was suggested that the combination of ritonavir and saquinavir (both 400 mg twice daily) could cancel out the effects of rifampicin on saquinavir, so therapeutic levels of all three drugs could be achieved. This assumption was successfully demonstrated in 2 HIV+ subjects.[11] The CDC state that rifampicin or rifabutin can probably be used in combination with saquinavir if ritonavir is included in the regimen.[12]

(e) Ritonavir

In a study where ritonavir 500 mg twice daily was given with 150 mg rifabutin daily to 5 healthy subjects for 8 days, the maximum serum level of rifabutin was increased threefold and the AUC was increased fourfold (and the AUC of its active metabolite (25-O-desacetylrifabutin) 35-fold).[13] Seven subjects had to be withdrawn due to leucopenia. The risk of uveitis is known to be increased by rises in rifabutin levels and for this reason concurrent use is considered by the makers to be contraindicated.[14]

(f) Saquinavir

The maximum plasma levels of saquinavir 600 mg three times daily were reduced by about 40% after concurrent administration of rifabutin 300 mg daily, in 12 HIV+ subjects.[15] Rifampicin decreases plasma levels of saquinavir by more than 50%. The combined use of either rifampicin or rifabutin with saquinavir is contraindicated.[16]

Mechanism

The rifamycins are potent inducers of the cytochrome P450 isoenzyme CYP3A, by which the protease inhibitors are at least partially metabolised. The protease inhibitors act as cytochrome P450 inhibitors. The effects of combined treatment are therefore dependent on the relative affinity of each drug for cytochrome P450.

1. Polk RE, Brophy DF, Israel DS, Patron R, Sadler BM, Chittick GE, Symonds WT, Lou Y, Kristoff D, Stein DS. Pharmacokinetic interaction between amprenavir and rifabutin or rifampin in healthy males. Antimicrob Agents Chemother (2001) 45, 502–508.

2. Agenerase (Amprenavir). Glaxo Wellcome. Summary of product characteristics, October 2001.

3. Jaruratanasirikul S, Sriwiriyajan S. Pharmacokinetics of rifampicin administered alone and with indinavir. J Antimicrob Chemother (1999) 44 (Suppl A), 58.

4. McCrea J, Wyss D, Stone J, Carides A, Kusma S, Kleinbloesem C, Al-Hamdan Y, Yeh K, Deutsch P. Pharmacokinetic interaction between indinavir and rifampin. Clin Pharmacol Ther (1997) 61, 152.

5. Crixivan (Indinavir). Merck Sharp & Dohme Limited. Summary of product characteristics, July 2001.

6. Winchell GA, McCrea JB, Carides A, Kusma SE, Chiou R, Deutsch P, Yeh KC, Waldman S, Bjornsson TD. Pharmacokinetic interaction between indinavir and rifabutin. Clin Pharmacol Ther (1997) 61, 153.

7. The indinavir (MK 639) pharmacokinetic study group. Indinavir (MK 639) drug interaction studies. 11th International Conference on AIDS, Vancouver, 1996. Abstract Mo.B.174.

8. Narita M, Stambaugh JJ, Hollender ES, Jones D, Pitchenik AE, Ashkin D. Use of rifabutin with protease inhibitors for human immunodeficiency virus-infected patients with tuberculosis. Clin Infect Dis (2000) 30, 779–83.

9. Kerr B, Yuep G, Daniels R, Quart B, Kravcik S, Sahai J, Anderson R. Strategic approach to nelfinavir mesylate (NFV) drug interactions involving CYP3A metabolism. 6th European Conference on Clinical Aspects and Treatment of HIV-infection, Hamburg, 1997, 256.

10. Viracept (Nelfinavir). Roche Product Limited. Summary of product characteristics, October 2001.
11. Veldkamp AI, Hoetelmans RMW, Beijnen JH, Mulder JW, Meenhorst PL. Ritonavir enables combined therapy with rifampicin and saquinavir. *Clin Infect Dis* (1999) 29, 1586.
12. Anon. CDC alters recommendations on rifamycin-antiretroviral drug use. *Am J Health-Syst Pharm* (2000) 57, 735.
13. Cato A, Cavanaugh J, Shi H, Hsu A, Leonard J, Granneman R. The effect of multiple doses of ritonavir on the pharmacokinetics of rifabutin. *Clin Pharmacol Ther* (1998) 63, 414–21.
14. Norvir (Ritonavir). Abbott Laboratories Limited. Summary of product characteristics, January 2001.
15. Sahai J, Stewart F, Swick L, Gallicano K, Graber G, Seguin I, Tucker A, Bristow N, Cameron W. Rifabutin (RBT) reduces saquinavir (SAQ) plasma levels in HIV-infected patients. *Intersci Conf Antimicrob Agents Chemother* (1996) 36, 6.
16. Fortovase (Saquinavir). Roche Products Limited. Summary of product characteristics, January 2001.

Protease inhibitors + St John's wort

St John's wort causes a marked reduction in the serum levels of indinavir which may result in HIV treatment failure. Other protease inhibitors (nelfinavir, ritonavir, saquinavir) are predicted to be interact similarly.

Clinical evidence

Eight healthy subjects were given three 800 mg oral doses of **indinavir** on day 1 of a single drug pharmacokinetic study to achieve steady-state serum levels, and then an 800 mg on day 2. For the next 14 days they were given 300 mg **St John's wort extract** three times daily. On day 15, three 800 mg oral doses of **indinavir** with a single 800-mg dose on day 16. It was found that the **St John's wort** reduced the mean AUC of **indinavir** by 57% and decreased the 8 hr **indinavir** trough serum level by 81%.[1]

Mechanism

Not fully understood, but it seems highly likely that the St John's wort induces the activity of cytochrome P450 isoenzyme CYP3A4, thereby increasing the metabolism and loss of the indinavir from the body.

Importance and management

Direct information seems to be limited to this study, but the interaction would appear to be established. Such a large reduction in the serum levels of indinavir is likely to result in treatment failures and therefore St John's wort should be avoided. There seems to be no direct information about other protease inhibitors (**nelfinavir**, **ritonavir**, **saquinavir**) but since they are also metabolised by the same cytochrome P450 isoenzyme CYP3A4 it is reasonable to expect that they will be similarly affected by St John's wort. The advice of the CSM is that patients on any of these protease inhibitors should avoid St John's wort and that anyone already taking both should stop the St John's wort and have the HIV RNA viral load measured.[2] Study is needed to confirm that other protease inhibitors interact like indinavir.

1. Piscitelli SC, Burstein AH, Chaitt D, Alfaro RM, Falloon J. Indinavir concentrations and St John's wort. *Lancet* (2000) 355, 547–8.
2. Committee on Safety of Medicines. Message from Professor A Breckenridge (Chairman of CSM) and Fact Sheet for Health Care Professionals, 29th February 2000.

Prothionamide + Rifampicin (Rifampin) and/or Dapsone

Prothionamide appears to be very hepatotoxic and this is possibly increased by the concurrent use of rifampicin or isopiperazinylrifamycin SV. Prothionamide does not affect the pharmacokinetics of either dapsone or rifampicin.

Clinical evidence

In a study of 39 patients with leprosy, 39% became jaundiced after 24 to 120 days treatment with **dapsone** 100 mg daily, prothionamide

300 mg daily and **isopiperazinylrifamycin SV** 300 to 600 mg monthly. Laboratory evidence of liver damage occurred in a total of 56% of patients and despite the withdrawal of the drugs from all the patients, 2 of them died.[1] All the patients except 2 had taken **dapsone** before, alone, for 3 to 227 months without reported problems.[1] In another group of leprosy patients 22% (11 of 50) showed liver damage after treatment with **dapsone** 100 mg and prothionamide 300 mg daily, with **rifampicin** 900 mg, prothionamide 500 mg and **clofazimine** 300 mg monthly for 30 to 50 days. One patient died.[1] Most of the patients recovered within 30 to 60 days after withdrawing the treatment.

Jaundice, liver damage and deaths have occurred in other leprosy patients given **rifampicin** and prothionamide or **ethionamide**.[2–4] Prothionamide does not affect the pharmacokinetics of either **dapsone** or **rifampicin**.[5]

Mechanism

Although not certain, it seems probable that the liver damage was primarily caused by the prothionamide, possibly exacerbated by the rifampicin or the isopiperazinylrifamycin SV.

Importance and management

This serious and potentially life-threatening hepatotoxic reaction to prothionamide is established, but the part played by the other drugs, particularly the rifampicin, is uncertain. Strictly speaking this may not be an interaction. If prothionamide is given the liver function should be very closely monitored in order to detect toxicity as soon as possible.

1. Baohong J, Jiakun C, Chenmin W, Guang X. Hepatotoxicity of combined therapy with rifampicin and daily prothionamide for leprosy. *Lepr Rev* (1984) 55, 283–9.
2. Lesobre R, Ruffino J, Teyssier L, Achard F, Brefort G. Les ictères au cours du traitement par la rifampicine. *Rev Tuberc Pneumol (Paris)* (1969) 33, 393–403.
3. Report of the Third Meeting of the Scientific Working Group on Chemotherapy of Leprosy (THELEP) of the UNDP/World Bank/WHO Special Programme for Research and Training in Tropical Diseases. *Int J Lepr* (1981) 49, 431–6.
4. Cartel J-L, Millan J, Guelpa-Lauras C-C, Grosset JH. Hepatitis in leprosy patients treated by a daily combination of dapsone, rifampin, and a thioamide. *Int J Lepr* (1983) 51, 461–5.
5. Mathur A, Venkatesan K, Girdhar BK, Bharadwaj VP, Girdhar A, Bagga AK. A study of drug interactions in leprosy — 1. Effect of simultaneous administration of prothionamide on metabolic disposition of rifampicin and dapsone. *Lepr Rev* (1986) 57, 33–7.

Pyrantel + Piperazine

Piperazine opposes the anthelmintic actions of pyrantel.

Clinical evidence, mechanism, importance and management

Pyrantel acts as an anthelmintic because it depolarises the neuromuscular junctions of some intestinal nematodes causing the worms to contract. This paralyses the worms so that they are dislodged by peristalsis and expelled in the faeces. **Piperazine** also paralyses nematodes but it does so by causing hyperpolarisation of the neuromuscular junctions. These two pharmacological actions oppose one another, as was shown in two *in vitro* pharmacological studies. Strips of whole *Ascaris lumbricoides*, which contracted when exposed to pyrantel failed to do so when also exposed to **piperazine**.[1] Parallel electrophysiological studies using *Ascaris* cells confirmed that the depolarisation due to pyrantel (which causes the paralysis) was opposed by **piperazine**.[1]

In practical terms this means that **piperazine** does not add to the anthelmintic effect of pyrantel on *Ascaris* as might be expected, but opposes it. For this reason it is usually recommended that concurrent use should be avoided, but direct clinical evidence confirming that combined use is ineffective seems to be lacking. It seems reasonable to extrapolate the results of these studies on *Ascaris lumbricoides* (roundworm) to the other gastrointestinal parasites for which pyrantel is used, i.e. *Enterobius vermicularis* (threadworm or pinworm),

Ancylostoma duodenale, Necator americanus (hookworm) and *Trichostrongylus* spp. However, no one seems to have checked on this directly.

1. Aubry ML, Cowell P, Davey MJ, Shevde S. Aspects of the pharmacology of a new anthelmintic: pyrantel. *Br J Pharmacol* (1970) 38, 332–44.

Pyrazinamide + Miscellaneous drugs

Allopurinol is unlikely to be effective against pyrazinamide-induced hyperuricaemia and may make things worse. The uricosuric effects of probenecid are reduced by pyrazinamide. The makers of pyrazinamide say that it is contraindicated in hyperuricaemia and should be stopped if gouty arthritis develops. Antacids and food alter the rate but not the extent of absorption of pyrazinamide. Pyrazinamide may possibly adversely affect the control of diabetes.

Clinical evidence, mechanism, importance and management

(a) Allopurinol

It is thought pyrazinamide is hydrolysed in the body to pyrazinoic acid, which appears to be responsible for the hyperuricaemic effect of pyrazinamide. Pyrazinoic acid is oxidised by the enzyme xanthine oxidase to 5-hydroxypyrazoic acid.[1] Since **allopurinol** is an inhibitor of xanthine oxidase, its presence would increase pyrazinoic acid concentrations thereby probably worsening the pyrazinamide-induced hyperuricaemia.[2] **Allopurinol** would therefore appear to be unsuitable for treating pyrazinamide-induced hyperuricaemia.

In addition it should be pointed out that the makers of pyrazinamide warn that hyperuricaemia is a contraindication for its use, and that if hyperuricaemia accompanied by acute gouty arthritis occurs during treatment, the pyrazinamide should be stopped and not restarted. They also say that pyrazinamide should not be given unless regular uric acid determinations can be made.[3]

(b) Antacids

Mylanta (**aluminium-magnesium hydroxide**) 30 ml, 9 h before, with and after a single 30 mg/kg dose of pyrazinamide decreased the time to peak absorption by 17%, but had no effect on other pharmacokinetics parameters.[4] Concurrent use is unlikely to cause significant problems.

(c) Food

A single 30 mg/kg dose of pyrazinamide taken with a **high-fat breakfast** increased the time to peak absorption by 80%, but had no effect on other pharmacokinetics parameters.[4]

(d) Hypoglycaemic agents

The control of diabetes mellitus may possibly be more difficult in some patients taking pyrazinamide.[3]

(e) Probenecid

The interactions of **probenecid** and pyrazinamide and their effects on the excretion of uric acid are complex and intertwined. **Probenecid** increases the secretion of uric acid into the urine apparently by inhibiting its reabsorption from the kidney tubules.[5] Pyrazinamide on the other hand decreases the secretion of uric acid into the urine by a third to a half,[6] resulting in a rise in the serum levels of urate in the blood, thereby causing hyperuricaemia.[6,7] The result of using **probenecid** and pyrazinamide together is not however merely the simple sum of these two effects because, firstly, pyrazinamide additionally decreases the metabolism of the **probenecid** so that the uricosuric effects of **probenecid** are prolonged, and the effect of pyrazinamide reduced. Secondly, **probenecid** inhibits the secretion of pyrazinamide so that the pyrazinamide effects are increased.[8]

The overall effect is that if **probenecid** were to be used to treat the hyperuricaemia caused by pyrazinamide, the normal uricosuric ef-

fects of **probenecid** would be diminished and larger doses would be required.

1. Weiner IM, Tinker JP. Pharmacology of pyrazinamide: metabolic and renal function studies related to the mechanism of drug-induced urate retention. *J Pharmacol Exp Ther* (1972) 180, 411–34.
2. Urban T, Maquarre E, Housset C, Chouaid C, Ðevin E, Lebeau B. Hypersensibilité à l'allopurinol. Une cause possible d'hépatite et d'éruption cutanéo-muqueuse chez un patient sous antituberculeux. *Rev Mal Respir* (1995) 12, 314–16.
3. Zinamide (pyrazinamide). Merck, Sharp & Dohme. Summary of product characteristics, January 1998.
4. Peloquin CA, Bulpitt AE, Jaresko GS, Jelliffe RW, James GT, Nix DE. Pharmacokinetics of pyrazinamide under fasting conditions, with food, and with antacids. *Pharmacotherapy* (1998) 18, 1205–11.
5. Meisel AD, Diamond HS. Mechanism of probenecid-induced uricosuria: inhibition of reabsorption of secreted urate. *Arthritis Rheum* (1977) 20, 128.
6. Cullen JH, LeVine M, Fiore JM. Studies of hyperuricemia produced by pyrazinamide. *Am J Med* (1957) 23, 587–95.
7. Shapiro M, Hyde L. Hyperuricemia due to pyrazinamide. *Am J Med* (1957) 23, 596–9.
8. Yü T-F, Perel J, Berger L, Roboz J, Israili ZH, Dayton PG. The effect of the interaction of pyrazinamide and probenecid on urinary uric acid excretion in man. *Am J Med* (1977) 63, 723–8.

Pyrimethamine + Artemether

Artemether raises pyrimethamine plasma levels, but this does not appear to cause an increase in adverse effects.

Clinical evidence, mechanism, importance and management

In a 3-way single-dose crossover study, 8 healthy subjects were given either **artemether** 300 mg, pyrimethamine 100 mg or both drugs together. Although there was large inter-individual variation in the pharmacokinetics, the maximum plasma level of pyrimethamine was significantly raised by 44%. As there was no corresponding increase in adverse effects the authors suggest that the interaction may be of benefit.[1] More study is warranted to confirm this result.

1. Tan-ariya P, Na-Bangchang K, Ubalee R, Thanavibul A, Thipawangkosol P, Karbwang J. Pharmacokinetic interaction or artemether and pyrimethamine in healthy male Thais. *Southeast Asian J Trop Med Public Health* (1998) 29, 18–23.

Pyrimethamine + Co-trimoxazole or Sulphonamides

Serious pancytopenia and megaloblastic anaemia have been described in patients under treatment with pyrimethamine and either co-trimoxazole or other sulphonamides.

Clinical evidence

A woman taking 50 mg pyrimethamine weekly as malaria prophylaxis, developed petechial haemorrhages and widespread bruising within 10 days of starting to take **co-trimoxazole** (320 mg **trimethoprim** + 800 mg **sulfamethoxazole** daily) for a urinary-tract infection. She was found to have gross megaloblastic changes and pancytopenia in addition to being obviously pale and ill. After withdrawal of the two drugs she responded rapidly to hydroxocobalamin and folic acid, with chloroquine cover.[1] Note that the **co-trimoxazole** used in this case had a drug:drug ratio of 1:2.5 where the usual ratio is 1:5.

Similar cases have been described in other patients taking pyrimethamine with **co-trimoxazole**[2-4] or **sulfafurazole** (**sulfisoxazole**).[5]

Mechanism

Uncertain, but a reasonable surmise can be made. Pyrimethamine and trimethoprim are both 2,4 diamino-pyrimidines and both selectively inhibit the actions of the enzyme dihydrofolate reductase, which is concerned with the eventual synthesis of the nucleic acids needed for the production of new cells. The sulphonamides inhibit another part of the same synthetic chain. The adverse reactions seen would seem to reflect a gross depression of the normal folate metabolism caused by the combined actions of both drugs. Megaloblastic anaemia and pancytopenia are among the adverse reactions of pyrimethamine and, more rarely, of co-trimoxazole taken alone. In theory this should not occur but in practice it clearly does so occasionally.

Importance and management

Information seems to be limited to the reports cited, but the interaction appears to be established. Its incidence is unknown. Concurrent use need not be avoided but caution should be used in prescribing the combination, especially in the presence of other drugs or disease states that may predispose to folate deficiency.

1. Fleming AF, Warrell DA, Dickmeiss H. Co-trimoxazole and the blood. *Lancet* (1974) ii, 284–5.
2. Ansdell VE, Wright SG, Hutchinson DBA. Megaloblastic anaemia associated with combined pyrimethamine and co-trimoxazole administration. *Lancet* (1976) ii, 1257.
3. Malfatti S, Piccini A. Anemia megaloblastica pancitopenica in corso di trattamento con pirimetamina, trimethoprim e sulfametossazolo. *Haematologica* (1976) 61, 349–57.
4. Borgstein A, Tozer RA. Infectious mononucleosis and megaloblastic anaemia associated with Daraprim and Bactrim. *Cent Afr J Med* (1974) 20, 185.
5. Waxman S, Herbert V. Mechanism of pyrimethamine-induced megaloblastosis in human bone marrow. *N Engl J Med* (1969) 280, 1316–19.

Pyrimethamine/Sulfadoxine (*Fansidar*) + Iron

Iron possibly delays the eradication of the malaria parasite by pyrimethamine/sulfadoxine (*Fansidar*).

Clinical evidence, mechanism, importance and management

Because malarial infection is associated with anaemia, the effect of iron supplements given with antimalarial treatment was investigated in 222 children under 5 years old who had sought treatment for malaria and who were divided into 3 groups. All were given 12.5 to 25 mg pyrimethamine plus 250 to 500 mg sulfadoxine (*Fansidar*) as a single dose. One group then received no iron, another was given iron weekly and the third group was given iron daily. Iron was given as a 1.2% **ferrous sulphate** solution at a dose of 2 ml/kg. It was found that the iron therapy enhanced the haematological recovery of patients but appeared to prolong their parasitaemias, although the difference was not statistically significant. The authors quote evidence that this trend has been seen elsewhere, and suggest that **iron supplements** should be delayed until the malarial infection has been cleared, especially as effective treatment of malaria often also treats the anaemia, independent of iron treatment.[1]

1. Nwanyanwu OC, Ziba C, Kazembe PN, Gamadzi G, Gondwe J, Redd SC. The effect of oral iron therapy during treatment for *Plasmodium falciparum* malaria with sulphadoxine-pyrimethamine on Malawian children under 5 years of age. *Ann Trop Med Parasitol* (1996) 90, 589–95.

Pyrimethamine/Sulfadoxine (*Fansidar*) + Zidovudine

A study in patients with AIDS found that 250 mg zidovudine four times daily did not adversely affect the prevention of toxoplasma encephalitis with *Fansidar* (pyrimethamine/sulfadoxine), one tablet twice weekly for up to 8 months.[1]

1. Eljaschewitsch J, Schürmann D, Pohle HD, Ruf B. Zidovudine does not antagonize Fansidar in preventing toxoplasma encephalitis in HIV infected patients. 7th International Conference on AIDS; Science Challenging AIDS, Florence, Italy, 1991. Abstract W.B.2334.

Quinine + Miscellaneous drugs

The loss of quinine from the body is reduced by the concurrent use of cimetidine, but not ranitidine. A single case report describes a reduction in the serum levels and therapeutic effects of quinine in a patient when rifampicin was given. Urinary alkalinizers can increase the retention of quinine in

man, and antacids can reduce the absorption in *animals*. Doxycycline and colestyramine do not appear to alter the pharmacokinetics of quinine. None of these interactions appears to be of general clinical importance.

Clinical evidence, mechanism, importance and management

(a) Antacids

Magnesium and **aluminium hydroxide** gel depresses the absorption of quinine from the gut of *rats* and reduces blood quinine levels by 50 to 70%.[1] The reason appears to be that **aluminium hydroxide** slows gastric emptying which reduces absorption, and **magnesium hydroxide** also forms an insoluble precipitate with quinine. However, there seem to be no clinical reports of a reduction in the therapeutic effectiveness of quinine due to the concurrent use of antacids.

(b) Cimetidine, Ranitidine

Cimetidine (200 mg three times daily and 400 mg at night) for a week reduced the clearance of quinine in 6 healthy subjects by 27% while its half-life was increased by 49% (from 7.6 to 11.3 h) and the AUC was increased by 42%. Peak levels were unchanged. No interaction was seen when **cimetidine** was replaced by **ranitidine** 150 mg twice daily.[2] The probable reason is that **cimetidine** (a recognised enzyme inhibitor) reduces the metabolism of the quinine by the liver so that it is lost from the body more slowly, whereas **ranitidine** does not. The clinical importance of this is uncertain, but prescribers should be alert for any evidence of quinine toxicity during concurrent use.

(c) Colestyramine

Colestyramine 8 g did not alter the pharmacokinetics of quinine 600 mg, given concurrently to 8 healthy subjects. The authors warn that this lack of interaction may have been because only single doses were used, and suggest continuing to separate the administration of the two drugs until a lack of interaction is demonstrated in a multiple dose study.[3]

(d) Doxycycline

The pharmacokinetics of quinine were found to be unchanged by **doxycycline** when two groups of 13 patients with acute falciparum malaria were compared,[4] although *in vitro*, **doxycycline** appears to be a potent inhibitor of quinine metabolism.[5] No special precautions would seem to be necessary.

(e) Rifampicin

An isolated report describes a patient with myotonia controlled with quinine, whose symptoms worsened within 3 weeks of starting to take **rifampicin** for the treatment of tuberculosis. Peak quinine levels were found to be low, but rose again when the **rifampicin** was stopped. Control of the myotonia was regained after 6 weeks.[6] The probable reason is that **rifampicin** (a potent liver enzyme-inducing agent) increases the metabolism of the quinine by the liver, thereby hastening its clearance from the body and reducing its effects. Information appears to be limited to this report but it is consistent with the way **rifampicin** affects a number of other drugs. The general importance of this interaction is uncertain, but monitor the effects of concurrent use and raise the quinine dosage if necessary. Reduce the dosage when the **rifampicin** is stopped.

(f) Urinary alkalinizers and acidifiers

The excretion of unchanged quinine in man is virtually halved (from 17.4 to 8.9%) if the urine is changed from acid to alkaline. The reason is that in alkaline urine more of the quinine exists in the non-ionised (lipid soluble) form which is more easily reabsorbed by the kidney tubules.[7] However there seem to be no reports of adverse effects arising from changes in excretion due to this interaction and no special precautions seem to be necessary.

1. Hurwitz A. The effects of antacids on gastrointestinal drug absorption. II. Effect of sulfadiazine and quinine. *J Pharmacol Exp Ther* (1971) 179, 485–9.
2. Wanwimolruk S, Sunbhanich M, Pongmarutai M and Patamasucon P. Effects of cimetidine and ranitidine on the pharmacokinetics of quinine. *Br J Clin Pharmacol* (1986) 22, 346–50.
3. Ridtitid W, Wongnawa M, Kleekaew A, Mahatthanatrakul W, Sunbhanich M. Cholestyramine does not significantly decrease the bioavailability of quinine in healthy volunteers. *Asia Pac J Pharmacol* (1998) 13, 123–7.

4. Couet W, Laroche R, Floch JJ, Istin B, Fourtillan JB, Sauniere JF. Pharmacokinetics of quinine and doxycycline in patients with acute falciparum malaria: a study in Africa. *Ther Drug Monit* (1991) 13, 496–501.
5. Zhao X-J, Ishizaki T. A further interaction study of quinine with clinically important drugs by human liver microsomes: determinations of inhibition constant (K i) and type of inhibition. *Eur J Drug Metab Pharmacokinet* (1999) 24, 272–8.
6. Osborn JE, Pettit MJ, Graham P. Interaction between rifampicin and quinine: case report. *Pharm J* (1989) 243, 704.
7. Haag HB, Larson PS and Schwartz JJ. The effect of urinary pH on the elimination of quinine in man. *J Pharmacol Exp Ther* (1943) 79, 136–9.

Quinine + Tobacco smoking

Smokers clear quinine from the body much more quickly than non-smokers. The clinical importance of this is as yet uncertain.

Clinical evidence

A comparative study in 10 **smokers** (averaging 17 cigarettes daily) and 10 **non-smokers** given single 600-mg doses of quinine sulphate found that the **smokers** had a reduced AUC (44%), an increased clearance (77%) and a shortened half-life 7.5 vs 12 h), when compared to the **non-smokers**.[1]

Mechanism

The reason appears to be that tobacco smoke contains polycyclic aromatic compounds and other substances which are potent inducers of the liver enzymes which metabolise quinine. As a result the quinine is metabolised and cleared from the body more quickly. It is not yet clear which cytochrome P450 isoenzymes are affected.

Importance and management

Information seems to be limited to this study but the interaction would appear to be established. These results suggest that heavy smokers may need an increased dosage to control malaria (possibly roughly doubled) but more study is needed to confirm the clinical importance of this interaction.

1. Wanwimolruk S, Wong SM, Coville PF, Viriyayudhakorn S, Thitiarchakul S. Cigarette smoking enhances the elimination of quinine. *Br J Clin Pharmacol* (1993) 36, 610–14.

Quinolone antibacterials + Antacids

The serum levels of many of the quinolone antibacterials can be reduced below therapeutic concentrations by aluminium and magnesium antacids. Calcium antacids interact to a lesser extent, and bismuth antacids only minimally. Separating the administration by 2 to 6 h where significant interactions occur reduces admixture in the gut and can minimise the effects. The details are shown in the table.

Clinical evidence

There is a wealth of information about the quinolone/antacid interactions[1-41] and this is summarised in Table 5.3. This table shows what happens to the maximum serum levels (C_{max}) and the relative bioavailabilities (%) when the quinolones listed have been given at the same time as antacids, and when separated by time intervals (e.g. –2 h, +4 h, etc.).

Mechanism

It is believed that certain functional groups (3-carboxyl and 4-oxo) on the antibacterials form insoluble chelates with aluminium and magnesium ions within the gut which reduces their absorption.[7,25,42] The stability of the chelate formed seems to be an important factor in determining the degree of interaction.[42] See also 'Quinolone antibacterials + Iron and Zinc preparations', p.212).

Importance and management

The quinolone antibacterial/antacid interactions are generally well documented, well established and, depending on the particular quinolone and antacid concerned, of clinical importance. The risk is that the serum levels of the antibacterial may fall below minimally inhibitory concentrations (i.e. subtherapeutic against organisms such as staphylococci and *Ps. aeruginosa*[3]) so that treatment failures can occur.[43] The overall picture is that the aluminium/magnesium antacids interact to a greater extent than the calcium antacids, and bismuth antacids hardly at all.

(a) Aluminium-magnesium antacids

Table 5.4 shows that the aluminium-magnesium antacids can reduce the bioavailabilities of the quinolones. Separating their administration to reduce the admixture of the two drugs in the gut increases the bioavailability of these quinolones, a very broad rule-of-thumb being that the quinolones should be taken at least 2 h before and not less than 4 to 6 h after the antacid.[7-9,18,30,38,44] The only obvious exception is **fleroxacin** which appears to interact minimally. The outcome of taking these precautions should be well monitored.

(b) Calcium carbonate antacids

Information about the interactions with calcium carbonate antacids is much more limited than with the aluminium-magnesium antacids, but the table shows that the bioavailabilities of the three quinolones listed can be reduced. These reductions are less than those seen with the aluminium-magnesium antacids but using ciprofloxacin as a guide[14,29] a very broad rule-of-thumb would be to separate the drug administration by about 2 h to minimise this interaction. This is clearly not necessary with **levofloxacin**,[22] **lomefloxacin**,[36] or **ofloxacin**,[45] nor probably with some of the other quinolones, but in the absence of direct information a 2 h separation errs on the safe side. The outcome of taking these precautions should be well monitored.

(c) Bismuth antacids

Bismuth subsalicylate reduces the relative bioavailability of **ciprofloxacin** to 83.8%. Information about other quinolones appears to be lacking, however using ciprofloxacin as the guide it would seem that any interaction is likely only to be of minimal clinical importance, and no action appears to be necessary. However good monitoring would be a prudent precaution.

(d) Sodium antacids

Sodium bicarbonate does not interact significantly with **norfloxacin**[10] but information about other quinolones appears to be lacking. However bear in mind that in the case of **ciprofloxacin** an excessive rise in pH caused by antacids like sodium bicarbonate may possibly result in urinary crystalluria and kidney damage.

Possible alternatives to the antacids which do not appear to interact at all with the quinolones or only to a clinically irrelevant extent, include the H_2-blockers and the proton pump inhibitors.

1. Fleming LW, Moreland TA, Stewart WK, Scott AC. Ciprofloxacin and antacids. *Lancet* (1986) ii, 294.
2. Höffken G, Borner K, Glatzel PD, Koeppe P, Lode H. Reduced enteral absorption of ciprofloxacin in the presence of antacids. *Eur J Clin Microbiol* (1985) 4, 345.
3. Preheim LC, Cuevas TA, Roccaforte JS, Mellencamp MA, Bittner MJ. Ciprofloxacin and antacids. *Lancet* (1986) ii, 48.
4. Vinceneux P, Weber P, Gaudin H, Boussougant Y. Diminution de l'absorption de la péfloxacine par les pansements gastriques. *Presse Med* (1986) 15, 1826.
5. Maesen FPV, Davies BI, Geraedts WH, Sumajow CA. Ofloxacin and antacids. *J Antimicrob Chemother* (1987) 19, 848–50.
6. Sahai J, Healy D, Stotka J, Polk R. Influence of chronic administration of calcium (CA) on the bioavailability (BA) of oral ciprofloxacin (CIP). *Intersci Conf Antimicrob Agents Chemother* (1990) 29, 136.
7. Nix DE, Watson WA, Lener ME, Frost RW, Krol G, Goldstein H, Lettieri J, Schentag JJ. Effects of aluminum and magnesium antacids and ranitidine on the absorption of ciprofloxacin. *Clin Pharmacol Ther* (1989) 46, 700–705.
8. Grasela TH, Schentag JJ, Sedman AJ, Wilton JH, Thomas DJ, Schultz RW, Lebsack ME, Kinkel AW. Inhibition of enoxacin absorption by antacids or ranitidine. *Antimicrob Agents Chemother* (1989) 33, 615–17.
9. Nix DE, Wilton JH, Ronald B, Distlerath L, Williams VC, Norman A. Inhibition of norfloxacin absorption by antacids. *Antimicrob Agents Chemother* (1990) 34, 432–5.
10. Okhamafe AO, Akerele JO, Chukuka CS. Pharmacokinetic interactions of norfloxacin with some metallic medicinal agents. *Int J Pharmaceutics* (1991) 68, 11–18.
11. Brouwers JRBJ, van der Kam HJ, Sijtsma J, Proost JH. Important reduction of ciprofloxacin absorption by sucralfate and magnesium citrate solution. *Drug Invest* (1990) 2, 197–9.
12. Stroshane RM, Brown RR, Cook JA, Wissel PS, Silverman MH. Effect of food, milk, and antacid on the absorption of orally administered amifloxacin. *Rev Infect Dis* (1989) 11 (Suppl 5), S1018–S1019.

Table 5.3 Quinolone antibacterial/antacid interactions

Quinolone (mg:time[a])	Antacid or other coadministered drug	C_{max} (µg/ml) alone	with	Relative bioavailability (%)[b]	Ref
Amifloxacin					
200: +0.16 h	$Mg(OH)_2 + Al(OH)_3$	2.33	0.34	14.6	12
Ciprofloxacin					
250	$Mg(OH)_2 + Al(OH)_3$	3.69	<1.25	NR	1
500	$Mg(OH)_2 + Al(OH)_3$	2.6	0.82	NR	3
500: +24 h	$Mg(OH)_2 + Al(OH)_3$	1.7	0.1	NR	2
500: +24 h	$Mg(OH)_2 + Al(OH)_3$	1.9	0.13	9.5	15
750: −2 h	$Mg(OH)_2 + Al(OH)_3$	3.01	3.96	107.0	7
+0.08 h		3.42	0.68	15.1	
+2 h		3.42	0.88	23.2	
+4 h		3.01	2.62	70.0	
+6 h		2.63	2.64	108.5	
750: +0.08 h	$Al(OH)_3$	3.2	0.6	15.0	13
750	$Al(OH)_3$	2.3	0.8	NR	17
200	$Al(OH)_3$	1.3	0.2	12.0	32
250	$CaCO_3$	3.69	3.42 (ns)	NR	1
500	$CaCO_3$	1.53	1.37 (ns)	94.0 (ns)	29
500	$CaCO_3$	2.9	1.8	58.8	26
750: 0.08 h	$CaCO_3$	3.2	1.7	64.5	13
500: +2 h	$CaCO_3$	1.25	1.44	102.4	14
500	$CaCO_3$	2.9	1.8	58.9	6
500	Mg citrate	2.4	0.6	21.0	11
500	Bismuth salicylate (subsalicylate)	3.8	2.9	83.8	33
750	Bismuth salicylate (subsalicylate)	2.95	2.57	87.0	23
Enoxacin					
200	$Al(OH)_3$	2.26	0.46	15.4	19
400: +0.5 h	$Mg(OH)_2 + Al(OH)_3$	3.17	0.95	26.8	8
+2 h		3.17	1.95	52.3	
+8 h		3.17	2.88	82.7	
200	$Al(OH)_3$	2.3	0.5	15.8	32
Fleroxacin					
200	$Al(OH)_3$	2.4	1.8	82.8	32
Gatifloxacin					
200	$Al(OH)_3$	1.71	0.75	45.9	40
400	$Mg(OH)_2 + Al(OH)_3$	3.8	1.2	35.6	38
400: −2 h		3.8	2.1	57.9	
+2 h		3.4	3.3	82.5	
+4 h		3.4	3.5 (ns)	100.0 (ns)	
Grepafloxacin					
200	$Al(OH)_3$	NR	NR	60.0	34
Levofloxacin					
100	$Al(OH)_3$	1.82	0.64	56.3	22
100	$Al(OH)_3$	1.8	0.6	54.8	32
100	MgO	1.82	1.13	78.2	22
100	$CaCO_3$	1.45	1.12	96.7	22
Lomefloxacin					
200	$Mg(OH)_2 + Al(OH)_3$	1.91	1.03	59.2	25
200	$Al(OH)_3$	2.2	1.0	65.2	32
NR: +2 h	$Mg(OH)_2 + Al(OH)_3$	2.85	2.67 (ns)	88.2	18
−2 h		2.85	2.16	80.4	
−4 h		2.85	2.67 (ns)	90.1	
400	$Mg(OH)_2 + Al(OH)_3$	3.25	1.31	52.1	41
+12 h		3.25	3.66 (ns)		
−4 h		3.25	3.69 (ns)		
400	$CaCO_3$	4.72	4.08	97.9 (ns)	36

Table 5.3 Quinolone antibacterial/antacid interactions (Continued)

Quinolone (mg:time[a])	Antacid or other coadministered drug	C_{max} (µg/ml) alone	with	Relative bioavailability (%)[b]	Ref
Moxifloxacin					
400	$Mg(OH)_2$ + $Al(OH)_3$	2.57	1.0	74.0	37
Norfloxacin					
200	$Al(OH)_3$	1.45	< 0.01	2.7	19
400: +0.08	$Mg(OH)_2$ + $Al(OH)_3$	1.64	0.08	9.0 (based on urinary recovery)	9
−2 h		1.64	1.25	81.3	
200	$Al(OH)_3$	1.5	< 0.10	3.0	32
400	$Al(OH)_3$	1.51	1.09	71.2 (from saliva)	10
400	Mg trisilicate	1.51	0.43	19.3 (from saliva)	10
400	$CaCO_3$	1.64	0.56	37.5	9
400	$CaCO_3$	1.51	1.08	52.8 (from saliva)	10
400	Bismuth salicylate (subsalicylate)			89.7 (ns)	21
400	Sodium bicarbonate	1.40	1.47	104.9 (ns)	10
Ofloxacin					
200	$Al(OH)_3$	3.23	1.31	52.1	19
200	$Al(PO)_4$			93.1 (ns)	39
200	MgO + $Al(OH)_3$	1.97	1.10	62.0	24
200: +24 h	$Mg(OH)_2$ + $Al(OH)_3$	2.6	0.7	30.8	15
400: +2 h	$Mg(OH)_2$ + $Al(OH)_3$	3.7	2.6	79.2	16
−2 h		3.7	3.8 (ns)	101.9 (ns)	
+24 h		3.7	3.5 (ns)	95.3 (ns)	
600	$Mg(OH)_2$ + $Al(OH)_3$	8.11	6.13	NR	5
200	$Al(OH)_3$	3.2	1.3	52.1	32
400: +2 h	$CaCO_3$	3.2	3.3 (ns)	103.6 (ns)	16
−2 h		3.2	3.3 (ns)	97.9 (ns)	
+24 h		3.2	3.5 (ns)	95.9 (ns)	
Pefloxacin					
400	$Mg(OH)_2$ + $Al(OH)_3$	5.14	1.95	44.2	20
400	$Mg(OH)_2$ + $Al(OH)_3$	3.95	1.25	NR	4
400	$Mg(OH)_2$ + $Al(OH)_3$	5.1	2.0	45.7	31
Rufloxacin					
400: +0.08 h	$Mg(OH)_2$ + $Al(OH)_3$	3.74	2.12	59.7	27
400: −4 h	$Mg(OH)_2$ + $Al(OH)_3$	3.74	3.97 (ns)	84.7	27
Sparfloxacin					
400: −2 h	$Mg(OH)_2$ + $Al(OH)_3$	1.09	0.77	74.4	30
+2 h		1.09	0.95	82.4	
+4 h		1.09	1.17	93.4	
200	$Al(OH)_3$	0.865	0.683	64.9	28, 32
Tosufloxacin					
150	$Al(OH)_3$	0.3	0.1	29.2	32
Trovafloxacin					
300: −2 h	$Mg(OH)_2$ + $Al(OH)_3$	2.8	2.5	71.7	35
+5 h		2.8	1.1	33.7	

[a]Time interval between intake of quinolone and the other agent: − and + indicate that the quinolone was administered before and after, respectively, intake of the other agent.
[b]Calculated from AUC data.
NR, not reported; h, hour.

13. Frost RW, Lettieri JT, Noe A, Shamblen EC, Lasseter K. Effect of aluminum hydroxide and calcium carbonate antacids on ciprofloxacin bioavailability. *Clin Pharmacol Ther* (1989) 45, 165.
14. Lomaestro BM, Bailie GR. Effect of staggered dose of calcium on the bioavailability of ciprofloxacin. *Antimicrob Agents Chemother* (1991) 35, 1004–1007.
15. Höffken G, Lode H, Wiley R, Glatzel TD, Sievers D, Olschewski T, Borner K, Koeppe T. Pharmacokinetics and bioavailability of ciprofloxacin and ofloxacin: effect of food and antacid intake. *Rev Infect Dis* (1988) 10 (Suppl 1), S138–S139.
16. Flor S, Guay DRP, Opsahl JA, Tack K, Matzke GR. Effects of magnesium-aluminum hydroxide and calcium carbonate antacids on bioavailability of ofloxacin. *Antimicrob Agents Chemother* (1990) 34, 2436–8.
17. Golper TA, Hartstein AI, Morthland VH, Christensen JM. Effects of antacids and dialysate dwell times on multiple-dose pharmacokinetics of oral ciprofloxacin in patients on continuous ambulatory peritoneal dialysis. *Antimicrob Agents Chemother* (1987) 31, 1787–90.
18. Forster T, Blouin R. The effect of antacid timing on lomefloxacin bioavailability. *Intersci Conf Antimicrob Agents Chemother* (1989) 29, 318.
19. Shiba K, Saito A, Miyahara T, Tachizawa H, Fujimoto T. Effect of aluminium hydroxide, an antacid, on the pharmacokinetics of new quinolones in humans. Proc 15th Int Congr Chemother, Istanbul 1987, 168–9.
20. Metz R, Jaehde U, Sörgel F, Wiesemann H, Gottschalk B, Stephan U, Schunack W. Pharmacokinetic interactions and non-interactions of pefloxacin. Proc 15th Int Congr Chemother, Istanbul, 1987, 997–9.
21. Campbell NRC, Kara M, Hasinoff BB, Haddara WM, McKay DW. Norfloxacin interaction with antacids and minerals. *Br J Clin Pharmacol* (1992) 33, 115–16.
22. Shiba K, Sakai O, Shimada J, Okazaki O, Aoki H, Hakusui H. Effects of antacids, ferrous sulfate, and ranitidine on absorption of DR-3355 in humans. *Antimicrob Agents Chemother* (1992) 36, 2270–4.
23. Rambout L, Sahai J, Gallicano K, Oliveras L, Garber G. Effect of bismuth subsalicylate on ciprofloxacin bioavailability. *Antimicrob Agents Chemother* (1994) 38, 2187–90.
24. Shiba K, Yoshida M, Kachi M, Shimada J, Saito A, Sakai N. Effects of peptic ulcer-healing drugs on the pharmacokinetics of new quinolone (OFLX). 17th Int Congr Chemother, June 1991, Berlin, Abstract 415.
25. Shimada J, Shiba K, Oguma T, Miwa H, Yoshimura Y, Nishikawa T, Okabayashi Y, Kitagawa T, Yamamoto S. Effect of antacid on absorption of the quinolone lomefloxacin. *Antimicrob Agents Chemother* (1992) 36, 1219–24.
26. Sahai J, Healey DP, Stotka J, Polk RE. The influence of chronic administration of calcium carbonate on the bioavailability of oral ciprofloxacin. *Br J Clin Pharmacol* (1993) 35, 302–4.
27. Lazzaroni M, Imbimbo BP, Bargiggia S, Sangaletti O, Dal Bo L, Broccali G, Bianchi Porro G. Effects of magnesium-aluminum hydroxide antacid on absorption of rufloxacin. *Antimicrob Agents Chemother* (1993) 37, 2212–16.
28. Shimada J, Saito A, Shiba K, Hojo T, Kaji M, Hori S, Yoshida M, Sakai O. Pharmacokinetics and clinical studies on sparfloxacin. *Chemotherapy (Tokyo)* (1991) 39 (Suppl 4), 234–44.
29. Lomaestro BM, Bailie GR. Effect of multiple staggered doses of calcium on the bioavailability of ciprofloxacin. *Ann Pharmacother* (1993) 27, 1325–8.
30. Wilson J, Johnson RD, Caille G, Talbot G, Dorr MB, Heald D. The effect of staggered dosing of Maalox® on the oral bioavailability of sparfloxacin. *Pharm Res* (1994) 11 (10 Suppl), S-429.
31. Jaehde U, Sörgel F, Stephan U, Schunack W. Effect of an antacid containing magnesium and aluminum on absorption, metabolism and mechanism of renal elimination of pefloxacin in humans. *Antimicrob Agents Chemother* (1994) 38, 1129–33.
32. Shiba K, Sakamoto M, Nakazawa Y, Sakai O. Effect of antacid on absorption and excretion of new quinolones. *Drugs* (1995) 49 (Suppl 2), 360–1.
33. Sahai J, Oliveras L, Garber G. Effect of bismuth subsalicylate (Peptobismol. PB) on ciprofloxacin (C) absorption: a preliminary investigation. 17th Int Congr Chemother, June 1991, Berlin, Abstract 414.
34. Koneru B, Bramer S, Bricmont P, Maroli A, Shiba K. Effect of food, gastric pH and co-administration of antacid, cimetidine and probenecid on the oral pharmacokinetics of the broad spectrum antimicrobial agent grepafloxacin. *Pharm Res* (1996) 13 (9 Suppl), S414.
35. Teng R, Dogolo LC, Willavize SA, Freidman HL, Vincent J. Effect of Maalox and omeprazole on the bioavailability of trovafloxacin. *J Antimicrob Chemother* (1997) 39 (Suppl B), 93–7.
36. Lehto P, Kivistö KT. Different effects of products containing metal ions on the absorption of lomefloxacin. *Clin Pharmacol Ther* (1994) 56, 477–82.
37. Stass H, Böttcher M-F, Ochmann K. Evaluation of the influence of antacids and H₂ antagonists on the absorption of moxifloxacin after oral administration of a 400-mg dose to healthy volunteers. *Clin Pharmacokinet* (2001) 40 (Suppl 1), 39–48.
38. Lober S, Ziege S, Rau M, Schreiber G, Mignot A, Koeppe P, Lode H. Pharmacokinetics of gatifloxacin and interaction with an antacid containing aluminum and magnesium. *Antimicrob Agents Chemother* (1999) 43, 1067–71.
39. Martínez Carbaga M, Sánchez Navarro A, Colino Gandarillas CI, Domínguez-Gil A. Effects of two cations on gastrointestinal absorption of ofloxacin. *Antimicrob Agents Chemother* (1999) 44 (Suppl A), 141.
40. Shiba K, Kusajima H, Momo K. The effects of aluminium hydroxide, cimetidine, ferrous sulfate, green tea and milk on pharmacokinetics of gatifloxacin in healthy humans. *J Antimicrob Chemother* (1999) 44 (Suppl A), 141.
41. Kunka RL, Wong YY, Lyon JL. Effect of antacid on the pharmacokinetics of lemofloxacin. *Pharm Res* (1988) 5 (Suppl), S-165.
42. Mizuki Y, Fujiwara I, Yamaguchi T. Pharmacokinetic interactions related to the chemical structures of fluoroquinolones. *J Antimicrob Chemother* (1996) 37 (Suppl), A41–A55.

Table 5.4 Herbs contained in some Chinese herbal remedies[1,2]

Herb (plant part)	Amounts of herbs in the medicines (mg/2.5 g)				
	Hotyu-ekki-to	Rikkunshi-to	Juzen-taiho-to	Sho-saiko-to	Sairei-to
Atractylodis lanceae (rhizome)	278	248	175		125
Ginseng (root)	278	248	175	188	125
Glycyrrhizae (root)	104	662	688	125	83
Aurantii nobilis (pericarp)	139	124			
Zizyphi (fruit)	139	124		188	125
Zingiberis (rhizome)	635	631		63	42
Astragali (root)	278		175		
Angelicae (root)	208		175		
Bupleuri (root)	139			438	292
Cimicifugae (rhizome)	669				
Hoelen		248	175		125
Pinelliae (tuber)		248		313	208
Cinnamomi (cortex)			175		83
Rehmanniae (root)			175		
Paeoniae (root)			175		
Cnidii (rhizome)			175		
Scutellariae (root)				188	125
Alismatis (rhizome)					208
Polyporus					125

43. Noyes M, Polk RE. Norfloxacin and absorption of magnesium-aluminium. *Ann Intern Med* (1988) 109, 168–9.
44. Misiak P, Toothaker R, Lebsack M, Sedman A, Colburn W. The effect of dosing-time intervals on the potential pharmacokinetic interaction between oral enoxacin and oral antacid. *Intersci Conf Antimicrob Agents Chemother* (1988) 28, 367.
45. Sánchez Navarro A, Martínez Cabarga M, Dominguez-Gil Hurlé A. Comparative study of the influence of Ca²⁺ on absorption parameters of ciprofloxacin and ofloxacin. *J Antimicrob Chemother* (1994) 34, 119–25.

Quinolone antibacterials + Cetraxate

A single dose study found that cetraxate (dose not stated) did not affect the pharmacokinetics of a single 200-mg dose of ofloxacin.[1] No special precautions would seem to be necessary.

1. Shiba K, Yoshida M, Kachi M, Shimada J, Saito A, Sakai N. Effects of peptic ulcer-healing drugs on the pharmacokinetics of new quinolone (OFLX). 17th Int Congr Chemother, June 1991, Berlin, Abstract 415.

Quinolone antibacterials + Chinese herbal medicines

Sho-saiko-to, Rikkunshi-to and Sairei-to do not interact with ofloxacin, and Hotyu-ekki-to, Rikkunshi-to and Juzen-taiho-to do not interact with levofloxacin.

Clinical evidence, mechanism, importance and management

The bioavailability and urinary recovery of single 200 mg oral doses of **ofloxacin** were found not to be significantly altered in 7 healthy subjects when taken with any of three Chinese OTC medicines (**Sho-saiko-to**, **Rikkunshi-to** or **Sairei-to**).[1] Eight healthy subjects were given single 200 mg oral doses of **levofloxacin** with single doses 2.5 g doses of **Hotyu-ekki-to**, **Rikkunshi-to** or **Juzen-taiho-to**. None of them had a significant effect on the bioavailability of the **levofloxacin** or on its renal excretion.[2] There would therefore seem to be no reason for avoiding concurrent use. Information about other quinolones is lacking. The ingredients of three of these herbal medicines are detailed in Table 5.4.

1. Hasegawa T, Yamaki K, Nadai M, Muraoka I, Wang L, Takagi K, Nabeshima T. Lack of effect of Chinese medicines on bioavailability of ofloxacin in healthy volunteers. *Int J Clin Pharmacol Ther* (1994) 32, 57–61.
2. Hasegawa T, Yamaki K-I, Muraoka I, Nadai M, Takagi K, Nabeshima T. Effects of traditional Chinese medicines on pharmacokinetics of levofloxacin. *Antimicrob Agents Chemother* (1995) 39, 2135–7.

Quinolone antibacterials + Cytotoxic agents

The absorption of ciprofloxacin and ofloxacin can be reduced by the concurrent use of some cytotoxic agents but this is probably clinically unimportant.

Clinical evidence

(a) Ciprofloxacin

Six patients with newly diagnosed haematological malignancies (5 with acute myeloid leukaemia and one with non-Hodgkin's lymphoma) were treated with 500 mg **ciprofloxacin** twice daily to control possible infections when neutropenic. It was found that after 13 days chemotherapy their mean maximum serum **ciprofloxacin** levels had fallen by 46% (from 3.7 to 2.0 mg/l) and the $AUC_{0—4h}$ by 47% (from 10.7 to 5.7 mg/l.h). There were large individual differences between the patients. The cytotoxic agents used were **cyclophosphamide**, **cytarabine**, **daunorubicin**, **doxorubicin**, **mitoxantrone** and **vincristine**.[1]

(b) Ofloxacin

Ten patients with non-Hodgkin's lymphoma, hairy cell leukaemia or acute myeloid leukaemia were given 400 mg **ofloxacin** at breakfast time for antibacterial prophylaxis during neutropenia. Blood samples were taken 3 days before chemotherapy began and 2 to 3, 5 to 7 and 8 to 10 days afterwards. The maximum serum **ofloxacin** levels were reduced significantly 2 to 3 days after the chemotherapy (by 18%) but none of the other pharmacokinetic measurements were changed by the cytotoxic treatment. The serum levels had returned to normal by days 5 to 7. At all times serum levels exceeded the expected MICs of the gram-negative potential pathogens. The cytotoxic agents used were **cyclophosphamide**, **cytarabine**, **doxorubicin**, **etoposide**, **ifosfamide** (with mesna), **vincristine**, and prednisolone.[2]

Mechanism

Uncertain. The interaction seems to result from a reduction in absorption of the quinolones by the small intestine, possibly related to the damaging effect these cytotoxic agents have on the rapidly dividing cells of the intestinal mucosa.

Importance and management

Direct information is limited, but these reports are consistent with the way cytotoxic agents can reduce the absorption of some other drugs. The authors of both reports suggest that these changes are probably clinically unimportant, because the serum levels of achieved are likely to be sufficient to treat most infections. It would seem nevertheless prudent to monitor concurrent use to confirm that their prediction is true. If the suggested mechanism of interaction is correct, no interaction should occur if quinolones are given parenterally. Nothing appears to be documented about any of the other quinolone antibacterials.

1. Johnson EJ, MacGowan AP, Potter MN, Stockley RJ, White LO, Slade RR, Reeves DS. Reduced absorption of oral ciprofloxacin after chemotherapy for haematological malignancy. *J Antimicrob Chemother* (1990) 25, 837–42.
2. Brown NM, White LO, Blundell EL, Chown SR, Slade RR, MacGowan AP, Reeves DS. Absorption of oral ofloxacin after cytotoxic chemotherapy for haematological malignancy. *J Antimicrob Chemother* (1993) 32, 117–22.

Quinolone antibacterials + Dairy products

Dairy products reduce the bioavailability of ciprofloxacin, gatifloxacin and norfloxacin, but not amifloxacin, enoxacin, lomefloxacin, ofloxacin and probably not fleroxacin.

Clinical evidence, mechanism, importance and management

(a) Evidence of an interaction

A study in 7 healthy subjects given single 500-mg doses of **ciprofloxacin** found that 300 ml **milk** or **yoghurt** reduced the peak plasma levels by 36% and 47%, and the AUC by 33% and 36% respectively.[1] **Milk** (300 ml) reduced the AUC of 500 mg **ciprofloxacin** by about 30%.[2] Another study found that 300 ml **milk** or **yoghurt** reduced the absorption and the peak plasma levels of a single 200-mg dose of **norfloxacin** by roughly 50%.[3] In a study with **gatifloxacin** 200 mg, 200 ml **milk** reduced the AUC by about 15%.[4]

The proposed reason for all these changes is that the calcium in the **milk** and **yoghurt** combines with the **ciprofloxacin** and **norfloxacin** to produce insoluble chelates. The effect of these changes on the control of infection is uncertain but until the situation is clear patients should be advised not to take these **dairy products** within 1 to 2 h of either **ciprofloxacin** or **norfloxacin** to prevent admixture in the gut.

(b) Evidence of no interaction

A study in 21 healthy subjects found that 8 oz (about 250 ml **milk** had no clinically significant effects on the absorption of 300 mg of **ofloxacin**.[5] Another study confirmed the lack of a significant interaction with both **milk** and **yoghurt**.[6] The bioavailability of **amifloxacin** is also minimally altered by **milk**.[7] In another study, a **fat and liquid**

calcium meal was not found to have a clinically significant effect on the pharmacokinetics of **fleroxacin**.[8] **Milk** had no effect on **fleroxacin**[2] or **lomefloxacin**[9] pharmacokinetics. Another study found no effect of **milk** and a **standard breakfast** on enoxacin absorption.[10]

Therefore the quinolones that do not interact significantly would appear to be **amifloxacin, enoxacin, lomefloxacin, ofloxacin** and probably **fleroxacin**. They may provide a useful alternative to the interacting quinolones (see (i) above).

1. Neuvonen PJ, Kivistö KT, Lehto P. Interference of dairy products with the absorption of ciprofloxacin. *Clin Pharmacol Ther* (1991) 50, 498–502.
2. Hoogkamer JFW, Kleinbloesem CH. The effect of milk consumption on the pharmacokinetics of fleroxacin and ciprofloxacin in healthy volunteers. *Drugs* (1995) 49 (Suppl 2), 346–8.
3. Kivistö KT, Ojala-Karlsson P, Neuvonen PJ. Inhibition of norfloxacin absorption by dairy products. *Antimicrob Agents Chemother* (1992) 36, 489–91.
4. Shiba K, Kusajima H, Momo K. The effects of aluminium hydroxide, cimetidine, ferrous sulfate, green tea and milk on pharmacokinetics of gatifloxacin in healthy humans. *J Antimicrob Chemother* (1999) 44 (Suppl A), 141.
5. Dudley MN, Marchbanks CR, Flor SC, Beals B. The effect of food or milk on the absorption kinetics of ofloxacin. *Eur J Clin Pharmacol* (1991) 41, 569–71.
6. Neuvonen PJ, Kivistö KT. Milk and yoghurt do not impair the absorption of -ofloxacin. *Br J Clin Pharmacol* (1992) 33, 346–8.
7. Stroshane RM, Brown RR, Cook JA, Wissel PS, Silverman MH. Effect of food, milk, and antacid on the absorption of orally administered amifloxacin. *Rev Infect Dis* (1989) 11 (Suppl 5), S1018–S1019.
8. Bertino JS, Nafziger AN, Wong M, Stragand L, Puleo C. Effects of a fat- and calcium-rich breakfast on pharmacokinetics of fleroxacin administered in single and multiple doses. *Antimicrob Agents Chemother* (1994) 38, 499–503.
9. Lehto PL, Kivistö KT. Different effects of products containing metal ions on the absorption of lomefloxacin. *Clin Pharmacol Ther* (1994) 56, 477–82.
10. Lehto P, Kivistö KT. Effects of milk and food on the absorption of enoxacin. *Br J Clin Pharmacol* (1995) 39, 194–6.

Quinolone antibacterials + Didanosine

An extremely marked reduction in the serum levels of ciprofloxacin occurs if it is given at the same time as didanosine, because of an interaction with the antacid buffers in the didanosine formulation. Taking the ciprofloxacin 2 h before or 6 h after the didanosine minimises this interaction.

Clinical evidence

When 12 healthy subjects were given 750 mg **ciprofloxacin** with two **didanosine-placebo** tablets (i.e. all of the antacid additives but no didanosine), the **ciprofloxacin** AUC and maximum serum levels were reduced by 98% and 93% respectively.[1] Other studies have looked at the effect of separating the administration times. When 16 HIV+ patients were given 1500 mg daily doses of **ciprofloxacin** 2 h before **didanosine**, the **ciprofloxacin** AUC was reduced by only 26%.[2] Another study found that when 500 mg **ciprofloxacin** was given 2 h after taking two **didanosine-placebo** tablets the **ciprofloxacin** serum levels were reduced below minimal inhibitory concentrations, but giving the **ciprofloxacin** 2 h before gave normal blood levels.[3]

Mechanism

Not fully established, but the reason is almost certainly because of an interaction between the buffering agents in the didanosine formulation and the ciprofloxacin. Didanosine is extremely acid labile at pH values below 3 so that it has to be formulated with buffering agents (such as aluminium and magnesium hydroxides) to keep the pH as high as possible to minimise the acid-induced hydrolysis. Ciprofloxacin forms insoluble non-absorbable chelates with these metallic ions in the buffer so that its bioavailability is markedly reduced. See 'Quinolone antibacterials + Antacids', p.205.

Importance and management

Direct information is limited to these reports but it appears to be a clinically important interaction. Such drastic reductions in serum ciprofloxacin levels mean that minimal inhibitory concentrations against a considerable number of organisms are unlikely to be achieved. The ciprofloxacin should be given at least 2 hours before or 6 hours after

the didanosine (see 'Quinolone antibacterials + Antacids', p.205). **Other quinolone antibacterials** that interact with **antacids** are also expected to interact with didanosine, but so far reports are lacking.

1. Sahai J, Gallicano K, Oliveras L, Khaliq S, Hawley-Foss N, Garber G. Cations in the didanosine tablet reduce ciprofloxacin bioavailability. *Clin Pharmacol Ther* (1993) 53, 292–7.
2. Knupp CA, Barbhaiya RH. A multiple-dose pharmacokinetic interaction study between didanosine (Videx®) and ciprofloxacin (Cipro®) in male subjects seropositive for HIV but asymptomatic. *Biopharm Drug Dispos* (1997) 18, 65–77.
3. Sahai J. Avoiding the ciprofloxacin-didanosine interaction. *Ann Intern Med* (1995) 123, 394–5.

Quinolone antibacterials + Enteral feeds or Food

The absorption of ciprofloxacin can be reduced by the concurrent use of enteral feeds such as *Ensure, Jevity, Osmolite, Pulmocare* and *Sustacal*. The interaction with ofloxacin is much smaller and probably of little clinical importance. Most foods delay but do not reduce the absorption of amifloxacin, ciprofloxacin, enoxacin, gemifloxacin, lomefloxacin, ofloxacin or sparfloxacin.

Clinical evidence

(a) Ciprofloxacin + Enteral Feeds

The oral bioavailability of 750 mg **ciprofloxacin** was reduced by 28% when given to 13 normal subjects with *Ensure* and the mean maximum serum **ciprofloxacin** levels were reduced by 48%. The fasted subjects were given 120 ml of the study liquid (*Ensure* or water) and this was repeated at 30 min intervals for 5 doses. The **ciprofloxacin** was crushed and mixed with the second dose of the study liquid and the cup rinsed with another 60 ml of the study liquid.[1]

Other enteral feeds (*Jevity, Osmolite, Pulmocare* and *Sustacal*) similarly reduce the bioavailability and maximum serum levels of **ciprofloxacin** by about one third,[2-5] and another enteral feed, *Resource*, reduced the bioavailability by 25%.[6] One comparative study found that *Ensure* reduced the AUC of ciprofloxacin by 40.2% in men but by only 14.5% in women.[7]

Ciprofloxacin bioavailability was reduced by 53% and 67% by *Jevity* or *Sustacal* when given via gastrostomy or jejunostomy tube in a study of 26 hospitalised patients. Despite this, serum levels achieved with gastrostomy tubes were roughly equivalent to those seen taking tablets orally.[5]

(b) Ofloxacin + Enteral Feeds

The oral bioavailability of 400 mg **ofloxacin** was reduced by 10% when given to 13 normal subjects with *Ensure*. The mean maximum serum **ofloxacin** levels were reduced by 36%. The same procedure as described in (a) was followed.[1] Only small reductions in the AUCs of **ofloxacin** were seen in another study (210.5% in men, 213.2% in women) using *Ensure*.[7]

(c) Quinolone antibacterials + Food

Food delayed the absorption of **ciprofloxacin** and **ofloxacin** in 10 subjects, but their bioavailabilities remained unchanged.[8] Other studies confirmed that a delay occurs with the absorption of **ofloxacin**[9] and **lomefloxacin**[10] but the bioavailability is unchanged. **Food** similarly has little effect on **amifloxacin**.[11] **Food** also has no effect on the absorption of **enoxacin**, but **high carbohydrate meals** cause a delay (almost an hour) in the achievement of peak serum levels.[12] No clinically significant effect was seen on the pharmacokinetics of 320 mg or 640 mg of **gemifloxacin**,[13] or 200 mg of **sparfloxacin**,[14] when they were given to healthy subjects with high fat or standard meals, although the absorption of **sparfloxacin** was slightly delayed. All of these changes are probably of minimal clinical importance.

Mechanism

The quinolone antibacterials can form insoluble chelates with divalent ions, which reduces their absorption from the gut. Enteral feeds such as those used above contain at least two divalent ions, calcium and magnesium. See also 'Quinolone antibacterials + Antacids', p.205, 'Quinolone antibacterials + Iron and Zinc preparations', p.212. The differences seen in men and women are possibly due to a slower gastric emptying rate in men which increases the exposure of the quinolone to the enteral feed.[7]

Importance and management

The ciprofloxacin/enteral feed interaction is established. No treatment failures have been reported but it is expected to be clinically important. For example, if patients were to be switched from parenteral to oral ciprofloxacin, there could be a significant reduction in serum ciprofloxacin levels. Be alert for any evidence that ciprofloxacin is less effective and raise the dosage as necessary. The ofloxacin/enteral food interaction is much smaller and probably not clinically important but this needs confirmation. There are no specific reports about other quinolones but you should be alert for this interaction with any of them. Quinolones can be given with food without any decrease in levels.

1. Mueller BA, Brierton DG, Abel SR, Bowman L. Effect of enteral feeding with *Ensure* on oral bioavailabilities of ofloxacin and ciprofloxacin. *Antimicrob Agents Chemother* (1994) 38, 2101–5.
2. Noer BL, Angaran DM. The effect of enteral feedings on ciprofloxacin pharmacokinetics. *Pharmacotherapy* (1990) 10, 254.
3. Yuk JH, Nightingale CH, Quintiliani R, Yeston NS, Orlando R, Dobkin ED, Kambe JC, Sweeney KR, Buonpane EA. Absorption of ciprofloxacin administered through a nasogastric tube or a nasoduodenal tube in volunteers and patients receiving enteral nutrition. *Diagn Microbiol Infect Dis* (1990) 13, 99–102.
4. Yuk JH, Nightingale CH, Sweeney KR, Quintiliani R, Lettieri JT, Frost RW. Relative bioavailability in healthy volunteers of ciprofloxacin administered through a nasogastric tube with and without enteral feeding. *Antimicrob Agents Chemother* (1989) 33, 1118–20.
5. Healy DP, Brodbeck MC, Clendening CE. Ciprofloxacin absorption is impaired in patients given enteral feedings orally and via gastrostomy and jejunostomy tubes. *Antimicrob Agents Chemother* (1996) 40, 6–10.
6. Piccolo ML, Toossi Z, Goldman M. Effect of coadministration of a nutritional supplement on ciprofloxacin absorption. *Am J Hosp Pharm* (1994) 51, 2697–9.
7. Effect of gender on relative oral bioavailability of ciprofloxacin and ofloxacin when administered with an enteral feeding product. *Pharmacotherapy* (1997) 17, 1112.
8. Höffken G, Lode H, Wiley R, Glatzel TD, Sievers D, Olschewski T, Borner K, Koeppe T. Pharmacokinetics and bioavailability of ciprofloxacin and ofloxacin: effect of food and antacid intake. *Rev Infect Dis* (1988) 10 (Suppl 1), S138–S139.
9. Dudley MN, Marchbanks CR, Flor SC, Beals B. The effect of food or milk on the absorption kinetics of ofloxacin. *Eur J Clin Pharmacol* (1991) 41, 569–71.
10. Hooper WD, Dickinson RG, Eadie MJ. Effect of food on absorption of lomefloxacin. *Antimicrob Agents Chemother* (1990) 34, 1797–9.
11. Stroshane RM, Brown RR, Cook JA, Wissel PS, Silverman MH. Effect of food, milk, and antacid on the absorption of orally administered amifloxacin. *Rev Infect Dis* (1989) 11 (Suppl 5), S1018–S1019.
12. Somogyi AA, Bochner F, Keal JA, Rolan PE, Smith M. Effect of food on enoxacin absorption. *Antimicrob Agents Chemother* (1987) 31, 638–9.
13. Allen A, Bygate E, Clark D, Lewis A, Pay V. The effect of food on the bioavailability of oral gemifloxacin in healthy volunteers. *Int J Antimicrob Agents* (2000) 16, 45–50.
14. Johnson RD, Dorr MB, Hunt TL, Jensen BK, Talbot GH. Effects of food on the pharmacokinetics of sparfloxacin. *Clin Ther* (1999) 21, 982–91.

Quinolone antibacterials + Furosemide (Frusemide)

Furosemide (frusemide) causes a small, almost certainly unimportant, rise in the serum levels of lomefloxacin. The pharmacokinetics and diuretic effects of the furosemide are not changed.

Clinical evidence, mechanism, importance and management

A study in 8 healthy subjects found that when single doses of 200 mg **lomefloxacin** and 40 mg **furosemide (frusemide)** were taken together, the AUC of **lomefloxacin** was increased by 12%. The maximum serum levels and the half-life were also increased, but not to a statistically significant extent.[1,2] The suggested reason for the interaction is that there is some competition between the two drugs for excretion by the kidney tubules. No significant changes were seen in the pharmacokinetics of the **furosemide** nor in its diuretic effects.[1] The small rise in the serum levels of **lomefloxacin** are almost certainly too small to be important and there would seem to be no reason for avoiding

concurrent use. Information about other quinolone antibacterials appears to be lacking.

1. Sudoh T, Fujimura A, Shiga T, Sasaki M, Harada K, Tateishi T, Ohashi K, Ebihara A. Renal clearance of lomefloxacin is decreased by furosemide. *Eur J Clin Pharmacol* (1994) 46, 267–9.
2. Sudoh T, Fujimura A. Effect of furosemide and ranitidine on renal clearance of lomefloxacin. *Clin Pharmacol Ther* (1997) 61, 218.

Quinolone antibacterials + H₂-blockers

Cimetidine can increase the serum levels of some quinolone antibacterials (intravenous enoxacin, fleroxacin and oral clinafloxacin and pefloxacin), famotidine can reduce the serum levels of norfloxacin, and ranitidine can reduce the absorption of enoxacin, but none of these interactions appears to be clinically important.

Clinical evidence, mechanism

(a) No significant changes

Neither **cimetidine**[1,2] nor **ranitidine**[3,4] appear to have a clinically important effect on the pharmacokinetics of **ciprofloxacin**, nor **ranitidine** on the pharmacokinetics of **levofloxacin**,[5] **lomefloxacin**,[6-8] or **moxifloxacin**.[9] **Cimetidine** also appears not to interact with **gatifloxacin**,[10] **ofloxacin**,[11] **sparfloxacin**,[12] **trovafloxacin**[13] or **grepafloxacin**.[14] **Ranitidine** 150 mg twice daily did not to affect the pharmacokinetics of a single 400 mg intravenous dose of **enoxacin**.[15] **Famotidine** infusion (up to 40 mg) had no effect on the pharmacokinetics of a 400-mg dose of **grepafloxacin**.[16]

(b) Increased serum levels

Cimetidine was found to increase the AUC of intravenous **pefloxacin** by about 40%. It increased the half-life from 10.3 to 15.3 h and the clearance was reduced by almost by 30%.[17] **Cimetidine** decreased the total clearance of **fleroxacin** by about 25%, without much effect on renal clearance, and increased its elimination half-life by 32%.[18] **Enoxacin** plasma levels following a 400 mg intravenous dose were higher when 300 mg **cimetidine** four times daily was given concurrently. Renal clearance and systemic clearance were reduced 26% and 20% respectively, and the elimination half-life was increased 30%.[15] **Cimetidine** 300 mg four times daily for 4 days increased the maximum serum levels of **clinafloxacin** by 15% and increased its AUC by 44%.[19]

(c) Reduced serum levels

Famotidine given 8 h before **norfloxacin** significantly reduced its maximum serum concentrations in 6 healthy subjects, but the bioavailability (AUC) and urinary recovery rate were unchanged.[20]

(d) Reduced absorption and reduced clearance

Ranitidine 50 mg given intravenously 2 h before a single 400 mg oral dose of **enoxacin** was found to have reduced the absorption by 26 to 40%,[21,22] which seemed to be related to changes in gastric pH caused by the **ranitidine**.[22] **Cimetidine** reduces the clearance of **levofloxacin** by about 25% and increases its AUC by almost 30%.[23]

Importance and management

Although the pharmacokinetic changes seen in some of these studies are not small, none has been shown to affect the outcome of treatment and they are probably only of minor clinical relevance.

1. Ludwig E, Graber H, Székely É, Csiba A. Metabolic interactions of ciprofloxacin. *Diagn Microbiol Infect Dis* (1990) 13, 135–41.
2. Prince RA, Liou W-S, Kasik JE. Effect of cimetidine on ciprofloxacin pharmacokinetics. *Pharmacotherapy* (1990) 10, 233.
3. Höffken G, Lode H, Wiley R, Glatzel TD, Sievers D, Olschewski T, Borner K, Koeppe T. Pharmacokinetics and bioavailability of ciprofloxacin and ofloxacin: effect of food and antacid intake. *Rev Infect Dis* (1988) 10 (Suppl 1), S138–9.
4. Nix DE, Watson WA, Lener ME, Frost RW, Krol G, Goldstein H, Letterei J, Schentag JJ. Effects of aluminum and magnesium antacids and ranitidine on the absorption of ciprofloxacin. *Clin Pharmacol Ther* (1989) 46, 700–5.
5. Shiba K, Sakai O, Shimada J, Okazaki O, Aoki H, Hakusui H. Effects of antacids, ferrous sulphate, and ranitidine on absorption of DR-3355 in humans. *Antimicrob Agents Chemother* (1992) 36, 2270–4.

6. Nix D, Schentag J. Lomefloxacin (L) absorption kinetics when administered with raniti-dine (R) and sucralfate (S). *Intersci Conf Antimicrob Agents Chemother* (1989) 29, 317.
7. Sudoh T, Fujimura A, Harada K, Sunaga A, Ohmori M, Sakamoto K, Kumagai Y. Effect of ranitidine on renal clearance of lomefloxacin (LFLX). *Jpn J Pharmacol* (1995) 67 (Suppl 1), 165P.
8. Sudoh T, Fujimura A, Harada K, Sunaga A, Ohmori M, Sakamoto K. Effect of ranitidine on renal clearance of lomefloxacin. *Eur J Clin Pharmacol* (1996) 51, 95–8.
9. Stass H, Böttcher M-F, Ochmann K. Evaluation of the influence of antacids and H₂ an-tagonists on the absorption of moxifloxacin after oral administration of a 400-mg dose to healthy volunteers. *Clin Pharmacokinet* (2001) 40 (Suppl 1), 39–48.
10. Shiba K, Kusajima H, Momo K. The effects of aluminium hydroxide, cimetidine, ferrous sulfate, green tea and milk on pharmacokinetics of gatifloxacin in healthy humans. *J An-timicrob Chemother* (1999) 44 (Suppl A), 141.
11. Shiba K, Yoshida M, Kachi M, Shimada J, Saito A, Sakai N. Effects of peptic ulcer-heal-ing drugs on the pharmacokinetics of new quinolone (OFLX). 17th International Con-gress on Chemotherapy, Berlin, June 1991. Abstract 415.
12. Gries JM, Honorato J, Taburet AM, Alvarez MP, Sadaba B, Azanza JR, Singlas E. Ci-metidine does not alter sparfloxacin pharmacokinetics. *Int J Clin Pharm Ther* (1995) 33, 585–7.
13. Purkins L, Oliver SD, Willavize SA. An open, controlled, crossover study on the effects of cimetidine on the steady-state pharmacokinetics of trovafloxacin. *Eur J Clin Micro-biol Infect Dis* (1998) 17, 431–3.
14. Koneru B, Bramer S, Bricmont P, Maroli A, Shiba K. Effect of food, gastric pH and co-administration of antacid, cimetidine and probenecid on the oral pharmacokinetics of the broad spectrum antimicrobial agent grepafloxacin. *Pharm Res* (1996) 13 (9 Suppl), S414.
15. Misiak PM, Eldon MA, Toothaker RD, Sedman AJ. Effects of oral cimetidine or raniti-dine on the pharmacokinetics of intravenous enoxacin. *J Clin Pharmacol* (1993) 33, 53–6.
16. Efthymiopoulos C, Bramer SL, Maroli A. Effect of food and gastric pH on the bioavail-ability of grepafloxacin. *Clin Pharmacokinet* (1997) 33 (Suppl 1), 18–24.
17. Sörgel F, Mahr G, Koch HU, Stephan U, Wiesemann HG, Malter U. Effects of cimeti-dine on the pharmacokinetics of pefloxacin in healthy volunteers. *Rev Infect Dis* (1988) 10 (Suppl 1), S137.
18. Portmann R. Influence of cimetidine on fleroxacin pharmacokinetics. *Drugs* (1993) 45 (Suppl 3), 471.
19. Randinitis EJ, Koup JR, Bron NJ, Hounslow NJ, Rausch G, Abel R, Vassos AB, Sedman AJ. Drug interaction studies with clinafloxacin and probenecid, cimetidine, phenytoin and warfarin. *Drugs* (1999) 58 (Suppl 2), 254–5.
20. Shimada J, Hori S. Effect of antiulcer drugs on gastrointestinal absorption of norfloxacin. *Chemotherapy (Tokyo)* (1992) 40, 1141–7.
21. Grasela TH, Schentag JJ, Sedman AJ, Wilton JH, Thomas DJ, Schultz RW, Lebsack ME, Kinkel AW. Inhibition of enoxacin absorption by antacids or ranitidine. *Antimicrob Agents Chemother* (1989) 33, 615–17.
22. Lebsack ME, Nix D, Ryerson B, Toothaker RD, Welage L, Norman AM, Schentag JJ, Sedman AJ. Effect of gastric acidity on enoxacin absorption. *Clin Pharmacol Ther* (1992) 52, 252–6.
23. Gaitonde MD, Mendes P, House ESA, Lehr KH. The effects of cimetidine and probene-cid on the pharmacokinetics of levofloxacin (LFLX). *Intersci Conf Antimicrob Agents Chemother* (1995) 35, 8.

Quinolone antibacterials + Iron and Zinc preparations

Ferrous fumarate, gluconate, sulphate and other prepara-tions containing elemental iron can reduce the absorption of **ciprofloxacin, gatifloxacin, levofloxacin, norfloxacin, ofloxacin and sparfloxacin** from the gut. Serum levels of the antibacterial may become subtherapeutic as a result. Fler-oxacin appears not to be affected and lomefloxacin only min-imally. Gemifloxacin does not appear to interact when given 2 h before or 3 h after ferrous sulphate. No interaction ap-pears to occur with iron-ovotransferrin. Zinc appears to in-teract like iron.

Clinical evidence

(a) Ciprofloxacin

The absorption of **ciprofloxacin** is markedly reduced by iron prepa-rations which contain elemental iron. Several studies have clearly demonstrated reductions in the AUC and maximum serum levels of 30 to 90% with **ferrous fumarate**,[1] **ferrous gluconate**,[2] **ferrous sul-phate**,[2-6] **iron-glycine sulphate**,[7] *Centrum Forte*[2] (a multi-mineral preparation containing iron, magnesium, zinc, calcium, copper and manganese) and with *Stresstabs 600-with-zinc*[5] (a multivitamin-with-zinc preparation). However **iron-ovotransferrin** has been found to have no significant effect on the absorption of **cipro-floxacin**.[8,9]

(b) Fleroxacin

A study in 12 volunteers found that **ferrous sulphate** (100 mg ele-mental iron) had no significant effect on the pharmacokinetics of **fler-oxacin**.[10]

(c) Gatifloxacin

A study in 6 healthy subjects found that **ferrous sulphate** 160 mg given with **gatifloxacin** 200 mg caused a decrease in the maximum serum levels and AUC of **gatifloxacin** by 49 and 29% respectively.[11]

(d) Gemifloxacin

Gemifloxacin 320 mg was given either 2 h after or 3 h before **fer-rous sulphate** 325 mg in a study in 27 healthy subjects. The pharma-cokinetics of **gemifloxacin** were not significantly altered in either case.[12]

(e) Levofloxacin

Ferrous sulphate has been found to reduce the bioavailability of **lev-ofloxacin** by 79%.[13]

(f) Lomefloxacin

When 400 mg **lomefloxacin** was given with **ferrous sulphate** (equivalent to 100 mg elemental iron), the **lomefloxacin** maximum serum levels were reduced by about 28% and the AUC by about 14%.[14]

(g) Norfloxacin

Ferrous sulphate reduced the AUC and maximum serum levels of a single 400-mg dose of **norfloxacin** in 8 normal subjects by 73 and 75% respectively.[6] **Ferrous sulphate** caused a 51% reduction in the **norfloxacin** AUC in another study,[15,16] and a 97% reduction in bioa-vailability in a further single dose study.[17] The same authors also found that both **ferrous sulphate** and **zinc sulphate** reduced the uri-nary recovery of **norfloxacin** by 55 and 56% respectively.[18]

(h) Ofloxacin

Ferrous sulphate (100 mg elemental iron) reduced the AUC and the maximum serum levels following a single 400-mg dose of **ofloxacin** in 8 healthy subjects by 25% and 36% respectively.[6] An 11% de-crease in absorption was seen when 9 healthy volunteers were given 200 mg **ofloxacin** with 1050 mg **ferrous sulphate**.[19] Elemental iron 200 mg (in the form of an **iron-glycine-sulphate** complex) reduced the bioavailability of **ofloxacin** 400 mg in 12 healthy subjects by 36%.[7]

(i) Sparfloxacin

In a single dose study in 6 subjects, 525 mg **ferrous sulphate** (170 mg elemental iron) reduced the AUC of 200 mg **sparfloxacin** by 27%.[15,16]

Mechanism

It is believed that the quinolones form a complex with iron and zinc (by chelation between the metal ion and the 4-oxo and adjacent car-boxyl groups) which is less easily absorbed by the gut. However, a study in *rats* using oral iron and intravenous ciprofloxacin suggested that the interaction may not be entirely confined to the gut.[20] This needs further study. Iron-ovotransferrin differs from other iron prep-arations in being able to combine directly with the transferrin recep-tors of intestinal cells, and appears to release little elemental iron into the gut to interact with the quinolones.

Importance and management

The quinolone/iron interactions are established and would appear to be of clinical importance because the serum antibacterial levels can become subtherapeutic. In descending order the extent of the interac-tion appears to be

norfloxacin>levofloxacin>ciprofloxacin>gati-floxacin>ofloxacin=sparfloxacin>lomefloxacin.

None of these should be taken at the same time as any iron prepara-tion which contains substantial amounts of elemental iron (e.g. all of those cited above except iron-ovotransferrin). Since the quinolones are rapidly absorbed, taking them 2 h before the iron should minimise the risk of admixture in the gut and largely avoid this interaction. In-formation about other quinolones seems to be lacking but the same precautions should be taken with all of them except fleroxacin, which appears not to interact, and lomefloxacin, which seems to interact only minimally.

Iron-ovotransferrin does not interact with ciprofloxacin and is not expected to interact with any of the quinolones (see 'Mechanism') but this awaits confirmation.

There seems to be very little data about the zinc/quinolone interactions, but zinc appears to interact like iron so that the same precautions suggested for iron should be followed.

1. Brouwers JRBJ, Van der Kam HJ, Sijtsma J, Proost JH. Decreased ciprofloxacin absorption with concomitant administration of ferrous fumarate. *Pharm Weekbl (Sci)* (1990) 12, 182–3.
2. Kara M, Hasinoff BB, McKay DW, Campbell NRC. Clinical and chemical interactions between iron preparations and ciprofloxacin. *Br J Clin Pharmacol* (1991) 31, 257–61.
3. Polk RE. Effect of ferrous sulfate and multivitamins with zinc on the absorption of ciprofloxacin in normal volunteers. Intersci Conf Antimicrob Agents Chemother (1989) 29, 136.
4. Le Pennec MP, Kitzis MD, Terdjman M, Foubard S, Garbarz E, Hanania G. Possible interaction of ciprofloxacin with ferrous sulphate. *J Antimicrob Chemother* (1990) 25, 184–5.
5. Polk RE, Healy DP, Sahai J, Drwal L, Racht E. Effect of ferrous sulfate and multivitamins with zinc on absorption of ciprofloxacin in normal volunteers. *Antimicrob Agents Chemother* (1989) 33, 1841–4.
6. Lehto P, Kivistö KT, Neuvonen PJ. The effect of ferrous sulphate on the absorption of norfloxacin, ciprofloxacin and ofloxacin. *Br J Clin Pharmacol* (1994) 37, 82–5.
7. Lode H, Stuhlert P, Deppermann KH, Mainz D, Borner K, Kotvas K, Koeppe P. Pharmacokinetic interactions between oral ciprofloxacin (CIP)/ofloxacin (OFL) and ferrosalts. *Intersci Conf Antimicrob Agents Chemother* (1989) 29,136.
8. Sirtori CR, Barbi S, Dorigotti F, Baldassarre D, Pazzucconi F. Iron-ovotransferrin preparation does not interfere with fluoroquinolone absorption. *Therapie* (1995) 50 (Suppl), Abstract 500.
9. Pazzucconi F, Barbi S, Baldassarre D, Colombo N, Dorigotti F, Sirtori CR. Iron-ovotransferrin preparation does not interfere with ciprofloxacin absorption. *Clin Pharmacol Ther* (1996) 59, 418–22.
10. Sörgel F, Naber KG, Kinzig M, Frank A, Birner B. Effect of ferrous sulfate on fleroxacin analyzed by the confidence interval (CI) approach. *Pharm Res* (1995) 12 (9 Suppl), S-422.
11. Shiba K, Kusajima H, Momo K. The effects of aluminium hydroxide, cimetidine, ferrous sulfate, green tea and milk on pharmacokinetics of gatifloxacin in healthy humans. *J Antimicrob Chemother* (1999) 44 (Suppl A), 141.
12. Allen A, Bygate E, Faessel H, Isaac L, Lewis A. The effect of ferrous sulphate and sucralfate on the bioavailability of oral gemifloxacin in healthy volunteers. *Int J Antimicrob Agents* (2000) 15, 283–9.
13. Shiba K, Okazaki O, Aoki H, Sakai O, Shimada J. Inhibition of DR-3355 absorption by metal ions. *Intersci Conf Antimicrob Agents Chemother* (1991) 31, 198.
14. Lehto P, Kivistö KT. Different effects of products containing metal ions on the absorption of lomefloxacin. *Clin Pharmacol Ther* (1994) 56, 477–82.
15. Kanemitsu K, Hori S, Yanagawa A, Shimada J. Effect of ferrous sulfate on the pharmacokinetics of sparfloxacin. *Chemotherapy (Japan)* (1994) 42, 6–13.
16. Kanemitsu K, Hori S, Yanagawa A, Shimada J. Effect of ferrous sulfate on the absorption of sparfloxacin in healthy volunteers and rats. *Drugs* (1995) 49 (Suppl 2), 352–6.
17. Okhamafe AO, Akerele JO, Chukuka CS. Pharmacokinetic interactions of norfloxacin with some metallic medicinal agents. *Int J Pharmaceutics* (1991) 68, 11–18.
18. Campbell NRC, Kara M, Hasinoff BB, Haddara WM, McKay DW. Norfloxacin interaction with antacids and minerals. *Br J Clin Pharmacol* (1992) 33, 115–16.
19. Martínez Cabarga M, Sánchez Navarro A, Colino Gandarillas CI, Domínguez-Gil A. Effects of two cations on gastrointestinal absorption of ofloxacin. *Antimicrob Agents Chemother* (1991) 35, 2102–5.
20. Wong PY, Zhu M, Li RC. Pharmacokinetic and pharmacodynamic interactions between intravenous ciprofloxacin and oral ferrous sulfate. *J Chemother* (2000) 12, 286–93.

Quinolone antibacterials + NSAIDs

A number of cases of convulsions have been seen in Japanese patients treated with fenbufen and enoxacin, and there is also one possible case involving ofloxacin. Use of these drugs together should be avoided, but normally no interaction seems to occur with most quinolones and NSAIDs. Isolated cases of convulsions or other neurological toxicity or skin eruptions have been seen with ciprofloxacin combined with indometacin, mefenamic acid or naproxen. These appear to be very rare events.

Clinical evidence

(a) Ciprofloxacin + Fenbufen, Indometacin, Mefenamic acid, Naproxen

As of 1995 the maker of ciprofloxacin had, on record, two confirmed spontaneous reports of convulsions in patients on ciprofloxacin and an NSAID, one with **mefenamic acid** and the other with **naproxen**.[1] These appear to be the only medically validated reports of ciprofloxacin/NSAID reactions to date.[1]

A woman on 250 mg chloroquine and 1 g **naproxen** daily developed dizziness, anxiety and tremors within a week of starting 1 g ciprofloxacin daily. The symptoms largely resolved when the chloroquine was stopped; it was not known if she also stopped the naproxen. Two months after chloroquine was discontinued, while she

was still taking ciprofloxacin, **indometacin** was started. This time she developed pain in her feet and became extremely tired. The pain partially subsided and the fatigue vanished when the ciprofloxacin was stopped. Later she was found to have some axonal demyelination, compatible with drug-induced polyneuropathy.[2]

A study in 8 healthy subjects found that the pharmacokinetics of ciprofloxacin were unaffected by 3 days treatment with **fenbufen**.[3] Another study found that combined single doses of ciprofloxacin and **fenbufen** in 12 healthy subjects produced no evidence of increased excitatory effects on CNS function using EEG recordings.[4]

(b) Enoxacin, Ofloxacin + Fenbufen

A total of 17 Japanese patients have been identified, with apparently no previous history of seizures, who in the 1986–7 period developed convulsions when treated with **fenbufen** (400–1200 mg daily) and **enoxacin** (200–800 mg). One other patient on 800 mg **fenbufen** had what are described as involuntary movements of the neck and upper extremities after taking 600 mg **ofloxacin**.[5] Other reports comment on this interaction.[6,7] Yet another report mentions 7 patients who had convulsions after taking **fenbufen** and **enoxacin**, but is not certain whether they are included in the 17 or not.[8] An 87-year-old Japanese woman on **enoxacin** (200 mg) also had convulsions when given a single intravenous dose of 50 mg flurbiprofen.[9]

(c) Ofloxacin, Pefloxacin + Aspirin, Diclofenac, Indometacin, Ketoprofen, Dipyrone (metamizole sodium)

The pharmacokinetics of **pefloxacin** and **ofloxacin** in 10 healthy subjects were found to be unchanged over 3 days by 100 mg **ketoprofen** daily.[10] The incidence of psychotic side-effects (euphoria, hysteria, psychosis) in 151 patients on **ofloxacin** was not increased by the concurrent use of NSAIDs (**aspirin**, **diclofenac**, **indometacin**, dipyrone).[11]

(d) Sparfloxacin + Mefenamic acid

A single case report describes drug eruptions (erythematous papules) attributed to sparfloxacin hypersensitivity induced by **mefenamic acid** in a 62-year-old woman.[12]

Mechanisms

Not fully understood. Convulsions have occurred in a few patients taking quinolones alone, some of whom were epileptic and some of whom were not (see 'Anticonvulsants + Quinolone antibacterials', p.317). Experiments in *mice* have shown that quinolones competitively inhibit the binding of gamma-amino butyric acid (GABA) to its receptors. GABA is an inhibitory transmitter in the CNS, which is believed to be involved in the control of convulsive activity. Enoxacin and fenbufen are known to affect the GABA receptor site in the hippocampus and frontal cortex of *mice*, which is associated with convulsive activity.[13] It could be that if and when an interaction occurs the NSAID simply lowers the amount of quinolone needed to precipitate convulsions in the susceptible individuals.

Importance and management

The enoxacin/fenbufen interaction is established but it seems to be uncommon. Its apparent incidence is possibly exaggerated (so it has been suggested) by the very wide use of fenbufen in Japan for conditions such as colds and influenza, which would probably be treated differently elsewhere. It would seem prudent to avoid fenbufen with enoxacin or any other quinolone antibacterial. There are very many alternatives.

Reports of adverse interactions between other quinolones and NSAIDs are rare. The general warning about convulsions with quinolones and NSAIDs issued by the CSM[14] seems to be an extrapolation from the enoxacin/fenbufen interaction, and from some *animal* experiments, to cover all quinolones and all NSAIDs. In addition to the data cited above relating to ciprofloxacin, an epidemiological study of 856 users of quinolones (ciprofloxacin, enoxacin, nalidixic acid) and a range of NSAIDs found no cases of convulsions.[15] The overall picture would therefore seem to be that although a potential for interaction exists, the risk is very small indeed and normally there would seem to be little reason for most patients on quinolones to avoid NSAIDs. Epileptic patients are a possible exception (see 'Anticonvulsants + Quinolone antibacterials', p.317).

1. Bomford J. Ciprofloxacin. *Pharm J* (1995) 255, 674.
2. Rollof J, Vinge E. Neurological adverse effects during concomitant treatment with ciprofloxacin, NSAIDS, and chloroquine: possible drug interaction. *Ann Pharmacother* (1993) 27, 1058–9.
3. Kamali F. Lack of a pharmacokinetic interaction between ciprofloxacin and fenbufen. *J Clin Pharm Ther* (1994) 19, 257–9.
4. Kamali F, Ashton CH, Marsh VR, Cox J. Is there a pharmacodynamic interaction between ciprofloxacin and fenbufen? *Br J Clin Pharmacol* (1997) 43, 545P–546P.
5. Lederle. Data on file. Personal Communication, January 1996.
6. Takeo G, Shibuya N, Motomura M, Kanazawa H, Shishido H. A new DNA gyrase inhibitor induces convulsions: a case report and animal experiments. *Chemotherapy (Tokyo)* (1989) 37, 1154–9.
7. Morita H, Maemura K, Sakai Y, Kaneda Y. A case with convulsion, loss of consciousness and subsequent acute renal failure caused by enoxacin and fenbufen. *Nippon Naika Gakkai Zasshi* (1988) 77, 744–5.
8. Hori S, Shimada J, Saito A, Matsuda M, Miyahara T. Comparison of the inhibitory effects of new quinolones on γ-aminobutyric acid receptor binding in the presence of anti-inflammatory drugs. *Rev Infect Dis* (1989) 11 (Suppl 5), S1397–S1398.
9. Mizuno J, Takumi Z, Kaneko A, Tsutsui T, Tsutsui T, Zushi N, Machida K. Convulsion following the combination of single preoperative oral administration of enoxacine and single postoperative intravenous administration of flurbiprofen axetil. *Jpn J Anesthsiol* (2001) 50, 425–8.
10. Fillastre JP, Leroy A, Borsa-Lebas F, Etienne I, Gy C, Humbert G. Effects of ketoprofen (NSAID) on the pharmacokinetics of pefloxacin and ofloxacin in healthy volunteers. *Drugs Exp Clin Res* (1992) 18, 487–92.
11. Jüngst G, Weidmann E, Breitstadt A, Huppertz E. Does ofloxacin interact with NSAIDs to cause psychotic side effects? 17th International Congress on Chemotherapy, Berlin, June 23–8, 1991. Abstract 412.
12. Oiso N, Taniguchi S, Goto Y, Hisa T, Mizuno N, Mochida K, Hamada T, Yorifuji T. A case of drug eruption due to sparfloxacin (SPFX) and mefenamic acid. *Skin Res* (1995) 37, 321–7.
13. Motomura M, Kataoka Y, Takeo G, Shibayama K, Ohishi K, Nakamura T, Niwa M, Tsujihata M, Nagataki S. Hippocampus and frontal cortex are the potential mediatory sites for convulsions induced by new quinolones and non-steroidal anti-inflammatory drugs. *Int J Clin Pharmacol Ther Toxicol* (1991) 29, 223–7.
14. Committee on Safety of Medicines. Convulsions due to quinolone antimicrobial agents. *Current Problems* (1991) 32, 2.
15. Mannino S, Garcia-Rodriguez LA, Jick SS. NSAIDs, quinolones and convulsions: an epidemiological approach. *Post Marketing Surveillance* (1992) 6, 119–28.

Quinolone antibacterials + Opioids

Trovafloxacin alters the pharmacokinetics of morphine and oxycodone alters the pharmacokinetics of levofloxacin, but neither change is clinically significant.

Clinical evidence, mechanism, importance and management

An intravenous infusion of **morphine** 0.15 mg/kg given with **trovafloxacin** 200 mg to 18 healthy subjects caused a 36% reduction in the **trovafloxacin** AUC and a 46% reduction in the maximum serum levels. These levels were considered sufficient for prophylaxis of infection, and remained above the MICs of the most likely organisms to cause post-surgical infections. Also, the bioavailability and effects of **morphine** were not significantly changed by concurrent **trovafloxacin**.[1]

The possibility of a similar interaction between **levofloxacin** and **oxycodone** was studied in 8 healthy subjects. The pharmacokinetics of **levofloxacin** 500 mg were not significantly altered by 4-hourly doses of **oxycodone** 5 mg.[2]

1. Vincent J, Hunt T, Teng R, Robarge L, Willavize SA, Friedman HL. The pharmacokinetic effects of coadministration of morphine and trovafloxacin in healthy subjects. *Am J Surg* (1998) 176 (Suppl 6A), 32S–38S.
2. Grant EM, Zhong MK, Fitzgerald JF, Nicolau DP, Nightingale C, Quintiliani R. Lack of interaction between levofloxacin and oxycodone: pharmacokinetics and drug disposition. *J Clin Pharmacol* (2001) 41, 206–9.

Quinolone antibacterials + Other antibacterials

Rifampicin (rifampin) appears not to have a clinically important effect on ciprofloxacin, fleroxacin, pefloxacin and possibly grepafloxacin. Azlocillin reduces the clearance of ciprofloxacin. Piperacillin, ceftazidime and tobramycin appear not to affect the pharmacokinetics of pefloxacin, nor amoxicillin the absorption of ofloxacin. Clindamycin appears not to affect the pharmacokinetics of ciprofloxacin but it may antagonise its effects on S. aureus.

Clinical evidence, mechanism, importance and management

(a) Quinolones + Rifampicin (Rifampin)

Ciprofloxacin 750 mg 12-hourly and **rifampicin** 300 mg 12-hourly for 2 weeks did not significantly affect the pharmacokinetics of either drug in 12 elderly patients (aged 67 to 95).[1] This is confirmed by other pharmacokinetic studies, one of which also reported that combined use provided excellent serum bactericidal activity against *S. aureus* strains, although activity was modestly lower than **rifampicin** alone.[2-4]

A study in 8 healthy subjects found that 900 mg **rifampicin** daily for 10 days decreased the half-life and $AUC_{0 \text{ to } 12}$ of **pefloxacin** 400 mg twice daily by about 30% due to a 35% increase in total plasma clearance.[5] Despite these changes the serum **pefloxacin** levels still remained well above the minimal inhibitory concentrations (0.50 mg/l) for 90% of strains of methicillin-sensitive strains of *S. aureus* and *S. epidermis*.[5] Another study in 13 healthy subjects found that after taking 600 mg **rifampicin** daily for a week, the clearance of **fleroxacin** 400 mg daily was increased by 15%. However, the **fleroxacin** levels remained above the MIC_{90} of methicillin-sensitive strains of *S. aureus* and *S. epidermis* for at least 24 h.[6,7] No special precautions would seem necessary if rifampicin is given with any of these quinolones.

(b) Quinolones + Clindamycin

One study found that the pharmacokinetics of **ciprofloxacin** (200 mg given intravenously) were not affected by **clindamycin** (600 mg given intravenously) and there is evidence that combined use may possibly enhance the antibacterial activity, particularly against *S. aureus* and *S. pneumoniae*.[8] However, another study found that the serum bactericidal activity of **ciprofloxacin** against *S. aureus* was completely antagonised by **clindamycin**, if the strains were susceptible to the latter.[3]

(c) Quinolones + Metronidazole

A study found that a single oral dose of **metronidazole** 400 mg had no effect on the pharmacokinetics of **pefloxacin**, and similarly **pefloxacin** did affect the pharmacokinetics of **metronidazole**.[9] Similar results were found with **ciprofloxacin** or **ofloxacin** (both 200 mg intravenously) and **metronidazole** 500 mg intravenously,[10] and **metronidazole/ciprofloxacin** orally.[11] A further study, investigating concurrent use of **metronidazole** 500 mg intravenously and **ciprofloxacin** 200 mg intravenously, again did not find any significant pharmacokinetic changes, although the **ciprofloxacin** volume of distribution was 20% lower during concurrent use of **metronidazole**.[8]

(d) Quinolones + Other antibacterials

Another study found that single intravenous doses of either 2 g **ceftazidime** or 100 mg **tobramycin** had no effect on the pharmacokinetics of **pefloxacin**, and **pefloxacin** did affect the pharmacokinetics of either of these antibacterials.[9] A study designed to assess the potential interaction between **trovafloxacin** and **azithromycin**, which may be used concurrently against STDs, found no significant alteration in the pharmacokinetics of either drug.[12]

(e) Quinolones + Penicillins

A single-dose study in 6 healthy subjects found that **azlocillin** (60 mg/kg by intravenous infusion) reduced the clearance of **ciprofloxacin** (4 mg/kg by intravenous infusion) by 35%. The pharmacokinetics of **azlocillin** were not affected.[13] Another study found that concurrent use of a single intravenous dose of 4 g **piperacillin**, and **pefloxacin** 400 mg did not affect the pharmacokinetics of either drug.[9] The absorption of **ofloxacin** 400 mg was not altered by **amoxicillin** 3 g when given to 6 healthy subjects.[14] In another study, in 12 healthy subjects, the serum bacterial activity of **ciprofloxacin** plus piperacillin against a variety of organisms was found to be additive, rather than antagonistic or synergistic, and also that the clearance of ciprofloxacin was reduced by 24%.[15,16]

1. Chandler MHH, Toler SM, Rapp RP, Muder RR, Korvick JA. Multiple-dose pharmacokinetics of concurrent oral ciprofloxacin and rifampin therapy in elderly patients. *Antimicrob Agents Chemother* (1990) 34, 442–7.

2. Polk RE. Drug-drug interactions with ciprofloxacin and other fluoroquinolones. *Am J Med* (1989) 87 (Suppl 5A), 76S–81S.

3. Weinstein MP, Deeter RG, Swanson KA, Gross JS. Crossover assessment of serum bactericidal activity and pharmacokinetics of ciprofloxacin alone and in combination in healthy elderly volunteers. *Antimicrob Agents Chemother* (1991) 35, 2352–8.

4. Jhaj R, Roy A, Uppal R, Behera D. Influence of ciprofloxacin on pharmacokinetics of rifampin. *Curr Ther Res* (1997) 58, 260–5.

5. Humbert G, Brumpt I, Montay G, Le Liboux A, Frydman A, Borsa-Lebas F, Moore N. Influence of rifampin on the pharmacokinetics of pefloxacin. *Clin Pharmacol Ther* (1991) 50, 682–7.

6. Schrenzel J, Dayer P, Weidekamm E, Portmann R, Lew DP. Influence of rifampin on the pharmacokinetics of fleroxacin. *Intersci Conf Antimicrob Agents Chemother* (1992) 32, 355.

7. Schrenzel J, Dayer P, Leemann T, Weidekamm E, Portmann R, Lew DP. Influence of rifampin on fleroxacin pharmacokinetics. *Antimicrob Agents Chemother* (1993) 37, 2132–8.

8. Deppermann K-M, Boeckh M, Grineisen S, Shokry F, Borner K, Koeppe P, Krasemann C, Wagner J, Lode H. Brief report: combination effects of ciprofloxacin, clindamycin, and metronidazole intravenously in volunteers. *Am J Med* (1989) 87 (Suppl 5A), 46S–48S.

9. Metz R, Jaehde U, Wiesemann H, Gottschalk B, Stephan U, Schunack W. Pharmacokinetic interactions and non-interactions of pefloxacin. Proc 15th Int Congr Chemother, Istanbul, 1987, 997–9.

10. Boeckh M, Grineisen S, Shokry F, Koeppe P, Borner K, Krasemann C, Lode H. Pharmacokinetics and serum bactericidal activity (SBA) of ciprofloxacin (CIP) and ofloxacin (OFL) alone and in combination with metronidazole (METRO) or clindamycin (CLINDA). *Intersci Conf Antimicrob Agents Chemother* (1988) 28, 246.

11. Ludwig E, Graber H, Székely É, Csiba A. Metabolic interactions of ciprofloxacin. *Diagn Microbiol Infect Dis* (1990) 13, 135–41.

12. Foulds G, Cohen MJ, Geffken A, Willavize S, Hunt T. Coadministration of azithromycin 1-g packet does not affect the bioavailability of trovafloxacin. *Intersci Conf Antimicrob Agents Chemother* (1998) 38, 31.

13. Barriere SL, Catlin DH, Orlando PL, Noe A, Frost RW. Alteration in the pharmacokinetic disposition of ciprofloxacin by simultaneous administration of azlocillin. *Antimicrob Agents Chemother* (1990) 34, 823–6.

14. Paintaud G, Alván G, Hellgren U, Nilsson-Ehle I. Lack of effect of amoxycillin on the absorption of ofloxacin. *Eur J Clin Pharmacol* (1993) 44, 207–9.

15. Strenkoski LC, Forrest A, Schentag JJ, Nix DE. Pharmacodynamic (PD) interactions of ciprofloxacin (C), piperacillin (P) and piperacillin/tazobactam (PT) in volunteer subjects. *Intersci Conf Antimicrob Agents Chemother* (1994) 34, 118.

16. Strenkoski-Nix LC, Forrest A, Schentag JJ, Nix DE. Pharmacodynamic interactions of ciprofloxacin, piperacillin, and piperacillin/tazobactam in healthy volunteers. *J Clin Pharmacol* (1998) 38, 1063–71.

Quinolone antibacterials + Pancreatic enzyme supplements

Ciprofloxacin is not affected by pancreatic enzyme supplements.

Clinical evidence, mechanism, importance and management

Six patients with cystic fibrosis, chronically infected with *P. aeruginosa* and treated with a range of drugs including ceftazidime, tobramycin, ticarcillin and salbutamol, demonstrated no significant changes in the pharmacokinetics of single 250-mg doses of ciprofloxacin when given standard doses of pancreatic enzymes (seven *Pancrease* capsules).[1] No special precautions would seem to be necessary during concurrent use.

1. Mack G, Cooper PJ, Buchanan N. Effects of enzyme supplementation on oral absorption of ciprofloxacin in patients with cystic fibrosis. *Antimicrob Agents Chemother* (1991) 35, 1484–5.

Quinolone antibacterials + Pirenzepine

Four doses of pirenzepine 50 mg delayed the absorption of ciprofloxacin and ofloxacin in 10 healthy subjects, but their bioavailabilities remained unchanged.[1] These changes are unlikely to be of clinical significance.

1. Höffken G, Lode H, Wiley R, Glatzel TD, Sievers D, Olschewski T, Borner K, Koeppe T. Pharmacokinetics and bioavailability of ciprofloxacin and ofloxacin: effect of food and antacid intake. *Rev Infect Dis* (1988) 10 (Suppl 1), S138–S139.

Quinolone antibacterials + Probenecid

The serum levels of cinoxacin, fleroxacin and nalidixic acid are increased by probenecid. The clearance of ofloxacin and the urinary excretion of ciprofloxacin, clinafloxacin, enoxacin and possibly fleroxacin are reduced by probenecid. The clinical importance of these changes is uncertain. Grepafloxacin, levofloxacin and moxifloxacin appear not to interact to a clinically relevant extent.

Clinical evidence

(a) Cinoxacin

A study in 6 healthy subjects found that while taking 500 mg probenecid three times daily the serum levels of cinoxacin (as an intravenous infusion) were approximately doubled.[1]

(b) Ciprofloxacin

Probenecid 1 g given 30 min before 500 mg ciprofloxacin was found to reduce the ciprofloxacin renal clearance by up to 50%. Other pharmacokinetic parameters (maximum serum levels, AUC) were unchanged and no accumulation of ciprofloxacin appeared to occur.[2] Another study confirmed that the renal clearance of ciprofloxacin is reduced by probenecid (in this study by 64%) but the distribution of the ciprofloxacin in tears, sweat and saliva is unchanged.[3]

(c) Clinafloxacin

Probenecid 1 g given 1 h before a single 400-mg dose of clinafloxacin reduced the total and renal clearance of the clinafloxacin by 24% and 36% respectively, the AUC was raised 32% and the elimination half-life was increased from 6.3 to 7 h.[4]

(d) Enoxacin

In one subject, the renal clearance of 600 mg enoxacin was approximately halved (from 374 to 171 ml/min) and the half life increased from 3.5 to 4.5 h after receiving 2.5 g probenecid.[5]

(e) Fleroxacin

A study in 6 healthy subjects given a single 200-mg dose of fleroxacin, followed by 500 mg probenecid 0.5, 12, 24 and 36 h later, found that the fleroxacin AUC was increased by 37% (from 32.6 to 44.7 mg.h/l), the maximal serum levels were slightly but not significantly increased, and its urinary excretion was decreased by 22%.[6] Another study found that probenecid had no significant effects of its urinary excretion.[7]

(f) Grepafloxacin

A study in 32 healthy subjects given a single 200-mg dose of grepafloxacin showed probenecid had no effects on grepafloxacin pharmacokinetics.[8] Similar results were found in another 6 healthy subjects.[9]

(g) Levofloxacin

A study in 12 healthy subjects given single 500 mg oral doses of levofloxacin found that although probenecid reduced its renal clearance by about a third and increased its AUC and half-life by similar amounts, the 72-hour urinary levofloxacin excretion was unaltered.[10]

(h) Moxifloxacin

A study in 12 healthy subjects given a single 400-mg dose of moxifloxacin showed that probenecid had no clinically significant effects on the pharmacokinetics of moxifloxacin.[11]

(i) Nalidixic acid

Two volunteers, acting as their own controls, ingested 500 mg nalidixic acid with and without 500 mg probenecid. Their peak serum nalidixic acid levels were unaffected at 2 h, but at 8 h the levels were increased threefold by the presence of **probenecid.**[12]

Another study in 5 women with urinary tract infections treated with **nalidixic acid** showed that the concurrent use of **probenecid** increased the maximal serum **nalidixic acid** concentrations and the AUC by 43% and 74% respectively.[13]

(j) Norfloxacin

The mean 12 h urinary recovery of 200 mg norfloxacin was reduced to about half in 5 subjects when given 1 g **probenecid.** Serum concentrations were unaffected.[14]

(k) Ofloxacin

A study in 8 healthy subjects given a single 200-mg dose of **ofloxacin** with or without 500 mg **probenecid** showed that the AUC of **ofloxacin** was increased by 16% and the total body clearance decreased by 14%. Other pharmacokinetic parameters were not significantly affected.[15]

(l) Sparfloxacin

Probenecid 1.5 g did not significantly affect the clearance, the AUC or the half-life of 200 mg **sparfloxacin** in 6 healthy subjects.[16]

Mechanism

The likely explanation is that probenecid successfully competes with these quinolones for tubular excretion so that renal elimination is reduced and they are retained in the body. Some quinolones are more dependent on glomerular filtration for excretion, and thus are unaffected by competition for tubular excretion.[7]

Importance and management

Established interactions, but their clinical importance seems not to have been assessed. There appears to be no reason for avoiding concurrent use. The increased bioavailability seen with ofloxacin, and the increased serum levels seen with cinoxacin, fleroxacin and nalidixic acid might possibly improve the treatment of systemic infections. However, the reduced levels in the urine seen with ciprofloxacin, enoxacin, norfloxacin and possibly fleroxacin might be expected to reduce their effectiveness for urinary tract infections. Monitoring would therefore seem to be appropriate. There seems to be no information about other quinolones except sparfloxacin, which appears not to interact, or levofloxacin and moxifloxacin, which appear not to be affected to a significant extent.

1. Rodriguez N, Madsen PO, Welling PG. Influence of probenecid on serum levels and urinary excretion of cinoxacin. *Antimicrob Agents Chemother* (1979) 15, 465–69.
2. Wingender W, Beerman D, Förster D, Graefe K-H, Kuhlmann J. Interactions of ciprofloxacin with food intake and drugs. *Curr Clin Pract Ser* (1986) 34, 136–40.
3. Jaehde U, Sörgel F, Reiter A, Sigl G, Naber KG, Schunack W. Effect of probenecid on the distribution and elimination of ciprofloxacin in humans. *Clin Pharmacol Ther* (1995) 58, 532–41.
4. Randinitis EJ, Koup JR, Bron NJ, Hounslow NJ, Rausch G, Abel R, Vassos AB, Sedman AJ. Drug interaction studies with clinafloxacin and probenecid, cimetidine, phenytoin and warfarin. *Drugs* (1999) 58 (Suppl 2), 254–5.
5. Wijnands WJA, Vree TB, Baars AM, van Herwaarden CLA. Pharmacokinetics of enoxacin and its penetration into bronchial secretions and lung tissue. *J Antimicrob Chemother* (1988) 21 (Suppl B), 67–77.
6. Shiba K, Saito A, Shimada J, Hori S, Kaji M, Miyahara T, Kusajima H, Kaneko S, Saito S, Uchida H. Interactions of fleroxacin with dried aluminium hydroxide gel and probenecid. *Rev Infect Dis* (1989) 11 (Suppl 5), S1097–S1098.
7. Weidekamm E, Portmann R, Suter K, Partos C, Dell D, Lücker PW. Single- and multiple dose pharmacokinetics of fleroxacin, a trifluorinated quinolone, in humans. *Antimicrob Agents Chemother* (1987) 31, 1909–14.
8. Koneru B, Bramer S, Bricmont P, Maroli A, Shiba K. Effect of food, gastric pH and co-administration of antacid, cimetidine and probenecid on the oral pharmacokinetics of the broad spectrum antimicrobial agent grepafloxacin. *Pharm Res* (1996) 13 (9 Suppl), S414.
9. Shiba K, Yoshida M, Hori S, Shimada J, Saito A, Sakai O. Pharmacokinetic interaction of OPC-17116 with probenecid in healthy volunteers. *Intersci Conf Antimicrob Agents Chemother* (1991) 31, 346.
10. Gaitonde MD, Mendes P, House ESA, Lehr KH. The effects of cimetidine and probenecid on the pharmacokinetics of levofloxacin (LVFX). *Intersci Conf Antimicrob Agents Chemother* (1995) 35, 8.
11. Stass H, Sachse R. Effect of probenecid on the kinetics of a single oral 400-mg dose of moxifloxacin in healthy male volunteers. *Clin Pharmacokinet* (2001) 40 (Suppl 1), 71–76.
12. Dash H, Mills J. Severe metabolic acidosis associated with nalidixic acid overdose. *Ann Intern Med* (1976) 84, 570–1.
13. Ferry N, Cuisinaud G, Pozet N, Zech PY, Sassard J. Influence du probénécide sur la pharmacocinétique de l'acide nalidixique. *Therapie* (1982) 37, 645–9.
14. Shimada J, Yamaji T, Ueda Y, Uchida H, Kusajima H, Irikura T. Mechanism of renal excretion of AM-715, a new quinolonecarboxylic acid derivative, in rabbits, dogs, and humans. *Antimicrob Agents Chemother* (1983) 23, 1–7.
15. Nataraj B, Rao Mamidi NVS, Krishna DR. Probenecid affects the pharmacokinetics of ofloxacin in healthy volunteers. *Clin Drug Invest* (1998) 16, 259–62.
16. Shimada J, Saito A, Shiba K, Hojo T, Kaji M, Hori S, Yoshida M, Sakai O. Pharmacokinetics and clinical studies of sparfloxacin. *Chemotherapy (Tokyo)* (1991) 39 (Suppl 4), 234–44.

Quinolone antibacterials + Proton pump inhibitors

Proton pump inhibitors do not appear to interact with quinolone antibacterials.

Clinical evidence, mechanism, importance and management

The maximum plasma concentration of **gemifloxacin** 320 mg, given to 13 healthy subjects who had taken 4 days of **omeprazole** 40 mg daily, was raised by 10% when compared to the levels obtained without pre-dosing with **omeprazole.**[1] Therefore no precautions would seem necessary if these drugs are taken together.

1. Allen A, Vousden M, Lewis A. Effect of omeprazole on the pharmacokinetics of oral gemifloxacin in healthy volunteers. *Chemotherapy* (1999) 45, 496–503.

Quinolone antibacterials + Sucralfate

Sucralfate causes only a modest reduction in fleroxacin levels whereas a marked reduction occurs in the absorption of ciprofloxacin, enoxacin, gemifloxacin, levofloxacin, lomefloxacin, moxifloxacin, ofloxacin, norfloxacin and sparfloxacin if taken together. The interaction is very much reduced or fails to occur if the sucralfate is given 2 to 6 h after the quinolone.

Clinical evidence

(a) Ciprofloxacin

The absorption of 500 mg **ciprofloxacin** in 8 healthy subjects was reduced by 88% (from 8.8 to 1.1 micrograms.h/ml) and the maximum serum concentration by 90% (from 2.0 to 0.2 micrograms/ml) while taking 1 g **sucralfate** four times daily.[1]

A patient given 1 g **sucralfate** four times daily had serum **ciprofloxacin** levels which were 85 to 90% lower than 5 other patients who were not taking **sucralfate.**[2] A single dose study found a 96% reduction in the AUC of **ciprofloxacin** following a 2 g dose of **sucralfate.**[3] A study in 12 healthy subjects found that a 1 g dose of **sucralfate** 6 and 2 h before a single 750-mg dose of **ciprofloxacin,** reduced the **ciprofloxacin** AUC by about 30%. Three of the subjects showed little or no changes but a decrease of more than 50% was seen in 4 others.[4] A related study in 12 healthy subjects found that the bioavailability of 750 mg **ciprofloxacin** was 4%, 80% and 93% respectively when given at the same time, 2 h and 6 h before the **sucralfate.**[5] The concurrent use of oral **sucralfate** does not affect the control, by intravenous **ciprofloxacin,** of aerobic bacteria in the gut.[6]

(b) Enoxacin

Sucralfate 1 g given to 8 normal subjects 2 h before or with 400 mg **enoxacin** reduced the bioavailability by 54% and 88% respectively. When **sucralfate** was given 2 h after the **enoxacin,** no changes occurred.[7]

(c) Fleroxacin

The bioavailability of 400 mg **fleroxacin** was reduced to 76% in 20 healthy subjects taking 1 g **sucralfate** 6-hourly.[8,9]

(d) Gemifloxacin

Gemifloxacin 320 mg was given either 2 h after or 3 h before **sucralfate** 2 g in a study in 27 healthy subjects. The pharmacokinetics of **gemifloxacin** were not significantly altered when **sucralfate** was given after the **gemifloxacin**, probably due to its rapid absorption. However, when **sucralfate** was given 3 h before **gemifloxacin**, the AUC was decreased by 53% and the maximum plasma levels by 69%.[10]

(e) Levofloxacin

The pharmacokinetics of **levofloxacin** are unaffected by **sucralfate** taken either 2 h afterwards.[11]

(f) Lomefloxacin

A study in 12 subjects found that when 400 mg **lomefloxacin** was given 2 h after 1 g **sucralfate** the **lomefloxacin** AUC was reduced by about 25% and the maximal serum concentration by 30%.[12] Another study in 8 healthy subjects found that when 400 mg **lomefloxacin** was given with 1 g **sucralfate**, the **lomefloxacin** AUC was reduced by 51%.[13]

(g) Moxifloxacin

A study in 12 healthy subjects given 1 g **sucralfate** at the same time and 5, 10, 15 and 24 h after a single dose of 400 mg **moxifloxacin**, found a reduction in the AUC and maximum serum concentration of **moxifloxacin** by 40% and 29% respectively.[14]

(h) Norfloxacin

A study in 8 normal subjects showed that while taking **sucralfate** 1 g four times daily the AUC of single 400 mg doses of **norfloxacin** was markedly reduced, by 98%, when taken with the **sucralfate**, and by 42% when taken 2 h afterwards.[15-17] Another study found a reduction of 91% when 400 mg **norfloxacin** was taken with 1 g **sucralfate**, but no reduction when the **norfloxacin** was taken 2 h before.[18]

(i) Ofloxacin

A single dose study found that **sucralfate** (dose not stated) reduced the maximum serum levels and the AUC of a single dose of **ofloxacin** 200 mg to about one-third.[19] Another study found a reduction of 61% when 400 mg **ofloxacin** was taken with 1 g **sucralfate**, but no reduction when the ofloxacin was taken 2 h before.[18] The interaction was reduced by the presence of food, but was still marked.[20]

(j) Sparfloxacin

In a study in 15 healthy subjects 1 g **sucralfate** four times daily reduced the maximum serum levels, the AUC and the relative bioavailability of 400 mg **sparfloxacin** daily by 39, 47 and 44% respectively.[21] In a study assessing staggered dosing of **sucralfate** 1.5 g on the pharmacokinetics of **sparfloxacin** 300 mg, the AUC was unaffected by giving **sucralfate** 4 h after the quinolone, but was decreased by 34% when given 2 h before, and 51% when given at the same time as **sucralfate**.[22]

Mechanism

Not fully established, but a likely explanation is that the aluminium hydroxide component of sucralfate (about 200 mg in each g) forms an insoluble chelate between the cation and the 4-keto and 3-carboxyl groups of the quinolone, which reduces its absorption. See also 'Quinolone antibacterials + Antacids', p.205.

Importance and management

Established and clinically important interactions. Because it seems probable that serum ciprofloxacin, enoxacin, gemifloxacin, levofloxacin, lomefloxacin, moxifloxacin, ofloxacin, norfloxacin and sparfloxacin levels will be reduced to subtherapeutic concentrations if given with the sucralfate, separate the dosages as much as possible (by 2 h or more), giving the quinolone first. The study with moxifloxacin suggested that sucralfate should not be given for 2 h before or 4 h after the quinolone, but more study is needed to confirm both these findings and the effectiveness of separating the dosages. The interaction with fleroxacin is only modest (bioavailability reduced 24%) and probably not clinically important, but some separation of the dosages might improve matters even further. This needs confirmation. Pefloxacin also interacts with antacids containing aluminium hydroxide (see 'Quinolone antibacterials + Antacids', p.205) and may therefore possibly interact with sucralfate. Alternatives to sucralfate are the H_2-blockers and proton pump inhibitors.

1. Garrelts JC, Godley PJ, Peterie JD, Gerlach EH, Yakshe CC. Sucralfate significantly reduces ciprofloxacin concentrations in serum. *Antimicrob Agents Chemother* (1990) 34, 931–3.
2. Yuk JH, Nightingale CN, Quintiliani R. Ciprofloxacin levels when receiving sucralfate. *JAMA* (1989) 262, 901.
3. Brouwers JRBJ, Van Der Kam HJ, Sijtsma J, Proost JH. Important reduction of ciprofloxacin absorption by sucralfate and magnesium citrate solution. *Drug Invest* (1990) 2, 197–9.
4. Nix DE, Watson WA, Handy L, Frost RW, Rescott DL, Goldstein HR. The effect of sucralfate pretreatment on the pharmacokinetics of ciprofloxacin. *Pharmacotherapy* (1989) 9, 377–80.
5. Van Slooten AD, Nix DE, Wilton JH, Love JH, Spivey JM, Goldstein HR. Combined use of ciprofloxacin and sucralfate. *DICP Ann Pharmacother* (1991) 25, 578–82.
6. Krueger WA, Ruckdeschel G, Unertl K. Influence of intravenously administered ciprofloxacin on aerobic intestinal microflora and fecal drug levels when administered simultaneously with sucralfate. *Antimicrob Agents Chemother* (1997) 41, 1725–30.
7. Ryerson B, Toothaker R, Schleyer I, Sedman A, Colburn W. Effect of sucralfate on enoxacin pharmacokinetics. *Intersci Conf Antimicrob Agents Chemother* (1989) 29, 136.
8. Lubowski TJ, NIghtingale CH, Sweeney K, Quintiliani R. An unusually marginal interaction between fleroxacin and sucralfate. *Intersci Conf Antimicrob Agents Chemother* (1992) 32, 355.
9. Lubowski TJ, Nightingale CH, Sweeney K, Quintiliani R. Effect of sucralfate on pharmacokinetics of fleroxacin in healthy volunteers. *Antimicrob Agents Chemother* (1992) 36, 2758–60.
10. Allen A, Bygate E, Faessel H, Isaac L, Lewis A. The effect of ferrous sulphate and sucralfate on the bioavailability of oral gemifloxacin in healthy volunteers. *Int J Antimicrob Agents* (2000) 15, 283–9.
11. Lee L-J, Hafkin B, Lee I-D, Hoh J, Dix R. Effect of food and sucralfate on a single oral dose of 500 milligrams of levofloxacin in healthy subjects. *Antimicrob Agents Chemother* (1997) 41, 2196–2200.
12. Nix D, Schentag J. Lomefloxacin (L) absorption kinetics when administered with ranitidine (R) and sucralfate (S). *Intersci Conf Antimicrob Agents Chemother* (1989) 29, 317.
13. Lehto P, Kivistö KT. Different effects of products containing metal ions on the absorption of lomefloxacin. *Clin Pharmacol Ther* (1994) 56, 477–82.
14. Stass H, Schühly U, Möller J-G, Delesen H. Effects of sucralfate on the oral bioavailability of moxifloxacin, a novel 8-methoxyfluoroquinolone, in healthy volunteers. *Clin Pharmacokinet* (2001) 40 (Suppl 1), 49–55.
15. Parpia SH, Nix DE, Hejmanowski LG, Wilton JH, Goldstein HR, Schentag JJ. The effect of sucralfate on the oral bioavailability of norfloxacin. *Pharmacotherapy* (1988) 8, 140.
16. Parpia SH, Nix DE, Hejmanowski LG, Goldstein HR, Witton JH, Schentag JJ. Sucralfate reduces the gastrointestinal absorption of norfloxacin. *Antimicrob Agents Chemother* (1989) 33, 99–102.
17. Nix DE, Wilton JH, Schentag JJ, Parpia SH, Norman A, Goldstein HR. Inhibition of norfloxacin absorption by antacids and sucralfate. *Rev Infect Dis* (1989) 11 (Suppl 5), S1096.
18. Lehto P, Kvistö KT. Effect of sucralfate on absorption of norfloxacin and ofloxacin. *Antimicrob Agents Chemother* (1994) 38, 248–51.
19. Shiba K, Yoshida M, Kachi M, Shimada J, Saito A, Sakai N. Effects of peptic ulcer-healing drugs on the pharmacokinetics of new quinolone (OFLX). 17th Int Congr Chemother, June 1991, Berlin, Abstract 415.
20. Kawakami J, Matsuse T, Kotaki H, Seino T, Fukuchi Y, Orimo H, Sawada Y, Iga T. The effect of food on the interaction of ofloxacin with sucralfate in healthy volunteers. *Eur J Clin Pharmacol* (1994) 47, 67–9.
21. Zix JA, Geerdes-Fenge HF, Rau M, Vöckler J, Borner K, Koeppe P, Lode H. Pharmacokinetics of sparfloxacin and interaction with cisapride and sucralfate. *Antimicrob Agents Chemother* (1997) 41, 1668–1672.
22. Kamberi M, Nakashima H, Ogawa K, Oda N, Nakano S. The effect of staggered dosing of sucralfate on oral bioavailability of sparfloxacin. *Br J Clin Pharmacol* (2000) 49, 98–103.

Quinolone antibacterials + Ursodeoxycholic acid (Ursodiol)

An isolated report describes a reduction in serum ciprofloxacin levels in a patient when treated with ursodeoxycholic acid (ursodiol).

Clinical evidence, mechanism, importance and management

A man with metastatic colon cancer had unusually low serum levels of **ciprofloxacin** when given orally, his only other medication being 300 mg **ursodeoxycholic acid** twice daily for gallstones. Despite the low antibacterial serum levels the bacteraemia cleared. Several months later when readmitted to hospital he was again given both drugs, but this time staggered, and then later both drugs together. When taken together the AUC of the **ciprofloxacin** was reduced by 50%.[1] The reason for this interaction is not understood.

This seems to be the first and only report of a quinolone antibacterial/**ursodeoxycholic acid** interaction and its importance is uncertain, but it would now seem prudent to be alert for this interaction with any quinolone. More study is needed to establish this interaction, its importance, and its mechanism.

1. Belliveau PP, Nightingale CH, Quintiliani R, Maderazo EG. Reduction in serum concentrations of ciprofloxacin after administration of ursodiol to a patient with hepatobiliary disease. *Clin Infect Dis* (1994) 19, 354–5.

Rifabutin (Ansamycin) + Azithromycin

Rifabutin and azithromycin seem not to affect the serum levels of each other, but a very high incidence of neutropenia and leucopenia was seen in one study.

Clinical evidence

A study in 12 healthy subjects was designed to investigate the safety and possible interactions between rifabutin 300 mg daily and **azithromycin** 250 mg daily or **clarithromycin**, 500 mg twice daily, for a course of 14 days. The subjects were matched against 18 healthy controls who received either of the macrolides or rifabutin alone. The study had to be abandoned after 10 days because 14 patients developed neutropenia, 2 taking rifabutin alone, and all 12 of those on a rifabutin/macrolide combination. Because of the early cessation of the study the pharmacokinetics of rifabutin/**azithromycin** and rifabutin/**clarithromycin** could not be fully assessed. However, from the limited information available it seems that **clarithromycin**, but not **azithromycin** affected the pharmacokinetics of rifabutin.[1]

Another group using rifabutin and **azithromycin** (500 mg daily) did not experience the problem of uveitis sometimes seen with other macrolide drugs (such as clarithromycin) when combined with rifabutin.[2] Yet another report attributed the development of uveitis to a possible rifabutin/**azithromycin** interaction, but what happened seems much more likely to have been due to the presence of **fluconazole**, which is known to interact with rifabutin.[3]

Mechanism

The reasons for the leucopenia are not known.

Importance and management

Information is very limited but what is known suggests that a very close watch should be kept on the white cell profile if the concurrent use of rifabutin and azithromycin is undertaken. More study is needed. Also see 'Clarithromycin + Rifamycins', p.148.

1. Apseloff G, Foulds G, LaBoy-Goral L, Willavize S, Vincent J. Comparison of azithromycin and clarithromycin in their interactions with rifabutin in healthy volunteers. *J Clin Pharmacol* (1998) 38, 830–5.
2. Kelleher P, Helbert M, Sweeney J, Anderson J, Parkin J, Pinching A. Uveitis associated with rifabutin and macrolide therapy for *Mycobacterium avium intracellulare* infection in AIDS patients. *Genitourin Med* (1996) 72, 419-21.
3. Havlir D, Torriani F, Dubé M. Uveitis associated with rifabutin prophylaxis. *Ann Intern Med* (1994) 121, 510–12.

Rifabutin (Ansamycin) + Miscellaneous drugs

The makers and the CSM in the UK warn that rifabutin may possibly reduce the effects of a number of drugs, but these predictions appear to be based on *in vitro* studies and theoretical considerations and not on direct clinical evidence.

Clinical evidence, mechanism, importance and management

In addition to the drugs listed with rifabutin in the Index which are more fully discussed in individual monographs, the makers say that rifabutin might reduce the activity of **analgesics**, **anticoagulants**, **corticosteroids**, **ciclosporin**, **digitalis** (although not **digoxin**), **dapsone**, **oral hypoglycaemics**, **opioids**, **phenytoin** and **quinidine**. They also say that the trough levels of **tacrolimus** may be reduced. The suggested reason is that rifabutin induces the activity of cytochrome P450 isoenzyme CYP3A, which is concerned with the metabolism of these drugs.[1] However, rifabutin does not have the equivalent potent enzyme inducing activity of rifampicin and any interactions are therefore likely to have a very much smaller effect.[2] The CSM has repeated the same warnings for **anticoagulants**, **ciclosporin**, **oral hypoglycaemics**, **phenytoin** and added **carbamazepine**,[3] but it needs to be made clear that this is not a list of drugs known to interact with rifabutin. These are predictions based on *in vitro* data and there appears as yet to be no direct clinical data or case reports to confirm that these potential interactions are of clinical relevance.

The makers also say that no significant interactions may be expected between rifabutin and **ethambutol**, **pyrazinamide**, **sulphonamides** or **zalcitabine**.

1. Mycobutin (Rifabutin). Pharmacia. Summary of product characteristics, July 1997.
2. Narang PK, Gupta S, Li RC, Strolin-Benedetti M, Bruna CD, Bianchine JR. Assessing dosing implications of enzyme inducing potential: rifabutin (RIF) vs. rifampicin (RFM). *Intersci Conf Antimicrob Agents Chemother* (1993) 33, 228.
3. Committee on the Safety of Medicines/Medicines Control Agency. Revised indication and drug interactions of rifabutin. *Current Problems* (1997) 23, 14.

Rifampicin (Rifampin) + Aminosalicylic acid (PAS)

The serum levels of rifampicin are approximately halved if aminosalicylic acid granules containing bentonite are used concurrently. This interaction may possibly be avoided by separating the dosages by 8 to 12 h or by using an aminosalicylic acid formulation that does not contain bentonite.

Clinical evidence

The serum rifampicin levels (doses 10 mg/kg) of 30 patients with tuberculosis were reduced more than 50% (from 6.06 to 2.91 micrograms/ml) at 2 h by the concurrent use of **aminosalicylate**.[1,2] Later studies on 6 healthy subjects showed that this interaction was not due to the **aminosalicylic acid** itself but to the **bentonite** which was the main excipient of the granules.[3] The rifampicin AUC was statistically unchanged in the presence of **sodium aminosalicylate** tablets (no **bentonite**), whereas it was reduced by more than 37% in the presence of **bentonite** from **aminosalicylate** granules.[3]

Other studies confirm this marked reduction in serum rifampicin levels in the presence of **bentonite** in **aminosalicylic acid granules**.[4]

Mechanism

The bentonite excipient in the aminosalicylic acid granules adsorbs the rifampicin onto its surface so that much less is available for absorption by the gut, resulting in reduced serum levels.[3] Bentonite is a naturally occurring mineral (montmorillonite) consisting largely of hydrate aluminium silicate, and is similar to kaolin.

Importance and management

A well documented and clinically important interaction. Separating the administration of the two drugs by 8 to 12 h to prevent their mixing in the gut has been suggested as an effective way to prevent this interaction.[1] An alternative is to give aminosalicylic acid preparations that do not contain bentonite or any other substances that can adsorb rifampicin.

1. Boman G, Hanngren Å, Malmborg A-S, Borgå O, Sjöqvist F. Drug Interaction: decreased serum concentrations of rifampicin when given with P.A.S. *Lancet* (1971) i, 800.

2. Boman G, Borgå O, Hanngren Å, Malmborg A-S and Sjöqvist F. Pharmacokinetic inter-actions between the tuberculostatics rifampicin, para-aminosalicylic acid and isoniazid. *Acta Pharmacol Toxicol* (1970) 28 (Suppl 1), 15.
3. Boman G, Lundgren P, Stjernström G. Mechanism of the inhibitory effect of PAS gran-ules on the absorption of rifampicin: adsorption of rifampicin by an excipient, bentonite. *Eur J Clin Pharmacol* (1975) 8, 293–9.
4. Boman G. Serum concentration and half-life of rifampicin after simultaneous oral admin-istration of aminosalicylic acid or isoniazid. *Eur J Clin Pharmacol* (1974) 7, 217–25.

Rifampicin (Rifampin) + Antacids

The absorption of rifampicin can be reduced up to about a third by the concurrent use of antacids, but the clinical im-portance of this is uncertain.

Clinical evidence

When single 600-mg doses of rifampicin were taken with different antacids and 200 ml of water by 5 healthy subjects, the absorption of the rifampicin was reduced. The antacids caused a fall in the urinary excretion of rifampicin as follows: with 15 or 30 ml **aluminium hy-droxide gel** 29 to 31%; with 2 or 4 g **magnesium trisilicate** 31 to 36%; and with 2 g **sodium bicarbonate** 21%.[1]

Three groups of 15 patients with tuberculosis were given single oral doses of rifampicin 10 to 12 mg/kg, isoniazid 300 mg and ethambutol 20 mg/kg either alone or with 4 teaspoonfuls of antacid. A significant number of patients had peak rifampicin concentrations below 6.5 micrograms/ml with *Aludrox* (**aluminium hydroxide**), but no significant effect was noted with *Gelusil* (**aluminium hydroxide plus magnesium trisilicate**).[2] However, in a further study in 14 healthy subjects, administration of 30 ml *Mylanta* (**aluminium-mag-nesium hydroxide**) 9 h before, with and after rifampicin had no ef-fect on the pharmacokinetics of rifampicin.[3]

Mechanism

The rise in the pH within the stomach caused by these antacids reduc-es the dissolution of the rifampicin thereby inhibiting its absorption. In addition aluminium ions may form less soluble chelates with ri-fampicin, and magnesium trisilicate can adsorb rifampicin, both of which would also be expected to reduce bioavailability.[1]

Importance and management

Direct information seems to be limited to these reports. No one seems to have assessed the effects of 20 to 35% reductions in absorption on rifampicin treatment, but if antacids are given it would be prudent to be alert for any evidence that treatment is less effective than expected. More study is needed.

1. Khalil SAH, El-Khordagui LK, El-Gholmy ZA. Effect of antacids on oral absorption of rifampicin. *Int J Pharmaceutics* (1984) 20, 99–106.
2. Gupta PR, Mehta YR, Gupta ML, Sharma TN, Jain D, Gupta RB. Rifampicin-aluminium antacid interaction. *J Assoc Physicians India* (1988) 36, 363–4.
3. Peloquin CA, Namdar R, Singleton MD, Nix DE. Pharmacokinetics of rifampin under fasting conditions, with food, and with antacids. *Chest* (1999) 115, 12–18.

Rifampicin (Rifampin) + Clofazimine

Rifampicin appears not to interact adversely with clofaz-imine.

Clinical evidence, mechanism, importance and management

The pharmacokinetics of rifampicin were not altered by multiple dos-es of **clofazimine**.[1] A single dose study similarly found that the bioa-vailability of **clofazimine** remained unaltered when rifampicin was given concurrently, although a reduction in the rate of absorption was seen.[2] No special precautions would seem to be necessary.

1. Venkatesan K, Mathur A, Girdhar BK, Bharadwaj VP. The effect of clofazimine on the pharmacokinetics of rifampicin and dapsone in leprosy. *J Antimicrob Chemother* (1986) 18, 715–18.

2. Mehta J, Gandhi IS, Sane SB, Wamburkar MN. Effect of clofazimine and dapsone on ri-fampicin (Lositril) pharmacokinetics in multibacillary and paucibacillary leprosy cases. *Indian J Lepr* (1985) 57, 297–310.

Rifampicin (Rifampin) + Co-trimoxazole

Co-trimoxazole can increase rifampicin serum levels.

Clinical evidence, mechanism, importance and management

Co-trimoxazole (two tablets each containing trimethoprim 160 mg and sulfamethoxazole 400 mg, given 12-hourly) for 5 to 10 days in 15 patients with tuberculosis, who had taken rifampicin 450 mg daily for at least 15 days, increased the median AUC of rifampicin by 62% and the peak levels by 31%. The reasons are not understood. No adverse effects were seen, but the authors of the report point out that while concurrent use may be beneficial there is also the risk that hepatotox-icity may be increased.[1] Good monitoring is advised.

1. Bhatia RS, Uppal R, Malhi R, Behera D, Jindal SK. Drug interaction between rifampicin and co-trimoxazole in patients with tuberculosis. *Hum Exp Toxicol* (1991) 10, 419–21.

Rifampicin (Rifampin) + Food

Food delays and reduces the absorption of rifampicin from the gut.

Clinical evidence

When a single 10 mg/kg dose of rifampicin was taken by 6 healthy subjects with a **standard Indian breakfast** (125 g wheat, 10 g visi-ble fat, 350 g vegetables) the absorption of the rifampicin was re-duced. The AUC after 8 h was reduced by 26% and the peak plasma levels were reduced by about 30% (from 11.84 micrograms/ml at 2 h to 8.35 micrograms/ml at 4 h).[1] In another study, where rifampicin 600 mg was administered with a **high-fat breakfast**, the maximum serum level was reduced by 36% and the absorption was delayed, but the AUC was not significantly altered.[2]

Mechanism

Not understood.

Importance and management

An established interaction. The recommendation is that rifampicin should be taken on an empty stomach or 30 min before a meal, or 2 h after a meal to ensure rapid and complete absorption.

1. Polasa K, Krishnaswamy K. Effect of food on bioavailability of rifampicin. *J Clin Phar-macol* (1983) 23, 433–7.
2. Peloquin CA, Namdar R, Singleton MD, Nix DE. Pharmacokinetics of rifampin under fasting conditions, with food, and with antacids. *Chest* (1999) 155, 12–18.

Rifampicin (Rifampin) + Probenecid

Whether or not the serum levels of rifampicin are increased by the concurrent use of probenecid seems uncertain and un-predictable.

Clinical evidence, mechanism, importance and management

A study in 6 healthy subjects given 2 g **probenecid** before and after taking single 300-mg doses of rifampicin showed that mean peak se-rum rifampicin levels were raised by 86%. At 4, 6 and 9 h the percent-age increases were 118, 90 and 102% respectively.[1] However, subsequent studies in patients taking either 600 mg rifampicin or 300 mg rifampicin plus 2 g **probenecid** taken 30 min before, showed that the latter group achieved serum rifampicin levels which were only about half those achieved by those on 600 mg rifampicin, suggesting no interaction occurred.[2] The reasons for these discordant results are not understood, although it has been suggested that erratic rifampicin absorption may have played a part.[2]

The response of patients to concurrent use of these two drugs is so inconsistent and unpredictable that these drugs should be used together with care, remembering that the occasional patient may show elevated rifampicin levels.

1. Kenwright S, Levi AJ. Impairment of hepatic uptake of rifamycin antibiotics by probenecid, and its therapeutic implications. *Lancet* (1973) ii, 1401–5.
2. Fallon RJ, Lees AW, Allan GW, Smith J, Tyrrell WF. Probenecid and rifampicin serum levels. *Lancet* (1975) ii, 792–4.

Rifampicin (Rifampin) + Ranitidine

Ranitidine appears not to interact with rifampicin.

Clinical evidence, mechanism, importance and management

A controlled study in 112 patients with pulmonary tuberculosis treated 2 groups, one with a daily regimen of rifampicin 10 mg/kg, isoniazid 300 mg and ethambutol 20 mg/kg and 150 mg **ranitidine** twice daily, and the other without the ranitidine. The pharmacokinetics of the rifampicin (as measured by the total and unchanged urinary excretion) were not affected by the concurrent use of **ranitidine**. No changes occurred in the incidence of adverse hepatic reactions, while gastrointestinal reactions were reduced.[1] There would seem to be no reason for avoiding the concurrent use of these drugs. **Ranitidine** also appears not to interact with isoniazid (see 'Isoniazid + Cimetidine or Ranitidine', p.162).

1. Purohit SD, Johri SC, Gupta PR, Mehta YR, Bhatnagar M. Ranitidine-rifampicin interaction. *J Assoc Physicians India* (1992) 40, 308–10.

Rifampicin (Rifampin) + Troleandomycin

Cholestatic jaundice has been attributed to the concurrent use of these two antibacterials.

Clinical evidence, mechanism, importance and management

Two cases of cholestatic jaundice have been reported in patients treated with both rifampicin and **troleandomycin**.[1,2] Both antibacterials are potentially hepatotoxic and it seems possible that their liver damaging effects can be additive. As a general rule, where possible, the concurrent use of hepatotoxic drugs should be avoided.

1. Piette F, Peyrard P. Ictère bénin médicamenteux lors d'un traitement associant rifampicine-triacétyloléandomycine. *Nouv Presse Med* (1979) 8, 368–9.
2. Givaudan JF, Gamby T, Privat Y. Ictère cholestatique après association rifampicine-troléandomycine: une nouvelle observation. *Nouv Presse Med* (1979) 8, 2357.

Rifapentine + Other drugs

Rifapentine is a derivative of rifampicin with a similar antibacterial spectrum, an approximately ten times greater potency, and a longer half-life. Like rifampicin it is a potent liver enzyme inducing agent.[1,2] Few clinically important interactions have been documented, but it would be expected to interact with many of the drugs with which rifampicin interacts. See Index.

1. Durand DV, Hampden C, Boobis AR, Park BK, Davies DS. Induction of mixed function oxidase activity in man by rifapentine (MDL 473), a long-acting rifamycin derivative. *Br J Clin Pharmacol* (1986) 21, 1–7.

2. Li AP, Reith MK, Rasmussen A, Gorski JC, Hall SD, Xu L, Kaminski DL, Cheng LK. Primary human hepatocytes as a tool for the evaluation of structure-activity relationship in cytochrome P450 induction potential of xenobiotics: evaluation of rifampin, rifapentine and rifabutin. *Chem Biol Interact* (1997) 107, 17–30.

Rimantadine + Cimetidine

Cimetidine causes a small but probably clinically unimportant rise in the serum levels of rimantadine.

Clinical evidence, mechanism, importance and management

After taking 300 mg **cimetidine** four times daily for 6 days, the AUC of a single 100-mg dose of rimantadine in 23 healthy subjects was increased by 20% and the apparent total clearance reduced by 18%. The authors of the study suggest that these changes are likely to have little, if any, clinical consequences.[1] However, this needs confirmation in patients.

1. Holazo AA, Choma N, Brown SY, Lee LF, Wills RJ.Effect of cimetidine on the disposition of rimantadine in healthy subjects. *Antimicrob Agents Chemother* (1989) 33, 820–3.

Sulfamethoxazole + Salbutamol (Albuterol)

Salbutamol reduces the rate but increases the extent of absorption of sulfamethoxazole.

Clinical evidence, mechanism, importance and management

Oral **salbutamol (albuterol)** 4 mg four times daily for 2 weeks had no effect on most of the pharmacokinetics of a single 400 mg oral dose of sulfamethoxazole (in co-trimoxazole) given to 6 healthy subjects. However, the absorption rate constant was reduced by about 40% and the extent of absorption over 72 h was increased by 22.6%.[1] A possible reason is that the stimulation of the beta-receptors by the **salbutamol** in the gut causes relaxation, which allows an increased contact time for the sulfamethoxazole.[1] The clinical significance of this interaction awaits assessment, but it seems unlikely to be of importance. No interaction would be expected with inhaled **salbutamol**.

1. Adebayo GI, Ogundipe TO. Effects of salbutamol on the absorption and disposition of sulphamethoxazole in adult volunteers. *Eur J Drug Metab Pharmacokinet* (1989) 14, 57–60.

Sulphonamides + Barbiturates

The anaesthetic effects of thiopental are increased but shortened by pretreatment with sulfafurazole (sulfisoxazole). Phenobarbital appears not to interact significantly with sulfafurazole or sulfisomidine. There seem to be no reports of any adverse sulphonamide/barbiturate interactions.

Clinical evidence

(a) Sulfafurazole + Thiopental

A study in 48 patients showed that the prior intravenous administration of **sulfafurazole** 40 mg/kg reduced the required anaesthetic dosage of **thiopental** by 36%, but the duration of action was shortened.[1] This interaction has also been observed in *animal* experiments.[2]

(b) Sulfafurazole or Sulfisomidine + Phenobarbital

A study in children showed that **phenobarbital** did not affect the pharmacokinetics of **sulfafurazole** or **sulfisomidine**.[3]

Mechanism

It is suggested that sulfafurazole successfully competes with the thiopental for the plasma protein binding sites,[4] the result being that more free and active barbiturate molecules remain in circulation to exert their anaesthetic effects and a smaller dose is therefore required.

Importance and management

The evidence for the sulfafurazole/thiopental interaction is limited, but it appears to be strong. Less thiopental than usual may be required to achieve adequate anaesthesia, but since the awakening time is shortened repeated doses may be needed. Information about other sulphonamide-barbiturate interactions is also very limited, but none of those reported so far seems to be of clinical importance.

1. Csögör SI, Kerek SF. Enhancement of thiopentone anaesthesia by sulphafurazole. *Br J Anaesth* (1970) 42, 988–90.
2. Csögör SI, Pálffy B, Feztz G, Papp J. Influence du sulfathiazol sur l'effet narcotique du thiopental et de l'hexobarbital. *Rev Roum Physiol* (1971) 8, 81–5.
3. Krauer B. Vergleichende Untersuchung der Eliminationskinetik zweier Sulfonamide bei Kindern mit und ohne Phenobarbitalmedikation. *Schweiz Med Wochenschr* (1971) 101, 668–71.
4. Csögör SI, Papp J. Competition between sulphonamides and thiopental for binding sites of plasma proteins. *Arzneimittelforschung* (1970) 20, 1925–7.

Sulphonamides + Local anaesthetics or Para-aminobenzoic acid

The para-aminobenzoic acid (PABA) derived from certain local anaesthetics can reduce the effects of the sulphonamides and allow the development of local and even generalised infections.

Clinical evidence

Four patients on **sulphonamides** developed local infections in areas where **procaine** had been injected prior to diagnostic taps in meningitis, or draining procedures in empyema. Extensive cellulitis of the lumbar region occurred in one case, and abscesses appeared at the puncture sites in another.[1]

A study demonstrated that the amount of **procaine** in pleural fluid after anaesthesia for thoracentesis was sufficient to inhibit the antibacterial activity of 0.005% **sulphapyridine** against type III pneumococci.[2] Other studies in *animals* confirm that antagonism can occur both in *vitro*[3-5] and in *vivo*[6] with local anaesthetics that are hydrolysed to **PABA**.

Mechanism

The ester type of local anaesthetic is hydrolysed within the body to produce PABA. **PABA** and the sulphonamides compete with one another to take part in the synthesis of folate by bacteria. The relative concentrations of each molecule are among the factors that determine the 'winner'. Hence the clinical importance of achieving adequate concentrations of the sulphonamide and of avoiding the introduction of additional **PABA** molecules.

Importance and management

Clinical examples of this interaction seem to be few, but the supporting evidence (human, *animal* and in *vitro* studies dating back to the mid-1940s) is strong. This would seem to be an interaction of clinical importance. Local anaesthetics of the ester type which are hydrolysed to PABA (e.g. tetracaine (amethocaine), procaine, benzocaine) should be avoided in patients using sulphonamides, whereas those of the amide type (bupivacaine, cinchocaine (dibucaine), lidocaine (lignocaine), mepivacaine and prilocaine) do not interact adversely.

1. Peterson OL, Finland M. Sulfonamide inhibiting action of procaine. *Am J Med Sci* (1944) 207, 166–75.
2. Boroff DA, Cooper A, Bullowa JGM. Inhibition of sulfapyridine by procaine in chest fluids after procaine anesthesia. *Proc Soc Exp Biol Med* (1941) 47,182–3.
3. Casten D, Fried JJ, Hallman FA. Inhibitory effect of procaine on the bacteriostatic activity of sulfathiazole. *Surg Gynecol Obstet* (1943) 76, 726–8.

4. Powell HM, Krahl ME, Clowes GHA. Inhibition of chemotherapeutic action of sulfapyridine by local anesthetics. *J Indiana State Med Ass* (1942) 35, 62–3.
5. Walker BS, Derow MA. The antagonism of local anesthetics against the sulfonamides. *Am J Med Sci* (1945) 210, 585–8.
6. Pfeiffer CC, Grant CW. The procaine-sulfonamide antagonism: an evaluation of local anesthetics for use with sulfonamide therapy. *Anesthesiology* (1944) 5, 605–14.

Terbinafine + Miscellaneous drugs

The serum levels of terbinafine are reduced by rifampicin. Terbinafine causes a small, clinically unimportant fall in ciclosporin serum levels. Two isolated reports describe increases in the serum levels of imipramine and nortriptyline. Terbinafine is reported not interact to a clinically relevant extent with astemizole, cimetidine, midazolam, nifedipine, oral contraceptives, ranitidine, terfenadine, tolbutamide or triazolam.

Clinical evidence, mechanism, importance and management

(a) Antihistamines

In a large scale post-marketing survey of 25,884 patients on terbinafine, over 40% were taking at least one other drug. From amongst this group, an unknown number of patients were taking **astemizole** or **terfenadine**. No adverse interactions were reported.[1] The makers of terbinafine state that studies undertaken in *vitro* and in healthy volunteers indicate that terbinafine does not inhibit or induce any cytochrome P450 isoenzyme other than CYP2D6 and thus may safely be given to patients taking **terfenadine**.[2] No special precautions would therefore appear to be necessary.

(b) Benzodiazepines

Terbinafine 250 mg daily for 4 days had no effect on the pharmacokinetics of a single 7.5-mg dose of **midazolam**[3] or a single 250 micrograms dose of **triazolam**[4] in 12 healthy subjects nor on their performance of a number of psychomotor tests. No special precautions would seem to be necessary.

(c) Ciclosporin

After taking 250 mg terbinafine daily for 6 to 7 days the mean AUC of single 300-mg doses of **ciclosporin** in 20 healthy subjects was decreased by 13% and the maximum blood concentration was reduced by 14%. It was suggested that as *Sandimmun* was used in the study, inter- and intra-individual variations in **ciclosporin** absorption caused these differences rather than any drug interaction.[5,6] Another study in 11 patients with kidney, heart or lung transplants found that 250 mg terbinafine daily for 12 weeks caused a small but clinically irrelevant decrease in serum **ciclosporin** levels.[7] These studies broadly confirm previous in *vitro* work with human liver microsomal enzymes which found that terbinafine either does not inhibit **ciclosporin** metabolism or it only causes modest inhibition.[8-10] The small changes in the pharmacokinetics of **ciclosporin** appear to be clinically unimportant. No special precautions appear to be necessary.

(d) Ethinylestradiol

An in *vitro* study in human livers showed that terbinafine did not alter the pharmacokinetics of **ethinylestradiol**.[8] However, the makers of terbinafine note that menstrual disturbances have occurred in patients on both **oral contraceptives** and terbinafine.[2] In a post-marketing survey which included 314 patients taking both **oral contraceptives** and terbinafine the rate of menstrual disorders was within the rate reported for patients on **oral contraceptives** alone.[11]

(e) H_2-blockers

Cimetidine 400 mg twice daily for 5 days increased the AUC of a single 250-mg dose of terbinafine in 12 healthy subjects by 34% and reduced its clearance by 30%.[12] The likely reason is that **cimetidine** (a known enzyme inhibitor) reduces the metabolism of the terbinafine by the liver so that it is cleared from the body more slowly. However, it seems that this modest increase in the serum levels of terbinafine is of little or no clinical relevance, because in a large scale post-marketing survey (see (a) above) no interactions in patients taking terbinafine with **cimetidine** or **ranitidine** were reported.[1] No special precautions would appear to be necessary.

(f) Hypoglycaemic agents

On the basis of studies with human liver microsomes,[8] the makers of terbinafine also suggest that an interaction with **tolbutamide** is unlikely.[2] This is supported by a large scale post-marketing survey (see (a) above) which identified no interaction on concurrent use of terbinafine and **tolbutamide**.[1] In a 154 patient subgroup of this survey no additional risk was noted due to co-administered oral **hypoglycaemics** and terbinafine.[11]

(g) Nifedipine

A study in 12 healthy subjects found no alteration in the pharmacokinetics of **nifedipine** 30 mg (as *Procardia XL*) when given with terbinafine 250 mg.[13]

(h) Other antifungals

An *in vitro* study designed to assess the efficacy of combination antifungal therapy, found that terbinafine, in combination with **amphotericin B**, **fluconazole** or **itraconazole**, enhanced the activity of the antifungals against *Candida albicans*. The authors conclude that this enhanced activity is likely to be reflected in clinical practice, but this has not yet been assessed and so further investigation is needed.[14]

(i) Rifampicin (Rifampin)

In 12 subjects 600 mg **rifampicin** daily for 6 days halved the AUC of terbinafine and approximately doubled its clearance.[12] **Rifampicin** is a potent enzyme inducing agent which increases the metabolism and loss from the body of many drugs. Be alert, therefore, for the need to increase the dosage of terbinafine if **rifampicin** is given. A broad estimate is that the dosage will need to be about doubled.

(j) Tricyclic antidepressants

A man aged 51 who had been on lithium carbonate and varying doses of **imipramine** 150 to 200 mg daily for 10 years was additionally started on 250 mg oral **terbinafine** daily for onychomycosis. About a week later he complained of dizziness, muscle twitching and excessive mouth dryness. His serum **imipramine** levels measured 5 days later had risen to 530 nanograms/ml from his usual range of 100 to 200 nanograms/ml. Within 10 days of reducing his daily **imipramine** dose from 200 to 75 mg daily, his serum levels had fallen to 229 nanograms/ml. His liver function was normal.[15] Another isolated report describes a marked increase in the serum levels of **nortriptyline** (about doubled) accompanied by evidence of toxicity (fatigue, vertigo, loss of energy and appetite, and falls) in a 74-year-old man taking 125 mg **nortriptyline** daily within 14 days of starting 250 mg terbinafine daily. His symptoms responded to a dose reduction to 75 mg daily. His serum levels showed a similar elevation when he was later re-challenged with terbinafine. His liver function was normal.[16]

This seems to be the first and only report of an adverse terbinafine/tricyclic antidepressant interaction so that there would seem to be little reason for avoiding concurrent use, but it would now seem prudent to monitor the outcome of giving these two together in any patient.

1. Hall M, Monka C, Krupp P, O'Sullivan D. Safety of oral terbinafine. Results of a post-marketing surveillance study in 25 884 patients. *Arch Dermatol* (1997) 133, 1213–19.
2. Lamisil (Terbinafine). Novartis Pharmaceuticals UK Ltd. Summary of product characteristics, November 2001.
3. Ahonen J, Olkkola KT, Neuvonen PJ. Effect of itraconazole and terbinafine on the pharmacokinetics and pharmacodynamics of midazolam in healthy volunteers. *Br J Clin Pharmacol* (1995) 40, 270–2.
4. Varhe A, Olkkola KT, Neuvonen PJ. Fluconazole, but not terbinafine, enhances the effects of triazolam by inhibiting its metabolism. *Br J Clin Pharmacol* (1996) 41, 319–23.
5. Long CC, Hill SA, Thomas RC, Holt DW, Finlay AY. The effect of terbinafine on the pharmacokinetics of cyclosporin in vivo. *Skin Pharmacol* (1992) 5, 200–1.
6. Long CC, Hill SA, Thomas RC, Johnston A, Smith SG, Kendall F, Finlay AY. Effect of terbinafine on the pharmacokinetics of cyclosporin in humans. *J Invest Dermatol* (1994) 102, 740–3.
7. Jensen P, Lehne G, Fauchald P, Simonsen S. Effect of oral terbinafine treatment on cyclosporin pharmacokinetics in organ transplant recipients with dermatophyte nail infection. *Acta Derm Venereol (Stockh)* (1996) 76, 280–1.
8. Back DJ, Stevenson P, Tjia JF. Comparative effects of two antimycotic agents, ketoconazole and terbinafine, on the metabolism of tolbutamide, ethinyloestradiol, cyclosporin and ethoxycoumarin by human liver microsomes *in vitro*. *Br J Clin Pharmacol* (1989) 28, 166–70.
9. Shah IA, Whiting PH, Omar G, Ormerod AD, Burke MD. The effects of retinoids and terbinafine on the human hepatic microsomal metabolism of cyclosporin. *Br J Dermatol* (1993) 129, 395–8.
10. Back DJ, Tjia JF, Abel SM. Azoles, allylamines and drug metabolism. *Br J Dermatol* (1992) 126 (Suppl 39), 14–18.
11. O'Sullivan DP, Needham CA, Bangs A, Atkin K, Kendall FD. Postmarketing surveillance of oral terbinafine in the UK: report of a large cohort study. *Br J Clin Pharmacol* (1996) 42, 559–65.
12. Jensen JC. Pharmacokinetics of Lamisil® in humans. *J Dermatol Treat* (1990) 1 (Suppl 2), 15–18.
13. Cramer JA, Robbins B, Barbeito R, Bedman TC, Dreisbach A, Meligeni JA. Lamisil®: interaction study with a sustained release nifedipine formulation. *Pharm Res* (1996) 13 (9 Suppl), S436.
14. Barchiesi F, Falconi Di Francesco L, Compagnucci P, Arzeni D, Giacometti A, Scalise G. In-vitro interaction of terbinafine with amphotericin B, fluconazole and itraconazole against clinical isolates of *Candida albicans*. *J Antimicrob Chemother* (1998) 41, 59–65.
15. Teitelbaum ML, Pearson VE. Imipramine toxicity and terbinafine. *Am J Psychiatry* (2001) 158, 2086.
16. van der Kuy P-HM, Hooymans PM, Verkaaik AJB. Nortriptyline intoxication induced by terbinafine. *BMJ* (1998) 316, 441.

Tetracyclines + Alcohol

Doxycycline serum levels may fall below minimum therapeutic concentrations in alcoholic patients, but tetracycline itself is not affected, and it seems likely that the other tetracyclines are also not affected. There is nothing to suggest that moderate amounts of alcohol have a clinically relevant effect on the serum levels of doxycycline or any other tetracycline in non-alcoholic subjects.

Clinical evidence

(a) Alcoholic patients

A study in to the effects of **alcohol** on tetracyclines found that the half-life of **doxycycline** was 10.5 h in 6 alcoholics compared with 14.7 h in 6 healthy volunteers. The serum **doxycycline** levels of 3 of the alcoholic patients fell below what is generally accepted as the minimum therapeutic concentration. The half-life of **tetracycline** was the same in both groups. All of them were given 100 mg **doxycycline** daily after a 200 mg loading dose, and 500 mg **tetracycline** twice daily after an initial 750 mg loading dose.[1]

(b) Non-alcoholic patients

Single 500-mg doses of **tetracycline** were given to 9 healthy subjects with water or an **alcoholic drink** (270 mg/kg of **alcohol**). The **alcohol** caused a 33% rise in the maximum serum **tetracycline** levels (from 9.3 to 12.4 micrograms/ml), and a 50% rise in the **tetracycline** AUC.[2] The clinical relevance of this rise is unknown.

Another study in healthy subjects found that **cheap red wine,** but **not whisky** (both 1 g/kg) postponed the absorption of **doxycycline**, probably because of the acetic acid content which slows gastric emptying. However, the total absorption was not affected. The authors concluded[3] that "the acute intake of **alcoholic beverages** generally does not interfere with the kinetics of **doxycycline** to an extent which would jeopardise therapeutic levels in tissues".

Mechanism

Heavy drinkers can metabolise some drugs much more quickly than non-drinkers due to the enzyme-inducing effects of alcohol,[4] and the interaction with doxycycline would seem to be due to this effect, possibly associated with some reduction in absorption from the gut.

Importance and management

Information is limited, but the doxycycline/alcohol interaction appears to be established and of clinical significance in alcoholics but not in non-alcoholic individuals. One possible solution to the problem of enzyme induction, suggested by epileptic patients, is to dose the alcoholic subjects twice daily instead of only once.[5] Alternatively tetracycline could be used because it appears not to be affected. There is nothing to suggest that moderate or even occasional heavy drinking has a clinically relevant effect on any of the tetracyclines in non-alcoholic subjects.

1. Neuvonen PJ, Penttilä O, Roos M, Tirkkonen J. Effect of long-term alcohol consumption on the half-life of tetracycline and doxycycline in man. *Int J Clin Pharmacol Biopharm* (1976) 14, 303–7.
2. Seitz C, Garcia J, Arancibia A. Influence of ethanol ingestion on tetracycline kinetics. *Int J Clin Pharmacol Ther* (1995) 33, 462–4.
3. Mattila MJ, Laisi U, Linnoila M, Salonen R. Effect of alcoholic beverages on the pharmacokinetics of doxycycline in man. *Acta Pharmacol Toxicol* (1982) 50, 370–3.
4. Misra PS, Lefèvre A, Ishii H, Rubin E, Lieber CS. Increase of ethanol, meprobamate and pentobarbital metabolism after chronic ethanol administration in man and rats. *Am J Med* (1971) 51, 346–51.
5. Neuvonen PJ, Penttilä O, Lehtovaara R and Aho K. Effect of antiepileptic drugs on the elimination of various tetracycline derivatives. *Eur J Clin Pharmacol* (1975) 9, 147–54.

Tetracyclines + Antacids

The serum levels and as a consequence the therapeutic effectiveness of the tetracycline antibacterials can be markedly reduced or even abolished by the concurrent use of antacids containing aluminium, bismuth, calcium or magnesium. Other antacids such as sodium bicarbonate that raise the gastric pH may also reduce the bioavailability of some tetracycline preparations. Even the serum levels of intravenous doxycycline can be reduced.

Clinical evidence

(a) Aluminium-containing antacids

Two teaspoonfuls of **aluminium hydroxide gel** (*Amphogel*) given with 500 mg **chlortetracycline** to 5 patients and 6 normal subjects every 6 h reduced the serum levels of the antibacterial by about 80 to 90% within 48 h of starting concurrent antacid. One patient had a recurrence of her urinary tract infection, which only subsided when the antacid was withdrawn, and one patient maintained **chlortetracycline** levels despite antacid treatment.[1] Similar results were obtained in other studies.[2,3]

Further studies showed that 30 ml **aluminium hydroxide** reduced **oxytetracycline** serum levels by more than 50%,[3] 20 ml caused a 75% reduction in **demeclocycline** serum levels,[4] 15 ml caused a 100% reduction in serum **doxycycline** levels,[5] and 30 ml **magnesium-aluminium hydroxide** (*Maalox*) caused a 90% reduction in **tetracycline** serum levels.[6] Other studies support this **doxycycline**/antacid interaction.[7] The mean serum levels of an intravenous dose of **doxycycline** were also found to be reduced by 36% when 30 ml **aluminium hydroxide** was taken four times daily, for 2 days before and after the antibacterial.[8]

(b) Calcium, magnesium or bismuth-containing antacids

Bismuth subsalicylate markedly reduces the absorption of **tetracycline** (by 34%)[9] and a 50% reduction in the maximum serum level of **doxycycline** occurred on concurrent administration.[10] It has been suggested the excipient *Veegum* (**magnesium aluminium silicate**) in some **bismuth subsalicylate** formulations enhances the reduction.[11] **Bismuth carbonate** similarly interacts with the **tetracyclines** *in vitro*.[12] **Magnesium sulphate** certainly interacts with **tetracycline**, but in the clinical study on record[13] the amount of **magnesium** was much higher than would normally be found in the usual dose of antacid. There seem to be no direct clinical studies with **calcium-containing antacids**, but a clinically important interaction seems almost a certainty, based on an *in vitro* study with **calcium carbonate**,[12] **calcium in milk**, (see 'Tetracyclines + Milk and Dairy products', p.226 **dicalcium phosphate**,[14] and **calcium** as an excipient in **tetracycline capsules**.[15]

(c) Sodium-containing antacids

Sodium bicarbonate 2 g reduced the absorption of a 250 mg capsule of **tetracycline hydrochloride** in 8 subjects by 50%. If however the **tetracycline** was dissolved before administration, the absorption was unaffected by the **sodium bicarbonate**.[16] Another study stated that 2 g **sodium bicarbonate** had an insignificant effect on **tetracycline** absorption.[6]

Mechanism

Work in the mid-1950s demonstrated that the tetracyclines bind with aluminium, bismuth, calcium, magnesium and other metallic ions to form compounds (chelates) which are much less soluble and therefore much less readily absorbed by the gut.[17] In addition the solubility of the tetracyclines is a hundred times greater at pH 1 to 3 than at pH 5 to 6, so that an antacid that raises the gastric pH above about 4 for 20 to 30 min could prevent up to 50% of the tetracycline from being fully dissolved in the stomach.[16] Once the undissolved drug is emptied out of the stomach, the pH in the duodenum (5 to 6) and in the rest of the gut are unfavourable for full dissolution, so it remains unavailable for absorption. This may also explain why sodium bicarbonate interacts with tetracycline. A third reason for the reduced absorption may be because the tetracyclines are adsorbed onto the antacid.[9]

Importance and management

Extremely well-documented, long and well-established interactions. Their clinical importance depends on how much the serum tetracycline levels are lowered, but with normal antacid dosages the reductions cited above (50 to 100%) are so large that many organisms will not be exposed to minimum inhibitory concentrations (MIC). As a general rule none of the aluminium, bismuth, calcium or magnesium containing antacids, or others such as sodium bicarbonate that can markedly alter gastric pH, should be given at the same time as the tetracycline antibacterials. If they must be used, separate the dosages maximally (2 to 3 h or more) to prevent their admixture in the gut. Sodium bicarbonate and other antacids which only affect the extent of absorption by altering gastric pH will only interact with tetracycline preparations which are not already dissolved before ingestion (e.g. those in capsule form). Patients should be warned about taking any OTC antacids and indigestion preparations.

Instead of using antacids to minimise the gastric irritant effects of the tetracyclines it is usually recommended that tetracyclines are taken after food, however it is not entirely clear how much this affects their absorption (see 'Tetracyclines + Food', p.225).

1. Waisbren BA, Hueckel JS. Reduced absorption of aureomycin caused by aluminum hydroxide gel (*Amphojel*). *Proc Soc Exp Biol Med* (1950) 73, 73–4.
2. Seed JC, Wilson CE. The effect of aluminum hydroxide on serum aureomycin concentrations after simultaneous oral administration. *Bull John Hopkins Hosp* (1950) 86, 415–8.
3. Michel JC, Sayer RJ, Kirby WMM. Effect of food and antacids on blood levels of aureomycin and terramycin. *J Lab Clin Med* (1950) 36, 632–4.
4. Scheiner J, Altemeier WA. Experimental study of factors inhibiting absorption and effective therapeutic levels of declomycin. *Surg Gynecol Obstet* (1962) 114, 9–14.
5. Rosenblatt JE, Barrett JE, Brodie JL, Kirby WMM. Comparison of in vitro activity and clinical pharmacology of doxycycline with other tetracyclines. *Antimicrob Agents Chemother* (1966) 6, 134–41.
6. Garty M, Hurwitz A. Effect of cimetidine and antacids on gastrointestinal absorption of tetracycline. *Clin Pharmacol Ther* (1980) 28, 203–7.
7. Deppermann K-M, Lode H, Höffken G, Tschink G, Kalz C, Koeppe P. Influence of ranitidine, pirenzepine, and aluminum magnesium hydroxide on the bioavailability of various antibiotics, including amoxicillin, cephalexin, doxycycline, and amoxicillin-clavulanic acid. *Antimicrob Agents Chemother* (1989) 33, 1901–7.
8. Nguyen VX, Nix DE, Gillikin S, Schentag JJ. Effect of oral antacid administration on the pharmacokinetics of intravenous doxycycline. *Antimicrob Agents Chemother* (1989) 33, 434–6.
9. Albert KS, Welch RD, De Sante KA, Disanto AR. Decreased tetracycline bioavailability caused by a bismuth subsalicylate antidiarrheal mixture. *J Pharm Sci* (1979) 68, 586–8.
10. Ericsson CD, Feldman S, Pickering LK, Cleary TG. Influence of subsalicylate bismuth on absorption of doxycycline. *JAMA* (1982) 247, 2266–7.
11. Healy DP, Dansereau RJ, Dunn AB, Clendening CE, Mounts AW, Deepe GS. Reduced tetracycline bioavailability caused by magnesium aluminum silicate in liquid formulations of bismuth subsalicylate. *Ann Pharmacother* (1997) 31, 1460–4.
12. Christensen EKJ, Kerckhoffs HPM, Huizinga T. De invloed van antacida op de afgifte in vitro van tetracyclinehydrochloride. *Pharm Weekbl* (1967) 102, 463–73.
13. Harcourt RS, Hamburger M. The effect of magnesium sulfate in lowering tetracycline blood levels. *J Lab Clin Med* (1957) 50, 464–8.
14. Boger WP, Gavin JJ. An evaluation of tetracycline preparations. *N Engl J Med* (1959) 261, 827–32.
15. Sweeney WM, Hardy SM, Dornbush AC, Ruegsegger JM. Absorption of tetracycline in human beings as affected by certain excipients. *Antibiot Med Clin Ther* (1957) 4, 642–56.
16. Barr WH, Adir J, Garrettson L. Decrease of tetracycline absorption in man by sodium bicarbonate. *Clin Pharmacol Ther* (1971) 12, 779–84.
17. Albert A, Rees CW. Avidity of the tetracyclines for the cations of metals. *Nature* (1956) 177, 433–4.

Tetracyclines + Anticonvulsants

The serum levels of doxycycline are reduced and may fall below the accepted therapeutic minimum in patients on long-term treatment with barbiturates, phenytoin or carbamazepine. Other tetracyclines do not appear to be affected.

Clinical evidence

A study in 14 patients taking **phenytoin** (200 to 500 mg daily), **carbamazepine** (300 to 1000 mg daily)or both found that the half-life of **doxycycline** was approximately halved (from 15.1 to 7.2, 8.4, and 7.4 h respectively) when compared to 9 other patients not taking anticonvulsants.[1]

Similar results were found in 16 other patients on anticonvulsant therapy with **phenytoin**, **carbamazepine**, **primidone** and **phenobarbital**. The serum **doxycycline** levels of almost all of them fell below 0.5 micrograms/ml during the 12 to 24 h period following their last dose of **doxycycline** 100 mg. **Tetracycline**, **methacycline**, **oxytetracycline**, **demeclocycline** and **chlortetracycline** were not significantly affected by these anticonvulsants.[2] Other studies confirm this interaction between some **barbiturates** (**amobarbital**, **pentobarbital**, **phenobarbital**) and **doxycycline**.[3,4]

Mechanism

Uncertain. These anticonvulsants are known enzyme-inducing agents and it seems probable that they increase the metabolism of the doxycycline by the liver, thereby hastening its clearance from the body.

Importance and management

The doxycycline/anticonvulsant interactions are established, but just how much treatment with doxycycline is affected seems not to have been studied. Serum doxycycline levels below 0.5 micrograms/ml are less than the accepted minimum inhibitory concentration (MIC) so that it seems likely that the antibacterial will fail to be effective. To accommodate this potential problem is has been suggested that doxycycline dosage could be doubled.[2] Alternatively other tetracyclines could be used which are reported not to be affected by the anticonvulsants (tetracycline, methacycline, oxytetracycline, demeclocycline and chlortetracycline).[2]

1. Penttilä O, Neuvonen PJ, Aho K, Lehtovaara R. Interaction between doxycycline and some antiepileptic drugs. *BMJ* (1974) 2, 470–2.
2. Neuvonen PJ, Penttilä O, Lehtovaara R, Aho K. Effect of antiepileptic drugs on the elimination of various tetracycline derivatives. *Eur J Clin Pharmacol* (1975) 9, 147–54.
3. Neuvonen PJ, Penttilä O. Interaction between doxycycline and barbiturates. *BMJ* (1974) 1, 535–6.
4. Alestig K. Studies on the intestinal excretion of doxycycline. *Scand J Infect Dis* (1974) 6, 265–71.

Tetracyclines + Coffee or Orange Juice

Orange juice and coffee do not interact with tetracycline.

Clinical evidence, mechanism, importance and management

A study in 9 healthy subjects found that 200 ml of **orange juice** or **coffee** (milk content, if any, unstated) did not significantly affect the bioavailability of a single 250 mg dose of **tetracycline**. This is despite the fact that **orange juice** contains 35 to 70 mg calcium per 100 ml, which might be expected to combine with **tetracycline** to produce poorly absorbable chelates (see 'Tetracyclines + Milk and Dairy products', p.226). The reason seems to be that at the relevant pH values in the gut, the calcium is bound to components within the **orange juice** (citric, tartaric and ascorbic acids) and is not free to combine with the **tetracycline**.[1] Nobody seems to have checked on other tetracyclines, but it seems likely that they will behave similarly.

1. Jung H, Rivera O, Reguero MT, Rodríguez JM, Moreno-Esparza R. Influence of liquids (coffee and orange juice) on the bioavailability of tetracycline. *Biopharm Drug Dispos* (1990) 11, 729–34.

Tetracyclines + Colestipol

Colestipol can markedly reduce the absorption of tetracycline.

Clinical evidence

Colestipol 30 g taken either in 180 ml water or orange juice reduced the absorption of a single 500-mg dose of oral **tetracycline hydrochloride** in 9 healthy subjects by 54 to 56%, as measured by recovery in the urine.[1]

Mechanism

Colestipol binds to bile acids in the gut and can also bind with some drugs, thereby reducing their availability for absorption. An *in vitro* study found a 30% binding.[2] The presence of citrate ions in the orange juice which can also bind to colestipol appears not to have a marked effect on the binding of the tetracycline.

Importance and management

An established interaction. Direct information seems to be limited to the reports cited, but it is consistent with the way colestipol interacts with other drugs. In practice colestipol is normally given in 15 to 30 g daily doses, divided into two or four doses, and tetracycline in 250 to 500-mg doses 6-hourly, which means that it is difficult to avoid some mixing in the gut. It seems very probable that a clinically important interaction will occur, but by how much the steady-state serum tetracycline levels are affected seems not to have been determined. Tell patients to separate the dosages as much as possible. Monitor the outcome well. It may be necessary to increase the dosage of tetracycline. Information about other tetracyclines is lacking but it also seems likely that they will interact similarly.

1. Friedman H, Greenblatt DJ, LeDuc BW. Impaired absorption of tetracycline by colestipol is not reversed by orange juice. *J Clin Pharmacol* (1989) 29, 748–51.
2. Ko H, Royer ME. *In vitro* binding of drugs to colestipol hydrochloride. *J Pharm Sci* (1974) 63, 1914–20.

Tetracyclines + Diuretics

It has been recommended that the concurrent use of tetracyclines and diuretics should be avoided because of their association with rises in blood urea nitrogen levels.

Clinical evidence, mechanism, importance and management

A retrospective study of patient records as part of the Boston Collaborative Drug Surveillance Program showed that an association existed between **tetracycline** administration with **diuretics** (not named) and rises in blood urea nitrogen (BUN) levels.[1] Both diuretics and **tetracycline** are known to cause rises in BUN levels.[2] The recommendation was made that tetracyclines should be avoided in patients on **diuretics** when alternative antibacterials could be substituted.[1] However, the results of this study have been much criticised as the authors could not exclude physician bias,[1,2] they did not define what was meant by 'clinically significant rise in BUN',[2] they did not state whether on not this rise affected the patients,[2] they did not also measure creatinine levels[3] and they did not specify which diuretics were involved.[2] The patients most affected also had the highest levels of BUN before starting tetracyclines. Tetracyclines alone are known to cause rises in BUN, especially where a degree of renal impairment exists, although it has been suggested that **doxycycline** is less prone to this effect.[4] It would seem that tetracyclines and diuretics may be used together safely, although it would be wise to give thought to the patient's renal function.

1. Boston Collaborative Drug Surveillance Program. Tetracycline and drug-attributed rises in blood urea nitrogen. *JAMA* (1972) 220, 377–9.
2. Tannenberg AM. Tetracyclines and rises in urea nitrogen. *JAMA* (1972) 221, 713.
3. Dijkhuis HJPM, van Meurs AJ. Tetracycline and BUN level. *JAMA* (1973) 223, 441.
4. Alexander MR. Tetracyclines and rises in urea nitrogen. *JAMA* (1972) 221, 713–14.

Tetracyclines + Food

The calcium in food can complex with tetracycline to reduce its absorption.

Clinical evidence, mechanism, importance and management

Tetracycline 250 mg was given to 9 healthy subjects with 200 ml **water** on a **empty stomach**. The **tetracycline** bioavailability was compared with its administration after taking a **standard meal** (two slices of bread, ham, tomato, and water – containing 145 mg calcium) and a **Mexican meal** (two tortillas, beans, two eggs, tomato and water – containing 235 mg calcium). The cumulative amounts of **tetracycline** excreted in the urine at 72 h were 151.2 mg (fasting), 90.05 mg (**standard meal**) and 68.47 mg (**Mexican meal**).[1] The reason for the reduced bioavailability is that these meals contain calcium, which combines with the tetracycline in the gut to produce a less easily absorbed chelate. The absorption of a 300-mg dose of **demeclocycline** was not affected when administered with a meal not containing dairy products.[2] These interactions are very well established and clinically important (see also 'Tetracyclines + Milk and Dairy products', p.226).

It is usual to recommend that tetracyclines are taken 1 h before food or 2 h afterwards, to minimise admixture in the gut and to reduce the effects of this interaction. The separation is something of a compromise, because food can help to minimise the gastric irritant effects of the tetracyclines. **Doxycycline** seems to be minimally affected by food.[3]

1. Cook HJ, Mundo CR, Fonseca L, Gasque L, Moreno-Esparza R. Influence of the diet on bioavailability of tetracycline. *Biopharm Drug Dispos* (1993) 14, 549–53.
2. Scheiner J, Altemeier WA. Experimental study of factors inhibiting absorption and effective therapeutic levels of declomycin. *Surg Gynecol Obstet* (1962) 114, 9–14.
3. Rosenblatt JE, Barrett JE, Brodie JL, Kirby WMM. Comparison of in vitro activity and clinical pharmacology of doxycycline with other tetracyclines. *Antimicrob Agents Chemother* (1966) 6, 134–41.

Tetracyclines + H₂-blockers

Cimetidine seems not to affect the serum levels of tetracycline. Ranitidine seems not to affect the serum levels of doxycycline.

Clinical evidence, mechanism, importance and management

A study in 5 subjects showed that 3 days of **cimetidine** (200 mg three times daily and 400 mg at bedtime) reduced the absorption of a single dose of **tetracycline** 500 mg in capsule form by about 30%, but not when the **tetracycline** was given in solution.[1] However when **tetracycline** in either tablet or suspension form was given to 6 subjects with 1200 mg **cimetidine** daily for 6 days, no changes in the serum levels of **tetracycline** were seen,[2] which was similar to the results in a third study.[3]

In 10 healthy subjects, the bioavailability of 200 mg **doxycycline** was not altered by 3 doses of 150 mg of **ranitidine**.[4]

No special precautions would seem necessary with either combination. Information about other tetracyclines seems to be lacking.

1. Cole JJ, Charles BG, Ravenscroft PJ. Interaction of cimetidine with tetracycline absorption. *Lancet* (1980) ii, 536.

2. Fisher P, House F, Inns P, Morrison PJ, Rogers HJ, Bradbrook ID. Effect of cimetidine on the absorption of orally administered tetracycline. *Br J Clin Pharmacol* (1980) 9, 153–8.
3. Garty M, Hurwitz A. Effect of cimetidine and antacids on gastrointestinal absorption of tetracycline. *Clin Pharmacol Ther* (1980) 28, 203–7.
4. Deppermann K-M, Lode H, Höffken G, Tschink G, Kalz C, Koeppe P. Influence of ranitidine, pirenzepine, and aluminium magnesium hydroxide on the bioavailability of various antibiotics, including amoxicillin, cephalexin, doxycycline, and amoxicillin-clavulanic acid. *Antimicrob Agents Chemother* (1989) 33, 1901–7.

Tetracyclines + Iron preparations

The absorption from the gut of both the tetracyclines and of iron salts is markedly reduced by concurrent use, leading to depressed drug serum levels. Their therapeutic effectiveness may be reduced or even abolished. If both must be given, their administration should be maximally separated to minimise mixing in the gut.

Clinical evidence

(a) Effect of iron on absorption of the tetracyclines

An investigation in 10 healthy subjects given single oral doses of tetracyclines (200 to 500 mg) showed that the concurrent use of 200 mg **ferrous sulphate** decreased the serum antibacterial levels as follows: **tetracycline** 40 to 50%; **oxytetracycline** 50 to 60%; **methacycline** and **doxycycline** 80 to 90%.[1] Another study in 2 groups of 8 healthy subjects found that 300 mg **ferrous sulphate** reduced the absorption of **tetracycline** by 81% and of **minocycline** by 77%.[2]

Other studies found that in some instances the **iron** caused the tetracycline serum levels to fall below minimum bacterial inhibitory concentrations (MIC).[3,4] If the **iron** was given 3 h before or 2 h after a **tetracycline** the serum levels were not significantly depressed,[3-5] with the exception of **doxycycline**.[5] Even when the **iron** was given up to 11 h after **doxycycline**, serum concentrations were still lowered 20 to 45%.[5]

(b) Effect of tetracyclines on the absorption of iron

When 250 mg **ferrous sulphate** (equivalent to 50 mg Fe^{2+}) was given with 500 mg **tetracycline**, the absorption of **iron** was reduced by up to 78% in normal subjects, and up to 65% in those with depleted iron stores.[6,7]

Mechanism

The tetracyclines have a strong affinity for iron and form poorly soluble tetracycline-iron chelates, which are much less readily absorbed by the gut, and as a result the serum tetracycline levels achieved are much lower.[8,9] There is also less free iron available for absorption. Separating the administration of the two prevents their admixture,[3,4] but in the case of doxycycline some of the antibacterial is returned into the gut in the bile which tends to thwart any attempt to keep the iron and antibacterial apart. Even when given intravenously the half-life of doxycycline is reduced.[5] The different extent to which iron salts interact with the tetracyclines appears to be a reflection of their ability to liberate ferrous and ferric ions, which are free to combine with the tetracycline.[10]

Importance and management

Well-documented and well-established interactions of clinical importance. Reductions in serum tetracycline levels of the order of 30 to 90% due to the presence of iron are so large that levels may fall below those which inhibit bacterial growth (MIC).[4] However, the extent of the reductions depends on a number of factors.

(a) The particular tetracycline used: tetracycline itself in the study cited above was affected the least.[1]

(b) the time-interval between the administration of the two drugs: giving the iron 3 h before or 2 to 3 h after the antibacterial is satisfactory with tetracycline itself,[3] but even 11 h is inadequate for doxycycline.

(c) the particular iron preparation used: with tetracycline the reduc-

tion in serum levels with ferrous sulphate was 80 to 90%, with ferrous fumarate, succinate and gluconate, 70 to 80%; with ferrous tartrate, 50%; and with ferrous sodium edetate, 30%. This was with doses containing equivalent amounts of elemental iron.[10]

The interaction can therefore be accommodated by separating the dosages as much as possible, avoiding the use of doxycycline, and choosing one of the iron preparations causing minimal interference.

One suggestion is a schedule in which 500 mg tetracycline is given 30 to 60 min before breakfast and dinner (total daily dose 1 g), and 50 mg Fe^{2+} 1 h before lunch and 2 to 4 h after dinner.[7] This provides the patient with bacteriostatic tetracycline serum concentrations and a daily iron absorption of 25 mg, sufficient to allow optimal haemoglobin regeneration.

Only tetracycline, oxytetracycline, methacycline, minocycline and doxycycline have been shown to interact with iron, but it seems reasonable to expect that the others will behave in a similar way.

1. Neuvonen PJ, Gothoni G, Hackman R, Björksten K. Interference of iron with the absorption of tetracyclines in man. *BMJ* (1970) 4, 532–4.
2. Leyden JJ. Absorption of minocycline hydrochloride and tetracycline hydrochloride. Effect of food, milk, and iron. *J Am Acad Dermatol* (1985) 12, 308–12.
3. Mattila MJ, Neuvonen PJ, Gothoni G, Hackman CR. Interference of iron preparations and milk with the absorption of tetracyclines. Excerpta Medica Int Congr Series No. 254 (1972). Toxicological problems of drug combinations, 128–33.
4. Gothoni G, Neuvonen PJ, Mattila M, Hackman R. Iron-tetracycline interaction: effect of time interval between the drugs. *Acta Med Scand* (1972) 191, 409–11.
5. Neuvonen PJ, Penttilä O. Effect of oral ferrous sulphate on the half-life of doxycycline in man. *Eur J Clin Pharmacol* (1974) 7, 361–3.
6. Heinrich HC, Oppitz KH, Gabbe EE. Hemmung der Eisenabsorption beim Menschen durch Tetracyclin. *Klin Wochenschr* (1974) 52, 493–8.
7. Heinrich HC, Oppitz KH. Tetracycline inhibits iron absorption in man. *Naturwissenschaften* (1973) 60, 524–5.
8. Albert A, Rees CW. Avidity of the tetracyclines for the cations of metals. *Nature* (1956) 177, 433–4.
9. Albert A, Rees C. Incompatibility of aluminium hydroxide and certain antibiotics. *BMJ* (1955) 2, 1027–8.
10. Neuvonen PJ, Turakka H. Inhibitory effect of various iron salts on the absorption of tetracycline in man. *Eur J Clin Pharmacol* (1974) 7, 357–60.

Tetracyclines + Kaolin-pectin

Kaolin-pectin reduces the absorption of tetracycline.

Clinical evidence, mechanism, importance and management

Healthy subjects were given 250 mg **tetracycline hydrochloride** as a solution or as a capsule, with and without 30 ml **kaolin-pectin** (*Kaopectate*). The absorption of both formulations was reduced by about 50% by the **kaolin-pectin**. Even when the **kaolin-pectin** was given 2 h before or after the **tetracycline**, the drug absorption was still reduced by about 20%.[1] A likely reason is that **tetracycline** becomes adsorbed onto the **kaolin-pectin** so that less is available for absorption.

If these two drugs are given together, consider separating the dosages more than 2 h to minimise admixture in the gut. It may even then be necessary to increase the **tetracycline** dosage. Information about other **tetracyclines** is lacking, but be alert for them to interact similarly.

1. Gouda MW. Effect of an antidiarrhoeal mixture on the bioavailability of tetracycline. *Int J Pharmaceutics* (1993) 89, 75–7.

Tetracyclines + Metoclopramide

20 mg metoclopramide were found to double the rate of absorption of tetracycline in four convalescent patients and slightly to reduce the maximum serum levels following a sin-
gle 500 mg dose.[1] This appears to be of little clinical importance.

1. Nimmo J. The influence of metoclopramide on drug absorption. *Postgrad Med J* (1973) 49 (July Suppl), 25–8.

Tetracyclines + Milk and Dairy products

The absorption of the tetracyclines can be markedly reduced (up to 70 to 80%) if they are allowed to come into contact with milk or other dairy products. As a result their therapeutic effects may be diminished or even abolished. Doxycycline and minocycline are less affected (25 to 30% reduction).

Clinical evidence

The **demeclocycline** serum levels were 70 to 80% lower when 300-mg doses were taken with dairy products than those in 4 subjects given the same amount of antibacterial but with a meal containing no dairy products. The dairy products used were either 8 oz (about 250 ml) of **fresh pasteurized milk**, 8 oz **buttermilk** or 4 oz **cottage cheese**, each given to 4 healthy subjects.[1] In another study a 50% reduction was seen in subjects given tetracycline (500 mg), **methacycline** or **oxytetracycline** with 300 ml of **milk**. Doxycycline was not affected.[2,3]

A 20% reduction in serum **doxycycline** levels (from 1.79 to 1.45 micrograms/ml) was found 2 h after a single 100 mg oral dose with 240 ml **milk**.[4] Another study in 9 healthy subjects found a 30% reduction in the absorption, and a 24% reduction in peak serum levels of 200 mg **doxycycline** when taken with 300 ml **fresh milk**.[5] About 180 ml (6 oz) **homogenised milk** reduced the absorption of 100 mg **minocycline** by 27% and 250 mg **tetracycline hydrochloride** by 65%.[6]

Mechanism

The tetracyclines have a strong affinity for the calcium ions which are found in abundance in milk and dairy products. The tetracycline/calcium chelates formed are much less readily absorbed from the gastrointestinal tract and as a result the serum levels achieved are much lower. Some tetracyclines have a lesser tendency to form chelates, which explains why their serum levels are reduced to a smaller extent than other tetracyclines.[7]

Importance and management

Well documented and very well established interactions of clinical importance. Reductions in serum tetracycline levels of 50 to 80% are so large that their antibacterial effects may become minimal or even nil. For this reason tetracyclines should not be taken with milk or dairy products such as yoghurt or cheese. Separate the ingestion of these foods and the administration of the tetracycline as much as possible. In the case of iron, which interacts by the same mechanism, 2 to 3 h is enough. The small amounts of milk in coffee appear not to matter[8], and this is probably true for tea as well. Doxycycline[5,9] and minocycline[6] are not affected as much by dairy products (reductions of about 25 to 30%) and in this respect have some advantages over other tetracyclines.

1. Scheiner J, Altemeier WA. Experimental study of factors inhibiting absorption and effective therapeutic levels of declomycin. *Surg Gynecol Obstet* (1962) 114, 9–14.
2. Neuvonen P, Matilla M, Gothoni H, Hackman R. Interference of iron and milk with absorption of tetracycline. *Scand J Clin Lab Invest* (1971) 116 (Suppl 27), 76.
3. Matilla MJ, Neuvonen PJ, Gothoni G, Hackman CR. Interference of iron preparations and milk with the absorption of tetracyclines. *Excerpta Medica Int Congr Series* (1972) 254, 128–33.
4. Rosenblatt JE, Barrett JE, Brodie JL, Kirby WMM. Comparison of in vitro activity and clinical pharmacology of doxycycline with other tetracyclines. *Antimicrob Agents Chemother* (1966) 6, 134–41.
5. Meyer FP, Specht H, Quednow B, Walther H. Influence of milk on bioavailability of doxycycline — new aspects. *Infection* (1989) 17, 245–6.
6. Leyden JJ. Absorption of minocycline hydrochloride and tetracycline hydrochloride. Effect of food, milk, and iron. *J Am Acad Dermatol* (1985) 12, 308–12.
7. Albert A, Rees CW. Avidity of the tetracyclines for the cations of metals. *Nature* (1956) 177, 433–4.

8. Jung H, Rivera O, Reguero MT, Rodríguez JM, Moreno-Esparza R. Influence of liquids (coffee and orange juice) on the bioavailability of tetracycline. *Biopharm Drug Dispos* (1990) 11, 729–34.

9. Siewert M, Blume H, Stenzhorn G, Kieferndorf U, Lenhard G. Zur Qualitätsbeurteilung von doxycyclinhaltigen ertigarzneimitteln. 3. Mitteilung: Vergleichende Bioverfügbarkeitsstudie unter Berücksichtigung einer Einnahme mit Milch. *Pharm Ztg* (1990) 3, 96–102.

Tetracyclines + Phenothiazines

An isolated report describes black galactorrhoea in a woman treated with minocycline, perphenazine, amitriptyline and diphenhydramine.

Clinical evidence, mechanism, importance and management

A woman taking 100 mg **minocycline** twice daily for 4 years to control pustulocystic acne, and also taking **perphenazine**, **amitriptyline** and **diphenhydramine**, developed irregular darkly pigmented macules in the areas of acne scarring and later began to produce droplets of darkly coloured milk. The milk was found to contain macrophages filled with positive iron-staining particles and assumed to be haemosiderin. The situation resolved when the drugs were withdrawn, the galactorrhoea within a week and the skin staining over 6 months.[1] Galactorrhoea is a known side-effect of the phenothiazines and is due to an elevation of serum prolactin levels caused by the blockade of dopamine receptors in the hypothalamus. The dark colour appeared to be a side-effect of the **minocycline**, which can cause haemosiderin to be deposited in cells, and in this instance to be scavenged by the macrophages that were then secreted in the milk.

1. Basler RSW, Lynch PJ. Black galactorrhoea as a consequence of minocycline and phenothiazine therapy. *Arch Dermatol* (1985) 121, 417–18.

Tetracyclines + Quinapril

The absorption of oral tetracycline is reduced by the magnesium carbonate excipient in the Parke Davis quinapril formulation.

Clinical evidence

The Parke Davis formulation of **quinapril** (*Accupro*) also contains **magnesium carbonate** (250 mg in a 40 mg **quinapril** capsule, 47 mg in a 5 mg capsule). A pharmacokinetic study in 12 healthy subjects of the potential interaction between the **magnesium carbonate** in these capsules and **tetracycline hydrochloride** found that single doses of both of these formulations of **quinapril** markedly reduced the **tetracycline** absorption. The 5 mg and 40 mg **quinapril** capsules reduced the **tetracycline** AUC by 28% and 37% respectively, and the maximum serum levels were reduced by 25% and 34% respectively.[1]

Mechanism

The reason for these reductions is that the magnesium carbonate and the tetracycline form a less soluble chelate in the gut which is less well absorbed (see 'Tetracyclines + Antacids', p.223).

Importance and management

An established interaction but the extent of the reduction is only moderate and its clinical importance is uncertain. However, the authors of the study recommend that the concurrent use of this formulation of **quinapril** and **tetracycline** should be avoided.[1] This is repeated in the makers drug datasheet.[2] Other tetracyclines would be expected to behave similarly. One possible way to accommodate this interaction (as with the tetracycline/antacid interaction) is to separate the dosages as much as possible (by about 2 to 3 h) to minimise admixture in the gut.

1. Parke Davis Ltd. Effect of magnesium-containing quinapril tablets on the single-dose pharmacokinetics of tetracycline in healthy volunteers, protocol 906-237. Data on file, Report RR 764–00872.

2. Accupro (Quinapril). Parke Davis. Summary of product characteristics, October 1998.

Tetracyclines + Rifampicin (Rifampin)

Some patients ('poor metabolisers') show a marked fall in serum doxycycline levels if given rifampicin. Treatment failure may result.

Clinical evidence

Rifampicin 10 mg/kg daily caused a considerable reduction in the serum **doxycycline** levels of 7 patients who were taking 200 mg of **doxycycline** daily. The reduction was very marked in 4 patients but not significant in the other 3. A mean fall of 36% (from 14.18 to 9.11 h) occurred in the **doxycycline** half-life, a 106% increase in clearance and a reduction in the AUC of 54%.[1,2]

Five patients with brucellosis on 200 mg **doxycycline** daily showed a fall in the **doxycycline** half-life from 14.52 h to 7.99 h when treated with 200 mg **rifampicin** daily.[3] Another study of 20 patients treated for brucellosis found that serum **doxycycline** levels were lower when combined with **rifampicin** than with **streptomycin**, and the mean AUCs were also nearly 60% lower. There were no treatment failures in the **doxycycline/streptomycin** group, but 2 out of 10 occurred in the **doxycycline/rifampicin** group.[4] A meta-analysis of 6 trials involving 544 patients with brucellosis found significantly higher numbers of relapses and lower numbers of initial cures with **doxycycline/rifampicin** than with **doxycycline/streptomycin**.[5]

Mechanism

Not established, but it seems almost certain that the rifampicin (a known potent enzyme inducing agent) increases the metabolism of the doxycycline thereby increasing its loss from the body.

Importance and management

The doxycycline/rifampicin interaction is established and of clinical importance, but only (apparently) in those who are 'poor metabolisers' of doxycycline. Monitor the effects of concurrent use and increase the doxycycline dosage as necessary. The study cited above[1,2] revealed that before the rifampicin was given, the doxycycline half-life in those patients who were affected by this interaction was longer (17.8 h) than in the others (9.2 h). This would seem to be a way of identifying those patients ('poor metabolisers') who are likely to be at risk. No clinically important adverse interaction appears to occur between doxycycline and streptomycin.

1. Garraffo R, Dellamonica P, Fournier JP, Lapalus P, Bernard E, Beziau H, Chichmanian RM. Effet de la rifampicine sur la pharmacocinétique de la doxycycline. *Path Biol (Paris)* (1987) 35, 746–9.

2. Garraffo R, Dellamonica P, Fourniuer JP, Lapalus P, Bernard E. The effect of rifampicin on the pharmacokinetics of doxycycline. *Infection* (1988) 16, 297–8.

3. Bessard G, Stahl JP, Dubois F, Gaillat J, Micoud M. Modification de la pharmacocinétique de la doxycycline par l'administration de rifampicine chez l'homme. *Med Maladies Infect* (1983) 13, 138–41.

4. Colmenero JD, Fernández-Gallardo LC, Agúndez JAG, Sedeño J, Benítez J, Valverde E. Possible implications of doxycycline-rifampin interaction for the treatment of brucellosis. *Antimicrob Agents Chemother* (1994) 38, 2798–2802.

5. Solera J, Martínez-Alfaro J, Sáez L. Metaánalisis sobre la eficacia de la combinación de rifampicina y doxiciclina en el tratamiento de la brucelosis humana. *Med Clin (Barc)* (1994) 102, 731–8.

Tetracyclines + Sucralfate

On theoretical grounds the absorption of tetracycline may possibly be reduced by sucralfate, but clinical confirmation of this appears to be lacking.

Clinical evidence, mechanism, importance and management

The makers of sucralfate, point out in the summary of product characteristics that **sucralfate** reduces the bioavailability of **tetracycline**, probably because the two become bound together in the gut, thereby reducing absorption. The suggestion is made that they should therefore possibly be given 2 hours apart to minimise their admixture in the gut.[1] There do not appear to be any clinical reports in the literature confirming this interaction, nor and none were known to the maker Wyeth,[2] so that this potential interaction has yet to be shown to be clinically relevant.

1. Antepsin (Sucralfate). Chugai Pharma UK Limited. Summary of product characteristics, December 1998.
2. Wyeth. Personal Communication, 1995.

Tetracyclines + Thiomersal

Patients being treated with tetracyclines who use contact lens solutions containing thiomersal (thimerosal) may experience an inflammatory ocular reaction.

Clinical evidence, mechanism, importance and management

The observation that 2 patients had ocular reactions (red eye, irritation, blepharitis) when they used a 0.004% **thiomersal**-containing contact-lens solution while taking a **tetracycline**, prompted further study of this interaction. A questionnaire revealed 9 other cases that suddenly began shortly after starting to use a **tetracycline**, in patients who had used **thiomersal** containing solutions for 6 months without problem. In each case the reaction cleared when the **thiomersal** or the **tetracycline** was stopped. The same reaction was also clearly demonstrated in *rabbits*.[1] The reasons are not understood. It would seem prudent to avoid the concurrent use of these compounds.

1. Crook TG, Freeman JJ. Reactions induced by the concurrent use of thimerosal and tetracycline. *Am J Optom Physiol Opt* (1983) 60, 759–61.

Tetracyclines + Zinc sulphate

The absorption of tetracycline can be reduced by as much as 50% if zinc sulphate is taken concurrently. Separating their administration as much as possible minimises the effects of this interaction. Doxycycline interacts minimally with zinc.

Clinical evidence

Tetracycline 500 mg was given to 7 subjects either alone or with **zinc sulphate** (200 mg containing 45 mg Zn^{2+}). The **tetracycline** serum concentrations were reduced by 30 to 40% by the presence of the **zinc**, and the **tetracycline** AUC was similarly reduced.[1] This study was repeated with **doxycycline** 200 mg. **Doxycycline** absorption was not affected by **zinc**.[1] A more than 50% reduction in **tetracycline** absorption has been seen in other studies when **zinc** was given concurrently.[2,3]

The reduction in serum **zinc** concentrations, on concurrent use with **tetracycline** was found to be minimal.[2]

Mechanism

Zinc (like iron, calcium, magnesium and aluminium) forms a relatively stable and poorly absorbed chelate with tetracycline within the gut which results in a reduction in the amount of antibacterial available for absorption.[4,5]

Importance and management

An established and moderately well documented interaction of clinical importance. Separate the administration of tetracycline and zinc sulphate as much as possible to minimise admixture in the gut. In the case of iron, which interacts by the same mechanism, 2 to 3 h is enough.[6] An alternative is to use doxycycline.[1] Other tetracyclines would be expected to interact like tetracycline itself, but this needs confirmation. The small reduction in serum zinc concentrations is likely to be of little practical importance.[2]

1. Penttilä O, Hurme H, Neuvonen PJ. Effect of zinc sulphate on the absorption of tetracycline and doxycycline in man. *Eur J Clin Pharmacol* (1975) 9, 131–4.
2. Andersson K-E, Bratt L, Dencker H, Kamme C, Lanner E. Inhibition of tetracycline absorption by zinc. *Eur J Clin Pharmacol* (1976) 10, 59–62.
3. Mapp RK, McCarthy TJ. The effect of zinc sulphate and of bicitropeptide on tetracycline absorption. *S Afr Med J* (1976) 50, 1829–30.
4. Albert A, Rees CW. Avidity of the tetracyclines for the cations of metals. *Nature* (1956) 177, 433–4.
5. Doluisio JT, Martin AN. Metal complexation of the tetracycline hydrochlorides. *J Med Chem* (1963) 16, 16.
6. Gothoni G, Neuvonen PJ, Mattila M, Hackman R. Iron-tetracycline interaction: effect of time interval between the drugs. *Acta Med Scand* (1972) 191, 409–11.

Tiliquinol + Tilbroquinol

A single case report describes acute hepatitis attributed to an interaction between tiliquinol and tilbroquinol.

Clinical evidence, mechanism, importance and management

A single case report describes acute hepatitis attributed to an interaction between **tiliquinol** and **tilbroquinol**. A 54-year-old woman being treated for amoebic dysentery with *Intétrix* (200 mg **tiliquinol** plus 800 mg **tilbroquinol**) developed acute hepatitis after 4 days treatment. Before starting *Intétrix* her liver function tests had been normal. The *Intétrix* was discontinued and the patient rapidly improved, regaining normal liver function tests over 3 weeks. Hepatitis was confirmed by biopsy, and infective causes were ruled out.[1] The general importance of this incident is unknown.

1. Caroli-Bosc F-X, Chichmanian R-M, Caumes É, Saint-Paul M-C, Marty P, Demarquay J-F, Hastier P, Delmont J-P. Hépatite aiguë due à l'association de tiliquinol et tilbroquinol (Intétrix®). *Gastroenterol Clin Biol* (1996) 20, 605–6.

Tinidazole + Cimetidine

Cimetidine reduces the loss of tinidazole from the body. The clinical importance of this is uncertain.

Clinical evidence, mechanism, importance and management

After taking 400 mg **cimetidine** twice daily for 7 days the peak serum levels of tinidazole in 6 healthy subjects following a single 600-mg dose were raised by 21%, the 24 h AUC was increased by 40% and the half-life increased by 47% (from 7.66 to 11.23 h).[1] The probable reason is that the **cimetidine** inhibits the metabolism of the tinidazole by the liver, thereby reducing its loss from the body. Some small increase in both the therapeutic and the toxic effects of tinidazole may possibly occur, but the clinical importance of this is uncertain. It appears not to have been studied.

1. Patel RB, Shah GF, Raval JD, Gandhi TP, Gilbert RN. The effect of cimetidine and rifampicin on tinidazole kinetics in healthy human volunteers. *Indian Drugs* (1986) 23, 338–41.

Tinidazole + Rifampicin (Rifampin)

Rifampicin increases the loss of tinidazole from the body. The clinical importance of this is uncertain.

Clinical evidence, mechanism, importance and management

After taking 600 mg **rifampicin** daily for 7 days the peak serum levels of tinidazole in 6 healthy subjects following a single 600-mg dose were reduced by 22%, the 24 h AUC was reduced by 30% and the half-life reduced by 27% (from 7.66 to 5.6 h).[1] The probable reason is that the **rifampicin** increases the metabolism of the tinidazole by the liver, thereby increasing its loss from the body. Some small reduction in the therapeutic effects of tinidazole would be expected, but the clinical importance of this is uncertain. It appears not to have been studied.

1. Patel RB, Shah GF, Raval JD, Gandhi TP, Gilbert RN. The effect of cimetidine and rifampicin on tinidazole kinetics in healthy human volunteers. *Indian Drugs* (1986) 23, 338–41.

Trimethoprim + Antacids

Magnesium trisilicate and kaolin-pectin reduce the bioavailability of trimethoprim in *rats*, but the clinical importance of this in man is uncertain.

Clinical evidence, mechanism, importance and management

A study in *rats* showed that **magnesium trisilicate** and **kaolin-pectin** reduced the peak serum levels (at 1 h) of oral trimethoprim by about 50 and 30% respectively, and the AUC by 30 and 21%.[1] Whether this interaction affects the clinical effectiveness of trimethoprim in man has not been assessed, but the possibility should be borne in mind.

1. Babhair SA, Tariq M. Effect of magnesium trisilicate and kaolin-pectin on the bioavailability of trimethoprim. *Res Commun Chem Pathol Pharmacol* (1983) 40, 165–8.

Trimethoprim + Guar gum or Food

Guar gum and food can reduce the absorption of trimethoprim from a suspension.

Clinical evidence, mechanism, importance and management

A study over a 24-h period, in 12 healthy subjects given a single 3 mg/kg oral dose of a trimethoprim suspension, showed that the mean peak serum levels were depressed by 21% and 15% by **food** and **food with** 5 g **guar gum** respectively. **Food**, both with **guar gum** and alone reduced the AUC by about 22%.[1] The greatest individual reductions in peak serum levels and AUC were 44% and 36% with **food**, and 48% and 38% with **food + guar gum**.[1] The reasons are not understood but it may be due to adsorption of the trimethoprim onto the **food and guar gum**.

The clinical importance of this interaction is still uncertain but since a marked reduction in absorption can occur in some individuals it would seem sensible to take trimethoprim suspension between meals. Whether the same interaction occurs with other trimethoprim formulations is not known.

1. Hoppu K, Tuomisto J, Koskimies O and Simell O. Food and guar decrease absorption of trimethoprim. *Eur J Clin Pharmacol* (1987) 32, 427–9.

Typhoid vaccine (Oral, live) + Mefloquine

Mefloquine and oral attenuated live typhoid vaccine should not be given at the same time.

Clinical evidence, mechanism, importance and management

Mefloquine may attenuate immunisation with oral typhoid vaccine. As mefloquine is rapidly absorbed it has been suggested that by 8 h after a dose, the levels of **mefloquine** will be insufficient to inhibit live oral typhoid vaccine.[1] The makers of **mefloquine** say that immunisation with vaccines like oral typhoid should be completed at least 3 days before the first dose of **mefloquine**.[2] The British National Formulary seem to agree that the 3-day gap is preferable, but they also say that **mefloquine** could be given 12 hours before or after vaccination with oral typhoid vaccine.[3] This is in agreement with the UK Department of Health advice.[4] It would therefore seem advisable to separate administration by 3 days where possible, bearing in mind that a 12-hour gap may be sufficient in more urgent cases.

1. Cryz SJ. Post-marketing experience with live oral Ty21a vaccine. *Lancet* (1993) 341, 49–50.
2. Lariam (Mefloquine). Roche Products Limited. Summary of product characteristics, August 2000.
3. British National Formulary (2002) 43, 593.
4. HMSO. Immunisation Against Infectious Disease (1996) 247.

Vaccines + Ciclosporin

Ciclosporin reduces the ability of the body to develop immunity when given influenza vaccine.

Clinical evidence

(a) Influenza vaccine + Ciclosporin

A comparative study on 59 kidney transplant patients found that 21 patients on **ciclosporin** and prednisone had a significantly lower immune response to **influenza vaccine** (inactivated trivalent) than 38 patients on azathioprine and prednisone or 29 healthy subjects taking no drugs. All of the immune response measurements made (mean antibody levels, fourfold or greater titre rise, seroconversion to protective titres, the effects of booster immunization in those who responded poorly to the first vaccination) were reduced by 20 to 30% in those on **ciclosporin**.[1]

Confirmation of the practical importance of this is described in a case report of a heart transplant patient on **ciclosporin** who failed to respond to **influenza vaccination** while receiving **ciclosporin** and prednisone. He had two episodes of influenza, one serologically confirmed and it was later shown that vaccination had not resulted in seroconversion.[2]

(b) Other vaccines + Ciclosporin

Since the effectiveness of influenza vaccination is reduced by **ciclosporin** it seems logical to expect that **other vaccines** will be similarly affected. It has been suggested that because **ciclosporin** can induce tolerance to antigens, a situation where the patient becomes more (instead of less) susceptible to the infections against which one is trying to provide protection could develop.[3]

Mechanism

Immunosuppression by ciclosporin diminishes the ability of the body to respond immunologically both to transplants and to influenza vaccination.

Importance and management

An established and clinically important interaction. The effectiveness of influenza vaccination may be reduced or abolished if ciclosporin is being used. One suggestion is that if patients remain unprotected after a single vaccination and a booster dose also fails to be effective, **amantadine** 200 mg daily should be given during an influenza epidemic. It will protect against influenza A but not B infection.[2]

1. Versluis DJ, Beyer WEP, Masurel N, Wenting GJ, Weimar W. Impairment of the immune response to influenza vaccination in renal transplant recipients by cyclosporine, but not azathioprine. *Transplantation* (1986) 42, 376–9.

2. Beyer WEP, Diepersloot RJA, Masurel N, Simoons ML, Weimar W. Double failure of influenza vaccination in a heart transplant patient. *Transplantation* (1987) 43, 319.
3. Grabenstein JD, Baker JR. Comment: cyclosporine and vaccination. *Drug Intell Clin Pharm* (1985) 19, 679–80.

Valaciclovir + Antacids

Valaciclovir does not interact with an aluminium/magnesium hydroxide antacid.

Clinical evidence, mechanism, importance and management

On three separate occasions, 18 healthy subjects were given a single 1 g oral dose of valaciclovir either alone, 65 min before, or 30 min after taking 30 ml *Maalox* (**aluminium hydroxide**, **magnesium hydroxide**). The pharmacokinetics of the **aciclovir** (which is produced from valaciclovir in the body) remained unchanged. It was concluded that no special precautions are needed if these drugs are taken together, and the authors of the report also suggest that it is unlikely that **other antacids** will interact.[1]

1. de Bony F, Bidault R, Peck R, Posner J. Lack of interaction between valaciclovir, the L-valyl ester of acyclovir, and Maalox antacid. *J Antimicrob Chemother* (1996) 37, 383–7.

Valaciclovir + Thiazide diuretics

Hydrochlorothiazide does not interact adversely with valaciclovir.

Clinical evidence, mechanism, importance and management

A study in a group of elderly subjects (65 to 83 years old) given 500 or 1000 mg valaciclovir three times daily for 8 days found that its safety profile, whether taking **hydrochlorothiazide** or not, was similar to that in young healthy subjects.[1,2] The pharmacokinetics of the active metabolite **aciclovir** following valaciclovir were not significantly different.[2] There would seem to be no reason for avoiding concurrent use.

1. Wang LH, Schultz M, Weller S, Smiley ML, Blum MR. Pharmacokinetics and safety of valaciclovir, an acyclovir prodrug, in geriatric volunteers with and without concomitant diuretic therapy. *J Am Geriatr Soc* (1993) 41 (10 Suppl), SA23.
2. Wang LH, Schultz M, Weller S, Smiley ML, Blum MR. Pharmacokinetics and safety of multiple-dose valaciclovir in geriatric volunteers with and without concomitant diuretic therapy. *Antimicrob Agents Chemother* (1996) 40, 80–5.

Vancomycin + Colestyramine or Colestipol

Colestyramine when used to bind the cytotoxin produced by *Clostridium difficile* within the gut may also bind with vancomycin, thereby reducing its antibacterial efficacy. Colestipol binds to vancomycin much less strongly.

Clinical evidence, mechanism, importance and management

Both vancomycin and **colestyramine** have been used together to treat antimicrobial-associated colitis. The reasoning behind this combined treatment is that oral vancomycin is active against the organism (*Clostridium difficile*), which is associated with this condition, and **colestyramine** binds to the cytotoxin which the organism produces.[1] In theory this two-pronged attack sounds a good idea, but one of the problems is that the **colestyramine** also binds with the vancomycin within the gut, thereby reducing its biological activity (about tenfold according to *in vitro* studies). **Colestipol** binds much less strongly so that the vancomycin is released from it much more easily. What is not entirely clear is whether, because of this interaction, vancomycin alone is as effective as vancomycin plus **colestyramine**. To overcome this potential problem it has been suggested that a vancomycin dosage of 2 g daily should be used, and that the administration of the vancomycin and **colestyramine** should be separated as much as possible to minimise their admixture in the gut.[2] More study is needed to confirm that this is successful and to assess the implications for intravenous vancomycin.

1. Gotz VP, Rand KH. Medical management of antimicrobial-associated diarrhea and colitis. *Pharmacotherapy* (1982) 2, 100–9.
2. Taylor NS, Bartlett JG. Binding of *Clostridium difficile* cytotoxin and vancomycin by anion-exchange resins. *J Infect Dis* (1980) 141, 92–7.

Vancomycin + Dobutamine, Dopamine, Furosemide

There is evidence from a study in patients in intensive care following cardiac surgery that dobutamine, dopamine and furosemide can markedly reduce vancomycin serum levels.

Clinical evidence, mechanism, importance and management

A retrospective evaluation of the records of 18 critically ill patients in intensive care units following cardiac surgery, suggested that drugs with important haemodynamic effects (**dopamine**, **dobutamine**, **furosemide**) may lower the serum levels of vancomycin. It was noted that withdrawal of the interacting drugs was followed by a substantial increase (50%) in the minimum steady-state serum levels of vancomycin (13.3 mg/l compared with 8.79 mg/l), despite no major changes in body weight or estimated renal clearance. This resulted in a mean dose reduction of 4.26 mg/kg/day. The suggested reason for this interaction is that by increasing cardiac output these drugs can increase the renal clearance of vancomycin, thereby reducing its serum levels.[1] The clinical implication is that in this particular situation creatinine clearance is a less good predictor of vancomycin clearance and consequently dose. Good therapeutic drug monitoring is needed to ensure that serum vancomycin levels are optimal and not subtherapeutic. More confirmatory study is needed.

1. Pea F, Porreca L, Baraldo M, Furlanut M. High vancomycin dosage regimens required by intensive care unit patients cotreated with drugs to improve haemodynamics following cardiac surgical procedures. *J Antimicrob Chemother* (2000) 45, 329–35.

Vancomycin + Indometacin (Indomethacin)

Indometacin reduces the loss of vancomycin from the body in premature babies.

Clinical evidence, mechanism, importance and management

The half-life of vancomycin (15 to 20 mg/kg iv given over 1 h) was found to be 24.6 h in 6 premature neonates with patent ductus arteriosus given **indometacin**, compared with only 7 h in 5 other premature neonates without patent ductus arteriosus and not given **indometacin**.[1] The reason is uncertain but it seems possible that the **indometacin** reduces the clearance of the vancomycin (and other drugs) by the kidneys. The authors of this report suggest that the usual vancomycin maintenance dosage should be halved if **indometacin** is also being used. It is not known whether **indometacin** has the same effect on vancomycin in adult patients.

1. Spivey JM, Gal P. Vancomycin pharmacokinetics in neonates. *Am J Dis Child* (1986) 140, 859.

Vancomycin + Nephrotoxic and Ototoxic drugs

The risk of nephrotoxicity and ototoxicity with vancomycin may possibly be increased if given with other drugs with similar toxic effects.

Clinical evidence, mechanism, importance and management

Vancomycin is both potentially nephrotoxic and ototoxic, and its makers therefore suggest that it should be used with particular care or avoided in patients with renal impairment or deafness.[1] They also advise the avoidance of other drugs which are nephrotoxic and which might therefore be additive. They list **amphotericin B**, **aminoglycosides**, **bacitracin**, **polymyxin B**, **colistin**, **viomycin** and **cisplatin**. They also list **etacrynic acid** and **furosemide (frusemide)** as potentially aggravating ototoxicity. The monograph 'Aminoglycosides + Vancomycin', p.134 in this chapter outlines some of the evidence that additive nephrotoxicity can occur with the **aminoglycosides**, but there seems to be no direct evidence about the other drugs. Even so, the general warning issued by the makers to monitor carefully is a reasonable precaution.

1. Vancomycin. Faulding Pharmaceuticals Plc. Summary of product characteristics, July 2000.

Vancomycin + Theophylline

Theophylline appears not to interact with vancomycin in infants.

Clinical evidence, mechanism, importance and management

Five low birth weight preterm infants with a mean gestational age of 25 weeks, weighing 1.1 kg and a mean age of 62 days, were treated with **theophylline** (serum levels of 6.6 mg/l) for apnoea of prematurity. It was found that the pharmacokinetics of vancomycin (20 mg/kg at 12 to 18 h intervals) given for suspected sepsis were unchanged by the presence of the **theophylline**, when compared with previously published reports about vancomycin in neonates.[1] There seems to be no other clinical reports about vancomycin with **theophylline**, and nothing to suggest that vancomycin has any effect on the serum levels of **theophylline**.

1. Ilagan NB, MacDonald JL, Liang K-C, Womack SJ. Vancomycin pharmacokinetics in low birth weight preterm neonates on therapeutic doses of theophylline. *Pediatr Res* (1996) 39, 74A.

Vidarabine + Allopurinol

There is evidence that if allopurinol and vidarabine (adenine arabinoside) are used concurrently the toxicity of vidarabine may be increased.

Clinical evidence

Two patients with chronic lymphocytic leukaemia treated with 300 mg **allopurinol** daily developed severe neurotoxicity (coarse rhythmic tremors of the extremities and facial muscles, and impaired mentation) 4 days after vidarabine was added for the treatment of viral infections.[1] A retrospective search to find other patients who had taken both drugs for 4 days revealed a total of 17 patients, 5 of whom had experienced adverse reactions including tremors, nausea, pain, itching and anaemia.[1]

Mechanism

Uncertain. One suggestion is that the allopurinol causes hypoxanthine arabinoside, the major metabolite of vidarabine, to accumulate by inhibiting xanthine oxidase. A study with *rat* liver cytosol showed that allopurinol greatly increased the half-life of this metabolite.[2]

Importance and management

Information seems to be limited to this study so that the general clinical importance of this possible interaction is uncertain, but it would be prudent to exercise particular care if these drugs are used together. More study is needed.

1. Friedman HM, Grasela T. Adenine arabinoside and allopurinolpossible adverse drug interaction. *N Engl J Med* (1981) 304, 423.
2. Drach JC, Rentea RG, Cowen ME. The metabolic degradation of 9-β-D-arabinofuranosyladenine (ara-A) *in vitro*. *Fedn Proc* (1973) 32, 777.

Zidovudine + Aciclovir or Famciclovir

Concurrent use normally appears to be uneventful, but an isolated report describes overwhelming fatigue in one patient when given zidovudine and iv aciclovir.

Clinical evidence

A study in 50 HIV+ men found no pharmacokinetic interaction between **zidovudine** 100 mg and **aciclovir** 200 or 400 mg, both 4-hourly, 5 times a day, and the combination was well tolerated over a 6-month period.[1] When 41 HIV+ patients on **zidovudine** were given **aciclovir**, no changes in the pharmacokinetics of the **zidovudine** occurred and the side-effects were unchanged.[2] In a group of AIDS patients on **zidovudine**, some of whom were also given **aciclovir**, no obvious problems developed that could be attributed to the use of the **aciclovir**.[3] In contrast, a man with herpes who had been treated with 250 mg **intravenous aciclovir** 8-hourly for 3 days, developed overwhelming fatigue and lethargy within about an hour of being given 200 mg **zidovudine**. This lessened slightly on changing to **oral aciclovir**, which was continued for 3 days, and resolved when the **aciclovir** was withdrawn. The symptoms developed again when **intravenous aciclovir** was given as a test.[4]

Only minimal changes in zidovudine pharmacokinetics were seen when 12 HIV+ patients stabilised on 400 to 1000 mg **zidovudine** daily were given a single dose of 500 mg **famciclovir**.[5]

Mechanism

The isolated case of fatigue is not understood.

Importance and management

The adverse interaction described with zidovudine and aciclovir appears to be rare. There would seem to be no reason for avoiding concurrent use.

1. Hollander H, Lifson AR, Maha M, Blum R, Rutherfod GW, Nusinoff-Lehrman S. Phase I study of low-dose zidovudine and acyclovir in asymptomatic human immunodeficiency virus seropositive individuals. *Am J Med* (1989) 87, 628–32.
2. Tartaglione TA, Collier AC, Opheim K, Gianola FG, Benedetti J, Corey L. Pharmacokinetic evaluations of low- and high-dose zidovudine plus high-dose acyclovir in patients with symptomatic human immunodeficiency virus infection. *Antimicrob Agents Chemother* (1991) 35, 2225–31.
3. Richman DD, Fischl MA, Grieco MH, Gottlieb MS, Volberding PA, Laskin OL, Leedom JM, Groopman JE, Mildvan D, Hirsch MS, Jackson GG, Durack DT, Nusinoff-Lehrman S and the AZT Collaborative Working Group. The toxicity of azidothymidine (AZT) in the treatment of patients with AIDS and AIDS-related complex. A double-blind, placebo-controlled trial. *N Engl J Med* (1987) 317, 192–7.
4. Bach MC. Possible drug interaction during therapy with azidothymidine and acyclovir for AIDS. *N Engl J Med* (1987) 316, 547.
5. Rousseau F, Scott S, Pratt S, Fowles S, Sparrow P, Lascoux C, Lehner V, Sereni D. Safe coadministration of famciclovir and zidovudine. *Intersci Conf Antimicrob Agents Chemother* (1994) 34, 83.

Zidovudine + Benzodiazepines

Oxazepam causes a modest increase in the bioavailability of zidovudine, and can increase the incidence of headaches. Lorazepam possibly behaves similarly.

Clinical evidence, mechanism, importance and management

A pharmacokinetic study in 6 HIV patients found that **oxazepam** did not significantly affect the bioavailability of zidovudine. All of them were sleepy and fatigued while taking **oxazepam**, and 5 of the 6 complained of headaches while taking both drugs, compared to only 1 of 6 while taking zidovudine only and none while taking **oxazepam** only. The authors of the report suggest that if headaches occur during concurrent use, the benzodiazepine should be stopped.[1] A previous *in vitro* study using human liver microsomes confirmed that **oxazepam** inhibits the metabolism of zidovudine to its glucuronide, and **lorazepam** behaves in the same way.[2] The same precautions suggested for **oxazepam** would therefore appear to apply to **lorazepam** as well.

1. Mole L, Israelski D, Bubp J, O'Hanley P, Merigan T, Blaschke T. Pharmacokinetics of zidovudine alone and in combination with oxazepam in HIV infected patients. *J Acquir Immune Defic Syndr* (1993) 6, 56–60.
2. Unadkat JD, Chien J. Lorazepam and oxazepam inhibit the metabolism of zidovudine (ZDV or azidothymidine) in an *in vitro* human liver microsomal system. *Pharm Res* (1988) 5 (Suppl), S177.

Zidovudine + Paracetamol (Acetaminophen)

Limited and unconfirmed evidence suggests that paracetamol possibly increases the bone marrow suppressant effects of zidovudine. A single case report describes severe liver toxicity.

Clinical evidence

A study of zidovudine use in 282 AIDS patients found that haematological abnormalities (anaemia, leucopenia, neutropenia) were very common indeed and 21% needed multiple red cell transfusions. Some of the patients also received **paracetamol**, which increased the haematological toxicity (neutropenia) by an unstated amount.[1] A patient on zidovudine and co-trimoxazole took 2g **paracetamol** over 24 h, then 1.3g **paracetamol** over the following 12 h. Within 2 days he developed severe hepatotoxicity, and as other causes were excluded the reaction was attributed to **paracetamol**.[2]

Short-term clinical studies using up to 650 mg **paracetamol** 4-hourly found that it had no clinically significant effects the pharmacokinetics of zidovudine[3-6] although in one case clearance was slightly increased.[7] An 8-month study in a single patient suggested that long-term concurrent use did not affect the pharmacokinetics of either drug. However, in this individual very rapid absorption and a high peak serum level of zidovudine were seen, so that for safety the zidovudine dosage was reduced to one third (100 mg 6-hourly instead of 200 mg 4-hourly).[8]

Mechanism

Not understood. Paracetamol does not increase the serum levels of zidovudine,[3-5,7] which might have provided an explanation for the apparent increased toxicity. One *in vitro* study found that paracetamol does not affect the glucuronidation of zidovudine[9] whereas another found that it did inhibit its metabolism to the glucuronide.[10]

Importance and management

There is very little hard evidence to go on at the moment, but it would clearly be prudent to monitor any patient taking both drugs for any evidence of bone marrow or liver toxicity. The short-term use of both drugs does not appear to alter the pharmacokinetics of either drug. More study is needed.

1. Richman DD, Fischl MA, Grieco MH, Gottlieb MS, Volberding PA, Laskin OL, Leedom JM, Groopman JE, Mildvan D, Hirsch MS, Jackson GG, Durack DT, Nusinoff-Lehrman S and the AZT Collaborative Working Group. The toxicity of azidothymidine (AZT) in the treatment of patients with AIDS and AIDS-related complex. A double-blind, placebo-controlled trial. *N Engl J Med* (1987) 317, 192–7.
2. Shriner K, Goetz MB. Severe hepatotoxicity in a patient receiving both acetaminophen and zidovudine. *Am J Med* (1992) 93, 94–6.
3. Steffe EM, King JH, Inciardi JF, Flynn NF, Goldstein E, Tonjes TS, Benet LZ. The effect of acetaminophen on zidovudine metabolism in HIV-infected patients. *J Acquir Immune Defic Syndr* (1990) 3, 691–4.
4. Ptachcinski J, Pazin G, Ho M. The effect of acetaminophen on the pharmacokinetics of zidovudine. *Pharmacotherapy* (1989) 9, 190.
5. Pazin GJ, Ptachcinski RJ, Sheehan M, Ho M. Interactive pharmacokinetics of zidovudine and acetaminophen. 5th International Conference on AIDS, Montreal, 1989. Abstract M.B.P.338.
6. Burger DM, Meenhorst PL, Underberg WJM, van der Heijde JF, Koks CHW, Beijnen JH. Short-term, combined use of paracetamol and zidovudine does not alter the pharmacokinetics of either drug. *Neth J Med* (1994) 44, 161–5.
7. Sattler FR, Ko R, Antoniskis D, Shields M, Cohen J, Nicoloff J, Leedom J, Koda R. Acetaminophen does not impair clearance of zidovudine. *Ann Intern Med* (1991) 114, 937–40.
8. Burger DM, Meenhorst PL, Koks CHW, Beijnen JH. Pharmacokinetics of zidovudine and acetaminophen in a patient on chronic acetaminophen therapy. *Ann Pharmacother* (1994) 28, 327–30.
9. Kamali F, Rawlins MD. Influence of probenecid and paracetamol (acetaminophen) on zidovudine glucuronidation in human liver *in vitro*. *Biopharm Drug Dispos* (1992) 13, 403–9.
10. Schumann L, Unadkat JD. Does acetaminophen potentiate the hematotoxicity of zidovudine (ZDV or AZT) by inhibition of its metabolism to the glucuronide? *Pharm Res* (1988) 5 (Suppl), S-177.

6

Anticoagulant drug interactions

The blood clotting process

When blood is shed or clotting is initiated in some other way, a complex cascade of biochemical reactions is set in motion which ends in the formation of a network or clot of insoluble protein threads enmeshing the blood cells. These threads are produced by the polymerization of the molecules of fibrinogen (a soluble protein present in the plasma) into threads of insoluble fibrin. The penultimate step in the chain of reactions requires the presence of an enzyme, thrombin, which is produced from its precursor prothrombin, already present in the plasma. Figure 6.1 is a highly simplified diagram to illustrate the final stages of this cascade of reactions.

Mode of action of the anticoagulants

The oral anticoagulants extend the time taken for blood to clot and, it is believed, also inhibit the pathological formation of blood clots within blood vessels by reducing the concentrations within the plasma of a number of components necessary for the cascade to proceed, namely factors VII, IX, X and II (prothrombin). The parts played by three of these four are not shown in the simplified diagram illustrated but they are essential for the production of the so-called 'thromboplastins'.

The synthesis of normal amounts of these four factors takes place within the liver with vitamin K as one of the essential ingredients, but, in the presence of an oral anticoagulant, the rate of synthesis of all four is retarded. One of the early theories to explain why this happens was based on the observed resemblance between the molecular shapes of vitamin K and the oral anticoagulants. It was suggested that the molecules were sufficiently similar for the anticoagulant actually to take part in the biochemical reactions by which all four are synthe-

sised, but sufficiently dissimilar to prevent the completion of these reactions. The term 'competitive antagonist' is used to describe this situation because vitamin K and the oral anticoagulants compete with one another to take part in the reactions, their relative concentrations being among the factors which determine the 'winner'. This theory is now known to be too simple, but the basic principle of a concentration competition between the two types of molecules remains perfectly valid. A reduction in the concentrations and activity of all four factors is embraced by the portmanteau term 'hypoprothrombinaemia'.

The therapeutic use of the oral anticoagulants

During anticoagulant therapy it is usual to depress the levels of the prothrombin and factors VII, IX and X to those which are believed to give protection against intravascular clotting, without running the risk of excessive depression which leads to bleeding. To achieve this each patient is individually titrated with doses of anticoagulant until the desired response is attained, a procedure which normally takes several days because the oral anticoagulants do not act directly on the blood clotting factors already in circulation, but on the rate of synthesis of new factors by the liver. The 'end point' of the titration is determined by one of a number of different but closely related laboratory *in vitro* tests which measure the extension in the time taken for the blood to clot (e.g. the so-called 'one-stage prothrombin time' or PT). The result of the test may be expressed, not in seconds, but as a ratio or a percentage of normal values. The normal plasma clotting time, using the Quick one-stage prothrombin time test, is about 12 s, an extension to about 24 to 30 s or so is usually regarded as adequate in anticoagulant therapy. Other tests include the thrombotest and the prothrombin-proconvertin (P-P) test.

The International Normalised Ratio (INR) was adopted by the WHO in 1982 to take into account the sensitivities of the different thromboplastins used in laboratories across the world, the formula for calculating the INR being as follows:

$$INR = \left(\frac{\text{patient's prothrombin time in seconds}}{\text{mean normal prothrombin time in seconds}} \right)^{ISI}$$

The WHO reference thromboplastin has an International Sensitivity Index (ISI) of 1.0, whereas other thromboplastins may have different sensitivities. The standard INR range for most clinical situations is 2 to 3, but for some patients who have had recurrent thromboses or heart prostheses the INR range may be 2.5 to 3.5 or even higher.

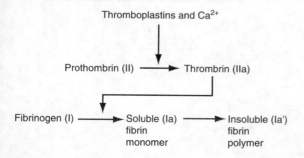

Fig. 6.1 A highly simplified flow diagram of the final stages of the blood clotting process.

Anticoagulant interactions

Therapeutically desirable prothrombin levels can be upset by a number of factors including diet, disease and the use of other drugs. In the case of drugs, either the addition or the withdrawal may upset the balance in a patient already well stabilised on the anticoagulant. Some drugs increase the activity of the anticoagulants and can cause bleeding if the dosage of the anticoagulant is not reduced appropriately. Others reduce the activity and return the prothrombin time to normal. If one believes in the therapeutic value of the oral anticoagulants, both situations are serious and may be fatal, although excessive hypoprothrombinaemia manifests itself more obviously and immediately as bleeding and is usually regarded as the more serious.

Bleeding and its treatment

When prothrombin times become excessive, bleeding can occur. In order of decreasing frequency the bleeding shows itself as ecchymoses, blood in the urine, uterine bleeding, black faeces, bruising, nose-bleeding, haematoma, gum bleeding, coughing and vomiting blood.

The British Society for Haematology has given advice on the appropriate course of action if bleeding occurs in patients taking anticoagulants, and this is readily available in summarised form in the British National Formulary.

This chapter is concerned with those drugs which affect the activity of the anticoagulants. When the anticoagulant is the affecting agent the interaction is dealt with elsewhere in this book. The Index should be consulted.

Table 6.1 Anticoagulants. Not all of the anticoagulants listed are mentioned in the text

Generic names	Proprietary names
Oral anticoagulants	
Coumarins	
Acenocoumarol (Nicoumalone)	*Mini-sintrom, Sinthrome, Sintrom*
Dic(o)umarol (Bishydroxycoumarin)	
Ethyl biscoumacetate	
Phenprocoumon	*Falithrom, Marcoumar, Marcumar, Marcuphen, Phenpro*
Tioclomarol	*Apegmone*
Warfarin potassium and sodium	*Aldocumar, Coumadin, Coumadine, Marevan, Orfarin, Varfine, Waran, Warfant, Warfilone*
Indanediones	
Anisindione	*Miradon*
Bromindione	
Diphenadione	
Phenindione	*Dindevan, Pindione*
Parenteral anticoagulants	
Heparin	*Ateroclar, Calcihep, Calciparin, Calciparina, Calciparine, Calcipor, Calparine, Canusal, Chemyparin, Clarisco, Croneparina, Demovarin, Depot-Thrombophob-N, Disebrin, Ecabil, Ecafast, Ecasolv, Emoklar, Eparical, Eparinlider, Eparinovis, Epsoclar, Essaven 60 000, Gelparine, Hemeran, Hemofluss, Hepacal, Hepaflex, HepaGel, Hepalean, Hepalean-Lok, Hepaplus, Hepathromb, Hepathrombin, Hepa-Gel, Hepa-Salbe, Hepflush, Heplok, Hepsal, Hep-Flush, Hep-Lock, Hep-Rinse, Inhepar, Isoclar, Lioton, Liquemin, Liquemin N, Liquemine, Menaven, Mica, Minihep, Monoparin, Multiparin, Normoparin, Nycoheparin, Perivar Venensalbe, Proparin, Pump-Hep, Reoflus, Sportino, Thrombareduct, Thrombophob, Thrombophob-S, Traumalitan, Trombofob, Trombolisin, Unihep, Uniparin, Venalitan, Venoruton Emulgel, Venoruton Heparin, Vetren, Zepac*
Dalteparin	*Boxol, Fragmin, Fragmine*
Enoxaparin	*Clexane, Decipar, Flunox, Klexane, Lovenox, Trombenox*
Lepirudin	*Refludan, Refludan , Refludin*
Tinzaparin	*Innohep*

Anticoagulants + ACE inhibitors

With the exception of a single, isolated and unexplained case of haemorrhage attributed to an acenocoumarol (nicoumalone)/fosinopril interaction, no other ACE-inhibitor has so far been shown to interact significantly with an oral anticoagulant.

Clinical evidence, mechanism, importance and management

Benazepril 20 mg daily has been found not affect the serum levels of either **warfarin** or **acenocoumarol (nicoumalone)**. The anticoagulant activity of **acenocoumarol** was not altered, but the effects of **warfarin** were slightly reduced, but not enough to be clinically important.[1] Cilazapril 2.5 mg daily for 3 weeks had no effect on the thrombotest times or coagulation factors II, VII and X in 28 patients on long-term **acenocoumarol** or **phenprocoumon** treatment.[2] Enalapril 20 mg for 5 days is reported not to have affected the anticoagulant effects of **warfarin** (2.5 to 7.5 mg daily).[3] Moexipril 15 mg daily for six days was found not to affect the pharmacokinetics or pharmacodynamics of 50 mg **warfarin**.[4] Ramipril 5 mg daily for 7 days in 8 subjects had no effect on the pharmacokinetics or anticoagulant effects of **phenprocoumon**.[5] Ramipril 5 mg daily for 3 weeks had no effect on the anticoagulant effects of **acenocoumarol** or **phenprocoumon** in groups of 10 subjects.[6] Temocapril 20 mg daily for 2 weeks had no effect on the pharmacokinetics of **warfarin** in 24 normal subjects.[7] The absence of a **warfarin/temocapril** interaction was confirmed in another study.[8] Trandolapril is also reported not to interact with **warfarin** (see Chapter 8).

Contrasting with all this evidence, there is a single, unexplained and isolated case of haemorrhage attributed to an interaction between **acenocoumarol** and **fosinopril**[9] but there seems to be no other evidence that **fosinopril** normally interacts with the oral anticoagulants.

No special precautions would therefore seem necessary if any of these anticoagulants and ACE-inhibitors are used concurrently (with the possible exception of **fosinopril**). There appears to be nothing documented about any of the other anticoagulants and ACE-inhibitors but it seems unlikely that a clinically relevant interaction will occur with any of them.

1. Van Hecken A, De Lepeleire I, Verbesselt R, Arnout J, Angehrn J, Youngberg C, De Schepper PJ. Effect of benazepril, a converting enzyme inhibitor, on plasma levels and activity of acenocoumarol and warfarin. *Int J Clin Pharmacol Res* (1988) 8, 315–19.
2. Boeijinga JK, Breimer DD, Kraaij CJ, Kleinbloesem CH. Absence of interaction between the ACE inhibitor cilazapril and coumarin derivatives in elderly patients on long term oral anticoagulants. *Br J Clin Pharmacol* (1992) 33, 553P.
3. Gomez HJ, Cirillo VJ, Irvin JD. Enalapril: a review of human pharmacology. *Drugs* (1985) 30 (Suppl 1), 13–24.
4. Van Hecken A, Verbesselt R, Depré M, Tjandramaga TB, Angehrn J, Cawello W, De Schepper PJ. Moexipril does not alter the pharmacokinetics of pharmacodynamics of warfarin. *Eur J Clin Pharmacol* (1993) 45, 291–3.
5. Verho M, Malerczyk V, Grötsch H, Zenbil I. Absence of interaction between ramipril, a new ACE-inhibitor, and phenprocoumon, an anticoagulant agent. *Pharmatherapeutica* (1989) 5, 392–9.
6. Boeijinga JK, Matroos AW, van Maarschalkerweerd MW, Jeletich-Bastiaanse A, Breimer DD. No interaction shown between ramipril and coumarine derivatives. *Curr Ther Res* (1988) 44, 902–8.
7. Siepmann M, Kirch W, Kleinbloesem CH. Non-interaction of temocapril, an ACE-inhibitor, with warfarin. *Clin Pharmacol Ther* (1996) 59, 214.
8. Lankhaar G, Eckenberger P, Ouwerkerk MJA, Dingemanse J. Pharmacokinetic-pharmacodynamic investigation of a possible interaction between steady-state temocapril and warfarin in healthy subjects. *Clin Drug Invest* (1999) 17, 399–405.
9. de Tomás ME, Sáez L, Beltrán S, Gato A. Probable interacción farmacológica entre fosinopril y acenocoumarol. *Med Clin (Barc)* (1997) 108, 757.

Anticoagulants + Acemetacin or Oxametacin

The anticoagulant effects of warfarin and acenocoumarol (nicoumalone) can be increased by the concurrent use of oxam-

etacin. An anticoagulant dosage reduction may be needed. Acemetacin does not interact with phenprocoumon.

Clinical evidence, mechanism, importance and management

Oxametacin (100 mg three times a day) for 14 days reduced the thrombotest percentages of 12 anticoagulated patients (11 on **warfarin** and one on **acenocoumarol (nicoumalone)**) from 11.2 to 7.8%. A third needed a reduction in their anticoagulant dosage or its withdrawal.[1] Concurrent use should be monitored, reducing the anticoagulant dosage if necessary. Apply the same precautions with any other anticoagulant but direct information is lacking. A study in 20 patients on **phenprocoumon** found no interaction with 60 mg **acemetacin** three times daily.[2]

1. Baele G, Rasquin K, Barbier F. Effects of oxametacin on coumarin anticoagulation and on platelet function in humans. *Arzneimittelforschung* (1983) 33, 149–52.
2. Hess H, Koeppen R. Kontrollierte Doppelblindestudie zur Frage von möglichen Interferenz von Acemetacin mit einer laufenden Antikoagulanzien-Therapie. *Arzneimittelforschung* (1980) 30, 1421–3.

Anticoagulants + Acitretin or Etretinate

A single case report describes reduced warfarin effects in a patient when given etretinate. Acitretin does not significantly alter the anticoagulant effects of phenprocoumon.

Clinical evidence

(a) Phenprocoumon + Acitretin

50 mg **acitretin** daily for 10 days slightly increased the prothrombin complex activity of 10 subjects on **phenprocoumon** (1.5 to 3.0 mg daily) from 22 to 24% (corresponding INRs of 2.91 and 2.71), but there were no important changes in Quick values.[1]

(b) Warfarin + Etretinate

A man with T-cell lymphoma who had recently had chemotherapy (cyclophosphamide, adriamycin, vincristine and prednisolone) was anticoagulated with **warfarin** after developing a pulmonary embolism. When he started 40 mg **etretinate** daily it was found necessary to increase his **warfarin** dosage from 7 to 10 mg daily. His liver function tests were normal.[2] This report is a little confused by the other drugs being taken concurrently (co-proxamol, tolbutamide, 8-methoxypsoralen, prednisone, brompheniramine, cimetidine), some of which can interact with **warfarin**.

Mechanism

Not understood.

Importance and management

Information appears to be limited to these reports. Monitor the concurrent use of warfarin and etretinate in any patient, increasing the anticoagulant dosage as necessary. Follow the same precautions with acitretin which is a metabolite of etretinate because of the possibility that it may interact similarly. No special precautions seem necessary if acitretin is given to patients on phenprocoumon but the outcome should be monitored. There seems to be no information about other anticoagulants.

1. Hartmann D, Mosberg H, Weber W. Lack of effect of acitretin on the hypoprothrombinemic action of phenprocoumon in healthy volunteers. *Dermatologica* (1989) 178, 33–6.
2. Ostlere LS, Langtry JAA, Jones S, Staughton RCD. Reduced therapeutic effect of warfarin caused by etretinate. *Br J Dermatol* (1991) 124, 505–10.

Anticoagulants + Alcohol

The effects of the oral anticoagulants are unlikely to be changed in those with normal liver function who drink small or moderate amounts of alcohol, but heavy drinkers or patients with some liver disease may show considerable fluctuations in their prothrombin times.

Clinical evidence

(a) Patients and subjects free from liver disease

20 oz (1 pint or 56.4 g ethanol) of a **Californian white table wine** daily given over a 3-week period at meal times to 8 normal subjects anticoagulated with **warfarin**, were found to have no significant effects on either the serum **warfarin** levels or the anticoagulant response.[1]

Other studies in both patients and normal subjects on either **warfarin** or **phenprocoumon** have very clearly confirmed the absence of an interaction with **alcohol**.[2-5] In one study the subjects were given almost 600 ml of a **table wine** (12% alcohol) or 300 ml of a **fortified wine** (20% alcohol).[4-6]

(b) Chronic alcoholics or those with liver disease

A study[7] in 15 alcoholics given a single dose of **warfarin** who had been drinking heavily (250 g ethanol or more daily) for at least 3 months, confirmed the results of a previous investigation that the half-life of **warfarin** was reduced from 40.1 to 26.5 h but, surprisingly, a comparison of their prothrombin times with those of normal subjects showed no differences.[8]

Other reports have shown that prothrombin times and **warfarin** levels of those with liver cirrhosis and other dysfunction can rise markedly after they have been on the binge, but restabilise soon afterwards when the drinking stops.[3,9]

Mechanism

It seems probable that in man, as in *rats*,[10] continuous heavy drinking stimulates the hepatic enzymes concerned with the metabolism of warfarin, leading to its more rapid elimination.[7] As a result the half-life shortens. The fluctuations in prothrombin times in those with liver dysfunction[3,9] may possibly occur because sudden large amounts of alcohol exacerbate the general malfunction of the liver and this affects the way it metabolises warfarin. It may also change the ability of the liver to synthesise the blood clotting factors.[11]

Importance and management

The absence of an alcohol/anticoagulant interaction in those free from liver disease is well documented and well established. It appears to be quite safe for patients on oral anticoagulants to drink small or moderate amounts of alcohol. Even much less conservative amounts (up to 8 oz/250 ml of spirits[2] or a pint of wine[1]) do not create problems with the anticoagulant control, so that there appears to be a good margin of safety even for the less than abstemious. Only warfarin and phenprocoumon have been investigated but other anticoagulants are expected to behave similarly. On the other hand those who drink heavily may possibly need above-average doses of the anticoagulant, while those with liver damage who continue to drink may experience marked fluctuations in their prothrombin times. This typically occurs in alcoholics after going on the binge over the weekend. An attempt to limit their intake of alcohol is desirable from this as well as from other points of view.

1. O'Reilly RA. Warfarin and wine. *Clin Res* (1978) 26, 145A.
2. Waris E. Effect of ethyl alcohol on some coagulation factors in man during anticoagulant therapy. *Ann Med Exp Biol Fenn* (1965) 115, 53.
3. Udall JA. Drug interference with warfarin therapy. *Clin Med* (1970) 77, 20–25.
4. O'Reilly RA. Lack of effect of mealtime wine on the hypoprothrombinemia of oral anticoagulants. *Am J Med Sci* (1979) 277, 189–94.
5. O'Reilly RA. Lack of effect of fortified wine ingested during fasting and anticoagulant therapy. *Arch Intern Med* (1981) 141, 458–9.
6. O'Reilly RA. Effect of wine during meals and fasting on the hypoprothrombinemia of oral anticoagulants. *Clin Pharmacol Ther* (1980) 27, 277.
7. Kater RMH, Roggin G, Tobon F, Zieve P, Iber FL. Increased rate of clearance of drugs from the circulation of alcoholics. *Am J Med Sci* (1969) 258, 35.
8. Kater RMH, Carruli N, Iber FL. Differences in the rate of ethanol metabolism in recently drinking alcoholic and nondrinking subjects. *Am J Clin Nutr* (1969) 22, 1608–17.
9. Breckenridge A, Orme M. Clinical implications of enzyme induction. *Ann N Y Acad Sci* (1971) 179, 421–31.
10. Rubin E, Hutterer F, Lieber CS. Ethanol increases hepatic smooth endoplasmic reticulum and drug metabolizing enzymes. *Science* (1968) 159, 1469–70.
11. Riedler G. Einfluß des Alkohols auf die Antikoagulantientherapie. *Thromb Diath Haemorrh* (1966) 16, 613–35.

Anticoagulants + Allopurinol

Most patients on oral anticoagulants given allopurinol do not develop an adverse interaction, but because excessive hypoprothrombinaemia and bleeding can occur quite unpredictably in a few individuals it is important to monitor the initial anticoagulant response in all patients.

Clinical evidence

An extensive multi-hospital study[1] of the adverse effects of **allopurinol** identified 3 patients who had developed excessive anticoagulation while concurrently taking **warfarin** and **allopurinol**. One of them developed extensive intrapulmonary haemorrhage and had a prothrombin time of 71 s.

A sharp increase in prothrombin times was seen in a very elderly woman on **warfarin** when given **allopurinol**.[2] Two patients on long-term treatment with **phenprocoumon** began to bleed when started on **allopurinol**.[3] A man on **warfarin** demonstrated a 42% increase in his prothrombin ratio after taking 100 mg **allopurinol** for 2 days.[4] Doses of 2.5 mg/kg **allopurinol** twice daily for 14 days increased the mean half-life of a single dose of **dicoumarol** in 6 normal subjects from 51 to 152 h,[5] whereas 3 other subjects showed an increase from only 13 to 17 h.[6] The disposition of **warfarin** remained unaltered.[6] No change was seen in the prothrombin ratios of 2 patients on **warfarin** who took **allopurinol** for 3 weeks,[7] whereas one out of 6 subjects taking **allopurinol** for a month demonstrated a 30% reduction in the elimination of **warfarin**.[7] There is another case report of an interaction.[8]

Mechanism

It has been suggested that, as in *rats*, allopurinol inhibits the metabolism of the anticoagulants by the liver, thereby prolonging their effects and half-lives.[4-6] There is a wide individual variability in the effects of allopurinol on drug metabolism in man,[7] so that only a few individuals are affected.

Importance and management

An established, clinically important but very uncommon interaction. Its incidence is not known precisely but it appears to be quite small. Since it is impossible to predict who is likely to be affected, monitor the prothrombin times of any patient on an anticoagulant when allopurinol is first added. The interaction has only been reported with warfarin, phenprocoumon and dicoumarol, but it would be prudent to apply the same precautions with any anticoagulant.

1. McInnes GT, Lawson DH, Jick H. Acute adverse reactions attributed to allopurinol in hospitalised patients. *Ann Rheum Dis* (1981) 40, 245–9.
2. Self TH, Evans WE, Ferguson T. Drug enhancement of warfarin activity. *Lancet* (1975) ii, 557–8.
3. Jähnchen E, Meinertz T, Gilfrich HJ. Interaction of allopurinol with phenprocoumon in man. *Klin Wochenschr* (1977) 55, 759–61.
4. Barry M, Feeley J. Allopurinol influences aminophenazone elimination. *Clin Pharmacokinet* (1990) 19, 167–9.
5. Vesell ES, Passananti GT, Greene FE. Impairment of drug metabolism in man by allopurinol and nortriptyline. *N Engl J Med* (1970) 283, 1484–8.
6. Pond SM, Graham GG, Wade DN, Sudlow G. The effect of allopurinol and clofibrate on the elimination of coumarin anticoagulants in man. *Aust N Z J Med* (1975) 5, 324–8.
7. Rawlins MD, Smith SE. Influence of allopurinol on drug metabolism in man. *Br J Pharmacol* (1973) 48, 693.
8. Weart CW. Coumarin and allopurinol. A drug interaction case report. 32nd Annual Meeting, American Society of Hospital Pharmacists (1975).

Anticoagulants + Aminoglutethimide

The anticoagulant effects of warfarin and acenocoumarol (nicoumalone) can be reduced by the concurrent use of

aminoglutethimide. **The extent of the reduction appears to be related to the aminoglutethimide dosage.**

Clinical evidence

A study in patients treated for breast cancer with **aminoglutethimide** and on **warfarin** found that a low dose **aminoglutethimide** regimen (125 mg twice daily) increased the clearance of **warfarin** by 41.2% whereas a high dose regimen (250 mg four times daily) increased the clearance by 90.8%. The effects of the interaction developed fully by 14 days. *(R)*-**warfarin** and *(S)*-**warfarin** were equally affected.[1]

Two patients needed a three to fourfold increase in **warfarin** dosage while taking 250 mg **aminoglutethimide** four times a day.[2] The increased requirement persisted for 2 weeks after the **aminoglutethimide** was stopped, and then declined. Brief mention of the need to take 'much larger doses' of **warfarin** while on **aminoglutethimide** is reported elsewhere.[3] Three patients on **acenocoumarol (nicoumalone)** needed a doubled dosage to maintain adequate anticoagulation while taking 250 mg **aminoglutethimide** four times daily for 3 to 4 weeks.[4]

Mechanism

Uncertain. The most likely explanation is that aminoglutethimide, like glutethimide, stimulates the activity of the liver enzymes concerned with the metabolism of the anticoagulants, thereby increasing their loss from the body. Some effect on blood steroid levels which might affect coagulation has also been suggested.[2]

Importance and management

An established and clinically important interaction. Monitor the effects of adding aminoglutethimide to patients already on warfarin or acenocoumarol (nicoumalone) and increase the anticoagulant dosage as necessary. Up to four times the dosage may be needed. The extent of the effects would appear to be related to the dosage of aminoglutethimide used. Reduce the anticoagulant dosage if aminoglutethimide is withdrawn. Information about other anticoagulants is lacking but it would be prudent to apply the same precautions with any of them.

1. Lønning PE, Ueland PM, Kvinnsland S. The influence of a graded dose schedule of aminoglutethimide on the disposition of the optical enantiomers of warfarin in patients with breast cancer. *Cancer Chemother Pharmacol* (1986) 17, 177–81.
2. Lønning PE, Kvinnsland S, Jahren G. Aminoglutethimide and warfarin. A new important drug interaction. *Cancer Chemother Pharmacol* (1984) 12, 10–12.
3. Murray RML, Pitt P, Jerums G. Medical adrenalectomy with aminoglutethimide in the management of advanced breast cancer. *Med J Aust* (1981) 1, 179–81.
4. Bruning PF, Bonfrer JGM. Aminoglutethimide and oral anticoagulant therapy. *Lancet* (1983) ii, 582.

Anticoagulants + Aminoglycoside antibacterials

If the intake of vitamin K is normal, either no interaction occurs or only a small and clinically unimportant increase in the effects of the oral anticoagulants takes place during concurrent treatment with neomycin, kanamycin or paromomycin. No interaction of any importance is likely with other aminoglycoside antibacterials administered parenterally.

Clinical evidence

Six out of 10 patients on **warfarin** who were given 2 g **neomycin** daily over a three-week period showed a gradual increase in their prothrombin times averaging 5.6 seconds.[1] The author of this report also describes another study on 10 patients taking **warfarin** given 4 g **neomycin** daily which produced essentially similar results.[2]

A small increase in the effects of an un-named anticoagulant was seen in 5 patients given **neomycin** with **bacitracin**, 3 patients on 1 g **streptomycin** daily, and 2 patients on 1 g **streptomycin** with 1 million units of **penicillin** daily.[3] No interaction was found in other long-term studies of **warfarin** with **neomycin**,[4,5] or **warfarin** or **dicoumarol** with **paromomycin**.[5]

Mechanism

Not understood. One idea is that these antibacterials increase the anticoagulant effects by decimating the bacterial population in the gut, thereby reducing their production of vitamin K. However this incorrectly supposes that the gut bacteria are normally an essential source of the vitamin.[5] Another suggestion is that these antibacterials decrease the vitamin K absorption as part of a general antibacterial-induced malabsorption syndrome.[6]

Importance and management

A sparsely documented interaction but common experience seems to confirm that normally no interaction of any significance occurs. Concurrent use need not be avoided. Occasionally vitamin K deficiency and/or spontaneous bleeding[7,8] is seen after the prolonged use of gut-sterilising antibacterials, a totally inadequate diet, starvation or some other condition in which the intake of vitamin K is very limited. Under these circumstances the effects of the oral anticoagulants would be expected to be significantly increased and appropriate precautions should be taken. Only warfarin and dicoumarol feature in the reports cited but it seems probable that the other anticoagulants will behave similarly. There is nothing to suggest that an adverse interaction occurs between the oral anticoagulants and aminoglycosides administered parenterally.

1. Udall JA. Drug interference with warfarin therapy. *Clin Med* (1970) 77, 20–25.
2. Udall JA. Human sources and absorption of vitamin K in relation to anticoagulation stability. *JAMA* (1965) 194, 107–9.
3. Magid E. Tolerance to anticoagulants during antibiotic therapy. *Scand J Clin Lab Invest* (1962) 14, 565–6.
4. Schade RWB, van't Laar A, Majoor CLH, Jansen AP. A comparative study of the effects of cholestyramine and neomycin in the treatment of type II hyperlipoproteinaemia. *Acta Med Scand* (1976) 199, 175–80.
5. Messinger WJ, Samet CM. The effect of bowel sterilizing antibiotic on blood coagulation mechanisms. The anti-cholesteric effect of paromomycin. *Angiology* (1965) 16, 29–36.
6. Faloon WW, Paes IC, Woolfolk D, Nankin H, Wallace K, Haro EN. Effect of neomycin and kanamycin upon intestinal absorption. *Ann N Y Acad Sci* (1966) 132, 879–87.
7. Haden HT. Vitamin K deficiency associated with prolonged antibiotic administration. *Arch Intern Med* (1957) 100, 986–8.
8. Frick PG, Riedler G, Brögli H. Dose response and minimal daily requirement for vitamin K in man. *J Appl Physiol* (1967) 23, 387–9.

Anticoagulants + Aminosalicylic acid (PAS) and/or Isoniazid

A report attributes a bleeding episode in a patient on warfarin to the concurrent use of isoniazid. Another report describes a markedly increased anticoagulant response in a patient when given aminosalicylic acid and isoniazid.

Clinical evidence

A man on **warfarin** and taking 300 mg **isoniazid** daily began to bleed (haematuria, bleeding gums, etc.) within 10 days of accidentally doubling his dosage of **isoniazid**. His prothrombin time had increased from 26.3 to 53.3 s.[1]

Another patient taking digoxin, potassium chloride, dioctyl calcium sulfosuccinate, diazepam and **warfarin**, was additionally given 12 g **aminosalicylic acid**, 300 mg **isoniazid** and 100 mg pyridoxine daily. His prothrombin time increased from 18 to 130 s over 20 days but no signs of haemorrhage were seen.[2] Two patients on **isoniazid, aminosalicylic acid** and **streptomycin** (but not taking anticoagulants) developed haemorrhage attributed to the anticoagulant effects of **isoniazid**.[3]

Mechanism

Not understood. The small depressant effect which aminosalicylic acid has on prothrombin formation in man is unlikely to have been responsible. Isoniazid can increase the anticoagulant effects of dicoumarol in *dogs*[4] but not of warfarin in *rabbits*.[5] In *dogs* the effect is thought to be due to inhibition by the isoniazid of the liver enzymes concerned with the metabolism of the anticoagulant, resulting in a slower clearance from the body.[4]

Importance and management

The interactions of warfarin with isoniazid and aminosalicylic acid are not established. Concurrent use need not be avoided, but prescribers should be aware of these cases and monitor the effects.

1. Rosenthal AR, Self TH, Baker ED, Linden RA. Interaction of isoniazid and warfarin. *JAMA* (1977) 238, 2177.
2. Self TH. Interaction of warfarin and aminosalicylic acid. *JAMA* (1973) 223, 1285.
3. Castell FA. Accion anticoagulante de la isoniazida. *Enfermedades de Torax* (1969) 69, 153–62.
4. Eade NR, McLeod PJ, MacLeod SM. Potentiation of bishydroxycoumarin in dogs by isoniazid and p-aminosalicylic acid. *Am Rev Respir Dis* (1971) 103, 792–9.
5. Kiblawi SS, Jay SJ, Bang NU, Rowe HM. Influence of isoniazid on the anticoagulant effect of warfarin. *Clin Ther* (1979) 2, 235–9.

Anticoagulants + Amiodarone

The anticoagulant effects of warfarin, phenprocoumon and acenocoumarol (nicoumalone) are increased by amiodarone and bleeding may occur if the dosage of the anticoagulant is not reduced appropriately. The onset of this interaction may be slow, and may persist long after the amiodarone has been withdrawn.

Clinical evidence

Five out of 9 patients who were well stabilised on **warfarin** showed signs of bleeding (4 had microscopic haematuria and one had diffuse ecchymoses) within 3 to 4 weeks of starting to take **amiodarone** (dosage not stated). All 9 showed increases in their prothrombin times averaging 21 s. It was necessary to decrease the **warfarin** dosage by an average of a third (range 16 to 45%) to return their prothrombin times to the therapeutic range. The effects of **amiodarone** persisted for 6 to 16 weeks in 4 of the patients from whom it was withdrawn.[1]

A prolongation in prothrombin times and/or bleeding has been described in other patients on **warfarin** given 200 to 800 mg **amiodarone** daily.[2-14] **Amiodarone** similarly interacts with **phenprocoumon**[15] and **acenocoumarol (nicoumalone)**.[16-21]

Mechanism

Experimental evidence suggests that amiodarone inhibits cytochrome P450 isoenzyme CYP2C9 (an enzyme concerned with the metabolism of (S)-warfarin) so that the loss of the anticoagulant from the body is decreased and its effects are thereby increased.[22]

Importance and management

A well documented, established and clinically important interaction. It appears to occur in most patients.[1,5,11,23] The dosage of warfarin and phenprocoumon should be reduced by one-third to two-thirds[1,8,11,15,24] if amiodarone is added to established anticoagulant treatment. One report suggests an average 35% warfarin reduction in a 70 kg patient on 200 mg amiodarone daily, 50% if on 400 mg and 65% if on 600 mg and above.[8] Another suggests slightly smaller reductions: a 21% in warfarin dosage if on 100 mg amiodarone daily, 26% if on 200 mg, 30% if on 300 mg and 35% if on 400 mg.[25] The dosage of acenocoumarol (nicoumalone) should be reduced by between one-third to one-half.[12,16,21] Some of these suggested reductions are very broad generalizations and individual patients may need more or less.[26] The interaction begins to develop within 2 weeks and may persist for many weeks after the withdrawal of the amiodarone because up to one-third of the amiodarone may still be present a month after treatment has ceased.[27] Prothrombin Times should be very closely monitored both during and following treatment. One study advises weekly monitoring for the first 4 weeks,[11] the importance of which was underlined by a case report of a patient who bled more than 2 weeks after it was thought that stability had been

achieved.[13] It would seem prudent to assume that other anticoagulants interact similarly, but so far there is no direct evidence that they do so.

1. Martinowitz U, Rabinovici J, Goldfarb D, Many A, Bank H. Interaction between warfarin sodium and amiodarone. *N Engl J Med* (1981) 304, 671–2.
2. Rees A, Dalal JJ, Reid PG, Henderson AH, Lewis MJ. Dangers of amiodarone and anticoagulant treatment. *BMJ* (1981) 282, 1756–7.
3. Serlin MJ, Sibeon RG, Green GJ. Dangers of amiodarone and anticoagulant treatment. *BMJ* (1981) 283, 58.
4. Simpson WT. A review of the therapeutic results and unwanted effects of amiodarone. In 'Amiodarone in Cardiac Arrhythmias'. Simpson WT and Caldwell ADS (eds). Roy Soc Med Int Congr Ser 16. Royal Society of Medicine/Academic Press/Grune and Stratton, London (1979) p. 45–52.
5. Hamer A, Peter T, Mandel WJ, Scheinman MM, Weiss D. The potentiation of warfarin anticoagulation by amiodarone. *Circulation* (1982) 65, 1025–29.
6. Ugovern B, Garan H, Kelly E, Ruskin JN. Adverse reactions during treatment with amiodarone. *BMJ* (1983) 287. 175–80.
7. Raeder EA, Podrid PJ, Lown B. Side effects and complications of amiodarone therapy. *Am Heart J* (1985) 109, 975–83.
8. Almog S, Shafran N, Halkin H, Weiss P, Farfel Z, Martinowitz U, Bank H. Mechanism of warfarin potentiation by amiodarone: dose- and concentration-dependent inhibition of warfarin elimination. *Eur J Clin Pharmacol* (1985) 28, 257–261.
9. Watt AH, Stephens MR, Buss DC, Routledge PA. Amiodarone reduces plasma warfarin clearance in man. *Br J Clin Pharmacol* (1985) 20, 707–9.
10. O'Reilly RA, Trager WF, Rettie AE, Goulart DA. Interaction of amiodarone with racemic warfarin and its separate enantiomorphs in humans. *Clin Pharmacol Ther* (1987) 42, 290–4.
11. Kerin NZ, Blevins RD, Goldman L, Faitel K, Rubenfire M. The incidence, magnitude, and time course of the amiodarone-warfarin interaction. *Arch Intern Med* (1988) 148, 1779–81.
12. Caraco Y, Chajek-Shaul T. The incidence and clinical significance of amiodarone and acenocoumarol interaction. *Thromb Haemost* (1989) 62, 906–8.
13. Cheung B, Lam FM, Kumana CR. Insidiously evolving, occult drug interaction involving warfarin and amiodarone. *BMJ* (1996) 312, 107–8.
14. Chan TYK. Drug interactions as a cause of overanticoagulation and bleedings in Chinese patients receiving warfarin. *Int J Clin Pharmacol Ther* (1998) 36, 403–5.
15. Broekmans AW, Meyboom RHB. Bijwerkingen van geneesmiddelen. Potentiëring van het cumarine-effect door amiodaron (Cordarone). *Ned Tijdschr Geneeskd* (1982) 126, 1415–17.
16. Arboix M, Frati ME, Laporte J-R. The potentiation of acenocoumarol anticoagulant effect by amiodarone. *Br J Clin Pharmacol* (1984) 18, 355–60.
17. El Allaf D, Sprynger M, Carlier J. Potentiation of the action of oral anticoagulants by amiodarone. *Acta Clin Belg* (1984) 39, 306–8.
18. Richard C, Riou B, Fournier C, Rimailho A, Auzepy P. Depression of vitamin K-dependent coagulation by amiodarone. *Circulation* (1983) 68 (Suppl III), 278.
19. Richard C, Riou B, Berdeaux A, Forunier C, Khayat D, Rimailho A, Giudicelli JF, Auzépy P. Prospective study of the potentiation of acenocoumarol by amiodarone. *Eur J Clin Pharmacol* (1985) 28, 625–9.
20. Pini M, Manotti C, Quintavalla R. Interaction between amiodarone and acenocoumarin. *Thromb Haemost* (1985) 54, 549.
21. Fondevila C, Meschengieser S, Lazzari MA. Amiodarone potentiates acenocoumarin. *Thromb Res* (1988) 53, 203–8.
22. Heimark LD, Wienkers L, Kunze K, Gibaldi M, Eddy AC, Trager WF, O'Reilly RA, Goulart DA. The mechanism of the interaction between amiodarone and warfarin in humans. *Clin Pharmacol Ther* (1992) 51, 398–407.
23. Kerin N, Blevins R, Goldman L, Faitel K, Rubenfire M. The amiodarone-warfarin interaction: incidence, time course and clinical significance. *J Am Coll Cardiol* (1986) 7, 91A.
24. Watt AH, Buss DC, Stephens MR, Routledge PA. Amiodarone reduced plasma warfarin clearance in man. *Br J Clin Pharmacol* (1985) 19, 591P.
25. Sanoski CA, Bauman JL. Long-term characterization of the amiodarone-warfarin drug interaction. *J Am Coll Cardiol* (1998) 31 (2 Suppl A), 507A–508A.
26. Fondevila C, Meschengieser S, Lazzari M. Amiodarone-acenocoumarin interaction. *Thromb Haemost* (1991) 65, 328.
27. Broekhuysen J, Laruel R, Sion R. Recherches dans la série des benzofurannes. XXXVII. Étude comparée du transit et du métabolisme de l'amiodarone chez diverses espèces animales et chez l'homme. *Arch Int Pharmacodyn Ther* (1969) 177, 340–59.

Anticoagulants + Anabolic steroids and related sex hormones

The anticoagulant effects of acenocoumarol (nicoumalone), bromindione, dicoumarol, phenindione, phenprocoumon and warfarin are markedly increased by the concurrent use of danazol, ethylestrenol (ethyloestrenol), oxymetholone, methandienone (methandrostenolone), methyltestosterone, norethandrolone and stanozolol. Bleeding may occur if the anticoagulant dosage is not reduced appropriately.

Clinical evidence

Six patients stabilised on **warfarin** or **phenindione** were started on 15 mg **oxymetholone** daily. One patient developed extensive subcutaneous bleeding and another had haematuria. After 30 days on **oxymetholone** all 6 patients had thrombotests of less than 5% which returned to the therapeutic range within a few days of its withdrawal.[1]

Similarly increased anticoagulant effects and bleeding have been described in studies and case reports involving **warfarin** with **danazol**,[2-5] **oxymetholone**,[6-8] **methandienone**[6,9-11] or **stanozolol**;[12-15] **dicoumarol** with **norethandrolone**[6] or **stanozolol**;[16] **bromindione** with **methandienone**;[6,9] **phenindione** with **ethylestrenol (ethyloestrenol)**;[17] **phenprocoumon** with **methyltestosterone**;[18] and **acenocoumarol (nicoumalone)** with **oxymetholone**.[19]

One report[8] says that 3 patients on **warfarin** given *Sustanon* (containing four combined esters of **testosterone**) developed no changes in their anticoagulant requirements, whereas another report[20] describes a woman who showed a 78% and a 65% increase in prothrombin times on two occasions when using a 2% **testosterone propionate** vaginal ointment twice daily. A 25% reduction in **warfarin** dosage was needed.

Mechanism

Not understood. Various theories have been put forward including increased metabolic destruction of the blood clotting factors, or decreased synthesis;[9,21] reduced levels of plasma triglycerides which might reduce vitamin-K availability (though this is disputed);[6,10] and increased concentrations of the anticoagulant at the receptor site or increased receptor affinity.

Importance and management

Well documented, well established and clinically important interactions which develop rapidly, possibly within 2 to 3 days. Most, if not all, patients are affected.[1,21] If concurrent use cannot be avoided, the dosage of the anticoagulant should be appropriately reduced. One recommendation is that the initial dosage of danazol[3] should be halved. One-third to one-half of the dosage of acenocoumarol (nicoumalone) was needed in one patient given oxymetholone,[19] however the size of the reduction with other steroids is uncertain. After withdrawal of the steroid the anticoagulant dosage will need to be increased. It seems probable that all the anticoagulants will interact with any 17-alkyl substituted steroid such as fluoxymesterone and oxandrolone, but as yet there is no direct evidence that they do so. The situation with testosterone and other non 17-alkylated steroids is not clear (see cases cited above).[8,20]

1. Longridge RGM, Gillam PMS, Barton GMG. Decreased anticoagulant tolerance with oxymetholone. *Lancet* (1971) ii, 90.
2. Goulbourne IA, MacLeod DAD. An interaction between danazol and warfarin. Case report. *Br J Obstet Gynaecol* (1981) 88, 950–1.
3. Small M, Peterkin M, Lowe GDO, McCune G, Thomson JA. Danazol and oral anticoagulants. *Scott Med J* (1982) 27, 331–2.
4. Meeks ML, Mahaffey KW, Katz MD. Danazol increases the anticoagulant effect of warfarin. *Ann Pharmacother* (1992) 26, 641–2.
5. Booth CD. A drug interaction between danazol and warfarin. *Pharm J* (1993) 250, 439.
6. Murakami M, Odake K, Matsuda T, Onchi K, Umeda T, Nishino T. Effects of anabolic steroids on anticoagulant requirements. *Jpn Circ J* (1965) 29, 243–50.
7. Robinson BHB, Hawkins JB, Ellis JE, Moore-Robinson M. Decreased anticoagulant tolerance with oxymetholone. *Lancet* (1971) i, 1356.
8. Edwards MS, Curtis JR. Decreased anticoagulant tolerance with oxymetholone. *Lancet* (1971) ii, 221.
9. Pyörälä K, Kekki M. Decreased anticoagulant tolerance during methandrostenolone therapy. *Scand J Clin Lab Invest* (1963) 15, 367–74.
10. Dresdale FC, Hayes JC. Potential dangers in the combined use of methandrostenolone and sodium warfarin. *J Med Soc New Jers* (1967) 64, 609–12.
11. McLaughlin GE, McCarty DJ, Segal BL. Hemarthrosis complicating anticoagulant therapy. A report of three cases. *JAMA* (1966) 196, 1020–1.
12. Acomb C, Shaw PW. A significant interaction between warfarin and stanozolol. *Pharm J* (1985) 234, 73–4.
13. Cleverly CR. Personal communication, March 1987.
14. Shaw PW, Smith AM. Possible interaction of warfarin and stanozolol. *Clin Pharm* (1987) 6, 500–2.
15. Elwin C-E, Törngren M. Samtidigt intag av warfarin och stanozolol orsak till blödningar hos patienten. *Lakartidningen* (1988) 85, 3290.
16. Howards CW, Hanson SG, Wahed MA. Anabolic steroids and anticoagulants. *BMJ* (1977) i, 1659.
17. Vere DW, Fearnley GR. Suspected interaction between phenindione and ethylœstrenol. *Lancet* (1968) ii, 281.
18. Husted S, Andreasen F, Foged L. Increased sensitivity to phenprocoumon during methyltestosterone therapy. *Eur J Clin Pharmacol* (1976) 10, 209–16.
19. de Oya JC, del Río A, Noya M, Villeneuva A. Decreased anticoagulant tolerance with oxymetholone in paroxysmal noctural hæmoglobinuria. *Lancet* (1971) ii, 259.
20. Lorentz SM, Weibert RT. Potentiation of warfarin anticoagulation by topical testosterone ointment. *Clin Pharm* (1985) 4, 332–4.
21. Schrogie JJ, Solomon HM. The anticoagulant response to bishydroxycoumarin. II. The effect of D-thyroxine, clofibrate, and norethandrolone. *Clin Pharmacol Ther* (1967) 8, 70–7.

Anticoagulants + Angiotensin II antagonists

Eprosartan, irbesartan and telmisartan do not interact to a clinically relevant extent with warfarin.

Clinical evidence, mechanism, importance and management

Eighteen normal subjects on **warfarin** with INRs between 1.3 and 1.6 showed no clinically relevant changes in anticoagulation when given 300 mg **eprosartan** twice daily.[1,2] Sixteen normal subjects were given 2.5 to 10 mg **warfarin** daily for 2 weeks, to which was added 300 mg **irbesartan** or a placebo daily for a further week. There was no evidence of any pharmacokinetic or pharmacodynamic interactions.[3,4] Twelve normal subjects stabilised on **warfarin** and with INRs between 1.2 and 1.8 were additionally given 120 mg **telmisartan** daily for 10 days. A small statistically significant decrease in the mean trough plasma **warfarin** concentrations occurred but the anticoagulation remained unchanged.[5,6]

There would therefore appear to be no reason for taking special precautions during the concurrent use of any of these angiotensin II receptor antagonists and **warfarin**. Information about other anticoagulants and other angiotensin II receptor antagonists seems to be lacking. See also 'Candesartan + Miscellaneous drugs', p.385, 'Losartan + Miscellaneous drugs', p.398 and 'Valsartan + Miscellaneous drugs', p.410.

1. Martin DE, Kazierad DJ, Ilson B, Zariffa N, Boike S, Jorasky D. Eprosartan (E), an angiotensin II antagonist, does not affect the anticoagulant activity of warfarin (W). *J Clin Pharmacol* (1996) 36, 849.
2. Kazierad DJ, Martin DE, ilson B, Boike S, Zariffa N, Forrest A, Jorasky DK. Eprosartan does not affect the pharmacodynamics of warfarin. *J Clin Pharmacol* (1998) 38, 649-53.
3. Gielsdorf W, Mangold B, Marion MR. Pharmacodynamics and pharmacokinetics of warfarin given with irbesartan. *Clin Pharmacol Ther* (1998) 63, 228.
4. Mangold B, Gielsdorf W, Marino MR. Irbesartan does not affect the steady-state pharmacodynamics and pharmacokinetics of warfarin. *Eur J Clin Pharmacol* (1999) 55, 593-8.
5. Su CAPF, van Lier JJ, Schwietert HR, Stangier J, Comelissen PJG, Jonkman JHG. Influence of telmisartan, a non-peptide angiotensin II (A II) receptor antagonist on steady state pharmacodynamics and pharmacokinetics of warfarin in healthy subjects. *Naunyn Schmiedebergs Arch Pharmacol* (1996) 353 (4 Suppl), R155.
6. Stangier J, Su C-APF, Hendricks MGC, van Lier JJ, Sollie FAE, Oosterhuis B, Jonkman JHG. Steady-state pharmacodyamics and pharmacokinetics of warfarin in the presence and absence of telmisartan in healthy male volunteers. *J Clin Pharmacol* (2000) 40, 1331-7.

Anticoagulants + Antacids

There is some evidence that the absorption of dicoumarol may be increased by magnesium hydroxide and warfarin by magnesium trisilicate, but there is no direct evidence that this is clinically important. Aluminium hydroxide does not interact with either warfarin or dicoumarol, and magnesium hydroxide does not interact with warfarin.

Clinical evidence

(a) Dicoumarol + aluminium or magnesium hydroxide

15 ml of **magnesium hydroxide** (*Milk of Magnesia*) taken with **dicoumarol**, and a further dose 3 h later, was found to raise serum **dicoumarol** levels of 6 subjects by 75% and the AUC by 50%. No interaction occurred with **aluminium hydroxide**.[1]

(b) Warfarin + aluminium or magnesium hydroxide, or magnesium trisilicate

30 ml **aluminium/magnesium hydroxide** (*Maalox*) given with **warfarin**, and four subsequent doses at 2 h intervals, had no effect on the plasma **warfarin** levels or on the anticoagulant response of 6 subjects.[2]

No interaction occurs with **warfarin** and **aluminium hydroxide** (*Amphogel*),[1] but an *in vitro* study suggests that the absorption of **warfarin** may be increased by **magnesium trisilicate**.[3]

Mechanism

It is suggested that dicoumarol forms a more readily absorbed chelate with magnesium so that its effects are increased.[2,4]

Importance and management

No special precautions need be taken if aluminium or magnesium hydroxide antacids are given to patients on warfarin, or if aluminium hydroxide is given to those on dicoumarol. Choosing these antacids avoids the possibility of an adverse interaction. Despite the evidence from the studies cited, there seems to be no direct clinical evidence of any important adverse interaction between any anticoagulant and an antacid.

1. Ambre JJ, Fischer LJ. Effect of coadministration of aluminum and magnesium hydroxides on absorption of anticoagulants in man. *Clin Pharmacol Ther* (1973) 14, 231–7.
2. Robinson DS, Benjamin DM, McCormack JJ. Interaction of warfarin and nonsystemic gastrointestinal drugs. *Clin Pharmacol Ther* (1971) 12, 491–5.
3. McElnay JC, Harron DWG, D'Arcy PF, Collier PS. Interaction of warfarin with antacid constituents. *BMJ* (1978) 2, 1166.
4. Akers MJ, Lach JL, Fischer LJ. Alterations in the absorption of dicoumarol by various excipient materials. *J Pharm Sci* (1973) 62, 391–5.

Anticoagulants + Ascorbic acid (Vitamin C)

Four controlled studies with large numbers of patients failed to demonstrate any interaction, although two isolated cases have been reported in which the effects of warfarin were reduced by ascorbic acid.

Clinical evidence

The prothrombin time of a woman, stabilised on 7.5 mg **warfarin** daily, who began to take regular amounts of **ascorbic acid** (dose not stated), fell steadily from 23 s to 19, 17 and then 14 s with no response to an increase in the dosage of **warfarin** to 10, 15 and finally 20 mg daily. The prothrombin time returned to 28 s within 2 days of stopping the **ascorbic acid**.[1] A woman who had been taking 16 g **ascorbic acid** daily proved to be unusually resistant to the actions of **warfarin** and required 25 mg daily before a significant increase in prothrombin times was achieved.[2]

In contrast, no changes in the effects of **warfarin** were seen in 5 patients given 1 g **ascorbic acid** daily for a fortnight,[3] in 84 patients given an unstated amount for 10 weeks,[4] in 11 patients given up to 4 g daily for 2 weeks,[5] or in 19 patients given up to 5 to 10 g daily for 1 or 2 weeks.[6] In this last study a mean fall of 17.5% in total plasma **warfarin** concentrations was seen.

Mechanism

Not understood. Some *animal* studies have demonstrated this interaction[7,8] and others have not,[9,10] but none of them has provided any definite clues about why it ever occurs, and then only rarely. One suggestion is that high doses of ascorbic acid can cause diarrhoea which might prevent adequate absorption of the anticoagulant.

Importance and management

Well-controlled clinical studies in large numbers of patients on warfarin have failed to confirm this interaction, even using very large doses of ascorbic acid (up to 10 g daily). There is no good reason for avoiding the concurrent use. Information about other anticoagulants is lacking, but it seems likely that they will behave similarly. However er check on any patient particularly resistant to the warfarin to confirm that ascorbic acid is not being taken.

1. Rosenthal G. Interaction of ascorbic acid and warfarin. *JAMA* (1971) 215, 1671.
2. Smith EC, Skalski RJ, Johnson GC, Rossi GV. Interaction of ascorbic acid and warfarin. *JAMA* (1972) 221, 1166.
3. Hume R, Johnstone JMS, Weyers E. Interaction of ascorbic acid and warfarin. *JAMA* (1972) 219, 1479.
4. Dedichen J. The effect of ascorbic acid given to patients on chronic anticoagulant therapy. *Boll Soc Ital Cardiol* (1973) 18, 690–2.
5. Blakely JA. Interaction of warfarin and ascorbic acid. 1st Florence Conference on Haemostasis and Thrombosis, May 1977. Abstracts p 99.

6. Feetam CL, Leach RH, Meynell MJ. Lack of a clinically important interaction between warfarin and ascorbic acid. *Toxicol Appl Pharmacol* (1975) 31, 544–7.
7. Sigell LT, Flessa HC. Drug interactions with anticoagulants. *JAMA* (1970) 214, 2035.
8. Sullivan WR, Gangstad EO, Link KP. Studies on the hemorrhagic sweet clover disease. XII. The effect of *l*-ascorbic acid on the hypoprothrombinemia induced by 3,3'-methylenebis (4-hydroxycoumarin) in the guinea pig. *J Biol Chem* (1943) 151, 477–85.
9. Weintraub M, Griner PF. Warfarin and ascorbic acid: lack of evidence for a drug interaction. *Toxicol Appl Pharmacol* (1974) 28, 53–6.
10. Deckert FW. Ascorbic acid and warfarin. *JAMA* (1973) 223, 440.

Anticoagulants + Aspirin or other Salicylates

500 mg aspirin daily increases the likelihood of bleeding 3 to 5 times in those taking anticoagulants, it damages the stomach wall, prolongs bleeding times and in 2 to 4-g daily doses can increase prothrombin times, whereas low-dose aspirin (75 to 100 mg daily) seems to be safer. Despite these potential problems some large scale studies have concluded that possibly the overall benefits of concurrent use may outweigh the risks. Increased warfarin effects have been seen when methyl salicylate or trolamine salicylate were used on the skin.

Clinical evidence

(a) Oral salicylates

A study in 534 patients with artificial heart valves found that three times as many bled (requiring blood transfusion or hospitalization) among those on 500 mg **aspirin** daily (14%) as among those on **warfarin** alone (5%). Bleeding was mainly gastrointestinal or cerebral. All of those with intracerebral bleeding died.[1]

This finding broadly confirms two other studies on a total of 270 patients in whom bleeding was found to be about five times more common in anticoagulated patients taking **aspirin** (0.5 to 1.0 g daily) than among those taking only the anticoagulant.[2,3] A further study found that 1 g **aspirin** daily increased the bleeding episodes in those on **unnamed anticoagulants** from 4.7 to 13.9 per 100 patients per year.[4] A 20% incidence of severe upper gastrointestinal bleeding was seen in a study of 138 coronary stent patients given **heparin** or **warfarin** with 325 mg **aspirin** daily. Ten of the patients needed a blood transfusion.[5] A study of 75 patients taking **acenocoumarol (nicoumalone)** and **aspirin** reported serious bleeding in 2.7% and mild bleeding in 33% but no fatalities.[6] Other studies in patients taking **dicoumarol**, **acenocoumarol** or **warfarin** found that 2 to 4 g **aspirin** daily increased the anticoagulant effects. The anticoagulant dosage could be reduced about 30%.[7,8] However another investigator using **warfarin** with 3 g **aspirin** daily failed to find any effect on prothrombin times.[9]

Low-dose aspirin (75 mg daily) doubles the normal blood loss from the gastric mucosa but it still remains very small (compared with the 14-fold increase with 2.4 g daily) and **warfarin** does not increase it.[10] Only minor episodes of bleeding (nose bleeds, bruising) occur with **low dose aspirin** and low intensity **warfarin** (INR 1.5).[11] Another study using **100 mg aspirin** daily found that although there was some increase in bleeding, the risk was more than offset by the overall reduction in mortality.[12]

(b) Topical salicylates

Methyl salicylate in form of **gel**, **oil** or **ointment** applied to the skin has been found to increase the effects of **warfarin**. Bleeding and bruising and/or raised INRs have been seen with both high[13-16] and low doses[17] of **methyl salicylate**. One report described the possible additive effects of **methyl salicylate oil** (*Kwan Loong Medicated Oil*) and a decoction of '*Danshen*' (the root of *Salvia miltiorrhiza*) on the response to **warfarin**.[18] A raised prothrombin time has also been reported with topical **trolamine salicylate**.[15]

Mechanism

Aspirin has a direct irritant effect on the stomach lining and can cause gastrointestinal bleeding. It also decreases platelet aggregation and prolongs bleeding times, all of which would seem to account for some of the bleeding episodes described.[1-3] In addition, large doses (2 to

4 g daily) of aspirin alone are known to have a direct hypoprothrom-binaemic effect, like the anticoagulants, which is reversible by vita-min K,[19-22] and which can be additive with the effects of the anticoagulant. Methyl and trolamine salicylate can also interact be-cause they are absorbed through the skin.

Importance and management

The anticoagulant/aspirin interaction is well documented and current wisdom regards it as clinically important, for which reason it is usual to avoid normal analgesic and anti-inflammatory doses while taking any anticoagulant, although only dicoumarol, acenocoumarol (nicou-malone) and warfarin appear to have been investigated. Patients should be told that many proprietary non-prescription analgesic, anti-pyretic, cold and influenza preparations may contain substantial amounts of aspirin. Tell them that it may be listed as acetylsalicylic acid. Paracetamol (acetaminophen) is a safer analgesic substitute (but not entirely without problems – see 'Anticoagulants + Paracetamol (Acetaminophen)', p.283. Low-dose aspirin (75 mg daily) used for its platelet anti-aggregant effects appears not to interact to a clinically relevant extent. Some of the other salicylates are less irritant and have a smaller effect on platelet function than aspirin so that, on theoretical grounds, the avoidance of concurrent use may be less important. Re-member too that topical methyl salicylate and trolamine salicylate can also interact.

However an alternative perspective on the anticoagulant/aspirin in-teraction is provided by a meta-analysis of four studies involving al-most 900 patients carried out between 1976 and 1993. It was concluded that the combined use of oral anticoagulants and aspirin (100 to 500 mg daily) significantly reduced mortality and embolic complications in patients with prosthetic heart valves, although this was partly offset by some increase in major bleeding episodes. Nev-ertheless the overall picture was that the benefits possibly outweighed the problems.[23] Another very large scale study which compared war-farin alone (INRs 4.2 to 2.5) with warfarin plus 150 mg aspirin daily (INRs 2.8 to 2.2) found that the aspirin group showed a higher inci-dence of minor bleeding (2.9% compared with 1.4%) but the inci-dence of serious and fatal bleeding was the same in the two groups.[24] Yet another study found no differences in bleeding rates in stroke pa-tients given heparin and/or warfarin with or without aspirin.[25] So per-haps there is now a case for some rethinking about our current belief in the hazards of the anticoagulant/aspirin interaction.

1. Chesebro JH, Fuster V, Elveback LR, McGoon DC, Pluth JR, Puga FJ, Wallace RB, Danielson GK, Orszulak TA, Piehler JM, Schaff HV. Trial of combined warfarin plus dipyridamole or aspirin therapy in prosthetic heart valve replacement: danger of aspirin compared with dipyridamole. Am J Cardiol (1983) 51, 1537–41.
2. Altman R, Boullon F, Rouvier J, Rada R, de la Fuente L, Favaloro R. Aspirin and proph-ylaxis of thromboembolic complications in patients with substitute heart valves. J Tho-rac Cardiovasc Surg (1976) 72, 127–9.
3. Dale J, Myhre E, Storstein O, Stormorken H, Efskind L. Prevention of arterial throm-boembolism with acetylsalicylic acid. A controlled clinical study in patients with aortic ball valves. Am Heart J (1977) 94, 101–111.
4. Dale J, Myhre E, Loew D. Bleeding during acetylsalicylic acid and anticoagulant therapy in patients with reduced platelet reactivity after aortic valve replacement. Am Heart J (1980) 99, 746–52.
5. Younossi ZM, Strum WB, Cloutier D, Teirstein PS, Schatz RA. Upper GI bleeding in postcoronary stent patients following aspirin and anticoagulant treatment. Gastroenter-ology (1995) 108 (4 Suppl), A265.
6. Sámóczi M, Farkas A, Sipos E, Tarján J. Acenocoumarol és acetylsalicylsav együttes al-kalmazásának szövedmenyei szívinfarktus után és instabil anginában. Orv Hetil (1995) 136, 177–9.
7. Watson RM, Pierson RN. Effect of anticoagulant therapy upon aspirin-induced gastroin-testinal bleeding. Circulation (1961) 24, 613.
8. O'Reilly RA, Sahud MA, Aggeler PM. Impact of aspirin and chlorthalidone on the phar-macodynamics of oral anticoagulants drugs in man. Ann N Y Acad Sci (1971) 179, 173.
9. Udall JA. Drug interference with warfarin therapy. Am J Cardiol (1969) 23, 143.
10. Prichard PJ, Kitchingman GK, Walt RP, Daneshmend TK, Hawkey CJ. Human gastric mucosal bleeding induced by low dose aspirin, but not warfarin. BMJ (1989) 298, 493–6.
11. Meade TW, Roderick PJ, Brennan PJ, Wilkes HC, Kelleher CC. Extra-cranial bleeding and other symptoms due to low dose aspirin and low intensity oral anticoagulation. Thromb Haemost (1992) 68, 1–6.
12. Turpie AGG, Gent M, Laupacis A, Latour Y, Gunstensen J, Basile F, Klimek M, Hirsh J. A comparison of aspirin with placebo in patients treated with warfarin after heart-valve replacement. N Engl J Med (1993) 329, 524–9.
13. Chow WH, Cheung KL, Ling HM, See T. Potentiation of warfarin anticoagulation by topical methylsalicylate ointment. J R Soc Med (1989) 82, 501–2.
14. Yip ASB, Chow WH, Tai YT, Cheung KL. Adverse effect of topical methylsalicylate ointment on warfarin anticoagulation: an unrecognized potential hazard. Postgrad Med J (1990) 66, 367–9.
15. Littleton F. Warfarin and topical salicylates. JAMA (1990) 263, 2888.
16. Ramanathan M. Warfarin-topical salicylate interactions: case reports. Med J Malaysia (1995) 50, 278–9.
17. Joss JD, LeBlond RF. Potentiation of warfarin anticoagulation associated with topical methyl salicylate. Ann Pharmacother (2000) 34, 729–33.
18. Tam LS, Chan TYK, Leung WK, Critchley JAJH. Warfarin interactions with Chinese traditional medicines: danshen and methyl salicylate medicated oil. Aust N Z J Med (1995) 25, 258.
19. Shapiro S. Studies on prothrombin. VI. The effect of synthetic vitamin K on the pro-thrombinopenia induced by salicylate in man. JAMA (1944) 125, 546–8.
20. Quick AJ, Clesceri L. Influence of acetylsalicylic acid and salicylamide on the coagula-tion of the blood. J Pharmacol Exp Ther (1960) 128, 95.
21. Meyer OO, Howard B. Production of hypoprothrombinaemia and hypocoagulability of the blood with salicylates. J Pharmacol Exp Ther (1943) 53, 251.
22. Park BK, Leck JB. On the mechanism of salicylate-induced hypoprothrombinaemia. J Pharm Pharmacol (1981) 33, 25–8.
23. Fiore L, Brophy M, Deykin D, Cappelleri J, Lau J. The efficacy and safety of the addition of aspirin in patients treated with oral anticoagulants after heart valve replacement: a meta-analysis. Blood (1993) 82 (10 Suppl 1), 409a.
24. Hurlen M, Erikssen J, Smith P, Arnesen H, Rollag A. Comparison of bleeding complica-tions of warfarin and warfarin plus acetylsalicylic acid: a study in 3166 outpatients. J In-tern Med (1994) 236, 299–304.
25. Fagan SC, Kertland HR, Tietjen GE. Safety of combination aspirin and anticoagulation in acute ischemic stroke. Ann Pharmacother (1994) 28, 441–3.

Anticoagulants + Azapropazone

The anticoagulant effects of warfarin are markedly increased by azapropazone. Bleeding will occur if the dosage of warfa-rin is not considerably reduced. The makers contraindicate concurrent use.

Clinical evidence

A woman on digoxin, furosemide (frusemide), spironolactone, allo-purinol, and stabilised on **warfarin** (prothrombin ratio 2.8) developed haematemesis within four days of starting to take 300 mg **azapropa-zone** four times a day. Her prothrombin ratio was found to have risen to 15.7 (prothrombin time of 220 s). Subsequent gastroscopic exami-nation revealed a benign ulcer, the presumed site of the bleeding.[1]

At least 12 other patients are reported to have developed this inter-action. Bruising or bleeding (melaena, epistaxis, haematuria, etc) and prolonged prothrombin times occurred within a few days of starting **azapropazone**.[2-7] Three died.[4-6] Another patient on **warfarin** and **az-apropazone** and also taking diclofenac and co-proxamol showed an increase in prothrombin times.[8] This interaction has been experimen-tally confirmed in two normal subjects.[9]

Mechanism

Not understood. Azapropazone displaces warfarin from its plasma protein binding sites[9-11] thereby increasing the amount of free and pharmacologically active molecules, but it is almost certain that this alone does not fully account for the clinical effects reported. Changes in the metabolism of the warfarin are probably mainly responsible.

Importance and management

The warfarin/azapropazone interaction is established and clinically important. The incidence is uncertain. Because of the risk of serious bleeding the makers of azapropazone say that it should not be used with warfarin or any other anticoagulant.

1. Powell-Jackson PR. Interaction between azapropazone and warfarin. BMJ (1977) 1, 1193.
2. Green AE, Hort JF, Korn HET, Leach H. Potentiation of warfarin by azapropazone. BMJ (1977) 1, 1532.
3. Beeley L. Bulletin of the West Midlands Adverse Drug Reaction Study Group. Univer-sity of Birmingham, England. January 1980, no 10.
4. Anon. Interactions. Doctors warned on warfarin dangers. Pharm J (1983) 230, 676.
5. Win N, Mitchell DC, Jones PAE, French EA. Azapropazone and warfarin. BMJ (1991) 302, 969–70.
6. Beeley L, Cunningham H, Carmichael AE, Brennan A. Bulletin of the West Midlands Centre for Adverse Drug Reaction Reporting (1991) 33, 19.
7. Beeley L, Magee P, Hickey FM. Bulletin of the West Midlands Centre for Adverse Drug Reaction Reporting (1989) 28, 34.
8. Beeley L, Stewart P and Hickey FL. Bulletin of the West Midlands Centre for Adverse Drug Reaction Reporting (1987) 27, 27.
9. McElnay JC, D'Arcy PF. Interaction between azapropazone and warfarin. BMJ (1977) 2, 773.
10. McElnay JC, D'Arcy PF. The effect of azapropazone on the binding of warfarin to hu-man serum proteins. J Pharm Pharmacol (1978) 30 (Suppl), 73P.
11. McElnay JC, D'Arcy PF. Interaction between azapropazone and warfarin. Experientia (1978) 34, 1320–1.

Anticoagulants + Azithromycin

Azithromycin does not usually interact with warfarin, but very occasionally and unpredictably raised INRs, hypoprothrombinaemia and bleeding have been seen.

Clinical evidence

(a) Warfarin effects unchanged

A very large scale study in patients treated with azithromycin found no evidence that 1.5 g for 5 days had any effect on the prothrombin time response to single doses of **warfarin**.[1] A retrospective study of 26 patients on warfarin found no evidence that treatment with azithromycin had any effect on their INRs.[2] A study in normal subjects found that azithromycin did not alter the anticoagulant effects of single 15 mg doses of **warfarin**.[3]

(b) Warfarin effects increased

A 41-year-old woman on haemodialysis and taking **warfarin** was given a short course of azithromycin (500 mg on day 1, reduced to 250 mg daily for the next 4 days). Three days after finishing the azithromycin the woman's INR was found to have risen to 4.88 from her normal range of 1.5 to 2.7.[4]

A 53-year-old man who had been taking **warfarin** for several years (INRs 2.0 to 2.8) following a mitral valve replacement, was hospitalised a couple of days after starting to cough blood and blood-streaked mucus. He had finished a 5-day course of azithromycin 2 days previously (500 mg on day 1, reduced to 250 mg for the next 4 days). His prothrombin time was found to have risen to 106 sec. The **warfarin** was stopped and phytonadione given, but he later died from cardiac arrest.[5]

A 71-year old man stabilised on **warfarin** with INRs between 2.5 and 3.6 developed an INR of 15.16 six days after starting a 5-day course of azithromycin.[6]

The makers[7] of azithromycin are quoted as having on their records 14 reports of ". . . a potential increase in the hypoprothrombinemic effect of **warfarin** during or immediately following a course of azithromycin." Two unconfirmed cases of possible interaction have been reported to the Medicines Control Agency (MCA) in the UK,[8] and 2 other cases have been reported from Australia.[9]

Mechanism

Not understood.

Importance and management

Normally no interaction occurs, but because very occasionally and unpredictably the effects of warfarin are increased, all patients should be well monitored when first given azithromycin, bearing in mind that because of azithromycin's long half-life the interaction may possibly not become apparent until a couple of days after a short course (i.e. 5 days) of azithromycin has been stopped. These precautions are in line with the maker's recommendations.[3] Information about other oral anticoagulants is lacking but it would be prudent to follow the same precautions suggested for warfarin.

1. Hopkins S. Clinical tolerance and safety of azithromycin. *Am J Med* (1991) 91 (Suppl 3A), 40S–45S.
2. Beckey N, Parra D, Colon A. Retrospective evaluation of a potential interaction between azithromycin and warfarin in patients stabilized on warfarin. *Pharmacotherapy* (2000) 20, 1055-9.
3. Zithromax (Azithromycin). Pfizer Limited. Summary of product characteristics, May 2001.
4. Lane G. Increased hypoprothrombinemic effect of warfarin possibly induced by azithromycin. *Ann Pharmacother* (1996) 30, 884–5.
5. Woldtveldt BR, Cahoon CL, Bradley LA, Miller SJ. Possible increased anticoagulant effect of warfarin induced by azithromycin. *Ann Pharmacother* (1998) 32, 269–70.
6. Foster DR, Milan NL. Potential interaction between azithromycin and warfarin. *Pharmacotherapy* (1999) 19, 902-8.
7. Gomes DF. Pfizer Laboratories, New York, USA. Quoted as personal communication, 1997 by Woldtveldt BR, Cahoon CL, Bradley LA, Miller SJ. Possible increased anticoagulant effect of warfarin induced by azithromycin. *Ann Pharmacother* (1998) 32, 269–70.
8. Pfizer Limited. Personal Communication, December 1998.
9. Wiese MD, Cosh DG. Raised INR with concurrent warfarin and azithromycin. *Aust J Hosp Pharm* (1999) 29, 159-161.

Anticoagulants + Aztreonam

Aztreonam occasionally causes a prolongation in prothrombin times which in theory might possibly be additive with the effects of conventional anticoagulants.

Clinical evidence, mechanism, importance and management

A few patients on **aztreonam** develop prolonged prothrombin times which respond to vitamin K treatment. The incidence is low. In three studies it ranged from 1 to 10%.[1-3] The partial thromboplastin time is also increased. There seem to be no confirmed adverse reports about patients taking **oral anticoagulants** and **aztreonam** together, but it seems possible that their hypoprothrombinaemic effects might be additive. If you add **aztreonam** to an established regimen with **warfarin** or **any other anticoagulant**, you should monitor the effects. Tell the patient to be alert for any evidence of otherwise unexplained bruising or bleeding.

1. Rusconi F, Assael BM, Boccazzi A, Colombo R, Crossignani RM, Garlaschi L, Rancilio L. Aztreonam in the treatment of severe urinary tract infections in pediatric patients. *Antimicrob Agents Chemother* (1986) 30, 310–14.
2. Giamarellou H, Galanakis N, Dendrinos CH, Kanellakopoulou K, Petrikkos G, Koratzanis G, Daikos GK. Clinical experience with aztreonam in a variety of gram-negative infections. *Chemioterapia* (1985) 4 (Suppl 1), 75–80.
3. Giamerellou H, Koratzanis G, Kanellakopoulou K, Galanakis N, Papoulis G, ElMessidi M, Daikos G. Aztreonam versus cefamandole in the treatment of urinary tract infections. *Chemioterapia* (1984) 3, 127–31.

Anticoagulants + Barbiturates

The effects of the anticoagulants are reduced by the concurrent use of barbiturates. Full therapeutic anticoagulation may only be achieved by raising the anticoagulant dosage about 30 to 60%. If the barbiturate is later withdrawn, the anticoagulant dosage should be reduced to avoid the risk of bleeding. Primidone is metabolised to phenobarbital (phenobarbitone) and is expected to interact similarly, but it is uncertain whether it does.

Clinical evidence

Two examples from many:

A study on 16 patients on long-term **warfarin** treatment showed that when they were also given 2 mg/kg **phenobarbital (phenobarbitone)**, their average daily **warfarin** requirements rose over a 4-week period by 25% (from 5.7 to 7.1 mg daily).[1]

An investigation on 12 patients taking either **warfarin** or **phenprocoumon** demonstrated that when concurrently given **secbutobarbital (secbutobarbitone) sodium**, 60 mg daily for the first week and 120 mg daily for the next two weeks, their anticoagulant requirements rose by 35 to 60%, reaching a maximum after 4 to 5 weeks.[2]

This interaction has been described in man between **warfarin** and **amobarbital (amylobarbitone)**,[3-6] **butobarbital (butobarbitone)**,[7] **heptabarb (heptabarbitone)**,[8,9] **phenobarbital (phenobarbitone)**,[10-14] **secobarbital (quinalbarbitone)**[3,4,6,14-17] and **secbutobarbital (secbutobarbitone)**;[2] between **dicoumarol** and **aprobarbitone (aprobarbital)**,[18] **heptabarb (heptabarbitone)**,[19,20] **phenobarbital (phenobarbitone)**[21-23] and **vinbarbital (vinbarbitone)**;[18] between **ethyl biscoumacetate** and **amobarbital (amylobarbitone)**,[19,24] **pentobarbital (pentobarbitone)**,[25] and **phenobarbital (phenobarbitone)**;[24] between **phenprocoumon** and **secbutobarbital (secbuto-**

barbitone);[2] and between **acenocoumarol (nicoumalone)** and **pentobarbital (pentobarbitone)**[26] and **heptabarb (heptabarbitone)**.[20]

Mechanism

Studies in man and *animals*[4,8,10,13,16] clearly show that the barbiturates are potent liver enzyme inducing agents which increase the metabolism and clearance of the anticoagulants from the body. They may also reduce the absorption of dicoumarol from the gut.[20]

Importance and management

The anticoagulant/barbiturate interactions are clinically important and very well documented. The reduced anticoagulant effects expose the patient to the risk of thrombus formation if the dosage is not increased appropriately. A very large number of anticoagulant/barbiturate pairs have been found to interact and the others may be expected to behave similarly. The only known exception is secobarbital (quinalbarbitone) which in daily doses of 100 mg appears to have little[14] or no[6,15,16] effect on dicoumarol or warfarin, but in daily doses of 200 mg interacts like the other barbiturates.[6,15] The barbiturates interact less with *R*-warfarin than *S*-warfarin, but in practice *R*-warfarin appears to have little advantage over the usual *RS*-racemic mixture.[27,28]

The reduction in the anticoagulant effects begins within a week, sometimes within 2 to 4 days, reaching a maximum after about 3 weeks, and it may still be evident up to 6 weeks after stopping the barbiturate.[2] Patients' responses can vary considerably. Stable anticoagulant control can be re-established[5] in the presence of the barbiturate by increasing the anticoagulant dosage by about 30 to 60%.[1,2,12,23] This may be necessary for epileptic patients.[5] Care must be taken not to withdraw the barbiturate without also reducing the anticoagulant dosage, otherwise bleeding will occur.[1,5,12] Alternative non-interacting sedative and hypnotic drugs which are safer (?) and easier to use include nitrazepam, chlordiazepoxide, diazepam, and flurazepam. See 'Anticoagulants + Benzodiazepines', p.244. Information is lacking about anticoagulants other than those cited, but they are expected to interact similarly.

Primidone is metabolised in the body to phenobarbital (phenobarbitone) and is therefore expected to interact like phenobarbital, although there seem to be no reports of **anticoagulant/primidone** interactions. Notwithstanding it would be prudent to be alert for reduced anticoagulant effects if primidone is given concurrently.

1. Robinson DS, MacDonald MG. The effect of phenobarbital administration on the control of coagulation achieved during warfarin therapy in man. *J Pharmacol Exp Ther* (1966) 153, 250–3.
2. Antlitz AM, Tolentino M, Kosai MF. Effect of butabarbital on orally administered anticoagulants. *Curr Ther Res* (1968) 10, 70–3.
3. Breckenridge A, Orme M. Clinical implications of enzyme induction. *Ann N Y Acad Sci* (1971) 179, 421–31.
4. Robinson DS, Sylwester D. Interaction of commonly prescribed drugs and warfarin. *Ann Intern Med* (1970) 72, 853–6.
5. Williams JRB, Griffin JP, Parkins A. Effect of concomitantly administered drugs on the control of long term anticoagulant therapy. *Q J Med* (1976) 45, 63.
6. Whitfield JB, Moss DW, Neale G, Orme M, Breckenridge A. Changes in plasma γ-glutamyl transpeptidase activity associated with alterations in drug metabolism in man. *BMJ* (1973) 1, 316–18.
7. MacGregor AG, Petrie JC and Wood RA. Therapeutic conferences. Drug interaction. *BMJ* (1971) 1, 389.
8. Levy G, O'Reilly RA, Aggeler PM, Keech GM. Pharmacokinetic analysis of the effect of barbiturate on the anticoagulant action of warfarin in man. *Clin Pharmacol Ther* (1970) 11, 372–7.
9. O'Reilly RA, Aggeler PM. Effect of barbiturates on oral anticoagulants in man. *Clin Res* (1969) 17, 153.
10. MacDonald MG, Robinson DS, Sylwester D, Jaffe JJ. The effects of phenobarbital, chloral betaine, and glutethimide administration on warfarin plasma levels and hypoprothrombinemic responses in man. *Clin Pharmacol Ther* (1969) 10, 80–4.
11. Seller K, Duckert F. Properties of 3-(1-phenyl-propyl)-4-oxycoumarin (Marcoumar) in the plasma when tested in normal cases and under the influence of drugs. *Thromb Diath Haemorrh* (1969) 19, 89.
12. MacDonald MG, Robinson DS. Clinical observations of possible barbiturate interference with anticoagulation. *JAMA* (1968) 204, 97–100.
13. Corn M. Effect of phenobarbital and glutethimide on biological half-life of warfarin. *Thromb Diath Haemorrh* (1966) 16, 606–12.
14. Udall JA. Clinical implications of warfarin interactions with five sedatives. *Am J Cardiol* (1975) 35, 67–71.
15. Feuer DJ, Wilson WR, Ambre JJ. Duration of effect of secobarbital on the anticoagulant effect and metabolism of warfarin. *Pharmacologist* (1974) 16, 195.
16. Breckenridge A, Orme ML'E, Davies L, Thorgeirsson SS, Davis DS. Dose-dependent enzyme induction. *Clin Pharmacol Ther* (1973) 14, 514–20.
17. Cucinell SA, Odessky L, Weiss M, Dayton PG. The effect of chloral hydrate on bishydroxycoumarin metabolism. A fatal outcome. *JAMA* (1966) 197, 144–6.
18. Johansson S-A. Apparent resistance to oral anticoagulant therapy and influence of hypnotics on some coagulation factors. *Acta Med Scand* (1968) 184, 297–300.
19. Dayton PG, Tarcan Y, Chenkin T, Weiner M. The influence of barbiturates on coumarin plasma levels and prothrombin response. *J Clin Invest* (1961) 40, 1797–1802.
20. Aggeler PM, O'Reilly RA. Effect of heptabarbital on the response to bishydroxycoumarin in man. *J Lab Clin Med* (1969) 74, 229–38.
21. Corn M, Rockett JF. Inhibition of bishydroxycoumarin activity by phenobarbital. *Med Ann Dist Columbia* (1965) 34, 578–9.
22. Cucinell SA, Conney AH, Sansur M, Burns JJ. Drug interactions in man. One lowering effect phenobarbital on plasma levels of bishydroxycoumarin (Dicumarol) and diphenylhydantoin (Dilantin). *Clin Pharmacol Ther* (1965) 6, 420.
23. Goss JE, Dickhaus DW. Increased bishydroxycoumarin requirements in patients receiving phenobarbital. *N Engl J Med* (1965) 273, 1094–5.
24. Avellaneda M. Interferencia de los barbituricos en la accion del Tromexan. *Medicina* (1955) 15, 109–15.
25. Reverchon F, Sapir M. Constatation clinique d'un antagonisme entre barbituriques et anticoagulants. *Presse Med* (1961) 69, 1570–1.
26. Kroon C, de Boer A, Hoogkamer JFW, Schoemaker HC, vd Meer FJM, Edelbroek PM, Cohen AF. Detection of drug interactions with single dose acenocoumarol: new screening method? *Int J Clin Pharmacol Ther Toxicol* (1990) 28, 355–60.
27. Orme M, Breckenridge A. Enantiomers of warfarin and phenobarbital. *N Engl J Med* (1976) 295, 1482–3.
28. O'Reilly RA, Trager WF, Motley CH, Howald W. Interaction of secobarbital with warfarin pseudoracemates. *Clin Pharmacol Ther* (1980) 28, 187–95.

Anticoagulants + Benfluorex

Benfluorex does not alter the anticoagulant effects of phenprocoumon.

Clinical evidence, mechanism, importance and management

Twenty-five patients on **phenprocoumon** showed no significant changes in their prothrombin times while taking 450 mg **benfluorex** daily for 9 weeks when compared with equivalent periods before and after while not taking **benfluorex**.[1] There seems to be no information about other anticoagulants.

1. De Witte P, Brems HM. Co-administration of benfluorex with oral anticoagulant therapy. *Curr Med Res Opin* (1980) 6, 478–80.

Anticoagulants + Benzbromarone

The anticoagulant effects of warfarin are increased by benzbromarone. Bleeding may occur if the warfarin dosage is not reduced by about one-third. Other anticoagulants (acenocoumarol (nicoumalone), ethyl biscoumacetate, phenindione) are said not to interact but the information available is very limited.

Clinical evidence

The observation that 2 patients bled (haematuria, gastrointestinal bleeding) when given warfarin and benzbromarone for gout, prompted a more detailed study in 7 other patients. The thrombotest values of these 7 averaged 24.7% while taking both warfarin and benzbromarone (average dosage 57.1 mg daily), but when the benzbromarone was stopped for a week they rose to 47.3%. On restarting the benzbromarone the thrombotest values fell back to 30.3%. The Factor II activity and PIVKA-II concentration changes ran in parallel with these thrombotest values. The total plasma warfarin levels fell during the period when the benzbromarone had been stopped.[1] Another later controlled study found that benzbromarone reduced the warfarin requirements of 13 patients by 36% (from 3.9 to 2.5 mg daily).[2] These two studies confirm observations on other patients with prosthetic valve replacements who showed haemorrhagic tendencies when given both drugs.[3]

In contrast it has been claimed that no increases in the anticoagulant effects of acenocoumarol (nicoumalone), ethyl biscoumacetate or phenindione were seen in a few patients given benzbromarone.[4]

Mechanism

Benzbromarone selectively inhibits the metabolism of *(S)*-warfarin so that its loss from the body is reduced and its effects are increased. The metabolism of the *(R)*-warfarin remains unchanged.[2]

Importance and management

The warfarin/benzbromarone interaction is established and clinically important. If benzbromarone is added to established warfarin treatment, be alert for the need to reduce the dosage by about one-third to prevent over-anticoagulation and possible bleeding. Information about other anticoagulants is very limited but what is known suggests that acenocoumarol (nicoumalone), ethyl biscoumacetate, phenindione do not interact, nevertheless it would be prudent to monitor the outcome when benzbromarone is first added to treatment with any of them. More study is needed.

1. Shimodaira H, Takahashi K, Kano K, Matsumoto Y, Uchida Y, Kudo T. Enhancement of anticoagulant action by warfarin-benzbromarone interaction. *J Clin Pharmacol* (1996) 36, 168–74.
2. Takahashi H, Sato T, Shimoyama Y, Shioda N, Shimizu T, Kubo S, TAmura N, Tainaka H, Yasumori T, Echizen H. Potentiation of anticoagulant effect of warfarin caused by enantioselective metabolic inhibition by the uricosuric agent benzbromarone. *Clin Pharmacol Ther* (1999) 66, 569-81.
3. Hadama T, Takasaki H, Mori Y, Oka K, Shigemitu O, Fujishima K. A study on optimization of coagulative function by warfarin and antiplatelet agents in patients with prosthetic valve replacement. *J Jpn Cardiovasc Surg Assoc* (1990) 19, 1264–6.
4. Masbernard A. Quoted as personal communication (1977) by Heel RC, Brogden RN, Speight TM, Avery GS. Benzbromarone: a review of its pharmacological properties and their use in gout and hyperuricaemia. *Drugs* (1977) 14, 349–66.

Anticoagulants + Benziodarone

The anticoagulant effects of acenocoumarol (nicoumalone), ethyl biscoumacetate, diphenadione and warfarin are increased by benziodarone. The dosage of anticoagulant should be reduced appropriately. Chlorindione, dicoumarol and indandione do not interact, but the situation with phenprocoumon is not clear.

Clinical evidence

90 patients on anticoagulants were given 200 mg **benziodarone** three times a day for two days and 100 mg three times a day thereafter. To maintain constant PP percentages the anticoagulant dosages were reduced as follows: **ethyl biscoumacetate** 17% (9 patients), **diphenadione** 42% (8 patients), **acenocoumarol (nicoumalone)** 25% (7 patients) and **warfarin** 46% (15 patients). No changes were needed in those taking **chlorindione** (5 patients), **dicoumarol** (9 patients), **phenindione** (10 patients) or **phenprocoumon** (8 patients). A parallel study on 12 normal subjects confirmed the interaction with **warfarin**.[1]

The absence of an interaction with **dicoumarol** confirms a previous study,[2] however another study found that 300 to 600 mg **benziodarone** daily increased the anticoagulant effects of **phenprocoumon** in 9 out of 29 patients and the ecchymoses observed were more frequent and larger.[3] The metabolism of **ethyl biscoumacetate** appears to be increased by **benziodarone**.[3]

Mechanism

Not understood. Benziodarone alone has no definite effect on the activity of prothrombin or factors VII, IX or X.

Importance and management

Information appears to be limited to the studies cited, but the interaction would seem to be established. The dosages of the interacting anticoagulants and possibly of phenprocoumon should be reduced appropriately to prevent bleeding. No particular precautions are necessary with the non-interacting anticoagulants.

1. Pyörälä K, Ikkala E, Siltanen P. Benziodarone (Amplivix®) and anticoagulant therapy. *Acta Med Scand* (1963) 173, 385–9.
2. Gillot P. Valeur therapeutique du L. 2329 dans l'angine de poitrine. *Acta Cardiol* (1959) 14, 494–515.

3. Verstraete M, Vermylen J, Claeys H. Dissimilar effect of two anti-anginal drugs belonging to the benzofuran group on the action of coumarin derivatives. *Arch Int Pharmacodyn Ther* (1968) 176, 33–41.

Anticoagulants + Benzodiazepines

The anticoagulant effects of warfarin are not affected by chlordiazepoxide, diazepam, flurazepam, nitrazepam or triazolam. The effects of phenprocoumon are not affected by nitrazepam or oxazepam, nor ethyl biscoumacetate by chlordiazepoxide. An interaction between any oral anticoagulant and a benzodiazepine is unlikely, but there are three unexplained and unconfirmed cases attributed to an interaction.

Clinical evidence

A number of studies on a very large number of patients given anticoagulants and benzodiazepines for extended periods confirm the lack of an interaction between **warfarin** and **chlordiazepoxide**,[1-5] **diazepam**,[1,4,5] **flurazepam**,[6] **nitrazepam**[1,4,7] or **triazolam**;[8] between **ethyl biscoumacetate** and **chlordiazepoxide**;[9] and between **phenprocoumon**, **oxazepam**[10] and **nitrazepam**.[11]

There are three discordant reports: A patient on **warfarin** showed an increased anticoagulant response when given **diazepam**.[12] A patient on **dicoumarol** developed multiple ecchymoses and a prothrombin time of 53 s within a fortnight of starting to take 20 mg **diazepam** daily.[13] And a patient showed a fall in serum **warfarin** levels and in the anticoagulant response when given **chlordiazepoxide**.[7] It is by no means certain that these responses were due to an interaction.

Mechanism

The three discordant reports are not understood. Enzyme induction is a possible explanation in one case[7] because increases in the urinary excretion of 6-beta-hydroxycortisol have been described during chlordiazepoxide use.[1,7]

Importance and management

Well documented and well established. The weight of evidence and common experience show that benzodiazepines do not normally interact with the anticoagulants. Not all of the anticoagulant/benzodiazepine pairs have been examined, but none of them would be expected to interact.

1. Orme M, Breckenridge A, Brooks RV. Interactions of benzodiazepines with warfarin. *BMJ* (1972) 3, 611–14.
2. Lackner H, Hunt VE. The effect of Librium on hemostasis. *Am J Med Sci* (1968) 256, 368–72.
3. Robinson DS, Sylwester D. Interaction of commonly prescribed drugs and warfarin. *Ann Intern Med* (1970) 72, 853–6.
4. Breckenridge A, Orme M. Interaction of benzodiazepines with oral anticoagulants. In 'The Benzodiazepines'. Garattini S, Mussini E and Randall LO (eds) Raven Press, NY. (1973) p. 647–54.
5. Solomon HM, Barakat MJ, Ashley CJ. Mechanisms of drug interaction. *JAMA* (1971) 216, 1997–9.
6. Robinson DS and Amidon EI. Interaction of benzodiazepines with warfarin in man. In 'The Benzodiazepines'. Garattini S, Mussini E and Randall LO (eds) Raven Press, NY. (1973) p. 641–3.
7. Breckenridge A, Orme M. Clinical implications of enzyme induction. *Ann N Y Acad Sci* (1971) 179, 421–31.
8. Cohon MS. (Upjohn) Quoted as In-house data in 'Triazolam human pharmacokinetic review, Halcion® tablets,' Drug Information Services Unit, January 1990, pp 24–5.
9. van Dam FE, Gribnau-Overkamp MJH. The effect of some sedatives (phenobarbital, glutethimide, chlordiazepoxide, chloral hydrate) on the rate of disappearance of ethyl biscoumacetate from the plasma. *Folia Med Neerl* (1967) 10, 141–5.
10. Schneider J, Kamm G. Beeinflußt Oxazepam (Adumbran®) die Antikoagulanzientherapie mit Phenprocoumon? *Med Klin* (1978) 73, 153–6.
11. Bieger R, De Jonge H, Loeliger EA. Influence of nitrazepam on oral anticoagulation with phenprocoumon. *Clin Pharmacol Ther* (1972) 13, 361–5.
12. McQueen EG. New Zealand Committee on Adverse Drug Reactions. 9th Annual Report 1974. *N Z Med J* (1974) 80, 305.
13. Taylor PJ. Hemorrhage while on anticoagulant therapy precipitated by drug interaction. *Ariz Med* (1967) 24, 697–9.

Anticoagulants + Benzydamine Hydrochloride

Benzydamine does not alter the anticoagulant effects of phenprocoumon.

Clinical evidence, mechanism, importance and management

Fourteen patients on **phenprocoumon** showed no significant changes in their anticoagulant response while taking 150 mg **benzydamine** daily for 2 weeks, although there was some evidence of a fall in blood levels of the anticoagulant.[1] No particular precautions would seem necessary during concurrent use. Information about other anticoagulants is lacking.

1. Duckert F, Widmer LK, Madar G. Gleichzeitige Behandlung mit oralen Antikoagulantien und Benzydamin. *Schweiz Med Wochenschr* (1974) 104, 1069–71.

Anticoagulants + Beta-blockers

The effects of the oral anticoagulants are not normally affected by the concurrent use of beta-blocking drugs although one or two isolated and unexplained cases have been reported.

Clinical evidence, mechanism, importance and management

No clinically important interactions were seen in 5 patients on **warfarin** and **acebutolol**,[1] in 8 subjects on **warfarin** and **betaxolol**,[2] in 6 subjects on **warfarin** and **bisoprolol**,[3] in 10 men on **warfarin** and **esmolol**,[4] in 15 patients on **phenprocoumon** and **pindolol**,[5] or in 9 patients on **acenocoumarol (nicoumalone)** or **warfarin** given **atenolol** or **metoprolol**.[6] A 15% rise in the serum **warfarin** levels of 6 subjects was seen after taking 80 mg **propranolol** twice daily,[7] but while this was statistically significant it is unlikely to be clinically relevant. Single dose studies in 6 subjects on **warfarin** and **propranolol**, **metoprolol** or **atenolol** also demonstrated no clinically significant interactions.[8] A transient increase in **phenprocoumon** levels was seen in single dose studies in subjects given **metoprolol**,[9] but not when given **atenolol**[9] or **carvedilol**.[10,11] **Carvedilol** is also reported not to alter the *in vitro* protein binding of **warfarin**.[12]

In contrast, a patient on **warfarin** showed a marked rise in his British Corrected Ratio when given **propranolol**.[13] Haemorrhagic tendencies without any changes in Quick time or any other impairment of coagulation has been described in 2 patients on **phenindione** and **propranolol**.[14]

These findings confirm the general clinical experience that the effects of the oral anticoagulants are not normally affected by beta-blockers, but very rarely and quite unpredictably some changes may be seen. Monitor if **propranolol** is used, but only clinically minor or trivial effects are expected to occur in most individuals.

1. Ryan JR. Clinical pharmacology of acebutolol. *Am Heart J* (1985) 109, 1131.
2. Thiercelin JF, Warrington SJ, Thenot JP, Orofiamma B. Lack of interaction of betaxolol on warfarin induced hypocoagulability. In Proc 2nd Eur. Cong Biopharm Pharmacokinet. Vol III: Clinical Pharmacokinetics (published by Imprimerie de l'Universite de Clermont Ferrant, 1984) edited by Aiache JM and Hirtz J, pp 73–80.
3. Warrington SJ, Johnston A, Lewis Y, Murphy M. Bisoprolol: studies of potential interactions with theophylline and warfarin in healthy volunteers. *J Cardiovasc Pharmacol* (1990) 16 (Suppl 5), S164–S168.
4. Lowenthal DT, Porter RS, Saris SD, Bies CM, Slegowski MB, Staudacher A. Clinical pharmacology, pharmacodynamics and interactions of esmolol. *Am J Cardiol* (1985) 56, 14F–17F.
5. Vinazzer H. Effect of the beta-receptor blocking agent Visken® on the action of coumarin. *Int J Clin Pharmacol Biopharm* (1975) 12, 458–60.
6. Mantero F, Procidano M, Vicariotto MA , Girolami A. Effect of atenolol and metoprolol on the anticoagulant activity of acenocoumarin. *Br J Clin Pharmacol* (1984) 17, 94S–96S.
7. Scott AK, Park BK, Breckenridge AM. Interaction between warfarin and propranolol. *Br J Clin Pharmacol* (1984) 17, 86S.
8. Bax NDS, Lennard MS, Tucker GT, Woods HF, Porter NR, Malia RG, Preston FE. The effect of β-adrenoceptor antagonists on the pharmacokinetics and pharmacodynamics of warfarin after a single dose. *Br J Clin Pharmacol* (1984) 17, 553–7.

9. Spahn H, Kirch W, Mutschler E, Ohnhaus EE, Kitteringham NR, Lögering HJ, Paar D. Pharmacokinetic and pharmacodynamic interactions between phenprocoumon and atenolol or metoprolol. *Br J Clin Pharmacol* (1984) 17, 97S–102S.
10. Caspary S, Merz P-G, Brei R, Harder S. Interaction profile of carvedilol: investigations with digitoxin and phenprocoumon. *Int J Clin Pharmacol Ther Toxicol* (1992) 30, 537–8.
11. Harder S, Brei R, Caspary S, Merz PG. Lack of a pharmacokinetic interaction between carvedilol and digitoxin or phenprocoumon. *Eur J Clin Pharmacol* (1993) 44, 583–6.
12. Data on file, database on carvedilol, SmithKline Beecham, quoted by Ruffolo RR, Boyle DA, Venuti RP, Lukas MA. Carvedilol (Kredex®): a novel multiple action cardiovascular agent. *Drugs Today* (1991) 27, 465–92.
13. Bax NDS, Lennard MS, Al-Asady S, Deacon CS, Tucker GT, Woods HF. Inhibition of drug metabolism by antagonists. *Drugs* (1983) 25 (Suppl 2), 121–6.
14. Neilson GH, Seldon WA. Propranolol in angina pectoris. *Med J Aust* (1969) 1, 856.

Anticoagulants + Bicalutamide

The suggestion that bicalutamide might interact with warfarin appears to be based largely on questionable theoretical considerations.

Clinical evidence, mechanism, importance and management

The makers say[1] that "*in vitro* studies have shown that **bicalutamide** can displace the coumarin anticoagulant, **warfarin**, from its protein binding sites. It is therefore recommended that if **Casodex** 150 mg is started in patients who are already receiving coumarin anticoagulants, prothrombin time should be closely monitored." It used to be thought that the displacement of **warfarin** from its protein binding sites by other drugs normally resulted in clinically important interactions, but that is now known not to be true. So if it eventually turns out that **bicalutamide** interacts with **warfarin**, it is not likely to do so solely by protein binding displacement. The makers say that they do not know of any reports of **warfarin/bicalutamide** interactions, apart from an isolated case of a raised INR in one patient on **warfarin** who had taken three times the recommended dose of **bicalutamide**, but no causal link with **bicalutamide** was established.[2] There would therefore seem little reason at the moment to believe that **bicalutamide** in normal doses interacts with **warfarin**, but until more is known it would seem prudent to monitor the effects if it is started.

1. Casodex (Bicalutamide). AstraZeneca. Summary of product characteristics, November 2001.
2. Zeneca. Personal Communication, October 1995.

Anticoagulants + Boldo or Fenugreek

A report describes a woman on warfarin whose INR rose modestly when she began to take boldo and fenugreek.

Clinical evidence, mechanism, importance and management

A woman treated with **warfarin** for atrial fibrillation whose INRs normally fell within the range 2 to 3 showed a modest rise in her INR to 3.4, apparently being due to the additional use of 10 drops of **boldo** after meals and one capsule of **fenugreek** before meals to help her liver. A week after stopping these two herbal medicines her INR had fallen to 2.6. When she restarted them, her INR rose to 3.1 after a week and to 3.4 after 2 weeks. Her INR was later restabilised in the normal range in the presence of these two medicines by reducing the **warfarin** dosage by 15%.[1] The mechanism of this apparent interaction remains unknown, and it is not known whether both herbs or just one was responsible for what happened. **Boldo** comes from *Peumas boldus* and **fenugreek** from *Trigonelle foenum-graecum*, neither of which is recognised as having either anticoagulant or antiplatelet activity.

This patient showed no undesirable reactions (e.g. bruising or bleeding), but this case serves to draw attention to the possibility of an interaction in other patients on anticoagulants if these herbal medicines are taken concurrently.

1. Lambert JP, Cormier A. Potential interaction between warfarin and boldo-fenugreek. *Pharmacotherapy* (2001) 21, 509–12.

Anticoagulants + Broxuridine

The anticoagulant effects of warfarin were markedly increased in a patient after receiving a number of courses of broxuridine.

Clinical evidence, mechanism, importance and management

A 65-year-old man with grade III anaplastic astrocytoma under treatment with **warfarin** was given a number of courses of 1400 mg **broxuridine** daily iintravenously as a radiosensitiser. His prothrombin times were unaffected by the first 4-day course of **broxuridine**, but they became more prolonged with successive courses and after the fourth course his prothrombin time climbed to about 45 s which was treated with 10 mg vitamin K. A significant increase also took place when a fifth cycle of 990 mg **broxuridine** was given so that the **warfarin** had to be stopped.[1] The reason for this reaction is not understood. Those using **broxuridine** should be aware that this adverse interaction has occurred.

1. Oster SE, Lawrence HJ. Potentiation of anticoagulant effect of coumadin by 5-bromo-2'-deoxyuridine (BUDR). *Cancer Chemother Pharmacol* (1988) 22, 181.

Anticoagulants + Bucolome

Bucolome increases the anticoagulant effects of warfarin. The warfarin dosage should be reduced.

Clinical evidence

A study in Japanese patients on **warfarin** found that the addition of 300 mg bucolome daily in 21 patients increased their INRs 1.5-fold (despite a 58% **warfarin** dosage reduction) when compared with another group of 34 patients on **warfarin** not receiving bucolome.[1] In another 7-day study, 25 Japanese patients with heart disease on **warfarin** and **bucolome** (300 mg daily) were compared with another control group of 30 taking **warfarin** alone. It was found that **bucolome** had no effect on the serum levels of *(R)*-warfarin but both the serum levels of *(S)*-warfarin and the prothrombin times rose. These changes were complete within 7 days. The report of this study presents its results in the form of serum concentration/dose ratios and prothrombin time/dose ratios which obscure the extent of these changes, but the authors of this report conclude that the dose of **warfarin** should be reduced by 30 to 60% if **bucolome** is added to established **warfarin** treatment.[2] The authors of this study[2] also say that **bucolome** ". . . has been widely used as an enhancer for the anticoagulatory effect of **warfarin** in Japan . . ."

Mechanism

In vitro studies show that the bucolome can inhibit the metabolism of the more potent enantiomer *(S)*-warfarin by cytochrome P450 isoenzyme CYP2C9, thereby reducing its clearance and increasing its effects.[1]

Importance and management

Information appears to be limited to the reports cited here but the interaction would seem to be established and clinically important. A reduced warfarin dosage (the study cited above suggests a 30 to 60% reduction)[2] will be needed if both drugs are used concurrently to avoid excessive anticoagulation and possible bleeding. Information about other anticoagulants is lacking but be alert for this interaction with any of them. More study is needed.

1. Takahashi H, Kashima T, Kimura S, Murata N, Takaba T, Iwade K, Abe T, Tainaka H, Yasumori T, Echizen H. Pharmacokinetic interaction between warfarin and a uricosuric agent, bucolome: application of in vitro approaches to predicting in vivo reduction of (S)-warfarin clearance. *Drug Metab Dispos* (1999) 27, 1179–86.
2. Matsumoto K, Ishida S, Ueno K, Hashimoto H, Takada M, Tanaka K, Kamacura S, Miyatake K, Shibakawa M. The stereoselective effects of bucolome on the pharmacokinetics and pharmacodynamics of racemic warfarin. *J Clin Pharmacol* (2001) 41, 459–64.

Anticoagulants + Calcium channel blockers

Amlodipine, diltiazem and felodipine appear not to affect the anticoagulant effects of warfarin significantly, nor prenylamine the effects of phenprocoumon.

Clinical evidence, mechanism, importance and management

The makers say that studies in normal subjects have shown that **amlodipine** does significantly alter the effect of **warfarin** on prothrombin times.[1] **Felodipine** 10 mg daily for 14 days was found not to alter the anticoagulant effects of **warfarin** in normal subjects.[2] In another study, 10 men were given racemic **warfarin**, 8 *(R)*-warfarin as single 1.5 mg/kg intravenous doses, and 10 were given *(S)*-warfarin as single 0.75 mg/kg intravenous doses. After taking 120 mg diltiazem three times a day for 4 days the clearance of *(R)*-warfarin was decreased by about 20% but the more potent *(S)*-warfarin remained unaffected. The total anticoagulant response remained unchanged.[3] Two related studies by the same authors found that 30 mg diltiazem three times daily for a week caused no clinically relevant changes in the anticoagulant effects of **warfarin** in 20 normal subjects.[4,5] The addition of 60 mg **prenylamine** three times daily for 3 weeks had no effect on the prothrombin times of 30 patients with angina taking **phenprocoumon**.[6]

No special precautions would therefore seem to be necessary during concurrent use of any of these anticoagulant/calcium channel blocker pairs. Information about other anticoagulants and other calcium channel blockers appears to be lacking, but the absence of adverse reports about these very widely used drugs suggests that concurrent use is normally uneventful.

1. Istin (Amlodipine). Pfizer Limited. Summary of product characteristics, March 2000.
2. Grind M, Murphy M, Warrington S, Åberg J. Method for studying drug-warfarin interactions. *Clin Pharmacol Ther* (1993) 54, 381–7.
3. Abernethy DR, Kaminsky LS, Dickinson TH. Selective inhibition of warfarin metabolism by diltiazem in humans. *J Pharmacol Exp Ther* (1991) 257, 411–15.
4. Lucas BD, Mohiuddin SM, Stoysich AM, Destache CJ, Hunter CB, Stading JA, Hilleman DE. Assessment of a possible pharmacokinetic interaction between diltiazem and warfarin. *Pharmacotherapy* (1992) 12, 259.
5. Stoysich AM, Lucas BD, Mohiuddin SM, Milleman DE. Further elucidation of pharmacokinetic interaction between diltiazem and warfarin. *Int J Clin Pharmacol Ther* (1996) 34, 56–60.
6. Böhm C, Denes G. Untersuchung zur Erfassung eventueller Klinischer Interaktionen zwichsen Phenprocoumon und Prenylamin (Ergebnisse einer Multizenterstudie). *Acta Ther* (1987) 13, 333–43.

Anticoagulants + Carbamazepine or Oxcarbazepine

The anticoagulant effects of warfarin can be markedly reduced by carbamazepine. Its dosage may need to be approximately doubled to accommodate this interaction. Oxcarbazepine appears not to interact. A reduction in the anticoagulant effects of phenprocoumon due to carbamazepine has also been described in two patients.

Clinical evidence

(a) Phenprocoumon + Carbamazepine

A man in his mid-twenties developed multiple thrombotic episodes due to hereditary resistance to activated protein C. Because of cerebral embolic strokes he developed epileptic seizures and was started on 400 mg **carbamazepine** daily, followed 6 days later by **phenprocoumon**. It was found that relatively large doses (8 mg daily) had to be given to achieve adequate anticoagulation (prothrombin time ratio of 50 to 60%) until the **carbamazepine** was withdrawn, whereupon the **phenprocoumon** dosage could be reduced to 1.5 mg daily with a prothrombin time ratio of 30 to 40%.[1] Another patient on **phenprocoumon** showed a dramatic increase in his prothrombin time ratio when given **carbamazepine**. The values returned to normal when the **carbamazepine** was stopped.[2]

(b) Warfarin + Carbamazepine

Two patients on **warfarin** given **carbamazepine** (200 mg daily for the first week, 400 mg daily for the second and 600 mg for the third) showed an approximately 50% fall in serum **warfarin** levels which was reflected in sharp rises in their PP percentages.[3] The half-life of **warfarin** in three other patients fell by 53, 11 and 60% respectively when similarly treated.[3]

This interaction has been described in 6 other reports.[4-9] One of them describes a patient stabilised on both drugs who developed widespread dermal ecchymoses and a prothrombin time of 70 s a week after stopping the **carbamazepine**. She was restabilised on approximately half the dose of **warfarin** in the absence of the **carbamazepine**.[9]

(c) Warfarin + Oxcarbazepine

A study in 10 subjects on **warfarin** found that 450 mg **oxcarbazepine** twice daily for a week increased the Quick values from 41 to only 46.[10] A very similar study by the same workers found a change in Quick values from 36.6 to 38.1% due to **oxcarbazepine**.[11]

Mechanism

Uncertain, but the available evidence suggests that carbamazepine increases the metabolism of warfarin by the liver, thereby increasing its loss from the body and reducing its effects.[3,4] This may also possibly explain the phenprocoumon interaction. Oxcarbazepine on the other hand has relatively little enzyme inducing activity.

Importance and management

The warfarin/carbamazepine interaction is moderately well-documented, established and clinically important. The incidence is uncertain but monitor the anticoagulant response if carbamazepine is added to established treatment with warfarin and anticipate the need to double the dosage. Oxcarbazepine appears to be a relatively non-interacting alternative.

Information about the phenprocoumon/carbamazepine interaction seems to be limited to the two reports cited, nevertheless it would now be prudent to monitor concurrent use in any patient, being alert for the need to increase the phenprocoumon dosage. The same precautions would seem sensible with any other oral anticoagulant but information appears to be lacking.

1. Böttcher T, Buchmann J, Zettl U-K, Benecke R. Carbamazepine-phenprocoumon interaction. *Eur Neurol* (1997) 38, 132–3.
2. Schlienger R, Kurmann M, Drewe J, Müller-Spahn F, Seifritz E. Inhibition of phenprocoumon anticoagulation by carbamazepine. *Eur Neuropsychopharmacol* (2000) 10, 219–21.
3. Hansen JM, Siersbæk-Nielsen K, Skovsted L. Carbamazepine-induced acceleration of diphenylhydantoin and warfarin metabolism in man. *Clin Pharmacol Ther* (1971) 12, 539–43.
4. Ross JRY, Beeley L. Interaction between carbamazepine and warfarin. *BMJ* (1980) 1, 1415–16.
5. Kendall AG, Boivin M. Warfarin-carbamazepine interaction. *Ann Intern Med* (1981) 94, 280.
6. Massey EW. Effect of carbamazepine on Coumadin metabolism. *Ann Neurol* (1983) 13, 691–2.
7. Penry JK, Newmark ME. The use of antiepileptic drugs. *Ann Intern Med* (1981) 94, 280.
8. Beeley L, Stewart P, Hickey FM. Bulletin of the West Midlands for Adverse Drug Reaction Reporting (1988) 26, 18.
9. Denbow CE, Fraser HS. Clinically significant hemorrhage due to warfarin-carbamazepine interaction. *South Med J* (1990) 83, 981.
10. Krämer G, Tettenborn B, Klosterkov-Jensen P, Stoll KD. Oxcarbazepine-warfarin drug interaction study in healthy volunteers. *Epilepsia* (1991) 32 (Suppl 1), 70.
11. Krämer G, Tettenborn B, Klosterkov Jensen P, Menge GP, Stoll KD. Oxcarbazepine does not affect the anticoagulant activity of warfarin. *Epilepsia* (1992) 33, 1145–8.

Anticoagulants + Carbon tetrachloride

A single case report describes an increase in the anticoagulant effects of dicoumarol in a patient who accidentally drank some carbon tetrachloride.

Clinical evidence, mechanism, importance and management

A patient, well stabilised on **dicoumarol**, accidentally drank 0.1 ml **carbon tetrachloride**. Next day his prothrombin time had risen to 41 s (prothrombin activity fall from 18 to 10%). These values were approximately the same next day although the **dicoumarol** had been withdrawn, and marked hypoprothrombinaemia persisted for another 5 days.[1]

The probable reason for this reaction is that **carbon tetrachloride** is very toxic to the liver, the changed anticoagulant response being a manifestation of this. **Carbon tetrachloride**, once used as an anthelmintic in man, is no longer used in human medicine, but is still employed as an industrial solvent and degreasing agent. On theoretical grounds it would seem possible for anticoagulated patients exposed to substantial amounts of the vapour to experience this interaction but this has not been reported.

1. Luton EF. Carbon tetrachloride exposure during anticoagulant therapy. Dangerous enhancement of hypoprothrombinemic effect. *JAMA* (1965) 194, 1386–7.

Anticoagulants + Carnitine

An isolated report describes gastrointestinal bleeding and a marked increase in the anticoagulant effects of acenocoumarol (nicoumalone) in a patient given L-carnitine.

Clinical evidence, mechanism, importance and management

A woman who had taken acenocoumarol (nicoumalone) for 17 years because of aortic and mitral prosthetic valves was admitted to hospital with melaena within 5 days of starting to take 1 g L-carnitine daily. Her INR had risen from 2.1 to 7. Endoscopy and colonoscopy revealed diffuse bleeding from superficial erosions in the gut. She was discharged 10 days later on the same dose of acenocoumarol with an INR of 2.1 without the carnitine.[1] The reason for this apparent interaction is not known.

This seems to the first and only recorded case of an interaction between an oral anticoagulant and carnitine, but it would now be prudent to monitor the outcome if carnitine is added to a stable regime with any oral anticoagulant, being alert for an increased response.

1. Martinez E, Domingo P, Roca-Cusachs A. Potentiation of acenocoumarol action by L-carnitine. *J Intern Med* (1993) 233, 94.

Anticoagulants + Celecoxib

There is good evidence that celecoxib does not normally interact with warfarin but a few isolated and rare cases of raised INRs accompanied by bleeding have been attributed to the concurrent use of warfarin and celecoxib.

Clinical evidence, mechanism, importance and management

24 normal subjects were given 2 to 5 mg **warfarin** daily to produce a stable prothrombin time of 1.2 to 1.7 times their pretreatment values for at least 3 consecutive days. They were then additionally given 200 mg **celecoxib** or placebo twice daily for a week. It was found that the pharmacokinetics of both the *S*- and *R*-enantiomers of **warfarin**

and the prothrombin times were unchanged by the presence of the **celecoxib**.[1,2]

However, in contrast, a report describes an increased INR and bleeding (haemoptysis), orthopnoea and dyspnoea on exercise which developed in a 73-year old woman on **warfarin** 5 weeks after **celecoxib** was added. This patient also had hypothyroidism and heart failure. Her INR restabilised when the **warfarin** and **celecoxib** were stopped and vitamin K was given.[3] What is not clear is whether the **celecoxib** alone was responsible for what happened. Another report describes a woman of 88 on **warfarin** who also showed an INR rise when 200 mg **celecoxib** was started. After several **warfarin** dosage adjustments she was later restabilised on a 25% lower **warfarin** dose.[4] The makers also report[5] that ". . . bleeding events have been reported, predominantly in the elderly, in association with increases in prothrombin time in patients receiving *Celebrex* (**celecoxib**) concurrently with **warfarin**."

These cases of interaction need to be set in the broad context of the 4 million prescriptions for **celecoxib** which were dispensed over the 18-month period from December 1998, approximately 1% of which it is estimated were for patients who would have been on **warfarin**,[5] so that the incidence of this adverse interaction is clearly very low indeed. Even so it would now seem prudent to monitor INRs in patients on **warfarin** if **celecoxib** is added or removed so that any rare cases of interaction can be identified and dealt with accordingly. Information about **other anticoagulants** appears to be lacking but the same precautions would seem appropriate.

1. Karim A, Tolbert D, Piergies A, Hunt T, Hubbard R, Harper K, Slater M, Geis GS. Celecoxib, a specific COX-2 inhibitor, lacks significant drug-drug interactions with methotrexate or warfarin. *Arthritis Rheum* (1998) 41 (9 Suppl), S315.
2. Karim A, Tolbert D, Piergies A, Hubbard RC, Harper K, Wallemark C-B, Slater M, Geis GS. Celecoxib does not significantly alter the pharmacokinetics or hypoprothrombinemic effect of warfarin in healthy subjects. *J Clin Pharmacol* (2000) 40, 655–63.
3. Mersfedler TL, Stewart LR. Warfarin and celecoxib interaction. *Ann Pharmacother* (2000) 34, 325–7.
4. Haase KK, Rojas-Fernandez CH, Lane L, Frank DA. Potential interaction between celecoxib and warfarin. *Ann Pharmacother* (2000) 34, 666–7.
5. FDA MedWatch Program, May 1999. Available at: http://www.fda.gov/medwatch/safety/1999/celebr.htm (accessed 21/12/2000).

Anticoagulants + Cephalosporins or Vancomycin

Most cephalosporins do not interact with oral anticoagulants, but those with an *N*-methylthiotetrazole side-chain and some others can occasionally cause enough hypoprothrombinaemia for bleeding to occur when used alone. These effects can be additive with those of conventional anticoagulants. See the text for the named drugs. Vancomycin possibly causes a small increase in the effects of warfarin.

Clinical evidence

A study of this interaction was prompted by 2 patients who developed unusually high prothrombin times (one of them bled) when given **warfarin** and **cefamandole** (**cephamandole**). Sixty other patients undergoing heart valve replacement surgery were given antibacterials prophylactically before the chest incision was made, and at six-hourly intervals thereafter for about 72 h. Those given 2 g **cefamandole** (44 patients) and to a lesser extent **cefazolin** (**cephazolin**) showed a much greater anticoagulant response than those given 500 mg **vancomycin** (16 patients).[1] A later study by the same workers confirmed these findings. After three days of concurrent use the prothrombin times as a percentage of activity were as follows: **cefamandole** 29%, **cefazolin** 38%, **vancomycin** 51%.[2]

Serious bleeding following the use of **cefamandole** (in the absence of an anticoagulant) has been described in 3 out of 37 patients in another report,[3] Seven other cases are described elsewhere.[4]

Other cephalosporins which when used *alone* have been reported to cause hypoprothrombinaemia include **cefoperazone**,[5-9] **cefotetan**,[10] **cefoxitin**,[11] **ceftriaxone**,[12] **cefalotin** (**cephalothin**),[13] **cefazolin**,[14-16] and **latamoxef** (**moxalactam**).[11,17] Extended prothrombin times are also said to occur with **cefaloridine** (**cephaloridine**).[18]

Cefixime with anticoagulants (**warfarin, phenindione**) has also been implicated in a handful of cases of bleeding and/or increased INRs, but the evidence is inconclusive[19] and no problems were found in another small study in which **cefixime** was used.[20] In the UK the CSM's 'Drug Analysis Print' covering the period 1979–97 very briefly records raised INRs in three patients on **acenocoumarol, warfarin** or an **unknown anticoagulant** when given **cefaclor**. When set against the extensive use of **cefaclor** over almost 30 years, these interactions are clearly very rare indeed.[21,22]

Severe haemorrhage has been reported in 3 patients on **acenocoumarol** (**nicoumalone**) when treated with **cefotiam.** One developed an abdominal haematoma and an INR of 10.4 within 2 days. Another had gastrointestinal bleeding and melaena after one day's use. The third died from intracranial haemorrhage on the day she started **cefotiam**.[23] A study in nine patients on **warfarin** failed to find a clinically relevant interaction with **cefonicid**,[24] however a later study identified 9 patients on **acenocoumarol** (**nicoumalone**) who showed increased INRs within 3 to 8 days of being given **cefonicid**. They needed a reduction in the anticoagulant dosage of betwen about one-third to one-half.[25] A patient on **acenocoumarol** bled after being additionally given **cefonicid**.[26]

Mechanism

Cephalosporins with an *N*-methylthiotetrazole side-chain can act like the oral anticoagulants as vitamin K antagonists to reduce the production of the blood clotting factors. They can therefore cause bleeding on their own and worsen the risk of bleeding by simple addition if given with conventional anticoagulants. In addition some of them may also inhibit platelet function.[27] Ceftriaxone seems to act similarly although it has an *N*-methylthiotriazine ring instead.

Importance and management

Most cephalosporins do not normally cause bleeding or interact with the oral anticoagulants. This is confirmed by general experience and by a small study in patients given **warfarin** and **cefuroxime**, **cefalexin** (**cephalexin**) or **cefradine** (**cephradine**)[20]. In contrast, the 'risky' cephalosporins are those cited in the 'Clinical Evidence' above, namely **cefaclor**, **cefaloridine** (**cephaloridine**), **cefalotin** (**cephalothin**), **cefazolin** (**cephazolin**), **cefixime**, **cefonicid**, **cefoperazone**, **cefotetan**, **cefotiam**, **cefoxitin**, **ceftriaxone**, **cephamandole** and **latamoxef** (**moxalactam**). All of these have sometimes caused bleeding alone or in the presence of an anticoagulant. The incidence is very variable: in some instances only isolated cases have been reported whereas a15% bleeding rate was found in one study with **latamoxef** alone, 22% in another, but only 8% with **cefoxitin** alone.[11,28] Patients most at risk seem to be those whose intake of vitamin K is restricted (poor diet, malabsorption syndromes, etc.) and those with renal failure. The use of an anticoagulant represents just another factor which may precipitate bleeding.

A possible solution to the problem is to use a non-interacting cephalosporin. Alternatively you should monitor the outcome closely, particularly in the early stages of treatment, adjusting the anticoagulant dosage if necessary. Excessive hypoprothrombinaemia can be controlled with vitamin K.

A number of cephalosporins which also possess the *N*-methylthiotetrazole side-chain are expected to behave similarly, but have not so far been reported to do so. These include **cefazeflur**, **cefmenoxime**, **cefmetazole**, **cefminox**, **ceforanide** and **cefpiramide**. The situation with **cefixime** is still uncertain.[19,20]

The study[1] cited above in which surgical patients were given warfarin with either a cephalosporin or **vancomycin** indicates that vancomycin interacts with **warfarin** but the increase in prothrombin times seems not to be large. There seem to be no reports of problems with vancomycin and **warfarin** or any other anticoagulant, but it would seem prudent to monitor prothrombin times if both drugs are used.

1. Angaran DM, Dias VC, Arom KV, Northrup WF, Kersten TE, Lindsay WG, Nicoloff DM. The influence of prophylactic antibiotics on the warfarin anticoagulation response in the postoperative prosthetic cardiac valve patient. *Ann Surg* (1984) 199, 107–111.

2. Angaran DM, Dias VC, Arom KV, Northrup WF, Kersten TG, Lindsay WG, Nicoloff DM. The comparative influence of prophylactic antibiotics on the prothrombin response to warfarin in the postoperative prothetic cardiac valve patients. *Ann Surg* (1987) 206, 155–61.
3. Hooper CA, Haney BB, Stone HH. Gastrointestinal bleeding due to vitamin K deficiency in patients on parenteral cefamandole. *Lancet* (1980) i, 39–40.
4. Rymer W, Greenlaw CW. Hypoprothrombinemia associated with cefamandole. *Drug Intell Clin Pharm* (1980) 14, 780–3.
5. Meisel S. Hypoprothrombinaemia due to cefoperazone. *Drug Intell Clin Pharm* (1984) 18, 316.
6. Cristiano P. Hypoprothrombinemia associated with cefoperazone treatment. *Drug Intell Clin Pharm* (1984) 18, 314–16.
7. Osborne JC. Hypoprothrombinemia and bleeding due to cefoperazone. *Ann Intern Med* (1985) 102, 721–2.
8. Freedy HR, Cetnarowski AB, Lumish RM, Schafer FJ. Cefoperazone-induced coagulopathy. *Drug Intell Clin Pharm* (1986) 20, 281–3.
9. Andrassy K, Kodersich J, Fritz S, Bechtold H, Sonntag H. Alteration of hemostasis associated with cefoperazone treatment. *Infection* (1986) 14, 27–31.
10. Conjura A, Bell W, Lipsky JJ. Cefotetan and hypoprothrombinemia. *Ann Intern Med* (1988) 108, 643.
11. Brown RB, Klar J, Lemeshow S, Teres D, Pastides H, Sands M. Enhanced bleeding with cefoxitin or moxalactam. Statistical analysis within a defined population of 1493 patients. *Arch Intern Med* (1986) 146, 2159–64.
12. Haubenstock A, Schmidt P, Zazgornik J, Balcke P, Kopsa H. Hypoprothrombinaemic bleeding associated with ceftriaxone. *Lancet* (1983) 1, 1215–16.
13. Natelson EA, Brown CH, Bradshaw MW. Influence of cephalosporin antibiotics on blood coagulation and platelet function. *Antimicrob Agents Chemother* (1976) 9, 91–3.
14. Lerner PI, Lubin A. Coagulopathy with cefazolin in uremia. *N Engl J Med* (1974) 290, 1324.
15. Khaleeli M, Giorgio AJ. Defective platelet function after cephalosporin administration. *Blood* (1976) 48, 971.
16. Dupuis LL, Paton TW, Suttie JW, Thiessen JJ, Rachlis A. Cefazolin-induced coagulopathy. *Clin Pharmacol Ther* (1984) 35, 237.
17. Beeley L, Beadle R and Lawrence R. Bulletin of the West Midlands Centre for Adverse Drug Reaction Reporting (1984) 19, 15.
18. Council on Drugs. Evaluation of a new antibacterial agent, cephaloridine (Loridine). *JAMA* (1986) 206, 1289.
19. Lederle Laboratories. Personal communication, December 1995.
20. Pharmacy Anticoagulant Clinic Study Group. A multicentre survey of the effect of antibiotics on the INR of anticoagulated patients. *Pharm J* (1996) 257 (Pharmacy Practice Suppl), R30.
21. Distaclor (Cefaclor). Dista Products Limited. Summary of product characteristics, May 1999.
22. Dista Products Limited. Personal communication, December 1997.
23. Gras-Champel V, Sauvé L, Perault MC, Laine P, Gouello JP, Decocq G, Masson H, Touzard M, Andréjak M. Association cefotiam et acenocoumarol: a propos de 3 cas d'hémorragies. *Therapie* (1998) 53, 191.
24. Angaran DM, Tschida VH, Copa AK. Effect of cefonicid (CN) on prothrombin time (PT) in outpatients (OP) receiving warfarin (W) therapy. *Pharmacotherapy* (1988) 8, 120.
25. Puente Garcia M, Bécares Martinez FJ, Merlo Arroyo J, García Sánchez G, García Díaz B, Cervero Jiménez M. Potenciación del efecto anticoagulante del acenocoumaril por cefonicid. *Rev Clin Esp* (1999) 199, 620–1.
26. Riancho JA, Olmos JM, Sedano C. Life-threatening bleeding in a patient being treated with cefonicid. *Ann Intern Med* (1995) 123, 472–3.
27. Bang NU, Tessler SS, Heidenreich RO, Marks CA, Mattler LE. Effects of moxalactam on blood coagulation and platelet function. *Rev Infect Dis* (1982) 4 (Suppl), S546–S554.
28. Morris DL. Fabricius PJ, Ambrose NS, Scammell B, Burdon DW, Keighley MRB. A high incidence of bleeding is observed in a trial to determine whether addition of metronidazole is neeeded with latamoxef for prophylaxis in colorectal surgery. *J Hosp Infect* (1984) 5, 398–408.

Anticoagulants + Cetirizine

An isolated report describes bleeding and a markedly raised INR in an old man on acenocoumarol (nicoumalone) when given cetirizine.

Clinical evidence, mechanism, importance and management

A man of 88 taking acenocoumarol (nicoumalone) for deep-vein thrombosis developed acute and severe epistaxis after a fall within 3 days of starting to take 10 mg cetirizine daily for allergic rhinitis.[1] He was also taking amitriptyline, amlodipine and spironolactone. His INR was found to have risen from 1.5 to 14. The authors of this report suggest that the cetirizine concentration may have been particularly high because of some renal impairment, and that it displaced the acenocoumarol from its plasma protein binding sites thereby increasing its effects, however it should be said that this mechanism of interaction on its own is now largely discredited as an explanation for interactions between anticoagulants and highly bound drugs. This appears to be the first and only report of an anticoagulant/cetirizine interaction and it seems unlikely to be of general importance.

1. Berod T, Mathiot I. Probable interaction between cetirizine and acenocoumarol. *Ann Pharmacother* (1997) 31, 122.

Anticoagulants + Chloral hydrate, Chloral betaine or Triclofos

The anticoagulant effects of warfarin are transiently increased by chloral hydrate, but this is normally of little or no clinical importance. Chloral betaine, petrichloral and triclofos may be expected to behave similarly.

Clinical evidence

A retrospective study on 32 patients just starting on **warfarin** showed that while the loading doses of **warfarin** in the control and **chloral hydrate**-treated groups were the same, the **warfarin** requirements of the **chloral** group during the first 4 days fell by about one-third, but rose again to normal by the fifth day.[1]

A study on 10 patients and 4 normal subjects taking **warfarin** showed that when given 1 g **chloral hydrate** each night, there was a minor, clinically unimportant and short-lived increase in the prothrombin times of 5 of them during the first few days of concurrent treatment, but no change in the overall long-term anticoagulant control occurred.[2]

Similar results have been described in other studies on large numbers of patients taking **warfarin** and **chloral hydrate**[3-8] or **triclofos**.[9] **Chloral betaine** appears to behave similarly.[10] An isolated and by no means fully explained case of fatal hypoprothrombinaemia in a patient on **dicoumarol** who was given **chloral** for 10 days, later replaced by secobarbital, has been reported.[11] Another patient on **dicoumarol** and **chloral** showed a reduction in prothrombin times.[11]

Mechanism

Chloral hydrate is mainly metabolised to trichloroacetic acid which then successfully competes with warfarin for its binding sites on plasma proteins.[6] As a result, free and active molecules of warfarin flood into plasma water by displacement so that the effects of the warfarin are increased. But this is only short-lived because the warfarin molecules become exposed to metabolism by the liver, so that their effects are reduced once more.

Importance and management

The warfarin/chloral interaction is well-documented and well understood, but normally of little or no clinical importance. There is very good evidence that concurrent use need not be avoided,[1-8] however the ultracautious might wish to keep an eye on the anticoagulant response during the first 4 to 5 days. It is not certain whether other anticoagulants behave in the same way because the evidence is sparse, indirect and inconclusive,[11-13] but what is known suggests that they probably do.

Triclofos[9] and **chloral betaine**[10] appear to behave like **chloral hydrate**, and **petrichloral** may also be expected to do so. **Dichloralphenazone** on the other hand interacts quite differently (see 'Anticoagulants + Dichloralphenazone', p.256).

1. Boston Collaborative Drug Surveillance Program. Interaction between chloral hydrate and warfarin. *N Engl J Med* (1972) 286, 53–5.
2. Udall JA. Warfarin-chloral hydrate interaction. Pharmacological activity and significance. *Ann Intern Med* (1974) 81, 341–4.
3. Griner PF, Raisz LG, Rickles FR, Wiesner PJ, Odoroff CL. Chloral hydrate and warfarin interaction: clinical significance? *Ann Intern Med* (1971) 74, 540–3.
4. Udall JA. Clinical implications of warfarin interactions with five sedatives. *Am J Cardiol* (1975) 35, 67–71.
5. Udall JA. Warfarin interactions with chloral hydrate and glutethimide. *Curr Ther Res* (1975) 17, 67–74.
6. Sellers EM, Koch-Weser J. Kinetics and clinical importance of displacement of warfarin from albumin by acidic drugs. *Ann N Y Acad Sci* (1971) 179, 213–25.
7. Breckenridge A, Orme ML'E, Thorgeirsson S, Davies DS, Brooks RV. Drug interactions with warfarin: studies with dichloralphenazone, chloral hydrate and phenazone (antipyrine). *Clin Sci* (1971) 40, 351–64.
8. Breckenridge A, Orme M. Clinical implications of enzyme induction. *Ann N Y Acad Sci* (1971) 179, 421–31.
9. Sellers EM, Lang M, Koch-Weser J, Colman RW. Enhancement of warfarin-induced hypoprothrombinemia by triclofos. *Clin Pharmacol Ther* (1972) 13, 911–15.
10. MacDonald MG, Robinson DS, Sylwester D, Jaffe JJ. The effects of phenobarbital, chloral betaine, and glutethimide administration on warfarin plasma levels and hypoprothrombinemic responses in man. *Clin Pharmacol Ther* (1969) 10, 80–4.
11. Cucinell SA, Odessky L, Weiss M, Dayton PG. The effect of chloral hydrate on bishydroxycoumarin metabolism. A fatal outcome. *JAMA* (1966) 197, 144–6.

12. Dayton PG, Tarcam Y, Chenkin T, Wiener M. The influence of barbiturates on coumarin plasma levels on prothrombin response. *J Clin Invest* (1961) 40, 1797.
13. van Dam FE, Gribnau-Overkamp MJH. The effect of some sedatives (phenobarbital, gluthetimide, chlordiazepoxide, chloral hydrate) on the rate of disappearance of ethyl biscoumacetate from the plasma. *Folia Med Neerl* (1967) 10, 141–5.

Anticoagulants + Chloramphenicol

There is some limited evidence that the anticoagulant effects of acenocoumarol (nicoumalone), dicoumarol and possibly ethyl biscoumacetate can be increased by the concurrent use of oral chloramphenicol. An isolated report attributes a marked INR rise in a patient on warfarin to the use of chloramphenicol eye drops.

Clinical evidence

A study in 4 patients showed that the half-life of **dicoumarol** was increased on average by a factor of three (from 8 to 25 h) when treated with 2 g **chloramphenicol** daily for 5 to 8 days.[1]

Three out of 9 patients taking an **unnamed anticoagulant** showed a fall in their Prothrombin-Proconvertin values from a range of 10 to 30% down to less than 6% when given 1 to 2 g **chloramphenicol** daily for 4 to 6 days. One patient showed a smaller reduction.[2] There is another report of an increased anticoagulant response involving **acenocoumarol (nicoumalone)**, and a brief comment implicating, but not confirming, an interaction involving **dicoumarol** and **ethyl biscoumacetate**.[3]

An isolated report describes a woman of 83 on **warfarin** who showed a rise in her INR to 8.92 from a normal range of 1.9 to 2.8 within 2 weeks of starting to use eye drops containing **chloramphenicol** 5 mg, dexamethasone sodium phosphate 1 mg and tetrahydrozoline hydrochloride 0.25 mg in each ml. She used one drop in each eye four times daily.[4] Hypoprothrombinaemia and bleeding have also been described in patients on **chloramphenicol** in the absence of an anticoagulant.[5,6]

Mechanism

Uncertain. One suggestion is that the chloramphenicol inhibits the liver enzymes concerned with the metabolism of the anticoagulants so that their effects are prolonged and increased.[1] Another is that the antibacterial decimates the gut bacteria thereby decreasing a source of vitamin K, but it is doubtful if these bacteria are normally an important source of the vitamin except in exceptional cases where dietary levels are very inadequate.[7] A third suggestion is that chloramphenicol blocks production of prothrombin by the liver.[5]

Importance and management

The documentation for the anticoagulant/oral chloramphenicol interaction is very sparse and poor (the best being the report about dicoumarol) so that this interaction is by no means adequately established. There would therefore appear to be little reason for avoiding concurrent use, but for complete safety it might be prudent to monitor prothrombin times if oral chloramphenicol is started in patients taking any anticoagulant, being alert for the need to reduce the anticoagulant dosage.

The report about an apparent warfarin/topical chloramphenicol interaction is very surprising because the amount of chloramphenicol absorbed from eye drops is relatively small and because, despite the very widespread use of warfarin and chloramphenicol for very many years, this report appears to be the only one implicating warfarin and chloramphenicol in any form. This suggests that any such interaction is very unlikely indeed, however the ultracautious may wish to monitor the outcome if topical chloramphenicol is used.

1. Christensen LK, Skovsted L. Inhibition of drug metabolism by chloramphenicol. *Lancet* (1969) ii, 1397.
2. Magid E. Tolerance to anticoagulants during antibiotic therapy. *Scand J Clin Lab Invest* (1962) 14, 565–6.
3. Johnson R, David A, Chartier Y. Clinical experience with G-23350 (Sintrom). *Can Med Assoc J* (1957) 77, 759–61.

4. Leone R, Ghiotto E, Conforti A, Velo G. Potential interaction between warfarin and ocular chloramphenicol. *Ann Pharmacother* (1999) 33, 114.
5. Klippel AP, Pitsinger B. Hypoprothrombinemia secondary to antibiotic therapy and manifested by massive gastrointestinal hemorrhage. *Arch Surg* (1968) 96, 266–8.
6. Matsaniotis N, Messaritikas J, Vlachou C. Hypoprothrombinaemic bleeding in infants associated with diarrhoea and antibiotics. *Arch Dis Child* (1970) 45, 586–7.
7. Udall JA. Human sources and absorption of vitamin K in relation to anticoagulant stability. *JAMA* (1965), 194, 107.

Anticoagulants + Cinchophen

The anticoagulant effects of dicoumarol, ethyl biscoumacetate and phenindione are markedly increased by cinchophen. Bleeding will occur if the anticoagulant dosage is not reduced appropriately.

Clinical evidence

A patient on an **un-named anticoagulant** was given a total of 4 g **cinchophen** over a period of 2 days, at the end of which his prothrombin levels were found to be less than 5%. The next day he had haematemeses and died. This prompted a study in three patients taking **phenindione**, **ethyl biscoumacetate** or **dicoumarol**. Within 2 days of starting 4 g **cinchophen** daily the prothrombin levels of two of them fell sharply from a range of 10 to 25% to less than 5%. A smaller fall occurred in the third patient.[1]

Mechanism

Cinchophen by itself appears to have a direct effect on the liver, like the oral anticoagulants, which reduces the synthesis of prothrombin.[2] There is a latent period similar to that of dicoumarol before the fall in blood prothrombin levels begins, and a short delay after its withdrawal before the prothrombin levels rise again.[1] Its effects can be reversed by the administration of vitamin K.[3] This interaction would therefore seem to result from the additive effects of two anticoagulant drugs.

Importance and management

Direct information about this interaction seems to be limited to the report cited,[1] but what is known suggests that it is of clinical importance. Its incidence is uncertain. Cinchophen should not be given to patients on any anticoagulant unless the prothrombin times can be well monitored and the dosage reduced appropriately.

1. Jarnum S. Cinchophen and acetylsalicylic acid in anticoagulant treatment. *Scand J Clin Lab Invest* (1954) 6, 91–3.
2. Hueper WC. Toxicity and detoxication of cinchophen. *Arch Pathol* (1946) 41, 592–600.
3. Rawls WB. Prevention of cinchophen toxicity by use of vitamin K. *N Y State J Med* (1942) 42, 2021–3.

Anticoagulants + Cisapride

Cisapride normally causes only a small increase in the anticoagulant effects of acenocoumarol (nicoumalone) and a small fall in the effects of warfarin, although an isolated report describes a marked increase in one patient on warfarin. Phenprocoumon appears not to interact.

Clinical evidence

(a) Acenocoumarol (Nicoumalone)

Twenty-two patients on **acenocoumarol** showed an increase in thrombotest values while on **cisapride** (10 mg three times daily for 3 weeks). These values fell when the **cisapride** was stopped.[1]

(b) Phenprocoumon

A study in 24 normal subjects found that 10 mg **cisapride** four times daily did not significantly affect the anticoagulant effects of **phenprocoumon**.[2]

(c) Warfarin

Twelve normal subjects on **warfarin** showed a small but statistically insignificant rise in their **warfarin** requirements (from 44.5 to 49 mg) when given 10 mg **cisapride** daily for 25 days.[3] This contrasts with a report of a 75-year-old man with a heart valve prothesis and well stabilised on **warfarin** whose INR rose from 2.2 to 2.5 to 10.7 within 3 weeks of stopping 10 mg **metoclopramide** four times daily and starting 10 mg **cisapride** four times daily. It seems doubtful if stopping the metoclopramide or any other factors were responsible.[4]

Mechanism

The increased acenocoumarol effects were attributed to an increase in gastrointestinal motility caused by cisapride which increased acenocoumarol absorption. The warfarin/cisapride interaction is not understood.

Importance and management

Information appears to be limited to the reports cited here which indicate that normally cisapride causes only very small changes in the anticoagulant effects of acenocoumarol (nicoumalone) and warfarin, except in one isolated case where a marked increase in warfarin effects occurred. However to be on the safe side it seems advisable to monitor the effects briefly after starting or stopping cisapride so that the anticoagulant dosage can be modified if needed (a maker's recommendation[5]). Phenprocoumon apparently does not interact. Information about other anticoagulants appears to be lacking.

1. Janssen Pharmacetica (Jonker JJC). Effect of cisapride on anticoagulant treatment with acenocoumarol. Data on file (Clinical Research Report, R 51619-NL), August 1985.
2. Wesemeyer D, Mönig H, Gaska T, Masuch S, Seiler KU, Huss H, Bruhn HD. Der Einfluß von Cisaprid und Metoclopramid auf die Bioverfügbarkeit von Phenprocoumon. Hamostaseologie (1991) 11, 95–102.
3. Daneshmend TK, Mahida YR, Bhaskar NK, Hawkey CJ. Does cisapride alter the anticoagulant effect of warfarin? A pharmacodynamic assessment. British Society of Gastroenterology Spring Meeting, 12–14 April 1989.
4. Darlington MR. Hypoprothrombinemia induced by warfarin sodium and cisapride. Am J Health-Syst Pharm (1997) 54, 320–1.
5. Prepulsid (Cisapride). Janssen-Cilag Ltd. ABPI Compendium of Datasheets and Summaries of Product Characteristics, 1999–2000, p 655–6.

Anticoagulants + Clarithromycin

A marked increase in the effects of warfarin with bleeding has been seen in a few patients when concurrently treated with clarithromycin. A marked increase in INRs occurred in six patients on acenocoumarol (nicoumalone) and in another on phenprocoumon when given clarithromycin.

Clinical evidence

(a) Acenocoumarol (Nicoumalone)

A woman of 75 on long-term treatment with **acenocoumarol** showed a rise in her INR from 2.1 to 9 within a week of starting to take 250 mg **clarithromycin** twice daily.[1] Five patients on **acenocoumarol** showed a mean increase in their INRs from 2.46 to 5.51 when treated with **clarithromycin**.[2] The largest increase was from 1.95 to 7.01.

(b) Phenprocoumon

A woman of 70 using **phenprocoumon** chronically developed a marked increase in prothrombin times but no bleeding within four days of starting 500 mg **clarithromycin** daily. The **phenprocoumon** was stopped and phytomenadione administered. When the antibacterial was withdrawn she was restabilised on the original dosage of **phenprocoumon**.[3]

(c) Warfarin

A man of 68 on **warfarin** for a heart valve replacement and also taking sertraline and metoprolol, was started on a 5-day course of **clarithromycin** (dose not stated). He very rapidly developed haematuria and was found to have a prothrombin time of 57 s. The **warfarin** was stopped and after two doses of vitamin K he was discharged on his usual 5-mg dose of **warfarin**. Another patient developed prothrombin times in the high 20s within a week of starting 1 g **clarithromycin** daily and his **warfarin** dosage was accordingly halved. When the **clarithromycin** was stopped and the **warfarin** dosage was raised again to its usual dose his prothrombin times fell again to their former values. A man on **warfarin** with INRs in the range 1.61 to 3.99 developed an INR of 16.8 within 17 days of starting 500 mg **clarithromycin** twice daily.[4] Two patients on **warfarin** showed marked increases in INRs (to 9.03 and 5.6) 5 days after starting clarithromycin.[5] A woman of 72 stabilised on **warfarin** developed an INR of 7.3 within 12 days of starting to take 500 mg **clarithromycin** three times daily.[6] Suprachoroidal haemorrhage occurred in a woman on **warfarin** after taking 500 mg **clarithromycin** daily for a week. Her INR had risen from 2.3 to 8.2.[7] One out of 12 patients on **warfarin** and **clarithromycin** in a clinical study showed a potential anticoagulant effect (purpura) which was not considered by the investigator to be related to the use of **clarithromycin**, however the manufacturers of **clarithromycin** have a number of individual case reports on record describing patients worldwide on **warfarin** who have shown elevated prothrombin times (sometimes accompanied by serious bleeding) when they were treated with clarithromycin.[8] In 1992 the CSM notified[9] prescribers in the UK of a case of a woman taking **warfarin** for mitral valve disease who suffered a fatal cerebrovascular bleed 3 days after starting to take **clarithromycin**. Her INR was above 10.

Mechanism

Not known. Clarithromycin is a macrolide related to erythromycin. It possibly binds in a similar way to cytochrome P450 to form inactive complexes which reduce the metabolism of these anticoagulants, resulting in a reduction in their clearance and an increase in their effects.

Importance and management

The warfarin/clarithromycin interaction is established and potentially serious, but unpredictable and uncommon. Far less is known about the interaction of clarithromycin with phenprocoumon and acenocoumarol (nicoumalone), limited apparently to the reports cited here, but these interactions are equally unpredictable and uncommon. Since it is not known who is likely to be affected, you should monitor prothrombin times in any patient when clarithromycin is first added because the reaction when it occurs can be rapid. Erythromycin is not a good alternative antibacterial because it appears to interact similarly, but there is good evidence that azithromycin and midecamycin diacetate (miocamycin) are normally non-interacting alternative macrolides, but see the individual monographs for details. Information about other oral anticoagulants seems to be lacking but it would seem prudent to use the same precautions with any of them.

1. Grau E, Real E, Pastor E. Interaction between clarithromycin and oral anticoagulants. Ann Pharmacother (1996) 30, 1495–6.
2. Sánchez B, Muruzábal MJ, Peralta G, Santiago G, Castilla A, Aguilera JP, Arjona R. Clarithromycin-oral anticoagulants interaction. Report of five cases. Clin Drug Invest (1997) 13, 220–2.
3. Meyboom RHB, Heere FJ, Egberts ACG, Lastdrager CJ. Vermoedelijke potentiëring van fenprocoumon door claritromycine en roxitromycine. Ned Tijdschr Geneeskd (1996) 140, 375–7.
4. Recker MW, Kier KL. Potential interaction between clarithromycin and warfarin. Ann Pharmacother (1997) 31, 996–8.
5. Oberg KC. Delayed elevation of international normalized ratio with concurrent clarithromycin and warfarin therapy. Pharmacotherapy (1998) 18, 386–91.
6. Gooderham MJ, Bolli P, Fernandez PG. Concomitant digoxin toxicity and warfarin interaction in a patient receiving clarithromycin. Ann Pharmacother (1999) 33, 796-9.
7. Dandekar SS, Laidlaw DAH. Suprachoroidal haemorrhage after addition of clarithromycin. J R Soc Med (2001) 94, 583-4.
8. Abbott Laboratories. Data on file, February 1995.
9. Committee on Safety of Medicines. Reminders: interaction between macrolide antibiotics and warfarin. Current Problems (1992) 35, 4.

Anticoagulants + Clindamycin

An isolated report describes bleeding and a markedly increased INR in a woman tentatively attributed to a warfa-

rin/clindamycin interaction. She had multiple medical conditions and was also taking a whole range of other drugs.

Clinical evidence, mechanism, importance and management

A woman of 47 with multiple medical problems on **warfarin** (and also taking azathioprine, captopril, furosemide (frusemide), insulin, captopril, prednisone, thyroxine, valproic acid and zolpidem) had all her teeth removed under the general anaesthetic. Sixteen days later she needed a dental abscess drained and was started on 300 mg oral **clindamycin** four times daily with 600 mg ibuprofen for any discomfort. On day 17 she needed a suture to stop some bleeding and her INR was found to be 3.5. By day 20 she had developed more severe oral bleeding which needed emergency room treatment. Her INR was found to have risen to 13 and her haematocrit 18%. She was treated successfully with a blood transfusion and vitamin K.[1]

This appears to be an isolated case from which no general conclusions should be drawn because the whole picture is so obscure and uncertain. This woman had a history of rheumatic fever, an artificial heart valve, hypertension, diabetes, arthritis, autoimmune haemolytic anaemia, a major and several minor strokes, peptic ulceration, hypothyroidism, renal vein thrombosis, a single kidney, seizures, systemic lupus erythematosus and partial liver dysfunction.

1. Aldous JA, Olson CJ. Managing patients on warfarin therapy: a case report. *Spec Care Dentist* (2001) 21, 109–112.

Anticoagulants + Colestyramine or Colestipol

The anticoagulant effects of phenprocoumon and warfarin can be reduced by colestyramine. Separating the dosages as much as possible may help to minimise the effects of this interaction. An isolated and unexplained report describes a paradoxical increase in the effects of warfarin. No important interaction occurs between phenprocoumon or warfarin and colestipol.

Clinical evidence

(a) Phenprocoumon or warfarin + colestipol

Phenprocoumon serum levels and the prothrombin response were unaffected in four normal subjects by the simultaneous administration of 8 g **colestipol**.[1] No changes in the absorption of single 10 doses of **warfarin** in the presence of 10 g **colestipol** were seen in another study.[2]

(b) Phenprocoumon or warfarin + colestyramine

10 subjects were treated for one-week periods either with warfarin alone or **warfarin** with 8 g **colestyramine** given three times a day. With warfarin alone peak serum levels reached 5.6 micrograms/ml and prothrombin times were prolonged by 11 s. With colestyramine given 30 min after the warfarin, peak levels were reduced to 2.7 micrograms/ml and the prothrombin times were prolonged by 8 s, whereas when the colestyramine was given 6 h after the warfarin, peak levels reached 4.7 micrograms/ml and prothrombin times were again prolonged by 11 .[3]

Comparable results have been found in other studies using single doses of **warfarin** or **phenprocoumon**.[4]

An isolated and unexplained report describes a very marked increase in the effects of **warfarin** (prothrombin time 78.9 s) in a very elderly patient with multiple pathologies when given colestyramine.[5]

Mechanism

Colestyramine binds to bile acids within the gut and also to anticoagulants, thereby preventing their absorption.[4,6-9] As both warfarin and phenprocoumon undergo enterohepatic recycling, continuous further contact with the colestyramine can occur.[10,11] Colestyramine also reduces the absorption of fat-soluble vitamins such as vitamin K so that

it can have some direct hypoprothrombinaemic effects of its own.[12,13] This may offset to some extent the full effects of its interaction with anticoagulants. Colestipol on the other hand appears not to bind to any great extent at the pH values in the gut.[1] The paradoxical increase in the effects of warfarin in the isolated case cited above remains unexplained.[5]

Importance and management

The phenprocoumon/colestyramine and warfarin/colestyramine interactions are established, but their magnitude and clinical importance is still uncertain. If concurrent use is thought necessary, prothrombin times should be monitored and the dosage of the anticoagulant increased appropriately. Giving the colestyramine 3 to 6 h after the anticoagulant has been shown to minimise the effects of this interaction.[3,14] Information about other anticoagulants is lacking but as colestyramine interacts with dicoumarol and ethylbiscoumacetate in *animals*[9] it would be prudent to expect them to interact similarly in man.

No special precautions appear necessary if warfarin or phenprocoumon and colestipol are given concurrently. There seems to be no information about other anticoagulants.

1. Harvengt C, Desager JP. Effects of colestipol, a new bile acid sequestrant, on the absorption of phenprocoumon in man. *Eur J Clin Pharmacol* (1973) 6, 19–21.
2. Heel RC, Brogden RN, Pakes GE, Speight TM, Avery GS. Colestipol: a review of its pharmacological properties and therapeutic effects in patients with hypercholesterolaemia. *Drugs* (1980) 19, 161–80.
3. Kuentzel WP, Brunk SF. Cholestyramine-warfarin interaction in man. *Clin Res* (1970) 18, 594.
4. Robinson DS, Benjamin DM, McCormack JJ. Interaction of warfarin and nonsystemic gastrointestinal drugs. *Clin Pharmacol Ther* (1971) 12, 491–5.
5. Lawler DP, Hyers TM. Extreme prolongation of the prothrombin time in a patient receiving warfarin and cholestyramine. *Cardiovasc Rev Rep* (1993) April, 72–4.
6. Benjamin D, Robinson DS, McCormack J. Cholestyramine binding of warfarin in man and in vitro. *Clin Res* (1970) 18, 336.
7. Hahn KJ, Eiden W, Schettle M, Hahn M, Walter E, Weber E. Effect of cholestyramine on the gastrointestinal absorption of phenprocoumon and acetylsalicylic acid in man. *Eur J Clin Pharmacol* (1972) 4, 142.
8. Gallo DG, Bailey KK, Sheffner AL. The interaction between cholestyramine and drugs. *Proc Soc Exp Biol Med* (1965) 120, 60.
9. Tembo AV, Bates TR. Impairment by cholestyramine of dicumarol and tromexan absorption in rats: a potential drug interaction. *J Pharmacol Exp Ther* (1974) 191, 53–9.
10. Jähnchen E, Meinertz T, Gilfrich H-J, Kersting F, Groth U. Enhanced elimination of warfarin during treatment with cholestyramine. *Br J Clin Pharmacol* (1978) 5, 437–40.
11. Meinertz T, Gilfrich H-J, Groth N, Jonen HG, Jahnchen E. Interruption of the enterohepatic circulation of phenprocoumon by cholestyramine. *Clin Pharmacol Ther* (1977) 21, 166.
12. Casdorph HR. Safe uses of cholestyramine. *Ann Intern Med* (1970) 72, 759.
13. Gross L, Brotman M. Hypoprothrombinemia and hemorrhage associated with cholestyramine therapy. *Ann Intern Med* (1970) 72, 95–6.
14. Cali TJ. Combined therapy with cholestyramine and warfarin. *Am J Pharm Sci Support Public Health* (1975) 147, 166–9.

Anticoagulants + Contraceptives (oral) and related sex hormones

The anticoagulant effects of dicoumarol and phenprocoumon can be decreased, and the effects of acenocoumarol (nicoumalone) increased by the concurrent use of oral contraceptives. A modest dosage adjustment may be necessary. Oral contraceptives should usually be avoided by those taking oral anticoagulants. An isolated report describes a marked INR increase in a woman on warfarin when given emergency contraception with levonorgestrel. A report describes a woman who needed more acenocoumarol when her HRT treatment with oral conjugated estrogens (oestrogens) was changed to transdermal estriol (oestriol).

Clinical evidence

(a) Acenocoumarol (Nicoumalone) + oral contraceptives or estrogens

A survey on 12 patients taking **acenocoumarol** showed that while taking **oral contraceptives**, over an average of 2 years their anticoagulant dosage requirements were reduced by about 20%. Even then they were anticoagulated to a higher degree (prothrombin ratio of 1.67 compared with 1.50) than with the anticoagulant alone. The contraceptives used were *Neogynona*, *Microgynon*, *Eugynon* (ethinylestradiol (ethinyloestradiol) with levonorgestrel) or *Topasel* (intramuscular ampoules of estradiol enantate with algestone).[1]

A postmenopausal woman of 53 needed an increase in her daily dose of acenocoumarol from 2.0 to 3.5 mg when her hormonal replacement treatment (HRT) was changed from 0.625 mg oral conjugated oestrogens daily to 50 micrograms transdermal oestriol daily. When the oral conjugated oestrogens were restarted, her acenocoumarol requirements fell to their former levels.[2]

(b) Dicoumarol + oral contraceptives

A study on 4 healthy subjects given single 150 or 200-mg doses of dicoumarol after a 20-day course of *Enovid* (norethynodrel and mestranol) showed that the anticoagulant effects were decreased in three of the four, although the dicoumarol half-life remained unaltered.[3]

(c) Phenprocoumon + oral contraceptives

A controlled study in 14 women showed that while taking combined oral contraceptives the clearance of a single 0.22 mg/kg dose of phenprocoumon was increased by 25% (from 1.61 to 1.96 ml/min/kg).[4]

(d) Un-named anticoagulants

Megestrol is reported to increase bleeding times with anticoagulants (un-named) in a very brief report about one patient.[5]

(e) Warfarin + Levonorgestrel

A woman of 39 with familial type 1 antithrombin deficiency and a history of extensive deep vein thrombosis and pulmonary embolism, treated with warfarin, was given levonorgestrel for emergency contraception. Within 3 days her INR had risen from 2.1 to 8.1. No bleeding occurred. Her INR fell to normal after stopping the warfarin for 2 days.[6] This appears thus far to be an isolated case so that its general importance is not known.

Mechanism

Not understood. The oral contraceptives increase plasma levels of some blood clotting factors (particularly factor X and fibrinogen) and reduce levels of antithrombin III.[7] They can apparently increase the metabolism (glucuronidation) of phenprocoumon.[4,8] The authors of the report about levonorgestrel suggest that it might have displaced the warfarin from its binding sites thereby increasing its activity, although this mechanism is now generally discounted.

Importance and management

Direct information seems to be limited to these reports. Oral contraceptives are normally contraindicated in those with thromboembolic disorders but if they must be used, be alert for any changes in the anticoagulant response if an oral contraceptive is started or stopped. One study suggests that the progestogen-only contraceptives may not affect the coagulability of the blood as much as the oestrogen/progestogen combined contraceptives, but whether this is reflected in an absence of an interaction with the oral anticoagulants is not documented.[9] The report about the apparent warfarin/levonorgestrel interaction seems thus far to be isolated so that its general importance is unknown. Information about an hormonal replacement treatment (HRT)/estrogen interaction appears to be limited to the report cited, but be alert for any changes in anticoagulant requirements if the route of administration is changed.

1. de Teresa E, Vera A, Ortigosa J, Alonso Pulpon L, Puente Arus A, de Artaza M. Interaction between anticoagulants and contraceptives: an unsuspected finding. *BMJ* (1979) 2, 1260.
2. Exner T, Kraus M. Interference with oral anticoagulant treatment by oestrogen - influence of oestrogen administration route. *Thromb Haemost* (1999) 81, 471–2.
3. Schrogie JJ, Solomon HM, Zieve PD. Effect of oral contraceptives on vitamin K-dependent clotting activity. *Clin Pharmacol Ther* (1967) 8, 670–5.
4. Mönig H, Baese C, Heidemann HT, Ohnhaus EE, Schulte HM. Effect of oral contraceptive steroids on the pharmacokinetics of phenprocoumon. *Br J Clin Pharmacol* (1990) 30, 115–18.
5. Beeley L, Stewart P, Hickey FM. Bulletin of the West Midlands Centre for Adverse Drug Reaction Reporting (1988) 27, 24.
6. Ellison J, Thomson AJ, Greer IA, Walker ID. Apparent interaction between warfarin and levonorgestrel used for emergency contraception. *BMJ* (2000) 321, 1382.
7. Robinson GE, Burren T, Mackie IJ, Bounds W, Walshe K, Faint R, Guillebaud J, Machin SJ. Changes in haemostasis after stopping the combined contraceptive pill: implications for major surgery. *BMJ* (1991) 302, 269–71.
8. Mönig H, Baese C, Heidemann HT, Schulte HM. The use of oral contraceptive steroids affects the pharmacokinetics of phenprocoumon. *Acta Endocrinol (Copenh)* (1989) 120 (Suppl), 180.
9. Poller L, Thomson JM, Tabiowo A, Priest CM. Progesterone oral contraception and blood coagulation. *BMJ* (1969) 1, 554–6.

Anticoagulants + Corticosteroids or Corticotropin (Corticotrophin, ACTH)

Only small changes (increases or decreases) in anticoagulation normally occur during concurrent treatment with oral anticoagulants and low-to-moderate doses of corticosteroids or corticotropin (corticotrophin, ACTH), but one patient bled severely when given corticotropin. Seven other patients have shown very marked prothrombin time increases when given high-dose corticosteroids.

Clinical evidence

(a) Increased anticoagulant effects

Ten out of 14 patients on long-term treatment with either dicoumarol or phenindione showed a small but definite increase in their anticoagulant responses when treated with corticotropin (corticotrophin, ACTH) for 4 to 9 days.[1] A patient controlled on ethyl biscoumacetate began to bleed severely from the gut and urinary tract within three days of starting treatment with corticotropin (10 mg in 500 ml of 5% dextrose intravenously twice daily).[2] A controlled study in 10 patients, 5 on fluindione or acenocoumarol (nicoumalone) and 5 without an anticoagulant, found that pulse high-dose intravenous methylprednisolone increased the mean INR of those taking an anticoagulant from a baseline of 2.75 to 8.04. Methylprednisolone alone did not increase the prothrombin time. All of the patients had antiphospholipid syndrome (APS).[3,4] Two patients on warfarin are also reported to have shown significant prolongations in their prothrombin times when given high-dose corticosteroids (methylprednisolone, dexamethasone) for the treatment of multiple sclerosis.[5]

(b) Decreased anticoagulant effects

A study on 24 patients anticoagulated for several days with dicoumarol showed that 2 h after receiving 10 mg prednisone their silicone coagulation time had decreased from 28 to 24 min, and 2 h later was down to 22 min.[6]

A decrease in the anticoagulant effects of ethyl biscoumacetate is described in 2 patients given corticotropin (corticotrophin, ACTH) and cortisone.[7]

Mechanism

Not understood. Corticosteroids can increase the coagulability of the blood in the absence of anticoagulants.[8,9] Increased effects have been described in *animals*.[2]

Importance and management

The interaction with low to moderate doses of corticosteroids is by no means well established and is very poorly documented. Very few serious reports seem to have been reported in the last 30 years suggesting that problems are rare. The most constructive thing that can be said is that if either corticotropin (corticotrophin, ACTH) or any corticosteroid is given to patients taking anticoagulants, the effects should be monitored, but it is impossible to predict whether any dosage adjustments will be upward or downward.

The situation with high dose methylprednisolone or dexamethasone is clearly different. Although the evidence is limited, marked INR increases have been reported and INRs should be closely monitored (daily has been recommended[3]) if these or other high-dose corticosteroids are added to established treatment with any oral anticoagulant. More study is needed.

1. Hellem AJ, Solem JH. The influence of ACTH on prothrombin-proconvertin values in blood during treatment with dicumarol and phenylindandione. *Acta Med Scand* (1954) 150, 389–93.

2. van Cauwenberge H, Jacques LB. Haemorrhagic effect of ACTH with anticoagulants. *Can Med Assoc J* (1958) 79, 536–40.
3. Costedoat-Chalumeau N, Amoura Z, Aymard G, Sevin O, Wechsler B, Cacoub P, Huong Du, Le Th, Diquet B, Ankri A, Piette J-C. Potentiation of vitamin K antagonists by high-dose intravenous methylprednisolone. *Ann Intern Med* (2000) 132, 631–5.
4. Costedoat-Chalumeau N, Amoura Z, Wechsler B, Ankri A, Piette J-C. Implications of interaction between vitamin K antagonists and high-dose intravenous methylprednisolone in the APS. *J Autoimmun* (2000) 15, A22.
5. Kaufman M. Treatment of sclerosis with high-dose corticosteroids may prolong the prothrombin time to dangerous levels in patients taking warfarin. *Multiple Sclerosis* (1997) 3, 248–9.
6. Menczel J, Dreyfuss F. Effect of prednisone on blood coagulation time in patients on dicumarol therapy. *J Lab Clin Med* (1960) 56, 14–20.
7. Chatterjea JB, Salomon L. Antagonistic effects of A.C.T.H. and cortisone on the anticoagulant activity of ethyl biscoumacetate. *BMJ* (1954) 2, 790–2.
8. Cosgriff SW, Diefenbach AF, Vogt W. Hypercoagulability of the blood associated with ACTH and cortisone therapy. *Am J Med* (1950) 9, 752–6.
9. Ozsoylu S, Strauss HS and Diamond LK. Effects of corticosteroids on coagulation of the blood. *Nature* (1962) 195, 1214–15.

Anticoagulants + Curbicin

The INRs of two patients increased after taking Curbicin. One of them was also taking warfarin.

Clinical evidence, mechanism, importance and management

A man of 73 who was taking 3 tablets of **Curbicin** daily was found to have an INR of 2.1 (normal 0.9 to 1.2) despite no anticoagulant treatment. His INR value improved (1.3 to 1.4) when he was given vitamin K, but did not normalize (to 1.0) until a week after stopping the **Curbicin**. Another patient on **warfarin** and simvastatin, with stable INR values around 2.4, showed an increase in his INR to 3.4 within 6 days of starting to take 5 tablets of **Curbicin** daily. Within a week of stopping the **Curbicin**, his INR had fallen to its previous value. **Curibicin** is a herbal remedy used for micturition problems which contains extracts from the fruit of *Serenoa repens* (Saw palmetto) and the seed of *Cucurbita pepo*.[1]

The authors of this report suggest that what happened was possibly due to the presence of vitamin E in the **Curbicin** preparation (each tablet also contains 10 mg), but vitamin E does not normally affect INRs (see 'Anticoagulants + Vitamin E', p.300). However, whether or not the mechanism is known it would now be prudent to monitor patients on **warfarin** or any other oral anticoagulant if **Curbicin** is taken concurrently.

1. Yue, Q-Y, Jansson K. Herbal drug Curbicin and anticoagulant effect with and without warfarin: possibly related to the vitamin E component. *J Am Geriatr Soc* (2001) 49, 838.

Anticoagulants + Cytotoxic (antineoplastic) agents

A number of case reports describe an increase in the effects of warfarin, accompanied by bleeding in some cases, caused by the concurrent use of cytotoxic drug regimens containing carboplatin, chlormethine (mustine), cyclophosphamide, doxorubicin, etoposide, 5-fluorouracil (5-FU), ftorafur, gemcitabine, ifosfamide/mesna, methotrexate, procarbazine, sulofenur, *Uftoral*, vincristine and vindesine. A decrease in the effects of warfarin has been seen with regimens of azathioprine, cyclophosphamide, mercaptopurine and mitotane, a decrease in the effects of phenprocoumon with azathioprine and a decrease in the effects of acenocoumarol (nicoumalone) with mercaptopurine.

Clinical evidence

(a) Anticoagulant effects increased

The INR of a man on **warfarin** increased from a baseline range of 1.15 to 2.11 to 12.6 within 16 days of a first course of chemotherapy with **carboplatin** and **etoposide**.[1]

A man on **warfarin** showed a progressive rise in prothrombin times when given a continuous infusion of **fluorouracil**.[2] Three out of 25 patients developed blood loss from the gut when treated with **warfarin** and rapid intravenous **fluorouracil** which was controlled by giving a transfusion and stopping the **warfarin**.[3] A man developed a prolonged prothrombin time with epistaxis, haematemesis, haematuria and haemtochezia attributed to an interaction between **warfarin** and **fluorouracil**.[4] The INR of an elderly man on **warfarin** increased from 3 to almost 40 after being given **fluorouracil** and **levamisole** for 4 weeks, and he again demonstrated increased **warfarin** effects when rechallenged with **fluorouracil**.[5] At least another 7 patients have been described who similarly showed increased INRs and needed warfarin dosage reductions while concurrently receiving fluorouracil.[6-8]

Increased INRs and bleeding (haemoptysis) were also seen in a patient on **warfarin** when treated with *Orzel* (uracil/ftorafur in a 4:1 molar ratio). **Ftorafur** is a pro-drug of **fluorouracil** to which it is metabolised in the body. This patient needed a 63% reduction in the warfarin dosage.[9] *Uftoral* (**tegafur/uracil**) is another prodrug of **fluorouracil** and the makers say that marked elevations in prothrombin times and INRs have been reported in patients on **warfarin** when *Uftoral* was added.[10]

A woman stabilised on **warfarin** developed an iliopsoas haematoma three weeks after starting treatment with **cyclophosphamide**, **methotrexate**, **fluorouracil**, **vincristine** and **prednisone**.[11] The prothrombin times of 2 women on **warfarin** approximately doubled, accompanied by bleeding, on day 15 of each cycle of adjuvant treatment with **CMF** (**cyclophosphamide**, **methotrexate** and **fluorouracil**).[12] The INR of a woman on **warfarin** rose from a range of 2.02–2.80 to 4.15–10 by day 23 of the first cycle of **CMF**.[13]

A man of 63 needed a reduction in his weekly **warfarin** dosage from 59.23 to 50.75 mg while receiving 2 cycles of **gemcitabine** in order to keep his INR within in the therapeutic range (about 2.5). When the **gemcitabine** treatment was over his **warfarin** dosage had to be increased again.[14] Another elderly man on **warfarin** showed a marked increase in prothrombin times (prolongation of 8 to 15 s) on two occasions when given 500 mg **etoposide** and 5 mg **vindesine**.[15] The prothrombin times of an elderly man given **warfarin** increased 50 to 100% in the middle of three cycles of treatment with **ProMace-Mopp** (**cyclophosphamide**, **doxorubicin**, **etoposide**, **methchlorethamine**, **vincristine**, **procarbazine**, **methotrexate** and **prednisone**), and he developed a subconjunctival haemorrhage during the first cycle.[15] Three patients on **warfarin** showed a marked and very rapid increase in INRs when treated with **ifosfamide/mesna**.[16] Three patients developed a marked increase in prothrombin times while receiving **warfarin** and **sulofenur (LY186641)**.[17]

(b) Anticoagulant effects decreased

A survey of 103 patients with the antiphospholipid syndrome found that **azathioprine** appeared to increase the warfarin requirements.[18] A woman who was resistant to **warfarin** (14 to 17 mg daily) while taking **azathioprine** began to bleed (epistaxes, haematemesis) when the **azathioprine** was stopped. She was restabilised on 5 mg **warfarin** daily.[19] Reduced **warfarin** effects were seen in 2 other patients while taking **azathioprine**,[20,21] one of whom showed a marked fall in serum warfarin levels during **azathioprine** treatment.[21] Two women with systemic lupus erythematosus on **phenprocoumon** showed marked falls in INRs during treatment with **azathioprine**,[22] and another woman showed **warfarin** resistance and needed an almost 4 times increase in the dose of **warfarin** when given **azathioprine**.[23] A man well stabilised on **warfarin** showed a marked reduction in his anticoagulant response on two occasions when treated with **mercaptopurine**,[24] but no changes occurred when given busulfan (**busulphan**), **cyclophosphamide**, **cytarabine** or **melphalan**. A woman needed a marked increase in her dosage of **acenocoumarol** (**nicoumalone**) – from 21 to 70 mg weekly – while under treatment with 100 mg **mercaptopurine** daily.[25] A woman on **warfarin** showed a marked rise in prothrombin times when her treatment with **cyclophosphamide** was withdrawn.[26] The anticoagulant effects of **warfarin** were progressively reduced in a woman while receiving **mitotane**.[27] Later this effect began to reverse.

Mechanisms, importance and management

Just why these responses occurred is not understood (except possibly with mercaptopurine which appears to increase the synthesis or activation of prothrombin[28]). It is not even possible in some cases to identify precisely the drug (or drugs) responsible. The absence of problems in many studies using warfarin as an adjunct to chemotherapy[29,30] and the small number of reports describing difficulties suggest that many of these interactions may be uncommon events. The concurrent use of most of these drugs need not be avoided but there is clearly a need to monitor the effects of warfarin closely both during and after treatment with these and other cytotoxic agents to ensure that prothrombin times are well controlled. The anticoagulant dosages may need adjustment. It has been suggested that subcutaneous heparin should be given rather than warfarin to patients on sulofenur.[17] Information about other anticoagulants appears to be lacking.

1. Le AT, Hasson NK, Lum BL. Enhancement of warfarin response in a patient receiving etoposide and carboplatin chemotherapy. *Ann Pharmacother* (1997) 31, 1006–8.
2. Wajima T, Mukhopadhyay P. Possible interactions between warfarin and 5-fluorouracil. *Am J Hematol* (1992) 40, 238–43.
3. Chelobowski RT, Gota CH, Chann KK, Weiner JM, Block JB, Batemen JR. Clinical and pharmacokinetic effects on combined warfarin and 5-fluorouracil in advanced colon cancer. *Cancer Res* (1982) 42, 4827–30.
4. Brown MC. Multisite mucous membrane bleeding due to a possible interaction between warfarin and 5-fluorouracil. *Pharmacotherapy* (1997) 17, 631–3.
5. Scarfe MA, Israel MK. Possible drug interaction between warfarin and combination of levamisole and fluorouracil. *Ann Pharmacother* (1994) 28, 464–7.
6. Brown MC. An adverse interaction between warfarin and 5-fluorouracil; a case report and review of the literature. *Chemotherapy* (1999) 45, 392–5.
7. Kolesar JM, Johnson CL, Freeberg BL, Berlin JD, Schiller JH. Warfarin-5-FU interaction – a consecutive case series. *Pharmacotherapy* (1999) 19, 1445–9.
8. Aki Z, Kotiloğlu G, Özyilkan Ö. A patient with a prolonged prothrombin time due to an adverse interaction between 5-fluorouracil and warfarin. *Am J Gastroenterol* (2000) 95, 1093–4.
9. Karwal MW, Schlueter AJ, Arnold MM, Davis RT. Presumed drug interaction between Orzel® and warfarin. *Blood* (1999) 94 (10 Suppl 1, part 2) 106b.
10. Uftoral (tegafur/uracil). Bristol-Myers Squibb Pharmaceuticals. Summary of product characteristics, January 2001.
11. Booth BW, Weiss RB. Venous thrombosis during adjuvant chemotherapy. *N Engl J Med* (1981) 305, 170.
12. Seifter EJ, Brooks BJ, Urba WJ. Possible interactions between warfarin and antineoplastic drugs. *Cancer Treat Rep* (1985) 69, 244–5.
13. Malacarne P, Maestri A. Possible interactions between antiblastic agents and warfarin inducing prothrombin time abnormalities. *Recenti Prog Med* (1996) 87, 135.
14. Kinikar SA, Kolesar JM. Identification of a gemcitabine-warfarin interaction. *Pharmacotherapy* (1999) 19, 1331-3.
15. Ward K, Bitran JD. Warfarin, etoposide, and vindesine interactions. *Cancer Treat Rep* (1984) 68, 817–18.
16. Hall G, Lind MJ, Huang M, Moore A, Gane A, Roberts JT, Cantwell BMJ. Intravenous infusions of ifosfamide/mesna and perturbation of warfarin anticoagulant control. *Postgrad Med J* (1990) 66, 860–1.
17. Fossella FV, Lippman SM, Seitz DE, Alberts DS, Taylor CW, Wiltshaw E, Hardy J, O'Brien M, Haynes TR, Wolen RL. Hypoprothrombinemia from coadministration of sulofenur (LY 186641) and warfarin: report of three cases. *Invest New Drugs* (1991) 9, 357–9.
18. Khamashta MA, Cuadrado MJ, Mujic F, Taub N, Hunt BJ, Hughes GRV. Effect of azathioprine on the anticoagulant activity of warfarin in patients with the antiphospholipid syndrome. *Lupus* (1998) 7 (Suppl 2), S227.
19. Singleton JD, Conyers L. Warfarin and azathioprine: an important drug interaction. *Am J Med* (1992) 92, 217.
20. Rivier G, Khamashta MA, Hughes GRV. Warfarin and azathioprine: a drug interaction does exist. *Am J Med* (1993) 95, 342.
21. Rotenberg M, Levy Y, Shoenfeld Y, Almog S, Ezra D. Effect of azathioprine on the anticoagulant activity of warfarin. *Ann Pharmacother* (2000) 34, 120-2.
22. Jeppesen U, Rasmussen JM, Brøsen K. Clinically important interaction between azathioprine (Imurel) and phenprocoumon (Marcoumar). *Eur J Clin Pharmacol* (1997) 52, 503–4.
23. Havrda DE, Rathburn S, Scheid D. A case report of warfarin resistance due to azathioprine and review of the literature. *Pharmacotherapy* (2001) 21, 355–7.
24. Spiers ASD, Mibashan RS. Increased warfarin requirement during mercaptopurine therapy: a new drug interaction. *Lancet* (1974) ii, 221–2.
25. Fernádez MA, Regadera A, Aznar J. Acenocoumarol and 6-mercaptopurine: an important drug interaction. *Haematologica* (1999) 84, 664–5.
26. Tashima CK. Cyclophosphamide effect on coumarin anticoagulation. *South Med J* (1979) 72, 633–4.
27. Cuddy PG, Loftus LS. Influence of mitotane on the hypoprothrombinemic effect of warfarin. *South Med J* (1986) 79, 387–8.
28. Martini A, Jähnchen E. Studies in rats on the mechanisms by which 6-mercaptopurine inhibits the anticoagulant effect of warfarin. *J Pharmacol Exp Ther* (1977) 201, 547–53.
29. Zacharski LR, Henderson WG, Rickles FR, Forman WB, Cornell CJ, Forcier RJ, Edwards RL, Headley E, Kim S-H, O'Donnell JF, O'Dell R, Tornyos K, Kwaan HC. Effect of warfarin anticoagulation on survival in carcinoma of the lung, colon, head and neck, and prostate. *Cancer* (1984) 53, 2046–52.
30. Zacharski LR, Henderson WG, Rickles FR, Forman WB, Cornell CJ, Forcier RJ, Edwards RL, Headley E, Kim S-H, O'Donnell JF, O'Dell R, Tornyos K, Kwaan HC. Effect of warfarin on survival in small cell carcinoma of the lung. *JAMA* (1981) 245, 831–5.

Anticoagulants + Danshen

Two case reports and some other evidence indicates that *Danshen*, a Chinese herbal remedy, can increase the effects of warfarin resulting in bleeding.

Clinical evidence

A woman who had had venous mitral valve valvuloplasty and who was taking furosemide (frusemide), digoxin and **warfarin,** began additionally to take ***Danshen*** (the root of *Salvia miltiorrhiza*) every other day for intermittent influenza-like symptoms. After about a month she was hospitalised with malaise, breathlessness and fever and was found to be both very anaemic and over-anticoagulated (prothrombin time > 60s, INR > 5.62). Her anaemia was attributed to occult gastrointestinal bleeding and the over-anticoagulation to an interaction with the ***Danshen.*** Later she was restabilised on the **warfarin** in the absence of the ***Danshen*** with a normal INR (2.5), and within 4 months her haemoglobin levels were normal.[1]

Another report describes a man on **warfarin** (and also on digoxin, captopril and frusemide) with an INR of about 3.0, who developed chest pain and breathlessness about 2 weeks after starting to take ***Danshen***. He was found to have a massive pleural effusion, later drained of blood, and an INR elevated to 8.4. He was later discharged on his usual dose of **warfarin** in the absence of the ***Danshen*** and with an INR stable again at 3.[2]

Mechanism

Not fully understood. Studies in *rats* show that Danshen can increase the bioavailabilty of both *(R)*- and *(S)*-warfarin thereby increasing its effects.[3]

It may also affect haemostasis by inhibiting platelet aggregation and by interfering with extrinsic coagulation, and it also has antithrombin III-like activity and can promote fibrinolytic activity. Acting in concert these activities might be expected to result in bleeding complications.

Importance and management

Clinical information appears to be limited to these two case reports and one other which also involved methylsalicylate (see 'Anticoagulants + Aspirin or other Salicylates', p.240)[4] which is also known to increase the effects of warfarin. This interaction is therefore not yet very well established but there is now enough evidence to suggest that normally *Danshen* should be avoided by patients on warfarin (although with very careful monitoring and warfarin dosage adjustments safe concurrent use might be possible). More study is needed. Information about other oral anticoagulants is lacking but it would seem sensible to take the same precautions if using any of them.

1. Yu CM, Chan JCN, Sanderson JE. Chinese herbs and warfarin potentiation by 'Danshen'. *J Intern Med* (1997) 241, 337–9.
2. Izzat MB, Yim APC, El-Zufari MH. A taste of Chinese medicine. *Ann Thorac Surg* (1998) 66, 941–2.
3. Lo ACT, Chan K, Yeung JHK, Woo KS. The effects of Danshen (*Salvia miltiorrhiza*) on pharmacokinetics and dynamics of warfarin in rats. *Eur J Drug Metab Pharmacokinet* (1992) 17, 257–62.
4. Tam LS, Chan TYK, Leung WK, Critchley JAJH. Warfarin interactions with Chinese traditional medicines: danshen and methyl salicylate medicated oil. *Aust N Z J Med* (1995) 25, 258.

Anticoagulants + Dextropropoxyphene (Propoxyphene) or Co-proxamol

Seven patients on warfarin have shown a marked increase in prothrombin times and/or bleeding when given Distalgesic (dextropropoxyphene/paracetamol (acetaminophen), co-

proxamol), but the interaction seems to be very uncommon. One unexplained death has occurred.

Clinical evidence

(a) Dextroproxyphene/paracetamol (Co-proxamol, Distalgesic)

A man on 6 mg **warfarin** daily developed marked haematuria within 6 days of starting to take two tablets of *Distalgesic* (**dextropropoxyphene** 32.5 mg, **paracetamol** (**acetaminophen**) 325 mg per tablet) three times a day. His plasma **warfarin** levels had risen by one-third (from 1.8 to 2.4 micrograms/ml).[1] A woman controlled for 6 weeks on **warfarin** showed gross haematuria within only 5 h of taking six tablets of *Distalgesic* over a 6-h period. Her prothrombin time increased from about 30–40 s to 130 s.[1]

This interaction has been seen in 5 other patients on **warfarin**.[2-6] The prothrombin time of one of them rose from 28—44 s to 80 s within 3 days of substituting **paracetamol** (**acetaminophen**) by two tablets of *Distalgesic* four times a day.[3] Another developed a prothrombin time of more than 50 s after taking 30 tablets of *Darvocet-N 100* (**dextropropoxyphene** 100 mg, **paracetamol** (**acetaminophen**) 650 mg) and possibly an unknown amount of ibuprofen over a 3-day period. Increased **warfarin** effects leading to severe retroperitoneal haemorrhage have also been briefly reported in a patient taking **co-proxamol** (**dextropropoxyphene + paracetamol**). **Methocarbamol** may have been a contributory factor.[5]

(b) Dextropropoxyphene

A double-blind trial on 23 patients anticoagulated with **un-named coumarol derivatives** and given 450 mg **dextropropoxyphene** daily for 15 days failed to show any change in prothrombin times.[7] Death due to unknown causes in a patient on **warfarin** and **dextropropoxyphene** has also been described.[8]

Mechanism

Not understood. It seems possible that in man, as in *animals*,[9] dextropropoxyphene inhibits or competes with the liver enzymes concerned with the metabolic clearance of warfarin, thereby prolonging and increasing its effects. There is also the possibility that the paracetamol (acetaminophen) component of the *Distalgesic* and *Darvocet-N* had some part to play (see also 'Anticoagulants + Paracetamol (Acetaminophen)', p.283. But just why only a few individuals are affected is not clear.

Importance and management

Information about this interaction is very sparse and seems to be limited to the reports cited. This suggests that only a few patients are likely to develop this interaction with warfarin and dextropropoxyphene/paracetamol or dextroproxyphene, but it is not possible to predict who will be affected. Concurrent use need not be avoided but it would be prudent initially to monitor the effects of adding these drugs, whether using warfarin or any other anticoagulant, because the occasional patient may show a marked response.

1. Orme M, Breckenridge A, Cook P. Warfarin and Distalgesic interaction. *BMJ* (1976) i, 200.
2. Jones RV. Warfarin and *Distalgesic* interaction. *BMJ* (1976) i, 460.
3. Smith R, Prudden D, Hawkes C. Propoxyphene and warfarin interaction. *Drug Intell Clin Pharm* (1984) 18, 822.
4. Justice JL, Kline SS. Analgesics and warfarin. A case that brings up questions and cautions. *Postgrad Med* (1988) 83, 217.
5. Beeley L, Magee P, Hickey FN. Bulletin of the West Midlands Centre for Adverse Drug Reaction Reporting (1990) 30, 32.
6. Pilszek FH, Moloney D, Sewell JR. Case report: increased anticoagulant effect of warfarin in patient taking a small dose of co-proxamol. Personal communication, 1994.
7. Franchimont P, Heynen G. Comparative study of ibuprofen and dextropropoxyphene in scapulo-humeral periarthritis following myocardial infarction. 13th International Congress of Rheumatol, Kyoto, Japan. 30th Sept–6th Oct 1973.
8. Udall JA. Drug interference with warfarin therapy. *Clin Med* (1970) 77, 20–5.
9. Breckenridge A, Orme ML'E, Thorgeirsson S, Davies DS, Brooks RV. Drug interactions with warfarin: studies with dichloralphenazone, chloral hydrate and phenazone (antipyrine). *Clin Sci* (1971) 40, 351.

Anticoagulants + Dichloralphenazone

The anticoagulant effects of warfarin are reduced by the concurrent use of dichloralphenazone. Other anticoagulants probably interact similarly.

Clinical evidence

Five patients on long-term **warfarin** treatment showed an approximately 50% (20.2 to 68.5%) reduction in plasma **warfarin** levels, and a fall in the anticoagulant response, when given 1.3 g doses of **dichloralphenazone** each night for two weeks. Another patient given the same doses nightly over a month showed a 70% fall in plasma **warfarin** levels and a thrombotest percentage rise from 9 to 55%. These values returned to normal when the hypnotic was withdrawn.[1] Similar results have been described in other reports.[2,3]

Mechanism

The phenazone (antipyrine) component of the hypnotic is a potent liver enzyme inducing agent which increases the metabolism and clearance of the warfarin, thereby reducing its effects.[1,3] The effects of the chloral appear to be minimal (see 'Anticoagulants + Chloral hydrate', p.249).

Importance and management

Information is limited, but it appears to be an established and clinically important interaction, probably affecting most patients. The dosage of warfarin will need to be increased to accommodate this interaction. Non-interacting alternatives for dichloralphenazone may be found among the benzodiazepines (see 'Anticoagulants + Benzodiazepines', p.244 in this chapter). If the dosage of warfarin has been disturbed by using dichloralphenazone, it may take up to a month for it to restabilise. It would be prudent to expect other oral anticoagulants to interact similarly, but there is no direct evidence as yet that they do so.

1. Breckenridge A, Orme ML'E, Thorgeirrson S, Davies DS, Brooks RV. Drug interaction with warfarin: studies with dichloralphenazone, chloral hydrate and phenazone (antipyrine). *Clin Sci* (1971) 40, 351.
2. Breckenridge A, Orme ML'E, Davies DS, Thorgeirsson S, Dollery CT. Induction of drug metabolising enzymes in man and rat by dichloralphenazone. 4th International Congress of Pharmacology. Basel, 1969.
3. Breckenridge A, Orme M. Clinical implications of enzyme induction. *Ann N Y Acad Sci* (1971) 179, 421–31.

Anticoagulants + Diflunisal

There is some limited evidence that diflunisal can increase the anticoagulant effects of acenocoumarol (nicoumalone) and possibly warfarin, but phenprocoumon appears not to be affected. Prothrombin times should be checked if diflunisal is added or withdrawn in patients taking any anticoagulant.

Clinical evidence

The serum **warfarin** levels of 5 normal subjects on subtherapeutic doses fell by about a third (from 741 to 533 ng/ml) when given 500 mg **diflunisal** for 2 weeks, but the anticoagulant response was unaffected. When the **diflunisal** was withdrawn, the serum **warfarin** levels rose once more while the anticoagulant response fell.[1] Another report very briefly describes an increased INR during concurrent use.[2]

A brief report states that 3 out of 6 subjects on **acenocoumarol** (**nicoumalone**) experienced significant increases in prothrombin times when given 750 mg **diflunisal** daily, but no interaction was seen in 2 subjects on **phenprocoumon**.[3]

Mechanism

Uncertain. Diflunisal can displace warfarin from its plasma protein binding sites[1] but this on its own is almost certainly not the full explanation.

Importance and management

This interaction is neither well defined nor well documented. Its importance is uncertain, however the reports cited and the manufacturers literature suggest that an increased anticoagulant effect should be looked for if diflunisal is added to established treatment with any anticoagulant. A decreased effect would be expected if diflunisal is withdrawn. Phenprocoumon is possibly an exception and appears not to interact. The risk of bleeding (because of changes in platelet activity or gastrointestinal irritation) appears to be less than with aspirin.[4]

1. Serlin MJ, Mossman S, Sibeon RG, Tempero KF, Breckenridge AM. Interaction between diflunisal and warfarin. *Clin Pharmacol Ther* (1980) 28, 493–8.
2. Beeley L, Cunningham H, Carmichael A, Brennan A. Bulletin of the West Midlands Centre for Adverse Drug Reporting (1992) 35, 13.
3. Caruso I et al. Unpublished observations quoted in ref. 2.
4. Tempero KF, Cirillo VJ, Steelman SL. Diflunisal: a review of pharmacokinetic and pharmacodynamic properties, drug interactions, and special tolerability studies in humans. *Br J Clin Pharmacol* (1977) 4, 31S.

Anticoagulants + Dipyridamole

Mild bleeding can sometimes occur if anticoagulants and dipyridamole are used concurrently, even though prothrombin times remain stable and well within the therapeutic range.

Clinical evidence

30 patients stabilised on either **warfarin** (28 patients) or **phenindione** (two patients) showed no significant changes in prothrombin times when given **dipyridamole** in doses up to 400 mg daily for a month, but 3 patients developed mild bleeding (epistaxis, bruising, haematuria) which resolved when either drug was withdrawn or the dosage reduced.[1]

Two other reports state that prothrombin ratios remain unaltered when **dipyridamole** is given with **warfarin**, and claim that there is no risk of bleeding.[2,3] No bleeding problems were described in a study of the value of combined use (300 mg **dipyridamole** daily) in patients with heart valve replacements.[4]

Mechanism

Uncertain. A reduction in platelet adhesiveness or aggregation induced by the dipyridamole may have been responsible.[1]

Importance and management

Information seems to be very limited. Since bleeding can sometimes occur even when prothrombin values are within the therapeutic range, some caution is appropriate. The authors of the study cited suggest that prothrombin activity should be maintained at the upper end of the therapeutic range as a precaution.[1] Only warfarin and phenindione have been implicated, but it would be sensible to apply the same precautions with any anticoagulant.

1. Kalowski S, Kincaid-Smith P. Interaction of dipyridamole with anticoagulants in the treatment of glomerulonephritis. *Med J Aust* (1973) 2, 164–6.
2. Rajah SM, Sreeharan N, Rao S, Watson D. Warfarin versus warfarin plus dipyridamole on the incidence of arterial thromboembolism in prosthetic heart valve patients. 7ᵗʰ International Congress of Thrombosis and Haemostasis, London (1979). Abstract 379.
3. Donaldson DR, Sreeharan N, Crow MJ, Rajah SM. Assessment of the interaction of warfarin with aspirin and dipyridamole. *Thromb Haemost* (1982) 47, 77.
4. Kawazoe K, Fujita T, Manabe H. Dipyridamole combined with anticoagulant in prevention of early postoperative thromboembolism after cardiac valve replacement. *Thromb Res* (1991) (Suppl 12), 27–33.

Anticoagulants + Disopyramide

The anticoagulant effects of warfarin are reduced to some extent by disopyramide in many patients, but there are two reports of patients who needed less warfarin while taking disopyramide.

Clinical evidence

(a) Reduced warfarin effects

A study in 10 patients with recent atrial fibrillation scheduled for electroconversion, maintained on **warfarin** and with a British Corrected Ratio of 2 to 3, found that **disopyramide** increased the clearance of **warfarin** by 21% (from 166.3 to 201.1 ml/h).[1] Another study found that 2 out of 3 patients needed a **warfarin** dosage increase of about 10% when concurrently treated with **disopyramide** (600 mg daily) for atrial fibrillation.[2]

(b) Increased warfarin effects

A report describes a patient who, following a myocardial infarction, was given 3 mg **warfarin** daily and 100 mg **disopyramide** six-hourly with digoxin, furosemide (frusemide) and potassium supplements. When the **disopyramide** was withdrawn his **warfarin** requirements doubled over a nine-day period.[3] An increased response to **warfarin** in the presence of **disopyramide** has been seen in another patient.[4]

Mechanism

Unknown. One idea is that when the disopyramide controls fibrillation, changes occur in cardiac output and in the flow of blood through the liver which might have an effect on the synthesis of the blood clotting factors.[2,5] But the discordant response in the 2 patients remains unexplained.

Importance and management

Very poorly documented and not established. The outcome of concurrent use is uncertain. It would be prudent to monitor the response to any anticoagulant if disopyramide is given or withdrawn, and appropriate dosage adjustments made if necessary.

1. Woo KS, Chan K, Pun CO. The mechanisms of warfarin-disopyramide interaction. *Circulation* (1987) 76 (Suppl 4), IV-520.
2. Sylvén C, Anderson P. Evidence that disopyramide does not interact with warfarin. *BMJ* (1983) 286, 1181.
3. Haworth E, Burroughs AK. Disopyramide and warfarin interaction. *BMJ* (1977) 2, 866–7.
4. Marshall J. Personal communication, 1987.
5. Ryll C, Davis LJ. Warfarin-disopyramide interaction? *Drug Intell Clin Pharm* (1979) 13, 260.

Anticoagulants + Disulfiram

The anticoagulant effects of warfarin are increased by disulfiram and bleeding can occur if the anticoagulant dosage is not reduced appropriately. Bad breath smelling of bad eggs has also been described during concurrent treatment.

Clinical evidence

Haemorrhage in a patient given **warfarin** and **disulfiram** prompted study of this interaction.[1] Eight normal subjects anticoagulated with **warfarin** were given 500 mg **disulfiram** daily for 21 days. The plasma **warfarin** levels of 7 of them rose by an average of 20% and their prothrombin activity fell by about 10%.

Other experiments with single doses of **warfarin** confirm these results,[2–4] and the interaction has been described in other reports.[5,6] Bad breath reminiscent of the smell of bad eggs has also been described in patients taking **warfarin** and **disulfiram**.[6]

Mechanism

Not fully understood. The suggestion[2-4] that disulfiram inhibits the liver enzymes concerned with the metabolism of warfarin has not been confirmed by later studies.[7] It is now postulated[7] that disulfiram may chelate with the metal ions necessary for the production of active thrombin from prothrombin, thereby augmenting the actions of warfarin.

Importance and management

An established interaction, although direct information about patients is very limited. What is known suggests that most individuals will demonstrate this interaction. If concurrent use is thought appropriate, the effects of warfarin or any other anticoagulant should be monitored and suitable dosage adjustments made when adding or withdrawing disulfiram. Patients already on disulfiram should be started on a small dose of anticoagulant.

1. Rothstein E. Warfarin effect enhanced by disulfiram. *JAMA* (1968) 206, 1051.
2. O'Reilly RA. Interaction of sodium warfarin and disulfiram (Antabuse®) in man. *Ann Intern Med* (1973) 78, 73–6.
3. O'Reilly RA. Potentiation of anticoagulant effect by disulfiram (Antabuse®). *Clin Res* (1971) 19, 180.
4. O'Reilly RA. Interaction of warfarin and disulfiram in man. *Fedn Proc* (1972) 31, 248.
5. Rothstein E. Warfarin effect enhanced by disulfiram (Antabuse). *JAMA* (1972) 221, 1052–3.
6. O'Reilly RA and Mothley CH. Breath odor after disulfiram. *JAMA* (1977) 238, 2600.
7. O'Reilly RA. Dynamic interaction between disulfiram and separated enantiomorphs of racemic warfarin. *Clin Pharmacol Ther* (1981) 29, 332–6.

Anticoagulants + Ditazole

Ditazole does not alter the anticoagulant effects of acenocoumarol (nicoumalone).

Clinical evidence, mechanism, importance and management

50 patients with artificial heart valves taking **acenocoumarol (nicoumalone)** showed no changes in their prothrombin times while taking 800 mg **ditazole** daily.[1] No special precautions are needed. There seems to be no information about other anticoagulants.

1. Jacovella G, Milazzotto F. Ricerca di interazioni fra ditazolo e anticoagulanti in portatori di protesi valvolari intracardache. *Clin Ter* (1977) 80, 425–31.

Anticoagulants + Diuretics

Diuretics in general appear not to interact significantly with anticoagulants. Bumetanide, chlortalidone (chlorthalidone), chlorothiazide, furosemide (frusemide), torasemide and spironolactone have been shown either not to interact or to cause only a small reduction in the effects of the anticoagulants of minimal or no clinical importance. The possible exceptions are etacrynic acid (ethacrynic acid) which on rare occasions has caused a marked increase in the effects of warfarin, and tienilic acid (ticrynafen) which can have a marked effect and cause bleeding.

Clinical evidence

(a) Acenocoumarol (nicoumalone), phenprocoumon or warfarin + chlortalidone (chlorthalidone)

Six normal subjects given single 1.5 mg/kg doses of **warfarin** showed reduced hypoprothrombinaemia (from 77 to 58 u) when also given 100 mg **chlortalidone** daily, although the plasma **warfarin** levels remained unaltered.[7] Similarly reduced anticoagulant effects have been described with **phenprocoumon**, and **clorindione** but no significant effects were seen on the activity of **acenocoumarol**.[8]

(b) Ethyl biscoumacetate, acenocoumarol (nicoumalone) and warfarin + tienilic acid

Two patients taking **ethyl biscoumacetate** began to bleed spontaneously (haematuria, ecchymoses of the legs and gastrointestinal bleeding) when they started to take 250 mg **tienilic acid** daily. The thrombotest percentage of one of them was found to have fallen below 10%.[1] Increased anticoagulant effects and/or bleeding, beginning within a few days, have been described in patients or subjects given **tienilic acid** while taking **ethyl biscoumacetate**,[1,2] **acenocoumarol**[3,4] or **warfarin**.[2,5,6]

(c) Phenprocoumon + furosemide (frusemide) or torasemide

A pharmacokinetic study in 17 normal subjects found that 40 mg **furosemide** twice daily had no effect on the pharmacokinetics of single oral doses of **phenprocoumon** (0.22 mg/kg).[9] Another study in 46 patients with congestive heart failure and found that 40 mg **furosemide** or 20 mg **torasemide** daily for 8 days did not alter the anticoagulant effects of **phenprocoumon**.[10]

(d) Warfarin + etacrynic acid (ethacrynic acid)

A case report describes a marked increase in the anticoagulant effects of **warfarin** in a woman on two occasions when administered doses of **etacrynic acid** ranging from 50 to 300 mg. She had hypoalbuminaemia.[11] A therapeutically significant interaction between **warfarin** and **etacrynic acid** is reported elsewhere, but no details are given.[12]

(e) Warfarin + furosemide (frusemide) or bumetanide

A study in 10 normal subjects showed that their response to single 0.8 mg/kg doses of **warfarin** were unaffected by taking 1 mg **bumetanide** daily for 14 days.[13] This confirms a previous study in 11 normal subjects given 2 mg daily.[14] A study on 6 normal subjects showed that **warfarin** plasma levels, half-lives and prothrombin times in response to a 50 mg oral dose were not significantly altered by the presence of **furosemide** (80 mg daily).[14] A 28% decrease in the INR of one patient on **warfarin** was seen when **furosemide** was given, attributed to volume depletion caused by the diuretic.[15]

(f) Warfarin + spironolactone

A study in 9 subjects given single 1.5 mg/kg doses of **warfarin** showed that the concurrent use of 200 mg **spironolactone** reduced the prothrombin time (expressed as a percentage of the control activity with warfarin alone) from 100 to 76%. Plasma **warfarin** levels remained unchanged.[16]

(g) Warfarin + thiazides

A study on 8 normal subjects given single 40 to 60-mg oral doses of **warfarin** and 1 g **chlorothiazide** daily showed that the mean half-life of the anticoagulant was increased slightly (from 39 to 44 h) but the prothrombin time was barely affected (from 18.9 to 18.6 s).[17]

Mechanism

It has been suggested that the diuresis induced by chlortalidone, furosemide and spironolactone reduces plasma water which leads to a concentration of the blood clotting factors.[7,15,16] Etacrynic acid can displace warfarin from its plasma protein binding sites,[18] but it is almost certain that this, on its own, does not explain the marked interaction described.[11,12] Tienilic acid reduces the metabolism of *S*-warfarin (but not *R*-warfarin) thereby prolonging its stay in the body and increasing its effects.[6] It was originally thought that this was a drug displacement interaction.[1,19,20]

Importance and management

The documentation relating to diuretics in general (other than tienilic acid) is very limited and seems to be confined to the reports cited here, most of which are single dose studies. I have been unable to trace any others. The evidence which is available suggests that these diuretics either do not interact at all with the anticoagulants, or only to an extent which is of little clinical relevance. This is in general agreement with common experience. No special precautions normally seem to be necessary, except possibly with etacrynic acid (ethacrynic acid) where it might be prudent to monitor the outcome particularly in those with hypoalbuminaemia or kidney dysfunction.

The anticoagulant/tienilic acid interaction is established and of clinical importance. The incidence is uncertain. Concurrent use should be avoided. If that is not possible, prothrombin times should be closely monitored and the anticoagulant dosage reduced as necessary. There seems to be no information about other anticoagulants not specifically cited here but it would be prudent to assume that they will interact with tienilic acid similarly. Tienilic acid has been withdrawn in many countries because of its hepatotoxicity.

1. Detilleux M, Caquet R, Laroche C. Potentialisation de l'effet des anticoagulants comariniques par un nouveaux diurétique, l'acide tiénilique. *Nouv Presse Med* (1976) 5, 2395.
2. Prandota J, Pankow-Prandota L. Klinicznie znamienna interakcja nowego leku moczopednego kwasu tienylowego z lekami przeciwzakrzepowymi pochodnymi kumaryny. *Przegl Lek* (1982) 39, 385–8.
3. Portier H, Destaing F, Chavve L. Potentialisation de l'effet des anticoagulantes coumariniques par l'acide tiénilique: une nouvelle observation. *Nouv Presse Med* (1977) 6, 468.
4. Grand A, Drouin B, Arche G-J. Potentialisation de l'action anticoagulante des anti-vitamines K par l'acide tiénilique. *Nouv Presse Med* (1977) 6, 2691.
5. McLain DA, Garriga FJ, Kantor OS. Adverse reactions associated with ticrynafen use. *JAMA* (1980) 243, 763–4.
6. O'Reilly RA. Ticrynafen-racemic warfarin interaction: hepatotoxic or stereoselective? *Clin Pharmacol Ther* (1982) 32, 356–61.
7. O'Reilly RA, Sahud MA, Aggeler PM. Impact of aspirin and chlorthalidone on the pharmacodynamics of oral anticoagulant drugs in man. *Ann N Y Acad Sci* (1971) 179, 173–86.
8. Vinazzer H. Die Beeinflussungen der Antikoagulantientherapie durch ein Diuretikum. *Wien Z Inn Med* (1963) 44, 323–7.
9. Mönig H, Böhm M, Ohnhaus EE, Kirch W. The effects of frusemide and probenecid on the pharmacokinetics of phenprocoumon. *Eur J Clin Pharmacol* (1990) 39, 261–5.
10. Piesche L, Bölke T. Comparative clinical trial investigating possible interactions of torasemide (20 mg o.d.) or furosemide (40 mg o.d.) with phenprocoumon in patients with congestive heart failure. 4th International Congress on Diuretics, Boca Raton, Florida Oct 11–16 1992. Eds. Puschett JB, Greenberg A. Int Congr Series 1023 (1993) 267–70.
11. Petrick RJ, Kronacher N, Alcena V. Interaction between warfarin and ethacrynic acid. *JAMA* (1975) 231, 843–4.
12. Koch-Weser J. Hemorrhagic reactions and drug interactions in 500 warfarin-treated patients. *Clin Pharmacol Ther* (1973) 14, 139.
13. Nipper H, Kirby S, Iber FL. The effect of bumetanide on the serum disappearance of warfarin sodium. *J Clin Pharmacol* (1981) 21, 654–6.
14. Nilsson CM, Horton ES, Robinson DS. The effect of furosemide and bumetanide on warfarin metabolism and anticoagulant response. *J Clin Pharmacol* (1978) 18, 91–4.
15. Laizure SC, Madlock L, Cyr M, Self T. Decreased hypoprothrombinemic effect of warfarin associated with furosemide. *Ther Drug Monit* (1997) 19, 361–3.
16. O'Reilly RA. Spironolactone and warfarin interaction. *Clin Pharmacol Ther* (1980) 27, 198–201.
17. Robinson DS, Sylwester D. Interaction of commonly prescribed drugs and warfarin. *Ann Intern Med* (1970) 72, 853–6.
18. Sellers EM, Koch-Weser J. Kinetics and clinical importance of displacement of warfarin from albumin by acidic drugs. *Ann N Y Acad Sci* (1971) 179, 213–25.
19. Slattery JT, Levy G. Ticrynafen effect on warfarin protein binding in human serum. *J Pharm Sci* (1979) 68, 393.
20. Prandota J, Albengres E, Tillement JP. Effect of tienilic acid (Diflurex) on the binding of warfarin 14C to human plasma proteins. *Int J Clin Pharmacol Ther Toxicol* (1980) 18, 158–62.

Anticoagulants + Dong quai (Angelica sinensis)

Two case reports describe a very marked increase in the anticoagulant effects of warfarin when dong quai was added.

Clinical evidence, mechanism, importance and management

A 46-year old African-American woman with atrial fibrillation and stabilised on **warfarin** showed a greater than twofold increase in her prothrombin time and INR after taking **dong quai** for 4 weeks. The prothrombin time and INR were back to normal 4 weeks after stopping the **dong quai**.[1] Another woman who had been taking **warfarin** for 10 years developed widespread bruising and an INR of 10, a month after starting to take **dong quai**.[2]

The reasons are not understood but **dong quai** is known to consist of natural coumarin derivatives which may possibly have anticoagulant properties and inhibit platelet aggregation.

These seem to be only reports of this apparent interaction, but patients on **warfarin** should be warned of the potential risks of also taking **dong quai**. For safety **dong qaui** should be avoided unless the effects on anticoagulation can be monitored. More study is needed. Information about other anticoagulants is lacking.

1. Page RL, Lawrence JD. Potentiation of warfarin by dong quai. *Pharmacotherapy* (1999) 19, 870-6.
2. Ellis GR, Stephens MR. Untitled report. *BMJ* (1999) 319, 650.

Anticoagulants + Erythromycin

A marked increase in the effects of warfarin with bleeding has been seen in a small number of patients when concurrently treated with erythromycin, but most patients are unlikely to develop a clinically important interaction. This interaction has also been seen in two patients on acenocoumarol (nicoumalone).

Clinical evidence

(a) Acenocoumarol (Nicoumalone)

Haemorrhage occurred in a patient on **acenocoumarol** when treated with **erythromycin**.[14] Another patient on **acenocoumarol** showed an INR rise from 3–4.5 to 15 within a week of starting to take 1.5 mg **erythromycin ethylsuccinate** but no bleeding was seen.[15]

(b) Warfarin

An elderly woman on **warfarin**, digoxin, hydrochlorothiazide and quinidine developed haematuria and bruising within a week of starting to take 2 g **erythromycin stearate** daily. Her prothrombin time had risen to 64 s.[1] At least 8 other cases of bleeding and/or hypoprothrombinaemia have been described in patients on **warfarin** when given **erythromycin** (as **ethylsuccinate**, **stearate**, **estolate**, **lactobionate** or **base**).[2-9]

A study in 12 normal subjects found that the clearance of a single dose of **warfarin** was reduced by an average of 14% (range zero to almost one-third) after taking 1 g **erythromycin** daily for 8 days.[10] **Erythromycin** caused only a small increase in the effects of **warfarin** in another study on 8 patients.[11,12] A single-dose study with warfarin in 15 normal subjects found that 5 day's treatment with 1 g **erythromycin** daily increased the AUC of (S)-warfarin by 11.2% and of (R)-warfarin by 11.9%. The INR increased by 10.2%.[13]

Mechanism

It is believed that erythromycin can stimulate the liver enzymes to produce metabolites which bind to cytochrome P450 to form inactive complexes, the result being that the metabolism of warfarin is reduced and its effects are thereby increased.[10] But why it only happens to any great extent in a few individuals is not clear.

Importance and management

An established and unpredictable interaction. The paucity of reports about problems suggests that its clinical relevance in most patients is very limited but in a few patients the effects are apparently considerable. Concurrent use need not be avoided but it would be prudent initially to monitor the effects closely, especially in those who clear warfarin and other anticoagulants slowly and who therefore only need low doses. The elderly in particular would seem to fall into this higher risk category. Reports of interactions between erythromycin and anticoagulants other than warfarin and acenocoumarol appear to be lacking, but the same precautions would seem advisable with any of them.

1. Bartle WR. Possible warfarin-erythromycin interaction. *Arch Intern Med* (1980) 140, 985–7.
2. Schwartz JI, Bachmann KA. Erythromycin-warfarin interaction. *Arch Intern Med* (1984) 144, 2094.
3. Husserl FE. Erythromycin-warfarin interaction. *Arch Intern Med* (1983) 143, 1831–6.
4. Sato RI, Gray DR, Brown SE. Warfarin interaction with erythromycin. *Arch Intern Med* (1984) 144, 2413–14.
5. Friedman HS, Bonventre MV. Erythromycin-induced digoxin toxicity. *Chest* (1982) 82, 202.
6. Hansten PD, Horn JR. Erythromycin and warfarin. *Drug Interactions Newsletter* (1985) 5, 37–40.
7. Hassell D, Utt JK. Suspected interaction: warfarin and erythromycin. *South Med J* (1985) 78, 1015–16.
8. Bussey HI, Knodel LC, Boyle DA. Warfarin-erythromycin interaction. *Arch Intern Med* (1985) 145, 1736–7.
9. O'Donnell D. Antibiotic-induced potentiation of oral anticoagulant agents. *Med J Aust* (1989) 150, 163–4.
10. Bachmann K, Schwartz JI, Forney R, Frogameni A, Jauregui LE. The effect of erythromycin on the disposition kinetics of warfarin. *Pharmacology* (1984) 28, 171–6.

11. Weibert RT, Lorentz SM, Townsend RJ, Cook CE, Klauber MR, Jagger PI. Effect of erythromycin in patients receiving long-term warfarin therapy. *Clin Pharmacol Ther* (1987) 41, 224.
12. Weibert RT, Lorentz SM, Townsend RJ, Cook CE, Klauber MR, Jagger PI. Effect of erythromycin in patients receiving long-term warfarin therapy. *Clin Pharm* (1989) 8, 210–14.
13. Ellsworth A, Horn JR, Wilkinson W, Black DJ, Church L, Sides GD, Harris J, Cullen PD. An evaluation of the effect of dirithromycin (D) and erythromycin (E) on the pharmacokinetics and pharmacodynamics of warfarin (W). *Intersci Conf Antimicrob Agents Chemother* (1995) 35, 9.
14. Grau E, Fontcuberta J, Félez J. Erythromycin-oral anticoagulants interaction. *Arch Intern Med* (1986) 146, 1639.
15. Grau E, Real E, Pastor E. Macrolides and oral anticoagulants: a dangerous association. *Acta Haematol (Basel)* (1999) 102, 113–14.

Anticoagulants + Ethchlorvynol

The anticoagulant effects of dicoumarol and warfarin are reduced by the concurrent use of ethchlorvynol.

Clinical evidence

Six patients on **dicoumarol** showed a rise in their Quick index from 38 to 55% while taking 1 g **ethchlorvynol** daily over an 18-day period. Another patient on **dicoumarol** became over-anticoagulated and developed haematuria on two occasions when the **ethchlorvynol** was withdrawn, once for 6 days and the other for 4 days.[1] A marked reduction in the anticoagulant effects of **warfarin** occurred in another patient when given **ethchlorvynol**.[2]

Mechanism

Uncertain. The idea that ethchlorvynol increases the metabolism of the anticoagulants by the liver is not confirmed by studies in *dogs* and *rats*.[3]

Importance and management

Information is very sparse and limited to dicoumarol and warfarin, but the interaction seems to be established. Be alert for other anticoagulants to behave similarly. Anticipate the need to alter the anticoagulant dosage if ethchlorvynol is started or stopped. An alternative non-interacting substitute for ethchlorvynol may be found among the benzodiazepines.

1. Johansson S-A. Apparent resistance to oral anticoagulant therapy and influence of hypnotics on some coagulation factors. *Acta Med Scand* (1968) 184, 297–300.
2. Cullen SI and Catalano PM. Griseofulvin-warfarin antagonism. *JAMA* (1967) 199, 582.
3. Martin YC. The effect of ethchlorvynol on the drug-metabolising enzymes of rats and dogs. *Biochem Pharmacol* (1967) 16, 2041–4.

Anticoagulants + Etodolac

Etodolac appears not to interact with warfarin.

Clinical evidence, mechanism, importance and management

Eighteen normal subjects were given **warfarin** (20 mg on day 1, 10 mg on days 2 and 3) or **etodolac** (200 mg 12-hourly) or both drugs together in a three-period crossover study, each period lasting 2.5 days. Although the median peak serum levels of the **warfarin** fell by 19% and the median total clearance fell by 13% while taking both drugs, the prothrombin time response remained unchanged. Another study in 16 normal subjects given **warfarin** (20 mg on day 1, 10 mg on days 2 and 3) with and without 200 mg etodolac (200 mg 12-hourly) found some small changes in the pharmacokinetics of **warfarin** but its effects were unchanged.[2]

There would therefore seem to be no reason for avoiding concurrent use although it would be prudent to monitor the response, firstly because all NSAIDs have some effect on platelet activity, and secondly

because clinical experience with **etodolac** is still fairly limited. There seems to be nothing documented about other anticoagulants.

1. Ermer JC, Hicks DR, Wheeler SC, Kraml M, Jusko WJ. Concomitant etodolac affects neither the unbound clearance nor the pharmacologic effect of warfarin. *Clin Pharmacol Ther* (1994) 55, 305–16.
2. Zvaifler N. A review of the antiarthritic efficacy and safety of etodolac. *Clin Rheumatol* (1989) 8 (Suppl 1), 43–53.

Anticoagulants + Felbamate

An isolated case report describes a marked increase in the effects of warfarin in a man attributed to the addition of felbamate.

Clinical evidence, mechanism, importance and management

A man of 62 with a seizure disorder and on **warfarin** had his antiepileptic treatment with carbamazepine, phenobarbital (phenobarbitone) and sodium valproate discontinued and replaced by 2.4 g **felbamate** daily and later 3.2 g daily. Within 14 days his INR had risen from a normal range of 2.5–3.5 to 7.8. After stopping and later restarting the **warfarin** his INR rose within about another 14 days to 18.2. He was eventually restabilised on about half his former **warfarin** dosage. The authors of the report suggest that the withdrawal of the carbamazepine and phenobarbital was an unlikely reason for this reaction (both are enzyme inducers which would be expected to reduce the effects of **warfarin**) because no increases in **warfarin** dosage had been needed when they were started. Suspicion therefore falls on the **felbamate**, but it is clearly difficult to be sure that the withdrawal of the anticonvulsants did not have some part to play. Just why **felbamate** should interact like this is not known, but it is suggested that it inhibits the metabolism of the **warfarin**.[1] A letter commenting on this report favours the idea that what occurred was in fact due to the withdrawal of the carbamazepine and phenobarbital.[2]

The general importance of this interaction (if such it is) is uncertain, but it would now seem prudent to monitor the INR if **felbamate** is started or stopped in any patient, being alert for the need to reduce the **warfarin** dosage. More study is needed.

1. Tisdel KA, Israel DS, Kolb KW. Warfarin-felbamate interaction: first report. *Ann Pharmacother* (1994) 28, 805.
2. Glue P, Banfield CR, Colucci RD, Perhach JL. Comment: warfarin-felbamate interaction. *Ann Pharmacother* (1994) 28, 1412–13.

Anticoagulants + Fenyramidol (Phenyramidol)

The anticoagulant effects of warfarin, dicoumarol and phenindione are increased by fenyramidol (phenyramidol). Bleeding can occur if the anticoagulant dosage is not reduced appropriately.

Clinical evidence

Two patients on **warfarin** showed a marked increase in their prothrombin times when given 1.2 to 1.6 g **fenyramidol (phenyramidol)** daily. One of them bled. Further study on 8 other patients taking **warfarin**, **dicoumarol**, or **phenindione** showed that a marked increase in their prothrombin times occurred within 3 to 7 days of starting to take 0.8 to 1.6 g **fenyramidol** daily. No marked change occurred in a patient on **phenprocoumon**, but he only took the **fenyramidol** for three days.[1]

Mechanism

Studies in man, *mice* and *rabbits* suggest that fenyramidol inhibits the metabolism of the anticoagulants so that they are cleared from the body more slowly and their effects are thereby increased and prolonged.[2]

Importance and management

An established interaction although the documentation is very limited. Monitor prothrombin times and reduce the anticoagulant dosage as necessary to avoid bleeding. Anticoagulants other than those cited may be expected to behave similarly. The failure to demonstrate an interaction with phenprocoumon may have been because the fenyramidol (phenyramidol) was given for such a short time.

1. Carter SA. Potentiation of the effect of orally administered anticoagulants by phenyramidol hydrochloride. *N Engl J Med* (1965) 273, 423–6.
2. Solomon HM, Schrogie JJ. The effect of phenyramidol on the metabolism of bishydroxycoumarin. *J Pharmacol Exp Ther* (1966) 154, 660–6.

Anticoagulants + Feprazone

The anticoagulant effects of warfarin are increased by feprazone which can lead to bleeding.

Clinical evidence

Five patients on long term **warfarin** treatment showed a mean prothrombin time rise from 29 to 38 s after 5 days' treatment with 300 mg **feprazone** daily, despite a 40% reduction in the **warfarin** dosage (from 5 to 3 mg daily). Four days after withdrawal of the **feprazone**, their prothrombin times were almost back to pretreatment levels.[1]

Mechanism

Unknown. Feprazone is highly bound to plasma proteins so that some displacement from plasma protein binding sites can occur, but this alone almost certainly does not explain this interaction.

Importance and management

Although information is limited to the study quoted, the interaction would appear to be established. Concurrent use should be avoided to prevent bleeding. If that is not possible, the anticoagulant response should be closely monitored and suitable reductions made to the warfarin dosage. Other anticoagulants may be expected to behave similarly.

1. Chierichetti S, Bianchi G, Cerri B. Comparison of feprazone and phenylbutazone interaction with warfarin in man. *Curr Ther Res* (1975) 18, 568–72.

Anticoagulants + Fibrates

The fibrates increase the effects of oral anticoagulants. This has been reported with bezafibrate and acenocoumarol (nicoumalone), phenprocoumon or warfarin; with ciprofibrate and warfarin; with clofibrate and dicoumarol, phenindione or warfarin; with fenofibrate and acenocoumarol or warfarin, and with gemfibrozil and warfarin. Bleeding is likely if the anticoagulant dosage is not reduced appropriately (between about one-third to one-half). There have been fatalities.

Clinical evidence

(a) Bezafibrate

A study on 15 patients with hyperlipidaemia on **phenprocoumon** found that it was necessary to reduce the anticoagulant dosage by 20% when given 450 mg **bezafibrate** daily, and by 33% when given 600 mg.[1] In another study in 22 patients taking 400 mg **bezafibrate** daily the dosage of **acenocoumarol (nicoumalone)** had to be reduced by 20% to maintain a constant INR.[2] Severe hypoprothrombinaemia and gastrointestinal bleeding occurred in a patient (with hypoalbuminaemia due to nephrotic syndrome and chronic renal failure) on **acenocoumarol** when **bezafibrate** was added without a suitable adjustment of the anticoagulant dosage.[3] A woman showed an increased response to **warfarin** while taking **bezafibrate**, and a man

showed a reduced response to **warfarin** when he stopped taking **bezafibrate**.[4]

(b) Ciprofibrate

A two-way randomised placebo-controlled crossover study in 12 young healthy men found that the anticoagulant effects of a single 25-mg dose of **racemic warfarin** were increased 50% when taken on day 21 of a 26-day course of 100 mg **ciprofibrate** daily. The **ciprofibrate** caused a 28% decrease in the apparent intrinsic clearance of *(S)*-warfarin, which is the more active enantiomer.[5]

(c) Clofibrate

A study in three hospitals of 42 patients taking either **pheninidone** or **warfarin** showed that when additionally given **clofibrate** it was necessary to reduce the dosages of the anticoagulants. Ten out of 15 in Belfast needed a 25% reduction and 5 of them bled. All 9 in Edinburgh needed a 33% reduction, and 14 out of 18 in Johannesburg also needed a reduction.[6]

This interaction has been confirmed in other studies on a considerable number of patients anticoagulated with **warfarin**,[7-12] **phenindione**[13-15] or **dicoumarol**.[16] Bleeding has been described frequently, and death due to haemorrhage has occurred in at least two cases.[10,15]

(d) Fenofibrate (procetofene)

Two patients on **acenocoumarol (nicoumalone)** needed a 30% reduction in their dosage to maintain the same prothrombin time when given 200 mg **fenofibrate** in the morning and 100 mg in the evening.[17]

A patient on **warfarin** showed a rise in his INR from a range of 2.0 to 2.5 to 8.5 within a week of starting 200 mg **fenofibrate** daily. His INRs later restabilised when the **warfarin** dosage was reduced by 27%. Another patient on **warfarin** similarly showed a marked INR rise (from a range of 2.8-3.5 to 5.6) within 10 days of starting **fenofibrate** (dosage not stated).[18] Six patients taking **coumarin anticoagulants** (not specifically named) needed an average dosage reduction of 12% (range 0 to 21%) when treated with **fenofibrate**.[19] Yet another patient on **warfarin** showed an INR rise to 18 and bled when gemfibrozil was replaced by **fenofibrate**.[20] In another study it was found that **fenofibrate** increased the effects of **un-named anticoagulants** in 4 patients by the same amount as that seen with **clofibrate** (i.e. by about one-third[21]). A patient on an **un-named anticoagulant** developed haematuria when treated with **fenofibrate**.[22]

(e) Gemfibrozil

A brief report describes bleeding (". . . menstrual cycle prolonged and lots of blood clots . . .") and much higher prothrombin times (values not given) in a woman on **warfarin** within two weeks of starting to take 1200 mg **gemfibrozil** daily. Halving the **warfarin** dosage resolved the problem.[23] A patient stabilised on **warfarin** developed severe hypoprothrombinaemia and bleeding 4 weeks after starting gemfibrozil.[24] **Gemfibrozil** causes haemostatic changes very similar to those seen with clofibrate.[25]

Mechanism

Uncertain. Clofibrate can displace warfarin from its plasma protein binding sites,[26-28] but this does not adequately explain the interaction. Another suggestion is that the fibrates increase the affinity of the anticoagulant for the receptor sites or possibly alter the metabolism.[1,5,16]

Importance and management

The interactions of clofibrate with dicoumarol, phenindione and warfarin are established, clinically important and potentially serious. Severe bleeding (fatal in some instances) has been seen. The incidence of the interaction is reported to be between 20 and 100%,[1,7] but it would be prudent to assume that all patients will be affected. The anticoagulant dosage should be reduced initially by between one-third to one-half to avoid the risk of bleeding, and adjusted appropriately thereafter. Information about other oral anticoagulants is lacking but it would be prudent to assume that they will interact with clofibrate in a similar way.

Less is known about fenofibrate and even less about bezafibrate, ciprofibrate and gemfibrozil (the reports cited here are all I have been able to find) but it would be prudent to follow the same precautions suggested for ciprofibrate if any of them is used with any oral anticoagulant. More study is needed.

1. Zimmermann R, Ehlers W, Walter E, Hoffrichter A, Lang PD, Andrassy K, Schlierf G. The effect of bezafibrate on the fibrinolytic enzyme system and the drug interaction with racemic phenprocoumon. *Atherosclerosis* (1978) 29, 477–85.
2. Manotti C, Quintavalla R, Pini M, Tomasini G, Vargiu G, Dettori AG. Interazione farmacologica tra bezafibrato in formulazione retard ed acenocoumarolo. Studio clinico. *G Arteriosclerosi* (1991) 16, 49–52.
3. Blum A, Seligman H, Livneh A, Ezra D. Severe gastrointestinal bleeding induced by a probable hydroxycoumarin-bezafibrate interaction. *Isr J Med Sci* (1992) 28, 47–9.
4. Beringer TRO. Warfarin potentiation with bezafibrate. *Postgrad Med J* (1997) 73, 657–8.
5. Sanofi Withrop Ltd. Personal communication, December 1997.
6. Oliver MF, Roberts SD, Hayes D, Pantridge JF, Suzman MM, Bersohn I. Effect of Atromid and ethyl chlorophenoxyisobutyrate on anticoagulant requirements. *Lancet* (1963) i, 143–4.
7. Udall JA. Drug interference with warfarin therapy. *Clin Med* (1970) 77, 20–5.
8. Eastham RD. Warfarin dosage, clofibrate, and age of patient. *BMJ* (1973) ii, 554.
9. Roberts SD, Pantridge JF. Effect of Atromid on requirements of warfarin. *J Atheroscler Res* (1963) 3, 655–7.
10. Solomon RB, Rosner F. Massive hemorrhage and death during treatment with clofibrate and warfarin. *N Y State J Med* (1973) 73, 2002.
11. Bjornsson TD, Meffin PJ, Blaschke TF. Interaction of clofibrate with the optical enantiomorphs of warfarin. *Pharmacologist* (1976) 18, 207.
12. Counihan TB, Keelan P. Atromid in high cholesterol states. *J Atherscler Res* (1963) 3, 580–3.
13. Williams GEO, Meynell MJ, Gaddie R. Atromid and anticoagulant therapy. *J Atheroscler Res* (1963) 3, 658–70.
14. Rogen AS, Ferguson JC. Clinical observations on patients treated with Atromid and anticoagulants. *J Atheroscler Res* (1963) 3, 671–6.
15. Rogen AS, Ferguson JC. Effect of Atromid on anticoagulant requirements. *Lancet* (1963) i, 272.
16. Schrogie JJ, Solomon HM. The anticoagulant response to bishydroxycoumarin. II. The effect of D-thyroxine, clofibrate, and norethandrolone. *Clin Pharmacol Ther* (1967) 8, 70–7.
17. Harvengt C, Heller F, Desager JP. Hypolipidemic and hypouricemic action of fenofibrate in various types of hyperlipoproteinemias. *Artery* (1980) 7, 73–82.
18. Ascah KJ, Rock GA, Wells PS. Interaction between fenofibrate and warfarin. *Ann Pharmacother* (1998) 32, 765–8.
19. Stähelin HB, Seiler W, Pult N. Erfahrungen mit dem Lipidsenker Procetofen (Lipanthyl®) *Schweiz Rundsch Med Prax* (1979) 68, 24–8.
20. Aldridge MA, Ito ML. Fenofibrate and warfarin interaction. *Pharmacotherapy* (2001) 21, 886–9.
21. Raynaud P. Un nouvel hypolipidemiant: le procetofene. *Rev Med Tours* (1977) 11, 325–30.
22. Lauwers PL. Effect of procetofene on blood lipids of subjects with essential hyperlipidaemia. *Curr Ther Res* (1979) 26, 30–8.
23. Ahmad S. Gemfibrozil interaction with warfarin sodium (Coumadin). *Chest* (1990) 98, 1041–2.
24. Rindone JP, Keng HC. Gemfibrozil-warfarin interaction resulting in profound hypoprothrombinaemia. *Chest* (1998) 114, 641–2.
25. Rasi VPO, Torstila I. The effect of gemfibrozil upon platelet function and blood coagulation. Preliminary report. *Proc R Soc Med* (1976) 69 (Suppl 2), 109–11.
26. Solomon HM, Schrogie JJ, Williams D. The displacement of phenylbutazone-C¹⁴ and warfarin-C¹⁴ from human albumin by various drugs and fatty acids. *Biochem Pharmacol* (1968) 17, 143.
27. Solomon HM, Schrogie JJ. The effect of various drugs on the binding of warfarin-¹⁴C to human albumin. *Biochem Pharmacol* (1967) 16, 1219–26.
28. Bjornsson TD, Meffin PJ, Swezey S, Blaschke TF. Clofibrate displaces warfarin from plasma proteins in man: an example of a pure displacement interaction. *J Pharmacol Exp Ther* (1979) 210, 316–21.

Anticoagulants + Floctafenine or Glafenine

The anticoagulant effects of acenocoumarol (nicoumalone) and phenprocoumon are increased by floctafenine. The anticoagulant effects of phenprocoumon are increased by glafenine but no interaction occurs with acenocoumarol, ethyl biscoumacetate or 'indanedione'.

Clinical evidence, mechanism, importance and management

(a) Floctafenine

A double-blind study[1] on 10 patients on **acenocoumarol (nicoumalone)** or **phenprocoumon** showed that concurrent treatment with 800 mg **floctafenine** daily prolonged their thrombotest times by an average of approximately one-third. The anticoagulant dosage of some of the patients was reduced. The reasons are not understood. The effects of concurrent use should be monitored and the anticoagulant dosage reduced as necessary. Information about other anticoagulants is lacking, but the same precautions would seem to be appropriate.

(b) Glafenine

A double-blind study on 20 patients stabilised on **phenprocoumon** showed that a significant increase in thrombotest times occurred within a week of starting to take 600 mg **glafenine** daily.[2] Another report states that five out of seven patients needed an anticoagulant dosage reduction while taking **glafenine**.[3] The reason is not understood. Monitor the effects of concurrent use and reduce the anticoagulant dosage appropriately. Ten subjects on **acenocoumarol (nicoumalone)**, **ethyl biscoumacetate** or '**indanedione**' showed no changes in their anticoagulant response when given 800 mg **glafenine** daily over a 4-week period.[4]

1. Boeijinga JK, van de Broeke RN, Jochemsen R, Breimer DD, Hoogslag MA, Jeletich-Bastiaanse A. De invloed van floctafenine (Idalon) op antistollingsbehandeling met coumarinederivaten. *Ned Tijdschr Geneeskd* (1981) 125, 1931–5.
2. Boeijinga JK, van der Vijgh WJF. Double blind study of the effect of glafenine (Glifanan®) on oral anticoagulant therapy with phenprocoumon (Marcumar®). *Eur J Clin Pharmacol* (1977) 12, 291–6.
3. Boeijinga JK, Bing GT, van der Meer J. De invloed van glafenine (Glifanan) op antistollingsbehandeling met coumarinederivaten. *Ned Tijdschr Geneeskd* (1974) 118, 1895–8.
4. Raby C. Recherches sur une éventuelle potentialisation de l'action des anticoagulants de synthèse par la glafénine. *Therapie* (1977) 32, 293–9.

Anticoagulants + Flosequinan

Flosequinan normally appears not to interact to a clinically significant extent with warfarin.

Clinical evidence, mechanism, importance and management

20 patients anticoagulated with **warfarin** showed statistically significant increases in INR, PTT and Prothrombin Times, and a decrease in factor VII when given 50 mg **flosequinan** twice daily for 2 weeks, but the values remained within acceptable clinical levels and none of the changes was considered to be clinically relevant.[1] Isolated reports of decreased **warfarin** requirements have been reported to the makers of **flosequinan**, but no causal link has been established.[2] No special precautions seem necessary during concurrent use except that it has been suggested that INRs should be well monitored in those with severe heart failure who are given **flosequinan** and **warfarin**. Flosequinan was withdrawn from general use in July 1993.

1. Boots Pharmaceuticals. Data on file (Study FN/89/132), 1993.
2. Boots Pharmaceuticals. Personal communication, August 1993.

Anticoagulants + Fluconazole

The anticoagulant effects of warfarin are increased by fluconazole. Bleeding may occur if the anticoagulant dosage is not reduced appropriately. Acenocoumarol (nicoumalone) also appears to interact.

Clinical evidence

(a) Acenocoumarol (Nicoumalone)

A patient on **acenocoumarol** suffered an intracranial haemorrhage (prothrombin time 170 s) 5 days after starting to take 200 mg **fluconazole** daily.[1]

(b) Warfarin

Seven patients on **warfarin** showed the following increases in prothrombin times when 100 mg **fluconazole** was added: 15.8 s on day 1, 18.9 s on day 5, and 21.9 s on day 8. The **fluconazole** was stopped early in 3 of the patients due to high prothrombin times, but none exceeded an increase of 9.7 s and no bleeding occurred.[2]

A crossover study in 13 subjects given 200 mg **fluconazole** daily for 7 days and then a single 15-mg dose of **warfarin** found that the changes in the prothrombin time curve over 168 h were increased about 10% in 10 subjects, by about 13% in 2 subjects, and doubled in one other. The last subject was given vitamin K.[3] 400 mg **fluconazole** daily for a week increased the prothrombin time AUC following a single dose of pseudoracemic **warfarin** in 6 subjects by 44%.[4] Increased prothrombin times and INRs have been reported in a number of other patients and subjects on **warfarin** when treated with **fluconazole**.[5-12] Four patients bled.[5,9,11,13]

Mechanism

In vitro studies using human liver microsomes clearly demonstrate that fluconazole inhibits cytochrome P450 isoenzymes CYP2C9, CYP3A4 and possibly others.[14] *In vivo* this results in the accumulation of warfarin and in an increase in its effects, possibly leading to bleeding.[12] Other anticoagulants are probably affected in the same way.

Importance and management

An established and clinically important interaction. If fluconazole is added to treatment with warfarin or acenocoumarol (nicoumalone), the prothrombin times should be very well monitored and the anticoagulant dosage reduced as necessary. On the basis of kinetic studies it has been predicted that an approximately 20% reduction in the warfarin dosage may be needed when using 50 mg fluconazole daily, ranging to about a 70% reduction when using 600 mg fluconazole daily.[15] However remember that individual variations between patients can be considerable. There seems to be no information about other anticoagulants, but it would be prudent to follow the same precautions with any of them.

1. Isalska BJ, Stanbridge TN. Fluconazole in the treatment of candidal prosthetic valve endocarditis. *BMJ* (1988) 297, 178–9.
2. Crussell-Porter LL, Rindone JP, Ford MA, Jaskar DW. Low-dose fluconazole therapy potentiates the hypoprothrombinemic response of warfarin sodium. *Arch Intern Med* (1993) 153, 102–4.
3. Lazar JD, Wilner KD. Drug interactions with fluconazole. *Rev Infect Dis* (1990) 12 (Suppl 3), S327–S333.
4. Black DJ, Gidal BE, Seaton TL, McDonnell ND, Kunze KL, Evans JS, Bauwens JE, Petersdorf SH, Trager WF. An evaluation of the effect of fluconazole on the stereoselective metabolism of warfarin (W). *Clin Pharmacol Ther* (1992) 51, 184.
5. Seaton TL, Celum CL, Black DJ. Possible potentiation of warfarin by fluconazole. *DICP Ann Pharmacother* (1990) 24, 1177–8.
6. Tett S, Carey D, Lee H-S. Drug interactions with fluconazole. *Med J Aust* (1992) 156, 365.
7. Beeley L, Cunningham H, Brennan A. Bulletin of the West Midlands Centre of Adverse Drug Reporting. (1993) 36, 17.
8. Rieth H, Sauerbrey N. Interaktionsstudien mit Fluconazol, einem neuen Triazolantimykotikum. *Wien Med Wochenschr* (1989) 139, 370–4.
9. Kerr HD. Case report: potentiation of warfarin by fluconazole. *Am J Med Sci* (1993) 305, 164–5.
10. Gericke KR. Possible interaction between warfarin and fluconazole. *Pharmacotherapy* (1993) 13, 508–9.
11. Baciewicz AM, Menke JJ, Bokar JA, Baud EB. Fluconazole-warfarin interaction. *Ann Pharmacother* (1994) 28, 1111.
12. Black DJ, Kunze KL, Wienkers LC, Gidal BE. Seaton TL, McDonnell ND, Evans JS, Bauwens JE, Trager WF. Warfarin-fluconazole II. A metabolically based drug interaction: in vivo studies. *Drug Metab Dispos* (1996) 24, 422–8.
13. Mootha VV, Schluter ML, Das A. Intraocular hemorrhages due to warfarin-fluconazole drug interaction in a patient with presumed Candida Endophthalmitis. *Arch Ophthalmol* (2002) 120, 94–5.
14. Kunze KL, Wienkers LC, Thummel KE, Trager WF. Warfarin-fluconazole I. Inhibition of the human cytochrome P450–dependent metablism of warfarin by fluconazole: in vitro studies. *Drug Metab Dispos* (1996) 24, 414–21.
15. Kunze KL, Trager WF. Warfarin-fluconazole III. A rational approach to management of a metabolically based drug interaction. *Drug Metab Dispos* (1996) 24, 429–35.

Anticoagulants + Fluoxetine

Normally fluoxetine appears not to interact with warfarin but very occasionally and unpredictably increased effects (raised INRs, bruising, bleeding) have been reported.

Clinical evidence

(a) Evidence of no interaction

Fluoxetine given as a single dose or in multiple doses over 8 days had no effect on the pharmacokinetics or the anticoagulant effects of 20 mg **warfarin**.[1] The half-life of **warfarin** was not significantly changed in 3 normal subjects by either a single 30-mg dose of **fluox-**etine given 3 h before the **warfarin**, or by 30 mg **fluoxetine** daily for a week.[2] Six patients anticoagulated with **warfarin** showed no significant changes in their prothrombin times while taking 20 mg **fluoxetine** daily for 21 days.[3]

(b) Evidence of an interaction

The INR of a man on **warfarin**, amiodarone, furosemide (frusemide), digoxin, ciprofloxacin and levothyroxine rose sharply from a range of 1.8-2.3 to 14.9 within 5 days of starting 20 mg **fluoxetine** daily. The INR of another man with metastatic carcinoma on **warfarin**, dexamethasone, bisacodyl and lactulose rose from a range of 2.5–3.5 to 15.5 within 2 weeks of starting 20 mg **fluoxetine** daily. He showed microscopic haematuria but no bleeding. Yet another man on **warfarin** developed a large spontaneous abdominal haematoma when given **fluoxetine**.[4] The INRs of 2 other patients on **warfarin** increased when **fluoxetine** was given, and fell again when it was withdrawn.[5] An elderly man on **warfarin** developed an elevated INR and died of a cerebral haemorrhage when given diazepam and **fluoxetine**.[6] A very brief report describes increased **warfarin** effects and small bowel haemorrhage in one patient on **fluoxetine**. The concurrent use of **mefenamic acid** may have been a contributory factor.[7,8] Another patient on **fluoxetine** developed severe bruising when given **warfarin**.[9] The CSM in the UK is also said to have 4 other similar cases on record.[5] Another retrospective study of patient records identified 8 patients on **warfarin** all of whom showed prolongation of prothrombin times (extent not stated) which was attributed to the concurrent use of **fluoxetine**.[10]

Mechanism

Not understood. One suggestion is that fluoxetine inhibits the metabolism of the warfarin by the liver, thereby causing its effects to be increased.[4] It is also known that large doses of fluoxetine in the absence of an anticoagulant can sometimes cause bruising and bleeding episodes.[11,12] What is not clear is just why this apparent interaction affects only a very few individuals.

Importance and management

Information appears to be limited to the reports cited. The overall picture seems to be that normally no clinically relevant interaction occurs but occasionally and unpredictably a few individuals develop raised INRs and possibly bleeding. Bearing in mind the now extremely wide use of both drugs these episodes would seem to be rare. The concurrent use of warfarin and fluoxetine need not be avoided but the outcome should be monitored so that any rare cases can be identified and dealt with accordingly. Information about other anticoagulants seems to be lacking.

1. Lemberger L, Bergstrom RF, Wolen RL, Farid NA, Enas GG, Aronoff GR. Fluoxetine: clinical pharmacology and physiologic disposition. *J Clin Psychiatry* (1985) 46, 14–19.
2. Rowe H, Carmichael R, Lemberger L. The effect of fluoxetine on warfarin metabolism in the rat and man. *Life Sci* (1978) 23, 807–12.
3. Ford MA, Anderson ML, Rindone JP, Jaskar DW. Lack of effect of fluoxetine on the hypoprothrombinemic response of warfarin. *J Clin Psychopharmacol* (1997) 17, 110–12.
4. Hanger HC, Thomas F. Fluoxetine and warfarin interactions. *N Z Med J* (1995), 108, 157.
5. Woolfrey S, Gammack NS, Dewar MS, Brown PJE. Fluoxetine-warfarin interaction. *BMJ* (1993) 307, 241.
6. Dent LA, Orrock MW. Warfarin-fluoxetine and diazepam-fluoxetine interaction. *Pharmacotherapy* (1997) 17, 170–2.
7. Beeley L, Magee P, Hickey FN. Bulletin of the West Midlands Centre for Adverse Drug Reaction Reporting (1990) 30, 32.
8. Dista Products Limited. Personal communication, May 1990.
9. Claire RJ, Servis ME, Cram DL. Potential interaction between warfarin sodium and fluoxetine. *Am J Psychiatry* (1991) 148, 1604.
10. Wu J-R, Li P-YY, Yang Y-HK. Concurrent use of fluoxetine and warfarin prolongs prothrombin time: a retrospective survey. *Pharmacotherapy* (1997) 17, 1080.
11. Aranth J, Lindberg C. Bleeding, a side effect of fluoxetine. *Am J Psychiatry* (1992) 149, 412.
12. Yaryura-Tobias JA, Kirschen H, Ninian P, Mosberg HJ. Fluoxetine and bleeding in obsessive-compulsive disorder. *Am J Psychiatry* (1991) 148, 949.

Anticoagulants + Flupirtine

Flupirtine does not interact with phenprocoumon.

Clinical evidence, mechanism, importance and management

12 normal subjects showed no significant changes in serum **phenprocoumon** levels while taking 1.5 mg daily when additionally given 100 mg **flupirtine** three times daily for 14 days. The prothrombin times were also not significantly changed.[1] There would therefore seem to be no reason for taking special precautions if these drugs are given concurrently. Information about other oral anticoagulants seems to be lacking.

1. Harder S, Thürmann P, Hermann R, Weller S, Mayer M. Effects of flupirtine coadministration on phenprocoumon plasma concentrations and prothrombin time. *Int J Clin Pharmacol Ther* (1994) 32, 577–581.

Anticoagulants + Flutamide

Flutamide can increase the anticoagulant effects of warfarin.

Clinical evidence

Five patients with prostatic cancer on **warfarin** showed increases in their prothrombin times when given **flutamide**. For example, one patient needed reductions in his **warfarin** dosage from 35 to 22.5 mg weekly over a 2-month period. Another showed a prothrombin time rise from 15 to 37 s within 4 days of starting 750 mg **flutamide** daily.[1]

Mechanism

Not understood. Flutamide sometimes causes liver dysfunction.

Importance and management

Information is very limited but the interaction would seem to be established. Monitor prothrombin times if flutamide is given to patients on warfarin, reducing the dosage when necessary. Nothing seems to be known about the effects on other anticoagulants but it would seem prudent to follow the same precautions.

1. Schering-Plough Ltd. Personal communication, February 1990.

Anticoagulants + Food & Drinks

The rate of absorption of dicoumarol can be increased by food. Grapefruit juice is reported not affect acenocoumarol (nicoumalone) but may possibly cause a modest INR rise in a few individuals on warfarin. Two reports describe antagonism of the effects of warfarin by ice-cream, and another report attributes an increase in prothrombin time to the use of aspartame. Avocado, soybean protein and soybean oil and other intravenous lipids may also reduce the effects of warfarin. See also 'Anticoagulants + Alcohol', p.235, 'Anticoagulants + Natto', p.279, and 'Anticoagulants + Vitamin K', p.300.

Clinical evidence

(a) Acenocoumarol (Nicoumalone), Warfarin + Grapefruit juice

No clinically important interaction was detected when 12 normal subjects were given a single 10-mg oral dose of **acenocoumarol** and 150 ml **grapefruit juice**.[1,2] Another two-way crossover study in 24 patients found that while taking 250 ml **grapefruit juice** over a 4-week period the frequency of the **warfarin** dosage adjustments which were needed by the group as a whole was the same as when taking the placebo (**orange juice**), but 4 individuals showed a clinically significant, progressive and sustained 12 to 25% decrease in the **warfarin**/INR ratio.[3]

(b) Dicoumarol + Food

A study with 10 normal subjects showed that the peak serum concentrations of **dicoumarol**, following a single 250 mg dose, were increased on average by 85% when taken with **food**. Two subjects showed increases of 242 and 206%.[4]

(c) Warfarin + aspartame, avocado, ice-cream, soy

A very brief report states that a patient on **warfarin** showed a raised prothrombin time, possibly due to the use of **aspartame**.[5] Two women on **warfarin** showed falls in their INRs (from 2.5 to 1.6 and from 2.7 to 1.6 respectively) when they started to eat 100 g **avocado** or more daily. Their INRs climbed again when the **avocado** was stopped.[6]

A woman taking 22.5 mg **warfarin** in single daily doses failed to show the expected prolongation of her prothrombin times. It was then discovered that she took the **warfarin** in the evening and she always ate **ice-cream** before going to bed. When the **warfarin** was taken in the mornings, the prothrombin times increased.[7] Another patient's **warfarin** requirements almost doubled when she started to eat very large quantities of **ice cream** (1 litre each evening) but not while taking normal amounts. She took the **warfarin** at 6 pm and the **ice cream** at about 10 pm.[8]

A study in 10 patients with hypercholesterolaemia found that two weeks' treatment with a **soy-protein** cholesterol-lowering diet caused a marked reduction (Quick time increase of 114%) in the anticoagulant effects of **warfarin**.[9] 'Warfarin resistance' was seen in two other patients, one when given a constant intravenous infusion of **soybean oil emulsion** (*Intralipid*),[10] and the other when given an emulsified infusion preparation of **propofol** containing 10% **soybean oil**, and later when given 20% *Liposyn II*.[11]

Mechanisms

Not understood. One suggestion for the dicoumarol/food reaction[4] is that prolonged retention of dicoumarol with food in the upper part of the gut, associated with increased tablet dissolution, may have been responsible for the increased absorption. Soy protein possibly increases the activity of vitamin K at its liver receptors, thereby reducing the effects of warfarin. Avocado contains too little vitamin K (8 micrograms/100 g) for it to affect warfarin by competitive inhibition. The 4 patients who showed some evidence of a grapefruit juice/warfarin may possibly have had an increased susceptibility to the inhibitory effects of grapefruit juice on cytochrome P450 isoenzyme CYP3A4 activity in the gut.[3]

Importance and management

None of these interactions is very well documented but they clearly demonstrate that some foods and drinks, and particularly intravenous lipid preparations, can affect the response to the oral anticoagulants and may account for the otherwise unexplained fluctuations or changes in the anticoagulant response which some patients show. There is not enough evidence to suggest that any of these foods, drinks or preparations should be avoided unless serious problems develop.

1. van Rooij J, van der Meer FJM, Schoemaker HC, Cohen AF. Comparison of the effect of grapefruit juice and cimetidine on pharmacokinetics and anticoagulant effect of a single dose of acenocoumarol. *Br J Clin Pharmacol* (1993) 35, 548P.
2. van der Meer FJM. Personal communication, April 1994.
3. Dresser GK, Munoz C, Cruikshank M, Kovacs M, Spence JD. Grapefruit juice-warfarin interaction in anticoagulated patients. *Clin Pharmacol Ther* (1999) 65, 193.
4. Melander A, Wahlin E. Enhancement of dicoumarol bioavailability by concomitant food intake. *Eur J Clin Pharmacol* (1978) 14, 441–4.
5. Beeley L, Beadle F, Lawrence R. Bulletin of the West Midlands Centre for Adverse Drug Reaction Reporting. (1984) 19, 9.
6. Plickstein D, Shaklai M, Inbal A. Warfarin antagonism by avocado. *Lancet* (1991) 337, 914–15.
7. Simon LS, Likes KE. Hypoprothrombinemic response due to ice cream. *Drug Intell Clin Pharm* (1978) 12, 121–2.
8. Blackshaw CA, Watson VA. Interaction between warfarin and ice cream. *Pharm J* (1990) 244, 318.
9. Gaddi A, Sangiorgi Z, Ciarrocchi A, Braiato A, Descovich GC. Hypocholesterolemic soy protein diet and resistance to warfarin therapy. *Curr Ther Res* (1989) 45, 1006–10.

10. Lutomski DM, Palascak JE, Bower RH. Warfarin resistance associated with intravenous lipid administration. *J Parenter Enteral Nutr* (1987) 11, 316–18.
11. MacLaren R, Wachsman BA, Swift DK, Kuhl DA. Warfarin resistance associated with intravenous lipid administration: discussion of propofol and review of the literature. *Pharmacotherapy* (1997) 17, 1331–7.

Anticoagulants + Ginger

Despite some claims that ginger can interact with warfarin, there seems to be no clinical evidence to support this idea.

Clinical evidence, mechanism, importance and management

Ginger (*Zingiber Officinale*) is sometimes listed as a herb which interacts with **warfarin**,[1,2] but there do not appear to be any clinical reports of such an interaction. No reports were also found by two authors who undertook a comprehensive literature search using MEDLINE and a whole range of abstracting services (International Bibliographic Information on Dietary Supplements, International Pharmaceutical Abstracts, Reactions, Natural Medicines Comprehensive Database, German Commission E Monographs, The Review of Natural Products, Drug Interaction Facts, AltMedDex, Drug Therapy Screening System).[3]

There is a case report suggesting that **ginger** can inhibit platelet aggregation but other studies failed to confirm this effect, and the evidence to date suggests that there is no real substance to the idea that a **warfarin/ginger** interaction can take place.

1. Argento A, Tiraferri E, Marzaloni M. Oral anticoagulants and medicinal plants. An emerging interaction. *Ann Ital Med Int* (2000) 15, 139-43
2. Braun L. Herb-drug interaction guide. *Aust Fam Physician* (2001) 30, 473-6.
3. Vaes LPJ, Chyka PA. Interactions of warfarin with garlic, ginger, ginkgo, or ginseng: nature of the evidence. *Ann Pharmacother* (2000) 34, 1478-82.

Anticoagulants + Ginseng

An isolated report describes a man on warfarin whose INR was halved within 2 weeks of starting to take ginseng. There seem to be no other reports of an oral anticoagulant/ginseng interaction.

Clinical evidence, mechanism, importance and management

A man on long-term **warfarin** treatment because of a heart valve prosthesis (he was also taking diltiazem, glyceryl trinitrate and salsalate) showed a fall in his INR from 3.1 to 1.5 within 2 weeks of starting to take **ginseng** capsules (*Ginsana*) three times daily. This preparation contains 100 mg of standardised concentrated **ginseng** in each capsule. Within 2 weeks of stopping the **ginseng** his INR had risen again to 3.3.[1] Apart from the **ginseng** there was no other identifiable cause for this reaction, the mechanism of which is not clear. A later study in *rats* failed to find any evidence of a **warfarin/ginseng** interaction.[2]

This seems to be the first and only report of a **warfarin/ginseng** interaction. Bearing in mind the now wide-spread use of **ginseng**, the absence of interaction reports suggests that concurrent use is normally without problems, however there have been handful of reports of spontaneous bleeding in patients using **ginseng** preparations in the absence of an anticoagulant.[3,4] Ginseng has been found to contain antiplatelet components which might explain why bleeding sometimes occurs.[5]

1. Janetzky K, Morreale AP. Probable interaction between warfarin and ginseng. *Am J Health-Syst Pharm* (1997) 54, 692–3.
2. Zhu M, Chan KW, Ng LS, Chang Q, Chang S, Li RC. Possible influences of ginseng on the pharmacokinetics and pharmacodynamics of warfarin in rats. *J Pharm Pharmacol* (1999) 51, 175–80.
3. Hopkins MP, Androff L, Benninghoff AS. Ginseng face cream and unexplained vaginal bleeding. *Am J Obstet Gynecol* (1988) 159, 1121–2.
4. Greenspan EM. Ginseng and vaginal bleeding. *JAMA* (1983) 249, 2018.
5. Kuo SC, Teng CM, Leed JC, Ko FN, Chen SC, Wu TS. Antiplatelet components in Panax ginseng. *Planta Med* (199) 56, 164–7.

Anticoagulants + Glucagon

The anticoagulant effects of warfarin are rapidly and markedly increased by glucagon in large doses (50 mg or more over 2 days) and bleeding can occur if the warfarin dosage is not reduced appropriately.

Clinical evidence

Eight out of 9 patients on **warfarin** showed a marked increase in the anticoagulant effects (prothrombin times of 30 to 50 s or more) when given 50 mg **glucagon** over 2 days. Three of them bled. Eleven other patients given a total of 30 mg **glucagon** over 1 to 2 days failed to show this interaction.[1]

Mechanism

Unknown. Changes in the production of blood clotting factors and an increase in the affinity of warfarin for its site of action have been proposed.[1] A study in *guinea pigs* using acenocoumarol (nicoumalone) suggested that changes in warfarin metabolism or its absorption from the gut are not responsible.[2]

Importance and management

This appears to be an established interaction of clinical importance, although direct information is limited to the report cited.[1] Its authors recommend that if 25 mg glucagon per day or more are given for 2 or more days, the dosage of warfarin should be reduced in anticipation and prothrombin times closely monitored. Smaller doses (total 30 mg) are reported not to interact.[1] Information about other anticoagulants is lacking, but it would be prudent to assume that they will interact similarly.

1. Koch-Weser J. Potentiation by glucagon of the hypoprothrombinemic action of warfarin. *Ann Intern Med* (1970) 72, 331—5.
2. Weiner M, Moses D. The effect of glucagon and insulin on the prothrombin response to coumarin anticoagulants. *Proc Soc Exp Biol Med* (1968) 127, 761–3.

Anticoagulants + Glutethimide

The anticoagulant effects of warfarin and ethyl biscoumacetate can be decreased by the concurrent use of glutethimide.

Clinical evidence

10 subjects on **warfarin** with prothrombin times of 18 to 22 s showed a mean reduction of 4 s in their prothrombin times after taking 500 mg **glutethimide** daily for 4 weeks.[1,2] Other studies have shown that 1 g **glutethimide** daily for 3 weeks reduces the half-life of **warfarin** by between one-third to one-half.[3,4] An unexplained report describes a paradoxical increase in prothrombin times and haemorrhage in a patient on **warfarin** after taking 3.5 g **glutethimide** over a 5-day period.[5]

750 mg **glutethimide** daily for 10 days reduced the half-life of **ethyl biscoumacetate** in one patient by about one-third,[6,7] whereas in contrast, an early study on 25 patients on **ethyl biscoumacetate** found no evidence of an interaction.[8]

Mechanism

Glutethimide is a liver enzyme inducing agent which increases the metabolism and clearance of the anticoagulants from the body, thereby reducing their effects.[1-4,6,7] There is no obvious explanation for the reports of 'no interaction'[8] and of an 'increased effect'[5] cited above.

Importance and management

The warfarin/glutethimide interaction is established, while the ethyl biscoumacetate/glutethimide interaction is uncertain. Information about both interactions is limited and there seems to be nothing documented about any other anticoagulant, however it would be prudent to monitor the effect of adding glutethimide to patients taking any oral anticoagulant, being alert for the need to increase the anticoagulant dosage. Other interactions due to enzyme induction can take several weeks to develop fully and persist after withdrawal, so good monitoring and dosage adjustment should continue until anticoagulant stability has been achieved. A non-interacting substitute for glutethimide may possibly be found among the benzodiazepines.

1. Udall JA. Clinical implications of warfarin interactions with five sedatives. *Am J Cardiol* (1975) 35, 67–71.
2. Udall JA. Warfarin interactions with chloral hydrate and glutethimide. *Curr Ther Res* (1975) 17, 67.
3. Corn M. Effect of phenobarbital and glutethimide on biological half-life of warfarin. *Thromb Diath Haemorrh* (1966) 16, 606–12.
4. MacDonald MG, Robinson DS, Sylwester D, Jaffe JJ. The effects of phenobarbital, chloral betaine, and glutethimide administration on warfarin plasma levels and hypoprothrombinemic responses in man. *Clin Pharmacol Ther* (1969) 10, 80–4.
5. Taylor PJ. Hemorrhage while on anticoagulant therapy precipitated by drug interaction. *Ariz Med* (1967) 24, 697–9.
6. van Dam FE, Overkamp MJH. The effect of some sedatives (phenobarbital, glutethimide, chlordiazepoxide, chloral hydrate) on the rate of disappearance of ethylbiscoumacetate from the plasma. *Folia Med Neerl* (1967) 10, 141.
7. van Dam FE, Overkamp M, Haanen C. The interaction of drugs. *Lancet* (1966) ii, 1027.
8. Grilli H. Glutethimida y tiempo de protrombina. Su aplicación en la terapéutica anticoagulante. *Prensa Med Argent* (1959) 46, 2867–9.

Anticoagulants + Griseofulvin

The anticoagulant effects of warfarin can be reduced by the concurrent use of griseofulvin in some but not all patients.

Clinical evidence

The anticoagulant effects of **warfarin** were markedly reduced in 3 out of 4 individuals (2 of them patients) when they were given 1 to 2 g **griseofulvin** daily. The fourth subject (a volunteer) showed no interaction, even when the **griseofulvin** dosage was raised to 4 g daily for 2 weeks.[1]

In another study[2] only 4 out of 10 patients on **warfarin** showed this interaction after taking 1 g **griseofulvin** daily for 2 weeks.[2] The average reduction in prothrombin time was 4.2 s. A very brief report describes a coagulation defect in a patient on **warfarin** and **griseofulvin**.[3] Yet another describes this interaction in man which took 12 weeks to develop fully.[4] He eventually needed a 41% increase in his daily dose of **warfarin**.

Mechanism

Not understood. It has been suggested that the griseofulvin acts as a liver enzyme inducer which increases the metabolism of the warfarin, thereby reducing its effects.[1,4]

Importance and management

An established interaction but not well documented. It affects some but not all patients (3 out of 4, and 4 out of 10).[1,2] Because of its unpredictability, the prothrombin times of all patients on warfarin who are given griseofulvin should be monitored, and suitable warfarin dosage increases made as necessary. Information about other anticoagulants is lacking, but it would be prudent to assume that they will interact similarly.

1. Cullen SI, Catalano PM. Griseofulvin-warfarin antagonism. *JAMA* (1967) 199, 582–3.
2. Udall JA. Drug interference with warfarin therapy. *Clin Med* (1970) 77, 20–5.
3. McQueen EG. New Zealand Committee on Adverse Drug Reactions: 14th Annual Report. *N Z Med J* (1980) 91, 226.
4. Okino K, Weibert RT. Warfarin-griseofulvin interaction. *Drug Intell Clin Pharm* (1986) 20, 291–3.

Anticoagulants + H₂-blockers

The anticoagulant effects of warfarin can be increased if cimetidine is given concurrently. Severe bleeding has occurred in a few patients but some show no interaction at all. Aceno-coumarol (nicoumalone) and phenindione seem to interact similarly but not phenprocoumon. Famotidine, nizatidine, ranitidine and roxatidine normally appear to be non-interacting alternative H₂-blockers but bleeding has been reported in a handful of cases.

Clinical evidence

(a) Cimetidine

A very brief report in 1978, published as a letter by the makers of **cimetidine**, stated that at that time they were aware of 17 cases worldwide indicating that 1 g **cimetidine** daily could cause a prothrombin time rise of about 20% in those stabilised on **warfarin**.[1]

A number of studies and case reports have confirmed this interaction with **warfarin**.[2-9] Serum **warfarin** levels are reported to rise 25—80%,[8] and prothrombin times can be increased >30 s. Severe bleeding (haematuria, internal haemorrhages, etc.) and very prolonged prothrombin times have been seen in few patients.[2,4,6,7,9] However one study found that only half of the group of 14 patients actually demonstrated this interaction,[10] and another on 27 patients found that although the AUC of **warfarin** increased by 21—39% and the clearance fell by 22—28%, prothrombin times only increased by 2—2.6 s.[11] A pharmacokinetic study on 6 normal subjects found that cimetidine did not affect *(S)*-warfarin but increased the serum levels of *(R)*-warfarin, however the overall clinical effect was minimal.[12] **Acenocoumarol (nicoumalone)** and **phenindione** appear to interact like **warfarin**,[3,13] but not **phenprocoumon**.[14]

(b) Famotidine

A study in 8 subjects taking subtherapeutic doses of **warfarin** (mean 4 mg daily) showed that 7 days' treatment with 40 mg **famotidine** did not affect prothrombin times, thrombotest coagulation times or steady-state serum warfarin levels.[15] No changes in prothrombin times were seen in 3 patients on **acenocoumarol (nicoumalone)** or **fluindione** when given **famotidine**.[16] However in another report 2 patients on **warfarin** are said to have bled and had prolonged prothrombin times attributed to the concurrent use of **famotidine**.[17]

(c) Nizatidine

Nizatidine appears to behave like **ranitidine** and normally does not interact with **warfarin**,[18,19] but an isolated case of bleeding and markedly prolonged prothrombin times have been seen.[17]

(d) Ranitidine

The concurrent use of 400 mg **ranitidine** daily for 2 weeks had no effect on **warfarin** concentrations or on prothrombin times in five subjects.[20] In another study with 11 subjects it was found that 300 mg **ranitidine** daily for 3 days had no effect on the pharmacodynamics or pharmacokinetics of a single dose of **warfarin**.[2] In contrast, a third study[21,22] on 5 subjects reported that 300 mg **ranitidine** daily for a week reduced the clearance of a single dose of **warfarin** by almost 30%, but the half-life was not significantly changed and prothrombin times were not measured. **Ranitidine** 750 mg daily given to 2 subjects was also reported to have reduced the **warfarin** clearance by more than 50%. A number of aspects of this last study are open to doubt and the validity of the results is questionable. There is however an isolated report where 600 mg **ranitidine** daily, but not 300 mg, appeared to have been the cause of hypoprothrombinaemia and bleeding in a patient on **warfarin**.[23]

(e) Roxatidine

Twelve normal subjects anticoagulated with **warfarin** showed no changes in pharmacokinetics of the **warfarin** or the prothrombin ratio when given 150 mg **roxatidine** daily for four days.[24]

Mechanism

Cimetidine can inhibit the liver enzymes concerned with the metabolism (phase one hydroxylation) and clearance of warfarin so that its effects are prolonged and increased.[25] This also appears to be true for acenocoumarol and phenindione, but not phenprocoumon which is metabolised by different enzymes using another biochemical pathway (phase two glucuronidation).[14] The warfarin/cimetidine interaction has been found to be stereoselective, that is to say the cimetidine interacts with the $R(+)$-isomer but not with the $S(-)$-isomer.[12,26-28] The other H_2-blockers normally do not act as enzyme inhibitors.

Importance and management

The warfarin/cimetidine interaction is well documented, well established and clinically important but for reasons which are not understood many patients (probably up to 50% or even more) may not develop this interaction. Because of this unpredictability and to avoid bleeding with certainty the response should be monitored well in every patient when cimetidine is first added, being alert for the need to reduce the warfarin dosage. Acenocoumarol (nicoumalone) and phenindione are reported to interact similarly but the documentation is much more limited. Expect other anticoagulants to behave in the same way, with the possible exception of phenprocoumon.

Famotidine, nizatidine, ranitidine and roxatidine normally appear not to interact with oral anticoagulants, but concurrent use should be monitored because quite unpredictably and rarely an extension of prothrombin times and bleeding have been seen.

1. Flind AC. Cimetidine and oral anticoagulants. *Lancet* (1978) ii, 1054.
2. Silver BA, Bell WR. Cimetidine potentiation of the hypoprothrombinemic effect of warfarin. *Ann Intern Med* (1979) 90, 348–9.
3. Serlin MJ, Sibeon RG, Mossman S, Breckenridge AM, Williams JRB, Atwood JL, Willoughby JMT. Cimetidine: interaction with oral anticoagulants in man. *Lancet* (1979) ii, 317–19.
4. Hetzel D, Birkett D, Miners J. Cimetidine interaction with warfarin. *Lancet* (1979) ii, 639.
5. Breckenridge AM, Challiner M, Mossman S, Park BK, Serlin MJ, Sibeon RG, Williams JRB, Willoughby JMT. Cimetidine increases the action of warfarin in man. *Br J Clin Pharmacol* (1979) 8, 392P–393P.
6. Wallin BA, Jacknowitz A, Raich PC. Cimetidine and effect of warfarin. *Ann Intern Med* (1979) 90, 993.
7. Kerley B, Ali M. Cimetidine potentiation of warfarin action. *Can Med Assoc J* (1982) 126, 116.
8. O'Reilly RA. Comparative interaction of cimetidine and ranitidine with racemic warfarin in man. *Arch Intern Med* (1984) 144, 989–91.
9. Devanesen S. Prolongation of prothrombin time with cimetidine. *Med J Aust* (1981) 1, 537.
10. Bell WR, Anderson KC, Noe DA, Silver BA. Reduction in the plasma clearance rate of warfarin induced by cimetidine. *Arch Intern Med* (1986) 146, 2325–8.
11. Sax MJ, Randolph WC, Peace KE, Chretien S, Frank WO, Braverman AJ, Gray DR, McCree LC, Wyle F, Jackson BJ, Beg MA, Young MD. Effect of two cimetidine regimens on prothrombin time and warfarin pharmacokinetics during long-term warfarin therapy. *Clin Pharm* (1987) 6, 492–5.
12. Niopas I, Toon S, Aarons L, Rowland M. The effect of cimetidine on the steady-state pharmacokinetics and pharmacodynamics of warfarin in humans. *Eur J Clin Pharmacol* (1999) 55, 399-404.
13. van Rooij J, van der Meer FJM, Schoemaker HC, Cohen AF. Comparison of the effect of grapefruit juice and cimetidine on pharmacokinetics and anticoagulant effect of a single dose of acenocoumarol. *Br J Clin Pharmacol* (1993) 35, 548P.
14. Harenberg J, Staiger C, de Vries JX, Walter E, Weber E, Zimmerman R. Cimetidine does not increase the anticoagulant effect of phenprocoumon. *Br J Clin Pharmacol* (1982) 14, 292–3.
15. De Lepeleire I, van Hecken A, Verbesselt R, Tjandra-Maga TB, Buntix A, Distlerath L, De Schepper PJ. Lack of interaction between famotidine and warfarin. *Int J Clin Pharmacol Res* (1990) 10,161–71.
16. Chichmanian RM, Mignot G, Spreux A, Jean-Girard C, Hofliger P. Tolérance de la famotidine. Étude due réseau médecins sentinelles en pharmacovigilance. *Therapie* (1992) 47, 239–43.
17. Shinn AF. Unrecognized drug interactions with famotidine and nizatidine. *Arch Intern Med* (1991) 151, 810–14.
18. Callaghan JT, Nyhart EH. Drug interactions between H_2-blockers and theophylline (T) or warfarin (W). *Pharmacologist* (1988) 30, A14.
19. Cournot A, Berlin I, Sallord JC, Singlas E. Lack of interaction between nizatidine and warfarin during concurrent use. *J Clin Pharmacol* (1988) 28, 1120–2.
20. Serlin MJ, Sibeon RG, Breckenridge AM. Lack of effect of ranitidine on warfarin action. *Br J Clin Pharmacol* (1981) 12, 791–4.
21. Desmond PV, Breen KJ, Harman PJ, Mashford ML, Morphett BJ. Decreased clearance of warfarin after treatment with cimetidine or ranitidine. *Aust N Z J Med* (1983) 13, 327.
22. Desmond PV, Mashford ML, Harman PJ, Morphett BJ, Breen KJ, Wang YM. Decreased oral warfarin clearance after ranitidine and cimetidine. *Clin Pharmacol Ther* (1984) 35, 338–41.
23. Baciewicz AM, Morgan PJ. Ranitidine-warfarin interaction. *Ann Intern Med* (1990) 112, 76–7.
24. Labs RA. Interaction of roxatidine acetate with antacids, food and other drugs. *Drugs* (1988) 35 (Suppl 3), 82–9.
25. Henry DA, MacDonald IA, Kitchingman G, Bell GD, Langman MJS. Cimetidine and ranitidine: comparison of effects on hepatic drug metabolism. *BMJ* (1980) 281, 775–7.
26. Choonara IA, Cholerton S, Haynes BP, Breckenridge AM, Park BK. Stereoselective interaction between the R enantiomer of warfarin and cimetidine. *Br J Clin Pharmacol* (1986) 21, 271–77.
27. Toon S, Hopkins KJ, Garstang FM, Diquet B, Gill TS, Rowland M. The warfarin-cimetidine interaction: stereochemical considerations. *Br J Clin Pharmacol* (1986) 21, 245–6.
28. Niopas J, Toon S, Rowland M. Further insight into the stereoselective interaction between warfarin and cimetidine in man. *Br J Clin Pharmacol* (1991) 32, 508–11.

Anticoagulants + Halofenate

An isolated case report describes a marked increase in the anticoagulant effects of warfarin caused by the concurrent use of halofenate.

Clinical evidence, mechanism, importance and management

A patient, controlled on 10 mg **warfarin** daily, showed a dramatic increase in his prothrombin time to 103 s when he was given 10 mg/kg **halofenate** daily. His prothrombin times returned to normal when the **warfarin** dosage was reduced to 2.5 mg daily.[1] A similar interaction has been seen in *dogs* and it is suggested that **halofenate** can affect both the synthesis and destruction of prothrombin, the net effect being a prolongation of the prothrombin time.[2] Although this interaction appears to be of little general importance, it should be borne in mind if these drugs are used together.

1. McMahon FG, Jain A, Ryan JR, Hague D. Some effects of MK 185 on lipid and uric acid metabolism in man. *Univ Mich Med Cent J* (1970) 36, 247.
2. Weintraub M, Griner PF. Alterations in the effects of warfarin in dogs by halofenate. An influence upon the kinetics of prothrombin. *Thromb Diath Haemorrh* (1975) 34, 445–54.

Anticoagulants + Haloperidol

A single case report describes a marked reduction in the anticoagulant effects of phenindione caused by the concurrent use of haloperidol.

Clinical evidence, mechanism, importance and management

A man, stabilised on 50 mg **phenindione** daily, was given **haloperidol** by injection (5 mg eight-hourly for 24 h) followed by 3 mg twice daily by mouth. Adequate anticoagulation was not achieved even when the **phenindione** dosage was increased to 150 mg. When the **haloperidol** dosage was halved, the necessary dose of anticoagulant was 100 mg, and only when the **haloperidol** was withdrawn was it possible to return to the original anticoagulant dosage.[1] The reasons for this are not understood. The general importance of this interaction is probably small and concurrent use need not be avoided, but prescribers should be aware of this case.

1. Oakley DP, Lautch H. Haloperidol and anticoagulant treatment. *Lancet* (1963) ii, 1231.

Anticoagulants + Heparinoids

An isolated case report describes bleeding in a patient on acenocoumarol (nicoumalone) after using a heparinoid-impregnated bandage. Some of the normal tests of anticoagulation are unreliable for a few hours after giving danaparoid to patients already on acenocoumarol.

Clinical evidence, mechanism, importance and management

A man who was well stabilised on **acenocoumarol (nicoumalone)** and also taking metoprolol, dipyridamole and isosorbide dinitrate began to bleed within about 3 days of starting to use a medicated bandage on an inflamed lesion on his hand, probably caused by a mosquito bite. His prothrombin percentage was found to have fallen to less than 10%. The bandage was impregnated with a semi-synthetic heparinoid compound based on **xylane acid polysulphate** [possibly pentosan polysulphate].[1] It would appear that enough of the heparinoid had been absorbed through his skin to increase his anticoagulation to the point where he began to bleed. This case is unusual but it illustrates the need to keep a close watch on patients who are given a range of drugs, some of which can potentially cause bleeding.

A study in 6 normal subjects, anticoagulated with **acenocoumarol** (steady-state thrombotest values of 10 to 15%), found that a single intravenous bolus injection of 3250 anti-Xa units of **danaparoid (Org 10172)** prolonged the Prothrombin time, activated partial thromboplastin time and Stypven time more than would have been expected by the simple addition of the effects of both drugs. These effects were seen up to 1 h. The thrombotest was affected up to 5 h.[2] The results of these clinical tests may therefore be unreliable during these periods. There is no suggestion that concurrent use should be avoided.

1. Potel G, Maulaz B, Pabœcuf C, Touze MD, Baron D. Potentialisation de l'acénocoumarol après application cutanée d'un héparinoide semi-synthétique. *Therapie* (1989) 44, 67–8.
2. Stiekema JCJ, de Boer A, Danhof M, Kroon C, Broekmans AW, van Dinther TG, Voerman J, Breimer DD. Interaction of the combined medication with the new low-molecular-weight heparinoid Iomoparan® (Org 10172) and acenocoumarol. *Haemostasis* (1990) 20,136–46.

Anticoagulants + Herbal remedies

Isolated reports described increases in the anticoagulant effects of warfarin in patients taking medicinal garlic or a herbal tea made from *Lycium barbarum*. Increased anticoagulation was also seen in a patient on acenocoumarol after using a melilot-containing topical cream. These and other herbal remedies such as PC-SPES and possibly also tonka beans and sweet woodruff contain naturally occurring anticoagulants which may be expected to be additive with the effects of conventional anticoagulant drugs.

Clinical evidence, mechanism, importance and management

(a) Garlic

The INR of a patient stabilised on **warfarin** more than doubled and haematuria occurred eight weeks after starting to take three *Höfels garlic pearles* daily. The situation resolved when the **garlic** was stopped. The INR rose on a later occasion while taking two *Kwai garlic tablets* daily. The INR of another patient also more than doubled while taking six *Kwai* **garlic tablets** daily.[1,2] The reasons are not known.

Information about an anticoagulant/**garlic** interaction seems to be limited to just these two anecdotal reports from one author. Bearing in mind the wide-spread use of **garlic** and **garlic** products, it seems most unlikely that an anticoagulant/**garlic** interaction is of general importance. However it is worth noting that **garlic** has been associated with decreased platelet aggregation and a few cases of spontaneous bleeding (in the absence of an anticoagulant).[3,4]

(b) Lycium barbarum

A 61-year-old Chinese woman stabilised on **warfarin** (INRs normally 2-3) showed an unexpected INR rise to 4.1 during a routine monthly check. No bleeding was seen. She was also taking atenolol, benazepril, digoxin and fluvastatin. It was found that 4 days before visiting the clinic she had started to take 3 or 4 glasses (about 6 oz) daily of a Chinese herbal tea made from the fruits of *Lycium barbarum* (also known as Chinese wolfberry, gou qi zi, Fructus Lycii Chinensis or *Lycium chinense*) to treat blurred vision caused by a sore eye. This herbal remedy is used to ". . . combat yin deficiences . . ." When the herbal treatment was stopped, her INRs rapidly returned to normal. Later *in vitro* studies showed that an infusion of *Lycium barbarum* caused some inhibition of cytochrome P450 isoenzyme CYP2C9 but too weak to explain why this interaction occurred.[5] So far this is an isolated case but it draws attention to the possibility of problems with this herbal remedy in other patients.

(c) PC-SPES

An isolated case report describes a 62-year-old man with hormone-refractory prostate cancer who was hospitalised after developing nose bleeding, abdominal pain, haematuria and maroon-coloured faeces. He was found to have extensive ecchymoses, a large retroperitoneal

haematoma and a prothrombin time of >106 s. He was not taking any prescribed **anticoagulant drugs**, but it turned out that he was taking 12 capsules daily (twice the makers recommendation) of a herbal preparation, **PC-SPES**, which has potent estrogenic and antineoplastic activity, and is used for treating prostate cancer. This preparation contains 8 herbs,[6] one of which is **Baikal skullcap** or **Huang-chin** (*Scutellaria baicalensis Georgi*) which is believed to contain a phytocoumarin that can act as an anticoagulant.[7] It would seem that the patient had inadvertently over-anticoagulated himself.

(d) Tonka, Melilot, Sweet Woodruff

A woman with unexplained abnormal menstrual bleeding was found to have a prothrombin time of 53 s, and laboratory tests showed that her blood clotting factors were abnormally low. When given parenteral vitamin K her prothrombin time rapidly returned to normal (suggesting that she was taking a vitamin K antagonist of some kind). She strongly denied taking any anticoagulant drugs, but it was eventually discovered that she had been drinking large quantities of a herbal tea containing among other ingredients **tonka beans**, **melilot** and **sweet woodruff**, all of which contain natural coumarins that can be converted into anticoagulants by moulds.[8] The anticoagulant effects of these compounds may possibly have been increased by the **paracetamol** (**acetaminophen**) and **dextropropoxyphene** (**propoxyphene**) which she was taking concurrently.

A woman of 66 on **acenocoumarol** (and also taking levothyroxine and prazepam) showed an increase in her INRs after massaging a proprietary topical cream (*Cyclo 3*) containing **melilot** and *ruscus aculeatus* on her legs three times daily. On the first occasion her INR rose from about 2 to 5.8 after 7 days' use, and on a later occasion it rose to 4.6 after 10 days' use.[9]

These cases are isolated but they show that herbal preparations of this kind can affect anticoagulation. No prescribed anticoagulant drug was being used by the first patient. In the second case, absorption through the skin was enough to upset the anticoagulant control.

1. Sunter W. Warfarin and garlic. *Pharm J* (1991) 246, 722.
2. Sunter W. Personal communication, July 1991.
3. German K, Kumar U, Blackford HN. Garlic and the risk of TURP bleeding. *Br J Urol* (1995) 76, 518.
4. Rose KD, Croissant PD, Parliament CF, Levin MP. Spontaneous spinal epidural hematoma with associated platelet dysfunction from excessive garlic ingestion: a case report. *Neurosurgery* (1990) 26, 880-2.
5. Lam AY, Elmer GW, Mohutsky M. Possible interaction between warfarin and *Lycium barbarum*. *Ann Pharmacother* (2001) 35, 1199-1201.
6. Ades T, Gansler T, Miller M, Rosenthal DS. PC-SPES: current evidence and remaining questions. *C A Cancer J Clin* (2001) 51, 199-204.
7. Weinrobe MC, Montgomery B. Acquired bleeding diathesis in a patient taking PC-SPEC. *N Engl J Med* (2001) 345, 1213-4.
8. Hogan RP. Hemorrhagic diathesis caused by drinking an herbal tea. *JAMA* (1983) 249, 2679–80.
9. Chiffoleau A, Huguenin H, Veyrac G, Argaiz V, Dupe D, Kayser M, Bourin M, Jolliet P. Interaction entre mélilot et acénocoumarol ? (mélilot-*ruscus aculeatus*). *Therapie* (2001) 56, 321-7.

Anticoagulants + Herbicides

An isolated report describes a marked increase in the anticoagulant effects of acenocoumarol (nicoumalone) with bleeding caused by use of a herbicide.

Clinical evidence, mechanism, importance and management

A 55-year-old patient with mitral and aortic prostheses, stabilised on 2 mg acenocoumarol (nicoumalone) daily and with a normal thrombotest of 6 to 7% (INR 3.6 to 4.2), was hospitalised because of severe and uncontrollable gum bleeding. He responded when given a transfusion of fresh plasma. The cause of the marked increase in the anticoagulant effects of the acenocoumarol was eventually identified as almost certainly being due to the use of a herbicide (SATURN-S) containing thiobenzcarb and molinate (two thiocarbamates) which the patient was using to spray his rice crop. The thiobenzcarb can be absorbed through the skin and the molinate by inhalation. Just how these two compounds interact with acenocoumarol is not known but the authors of the report suggest the possibility that these herbicides may have inhibited the metabolism of the anticoagulant, thereby increasing its effects. The patient was later restabilised on his former dose of acenocoumarol.[1]

This seems to be the first and only report of this interaction but it highlights one of the possible risks of using chemical sprays (herbicides, pesticides etc) which have never been formally tested for their potential to interact with drugs.

1. Fernández MA, Aznar J. Potenciación del efecto anticoagulante del acenocoumarol por un herbicida. *Rev Iberoamer Tromb Hemostasia* (1988) 1, 40–1.

Anticoagulants + Hydrocodone

The anticoagulant effects of warfarin have been shown to be increased by hydrocodone in a patient and in a normal subject.

Clinical evidence, mechanism, importance and management

A patient, well stabilised on **warfarin** (and also taking digoxin, propranolol, clofibrate and spironolactone) showed a rise in his prothrombin time from about twice to three times his control value when he began to take *Tussionex* (**hydrocodone + phenyltoloxamine**) for a chronic cough. When the cough syrup was discontinued, his prothrombin time fell again. In a subsequent study in a volunteer the equivalent dosage of **hydrocodone** increased the elimination half-life of **warfarin** from 30 to 42 h.[1] The reason is not known. Concurrent use need not be avoided but monitor the effects and reduce the **warfarin** dosage if necessary.

1. Azarnoff DL. Drug interactions: the potential for adverse effects. *Drug Inf J* (1972) 6, 19–25.

Anticoagulants + Indinavir or Ritonavir

Ritonavir has been predicted to raise warfarin levels and INRs. This was confirmed by one case report whereas two others found entirely the opposite. One of these latter reports also suggests that indinavir might cause a moderate reduction in anticoagulation.

Clinical evidence

(a) Warfarin effects increased

In vitro and *in vivo* studies have shown that **ritonavir** is a potent inhibitor of cytochrome P450 isoenzymes CYP3A4, CYP2D6 and to a lesser extent CYP2C9, enzymes which are concerned with the metabolism of a large number of drugs. This means that **ritonavir** might be expected to increase the serum levels of the drugs metabolised by these cytochromes, leading in some cases to toxicity. Based primarily on a review of the literature, the makers of **ritonavir** have therefore assembled lists of drugs which they predict may interact, one of which is **warfarin**.[1,2] The following case is consistent with this prediction:

A man with deep vein thrombosis on 10 mg **warfarin** daily and INRs in the range 2.4 to 3.0 had his treatment for HIV changed from efavirenz and abacavir to **ritonavir**, nelfinavir and combivir. Within 5 days his INR had risen to 10.4 without any sign of bleeding. It proved difficult to achieve acceptable and steady INRs both while in hospital and after discharge, but eventually it was discovered that the patient could not tolerate liquid **ritonavir** because of nausea and vomiting, so that he had sometimes skipped or lowered the **ritonavir** dose or even refused to take it, and on those occasions the INRs had been low, whereas when he took the full dose of **ritonavir** the INRs were high.[3]

(b) Warfarin effects reduced

A man of 50 with HIV, stabilised on **warfarin**, was additionally started on 800 mg **indinavir** 8-hourly, but it had to be withdrawn after 12 days because of a generalised skin rash. It was then found that the **indinavir** had caused a moderate reduction in his level of anticoagulation (as measured by the prothrombin complex activity – PCA). His PCA rose from a range of 20-38% at 10 days after **indinavir** had been stopped and to 53% after 25 days When **ritonavir** (escalating doses up to 600 mg 12 hourly) was started instead, the **warfarin** dosage had to be raised from 6.25 to 8.75 mg daily to achieve PCAs in the range 31 to 33%.[4]

The INR of a 27-year-old woman with HIV and taking **warfarin** fell when she was additionally given **ritonavir**, clarithromycin and zidovudine. It was necessary almost to double the warfarin dosage to maintain satisfactory INRs. 3 Months later when the **ritonavir** was withdrawn, her INR more than tripled within a week. Her final warfarin maintenance dose was half of that needed before the **ritonavir** was started, and a quarter of the dose just before stopping the **ritonavir**. This case was complicated by the use or withdrawal of a number of other drugs (co-trimoxazole, didanosine, rifabutin, an oral contraceptive, megestrol) some of which can interact with warfarin.[5]

Mechanism

The increase in the anticoagulant effects seen in (a) above is consistent with the makers prediction that warfarin levels are expected to be increased by the inhibitory effects of ritonavir on the metabolism of warfarin, leading to increased warfarin effects, however the second two cases (b) suggest just the opposite and are unexplained.

Importance and management

The warfarin/ritonavir interaction is not established, but until more is known it would be prudent to monitor the prothrombin times and INRs of any patient if ritonavir is added, being alert for the need to modify the warfarin dosage, – but whether up or down is still uncertain. Information about other anticoagulants is lacking but the same precautions would seem sensible.

Information about a warfarin/indinavir interaction so far seems to be limited to the report cited, but the same precautions suggested for ritonavir would be appropriate.

1. Norvir (Ritonavir). Abbott Laboratories Limited. Summary of product characteristics, January 2001.
2. Norvir (Ritonavir). Product information. Physicians Desk Reference, 2002.
3. Newshan G, Tsang P. Ritonavir and warfarin interaction. *AIDS* (1999) 13, 1788-9.
4. Gatti G, Alessandrini A, Camera M, Di Biagnio A, Bassetti M, Rizzo F. Influence of indinavir and ritonavir on warfarin anticoagulant activity. *AIDS* (1998) 12, 825-6.
5. Knoell KR, Young TM, Cousins ES. Potential interaction involving warfarin and ritonavir. *Ann Pharmacother* (1998) 32, 1299-1302.

Anticoagulants + Indometacin (Indomethacin)

The anticoagulant effects of acenocoumarol (nicoumalone), clorindione, phenprocoumon and warfarin are not normally affected by the concurrent use of indometacin (indomethacin). However some caution is still necessary because indometacin can irritate the gut. In a handful of cases bleeding, attributed to an interaction, has been reported.

Clinical evidence

100 mg **indometacin (indomethacin)** daily for five days had no effect on the anticoagulant effects of **warfarin** in 16 normal subjects. When taken for 11 days by 19 normal subjects, neither the anticoagulant effects nor the half-life of **warfarin** were affected.[1]

Other studies in normal subjects and patients anticoagulated with **clorindione**,[2] **acenocoumarol (nicoumalone)**[3] or **phenprocoumon**[2,4,5] similarly showed that the anticoagulant effects were not changed by **indometacin**.

In contrast, a handful of somewhat equivocal reports describe possible interactions in patients taking **warfarin**. Two patients were also taking **allopurinol** which is known to interact occasionally with anticoagulants.[6,7] Another patient appeared to be inadequately stabilised on the anticoagulant before the **indometacin** was given.[8] No details are given in the third case,[9] and four other isolated and equivocal cases appear to result from unexplained interactions.[7,10-12] The validity of one[12] of these has been questioned.[13]

Mechanism

None. Indometacin reduces platelet aggregation and thereby prolongs bleeding when it occurs.

Importance and management

It is well established that normally indometacin (indomethacin) does not alter the anticoagulant effects acenocoumarol (nicoumalone), clorindione, phenprocoumon or warfarin. Other anticoagulants are expected to behave similarly. Concurrent use need not be avoided but good monitoring is still appropriate, firstly because indometacin, like other NSAIDs, can cause gastrointestinal irritation, ulceration and bleeding which may be prolonged (with a fatal outcome in one case[10]), and secondly because the handful of cases of unexplained and unconfirmed possible interactions cannot be dismissed entirely.

1. Vesell ES, Passananti GT, Johnson AO. Failure of indomethacin and warfarin to interact in normal human volunteers. *J Clin Pharmacol* (1975) 15, 486–95.
2. Müller G, Zollinger W. The influence of indomethacin on blood coagulation, particularly with regard to the interference with anticoagulant treatment. Die Entzundung-Grundlagen und Pharmakologische Beeinflussung. International Symposium on Inflammation. Freiburg, Breisgau, May 4–6, 1966. Heister R and Hofmann HF (eds), Urban and Schwarzenburg, Munich (1966).
3. Gáspárdy von G, Bálint G, Gáspárdy G. Wirkung der Kombination Indomethacin und Syncumar (Acenocumaral) auf den Prothrombinspiegel im Blutplasma. *Z Rheumaforsch* (1967) 26, 332–5.
4. Frost H, Hess H. Concomitant administration of indomethacin and anticoagulants. Die Entzundung-Grundlagen und Pharmakologische Beeinflussung. International Symposium on Inflammation. Freiburg, Breisgau, May 4–6, 1966. Heister R and Hofmann HF (eds), Urban and Schwarzenburg, Munich (1966).
5. Muller KH, Herrmann K. Is simultaneous therapy with anticoagulants and indomethacin feasible? *Med Welt* (1966) 17, 1553–4.
6. Ødegaard AE. Undersøkelse av interaksjon mellom antikoagulantia og indometacin. *Tidsskr Nor Laegeforen* (1974) 94, 2313–14.
7. Chan TYK. Prolongation of prothrombin time with the use of indomethacin and warfarin. *Br J Clin Pract* (1997) 51, 177-8.
8. Koch-Weser J. Haemorrhagic reactions and drug interactions in 500 warfarin-treated patients. *Clin Pharmacol Ther* (1973) 14, 139.
9. McQueen EG. New Zealand Committee on Adverse Reactions. *N Z Med J* (1980) 91, 226.
10. Self TH, Soloway MS, Vaughn D. Possible interaction of indomethacin and warfarin. *Drug Intell Clin Pharm* (1978) 12, 580–1.
11. Beeley L, Stewart P. Bulletin of the West Midlands Centre for Adverse Drug Reaction Reporting (1987) 25, 28.
12. Chan TYK, Lui SF, Chung SY, Luk S, Critchley JAJH. Adverse interaction between warfarin and indomethacin. *Drug Safety* (1994) 10, 267–9.
13. Day R, Quinn D. Adverse interaction between warfarin and indomethacin. *Drug Safety* (1994) 11, 213–14.

Anticoagulants + Influenza vaccines

The concurrent use of warfarin and influenza vaccine is usually safe and uneventful, but there are reports of bleeding in a handful of patients (life-threatening in one case) attributed to an interaction. Acenocoumarol (nicoumalone) also does not normally interact.

Clinical evidence

(a) Evidence of no interaction

After vaccination with **1982/3 Trivalent influenza vaccines**, **Types A and B**, the prothrombin times of 21 men on long-term **warfarin** treatment were not significantly altered.[1]

Other studies[2,3] on 13 and 19 elderly men and women, 24, 26 and 33 other patients,[4-6] found no evidence of an adverse **warfarin/influenza vaccine** interaction, although a small increase in the prothrombin ratio (from 1.68 to 1.81) was seen in one study[5] and a small prothrombin time decrease in another.[6] No interaction was seen in

other studies on four volunteer subjects[7] or on 7 and 33 residents in nursing homes.[8,9] One case of gross but transient haematuria occurred, but it was not possible to link this firmly with the vaccination.[8] **Trivalent influenza vaccine** has also been shown not to affect anticoagulation with **acenocoumarol** (**nicoumalone**).[10,11]

(b) Evidence of an interaction

A very brief report[12] describes a patient on long-term **warfarin** treatment who ". . . almost bled to death after receiving a '**flu shot**'. . ." No further details are given.[12] An elderly man on long-term **warfarin** treatment developed bleeding (haematemesis and melaena) shortly after being given an **influenza vaccine**. His prothrombin time was found to be 36 s. A subsequent study on eight patients showed that vaccination (with **Trivalent types A and B**) prolonged their prothrombin times by 40%, but no signs of bleeding were seen.[13] A man well-stabilised on **warfarin** developed diffuse gastric bleeding and a massive gastrointestinal haemorrhage (prothrombin time of 48 s) within 10 days of **influenza vaccination**.[14] Another patient on **warfarin** showed INR increases from 2.5 to 6.0 and 7.0 on two successive years when vaccinated against influenza.[15]

Mechanism

Not understood. One suggestion is that when an interaction occurs the synthesis of the blood clotting factors is altered.[13] There is no evidence that the vaccine changes the metabolism of the warfarin[13] although the metabolism of aminopyrine (used as an indicator of changes in metabolism) is reduced.[14]

Importance and management

A well-investigated interaction. The weight of evidence shows that influenza vaccination in those taking warfarin is normally safe and uneventful, nevertheless it would be prudent to be on the alert because very occasionally and unpredictably bleeding may occur. Acenocoumarol (nicoumalone) appears to behave like warfarin. Information about other anticoagulants is lacking but it seems probable that they too will not normally interact.

1. Lipsky BA, Pecoraro RE, Roben NJ, de Blaquiere P, Delaney CJ. Influenza vaccination and warfarin anticoagulation. *Ann Intern Med* (1984) 100, 835–7.
2. Gomolin IH, Chapron DJ and Luhan PA. Effects of influenza virus vaccine on theophylline and warfarin clearance in institutionalized elderly. *J Am Geriatr Soc* (1984) 32 (April Suppl), S21.
3. Gomolin IH, Chapron DJ, Luhan PA. Lack of effect of influenza vaccine on theophylline levels and warfarin anticoagulation in the elderly. *J Am Geriatr Soc* (1985) 33, 269–72.
4. Bussey HI, Saklad JJ. Influence of influenza vaccine on warfarin therapy. *Drug Intell Clin Pharm* (1986) 20, 460.
5. Weibert RT, Lorentz SM, Norcross WA, Klauber MR, Jagger PI. Effect of influenza vaccine in patients receiving long-term warfarin therapy. *Clin Pharm* (1986) 5, 499–503.
6. Bussey HI, Saklad JJ. Effect of influenza vaccine on chronic warfarin therapy. *Drug Intell Clin Pharm* (1988) 22, 198–201.
7. Scott AK, Cannon J and Breckenridge AM. Lack of effect of influenza vaccination on warfarin in healthy volunteers. *Br J Clin Pharmacol* (1985) 19, 144P.
8. Patriara PA, Kendal AP, Stricof RL, Weber JA, Meissner MK, Dateno B. Influenza vaccination and warfarin or theophylline toxicity in nursing home residents. *N Engl J Med* (1983) 308, 1601–2.
9. Gomolin IH. Lack of effect of influenza vaccine on warfarin anticoagulation in the elderly. *Can Med Assoc J* (1986) 135, 39–41.
10. Souto JC, Oliver A, Montserrat I, Mateo J, Sureda A, Fontcurberta J. Lack of effect of influenza vaccine on anticoagulation by acenocoumarol. *Ann Pharmacother* (1993) 27, 365–8.
11. Souto JC, Garí M, Borrell M, Fontcuberta J. Ausencia de interacción entre los anticoagulantes orales y las vacuna antigripal. *Med Clin (Barc)* (1993) 101, 637.
12. Sumner HW, Holtzman JL, McClain CJ. Drug-induced liver disease. *Geriatrics* (1981) 36, 83–96.
13. Kramer P, Tsuru M, Cook CE, McClain CJ, Holtzman JL. Effect of influenza vaccine on warfarin anticoagulation. *Clin Pharmacol Ther* (1984) 35, 416–18.
14. Kramer P, McClain CJ. Depression of aminopyrine metabolism by influenza vaccine. *N Engl J Med* (1981) 305, 1262–4.
15. Beeley L, Cunningham H, Carmichael AE, Brennan A. Newsletter of the West Midlands Centre for Adverse Drug Reaction Reporting (1991), 33, 19.

Anticoagulants + Insecticides

A patient showed a marked increase in his response to acenocoumarol when exposed to insecticides containing ivermectin and metidation. Another patient totally failed to respond to warfarin after very heavy exposure to a camphechlor/lindane insecticide.

Clinical evidence

(a) Acenocoumarol + Ivermectin and Metidation

A farmer in Spain, normally well stabilised on **acenocoumarol** (**nicoumalone**) and amiodarone, showed marked rises in his INRs (from 3.5 up to 7.9) requiring a reduction in his anticoagulant dosage (from 12 mg to 8 mg weekly) which occurred during the Summer months. It was then discovered that he was using insecticides containing **ivermectin** and **metidation** on his trees without any protective clothing. No bleeding occurred.[1]

(b) Warfarin + Camphechlor/Lindane

A rancher in the USA on **warfarin** showed a very marked reduction in his anticoagulant response after dusting his sheep with an insecticide containing 5% **camphechlor** (**toxaphene**) and 1% **lindane** (**gamma-benzene hexachloride**). Over a 2-year period he showed periods of considerable 'warfarin resistance' which were linked to the use of this insecticide. Normally 7.5 mg **warfarin** daily maintained his prothrombin time in the therapeutic range, but after exposure to the insecticide even 15 mg daily failed to have any effect at all.[2] The dusting was done by putting the insecticide in a sack and hitting the sheep with it in an enclosed barn.[2]

Mechanisms

The acenocoumarol/ivermectin and metidation interaction is not understood. Ivermectin used for onchocerciasis normally has no effect on prothrombin times when used alone,[3,4] but two unexplained cases of prolonged prothrombin times associated with the development of haematomas have been reported.[5] Metidation is an organophosphate. Camphechlor and lindane are known liver enzyme inducing agents[6] which increase the metabolism and clearance of the warfarin, thereby reducing and even abolishing its effects.

Importance and management

Information about these interactions appears to be limited to these isolated case reports. Neither interaction is well established and neither would appear not to be of general clinical importance. The chlorinated hydrocarbon insecticides have been withdrawn from general use in most countries so that the possibility of an interaction with any anticoagulant is now very small. No other cases of interaction between an anticoagulant and ivermectin, whether used as an insecticide or for the treatment of onchocerciasis, appear to have been reported.

As a general rule farm workers and others should use proper protection (gloves, masks, protective clothing) if they are exposed to substantial amounts of any insecticide because they can be both directly toxic and can also apparently interact with some prescribed drugs, including the anticoagulants, even if only very rarely.

1. Fernandéz MA, Ballasteros S, Aznar J. Oral anticoagulants and insecticides. *Thromb Haemost* (1998) 80, 724.
2. Jeffery WH, Ahlin TA, Goren C, Hardy WR. Loss of warfarin effect after occupational insecticide exposure. *JAMA* (1976) 236, 2881–2.
3. Richards FO, McNeeley MB, Bryan RT, Eberhard ML, McNeeley DF, Lammie PJ, Spencer HC. Ivermectin and prothrombin time. *Lancet* (1989) i, 1139-40.
4. Pacque MC, Munoz B, White AT, Williams PN, Greene BM, Taylor HR. Ivermectin and prothrombin time. *Lancet* (1989) i, 1140.
5. Homeida MMA, Bagi IA, Ghalib HW, El Sheikh H, Ismail A, Yousif MA, Sulieman S, Ali HM, Bennett JL, Williams J. Prolongation of prothrombin time with ivermectin. *Lancet* (1988) i, 1346-7.
6. Conney AH. Environmental factors influencing drug metabolism. In Fundamentals of Drug Metabolism and Disposition. LaDu BN, Mandel HG and Way EL (eds). Williams and Wilkins Co (1971) 253.

Anticoagulants + Interferon

Preliminary evidence indicates that the effects of nicoumalone (acenocoumarol) and warfarin may be increased by interferon.

Clinical evidence

A woman on long-term **warfarin** treatment (2.5 to 3.5 mg daily) showed a Prothrombin Time rise from 16.7 to 20.4 s after taking 6.0 MU **interferon-alfa** for 10 days. Her serum **warfarin** levels rose from about 0.8 to 5.2 micrograms/ml. She responded to a reduction in the **warfarin** dosage (2.5 mg daily for 10 days and then 2.0 mg daily). The authors of the report also say that they have seen four other patients on **warfarin** who needed a dosage reduction when given interferon, two of them while taking **interferon beta** and the other two while taking **interferon alfa-2b**.[1] A woman on **nicoumalone** (**acenocoumarol**) showed gingival bleeding and a thrombotest rise from 35% to 19% within 6 weeks of starting treatment with 3 million units of **interferon-alpha 2b** three times weekly. Her thrombotest percentages stabilised between 25 and 40% when the **nicoumalone** dosage was reduced to 1 mg daily from the previous dosage of 1 and 2 mg on alternate days. The extent of the anticoagulation increased when the **interferon** was reduced to twice weekly.[2]

Mechanism

Not understood. The authors of both reports postulate that the interferon reduces the metabolism of the anticoagulants by the liver, thereby reducing their clearance and increasing their effects.[1,2]

Importance and management

These reports seem to be the only ones to describe this interaction so the interaction is not yet well established, however it would seem prudent to monitor the effects if interferon is added to nicoumalone or warfarin treatment, reducing the dosage if necessary. Information about other anticoagulants is lacking, but the same precautions would be appropriate with any of them.

1. Adachi Y, Yokoyama Y, Nanno T, Yamamoto T. Potentation of warfarin by interferon. *BMJ* (1995) 311, 292.
2. Serratrice J, Durand J-M, Morange S. Interferon-alpha 2b interaction with acenocoumarol. *Am J Hematol* (1998) 57, 89–92.

Anticoagulants + Isoxicam, Meloxicam or Piroxicam

Piroxicam can increase the effects of warfarin and acenocoumarol (nicoumalone). Bleeding may occur if the anticoagulant dosage is not reduced. Isoxicam appears to act similarly. Meloxicam does not interact with warfarin or affect platelets and appears to irritate the gut less than many other NSAIDs.

Clinical evidence

(a) Isoxicam

Six patients stabilised on **warfarin** needed a reduction in their **warfarin** dosage, averaging 20% (range 10 to 30%), when given 200 mg **isoxicam** daily over a 6-week period. The effects of the interaction appeared in the second week and almost reached a maximum after 4 weeks.[1]

(b) Meloxicam

Meloxicam 15 mg daily for 7 days did not significantly affect the pharmacokinetics of **warfarin** or INR values in a group of 14 normal subjects stabilised at 1.2–1.8.[2]

(c) Piroxicam

A man stabilised on **warfarin** showed a fall in his prothrombin time from 1.7 to 1.9 times his control value to a value of 1.3 when he stopped taking 20 mg **piroxicam** daily. The prothrombin times rose again when he re-started the **piroxicam**, and fell and rose again when the **piroxicam** was again stopped and re-started.[3] Another patient on **warfarin** showed increases and then decreases in prothrombin times when 20 mg **piroxicam** daily was started and then stopped.[4] Two Chinese patients showed INR rises up to 4.5 after being treated with 20 mg oral **piroxicam** daily and 0.5% topical **piroxicam** gel. One of them showed bruises over the legs within 3 days.[5] (Note that Chinese patients are more sensitive to the anticoagulant effects of **warfarin** than some other races).

A woman who spread **warfarin rat poison** with bare hands developed intracerebral bleeding, possibly exacerbated by the **piroxicam** she was taking.[6]

Piroxicam 20 mg daily increased the effects of **acenocoumarol (nicoumalone)** in 4 out of 11 subjects, 3 being considered mild and one being significant.[7] An increased prothrombin ratio has been seen in another patient.[8] A further patient on **acenocoumarol** developed gastrointestinal bleeding 3 days after starting to take 20 mg **piroxicam** daily. His INR rose from 2.2 to 6.5.[9] A single dose clinical study found that 40 mg **piroxicam** caused major changes in the pharmacokinetics of racemic **acenocoumarol**. The AUC of the more active **acenocoumarol** *(R)*-isomer was found to be increased by 51% and its maximum serum levels increased by 27%.[10] Similar (or the same) findings by the same group of workers are described elsewhere.[11]

Mechanism

What is known suggests that piroxicam inhibits the metabolism of these anticoagulants by the liver, thereby increasing their anticoagulant effects.[10] In addition isoxicam and piroxicam have antiplatelet effects.

Importance and management

The acenocoumarol piroxicam and warfarin/piroxicam interactions are established but the documentation is only moderate. Concurrent use need not be avoided but monitor the outcome well and anticipate the need to reduce the anticoagulant dosage. Remember that piroxicam can cause gastrointestinal irritation and reduce platelet aggregation. It is probably easier to use alternative non-interacting NSAIDs. Information about other anticoagulants not cited is lacking but it would be prudent to assume that they will interact similarly. Isoxicam interacts like piroxicam but has been withdrawn worldwide because of its toxicity.

Meloxicam does not interact with warfarin. It does not affect platelets and thereby prolong the bleeding times, and does not irritate the gut mucosa as much as many other NSAIDs, nevertheless the makers still advise good monitoring if used concurrently. Information about other anticoagulants is lacking.

1. Farnham DJ. Studies of isoxicam in combination with aspirin, warfarin sodium and cimetidine. *Semin Arthritis Rheum* (1983) 12 (Suppl 2), 179–83.
2. Türck D, Su CAPF, Heinzel G, Busch U, Bluhmki E, Hoffman J. Lack of interaction between meloxicam and warfarin in healthy volunteers. *Eur J Clin Pharmacol* (1997) 51, 421–5.
3. Rhodes RS, Rhodes PJ, Klein C, Sintek CD. A warfarin-piroxicam drug interaction. *Drug Intell Clin Pharm* (1985) 19, 556–8.
4. Mallet L, Cooper JW. Prolongation of prothrombin time with the use of piroxicam and warfarin. *Can J Hosp Pharm* (1991) 44, 93–4.
5. Chan TYK. Drug interactions as a cause of overanticoagulation and bleedings in Chinese patients receiving warfarin. *Int J Clin Pharmacol Ther* (1998) 36, 403–5.
6. Abell TL, Merigian KS, Lee JM, Holbert JM, McCall JW. Cutaneous exposure to warfarin-like anticoagulant causing an intracerebral hemorrhage: a case report. *Clin Toxicol* (1994) 32, 69–73.
7. Jacotot B. Interaction of piroxicam with oral anticoagulants. 9th European Congress of Rheumatology, Wiesbaden, September 1979, pp 46–48.
8. Beeley L, Stewart P. Bulletin of the West Midlands Centre for Adverse Drug Reaction Reporting (1987) 25, 28.
9. Desprez D, Blanc P, Larrey D, Michel H. Hémorragie digestive favorisée par une hypocoagulation excessive due à une interaction médicamenteuse piroxicam — antagonisme de la vitamine K. *Gastroenterol Clin Biol* (1992) 16, 906–7.
10. Bonnabry P, Desmeules J, Leemann T, Dayer P. Stereoselective inhibition of acenocoumarol metabolism by piroxicam. *Clin Pharmacol Ther* (1996) 59, 151.
11. Bonnabry P, Desmeules J, Rudaz S, Leeman T, Veuthey J-L, Dayer P. Stereoselective interaction between piroxicam and acenocoumarol. *Br J Clin Pharmacol* (1996) 41, 525–30.

Anticoagulants + Itraconazole

An isolated report describes a very marked increase in the anticoagulant effects of warfarin, accompanied by bruising and bleeding, in a patient when given itraconazole.

Clinical evidence, mechanism, importance and management

A woman stabilised on **warfarin** (5 mg daily) and also taking ipratropium bromide, salbutamol, budesonide, quinine sulphate and omeprazole, was additionally started on 200 mg **itraconazole** twice daily for oral candidiasis caused by the inhaled steroid. Within 4 days she developed generalised bleeding and recurrent nose bleeds. Her INR had risen to more than 8. The **warfarin** and **itraconazole** were stopped, but next day she had to be admitted to hospital for intractable bleeding and increased bruising, for which she was treated with fresh frozen plasma. Two days later when the bleeding had stopped and her INR had returned to 2.4, she was restarted on **warfarin** and later re-stabilised on her original dosage.[1] The reasons for this reaction are not understood but it is possible that the **itraconazole** inhibited the metabolism of the **warfarin**. The quinine and the omeprazole may also have had some minor part to play in what happened.

This seems to be the first and only report of this interaction so that its general importance is uncertain, but it would clearly be sensible to monitor the effects of adding **itraconazole** to a stabilised regimen of **warfarin**. Warn patients to seek informed advice if any unexplained bruising or bleeding occurs. Information about other anticoagulants is lacking.

1. Yeh J, Soo S-C, Summerton C, Richardson C. Potentiation of action of warfarin by itraconazole. *BMJ* (1990) 301, 669.

Anticoagulants + Ketoconazole

Three elderly patients showed an increase in the anticoagulant effects of warfarin when given ketoconazole. There is other evidence which shows that not all individuals will demonstrate this interaction.

Clinical evidence

An elderly woman, stabilised on **warfarin** for 3 years, complained of spontaneous bruising 3 weeks after starting a course of **ketoconazole** (200 mg twice daily). Her British comparative ratio was found to have risen from 1.9 to 5.4. Her liver function was normal. She was re-stabilised on her previous **warfarin** dosage 3 weeks after the **ketoconazole** was withdrawn.

The CSM in the UK has a report of a man of 84 taking **warfarin** whose British comparative ratio rose to 4.8 when given **ketoconazole**, and fell to 1.4 when it was withdrawn.[1] Janssen, the makers of **ketoconazole**, also have a report of an elderly man on **warfarin** whose prothrombin time climbed from 26–39 s to over 60 s when given 400 mg **ketoconazole** daily.[2] In contrast, 2 volunteers showed no changes in their anticoagulant response to **warfarin** when concurrently treated with **ketoconazole** (200 mg daily) over a 3-week period.[3]

Mechanism

Uncertain. It has been suggested[4] that in humans, as in *rats*,[5] ketoconazole may inhibit liver enzymes concerned with the metabolism of warfarin so that its effects are increased. It is perhaps noteworthy that all of the cases involved elderly patients whose liver function may already have been poor.

Importance and management

Information about this interaction seems to be limited to the reports cited. Its general importance and incidence is therefore uncertain, but it is probably quite small, however it would now seem prudent to monitor the anticoagulant response of any patient when first given both drugs, particularly the elderly, to ensure that excessive hypoprothrombinaemia does not occur. Information about other anticoagulants is lacking.

1. Smith AG, Potentiation of oral anticoagulants by ketoconazole. *BMJ* (1984) 288, 188–9.
2. Janssen Pharmaceutical Limited. Personal communication, April 1986.
3. Stevens DA, Stiller RL, Williams PL, Sugar AM. Experience with ketoconazole in three major manifestations of progressive coccidioidomycosis. *Am J Med* (1983) 74, 58–63.
4. Simpson JG, Cunningham C, Whiting P. Potentiation of oral anticoagulants by ketoconazole. *BMJ* (1984) 288, 646.
5. Niemegeers CJE, Levron JC, Awouters F, Janssen PAJ. Inhibition and induction of microsomal enzymes in the rat. A comparative study of four antimycotics: miconazole, econazole, clotrimazole and ketoconazole. *Arch Int Pharmacodyn Ther* (1981) 251, 26–38.

Anticoagulants + Ketorolac

Ketorolac appears not to interact with warfarin, but it may possibly cause serious gastrointestinal bleeding and is considered by the CSM and its makers as contraindicated in patients taking oral anticoagulants. However intramuscular ketorolac and subcutaneous enoxaparin appear not to interact adversely.

Clinical evidence, mechanism, importance and management

After taking 10 mg ketorolac four times daily for 6 days, no major changes occurred in the pharmacokinetics of *(R)-* or *(S)-*warfarin, nor in the pharmacokinetic profile of a single 25-mg dose of racemic warfarin in 12 normal subjects.[1] This suggests that ketorolac is normally unlikely to affect the anticoagulant response of patients taking warfarin chronically, but this needs confirmation. However the CSM in the UK has had five reports of post-operative haemorrhage and four reports of gastrointestinal haemorrhage (one fatal) in patients taking ketorolac. A US study also identified an increased risk of gastrointestinal bleeding with ketorolac. On the basis of this and other evidence the CSM and the makers say that ketorolac is contraindicated with anticoagulants, including **low doses of heparin.**[2,3] However a study in hip replacement patients given once daily subcutaneous **enoxaparin** (40 mg to 4000 iu) found that there were no significant differences between two groups of patients, one also given 30 mg intramuscular **ketorolac** (34 patients) and the other group given **unnamed opioids** (26 patients), in terms of intraoperative blood loss, post-operative drainage, transfusion requirements, bruising, wound oozing, and leg swelling.[4]

1. Toon S, Holt BL, Mullins FGP, Bullingham R, Aarons L, Rowland M. Investigations into the potential effects of multiple dose ketorolac on the pharmacokinetics and pharmacodynamics of racemic warfarin. *Br J Clin Pharmacol* (1990) 30, 743–50.
2. Committee on the Safety of Medicines. *Current Problems* (1993) 19, 5–6.
3. Toradol (Ketorolac). Roche Products Limited. Summary of product characteristics, October 2000.
4. Weale AE, Warwick DJ, Durant N, Protheroe D. Is there a clinically significant interaction between low molecular weight heparin and non-steroidal analgesics after total hip replacement? *Ann R Coll Surg Engl* (1995) 77, 35–7.

Anticoagulants + Lansoprazole

Lansoprazole does not normally interact with warfarin, but two isolated cases of increased warfarin effects have been attributed to an interaction.

Clinical evidence, mechanism, importance and management

A study on 24 subjects found that 60 mg **lansoprazole** daily for nine days had no effect on the pharmacokinetics of either *(S)-* or *(R)-*warfarin, and no significant changes were seen in their prothrombin times.[1]

In contrast the makers of **lansoprazole** have in their records two reports of possible interactions. An elderly patient on **warfarin** with an aortic valve replacement developed an INR of 7 when **lansoprazole** was added. Despite a **warfarin** dosage adjustment he had a gastrointestinal haemorrhage, a myocardial infarction and died after 3 weeks. Another man on **warfarin** (as well as amiodarone, furosemide (frusemide) and lisinopril) experienced confusion, hallucinations and an increased INR (value not known) when given **lansoprazole**. When the **lansoprazole** was stopped after 4 days he recovered. It is uncertain whether this was an interaction or whether he had had an incorrect **warfarin** dosage.[2]

The overall picture is that no adverse interaction with warfarin would be expected, but because these isolated cases have occurred it would be prudent to monitor the outcome when lansoprazole is first added. This is the underlying reason for the warning issued by the makers[3] of lansoprazole: ". . . caution should be exercised when . . . warfarin is taken concomitantly with the administration of *Zoton*." Information about other anticoagulants is lacking but the same precautions would seem appropriate with any of them.

1. Cavanaugh JH, Winters EP, Cohen A, Locke CS, Braeckman R. Lack of effect of lansoprazole on steady state warfarin metabolism. *Gastroenterology* (1991) 100, A40.
2. Wyeth. Personal communication, January 1998.
3. Zoton (Lansoprazole). Wyeth Laboratories. Summary of product characteristics, September 2001.

Anticoagulants + Laxatives, Liquid paraffin or Psyllium

The theoretical possibility that laxatives or liquid paraffin might affect the response to oral anticoagulants appears to be unconfirmed. Psyllium (ispaghula) has been shown not to affect either the absorption or the anticoagulant effects of warfarin.

Clinical evidence, mechanism, importance and management

A study in 6 normal subjects showed that **psyllium**, given as a 14 g dose of colloid (*Metamucil*) in a small amount of water with a single 40-mg dose of **warfarin**, and three further doses of **psyllium** at 2 h intervals thereafter, did not affect either the absorption or the anticoagulant effects of the **warfarin**.[1] In theory, **laxatives** and **liquid paraffin (mineral oil)** which shorten the transit time along the gut might be expected to decrease the absorption of both vitamin K and the oral anticoagulants. **Liquid paraffin** might also be expected to impair the absorption of the lipid-soluble vitamin, but despite warnings in various books, reviews and lists of drug interactions, there appears to be no direct evidence, as yet, that this is an interaction of any practical importance.

1. Robinson DS, Benjamin DM, McCormack JJ. Interaction of warfarin and nonsystemic gastrointestinal drugs. *Clin Pharmacol Ther* (1971) 12, 491–5.

Anticoagulants + Lornoxicam (Chlortenoxicam)

Lornoxicam can raise serum warfarin levels to a moderate extent and increase its anticoagulant effects but appears not to interact with acenocoumarol (nicoumalone) and only interacts slightly with phenprocoumon.

Clinical evidence

(a) Acenocoumarol (Nicoumalone)

An open crossover study in 6 normal subjects found that 8 mg lornoxicam twice daily had no effect on the pharmacokinetics or the anticoagulant activity of 10 mg racemic **acenocoumarol**.[1]

(b) Phenprocoumon

An open crossover study in 6 normal subjects given a single 9 mg dose of racemic **phenprocoumon** found that lornoxicam increased the bioavailabilities of *(S)*- and *(R)*-**phenprocoumon** by 14 and 6% respectively, and decreased their clearances by 15 and 6%. Statistically significant reductions in the activities of factors II and VII were seen.[2]

(c) Warfarin

12 normal subjects were firstly given 4 mg **lornoxicam** twice daily for 5 days, then **warfarin** was added until a stable prothrombin time, averaging 23.58 s, was achieved. The period to achieve this varied from 9 to 24 days, depending on the subject. The **warfarin** was continued but the **lornoxicam** withdrawn, whereupon the mean prothrombin time fell to 19.5 s and the serum **warfarin** levels fell by 25% (from 1.02 to 0.77 micrograms/ml). The INR fall was from 1.48 to 1.23.[3,4]

Mechanisms

Not known but it is possible that the **lornoxicam** inhibits the liver metabolism and loss of **warfarin** from the body.

Importance and management

Information seems to be limited to these studies, but it would now be prudent to monitor the outcome if lornoxicam is added to warfarin, reducing the warfarin dosage as necessary. Lornoxicam appears not to interact with acenocoumarol, and only interacts to a clinically irrelevant extent with phenprocoumon. Information about other anticoagulants is lacking but to be on the safe side it would be prudent to monitor well.

1. Masche UP, Rentasch KM, Von Felten A, Meier PJ, Fattinger KE. No clinically relevant effect of lornoxicam intake on acenocoumarol pharmacokinetics and pharmacodynamics. *Eur J Clin Pharmacol* (1999) 54, 856–8.
2. Masche UP, Rentasch KM, Von Felten A, Meier PJ, Fattinger KE. Opposite effects of lornoxicam co-administration on phenprocoumon pharmacokinetics and pharmacodynamics. *Eur J Clin Pharmacol* (1999) 54, 857–64.
3. Ravic M, Turner P. Study of a potential effect of chlortenoxicam on the anticoagulant activity of warfarin. *Eur J Pharmacol* (1990) 183, 1030.
4. Ravic M, Johnston A, Turner P, Ferber HP. A study of the interaction between lornoxicam and warfarin in healthy volunteers. *Hum Exp Toxicol* (1990) 9, 413–14.

Anticoagulants + Lovastatin

The anticoagulant effects of warfarin can be increased by lovastatin in some patients. Bleeding may occur unless the anticoagulant dosage is reduced.

Clinical evidence

Two patients on **warfarin** approximately doubled their prothrombin times (from 18–24 s to 42–48 s) within 10 to 21 days of starting to take 20 mg **lovastatin** daily. One developed minor rectal bleeding and the other had haematuria and epistaxes. The problem rapidly resolved when the **warfarin** dosage was reduced from 5 to 2 mg daily.[1] A prothrombin time increase from 15 to 24 s occurred in another patient on **warfarin** after taking 20 mg **lovastatin** daily for 2 weeks.[2]

The makers of **lovastatin** have 10 other reports of bleeding and/or increased prothrombin times in patients on **warfarin** when given **lovastatin**, but no details are given.[3,4] A study in 8 patients on **warfarin** found that 40 mg **lovastatin** for 7 days increased the INR by 17%.[5]

Mechanism

Uncertain. Inhibition of the metabolism of the warfarin which results in its accumulation has been suggested.[1]

Importance and management

Information seems to be limited to these reports but the interaction is established. The incidence and extent are uncertain but prothrombin times should be monitored in all patients if warfarin or any other anticoagulant is started, stopped or its dosage changed. A 60% dosage reduction was effective in one case.[1]

1. Ahmad S. Lovastatin. Warfarin interaction. *Arch Intern Med* (1990) 150, 2407.
2. Hoffman HS. The interaction of lovastatin and warfarin. *Conn Med* (1992) 56, 107.

3. Tobert JA, Shear CL, Chremos AN, Mantell GE. Clinical experience with lovastatin. *Am J Cardiol* (1990) 65, 23F–26F.
4. Tobert JA. Efficacy and long-term adverse effect pattern of lovastatin. *Am J Cardiol* (1988) 62, 28J–34J.
5. O'Rangers EA, Ford M, Hershey A. The effect of HMG-coA reductase inhibitors on the anticoagulant response to warfarin. *Pharmacotherapy* (1994) 14, 349.

Anticoagulants + Lysine clonixinate

Lysine clonixinate does not alter the anticoagulant effects of phenprocoumon.

Clinical evidence, mechanism, importance and management

An open, randomised, twofold, crossover controlled study in 12 healthy men found that the pharmacokinetics and the anticoagulant activity of single 18-mg doses of **phenprocoumon** were unchanged by the concurrent use of **lysine clonixinate**. The subjects were given 125 mg **lysine clonixinate** five times daily for 3 days before and for 13 days after the single doses of **phenprocoumon**.[1] No special precautions would therefore seem to be required if these two drugs are taken concurrently, over and above the general precautions needed with most NSAIDs which can cause some gastrointestinal bleeding. Information about other anticoagulants seems to be lacking.

1. Russmann S, Dilger K, Trenk D, Nagyivanyi P, Jänchen E. Effect of lysine clonixate on the pharmacokinetics and anticoagulant activity of phenprocoumon. *Arzneimittelforschung* (2001) 51, 891–895.

Anticoagulants + Macrolide antibacterials

Midecamycin diacetate (miocamycin, ponsinomycin) appears not to interact with acenocoumarol (nicoumalone) nor dirithromycin with warfarin, but increased warfarin effects have been seen in some patients given roxithromycin, and there are isolated cases with acenocoumarol (nicoumalone) and phenprocoumon. See also 'Anticoagulants + Clarithromycin', p.251 and 'Anticoagulants + Erythromycin', p.259.

Clinical evidence, mechanism, importance and management

(a) Acenocoumarol (Nicoumalone) + Midecamycin diacetate

The pharmacokinetics of a single oral dose of **acenocoumarol** were not significantly changed in 6 subjects after taking 800 mg **midecamycin diacetate** twice daily for 4 days.[1] This suggests that no interaction is likely in patients but confirmation of this is needed. There seems to be no information as yet about other anticoagulants.

(b) Acenocoumarol, Phenprocoumon, Warfarin + Roxithromycin

A woman of 79 on long-term **acenocoumarol (nicoumalone)** treatment developed a large abdominal wall haematoma shortly after starting to take 150 mg **roxithromycin** twice daily for a lung infection.[2] Her INR had risen to 5.9.

A man of 75 taking **phenprocoumon** chronically developed a marked increase in prothrombin times but no bleeding when given **roxithromycin**. The **phenprocoumon** was stopped and phytomenadione administered. When the antibacterial was withdrawn he was re-stabilised on the original dosage of **phenprocoumon**.[3]

Roxithromycin 150 mg twice daily for 2 weeks had no significant effect on the thrombotest percentages of 21 normal subjects given enough **warfarin** to maintain the values at 10 to 20%. Serum **roxithromycin** levels also remained unchanged.[4] However during the 1991–5 period The Centre for Adverse Reactions Monitoring of New Zealand (CARM) received seven reports of a possible interaction with **roxithromycin** resulting in increased **warfarin** effects, and the Adverse Drug Reactions Advisory Committee of Australia (ADRAC) received nine similar reports during the same period.[5]

These reports suggest that it would be prudent to monitor the outcome when **roxithromycin** is first added to established treatment with any oral anticoagulant because the interaction is unpredictable and potentially serious. More study is needed.

(c) Warfarin + Dirithromycin

The pharmacokinetic and pharmacodynamics of single oral doses of racemic **warfarin** (0.5 mg/kg) in 15 normal subjects were not altered by 500 mg **dirithromycin** daily for 5 days.[6] No special precautions would therefore seem necessary if both drugs are used concurrently.

1. Couet W, Istin B, Decourt JP, Ingrand I, Girault J, Fourtillan JB. Lack of effect of ponsinomycin on the pharmacokinetics of nicoumalone enantiomers. *Br J Clin Pharmacol* (1990) 30, 616–20.
2. Chassany O, Logeart I, Choulika S, Caulin C. Hématome pariétal abdominal lors d'un traitement associant acénocoumarol et roxithromycine. *Presse Med* (1998) 27, 1103.
3. Meyboom RHB, Heere FJ, Egberts ACG, Lastdrager CJ. Vermoedelijke potentiëring van fenprocoumon door claritromycine en roxithromycine. *Ned Tijdschr Geneeskd* (1996) 140, 375–7.
4. Paulsen O, Nilsson L-G, Saint-Salvi B, Manuel C, Lunell E. No effect of roxithromycin on pharmacokinetic or pharmacodynamic properties of warfarin and its enantiomers. *Pharmacol Toxicol* (1988) 63, 215–20.
5. Ghose K, Ashton J, Rohan A. Possible interaction of roxithromycin with warfarin; updated review of ADR reports. *Clin Drug Invest* (1995) 10, 303–9.
6. Ellsworth A, Horn JR, Wilkinson W, Black DJ, Church L, Sides GD, Harris J, Cullen PD. An evaluation of the effect of dirithromycin (D) and erythromycin (E) on the pharmacokinetics and pharmacodynamics of warfarin (W). *Intersci Conf Antimicrob Agents Chemother* (1995) 35, 9.

Anticoagulants + Mango fruit (*Mangifera indica*)

There is evidence that eating mango fruit can moderately increase the anticoagulant effects of warfarin. None of the patients in whom this interaction was seen showed any evidence of bleeding.

Clinical evidence, mechanism, importance and management

A study in 13 patients on **warfarin** found evidence that eating **mango fruit** (*Mangifera indica*) increased their INRs by an average of 38% (from 2.79 to 3.85) but no bleeding occurred. No other explanation for the increased INRs could be identified. The patients were reported to have eaten 1 to 6 **mangos** daily for 2 days to 1 month before attending the anticoagulant clinic. When **mango** was identified as a possible cause for their increased INRs, the patients were told to stop eating **mango**, whereupon their mean INRs fell within 2 weeks by almost 18%. When 2 of the patients whose mean INRs had originally risen by 13% were later rechallenged with **mango** (rather less than before), their mean INRs rose by 9%.[1]

The reason for this apparent interaction is not known but the authors of the report speculate about the possible role of vitamin A (reported to be 8061 IU in an average sized **mango** of 130 g, without seed). In practical terms this increase in INRs would not seem to represent a serious problem because none of the patients studied showed any evidence of bleeding although one patient's INR rose to 5.1 (a 54% increase). There appear to be no other reports in the literature of a **warfarin/mango** interaction, nor of interactions between **mango** or any other oral anticoagulant. More study of this interaction is needed but at the present time there insufficient reason to suggest that patients on **warfarin** should avoid **mango fruit**.

1. Monterrey-Rodríguez J, Feliú JF, Rivera-Miranda GC. Interaction between warfarin and mango fruit. *Ann Pharmacother* (2002) 36, 940-1.

Anticoagulants + Meclofenamic acid or Mefenamic acid

The anticoagulant effects of warfarin are increased to some extent by meclofenamic acid and a moderate reduction in the

warfarin dosage may be needed. Mefenamic acid appears not to interact significantly.

Clinical evidence

(a) Meclofenamic acid

After taking **sodium meclofenamate** (200—300 mg daily) for 7 days, the average dose of **warfarin** required by 7 patients fell from 6.5 to 4.25 mg daily, and by the end of 4 weeks it was 5.5 mg (a 16% reduction with a 0—25% range).[1]

(b) Mefenamic acid

After taking 2 g **mefenamic acid** daily for a week the mean prothrombin concentrations (20.03%) of 12 normal subjects on **warfarin** fell by 3.49%.[2] Microscopic haematuria were seen in 3 of them, but no overt haemorrhage. Their prothrombin concentrations were 15 to 25% of normal, well within the accepted anticoagulant range.

Mechanisms

Uncertain. Mefenamic acid can displace warfarin from its plasma protein binding sites,[3-5] and *in vitro* studies have shown that therapeutic concentrations (equivalent to 4 g daily) can increase the unbound and active warfarin concentrations by 140 to 340%.[3,4] But this interaction mechanism alone is only likely to have a transient effect.

Importance and management

The warfarin/meclofenamic acid interaction is established but of only moderate clinical importance. A small reduction in warfarin dosage may be needed. Mefenamic acid appears not to interact significantly, but bear in mind that both of these NSAIDs may irritate the gut. There seems to be no information about other anticoagulants.

1. Baragar FD, Smith TC. Drug interaction studies with sodium meclofenamate (Meclomen®). *Curr Ther Res* (1978) 23 (April Suppl), S51–S59.
2. Holmes EL. Pharmacology of the fenamates: IV. Toleration by normal human subjects. *Ann Phys Med* (1966) 9 (Suppl), 36–49.
3. Sellers EM, Koch-Weser J. Displacement of warfarin from human albumin by diazoxide and ethacrynic, mefenamic and nalidixic acids. *Clin Pharmacol Ther* (1970) 11, 524–9.
4. Sellers EM, Koch-Weser J. Kinetics and clinical importance of displacement of warfarin from albumin by acidic drugs. *Ann N Y Acad Sci* (1971) 179, 213.
5. McElnay JC, D'Arcy PFD. Displacement of albumin-bound warfarin by anti-inflammatory agent *in vitro*. *J Pharm Pharmacol* (1980) 32, 709.

Anticoagulants + Meprobamate

The anticoagulant effects of warfarin are not altered to a clinically relevant extent by the concurrent use of meprobamate.

Clinical evidence, mechanism, importance and management

Nine men stabilised on **warfarin** were given 1600 mg **meprobamate** daily for two weeks. Three of them showed a small increase in prothrombin times, five a small decrease and one remained unaffected.[1] 10 other patients on **warfarin** showed only a small clinically unimportant reduction in prothrombin times when given 2400 mg **meprobamate** daily for 4 weeks.[2] Similar results were found in another study.[3] No particular precautions would therefore seem to be needed if **meprobamate** is added to established treatment with **warfarin.** Other anticoagulants would be expected to behave similarly, but this requires confirmation.

1. Udall JA. Warfarin therapy not influenced by meprobamate. A controlled study in nine men. *Curr Ther Res* (1970) 12, 724–8.
2. Gould L, Michael A, Fisch S, Gomprecht RF. Prothrombin levels maintained with meprobamate and warfarin. A controlled study. *JAMA* (1972) 220, 1460-2.
3. DeCarolis PP, Gelfand ML. Effect of tranquillizers on prothrombin times response to coumarin. *J Clin Pharmacol* (1975) 15, 557.

Anticoagulants + Meptazinol

The anticoagulant effects of warfarin are not altered by meptazinol.

Clinical evidence, mechanism, importance and management

800 mg **meptazinol** daily for 7 days had no significant effect on the prothrombin times of 6 elderly patients on **warfarin** (approximately 5 mg daily).[1] No special precautions seem to be necessary. Information about other anticoagulants is lacking.

1. Ryd-Kjellen E, Alm A. Effect of meptazinol on chronic anticoagulant therapy. *Hum Toxicol* (1986) 5, 101–2.

Anticoagulants + Mesalazine (Mesalamine)

A single case report describes reduced warfarin effects in a patient when given mesalazine (mesalamine).

Clinical evidence

A woman on 5 mg warfarin daily, with INRs between 2 and 3, was additionally started on 800 mg mesalazine (mesalamine) three times daily for the treatment of a caecal ulcer. Four weeks later she presented in hospital with left leg pain which was diagnosed as an acute popliteal vein thrombosis, and at the same time it was found that her Prothrombin Time and INR had fallen to 1.3 s and 0.9 respectively. Over the next 10 days Prothrombin Times of up to 1.7 s were achieved by increasing the doses of warfarin up to 10 mg daily, but a satisfactory INR (2.1) was only reached when the mesalazine was stopped. The report says that serum warfarin levels were not detectable during the use of mesalazine.[1]

Mechanism

Not understood. None of the other drugs being taken by this patient (lorazepam, isradipine, lisinopril and famotidine) are known to interact.

Importance and management

This appears to be the first and only report of a warfarin/mesalazine interaction which suggests that it is unlikely to be of general importance, but to be on the safe side the prothrombin times should be monitored if mesalazine is added to established treatment with warfarin. Information about other oral anticoagulants is lacking.

1. Marinella MA. Mesalamine and warfarin therapy resulting in decreased warfarin effect. *Ann Pharmacother* (1998) 32, 841-2.

Anticoagulants + Metamizole sodium (Dipyrone)

One report claims that no interaction occurs with phenprocoumon or ethyl biscoumacetate, whereas another describes a rapid but transient increase in the effects of ethyl biscoumacetate.

Clinical evidence, mechanism, importance and management

The concurrent use of 1 g **metamizole sodium (dipyrone)** daily did not alter the anticoagulant effects of either **phenprocoumon** (5 subjects) or **ethyl biscoumacetate** (6 subjects).[1] Another report describes a short-lived but rapid increase (within 4 h) in the effects of **ethyl biscoumacetate** caused by **metamizole sodium**.[2] The reasons are not understood. Monitor the effects if concurrent use is thought

appropriate. **Metamizole sodium** is believed to cause serious blood dyscrasias including agranulocytosis so that the advisability of its use is uncertain.

1. Badian M, Le Normand Y, Rupp W, Zapf R. There is no interaction between dipyrone (metamizol) and the anticoagulants, phenprocoumon and ethylbiscoumacetate, in normal caucasian subjects. *Int J Pharmaceutics* (1984) 18, 9–15.
2. Mehvar SR, Jamali F. Dipyrone-ethylbiscoumacetate interaction in man. *Indian J Pharm* (1981) 7, 293–9.

Anticoagulants + Methaqualone

Methaqualone may cause a very small and clinically unimportant reduction in the anticoagulant effects of warfarin.

Clinical evidence, mechanism, importance and management

The average prothrombin times of 10 patients on **warfarin** were 20.9 s before, 20.4 s during, and 19.6 s after taking 300 mg **methaqualone** at bedtime for 3 weeks.[1] The plasma **warfarin** levels of another patient were unaffected by **methaqualone**, although there was some evidence that enzyme induction had occurred.[2] **Methaqualone** has some enzyme-inducing effects so that any small changes in prothrombin times reflect a limited increase in the metabolism and clearance of **warfarin**, but too small to matter.[2,3] No special precautions seem to be necessary. Other anticoagulants are expected to behave like warfarin.

1. Udall JA. Clinical implications of warfarin interactions with five sedatives. *Am J Cardiol* (1975) 35, 67–71.
2. Whitfield JB, Moss DW, Neale G, Orme M, Breckenridge A. Changes in plasma γ-glutamyl transpeptidase activity associated with alterations in drug metabolism in man. *BMJ* (1973) i, 316–18.
3. Nayak RK, Smyth RD, Chamberlain AP. Methaqualone pharmacokinetics after single and multiple dose administration in man. *J Pharmacokinet Biopharm* (1974) 2, 107.

Anticoagulants + Methylphenidate

Methylphenidate appears not to interact with ethyl biscoumacetate. There appears to be no information about other anticoagulants.

Clinical evidence, importance and management

One study found that the half-life of **ethyl biscoumacetate** in 4 normal subjects was approximately doubled after taking 20 mg **methylphenidate** daily for 3 to 5 days, due, it was suggested, to the enzyme inhibitory effects of the methylphenidate,[1] but a later double-blind study on 12 subjects failed to confirm this interaction.[2] There seem to be no other reports of an interaction between **methylphenidate** and an anticoagulant, and no obvious reasons for avoiding concurrent use.

1. Garrettson LK, Perel JM, Dayton PG. Methylphenidate interaction with both anticonvulsants and ethyl biscoumacetate. *JAMA* (1969) 207, 2053.
2. Hague DE, Smith ME, Ryan JR, McMahon FG. The interaction of methylphenidate and prolintane with ethyl biscoumacetate metabolism. *Fedn Proc* (1971) 30, 336Abs.

Anticoagulants + Metoclopramide

Metoclopramide causes a small change in the pharmacokinetics of phenprocoumon, but no important changes in the anticoagulant effects seem to occur.

Clinical evidence, mechanism, importance and management

10 days' treatment with 30 mg metoclopramide daily reduced the AUC of a single dose of phenprocoumon in 12 normal subjects by 16%, but no significant changes in the anticoagulant effects were

seen.[1] There seems to be no other information about phenprocoumon or any other anticoagulant.

1. Wesermeyer D, Mönig H, Gaska T, Masuch S, Seiler KU, Huss H, Bruhn HD. Der Einflu(E1) von Cisaprid und Metoclopramid auf die Bioverfügbarkeit von Phenprocoumon. *Hamostaseologie* (1991) 11, 95–102.

Anticoagulants + Metrifonate (Metriphonate)

Metrifonate appears not to interact with warfarin.

Clinical evidence, mechanism, importance and management

A double-blind, placebo-controlled two-period and two-treatment crossover study found that the pharmacokinetics and pharmacodynamics of a single 25-mg dose of warfarin were unchanged when given to 14 normal subjects on day 4 of an 8-day course of 50 mg metrifonate daily. Plasma warfarin levels and prothrombin times remained unchanged.[1] This suggests that no special precautions are needed if these two drugs are used concurrently. Information about other anticoagulants is lacking.

1. Heinig R, Kitchin N, Rolan P. Disposition of a single dose of warfarin in healthy individuals after pretreatment with metrifonate. *Clin Drug Invest* (1999) 18, 151–9.

Anticoagulants + Metronidazole

The anticoagulant effects of warfarin are markedly increased by metronidazole. Bleeding can occur if the dosage of warfarin is not reduced appropriately.

Clinical evidence

Metronidazole 750 mg daily for a week increased the half-life of **racemic warfarin** (i.e. the normal ordinary mixture of $R(+)$ and $S(-)$) by about one-third (from 35 to 46 h) in 8 normal subjects. The anticoagulant effects of $S(-)$**-warfarin** were virtually doubled and the half-life increased by 60%, but no change in the response to $R(+)$ was seen (except in one subject).[1]

Bleeding has been seen in 2 patients taking **warfarin** and **metronidazole**.[2,3] One of them had severe pain in one leg, ecchymoses and haemorrhage of both legs, and an increase in her prothrombin time from 17/19 s to 147 s within 17 days of starting the **metronidazole**.[2]

Mechanism

Metronidazole appears to inhibit the activity of the enzymes responsible for the metabolism (ring oxidation) of the $S(-)$-warfarin, but not the $R(+)$-warfarin.[1] As a result the racemate with the more potent activity is retained within the body, and its actions are increased and prolonged.

Importance and management

An established and clinically important interaction, although the documentation is small. If concurrent use cannot be avoided, reduce the warfarin dosage appropriately (by between about one-third to one-half). Nothing seems to be documented about other anticoagulants but it would be prudent to expect them to behave similarly, although some indirect evidence suggests that no interaction possibly occurs with **phenprocoumon**.[4]

1. O'Reilly RA. The stereoselective interaction of warfarin and metronidazole in man. *N Engl J Med* (1976) 295, 354–7.
2. Kazmier FJ. A significant interaction between metronidazole and warfarin. *Mayo Clin Proc* (1976) 51, 782–4.
3. Dean RP, Talbert RL. Bleeding associated with concurrent warfarin and metronidazole therapy. *Drug Intell Clin Pharm* (1980) 14, 864–6.
4. Staiger C, Wang NS, de Vries J, Weber E. Untersuchungen zur Wirkung von Metronidazol auf den Phenazon-Metabolismus. *Arzneimittelforschung* (1984) 34, 89–91.

Anticoagulants + Miconazole

The anticoagulant effects of acenocoumarol (nicoumalone), ethyl biscoumacetate, fluindione, phenindione, phenprocoumon, tioclomarol and warfarin can be markedly increased if miconazole is given orally. Bleeding can occur if the anticoagulant dosage is not reduced appropriately (probably to about half). The interaction can occur with buccal gel formulations and has also been seen in a few middle-aged and elderly women using intravaginal miconazole, and in one elderly man using a miconazole cream on his skin.

Clinical evidence

Two patients with prosthetic heart valves on **warfarin** developed haemorrhagic complications within 10 days of starting **miconazole** (250 g four times a day). One of them developed blood blisters and bruised easily. Her prothrombin ratio had risen from 2–3 to 16. The other patient had a prothrombin ratio of 23.4. He developed two haematomas soon after both drugs were withdrawn. Both patients were subsequently restabilised in the absence of **miconazole** on their former doses of **warfarin**.[1]

The Centres de Pharmacovigilance Hospitaliere in Bordeaux have on record 5 cases where **miconazole** (500 g daily) was responsible for a marked increase in prothrombin times and/or bleeding (haematomas, haematuria, gastrointestinal bleeding) in patients taking **acenocoumarol (nicoumalone)** (2 cases), **ethyl biscoumacetate** (1 case), **tioclomarol** (1 case) and **phenindione** (1 case).[2] Other cases and reports of this interaction have been described elsewhere involving **acenocoumarol, phenprocoumon** and **warfarin**.[2-9]

The New Zealand Centre for Adverse Reactions Monitoring reported 5 patients on **warfarin** whose INRs rose from normal values to 7.5 to 18.0 within 7 to 15 days of starting to take **miconazole oral gel**.[10] Other reports confirm that this interaction takes place between **acenocoumarol (nicoumalone)**,[11-14] **fluindione**,[15] or **warfarin**[16-21] and **miconazole oral gel**.

The Netherlands Pharmacovigilance Foundation Lareb reported 2 elderly women patients on **acenocoumarol** whose INRs rose sharply and rapidly when given a short (3-day) course of 400 mg capsules of **intravaginal miconazole**.[22] Another report describes the development of ecchymoses and an INR of 9.77 in a woman of 55 on **warfarin** on the third day after starting to use 200 mg **miconazole vaginal suppositories**. She showed increased INRs on two subsequent occasions attributed to this interaction.[23] Yet another report describes haemorrhage of the kidney in a 52-year old woman on **warfarin** after using **vaginal miconazole** for 12 days.[24] A man of 80 stabilised on long term **warfarin** showed a rise in his INR to 21.4 after using a **miconazole cream** for a fungal infection on his groin for 2 weeks. He showed no evidence of bruising or bleeding.[25]

Mechanism

There is evidence that miconazole inhibits the metabolism of warfarin by the liver (inhibition of cytochrome P450 isoenzyme CYP2C9) thereby reducing its loss from the body and increasing its effects.[7] Just why other anticoagulants are affected is still uncertain. Absorption from the gut, or very unusually from the vagina in some postmenopausal women (see also comments below) and even exceptionally through the skin, can result in increased anticoagulant effects.

Importance and management

A very well established and potentially serious interaction of clinical importance. Many of the reports are about **warfarin** but most of the common oral anticoagulants in current use (**acenocoumarol, ethyl biscoumacetate, fluindione, phenindione, phenprocoumon, tioclomarol**) have been implicated. In some cases the bleeding has taken 7 to 15 days to develop[1,2,8] whereas others have bled within only 3 days.[4,23] Raised INRs have been seen even sooner. **Oral miconazole** should therefore not be given to patients on any oral anticoagulant unless the prothrombin times can be closely monitored and suitable dosage reductions made. Two reports indicate that halving the dose may be sufficient[2,5] but in some instances the reduction needed may be much greater. One patient required an increase in her **acenocoumarol (nicoumalone)** dosage from 2 mg twice weekly to 3 to 4 mg daily when miconazole (dose not stated) was withdrawn.[3]

The interaction can also occur with **miconazole oral gel** because much of it is swallowed. Patients have bled or showed prolonged prothrombin times as a result of this interaction.[6,8,11-17,19,20]

An interaction with **intravaginal miconazole** would not normally be expected because its systemic absorption is usually very low (less than 2%) in healthy women of child-bearing age,[26] however the reports cited above[22-24] show that significant absorption can apparently occur in a few patients with particular conditions (possibly inflamed postmenopausal vaginal tissue) which allows an interaction to occur. Appropriate monitoring is therefore needed even with this route of administration in potentially at-risk women. **Topical miconazole** would also not be expected to interact, but the single report cited shows that sometimes it can.[25]

Nystatin is a possible alternative antifungal which has not been reported to interact with the oral anticoagulants.

1. Watson PG, Lochan RG, Redding VJ. Drug interaction with coumarin derivative anticoagulants. *BMJ* (1982) 285, 1044–5.
2. Loupi E, Descotes J, Lery N, Evreux J Cl. Interactions medicamenteuses et miconazole. *Therapie* (1982) 37, 437–41.
3. Anon. New possibilities in the treatment of systemic mycoses. Reports on the experimental and clinical evaluation of miconazole. Round table discussion and Chairman's summing up. *Proc R Soc Med* (1977), 70 (Suppl l), 52.
4. Ponge T, Barrier J, Spreux A, Guillou B, Larousse C, Grolleau JY. Potentialisation des effets de l'acénocoumarol par le miconazole. *Therapie* (1982) 37, 221–2.
5. Goenen M, Reynaert M, Jaumin P, Chalant CH, Tremouroux J. A case of candida albicans endocarditis three years after an aortic valve replacement. *J Cardiovasc Surg* (1977) 18, 391–6.
6. Beeley L, Magee P, Hickey FM. Bulletin of the West Midlands Centre for Adverse Drug Reaction Reporting (1989) 29, 33.
7. O'Reilly RA, Goulart DA, Kunze KL, Neal J, Gibaldi M, Eddy AC, Trager WF. Mechanisms of the stereoselective interaction between miconazole and racemic warfarin in human subjects. *Clin Pharmacol Ther* (1992) 51, 656–67.
8. Bailey GM, Magee P, Hickey FM, Beeley L. Miconazole and warfarin interaction. *Pharm J* (1989) 242, 183.
9. Marco M, Guy AJ. Retroperitoneal haematoma and small bowel intramural haematoma caused by warfarin and miconazole interaction. *Int J Oral Maxillofac Surg* (1997) 27, 485.
10. Pillans P, Woods DJ. Interaction between miconazole oral gel (Daktarin) and warfarin. *N Z Med J* (1996) 109, 346.
11. Ducroix JP, Smail A, Sevenet F, Andrejak M, Baillet J. Hématome oesophagien secondaire à une potentialisation des effets de l'acénocoumarol par le gel buccal de miconazole. *Rev Med Interne* (1989) 10, 557–9.
12. Marotel C, Cerisay D, Vasseur P, Rouvier B, Chabanne JP. Potentialisation des effets de l'acénocoumarol par le gel buccal de miconazole. *Presse Med* (1986) 15, 1684–5.
13. Gutierrez MA, Olalla I, Muruzábal MJ, Ortín M, Peralta FG. Miconazole oral gel enhances acenocoumarol anticoagulant activity. Report of three cases. *Eur J Clin Pharmacol* (1997) 52 (Suppl), A132.
14. Ortín M, Olalla JI, Muruzábal MJ, Peralta FG, Gutiérrez MA. Miconazole oral gel enhances acenocoumarol anticoagulant activity: a report of three cases. *Ann Pharmacother* (1999) 33, 175–77.
15. Ponge T, Rapp MJ, Fruneau P, Ponge A, Wassen-Hove L, Larousse C, Cottin S. Interaction médicamenteuse impliquant le miconazole en gel et la fluindione. *Therapie* (1987) 42, 412–13.
16. Colquhoun MC, Daly M, Stewart P, Beeley L. Interaction between warfarin and miconazole oral gel. *Lancet* (1987) i, 695–6.
17. Shenfield GM, Page M. Potentiation of warfarin action by miconazole oral gel. *Aust N Z J Med* (1991) 21, 928.
18. Ariyaratnam S, Thakker NS, Sloan P, Thornhill MH. Potentiation of warfarin anticoagulant activity by miconazole oral gel. *BMJ* (1997) 314, 349.
19. Evans N, Orme DS, Sedgwick ML, Youngs GR. Treating oral candidiasis: potentially fatal. *Br Dent J* (1997) 182, 452.
20. Pemberton MN, Sloan P, Ariyaratnam S, Thakker NS, Thornhill MH. Derangement of warfarin anticoagulation by miconazole oral gel. *Br Dent J* (1998) 184, 68–9.
21. Øgard CG, Vestergaad H. Interaktion mellem warfarin og oral miconazol-gel. *Ugeskr Laeger* (2000) 162, 5511.
22. Lansdorp D, Bressers HPHM, Dekens-Konter JAM, Meyboom RHB. Potentiation of acenocoumarol during vaginal administration of miconazole. *Br J Clin Pharmacol* (1999) 47, 225–6.
23. Thirion DJ, Zanetti LAF. Potentiation of warfarin's hypoprothrombinemic effect with miconazole vaginal suppositories. *Pharmacotherapy* (2000) 20, 98–9.
24. Anon. Miconazole-warfarin interaction: increased INR. Canadian Adverse Drug Reaction Newsletter (2001) 11, reproduced in *Can Med Assoc J* (2001) 165, 81.
25. Devaraj A, O'Beirne JPO, Veasey R, Dunk AA. Interaction between warfarin and topical miconazole cream. *BMJ* (2002) 325, 77.
26. Daneshmend TK. Systemic absorption of miconazole from the vagina. *J Antimicrob Chemother* (1986) 18, 507–11.

Anticoagulants + Miglitol

Miglitol appears not to interact with warfarin.

Clinical evidence, mechanism, importance and management

Twenty-four normal subjects were given 100 mg **miglitol** or a placebo three times daily for 7 days in a double-blind, randomised, placebo-controlled crossover study. On day 4 they were also given a single 25 mg oral dose of **warfarin**. Neither the pharmacokinetics nor the pharmacodynamics of *(R)*- or *(S)*-**warfarin** were affected by the **miglitol**,[1] and there would therefore seem to be no reason for avoiding concurrent use. Information about other anticoagulants is lacking.

1. Schall R, Müller FO, Hundt HKL, Duursema L, Groenewoud G, Middle MV. Study of the effect of miglitol on the pharmacokinetics and pharmacodynamics of warfarin in healthy males. *Arzneimittelforschung* (1996) 46, 41–6.

Anticoagulants + Misoprostol

A reduction in the anticoagulant effects of acenocoumarol (nicoumalone) has been attributed to the use of misoprostol in an isolated case report.

Clinical evidence, mechanism, importance and management

A woman of 39 on **acenocoumarol (nicoumalone)** and also taking celiprolol, triamterene, cyclothiazide, pravastatin and diosmin showed a rise in her prothrombin levels from 0.3 to 1.0 within 8 days of starting diclofenac and 400 micrograms **misoprostol** daily. A day after these two drugs had been withdrawn her prothrombin level had fallen to 0.67, and after another 3 days to 0.32.[1] The reasons for this reaction is not known, but suspicion falls on the **misoprostol** because diclofenac, if and when it interacts with anticoagulants, increases rather than reduces their effects (see 'Anticoagulants + NSAIDs', p.280). But just why **misoprostol** should cause these changes is not clear.

This is an isolated case, complicated by the presence of a number of other drugs, nevertheless it would now seem prudent to monitor prothrombin times if **misoprostol** is added to established treatment with any anticoagulant. More study is needed.

1. Martin MP, Jonville-Bera AP, Bera F, Caillard X, Autret E. Interaction entre le misoprostol et l'acénocoumarol. *Presse Med* (1995) 24, 195.

Anticoagulants + Monoamine oxidase inhibitors (MAOIs)

The theoretical possibility that the concurrent use of an MAOI might increase the effects of the oral anticoagulants has not been confirmed in man. Moclobemide does not interact with phenprocoumon nor brofaromine with warfarin.

Clinical evidence, mechanism, importance and management

A number of studies[1-4] have shown that the **monoamine oxidase inhibitors** can increase the effects of some **oral anticoagulants** in *animals*, but reports of this interaction in man are lacking and no special precautions seem to be necessary. A study in normal subjects found that 200 mg **moclobemide** three times daily for 7 days had no effect on the anticoagulant effects of **phenprocoumon**.[5,6] Another study in 12 normal subjects also found no evidence that **brofaromine** alters the anticoagulant effects of **warfarin**.[7]

1. Fumarola D, De Rinaldis P. Ricerche sperimentali sugli inibitori della mono-aminossidasi. Influenza della nialmide sulla attività degli anticoagulanti indiretti. *Haematologica* (1964) 49, 1248–66.

2. Reber K, Studer A. Beeinflussung der Wirkung einiger indirekter Antikoagulantien durch Monoaminoxydase-Hemmer. *Thromb Diath Haemorrh* (1965) 14, 83–7.
3. de Nicola P, Fumarola D, de Rinaldis P. Beeinflussung der gerinnungshemmenden Wirkung der indirekten Antikoagulantien durch die MAO-Inhibitoren. *Thromb Diath Haemorrh* (1964) 12 (Suppl), 125–7.
4. Hrdina P, Rusnáková M, Kovaléčk V. Changes of hypoprothrombinaemic activity of indirect anticoagulants after MAO inhibitors and reserpine. *Biochem Pharmacol* (1953) 12 (Suppl), 241.
5. Zimmer R, Gieschke R, Fischbach R, Gasic S. Interaction studies with moclobemide. *Acta Psychiatr Scand* (1990) (Suppl 360), 84–6.
6. Amrein R, Güntert TW, Dingemanse J, Lorscheid T, Stabl M, Schmid-Burgk W. Interactions of moclobemide with concomitantly administered medication: evidence from pharmacological and clinical studies. *Psychopharmacology (Berl)* (1992) 106, S24–S31.
7. Harding SR, Conly J, Lawrin-Workewych M, D'Souza J. A study of the interaction between brofaromine and warfarin in healthy volunteers. *Clin Invest Med* (1992) 15 (Suppl), A18.

Anticoagulants + Moracizine

An isolated report describes bleeding in a patient on warfarin when given moracizine, but most patients do not seem to be affected.

Clinical evidence

The prothrombin time of a woman on **warfarin**, digoxin, captopril and prednisone rose from 15–20 s to 41 s within 4 days of starting 300 mg **moracizine** three times daily. She bled (haematemesis, haematuria), but responded rapidly to withdrawal of the **warfarin** and **moracizine**, and the administration of phytonadione.[1]

This report contrasts with two others: 250 mg **moracizine** 8-hourly for 14 days caused little or no change in the pharmacokinetics of single 25-mg doses of **warfarin** in 12 normal subjects. There was only a slight decrease in the warfarin elimination half-life (from 37.6 to 34.2 h) and no change in prothrombin times.[2,3] In 51 patients receiving **warfarin** chronically, no significant changes in **warfarin** dosage requirements were needed after **moracizine** was started.[2]

Mechanism

Not understood.

Importance and management

Information appears to be limited to these reports. Although most patients seem unlikely to be affected, it would be prudent to monitor the outcome of giving moracizine to patients receiving warfarin. As yet information about other anticoagulants does not appear to be available.

1. Serpa MD, Cosslias J, McGreevy MJ. Moricizine-warfarin: a possible interaction. *Ann Pharmacother* (1992) 26, 127.
2. Quoted as data on file, Du Pont Pharmaceuticals, by Siddoway LA, Schwartz SL, Barbey JT, Woosley RL. Clinical pharmacokinetics of moricizine. *Am J Cardiol* (1990) 65, 21D–25D.
3. Benedek IH, King S-YP, Powell RJ, Agra AM, Schary WL, Pieniaszek HJ. Effect of moricizine on the pharmacokinetics and pharmacodynamics of warfarin in healthy volunteers. *J Clin Pharmacol* (1992) 32, 558–63.

Anticoagulants + Natto

Natto, a Japanese food made from fermented soya bean, can reduce the effects of warfarin.

Clinical evidence

A retrospective study of 10 patients on **warfarin** who had received heart valve replacements found that eating **natto** caused the thrombotest values to rise from a range of 12–25% to 33–100%. The extent of the rise appeared to be related to the amount eaten. The values fell again when the **natto** was stopped. A healthy subject on **warfarin** with a thrombotest value of 40%, showed no changes 5 h after eating 100 g **natto**, but demonstrated a rise to 86% after 24 h and to 90% after 48 h.[1] Similar rises were seen in *animals*.[1]

Mechanism

Not fully established. Natto appears not to contain significant amounts of vitamin K, but there is evidence that after ingestion, the activity of *Bacillus natto* on the natto in the gut causes a marked increase in the synthesis and subsequent absorption of vitamin K.[1] This would oppose the actions of the warfarin (see 'Anticoagulants + Vitamin K', p.300).

Importance and management

Information appears to be limited to this study[1] and a previous one by the same author,[2] however the interaction appears to be established. Patients on warfarin should be advised to avoid natto. Other oral anticoagulants would be expected to be similarly affected (assuming that the proposed mechanism of interaction is correct).

1. Kudo T. Warfarin antagonism of natto and increase in serum vitamin K by intake of natto. *Artery* (1990) 17, 189–201.
2. Kudo T, Uchibori Y, Astumi K, Numao K, Miura M, Shigara M, Hashimoto A. Warfarin antagonism by intake of natto under anticoagulant therapy. *Igaku No Ayumi* (1978) 104, 36.

Anticoagulants + Nevirapine

Three cases suggest that warfarin requirements are increased (approximately doubled) if nevirapine is given concurrently.

Clinical evidence, mechanism, importance and management

A man taking 2.5 mg **warfarin** daily and with an INR in the range of 2.1 to 2.4 needed a doubled daily dose when his treatment with zidovudine and didanosine was replaced by stavudine, lamivudine and nevirapine. A few days later when his treatment was again changed (to stavudine, lamivudine and saquinavir) his original **warfarin** dosage was found to be adequate. Another patient was resistant to doses of **warfarin** of up to 17 mg daily while taking zidovudine, lamivudine and nevirapine, but he responded to 5 mg **warfarin** daily when the nevirapine was withdrawn. The warfarin dosage had to be raised up to 12 mg daily when nevirapine was restarted. Yet another patient showed resistance to **warfarin** while taking nevirapine.[1]

The reasons for this **warfarin**/nevirapine interaction are not known but it is suggested that nevirapine possibly induces the enzymes concerned with the metabolism of the **warfarin** so that it is cleared from the body more quickly. Information seems to be limited to these three cases, but it would now be prudent to monitor prothrombin times and INRs in any patient if **warfarin** and nevirapine are used concurrently, being alert for the need to increase the **warfarin** dosage (about doubled these reports indicate). Information about other oral anticoagulants seems to be lacking but it would now seem sensible to monitor well if nevirapine is used with any of them.

1. Dionisio D, Mininni S, Bartolozzi D, Esperti F, Vivarelli A, Leoncini F. Need for increased dose of warfarin in HIV patients taking nevirapine. *AIDS* (2001) 15, 277-8.

Anticoagulants + Nizatidine

Nizatidine does not interact with warfarin.

Clinical evidence, mechanism, importance and management

Seven normal subjects given enough **warfarin** (about 5 to 6 mg daily) to increase prothrombin times from 11.5 to 17.6 s showed no significant changes in their prothrombin times, kaolin-cephalin clotting times, the activity of factors II, VII, XI and X, or on their steady-state serum **warfarin** levels when given 300 mg **nizatidine** daily for 2 weeks.[1] This failure of **nizatidine** to affect **warfarin** levels is consistent with its lack of enzyme inhibitory activity, unlike cimetidine.

No particular precautions appear to be necessary during concurrent use. Other anticoagulants would be expected to behave similarly.

1. Cournot A, Berlin I, Sallord JC, Singlas E. Lack of interaction between nizatidine and warfarin during concurrent use. *J Clin Pharmacol* (1988) 28, 1120–2.

Anticoagulants + NSAIDs

No interaction normally occurs with ibuprofen in normal doses, and this also would appear to be true for bromfenac, diclofenac, fenbufen, indoprofen, ketoprofen, naproxen, oxaprozin, pirprofen and tolmetin, but isolated cases have been described with diclofenac, ibuprofen, ketoprofen, tiaprofenic acid and tolmetin. The effects of the anticoagulants can be increased by flurbiprofen in a few patients and they may bleed. The makers of fenoprofen say that an interaction is possible, but there seems to be no direct clinical evidence that it actually occurs. All NSAIDs cause some gastrointestinal irritation and possible bleeding, and should be used with care in patients taking oral anticoagulants. Other NSAIDs are discussed individually elsewhere. See Index.

Clinical evidence

(a) Bromfenac

50 mg **bromfenac** three times daily had no effect on the anticoagulant effects of **warfarin** in 15 normal subjects.[1]

(b) Diclofenac

Studies in 32 patients and a further 20 patients on **acenocoumarol (nicoumalone)** showed that the concurrent use of 100 mg **diclofenac** daily normally does not alter its anticoagulant effects.[2] Other studies similarly confirm that **diclofenac** normally does not interact with either **acenocoumarol, phenprocoumon** or **warfarin.**[3-6] However an unexplained case of pulmonary haemorrhage associated with a very prolonged prothrombin time has been described,[7] and another report states that the INR of a patient on **warfarin** rose from 2.8 to 5.8 after only three doses of **diclofenac.**[8] A Chinese patient on **warfarin** developed an INR of 4 within 4 days of using a 1% **diclofenac** topical gel for joint pain.[9] Note that Chinese patients are particularly sensitive to the anticoagulant effects of warfarin.

(c) Fenbufen

A study in 5 subjects on **warfarin** showed that when given 800 mg **fenbufen** daily for a week, their prothrombin times within 2 days were increased by 1.9 s, and the serum **warfarin** levels fell by 14%.[10] These changes are unlikely to be clinically significant but this needs confirmation.

(d) Fenoprofen

In vitro evidence shows that the phenylalkanoic acid derivatives can displace anticoagulants from plasma protein binding sites, but there is no direct clinical evidence that this results in a clinically important interaction with **fenoprofen.**

(e) Flurbiprofen

Nineteen patients on **phenprocoumon** given 150 mg **flurbiprofen** daily showed a small but significant fall in prothrombin times. Two patients bled (haematuria, epistaxis, haemorrhoidal bleeding) and three patients showed a fall in prothrombin times below the therapeutic range. The authors concluded that concurrent use is compatible with anticoagulation, but suggested good monitoring in the early stages.[11]

Two patients on **acenocoumarol (nicoumalone)** showed a rise in thrombotest times and bled (haematuria, melaena, haematomas) within 2 to 3 days of starting to take 150 to 300 mg **flurbiprofen** daily.[12] A necrotising purpuric rash accompanied by an increase in the thrombotest values was seen in 2 patients on **warfarin** treated with **flurbiprofen.**

(f) Ibuprofen

Studies with 19 patients[13,14] and 24 patients[15] on **phenprocoumon**, and 36 subjects,[16] 50 patients and 30 subjects,[17] and 40 patients[18] on **warfarin** showed that the effects of these anticoagulants were not altered while concurrently taking 600 to 2400 mg **ibuprofen** daily for 7 to 14 days. However one study on 20 patients taking **warfarin** showed that 1800 mg **ibuprofen** daily significantly prolonged bleeding times (4 cases above the normal range) and microscopic haematuria and haematoma were seen.[19] A raised INR occurred in one patient on **warfarin** who used topical **ibuprofen**,[8] and subclinical bleeding with a raised INR in a woman of 74 with multiple medical problems when treated with **warfarin** and **ibuprofen.**[20]

(g) Indoprofen

A study on 18 patients on **warfarin** given 600 mg **indoprofen** daily for 7 days showed that no changes occurred in any of the blood coagulation measurements made.[21]

(h) Ketoprofen

A study in 15 normal subjects stabilised on **warfarin** found that 100 mg **ketoprofen** twice daily for 7 days had no effect on their prothrombin times or coagulation cascade parameters, and there was no evidence of bleeding.[22] This contrasts with an isolated case of bleeding in a patient on **warfarin** (prothrombin time increased from 18 to 41 s) a week after starting to take 75 mg **ketoprofen** daily.[23]

(i) Naproxen

A study on 10 subjects showed that 17 days treatment with **naproxen** (750 mg daily) did not alter the pharmacokinetics of a single dose of **warfarin**, or its anticoagulant effects.[24] Similar results were found in another study.[25] Yet another study in patients on **phenprocoumon** showed that 500 mg **naproxen** daily transiently increased the anticoagulant effects and caused an unimportant change in primary bleeding time.[26]

(j) Oxaprozin

A study in 10 normal subjects stabilised on **warfarin** for an average of 13 days showed that while taking 1200 mg **oxaprozin** daily for 7 days their prothrombin times were not significantly altered.[27]

(k) Pirprofen

A study in 18 patients on long-term treatment with **phenprocoumon** showed that there was no change in the anticoagulant effects while taking 600 mg **pirprofen** daily. Bleeding time was prolonged by about 50%.[28]

(l) Tiaprofenic acid

A study in 6 subjects on **phenprocoumon** showed that while taking 800 mg **tiaprofenic acid** daily for 2 days the anticoagulant effects and the pharmacokinetic profiles of both drugs remained unchanged.[29,30] No significant interaction occurred in nine patients on **acenocoumarol (nicoumalone)** given 600 mg **tiaprofenic acid** daily for 2 weeks, but a 'rebound' rise in prothrombin percentages occurred following its withdrawal.[31] However an elderly man on **acenocoumarol** had severe epistaxis and bruising 4 to 6 weeks after starting to take 600 mg **tiaprofenic acid** daily. His prothrombin time had risen to 129 s.[32]

(m) Tolmetin

Fifteen subjects on **warfarin** showed no changes in prothrombin times while taking 1200 mg **tolmetin** daily over a 3-week period.[33] Fifteen subjects on **phenprocoumon** similarly showed no changes in prothrombin times when given 800 mg **tolmetin** daily for 10 days.[34] Bleeding times are also reported not to be significantly altered in subjects or patients on **phenprocoumon**[34] or **acenocoumarol (nicoumalone)**[35] when given 800 mg **tolmetin** daily. However there is a single unexplained case report of a diabetic patient on insulin, digoxin, theophylline, ferrous sulphate, furosemide (frusemide) and sodium polystyrene sulphonate who bled after taking three 400-mg doses of **tolmetin**. His prothrombin time had risen from 15–22 s to 70 s.[36] The manufacturers of **tolmetin** and the FDA also have 10 other cases on record.[36,37] However the manufacturers of **tolmetin** point out that over a 10-year period approximately 10 million patients have received **tolmetin** so that the risk of an interaction appears to be very small indeed.[37]

Mechanism

Drug displacement and enzyme inhibition do not seem to explain the anticoagulant/flurbiprofen interactions.[11] Most of the phenylalkanoic acid derivatives can displace the anticoagulants from plasma protein binding sites to some extent, but this mechanism on its own is rarely, if ever, responsible for a clinically important drug interaction.

Importance and management

It is well established that no adverse interaction normally occurs between ibuprofen and either warfarin or phenprocoumon, (although isolated and unexplained cases have occurred but only very rarely). Other anticoagulants would be expected to behave similarly. The absence of a clinically relevant interaction also appears to be true for bromfenac, indoprofen, fenbufen, ketoprofen, naproxen, oxaprozin and pirprofen although the documentation is more limited. However a few patients have bled when given diclofenac, flurbiprofen or tolmetin. As this is unpredictable and occasionally serious it is important to monitor the effects of concurrent use of these three NSAIDs in all patients. There also seems to be a slight possibility of an interaction with tiaprofenic acid, but with fenoprofen it appears at present to be only theoretical.

Some care is still needed with every NSAID because, to a greater or lesser extent, they irritate the stomach lining and have effects on platelet activity which can affect bleeding times and result in gastrointestinal bleeding and ulceration. One very extensive study found a nearly 13-fold increase in the risk of developing haemorrhagic peptic ulcer disease in the elderly taking oral anticoagulants and NSAIDs.[38] See the Index for the interactions of anticoagulants with other NSAIDs not dealt with in this monograph.

1. Korth-Bradley JM, Cevallos WH, McPherson MK, Decleene SA, Neefe DL. PK/PD evaluation of the potential interaction between bromfenac and warfarin. *Clin Pharmacol Ther* (1994) 55, 124.
2. Michot F, Ajdacic K, Glaus L. A double-blind clinical trial to determine if an interaction exists between diclofenac sodium and the oral anticoagulant acenocoumarol (nicoumalone). *J Int Med Res* (1975) 3, 153–7.
3. Wagenhäuser F. Research findings with a new, non-steroidal antirheumatic agent. *Scand J Rheumatol* (1975) 4 (Suppl 8), S05-01.
4. Krzywanek HJ, Breddin K. Beeinflußt Diclofenac die orale Antikoagulantientherapie und die Plättchenaggregation? *Med Welt* (1977) 28, 1843–5.
5. Breddin K (1975) Cited as personal communication in Michot F, Ajdacic K, Glaus L. A double-blind clinical trial to determine if an interaction exists between diclofenac sodium and the oral anticoagulant acenocoumarol (nicoumalone). *J Int Med Res* (1975) 3, 153–7.
6. Fitzgerald DE, Russell JG. Voltarol and warfarin, an interaction? In Current Themes in Rheumatology, Chiswell RJ and Birdwood GFB (Eds). Cambridge Medical Publications p 26–7.
7. Cuadrado Gómez LM, Palau Beato E, Pérez Venegas J, Pérez Moro E. Hemorragia pulmonar debido a la interacción de acenocoumarina y diclofenac sódico. *Rev Clin Esp* (1987) 181, 227–8.
8. Beeley L, Cunningham H, Carmichael AE, Brennan A. Newsletter of the West Midlands Centre for Adverse Drug Reaction Reporting (1991), 33, 18.
9. Chan TYK. Drug interactions as a cause of overanticoagulation and bleedings in Chinese patients receiving warfarin. *Int J Clin Pharmacol Ther* (1998) 36, 403-5.
10. Savitsky JP, Terzakis T, Bina P, Chiccarelli F, Haynes J. Fenbufen-warfarin interaction in healthy volunteers. *Clin Pharmacol Ther* (1980) 27, 284.
11. Marbet GA, Duckert F, Walter M, Six P, Airenne H. Interaction study between phenprocoumon and flurbiprofen. *Curr Med Res Opin* (1977) 5, 26.
12. Stricker BHC, Delhez JL. Interaction between flurbiprofen and coumarins. *BMJ* (1982) 285, 812–13.
13. Thilo D, Nyman F, Duckert F. A study of the effects of the anti-rheumatic drug ibuprofen (Brufen) on patients being treated with the oral anti-coagulant phenprocoumon (Marcoumar). *J Int Med Res* (1974) 2, 276–8.
14. Duckert F. The absence of effect of the antirheumatic drug ibuprofen on oral anticoagulation with phenprocoumon. *Curr Med Res Opin* (1975) 3, 556–7.
15. Boekhout-Mussert MJ, Loeliger EA. Influence of ibuprofen on oral anti-coagulation with phenprocoumon. *J Int Med Res* (1974) 2, 279–83.
16. Penner JA, Abbrecht PH. Lack of interaction between ibuprofen and warfarin. *Curr Ther Res* (1975) 18, 862–71.
17. Goncalves L. Influence of ibuprofen on haemostasis in patients on anticoagulant therapy. *J Int Med Res* (1973) 1, 180–3.
18. Marini U, Cecchi A, Venturino M. Mancanza di interazione tra ibuprofen lisinato e anticoagulanti orali. *Clin Ter* (1985) 112, 25–9.
19. Schulman S, Henriksson K. Interaction of ibuprofen and warfarin on primary haemostasis. *Br J Rheumatol* (1989) 28, 46–9.
20. Ernst ME, Buys LM. Re-evaluating the safety of concurrent warfarin and ibuprofen. *J Pharm Technol* (1997) 13, 244–7.
21. Jacono A, Caso P, Gualtieri S, Raucci D, Bianchi A, Vigorito C, Bergamini N, Iadevaia V. Clinical study of the possible interactions between indoprofen and oral anticoagulants. *Eur J Rheumatol Inflamm* (1981) 4, 32–5.
22. Mieszczak C, Winther K. Lack of interaction of ketoprofen with warfarin. *Eur J Clin Pharmacol* (1993) 44, 205–6.
23. Flessner MF, Knight H. Prolongation of prothrombin time and severe gastrointestinal bleeding associated with combined use of warfarin and ketoprofen. *JAMA* (1988) 259, 353.
24. Slattery JT, Levy G, Jain A, McMahon FG. Effect of naproxen on the kinetics of elimination and anticoagulant activity of a single dose of warfarin. *Clin Pharmacol Ther* (1979) 25, 51–60.
25. Jain A, McMahon FG, Slattery JT, Levy G. Effect of naproxen on the steady-state serum concentration and anticoagulant activity of warfarin. *Clin Pharmacol Ther* (1979) 25, 61–6.
26. Angelkort B. Zum einfluß von Naproxen auf die thrombozytäre Blutstillung und die Antikoagulantien-Behandlung mit Phenprocoumon. *Fortschr Med* (1978) 96, 1249–52.
27. Davis LJ, Kayser SR, Hubscher J, Williams RL. Effect of oxaprozin on the steady-state anticoagulant activity of warfarin. *Clin Pharm* (1984) 3, 295–7.
28. Marbet GA, Duckert F, Schönenberger PM. Eine Untersuchung über Wechselwirkungen zwischen Pirprofen und Phenprocoumon. *Fortschr Med* (1985) 103, 207–9.
29. von Durr J, Pfeiffer MH, Wetzelsberger K, Lucker PW. Untersuchung zur Frage einer Interaktion von Tiaprofensaure und Phenprocoumon. *Arzneimittelforschung* (1981) 31, 2163–7.
30. Lücker PW, Penth B, Wetzelsberger K. Pharmacokinetic interaction between tiaprofenic acid and several other compounds for chronic use. *Rheumatology* (1982) 7, 99–106.
31. Meurice J. Interaction of tiaprofenic acid and acenocoumarol. *Rheumatology* (1982) 7, 111–17.
32. Whittaker SJ, Jackson CW, Whorwell PJ. A severe, potentially fatal, interaction between tiaprofenic acid and nicoumalone. *Br J Clin Pract* (1986) 40, 440.
33. Whitsett TL, Barry JP, Czerwinski AW, Hall WH, Hampton JW. Tolmetin and warfarin: a clinical investigation to determine if interaction exists. In 'Tolmetin, A New Non-steroidal Anti-Inflammatory Agent.' Ward JR (ed). Proceedings of a Symposium, Washington DC, April 1975, Excerpta Medica, Amsterdam, New York, p. 160.
34. Rüst O, Biland L, Thilo D, Nyman D, Duckert F. Prüfung des Antirheumatikums Tolmetin auf Interaktionen mit oralen Antikoagulantien. *Schweiz Med Wochenschr* (1975) 105, 752–3.
35. Malbach E. Über die Beeinflussung der Blutungszeit durch Tolectin. *Schweiz Rundsch Med Prax* (1978) 67, 161–3.
36. Koren JF, Cochran DL, Janes RL. Tolmetin-warfarin interaction. *Am J Med* (1987) 82, 1278–9.
37. Santopolo AC. Tolmetin-warfarin interaction. *Am J Med* (1987) 82, 1279–80.
38. Shorr RI, Ray WA, Daugherty JR, Griffin MR. Concurrent use of nonsteroidal anti-inflammatory drugs and oral anticoagulants places elderly persons at high risk for hemorrhagic peptic ulcer disease. *Arch Intern Med* (1993) 153, 1665–70.

Anticoagulants + Omapatrilat

Omapatrilat does not interact with warfarin.

Clinical evidence, mechanism, importance and management

Sixteen normal men were given 2.5 to 10 mg **warfarin** daily for 14 days, to which was then added either 25 mg omapatrilat or a placebo daily for a further 7 days. No changes in prothrombin time or trough serum **warfarin** levels were found while taking omapatrilat, and concurrent use was well tolerated.[1] There would therefore appear to be no reason for avoiding the concurrent use of these drugs.

1. Mangold B, Gielsdorf W, Norton J, Liao W. Omapatrilat does not affect the steady-state of warfarin. *Clin Pharmacol Ther* (1999) 65, 131.

Anticoagulants + Omeprazole

Omeprazole normally causes only a small and clinically trivial change in the anticoagulant effects of warfarin, and normally does not interact with acenocoumarol (nicoumalone), but one patient on warfarin developed a prolonged prothrombin time and bled, and another on acenocoumarol did the same. An isolated case report describes a decrease in the prothrombin time in a patient given heparin and omeprazole.

Clinical evidence

(a) Acenocoumarol (Nicoumalone)

A comparative retrospective study of 118 patients given **acenocoumarol** with **omeprazole** and 299 age- and sex-matched patients on **acenocoumarol** without omeprazole, found no evidence that an interaction occurs.[1] Eight normal subjects were given a single 10-mg dose of **acenocoumarol** on day 2 of a 3-day study while taking 40 mg **omeprazole** or a placebo daily. The presence of the **omeprazole** had no effect on the pharmacokinetics or anticoagulant effects of the **acenocoumarol**.[2]

In contrast, an isolated case report describes a 78-year-old woman stabilised on **acenocoumarol** for 60 days who developed gross haematuria within five days of starting 20 mg **omeprazole** daily. Her INR had risen from 2.5/3.0 to 5.7, and it fell once again when the **omeprazole** was stopped.[3]

(b) Heparin

An isolated report very briefly describes a decrease in the prothrombin time of a patient treated with **heparin** and **omeprazole**. No details are given.[4]

(c) Warfarin

Twenty-one normal subjects anticoagulated with **warfarin** had a statistically significant though small decrease in their mean thrombotest percentage (from 21.1 to 18.7%) after taking 20 mg **omeprazole** daily for two weeks. (S)-**warfarin** serum levels remained unchanged but a slight (12%) rise in (R)-**warfarin** levels was seen.[5] Twenty-eight patients anticoagulated with **warfarin** given 20 mg **omeprazole** daily for 3 weeks had no significant changes in their coagulation times or thrombotest values. (S)-**warfarin** levels were unchanged while a 9.5% increase in (R)-**warfarin** levels occurred.[6]

In contrast, a man well controlled on 5 mg **warfarin** daily developed widespread bruising and haematuria 2 weeks after starting to take 20 mg **omeprazole** daily. His prothrombin time was found to have risen to 48 s. He was later restabilised on 20 mg **omeprazole** daily with the **warfarin** dosage reduced to 2 mg daily.[7]

Mechanism

It seems possible that omeprazole causes a slight to moderate inhibition of the metabolism of oral anticoagulants by the liver in a stereoselective manner, but just why just one patient on warfarin and one on acenocoumarol should show such marked effects is not known. One postulate is that the latter occurred because the patient was a poor metaboliser.[2]

Importance and management

Normally no clinically relevant interaction appears to occur between acenocoumarol or warfarin and omeprazole but it seems that rarely and unpredictably a more marked and clinically important interaction can take place. For this reason the response of patients on either of these two anticoagulants should be monitored when omeprazole is first added. There seems to be no information about other oral anticoagulants but the same precautions would seem appropriate. The general importance of the heparin/omeprazole interaction is uncertain. More study is needed.

1. Vreeburg EM, De Vlaam-Schluter GM, Trienekens PH, Snel P, Tytgat GNJ. Lack of effect of omeprazole in oral acenocoumarol anticoagulant therapy. *Scand J Gastroenterol* (1997) 32, 991–4.

2. de Hoon JNJM, Thijssen HHW, Beysens AJMM, Van Bortel LMAB. No effect of short-term omeprazole intake on acenocoumarol pharmacokinetics and pharmacodynamics. *Br J Clin Pharmacol* (1997) 44, 399–401.

3. García B, Lacambra C, Garrote F, García-Plaza I, Solis J. Possible potentiation of anticoagulant effect of acenocoumarol by omeprazole. *Pharm World Sci* (1994) 16, 231–2.

4. Beeley L, Cunningham H, Brennan A. Bulletin of the West Midlands Centre for Adverse Drug Reaction Reporting (1993) 36, 9.

5. Sutfin T, Balmer K, Boström H, Eriksson S, Höglund P, Paulsen O. Stereoselective interaction of omeprazole with warfarin in healthy men. *Ther Drug Monit* (1989) 11, 176–84.

6. Unge P, Svedberg L-E, Nordgren A, Blom H, Andersson T, Lagerström P-O, Idström J-P. A study of the interaction of omeprazole and warfarin in anticoagulated patients. *Br J Clin Pharmacol* (1992) 34, 509–12.

7. Ahmad S. Omeprazole-warfarin interaction. *South Med J* (1991) 84, 674–5.

Anticoagulants + Orlistat

Orlistat does not interact with warfarin.

Clinical evidence, mechanism, importance and management

In a three-party blind, placebo-controlled, randomised and two-way crossover study, 12 normal subjects were given 120 mg **orlistat** three times daily for 16 days, and a single 30 mg dose of racemic **warfarin** on day 11. The pharmacokinetics and pharmacodynamics of the **warfarin** were not altered by the **orlistat**, and the absorption of vitamin K from regular diets was not affected.[1,2] No special precautions would seem necessary if **warfarin** and **orlistat** are given concurrently. Information about other anticoagulants is lacking.

1. Zhi J, Melia AT, Koss-Twardy S, Passe S, Rakhit A. The effect of orlistat on the pharmacokinetics (PK) and pharmacodynamics (PD) of warfarin and on the absorption of vitamin K (V_K) in healthy volunteers. *Pharm Res* (1995) 12 (9 Suppl), S-410.

2. Zhi J, Melia AT, Guerciolini R, Koss-Twardy SG, Passe SM, Rakhit A, Sadowski JA. The effect of orlistat on the pharmacokinetics and pharmacodynamics of warfarin in healthy volunteers. *J Clin Pharmacol* (1996) 36, 659–666.

Anticoagulants + Oxaceprol

An isolated report describes a marked fall in the response to fluindione in a patient when given oxaceprol.

Clinical evidence, mechanism, importance and management

A woman of 77 with hypertension and atrial fibrillation, under treatment with propafenone, furosemide (frusemide), enalapril and **fluindione** (15 mg daily), was additionally started on 300 mg **oxaceprol** daily. Within 2 days her Quick Time had risen from 26 to 57% and by the end of the week to 65%. When the **oxaceprol** was withdrawn, her Quick Time returned to its previous values (23 to 30%).[1] The mechanism is not understood. The general importance of this interaction is not known but the concurrent use of **oxaceprol** and any anticoagulant should be well monitored; be alert for the need to modify the anticoagulant dosage.

1. Bannwarth B, Tréchot P, Mathieu J, Froment J, Netter P. Interaction oxacéprol-fluindione. *Therapie* (1990) 45, 162–3.

Anticoagulants + Oxyphenbutazone

The anticoagulant effects of warfarin are markedly increased by oxyphenbutazone which can lead to serious bleeding.

Clinical evidence, mechanism, importance and management

A man on **warfarin** developed gross haematuria within 9 days of starting to take 400 mg **oxyphenbutazone** daily. His prothrombin time had increased to 68 s. A subsequent study on him confirmed that the hypoprothrombinaemia was due to the **oxyphenbutazone**.[1] Two similar cases have been described elsewhere.[2,3] A clinical study has also shown that **oxyphenbutazone** slows the clearance of **dicoumarol**.[4]

Oxyphenbutazone is the major metabolite of phenylbutazone within the body and it may be presumed that the explanation for the anticoagulant/phenylbutazone interaction equally applies to **oxyphenbutazone** (see 'Anticoagulants + Phenylbutazone', p.285). Direct evidence of this interaction seems to be limited to the reports cited here, but it would appear to be established and of clinical importance. It would be prudent to apply all the precautions suggested for phenylbutazone.

1. Hobbs CB, Miller AL, Thornley JH. Potentiation of anticoagulant therapy by oxyphenylbutazone. A probable case. *Postgrad Med J* (1965) 41, 563–5.

2. Fox SL. Potentiation of anticoagulants caused by pyrazole compounds. *JAMA* (1964) 188, 320–1.
3. Taylor PJ. Hemorrhage while on anticoagulant therapy precipitated by drug interaction. *Ariz Med* (1967) 24, 697.
4. Weiner M, Siddiqui AA, Bostanci N, Dayton PG. Drug interactions: the effect of combined administration on the half-life of coumarin and pyrazolone drugs in man. *Fedn Proc* (1965) 24, 153.

Anticoagulants + Paracetamol (Acetaminophen)

The anticoagulant effects of acenocoumarol (nicoumalone), anisindione, dicoumarol, phenprocoumon and warfarin are normally not affected, or only increased to a small extent, by small occasional doses of paracetamol (acetaminophen), but a reduction in the anticoagulant dosage may be needed if larger doses are taken regularly for longer periods. There is good evidence from large-scale studies that concurrent use increases the incidence of upper gastrointestinal bleeding.

Clinical evidence

(a) Prothrombin times unchanged

Ten patients on **warfarin** showed no changes in their prothrombin times when given 3 g **paracetamol** (**acetaminophen**) daily for 2 weeks.[1] A further study on 10 patients given **warfarin** or **phenprocoumon** found that two 650-mg doses of **paracetamol** similarly had no effect on prothrombin times measured over the following 48 h.[2]

Twenty normal subjects showed no significant changes in the pharmacokinetics of single 20-mg doses of **warfarin**, or in prothrombin times, after taking 4.0 g **paracetamol** daily for 2 weeks.[3]

(b) Prothrombin times increased

The prothrombin times of 50 patients taking **anisindione, dicoumarol, phenprocoumon** or **warfarin** were increased by an average of 3.7 s after taking 2.6 g **paracetamol** (**acetaminophen**) daily for 2 weeks.[4] **Paracetamol** 2 g daily for 3 weeks increased the thrombotest times of 10 patients on coumarin anticoagulants (6 on **phenprocoumon** and 4 on **acenocoumarol** (**nicoumalone**)) by approximately 20%. The anticoagulant dosage was reduced in 5 out of the 10 patients and in one of the 10 control patients.[5,6] Fifteen normal subjects, given enough **warfarin** to increase their prothrombin times by 1.35 to 1.50, were additionally given 4.0 g **paracetamol** daily for 2 weeks. The prothrombin times of 7 rose by more than 20% (to 1.75) compared with one subject taking placebo, and by more than 33% (to 2.0) in 5 others. The increases were seen from about day 7 and were maximal after 12.5 days.[7] A retrospective study of the factors which increased the risk of excessive anticoagulation with **warfarin** found that taking 9 g **paracetamol** or more weekly increased by tenfold the odds of having an INR greater than 6.0.[8] The increases occurred in a dose-dependent manner.[8]

A woman on **warfarin** developed a retroperitoneal haematoma after taking 8 to 10 tablets (400 to 500 mg) **paracetamol** over the previous 4 days. Her INR had risen to 7.5.[9] A report describes bleeding (haematuria, gum bleeding) in a woman on **warfarin** after taking about 1.6 g **paracetamol** daily for 10 days in a compound **paracetamol/codeine** preparation. Her prothrombin time rose to 96 s.[10,11] Another report describes bleeding from the gums and bruising and increased INRs (up to 12.0) in a woman on **warfarin** after taking 14 g **paracetamol** (in **co-dydramol**) over 7 days on one occasion and 14 g (in *Tylex*) over 8 days on another.[12] A very large-scale study in Denmark found that the incidence of hospitalisation for upper gastrointestinal bleeding in patients on **warfarin** or **phenprocoumon** rose from a standard incidence ratio (SRI) of 2.8 to 4.4 when paracetamol was taken concurrently.[13]

See also 'Anticoagulants + Dextropropoxyphene', p.255 because **paracetamol** is a component of co-proxamol, *Distalgesic* and *Darvocet*.

Mechanism

Not understood.

Importance and management

An established interaction although there are unexplained inconsistencies in the evidence. The weight of clinical evidence and common experience indicates that occasional small doses of paracetamol (acetaminophen) — no more than about five tablets (5 x 500 mg) weekly[8] — are unlikely to cause important INR rises in patients on oral anticoagulants, but if larger amounts are taken the risk of getting INRs above 6 steadily rises in a dose-dependent manner, and only 2 to 3 tablets daily for a week can increase the risks up to 10-fold.[8] This means that if more than occasional doses are taken for longer than a few days it would be prudent to monitor prothrombin times so that any anticoagulant dosage reductions can be made.[14] INRs should normally not exceed 4.0. Anticoagulants other than those specifically cited above would be expected to interact similarly. Paracetamol is generally safer than aspirin as an analgesic in the presence of an anticoagulant because it does not affect platelets or cause gastric bleeding.

1. Udall JA. Drug interference with warfarin therapy. *Clin Med* (1978) 77, 20–5.
2. Antlitz AM, Awalt LF. A double blind study of acetaminophen used in conjunction with oral anticoagulant therapy. *Curr Ther Res* (1969) 11, 360–1.
3. Kwan D, Bartle WR, Walker SE. The effects of acute and chronic acetaminophen dosing on the pharmacodynamics and pharmacokinetics of (R)- and (S) warfarin. *Clin Pharmacol Ther* (1995) 57, 212.
4. Antlitz AM, Mead JA ,Tolentino MA. Potentiation of oral anticoagulant therapy by acetaminophen. *Curr Ther Res* (1968) 10, 501–7.
5. Boeijinga JJ, Boerstra EE, Ris P, Breimer DD, Jeletich-Bastiaanse A. Interaction between paracetamol and coumarin anticoagulants. *Lancet* (1982) i, 506.
6. Boeijinga JK, Boerstra EE, Ris P, Breimer DD, Jeletich-Bastiaanse A. De invloed van paracetamol op antistollingsbehandeling met coumarinederivaten. *Pharm Weekbl* (1983) 118, 209–12.
7. Rubin RN, Mentzer RL, Budzynski AZ. Potentiation of anticoagulant effect of warfarin by acetaminophen (Tylenol[R]). *Clin Res* (1984) 32, 698A.
8. Hylek EM, Heiman H, Skates SJ, Sheehan MA, Singer DE. Acetaminophen and other risk factors for excessive warfarin anticoagulation. *JAMA* (1998) 279, 657–62.
9. Andrews FJ. Retroperitoneal haematoma after paracetamol increased anticoagulation. *Emerg Med J* (2002) 19. 84–5.
10. Kwan D, Bartle WR. Drug interactions with warfarin. *Med J Aust* (1993) 158, 574.
11. Bartle WR, Blakey JA. Potentiation of warfarin anticoagulation by acetaminophen. *JAMA* (1991) 265, 1260.
12. Fitzmaurice DA, Murray JA. Potentiation of anticoagulant effect of warfarin. *Postgrad Med J* (1997) 73, 439–40.
13. Johnsen P, Sorensen HT, Mellemkjoer L, Blot WJ, Nielsen GL, McLaughlin JK, Olsen JH. Hospitalisation for upper gastrointestinal bleeding associated with the use of oral anticoagulants. *Thromb Haemost* (2001) 86, 563–8.
14. Bell WR. Acetaminophen and Warfarin: an undesirable synergy. *JAMA* (1998) 279, 702–3.

Anticoagulants + Penicillins

The effects of the oral anticoagulants are not normally altered by the penicillins but isolated cases of increased prothrombin times and/or bleeding have been seen in patients given amoxicillin (amoxycillin), ampicillin/flucloxacillin, benzylpenicillin or talampicillin. Carbenicillin in the absence of an anticoagulant can prolong prothrombin times and might therefore also do so in the presence of an anticoagulant. In contrast, a handful of cases of reduced warfarin effects have been seen with dicloxacillin and nafcillin, and possibly with amoxicillin.

Clinical evidence

(a) Increased anticoagulant effects

A woman on **acenocoumarol** (**nicoumalone**) developed bruising and an increased INR (7.1) within a week of starting 500 mg **amoxicillin** (**amoxycillin**) 8-hourly.[1] The prothrombin time of a patient on **warfarin** increased when treated with **ampicillin/flucloxacillin**, and both bleeding and an increase in the prothrombin ratio has been described in a patient on **warfarin** given **talampicillin**.[2] Hypoprothrombinaemia has been described in one patient on **warfarin** given 24 million units of **benzylpenicillin** daily intravenously.[3] **Benzylpenicillin** is also known to be able to increase bleeding times and cause bleeding in the absence of an anticoagulant.[4] Increases in bleeding times, bleeding,[4-9] and extended prothrombin times[8,9] have been described with **carbenicillin** in the absence of an anticoagulant. **Ampicillin**, **methicillin** and **ticarcillin** are also reported to prolong bleeding times,[10-13] and in theory might also increase the effects of both **heparin** and the oral anticoagulants, but reports of such interactions seem to be lacking (except with **ampicillin/flucloxacillin** mentioned above).

(b) Decreased anticoagulant effects

The prothrombin time of a patient stabilised on **warfarin** fell from a range of 20–25 s down to 14–17 s (despite a doubling of the **warfarin** dosage) when given 12 g **nafcillin** daily intravenously.[14] A few months after the **nafcillin** was discontinued, the half-life of the **warfarin** was found to have climbed from 11 to 44 h. Nine other cases of this 'warfarin resistance' with **high dose nafcillin** have been reported.[15-21] Seven days' treatment with 500 mg **dicloxacillin sodium** four times daily and at bedtime reduced the mean prothrombin times of 7 patients on **warfarin** by 1.9 s. One patient showed a 5.6 s reduction.[22] Another patient on **warfarin** showed a 17% fall in prothrombin times within 4 to 5 days of starting 500 mg **dicloxacillin** four times daily, and 7 other patients out of 26 similarly treated were also identifed as having shown a 17% fall in prothrombin times.[23] Yet another case involving **dicloxacillin** is described elsewhere.[20] A very brief report states that **amoxicillin (amoxycillin)** caused an unspecified decrease in prothrombin times in 5 patients, but by implication it was small and of limited clinical importance.[24]

Mechanisms

Not understood. The nafcillin-warfarin interaction is possibly due to increases in the metabolism of warfarin by the liver. Changes in bleeding times caused by the other penicillins appear to result from changes in antithrombin III activity, blood platelet changes and alterations in the fibrinogen-fibrin conversion. Dicloxacillin possibly reduces serum warfarin levels.[23]

Importance and management

Documented reports of oral anticoagulant/penicillin interactions are relatively rare, bearing in mind how frequently these drugs are used, so that the broad picture is that no clinically relevant interaction normally occurs with most penicillins. This lack of interaction was confirmed by a fairly limited clinical study with **phenoxymethylpenicillin**, **amoxicillin (amoxycillin)**, **ampicillin**, **co-amoxiclav** and **flucloxacillin**).[25] The two possible exceptions are warfarin with **dicloxacillin** and particularly **high dose nafcillin** which may possibly call for an increased warfarin dosage in some patients.

Even though the general picture is of 'no interaction', some individual physicians say that they have seen changes with otherwise normally non-interacting penicillins and this is reflected in a statement in the British National Formulary which says that ". . . common experience in anticoagulant clinics is that INR can be prolonged by a few seconds following a course of broad-spectrum antibiotic e.g. ampicillin . . ." For this reason concurrent use should be monitored so that the very occasional and unpredictable cases (increases or decreases in the anticoagulant effects) can be identified and handled accordingly.

1. Soto J, Sacristan JA, Alsar MJ, Fernandez-Viadero C, Verduga R. Probable acenocoumarol-amoxycillin interaction. *Acta Haematol (Basel)* (1993) 90, 195–7.
2. Beeley L, Daly M. Bulletin of the West Midlands Centre for Adverse Drug Reaction Reporting (1986) 23, 13.
3. Brown MA, Korschinski ED, Miller DR. Interaction of penicillin-G and warfarin? *Can J Hosp Pharm* (1979) 32, 18–19.
4. Roberts PL. High dose penicillin and bleeding. *Ann Intern Med* (1974) 81, 267–8.
5. Brown CH, Natelson EA, Bradshaw MW, Williams TW, Alfrey CP. The hemostatic defect produced by carbenicillin *N Engl J Med* (1974) 291, 265–70.
6. McClure PD, Casserly JG, Monsier C, Crozier D. Carbenicillin-induced bleeding disorder. *Lancet* (1970) ii, 1307–8.
7. Waisbren BA, Evani SV, Ziebert AP. Carbenicillin and bleeding. *JAMA* (1971) 217, 1243.
8. Yudis M, Mahood WH, Maxwell R. Bleeding problems with carbenicillin. *Lancet* (1972) ii, 599.
9. Lurie A, Ogilvie M, Townsend R, Gold C, Meyers AM, Goldberg B. Carbenicillin-induced coagulopathy. *Lancet* (1970) i, 1114–15.
10. Andrassy K, Ritz E, Weisschedel E. Bleeding after carbenicillin administration. *N Engl J Med* (1975) 292, 109–10.
11. Brown CH, Bradshaw MW, Natelson EA, Alfrey CP, Williams TW. Defective platelet function following the administration of penicillin compounds. *Blood* (1976) 47, 949–56.
12. Brown CH, Natelson EA, Bradshaw MW, Alfrey CP, Williams TW. Study of the effects of ticarcillin on blood coagulation and platelet function. *Antimicrob Agents Chemother* (1975) 7, 652.
13. Beeley L, Stewart P. Bulletin of the West Midland Centre for Adverse Drug Reaction Reporting (1987) 25, 16.
14. Qureshi GD, Reinders TP, Somori GJ, Evans HJ. Warfarin resistance with nafcillin therapy. *Ann Intern Med* (1984) 100, 527–9.
15. Fraser GL, Miller M, Kane K. Warfarin resistance associated with nafcillin therapy. *Am J Med* (1989) 87, 237–8.
16. Du Pont Pharmaceuticals (1988). Quoted as personal communication in Fraser GL, Miller M, Kane K. Warfarin resistance associated with nafcillin therapy. *Am J Med* (1989) 87, 237–8.
17. Davis RL, Berman W, Wernly JA, Kelly HW. Warfarin-nafcillin interaction. *J Pediatr* (1991) 118, 300–3.
18. Shovick VA, Rihn TL. Decreased hypoprothrombinemic response to warfarin secondary to the warfarin-nafcillin interaction. *DICP Ann Pharmacother* (1991) 25, 598–9.
19. Heilker GM, Fowler JW, Self TH. Possible nafcillin-warfarin interaction. *Arch Intern Med* (1994) 154, 822–4.
20. Taylor AT, Pritchard DC, Goldstein AO, Fletcher JL. Continuation of warfarin-nafcillin interaction during dicloxacillin therapy. *J Fam Pract* (1994) 39, 182–5.
21. Baciewicz AM, Heugel AM, Rose PG. Probable nafcillin-warfarin interaction. *J Pharm Technol* (1999) 15, 5–7.
22. Krstenansky PM, Jones WN, Garewal HS. Effect of dicloxacillin sodium on the hypoprothrombinemic response to warfarin sodium. *Clin Pharm* (1987) 6, 804–6.
23. Mailloux AT, Gidal BE, Sorkness CA. Potential interaction between warfarin and dicloxacillin. *Ann Pharmacother* (1996) 30, 1402–7.
24. Radley AS, Hall J. Interactions. *Pharm J* (1992) 249, 81.
25. Pharmacy Anticoagulant Clinic Study Group. A multicentre survey of antibiotics on the INR of anticoagulated patients. *Pharm J* (1996) 257 (Pharmacy Practice Suppl), R30.

Anticoagulants + Pentoxifylline (Oxpentifylline)

The anticoagulant effects of phenprocoumon were not significantly altered by the concurrent use of pentoxifylline (oxpentifylline) in one study, but serious bleeding has been seen with pentoxifylline alone and in the presence of acenocoumarol (nicoumalone).

Clinical evidence, mechanism, importance and management

The anticoagulant effects of **phenprocoumon** were slightly but not significantly altered by the concurrent use of 1600 mg **pentoxifylline (oxpentifylline)** daily for 27 days in 10 patients.[1] However another report describes 3 major haemorrhagic problems (2 fatal cerebral, 1 gastrointestinal bleeding) in a group of patients taking **acenocoumarol (nicoumalone)** with **pentoxifylline** (400 mg three times daily) for the treatment of intermittent claudication.[2] Yet another describes acute gastrointestinal bleeding in a woman after being given 400 mg **pentoxifylline** three times daily for 2 days, in the absence of an anticoagulant,[3] clearly indicating that bleeding may not necessarily be the result of an interaction.

Since there is some risk of bleeding, possibly serious, with **pentoxifylline**, it would be prudent to monitor its use, whether an anticoagulant is present or not.

1. Ingerslev J, Mouritzen C, Stenbjerg S. Pentoxifylline does not interfere with stable coumarin anticoagulant therapy: a clinical study. *Pharmatherapeutica* (1986) 4, 595–600.
2. Dettori AG, Pini M, Moratti A, Paolicelli M, Basevi P, Qintavalla R, Manotti C, Di Lecce C and The APIC Study Group. Acenocoumarol and pentoxifylline in intermittent claudication. A controlled clinical study. *Angiology* (1989) 40, 237–48.
3. Oren R, Yishar U, Lysy J, Livshitz T, Ligumsky M. Pentoxifylline-induced gastrointestinal bleeding. *DICP Ann Pharmacother* (1991) 25, 315–16.

Anticoagulants + Phenazone (Antipyrine)

The anticoagulant effects of warfarin are reduced by the concurrent use of phenazone.

Clinical evidence

The plasma **warfarin** concentrations of 5 patients were halved (from 2.93 to 1.41 micrograms/ml) and the anticoagulant effects accordingly reduced after taking 600 mg **phenazone** daily for 50 days.[1] The prothrombin percentage of one patient rose from 5 to 50%. In an associated study it was found that 600 mg **phenazone** daily for 30 days caused falls in the **warfarin** half-lives in 2 patients from 47 to 27 h and from 69 to 39 h respectively.[1-3]

Mechanism

Phenazone is an enzyme inducing agent which increases the metabolism and clearance of warfarin from the body, thereby reducing its effects.[1-3]

Importance and management

An established interaction. The effects of concurrent use should be monitored and the dosage of warfarin increased appropriately. Other anticoagulants may be expected to behave similarly.

1. Breckenridge A, Orme M. Clinical implication of enzyme induction. *Ann N Y Acad Sci* (1971) 179, 421.
2. Breckenridge A, Orme ML'E, Thorgeirsson S, Davies DS, Brooks RV. Drug interactions with warfarin: studies with dichloralphenazone, chloral hydrate and phenazone (Antipyrine). *Clin Sci* (1971) 40, 351.
3. Breckenridge A, Orme ML'E, Thorgeirsson S, Dollery CT. Induction of drug metabolising enzymes in man and rat by dichloralphenazone. 4th International Congress of Pharmacology, Basel, July 14–18 (1969) 182.

Anticoagulants + Phenothiazines

Chlorpromazine does not interact significantly with acenocoumarol (nicoumalone).

Clinical evidence, mechanism, importance and management

Although **chlorpromazine** in doses of 40 to 100 mg is said to have ". . . played a slightly sensitising role . . ." in 2 out of 8 patients on **acenocoumarol (nicoumalone)**[1] and is reported to increase its anticoagulant effects in *animals*,[2] there is nothing to suggest that special precautions are need during concurrent use in man. No important interactions appear to occur between any of the oral anticoagulants and phenothiazines.

1. Johnson R, David A, Chartier Y. Clinical experience with G-23350 (Sintrom). *Can Med Assoc J* (1957) 77, 760.
2. Weiner M. Effect of centrally active drugs on the action of coumarin anticoagulants. *Nature* (1966) 212, 1599–1600.

Anticoagulants + Phenylbutazone

The anticoagulant effects of warfarin are markedly increased by phenylbutazone. Concurrent use should be avoided because serious bleeding can occur. Bleeding has been seen in patients on phenindione or phenprocoumon when given phenylbutazone, but successful concurrent use has been achieved with both phenprocoumon and acenocoumarol (nicoumalone) apparently because the anticoagulant dosage was carefully reduced.

Clinical evidence

(a) Phenylbutazone added to stabilised warfarin treatment

A man, stabilised on **warfarin** following mitral valve replacement, was later given **phenylbutazone** for back pain by his general practitioner. On admission to hospital a week later he had epistaxis, and his face, legs and arms had begun to swell. He showed extensive bruising of the jaw, elbow and calves, some evidence of gastrointestinal bleeding, and a prothrombin time of 98 s.[1]

(b) Warfarin added to treatment with phenylbutazone

A man, hospitalised following a myocardial infarction, was given a single 600-mg dose of **phenylbutazone**. Next day, when coagulation studies were done, his prothrombin time was 12 s and he was given 40 mg **warfarin** to initiate anticoagulant therapy. Within 48 h he developed massive gastrointestinal bleeding and was found to have a prothrombin time exceeding 100 s.[2]

There are numerous other reports of this interaction in man involving **warfarin**,[3-10] **phenprocoumon**[11-13] and **acenocoumarol (nicoumalone)**.[14] A single unconfirmed report describes this interaction in two patients taking **phenindione**.[15]

Mechanism

Phenylbutazone inhibits the metabolism of $S(-)$-warfarin (the more potent of the two isomers) so that it is cleared from the body more slowly and its effects are increased and prolonged.[16,17] Phenylbutazone also very effectively displaces the anticoagulants from their plasma protein binding sites, thereby increasing the concentrations of free and active anticoagulant molecules in plasma water,[3,8,18-20] but the importance of this latter mechanism is probably small.

Importance and management

The **warfarin**/phenylbutazone interaction is very well established and clinically important. Serious bleeding can occur and concurrent use should be avoided. Much less is known about **phenindione** with phenylbutazone but it is probably equally unsafe.[15] Direct evidence of a serious **phenprocoumon**/phenylbutazone interaction seems to be limited to two reports,[11,13] and there is good evidence[21] that successful and apparently uneventful concurrent use is possible, presumably because in the case cited the response and the anticoagulant dosages were carefully controlled. A study in 357 patients given 600 mg phenylbutazone to which was added **acenocoumarol (nicoumalone)** from day 5 onwards found that 25% less acenocoumarol was needed than in control group on acenocoumarol alone. Evidently concurrent use is possible. Information about **other anticoagulants** is lacking, but until there is clear evidence to the contrary, expect them to behave like warfarin. Remember too that phenylbutazone affects platelet aggregation and can cause gastrointestinal bleeding, whether an anticoagulant is present or not. Alternative non-interacting NSAIDs include ibuprofen and naproxen. See Index.

1. Bull J, Mackinnon J. Phenylbutazone and anticoagulant control. *Practitioner* (1975) 215, 767–9.
2. Robinson DS. The application of basic principles of drug interaction to clinical practice. *J Urol (Baltimore)* (1975) 113, 100.
3. Aggeler PM, O'Reilly RA, Leong I, Kowitz PE. Potentiation of anticoagulant effect of warfarin by phenylbutazone. *N Engl J Med* (1967) 276, 496–501.
4. Udall JA. Drug interference with warfarin therapy. *Clin Med* (1970) 77, 20–5.
5. McLaughlin GE, McCarty DJ, Segal BL. Hemarthrosis complicating anticoagulant therapy. Report of three cases. *JAMA* (1966) 196, 1020–1.
6. Hoffbrand BI, Kininmonth DA. Potentiation of anticoagulants. *BMJ* (1967) 2, 838.
7. Eisen MJ. Combined effect of sodium warfarin and phenylbutazone. *JAMA* (1964) 189, 64–5.
8. O'Reilly RA. The binding of sodium warfarin to plasma albumin and its displacement by phenylbutazone. *Ann N Y Acad Sci* (1973) 226, 293–308.
9. Schary WL, Lewis RJ, Rowland M. Warfarin-phenylbutazone interaction in man: a long-term multiple-dose study. *Res Commun Chem Pathol Pharmacol* (1975) 10, 663–72.
10. Chierichetti S, Bianchi G, Cerri B. Comparison of feprazone and phenylbutazone interaction with warfarin in man. *Curr Ther Res* (1975) 18, 568–72.
11. Sigg A, Pestalozzi H, Clauss A, Koller F. Verstärkung der Antikoagulantienwirkung durch Butazolidin. *Schweiz Med Wochenschr* (1956) 42, 1194–5.
12. Seiler K, Duckert F. Properties of 3-(1-phenyl-propyl)-4-oxycoumarin (Marcoumar®) in the plasma when tested in normal cases under the influence of drugs. *Thromb Diath Haemorrh* (1968) 19, 389–96.
13. O'Reilly RA. Phenylbutazone and sulfinpyrazone interaction with oral anticoagulant phenprcoumon. *Arch Intern Med* (1982) 142, 1634.
14. Guggisberg W, Montigel C. Erfahrungen mit kombinierter Butazolidin-Sintrom-Prophylaxe und Butazolidin-prophylaxe thromboembolischer Erkrankungen. *Ther Umsch* (1958) 15, 227.
15. Kindermann A. Vasculäres Allergid nach Butalidon und Gefahren Kombinierter Anwendung mit Athrombon (Phenylindandion). *Dermatol Wochenschr* (1961) 143, 172–8.
16. Lewis RJ, Trager WF, Chan KK, Breckenridge A, Orme M, Rowland M, Schary W. Warfarin. Stereochemical aspects of its metabolism and the interaction with phenylbutazone. *J Clin Invest* (1974) 53, 1607–17.
17. O'Reilly RA, Trager WF, Motley CH, Howald W. Stereoselective interaction of phenylbutazone with [^{12}C/^{13}C] warfarin pseudoracemates in man. *J Clin Invest* (1980) 65, 746–53.
18. Tillement J-P, Zini R, Mattei C, Singlas E. Effect of phenylbutazone on the binding of vitamin K antagonists to albumin. *Eur J Clin Pharmacol* (1973) 6, 15–18.
19. Solomon HM, Schrogie JJ. The effect of various drugs on the binding of warfarin-^{14}C to human albumin. *Biochem Pharmacol* (1967) 16, 1219–26.

20. O'Reilly RA. Interaction of several coumarin compounds with human and canine plasma albumin. *Mol Pharmacol* (1971) 7, 209–18.
21. Kaufmann P. Vergleich zwischen einer Thromboembolieprophylaxe mit Antikoagulantien und mit Butazolidin. *Schweiz Med Wochenschr* (1957) 87 (Suppl 24), 755–9.

Anticoagulants + Picotamide

Picotamide does not alter the anticoagulant effects of warfarin.

Clinical evidence, mechanism, importance and management

300 mg **picotamide** daily for 10 days had no effect on the serum levels of **warfarin** or its anticoagulant effects in 10 patients with aortic or mitral valve prostheses.[1] No special precautions would seem necessary. There seems to be no information about other anticoagulants.

1. Parise P, Gresele P, Viola E, Ruina A, Migliacci R, Nenci GG. La picotamide non interferisce con l'attività antiacoagulante del warfarin in pazienti portatori di protesi valvolari cardiache. *Clin Ter* (1990) 135, 479–82.

Anticoagulants + Piracetam

A single case report describes a woman on warfarin who began to bleed within a month of starting to take piracetam.

Clinical evidence, mechanism, importance and management

A woman patient on regular treatment with **warfarin**, insulin, levothyroxine and digoxin began to bleed (menorrhagia) within a month of starting to take 600 mg **piracetam** (*Nootropil*) daily. Her British Corrected Ratio (BCR) was found to have risen to 4.1 (normal range 2.3 to 2.8). Within 2 days of withdrawing both the **warfarin** and **piracetam** her BCR had fallen to 2.07.[1] The reason for this apparent interaction is not known. There is far too little evidence to forbid concurrent use, but be alert for this reaction if both drugs are used.

1. Pan HYM, Ng RP. The effect of Nootropil in a patient on warfarin. *Eur J Clin Pharmacol* (1983) 24, 711.

Anticoagulants + Pirmenol

The anticoagulant effects of warfarin are not changed by pirmenol.

Clinical evidence, mechanism, importance and management

The prothrombin time response to a single 25-mg dose of **warfarin** was reduced by 0.2 to 1.3 sec in an experimental study in 12 normal subjects who had taken 150 mg **pirmenol** twice daily for 7 days.[1] This suggested that some changes in the dosage of **warfarin** might be required in clinical practice, but a later study found that the prothrombin times of 10 patients on **warfarin** were not significantly changed when they were additionally given 150 mg **pirmenol** twice daily by mouth for 14 days.[2] No special precautions would therefore seem to be necessary. There seems as yet to be no information about other anticoagulants.

1. Janiczek N, Bockbrader HN, Lebsack ME, Sedman AJ, Chang T. Effect of pirmenol (CI-845) on prothrombin (PT) time following concomitant administration of pirmenol and warfarin to healthy volunteers. *Pharm Res* (1988) 5, S-155.
2. Stringer KA, Switzer DF, Abadier R, Lebsack ME, Sedman A, Chrymko M. The effect of pirmenol administration on the anti-coagulant activity of warfarin. *J Clin Pharmacol* (1991) 31, 607–10.

Anticoagulants + Ponalrestat

Ponalrestat does not alter the anticoagulant effects of warfarin.

Clinical evidence, mechanism, importance and management

Twelve diabetics stabilised on **warfarin** showed no changes in **warfarin** serum levels or prothrombin ratios when concurrently treated with 600 mg **ponalrestat** daily for 2 weeks.[1] No special precautions seem necessary. There seems to be no information about other anticoagulants.

1. Moulds RFW, Fullinfaw RO, Bury RW, Plehwe WE, Jacka N, McGrath KM, Martin FIR. Ponalrestat does not cause a protein binding interaction with warfarin in diabetic patients. *Br J Clin Pharmacol* (1991) 31, 715–18.

Anticoagulants + Pravastatin

Pravastatin appears not to interact with warfarin but an isolated case of bleeding has been seen in a patient taking fluindione.

Clinical evidence

(a) Fluindione

A woman with atrial fibrillation on **fluindione** and with an INR between 2.5 and 3.5, developed haematuria within 5 days of starting 10 mg **pravastatin** daily. Her INR had climbed to 10.2. Treatment was stopped and her INR then fell to 3.8 within 72 h.[1]

(b) Warfarin

Ten normal subjects were given 20 mg pravastatin alone twice daily for three-and-a-half days, 5 mg **warfarin** alone twice daily for 6 days, and then both pravastatin and **warfarin** together for 6 days. The **warfarin** did not alter the pharmacokinetics of pravastatin, nor were the anticoagulant effects or the plasma protein binding of the **warfarin** significantly changed.[2] Pravastatin 20 mg for 7 days had no effect on the INRs of 8 patients on **warfarin**.[3] No changes in prothrombin times were seen in extensive clinical trials in patients, some of whom were on **warfarin** and pravastatin.[4] No interaction was seen in another 46 patients on **warfarin** and pravastatin.[5]

Mechanism

None with warfarin. The fluindione/pravastatin interaction is not understood.

Importance and management

The picture presented by these studies and reports is that no interaction is likely with warfarin and pravastatin, but the isolated case involving fluindione suggests that it might be prudent to monitor the outcome when pravastatin is first added to treatment with this anticoagulant. There appears to be nothing documented about any of the other anticoagulants.

1. Trenque T, Choisy H, Germain M-L. Pravastatin: interaction with oral anticoagulant? *BMJ* (1996) 312, 886.
2. Light RT, Pan HY, Glaess SR, Bakry D (ER Squibb). A report on the pharmacokinetic and pharmacodynamic interaction of pravastatin and warfarin in healthy male volunteers. Data on file, (Protocol No 27, 201-59), 1988.
3. O'Rangers EA, Ford M, Hershey A. The effect of HMG-coA reductase inhibitors on the anticoagulant response to warfarin. *Pharmacotherapy* (1994) 14, 349.
4. Catalano P. Pravastatin safety: an overview. In: Wood C, (ed). Lipid management: pravastatin and the differential pharmacology of HMG-CoA reductase inhibitors. Roy Soc Med Round Table Ser No.16. Oxford, Alden Press (1990) 26–31.
5. Lin JC, Stolley SN, Morreale AP, Marcus DB. The effect of converting from pravastatin to simvastatin on the pharmacodynamics of warfarin. *J Clin Pharmacol* (1999) 39, 86-90.

Anticoagulants + Probenecid

Some preliminary evidence suggests that probenecid increases the loss of phenprocoumon from the body. The anticoagulant effects would be expected to be decreased.

Clinical evidence, mechanism, importance and management

Probenecid 500 mg four times daily for 7 days reduced the AUC of a single 0.22 mg/kg dose of phenprocoumon in 17 normal subjects by 48%.[1] The reasons are not understood, but one possibility is that while probenecid inhibits the glucuronidation of phenprocoumon (its normal route of metabolism) it may also increase the formation of hydroxylated metabolites so that its overall loss is increased.[1] This study suggests that, in the presence of probenecid, the dosage of phenprocoumon may need to be increased, but this awaits formal clinical confirmation in patients. There seems to be nothing documented about other anticoagulants.

1. Mönig H, Böhm M, Ohnhaus EE, Kirch W. The effects of frusemide and probenecid on the pharmacokinetics of phenprocoumon. *Eur J Clin Pharmacol* (1990) 39, 261–5.

Anticoagulants + Proguanil

An isolated report describes bleeding in a woman patient on warfarin after taking proguanil for about 5 weeks.

Clinical importance, mechanism, importance and management

A woman stabilised on warfarin developed haematuria, bruising and abdominal and flank discomfort about 5 weeks after starting to take 200 mg proguanil daily. Her prothrombin ratio was found to be 8.6. Within 12 h of being treated with fresh frozen plasma and vitamin K her prothrombin ratio had fallen to 2.3.[1] The mechanism of this interaction is unknown. Its general importance is uncertain, but it would now seem prudent to monitor the response to any anticoagulant when proguanil is first added.

1. Armstrong G, Beg MF, Scahill S. Warfarin potentiation by proguanil. *BMJ* (1991) 303, 789.

Anticoagulants + Prolintane

The anticoagulant effects of ethyl biscoumacetate are not affected by the concurrent use of prolintane.

Clinical evidence, mechanism, importance and management

The responses to single 20-mg/kg doses of ethyl biscoumacetate were examined in 12 subjects before and after 4 days' treatment with 20 mg prolintane daily. The mean half-life of the anticoagulant and prothrombin times remained unchanged.[1] Other anticoagulants probably behave similarly, but this requires confirmation. There would seem to be no reason for avoiding concurrent use.

1. Hague DE, Smith ME, Ryan JR, McMahon FG. The effect of methylphenidate and prolintane on the metabolism of ethyl biscoumacetate. *Clin Pharmacol Ther* (1971) 12, 259–62.

Anticoagulants + Propafenone

The anticoagulant effects of warfarin and possibly fluindione and phenprocoumon are increased by the concurrent use of propafenone. A reduction in the anticoagulant dosage may be necessary.

Clinical evidence

The mean steady-state serum levels of warfarin in eight normal subjects taking 5 mg daily rose by 38% (from 0.98 to 1.36 micrograms/ml) after taking 225 mg propafenone three times daily for a week. Five of the 8 showed prothrombin time increases of 4 to 6 s.[1] Two further reports describe marked increases in the anticoagulant effects of fluindione and phenprocoumon in 2 patients treated with propafenone.[2,3]

Mechanism

A possible reason is that the propafenone reduces the metabolism and loss from the body of these anticoagulants, thereby increasing their effects.

Importance and management

Information seems to be limited to these reports but they show that prothrombin times should be well monitored if propafenone is given to patients on fluindione, warfarin or phenprocoumon. The anticoagulant dosage should be reduced where necessary. It would be prudent to apply the same precautions with any other anticoagulant.

1. Kates RE, Yee Y-G, Kirsten EB. Interaction between warfarin and propafenone in healthy volunteer subjects. *Clin Pharmacol Ther* (1987) 42, 305–11.
2. Körst HA, Brandes J-W, Littmann K-P. Cave: Propafenon potenziert Wirkung von oralen Antikoagulantien. *Med Klin* (1981) 76, 349–50.
3. Welsch M, Heitz C, Stephan D, Imbs JL. Potentialisation de l'effet anticoagulant de la fluindione par la propafénone. *Therapie* (1991) 46, 253–5.

Anticoagulants + Proquazone

The anticoagulant effects of phenprocoumon are not affected by the concurrent use of proquazone.

Clinical evidence, mechanism, importance and management

Proquazone 300 mg daily for 14 days had no effect on the plasma levels of factors II, VII, X, or prothrombin times or platelet aggregation in 20 patients on phenprocoumon.[1] Other anticoagulants probably behave similarly but this requires confirmation.

1. Vinazzer H. On the interaction between the anti-inflammatory substance proquazone (RU 43-715) and phenprocoumone. *Int J Clin Pharmacol Biopharm* (1977) 15, 214–16.

Anticoagulants + Quinidine

The anticoagulant effects of warfarin can be increased (bleeding has been seen), decreased or remain unaltered when quinidine is given concurrently. A decrease in the effects of dicoumarol has also been reported.

Clinical evidence

(a) Anticoagulant effects increased

Three patients stabilised on warfarin with prothrombin levels within the range 18 to 25% began to bleed within 7 to 10 days of starting to take 800 to 1400 mg quinidine daily. Their prothrombin levels were found to have fallen to 6–8%. Bleeding ceased when the warfarin was withdrawn.[1]

There are other reports of haemorrhage associated with the concurrent use of warfarin and quinidine.[2-4]

(b) Anticoagulant effects decreased

Four patients on warfarin or dicoumarol needed dosage increases of 7 to 23% to maintain adequate anticoagulation while receiving 1200 mg quinidine daily.[5]

(c) Anticoagulant effects unaltered

10 patients on long-term treatment with **warfarin** (2.5 to 12.5 mg daily) showed no significant alteration in their prothrombin times when given 800 mg **quinidine** daily for 2 weeks.[6-8] Another study on 8 patients also failed to find evidence of an interaction.

Mechanism

Quinidine can depress the synthesis of the vitamin-K dependent blood clotting factors and has a direct hypoprothrombinaemic effect of its own.[2] This would account for its additive effects with warfarin,[1] but does not explain why it can apparently also have antagonistic effects,[5] or no effect at all.[6-8]

Importance and management

Since increases[1-3,9] (with subsequent bleeding) and decreases[5] in the effects of warfarin, as well as the absence of an interaction[4,6-8] have been described, the outcome of concurrent use is clearly very uncertain. It would therefore be prudent to monitor the effects of quinidine closely to ensure that prothrombin times remain within the therapeutic range. The same precautions should apply with all the other anticoagulants, although nothing seems to be documented about any but dicoumarol, cited above.[5]

1. Gazzaniga AB, Stewart DR. Possible quinidine-induced hemorrhage in a patient on warfarin sodium. *N Engl J Med* (1969) 280, 711–12.
2. Beaumont JL, Tarrit A. Les accidents hémorrhagiques survenus au cours de 1500 traitements anticoagulants. *Sang* (1955) 26, 680–95.
3. Koch-Weser J. Quinidine-induced hypoprothrombinemic hemorrhage in patients on chronic warfarin therapy. *Ann Intern Med* (1968) 68, 511–17.
4. Jones FL. More on quinidine induced hypoprothrombinaemia. *Ann Intern Med* (1986) 69, 1074.
5. Sylven C, Anderson P. Evidence that disopyramide does not interact with warfarin. *BMJ* (1983) 286, 1181.
6. Udall JA. Quinidine and hypoprothrombinemia. *Ann Intern Med* (1968) 69, 403–4.
7. Udall JA. Drug interference with warfarin therapy. *Am J Cardiol* (1969) 23, 143.
8. Udall J. Drug interference with warfarin therapy. *Clin Med* (1970) 77, 20–5.
9. Sopher IM, Ming SC. Fatal corpus luteum haemorrhage during anticoagulant therapy. *Obstet Gynecol* (1971) 37, 695–7.

Anticoagulants + Quinine

Normally no clinically significant interaction occurs but isolated reports describe increased warfarin effects in two women after drinking large amounts of quinine-containing tonic water, and increased phenprocoumon effects and bleeding in a man.

Clinical evidence

A woman on **warfarin** needed a dosage reduction from 6 to 4 mg daily when she started to drink 1 to 1.5 litres of **tonic water** containing **quinine** each day. Her **warfarin** requirements rose again when the **tonic water** was stopped. Another woman needed a **warfarin** dosage reduction from 4 to 2 mg daily when she started to drink over 2 litres of **tonic water** daily. They were probably taking about 80—180 mg **quinine** daily.[1] A patient on chronic **phenprocoumon** treatment repeatedly developed extensive haematuria within 24 h of drinking 1 litres of 'Indian tonic water' containing 30 mg **quinine**.[2]

Mechanism

Not understood. Two studies[3,4] using the Page method[5] to measure prothrombin times showed that marked increases (up to 12 s) could occur when 330-mg doses of quinine were given in man in the absence of an anticoagulant, but other studies[4,6] using the conventional Quick method found that the prothrombin times were only prolonged by 0 to 2.1 s. The changes in prothrombin times could be completely reversed by vitamin K (menadiol sodium diphosphate)[3,4] which suggests that quinine, like the oral anticoagulants, is a competitive inhibitor of vitamin K. The increase in prothrombin times and their decrease in response to vitamin K took several days, which is consistent with a pharmacological action involving changes in the synthesis by the liver of blood clotting factors.

Importance and management

Common experience would seem to confirm that any increase in the effects of oral anticoagulants is normally very small and of little or no clinical importance. Concurrent use need not be avoided, however the isolated cases cited show that very exceptionally much larger changes and even bleeding can occur even with quite a small doses (30 mg). Quinine can be given in doses of up to 2 g daily for the treatment of malaria.

1. Clark DJ. Clinical curio: warfarin and tonic water. *BMJ* (1983) 286, 1258.
2. Iven H, Lerche L, Kaschube M. Influence of quinine and quinidine on the pharmacokinetics of phenprocoumon in rat and man. *Eur J Pharmacol* (1990) 183, 662.
3. Pirk LA, Engelberg R. Hypoprothrombinemic action of quinine sulfate. *JAMA* (1945) 128, 1093–5.
4. Pirk LA, Engelberg R. Hypoprothrombinemic action of quinine sulfate. *Am J Med Sci* (1947) 213, 593–7.
5. Page RC, de Beer EJ, Orr ML. Prothrombin studies using Russell viper venom. II. Relation of clotting time to prothrombin concentration in human plasma. *J Lab Clin Med* (1941) 27, 197–201.
6. Quick AJ. Effect of synthetic vitamin K and quinine sulfate on the prothrombin level. *J Lab Clin Med* (1946) 31, 79–84.

Anticoagulants + Quinolone antibacterials

The quinolone antibacterials normally appear not to increase the effects of anticoagulants in most patients, but increased effects and even bleeding have been seen quite unpredictably in some patients on warfarin when given nalidixic acid, levofloxacin, norfloxacin, ofloxacin or particularly ciprofloxacin; or while taking acenocoumarol (nicoumalone) when given nalidixic acid or pefloxacin. A very small and probably clinically irrelevant increase has been seen with clinafloxacin.

Clinical evidence

(a) Ciprofloxacin

Bayer, the UK manufacturers of **ciprofloxacin**, have in their records reports of no significant changes in prothrombin times in 40 patients chronically treated with **ethyl biscoumacetate** or **acenocoumarol (nicoumalone)** when **ciprofloxacin** was used concurrently.[1] No clinically relevant effects on **warfarin** anticoagulation were seen in studies in 9 and 16 patients given 500 mg **ciprofloxacin** twice daily for 7 or 10 days,[2,3] or in 13 and 33 patients given 750 mg twice daily for 12 to 14 days.[4-6]

In contrast, there are many scattered reports where **ciprofloxacin** has apparently been responsible for increased prothrombin times and/or bleeding in patients on **warfarin**. The FDA has on its Spontaneous Reporting System (SDS) database a total of 66 such cases over the 10 year period 1987–97. Those cases where details were available showed that the median prothrombin was 38.0, the INR 10, and the mean time when the problem was identified was 5.5 days. Hospitalization was reported in 15 cases, bleeding in 25 cases and death on one case.[7] There are a number of other individual case reports describing moderate to marked increases in prothrombin times and/or bleeding in patients on **warfarin** associated with taking **ciprofloxacin**.[1,7-14]

(b) Clinafloxacin

Clinafloxacin 200 mg twice daily for 14 days had no effect on the steady-state (*S*)-**warfarin** levels in normal healthy subjects but the levels of the less active enantiomer (*R*)-**warfarin** were increased 32% and the mean INR was increased by 13%. The reason is not known but the authors of the report attributed it to changes in gut flora caused by the **clinafloxacin**.[15]

(c) Enoxacin

Enoxacin 400 mg twice daily did not affect the pharmacokinetics of (*S*)-**warfarin** in 6 normal subjects, whereas the clearance of (*R*)-**warfarin** was decreased from 0.22 to 0.15 l/h and its elimination half-life was prolonged from 36.8 to 52.2 h. The overall anticoagulant (hypoprothrombinaemic) response to the **warfarin** was unaltered.[16] Another report about one patient is in agreement with these findings.[17]

(d) Fleroxacin

The pharmacokinetics and pharmacodynamics (prothrombin time and factor VII clotting time) of single 25-mg doses of **racemic warfarin** were unaffected in 12 normal subjects after taking 400 mg **fleroxacin** four times daily for nine days.[18]

(e) Gemifloxacin

A double-blind, randomised and placebo controlled study found that normal subjects on fixed doses of **warfarin** and with INRs in the range 1.3 to 1.8 showed no INR changes when additionally given 320 mg **gemifloxacin** daily for 7 days.[19]

(f) Grepafloxacin

Sixteen normal subjects on a fixed dose of **warfarin** and with INRs in the range 1.5 to 2.5 showed no INR changes when concurrently given 600 mg **grepafloxacin** daily for 10 days. The pharmacokinetics of the **grepafloxacin** were unchanged by the **warfarin**.[20,21]

(g) Levofloxacin

Levofloxacin 500 mg twice daily for 6 days had no effect on the pharmacokinetics or pharmacodynamics of $R(+)$- and $S(-)$-warfarin in 16 normal subjects given single 30 mg oral doses.[22] However two 75-year-old patients on **warfarin** were found to have increases in their INRs to 5.7 and to 7.9 respectively shortly after stopping 500 mg **levofloxacin** daily.[23]

(h) Nalidixic acid

A patient, well stabilised on **warfarin** (prothrombin ratio 2.0), developed a purpuric rash and bruising within six days of starting 2 g **nalidixic** acid daily. Her prothrombin time had risen to 45 s.[24] Another patient, previously well controlled on **warfarin**, developed a prothrombin time of 60 s 10 days after starting 3 g **nalidixic** acid daily.[25] The INR of woman of 84 on **warfarin** rose from 1.9 to 9.6 when **nalidixic** acid was added.[26] Yet another patient on **acenocoumarol (nicoumalone)** developed hypoprothrombinaemia after receiving 1 g **nalidixic acid** daily.[27]

(i) Norfloxacin

Six days' treatment with 400 mg **norfloxacin** twice daily was found not to alter either the pharmacokinetics or anticoagulant effects of **warfarin** in 10 normal subjects.[28]

In contrast, a 91-year-old woman on **warfarin** and digoxin developed a serious brain haemorrhage within 11 days of starting to take **norfloxacin** (precise dose not stated but said to be 'full'). Her prothrombin times had risen from 21.6 to 36.5 s. The manufacturers of **norfloxacin** (MSD) are said to have other reports of a **warfarin/norfloxacin** interaction but no details are given.[29] The FDA also has on record 3 cases of increased prothrombin times in patients on **warfarin** (2 of them bled) when given 800 mg **norfloxacin** daily.[7]

(j) Ofloxacin

Ofloxacin 200 mg daily for week did not significantly affect the prothrombin times of 7 subjects on **phenprocoumon**.[30] However a woman with a mitral valve replacement and under treatment with digoxin, furosemide (frusemide), spironolactone, verapamil and 5 mg **warfarin** daily, showed a marked increase in her international normalised ratio (from 2.5 to 4.4) within 2 days of starting to take 200 mg **ofloxacin** three times daily. Two days later the ratio had risen to 5.8.[31] An increased INR has been briefly described in another patient.[4] Yet another on **warfarin** developed gross haematuria and a prothrombin time of 78 s 5 days after starting to take 800 mg **ofloxacin** daily.[32]

(k) Pefloxacin

A patient showed a marked increase in the effects of **acenocoumarol (nicoumalone)** (Quick time reduced from 26 to less than 5%) within 5 days of starting to take **pefloxacin** (800 mg daily) and rifampicin (1200 mg daily).[33] Rifampicin is an enzyme inducer which normally causes a reduction in the effects of the anticoagulants, which would suggest that the **pefloxacin** was responsible for this reaction.

(l) Temafloxacin

Temafloxacin 600 mg twice daily was found to have no effect on the pharmacokinetics of **warfarin** at steady-state in normal healthy subjects.[34] Temafloxacin has been withdrawn because of toxicity.

(m) Trovafloxacin

Normal subjects stabilised on **warfarin** and with INRs in the range 1.3 to 1.7 were additionally given 200 mg **trovafloxacin** daily for 7 days. No changes in the pharmacokinetics of either *(S)*- or *(R)*-**warfarin** occurred and no significant changes in mean INRs were seen.[35]

Mechanism

Uncertain. It is not clear what other factors might have been responsible in those cases where the effects of the anticoagulants were increased. *In vitro* experiments[36,37] have shown that nalidixic acid can displace warfarin from its binding sites on human plasma albumin, but this mechanism on its own is almost certainly not the full explanation.

Importance and management

The extent of the documentation is variable depending on the quinolone in question but generally moderate. The overall picture is that no adverse interaction normally occurs between these quinolones and oral anticoagulants, but rarely and unpredictably increased anticoagulant effects and even bleeding can occur with some of them. It is difficult to know whether the relatively large number of cases seen with ciprofloxacin are because this quinolone interacts more frequently than the others or whether the figure is boosted by the very widespread use of this antibacterial. Whatever the answer, there is no need to avoid using any of the quinolones with oral anticoagulants but it would be prudent to monitor the effects when any quinolone antibacterial is first added to treatment with any oral anticoagulant so that any problems can be quickly identified. So far there appears to be no information about any of the other quinolones or oral anticoagulants not cited here.

1. Bayer UK Limited. Personal communication, 1988.
2. Rindone JP, Keuey CL, Jones WN, Garewal HS. Hypoprothrombinemic effect of warfarin not influenced by ciprofloxacin. *Clin Pharm* (1991) 10, 136–8.
3. Bianco TM, Bussey HI, Farnett LE, Linn WD, Roush MK, Wong YWJ. Potential warfarin-ciprofloxacin interaction in patients receiving long-term anticoagulation. *Pharmacotherapy* (1992) 12, 435–9.
4. Israel DS, Stotka JL, Rock WL, Polk RE. Effect of ciprofloxacin (C) administration on warfarin (W) response in adult subjects. *Intersci Conf Antimicrob Agents Chemother* (1991) 31, 199.
5. Polk RE, Israel D, Sintek C, Klein C, Swaim WR, Pluhar R, Lettieri J, Heller AH. Effect of ciprofloxacin (C) on response to warfarin (W) in anticoagulated adults. *Intersci Conf Antimicrob Agents Chemother* (1994) 34, 3.
6. Israel DS, Stotka J, Rock W, Sintek CD, Kamada AK, Klein C, Swaim WR, Pluhar RE, Toscano JP, Lettieri JT, Heller AH, Polk RE. Effect of ciprofloxacin on the pharmacokinetics and pharmacodynamics of warfarin. *Clin Infect Dis* (1996) 22, 251–6.
7. Ellis RJ, Mayo MS, Bodensteiner DM. Ciprofloxacin-warfarin coagulopathy: a case series. *Am J Hematol* (2000) 63, 28–31.
8. Mott FE, Murphy S, Hunt V. Ciprofloxacin and warfarin. *Ann Intern Med* (1989) 111, 542–3.
9. Linville D, Emory C, Graves L. Ciprofloxacin and warfarin interaction. *Am J Med* (1991) 90, 765.
10. Beeley L, Cunningham H, Carmichael AE, Brennan A. Newsletter of the West Midlands Centre for Adverse Drug Reaction Reporting (1991), 33, 36
11. Kamada AK. Possible interaction between ciprofloxacin and warfarin. *DICP Ann Pharmacother* (1990) 24, 27–8.
12. Johnson KC, Joe RH, Self TH. Drug interaction. *J Fam Pract* (1991) 33, 338.
13. Renzi R, Finkbeiner S. Ciprofloxacin interaction with warfarin: a potentially dangerous side-effect. *Am J Emerg Med* (1991) 9, 551–2.
14. Dugoni-Kramer BM. Ciprofloxacin-warfarin interaction. *DICP Ann Pharmacother* (1991) 25, 1397.
15. Randinitis EJ, Koup JR, Bron NJ, Hounslow NJ, Rausch G, Abel R, Vassos AB, Sedman AJ. Drug interaction studies with clinafloxacin and probenecid, cimetidine, phenytoin and warfarin. *Drugs* (1999) 58 (Suppl 2), 254-5.
16. Toon S, Hopkins KJ, Garstang FM, Aarons L, Sedman A, Rowland M. Enoxacin-warfarin interaction: pharmacokinetic and stereochemical aspects. *Clin Pharmacol Ther* (1987) 42, 33–41.
17. McLeod AD, Burgess C. Drug interaction with warfarin and enoxacin. *N Z Med J* (1988) 101, 216.
18. Holazo AA, Soni PP, Kachevsky V, Min BH, Townsend L, Patel IH. Fleroxacin-warfarin interaction in humans. *Intersci Conf Antimicrob Agents Chemother* (1990) 30, 253.
19. Davy M, Bird N, Rost KL, Fuder H. Lack of effect of gemifloxacin on the steady-state pharmacodynamics of warfarin in healthy volunteers. *Chemotherapy* (1999) 45, 491-5.
20. Koneru B, Bramer S, Bricmont P, Maroli A. A pharmacokinetic and pharmacodynamic study of the potential drug interaction between grepafloxacin and warfarin in normal volunteers. *Pharm Res* (1996) 13 (9 Suppl), S-346.
21. Efthymiopoulos C, Bramer SL, Maroli A, Blum B. Theophylline and warfarin interaction studies with grepafloxacin. *Clin Pharmacokinet* (1997) 33 (Suppl 1), 39–46.

22. Liao S, Palmer M, Fowler C, Nayak RK. Absence of an effect of levofloxacin on warfarin pharmacokinetics and anticoagulation in male volunteers. *J Clin Pharmacol* (1996) 36, 1072–7.
23. Ravnan SL, Locke C. Levofloxacin and warfarin interaction. *Pharmacotherapy* (2001) 21, 884-5.
24. Hoffbrand BI. Interaction of nalidixic acid and warfarin. *BMJ* (1974) 2, 666.
25. Leor J, Levartowsky D, Sharon C. Interaction between nalidixic acid and warfarin. *Ann Intern Med* (1987) 107, 601.
26. Gullov AL, Koefoed BG, Petersen P. Interaktion mellem warfarin og nalidinsyre. *Ugeskr Laeger* (1996) 158, 5174–5.
27. Potasman I, Bassan H. Nicoumalone and nalidixic acid interaction. *Ann Intern Med* (1980) 92, 571.
28. Rocci ML, Vlasses PH, Distlerath LM, Gregg MH, Wheeler SC, Zing W, Bjornsson TD. Norfloxacin does not alter warfarin's disposition or anticoagulant effect. *J Clin Pharmacol* (1990) 30, 728–32.
29. Linville T, Matanin D. Norfloxacin and warfarin. *Ann Intern Med* (1989) 110, 751–2.
30. Verho M, Malerczyk V, Rosenkrantz B, Grötsch H. Absence of interaction between ofloxacin and phenprocoumon. *Curr Med Res Opin* (1987) 10, 474–9.
31. Leor J, Matetzki S. Ofloxacin and warfarin. *Ann Intern Med* (1988) 109, 761.
32. Baciewicz AM, Ashar BH, Locke TW. Interaction of ofloxacin and warfarin. *Ann Intern Med* (1993) 119, 1223.
33. Pertek JP, Helmer J, Vivin P, Kipper R. Potentialisation d'une antivitamine K par l'association péfloxacine-rifampicine. *Ann Fr Anesth Reanim* (1986) 5, 320–1.
34. Millar E, Coles S, Wyld P, Nimmor W. Temafloxacin does not potentiate the anticoagulant effect of warfarin in healthy subjects. *Clin Pharmacokinet* (1992) 22 (Suppl 1), 102–6.
35. Teng R, Apelsoff G, Vincent J, Pelletier SM, Willavize SA, Friedman JL. Effect of trovafloxacin (CP-99,219) on the pharmacokinetics and pharmacodynamics of warfarin in healthy male subjects. *Intersci Conf Antimicrob Agents Chemother* (1996) 36, A2.
36. Sellers EM and Koch-Weser J. Kinetics and clinical importance of displacement of warfarin from albumin by acidic drugs. *Ann N Y Acad Sci* (1971) 179, 213.
37. Sellers EM, Koch-Weser J. Displacement of warfarin from human albumin by diazoxide and ethacrynic, mefenamic, and nalidixic acids. *Clin Pharmacol Ther* (1970) 11, 524–9.

Anticoagulants + Rifampicin (Rifampin)

The anticoagulant effects of acenocoumarol (nicoumalone), phenprocoumon and warfarin are markedly reduced by the concurrent use of rifampicin. The anticoagulant dosage will need to be increased (possibly two to threefold) to accommodate this interaction.

Clinical evidence

The dosage of **acenocoumarol (nicoumalone)** needed to be markedly increased in 18 patients to maintain the Quick value within the therapeutic range after being given 900 mg **rifampicin** daily for 7 days.[1] There are numerous reports and studies of this interaction in man involving a considerable number of patients and subjects on **acenocoumarol**,[2] **phenprocoumon**[3,4] or **warfarin**.[5-14]

Mechanism

Rifampicin is a potent liver enzyme inducing agent which increases the metabolism and clearance of the anticoagulants from the body, thereby reducing their effects.[15] Other mechanisms may also be involved.[13] One study found that the serum levels of warfarin and the prothrombin response were approximately halved.[6]

Importance and management

A very well documented and clinically important interaction which will occur in most patients. A marked reduction in the anticoagulant effects may be expected within 5 to 7 days of starting the rifampicin,[1,5] persisting for about the same length of time or longer after the rifampicin has been withdrawn. With warfarin there is evidence that the dosage may need to be doubled[5] or tripled[9] to accommodate this interaction, and reduced by an equivalent amount following withdrawal of the rifampicin.[5,8,13] Other anticoagulants are expected to behave similarly.

1. Michot F, Bürgi M, Büttner J. Rimactan (Rifampizin) und Antikoagulantientherapie. *Schweiz Med Wochenschr* (1970) 100, 583–4.
2. Sennwald G. Etude de l'influence de la rifampicine sur l'effet anticoagulant de l'acénocoumarol. *Rev Med Suisse Romande* (1974) 94, 945–54.
3. Boekhout-Mussert RJ, Bieger R, van Brummelen A, Lemkes HHPJ. Inhibition by rifampin of the anticoagulant effect of phenprocoumon. *JAMA* (1974) 229, 1903–4.
4. Ohnhaus EE, Kampschulte J, Mönig H. Effect of propranolol and rifampicin on liver blood flow and phenoprocoumon elimination. *Acta Pharmacol Toxicol* (1986) 59 (Suppl 4), 92.
5. Romankiewicz JA, Ehrman M. Rifampin and warfarin: a drug interaction. *Ann Intern Med* (1975) 82, 224–5.

6. O'Reilly RA. Interaction of sodium warfarin and rifampin. Studies in man. *Ann Intern Med* (1974) 81, 337–40.
7. O'Reilly RA. Interaction of rifampin and warfarin in man. *Clin Res* (1973) 21, 207.
8. Self TH, Mann RB. Interaction of rifampicin and warfarin. *Chest* (1975) 67, 490–1.
9. Fox P. Warfarin-rifampicin interaction. *Med J Aust* (1982) 1, 60.
10. O'Reilly RA. Interaction of chronic daily warfarin therapy and rifampin. *Ann Intern Med* (1975) 83, 506–8.
11. Felty P. Warfarin-rifampicin interaction. *Med J Aust* (1952) 62, 60.
12. Beeley L, Daly M, Stewart P. Bulletin of the West Midlands Centre for Adverse Drug Reaction Reporting (1987) 24, 23.
13. Almog S, Martinowitz U, Halkin H, Bank HZ, Farfel Z. Complex interaction of rifampin and warfarin. *South Med J* (1988) 81, 1304–6.
14. Casner PR. Inability to attain oral anticoagulation: warfarin-rifampin interaction revisited. *South Med J* (1996) 89, 1200–3.
15. Heimark LD, Gibaldi M, Trager WF, O'Reilly RA, Goulart DA. The mechanism of the warfarin-rifampicin drug interaction in humans. *Clin Pharmacol Ther* (1987) 42, 388–94.

Anticoagulants + Rioprostil

Rioprostil can reduce the effects of the oral anticoagulants to some extent but the clinical importance of this is uncertain.

Clinical evidence, mechanism, importance and management

The effects of 7 days' pretreatment with **rioprostil** (0.3 mg twice daily) on the anticoagulant effects of single doses of **acenocoumarol (nicoumalone)** (10 mg) or **phenprocoumon** (0.2 mg/kg) were examined on 13 subjects. The pharmacokinetics of these anticoagulants remained unchanged but their effects were reduced. The thrombotest and Factor VII activity percentages rose for reasons which are not understood. For example, those on **phenprocoumon** showed a rise in the thrombotest percentages on day 3 from a range of 18 to 50% (with **rioprostil**) to 26 to 100% (without **rioprostil**). However the authors of this report[1] say that ". . . the observed interaction can be classed with the pharmacological curiosities because there is poor clinical relevancy." Until this is confirmed the effects of the concurrent use of **rioprostil** and any anticoagulant should be monitored for evidence of a reduced anticoagulant effect, but there would seem to be no reason for avoiding **rioprostil**.

1. Thijssen HHW, Hamulyàk K. The interaction of the prostaglandin E derivative rioprostil with oral anticoagulant agents. *Clin Pharmacol Ther* (1989) 46, 110–16.

Anticoagulants + Saquinavir

An isolated report describes a gradual INR rise in an elderly patient on warfarin when given saquinavir.

Clinical evidence, mechanism, importance and management

A man of 73 year who was HIV positive and who had been on warfarin, co-trimoxazole, nizatidine, stavudine and lamivudine for 7 months was additionally started on 600 mg saquinavir three times daily. His INR, which had been stable at around 2 for 5 months, rose to 2.46 after 4 weeks, and to 4.24 after 8 weeks, which the authors of the report attributed to an interaction with the saquinavir, tentatively suggesting that it might have reduced the metabolism of the warfarin by inhibiting cytochrome P450 isoenzyme CYP3A4.[1] The situation was solved by reducing the warfarin dosage by 20%.[1] This is the first and only report of this possible interaction and its general importance is not known, but it would now be prudent to monitor the effect of adding saquinavir to established warfarin treatment in any patient. Information about other anticoagulants is lacking, but the same precautions would seem to be reasonable.

1. Darlington MR. Hypoprothrombinemia during concomitant therapy with warfarin and saquinavir. *Ann Pharmacother* (1997) 31, 647.

Anticoagulants + Simvastatin

Simvastatin normally causes only a small, clinically irrelevant increase in the anticoagulant effects of warfarin. More marked effects have been seen in just one patient on warfarin and another on acenocoumarol (nicoumalone).

Clinical evidence

Twenty normal subjects on 5 to 13 mg **warfarin** daily and with prothrombin times averaging 19 s, had an increase in their prothrombin times of less than 2 s after taking 40 mg **simvastatin** daily for 7 days.[1] 23 patients anticoagulated with **warfarin** showed only small INR increases (a mean of +0.8 with 20 or 40 mg **simvastatin** daily). No **warfarin** dose changes were needed and no problems with anticoagulation occurred.[2] The UK Summary of Product Characteristics for *Zocor* (**simvastatin**)[3] says that ". . . in two clinical studies, one in normal volunteers and the other in hypercholesterolaemic patients, **simvastatin** 20 to 40 mg daily modestly potentiated the effect of **coumarin anticoagulants**: the . . . INR increased from a baseline of 1.7 to 1.8 and from 2.6 to 3.4 in the volunteer and patient studies, respectively . . ." A patient on **warfarin** with Type III hyperlipoproteinaemia showed no changes in her INR over 20 weeks when concurrently treated with 20 mg **simvastatin** daily.[4] A study in 46 patients on warfarin found that when their treatment for hyperlipidaemia was changed from **pravastatin** to **simvastatin**, no important warfarin dosage changes were needed and no unusual bleeding was seen.[5]

In contrast a single very brief case report describes bruising, haematuria and a raised INR in one patient given **simvastatin** and **warfarin**.[6] Another single report describes a patient on **acenocoumarol (nicoumalone)** whose INR rose from a range of 2–3.5 to 9 within 3 weeks of starting to take 20 mg **simvastatin** daily.[7]

Mechanism

Not understood. Simvastatin has been found not to have a significant effect on the protein binding of warfarin in hypercholesterolaemic patients,[8] but even if it were to take place, protein binding displacement as a major mechanism of interaction has now been largely discredited as a valid explanation for most clinically significant interactions between highly bound drugs.

Importance and management

Information appears to be limited to these reports. No clinically relevant interaction would normally seem to occur with warfarin, however it would be prudent to monitor concurrent use in the early stages, or if the simvastatin dosage is changed, so that any rare and unpredictable cases can be safely managed. Information about anticoagulants other than acenocoumarol (nicoumalone) and warfarin is lacking but the same simple precautions would seem appropriate with any oral anticoagulant.

1. Zocor (Simvastatin). Product information. Physician's Desk Reference, 2001.

2. Keech A, Collins R, MacMahon S, Armitage J, Lawson A, Wallendszus K, Fatemian M, Kearney E, Lyon V, Mindell J, Mount J, Painter R, Parish S, Slavin B, Sleight P, Youngman L, Peto R. Three-year follow-up of the Oxford cholesterol study: assessment of the efficacy and safety of simvastatin in preparation for a large mortality study. *Eur Heart J* (1994) 15, 255–69.

3. Zocor (Simvastatin). Merck Sharp & Dohme Limited. Summary of product characteristics, March 2000.

4. Gaw A, Wosornu D. Simvastatin during warfarin therapy in hyperlipoproteinaemia. *Lancet* (1992) 340, 979–80.

5. Lin JC, Stolley SN, Morreale AP, Marcus DB. The effect of converting from pravastatin to simvastatin on the pharmacodynamics of warfarin. *J Clin Pharmacol* (1999) 39, 86–90.

6. Beeley L, Cunningham H, Carmichael AE, Brennan A. Newsletter of the West Midlands Centre for Adverse Drug Reaction Reporting, July 1991, p 3.

7. Grau E, Perella M, Pastor E. Simvastatin-oral anticoagulant interaction. *Lancet* (1996) 347, 405–6.

8. Feely J, O'Connor P. Effects of HMG Co A reductase inhibitors on warfarin binding. *Drug Invest* (1991) 3, 315–16.

Anticoagulants + Sodium valproate

Sodium valproate appears not to interact with the oral anticoagulants to a clinically relevant extent.

Clinical evidence, mechanism, importance and management

The makers of **sodium valproate** recommend caution with vitamin K dependent **anticoagulants** as **sodium valproate** may displace them from protein binding sites.[1] There is certainly some *in vitro* evidence that the serum binding of **warfarin** is decreased by **sodium valproate** so that free **warfarin** levels rise[2-4] (by 32% according to one study[3]). Linked with this last study is a report of a woman on **warfarin** whose prothrombin times and INRs were briefly raised when **sodium valproate** was added.[3] The report says that the ". . . **warfarin** regimen underwent numerous adjustments to maintain her PT ratio and INR within the desired range . . ." but when she was later discharged her **warfarin** dosage was just the same as before the **sodium valproate** was started.[3] It may be that, as with the warfarin/chloral hydrate interaction (see 'Anticoagulants + Chloral hydrate, Chloral betaine or Triclofos', p.249), any interaction occurs only transiently when the **sodium valproate** is added, and the situation rapidly restabilises without any real need to adjust the **warfarin** dosage. There seem to be no other reports of problems associated with concurrent use nor any other direct evidence that an interaction of clinical importance normally occurs. A report about one patient found that **sodium valproate** did not alter the anticoagulant effects of **phenprocoumon**.[5]

The makers also point out that **sodium valproate** inhibits the second stage of platelet aggregation, and that a reversible prolongation of bleeding times and thrombocytopenia has been reported with doses above those recommended.[1] But there seems to be little reason for particular precautions when using **sodium valproate**, over and above those normally taken with the oral anticoagulants.

1. Epilim (Sodium valproate). Sanofi Synthelabo. Summary of product characteristics, March 2001.

2. Urien S, Albengres E, Tillement J-P. Serum protein binding of valproic acid in healthy subjects and in patients with liver disease. *Int J Clin Pharmacol Ther Toxicol* (1981) 19, 319–25.

3. Guthrie SK, Stoysich AM, Bader G, Hilleman DE. Hypothesized interaction between valproic acid and warfarin. *J Clin Psychopharmacol* (1995) 15, 138–9.

4. Panjehshahin MR, Bowmer CJ, Yates MS. Effect of valproic acid, its unsaturated metabolites and some structurally related fatty acids on the binding of warfarin and dansylsarcosine to human albumin. *Biochem Pharmacol* (1991) 41, 1227–33.

5. Schlienger R, Kurmann M, Drewe J, Müller-Spahn F, Seifritz E. Inhibition of phenprocoumon anticoagulation by carbamazepine. *Eur Neuropsychopharmacol* (2000) 10, 219-21.

Anticoagulants + St John's wort (*Hypericum perforatum*)

St John's wort can cause a moderate reduction in the anticoagulant effects of phenprocoumon and warfarin, but an isolated and unexplained report also describes an increased anticoagulant effect in one patient on phenprocoumon.

Clinical evidence

(a) Phenprocoumon

A randomised, single blind placebo-controlled cross-ver study in 10 normal men found that after taking 900 mg **St John's wort** extract (*LI 160, Lichtwer Pharma*) daily for 11 days, the AUC of a single 12 mg dose of **phenprocoumon** was reduced by 17.4%. This study contrasts with another report about a 75-year old woman on **phenprocoumon** who showed an *increased* anticoagulant response (a rise in the Quick time) 2 months after starting to take **St John's wort**.[1]

(b) Warfarin

The Swedish Medical Products Agency received seven case reports over the 1998–99 period of patients stabilised on **warfarin** who showed decreased INRs when **St John's wort** was added. Their INRs fell from the normal therapeutic range about 2 to 4 to about 1.5. Two patients are described who needed **warfarin** dosage increases of 6.6% and 15% when the **St John's wort** was added. The INRs of 4 of the patients returned to their former values when the **St John's wort** was stopped.[2]

Mechanism

Not know, but it is suggested that the St John's wort increases the metabolism and clearance of the anticoagulants[2,3] possibly by induction of cytochrome P450 isoenzyme CYP2C9, or it inhibits its absorption from the gut.[3] Just why one patient showed a paradoxical increase in anticoagulant effects is not known.

Importance and management

Information seems to be limited to these brief reports, the picture being that these interactions are of moderate clinical importance. It would be prudent to monitor the INRs of patients on phenprocoumon, warfarin or any other anticoagulant if they start taking St John's wort, being alert for the need to raise the anticoagulant the dosage. The 2 patients described above needed warfarin increases of 6.6 and 15%. The advice of the Committee on the Safety of Medicines in the UK is to stop St John's wort and then adjust the anticoagulant dosage as necessary.[4] More study is needed.

1. Bon S, Hartmann, Kubn M. Johanniskraut: Ein Enzyminduktor? *Schweiz Apothekerzeitung* (1999) 16, 535-6.
2. Yue Q-Y, Bergquist C, Gérden B. Safety of St John's wort (*Hypericum perforatum*). *Lancet* (2000) 355, 576-7.
3. Maurer A, Johne A, Bauer S, Brockmöller J, Donath F, Roots I, Langheinrich M, Hübner W-D. Interaction of St John's wort extract with phenprocoumon. *Eur J Clin Pharmacol* (1999) 55, A22.
4. Committee on the Safety of Medicines (UK). Message from Professor A Breckenridge (Chairman of CSM) and Fact Sheet for Health Care Professionals, 29th February 2000.

Anticoagulants + Sucralfate

Four case reports describe a marked reduction in the effects of warfarin in four patients given sucralfate. Other evidence suggests that this interaction is uncommon.

Clinical evidence

A man on multiple therapy (digoxin, furosemide (frusemide), chlorpropamide, potassium chloride) showed serum **warfarin** levels which were depressed about two-thirds when given **sucralfate**. When the **sucralfate** was withdrawn, his serum **warfarin** levels rose to their former levels accompanied by the expected prolongation of prothrombin times.[1] Another patient's prothrombin times remained subtherapeutic while taking **sucralfate**, despite **warfarin** doses of up to 17.5 mg daily. When the **sucralfate** was stopped his prothrombin time rose to 1.5 times his control, even though the **warfarin** dose was reduced to 10 mg daily.[2] Two other patients showed reduced responses to **warfarin** while taking **sucralfate**.[3,4]

In contrast, an open crossover study on 8 elderly patients taking **warfarin** found that their anticoagulant response and serum **warfarin** levels remained unchanged while taking **sucralfate** (1 g three times a day) over a 2-week period.[5] No interaction was found in another study.[6]

Mechanism

Unknown. It is suggested that the sucralfate may possibly adsorb the warfarin so that its bioavailability is reduced.[2]

Importance and management

The documentation appears to be limited to the reports cited. Any interaction would therefore seem to be uncommon. Concurrent use need not be avoided but be alert for evidence of a reduced anticoagulant response to warfarin. Information about other anticoagulants is lacking, but it would seem prudent to take the same precautions. Ranitidine is an alternative non-interacting anti-ulcer agent.

1. Mungall D, Talbert RL, Phillips C, Jaffe D, Ludden TM. Sucralfate and warfarin. *Ann Intern Med* (1983) 98, 557.
2. Braverman SE, Marino MT. Sucralfate-warfarin interaction. *Drug Intell Clin Pharm* (1988) 22, 913.
3. Rey AM, Gums JG. Altered absorption of digoxin, sustained-release quinidine, and warfarin with sucralfate absorption. *DICP Ann Pharmacother* (1991) 25, 745–6.
4. Parrish RH, Waller B, Gondalia BG. Sucralfate-warfarin interaction. *Ann Pharmacother* (1992) 26, 1015–16.
5. Neuvonen PJ, Jaakkola A, Tötterman J, Penttilä O. Clinically significant sucralfate-warfarin interaction is not likely. *Br J Clin Pharmacol* (1985) 20, 178–80.
6. Talbert RL, Dalmady-Israel C, Bussey HI, Crawford MH, Ludden TM. Effect of sucralfate on plasma warfarin concentration in patients requiring chronic warfarin therapy. *Drug Intell Clin Pharm* (1985) 19, 456–7.

Anticoagulants + Sulfasalazine

An isolated case report describes a marked reduction in the response to warfarin when sulfasalazine was started.

Clinical evidence, mechanism, importance and management

A woman of 37 on long-term **warfarin** treatment (and also taking albuterol, aspirin, azathioprine, ethinyloestradiol/norgestrel) had her treatment for arthritis and ulcerative colitis changed from 5-aminosalicylic acid to 1000 mg **sulfasalazine** four times daily. The day after the change her INR was found to be subtherapeutic (1.5 compared with the usual 2 to 3) and she needed numerous increases in the **warfarin** doses over the next 6 weeks, eventually increased to 250% (from 30 to 75 mg weekly), before acceptable INRs were achieved. During this period she developed a new deep vein thrombosis requiring treatment with dalteparin. When the **sulfasalazine** was later stopped and the 5-aminosalicylate restarted, her **warfarin** dosage requirements dropped to 45 mg weekly.[1]

This is an unexplained and isolated case, and its validity has been challenged.[2] There are no other reports in the literature and this possible interaction it is not therefore of general importance, nevertheless prescribers should be aware of it if **sulfasalazine** is added to **warfarin** treatment. Information about other oral anticoagulants is lacking.

1. Teefy AM, Martin JE, Kovacs MJ. Warfarin resistance due to sulfasalazine. *Ann Pharmacother* (2000) 34, 1265–8.
2. Sherman JJ. Comment: other factors should be considered in a possible warfarin and sulfasalazine interaction. *Ann Pharmacother* (2001) 35, 506.

Anticoagulants + Sulfinpyrazone (Sulphinpyrazone)

The anticoagulant effects of warfarin and acenocoumarol (nicoumalone) are markedly increased by sulfinpyrazone (sulphinpyrazone). Serious bleeding can occur if the anticoagulant dosage is not reduced appropriately. Phenprocoumon does not interact significantly.

Clinical evidence

The prothrombin ratios of 5 patients on **warfarin** rose rapidly over 2 to 3 days after 800 mg **sulfinpyrazone (sulphinpyrazone)** was added. The average **warfarin** requirements fell by 46% and 2 patients needed vitamin K to combat the excessive hypoprothrombinaemia. When the **sulfinpyrazone** was withdrawn, the **warfarin** requirements rose to their former levels within 1 to 2 weeks.[1]

This interaction has been described in numerous studies and case reports in those taking **warfarin**[2-11] and **acenocoumarol (nicoumalone)**.[12] Severe bleeding occurred in some instances. An increased effect followed by an unexplained reduced effect has been described in one report.[6] In a trial using **acenocoumarol** it was found possible to reduce the anticoagulant dosage by an average of 20% while taking 800 mg **sulfinpyrazone** daily.[12] **Phenprocoumon** is reported not to interact.[13,14]

Mechanism

Some early *in vitro* evidence[15,16] suggested that plasma protein binding displacement might explain this interaction, but more recent clinical studies[1,17-19] indicate that sulfinpyrazone also inhibits the metabolism of the anticoagulants (the more potent $S(-)$-isomer in the case of warfarin) so that the anticoagulant is cleared from the body more slowly and its effects are increased and prolonged.

Importance and management

A well established interaction of clinical importance. If sulfinpyrazone (sulphinpyrazone) is added, the prothrombin time should be well monitored and suitable anticoagulant dosage reductions made. Halving the dosage of warfarin[1,11,15] and reducing the acenocoumarol (nicoumalone) dosage by 20%[12] proved to be adequate in patients taking 600 to 800 mg sulfinpyrazone daily. Phenprocoumon is reported not to interact,[13,14] but it would be prudent to expect other anticoagulants to behave like warfarin and acenocoumarol. It has been recommended that because of the difficulties of monitoring this interaction and of making the necessary dosage adjustments, concurrent use should not be undertaken unless the patient is hospitalised.[3]

1. Miners JO, Foenander T, Wanwimolruk S, Gallus AS, Birkett DJ. Interaction of sulphinpyrazone with warfarin. *Eur J Clin Pharmacol* (1982) 22, 327–31.
2. Weiss M. Potentiation of coumarin effect by sulphinpyrazone. *Lancet* (1979) i, 609.
3. Mattingly D, Bradley M, Selley PJ. Hazards of sulphinpyrazone. *BMJ* (1978) 2, 1786–9.
4. Davis JW, Johns LE. Possible interaction of sulphinpyrazone with coumarins. *N Engl J Med* (1978) 299, 955.
5. Bailey RR, Reddy J. Potentiation of warfarin action by sulphinpyrazone. *Lancet* (1980) i, 254.
6. Nenci GG, Agnelli G, Berretini M. Biphasic sulphinpyrazone-warfarin interaction. *BMJ* (1981) 282, 1361–2.
7. Gallus A, Birkett D. Sulphinpyrazone and warfarin: a probable drug interaction. *Lancet* (1980) i, 535.
8. Jamil A, Reid JM, Messer M. Interaction between sulphinpyrazone and warfarin. *Chest* (1981) 79, 375.
9. Girolami A, Schivazappa L, Fabris F, Randi ML. Biphasic sulphinpyrazone-warfarin interaction. *BMJ* (1981) 283, 1338.
10. Thompson PL, Serjeant C. Potentially serious interaction of warfarin with sulphinpyrazone. *Med J Aust* (1981) 1, 41.
11. Girolami A, Fabris F, Casonata A, Randi ML. Potentiation of anticoagulant response to warfarin by sulphinpyrazone: a double-blind study in patients with prosthetic heart valves. *Clin Lab Haematol* (1982) 4, 23–6.
12. Michot F, Holt NF, Fontanilles F. Über die beeinflussung der gerinnungshemmenden Wirkungen von Acenocoumarol durch Sulphinpyrazon. *Schweiz Med Wochenschr* (1981) 111, 255–60.
13. O'Reilly RA. Phenylbutazone and sulphinpyrazone interaction with oral anticoagulant phenprocoumon. *Arch Intern Med* (1982) 142, 1634–7.
14. Heimark LD, Toon S, Gibaldi M, Trager WF, O'Reilly RA, Goulart DA. The effect of sulfinpyrazone on the disposition of pseudoracemic phenprocoumon in humans. *Clin Pharmacol Ther* (1987) 42, 312–19.
15. Tulloch JA, Marr TCK. Sulphinpyrazone and warfarin after myocardial infarction. *BMJ* (1979) ii, 133.
16. Seiler K, Duckert F. Properties of 3-(1-phenyl-propyl)-4-oxycoumarin (Marcoumar®) in the plasma when tested in normal cases and under the influence of drugs. *Thromb Diath Haemorrh* (1968) 19, 389–96.
17. O'Reilly RA, Goulart DA. Comparative interaction of sulphinpyrazone and phenylbutazone with racemic warfarin: alteration *in vivo* of free fraction of plasma albumin. *J Pharmacol Exp Ther* (1981) 219, 691–4.
18. O'Reilly RA. Stereoselective interaction of sulfinpyrazone with racemic warfarin and its separated enantiomorphs in man. *Circulation* (1982) 65, 202–7.
19. Toon S, Low LK, Gibaldi M, Trager WF, O'Reilly RA, Motley CH, Goulart DA. The warfarin-sulfinpyrazone interaction: stereochemical considerations. *Clin Pharmacol Ther* (1986) 39, 15–24.

Anticoagulants + Sulindac

Five patients have shown a marked increase in the anticoagulant effects of warfarin when given sulindac (two of them bled), but it seems probable that only the occasional patient will develop this interaction.

Clinical evidence

A patient on **warfarin**, ferrous sulphate, phenobarbital (phenobarbitone) and sulfasalazine (sulphasalazine) showed a marked increase in his prothrombin times (more than three times the control value) after taking 200 mg **sulindac** daily for 5 days.[1-3] There are 4 similar cases of this interaction on record.[3-5] Two of the patients bled, one of whom did so after taking only three 100-mg doses of **sulindac**.[4]

In contrast, studies in patients and normal subjects on **warfarin** or **phenprocoumon** and given **sulindac** failed to demonstrate this interaction.[3,6,7]

Mechanism

Not understood.

Importance and management

An established but uncommon and unpredictable interaction affecting only the occasional patient.[3,6] Monitor the effects if sulindac is added to warfarin or any other anticoagulant, bearing in mind that all NSAIDs can irritate the gastric mucosa, affect platelet activity and cause gastrointestinal bleeding. Alternative anti-inflammatory drugs which do not interact include ibuprofen and naproxen (see Index).

1. Beeley L. Bulletin of the West Midlands Adverse Reaction Reporting Group (1978) No. 6.
2. Beeley L, Baker S. Personal communication, 1978.
3. Ross JRY, Beeley L. Sulindac, prothrombin time, and anticoagulants. *Lancet* (1979) ii, 1075.
4. Carter SA. Potential effect of sulindac on response of prothrombin-time to oral anticoagulants. *Lancet* (1979) ii, 698–9.
5. McQueen EG. New Zealand Committee on Adverse Drug Reactions. 17th Annual Report 1982. *N Z Med J* (1983) 96, 95–9.
6. Loftin JP, Vesell ES. Interaction between sulindac and warfarin: different results in normal subjects and in an unusual patient with a potassium-losing renal tubular defect. *J Clin Pharmacol* (1979) 19, 733–42.
7. Schenk H, Klein G, Haralambus J, Goebel R. Coumarintherapie unter dem antirheumaticum sulindac. *Z Rheumatol* (1980) 39, 102–8.

Anticoagulants + Suloctidil or Zomepirac

Suloctidil does not significantly alter the anticoagulant effects of phenprocoumon, nor zomepirac the effects of warfarin.

Clinical evidence, mechanism, importance and management

Eight patients showed no significant changes in the anticoagulant effects of **phenprocoumon** when treated with 300 mg **suloctidil** three times a day.[1] The anticoagulant effects of **warfarin** were similarly unaltered in 16 subjects given 150 mg **zomepirac** four times a day.[2] No special precautions would therefore seem to be necessary. Information about other anticoagulants is lacking.

1. Verhaeghe R, Vanhoof A. The concomitant use of suloctidil and a long-acting oral anticoagulant. *Acta Clin Belg* (1977) 32, 36–8.
2. Minn FL, Zinny MA. Zomepirac and warfarin: a clinical study to determine if interaction exists. *J Clin Pharmacol* (1980) 20 (5-6 part 2), 418–21.

Anticoagulants + Sulphonamides

The anticoagulant effects of warfarin are increased by co-trimoxazole (sulfamethoxazole (sulphamethoxazole)/trimethoprim). Bleeding may occur if the dosage of the warfarin is not reduced appropriately. Phenindione does not interact with co-trimoxazole. There is also evidence that sulfaphenazole (sulphaphenazole), sulfafurazole (sulphafurazole, sulfisoxazole) and sulfamethizole (sulphamethizole) may interact like co-trimoxazole.

Clinical evidence

(a) Co-trimoxazole (sulfamethoxazole (sulphamethoxazole)/trimethoprim)

Six out of 20 patients taking **warfarin** showed an increase in their prothrombin ratios within 2 to 6 days of starting to take two tablets of **co-trimoxazole** daily (each tablet contains 400 mg **sulfamethoxazole** and 80 mg **trimethoprim**).[1] One patient bled and needed to be given vitamin K. The **warfarin** was temporarily withdrawn from 4 patients and the dosage was reduced in the last patient to control excessive hypoprothrombinaemia.[1]

An increase in the effects of **warfarin** caused by **co-trimoxazole** has been described in numerous other reports.[2-18] In some cases bleeding occurred. **Phenindione** is reported not to interact.[19]

(b) Sulfafurazole (sulphafurazole)

A man taking digitalis, diuretics, antacids and **warfarin** was later started on 500 mg **sulfafurazole** six-hourly. After 9 days his pro-thrombin time had risen from 20 to 28 s, and after 14 days he bled (haematuria, haemoptysis, gum bleeding). His prothrombin time had risen to 60 s.[20]

Two other patients bled and demonstrated prolonged prothrombin times when given **warfarin** and **sulfafurazole**.[21,22]

(c) Sulfamethizole (sulphamethizole)

The half-life of **warfarin** was increased over 40% (from 65 to 93 h) in 2 patients after taking 4 g **sulfamethizole** daily for a week.[23]

(d) Sulfaphenazole (sulphaphenazole)

Sixteen patients given single oral doses of **phenindione** and 500 mg **sulfaphenazole** showed prothrombin time increases after 24 h of 16.8 s compared with 10.3 s in 12 other patients who had only had **phenindione**.[24] These patients almost certainly had some hypoalbu-minaemia.

Mechanism

Not fully understood. Plasma protein binding displacement can oc-cur, but on its own it does not provide an adequate explanation.[25,26] Sulphonamides can drastically reduce the intestinal bacterial synthe-sis of vitamin K, but this is not normally an essential source of the vi-tamin unless dietary sources are exceptionally low.[27] Evidence suggesting that the metabolism of the anticoagulants is decreased ap-pears not to be fully established.[23,25] It has been shown that co-tri-moxazole largely affects the more potent (S)-warfarin.[13]

Importance and management

The warfarin/co-trimoxazole interaction is well documented and well established. The incidence appears to be high. If bleeding is to be avoided the warfarin dosage should be reduced and prothrombin times well monitored. Information about other anticoagulants is lack-ing, apart from phenindione which is said not to interact.

The phenindione/sulfaphenazole, warfarin/sulfafurazole and warfa-rin/sulfamethizole interactions are poorly documented, but it would seem prudent to follow the precautions suggested for co-trimoxazole if any of these sulphonamides is given. Some caution would be appro-priate with any sulphonamide, but direct information about interac-tions is lacking.

1. Hassall C, Feetam CL, Leach RH, Meynell MJ. Potentiation of warfarin by co-trimoxa-zole. *Lancet* (1975) ii, 1155–6.
2. Barnett DB, Hancock BW. Anticoagulant resistance: an unusual case. *BMJ* (1975) i, 608–9.
3. O'Reilly RA, Motley CH. Racemic warfarin and trimethoprim-sulfamethoxazole inter-action in humans. *Ann Intern Med* (1979) 91, 34–6.
4. Hassal C, Feetam CL, Leach RH, Meynell MJ. Potentiation of warfarin by co-trimoxa-zole. *BMJ* (1975) 2, 684.
5. Tilstone WJ, Gray JMB, Nimmo-Smith RH, Lawson DH. Interaction between warfarin and sulphamethoxazole. *Postgrad Med J* (1977) 53, 388–90.
6. Kaufman JM, Fauver HE. Potentiation of warfarin by trimethoprim-sulfamethoxazole. *Urology* (1980) 16, 601–3.
7. Beeley L, Ballantine N, Beadle F. Bulletin of the West Midlands Centre for Adverse Drug Reaction Reporting (1983) 16, 7.
8. McQueen EG. New Zealand Committee on Adverse Drug Reactions. 17th Annual Re-port 1982. *N Z Med J* (1983) 96, 95–9.
9. Greenlaw CW. Drug interaction between co-trimoxazole and warfarin. *Am J Hosp Pharm* (1979) 36, 1155.
10. Errick JK, Keys PW. Co-trimoxazole and warfarin: case report of an interaction. *Am J Hosp Pharm* (1979) 35, 1399–1401.
11. O'Donnell D. Antibiotic-induced potentiation of oral anticoagulant agents. *Med J Aust* (1989) 150, 163–4.
12. Keys PW. Drug interaction between co-trimoxazole and warfarin. *Am J Hosp Pharm* (1979) 36, 1155–6.
13. O'Reilly RA. Stereoselective interaction of trimethoprim-sulfamethoxazole with the separated enantiomorphs of racemic warfarin in man. *N Engl J Med* (1980) 302, 33–5.
14. Beeley L, Magee P, Hickey FM. Bulletin of the West Midlands Centre for Adverse Drug Reaction Reporting (1989) 28, 29.
15. Wolf R, Elman M, Brenner S. Sulfonamide-induced bullous hemorrhagic eruption in a patient with low prothrombin time. *Isr J Med Sci* (1992) 28, 882–4.
16. Erichsen C, Sndenaa K, Sreidge JA, Andersen E, Tysvoer A. Spontaneous liver haemato-mas induced by anti-coagulation therapy. A case report and review of the literature. *Hepatogastroenterology* (1993) 40, 402–6.
17. Cook DE, Ponte CD. Suspected trimethoprim/sulfamethoxazole-induced hypoprothrom-binemia. *J Fam Pract* (1994) 39, 589–91.
18. Chafin CC, Ritter BA, James A, Self TH. Hospital admission due to warfarin potentiation by TMP-SMX. *Nurse Pract* (2000) 25, 73-75.
19. De Swiet J. Potentiation of warfarin by co-trimoxazole. *BMJ* (1975) 3, 491.
20. Self TH, Evans W, Ferguson T. Interaction of sulfisoxazole and warfarin. *Circulation* (1975) 52, 528.
21. Sioris LJ, Weibert RT, Pentel PR. Potentiation of warfarin anticoagulation by sulfisoxa-zole. *Arch Intern Med* (1980) 140, 546–7.
22. Kayser S. Warfarin-sulfonamide interaction. Hospital Pharmacy Bulletin, University of California at San Francisco Hospitals 1978.
23. Lumholtz B, Siersbaek-Nielsen K, Skovsted L, Kampmann J, Hansen JM. Sulphame-thizole-induced inhibition of diphenylhydantoin, tolbutamide and warfarin metabolism. *Clin Pharmacol Ther* (1975) 17, 731.
24. Varma DR, Gupta RK, Gupta S, Sharma KK. Prothrombin response to phenindione dur-ing hypoalbuminaemia. *Br J Clin Pharmacol* (1975) 2, 467–8.
25. Seiler K, Duckert F. Properties of 3-(1-phenyl-propyl)-4-oxycoumarin (Marcoumar®) in the plasma when tested in normal cases and under the influence of drugs. *Thromb Diath Haemorrh* (1968) 19, 389–96.
26. Solomon HM, Schrogie JJ. The effect of various drugs on the binding of warfarin-^{14}C to human albumin. *Biochem Pharmacol* (1967) 16, 1219–26.
27. Udall JA. Human sources and absorption of vitamin K in relation to anticoagulation sta-bility. *JAMA* (1965) 194, 107–9.

Anticoagulants + Tamoxifen

The anticoagulant effects of acenocoumarol (nicoumalone) and warfarin are markedly increased by tamoxifen. A dosage reduction (about one-half, or even more) may be needed to avoid bleeding.

Clinical evidence

A woman on **warfarin** needed a dosage reduction from 5 to 1 mg dai-ly to keep her prothrombin time within the range 20 to 25 s when giv-en 40 mg **tamoxifen** daily. A retrospective study of the records of 5 other patients on **tamoxifen** revealed that 2 had shown marked in-creases in prothrombin times and bleeding shortly after starting war-farin. The other 3 needed **warfarin** doses which were about one-third of those taken by other patients not on **tamoxifen**.[1]

This confirms the first report of this interaction in a woman on **war-farin** who developed haematemesis, abdominal pain and haematuria 6 weeks after starting 20 mg **tamoxifen** daily. Her prothrombin time had risen from 39 to 206 s. She was restabilised on a little over half the **warfarin** dosage while continuing to take the **tamoxifen**.[2] The Aberdeen Hospitals Drug File has on record 22 patients given both drugs. Seventeen of them had no problems but 2 developed grossly elevated **warfarin** levels and 3 haemorrhaged.[3] The manufacturers of **tamoxifen** have another report of this interaction on their files.[2] A woman on **acenocoumarol (nicoumalone)** died after a massive brain haemorrhage about 3 weeks after starting to take 20 mg **tamoxifen** daily.[4]

Mechanism

Uncertain. It seems possible that these drugs compete for the same metabolizing systems in the liver, the result being that the loss of the anticoagulant is reduced and its effects are increased and prolonged.

Importance and management

An established and clinically important interaction which apparently affects some but not all patients. Monitor the effects closely if tamoxifen is added to treatment with warfarin or acenocoumarol (ni-coumalone) and reduce the dosage as necessary. The reports cited here indicate a reduction of between one-half to two-thirds for warfa-rin but some patients may need much larger reductions. The dosage reduction needed for acenocoumarol is not known but it is likely to be similar. The dosage will need to be increased if the tamoxifen is later withdrawn. The authors of one of the reports[1] postulate that the anti-tumour effects of the tamoxifen may also possibly be reduced. This needs further study. The effect of tamoxifen on other anticoagulants is uncertain but be alert for the same interaction to occur.

1. Tenni P, Lalich DL, Byrne MJ. Life threatening interaction between tamoxifen and war-farin. *BMJ* (1989) 298, 93.
2. Lodwick R, McConkey B, Brown AM, Beeley L. Life threatening interaction between tamoxifen and warfarin. *BMJ* (1987) 295, 1141.

3. Ritchie LD, Grant SMT. Tamoxifen-warfarin interaction: the Aberdeen hospitals drug file. *BMJ* (1989) 298, 1253.
4. Gustovic P, Baldin B, Tricoire MJ, Chichmanian RM. Interaction tamoxifène-acénocoumarol. Une interaction potentiellement dangereuse. *Therapie* (1994) 49, 55–6.

Anticoagulants + Tamsulosin

There is evidence that acenocoumarol (nicoumalone) and tamsulosin do not interact adversely.

Clinical evidence, mechanism, importance and management

A double-blind, placebo-controlled, crossover study in 15 normal subjects found that **tamsulosin** (dose not stated) had no effect on the pharmacokinetics or anticoagulant effects of a single dose of **acenocoumarol (nicoumalone)** (dose not stated but said to be high).[1] There would therefore appear to be no reason for taking special precautions if these drugs are used concurrently. Information about other anticoagulants seems to be lacking.

1. Rolan P, Clarke C, Mullins F, Terpstra IJ. Assessment of potential effects of tamsulosin (Omnic®) on the pharmacokinetics and pharmacodynamics of nicoumalone; are there interactions between tamsulosin (Omnic®) and nicoumalone. *J Urol (Baltimore)* (1999) 161 (4 Suppl), 235.

Anticoagulants + Teicoplanin

An isolated case report describes a marked reduction in the effects of warfarin attributed to teicoplanin.

Clinical evidence, mechanism, importance and management

A woman of 60 on digoxin, furosemide (frusemide) and **warfarin** (INR 3.5 to 5) developed a fever after mitral valve replacement surgery and was put on 900 mg **rifampicin** and 800 mg **teicoplanin** daily. Within 3 days her INR began to fall and by day 6 it was down to 1. Despite progressive **warfarin** increases to 10, 15 and 20 mg daily, her INR stayed between 1.2 and 1.6, even when the **rifampicin** was stopped after about 20 days treatment, and remained low for a further 20 days until the **teicoplanin** was also stopped.[1]

Some of this resistance to **warfarin** was undoubtedly due to the **rifampicin** (a known and potent inducer of **warfarin** metabolism) but the INRs remained depressed for a further 20 days after it was withdrawn suggesting that the **teicoplanin** had its own part to play. The reasons are not known. This is an isolated case and its general importance is not known, but it would now be prudent to monitor the INRs closely in any patient on **warfarin** who is given **teicoplanin**. Information about other anticoagulants is lacking.

1. Agosta FG, Liberato NL, Chiofalo F. Warfarin resistance induced by teicoplanin. *Haematologica* (1997) 82, 637–40.

Anticoagulants + Tenoxicam

Tenoxicam does not alter the anticoagulant effects of warfarin. Preliminary data also indicate that it does not interact with phenprocoumon.

Clinical evidence, mechanism, importance and management

Single-dose and steady-state studies in 14 subjects found that 20 mg **tenoxicam** daily for 14 days had no significant effect on the anticoagulant effects of **warfarin** or on bleeding times.[1] Case studies in a small number of patients and subjects similarly found no significant effect on the anticoagulant effects of **phenprocoumon**.[2] No special precautions would seem to be necessary.

1. Eichler H-G, Jung M, Kyrle PA, Rotter M, Korn A. Absence of interaction between tenoxicam and warfarin. *Eur J Clin Pharmacol* (1992) 42, 227–9.
2. Quoted as data on file, Hoffmann-La Roche & Co, by Eichler H-G, Jung M, Kyrle PA, Rotter M, Korn A. Absence of interaction between tenoxicam and warfarin. *Eur J Clin Pharmacol* (1992) 42, 227–9.

Anticoagulants + Terbinafine

Terbinafine does not normally interact with warfarin, but one isolated case describes reduced anticoagulation and another describes increased anticoagulation.

Clinical evidence

A randomised, double-blind, placebo-controlled trial in 16 normal subjects, given 250 mg **terbinafine** or a placebo daily for 14 days, found that the pharmacokinetics and anticoagulant effects of a single oral dose of 30 mg **warfarin** given on day 8 remained unchanged.[1] A large scale post-marketing surveillance study involving 10,361 patients treated with **terbinafine** identified a total of 26 who had also been given **warfarin**. Only 4 showed any adverse effects, none of which suggested a **terbinafine/warfarin** interaction.[2,3] Other *in vivo* and *in vitro* studies (see 'Mechanism') provide further evidence that no interaction would be expected.[4,5]

In contrast, an isolated report describes a 68-year-old woman on long term **warfarin** treatment whose INR fell from 2.1 to 1.1 within a month of starting a 3-month course of treatment with 250 mg **terbinafine** daily for tinea unguium. It was necessary to raise her **warfarin** dosage from 5.5 to 7.5–8.0 mg daily while taking the **terbinafine**, and to reduce it stepwise to 5.5 mg over the 4 weeks after the **terbinafine** treatment was over.[6] Another isolated case report describes and elderly woman on **warfarin** and cimetidine who developed gastrointestinal bleeding about a month after starting **terbinafine**.[7]

Mechanism

Normally none. *In vivo* studies with antipyrine show that terbinafine has little or no effect as an enzyme inducer, and this is confirmed by *in vitro* studies using human liver microsomes.[4,5] The isolated cases are not understood.

Importance and management

Normally no interaction occurs between warfarin and terbinafine – this is well established and adequately documented – while the two isolated cases cited are rarities, and unexplained. There appears therefore to be no reason for avoiding concurrent use, but if terbinafine is added to established treatment with warfarin it would be prudent to monitor the outcome so that in the very unlikely event of an interaction happening it can identified and dealt with appropriately. Information about other anticoagulants is lacking.

1. Guerret M, Francheteau P, Hubert M. Evaluation of effects of terbinafine on single oral dose pharmacokinetics and anticoagulant actions of warfarin in healthy volunteers. *Pharmacotherapy* (1997) 17, 767–73.
2. Novartis. Personal communication, February 1998.
3. O'Sullivan DP, Needham CA, Bangs A, Atkin K, Kendall FD. Postmarketing surveillance of oral terbinafine in the UK; report of a large cohort study. *Br J Pharmacol* (1996) 42, 559–65.
4. Back DJ, Tjia JF. Comparative effects of the antimycotic drugs ketoconazole, fluconazole, itraconazole and terbinafine on the metabolism of cyclosporin by human liver microsomes. *Br J Clin Pharmacol* (1991) 32, 624–6.
5. Seyffer R, Eichelbaum M, Jensen JC, Klotz U. Antipyrine metabolism is not affected by terbinafine, a new antifungal agent. *Eur J Clin Pharmacol* (1989) 37, 3231–3.
6. Warwick JA, Corrall RJ. Serious interaction between warfarin and oral terbinafine. *BMJ* (1998) 316, 440.
7. Gupta AK, Ross GS. Interaction between terbinafine and warfarin. *Dermatology* (1998) 196, 266–7.

Anticoagulants + Terodiline

Terodiline does not alter the anticoagulant effects of warfarin.

Clinical evidence, mechanism, importance and management

Twenty-two normal subjects were given enough warfarin (2.5 to 9.4 mg daily) to achieve thrombotest percentages within the 10 to 20% range. When additionally given 25 mg terodiline twice daily for 2 weeks, the serum levels and anticoagulant effects of the warfarin were unchanged.[1] No special precautions would seem necessary during concurrent use. There seems to be nothing documented about other anticoagulants.

1. Höglund P, Paulsen O, Bogentoft S. No effect of terodiline on anticoagulation effect of warfarin and steady-state plasma levels of warfarin enantiomers in healthy volunteers. *Ther Drug Monit* (1989) 11, 667–73.

Anticoagulants + Tetracyclic, Tricyclic and other antidepressants

Amitriptyline and possibly other tricyclics can cause unpredictable increases or decreases in prothrombin times which can make stable anticoagulation difficult. Maprotiline and mianserin do not usually interact, but isolated cases have been reported with both mianserin and lofepramine.

Clinical evidence

A study[1,2] in 6 volunteers given nortriptyline (0.6 mg/kg daily) for 8 days indicated that the mean half-life of dicoumarol was increased from 35 to 106 h, but a later study failed to find a consistent effect of either nortriptyline (40 mg daily) or amitriptyline (75 mg daily) taken over 9 days on the half-lives or elimination of either dicoumarol or warfarin in 12 normal subjects. The half-lives were shortened, prolonged or remained unaffected.[3]

Three reports have noted that the control of anticoagulation may be more difficult in patients taking amitriptyline and other tricyclic antidepressants.[4-6] One of them found that amitriptyline caused unpredictable and ". . . massive fluctuations . . ." in prothrombin times (increases and decreases) in 7 patients given phenprocoumon which made it difficult to establish stable anticoagulation, when compared with 7 other patients not taking amitriptyline.[7,8]

Another very brief report suggests the possibility of increased warfarin effects in patients given lofepramine.[9]

The anticoagulant effects of acenocoumarol (nicoumalone) (20 patients) have been shown to be unaffected by the use of maprotiline (150 mg daily),[10] and the effects of phenprocoumon (60 patients) were not affected by mianserin (30–60 mg daily).[11] A single case report describes a man on warfarin whose prothrombin time rose from 20 to 25 s after taking 10 mg mianserin daily for 7 days.[12] However a man on acenocoumarol and amiodarone needed an increase in his acenocoumarol dosage when given mianserin.[13]

Mechanism

Not understood. One suggestion is that the tricyclic antidepressants inhibit the metabolism of the anticoagulant (seen in *animals* with nortriptyline and amitriptyline on warfarin,[14] but not with desipramine on acenocoumarol[15]). Another idea is that the tricyclics slow intestinal motility thereby increasing the time available for the dissolution and absorption of dicoumarol.

Importance and management

Information about interactions between anticoagulants and tricyclic antidepressant is limited, patchy and inconclusive, but some difficulty in maintaining stable anticoagulation seems possible although

there would seem to be no strong reasons for totally avoiding concurrent use. Good monitoring is advisable. Maprotiline and mianserin do not usually interact, but monitor the outcome because some changes have been seen in individual patients.

1. Vesell ES, Passananti GT, Greene FE. Impairment of drug metabolism in man by allopurinol and nortriptyline. *N Engl J Med* (1970) 283, 1484–8.
2. Vesell ES, Passananti GT, Aurori KC. Anomalous results of studies on drug interaction in man. *Pharmacology* (1975) 13, 101–111.
3. Pond SM, Graham GG, Birkett DJ, Wade DN. Effects of tricyclic antidepressants on drug metabolism. *Clin Pharmacol Ther* (1975) 18, 191.
4. Koch-Weser J. Haemorrhagic reactions and drug interactions in 500 warfarin treated patients. *Clin Pharmacol Ther* (1973) 14, 139.
5. Williams JRB, Griffin JP, Parkins A. Effect of concomitantly administered drugs on the control of long term anticoagulant therapy. *Q J Med* (1976) 45, 63.
6. Hampel H, Berger C, Müller-Spahn F. Modified anticoagulant potency in an amitriptyline-treated patient? *Acta Haematol (Basel)* (1996) 96, 178–80.
7. Hampel H, Berger C, Kuss H-J, Hock C, Kurtz G, Müller-Spahn F. Modified anticoagulant potency of phenprocoumon during tricyclic antidepressant treatment: a potential drug-drug interaction. *Pharmacopsychiatry* (1995) 28, 183.
8. Hampel H, Berger C, Kuss H-J, Müller-Spahn F. Unstable anticoagulation in the course of amitriptyline treatment. *Pharmacopsychiatry* (1996) 29, 33–7.
9. Beeley L, Stewart P, Hickey FM. Bulletin of the West Midlands Centre for Adverse Drug Reaction Reporting (1988) 26, 21.
10. Michot F, Glaus K, Jack DB, Theobald W. Antikoagulatorische Wirkung von Sintrom® und Konzentration von Ludiomil® im Blut bei gleichzeitiger Verabreichung beider Präparate. *Med Klin* (1975) 70, 626–9.
11. Kopera H, Schenk H, Stulemeijer S. Phenprocoumon requirement, whole blood coagulation time, bleeding time and plasma γ-GT in patients receiving mianserin. *Eur J Clin Pharmacol* (1978) 13, 351–6.
12. Warwick HMC, Mindham RHS. Concomitant administration of mianserin and warfarin. *Br J Psychiatry* (1983) 143, 308–12.
13. Baettig D, Tillement J-P, Baumann P. Interaction between mianserin and acenocoumarin: a single case study. *Int J Clin Pharmacol Ther* (1994) 32, 165–7.
14. Loomis CW, Racz WJ. Drug interactions of amitriptyline and nortriptyline with warfarin in the rat. *Res Commun Chem Pathol Pharmacol* (1980) 30, 41–58.
15. Weiner M. Effect of centrally active drugs on the action of coumarin anticoagulants. *Nature* (1966) 212, 1599–1600.

Anticoagulants + Tetracyclines

The effects of the anticoagulants are not usually altered to a clinically relevant extent by concurrent treatment with tetracycline antibacterials, but a few patients have shown increases and a handful have bled.

Clinical evidence

Six out of 9 patients on an un-named anticoagulant showed a fall in their PP% from a range of 10 to 30% to less than 6% when treated with 250 mg chlortetracycline four times a day for 4 days.[1] A woman on warfarin bled (menorrhagia) after taking 200 mg doxycycline daily for eight days.[2] Two patients on acenocoumarol (nicoumalone) or warfarin developed markedly increased prothrombin ratios with bruising, haematomas and bleeding when treated with doxycycline.[3] Another patient with multiple medical problems and on warfarin and a range of drugs (alendronate, atorvastatin, albuterol, diltiazem, fluticasone) developed peritoneal bleeding and an INR of 7.2 (previously 2.6) 6 days after starting 200 mg doxycycline daily.[4] One patient out of 20 on dicoumarol bled when given tetracycline.[5] A patient on warfarin showed a marked increase in INR (from about 2.0 to 7.66) 6 weeks after starting to take 250 mg tetracycline four times daily, with INR changes over the following months which broadly paralleled the decreases in the tetracycline dosage.[6] An increased anticoagulant effect is briefly mentioned in 2 other reports,[7,8] A patient on warfarin bled (right temporal lobe haematoma) and had an extended prothrombin time a week after starting to take tetracycline/nystatin.[9] Another patient on warfarin also bled (epistaxis, haematemesis, melaena) 3 weeks after starting to take tetracycline/nystatin.[9] A clinical study on 9 patients on warfarin found an estimated 0.528 increase in the INR when given un-named tetracyclines.[10]

Mechanism

Not understood. Tetracyclines in the absence of anticoagulants can reduce prothrombin activity,[11,12] and both hypoprothrombinaemia and bleeding have been described.[13,14] It seems possible that very occasionally the anticoagulant and the tetracycline have additive hypoprothrombinaemic effects. The idea that antibacterials can decimate the intestinal flora of the gut thereby depleting the body of an essential source of vitamin K has been shown to be incorrect, apart from exceptional cases where normal dietary sources are extremely low.[15,16]

Importance and management

A relatively sparsely documented interaction, bearing in mind that the tetracyclines have been in very wide-spread use for many years. It can therefore reasonably be concluded that normally any changes are of little clinical relevance so that concurrent use need not be avoided, nevertheless because a few patients have unpredictably shown increased anticoagulant effects and even bleeding, the effects should be monitored when a tetracycline is first added to established anticoagulant treatment.

1. Magid E. Tolerance to anticoagulants during antibiotic therapy. *Scand J Clin Lab Invest* (1962) 14, 565–6.
2. Westfall LK, Mintzer DL, Wiser TH. Potentiation of warfarin by tetracycline. *Am J Hosp Pharm* (1980) 37, 1620, 1625.
3. Caraco Y, Rubinow A. Enhanced anticoagulant effect of coumarin derivatives induced by doxycycline coadministration. *Ann Pharmacother* (1992) 26, 1084–6.
4. Baciewicz AM, Bal BS. Bleeding associated with doxycycline and warfarin treatment. *Arch Intern Med* (2001) 161, 1231.
5. Chiavazza F, Merialdi A. Sulle interferenze fra dicumarolo e antibiotici. *Minerva Ginecol* (1973) 25, 630–1.
6. Danos EA. Apparent potentiation of warfarin activity by tetracycline. *Clin Pharm* (1992) 11, 806–8.
7. Wright IS. The pathogenesis and treatment of thrombosis. *Circulation* (1952) 5, 161–88.
8. Scarrone LA, Beck DF, Wright IS. A comparative evaluation of Tromexan and dicoumarol in the treatment of thromboembolic conditions — based on experience with 514 patients. *Circulation* (1952) 6, 489.
9. O'Donnell D. Antibiotic-induced potentiation of oral anticoagulant agents. *Med J Aust* (1989) 150, 163–4.
10. Pharmacy Anticoagulant Clinic Study Group. A multicentre survey of antibiotics on the INR of anticoagulated patients. *Pharm J* (1996) 257 (Pharmacy Practice Suppl), A30.
11. Searcy RL, Craig RG, Foreman JA. Blood clotting anomalies associated with intensive tetracycline therapy. *Clin Res* (1964) 12, 230.
12. Searcy RL, Simms NM, Foreman JA, Bergquist LM. Evaluation of the blood-clotting mechanism in tetracycline-treated patients. *Antimicrob Agents Chemother* (1964) 4, 179–83.
13. Rios JF. Hemorrhagic diathesis induced by antimicrobials. *JAMA* (1968) 205, 142.
14. Kippel AP, Pitsinger B. Hypoprothrombinaemia secondary to antibiotic therapy and manifested by massive gastrointestinal haemorrhage. *Arch Surg* (1968) 96, 266.
15. Udall JA. Human sources and absorption of vitamin K in relation to anticoagulation stability. *JAMA* (1965) 194, 107–9.
16. Pineo GF, Gallus AS, Hirsh J. Unexpected vitamin K deficiency in hospitalized patients. *Can Med Assoc J* (1973) 109, 880–3.

Anticoagulants + Thyroid or Antithyroid compounds

The anticoagulant effects of warfarin, dicoumarol, acenocoumarol (nicoumalone) and phenindione are increased by the concurrent use of thyroid compounds. Bleeding can occur if the anticoagulant is not reduced appropriately. A reduction in the anticoagulant effects may be expected if antithyroid compounds are used.

Clinical evidence

Hypothyroidic patients are relatively resistant to the effects of the oral anticoagulants and need larger doses than hyperthyroidic patients who are relatively sensitive.[1-5] Drug-induced changes in thyroid status (even in those who are euthyroidic but who are taking **dextrothyroxine** for hypercholesterolaemia) will alter the response to the oral anticoagulants.

(a) Thyroid compounds

A patient with myxoedema required a gradual reduction in his dosage of **phenindione** from 200 to 75 mg daily as his thyroid status was restored by the administration of **liothyronine**.[6] Seven out of 11 euthyroidic patients on **warfarin** showed lengthening prothrombin times and needed a small weekly dosage reduction in **warfarin** (by 2.5 mg to 30 mg) during the first 4 weeks of treatment with 4 to 8 mg **dextrothyroxine** daily for hypercholesterolaemia. One patient bled.[7] Hypoprothrombinaemia and bleeding have been described in 2 patients

on **warfarin** when their **thyroid** replacement therapy was started or increased.[8] Similar responses have been described in other reports and studies involving **warfarin**,[5,9-11] **dicoumarol**[12] or **acenocoumarol (nicoumalone)**.[6]

(b) Antithyroid compounds

A hyperthydroidic patient on **warfarin** showed a marked increase in his prothrombin times on two occasions when his treatment with **thiamazole (methimazole)** was stopped and he became hyperthyroidic again.[1]

Mechanism

In hypothyroidic patients the catabolism (destruction) of the blood clotting factors (II, VII, IX and X) is low and this tends to cancel to some extent the effects of the anticoagulants which reduce blood clotting factor synthesis. Conversely, in hyperthyroidic patients in whom the catabolism is increased, the net result is an increase in the effects of the anticoagulants.[13] It has also been suggested that the thyroid hormones may increase the affinity of the anticoagulants for its receptor sites.[9,14]

Importance and management

A well documented and clinically important interaction occurs if oral anticoagulants and thyroid compounds are taken concurrently.

Hypothyroidic patients taking an anticoagulant who are subsequently treated with thyroid as replacement therapy will need a changing downward adjustment of the anticoagulant dosage as treatment proceeds if excessive hypoprothrombinaemia and bleeding are to be avoided. Some adjustment may be necessary with euthyroidic (normal) patients given **dextrothyroxine** for hypercholesterolaemia. All of the oral anticoagulants may be expected to behave similarly.

As the thyroid status of hyperthyroidic patients returns to normal by the use of antithyroid drugs (e.g. carbimazole, thiamazole (methimazole), propylthiouracil) an increase in the anticoagulant requirements would be expected. Propylthiouracil in the absence of an anticoagulant has very occasionally been reported to cause hypoprothrombinaemia and bleeding.[15,16]

1. Vagenakis AG, Cote R, Miller ME, Braverman LE, Stohlman F. Enhancement of warfarin-induced hypoprothrombinemia by thyrotoxicosis. *Johns Hopkins Med J* (1972) 131, 69–73.
2. Self TH, Straughn AB, Weisburst MR. Effect of hyperthyroidism on hypoprothrombinemic response to warfarin. *Am J Hosp Pharm* (1976) 33, 387–9.
3. McIntosh TJ, Brunk SF, Kölln I. Increased sensitivity to warfarin in thyrotoxicosis. *J Clin Invest* (1970) 49, 63a.
4. Rice AJ, McIntosh TJ, Fouts JR, Brunk SF, Wilson WR. Decreased sensitivity to warfarin in patients with myxedema. *Am J Med Sci* (1971) 262, 211–15.
5. Chute JP, Dahut WL, Shakir KM, Georgiadis MS, Frame JN. Enhancement of warfarin induced hypoprothrombinemia by hyperthyroidism. *Blood* (1994) 84 (10 Suppl 1), 674a.
6. Walters MB. The relationship between thyroid function and anticoagulant therapy. *Am J Cardiol* (1963) 11, 112.
7. Owens JC, Neeley WB, Owen WR. Effect of sodium dextrothyroxine in patients receiving anticoagulants. *N Engl J Med* (1962) 266, 76.
8. Hansten PD. Oral anticoagulants and drugs which alter thyroid function. *Drug Intell Clin Pharm* (1980) 14, 331.
9. Solomon HM, Schrogie JJ. Change in receptor site affinity: a proposed explanation for the potentiating effect of D-thyroxine on the anticoagulant response to warfarin. *Clin Pharmacol Ther* (1967) 8, 797–9.
10. Winters WL, Soloff LA. Observations on sodium d-thyroxine as a hypocholesterolemic agent in persons with hypercholesterolemia with and without ischemic heart disease. *Am J Med Sci* (1962) 243, 458.
11. Costigan DC, Freedman MH, Ehrlich RM. Potentiation of oral anticoagulant effect by L-thyroxine. *Clin Pediatr (Phila)* (1984) 23, 172–4.
12. Jones RJ, Cohen L. Sodium dextro-thyroxine in coronary disease and hypercholesterolemia. *Circulation* (1961) 24, 164–70.
13. Loeliger EA, van der Esch B, Mattern MJ, Hemker HC. The biological disappearance rate of prothrombin, factors VII, IX and X from plasma in hypothyroidism, hyperthyroidism and during fever. *Thromb Diath Haemorrh* (1964) 10, 267–77.
14. Schrogie JJ, Solomon HM. The anticoagulant response to bishydroxycoumarin. II. The effect of D-thyroxine, clofibrate and norethandrolone. *Clin Pharmacol Ther* (1967) 8, 70–7.
15. D'Angelo G, LeGresley L. Severe hypoprothrombinemia after propylthiouracil therapy. *Can Med Assoc J* (1959) 71, 479.
16. Gotta AW, Sullivan CA, Seaman J, Jean-Gilles B. Prolonged intraoperative bleeding caused by propylthiouracil-induced hypoprothrombinemia. *Anesthesiology* (1972) 37, 562–3.

Anticoagulants + Tiabendazole (Thiabendazole)

An isolated case report describes a marked increase in the anticoagulant effects of acenocoumarol (nicoumalone) in a patient given tiabendazole (thiabendazole).

Clinical evidence, mechanism, importance and management

An increase in the anticoagulant effects of acenocoumarol (nicoumalone) occurred in a patient with nephrotic syndrome undergoing dialysis when given 8 g tiabendazole (thiabendazole) daily for three days. His INR rose from 2.9 to more than 5.[1] The reasons are not understood, nor is the general importance of this interaction known. There seem to be no other reports.

1. Henri P, Mosquet B, Hurault de Ligny B, Lacotte J, Cardinau E, Moulin M, Ryckelinck JP. Imputation d'une hypocoagulabilité à l'interaction tiabendazole-acénocoumarol. *Therapie* (1993) 48, 500–501.

Anticoagulants + Ticlopidine

The anticoagulant effects of acenocoumarol (nicoumalone) are modestly reduced by ticlopidine, but the anticoagulant effects of warfarin are unchanged. The makers of ticlopidine strongly advise avoidance of concurrent use because of the possible increased bleeding risks. There is some evidence that liver damage may occur in a small number of patients given warfarin and ticlopidine.

Clinical evidence

(a) Acenocoumarol (Nicoumalone)

A retrospective study of 36 patients with heart valve prostheses found that when concurrently treated with 250 mg **ticlopidine** daily, 29 of them had needed a mean 13% increase in **acenocoumarol** dosage (from 15.5 to 17.5 mg weekly), accompanied by a small INR rise (from 3.05 to 3.13). One patient detailed needed a dosage increase from 14 to 21 mg weekly. INR changes were detectable with a week of starting the **ticlopidine**.[1]

(b) Warfarin

Ten men on chronic **warfarin** treatment showed a significant increase in their mean *(R)*-**warfarin** levels (+29.8%) when given 250 mg **ticlopidine** twice daily for two weeks, but no changes in their *(S)*-**warfarin** levels occurred and no significant changes in their INRs were seen.[2,3] *(R)*-**warfarin** is very much the less active of the two enantiomers.

A Japanese study found evidence that **warfarin** and **ticlopidine** together can very occasionally cause cholestatic liver injury and severe jaundice. Four out of 132 patients (3%) given both drugs after cardiovascular surgery demonstrated this toxicity.[4]

Mechanism

Not understood. It seems possible that ticlopidine inhibits the metabolism of *(R)*-warfarin, but just why concurrent use very occasionally cause liver injury is not known. The interaction with acenocoumarol is not understood.

Importance and management

Information seems to be limited to the reports cited. A small to moderate increase in the acenocoumarol (nicoumalone) dosage may be needed if ticlopidine is added, but none seems to be necessary with warfarin, although it might be prudent to monitor for any evidence of liver damage if both drugs are used. There appears to be no information about other anticoagulants. However, the makers of ticlopidine strongly advise[5] the avoidance of ticlopidine with any anticoagulant because of the increased risk of bleeding (a combination of anticoagulant and platelet anti-aggregant activity). If exceptionally both drugs are used ". . . close clinical and laboratory monitoring (APPT) is required."

1. Salar A, Domenech P, Martinéz F. Ticlopidine antagonizes acencoumarol treatment. *Thromb Haemost* (1997) 77, 223–4.
2. Gidal BE, Sorkness CA, McGill KA, Larsen RL, Pitterle ME, Levine RF. Evaluation of a potential enantioselective interaction between warfarin (W) and ticlopidine (T) in chronically anticoagulated patients. *Clin Pharmacol Ther* (1994) 55, 164.
3. Gidal BE, Sorkness CA, McGill KA, larson R, Levine RR. Evaluation of a potential enantioselective interaction between ticlopidine and warfarin in chronically anticoagulated patients. *Ther Drug Monit* (1995) 27, 33–8.
4. Takase K, Fujioka H, Ogasawara M, Aonuma H, Tameda Y, Nakano T, Kosaka Y. Drug-induced hepatitis during combination therapy of warfarin potassium and ticlopidine hydrochloride. *Mie Med J* (1990) 40, 27–32.
5. Ticlid (Ticlopidine). Sanofi-Synthelabo. Summary of product characteristics, May 2000.

Anticoagulants + Tobacco smoking

Tobacco smoking slightly reduces the response to warfarin, but this appears not be clinically relevant in most patients.

Clinical evidence, mechanism, importance and management

When 9 smokers who normally **smoked** at least one pack daily stopped smoking, they showed a 13% increase in their average steady-state **warfarin** levels, a 13% decrease in **warfarin** clearance and a 23% increase in the **warfarin** half-life but no changes in prothrombin times.[1] A man of 80 on **warfarin** showed a steady rise in his INR (from about 2 to 3.7) over a 3-month period when he gave up smoking up to 2 packs per day. No bleeding occurred.[2]

The reason for these changes appears to be that some of the components of **tobacco smoke** act as liver enzyme inducing (stimulating) agents which cause a small increase in the metabolism of the warfarin. When smoking stops, the enzymes are therefore no longer stimulated, the metabolism of the **warfarin** falls slightly and its effects are correspondingly slightly increased. A later retrospective study of 200 patients who had undergone cardiac valve replacement found no statistically significant differences between the **warfarin** dosage requirements of **non-smokers**, **light smokers** (< 20 cigarettes daily) or **heavy smokers** (> 20 cigarettes daily).[3]

The overall picture seems to be that smoking (or giving up smoking) only has a slight to moderate effect on the response to **warfarin**, and only the occasional patient will need a small dosage alteration. This should easily be detected in the course of routine INR checks. Information about other anticoagulants seems to be lacking.

1. Bachmann K, Shapiro R, Fulton R, Carroll FT, Sullivan TJ. Smoking and warfarin disposition. *Clin Pharmacol Ther* (1979) 25, 309–15.
2. Colucci VJ. Increase in international normalized ratio associated with smoking cessation. *Ann Pharmacother* (2001) 35, 385–6.
3. Weiner B, Faraci PA, Fayad R, Swanson L. Warfarin dosage following prosthetic valve replacement: effect of smoking history. *Drug Intell Clin Pharm* (1984) 18, 904–6.

Anticoagulants + Tolfenamic acid

Tolfenamic acid has a small, clinically irrelevant effect on bleeding time when given alone,[1,2] but it is not entirely clear whether it is safe with anticoagulants or not. To be on the safe side the makers suggest good monitoring during concurrent use.[2]

1. Vapaatalo H, Österman T, Tokola O, Tokola R. Acute effects of tolfenamic acid on hemostatic functions and arachidonic acid metabolism. *Curr Ther Res* (1986) 39, 250–9.
2. Thames Laboratories. Personal communication, November 1996.

Anticoagulants + Tolrestat

Tolrestat appears not to interact with warfarin.

Clinical evidence, mechanism, importance and management

Thirteen normal subjects were given single 30-mg doses of warfarin before and after taking 400 mg tolrestat daily for 10 days. The pharmacokinetics of both drugs and the prothrombin times remained largely unchanged, although the prothrombin response to the warfarin was a little delayed and shortened.[1] No special precautions seem necessary if both drugs are used concurrently.

1. Meng X, Parker V, Turner M, Hicks D, Boxenbaum H, Chiang S. Effect of tolrestat (T) on pharmacokinetics (PK) and pharmacodynamics of warfarin (W). *Clin Pharmacol Ther* (1994) 55, 200.

Anticoagulants + Trazodone

A handful of case reports describe a moderate reduction in the anticoagulant effects of warfarin caused by trazodone whereas one small formal study found no interaction.

Clinical evidence, mechanism, importance and management

A woman needed a 17% increase (from 6.4 to 7.5 mg) in her daily dosage of warfarin when given 300 mg trazodone daily in order to maintain her prothrombin time at 20 s. Her warfarin requirements fell when the trazodone was later withdrawn.[1] A retrospective chart review study identified three other patients whose INRs also fell when trazodone was added to treatment with warfarin but no adverse effects were seen. One of the patients needed a 25% increase in the warfarin dosage.[2] The reasons for this reaction are not understood. In contrast, six anticoagulated patients on heparin or an unnamed coumarin anticoagulant showed no significant changes in prothrombin times when given 75 mg trazodone daily.[3]

The incidence of this interaction is unknown. All the evidence suggests that it is uncommon but because quite unpredictably the occasional patient may show an interaction, check the prothrombin times of all patients on warfarin if trazodone is started or stopped and adjust the dosage if necessary. The interaction can occur within a few days. Information about other anticoagulants seems to be lacking.

1. Hardy J-L, Sirois A. Reduction of prothrombin and partial thromboplastin times with trazodone. *Can Med Assoc J* (1986) 135, 1372.
2. Small NL, Giamonna KA. Interaction between warfarin and trazodone. *Ann Pharmacother* (2000) 34, 734-6.
3. Cozzolino G, Pazzaglia I, De Gaetano V, Macri M. Clinical investigation on the possible interaction between anti-coagulants and a new psychotropic drug (Trazodone). *Clin Europea* (1972) 11, 593.

Anticoagulants + Trimethoprim

Trimethoprim can cause a small increase in the effects of warfarin which appears to be of little or no clinical importance.

Clinical evidence, mechanism, importance and management

Some books, charts and reviews of interactions say that trimethoprim interacts with the oral anticoagulants to increase their effects, the implication being that it is clinically important, but there appears to only one published study of this interaction, which identified 12 patients on warfarin who showed a very small INR increase (+0.363) when given trimethoprim, but this was not statistically significant.[1] There do not appear to be any other reports, and none describing real clinical problems during concurrent use (except when combined with sulfamethoxazole (sulphamethoxazole) in co-trimoxazole). A literature search undertaken in 1992 by the makers of trimethoprim similarly failed to find any reports of a clinically important anticoagulant/trimethoprim interaction.[2] This relative silence in the literature would therefore suggest that in practice any interaction, if it occurs, is of only minor importance, and the anticoagulant dosage probably needs little or no adjustment.

1. Pharmacy Anticoagulant Clinic Study Group. A multicentre survey of antibiotics on the INR of anticoagulated patients. *Pharm J* (1996) 257 (Pharmacy Practice Suppl), R30.
2. Bristol-Myers Squibb Pharmaceuticals Ltd. Personal Communication, January 1997.

Anticoagulants + Ubidecarenone (Coenzyme Q10)

The anticoagulant effects of warfarin are reported to have been reduced in four patients by ubidecarenone but transiently increased in another.

Clinical evidence, mechanism, importance and management

Two patients on warfarin showed INR falls from about 2.5 to 1.4/1.3 after taking 30 mg ubidecarenone daily for 2 weeks. The INRs rapidly returned to normal when the ubidecarenone was stopped. Another patient on warfarin similarly showed INR falls on two occasions while taking ubidecarenone.[1] Yet another patient showed a reduced response to warfarin while taking ubidecarenone, but responded normally when it was stopped.[2]

In contrast 1 of 2 other patients taking ubidecarenone to treat alopecia caused by long-term warfarin treatment showed a transient INR *increase* when the ubidecarenone was introduced.[3] The reasons for these INR changes is not known but it may be that ubidecarenone has some Vitamin K-like activity, and there is also evidence from *animal* studies that ubidecarenone may alter the metabolism of *(R)*-warfarin.[4]

Direct information seems to be limited to these reports, but they act as a useful warning about the possibility of an interaction. Monitor the outcome if ubidecarenone is added to established warfarin treatment. Information about other oral anticoagulants is lacking.

1. Spigset O. Reduced effect of warfarin caused by ubidecarenone. *Lancet* (1994) 344, 1372–3.
2. Landbo C, Almdal TP. Interaction mellem warfarin og coenzym Q10. *Ugeskr Laeger* (1998) 160, 3226–7.
3. Nagao T, Ibayashi S, Fujii K, Sugimori H, Sadoshima S, Fujishima M. Treatment of warfarin-induced hair loss with ubidecarenone. *Lancet* (1995) 346, 1104–5.
4. Zhou S, Chan E. Effect of ubidearenone on warfarin anticoagulation and pharmacokinetics of warfarin enantiomers in rats. *Drug Metab Drug Interact* (2001) 18, 99–122.

Anticoagulants + Viloxazine

The anticoagulant effects of acenocoumarol (nicoumalone) and fluindione are increased by viloxazine.

Clinical evidence

A woman of 82 who was taking acenocoumarol (nicoumalone), molsidomine and flunitrazepam for angina, hypertension and atrial fibrillation showed a rise in her INR from 3.3 to 7.9 when she started to take viloxazine (dose not stated) for depression. Five days after stopping the viloxazine her INR had fallen to 2.6.[1]

This report briefly describes 3 other cases where viloxazine caused an increase in the anticoagulant effects of acenocoumarol and fluindione.[1]

Mechanism

Not understood. The authors of the report suggest that viloxazine possibly inhibits cytochrome P450 within the liver, resulting in a reduction in the metabolism and loss of the anticoagulants from the body.[1]

Importance and management

Information seems to be limited to this report so that its general importance is uncertain. Be alert for the need to reduce the dosage of acenocoumarol (nicoumalone) and fluindione if viloxazine is added to established anticoagulant treatment to avoid possible bleeding. Take the same precautions with any of the other oral anticoagulants but so far there seems to be no direct evidence that they interact.

1. Chiffoleau A, Delavaud P, Spreux A, Fialip J, Kergueris MF, Chichmanian RM, Lavarenne J, Bourin M, Larousse C. Existe-t-il une interaction métabolique entre la viloxazine et les antivitamines K? *Therapie* (1993) 48, 492–3.

Anticoagulants + Vinpocetine

Preliminary evidence suggests that the anticoagulant effects of warfarin may possibly be reduced to a small extent by vinpocetine.

Clinical evidence, mechanism, importance and management

A study in 18 normal subjects compared the effects of single 25 mg doses of warfarin before and while taking 10 mg vinpocetine daily.[1] A small reduction in the anticoagulant effects occurred, but more study is needed to find out whether this is clinically important. Monitor the effects of concurrent use.

1. Hitzenberger G, Sommer W, Grandt R. Influence of vinpocetine on warfarin-induced inhibition of coagulation. *Int J Clin Pharmacol Ther Toxicol* (1990) 28, 323–8.

Anticoagulants + Vitamin E

The anticoagulant effects of warfarin normally appear to be unchanged by vitamin E, although there is an isolated case of bleeding attributed to concurrent use. The effects of dicoumarol may possibly be reduced by vitamin E.

Clinical evidence

(a) Warfarin effects unchanged

A double-blind placebo controlled study in 25 patients on **warfarin** found that 800 or 1200 IU of **vitamin E** daily for a month caused no clinically relevant changes in their prothrombin times and INRs.[1] Another study on 12 anticoagulated patients also found that the anticoagulant effects of **warfarin** were unchanged by the administration of 100 or 400 IU **vitamin E** daily for 4 weeks.[2]

(b) Warfarin effects increased

A patient on **warfarin** (and also taking digoxin, furosemide (frusemide), clofibrate, potassium chloride and phenytoin, later substituted by quinidine) began to bleed apparently as a result of secretly taking 1200 IU **vitamin E** daily over a 2-month period. His prothrombin time was found to be 36 s. A later study showed that 800 IU **vitamin E** daily reduced his blood clotting factor levels and caused bleeding.[3]

(c) Dicoumarol effects reduced

A study on 3 normal subjects found that 42 IU **vitamin E** daily for a month reduced the response to a single dose of **dicoumarol** after 36 h from 52 to 33%.[4]

Mechanism

Not understood. The suggested explanations are that vitamin E interferes with the activity of vitamin K in producing the blood clotting factors,[3] and increases in the dietary requirements of vitamin K.[5,6]

Importance and management

Information is limited but the evidence suggests that most patients on warfarin are unlikely to have problems if given even quite large daily

doses (up to 1200 IU) of vitamin E, nevertheless the isolated case cited here shows that occasionally and unpredictably the warfarin effects can be changed. For this reason prothrombin times should be monitored when vitamin E is first added (within 1 to 2 weeks has been recommended).[1] The same precautions would also seem appropriate with dicoumarol as well. Information about other oral anticoagulants is lacking.

1. Kim JM, White RH. Effect of vitamin E on the anticoagulant response to warfarin. *Am J Cardiol* (1996) 77, 545–6.
2. Corrigan JJ, Ulfers LL. Effect of vitamin E on prothrombin levels in warfarin-induced vitamin K deficiency. *Am J Clin Nutr* (1981) 34, 1701–5.
3. Corrigan JJ, Marcus FI. Coagulopathy associated with vitamin E ingestion. *JAMA* (1974) 230, 1300–1.
4. Schrogie JJ. Coagulopathy and fat-soluble vitamins. *JAMA* (1975) 232, 19.
5. Anon. Vitamin K, vitamin E and the coumarin drugs. *Nutr Rev* (1982) 40, 180–2.
6. Anon. Megavitamin E supplementation and vitamin K-dependent carboxylation. *Nutr Rev* (1983) 41, 268–70.

Anticoagulants + Vitamin K

The effects of the anticoagulants can be reduced or abolished by the concurrent use of vitamin K. This can be used as an effective antidote for anticoagulant overdosage, but unintentional and unwanted antagonism has occurred in patients after taking some proprietary chilblain preparations, health foods, food supplements, enteral feeds or exceptionally large amounts of some green vegetables (such as spinach, brussel sprouts or broccoli) or green tea which can contain significant amounts of vitamin K. See also 'Anticoagulants + Food', p.264 and 'Anticoagulants + Natto', p.279.

Clinical evidence

A woman on **acenocoumarol (nicoumalone)** showed a fall in her British corrected anticoagulant ratio to 1.2 (normal range 1.8 to 3.0) within two days of starting to take an OTC chilblain preparation (**Gon**) containing 10 mg **acetomenaphthone** per tablet. She took a total of 50 mg vitamin K over 48 h.[1]

Similar antagonism has been described in patients on **warfarin** taking liquid dietary supplements such as **Ensure**,[2-6] **Ensure-Plus**,[7,8] **Isocal**,[9] **Nutrilite 330**[10] and **Osmolite**.[11-14] A reduction in the effects of **dicoumarol**, **acenocoumarol** and **warfarin** (described as 'warfarin resistance') has been seen in those whose diets contained large amounts of **green vegetables** (up to 0.75 to 1.1 lbs daily)[15-17] such as **spinach**,[18,19] **brussel sprouts**,[20] or **broccoli**,[19,21] or **liver**[21,22] which are rich in vitamin K. A formal study of the effects of vitamin K-rich vegetables (**brussel sprouts, broccoli, lettuce, spinach**) clearly demonstrated a disturbance of the control of anticoagulation in 37 patients on **warfarin**.[23]

A patient on **warfarin** showed a fall in his INRs from over 3 (ranged 3.20 to 3.79) to 1.37 attributed to the ingestion of very large quantities of **green tea** (0.5 to 1.0 gallon (US) (about 2 to 4 L) each day for a week.[24]

Mechanism

The oral anticoagulants compete with the normal supply of vitamin K from the gut to reduce the synthesis by the liver of blood clotting factors. If this supply is boosted by an unusually large intake of vitamin K, the competition swings in favour of the vitamin and the synthesis of the blood clotting factors begins to return to normal. As a result the prothrombin time also begins to fall to its normal value. Brussel sprouts increase the metabolism of warfarin to a small extent which would also decrease its effects.[20] There is also some evidence that a physico-chemical interaction (possibly binding to protein) may possibly occur between warfarin and enteral foods in the gut.[14,25]

Importance and management

A very well established, well documented and clinically important interaction expected to occur with every oral anticoagulant because they have a common mode of action. The drug intake and diet of any patient who shows 'warfarin resistance' should be investigated for the possibility of this interaction. It can be accommodated either by increasing the anticoagulant dosage, or by reducing the intake of vitamin K. In one case separating the administration of the warfarin and an enteral food by 3 h or more was effective.[14] However patients on vitamin K-rich diets should not change their eating habits without at the same time reducing the anticoagulant dosage because excessive anticoagulation and bleeding may occur.[21] It is estimated that a normal Western diet contains 300 to 500 micrograms vitamin K daily, and that the minimum daily requirement is 0.30 to 1.50 micrograms/kg body weight (about 100 micrograms in a 10 stone/140 lb/63 kg individual). Table 6.2 gives the vitamin K content of some foods. Other tables listing the vitamin K content of the enteral feeds have been published,[4,9,10,12,26] but the situation is continually changing as manufacturers reformulate their products, in some instances to accommodate the problem of this interaction.

1. Heald GE, Poller L. Anticoagulants and treatment for chilblains. *BMJ* (1974) 1, 455.
2. O'Reilly RA, Rytand DA. 'Resistance' to warfarin due to unrecognized vitamin K supplementation. *N Engl J Med* (1980) 303, 160–1.
3. Westfall LK. An unrecognized cause of warfarin resistance. *Drug Intell Clin Pharm* (1981) 15, 131.
4. Howard PA, Hannaman KN. Warfarin resistance linked to enteral nutrition products. *J Am Diet Assoc* (1985) 85, 713–15.
5. McIntire B, Wright RA. Enteral alimentation: an update on new products. *Nutr Supp Serv* (1981) 1, 7.
6. Bridgen ML. When bleeding complicates oral anticoagulant therapy. *Postgrad Med* (1995) 98, 153–68.
7. Zallman JA, Lee DP, Jeffrey PL. Liquid nutrition as a cause of warfarin resistance. *Am J Hosp Pharm* (1981) 38, 1174.
8. Michaelson R, Kempin SJ, Navia B, Gold JWM. Inhibition of the hypoprothrombinemic effect of warfarin (Coumadin®) by Ensure-Plus, a dietary supplement. *Clin Bull* (1980) 10, 171–2.
9. Watson AJM, Pegg M, Green JRB. Enteral feeds may antagonise warfarin. *BMJ* (1984) 288, 557.
10. Oren B, Shvartzman P. Unsuspected source of vitamin K in patients treated with anticoagulants: a case report. *Fam Pract* (1989) 6, 151–2.
11. Lader EW, Yang L, Clarke A. Warfarin dosage and vitamin K in Osmolite. *Ann Intern Med* (1980) 93, 373–4.
12. Parr MD, Record KE, Griffith GL, Zeok JV, Todd EP. Effect of enteral nutrition on warfarin therapy. *Clin Pharm* (1982) 1, 274–6.
13. Lee M, Schwartz RN, Sharifi R. Warfarin resistance and vitamin K. *Ann Intern Med* (1981) 94, 140–1.
14. Petretich DA. Reversal of Osmolite-warfarin interaction by changing warfarin administration time. *Clin Pharm* (1990) 9, 93.
15. Anon. Leafy vegetables in diet alter prothrombin time in patients taking anticoagulant drugs. *JAMA* (1964) 187, 27.
16. Qureshi GD, Reinders P, Swint JJ, Slate MB. Acquired warfarin resistance and weight-reducing diet. *Arch Intern Med* (1981) 141, 507–9.
17. Kempin SJ. Warfarin resistance caused by broccoli. *N Engl J Med* (1983) 308, 1229–30.
18. Udall JA, Krock LB. A modified method of anticoagulant therapy. *Curr Ther Res* (1968) 10, 207.

19. Karlson B, Leijd B, Hellström A. On the influence of vitamin K-rich vegetables and wine on the effectiveness of warfarin treatment. *Acta Med Scand* (1986) 220, 347–50.
20. Ovesen L, Lyduch S, Idorn ML. The effect of a diet rich in brussel sprouts on warfarin pharmacokinetics. *Eur J Clin Pharmacol* (1988) 33, 521–3.
21. Chow WH, Chow TC, Tse TM, Tai YT, Lee WT. Anticoagulation instability with life-threatening complication after dietary modification. *Postgrad Med J* (1990) 66, 855–7.
22. Kalra PA, Cooklin M, Wood G, O'Shea GM, Holmes AM. Dietary modification as a cause of anticoagulation instability. *Lancet* (1988) ii, 803.
23. Pedersen FM, Hamberg O, Hess K, Ovesen L. The effect of dietary vitamin K on warfarin-induced anticoagulation. *J Intern Med* (1991) 229, 517–20.
24. Taylor JR, Wilt VM. Probable antagonism of warfarin by green tea. *Ann Pharmacother* (1999) 33, 426–8.
25. Allen JB, Penrod LE, Vickery WE. Warfarin resistance and enteral feedings: an in vitro study. *Arch Phys Med Rehabil* (1991) 72, 832.
26. Kutsop JJ. Update on vitamin K$_1$ content of enteral products. *Am J Hosp Pharm* (1984) 41, 1762.

Anticoagulants + Zafirlukast

Zafirlukast increases the anticoagulant effects of warfarin. A reduction in the warfarin dosage will be needed to avoid over-anticoagulation.

Clinical evidence

16 normal subjects taking 80 mg **zafirlukast** or a placebo twice daily for 10 days were additionally given a single 25 mg dose of racemic **warfarin** on day 5. The mean AUC of the *(S)*-warfarin was increased by 63% and the half life by 36%. but the pharmacokinetics of the *(R)*-warfarin were not significantly changed. The mean prothrombin time increased by 35%.[1]

An 85-year-old woman on **warfarin** and other drugs (salbutamol (albuterol), diltiazem, digoxin, furosemide (frusemide) and potassium) was admitted to hospital with various cardiac-related problems and bleeding (epistaxis, melaena, multiple bruising) attributed to the use of **zafirlukast**, 20 mg twice daily. Her INR had risen from 1.1 (measured 6 months previously) to 4.5. The report does not say how long she had been taking the both drugs together.[2]

Mechanism

The reason for the interaction is thought to be that the zafirlukast inhibits cytochrome P450 isoenzyme CYP2C9 which is concerned with the metabolism of warfarin, as a result its serum levels and its effects are increased.[1,3]

Importance and management

Information appears to be limited to these reports but the interaction would seem to be established. If zafirlukast is given to patients stabilised on warfarin, you should monitor prothrombin times well and be alert for the need to reduce the warfarin dosage (the extent awaits assessment) to avoid over-anticoagulation. Information about other oral anticoagulants is lacking but phenprocoumon would not be expected to interact in this way because it is metabolised differently (mainly by conjugation to a glucuronide), but this needs confirmation.

1. Suttle AB, Vargo DL, Wilkinson LA, Birmingham BK, Lasseter K. Effect of zafirlukast on the pharmacokinetics of R- and S-warfarin in healthy men. *Clin Pharmacol Ther* (1997) 61, 186.
2. Morkunas A, Graeme K. Zafirlukast-warfarin drug interaction with gastrointestinal bleeding. *J Toxicol Clin Toxicol* (1997) 35, 501.
3. Accolate (Zafirlukast). Professional information brochure, Zeneca Pharmaceuticals, Wilmington, DE, USA, April 1997.

Anticoagulants + Zileuton

Zileuton increases the anticoagulant effects of warfarin.

Clinical evidence

Twenty-four normal subjects who had been titrated with racemic **warfarin** to achieve prothrombin times of 14 to 18 s for a week, were additionally given 600 mg **zileuton** or a placebo six-hourly for a further week. The **zileuton** had no effect on the pharmacokinetics of *(S)*-

Table 6.2 Vitamin K content of some meat and vegetables

Foods	Vitamin K content (μg/100 g)
Turnip greens	650
Beetroot	650
Broccoli	200
Cabbage	125
Green beans	14
Lettuce	129
Liver, pig	25
Liver, beef	92
Potatoes	3
Spinach	89

Data from:
1. Olson RE. Vitamin K. In: Modern nutrition in health and disease. Goodhart RS and Shils ME (eds.) Lea and Febiger, Philadelphia (1980) p. 170–80.
2. Chow WH, Chow TC, Tse TM, Tai YT, Lee WT. Anticoagulation instability with life-treatening complication after dietary modification. *Postgrad Med J* (1990) 66, 855–7.

warfarin, but the *(R)*-**warfarin** serum levels rose and its clearance fell (by 15%). The mean prothrombin times in the mornings before taking the **warfarin** rose from 17.5 to 19.8 s, and in the evenings 12 h later they rose from 17.1 to 19.1 s. The corresponding changes in the placebo group were from 18.1 to 18.8 s and 17.3 to 17.5 s.[1]

Mechanism

Not yet established but it seems likely that the zileuton inhibits the metabolism of the *(R)*-warfarin (probably by cytochrome P450 isoenzyme CYP1A2) causing it to accumulate, thereby increasing its effects.

Clinical importance and management

Information seems to be limited to this study, but the interaction appears to be established. If zileuton is added to established treatment with warfarin, be alert for the need to reduce the warfarin dosage. Monitor well. Information about other anticoagulants is as yet lacking, but it would now be prudent to monitor their concurrent use.

1. Awni WM, Hussein Z, Granneman GR, Patterson KJ, Dube LM, Cavanaugh JH. Pharmacodynamic and stereoselective pharmacokinetic interactions between zileuton and warfarin in humans. *Clin Pharmacokinet* (1995) 29 (Suppl 2), 67–76.

Heparin + Aprotinin

Aprotinin-treated patients also given protamine may subsequently need increased doses of heparin.

Clinical evidence, mechanism, importance and management

One report suggested that patients who had been treated with aprotinin needed considerably more heparin than usual, the suggested reason being that aprotinin has an effect on antithrombin III.[1] A later report however pointed out that the more likely reason was that these aprotinin-treated patients had also been given protamine which would oppose the effects of the heparin.[2] Whatever the explanation, be alert for the need to use more heparin after aprotinin has been used.

1. Fisher AR, Bailey CR, Shannon CN, Wielogorski AK. Heparin resistance after aprotinin. *Lancet* (1992) 340, 1230–1.
2. Hunt BJ, Murkin JM. Heparin resistance after aprotinin. *Lancet* (1993) 341, 126.

Heparin + Aspirin

Although concurrent use is effective in the prevention of post-operative thromboembolism, the risk of bleeding in patients receiving heparin is increased almost two-and-a-half times by the use of aspirin.

Clinical evidence

Eight out of 12 patients developed serious bleeding when treated with heparin (5000 units subcutaneously every 12 h) and **aspirin** (600 mg twice daily) as prophylaxis for deep vein thrombosis following operations for fracture of the hip. Haematomas of the hip and thigh occurred in 3 patients, bleeding through the wound in 4, and uterine bleeding in the other patient.[1]

An epidemiological study of 2656 patients given heparin and **aspirin** (doses not stated) revealed that the incidence of bleeding was almost 2.5 times that which was seen in patients not given **aspirin**.[2] A striking prolongation of bleeding times is described elsewhere[3] in patients on heparin after treatment with **aspirin**. Yet another study confirms that **aspirin** increases the risk of severe upper gastrointestinal bleeding in patients given heparin.[4]

Mechanism

Heparin suppresses the normal blood clotting mechanisms and prolongs bleeding times.[3] Aspirin decreases platelet aggregation so that any heparin-induced bleeding is exaggerated and prolonged.[3]

Importance and management

An established and important interaction. Although concurrent use is effective in the prevention of post-operative thromboembolism,[5] the risks of this interaction need to be very carefully considered, and the advantages and disadvantages carefully weighed. The assertion[6] made in 1969 that aspirin "... should be scrupulously avoided in patients on heparin ..." is an overstatement, but it emphasises the need for care. Concurrent use should certainly be carefully monitored. If an analgesic is required, paracetamol (acetaminophen) is a safer substitute for aspirin.

1. Yett HS, Skillman JJ, Salzman EW. The hazards of aspirin plus heparin. *N Engl J Med* (1978) 298, 1092.
2. Walker AM, Jick H. Predictors of bleeding during heparin therapy. *JAMA* (1980) 244, 1209.
3. Heiden D, Rodvien R, Mielke CH. Heparin bleeding, platelet dysfunction, and aspirin. *JAMA* (1981) 246, 330.
4. Younossi ZM, Strum WB, Cloutier D, Teirstein PS, Schatz RA. Upper GI bleeding in postcoronary stent patients following aspirin and anticoagulant treatment. *Gastroenterology* (1995) 108 (4 Suppl), A265.
5. Vinazzer H, Loew D, Simma W, Brücke P. Prophylaxis of postoperative thromboembolism by low dose heparin and by acetylsalicylic acid given simultaneously. A double blind study. *Thromb Res* (1980) 17, 177–84.
6. Deykin D. The use of heparin. *N Engl J Med* (1976) 294, 1122.

Heparin + Dextran

Although concurrent use can be successful and uneventful, there is evidence that the anticoagulant effects of heparin can be increased by some dextrans. It has been suggested that the heparin dosage may need to be reduced by up to a half during concurrent use to prevent bleeding.

Clinical evidence

A study on 9 patients with peripheral vascular disease showed that the mean clotting time 1 h after the infusion of 10,000 u heparin was increased from 36 to 69 s when given at the same time as 500 ml **dextran**. **Dextran** alone had no effect, but the mean clotting time after 5,000 u heparin with **dextran** was almost the same as after 10,000 u heparin alone.[1,2]

The abstract quoted[1] contains some confusing typographical errors but the correct text has been confirmed.[2] This study would seem to explain two other reports of an increase in the incidence of bleeding in those given both heparin and **dextran**.[3,4]

Mechanism

Both heparin and dextran prolong coagulation time, but by a number of different and independent mechanisms. When given together their effects would seem to be additive.[3]

Importance and management

Direct documentation is limited, but the interaction seems to be established. Uneventful concurrent use[5,6] has been described with dextran 40 which suggests that the interaction may possibly be confined to the use of dextran 70, but this requires confirmation. If concurrent use is undertaken the effects should be very closely monitored and the dosage of heparin reduced as necessary (between one-third to one-half has been recommended[1]).

1. Atik M. Potentiation of heparin by dextran and its clinical implication. *Thromb Haemorrh* (1977) 38, 275.
2. Atik M. Personal communication, April 1980.
3. Bloom WL, Brewer SS. The independent yet synergistic effects of heparin and dextran. *Acta Chir Scand* (1968) 387 (Suppl), 53–7.
4. Morrison ND, Stephenson CBS, Maclean D, Stanhope JM. Deep vein thrombosis after femoropopliteal bypass grafting with observations on the incidence of complications following the use of dextran 70. *N Z Med J* (1976) 84, 233–7.

5. Schöndorf TH, Weber V. Prevention of deep venous thrombosis in orthopedic surgery with the combination of low dose heparin plus either dihydroergotamine or dextran. *Scand J Haematol* (1980) 36 (Suppl), 126–40.

6. Serjeant JCB. Mesenteric embolus treated with low-molecular weight dextran. *Lancet* (1965) i, 139.

Heparin + Glyceryl trinitrate (Nitroglycerin) or Isosorbide dinitrate

Some studies claim that the effects of heparin are reduced by the concurrent infusion of nitrates, but others have failed to confirm this interaction.

Clinical evidence

(a) Heparin effects reduced

While receiving intravenous **glyceryl trinitrate**, 7 patients with coronary artery disease needed an increased dose of intravenous heparin to achieve satisfactory anticoagulation (activated partial thromboplastin times (APTT) of 1.5 to 2.53 × control values). When the **glyceryl trinitrate** was stopped 6 out of the 8 showed an marked increase in APTT values to 3.5. One patient had transient haematuria.[1]

This study confirms a previous report, the authors of which attributed this response to an interaction with the propylene glycol diluent of the **glyceryl trinitrate** infusion.[2] However it still occurred when **glyceryl trinitrate** was given without propylene glycol.[1] The partial thromboplastin time (PTT) of 27 patients given heparin was approximately halved (from 130 to about 60 s) when additionally given 2 to 5 mg/h **glyceryl trinitrate** intravenously. The heparin levels measured in nine patients were unchanged. The PTT rose again when the **glyceryl trinitrate** was stopped.[3,4] The PTT in 8 out of 10 patients treated with heparin was reduced by 2 to 5 mg/h **glyceryl trinitrate**.[5] Yet another study found that concurrent use had no effect at 2 h, but heparin levels were markedly reduced (by 56%) at 4 h, and the APTT ratio was accordingly lower.[6] Reduced heparin effects have been described in other studies.[7-9]

(b) Heparin effects unchanged

A study in 10 patients following angioplasty found no significant APTT changes over a 30 min period following the addition of intravenous **glyceryl trinitrate** (41 to 240 micrograms/ml) to infusions of heparin.[10] A 60-minute infusion of 5 mg **glyceryl trinitrate** in eight normal subjects had no effect on the APTT or prothrombin time following a 5000-U intravenous injection of heparin.[11] A further study in 24 patients failed to find any effects on APTT in 17 of the patients on heparin infused with 1 to 5 mg **glyceryl trinitrate** or **isosorbide dinitrate**, and only 3 had increases of more than 17 s when the nitrate was stopped.[12] No evidence of any change in the anticoagulant effect of a 40 U.kg^{-1} bolus of heparin by 100 micrograms.min^{-1} infusion of **glyceryl trinitrate** was found in 7 normal subjects.[13] Another study in 22 patients failed to find a significant change in APTT due to heparin and **glyceryl trinitrate**.[14] The authors of another brief report also question the existence of this interaction.[15] Yet another study found that a **glyceryl trinitrate** infusion of 1 micrograms/kg/min had no effect on the activity of heparin (40 to 180 units/kg) in 13 patients on chronic **nitrate** treatment.[16] No inhibition of heparin anticoagulation was seen in 45 patients with acute angina or myocardial infarction on low-dose (5 to 20 micrograms/min) or 13 on high dose (80 to 240 micrograms/min) **glyceryl trinitrate**.[17] No reduction in the anticoagulant effects of heparin were seen a controlled study 42 patients on low dose intravenous nitrates (**glyceryl trinitrate** or **isosorbide**).[18] No clinically significant changes in heparin requirements (1000 units/h) were seen in yet another study in patients given **glyceryl trinitrate** (100 micrograms/min).[19]

Mechanism

Not understood. One study suggests that what occurs is related to a glyceryl trinitrate-induced antithrombin III abnormality.[5] Another says that heparin levels are lowered.[6]

Importance and management

The discord between these reports is not understood. Until the situation is resolved it would clearly be prudent to monitor the effects of concurrent use, being alert for the need to use higher doses of heparin in the presence of glyceryl trinitrate. If this interaction occurs, remember to reduce the heparin dosage when the glyceryl trinitrate or isosorbide infusion is stopped. More study is needed.

1. Habbab MA, Haft JI. Heparin resistance induced by intravenous nitroglycerin. A word of caution when both drugs are used concomitantly. *Arch Intern Med* (1987) 147, 857–60.

2. Col J, Col-Debeys C, Lavenne-Pardonge E, Meert P, Hericks L, Broze MC, Moriau M. Propylene glycol-induced heparin resistance during nitroglycerin infusion. *Am Heart J* (1985) 110, 171–3.

3. Pizzulli L, Nitsch J, Luederitz B. Nitroglycerin inhibition of the heparin effect. *Eur Heart J* (1989) 10 (Abstract Suppl), 116.

4. Pizzulli L, Nitsch J, Lüederitz B. Hemmung der Heparinwirkung durch Glyceroltrinitrat. *Dtsch Med Wochenschr* (1988) 113, 1837–40.

5. Becker RC, Corrao JM, Bovill EG, Gore JM, Baker SP, Miller ML, Lucas FV, Alpert JA. Intravenous nitroglycerin-induced heparin resistance: a qualitative antithrombin III abnormality. *Am Heart J* (1990) 119, 1254–61.

6. Brack MJ, Gershlick AH. Nitrate infusion even in low dose decreases the anticoagulant effect of heparin through a direct effect on heparin levels. *Eur Heart J* (1991) 12 (Abstract Suppl), 80.

7. Dascalov TN, Chaushev AG, Petrov AB, Stancheva LG, Stanachcova SD, Ivanov AA. Nitroglycerin inhibition of the heparin effect in acute myocardial infarction patients. *Eur Heart J* (1990) 11 (Abstract Suppl), 321.

8. Pizzulli L, Nitsch J, Lüderitz B. Nitroglycerin inhibition of the heparin effect. *Eur Heart J* (1989) 10 (Abstract Suppl), 116.

9. Brack MJ, More RS, Hubner PJB, Gerschlick AH. The effect of low dose nitroglycerine on plasma heparin concentrations and activated partial thromboplastin times. *Blood Coag Fibrinol* (1993) 4, 183–6.

10. Lepor NE, Amin DK, Berberian L, Shah PK. Does nitroglycerin induce heparin resistance? *Clin Cardiol* (1989) 12, 432–4.

11. Bode V, Welzel D, Franz G, Polensky V. Absence of drug interaction between heparin and nitroglycerin. *Arch Intern Med* (1990) 150, 2117–19.

12. Pye M, Olroyd KG, Conkie J, Hutton I, Cobbe SM. Is there an interaction between IV nitrate therapy and heparin anticoagulation? A clinical and in virto study. *Eur Heart J* (1991) 12 (Abstract Suppl), 80.

13. Schoenenberger RA, Ménat L, Weiss P, Marbett GA, Ritz R. Absence of nitroglycerin-induced heparin resistance in healthy volunteers. *Eur Heart J* (1992) 13, 411–14.

14. Gonzalez ER, Jones HD, Graham S, Elswick RK. Assessment of the drug interaction between intravenous nitroglycerin and heparin. *Ann Pharmacother* (1992) 26, 1512–14.

15. Day MW, Absher RK. We don't observe the same heparin-nitroglycerin reactions. *Critical Care Nurse* (1992) 12, 18.

16. Reich DL, Hammerschlag BC, Rand JH, Perucho-Powell MH, Thys DM. Modest doses of nitroglycerin do not interfere with beef lung heparin anticoagulation in patients taking nitrates. *J Cardiothorac Vasc Anesth* (1992) 6, 677–9.

17. Nottestad SY, Mascette AM. Nitroglycerin-induced resistance: absence of interaction at clinically relevant doses. *Mil Med* (1994) 159, 569–71.

18. Bechtold H, Kleist P, Landgraf K, Möser K. Einfluß einer niedrigdosierten intravenösen Nitrattherpie auf die antikagulatorische Wirkung von Heparin. *Med Klin* (1994) 89, 360–6.

19. Berk SI, Grunwald A, Pal S, Bodenheimer MM. Effect of intravenous nitroglycerin on heparin dosage requirements in coronary artery disease. *Am J Cardiol* (1993) 72, 393-6.

Heparin + Miscellaneous drugs

Changes in the protein binding of several drugs (diazepam, propranolol, quinidine and verapamil) by heparin appears not to be of clinical importance. Patients who smoke may possibly need fractionally more heparin than non-smokers.

Clinical evidence, mechanism, importance and management

(a) Diazepam, Propranolol, Quinidine and Verapamil

A number of studies have found that heparin reduces the plasma protein binding in man and *animals* of several drugs including **diazepam**,[1,2] **propranolol**,[1] **quinidine**[3] and **verapamil**.[4] For example, 3 patients on oral **propranolol** and 3 given 10 mg **diazepam** intramuscularly were given 3000 IU heparin just before cardiac catheterization. Five minutes after the heparin, the free fraction of **diazepam** was found to have risen fourfold (from 1.8 to 7.9%) while the free levels had risen from 2.0 to 8.4 ng/ml. The free fraction of the **propranolol** rose from 7.4 to 12.5% and the free levels rose from 1.7 to 2.7 ng/ml.[1]

The postulated reason for these changes is that the heparin displaces these drugs from their binding sites on the plasma albumins with additionally some changes in free fatty acid levels. It was also suggested that these changes in protein binding might possibly have some clinical consequences. For example, would there be sudden increases in sedation or respiratory depression because of the rapid increase in the active (free) fraction of **diazepam**?

The answer seems to be these changes are not likely to be of clinical importance. One study even suggested that the heparin-induced protein binding changes are an artefact of the study methods used,[5] and this would seem to be supported by an experimental study which failed to find that heparin had any effect on the beta-blockade of **propranolol**.[6] Moreover there seem to be no other reports confirming that these interactions are of real clinical importance. No special precautions would seem to be necessary.

(b) Tobacco smoking

A study of the factors affecting the sensitivity of individuals to heparin found that its half-life in **smokers** was 0.62 compared with 0.97 h in non-smokers. The dosage requirements of the smokers was slightly increased (18.8 compared with 16.0 U/h/lean body weight).[7] These differences would seem to be too small to be of much practical importance.

1. Wood AJJ, Robertson D, Robertson RM, Wilkinson GR, Wood M. Elevated plasma free drug concentrations of propranolol and diazepam during cardiac catheterization. *Circulation* (1980) 62, 1119–22.
2. Routledge PA, Kitchell BB, Bjornsson TD, Skinnner T, Linnoila M, Shand DG. Diazepam and *N*-desmethyldiazepam redistribution after heparin. *Clin Pharmacol Ther* (1980) 27, 528–32.
3. Kessler KM, Leech RC, Spann JF. Blood collection techniques, heparin and quinidine protein binding. *Clin Pharmacol Ther* (1979) 25, 204–10.
4. Keefe DL, Yee YG, Kates RE. Verapamil protein binding in patients and normal subjects. *Clin Pharmacol Ther* (1981) 29, 21–6.
5. Brown JE, Kitchell BB, Bjornsson TD, Shand DG. The artifactual nature of heparin-induced drug protein-binding alterations. *Clin Pharmacol Ther* (1981) 30, 636–43.
6. DeLeve LD, Piafsky KM. Lack of heparin effect on propranolol-induced beta-adrenoceptor blockade. *Clin Pharmacol Ther* (1982) 31, 216.
7. Cipolle RJ, Seifert RD, Neilan BA, Zaske DE, Haus E. Heparin kinetics: variables related to disposition and dosage. *Clin Pharmacol Ther* (1981) 29, 387–93.

Heparin + Molsidomine

Molsidomine appears not to interact adversely with heparin.

Clinical evidence, mechanism, importance and management

A comparative study in patients treated with intravenous heparin and glyceryl trinitrate (27 patients) or 2 mg molsidomine (15 patients) found that while the glyceryl trinitrate reduced the partial thromboplastin times (PTTs) due to the heparin (see also 'Heparin + Glyceryl trinitrate (Nitroglycerin) or Isosorbide dinitrate', p.303) no such interaction occurred with the molsidomine.[1] No special precautions would therefore appear to be needed if both drugs are used.

1. Wiemer M, Pizzulli L, Reichert H, Lüderitz B. Gibt es eine Wechselwirkung zwischen Heparin und Moldisomin?. *Med Klin* (1994) 89, 45-6.

Heparin + Probenecid

Some very limited evidence suggests that the effects of heparin may be possibly increased by probenecid and bleeding may occur.

Clinical evidence, mechanism, importance and management

In 1950 (but not reported[1] until 1975) a woman with subacute bacterial endocarditis was treated with **probenecid** orally and penicillin by intravenous drip, kept open with minimal doses of heparin. After a total of 215 mg (about 20,000 u) heparin had been given over a 3-week period, increasing epistaxes developed and the clotting time was found to be 24 min (normal 5 to 60). This was controlled with protamine. It had previously been observed that **carinamide**, the predecessor of **probenecid**, prolonged clotting times in the presence of heparin.[2] The general importance of this possible interaction is uncertain, but it would seem prudent to monitor the effects of concurrent use.

1. Sanchez G. Enhancement of heparin effect by probenecid. *N Engl J Med* (1975) 292, 48.
2. Sirka HD, McCleery RS, Artz CP. The effect of carinamide with heparin on the coagulation of human blood: a preliminary report. *Surgery* (1948) 24, 811.

Heparin + Streptokinase

Patients previously treated with streptokinase appear to be partially resistant to the anticoagulant effects of heparin.

Clinical evidence, mechanism, importance and management

50 patients given streptokinase (750,000 to 1,500,000 U) for acute myocardial infarction needed approximately 24% more heparin (37755 compared with 30294 u daily) in order to achieve the desired activated partial thromboplastin time (APTT) than other patients who had not had streptokinase. Even then their APTTs were 15% lower. Anticoagulation was also delayed (5 days compared with 3). The reasons are not understood. On the basis of this study, anticipate the need to use higher heparin doses and to make more frequent dosage adjustments if streptokinase has been given.[1] These patients also needed more warfarin (+12%) but this value was not statistically significant.[1] More study is needed.

1. Zagher D, Maaravi Y, Matzner Y, Gilon D, Gotsman MS, Weiss T. Partial resistance to anticoagulation after streptokinase treatment for acute myocardial infarction. *Am J Cardiol* (1990) 66, 28–30.

Lepirudin + Miscellaneous drugs

The makers warn of the increased bleeding risks if lepirudin is used with other thrombolytics or oral anticoagulants.

Clinical evidence, mechanism, importance and management

The makers say that no formal interaction studies have been done but they reasonably warn that the concurrent use of lepirudin and other thrombolytics (they name **alteplase** and **streptokinase**) may ". . . increase the risk of bleeding complications and considerably enhance the effect of *Refludan* (lepirudin) on a PTT prolongation." They also warn about the increased risks of bleeding if coumarin derivatives (**warfarin and other oral anticoagulants**) are used concurrently. Their recommendation for exchanging lepirudin treatment with an **oral anticoagulant** is to reduce the lepirudin dosage gradually to reach a PTT ratio just above 1.5 before beginning the **oral anticoagulant**, and to stop the lepirudin as soon as the INR reaches 2.0.[1]

1. Refludan (Lepirudin). Hoechst Marion Roussel Limited, Summary of product characteristics, March 1997.

7

Anticonvulsant drug interactions

The anticonvulsant drugs listed in Table 7.1 find their major application in the treatment of various kinds of epilepsy, although some of them are also used for other conditions. The list is not exclusive by any means, but it contains the anticonvulsant drugs that are discussed either in this chapter or elsewhere in this book. In addition, some of the barbiturates that are not used as anticonvulsants are also included in this chapter. The Index should be consulted for a full list of interactions involving all of these drugs.

Table 7.1 Anticonvulsant drugs

Generic names	Proprietary names
Acetazolamide	Acetadiazol, Azomid, Carbinib, Dazamide, Defiltran, Diamox, Diuramid, Edemox, Glaupax, Odemin, Uramox
Carbamazepine	Antafit, Atretol, Bioneuryl, Bioreunil, Carba, Carbabeta, Carbaflux, Carbagamma, Carbagen, Carbalan, Carbatrol, Carbaval, Carbazene, Carbazep, Carbazina, Carbi, Carbium, Carmapine, Carpaz, Carpin, Carpine, Carzepine, Clostedal, Degranol, Deleptin, Epimaz, Epitol, espa-lepsin, Finlepsin, Fitzecalm, Fokalepsin, Gericarb, Hermolepsin, Karbac, Mapezine, Neugeron, Neurotol, Neurotop, Nordotol, Novo-Carbamaz, Panitol, Sirtal, Taver, Tegretal, Tegretard, Tegretol, Temporol, Teril, Timonil, Trimonil, Voluto
Clobazam	Castilium, Frisium, Noiafren, Urbanil, Urbanol, Urbanyl
Clonazepam	Antelepsin, Clonapam, Clonex, Iktorivil, Kenoket, Klonopin, Kriadex, Paxam, Rivatril, Rivotril
Ethosuximide	Emeside, Petinimid, Petnidan, Suxilep, Suxinutin, Zarondan, Zarontin
Ethylphenacemide (Pheneturide)	Laburide
Felbamate	Felbatol, Taloxa
Flunarizine	Amalium, Axilin, Cedelate, Fasolan, Flerudin, Floxin, Fludan, Flugeral, Flulium, Flunagen, Flunarin, Flunarium, Flunavert, Flunaza, Flunazine, Fluricin, Flurpax, Fluvert, Fluxarten, FNZ, Gradient, Hexilium, Issium, Liberal, Medilium, Nafluryl, Poli-Flunarin, Sibelium, Simoyiam, Sobelin, Vasculene, Vasilium, Vertix, Zelium, Zinasen
Gabapentin	Aclonium, Equipax, Neurontin, Progresse
Lamotrigine	Labileno, Lamicitin, Lamictal, Neurium
Losigamone	
Mesuximide (Methsuximide)	Celontin, Petinutin
Methylphenobarbital (Methylphenobarbitone)	Mebaral, Prominal
Oxcarbazepine	Apydan, Auram, Trileptal, Trileptin
Phenobarbital (Phenobarbitone)	Alepsal, Aparoxal, Aphenylbarbit, Bialminal, Comizial, Edhanol, Fenemal, Fenocris, Gardenal, Gardenale, Gratusminal, Kaneuron, Lepinal, Lepinaletten, Lethyl, Luminal, Luminale, Luminaletas, Luminalette, Luminaletten, Neurobiol, Phenaemal, Phenaemaletten, Phenotal, Sedabarb, Sevrium, Solfoton
Phenytoin (Diphenylhydantoin)	Aurantin, Dilantin, Dintoina, Diphantoine, Ditoin, Ditomed, Di-Hydan, Epamin, Epanutin, Epelin, Epilantine, Epilan-D, Epinat, Fenantoin, Fenidantal, Fenidantoin S, Fenital, Fenitron, Hidantal, Hidantina, Hidantoina, Hydantin, Lehydan, Neosidantoina, Nuctane, Pepsytoin, Phenhydan, Phenytek, Sinergina, Zentropil
Primidone	Cyral, Liskantin, Mylepsinum, Mysoline, Prysoline, Resimatil
Progabide	
Sodium valproate (Valproic acid)	Absenor, Atemperator, Convulex, Convulsofin, Criam, Delepsine, Depacon, Depakene, Depakin, Depakine, Depakote, Depalept, Depamag, Deprakine, Deproic, Diplexil, Encorate, Epiject, Epilenil, Epilim, Epival, Ergenyl, Leptilan, Leptilanil, Mylproin, Orfiril, Orlept, Pimiken, Valpakine, Valparin, Valporal, Valpro, Valprosid
Stiripentol	
Sulthiame	
Tiagabine	Gabatril, Gabitril
Topiramate	Epitomax, Topamax, Topimax
Valpromide (Dipropylacetamide)	Depamide
Vigabatrin	Sabril, Sabrilan, Sabrilex

Anticonvulsants + Acetazolamide

Severe osteomalacia and rickets have been seen in patients on phenytoin, phenobarbital and primidone when concurrently treated with acetazolamide. A marked reduction in serum primidone levels with a loss in seizure control, and rises in serum carbamazepine levels with toxicity have also been described in a very small number of patients.

Clinical evidence

(a) Osteomalacia

Severe osteomalacia developed in 2 young women on phenytoin, primidone or phenobarbital while taking 750 mg acetazolamide daily, despite a normal intake of calcium. When the acetazolamide was withdrawn, the hyperchloraemic acidosis shown by both patients abated and their high urinary excretion of calcium fell by 50%.[1]

This interaction has been described in 2 adults[2] and 3 children,[3] who developed rickets.

(b) Reduced serum primidone levels

A patient on primidone showed an increased fit-frequency and a virtual absence of primidone (or phenobarbital) in the serum when treated with 250 mg acetazolamide daily. Primidone levels rose when the acetazolamide was withdrawn, probably due to improved absorption. A subsequent study in 2 other patients found that acetazolamide had a small effect on the primidone in one, and no effect in the other.[4]

(c) Increased serum carbamazepine levels

A girl of 9 and two teenage boys of 14 and 19, all of them on the highest dosages of carbamazepine tolerable without side-effects, developed signs of toxicity after taking acetazolamide (250 to 750 mg daily). They were also found to have elevated serum carbamazepine levels (by about 25 to 50%). In one instance toxicity appeared within 48 h.[5]

The seizure control of 54 children with grand mal and temporal lobe epilepsy was improved when acetazolamide (10 mg/kg daily) was added to carbamazepine. Serum carbamazepine levels rose by 1 to 6 mg/l in 60% of the 33 patients sampled. Side effects developed in 10 children, and in 8 children this was within 1 to 10 days of starting the acetazolamide. The side effects responded to a reduction in the carbamazepine dosage.[6]

Mechanisms

Uncertain. (a) Mild osteomalacia induced by anticonvulsants is a recognised phenomenon.[7] It seems that this is exaggerated by acetazolamide, which increases urinary calcium excretion, possibly by causing systemic acidosis, which results from the reduced absorption of bicarbonate by the kidney. (b) and (c) Not understood.

Importance and management

The documentation of all of these interactions is very limited, and their incidence uncertain. Concurrent use should be monitored for the possible development of these adverse interactions and steps taken to accommodate them. Withdraw the acetazolamide if necessary, or adjust the dosage of anticonvulsants appropriately. In the case of the children with rickets[3] the acetazolamide was withdrawn and high doses of vitamin D was given. It seems possible that other carbonic anhydrase inhibitors may behave like acetazolamide.

1. Mallette LE. Anticonvulsants, acetazolamide and osteomalacia. *N Engl J Med* (1975) 292, 668.
2. Mallette LE. Acetazolamide-accelerated anticonvulsant osteomalacia. *Arch Intern Med* (1977) 137, 1013–17.
3. Matsuda I, Takekoshi Y, Shida N, Fujieda K, Nagai B, Arashima S, Anakura M, Oka Y. Renal tubular acidosis and skeletal demineralization in patients on long-term anticonvulsant therapy. *J Pediatr* (1975) 87, 202–5.
4. Syversen GB, Morgan JP, Weintraub M, Myers GJ. Acetazolamide-induced interference with primidone absorption. *Arch Neurol* (1977) 34, 80–4.
5. McBride MC. Serum carbamazepine levels are increased by acetazolamide. *Ann Neurol* (1984) 16, 393.
6. Forsythe WI, Owens JR, Toothill C. Effectiveness of acetazolamide in the treatment of carbamazepine-resistant epilepsy in children. *Dev Med Child Neurol* (1981) 23, 761–9.
7. Anast CS. Anticonvulsant drugs and calcium metabolism. *N Engl J Med* (1975) 292, 567–8.

Anticonvulsants + Aciclovir

An isolated report describes a marked reduction in serum phenytoin and sodium valproate levels in a child given aciclovir. Seizure frequency increased.

Clinical evidence, mechanism, importance and management

A 7-year-old boy with epilepsy on phenytoin, sodium valproate and nitrazepam was started on 1 g oral aciclovir daily for 6 days. After 4 days his trough serum phenytoin levels had fallen from 17 to 5 micrograms/ml, and his trough sodium valproate levels from 32 to 22 micrograms/ml. When the aciclovir treatment was over, the serum levels of both anticonvulsants rose again, over 3 to 6 days. During the period when the anticonvulsant levels were restabilising, the seizure frequency markedly increased and his EEG worsened. The reason for this apparent interaction is not known, but the authors of the report suggest that the aciclovir may possibly have reduced the absorption of the anticonvulsants, in some way not understood.[1]

This appears to be the first and only report of an interaction between these drugs. Its general clinical importance is not known, but it would now seem prudent to be alert to the possibility of this interaction in any patient on either anticonvulsant if aciclovir is given. More study is needed.

1. Parmeggiani A, Riva R, Posar A, Rossi PG. Possible interaction between acyclovir and antiepileptic treatment. *Ther Drug Monit* (1995) 17, 312–15.

Anticonvulsants + Alcohol

Moderate social drinking appears not to affect the serum levels of carbamazepine, ethosuximide or phenytoin. Some small changes are seen in serum phenobarbital and sodium valproate levels, but no changes in the control of epilepsy seem to occur.

Clinical evidence, mechanism, importance and management

A study in 29 non-drinking epileptics found that when they drank 1 to 3 glasses of an alcoholic beverage (1 to 3 units) over a 2-h period, twice a week, for 16 weeks, the serum levels of carbamazepine, ethosuximide and phenytoin were unchanged when compared with those from a control group of 23 epileptics given drinks without alcohol. There was a marginal change in phenobarbital levels, and some increase in serum sodium valproate levels. However, this effect is hard to interpret as valproate levels are known fluctuate and are hard to reproduce. Other anticonvulsants used were clonazepam, primidone and sulthiame, but too few patients used these for a valid statistical analysis to be carried out. Maximum blood alcohol levels ranged from 5 to 33 mg%. More important than any changes which occurred in serum anticonvulsant levels, was the finding that this social drinking had no effect on the frequency of tonic-clonic convulsions, partial complex seizures, or on the epileptic activity as measured by EEGs.[1] There would therefore seem to be no reason for epileptics to avoid alcohol in moderate social amounts, but heavy drinking should be avoided as it may increase seizure frequency. See also 'Phenytoin + Alcohol', p.338, 'Alcohol + Barbiturates', p.19 and 'Topiramate + Alcohol', p.362.

1. Höppener RJ, Kuyer A, van der Lugt PJM. Epilepsy and alcohol: the influence of social alcohol on seizures and treatment in epilepsy. *Epilepsia* (1983) 24, 459–71.

Anticonvulsants + Aspartame

Aspartame can cause convulsions in some susceptible individuals.

Clinical evidence, mechanism, importance and management

Grand mal seizures have been reported in 80 people associated with the consumption of **aspartame** (*NutraSweet*®). Three of them were taking **phenytoin**. Petit mal and psychomotor attacks were also seen in another 18 subjects taking **aspartame**.[1] The authors note that another 149 cases of **aspartame**-associated convulsions had been reported to the FDA.[1] The reasons for this adverse reaction are not understood. It would seem prudent for patients taking anticonvulsants to avoid **aspartame**.

1. Roberts HJ. Aspartame (Nutrasweet®)-associated epilepsy. *Clin Res* (1988) 36, 349A.

Anticonvulsants + Aspirin or NSAIDs

Carbamazepine is unaffected by aspirin or tolfenamic acid. Phenytoin toxicity has been seen in two patients, one on aspirin, the other on ibuprofen, but other evidence suggests that these reactions are very rare. Serum phenytoin levels can be markedly increased by the concurrent use of azapropazone and toxicity can develop rapidly. It is inadvisable for patients to take these drugs concurrently. Phenytoin serum levels can be increased by phenylbutazone. Toxicity may occur if the phenytoin dosage is not reduced appropriately. It seems likely that oxyphenbutazone will interact similarly. No clinically significant interaction occurs with phenytoin and bromfenac of tolfenamic acid. Sodium valproate toxicity developed in three patients when given large and repeated doses of aspirin. Naproxen appears not to interact with sodium valproate.

Clinical evidence, mechanism, importance and management

(a) Carbamazepine + Aspirin

No changes in **carbamazepine** serum levels were seen in 10 patients while taking 1500 mg **aspirin** for 3 days.[1] It would appear no precautions are necessary if aspirin is used in patients on carbamazepine.

(b) Carbamazepine + Tolfenamic acid

Tolfenamic acid 300 mg for 3 days had no significant effect on the serum levels of **carbamazepine** in 11 patients.[1] No special precautions seem necessary if these drugs are taken concurrently.

(c) Phenytoin + Aspirin

It has been claimed that if a patient has been taking large quantities of **aspirin** for headache **phenytoin** is potentiated.[2] This comment remains unconfirmed, although a study in 10 healthy subjects did find that a 975-mg dose of **aspirin** caused protein binding displacement of **phenytoin**. However, the extent of the displacement was considered unlikely to be clinically significant, and doses of 325 and 650 mg showed no appreciable effect.[3] Similar effects on protein binding displacement have been seen in other studies.[4-8] However, although the ratios of free and bound **phenytoin** may change, there does not appear to be a clinical effect, possibly because the extra free **phenytoin** is metabolised by the liver.[7] A study in 10 epileptics on **phenytoin** found that when given 500 mg **aspirin** three times daily for 3 days, no significant changes in serum **phenytoin** levels or anticonvulsant effects occurred.[1] Bearing in mind the extremely common use of **aspirin**, the almost total silence in the literature about an adverse **phenytoin/aspirin** interaction implies that no special precautions are normally needed.

(d) Phenytoin + Azapropazone

When a patient developed phenytoin toxicity within 2 weeks of starting 600 mg **azapropazone** twice daily, further study was made in 5 healthy subjects given 125 to 250 mg phenytoin daily. When additionally given 600 mg **azapropazone** twice daily, their mean serum phenytoin levels fell briefly from 5 to 3.7 micrograms/ml before rising steadily over the next 7 days to 10.5 micrograms/ml.[9,10] An extension of this study is described elsewhere.[11]

Another report describes phenytoin toxicity in a woman when fenclofenac was replaced by 1200 mg **azapropazone** daily.[12]

The most likely explanation is that **azapropazone** inhibits the liver enzymes concerned with the metabolism of phenytoin, resulting in its accumulation in the body. It also seems possible that **azapropazone** displaces phenytoin from its plasma protein binding sites so that levels of unbound (and active) phenytoin are increased. This means that toxicity might occur at serum levels which would be well tolerated in the absence of **azapropazone**. Information seems to be limited to the reports cited, but it appears to be a clinically important interaction. The incidence is uncertain, but it was demonstrated in all of the 5 subjects examined in the study cited.[9,11] As toxicity may possibly occur at serum levels that would be well tolerated in the absence of azapropazone, concurrent use is potentially hazardous and the makers state that azapropazone should not be given to patients taking phenytoin.

(e) Phenytoin + Bromfenac

Twelve healthy subjects were given 50-mg doses oral **bromfenac** three times daily for 4 days and then 300 to 330 mg phenytoin for up to 14 days (to achieve stable levels), and then both drugs for 8 days. It was found that the peak phenytoin serum levels and AUC were increased by 9% and 11% respectively, while the **bromfenac** peak levels and its AUC fell by 42%. The suggested reason for the fall in **bromfenac** levels is that the phenytoin increases its metabolism by the liver.[13] In practical terms these results indicate that there is no need to adjust the dosage of phenytoin if **bromfenac** is added, nor any need to increase the **bromfenac** dosage unless there is any evidence that its efficacy is diminished.

(f) Phenytoin + Ibuprofen

Studies in healthy subjects have shown that the pharmacokinetics of single doses of **phenytoin** 300 or 900 mg are not significantly altered by 300 or 400 mg **ibuprofen** 6-hourly.[14,15] However, a single report describes a woman stabilised on 300 mg **phenytoin** daily who developed **phenytoin** toxicity within a week of starting to take 400 mg **ibuprofen** four times daily.[16] Her serum **phenytoin** levels had risen to 101 mmol/l. The phenytoin was stopped for 3 days and the ibuprofen withdrawn, and within 10 days the phenytoin level had dropped to 68 mmol/l. The reasons for this interaction are not understood.

Both **phenytoin** and **ibuprofen** have been available for a number of years and this case seems to be the first and only report of an adverse interaction. No special precautions would normally seem to be necessary.

(g) Phenytoin + Oxyphenbutazone or Phenylbutazone

Six epileptics on phenytoin (200 to 350 mg daily) given 100 mg **phenylbutazone** three times daily showed a mean fall in their phenytoin serum levels from 15 to 13 micrograms/ml over the first 3 days, after which the levels climbed steadily to 19 micrograms/ml over the next 11 days. One patient developed signs of toxicity. His levels of free phenytoin more than doubled.[1]

The predominant effect of phenylbutazone seems to be the inhibition of the enzymes concerned with the metabolism of phenytoin[17] (steady-state half-life increased from 13.7 to 22 h), leading to its accumulation in the body and a rise in its serum levels. The initial transient fall may possibly be related in some way to the displacement by the phenylbutazone of the phenytoin from its plasma protein binding sites.[18] An established interaction, although the documentation is very limited. Monitor the outcome of adding phenylbutazone and reduce the phenytoin dosage as necessary. There is no direct evidence that **oxyphenbutazone** interacts like phenylbutazone, but since it is the main metabolic product of phenylbutazone in the body and has been shown to prolong the half-life of phenytoin in *animals*[19] it would be expected to interact similarly.

(h) Phenytoin + Tolfenamic acid

Tolfenamic acid 300 mg for 3 days had no significant effect on the serum levels of **phenytoin** in 11 patients.[1] No special precautions seem necessary if these drugs are taken concurrently.

(i) Sodium valproate + Aspirin

A girl of 17 taking 21 mg/kg sodium valproate daily was prescribed 18 mg/kg of **aspirin** daily for lupus arthritis. Within a few days she developed a disabling tremor which disappeared when the **aspirin** was stopped. Total serum valproate levels were not significantly changed, but the free fraction fell from 24 to 14% when the **aspirin** was withdrawn. Similar toxic reactions (tremor, nystagmus, drowsiness, ataxia) were seen in 2 children, aged 6 and 4 years, given 12 and 20 mg/kg **aspirin** four-hourly while taking sodium valproate.[20] Aspirin displaces sodium valproate from its protein binding sites[21] and also alters its metabolism by the liver[22] so that the levels of free (and pharmacologically active) sodium valproate rise. This could temporarily increase both the therapeutic and toxic effects of the sodium valproate. However, there is evidence that increased hepatic elimination of sodium valproate counterbalances this effect.

Direct information seems to be limited to the studies cited. Clinically relevant interactions appear rare, probably because in most cases the effects of aspirin on free valproate levels cancel each other out. The combination need not necessarily be avoided, but it would seem prudent to be aware of this interaction if both drugs are used. More study is needed.

(j) Sodium valproate + Naproxen

A study in 6 healthy subjects found that 500 mg **naproxen** moderately displaces sodium valproate from its protein binding sites, but not enough to have any clinical relevance.[23] No clinically important interaction seems to occur between sodium valproate and naproxen.

1. Neuvonen PJ, Lehtovaara R, Bardy A, Elomaa E. Antipyretic analgesics in patients on anti-epileptic drug therapy. *Eur J Clin Pharmacol* (1979) 15, 263–8.
2. Toakley JG. Dilantin overdosage. *Med J Aust* (1968) 2, 640.
3. Leonard RF, Knott PJ, Rankin GO, Robinson DS, Melnick DE. Phenytoin-salicylate interaction. *Clin Pharmacol Ther* (1981) 29, 56–60.
4. Ehrnebo M, Odar-Cederlöf I. Distribution of pentobarbital and diphenylhydantoin between plasma and cells in blood: effect of salicylic acid, temperature and total drug concentration. *Eur J Clin Pharmacol* (1977) 11, 37–42.
5. Fraser DG, Ludden TM, Evens RP, Sutherland EW. Displacement of phenytoin from plasma binding sites by salicylate. *Clin Pharmacol Ther* (1980) 27, 165–9.
6. Paxton JW. Effects of aspirin on salivary and serum phenytoin kinetics in healthy subjects. *Clin Pharmacol Ther* (1980) 27, 170–8.
7. Olanow CW, Finn A, Prussak C. The effect of salicylate on phenytoin pharmacokinetics. *Trans Am Neurol Assoc* (1979) 104, 109–10.
8. Inoue F, Walsh RJ. Folate supplements and phenytoin-salicylate interaction. *Neurology* (1983) 33, 115–16.
9. Geaney DP, Carver JG, Aronson JK, Warlow CP. Interaction of azapropazone with phenytoin. *BMJ* (1982) 284, 1373.
10. Aronson JK, Hardman M, Reynolds DJM. ABC of monitoring drug therapy. Phenytoin. *BMJ* (1992) 305, 1215–18.
11. Geaney DP, Carver JG, Davies CL, Aronson JK. Pharmacokinetic investigation of the interaction of azapropazone with phenytoin. *Br J Clin Pharmacol* (1983) 15, 727–34.
12. Roberts CJC, Daneshmend TK, Macfarlane D, Dieppe PA. Anticonvulsant intoxication precipitated by azapropazone. *Postgrad Med J* (1981) 57, 191–2.
13. Gumbhir-Shah K, Cevallos WH, DeCleene SA, Korth-Bradley JM. Evaluation of pharmacokinetic interaction between bromfenac and phenytoin in healthy males. *J Clin Pharmacol* (1997) 37, 160–8.
14. Bachmann KA, Schwartz JI, Forney RB, Jauregui L, Sullivan TJ. Inability of ibuprofen to alter single dose phenytoin disposition. *Br J Clin Pharmacol* (1986) 21, 165–9.
15. Townsend RJ, Fraser DG, Scavone JM, Cox SR. The effects of ibuprofen on phenytoin pharmacokinetics. *Drug Intell Clin Pharm* (1985) 19, 447–8.
16. Sandyk R. Phenytoin toxicity induced by interaction with ibuprofen. *S Afr Med J* (1982) 62, 592.
17. Andreasen PB, Frøland A, Skovsted L, Andersen SA, Hague M. Diphenylhydantoin half-life in man and its inhibition by phenylbutazone: the role of genetic factors. *Acta Med Scand* (1973) 193, 561–4.
18. Lunde PKM, Rane A, Yaffe SJ, Lund L, Sjöqvist F. Plasma protein binding of diphenylhydantoin in man. Interaction with other drugs and the effect of temperature and plasma dilution. *Clin Pharmacol Ther* (1970) 11, 846–55.
19. Soda DM, Levy G. Inhibition of drug metabolism by hydroxylated metabolites: cross-inhibition and specificity. *J Pharm Sci* (1975) 64, 1928–31.
20. Goulden KJ, Dooley JM, Camfield PR, Fraser AD. Clinical valproate toxicity induced by acetylsalicylic acid. *Neurology* (1987) 37, 1392–4.
21. Orr JM, Abbott FS, Farrell K, Ferguson S, Sheppard I, Godolphin W. Interaction between valproic acid and aspirin in epileptic children: serum protein binding and metabolic effects. *Clin Pharmacol Ther* (1982) 31, 642–9.
22. Abbott FS, Kassam J, Orr JM, Farrell K. The effect of aspirin on valproic acid metabolism. *Clin Pharmacol Ther* (1986) 40, 94–100.
23. Grimaldi R, Lecchini S, Crema F, Perucca E. In vivo plasma protein binding interaction between valproic acid and naproxen. *Eur J Drug Metab Pharmacokinet* (1984) 9, 359–63.

Anticonvulsants + Calcium Carbimide or Disulfiram

Phenytoin serum levels are markedly and rapidly increased by the concurrent use of disulfiram. Phenytoin toxicity can develop. There is evidence that phenobarbital and carbamazepine are not affected by disulfiram, and that phenytoin is not affected by calcium carbimide.

Clinical evidence

The serum **phenytoin** levels of 4 patients on long-term treatment showed rises of 100 to 500% over a 9-day period when concurrently treated with 400 mg **disulfiram** daily, with no signs of levelling off even 3 to 4 days after the **disulfiram** was withdrawn. Levels had still not returned to normal 14 days after the disulfiram was withdrawn. Two patients developed signs of mild **phenytoin** toxicity.[1] In a follow-up study on 2 patients, one of them developed ataxia and both showed a rise in serum **phenytoin** levels of 25 and 50% over 5 days of concurrent disulfiram treatment.[2]

Disulfiram increased the half-life of **phenytoin** in 10 healthy subjects from 11 to 19 h.[3] There are also other case reports describing this interaction.[4-7]

Phenobarbital levels (from primidone in 3 patients and phenobarbital in one patient) showed only minor serum level fluctuations of about 10% when given concurrently with **disulfiram** for 9 days.[1,2]

Carbamazepine also appears not to interact. Signs of toxicity disappeared in a patient when **phenytoin** was replaced by **carbamazepine**,[6] and the observation, that **disulfiram** does not interact with **carbamazepine**, was confirmed in a study of 5 epileptic, non-alcoholic patients.[8]

A study in 4 patients showed that **calcium carbimide** 50 mg daily for a week followed by 100 mg for 2 weeks had no effect on serum **phenytoin** levels.[2]

Mechanism

Disulfiram inhibits the liver enzymes concerned with the metabolism of phenytoin thereby prolonging its stay in the body and resulting in a rise in its serum levels, to toxic concentrations in some instances. One study concluded that the inhibition was non-competitive.[7]

Importance and management

An established, moderately well documented, clinically important and potentially serious interaction. It seems to occur in most patients and develops rapidly. Recovery may take 2 to 3 weeks after the **disulfiram** is withdrawn. It has been suggested that the dosage of **phenytoin** could be reduced to accommodate the interaction, but it would be difficult to maintain the balance required. Monitor very closely if both drugs are given.[2]

Alternative anticonvulsants include **phenobarbital** or **carbamazepine**.

Unlike **disulfiram**, **calcium carbimide** appears not to interact.

1. Olesen OV. Disulfiramum (Antabuse®) as inhibitor of phenytoin metabolism. *Acta Pharmacol Toxicol* (1966) 24, 317–22.
2. Olesen OV. The influence of disulfiram and calcium carbimide on the serum diphenylhydantoin excretion of HPPH in the urine. *Arch Neurol* (1967) 16, 642–4.
3. Svendsen TL, Kristensen MB, Hansen JM, Skovsted L. The influence of disulfiram on the half-life and metabolic clearance rate of diphenylhydantoin and tolbutamide in man. *Eur J Clin Pharmacol* (1976) 9, 439–41.
4. Kiørboe E. Phenytoin intoxication during treatment with Antabuse®. *Epilepsia* (1966) 7, 246–9.
5. Kiørboe E. Antabus som årsag til forgiftning med fenytoin. *Ugeskr Laeger* (1966) 128, 1531–6.
6. Dry J, Pradalier A. Intoxication par la phénytoïne au cours d'une association thérapeutique avec le disulfirame. *Therapie* (1973) 28, 799–802.
7. Taylor JW, Alexander B, Lyon LW. Mathematical analysis of a phenytoin-disulfiram interaction. *Am J Hosp Pharm* (1981) 38, 93–5.
8. Krag B, Dam M, Angelo H, Christensen JM. Influence of disulfiram on the serum concentration of carbamazepine in patients with epilepsy. *Acta Neurol Scand* (1981) 63, 395–8.

Anticonvulsants + Calcium channel blockers

(A) Anticonvulsant and toxic effects increased: both diltiazem and verapamil can increase serum carbamazepine levels causing toxicity. Diltiazem can also increase serum phenytoin levels. A single case report describes phenytoin toxicity with nifedipine but, like amlodipine, usually it appears not to interact.

(B) Calcium channel blocker effects altered: the serum levels of felodipine and nimodipine are very markedly reduced by carbamazepine, phenobarbital and phenytoin, but felodipine levels are only modestly reduced by oxcarbazepine. Verapamil levels may also be very much reduced by phenobarbital and phenytoin. Phenytoin reduces nisoldipine levels. Nimodipine levels are raised by sodium valproate, but not carbamazepine, phenobarbital or phenytoin.

Clinical evidence

(A) Anticonvulsant and toxic effects increased

(a) Carbamazepine + Amlodipine, Diltiazem or Nifedipine

An epileptic patient on 1 g **carbamazepine** daily (400 mg in the morning, 600 mg in the evening) developed signs of toxicity (dizziness, nausea, ataxia and diplopia) within 2 days of starting to take 60 mg **diltiazem** three times a day. His serum **carbamazepine** levels had risen by about 40% (to 21 mg/l), but fell once again when the **diltiazem** was stopped. No interaction occurred when the **diltiazem** was replaced by **nifedipine** 20 mg three times a day.[1] Other reports describe **carbamazepine** toxicity and a rise in serum levels of up to fourfold in a total of 10 patients given **diltiazem**.[2-6] One patient required a 62% reduction in **carbamazepine** dose.[2] Another patient showed a marked fall in serum **carbamazepine** levels of 54% when **diltiazem** was stopped.[7] A retrospective study of 5 patients suggested that **nifedipine** does not usually interact with **carbamazepine**.[4] A man showed a marked rise in serum carbamazepine levels when **nifedipine** was replaced by **diltiazem.** When **diltiazem** was replaced by **amlodipine**, his carbamazepine levels returned to normal, suggesting neither **nifedipine** nor **amlodipine** interact.[8]

(b) Carbamazepine or Oxcarbazepine + Verapamil

Carbamazepine toxicity developed in 6 epileptic patients within 36 to 96 h of starting 120 mg **verapamil** three times a day. The symptoms disappeared when the **verapamil** was withdrawn. Total **carbamazepine** serum levels had risen by 46% (33% in free plasma **carbamazepine** concentrations). Rechallenge of 2 of the patients who only showed mild toxicity with a lower dose of **verapamil** (120 mg twice a day) caused a similar rise in serum **verapamil** levels, again with mild toxicity. This report also describes another patient with elevated serum **carbamazepine** levels while taking **verapamil**.[9]

Carbamazepine toxicity is described in 3 other patients, again caused by **verapamil**.[10,11] The **verapamil** was successfully replaced by **nifedipine** in one patient.[10] **Oxcarbazepine** 450 mg twice daily was given to 10 healthy subjects who were then additionally given 120 mg **verapamil** twice daily for 5 days. The AUC of the monohydroxy derivative of the **oxcarbazepine** (the active metabolite) fell by about 20% but **oxcarbazepine** levels were unaltered.[12]

(c) Phenytoin + Diltiazem

Elevated serum phenytoin levels and signs of toxicity developed in 2 out of 14 patients on phenytoin when they were additionally given **diltiazem**.[4] A patient taking 250 mg **phenytoin** twice daily developed signs of toxicity within 2 weeks of starting 240 mg **diltiazem** 8-hourly.[13]

(d) Phenytoin + Nifedipine

An isolated report describes phenytoin toxicity in a man on **phenytoin,** 3 weeks after starting to take 30 mg **nifedipine** daily. His serum **phenytoin** level was 30.4 micrograms/ml. The nifedipine was stopped, and over the next 2 weeks his serum **phenytoin** levels fell to 10.5 micrograms/ml. A further 2 weeks later all the symptoms had

gone.[14] A retrospective study of patients suggested that **nifedipine** does not usually interact.[4]

(B) Calcium channel blocker effects altered

(a) Felodipine + Carbamazepine, Oxcarbazepine, Phenobarbital or Phenytoin

After taking 10 mg **felodipine** daily for 4 days, 10 epileptics on **carbamazepine** or **phenytoin** or **phenobarbital**, or **carbamazepine** with **phenytoin**, had markedly reduced serum **felodipine** levels (peak levels of 1.6 nmol/l compared with 8.9 nmol/l in 12 control subjects). The bioavailability was reduced to 6.6%.[15] Another study in 8 subjects found that the AUC of **felodipine** was reduced by much less (28%) while taking 600 to 900 mg **oxcarbazepine** daily for a week.[16]

(b) Nifedipine + Carbamazepine

A study in 12 epileptics on long-term treatment with **carbamazepine** found that the bioavailability of 20 mg nifedipine was only 22% of the values seen in 12 healthy subjects not taking **carbamazepine**.[17]

(c) Nifedipine + Phenobarbital

After taking 100 mg **phenobarbital** daily for 2 weeks the clearance of a single 20-mg dose of **nifedipine** in a 'cocktail' also containing sparteine, mephenytoin and antipyrine was increased almost threefold in 15 healthy subjects. The **nifedipine** AUC was reduced by about 60%.[18]

(d) Nimodipine + Carbamazepine, Phenobarbital, Phenytoin or Sodium valproate

A study in 8 epileptic patients on long-term treatment with **phenobarbital**, **carbamazepine** with **phenobarbital**, **carbamazepine** with **clobazam,** or **carbamazepine** with **phenytoin** found that the AUC of a single 60-mg oral dose of **nimodipine** was only about 15% of that obtained from a group of healthy subjects. In another group of epileptic patients on **sodium valproate**, the AUC of **nimodipine** was about 50% higher than in the control group.[19]

(e) Nisoldipine + Phenytoin, Phenobarbital or Carbamazepine

Twelve epileptic patients on long-term **phenytoin** treatment and 12 healthy subjects were given single 40- or 20-mg doses of **nisoldipine**. The mean **nisoldipine** AUCs (normalised for a 20-mg dose) were 1.6 micrograms/l/h for the epileptics, and 15.2 micrograms/l/h for the healthy subjects.[20] The authors of this study predict that **carbamazepine** and **phenobarbital** will interact similarly, because like **phenytoin**, they also induce the same enzyme system (cytochrome P450 isoenzyme CYP3A4) but this needs confirmatory clinical studies.

(f) Verapamil + Phenobarbital

A study in 7 healthy subjects showed that after taking 100 mg **phenobarbital** daily for 3 weeks the clearance of **verapamil** 80 mg sixhourly) was increased fourfold and the bioavailability was reduced fivefold.[21]

(g) Verapamil + Phenytoin

A woman on **phenytoin** showed persistently subnormal serum **verapamil** levels (less than 50 nanograms/ml) despite increases in the verapamil dosage from 80 mg twice daily to 160 mg three times daily. When the **phenytoin** was stopped, her serum **verapamil** levels rose to expected concentrations.[22]

Mechanism

It would appear that the calcium channel blockers inhibit the metabolism of carbamazepine and phenytoin by the liver, thereby reducing their loss from the body and increasing serum levels. In contrast, the anticonvulsants are well recognised as enzyme inducers, which can increase the metabolism of the calcium channel blockers by the liver, resulting in a very rapid loss from the body.

Importance and management

(A) Anticonvulsant and toxic effects increased

Information about the effects of calcium channel blockers on anticonvulsants is limited, but what is known indicates that if verapamil or diltiazem are given with carbamazepine, or diltiazem is given with phenytoin, the anticonvulsant dosage may possibly need to be reduced to avoid toxicity. A 50% reduction in the dose of carbamazepine has been suggested if diltiazem is to be used.[5] Nifedipine and amlodipine normally appear to be non-interacting alternatives, but there is an isolated case of a nifedipine interaction with phenytoin. Oxcarbazepine appears to be a non-interacting alternative for carbamazepine. There appears to be no information about the effects of calcium channel blockers on other anticonvulsants.

(B) Calcium channel blocker effects altered

Carbamazepine, phenobarbital and phenytoin markedly reduce felodipine and nimodipine levels, and both phenobarbital and phenytoin can have the same effect on verapamil, and possibly nifedipine. Nisoldipine levels are reduced by phenytoin, and are predicted to be reduced by carbamazepine and phenobarbital. A considerable increase in the dosage of these calcium channel blockers will probably be needed in epileptic patients taking these drugs, but oxcarbazepine has only a moderate effect. The nimodipine dosage may need to be reduced with sodium valproate. There is no direct information of interactions with other calcium channel blockers, but be alert for evidence of reduced effects with others metabolised in a similar way.

1. Brodie MJ, Macphee GJA. Carbamazepine neurotoxicity precipitated by diltiazem. *BMJ* (1986) 292, 1170–1.
2. Eimer M, Carter BL. Elevated serum carbamazepine concentrations following diltiazem initiation. *Drug Intell Clin Pharm* (1987) 21, 340–2.
3. Ahmad S. Diltiazem-carbamazepine interaction. *Am Heart J* (1990) 120, 1485.
4. Bahls FH, Ozuna J, Ritchie DE. Interactions between calcium channel blockers and the anticonvulsants carbamazepine and phenytoin. *Neurology* (1991) 41, 740–2.
5. Shaughnessy AF, Mosley MR. Elevated carbamazepine levels associated with diltiazem use. *Neurology* (1992) 42, 937–8.
6. Maoz E, Grossman E, Thaler M, Rosenthal T. Carbamazepine neurotoxic reaction after administration of diltiazem. *Arch Intern Med* (1992) 152, 2503–4.
7. Gadde K, Calabrese JR. Diltiazem effect on carbamazepine levels in manic depression. *J Clin Psychopharmacol* (1990) 10, 378–9.
8. Cuadrado A, Sánchez MB, Peralta G, González M, Verdejo A, Amat G, Bravo J, Fdez Cortizo MJ, Adín J, De Cos MA, Mediavilla A, Armijo JA. Carbamazepine-amlodipine: a free interaction association? *Methods Find Exp Clin Pharmacol* (1996) 18 (Suppl C), 65.
9. Macphee GJA, McInnes GT, Thompson GG, Brodie MJ. Verapamil potentiates carbamazepine neurotoxicity: a clinically important inhibitory interaction. *Lancet* (1986) i, 700–3.
10. Beattie B, Biller J, Mehlhaus B, Murray M. Verapamil-induced carbamazepine neurotoxicity. *Eur Neurol* (1988) 28, 104–5.
11. Price WA, DiMarzio LR. Verapamil-carbamazepine neurotoxicity. *J Clin Psychiatry* (1988) 49, 80.
12. Krämer G, Tettenborn B, Flesch G. Oxcarbazepine-verapamil drug interaction in healthy volunteers. *Epilepsia* (1991) 32 (Suppl 1), 70–1.
13. Clarke WR, Horn JR, Kawabori I, Gurtel S. Potentially serious drug interactions secondary to high-dose diltiazem used in the treatment of pulmonary hypertension. *Pharmacotherapy* (1993) 13, 402–5.
14. Ahmad S. Nifedipine-phenytoin interaction. *J Am Coll Cardiol* (1984) 3, 1582.

Table 7.2 Cases of anticonvulsant and cytotoxic drug interactions

Anticonvulsant	Cytotoxic agents	Malignancy	Outcome	Ref
Phenytoin (Diphenylhydantoin)	Cisplatin Vinblastine Bleomycin	Metastatic germ cell tumour	Estimated phenytoin level 15 micrograms/ml, but level only reached 2 micrograms/ml. Patient fitted.	2
Phenytoin (Diphenylhydantoin) Primidone	Cisplatin Vinblastine Bleomycin	Metastatic embryonal cell cancer	Phenytoin 800 mg daily gave a level of 15 micrograms/ml whilst on chemotherapy. After chemotherapy the same dose produced a toxic level of 42.8 micrograms/ml. Phenobarbital levels unaffected.	3
Phenytoin (Diphenylhydantoin) Phenobarbital (Phenobarbitone)	Vinblastine Carmustine Methotrexate	Lung cancer with brain metastases	Phenytoin levels fell from 9.4 to 5.6 micrograms/ml 24 h after vinblastine. Patient fitted. Phenytoin levels returned to normal 2 weeks after chemotherapy. Phenobarbital levels unaffected.	4
Phenytoin (Diphenylhydantoin) Carbamazepine Sodium valproate	Doxorubicin (Adriamycin) Cisplatin Cyclophosphamide Altretamine	Papillary adenocarcinoma of the ovaries	Seizures occurred 2 to 3 days after starting chemotherapy. All drug levels dropped to one-third or lower. Doses increased to compensate, which led to phentoin toxicity when the chemotherapy finished.	5
Phenytoin (Diphenylhydantoin)	Carboplatin	Small cell lung cancer with brain metastases	Phenytoin level dropped from 9.7 micrograms/ml 10 days into chemotherapy, resulting in seizures. Phenytoin dose had to be increased by 35% to achieve a level of 10.7 micrograms/ml.	8
Phenytoin (Diphenylhydantoin)	Dacarbazine Carmustine Cisplatin Tamoxifen	Malignant melanoma with brain metastases	Phenytoin level of only 2.5 micrograms/ml despite a loading 1 g dose and a daily dose of 500 mg phenytoin.	9
Phenytoin (Diphenylhydantoin) followed by Carbamazepine	Vincristine Cytarabine Hydroxycarbamide (Hydroxyurea) Duanorubicin Methotrexate Tioguanine (Thioguanine) Cyclophosphamide Carmustine	Stage IV T-cell lymphoma	Phenytoin failed to reach therapeutic levels and so was substituted with carbamazepine. Chemotherapy caused carbamazepine levels to drop below therapeutic resulting in seizures. Increasing the dose from 30 to 50 mg/kg/day prevented subtherapeutic levels.	6
Phenytoin (Diphenylhydantoin)	Methotrexate 6-Mercaptopurine Vincristine	Acute lymphoblastic leukaemia	Phenytoin levels dropped from 19.8 micrograms/ml on the day before chemotherapy to 3.6 micrograms/ml on the 6th day of chemotherapy.	7

15. Capewell S, Freestone S, Critchley JAJH, Pottage A, Prescott LF. Reduced felodipine bioavailability in patients taking anticonvulsants. *Lancet* (1988) ii, 480–2.
16. Zaccara G, Galimberti PW, Bendoni L, Menge GP, Schwabe S, Monza GC. Influence of single and repeated doses of oxcarbazepine on the pharmacokinetic profile of felodipine. *Ther Drug Monit* (1993) 15, 39–42.
17. Routledge PA, Soryal I, Eve MD, Williams J, Richens A, Hall R. Reduced bioavailability of nifedipine in patients with epilepsy receiving anticonvulsants. *Br J Clin Pharmacol* (1998) 45, 196P.
18. Schellens JHM, van der Wart JHF, Brugman M, Breimer DD. Influence of enzyme induction and inhibition on the oxidation of nifedipine, sparteine, mephenytoin and antipyrine in humans assessed by a cocktail study design. *J Pharmacol Exp Ther* (1989) 249, 638–45.
19. Tartara A, Galimberti CA, Manni R, Parietti L, Zucca C, Baasch H, Caresia L, Mück W, Barzaghi N, Gatti G, Perucca E. Differential effects of valproic acid and enzyme-inducing anticonvulsants on nimodipine pharmacokinetics in epileptic patients. *Br J Clin Pharmacol* (1991) 32, 335–40.
20. Michelucci R, Cipolla G, Passarelli D, Gatti G, Ochan M, Heinig R, Tassinari CA, Perucca E. Reduced plasma nisoldipine concentrations in phenytoin-treated patients with epilepsy. *Epilepsia* (1996) 37, 1107–10.
21. Rutledge DR, Pieper JA, Sirmans SM, Mirvis DM. Verapamil disposition after phenobarbital treatment. *Clin Pharmacol Ther* (1987) 41, 245.
22. Woodcock BG, Kirsten R, Nelson K, Rietbrock S, Hopf R, Kaltenbach M. A reduction in verapamil concentrations with phenytoin. *N Engl J Med* (1991) 325, 1179.

Anticonvulsants + Cytotoxic drugs

Carbamazepine, phenytoin and sodium valproate serum levels can fall during concurrent treatment with several cytotoxic drug regimens and seizures can occur if the anticonvulsant dosages are not raised appropriately. In contrast tegafur has been responsible for causing acute phenytoin toxicity. The effects of some cytotoxics are reduced or changed by anticonvulsants.

Clinical evidence

(a) Anticonvulsant levels reduced

A retrospective study reviewed the effects of 3 to 4 week cycles of 72 h of **carmustine** and **cisplatin** chemotherapy on the **phenytoin** levels of patients with brain tumours. Patients that vomited because of the chemotherapy were excluded, leaving 19 patients for assessment. A **phenytoin** dose increase was required in three-quarters of patients, which was, on average, 40% of the original dose (range 20 to 100%). The effect on phenytoin levels persisted after the chemotherapy had finished, with levels returning to normal 2 to 3 weeks later.[1]

There are many other case reports[2-9] of a variety of types of chemotherapy having a similar effect. See Table 7.2 for details.

(b) Anticonvulsant levels raised

Three patients with malignant brain tumours developed acute **phenytoin** toxicity associated with raised serum phenytoin levels when concurrently treated with *UFT* (**uracil** and **tegafur**, a prodrug of **fluorouracil**). One of the patients showed no interaction when the *UFT* was replaced by **fluorouracil**.[10] Acute **phenytoin** toxicity has also been described with **tegafur** alone.[11]

(c) Cytotoxic effects reduced or altered

See 'Doxorubicin (Adriamycin) + Barbiturates', p.500, 'Ifosfamide + Barbiturates', p.505, 'Streptozocin + Phenytoin', p.522, 'Teniposide + Anticonvulsants', p.523.

Mechanisms

Not fully understood, but a suggested reason for the fall in serum anticonvulsant levels is that these cytotoxic drugs damage the intestinal wall, which reduces the absorption of the anticonvulsants. Other mechanisms may also have some part to play. The raised serum phenytoin levels possibly occur because the liver metabolism of the phenytoin is reduced by these cytotoxics. Changes in plasma protein binding may also have been involved.

Importance and management

Information is scattered and incomplete. Serum anticonvulsant levels should be closely monitored during treatment with any of these cytotoxics, making dosage adjustments as necessary. It is not always easy to know which of the individual cytotoxic drugs was responsible for the changed serum anticonvulsant levels.

1. Grossman SA, Sheidler VR, Gilbert MR. Decreased phenytoin levels in patients receiving chemotherapy. *Am J Med* (1989) 87, 505–10.
2. Sylvester RK, Lewis FB, Caldwell KC, Lobell M, Perri R, Sawchuk RA. Impaired phenytoin bioavailability secondary to cisplatinum, vinblastine, and bleomycin. *Ther Drug Monit* (1984) 6, 302–5.
3. Fincham RW, Schottelius DD. Case report. Decreased phenytoin levels in antineoplastic therapy. *Ther Drug Monit* (1979) 1, 277–83.
4. Bollini P, Riva R, Albani F, Ida N, Cacciari L, Bollini C, Baruzzi A. Decreased phenytoin level during antineoplastic therapy: a case report. *Epilepsia* (1983) 24, 75–8.
5. Neef C, de Voogd-van der Straaten I. An interaction between cytostatic and anticonvulsant drugs. *Clin Pharmacol Ther* (1988) 43, 372–5.
6. Nahum MP, Ben Arush MW, Robinson E. Reduced plasma carbamazepine level during chemotherapy in a child with malignant lymphoma. *Acta Paediatr Scand* (1990) 79, 873–5.
7. Jarosinski PF, Moscow JA, Alexander MS, Lesko LJ, Balis FM, Poplack DG. Altered phenytoin clearance during intensive treatment for acute lymphoblastic leukemia. *J Pediatr* (1988) 112, 996–9.
8. Dofferhoff ASM, Berensen HH, Naalt Jvd, Haaxma-Reiche H, Smit EF, Postmus PE. Decreased phenytoin level after carboplatin treatment. *Am J Med* (1990) 89, 247–8.
9. Gattis WA, May DB. Possible interaction involving phenytoin, dexamethasone, and antineoplastic agents: a case report and review. *Ann Pharmacother* (1996) 30, 520–6.
10. Wakisaka S, Shimauchi M, Kaji Y, Nonaka A, Kinoshita K. Acute phenytoin intoxication associated with the antineoplastic agent UFT. *Fukuoka Igaku Zasshi* (1990) 81, 192–6.
11. Hara T, Ichimiya A. Acute phenytoin intoxication caused by drug interaction with an antitumour agent, tegafur. 20th Jpn Conf Epilepsia, Tokyo, Nov 1986.

Anticonvulsants + Dextromethorphan

Dextromethorphan appears not to affect the serum levels of carbamazepine or phenytoin.

Clinical evidence, mechanism, importance and management

A double-blind crossover study in epileptic patients with severe complex partial seizures, 5 on **carbamazepine** and 4 on **phenytoin**, found that the concurrent use of **dextromethorphan** 120 mg daily in liquid form (*Delsym*) over 3 months had no effect on the serum anticonvulsant levels. There was a non-significant alteration in the complex partial seizure and tonic-clonic seizure frequency.[1]

1. Fisher RS, Cysyk BJ, Lesser RP, Pontecorvo MJ, Ferkany JT, Schwerdt PR, Hart J, Gordon B. Dextromethorphan for treatment of complex partial seizures. *Neurology* (1990) 40, 547–9.

Anticonvulsants + Dextropropoxyphene (Propoxyphene)

Carbamazepine serum levels can be raised by the concurrent use of dextropropoxyphene. Toxicity may develop unless suitable dosage reductions are made. A trivial or only modest rise in serum phenytoin or phenobarbital levels may occur so that the development of toxicity is unlikely in most patients. Oxcarbazepine appears not to interact with dextropropoxyphene.

Clinical evidence

(a) Carbamazepine

The observation of toxicity (headache, dizziness, ataxia, nausea, tiredness) in patients during the concurrent use of **carbamazepine** and **dextropropoxyphene** (**propoxyphene**) prompted further study. Five **carbamazepine**-treated patients given 65 mg **dextropropoxyphene** three times daily showed a mean rise in serum **carbamazepine** levels of 65%, and 3 showed evidence of **carbamazepine** toxicity. **Carbamazepine** levels were not taken in a further 2 patients because they withdrew after 2 days of treatment due to side effects.[1,2] In a further study a 66% rise in **carbamazepine** levels was seen after 6 days treatment with **dextropropoxyphene**.[3]

Carbamazepine toxicity due to this interaction is reported elsewhere,[4-7] and rises in trough serum **carbamazepine** levels of 69 to 600% have been described.[8] A study in the elderly compared groups of patients taking either **carbamazepine** or **dextropropoxyphene** alone, with patients on both drugs (21 subjects). The **carbamazepine** dose was about a third lower in those receiving combined treatment, yet the mean serum **carbamazepine** levels were still 25% higher than in the patients not taking **dextropropoxyphene**. The prevalence of side-effects was also higher in patients on both drugs.[9]

(b) Oxcarbazepine

Dextropropoxyphene 65 mg three times daily for 7 days did not affect the steady-state levels of the active metabolite of **oxcarbazepine** in 7 patients with epilepsy or trigeminal neuralgia.[10]

(c) Phenobarbital

An average rise in the serum **phenobarbital** levels of 20% was seen in 4 epileptic patients after taking **dextropropoxyphene** 65 mg three times a day for a week.[3]

(d) Phenytoin

Only a very small rise in serum **phenytoin** levels occurred in 6 patients when concurrently treated with **dextropropoxyphene** 65 mg three times daily for 6 to 13 days.[3] In contrast, a review briefly mentions one patient who developed toxic serum **phenytoin** levels while taking **dextropropoxyphene** (up to 600 mg daily) on an as required basis.[11]

Mechanism

Uncertain. It is suggested that the dextropropoxyphene inhibits the metabolism of the carbamazepine by the liver enzymes, leading to its accumulation in the body.[1,2] This may also be true to a much lesser extent for the phenobarbital.

Importance and management

The carbamazepine/dextropropoxyphene interaction is very well established and clinically important. If concurrent use is necessary reduce the dosage of carbamazepine appropriately (by about one-third, or more) to prevent the development of toxicity. In many cases it may be simpler to use a non-interacting analgesic, although the occasional single dose of dextropropoxyphene probably does not matter. The concurrent use of dextropropoxyphene and either phenytoin or phenobarbital need not be avoided, but since rises in the serum levels of both anticonvulsants can occur it would be prudent to monitor the outcome. It is probably sufficient just to monitor for increased side-effects. No special precautions seem necessary with oxcarbazepine.

1. Dam M, Christiansen J. Interaction of propoxyphene with carbamazepine. *Lancet* (1977) ii, 509.
2. Dam M, Kristensen CB, Hansen BS, Christiansen J. Interaction between carbamazepine and propoxyphene in man. *Acta Neurol Scand* (1977) 56, 603–7.
3. Hansen BS, Dam M, Brandt J, Hvidberg EF, Angelo H, Christensen JM, Lous P. Influence of dextropropoxyphene on steady state serum levels and protein binding of three anti-epileptic drugs in man. *Acta Neurol Scand* (1980) 61, 357–67.
4. Yu YL, Huang CY, Chin D, Woo E, Chang CM. Interaction between carbamazepine and dextropropoxyphene. *Postgrad Med J* (1986) 62, 231–3.
5. Kubacka RT, Ferrante JA. Carbamazepine-propoxyphene interaction. *Clin Pharm* (1983) 2, 104.
6. Risinger MW. Carbamazepine toxicity with concurrent use of propoxyphene: a report of five cases. *Neurology* (1987) 37 (Suppl 1), 87.
7. Allen S. Cerebellar dysfunction following dextropropoxyphene-induced carbamazepine toxicity. *Postgrad Med J* (1994) 70, 764.
8. Oles KS, Mirza W, Penry JK. Catastrophic neurologic signs due to drug interaction: Tegretol and Darvon. *Surg Neurol* (1989) 32, 144–51.
9. Bergendal L, Friberg A, Schaffrath AM, Holmdahl M, Landahl S. The clinical relevance of the interaction between carbamazepine and dextropropoxyphene in elderly patients in Gothenburg, Sweden. *Eur J Clin Pharmacol* (1997) 53, 203–6.
10. Mogensen PH, Jorgensen L, Boas J, Dam M, Vesterager A, Flesch G, Jensen PK. Effects of dextropropoxyphene on the steady-state kinetics of oxcarbazepine and its metabolites. *Acta Neurol Scand* (1992) 85, 14–17.
11. Kutt H. Biochemical and genetic factors regulating Dilantin metabolism in man. *Ann N Y Acad Sci* (1971) 179, 704–22.

Anticonvulsants + Erythromycin

Carbamazepine serum levels can very rapidly rise to toxic concentrations if erythromycin is given concurrently. Toxicity has been described in many reports. See also 'Carbamazepine + Macrolide antibacterials', p.328. An isolated report describes sodium valproate intoxication in a woman given erythromycin. Erythromycin appears not to interact with oxcarbazepine or phenytoin.

Clinical evidence

(a) Carbamazepine

A girl of 8 on 50 mg **phenobarbital** and 800 mg **carbamazepine** daily was additionally given 500 mg and later 1000 mg **erythromycin** daily. Within 2 days she began to experience balancing difficulties and ataxia which were eventually attributed to **carbamazepine** toxicity. Her serum **carbamazepine** levels were found to have risen from a little below 10 micrograms/ml to over 25 micrograms/ml (therapeutic range 2 to 10 micrograms/ml). The levels rapidly returned to normal after **carbamazepine** was withheld for 24 h and the erythromycin stopped.[1]

A study in 7 healthy subjects confirmed that erythromycin can cause significant increases in carbamazepine levels,[2] and a study in 8 healthy subjects showed that the clearance of **carbamazepine** is reduced by an average of 20% (range 5 to 41%) by concurrent use of erythromycin 1g daily for 5 days.[3]

Marked rises in serum **carbamazepine** levels (up to fivefold in some cases) and/or toxicity (including cases of hepatorenal failure and AV block as well as more typical signs of carbamazepine toxicity) have been described in over 30 cases involving both children and adults. Symptoms commonly began within 24 to 72 h of starting **erythromycin**, although in some cases it was as early as 8 h. In most cases toxicity resolved within 3 to 5 days of stopping the **erythromycin**.[4-23]

(b) Oxcarbazepine

The pharmacokinetics of single 600-mg doses of **oxcarbazepine** in 8 healthy subjects were unaffected by 7 days' treatment with 500 mg **erythromycin** twice daily.[24]

(c) Phenytoin

A single-dose study showed that the mean clearance of **phenytoin** was unchanged by 7 days of **erythromycin** treatment in 8 healthy subjects. However, there were occasional large changes in phenytoin clearance.[25]

(d) Sodium valproate

A woman taking lithium and high-dose **sodium valproate** (3500 mg daily) developed fatigue and walking difficulties a day after starting 250 mg **erythromycin** four times daily. Within a week she had also developed slurred speech, confusion, difficulty in concentrating and a worsening gait. Her serum **valproate** levels had risen from 88 mg/l (measured 2 months before) to 260 mg/l. She recovered within 24 h of the **valproate** and **erythromycin** being withdrawn. Her serum lithium levels remained unchanged.[26] This case report contrasts with another study in a 10-year-old boy taking 375 mg **sodium valproate** twice daily who showed only very small and clinically unimportant changes in the pharmacokinetics of the valproate, consistent with inhibition of cytochrome P450 metabolism, when given 250 mg **erythromycin** four times daily.[27]

Mechanism

It is suggested[28] that erythromycin has a high affinity for the active site on the cytochrome P450 isoenzyme CYP3A4 which is concerned with the metabolism of the carbamazepine. Consequently the metabolism of carbamazepine is rapidly and markedly inhibited, resulting in its rapid accumulation which leads to toxicity.

Importance and management

The carbamazepine/erythromycin interaction is very well documented, well established and of clinical importance. Its incidence is uncertain but concurrent use should be avoided unless the effects can be very closely monitored by measurement of serum carbamazepine levels and suitable dosage reductions made. Toxic symptoms (ataxia, vertigo, drowsiness, lethargy, confusion, diplopia) can develop within 24 h, but serum carbamazepine levels can return to normal within

8 to 12 h of withdrawing the antibacterial.[11] Some other macrolide antibacterials interact similarly — see 'Carbamazepine + Macrolide antibacterials', p.328. There is only a single case report of erythromycin interacting with sodium valproate, and erythromycin appears not to interact with oxcarbazepine or phenytoin.

1. Amedee-Manesme O, Rey E, Brussieux J, Goutieres F and Aicardi J. Antibiotiques à ne jamais associer à la carbamazépine. *Arch Fr Pediatr* (1982) 39, 126.
2. Miles MV, Tennison MB. Erythromycin effects on multiple-dose carbamazepine kinetics. *Ther Drug Monit* (1989) 11, 47–52.
3. Wong YY, Ludden TM, Bell RD. Effect of erythromycin on carbamazepine kinetics. *Drug Intell Clin Pharm* (1982) 16, 484.
4. Straughan J. Erythromycin-carbamazepine interaction? *S Afr Med J* (1982) 61, 420–1.
5. Mesdjian E, Dravet C, Cenraud B, Roger J. Carbamazepine intoxication due to triacetyloleandomycin administration in epileptic patients. *Epilepsia* (1980) 21, 489–96.
6. Vajda FJE, Bladin PF. Carbamazepine-erythromycin-base interaction. *Med J Aust* (1984) 140, 81.
7. Hedrick R, Williams F, Morin R, Lamb WA, Cate JC. Carbamazepine-erythromycin interaction leading to carbamazepine toxicity in four epileptic children. *Ther Drug Monit* (1983) 5, 405–7.
8. Miller SL. The association of carbamazepine intoxication and erythromycin use. *Ann Neurol* (1985) 18, 413.
9. Berrettini WH. A case of erythromycin-induced carbamazepine toxicity. *J Clin Psychiatry* (1986) 47, 147.
10. Carranco E, Kareus J, Co S, Peak V, Al-Rajeh S. Carbamazepine toxicity induced by concurrent erythromycin therapy. *Arch Neurol* (1985) 42, 187–8.
11. Goulden KJ, Camfield P, Dooley JM, Fraser A, Meek DC, Renton KW, Tibbles JAR. Severe carbamazepine intoxication after coadministration of erythromycin. *J Pediatr* (1986) 109, 135–8.
12. Wroblewski BA, Singer WD, Whyte J. Carbamazepine-erythromycin interaction. Case studies and clinical significance. *JAMA* (1986) 255, 1165–7.
13. Kessler JM. Erythromycin-carbamazepine interaction. *S Afr Med J* (1985) 67, 1038.
14. Jaster PJ, Abbas D. Erythromycin-carbamazepine interaction. *Neurology* (1986) 36, 594–5.
15. Loiseau P, Guyot M, Pautrizel B, Vincon G, Albin H. Intoxication par la carbamazépine due à l'interaction carbamazepine-érythromycine. *Presse Med* (1985) 14, 162.
16. Zitelli BJ, Howrie DL, Altman H, Marcon TJ. Erythromycin-induced drug interactions. *Clin Pediatr (Phila)* (1987) 26, 117–19.
17. Goldhoorn PB, Hofstee N. Een interactie tussen erytromycine en carbamazepine. *Ned Tijdschr Geneeskd* (1989) 133, 1944.
18. Mitsch RA. Carbamazepine toxicity precipitated by intravenous erythromycin. *DICP Ann Pharmacother* (1989) 23, 878–9.
19. Macnab AJ, Robinson JL, Adderly RJ, D'Orsogna L. Heart block secondary to erythromycin-induced carbamazepine toxicity. *Pediatrics* (1987) 80, 951–3.
20. Woody RC, Kearns GL, Bolyard KJ. Carbamazepine intoxication following the use of erythromycin in children. *Pediatr Infect Dis J* (1987) 6, 578–9.
21. Stafstrom CE, Nohria V, Loganbill H, Nahouraii R, Boustany R-M, DeLong GR. Erythromycin-induced carbamazepine toxicity: a continuing problem. *Arch Pediatr Adolesc Med* (1995) 149, 99–101.
22. Mota CR, Carvalho C, Mota C, Ferreira P, Vilarinho A, Pereira E. Severe carbamazepine toxicity induced by concurrent erythromycin therapy. *Eur J Pediatr* (1996) 155, 345–8.
23. Viani F, Claris-Appiani A, Rossi LN, Giani M, Romeo A. Severe hepatorenal failure in a child receiving carbamazepine and erythromycin. *Eur J Pediatr* (1992) 151, 715–16.
24. Keränen T, Jolkkonen J, Jensen PK, Menge GP, Andersson P. Absence of interaction between oxcarbazepine and erythromycin. *Acta Neurol Scand* (1992) 86, 120–3.
25. Bachmann K, Schwartz JI, Forney RB, Jauregui L. Single dose phenytoin clearance during erythromycin treatment. *Res Commun Chem Pathol Pharmacol* (1984) 46, 207–17.
26. Redington K, Wells C, Petito F. Erythromycin and valproate interaction. *Ann Intern Med* (1992) 116, 877–8.
27. Gopaul SV, Farrell K, Rakshi K, Abbott FS. A case study of erythromycin interaction with valproic acid. *Pharm Res* (1996) 13 (9 Suppl), S434.
28. Levy RH, Johnson CM, Thummel KE, Kerr BM, Kroetz DL, Korzecwa KR, Gonzales FJ. Mechanism of the interaction between carbamazepine and erythromycin. *Epilepsia* (1993) 34 (Suppl 6), 37–8.

Anticonvulsants + Folic acid

If folic acid supplements are given to treat folate deficiency, which can be caused by the use of anticonvulsants (phenytoin, phenobarbital, primidone and possibly pheneturide), the serum anticonvulsant levels may fall, leading to decreased seizure control in some patients.

Clinical evidence

A study on 50 folate-deficient epileptics (taking **phenytoin, phenobarbital** and **primidone** in various combinations) found that after one months' treatment with 5 mg **folic acid** daily, the serum **phenytoin** levels of one group of 10 patients had fallen from 20 to 10 micrograms/ml. In another group of patients taking 15 mg folic acid daily the levels of **phenytoin** fell from 14 to 11 micrograms/ml. Only one patient (in the 5 mg folic acid group) showed a marked increase in fit frequency and severity. No alterations were seen in the phenobarbital levels.[1]

Another long-term study was conducted in 26 patients with folic acid deficiency (serum folate less than 5 ng/ml), and treated with two

or more drugs (**phenytoin, phenobarbital, primidone**). The mental state of 22 of them (as shown by increased alertness, concentration, sociability etc) improved to a variable degree when they were given 5 mg **folic acid** three times daily. However, the frequency and severity of fits in 13 patients (50%) increased to such an extent that the vitamin had to be withdrawn from 9 of them.[2]

Similar results both of increased seizure activity and decreased serum folate levels have been described in other studies and reports.[3-5]

Mechanism

Patients on anticonvulsants may have subnormal serum folic acid levels and frequencies of 27 to 76% have been reported.[6] It is believed that this is due to the enzyme-inducing characteristics of the anticonvulsants, which make excessive demands on folate for the synthesis of the cytochromic enzymes concerned with drug metabolism. Ultimately drug metabolism becomes limited by the lack of folate, and patients may also develop a depression in their general mental health[2] and even frank megaloblastic anaemia.[6,7] If folic acid is then given to treat this deficiency, the metabolism of the anticonvulsant increases once again,[8] resulting in a reduction in serum anticonvulsant levels, which in some instances may become so low that seizure control is partially or totally lost.

Importance and management

A very well documented and clinically important interaction (only a few references are listed here). Reductions in serum phenytoin levels of 16 to 50% after taking 5 to 15 mg folic acid daily for 2 to 4 weeks have been described.[1,3,9] The incidence is uncertain. If folic acid supplements are given to folate-deficient epileptics taking phenytoin, phenobarbital, primidone and possibly pheneturide, their serum anticonvulsant levels should be well monitored so that suitable dosage increases can be made.

1. Baylis EM, Crowley JM, Preece JM, Sylvester PE, Marks V. Influence of folic acid on blood-phenytoin levels. *Lancet* (1971) i, 62–4.
2. Reynolds EH. Effects of folic acid on the mental state and fit-frequency of drug-treated epileptic patients. *Lancet* (1967) i, 1086–9.
3. Strauss RG, Bernstein R. Folic acid and Dilantin antagonism in pregnancy. *Obstet Gynecol* (1974) 44, 345–8.
4. Latham AN, Millbank L, Richens A, Rowe DJF. Liver enzyme induction by anticonvulsant drugs, and its relationship to disturbed calcium and folic acid metabolism. *J Clin Pharmacol* (1973) 13, 337–42.
5. Berg MJ, Fincham RW, Ebert BE, Schottelius DD. Phenytoin pharmacokinetics: before and after folic acid administration. *Epilepsia* (1992) 33, 712–20.
6. Davis RE, Woodliff HJ. Folic acid deficiency in patients receiving anticonvulsant drugs. *Med J Aust* (1971) 2, 1070–2.
7. Ryan GMS, Forshaw JWB. Megaloblastic anaemia due to phenytoin sodium. *BMJ* (1955) 11, 242–3.
8. Berg MJ, Fischer LJ, Rivey MP, Vern BA, Lantz RK, Schottelius DD. Phenytoin and folic acid interaction: a preliminary report. *Ther Drug Monit* (1983) 5, 389–94.
9. Furlanut M, Benetello P, Avogaro A, Dainese R. Effects of folic acid on phenytoin kinetics in healthy subjects. *Clin Pharmacol Ther* (1978) 24, 294–7.

Anticonvulsants + Gabapentin

Gabapentin does not normally affect the pharmacokinetics of carbamazepine, phenytoin, phenobarbital or sodium valproate, and no dosage adjustments are needed if it is used concurrently. However, an isolated report describes increased phenytoin levels and toxicity in one patient when given gabapentin.

Clinical evidence, mechanism, importance and management

The pharmacokinetics of both **phenytoin** and **gabapentin** remained unchanged in 8 epileptics who were given 400 mg **gabapentin** three times daily for 8 days, in addition to their normal phenytoin treatment, which they had been taking for at least 2 months.[1] Other studies confirm that the steady-state pharmacokinetics of **phenytoin** are unaffected by **gabapentin**, and that the pharmacokinetics of **gabapentin** are similarly unaffected by **phenytoin**.[2-4] These reports contrast with an isolated report of a patient on **phenytoin, carbamazepine** and **clobazam** whose serum **phenytoin** levels increased three to fourfold, with symptoms of toxicity on two occasions when given 300 to 600 mg **gabapentin** daily. **Carbamazepine** serum levels remained unchanged. The author suggests that this differing reaction may be because the patient was on more than one anti-epileptic drug, unlike previous studies where only single agents had been used.[5]

Gabapentin does not affect **phenobarbital** levels, nor is it affected by **phenobarbital**.[2,3,6] Other studies confirm that the steady-state pharmacokinetics of **carbamazepine** and **sodium valproate** are unaffected by **gabapentin**, and that the pharmacokinetics of **gabapentin** are similarly unaffected by these anticonvulsants.[2-4]

It would seem therefore that no dosage adjustments are normally needed if **gabapentin** is added to treatment with most of these anticonvulsants. However, if **gabapentin** is added to **phenytoin** it may be wise to bear the possibility of raised **phenytoin** levels in mind. See also 'Felbamate + Gabapentin', p.335.

1. Anhut H, Leppik I, Schmidt B, Thomann P. Drug interaction study of the new anticonvulsant gabapentin with phenytoin in epileptic patients. *Naunyn Schmiedebergs Arch Pharmacol* (1988) 337 (Suppl), R127.
2. Brockbrader HN, Radulovic LL, Loewen G, Chang T, Welling PG, Reece PA, Underwood B, Sedman AJ. Lack of drug-drug interactions between Neurontin (gabapentin) and other antiepileptic drugs. 20th International Epilepsy Congress, Oslo, Norway. July 1993 (Abstract).
3. Richens A. Clinical pharmacokinetics of gabapentin.New Trends in Epilepsy Management: The Role of Gabapentin International Congress and Symposium Series No 198, Royal Society of Medicine Services, London, NY 1993, 41–6.
4. Radulovic LL, Wilder BJ, Leppik IE, Bockbrader HN, Chang T, Posvar EL, Sedman AJ, Uthman BM, Erdman GR. Lack of interaction of gabapentin with carbamazepine or valproate. *Epilepsia* (1994) 35, 155–61.
5. Tyndel F. Interaction of gabapentin with other antiepileptics. *Lancet* (1994) 343, 1363–4.
6. Hooper WD, Kavanagh MC, Herkes GK, Eadie MJ. Lack of a pharmacokinetic interaction between phenobarbitone and gabapentin. *Br J Clin Pharmacol* (1991) 31, 171–4.

Anticonvulsants + Mefloquine

An epileptic woman controlled on sodium valproate developed convulsions when given mefloquine. Mefloquine is normally contraindicated in epileptics.

Clinical evidence, mechanism, importance and management

An isolated report describes a woman of 20, with a 7-year history of epilepsy (bilateral myoclonus and generalised tonic-clonic seizures) treated with 1300 mg **sodium valproate** daily, who developed tonic-clonic seizures 8 h after taking the second of 3 prophylactic doses of 250 mg **mefloquine**.[1] It is not clear whether this resulted from a drug-drug or a drug-disease interaction. The makers of **mefloquine** advise its avoidance in those with a history of convulsions as it may increase the risk of convulsions. In these patients **mefloquine** should be used only for curative treatment if compelling reasons exist.[2]

1. Besser R, Krämer G. Verdacht auf anfallfördernde Wirkung von Mefloquin (Lariam®). *Nervenarzt* (1991) 62, 760–1.
2. Lariam (Mefloquine). Roche Products Limited. Summary of product characteristics, August 2000.

Anticonvulsants + Oxcarbazepine

Oxcarbazepine appears not to affect the pharmacokinetics of carbamazepine, phenytoin or sodium valproate. Phenytoin and phenobarbital can increase the loss of the active metabolite of oxcarbazepine. However, in practical terms there appear to be no clinically relevant adverse interactions if oxcarbazepine is given with any of these anticonvulsants.

Clinical evidence

(a) Effects of oxcarbazepine on other anticonvulsants

A double-blind crossover comparison of **oxcarbazepine** and **carbamazepine** in 42 epileptics found that when **carbamazepine** was replaced by **oxcarbazepine**, the serum levels of concurrent **sodium valproate** rose by 32%, and the serum levels of **phenytoin** rose by 23%. In patients taking both **sodium valproate** and **phenytoin** to-

gether, **oxcarbazepine** caused a rise in the serum levels of 21 and 25% respectively. The trial extended over 12 weeks to establish steady-state levels.[1] Another study in 4 young epileptics (aged 13 to 17) found that the level to dose ratio of free **sodium valproate** rose when switched from **carbamazepine** to **oxcarbazepine**, with an increase in sodium valproate side-effects, which resolved when the valproate dose was decreased.[2]

A later study in 35 epileptic patients found that 300 mg **oxcarbazepine** three times daily added to treatment with **carbamazepine**, **sodium valproate** or **phenytoin** for 3 weeks caused no clinically relevant changes in the pharmacokinetics of any of these anticonvulsants.[3]

(b) Effects of other anticonvulsants on oxcarbazepine

The pharmacokinetics of **oxcarbazepine** and its active metabolite (**10-hydroxy-carbazepine**) were not significantly affected by **sodium valproate**, but the AUCs of both were reduced (by 43% and 25%) by **phenobarbital**.[4] Similarly a study found a 29% reduction in the AUC of **10-hydroxy-carbazepine** with **phenytoin**.[3] Another study also showed that the serum levels of the active metabolite **10-hydroxy-carbazepine** were not affected by **phenobarbital** or **phenytoin** but the further conversion of the **10-hydroxy-carbazepine** to *trans*-10,11-dihydroxy-10,11-dihydrocarbamazepine was increased.[5] Since the conversion to *trans*-10,11-dihydroxy-10,11-dihydrocarbamazepine is a minor step in the metabolism of **10-hydroxy-carbazepine**, the overall anti-epileptic action of oxcarbazepine is unlikely to be changed. Correspondingly, a study found that **phenytoin** (100 to 375 mg daily) increased the clearance of the active **oxcarbazepine** metabolite by almost 40%.[6] The AUC of **10-hydroxy-carbazepine** was also 40% lower in the presence of **carbamazepine**.[3]

Mechanism

Unlike carbamazepine, oxcarbazepine appears not to have marked enzyme-inducing properties so that it would not be expected to affect the metabolism of other anticonvulsants. However, other anticonvulsants can increase the metabolism of the active metabolite of oxcarbazepine, 10-hydroxy-carbazepine.

Importance and management

Information about the concurrent use of oxcarbazepine and other anticonvulsants is limited, but growing. The overall picture seems to be that, unlike carbamazepine, oxcarbazepine is not a potent enzyme inducer and therefore it does not markedly affect the serum levels of other anticonvulsants. Any changes in the pharmacokinetics of oxcarbazepine brought about by other anticonvulsants seem to be of minimal clinical relevance. There appears to be no reason for avoiding concurrent use, but good monitoring would still seem advisable. There is the theoretical risk that 10-hydroxy-carbazepine levels might rise to toxic levels if carbamazepine or phenytoin are withdrawn.[3]

1. Houtkooper MA, Lammertsma A, Meyer JWA, Goedhart DM, Meinardi H, van Oorschot CAEH, Blom GF, Höppener RJEA, Hulsman JARJ. Oxcarbazepine (GP 47.680): a possible alternative to carbamazepine? *Epilepsia* (1987) 28, 693–8.
2. Battino D, Croci D, Granata T, Bernadi G, Monza G. Changes in unbound and total valproic acid concentrations after replacement of carbamazepine with oxcarbazepine. *Ther Drug Monit* (1992) 14, 376–9.
3. McKee PJW, Blacklaw J, Forrest G, Gillham RA, Walker SM, Connelly D, Brodie MJ. A double blind, placebo-controlled interaction study between oxcarbazepine and carbamazepine, sodium valproate and phenytoin in epileptic patients. *Br J Clin Pharmacol* (1994) 37, 27–32.
4. Tartara A, Galimberti CA, Manni R, Morini R, Limido G, Gatti G, Bartoli A, Strad G, Perucca E. The pharmacokinetics of oxcarbazepine and its active metabolite 10-hydroxy-carbazepine in healthy subjects and in epileptic patients taking phenobarbitone or valproic acid. *Br J Clin Pharmacol* (1993) 36, 366–8.
5. Kumps A, Wurth C. Oxcarbazepine disposition: preliminary observations in patients. *Biopharm Drug Dispos* (1990) 11, 365–70.
6. Arnoldussen W, Hulsman J, Rentmeester T. Interaction between oxcarbazepine and phenytoin. *Epilepsia* (1993) 34 (Suppl 6), 37.

Anticonvulsants + Oxiracetam

Oxiracetam does not affect the serum levels of sodium valproate, carbamazepine or clobazam, but the loss of oxira-

cetam from the body may be increased by these drugs, so that some change in its dosage may possibly be needed.

Clinical evidence, mechanism, importance and management

Oxiracetam 800 mg twice daily for 14 days did not affect the serum levels of **sodium valproate**, **carbamazepine**, **clobazam** and their metabolites when given to 4 epileptics.[1] However, it was noted that the **oxiracetam** half-life was shorter (2.8 to 7.56 h)[1] than in a previous study (5.6 to 11.7 h) in healthy subjects who had been given 2 g **oxiracetam**.[2] There would seem to be no reason for avoiding concurrent use in patients taking these anticonvulsants, but it may be necessary to raise the **oxiracetam** dosage or give it more frequently. More study is needed to confirm these findings.

1. van Wieringen A, Meijer JWA, van Emde Boas W, Vermeij TAC. Pilot study to determine the interaction of oxiracetam with antiepileptic drugs. *Clin Pharmacokinet* (1990) 18, 332–8.
2. Perucca E, Albrici A, Gatti G, Spalluto R, Visconti M, Crema A. Pharmacokinetics of oxiracetam following intravenous and oral administration in healthy volunteers. *Eur J Drug Metab Pharmacokinet* (1984) 9, 267–74.

Anticonvulsants + Progabide

Serum phenytoin levels can rise if progabide is used concurrently so that a reduced phenytoin dosage may be required. Changes in the serum levels of other anticonvulsants (carbamazepine, clonazepam, phenobarbital, sodium valproate) caused by progabide and their effects on serum progabide levels appear to be only moderate or small.

Clinical evidence

(a) Carbamazepine, clonazepam, phenobarbital or sodium valproate

Information about these anticonvulsants is limited, but **progabide** is reported to minimally reduce,[1-3] minimally increase[3] or not to change **carbamazepine**[4-8] serum levels. An increase in **carbamazepine-epoxide** levels of up to 24% has also been reported.[2,7] **Sodium valproate**,[5-8] and **clonazepam**[9] serum levels were not significantly affected. Progabide appears to cause a small increase in serum **phenobarbital** levels which is of little clinical importance.[3,5-7]

(b) Phenytoin

Marked increases in serum **phenytoin** levels have been seen in a few patients given **progabide** concurrently[3,4,8,10] while smaller changes have been described in some studies,[6,7] and negligible changes in others.[5]

In one study, 17 out of 26 epileptics needed a reduction in **phenytoin** dosage to keep the levels within 25% of the serum levels before **progabide** was given. Over half the patients needed a dose reduction within 4 weeks of starting concurrent treatment. Most of those needing a dosage reduction showed a maximum increase in the serum level of 40% or more, which was sometimes accompanied by toxicity.[4,11] In a later report of this study in a total of 32 epileptics taking carbamazepine plus **phenytoin**, 22 needed a reduction in **phenytoin** dosage to maintain serum levels within 25%, when **progabide** was given. In addition, it appeared this effect on **phenytoin** serum levels continued for a while after **progabide** treatment ended.[10]

Mechanism

Uncertain.

Importance and management

Some small to moderate changes in the serum levels of carbamazepine, phenobarbital, sodium valproate and clonazepam can apparently occur in the presence of progabide, but only the phenytoin/progabide interaction appears to be clinically relevant. Be alert for the need to reduce the dosage of phenytoin if progabide is used

concurrently. The minor effects of the antiepileptics on progabide levels are of unknown significance.

1. Dam M, Gram L, Philbert A, Hansen BS, Blatt Lyon B, Christensen JM, Angelo HR. Progabide: a controlled trial in partial epilepsy. *Epilepsia* (1983) 24, 127–34.
2. Graves NM, Fuerst RH, Cloyd JC, Brundage RC, Welty TE, Leppik IE. Progabide-induced changes in carbamazepine metabolism. *Epilepsia* (1988) 29, 775–80.
3. Schmidt D, Utech K. Progabide for refractory partial epilepsy: a controlled add-on trial. *Neurology* (1986) 36, 217–221.
4. Cloyd JC, Brundage RC, Leppik IE, Graves NM, Welty TE. Effect of progabide on serum phenytoin and carbamazepine concentrations: a preliminary report. In: LERS Monograph series, volume 3. Edited by Bartholini G et al. Epilepsy and GABA receptor agonists: basic and therapeutic research. Meeting, Paris, March 1984. Raven Press, New York. (1985) pp 271–8.
5. Thénot JP, Bianchetti G, Abriol C, Feuerstein J, Lambert D, Thébault JJ, Warrington SJ, Rowland M. Interactions between progabide and antiepileptic drugs. In: LERS Monograph series, volume 3. Edited by Bartholini G et al. Epilepsy and GABA receptor agonists: basic and therapeutic research. Meeting, Paris, March 1984. Raven Press, New York. (1985) pp 259–69.
6. Bianchetti G, Thiercelin JF, Thenot JP, Feuerstein J, Lambert D, Rulliere R, Thebault JJ, Morselli PL. Effect of progabide on the pharmacokinetics of various antiepileptic drugs. *Neurology* (1984) 34 (Suppl 1), 213.
7. Bianchetti G, Padovani P, Thénot JP, Thiercelin JF, Morselli PL. Pharmacokinetic interactions of progabide with other antiepileptic drugs. *Epilepsia* (1987) 28, 68–73.
8. Crawford P, Chadwick D. A comparative study of progabide, valproate and placebo as add-on therapy in patients with refractory epilepsy. *J Neurol Neurosurg Psychiatry* (1986) 49, 1251–7.
9. Warrington SJ, O'Brien C, Thiercelin JF, Orofiamma B and Morselli PL. Evaluation of pharmacodynamic interaction between progabide and clonazepam in healthy men. In: LERS Monograph series, volume 3. Edited by Bartholini G et al. Epilepsy and GABA receptor agonists: basic and therapeutic research. Meeting, Paris, March 1984. Raven Press, New York. (1985) pp 279–86.
10. Brundage RC, Cloyd JC, Leppik IE, Graves NM and Welty TE. Effect of progabide on serum phenytoin and carbamazepine concentrations. *Clin Neuropharmacol* (1987) 10, 545–54.
11. Brundage RC, Leppik IE, Cloyd JC, Graves NM. Effect of progabide on phenytoin pharmacokinetics. *Epilepsia* (1984) 25, 656–7.

Anticonvulsants + Pyridoxine (Vitamin B$_6$)

Daily doses of pyridoxine of 200 mg can cause reductions of 40 to 50% in the serum phenytoin and phenobarbital levels of some patients.

Clinical evidence

Pyridoxine 200 mg daily for 4 weeks reduced the **phenobarbital** serum levels of 5 epileptics by about 50%. Reductions in serum **phenytoin** levels of about 35% (range 17 to 70%) were also seen when patients were given **pyridoxine** (80 to 400 mg daily) for 2 to 4 weeks. A number of other patients were not affected.[1]

Mechanism

It is suggested that the pyridoxine increases the activity of the liver enzymes concerned with the metabolism of these anticonvulsants.[1]

Importance and management

Information seems to be limited to just one report, but what is known suggests that concurrent use should be monitored if large doses of pyridoxine like this are used, being alert for the need to increase the anticonvulsant dosage. It seems unlikely that small doses (as in multivitamin preparations) will interact to any great extent.

1. Hansson O, Sillanpaa M. Pyridoxine and serum concentration of phenytoin and phenobarbitone. *Lancet* (1976) i, 256.

Anticonvulsants + Quinine

Preliminary evidence suggests that the effects of carbamazepine and phenobarbital may be increased by quinine,

possibly leading to toxicity. **Phenytoin** appears not to be affected.

Clinical evidence, mechanism, importance and management

Single doses of 200 mg **carbamazepine**, 120 mg **phenobarbital** or 200 mg **phenytoin** were given to 3 groups of 6 healthy subjects with and without a single 600-mg dose of **quinine sulphate**. The AUC and peak plasma level were increased by 104% and 57% for **carbamazepine**, and by 81% and 53% for **phenobarbital**. **Phenytoin** was not significantly affected. The reasons are not known but the authors suggest that **quinine** inhibits the metabolism of **carbamazepine** and **phenobarbital** (but not **phenytoin**) by the liver, so that they are lost from the body more slowly.[1]

Information seems to be limited to this study. The importance of these interactions awaits assessment in a clinically realistic situation (i.e. in patients under treatment taking multiple doses) but in the meantime it would seem prudent to monitor the effects of **carbamazepine** or **phenobarbital** for evidence of increased effects and possible toxicity if **quinine** is added. Be alert for increased sedation, nausea and ataxia with **phenobarbital**, and diplopia, nausea and ataxia with **carbamazepine**. **Phenytoin** appears not to interact.

1. Amabeoku GJ, Chikuni O, Akino C, Mutetwa S. Pharmacokinetic interaction of single doses of quinine and carbamazepine, phenobarbitone and phenytoin in healthy volunteers. *East Afr Med J* (1993) 70, 90–3.

Anticonvulsants + Quinolone antibacterials

Quinolone antibacterials very occasionally cause convulsions, therefore they should generally be avoided in patients with epilepsy. Four individuals have shown a marked fall in serum phenytoin levels when ciprofloxacin was started, whereas another showed a rise. Phenytoin levels may rise if clinafloxacin is given.

Clinical evidence, mechanism, importance and management

(a) Ciprofloxacin

The makers suggest that **ciprofloxacin** should be used with caution or avoided in epileptics because a very small number of patients have developed convulsions.[1] Ciprofloxacin has been associated with convulsions in both epileptic[2-4] and non-epileptic patients.[2,3,5-7] Two of the patients were also being treated with **theophylline**.[4,6]

In a study of the effect of ciprofloxacin on **phenytoin** levels, only one of 4 healthy subjects experienced a decrease in the phenytoin maximum serum levels when ciprofloxacin was added.[8] Case reports show a variety of effects. In one report blood levels of **phenytoin** and **valproic acid** were not affected by **ciprofloxacin**.[2] However, three other case reports describe falls of about 50% in **phenytoin** serum levels when **ciprofloxacin** was added, accompanied by seizures in two instances.[9-11] Conversely, another report describes a rise in **phenytoin** levels in an elderly woman, possibly caused by ciprofloxacin.[12] The implications of these **phenytoin/ciprofloxacin** interactions are discussed in two published letters, where care is recommended.[13,14]

(b) Clinafloxacin

Phenytoin 300 mg daily was given to healthy subjects for 10 days, then 400 mg **clinafloxacin** twice daily was added for a further 2 weeks. The maximum serum **phenytoin** levels rose by 18% (from 6.74 to 7.95 mg/l), the AUC rose by 20% and the clearance fell by 17%.[15] It would therefore be prudent to monitor **phenytoin** levels if **ciprofloxacin** is added, being alert for the need to reduce the **phenytoin** dosage.

(c) Enoxacin

Enoxacin may possibly lower the convulsive threshold in patients predisposed to seizures,[16] but it appears not to interact directly with **phenytoin** to alter its serum levels nor are serum **enoxacin** levels significantly altered by **phenytoin**.[17]

(d) Nalidixic acid

During the period 1964 to 1975 the CSM in the UK received 8 reports of convulsions associated with **nalidixic acid**. Another case was reported in 1977, and three had been described in Australia by 1971.[18]

(e) Norfloxacin

Norfloxacin may possibly lower the convulsive threshold in patients with or without a history of seizures.[7,19]

(f) Ofloxacin

Ofloxacin may possibly lower the convulsive threshold in patients with or without a history of seizures.[7]

These reports suggest that quinolone antibacterials should either be avoided in epileptics, or only used when the benefits of treatment outweigh the potential risks of seizures. Most of the reactions seem to be disease/drug interactions rather than drug/drug interactions, the usual outcome being that the control of epilepsy is worsened.

1. Ciproxin (Ciprofloxacin). Bayer plc. Summary of product characteristics, November 2001.
2. Slavich IL, Gleffe R, Haas EJ. Grand mal epileptic seizures during ciprofloxacin therapy. *JAMA* (1989) 261, 558–9.
3. Schacht P, Arcieri G, Branolte J, Bruck H, Chyský V, Griffith E, Gruenwaldt G, Hullmann R, Konopka CA, O'Brien B, Rahm V, Ryoki T, Westwood A, Weuta H. Worldwide clinical data on efficacy and safety of ciprofloxacin. *Infection* (1988) 16 (Suppl 1), S29–S43.
4. Karki SD, Bentley DW, Raghavan M. Seizure with ciprofloxacin and theophylline combined therapy. *DICP Ann Pharmacother* (1990) 24, 595–6.
5. Beeley L, Magee P, Hickey F. Newsletter of West Midlands Centre for Adverse Drug Reaction Reporting, January 1989.
6. Arcieri G, Griffith E, Gruenwaldt G, Heyd A, O'Brien B, Becker N, August R. Ciprofloxacin: an update on clinical experience. *Am J Med* (1987) 82 (Suppl 4A), 381–6.
7. Committee on Safety of Medicines/Medicines Control Agency. Convulsions due to quinolone antimicrobial agents. *Current Problems* (1991) 32, 2.
8. Job ML, Arn SK, Strom JG, Jacobs NF, D'Souza MJ. Effect of ciprofloxacin on the pharmacokinetics of multiple-dose phenytoin serum concentrations. *Ther Drug Monit* (1994) 16, 427–31.
9. Dillard ML, Fink RM, Parkerson R. Ciprofloxacin-phenytoin interaction. *Ann Pharmacother* (1992) 26, 263.
10. Pollak PT, Slayter KL. Hazards of doubling phenytoin dose in the face of an unrecognized interaction with ciprofloxacin. *Ann Pharmacother* (1997) 31, 61–4.
11. Brouwers PJ, DeBoer LE, Guchelaar H-J. Ciprofloxacin-phenytoin interaction. *Ann Pharmacother* (1997) 31, 498.
12. Hull RL. Possible phenytoin-ciprofloxacin interaction. *Ann Pharmacother* (1993) 27, 1283.
13. Pollak PT, Slayter KL. Comment: ciprofloxacin-phenytoin interaction. *Ann Pharmacother* (1997) 31, 1549–50.
14. Brouwers PJ, de Boer LE, Guchelaar H-J. Comment: ciprofloxacin-phenytoin interaction. *Ann Pharmacother* (1997) 31, 1550.
15. Randinitis EJ, Koup JR, Bron NJ, Hounslow NJ, Rausch G, Abel R, Vassos AB, Sedman AJ. Drug interaction studies with clinafloxacin and probenecid, cimetidine, phenytoin and warfarin. *Drugs* (1999) 58 (Suppl 2), 254–5.
16. Simpson KJ, Brodie MJ. Convulsions related to enoxacin. *Lancet* (1985) 2, 161.
17. Thomas D, Humphrey G, Kinkel A, Sedman A, Rowland M, Toon S, Aarons L, Hopkins K. A study to evaluate the potential pharmacokinetic interaction between oral enoxacin (ENX) and oral phenytoin (PHE). *Pharm Res* (1986) 3 (Suppl), 99S.
18. Fraser AG, Harrower ADB. Convulsions and hyperglycaemia associated with nalidixic acid. *BMJ* (1977) 2, 1518.
19. Anastasio GD, Menscer D, Little JM. Norfloxacin and seizures. *Ann Intern Med* (1988) 109, 169–70.

Anticonvulsants + Remacemide

Remacemide causes modest increases in carbamazepine and phenytoin serum levels: dose reductions of carbamazepine, but not phenytoin may be necessary. Carbamazepine and phenytoin moderately reduce remacemide serum levels. Sodium valproate does not appear to interact with remacemide.

Clinical evidence

(a) Carbamazepine

A group of 10 patients on **carbamazepine** were additionally given up to 300 mg **remacemide** twice daily for 2 weeks. Small increases in **carbamazepine** minimum serum levels and AUC of 20% and of 22% respectively were found. No patients showed symptoms of **car-**

bamazepine toxicity.[1] Another study of 11 patients on **car-bamazepine** showed a similar increase in **carbamazepine** AUC (20 to 30%) caused by **remacemide**, again without signs of toxicity. No consistent changes in the AUC for the main metabolite of **carbamazepine** were seen.[2] Another study has reported a slight inhibitory effect of **remacemide** on **carbamazepine** metabolism, which is in line with these other findings.[3] One of these studies also reported that the AUC of **remacemide** was decreased by 40 to 50% and its main metabolite by about 70% when compared with healthy subjects (presumably not taking carbamazepine).[2]

However, a further trial of the efficacy of remacemide and carbamazepine in combination found that about two-thirds of the 120 patients treated needed 14 to 50% reductions in their carbamazepine dose, to ensure levels remained in the therapeutic range.[4]

(b) Phenytoin

A group of 10 patients on **phenytoin** were additionally given up to 300 mg **remacemide** twice daily for 2 weeks. On average the **remacemide** did not affect **phenytoin** pharmacokinetics but 5 patients showed an increase in minimum serum levels of 30% or more. No patients showed symptoms of **phenytoin** toxicity.[1] In another study 10 epileptics, who had been on **phenytoin** for at least 3 months, were given 300 mg **remacemide** twice daily for 12 days. **Phenytoin** maximum serum levels were increased by 13.7% and the AUC was raised by 11.5%. Average concentrations of **remacemide** and its main metabolite were around only 40 and 30% of those achieved in healthy volunteers taking **remacemide** alone, at the same dosage.[5] Another study reported a slight inhibitory effect of **remacemide** on **phenytoin** metabolism, which is in line with these other findings.[3]

(c) Sodium valproate

A group of 10 patients on **sodium valproate** were additionally given **remacemide** up to 300 mg twice daily for 14 days. The pharmacokinetics of **sodium valproate** remained unchanged.[1] Another study in 17 patients confirmed these findings,[6] and an earlier study by the same authors also noted no effect of **remacemide** on **valproate** metabolism.[3]

Mechanism

Not fully understood, but *in vitro* studies indicate that remacemide inhibits the cytochrome P450 isoenzyme CYP3A4 which *in vivo* would be expected to result in a reduction in the metabolism of the carbamazepine resulting in an increase in its serum levels. Remacemide appears to inhibit CYP2C9 to a lesser extent, which is reflected in a smaller interaction with phenytoin. Sodium valproate is metabolised by glucuronidation and is therefore unaffected.[1]

Carbamazepine and phenytoin also seem to increase the metabolism of the remacemide.[5]

Importance and management

Information is limited but the remacemide/carbamazepine and remacemide/phenytoin interactions appear to be established, but so far only the carbamazepine interaction seems to be of clinical importance. Even so, until more experience has been gained, monitor the effects of concurrent use with phenytoin. No interaction occurs between remacemide and sodium valproate.

1. Riley RJ, Slee D, Martin CA, Webborn PJH, Wattam DG, Jones T, Logan CJ. *In vitro* evaluation of pharmacokinetic interactions between remacemide hydrochloride and established anticonvulsants. *Br J Clin Pharmacol* (1996) 41, 461P.
2. Leach JP, Blacklaw J, Stewart M, Jamieson V, Jones T, Oxley R, Richens A, Brodie MJ. Mutual pharmacokinetic interactions between remacemide hydrochloride and carbamazepine. *Epilepsia* (1995) 36 (Suppl 3), S163.
3. Leach JP, Blacklaw J, Stewart M, Jamieson V, Oxley R, Richens A, Brodie MJ. Interactions between remacemide and the established antiepileptic drugs. *Epilepsia* (1994) 35 (Suppl 7), 75.
4. Mawer GE, Jamieson V, Lucas SB, Wild JM. Adjustment of carbamazepine dose to offset the effects of the interaction with remacemide hydrochloride in a double-blind, mutlicentre, add-on drug trial (CR2237) in refractory epilepsy. *Epilepsia* (1999) 40, 190–6.
5. Leach JP, Girvan J, Jamieson V, Jones T, Richens A, Brodie MJ. Mutual interaction between remacemide hydrochloride and phenytoin. *Epilepsy Res* (1997) 26, 381–8.
6. Leach JP, Girvan J, Jamieson V, Jones T, Richens A, Brodie MJ. Lack of pharmacokinetic interaction between remacemide hydrochloride and sodium valproate in epileptic patients. *Seizure* (1997) 6, 179–84.

Anticonvulsants + Stiripentol

Stiripentol causes marked rises in the serum levels of carbamazepine, phenobarbital and phenytoin. Reduce their dosages to avoid the development of toxicity. Stiripentol causes only a small rise in the serum levels of sodium valproate and dosage adjustments are not needed.

Clinical evidence

Epileptic patients taking two or three anticonvulsants (**phenytoin, phenobarbital, carbamazepine, clobazam, primidone, nitrazepam**) were additionally given stiripentol (increasing from 600 to 2400 mg daily). All 5 patients on **phenytoin** showed an average 37% reduction in the **phenytoin** clearance while taking 1200 mg **stiripentol** daily, and a 78% reduction while on 2400 mg **stiripentol** daily. These changes in clearance were reflected in marked rises in the steady-state serum levels of the anticonvulsants: for example the serum **phenytoin** levels of one patient rose from 14.4 mg/l to 27.4 mg/l over 30 days while he was taking **stiripentol**, despite a 50% reduction in his **phenytoin** dosage. **Phenytoin** toxicity was seen in another two subjects.[1] The clearance of **carbamazepine** in one subject fell by 39% while on 1200 mg **stiripentol** daily and by 71% while on 2400 mg **stiripentol** daily. **Phenobarbital** clearance in two subjects fell by about 30 to 40% while taking 2400 mg **stiripentol** daily.[1] Three other studies in adults and children confirmed that **stiripentol** reduces the clearance of **carbamazepine** by between one-half to two-thirds,[2-4] and significantly increases carbamazepine levels.[5]

Sodium valproate 1 g daily was given to 8 subjects with or without 1200 mg **stiripentol** daily. The **stiripentol** caused a 14% increase in peak serum levels of the **valproate**.[6] No adverse effects on motor, perceptual or attention tests were seen in another 11 patients when **stiripentol** was combined with other antiepileptic drugs, but the doses of phenobarbital, phenytoin and carbamazepine were reduced before the combination was taken.[7]

Mechanism

Stiripentol inhibits the activity of various cytochrome P450 liver isoenzymes including CYP1A2, CYP2C9, CYP2C19, CYP2D6 and CYP3A4, some of which are concerned with the metabolism of the anticonvulsants. As a result the loss of the anticonvulsant from the body is reduced and the serum levels rise accordingly.[3,8] In the case of sodium valproate, cytochrome P450-mediated metabolism is only involved in minor valproate metabolic pathways and therefore only a small rise in serum levels occurs.[6]

Importance and management

Established and clinically important interactions. The phenytoin, phenobarbital and carbamazepine dosages should be reduced to avoid the development of elevated serum levels and possible toxicity during the concurrent use of stiripentol. In the case of phenytoin, halving the dose may not be enough. One study[3] suggests that the carbamazepine dosage should be decreased incrementally over 7 to 10 days, beginning as soon as the stiripentol is started and, regardless of age, the maintenance dose of carbamazepine should aim to give serum levels of 5 to 10 micrograms/ml. Stiripentol causes only small changes in the serum levels of sodium valproate and dosage adjustments are unlikely to be needed in this combination.

1. Levy RH, Loiseau P, Guyot M, Blehaut HM, Tor J, Morland TA. Stiripentol kinetics in epilepsy: nonlinearity and interactions. *Clin Pharmacol Ther* (1984) 36, 661–9.
2. Levy RH, Kerr BM, Farwell J, Anderson GD, Martinez-Lage JM, Tor J. Carbamazepine/stiripentol interaction in adult and pediatric patients. *Epilepsia* (1989) 30, 701.
3. Kerr BM, Martinez-Lage JM, Viteri C, Tor J, Eddy AC, Levy RH. Carbamazepine dose requirements during stiripentol therapy: influence of cytochrome P-450 inhibition by stiripentol. *Epilepsia* (1991) 32, 267–74.
4. Levy RH, Martinez-Lage JM, Tor J, Blehaut H, Gonzalez I, Bainbridge B. Stiripentol level-dose relationship and interaction with carbamazepine in epileptic patients. *Epilepsia* (1985) 26, 544–5.

5. Tran A, Vauzelle-Kervroedan F, Rey E, Pons G. d'Athis P, Chiron C, Dulac O, Renard F, Olive G. Effect of stiripentol on carbamazepine plasma concentration and metabolism in epileptic children. *Eur J Clin Pharmacol* (1996) 50, 497–500.

6. Levy RH, Loiseau P, Guyot M, Acheampong A, Tor J, Rettenmeier AW. Effects of stiripentol on valproate plasma level and metabolism. *Epilepsia* (1987) 28, 605.

7. Loiseau P, Strube E, Tor J, Levy RH, Dodrill C. Evaluation neuropsychologique et thérapeutique du stiripentol dans l'épilepsie. *Rev Neurol (Paris)* (1988) 144, 165–72.

8. Mather GG, Bishop FE, Trager WF, Kunze KK, Thummel KE, Shen DD, Roskos LK, Lepage F, Gillardin JM, Levy RH. Mechanisms of stiripentol interactions with carbamazepine and phenytoin. *Epilepsia* (1995) 36 (Suppl 3), S162.

Anticonvulsants + Tamoxifen

Some preliminary evidence suggests that high dose tamoxifen can cause the serum levels of phenytoin to rise, causing toxicity. Carbamazepine may possibly not interact.

Clinical evidence, mechanism, importance and management

A man who had undergone an operation 10 years previously for a brain tumour and had since remained seizure-free on **phenytoin** 200 mg twice daily began to have breakthrough seizures. It was established that his brain tumour had recurred and so **tamoxifen** was started as experimental treatment. The dose of **tamoxifen** was slowly titrated to 200 mg daily over a 6-week period. He continued to receive **phenytoin** and was also given **carbamazepine** as his seizures were not controlled, but when the maximum dosage of **tamoxifen** (200 mg daily) was reached he began to develop signs of **phenytoin** toxicity with a serum level of 28 micrograms/ml. The toxicity disappeared and the **phenytoin** levels decreased when the **phenytoin** dosage was reduced. The **carbamazepine** serum levels remained unchanged throughout.[1]

The authors of this report say that other patients of theirs similarly treated with **tamoxifen** also developed **phenytoin** toxicity, which disappeared when the **phenytoin** dosage was reduced 15 to 20%. The reasons for this interaction are not known, but it could be that the **tamoxifen** reduces the metabolism of the **phenytoin** by the liver because they both compete for the same metabolising enzymes.

The evidence for this interaction is very slim indeed and it may possibly only occur with high dose **tamoxifen**. Nevertheless it would now seem prudent to monitor **phenytoin** levels if **tamoxifen** is added, especially in high dose.

1. Rabinowicz AL, Hinton DR, Dyck P, Couldwell WT. High-dose tamoxifen in treatment of brain tumors: interaction with antiepileptic drugs. *Epilepsia* (1995) 36, 513–15.

Anticonvulsants + Terbinafine

An isolated report describes the development of fatal toxic epidermal necrolysis in a patient on long-term phenobarbital and carbamazepine shortly after starting to take terbinafine.

Clinical evidence, mechanism, importance and management

An isolated report describes a 26-year-old woman with cerebral palsy who had been taking 15 mg **phenobarbital** plus 400 mg **carbamazepine** daily for 12 years to control epilepsy, and who developed fatal toxic epidermal necrolysis 2 weeks after starting oral **terbinafine** 250 mg daily for tinea corporis. The reasons are not understood, but the authors point out all three drugs can cause adverse skin reactions (erythema multiforme) and suggest that some synergism may have occurred.[1] It is uncertain whether this was a true interaction or a **terbinafine** adverse effect, but prescribers should be aware of this case if these drugs are used together.

1. White SI, Bowen-Jones D. Toxic epidermal necrolysis induced by terbinafine in a patient on long-term anti-epileptics. *Br J Dermatol* (1996) 134, 188–9.

Anticonvulsants + Terfenadine

Carbamazepine toxicity attributed to the use of terfenadine has been described in one case report but the interaction is not established. Terfenadine does not alter the pharmacokinetics of phenytoin.

Clinical evidence, mechanism, importance and management

(a) Carbamazepine

A woman of 18 taking **carbamazepine** after treatment for brain metastases, developed confusion, disorientation, visual hallucinations, nausea and ataxia shortly after starting 60 mg **terfenadine** twice daily for rhinitis. The symptoms were interpreted as **carbamazepine** toxicity, however her total **carbamazepine** serum levels of 8.9 mg/l were within the normal range. An interaction due to protein binding displacement was suspected, so free **carbamazepine** was measured. The levels of free **carbamazepine** were found to be 6 mg/l, almost three times the upper limit of normal. All the symptoms disappeared when the **terfenadine** was stopped. The authors speculate that the **terfenadine** had displaced the **carbamazepine** from its plasma protein binding sites, thereby increasing the levels of free and active **carbamazepine**.[1] The report is very brief and does not say whether any other drugs were being taken concurrently, so that this interaction is not established.

(b) Phenytoin

A one-day and a 2-week course of 60 mg **terfenadine** twice daily had no effect on the pharmacokinetics of **phenytoin** in 12 epileptics.[2] No special precautions are needed if both drugs are used.

1. Hirschfeld S, Jarosinski P. Drug interaction of terfenadine and carbamazepine. *Ann Intern Med* (1993) 118, 907–8.
2. Coniglio AA, Garnett WR, Pellock JH, Tsidonis O, Hepler CD, Serafin R, Small RE, Driscoll SM, Karnes HT. Effect of acute and chronic terfenadine on free and total serum phenytoin concentrations in epileptic patients. *Epilepsia* (1989) 30, 611–16.

Anticonvulsants + Tobacco smoking

Smoking appears to have no important effect on the serum levels of phenytoin, phenobarbital or carbamazepine.

Clinical evidence, mechanism, importance and management

A comparative study in 88 epileptic patients taking anticonvulsants (**phenobarbital**, **phenytoin** and **carbamazepine** alone and in combination) found that although **smoking** had a tendency to lower the steady-state serum concentrations of these drugs, a statistically significant effect was only shown on the concentration–dose ratios of the **phenobarbital**-treated patients.[1] In practical terms **smoking** appears to have only a negligible effect on the serum levels of these anticonvulsants and epileptics who smoke are unlikely to need higher doses than non-smokers.

1. Benetello P, Furlanut M, Pasqui L, Carmillo L, Perlotto N, Testa G. Absence of effect of cigarette smoking on serum concentrations of some anticonvulsants in epileptic patients. *Clin Pharmacokinet* (1987) 12, 302–4.

Anticonvulsants + Vigabatrin

Vigabatrin appears to interact minimally with most other anticonvulsants. It causes a small to moderate fall in serum

phenytoin levels and trivial falls in phenobarbital) and primidone levels. No interaction appears to occur with carbamazepine or sodium valproate.

Clinical evidence

Vigabatrin 2 to 3 g daily did not change the serum levels of **phenobarbital** in 26 patients, of **carbamazepine** in 12 patients or of **sodium valproate** in 2 patients. However, the mean serum **phenytoin** levels in 19 patients were about 30% lower during concurrent use, and in 2 patients they fell below the therapeutic range. Seizure-frequency generally remained unaltered.[1] A later study found only a small mean fall in the serum **phenytoin** levels of 21 patients, but a subset of 7 patients showed a 25 to 50% fall. **Carbamazepine**, **phenobarbital** and **primidone** levels were not significantly altered.[2] Another study found that vigabatrin caused serum level reductions of 20% with **phenytoin**, 7% with **phenobarbital** and 11% with **primidone**. The frequency of complex partial seizures was halved, but in this study seizure frequency increased with **phenytoin** and its dosage had to be increased.[3] Four other studies have shown roughly similar results.[4-7]

The combined use of **vigabatrin** and **sodium valproate** in 16 children with refractory epilepsy was found not to affect the steady-state serum levels of either drug and it reduced the frequency of seizures.[8]

Mechanisms

Not understood.

Importance and management

Vigabatrin appears to interact either minimally or not at all with most other anticonvulsants. A small increase in the dosage of phenytoin may possibly be needed in some patients but no dosage changes seem necessary with the other anticonvulsants cited.

1. Tassinari CA, Michelucci R, Ambrosetto G, Salvi F. Double-blind study of vigabatrin in the treatment of drug-resistant epilepsy. *Arch Neurol* (1987) 44, 907–10.
2. Gatti G, Bartoli A, Marchiselli R, Michelucci R, Tassinari CA, Pisani F, Zaccara G, Timmings P, Richens A, Perucca E. Vigabatrin-induced decrease in serum phenytoin concentration does not involve a change in phenytoin bioavailability. *Br J Clin Pharmacol* (1993) 36, 603–6.
3. Browne TR, Mattson RH, Penry JK, Smith DB, Treiman DM, Wilder BJ, Ben-Menachem E, Miketta RM, Sherry KM, Szabo GK. A multicentre study of vigabatrin for drug-resistant epilepsy. *Br J Clin Pharmacol* (1989) 95S–100S.
4. Rimmer EM, Richens A. Double-blind study of γ-vinyl GABA in patients with refractory epilepsy. *Lancet* (1984) i, 189–90.
5. Browne TR, Mattson RH, Penry JK, Smith DB, Treiman DM, Wilder BJ, Ben-Menachem E, Napoliello MJ, Sherry KM, Szabo GK. Vigabatrin for refractory complex partial seizures: multicenter single-blind study with long-term follow up. *Neurology* (1987) 37, 184–9.
6. Rimmer EM, Richens A. Interaction between vigabatrin and phenytoin. *Br J Clin Pharmacol* (1989) 27, 27S–33S.
7. Bernardina BD, Fontana E, Vigevano F, Fusco L, Torelli D, Galeone D, Buti D, Cianchetti C, Gnanasakthy A, Iudice A. Efficacy and tolerability of vigabatrin in children with refractory partial seizures: a single-blind dose-increasing study. *Epilepsia* (1995) 36, 687–91.
8. Armijo JA, Arteaga R, Valdizán EM, Herranz JL. Coadministration of vigabatrin and valproate in children with refractory epilepsy. *Clin Neuropharmacol* (1992) 15, 459–69.

Anticonvulsants + Viloxazine

Viloxazine can cause a marked rise in serum carbamazepine levels. Toxicity may occur if the carbamazepine dosage is not reduced appropriately. Viloxazine can also raise serum phenytoin to toxic levels. Oxcarbazepine appears not to interact with viloxazine.

Clinical evidence

(a) Carbamazepine

A 50% rise in serum carbamazepine levels (from 8.1 to 12.1 micrograms/ml) was seen in 7 patients after taking 100 mg **viloxazine** three times daily for 3 weeks.[1] Signs of mild intoxication (dizziness, ataxia, fatigue, drowsiness) developed in 5 of them. These symptoms disappeared and the serum **carbamazepine** levels fell when the **viloxazine** was withdrawn.[1] Another report found a 2.5-fold

increase in serum **carbamazepine** levels in one patient within 2 weeks of adding 300 mg **viloxazine** daily.[2] Another report found an average 55% rise in plasma carbamazepine levels and toxicity was seen in 4 of the 7 patients studied.[3] Yet another patient developed choreoathetosis and increased serum **carbamazepine** levels, which was attributed to the addition of **viloxazine**.[4] In one study, the pharmacokinetics of a single dose of **viloxazine** were reported to be unaffected by **carbamazepine**,[5] but in the case report cited above, which was at steady state, the **viloxazine** levels were found to be reduced.[2]

(b) Oxcarbazepine

The steady-state serum **oxcarbazepine** levels of 6 patients with simple or partial seizures on an average dose of 1500 mg **oxcarbazepine** daily were unaffected by the addition of 100 mg **viloxazine** twice daily for 10 days. No adverse side effects were seen.[6,7]

(c) Phenytoin

A 37% rise in serum **phenytoin** levels (from 18.8 to 25.7 micrograms/ml) was seen in 10 epileptic patients taking **phenytoin** over the 3 weeks following the addition of 150 to 300 mg **viloxazine** daily. The rise ranged from 7 to 94%. Signs of toxicity (ataxia, nystagmus) developed in 4 of the patients 12 to 16 days after starting the **viloxazine**. Their serum **phenytoin** levels had risen to between 32.3 and 41 micrograms/ml.[8] The symptoms disappeared and **phenytoin** levels fell when the **viloxazine** was withdrawn.[8] The pharmacokinetics of **viloxazine** were unaffected by **phenytoin**.[5]

Mechanism

Uncertain. What is known suggests that the viloxazine inhibits the metabolism of some anticonvulsants, thereby reducing their clearance from the body and raising their serum levels.

Importance and management

Information seems to be limited to the reports cited. If concurrent use is undertaken, both serum carbamazepine and phenytoin levels should be monitored closely and suitable dosage reductions made as necessary to avoid the possible development of toxicity. No special precautions seem necessary with oxcarbazepine.

1. Pisani F, Narbone MC, Fazio A, Crisafulli P, Primerano G, Amendola D'Angostino A, Oteri G, Di Perri R. Effect of viloxazine on serum carbamazepine levels in epileptic patients. *Epilepsia* (1984) 25, 482–5.
2. Odou P, Geronimi-Ferret D, Degen P, Robert H. Viloxazine-carbamazépine. Double interaction dangereuse? A propos d'un cas. *J Pharm Clin* (1996) 15, 157–60.
3. Pisani F, Fazio A, Oteri G, Perucca E, Russo M, Trio R, Pisani B, Di Perri R. Carbamazepine-viloxazine interaction in patients with epilepsy. *J Neurol Neurosurg Psychiatry* (1986) 49, 1142–5.
4. Mosquet B, Starace J, Madelaine S, Simon JY, Lacotte J, Moulin M. Syndrome choréo-athétosique sous carbamazépine et viloxazine. *Therapie* (1994) 49, 513–22.
5. Pisani F, Fazio A, Spina E, Artesi C, Pisani B, Russo M, Trio R, Perucca E. Pharmacokinetics of the antidepressant drug viloxazine in normal subjects and in epileptic patients receiving chronic anticonvulsant treatment. *Psychopharmacology (Berl)* (1986) 90, 295–8.
6. Pisani F, Oteri G, Russo M, Trio R, Amendola D'Agostino A, Di Perri R, Flesch G, Monza GC. Double-blind, within-patient study to evaluate the influence of viloxazine on the steady-state plasma levels of oxcarbazepine and its metabolites. *Epilepsia* (1991) 32 (Suppl 1), 70.
7. Pisani F, Fazio A, Oteri G, Artesi C, Xiao B, Perucca E, Di Perri R. Effects of the antidepressant drug viloxazine on oxcarbazepine and its hydroxylated metabolites in patients with epilepsy. *Acta Neurol Scand* (1994) 90, 130–2.
8. Pisani F, Fazio A, Artesi C, Russo M, Trio R, Oteri G, Perucca E, Di Perri R. Elevation of plasma phenytoin by viloxazine in epileptic patients: a clinically significant interaction. *J Neurol Neurosurg Psychiatry* (1992) 55, 126–7.

Barbiturates + Caffeine

The hypnotic effects of pentobarbital are reduced or abolished by the concurrent use of caffeine. Caffeine-containing drinks or analgesics should be avoided at bedtime if satisfactory hypnosis is to be achieved.

Clinical evidence

A placebo, or 250 mg **caffeine**, or 100 mg **pentobarbital**, or both **caffeine** and **pentobarbital** were given to 34 patients. It was found that the hypnotic effects of the **pentobarbital/caffeine** combination were indistinguishable from the placebo.[1]

Mechanism

Caffeine stimulates the cerebral cortex and impairs sleep, whereas pentobarbital depresses the cortex and promotes sleep. These mutually opposing actions would seem to explain this interaction.

Importance and management

This seems to be only direct study of this interaction, but it is well supported by common experience and the numerous studies of the properties of each of these compounds. Patients given barbiturate hypnotics should avoid caffeine-containing drinks (tea, coffee, *Coca-Cola*, etc.) or analgesics at or near bedtime if the hypnotic is to be effective. The same is probably true for other non-barbiturate hypnotics, but this needs confirmation.

1. Forrest WH, Bellville JW, Brown BW. The interaction of caffeine with pentobarbital as a nighttime hypnotic. *Anesthesiology* (1972) 36, 37–41.

Barbiturates + Cimetidine or Ranitidine

Phenobarbital reduces the absorption of cimetidine, while cimetidine increases the metabolism of pentobarbital, but both interactions seem to be of very limited clinical importance. Ranitidine appears not to interact.

Clinical evidence

In vitro studies with human liver microsomes showed that **cimetidine** in above clinical concentrations reduced the metabolism of **pentobarbital**, whereas **ranitidine** did not interact.[1] **Phenobarbital** 100 mg daily for 3 weeks reduced the AUC of a single 400 mg oral dose of **cimetidine** in 8 healthy subjects by 15%, and the time during which the plasma concentrations of the **cimetidine** exceeded 0.5 micrograms/ml (regarded as therapeutically desirable) was reduced by 11%.[2]

Mechanism

Cimetidine is an enzyme inhibitor which reduces the rate of metabolism of pentobarbital. Phenobarbital apparently stimulates the enzymes in the gut wall so that the metabolism of the cimetidine is increased. Thus the amount of cimetidine absorbed and released into the circulation is reduced. Ranitidine is not an enzyme inhibitor and therefore would not be expected to interact like cimetidine.

Importance and management

Direct information is very limited, but the effects of these mutual interactions are small and unlikely to be clinically important. No special precautions seem to be necessary. Direct information about other barbiturates is lacking but it seems probable that they will behave similarly. Ranitidine does not interact.

1. Knodell RG, Holtzmann JL, Crankshaw DL, Steele NM, Stanley LN. Drug metabolism by rat and human hepatic microsomes in response to interaction with H₂-receptor antagonists. *Gastroenterology* (1982) 82, 84–8.
2. Somogyi A, Thielscher S, Gugler R. Influence of phenobarbital treatment on cimetidine kinetics. *Eur J Clin Pharmacol* (1981) 19, 343–7.

Barbiturates + Codeine

A study in patients found that 60 mg codeine increased the hypnotic actions of 100 mg secobarbital resulting in synergism in the sedative effects.[1]

1. Bellville JW, Forrest WH, Shroff P, Brown BW. The hypnotic effects of codeine and secobarbital and their interaction in man. *Clin Pharmacol Ther* (1971) 12, 607–12.

Barbiturates + Felbamate

Felbamate normally causes a moderate increase in serum phenobarbital levels, however phenobarbital toxicity occurred in one patient when felbamate was added.

Clinical evidence

When 24 healthy subjects on 100 mg **phenobarbital** daily were additionally given 1200 mg **felbamate** twice daily for 10 days, the AUC and the maximum serum levels of **phenobarbital** were raised 22 and 24% respectively. Concurrent use was said to be safe and well tolerated.[1,2] A 30% increase in phenobarbital plasma concentrations were seen in another 19 patients on **phenobarbital** or **primidone** (which is metabolised to **phenobarbital**) when given **felbamate** (average dose 2458 mg daily).[3] A **phenobarbital** dosage reduction of about 30% was needed in another 6 patients when started on **felbamate**.[4] A man on sodium valproate showed an almost 50% increase in **phenobarbital** serum levels over a 5-week period after 50 mg/kg **felbamate** was added, despite an initial **phenobarbital** dosage reduction from 230 mg to 200 mg daily. He was hospitalised because of increased lethargy, anorexia and ataxia and was eventually discharged with a **phenobarbital** dosage of 150 mg daily.[5]

Barbiturates apparently have little or no effect on the pharmacokinetics of **felbamate**.[2,6,7]

Mechanism

Not established. It seems possible that the felbamate may inhibit more than one pathway for the metabolism of the phenobarbital, resulting in a reduction in its loss from the body. The cytochrome P450 isoenzyme CYP2C19 may be involved.[1,2,8]

Importance and management

An established interaction. If you add felbamate to established treatment with phenobarbital or primidone, particularly in patients already taking substantial doses, monitor well for any evidence of increased side-effects (drowsiness, lethargy, anorexia, ataxia) and reduce the dosages of the phenobarbital or primidone if necessary.

1. Reidenberg P, Glue P, Banfield C, Colucci R, Meehan J, Radwanski E, Mojavarian P, Lin C, Affime MB. Effects of felbamate on the multiple dose pharmacokinetics of phenobarbital. *J Clin Pharmacol* (1994) 34, 1016.
2. Reidenberg P, Glue P, Banfield CR, Colucci RD, Meehan JW, Radwanski E, Mojavarian P, Lin C-C, Nezamis J, Guillaume M, Affime MB. Effects of felbamate on the pharmacokinetics of phenobarbital. *Clin Pharmacol Ther* (1995) 58, 279–87.
3. Kerrick JM, Wolff DL, Risinger MW, Graves NM. Increased phenobarbital plasma concentrations after felbamate initiation. *Epilepsia* (1994) 35 (Suppl 8), 96.
4. Sachdeo RC, Padela MF. The effect of felbamate on phenobarbital serum concentrations. *Epilepsia* (1994) 35 (Suppl 8), 94.
5. Gidal BE, Zupanc ML. Potential pharmacokinetic interaction between felbamate and phenobarbital. *Ann Pharmacother* (1994) 28, 455–8.
6. Kelley MT, Walson PD, Cox S, Dusci LJ. Population pharmacokinetics of felbamate in children. *Ther Drug Monit* (1997) 19, 29–36.
7. Kelley MT, Watson PD, Cox S. Population kinetics of felbamate in children. *Clin Pharmacol Ther* (1996) 59, 213.
8. Glue P, Banfield CR, Perhach JL, Mather GG, Racha JK, Levy RH. Pharmacokinetic interactions with felbamate. *Clin Pharmacokinet* (1997) 33, 214–24.

Barbiturates + Influenza vaccines

Influenza vaccine can cause a moderate rise in serum phenobarbital levels.

Clinical evidence, mechanism, importance and management

Serum **phenobarbital** levels rose by about 30% in 11 out of 27 children when given 0.5 ml of a **whole virus influenza vaccine USP, types A and B**, (Squibb). Levels remained elevated 28 days after vaccination.[1]

The suggested reason is the **vaccine** inhibits the liver enzymes concerned with the metabolism of **phenobarbital**, thereby reducing its loss from the body. Information is very limited but it seems unlikely that such a moderate increase in serum **phenobarbital** levels will have much clinical relevance.

1. Jann MW, Fidone GS. Effect of influenza vaccine on serum anticonvulsant concentrations. *Clin Pharm* (1986) 5, 817–20.

Barbiturates + Miconazole

Miconazole increases serum pentobarbital levels.

Clinical evidence, mechanism, importance and management

Pentobarbital was given to 5 patients in intensive care to decrease intracranial pressure. When **miconazole** was added to treatment, all patients showed marked rises in serum **pentobarbital** levels, and falls in total plasma clearance of 50 to 90%. The reason is thought to be that **miconazole** inhibits the liver enzymes concerned with the metabolism of the barbiturate, thereby reducing its clearance from the body.[1] It would be prudent to monitor the effects of concurrent use to ensure that serum barbiturate levels do not rise too high. There seems to be no information about other barbiturates.

1. Heinemeyer G, Roots I, Schulz H, Dennhardt R. Hemmung der Pentobarbital-Elimination durch Miconazol bei Intesivtherapie des erhöhten intracraniellen Druckes. *Intensivmed* (1985) 22, 164–7.

Barbiturates + Rifampicin (Rifampin)

Rifampicin markedly increases the clearance of hexobarbital from the body, and phenobarbital possibly increases the clearance of rifampicin.

Clinical evidence

(a) Effect of rifampicin on hexobarbital

Rifampicin 1200 mg daily for 8 days decreased the average elimination half-life of a single intravenous dose of **hexobarbital** in 6 healthy subjects from 407 to 171 min, and increased the metabolic clearance threefold.[1]

Similar results have been found in other studies in healthy subjects[2] and patients with cirrhosis or cholestasis.[3] Further studies with **hexobarbital** enantiomers found that 600 mg **rifampicin** daily for 14 days caused a sixfold increase in the clearance of *S(+)*-**hexobarbital** in both young (average 29 years) and old (average 71 years) subjects. However, the clearance of *R(−)*-**hexobarbital** was increased 89-fold in the young and only 19-fold in the old. The reasons for these stereoselective differences are unclear.[4]

(b) Effect of phenobarbital on rifampicin

Conflicting evidence. One study showed no significant effect[5] whereas another indicated that the serum levels of **rifampicin** were reduced.[6]

Mechanism

Rifampicin is a potent liver enzyme inducing agent which accelerates the metabolism of the hexobarbital. Whether phenobarbital (also a potent enzyme inducing agent) can affect the metabolism of rifampicin in a similar way is not clear.

Importance and management

The documentation for both of these interactions is very limited, but the effects seen are consistent with what is known about these drugs. Concurrent use need not be avoided, but be alert for a reduced response to both drugs. Be aware of the differences between old and

young patients and increase the dosages as necessary. Whether rifampicin interacts with other barbiturates is uncertain.

1. Breimer DD, Zilly W, Richter E. Influence of rifampicin on drug metabolism: differences between hexobarbital and antipyrine. *Clin Pharmacol Ther* (1977) 21, 470–81.
2. Zilly W, Breimer DD, Richter E. Induction of drug metabolism in man after rifampicin treatment measured by increased hexobarbital and tolbutamide clearance. *Eur J Clin Pharmacol* (1975) 9, 219–27.
3. Zilly W, Breimer DD, Richter E. Stimulation of drug metabolism by rifampicin in patients with cirrhosis or cholestasis measured by increased hexobarbital and tolbutamide clearance. *Eur J Clin Pharmacol* (1977) 11, 287–93.
4. Smith DA, Chandler MHH, Shedlofsky SI, Wedlund PJ, Blouin RA. Age-dependent stereoselective increase in the oral clearance of hexobarbitone isomers caused by rifampicin. *Br J Clin Pharmacol* (1991) 32, 735–9.
5. Acocella G, Bonollo L, Mainardi M, Margaroli P, Nicolis FB. Kinetic studies on rifampicin. III. Effect of phenobarbital on the half-life of the antibiotic. *Tijdschr Gastroenterol* (1974) 17, 151–8.
6. de Rautlin de la Roy Y, Beauchant G, Breuil K, Patte F. Diminution du taux sérique de rifampicine par le phénobarbital. *Presse Med* (1971) 79, 350.

Barbiturates + Sodium valproate

Serum phenobarbital levels can be increased by the concurrent use of sodium valproate, which may result in excessive sedation and lethargy. A reduction in the dosage of the phenobarbital by between one-third to one-half can be safely carried out without loss of seizure control. Small reductions in sodium valproate levels have also been reported.

Clinical evidence

A 6-month study in 11 epileptics on **phenobarbital** 90 to 400 mg daily showed that when they were additionally given **sodium valproate** 11.2 to 42.7 mg/kg daily sedation developed. On average the dosage of **phenobarbital** was reduced to 54% of the original dose with continued good seizure control. Another 2 patients who did not have their **phenobarbital** dose reduced showed significantly increased **phenobarbital** levels of 12 and 48% when **sodium valproate** was added.[1]

Another study showed that 1200 mg **sodium valproate** daily raised serum **phenobarbital** levels in 20 patients by an average of 27%. Signs of toxicity occurred in 13 patients, but the dose only needed to be reduced in 3 patients.[2] This interaction has been described in numerous other reports and dose reductions of the **phenobarbital** were almost always necessary to avoid excessive drowsiness.[3-16] In one study the rise in **phenobarbital** levels was much greater in children (over 100%) than in adults (about 50%).[17]

A reduction in **sodium valproate** levels of about 25% has also been reported, but the effect on seizure control was not mentioned.[18] Another reduction in valproate levels has been reported elsewhere.[19]

Mechanism

The evidence indicates that sodium valproate inhibits three steps in the metabolism of phenobarbital by the liver, leading to its accumulation in the body. The formation of *p*-hydroxyphenobarbital by the cytochrome P450 isoenzyme CYP2C9,[20] the *N*-glucosidation of phenobarbital[21] and the *O*-glucuronidation of *p*-hydroxyphenobarbital[21] appear to be inhibited by valproate.

Importance and management

An extremely well documented and well established interaction of clinical importance. The incidence seems to be high. The effects of concurrent use should be well monitored and suitable phenobarbital dosage reductions made as necessary to avoid toxicity. It would seem that the dosage can be safely reduced by a third to a half with full seizure control.[1] The significance of the reduction in sodium valproate levels is not clear, especially as valproate levels do not correlate well with efficacy of treatment.

1. Wilder BJ, Willmore LJ, Bruni J, Villarreal HJ. Valproic acid: interaction with other anticonvulsant drugs. *Neurology* (1978) 28, 892–6.
2. Richens A, Ahmad S. Controlled trial of sodium valproate in severe epilepsy. *BMJ* (1975) 4, 255–6.
3. Schobben F, van der Kleijn E and Gabreëls FJM. Pharmacokinetics of di-n-propylacetate in epileptic patients. *Eur J Clin Pharmacol* (1975) 8, 97–105.

4. Gram L, Wulff K, Rasmussen KE, Flachs H, Würtz-Jørgensen A, Sommerbeck KW, Løhren V. Valproate sodium: a controlled clinical trial including monitoring of drug levels. *Epilepsia* (1977) 18, 141–8.
5. Jeavons PM, Clark JE. Sodium valproate in treatment of epilepsy. *BMJ* (1974) 2, 584–6.
6. Völzke E, Doose H. Dipropylacetate (Dépakine®, Ergenyl®) in the treatment of epilepsy. *Epilepsia* (1973) 14, 185–93.
7. Millet Y, Sainty JM, Galland MC, Sidoine R, Jouglard J. Problèmes posés par l'association thérapeutique phénobarbital-dipropylacétate de sodium. A propos d'un cas. *Eur J Toxicol Environ Hyg* (1976) 9, 381–3.
8. Jeavons PM, Clark JE, Maheshwari MC. Treatment of generalized epilepsies of childhood and adolescence with sodium valproate ('Epilim'). *Dev Med Child Neurol* (1977) 19, 9–25.
9. Vakil SD, Critchley EMR, Phillips JC, Fahim Y, Haydock C, Cocks A, Dyer T. The effect of sodium valproate (Epilim) on phenytoin and phenobarbitone blood levels. Clinical and Pharmacological Aspects of Sodium Valproate (Epilim) in the Treatment of Epilepsy. Proceedings of a Symposium held at Nottingham University, September 1975, 75–7.
10. Scott DF, Boxer CM, Herzberg JL. A study of the hypnotic effects of Epilim and its possible interaction with phenobarbitone. Clinical and Pharmacological Aspects of Sodium Valproate (Epilim) in the Treatment of Epilepsy. Proceedings of a Symposium held at Nottingham University, September 1975.
11. Richens A, Scoular IT, Ahmad S, Jordan BJ. Pharmacokinetics and efficacy of Epilim in patients receiving long-term therapy with other antiepileptic drugs. Clinical and Pharmacological Aspects of Sodium Valproate (Epilim) in the Treatment of Epilepsy. Proceedings of a Symposium held at Nottingham University, September 1975, 78–88.
12. Loiseau P, Orgogozo JM, Brachet-Liermain A, Morselli PL. Pharmacokinetic studies on the interaction between phenobarbital and valproic acid. In Adv Epileptol Proc Cong Int League Epilepsy 13th. Edited by Meinardi H and Rowan A. (1977/8) p 261–5.
13. Fowler GW. Effect of dipropylacetate on serum levels of anticonvulsants in children. *Proc West Pharmacol Soc* (1978) 21, 37–40.
14. Patel IH, Levy RH, Cutler RE. Phenobarbital-valproic acid interaction. *Clin Pharmacol Ther* (1980) 27, 515–21.
15. Coulter DL, Wu H, Allen RJ. Valproic acid therapy in childhood epilepsy. *JAMA* (1980) 244, 785–8.
16. Kapetanovic IM, Kupferberg HJ, Porter RJ, Theodore W, Schulman E, Penry JK. Mechanism of valproate-phenobarbital interaction in epileptic patients. *Clin Pharmacol Ther* (1981) 29, 480–6.
17. Fernandez de Gatta MR, Alonso Gonzalez AC, Garcia Sanchez MJ, Dominguez-Gil Hurle A, Santos Borbujo J, Monzon Corral L. Effect of sodium valproate on phenobarbital serum levels in children and adults. *Ther Drug Monit* (1986) 8, 416–20.
18. May T, Rambeck B. Serum concentrations of valproic acid: influence of dose and comedication. *Ther Drug Monit* (1985) 7, 387–90.
19. Meinardi H, Bongers E. Analytical data in connection with the clinical use of di-n-propylacetate. In Clinical Pharmacology of Antiepileptic Drugs, edited by Schneider H et al. Springer-Verlag, NY and Berlin (1975) 235–41.
20. Hurst SI, Hargreaves JA, Howald WN, Racha JK, Mather GG, Labroo R, Carlson SP, Levy RH. Enzymatic mechanism for the phenobarbital-valproate interaction. *Epilepsia* (1997) 38 (Suppl 8), 111–12.
21. Bernus I, Dickinson RG, Hooper WD, Eadie MJ. Inhibition of phenobarbitone *N*-glucosidation by valproate. *Br J Clin Pharmacol* (1994) 38, 411–16.

Barbiturates + Troleandomycin

A patient showed a fall in his serum phenobarbital levels when concurrently treated with troleandomycin.

Clinical evidence, mechanism, importance and management

A patient on **phenobarbital** as well as **carbamazepine** showed a fall in serum **phenobarbital** levels from about 40 to 31 micrograms/ml and a rise in carbamazepine levels, when treated with **troleandomycin**.[1] The general importance of this single report is uncertain, but it would now seem prudent to be alert for changes in seizure control if this antibacterial is used. See also 'Carbamazepine + Macrolide antibacterials', p.328.

1. Dravet C, Mesdjian E, Cenraud B and Roger J. Interaction between carbamazepine and triacetyloleandomycin. *Lancet* (1977) i, 810.

Carbamazepine + Allopurinol

Allopurinol can gradually raise serum carbamazepine levels by about a third. Some reduction in the carbamazepine dosage may eventually be needed.

Clinical evidence

In a 6-month study, 7 epileptic patients on anticonvulsants, which included carbamazepine, were also given allopurinol (100 mg three times daily for 3 months then 200 mg three times daily for 3 months). The mean trough steady-state serum carbamazepine levels of 6 of the

patients rose by 30% or more and the carbamazepine clearance fell by 32% during the second 3-month period. A reduction in carbamazepine dosage was needed in 3 patients because of the symptoms that developed.[1]

Mechanism

Uncertain. A possible explanation is that allopurinol can act as a liver enzyme inhibiting agent which reduces the metabolism and clearance of other drugs by the liver.

Importance and management

Information is limited to this study, but be alert for the need to reduce the dosage of carbamazepine if allopurinol is added. This interaction apparently takes several weeks or even months to develop fully. More study is needed.

1. Mikati M, Erba G, Skouteli H, Gadia C. Pharmacokinetic study of allopurinol in resistant epilepsy: evidence for significant drug interactions. *Neurology* (1990) 40 (Suppl 1), 138.

Carbamazepine + Amiodarone

Carbamazepine pharmacokinetics appear not to be affected by amiodarone.

Clinical evidence, mechanism, importance and management

A single 400-mg dose of carbamazepine was given to 9 patients with cardiac disease (premature ventricular contractions, supraventricular tachycardia, sinus arrhythmia) before and after taking 200 mg **amiodarone** twice daily for a month. The pharmacokinetics of carbamazepine were found to be unchanged by the **amiodarone** treatment. This certainly suggests that no clinically important interaction occurs, but it needs confirmation in patients who are treated with both drugs long term. The authors postulate that the **amiodarone** dosage may have been too low to inhibit the metabolism of the carbamazepine by the liver.[1]

1. Leite SAO, Leite PJM, Rocha GA, Routledge PA, Bittencourt PRM. Carbamazepine kinetics in cardiac patients before and during amiodarone. *Arq Neuropsiquiatr* (1994) 52, 210–15.

Carbamazepine + Antipsychotics

Toxicity, due to an increase in the serum levels of carbamazepine-epoxide, has been reported in 3 patients on carbamazepine when given loxapine, or chlorpromazine with amoxapine. Thioridazine however, appears not to interact. Carbamazepine can lower fluphenazine serum levels. Some preliminary evidence also suggests that the use of antipsychotics with carbamazepine may possibly increase the risk of developing Stevens-Johnson syndrome.

Clinical evidence, mechanism, importance and management

(a) Raised carbamazepine-epoxide levels

Two patients, one on 500 mg **loxapine** daily and the other on 350 mg **chlorpromazine** and 300 mg **amoxapine** daily, developed toxicity (ataxia, nausea, anxiety) when given 600 to 900 mg carbamazepine daily, even though their serum carbamazepine levels were low to normal.[1] In another case, neurotoxicity (ataxia, lethargy, visual disturbances) developed in a man given carbamazepine and **loxapine**.[2] In all 3 cases, the toxicity appeared to be due to elevated carbamazepine-epoxide levels (the metabolite of carbamazepine).[1,2] The problem resolved when the carbamazepine dosages were reduced. The authors of both reports advise monitoring the serum levels of both carbamazepine and its metabolite if toxicity develops.[1,2]

(b) No changes to carbamazepine-epoxide levels

Thioridazine 100 to 200 mg daily was found to have no effect on the steady-state levels of carbamazepine or carbamazepine-epoxide in 8 epileptic patients,[3] and also carbamazepine had no significant effect on **thioridazine** serum levels.[4]

(c) Reduced fluphenazine levels

A patient on 37.5 mg **fluphenazine decanoate** weekly showed a serum level rise from 0.6 nanograms/ml to 1.17 nanograms/ml 6 weeks after stopping 800 mg carbamazepine daily. A moderate improvement in his schizophrenic condition occurred.[5]

(d) Stevens-Johnson syndrome

Three patients on various antipsychotics (**fluphenazine, haloperidol, trifluoperazine, chlorpromazine**) developed Stevens-Johnson syndrome within 8 to 14 days of starting to take carbamazepine. All 3 had erythema multiforme skin lesions and involvement of at least two mucous membranes. After treatment, all 3 were restarted on all their previous drugs, except carbamazepine, without problems.[6] Another case has been reported in a patient on carbamazepine, **lithium carbonate, haloperidol** and **trihexyphenidyl (benzhexol)**.[7] The reasons are not understood. Stevens-Johnson syndrome with carbamazepine is rare and appears only to have been described in two patients on carbamazepine alone.[8,9] It is not yet clear whether the concurrent use of antipsychotics increases the risk of its development, but until more is known it would be prudent to monitor the outcome, particularly during the first 2 weeks of combined use. More study is needed.

1. Pitterle ME, Collins DM. Carbamazepine-10,11-epoxide evaluation associated with coadministration of loxitane or amoxapine. *Epilepsia* (1988) 29, 654.
2. Collins DM, Gidal BE, Pitterle ME. Potential interaction between carbamazepine and loxapine: case report and retrospective review. *Ann Pharmacother* (1993) 27, 1180–3.
3. Spina E, Amendola D'Agostino AM, Ioculano MP, Oteri G, Fazio A, Pisani F. No effect of thioridazine on plasma concentrations of carbamazepine and its active metabolite carbamazepine-10,11-epoxide. *Ther Drug Monit* (1990) 12, 511–13.
4. Tiihonen J, Vartiainen H, Hakola P. Carbamazepine-induced changes in plasma levels of neuroleptics. *Pharmacopsychiatry* (1995) 28, 26–8.
5. Jann MW, Fidone GS, Hernandez JM, Amrung S, Davis CM. Clinical implications of increased antipsychotic plasma concentrations upon anticonvulsant cessation. *Psychiatry Res* (1989) 28, 153–9.
6. Wong KE. Stevens-Johnson Syndrome in neuroleptic-carbamazepine combination. *Singapore Med J* (1990) 31, 432–3.
7. Fawcett RG. Erythema multiforme major in a patient treated with carbamazepine. *J Clin Psychiatry* (1987) 48, 416–17.
8. Coombes BW. Stevens-Johnson syndrome associated with carbamazepine ("Tegretol"). *Med J Aust* (1965) 1, 895–6.
9. Patterson JF. Stevens-Johnson syndrome associated with carbamazepine. *Clin Psychopharmacol* (1985) 5, 185.

Carbamazepine + Azole antifungals

Ketoconazole causes a small to moderate rise in serum carbamazepine levels, and adverse effects have been seen when carbamazepine was used concurrently with fluconazole or miconazole.

Clinical evidence

(a) Fluconazole

A 33-year-old man who was stabilised on carbamazepine for seizures became extremely lethargic after taking 150 mg of **fluconazole** for 3 days. His carbamazepine level was found to have risen from 11.1 to 24.5 micrograms/ml. Symptoms resolved when both drugs were stopped, and carbamazepine was later reintroduced without problem.[1]

(b) Ketoconazole

A study in 8 patients with epilepsy taking carbamazepine found that the addition of 200 mg oral **ketoconazole** for 10 days increased their serum carbamazepine levels by 28.6% (from 5.6 to 7.2 micrograms/ml) whereas the carbamazepine-epoxide levels were unchanged. When the **ketoconazole** was stopped the serum carbamazepine levels fell to their former levels.[2]

(c) Miconazole

A patient on long-term treatment with carbamazepine 400 mg daily developed malaise, myoclonia and tremor within 3 days of being given 1125 mg **miconazole**. The same reaction occurred on each subsequent occasion when the patient was again given **miconazole**. These toxic effects disappeared when the **miconazole** was withdrawn.[3]

Mechanism

The reason for the carbamazepine serum level rise is though to be that the azole antifungals inhibit cytochrome P450 isoenzyme CYP3A4 to varying degrees, and this isoenzyme is concerned with the metabolism of carbamazepine.

Importance and management

The rise in carbamazepine serum levels seen in the studies with ketoconazole is only moderate, but the case reports with fluconazole and miconazole indicate that larger, potentially more serious interactions are possible. It would seem prudent to monitor the outcome of adding azole antifungals to established carbamazepine treatment, being alert for any evidence of increased carbamazepine side-effects.

1. Nair DR, Morris HH. Potential fluconazole-induced carbamazepine toxicity. *Ann Pharmacother* (1999) 33, 790–2.
2. Spina E, Arena D, Scordo MG, Fazio A, Pisani F, Perucca E. Elevation of plasma carbamazepine concentrations by ketoconazole in patients with epilepsy. *Ther Drug Monit* (1997) 19, 535–8.
3. Loupi E, Descotes J, Lery N, Evreux JC. Interactions medicamenteuses et miconazole. A propos de 10 observations. *Therapie* (1982) 37, 437–41.

Carbamazepine or Oxcarbazepine + Cimetidine or Ranitidine

Epileptic patients and subjects chronically treated with carbamazepine show a transient increase in serum levels, possibly accompanied by an increase in side-effects, for the first few days after starting to take cimetidine, but these side-effects rapidly disappear. This does not occur with oxcarbazepine. Ranitidine appears not to interact with carbamazepine.

Clinical evidence

(a) Carbamazepine

The steady-state carbamazepine levels of 8 healthy subjects on carbamazepine 300 mg twice daily increased by 17% within 2 days of starting 400 mg **cimetidine** three times daily. Side-effects occurred in 6 patients, but after 7 days treatment the carbamazepine levels had fallen again and the side effects disappeared.[1]

The steady-state carbamazepine levels of 7 epileptic patients on chronic treatment remained unaltered when given 1 g **cimetidine** daily for a week.[2] Another study also showed a lack of an interaction in 11 epileptic patients.[3] A very elderly woman, aged 89, developed signs of carbamazepine toxicity within 2 days of starting to take 400 mg **cimetidine** daily, and showed a rise in serum carbamazepine levels, which fell when the cimetidine was withdrawn.[4]

The results of these studies in patients and subjects taking carbamazepine long term differ from single-dose studies and short-term studies in healthy subjects. For example, a 33% rise in serum carbamazepine levels,[5] a 20% fall in clearance[6] and a 26% increase in the AUC[7] have been reported, which would indicate potential for a clinically significant interaction (see 'Mechanism').

Ranitidine 300 mg daily did not affect the pharmacokinetics of a single 600-mg dose of carbamazepine when given to 8 healthy subjects.[8]

(b) Oxcarbazepine

No changes in the pharmacokinetics of a single 600-mg oral dose of oxcarbazepine were seen in 8 healthy subjects after taking 400 mg **cimetidine** twice daily for 7 days.[9]

Mechanism

Not fully understood. It is thought that cimetidine can inhibit the activity of the liver enzymes concerned with the metabolism of carbamazepine, resulting in its reduced clearance from the body, but the effect is short-lived because the auto-inducing effects of the carbamazepine oppose it. This would possibly explain why the single-dose and short-term studies in healthy subjects suggest that a clinically important interaction could occur, but in practice the combination causes few problems in patients on long-term treatment.

Importance and management

The carbamazepine/cimetidine interaction is established but of minimal importance. Patients on long-term treatment with carbamazepine should be warned that for the first few days after starting to take cimetidine they may possibly experience some increase in the carbamazepine side-effects (nausea, headache, dizziness, fatigue, drowsiness, ataxia, an inability to concentrate, a bitter taste). However, because the serum levels are only transiently increased, these side-effects normally subside and disappear by the end of a week. **Ranitidine** appears to be a non-interacting alternative to cimetidine. Oxcarbazepine appears not to interact with cimetidine.

1. Dalton MJ, Powell JR, Messenheimer JA, Clark J. Cimetidine and carbamazepine: a complex drug interaction. *Epilepsia* (1986) 27, 553–8.
2. Sonne J, Lühdorf K, Larsen NE and Andreasen PB. Lack of interaction between cimetidine and carbamazepine. *Acta Neurol Scand* (1983) 68, 253–6.
3. Levine M, Jones MW, Sheppard I. Differential effect of cimetidine on serum concentrations of carbamazepine and phenytoin. *Neurology* (1985) 35, 562–5.
4. Telerman-Topet N, Duret ME, Coërs C. Cimetidine interaction with carbamazepine. *Ann Intern Med* (1981) 94, 544.
5. Macphee GJA, Thompson GG, Scobie G, Agnew E, Park BK, Murray T, McColl KEL, Brodie MJ. Effects of cimetidine on carbamazepine auto- and hetero-induction in man. *Br J Clin Pharmacol* (1984) 18, 411–19.
6. Webster LK, Mihaly GW, Jones DB, Smallwood RA, Phillips JA, Vajda FJ. Effect of cimetidine and ranitidine on carbamazepine and sodium valproate pharmacokinetics. *Eur J Clin Pharmacol* (1984) 27, 341–3.
7. Dalton MJ, Powell JR, Messenheimer JA. The influence of cimetidine on single-dose carbamazepine pharmacokinetics. *Epilepsia* (1985) 26, 127–30.
8. Dalton MJ, Powell JR, Messenheimer JA. Ranitidine does not alter single-dose carbamazepine pharmacokinetics in healthy adults. *Drug Intell Clin Pharm* (1985) 19, 941–4.
9. Keränen T, Jolkkonen J, Klosterskov-Jensen P, Menge GP. Oxcarbazepine does not interact with cimetidine in healthy volunteers. *Acta Neurol Scand* (1992) 85, 239–42.

Carbamazepine + Colestyramine or Colestipol

Colestipol causes a minor reduction in the absorption of carbamazepine which is unlikely to be clinically significant. Cholestyramine does not appear to interact.

Clinical evidence, mechanism, importance and management

Colestyramine 8 g did not affect the absorption of 400 mg carbamazepine in 6 healthy subjects, whereas 10 g **colestipol** reduced it by 10%. Both **colestyramine** and **colestipol** were given as a single dose 5 min after the carbamazepine.[1] This small reduction is unlikely to be clinically important, but concurrent use should nonetheless be monitored.

1. Neuvonen PJ, Kivistö K, Hirvisalo EL. Effects of resins and activated charcoal on the absorption of digoxin, carbamazepine and frusemide. *Br J Clin Pharmacol* (1988) 25, 229–33.

Carbamazepine + Danazol

Serum carbamazepine levels can be doubled by the concurrent use of danazol. Carbamazepine toxicity may occur unless the dosage is reduced appropriately.

Clinical evidence

The serum carbamazepine levels of 6 epileptics approximately doubled within 7 to 30 days of being treated with **danazol** 400 to 600 mg daily. Acute carbamazepine toxicity (dizziness, drowsiness, blurred vision, ataxia, nausea) was experienced by 5 out of the 6 patients.[1]

Other reports similarly describe rises in serum carbamazepine levels of 50 to 100% (with toxicity seen in some instances) when **danazol** was added.[2-4]

Mechanism

Danazol inhibits the metabolism (by the epoxide-trans-diol pathway) of carbamazepine by the liver, thereby reducing its loss from the body.[2,5] During danazol treatment the clearance of carbamazepine has been found to be reduced by 60%, and the half-life more than doubled.[2]

Importance and management

An established and clinically important interaction. If concurrent use is necessary carbamazepine serum levels should be monitored and the dosage reduced as necessary.

1. Zeilinski JJ, Lichten EM, Haidukewych D. Clinically significant danazol-carbamazepine interaction. *Ther Drug Monit* (1987) 9, 24–7.
2. Krämer G, Theisohn M, von Unruh GE, Eichelbaum M. Carbamazepine-danazol drug interaction: its mechanism examined by a stable isotope technique. *Ther Drug Monit* (1986) 8, 387–92.
3. Hayden M, Buchanan N. Danazol-carbamazepine interaction. *Med J Aust* (1991) 155, 851.
4. Nelson MV. Interaction of danazol and carbamazepine. *Am J Psychiatry* (1988) 145, 768–9.
5. Krämer G, Besser R, Theisohn M, Eichelbaum M. Carbamazepine-danazol drug interaction: mechanism and therapeutic usefulness. *Acta Neurol Scand* (1984) 70, 249.

Carbamazepine + Diuretics

Two patients on carbamazepine developed hyponatraemia when given hydrochlorothiazide or furosemide (frusemide).

Clinical evidence, mechanism, importance and management

Two epileptic patients developed symptomatic hyponatraemia while on carbamazepine, one while taking **hydrochlorothiazide** and the other while taking **furosemide (frusemide)**.[1] The reasons are uncertain but all three drugs can cause sodium to be lost from the body. This seems to be an uncommon interaction, but be aware that it can occur.

1. Ramzy Y, Nastase C, Camille Y, Henderson M, Belzile L and Beland F. Carbamazepine, diuretics and hyponatremia: a possible interaction. *J Clin Psychiatry* (1987) 48, 281–3.

Carbamazepine + Felbamate

Felbamate reduces serum carbamazepine levels but increases serum levels of the active metabolite, carbamazepine-epoxide. Felbamate levels may fall. The importance of these changes is uncertain but it is likely to be small.

Clinical evidence

The serum carbamazepine levels of 22 patients, with doses adjusted to keep levels in the range of 4 to 12 micrograms/ml, fell by 25%

(range 10 to 42%) when additionally given **felbamate** 3000 mg daily. The decrease occurred within a week, reaching a plateau after 2 to 4 weeks, and returning to the original levels within 2 to 3 weeks of stopping the felbamate.[1] Other studies in epileptics have found reductions in carbamazepine levels of between 18 and 31% when **felbamate** was given concurrently.[2-7] Some of these studies also found that the serum levels of the active carbamazepine metabolite carbamazepine-epoxide rose by 33% to 57%.[1,4,5]

Carbamazepine increased the clearance of **felbamate** by up to 49%.[8-11]

Mechanism

Not established. It is thought that the felbamate increases the metabolism of the carbamazepine.[1]

Importance and management

This interaction is established, but its clinical importance is uncertain because the modest fall in serum carbamazepine levels would seem to be offset by the rise in levels of its metabolite, carbamazepine-epoxide, which also has anticonvulsant activity. There is probably no need to alter the carbamazepine dosage initially, but monitor carbamazepine levels carefully and be alert for any changes in the anticonvulsant control. The importance of the increased felbamate clearance is uncertain. More study is needed.

1. Albani F, Theodore WH, Washington P, Devinsky O, Bromfield E, Porter RJ, Nice FJ. Effect of Felbamate on plasma levels of carbamazepine and its metabolites. *Epilepsia* (1991) 32, 130–2.
2. Fuerst RH, Graves NM, Leppik IE, Remmel RP, Rosenfeld WE, Sierzant TL. A preliminary report on alteration of carbamazepine and phenytoin metabolism by felbamate. *Drug Intell Clin Pharm* (1986) 20, 465–6.
3. Fuerst RH, Graves NM, Leppik IE, Brundage RC, Holmes GB, Remmel RP. Felbamate increases phenytoin but decreases carbamazepine concentrations. *Epilepsia* (1988) 29, 488–91.
4. Howard JR, Dix RK, Shumaker RC, Perhach JL. The effect of felbamate on carbamazepine pharmacokinetics. *Epilepsia* (1992) 33 (Suppl 3), 84–5.
5. Wagner ML, Remmel RP, Graves NM, Leppik IE. Effect of felbamate on carbamazepine and its major metabolites. *Clin Pharmacol Ther* (1993) 53, 536–43.
6. Theodore WH, Raubertas RF, Porter RJ, Nice F, Devinsky O, Reeves P, Bromfield E, Ito B, Balish M. Felbamate: a clinical trial for complex partial seizures. *Epilepsia* (1991) 32, 392–7.
7. Leppik IE, Dreifuss FE, Pledger GW, Graves NM, Santilli N, Drury I, Tsay JY, Jacobs MP, Bertram E, Cereghino JJ, Cooper G, Sahlroot JT, Sheridan P, Ashworth M, Lee SI, Sierzant TL. Felbamate for partial seizures: results of a controlled clinical trial. *Neurology* (1991) 41, 1785–9.
8. Wagner ML, Graves NM, Marienau K, Holmes GB, Remmel RP, Leppik IE. Discontinuation of phenytoin and carbamazepine in patients receiving felbamate. *Epilepsia* (1991) 32, 398–406.
9. Kelley MT, Walson PD, Cox S, Dusci LJ. Population pharmacokinetics of felbamate in children. *Ther Drug Monit* (1997) 19, 29–36.
10. Kelley MT, Walson PD, Cox S. Population kinetics of felbamate in children. *Clin Pharmacol Ther* (1996) 59, 213.
11. Banfield CR, Zhu G-RR, Jen JF, Jensen PK, Schumaker RC, Perhach JL Affrime MB, Glue P. The effect of age on the apparent clearance of felbamate: a retrospective analysis using nonlinear mixed-effects modeling. *Ther Drug Monit* (1996) 18, 19–29.

Carbamazepine + Influenza vaccines

Carbamazepine levels rose modestly 14 days after influenza vaccination.

Clinical evidence, mechanism, importance and management

A 47% rise in the serum **carbamazepine** levels (6.17 to 9.04 micrograms/ml) of 20 children occurred 14 days after being given 0.5 ml of an **influenza vaccine USP, types A and B, whole virus** (Squibb). Levels remained elevated on day 28.[1]

The suggested reason is the **vaccine** inhibits the liver enzymes concerned with the metabolism of **carbamazepine**, thereby reducing its loss from the body. Information is very limited but it seems unlikely that this moderate increase in serum **carbamazepine** levels will have much clinical relevance.

1. Jann MW, Fidone GS. Effect of influenza vaccine on serum anticonvulsant concentrations. *Clin Pharm* (1986) 5, 817–20.

Carbamazepine + Gemfibrozil

Two patients with hyperlipoproteinaemia showed rises in carbamazepine serum levels when gemfibrozil was added.

Clinical evidence, mechanism, importance and management

When 2 patients stabilised on carbamazepine were treated for type IV hyperlipoproteinaemia with **gemfibrozil** they showed rises in their serum carbamazepine levels. One patient showed a rise from 8.8 to 11.4 micrograms/ml within 4 days of starting **gemfibrozil** 300 mg daily, while a rise from 8.3 to 13.7 micrograms/ml was found in the other patient 3 months after starting to take 300 mg **gemfibrozil** twice daily.[1] The suggested reason is that the clearance of carbamazepine is increased in those with elevated cholesterol and total lipids, thus when the condition is treated with **gemfibrozil**, the clearance becomes more normal, which results in a rise in the serum carbamazepine levels.[2] The clinical importance of this interaction is uncertain but be alert for any evidence of carbamazepine toxicity if **gemfibrozil** is added.

1. Denio L, Drake ME, Pakalnis A. Gemfibrozil-carbamazepine interaction in epileptic patients. *Epilepsia* (1988) 29, 654.
2. Wichlinski LM, Sieradzki E, Gruchala M. Correlation between the total cholesterol serum concentration data and carbamazepine steady-state blood levels in humans. *Drug Intell Clin Pharm* (1983) 17, 812–14.

Carbamazepine + Isoniazid

Carbamazepine serum levels are markedly and very rapidly increased by the concurrent use of isoniazid. Toxicity can occur if the carbamazepine dosage is not reduced appropriately.

Clinical evidence

Disorientation, listlessness, aggression, lethargy and, in one case, extreme drowsiness developed in 10 out of 13 patients stabilised on carbamazepine when concurrently treated with 200 mg **isoniazid** daily. Serum carbamazepine levels were measured in 3 of the patients and they were found to have risen above the normal therapeutic range (initial level not stated).[1]

Carbamazepine toxicity, associated with marked rises in serum carbamazepine levels, has been described in other reports.[2-6] Some of the patients were also taking **sodium valproate**, which does not seem to be implicated in the interaction, and in one case **cimetidine**, which was thought to have potentiated the interaction.[6] One report describes carbamazepine toxicity in a patient when given **isoniazid** but only when **rifampicin** was present as well. Usually the enzyme inducing effects of rifampicin would be expected to counteract any enzyme inhibition by isoniazid, so this report is somewhat inexplicable.[7]

There is also some limited evidence that carbamazepine may increase the hepatotoxicity of **isoniazid**.[8]

Mechanism

It seems probable that the isoniazid inhibits the activity of the liver enzymes concerned with the metabolism and clearance of carbamazepine, so that it accumulates in the body.

Importance and management

The documentation is not large, but a clinically important and potentially serious interaction is established. Toxicity can develop quickly (within 1 to 5 days) and also seems to disappear quickly if the isoniazid is withdrawn. Concurrent use should not be undertaken unless the effects can be closely monitored and suitable downward dosage adjustments made (a reduction to between one-half or one-third was effective in 3 patients[1]). It seems probable that those who are 'slow' metabolisers of isoniazid may show this interaction more quickly and to a greater extent than fast metabolisers.[2]

1. Valsalan VC, Cooper GL. Carbamazepine intoxication caused by interaction with isoniazid. *BMJ* (1982) 285, 261–2.
2. Wright JM, Stokes EF, Sweeney VP. Isoniazid-induced carbamazepine toxicity and vice versa: a double drug interaction. *N Engl J Med* (1982) 307, 1325–7.
3. Block SH. Carbamazepine-isoniazid interaction. *Pediatrics* (1982) 69, 494–5.
4. Poo Argüelles P, Samarra Riera JM, Gairí Tahull JM, Vernet Bori A. Interacción carbamacepina-tuberculostáticos. *Med Clin (Barc)* (1984) 83, 867–8.
5. Beeley L, Ballantine N. Bulletin of the West Midlands Adverse Drug Reaction Study Group (1981) 13, 8.
6. García B, Zaborras E, Areas V, Obeso G, Jiménez I, de Juana P, Bermejo T. Interaction between isoniazid and carbamazepine potentiated by cimetidine. *Ann Pharmacother* (1992) 26, 841–2.
7. Fleenor ME, Harden JW, Curtis G. Interaction between carbamazepine and antituberculous agents. *Chest* (1991) 99, 1554.
8. Barbare JC, Lallement F, Vorhauer W, Veyssier P. Hépatotoxicité de l'isoniazide: influence de la carbamazépine? *Gastroenterol Clin Biol* (1986) 10, 523–4.

Carbamazepine + Isotretinoin

A study in one patient found that isotretinoin modestly reduced the serum levels of carbamazepine and its active metabolite. Another study found that no interaction occurs between isotretinoin and phenytoin.

Clinical evidence, mechanism, importance and management

The carbamazepine AUC in an epileptic patient taking carbamazepine 600 mg daily was reduced by 11% while taking 500 micrograms/kg daily of **isotretinoin**, and by 24% when taking 1000 micrograms/kg daily. The AUC of carbamazepine-epoxide (the active metabolite of carbamazepine) was reduced by 21 and 44% by the small and large doses of isotretinoin respectively. The patient showed no adverse effects but the author of the report suggests that concurrent use should be monitored.[1] A study in 7 healthy subjects taking 300 mg **phenytoin** daily found that the addition of 40 mg **isotretinoin** twice daily for 11 days had no effect on the steady-state pharmacokinetics of **phenytoin**.[2] No special precautions would seem to be needed if these drugs are given concurrently.

1. Marsden JR. Effect of isotretinoin on carbamazepine pharmacokinetics. *Br J Dermatol* (1988) 119, 403–4.
2. Oo C, Barsanti F, Zhang R. Lack of effect of isotretinoin on the pharmacokinetics of phenytoin at steady-state. *Pharm Res* (1997) 14 (11 Suppl), S-561.

Carbamazepine or Oxcarbazepine + Lamotrigine

Some but not all studies have found that lamotrigine raises the serum levels of the active metabolite of carbamazepine. Toxicity has been seen. A case report describes similar toxicity with oxcarbazepine and lamotrigine.

Clinical evidence

(a) Evidence of changes in carbamazepine metabolism

The addition of **lamotrigine** increased the serum levels of the active metabolite of carbamazepine (carbamazepine-epoxide) in 3 epileptic patients, but carbamazepine levels remained unchanged. One of the patients had carbamazepine epoxide serum levels of 2.0 to 2.2 micrograms/ml while taking 1100 mg carbamazepine daily. The levels rose to 4.7 to 8.7 micrograms/ml when **lamotrigine** was added. Symptoms of toxicity occurred in 2 patients (dizziness, double vision, sleepiness, nausea).[1] In another study in 10 patients, the addition of 200 mg **lamotrigine** increased the mean serum carbamazepine-epoxide levels by 47%. Toxicity was seen in 6 patients (dizziness, nausea, diplopia).[2,3] Cerebellar toxicity (nausea, vertigo, nystagmus, ataxia) developed in 8 out of 9 patients on subtoxic and just-tolerated doses of carbamazepine when **lamotrigine** was added. Analysis showed

that in all 8 cases at least one of the three levels of carbamazepine, carbamazepine-epoxide or **lamotrigine** had become unusually high.[4]

(b) Evidence of no changes in carbamazepine metabolism

The studies cited in (a) contrast with others that failed to find pharmacokinetic effects. No changes in carbamazepine levels were seen in two studies,[5,6] and another found that 200 to 300 mg **lamotrigine** daily had no effect on the disposition of orally administered carbamazepine-epoxide.[7] Another study in 47 patients on carbamazepine, to which **lamotrigine** was added, found no significant changes in carbamazepine or carbamazepine-epoxide levels, but despite this 9 cases of diplopia or dizziness were recorded, predominantly in those whose carbamazepine levels were already high before the **lamotrigine** was added.[8] A further well-designed study found that **lamotrigine** 100 mg twice daily for a week had no effect on the pharmacokinetics of carbamazepine or carbamazepine-epoxide after a single 200-mg dose of carbamazepine in healthy subjects.[9]

Mechanisms

The apparent contradiction between the results described in (a) and (b) is not understood. One suggestion to account for the toxic symptoms seen in some patients is that it occurs at the site of action (a pharmacodynamic interaction) rather than because lamotrigine increases the carbamazepine-epoxide serum levels.[8]

A case report of severe toxicity that occurred with **oxcarbazepine** plus **lamotrigine** would appear to support this idea, because oxcarbazepine is not metabolised to epoxides.[10]

Importance and management

A confusing situation, but in practical terms it means that carbamazepine serum drug levels and the response to treatment should be well monitored if lamotrigine is added. The carbamazepine dosage may need to be reduced, especially if serum levels are already high. More study is needed. Information about oxcarbazepine plus lamotrigine is very limited, but good monitoring would also be advisable.

1. Graves NM, Ritter FJ, Wagner ML, Floren KL, Alexander BJ, Campbell JI, Leppik IE. Effect of lamotrigine on carbamazepine epoxide concentrations. *Epilepsia* (1991) 32 (Suppl 3), 13.
2. Warner T, Patsalos PN, Prevett M, Elyas AA, Duncan JS. Lamotrigine-induced carbamazepine toxicity: a pharmacokinetic interaction. *Epilepsia* (1991) 32 (Suppl 1), 95.
3. Warner T, Patsalos PN, Prevett M, Elyas AA, Duncan JS. Lamotrigine-induced carbamazepine toxicity: an interaction with carbamazepine-10,11-epoxide. *Epilepsy Res* (1992) 11, 147–50.
4. Wolf P. Lamotrigine: preliminary clinical observations on pharmacokinetics and interactions with traditional antiepileptic drugs. *J Epilepsy* (1992) 5, 73–9.
5. Jawad S, Richens A, Goodwin G, Yuen WC. Controlled trial of lamotrigine (Lamictal) for refractory partial seizures. *Epilepsia* (1989) 30, 356–63.
6. Eriksson A-S, Hoppu K, Nergårdh A, Boreus L. Pharmacokinetic interactions between lamotrigine and other antiepileptic drugs in children with intractable epilepsy. *Epilepsia* (1996) 37, 769–73.
7. Pisani F, Xiao B, Fazio A, Spina E, Perucca E, Tomson T. Single dose pharmacokinetics of carbamazepine-10,11-epoxide in patients on lamotrigine monotherapy. *Epilepsy Res* (1994) 19, 245–8.
8. Besag FMC, Subel B, Pool F, Berry D, Newbery JE. Carbamazepine toxicity with lamotrigine: a pharmacokinetic or pharmacodynamic interaction? *Epilepsia* (1994) 35 (Suppl 7), 73.
9. Malminiemi K, Keränen T, Kerttula T, Moilanen E, Ylitalo P. Effects of short-term lamotrigine treatment on pharmacokinetics of carbamazepine. *Int J Clin Pharmacol Ther* (2000) 38, 540–5.
10. Alving J. Case of severe acute intoxication with oxcarbazepine combined with lamotrigine. *Epilepsia* (1994) 35 (Suppl 7), 72.

Carbamazepine + Lansoprazole

Some anecdotal reports suggest that carbamazepine serum levels may possibly be reduced by lansoprazole in a few patients.

Clinical evidence, mechanism, importance and management

The makers of **lansoprazole** have on record 5 undetailed case reports of apparent interaction between **lansoprazole** and carbamazepine. One of them describes the development of carbamazepine toxicity when **lansoprazole** was added, but there is some doubt about this case because it is thought that the patient may have started to take higher doses of carbamazepine.

The other 4 cases however are consistent in that carbamazepine levels fell shortly after **lansoprazole** was added and/or the control of seizures suddenly worsened. One patient showed a fall in carbamazepine serum levels from 11.5 to 7.7 mg/l. The carbamazepine levels of another patient returned to normal when the **lansoprazole** was stopped.[1] One suggested reason is that the lowered gastric pH due to the **lansoprazole** may have reduced the absorption of the carbamazepine, resulting in reduced seizure control,[1] although other proton pump inhibitors, which also lower the gastric pH seem not to have been reported to interact like this.

Information seems to be limited to this handful of reports from which no broad general conclusions can be drawn, but they do suggest that patients should be monitored if **lansoprazole** is added to established treatment with carbamazepine.

1. Wyeth (UK). Personal communication, September 2001.

Carbamazepine + Macrolide antibacterials

Carbamazepine serum levels are markedly and rapidly increased by the concurrent use of clarithromycin or troleandomycin. Toxicity can often develop within 1 to 3 days. Flurithromycin, josamycin and midecamycin diacetate appear to interact to a lesser extent and roxithromycin not at all. See also 'Anticonvulsants + Erythromycin', p.313.

Clinical evidence

(a) Clarithromycin

A pharmacokinetic study[1] in healthy subjects found that **clarithromycin** 500 mg 12-hourly for 5 days increased the AUC of a single 400-mg dose of carbamazepine by 26%. A retrospective study of 5 epileptic patients found that when they were given **clarithromycin** (dosage not stated) their serum carbamazepine levels rose by 20 to 50% within 3 to 5 days, despite 30 to 40% reductions in the carbamazepine dosage in 4 of them. Carbamazepine levels in the toxic range were seen in 3 of them, and their carbamazepine dosages were then even further reduced.[2] A number of case reports have described **carbamazepine** toxicity after the addition of **clarithromycin** in adults,[3,4] and children.[5,6] Two other epileptic patients showed marked rises in serum carbamazepine levels when given 500 mg **clarithromycin** three times daily and omeprazole.[7] It is not clear whether the omeprazole also had some part to play.[8,9]

(b) Flurithromycin

Flurithromycin 500 mg three times daily for a week has been found to increase the AUC of a single 400-mg dose of carbamazepine by about 20%.[10]

(c) Josamycin

Josamycin 2 g daily for a week has been found to reduce the clearance of carbamazepine by about 20%.[11,12]

(d) Midecamycin diacetate (miocamycin; ponsinomycin)

A single dose study in 14 subjects found that after taking 800 mg **midecamycin diacetate** twice daily for 8 days the AUC of a single 200-mg dose of carbamazepine was increased by 15%, and the AUC of its active metabolite (10,11 epoxycarbamazepine) was reduced 26%.[13] Another study in patients on carbamazepine found that the addition of 600 mg **midecamycin diacetate** twice daily caused a small increase in the trough serum levels of carbamazepine, and only an 11.6% increase in the AUC.[14]

(e) Roxithromycin

Roxithromycin 150 mg twice daily for 8 days did not affect the pharmacokinetics of a single 200-mg dose of carbamazepine.[15]

(f) Troleandomycin

Signs of carbamazepine toxicity (dizziness, nausea, vomiting, excessive drowsiness) developed in 8 epileptic patients on carbamazepine within 24 h of starting to take **troleandomycin**. The only 2 patients available for examination showed a sharp rise in serum carbamazepine levels (from about 5 to 28 micrograms/ml) over 3 days, and a rapid fall following withdrawal.[16,17]

Another report by the same authors describes a total of 17 similar cases of toxicity caused by **troleandomycin**.[18] Some of the patients demonstrated three or fourfold increases in serum carbamazepine levels. Another case has been described elsewhere.[19] In most instances the serum carbamazepine levels returned to normal within about 3 to 5 days of withdrawing the macrolide.[18]

Mechanism

It seems probable that clarithromycin and troleandomycin, and to a much lesser extent some of the other macrolides, slow the rate of metabolism of the carbamazepine by the liver enzymes so that the anticonvulsant accumulates within the body. Troleandomycin forms an inactive complex with cytochrome P450 in the liver.[20]

Importance and management

The carbamazepine/troleandomycin interaction is established, clinically important and potentially serious. The incidence is high. The rapidity of its development (24 h in some cases) and the extent of the rise in serum carbamazepine levels suggest that it would be difficult to control carbamazepine levels by reducing the dosage. Concurrent use should be avoided if possible.

The carbamazepine/clarithromycin interaction is also established, clinically important and potentially serious. It has been recommended that carbamazepine dosages should be reduced 30 to 50% during treatment with clarithromycin; that monitoring should be done within 3 to 5 days, and patients should be told to tell their doctor of any signs of toxicity (dizziness, diplopia, ataxia, mental confusion).

Josamycin, flurithromycin and midecamycin diacetate appear to be safer alternatives to either clarithromycin, erythromycin or troleandomycin, nevertheless a small or moderate reduction in the dosage of the carbamazepine may be needed, with subsequent good monitoring. Pharmacokinetic data suggest roxithromycin does not interact. See also 'Anticonvulsants + Erythromycin', p.313.

1. Richens A, Chu S-Y, Sennello LT, Sonders RC. Effect of multiple doses of clarithromycin (C) on the pharmacokinetics (Pks) of carbamazepine (Carb). Intersci Conf Antimicrob Agents Chemother (1990) 30, 213.
2. O'Connor NK, Fris J. Clarithromycin-carbamazepine interaction in a clinical setting. J Am Board Fam Pract (1994) 7, 489–92.
3. Albani F, Riva R, Baruzzi A. Clarithromycin-carbamazepine interaction: a case report. Epilepsia (1993) 34, 161–2.
4. Yasui N, Otani K, Kaneko S, Shimoyama R, Ohkubo T, Sugawara K. Carbamazepine toxicity induced by clarithromycin coadministration in psychiatric patients. Int Clin Psychopharmacol (1997) 12, 225–9.
5. Stafstrom CE, Nohria V, Loganbill H, Nahouraii R, Boustany R-M, DeLong GR. Erythromycin-induced carbamazepine toxicity: a continuing problem. Arch Pediatr Adolesc Med (1995) 149, 99–101.
6. Carmona Ibáñez G, Guevara Serrano J, Gisbert González S. Toxicidad de carbamacepina inducida por eritromicina. Un problema frecuente. Farm Clin (1996) 13, 698–700.
7. Metz DC, Getz HD. Helicobacter pylori gastritis therapy with omeprazole and clarithromycin increases serum carbamazepine levels. Dig Dis Sci (1995) 40, 912–15.
8. Dammann H-G. Therapy with omeprazole and clarithromycin increases serum carbamazepine levels in patients with H.pylori gastritis. Dig Dis Sci (1996) 41, 519.
9. Metz DC, Getz HD. Therapy with omeprazole and clarithromycin increases serum carbamazepine levels in patients with H.pylori gastritis. Dig Dis Sci (1996) 41, 519–20.
10. Barzaghi N, Gatti G, Crema F, Faja A, Monteleone M, Amione C, Leone L, Perucca E. Effect of flurithromycin, a new macrolide antibiotic, on carbamazepine disposition in normal subjects. Int J Clin Pharmacol Res (1988) 8, 101–5.
11. Albin H, Vincon G, Pehourcq F, Dangoumau J. Influence de la josamycine sur la pharmacocinétique de la carbamazépine. Therapie (1982) 37, 151–6.
12. Vincon G, Albin H, Demotes-Mainard F, Guyot M, Brachet-Liermain A, Loiseau P. Pharmacokinetic interaction between carbamazepine and josamycin. Proc Eur Congr Biopharmaceutics Pharmacokinetics vol III: Clinical Pharmacokinetics. Edited by Aiache JM and Hirtz J. Published by Imprimerie de l'Universite de Clermont-Ferrand. (1984) pp 270–6.
13. Couet W, Istin B, Ingrand I, Girault J, Fourtillan J-B. Effect of ponsinomycin on single-dose kinetics and metabolism of carbamazepine. Ther Drug Monit (1990) 12, 144–9.
14. Zagnoni PG, DeLuca M, Casini A. Carbamazepine-miocamycin interaction. Epilepsia (1991) 32 (Suppl 1), 28.
15. Saint-Salvi B, Tremblay D, Surjus A, Lefebvre MA. A study of the interaction of roxithromycin with theophylline and carbamazepine. J Antimicrob Chemother (1987) 20 (Suppl B), 121–9.
16. Dravet C, Mesdjian E, Cenraud B, Roger J. Interaction between carbamazepine and triacetyloleandomycin. Lancet (1977) i, 810–11.
17. Dravet C, Mesdjian E, Cenraud B, Roger J. Interaction carbamazépine triacétyloléandomycine: une nouvelle interaction médicamenteuse? Nouv Presse Med (1977) 6, 467.
18. Mesdjian E, Dravet C, Cenraud B, Roger J. Carbamazepine intoxication due to triacetyloleandomycin administration in epileptic patients. Epilepsia (1980) 21, 489–96.

19. Amedee-Manesme O, Rey E, Brussieux J, Goutieres F, Aicardi J. Antibiotiques à ne jamais associer à la carbamazépine. *Arch Fr Pediatr* (1982) 39, 126.
20. Pessayre D, Larrey D, Vitaux J, Breil P, Belghiti J, Benhamou J-P. Formation of an inactive cytochrome P-450 Fe(II)-metabolite complex after administration of troleandomycin in humans. *Biochem Pharmacol* (1982) 31, 1699–1704.

Carbamazepine + Metronidazole

An isolated report describes increased serum carbamazepine levels and toxicity in a patient additionally given metronidazole.

Clinical evidence, mechanism, importance and management

A woman on 1 g carbamazepine daily was additionally started on co-trimoxazole twice daily and 250 g **metronidazole** three times daily for diverticulitis. After 2 days the co-trimoxazole was stopped, the **metronidazole** dosage was doubled, and given intravenously, and 500 mg **cefazolin** 8-hourly added. After 2 days she complained of diplopia, dizziness and nausea, and her serum carbamazepine levels were found to have risen from 9.0 to 14.3 micrograms/ml. A month later (presumably after the **metronidazole** had been withdrawn) her serum carbamazepine levels had fallen to 7.1 micrograms/ml. The reasons for this reaction are not understood.[1]

This appears to be the first and only report of an interaction between carbamazepine and **metronidazole**, so its general importance is uncertain. Be aware of this interaction if concurrent use is necessary. More study is needed.

1. Patterson BD. Possible interaction between metronidazole and carbamazepine. *Ann Pharmacother* (1994) 28, 1303–4.

Carbamazepine + Monoamine oxidase inhibitors (MAOIs)

Phenelzine, moclobemide and tranylcypromine appear not to interact adversely with carbamazepine.

Clinical evidence, mechanism, importance and management

There appear to be no reports of adverse reactions during concurrent treatment with MAOIs and carbamazepine. However, the makers of carbamazepine say that concurrent use should be avoided because of the close structural similarity between carbamazepine and the tricyclic antidepressants (and therefore the theoretical risk of an adverse interaction). Several reports describe successful use of carbamazepine and MAOIs, namely **tranylcypromine**,[1,2] **phenelzine**,[3] and **moclobemide**.[4] Bearing in mind that the MAOIs and the tricyclics can be administered together under certain well controlled conditions without problems (see 'Monoamine oxidase inhibitors (MAOIs) + Tricyclic antidepressants', p.682), the warning about the risks may possibly prove to be overcautious. As yet there seems to be no direct information about other MAOIs.

1. Lydiard RB, White D, Harvey B, Taylor A. Lack of pharmacokinetic interaction between tranylcypromine and carbamazepine. *J Clin Psychopharmacol* (1987) 7, 360.
2. Joffe RT, Post RM, Uhde TW. Lack of pharmacokinetic interaction of carbamazepine with tranylcypromine. *Arch Gen Psychiatry* (1985) 42, 738.
3. Yatham LN, Barry S, Mobayed M, Dinan TG. Is the carbamazepine-phenelzine combination safe? *Am J Psychiatry* (1990) 147, 367.
4. Amrein R, Güntert TW, Dingemanse J, Lorscheid T, Stabl M, Schmid-Burgk W. Interactions of moclobemide with concomitantly administered medication: evidence from pharmacological and clinical studies. *Psychopharmacology (Berl)* (1992) 106, S24–S31.

Carbamazepine + Nefazodone

Five patients developed elevated serum carbamazepine levels and toxicity when nefazodone was added, but a study in healthy subjects using lower carbamazepine doses found the combination was well tolerated. Carbamazepine markedly reduced nefazodone levels.

Clinical evidence

A patient on 1000 mg carbamazepine daily developed evidence of toxicity (light-headedness, ataxia) within 15 days of starting to take **nefazodone** (initially 100 mg twice daily increasing to 150 mg twice daily after a week). Her serum carbamazepine levels had risen from a range of 7.0 to 8.3 micrograms/ml to 10.8 micrograms/ml. It was found necessary to reduce the carbamazepine dosage to 600 mg daily to eliminate these side effects and to achieve serum levels of 7.4 micrograms/ml.[1] In 4 other patients on carbamazepine 800 or 1000 mg daily the addition of **nefazodone** caused up to threefold rises in carbamazepine levels. The carbamazepine dose was reduced by 25 to 60%.[1,2] These cases are in contrast to a study in 12 healthy subjects in which 5 days of carbamazepine and **nefazodone** were well tolerated. However, the levels of carbamazepine were slightly increased (23% increase in AUC) and the levels of nefazodone markedly decreased (93% decrease in AUC). The difference may be because only 400 mg of carbamazepine was used, and the authors suggest that there may be a greater effect with higher doses.[3]

Mechanism

Both drugs are metabolised by the cytochrome P450 isoenzyme CYP3A4, so it would seem that nefazodone can inhibit carbamazepine metabolism, while carbamazepine can induce nefazodone metabolism.

Importance and management

Information is limited, but it would seem prudent to monitor for signs of carbamazepine toxicity if nefazodone is added to established treatment, especially with doses of carbamazepine above 800 mg. The nefazodone dosage may need to be increased in the presence of carbamazepine, so be alert for a reduced effect. Further study is needed.

1. Ashton AK, Wolin RE. Nefazodone-induced carbamazepine toxicity. *Am J Psychiatry* (1996) 153, 733.
2. Roth L, Bertschy G. Nefazodone may inhibit the metabolism of carbamazepine: three case reports. *Eur Psychiatry* (2001) 16, 320–1.
3. Laroudie C, Salazar DE, Cosson J-P, Cheuvart B, Istin B, Girault J, Ingrand I, Decourt J-P. Carbamazepine-nefazodone interaction in healthy subjects. *J Clin Psychopharmacol* (2000) 20, 46–53.

Carbamazepine + Omeprazole or Pantoprazole

No clinically relevant interaction appears to occur between carbamazepine and omeprazole or pantoprazole.

Clinical evidence, mechanism, importance and management

(a) Omeprazole

Omeprazole 20 mg daily for 14 days was found to increase the AUC of a single 400-mg dose of carbamazepine in 7 patients by 75%. The clearance was reduced by 40% and the elimination half-life was more than doubled (from 17.2 to 37.3 h).[1] However, a retrospective study of the records of 10 patients on **omeprazole** and continuous treatment with carbamazepine (rather than a single dose) found a non-significant reduction in carbamazepine serum levels.[2] The reason for these contradictory results seems to be that while **omeprazole** can inhibit the oxidative metabolism of single doses of carbamazepine, when the carbamazepine is taken continuously it induces its own metabolism through the cytochrome P450 isoenzyme CYP3A4, thereby opposing the effects of this interaction.[2] It seems therefore that in practice no clinically relevant interaction is likely to occur.

(b) Pantoprazole

Pantoprazole 40 mg daily for 5 days had no effect on the AUC of carbamazepine or carbamazepine epoxide after a single 400-mg dose of carbamazepine in healthy subjects. No special precautions appear to be necessary during concurrent use.[3]

1. Naidu MUR, Shoba J, Dixit VK, Kumar A, Kumar TR, Sekhar KR, Sekhar EC. Effect of multiple dose omeprazole on the pharmacokinetics of carbamazepine. *Drug Invest* (1994) 7, 8–12.
2. Böttiger Y, Bertilsson L. No effect on plasma carbamazepine concentration with concomitant omeprazole treatment. *Drug Invest* (1995) 9, 180–1.
3. Huber R, Bliesath H, Hartmann M, Steinijans VW, Koch H, Mascher H, Wurst W. Pantoprazole does not interact with the pharmacokinetics of carbamazepine. *Int J Clin Pharmacol Ther* (1998) 36, 521–4.

Carbamazepine + Phenobarbital

Carbamazepine serum levels are reduced to some extent by the concurrent use of phenobarbital, but seizure control remains unaffected.

Clinical evidence

A comparative study showed that on average patients taking both carbamazepine and **phenobarbital** (44 patients) had carbamazepine serum levels which were 18% lower than those taking carbamazepine alone (43 patients).[1]

Similar results were found in other studies in both adult and child patients treated with both drugs.[2,3] The seizure control remained unaffected. Carbamazepine-epoxide levels were increased.[3,4]

Mechanism

It seem probable that phenobarbital stimulates the liver enzymes concerned with the metabolism of the carbamazepine, resulting in its more rapid clearance from the body.

Importance and management

An established interaction, but of little practical importance since the seizure control is not diminished, despite the small fall in serum carbamazepine levels. This is because its metabolite (carbamazepine-epoxide) also has anticonvulsant activity. See also 'Carbamazepine + Primidone', p.330.

1. Christiansen J, Dam M. Influence of phenobarbital and diphenylhydantoin on plasma carbamazepine levels in patients with epilepsy. *Acta Neurol Scand* (1973) 49, 543–6.
2. Cereghino JJ, Brock JT, Van Meter JC, Penry JK, Smith LD, White BG. The efficacy of carbamazepine combinations in epilepsy. *Clin Pharmacol Ther* (1975) 18, 733–41.
3. Rane A, Höjer B, Wilson JT. Kinetics of carbamazepine and its 10,11-epoxide metabolite in children. *Clin Pharmacol Ther* (1976) 19, 276–83.
4. Dam M, Jensen A, Christiansen J. Plasma level and effect of carbamazepine in grand mal and psychomotor epilepsy. *Acta Neurol Scand* (1975) 75 (Suppl 51), 33–8.

Carbamazepine + Primidone

A single case report suggests that primidone can reduce the effects of carbamazepine. There is other evidence that carbamazepine may reduce primidone serum levels.

Clinical evidence

The complex partial seizures of a 15-year-old boy failed to be controlled despite treatment with **primidone** (12 mg/kg daily in three doses) and carbamazepine (10 mg/kg daily in three doses). Even when the carbamazepine dosage was increased from 10 to 20 and then to 30 mg/kg daily his serum carbamazepine levels only rose from 3.5 to 4.0 and then to 4.8 micrograms/ml, and his seizures continued. When the **primidone** was gradually withdrawn his serum carbamazepine levels climbed to 12 micrograms/ml and his seizures completely disappeared.[1]

An analysis of serum levels of anticonvulsants in children found that the serum levels of **primidone** tended to be lower in those on carbamazepine, but no details were given.[2]

Mechanism

When the primidone was stopped in the single case cited, the clearance of the carbamazepine decreased by about 60%.[1] This is consistent with the known enzyme-inducing effects of primidone (converted in the body to phenobarbital) which can increase the metabolism of other drugs by the liver.

Importance and management

Direct information seems to be limited to these reports so that their general importance is uncertain, but be alert for evidence of reduced anticonvulsant control if either drug is added to treatment with the other. See also 'Carbamazepine + Phenobarbital', p.330. More study is needed.

1. Benetello P, Furlanut M. Primidone-carbamazepine interaction: clinical consequences. *Int J Clin Pharmacol Res* (1987) 7, 165–8.
2. Windorfer A, Sauer W. Drug interactions during anticonvulsant therapy in childhood: diphenylhydantoin, primidone, phenobarbitone, clonazepam, nitrazepam, carbamazepin and dipropylacetate. *Neuropadiatrie* (1977) 8, 29–41.

Carbamazepine + Protease inhibitors

Four patients developed carbamazepine toxicity when concurrently treated with ritonavir. Limited evidence suggests indinavir may not interact, whereas nelfinavir may.

Clinical evidence, mechanism, importance and management

An HIV+ patient with epilepsy was concurrently treated with **ritonavir** and carbamazepine, which resulted in a rise in the carbamazepine serum levels, accompanied by vomiting, vertigo and transient liver dysfunction. When the **ritonavir** was stopped and the carbamazepine dosage reduced, the toxic symptoms subsided and the liver function returned to normal.[1] Three other cases also document two to threefold rises in carbamazepine levels with associated toxicity, caused by the addition of **ritonavir**.[2-4] Interestingly, in these latter 3 cases, all the patients had previously been treated with **indinavir** and carbamazepine without carbamazepine toxicity. In one case a carbamazepine dose reduction from 600 to 100 mg daily was needed to keep the levels within the therapeutic range.[3] **Nelfinavir** may also have interacted with carbamazepine in one of these cases.[4]

Mechanism

Ritonavir is a potent inhibitor of the cytochrome P450 isoenzyme CYP3A4, which is concerned with the metabolism of carbamazepine. Such inhibition would result in a rise in the serum levels of the carbamazepine leading to the development of toxicity.[1-4] In one case,[3] efavirenz, a known CYP3A4 inducer was used concurrently, yet did not seem to attenuate the effects of ritonavir.

Importance and management

Although the information is fairly limited, the effects of the interaction with ritonavir can be dramatic. It would now be prudent to monitor the concurrent use of these two drugs, being alert for the need to reduce the dosage of the carbamazepine. Nelfinavir may also interact, but indinavir possibly does not.

1. Kato Y, Fujii T, Mizoguchi N, Takata N, Ueda K, Feldman MD, Kayser SR. Potential interaction between ritonavir and carbamazepine. *Pharmacotherapy* (2000) 20, 851-4.
2. Berbel Garcia A, Latorre Ibarra A, Porta Etessam J, Martinez Salio A, Perez Martinez DA, Saiz Diaz R, Toledo Heras M. Protease inhibitor-induced carbamazepine toxicity. *Clin Neuropharmacol* (2000) 23, 216–18.
3. Burman W, Orr L. Carbamazepine toxicity after starting combination antiretroviral therapy including ritonavir and efavirenz. *AIDS* (2000) 14, 2793–4.
4. Mateu-de-Antonio J, Grau S, Gimeno-Bayón J-L, Carmona A. Ritonavir-induced carbamazepine toxicity. *Ann Pharmacother* (2001) 35, 125–6.

Carbamazepine + Selective serotonin re-uptake inhibitors (SSRIs)

Some, but not all, reports indicate that carbamazepine serum levels can be increased by fluoxetine and fluvoxamine. Toxicity may develop. Sertraline normally appears not to affect carbamazepine, but sertraline levels may be reduced by carbamazepine. Isolated cases of a Parkinson-like and serotonin syndrome have occurred with fluoxetine and carbamazepine, while an isolated case of pancytopenia has been reported with sertraline and carbamazepine. Consideration should be given to the fact that SSRIs have been known to cause seizures.

Clinical evidence

(a) Fluoxetine

Two patients developed carbamazepine toxicity (diplopia, blurred vision, tremor, vertigo, nausea, tinnitus etc.) within 7 and 10 days of starting to take 20 mg fluoxetine daily. Their serum carbamazepine levels were found to have risen by about 33 and 60%. The problem was resolved in one of them by reducing the carbamazepine dosage from 1000 mg to 800 mg daily, and in the other by stopping the fluoxetine.[1] The effects seen in these cases are supported by a study in 6 healthy patients, where adding fluoxetine 20 mg daily to steady-state carbamazepine caused a rise in the carbamazepine AUC of about 25 to 50% and also of its active epoxide metabolite.[2,3]

In contrast, 20 mg fluoxetine daily for 3 weeks was found to have no effect on the serum levels of carbamazepine or its active epoxide metabolite in 8 epileptic patients stabilised on carbamazepine.[4]

Besides these pharmacokinetic changes, two cases of Parkinsonism have been seen, within 3 and 9 days of adding fluoxetine to carbamazepine treatment. In neither case were the carbamazepine levels affected.[5] A case of the serotonin syndrome (shivering, agitation, myoclonic-like leg contractions, diaphoresis etc.) has also been seen, in a woman on 200 mg carbamazepine daily and fluoxetine 20 mg daily.[6]

(b) Fluvoxamine

Increased serum levels and signs of carbamazepine toxicity (nausea, vomiting) were seen in 3 patients on long-term carbamazepine when the were additionally given fluvoxamine. The carbamazepine level almost doubled in one of them within 10 days of starting 50 to 100 mg fluvoxamine daily. The interaction was accommodated by reducing the carbamazepine dosage by 200 mg daily in all three (from 1000 to 800 in one of them, and from 800 to 600 mg daily in the other two).[7,8] An approximate doubling of carbamazepine levels has also been seen in other patients given fluvoxamine.[9-12]

In contrast, 100 mg fluvoxamine daily for 3 weeks was found to have no effect on the serum levels of carbamazepine or its active epoxide metabolite in 7 epileptic patients stabilised on carbamazepine.[4]

(c) Sertraline

A double blind, placebo-controlled, parallel group study in 13 healthy subjects (7 on sertraline, 6 on placebo) found that 200 mg sertraline daily for 17 days had no effect on the pharmacokinetics of carbamazepine 200 mg twice daily, nor on the pharmacokinetics of carbamazepine-epoxide. In addition, sertraline did not potentiate the cognitive effects of carbamazepine.[13]

However, an isolated report describes a woman stabilised for 2 years on 600 mg carbamazepine and 100 mg flecainide daily, who showed a rise in trough serum carbamazepine levels from 4.7 to 8.5 micrograms/ml within 4 weeks of starting 100 mg sertraline daily. After 3 months of treatment, carbamazepine levels were 11.9 micrograms/ml. At the same time she developed pancytopenia (interpreted as a toxic bone marrow reaction to the increased carbamazepine), which improved when the carbamazepine and sertraline were stopped.[14]

An isolated report describes a woman with schizoaffective disorder successfully treated for 3 years with haloperidol and carbamazepine

who was additionally given 50 mg sertraline daily for depression. When she failed to respond, the sertraline dosage was progressively increased to 300 mg daily but her sertraline serum levels remained low (about 17 to 25% of those predicted). Another patient on carbamazepine similarly failed to respond to the addition of sertraline and had low sertraline levels.[15]

Mechanisms

The evidence suggests that fluoxetine and fluvoxamine inhibit the metabolism of carbamazepine by the liver (presumably inhibition of cytochrome P450 isoenzyme CYP2D6) so that its loss from the body is reduced, leading to a rise in its serum levels.[2,3,7,9,10]

Sertraline serum levels may be reduced because carbamazepine is an inducer of cytochrome CYP3A4, which would increase its metabolism and clearance from the body.

Importance and management

Information appears to be limited to these reports. It is not clear why they are inconsistent, but be alert for an increase in carbamazepine serum levels and toxicity if fluoxetine, fluvoxamine or possibly sertraline is added. The interaction appears rare. A literature search[16] by the makers of fluvoxamine only identified 9 cases of fluvoxamine/sertraline interaction up until 1995. However, because of the unpredictability of this interaction it would be prudent to monitor concurrent use, particularly in the early stages, so that any patient affected can be identified. Be alert for the need to reduce the carbamazepine dosage.

The makers of fluoxetine suggest that carbamazepine should be started at or adjusted towards the lower end of the dosage range in those on fluoxetine. They additionally suggest caution if fluoxetine has been taken during the previous 5 weeks.[17]

Note that SSRIs may increase seizure frequency and should therefore be used with caution in patients with epilepsy, and avoided in those with unstable epilepsy.

1. Pearson HJ. Interaction of fluoxetine with carbamazepine. *J Clin Psychiatry* (1990) 51, 126.
2. Grimsley SR, Jann MW, D'Mello AP, Carter GC, D'Souza MJ. Pharmacodynamics and pharmacokinetics of fluoxetine/carbamazepine interaction. *Clin Pharmacol Ther* (1991) 49, 135.
3. Grimsley SR, Jann MW, Carter JG, D'Mello AP, D'Souza MJ. Increased carbamazepine plasma concentrations after fluoxetine coadministration. *Clin Pharmacol Ther* (1991) 50, 10–15.
4. Spina E, Avenoso A, Pollicino AM, Caputi AP, Fazio A, Pisani F. Carbamazepine coadministration with fluoxetine or fluvoxamine. *Ther Drug Monit* (1993) 15, 247–50.
5. Gernaat HBPE, van de Woude J, Touw DJ. Fluoxetine and parkinsonism in patients taking carbamazepine. *Am J Psychiatry* (1991) 148, 1604–5.
6. Dursun SM, Mathew VM, Reveley MA. Toxic serotonin syndrome after fluoxetine plus carbamazepine. *Lancet* (1993) 342, 442–3.
7. Fritze J, Unsorg B, Lanczik M. Interaction between carbamazepine and fluvoxamine. *Acta Psychiatr Scand* (1991) 84, 583–4.
8. Fritze J, Lanczik M. Pharmacokinetic interactions of carbamazepine and fluvoxamine. *Pharmacopsychiatry* (1993) 26, 153.
9. Bonnet P, Vandel S, Nezelof S, Sechter D, Bizouard P. Carbamazepine, fluvoxamine. Is there a pharmacokinetic interaction? *Therapie* (1992) 47, 165.
10. Martinelli V, Bocchetta A, Palmas AM, del Zompo M. An interaction between carbamazepine and fluvoxamine. *Br J Clin Pharmacol* (1993) 36, 615–16.
11. Debruille C, Robert H, Cottencin O, Regnaut N, Gignac C. Interaction carbamazépine/fluvoxamine: à propos de deux observations. *J Pharm Clin* (1994) 13, 128–30.
12. Cottencin O, Regnaut N, Thevenon Gignac C, Thomas P, Goudemand M, Debruille C, Robert H. Interaction carbamazepine-fluvoxamine sur le taux plasmatique de carbamazepine. *Encephale* (1995) 21, 141–5.
13. Rapeport WG, Williams SA, Muirhead DC, Dewland PM, Tanner T, Wesnes K. Absence of a sertraline-mediated effect on the pharmacokinetics and pharmacodynamics of carbamazepine. *J Clin Psychiatry* (1996) 57 (Suppl 1), 20–3.
14. Joblin M, Ghose K. Possible interaction of sertraline with carbamazepine. *N Z Med J* (1994) 107, 43.
15. Khan A, Shad MU, Preskorn SH. Lack of sertraline efficacy probably due to an interaction with carbamazepine. *J Clin Psychiatry* (2000) 61, 526–7.
16. Wagner W, Vause EW. Fluvoxamine. A review of global drug-drug interaction data. *Clin Pharmacokinet* (1995) 29 (Suppl 1), 26–32.
17. Prozac (Fluoxetine). Eli Lilly and Company Limited. Summary of product characteristics, July 2000.

Carbamazepine + Sodium valproate

The serum levels of carbamazepine may fall by 20 to 25% (or remain unaffected) during concurrent use with sodium valproate, and those of sodium valproate may fall by 60% or

more. However, the rise in the levels of carbamazepine-epoxide, which also has anticonvulsant activity, may possibly offset the effects of this interaction (but also cause side-effects). Concurrent use may possibly increase the incidence of sodium valproate induced hepatotoxicity.

Clinical evidence

(a) Serum carbamazepine levels reduced, unchanged

A study in 7 adult epileptics who had been taking carbamazepine (8.3 to 13.3 mg/kg) for more than 2 months showed that their steady-state serum carbamazepine levels fell by an average of 24% (range 3 to 59%) over a 6-day period when concurrently treated with **sodium valproate** 1 g twice daily. The carbamazepine levels fell in 6 of the patients and remained unchanged in one. The levels of the active metabolite, carbamazepine-10,11-epoxide increased by a mean of 38%, with small decreases or no change in 4 patients and 24 to 150% increases in the remaining 3 patients.[1,2]

Other reports state that falls,[3,4] no changes[3,5-7] and even a slight rise[4] in carbamazepine levels have been seen in some patients concurrently treated with sodium valproate. Rises in the serum levels of carbamazepine-10,11-epoxide of about 50 to 100% have also been described.[6,8] This active metabolite may cause the development of marked side-effects such as blurred vision, dizziness, vomiting, tiredness and even nystagmus.[6-9] Acute psychosis occurred in one patient when carbamazepine was added to **sodium valproate** treatment, which was tentatively attributed to elevated epoxide levels.[10]

(b) Serum sodium valproate levels reduced

A study on the kinetics of **sodium valproate** in 6 healthy subjects showed that the concurrent use of carbamazepine, 200 mg daily, over a 17-day period increased the **sodium valproate** clearance by 30%.[11]

Other reports have described reductions in serum **sodium valproate** levels of 34 to 38% when carbamazepine was added,[12,13] and rises of 50 to 65% when the carbamazepine was withdrawn.[14,15] The rise appears to reach a plateau after about 4 weeks.[15]

(c) Increased sodium valproate-induced hepatotoxicity or neurological effects

Evidence from epidemiological studies suggests that the risk of fatal hepatotoxicity is higher when **sodium valproate** is given with other anticonvulsants than when it is given alone, especially in infants.[16,17] A single case report describes hepatocellular and cholestatic jaundice and a reversible Parkinsonian syndrome in a woman on **sodium valproate** when carbamazepine was added, which reversed when carbamazepine was withdrawn. Levels of both drugs did not exceed the therapeutic range at any stage. The Parkinsonian syndrome was attributed to a drug interaction, whereas the hepatic toxicity was considered most likely to be due to the carbamazepine, although the valproate may have contributed.[18]

Mechanism

The evidence suggests that each drug increases the metabolism of the other, so that both are cleared from the body more quickly. However, the latter stages of carbamazepine metabolism appear to be inhibited. The levels of the metabolite carbamazepine-epoxide increase during concurrent use, probably by inhibition of its metabolism to carbamazepine-10,11-trans-diol.[19,20] This metabolite is then further converted by glucuronidation and it seems that this step is also inhibited.[20] Carbamazepine may also possibly increase the formation of a minor but hepatotoxic metabolite of sodium valproate (2-propyl-4-pentenoic acid or 4-ene-VPA).[21]

Importance and management

Moderately well documented interactions, both of which seem to be established. Be alert for falls in the serum levels of both drugs. However, the clinical importance of this is uncertain because the metabolite of carbamazepine (carbamazepine-epoxide) also has anticonvulsant activity so that it may not be necessary to increase the dosages of the drugs to maintain adequate seizure control. Be alert for evidence of high levels of carbamazepine-epoxide and its associated

toxicity. Also bear in mind the evidence that concurrent use may possibly increase the incidence of sodium valproate induced liver toxicity.

1. Levy RH, Morselli PL, Bianchetti G, Guyot M, Brachet-Liermain A, Loiseau P. Interaction between valproic acid and carbamazepine in epileptic patients. Metabolism of Antiepileptic Drugs edited by RH Levy et al. Raven Press, New York (1984) 45–51.
2. Levy RH, Moreland TA, Morselli PL, Guyot M, Brachet-Liermain A, Loiseau P. Carbamazepine/valproic acid interaction in man and rhesus monkey. Epilepsia (1984) 25, 338–45.
3. Wilder BJ, Willmore LJ, Bruni J, Villarreal HJ. Valproic acid: interaction with other anticonvulsant drugs. Neurology (1978) 28, 892–6.
4. Varma R, Michos GA, Varma RS, Hoshino AY. Clinical trials of Depakene (valproic acid) coadministered with other anticonvulsants in epileptic patients. Res Commun Psychol Psychiatr Behav (1980) 5, 265–73.
5. Fowler GW. Effects of dipropylacetate on serum levels of anticonvulsants in children. Proc West Pharmacol Soc (1978) 21, 37–40.
6. Pisani F, Fazio A, Oteri G, Ruello C, Gitto C, Russo R, Perucca E. Sodium valproate and valpromide: differential interactions with carbamazepine in epileptic patients. Epilepsia (1986) 27, 548–52.
7. Sunaoshi W, Miura H, Takanashi S, Shira H, Hosoda N. Influence of concurrent administration of sodium valproate on the plasma concentrations of carbamazepine and its epoxide and diol metabolites. Jpn J Psychiatry Neurol (1991) 45, 474–7.
8. Kutt H, Solomon G, Peterson H, Dhar A, Caronna J. Accumulation of carbamazepine epoxide caused by valproate contributing to intoxication syndromes. Neurology (1985) 35 (Suppl 1), 286.
9. Rambeck B, Sälke-Treumann A, May T, Boenigk HE. Valproic acid-induced carbamazepine-10,11-epoxide toxicity in children and adolescents. Eur Neurol (1990) 30, 79–83.
10. McKee RJW, Larkin JG, Brodie MJ. Acute psychosis with carbamazepine and sodium valproate. Lancet (1989) i, 167.
11. Bowdle TA, Levy RH, Cutler RE. Effects of carbamazepine on valproic acid kinetics in normal subjects. Clin Pharmacol Ther (1979) 26, 629–34.
12. Reunanen MI, Luoma P, Myllylä VV, Hokkanen E. Low serum valproic acid concentrations in epileptic patients on combination therapy. Curr Ther Res (1980) 28, 456–62.
13. May T, Rambeck B. Serum concentrations of valproic acid: influence of dose and comedication. Ther Drug Monit (1985) 7, 387–90.
14. Henriksen O, Johannessen SI. Clinical and pharmacokinetic observations on sodium valproate – a 5 year follow-up study in 100 children with epilepsy. Acta Neurol Scand (1982) 65, 504–23.
15. Jann MW, Fidone GS, Israel MK, Bonadero P. Increased valproate serum concentrations upon carbamazepine cessation. Epilepsia (1988) 29, 578–81.
16. Dreifuss FE, Santilli N, Langer DH, Sweeney KP, Moline KA, Menander KB. Valproic acid fatalities: a retrospective review. Neurology (1987) 37, 379–85.
17. Dreifuss FE, Langer DH, Moline KA, Maxwell DE. Valproic acid hepatic fatalities. II. US experience since 1984. Neurology (1989) 39, 201–7.
18. Froomes PR, Stewart MR. A reversible Parkinsonian syndrome and hepatotoxicity following addition of carbamazepine to sodium valproate. Aust N Z J Med (1994) 24, 413–14.
19. Pisani F, Caputo M, Fazio A, Oteri G, Russo M, Spina E, Perucca E, Bertilsson L. Interaction of carbamazepine-10,11-epoxide, an active metabolite of carbamazepine, with valproate: a pharmacokinetic study. Epilepsia (1990) 31, 339–42.
20. Bernus I, Dickinson RG, Hooper WD, Eadie MJ. The mechanism of the carbamazepine-valproate interaction in humans. Br J Clin Pharmacol (1997) 44, 21–27.
21. Levy RH, Rettenmeier AW, Anderson GD, Wilensky AJ, Friel PN, Baillie TA, Acheampong A, Tor J, Guyot M, Loiseau P. Effects of polytherapy with phenytoin, carbamazepine, and stiripentol on formation of 4-ene-valproate, a hepatotoxic metabolite of valproic acid. Clin Pharmacol Ther (1990) 48, 225–35.

Carbamazepine + Trazodone

A single case report describes a moderate rise in serum carbamazepine levels in a patient when given trazodone.

Clinical evidence, mechanism, importance and management

A man of 53 was treated with 600 mg carbamazepine daily, later increased to 700 mg. Two months after starting 100 mg **trazodone** daily his serum carbamazepine levels and the concentration/dose ratio had increased by about 26%, but no signs or symptoms of carbamazepine toxicity were seen. The reasons for this interaction are not known but the authors suggest that it might be because the **trazodone** inhibits cytochrome P450 isoenzyme CYP3A4 resulting in a reduction in the metabolism of the carbamazepine.[1]

This seems to be the first and only report of a carbamazepine/**trazodone** interaction and its general importance is unknown. The rise was only moderate and in this case was clinically irrelevant, but a carbamazepine serum rise of 26% might possibly be of importance in those patients with serum levels already near the top end of the therapeutic range. Monitoring would now seem to be appropriate in any patient given both drugs.

1. Romero AS, Delgado RG, Peña MF. Interaction between trazodone and carbamazepine. Ann Pharmacother (1999) 33, 1370.

Carbamazepine + Valnoctamide

Carbamazepine toxicity may develop if valnoctamide is taken concurrently.

Clinical evidence, mechanism, importance and management

A study in 6 epileptics on carbamazepine 800 to 1200 mg daily found that **valnoctamide** 200 mg three times daily for 7 days caused a 1.5 to 6.5-fold increase in the serum levels of carbamazepine-epoxide (an active metabolite). Clinical signs of carbamazepine toxicity (drowsiness, ataxia, nystagmus) were seen in 4 of them. One patient who was also taking **phenytoin** and one patient who was also taking **phenobarbital** showed no changes in the serum levels of either of these anticonvulsants.[1] A further study in 6 healthy subjects found that 600 mg **valnoctamide** daily for 8 days increased the half-life of a single 100-mg dose of carbamazepine-epoxide threefold (from 6.7 to 19.7 h) and decreased its oral clearance fourfold.[2]

Mechanism

The reason appears to be that the valnoctamide inhibits the enzyme epoxide hydrolase, which is concerned with the metabolism and elimination of carbamazepine and its metabolite.[1,2]

Importance and management

Information is limited but the interaction appears to be established. Patients on carbamazepine who additionally take valnoctamide (available as a non-prescription tranquilliser in some countries) could rapidly develop carbamazepine toxicity because the metabolism of its major metabolite, carbamazepine-epoxide, is inhibited. This interaction is very similar to the interaction which can occur between carbamazepine and valpromide (an isomer of valnoctamide). See 'Carbamazepine + Valpromide', p.333. Valnoctamide should be avoided unless the carbamazepine dosage can be reduced appropriately.

1. Pisani F, Fazio A, Artesi C, Oteri G, Spina E, Tomson T, Perucca E. Impairment of carbamazepine-10,11-epoxide elimination by valnoctamide, a valpromide isomer, in healthy subjects. Br J Clin Pharmacol (1992) 34, 85–7.
2. Pisani F, Haj-Yehia A, Fazio A, Artesi C, Oteri G, Perucca E, Kroetz DL, Levy RH, Bialer M. Carbamazepine-valnoctamide interaction in epileptic patients: in vitro/in vivo correlation. Epilepsia (1993) 34, 954–9.

Carbamazepine + Valpromide

Carbamazepine toxicity can occur if valpromide is substituted for sodium valproate in patients taking carbamazepine. The serum levels of carbamazepine may not rise but the levels of its active metabolite, carbamazepine-epoxide, can be markedly increased. The dose of carbamazepine may need to be reduced.

Clinical evidence

Symptoms of carbamazepine toxicity developed in 5 out of 7 epileptic patients on carbamazepine when concurrent treatment with sodium valproate was replaced by **valpromide**, despite the fact that their serum carbamazepine levels did not increase.[1] The toxicity appeared to be connected with a fourfold increase in the serum levels of the metabolite of carbamazepine (carbamazepine-10,11-epoxide), which rose to 8.5 micrograms/ml.[1]

In another study in 6 epileptic patients the serum levels of this metabolite rose 330% (range 110 to 864%) within a week of concurrent use, and two of the patients developed confusion, dizziness and vomiting. The symptoms disappeared and serum carbamazepine-epoxide levels fell when the **valpromide** dosage was reduced to two-thirds.[2]

Mechanism

Valpromide reduces the metabolism by the liver of carbamazepine and its metabolite, carbamazepine-epoxide, because it inhibits epoxide hydrolase.[3] This metabolite has anticonvulsant activity but it may also be toxic if its serum levels become excessive.[2,4]

Importance and management

An established interaction. It is suggested that both carbamazepine and carbamazepine-epoxide serum levels should be monitored during concurrent use.[2] The dosages should be reduced appropriately if necessary. There is also some debate about whether this combination should be avoided, not only because of the risk of toxicity but also because inhibition of epoxide hydrolase may be undesirable.[1] This enzyme is possibly important for the detoxification of a number of teratogenic, mutagenic and carcinogenic epoxides.[1,2] More study is needed.

1. Meijer JWA, Binnie CD, Debets RMChr, Van Parys JAP and de Beer-Pawlikowski NKB. Possible hazard of valpromide-carbamazepine combination therapy in epilepsy. Lancet (1984) i, 802.
2. Pisani F, Fazio A, Oteri G, Ruello C, Gitto C, Russo R, Perucca E. Sodium valproate and valpromide: differential interactions with carbamazepine in epileptic patients. Epilepsia (1986) 27, 548–52.
3. Pisani F, Fazio A, Oteri G, Spina E, Perucca E and Bertilsson L. Effect of valpromide on the pharmacokinetics of carbamazepine-10,11-epoxide. Br J Clin Pharmacol (1988) 25, 611–13.
4. Levy RH, Kerr BM, Loiseau P, Guyot M and Wilensky AJ. Inhibition of carbamazepine epoxide elimination by valpromide and valproic acid. Epilepsia (1986) 27, 592.

Clonazepam + Felbamate

No significant changes in the pharmacokinetics of clonazepam occurred in 18 healthy subjects when concurrently treated with 1 mg clonazepam and 1200 mg felbamate 12-hourly for 10 days.[1,2] No serious adverse reactions were seen. There would therefore seem to be no reason for avoiding concurrent use.

1. Colucci R, Glue P, Banfield C, Reidenberg P, Meehan J, Lin C, Radwanski E, Korduba C, Affrime MB. Effects of felbamate on the pharmacokinetics of clonazepam. J Clin Pharmacol (1994) 34, 1015.
2. Colucci R, Glue P, Banfield C, Reidenberg P, Meehan J, Radwanski E, Korduba C, Lin C, Dogterom P, Ebels T, Hendricks G, Jonkman JHG, Affrime M. Effect of felbamate on the pharmacokinetics of clonazepam. Am J Ther (1996) 3, 294–7.

Ethosuximide + Isoniazid

A single report describes a patient who developed psychotic behaviour and signs of ethosuximide toxicity when concurrently treated with isoniazid.

Clinical evidence, mechanism, importance and management

An epileptic patient, well controlled on ethosuximide and sodium valproate for 2 years, developed persistent hiccuping, nausea, vomiting, anorexia and insomnia within a week of starting to take 300 mg **isoniazid** daily. Psychotic behaviour gradually developed over the next 5 weeks and so the isoniazid was stopped. The appearance of these symptoms appeared to be related to the sharp rise in serum ethosuximide levels (from about 50 up to 198 micrograms/ml).[1] It is suggested that the **isoniazid** may have inhibited the metabolism of the ethosuximide, leading to accumulation and toxicity. The general importance of this reaction is uncertain, but it would now seem prudent to monitor concurrent use in any patient.

1. van Wieringen A, Vrijlandt CM. Ethosuximide intoxication caused by interaction with isoniazid. Neurology (1983) 33, 1227–8.

Ethosuximide + Other anticonvulsants

Falls in serum ethosuximide levels can occur if carbamazepine, primidone or phenytoin are used concurrently, whereas methylphenobarbital or sodium valproate may cause a rise. The effect of all these changes on seizure control is uncertain.
Ethosuximide is reported to have caused phenytoin toxicity, and it appears that ethosuximide can reduce valproate serum levels.

Clinical evidence

(a) Barbiturates

A study in 29 epileptic patients showed that the concurrent use of **primidone** depressed serum ethosuximide levels,[1] whereas another report described a rise in ethosuximide levels when **methylphenobarbital** was used.[2] In another study, which compared the pharmacokinetics of a single dose of ethosuximide in 10 epileptic patients on phenobarbital, **phenytoin** and/or carbamazepine with 12 healthy controls, the epileptic group showed markedly shorter ethosuximide half-lives.[3] Phenobarbital levels (from **primidone**) do not appear to be affected by ethosuximide.[4]

(b) Carbamazepine

A study in 6 healthy subjects taking 500 mg ethosuximide daily showed that the mean serum levels of ethosuximide were reduced by 17% (from 32 to 27 mg/ml) after taking 200 mg **carbamazepine** daily for 18 days. One individual showed a 35% reduction in ethosuximide levels.[5] Another study, which compared 10 epileptic patients (taking enzyme-inducing antiepileptic drugs, including 4 taking **carbamazepine**) with 12 healthy controls found that the epileptic group showed markedly shorter ethosuximide half-lives.[3]

In contrast, no interaction was seen in another study in epileptic patients on ethosuximide and other anticonvulsants, although the effects of individual drugs were not able to be assessed.[2]

(c) Phenytoin

A study compared the pharmacokinetics of a single dose of ethosuximide in 10 epileptic patients on **phenobarbital**, **phenytoin** and/or carbamazepine with 12 healthy controls. The epileptic group showed markedly shorter ethosuximide half-lives.[3] Three cases have occurred in which ethosuximide appeared to have been responsible for increasing phenytoin levels,[6-8] leading to the development of **phenytoin** toxicity in 2 patients.[7,8]

(d) Sodium valproate

Four out of 5 patients taking ethosuximide (average dose 27 mg/kg) showed an approximately 50% increase in serum levels from 73 to 112 micrograms/ml within 3 weeks of starting to take **sodium valproate** (adjusted to the maximum tolerated dose). Sedation occurred and ethosuximide dose reductions were necessary.[9] In a single-dose study in 6 healthy subjects, 9 days treatment with **sodium valproate** was reported to have increased the ethosuximide half-life and reduced the clearance by 15%.[10] However, other studies have described no changes[11,12] or even reduced serum levels.[1]

One study in 13 children showed ethosuximide can lower **valproate** serum levels. In combination the **valproate** serum levels were lower than with ethosuximide alone (87 versus 120 micrograms/ml). After stopping ethosuximide the **valproate** levels rose by about 40% and when combined they fell by about 25%.[13]

Mechanism

The most probable explanation for the fall in ethosuximide levels is that the **carbamazepine** and the other enzyme inducing anticonvulsants increase the metabolism and clearance of ethosuximide, which is known to be metabolised by the cytochrome P450 isoenzyme CYP3A.[3]

Importance and management

The concurrent use of anticonvulsant agents is common and often advantageous. Information on these interactions is sparse and even contradictory and their clinical importance is uncertain. Nevertheless, good monitoring would clearly be appropriate if these drugs are used with ethosuximide to monitor for potential toxicity and to ensure adequate seizure control.

1. Battino D, Cusi C, Franceschetti S, Moise A, Spina S, Avanzini G. Ethosuximide plasma concentrations: influence of age and associated concomitant therapy. *Clin Pharmacokinet* (1982) 7, 176–80.
2. Smith GA, McKauge L, Dubetz D, Tyrer JH, Eadie MJ. Factors influencing plasma concentrations of ethosuximide. *Clin Pharmacokinet* (1979) 4, 38–52.
3. Giaccone M, Bartoli A, Gatti G, Marchiselli R, Pisani F, Latella MA, Perucca E. Effect of enzyme inducing anticonvulsants on ethosuximide pharmacokinetics in epileptic patients. *Br J Clin Pharmacol* (1996) 41, 575–9.
4. Schmidt D. The effect of phenytoin and ethosuximide on primidone metabolism in patients with epilepsy. *J Neurol* (1975) 209, 115–23.
5. Warren JW, Benmaman JD, Wannamaker BB, Levy RH. Kinetics of a carbamazepine-ethosuximide interaction. *Clin Pharmacol Ther* (1980) 28, 646–51.
6. Lander CM, Eadie MJ, Tyrer JH. Interactions between anticonvulsants. *Proc Aust Assoc Neurol* (1975) 12, 111–16.
7. Dawson GW, Brown HW, Clark BG. Serum phenytoin after ethosuximide. *Ann Neurol* (1978) 4, 583–4.
8. Frantzen E, Hansen JM, Hansen OE, Kristensen M. Phenytoin (Dilantin) intoxication. *Acta Neurol Scand* (1967) 43, 440–6.
9. Mattson RH, Cramer JA. Valproic acid and ethosuximide interaction. *Ann Neurol* (1980) 7, 583–4.
10. Pisani F, Narbone MC, Trunfio C, Fazio A, La Rosa G, Oteri G, Di Perri R. Valproic acid-ethosuximide interaction: a pharmacokinetic study. *Epilepsia* (1984) 25, 229–33.
11. Fowler GW. Effect of dipropylacetate on serum levels of anticonvulsants in children. *Proc West Pharmacol Soc* (1978) 21, 37–40.
12. Bauer LA, Harris C, Wilensky AJ, Raisys VA, Levy RH. Ethosuximide kinetics: possible interaction with valproic acid. *Clin Pharmacol Ther* (1982) 31, 741–5.
13. Sälke-Kellermann RA, May T, Boenigk HE. Influence of ethosuximide on valproic acid serum concentrations. *Epilepsy Res* (1997) 26, 345–349.

Felbamate + Antacids

Maalox Plus has no effect on the absorption of felbamate.

Clinical evidence, mechanism, importance and management

Felbamate 2400 mg daily was given to 9 epileptic women for 2 weeks. For a third week the felbamate was taken with **Maalox Plus** (aluminium/magnesium hydroxides). No significant changes in the serum levels or AUC were seen.[1] No special precautions would seem to be needed if felbamate is taken with this or any other similar **antacid**.

1. Sachdeo RC, Narang-Sachdeo SK, Howard JR, Dix RK, Shumaker RC, Perhach JL, Rosenberg A. Effect of antacid on the absorption of felbamate in subjects with epilepsy. *Epilepsia* (1993) 34 (Suppl 6), 79–80.

Felbamate + Erythromycin

Erythromycin does not alter felbamate pharmacokinetics.

Clinical evidence, mechanism, importance and management

In a randomised two-period crossover study, 12 epileptics were given 3000 or 3600 mg felbamate daily, either alone or with 333 mg **erythromycin** 8-hourly for 10 days. The pharmacokinetics of the felbamate were unchanged by the **erythromycin**.[1] There would therefore seem no reason for avoiding **erythromycin** in patients taking felbamate.

1. Montgomery PA, Sachdeo RJ, Narang-Sachdeo SK, Rosenberg A, Perhach JL. Felbamate pharmacokinetics after coadministration of erythromycin. *Epilepsia* (1994) 35 (Suppl 8), 113.

Felbamate + Gabapentin

There is evidence that the half-life of felbamate may be prolonged by gabapentin.

Clinical evidence, mechanism, importance and management

In a retrospective examination of the clinical data from patients taking felbamate, its half-life was found to be 24 h in 40 patients taking felbamate alone, whereas in 18 other patients taking **gabapentin** as well (including 7 taking a third drug), the half-life was extended to 32.7 h.[1] The practical clinical importance of this is uncertain but be alert for the need to reduce the felbamate dosage. More study is needed

1. Hussein G, Troupin AS, Montouris G. Gabapentin interaction with felbamate. *Neurology* (1996) 47, 1106.

Flunarizine + Anticonvulsants

Limited evidence suggests that anticonvulsants can reduce serum flunarizine levels.

Clinical evidence, mechanism, importance and management

A study of the value of flunarizine in treating epilepsy found that flunarizine levels were lower in patients receiving multiple anticonvulsants than in those receiving only one anticonvulsant (statistically significant only for the 10 mg flunarizine dose). Anticonvulsants received were **carbamazepine**, **phenytoin**, and **sodium valproate**. Flunarizine did not affect the serum levels of these other anticonvulsants.[1] There would seem to be no reason for avoiding concurrent use, but the outcome should be monitored.

1. Binnie CD, de Beukelaar F, Meijer JWA, Meinardi H, Overweg J, Wauquier A, van Wieringen A. Open dose-ranging trial of flunarizine as add-on therapy in epilepsy. *Epilepsia* (1985) 26, 424–8.

Fosphenytoin + Miscellaneous drugs

Fosphenytoin is a prodrug of phenytoin, which is rapidly and completely hydrolysed to phenytoin in the body. It is predicted to interact with other drugs just like phenytoin.[1]

1. Fierro LS, Savulich DH, Benezra DA. Safety of fosphenytoin sodium. *Am J Health-Syst Pharm* (1996) 53, 2707–12.

Gabapentin + Miscellaneous drugs

Cimetidine, *Maalox*, and probenecid do not interact to a clinically important extent with gabapentin. Gabapentin does not interact with combined oral contraceptives.

Clinical evidence, mechanism, importance and management

Gabapentin has been found not to induce or inhibit hepatic mixed function enzymes (as determined by its lack of effect on **antipyrine** (**phenazone**)), and is not metabolised, so it is therefore unlikely to interact with drugs which are affected by enzyme inducers or inhibitors.[1]

The steady-state pharmacokinetics of **ethinylestradiol** and **norethisterone** (in *Norlestrin*) were unaffected by repeated administration of gabapentin so that the reliability of **combined oral**

contraceptives of this type would not be expected to be altered.[1] *Maalox TC* 30 ml (magnesium and aluminium hydroxide) reduced the bioavailability of 400 mg gabapentin by less than 20% when given either at the same time or 2 h afterwards. When the antacid was given 2 h before, the bioavailability was reduced by 10%.[2] **Cimetidine** decreased the renal clearance of gabapentin by 12%, whereas **probenecid** had no effect on renal clearance.[1] None of these modest changes is expected to be of clinical importance. There would seem to be no need to take special precautions if any of these drugs is used concurrently

1. Busch JA, Bockbrader HN, Randinitis EJ, Chang T, Welling PG, Reece PA, Underwood B, Sedman AJ, Vollmer KO, Türck D. Lack of clinically significant drug interactions with Neurontin (Gabapentin). 20ᵗʰ International Epilepsy Congress. Oslo, Norway, July 1993. Abstract 013958.
2. Busch JA, Radulovic LL, Bockbrader HN, Underwood BA, Sedman AJ, Chang T. Effect of *Maalox TC®* on single-dose pharmacokinetics of gabapentin capsules in healthy subjects. *Pharm Res* (1992) 9 (10 Suppl), S-315.

Lamotrigine + Antituberculars

A case report describes a marked reduction in serum lamotrigine levels after a patient started treatment with rifampicin (rifampin), isoniazid and pyrazinamide.

Clinical evidence, mechanism, importance and management

A case report describes a 56 year-old woman taking 150 mg lamotrigine daily who showed unexpectedly low serum lamotrigine levels (1.3 mg/l) after starting **rifampicin (rifampin)**, **isoniazid** and **pyrazinamide** for tuberculous adenitis. This was thought to be due to potent enzyme inducing effects of the **rifampicin** on the lamotrigine metabolism. The lamotrigine dosage was therefore increased to 250 mg daily. After the antitubercular treatment was changed to **isoniazid** and **ethambutol**, the lamotrigine serum levels rose to 12.4 mg/l. The authors suggest that **isoniazid** possibly also inhibited the lamotrigine metabolism . No toxicity was seen.[1]

Information appears to be limited to this report, but it raises the possibility of a lamotrigine/**rifampicin** and a lamotrigine/**isoniazid** interaction. If either of these drugs is added to or withdrawn from lamotrigine treatment, be alert for the need to adjust the lamotrigine dosage. More study is needed to confirm these suspected effects.

1. Armijo JA, Sánchez B, Peralta FG, Cuadrado A, Leno C. Lamotrigine interaction with rifampicin and isoniazid. A case report. *Methods Find Exp Clin Pharmacol* (1996) 18 (Suppl C), 59.

Lamotrigine + Miscellaneous anticonvulsants

Phenobarbital and phenytoin have been associated with reduced lamotrigine serum levels. Clonazepam levels fell in four children when lamotrigine was added. Felbamate appears not to affect the pharmacokinetics of lamotrigine.

Clinical evidence, mechanism, importance and management

Phenobarbital and especially **phenytoin** were associated with decreased lamotrigine serum levels in a survey of patients.[1] Both of these drugs are known hepatic enzyme inducers and this may have lead to an increased clearance of lamotrigine.

No changes in the serum levels of **phenobarbital, phenytoin, primidone** were seen in another study in patients concurrently treated with 75 to 400 mg lamotrigine daily.[2] Lamotrigine had no effect on **ethosuximide** or **phenobarbital** serum levels in a group of children but the serum **clonazepam** levels fell about 38% in 4 of 8 patients when lamotrigine was added.[3] In two studies, **felbamate** did not appear to significantly affect the pharmacokinetics of lamotrigine.[4,5]

The clinical importance of these findings is not yet known, but no special precautions would seem necessary when adding lamotrigine to these anticonvulsants, except perhaps **clonazepam**, where monitoring would seem advisable. There may be a need to reduce the lamotrigine dosage if **phenobarbital** or **phenytoin** is withdrawn. See also 'Carbamazepine or Oxcarbazepine + Lamotrigine', p.327 and 'Lamotrigine + Sodium valproate', p.336.

1. May TW, Rambeck B, Jürgens U. Serum concentrations of lamotrigine in epileptic patients: the influence of dose and comedication. *Ther Drug Monit* (1996) 18, 523–31.
2. Jawad S, Richens A, Goodwin G, Yuen WC. Controlled trial of lamotrigine (Lamictal) for refractory partial seizures. *Epilepsia* (1989) 30, 356–63.
3. Eriksson A-S, Hoppu K, Nergårdh A, Boreus L. Pharmacokinetic interactions between lamotrigine and other antiepileptic drugs in children with intractable epilepsy. *Epilepsia* (1996) 37, 769–73.
4. Colucci R, Glue P, Holt B, Banfield C, Reidenberg P, Meehan JW, Pai S, Nomeir A, Lim J, Lin C-C, Affrime MB. Effect of felbamate on the pharmacokinetics of lamotrigine. *J Clin Pharmacol* (1996) 36, 634–8.
5. Gidal BE, Kanner A, Maly M, Rutecki P, Lensmeyer GL. Lamotrigine pharmacokinetics in patients receiving felbamate. *Epilepsy Res* (1997) 27, 1–5.

Lamotrigine + Sodium valproate

The serum levels of lamotrigine can be increased by sodium valproate. Concurrent use has been associated with skin rashes and other toxic reactions. Small increases, decreases or no changes in sodium valproate levels have been seen with lamotrigine.

Clinical evidence

(a) Increased lamotrigine serum levels

Sodium valproate 200 mg 8-hourly reduced the clearance of lamotrigine in 6 healthy subjects by 20%, and increased the AUC by 30%.[1,2] In another study in 18 healthy subjects receiving 500 mg **valproate** twice daily, the clearance of lamotrigine 50, 100 or 150 mg daily was also markedly reduced, and the half-life increased.[3,4] Meta-analysis of large numbers of epileptics found that although patients on both lamotrigine and **sodium valproate** tended to be taking lower doses of lamotrigine than other patients, the mean serum lamotrigine levels achieved were roughly doubled.[5] If at the same time they were also taking enzyme-inducing anticonvulsants, their serum levels of lamotrigine were only raised about 40%.[5] Similar results were found in another study.[6]

(b) Decreased and unchanged serum valproate levels

In a study 18 healthy subjects received 500 mg **valproate** twice daily. The addition of lamotrigine 50, 100 or 150 mg daily caused a 25% decrease in **valproate** serum levels and a 25% increase in **valproate** oral clearance.[3,7] A study in 31 children noted that the lamotrigine half-life was prolonged in those also taking **valproate**, however, in this study no clinically important changes in **valproate** serum levels were seen.[8]

(c) Toxic reactions

Severe and disabling tremor (sometimes preventing them from feeding themselves) was seen in 3 patients when they were treated with lamotrigine and **sodium valproate**. The problem resolved when the dosages were reduced.[9] Severe multiorgan dysfunction and disseminated intravascular coagulation was seen in 2 children when taking lamotrigine and **sodium valproate**.[10] In a study of 10 adult patients, all developed upper limb tremor during lamotrigine and **sodium valproate** comedication, which could be minimised by reducing the dosage of either or both drugs.[11] In a survey of 102 adult epileptics who had lamotrigine added to their therapy, 32 were also taking **valproate**. Of these, 9 patients (28%) developed a rash, whereas only 4 of the other 70 (6%) did so.[12] Another study successfully reintroduced lamotrigine in 3 patients, despite previous rashes.[13] The formation of toxic metabolites of **valproate** was unaffected by lamotrigine.[7]

Mechanisms

Not fully understood. It is thought that the two drugs compete for glucuronidation by the liver, which results in a decreased lamotrigine clearance.[1,2,14] Increased valproate clearance may be due to enzyme induction. A pharmacodynamic interaction has also been suggested.[11,15]

Importance and management

A moderately well documented interaction. Concurrent use can be therapeutically valuable, but the lamotrigine dosage may possibly need to be reduced (about halved) to avoid possible toxicity (sedation, tremor, ataxia, fatigue).[3,9,16] The outcome should be very well monitored. The effect on valproate levels seems to be variable and normally not great, however, be aware that changes may occur. The CSM in the UK has suggested that the concurrent use of sodium valproate is one of the main risk factors for the development of serious skin reactions to lamotrigine.[17] The reports cited above[9,10] also suggest that sometimes other serious reactions (disabling tremor, multiorgan dysfunction) can occur.

1. Yuen AWC, Land G, Weatherley BC, Peck AW. Sodium valproate inhibits lamotrigine metabolism. *Fundam Clin Pharmacol* (1991) 5, 468.
2. Yuen AWC, Land G, Weatherley BC, Peck AW. Sodium valproate acutely inhibits lamotrigine metabolism. *Br J Clin Pharmacol* (1992) 33, 511–13.
3. Anderson GD, Yau MK, Gidal BE, Harris SJ, Levy RH, Lai AA, Wolf KB, Wargin WA, Dren AT. Bidirectional interaction of valproate and lamotrigine in healthy subjects. *Clin Pharmacol Ther* (1996) 60, 145–56.
4. Yau MK, Wargin WA, Wolf KB, Lai AA, Dren AT, Harris SI, Morse IS. Effect of valproate on the pharmacokinetics of lamotrigine (Lamictal) at steady state. *Epilepsia* (1992) 33, (Suppl 3) 82.
5. Betts T, Goodwin G, Withers RM, Yuen AWC. Human safety of lamotrigine. *Epilepsia* (1991) 32 (Suppl 2), S17–S21.
6. May TW, Rambeck B, Jürgens U. Serum concentrations of lamotrigine in epileptic patients: the influence of dose and comedication. *Ther Drug Monit* (1996) 18, 523–31.
7. Anderson GD, Gidal BE, Levy RH, Yau MK, Wolf KB, Lai AA. Dren AT. Effect of lamotrigine (LTG, Lamictal) on the pharmacokinetics and biotransformation of valproate. *Epilepsia* (1992) 33 (Suppl 3), 82.
8. Eriksson A-S, Hoppu K, Nergårdh A, Boreus L. Pharmacokinetic interactions between lamotrigine and other antiepileptic drugs in children with intractable epilepsy. *Epilepsia* (1996) 37, 769–73.
9. Reutens DC, Duncan JS, Patsalos PN. Disabling tremor after lamotrigine with sodium valproate. *Lancet* (1993) 342, 185–6.
10. Chattergoon DS, McGuigan M, Koren G, Hwang P, Ito S. Multiorgan dysfunction and disseminated intravascular coagulation (DIC) in two children following lamotrigine and valproic acid. *Clin Invest Med* (1996) 19 (4 Suppl), S12.
11. Pisani F, Oteri G, Russo M, Trio R, Di Perri R, Perucca E, Richens A. Effects of lamotrigine-valproate comedication on seizure frequency and upper limb tremor: A pharmacodynamic interaction? *Epilepsia* (1995) 36 (Suppl 3), S264.
12. Russo M, Li LM, O'Donoghue MF, Sander JWAS, Duncan JS. Cutaneous rash with lamotrigine and concomitant valproate therapy. *Epilepsia* (1994) 35 (Suppl 7), 72.
13. Tavernor SJ, Newton ER, Brown SW. Rechallenge with lamotrigine after initial rash. *Epilepsia* (1994) 35 (Suppl 7), 72.
14. Panayiotopoulos CP, Ferrie CD, Knott C, Robinson RO. Interaction of lamotrigine with sodium valproate. *Lancet* (1993) 341, 445.
15. Ferrie CD, Panayiotopoulos CP. Therapeutic interaction of lamotrigine and sodium valproate in intractable myoclonic epilepsy. *Seizure* (1994) 3, 157–9.
16. Pisani F, Di Perri R, Perucca E, Richens A. Interaction of lamotrigine with sodium valproate. *Lancet* (1993) 341, 1224.
17. Committee on the Safety of Medicines/Medicines Control Agency. *Current Problems* (1996) 22, 12.

Levetiracetam + Miscellaneous drugs

Levetiracetam appears not to interact adversely with a range of other antiepileptic drugs (carbamazepine, gabapentin, lamotrigine, phenobarbital, phenytoin or primidone) nor with digoxin, food, oral contraceptives, probenecid or warfarin.

Clinical evidence, mechanism, importance and management

(a) Antiepileptics

There is good evidence that levetiracetam does not affect the serum levels of **carbamazepine, gabapentin, lamotrigine, phenobarbital, phenytoin** or **primidone**, and that none of these antiepileptic drugs affects the pharmacokinetics of levetiracetam.[1,2] No dosage adjustments would therefore seem to be needed if levetiracetam is used as add-on therapy with any of these drugs.

(b) Contraceptives

The pharmacokinetics of an **oral contraceptive (ethinylestradiol + levonorgestrel)** were found not to be affected by 1 g levetiracetam daily, nor were there any changes in LH or progesterone levels. The pharmacokinetics of levetiracetam also remained unaffected.[1] These findings indicate that no special or additional precautions are needed if **oral contraceptives** and levetiracetam are used concurrently.

(c) Digoxin, Warfarin

A randomised double-blind placebo-controlled trial in 42 healthy subjects given **warfarin** found that 1000 mg levetiracetam twice daily had no significant effect on the pharmacokinetics of either drug and the INRs were not significantly altered.[3,4] A double-blind, placebo-controlled, two-way crossover study in 11 healthy subjects on digoxin found that 1000 mg levetiracetam twice daily had no significant effect on the pharmacokinetics or pharmacodynamics of **digoxin**.[5] No special precautions are therefore needed if either of these drugs is used concurrently with levetiracetam.

(d) Probenecid, Food

500 mg **probenecid** four times daily was found not to affect the renal excretion of levetiracetam whereas that of its primary and pharmacologically inactive metabolite (ucb L057) was reduced, but its concentrations remained low. There is nothing to suggest that a clinically relevant adverse interaction takes place between **probenecid** and levetiracetam. The extent of absorption of levetiracetam is not affected by **food**, but the rate is slightly reduced.[1]

In vitro studies have shown that levetiracetam and its primary metabolite do not inhibit the major human liver cytochrome P450 isoenzymes (CYP1A2, 2A6, 2C8/9/10/19, 2D6, 2E1 or 3A4) or glucuronyl transferase, nor does levetiracetam cause enzyme induction.[1,3] It is therefore unlikely that levetiracetam will take part in interactions due to either enzyme induction or inhibition.

1. Levetiracetam (Keppra), UCB Pharma. Summary of Product Characteristics, September 2000.
2. Browne TR, Szabo GK, Josephs EG, Paz AJ. Absence of pharmacokinetic drug interaction of ucb L059 (levetiracetam) with phenytoin determined by simplified stable isotope tracer technique. *Epilepsia* (1998) 39 (Suppl 6), 58–9.
3. Nicolas J-M, Collart P, Gerin B, Mather G, Trager W, Levy R, Roba J. In vitro evaluation of potential drug interactions with levetiracetam, a new antiepileptic agent. *Drug Metab Dispos* (1999) 27, 250-4.
4. Ragueneau-Majlessi I, Levy RH, Meyerhoff C. Lack of effect of repeated administration of levetiracetam on the pharmacodynamic and pharmacokinetic profiles of warfarin. *Epilepsy Res* (2001) 47, 55–63.
5. Levy RH, Ragueneau-Majlessi I, Baltes E. Repeated administration of the novel antiepileptic agent levetiracetam does not alter digoxin pharmacokinetics and pharmacodyamics in healthy volunteers. *Epilepsia* (2000) 41 (Suppl 7), 227.

Losigamone + Phenytoin

There is evidence that the clearance of losigamone may be increased by phenytoin. The clinical importance of this is uncertain.

Clinical evidence, mechanism, importance and management

A placebo-controlled, double blind study over a 6 week period in 12 healthy subjects on the possible interactions of 500 mg losigamone twice daily and 100 mg **phenytoin** daily found that the steady state pharmacokinetics (AUC, maximum serum levels) of the **phenytoin** were unaffected by the losigamone. However, the AUC, clearance and half-life of the losigamone were decreased (no values given).[1] This suggests that the **phenytoin** induces the metabolism of the losigamone, but the clinical relevance of this remains to be assessed.

1. Krämer G, Wad N, Bredel-Geißler, Biber A, Dienel A. Losigamone-phenytoin interaction: a placebo-controlled, double-blind study in healthy volunteers. *Epilepsia* (1995) 36 (Suppl 3), S163.

Mesuximide + Other anticonvulsants

Phenobarbital, phenytoin, and possibly felbamate increase the levels of the active metabolite of mesuximide. Mesuximide increases the serum levels of phenobarbital and phenytoin.

Clinical evidence

A study in 94 hospitalised patients with petit mal epilepsy found that when mesuximide was given to patients on **phenobarbital** or **primidone**, the mean serum levels of **phenobarbital** rose by 38 and 40% respectively. Dose reductions were needed in 50% and 62% of patients, respectively. Mesuximide was also given to patients on **phenytoin**, which resulted in a 78% rise in the **phenytoin** serum levels requiring dose reductions in about 30% of the patients. It was also found that the concurrent use of either **phenobarbital** or **phenytoin** increased the serum levels of the active anticonvulsant metabolite of mesuximide.[1] Three adolescent epileptics on mesuximide developed mild side effects within 3 days of starting to take **felbamate**, which became more serious by the end of a month (decreased appetite, nausea, weight loss, insomnia, dizziness, hiccups, slurred speech). During this time the normethsuximide levels in 2 patients rose 26 and 46% respectively. The adverse effects disappeared and the normethsuximide levels fell when the mesuximide dosage was reduced. Other anticonvulsants being taken were **carbamazepine**, **ethotoin** and **sodium valproate**.[2]

Mechanism

The suggested reason is that all of these drugs compete for the same metabolic mechanisms (hydroxylation) in the liver. As a result each one is metabolised more slowly and is therefore is lost from the body more slowly.

Importance and management

Information about these interactions is limited. Nevertheless, concurrent therapy should be monitored. Anticipate the need to reduce the dose of phenytoin, phenobarbital or primidone if methsuximide is given. It has been suggested that levels of normethsuximide should also be monitored.[1] Anticipate the need to reduce the dose of methsuximide if felbamate is added.

1. Rambeck B. Pharmacological interactions of mesuximide with phenobarbital and phenytoin in hospitalized epileptic patients. *Epilepsia* (1979) 20, 147–56.
2. Patrias J, Espe-Lillo J, Ritter FJ. Felbamate-methsuximide interaction. *Epilepsia* (1992) 33 (Suppl 3) 84.

Oxcarbazepine + Antipyrine (Phenazone)

From studies with antipyrine (phenazone) it appears that oxcarbazepine can act as a liver enzyme inducer at high but not low dosage.

Clinical evidence, mechanism, importance and management

Antipyrine (phenazone) is used as a marker for possible changes in hepatic oxidase activity, so that the effects of oxcarbazepine on **antipyrine** pharmacokinetics have been investigated. Single and repeated doses of 300 mg oxcarbazepine twice daily did not affect **antipyrine** half-life or clearance.[1] In contrast **antipyrine** testing in 4 patients with neuralgia taking oxcarbazepine suggested that dose-dependent induction by oxcarbazepine may occur.[2] In another study of 13 healthy subjects 1800 mg oxcarbazepine daily reduced the half-life of **antipyrine** by 22%.[3] These studies suggest that at higher dosage oxcarbazepine may show some hepatic enzyme induction, whereas at lower dosages it does not.

1. Larkin JG, McKee PJW, Forrest G, Beastall GH, Park BK, Lowrie JI, Lloyd P, Brodie MJ. Lack of enzyme induction with oxcarbazepine (600 mg daily) in healthy subjects. *Br J Clin Pharmacol* (1991) 31, 65–71.

2. Patsalos PN, Zakrzewska JM, Elyas AA. Dose dependent enzyme induction by oxcarbazepine. *Eur J Clin Pharmacol* (1990) 39, 187–8.
3. Saano V, Schurr-Eisinger S, Möbius HJ, Menge G, Ezzet F, Andersson P, Schwabe S. Effect of oxcarbazepine on antipyrine metabolism in healthy volunteers. *Epilepsia* (1995) 36 (Suppl 3), S161.

Oxcarbazepine + Felbamate

No clinically relevant pharmacokinetic interaction occurs with oxcarbazepine and felbamate, but the incidence of side effects is increased.

Clinical evidence, mechanism, importance and management

A double-blind randomised study in 8 healthy subjects found that oxcarbazepine 300 to 600 mg 12 hourly with 600 to 1200 mg **felbamate** 12-hourly for 10 days had no effect on the plasma levels of the major active metabolite of oxcarbazepine (monohydroxyoxcarbazepine). However, the levels of dihydroxycarbazepine (a minor, inactive metabolite) were reduced, and the maximum serum levels of oxcarbazepine were reduced, by about 20%. These changes were considered to be clinically irrelevant, however, the incidence of some side effects (dizziness, somnolence, nausea, diplopia) rose during concurrent use.[1] See 'Anticonvulsants + Oxcarbazepine', p.315.

1. Hulsman JARJ, Rentmeester TW, Banfield CR, Reidenberg P, Colucci RD, Meehan JW, Radwanski E, Mojaverian P, Lin C-C, Nezamis J, Affrime MB, Glue P. Effects of felbamate on the pharmacokinetics of the monohydroxy and dihydroxy metabolites of oxcarbazepine. *Clin Pharmacol Ther* (1995) 58, 383–9.

Phenytoin + Alcohol

Chronic heavy drinking reduces serum phenytoin concentrations so that above-average doses of phenytoin may be needed to maintain adequate levels. Excessive drinking also seems to increase the frequency of seizures in epileptics, but moderate and occasional drinking has no effect.

Clinical evidence

(a) Acute alcohol ingestion

In a study designed to test the effects of acute **alcohol** intoxication in epileptics, 25 patients were given a 12 oz (about 340 ml drink of 25% **alcohol**. Blood alcohol levels ranged from 39 to 284 mg%. All patients showed signs of alcohol intoxication without any effect on seizure frequency.[1] The metabolism of a single dose of phenytoin was not affected by acute ingestion of **alcohol** in healthy subjects.[2]

(b) Heavy drinking

Blood phenytoin levels measured 24 h after the last dose of phenytoin in a group of 15 drinkers (consuming a minimum of 200 g **ethanol** daily for at least 3 months) were approximately half those of 76 non-drinkers. The phenytoin half-life was reduced by 30%.[3]

Another study confirmed that alcoholics without liver disease have lower than usual plasma levels of phenytoin after taking standard doses while drinking.[4] A report describes a chronic alcoholic who was resistant to large doses of phenytoin,[5] and another describes a reduction in serum phenytoin levels accompanied by seizures in a man when his consumption of **alcohol** increased.[6]

(c) Moderate social drinking

A study in non-drinking epileptics (17 in the experimental group, 14 in the control group) found that the serum levels of phenytoin were unchanged by moderate drinking, and there was no influence on tonic-clonic convulsions or partial complex seizures. The experimental group drank 1 to 3 glasses of an alcoholic beverage (equivalent to a glass of **beer** containing 9.85 g **ethanol**) twice a week, over a 2-h period for 16 weeks, and their maximum blood alcohol levels ranged from 5 to 33 mg%.[7]

Mechanism

Supported by *animal* data,[8] the evidence suggests that repeated exposure to large amounts of alcohol induces liver microsomal enzymes so that the rate of metabolism and clearance of phenytoin from the body is increased.

Importance and management

An established and clinically important interaction although the documentation is limited. Heavy drinkers may need above-average doses of phenytoin to maintain adequate serum levels. However, be aware that patients with liver impairment usually need lower doses of phenytoin, so the picture may be more complicated. Epileptics should be encouraged to limit their drinking because heavy drinking possibly increases the frequency of seizures,[9] and when intoxicated they may be less alert for any signs of an impending seizure. Moderate drinking appears to be safe.[1,7] See also 'Anticonvulsants + Alcohol', p.307.

1. Rodin EA, Frohman CE, Gottlieb JS. Effect of acute alcohol intoxication on epileptic patients. *Arch Neurol* (1961) 4, 115–18.
2. Schmidt D. Effect of ethanol intake on phenytoin metabolism in volunteers. *Experientia* (1975) 31, 1313–14.
3. Kater RMH, Roggin G, Tobon F, Zieve P, Iber FL. Increased rate of clearance of drugs from the circulation of alcoholics. *Am J Med Sci* (1969) 258, 35–9.
4. Sandor P, Sellers EM, Dumbrell M, Khouw V. Effect of short- and long-term alcohol use on phenytoin kinetics in chronic alcoholics. *Clin Pharmacol Ther* (1981) 30, 390–7.
5. Birkett DJ, Graham GG, Chinwah PM, Wade DN, Hickie JB. Multiple drug interactions with phenytoin. *Med J Aust* (1977) 2, 467–8.
6. Bellibas SE, Tuglular I. A case of phenytoin-alcohol interaction. *Therapie* (1995) 50, 487–8.
7. Höppener RJ, Kuyer A, van der Lugt PJM. Epilepsy and alcohol: the influence of social alcohol intake on seizures and treatment in epilepsy. *Epilepsia* (1983) 24, 459–71.
8. Rubin E, Lieber CS. Hepatic microsomal enzymes in man and rat: induction and inhibition by ethanol. *Science* (1968) 162, 690–1.
9. Lambie DG, Stanaway L, Johnson RH. Factors which influence the effectiveness of treatment of epilepsy. *Aust N Z J Med* (1986) 16, 779–84.

Phenytoin + Allopurinol

A single case report describes phenytoin toxicity in a boy when given allopurinol.

Clinical evidence, mechanism, importance and management

A 13-year-old boy with Lesch-Nyhan syndrome who was taking phenobarbital, clonazepam, sodium valproate and phenytoin (200 mg daily) became somnolent within 7 days of starting to take **allopurinol** 150 mg daily. His serum phenytoin levels were found to have almost tripled (from 7.5 to 20.8 micrograms/ml).[1] The reason for this reaction is not known (possibly inhibition of liver enzymes?) and its general importance is uncertain — but probably very small.

1. Yokochi K, Yokochi A, Chiba K, Ishizaki T. Phenytoin-allopurinol interaction: Michaelis-Menten kinetic parameters of phenytoin with and without allopurinol in a child with Lesch-Nyhan syndrome. *Ther Drug Monit* (1982) 4, 353–7.

Phenytoin + Amiodarone

Serum phenytoin levels can be raised, markedly so in some individuals, by the concurrent use of amiodarone. Phenytoin toxicity may occur if the dosage of phenytoin is not reduced appropriately. Amiodarone serum levels are reduced by phenytoin.

Clinical evidence

(a) Phenytoin serum levels increased

Three patients showed a marked rise in serum phenytoin levels 10 days to 4 weeks after being given **amiodarone** (400 to 1200 mg daily). One of them developed phenytoin toxicity (ataxia, lethargy, vertigo) within 4 weeks of starting to take **amiodarone** and had a serum phenytoin level of 40 micrograms/ml, representing a three to fourfold rise. Levels restabilised when the phenytoin dosage was withheld and then reduced from 300 to 200 mg daily. The serum phenytoin levels of the other 2 patients were approximately doubled by the **amiodarone**.[1]

A study in healthy subjects showed that after taking 200 mg **amiodarone** daily for 3 weeks the AUC of phenytoin was increased by 31%.[2] A pharmacokinetic study found that 200 mg **amiodarone** daily for 6 weeks raised the peak serum phenytoin levels by 33% and the AUC by 40%.[3] Other case reports describe two to threefold rises in serum phenytoin levels with toxicity 2 to 6 weeks after starting **amiodarone** in 3 patients.[4-6]

(b) Amiodarone serum levels reduced

A study in 5 healthy subjects given 200 mg **amiodarone** daily showed that over a 5-week period the serum amiodarone levels gradually increased. When phenytoin (3 to 4 mg/kg daily) was added for a period of 2 weeks, the serum **amiodarone** levels fell to concentrations that were between about one-half to two-thirds of those predicted.[7,8]

Mechanisms

Uncertain. (a) It seems possible that amiodarone inhibits the liver enzymes concerned with the metabolism of phenytoin, resulting in a rise in its serum levels.[3] It seems unlikely that drug displacement from protein binding sites had a part to play as free and bound levels of phenytoin remained constant.[3] (b) Phenytoin is an enzyme-inducing agent which possibly increases the metabolism of the amiodarone by the liver.

Importance and management

Information seems to be limited to the reports cited, but both interactions appear to be clinically important. Concurrent use should not be undertaken unless the effects can be well monitored.

(a) The phenytoin dosage should be reduced as necessary. A 25 to 30% reduction has been recommended for those taking 2 to 4 mg/kg daily, but it should be remembered that small alterations in phenytoin dose may result in a large change in phenytoin levels, as phenytoin kinetics are non-linear.[3,9,10] Note that the phenytoin levels in some individuals were doubled after only 10 days concurrent use.[1] Amiodarone is cleared from the body very slowly so that this interaction will persist for weeks after its withdrawal. Continued monitoring is important. Be aware that ataxia due to phenytoin toxicity may be confused with amiodarone-induced ataxia.[1,5]

(b) It is not clear whether the amiodarone dosage should be increased or not to accommodate this interaction because the metabolite of amiodarone (*N*-desmethylamiodarone) also has important antiarrhythmic effects.[8]

1. McGovern B, Geer VR, LaRaia PJ, Garan H, Ruskin JN. Possible interaction between amiodarone and phenytoin. *Ann Intern Med* (1984) 101, 650–1.
2. Nolan PE, Marcus FI, Hoyer G, Bliss M, Mayersohn MP, Gear K. Pharmacokinetic interaction between amiodarone and phenytoin. *J Am Coll Cardiol* (1987) 9 (2 Suppl A), 47A.
3. Nolan PE, Erstad BL, Hoyer GL, Bliss M, Gear K, Marcus FI. Steady-state interaction between amiodarone and phenytoin in normal subjects. *Am J Cardiol* (1990) 65, 1252–7.
4. Gore JM, Haffajee CI, Alpert JS. Interaction of amiodarone and diphenylhydantoin. *Am J Cardiol* (1984) 54, 1145.
5. Shackleford EJ, Watson FT. Amiodarone-phenytoin interaction. *Drug Intell Clin Pharm* (1987) 21, 921.
6. Ahmad S. Amiodarone and phenytoin: interaction. *J Am Geriatr Soc* (1995) 43, 1449–50.
7. Nolan PE, Marcus FI, Karol MD, Hoyer GL, Gear K. Evidence for an effect of phenytoin on the pharmacokinetics of amiodarone. *Pharmacotherapy* (1988) 8, 121.
8. Nolan PE, Marcus FI, Karol MD, Hoyer GL, Gear K. Effect of phenytoin on the clinical pharmacokinetics of amiodarone. *J Clin Pharmacol* (1990) 30, 1112–19.
9. Nolan PE, Erstad BL, Hoyer GL, Bliss M, Gear K, Marcus FI. Interaction between amiodarone and phenytoin. *Am J Cardiol* (1991) 67, 328–9.
10. Duffal SB, McKenzie SK. Interaction between amiodarone and phenytoin. *Am J Cardiol* (1991) 67, 328.

Phenytoin + Antacids

Some, but not all studies have shown that antacids can reduce phenytoin serum levels and this may have been responsible for some loss of seizure control in a few patients, but usually no clinically important interaction occurs.

Clinical evidence

(a) Evidence of an interaction

Three patients taking phenytoin were found to have low serum phenytoin levels (2 to 4 micrograms/ml) when given phenytoin and unnamed **antacids** at the same time, but when the **antacid** administration was delayed by 2 to 3 h the serum phenytoin levels rose two to threefold.[1]

A controlled study in 6 epileptics showed that *Gelusil* (**magnesium trisilicate** and **aluminium hydroxide**) caused a 12% reduction in serum phenytoin levels, although seizure frequency was not affected.[2] Elsewhere, 2 epileptics are reported to have shown inadequate seizure control, which coincided with their ingestion of **aluminium** and **magnesium hydroxide** antacids for dyspepsia.[3] Reduced levels of phenytoin (AUC reduced about one-third) occurred in 8 subjects given either **aluminium/magnesium hydroxide** or **calcium carbonate**,[4] and in 3 subjects given *Asilone* (**dimeticone, aluminium hydroxide**, and **magnesium oxide**).[5]

(b) Evidence of no interaction

A study in 6 healthy subjects given **aluminium hydroxide** or **magnesium hydroxide** failed to show any change in the rate or extent of absorption of a single dose of phenytoin,[3] and a similar study found **calcium carbonate** also had no effect on the absorption of phenytoin.[2] A study in 2 subjects found no alteration in the absorption of phenytoin due to **magnesium hydroxide, aluminium hydroxide-magnesium trisilicate** mixture or **calcium carbonate**.[6] In another study, no statistically significant decrease in absorption was seen in 6 subjects given *Asilone*.[5]

Mechanism

Not understood. One suggestion is that diarrhoea and a general increase in peristalsis caused by some antacids may cause a reduction in phenytoin absorption. Another is that antacids may cause changes in gastric acid secretion, which could affect phenytoin solubility.

Importance and management

This possible interaction is fairly well documented, but the results are conflicting. In practice it appears not to be important in most patients, although some loss of seizure control has been seen to occur in a few. The interaction is unpredictable because it seems to depend on the individual patient and the antacid being taken. Concurrent use need not be avoided but if there is any hint that an epileptic patient is being affected, separation of the dosages by 2 to 3 h may minimise the effects.

1. Pippinger L. Personal communication quoted by Kutt H in Interactions of antiepileptic drugs. *Epilepsia* (1975) 16, 393–402.
2. Kulshreshtha VK, Thomas M, Wadsworth J, Richens A. Interaction between phenytoin and antacids. *Br J Clin Pharmacol* (1978) 6, 177–9.
3. O'Brien LS, Orme ML'E, Breckenridge AM. Failure of antacids to alter the pharmacokinetics of phenytoin. *Br J Clin Pharmacol* (1978) 6, 176–7.
4. Carter BL, Garnett WR, Pellock JM, Stratton MA, Howell JR. Effect of antacids on phenytoin bioavailability. *Ther Drug Monit* (1981) 3, 333–40.
5. McElnay JC, Uprichard G, Collier PS. The effect of activated dimethicone and a proprietary antacid preparation containing this agent on the absorption of phenytoin. *Br J Clin Pharmacol* (1982) 13, 501–5.
6. Chapron DJ, Kramer PA, Mariano SL, Hohnadel DC. Effect of calcium and antacids on phenytoin bioavailability. *Arch Neurol* (1979) 36, 436–8.

Phenytoin + Anticoagulants

The serum levels of phenytoin can be increased by dicoumarol (toxicity seen) and phenprocoumon, but they are usually unchanged by warfarin and phenindione. However, a
single case of phenytoin toxicity has been seen with warfarin.
Phenytoin can reduce the anticoagulant effects of dicoumarol
and increase the effects of warfarin, whereas the effects of
phenprocoumon normally appear to be unaltered. A single
case of severe bleeding has been described with acenocoumarol (nicoumalone) and phenytoin.

Clinical evidence

See also Table 7.3.

(a) Acenocoumarol (Nicoumalone)

A 68-year-old woman with a double mitral valve lesion, atrial fibrillation and hypertension, on digoxin and diuretics, was stabilised on
acenocoumarol and paroxetine. Phenytoin was started because of a
seizure, and within 11 days she developed ataxia, lethargy and nystagmus (serum phenytoin levels of 125.9 micromol/l). At the same
time her INR was found to have climbed from a range of 2 to 4, up to
14.5 and a huge retroperitoneal haematoma was discovered. After appropriate treatment she was discharged on a reduced dosage of acenocoumarol and half the phenytoin dosage.[1]

(b) Dicoumarol

Phenytoin 300 mg daily was given to 6 subjects on constant daily
doses of dicoumarol (40 to 160 mg) for a week. No significant
changes in the prothrombin-proconvertin concentration occurred until 3 days after stopping the phenytoin. In the following 5 days it
climbed from 20 to 50%, with an accompanying drop in the serum dicoumarol levels.[2] Four other subjects on 60 mg dicoumarol daily
were also given 300 mg phenytoin daily for the first week of treatment, and then 100 mg daily for 5 more weeks. The prothrombin-proconvertin concentration had risen from 20 to 70% after 2 weeks of
concurrent treatment, and only fell to previous levels five and a half
weeks after stopping the phenytoin.[2]

A study in 6 subjects taking 300 mg phenytoin daily showed that
when additionally given dicoumarol (doses adjusted to give prothrombin values of about 30%) their serum phenytoin levels rose on
average over 7 days by almost 10 micrograms/ml (126%).[3] In another
study the half-life of phenytoin in 3 patients increased approximately
fivefold during dicoumarol treatment.[4]

A patient on dicoumarol developed phenytoin toxicity within a
few days of starting to take 300 mg phenytoin daily (dose based on a
weight of 62 kg). Phenytoin was withdrawn, and reintroduced at
200 mg daily, which gave satisfactory phenytoin levels.[5]

(c) Phenindione

A study in 4 patients on 300 mg phenytoin daily showed that when
additionally given phenindione their serum phenytoin levels were
not affected.[4]

(d) Phenprocoumon + Phenytoin

An investigation in patients on long-term phenprocoumon treatment
showed that in the majority of cases phenytoin had no significant effect on either serum phenprocoumon levels or the anticoagulant
control, although a few patients showed a fall and others a rise in serum anticoagulant levels.[6]

A study in 4 patients on 300 mg phenytoin daily showed that when
additionally given phenprocoumon their serum phenytoin levels
rose from about 10 to 14 micrograms/ml over 7 days.[4] The phenytoin
half-life increased from 9.9 to 14 h.

(e) Warfarin + Phenytoin

The prothrombin time of a patient on warfarin increased from 21 to
32 s over a month when given 300 mg phenytoin daily, despite a 22%
reduction in the warfarin dosage. He was restabilised on the original
warfarin dosage when the phenytoin was withdrawn. Another patient is said to have shown this interaction but no details are given.[7]
Four other reports describe this interaction.[8-11] One of them describes
a patient who had an increased anticoagulant response to warfarin for
the first 6 days after phenytoin was added. The anticoagulant effect
then declined to less than the level seen before the addition of phenytoin.[10]

A study in 2 patients on 300 mg phenytoin daily found that serum
phenytoin levels were unaffected by the concurrent use of warfarin
over 7 days, and the half-life of phenytoin in 4 other patients was unaffected.[4] However, a patient on 300 mg phenytoin daily has been described who developed signs of toxicity within a short time of starting
to take warfarin.[12]

Mechanisms

Multiple, complex and poorly understood. Dicoumarol and phenprocoumon (but not normally warfarin) appear to inhibit the metabolism
of phenytoin by the liver, so that its loss from the body is reduced.
Phenytoin appears to increase the metabolism of dicoumarol, reduce
the metabolism of warfarin, but has no effect on the metabolism of
phenprocoumon. Phenytoin possibly also has a diverse depressant effect on the liver which lowers blood clotting factor production.[13]

Importance and management

None of these interactions has been extensively studied nor are they
well established, but what is known suggests that the use of dicoumarol with phenytoin should be avoided. Serum phenytoin levels
should be well monitored if phenprocoumon is used, and both the
phenytoin levels and anticoagulant control should be monitored if
acenocoumarol (nicoumalone) or warfarin is given. Dosage adjustments may be needed to accommodate these interactions. Informa-

Table 7.3 Summary of interactions between phenytoin and anticoagulants

Concurrent treatment with phenytoin and anticoagulant	Effect on serum anticoagulant levels	Effect on serum phenytoin levels
Dicoumarol level	Reduced[2]	Markedly increased[3-5]
Phenprocoumon effect	Usually unchanged[6]	Increased[4]
Acenocoumarol (Nicoumalone) effect	Single case of increase[1]	Uncertain
Warfarin effect	Increased[7-11] Single case of increase followed by decrease[10]	Usually unchanged[4] Single case of increase[12]
Phenindione	Not documented	Usually unchanged[3,4]
Other anticoagulants	Not documented	Not documented

tion about other anticoagulants (apart from phenindione, see (c) above) appears to be lacking, but it would clearly be prudent to monitor the effects of concurrent use.

1. Abad-Santos F, Carcas AJ, F-Capitán C, Frias J. Case report. Retroperitoneal haematoma in a patient treated with acenocoumarol, phenytoin and paroxetine. *Clin Lab Haematol* (1995) 17, 195–7.
2. Hansen JM, Siersbæk-Nielsen K, Kristensen M, Skovsted L,Christensen LK. Effect of diphenylhydantoin on the metabolism of dicoumarol in man. *Acta Med Scand* (1971) 189, 15–19.
3. Hansen JM, Kristensen M, Skovsted L, Christensen LK. Dicoumarol-induced diphenyl-hydantoin intoxication. *Lancet* (1966) ii, 265–6.
4. Skovsted L, Kristensen M, Hansen JM, Siersbæk-Nielsen K. The effect of different oral anticoagulants on diphenylhydantoin (DPH) and tolbutamide metabolism. *Acta Med Scand* (1976) 199, 513–15.
5. Franzten E, Hansen JM, Hansen OE, Kristensen M. Phenytoin (Dilantin®) intoxication. *Acta Neurol Scand* (1967) 43, 440–6.
6. Chrishe HW, Tauchert M, Hilger HH. Effect of phenytoin on the metabolism of phen-procoumon. *Eur J Clin Invest* (1974) 4, 331.
7. Nappi JM. Warfarin and phenytoin interaction. *Ann Intern Med* (1979) 90, 852.
8. Koch-Weser J. Haemorrhagic reactions and drug interactions in 500 warfarin treated patients. *Clin Pharmacol Ther* (1973) 14, 139.
9. Taylor JW, Alexander B, Lyon LW. A comparative evaluation of oral anticoagulant-phenytoin interactions. *Drug Intell Clin Pharm* (1980) 14, 669–73.
10. Levine M, Sheppard I. Biphasic interaction of phenytoin with warfarin. *Clin Pharm* (1984) 3, 200–3.
11. Panegyres PK, Rischbieth RH. Fatal phenytoin warfarin interaction. *Postgrad Med J* (1991) 67, 98.
12. Rothermich NO. Diphenylhydantoin intoxication. *Lancet* (1966) ii, 640.
13. Solomon GE, Hilgartner MW, Kutt H. Coagulation defects caused by diphenylhydanto-in. *Neurology* (1972) 22, 1165–71.

Phenytoin + Antitubercular drugs

Serum phenytoin levels are markedly reduced by the concurrent use of rifampicin. If both rifampicin and isoniazid are given, serum phenytoin levels may fall in patients who are fast acetylators of isoniazid, but may occasionally rise in those who are slow acetylators. Phenytoin serum levels can be raised by the concurrent use of isoniazid alone. Those who are 'slow metabolisers' of isoniazid may develop phenytoin toxicity if the dosage of phenytoin is not reduced appropriately.

Clofazimine may reduce serum phenytoin levels.

Clinical evidence

(a) Phenytoin + Isoniazid

A study in 32 patients on phenytoin 300 mg daily showed that within a week of starting to take **isoniazid** 300 mg daily and para-aminosalicylic acid 15 g daily, 6 of them had phenytoin levels almost 5 micrograms/ml higher than the rest of the group. On the following days when levels of these 6 patients climbed above 20 micrograms/ml the typical signs of phenytoin toxicity were seen. All 6 had unusually high serum **isoniazid** serum levels and were identified as slow metabolisers of isoniazid.[1]

Rises in serum phenytoin levels and toxicity induced by the concurrent use of **isoniazid** has been described in numerous other reports[2-15] involving large numbers of patients, one of which describes a fatality.[8]

(b) Phenytoin + Rifampicin

A study in 6 patients showed that the clearance of phenytoin (100 mg given intravenously) doubled from 46.7 to 97.8 ml/min after 450 mg **rifampicin** daily was taken for 2 weeks.[16]

A man on phenytoin needed a dosage reduction from 375 to 325 mg daily to keep his serum phenytoin levels within the therapeutic range when his treatment with **rifampicin** came to an end.[17]

(c) Phenytoin + Rifampicin/Clofazimine

A man with AIDS taking a number of drugs (**rifampicin, clofazimine**, ciprofloxacin, ethambutol, clarithromycin, diphenoxylate, bismuth, octreotide, co-trimoxazole, amphotericin, 5-flucytosine, amikacin, zalcitabine) was additionally given phenytoin to control a right-sided seizure disorder. Despite taking 1600 mg of phenytoin daily, and a trial of intravenous treatment his trough phenytoin plasma levels remained almost undetectable until the **rifampicin** was withdrawn, when they rose to 5 micrograms/ml with the oral dose.

When the **clofazimine** was withdrawn the levels rose even further to 10 micrograms/ml.[18]

(d) Phenytoin + Rifampicin/Isoniazid

A patient on 300 mg phenytoin daily developed progressive drowsiness (a sign of phenytoin toxicity) during the first week of starting treatment with **isoniazid**, **rifampicin** and ethambutol. His serum phenytoin levels climbed to 46.1 micrograms/ml. He slowly recovered when the phenytoin was stopped. He was later stabilised on only 200 mg phenytoin daily. He proved to be a slow acetylator of isoniazid.[19] Another patient on 300 mg phenytoin daily was also started on **isoniazid**, **rifampicin** and ethambutol but, in anticipation of the response seen in the previous patient, his phenytoin dosage was reduced to 200 mg daily. Within 3 days he developed seizures because his serum phenytoin levels had fallen to only 8 micrograms/ml. He needed a daily dosage of 400 mg phenytoin to keep the serum levels within the therapeutic range. He was a fast acetylator of **isoniazid**.[19]

The clearance of phenytoin also doubled in 14 patients given 450 mg **rifampicin**, 300 mg **isoniazid** and 900 to 1200 mg ethambutol daily for 2 weeks. No further changes occurred in the kinetics of phenytoin after 3 months of antitubercular treatment. In this study, the interaction was of a similar magnitude in both the 8 slow and the 6 fast acetylators.[16]

Mechanism

Rifampicin (a known potent liver enzyme-inducing agent) increases the metabolism and clearance of the phenytoin from the body so that a larger dose is needed to maintain adequate serum levels. Isoniazid inhibits the liver microsomal enzymes which metabolise phenytoin, and as a result the phenytoin accumulates and its serum levels rise.[16,17] Only those who are 'slow metabolisers' of isoniazid (this is genetically determined) normally attain blood levels of isoniazid that are sufficiently high to cause extensive inhibition of the phenytoin metabolism. 'Fast metabolisers' remove the isoniazid too quickly for this to occur. Thus some individuals will show a rapid rise in phenytoin levels, which eventually reaches toxic concentrations, whereas others will show only a relatively slow and unimportant rise to a plateau within, or only slightly above the therapeutic range.

If isoniazid and rifampicin are given together, the enzyme inhibitory effects of isoniazid may oppose the effects of rifampicin in those who are slow acetylators of isoniazid, but in those who are fast acetylators, the isoniazid will be cleared too quickly for it effectively to oppose the rifampicin effects. However, in one study isoniazid did not counter the effects of rifampicin in slow acetylators.[16]

The interaction involving clofazimine is not understood.

Importance and management

Direct information seems to be limited to these reports, but the interactions appear to be of clinical importance. Monitor the serum phenytoin levels and increase the dosage appropriately if rifampicin alone is started. Reduce the dosage if the rifampicin is stopped. If both rifampicin and isoniazid are given, the outcome may depend on the isoniazid acetylator status of the patient. Those who are fast acetylators will probably also need an increased phenytoin dosage. Those who are slow acetylators may need a smaller phenytoin dosage if toxicity is to be avoided. All patients should be monitored very closely as the outcome is unpredictable. The interaction with phenytoin and isoniazid alone is well-documented, well-established, clinically important and potentially serious interaction. About 50% of the population are slow or relatively slow metabolisers of isoniazid,[1] but not all of them develop serum phenytoin levels in the toxic range. The reports indicate that somewhere between 10 and 33% of patients are at risk.[1-4,10] This adverse interaction may take only a few days to develop fully in some patients, but several weeks in others. Therefore concurrent use should be very closely monitored, making suitable dosage reductions as necessary. One patient was reported to have had better seizure control with fewer side-effects while taking both drugs than with phenytoin alone.[20]

Information about clofazimine seems to be limited to one report.

Monitor concurrent use, anticipating the need to increase the phenytoin dosage.

1. Brennan RW, Dehejia H, Kutt H, Verebely K, McDowell F. Diphenylhydantoin intoxication attendant to slow inactivation of isoniazid. *Neurology* (1970) 20, 687–93.
2. Kutt H, Brennan R, Dehejia H, Verebely K. Diphenylhydantoin intoxication. A complication of isoniazid therapy. *Am Rev Respir Dis* (1970) 101, 377–84.
3. Murray FJ. Outbreak of unexpected reactions among epileptics taking isoniazid. *Am Rev Respir Dis* (1962) 86, 729–32.
4. Kutt H, Winters W, McDowell FH. Depression of parahydroxylation of diphenylhydantoin by antituberculosis chemotherapy. *Neurology* (1966) 16, 594–602.
5. Manigand G, Thieblot P, Deparis M. Accidents de la diphénylhydantoïne induits par les traitements antituberculeux. *Presse Med* (1971) 79, 815–16.
6. Beauvais P, Mercier D, Hanoteau J, Brissand H-E. Intoxication a la diphenylhydantoine induite par l'isoniazide. *Arch Fr Pediatr* (1973) 30, 541–6.
7. Johnson J. Epanutin and isoniazid interaction. *BMJ* (1975) 1, 152.
8. Johnson J, Freeman HL. Death due to isoniazid (INH) and phenytoin. *Br J Psychiatry* (1975) 129, 511.
9. Geering JM, Ruch W, Dettli L. Diphenylhydantoin-Intoxikation durch Diphenylhydantoin-Isoniazid-Interaktion. *Schweiz Med Wochenschr* (1974) 104, 1224–8.
10. Miller RR, Porter J, Greenblatt DJ. Clinical importance of the interaction of phenytoin and isoniazid. A report from the Boston Collaborative Drug Surveillance Program. *Chest* (1979) 75, 356–8.
11. Witmer DR, Ritschel WA. Phenytoin-isoniazid interaction: a kinetic approach to management. *Drug Intell Clin Pharm* (1984) 18, 483–6.
12. Perucca E and Richens A. Anticonvulsant drug interactions. In: Tyrer J (ed) The treatment of epilepsy. MTP Lancaster. (1980) pp 95–128.
13. Sandyk R. Phenytoin toxicity induced by antituberculosis drugs. *S Afr Med J* (1982) 61, 382.
14. Yew WW, Lau KS, Ling MHM. Phenytoin toxicity in a patient with isoniazid-induced hepatitis. *Tubercle* (1991) 72, 309–10.
15. Walubo A, Aboo A. Phenytoin toxicity due to concomitant antituberculosis therapy. *S Afr Med J* (1995) 85, 1175–6.
16. Kay L, Kampmann JP, Svendsen TL, Vergman B, Hansen JEM, Skovsted L, Kristensen M. Influence of rifampicin and isoniazid on the kinetics of phenytoin. *Br J Clin Pharmacol* (1985) 20, 323–6.
17. Abajo FJ. Phenytoin interaction with rifampicin. *BMJ* (1988) 297, 1048.
18. Cone LA, Woodard DR, Simmons JC, Sonnenshein MA. Drug interactions in patients with AIDS. *Clin Infect Dis* (1992) 15, 1066–8.
19. O'Reilly D, Basran GS, Hourihan B, Macfarlane JT. Interaction between phenytoin and antituberculous drugs. *Thorax* (1987) 42, 736.
20. Thulasimnay M, Kela AK. Improvement of psychomotor epilepsy due to interaction of phenytoin-isoniazid. *Tubercle* (1984) 65, 229–30.

Phenytoin + Barbiturates

Concurrent use is common, advantageous and normally uneventful. Changes in serum phenytoin levels (often decreases but sometimes increases) can occur if phenobarbital is added, but seizure control is not usually affected. Phenytoin toxicity following barbiturate withdrawal has been seen. Increased phenobarbital levels and possibly toxicity may result from the addition of phenytoin to phenobarbital treatment.

Clinical evidence

(a) Phenytoin treatment to which phenobarbital is added

A study in 10 epileptics treated with phenytoin (2.8 to 6.8 mg/kg daily) showed that while taking **phenobarbital** (1.1 to 2.5 mg/kg daily) their serum phenytoin levels were depressed. Five patients showed a mean reduction of two-thirds (from 15.7 to 5.7 micrograms/ml). In most cases phenytoin levels rose again when the **phenobarbital** was withdrawn. In one patient this was so rapid and steep that he developed ataxia and a cerebellar syndrome with phenytoin levels up to 60 micrograms/ml, despite a reduction in phenytoin dosage.[1]

This depression of phenytoin levels by **phenobarbital** has been described in other reports.[2-5] However some of these also described a very transient and small rise[4] or no alteration[4,5] in serum phenytoin levels in individual patients. Three other studies have shown no alteration in phenytoin levels by **phenobarbital**.[6-8]

(b) Phenobarbital treatment to which phenytoin is added

Elevated serum **phenobarbital** levels occurred in epileptic children when they were additionally given phenytoin. In 5 patients illustrated, the **phenobarbital** levels approximately doubled. In some cases mild ataxia was seen but the relatively high barbiturate levels were well tolerated.[1] A long-term study in 6 adult epileptics found that when phenytoin was added to **phenobarbital**, the level/dose ratio of the **phenobarbital** gradually rose from an average of 8.66 to a maximum of 13.8 day.kg.l for one year, and then gradually fell again over the next 2 years.[9]

Mechanism

Phenobarbital can have a dual effect on phenytoin metabolism: it may cause enzyme induction, which results in a more rapid clearance of the phenytoin from the body, or with large doses it may inhibit metabolism by competing for enzyme systems. The total effect will depend on the balance between the two drugs. The reason for the elevation of serum phenobarbital levels is not fully understood.

Importance and management

Concurrent use is common and can be therapeutically valuable. Changes in dosage or the addition or withdrawal of either drug need to be monitored to ensure that drug toxicity does not occur, or that seizure control is worsened. The contradictory reports cited here do not provide a clear picture of what is likely to happen. Other barbiturates are also enzyme-inducing agents and may be expected to interact similarly.

1. Morselli PL, Rizzo M, Garattini S. Interaction between phenobarbital and diphenylhydantoin in animals and in epileptic patients. *Ann N Y Acad Sci* (1971) 179, 88–107.
2. Cucinell SA, Conney AH, Sansur M, Burns JJ. Drug interactions in man. I. Lowering effect of phenobarbital on plasma levels of bishydroxycoumarin (Dicumarol) and diphenylhydantoin (Dilantin). *Clin Pharmacol Ther* (1965) 6, 420–9.
3. Buchanan RA, Heffelfinger JC, Weiss CF. The effect of phenobarbital on diphenylhydantoin metabolism in children. *Pediatrics* (1969) 43, 114–16.
4. Kutt H, Haynes J, Verebely K, McDowell F. The effect of phenobarbital on plasma diphenylhydantoin level and metabolism in man and rat liver microsomes. *Neurology* (1969) 19, 611–16.
5. Garrettson LK, Dayton PG. Disappearance of phenobarbital and diphenylhydantoin from serum of children. *Clin Pharmacol Ther* (1970) 11, 674–9.
6. Diamond WD, Buchanan RA. A clinical study of the effect of phenobarbital on diphenylhydantoin plasma levels. *J Clin Pharmacol* (1970) 10, 306–11.
7. Booker HE, Tormey A, Toussaint J. Concurrent administration of phenobarbital and diphenylhydantoin: lack of interference effect. *Neurology* (1971) 21, 383–5.
8. Browne TR, Szabo GK, Evans J, Evans BA, Greenblatt DJ, Mikati MA. Phenobarbital does not alter phenytoin steady-state serum concentration or pharmacokinetics. *Neurology* (1988) 38, 639–42.
9. Encinas MP, Santos Buelga D, Alonso González AC, García Sánchez MJ, Domínguez-Gil Hurlé A. Influence of length of treatment on the interaction between phenobarbital and phenytoin. *J Clin Pharm Ther* (1992) 17, 49–50.

Phenytoin + Benzodiazepines

Reports are inconsistent: benzodiazepines can cause serum phenytoin levels to rise (toxicity has been seen), fall, or remain unaltered. In addition phenytoin may cause clonazepam, oxazepam and diazepam serum levels to fall.

Clinical evidence

(a) Serum phenytoin levels increased

The observation of toxicity in patients on phenytoin when given **chlordiazepoxide** or **diazepam** prompted more detailed study. The serum phenytoin levels of 25 patients on 300 or 400 mg phenytoin daily and one of these two benzodiazepines were 80 to 90% higher than those of 99 subjects not taking a benzodiazepine.[1]

Increased phenytoin serum levels and phenytoin toxicity have also been attributed in other reports to the concurrent use of **diazepam**[2,3] **clonazepam**,[4-7] and **chlordiazepoxide**.[8]

(b) Serum phenytoin levels decreased

The serum phenytoin levels of 12 patients given phenytoin and 1.5 to 12 mg **clonazepam** daily over a two-month period in a double-blind study showed a mean fall of about 30%. When data from 12 additional patients were combined, the mean fall was 18%.[9] Other studies describe similar findings with **clonazepam**[5,10] and **diazepam**.[11,12]

(c) Serum phenytoin levels unaltered and/or serum benzodiazepine levels reduced

Clonazepam did not alter serum phenytoin levels in one study,[13] and another concluded it produced no predictable change in phenytoin levels.[5] In addition, a study in 5 patients given 250 to 400 mg phenytoin daily showed that serum **clonazepam** levels were reduced by more than 50%.[14] **Diazepam**[15] and **oxazepam**[16] may be similarly affected in epileptic patients given phenytoin. **Alprazolam** did not affect serum phenytoin levels in healthy subjects.[17]

Mechanisms

The inconsistency of these reports is not understood. Benzodiazepine-induced changes in the metabolism of the phenytoin, both enzyme induction and inhibition,[2,8,12] as well as alterations in the apparent volume of distribution have been discussed. Enzyme induction may possibly account for the fall in serum benzodiazepine levels.

Importance and management

A confusing picture. Concurrent use certainly need not be avoided (it has proved to be valuable in many cases) but the serum phenytoin levels should be monitored so that undesirable changes can be detected. Only diazepam, chlordiazepoxide and clonazepam have been implicated, but it seems possible that other benzodiazepines could also interact.

1. Vajda FJE, Prineas RJ, Lovell RRH. Interaction between phenytoin and the benzodiazepines. *Lancet* (1971) i, 346.
2. Rogers HJ, Haslam RA, Longstreth J, Lietman PS. Phenytoin intoxication during concurrent diazepam therapy. *J Neurol Neurosurg Psychiatry* (1977) 40, 890–5.
3. Kariks J, Perry SW, Wood D. Serum folic acid and phenytoin levels in permanently hospitalized patients receiving anticonvulsant therapy. *Med J Aust* (1971) 2, 368–71.
4. Eeg-Olofsson O. Experiences with Rivotril in treatment of epilepsy — particularly minor motor epilepsy — in mentally retarded children. *Acta Neurol Scand* (1973) 49 (Suppl 53), 29–31.
5. Huang CY, McLeod JG, Sampson D, Hensley WJ. Clonazepam in the treatment of epilepsy. *Med J Aust* (1974) 2, 5–8.
6. Janz D, Schneider H. Bericht über Wodadiboff II (Workshop on the determination of anti-epileptic drugs in body fluids). In 'Antiepileptische Langzeitmedikation'. *Bibl Psychiatr* (1975) 151, 55–7.
7. Windorfer A, Sauer W. Drug interactions during anticonvulsant therapy in childhood: diphenylhydantoin, primidone, phenobarbitone, clonazepam, nitrazepam, carbamazepin and dipropylacetate. *Neuropaediatrie* (1977) 8, 29–41.
8. Kutt H, McDowell F. Management of epilepsy with diphenylhydantoin sodium. *JAMA* (1968) 203, 969–72.
9. Edwards VE, Eadie MJ. Clonazepam — a clinical study of its effectiveness as an anticonvulsant. *Proc Aust Assoc Neurol* (1973) 10, 61–6.
10. Saavedra IN, Aguilera LI, Faure E, Galdames DG. Case report. Phenytoin/clonazepam interaction. *Ther Drug Monit* (1985) 7, 481–4.
11. Siris JH, Pippenger CE, Werner WL, Masland RL. Anticonvulsant drug-serum levels in psychiatric patients with seizure disorders. *N Y State J Med* (1974) 74, 1554–6.
12. Houghton GW, Richens A. The effect of benzodiazepines and pheneturide on phenytoin metabolism in man. *Br J Clin Pharmacol* (1974) 1, P344–P345.
13. Johannessen SI, Strandjord RE, Munthe-Kaas AW. Lack of effect of clonazepam on serum levels of diphenylhydantoin, phenobarbital and carbamazepine. *Acta Neurol Scand* (1977) 55, 506–12.
14. Sjö O, Hvidberg EF, Naestoft J, Lund M. Pharmacokinetics and side-effects of clonazepam and its 7-amino metabolite in man. *Eur J Clin Pharmacol* (1975) 8, 249–54.
15. Hepner GW, Vesell ES, Lipton A, Harvey HA, Wilkinson GR, Schenker S. Disposition of aminopyrine, antipyrine, diazepam, and indocyanine green in patients with liver disease or on anticonvulsant therapy: diazepam breath test and correlations in drug elimination. *J Lab Clin Med* (1977) 90, 440–56.
16. Scott AK, Khir ASM, Steele WH, Hawksworth GM, Petrie JC. Oxazepam pharmacokinetics in patients with epilepsy treated long-term with phenytoin alone or in combination with phenobarbitone. *Br J Clin Pharmacol* (1983) 16, 441–4.
17. Patrias JM, DiPiro JT, Cheung RPF, Townsend RJ. Effect of alprazolam on phenytoin pharmacokinetics. *Drug Intell Clin Pharm* (1987) 21, 2A.

Phenytoin + Carbamazepine

The reports are inconsistent. Some describe rises in serum phenytoin levels (with toxicity) whereas others describe falls in both phenytoin and carbamazepine serum levels. Concurrent use should be monitored.

Clinical evidence

(a) Reduced serum phenytoin levels

Carbamazepine 600 mg daily for 4 to 14 days reduced the serum phenytoin levels of 3 out of 7 patients from 15 to 7 micrograms/ml, 18 to 12 micrograms/ml and 16 to 10 micrograms/ml respectively. Phenytoin serum levels rose again 10 days after withdrawal of the **carbamazepine**.[1]

Reduced serum phenytoin levels have been described in other reports.[2-5]

(b) Raised serum phenytoin levels

A study in 6 epileptics treated with phenytoin 350 to 600 mg daily showed that the addition of **carbamazepine** 600 to 800 mg daily increased the phenytoin serum levels by 35%, increased its half-life by 41% and reduced its clearance by 36.5% over a 12-week period. Neurotoxicity increased by 204%, with additional signs of toxicity (sedation, ataxia, nystagmus, etc.) developing in 5 of the 6 patients. The phenytoin dosage remained unchanged throughout the period of the study.[6]

Other reports have also described increases in serum phenytoin levels,[7-13] which were as large as 81%, and even up to 100% in some cases.[8,11]

(c) Reduced serum carbamazepine levels

A series of multiple regression analyses on data from a large number of patients (the precise number is not clear from the report), showed that phenytoin reduced serum **carbamazepine** on average by 0.9 micrograms/ml for each 2 mg/kg phenytoin taken each day.[7]

Reduced serum **carbamazepine** levels have been described in other studies and reports.[3,12,14-17] Two studies found that phenytoin markedly increased the levels of the active metabolite of **carbamazepine**, the 10,11-epoxide.[18,19]

Mechanisms

Not understood. It has been suggested that the interaction with carbamazepine may differ, depending on whether phenytoin metabolism is saturated. A reduction in phenytoin metabolism and increases in carbamazepine metabolism have been proposed.[13,18]

Importance and management

These contradictory reports make assessment of this interaction difficult. What is known indicates that it would be wise to monitor anticonvulsant levels during concurrent use (including the active metabolite of carbamazepine, carbamazepine-epoxide) so that steps can be taken to avoid the development of toxicity. Not all patients appear to demonstrate an adverse interaction, and it does not seem possible to identify those potentially at risk. The risk of carbamazepine-induced water intoxication is reported to be reduced in patients concurrently taking phenytoin.[15]

1. Hansen JM, Siersbæk-Nielsen K, Skovsted L. Carbamazepine-induced acceleration of diphenylhydantoin and warfarin metabolism in man. *Clin Pharmacol Ther* (1971) 12, 539–43.
2. Cereghino JJ, Van Meter JC, Brock JT, Penry JK, Smith LD, White BG. Preliminary observations of serum carbamazepine concentration in epileptic patients. *Neurology* (1973) 23, 357–66.
3. Hooper WD, Dubetz DK, Eadie MJ, Tyrer JH. Preliminary observations on the clinical pharmacology of carbamazepine ('Tegretol'). *Proc Aust Assoc Neurol* (1974) 11, 189–98.
4. Lai M-L, Lin T-S, Huang JD. Effect of single- and multiple-dose carbamazepine on the pharmacokinetics of diphenylhydantoin. *Eur J Clin Pharmacol* (1992) 43, 201–3.
5. Windorfer A, Sauer W. Drug interactions during anticonvulsant therapy in childhood: diphenylhydantoin, primidone, phenobarbitone, clonazepam, nitrazepam, carbamazepin and dipropylacetate. *Neuropaediatrie* (1977) 8, 29–41.
6. Browne TR, Szabo GK, Evans JE, Evans BA, Greenblatt DJ, Mikati MA. Carbamazepine increases phenytoin serum concentration and reduces phenytoin clearance. *Neurology* (1988) 38, 1146–50.
7. Lander CM, Eadie MJ, Tyrer JH. Interactions between anticonvulsants. *Proc Aust Assoc Neurol* (1975) 12, 111–16.
8. Gratz ES, Theodore WH, Newmark ME, Kupferberg HJ, Porter RJ, Qu Z. Effect of carbamazepine on phenytoin clearance in patients with complex partial seizures. *Neurology* (1982) 32, A223.
9. Browne TR, Evans JE, Szabo GK, Evans BA, Greenblatt DJ. Effect of carbamazepine on phenytoin pharmacokinetics determined by stable isotope technique. *J Clin Pharmacol* (1984) 24, 396.
10. Leppik IE, Pepin SM, Jacobi J, Miller KW. Effect of carbamazepine on the Michaelis-Menten parameters of phenytoin. In Metabolism of Antiepileptic Drugs (ed Levy RH et al) Raven Press, New York. (1984) pp 217–22.
11. Zielinski JJ, Haidukewych D, Leheta BJ. Carbamazepine-phenytoin interaction: elevation of plasma phenytoin concentrations due to carbamazepine comedication. *Ther Drug Monit* (1985) 7, 51–3.
12. Hidano F, Obata N, Yahaba Y, Unno K, Fukui R. Drug interactions with phenytoin and carbamazepine. *Folia Psychiatr Neurol Jpn* (1983) 37, 342–4.
13. Zielinski JJ, Haidukewych D. Dual effects of carbamazepine-phenytoin interaction. *Ther Drug Monit* (1987) 9, 21–3.
14. Cereghino JJ, Brock JT, Van Meter JC, Penry JK, Smith LD, White BG. The efficacy of carbamazepine combinations in epilepsy. *Clin Pharmacol Ther* (1975) 18, 733–41.
15. Perucca E, Richens A. Reversal by phenytoin of carbamazepine-induced water intoxication: a pharmacokinetic interaction. *J Neurol Neurosurg Psychiatry* (1980) 43, 540–5.
16. Ramsay RE, McManus DQ, Guterman A, Briggle TV, Vazquez D, Perchalski R, Yost RA, Wong P. Carbamazepine metabolism in humans: effect of concurrent anticonvulsant therapy. *Ther Drug Monit* (1990) 12, 235–41.
17. Chapron DJ, LaPierre BA, Abou-Elkair M. Unmasking the significant enzyme-inducing effects of phenytoin on serum carbamazepine concentrations during phenytoin withdrawal. *Ann Pharmacother* (1993) 27, 708–11.
18. Hagiwara M, Takahashi R, Watabe M, Amanuma I, Kan R, Takahashi Y, Kumashiro H. Influence of phenytoin on metabolism of carbamazepine. *Neurosciences* (1989) 15, 303–9.
19. Dam M, Jensen A, Christiansen J. Plasma level and effect of carbamazepine in grand mal and psychomotor epilepsy. *Acta Neurol Scand* (1975) 75 (Suppl 51), 33–8.

Phenytoin + Chloramphenicol

Serum phenytoin levels can be raised by the concurrent use of chloramphenicol. Phenytoin toxicity may occur unless the phenytoin dosage is reduced appropriately. Other evidence indicates that phenytoin may reduce or raise serum chloramphenicol levels in children.

Clinical evidence

(a) Serum phenytoin levels increased

A man on phenytoin 100 mg four times daily developed signs of toxicity within a week of additionally taking **chloramphenicol** (four six-hourly doses of 1 g intravenously followed by 2 g six-hourly). His serum phenytoin levels had risen approximately threefold, from about 7 to 24 micrograms/ml.[1]

This interaction has been described in a number of other reports.[2-10] One study showed that **chloramphenicol** more than doubled the half-life of phenytoin.[2]

(b) Serum chloramphenicol levels reduced or increased

A child on a 6-week course of **chloramphenicol** (100 mg/kg daily intravenously in four divided doses) showed a reduction in peak and trough serum levels of 46 and 74% respectively within 2 days of beginning additional treatment with phenytoin 4 mg/kg daily. Levels were further reduced by 63 and 87% respectively when additionally treated with phenobarbitone 4 mg/kg daily.[11]

In contrast, 6 children (aged 1 month to 12 years) developed raised, toxic **chloramphenicol** levels while concurrently receiving phenytoin.[12]

Mechanisms

It seems probable that chloramphenicol, a known enzyme inhibitor,[13] depresses the liver enzymes concerned with the metabolism of phenytoin thereby reducing its rate of clearance from the body. The changes in the pharmacokinetics of chloramphenicol in children are not understood.

Importance and management

The rise in serum phenytoin levels (a) in adults is well documented and clinically important. A two to fourfold rise can occur within a few days of beginning concurrent treatment. Concurrent use should be avoided unless the effects can be closely monitored and appropriate phenytoin dosage reductions made as necessary.

The general clinical importance of the changes in serum chloramphenicol levels in children (b) is uncertain, but the effects of concurrent use should certainly be monitored. More study is needed. It seems very doubtful if enough chloramphenicol is absorbed from eye-drop solutions or ointments for an interaction to occur, but this needs confirmation.

1. Ballek RE, Reidenberg MM, Orr L. Inhibition of diphenylhydantoin metabolism by chloramphenicol. *Lancet* (1973) i, 150.
2. Christensen LK, Skovsted L. Inhibition of drug metabolism by chloramphenicol. *Lancet* (1969) ii, 1397–9.
3. Houghton GW, Richens A. Inhibition of phenytoin metabolism by other drugs used in epilepsy. *Int J Clin Pharmacol Biopharm* (1975) 12, 210–16.
4. Rose JQ, Choi HK, Schentag JJ, Kinkel WR, Jusko WJ. Intoxication caused by interaction of chloramphenicol and phenytoin. *JAMA* (1977) 237, 2630–1.
5. Koup JR, Gibaldi M, McNamara P, Hilligoss DM, Colburn WA, Bruck E. Interaction of chloramphenicol with phenytoin and phenobarbital. *Clin Pharmacol Ther* (1978) 24, 571–5.
6. Vincent FM, Mills L, Sullivan JK. Chloramphenicol-induced phenytoin intoxication. *Ann Neurol* (1978) 3, 469.
7. Harper JM, Yost RL, Stewart RB, Ciezkowski J. Phenytoin-chloramphenicol interaction. *Drug Intell Clin Pharm* (1979) 13, 425–9.
8. Greenlaw CW. Chloramphenicol-phenytoin drug interaction. *Drug Intell Clin Pharm* (1979) 13, 609–10.
9. Saltiel M, Stephens NM. Phenytoin-chloramphenicol interaction. *Drug Intell Clin Pharm* (1980) 14, 221.
10. Cosh DG, Rowett DS, Lee PC, McCarthy PJ. Case report — phenytoin therapy complicated by concurrent chloramphenicol and enteral nutrition. *Aust J Hosp Pharm* (1987) 17, 51–3.
11. Powell DA, Nahata M, Durrell DC, Glazer JP and Hilty MD. Interactions among chloramphenicol, phenytoin and phenobarbitone in a pediatric patient. *J Pediatr* (1981) 98, 1001.
12. Krasinski K, Kusmiesz H, Nelson JD. Pharmacologic interactions among chloramphenicol, phenytoin and phenobarbital. *Pediatr Infect Dis* (1982) 1, 232–5.
13. Dixon RL, Fouts JR. Inhibition of microsomal drug metabolism pathway by chloramphenicol. *Biochem Pharmacol* (1962) 11, 715–20.

Phenytoin + Chlorphenamine

Phenytoin toxicity in two patients has been attributed to the concurrent use of chlorphenamine.

Clinical evidence, mechanism, importance and management

A week or so after starting to take **chlorphenamine** 4 mg three times daily, a woman on phenytoin and phenobarbital developed phenytoin toxicity with serum phenytoin levels of about 65 micrograms/ml. The toxic symptoms disappeared and phenytoin levels fell when the **chlorphenamine** was withdrawn.[1] Another woman on anticonvulsants, including phenytoin, developed slight grimacing of the face and involuntary jaw movements (but no speech slurring, ataxia or nystagmus) within 12 days of starting to take 12 to 16 mg **chlorphenamine** daily. Her serum phenytoin level had risen to 30 micrograms/ml but it fell when the **chlorphenamine** was withdrawn.[2]

The reason for these reactions is not clear but it has been suggested that **chlorphenamine** may have inhibited the metabolism of phenytoin by the liver. These are isolated cases so there would seem to be no good reason for avoiding concurrent use in all patients, but it would be reasonable to monitor the effects. There seem to be no reports of interactions between phenytoin and other antihistamines.

1. Pugh RNH, Geddes AM, Yeoman WB. Interaction of phenytoin with chlorpheniramine. *Br J Clin Pharmacol* (1975) 2, 173–5.
2. Ahmad S, Laidlaw J, Houghton GW, Richens A. Involuntary movements caused by phenytoin intoxication in epileptic patients. *J Neurol Neurosurg Psychiatry* (1975) 38, 225–31.

Phenytoin + Clarithromycin

Preliminary evidence suggests that clarithromycin may possibly raise serum phenytoin levels.

Clinical evidence, mechanism, importance and management

A retrospective study of serum phenytoin levels in a group of 21 patients with AIDS and a large control group of 557 subjects suggested that concurrent **clarithromycin** use (a total of 22 samples from at least 10 patients) was associated with higher serum phenytoin levels. The concentration/dose ratio of the phenytoin was 1.6 without **clarithromycin** and 3.9 with **clarithromycin**.[1] The reason is not known but it could be that **clarithromycin** inhibits the metabolism of the phenytoin by the liver.

This seems to be the first and only evidence that **clarithromycin** possibly interacts like this, but it would now seem prudent to check for any evidence of phenytoin toxicity if **clarithromycin** is added. More study is needed to clarify this situation.

1. Burger DM, Meenhorst PL, Mulder JW, Kraaijeveld CL, Koks CHW, Bult A, Beijnen JH. Therapeutic drug monitoring of phenytoin in patients with the acquired immunodeficiency syndrome. *Ther Drug Monit* (1994) 16, 616–20.

Phenytoin + Cloxacillin

A marked reduction in serum phenytoin levels in one patient has been attributed to the concurrent use of cloxacillin.

Clinical evidence, mechanism, importance and management

An epileptic woman taking 400 mg phenytoin daily, hospitalised for second degree burns sustained during a generalised seizure, showed an 'astonishing drop' in serum phenytoin levels (from 21.8 to 3.5 micrograms/ml) which was attributed to the concurrent use of **cloxacillin** 500 mg six-hourly. Serum phenytoin values within the original range and using the original dosage were only satisfactorily restored when the **cloxacillin** was withdrawn. The authors of the report advise a 'watchful awareness' if both drugs are used.[1] This seems to be the only report of an adverse interaction between phenytoin and a penicillin. Its incidence and general importance would seem to be very small if viewed against the very wide-spread use of the penicillins.

1. Fincham RW, Wiley DE, Schottelius DD. Use of phenytoin levels in a case of status epilepticus. *Neurology* (1976) 26, 879–81.

Phenytoin + Colestyramine or Colestipol

Neither colestyramine nor colestipol affect the absorption of phenytoin from the gut.

Clinical evidence, mechanism, importance and management

Neither **colestyramine** 5 g nor **colestipol** 10 g had a significant effect on the absorption of a single 500-mg dose of phenytoin in 6 healthy subjects. The resins were given 2 min before and 6 and 12 h after the phenytoin.[1] Another study in 6 healthy subjects found that 4 g **colestyramine** four times daily for 5 days had no significant effect on the extent of the absorption of 400 mg phenytoin.[2] No special precautions would seem to be necessary if either of these drugs and phenytoin is taken concurrently.

1. Callaghan JT, Tsuru M, Holtzman JL, Hunningshake DB. Effect of cholestyramine and colestipol on the absorption of phenytoin. *Eur J Clin Pharmacol* (1983) 24, 675–8.
2. Barzaghi N, Monteleone M, Amione C, Lecchini S, Perucca E, Frigo GM. Lack of effect of cholestyramine on phenytoin bioavailability. *J Clin Pharmacol* (1988) 28, 1112–14.

Phenytoin + Diazoxide

Three children and one adult showed very marked reductions in serum phenytoin levels when diazoxide was given, and in one case seizure control was lost. There is also some evidence that the effects of diazoxide may also be reduced.

Clinical evidence

A child receiving 29 mg/kg and an adult receiving 1000 mg phenytoin daily failed to achieve therapeutic phenytoin serum levels when given **diazoxide**. When the **diazoxide** was withdrawn, satisfactory serum phenytoin levels were achieved with dosages of only 6.6 mg/kg and 400 mg daily. When **diazoxide** was restarted experimentally in the adult, the serum phenytoin fell over 4 days to undetectable levels, and seizures occurred.[1] Two other reports describe this interaction.[2,3] In addition it appears that the effects of the **diazoxide** can also be reduced.[2,4]

Mechanism

What is known suggests that diazoxide increases the metabolism and the clearance of phenytoin from the body.[1,2] The half-life of diazoxide is possibly reduced by phenytoin.[4]

Importance and management

Information is limited to these reports, but the interaction would appear to be established. Monitor the effects of concurrent use, being alert for the need to increase the phenytoin dosage. The clinical importance of the reduced diazoxide effects is uncertain.

1. Roe TF, Podosin RL, Blaskovics ME. Drug Interaction: diazoxide and diphenylhydantoin. *J Pediatr* (1975) 87, 480–4.
2. Petro DJ, Vannucci RC, Kulin HE. Diazoxide-diphenylhydantoin interaction. *J Pediatr* (1976) 89, 331–2.
3. Turck D, Largilliere C, Dupuis B, Farriaux JP. Interaction entre le diazoxide et la phénytoïne. *Presse Med* (1986) 15, 31.
4. Pruitt AW, Dayton PG, Patterson JH. Disposition of diazoxide in children. *Clin Pharmacol Ther* (1973) 14, 73–82.

Phenytoin + Dichloralphenazone

Serum phenytoin levels may be reduced by the concurrent use of dichloralphenazone. Some loss in seizure control is possible.

Clinical evidence, mechanism, importance and management

After taking 1.3 g **dichloralphenazone** each night for 13 nights the total body clearance of phenytoin (single dose given intravenously) in 5 healthy subjects was doubled.[1] The phenazone component of **dichloralphenazone** is a known enzyme-inducer and the increased clearance of phenytoin is probably due to an enhancement of its metabolism by the liver. There seem to be no additional reports of adverse effects in patients given both drugs, so that the clinical importance of this interaction is uncertain. However, it would seem prudent to watch for falling serum phenytoin levels if **dichloralphenazone** is added to established treatment with phenytoin.

1. Riddell JG, Salem SAM, McDevitt DG. Interaction between phenytoin and dichloralphenazone. *Br J Clin Pharmacol* (1980) 9, 118P.

Phenytoin + Felbamate

Felbamate causes a moderate increase in serum phenytoin levels. Felbamate serum levels are reduced but the importance of this is uncertain.

Clinical evidence

A pilot study in 4 patients noted that **felbamate** increased serum phenytoin levels.[1] Therefore, in a further study the phenytoin dose was automatically reduced by 20% when felbamate was given. Of 5 patients, one needed a slight increase in phenytoin dosage, whereas 2 others needed a further reduction in their phenytoin dosage.[2] In a later full report of this study, it was noted that phenytoin dosage decreases of 10 to 30% were required to maintain stable levels.[3] Other studies in epileptic patients showed that **felbamate** increased serum phenytoin levels by about 20% (range 5 to 100%).[4,5] Studies in children and adults have found that phenytoin increased the clearance of **felbamate** by about 40%,[6,7] and decreased felbamate levels by 5 to 20%.[8] Another report says that **felbamate** clearance is reduced if the dosage of phenytoin is reduced.[9]

Mechanism

Uncertain but felbamate probably inhibits the metabolism of the phenytoin, thereby reducing its loss from the body and increasing its serum levels,[2,4] whereas phenytoin induces felbamate metabolism, thereby increasing its clearance.[9]

Importance and management

Established interactions but the changes are only moderate. You may need to reduce the phenytoin dosage (a 20% reduction seems to be about right[2,4] if felbamate is added, and to increase it if felbamate is withdrawn. The importance of the reduced felbamate levels is uncertain.

1. Sheridan PH, Ashworth M, Milne K, White BG, Santilli N, Lothman EW, Dreifuss FE, Jacobs MP, Martinez P, Leppik IE. Open pilot study of felbamate (ADD 03055) in partial seizures. *Epilepsia* (1986) 27, 649.
2. Fuerst RH, Graves NM, Leppik IE, Remmel RP, Rosenfeld WE, Sierzant TL. A preliminary report on alteration of carbamazepine and phenytoin metabolism by felbamate. *Drug Intell Clin Pharm* (1986) 20, 465–6.
3. Leppik IE, Dreifuss FE, Pledger GW, Graves NM, Santilli N, Drury I, Tsay JY, Jacobs MP, Bertram E, Cereghino JJ, Cooper G, Sahlroot JT, Sheridan P, Ashworth M, Lee SI, Sierzant TL. Felbamate for partial seizures: results of a controlled clinical trial. *Neurology* (1991) 41, 1785–9.
4. Fuerst RH, Graves NM, Leppik IE, Brundage RC, Holmes GB, Remmel RP. Felbamate increases phenytoin but decreases carbamazepine concentrations. *Epilepsia* (1988) 29, 488–91.
5. Sachedo R, Wagner M, Sachedo S, Schumaker RC, Perhach JL, Ward DL. Steady-state pharmacokinetics of phenytoin when coadministered with felbamate (Felbatol). *Epilepsia* (1992) 33 (Suppl 3), 84.
6. Kelley MT, Walson PD, Cox S, Dusci LJ. Population pharmacokinetics of felbamate in children. *Ther Drug Monit* (1997) 19, 29–36.
7. Banfield CR, Zhu G-RR, Jen JF, Jensen PK, Schumaker RC, Perhach JL Affrime MB, Glue P. The effect of age on the apparent clearance of felbamate: a retrospective analysis using nonlinear mixed-effects modeling. *Ther Drug Monit* (1996) 18, 19–29.
8. Sachedo R, Sachedo S, Wagner M, Reitz J, Schumaker RC, Perhach JL, Ward DL. Steady-state pharmacokinetics of felbamate (Felbatol) when coadministered with phenytoin. *Epilepsia* (1992) 33 (Suppl 3), 84.
9. Wagner ML, Graves NM, Marienau K, Holmes GB, Remmel RP, Leppik IE. Discontinuation of phenytoin and carbamazepine in patients receiving felbamate. *Epilepsia* (1991) 32, 398–406.

Phenytoin + Fenyramidol

Serum phenytoin levels can be markedly increased (by as much as twofold) by the concurrent use of fenyramidol. Phenytoin toxicity may occur unless the phenytoin dosage is reduced appropriately.

Clinical evidence

The observation that poorly controlled epileptics taking phenytoin improved when given **fenyramidol** prompted more detailed study. The mean serum concentrations of 5 subjects given phenytoin (100 mg three times daily) were doubled, increasing from 6.6 to 12.1 micrograms/ml after the addition of 400 mg **fenyramidol** three times daily for 6 days. All 5 subjects demonstrated an increase in levels, which ranged from about 40 to 200%.[1]

Mechanism

The evidence suggests that fenyramidol inhibits the liver microsomal enzymes concerned with the metabolism of the phenytoin, thereby prolonging its presence in the body.[1]

Importance and management

Information seems to be limited to this study, but the interaction would seem to be established. The incidence is uncertain, but all 5 subjects demonstrated rises in serum levels. Phenytoin serum levels should be closely monitored if fenyramidol is added and the phenytoin dosage reduced appropriately to ensure that toxicity does not occur.

1. Solomon HM, Schrogie JJ. The effect of phenyramidol on the metabolism of diphenylhydantoin. *Clin Pharmacol Ther* (1967) 8, 554–6.

Phenytoin + Fluconazole

Phenytoin serum levels can rise rapidly if fluconazole is given. Toxicity may develop unless the phenytoin dosage is reduced

appropriately. **There is also some limited evidence that fluconazole levels are reduced.**

Clinical evidence

In a randomised placebo-controlled study, 10 subjects given 200 mg phenytoin daily for the last 3 days of a 14-day course of **fluconazole** 200 mg daily were compared with 10 other subjects on phenytoin alone. The **fluconazole** caused the phenytoin AUC to rise by 75%, and the trough phenytoin serum levels to rise by 128%. Phenytoin appeared not to affect **fluconazole** trough serum levels.[1,2]

At least 7 cases of phenytoin toxicity caused by **fluconazole** have been documented.[3-6] A study in 9 healthy subjects found that 400 mg **fluconazole** daily for 6 days raised the AUC of a single dose of phenytoin by 33%.[7,8] Another study in 19 healthy subjects found a 75% rise in the AUC of phenytoin.[9] A brief report noted that 3 of 9 patients on fluconazole and phenytoin required an increase in fluconazole dose or the substitution of another antifungal. It was suggested that phenytoin may reduce **fluconazole** levels in some patients[10] although in the reports cited above[1,2,9] the **fluconazole** serum levels were unaltered.

Mechanism

Not fully established. It is thought that the fluconazole reduces the metabolism and clearance of the phenytoin by the liver, so that it accumulates.[2,3] It has been suggested that the fluconazole affects cytochrome P450 (possibly the cytochrome P450 isoenzymes CYP2C9 or CYP2C10).[8]

Importance and management

The increase in serum phenytoin levels is established and clinically important. Toxicity can develop within 2 to 7 days unless the phenytoin dosage is reduced. Monitor serum phenytoin levels closely and reduce the dosage appropriately. In two of the cases reported a reduction from 300 to 200 mg phenytoin daily controlled this interaction.[3,6] Also be alert for any evidence of reduced fluconazole effects.

1. Blum RA, Wilton JH, Hilligoss DM, Gardner MJ, Chin EB, Schentag JJ. Effect of fluconazole (F) on the disposition of phenytoin (P). *Clin Pharmacol Ther* (1990) 47, 182.
2. Blum RA, Wilton JH, Hilligoss DM, Gardner MJ, Henry EB, Harrison NJ, Schentag JJ. Effect of fluconazole on the disposition of phenytoin. *Clin Pharmacol Ther* (1991) 49, 420–5.
3. Mitchell AS, Holland JT. Fluconazole and phenytoin: a predictable interaction. *BMJ* (1989) 298, 1315.
4. Howitt KM, Oziemski MA. Phenytoin toxicity induced by fluconazole. *Med J Aust* (1989) 151, 603–4.
5. Sugar AM. Quoted as Personal Communication by Grant SM, Clissold SP. Fluconazole. A review of its pharmacodynamic and pharmacokinetic properties, and therapeutic potential in superficial and system mycoses. *Drugs* (1990) 39, 877–916.
6. Cadle RM, Zenon GJ, Rodriguez-Barradas MC, Hamill RJ. Fluconazole-induced symptomatic phenytoin toxicity. *Ann Pharmacother* (1994) 28, 191–5.
7. Touchette MA, Chandrasekar PH, Millad MA, Edwards DJ. Differential effects of ketoconazole and fluconazole on phenytoin and testosterone concentrations in man. *Pharmacotherapy* (1991) 11, 275.
8. Touchette MA, Chandrasekar PH, Millad MA, Edwards DJ. Contrasting effects of fluconazole and ketoconazole on phenytoin and testosterone disposition in man. *Br J Clin Pharmacol* (1992) 34, 75–8.
9. Lazar JD, Wilner KD. Drug interactions with fluconazole. *Rev Infect Dis* (1990) 12 (Suppl 3), S327–S333.
10. Tett S, Carey D, Lee H-S. Drug interactions with fluconazole. *Med J Aust* (1992) 156, 365.

Phenytoin + Food

The absorption of phenytoin can be affected by some foods. A very marked reduction in phenytoin absorption has been described when given with enteral feeds (e.g. Isocal, Osmolite) administered by nasogastric or jejunostomy tubes.

Clinical evidence

(a) Phenytoin + food and enteral feeds by mouth

A study showed that serum drug levels were lower than expected when phenytoin was disguised in **vanilla pudding** and given to mentally retarded children. However, when the phenytoin was mixed with

apple sauce, 3 out of 10 patients developed serum phenytoin levels within the toxic range, and the mean levels were twice those seen when the tablets were mixed with the vanilla pudding.[1] An epileptic showed a marked fall in his serum phenytoin levels accompanied by an increased seizure frequency when the phenytoin was given at bedtime with 8 oz of a food supplement (*Ensure*).[2] Another patient showed reduced phenytoin serum levels when given phenytoin as an oral suspension and oral *Fresubin liquid food concentrate*.[3] In contrast however a study in 10 healthy subjects found that when given *Ensure* or *Vivonex TEN* four-hourly for 24 h, the absorption of single 400 mg doses of phenytoin was unaffected.[4] Absorption of phenytoin as the acid in a micronised form (*Fenantoin*, ACO, Sweden) was faster and peak serum levels averaged 40% higher when given after **food**.[5] One single dose study found that when taken with **a meal** the total absorption of phenytoin was not affected, although it was slightly delayed.[6]

(b) Phenytoin + food by nasogastric tube

A patient on 300 mg phenytoin daily who was being fed with *Fortison* through a nasogastric tube achieved a phenytoin serum level of only 1.0 mg/l. When 420 mg phenytoin was given diluted in water and separated from the food by 2 h a serum level of 6 mg/l was achieved.[7] This report describes a similar reaction in another patient.[7]

A study in 20 patients and 5 healthy subjects found that about a 70% reduction in phenytoin absorption occurred when it was given by nasogastric tube with an **enteral feed** product (*Isocal*) at a rate of 100 to 125 ml/h.[8] Other reports describe the same interaction in patients given *Ensure*,[9] *Isocal*,[10,11] or *Osmolite*.[9,12-14]

(c) Phenytoin + food by jejunostomy tube

A woman with a history of seizures had acceptable serum phenytoin levels when phenytoin was given intravenously, but they fell from 19.1 to less than 2.5 micrograms/ml when a comparable dose of phenytoin suspension was given in the presence of an **enteral feed** product (*Jevity*) by jejunostomy tube.[15]

Mechanism

Not fully resolved. Phenytoin can bind to some food substances which reduces its absorption.[16,17] It can also become bound to the nasogastric tubing[18] and may also be poorly absorbed if the tubing empties into the duodenum rather than the stomach.[18] Delivery into the jejunum apparently makes matters even worse, because there is even less time for adequate absorption.[15]

Importance and management

(a). Phenytoin is often taken orally with water or food to reduce gastric irritation. This normally appears not to have a marked effect on absorption but the studies cited above show that some formulations and some foods can interact. If there are problems with the control of convulsions or evidence of toxicity, review how and when the patient is taking the phenytoin.

(b) & (c). The interaction between phenytoin and enteral foods given by nasogastric tube is well established and clinically important. The markedly reduced bioavailability has been successfully managed by giving the phenytoin diluted in water 2 h after stopping the feed, flushing with 60 ml of water, and waiting another 2 h before restarting the feed,[7,8] However, one limited study failed to confirm that this method is successful,[9] and some sources suggest waiting 6 h after the phenytoin dose before restarting the feed.[10] Some increase in the phenytoin dosage may also be needed. Monitor concurrent use closely. The same problem can clearly also occur when jejunostomy tube delivery is used but its management is not yet established.

1. Jann MW, Bean J, Fidone G. Interaction of dietary pudding with phenytoin. *Pediatrics* (1986) 78, 952–3.
2. Longe RL, Smith OB. Phenytoin interaction with an oral feeding results in loss of seizure control. *J Am Geriatr Soc* (1988) 36, 542–4.
3. Taylor DM, Massey CA, Willson WD, Dhillon S. Lowered serum phenytoin concentrations during therapy with liquid food concentrates. *Ann Pharmacother* (1993) 27, 369.
4. Marvel ME, Bertino JS. Comparative effects of an elemental and a complex enteral feeding formulation on the absorption of phenytoin suspension. *J Parenter Enteral Nutr* (1991) 15, 316–8.
5. Melander A, Brante G, Johansson Ö, Lindberg T, Wåhlin-Boll E. Influence of food on the absorption of phenytoin in man. *Eur J Clin Pharmacol* (1979) 15, 269–74.

6. Kennedy MC, Wade DN. The effect of food on the absorption of phenytoin. *Aust N Z J Med* (1982) 12, 258–61.
7. Summers VM, Grant R. Nasogastric feeding and phenytoin interaction. *Pharm J* (1989) 243, 181.
8. Bauer LA. Interference of oral phenytoin absorption by continuous nasogastric feedings. *Neurology* (1982) 32, 570–2.
9. Ozuna J, Friel P. Effect of enteral tube feeding on serum phenytoin levels. *J Neurosurg Nurs* (1984) 16, 289–91.
10. Pearce GA. Apparent inhibition of phenytoin absorption by an enteral nutrient formula. *Aust J Hosp Pharm* (1988) 18, 289–92.
11. Worden JP, Wood CA, Workman CH. Phenytoin and nasogastric feedings. *Neurology* (1984) 34, 132.
12. Hatton RC. Dietary interaction with phenytoin. *Clin Pharm* (1984) 3, 110–11.
13. Weinryb J, Cogen R. Interaction of nasogastric phenytoin and enteral feeding solution. *J Am Geriatr Soc* (1989) 37, 195–6.
14. Maynard GA, Jones KM, Guidry JR. Phenytoin absorption from tube feedings. *Arch Intern Med* (1987) 147, 1821.
15. Rodman DP, Stevenson TL, Ray TR. Phenytoin malabsorption after jejunostomy tube delivery. *Pharmacotherapy* (1995) 15, 801–5.
16. Millar SW, Strom JG. Stability of phenytoin in three enteral nutrient formulas. *Am J Hosp Pharm* (1988) 45, 2529–32.
17. Hooks MA, Longe RL, Taylor AT, Francisco GE. Recovery of phenytoin from an enteral nutrient formula. *Am J Hosp Pharm* (1986) 43, 685–8.
18. Fleisher D, Sheth N, Kou JH. Phenytoin interaction with enteral feedings administered through nasogastric tubes. *J Parenter Enteral Nutr* (1990) 14, 513–16.

Phenytoin + Immunoglobulins

An isolated report describes an epileptic patient on phenytoin who died two days after receiving immunoglobulin for Guillain-Barré syndrome.

Clinical evidence, mechanism, importance and management

A man on long-term phenytoin treatment (8 years) was diagnosed as having Guillain-Barré syndrome for which intravenous **immunoglobulin** was started at 0.4 g/kg daily. On day 2 the patient complained of abdominal pain, aching shoulders and backache. He subsequently developed hypotension and died, despite resuscitation attempts. A post-mortem suggested that he had died from hypersensitivity myocarditis, which the authors of the report suggest might have resulted from the long-term use of the phenytoin.[1] This hypersensitivity with phenytoin has been reported before.[2] Because this complication is so serious, the authors of this report suggest that leukocyte counts, in particular eosinophils, should be carried out before these two drugs are given concurrently.[1] The general importance of this alleged interaction is not known.

1. Koehler PJ, Koudstaal J. Lethal hypersensitivity myocarditis associated with the use of intravenous gammaglobulin for Guillain-Barré syndrome, in combination with phenytoin. *J Neurol* (1996) 243, 366–7.
2. Fenoglio JJ, McAllister HA, Mullick FG. Drug related myocarditis.I. Hypersensitivity myocarditis. *Hum Pathol* (1981) 12, 900–7.

Phenytoin + H$_2$-blockers

Phenytoin serum levels are raised by the use of cimetidine. Toxicity may occur if the phenytoin dosage is not reduced appropriately. Very rarely bone marrow depression develops with concurrent use. Famotidine, nizatidine and ranitidine do not normally interact with phenytoin but they appear to do so on rare occasions.

Clinical evidence

(a) Cimetidine

A 60% rise (from 5.7 to 9.1 micrograms/ml) was seen in the serum phenytoin levels of 9 patients when they were given **cimetidine**, 200 mg three times daily and 400 mg at night, for 3 weeks. The serum phenytoin fell to its former levels within 2 weeks of stopping the cimetidine.[1-3]

This interaction has been described in many reports and studies involving numerous patients[4-9] and healthy subjects.[10-14] Phenytoin toxicity developed in some individuals. The extent of the rise in serum levels is very variable being quoted as 13 to 33% over about

6 days in one report[4] and 22 to 280% over 3 weeks in another.[6,15] Severe and life-threatening agranulocytosis in 2 patients[16,17] and thrombocytopenia in 6 others[18-20] have also been attributed to concurrent use.

(b) Famotidine, nizatidine or ranitidine

A study in 4 patients given **ranitidine** for 2 weeks found that no interaction occurred,[6,15] and a study in 10 subjects given **famotidine** demonstrated that the phenytoin pharmacokinetics remained unaltered.[21,22] A double-blind crossover study in healthy subjects found that 150 mg **ranitidine** twice daily for 6 days had no significant effect on their steady state phenytoin levels.[23] However, a single case report describes phenytoin toxicity and a doubled serum level (from 18 to 33 micrograms/ml) in a patient when given **famotidine**.[24] A patient showed a 40% increase in serum phenytoin levels over a month when treated with 150 mg **ranitidine** twice daily,[25] and another also developed elevated serum phenytoin levels and signs of toxicity attributed to the use of **ranitidine**.[26] A single dose study found no evidence that **nizatidine** affects the metabolism of phenytoin.[27]

Mechanism

Cimetidine is a potent enzyme inhibitor which depresses the activity of the liver enzymes concerned with the metabolism of phenytoin, thus allowing it to accumulate in the body and, in some instances, to reach toxic concentrations. Famotidine, nizatidine and ranitidine normally do not affect these enzymes. Agranulocytosis and thrombocytopenia are relatively rare manifestations of bone marrow depression caused by these drugs.

Importance and management

The phenytoin/cimetidine interaction is well documented and clinically important. It is not possible to identify individuals who will show the greatest response, but those with serum levels at the top end of the therapeutic range are most at risk. Do not give cimetidine to patients already taking phenytoin unless the serum levels can be monitored and suitable dosage reductions made as necessary. Famotidine, nizatidine and ranitidine normally do not interact like cimetidine, but the rare isolated cases cited show that monitoring is advisable even with these H$_2$-blockers when they are first added to established treatment with phenytoin.

1. Neuvonen PJ, Tokola R, Kaste M. Cimetidine-phenytoin interaction: effect of serum phenytoin concentration and antipyrine test in man. *Naunyn Schmiedebergs Arch Pharmacol* (1980) 313 (Suppl), R60.
2. Neuvonen PJ, Tokola R, Kaste M. Cimetidine interaction with phenytoin. *BMJ* (1981) 283, 501.
3. Neuvonen PJ, Tokola R, Kaste M. Cimetidine-phenytoin interaction: effect of serum phenytoin concentration and antipyrine test. *Eur J Clin Pharmacol* (1981) 21, 215–20.
4. Hetzel DJ, Bochner F, Hallpike JF, Shearman DJC, Hann CS. Cimetidine interaction with phenytoin. *BMJ* (1981) 282, 1512.
5. Algozzine GJ, Stewart RB, Springer PK. Decreased clearance of phenytoin with cimetidine. *Ann Intern Med* (1981) 95, 244–5.
6. Watts RW, Hetzel DJ, Bochner F, Hallpike JF, Hann CS, Shearman DJC. Lack of interaction between ranitidine and phenytoin. *Br J Clin Pharmacol* (1983) 15, 499–500.
7. Phillips P, Hansky J. Phenytoin toxicity secondary to cimetidine administration. *Med J Aust* (1984) 141, 602.
8. Griffin JW, May JR, DiPiro JT. Drug interactions: theory versus practice. *Am J Med* (1984) 77 (Suppl 5B), 85–9.
9. Iteogu MO, Murphy JE, Shleifer N, Davis R. Effect of cimetidine on single-dose phenytoin kinetics. *Clin Pharm* (1983) 2, 302–4.
10. Bartle WR, Walker SE, Shapero T. Effect of cimetidine on phenytoin metabolism. *Clin Pharmacol Ther* (1982) 31, 202.
11. Bartle WR, Walker SE, Shapero T. Dose-dependent effect of cimetidine on phenytoin kinetics. *Clin Pharmacol Ther* (1983) 33, 649–55.
12. Frigo GM, Lecchini S, Caravaggi M, Gatti G, Tonini M, D'Angelo L, Perucca E, Crema A. Reduction of phenytoin clearance caused by cimetidine. *Eur J Clin Pharmacol* (1983) 25, 135–7.
13. Salem RB, Breland BD, Mishra SK, Jordan JE. Effect of cimetidine on phenytoin serum levels. *Epilepsia* (1983) 24, 284–8.
14. Hsieh Y-Y, Huang J-D, Lai M-L, Lin M-S, Liu R-T, Wan EC-J. The complexity of cimetidine-phenytoin interaction. *Taiwan Yi Xue Hui Za Zhi* (1986) 85, 395–402.
15. Hetzel DJ, Watts RW, Bochner F, Shearman DJC. Ranitidine, unlike cimetidine, does not interact with phenytoin. *Aust N Z J Med* (1983) 13, 324.
16. Sazie E, Jaffe JP. Severe granulocytopenia with cimetidine and phenytoin. *Ann Intern Med* (1980) 93, 151–2.
17. Al-Kawas FH, Lenes BA, Sacher RA. Cimetidine and agranulocytosis. *Ann Intern Med* (1979) 90, 992–3.
18. Wong YY, Lichtor T, Brown FD. Severe thrombocytopenia associated with phenytoin and cimetidine therapy. *Surg Neurol* (1985) 23, 169–72.
19. Yue CP, Mann KS, Chan KH. Severe thrombocytopenia due to combined cimetidine and phenytoin therapy. *Neurosurgery* (1987) 20, 963–5.
20. Arbiser JL, Goldstein AM, Gordon D. Thrombocytopenia following administration of phenytoin, dexamethasone and cimetidine: a case report and a potential mechanism. *J Intern Med* (1993) 234, 91–4.
21. Sambol NC, Upton RA, Chremos AN, Lin ET, Williams RL. A comparison of the influence of famotidine and cimetidine on phenytoin elimination and hepatic blood flow. *Br J Clin Pharmacol* (1989) 27, 83–7.
22. Sambol NC, Upton RA, Chremos AN, Lin E, Gee W, Williams RL. Influence of famotidine (Fam) and cimetidine (Cim) on the disposition of phenytoin (Phe) and indocyanine green (ICG). *Clin Pharmacol Ther* (1986) 39, 225.
23. Mukherjee S, Wicks JFC, Dixon JS, Richens A. Absence of a pharmacokinetic interaction between ranitidine and phenytoin. *Gastroenterology* (1996) 110 (Suppl), A202.
24. Shinn AF. Unrecognized drug interactions with famotidine and nizatidine. *Arch Intern Med* (1991) 151, 810,814.
25. Bramhall D, Levine M. Possible interaction of ranitidine with phenytoin. *Drug Intell Clin Pharm* (1988) 22, 979–80.
26. Ted Tse CS, Akinwande KI, Biallowons K. Phenytoin concentration elevation subsequent to ranitidine administration. *Ann Pharmacother* (1993) 27, 1448–51.
27. Bachmann KA, Sullivan TJ, Jaureq L, Reese JH, Miller K, Levine L. Absence of an inhibitory effect of omeprazole and nizatidine on phenytoin disposition, a marker of CYP2C activity. *Br J Clin Pharmacol* (1993) 36, 380–2.

Phenytoin + Hypoglycaemic agents

Large and toxic doses of phenytoin have been observed to cause hyperglycaemia, but normal therapeutic doses do not usually affect the control of diabetes. Two isolated cases of phenytoin toxicity have been attributed to the use of tolazamide or tolbutamide.

Clinical evidence

(a) The effect of phenytoin on the response to hypoglycaemic agents

Phenytoin has been shown in a number of reports[1-6] to raise the blood sugar levels of both diabetics and non-diabetics. However, in all but one of the cases quoted here the phenytoin dosage was large (at least 8 mg/kg) or even in the toxic range (70 to 80 mg/kg). There is little evidence that a hyperglycaemic response to usual doses of phenytoin is normally large enough to interfere with the control of diabetes either with diet alone or with conventional hypoglycaemic agents. In the case excepted above, where the patient received 1200 mg phenytoin in the 24 h following status epilepticus, the situation was complicated by the use of many other drugs and by kidney impairment.[2]

(b) The effect of hypoglycaemic agents on the response to phenytoin

Tolbutamide 500 mg two or three times daily was given to 17 patients on phenytoin 100 to 400 mg daily.[7] The patients showed a transient 45% rise in the amount of non-protein-bound phenytoin by day 2, which had disappeared by day 4. The introduction to this report briefly mentions a man given phenytoin and **tolazamide** who developed phenytoin toxicity, which disappeared when the **tolazamide** was replaced by **insulin**.[7] A woman previously successfully treated with phenytoin and **tolbutamide** developed toxicity on a later occasion when again given **tolbutamide**, but this time with twice the dose of phenytoin.[8]

Mechanisms

Studies in *animals* and man[9-11] suggest that phenytoin-induced hyperglycaemia occurs because the release of insulin from the pancreas is impaired. This implies that no interaction is possible without functional pancreatic tissue. Just why the phenytoin/tolazamide and phenytoin/tolbutamide interactions occurred is uncertain, but it is possible that they competitively inhibit phenytoin hydroxylation[12] by cytochrome P450 isoenzyme CYP2C9.[13]

Importance and management

The weight of evidence shows that no interaction of clinical importance normally occurs between phenytoin and the hypoglycaemic agents. No special precautions seem normally to be necessary. There appear to be only two unexplained cases on record of a sulphonylurea/phenytoin interaction.

1. Klein JP. Diphenylhydantoin intoxication associated with hyperglycaemia. *J Pediatr* (1966) 69, 463–5.
2. Goldberg EM, Sanbar SS. Hyperglycaemic, non-ketotic coma following administration of Dilantin (diphenylhydantoin). *Diabetes* (1969) 18, 101–6.

3. Peters BH, Samaan NA. Hyperglycaemia with relative hypoinsulinemia in diphenylhydantoin toxicity. *N Engl J Med* (1969) 281, 91–2.
4. Millichap JG. Hyperglycaemic effect of diphenylhydantoin. *N Engl J Med* (1969) 281, 447.
5. Fariss BL, Lutcher CL. Diphenylhydantoin-induced hyperglycaemia and impaired insulin release. *Diabetes* (1971) 20, 177–81.
6. Treasure T, Toseland PA. Hyperglycaemia due to phenytoin toxicity. *Arch Dis Child* (1971) 46, 563–4.
7. Wesseling H, Mols-Thürkow I. Interaction of diphenylhydantoin (DPH) and tolbutamide in man. *Eur J Clin Pharmacol* (1975) 8, 75–8.
8. Beech E, Mathur SVS, Harrold BP. Phenytoin toxicity produced by tolbutamide. *BMJ* (1988) 297, 1613–14.
9. Kizer JS, Vargas-Cordon M, Brendel K, Bressler R. The *in vitro* inhibition of insulin secretion by diphenylhydantoin. *J Clin Invest* (1970) 49, 1942–8.
10. Levin SR, Booker J, Smith DF, Grodsky M. Inhibition of insulin secretion by diphenylhydantoin in the isolated perfused pancreas. *J Clin Endocrinol Metab* (1970) 30, 400–1.
11. Malherbe C, Burrill KC, Levin SR, Karam JH, Forsham PH. Effect of diphenylhydantoin on insulin secretion in man. *N Engl J Med* (1972) 286, 339–42.
12. Wesseling H, Thurkow I and Mulder GJ. Effect of sulphonylureas (tolazamide, tolbutamide and chlorpropamide) on the metabolism of diphenylhydantoin in the rat. *Biochem Pharmacol* (1973) 22, 3033–40.
13. Tassaneeyakul W, Veronese ME, Birkett DJ, Doecke CJ, McManus ME, Sansom LN, Miners JO. Co-regulation of phenytoin and tolbutamide metabolism in humans. *Br J Clin Pharmacol* (1992) 34, 494–8.

Phenytoin + Influenza vaccines

Influenza vaccine is reported to increase, decrease or to have no effect on the serum levels of phenytoin. The efficacy of the vaccine remains unchanged.

Clinical evidence

(a) Phenytoin serum levels increased

About a 50% increase in the serum phenytoin levels (from 9.5 to 15.16 micrograms/ml) was seen 7 days after 8 epileptic children on phenytoin were given 0.5 ml **influenza virus vaccine USP, types A and B, whole virus** (Squibb). The levels returned to baseline over the following 7 days.[1] In another study, 4 patients whose phenytoin levels were only slightly raised 7 and 14 days after immunisation, showed serum phenytoin increases ranging from 46 to 170%, which returned to baseline over weeks 4 to 17 after being immunised with 0.5 ml **inactivated whole-viron trivalent vaccine**.[2] Temporary rises in serum phenytoin levels in 3 patients, related to **influenza vaccination**, are briefly described in another report.[3]

(b) Phenytoin serum levels decreased

Within 4 days of receiving 0.5 ml **subviron, trivalent influenza vaccine** the serum phenytoin levels of 7 patients were reduced by 11 to 14%, which is unlikely to have much clinical significance.[4]

(c) Phenytoin serum levels unchanged

A study in 16 patients given 0.5 ml **inactivated whole-viron trivalent influenza vaccine** showed that 7 and 14 days later their mean serum phenytoin levels were not significantly altered, although 4 of them showing a trend towards raised levels were investigated further (see (a) above).[2]

(d) Vaccine efficacy

The efficacy of **influenza vaccine** is reported to be unchanged by phenytoin.[5]

Mechanism

Where an interaction occurs it is suggested that it may be due to the inhibitory effect of the vaccine on the liver enzymes concerned with the metabolism of the phenytoin, resulting in a reduced clearance from the body.[1]

Importance and management

The outcome of immunisation with influenza vaccine on phenytoin levels is uncertain. Concurrent use need not be avoided but it would be prudent to monitor the effects closely. Be aware that any alteration in levels may take several weeks to develop.

1. Jann MW, Fidone GS. Effect of influenza vaccine on serum anticonvulsant concentrations. *Clin Pharm* (1986) 5, 817–20.

2. Levine M, Jones MW, Gribble M. Increased serum phenytoin concentration following influenza vaccination. *Clin Pharm* (1984) 3, 505–9.
3. Mooradian AD, Hernandez L, Tamai IC, Marshall C. Variability of serum phenytoin concentrations in nursing home patients. *Arch Intern Med* (1989) 149, 890–2.
4. Sawchuk RJ, Rector TS, Fordice JJ, Leppik IE. Case report. Effect of influenza vaccination on plasma phenytoin concentrations. *Ther Drug Monit* (1979) 1, 285–8.
5. Levine M, Beattie BL, McLean DM, Corman D. Phenytoin therapy and immune response to influenza vaccine. *Clin Pharm* (1985) 4, 191–4.

Phenytoin + Loxapine

A single case report describes depressed serum phenytoin levels during concurrent treatment with loxapine.

Clinical evidence, mechanism, importance and management

The serum phenytoin levels of an epileptic were depressed by the concurrent use of **loxapine**, and showed a marked rise when it was withdrawn.[1] The general importance of this is uncertain, but it would now seem prudent to monitor the effects in any patient, particularly as **loxapine** can lower the convulsive threshold. More study is needed.

1. Ryan GM, Matthews PA. Phenytoin metabolism stimulated by loxapine. *Drug Intell Clin Pharm* (1977) 11, 428.

Phenytoin + Methylphenidate

Raised serum phenytoin levels and phenytoin toxicity have been seen in three patients when given methylphenidate, but it is an uncommon reaction. One of the patients also showed raised serum primidone and phenobarbital levels.

Clinical evidence

A hyperkinetic epileptic boy of 5 taking 8.9 mg/kg phenytoin and 17.7 mg/kg primidone daily, developed ataxia without nystagmus when additionally treated with 40 mg **methylphenidate** daily. Serum levels of the anticonvulsants were found to be at toxic concentrations and only began to fall when the **methylphenidate** dosage was reduced.[1]

A further case of phenytoin toxicity occurred in another child when given **methylphenidate**.[2] Only one other case has been seen, but when later rechallenged with the two drugs this patient failed to demonstrate phenytoin toxicity.[3]

Conversely, this interaction has not been seen in clinical studies and observations of 3 healthy subjects[3] and over 11 patients[4] taking phenytoin and **methylphenidate**.

Mechanism

Not fully understood. The suggestion is that methylphenidate acts as an enzyme inhibitor, slowing the metabolism of the phenytoin by the liver and leading to its accumulation in those few individuals whose drug metabolising system is virtually saturated by phenytoin.

Importance and management

An uncommon interaction. Concurrent use need not be avoided but be alert for any evidence of phenytoin toxicity, particularly if the phenytoin dosage is high.

1. Garrettson LK, Perel JM, Dayton PG. Methylphenidate interaction with both anticonvulsants and ethyl biscoumacetate. A new action of methylphenidate. *JAMA* (1969) 207, 2053–6.
2. Ghofrani M. Possible phenytoin-methylphenidate interaction. *Dev Med Child Neurol* (1988) 30, 267–8.
3. Mirkin BL, Wright F. Drug interactions: effect of methylphenidate on the disposition of diphenylhydantoin in man. *Neurology* (1971) 21, 1123–8.
4. Kupferberg HJ, Jeffery W, Hunninghake DB. Effect of methylphenidate on plasma anticonvulsant levels. *Clin Pharmacol Ther* (1972) 13, 201–4.

Phenytoin + Metronidazole

A small and usually clinically unimportant rise in serum phenytoin levels may occur if metronidazole is used concurrently although a few patients have developed toxic levels.

Clinical evidence, mechanism, importance and management

A pharmacokinetic study[1] in 7 healthy subjects found that **metronidazole** 250 mg three times daily increased the half-life of a single 300 mg intravenous dose of phenytoin by about 40% (from 16 to 23 h) and reduced the clearance by 15%. In another study in 5 healthy subjects the pharmacokinetics of a single 300 mg oral dose of phenytoin were unaffected by 400 mg **metronidazole** twice daily for 6 days.[2] An anecdotal report describes 'several patients' who developed toxic phenytoin serum levels when given **metronidazole**.[3] The reason for these discordant reports is not clear, but if and when **metronidazole** affects serum phenytoin levels the rise seems to be relatively small and usually of minimal clinical importance. More study is needed.

1. Blyden GT, Scavone JM, Greenblatt DJ. Metronidazole impairs clearance of phenytoin but not of alprazolam or lorazepam. *J Clin Pharmacol* (1988) 28, 240–5.
2. Jensen JC, Gugler R. Interaction between metronidazole and drugs eliminated by oxidative metabolism. *Clin Pharmacol Ther* (1985) 37, 407–10.
3. Picard EH. Side effects of metronidazole. *Mayo Clin Proc* (1983) 58, 401.

Phenytoin + Miconazole

Two reports describe phenytoin toxicity in two patients when concurrently treated with miconazole.

Clinical evidence, mechanism, importance and management

An epileptic man, well controlled on phenytoin, developed signs of toxicity within a day of starting treatment with intravenous **miconazole** 500 mg eight-hourly and flucytosine. After a week of concurrent treatment his serum phenytoin levels had climbed by 50% (from 29 to 43 micrograms/ml). He had some signs of very mild phenytoin toxicity even before the antifungal treatment was started.[1] Another patient developed signs of toxicity (nystagmus, ataxia) within 5 days of starting to take 500 mg **miconazole** daily. His serum phenytoin climbed to 40.8 micrograms/ml. After discontinuation of the miconazole the same dose of phenytoin resulted in a level of 14.5 micrograms/ml.[2]

A probable explanation is that the **miconazole** can depress the metabolism and clearance of the phenytoin by the liver, resulting in its accumulation in the body. Evidence for this interaction seems to be limited to these reports, even so it would be prudent to avoid concurrent use unless serum phenytoin levels can be monitored and appropriate reductions made in the phenytoin dosage if necessary.

1. Rolan PE, Somogyi AA, Drew MJR, Cobain WG, South D, Bochner F. Phenytoin intoxication during treatment with parenteral miconazole. *BMJ* (1983) 287, 1760.
2. Loupi E, Descotes J, Lery N, Evreux JC. Interactions medicamenteuses et miconazole. A propos de 10 observations. *Therapie* (1982) 37, 437–41.

Phenytoin + Nitrofurantoin

An isolated report describes a reduction in serum phenytoin levels and poor seizure control in a patient when given nitrofurantoin.

Clinical evidence, mechanism, importance and management

A patient with seizures due to a brain tumour was treated with 300 mg phenytoin daily. He had a seizure within a day of starting additional treatment with 200 mg **nitrofurantoin** for a urinary tract infection and, despite a recent increase in the phenytoin dose to 350 mg, his serum phenytoin levels were found to be modestly reduced (from 36 to 30 micromol/l). They continued to fall to 25 micromol/l despite a further increase in the phenytoin dosage to 400 mg daily. When the **nitrofurantoin** was stopped he was restabilised on his original dosage of phenytoin. The reasons are not understood but, on the basis of a noted rise in serum gamma GT levels during the use of the **nitrofurantoin**, the authors speculate that it increased the metabolism of the phenytoin by the liver.[1] The general importance of this interaction is uncertain, but probably small.

1. Heipertz R, Pilz H. Interaction of nitrofurantoin with diphenylhydantoin. *J Neurol* (1978) 218, 297–301.

Phenytoin + Omeprazole or Lansoprazole

A study in patients found that 20 mg omeprazole daily did not affect the serum levels of phenytoin, whereas earlier studies in healthy subjects suggested that phenytoin levels might be raised by 40 mg omeprazole daily. Lansoprazole does not normally interact with phenytoin, but an isolated case report of toxicity is tentatively attributed to an interaction.

Clinical evidence

(a) Lansoprazole

Lansoprazole 60 mg daily for 7 days caused only a very small and clinically irrelevant rise (<3%) in the AUC of a single intravenous dose of phenytoin in a group of 12 healthy subjects.[1,2] In contrast the maker has an isolated report of the development of blurred vision, diarrhoea, muscle pain, dizziness, abdominal pain, salivary hypersecretion, increased sweating and incoordination in a man on phenytoin within a day of stopping 80 mg SR propranolol and starting **lansoprazole**.[3] The phenytoin serum levels were not measured but the symptoms might possibly have been due to phenytoin toxicity, although it should be said that if an interaction with **lansoprazole** was responsible, it developed unusually quickly.

(b) Omeprazole

Omeprazole 20 mg daily for 3 weeks caused no changes in the mean steady-state serum phenytoin levels in 8 epileptic patients.[4] Four patients had unchanged levels, 2 had falls and 2 had rises, but none of them was adversely affected by the **omeprazole** treatment.[4]

After taking 40 mg **omeprazole** daily for 7 days the AUC of a single 300-mg dose of phenytoin in 10 healthy subjects was increased by 25%.[5] In another study the clearance of a 250-mg intravenous dose of phenytoin was reduced by 15% by 40 mg **omeprazole** given for 7 days.[6] A further study found that 3 doses of **omeprazole** 40 mg had no effect on the pharmacokinetics of a single dose of phenytoin.[7]

Mechanism

Not understood. A possible explanation is that if the dosage of omeprazole is high enough, it may possibly reduce the metabolism of phenytoin thereby reducing its loss from the body. With lansoprazole, the overall picture is that it does not act as an enzyme inducer or inhibitor[8] (or it is only very weak) so that it would not be expected to interact with phenytoin to a clinically relevant extent (confirmed by the study cited above[1]).

Importance and management

Information is very limited but it seems that 20 mg omeprazole daily does not affect serum phenytoin levels, whereas 40 mg daily may possibly do so. The isolated report[3] of an interaction involving lansoprazole remains unexplained. No special precautions would normally seem necessary if lansoprazole or omeprazole is given with phenytoin, but until more is known it would be prudent to be aware of this possible interaction if concurrent use is necessary. More study is needed.

1. Karol MD, Mukherji D, Cavanaugh JH. Lack of effect of concomitant multi-dose lansoprazole on single-dose phenytoin pharmacokinetics in subjects. *Gastroenterology* (1994) 106, A103.
2. Karol MD, Locke CS, Cavanaugh JH. Lack of a pharmacokinetic interaction between lansoprazole and intravenously administered phenytoin. *J Clin Pharmacol* (1999) 39, 1283–9.
3. Wyeth, personal communication, January 1998.
4. Andersson T, Lagerström P-O, Unge P. A study of the interaction between omeprazole and phenytoin in epileptic patients. *Ther Drug Monit* (1990) 12, 329–33.
5. Prichard PJ, Walt RP, Kitchingman GK, Somerville KW, Langman MJS, Williams J, Richens A. Oral phenytoin pharmacokinetics during omeprazole therapy. *Br J Clin Pharmacol* (1987) 24, 543–5.
6. Gugler R, Jensen JC. Omeprazole inhibits oxidative drug metabolism. *Gastroenterology* (1985) 89, 1235–41.
7. Bachmann KA, Sullivan TJ, Jauregui L, Reese JH, Miller K, Levine L. Absence of an inhibitory effect of omeprazole and nizatidine on phenytoin disposition, a marker of CYP2C activity. *Br J Clin Pharmacol* (1993) 36, 380–2.
8. Cavanaugh JH, Park YK, Awni WM, Mukherjee DX, Karol MD, Granneman GR. Effect of lansoprazole on antipyrine and ICG pharmacokinetics. *Gastroenterology* (1991) 100, A40.

Phenytoin + Orlistat

Orlistat does not alter phenytoin pharmacokinetics.

Clinical evidence, mechanism, importance and management

In a placebo-controlled, randomised, two-day crossover study, 12 healthy subjects were given a single 300-mg dose of **phenytoin** or a placebo on day 4 of a 7-day course of 120 mg orlistat three times daily. It was found that the pharmacokinetics of the **phenytoin** were unchanged by the orlistat[1] and no special precautions are therefore thought to be needed if these two drugs are given concurrently.

1. Melia AT, Mulligan TE, Zhi J. The effect of orlistat on the pharmacokinetics of phenytoin in healthy volunteers. *J Clin Pharmacol* (1996) 36, 654–8.

Phenytoin + Pheneturide (Ethylphenacemide)

Phenytoin serum levels can be increased by about 50% if pheneturide (ethylphenacemide) is used concurrently.

Clinical evidence, mechanism, importance and management

The steady-state half-life of phenytoin was prolonged from 32 to 47 h by **pheneturide (ethylphenacemide)** in 9 patients. Mean serum levels were raised by about 50% but fell rapidly over the 2 weeks after **pheneturide** was withdrawn.[1] This study confirms a previous report of this interaction.[2] The reason for this reaction is uncertain, but since the two drugs have a similar structure it is possible that they compete for the same metabolising enzymes in the liver, thereby resulting, at least initially, in a reduction in the metabolism of the phenytoin. If concurrent use is undertaken the outcome should be well monitored. Reduce the phenytoin dosage as necessary.

1. Houghton GW, Richens A. Inhibition of phenytoin metabolism by other drugs used in epilepsy. *Int J Clin Pharmacol Biopharm* (1975) 12, 210–16.
2. Hulsman JW, van Heycop Ten Ham MW and van Zijl CHW. Influence of ethylphenacemide on serum levels of other anticonvulsant drugs. *Epilepsia* (1970) 11, 207.

Phenytoin + Phenothiazines

The serum levels of phenytoin can be raised or lowered by the use of chlorpromazine, prochlorperazine or thioridazine.

Clinical evidence

(a) Chlorpromazine

A patient stabilised on phenytoin, primidone and sulthiame showed a doubling in his serum phenytoin levels after taking 50 mg **chlorpromazine** daily for a month.[1] However, another 4 patients on 50 to 100 mg daily of **chlorpromazine** showed no interaction.[1] In another report one out of 3 patients treated with phenytoin and phenobarbital showed a fall in serum phenytoin levels when given **chlorpromazine**.[2] A further report states (without giving details) that in rare instances **chlorpromazine** has been noted to impair phenytoin metabolism.[3]

In a large study in patients on phenytoin taking various phenothiazines (**chlorpromazine, thioridazine** or **mesoridazine**), phenytoin levels were decreased by 44% and 33% when phenothiazines were started or the dose increased, respectively. A number of patients experienced an increased frequency of seizures. In patients who had these phenothiazines discontinued or the dosage decreased, phenytoin levels increased by 55% and 71%, respectively, and toxic levels occurred in some patients.[4]

(b) Prochlorperazine

A single report states (without giving details) that in rare instances **prochlorperazine** has been noted to impair phenytoin metabolism.[3]

(c) Thioridazine

One out of 6 patients on phenytoin and phenobarbital showed a marked rise in serum phenytoin levels when **thioridazine** was added, whereas 4 others showed a fall.[2] Phenytoin toxicity has also been described in 2 patients after about 2 weeks of concurrent treatment with **thioridazine**.[5] A retrospective study in 27 patients on phenytoin showed that 4 had an increase of at least 4 micrograms/ml, 2 had a decrease of at least 4 micrograms/ml, and the rest demonstrated no changes in phenytoin serum levels when given **thioridazine**.[6] Another retrospective study comparing 28 patients taking both phenytoin and thioridazine with patients taking either drug alone found no evidence that **thioridazine** increased the risk of phenytoin toxicity.[7] A further study found no changes in serum phenytoin or **thioridazine** levels in patients given both drugs, but serum levels of **mesoridazine** (the active metabolite of **thioridazine**) were reduced, suggesting higher doses of **thioridazine** may be necessary to achieve the same effect.[8] See also the study[4] in section (a), which showed a decrease in phenytoin levels and an increase in seizure frequency with phenothiazines including **thioridazine**.

Mechanism

Uncertain, but it may be related to changes in the metabolism of the phenytoin caused by the phenothiazines.

Importance and management

A confusing situation as the results are inconsistent. The concurrent use of phenytoin and the phenothiazines cited need not be avoided, but it would be prudent to watch for any signs of changes in serum phenytoin levels that would affect anticonvulsant control. It is also worth remembering that phenothiazines may decrease the seizure threshold. In one study a trend towards increased seizure frequency was noted after phenothiazines were added, or doses increased.[4] Whether all phenothiazines interact similarly is uncertain.

1. Houghton GW, Richens A. Inhibition of phenytoin metabolism by other drugs used in epilepsy. *Int J Clin Pharmacol Biopharm* (1975) 12, 210–16.
2. Siris JH, Pippenger CE, Werner WL, Masland RL. Anticonvulsant drug-serum levels in psychiatric patients with seizure disorders. Effects of certain psychotropic drugs. *N Y State J Med* (1974) 74, 1554–6.
3. Kutt H, McDowell F. Management of epilepsy with diphenylhydantoin sodium. Dosage regulation for problem patients. *JAMA* (1968) 203, 969–72.
4. Haidukewych D, Rodin EA. Effect of phenothiazines on serum antiepileptic drug concentrations in psychiatric patients with seizure disorder. *Ther Drug Monit* (1985) 7, 401–4.

5. Vincent FM. Phenothiazine-induced phenytoin intoxication. *Ann Intern Med* (1980) 93, 56–7.
6. Sands CD, Robinson JD, Salem RB, Stewart RB, Muniz C. Effect of thioridazine on phenytoin serum concentration: a retrospective study. *Drug Intell Clin Pharm* (1987) 21, 267–72.
7. Gotz VP, Yost RL, Lamadrid ME, Buchanan CD. Evaluation of a potential interaction: thioridazine-phenytoin — negative findings. *Hosp Pharm* (1984) 19, 555–7.
8. Linnoila M, Viukari M, Vaisanen K, Auvinen J. Effect of anticonvulsants on plasma haloperidol and thioridazine levels. *Am J Psychiatry* (1980) 137, 819–21.

Phenytoin + Protease inhibitors

Ritonavir was used to increase serum phenytoin levels to control status epilepticus in one patient, but there seem to be no reports of adverse reactions in other patients due to this interaction. Another isolated case describes unexpectedly reduced phenytoin serum levels and an increased fit-frequency, attributed to the use of nelfinavir.

Clinical evidence

(a) Nelfinavir

An isolated case report describes a patient on phenytoin who developed seizures when **nelfinavir** was added, associated with reduced serum phenytoin levels.[1]

(b) Ritonavir

A boy of 14 with cryptogenic partial epilepsy developed status epilepticus which was largely unresponsive to high dose phenytoin (20 mg/kg daily), with inadequate plasma levels. When his treatment was changed to 10 mg/kg phenytoin daily and 600 mg **ritonavir** twice daily (to act as a fast acting cytochrome P450 inhibitor) his serum phenytoin levels rose to 80 micromol/l and his fit-frequency fell from 30 to 4 seizures per day. When the **ritonavir** was withdrawn his fit-frequency rose again (to 60 seizures per day) despite high doses of phenytoin (30 mg/kg daily), and only fell again, quite dramatically, when the **ritonavir** was re-started. He was later stabilised on cimetidine and phenytoin[2] (see also 'Phenytoin + H$_2$-blockers', p.347).

Mechanism

Phenytoin is metabolised within the body by hydroxylation, a reaction catalysed by cytochrome P450 isoenzymes CYP2C9/10 of which ritonavir is an inhibitor. As a result of this inhibition the phenytoin levels were markedly raised. Nelfinavir, also an inhibitor, would have been expected to increase phenytoin levels, but in the case cited the levels fell, for reasons which are not understood.

Importance and management

Direct information about the phenytoin/ritonavir interaction appears to be limited to this single report which describes the deliberate and advantageous use of ritonavir to raise phenytoin levels. The question is whether unwanted and potentially toxic serum phenytoin levels might develop in other patients additionally given ritonavir? The answer seems to be that so far nothing appears to have been reported in the literature, but this interaction seems a possibility. If therefore ritonavir is added to established treatment with phenytoin it would be prudent to monitor the outcome, being alert for any evidence of toxicity. More study of this interaction is needed.

The phenytoin/nelfinavir report is paradoxical because increased rather than reduced phenytoin levels would have been expected because of nelfinavir's enzyme inhibitory effects. The case cited is isolated so that its general importance is unknown, but it would now be prudent to monitor concurrent use. The makers prediction is that phenytoin (and also **carbamazepine** and **phenobarbital**) will reduce nelfinavir serum levels because they are known inducers of cytochrome P450 isoenzyme CYP3A4 which is partially responsible for the metabolism of nelfinavir. For this reason they recommend considering alternative anticonvulsants,[3] but clinical confirmation of these predictions is as yet lacking.

Information about interactions between **other protease inhibitors** and phenytoin appear to be lacking.

1. Honda M, Yasuoka A, Aoki M, Oka S. A generalized seizure followed initiation of nelfinavir in a patient with human deficiency virus type 1 infection, suspected due to interaction between nelfinavir and phenytoin. *Intern Med* (1999) 38, 302–3.
2. Broderick A, Webb DW, McMenamin J, Butler K. A novel use of ritonavir. *AIDS* (1998) 12 (Suppl 4), S29.
3. Viracept (Nelfinavir). Roche Products Limited. Summary of product characteristics, October 2001.

Phenytoin + Shankhapushpi (SRC)

A case report, and an *animal* study, indicate that an anticonvulsant Ayurvedic herbal preparation, SRC (Shankhapushpi), can markedly reduce serum phenytoin levels, leading to an increased seizure frequency if the phenytoin dosage is not raised.

Clinical evidence

An epileptic man on phenobarbital 120 mg daily and phenytoin 500 mg daily developed an increased seizure frequency when **SRC** three times a day was added. His serum phenytoin levels were found to have fallen from 18.2 to 9.3 micrograms/ml whereas his phenobarbital levels were little changed. When the **SRC** was stopped the phenytoin serum levels climbed to 30.3 micrograms/ml, and toxicity was seen. A reduction in the dose of phenytoin to 400 mg daily resulted in levels of 16.2 micrograms/ml. Another possible case was reported.[1,2]

Subsequent studies in *rats* showed that **SRC** approximately halves the serum levels of phenytoin.[3] These pharmacokinetic effects were only seen after multiple doses, not single doses of phenytoin. A pharmacodynamic interaction, resulting in reduced antiepileptic activity was also noted.[1,3,4]

Mechanism

Not understood. There is evidence from animal studies that SRC may affect the pharmacokinetics of the phenytoin and possibly its pharmacodynamics as well,[1,3] thereby reducing its anticonvulsant activity. It is also suggested that one of the ingredients of SRC may have some convulsant activity.[3]

Importance and management

Information about this interaction appears to be limited to these reports. *SRC* is given because it has some anticonvulsant activity (demonstrated in *animal* studies[3,4]), but there is little point in combining it with phenytoin if the outcome is a fall in serum phenytoin levels, accompanied by an increase in fit-frequency. For this reason concurrent use should be avoided. *SRC* (*Shankhapushpi*) is a syrup containing *Convolvulus pluricaulis* leaves, *Nardostachys jatamansi* rhizomes, *Onosma bracteatum* leaves and flowers and the whole plant of *Centella asiatica*, *Nepeta hindostana* and *Nepeta elliptica*.[3] The first two of these plants appear to contain compounds with anticonvulsant activity.[5,6]

1. Kshirsagar NA, Personal communication 1991.
2. Kshirsagar NA, Dalvi SS, Joshi MV, Sharma SS, Sant HM, Shah PU, Chandra RS. Phenytoin and ayurvedic preparation – clinically important interaction in epileptic patients. *J Assoc Physicians India* (1992) 40, 354–5.
3. Dandekar UP, Chandra RS, Dalvi SS, Joshi MV, Gokhale PC, Sharma AV, Shah PU, Kshirsagar NA. Analysis of a clinically important interaction between phenytoin and Shankhapushpi, an Ayurvedic preparation. *J Ethnopharmacol* (1992) 35, 285–8.
4. Kshirsagar NA, Chandra RS, Dandekar UP, Dalvi SS, Sharma AV, Joshi MV, Gokhale PC, Shah PU. Investigation of a novel clinically important interaction between phenytoin and Ayurvedic preparation. *Eur J Pharmacol* (1990) 183, 519.
5. Sharma VN, Barar FSK, Khanna NK, Mahawar MM. Some pharmacological actions of *convolvulus pluricaulis* chois — an Indian indigenous herb. *Indian J Med Res* (1965) 53, 871–6.
6. Arora RB. In: Nardostachys jatamansi: a chemical, pharmacological and clinical appraisal. Pharmacological actions of Jatamansi. Indian Council of Medical Research Publications, Delhi (1965), 136.

Phenytoin + Sodium valproate

Concurrent use is common and usually uneventful. Initially total serum phenytoin levels may fall but this is offset by a rise in the levels of free (and active) phenytoin, which may very occasionally cause some toxicity. After continued use the total serum phenytoin levels rise once again. There is also some very limited evidence that concurrent use possibly increases the incidence of sodium valproate hepatotoxicity.

Clinical evidence

A number of reports clearly show that total serum levels fall during early concurrent use, while the concentrations of free phenytoin rise.[1-6] In one report it was noted that within 4 to 7 days the total serum phenytoin levels had fallen from 19.4 to 14.6 micrograms/ml.[1] A study extending over a year in 8 patients taking phenytoin and **sodium valproate**, showed that by the end of 8 weeks the serum phenytoin levels of 6 of them had fallen by almost as much as 50%, but had returned to their original levels in all but one patient by the end of the year.[7] Similar results were found in another study.[8] The occasional patient may show signs of phenytoin toxicity during this period and the dosage may need to be reduced.[9] Delirium was seen in one patient on **sodium valproate** when given phenytoin.[4]

Sodium valproate levels are reduced by the presence of phenytoin.[10,11] Very occasionally (and inexplicably) the fit-frequency has increased in patients on phenytoin given **sodium valproate**. Epidemiological studies suggest that the risk of fatal hepatotoxicity is higher when **sodium valproate** is given as polytherapy with enzyme inducers such as phenytoin than when it is given as monotherapy, especially in infants.[12,13] Hence concurrent use apparently carries some small risk.

Mechanism

The initial fall in serum phenytoin levels appears to result from the displacement of phenytoin by the sodium valproate from its protein binding sites,[1-6] the extent being subject to the diurnal variation in valproate levels.[14] This allows more of the unbound drug to be exposed to metabolism by the liver and the total phenytoin levels fall. After several weeks the metabolism of the phenytoin is inhibited by the valproate and its levels rise.[2,5] Phenytoin reduces sodium valproate levels, probably because it increases its metabolism by the liver. Because phenytoin is an enzyme inducer it may also possibly increase the formation of a minor but hepatotoxic metabolite of sodium valproate (2-propyl-4-pentenoic acid or 4-ene-VPA).[15]

Importance and management

An extremely well-documented interaction (only a selection of the references being listed here). Concurrent use is common and usually advantageous, the adverse effects of the interactions between the drugs usually being of only minor practical importance. However, the outcome should still be monitored. A few patients may experience mild and transient toxicity if sodium valproate is started, but most patients on phenytoin do not need a dosage change. During the first few weeks total serum phenytoin levels may fall by 20 to 50%, but usually no increase in the dosage is needed, because it is balanced by an increase in the levels of free (active) phenytoin levels. In the following period, the phenytoin levels may rise again 40 to 50%.

When monitoring concurrent use it is important to understand fully the implications of changes in 'total' and 'free' or 'unbound' serum phenytoin concentrations. A nomogram has been designed for predicting unbound phenytoin concentrations during concurrent use.[16] Various equations are also available.[17] The resulting prediction varies according to the method used. Saliva sampling, which measures free phenytoin is more reliable in this situation than total serum levels.[18]

Bear in mind the evidence that the incidence of sodium valproate induced liver toxicity may be increased, especially in infants.

1. Mattson RH, Cramer JA, Williamson PD, Novelly RA. Valproic acid in epilepsy: clinical and pharmacological effects. *Ann Neurol* (1978) 3, 20–5.
2. Perucca E, Hebdige S, Frigo GM, Gatti G, Lecchini S, Crema A. Interaction between phenytoin and valproic acid: plasma protein binding and metabolic effects. *Clin Pharmacol Ther* (1980) 28, 779–89.
3. Tsanaclis LM, Allen J, Perucca E, Routledge PA, Richens A. Effect of valproate on free plasma phenytoin concentrations. *Br J Clin Pharmacol* (1984) 18, 17–20.
4. Tollefson GD. Delirium induced by the competitive interaction between phenytoin and dipropylacetate. *J Clin Psychopharmacol* (1981) 1, 154–8.
5. Bruni J, Gallo JM, Lee CS, Pershalski RJ, Wilder BJ. Interactions of valproic acid with phenytoin. *Neurology* (1980) 30, 1233–6.
6. Friel PN, Leal KW, Wilensky AJ. Valproic acid-phenytoin interaction. *Ther Drug Monit* (1979) 1, 243–8.
7. Bruni J, Wilder BJ, Willmore LJ, Barbour B. Valproic acid and plasma levels of phenytoin. *Neurology* (1979) 29, 904–5.
8. Vakil SD, Critchley EMR, Philips JC, Fahim Y, Haydock D, Cocks A, Dyer T. The effect of sodium valproate (Epilim) on phenytoin and phenobarbitone blood levels. In 'Clinical and Pharmacological Aspects of Sodium Valproate (Epilim) in the Treatment of Epilepsy'. Proceedings of a symposium held at Nottingham University, September 1975, MCS Consultants, England, p 75–7.
9. Haigh D, Forsythe WI. The treatment of childhood epilepsy with sodium valproate. *Dev Med Child Neurol* (1975) 17, 743–8.
10. Rambeck B, May T. Serum concentrations of valproic acid: influence of dose and co-medication. *Ther Drug Monit* (1985) 7, 387–90.
11. Sackellares JC, Sato S, Dreifuss FE, Penry JK. Reduction of steady-state valproate levels by other antiepileptic drugs. *Epilepsia* (1981) 22, 437–41.
12. Dreifuss FE, Santilli N, Langer DH, Sweeney KP, Moline KA, Menander KB. Valproic acid fatalities: a retrospective review. *Neurology* (1987) 37, 379–85.
13. Dreifuss FE, Langer DH, Moline KA, Maxwell JE. Valproic acid hepatic fatalities. II. US experience since 1984. *Neurology* (1989) 39, 201–7.
14. Riva R, Albani F, Contin M, Perucca E, Ambrosetto G, Gobbi G, Santucci M, Procaccianti G, Baruzzi A. Time-dependent interaction between phenytoin and valproic acid. *Neurology* (1985) 35, 510–15.
15. Levy RH, Rettenmeier AW, Anderson GD, Wilensky AJ, Friel PN, Baillie TA, Acheampong A, Tor J, Guyot M, Loiseau P. Effects of polytherapy with phenytoin, carbamazepine, and stiripentol on formation of 4-ene-valproate, a hepatotoxic metabolite of valproic acid. *Clin Pharmacol Ther* (1990) 48, 225–35.
16. May TW, Rambeck B, Nothbaum N. Nomogram for the prediction of unbound phenytoin concentrations in patients on a combined treatment of phenytoin and valproic acid. *Eur Neurol* (1991) 31, 57–60.
17. Kerrick JM, Wolff DL, Graves NM. Predicting unbound phenytoin concentrations in patients receiving valproic acid: a comparison of two predicting methods. *Ann Pharmacother* (1995) 29, 470–4.
18. Knott C, Hamshaw-Thomas A, Reynolds F. Phenytoin-valproate interaction: importance of saliva monitoring in epilepsy. *BMJ* (1982) 284, 13–16.

Phenytoin + Selective serotonin re-uptake inhibitors (SSRIs)

Phenytoin serum levels can be increased in some patients by fluoxetine. Toxicity may occur. There are isolated reports of phenytoin toxicity with the concurrent use of fluvoxamine. Phenytoin and sertraline do not normally interact, nevertheless two patients have shown increased serum phenytoin levels. Note that SSRIs should be avoided in unstable epilepsy and used with care in other epileptics.

Clinical evidence

(a) Fluoxetine

An epileptic on 370 mg phenytoin, 4 mg diazepam and 6 mg clonazepam daily was started on 20 mg **fluoxetine** for depression.[1] Five days later her serum phenytoin levels had climbed from 18 to 26.5 mg/l, and a further 9 days later to 30 mg/l, accompanied by signs of toxicity (tremor, headache, abnormal thinking, increased partial seizure activity). Seven days after stopping the phenytoin the serum levels had fallen to 22 mg/l.

Two other patients, on 300 and 400 mg phenytoin daily respectively, showed marked rises in serum phenytoin levels (from 15 to 35 micrograms/ml and from 11.5 to 47 micrograms/ml), accompanied by signs of phenytoin toxicity, within 5 to 10 days of starting 20 or 40 mg **fluoxetine** daily. The problem resolved when the **fluoxetine** was stopped or the phenytoin dosage reduced.[2] Another patient only developed this interaction after taking **fluoxetine** for about 9 months.[3]

A review initiated by the FDA and the makers of fluoxetine briefly describes another 23 anecdotal observations of suspected phenytoin/**fluoxetine** interactions (most of them incompletely documented). These suggest that a marked increase in serum phenytoin levels (one and a half-fold), with accompanying toxicity, can occur within 1 to 42 days (mean onset time of 2 weeks) after starting **fluoxetine**.[4]

(b) Fluvoxamine

A report describes phenytoin intoxication (serum levels of 48 mg/l) in an 86-year-old woman after being additionally treated with 100 to 200 mg **fluvoxamine** daily for 10 days which the authors of the report attributed to inhibition of the metabolism of the phenytoin by the **fluvoxamine**.[5] However the **fluvoxamine** was started only 2 days after the phenytoin (200 mg twice daily) had been started, and the serum phenytoin levels were not checked until the intoxication had actually developed. Both drugs were then stopped and the phenytoin later successfully reinstated without the fluvoxamine. A world-wide analysis of data up to 1995 by the makers of fluvoxamine identified only 2 reported cases of drug-drug interactions (clinical symptoms only) between phenytoin and **fluvoxamine**.[6] Another case of a three-fold rise in phenytoin levels with toxicity has been reported in a woman given fluvoxamine.[7]

(c) Sertraline

A double-blind, randomised, placebo-controlled study in 30 healthy subjects taking 100 mg phenytoin three times daily, found that 50 to 200 mg **sertraline** daily did not affect the steady-state trough serum levels of phenytoin, nor was there any evidence that concurrent use impaired cognitive function.[8] However, another report describes 2 elderly patients whose serum phenytoin levels rose when given **sertraline**, but without evidence of toxicity. One of them showed an almost fourfold rise in serum phenytoin levels whereas the other showed a rise of only about one-third.[9]

Mechanism

An *in vitro* investigation showed that fluoxetine and fluvoxamine inhibited the metabolism of phenytoin by the cytochrome P450 isoenzyme CYP2C9 in human liver tissue.[10] This would presumably lead to a rise in serum phenytoin levels. In this study, **sertraline** was a weaker inhibitor of CYP2C9, and was considered less likely to interact with phenytoin.[10]

Importance and management

The interaction between phenytoin and fluoxetine appears to be established but its incidence is not known. Because of the unpredictable nature of this interaction, if fluoxetine is added to treatment with phenytoin in any patient be alert for the need to reduce the phenytoin dosage. Ideally the phenytoin serum levels should be monitored. There are fewer reports of a phenytoin/fluvoxamine interaction, so this interaction can be considered to be rare. However to be on the safe side you should monitor the effects when fluvoxamine is first added to treatment with phenytoin so that any patient affected can be identified. Similarly, be alert for any evidence of an increase in phenytoin side-effects if sertraline is used with phenytoin. More study of these interactions is needed. Note that SSRIs should be avoided in patients with unstable epilepsy, and those with controlled epilepsy should be carefully monitored, because of the potential increased seizure risk.

1. Woods DJ, Coulter DM, Pillans P. Interaction of phenytoin and fluoxetine. *N Z Med J* (1994) 107, 19.
2. Jalil P. Toxic reaction following the combined administration of fluoxetine and phenytoin: two case reports. *J Neurol Neurosurg Psychiatry* (1992) 55, 412–13.
3. Darley J. Interaction between phenytoin and fluoxetine. *Seizure* (1994) 3, 151–2.
4. Shader RI, Greenblatt DJ, von Moltke LL. Fluoxetine inhibition of phenytoin metabolism. *J Clin Psychopharmacol* (1994) 14, 375–6.
5. Feldman D, Claudel B, Feldman F, Allilaire JF, Thuillier A. Cas clinique d'interaction médicamenteuse entre phénytoïne et fluvoxamine. *J Pharm Clin* (1995) 14, 296–7.
6. Wagner W, Vause EW. Fluvoxamine. A review of global drug-drug interaction data. *Clin Pharmacokinet* (1995) 29 (Suppl 1), 26–32.
7. Mamiya K, Kojima K, Yukawa E, Higuchi S, Ieiri I, Ninomiya H, Tashiro N. Case report. Phenytoin intoxication induced by fluvoxamine. *Ther Drug Monit* (2001) 23, 75–7.
8. Rapeport WG, Muirhead DC, Williams SA, Cross M, Wesnes K. Absence of effect of sertraline on the pharmacokinetics and pharmacodynamics of phenytoin. *J Clin Psychiatry* (1996) 57 (Suppl 1), 24–8.
9. Haselberger MB, Freedman LS, Tolbert S. Elevated serum phenytoin concentrations associated with coadministration of sertraline. *J Clin Psychopharmacol* (1997) 17, 107–9.
10. Schmider J, Greenblatt DJ, von Moltke LL, Karsov D, Shader RI. Inhibition of CYP2C9 by selective serotonin reuptake inhibitors *in vitro*: studies of phenytoin p-hydroxylation. *Br J Clin Pharmacol* (1997) 44, 495–8.

Phenytoin + Sucralfate

The absorption of phenytoin can be reduced by about 7 to 20% by the concurrent use of sucralfate. There is indirect evidence that the interaction can be avoided by giving the phenytoin 2 h after the sucralfate.

Clinical evidence

Sucralfate 1 g was found to reduce the absorption of a single 300-mg dose of phenytoin in 8 healthy subjects by 20%, measured over a 48 h period.[1] Peak serum phenytoin levels were also reduced, but this was said to be statistically significant.

Another study demonstrated an absorption reduction of 7.7 to 9.5%, which was not thought to be clinically significant.[2] A similar interaction was demonstrated earlier in *dogs*.[3]

Mechanism

Uncertain, although it is likely that the sucralfate binds to the phenytoin and thus impairs absorption.

Importance and management

Information is limited, but this interaction would appear to be established. However, it should be noted that due to the nature of phenytoin pharmacokinetics, there may be a large margin of error in extrapolating the data from single dose studies to multiple dose studies. The reduction in absorption is quite small, but it might be enough to reduce the steady-state serum concentrations of phenytoin in some patients to levels where seizure control is lost. Concurrent use should be monitored. The study in *dogs*[3] showed that no change in absorption occurred if the phenytoin was given 2 h after the sucralfate, so it seems possible that the same precaution might prevent this interaction in man.

1. Smart HL, Somerville KW, Williams J, Richens A, Langman MJS. The effects of sucralfate upon phenytoin absorption in man. *Br J Clin Pharmacol* (1985) 20, 238–40.
2. Hall TG, Cuddy PG, Glass CJ, Melethil S. Effect of sucralfate on phenytoin bioavailability. *Drug Intell Clin Pharm* (1986) 20, 607–11.
3. Lacz JP, Groschang AG, Giesing DH, Browne RK. The effect of sucralfate on drug absorption in dogs. *Gastroenterology* (1982) 82, 1108.

Phenytoin + Sulfinpyrazone

Some limited evidence indicates that phenytoin serum levels may be markedly increased by the concurrent use of sulfinpyrazone. Toxicity may possibly occur unless the phenytoin dosage is reduced appropriately.

Clinical evidence

A review of the drug interactions of sulfinpyrazone identified two studies that demonstrated drug interactions with phenytoin.[1] In the first, the serum phenytoin levels of 2 out of 5 patients on phenytoin 250 to 350 mg daily were doubled from approximately 10 to 20 micrograms/ml within 11 days of starting to take 800 mg **sulfinpyrazone** daily. One of the remaining patients showed a small increase in phenytoin levels, but the other 2 showed no changes at all. When the **sulfinpyrazone** was withdrawn, the serum phenytoin concentrations fell to their former levels. The second was a clinical study in epileptic patients that showed that 800 mg **sulfinpyrazone** daily for a week increased the phenytoin half-life from 10 to 16.5 h and reduced the metabolic clearance from 59 to 32 ml/min.

Mechanism

Uncertain. It seems probable that sulfinpyrazone inhibits the metabolism of the phenytoin by the liver, thereby allowing it to accumulate in the body and leading to a rise in its serum levels. Displacement of phenytoin from its plasma protein binding sites may also have a small part to play.

Importance and management

Information seems to be limited to these studies, which await confirmation. A similar interaction is reported with phenylbutazone with which sulfinpyrazone has a very close chemical relationship (see 'Anticonvulsants + Aspirin or NSAIDs', p.308). Thus what is known suggests that concurrent use should be monitored and suitable phenytoin dosage reductions made where necessary. More study is needed.

1. Pedersen AK, Jacobsen P, Kampmann JP, Hansen JM. Clinical pharmacokinetics and potentially important drug interactions of sulphinpyrazone. *Clin Pharmacokinet* (1982) 7, 42–56.

Phenytoin + Sulphonamides and/or Trimethoprim

Phenytoin serum levels can be raised by the concurrent use of co-trimoxazole, sulfamethizole, sulfamethoxazole, sulfaphenazole, sulfadiazine and trimethoprim. Phenytoin toxicity may develop in some cases. Sulfadimethoxine, sulfamethoxypyridazine, sulfametoxydiazine and sulfafurazole (sulfisoxazole) are reported not to interact.

Clinical evidence

(a) Phenytoin + Co-trimoxazole or Trimethoprim

A patient on 400 mg phenytoin daily developed signs of toxicity (ataxia, nystagmus, loss of balance) within 2 weeks of starting to take 960 mg **co-trimoxazole** twice daily. His serum levels were found to have climbed to 152 micromol/l (normal range 40 to 80 micromol/l).[1]

A child developed phenytoin toxicity within 48 h of starting **co-trimoxazole**. Toxicity resolved when treatment was changed to amoxicillin. She was also taking sulthiame.[2] A clinical study showed that **co-trimoxazole** and **trimethoprim** can increase the phenytoin half-life by 39 and 51%, and decrease the mean metabolic clearance by 27 and 30%, respectively.[3] **Sulfamethoxazole** alone had only a small effect on the half-life and did not affect the clearance of phenytoin.[3]

(b) Phenytoin + Sulfamethizole

The development of phenytoin toxicity in a patient given **sulfamethizole** prompted a study of this interaction in 8 patients. After 7 days treatment with **sulfamethizole** (1 g four times daily) the phenytoin half-life had lengthened from 11.8 to 19.6 h. Of 4 further patients on long-term treatment, 3 showed rises in serum phenytoin levels from 22 to 33, from 19 to 23 and from 4 to 7 micrograms/ml respectively. The fourth patient was not affected.[4,5]

Another single-dose study showed that the half-life of phenytoin was similarly increased and the mean metabolic clearance reduced by 36%.[3]

(c) Phenytoin + Sulfaphenazole or Sulfadiazine

After taking 2 g **sulfaphenazole** (13 patients) or 4 g **sulfadiazine** (8 patients) daily for a week, the half-life of single intravenous doses of phenytoin were found to have increased by 237 and 80% respectively. The mean metabolic clearance decreased by 67 and 45% respectively.[3]

(d) Phenytoin + other sulphonamides

Sulfadimethoxine, sulfamethoxypyridazine, sulfametoxydiazine and sulfafurazole have been found not to interact significantly with phenytoin.[3]

Mechanism

The sulphonamides that interact appear to do so by inhibiting the metabolism of the phenytoin by the liver, resulting in its accumulation in the body. This would also seem to be true for trimethoprim.

Importance and management

The documentation seems to be limited to the reports cited, but the interaction is established. Co-trimoxazole, sulfamethizole, sulfadiazine, sulfaphenazole and trimethoprim can increase serum phenytoin levels. It probably occurs in most patients, but the small number of adverse reaction reports suggests that the risk of toxicity is small. It is clearly most likely in those with serum phenytoin levels at the top end of the range. If concurrent use is thought appropriate, the serum phenytoin levels should be closely monitored and the phenytoin dosage reduced if necessary. Alternatively use a non-interacting sulphonamide (see (d) above). There seems to be no information about other sulphonamides but it would be prudent to be alert for this interaction with any of them.

1. Wilcox JB. Phenytoin intoxication and co-trimoxazole. *N Z Med J* (1981) 94, 235–6.
2. Gillman MA, Sandyk R. Phenytoin toxicity and co-trimoxazole. *Ann Intern Med* (1985) 102, 559.
3. Mølholm Hansen J, Kampmann JP, Siersbæk-Nielsen K, Lumholtz B, Arrøe M, Abildgaard U, Skovsted L. The effect of different sulphonamides on phenytoin metabolism in man. *Acta Med Scand* (1979) (Suppl 624), 106–10.
4. Lumholtz B, Siersbaek-Nielsen K, Skovsted L, Kampmann J, Mølholm Hansen J. Sulfamethizole-induced inhibition of diphenylhydantoin, tolbutamide and warfarin metabolism. *Clin Pharmacol Ther* (1975) 17, 731–4.
5. Siersbaek-Nielsen K, Mølholm Hansen J, Skovsted L, Lumholtz B, Kampmann J. Sulphamethizole-induced inhibition of diphenylhydantoin and tolbutamide metabolism in man. *Clin Pharmacol Ther* (1973) 14, 148.

Phenytoin + Sulthiame

Serum phenytoin levels can be approximately doubled by the concurrent use of sulthiame. Phenytoin toxicity may occur unless suitable phenytoin dosage reductions are made.

Clinical evidence

The serum phenytoin levels in 6 out of 7 epileptic patients approximately doubled within about 5 to 25 days of starting to take 400 mg **sulthiame** daily. All experienced an increase in side effects and definite phenytoin toxicity occurred in 2 of them. In most of the patients, phenytoin serum levels fell back to baseline over the 2 months following the withdrawal of **sulthiame**.[1] All of the patients were also taking phenobarbital and greater variations in serum phenobarbital were seen, but this was not clinically important.[1]

A number of other reports confirm this interaction,[2-8] some of which describe the development of phenytoin toxicity.

Mechanism

The evidence suggests that sulthiame interferes with the metabolism of the phenytoin by the liver, leading to its accumulation in the body.

Importance and management

A reasonably well-documented, established and clinically important interaction. The incidence seems to be high. If sulthiame is added to established treatment with phenytoin, increases in serum phenytoin levels of up to 75% or more may be expected.[3,7] Phenytoin serum levels should be closely monitored and appropriate dosage reductions made to prevent the development of toxicity. The changes in phenobarbital levels appear to be unimportant.

1. Olesen OV, Jensen ON, Drug-interaction between sulthiame (Ospolot (R)) and phenytoin in the treatment of epilepsy. *Dan Med Bull* (1969) 16, 154–8.
2. Houghton GW, Richens A. Inhibition of phenytoin metabolism by sulthiame. *Br J Pharmacol* (1973) 49, 157P–158P.
3. Houghton GW, Richens A. Inhibition of phenytoin metabolism by sulthiame in epileptic patients. *Br J Clin Pharmacol* (1974) 1, 59–66.
4. Richens A, Houghton GW. Phenytoin intoxication caused by sulthiame. *Lancet* (1973) ii, 1442–3.
5. Houghton GW, Richens A. Inhibition of phenytoin metabolism by other drugs used in epilepsy. *Int J Clin Pharmacol Biopharm* (1975) 12, 210–16.
6. Frantzen E, Mølholm Hansen J, Hansen OE, Kristensen M. Phenytoin (Dilantin®) intoxication. *Acta Neurol Scand* (1967) 43, 440–6.
7. Houghton GW, Richens A. Phenytoin intoxication induced by sulthiame in epileptic patients. *J Neurol Neurosurg Psychiatry* (1974) 37, 275–81.
8. Mølholm Hansen J, Kristensen M and Skovsted L. Sulthiame (Ospolot®) as inhibitor of diphenylhydantoin metabolism. *Epilepsia* (1968) 9, 17–22.

Phenytoin + Tacrolimus

An isolated report describes an increase in serum phenytoin levels attributed to the use of tacrolimus.

Clinical evidence, mechanism, importance and management

A kidney transplant patient on 500 and 600 mg **phenytoin** on alternate days (and also taking azathioprine, bumetanide, digoxin, diltiazem, heparin, insulin and prednisone) had his immunosuppressant treatment changed from ciclosporin to tacrolimus 14 to 16 mg daily. About 7 weeks later he presented in hospital because of a fainting episode and was found to have raised serum **phenytoin** levels (increased from 18.4 to 36.2 micrograms/ml). The **phenytoin** was temporarily stopped until his serum levels had fallen again, and he was then discharged on a reduced **phenytoin** dosage of 400 and 500 mg on alternate days and had no further problems.[1]

The presumption is that the fainting episode was due to the raised serum phenytoin levels, possibly caused by inhibition of the metabolism of the phenytoin by the tacrolimus, although other factors may have had some part to play.[1] This is an isolated case and it is not known whether this interaction is likely to occur in other patients.

1. Thompson PA, Mosley CA. Tacrolimus-phenytoin interaction. *Ann Pharmacother* (1996) 30, 544.

Phenytoin + Theophylline

The serum levels of each drug and their therapeutic effects can be markedly reduced by the presence of the other. Dosage increases may be needed to maintain adequate concentrations. Separating the oral dosage by 1 to 2 h appears to minimise the effects of theophylline on phenytoin.

Clinical evidence

(a) Reduced phenytoin serum levels

The seizure frequency of an epileptic woman on phenytoin 100 mg four times daily increased when she was given intravenous and later oral **theophylline**. Her serum phenytoin levels had more than halved, from 15.7 to around 5 to 8 micrograms/ml. An increase in the phenytoin dosage to 200 mg three times daily raised her serum phenytoin levels to only 7 to 11 micrograms/ml until the drugs were given 1 to 2 h apart. The patient then developed phenytoin toxicity with a serum level of 33 micrograms/ml. A subsequent study in 4 healthy subjects confirmed that separating the dosages raised the serum levels of both drugs.[1]

A study in 14 subjects showed that, after 2 weeks of concurrent use, withdrawal of the **theophylline** resulted in a rise of greater than 40% in the mean serum phenytoin levels of 5 of the subjects and a mean rise of about 30% in the total group.[2]

(b) Reduced theophylline serum levels

The observation that a patient on phenytoin had lower than expected levels of **theophylline** prompted a study in 10 healthy subjects. After taking phenytoin for 10 days the clearance of **theophylline** was increased by 73%, and both the AUC and the half-life were reduced by about 50%.[3] A study in 6 healthy subjects showed that after taking 300 mg phenytoin daily for 3 weeks the mean clearance of **theophylline** was increased by 45% (range 31 to 65%).[4] Other reports on individual asthmatic patients and healthy subjects have shown that phenytoin can cause about a two to threefold increase in the clearance of **theophylline**.[5-8] Another study[9] and a case report[10] show that the effects of phenytoin (and phenobarbital) on **theophylline** can be additive with the effects of smoking.

Mechanisms

(a). Uncertain. The evidence suggests that theophylline inhibits the absorption of phenytoin from the gut.

(b). It seems probable that phenytoin, a known enzyme-inducing agent, increases the metabolism of theophylline by the liver, thereby hastening its clearance from the body.

Importance and management

These mutual interactions are established and of clinical importance. Patients given both drugs should be monitored to confirm that therapy remains effective. Ideally the serum levels should be measured to confirm that they remain within the therapeutic range. Dosage increases of theophylline of up to 50% or more may be required.[11] Separating the oral dosages by 1 to 2 h apparently minimises the effects of theophylline on phenytoin.[1]

1. Fincham RW, Schottelius DD, Wyatt R, Hendeles L, Weinberger M. Phenytoin-theophylline interaction: a case report. In Advances in Epileptology. Xth Epilepsy Int Symp. Wada JA and Perry JK (eds) Raven Press, NY (1980) p 505.
2. Taylor JW, Hendeles L, Weinberger M, Lyon LW, Wyatt R, Riegelman S. The interaction of phenytoin and theophylline. *Drug Intell Clin Pharm* (1980) 14, 638.
3. Marquis J-F, Carruthers SG, Spense JD, Brownstone YS, Toogood JH. Phenytoin-theophylline interaction. *N Engl J Med* (1982) 307, 1189–90.
4. Miller M, Cosgriff J, Kwong T, Morken DA. Influence of phenytoin on theophylline clearance. *Clin Pharmacol Ther* (1984) 35, 666–9.
5. Sklar SJ, Wagner JC. Enhanced theophylline clearance secondary to phenytoin therapy. *Drug Intell Clin Pharm* (1985) 19, 34–6.
6. Reed RC, Schwartz HJ. Phenytoin-theophylline-quinidine interaction. *N Engl J Med* (1983) 308, 724–5.
7. Landsberg K, Shalansky S. Interaction between phenytoin and theophylline. *Can J Hosp Pharm* (1988) 41, 31–2.
8. Adebayo GI. Interaction between phenytoin and theophylline in healthy volunteers. *Clin Exp Pharmacol Physiol* (1988) 15, 883–7.
9. Crowley JJ, Cusack BJ, Jue SG, Koup JR, Vestal RE. Cigarette smoking and theophylline metabolism: effects of phenytoin. *Clin Pharmacol Ther* (1987) 42, 334–40.
10. Nicholson JP, Basile SA, Cury JD. Massive theophylline dosing in a heavy smoker receiving both phenytoin and phenobarbital. *Ann Pharmacother* (1992) 26, 334–6.
11. Slugg PH, Pippenger CE. Theophylline and its interactions. *Cleve Clin Q* (1985) 52, 417–24.

Phenytoin + Ticlopidine

Four patients on phenytoin developed toxicity when ticlopidine was added. The makers of ticlopidine have other unpublished reports of increases in serum phenytoin levels associated with ticlopidine use.

Clinical evidence

A 71-year-old man on phenytoin, phenobarbital and colestyramine developed difficulty in walking and leg stiffness within a month of starting 250 mg **ticlopidine** twice daily. His serum phenytoin levels were found to have risen from 15 to 40 mg/l. When his phenytoin dosage was reduced from 350 to 200 mg daily, the serum levels fell to a range of 10 to 15 mg/l and the phenytoin toxicity disappeared. The **ticlopidine** appeared not to have a clinically relevant effect on the serum levels of the phenobarbital.[1] A man with history of complex partial seizures on phenytoin and clobazam developed signs of phenytoin toxicity (vertigo, ataxia, somnolence) within a week of starting 250 mg **ticlopidine** daily. His serum phenytoin levels had risen from 18 to 34 mg/l. When the phenytoin dosage was reduced from 250 to 200 mg daily the toxic signs disappeared within a few days and his serum phenytoin levels fell to 18 mg/l. To test whether an interaction had occurred, the **ticlopidine** was stopped, whereupon the serum phenytoin levels fell within about 3 weeks to 8 mg/l, during which time the patient experienced the first seizure he had had for 2 years. When the **ticlopidine** was restarted, his serum phenytoin levels rose again within a month to 19 mg/l.[2] A man developed acute phenytoin toxicity and showed a rise in serum phenytoin levels from around 18 mg/l to 35 mg/l within 3 weeks of starting 250 mg **ticlopidine** twice daily.[3] Another man also developed acute phenytoin toxicity and was found to have phenytoin serum levels of 46.5 mg/l, 25 days after starting to take 250 mg **ticlopidine** twice daily.[4]

The makers of **ticlopidine** are reported to have other unpublished cases of elevated phenytoin serum levels associated with **ticlopidine** use.[5]

Mechanism

Uncertain, but it is suggested that the metabolism of the phenytoin (possibly by the cytochrome P450 isoenzyme CYP2C19) in the liver was inhibited by the ticlopidine, resulting in its accumulation.[2-4]

Importance and management

Information appears to be limited to these reports. The general importance of this interaction is therefore not known, but it would now be prudent to monitor serum phenytoin levels very closely in any patient if ticlopidine is added to established treatment, being alert for the need to reduce the phenytoin dosage. More study is needed.

1. Rindone JP, Bryan G. Phenytoin toxicity associated with ticlopidine administration. *Arch Intern Med* (1996) 156, 1113.
2. Riva R, Cerullo A, Albani F, Baruzzi A. Ticlopidine impairs phenytoin clearance: a case report. *Neurology* (1996) 46, 1172–3.
3. Privitera M, Welty TE. Acute phenytoin toxicity followed by seizure breakthrough from a ticlopidine-phenytoin interaction. *Arch Neurol* (1996) 53, 1191–2.
4. Donahue SR, Flockhart DA, Abernethy DR, Ko J-W. Ticlopidine inhibition of phenytoin metabolism mediated by potent inhibition of CYP2C19. *Clin Pharmacol Ther* (1997) 62, 572–7.
5. Physicians' Desk Reference 1996. Montvale, NJ. Medical Economics (1996) 2156–9.

Phenytoin + Trazodone

A single case report describes phenytoin toxicity in a patient when given trazodone.

Clinical evidence, mechanism, importance and management

A patient taking 300 mg phenytoin daily developed progressive signs of phenytoin toxicity after taking 500 mg **trazodone** daily for 4 months. His serum phenytoin levels had risen from 17.8 to 46 micrograms/ml.[1] Therapeutic phenytoin serum levels were restored by reducing the phenytoin dosage to 200 mg daily and the **trazodone** to 400 mg daily. The reasons for this apparent interaction are not understood. Concurrent use need not be avoided but until more is known, patients should be monitored if given both drugs.

1. Dorn JM. A case of phenytoin toxicity possibly precipitated by trazodone. *J Clin Psychiatry* (1986) 47, 89–90.

Phenytoin + Tricyclic antidepressants

Some very limited evidence suggests that imipramine can raise serum phenytoin levels but nortriptyline and amitriptyline appear not to do so. Phenytoin possibly reduces serum desipramine levels. The tricyclics also lower the convulsive threshold.

Clinical evidence

(a) Serum phenytoin levels increased or unchanged

The serum phenytoin levels of 2 patients rose over a 3-month period when concurrently given **imipramine** 75 mg daily. One of them showed an increase in phenytoin levels from 30 to 60 micromol/l and developed mild toxicity (drowsiness and uncoordination). These signs disappeared and the phenytoin serum levels of both patients fell when the **imipramine** was withdrawn. One of them was also taking **nitrazepam** and **clonazepam**, and the other **sodium valproate** and **carbamazepine**, but were stable on these combinations before the addition of imipramine.[1]

Other studies have shown that **nortriptyline** 75 mg daily had an insignificant effect on the serum phenytoin levels of 5 patients,[2] and

that **amitriptyline** had no effect on the elimination of phenytoin in 3 subjects.[3]

(b) Serum tricyclic antidepressant levels reduced

A report describes 2 patients who had low serum **desipramine** levels, despite taking standard dosages, while concurrently taking phenytoin.[4]

Mechanisms

One suggestion is that imipramine inhibits the metabolism of the phenytoin by the liver, which results in its accumulation in the body. The reduced desipramine levels may be a result of enzyme induction by the phenytoin.

Importance and management

The documentation is very limited indeed and none of these interactions is adequately established. The tricyclic antidepressants as a group lower the seizure threshold,[5] which suggests extra care should be taken anyway, if deciding to use them in epileptic patients. If concurrent use is undertaken the effects should be very well monitored.

1. Perucca E, Richens A. Interaction between phenytoin and imipramine. *Br J Clin Pharmacol* (1977) 4, 485–6.
2. Houghton GW, Richens A. Inhibition of phenytoin metabolism by other drugs used in epilepsy. *Int J Clin Pharmacol Biopharm* (1975) 12, 210–16.
3. Pond SM, Graham GG, Birkett DJ, Wade DN. Effects of tricyclic antidepressants on drug metabolism. *Clin Pharmacol Ther* (1975) 18, 191–9.
4. Fogel BS, Haltzman S. Desipramine and phenytoin: a potential drug interaction of therapeutic relevance. *J Clin Psychiatry* (1987) 48, 387–8.
5. Dallos V, Heathfield K. Iatrogenic epilepsy due to antidepressant drugs. *BMJ* (1969) 4, 80–2.

Phenytoin + Zidovudine

Although one study found that zidovudine did not alter the pharmacokinetics of phenytoin, there is other evidence suggesting that some changes possibly occur, but these may be due to HIV infection.

Clinical evidence, mechanism, importance and management

Although there are said to have been 13 cases of a possible interaction between **zidovudine** and phenytoin, the details are not described in the report.[1] No significant changes in the pharmacokinetics of phenytoin 300 mg orally were seen in 12 asymptomatic HIV+ patients who were taking 200 mg **zidovudine** every 4 hours.[1] Another study found that the mean phenytoin dose was higher in HIV+ patients when compared to epileptic subjects without the virus, while the mean phenytoin levels in the HIV+ group were lower (i.e. a higher dose resulted in lower serum levels in HIV+ subjects). **Zidovudine** did not appear to affect the levels.[2,3] The current evidence would suggest that it is HIV infection, rather than **zidovudine** that affects phenytoin levels, but more study is needed to confirm this.

1. Sarver P, Lampkin TA, Dukes GE, Messenheimer JA, Kirby MG, Dalton MJ, Hak LJ. Effect of zidovudine on the pharmacokinetic disposition of phenytoin in HIV positive asymptomatic patients. *Pharmacotherapy* (1991) 11, 108–9.
2. Burger DW, Meerhorst PL, Koks CHW, Beijnen JH. Phenytoin (PH) monitoring in HIV (+) individuals: is there an interaction with zidovudine (ZDV)? 9th International Conference on AIDS & 5th World Congress on Sexually Transmitted Diseases, Berlin. June 6–11, 1993. Abstract PO-B31-2214.
3. Burger DM, Meerhorst PL, Mulder JW, Kraaijeveld CL, Koks CHW, Bult A, Beijnen JH. Therapeutic drug monitoring of phenytoin in patients with the acquired immunodeficiency syndrome. *Ther Drug Monit* (1994) 16, 616–20.

Phenytoin + Zileuton

The metabolism of phenytoin is unchanged by zileuton.

Clinical evidence, mechanism, importance and management

A controlled study in 20 healthy subjects found that the metabolism of single 300-mg doses of phenytoin was unaltered after taking 600 mg **zileuton** 6-hourly for 5 days.[1,2] More study is needed to confirm that these two drugs do not interact in practice, in patients.

1. Samara E, Granneman R, Dube L. Michaelis-Menten kinetics determine metabolic interaction between zileuton and phenytoin: a population approach. *Clin Pharmacol Ther* (1994) 55, 140.

2. Samara E, Cavanaugh JH, Mukherjee D, Granneman GR. Lack of pharmacokinetic interaction between zileuton and phenytoin in humans. *Clin Pharmacokinet* (1995) 29 (Suppl 2), 84–91.

Primidone + Barbiturates

Elevated serum phenobarbital levels may develop if primidone and phenobarbital are given concurrently.

Clinical evidence, mechanism, importance and management

Primidone is substantially converted into **phenobarbital** within the body. For example, a group of patients on long-term primidone without phenobarbital developed serum primidone levels of 9 micrograms/ml and serum **phenobarbital** levels of 31 micrograms/ml.[1] If **phenobarbital** is given at the same time the serum phenobarbital levels may become excessive. This effect may be possibly exacerbated if phenytoin is also being given (see also 'Primidone + Phenytoin', p.358). If concurrent use is undertaken be particularly alert for any evidence of **phenobarbital** intoxication.

1. Booker HE, Hosokowa K, Burdette RD, Darcey B. A clinical study of serum primidone levels. *Epilepsia* (1970) 11, 395–402.

Primidone + Clonazepam or Clorazepate

Clonazepam is reported to raise serum primidone levels. Clorazepate with primidone may possibly cause personality changes.

Clinical evidence, mechanism, importance and management

An analysis of serum levels of anticonvulsants in children found that those on concurrent **clonazepam** had markedly higher concentrations of primidone, and toxicity was seen.[1] Another report suggested that the concurrent use of primidone and **clorazepate** may have been responsible for the development of irritability, aggression and depression in 6 of 8 patients.[2] None of these effects appears to be well documented or confirmed but some caution would seem appropriate during concurrent use.

1. Windorfer A, Sauer W. Drug interactions during anticonvulsant therapy in childhood: diphenylhydantoin, primidone, phenobarbitone, clonazepam, nitrazepam, carbamazepin and dipropylacetate. *Neuropadiatrie* (1977) 8, 29–41.

2. Feldman RG. Clorazepate in temporal lobe epilepsy. *JAMA* (1976) 236, 2603.

Primidone + Isoniazid

A single case report describes elevated serum primidone levels and reduced phenobarbital levels during concurrent treatment with primidone and isoniazid.

Clinical evidence, mechanism, importance and management

A patient on primidone showed raised serum primidone levels and reduced serum phenobarbital levels due, it was demonstrated, to the concurrent use of **isoniazid**, which inhibited the metabolism of the primidone by the liver. The half-life of primidone rose from 8.7 to 14 h while taking **isoniazid** and steady-state primidone levels rose by 83%. The importance of this interaction is uncertain but prescribers should be aware that it can occur if concurrent treatment is undertaken.[1]

1. Sutton G, Kupferberg HJ. Isoniazid as an inhibitor of primidone metabolism. *Neurology* (1975) 25, 1179–81.

Primidone + Phenytoin

Serum phenobarbital levels are increased in patients on primidone when concurrently treated with phenytoin. This is normally an advantageous interaction, but phenobarbital toxicity occurs occasionally.

Clinical evidence

A study in 44 epileptic patients taking primidone and **phenytoin** showed that their serum phenobarbital:primidone ratio was high (4.35) compared with a ratio of 1.05 in 15 other patients who were only taking primidone.[1]

Similar results are described in other studies.[2-5] A few patients may develop toxicity.[6]

Mechanism

Phenytoin increases the metabolic conversion of primidone to phenobarbital while possibly depressing the subsequent metabolic destruction (hydroxylation) of the phenobarbital. The net effect is a rise in phenobarbital levels.[7]

Importance and management

Well documented. Concurrent use is common. This is normally an advantageous interaction since a metabolic product of primidone is phenobarbital, which is itself an active anticonvulsant. However, it should be borne in mind that phenobarbital serum levels can sometimes reach toxic concentrations,[6] even if only a small dose of phenytoin is added.

1. Fincham RW, Schottelius DD, Sahs AL. The influence of diphenylhydantoin on primidone metabolism. *Arch Neurol* (1974) 30, 259–62.

2. Fincham RW, Schottelius DD, Sahs AL. The influence of diphenylhydantoin on primidone metabolism. *Trans Am Neurol Assoc* (1973) 98, 197–9.

3. Schmidt D. The effect of phenytoin and ethosuximide on primidone metabolism in patients with epilepsy. *J Neurol* (1975) 209, 115–23.

4. Reynolds EH, Fenton G, Fenwick P, Johnson AL, Laundy M. Interaction of phenytoin and primidone. *BMJ* (1975) 2, 594–5.

5. Callaghan N, Feeley M, Duggan F, O'Callaghan M, Seldrup J. The effect of anticonvulsant drugs which induce liver microsomal enzymes on derived and ingested phenobarbitone levels. *Acta Neurol Scand* (1977) 56, 1–6.

6. Galdames D, Ortiz M, Saavedra I, Aguilera L. Interaccion fenitoina-primidona: intoxicacion por fenobarbital, en un adulto tratado con ambas drogas. *Rev Med Chil* (1980) 108, 716–20.

7. Porro MG, Kupferberg HJ, Porter RJ, Theodore WH, Newmark ME. Phenytoin: an inhibitor and inducer of primidone metabolism in an epileptic patient. *Br J Clin Pharmacol* (1982) 14, 294–7.

Primidone + Sodium valproate

Increases, decreases, and no change in serum primidone levels due to sodium valproate have been reported. Primidone-derived phenobarbital levels appear to be increased.

Clinical evidence

In a number of cases, patients taking primidone required a decrease in the primidone dosage after **sodium valproate** was added.[1-4] In 6 cases this was due to an increase in the primidone-derived phenobarbital level,[1] and in the other cases phenobarbital levels weren't measured, but the dosage reduction was needed to overcome the sedation which occurred when the **sodium valproate** was added.[2-4] Primidone levels were not measured in any of these cases.[1-4] In two other studies, primidone levels either decreased,[5] or did not change when **sodium valproate** was added.[6] However, phenobarbital levels, where measured, had increased.[6]

The serum primidone levels of 7 children taking 10 to 18 mg/kg daily rose two to threefold when **sodium valproate** (dosage not stated) was given concurrently. After 1 to 3 months of continued therapy the serum primidone levels fell in 3 of the patients but persisted in one. Follow-up primidone levels were not taken in the other 3 patients, and no patient had phenobarbital levels measured.[7]

In contrast, in a further study, neither phenobarbital levels nor primidone levels were significantly altered when sodium valproate was added to treatment.[8]

Mechanism

It has been suggested that sodium valproate decreases the conversion of primidone to phenobarbital, and decreases the metabolism of phenobarbital (see also 'Barbiturates + Sodium valproate', p.322). This would result in increased primidone and phenobarbital levels. However, increased renal clearance of primidone may occur, resulting in no overall change to the primidone levels. Depending on the balance between these various effects a variety of levels may result.[8] The results of one study suggest that proposed inhibition of primidone caused by sodium valproate may diminish over the first few months of concurrent use.[7]

Importance and management

There seems to be little consistency about the effect of sodium valproate on primidone levels. However, in the majority of cases phenobarbital levels seem to be raised (see also 'Barbiturates + Sodium valproate', p.322). Why this happens in only a selection of patients is not clear. It would seem prudent not to measure primidone levels without corresponding phenobarbital levels. Monitor the patient for increased signs of sedation, which may be resolved by a reduction in the primidone dose.

1. Wilder BJ, Willmore LJ, Bruni J, Villarreal HJ. Valproic acid: interaction with other anticonvulsant drugs. *Neurology* (1978) 28, 892–6.
2. Haigh D, Forsythe WI. The treatment of childhood epilepsy with sodium valproate. *Dev Med Child Neurol* (1975) 17, 743–8.
3. Richens A, Ahmad S. Controlled trial of sodium valproate in severe epilepsy. *BMJ* (1975) 4, 255–6.
4. Völzke E, Doose H. Dipropylacetate (Dépakine®, Ergenyl®) in the treatment of epilepsy. *Epilepsia* (1973) 14, 185–93.
5. Varma R, Michos GA, Varma RS, Hoshino AY. Clinical trials of Depakene (valproic acid) coadministered with other anticonvulsants in epileptic patients. *Res Commun Psychol Psychiatr Behav* (1980) 5, 265–73.
6. Yukawa E, Higuchi S, Aoyama T. The effect of concurrent administration of sodium valproate on serum levels of primidone and its metabolite phenobarbital. *J Clin Pharm Ther* (1989) 14, 387–92.
7. Windorfer A, Sauer W, Gädeke R. Elevation of diphenylhydantoin and primidone serum concentration by addition of dipropylacetate, a new anticonvulsant drug. *Acta Paediatr Scand* (1975) 64, 771–2.
8. Bruni J. Valproic acid and plasma levels of primidone and derived phenobarbital. *Can J Neurol Sci* (1981) 8, 91–2.

Sodium valproate + Antacids

The absorption of sodium valproate is slightly, but not significantly increased by *Maalox* (aluminium-magnesium hydroxide) but not by magnesium trisilicate or calcium carbonate suspension.

Clinical evidence, mechanism, importance and management

The AUC of a single 500-mg dose of sodium valproate (given 1 h after breakfast) was increased by 12% (range 3 to 28%) in 7 healthy subjects given 62 ml *Maalox* 1 h and 3 h after breakfast and at bedtime. Neither **magnesium trisilicate** suspension (*Trisogel*) nor **calcium carbonate** suspension (*Titralac*) had a significant effect on absorption.[1] No special precautions would seem necessary during concurrent use.

1. May CA, Garnett WR, Small RE, Pellock JM. Effects of three antacids on the bioavailability of valproic acid. *Clin Pharm* (1982) 1, 244–7.

Sodium valproate + Benzodiazepines

The concurrent use of sodium valproate and clonazepam may cause an increase in side effects, but seizure frequency in some patients is reduced. Diazepam and lorazepam serum levels may be raised by sodium valproate.

Clinical evidence

The addition of **clonazepam** to sodium valproate increased the unwanted effects (drowsiness, absence status) in 9 out of 12 children and adolescent patients.[1] Enhanced sedation has been briefly described during the concurrent use of sodium valproate and other unnamed **benzodiazepines**.[2]

Sodium valproate increased the serum levels of **diazepam** in healthy subjects.[3] A 40% decrease in the clearance of 2 mg **lorazepam** was seen in 6 out of 8 healthy subjects when they were given an intravenous bolus of **lorazepam** while taking 250 mg sodium valproate twice daily.[4] Another 16 healthy subjects, given 500 mg sodium valproate twice daily and 1 mg **lorazepam** 12-hourly, showed a 20% increase in the **lorazepam** AUC and a 17% reduction in clearance.[5]

Mechanism

It seems that sodium valproate reduces the glucuronidation of **lorazepam**,[4,5] and some other benzodiazepines may therefore be similarly affected.

Importance and management

It has been suggested that the combination of clonazepam and sodium valproate should be avoided.[1] However, a very brief letter points out that neither drug affects the serum concentrations of the other and that **clonazepam** and valproic acid can be given together in patients with absence seizures since some patients have an excellent response to the combination.[6] The clinical importance of the raised serum diazepam and lorazepam levels is not clear, but be alert for any evidence of increased effects and side-effects (drowsiness, ataxia) with all benzodiazepines if sodium valproate is used concurrently.

1. Jeavons PM, Clark JE, Maheshwari MC. Treatment of generalized epilepsies of childhood and adolescence with sodium valproate ('Epilim'). *Dev Med Child Neurol* (1977) 19, 9–25.
2. Völzke E, Doose H. Dipropylacetate (Dépakine®, Ergenyl®) in the treatment of epilepsy. *Epilepsia* (1973) 14, 185–93.
3. Dhillon S, Richens A. Valproic acid and diazepam interaction *in vivo*. *Br J Clin Pharmacol* (1982) 13, 553–60.
4. Anderson GD, Gidal BE, Kantor ED, Wilensky AJ. Lorazepam-valproate interaction: studies in normal subjects and isolated perfused rat liver. *Epilepsia* (1994) 35, 221–5.

5. Samara E, Granneman R, Saulis R, Witt G, Cavanaugh J. Pharmacokinetic-pharmacodynamic interaction between valproate and lorazepam. *Clin Pharmacol Ther* (1995) 57, 153.
6. Browne TR. Interaction between clonazepam and sodium valproate. *N Engl J Med* (1979) 300, 678.

Sodium valproate + Chlorpromazine

Sodium valproate serum levels are slightly raised in patients given chlorpromazine, but this appears to be of minimal clinical importance. An isolated report describes severe hepatotoxicity with concurrent use.

Clinical evidence, mechanism, importance and management

The sodium valproate steady-state trough serum levels of 6 patients taking 400 mg daily rose by 22% when given 100 to 300 mg **chlorpromazine** daily. The half-life increased by 14% and the clearance fell by 14% (possibly due to some reduction in the metabolism by the liver)[1]. This interaction would normally seem to be of minimal importance. Severe hepatotoxicity occurred in another patient when given both drugs,[2] but remember that both drugs independently, can be hepatotoxic.

1. Ishizaki T, Chiba K, Saito M, Kobayashi K, Iizuka R. The effects of neuroleptics (haloperidol and chlorpromazine) on the pharmacokinetics of valproic acid in schizophrenic patients. *J Clin Psychopharmacol* (1984) 4, 254–61.
2. Bach N, Thung SN, Schaffner F, Tobias H. Exaggerated cholestasis and hepatic fibrosis following simultaneous administration of chlorpromazine and sodium valproate. *Dig Dis Sci* (1989) 34, 1303–7.

Sodium valproate + Cimetidine or Ranitidine

Ranitidine does not interact with sodium valproate, and cimetidine interacts only minimally.

Clinical evidence, mechanism, importance and management

The clearance of a single oral dose of sodium valproate was reduced in 6 patients to a small extent (2 to 17%) after a 4 week course of **cimetidine**, but not by **ranitidine**.[1] It seems doubtful if the sodium valproate/**cimetidine** interaction is of clinical importance.

1. Webster LK, Mihaly GW, Jones DB, Smallwood RA, Phillips JA, Vajda FJ. Effect of cimetidine and ranitidine on carbamazepine and sodium valproate pharmacokinetics. *Eur J Clin Pharmacol* (1984) 27, 341–3.

Sodium valproate + Colestyramine

Colestyramine causes a very small reduction in the absorption of sodium valproate. No interaction occurs if the administration of the drugs is separated by 3 h.

Clinical evidence

Single 250-mg doses of sodium valproate were given to 6 healthy subjects either alone, at the same time as 4 g **colestyramine** (twice daily), or with the **colestyramine** taken 3 h after the sodium valproate. The bioavailability of sodium valproate taken alone and when separated from the **colestyramine** by 3 h remained the same. When the sodium valproate was taken at the same time as the **colestyramine** the sodium valproate AUC fell by 15% and the maximum serum levels fell by 21%.[1,2]

Mechanism

Colestyramine is a ion-exchange resin intended to bind with bile acids in the gut, but it can also bind with drugs as well, leading to a reduction in their absorption. This apparently occurs to a limited extent with sodium valproate.

Importance and management

Direct information appears to be limited to this single study, but what happened is consistent with the way colestyramine interacts with a number of other drugs. The fall in the bioavailability is small and probably of very limited clinical importance, but the interaction can be totally avoided by separating the dosages by 3 hours so that admixture in the gut is minimised.

1. Pennell AT, Ravis WR, Malloy MJ, Sead A, Diskin C. Cholestyramine decreases valproic acid serum concentrations. *J Clin Pharmacol* (1992) 32, 755.
2. Malloy MJ, Ravis WR, Pennell AT, Diskin CJ. Effect of cholestyramine resin on single dose valproate pharmacokinetics. *Int J Clin Pharmacol Ther* (1996) 34, 208–11.

Sodium valproate + Felbamate

Felbamate can raise sodium valproate serum levels causing toxicity (nausea, drowsiness, headaches, low platelet count, cognitive disturbances).

Clinical evidence

(a) Effect on sodium valproate

The average steady-state sodium valproate serum levels in 7 epileptics were raised 28% (from 66.9 to 85.4 micrograms/ml) by 1200 mg **felbamate** daily, and 54% (from 66.9 to 103.0 micrograms/ml) by 2400 mg daily. The AUCs using these two dosages were raised 28% and 54% respectively.[1,2] Valproate clearance was correspondingly reduced by **felbamate**.[1-3] Similar effects were seen in other studies.[4,5] It was suggested that in children the interaction may be more marked.[5] Many of the patients experienced nausea. Other toxic effects included lethargy, drowsiness, headaches, cognitive disturbances and low platelet counts.[1-4]

(b) Effect on felbamate

The clearance of **felbamate** was decreased 21% by sodium valproate in one study,[6] and another reported significantly lower **felbamate** clearance when taken with valproate.[7] Yet another noted only a minimal effect of sodium valproate on **felbamate** clearance.[8]

Mechanism

It is not clear whether the adverse side effects were due to the increased sodium valproate levels, or simply due to the additive side effects of both drugs. The mechanisms have been investigated but are not established.[9,10]

Importance and management

An established interaction. It may be necessary to reduce the sodium valproate dosage to avoid toxicity if felbamate is given. The authors of one report suggest a 30 to 50% reduction. It may also be necessary to reduce the felbamate dosage as well. Monitor concurrent use closely, particularly during the initial stages.

1. Wagner ML, Graves NM, Leppik IE, Remmel RP, Ward DL, Shumaker RC. The effect of felbamate on valproate disposition. *Epilepsia* (1991) 32 (Suppl 3), 15.
2. Wagner ML, Graves NM, Leppik IE, Remmel RP, Ward DL, Perhach JL. The effect of felbamate on valproic acid disposition. *Clin Pharmacol Ther* (1994) 56, 494–502.
3. Ward DL, Wagner ML, Perhach JL, Kramer L, Graves N, Leppik I, Shumaker RC. Felbamate steady-state pharmacokinetics during coadministration of valproate. *Epilepsia* (1991) 32 (Suppl 3), 8.
4. Liu H, Delgado MR. Significant drug interaction between valproate and felbamate in epileptic children. *Epilepsia* (1995) 36 (Suppl 3), S160.
5. Delgado MR. Changes in valproic acid concentrations and dose/level ratios by felbamate coadministration in children. *Ann Neurol* (1994) 36, 538.
6. Kelley MT, Walson PD, Cox S, Dusci LJ. Population pharmacokinetics of felbamate in children. *Ther Drug Monit* (1997) 19, 29–36.
7. Wagner ML, Leppik IE, Graves NM, Remme RP, Campbell JI. Felbamate serum concentrations: effect of valproate, carbamazepine, phenytoin and phenobarbital. *Epilepsia* (1990) 31, 642.
8. Banfield CR, Zhu G-RR, Jen JF, Jensen PK, Schumaker RC, Perhach JL Affrime MB, Glue P. The effect of age on the apparent clearance of felbamate: a retrospective analysis using nonlinear mixed-effects modeling. *Ther Drug Monit* (1996) 18, 19–29.

9. Bernus I, Dickinson RG, Hooper WD, Franklin ME, Eadie MJ. Effect of felbamate on the plasma protein binding of valproate. *Clin Drug Invest* (1995) 10, 288–95.

10. Hooper WD, Franklin ME, Glue P, Banfield CR, Radwanski E, McLaughlin DB, McIntyre ME, Dickinson RG, Eadie MJ. Effect of felbamate on valproic acid disposition in healthy volunteers: inhibition of ß-oxidation. *Epilepsia* (1996) 37, 91–7.

Sodium valproate or Semisodium valproate + Fluoxetine or Fluvoxamine

Isolated reports describe increases or decreases in serum valproate levels in a small number of patients when given fluoxetine. Some limited evidence suggests that sodium valproate may usefully augment the effects fluoxetine and fluvoxamine.

Clinical evidence

A mentally retarded patient with an atypical bipolar disorder on 3 g semisodium valproate (divalproex sodium) daily showed a rise in serum valproic acid levels from 93.5 to 152 mg/l within 2 weeks of starting to take 20 mg **fluoxetine** daily. The valproate dosage was reduced to 2.25 g daily and 2 weeks later the serum valproic acid levels had fallen to 113 mg/l. No adverse effects were seen.[1] A woman developed elevated serum sodium valproate levels (a rise from 78 to 126 mg/l) within 1 month of starting to take 20 mg **fluoxetine** daily. They fell again when the **fluoxetine** was stopped.[2]

In contrast 2 cases of reduced valproate levels with **fluoxetine** have also been reported. In the first case, a 67-year-old woman taking 2 g sodium valproate and 20 mg **fluoxetine** daily had a serum valproate level of 51.9 mg/l. This increased to 64.9 mg/l 9 days after **fluoxetine** was discontinued and fell to 32.6 mg/l 6 days after it was re-started. In the second case, an 81-year-old woman was taking 1 g sodium valproate plus 20 mg **fluoxetine** daily and had serum valproate levels of 41.9 mg/l. The fluoxetine was stopped, and 6 days later valproate serum levels had risen to 56.2 mg/l. After re-introduction of **fluoxetine** her valproate levels fell to 45.6 mg/l.[3]

Another report describes a woman with a history of panic attacks and depression who improved when sodium valproate was added to her treatment with **fluoxetine**. Yet another improved when sodium valproate was added to **fluvoxamine**, but 3 others who initially showed an improvement later relapsed.[4]

Mechanisms

Not understood.

Importance and management

These reports are somewhat confusing and inconsistent, but the overall picture is that concurrent use need not be avoided, but the outcome needs to be well monitored. More study is needed.

1. Sovner R, Davis JM. A potential drug interaction between fluoxetine and valproic acid. *J Clin Psychopharmacol* (1991) 11, 389.

2. Lucena MI, Blanco E, Corrales MA, Berthier ML. Interaction of fluoxetine and valproic acid. *Am J Psychiatry* (1998) 155, 575.

3. Droulers A, Bodak N, Oudjhani M, Lefevre des Noettes V, Bodak A. Decrease of valproic acid concentration in the blood when coprescribed with fluoxetine. *J Clin Psychopharmacol* (1997) 17, 139–40.

4. Corrigan FM. Sodium valproate augmentation of fluoxetine or fluvoxamine effects. *Biol Psychiatry* (1992) 31, 1178–9.

Sodium valproate + Isoniazid

An isolated report describes the development of raised serum sodium valproate levels and toxicity in a child when concurrently treated with isoniazid.

Clinical evidence, mechanism, importance and management

A girl of 5 with left partial seizures, successfully controlled on 600 mg sodium valproate daily and clonazepam for 7 months, developed signs of sodium valproate toxicity (drowsiness, asthenia) shortly after starting to take 200 mg **isoniazid** daily (because of a positive tuberculin reaction). Her serum valproate levels were found to have risen to around 121 to 139 mg/l (normal therapeutic range 50 to 100 mg/l).[1] Over the next few months various changes were made in her treatment, the most significant being a 62% reduction in the dosage of sodium valproate, to maintain satisfactory therapeutic levels. Later when the **isoniazid** was stopped her valproate levels fell below therapeutic levels and seizures re-occurred. It was then found necessary to increase the valproate to its former dosage. The suggested explanation is that the **isoniazid** inhibited the metabolism (oxidation) of the sodium valproate by the liver so that it accumulated and, in effect, became an overdose. The child was found to be a very slow acetylator of isoniazid.[1]

The general importance of this interaction is uncertain, but it would clearly be prudent to monitor sodium valproate levels if **isoniazid** is added, reducing the dosage where necessary.

1. Jonville AP, Gauchez AS, Autret E, Billard C, Barbier P, Nsabiyumva F, Breteau M. Interaction between isoniazid and valproate: a case of valproate overdosage. *Eur J Clin Pharmacol* (1991) 40, 197–8.

Sodium valproate + Losigamone

Losigamone appears to reduce sodium valproate serum levels.

Clinical evidence, mechanism, importance and management

A preliminary report of a study in 9 male subjects found that the serum levels and AUC of sodium valproate 600 mg daily were significantly reduced by the addition of 500 mg **losigamone** twice daily for 2 weeks, but no precise figures were reported. The **losigamone** serum levels and AUC were unchanged.[1] The clinical significance of this interaction is unknown, but it would clearly be prudent to monitor the outcome of concurrent use.

1. Krämer G, Wad N, Bredel-Geißler, Biber A, Dienel A. Losigamone-valproate-interaction: a placebo-controlled, double-blind study in healthy volunteers. *Epilepsia* (1995) 36 (Suppl 4), 53.

Sodium valproate + Methotrexate

An isolated report describes a seizure in a child following high dose methotrexate treatment, accompanied by a marked fall in serum sodium valproate levels.

Clinical evidence, mechanism, importance and management

A child with acute lymphoblastic leukaemia, who had been treated with sodium valproate for several months because of epileptic symptoms, was additionally given a high-dose 24-h infusion of **methotrexate** (5 g/m^2). A few hours later the child had a tonic-clonic seizure. During this and a subsequent high-dose **methotrexate** infusion, the serum sodium valproate levels were seen to fall sharply to about 25% of their usual level.[1] Following cycles of chemotherapy were managed by increasing the dose of sodium valproate and adding clonazepam. The patient had previously received **methotrexate** 1 g/m^2 without incident. The reasons for this interaction are not known but the authors of the report put forward a number of possible explanations: increased metabolism of unbound valproate, increased urinary excretion due to alkalinization, and decreased valproate absorption from the gut. This appears to be the first and only report of this interaction so that its general importance is not known. It is probably small. However it would clearly now be prudent to monitor sodium valproate levels if high dose **methotrexate** is given to any patient.

1. Schröder H, Østergaard JR. Interference of high-dose methotrexate in the metabolism of valproate? *Pediatr Hematol Oncol* (1994) 11, 445–9.

Sodium valproate + Panipenem/betamipron

Panipenem/betamipron dramatically reduced the valproate serum levels of 6 patients. Carbamazepine levels were unchanged.

Clinical evidence, mechanism, importance and management

A report describes 3 cases of Japanese children on anticonvulsant therapy who showed marked reductions in valproate serum levels while receiving **panipenem/betamipron** for serious chest infections.[1] An increased fit-frequency occurred in 2 of the patients. In one case the serum valproate levels fell from 30.1 to 1.53 mg/l within 4 days of starting the antimicrobial treatment, and rose again when it was stopped. All 3 patients were also taking **carbamazepine** but its serum levels were unchanged by the **panipenem/betamipron**. A further 3 cases of 60 to 100% reductions in valproate levels, within 2 days of starting concurrent treatment have been reported. Increased seizure frequency occurred in 2 cases.[2]

Information appears to be limited to these reports but it would now be prudent to monitor the valproate levels in any patient given this antimicrobial treatment, being alert for the need to increase the valproate dosage, or to use another antibacterial where possible.

1. Nagai K, Shimizu T, Togo A, Takeya M, Yokomizo Y, Sakata Y, Matsuishi T, Kato H. Decrease in serum levels of valproic acid during treatment with a new carbapenem, panipenem/betamipron. *J Antimicrob Chemother* (1997) 39, 295–6.
2. Yamagata T, Momoi MY, Murai K, Ikematsu K, Suwa K, Sakamoto K, Fujimura A. Panipenem—Betamipron and decreases in serum valproic acid concentration. *Ther Drug Monit* (1998) 20, 396–400.

Sodium valproate + Propranolol

No adverse interaction normally occurs, but one patient showed a 35% reduction in sodium valproate clearance when given propranolol.

Clinical evidence, mechanism, importance and management

An isolated report describes a fall in sodium valproate clearance from 1.66 to 1.19 L/h in a patient when given 40 mg **propranolol**, and a further fall to 1.08 L/h when given 80 mg. However 12 other patients on sodium valproate showed no changes in clearance, serum levels or half-life when given 60 or 120 mg **propranolol** daily for three weeks.[1] This interaction would therefore not appear to be of general importance. No special precautions would seem necessary.

1. Nemire RE, Toledo CA, Ramsay RE. A pharmacokinetic study to determine the drug interaction between valproate and propranolol. *Pharmacotherapy* (1996) 16, 1059–62.

Sodium valproate + Theophylline

A study in healthy subjects found that aminophylline did not affect the pharmacokinetics of a single 400-mg dose of sodium valproate.[1]

1. Kulkarni C, Vaz J, David J, Joseph T. Aminophylline alters pharmacokinetics of carbamazepine but not that of sodium valproate — a single dose pharmacokinetic study in human volunteers. *Indian J Physiol Pharmacol* (1995) 39, 122–6.

Tiagabine + Miscellaneous drugs

Tiagabine appears to cause a slight reduction in sodium valproate levels, and tiagabine serum levels are reduced by carbamazepine, phenytoin, phenobarbital and primidone. No interactions occur with alcohol, antipyrine (phenazone), cimetidine, digoxin, theophylline, triazolam or warfarin.

Clinical evidence, mechanism, importance and management

Tiagabine had no effect on the pharmacokinetics of **antipyrine** (**phenazone**) and therefore appears not induce or inhibit liver microsomal enzymes.[1] It does not alter the serum levels of most other anticonvulsant drugs[2,3] except for **sodium valproate**, but the reduction in levels seen was not expected to be clinically significant.[3]

The half-life of tiagabine is reduced from 5–8 h to 2–3 h in the presence of **carbamazepine** or **phenytoin**, which are enzyme inducers.[4] Studies in patients taking 1 to 3 other anticonvulsants (**phenobarbital, phenytoin, carbamazepine, primidone**) found that tiagabine half-lives were reduced when compared with normal subjects taking only tiagabine.[5] The makers say that the plasma concentrations of tiagabine may be reduced 1.5 to 3-fold by these enzyme inducing anticonvulsants.[6]

Volunteer studies have excluded any clinically relevant pharmacokinetic interactions between tiagabine and **cimetidine, digoxin, theophylline, warfarin** or **oral contraceptives** (see 'Oral contraceptives + Tiagabine', p.481), or any pharmacodynamic interactions between tiagabine and **alcohol**, and **triazolam**.[6-10]

1. Gustavson LE, Mengel HB. Pharmacokinetics of tiagabine, a γ-aminobutyric acid-uptake inhibitor, in healthy subjects after single and multiple doses. *Epilepsia* (1995) 36, 605–11.
2. Richens A, Chadwick DW, Duncan JS, Dam M, Gram L, Mikkelsen M, Morrow J, Mengel H, Shu V, McKelvy JF, Pierce MW. Adjunctive treatment of partial seizures with tiagabine: a placebo-controlled trial. *Epilepsy Res* (1995) 21, 37–42.
3. Gustavson LE, Cato A, Guenther HJ, Carlson GF, Witt GF, Cao GX, Qian JX, Boellner SW, Sommerville KW. Lack of clinically important drug interactions between tiagabine and carbamazepine, phenytoin, or valproate. *Epilepsia* (1995) 36 (Suppl 3), S159–S160.
4. Brodie MJ. Tiagabine pharmacology profile. *Epilepsia* (1995) 36 (Suppl 6), S7–S9.
5. So EL, Wolff D, Graves NM, Leppik IE, Cascino GD, Pixton GC, Gustavson LE. Pharmacokinetics of tiagabine as add-on therapy in patients taking enzyme-inducing drugs. *Epilepsy Res* (1995) 22, 221–6.
6. Gabitril (Tiagabine). Sanofi Synthelabo. Summary of product characteristics, July 2001.
7. Kastberg H, Jansen JA, Cole G, Wesnes K. Tiagabine: absence of kinetic or dynamic interactions with ethanol. *Drug Metabol Drug Interact* (1998) 14, 259–73.
8. Mengel H, Jansen JA, Sommerville K, Jonkman JHG, Wesnes K, Cohen A, Carlson GF, Marshall R, Snel S, Dirach J, Kastberg H. Tiagabine: evaluation of the risk of interaction with theophylline, warfarin, digoxin, cimetidine, oral contraceptives, triazolam, or ethanol. *Epilepsia* (1995) 36 (Suppl 3), S160.
9. Richens A, Marshall RW, Dirach J, Jansen JA, Snel S, Pedersen PC. Absence of interaction between tiagabine, a new antiepileptic drug, and the benzodiazepine triazolam. *Drug Metabol Drug Interact* (1998) 14, 159–77.
10. Mengel HB, Houston A, Back DJ. Tiagabine: evaluation of the risk of interaction with oral contraceptive pills in female volunteers. *Epilepsia* (1993) 34 (Suppl 2), 157.

Topiramate + Alcohol or CNS depressants

Topiramate may cause drowsiness, which is expected be additive with the effects of other CNS depressants.

Clinical evidence, mechanism, importance and management

The concurrent use of topiramate and **alcohol** or any other **CNS depressant** does not seem to have been studied, but during the clinical trials of topiramate it was noted that the incidence of drowsiness, confusion, impaired concentration, dizziness and fatigue was increased.[1] This would seem to be the basis of the statement by the makers of topiramate[2] that ". . . drowsiness is likely and *Topamax* may be more sedating than other antiepileptic drugs. These adverse events could potentially be dangerous in patients driving a vehicle or operating machinery."

It would therefore seem prudent to warn patients about this side-effect, and to suggest caution with alcohol and any other drug which has CNS depressant effects which could possibly be additive.

1. Topamax (Topiramate). Product monograph. Janssen-Cilag, September 1995.
2. Topamax (Topiramate). Janssen-Cilag Ltd. Summary of product characteristics, September 2001.

Topiramate + Anticonvulsants

The serum levels of phenytoin in some patients are slightly raised by topiramate, and topiramate serum levels may be reduced by carbamazepine or phenytoin. Topiramate appears not to interact adversely with phenobarbital, primidone or sodium valproate.

Clinical evidence

(a) Carbamazepine

Topiramate had no effect on the serum levels of the **carbamazepine** or on its main metabolite, but topiramate serum levels and AUC were about 40% lower when taken with **carbamazepine** compared with topiramate alone in a study in 12 epileptic patients.[1-3] Another study in epileptic patients confirmed that topiramate does not affect the pharmacokinetics of **carbamazepine**. However, in contrast, this study found that **carbamazepine** did not have a significant effect on the pharmacokinetics of topiramate.[4]

(b) Phenytoin

Topiramate was given to 12 epileptics stabilised on 260 to 600 mg **phenytoin** daily. The **phenytoin** increased the clearance of topiramate two to threefold. Half of the patients showed a decreased **phenytoin** clearance and an increased **phenytoin** AUC (raised about 25%) due to the topiramate, but the other half showed no changes.[5,6] This slight increase is said not to be clinically significant based on analyses from 6 add-on trials.[7]

(c) Phenobarbital or Primidone

A double blind, placebo-controlled study in 5 centres found that over periods of 8 to 12 weeks the serum levels of **phenobarbital** or **primidone** in outpatients (number not stated) with partial seizures remained unchanged while concurrently taking topiramate.[8]

(d) Sodium valproate

In a study in 12 epileptic patients, the pharmacokinetics of both topiramate and **sodium valproate** were slightly changed by concurrent treatment (topiramate AUC raised about 18%, **sodium valproate** AUC reduced 11.3%) but no clinically relevant changes occurred in a study in 12 epileptic patients.[9,10]

Mechanism

An *in vitro* study using human liver microsomes found that topiramate does not inhibit most hepatic cytochrome P450 isoenzymes, except for CYP2C19.[11] Since this isoenzyme is concerned with phenytoin but not carbamazepine metabolism, the interaction with phenytoin but not with carbamazepine would appear to be explained. The effect of carbamazepine and phenytoin on topiramate serum levels would possibly be caused by hepatic enzyme induction.

Importance and management

The topiramate/carbamazepine interaction, which possibly results in a moderate reduction in topiramate serum levels, appears to be established, but of limited clinical importance. The topiramate/phenytoin interaction also appears to be established. In both cases concurrent use seems largely to be advantageous, but check on the need to raise the topiramate dosage. No reduction in the phenytoin dosage seems necessary. There seems to be nothing to suggest that any adverse interaction occurs between topiramate and phenobarbital, primidone or sodium valproate.

1. Sachdeo S, Sachdeo R. Topiramate-Tegretol interaction. *Neurology* (1994) 44 (Suppl 2), A205.
2. Doose DR, Walker SA, Sachdeo R, Kramer LD, Nayak RK. Steady-state pharmacokinetics of Tegretol® (carbamazepine) and Topamax™ (topiramate) in patients with epilepsy on monotherapy and during combination therapy. *Epilepsia* (1994) 35 (Suppl 8), 54.
3. Sachdeo RC, Sachdeo SK, Walker SA, Kramer LD, Nayak RK, Doose DR. Steady-state pharmacokinetics of topiramate and carbamazepine in patients with epilepsy during monotherapy and concomitant therapy. *Epilepsia* (1996) 37, 774–80.
4. Wilensky AJ, Ojemann LM, Chemelir T, Margul BL, Doose DR. Topiramate pharmacokinetics in epileptic patients receiving carbamazepine. *Epilepsia* (1989) 30, 645–6.
5. Gisclon LG, Curtin CR, Kramer LD. A comparative study of the steady-state pharmacokinetics of phenytoin (Dilantin® Kapseals® brand) and topiramate (Topamax®) in male and female epileptic patients on monotherapy, and during combination therapy. *Pharm Res* (1994) 11 (10 Suppl), S-445.
6. Gisclon LG, Curtin CR, Kramer LD. The steady-state (SS) pharmacokinetics (PK) of phenytoin (Dilantin®) and topiramate (Topamax®) in epileptic patients on monotherapy and during combination therapy. *Epilepsia* (1994) 35 (Suppl 8), 54.
7. Johannessen SI. Pharmacokinetics and interaction profile of topiramate: review and comparison with other newer antiepileptic drugs. *Epilepsia* (1997) 38 (Suppl 1), S18–S23.
8. Doose DR, Walker SA, Pledger G, Lim P, Reife RA. Evaluation of phenobarbital and primidone/phenobarbital (primidone's active metabolite) plasma concentrations during administration of add-on topiramate therapy in five multicenter, double-blind, placebo-controlled trials in outpatients with partial seizures. *Epilepsia* (1995) 36 (Suppl 3), S158.
9. Liao S, Rosenfeld WE, Palmer M, Schaefer P, Pace K, Kramer LD, Nayak RK. The steady-state pharmacokinetics of Topamax™ (topiramate) and valproic acid in patients with epilepsy on monotherapy, and during combination therapy. *Pharm Res* (1994) 11 (10 Suppl), S-444.
10. Rosenfeld WE, Liao S, Kramer LD, Anderson G, Palmer M, Levy RH, Nayak RK. Comparison of the steady-state pharmacokinetics of topiramate and valproate in patients with epilepsy during monotherapy and concomitant therapy. *Epilepsia* (1997) 38, 324–33.
11. Levy RH, Bishop F, Streeter AJ, Trager WF, Kunze KL, Thummel KT, Mather GG. Explanation and prediction of drug interactions with topiramate using a CYP450 inhibition spectrum. *Epilepsia* (1995) 36 (Suppl 4), 47.

Valproate semisodium + Miscellaneous drugs

Valproate semisodium (semisodium valproate, divalproex sodium) is a coordination compound of sodium valproate and valproic acid in a 1:1 molar ratio. There is nothing to suggest that the interactions of this compound will not be the same as those seen with sodium valproate. See the Index.

Vigabatrin + Clomipramine

An isolated case report describes mania in an epileptic patient on vigabatrin attributed to the addition of clomipramine.

Clinical evidence, mechanism, importance and management

An isolated report describes an epileptic man on carbamazepine and clobazam who was started on 2 g vigabatrin daily for better seizure control. About a month after 35 mg **clomipramine** daily was started for depression the patient developed mania. The authors of the report attributed the mania to an interaction between the vigabatrin and the **clomipramine**.[1] No general conclusions can be based this single report.

1. Sastre-Garau P, Thomas P, Beaussart M, Goudemand M. Accès maniaque consécutif à une association vigabatrin-clomipramine. *Encephale* (1993) 19, 351–2.

Vigabatrin + Felbamate

No clinically relevant pharmacokinetic interactions appear to occur between vigabatrin and felbamate.

Clinical evidence, mechanism, importance and management

In a study of 16 subjects, 2400 mg **felbamate** daily increased the AUC of 2000 mg vigabatrin daily by 13%, which is unlikely to be clinically significant. In a second study using a further 18 subjects, no changes were detected in **felbamate** pharmacokinetics.[1] There would therefore seem to be no reason for avoiding concurrent use.

1. Reidenberg P, Glue P, Banfield C, Colucci R, Meehan J, Rey E, Radwanski E, Nomeir A, Lim J, Lin C, Guillaume M, Affrime MB. Pharmacokinetic interaction studies between felbamate and vigabatrin. *Br J Clin Pharmacol* (1995) 40, 157–60.

Zonisamide + Anticonvulsants

Phenobarbital, phenytoin and carbamazepine can cause a small to moderate reduction in the serum levels of zonisamide, while zonisamide shows variable effects on carbamazepine serum levels, but no important adverse interactions appear to occur. Clonazepam and sodium valproate appear not to interact.

Clinical evidence

(a) Effect of other anticonvulsants on zonisamide

The concurrent administration of **phenobarbital**, **phenytoin** or **carbamazepine** significantly reduced the ratio of serum level to administered dose of zonisamide (i.e. zonisamide serum levels were reduced) in one study, whereas **clonazepam** and **sodium valproate** were found not to interact.[1] In another study in 12 epileptic children taking 8.6 to 13.6 mg/kg zonisamide daily, 12.1 to 18.1 mg/kg daily **carbamazepine** reduced zonisamide serum levels by about 35 to 37%.[2] Another study found that **phenobarbital** increased the clearance of zonisamide from the body approximately twofold.[3]

In an early study in 2 groups of patients, one taking **carbamazepine** and the other **phenytoin**, it was noted that the zonisamide AUC following a single 400-mg dose was higher in the **carbamazepine** group than the **phenytoin** group.[4] The plasma protein binding of zonisamide is unaffected by other anticonvulsants (**phenobarbital**, **phenytoin**, **carbamazepine**, **sodium valproate**).[5]

(b) Effect of zonisamide on other anticonvulsants

In one study the proportion of the major metabolite of **carbamazepine**, carbamazepine-10,11-epoxide, in the serum was decreased when zonisamide was used concurrently, suggesting that zonisamide reduces **carbamazepine** metabolism.[1] An early pilot study in 10 patients had also noted a consistent rise in **carbamazepine** serum levels following initiation of zonisamide therapy.[6] The opposite effect was seen in a study of 16 paediatric patients in whom zonisamide reduced the ratio of **carbamazepine** serum levels to dose and increased the relative amount of its major metabolite in the serum, suggesting that zonisamide increases the metabolism of **carbamazepine**. However, the free fraction of carbamazepine remained unaltered.[7] Contrasting with all of these studies are two others which found no changes in the serum levels of **carbamazepine** or its metabolite when zonisamide was used.[2,8]

When 10 patients on **phenytoin** additionally took 300 to 600 mg zonisamide daily, the **phenytoin** serum levels were unaffected.[8] Another study in 21 paediatric patients found that zonisamide did not affect the serum levels (or protein binding) of **phenytoin** or **sodium valproate**.[9] A further study in 139 patients similarly found no marked changes in the serum levels of existing antiepileptic drugs (**carbamazepine**, **phenytoin**, **phenobarbital**, **primidone**, **valproic acid**)

when giving zonisamide as an add-on therapy but reported that the incidence of adverse effects, mainly fatigue, somnolence, dizziness and ataxia was higher with zonisamide (59.2%) than with the placebo (27.9%).[10]

Mechanism

Uncertain. It seems possible that phenobarbital, phenytoin and carbamazepine can induce the metabolism of zonisamide thereby reducing its serum levels.

Importance and management

None of these studies reported any major problems during concurrent use of zonisamide and these other antiepileptic drugs. There is the possibility of serum level alterations with phenobarbital, phenytoin and carbamazepine so that it would be prudent to monitor patients taking any of these combinations.

1. Shinoda M, Akita M, Hasegawa M, Hasegawa T, Nabeshima T. The necessity of adjusting the dosage of zonisamide when coadministered with other anti-epileptic drugs. *Biol Pharm Bull* (1996) 19, 1090–2.
2. Abo J, Miura H, Takanashi S, Shirai H, Sunaoshi W, Hosoda N, Abo K, Takei K. Drug interaction between zonisamide and carbamazepine: a pharmacokinetic study in children with cryptogenic localization-related epilepsies. *Epilepsia* (1995) 36 (Suppl 3), S162.
3. Schentag JJ, Gengo FM, Wilton AJ, Sedman AJ, Grasela TH, Bockbrader HN. Influence of phenobarbital, cimetidine, and renal disease on zonisamide kinetics. *Pharm Res* (1987) 4 (Suppl), S-79.
4. Ojemann LM, Shastri RA, Wilensky AJ, Friel PN, Levy RH, McLean JR, Buchanan RA. Comparative pharmacokinetics of zonisamide (CI-912) in epileptic patients on carbamazepine or phenytoin monotherapy. *Ther Drug Monit* (1986) 8, 293–6.
5. Kimura M, Tanaka N, Kimura Y, Miyake K, Kitaura T, Fukuchi H, Harada Y. Factors influencing serum concentration of zonisamide in epileptic patients. *Chem Pharm Bull (Tokyo)* (1992) 40, 193–5.
6. Sackellares JC, Donofrio PD, Wagner JG, Abou-Khalil B, Berent S, Aasved-Hoyt K. Pilot study of zonisamide (1,2-Benzisoxazole-3-methanesulfonamide) in patients with refractory partial seizures. *Epilepsia* (1985) 26, 206–11.
7. Minami T, Ieiri I, Ohtsubo K, Hirakawa Y, Ueda K, Higuchi S, Aoyama T. Influence of additional therapy with zonisamide (Excegran) on protein binding and metabolism of carbamazepine. *Epilepsia* (1994) 35, 1023–5.
8. Browne TR, Szabo GK, Kres J, Pylilo RJ. Drug interactions of zonisamide (CI–912) with phenytoin and carbamazepine. *J Clin Pharmacol* (1986) 26, 555.
9. Tasaki K, Minami T, Ieiri I, Ohtsubo K, Hirakawa Y, Ueda K, Higuchi S. Drug interactions of zonisamide with phenytoin and sodium valproate: serum concentrations and protein binding. *Brain Dev* (1995) 17, 182–5.
10. Schmidt D, Jacob R, Loiseau P, Deisenhammer E, Klinger D, Despland A, Egli M, Bauer G, Stenzel E, Blankenhorn V. Zonisamide for add-on treatment of refractory partial epilepsy: a European double-blind trial. *Epilepsy Res* (1993) 15, 67–73.

Zonisamide + Cimetidine

Cimetidine does not appear to alter zonisamide pharmacokinetics.

Clinical evidence, mechanism, importance and management

When single oral doses of 300 mg zonisamide were given to healthy subjects, it was found that **cimetidine** (dose not stated) did not affect the zonisamide clearance, half-life, apparent volume of distribution or the amount of drug recovered from the urine. The drugs were well tolerated.[1] No special precautions would seem to be needed if both drugs are used.

1. Schentag JJ, Gengo FM, Wilton JH, Sedman AJ, Grasela TH, Brockbrader HN. Influence of phenobarbital, cimetidine, and renal disease on zonisamide kinetics. *Pharm Res* (1987) 4 (Suppl), S-79.

8

Antihypertensive drug interactions

Hypertension (elevated blood pressure) can be controlled by the use of a very wide spectrum of drugs acting either centrally within the brain or peripherally. The drugs dealt with in this chapter include the centrally acting drugs (clonidine, methyldopa), adrenergic neurone blockers (guanethidine), vasodilators (alpha-1 blockers such as prazosin, indoramin and others whose mode of action is uncertain — e.g. hydralazine, diazoxide), angiotensin converting enzyme (ACE) in-

hibitors, angiotensin II antagonists and diuretics. The beta-blockers, calcium channel blockers, and pargyline (MAOI) are dealt with in separate chapters. Table 8.1 lists the drugs dealt with in this chapter and some of their proprietary names. Where these drugs are the affecting agent rather than the drug affected, the interactions are described elsewhere. The Index must be consulted for a full listing of all the interactions.

Table 8.1 Antihypertensive drugs

Generic names	Proprietary names
ACE inhibitors	
Benazepril	Briem, Cibace, Cibacen, Cibacene, Labopal, Lotensin, Tensanil, Zinadril
Captopril	Acenorm, Aceomel, Acepress, Acepril, Aceril, ACE-Hemmer, Actopril, Adocor, Alopresin, Aorten, Apocapen, Apo-Capto, Atrisol, Biodezil, Bugazon, Calpix, Capace, Capoten, Capotena , Capti, Captil, Captirex, Capto, Captobeta, Captodan, Captodoc, Captoflux, Captogamma, Captohexal, Captol, Captolane, Captomax, Captomed, Captomerck, Captomin, Captor, Captoser, Captosol, Captostad, Captotec, Captotyrol, Capto-basan, Capto-dura M, Captral, Captril, Captrizin, Cardiace, Cardiagen, Cardipril, Carencil, Catona, Catonet, Catoprol, Cesplon, Convertal, Cor tensobon, Coronorm, Cryopril, Dardex, Debax, Dilabar, Ecapresan, Ecaten, Ecopace, Enzace, Epicordin, Epsitron, Garanil, Gemzil, Geroten, Hipertex, Hipertil, Hipocatril, Hipotensil, Inhibace, Kaplon, Katopril, Kenolan, Ketanine, Keyerpril, Kimafan, Lenpryl, Lopirin, Lopril, Mereprine, Midrat, Mundil, Novapres, Nu-Capto, Oltens, Prilovase, Reductel, Rilcapton, Romir, Sansanal, Sigacap Cor, Tensiomin, Tensobon, Tensoprel, Tensopril, Tensostad, Toprilem, Vidapril, Zapto
Cilazapril	Dynorm, Inhibace, Inibace, Initiss, Inocar, Justor, Vascase
Delapril	Adecut, Cupressin, Delaket, Delakete
Enalapril/Enalaprilat	Acepril, Aceren, Acetensil, Alacor, Alphapril, Amprace, Anapril, Angiopril, Atens, Balpril, Baripril, Benalapril, Bionafil, Bitensil, Blocatril, Blootec, Cetampril, Clipto, Controlvas, Converten, Convertin, Corodil, Corprilor, Crinoren, Dabonal, Daren, Denapril, Ditensor, Ednyt, Enac, Enacard, Enadil, Enadura, Enahexal, Enalabene, Enaladil, Enalagamma, Enaloc, Enam, Enap, Enapren, Enapress, Enapril, Enaprotec, Enaran, Enaril, Enasifar, Enatec, Enatyrol, Enoval, Epril, Eupressin, Feliberal, Glioten, Herten, Hipoartel, Hypace, Iecatec, Imotoran, Innomel, Innovace, Insup, Invoril, Istopril, Kenopril, Korandil, Lapril, Linatil, Lipraken, Maleapril, Mepril, Nacor, Nalopril, Naprilene, Narapril, Naritec, Neolapril, Neotensin, Norpril, Palane, Pharmapress, Pralenal, Pres, Pressel, Pressitan, Pressotec, Pulsol, Quimalan, Reca, Renaton, Renipril , Renistad, Renitec, Reniten, Ristalen, Tensazol, Vasopril, Vasotec, Xanef
Fosinopril	Dynacil, Eliten, Fosinil, Fosinorm, Fosipres, Fositen, Fositens, Fozitec, Hicarlex, Hiperlex, Monopril, NewAce, Staril, Tenso Stop, Tensocardil, Tensogard, Vasopril
Imidapril	Tranatril
Lisinopril	Acemin, Acepril, Acerbon, Acetan, Alapril, Alfaken, Carace, Coric, Doneka, Farpresse, Fibsol, Hypomed, Iricil, Lanatin, Likenil, Linopril, Lipril, Lisigamma, Lisihexal, Lisinotyrol, Lisipril, Lisodur, Lisodura, Lispril, Novatec, Prinil, Prinivil, Secubar, Tensikey, Tensopril, Vasojet, Vivatec, Zestomax, Zestril
Moexipril	Femipres, Fempress, Moex, Perdix, Primoxil, Univasc
Pentopril	
Perindopril	Aceon, Acertil, Coversum, Coversyl, Procaptan

continued overleaf

Table 8.1 Antihypertensive drugs *(continued)*

Generic names	Proprietary names
Quinapril	*Accupril, Accuprin, Accupro, Acequin, Acuitel, Acuprel, Acupril, Acuretic, Asig, Ectren, Korec, Lidaltrin, Quinazil*
Ramipril	*Acovil, Altace, Carasel, Cardace, Delix, Hypren, Naprix, Pramace, Quark, Ramace, Triatec, Tritace, Unipril, Vesdil*
Spirapril	*Cardiopril, Quadropril, Renormax, Renpress, Setrilan*
Trandolapril	*Gopten, Mavik, Odric, Odrik, Preran, Udrik*

Adrenergic neurone blockers

Betanidine (Bethanidine)	
Debrisoquine	*Declinax*
Guanadrel	*Hylorel*
Guanethidine	*Ismelin*

Alpha-blocking agents

Alfuzosin	*Alfetim, Benestan, Dalfaz, Mittoval, Urion, UroXatral, Xatral*
Bunazosin	*Andante, Detantol*
Doxazosin	*Alfadil, Benur, Cadex, Cardoral, Cardoxan, Cardular PP, Cardura, Carduran, Dedralen, Diblocin, Doxacor, Doxagamma, Doxaloc, Doxazobene, Doxazomerck, Doxa-Puren, Normothen, Prodil, Progandol, Prostadilat, Supressin, Unoprost, Zoflux*
Indoramin	*Baratol, Doralese, Vidora, Wydora, Wypresin*
Phenoxybenzamine	*Dibenyline, Dibenzyline, Dibenzyran*
Phentolamine	*Herivyl, Q-Tech, Regitin, Regitina, Regitine, Rogitine, Vasomax, Z-Max*
Prazosin	*Adversuten, Alphavase, Alpress, Anapres, Apo-Prazo, Atodel, duramipress, Eurex, Hexapress, Hypotens, Hypovase, Hyprosin, Lopress, Minima, Minipres, Minipress, Mipraz, Mysial, Novo-Prazin, Nu-Prazo, Parabowl, Peripress, Polypress, Prasig, Pratsiol, Prazac, Prazohexal, Pressin, Sinozzard*
Tamsulosin	*Alna, Expros, Flomax, Harnal, Josir, Omix, Omnic, Pradif, Secotex, Urolosin*
Terazosin	*Adecur, Deflox, Dysalfa, Ezosina, Flotrin, Heitrin, Hytrin, Hytrin BPH, Hytrine, Hytrinex, Itrin, Magnurol, Sinalfa, Teraprost, Unoprost, Urodie, Uroflo, Vicard*
Urapidil	*Ebrantil, Elgadil, Eupressyl, Mediatensyl*

Angiotensin II antagonists

Candesartan	*Amias, Atacand, Blopress, Kenzen, Parapres, Ratacand*
Eprosartan	*Teveten, Tevetens*
Irbesartan	*Aprovel, Avapro, Irban, Karvea*
Losartan	*Corus, Cosaar, Cozaar, Loortan, Lortaan, Lorzaar, Losaprex, Losatal, Neo-Lotan, Nu-Lotan, Ocsaar, Redupress*
Telmisartan	*Micardis, Pritor*
Valsartan	*Diovan, Diovane, Kalpress, Nisis, Provas, Tareg, Valpression, Vals*

Beta-blockers

see Tables 10.1 to 10.4 in Chapter 10	

Calcium channel blockers

see Table 11.1 in Chapter 11	

Centrally-acting agents

Clonidine	*Adesipress-TTS, Aruclonin, Atensina, Catapres, Catapresan, Catapressan, Clonid-Ophtal, Clonistada, Clonnirit, Dispaclonidin, Dixarit, Duraclon, Edolglau, Epiclodina, Glausine, Haemiton, Isoglaucon, Mirfat, Normopresan, Paracefan*
Guanfacine	*Akfen, Estulic, Tenex*
Methyldopa	*Aldomet, Aldometil, Aldomin, Aldopren, Amender, Biotenzol, Dopamed, Dopamet, Dopasian, Dopegyt, Hydopa, Hy-Po-Tone, Isomet, Medomet, Medopa, Medopate, Medopren, Mefba, Meldopa, Normopress, Novo-Medopa, Nu-Medopa, Presinol, Prodopa, Servidopa, Siamdopa, Sinepress, Toparal*
Moxonidine	*Cynt, Moxon, Normatens, Normoxin, Physiotens*
Rilmenidine	*Hyperium, Iterium*

Table 8.1 Antihypertensive drugs *(continued)*

Generic names	Proprietary names
Directly-acting vasodilators	
Diazoxide	Eudemine, Glicemin, Hyperstat, Hypertonalum, Proglicem, Proglycem, Sefulken, Tensuril
Hydralazine	Alphapress, Apresolin, Apresolina, Apresoline, Bionobal, Cesoline, Hydrapres, Hyperphen, Novo-Hylazin, Nu-Hydral, Rolazine
Minoxidil	Alopexy, Alostil, Aloxidil, Apohair, Apo-Gain, Folcress, Hairgaine, Headway, Lacovin, Loniten, Lonnoten, Lonolox, Lonoten, Mantai, Minocalve, Minovital, Minox, Minoxi, Minoximen, Minoxitrim, Modil, Moxiral, Neocapil, Neoxidil, Normoxidil, Noxidil, Nuhair, Piloxil , Recrea, Regaine, Regro, Riteban, Rogaine, Tricovivax, Tricoxidil, Unipexil
Tolazoline	Priscol, Priscoline, Vaso-Dilatan
Diuretics	
see also Table 14.2 in Chapter 14	
Acetazolamide	Acetadiazol, Azomid, Carbinib, Dazamide, Defiltran, Diamox, Diuramid, Edemox, Glaupax, Odemin, Uramox
Potassium depleters	
Azosemide	Luret
Bumetanide	Betinex, Bumedyl, Bumex, Burinax, Burinex, Drenural, Farmadiuril, Fontego, Fordiuran, Miccil
Chlortalidone (Chlorthalidone)	Aquadon, Bioralin, Clortalil, Hidrona, Higroton, Higrotona, Hydro-long, Hygroton, Igroton, Thalitone
Etacrynic acid (Ethacrynic acid)	Edecril, Edecrin, Hydromedin, Reomax
Furosemide (Frusemide)	Aldic, Aquarid, Aquedux, Beurises, Biomisen, Butosali, Dirine, Diural, Diurapid, Diuret, Diurex, Diurin, Diurit, Diurix, Dryptal, Durafurid, Edenol, Froop, Frusehexal, Frusid, Frusol, Fudirine, Fural, Furanthril, Furese , Furesin, Furesis, Furetic, Furide, Furix, Furo, Furobeta, Furodrix, Furohexal, Furomed, Furomin, Furon, Furorese, Furosal, Furosan, Furosifar, Furostad, Furotyrol, Furovite, Furo-basan, Furo-BASF, Furo-Puren, Fursol, Fusid, Hawkmide, Henexal, Hydrex, Hydro-rapid, H-Mide, Impugan, Lasiletten, Lasilix, Lasix, Mediuresix, Miphar, Odemase, Oedemex, Osemin, Puresis, Rusyde, Salurin, Seguril, Selectofur, Sigasalur, Tenkafruse, Urasin, Uremide, Urex, Vesix, Zafimida
Metolazone	Diulo, Metenix 5, Mykrox, Zaroxolyn, Zaroxolyne
Piretanide	Arelix, Diural, Eurelix, Perbilen, Tauliz
Thiazides	
Torasemide (Torsemide)	Demadex, Dilutol, Diuremid, Diuresix, Isodiur, Sutril, Toradiur, Torem, Torrem, Unat
Potassium sparers	
Amiloride	Amikal, Amilamont, Berkamil, Kaluril, Medamor, Midamor, Midoride, Modamide, Nirulid
Canrenoate	Aldactone, Canrenol, Kalium-Can, Kanrenol, Luvion, Osyrol, Soldactone, Soludactone, Venactone
Spironolactone	Aldactone, Aldonar, Aldopur, Aldospirone, Altone, Aquareduct, Berlactone, Biolactona, duraspiron, Flumach, Hexalacton, Jenaspiron, Laractone, Nefrolactona, Novo-Spiroton, Osyrol, Practon, Primacton, Quimolactona, Spiractin, Spiresis, Spiretic, Spiridon, Spirix, Spiro, Spirobene, Spiroctan, Spiroderm, Spirohexal, Spirolang, Spiron, Spironex, Spirono, Spironol, Spironone, Spiropal, Spiroscand, Spirospare, Spirotone, Tensin, Uractone, Uractonum, Verospiron, Xenalon
Triamterene	Dyrenium, Dytac, Urocaudal
Rauwolfia alkaloids	
Reserpine	Rauserpin, Reserpina
Serotonin blockers	
Ketanserin	Ketensin, Perketan, Serepress, Sufrexal

ACE inhibitors + Albumin Solution

Acute hypotension has been seen in patients taking enalapril when rapidly infused with a stable plasma protein solution (SPPS).

Clinical evidence

A woman on **enalapril** (10 mg in the morning) underwent surgery for groin lymph node resection under spinal and general anaesthesia. When rapidly infused with 500 ml of the human albumin solution, **stable plasma protein solution** (*SPPS, Commonwealth Serum Laboratories, Melbourne, Australia*), her pulse rose to 90 to 100 bpm and systolic blood pressure fell from 100 to 60 mmHg and a red flush was noted on all exposed skin. The blood pressure was controlled with metaraminol (4.5 mg over 10 min) at 90 to 95 mmHg. When the *SPPS* was finished, the blood pressure and pulse rate spontaneously restabilised.[1]

Two very similar cases involving patients on **enalapril** when given *SPPS* have been recorded by the same author.[2,3]

Mechanism

Not fully established, but it is believed that *SPPS* contains low levels of pre-kallikrein activator which stimulates the production of bradykinin and other kinases which can cause vasodilatation and hypotension. Normally they are destroyed by kininase II (ACE), but with the ACE inhibited by the enalapril, their inactivation appear to be delayed so that their hypotensive effects are exaggerated and prolonged.[3,4]

Importance and management

An established interaction of clinical importance. The authors of one report suggest that if rapid expansion of intravascular volume is needed in patients taking ACE inhibitors, an artificial colloid might be a safer choice than *SPPS*.[1] The maker of *SPPS* also recommends an alternative plasma volume expander, including other albumin solutions.[5] There appear to be no reports about other ACE inhibitors but they would be expected to interact similarly.

1. McKenzie AJ. Possible interaction between SPPS and enalapril. *Anaesth Intensive Care* (1990) 18, 124–6.
2. Young K. Enalapril and SPPS. *Anesth Intensive Care* (1990) 18, 583.
3. Young K. Hypotension from the interaction of ACE inhibitors with stable plasma protein solution. *Anaesthesia* (1993) 48, 356.
4. Bonner G, Preis S, Schunk U, Toussaint C, Kaufman W. Haemodynamic effects of bradykinin on systemic and pulmonary circulation in healthy and hypertensive patients. *J Cardiovasc Pharmacol* (1990) 15, S46–S56.
5. Schiff P. SPPS, hypotension, and ACE inhibitors. *Med J Aust* (1992) 156, 363.

ACE inhibitors + Allopurinol

Three cases of serious Stevens-Johnson syndrome (one fatal) and two cases of hypersensitivity have been attributed to the concurrent use of captopril and allopurinol. Neutropenia and serious infection has also occurred. Anaphylaxis and myocardial infarction occurred in one man on enalapril when given allopurinol.

Clinical evidence

An elderly man with hypertension, chronic renal failure, congestive heart failure and mild polyarthritis on multiple drug treatment, which included **captopril** (50 mg daily) and diuretics, developed fatal Stevens-Johnson syndrome within 5 weeks of starting to take **allopurinol** 100 mg twice daily.[1] It was noted that the maker of **captopril** was aware of 2 other patients on **captopril** who developed the syndrome 3 to 5 weeks after **allopurinol** was started.[1] A later report describes fever, arthralgia and myalgia in a man chronic renal failure similarly treated. He improved when the **captopril** was withdrawn.[2] Exfoliatory facial dermatitis was seen in another patient with renal failure.[3] No significant pharmacokinetic changes were seen in 12 normal subjects

given 50 mg **allopurinol** twice daily and 300 mg **captopril** daily for three and a half days.[4] A man on **enalapril** had an acute anaphylactic reaction with severe coronary spasm, culminating in myocardial infarction, within 20 min of taking 100 mg **allopurinol**. He recovered.[5]

The maker of **captopril** also warns that neutropenia, resulting in serious infection, has occurred in patients on **captopril**, and that concurrent treatment with **allopurinol** may be a complicating factor, especially in those with renal impairment.[6]

Mechanism

Not understood. It is uncertain whether these are interactions, because allopurinol alone can cause severe hypersensitivity reactions, particularly in the presence of renal failure and the use of diuretics. Captopril can also induce a hypersensitivity reaction.

Importance and management

These interactions are not clearly established, and what happened is rare and unpredictable. All that can be constructively said is that patients on both drugs should be very closely monitored for any signs of hypersensitivity (e.g. skin reactions) or infection (sore throat, fever), especially if they have renal impairment. The maker of captopril recommends that differential white blood cell counts should be performed prior to therapy, every 2 weeks during the first 3 months of captopril, and periodically thereafter.[6] No pharmacokinetic interaction seems to occur. The makers of a number of other ACE inhibitors (e.g. **cilazapril**, **enalapril**, **imidapril**, **moexipril**, **trandolapril**) now state in their prescribing information that concomitant administration of ACE inhibitors and allopurinol may lead to an increased risk of leucopenia.[7-11] See also 'ACE inhibitors + Azathioprine', p.372 and 'Captopril + Procainamide', p.386.

1. Pennell DJ, Nunan TO, O'Doherty MJ, Croft DN. Fatal Stevens-Johnson syndrome in a patient on captopril and allopurinol. *Lancet* (1984) i, 463.
2. Samanta A, Burden AC. Fever, myalgia and arthralgia in a patient on captopril and allopurinol. *Lancet* (1984) i, 679.
3. Beeley L, Daly M, Stewart P. Bulletin West Midlands Centre for Adverse Drug Reaction Reporting (1987) 24, 9.
4. Levinson B, Sugarman AA, Stern M, Waclawski A, Manning J. Lack of kinetic interaction of captopril and allopurinol in healthy subjects. Proc Am Soc Hypertension (New York) 1987, p 129.
5. Ahmad S. Allopurinol and enalapril. Drug induced anaphylactic coronary spasm and acute myocardial infarction. *Chest* (1995) 108, 586.
6. Capoten (Captopril). E. R. Squibb & Sons Limited. Summary of product characteristics, July 2001.
7. Vascace (Cilazapril). Roche Products Ltd. Summary of product characteristics, December 2001.
8. Innovace (Enalapril). Merck Sharp & Dohme Ltd. Summary of product characteristics, May 2002.
9. Tanatril (Imidapril). Trinity Pharmaceuticals Ltd. Summary of product characteristics, March 2001.
10. Perdix (Moexipril). Schwarz Pharma Ltd. Summary of product characteristics, November 2001.
11. Gopten (Trandolapril). Abbot Laboratories Limited. Summary of product characteristics, December 2001.

ACE inhibitors + Antacids

Antacids have been found to reduce the absorption of captopril and fosinopril by about one-third, but this is unlikely to be clinically important. Antacids did not affect the pharmacokinetics of ramiprilat.

Clinical evidence, mechanism, importance and management

An antacid containing **aluminium hydroxide**, **magnesium carbonate** and **magnesium hydroxide** reduced the AUC of 50 mg **captopril** in 10 healthy subjects by about 40%. However, this did not alter the extent of the reduction in blood pressure.[1] Another study found that *Mylanta* (**aluminium and magnesium hydroxides**) similarly reduced the bioavailability of **fosinopril** 20 mg by about one-third.[2] The mechanism of this interaction is uncertain, but is unlikely to be due to elevated gastric pH since cimetidine did not have a similar effect.[2] Note that greater decreases in **captopril** bioavailability (caused by food) where found not to be clinically relevant (see 'Antihypertensives + Food', p.383), therefore, it is unlikely these changes will be clinically important. However, the makers of **fosinopril** suggest[3] separating administration of **fosinopril** and **antacids** by at least 2 h. It is briefly noted in a review that **antacid** administration did not affect the pharmacokinetics of ramiprilat, the active metabolite of **ramipril**.[4]

1. Mäntylä R, Männistö PT, Vuorela A, Sundberg S, Ottoila P. Impairment of captopril bioavailability by concomitant food and antacid intake. *Int J Clin Pharmacol Ther Toxicol* (1984) 22, 626–9.
2. Moore L, Kramer A, Swites B, Kramer P, Tu J. Effect of cimetidine and antacid on the kinetics of the active diacid of fosinopril in healthy subjects. *J Clin Pharmacol* (1988) 28, 946.
3. Staril (Fosinopril), E. R. Squibb & Sons Ltd. Summary of product characteristics, August 2001.
4. Todd PA, Benfield P. Ramipril. A review of its pharmacological properties and therapeutic efficacy in cardiovascular disorders. *Drugs* (1990) 39, 110–35.

ACE inhibitors + Aspirin and NSAIDs

The antihypertensive effects of captopril, enalapril, lisinopril and possibly cilazapril and perindopril can be reduced by indometacin. Low-dose aspirin (<300 mg daily) appears to have little effect on the antihypertensive efficacy of captopril and enalapril, but high-dose aspirin may reduce it in about 50% of patients. Ibuprofen reduced the antihypertensive efficacy of captopril. Lornoxicam caused a small rise in diastolic pressure in those on enalapril. Celecoxib had a minor effect on the efficacy of lisinopril in a single study. However, a case report describes an increase in blood pressure with rofecoxib and lisinopril. Sulindac had little or no effect on blood pressure in those on captopril or enalapril.

It is unclear whether aspirin attenuates the benefits of ACE inhibitors in coronary artery disease and heart failure. The likelihood of an interaction may depend on disease state. The combination of NSAID and ACE inhibitor may increase the risk of renal impairment. Rarely, hyperkalaemia has been associated with the combination.

Clinical evidence

(A) Effects on blood pressure

(a) Aspirin

(i) Captopril. In 8 patients with essential hypertension, **aspirin** 600 mg six-hourly for 5 doses did not significantly alter the blood pressure response to a single dose of **captopril** (25 to 100 mg), but 4 of the 8 did show a 35% reduction in the response to captopril.[1,2] In another study, **aspirin** 75 mg daily did not alter the antihypertensive effects of **captopril** 25 mg twice daily in 15 patients with hypertension.[3]

(ii) Enalapril. Two groups of 26 patients, one with mild to moderate hypertension on 20 mg **enalapril** twice daily and the other with severe primary hypertension on 20 mg **enalapril** twice daily (plus 30 mg nifedipine and 50 mg atenolol daily), were additionally given test doses of 100 and 300 mg **aspirin** daily. The 100-mg dose of **aspirin** did not alter the efficacy of the antihypertensive drugs, but the 300-mg dose reduced the antihypertensive efficacy in about half the patients in both groups. In these patients, the antihypertensive effects were diminished by 63% in the first group and by 91% in the second.[4] In contrast, another study in 7 patients with hypertension taking **enalapril** (mean daily dose 12.9 mg) found that neither **aspirin** 81 mg nor 325 mg daily had any significant effect on blood pressure.[5] A further study also found that **aspirin** 100 mg daily for 2 weeks did not alter the antihypertensive effect of **enalapril** in 18 patients.[6]

(b) Indometacin (Indomethacin)

(i) Captopril. In a randomised double-blind study, 105 patients with hypertension received captopril 25 to 50 mg twice daily for 6 weeks, which reduced their blood pressure by a mean of 8.6/5.6 mmHg. Indometacin 75 mg once daily was then added for one week, which caused a rise in blood pressure in the group as a whole of 4.6/2.7 mmHg (an attenuation of the effect of captopril of about 50%). Clear attenuation was seen in 67% of the patients, and occurred

regardless of baseline blood pressure.[7] This same interaction has been described in numerous earlier studies in patients with hypertension and in healthy subjects given **indometacin**.[1,2,8-14] A case is described of a man whose blood pressure was well controlled on captopril 75 mg daily (145/80 mmHg). This then rose to 220/120 mmHg when he self-medicated with indometacin 200 mg daily.[15] In contrast, a randomised crossover study in 11 patients found that indometacin 50 mg twice daily did not alter the antihypertensive efficacy of captopril 50 mg twice daily.[16]

(ii) Enalapril. **Indometacin** 50 mg twice daily for 1 week significantly reduced the antihypertensive effect of enalapril 20 to 40 mg once daily by about 18 to 22% in 9 patients with hypertension.[17] In another study in 18 patients, **indometacin** 25 mg three times daily attenuated the antihypertensive effect of **enalapril** 20 to 40 mg daily by about 45% when assessed by 24-hour ambulatory blood-pressure monitoring (9.4/4.1 mm/Hg increase in BP with indometacin), and by 12 to 23% when assessed by clinic blood pressure values.[6] Similar results were found in other studies.[18-21] A single case report describes a patient on **enalapril** 10 mg daily whose hypertension failed to be controlled when 100 mg **indometacin** daily in divided doses was added.[22] However other studies found **indometacin** did not significantly alter the blood pressure response to **enalapril**.[13,16,23,24]

(iii) Lisinopril. **Indometacin** 50 mg three times daily for 2 weeks produced mean blood pressure increases of 5.5/3.2 mmHg in patients on **lisinopril** 10 to 20 mg daily, in a crossover study.[25] Similarly, preliminary results of an earlier study found **indometacin** increased the blood pressure of 9 patients on lisinopril.[19] In contrast, **indometacin** 50 mg twice daily for 4 weeks was found to have little effect on the antihypertensive efficacy of **lisinopril** 40 mg daily in 16 patients in a preliminary report of another study.[26]

(iv) Other ACE inhibitors. A study in 16 hypertensive patients found that 50 mg **indometacin** twice daily reduced the blood pressure lowering effects of 2.5 mg **cilazapril** daily. The reduction was greater when cilazapril was added to indometacin therapy than when indometacin was added to cilazapril therapy (approximately 60% vs 30% reduction).[27] The antihypertensive effects of **perindopril** (4 to 8 mg daily) were found to be reduced by 30% by 50 mg **indometacin** twice daily in 10 hypertensive patients.[28] A brief mention is made in a review that the pharmacodynamics of **ramipril** were unaffected by 3 days of **indometacin** (dosage not stated) in healthy subjects.[29] **Indometacin** 25 mg three times daily did not alter the hypotensive effects of **trandolapril** 2 mg daily in 17 hypertensive patients.[30]

(c) Rofecoxib and other cox-2 selective NSAIDs

A case is described of a patient on **lisinopril** 10 mg daily whose blood pressure rose from 127/78 to 143/89 mmHg when given **rofecoxib** 25 mg daily. His blood pressure was controlled by increasing the dose of **lisinopril** to 20 mg daily.[31] In a double-blind study in hypertensive patients treated with **lisinopril** 10 to 40 mg daily, daytime blood pressure was 2.3/1.6 mmHg higher in 91 patients treated with **celecoxib** 200 mg twice daily for 4 weeks than in 87 patients receiving placebo. **Celecoxib** had no effect on blood pressure during sleep.[32]

(d) Sulindac

In one study, 200 mg **sulindac** twice daily given to patients taking **captopril** caused only a small rise in blood pressure: from 132/92 to 137/95 mmHg.[8] **Sulindac** 150 mg twice daily did not attenuate the blood pressure response to **captopril** when substituted for ibuprofen in an elderly women.[33] **Sulindac** 200 mg twice daily did not blunt the antihypertensive effect of **enalapril** in 9 patients with hypertension.[23,24]

(e) Other NSAIDs

In one single-dose study, **ibuprofen** 800 mg abolished the hypotensive effect of 50 mg **captopril** in 4 healthy subjects when they were on a high sodium diet, but not when they were on a low sodium diet.[11] A case report describes attenuation of the hypertensive effects of **captopril** by ibuprofen in an elderly woman.[33]

A single dose of **lornoxicam** 8 mg was found to have no effect on the systolic blood pressure of 6 hypertensive patients on **enalapril**, but a small rise in diastolic pressure (from 88.2 to 93.3 mmHg) occurred after 2 h.[18] **Oxaprozin** 1200 mg daily for 3 weeks did not affect the pharmacodynamics of **enalapril** 10 to 40 mg daily in 29 patients with hypertension.[34]

(B) Effects in coronary artery disease and heart failure

Various studies have looked at the short-term effects of the combination of ACE inhibitors and aspirin on haemodynamic parameters. Two of the 8 studies reviewed[35] showed aspirin adversely altered the haemodynamic effects of ACE inhibitors whereas the remaining 6 did not. In one of the studies showing an adverse interaction between aspirin and enalapril, **ticlopidine** did not interact adversely.[36] In a study on pulmonary function, **aspirin** 350 mg daily worsened pulmonary diffusion capacity and made the ventilatory response to exercise less effective in patients taking **enalapril** 20 mg daily, but did not exert this effect in the absence of ACE inhibitors.[37]

A number of large trials have used ACE inhibitors with aspirin. There have been sub-group analyses or retrospective reviews of these trials to examine the potential interaction.[38-49] The results are summarised in Table 8.2. However, an editorial[50] disputes the findings of one of these studies.[49]

(C) Effects on renal function

In a retrospective analysis, 3 of 162 patients who had been treated with ACE inhibitors and NSAIDs developed reversible renal failure compared with none of 328 treated with just ACE inhibitors and none of 2278 treated with just NSAIDs. One patient was treated sequentially with **naproxen** then **salsalate** and had a progressive decline in renal function over 19 months after **captopril** was started. Acute renal failure developed in another woman on **captopril** when she started to take **aspirin** for arthritis. Kidney function improved when both were stopped. Another man treated with unnamed **NSAIDs** developed reversible renal failure 4 days after starting to take **captopril**.[51] In another similar analysis in patients aged over 75 years, 2 out of 12 patients given an **ACE inhibitor** and an **NSAID** developed acute renal failure (1 died) and a further 4 showed deterioration in renal function.[52] In contrast, another retrospective analysis found no evidence that the adverse effects of **ACE inhibitors** on renal function were greater in those taking **NSAIDs**.[53] Another study found that **indometacin** 25 mg three times daily did not adversely affect renal function when used concomitantly with **trandolapril** 2 mg daily for 3 weeks in 17 hypertensive patients with normal baseline renal function.[54]

Table 8.2 Sub-group analyses of clinical trials assessing the interaction between aspirin and ACE inhibitors

Aspirin dose	ACE inhibitor	Indication	Finding	Refs
Evidence for an interaction				
Not reported	Enalapril	Heart failure	Combined treatment associated with reduced benefits compared with enalapril alone.	38
Not reported	Enalapril	Post-MI	Effect of enalapril less favourable in those taking aspirin at baseline.	39
Not reported	Not reported	Acute MI	Combined use associated with higher mortality than aspirin alone.	40
325 mg daily	Not reported	Post coronary angioplasty	Combined use associated with higher mortality than aspirin alone.	40
Not reported	Ramipril 5 to 10 mg daily	Acute MI with heart failure	Trend towards greater benefit of ramipril in those not receiving aspirin.	41
Not reported	Trandolapril 1 to 4 mg daily	Left ventricular dysfunction after acute MI	Trend towards greater benefit of trandolapril in those not receiving aspirin.	42
No evidence for an interaction				
250 mg daily	Captopril or enalapril	Secondary prevention of MI	Lower death rate in those on combined therapy than those on ACE inhibitor alone.	43
Not reported	Captopril 75 to 150 mg daily	Left ventricular dysfunction after MI	Trend towards greater benefit of captopril when taken with aspirin.	44
Not reported	Ramipril 10 mg daily	Prevention of MI (no left ventricular dysfunction or heart failure)	Benefits of ramipril not affected by aspirin.	45
80 to 100 mg daily	Captopril	Early treatment of acute MI	Benefits of captopril not affected by aspirin.	46
Not reported	Captopril 100 mg daily	Early treatment of acute MI	Benefits of captopril not affected by aspirin.	47
Not reported	Captopril, enalapril, ramipril, trandolapril	Left ventricular dysfunction or heart failure with or without MI	Benefits of ACE inhibitors not affected by aspirin.	48
160 to 325 mg daily	Captopril, enalapril, lisinopril	Early treatment of acute MI	30-day mortality of combined treatment similar to ACE inhibitor alone.	49

(D) Hyperkalaemia

Hyperkalaemia, resulting in marked bradycardia, was attributed to the use of **loxoprofen** in an elderly women on **imidapril**.[55]

(E) Pharmacokinetic studies

A single-dose study in 12 healthy subjects found that the pharmacokinetics of 20 mg **benazepril** and 325 mg **aspirin** were not affected by concurrent use.[56] The maker of **spirapril** briefly noted in a review that there was no relevant pharmacokinetic interaction between **spirapril** and **diclofenac**.[57] **Oxaprozin** did not affect the pharmacokinetics of **enalapril** in 29 patients with hypertension.[34] A brief mention is made in a review that the pharmacokinetics of **ramipril** were unaffected by 3 days **indometacin** administration (dosage not stated) in healthy subjects.[29]

Mechanism

(A). Some, but not all the evidence suggests that prostaglandins may be involved in the hypotensive action of ACE inhibitors, and that NSAIDs, by inhibiting prostaglandin synthesis, may antagonise the effect of ACE inhibitors. This effect may be dependent on sodium status and on plasma renin, therefore, it does not occur in all patients. It may also depend on the NSAID, with indometacin being frequently implicated, and aspirin and sulindac less so.

(B). Uncertain. The beneficial effects of ACE inhibitors in heart failure and ischaemic heart disease are due, in part, to the inhibition of the breakdown of kinins, which are important regulators of prostaglandin and nitric oxide synthesis. Such inhibition promotes vasodilation and afterload reduction. Aspirin may block these beneficial effects by inhibiting cyclo-oxygenase (COX) and prostaglandin synthesis to cause vasoconstriction, decreased cardiac output and worsening heart failure.[35,58]

(C). Both NSAIDs and ACE inhibitors alone can cause renal impairment. In patients whose kidneys are underperfused, they may cause further deterioration in renal function when used together.[59]

(D). Both ACE inhibitors and NSAIDs (rarely) can cause hyperkalaemia, often with associated renal impairment. The risk may be increased when both drugs are used together.

Importance and management

The interaction between indometacin and ACE inhibitors is well established, with a number of studies showing that indometacin can reduce the antihypertensive effect of captopril, enalapril, and lisinopril, and single studies showing it can reduce the antihypertensive effect of cilazapril and perindopril. A single study reported that trandolapril did not interact, but this requires confirmation. Note that the interaction may not occur in all patients. If indometacin is clearly required in a patient on any ACE inhibitor, it would be prudent to monitor blood pressure carefully. In comparative studies, indometacin has been shown to have less effect on the calcium channel blockers amlodipine, felodipine, and nifedipine, than on enalapril.[6,20,21] See also, 'Calcium channel blockers + NSAIDs', p.461. Therefore, a calcium channel blocker may be an alternative to an ACE inhibitor in a patient requiring indometacin.

Low-dose aspirin (<100 mg daily) does not alter the antihypertensive efficacy of captopril and enalapril. No special precautions are therefore required with ACE inhibitors and these low doses of aspirin. A high dose of aspirin (2.4g daily) has been reported to interact in 50% of patients in a single study. Aspirin 300 mg daily has been reported to interact in about 50% of patients in another study, whereas 325 mg daily did not interact in further study. Thus, at present, it appears that if an ACE inhibitor is used with aspirin in doses higher than 300 mg daily, blood pressure should be monitored more closely, and the ACE inhibitor dosage raised if necessary.

There is limited information about other NSAIDs with ACE inhibitors. Ibuprofen interacted with captopril in a single study. Isolated cases describe increases in blood pressure with rofecoxib and lisinopril, and ibuprofen and captopril. Single studies indicate that lornoxicam and oxaprozin have little or no effect on enalapril, and that celecoxib has little effect on lisinopril. Limited information also suggests that sulindac has little or no effect on ACE inhibitors. Until more is known, it may be prudent to increase blood pressure monitoring when any NSAID is added or discontinued in a patient on any ACE inhibitor. Intermittent use of NSAIDs should be considered as a possible cause of erratic control of blood pressure in patients on ACE inhibitors.

(B). In coronary artery disease and heart failure both ACE inhibitors and aspirin are used, and the information about a possible interaction is conflicting. This may be due to much of the clinical information being obtained from retrospective non-randomised analyses.[58] It may also be a factor of different disease states. For example an interaction may be less likely in patients with heart failure with an ischaemic aetiology than those with non-ischaemic causes because of the added benefits of aspirin in ischaemic heart disease.[60] The available data, and its implications, have been extensively reviewed.[35,50,58,60,61] One commentator has advised that, if possible, aspirin should be avoided in patients requiring long-term treatment for heart failure, particularly if heart failure is severe.[50] Others suggest avoiding aspirin and other NSAIDs in heart failure unless there are clear indications such as atherosclerosis.[35,58] The antiplatelet agents, ticlopidine or clopidogrel are possible alternatives to aspirin.[50,58,61] The use of lower doses of aspirin (80 to 100 mg daily rather than ≥325 mg daily) in those with heart failure on ACE inhibitors has also been suggested.[61] Conversely, an advisory council in the USA has stated that the available evidence supporting an interaction is not sufficiently compelling to justify altering the current practice of prescribing ACE inhibitors and aspirin together,[62] and others are in general agreement with this.[40,60] Data from ongoing randomised trials may provide further insight. Until these are available, combined low-dose aspirin and ACE inhibitors may continue to be used where there is a clear indication for both.

(C/D). Deterioration in renal function or acute renal failure are rare occurrences with the combination of NSAIDs and ACE inhibitors, and poor renal perfusion is a risk factor. Renal function should be monitored periodically in patients on ACE inhibitors and NSAIDs. Combined use may increase the risk of hyperkalaemia, but this appears to be rare.

1. Moore TJ, Crantz FR, Hollenberg NK, Koletsky RJ, Leboff MS, Swartz SL, Levine L, Podolsky S, Dluhy RG, Williams GH. Contribution of prostaglandins to the antihypertensive action of captopril in essential hypertension. *Hypertension* (1981) 3, 168–73.
2. Swartz SL, Williams GH. Angiotensin-converting enzyme inhibition and prostaglandins. *Am J Cardiol* (1982) 49, 1405–9.
3. Smith SR, Coffman TM, Svetkey LP. Effect of low-dose aspirin on thromboxane production and the antihypertensive effect of captopril. *J Am Soc Nephrol* (1993) 4, 1133–9.
4. Guazzi MD, Campodonico J, Celeste F, Guazzi M, Santambrogio G, Rossi M, Trabattoni D, Alimento M. Antihypertensive efficacy of angiotensin converting enzyme inhibition and aspirin counteraction. *Clin Pharmacol Ther* (1998) 63, 79–86.
5. Nawarskas JJ, Townsend RR, Cirigliano MD, Spinler SA. Effect of aspirin on blood pressure in hypertensive patients taking enalapril or losartan. *Am J Hypertens* (1999) 12, 784–9.
6. Polónia J, Boaventura I, Gama G, Camões I, Bernardo F, Andrade P, Nunes JP, Brandão F, Cerqueira-Gomes M. Influence of non-steroidal anti-inflammatory drugs on renal function and 24 h ambulatory blood pressure-reducing effects of enalapril and nifedipine gastrointestinal therapeutic system in hypertensive patients. *J Hypertens* (1995) 13, 925–31.
7. Conlin PR, Moore TJ, Swartz SL, Barr E, Gazdick L, Fletcher C, DeLucca P, Demopoulos L. Effect of indomethacin on blood pressure lowering by captopril and losartan in hypertensive patients. *Hypertension* (2000) 36, 461–5.
8. Salvetti A, Pedrinelli R, Magagna A, Ugenti P. Differential effects of selective and non-selective prostaglandin-synthesis inhibition on the pharmacological responses to captopril in patients with essential hypertension. *Clin Sci* (1982) 63, 261S–263S.
9. Silberbauer K, Stanek B, Templ H. Acute hypotensive effect of captopril in man modified by prostaglandin synthesis inhibition. *Br J Clin Pharmacol* (1982) 14, 87S–93S.
10. Witzgall H, Hirsch F, Scherer B, Weber PC. Acute haemodynamic and hormonal effects of captopril are diminished by indomethacin. *Clin Sci* (1982) 62, 611–15.
11. Goldstone R, Martin K, Zipser R, Horton R. Evidence for a dual action of converting enzyme inhibitor on blood pressure in normal man. *Prostaglandins* (1981) 22, 587–98.
12. Ogihara T, Maruyama A, Hata T, Mikami H, Nakamaru M, Naka T, Ohde H, Kumahara Y. Hormonal responses to converting enzyme inhibition in hypertensive patients. *Clin Pharmacol Ther* (1981) 30, 328–35.
13. Koopmans PP, Van Megen T, Thien T, Gribnau FWJ. The interaction between indomethacin and captopril or enalapril in healthy volunteers. *J Intern Med* (1989) 226, 139–42.
14. Fujita T, Yamashita N, Yamashita K. Effect of indomethacin on antihypertensive actions of captopril in hypertensive patients. *Clin Exp Hypertens* (1981) 3, 939–52.
15. Robles Iniesta A, Navarro de León MC, Morales Serna JC. Bloqueo de la acción antihipertensiva del captoprilo por indometacina. *Med Clin (Barc)* (1991) 96, 438.
16. Gerber JG, Franca G, Byyny RL, LoVerde M, Nies AS. The hypotensive action of captopril and enalapril is not prostacyclin dependent. *Clin Pharmacol Ther* (1993) 54, 523–32.
17. Salvetti A, Abdel-Haq B, Magagna A, Pedrinelli R. Indomethacin reduces the antihypertensive action of enalapril. *Clin Exp Hypertens A* (1987) 9, 559–67.
18. Walden RJ, Owens CWI, Graham BR, Snape A, Nutt J, Prichard BNC. NSAIDs and the control of hypertension: a pilot study. *Br J Clin Pharmacol* (1991) 33, 241P.

19. Duffin D, Leahey W, Brennan G, Johnston GD. The effects of indomethacin on the antihypertensive responses to enalapril and lisinopril. *Br J Clin Pharmacol* (1992) 34, 456P.
20. Morgan T, Anderson A. Interaction of indomethacin with felodipine and enalapril. *J Hypertens* (1993) 11 (Suppl 5), S338–S339.
21. Morgan TO, Anderson A, Bertram D. Effect of indomethacin on blood pressure in elderly people with essential hypertension well controlled on amlodipine or enalapril. *Am J Hypertens* (2000), 13, 1161–3.
22. Ahmad S. Indomethacin-enalapril interaction: an alert. *South Med J* (1991) 84, 411–2.
23. Oparil S, Horton R, Wilkins LH, Irvin J, Hammett DK, Dustan HP. Antihypertensive effect of enalapril (MK-421) in low renin essential hypertension: role of vasodilatory prostaglandins. *Clin Res* (1983) 31, 538A.
24. Oparil S, Horton R, Wilkins LH, Irvin J, Hammett DK. Antihypertensive effect of enalapril in essential hypertension: role of prostacyclin. *Am J Med Sci* (1987) 294, 395–402.
25. Fogari R, Zoppi A, Carretta R, Veglio F, Salvetti A: Italian Collaborative Study Group. Effect of indomethacin on the antihypertensive efficacy of valsartan and lisinopril: a multicentre study. *J Hypertens* (2002) 20: 1007–14.
26. Shaw W, Shapiro D, Antonello J, Cressman M, Vlasses P, Oparil S. Indomethacin does not blunt the antihypertensive effect of lisinopril. *Clin Pharmacol Ther* (1987) 41, 219.
27. Kirch W, Stroemer K, Hoogkamer JFW, Kleinbloesem CH. The influence of prostaglandin inhibition by indomethacin on blood pressure and renal function in hypertensive patients treated with cilazapril. *Br J Clin Pharmacol* (1989) 27, 297S–301S.
28. Abdel-Haq B, Magagna A, Favilla S, Salvetti A. Hemodynamic and humoral interaction between perindopril and indomethacin in essential hypertensive subjects. *J Cardiovasc Pharmacol* (1991) 18 (Suppl 7), S33–S36.
29. Quoted as data on file (Hoechst) by Todd PA, Benfield P. Ramipril. A review of its pharmacological properties and therapeutic efficacy in cardiovascular disorders. *Drugs* (1990) 39, 110–35.
30. Pritchard G, Lyons D, Webster J, Petrie JC, MacDonald TM. Indomethacin does not attenuate the hypotensive effect of trandolapril. *J Hum Hypertens* (1996) 10, 763–7.
31. Brown CH. Effect of rofecoxib on the antihypertensive effect of lisinopril. *Ann Pharmacother* (2000) 34, 1486.
32. White WB, Whelton A, Kent J, Verburg K. Effects of the cox-2 specific inhibitor celecoxib on ambulatory blood pressure in hypertensive patients on ACE inhibition. *Am J Hypertens* (2001) 14, 183A.
33. Espino DV, Lancaster MC. Neutralization of the effects of captopril by the use of ibuprofen in an elderly woman. *J Am Board Fam Pract* (1992) 5, 319–21.
34. Noveck RJ, McMahon FG, Bocanegra T, Karem A, Sugimoto D, Smith M. Effects of oxaprozin on enalapril and enaprilat pharmacokinetics, pharmacodynamics, blood pressure, heart rate, plasma renin activity, aldosterone and creatinine clearances in hypertensive patients. *Clin Pharmacol Ther* (1997), 61, 208.
35. Mahé I, Meune C, Diemer M, Caulin C, Bergmann J-F. Interaction between aspirin and ACE inhibitors in patients with heart failure. *Drug Safety* (2001) 24, 167–82.
36. Spaulding C, Charbonnier B, Cohen-Solal A, Juilliere Y, Kromer EP, Benhamda K, Cador R, Weber S. Acute hemodynamic interaction of aspirin and ticlopidine with enalapril: results of a double-blind, randomized comparative trial. *Circulation* (1998) 98, 757–65.
37. Guazzi M, Pontone G, Agostoni P. Aspirin worsens exercise performance and pulmonary gas exchange in patients with heart failure who are taking angiotensin-converting enzyme inhibitors. *Am Heart J* (1999) 138, 254–60.
38. Al-Khadra AS, Salem DN, Rand WM, Udelson JE, Smith JJ, Konstam MA. Antiplatelet agents and survival: a cohort analysis from the Studies of Left Ventricular Dysfunction (SOLVD) trial. *J Am Coll Cardiol* (1998) 31, 419–25.
39. Nguyen KN, Aursnes I, Kjekshus J. Interaction between enalapril and aspirin on mortality after acute myocardial infarction: subgroup analysis of the Cooperative New Scandanavian Enalapril Survival Study II (CONSENSUS II). *Am J Cardiol* (1997) 79, 115–19.
40. Peterson JG, Topol EJ, Sapp SK, Young JB, Lincoff AM, Lauer MS. Evaluation of the effects of aspirin combined with angiotensin-converting enzyme inhibitors in patients with coronary artery disease. *Am J Med* (2000) 109, 371–7.
41. The Acute Infarction Ramipril Efficacy (AIRE) Study Investigators. Effect of ramipril on mortality and morbidity of survivors of acute myocardial infarction with clinical evidence of heart failure. *Lancet* (1993) 342, 821–8.
42. Køber L, Torp-Pedersen C, Carlsen JE, Bagger H, Eliasen P, Lyngborg K, Videbæk J, Cole DS, Auclert L, Pauly NC, Aliot E, Persson S, Camm AJ, for the Trandolapril Cardiac Evaluation (TRACE) Study Group. A clinical trial of the angiotensin-converting-enzyme inhibitor trandolapril in patients with left ventricular dysfunction after myocardial infarction. *N Engl J Med* (1995) 333, 1670–6.
43. Leor J, Reicher-Reiss H, Goldbourt U, Boyko V, Gottlieb S, Battler A, Behar S. Aspirin and mortality in patients treated with angiotensin-converting enzyme inhibitors. A cohort study of 11,575 patients with coronary artery disease. *J Am Coll Cardiol* (1999) 33, 1920–5.
44. Pfeffer MA, Braunwald E, Moyé LA, Basta L, Brown EJ, Cuddy TE, Davis BR, Geltman EM, Goldman S, Flaker GC, Klein M, Lamas GA, Packer M, Rouleau J, Rouleau JL, Rutherford J, Wertheimer JH, Hawkins CM, on behalf of the SAVE Investigators. Effect of captopril on mortality and morbidity in patients with left ventricular dysfunction after myocardial infarction. Results of the survival and ventricular enlargement trial. *N Engl J Med* (1992) 327, 669–77.
45. The Heart Outcomes Prevention Evaluation Study Investigators. Effect of an angiotensin-converting-enzyme inhibitor, ramipril, on cardiovascular events in high-risk patients. *N Engl J Med* (2000) 342, 145–53.
46. Oosterga M, Anthonio RL, de Kam PJ, Kingma JH, Crijns HJ, van Gilst WH. Effects of aspirin on angiotensin-converting enzyme inhibition and left ventricular dilation one year after myocardial infarction. *Am J Cardiol* (1998) 81, 1178–81.
47. ISIS-4 (Fourth International Study of Infarct Survival) Collaborative Group. ISIS-4: a randomised factorial trial assessing early oral captopril, oral mononitrate, and intravenous magnesium sulphate in 58,050 patients with suspected acute myocardial infarction. *Lancet* (1995) 345, 669–85.
48. Flather MD, Yusuf S, Køber L, Pfeffer M, Hall A, Murray G, Trop-Pedersen C, Ball S, Pogue J, Moyé L, Braunwald E, for the ACE-inhibitor Myocardial Infarction Collaborative. Long-term ACE-inhibitor therapy in patients with heart failure or left-ventricular dysfunction: a systematic overview of data from individual patients. *Lancet* (2000) 335, 1575–81.
49. Latini R, Tognoni G, Maggioni AP, Baigent C, Braunwald E, Chen Z-M, Collins R, Flather M, Franzosi MG, Kjekshus J, Køber L, Liu L-S, Peto R, Pfeffer M, Pizzetti F, Santoro E, Sleight P, Swedberg K, Tavazzi L, Wang W, Yusuf S. Clinical effects of early angiotensin-converting enzyme inhibitor treatment for myocardial infarction are similar in the presence and absence of aspirin. *J Am Coll Cardiol* (2000) 35 1801–7.

50. Hall D. The aspirin—angiotensin-converting enzyme inhibitor tradeoff: to halve and halve not. *J Am Coll Cardiol* (2000) 35, 1808–12.
51. Seelig CB, Maloley PA, Campbell JR. Nephrotoxicity associated with concomitant ACE inhibitor and NSAID therapy. *South Med J* (1990) 83, 1144–8.
52. Adhiyaman V, Asghar M, Oke A, White AD, Shah IU. Nephrotoxicity in the elderly due to co-prescription of angiotensin converting enzyme inhibitors and nonsteroidal anti-inflammatory drugs. *J R Soc Med* (2001) 94, 512–14.
53. Sturmer T, Erb A, Keller F, Gunther KP, Brenner H. Determinants of impaired renal function with use of nonsteroidal anti-inflammatory drugs: the importance of half-life and other medications. *Am J Med* (2001) 111, 521–7.
54. Pritchard G, Lyons D, Webster J, Petrie JC, MacDonald TM. Do trandolapril and indomethacin influence renal function and renal function reserve in hypertensive patients? *Br J Clin Pharmacol* (1997) 44, 145–9.
55. Kurata C, Uehara A, Sugi T, Yamazake K. Syncope caused by nonsteroidal anti-inflammatory drugs and angiotensin-converting enzyme inhibitors. *Jpn Circ J* (1999) 63, 1002–3.
56. Sioufi A, Pommier F, Gauducheau N, Godbillon J, Choi L, John V. The absence of a pharmacokinetic interaction between aspirin and the angiotensin-converting enzyme inhibitor benazepril in healthy volunteers. *Biopharm Drug Dispos* (1994) 15, 451–61.
57. Grass P, Gerbeau C, Kutz K. Spirapril: pharmacokinetic properties and drug interactions. *Blood Pressure Suppl* (1994) 2, 7–13.
58. Massie BM, Teerlink JR. Interaction between aspirin and angiotensin-converting enzyme inhibitors: real or imagined. *Am J Med* (2000) 109, 431–3.
59. Sturrock ND, Struthers AD. Non-steroidal anti-inflammatory drugs and angiotensin-converting enzyme inhibitors: a commonly prescribed combination with variable effects on renal function. *Br J Clin Pharmacol* (1993) 35, 343–8.
60. Nawarskas JJ, Spinler SA. Update on the interaction between aspirin and angiotensin-converting enzyme inhibitors. *Pharmacotherapy* (2000) 20, 698–710.
61. Stys T, Lawson WE, Smaldone GC, Stys A. Does aspirin attenuate the beneficial effects of angiotensin-converting enzyme inhibition in heart failure? *Arch Intern Med* (2000) 160, 1409–13.
62. Consensus recommendations for the management of chronic heart failure. On behalf of the membership of the advisory council to improve outcomes nationwide in heart failure. *Am J Cardiol* (1999) 83, 1A–38A.

ACE inhibitors + Azathioprine

Anaemia has been seen in patients given azathioprine and enalapril or captopril. Leucopenia occasionally occurs with captopril and azathioprine.

Clinical evidence

(a) Anaemia

Nine out of 11 kidney transplant patients taking ACE inhibitors (**enalapril** or **captopril**) showed a haematocrit fall from 34 to 27%, and a haemoglobin fall from 11.6 to 9.5 g/dl when **ciclosporin** was replaced by **azathioprine**. Two patients were switched back to **ciclosporin**, and had a prompt rise in their haematocrit. Another 10 patients on both drugs similarly showed some anaemia when compared with 10 others not taking an ACE-inhibitor (haematocrit of 33 compared with 41%, and haemoglobin 11.5 compared with 14 g/dl).[1] A later study by the same group of workers (again in patients on **enalapril** and **captopril**) confirmed and extended these findings. No pharmacokinetic interaction between the ACE-inhibitors and **azathioprine** was found.[2]

(b) Leucopenia

A patient whose white cell count fell sharply when treated with **captopril** and **azathioprine** together, showed no leucopenia when given each drug separately.[3] Another patient who was given **captopril** (increased to 475 mg daily then reduced to 100 mg daily) immediately after discontinuing **azathioprine**, developed leucopenia. She was later successfully treated with **captopril** 4 to 6 mg daily.[4] Other patients have similarly shown leucopenia when given both drugs;[5,6] in one case this did not recur when rechallenged with captopril alone (at a lower dose).[6]

Mechanisms

(a). The anaemia appears to be due to suppression of erythropoietin by the ACE inhibitors, and azathioprine may cause patients to be more susceptible to this effect.[2]

(b). Uncertain. Additive bone marrow suppression?

Importance and management

The anaemia caused by captopril and enalapril in kidney transplant patients has been seen (see also 'Epoetin (recombinant human erythropoietin) + ACE inhibitors or Angiotensin II antagonists', p.887). The evidence that this effect can be potentiated by concomitant azathioprine is limited, but it would be prudent to monitor well if these drugs are used together. The evidence that concomitant use of ACE inhibitors and azathioprine increases the risk of leucopenia is also limited. However, the maker of captopril recommends that if captopril is used in patients on immunosuppressant therapy, differential white blood cell counts should be monitored regularly in the first 3 months of captopril therapy, especially if there is renal impairment.[7] The makers of a number of other ACE inhibitors (e.g. **cilazapril, imidapril, moexipril, trandolapril**) now state in their prescribing information that concomitant administration of ACE inhibitors and **cytostatic** or **immunosuppressive agents** may lead to an increased risk of leucopenia.[8-11] See also 'ACE inhibitors + Allopurinol', p.368 and 'Captopril + Procainamide', p.386.

1. Gossmann J, Kachel H-G, Schoeppe W, Scheuermann E-H. Anemia in renal transplant recipients caused by concomitant therapy with azathioprine and angiotensin-converting enzyme inhibitors. *Transplantation* (1993) 56, 585–9.
2. Gossmann J, Thürmann P, Bachmann T, Weller S, Kachel H-G, Schoeppe W, Scheuermann E-H. Mechanism of angiotensin converting enzyme inhibitor-related anemia in renal transplant recipients. *Kidney Int* (1996) 50, 973–8.
3. Kirchetz EJ, Gröne HJ, Rieger J, Hölscher M, Scheler F. Successful low dose captopril rechallenge following drug-induced leucopenia. *Lancet* (1981) i, 1363.
4. Case DB, Whitman HH, Laragh JH, Spiera H. Successful low dose captopril rechallenge following drug-induced leucopenia. *Lancet* (1981) i, 1362–3.
5. Elijovisch F, Krakoff LR. Captopril associated granulocytopenia in hypertension after renal transplantation. *Lancet* (1980), i, 927–8.
6. Edwards CRW, Drury P, Penketh A, Damluji SA. Successful re-introduction of captopril following neutropenia. *Lancet* (1981) i, 723.
7. Capoten (Captopril). E. R. Squibb & Sons Limited. Summary of product characteristics, July 2001.
8. Vascace (Cilazapril). Roche Products Ltd. Summary of product characteristics, December 2001.
9. Tanatril (Imidapril). Trinity Pharmaceuticals Ltd. Summary of product characteristics, March 2001.
10. Perdix (Moexipril). Schwarz Pharma Ltd. Summary of product characteristics, November 2001.
11. Gopten (Trandolapril). Abbot Laboratories Limited. Summary of product characteristics, December 2001.

ACE inhibitors + Beta-blockers

No clinically important adverse interactions have been seen between propranolol and cilazapril, quinapril, or ramipril, and between trandolapril and unnamed beta-blockers.

Clinical evidence, mechanism, importance and management

Propranolol 80 mg three times daily did not affect the pharmacokinetics of a single 20-mg dose of **quinapril** in 10 healthy subjects.[1,2] The pharmacokinetics of **ramipril** 5 mg daily were unaffected by **propranolol** 40 mg twice daily.[3] No significant pharmacokinetic interaction occurred between **cilazapril** 2.5 mg daily and **propranolol** 120 mg daily, but the reductions in blood pressure were more pronounced and long-lasting.[4,5]

The maker of trandolapril notes that in patients with left ventricular dysfunction after myocardial infarction, no clinical interactions have been found between **trandolapril** and **beta-blockers** (not named).[6]

No important adverse interaction seems to occur, and the combination of these ACE inhibitors and propranolol may be clinically useful.

1. Horvath AM, Blake DS, Ferry JJ, Sedman AJ, Colburn WA. Propranolol does not influence quinapril pharmacokinetics in healthy volunteers. *J Clin Pharmacol* (1987) 27, 719.
2. Horvath AM, Pilon D, Caillé G, Colburn WA, Ferry JJ, Frank GJ, Lacasse Y, Olson SC. Multiple-dose propranolol does not influence the single dose pharmacokinetics of quinapril and its active metabolite (quinaprilat). *Biopharm Drug Dispos* (1990) 11, 191–6.
3. van Griensven JMT, Seibert-Grafe M, Schoemaker HC, Frölich M, Cohen AF. The pharmacokinetic and pharmacodynamic interactions of ramipril with propranolol. *Eur J Clin Pharmacol* (1993) 45, 255–60.
4. Belz GG, Essig J, Kleinbloesem CH, Hoogkamer JFW, Wiegand UW, Wellstein A. Interactions between cilazapril and propranolol in man; plasma drug concentrations, hormone and enzyme responses, haemodynamics, agonist dose-effect curves and baroreceptor reflex. *Br J Clin Pharmacol* (1988) 26, 547–56.
5. Belz GG, Essig J, Erb K, Breithaupt K, Hoogkamer JFW, Kneer J, Kleinbloesem CH. Pharmacokinetic and pharmacodynamic interactions between the ACE inhibitor cilazapril and β-adrenoceptor antagonist propranolol in healthy subjects and in hypertensive patients. *Br J Clin Pharmacol* (1989) 27, 317S–322S.
6. Gopten (Trandolapril). Abbot Laboratories Ltd. Summary of product characteristics, December 2001.

ACE inhibitors + Calcium channel blockers

No clinically important adverse interactions have been seen between lisinopril, moexipril, or trandolapril and nifedipine; between benazepril or captopril and amlodipine; between ramipril and felodipine; or between spirapril and nicardipine.

Clinical evidence, mechanism, importance and management

No evidence of either a pharmacokinetic or adverse pharmacodynamic interaction was seen in 12 healthy subjects given single doses of **nifedipine** 20 mg and **lisinopril** 20 mg.[1] The maker notes that no clinically important pharmacokinetic interaction occurred between **moexipril** and **nifedipine** in healthy subjects, but that the antihypertensive effect was enhanced in patients. If **moexipril** is added to **nifedipine**, they recommend a reduced starting dose of **moexipril**.[2] The maker of **trandolapril** has data on file showing that there is no interaction between single doses of **trandolapril** and **nifedipine** in healthy subjects.[3] They also note that in patients with left ventricular dysfunction after myocardial infarction, no clinical interactions have been found between **trandolapril** and **calcium channel blockers** (not named).[4] No pharmacokinetic interaction occurred between single doses of **felodipine** 10 mg and **ramipril** 5 mg in healthy subjects. The blood pressure lowering effect of the combination was greater, and **ramipril** attenuated the reflex tachycardia caused by **felodipine**.[5] Preliminary findings suggest there was no pharmacokinetic interaction between single doses of **benazepril** and **amlodipine**.[6] No adverse interactions were seen in 29 hypertensive patients on **captopril** 25 mg twice daily when given **amlodipine** 10 mg daily. Blood pressure control was significantly improved.[7] The maker says that **amlodipine** has been safely administered with ACE inhibitors and that no **amlodipine** dosage changes are needed.[8] The maker of **spirapril** briefly noted in a review that **nicardipine** increased **spirapril** plasma concentrations by 25% and those of its active metabolite **spiraprilat** by 45%, and reduced **nicardipine** bioavailability by 30%. It was assumed that the interaction took place at the absorption site. However, the changes were not considered clinically relevant.[9]

A number of products combining an ACE inhibitor with a calcium channel blocker are available. In the UK, the British National Formulary states that use of such combinations may increase the range of adverse effects, and that they should be used only for those patients stabilised on the individual components in the same proportions.[10]

1. Lees KR, Reid JL. Lisinopril and nifedipine: no acute interaction in normotensives. *Br J Clin Pharmacol* (1988) 25, 307–13.
2. Perdix (Moexipril). Schwarz Pharma Ltd. Summary of product characteristics, March 2000.
3. New Horizons in Antihypertensive therapy. Gopten® Trandolapril. Knoll AG 1992.
4. Gopten (Trandolapril). Abbot Laboratories Ltd. Summary of product characteristics, December 2001.
5. Bainbridge AD, MacFadyen RJ, Lees KR, Reid JL. A study of the acute pharmacodynamic interaction of ramipril and felodipine in normotensive subjects. *Br J Clin Pharmacol* (1991) 31, 148–53.
6. Sun JX, Cipriano A, Kern JC, Chan K, John VA. Drug interaction study of benazepril and amlodipine in healthy subjects. *Pharm Res* (1992) 9 (10 Suppl), S313.
7. Maclean D, Mitchell ET, Wilcox RG, Walker P, Tyler HM. A double-blind cross-over comparison of amlodipine and placebo added to captopril in moderate to severe hypertension. *J Cardiovasc Pharmacol* (1988) 12 (Suppl 7), S85–S88.
8. Istin (Amlodipine). Pfizer Ltd. Summary of product characteristics, March 2000.
9. Grass P, Gerbeau C, Kutz K. Spirapril: pharmacokinetic properties and drug interactions. *Blood Press Suppl* (1994) 2, 7–13.
10. British National Formulary. 43rd ed. London: The British Medical Association and The Pharmaceutical Press; 2002. p. 92.

ACE inhibitors + Capsaicin

An isolated report describes cough in a woman taking an ACE inhibitor each time she used a topical cream containing capsaicin.

Clinical evidence, mechanism, importance and management

A woman of 53 who had been maintained on an **unnamed ACE inhibitor** for several years, complained of cough each time she applied *Axsain*, a cream containing 0.075% **capsaicin**, to her lower extremities. Whether this reaction would have occurred without the ACE inhibitor was not determined,[1] but pre-treatment with an ACE inhibitor is known to enhance the cough caused by inhaled **capsaicin**.[1] This potential interaction is probably of little general clinical importance.

1. Hakas JF. Topical capsaicin induces cough in patient receiving ACE inhibitor. *Ann Allergy* (1990) 65, 322.

ACE inhibitors + Cimetidine

No clinically important adverse interactions have been seen between cimetidine and captopril, enalapril, fosinopril, moexipril, quinapril or spirapril. Cimetidine modestly reduced the absorption of temocapril.

Clinical evidence, mechanism, importance and management

Cimetidine in healthy subjects did not appear to alter the pharmacokinetics or pharmacological effects of **captopril**[1] or **enalapril**,[2] or the pharmacokinetics of **quinapril**[3] or **fosinopril**.[4] The makers of **moexipril** say that no important pharmacokinetic interaction occurred with **cimetidine**.[5] The makers of **spirapril** briefly note in a review that **cimetidine** did not alter the plasma concentrations of **spirapril** or its active metabolite **spiraprilat**.[6] None of these pairs of drugs appears to interact to a clinically relevant extent, and no special precautions appear to be necessary.

Preliminary findings suggest cimetidine 400 mg twice daily had no effect on the metabolism of **temocapril** 20 mg daily in 18 healthy subjects, but the absorption was reduced 26%.[7] The clinical relevance of this is uncertain, but check that the effects of **temocapril** remain adequate if **cimetidine** is added.

1. Richer C, Bah M, Cadilhac M, Thuillez C, Giudicelli JF. Cimetidine does not alter free unchanged captopril pharmacokinetics and biological effects in healthy volunteers. *J Pharmacol* (1986) 17, 338–42.
2. Ishizaki T, Baba T, Murabayashi S, Kubota K, Hara K, Kurimoto F. Effect of cimetidine on the pharmacokinetics and pharmacodynamics of enalapril in normal volunteers. *J Cardiovasc Pharmacol* (1988) 12, 512–9.
3. Ferry JJ, Cetnarowski AB, Sedman AJ, Thomas RW, Horvath AM. Multiple-dose cimetidine administration does not influence the single-dose pharmacokinetics of quinapril and its active metabolite (CI-928). *J Clin Pharmacol* (1988) 28, 48–51.
4. Moore L, Kramer A, Swites B, Kramer P, Tu J. Effect of cimetidine and antacid on the kinetics of the active diacid of fosinopril in healthy subjects. *J Clin Pharmacol* (1988) 28, 946.
5. Perdix (Moexipril), Schwarz Pharma Ltd. Summary of product characteristics, November 2001.
6. Grass P, Gerbeau C, Kutz K. Spirapril: pharmacokinetic properties and drug interactions. *Blood Pressure* (1994) 3 (Suppl 2), 7–13.
7. Trenk D, Schaefer A, Eberle E, Jähnchen E. Effect of cimetidine on the pharmacokinetics of the ACE-inhibitor temocapril. *Eur J Clin Pharmacol* (1996) 50, 556.

ACE inhibitors + Clonidine

There is some evidence that the effects of captopril may be delayed when patients are switched from clonidine.[1] Note that sudden withdrawal of clonidine may cause rebound hypertension.

1. Gröne H-J, Kirchertz EJ, Rieger J. Mögliche Komplikationen und Probleme der Captopriltherapie bei Hypertonikern mit ausgeprägten Gefässchäden. *Therapiewoche* (1981) 31, 5280–7.

ACE inhibitors + Garlic

An isolated report describes marked hypotension and faintness in a patient on lisinopril when garlic was added.

Clinical evidence, mechanism, importance and management

A man whose blood pressure was 135/90 mmHg while on 15 mg **lisinopril** daily began to take 4 mg **garlic** daily (*Boots odourless garlic oil capsules*). Within 3 days he became faint on standing and was found to have a blood pressure of 90/60 mmHg. Stopping the **garlic** restored his blood pressure to 135/90 mmHg within a week. The **garlic** on its own did not lower his blood pressure. The reasons are not known.[1] This seems to be the first and only report of this reaction, so its general importance is small. There seems to be nothing documented about garlic and any of the other ACE inhibitors.

1. McCoubrie M. Doctors as patients: lisinopril and garlic. *Br J Gen Pract* (1996) 46, 107.

ACE inhibitors + Haemodialysis membranes

An anaphylactoid reaction (facial swelling, flushing, hypotension and dyspnoea) can occur in patients on ACE inhibitors within a few minutes of starting haemodialysis using high-flux polyacrylonitrile membranes ('AN69 Hospal').[1,2] The reasons are not known. Use an alternative membrane or an alternative hypotensive agent.[3]

1. Tielemans C, Madhoun P, Lenaers M, Schandene L, Goldman M, Vanherweghem JL. Anaphylactoid reactions during hemodialysis on AN69 membranes in patients receiving ACE inhibitors. *Kidney Int* (1990) 38, 982–4.
2. Verrsen L, Waer M, Vanrenterghem Y, Michielsen P. Angiotensin-converting-enzyme inhibitors and anaphylactoid reactions to high-flux membrane dialysis. *Lancet* (1990) 336, 1360–2.
3. Committee on Safety of Medicines. Anaphylactoid reactions to high-flux polyacrylonitrile membranes in combination with ACE inhibitors. *Current Problems* (1992) 33, 2.

ACE inhibitors + Interleukin-3

Preliminary evidence indicates that marked hypotension can occur in patients on ACE inhibitors if given interleukin-3.

Clinical evidence, mechanism, importance and management

Twenty-six patients with ovarian or small-cell undifferentiated cancers were treated with chemotherapy followed by **recombinant human interleukin-3**. Three of the 26 were taking ACE inhibitors (not named) and all three developed marked hypotension (WHO toxicity grade 2 or 3) within 1 to 4 h of the first **interleukin-3** injection. Their blood pressures returned to normal when the ACE inhibitors were stopped while continuing the **interleukin-3**. When the **interleukin-3** was stopped, they once again needed the ACE inhibitors to control their blood pressure. None of the other 23 patients showed hypotension except one who did so during a period of neutropenic fever.[1] The authors of the report suggest (and present some supporting evidence) that the drugs act synergistically to generate large amounts of NO in the blood vessel walls. This relaxes the smooth muscle in the blood vessel walls causing vasodilatation and consequent hypotension.[1] Information seems to be limited to this single report, but the interaction would appear to be established. Be alert for this reaction if inter-leukin-3 is used in any patient taking ACE inhibitors. More study is needed.

1. Dercksen MW, Hoekman K, Visser JJ, ten Bokkel Huinink WW, Pinedo HM, Wagstaff J. Hypotension induced by interleukin-3 in patients on angiotensin-converting enzyme inhibitors. *Lancet* (1995) 345, 448.

ACE inhibitors + Iron

Serious systemic reactions occurred in three patients given infusions of ferric sodium gluconate while taking enalapril. Oral ferrous sulphate may decrease absorption of captopril, but this is probably of little clinical importance.

Clinical evidence

(a) Intravenous iron

A man with iron-deficiency anaemia on furosemide (frusemide) and digoxin was given 125 mg **ferric sodium gluconate (*Ferlixit*)**[1] intravenously in 100 ml saline daily. Four days later, **enalapril** 5 mg daily was started. After the infusion of only a few drops of his next dose of **ferric sodium gluconate**, he developed diffuse erythema, abdominal cramps, hypotension, nausea and vomiting. He recovered after being given 200 mg hydrocortisone hemisuccinate. Three days later, in the absence of the **enalapril**, he recommenced the **iron infusions** for a further 10 days without problems, and was later treated uneventfully with the **enalapril**. Two other patients taking **enalapril** reacted similarly when given intravenous infusions of **ferric sodium gluconate**. Neither was given any more **intravenous iron** and later had no problems while taking **enalapril**.[2]

(b) Oral iron

A double-blind study in 7 healthy subjects, given single doses of **ferrous sulphate** 300 mg or placebo with **captopril** 25 mg, found that the AUC of unconjugated plasma captopril (the active form) was reduced by 37% although the maximum plasma levels were not substantially changed. The AUC of total plasma captopril was increased 43%, although this was not statistically significant. There were no significant differences in blood pressure between treatment and placebo groups.[3]

Mechanism

(a). Uncertain. Intravenous iron causes a variety of systemic reactions including fever, myalgia, arthralgia, hypotension, nausea and vomiting which are believed to be due to the release of various inflammatory mediators such as bradykinin and substance P from tissues caused by toxic free radicals. The authors of the report suggest that ACE inhibitors like enalapril decrease the breakdown of these kinins so that the toxic effects of the iron become exaggerated.[2]

(b). Reduced levels of unconjugated captopril in the plasma are probably due to reduced absorption resulting from a chemical interaction between ferric ions and captopril in the gastrointestinal tract.[3]

Importance and management

(a). The interaction with intravenous iron is not firmly established because about 25% of all patients given iron by this route develop a variety of systemic reactions, ranging from mild to serious anaphylactoid reactions. However the authors of the report point out that in a 13-month period in their clinic in which these three cases occurred, all of them involved enalapril, whereas there were none at all in another 15 patients not taking ACE inhibitors. Their recommendation is to use even more caution if intravenous iron is given to patients taking any ACE inhibitor.[2]

(b). There is limited evidence that orally administered iron may reduce the absorption of captopril. The clinical relevance of this is unknown, but probably small. Information about the effect of oral iron on other ACE inhibitors is lacking.

1. Rolla G. Personal communication, 1994.
2. Rolla G, Bucca C, Brussino L. Systemic reactions to intravenous iron therapy in patients receiving angiotensin converting enzyme inhibitor. *J Allergy Clin Immunol* (1994) 93, 1074–5.
3. Schaefer JP, Tam Y, Hasinoff BB, Tawfik S, Peng Y, Reimche L, Campbell NRC. Ferrous sulphate interacts with captopril. *Br J Clin Pharmacol* (1998) 46, 377–81.

ACE inhibitors + Loop or thiazide or related diuretics

The combination of captopril or other ACE inhibitors and loop or thiazide or related diuretics is normally safe and effective but 'first dose hypotension' (dizziness, lightheadedness, fainting,) can occur, particularly if the dose of diuretic is high and often associated with various predisposing conditions. A few cases of renal insufficiency, and even acute renal failure, have been reported in patients without renovascular disease when taking ACE inhibitors and diuretics, possibly associated with sodium depletion. Hypokalaemia may occur.

Clinical evidence

(a) First dose hypotensive reaction

The concurrent use of **captopril** and **loop** or **thiazide** or **related diuretics** is normally safe and effective, but some patients experience 'first dose hypotension' (i.e. dizziness, lightheadedness, fainting) after taking the first one or two doses of **captopril**. This appears to be associated with, and exaggerated by, certain conditions (congestive heart failure, renovascular hypertension, renal dialysis, high levels of renin and angiotensin, diarrhoea or vomiting, etc.) and/or hypovolaemia and sodium depletion caused by **diuretics**, particularly in high doses. A study describes one case of a woman whose blood pressure failed to respond to **furosemide (frusemide)** 10 mg intravenously. After 30 min she was given **captopril** 50 mg and within 45 min her blood pressure fell from 290/150 to 135/60 mmHg, and she required an infusion of saline.[1] In another study, a man developed severe postural hypotension shortly after **furosemide** was added to **captopril** 150 mg daily.[2]

Starting with a low dose of ACE inhibitor reduces the risk of important hypotension. In a study in 8 patients with hypertension on **hydrochlorothiazide** or **furosemide** for at least 4 weeks, **captopril** was started in small increasing doses from 6.25 mg. Symptomatic postural hypotension was seen in 2 of the 8 patients, but was only mild and transient.[3]

Hypotension is more common in patients with heart failure who are receiving large doses of diuretics. In a study in 124 patients with severe heart failure on **furosemide** (mean 170 mg daily) and spironolactone, the addition of **captopril** caused transient symptomatic hypotension in 44%. The **captopril** dose had to be reduced in 8 patients, and was later discontinued. A further 4 patients developed symptomatic hypotension after 1 to 2 months and **captopril** was discontinued.[4]

There is some evidence in patients with heart failure that the incidence of marked orthostatic hypotension requiring treatment discontinuation in the first 36 h was lower with **perindopril** 2 mg once daily than **captopril** 6.25 mg three times daily (6 cases versus 16 cases).[5]

(b) Hypokalaemia

Although ACE inhibitors can maintain body potassium, the concurrent use of **loop** and **thiazide** and **related diuretics** can result in hypokalaemia. In one analysis, 7 of 21 patients on diuretics given ACE inhibitors for heart failure developed hypokalaemia. This was corrected by potassium supplementation in 2 cases, an increase in the ACE inhibitor dose in 3 cases, and use of a potassium-sparing diuretic in the remaining 2 cases.[6]

(c) Impairment of renal function

The risk of ACE-inhibitor-induced renal impairment in patients with renovascular disease can be potentiated by **diuretics**.[7,8] Renal impairment in patients on **ACE-inhibitors** and **diuretics** has also been described in other conditions. A patient with congestive heart failure and moderate renal insufficiency developed acute non-oliguric renal failure while on **enalapril** 20 mg daily and **furosemide** 60 mg daily, which resolved when the sodium balance was restored.[9] Acute fatal renal failure developed in 2 patients within 4 weeks of being treated with **enalapril** and **furosemide** and in 2 other patients renal impairment developed over a longer period.[10] Reversible renal failure has been also been described in a patient with congestive heart failure when treated with **captopril** and **metolazone**.[11] In an analysis of 74 patients who had been treated with an **ACE inhibitor**, reversible acute renal failure was more common in those who were also treated with a **diuretic** than those who were not (11 of 33 patients compared with 1 of 41 patients).[12] In a prescription-event monitoring study, **enalapril** was thought to have contributed to deterioration in renal function which contributed to the subsequent deaths of 10 out of 75 patients. Nine of these 10 were receiving **loop** or **thiazide diuretics**, sometimes in high doses.[13] A controlled study in 34 patients with hypertensive nephrosclerosis identified 8 patients who developed reversible renal insufficiency when treated with **enalapril** and various other antihypertensives including a diuretic (**furosemide** or **hydrochlorothiazide**). In contrast, none out of 23 patients treated with placebo and various other antihypertensives developed renal insufficiency.[14] Subsequently, one of these patients was retreated with **enalapril** with recurrence of renal dysfunction. Discontinuation of the diuretics (**furosemide, hydrochlorothiazide,** and **triamterene**) led to an improvement in renal function despite the continuation of **enalapril**.[15]

(d) Pharmacokinetic and diuresis studies

A study in healthy subjects given single doses of **enalapril** and **furosemide** found no evidence of any pharmacokinetic interaction between these drugs.[16] Another study found that **captopril** did not affect the urinary excretion of **furosemide** and its subsequent diuretic effects.[17] However, a further study showed that, although **captopril** did not alter urinary excretion of furosemide, it did reduce diuresis.[18] Yet another study found that **captopril** reduced the urinary excretion of furosemide, and reduced the diuretic response during the first collecting period to 50%, and the natriuretic response to almost 30%, whereas **enalapril** and **ramipril** did not significantly alter the diuretic effects of **furosemide**.[19] **Lisinopril** did not alter plasma levels or urinary excretion of **furosemide**, nor did it alter urinary electrolyte excretion.[20]

Neither **captopril** nor **ramipril** altered the diuresis induced by **hydrochlorothiazide**.[19] The maker of **spirapril** briefly noted in a review that there was no relevant pharmacokinetic interaction between **spirapril** and **hydrochlorothiazide**.[21] The maker of **moexipril** notes that there was no clinically important pharmacokinetic interaction when moexipril was administered with hydrochlorothiazide in healthy subjects.[22]

Mechanisms

(a). The first dose hypotension interaction is not fully understood. One suggestion is that if considerable amounts of salt and water have already been lost as a result of using a diuretic, the resultant depletion in the fluid volume (hypovolaemia) transiently exaggerates the hypotensive effects of the ACE inhibitor.

(b). The cases of hypokalaemia are simply a result of the potassium-depleting effects of the diuretics.

(c). Diuretic-induced sodium depletion may be a factor in the renal insufficiency and failure sometimes observed with ACE inhibitors.

Importance and management

(a). The 'first dose hypotension' interaction between **ACE inhibitors** and **loop** or **thiazide** or **related diuretics** is well established. The risk is higher when the dose of diuretic is greater than furosemide (frusemide) 80 mg or equivalent, and in those with various conditions (see 'Clinical Evidence').[23] In patients on these doses of diuretic, consideration should be given to temporarily stopping the diuretic or reducing its dosage a few days before the **ACE inhibitor** is added. If this is not considered clinically appropriate, the first dose of the **ACE inhibitor** should be given under close specialist supervision. If marked

hypotension occurs, an infusion of saline may be required. In all patients on diuretics, therapy with **ACE inhibitors** should be started with a very low dose. Even in patients at low risk (e.g. those with uncomplicated essential hypertension on low-dose thiazides), to be on the safe side you should give all patients a simple warning about what can happen and what to do when they first start concurrent use. The immediate problem (dizziness, lightheadedness, faintness), if it occurs, can usually be solved by the patient lying down. Taking the first dose of the **ACE inhibitor** just before bedtime is also preferable.[24] Any marked hypotension is normally transient, but if problems persist it may be necessary temporarily to reduce the diuretic dosage. There is usually no need to avoid the combination just because an initially large hypotensive response has occurred. The **loop diuretics** and the **thiazide** or **related diuretics,** which are potential candidates for this interaction, are listed in Table 14.2.

A number of products combining an ACE inhibitor with a thiazide diuretic are available for the treatment of hypertension. These products should be used only in those patients who have been stabilised on the individual components in the same proportions.

(b). The use of ACE inhibitors in patients on potassium-depleting diuretics does not always prevent hypokalaemia developing. Serum potassium should be monitored.

(c). Renal failure appears to be uncommon, but the cases cited emphasise the need to monitor renal function in patients on **ACE inhibitors** and **diuretics**. If increases in blood urea and creatinine occur, a reduction in the dose of the ACE inhibitor and/or discontinuation of the diuretic may be required. The possibility of undiagnosed renal artery stenosis should be considered.

(d). None of the pharmacokinetic changes observed appear to be clinically significant.

1. Case DB, Atlas SA, Laragh JH, Sealey JE, Sullivan PA, McKinstry DN. Clinical experience with blockade of the renin-angiotensin-aldosterone system by an oral converting-enzyme inhibitor (SQ 14,225, captopril) in hypertensive patients. *Prog Cardiovasc Dis* (1978) 21, 195–206.
2. Ferguson RK, Vlasses PH, Koplin JR, Shirinian A, Burke JF, Alexander JC. Captopril in severe treatment-resistant hypertension. *Am Heart J* (1980) 99, 579–85.
3. Koffer H, Vlasses PH, Ferguson RK, Weis M, Adler AG. Captopril in diuretic-treated hypertensive patients. *JAMA* (1980) 244, 2532–5.
4. Dahlström U, Karlsson E. Captopril and spironolactone therapy for refractory congestive heart failure. *Am J Cardiol* (1993) 71, 29A–33A.
5. Haiat R, Piot O, Gallois H, Hanania G. Blood pressure response to the first 36 hours of heart failure therapy with perindopril versus captopril. French General Hospitals National College of Cardiologists. *J Cardiovasc Pharmacol* (1999) 33, 953–9.
6. D'Costa DF, Basu SK, Gunasekera NPR. ACE inhibitors and diuretics causing hypokalaemia. *Br J Clin Pract* (1990) 44, 26–7.
7. Watson ML, Bell GM, Muir AL, Buist TAS, Kellet RJ, Padfield PL. Captopril/diuretic combinations in severe renovascular disease: a cautionary note. *Lancet* (1983) ii, 404–5.
8. Hoefnagels WHL, Strijk SP, Thien T. Reversible renal failure following treatment with captopril and diuretics in patients with renovascular hypertension. *Neth J Med* (1984) 27, 269–74.
9. Funck-Brentano C, Chatellier G, Alexandre J-M. Reversible renal failure after combined treatment with enalapril and frusemide in a patient with congestive heart failure. *Br Heart J* (1986) 55, 596–8.
10. Stewart JT, Lovett D, Joy M. Reversible renal failure after combined treatment with enalapril and frusemide in a patient with congestive heart failure. *Br Heart J* (1986) 56, 489–90.
11. Hogg KJ, Hillis WS. Captopril/metolazone induced renal failure. *Lancet* (1986) 1, 501–2.
12. Mandal AK, Market RJ, Saklayen MG, Manjus RA, Yokokawa K. Diuretics potentiate angiotensin converting enzyme inhibitor-induced acute renal failure. *Clin Nephrol* (1994) 42, 170–4.
13. Speirs CJ, Dollery CT, Inman WHW, Rawson NSB, Wilton LV. Postmarketing surveillance of enalapril. II: Investigation of the potential role of enalapril in deaths with renal failure. *BMJ* (1988) 297, 830–2.
14. Toto RD, Mitchell HC, Lee HC, Milam C, Pettinger WA. Reversible renal insufficiency due to angiotensin converting enzyme inhibitors in hypertensive nephrosclerosis. *Ann Intern Med* (1991) 115, 513–19.
15. Lee H-C. Pettinger WA. Diuretics potentiate the angiotensin converting-enzyme inhibitor-associated acute renal dysfunction. *Clin Nephrol* (1992) 38, 236–7.
16. Van Hecken AM, Verbesselt R, Buntinx A, Cirillo VJ, De Schepper PJ. Absence of a pharmacokinetic interaction between enalapril and furosemide. *Br J Clin Pharmacol* (1987) 23, 84–7.
17. Fujimura A, Shimokawa Y, Ebihara A. Influence of captopril on urinary excretion of furosemide in hypertensive subjects. *J Clin Pharmacol* (1990) 30, 538–42.
18. Sommers De K, Meyer EC, Montcrieff J. Acute interaction of furosemide and captopril in healthy salt-replete man. *SA Tydskr Wet* (1991) 87, 375–7.
19. Toussaint C, Masselink A, Gentges A, Wambach G, Bönner G. Interference of different ACE -inhibitors with the diuretic action of furosemide and hydrochlorothiazide. *Klin Wochenschr* (1989) 67, 1138–46.
20. Sudoh T, Fujimura A, Shiga T, Tateishi T, Sunaga K, Ohashi K, Ebihara A. Influence of lisinopril on urinary electrolytes excretion after furosemide in healthy subjects. *J Clin Pharmacol* (1993) 33, 640–3.
21. Grass P, Gerbeau C, Kutz K. Spirapril: pharmacokinetic properties and drug interactions. *Blood Press Suppl* (1994) 2, 7–13.

22. Perdix (Moexipril). Schwarz Pharma Ltd. Summary of product characteristics, March 2000.
23. British National Formulary. 43rd ed. London: The British Medical Association and The Pharmaceutical Press; 2002. p. 90–2.
24. Captopril. Lagap Pharmaceuticals Ltd. Summary of product characteristics, July 1997.

ACE inhibitors + Minoxidil or Sodium nitroprusside

The hypotensive effects of captopril and either minoxidil or sodium nitroprusside appear to be synergistic.

Clinical evidence, mechanism, importance and management

In healthy subjects, **sodium nitroprusside** infusion caused a greater fall in blood pressure (mean arterial pressure 8 mmHg lower) when given with oral **captopril**.[1] In 4 patients on a beta-blocker and a diuretic, the addition of both **minoxidil** and **captopril** produced satisfactory control of blood pressure, when the addition of each drug individually was not effective. Moreover, the minoxidil dose needed to be reduced.[2] It has been suggested that captopril blunts the rise in plasma renin activity caused by the vasodilators.[1,2] Care should be taken when combining these drugs to avoid excessive hypotension.

1. Jennings GL, Gelman JS, Stockigt JR, Korner PI. Accentuated hypotensive effect of sodium nitroprusside in man after captopril. Clin Sci (1981) 61, 521–6.
2. Traub YM, Levey BA. Combined treatment with minoxidil and captopril in refractory hypertension. Arch Intern Med (1983) 143, 1142–4.

ACE inhibitors + Moracizine

Moracizine causes some moderate alterations in the pharmacokinetics of free captopril, but these are unlikely to be clinically important.

Clinical evidence, mechanism, importance and management

In a preliminary report, 19 normal subjects were given 250 mg **moracizine** 8-hourly or 50 mg **captopril** 8-hourly, either alone or together, for a total of 22 doses. When taken together the pharmacokinetics of the **moracizine** and total **captopril** remained unchanged, but the maximum serum levels of the free **captopril** and its AUC decreased by 32 and 14% respectively. The half-life of the free **captopril** was shorted by 44%.[1] These modest changes are unlikely to be clinically relevant. There seem to be no reports of adverse reactions when both drugs have been used together.

1. Pieniaszek HJ, Shum L, Widner P, Garner DM, Benedek IH. Pharmacokinetic interaction of moricizine and captopril in healthy volunteers. J Clin Pharmacol (1993) 33, 1005.

ACE inhibitors + Pergolide

An isolated report describes severe hypotension in a patient on lisinopril when given pergolide.

Clinical evidence, mechanism, importance and management

A man successfully treated for hypertension with 10 mg **lisinopril** daily experienced a severe hypotensive reaction within four hours of taking a single 0.05-mg dose of **pergolide** for periodic leg movements during sleep. He needed hospitalisation and treatment with intravenous fluids. It is not clear whether this patient was extremely sensitive to the **pergolide** or whether what occurred was due to an interaction, but it would now seem prudent to monitor the concurrent use of **pergolide** and ACE inhibitors, or other antihypertensives. The authors of this report suggest that the initial dose of **pergolide** should be 0.025 mg.[1]

1. Kando JC, Keck PE, Wood PA. Pergolide-induced hypotension. Ann Pharmacother (1990) 24, 543.

ACE inhibitors + Potassium-sparing diuretics

Combining ACE inhibitors with potassium-sparing diuretics (amiloride, spironolactone, triamterene) can result in clinically relevant or severe hyperkalaemia, particularly if other important risk factors are present.

Clinical evidence

(a) Hyperkalaemia

(i) Spironolactone. Twenty-five of 262 patients treated with ACE-inhibitors and **spironolactone** and admitted to hospital for medical emergencies were found to have serious hyperkalaemia (mean serum potassium 7.7 mmol/l and at least 8 mmol/l in 11 patients). These 25 patients were elderly (mean age 74 years) and being treated for hypertension, heart failure, diabetic nephropathy, proteinuria, or nephrotic syndrome: 22 had associated renal impairment. Combined treatment had been started an average of 22 weeks prior to the admission. The ACE inhibitors involved were **enalapril, captopril, lisinopril** or **perindopril**, and the average dose of **spironolactone** was 57 daily: 11 were also receiving a loop or thiazide diuretic. Nineteen had ECG changes associated with hyperkalaemia and 2 of then died, 2 required temporary pacing for third-degree heart block and 2 survived after sustained ventricular tachycardia and fibrillation; 17 required at least one haemodialysis session and 12 were admitted to intensive care.[1] A number of other cases of serious hyperkalaemia have been described in patients on ACE inhibitors (**captopril, enalapril, lisinopril**), **spironolactone**, and loop (furosemide or bumetanide) or thiazide (hydroflumethiazide) diuretics in 6 earlier reports.[2-5] Many of the patients were receiving greater than 75 mg spironolactone daily,[2,3] but one patient with moderate renal impairment was receiving just 25 mg daily.[5] In one report, the 4 cases had associated enalapril-induced deterioration in renal impairment and died.[2] Another patient died from complete heart block.[3]

(ii) Other potassium-sparing diuretics. The serum potassium levels of two patients taking furosemide and **unnamed potassium-sparing diuretics** and potassium supplements showed rises of 18% and 24% when given **captopril**. The rises occurred within one or two days. No clinical signs or symptoms of hyperkalaemia were seen but one of the patients had rise above the upper limits of normal for the laboratory.[6] In a postmarketing survey, 2 patients who had **enalapril**-associated renal impairment and died were also receiving **amiloride** and furosemide; one was also taking potassium supplements.[2] Five diabetic patients, 4 with some renal impairment, and taking **enalapril** or **captopril**, developed rapid and life-threatening hyperkalaemia within 8 to 18 days of having an **amiloride**/hydrochlorothiazide diuretic added to their treatment. Four of them showed severe cardiac dysrhythmias. Two suffered cardiac arrest and both died. Potassium levels were between 9.4 and 11 mmol/l in 4 of the patients.[7] In a preliminary report, the makers of enalapril noted that, of 47 serious cases of hyperkalaemia, 25 patients were on one or more (unnamed) potassium-sparing agents.[8]

(b) Serum potassium levels unchanged

A retrospective comparison of 35 patients treated for congestive heart failure found no differences in the plasma potassium levels of 16 patients already on furosemide, **amiloride** and **enalapril** when compared with another group of 19 patients on furosemide and **amiloride** alone. Patients were excluded from the comparison if they had significant renal impairment or were taking other drugs likely to affect serum potassium.[9] Another retrospective analysis found that giving **captopril** to 6 patients on *Dyazide* (hydrochlorothiazide/triamterene) had not increased the levels of serum potassium.[10]

Mechanism

ACE inhibitors reduce the levels of aldosterone, which results in the retention of potassium. This would be expected to be additive with the potassium-retaining effects of amiloride, spironolactone and triamterene leading to hyperkalaemia, but usually only if other risk factors are present (see 'Importance and management' below).

Importance and management

The interaction is fairly well documented and well established. Its incidence is uncertain, but if it occurs it can be serious and potentially life-threatening. Important hyperkalaemia appears to develop usually only if one or more other risk factors are also present, particularly renal impairment.

Because ACE inhibitors have potassium-sparing effects, potassium-sparing diuretics such as **amiloride** and **triamterene** should normally not be given concurrently. If, however, the use of both drugs is thought to be appropriate the serum potassium levels should be closely monitored so that any problems can be quickly identified. Note that the concurrent use of a potassium-depleting diuretic (a loop diuretic or a thiazide) with the potassium-sparing diuretic may not necessarily prevent the development of hyperkalaemia. The combination of an ACE inhibitor and **spironolactone** in heart failure is beneficial, but close monitoring of serum potassium is needed, especially with any changes in treatment or in the patients' clinical condition.

1. Schepkens H, Vanholder R, Billiouw J-M, Lameire N. Life-threatening hyperkalemia during combined therapy with angiotensin-converting enzyme inhibitors and spironolactone: an analysis of 25 cases. *Am J Med* (2001) 110, 438–41.
2. Speirs CJ, Dollery CT, Inman WHW, Rawson NSB, Wilton LV. Postmarketing surveillance of enalapril. II: Investigation of the potential role of enalapril with renal failure. *BMJ* (1988) 297, 830–2.
3. Lakhani M. Complete heart block induced by hyperkalaemia associated with treatment with a combination of captopril and spironolactone. *BMJ* (1986) 293, 271.
4. Lo TCN, Cryer RJ. Complete heart block induced by hyperkalaemia associated with treatment with a combination of captopril and spironolactone. *BMJ* (1986) 292, 1672.
5. Odawara M, Asano M, Yamashita K. Life-threatening hyperkalaemia caused by angiotensin-converting enzyme inhibitors and diuretics. *Diabetic Med* (1997) 14, 169–70.
6. Burnakis TG, Mioduch HJ. Combined therapy with captopril and potassium supplementation. A potential for hyperkalemia. *Arch Intern Med* (1984) 144, 2371–2.
7. Chiu T-F, Bullard MJ, Chen J-C, Liaw S-J, Ng C-J. Rapid life-threatening hyperkalemia after addition of amiloride HCl/hydrochlorothiazide to angiotensin-converting enzyme inhibitor therapy. *Ann Emerg Med* (1997) 30, 612–5.
8. Brown C, Rush J. Risk factors for the development of hyperkalemia in patients treated with enalapril for heart failure. *Clin Pharmacol Ther* (1989) 45, 167.
9. Radley AS, Fitzpatrick RW. An evaluation of the potential interaction between enalapril and amiloride. *J Clin Pharm Ther* (1987) 12, 319–23.
10. Schuna AA, Schmidt GR, Pitterle ME. Serum potassium concentrations after initiation of captopril therapy. *Clin Pharm* (1986) 5, 920–3.

ACE inhibitors + Potassium supplements and salt substitutes

ACE inhibitors maintain serum potassium levels so that potassium supplements are not normally needed. Hyperkalaemia is therefore a possibility if potassium supplements or potassium-containing salt substitutes are given, particularly in those patients where other risk factors are present such as decreased renal function.

Clinical evidence

(a) Potassium levels increased by concurrent use

(i) Potassium supplements. The serum potassium levels of a patient on a **potassium supplement** rose by 66% when **captopril** was added, with signs of a deterioration in renal function. Four others taking **potassium supplements** and furosemide (frusemide) (2 also taking unnamed potassium-sparing diuretics) showed rises of only 8 to 24% when given **captopril**. The rises occurred within 1 or 2 days. No clinical signs or symptoms of hyperkalaemia were seen, but 3 of the patients had rises above the upper limits of normal for the laboratory.[1] A postmarketing survey identified 10 patients in whom enalapril appeared to have been associated with renal function impairment and

death. Seven of them were also taking **potassium supplements** and/or potassium-sparing diuretics, and hyperkalaemia appeared to have been the immediate cause of death in 2 of them.[2] In 53 patients on ACE inhibitors who had hyperkalaemia in the absence of significant renal impairment, 5% were taking a potassium supplement.[3]

(ii) Dietary potassium. Two patients with renal impairment, one on **lisinopril** and the other on **enalapril**, developed marked hyperkalaemia shortly after starting to take *'Lo salt'* (a **salt substitute** containing 34.6 g **potassium** in every 100 g). One developed a life-threatening arrhythmia.[4] In 53 patients on ACE inhibitors who had hyperkalaemia in the absence of significant renal impairment, 30% were using a salt substitute, and 70% were eating a diet high in potassium-rich foods.[3]

(b) Potassium levels unaltered by concurrent use

A retrospective analysis of serum potassium before and after the addition of **captopril** to 14 patients without renal impairment on **potassium supplements** and either a loop diuretic, furosemide (frusemide) or hydrochlorothiazide found that the levels of serum potassium had not increased.[5] Another study in 6 healthy subjects found that intravenous **potassium chloride** caused virtually the same rise in serum potassium levels in those given **enalapril** as in those given a placebo.[6]

Mechanism

The potassium-retaining effects of ACE inhibitors (due to reduced aldosterone levels) are additive with increased intake of potassium, particularly when there are other contributory factors such as poor renal function.

Importance and management

The documentation of this interaction appears to be limited, but it is well established. In practice, a clinically relevant rise in potassium levels usually occurs only if other factors are also present, the most important of which is impaired renal function. To be practical: because ACE inhibitors have potassium-sparing effects, potassium supplements should normally not be given concurrently. If a supplement is needed serum potassium should be closely monitored. This is especially important where other possible contributory risk factors are known to be present.

Patients with heart disease and hypertension are often told to reduce their salt (sodium) intake. One way of doing this is to use potassium-containing salt substitutes. However, it appears that these may not be appropriate in patients taking ACE inhibitors.

1. Burnakis TG, Mioduch HJ. Combined therapy with captopril and potassium supplementation: a potential for hyperkalemia. *Arch Intern Med* (1984) 144, 2371–2.
2. Speirs CJ, Dollery CT, Inman WHW, Rawson NSB, Wilton LV. Postmarketing surveillance of enalapril. II: Investigation of the potential role of enalapril in deaths with renal failure. *BMJ* (1988) 297, 830–2.
3. Good CB, McDermott L, McCloskey B. Diet and serum potassium in patients on ACE inhibitors. *JAMA* (1995) 274, 538.
4. Ray KK, Dorman S, Watson RDS. Severe hyperkalaemia due to the concomitant use of salt substitutes and ACE inhibitors in hypertension: a potentially life-threatening interaction. *J Hum Hypertens* (1999) 13, 717–20.
5. Schuna AA, Schmidt GR, Pitterle ME. Serum potassium concentrations after initiation of captopril therapy. *Clin Pharm* (1986) 5, 920–3.
6. Scandling JD, Izzo JL, Pabico RC, McKenna BA, Radke KJ, Ornt DB. Potassium homeostasis during angiotensin-converting enzyme inhibition with enalapril. *J Clin Pharmacol* (1989) 29, 916–21.

ACE inhibitors + Probenecid

Probenecid decreases the renal clearance of captopril, but this is probably not clinically important. Enalapril serum levels are raised by probenecid.

Clinical evidence, mechanism, importance and management

Steady-state levels of unchanged and total **captopril** were slightly increased (14% and 36%) by the use of **probenecid** in healthy subjects. Renal clearance of unchanged **captopril** decreased by 44%, but total clearance was reduced by only 19%.[1] These moderated changes are unlikely to be clinically important. **Probenecid** 1 g twice daily for 5 days increased the AUC of **enalapril** and enalaprilat by about 50% after a single 20-mg dose in 12 healthy subjects. Renal clearance of **enalapril** decreased 73%.[2] A moderate increase in the hypotensive effects might be expected, but there do not appear to be any reports of adverse effects.

1. Singhvi SM, Duchin KL, Willard DA, McKinstry DN, Migdalof BH. Renal handling of captopril: effect of probenecid. *Clin Pharmacol Ther* (1982) 32, 182–9.

2. Noormohamed FH, McNabb WR, Lant AF. Pharmacokinetic and pharmacodynamic actions of enalapril in humans: effect of probenecid pretreatment. *J Pharmacol Exp Ther* (1990) 253, 362–8.

ACE Inhibitors + Rifampicin (Rifampin)

An isolated report describes a rise in blood pressure in one hypertensive patient attributed to an interaction between enalapril and rifampicin. Rifampicin may reduce the plasma levels of the active metabolites of imidapril and spirapril.

Clinical evidence, mechanism, importance and management

A man on **enalapril** and a variety of other drugs (warfarin, acebutolol, bendroflumethiazide (bendrofluazide), dipyridamole, metoclopramide and *Gaviscon*) developed a fever (38°C). Because of a probable *Brucella abortus* infection, he was additionally given streptomycin, oxytetracycline and **rifampicin** (**rifampin**), whereupon his blood pressure rose over the next 5 to 6 days from 164/104 to 180/115 mmHg. It was suspected that an interaction with the **rifampicin** was possibly responsible. Subsequent studies in the same patient showed that after stopping and then restarting the **rifampicin**, the 7 h AUC of **enalaprilat**, the active metabolite of the **enalapril**, was reduced by 31%, although the AUC of **enalapril** was unchanged.[1] There is also the hint of this interaction in another report, where **enalapril** failed to control blood pressure in a patient on **rifampicin**.[2] The maker of **spirapril** briefly noted in a review that coadministration of **rifampicin** and **spirapril** modestly decreased plasma **spirapril** concentrations and those of its active metabolite **spiraprilat**.[3] The maker of **imidapril** notes that **rifampicin** may reduce plasma levels of **imidaprilat**, the active metabolite of **imidapril**.[4]

The mechanism of this interaction is not clear because **rifampicin** is a potent liver enzyme inducing agent which might have been expected to cause the production of more, rather than less, of the active metabolites of these ACE inhibitors. However the authors of one of the reports postulate that the **rifampicin** might have increased the loss of the **enalaprilat** in the urine,[1] and others suggested that rifampicin stimulates the elimination of **spiraprilat** non-specifically.[3]

The general importance of these interactions is uncertain. The isolated reports with **enalapril** suggest minor clinical relevance. The makers of **spirapril** did not consider the modest pharmacokinetic changes to be clinically relevant.[3] However, the makers of **imidapril** state that **rifampicin** might reduce the antihypertensive efficacy of **imidapril**,[4] but this awaits clinical assessment.

1. Kandiah D, Penny WJ, Fraser AG, Lewis MJ. A possible drug interaction between rifampicin and enalapril. *Eur J Clin Pharmacol* (1988) 35, 431–2.

2. Tada Y, Tsuda Y, Otsuka T, Nagasawa K, Kimura H, Kusaba T, Sakata T. Case report: nifedipine-rifampicin interaction attenuates the effect on blood pressure in a patient with essential hypertension. *Am J Med Sci* (1992) 303, 25–7.

3. Grass P, Gerbeau C, Kutz K. Spirapril: pharmacokinetic properties and drug interactions. *Blood Pressure* (1994) 3 (Suppl 2), 7–13.

4. Tanatril (Imidapril) Trinity Pharmaceuticals Ltd. Summary of product characteristics, March 2001.

ACE inhibitors + Trimethoprim

Two reports describe serious hyperkalaemia apparently caused by trimethoprim and enalapril or quinapril, associated with impairment of renal function.

Clinical evidence

A 40-year-old woman with transplanted lungs (immunosuppressive treatment with ciclosporin, azathioprine, prednisolone) developed life-threatening hyperkalaemia (6.8 mmol/l) when treated with high dose **co-trimoxazole** 20/100 mg per kg daily for suspected *Pneumocystis carinii* pneumonia. She was also taking **enalapril**, gentamicin inhalation, salbutamol and *N*-acetylcysteine. She began to recover over a period of a week when the **co-trimoxazole** and **enalapril** were stopped, but she then developed fatal septic shock with multi-organ failure.[1] In another case, an elderly man treated with **quinapril** 20 mg daily for essential hypertension was found to have hyperkalaemia (serum potassium 7 to 7.4 mmol/l) and azotaemia after 20 days treatment with **co-trimoxazole** for mild acute pyelonephritis. **Co-trimoxazole** and **quinapril** were stopped, and nifedipine was given to control blood pressure. After treatment with dextrose, insulin, sodium polystyrene sulfonate and calcium gluconate, the azotaemia and hyperkalaemia resolved over 36 h.[2]

Mechanism

Hyperkalaemia has been reported in patients receiving co-trimoxazole alone. This is attributed to the **trimethoprim** component, which can have an amiloride-like (potassium-sparing) effect on the distal part of the kidney tubules. ACE inhibitors reduce aldosterone synthesis, which results in reduced renal loss of potassium. The interaction is probably due to the additive effects of these two mechanisms, compounded by impaired renal function.[1,2]

Importance and management

Clinical examples of this interaction seem to be few, but the possibility of hyperkalaemia with either trimethoprim or ACE inhibitors alone, particularly with other factors such as renal impairment, is well documented. Thus it may be prudent to monitor potassium levels if this combination is used. It has been suggested that trimethoprim should probably be avoided in elderly patients with chronic renal impairment taking ACE inhibitors, and that patients with AIDS taking an ACE inhibitor for associated nephropathy should probably discontinue this treatment during high-dose co-trimoxazole therapy.[2]

1. Bugge JF. Severe hyperkalaemia induced by trimethoprim in combination with an angiotensin-converting enzyme inhibitor in a patient with transplanted lungs. *J Intern Med* (1996) 240, 249–52.

2. Thomas RJ. Severe hyperkalemia with trimethoprim-quinapril. *Ann Pharmacother* (1996) 30, 413–14.

Acetazolamide + Beta-blockers

The concurrent use of acetazolamide and timolol eye-drops resulted in severe mixed acidosis in a patient with chronic obstructive lung disease.

Clinical evidence, mechanism, importance and management

An elderly man with severe chronic obstructive pulmonary disease was given 750 mg acetazolamide daily orally and 0.5% **timolol maleate eye-drops**, one drop in each eye twice daily, as premedication to reduce ocular hypertension before surgery for glaucoma. Five days later a progressive worsening of dyspnoea was seen and he was found to have a severe mixed acidosis.[1] The reason seems to have been the additive effects of acetazolamide, which blocked the excretion of hydrogen ions in the kidney, and the bronchoconstrictor effects of the **timolol**, which was sufficiently absorbed systemically to exacerbate the airway obstruction in this patient and thereby reduced the respiration. This isolated case emphasises the potential risks of using beta-blockers in patients with obstructive lung disease and of concurrent use with acetazolamide even if kidney function is normal.

1. Boada JE, Estopa R, Izquierdo J, Dorca J, Manresa F. Severe mixed acidosis by combined therapy with acetazolamide and timolol eyedrops. *Eur J Respir Dis* (1986) 68, 226–8.

Acetazolamide + Sodium bicarbonate

Acetazolamide is associated with development of renal calculi and it is claimed that sodium bicarbonate, even on alternate days, potentiates the risk of calculus formation.[1] The basis for this claim is not clear.

1. Rubenstein MA, Bucy JG. Acetazolamide-induced renal calculi. *J Urol (Baltimore)* (1975) 114, 610–12.

Alfuzosin + Miscellaneous drugs

Profound hypotension may occur in patients on alfuzosin during general anaesthesia. No important interactions are reported to occur with cimetidine, digoxin, or warfarin.

Clinical evidence, mechanism, importance and management

The makers of alfuzosin note that administration of **general anaesthetics** to patients receiving alfuzosin may cause profound hypotension, and they recommend that alfuzosin be withdrawn 24 hours before surgery. They report that no pharmacodynamic or pharmacokinetic interactions were observed in studies in healthy subjects given alfuzosin with **digoxin** or **warfarin**.[1]

Cimetidine 1 g daily in divided doses for 20 days was found to have minimal effects on the pharmacokinetics of single 5-mg doses of alfuzosin in 10 healthy subjects. The maximum serum levels and the AUC were increased by up to 24%, (not statistically significant) and the half-life was shortened by 14%. **Cimetidine** did not appear to increase the incidence of postural hypotension seen with **alfuzosin**.[2] These changes are not clinically relevant, and there would seem to be no reason for avoiding concurrent use.

1. Xatral (Alfuzosin). Sanofi Synthelabo. Summary of product characteristics, August 1998.
2. Desager JP, Harvengt C, Bianchetti G, Rosenzweig P. The effect of cimetidine on the pharmacokinetics of single oral doses of alfuzosin. *Int J Clin Pharmacol Ther Toxicol* (1993) 31, 568–71.

Alpha blockers + ACE inhibitors

Severe first-dose hypotension occurred in a patient on enalapril when given bunazosin, and synergistic hypotensive effects occurred with single doses of the two drugs in healthy subjects. The first-dose effect seen with some alpha₁-blockers (e.g. alfuzosin, prazosin, terazosin) is also likely to be potentiated by ACE-inhibitors. Tamsulosin did not have any clinically relevant effects on blood pressure in patients on maintenance enalapril.

Clinical evidence

When a patient on **enalapril** developed severe first-dose hypotension when given **bunazosin**, a further study of this interaction was made in 6 healthy subjects. When given 10 mg **enalapril** or 2 mg **bunazosin**, their systolic/diastolic pressures over 6 h were reduced by 9.5/6.7 mmHg. When given the **enalapril** followed by the **bunazosin** an hour later, the pressure falls were 27/28 mmHg. Even with a much smaller dose of **enalapril** (2.5 mg) the fall when given both drugs was 19/22 mmHg.[1] In a placebo-controlled study in 12 men with hyper-

tension on maintenance **enalapril,** the addition of **tamsulosin** 0.4 mg daily for 7 days then 0.8 mg daily for a further 7 days had no clinically relevant effects on blood pressure (assessed after 6 and 14 days of tamsulosin: blood pressure was not assessed on the first day of tamsulosin). The dose of **enalapril** did not need to be reduced.[2,3]

Mechanism

The first-dose effect seen with some alpha₁-blockers (e.g. alfuzosin, bunazosin, prazosin, terazosin) may be potentiated by ACE-inhibitors. Tamsulosin possibly has less effect on blood pressure since it has some selectivity for alpha₁A-receptors.

Importance and management

Direct information is limited. Acute hypotension (dizziness, fainting) sometimes occurs unpredictably with the first dose of some other alpha₁-blockers (e.g. alfuzosin, prazosin, terazosin), and it is well documented that this can be exaggerated if the patient is given or is already taking a beta-blocker or a calcium channel blocker (see 'Alpha blockers + Beta-blockers', p.380, and 'Alpha blockers + Calcium channel blockers', p.381). It would therefore seem prudent to apply the same precautions to ACE inhibitors, namely to give test doses of the drugs and to monitor the effects. Giving the first dose of these alpha₁-blockers at bedtime is recommended. Note that the acute hypotensive reaction appears to be short-lived. The maker of terazosin notes that the incidence of dizziness in patients with benign prostatic hyperplasia treated with terazosin was higher when they were also receiving an ACE inhibitor.[4] The makers of alfuzosin and prazosin warn that patients receiving antihypertensive drugs are at particular risk of developing postural hypotension after the first dose of alfuzosin or prazosin.[5,6] Tamsulosin may possibly have less effect on blood pressure, but this requires further study.

1. Baba T, Tomiyama T, Takebe K. Enhancement by an ACE inhibitor of first-dose hypotension caused by an alpha₁-blocker. *N Engl J Med* (1990) 322, 1237.
2. Lowe FC. Concomitant administration of tamsulosin and common antihypertensives: minimal potential for adverse interactions. *J Urol* (1997) 157 (4 Suppl), 138.
3. Lowe FC. Coadministration of tamsulosin and three antihypertensive agents in patients with benign prostatic hyperplasia: pharmacodynamic effect. *Clin Ther* (1997) 19, 730–42.
4. Hytrin (Terazosin). Abbott Laboratories Limited. Summary of product characteristics, October 2000.
5. Xatral (Alfuzosin). Sanofi Synthelabo. Summary of product characteristics, July 2001.
6. Hypovase (Prazosin). Pfizer Ltd. Summary of product characteristics, August 1998.

Alpha blockers + Beta-blockers

The risk of first-dose hypotension with prazosin is higher if the patient is already taking a beta-blocker. This is likely to be true of other alpha₁-blockers that have a first-dose effect (e.g. alfuzosin, bunazosin, terazosin). Tamsulosin did not have any clinically relevant effects on blood pressure in patients on maintenance atenolol.

Clinical evidence

Three out of 6 hypertensive patients on 400 mg **alprenolol** twice daily experienced a marked hypotensive reaction (dizziness, pallor, sweating) when given the first dose of 0.5 mg **prazosin**. All 6 patients had a greater reduction in blood pressure after the first prazosin dose than after 2 weeks of treatment with 0.5 mg three times daily (mean reduction 22/11 mmHg vs 4/4 mmHg). Three other patients taking **prazosin** 0.5 mg three times daily had no unusual fall in blood pressure when given the first dose of **alprenolol** 200 mg.[1] The severity and the duration of the 'first dose' response to **prazosin** was also found to be increased in healthy subjects given a single dose of **propranolol** or **primidolol** concurrently.[2] The pharmacokinetics of **prazosin** were not affected by either **alprenolol**[1] or **propranolol**.[3] In a placebo-controlled study in 12 men with hypertension on maintenance **atenolol**, the addition of **tamsulosin** 0.4 mg daily for 7 days then 0.8 mg daily for a further 7 days had no clinically relevant effect on blood pressure (assessed after 6 and 14 days of tamsulosin: blood pressure was not assessed on the first day of tamsulosin).[4] The maker of **alfuzosin** states that no pharmacodynamic or pharmacokinetic interaction occurred between **alfuzosin** and **atenolol** in healthy subjects, but also says that postural hypotension may occur in patients receiving antihypertensive medications when they start **alfuzosin**.[5] The maker of **doxazosin** notes that no adverse drug interaction has been observed between **doxazosin** and **beta-blockers**.[6]

Mechanism

The normal cardiovascular response (a compensatory increased heart output and rate) which should follow the first dose hypotensive reaction to some alpha₁-blockers is apparently compromised by the presence of a beta-blocker. The problem is usually only short-lasting because, within hours or days, some physiological compensation occurs which allows the blood pressure to be lowered without falling precipitously. Tamsulosin possibly has less effect on blood pressure since it has some selectivity for alpha$_{1A}$ receptors.

Importance and management

An established interaction. Some patients experience acute postural hypotension, tachycardia and palpitations when they begin to take prazosin or some other alpha₁-blockers (e.g. alfuzosin, bunazosin, terazosin). A few even collapse in a sudden faint within 30 to 90 min, and this can be exacerbated if they are already taking a beta-blocker. It is recommended that those already on beta-blockers should begin with a low-dose of these alpha₁-blockers, and that the first dose should be taken just before going to bed. They should also be told what may happen and what to do. No particular precautions seem necessary in patients already taking these alpha₁-blockers who are then additionally given a beta-blocker. Other alpha₁-blockers not associated with a first-dose effect include doxazosin, indoramin, and tamsulosin. Of these, tamsulosin may possibly have less effect on blood pressure, but this requires further study.

1. Seideman P, Grahnén A, Haglund K, Lindström B, von Bahr C. Prazosin first dose phenomenon during combined treatment with a β-adrenoceptor in hypertensive patients. *Br J Clin Pharmacol* (1982) 13, 865–70.
2. Elliott HL, McLean K, Sumner DJ, Meredith PA, Reid JL. Immediate cardiovascular responses to oral prazosin-effects of β-blockers. *Clin Pharmacol Ther* (1981) 29, 303–9.
3. Rubin P, Jackson G, Blaschke T. Studies on the clinical pharmacology of prazosin. II: The influence of indomethacin and of propranolol on the action and the disposition of prazosin. *Br J Clin Pharmacol* (1980) 10, 33–9.
4. Lowe FC. Coadministration of tamsulosin and three antihypertensive agents in patients with benign prostatic hyperplasia: pharmacodynamic effect. *Clin Ther* (1997) 19, 730–42.
5. Xatral (Alfuzosin). Sanofi Synthelabo. Summary of product characteristics, November 2000.
6. Cardura (Doxazosin). Pfizer Ltd. Summary of product characteristics. March 1999.

Alpha blockers + Calcium channel blockers

Blood pressure may fall sharply when calcium channel blockers are first given to patients already taking alpha₁-blockers that cause a first-dose effect (e.g. prazosin, terazosin), and vice versa. This appears to be less of a problem with those alpha₁-blockers that do not cause a first-dose effect, such as doxazosin. Tamsulosin did not have any clinically relevant effects on blood pressure in patients on maintenance nifedipine.

Clinical evidence

(a) Nifedipine

No serious adverse events or postural symptoms were seen in 6 normotensive subjects given 20 mg **nifedipine** twice daily for 10 days, to which was added 2 mg **doxazosin** once daily for 10 days. The same results were noted in 6 other normotensive subjects given 2 mg **doxazosin** once daily for 10 days, then additionally 20 mg **nifedipine** twice daily for 10 days. No pharmacokinetic interactions were found. There was a tendency for a first-dose hypotensive response when the second drug was added to the first, but no symptomatic orthostatic hypotension occurred.[1]

Two patients with severe hypertension given **prazosin** (4 or 5 mg) experienced a sharp fall in blood pressure shortly after being given **nifedipine** *sublingually*. One of them had a fall in standing blood pressure from 232/124 to 88/48 mmHg about 20 min after 10 mg **nifedipine**. He complained of dizziness. Eight other patients with hypertension were given a dose of **prazosin**, and blood pressure remained unchanged 1 h later. They were then given *sublingual* **nifedipine** or a placebo; 20 min after **nifedipine** they had less reduction in blood pressure than the earlier 2 patients (mean reduction of 25/12 mmHg when lying and 24/17 mmHg when standing).[2] However, it is not clear what contribution **prazosin** had to the effect seen with *sublingual* **nifedipine**, since the experiment was not repeated using a **prazosin** placebo. Note that *sublingual* **nifedipine** alone may cause dangerous falls in blood pressure.

In a placebo-controlled study in 12 men with hypertension on maintenance **nifedipine**, the addition of **tamsulosin** 0.4 mg daily for 7 days then 0.8 mg daily for a further 7 days had no clinically relevant effect on blood pressure (assessed after 6 and 14 days of tamsulosin: blood pressure was not assessed on the first day of tamsulosin). The dose of **nifedipine** did not need to be reduced.[3,4]

(b) Verapamil

A study in 8 normotensive subjects given single 1-mg doses of **prazosin** showed that the peak serum **prazosin** levels were raised 85% (from 5.2 to 9.6 nanograms/ml) when given with a single 160-mg dose of **verapamil**. The **prazosin** AUC increased by 62%. The standing blood pressure did not change after **verapamil** alone, fell from 114/82 to 99/81 mmHg after the **prazosin** alone, and, after both drugs, to 89/68 mmHg.[5,6]

When **verapamil** 120 mg twice daily was added to **terazosin** 5 mg daily in 12 hypertensive patients, the peak plasma levels and the AUC of the **terazosin** were increased by about 25%. In contrast, no changes in verapamil pharmacokinetics occurred when **terazosin** (1 mg increased to 5 mg daily) was added to **verapamil** 120 mg twice daily in another 12 patients.[7,8] Both groups of patients had significant falls in standing blood pressure when the combination therapy was first started. Symptomatic orthostatic hypotension occurred in 4 patients when **verapamil** was first added to **terazosin**, and in 2 when terazosin was first added to verapamil. Within about 3 weeks this had reduced.[8,9]

Mechanism

Not fully understood. It would seem to be that the vasodilatory effects of the alpha blockers and the calcium channel blockers can be additive or synergistic, particularly after the first dose.[1,5,10] The fall in blood pressure seen with prazosin and verapamil may, in part, result from a pharmacokinetic interaction.[10] Tamsulosin possibly has less effect on blood pressure since it has some selectivity for alpha$_{1A}$ receptors.

Importance and management

The interaction between calcium channel blockers and alpha₁-blockers that cause a first-dose effect (e.g. alfuzosin, bunazosin, prazosin, terazosin) would appear to be established and of clinical importance although the documentation is limited. Marked additive hypotensive effects can occur when concurrent therapy is started. It is recommended that patients already on calcium channel blockers should begin with a low-dose of these alpha₁-blockers, and that the first dose should be taken just before going to bed. Caution should also be exercised when calcium channel blockers are added to established alpha-blocker therapy. Patients should be warned about the possibilities of exaggerated hypotension, and told what to do if they feel faint and dizzy. The interaction appears less likely with alpha₁-blockers that are not associated with a first-dose effect (e.g. doxazosin, indoramin, tamsulosin). Of these, tamsulosin may possibly have less effect on blood pressure, but this requires further study.

1. Donnelly R, Elliott HL, Meredith PA, Howie CA, Reid JL. The pharmacodynamics and pharmacokinetics of the combination of nifedipine and doxazosin. *Eur J Clin Pharmacol* (1993) 44, 279–82.
2. Jee LD, Opie LH. Acute hypotensive response to nifedipine added to prazosin in treatment of hypertension. *BMJ* (1983) 287, 1514.
3. Lowe FC. Concomitant administration of tamsulosin and common antihypertensives: minimal potential for adverse interactions. *J Urol* (1997) 157 (4 Suppl), 138.
4. Lowe FC. Coadministration of tamsulosin and three antihypertensive agents in patients with benign prostatic hyperplasia: pharmacodynamic effect. *Clin Ther* (1997) 19, 730–42.

5. Pasanisi F, Meredith PA, Elliott HL, Reid JL. Verapamil and prazosin: pharmacodynamic and pharmacokinetic interactions in normal man. *Br J Clin Pharmacol* (1984) 18, 290P.
6. Pasanisi F, Elliott HL, Meredith PA, McSharry DR, Reid JL. Combined alpha adrenoceptor antagonism and calcium channel blockade in normal subjects. *Clin Pharmacol Ther* (1984) 36, 716–23.
7. Varghese A, Lenz M, Locke C, Granneman R, Laddu A, Pool J, Piwinski S, Taylor A. Combined terazosin and verapamil therapy in essential hypertension: pharmacokinetic interactions. *Clin Pharmacol Ther* (1991) 49, 130.
8. Lenz ML, Pool JL, Laddu AR, Varghese A, Johnston W, Taylor AA. Combined terazosin and verapamil therapy in essential hypertension. Hemodynamic and pharmacodynamic interactions. *Am J Hypertens* (1995) 8, 133–45.
9. Lenz M, Varghese A, Pool J, Laddu A, Johnston W, Piwinski S, Taylor A. Combined terazosin and verapamil therapy in essential hypertension: hemodynamic interactions. *Clin Pharmacol Ther* (1991) 49, 146.
10. Meredith PA, Elliott HL, Pasanisi F, Reid JL. Prazosin and verapamil: a pharmacokinetic and pharmacodynamic interaction. *Br J Clin Pharmacol* (1986) 21, 85P.

Alpha blockers + Diuretics

Patients with congestive heart failure who have had large doses of diuretics should start prazosin treatment with low doses. An increased incidence of dizziness was seen with the combination of terazosin and a diuretic.

Clinical evidence, mechanism, importance and management

The acute first-dose hypotension that can occur with some alpha blockers such as **prazosin** can be exacerbated by beta-blockers and calcium channel blockers (see 'Alpha blockers + Beta-blockers', p.380 and 'Alpha blockers + Calcium channel blockers', p.381), but there seems to be no direct evidence that **diuretics** normally do the same. However the maker of **prazosin** suggests that it is particularly important that patients with congestive heart failure who have undergone vigorous diuretic treatment should be given the initial dose at bedtime and the lowest dose (500 micrograms two to four times daily) to start with. The reason is that these patients may develop a decrease in left ventricular filling pressure with a resultant fall in cardiac output and systemic blood pressure.[1,2] There seems to be no reason for avoiding concurrent use if these precautions are taken. The maker of **terazosin** notes that the incidence of dizziness in patients with benign prostatic hyperplasia treated with **terazosin** was higher when they were also receiving a diuretic. They state that when **terazosin** is added to a diuretic, dose reduction and re-titration may be necessary.[3] The maker of **alfuzosin** states that no pharmacodynamic or pharmacokinetic interaction occurred between **alfuzosin** and **hydrochlorothiazide** in healthy subjects, but also says that postural hypotension may occur in patients receiving antihypertensive medications when they start **alfuzosin**.[4] The maker of **doxazosin** notes that no adverse drug interaction has been observed between **doxazosin** and **thiazide diuretics**.[5]

1. Invicta Pharmaceuticals. Personal communication, 1995.
2. Hypovase (Prazosin). Pfizer Ltd. Summary of product characteristics, August, 1998.
3. Hytrin (Terazosin). Abbott Laboratories Ltd. Summary of product characteristics, October 2000.
4. Xatral (Alfuzosin). Sanofi Synthelabo. Summary of product characteristics, July 2001.
5. Cardura (Doxazosin). Pfizer Ltd. Summary of product characteristics, March 1999.

Alpha blockers + NSAIDs

Indometacin (indomethacin) reduces the blood-pressure lowering effects of prazosin in some individuals.

Clinical evidence

A study in 9 healthy subjects found that 50 mg **indometacin (indomethacin)** twice daily for 3 days had no statistically significant effect on the hypotensive effect of a single 5-mg dose of **prazosin**. However, in 4 of the subjects it was noted that the maximum fall in the mean standing blood pressure due to the **prazosin** was 20 mmHg less when they were taking **indometacin**. Three of these 4 felt faint when given **prazosin** alone, but not while taking the **indometacin** as well.[1]

Mechanism

Not established. It seems probable that indometacin inhibits the production of hypotensive prostaglandins by the kidney.

Importance and management

Direct information seems to be limited to this study but what occurred is consistent with the way indometacin reduces the effects of many other different antihypertensives. It apparently does not affect every subject. If indometacin is added to established treatment with prazosin, be alert for a reduced antihypertensive response, although it is not known exactly what happens in patients taking both drugs chronically. However, in their datasheet, the makers say that prazosin has been given with indometacin (and also **aspirin** and **phenylbutazone**) without any adverse interaction in clinical experience to date.[2] Other makers also note that no adverse interaction has been seen between NSAIDs (unspecified) and doxazosin or terazosin.[3,4]

1. Rubin P, Jackson G, Blaschke T. Studies on the clinical pharmacology of prazosin. II: The influence of indomethacin and of propranolol on the action and disposition of prazosin. *Br J Clin Pharmacol* (1980) 10, 33–9.
2. Hypovase (Prazosin). Pfizer Ltd. Summary of product characteristics. August 1998.
3. Cardura (Doxazosin). Pfizer Ltd. Summary of product characteristics, March 1999.
4. Hytrin (Terazosin). Abbott Laboratories Ltd. Summary of product characteristics, October 2000.

Alpha blockers + Rifampicin (Rifampin)

Rifampicin markedly reduces bunazosin serum levels.

Clinical evidence, mechanism, importance and management

A 7-day course of 600 mg **rifampicin (rifampin)** daily reduced the mean maximum **bunazosin** serum levels of 15 healthy subjects taking 6 mg daily by 82% (from 11.6 to 2.1 nanograms/ml). The **bunazosin** AUC was reduced more than sevenfold (from 151 to 20 micrograms/l). The duration of blood-pressure lowering effect was shortened, the heart rate increase was less pronounced, and some side-effects of **bunazosin** treatment (fatigue, headache) disappeared.[1,2] The probable reason is that the **rifampicin** (a recognised, potent liver-enzyme inducing agent) increases the metabolism of the **bunazosin** by the liver so that it is lost from the body much more quickly.

The evidence seems to be limited to this study, but anticipate the need to raise **bunazosin** dosage levels if **rifampicin** is added. Information about other alpha-blockers does not seem to be available.

1. Al-Hamdan Y, Otto U, Kirch W. Interaction of rifampicin with bunazosin, an alpha$_1$-adrenoceptor antagonist. *J Clin Pharmacol* (1993) 33, 998.
2. Nokhodian A, Halabi A, Ebert U, Al-Hamdan Y, Kirch W. Interaction of rifampicin with bunazosin, an α$_1$-adrenoceptor antagonist, in healthy volunteers. *Drug Invest* (1993) 6, 362–4.

Amiloride + Cimetidine

Cimetidine does not alter serum amiloride levels or its diuretic effects, but amiloride can cause some minor reduction in the cimetidine levels.

Clinical evidence, mechanism, importance and management

A study in 8 healthy subjects given 5 mg amiloride daily found that the concurrent use of 400 mg **cimetidine** twice daily for 12 days reduced the renal clearance of amiloride by 17% and the urinary excretion of amiloride from 65 to 53% of the administered dose. The amiloride also reduced the excretion of the **cimetidine** from 43 to

32% of the dose and the AUC was reduced by 14%.[1] No changes in the diuretic effects (urinary volume, Na^+ or K^+ excretion) occurred. It seems that each drug reduces the gastrointestinal absorption of the other drug by as yet unidentified mechanisms. The overall serum levels of the amiloride remain unchanged because the reduced absorption is offset by a reduction in its renal excretion. These mutual interactions seem to be clinically unimportant.

1. Somogyi AA, Hovens CM, Muirhead MR, Bochner F. Renal tubular secretion of amiloride and its inhibition by cimetidine in humans and in an animal model. *Drug Metab Dispos* (1989) 17, 190–6.

Antihypertensives + Alcohol

Chronic moderate to heavy drinking raises the blood pressure and reduces, to some extent, the effectiveness of antihypertensive drugs. A few patients may experience postural hypotension, dizziness and fainting shortly after having a drink. Alpha blockers may enhance the hypotensive effect of alcohol in subjects susceptible to the alcohol flush syndrome.

Clinical evidence, mechanisms, importance and management

(a) Hypertensive reaction

A study in 40 men with essential hypertension (treated with **diuretics**, **beta-blockers**, **verapamil**, **prazosin**, **captopril** or **methyldopa**) who were moderate to heavy drinkers, showed that when they reduced their drinking over a six-week period from an average of 450 ml **ethanol** weekly (about 6 drinks daily) to 64 ml **ethanol** weekly, their average blood pressure fell by 5/3 mmHg.[1] The reasons are uncertain. These findings are consistent with those of other studies in hypertensive[2] and normotensive[3] men. It seems likely that this effect will occur with any antihypertensive. Patients with hypertension should be encouraged to reduce their intake of **alcohol**. It may then become possible to reduce the dosage of the antihypertensive.

(b) Hypotensive reaction

A few patients taking some antihypertensives feel dizzy or begin to 'black out' or faint if they stand up quickly or after exercise. This orthostatic and exertional hypotension may be exaggerated in some patients shortly after drinking **alcohol**, possibly because it can lower the output of the heart (noted in patients with various types of heart disease[4,5]). Patients just beginning antihypertensive treatment should be warned.

A study in 10 Japanese hypertensive patients found that **alcohol** 1 ml/kg decreased blood pressure for several hours. Treatment with **prazosin** 1 mg three times daily caused a significant reduction in blood pressure and enhanced alcohol-induced hypotension.[6] These effects may be restricted to Orientals. The reason being that the alcohol flush syndrome, caused by accumulation of vasodilative acetaldehyde due to a genetic alteration in aldehyde dehydrogenase, is rare in whites and blacks.[6] The clinical significance is uncertain as the dose of prazosin in the study was relatively small. Also the dose of alcohol was relatively large and the findings may not apply to more moderate drinking.

(c) CNS effects

For mention of the possibility of increased sedation with indoramin and alcohol, see 'Indoramin + Alcohol', p.397. For mention of the disulfiram-like reaction when tolazoline is given with alcohol, see 'Alcohol + Tolazoline', p.37. For the possible CNS effects of other antihypertensives and alcohol, see 'Alcohol + Calcium channel blockers', p.22 and 'Beta-blockers + Alcohol', p.432.

1. Puddey IB, Beilin LJ, Vandongen R. Regular alcohol use raises blood pressure in treated hypertensive subjects. A randomised controlled trial. *Lancet* (1987) i, 647–51.
2. Potter JF, Beevers DG. Pressor effect of alcohol in hypertension. *Lancet* (1984) i, 119–22.
3. Puddey IB, Beilin LJ, Vandongen R, Rouse IL, Rogers P. Evidence for a direct effect of alcohol on blood pressure in normotensive men — a randomized controlled trial. *Hypertension* (1985) 7, 707–13.
4. Gould L, Zahir M, DeMartino A, Gomprecht RF. Cardiac effects of a cocktail. *JAMA* (1971) 218, 1799–1802.
5. Conway N. Haemodynamic effects of ethyl alcohol in patients with coronary heart disease. *Br Heart J* (1968) 30, 638–44.
6. Kawano Y, Abe H, Kojima S, Takishita S, Omae T. Interaction of alcohol and an α_1-blocker on ambulatory blood pressure in patients with essential hypertension. *Am J Hypertens* (2000) 13, 307–12.

Antihypertensives + Fenfluramine

Fenfluramine can cause a small additional drop in blood pressure when used with antihypertensive agents.

Clinical evidence, mechanism, importance and management

Fenfluramine alone has some slight hypotensive activity.[1] In a trial in obese hypertensive patients, **fenfluramine** 60 mg daily modestly potentiated the antihypertensive effect of **betanidine (bethanidine)**, **guanethidine**, **methyldopa**, **reserpine**, and/or **diuretics**, but not of **debrisoquine**.[2,3] Four patients developed hypotension.[2] However note that **fenfluramine** was withdrawn in 1997 because its use was found to be associated with the development of valvular heart disease.

1. General Practitioner Clinical Trials. Hypotensive effect of fenfluramine in the treatment of obesity. *Practitioner* (1971) 207, 101–5.
2. Waal-Manning HJ, Simpson FO. Fenfluramine in obese patients on various antihypertensive drugs. Double-blind controlled trial. *Lancet* (1969) ii, 1392–5.
3. Simpson FO, Waal-Manning HJ. Use of fenfluramine in obese patients on antihypertensive therapy. *S Afr Med J* (1971) 45 (Suppl), 47–9.

Antihypertensives + Food

Food has little or no effect on the absorption of the ACE inhibitors cilazapril, enalapril, fosinopril, lisinopril, quinapril, spirapril, and trandolapril. Although food may reduce the absorption of captopril, moexipril, and possibly perindopril, this does not appear to be clinically important. Food reduced the absorption of imidapril, and the maker recommends it be administered 15 minutes before food. Food may increase the plasma levels of spironolactone, but again, this is probably not clinically important. The situation with hydralazine is unclear: increased, reduced and unchanged bioavailability has been reported.

Clinical evidence, mechanism, importance and management

(a) ACE inhibitors

Although **food** reduced the AUC of **captopril** (25 to 100 mg) by up to 56%[1-4] this had no effect on the maximum decrease in blood pressure.[1,3,4] One study reported a one-hour delay in the maximum hypotensive effect.[1] In another study, the extent and duration of antihypertensive efficacy of **captopril** 50 mg twice daily for one month was not affected by whether the drug was taken before or after food.[5] This study suggests that any pharmacokinetic changes are not clinically significant. However, decreasing the dose of an ACE inhibitor reduces the duration of the hypotensive effect and it has been suggested that these results should be confirmed with lower doses of **captopril**.[5]

Other studies have shown that **food** had no effect on the pharmacokinetics of **enalapril** and its active metabolite,[6] **quinapril** and its active metabolite,[7] and **lisinopril**.[8] Similarly, **food** had minimal effects of the pharmacokinetics of **cilazapril** (AUC decreased 14%).[9] The makers of **spirapril** briefly mention in a review that food delayed the absorption of **spirapril** by 1h, but did not affect the extent of absorption.[10] The makers state that food had no effect on the absorption of **fosinopril**[11] and **trandolapril**.[12]

Although **food** did not affect the pharmacokinetics of **perindopril**, the AUC of its active metabolite **perindoprilat** was reduced by 44%.[13,14] The blood-pressure lowering effects were not assessed, but it seems likely that they would not be affected (see captopril, above).

Food reduced the AUC of moexipril by 40 to 50%.[15] However, the reduced bioavailability is not expected to be clinically significant.[16] The maker of **imidapril** states that a fat-rich meal significantly reduces the absorption of **imidapril**, and they recommend that the drug be taken at the same time of day about 15 minutes before a meal.[17]

(b) Hydralazine

Food markedly enhanced the bioavailability of single doses of **hydralazine** 50 mg in healthy subjects in one study.[18] Similar findings were reported by the same research group with conventional **hydralazine** tablets, but not slow-release tablets.[19] In contrast, others found that **food** had no effect on the AUC of **hydralazine** in healthy subjects.[20] In contrast other studies have found that **food** decreases the AUC of **hydralazine** by 46% after administration of oral solution,[21] by 44% after conventional tablets,[22] and by 29% (not significant) after a slow-release preparation.[22] A reduction in antihypertensive effect was noted in the first study,[21] but no significant alteration in antihypertensive effect was seen in the second.[22] Similarly, others have reported a 55% decrease in **hydralazine** AUC when administered with a **meal** or 62% with a bolus dose of **enteral feed**, but no significant change when administered during an enteral infusion.[23] The widely different findings of these studies may be related to the problems in analysing hydralazine and its metabolites, all of which are unstable. All these studies were single-dose, and no studies have adequately assessed the possible clinical importance of any pharmacokinetic changes in long-term clinical use.

(c) Spironolactone

Food increased the plasma concentrations of **canrenone** (the major active metabolite of **spironolactone**) after a single dose of **spironolactone** 100 mg in healthy subjects.[24] However, the same research group later found that the steady-state **canrenone** levels did not differ when **spironolactone** 100 mg daily was taken at least 30 min before eating for 60 days compared with immediately after eating for 60 days, nor was antihypertensive efficacy altered. They suggest that the difference is due to a more specific drug assay in the second study.[25] In contrast, other authors reported that **food** increased the AUC of **spironolactone** by 71%, and of 3 of its metabolites (including canrenone) by 32% after a single dose in healthy subjects, but they did not assess whether this affected the hypotensive effect.[26] It appears from the long-term study, that food does not alter the antihypertensive efficacy of **spironolactone**.

1. Mäntylä R, Männistö PT, Vuorela A, Sundberg S, Ottoila P. Impairment of captopril bioavailability by concomitant food and antacid intake. *Int J Clin Pharmacol Ther Toxicol* (1984) 22, 626–9.
2. Singhvi SM, McKinstry DN, Shaw JM, Willard DA, Migdalof BH. Effect of food on the bioavailability of captopril in healthy subjects. *J Clin Pharmacol* (1982) 22, 135–40.
3. Ohman KP, Kagedal B, Larsson R, Karlberg BE. Pharmacokinetics of captopril and its effect on blood pressure during acute and chronic administration and in relation to food intake. *J Cardiovasc Pharmacol* (1985) 7 (Suppl), S20–S24.
4. Muller HM, Overlack A, Heck I, Kolloch R, Stumpe KO. The influence of food intake on pharmacodynamics and plasma concentration of captopril. *J Hypertens* (1985) 3 (Suppl), S135–S136.
5. Salvetti A, Pedrinelli R, Magagna A, Abdel-Haq B, Graziadei L. Influence of food on acute and chronic effects of captopril in essential hypertensive patients. *J Cardiovasc Pharmacol* (1985) 7 (Suppl), S25–S29.
6. Swanson BN, Vlasses PH, Ferguson RK, Bergquist PA, Till AE, Irvin JD, Harris K. Influence of food on the bioavailability of enalapril. *J Pharm Sci* (1984) 73, 1655–7.
7. Ferry JJ, Horvath AM, Sedman AJ, Latts JR, Colburn WA. Influence of food on the pharmacokinetics of quinapril and its active diacid metabolite, CI-928. *J Clin Pharmacol* (1987) 27, 397–9.
8. Mojaverian P, Rocci ML, Vlasses PH, Hoholick C, Clementi RA, Ferguson RK. Effect of food on the bioavailability of lisinopril, a nonsulfhydryl angiotensin-converting enzyme inhibitor. *J Pharm Sci* (1986) 75, 395–7.
9. Massarella JW, DeFeo TM, Brown AN, Lin A, Wills RJ. The influence of food on the pharmacokinetics and ACE inhibition of cilazapril. *Br J Clin Pharmacol* (1989) 27, 205S–209S.
10. Grass P, Gerbeau C, Kutz K. Spirapril: pharmacokinetic properties and drug interactions. *Blood Pressure* (1994) 3 (Suppl 2), 7–13.
11. Staril (Fosinopril). E. R. Squibb & Sons Ltd. Summary of product characteristics, November 1995.
12. Gopten (Trandolapril). Abbot Laboratories Ltd. Summary of product characteristics, December 2001.
13. Funck-Brentano C, Lecocq B, Jaillon P, Devissaguet M. Effects of food on the pharmacokinetics and ACE-inhibition of perindopril in healthy volunteers. *Excerpta Medica Int Congr Series* (1989) 839, 277–80.
14. Lecocq B, Funck-Brentano C, Lecocq V, Ferry A, Gardin M-E, Devissaguet M, Jaillon P. Influence of food on the pharmacokinetics of perindopril and the time course of angiotensin-converting enzyme inhibition in serum. *Clin Pharmacol Ther* (1990) 47, 397–402.
15. Perdix (Moexipril). Schwarz Pharma. Product Monograph, October 1995.
16. Stimpel M, Cawello W. Pharmacokinetics and ACE-inhibition of the new ACE-inhibitor moexipril: is coadministration with food of clinical relevance? *Hypertension* (1995) 25, 1384.
17. Tanatril (Imidapril). Trinity Pharmaceuticals Ltd. Summary of product characteristics, March 2001.
18. Melander A, Danielson K, Hanson A, Rudell B, Schersten B, Thulin T, Wåhlin E. Enhancement of hydralazine bioavailability by food. *Clin Pharmacol Ther* (1977) 22, 104–7.
19. Liedholm H, Wåhlin-Boll E, Hanson A, Melander A. Influence of food on the bioavailability of 'real' and 'apparent' hydralazine from conventional and slow-release preparations. *Drug Nutr Interact* (1982) 1, 293–302.
20. Walden RJ, Hernadez R, Witts D, Graham BR, Prichard BN. Effect of food on the absorption of hydralazine in man. *Eur J Clin Pharmacol* (1981) 20, 53–8.
21. Shepherd AM, Irvine NA, Ludden TM. Effect of food on blood hydralazine levels and response in hypertension. *Clin Pharmacol Ther* (1984) 36, 14–18.
22. Jackson SHD, Shepherd AMM, Ludden TM, Jamieson MJ, Woodworth J, Rogers D, Ludden LK, Muir KT. Effect of food on oral bioavailability of apresoline and controlled release hydralazine in hypertensive patients. *J Cardiovasc Pharmacol* (1990) 16, 624–8.
23. Semple HA, Koo W, Tam YK, Ngo LY, Coutts RT. Interactions between hydralazine and oral nutrients in humans. *Ther Drug Monit* (1991) 13, 304–8.
24. Melander A, Danielson K, Schersten B, Thulin T, Wåhlin E. Enhancement by food of canrenone bioavailability from spironolactone. *Clin Pharmacol Ther* (1977) 22, 100–3.
25. Thulin T, Wåhlin-Boll E, Liedholm H, Lindholm L, Melander A. Influence of food intake on antihypertensive drugs: spironolactone. *Drug Nutr Interact* (1983) 2, 169–73.
26. Overdiek HW, Merkus FW. Influence of food on the bioavailability of spironolactone. *Clin Pharmacol Ther* (1986) 40, 531–6.

Antihypertensives + Orlistat

Orlistat has been found in a handful of cases to oppose the effects of antihypertensive drugs (amlodipine, atenolol, enalapril, hydrochlorothiazide, losartan) resulting in marked increases in blood pressure, hypertensive crises and, one case, intracranial haemorrhage.

Clinical evidence, mechanism, importance and management

(a) Antihypertensive effects opposed

The Argentinian System of Pharmacovigilance identified the following 3 cases. An obese man whose hypertension was controlled at 120/80 mmHg with daily doses of **atenolol** 100 mg, **losartan** 100 mg and **hydrochlorothiazide** 12.5 mg developed a hypertensive crisis (260/140 mmHg) 7 days after starting to take 120 mg **orlistat** three times daily. The **orlistat** was stopped and the crisis was controlled. When later rechallenged with **orlistat**, his diastolic blood pressure rose to 100 to 110 mmHg within 5 days but the systolic increased only slightly. His blood pressure returned to baseline values 3 days after stopping the **orlistat**.[1]

Two other patients reacted similarly. One whose blood pressure was controlled at 130/85 mmHg on daily doses of **enalapril** 20 mg and **losartan** 50 mg developed hypertension (160/100 mmHg) and occasional systolic peaks of around 200 mmHg one week after starting 120 mg **orlistat** three times daily. The other patient was stable on daily doses of **enalapril** 20 mg and **amlodipine** 5 mg began to develop hypertensive peaks (180/120 mmHg) 60 days after starting 120 mg **orlistat** daily. He developed an intracranial haemorrhage. The hypertension responded to a change to **losartan/hydrochlorothiazide**, but 20 days later new hypertensive peaks developed (180/110–120 mmHg). When the orlistat was withdrawn, the hypertension was controlled within 48 h.[1]

The Uppsala Adverse Drug Reaction database has two reports of aggravated hypertension in women on antihypertensives and **orlistat**.[2] Transitory hypertension has also been reports in previously normotensive healthy individuals on 120 mg **orlistat** three times daily.[3,4]

(b) Antihypertensive pharmacokinetics unchanged

Healthy male subjects were given 50 mg **orlistat** three times daily for 7 to 8 days before and after being given single doses of 100 mg **atenolol**, 50 mg **captopril**, 40 mg **furosemide (frusemide)** or 20 mg slow-release **nifedipine**. The half-life of the **furosemide** and the time to peak serum levels of the **nifedipine** were slightly longer in the presence of the **orlistat**, but no other pharmacokinetic parameters were changed.[5]

Mechanism

Not understood. Suggestions include a decrease in the absorption of the drugs due to accelerated gastrointestinal transit, increased defaecation, diarrhoea, or an increase in the amount of fat in the chyme.[1] An explanation for the difference between (a) and (b) may be that the latter only looked at the single dose pharmacokinetics of the antihypertensives in normotensive subjects using only a small orlistat dosage (50 mg three times daily) whereas the reports (a) are about obese hypertensive patients taking 120 mg three times daily.

Importance and management

The antihypertensive/orlistat interaction seems to be confined to the reports cited here, but it appears to be an established, clinically important and potentially serious interaction. Just why only a handful of cases has been reported is unknown.

In practical terms, because the incidence of this interaction is quite unknown and because the outcome can be serious (hypertensive crises, intracranial haemorrhage), it would now seem important to monitor patients taking amlodipine, atenolol, enalapril, hydrochlorothiazide and losartan given orlistat to confirm that the antihypertensive treatment remains effective. What is not known is whether this is adverse reaction is confined to these named antihypertensives or whether it is a more general reaction. More study is needed to clarify the situation.

1. Valsecia ME, Malgor LA, Farfas EF, Figueras A, Laporte J-R. Interaction between orlistat and antihypertensive drugs. *Ann Pharmacother* (2001) 35, 1495-6.
2. *Who Pharmaceuticals Newsletter prepared in collaboration with the WHO Collaborating Centre for International Drug Monitoring* (2000) No 2. Also available at http://www.who.int/medicines/library/pnewslet/npn2-2000.html (Accessed 15/08/02).
3. Persson M, Vitols S, Yue QY. Orlistat associated with hypertension. *BMJ* (2000) 321, 87.
4. Persson M, Vitols S, Yue QY. Orlistat associated with hypertension. Author's reply. *BMJ* (2001) 322, 111.
5. Weber C, Tam YK, Schmidtke-Schrezenmeier G, Jonkmann JHG, van Brummelen P. Effect of the lipase inhibitor orlistat on the pharmacokinetics of four different antihypertensive drugs in healthy volunteers. *Eur J Clin Pharmacol* (1996) 51, 87–90.

Antihypertensives + Phenothiazines

The hypotensive side-effects of chlorpromazine and other phenothiazines may be additive with the effects of antihypertensives. Patients may feel faint and dizzy if they stand up quickly. Guanethidine-like drugs are the probable exception because their effects are opposed by the phenothiazines (see 'Guanethidine and related drugs + Phenothiazines', p.393). An isolated report describes paradoxical hypertension in a patient given methyldopa and trifluoperazine.

Clinical evidence

In one study, 8 normotensive patients given **methyldopa** (500 to 1000 mg daily) with **chlorpromazine** (200 to 400 mg daily) for schizophrenia experienced orthostatic dizziness and had reductions in their standing systolic blood pressure.[1] In another report, one patient experienced dizziness and hypotension (systolic pressure 76 mmHg) about an hour after being given 100 mg **chlorpromazine**, 0.1 mg **clonidine** and 40 mg **furosemide** (frusemide), and another, 2 hours after being given 0.1 mg **clonidine** and 1 mg intramuscular **haloperidol** (a butyrophenone with general properties similar to phenothiazines).[2] Another patient experienced fainting and marked orthostatic hypotension (blood pressure 66/48 mmHg) when given 6.25 mg **captopril** twice daily and 200 mg **chlorpromazine** three times daily. He had previously taken **chlorpromazine** with **nadolol**, **prazosin** and **hydrochlorothiazide** without any problems, although his blood pressure was poorly controlled on this therapy.[3] A patient on **chlorpromazine** given **nifedipine** for 2 days prior to surgery developed marked hypotension during surgery, which was eventually controlled with norepinephrine (noradrenaline).[4] In contrast, an isolated report describes a paradoxical rise in blood pressure in a patient with systemic lupus erythematosus and renal failure when treated with **methyldopa** and **trifluoperazine**. When the trifluoperazine was stopped, blood pressure fell.[5]

There is also an isolated and unexplained case of a psychotic patient on **fluphenazine decanoate** who began to demonstrate delirium, agitation disorientation, short-term memory loss, confusion and cloud-

ed consciousness within 10 days of starting to take 0.2 mg **clonidine** daily. These symptoms disappeared when the **clonidine** was stopped and returned when it was re-started. He had previously been successfully treated with **haloperidol** and **clonidine**.[6]

Mechanism

Simple addition of the hypotensive effects of both drugs seems to be the explanation for the increased hypotension and orthostasis. The suggested explanation for the methyldopa/trifluoperazine hypertensive interaction is that the phenothiazine blocked the reuptake of the 'false transmitter' (alpha-methyl noradrenaline) produced during therapy with methyldopa.[5]

Importance and management

The increased hypotension and orthostasis that can occur if chlorpromazine or other phenothiazines are used with antihypertensive drugs is established. Note that, of the phenothiazines, levomepromazine (methotrimeprazine) is particularly associated with postural hypotension. Monitor the reaction, particularly during the first period of treatment and warn patients what to do if they feel faint and dizzy. Dosage adjustment may be necessary. See also 'Beta-blockers + Phenothiazines', p.445. Guanethidine-like drugs behave differently because their antihypertensive actions can be opposed to some extent by the phenothiazines (see 'Guanethidine and related drugs + Phenothiazines', p.393).

1. Chouinard G, Pinard G, Prenoveau Y, Tetreault L. Alpha methyldopa-chlorpromazine interaction in schizophrenic patients. *Curr Ther Res* (1973) 15, 60–72.
2. Fruncillo RJ, Gibbons WJ, Vlasses PH, Ferguson RK. Severe hypotension associated with concurrent clonidine and antipsychotic medication. *Am J Psychiatry* (1985) 142, 274.
3. White WB. Hypotension with postural syncope secondary to the combination of chlorpromazine and captopril. *Arch Intern Med* (1986) 146, 1833–4.
4. Stuart-Taylor ME, Crosse MM. A plea for noradrenaline. *Anaesthesia* (1989) 44, 916–7.
5. Westhervelt FB, Atuk NO. Methyldopa-induced hypertension. *JAMA* (1974) 227, 557.
6. Allen RM, Flemenbaum A. Delirium associated with combined fluphenazine-clonidine therapy. *J Clin Psychiatry* (1979) 40, 236–7.

Antihypertensives + Phenylpropanolamine

A sustained-release preparation of phenylpropanolamine and brompheniramine was found to cause a minor and clinically insignificant rise in the blood pressures of patients on various antihypertensives.

Clinical evidence, mechanism, importance and management

A randomised double-blind crossover study in 13 patients with hypertension controlled with **unnamed diuretics** (7), **ACE inhibitors** (6), **beta-blockers** (5), **calcium channel blockers** (1) **and a centrally acting alpha-agonist** (1) found that a single dose of *Dimetapp Extentabs* (75 mg **phenylpropanolamine** + 12 mg **brompheniramine**) caused only a minor systolic/diastolic blood pressure rise (+1.7/+0.9 mmHg) over 4 h.[1] This sustained release preparation in this dosage has therefore no clinically important effect on the blood pressure, but (as the authors point out) these results do not necessarily apply to different doses and immediate-release preparations. A marked rise in blood pressure was seen in one patient on **methyldopa** and **oxprenolol** when given **phenylpropanolamine**, see 'Methyldopa + Sympathomimetics (indirectly-acting)', p.403. See also 'Beta-blockers + Sympathomimetics (indirectly-acting)', p.450.

1. Petrulis AS, Imperiale TF, Speroff T. The acute effect of phenylpropanolamine and brompheniramine on blood pressure in controlled hypertension. *J Gen Intern Med* (1991) 6, 503–6.

Candesartan + Miscellaneous drugs

No clinically relevant pharmacokinetic interactions occur between candesartan cilexetil and combined oral contra-

ceptives, hydrochlorothiazide, glibenclamide (glyburide), nifedipine or warfarin. Candesartan cilexetil did not alter the anticoagulant effect of warfarin There may be a risk of hyperkalaemia if candesartan is co-administered with potassium-sparing diuretics or potassium supplements. The makers suggest that co-administration of candesartan with lithium may result in elevated serum lithium. They also note that symptomatic hypotension may occur when candesartan cilexetil is given to those on high-dose diuretics.

Clinical evidence, mechanism, importance and management

The addition of candesartan cilexetil 16 mg daily for 10 days to **warfarin** therapy reduced the trough serum levels of **warfarin** by 7%, but this had no effect on prothrombin times.[1] The concurrent use of **hydrochlorothiazide** 25 mg daily and candesartan cilexetil 12 mg daily for 7 days increased the AUC and maximum serum levels of candesartan by 18 and 25% respectively, and reduced the AUC of hydrochlorothiazide by 14%, but these changes were not considered to be clinically relevant.[1] Neither **glibenclamide (glyburide)** 3.5 mg daily nor **nifedipine** 30 mg daily significantly affected the pharmacokinetics of candesartan cilexetil 16 mg daily, and their serum levels were not altered by the candesartan.[1] Candesartan cilexetil 8 mg daily had no effect on the pharmacokinetics of ethinylestradiol and levonorgestrel in a **combined oral contraceptive**, and no ovulation occurred during concurrent treatment.[1] No special precautions would therefore appear to be needed if any of these drugs is given with candesartan.

Based on evidence from other drugs that affect the renin-angiotensin system, the maker of candesartan cilexetil notes that concomitant use of potassium-sparing diuretics (e.g. **amiloride**, **spironolactone**, **triamterene**), **potassium supplements**, **salt substitutes** or other drugs that increase potassium levels may increase serum potassium.[2] It would be prudent to monitor potassium levels if concurrent use is required, particularly in those with renal impairment. Similarly, they also note that symptomatic hypotension may occur when candesartan cilexetil is started in patients with intravascular volume depletion such as those on **high-dose diuretics**. They recommend that volume depletion be corrected before candesartan cilexetil is given.[2] Based on reports of increases in serum lithium during concomitant use of **lithium** and ACE inhibitors (see 'Lithium carbonate + ACE inhibitors', p.652), the maker says this could also occur during co-administration of **lithium** and candesartan. Careful monitoring of serum lithium is advised.[2]

1. Jonkman JHG, van Lier JJ, van Heiningen PNM, Lins R, Sennewald R, Högemann A. Pharmacokinetic drug interaction studies with candesartan cilexetil. *J Hum Hypertens* (1997) 11 (Suppl 2), S31–S35.

2. Amias (Candesartan cilexetil). Takeda UK Ltd. Summary of product characteristics, January 2001.

Captopril + Procainamide

The combination of captopril and procainamide possibly increases the risk of neutropenia. No pharmacokinetic interaction occurs.

Clinical evidence, mechanism, importance and management

The pharmacokinetics of **captopril** 50 mg twice daily and **procainamide** 250 mg three-hourly were unaffected by concurrent use in healthy subjects.[1] However, the maker of **captopril** notes that neutropenia and serious infection have occurred in patients on **captopril** treated with **procainamide**. They recommend the combination be used with caution, especially in patients with impaired renal function. They suggest regular monitoring of differential white blood cell counts in the first 3 months of **captopril** therapy.[2] The makers of a number of other ACE inhibitors (e.g. cilazapril, enalapril, imidapril,

moexipril, trandolapril) now state in their prescribing information that concomitant administration of ACE inhibitors and procainamide may lead to an increased risk of leucopenia.[3-7] See also 'ACE inhibitors + Allopurinol', p.368 and 'ACE inhibitors + Azathioprine', p.372.

1. Sugerman AA, McKown J. Lack of kinetic interaction of captopril (CP) and procainamide (PA) in healthy subjects. *J Clin Pharmacol* (1985) 25, 460.

2. Capoten (Captopril). E. R. Squibb & Sons Ltd. Summary of product characteristics, July 2001.

3. Vascace (Cilazapril). Roche Products Ltd. Summary of product characteristics, December 2001.

4. Innovace (Enalapril). Merck Sharp & Dohme Ltd. Summary of product characteristics, February 2001.

5. Tanatril (Imidapril). Trinity. Summary of product characteristics, March 2001.

6. Perdix (Moexipril), Schwarz Pharma Ltd. Summary of product characteristics, March 2000.

7. Gopten (Trandolapril). Abbot Laboratories Ltd. Summary of product characteristics, December 2001.

Clonidine + Beta-blockers

Concurrent use can be therapeutically valuable, but a sharp and serious rise in blood pressure ('rebound hypertension') can follow sudden withdrawal of the clonidine, which may be worsened by the presence of a beta-blocker. Isolated cases of marked bradycardia and hypotension have been seen with clonidine and esmolol. There are also two reports describing paradoxical hypertension with the combination of clonidine and beta-blockers.

Clinical evidence

(a) Exacerbation of the clonidine-withdrawal hypertensive rebound

A woman with a blood pressure of 180/140 mmHg was treated with clonidine and **timolol**. When the clonidine was stopped in error, she developed a violent throbbing headache and became progressively confused, ataxic and semicomatose during which she also had a grand mal convulsion. Her blood pressure was found to have risen to 300+/185 mmHg.[1]

A number of other reports describe similar cases of hypertensive rebound (a sudden and serious rise in blood pressure) within 24 and 72 h of stopping the clonidine, apparently worsened by the presence of **propranolol**.[2-6] The symptoms resemble those of phaeochromocytoma and include tremor, apprehension, flushing, nausea, vomiting, severe headache and a serious rise in blood pressure. One patient died from a cerebellar haemorrhage.[5]

(b) Bradycardia and hypotension

A man anaesthetised with thiopental and diamorphine, with oxygen, nitrous oxide, enflurane and atracurium was given 50 micrograms clonidine to control hypertension. After 15 min he became tachycardic with rates up to 170 bpm. **Esmolol** 75 mg was given by slow infusion, whereupon his heart rate fell to 20. He responded to 1.2 mg atropine, 1 mg epinephrine (adrenaline) and 10 ml calcium chloride with a stable heart rate of 110 bpm.[7] Of 32 patients receiving **esmolol** during surgery in a clinical trial, one patient developed marked hypotension and bradycardia, which responded to 10 mg ephedrine. It was noted that this patient had been receiving clonidine.[8]

(c) Antagonism of the hypotensive effects

The combination of **sotalol** in daily doses of 160 mg and 0.45 mg clonidine daily caused a marked rise in blood pressure in 6 of 10 patients compared with either clonidine alone (3 patients) or sotalol alone (3 patients). Two of the 10 had blood pressures which were lower than with either drug alone, and the remaining 2 patients had no appreciable change in blood pressure.[9] Two cases of hypertension involving clonidine with **propranolol** have also been described.[10]

Mechanism

The normal additive hypotensive effects of these drugs result from the two acting in concert at different but complementary sites in the cardiovascular system. Just why antagonism sometimes occurs is unexplained. The reliability of one of the reports[9] has been questioned. The hypertensive rebound following clonidine withdrawal is thought to be due to an increase in the levels of circulating catecholamines. With the beta (vasodilator) effects blocked by a beta-blocker, the alpha (vasoconstrictor) effects of the catecholamines are unopposed and the hypertension is further exaggerated.

Importance and management

The rebound hypertension following clonidine withdrawal, seriously worsened by the presence of a beta-blocker, is well established. Control this adverse effect by stopping the beta-blocker several days before withdrawing the clonidine gradually.[11] A successful alternative is to replace the clonidine and the beta-blocker with labetalol[12] which is both an alpha- and a beta-blocker. If this is done, the blood catecholamine levels still rise markedly (20-fold) and the patient may experience tremor, nausea, apprehension and palpitations, but no serious blood pressure rise or headaches occur.[12] The dosage of labetalol will need to be titrated for the patient, with regular checks on the blood pressure over 2 to 3 days. If a hypertensive episode develops, control it with an alpha-blocking agent such as phentolamine.[2] Diazoxide is effective.[1,5] Re-introduction of the clonidine, given orally or intravenously, should also stabilise the situation. It is clearly important to emphasise to patients taking clonidine and beta-blockers that they must keep taking their drugs.

What are the advantages and disadvantages of combined treatment? Patients given clonidine and either propranolol[13] or atenolol[14] (non-selective blockers) showed additive hypotensive effects and smaller doses of clonidine could be used which decreased its troublesome side-effects (sedation and dry mouth). In contrast, with nadolol[14] (cardio-selective) the blood pressure reductions were the same as with either drug alone. The weight of evidence is that paradoxical hypertension is rare.[9,10]

1. Bailey RR, Neale TJ. Rapid clonidine withdrawal with blood pressure overshoot exaggerated by beta-blockade. *BMJ* (1976) i, 942–3.
2. Bruce DL, Croley TF, Less JS. Preoperative clonidine withdrawal syndrome. *Anesthesiology* (1979) 51, 90–2.
3. Cairns SA, Marshall AJ. Clonidine withdrawal. *Lancet* (1976) i, 368.
4. Strauss FG, Franklin SS, Lewin AJ, Maxwell MH. Withdrawal of antihypertensive therapy. Hypertensive crisis in renovascular hypertension. *JAMA* (1977) 238, 1734–6.
5. Vernon C, Sakula A. Fatal rebound hypertension after abrupt withdrawal of clonidine and propranolol. *Br J Clin Pract* (1979) 33, 112,121.
6. Reid JL, Wing LMH, Dargie HJ, Hamilton CA, Davies DS, Dollery CT. Clonidine withdrawal in hypertension. Changes in blood pressure and plasma and urinary noradrenaline. *Lancet* (1977) i, 1171–4.
7. Perks D, Fisher GC. Esmolol and clonidine — a possible interaction. *Anaesthesia* (1992) 47, 533–4.
8. Kanitz DD, Ebert TJ, Kampine JP. Intraoperative use of bolus doses of esmolol to treat tachycardia. *J Clin Anesth* (1990) 2, 238–42.
9. Saarimaa H. Combination of clonidine and sotalol in hypertension. *BMJ* (1976) i, 810.
10. Warren SE, Ebert E, Swerdlin A-H, Steinberg SM, Stone R. Clonidine and propranolol paradoxical hypertension. *Arch Intern Med* (1979) 139, 253.
11. Harris AL. Clonidine withdrawal and blockade. *Lancet* (1976) i, 596.
12. Rosenthal T, Rabinowitz B, Boichis H, Elazar E, Brauner A, Neufeld HN. Use of labetalol in hypertensive patients during discontinuation of clonidine therapy. *Eur J Clin Pharmacol* (1981) 20, 237–40.
13. Lilja M, Jounela AJ, Juustila H, Mattila MJ. Interaction of clonidine and β-blockers. *Acta Med Scand* (1980) 207, 173–6.
14. Fogari R, Corradi L. Interaction of clonidine and beta blocking agents in the treatment of essential hypertension. In 'Low dose oral and transdermal therapy of hypertension' (Proceedings of Conference 1984), edited by Weber MA, Drayer JIM, Kolloch R. Springer-Verlag, 1985, pp. 118–21.

Clonidine + Bupropion (Amfebutamone)

Bupropion did not reduce the hypotensive effect of clonidine in healthy subjects.[1]

1. Cubeddu LX, Cloutier G, Gross K, Grippo R, Tanner L, Lerea L, Shakarjian M, Knowlton G, Harden TK, Arendshorst W and Rogers JF. Bupropion does not antagonize cardiovascular actions of clonidine in normal subjects and spontaneously hypertensive rats. *Clin Pharmacol Ther* (1984) 35, 576–84.

Clonidine or Apomorphine + Oral Contraceptives

The sedative effects of clonidine are increased by the concurrent use of oral contraceptives, but those of apomorphine are decreased.

Clinical evidence, mechanism, importance and management

A study[1] in a group of women showed that the sedative effects of clonidine and of apomorphine were increased and decreased respectively while taking an oral contraceptive (ethinylestradiol 30 micrograms, levonorgestrel 150 or 250 micrograms). The clinical importance of this is uncertain.

1. Chalmers JS, Fulli-Lemaire I, Cowen PJ. Effects of the contraceptive pill on sedative responses to clonidine and apomorphine in normal women. *Psychol Med* (1985) 15, 363–7.

Clonidine + Prazosin

There is some evidence that prazosin may possibly reduce the antihypertensive effects of clonidine whereas other evidence suggests that this does not occur.

Clinical evidence, mechanism, importance and management

The hypotensive effects of an intravenous dose of clonidine were reduced in 18 patients with essential hypertension by the presence of prazosin.[1] A later crossover study by the same group with 17 patients with essential hypertension (mean blood pressures 170/103 mmHg) found that 0.3 mg clonidine for 4 days reduced pressures to 132/85 mmHg, whereas 6 mg prazosin daily for 3 days reduced the pressures to 160/99 mmHg. However when given together the pressures were only reduced to 158/97 mmHg.[2] Other studies using the combination have not reported a reduced antihypertensive effect.[3,4] In the presence of prazosin the rebound hypertension following clonidine withdrawal is only moderate (a rise from 145/85 to 169/104 mmHg).[4] More work is needed to establish what happens with certainty but it seems possible that concurrent use may not always be favourable. Monitor the effects.

1. Kapocsi J, Farsang C, Vizi ES. Prazosin partly blocks clonidine-induced hypotension in patients with essential hypertension. *Eur J Clin Pharmacol* (1987) 32, 331–4.
2. Farsang C, Varga K, Kapocsi J. Prazosin-clonidine and prazosin-guanfacine interactions in hypertension. *Pharmacol Res Commun* (1988) 20 (Suppl 1), 85–6.
3. Stokes GS, Gain JM, Mahoney JE, Raaftos J, Steward JH. Long term use of prazosin in combination or alone for treating hypertension. *Med J Aust* (1977) 2 (Suppl), 13–16.
4. Andréjak M, Fievet P, Makdassi R, Comoy E, de Fremont JF, Coevoet B, Fournier A. Lack of antagonism in the antihypertensive effects of clonidine and prazosin in man. *Clin Sci* (1981) 61, 453S–455S.

Clonidine + Rifampicin (Rifampin)

Rifampicin does not interact with clonidine.

Clinical evidence, mechanism, importance and management

Rifampicin 600 mg twice daily for 7 days had no effect on the elimination kinetics of clonidine nor on the pulse rates or blood pressures of 6 normal subjects taking 0.2 mg clonidine twice daily.[1] No special precautions would seem necessary.

1. Affrime MB, Lowenthal DT, and Rufo M. Failure of rifampin to induce the metabolism of clonidine in normal volunteers. *Drug Intell Clin Pharm* (1981) 15, 964–6.

Clonidine + Tricyclic and tetracyclic antidepressants

The tricyclic antidepressants, clomipramine, desipramine and imipramine reduce or abolish the antihypertensive effects of clonidine. Other tricyclics are expected to behave similarly. Hypertensive crisis developed in a woman on clonidine when given imipramine, and severe pain occurred in a man on amitriptyline and diamorphine when given clonidine intrathecally. Conversely, the tetracyclics, maprotiline and mianserin do not appear to alter the antihypertensive effects of clonidine. An isolated case report describes hypertensive crisis in a patient on mirtazapine and clonidine.

Clinical evidence

(a) Tricyclic antidepressants

Four out of 5 hypertensive patients on 600 to 1800 micrograms clonidine daily (with chlortalidone or hydrochlorothiazide) showed blood pressure rises averaging 22/15 mmHg when lying and 12/10 mmHg when standing after taking 75 mg **desipramine** daily for 2 weeks.[1]

This interaction has been seen in other patients taking **clomipramine, desipramine** and **imipramine**.[1-6] The antihypertensive effects of a single intravenous dose of clonidine were reduced about 50% in 6 patients given **desipramine** for 3 weeks,[3] and by 40 to 50% in 8 normal subjects given 25 mg **imipramine** three times daily and single 300 micrograms doses of clonidine before and on day 9 of **imipramine** treatment.[7] A man on 800 micrograms clonidine daily showed a blood pressure rise from 150/90 to 220/130 mmHg within 4 days of starting 75 mg **clomipramine** daily.[4] An elderly woman on 200 micrograms clonidine daily developed severe frontal headache, dizziness, chest and neck pain and tachycardia (120 bpm) with hypertension (230/124–130 mmHg) on the second day of taking 50 mg **imipramine** for incontinence.[8]

The effects of the withdrawal of clonidine from an elderly patient may have been made worse by the presence of **amitriptyline**.[9] A man with severe pain, well controlled with **amitriptyline**, sodium valproate and intrathecal boluses of diamorphine, experienced severe pain within 5 min of an intrathecal test dose of 75 micrograms clonidine.[10]

(b) Tetracyclic and related antidepressants

Maprotiline (100 mg in 4 divided doses over 22 hours) did not alter the effect of a single dose of clonidine on blood pressure or heart rate in 8 healthy subjects.[11] **Mianserin** 20 mg three times daily for 2 weeks had no effect on the control of blood pressure in 5 patients receiving clonidine.[12,13] Similarly, **mianserin** pretreatment did not significantly alter the hypotensive action of a single dose of clonidine in healthy subjects.[12,14] In contrast, an isolated report describes hypertensive urgency in a man with end-stage renal disease on clonidine, metoprolol and losartan when **mirtazapine** (a mianserin analogue) was added for depression.[15]

Mechanism

Not understood. One idea is that the tricyclics desensitise or block central alpha-2-receptors.[16] This would explain the interaction with mirtazapine (a mianserin analogue), which also has alpha-blocking properties.[15] However, mianserin (also an alpha-blocker) did not interact.[12] Another idea is that tricyclics block noradrenaline uptake. However, maprotiline, which also blocks noradrenaline uptake, did not interact.[11]

Importance and management

The clonidine/tricyclics interaction is established and clinically important. The incidence is uncertain but it is not seen in all patients.[1] Avoid concurrent use unless the effects can be monitored. Increasing the dosage of clonidine may possibly be effective. 'Titration' of the clonidine dosage was apparently done successfully in 10 out of 11 hypertensive patients already on amitriptyline or imipramine.[17] Only clomipramine, desipramine and imipramine have been implicated so far, but other tricyclics would be expected to behave similarly (seen in *animals* with amitriptyline, nortriptyline and protriptyline[18]). The tetracyclic antidepressants maprotiline and mianserin do not appear to interact with clonidine, but an isolated report describes hypertension with **mirtazapine**.

1. Briant RH, Reid JL, Dollery CT. Interaction between clonidine and desipramine in man. *BMJ* (1973) i, 522–3.
2. Coffler DE. Antipsychotic drug interaction. *Drug Intell Clin Pharm* (1976) 10, 114–15.
3. Checkley SA, Slade AP, Shur E, Dawling S. A pilot study of the mechanism of action of desipramine. *Br J Psychiatry* (1981) 138, 248–51.
4. Andrejak M, Fournier A, Hardin J-M, Coevoet B, Lambrey G, De Fremont J-F, Quichaud J. Suppression de l'effet antihypertenseur de la clonidine par la prise simultanée d'un antidépresseur tricyclique. *Nouv Presse Med* (1977) 6, 2603.
5. Lacomblez L, Warot D, Bouche P, Derouesne C. Suppression de l'effet antihypertenseur de la clonidine par la clomipramine. *Rev Med Interne* (1988) 9, 291–3.
6. Manchon ND, Bercoff E, Lemarchand P, Chassagne P, Senant J, Bourreille J. Fréquence et gravité des interactions médicamenteuses dan une population âgée: étude prospective concernant 63 malades. *Rev Med Interne* (1989) 10, 521–5.
7. Cubeddu LX, Cloutier G, Gross K, Grippo PA-CR, Tanner L, Lerea L, Shakarjian M, Knowlton G, Harden TK, Arendshorst W, Rogers JF. Bupropion does not antagonize cardiovascular actions of clonidine in normal subjects and spontaneously hypertensive rats. *Clin Pharmacol Ther* (1984) 35, 576–84.
8. Hui KK. Hypertensive crisis induced by interaction of clonidine with imipramine. *J Am Geriatr Soc* (1983) 31, 164–5.
9. Stiff JL, Harris DB. Clonidine withdrawal complicated by amitriptyline therapy. *Anesthesiology* (1983) 59, 73–4.
10. Hardy PAJ, Wells JCD. Pain after spinal intrathecal clonidine. An adverse interaction with tricyclic antidepressants? *Anaesthesia* (1988) 43, 1026–7.
11. Gundert-Remy U, Amann E, Hildebrandt R, Weber E. Lack of interaction between the tetracyclic antidepressant maprotiline and the centrally acting antihypertensive drug clonidine. *Eur J Clin Pharmacol* (1983) 25, 595–9.
12. Elliott HL, Whiting B, Reid JL. Assessment of the interaction between mianserin and centrally-acting antihypertensive drugs. *Br J Clin Pharmacol* (1983) 15, 323S–328S.
13. Elliott HL, McLean K, Sumner DJ, Reid JL. Absence of an effect of mianserin on the actions of clonidine or methyldopa in hypertensive patients. *Eur J Clin Pharmacol* (1983) 24, 15–19.
14. Elliott HL, McLean K, Reid JL, Sumner DJ. Pharmacodynamic studies on mianserin and its interaction with clonidine. *Br J Clin Pharmacol* (1981) 11, 122P.
15. Abo-Zena RA, Bobek MB, Dweik RA. Hypertensive urgency induced by an interaction of mirtazepine and clonidine. *Pharmacotherapy* (2000) 20, 476–8.
16. van Spanning HW, van Zwieten PA. The interference of tricyclic antidepressants with the central hypotensive effect of clonidine. *Eur J Pharmacol* (1973) 24, 402–4.
17. Raftos J, Bauer GE, Lewis RG, Stokes GS, Mitchell AS, Young AA, Maclachlan I. Clonidine in the treatment of severe hypertension. *Med J Aust* (1973) 1, 786–93.
18. van Zwieten PA. Interaction between centrally active hypotensive drugs and tricyclic antidepressants. *Arch Int Pharmacodyn Ther* (1975) 214, 12–30.

Cyclothiazide/triamterene + Pravastatin

Reversible diabetes mellitus developed in a woman taking cyclothiazide/triamterene when she was additionally given pravastatin.

Clinical evidence, mechanism, importance and management

A woman of 63 who had been on cyclothiazide/triamterene and acebutolol for 4 years, developed polyuria and polydipsia within 3 weeks of starting 20 mg **pravastatin** daily, which gradually worsened. After another 4 months she was hospitalised for hyperglycaemia which was treated with insulin and later glibenclamide (glyburide). The cyclothiazide/triamterene and **pravastatin** were stopped and gradually the diabetic symptoms began to abate. Five weeks after admission she was discharged without the need for any hypoglycaemic agent with the diabetes fully resolved.[1] The detailed reasons for this reaction are not understood, but it would seem that the **pravastatin** increased the hyperglycaemic potential of the thiazide diuretic to the point where frank diabetes developed. This is an isolated case and there would seem to be little reason normally to avoid the concurrent use of these drugs.

1. Jonville-Bera A-P, Zakian A, Bera FJ, Carré P, Autret E. Possible pravastatin and diuretics-induced diabetes mellitus. *Ann Pharmacother* (1994) 28, 964–5.

Diazoxide + Chlorpromazine and/or Thiazides

Excessive hyperglycaemia is possible if diazoxide is given with other drugs with hyperglycaemic activity (e.g. the thiazides, chlorpromazine).

Clinical evidence, mechanism, importance and management

An isolated report[1] describes a child on long-term treatment for hypoglycaemia with diazoxide, 8 mg/kg daily in divided doses, and **bendroflumethiazide (bendrofluazide)** 1.25 mg daily, who developed a diabetic precoma and severe hyperglycaemia after a single 30-mg dose of **chlorpromazine**. The reason is not understood but one idea is that all three drugs had additive hyperglycaemic effects. Enhanced hyperglycaemia has been seen in other patients given diazoxide and **trichlormethiazide**.[2] Caution is clearly needed to ensure that the hyperglycaemic effects do not become excessive.

1. Aynsley-Green A, Illig R. Enhancement by chlorpromazine of hyperglycaemic action of diazoxide. *Lancet* (1975) ii, 658–9.

2. Seltzer HS, Allen EW. Hyperglycemia and inhibition of insulin secretion during administration of diazoxide and trichlormethiazide in man. *Diabetes* (1969) 18, 19–28.

Diazoxide + Hydralazine

Severe hypotension, in some cases fatal, has followed the administration of diazoxide before or after hydralazine.

Clinical evidence

A previously normotensive 25-year-old woman had a blood pressure of 250/150 mmHg during the 34th week of pregnancy which failed to respond to magnesium sulphate given intravenously. It fell transiently to 170/120 mmHg when given 15 mg **hydralazine**. One hour later intravenous diazoxide, 5 mg/kg resulted in a blood pressure fall to 60/0 mmHg. Despite large doses of norepinephrine (noradrenaline), the hypotension persisted and the woman died.[1]

Other cases of severe hypotension are described in this and other studies and reports.[1-7] In some instances the patients had also had other antihypertensive agents such as **methyldopa**[1] or **reserpine**.[1,7] At least three of the cases had a fatal outcome.[7]

Mechanism

Not fully understood. The hypotensive effects (vasodilatory) of the two drugs are additive, and it would seem that in some instances the limit of the normal compensatory responses of the cardiovascular system to maintain an adequate blood pressure is reached.

Importance and management

An established, adequately documented and clinically important interaction. Concurrent use should be extremely cautious and thoroughly monitored. The authors of one of the reports cited[1] warn that ". . . diazoxide should be administered with caution to patients being concurrently treated with other potential vasodilatory or catecholamine depleting agents."

1. Henrich WL, Cronin R, Miller PD, Anderson RJ. Hypotensive sequelae of diazoxide and hydralazine therapy. *JAMA* (1977) 237, 264–5.

2. Miller WE, Gifford RW, Humphrey DC, Vidt DG. Management of severe hypertension with intravenous injections of diazoxide. *Am J Cardiol* (1969) 24, 870–5.

3. Kumar GK, Dastoor FC, Robayo JR, Razzaque MA. Side effects of diazoxide. *JAMA* (1976) 235, 275–6.

4. Tansey WA, Williams EG, Landesman RH and Schwarz MJ. Diazoxide. *JAMA* (1973) 225, 749.

5. Saker BM, Mathew TH, Eremin J, Kincaid-Smith P. Diazoxide in the treatment of the acute hypertensive emergency. *Med J Aust* (1968) 1, 592–3.

6. Finnerty FA. Hypertensive encephalopathy. *Am J Med* (1972) 52, 672–8.

7. Davey M, Moodley J, Soutter P. Adverse effects of a combination of diazoxide and hydrallazine therapy. *S Afr Med J* (1981) 59, 496–7.

Diuretics (potassium-sparing) + Potassium supplements and salt substitutes

The concurrent use of potassium-sparing diuretics (spironolactone, triamterene, amiloride) and potassium supplements can result in severe and even life-threatening hyperkalaemia unless potassium levels are well monitored and controlled. Potassium-containing salt substitutes can be equally hazardous.

Clinical evidence

In a retrospective analysis of hospitalised patients who had received spironolactone, hyperkalaemia had developed in 5.7% patients on **spironolactone** alone and 15.4% in those also taking a **potassium chloride supplement**. The incidence was 42% in those with severe azotaemia given **spironolactone** and a **potassium chloride supplement**.[1] A retrospective survey of another group of 25 patients on **spironolactone** and oral **potassium chloride supplements** found that half of them had developed hyperkalaemia.[2] The pacemaker of a patient failed because of hyperkalaemia caused by the concurrent use of **triamterene + hydrochlorothiazide** (*Dyazide*) and **potassium chloride** (*Slow-K*).[3] Another patient developed severe hyperkalaemia and cardiotoxicity as a result of treatment with **spironolactone** and a **potassium supplement**.[4] Three patients on **furosemide (frusemide)** and **spironolactone** became hyperkalaemic[5,6] because they took **potassium-containing salt substitutes** (*No Salt* in one case[5]). Two developed heart arrhythmias.[6]

Mechanism

The effects of these potassium-conserving diuretics and the potassium supplements are additive, resulting in hyperkalaemia.

Importance and management

The interaction with spironolactone is established and of clinical importance. **Triamterene** and **amiloride** would be expected to behave similarly. Avoid potassium supplements in patients on potassium-sparing diuretics except in cases of marked potassium depletion and where the effects can be closely monitored. Warn patients about the risks of salt substitutes containing potassium, which may increase the potassium intake by 50 to 60 mmol daily.[6] The signs and symptoms of hyperkalaemia include muscular weakness, fatigue, paraesthesia, flaccid paralysis of the extremities, bradycardia, shock and ECG abnormalities which may develop slowly and insidiously.

1. Greenblatt DJ, Koch-Weser J. Adverse reactions to spironolactone. A report from the Boston Collaborative Drug Surveillance Program. *Clin Pharmacol Ther* (1973) 14, 136–7.

2. Simborg DN. Medication prescribing on a university medical service — the incidence of drug combinations with potential adverse interactions. *Johns Hopkins Med J* (1976) 139, 23–6.

3. O'Reilly MV, Murnaghan DP, Williams MB. Transvenous pacemaker failure induced by hyperkalemia. *JAMA* (1974) 228, 336–7.

4. Kalbian VV. Iatrogenic hyperkalemic paralysis with electrocardiographic changes. *South Med J* (1974) 67, 342–5.

5. McCaughan D. Hazards of non-prescription potassium supplements. *Lancet* (1984) i, 513–14.

6. Yap V, Patel A, Thomsen J. Hyperkalemia with cardiac arrhythmia. Induction by salt substitutes, spironolactone, and azotemia. *JAMA* (1976) 236, 2775–6.

Diuretics + Trimethoprim

Excessively low serum sodium levels have been seen in a few patients taking thiazides with potassium-depleting diuretics when given trimethoprim or co-trimoxazole.

Clinical evidence

A 75-year-old woman with multiple medical conditions and taking **methyldopa**, **levothyroxine** and *Moduretic* (**hydrochlorothiazide + amiloride**) developed nausea and anorexia and was found to have hyponatraemia (107 mmol/l) within 4 days of starting to take **trimethoprim** 200 mg twice daily. The problem resolved when the *Moduretic* and **trimethoprim** were stopped. She was later discharged on methyldopa, levothyroxine and *Moduretic*. When rechallenged 4 months later with **trimethoprim** in the absence of *Moduretic* no hyponatraemia occurred, but it developed rapidly when the *Moduretic* was restarted.[1] The authors of this report say that they have seen several other patients who developed hyponatraemia within 4 to 12 days of taking **trimethoprim** or **co-trimoxazole** (**sulfamethoxazole + trimethoprim**), all of whom were elderly and all but one was taking a **diuretic**.[1]

Two other patients are described in another report who developed hyponatraemia when **co-trimoxazole** was added to treatment with *Moduret* (**hydrochlorothiazide + amiloride**) or **hydrochlorothiazide/triamterene**.[2]

Mechanism

Not established. Thiazides combined with potassium-sparing diuretics are said to be particularly liable to cause hyponatraemia.[3] Trimethoprim can also cause sodium loss, and it seems likely that this can be additive with the effects of other drugs.

Importance and management

Information is very limited but it would seem prudent to be on the alert for any signs of hyponatraemia (nausea, anorexia, etc.) in any patient while taking these drugs.

1. Eastell R, Edmonds CJ. Hyponatraemia associated with trimethoprim and a diuretic. *BMJ* (1984) 289, 1658–9.
2. Hart TL, Johnston LJ, Edmonds MW, Brownscombe L. Hyponatremia secondary to thiazide-trimethoprim interaction. *Can J Hosp Pharm* (1989) 42, 243–6.
3. Hornick P. Severe hyponatraemia in elderly patients: cause for concern. *Ann R Coll Surg Engl* (1996) 78, 230–1.

Eprosartan + Miscellaneous drugs

Fluconazole, ketoconazole, hydrochlorothiazide and ranitidine, do not alter the pharmacokinetics of eprosartan. Lipid lowering agents and calcium channel blockers have been administered safely with eprosartan. There may be a risk of hyperkalaemia if eprosartan is co-administered with potassium-sparing diuretics or potassium supplements. There may be a risk of symptomatic hypotension when eprosartan is started in patients on high-dose diuretics. Food modestly increases the bioavailability of eprosartan.

Clinical evidence, mechanism, importance and management

Sixteen healthy subjects were given 300 mg eprosartan twice daily for 20 days to which was added 200 mg **fluconazole** daily on days 11 to 20. **Fluconazole** had no effect on either the AUC or the maximum serum levels of eprosartan.[1,2] In a similar study, **ketoconazole** 200 mg daily was also found to have no effect on eprosartan pharmacokinetics.[2]

Seventeen healthy subjects were given a single 400-mg dose of eprosartan before and after taking 150 mg **ranitidine** twice daily for 3 days. The **ranitidine** caused some slight, statistically insignificant

and clinically irrelevant changes in the pharmacokinetics of the eprosartan.[2,3]

Eprosartan 800 mg decreased the AUC of **hydrochlorothiazide** 25 mg by 20% in healthy subjects, which is not clinically important. Conversely **hydrochlorothiazide** had no effect on eprosartan pharmacokinetics.[2] The maker notes that eprosartan has been safely co-administered with thiazide diuretics (e.g. **hydrochlorothiazide**) calcium channel blockers (e.g. **nifedipine**) and hypolipidaemic agents (e.g. **lovastatin, simvastatin, pravastatin, fenofibrate, gemfibrozil, niacin**).[4] No special precautions would therefore appear to be necessary if any of these drugs is given with eprosartan. However, the maker also states that symptomatic hypotension may occur when eprosartan is started in patients with sodium and/or volume depletion (e.g. **high-dose diuretic** therapy). If possible, the dose of **diuretic**[4] should be reduced prior to starting eprosartan.[4]

In clinical trials, significantly elevated serum potassium concentrations were noted in 0.9% of patients treated with eprosartan. The makers recommend that serum potassium is regularly monitored if eprosartan is used with potassium-sparing diuretics (e.g. **amiloride, spironolactone, triamterene**), **potassium supplements, salt substitutes** or other drugs that increase potassium levels in patients with renal impairment.[4] **Food** delays eprosartan absorption, and increases the AUC and maximum serum concentrations by <25%. The maker recommends that eprosartan is administered with food.[4]

1. Kazierad DJ, Martin DE, Tenero D, Boike SC, Ilson B, Freed MI, Etheredge R, Jorkasky DK. Fluconazole significantly alters the pharmacokinetics of losartan but not eprosartan. *Clin Pharmacol Ther* (1997) 61, 203.
2. Blum RA, Kazierad DJ, Tenero DM. A review of eprosartan pharmacokinetic and pharmacodynamic interaction studies. *Pharmacotherapy* (1999) 19, 79S–85S.
3. Tenero DM, Martin DE, Ilson BE, Boyle DA, Boike SC, Carr AM, Lundberg DE, Jorkasky DK. Effect of ranitidine on the pharmacokinetics of orally administered eprosartan, an angiotensin II antagonist, in healthy male volunteers. *Ann Pharmacother* (1998) 32, 304–8.
4. Teveten (Eprosartan). Solvay Healthcare Ltd. Summary of product characteristics, January 2002.

Furosemide (Frusemide) + Chloral hydrate

The intravenous injection of furosemide (frusemide) after treatment with chloral hydrate occasionally causes sweating, hot flushes, a variable blood pressure and tachycardia.

Clinical evidence

Six patients in a coronary care unit given an intravenous bolus of 40 to 120 mg furosemide (frusemide) and who had received **chloral hydrate** during the previous 24 h developed sweating, hot flushes, variable blood pressure, and tachycardia. The reaction was immediate and lasted about 15 min. No special treatment was given.[1]

A retrospective study of hospital records revealed that out of 43 patients who had received both drugs, one patient developed this reaction and two others may have done so.[2] The interaction has also been described in an 8-year-old boy.[3]

Mechanism

Not understood. One suggestion is that furosemide displaces trichloroacetic acid (the metabolite of chloral hydrate) from its protein binding sites, which in turn displaces levothyroxine or alters the serum pH so that the levels of free levothyroxine rise.[1] There is no experimental confirmation of this idea.

Importance and management

An established interaction, but information is limited to three reports. The incidence is uncertain but probably low. Concurrent use need not be avoided, but it would be prudent to given intravenous furosemide (frusemide) cautiously if chloral hydrate has been given recently. It seems possible that derivatives of chloral hydrate that break down in the body to release chloral hydrate (e.g. **dichloralphenazone, chloral betaine**) might interact similarly. There is no evidence that furosemide given orally or chloral hydrate given to patients already on furosemide initiates this reaction.[2]

1. Malach M, Berman N. Furosemide and chloral hydrate. Adverse drug interaction. *JAMA* (1975) 232, 638–9.
2. Pevonka MP, Yost RL, Marks RG, Howell WS, Stewart RB. Interaction of chloral hydrate and furosemide. A controlled retrospective study. *Drug Intell Clin Pharm* (1977) 11, 332–5.
3. Dean RP, Rudinsky BF, Kelleher MD. Interaction of chloral hydrate and intravenous furosemide in a child. *Clin Pharm* (1991) 10, 385–7.

Furosemide (Frusemide) or Bendroflumethiazide + Clofibrate

Treatment with clofibrate in patients with nephrotic syndrome receiving furosemide (frusemide) has sometimes led to marked diuresis and severe and disabling muscular symptoms.

Clinical evidence

Three patients with hyperlipoproteinaemia secondary to nephrotic syndrome, receiving 80 to 500 mg furosemide (frusemide) daily, developed severe muscle pain, low lumbar backache, stiffness and general malaise with pronounced diuresis within 3 days of receiving additional treatment with 1 to 2 g **clofibrate** daily. Similarly, muscle symptoms occurred within 3 days of starting **clofibrate** in a patient on bendroflumethiazide 10 mg daily. Three of these patients had documented raised serum transaminases or creatine phosphokinase. Two other patients had raised levels of serum transaminases or creatine phosphokinase during treatment with **clofibrate** and **furosemide**. In a further study in 4 of these patients and 4 healthy controls, free serum **clofibrate** was markedly higher in the patients, and this correlated with low serum albumin, and urinary **clofibrate** excretion was markedly delayed.[1]

Mechanism

Not understood. The marked diuresis may have been due to competition and displacement of the furosemide by the clofibrate from its plasma protein binding sites. Clofibrate occasionally causes a muscular syndrome which could have been exacerbated by (a) the urinary loss of Na^+ and K^+ and (b) the increase in the half-life of clofibrate.

Importance and management

The clinical documentation seems to be limited to this report. It appears to be a combination of a drug-drug interaction (clofibrate/furosemide) and a drug-disease interaction (clofibrate/nephrotic syndrome). The authors of this report suggest that serum proteins and renal function should be checked before giving clofibrate. If serum albumin is low, the total daily dosage of clofibrate should not exceed 0.5 g for each 1 g per 100 ml of the albumin concentration. More study is needed. See also 'Bezafibrate + Furosemide', p.870.

1. Bridgman JF, Rosen SM, Thorp JM. Complications during clofibrate treatment of nephrotic-syndrome hyperlipoproteinaemia. *Lancet* (1972) ii, 506–9.

Furosemide (Frusemide) + Colestyramine or Colestipol

Colestyramine and colestipol markedly reduce the absorption and diuretic effects of furosemide (frusemide). Giving the furosemide 2 to 3 h before either of these other drugs should minimise the effects of this interaction.

Clinical evidence

Colestyramine 8 g reduced the absorption of a single 40-mg dose of furosemide (frusemide) in 6 healthy subjects by 95%. The 4 h diuretic response was reduced by 77% (from 1510 to 350 ml. **Colestipol** 10 g

reduced the furosemide absorption by 80% and the 4 h diuretic response by 58% (from 1510 to 630 ml).[1]

Mechanism

Both colestyramine and colestipol are anionic exchange resins which can bind furosemide within the gut, thereby by reducing its absorption and its effects.

Importance and management

An established interaction, although direct evidence seems to be limited to this study. The absorption of furosemide (frusemide) is relatively rapid so that giving it 2 to 3 h before either the colestyramine or colestipol should be an effective way of overcoming this interaction. This needs confirmation.

1. Neuvonen PJ, Kivistö K, Hirvisalo EL. Effects of resins and activated charcoal on the absorption of digoxin, carbamazepine and frusemide. *Br J Clin Pharmacol* (1988) 25, 229–33.

Furosemide (Frusemide) + Epoprostenol

Epoprostenol infusion did not significantly alter the pharmacokinetics of furosemide (frusemide) in a study modelling the data from 23 patients with heart failure.[1]

1. Carlton LD, Patterson JH, Mattson CN, Schmith VD. The effects of epoprostenol on drug disposition II: a pilot study of the pharmacokinetics of furosemide with and without epoprostenol in patients with congestive heart failure. *J Clin Pharmacol* (1996) 36, 257–64.

Furosemide (Frusemide) or Bumetanide + Food

Food modestly reduces the bioavailability of furosemide (frusemide) and its diuretic effects. The bioavailability of bumetanide is not significantly affected by food.

Clinical evidence

Ten healthy subjects were given 40 mg **furosemide (frusemide)** with and without a **standard breakfast**. The **food** reduced the peak serum levels by 55% and the bioavailability by approximately 30%.[1] The results were almost identical when 5 of the subjects were given a **heavy meal**.[1] The diuresis over 10 h was reduced by 21% (from 2072 to 1640 ml and over 24 h by 15% (from 2668 to 2270 ml by administration of furosemide with breakfast.[1] A comparative study in 9 and 8 healthy subjects found that the absorption of both **bumetanide** 2 mg and **furosemide** 40 mg (administered as solutions), respectively were delayed and peak plasma levels reduced after a **standard breakfast**.[2] However, although the oral bioavailability of **furosemide** was reduced by about one-third by food (from 76% to 42%), the bioavailability of **bumetanide** was not significantly reduced by **food** (74% with food and 83% fasting). Conversely, food did not significantly alter the bioavailability of furosemide in an earlier study.[3]

Mechanism

Not understood.

Importance and management

Information is limited. It appears that the bioavailability of furosemide can be reduced by food, but in the one study assessing this, there was only a modest reduction in the diuretic effect. The authors of this study say that furosemide (frusemide) should not be given with food, but this is not standard clinical practice. Food does not affect the bioavailability of bumetanide administered as solution.

1. Beermann B, Midskov C. Reduced bioavailability and effect of furosemide given with food. *Eur J Clin Pharmacol* (1986) 29, 725–7.

2. McCrindle JL, Li Kam Wa TC, Nimmo WS, Prescott LF. Influence of food on the absorption of frusemide and bumetanide in man. *Br J Clin Pharmacol* (1994) 37, 478P.

3. Hammarlund MM, Paalzow LK, Odlind B. Pharmacokinetics of furosemide in man after intravenous and oral administration. Application of moment analysis. *Eur J Clin Pharmacol* (1984) 26, 197–207.

Furosemide (Frusemide) + Phenytoin

The diuretic effects of furosemide (frusemide) can be reduced as much as 50% if phenytoin is used concurrently.

Clinical evidence

The observation that dependent oedema in a group of epileptics was higher than expected, and the response to diuretic treatment seemed to be reduced, prompted further study. In 30 patients taking 200 to 400 mg **phenytoin** daily with 60 to 180 mg **phenobarbital** the maximal diuresis in response to 20 or 40 mg furosemide (frusemide) occurred after 3 to 4 h instead of the usual 2 h, and the total diuresis was reduced 68 and 51% respectively. When given 20 mg furosemide intravenously the total diuresis was reduced 50%. Some of the patients were also taking carbamazepine, pheneturide (ethylphenacemide), ethosuximide, diazepam or chlordiazepoxide.[1]

Another study in 5 healthy subjects given 100 mg **phenytoin** three times daily for 10 days showed that the maximal serum furosemide levels when given 20 mg furosemide, orally or intravenously, were reduced by 50%.[2]

Mechanism

Not fully understood. One suggestion is that the phenytoin causes changes in the jejunal Na^+ pump activity which reduces the absorption of the furosemide,[2] but this is not the whole story because an interaction also occurs when furosemide is given intravenously.[1] Another suggestion is that the phenytoin generates a 'liquid membrane' which blocks the transport of the furosemide to its active site.[3]

Importance and management

Information is limited but the interaction is established. A reduced diuretic response should be expected in the presence of phenytoin. A dosage increase may be needed.

1. Ahmad S. Renal insensitivity to frusemide caused by chronic anticonvulsant therapy. *BMJ* (1974) 3, 657–9.

2. Fine A, Henderson JS, Morgan DR, Tilstone WJ. Malabsorption of frusemide caused by phenytoin. *BMJ* (1977) 2, 1061–2.

3. Srivastava RC, Bhise SB, Sood R, Rao MNA. On the reduced furosemide response in the presence of diphenylhydantoin. *Colloids and Surfaces* (1986) 19, 83–8.

Furosemide (Frusemide) or Bumetanide + Probenecid

Probenecid decreases the renal clearance of furosemide (frusemide), but it appears not to alter its overall diuretic effect. Probenecid appears not to affect bumetanide.

Clinical evidence, mechanism, importance and management

(a) Furosemide (Frusemide)

Concurrent use has been closely studied to sort out renal pharmacological mechanisms of loop diuretics. One study in patients given 40 mg **furosemide** daily found that the addition of 0.5 g **probenecid** twice daily for 3 days reduced their urinary excretion of sodium by about 36% (from 56.3 to 35.9 mmol daily).[1] Other studies have also found some changes in overall diuresis (a fall in some studies,[2] a rise in others,[3] and no change in others[4,5]), and a reduction (35 to 80%) in the renal clearance of **furosemide**.[2,4-7] One study found that 1 g

probenecid increased the half-life of **furosemide** by 70% and decreased its oral clearance by 65%.[6] The clinical importance of these changes is uncertain, but probably small.

(b) Bumetanide

Probenecid 1 g did not affect the response of 8 normal subjects to 0.5 and 1 mg intravenous **bumetanide**.[8] Another study reported a fall in natriuresis and in the clearance of **bumetanide**, but of minimal clinical importance.[9]

1. Hsieh Y-Y, Hsieh B-S, Lien W-P, Wu T-L. Probenecid interferes with the natriuretic action of furosemide. *J Cardiovasc Pharmacol* (1987) 10, 530–4.

2. Honari J, Blair AD, Cutler RE. Effects of probenecid on furosemide kinetics and natriuresis in man. *Clin Pharmacol Ther* (1977) 22, 395–401.

3. Brater DC. Effects of probenecid on furosemide response. *Clin Pharmacol Ther* (1978) 24, 548–54.

4. Homeida M, Roberts C, Branch RA. Influence of probenecid and spironolactone on furosemide kinetics and dynamics in man. *Clin Pharmacol Ther* (1977) 22, 402–9.

5. Smith DE, Gee WL, Brater DC, Lin ET, Benet LZ. Preliminary evaluation of furosemide-probenecid interaction in humans. *J Pharm Sci* (1980) 69, 571–5.

6. Vree TB, van den Biggelaar-Martea M, Verwey-van Wissen CPWGM. Probenecid inhibits the renal clearance of frusemide and its acyl glucuronide. *Br J Clin Pharmacol* (1995) 39, 692–5.

7. Sommers DK, Meyer EC, Moncrieff J. The influence of co-administered organic acids on the kinetics and dynamics of frusemide. *Br J Clin Pharmacol* (1991) 32, 489–93.

8. Brater DC, Chennavasin P. Effect of probenecid on response to bumetanide in man. *J Clin Pharmacol* (1981) 21, 311–15.

9. Lant AF. Effects of bumetanide on cation and anion transport. *Postgrad Med J* (1975) 51 (Suppl 6), 35–42.

Furosemide (Frusemide) + Ranitidine

Ranitidine causes a moderate increase in the bioavailability of furosemide (frusemide).

Clinical evidence, mechanism, importance and management

Eighteen healthy subjects were given 40 mg furosemide (frusemide) orally 1 h after 50 mg intravenous **ranitidine** or saline. The **ranitidine** increased the AUC of the furosemide by 28% and the maximum serum levels by 37%.[1] The effects of furosemide are therefore expected to be moderately increased by **ranitidine**, but the clinical importance of this is probably small. No special precautions seem necessary.

1. Müller FO, De Vaal AC, Hundt KL, Luus HG. Intravenous ranitidine enhances furosemide bioavailability. *Klin Pharmakol Ak* (1993) 4, 26.

Guanethidine and related drugs + Haloperidol or Thiothixene

The antihypertensive effects of guanethidine can be reduced by the concurrent use of haloperidol or thiothixene.

Clinical evidence

Three hypertensive patients taking 60 to 150 mg **guanethidine** daily showed rises in their blood pressures when **haloperidol** (6 to 9 mg daily) was added: from 132/95 to 149/99 mmHg in the first patient; from 125/84 to 148/100 mmHg in the second; and from 138/91 to 154/100 mmHg in the third. One of the patients later tested with 60 mg **thiothixene** daily showed a rise from 126/87 to 156/110 mmHg.[1] These results have been reported elsewhere.[2,3]

Mechanism

Haloperidol and thiothixene prevent the entry of guanethidine into the adrenergic neurones of the sympathetic nervous system so that its blood pressure lowering effects are reduced or lost. This is essentially the same mechanism of interaction as that seen with the tricyclic antidepressants and chlorpromazine.

Importance and management

Information seems to be limited to this report, but it is supported by the well-documented pharmacology of these drugs. It appears to be clinically important. If haloperidol or thiothixene are given to patients on guanethidine, monitor their blood pressures and raise the guanethidine dosage as necessary.[3] There is no direct evidence of an interaction between guanethidine or related drugs and other butyrophenones or thioxanthenes but it would be prudent to adopt the same precautions.

1. Janowsky DS, El-Yousef MK, Davis JM, Fann WE, Oates JA. Guanethidine antagonism by antipsychotic drugs. *J Tenn Med Assoc* (1972) 65, 620–2.
2. Davis JM. Psychopharmacology in the aged. Use of psychotropic drugs in geriatric patients. *J Geriatr Psychiatry* (1974) 7, 145–59.
3. Janowsky DS, El-Yousef MK, Davis JM, Fann WE. Antagonism of guanethidine by chlorpromazine. *Am J Psychiatry* (1973) 130, 808–12.

Guanethidine and related drugs + Levodopa

When additionally given levodopa it was possible to reduce the dosage of guanethidine in one patient, and another was able to stop using a diuretic.

Clinical evidence, mechanism, importance and management

A brief report describes a patient on **guanethidine** and a diuretic who, when given **levodopa** (dose not stated but said to be within the ordinary therapeutic range) required a reduction in his daily dose of **guanethidine** from 60 to 20 mg. Another patient similarly treated was able to discontinue the diuretic.[1] The suggested reason is that the hypotensive side-effects of the **levodopa** are additive with the effects of the **guanethidine**. Direct information seems to be limited to this report but it would be wise to confirm that excessive hypotension does not develop if **levodopa** is added to treatment with **guanethidine** or guanethidine-like drugs.

1. Hunter KR, Stern GM, Laurence DR. Use of levodopa with other drugs. *Lancet* (1970) ii, 1283–5.

Guanethidine and related drugs + Monoamine oxidase inhibitors (MAOIs)

The antihypertensive effects of guanethidine can be reduced by nialamide.

Clinical evidence, mechanism, importance and management

Four out of 5 hypertensive patients on **guanethidine** (25 to 35 mg daily) showed a blood pressure rise from 140/85 to 165/100 mmHg 6 h after being given a single 50-mg dose of **nialamide**.[1] The reason is not understood but one idea is that MAOIs possibly oppose the **guanethidine**-induced loss of norepinephrine (noradrenaline) from sympathetic neurones. Direct information seems to be limited to this single dose study so that the outcome of long-term use is uncertain, but it would be prudent to monitor the effects if any **MAOI** is given to patients taking any **guanethidine**-like drug.

1. Gulati OD, Dave BT, Gokhale SD, Shah KM. Antagonism of adrenergic neuron blockade in hypertensive subjects. *Clin Pharmacol Ther* (1966) 7, 510–4.

Guanethidine and related drugs + Phenothiazines

Large doses of chlorpromazine may reduce or even abolish the antihypertensive effects of guanethidine although in some patients the inherent hypotensive effects of the chlorpromazine may possibly predominate.

Clinical evidence

Two severely hypertensive patients, well controlled on 80 mg **guanethidine** daily, were additionally given 200 to 300 mg **chlorpromazine** daily. The diastolic blood pressure of one rose over 10 days from 94 to 112 mmHg and continued to climb to 116 mmHg even when the **chlorpromazine** was withdrawn. The diastolic pressure of the other rose from 105 to 127 mmHg, and then on to 150 mmHg even after the **chlorpromazine** had been withdrawn.[1]

Other reports similarly describe marked rises in blood pressure in patients on **guanethidine** when given **chlorpromazine** 100 to 400 mg daily.[2-4]

Mechanism

Chlorpromazine prevents the entry of guanethidine into the adrenergic neurones of the sympathetic nervous system so that its blood pressure lowering effects are lost. This is essentially the same mechanism of interaction as that seen with the tricyclic antidepressants.

Importance and management

Direct information is limited but the interaction is established and can be clinically important. It may take several days to develop. Not all patients may react to the same extent.[2,5] Monitor concurrent use and raise the guanethidine dosage if necessary. It is uncertain how much chlorpromazine is needed before a significant effect occurs but the smallest dose of chlorpromazine used in the documented studies was 100 mg with 90 mg guanethidine which raised the blood pressure from 113/82 to 153/105 mmHg.[2] The inherent hypotensive effects of the chlorpromazine may possibly reduce the effects of this interaction. Other guanethidine-like antihypertensives (**betanidine**, **debrisoquine**, **guanadrel** etc.) would be expected to interact similarly but nobody seems to have checked on this, nor on the effects of phenothiazines other than chlorpromazine. The effects should be monitored. **Molindone** is reported not to interact.[6]

1. Fann WE, Janowsky DS, Davis JM, Oates JA. Chlorpromazine reversal of the antihypertensive action of guanethidine. *Lancet* (1971) ii, 436–7.
2. Janowsky DS, El-Yousef MK, Davis JM, Fann WE, Oates JA. Guanethidine antagonism by antipsychotic drugs. *J Tenn Med Assoc* (1972) 65, 620–2.
3. Janowsky DS, El-Yousef MK, Davis JM, Fann WE. Antagonism of guanethidine by chlorpromazine. *Am J Psychiatry* (1973) 130, 808–12.
4. Davis JM. Psychopharmacology in the aged. Use of psychotropic drugs in geriatric patients. *J Geriatr Psychiatry* (1974) 7, 145–59.
5. Tuck D, Hamberger B and Sjoqvist F. Drug interactions: effect of chlorpromazine on the uptake of monoamines into adrenergic neurones in man. *Lancet* (1972) ii, 492.
6. Simpson LL. Combined use of molindone and guanethidine in patients with schizophrenia and hypertension. *Am J Psychiatry* (1979) 136, 1410–14.

Guanethidine + Phenylbutazone

Phenylbutazone and kebuzone reduce the antihypertensive effects of guanethidine.

Clinical evidence, mechanism, importance and management

Twenty patients on 75 mg **guanethidine** daily showed a mean systolic blood pressure rise of 20 mmHg (from 169 to 189 mmHg) when concurrently treated with 750 mg **phenylbutazone** or **kebuzone** daily.[1] This rise represents about a 35% reduction in the antihypertensive effect of **guanethidine**. The mechanism of this interaction is uncertain but it is probably due to salt and water retention by these pyrazolone compounds. Direct evidence seems to be limited to this report, but it is in line with what is known about these anti-inflammatory compounds. Patients taking guanethidine should be monitored if **phenylbutazone**, **kebuzone** or **oxyphenbutazone** are given concurrently. There does not appear to be any information on guanethidine and other NSAIDs.

1. Polak F. Die hemmende Wirkung von Phenylbutazon auf die durch einige Antihypertonika hervorgerufene Blutdrucksenkung bei Hypertonikern. *Z Gesamte Inn Med* (1967) 22, 375–6.

Guanethidine and related drugs + Pizotifen

An isolated report describes the abolition of the antihypertensive effects of debrisoquine by pizotifen.

Clinical evidence, mechanism, importance and management

A man with severe focal glomerulonephritis and hypertension, well controlled on **debrisoquine**, 30 mg eight-hourly, **timolol** 10 mg eight-hourly and **furosemide (frusemide)** 40 mg in the morning, was additionally given **pizotifen** (*Sanomigran*) as a prophylactic for migraine. Over the next few weeks his blood pressure climbed from 130/90 to 195/145 mmHg. It was found impossible to lower the pressure with either **diazoxide** or **prazosin**, but within 48 h of withdrawing the **pizotifen** the pressure had fallen to 105/82 mmHg and later stabilised at 140/90 mmHg.[1] The reason is not known but the makers of **pizotifen**, suggest that as it is structurally similar to the tricyclic antidepressants, it may possibly oppose the actions of **debrisoquine** in a similar way by blocking the entry of the antihypertensive into the adrenergic neurones of the sympathetic nervous system.[1] Information is limited to this report but it would be wise to check for this interaction in any patient on **debrisoquine** or any other guanethidine-like hypertensive if **pizotifen** is given.

1. Bailey RR. Antagonism of debrisoquine sulphate by pizotifen (*Sandomigran*). *N Z Med J* (1976) 83, 449.

Guanethidine and related drugs + Sympathomimetics (directly-acting)

The pressor effects of norepinephrine (noradrenaline), phenylephrine, metaraminol and similar drugs can be increased two- to fourfold in the presence of guanethidine and related drugs (betanidine, debrisoquine, guanadrel, etc.). The mydriatic effects are similarly enhanced and prolonged.

Clinical evidence

(a) Pressor responses

A study in 6 normal subjects, given 200 mg **guanethidine** on the first day of study and 100 mg daily for the next 2 days, showed that their pressor responses (one third pulse pressure + diastolic pressure) when infused with **norepinephrine (noradrenaline)** in a range of doses were enhanced two-and-a-half to four times. Moreover cardiac arrhythmias appeared at lower doses of **norepinephrine** and with greater frequency than in the absence of **guanethidine**, and were more serious in nature.[1]

There are reports of this enhanced pressor response involving **debrisoquine** with oral **phenylephrine**,[2-4] **bretylium** with **norepinephrine**,[5] and **guanethidine** with **metaraminol**.[6] In the latter instance, 10 mg **metaraminol** given intravenously rapidly caused a blood pressure rise to 220/130 mmHg accompanied by severe headache and extreme angina. An increased blood pressure (from 165/92 to 210/120 mmHg) was also seen in a patient on **guanethidine** who, prior to surgery, was treated with **phenylephrine eye drops**.[7]

(b) Mydriatic responses

The mydriasis due to **phenylephrine** administered as a 10% **eye drop** solution was observed to be prolonged for up to 10 h in a patient concurrently receiving **guanethidine** for hypertension.[8] This enhanced mydriatic response has been described in other studies involving

guanethidine with **epinephrine (adrenaline), phenylephrine** or **methoxamine**;[9] and **debrisoquine** with **phenylephrine**[4] or **ephedrine**.[9]

Mechanism

If sympathetic nerves are cut surgically, the receptors which they normally stimulate become hypersensitive. By preventing the release of norepinephrine from adrenergic neurones, guanethidine and other adrenergic neurone blockers cause a temporary 'drug-induced sympathectomy' which is also accompanied by hypersensitivity of the receptors. Hence the increased response to the stimulation of the receptors by directly acting sympathomimetics.

Importance and management

An established, well-documented and potentially serious interaction. Since the pressor effects are grossly exaggerated, dosages of directly-acting sympathomimetics (alpha-agonists) should be reduced appropriately. The pressor effects of norepinephrine (noradrenaline) are increased two- to fourfold, and of phenylephrine twofold. In addition it should be remembered that the incidence and severity of heart arrhythmias is increased.[1,3] Considerable care is required. Direct evidence seems to be limited to norepinephrine, phenylephrine and metaraminol, but dopamine and methoxamine possess direct sympathomimetic activity and may be expected to interact similarly. No interaction would be expected with the beta-agonist drugs used for the treatment of asthma (such as terbutaline, salbutamol). Betanidine and other guanethidine-like drugs (debrisoquine, guanadrel, etc.) are also expected to behave like guanethidine. If as a result of this interaction the blood pressure becomes grossly elevated, it can be controlled by the administration of an alpha-adrenergic blocker such as phentolamine.[2,4] Oral nifedipine (sustained release) may also be effective.

Phenylephrine is contained in a number of OTC cough and cold preparations, a few of which contain up to 10 mg in a dose. This dose is only likely to cause a moderate blood pressure rise, compared with the marked rise seen in subjects on debrisoquine given phenylephrine 0.75 mg/kg (roughly 45 mg in a 10-stone individual).[3,10] However this requires confirmation.

An exaggerated pressor response is clearly much more potentially serious than enhanced and prolonged mydriasis, but the latter is also possible and undesirable. The same precautions apply about using smaller amounts of the sympathomimetic drugs.

1. Mulheims GH, Entrup RW, Palewonsky D, Mierzwiak DS. Increased sensitivity of the heart to catecholamine-induced arrhythmias following guanethidine. *Clin Pharmacol Ther* (1965) 6, 757.
2. Aminu J, D'Mello A, Vere DW. Interaction between debrisoquine and phenylephrine. *Lancet* (1970) ii, 935–6.
3. Allum W, Aminu J, Bloomfield TH, Davies C, Scales AH, Vere DW. Interaction between debrisoquine and phenylephrine in man. *Br J Pharmacol* (1973) 47, 675P–676P.
4. Allum W, Aminu J, Bloomfield TH, Davies C, Scales AH, Vere DW. Interaction between debrisoquine and phenylephrine in man. *Br J Clin Pharmacol* (1974) 1, 51–7.
5. Laurence DR, Nagle RE. The interaction of bretylium with pressor agents. *Lancet* (1961) i, 593–4.
6. Stevens FRT. A danger of sympathomimetic drugs. *Med J Aust* (1966) 2, 576.
7. Kim JM, Stevenson CE, Matthewson HS. Hypertensive reactions to phenylephrine eyedrops in patients with sympathetic denervation. *Am J Ophthalmol* (1978) 85, 862–8.
8. Cooper B. Neo-synephrine (10%) eye drops. *Med J Aust* (1968) 55,420.
9. Sneddon JM, Turner P. The interactions of local guanethidine: tolerance and effects on adrenergic nerve function and response to sympathomimetic amines. *Br J Pharmacol* (1962) 19, 13.
10. Boura ALA, Green AF. Comparison of bretylium and guanethidine; tolerance and effects on adrenergic nerve function and responses to sympathomimetic amines. *Br J Pharmacol* (1962) 19, 13–41.

Guanethidine and related drugs + Sympathomimetics (indirectly-acting) and related drugs

The antihypertensive effects of guanethidine and guanethidine-like drugs (betanidine, debrisoquine, guanadrel, etc.) can be reduced or abolished by the concurrent use of indirectly-acting sympathomimetics and related drugs, which are

contained in cough, cold and influenza remedies or are used as appetite suppressants (amphetamines, ephedrine, pseudoephedrine, phenylpropanolamine, mazindol, methylphenidate, etc.). The blood pressure may even rise higher than before treatment with the antihypertensive.

Clinical evidence

When 16 hypertensive patients on 25 to 35 mg **guanethidine** daily were additionally given **dexamfetamine (dextroamphetamine)** (10 mg orally), **ephedrine** (90 mg orally), **metamfetamine** (30 mg intramuscularly) or **methylphenidate** (20 mg orally), the effects of the **guanethidine** were completely abolished and in some instances the blood pressures rose higher than before treatment with **guanethidine**.[1]

Other reports describe the same interaction between **guanethidine** and dexamfetamine;[2] **betanidine** and **phenylpropanolamine**[3] or **mazindol**;[4] **bretylium** and **amfetamine**;[5] **debrisoquine** and **mazindol**;[6] and an unnamed adrenergic blocker and **ephedrine**.[7]

Mechanism

Indirectly acting sympathomimetic amines not only prevent guanethidine-like drugs from entering the adrenergic neurones of the sympathetic nervous system, but they can also displace the antihypertensive drug already there.[8] As a result the blood pressure lowering effects are lost. In addition these amines release norepinephrine (noradrenaline) from the neurones which raises the blood pressure. Thus the antihypertensive effects are not only opposed, but the pressure may even be raised higher than before treatment.[8-13] Mazindol is related to the tricyclic antidepressants and probably interacts solely by blocking the entry of the guanethidine-like drugs into adrenergic neurones.

Importance and management

Well documented, well established and clinically important interactions. Patients taking guanethidine or related drugs (bretylium, betanidine, debrisoquine, guanadrel, etc.) should avoid indirectly-acting sympathomimetics (named above). Warn them against the temptation to use proprietary OTC nasal decongestants containing any of these amines to relieve the nasal stuffiness commonly associated with the use of guanethidine and related drugs. The same precautions apply to the sympathomimetics used as appetite suppressants. However **amfepramone (diethylpropion)** has been used with guanethidine and betanidine without any adverse events.[14] Not every guanethidine-like antihypertensive-sympathomimetic combination has been investigated in man, but from their well-understood pharmacology they are expected to behave similarly.

1. Gulati OD, Dave BT, Gokhale SD, Shah KM. Antagonism of adrenergic neurone blockade in hypertensive subjects. *Clin Pharmacol Ther* (1966) 7, 510–4.
2. Ober KF, Wang RIH. Drug interactions with guanethidine. *Clin Pharmacol Ther* (1973) 14, 190–5.
3. Misage JR, McDonald RH. Antagonism of hypotensive action of bethanidine by 'common cold' remedy. *BMJ* (1970) 4, 347.
4. Boakes AJ. Antagonism of bethanidine by mazindol. *Br J Clin Pharmacol* (1977) 4, 486–7.
5. Wilson R, Long C. Action of bretylium antagonised by amphetamine. *Lancet* (1960) ii, 262.
6. Parker J. Wander Pharmaceuticals, England. Personal communication (1976).
7. Starr KJ, Petrie JC. Drug interactions in patients on long-term oral anticoagulant and antihypertensive adrenergic neurone-blocking drugs. *BMJ* (1972) 4, 133–5.
8. Flegin OT, Morgan DH, Oates JA, Shand DG. The mechanism of the reversal of the effect of guanethidine by amphetamines in cat and man. *Br J Pharmacol* (1970) 39, 253P–254P.
9. Day MD, Rand MJ. Antagonism of guanethidine and bretylium by various agents. *Lancet* (1962) 2, 1282–3.
10. Day MD, Rand MJ. Evidence for a competitive antagonism of guanethidine by dexamphetamine. *Br J Pharmacol* (1963) 20, 17–28.
11. Day MD. Effect of sympathomimetic amines on the blocking action of guanethidine, bretylium and xylocholine. *Br J Pharmacol* (1962) 18, 421–39.
12. Starke K. Interactions of guanethidine and indirectly-acting sympathomimetic amines. *Arch Int Pharmacodyn Ther* (1972) 195, 309–14.
13. Boura ALA, Green AF. Comparison of bretylium and guanethidine: tolerance effects on adrenergic nerve function and responses to sympathomimetic amines. *Br J Pharmacol* (1962) 19, 13–41.
14. Seedat YK, Reddy J. Diethylpropion hydrochloride (Tenuate Dospan) in the treatment of obese hypertensive patients. *S Afr Med J* (1974) 48, 569.

Guanethidine and related drugs + Tricyclic and tetracyclic antidepressants

The antihypertensive effects of guanethidine, betanidine, bretylium and debrisoquine are reduced or abolished by the concurrent use of tricyclic antidepressants such as amitriptyline, desipramine, imipramine, nortriptyline and protriptyline. Doxepin in doses of more than 200 to 250 mg daily interacts similarly, but in smaller doses appears not to do so. Maprotiline only interacts in a few individuals. Mianserin appears not to interact.

Clinical evidence

(a) Tricyclic antidepressants

Five hypertensive patients, controlled on 50 to 150 mg **guanethidine** daily, showed a blood pressure rise of 27 mmHg (diastolic pressure + one-third pulse pressure) when given 50 to 75 mg **desipramine** or 20 mg **protriptyline** daily for 1 to 9 days. The full antihypertensive effects of the guanethidine were not re-established until 5 days after the antidepressants were withdrawn.[1]

The same interaction has been described in other reports between **guanethidine** and **desipramine**,[2,3] **imipramine**,[4] **amitriptyline**,[5-7] **protriptyline**[3] and **nortriptyline**;[8] between **betanidine** and **desipramine**,[1-3,9] **imipramine**,[7,10] **amitriptyline**,[10] and **nortriptyline**;[10,11] and between **debrisoquine** and **desipramine**[3] and **amitriptyline**.[7,10] In some cases the interaction develops rapidly and fully within a few hours and lasts for many days (e.g. two 25-mg doses of **desipramine** – less than a day's dosage – completely abolished the effects of **betanidine** for an entire week[2]), whereas the interaction with **guanethidine** may take several days to develop fully. **Doxepin** does not interact until doses of about 200 to 250 mg daily are used, but with 300 mg or more daily it interacts to the same extent as other tricyclics.[9,12-17] An experimental study has shown that **tricyclic antidepressants** can return the blood pressure to normal in patients taking **bretylium**, without reducing its antiarrhythmic efficacy.[18]

(b) Tetracyclic and related antidepressants

A rise in blood pressure occurred in 1 of 6 patients on **betanidine** and **maprotiline** in one study,[19] and in 1 of 4 patients receiving **maprotiline** with **guanethidine**, **debrisoquine**, or **betanidine** in another.[7] In a study in 3 patients, **mianserin** did not alter the antihypertensive efficacy of **guanethidine** or **betanidine**.[20] Similar results were reported in a 2-week study in 6 patients on **betanidine**.[21]

Mechanism

The guanethidine-like drugs exert their hypotensive actions firstly by entering the adrenergic nerve endings associated with blood vessels using the norepinephrine (noradrenaline) uptake mechanism. The tricyclics successfully compete for the same mechanism so that the antihypertensives fail to reach their site of action and, as a result, the blood pressure rises once again.[22] The differences in the rate of development, duration and extent of the interactions reflect the differences between the various guanethidine-like drugs and the various tricyclics, as well as individual differences between patients.

Importance and management

A very well documented and well established interaction of clinical importance. Not every combination of guanethidine-like drug and tricyclic antidepressant has been studied but all are expected to interact similarly. Concurrent use should be avoided unless the effects are very closely monitored and the interaction balanced by raising the dosage of the antihypertensive. Note that the use of guanethidine and related adrenergic neurone blockers has largely been superseded by other antihypertensive drug classes.

1. Mitchell JR, Arias L, Oates JA. Antagonism of the antihypertensive actions of guanethidine sulfate by desipramine hydrochloride. *JAMA* (1967) 202, 973–6.

2. Oates JA, Mitchell JR, Feagin OT, Kaufmann JS, Shand DG. Distribution of guanidinium antihypertensives-mechanism of their selective action. *Ann N Y Acad Sci* (1971) 179, 302–9.
3. Mitchell JR, Cavanaugh JH, Arias L, Oates JA. Guanethidine and related agents. III. Antagonism by drugs which inhibit the norepinephrine pump in man. *J Clin Invest* (1970) 49, 1596.
4. Leishman AWD, Matthews HL, Smith AJ. Antagonism of guanethidine by imipramine. *Lancet* (1963) i, 112.
5. Meyer JF, McAllister CK, Goldberg LI. Insidious and prolonged antagonism of guanethidine by amitriptyline. *JAMA* (1970) 213, 1487–8.
6. Ober KF, Wang RIH. Drug interactions with guanethidine. *Clin Pharmacol Ther* (1973) 14, 190–5.
7. Smith AJ, Bant WP. Interactions between post-ganglionic sympathetic blocking drugs and anti-depressants. *J Int Med Res* (1975) 3 (Suppl 2), 55–60.
8. McQueen EG. New Zealand Committee on Adverse Reactions: Ninth Annual Report 1974. *N Z Med J* (1974) 80, 305–11.
9. Oates JA, Fann WE, Cavanaugh JH. Effect of doxepin on the norepinephrine pump. A preliminary report. *Psychosomatics* (1969) 10 (Suppl), 12.
10. Skinner C, Coull DC, Johnston AW. Antagonism of the hypotensive action of bethanidine and debrisoquine by tricyclic antidepressants. *Lancet* (1969) ii, 564–6.
11. LaCorte WStJ, Ryan JR, McMahon FG, Jain AK, Ginzler F, Duncan W, Morley E. Titrating nortriptyline with bethanidine to eliminate the hypotensive effects in normal males. *Clin Pharmacol Ther* (1982) 31, 241.
12. Fann WE, Cavanaugh JH, Kaufmann JS, Griffith JD, Davis JM, Janowsky DS, Oates JA. Doxepin: effects on transport of biogenic amines in man. *Psychopharmacologia* (1971) 22, 111.
13. Gerson IM, Friedman R, Unterberger H. Non-antagonism of anti-adrenergic agents by dibenzoxepine (preliminary report). *Dis Nerv Syst* (1970) 31, 780–2.
14. Ayd FJ. Long-term administration of doxepin (Sinequan). *Dis Nerv Syst* (1971) 32, 617–22.
15. Ayd FJ. Doxepin with other drugs. *South Med J* (1973) 66, 465–71.
16. Ayd FJ. Maintenance doxepin (Sinequan) therapy for depressive illness. *Dis Nerv Syst* (1975) 36, 109–14.
17. Poe TE, Edwards JL, Taylor RB. Hypertensive crisis possibly due to drug interaction. *Postgrad Med* (1979) 66, 235–7.
18. Woosley RL, Reele SB, Roden DM, Nies AS, Oates JA. Pharmacological reversal of hypotensive effect complicating antiarrhythmic therapy with bretylium. *Clin Pharmacol Ther* (1982) 32, 313–21.
19. Briant RH, George CF. The assessment of potential drug interaction with a new tricyclic antidepressant drug. *Br J Clin Pharmacol* (1974) 1, 113.
20. Burgess CD, Turner P, Wadsworth J. Cardiovascular responses to mianserin hydrochloride: a comparison with tricyclic antidepressant drugs. *Br J Clin Pharmacol* (1978) 5, 21S–28S.
21. Coppen A, Ghose K, Swade C, Wood K. Effect of mianserin hydrochloride on peripheral uptake mechanisms for noradrenaline and 5-hydroxytryptamine in man. *Br J Clin Pharmacol* (1978) 5, 13S–17S.
22. Cairncross KD. On the peripheral pharmacology of amitriptyline. *Arch Int Pharmacodyn Ther* (1965) 154, 438–48.

Guanethidine and related drugs + Tyramine-rich foods

One study found no interaction between debrisoquine and tyramine, but a single case report describes a serious hypertensive reaction in a patient who ate 50 g Gruyère cheese.

Clinical evidence

A study in 4 hypertensive patients taking 40 to 60 mg **debrisoquine** daily showed that when they were given oral doses of **tyramine** in water only a moderate and unimportant increase in their sensitivity occurred. Intestinal MAO-activity remained unchanged.[1] These results contrast with those found in a hypertensive woman, treated for a week with doses of **debrisoquine** progressively increased to 70 mg daily, who was given 50 g **Gruyère cheese** to eat. Within 5 min her blood pressure had risen from 135/85 mmHg to 170/90 mmHg, and by the end of an hour it had climbed to 195/165 mmHg. It fell to 160/95 mmHg when 2 mg phentolamine was given, but rose again to 200/110 mmHg during the next hour.[2]

Mechanism

Not understood. Debrisoquine has some MAO-inhibitory activity but (unlike the antidepressant MAO-inhibitors) it appears not to affect the MAO in the gut wall so that tyramine is metabolised normally.[1,3] For a detailed account of the MAO-tyramine interaction see 'Monoamine oxidase inhibitors (MAOIs) + Tyramine-rich foods', p.685. In the isolated case cited it may have been that the cheese contained particularly large amounts of tyramine which were absorbed through the mucosal lining of the mouth while being chewed. If this is what happened, the tyramine by-passed the liver and was able to release the norepinephrine (noradrenaline) from the adrenergic sympathetic neurones resulting in a rise in blood pressure.

Importance and management

Information seems to be limited to the reports cited. The absence of other reports of a hypertensive reaction would seem to be a measure of its rarity. Prescribers may feel it prudent to warn their patients about tyramine-rich foods. A list of these is to be found in the monograph 'Monoamine oxidase inhibitors (MAOIs) + Tyramine-rich foods', p.685. No interaction would be expected with the other guanethidine-like drugs.

1. Pettinger WA, Korn A, Spiegel H, Solomon HM, Pocelinko R, Abrams WB. Debrisoquin, a selective inhibitor of intraneuronal monoamine oxidase in man. *Clin Pharmacol Ther* (1969) 10, 667–74.
2. Amery A, Deloof W. Cheese reaction during debrisoquine treatment. *Lancet* (1970) ii, 613.
3. Pettinger WA, Horst WD. Quantifying metabolic effects of antihypertensive and other drugs at the sympathetic neuron level: clinical and basic correlations. *Ann N Y Acad Sci* (1971) 179, 310–21.

Guanfacine + Tricyclic antidepressants

A single report describes a reduced antihypertensive response to guanfacine in a patient given amitriptyline and later imipramine.

Clinical evidence

A woman of 38 with hypertension, well controlled with 2 mg guanfacine daily, showed a rise in her blood pressure from 138/89 mmHg to 150/100 mmHg after taking 75 mg **amitriptyline** daily for 7 to 14 days. The pressure fell again when the **amitriptyline** was stopped. A month later her blood pressure rose to 142/98 mmHg after taking 50 mg **imipramine** daily for two days, and fell again when it was stopped.[1]

Mechanism

Uncertain. A possible reason is, that like clonidine (another alpha-2 agonist), the uptake of guanfacine into neurones within the brain is blocked by tricyclic antidepressants, thereby reducing its effects.

Importance and management

Direct information is limited to this report, but it is supported by *animal* studies[2] and consistent with the way another alpha-2 agonist (clonidine) interacts with tricyclic antidepressants (see 'Clonidine + Tricyclic and tetracyclic antidepressants', p.388). Be alert for this interaction in any patient given guanfacine and any tricyclic antidepressant. **Guanabenz** is another alpha-2 agonist which might interact similarly, but as yet there is no direct clinical evidence that it does so.

1. Buckley M, Feeley J. Antagonism of antihypertensive effect of guanfacine by tricyclic antidepressants. *Lancet* (1991) 337, 1173–4.
2. Ohkubo K, Suzuki K, Oguma T, Otorii T. Central hypotensive effects of guanfacine in anaesthetised rabbits. *Nippon Yakurigaku Zasshi* (1982) 79, 263–74.

Hydralazine + Indometacin (Indomethacin) or Diclofenac

It is uncertain whether indometacin does or does not reduce or abolish the hypotensive effects of hydralazine, whereas diclofenac appears to oppose dihydralazine.

Clinical evidence, mechanism, importance and management

After taking 200 mg **indometacin** (**indomethacin**), the hypotensive response to 0.15 mg/kg hydralazine given intravenously to healthy subjects was abolished, and the subjects only responded when given another dose 30 min later.[1] In contrast another study, also in healthy subjects, found that 100 mg **indometacin** daily did not affect the hypotensive response to a single 0.2-mg/kg dose of hydralazine given intravenously.[2] Thus it is not clear if **indometacin** interacts with hydralazine given intravenously, and equally uncertain if an interaction occurs when hydralazine is given orally. On the other hand a single-dose study in 4 hypertension subjects found that the actions of intravenous **dihydralazine** (hypotensive, effects on urinary excretion, heart rate and sodium clearance) were reduced by intravenous **diclofenac**.[3] It would be prudent to monitor concurrent use of hydralazine and related drugs and these NSAIDs.

1. Cinquegrani MP, Liang C-S. Indomethacin attenuates the hypotensive action of hydralazine. *Clin Pharmacol Ther* (1986) 39, 564–70.
2. Jackson SHD, Pickles H. Indomethacin does not attenuate the effects of hydralazine in normal subjects. *Eur J Clin Pharmacol* (1983) 25, 303–5.
3. Reimann IW, Ratge D, Wisser H, Fröhlich JC. Are prostaglandins involved in the antihypertensive effect of dihydralazine? *Clin Sci* (1981) 61, 319S–321S.

Imidapril + Miscellaneous

The makers advise caution if imidapril is given with lithium. Imidapril may enhance insulin sensitivity. The antihypertensive effects may be reduced by sympathomimetics, and the bioavailability may be reduced by antacids.

Clinical evidence, mechanism, importance and management

Co-administration of imidapril and **lithium** may result in reduced **lithium** excretion. Monitoring of serum **lithium** is advised.[1] See also 'Lithium carbonate + ACE inhibitors', p.652. Hypoglycaemia may occur during co-administration of imidapril and **insulin** or **oral hypoglycaemic drugs** (see also 'Hypoglycaemic agents + ACE inhibitors', p.564). The bioavailability of imidapril may be reduced by **antacids**. The antihypertensive effects of imidapril may be reduced by **sympathomimetics**.[1]

1. Tanatril (Imidapril). Trinity Pharmaceuticals Ltd. Summary of product characteristics, March 2001.

Indoramin + Alcohol

The serum levels of both indoramin and alcohol may be raised by concurrent use. The increased drowsiness may possibly increase the risks when driving.

Clinical evidence

When 10 healthy subjects were given a single 50-mg oral dose of indoramin together with 0.5 g/kg **alcohol** in 600 ml alcohol-free lager, the AUC of indoramin was increased by 25% and the peak levels raised by 58%.[1,2] When given a single 0.175 mg/kg intravenous dose of indoramin together with the same oral dose of **alcohol**, a 26% rise in blood **alcohol** levels occurred during the first 1.25 h after dosing, but no change in indoramin pharmacokinetics were seen. The combination of **alcohol** and indoramin caused more sedation than either drug alone.[2]

Mechanism

Uncertain. Increased absorption of the indoramin from the gut or reduced liver metabolism may be responsible for the raised indoramin serum levels. The increase in sedation would appear additionally to be due to the additive sedative effects of the two drugs.

Importance and management

Information is limited but the interaction appears to be established. The clinical importance of the raised serum indoramin and alcohol levels is uncertain, however since indoramin sometimes causes drowsiness when it is first given, there is the possibility that alertness will be reduced, which could increase the risks of driving or handling other machinery. Patients should be warned. More study is needed. For mention of the effect of moderate to heavy drinking on the efficacy of antihypertensives in general, see 'Antihypertensives + Alcohol', p.383.

1. Abrams SML, Pierce DM, Franklin RA, Johnston A, Marrott PK, Cory EP, Turner P. Effect of ethanol on indoramin pharmacokinetics. *Br J Clin Pharmacol* (1984) 18, 294P–295P.
2. Abrams SML, Pierce DM, Johnston A, Hedges A, Franklin RA, Turner P. Pharmacokinetic interaction between indoramin and ethanol. *Hum Toxicol* (1989) 8, 237–41.

Irbesartan + Miscellaneous drugs

Irbesartan appears not to interact to a clinically relevant extent with beta-blockers and calcium channel blockers. It may have useful additive hypotensive effects with hydrochlorothiazide. There may be a risk of hyperkalaemia if irbesartan is co-administered with potassium-sparing diuretics or potassium supplements. Co-administration of irbesartan with lithium may result in elevated serum lithium. Fluconazole may inhibit the metabolism of irbesartan.

Clinical evidence, mechanism, importance and management

No pharmacokinetic interactions were found between irbesartan 150 mg daily and **hydrochlorothiazide** 25 mg daily in patients with mild to moderate hypertension, and the blood pressure lowering effects were additive.[1] The makers say that irbesartan has been safely given with **thiazides** and other antihypertensives such as **beta-blockers** and long-acting **calcium channel blockers**, but they warn that **high-dose diuretics** may result in volume depletion and the risk of hypotension when irbesartan is first started.[2]

A study in healthy subjects found that a **high fat breakfast** had no clinically relevant effects on the bioavailability of a single 300-mg dose of irbesartan.[3]

The makers of irbesartan point out that other drugs that affect the renin-angiotensin system (e.g. ACE inhibitors) can cause hyperkalaemia, especially in renal impairment and/or heart failure and if given with **potassium supplements, salt substitutes, potassium-sparing diuretics,** or other drugs that may increase serum potassium. They recommend that serum potassium should be monitored in patients given irbesartan with any of these risk factors.[2] Similarly, since ACE inhibitors can raise serum **lithium** levels (see 'Lithium carbonate + ACE inhibitors', p.652), they recommend close monitoring of lithium levels in patients on **lithium** and irbesartan.[2]

Based on *in vitro* data, no interaction would be expected between irbesartan and drugs whose metabolism depends on cytochrome P450 isoenzymes CYP1A1, CYP1A2, CYP2A6, CYP2B6, CYP2D6, CYP2E1 or CYP3A4.[2,4] Irbesartan itself is primarily metabolised by CYP2C9,[2,4] and a study in 15 healthy subjects given 150 mg irbesartan daily found that the steady-state AUC was increased 63% and maximum blood levels 19% by concomitant **fluconazole** 200 mg daily for 10 days, probably as a result of CYP2C9 inhibition.[5] However, the maker considers these changes are unlikely to be clinically relevant.[6] Despite **nifedipine** being considered an inhibitor of CYP2C9, a study in 12 healthy subjects given 300 mg irbesartan daily for 4 days followed by the addition of 30 mg **nifedipine** daily for a further 4 days found that **nifedipine** did not alter the pharmacokinetics of irbesartan.[7]

1. Marino MR, Langenbacher KM, Ford NF, Beierle F, Shamblen EC, Lasseter KC. Effect of hydrochlorothiazide on the pharmacokinetics and pharmacodynamics of irbesartan. *Clin Pharmacol Ther* (1997) 61, 207.
2. Aprovel (Irbesartan), Sanofi Synthelabo. Summary of product characteristics, April 2002.
3. Vachharajani NN, Shyu WC, Mantha S, Park J-S, Greene DS, Barbhaiya RH. Lack of effect of food on the oral bioavailability of irbesartan in healthy male volunteers. *J Clin Pharmacol* (1998) 38, 433–6.
4. Taavitsainen P, Kiukaanniemi K, Pelkonen O. In vitro inhibition screening of human hepatic P450 enzymes by five angiotensin-II receptor antagonists. *Eur J Clin Pharmacol* (2000) 56, 135–40.
5. Kovacs SJ, Wilton JH, Blum RA. Steady state pharmacokinetics of irbesartan alone and in combination with fluconazole. *Clin Pharmacol Ther* (1999) 65, 132.
6. Marino MR, Vachharajani NN. Drug interactions with irbesartan. *Clin Pharmacokinet* (2001) 40, 605–14.
7. Marino MR, Hammett JL, Perreira II, Ford NF, Uderman HD. Effect of nifedipine on the steady-state pharmacokinetics and pharmacodynamics of irbesartan in healthy subjects. *J Cardiovasc Pharmacol Ther* (1998) 3, 111–18.

Ketanserin + Beta-blockers

The pharmacokinetics of neither drug appears to be affected by the presence of the other but additive hypotensive effects may occur. Very marked and acute hypotension has been seen in two patients on atenolol when first given ketanserin.

Clinical evidence, mechanism, importance and management

A study in 6 patients and 2 healthy subjects given ketanserin (40 mg twice daily for three weeks) showed that the concurrent use of **propranolol** (80 mg twice daily for 6 days) did not significantly alter the steady-state plasma levels of ketanserin.[1] Another study on healthy subjects, using single doses of both drugs, showed that the pharmacokinetics of neither drug was affected by the presence of the other.[2] The hypotensive effects of the ketanserin were slightly increased by the **propranolol** in the study already cited[1] and additive hypotensive effects were seen in a study in patients with essential hypertension.[3] Acute hypotension is reported to have occurred in two patients taking **atenolol** within an hour of additionally being given a 40-mg oral dose of ketanserin. One of them briefly lost consciousness.[4] Concurrent use can be valuable and uneventful but a few patients may experience marked hypotensive effects when first given ketanserin. Patients should be warned. Information about the concurrent use of other beta-blockers seems not to be available.

1. Trenk D, Lühr A, Radkow N, Jähnchen E. Lack of effect of propranolol on the steady-state plasma levels of ketanserin. *Arzneimittelforschung* (1985) 35, 1286–8.
2. Williams FM, Leeser JE, Rawlins MD. Pharmacodynamics and pharmacokinetics of single doses of ketanserin and propranolol alone and in combination in healthy volunteers. *Br J Clin Pharmacol* (1986) 22, 301–8.
3. Hedner T, Persson B. Antihypertensive properties of ketanserin in combination with β-adrenergic blocking agents. *J Cardiovasc Pharmacol* (1985) 7 (Suppl 7), S161–S163.
4. Waller PC, Cameron HA, Ramsey LE. Profound hypotension after the first dose of ketanserin. *Postgrad Med J* (1987) 63, 305–7.

Ketanserin + Diuretics

Sudden deaths, probably from heart rhythm abnormalities, are markedly increased in patients taking potassium-losing diuretics if they are concurrently treated with high doses of ketanserin. Potassium-sparing diuretics do not appear to interact in this way and no interaction seems to occur with low doses of ketanserin.

Clinical evidence, mechanism, importance and management

A large multi-national study[1] involving 3899 patients found that a harmful and potentially fatal interaction could occur in those given ketanserin (40 mg three times daily) and **potassium-losing diuretics**. Of 249 patients on both drugs, 35 died (16 suddenly) compared with only 15 of 260 (5 suddenly) taking a placebo and **potassium-losing diuretics**. No significant increase in the number of deaths occurred in those on ketanserin and **potassium-sparing diuretics**.

The reason for the deaths seems to be that the ketanserin accentuates and exaggerates the harmful effects of the **potassium-losing diuretics** on the heart which can worsen arrhythmias. It was found that the corrected QT interval of the heart was prolonged as follows: **ketanserin alone** (18 ms), **ketanserin + potassium-sparing diuretics** (24 ms), **ketanserin + potassium-losing diuretics** (30 ms). In some individuals this can apparently have a fatal outcome. Preliminary results of a later study on 33 patients using a smaller dose of ketanserin (20 mg twice daily) with **potassium-losing diuretics** (**furosemide (frusemide), thiazides**) found no evidence that this dose prolonged the QT_c interval.[2] The pharmacokinetics of single doses of ketanserin 20 mg were not altered by single 25-mg doses of **hydrochlorothiazide**.[3]

Potassium-losing diuretics (**thiazides, furosemide**, etc.) with relatively high doses of ketanserin (40 mg three times daily) should be avoided but lower doses seem to be safe. **Potassium-sparing diuretics** (**amiloride, triamterene**, etc.) also seem to be safe even with the higher dose of ketanserin.

1. Prevention of Atherosclerotic Complications with Ketanserin Trial Group. Prevention of atherosclerotic complications: controlled trial of ketanserin. *BMJ* (1989) 298, 424–30.
2. Van Gool R, Symoens J. Ketanserin in combination with diuretics: effect on QTc-interval. *Eur Heart J* (1990) 11 (Suppl), 57.
3. Botha JH, McFadyen ML, Leary WPP, Janssens M. No effect of single-dose hydrochlorothiazide on the pharmacokinetics of single-dose ketanserin. *Curr Ther Res* (1991) 49, 225–30.

Ketanserin + Miscellaneous drugs

Ketanserin should not be given with certain antiarrhythmics, naftidrofuryl or tricyclic antidepressants because of the risk of potentially fatal cardiac arrhythmias. Drowsiness and dizziness are common side-effects which may possibly be additive with the effects of other CNS depressants.

Clinical evidence, mechanism, importance and management

Ketanserin has weak class-III antiarrhythmic activity and can prolong the QT_c interval. For safety reasons it has therefore been advised that it should be avoided in patients with existing QT_c prolongation, atrioventricular or sinoauricular block of higher degree, or severe bradycardia (<50 bpm).[1] For the same reason the concurrent use of drugs which affect repolarisation (**antiarrhythmics of classes Ia, Ic, III**) or those which cause conduction disturbances (**naftidrofuryl, tricyclic antidepressants**) should be avoided.[1] See also 'Drugs that prolong the QT interval + Other drugs that prolong the QT interval', p.103.

Dizziness and drowsiness are common side effects and therefore it seems likely that these will be additive with other **CNS depressants** and **alcohol** which may possibly make driving more hazardous. This needs confirmation.

1. Distler A. Clinical aspects during therapy with the serotonin antagonist ketanserin. *Clin Physiol Biochem* (1990) 8 (Suppl 3), 64–80.

Ketanserin + Nifedipine

A few elderly patients given ketanserin and nifedipine may experience an increase in heart arrhythmias.

Clinical evidence, mechanism, importance and management

A study in 20 subjects aged 60 or more, with normal or slightly raised blood pressures, found that the concurrent use of ketanserin and **nifedipine** for a week did not, on average, affect their blood pressures, heart rates, or the QT intervals, but 2 of the subjects monitored over 24 h showed a marked increase in the frequency of ectopic beats, couplets and ventricular tachycardia.[1] The reasons are not understood. The authors of this study say that their findings do not exclude the possibility that the combined use of these two drugs might therefore increase arrhythmia in some elderly patients.[1] Concurrent use in the elderly should be monitored.

1. Alberio L, Beretta-Piccoli C, Tanzi F, Koch P, Zehender M. Kardiale Interaktionen zwischen Ketanserin und dem Calcium-Antagonisten Nifedipin. *Schweiz Med Wochenschr* (1992) 122, 1723–7.

Losartan + Miscellaneous drugs

Losartan appears not to interact to a clinically relevant extent with warfarin. The pharmacokinetics and blood-pressure lowering effect of losartan were not affected by cimetidine, erythromycin and itraconazole. Fluvastatin, grapefruit juice, hydrochlorothiazide, ketoconazole and phenobarbital have a

minor or no effect on the pharmacokinetics of losartan and its
active metabolite E3174. The clearance of losartan is increased by rifampicin (rifampin), reducing its blood-pressure
lowering effect. Indometacin may attenuate the antihypertensive effect of losartan, but low-dose aspirin does not. There
may be a risk of hyperkalaemia if losartan is co-administered
with potassium-sparing diuretics or potassium supplements.
There may be a risk of symptomatic hypotension when losartan is started in patients on high-dose diuretics. There is a report of acute renal failure in a diabetic patient on losartan
when given intravenous mannitol.

Clinical evidence, mechanism, importance and management

(a) Aspirin

A study in 10 patients with hypertension taking losartan (mean daily
dose 47.5 mg) found that neither aspirin 81 mg nor 325 mg daily had
any significant effect on blood pressure.[1]

(b) Cimetidine

A 2-period, randomised, crossover study in 8 healthy subjects given
100 mg losartan before and after taking 400 mg cimetidine four
times daily for 6 days found that the pharmacokinetics and pharmacodynamics of the losartan and its active metabolite (E3174) were not
changed to a clinically relevant extent by the cimetidine.[2] No special
precautions are needed if these drugs are used concurrently.

(c) Erythromycin

When 10 healthy subjects were given 50 mg losartan alone daily for
a week and then after a 6-day washout period, 50 mg losartan daily
plus 500 mg erythromycin four times daily for a week, it was found
that the erythromycin had no significant effect on the pharmacokinetics of the losartan or its active metabolite (E3174). In addition,
erythromycin did not alter the blood pressure lowering effect of losartan.[3] Inhibition of cytochrome P450 isoenzyme CYP3A4 alone does not
appear to prevent the conversion of losartan to E3174. There
would therefore appear to be no reason to take any special precautions
if both drugs used concurrently.

(d) Fluconazole

Sixteen healthy subjects were given 100 mg losartan daily for 20
days, to which was added 200 mg fluconazole daily on days 11 to 20.
Preliminary results showed the AUC and maximum plasma levels of
losartan were increased by 69 and 31% respectively by fluconazole,
and those of losartan's active metabolite (E1374) were reduced by 41
and 54% respectively.[4] In another study, 11 healthy subjects were
given a single dose of 50 mg losartan before after 4 days of fluconazole (400 mg on day 1 and 200 mg daily on days 2 to 4). The AUC of
losartan was increased by 27% while its maximum plasma level was
reduced by 23% by fluconazole. The AUC and the maximum plasma
levels of E3174 were reduced by 47% and 77% respectively. However, no significant changes in the hypotensive effect of losartan were
noted.[5,6]

It was presumed that fluconazole inhibits the conversion of losartan
to its active metabolite by inhibiting cytochrome P450 isoenzyme
CYP2C9 (but see also Fluvastatin below)[4,6] The lack of pharmacodynamic changes suggests that this pharmacokinetic interaction may not
be clinically important, but this requires confirmation in the clinical
setting.

(e) Fluvastatin

A crossover study was carried out in 12 healthy subjects given 50 mg
losartan in the morning for 7 days, followed by 7 days of 40 mg fluvastatin at bedtime, and finally both drugs together for another 7
days. It was found that the steady-state pharmacokinetics of losartan
and its active metabolite E3174 were not significantly altered by the
fluvastatin.[7,8] The authors concluded that inhibition of cytochrome
P450 isoenzyme CYP2C9 alone does not appear to prevent the conversion of losartan to E3174, and that CYP3A4 inhibition may be required as well. There would therefore appear to be no need to take any
special precautions if these drugs are used concurrently.

(f) Grapefruit juice

A study in 9 healthy subjects found that administration of grapefruit
juice with a single dose of losartan 50 mg increased the time for losartan to be detected in the serum by 50% and reduced the AUC of the
active metabolite E3174 by 26%. These effects may be due to inhibition of cytochrome P450 isoenzyme CYP3A4 and activation of P-
glycoprotein.[9] However, the changes seen are unlikely to be clinically
relevant.

(g) Hydrochlorothiazide

Twelve patients with mild or moderate hypertension were given
50 mg losartan alone or with 12.5 mg hydrochlorothiazide daily for
7 days. The AUC of hydrochlorothiazide decreased 17% during
concurrent use (not considered clinically significant) while the pharmacokinetics of losartan were unchanged.[10] Another study has shown
that these drugs have useful additive effects in the control of hypertension.[11] The maker notes that symptomatic hypotension may occur
when losartan is started in patients with intravascular volume depletion such as those on high-dose diuretics. In these patients volume
depletion should be corrected, or a lower starting dose of losartan
should be used.[12]

(h) Indometacin (Indomethacin)

In a randomised double-blind study, 111 patients with hypertension
received losartan 50 mg once daily for 6 weeks, and this reduced their
blood pressure by a mean of 7.9/5.3 mmHg. Indometacin 75 mg
once daily was then added for one week, and this caused a rise in
blood pressure in the group as a whole of 3.8/2.2 mmHg (an 45% reduction in the effect of losartan). A clear reduction in the effect of
losartan was seen in 69% of the patients.[13] In contrast, a much smaller
study in 10 patients with essential hypertension treated with losartan
found that indometacin 50 mg twice daily caused sodium retention
but did not significantly attenuate the antihypertensive effects of losartan.[14] Patients on losartan who require indometacin should be monitored for alterations in blood pressure control.

(i) Itraconazole

The pharmacokinetics and pharmacodynamics (blood pressures,
heart rates) of losartan and its active metabolite E3174 following a
50 mg dose of losartan were not significantly affected by 200 mg
itraconazole daily for 4 days in 11 healthy subjects.[5,6] Inhibition of
cytochrome P450 isoenzyme CYP3A4 alone does not appear to prevent the conversion of losartan to E3174. No special precautions
would appear to be needed if these drugs are used concurrently.

(j) Ketoconazole

Preliminary results of a study in 11 healthy subjects found that ketoconazole 400 mg daily for 4 days did not affect the conversion of
losartan to its active metabolite, E3174, or the plasma clearances of
losartan and E3174 after a single intravenous dose of losartan
30 mg.[15] Inhibition of cytochrome P450 isoenzyme CYP3A4 alone
does not appear to prevent the conversion of losartan to E3174. No
special precautions would appear to be needed if these drugs are used
concurrently.

(k) Mannitol

A man with diabetic nephropathy receiving losartan 25 mg twice daily for hypertension developed acute renal failure after being given a
total of 420 g mannitol intravenously over 4 days for haemorrhagic
glaucoma. His mental state and renal status improved following
haemodialysis and stopping both mannitol and losartan.[16] The mechanism is not fully understood but the combination may result in a
marked decrease in glomerular filtration rate. Caution is recommended.

(l) Phenobarbital

Pharmacokinetic studies have not found a clinically significant interaction between losartan and phenobarbital.[12]

(m) Potassium-sparing diuretics or potassium supplements

Losartan can cause hyperkalaemia (incidence of 1.5% in clinical trials).[12] The makers of losartan advise against the concomitant use of
other drugs that may increase potassium levels including potassium-
sparing diuretics (e.g. amiloride, spironolactone, triamterene), po-

tassium supplements, salt substitutes.[12] If these are necessary it would be prudent to monitor potassium levels closely.

(n) Rifampicin (Rifampin)

Ten healthy subjects were given 50 mg losartan alone daily for a week and then after a 6-day washout period, 50 mg losartan daily plus 300 mg **rifampicin** twice daily for a week. It was found that the **rifampicin** reduced the losartan AUC by 35%, reduced its half-life from 2 to 0.9 h, and increased its clearance by 60%. The AUC of the active metabolite E3174 was reduced by 41% and its half-life was reduced from 5.1 to 2.5 h. Diastolic blood pressure was significantly reduced by losartan alone, but not by the combination.[3] The presumed reason is that the **rifampicin** (a recognised enzyme-inducer) increases the metabolism of the losartan by the liver (by cytochrome P450 isoenzymes CYP2C9 and CYP3A4). The clinical importance of this interaction still awaits assessment, but it would seem likely that the antihypertensive effects of the losartan would be reduced by **rifampicin**. If both drugs are used, be alert for the need to increase the losartan dosage. More study is needed.

(o) Warfarin

In a two-period placebo-controlled, randomised crossover study, 10 healthy subjects were given 100 mg losartan daily for 13 days to which was added on day 7 a single 30 mg oral dose of **warfarin**. The pharmacokinetics of the **warfarin** (both *R*- and *S*-) and its anticoagulant effects were not altered by the losartan. Losartan alone for a week also had no effect on prothrombin times.[17] This evidence suggests that no interaction is likely if both drugs are used concurrently. Information about other anticoagulants is lacking.

1. Nawarskas JJ, Townsend RR, Cirigliano MD, Spinler SA. Effect of aspirin on blood pressure in hypertensive patients taking enalapril or losartan. *Am J Hypertens* (1999) 12, 784–9.
2. Goldberg MR, Lo M-W, Bradstreet TE, Ritter MA, Höglund P. Effects of cimetidine on pharmacokinetics and pharmacodynamics of losartan, an AT₁-selective non-peptide angiotensin II receptor antagonist. *Eur J Clin Pharmacol* (1995) 49, 115–19.
3. Williamson KM, Patterson JH, McQueen RH, Adams KF, Pieper JA. Effects of erythromycin or rifampin on losartan pharmacokinetics in healthy volunteers. *Clin Pharmacol Ther* (1998) 63, 316–23.
4. Kazierad DJ, Martin DE, Tenero D, Boike SC, Ilson B, Freed MI, Etheredge R, Jorkasky DK. Fluconazole significantly alters the pharmacokinetics of losartan but not eprosartan. *Clin Pharmacol Ther* (1997) 61, 203.
5. Kaukonen K-M, Olkkola KT, Neuvonen PJ. Fluconazole but not itraconazole decreases the metabolism of losartan to E-3174. *Clin Pharmacol Ther* (1998) 63, 151.
6. Kaukonen KM, Olkkola KT, Neuvonen PJ. Fluconazole but not itraconazole decreases the metabolism of losartan to E-3174. *J Clin Pharmacol* (1998) 53, 445–9.
7. Meadowcroft AM, Williamson KM, Patterson JH, Hinderliter AL, Pieper JA. The effects of fluvastatin, a CYP2C9 inhibitor, on losartan pharmacokinetics. *Clin Pharmacol Ther* (1998) 63, 213.
8. Meadowcroft AM, Williamson KM, Patterson JH, Hinderliter AL, Pieper JA. The effects of fluvastatin, a CYP2C9 inhibitor, on losartan pharmacokinetics in healthy volunteers. *J Clin Pharmacol* (1999) 39, 418–24.
9. Zaidenstein R, Sobak S, Gips M, Avni B, Dishi V, Weissgarten Y, Golik A, Scapa E. Effect of grapefruit juice on the pharmacokinetics of losartan and its active metabolite E3174 in healthy volunteers. *Ther Drug Monit* (2001) 23, 369–73.
10. McCrea JB, Lo M-W, Tomasko L, Lin CC, Hsieh JY-K, Capra NL, Goldberg MR. Absence of a pharmacokinetic interaction between losartan and hydrochlorothiazide. *J Clin Pharmacol* (1995) 35, 1200–6.
11. MacKay JH, Arcuri K, Goldberg AI, Snapinn S, Sweet CS. Losartan and low-dose hydrochlorothiazide in patients with essential hypertension. A double-blind, placebo-controlled trial of concomitant administration compared with individual components. *Arch Intern Med* (1996) 156, 278–85.
12. Cozaar (Losartan) Merck Sharp & Dohme Ltd. Summary of product characteristics. December 2001.
13. Conlin PR, Moore TJ, Swartz SL, Barr E, Gazdick L, Fletcher C, DeLucca P, Demopoulos L. Effect of indomethacin on blood pressure lowering by captopril and losartan in hypertensive patients. *Hypertension* (2000) 36, 461–5.
14. Olsen ME, Thomsen T, Hassager C, Ibsen H, Dige-Petersen H. Hemodynamic and renal effects of indomethacin in losartan-treated hypertensive individuals. *Am J Hypertens* (1999) 12, 209–16.
15. McCrea JB, Lo MW, Furtek CI, Ritter MA, Carides A, Waldman SA, Bjornsson TD, Goldberg MR. Ketoconazole does not affect the systemic conversion of losartan to E-3174. *Clin Pharmacol Ther* (1996) 59, 169.
16. Matsumura M. Mannitol-induced toxicity in a diabetic patient receiving losartan. *Am J Med* (2001) 110, 331.
17. Kong A-N T, Tomasko P, Waldman SA, Osborne B, Deutsch PJ, Goldberg MR, Bjornsson TD. Losartan does not affect the pharmacokinetics and pharmacodynamics of warfarin. *J Clin Pharmacol* (1995) 35, 1008–15.

Loop diuretics + NSAIDs or Aspirin or Paracetamol

The antihypertensive and diuretic effects of furosemide (frusemide) can be reduced or even abolished by the concur-rent use of indometacin (indomethacin). Diclofenac, diflunisal, flurbiprofen, ketorolac, lornoxicam, naproxen, piroxicam and tolfenamic acid also appear to interact similarly although much less information is available. Azapropazone, flupirtine, ibuprofen, ketoprofen, meloxicam, metamizole sodium (dipyrone), mofebutazone, oxindanac, paracetamol (acetaminophen), pirprofen, sulindac and tenoxicam may possibly not interact at all or may do so to a much lesser extent. Bumetanide and torasemide appear to be affected in the same way as furosemide.

Clinical evidence

(a) Bumetanide + Aspirin

Aspirin 640 mg four times daily reduced the 24-h urinary output in response to 1 mg **bumetanide** in eight healthy subjects by 18%.[1]

(b) Furosemide (Frusemide) + Azapropazone

Ten healthy subjects showed no change in their urinary excretion caused by **furosemide** (40 mg daily) when they were concurrently given **azapropazone** (600 mg twice daily). The **furosemide** did not antagonise the uricosuric effects of the **azapropazone**.[2]

(c) Furosemide (Frusemide) + Diclofenac

A study in patients with heart failure and cirrhosis showed that 150 mg **diclofenac** daily reduced the **furosemide-**induced excretion of sodium by 38%, but the excretion of potassium was unaltered.[3]

(d) Furosemide (Frusemide) + Diflunisal

A study in 12 healthy subjects showed that 500 mg **diflunisal** twice daily interacted with **furosemide** like indometacin: sodium excretion was reduced 59% but potassium excretion remained unchanged.[4]

In patients with heart failure and cirrhosis treated with **furosemide**, 500 to 700 mg **diflunisal** daily decreased the sodium excretion by 36% and the potassium excretion by 47%.[3] However another study failed to find an interaction.[5]

(e) Furosemide (Frusemide) + Flurbiprofen

A study in 7 healthy subjects showed that the increase in renal osmolal clearance of a standard water load, in response to 40 mg **furosemide** given orally or 20 mg intravenously, fell from 105 to 19% and from 140 to 70% respectively following concurrent treatment with 100 mg **flurbiprofen**.[6]

A single-dose study in 10 healthy subjects showed that 100 mg **flurbiprofen** reduced the urinary volume by 10% and sodium and potassium excretion by 9% and 12% respectively following 80 mg **furosemide** orally.[7]

(f) Furosemide (Frusemide) + Flupirtine

A study in healthy subjects found that a single 200-mg dose of **flupirtine** did not affect the overall **furosemide** diuresis, but it was slightly delayed.[8]

(g) Furosemide (Frusemide) + Ibuprofen

An elderly man with cardiac failure treated with digoxin, isosorbide dinitrate and 80 mg **furosemide** daily, developed congestive heart failure with ascites when given 400 mg **ibuprofen** three times daily. His serum urea and creatinine levels climbed and no diuresis occurred even when the **furosemide** dosage was doubled. Two days after withdrawing the **ibuprofen**, brisk diuresis took place, renal function returned to normal and his condition improved steadily.[9] Another elderly patient similarly showed a poor response to **furosemide** (and later to metolazone as well) until **ibuprofen** (600 mg four times daily) and at least two **aspirin** daily were stopped.[10] This was due to hyponatraemic hypovolaemia.

(h) Furosemide (Frusemide), Bumetanide or Torasemide + Indometacin (Indomethacin)

A study in 4 normal subjects and 6 patients with essential hypertension showed that **furosemide** alone (80 mg three times daily) reduced the mean blood pressure by 13 mmHg, but when given with **indometacin** (50 mg four times daily) the blood pressures returned to virtually pretreatment levels. Moreover the normal urinary sodium loss induced by the **furosemide** was significantly reduced.[11]

A study in healthy subjects and patients with congestive heart failure given **furosemide** showed that 100 mg **indometacin** reduced the urinary output by 53% and also reduced the excretion of Na⁺, K⁺ and Cl⁻ by 64%, 49% and 62% respectively.[12] Another study found a 20 to 30% reduction in urinary output.[13] A single 100-mg dose of **indometacin** was also found to reduce the **bumetanide**-induced output of urine, Na⁺ and Cl⁻ (but not K⁺) by about 25%.[14-16] There are other reports confirming the interaction between **furosemide** or **bumetanide** and **indometacin**, some of which are detailed clinical studies whereas others describe individual patients who have developed cardiac failure as a result of this interaction.[1,17-21] An early study in healthy subjects suggested that **torasemide** was not affected by **indometacin**,[22] but on the basis of later work the same workers now say that pathological factors in patients may allow the same interaction to occur.[23]

(i) Furosemide (Frusemide) + Ketoprofen

A study in 12 healthy subjects given 40 mg **furosemide** daily found that 100 mg **ketoprofen** twice daily reduced the 6 h urine output by 67 ml, and the 24 h output by 651 ml on the first day of treatment. However no significant differences were seen after 5 days treatment.[24]

(j) Furosemide (Frusemide) + Ketorolac

Twelve healthy subjects were given 30 mg oral **ketorolac** four times daily, and then a single 30-mg intramuscular dose 30 min before 40 mg **furosemide** intravenously. No precise figures are given in the abstract but the maximum serum level of the **furosemide**, its diuretic effect and the electrolyte loss were said to be significantly reduced by the **ketorolac**.[25] The makers say that the diuretic response of **furosemide** is reduced about 20%.[26] Another study in healthy elderly people found when given 40 mg **furosemide** after taking 120 mg oral **ketorolac** the day before and 30 mg intramuscularly half-an-hour before, the urine output fell by 16% and the sodium output by 26% over the next 8 h.[27]

(k) Furosemide (Frusemide) + Lornoxicam

A study in 12 normal subjects found that 4 mg **lornoxicam** significantly antagonised the diuretic and natriuretic effects of **furosemide**.[28]

(l) Furosemide (Frusemide) + Meloxicam

Meloxicam 15 mg daily for 3 days had no significant effect on the pharmacokinetics of 40 mg **furosemide** in 12 healthy subjects. The **furosemide**-induced diuresis was unchanged while the cumulative urinary electrolyte excretion was somewhat lower, but this was considered to be clinically irrelevant.[29]

(m) Furosemide (Frusemide) + Metamizole sodium (Dipyrone)

A study in 9 healthy subjects found that while taking 3 g **metamizole sodium** daily for 3 days, the clearance of 20 mg **furosemide** intravenously was reduced (from 175 to 141 ml/min) but the diuretic effects of the **furosemide** were unchanged.[30]

(n) Furosemide (Frusemide) + Mofebutazone

A study in 10 healthy subjects showed that 600 mg **mofebutazone** had no effect on the diuretic effects of 40 mg **furosemide**. The urinary volume and excretion of sodium, potassium and chloride were unchanged.[31]

(o) Furosemide (Frusemide) + Naproxen

Two elderly women with congestive heart failure failed to respond to treatment with **furosemide** and digoxin until the **naproxen** they were taking was withdrawn.[9]

A single-dose study in patients with cardiac failure showed that the volume of urine excreted in response to **furosemide** was reduced about 50% by **naproxen**.[13]

(p) Furosemide (Frusemide) + Oxindanac

A study in 8 healthy subjects found that 300 mg **oxindanac** twice daily did not affect the natriuresis of 40 mg **furosemide** twice daily.[32]

(q) Furosemide (Frusemide) + Paracetamol (Acetaminophen)

Paracetamol 1 g four times daily for 2 days was found to have no effect on the diuresis or natriuresis of 20 mg intravenous **furosemide** in 10 healthy women.[33]

(r) Furosemide (Frusemide) + Piroxicam

A 96-year-old woman with congestive heart failure failed to respond adequately to **furosemide** until the dosage of **piroxicam** she was taking was reduced from 20 to 10 mg daily.[34]

(s) Furosemide (Frusemide) + Pirprofen

A study in 8 patients showed that 800 mg **pirprofen** did not significantly affect the diuresis induced by **furosemide** or the urinary excretion of sodium.[35]

(t) Furosemide (Frusemide) or Bumetanide + Sulindac or Tolfenamic acid

A study in 8 healthy subjects showed that **tolfenamic acid** (300 mg) reduced the diuretic response (volume, sodium, potassium and chloride) to a single 1-mg dose of **bumetanide** by 34% at 2 h, whereas the effects of 300 mg **sulindac** were smaller and not statistically significant.[36]

Another study showed that in patients with cirrhosis and ascites that 150 mg **sulindac** reduced the diuretic effects (volume, sodium, potassium) of 80 mg **furosemide** given intravenously by 76%, 85% and 43% respectively.[37]

(u) Furosemide (Frusemide) + Tenoxicam

A study in 12 patients showed that 20 to 40 mg **tenoxicam** daily had no significant effect on the urinary excretion of sodium or chloride due to 40 mg **furosemide**, and blood pressure, heart rate and body weight also were not affected.[38]

Mechanism

Uncertain and complex. It seems almost certain that a number of different mechanisms come into play. One probable mechanism is concerned with the synthesis of renal prostaglandins which occurs when the loop diuretics cause sodium excretion. If this synthesis is blocked by drugs such as the NSAIDs, then renal blood flow and diuresis will be altered.[39] Indometacin is a non-specific inhibitor of cyclo-oxygenase, whereas sulindac selectively inhibits cyclo-oxygenase outside the kidney and meloxicam is selective for cyclo-oxygenase-2 which may explain why their interactions are small or non-existent.

Importance and management

The furosemide (frusemide)/indometacin interaction is very well documented and of clinical importance, whereas far less is known about the interactions with other NSAIDs. Concurrent use often need not be avoided but the effects should be checked and the furosemide dosage raised as necessary. Patients at greatest risk are likely to be the elderly with cirrhosis, cardiac failure and/or renal insufficiency. Some of the data comes from studies in healthy subjects rather than patients so that the total picture is still far from clear. Diclofenac, diflunisal, flurbiprofen, ketoprofen, ketorolac, naproxen, piroxicam and tolfenamic acid are known to interact in some individuals, but not necessarily to the same extent as indometacin. If raising the diuretic dosage is ineffective, another NSAID such as azapropazone, flupirtine, ibuprofen, metamizole sodium (dipyrone), oxindanac, meloxicam, paracetamol (acetaminophen), pirprofen, sulindac or tenoxicam may not interact significantly (this is not necessarily true for patients with cirrhosis and ascites[37]). Not every NSAID seems to have been investigated but be alert for this interaction with any of them. Phenylbutazone and oxyphenbutazone would be expected to interact because they cause sodium retention and oedema.

Much less is known about bumetanide, and even less about torasemide, but the evidence suggests that they interact like furosemide with indometacin. It would therefore seem prudent to be alert for interactions with any of the NSAIDs with which furosemide interacts. More study is needed.

1. Kaufman J, Hamburger R, Matheson J, Flamenbaum W. Bumetanide-induced diuresis and natriuresis: effect of prostaglandin synthetase inhibition. *J Clin Pharmacol* (1981) 21, 663–7.

2. Williamson PJ, Ene MD, Roberts CJC. A study of the potential interactions between az-apropazone and frusemide in man. *Br J Clin Pharmacol* (1984) 18, 619–23.
3. Jean G, Meregalli G, Vasilocò M, Silvani A, Scapaticci R, Della Ventura GF, Baiocchi C, Thiella G. Interazioni tra terapia diuretica e farmaci antiinfiammatori non steroidei. *Clin Ter* (1983) 105, 471–5.
4. Favre L, Glasson PH, Riondel A, Vallotton MB. Interaction of diuretics and non-steroi-dal anti-inflammatory drugs in man. *Clin Sci* (1983) 64, 407–15.
5. Tobert JA, Ostaszewski T, Reger B, Mesinger MAP, Cook TJ. Diflunisal-furosemide in-teraction. *Clin Pharmacol Ther* (1980) 27, 289–90.
6. Rawles JM. Antagonism between non-steroidal anti-inflammatory drugs and diuretics. *Scott Med J* (1982) 27, 37–40.
7. Symmons D, Kendall MJ. Non-steroidal anti-inflammatory drugs and frusemide-induced diuresis. *BMJ* (1981) 283, 988–9.
8. Johnston A, Warrington SJ, Turner P, Riethmuller-Winzen H. Comparison of flupritine and indomethacin on frusemide-induced diuresis. *Postgrad Med J* (1987) 63, 959–61.
9. Laiwah ACY, Mactier RA. Antagonistic effect of non-steroidal anti-inflammatory drugs on frusemide-induced diuresis in cardiac failure. *BMJ* (1981) 283, 714.
10. Goodenough GK, Lutz LJ. Hyponatremic hypervolemia caused by a drug-drug interac-tion mistaken for syndrome of inappropriate ADH. *J Am Geriatr Soc* (1988) 36, 285–6.
11. Patak RV, Mookerjee BK, Bentzel CJ, Hysert PE, Babej M, Lee JB. Antagonism of the effects of furosemide by indomethacin in normal and hypertensive man. *Prostaglandins* (1975) 10, 649–59.
12. Sörgel F, Koob R, Gluth WP, Krüger B, Lang E. The interaction of indomethacin and furosemide in patients with congestive heart failure. *Clin Pharmacol Ther* (1985) 37, 231.
13. Faunch R. Non-steroidal anti-inflammatory drugs and frusemide-induced diuresis. *BMJ* (1981) 283, 989.
14. Aggernæs KH. Indometacinhæmning af bumetaniddiurese. *Ugeskr Laeger* (1980) 142, 691–3.
15. Brater C, Chennavasin P. Indomethacin and the response to bumetanide. *Clin Pharmacol Ther* (1980) 27, 421–5.
16. Brater DC, Fox WR, Chennavasin P. Interaction studies with bumetanide and furosem-ide. Effects of probenecid and of indomethacin on response to bumetanide in man. *J Clin Pharmacol* (1981) 21, 647–53.
17. Allan SG, Knox J, Kerr F. Interaction between diuretics and indomethacin. *BMJ* (1981) 283, 1611.
18. Ahmad S. Indomethacin-bumetanide interaction: an alert. *Am J Cardiol* (1984) 54, 246–7.
19. Poe TE, Scott RB, Keith JF. Interaction of indomethacin with furosemide. *J Fam Pract* (1983) 16, 610–16.
20. Ritland S. Alvorlig interaksjon mellom indometacin og furosemid. *Tidsskr Nor Laege-foren* (1983) 103, 2003.
21. Nordrehaug JE. Alvorlig interaksjon mellom indometacin og furosemid. *Tidsskr Nor Laegeforen* (1983) 103, 1680–1.
22. Van Ganse E, Douchamps J, Deger F, Staroukine M, Vernioy A, Herchuelz A. Failure of indomethacin to impair the diuretic and natriuretic effects of the loop diuretic torasem-ide in healthy volunteers. *Eur J Clin Pharmacol* (1986) 31 (Suppl), 43–7.
23. Herschuelz A, Derenne F, Deger F, Juvent M, van Ganse E. Staroutkine M, Vernioy A, Boeynaems JM, Douchamps J. Interaction between nonsteroidal anti-inflammatory drugs and loop diuretics: modulation by sodium balance. *J Pharmacol Exp Ther* (1989) 248, 1175–81.
24. Li Kam Wa TC, Lawson M, Jackson SHD, Hitoglou-Makedou A, Turner P. Interaction of ketoprofen and frusemide in man. *Postgrad Med J* (1991) 67, 655–8.
25. Shah J, Bullingham R, Jonkman J, Curd J, Taylor R, Fratis A. PK-PD interaction of ketorolac and furosemide in healthy volunteers in a normovolemic state. Clin Pharmacol Ther (1994) 55, 198.
26. Toradol (Ketorolac trometamol), Roche Products Limited. Summary of product charac-teristics, October 2000.
27. Jones RW, Notarianni LJ, Parker G. The effect of ketorolac tromethamine on the diuretic response of frusemide in healthy elderly people. *Therapie* (1995) 50 (Suppl), Abstract 98.
28. Ravic M, Johnston A, Turner P. clinical pharmacological studies of some possible inter-actions of lornoxicam with other drugs. *Postgrad Med J* (1990) 66 (Suppl 4), S30–S34.
29. Müller FO, Schall R, de Vaal AC. Groenewoud G, Hundt HKL, Middle MV. Influence of meloxicam on furosemide pharmacokinetics and pharmacodynamics in healthy vol-unteers. *Eur J Clin Pharmacol* (1995) 48, 247–51.
30. Rosenkranz B, Lehr K-H, Mackert G, Seyberth HW. Metamizole-furosemide interaction study in healthy volunteers. *Eur J Clin Pharmacol* (1992) 42, 593–8.
31. Matthei U, Grabensee B, Loew D. The interaction of mofebutazone with furosemide. *Curr Med Res Opin* (1987) 10, 638–44.
32. Tamm C, Favre L, Spence S, Pfister S, Vallotton MB. Interaction of oxindanac and fruse-mide in man. *Eur J Clin Pharmacol* (1989) 37, 17–21.
33. Martin U, Prescott LF. The interaction of paracetamol with frusemide. *Br J Clin Phar-macol* (1994) 37, 464–7.
34. Baker DE. Piroxicam-furosemide drug interaction. *Drug Intell Clin Pharm* (1988) 22, 505–6.
35. Sorgel F, Hemmerlein M and Lang E. Wirkung von Pirprofen und Indometacin auf die Effekte von Oxprenolol und Furosemid. *Arzneimittelforschung* (1984) 34, 1330–2.
36. Pentikäinen PJ, Tokola O and Vapaatalo H. Non-steroidal anti-inflammatory drugs and bumetanide response in man. Comparison of tolfenamic acid and sulindac. *Clin Pharma-col Ther* (1986) 39, 219.
37. Kronborg I, Daskalopoulos D, Katkov W, Zipser RD. The influence of sulindac and in-domethacin on renal function and furosemide-induced diuresis in patients with cirrhosis and ascites. *Clin Res* (1984) 32, 14A.
38. Hartmann D, Kleinbloesem CH, Lücker PW, Vetter G. Study on the possible interaction between tenoxicam and furosemide. *Arzneimittelforschung* (1987) 37, 1072–6.
39. Passmore AP, Copeland CS, Johnston GD. The effects of ibuprofen and indomethacin on renal function in the presence and absence of frusemide in healthy volunteers on a re-stricted sodium diet. *Br J Clin Pharmacol* (1990) 29, 311–19.

Methyldopa + Barbiturates

The effects of methyldopa are not altered by the use of pheno-barbital.

Clinical evidence, mechanism, importance and management

Indirect evidence from one study in hypertensive subjects suggested that **phenobarbital** could reduce methyldopa levels,[1] but later work which directly measured the blood levels of methyldopa failed to find any evidence of an interaction.[2]

1. Káldor A, Juvancz P, Demeczky M, Sebestyen, Palotas J. Enhancement of methyldopa metabolism with barbiturate. *BMJ* (1971) 3, 518–19.
2. Kristensen M, Jørgensen M, Hansen T. Plasma concentration of alfamethyldopa and its main metabolite, methyldopa-O-sulphate, during long term treatment with alfamethyl-dopa with special reference to possible interaction with other drugs given simultaneously. *Clin Pharmacol Ther* (1973) 14, 139–40.

Methyldopa + Cephalosporins

Two reports describe the development of pustular eruptions in two women taking methyldopa when they were given ce-fradine or cefazolin. Use of methyldopa may have been coin-cidental.

Clinical evidence, mechanism, importance and management

A 74-year-old black woman on methyldopa and insulin developed pruritus on her arms and legs within 2 h of starting to take **cefradine** 250 mg six-hourly. Cefradine was stopped after 7 doses. Over the next 2 days fever and a widespread pustular eruption developed.[1] An-other black woman of 65 on methyldopa and furosemide (frusemide) experienced severe pruritus within 8 h of starting to receive 1 g **ce-fazolin sodium** intravenously every 12 h. Over the next two days su-perficial and coalescing pustules appeared on her trunk, arms and legs.[2] The authors of the first report attributed the reaction to cefra-dine. The authors of the second report note that the concurrent use of methyldopa may or may not have been a contributing factor in both reports.[2] There seem to be no other reports of this reaction.

1. Kalb RE, Grossman ME. Pustular eruption following administration of cephradine. *Cutis* (1986) 38, 58–60.
2. Stough D, Guin JD, Baker GF, Haynie L. Pustular eruptions following administration of cefazolin: a possible interaction with methyldopa. *J Am Acad Dermatol* (1987) 16, 1051–2.

Methyldopa + Disulfiram

An isolated report describes a patient whose hypertension failed to respond to methyldopa in the presence of disulfiram.

Clinical evidence, mechanism, importance and management

The hypertension of an alcoholic patient on **disulfiram** failed to re-spond to moderate to high doses of intravenous methyldopa, but did so when given oral low-dose clonidine. The postulated reason is that **disulfiram** blocks the activity of dopamine beta-hydroxylase, the en-zyme responsible for the conversion of the methyldopa to its active form.[1] The general importance of this alleged interaction is uncertain.

1. McCord RW, LaCorte WS. Hypertension refractory to methyldopa in a disulfiram-treated patient. *Clin Res* (1984) 32, 923A.

Methyldopa + Haloperidol

Three cases of dementia have been attributed to the use of methyldopa and haloperidol, but concurrent use without serious problems has also been described.

Clinical evidence

Two patients on long term treatment with methyldopa (1 to 1.5 g daily) without problems developed a dementia syndrome (mental retardation, loss of memory, disorientation, etc.) within 3 days of starting to take 6 to 8 mg **haloperidol** daily. The symptoms cleared within 72 h of stopping the **haloperidol**.[1] Another patient treated with these drugs showed severe irritability and aggressive behaviour.[2]

Mechanism

Not understood. Among the side-effects of methyldopa relevant to this interaction are sedation, depression and dementia; and of haloperidol, drowsiness, dizziness and depression.

Importance and management

These 3 cases must be viewed alongside another report of a 4-week trial in 10 schizophrenics given 500 mg methyldopa and 10 mg haloperidol daily. Among the important side-effects were somnolence (8 patients) and dizziness (6 patients), but no serious interaction of the kind described above.[3] Concurrent use need not be avoided but it would be prudent to be on the alert for the development of adverse effects.

1. Thornton WE. Dementia induced by methyldopa with haloperidol. *N Engl J Med* (1976) 294, 1222.
2. Nadel I, Wallach M. Drug interaction between haloperidol and methyldopa. *Br J Psychiatry* (1979) 135, 484.
3. Chouinard G, Pinard G, Serrano M, Tetreault L. Potentiation of haloperidol by α-methyldopa in the treatment of schizophrenic patients. *Curr Ther Res* (1973) 15, 473–83.

Methyldopa + Iron salts

The antihypertensive effects of methyldopa can be reduced by the concurrent use of ferrous sulphate. Ferrous gluconate appears to interact similarly.

Clinical evidence

Arising out of a metabolic study of the interaction between methyldopa and **ferrous sulphate**, 5 hypertensive patients who had been taking 250 to 1500 mg methyldopa daily for more than a year were additionally given 325 mg **ferrous sulphate** three times daily. After 2 weeks the blood pressures of all of them had risen. The systolic pressures of 3 of them had risen by more than 15 mmHg. Four had diastolic pressure rises, two of them exceeding 10 mmHg.[1] Reductions of 88% and 79% in the renal excretion of unmetabolised methyldopa were seen when methyldopa was given with **ferrous sulphate** and **ferrous gluconate** respectively.[1] A further study found that if the **ferrous sulphate** was given at the same time, or 1 h or 2 h before the methyldopa, the bioavailability of the methyldopa was reduced 83%, 55% and 42% respectively.[2]

Mechanism

Uncertain. One suggestion is that the iron chelates or complexes with the methyldopa in the gut, thereby reducing its absorption (reduced 50%).[1,3] The increase in the metabolic sulphonation of the methyldopa also seems to have a part to play.

Importance and management

Information is limited and this interaction is as yet unconfirmed but it appears to be clinically important. Monitor the effects of concurrent use and increase the methyldopa dosage as necessary. Separating the dosages by up to 2 h apparently only partially reduces the effects of this interaction. Ferrous gluconate appears to interact like ferrous sulphate.

1. Campbell N, Paddock V, Sundaram R. Alteration of methyldopa absorption, metabolism, and blood pressure control caused by ferrous sulfate and ferrous gluconate. *Clin Pharmacol Ther* (1988) 43, 381–6.
2. Campbell NRC, Hasinoff BB. Iron supplements: a common cause of drug interactions. *Br J Clin Pharmacol* (1991) 31, 251–55.
3. Campbell NRC, Campbell RRA, Hasinoff BB. Ferrous sulfate reduces methyldopa absorption: methyldopa: iron complex formation as a likely mechanism. *Clin Invest Med* (1990) 13, 329–32.

Methyldopa + Oxazepam

A single case report suggests that blood pressure control in essential hypertension with methyldopa may possibly be made more difficult in the presence of oxazepam.

Clinical evidence, mechanism, importance and management

A 54-year-old woman with insomnia and essential hypertension had unexplained variability in blood pressure on 750 mg methyldopa three times daily and a thiazide diuretic. Within a week of stopping 60 mg **oxazepam** nightly, she developed grand mal convulsions and hypertension (190/90 mmHg standing, 240/140 mmHg lying). Her hypertension was then successfully controlled by switching to atenolol and prazosin. The authors of this report suggest that short-acting benzodiazepines such as **oxazepam** can cause transient hypotension after a dose, but that hypertension may occur on withdrawal. These effects may complicate the management of hypertension.[1] The general importance of this possible interaction is not established.

1. Stokes GS. Can short-acting benzodiazepines exacerbate essential hypertension? *Cardiovasc Rev Rep* (1989) 10, 60–1.

Methyldopa + Phenoxybenzamine

An isolated case report describes total urinary incontinence in a patient treated with methyldopa and phenoxybenzamine after bilateral lumbar sympathectomy.

Clinical evidence, mechanism, importance and management

A woman who had previously had bilateral lumbar sympathectomy for Raynaud's disease developed total urinary incontinence when given 500 to 1500 mg methyldopa and 12.5 mg **phenoxybenzamine** daily, but not with either drug alone. This would seem to be the outcome of the additive effects of the sympathectomy and the two drugs on the sympathetic control of the bladder sphincters.[1] Stress incontinence has previously been described with these drugs. The general importance of this interaction is probably small.

1. Fernandez PG, Sahni S, Galway BA, Granter S, McDonald J. Urinary incontinence due to interaction of phenoxybenzamine and α-methyldopa. *Can Med Assoc J* (1981) 124, 174.

Methyldopa + Sympathomimetics (indirectly-acting)

Indirectly-acting sympathomimetics might be expected to cause a blood pressure rise in patients taking methyldopa, and an isolated case report describes such a reaction in a patient taking methyldopa and oxprenolol when he took a decongestant containing phenylpropanolamine, but in practice

this interaction normally seems to be of little or no general practical importance. The mydriatic effects of ephedrine are reported to be depressed by methyldopa.

Clinical evidence, mechanism, importance and management

In a study in 5 hypertensive subjects taking 2 to 3 g methyldopa daily, the pressor (rise in blood pressure) effects of **tyramine** were doubled.[1] In another study the pressor effect of tyramine was 50/16 mmHg compared with 18/10 mmHg before methyldopa treatment.[2]

A man with renal hypertension, whose blood pressure was well controlled with 250 mg methyldopa twice daily and 160 mg oxprenolol three times daily, showed a rise in blood pressure from about 120–140/70–80 mmHg to 200/150 mmHg within 2 days of starting to take two tablets of **Triogesic** (**phenylpropanolamine** 12.5 mg and **paracetamol** 500 mg) three times a day. His blood pressure fell when the **Triogesic** was withdrawn.[3] The reason for this is uncertain. One suggestion is that the methyldopa causes the replacement of norepinephrine (noradrenaline) at adrenergic nerve endings by methylnoradrenaline which has weaker pressor (alpha) activity but greater vasodilator (beta) activity. With the vasodilator activity blocked by the oxprenolol, the vasoconstrictor activity (pressor) of the **phenylpropanolamine** would be unopposed and exaggerated. Alternatively it could have been that he was unusually sensitive to the pressor effects of **phenylpropanolamine**.

Despite the information derived from the studies outlined above[1,2] and the single report cited, there seems to be nothing else in the literature to suggest that indirectly-acting sympathomimetics normally cause an adverse reaction (rise in blood pressure) with methyldopa. In fact the antihypertensive effects of methyldopa were found not to be affected by **amfepramone (diethylpropion)** in a group of patients treated with both drugs.[4]

One report states that the normal mydriatic effects of **ephedrine** are depressed by methyldopa.[5]

1. Pettinger W, Horwitz D, Spector S, Sjoerdsma A. Enhancement by methyldopa of tyramine sensitivity in man. *Nature* (1963) 200, 1107–8.
2. Dollery CT, Harington M, Hodge JV. Haemodynamic studies with methyldopa: effect on cardiac output and response to pressor amines. *Br Heart J* (1963) 25, 670–6.
3. McLaren EH. Severe hypertension produced by interaction of phenylpropanolamine with methyldopa and oxprenolol. *BMJ* (1976) 3, 283–4.
4. Seedat YK, Reddy J. Diethylpropion hydrochloride (Tenuate, Dospan) in the treatment of obese hypertensive patients. *S Afr Med J* (1974) 48, 569.
5. Sneddon JM, Turner P. Ephedrine mydriasis in hypertension and the response to treatment. *Clin Pharmacol Ther* (1969) 10, 64–71.

Methyldopa + Tricyclic and related antidepressants

The antihypertensive effects of methyldopa are not normally adversely affected by the concurrent use of desipramine but an isolated report describes hypertension, tachycardia, tremor and agitation in man on methyldopa when additionally treated with amitriptyline. The tetracyclic mianserin appears not to interact.

Clinical evidence

A hypertensive man, controlled on 700 mg methyldopa daily with a diuretic, experienced tremor, agitation, tachycardia (148 bpm) and hypertension (a rise from 120–150/80–90 mmHg to 170/110 mmHg) within 10 days of starting to take 75 mg **amitriptyline** daily. A week after stopping the **amitriptyline** his pulse rate was 100 and his blood pressure 160/90 mmHg.[1] In contrast, a double-blind crossover study in 5 subjects (one with mild hypertension) found that 25 mg **desipramine** three times daily for 3 days had no significant effect on the hypotensive effects of single 750-mg doses of methyldopa.[2] Another study in 3 hypertensive patients on methyldopa (2.5 to 3 g daily) found that when given 75 mg **desipramine** daily for 5 to 6 days, the blood pressure (diastolic + one-third pulse pressure) fell by

5 mmHg.[3] **Mianserin** (a tetracyclic) 20 mg three times daily for 2 weeks had no effect on the control of blood pressure in 6 patients receiving methyldopa, although 2 patients developed symptomatic hypotension after the first dose of **mianserin**.[4,5]

Mechanism

Not understood. Antagonism of the antihypertensive actions of methyldopa by tricyclic antidepressants is seen in *animals* and it seems to occur within the brain.[6,7]

Importance and management

Normally no adverse interaction occurs, nevertheless it would seem prudent to monitor the effects of concurrent use if amitriptyline or any other tricyclic antidepressant is given to patients on methyldopa. Methyldopa sometimes induces depression so it is generally considered contra-indicated in depressed patients anyway.

1. White AG. Methyldopa and amitriptyline. *Lancet* (1965) ii, 441.
2. Reid JL, Porsius AJ, Zamboulis C, Polak G, Hamilton CA, Dean CR. The effects of desmethylimipramine on the pharmacological actions of alpha methyldopa in man. *Eur J Clin Pharmacol* (1979) 16, 75–80.
3. Mitchell JR, Cavanaugh JH, Arias L, Oates JA. Guanethidine and related agents. III. Antagonism by drugs which inhibit the norepinephrine pump in man. *J Clin Invest* (1970) 49, 1596.
4. Elliott HL, Whiting B, Reid JL. Assessment of the interaction between mianserin and centrally-acting antihypertensive drugs. *Br J Clin Pharmacol* (1983) 15, 323S–328S.
5. Elliott HL, McLean K, Sumner DJ, Reid JL. Absence of an effect of mianserin on the actions of clonidine or methyldopa in hypertensive patients. *Eur J Clin Pharmacol* (1983) 24, 15–19.
6. van Spanning HW, van Zwieten PA. The interaction between alpha-methyl-dopa and tricyclic antidepressants. *Int J Clin Pharmacol Biopharm* (1975) 11, 65–7.
7. van Zwieten PA. Interaction between centrally acting hypotensive drugs and tricyclic antidepressants. *Arch Int Pharmacodyn Ther* (1975) 214, 12–30.

Metolazone + NSAIDs

The excretion of urinary sodium and potassium by metolazone is reduced by indometacin (indomethacin) and to a lesser extent by sulindac.

Clinical evidence, mechanism, importance and management

Indometacin (**indomethacin**) was found to reduce the urinary sodium excretion due to metolazone by 34% in 6 healthy subjects, whereas **sulindac** reduced it by 19%. The excretion of total potassium fell by 30% when given with **indometacin** and by 16% with **sulindac**.[1] A possible reason is that these NSAIDs block prostaglandin synthesis in the kidneys. The clinical importance of these changes is uncertain but the authors of the report suggest[1] caution in those ". . . whose renal function may be prostaglandin sensitive and/or those whose volume status is tentative, such as patients with chronic renal failure, volume depletion or congestive heart failure."

1. Ripley EBD, Gehr TWB, Wallace H, Wade J, Kish C, Sica DA. The effect of nonsteroidal agents (NSAIDs) on the pharmacokinetics and pharmacodynamics of metolazone. *Int J Clin Pharmacol Ther* (1994) 32, 12–18.

Minoxidil + Glibenclamide (Glyburide)

Doses of glibenclamide (glyburide) 5 mg, but not 2.5 mg, can reduce the hypotensive effects of minoxidil to some extent, but the clinical importance of this is not yet known.

Clinical evidence, mechanism, importance and management

A single-dose study in 9 healthy subjects found that 2.5 mg **glibenclamide** (**glyburide**) did not alter the hypotensive effect of 5 mg minoxidil, but, in a further 4 subjects a larger dose of **glibenclamide**, 5 mg caused some loss in its hypotensive effects. The suggested reason is that these two drugs have opposing effects on the potassium channels of the smooth muscle of blood vessels.[1] What is not yet clear is whether this interaction is clinically relevant or not. More study is needed.

1. Stein CM, Brown N, Carlson MG, Campbell P, Wood AJJ. Coadministration of glyburide and minoxidil, drugs with opposing effects on potassium channels. *Clin Pharmacol Ther* (1997) 61, 662–8.

Moexipril + Miscellaneous drugs

Moexipril is reported not to interact adversely with cholesterol-lowering agents, digoxin, hormone replacement therapy or oral hypoglycaemic agents. The makers warn about the potential risks of toxicity with lithium. See the Index for other interactions with Moexipril.

Clinical evidence, mechanism, importance and management

The makers say that no important pharmacokinetic interaction was seen when moexipril was given with **digoxin**, in healthy subjects.[1] They also have clinical trials showing there was no evidence of clinically important adverse interactions when moexipril was used with **cholesterol-lowering agents**, **digoxin** or **oral hypoglycaemic agents**. None of these drugs was specifically named.[2]

A study in 95 hypertensive postmenopausal women treated with **hormone replacement therapy** found that **moexipril** did not affect metabolic parameters associated with cardiovascular disease and coadministration was considered safe and effective.[3]

No interaction with **lithium** has been reported, but on the basis of adverse reports involving other ACE inhibitors (see 'Lithium carbonate + ACE inhibitors', p.652) the makers warn about the risk of increased serum lithium levels and possible toxicity if given with **lithium**.[1]

1. Perdix (Moexipril), Schwarz Pharma Ltd. Summary of product characteristics, March 2000.
2. Perdix (Moexipril). Schwarz Pharma. Product Monograph. Data on file, October 1995.
3. Koch B, Oparil S, Stimpel M. Co-administration of an ACE-inhibitor (moexipril) and hormonal replacement therapy in postmenopausal women. *J Hum Hypertens* (1999) 13, 337–42.

Moxonidine + Miscellaneous drugs

On theoretical grounds the makers of moxonidine advise withdrawal of beta-blockers before withdrawal of moxonidine. They advise the avoidance of alcohol and tricyclic antidepressants. They also suggest care with benzodiazepines, hypnotics and sedatives because of possible increased sedation. No relevant pharmacokinetic interactions occur with digoxin, glibenclamide (glyburide), moclobemide or hydrochlorothiazide.

Clinical evidence, mechanism, importance and management

The presence of a beta-blocker can exacerbate the rebound hypertension which follows the withdrawal of clonidine (see 'Clonidine + Beta-blockers', p.386). Although no such rebound hypertension has actually been seen when moxonidine is withdrawn, for safety's sake the makers currently advise that any **beta-blocker** should be stopped first, followed by the moxonidine a few days later.[1,2] The cognitive function of 24 healthy subjects was not impaired by 0.4 mg moxonidine daily, but the presence of moxonidine was found to increase the impairment caused by 1 mg **lorazepam** daily.[3,4] For this reason the makers warn that the sedative effects of the **benzodiazepines** may possibly be enhanced by moxonidine.[2] Drowsiness and dizziness have been reported with moxonidine which, the makers suggest, may be additive with the effects of **sedatives** and **hypnotics**.[1] They also advise the avoidance of **alcohol** and **tricyclic antidepressants**, although clinical experience is said to be lacking and there are no obvious theoretical reasons for avoiding the latter.[1] A study in healthy subjects given moxonidine 0.4 mg daily and single doses of **moclobemide** 300 mg found no pharmacokinetic interaction. Moxonidine alone or with moclobemide did not significantly affect cognitive function.[4]

No clinically relevant pharmacokinetic interactions were seen in steady-state studies with 0.2 mg moxonidine twice daily and 0.2 mg **digoxin** daily or 25 mg **hydrochlorothiazide** twice daily or 2.5 mg **glibenclamide (glyburide)** daily.[5-7]

1. Solvay Healthcare. Personal communication, September 1996.
2. Moxonidine (Physiotens). Solvay Healthcare, Summary of Product Characteristics, March 2002.
3. Grahnen A, Weimann HJ, Wesnes K, Jansson B, Küppers H. Acute cognitive effects following addition of single doses of lorazepam to moxonidine/placebo maintenance treatment. *J Hypertens* (1996) 14 (Suppl 1), S228.
4. Wesnes K, Simpson PM, Jansson B, Grahnén A, Wemann H-J, Küppers H. Moxonidine and cognitive function: interactions with moclobemide and lorazepam. *Eur J Clin Pharmacol* (1997) 52, 351–8.
5. Weimann H-J, Rudolph M. Clinical pharmacokinetics of moxonidine. *J Cardiovasc Pharmacol* (1992) 20 (Suppl 4), S37–S41.
6. Pabst G, Weimann H-J, Weber W. Lack of pharmacokinetic interactions between moxonidine and digoxin. *Clin Pharmacokinet* (1992) 23, 477–81.
7. Muller M, Weimann H-J, Eden G, Weber W, Michaelis K, Dilger C, Achtert G. Steady state investigation of possible pharmacokinetic interactions of moxonidine and glibenclamide. *Eur J Drug Metab Pharmacokinet* (1993) 18, 277–83.

Sodium nitroprusside + Diltiazem

Diltiazem possibly reduces the amount of sodium nitroprusside needed during surgery to control hypotension.

Clinical evidence, mechanism, importance and management

Twenty patients were given a sodium nitroprusside infusion to reduce mean arterial blood pressure to 55 to 60 mmHg during surgery lasting on average 200 min. Half were also given **diltiazem** by infusion to achieve plasma levels of 70 to 90 nanograms/ml. The **diltiazem** allowed a 55% reduction in the amount of sodium nitroprusside used. Tachyphylaxis, tachycardia and an increase in thiocyanate levels were only seen in the group without **diltiazem**.[1] There would therefore appear to be advantages in using these drugs in combination. The inference to drawn is that patients already taking **diltiazem** orally will possibly need lower doses of sodium nitroprusside.

1. Bernard J-M, Moren J, Demeure D, Hommeril J-L, Pinaud M. Diltiazem reduces the nitroprusside doses for deliberate hypotension. *Anesthesiology* (1992) 77, A427.

Omapatrilat + Atenolol or Furosemide

Omapatrilat appears not to interact to a clinically relevant extent with atenolol or furosemide (frusemide).

Clinical evidence, mechanism, importance and management

A study in healthy subjects found that omapatrilat 10 or 25 mg daily for 5 days did not alter the diuretic properties of concurrent **furosemide (frusemide)** 20 mg daily. **Furosemide** did not alter the effect of omapatrilat on urinary excretion of atrial natriuretic peptide (which is involved in reducing blood pressure).[1] No special precautions would seem necessary.

A single-dose study in 24 healthy subjects found that although the AUC and peak plasma levels of **atenolol** 50 mg were reduced by 30% by omapatrilat 40 mg the effects of **atenolol** on minimum and average resting heart rate were unaltered. **Atenolol** had no significant effects on the pharmacokinetics of omapatrilat.[2] Information seems limited to this single dose study but clinical significance of the effects is probably small.

1. Uderman HD, Delaney CL, Catanzariti PA, Vesterqvist O, Ferreira IM, Liao W. Coadministration of omapatrilat does not alter furosemide induced diuresis. *Am J Hypertens* (2000) 13, 135A–136A.
2. Hammett J, Hutman HW, Malhotra B, Ferreira I, Slugg P. The pharmacodynamics and pharmacokinetics of coadministration of omapatrilat and atenolol. *Clin Pharmacol Ther* (2000) 67, 124.

Piretanide + Miscellaneous drugs

The urinary excretion of sodium due to piretanide is reduced by probenecid and indometacin (indomethacin), but not by piroxicam.

Clinical evidence, mechanism, importance and management

A comparative study into the pharmacological mechanisms underlying the way drugs interfere with the actions of loop diuretics found that 1 g **probenecid**, 50 mg **indometacin (indomethacin)** and 20 mg **piroxicam** reduced the peak fractional excretion of sodium due to piretanide 6 mg orally by 65%, 35% and 0% respectively.[1] Another study confirmed that **probenecid** reduces the natriuretic effects of piretanide.[2] The clinical importance of these changes was not studied, but it would now seem prudent to check the effectiveness of piretanide in the presence of either **probenecid** or **indometacin**.

1. Dixey JJ, Noormohamed FH, Pawa JS, Lant AF, Brewerton DA. The influence of nonsteroidal anti-inflammatory drugs and probenecid on the renal response to and kinetics of piretanide in man. *Clin Pharmacol Ther* (1988) 44, 531–9.
2. Noormohamed FH, Lant AF. Analysis of the natriuretic action of a loop diuretic, piretanide, in man. *Br J Clin Pharmacol* (1991) 31, 463–9.

Prazosin + Miscellaneous drugs

The makers of prazosin say in their datasheet that it has been administered without any adverse interactions in clinical experience with the following drugs: antiarrhythmics (procainamide, quinidine), antigout agents (allopurinol, colchicine, probenecid), benzodiazepines (diazepam, chlordiazepoxide), dextropropoxyphene (propoxyphene), hypoglycaemic agents (insulin, chlorpropamide, phenformin, tolazamide, tolbutamide) and phenobarbital.[1]

1. Hypovase (Prazosin), Pfizer Ltd. Summary of Product Characteristics, August 1998.

Rauwolfia alkaloids + Tricyclic antidepressants

The rauwolfia alkaloids cause depression and are not usually used in patients needing treatment for depression, but there are a few reports of their successful use in some resistant forms of depression when combined with the tricyclic antidepressants.

Clinical evidence, mechanism, importance and management

Depression and sedation are among the very well-recognised side effects of rauwolfia treatment. For example, out of a total of 270 patients given treatment for hypertension with **rauwolfia**, 23% developed depressive episodes within 7 months of starting treatment.[1] *Animals* treated with **reserpine** have been widely used by pharmacologists as experimental models of depression when testing the effectiveness of new compounds with potential antidepressant activity. The rauwolfia alkaloids cause adrenergic (norepinephrine-releasing) and serotoninergic (5-HT-releasing) neurones to become depleted of their normal stores of neurotransmitter, the result being that very reduced amounts are available for release by nerve impulses. Because of this action at adrenergic sympathetic nerve endings the blood pressure falls. The brain possesses both types of neurone and failure in transmission is believed to be responsible for the sedation and depression which can occur. However one study describes 14 out of 15 patients with endogenous depression resistant to **imipramine** who responded well when 7.5 to 10 mg **reserpine** daily for 2 days

was added to **imipramine** (after an initial manic response): in 6 of these improvement was maintained throughout the 6-month follow-up.[2] Other reports describe the use of **reserpine** with **desipramine**[3,4] and **imipramine**[3,5] although the authors of the latter question the advantages claimed by other workers. However, in general, concurrent use should be avoided. Only in well-controlled situations and with patients unresponsive to other forms of treatment should this combination be used.

1. Bolte E, Marc-Aurele J, Brouillet J, Beauregard P, Verdy M, Genest J. Mental depressive episodes during rauwolfia therapy for arterial hypertension with special reference to dosage. *Can Med Assoc J* (1959) 80, 291.
2. Haškovec L, Ryšánek K. The action of reserpine in imipramine-resistant depressive patients. A clinical and biochemical study. *Psychopharmacologia* (1967) 11, 18–30.
3. Pöldinger W. Combined administration of desipramine and reserpine or tetrabenazine in depressed patients. *Psychopharmacologia* (1963) 4, 308–10.
4. Amsterdam JD, Berwish N. Treatment of refractory depression with combination reserpine and tricyclic antidepressant therapy. *J Clin Psychopharmacol* (1987) 7, 238–42.
5. Carney MWP, Thakurdas H, Sebastian J. Effects of imipramine and reserpine in depression. *Psychopharmacologia* (1969) 14, 349–50.

Spirapril + Glibenclamide

The makers of spirapril briefly note in a review that there was no pharmacokinetic interaction between spirapril and glibenclamide (glyburide).[1] See also 'Hypoglycaemic agents + ACE inhibitors', p.564.

1. Grass P, Gerbeau C, Kutz K. Spirapril: pharmacokinetic properties and drug interactions. *Blood Press Suppl* (1994) 2, 7–13.

Spironolactone + Aspirin

The antihypertensive effects of spironolactone are unaffected by the concurrent use of aspirin in patients with hypertension, although there is evidence that the spironolactone-induced loss of sodium in the urine is reduced in healthy subjects.

Clinical evidence

(a) Effects in hypertensive patients

Five patients with low-renin essential hypertension, well-controlled for 4 months or more with 100 to 300 mg spironolactone daily, were examined in a double-blind crossover trial. Daily doses of **aspirin** of 2.4 to 4.8 g given over 6-week periods had no effect on blood pressure, serum electrolytes, body weight, urea nitrogen or plasma renin activity.[1]

(b) Effects in healthy subjects

In 10 healthy subjects given single 25-, 50- and 100-mg doses of spironolactone, a single 600-mg dose of **aspirin** reduced the urinary excretion of electrolytes. In a further study, the effectiveness of the spironolactone was reduced 70%, and the overnight sodium excretion reduced by a third in 7 of these subjects given 25 mg spironolactone four times daily for one week then a single 600-mg dose of **aspirin**.[2]

Reductions in sodium excretion are described in other studies.[3,4] In one of these the sodium excretion was completely abolished when **aspirin** was given one-and-a-half hours after the spironolactone, but when administered in the reverse order the inhibition of sodium excretion by **aspirin** was not completely abolished by spironolactone.[4]

Mechanism

Uncertain. There is evidence that the active secretion of canrenone (the active metabolite of spironolactone) is blocked by aspirin, but the significance of this is not entirely clear.[3]

Importance and management

An adequately but not extensively documented interaction. Despite the results of the studies in healthy subjects, the study in hypertensive patients shows that the blood pressure lowering effects of spironolactone are not affected by aspirin. Concurrent use need not be avoided, but it would be prudent nonetheless to monitor the response to confirm that no adverse interaction is taking place.

1. Hollifield JW. Failure of aspirin to antagonize the antihypertensive effect of spironolactone in low-renin hypertension. *South Med J* (1976) 69, 1034–6.
2. Tweeddale MG, Ogilvie RI. Antagonism of spironolactone-induced natriuresis by aspirin in man. *N Engl J Med* (1973) 289, 198.
3. Ramsay LE, Harrison IR, Shelton JR, Vose CW. Influence of acetylsalicylic acid on the renal handling of a spironolactone metabolite in healthy subjects. *Eur J Clin Pharmacol* (1976) 10, 43–8.
4. Elliott HC. Reduced adrenocortical steroid excretion rates in man following aspirin administration. *Metabolism* (1962) 11, 1015–18.

Spironolactone + Dextropropoxyphene (Propoxyphene)

A single case report describes the development of gynaecomastia and a rash in a man on spironolactone when he was given dextropropoxyphene.

Clinical evidence, mechanism, importance and management

A patient who had been taking spironolactone uneventfully for 4 years developed swollen and tender breasts and a rash on his chest and neck a fortnight after starting to take *Darvon*, a compound preparation containing **dextropropoxyphene (propoxyphene)**, **aspirin**, **phenacetin** and **caffeine**. The problem disappeared when both drugs were withdrawn but the rash reappeared when the *Darvon* alone was given. It disappeared again when it was withdrawn. No problems occurred when the spironolactone was given alone, but both the rash and the gynaecomastia recurred when the *Darvon* was added.[1] The reasons for this reaction are not understood. Gynaecomastia is a known side-effect of spironolactone (incidence 1.2%). The authors of this report reasonably surmise that the **dextropropoxyphene** component of *Darvon* was largely responsible in some way. Concurrent use need not be avoided but prescribers should be aware of this case.

1. Licata AA, Bartter FC. Spironolactone-induced gynecomastia related to allergic reaction to 'darvon compound'. *Lancet* (1976) ii, 905.

Telmisartan + Miscellaneous drugs

No clinically relevant pharmacokinetic interactions occur between telmisartan and hydrochlorothiazide, glibenclamide, ibuprofen, paracetamol (acetaminophen), or amlodipine. There may be a risk of hyperkalaemia if telmisartan is co-administered with potassium-sparing diuretics, potassium supplements or other drugs that may increase plasma potassium levels. It is possible that co-administration of telmisartan with lithium may result in elevated serum lithium. There may be a risk of symptomatic hypotension when eprosartan is started in patients on high-dose diuretics.

Clinical evidence, mechanism, importance and management

When telmisartan 160 mg daily and **hydrochlorothiazide** 25 mg daily were co-administered for 7 days, there was no difference in AUC and maximum plasma concentrations of either drug compared with when they were given alone in a study in 13 healthy subjects. Transient dizziness associated with postural hypotension was the most common adverse event.[1] The maker states that symptomatic hypotension may occur when telmisartan is started in patients with sodium and/or volume depletion (e.g. those on **high-dose diuretic** therapy).[2]

In another study in healthy subjects, telmisartan 120 mg daily had no effect on the pharmacokinetics of **amlodipine** 10 mg daily, and there were no adverse events of note.[3] Telmisartan 120 mg had no effect on the pharmacokinetics of **paracetamol (acetaminophen)** 1 g in a single-dose study in healthy subjects, or on the pharmacokinetics of **ibuprofen** 400 mg three times a day in a multiple-dose study.[4] The maker also notes that, in a pharmacokinetic study telmisartan did not interact with **glibenclamide**.[2]

Based on evidence from other drugs which affect the renin-angiotensin system, the makers of telmisartan warn that concomitant use of **potassium-sparing diuretics** (e.g. **amiloride**, **spironolactone**, **triamterene**), **potassium supplements**, **salt substitutes** or other drugs that increase potassium levels may increase serum potassium. They recommend that the combinations be used cautiously. The maker also recommends that because increases in serum lithium have been noted during concomitant use of **lithium** and ACE inhibitors (see 'Lithium carbonate + ACE inhibitors', p.652), serum lithium levels should be carefully monitored during co-administration of **lithium** and telmisartan.[2]

1. Young CL, Dias VC, Stangier J. Multiple-dose pharmacokinetics of telmisartan and of hydrochlorothiazide following concurrent administration in healthy subjects. *J Clin Pharmacol* (2000) 40, 1323–30.
2. Micardis (Telmisartan). Boehringer Ingelheim Limited. Summary of product characteristics. December 1999.
3. Stangier J, Su CA. Pharmacokinetics of repeated oral doses of amlodipine and amlodipine plus telmisartan in healthy volunteers. *J Clin Pharmacol* (2000) 40, 1347–54.
4. Stangier J, Su CA, Fraunhofer A, Tetzloff W. Pharmacokinetics of acetaminophen and ibuprofen when coadministered with telmisartan in healthy volunteers. *J Clin Pharmacol* (2000) 40, 1338–46.

Thiazides + Colestyramine or Colestipol

The absorption of hydrochlorothiazide from the gut can be reduced by a third if colestipol is given concurrently, and two-thirds by colestyramine. The diuretic effects are reduced accordingly. Separating the dosages of the thiazide and the colestyramine by 4 h can reduce but not totally overcome the effects of this interaction.

Clinical evidence

The blood levels of the **hydrochlorothiazide** were reduced to about one-third in 6 healthy subjects taking 8 g **colestyramine** 2 min before and 6 and 12 h after a single 75-mg oral dose. Total urinary excretion fell to 15%. In a parallel study with 10 g **colestipol**, the blood levels of the thiazide fell to about two-thirds and the total urinary excretion fell to 57%.[1] A further study showed that giving the **colestyramine** 4 h after the **hydrochlorothiazide** reduced the effects of the interaction but the absorption was still reduced by one-third.[2] Another study demonstrated a 42% reduction when using **chlorothiazide** and **colestipol**.[3]

Mechanism

Hydrochlorothiazide becomes bound to these non-absorbable anionic exchange resins within the gut, and less is available for absorption.

Importance and management

Established interactions of clinical importance. The best dosing schedule would appear to be to give the hydrochlorothiazide 4 h before the colestyramine to minimise mixing in the gut. Even so a one-third reduction in thiazide absorption occurs.[2] The optimum time-interval with colestipol has not been investigated but it would be reasonable to take similar precautions. Information about other thiazides is lacking although it seems likely that they will interact similarly.

1. Hunninghake DB, King S, La Croix K. The effect of cholestyramine and colestipol on the absorption of hydrochlorothiazide. *Int J Clin Pharmacol Ther Toxicol* (1982) 20, 151–4.
2. Hunninghake DB, Hibbard DM. Influence of time intervals for cholestyramine dosing on the absorption of hydrochlorothiazide. *Clin Pharmacol Ther* (1986) 39, 329–34.
3. Kauffmann RE, Azarnoff DL. Effect of colestipol on gastrointestinal absorption of chlorothiazide in man. *Clin Pharmacol Ther* (1973) 14, 886.

Thiazides + NSAIDs

The antihypertensive effects of the thiazides can be reduced to some extent by indometacin (indomethacin), but it appears to be of only moderate clinical importance and may possibly only be a transient interaction. Ibuprofen appears to interact to a lesser extent or not at all. Piroxicam, naproxen and phenylbutazone may interact. No adverse interaction appears to occur with diclofenac, diflunisal, or sulindac.

Clinical evidence

(a) Thiazides + Indometacin

A double-blind controlled trial in 7 patients with hypertension on 5 to 10 mg **bendroflumethiazide** (**bendrofluazide**) or **amiloride** 5 to 10 mg + **hydrochlorothiazide** 50 to 100 mg, found that additional treatment with 100 mg **indometacin** daily for 3 weeks raised their systolic/diastolic blood pressures by 13/9 mmHg when lying and by 16/9 mmHg when standing. Body weight increased by 1.1 kg.[1] A later study in patients on **hydrochlorothiazide** found a 6/3 mmHg blood pressure rise after 2 weeks of **indometacin**, which had gone after 4 weeks.[2] Only a 5/1 mmHg blood pressure rise was seen in another study in hypertensive patients on **hydrochlorothiazide** given 100 mg **indometacin** (**indomethacin**) daily,[3] whereas no significant changes in blood pressure were seen in healthy subjects.[4] **Indometacin** 100 mg was found to reduce the urinary excretion of sodium and chloride caused by **bemetizide** by 47 and 44% respectively in healthy subjects,[5] but it had no effect on the sodium excretion caused by **hydrochlorothiazide**.[6] **Indometacin** did not affect the pharmacokinetics of **hydrochlorothiazide**.[4,6]

(b) Thiazides + Other NSAIDs

Diflunisal 375 mg twice daily caused the plasma levels of **hydrochlorothiazide** to rise by 25 to 30%, but this appears to be clinically unimportant.[7,8] **Diflunisal** also has uricosuric activity, which counteracts the uric acid retention that occurs with **hydrochlorothiazide**. **Diclofenac** and **sulindac** do not reduce either the hypotensive or diuretic effects of **hydrochlorothiazide**, and may even slightly enhance the antihypertensive effects.[2,3,9-11] Another study found that **diclofenac** and **sulindac** did not alter the antihypertensive efficacy of *Moduretic* (**hydrochlorothiazide** + **amiloride**) and beta-blockers.[12] One study[2] found that **naproxen** had no clinically relevant interaction with **hydrochlorothiazide** alone, while another found that **naproxen**, and also **piroxicam**, attenuated antihypertensive efficacy of **hydrochlorothiazide** plus **timolol**.[11]

Ibuprofen (400 mg or 600 mg three times daily for 4 weeks) caused a small rise in systolic but not in diastolic pressures in 2 studies in patients on **hydrochlorothiazide**,[10,13] but not in another involving **bendroflumethiazide** (**bendrofluazide**).[14] Another study found that 400 mg **ibuprofen** three times daily had no effect on blood pressures controlled by **triamterene-hydrochlorothiazide**, although one patient showed a marked fall in kidney function.[15] **Ibuprofen** 800 mg four times daily for a week had little effect on blood pressures controlled with **hydrochlorothiazide** in yet another study.[16] Both **ibuprofen** and **diclofenac** can cause a weight rise.[10] In 15 patients on **hydrochlorothiazide** 50 mg daily, a mean systolic blood pressure rise of 18 mmHg (from 171 to 189 mmHg) occurred when they were treated with 750 mg **phenylbutazone** or **kebuzone** daily. This rise represents about a 35% reduction in the antihypertensive effect of **hydrochlorothiazide**.[17]

Mechanism

Not understood. Since the prostaglandins have a role to play in kidney function, drugs such as the NSAIDs, which inhibit their synthesis, might be expected to have some effect on the actions of diuretics whose effects also depend on the activity of the prostaglandins. A study in *rats* suggested that indometacin may oppose the thiazides by reducing chloride delivery to the site of thiazide action in the distal tubule.[18] The lack of effect with sulindac may be due to the absence of renal excretion of its active sulfide metabolite.[11]

Importance and management

The thiazide/indometacin interaction is well documented although the findings are not entirely consistent. It seems to be of only moderate clinical importance, but the effects of concurrent use should be monitored and the thiazide dosage modified if necessary. Ibuprofen interacts to a lesser extent or not at all. Piroxicam, naproxen, and phenylbutazone may interact. No adverse interaction appears to occur with diclofenac, sulindac or diflunisal. The uricosuric effects of diflunisal may be usefully exploited to counteract the uric acid retention which occurs with hydrochlorothiazide. The effects of other NSAIDs do not seem to have been studied.

1. Watkins J, Abbott EC, Hensby CN, Webster J, Dollery CT. Attenuation of hypotensive effect of propranolol and thiazide diuretics by indomethacin. *BMJ* (1980) 281, 702–5.
2. Koopmans PP, Thien Th, Gribnau FWJ. Influence of non-steroidal anti-inflammatory drugs on diuretic treatment of mild to moderate essential hypertension. *BMJ* (1984) 289, 1492–4.
3. Koopmans PP, Thien Th, Thomas CMG, van den Berg RJ, Gribnau FWJ. The effects of sulindac and indomethacin on the antihypertensive and diuretic action of hydrochlorothiazide in patients with mild to moderate essential hypertension. *Br J Clin Pharmacol* (1986) 21, 417–23.
4. Koopmans PP, Kateman WGPM, Tan Y, van Ginneken CAM, Gribnau FWJ. Effects of indomethacin and sulindac on hydrochlorothiazide kinetics. *Clin Pharmacol Ther* (1985) 37, 625–8.
5. Düsing R, Nicolas V, Glatte B, Glänzer K, Kipnowski J, Kramer HJ. Interaction of bemetizide and indomethacin in the kidney. *Br J Clin Pharmacol* (1983) 16, 377–84.
6. Williams RL, Davies RO, Berman RS, Holmes GI, Huber P, Gee WL, Lin ET, Benet LZ. Hydrochlorothiazide pharmacokinetics and pharmacologic effect: the influence of indomethacin. *J Clin Pharmacol* (1982) 22, 32–41.
7. Tempero KF, Cirillo VJ, Steelman SL. Diflunisal: a review of the pharmacokinetic and pharmacodynamic properties, drug interactions and special tolerability studies in humans. *Br J Clin Pharmacol* (1977) 4, 31S.
8. Tempero KF, Cirillo VJ, Steelman SL, Besselaar GH, Smit Sibinga CTh, De Schepper P, Tjandramaga TB, Dresse A, Gribnau FWJ. Special studies on diflunisal, a novel salicylate. *Clin Res* (1975) 23, 224A.
9. Steiness E, Waldorff S. Different interactions of indomethacin and sulindac with thiazides in hypertension. *BMJ* (1982) 285, 1702–3.
10. Koopmans PP, Thien Th, Gribnau FWJ. The influence of ibuprofen, diclofenac and sulindac on the blood pressure lowering effect of hydrochlorothiazide. *Eur J Clin Pharmacol* (1987) 31, 553–7.
11. Wong DG, Spence JD, McDonald JWD, Lamki LM. Non-steroidal antiinflammatory drugs (NSAID) vs placebo in hypertension treated with diuretic and β-blocker. *Clin Pharmacol Ther* (1984) 35, 284.
12. Stokes GS, Brooks PM, Johnson HJ, Monaghan JC, Okoro EO, Kelly D. The effects of sulindac and diclofenac in essential hypertension controlled by treatment with a beta-blocker and/or diuretic. *Clin Exp Hypertens A* (1991) 13, 1169–78.
13. Gurwitz JH, Everitt DE, Monane M, Glynn RJ, Choodnovskiy I, Beaudet MP, Avorn J. The impact of ibuprofen on the efficacy of antihypertensive treatment with hydrochlorothiazide in elderly persons. *J Gerontol* (1996) 51A, M74–M79.
14. Davies JG, Rawlins DC, Busson M. Effect of ibuprofen on blood pressure control by propranolol and bendrofluazide. *J Int Med Res* (1988) 16, 173–81.
15. Gehr TWB, Sica DA, Steiger BW, Marshall C. Interaction of triamterene-hydrochlorothiazide and ibuprofen. *Clin Pharmacol Ther* (1990) 47, 200.
16. Wright JT, McKenney JM, Lehany AM, Bryan DL, Cooper LW, Lambert CM. The effect of high-dose short-term ibuprofen on antihypertensive control with hydrochlorothiazide. *Clin Pharmacol Ther* (1989) 46, 440–4.
17. Polak F. Die hemmende Wirkung von Phenylbutazon auf die durch einige Antihypertonika hervorgerufene Blutdrucksenkung bei Hypertonikern. *Z Gesamte Inn Med* (1976) 22, 375–6.
18. Kirchner KA, Brandon S, Mueller RA, Smith MJ, Bower JD. Mechanism of attenuated hydrochlorothiazide response during indomethacin administration. *Kidney Int* (1987) 31, 1097–1103.

Thiazides + Propantheline

Propantheline can increase the absorption of hydrochlorothiazide from the gut.

Clinical evidence, mechanism, importance and management

The absorption of **hydrochlorothiazide** 75 mg in 6 healthy fasting subjects was delayed and increased (AUC +23% and urinary recovery +36%) by the concurrent use of 60 mg **propantheline**, due, it is suggested, to a slower delivery of the drug to its areas of absorption.[1] The clinical importance of this is uncertain, but is likely to be small.

1. Beermann B, Groschinsky-Grind M. Enhancement of the gastrointestinal absorption of hydrochlorothiazide by propantheline. *Eur J Clin Pharmacol* (1978) 13, 385–7.

Tolazoline + H₂-blockers

Cimetidine and ranitidine can reduce or abolish the effects of tolazoline when used as a pulmonary vasodilator in children.

Clinical evidence

A newborn infant with persistent foetal circulation was given a continuous infusion of tolazoline to reduce pulmonary hypertension. The oxygenation improved but gastrointestinal bleeding occurred. When **cimetidine** was given, the condition of the child deteriorated with a decrease in oxygen saturation and arterial pO_2 values.[1]

This report is similar to another in which the fall in pulmonary arterial pressure in a child due to tolazoline was reversed when **cimetidine** was given for acute gastrointestinal haemorrhage.[2] Another study found that **ranitidine** (3 mg/kg intravenously) abolished the fall in pulmonary and systemic vascular resistance in 12 children who had been treated with tolazoline (1 to 2 mg/kg) as a pulmonary vasodilator.[3]

Mechanism

Tolazoline dilates the pulmonary vascular system by stimulating both H_1- and H_2-receptors. Cimetidine and ranitidine block H_2-receptors so that at least part of the tolazoline effects are abolished. It has been suggested that this interaction is confined to children.[2]

Importance and management

An established interaction. Cimetidine and ranitidine are not suitable agents against the gastrointestinal side-effects of tolazoline in children. Other H₂-blockers would be expected to behave similarly. Antacids have been used, and omeprazole is a possible alternative but this needs confirmation.

1. Roll C, Hanssler L. Interaktion von Tolazolin und Cimetidin bei persistierender fetaler Zirkulation des Neugeborenen. *Monatsschr Kinderheilkd* (1993) 141, 297–9.
2. Jones ODH, Shore DF, Rigby ML. The use of tolazoline hydrochloride as a pulmonary vasodilator in potentially fatal episodes of pulmonary vasoconstriction after cardiac surgery in children. *Circulation* (1981) 64 (Suppl II), 134–9.
3. Bush A. Busst CM, Knight WB, Shinebourne EA. Cardiovascular effects of tolazoline and ranitidine. *Arch Dis Child* (1987) 62, 241–6.

Torasemide + Miscellaneous drugs

No adverse interaction occurs if torasemide and cimetidine or glibenclamide (glyburide) are taken concurrently.

Clinical evidence, mechanism, importance and management

Cimetidine 300 mg four times daily for 3 days was found to have no effect on the pharmacokinetics of single 10 mg oral doses of torasemide in 11 healthy subjects, nor were there any changes in the volume of urine or the excretion of sodium, potassium or chloride.[1] A three month trial in 32 patients with congestive heart failure and type II (NIDDM) diabetes mellitus on **glibenclamide (glyburide)** found that 5 mg torasemide daily caused a small but not clinically relevant fall in blood glucose levels.[2] There would seem to be no reason for avoiding torasemide in patients taking either **cimetidine** or **glibenclamide (glyburide)**.

1. Kramer WG. Lack of effect of cimetidine on torasemide pharmacokinetics and pharmacodynamics in healthy subjects. 4th Int Congr Diuretics, Boca Raton, Florida Oct 11–16th 1992. Eds. Puschett JB, Greenberg A. *Int Congr Series 1023* (1993), 361–4.
2. Lehnert H, Schmitz H, Beyer J, Wilmbusse H, Piesche L. Controlled clinical trial investigating the influence of torasemide and furosemide on carbohydrate metabolism in patients with cardiac failure and concomitant type II diabetes. 4th Int Congr Diuretics, Boca Raton, Florida Oct 11–16th 1992. Eds. Puschett JB, Greenberg A. *Int Congr Series 1023* (1993), 271–4.

Trandolapril + Miscellaneous drugs

Trandolapril appears not to interact adversely with aspirin, thrombolytics, nitrates, digoxin or warfarin. Based on the risk of orthostatic hypotension with other antihypertensives, the makers of trandolapril advise caution with some neuroleptics and antidepressants. Based on other ACE inhibitors, lithium toxicity is also a possibility.

Clinical evidence, mechanism, importance and management

The maker of trandolapril has data on file showing that there was no significant pharmacokinetic interaction between trandolapril and **digoxin** in healthy subjects.[1] They also note that in patients with left ventricular dysfunction after myocardial infarction, no clinical interactions have been found between trandolapril and **digoxin**, **aspirin**, or unnamed **thrombolytics** and **nitrates**.[2,3] See also 'Digitalis glycosides + ACE inhibitors', p.528, and 'ACE inhibitors + Aspirin and NSAIDs', p.369. Other studies (also quoted by the makers) identified no problems when trandolapril was given to **diabetic patients** and others with glucose intolerance,[1] but as a precaution they recommend monitoring blood glucose levels.[2,3] You should be aware that very rarely marked hypoglycaemia has been seen in diabetic patients on insulin or sulfonylurea oral hypoglycaemic agents when given other ACE inhibitors (see 'Hypoglycaemic agents + ACE inhibitors', p.564). The makers also point out the risk of orthostatic hypotension in those taking **neuroleptics** or **tricyclic antidepressants**, and note that reduced elimination of **lithium** may occur (serum lithium should be monitored).[2,3] These warnings are based, not unreasonably, on the adverse reactions seen with other antihypertensives (see 'Antihypertensives + Phenothiazines', p.385) and ACE inhibitors (see 'Lithium carbonate + ACE inhibitors', p.652), but not apparently on direct observations with trandolapril.[4] Trandolapril 2 mg daily for 13 days did not affect the pharmacodynamics of a single dose of warfarin 25 mg administered on day 8 in a study in 19 healthy subjects.[5] See also 'Anticoagulants + ACE inhibitors', p.235.

1. New Horizons in Antihypertensive therapy. Gopten® Trandolapril. Knoll AG 1992.
2. Gopten (Trandolapril). Abbott Laboratories Ltd. Summary of product characteristics, December 2001.
3. Odrik (Trandolapril). Hoechst Marion Roussel Ltd. Summary of product characteristics, September 1999.
4. Knoll Ltd. Personal communication, 1993.
5. Meyer BH, Muller FO, Badenhorst PN, Luus HG, De La Rey N. Multiple doses of trandolapril do not affect warfarin pharmacodynamics. *S Afr Med J* (1995) 85, 768–70.

Triamterene + Cimetidine or Ranitidine

Ranitidine reduces the absorption and the diuretic effects of triamterene but the clinical importance of this is uncertain. Cimetidine appears not to interact with triamterene significantly.

Clinical evidence

(a) Cimetidine

A study in 6 healthy subjects given 100 mg triamterene daily for 4 days showed that, although 400 mg **cimetidine** twice daily increased the triamterene AUC by 22%, reduced its metabolism (hydroxylation) by 32% and its renal clearance by 28% as well as its absorption, the loss of sodium in the urine was not significantly changed nor were its potassium-sparing effects altered.[1]

(b) Ranitidine

Ranitidine 150 mg twice daily for 4 days approximately halved the absorption of 100 mg triamterene daily (as measured by its renal clearance) in 8 healthy subjects. Its metabolism was also reduced, the total effect being a 21% reduction in the AUC. As a result of the reduced serum triamterene levels the urinary sodium loss was reduced to some extent but potassium excretion remained unchanged.[2]

Mechanism

These changes are due to reduced triamterene absorption from the gut and reduced liver metabolism and renal excretion caused by the these H_2-blockers.

Importance and management

Information about the triamterene/ranitidine interaction is limited and the clinical importance remains uncertain. Nobody seems to have measured whether this interaction significantly reduces the diuretic effects of triamterene in patients. The outcome of concurrent use should therefore be monitored. Cimetidine also interacts with triamterene but this appears to be clinically unimportant because its diuretic effects are minimally changed.[1] No dosage changes are likely to be necessary.

1. Muirhead MR, Somogyi AA, Rolan PE, Bochner F. Effect of cimetidine on renal and hepatic drugs elimination: studies with triamterene. *Clin Pharmacol Ther* (1986) 40, 400–7.
2. Muirhead M, Bochner F, Somogyi A. Pharmacokinetic drug interactions between triamterene and ranitidine in humans: alterations in renal and hepatic clearances and gastrointestinal absorption. *J Pharmacol Exp Ther* (1988) 244, 734–9.

Triamterene + NSAIDs

Concurrent use of triamterene and indometacin (indomethacin) may rapidly lead to acute renal failure. An isolated case of renal impairment with diclofenac has been reported.

Clinical evidence

A study in 4 healthy subjects showed that the concurrent use of **indometacin** (**indomethacin**) (150 mg daily) and triamterene (200 mg daily) over a 3-day period reduced the creatinine clearance of two of them by 62 and 72% respectively. Kidney function returned to normal after a month. **Indometacin** alone caused an average 10% fall in creatinine clearance, but triamterene alone caused no consistent change in kidney function. No adverse reactions were seen in 18 other subjects treated in the same way with indometacin and three other diuretics (**furosemide** (**frusemide**), **hydrochlorothiazide**, **spironolactone**).[1,2] Five patients have been described who rapidly developed acute renal failure after receiving **indometacin** and triamterene either concurrently or sequentially.[3-6]

A patient receiving **triamterene** 100 mg plus **trichlormethiazide** 2 mg daily was given 75 mg **diclofenac** intramuscularly before admission to hospital with breast pain. On admission serum creatinine was 91 micromol/l and after 2 days had increased to 248 micromol/l. It returned to normal over 2 weeks. Subsequent **diclofenac** by mouth produced no adverse effects. The observed deterioration in renal function was attributed to an interaction between triamterene and **diclofenac**.[7]

One report found that **diflunisal** had no effects on the pharmacokinetics of triamterene itself in healthy volunteers, but the plasma AUC of an active metabolite, *p*-hydroxytriamterene was increased more than fourfold.[8]

Mechanism

Uncertain. One suggestion is that triamterene causes renal ischaemia for which the kidney compensates by increasing prostaglandin (PGE$_2$) production, thereby preserving renal blood flow. Indometacin opposes this by inhibiting prostaglandin synthesis, so that the damaging effects of triamterene on the kidney continue unchecked. Increases in pharmacologically active metabolites of triamterene due to competition for renal excretory pathways may occur but the clinical significance is uncertain.

Importance and management

Information is limited to these reports, but the interaction with indometacin is established. The incidence is uncertain but it occurred in two of the four healthy subjects in the study cited.[1,2] Since acute renal failure can apparently develop unpredictably and very rapidly it

would seem prudent to avoid concurrent use of triamterene and indometacin where possible. The authors of the report with diclofenac suggest caution with the use of any NSAID with triamterene.[7]

1. Favre L, Glasson P, Vallotton MB. Reversible acute renal failure from combined triamterene and indomethacin. A study in healthy subjects. *Ann Intern Med* (1982) 96, 317–20.
2. Favre L, Glasson PH, Riondel A, Vallotton MB. Interaction of diuretics and non-steroidal anti-inflammatory drugs in man. *Clin Sci* (1983) 64, 407–15.
3. McCarthy JT, Torres VE, Romero JC, Wochos DN, Velosa JA. Acute intrinsic renal failure induced by indomethacin: role of prostaglandin synthetase inhibition. *Mayo Clin Proc* (1982) 57, 289–96.
4. McCarthy JT. Drug induced renal failure. *Mayo Clin Proc* (1982) 57, 463.
5. Weinberg MS, Quigg RJ, Salant DJ, Bernard DB. Anuric renal failure precipitated by indomethacin and triamterene. *Nephron* (1985) 40, 216–18.
6. Mathews A, Baillie GR. Acute renal failure and hyperkalemia associated with triamterene and indomethacin. *Vet Hum Toxicol* (1986) 28, 224–5.
7. Härkönen M, Ekblom-Kullberg S. Reversible deterioration of renal function after diclofenac in patient receiving triamterene. *BMJ* (1986) 293, 698–9.
8. Jacob SS, Franklin ME, Dickinson RG, Hooper WD. The effect of diflunisal on the elimination of triamterene in human volunteers. *Drug Metabol Drug Interact* (2000) 16, 159–71.

Valsartan + Miscellaneous drugs

Glibenclamide (glyburide) causes a small reduction in valsartan serum levels while cimetidine causes a small rise, but neither seems to be of any clinical relevance. The makers warn about the concurrent use of potassium-depleting diuretics and potassium supplements. They also note that symptomatic hypotension may occur when valsartan is started in patients with severe sodium or volume depletion such as those on high-dose diuretics. Indometacin (indomethacin) may attenuate the antihypertensive effect of valsartan. There is no pharmacokinetic interaction between valsartan and amlodipine, atenolol, or furosemide (frusemide). Valsartan does not significantly alter the activity of warfarin. Valsartan may modestly reduce the availability of hydrochlorothiazide, but the combination is clinically useful.

Clinical evidence, mechanism, importance and management

In a series of studies with groups of 12 healthy subjects, the possible pharmacokinetic interactions of single 160-mg doses of valsartan with single doses of the following drugs were examined: **amlodipine** (5 mg),[1] **atenolol** (100 mg),[2] **cimetidine** (800 mg),[3] **furosemide** (**frusemide**) (40 mg),[4] **glibenclamide** (**glyburide**) (1.75 mg),[1] **hydrochlorothiazide** (25 mg)[1] and **indometacin** (**indomethacin**) (100 mg).[1] For most of these combinations, no changes in the pharmacokinetics of either drug were found, although the pharmacokinetics of valsartan showed wide variations between subjects.[1] **Cimetidine** increased the rate of absorption of valsartan (by increasing gastric pH) resulting in a higher maximum plasma concentration (increased about 50%), but only marginally increased the extent of absorption (7% increase in AUC).[3] **Glibenclamide** appeared to decrease plasma concentrations of valsartan (16% decrease in AUC).[1] Valsartan reduced the systemic availability of **hydrochlorothiazide** (AUC decreased 31%).[1] The changes in valsartan pharmacokinetics seen with **glibenclamide** and **cimetidine** appear to have little or no clinical relevance but the makers[5] cautiously say that **glibenclamide** ". . . may cause a decrease in the systemic exposure to valsartan . . .", and if valsartan is ". . . used together with **cimetidine** the systemic exposure to valsartan may be marginally increased . . ." The changes in **hydrochlorothiazide** pharmacokinetics appear to be of no practical importance, and the combination produces a significant and useful additional reduction in blood pressure.

Despite there being no pharmacokinetic interaction with **indometacin**, a pharmacodynamic interaction has been seen. **Indometacin** 50 mg three times daily for 2 weeks produced an increase in mean blood pressure (2.1/1.9 mmHg) in patients on **valsartan** 80 to 160 mg daily, in a crossover study.[6]

Warfarin 10 mg daily for 3 days had no effect on the pharmacokinetics of a single 160-mg dose of valsartan in 12 healthy subjects. Valsartan caused a small increase in prothrombin time of about 12%, which was not considered clinically important. No dosage adjustment of either drug is required when they are co-administered.[1,7]

The makers say that the concurrent use of valsartan with potassium-sparing diuretics (**amiloride**, **spironolactone**, **triamterene**), **potassium supplements** or **potassium-containing salt substitutes** may increase serum potassium levels and comedication is therefore inadvisable.[5] If comedication is required, serum potassium should be monitored, especially in those with renal impairment. The maker also notes that symptomatic hypotension may occur when valsartan is started in patients with severe sodium or volume depletion such as those on **high-dose diuretics**. In the diuretic dose cannot be reduced, a lower starting dose of valsartan is recommended.[5]

1. Novartis Pharmaceuticals Ltd. Data on file, Protocols 07,37,40,43, 52.
2. Czendlik CH, Sioufi A, Preiswerk G, Howald H. Pharmacokinetic and pharmacodynamic interaction of single doses of valsartan and atenolol. *Eur J Clin Pharmacol* (1997) 52, 451–9.
3. Schmidt EK, Antonin KH, Flesch G, Racine-Poon A. An interaction study with cimetidine and the new angiotensin II antagonist valsartan. *Eur J Clin Pharmacol* (1998) 53, 451–8.
4. Bindschedler M, Degen P, Flesch G, de Gasparo M, Preiswerk G. Pharmacokinetic and pharmacodynamic interaction of single oral doses of valsartan and furosemide. *Eur J Clin Pharmacol* (1997) 52, 371–8.
5. Diovan (Valsartan) Novartis Pharmaceuticals Ltd. Summary of product characteristics, November 2001.
6. Fogari R, Zoppi A, Carretta R, Veglio F, Salvetti A: Italian Collaborative Study Group. Effect of indomethacin on the antihypertensive efficacy of valsartan and lisinopril: a multicentre study. *J Hypertens* (2002) 20: 1007–14.
7. Knight H, Flesch G, Prasad P, Lloyd P, Douglas J. Lack of pharmacokinetic and pharmacodynamic interaction between valsartan and warfarin. *J Hypertens* (2000) 18 (Suppl 4), S89.

9

Antiparkinsonism and related drug interactions

The drugs in this chapter are classified together because their major therapeutic application is in the treatment of Parkinson's disease, although some of the related anticholinergic (antimuscarinic) drugs included here are used for totally different conditions. Parkinson's disease is named after Dr James Parkinson who a century-and-a-half ago described the four main signs of the disease, namely muscle rigidity, tremor, muscular weakness and hypokinesia. Similar symptoms may also be displayed as the unwanted side-effects of therapy with certain drugs.

The basic cause of the disease lies in the basal ganglia of the brain, particularly the corpus striatum and the substantia nigra, where the normal balance between dopaminergic nerve fibres (those which use dopamine as the chemical transmitter) and the cholinergic nerve fibres (acetylcholine as the transmitter) is lost because the dopaminergic fibres degenerate. As a result the cholinergic fibres come to be in dominant control. Much of the treatment of Parkinson's disease is based on an attempt to redress the balance, either by limiting the activity of the cholinergic fibres with anticholinergic (atropine-like) drugs, and/or by 'topping up' the dopaminergic system with dopamine in the form of levodopa, or with other agents such as amantadine or bromocriptine which increase dopaminergic activity in the brain. Dopamine cannot penetrate the blood-brain barrier so that its precursor, dopa, is given instead. These days it is common to include with dopa an enzyme-inhibitor such as carbidopa (in *Sinemet*) or benserazide (in *Madopar*) which prevents the 'wasteful' enzymic metabolism of the levo-dopa outside the brain and thereby allows the use of lower oral doses which have fewer side-effects.

In addition to the interactions discussed in this chapter, some of the drugs are involved in interactions described elsewhere. Selegiline is also not discussed here (but in Chapter 18) because it is a monoamine oxidase inhibitor. Consult the Index for a full listing.

Table 9.1 Antiparkinsonian drugs

Generic names	Proprietary names
Anticholinergics	
Benztropine	*Cogentin, Cogentinol, Phatropine*
Biperiden	*Akineton, Cinetol, Dekinet, Ipsatol, Kinex, Norakin N*
Bornaprine	*Sormodren*
Caramiphen	
Chlorphenoxamine	*Clorevan, Systral*
Dexetimide	*Tremblex*
Diethazine	
Ethopropazine (Profenamine)	*Parsitan*
Ethybenztropine	
Metixene (Methixene)	*Metixen, Tremaril, Tremarit, Tremoquil*
Orphenadrine (Mephenamine)	*Banflex, Biorphen, Disipal, Flexin, Flexoject, Flexon, Lysantin, Norflex, Orfenace, Orfenal*
Procyclidine	*Arpicolin, Kemadren, Kemadrin, Muscinil, Osnervan, Procyclid*
Trihexiphenidyl (Benzhexol)	*Aca, Acamed, Apo-Trihex, Artandyl, Artane, Broflex, B-Hex, Hipokinon, Pargitan, Parkinane, Parkopan, Partane, Peragit, Pozhexol, Tridyl, Triexidyl, Trihexy*
Tropatepine	*Lepticur*
Other drugs possessing anticholinergic (antimuscarinic) activity are listed in Table 9.2	
Amantadine	*Adekin, Aman, Amanta, Amantagamma, Amantan, Amixx, Atarin, A-Parkin, Cerebramed, Endantadine, Hofcomant, InfectoFlu, Infex, Lysovir, Mantadan, Mantadix, Mantidan, Noctal, Paritrel, Parkadina, PK-Merz, Profil, Symmetrel, Tregor, Virucid*
Bromocriptine	*Antiprotin, Bromed, Bromergon, Bromocrel, Bromohexal, Bromolactin, Bromopar, Bromo-Kin, Bromtine, Broptin, Cehapark, Crilem, Cryocriptina, Kirim, Kriptiser, Kripton, Medocriptine, Parilac, Parlodel, Pravidel, Serocryptin, Suplac, Umprel, Zolac*
Levodopa (L-Dopa)	*Dopaflex, Dopar, Larodopa, Levomet*
Levodopa + Benserazide	*Aktipar, Dopamed, Levobens, Levopar, PK-Levo, Madopar, Modopar, Prolopa*
Levodopa + Carbidopa	*Apo-Lovocarb, Atamet, Carbilev, Cloisone, Cronomet, Dopicar, Isicom, Kardopal, Kinson, Lemdopa, Levocarb, Levomed, Nacom, Nu-Levocarb, Racovel, Sinemet, Striaton*
Pergolide	*Celance, Nopar, Parkotil, Permax, Pharken*
Piribedil	*Trivastal, Trivastan*
Pramipexole	*Mirapex, Mirapexin, Sifrol*
Selegiline	*Amboneural, Amindan, Antiparkin, Apomex, Atapryl, Carbex, Clondepryl, Cognitiv, Deprenyl, Deprilan, Egibren, Eldepryl, Elegelin, Elepril, Julab, Jumex, Jumexal, Jumexil, Kinline, MAOtil, Movergan, Niar, Plurimen, Regepar, Sefmex, Selecim, Seledat, Selegam, Selegos, Selemerck, Selepark, Selgene, Selgimed, Seline, Tremorex, Zelapar*

Amantadine + Co-trimoxazole

An elderly patient on amantadine developed acute mental confusion when given co-trimoxazole (sulfamethoxazole (sulphamethoxazole) + trimethoprim).

Clinical evidence, mechanism, importance and management

An 84-year-old with parkinsonism, chronic obstructive pulmonary disease and chronic atrial fibrillation, was treated with 100 mg amantadine twice daily and digoxin for at least 2 years. Within 72 h of starting **co-trimoxazole** (*Septra DS*) twice daily for bronchitis he became mentally confused, incoherent and combative. He also showed cogwheel rigidity and a resting tremor. Within 24 h of stopping the amantadine and **co-trimoxazole**, the patient's mental status returned to normal.[1] The reasons for this reaction are not understood but, on the basis of *animal* studies, the authors suggest that the **trimethoprim** component of the **co-trimoxazole** may have competed with the amantadine for renal secretion, resulting in an accumulation of amantadine with its toxic effects.[1] In fact both drugs can cause some mental confusion. This interaction is more likely in the elderly because ageing results in a decrease in the clearance of these and many other drugs.

The general importance of this interaction is uncertain, but it would now seem prudent to monitor the effects of concurrent use in any patient, particularly the elderly.

1. Speeg KV, Leighton JA, Maldonado AL. Case report: toxic delirium in a patient taking amantadine and trimethoprim-sulfamethoxazole. *Am J Med Sci* (1989) 298, 410–12.

Amantadine + Miscellaneous drugs

The use of amantadine in patients taking phenylpropanolamine, other CNS stimulants, or having treatment with other drugs for epilepsy, gastrointestinal ulceration, parkinsonism or congestive heart failure may cause problems. Quinine and quinidine can reduce the loss of amantadine in the urine. A single report describes the aggravation of tremor in two patients when given cisapride, but no interaction apparently occurs with paracetamol (acetaminophen).

Clinical evidence, mechanism, importance and management

The US makers of amantadine recommend that amantadine should be given with caution if **CNS stimulants** are being used.[1] Two patients on amantadine experienced aggravation of tremor while taking **cisapride** but the general importance of this is uncertain.[2] An isolated report describes the development of severe psychosis in a woman within 7 to 8 days of starting 100 mg amantadine and 80 mg **phenylpropanolamine** daily. The reasons are not known but both drugs alone in high doses sometimes cause psychosis.[3] The UK makers[4] of amantadine also say that it should be avoided by those who are subject to **convulsions** or with a history of **gastric ulceration**. They warn that amantadine can aggravate the CNS, gastrointestinal and other side-effects of drugs used in the treatment of Parkinson's disease (**anticholinergics**, **levodopa**).[4] Tables 9.1 and 9.2 in this chapter contain lists of drugs with anticholinergic activity. Amantadine sometimes causes peripheral oedema which may possibly have an adverse effect on the control of congestive heart failure. No pharmacokinetic interaction was seen in a study using 200 mg amantadine daily and a single 650-mg dose of **paracetamol** (**acetaminophen**).[5]

Single dose studies of renal cationic drug excretion in human volunteers found that **quinine** (200 mg) and **quinidine** (200 mg) reduced the renal clearance of amantadine (3 mg/kg) by 36% and 48% respectively, but only in male subjects.[6] Whether long-term use of these drugs would therefore cause a clinically relevant rise in serum

amantadine serum levels is uncertain; be alert for any evidence of amantadine toxicity (headache, nausea, dizziness, etc.) if either of these two drugs is used concurrently.

1. Symmetrel (Amantadine). Endo Pharmaceutical Inc. US prescribing information, February 1998.
2. Sempere AP, Duarte J, Cabezas C, Clavería LE, Coria F. Aggravation of parkinsonian tremor by cisapride. *Clin Neuropharmacol* (1995) 18, 76–8.
3. Stroe AE, Hall J, Amin F. Psychotic episode related to phenylpropanolamine and amantadine in a healthy female. *Gen Hosp Psychiatry* (1995) 17, 457–8.
4. Symmetrel (Amantadine). Alliance Pharmaceuticals. Summary of product characteristics, October 1999.
5. Aoki FY, Sitar DS. Effects of chronic amantadine hydrochloride ingestion on its and acetaminophen pharmacokinetics in young adults. *J Clin Pharmacol* (1992) 32, 24–7.
6. Gaudry SE, Sitar DS, Smyth DD, McKenzie JK, Aoki FY. Gender and age as factors in the inhibition of renal clearance of amantadine by quinine and quinidine. *Clin Pharmacol Ther* (1993) 54, 23–7.

Amantadine + Thiazides

Concurrent use can be successful and uneventful but two patients have been described who developed amantadine toxicity when given hydrochlorothiazide-triamterene or cyclopenthiazide-K.

Clinical evidence

Amantadine toxicity (ataxia, agitation, hallucinations) developed in a patient within a week of starting to take two tablets of *Dyazide* (**hydrochlorothiazide-triamterene**) daily. The symptoms rapidly disappeared when all the drugs were withdrawn. In a later study this patient showed a 50% rise in amantadine serum levels (from 156 to 243 ng/ml) after taking the diuretic for 7 days.[1]

Confusion and hallucinations are briefly described in another patient given amantadine and **cyclopenthiazide-K**.[2] In contrast, the successful and apparently uneventful concurrent use of amantadine and diuretics (one of them named as a **thiazide**)[3] has also been described.[3,4]

Mechanism

Uncertain. Amantadine is largely excreted unchanged in the urine and it seems probable that these diuretics reduce the renal clearance.[1]

Importance and management

Information about an adverse interaction appears to be limited to these 2 reports. Its incidence is uncertain. There seems to be little reason for avoiding concurrent use, but the effects should be well monitored.

1. Wilson TW, Rajput AH. Amantadine–Dyazide interaction. *Can Med Assoc J* (1983) 129, 974–5.
2. New Zealand Committee on Adverse Drug Reactions. 11th year. April 1975-March 1976. Serial no 5476.
3. Birdwood GFB, Gilder SSB, Wink CAS (eds). Parkinson's Disease. A new approach to treatment. Int Clin Symp Report on Symmetrel in Parkinsonism. London June 1971. Academic Press (1971) p 66.
4. Parkes JD, Marsden CD, Price P. Amantadine-induced heart-failure. *Lancet* (1977) i, 904.

Anticholinergics + Anticholinergics

Additive anticholinergic (antimuscarinic) effects, both peripheral and central, can develop if drugs with anticholinergic effects are used together. The outcome may be harmful.

Clinical evidence, mechanism, importance and management

The anticholinergic (antimuscarinic) effects of some drugs are exploited therapeutically. These include atropine and drugs such as trihexyphenidyl (benzhexol) and benztropine (Table 9.1) which are used for the control of parkinsonian symptoms. Other drugs with a broader spectrum of activity (Table 9.2) may also possess some anticholinergic side-effects which are unwanted and troublesome but

Table 9.2 Drugs with anticholinergic effects (main or side-effects)

Drug group	Individual drugs
Antiarrhythmics	Disopyramide, Propafenone
Antiemetics	Cyclizine, Dimenhydrinate, Hyoscine (scopolamine), Meclozine
Antihistamines	Brompheniramine, Chlorphenamine (chlorpheniramine), Cyproheptadine, Diphenhydramine, Hydroxyzine, Triprolidine
Antiparkinson agents (anticholinergics)	see Table 9.1
Antispasmodics	Anisotropine, Atropine, Belladonna alkaloids, Dicycloverine (dicyclomine), Flavoxate, Hyoscine (scopolamine), Hyoscyamine, Isopropamide, Oxybutynin, Propantheline, Tolterodine
Antiulcer drugs	Clidinium, Hexocyclium, Isopropamide, Mepenzolate, Methanthelinium (Methantheline), Oxyphencyclimine, Pirenzepine, Tridihexethyl
Cycloplegic mydriatics	Atropine, Cyclopentolate, Homatropine, Hyoscine (scopolamine), Tropicamide
Muscle relaxants	Baclofen, Cyclobenzaprine, Orphenadrine
Neuroleptics	Chlorpromazine, Chlorprothixene, Clozapine, Loxapine, Perphenazine, Pimozide, Mesoridazine, Trifluoperazine, Thioridazine
Peripheral vasodilator	Papaverine
Tricyclic and related antidepressants	Amitriptyline, Amoxapine, Clomipramine, Desipramine, Doxepin, Imipramine, Maprotiline, Nortriptyline, Protriptyline, Trimipramine

After Barkin RL, Stein ZLG. *South Med J* (1989) 82, 1547, and others. The categorisation is not exclusive; some of these drugs are used for a range of effects. There are many other anticholinergic drugs.

usually not serious, unless they are worsened by the addition of another drug with similar properties.

The easily recognised and common peripheral anticholinergic effects are blurred vision, dry mouth, constipation, difficulty in urination, reduced sweating, tachycardia and possibly exacerbation of narrow angle glaucoma. Central effects include confusion, disorientation, visual hallucinations, agitation, irritability, delirium, memory problems, belligerence and even assaultiveness. Problems are most likely to arise with patients with particular physical conditions such as glaucoma (drainage worsened), prostatic hypertrophy (urination made even more difficult) or constipation. It has been pointed out that these anticholinergic side-effects can mimic old age conditions.

Tables 9.1 and 9.2 list many of the drugs with anticholinergic effects which may be expected to be additive if used together, but apart from some reports describing life-threatening reactions (see 'Antipsychotics + Anticholinergics', p.692) there are very few reports describing this simple additive interaction, probably because the outcome is so obvious. Many of these interactions, unlike virtually all of the other interactions described in this book, are therefore 'theoretical' but their probability is high.

Some drugs with only minimal anticholinergic properties some-

times cause difficulties if given with other anticholinergics. A patient on **isopropamide iodide** (an anticholinergic antispasmodic) only developed urinary retention needing catheterization when additionally given 75 mg **trazodone** daily, but not with either drug alone.[1] **Trazodone** is usually regarded as having little or no anticholinergic effects.

If the central anticholinergic syndrome caused by the use of anticholinergic drugs is not clearly recognised for what it is, there is the risk that **neuroleptic (antipsychotic) agents** will be additionally prescribed. Many of these also have anticholinergic side-effects so that matters are simply made worse. If the patient then demonstrates dystonias, akathisia, tremor and rigidity, even more anticholinergics may be added to control the extrapyramidal effects, which merely adds to the continuing downward spiral of drug-induced problems.

In addition to the obvious and very well recognised drugs with anticholinergic effects, a study of the 25 drugs most commonly prescribed for the elderly identified detectable anticholinergic activity (using an anticholinergic radioreceptor assay) in 14 of them, 9 of which (**ranitidine, codeine, dipyridamole, warfarin, isosorbide, theophylline, nifedipine, digoxin,** and **prednisolone**) have been shown to cause significant impairment in tests of memory and attention in the elderly.[2] Thus the problem may not necessarily be confined to those drugs which have well recognised anticholinergic properties. See also 'Antipsychotics + Anticholinergics', p.692.

1. Chan CH, Ruskiewicz RJ. Anticholinergic side effects of trazodone combined with another pharmacological agent. *Am J Psychiatry* (1990) 147, 533.
2. Tune L, Carr S, Hoag E, Cooper T. Anticholinergic effects of drugs commonly prescribed for the elderly: potential means for assessing risk of delirium. *Am J Psychiatry* (1992) 149, 1393–4.

Anticholinergics + Betel nuts (Areca)

The control of the extrapyramidal (parkinsonian) side-effects of fluphenazine and flupenthixol with procyclidine was lost in two patients when they began to chew betel nuts.

Clinical evidence

An Indian patient on depot **fluphenazine** (50 mg every three weeks) for schizophrenia, and with mild parkinsonian tremor controlled with **procyclidine** (5 mg twice daily), developed marked rigidity, bradykinesia and jaw tremor when he began to chew **betel nuts**. The symptoms were so severe he could barely speak. When he stopped chewing the nuts his stiffness and abnormal movements disappeared. Another patient on **flupenthixol** developed marked stiffness, tremor and akathisia, despite taking up to 20 mg **procyclidine** daily, when he began to chew **betel nuts**. The symptoms vanished within 4 days of stopping the nuts.[1]

Mechanism

Betel nuts contain arecoline which mimics the actions of acetylcholine. It seems that the arecoline opposed the actions of the anticholinergic procyclidine which was being used to control the extrapyramidal side-effects of the two antipsychotics, thereby allowing these side-effects to emerge.

Importance and management

Direct information seems to be limited to this report but the interaction would seem to be established and clinically important. Patients taking anticholinergic drugs for the control of drug-induced extrapyramidal (Parkinson-like) symptoms or Parkinson's disease should avoid betel nuts. The authors of this report suggest that a dental inspection for the characteristic red stains of the betel may possibly provide a simple explanation for the sudden and otherwise mysterious deterioration in the symptoms of patients from Asia and the East Indies.

1. Deahl M. Betel nut-induced extrapyramidal syndrome: an unusual drug interaction. *Mov Disord* (1989) 4, 330–3.

Apomorphine + Miscellaneous drugs

The hypotensive side-effects of apomorphine may possibly be increased by nitrates or alcohol. The concurrent use of other drugs used for erectile dysfunction or dopamine agonists or antagonists is not recommended. There is evidence that ACE inhibitors, alpha blockers, antidepressants, anticonvulsants, beta-blockers, calcium channel blockers, domperidone, ondansetron and prochlorperazine do not interact adversely. See also 'Levodopa + Apomorphine', p.418.

Clinical evidence, mechanism, importance and management

Apomorphine is a non-analgesic morphine derivative which stimulates dopamine receptors (predominantly D_2) and is used for parkinsonism and also for erectile dysfunction. In both situations it acts on dopamine receptors within the brain. For parkinsonism the apomorphine is usually given subcutaneously,[1] while for erectile dysfunction there is a sublingual preparation.[2] There appear to be no clinical reports of severe adverse interactions but the makers of apomorphine preparations for both conditions issue warnings about possible interactions and some information about drugs which do not interact.

(a) Alcohol

The makers say that interaction studies in volunteers given apomorphine for erectile dysfunction found that **alcohol** increased the incidence and extent of hypotension (one of the side-effects of apomorphine). They also point out that alcohol can diminish sexual performance.[2]

(b) Antidepressants, Anticonvulsants

The makers say that there are no adverse reports about interactions between apomorphine and either **antidepressants** or **anticonvulsants**, and no studies have been undertaken, but clinical experience suggests that no interaction occurs.[2]

(c) Antinauseants

It is standard practice to give **domperidone** (usually 20 mg three times daily) as an antinauseant for 2–3 days before giving apomorphine (usually subcutaneously in doses of 3–30 mg) for the treatment of the disabling motor fluctuations which can occur in Parkinson's disease.[1] The need for the antinauseant is because apomorphine can trigger the chemoreceptors within the vomiting centre in the brain. The smaller doses of apomorphine used for erectile dysfunction (2 to 3 mg) do not normally cause vomiting, but nausea does occur in about 7% of patients and the makers say that interaction studies and/or clinical experience show that **domperidone**, **ondansetron** or **prochlorperazine** may safely be given concurrently as antinauseants.[2] Studies with other antinauseants have not been carried out so at the moment concurrent use is not recommended.[2]

(d) Nitrates and antihypertensives

The makers report that in a group of 40 patients given 5 mg apomorphine sublingually for erectile dysfunction and given **nitrates** (not specifically named), 4 of them experienced vasovagal symptoms and significant standing blood pressure decreases (i.e. they felt faint and dizzy). The dose used was slightly higher than the recommended 2- to 3-mg dose. On the basis of this study the makers suggest ". . . caution . . ." which in practice means telling patients what may possibly happen and what to do (to lie down).[2] Parallel studies in patients taking **ACE inhibitors**, **alpha blockers**, **beta-blockers** or **calcium channel blockers** found no significant interactions.[2]

(e) Other dopamine agonists or antagonists

The makers say that apomorphine should not be given with other centrally-acting dopamine agonists and antagonists[2] because potentially they may interact at dopamine receptors. Such drugs would include some **antipsychotics** but thus far clinical reports of problems seem to be lacking.

(f) Other drugs used for erectile dysfunction

The makers say that no formal studies have been done with a combination of apomorphine and other drugs used for erectile dysfunction but there seems to be no evidence of problems, nevertheless they do not recommend concurrent use.[2] The other drugs used for this condition would include **alprostadil, moxisylyte, papaverine/phentolamine** and **sildenafil**.

1. APO-go (Apomorphine). Britannia Pharmaceuticals Ltd. Summary of Product Characteristics, January 2000.
2. Uprima (Apomorphine). Abbott Laboratories Ltd. Summary of Product Characteristics, May 2001.

Bromocriptine + Alcohol

There is some very limited evidence that the adverse effects of bromocriptine may possibly be increased by alcohol.

Clinical evidence, mechanism, importance and management

Intolerance to **alcohol** has been briefly mentioned in a report about patients taking bromocriptine for acromegaly.[1] In another report 2 patients with high prolactin levels were said to have developed the side-effects of bromocriptine, even in low doses, while continuing to drink.[2] When they abstained, the frequency and the severity of the side-effects fell, even with higher doses of bromocriptine. This, it is suggested, may be due to some **alcohol**-induced increase in the sensitivity of dopamine receptors.[1] No other reports of this interaction have been traced.[3] There would seem to be little reason, on the basis of this extremely sparse evidence, to tell all patients on bromocriptine not to drink, but it would be reasonable to warn them to avoid **alcohol** if side-effects develop.

1. Wass JAH, Thorner MO, Morris DV, Rees LH, Mason AE, Besser EM. Long-term treatment of acromegaly with bromocriptine. *BMJ* (1977) 1, 875.
2. Ayres J, Maisey MN. Alcohol increases bromocriptine's side effects. *N Engl J Med* (1980) 302, 806.
3. Hunt M (Sandoz). Personal communication (1990).

Bromocriptine + Griseofulvin

Evidence from a single case where bromocriptine was being used for acromegaly suggests that its effects can be opposed by griseofulvin.

Clinical evidence, mechanism, importance and management

The effects of bromocriptine, used for the treatment of acromegaly, were blocked when a patient was given **griseofulvin** for the treatment of a mycotic infection.[1] The mechanism of this interaction and its general importance are unknown, but prescribers should be aware of it when treating patients with bromocriptine.

1. Schwinn G, Dirks H, McIntosh C, Köbberling J. Metabolic and clinical studies on patients with acromegaly treated with bromocriptine over 22 months. *Eur J Clin Invest* (1977) 7, 101–7.

Bromocriptine + Levodopa/Carbidopa

An isolated report describes a patient who developed the serotonin syndrome when levodopa/carbidopa was added to treatment with bromocriptine.

Clinical evidence

A patient with parkinsonism who had been taking 60 mg bromocriptine daily for nearly 3 years, was additionally started on **levodopa/carbidopa** (25/250 mg daily increasing over a week to 75/750 mg) while the bromocriptine dose was reduced to 20 mg daily. On the seventh day he developed shivering, myoclonus, hyper-reflexia, clonus, tremor, diaphoresis, anxiety, diarrhoea, tachycardia and had a temperature of 37.9°C with a blood pressure of 180/100 mmHg. Serotonin syndrome was suspected and the patient was treated with the 5-HT antagonist methysergide to which he responded.[1]

Mechanism

Not understood. The serotonin syndrome is thought to occur because of increased stimulation of the 5-HT receptors in the brainstem and spinal cord. A similar clinical picture occurs with neuroleptic malignant syndrome which can occur when a dopamine agonist like bromocriptine is withdrawn, however had this been the case the addition of a 5-HT antagonist would have been expected to worsen the condition.

Importance and management

This appears to be an isolated incident and not of general importance, but good monitoring is clearly important if these drugs are given concurrently.

1. Sandyk R. L-Dopa induced "serotonin syndrome" in a parkinsonian patient on bromocriptine. J Clin Psychopharmacol (1986) 6, 194–5.

Bromocriptine + Macrolide antibacterials

Bromocriptine toxicity occurred in an elderly man when given josamycin and in an elderly woman given erythromycin. Two reports found that erythromycin causes an increase in serum bromocriptine levels.

Clinical evidence

(a) Erythromycin

250 mg **erythromycin estolate** four times daily for 4 days caused a marked change in the pharmacokinetics of a single 5-mg oral dose of bromocriptine in 5 normal subjects. The clearance of the bromocriptine was decreased by 70.6%, the peak serum levels were raised by 460% and the AUC was increased by 268%.[1,2]

Another report describes 2 women on levodopa and bromocriptine for parkinsonism which was better controlled when **erythromycin** was added. Bromocriptine serum levels were found to be 40–50% higher.[3] An elderly woman on levodopa and bromocriptine developed psychotic symptoms which were attributed to bromocriptine toxicity when treated with **erythromycin**.[4]

(b) Josamycin

An elderly man with Parkinson's disease, well-controlled for 10 months on daily treatment with levodopa (and benserazide) 200 mg, bromocriptine 70 mg and domperidone 60 mg, was additionally given 2 g **josamycin** daily for a respiratory infection. Shortly after the first dose he became drowsy with visual hallucinations, and began to show involuntary movements of his limbs similar to the dystonic and dyskinetic movements seen in choreoathetosis. These adverse effects (interpreted as bromocriptine toxicity) disappeared within a few days of withdrawing the antibacterial.[5]

Mechanism

Not understood. One suggestion is that these macrolides inhibit the metabolism of the bromocriptine by the liver, thereby reducing its loss from the body and raising its serum levels.[5]

Importance and management

Information seems to be limited to these reports. Concurrent use should be well monitored if either of these macrolide antibacterials is added to bromocriptine treatment. Moderately increased bromocriptine levels may be therapeutically advantageous, but grossly elevated levels can be toxic. There seems to be no direct evidence about any other macrolides, but some of them certainly inhibit liver metabolism and can raise the serum levels of other drugs.

1. Nelson MV, Berchou RC, Kareti D, LeWitt PA. Pharmacokinetic evaluation of erythromycin and caffeine administered with bromocriptine in normal subjects. Clin Pharmacol Ther (1990), 47,166.
2. Nelson MV, Berchou RC, Kareti D, LeWitt PA. Pharmacokinetic evaluation of erythromycin and caffeine administered with bromocriptine. Clin Pharmacol Ther (1990) 47, 694–7.
3. Sibley WA, Laguna JF. Enhancement of bromocriptine clinical effect and plasma levels with erythromycin. Excerpta Med (1981) 548, 329–30.
4. Alegre M, Noé E, Martínez Lage JM. Psicosis por interacción de eritromicina con bromocriptina en enfermedad de Parkinson. Neurologia (1997) 12, 429.
5. Montastruc JL, Rascol A. Traitement de la maladie de Parkinson par doses élevées de bromocriptine: interaction possible avec la josamycine. Presse Med (1984) 13, 2267–8.

Bromocriptine + Sympathomimetics

A healthy woman taking bromocriptine developed very severe headache and marked hypertension after additionally taking phenylpropanolamine. Another woman developed seizures with cerebral vasospasm, and a third developed a severe headache, hypertension and severe cardiac dysfunction after additionally taking isometheptene. Yet another developed psychosis when pseudoephedrine was added.

Clinical evidence

Two normal healthy women who had given birth 3–4 days previously, developed severe headaches while taking bromocriptine (2.5 mg twice daily) for milk suppression. After additionally taking three one-hourly 65-mg doses of **isometheptene mucate** (a sympathomimetic), the headache of one of them markedly worsened, and hypertension with life-threatening ventricular tachycardia and cardiac dysfunction developed. The other developed seizures and cerebral vasospasm after taking two 75-mg doses of **phenylpropanolamine**.[1]

A woman of 32 uneventfully took two 5-mg doses of bromocriptine for milk suppression following the birth of a child. Within 2 h of taking a third dose with two tablets of *Neozep* (**phenylpropanolamine** 25 mg, paracetamol (acetaminophen) 150 mg, salicylamide 150 mg, chlorphenamine (chlorpheniramine) 2 mg, ascorbic acid 25 mg in each tablet) for allergic rhinitis, she awoke with a very severe headache and was found to have a blood pressure of 240/140 mmHg. She was given 5 mg intramuscular morphine and her blood pressure became normal within 24 h. Another 5-mg dose of bromocriptine taken 48 h later had the same effect (this time no *Neozep* was taken) but the blood pressure rise was less severe (160/120 mmHg).[2]

A woman who had recently given birth and who had taken bromocriptine 2.5 mg twice daily for 9 days without problems became psychotic shortly after starting 60 mg **pseudoephedrine** four times daily.[3]

Mechanisms

Not understood. Severe hypertension occasionally occurs with both bromocriptine and phenylpropanolamine when given alone. Shortly after giving birth some individuals also show increased vascular reactivity, and it could be that all of these factors conspired together to cause these adverse effects.[2] Psychosis occasionally occurs after giving birth or on bromocriptine alone, so that the addition of pseudoephedrine may have been coincidental.[3]

Importance and management

Direct information seems to be limited to these four cases, but the severity of the reactions suggests that it might be prudent for other patients to avoid sympathomimetics like these while taking bromocriptine. More study is needed.

1. Kulig K, Moore LL, Kirk M, Smith D, Stallworth J, Rumack B. Bromocriptine-associated headache: possible life-threatening sympathomimetic interaction. Obstet Gynecol (1991) 78, 941–3.
2. Chan JCN, Critchley JAJH, Cockram CS. Postpartum hypertension, bromocriptine and phenylpropanolamine. Drug Invest (1994) 8, 254–6.
3. Reeves RR, Pinkofsky HB. Postpartum psychosis induced by bromocriptine and pseudoephedrine. J Fam Pract (1997) 45, 164–6.

Levodopa + Antacids

Antacids appear not to interact significantly with levodopa, except possibly with one slow-release preparation, the bioavailability of which is reduced.

Clinical evidence, mechanism, importance and management

Levodopa can be metabolised in the stomach so that, in theory at least, antacids which increase gastric emptying might decrease this 'wasteful' metabolism and increase the amounts available for absorption. This would seem to be confirmed by one study which found that an **aluminium-magnesium hydroxide** antacid raised peak serum levodopa levels and they occurred sooner.[1,2] However no interaction was seen when **magaldrate** was used,[3] nor in a study in 15 parkinsonian patients taking bromocriptine, levodopa and carbidopa who were given six 30-ml doses of **aluminium hydroxide** (*Mylanta*) daily. No effect was seen on the fluctuations in response to levodopa which normally occur.[4] However in another study using *Madopar HBS*, a sustained release preparation of levodopa and benserazide, the concurrent use of an **un-named antacid** reduced the bioavailability by about one-third.[5] The overall picture is that concurrent use need not be avoided, but the outcome should be monitored.

1. Rivera-Calimlim L, Dujovne CA, Morgan JP, Lasagna L, Bianchine JR. Absorption and metabolism of L-dopa by the human stomach. *Eur J Clin Invest* (1971) 1, 313–20.
2. Pocelinko GBT, Solomon HM. The effect of an antacid on the absorption and metabolism of levodopa. *Clin Pharmacol Ther* (1972) 13, 149.
3. Leon AS, Spiegel HE. The effect of antacid administration on the absorption and metabolism of levodopa. *J Clin Pharmacol* (1972) 12, 263.
4. Lau E, Waterman K, Glover R, Schulzer M, Calne DB. Effect of antacid on levodopa therapy. *Clin Neuropharmacol* (1986) 9, 477–9.
5. Malcolm SL, Allen JG, Bird H, Quinn NP, Marion MH, Marsden CD, O'Leary CG. Single dose pharmacokinetics of Madopar HBS in patients and effect of food and antacid on the absorption of Madopar HBS in volunteers. *Eur Neurol* (1987) 27 (Suppl 1), 28–35.

Levodopa + Anticholinergics

Although anticholinergic drugs are very widely used in conjunction with levodopa, they may reduce the absorption of levodopa and reduce its therapeutic effects to some extent.

Clinical evidence

A study in 6 normal subjects and 6 patients with Parkinson's disease showed that the administration of **trihexyphenidyl (benzhexol)** lowered the peak serum levels and reduced the absorption of levodopa in about half of the subjects by an average of 16–20%.[1]

A patient who needed 7 g levodopa daily while taking **homatropine** developed levodopa toxicity when the **homatropine** was withdrawn, and he was subsequently restabilised on 4 g levodopa daily.[2] This interaction is described in another report.[3]

Mechanism

Anticholinergics delay gastric emptying which gives the gastric mucosa more time to metabolise the levodopa 'wastefully' so that less is available for absorption in the small intestine.[4]

Importance and management

Anticholinergics are almost certainly the most commonly co-administered drugs with levodopa (one study[1] suggests that the incidence may be as much as 50%), but be alert for any evidence of a reduced levodopa response if anticholinergics are added, or for levodopa toxicity if they are withdrawn.

1. Algeri S, Cerletti C, Curcio M, Morselli PL, Bonollo L, Buniva G, Minazzi M, Minoli G. Effect of anticholinergic drugs on gastro-intestinal absorption of L-dopa in rats and in man. *Eur J Pharmacol* (1976) 35, 293–9.

2. Fermaglich J, O'Doherty DS. Effect of gastric motility on levodopa. *Dis Nerv Syst* (1972) 33, 624–5.
3. Birket-Smith E. Abnormal involuntary movements in relation to anticholinergics and levodopa therapy. *Acta Neurol Scand* (1975) 52, 158–60.
4. Rivera-Calimlim L, Dujovne CA, Morgan JP, Lasagna L, Bianchine JR. Absorption and metabolism of L-dopa by the human stomach. *Eur J Clin Invest* (1971) 1, 313–20.

Levodopa + Apomorphine

A pharmacokinetic study on one patient suggests that for the best control of parkinsonism the levodopa should be given when the 'on' period following apomorphine is over, and not before.

Clinical evidence

Subcutaneous **apomorphine** can be given on an 'on-demand' basis for the wearing off motor fluctuations in patients with parkinsonism, but because it can sometimes appear to be ineffective or delayed, a pharmacokinetic study was carried out in one patient to find out the optimum time to take the next dose of levodopa/carbidopa.

On 4 randomly assigned days the patient was given half of a 25/100 *Sinemet* tablet (levodopa/carbidopa) during the last third of an 'on' period following a 3 mg subcutaneous dose of **apomorphine**. Or the *Sinemet* was given after the end of the 'on' period. The levodopa AUC was 42.3 mg/l.min during the 'on' period, and 100.2 mg/l.min after the end of the 'on' period. The maximum serum levels of the levodopa were correspondingly approximately doubled and the time to reach maximum serum concentrations was about halved. The pharmacokinetics of the **carbidopa** were similar to those of levodopa.[1]

Mechanism

Uncertain, but the evidence points to a reduction in the absorption of the *Sinemet* from the gut caused by the apomorphine.

Importance and management

This study was carried out on just one patient, but the tentative conclusion was reached that when trying to maintain a patient in an 'on' state all day it would seem best to give the *Sinemet* after the end of the previous 'on' period with apomorphine, and not before. More study is needed.

1. Sampaio C, Branco MC, Rosa MM, Passarinho M, Castro-Caldas A. A pharmacokinetic interaction between subcutaneous apomorphine and levodopa/carbidopa (Sinemet®). *Clin Drug Invest* (1995) 9. 363–6.

Levodopa + Baclofen

Unpleasant side-effects have been seen (hallucinations, confusion, headache, nausea) in those on levodopa when given baclofen, and the symptoms of parkinsonism were worsened.

Clinical evidence

Twelve patients with parkinsonism on levodopa were additionally given **baclofen**. The eventual **baclofen** dosage was intended to be 90 mg daily but the side-effects were considerable (visual hallucinations, a toxic confusional state, headaches, nausea) so that only 2 reached this dosage, and 2 patients withdrew because they could not tolerate these side-effects. The mean dosage for those who continued was 45 mg daily. Rigidity was aggravated by an average of 46% and functional capacity deteriorated by 21%.[1]

A patient with paralysis agitans on *Sinemet* (levodopa + carbidopa), orphenadrine and diazepam became acutely confused, agitated, incontinent and hallucinated when given a third dose of **baclofen** (in all 15 mg). The **baclofen** was stopped but on the following night she again hallucinated and became confused. The next day she was given two 2.5-mg doses of **baclofen** but she became anxious and hallucinated with paranoid ideas.[2]

Mechanism

Not understood. One suggestion is that the baclofen deranges the dopamine metabolism.[2] The toxicity seen appears to be an exaggeration of the known side-effects of baclofen.

Importance and management

Information appears to be limited to these reports, but they suggest that baclofen is probably best avoided in patients taking levodopa.

1. Lees AJ, Shaw KM, Stern GM. Baclofen in Parkinson's disease. *J Neurol Neurosurg Psychiatry* (1978) 41, 707–8.
2. Skausig OB, Korsgaard S. Hallucinations and baclofen. *Lancet* (1977) 1, 1258.

Levodopa + Benzodiazepines

The therapeutic effects of levodopa can be reduced or abolished in some patients by the concurrent use of chlordiazepoxide, diazepam or nitrazepam.

Clinical evidence

Eight patients on levodopa were given various benzodiazepines, mostly in unstated doses, but said to be within the normal therapeutic range. No adverse interaction occurred in 3 given **chlordiazepoxide** or one given **oxazepam**, but a dramatic deterioration in the control of parkinsonism was seen in a man given 5 mg **diazepam** twice daily, from which he spontaneously recovered. Two out of 3 given **nitrazepam** also showed marked deterioration but failed to react in the same way when rechallenged with **nitrazepam** in 3 further tests.[1]

There are other reports of a loss in the control of the parkinsonism in 9 patients given **chlordiazepoxide**[2-6] and 3 patients given **diazepam**.[5] However another report says that **diazepam**, and especially **flurazepam**, are valuable for sleep induction and maintenance in patients on levodopa.[7]

Mechanism

Not understood.

Importance and management

Established and clinically important interactions but the incidence is uncertain. Apparently it only affects some patients. Concurrent use need not be avoided but monitor the outcome closely for any sign of deterioration in the control of the parkinsonism. Information about other benzodiazepines is lacking but it would seem reasonable to apply the same precautions. 75 mg **hydroxyzine** daily was found to be a non-interacting substitute for chlordiazepoxide in one patient.[6]

1. Hunter KR, Stern GM, Laurence DR. Use of levodopa with other drugs. *Lancet* (1970) ii, 1283.
2. Mackie L. Drug antagonism. *BMJ* (1971) 2, 651.
3. Schwartz GA, Fahn S. Newer medical treatments in parkinsonism. *Med Clin North Am* (1970) 54, 773.
4. Brogden RN, Speight TM, Avery GS. Levodopa: a review of its pharmacological properties and therapeutic use with particular reference to Parkinsonism. *Drugs* (1971) 2, 262.
5. Wodak J, Gilligan BS, Veale JL, Dowty BJ. Review of 12 months' treatment with L-dopa in Parkinson's disease with remarks on unusual side-effects. *Med J Aust* (1972) 2, 1277–82.
6. Yosselson-Superstine S, Lipman AG. Chlordiazepoxide interaction with levodopa. *Ann Intern Med* (1982) 96, 259–60.
7. Kales A, Ansel RD, Markham CH, Scharf MB, Tan T-L. Sleep in patients with Parkinson's disease and normal subjects prior to and following levodopa administration. *Clin Pharmacol Ther* (1971) 12, 397–406.

Levodopa + Beta-blockers

Concurrent use normally appears to be favourable, but the long-term effects of the elevated growth hormone levels are uncertain.

Clinical evidence, mechanism, importance and management

Most of the effects of combined use seem to be favourable. Dopamine derived from levodopa stimulates beta-receptors in the heart which can cause heart arrhythmias. These receptors are blocked by **propranolol**.[1] An enhancement of the effects of levodopa and a reduction in tremor in some[2] but not all patients taking oxprenolol or propranolol[3,4] have been described. However there is evidence that growth hormone levels are substantially raised,[5] but to what extent this might prove to be an adverse response during long-term treatment appears not to have been assessed.

1. Goldberg LI, Whitsett TL. Cardiovascular effects of levodopa. *Clin Pharmacol Ther* (1971) 12, 376.
2. Kissel P, Tridon P, Andre JM. Levodopa-propranolol therapy in parkinsonian tremor. *Lancet* (1974) ii, 403.
3. Sandler M, Fellows LE, Calne DB, Findley LJ. Oxprenolol and levodopa in parkinsonian patients. *Lancet* (1975) i, 168.
4. Marsden CD, Parkes JD, Rees JE. Propranolol in Parkinson's disease. *Lancet* (1974) ii, 410.
5. Camanni F, Massara F. Enhancement of levodopa-induced growth hormone stimulation by propranolol. *Lancet* (1974) i, 942.

Levodopa or Piribedil + Clonidine

Clonidine is reported to oppose the effects of levodopa or piribedil used to control Parkinson's disease.

Clinical evidence

A study in 7 patients (5 taking **piribedil** and 2 taking **levodopa with benserazide**) found that concurrent treatment with 1.5 mg **clonidine** daily for 10–24 days caused a worsening of the parkinsonism (an exacerbation of rigidity and akinesia). The concurrent use of anticholinergic drugs reduced the effects of this interaction.[1]

Another report on 10 hypertensive and 3 normotensive patients with Parkinson's disease, some of them taking **levodopa** and some of them not, claimed that concurrent treatment with **clonidine** did not affect the control of the parkinsonism, although 2 patients stopped taking the **clonidine** because of an increase in tremor and gait disturbance.[2]

Mechanism

Not understood. A suggestion is that the clonidine opposes the antiparkinson effects by stimulating alpha-receptors in the brain. Another idea is that the clonidine directly stimulates post-synaptic dopaminergic receptors.

Importance and management

Information seems to be limited to these reports. Be alert for a reduction in the control of the Parkinson's disease during concurrent use. The effects of this interaction appear to be reduced if anticholinergic drugs are also being used.

1. Shoulson I, Chase TN. Clonidine and the anti-parkinsonian response to L-dopa or piribedil. *Neuropharmacology* (1976) 15, 25–7.
2. Tarsy D, Parkes JD, Marsden CD. Clonidine in Parkinson disease. *Arch Neurol* (1975) 32, 134–6.

Levodopa + Dacarbazine

An isolated report describes a reduction in the effects of levodopa caused by dacarbazine.

Clinical evidence, mechanism, importance and management

A patient who had been treated surgically for melanoma in 1973, continued to have **dacarbazine** treatment (200 mg intravenously daily) for sporadic positive melanuria. He developed Parkinson's disease in 1978 for which levodopa was started in 1985, but he complained that its effects were reduced each time he was treated with **dacarbazine**: his daily living Schwab and England activities score fell by as much as 25%. A subsequent double-blind study on the patient using a modified Columbia Score confirmed that this was so.[1] The reasons are not understood, but since the serum dopamine levels remained unchanged it is suggested that competition between the two drugs at the blood-brain barrier may be the explanation.[1] Be alert for the need to increase the levodopa dosage if **dacarbazine** is used concurrently.

1. Merello M, Esteguy M, Perazzo F, Leiguarda R. Impaired levodopa response in Parkinson's disease during melanoma therapy. *Clin Neuropharmacol* (1992) 15, 69–74.

Levodopa or Bromocriptine + Domperidone

Domperidone be used to prevent nausea and vomiting caused by levodopa or bromocriptine used for parkinsonism, but it seems possible that it will oppose the effects of bromocriptine when used to reduce prolactin levels.

Clinical evidence, mechanism, importance and management

Domperidone is a dopamine antagonist, similar to metoclopramide, which can be used to control the nausea and vomiting associated with the treatment of Parkinson's disease with **levodopa** or **bromocriptine**. It acts on the dopamine receptors in the stomach wall and normally appears not to oppose the effects of **levodopa** within the brain because it does not readily cross the blood-brain barrier, although some extrapyramidal symptoms have been observed. It may even slightly increase the bioavailability and effects of **levodopa**.[1]

Domperidone raises prolactin levels, sometimes causing galactorrhoea,[2-4] gynaecomastia or mastalgia,[3,5] and may therefore be inappropriate for patients being treated with **bromocriptine** to reduce prolactin levels. This needs confirmation.

1. Shindler JS, Finnerty GT, Towlson K, Dolan AL, Davies CL, Parkes JD. Domperidone and levodopa in Parkinson's disease. *Br J Clin Pharmacol* (1984) 18, 959–62.
2. Cann PA, Read NW, Holdsworth CD. Galactorrhoea as a side effect of domperidone. *BMJ* (1983) 286, 1395–6.
3. Cann PA, Read NW, Holdsworth CD. Oral domperidone: double blind comparison with placebo in irritable bowel syndrome. *Gut* (1983) 24. 1135–40.
4. Moriga M. A multicentre double-blind study of domperidone and metoclopramide in the symptomatic control of dyspepsia. *Roy Soc Med Int Congr Symp Ser* (1981) 36, 77–9.
5. Van der Steen M, Du Caju MVL, Van Acker KJ. Gynaecomastia in a male infant given domperidone. *Lancet* (1982) 2, 884–5.

Levodopa + Entacapone

Entacapone increases the serum levels of levodopa. An apparently useful interaction.

Clinical evidence, mechanism, importance and management

A single 200-mg oral dose of **entacapone** given to 8 patients with parkinsonism on long-term treatment with levodopa/carbidopa raised the levodopa AUC by 46% and extended its elimination half-life from 1.5 to 2.0 h. The peak serum levels were not increased, but the overall serum levels remained higher for several hours. The cardiovascular autonomic responses to sympathetic and parasympathetic stimuli were unchanged.[1] The AUC of levodopa was increased up to 65% in another study in normal subjects, depending on the dosage of **entacapone** used (50–400 mg).[2] There would seem to be no reason for avoiding concurrent use, and the higher serum levodopa levels may possibly help parkinsonism patients with clinically fluctuating motor responses.

1. Myllylä VV, Sotaniemi KA, Illi A, Suominen K, Keränen T. Effect of entacapone, a COMT inhibitor, on the pharmacokinetics of levodopa and on cardiovascular responses in patients with Parkinson's disease. *Eur J Clin Pharmacol* (1993) 45, 419–23.
2. Keränen T, Gordin A, Harjola V-P, Karlsson M, Korpela K, Pentikäinen PJ, Rita H, Seppälä L, Wikberg T. The effect of catechol-*O*-methyl transferase inhibition by entacapone on the pharmacokinetics and metabolism of levodopa in healthy volunteers. *Clin Neuropharmacol* (1993) 16, 145–56.

Levodopa/Carbidopa + Ferrous sulphate

Ferrous sulphate can reduce the bioavailability of levodopa and carbidopa, and may possibly reduce the control of Parkinson's disease.

Clinical evidence

A study in 9 patients with Parkinson's disease showed that a single 325-mg dose of **ferrous sulphate** reduced the AUC of levodopa by 30% and of carbidopa by more than 75%. Some, but not all, of the patients showed some worsening in the control of their disease.[1]

In a previous study 8 normal subjects were given a single 250-mg dose of levodopa, with and without a single 325-mg dose of **ferrous sulphate**, and the serum levodopa levels were measured for the following 6 h. Peak serum levodopa levels were reduced by 55% (from 3.6 to 1.6 nmol/l) and the AUC was reduced by 51% (from 257 to 125 nmol.min/ml). Those subjects who had the highest peak levels and greatest absorption showed the greatest reductions when given **ferrous sulphate**.[2]

This interaction has also been demonstrated in *animal* experiments.[3]

Mechanism

Ferrous iron rapidly oxidizes to ferric iron at the pH values found in the gastrointestinal tract which then binds strongly to carbidopa and levodopa to form chelation complexes which are poorly absorbed.[2,4]

Importance and management

Information appears to be limited to these studies. The importance of this interaction in patients taking both drugs chronically awaits further study, but the extent of the reductions in absorption (30–50%) and the hint of worsening control[1] suggests that this interaction may be of clinical importance. Be alert for any evidence of this. Increasing the levodopa or carbidopa dosage or separating the administration of the iron as much as possible may prove to be effective. More study is needed.

1. Campbell NRC, Rankine D, Goodridge AE, Hasinoff BB, Kara M. Sinemet-ferrous sulphate interaction in patients with Parkinson's disease. *Br J Clin Pharmacol* (1990) 30, 599–605.
2. Campbell NRC, Hasinoff B. Ferrous sulfate reduces levodopa bioavailability: chelation as a possible mechanism. *Clin Pharmacol Ther* (1989) 45, 220–5.
3. Campbell RRA, Hasinoff B, Chernenko G, Barrowman J, Campbell NRC. The effect of ferrous sulfate and pH on L-dopa absorption. *Can J Physiol Pharmacol* (1990) 68, 603–7.
4. Greene RJ, Hall AD, Hider RC. The interaction of orally administered iron with levodopa and methyldopa therapy. *J Pharm Pharmacol* (1990) 42, 502–4.

Levodopa and Amantadine + Fluoxetine

Concurrent use can be beneficial although sometimes parkinsonian symptoms are worsened.

Clinical evidence

Four patients on levodopa (440–990 mg daily), a dopamine decarboxylase inhibitor (drug and dose not stated) and amantadine (dose not stated), showed a deterioration in the control of their parkinsonism when additionally given 20 mg **fluoxetine** daily. The **fluoxetine** was withdrawn and their motor performance was restored. The antidepressant efficacy of **fluoxetine** was however found to be substantial in all 4 patients.[1] In a retrospective survey of 23 parkinsonian patients who were given **fluoxetine** (up to 40 mg daily), 20 showed no worsening of their parkinsonism but in 3 others it worsened to a mild degree.[2]

Mechanism

Not understood. Extrapyramidal effects are recognised side effects of fluoxetine.

Importance and management

Although the information is limited it seems that fluoxetine can be of benefit in treating depression in patients with Parkinson's disease, but in some cases parkinsonism is worsened. Monitor the outcome and withdraw the fluoxetine if necessary.

1. Jansen Steur ENH. Increase of Parkinson disability after fluoxetine medication. *Neurology* (1993) 43, 211–3.
2. Caley CF, Freiman JH. Does fluoxetine exacerbate Parkinson's disease? *J Clin Psychiatry* (1992) 53, 278–282.

Levodopa + Food

The fluctuations in response to levodopa experienced by some patients may be due to timing of meals and the kind of diet, particularly the protein content, both of which can reduce the effects of levodopa.

Clinical evidence

(a) Changes in absorption

A study[1] in patients with Parkinson's disease treated with levodopa showed that if taken with a **meal**, the mean absorption of the levodopa from the gut and the peak plasma levels were reduced by 27 and 29% respectively, and the peak serum level was delayed by 34 min. Another study showed that peak serum levodopa levels were reduced if taken with **food** rather than when fasting.[2] A study in normal subjects found that a **low protein meal** caused a small reduction in absorption.[3]

(b) Changes in response

A study showed that **glycine** and **lysine** given to 4 patients receiving levodopa as a constant intravenous infusion had no effect, but **phenylalanine**, **leucine** and **isoleucine** reduced the clinical response although the serum levodopa levels remained unchanged.[1]

Other studies have shown that a high daily intake of **protein** reduces the effects of levodopa, compared with the situation when the intake of **protein** is low.[4-6]

Mechanisms

(a) Meals which delay gastric emptying allow the levodopa to be exposed to 'wasteful' metabolism in the gut which reduces the amount available for absorption. In addition (b) some large neutral amino acids arising from the digestion of proteins can compete with levodopa for transport into the brain so that the therapeutic response may be reduced, whereas other amino acids do not have this effect.[1,3,5]

Importance and management

An established interaction, but unpredictable. Since the fluctuations in the response of patients to levodopa may be influenced by what is eaten, and when, a change in the pattern of drug and food administration on a trial-and-error basis may be helpful. Multiple small doses of levodopa and distributing the intake of proteins may also iron out the effects of these interactions. Diets which conform to the recommended daily allowance of protein (0.8 g/kg body weight) are reported to eliminate this adverse drug-food interaction.[5]

1. Anon. Timing of meals may affect clinical response to levodopa. *Am Pharm* (1985) 25, 34–5.
2. Morgan JP, Bianchine JR, Spiegel HE, Nutley NJ, Rivera-Calimlim L, Hersey RM. Metabolism of levodopa in patients with Parkinson's disease. *Arch Neurol* (1971) 25, 39–44.
3. Robertson DRC, Higginson I, Macklin BS, Renwick AG, Waller DG, George CF. The influence of protein containing meals on the pharmacokinetics of levodopa in healthy volunteers. *Br J Clin Pharmacol* (1991) 31, 413–7.
4. Gillespie NG, Mena I, Cotzias GC, Bell MA. Diets affecting treatment of parkinsonism with levodopa. *J Am Diet Assoc* (1973) 62, 525–8.
5. Juncos JL, Fabbrini G, Mouradian MM, Serrati C, Chase TN. Dietary influences on the antiparkinsonian response to levodopa. *Arch Neurol* (1987) 44, 1003–5.
6. Carter JH, Nutt JG, Woodward WR, Hatcher LF, Trotman TL. Amount and distribution of dietary protein affects clinical response to levodopa in Parkinson's disease. *Neurology* (1989) 39, 552–6.

Levodopa + Isoniazid

There is evidence that isoniazid can reduce the control of Parkinson's disease with levodopa, apparently by reducing its serum levels. An isolated case report describes hypertension, tachycardia, flushing and tremor in a patient attributed to concurrent use.

Clinical evidence

Following the observation that the levodopa-induced choreic dyskinesias of one patient were reduced by **isoniazid**, a further study was made in 20 others. It was found that **isoniazid** (average dose 290 mg) reduced the dyskinesias of 18 of them, but it was accompanied by an intolerable worsening of the parkinsonism. Control of the parkinsonism was restored when the **isoniazid** was stopped.[1] Another patient similarly showed a deterioration in the control of parkinsonism when given **isoniazid**/rifampicin (*Rifinah*). When the antituberculars were stopped, the patient's motor performance improved (lengthened by 75%), the levodopa AUC rose by 37%, its half-life lengthened by 103% while the maximum serum levels fell by 33%.[2]

An isolated report describes a patient on levodopa who developed hypertension, agitation, tachycardia, flushing and severe non-parkinsonian tremor after starting to take **isoniazid**. He recovered when the **isoniazid** was stopped.[3]

Mechanism

Not understood. Metabolic studies in one patient suggest that isoniazid inhibits dopa-decarboxylase.[2] The isolated case of hypertension and tachycardia is also not understood.

Importance and management

Information seems to be limited to the reports cited, which is somewhat surprising bearing in mind how long both drugs have been available. If concurrent use is thought to be necessary, be alert for any evidence of a reduction in the control of the parkinsonism. It would seem logical to accommodate this interaction by increasing the levodopa dosage, but nobody seems to have tried this. More study is needed. The isolated case seems not to be of general importance.

1. Gershanik DS, Luquin MR, Scipioni O, Obeso JA. Isoniazid therapy in Parkinson's disease. *Mov Disord* (1988) 3, 133–9.
2. Wenning GK, O'Connell MT, Patsalos PN, Quinn NP. A clinical and pharmacokinetic case study of an interaction of levodopa and antituberculous therapy in Parkinson's disease. *Mov Disord* (1995) 10, 644–7.
3. Morgan JP. Isoniazid and levodopa. *Ann Intern Med* (1980) 92, 434.

Levodopa + Methionine

The effects of levodopa can be reduced by methionine.

Clinical evidence

Fourteen patients with Parkinson's disease and treated with levodopa were given a **low-methionine** diet for a period of 8 days. Five out of 7 then given 4.5 g **methionine** daily showed a definite worsening of the symptoms (gait, tremor, rigidity, etc.) which ceased when the **methionine** was withdrawn. Three out of 7 given a placebo showed some subjective improvement.[1] This report confirms the results of a previous study.[2]

Mechanism

Uncertain. One idea is that the methionine competes with the levodopa for active transport into the brain so that its effects are reduced.

Importance and management

Information is very limited but it indicates that large doses of methionine should be avoided in patients being treated with levodopa.

1. Pearce LA, Waterbury LD. L-methionine: a possible levodopa antagonist. *Neurology* (1974) 24, 640–1.
2. Pearce LA, Waterbury LD. L-methionine: a possible levodopa antagonist. *Neurology* (1971) 21, 410.

Levodopa + Methyldopa

Methyldopa can increase the effects of levodopa and permit a reduction in the dosage in some patients, but it can also worsen dyskinesias in others. A small increase in the hypotensive actions of methyldopa may also occur.

Clinical evidence

(a) Effects on the response to levodopa

A double-blind crossover trial in 10 patients with Parkinson's disease who had been taking levodopa for 12–40 months, showed that the optimum daily dose of levodopa, 5.5 g, fell by 78% when using the highest doses of **methyldopa** studied (1920 mg daily) and by 50% with 800 mg **methyldopa** daily.[1]

A one-third[2] and a two-thirds[3] reduction in the levodopa dosage during concurrent treatment with **methyldopa** have been described in other reports. Another report states that the control of Parkinson's disease in some patients improved during concurrent use, but worsened the dyskinesias in others.[4] **Methyldopa** on its own can cause a reversible parkinsonian-like syndrome.[5-7]

(b) Effects on the response to methyldopa

A study in 18 patients with Parkinson's disease showed that levodopa and **methyldopa** taken together lowered the blood pressure in doses which, when given singly, did not alter the pressure. Daily doses of 1–2.5 g levodopa with 500 mg **methyldopa** caused a 12/6 mmHg fall in blood pressure. No change in the control of the Parkinson's disease was seen, but the study lasted only a few days.[8]

Mechanism

Not understood.[9] (a) One idea is that the methyldopa inhibits the enzymic destruction of levodopa outside the brain so that more is available to exert its therapeutic effects. Another is that a false neurotransmitter produced from methyldopa opposes the effects of levodopa. (b) The increased hypotension may simply be due to the additive effects of the two drugs.

Importance and management

Well documented, but the picture presented is a little confusing. Concurrent use need not be avoided but the outcome should be well monitored. The use of methyldopa may allow a reduction in the dosage of the levodopa (the reports cited[1-3] quote figures of between 30 and 78%) and may enhance the control of Parkinson's disease, but it should also be borne in mind that in some patients the control may be worsened. The increased hypotensive effects seem to be small but they too should be checked.

1. Fermaglich J, Chase TN. Methyldopa or methyldopahydrazine as levodopa synergists. *Lancet* (1973) i, 1261–2.
2. Mones KJ. Evaluation of alpha methyl dopa and alpha methyl dopa hydrazine with L-dopa therapy. *N Y State J Med* (1974) 74, 47–51.
3. Fermaglich J, O'Doherty DS. Second generation of L-dopa therapy. *Neurology* (1971) 21, 408.
4. Sweet RD, Lee JE, McDowell FH. Methyldopa as an adjunct to levodopa treatment of Parkinson's disease. *Clin Pharmacol Ther* (1972) 13, 23–7.
5. Groden BM. Parkinsonism occurring with methyldopa treatment. *BMJ* (1963) 2, 1001.
6. Peaston MJT. Parkinsonism associated with alpha-methyldopa therapy. *BMJ* (1964) 2, 168.
7. Strang RR. Parkinsonism occurring during methyldopa therapy. *Can Med Assoc J* (1966) 95, 928.
8. Gibberd FB, Small E. Interaction between levodopa and methyldopa. *BMJ* (1973) 2, 90–1.
9. Smith SE. The pharmacological actions of 3,4-dihydroxy-phenyl-alpha-methylalanine (alpha-methyldopa), an inhibitor of 5-hydroxytryptophan decarboxylase. *Br J Pharmacol* (1960) 15, 319.

Levodopa + Metoclopramide

Some of the effects of levodopa are increased by metoclopramide and other effects are opposed. The outcome of concurrent use is uncertain.

Clinical evidence, mechanism, importance and management

Metoclopramide is a dopamine antagonist and occasionally it causes extrapyramidal disturbances (Parkinson-like symptoms) especially in children.[1] On the other hand **metoclopramide** opposes the effects of levodopa on stomach emptying which can result in an increase in the bioavailability of levodopa.[2,3] The outcome of these two opposite effects (reduced effects and increased bioavailability) is uncertain, but it would be prudent to monitor concurrent use. There seem to be no clinical reports describing an adverse interaction.

1. Castells-Van Daele M, Jaeken J, Van der Schueren P. Dystonic reactions in children caused by metoclopramide. *Arch Dis Child* (1970) 45, 130–3.
2. Berkowitz DM, McCallum RW. Interaction of levodopa and metoclopramide on gastric emptying. *Clin Pharmacol Ther* (1980) 27, 414–20.
3. Mearrick PT, Wade DN, Birkett DJ, Morris J. Metoclopramide, gastric emptying and L-dopa absorption. *Aust NZ J Med* (1974) 4, 144–8.

Levodopa + Mirtazapine

An isolated report describes the development of serious psychosis attributed to a levodopa/mirtazapine interaction.

Clinical evidence, mechanism, importance and management

A 44-year old woman with Parkinson's disease under treatment with levodopa, pergolide, selegiline and memantine was additionally started on **mirtazapine** in increasing doses rising from 15 to 60 mg over 24 days for moderate depression, labile mood, anxiety, social withdrawal and sleep disturbance. She initially improved but then major depression developed and on day 26 she attempted self-strangulation. She recovered when the **mirtazapine**, memantine and selegiline were stopped and low-dose clozapine started.[1]

1. Normann C, Hesslinger B, Frauenknecht S, Berger M, Walden J. Psychosis during chronic levodopa therapy triggered by the new antidepressant drug mirtazapine. *Pharmacopsychiatry* (1997) 30, 263–5.

Levodopa or Whole broad beans + Monoamine oxidase inhibitors (MAOIs)

A rapid, serious and potentially life-threatening hypertensive reaction can occur in patients on non-selective, irreversible MAOIs if given levodopa or if they eat whole broad beans which contain dopa, but no serious hypertensive reaction occurs with selective MAO-A inhibitors such as moclobemide (although the side effects may worsen). An interaction with compound levodopa preparations containing carbidopa or benserazide (*Sinemet, Madopar*) is unlikely. No serious acute interaction occurs with selegiline, a selective MAO-B inhibitor used as an adjunct to levodopa, but there is some evidence that chronic concurrent use may be associated with increased mortality.

Clinical evidence

(a) Levodopa + Non-selective, irreversible MAOIs

A patient who had been taking **phenelzine** daily for 10 days was given 50 mg **levodopa** by mouth. Within an hour his blood pressure had risen from 135/90 to about 190/130 mmHg, and despite the intravenous injection of 5 mg phentolamine it continued to rise over the next 10 min to 200/135 mmHg, before falling in response to a further 4 mg injection of phentolamine. Next day the experiment was repeated with 25 mg **levodopa** but no blood pressure changes were seen. Three weeks after withdrawal of the **phenelzine** even 500 mg **levodopa** had no effect on the blood pressure.[1]

Similar cases of severe and acute hypertension, accompanied in most instances by flushing, throbbing and pounding in the head, neck and chest, and lightheadedness have been described in other case reports and studies involving the concurrent use of **levodopa** with **pargyline**,[2] **nialamide**,[3,4] **tranylcypromine**,[4-6] **phenelzine**[7,8] and **isocarboxazid**.[9]

(b) Whole broad beans + Non-selective, irreversible MAOIs

A hypertensive reaction similar to the one described (a) above can occur in patients taking non-selective, irreversible **MAOIs** who have eaten **WHOLE cooked broad beans** (*Vicia faba L*), that is to say the beans with pods, the latter normally containing dopa.[10] The reports of this interaction involved **pargyline**[11] and **phenelzine**.[12]

(c) Levodopa + Selective MAO-A inhibitors (Moclobemide)

A study in 12 normal subjects given a single dose of *Madopar* (**levodopa + benserazide**) with 400 mg **moclobemide** daily found that headache, nausea and insomnia were increased, but no hypertensive reaction was seen.[13]

(d) Levodopa + Selective MAO-B inhibitors (Selegiline)

The combination of **levodopa** and **selegiline** has been very extensively used. No serious hypertensive reactions of the kind seen with non-selective MAOIs occurs, no adverse pharmacokinetic interactions take place,[14,15] any serious adverse interactions are said to be lacking,[16,17] the combination is claimed to be beneficial in modifying the fluctuating response to levodopa[18-21] and one large scale study of 941 patients over a 10 year period on **levodopa/benserazide** concluded that its combination with **selegiline** gave an improvement and a prolongation of life-expectancy.[22,23]

However in contrast, other studies of long-term combined treatment in very large numbers of patients reported minimal benefits,[19,24] that mortality was significantly greater,[24] and that **selegiline** actually accentuated the patient deterioration in early parkinsonism.[25] Urinary retention has also been suggested as being associated with this drug combination.[26]

Mechanism

Not fully understood. Levodopa is enzymically converted in the body, firstly to dopamine and then to norepinephrine (noradrenaline), both of which are normally under enzymic attack by monoamine oxidase. But in the presence of a MAOI this attack is suppressed which means that the total levels of dopamine and norepinephrine are increased. Precisely how this then leads to a sharp rise in blood pressure is not clear, but either dopamine or norepinephrine, or both, directly or indirectly stimulate the alpha-receptors of the cardiovascular system.

Importance and management

The interaction between the irreversible, older, non-selective MAOIs (listed in Table 18.1 in Chapter 18) and levodopa or whole broad beans is well documented, serious and potentially life-threatening. Patients should not be given levodopa during treatment with any of these MAOIs, whether used for depression or hypertension, and for a period of 2–3 weeks after their withdrawal. The same precautions apply to the eating of WHOLE cooked broad beans, the dopa being in the pods but not in the beans. If accidental ingestion occurs the hypertensive reaction can be controlled by the intravenous injection of an alpha-blocker such as phentolamine, or by chewing and swallowing with water the contents of a 10-mg nifedipine capsule. This interaction is inhibited in man by the presence of dopa decarboxylase inhibitors[5] such as carbidopa and benserazide (in *Sinemet* and *Madopar*) so that a serious interaction is unlikely to occur with these preparations, even so the makers continue to list the MAOIs among their contraindications.

No important acute adverse interaction appears to occur between levodopa and moclobemide but some side-effects can apparently occur.

No acute adverse interactions occur if levodopa and selegiline are given concurrently, but the makers say that if maximal doses of levodopa are used, involuntary movements and agitation may occur which will disappear if the levodopa dosage is reduced (about 30% is suggested). The evidence about chronic use is contradictory but clearly some doubts now exist about the benefits of combined use so that prescribers should bear this in mind before initiating therapy.

1. Hunter KR, Boakes AJ, Laurence DR, Stern GM. Monoamine oxidase inhibitors and L-dopa. *BMJ* (1970) 3, 388.
2. Hodge JV. Use of monoamine-oxidase inhibitors. *Lancet* (1965) i, 764–5.
3. Friend DG, Bell WR, Kline NS. The action of L-dihydroxyphenylalanine in patients receiving nialamide. *Clin Pharmacol Ther* (1965) 6, 362–6.
4. Horwitz D, Goldberg LI, Sjoerdsma A. Increased blood pressure responses to dopamine and norepinephrine produced by monoamine oxidase inhibitors in man. *J Lab Clin Med* (1960) 56, 747–53.
5. Teychenne PF, Calne DB, Lewis PJ, Findley LJ. Interactions of levodopa with inhibitors of monoamine oxidase and L-aromatic amino acid decarboxylase. *Clin Pharmacol Ther* (1975) 18, 273.
6. Sharpe J, Marquez-Julio A, Ashby P. Idiopathic orthostatic hypotension treated with levodopa and MAO inhibitor: a preliminary report. *Can Med Assoc J* (1972) 107, 296.
7. Schildkraut JJ, Klerman GL, Friend DG, Greenblatt M. Biochemical and pressor effects of oral D,L-dihydroxyphenylalanine in patients pretreated with antidepressant drugs. *Ann N Y Acad Sci* (1963) 107, 1005–15.
8. Kassirer JP, Kopelman RI. A modern medical Descartes. *Hosp Pract* (1987) September 15th, 17–25.
9. Birkmayer W, Hornykiewicz O. Archiv fur Psychiatrie und der Nervenkrankheiten vereinigt mit Zeitschrift fur die gasamte Psychiatrie und Neurologie (1962) 203, 560. Quoted in ref 1.
10. McQueen EG. Interactions with monoamine oxidase inhibitors. *BMJ* (1975) 3, 101.
11. Hodge JV, Nye ER, Emerson GW. Monoamine-oxidase inhibitors, broad beans, and hypertension. *Lancet* (1964) i, 1108.
12. Bromley DJ. Monoamine oxidase inhibitors. *Lancet* (1964) i, 1181.
13. Dingemanse J. An update of recent moclobemide interaction data. *Int Clin Psychopharmacol* (1993) 7, 167–80.
14. Roberts J, Waller DG, O'Shea NO, Macklin BS, Renwick AG. The effect of selegiline on the peripheral pharmacokinetics of levodopa in young volunteers. *Br J Clin Pharmacol* (1995) 40, 404–6.
15. Cedarbaum JM, Silvestri M, Clark M, Harts A, Kutt H. L-Deprenyl pharmacokinetics, and response fluctuations in Parkinson's disease. *Clin Neuropharmacol* (1990) 13, 29–35.
16. Birkmayer W, Riederer P, Ambrozi I, Youdim MBH. Implications of combined treatment with 'Madopar' and L-deprenil in Parkinson's disease. *Lancet* (1977) i, 439.
17. Elsworth JD, Glover V, Reynolds GP, Sandler M, Lees AJ, Phuapradit P, Shaw KM, Stern GM, Kumar P. Deprenyl administration in man: a selective monoamine oxidase B inhibitor without a 'cheese effect'. *Psychopharmacology (Berl)* (1978) 57, 33.
18. Shan DE, Yeh SI. An add-on study of selegiline to Madopar in the treatment of parkinsonian patients with dose-related fluctuations: comparison between Jumexal and Parkryl. *Zhonghua Yi Xue Za Zhi (Taipei)* (1996), 58, 264–8.
19. Brannan T, Yahr MD. Comparative-study of selegiline plus L-dopa–carbidopa versus L-dopa–carbidopa alone in the treatment of Parkinson's disease. *Ann Neurol* (1995) 37, 95–8.
20. Golbe LI, Lieberman AN, Muenter MD, Ahlslog JE, Gopinathan G, Neophytides AN, Foo SH, Duvoisin RC. Deprenyl in the treatment of symptom fluctuations in advanced Parkinson's disease. *Clin Neuropharmacol* (1988) 11, 45–55.

21. Presthus J, Berstad J, Lien K. Selegiline (l-deprenyl) and low-dose levodopa treatment of Parkinson's disease. *Acta Neurol Scand* (1987) 76, 200–3.

22. Birkmayer W, Birkmayer GD. Effect of (–)deprenyl in long-term treatment of Parkinson's disease. A 10-years experience. *J Neural Transm* (1986) 22 (Suppl), 219–25.

23. Birkmayer W, Knoll J, Riederer P, Youdim MBH, Hars V, Marton J. Increased life expectancy resulting from addition of L-deprenyl to Madopar® treatment in Parkinson's disease: a longterm study. *J Neural Transm* (1985) 64, 113–127.

24. Parkinson's Disease Research Group of the United Kingdom. Comparison of therapeutic effects and mortality data of levodopa and levodopa combined with selegiline in patients with early, mild Parkinson's disease. *BMJ* (1995) 311, 1602–7.

25. Olanow CW, Hauser RA, Gauger L, Malapira T, Koller W, Hubble J, Bushenbark K, Lilienfeld D, Esterlitz J. The effect of deprenyl and levodopa on the progression of Parkinson's disease. *Ann Neurol* (1995) 38, 771–7.

26. Waters H. Side effects of selegiline. *Geriatr Psychiatry Neurol* (1992) 5, 31–34.

Levodopa + Papaverine

There are case reports of a deterioration in the control of parkinsonism in patients treated with levodopa when given papaverine, but a controlled trial failed to confirm this interaction.

Clinical evidence

(a) Levodopa effects reduced

A woman with long-standing parkinsonism, well controlled on levodopa and later levodopa with benserazide, began to show a steady worsening of her parkinsonism within a week of additionally starting 100 mg **papaverine** daily. The deterioration continued until the **papaverine** was withdrawn. The normal response to levodopa returned within a week. Four other patients showed a similar response.[1]

Two other similar cases have been described in another report.[2]

(b) Levodopa effects unchanged

A double-blind crossover trial was carried out on 9 patients with parkinsonism being treated with levodopa (range 100–750 mg daily) plus a decarboxylase inhibitor. Two of them were also taking bromocriptine (40 mg daily) and two trihexyphenidyl (benzhexol) (15 mg daily). No changes in the control of their disease were seen when they were concurrently treated with 150 mg **papaverine** hydrochloride daily for three weeks.[3]

Mechanism

Not understood. One suggestion is that papaverine blocks the dopamine receptors in the striatum of the brain, thereby inhibiting the effects of the levodopa.[1,4] Another is that papaverine may have a reserpine-like action on the vesicles of adrenergic neurones.[1,5]

Importance and management

Direct information seems to be limited to the reports cited. Concurrent use can apparently be uneventful, however in the light of the reports of adverse interactions it would be prudent to monitor the outcome closely. Carefully controlled trials can provide a good picture of the general situation, but may not necessarily pick out the occasional patient who may be affected by an interaction.

1. Duvoisin RC. Antagonism of levodopa by papaverine. *JAMA* (1975) 231, 845.

2. Posner DM. Antagonism of levodopa by papaverine. *JAMA* (1975) 233, 768.

3. Montastruc JL, Rascol O, Belin J, Ane M, Rascol A. Does papaverine interact with levodopa in Parkinson's disease? *Ann Neurol* (1987) 22, 558–9.

4. Gonzalez-Vegas JA. Antagonism of dopamine-mediated inhibition in the nigro-striatal pathway: a mode of action of some catatonia-inducing drugs. *Brain Res* (1974) 80, 219–28.

5. Cebeddu LX and Weiner JA. Relationship between a granular effect and exocytic release of norepinephrine by nerve stimulation. *Pharmacologist* (1974) 16, 190.

Levodopa + Penicillamine

Penicillamine can raise serum levodopa levels in a few patients, and improve the control of the Parkinsonism, but the adverse effects of levodopa may be also be increased.

Clinical evidence, mechanism, importance and management

600 mg **penicillamine** daily increased the serum levodopa levels of a patient by almost 60% (from 3015 to 4760 ng/ml/h), and improved the control of the parkinsonian symptoms, but increased dyskinesia was also seen.[1] This patient[1] and two others[2] who also showed improvement, had low levels of serum copper and ceruloplasmin. It is not understood why **penicillamine** should have this effect on levodopa. Other patients with normal levels were found not to be affected by this interaction.[2]

This limited evidence therefore suggests that the concurrent use of levodopa and **penicillamine** need not be avoided, and some patients may be improved, but there does not seem to be any, or much, advantage in deliberately giving **penicillamine** if the same end can be achieved by raising the levodopa dosage. However if you give both drugs, monitor the effects.

1. Mizuta E, Kuno S. Effect of D-penicillamine on pharmacokinetics of levodopa in Parkinson's disease. *Clin Neuropharmacol* (1993) 16, 448–50.

2. Sato M, Yamane K, Oosawa Y, Tanaka H, Shirata A, Nagayama T, Maruyama S. Two cases of Parkinson's disease whose symptoms were markedly improved by D-penicillamine: a study on cases displaying a slightly low level of serum copper and ceruloplasmin. *Neurol Therap (Chiba)* (1992) 9, 555–9.

Levodopa + Phenothiazines or Butyrophenones

Phenothiazines and butyrophenones can oppose the effects of levodopa. The antipsychotic effects and extrapyramidal side-effects of the phenothiazines can be opposed by levodopa.

Clinical evidence, mechanism, importance and management

Phenothiazines (e.g. **chlorpromazine**) and **butyrophenones** (e.g. **haloperidol, droperidol**) block the dopamine receptors in the brain and can therefore upset the balance between cholinergic and dopaminergic components within the corpus striatum and substantia nigra. As a consequence they may not only induce the development of extrapyramidal (Parkinson-like) symptoms, but they can aggravate parkinsonism and antagonise the effects of levodopa used in its treatment.[1-3] Antiemetics such as **prochlorperazine**[1,2] and **trifluoperazine**[2] can behave in this way. For this reason drugs of this kind are generally regarded as contraindicated in patients under treatment for Parkinson's disease, or only used with great caution in carefully controlled conditions. Non-phenothiazine antiemetics which do not antagonise the effects of levodopa include **cyclizine** (*Marzine*) and **difenidol** (*Vontrol*).

The extrapyramidal symptoms which frequently occur with the **phenothiazines** have been treated with varying degrees of success with levodopa, but the levodopa may also antagonise the antipsychotic effects of the **phenothiazines**.[4,5]

1. Duvoisin R.C. Diphenidol for levodopa-induced nausea and vomiting. *JAMA* (1972) 221, 1408.

2. Campbell JB. Long-term treatment of Parkinson's disease with levodopa. *Neurology* (1970) 20, 18–22.

3. Klawans HL, Weiner WJ. Attempted use of haloperidol in the treatment of L-dopa induced dyskinesias. *J Neurol Neurosurg Psychiatry* (1974) 37, 427–30.

4. Yaryura-Tobias JA, Wolpert A, Dona L, Merlis S. Action of L-dopa in drug-induced extrapyramidalism. *Dis Nerv Syst* (1970) 1, 60–3.

5. Hunter KR, Stern GM, Laurence DR. Use of levodopa and other drugs. *Lancet* (1970) ii, 1283.

Levodopa + Phenylbutazone

A single case report describes antagonism of the effects of levodopa by phenylbutazone.

Clinical evidence, mechanism, importance and management

A patient who was very sensitive to levodopa found that only by taking frequent small doses (125 mg) was he able to prevent the involuntary movements of his tongue, jaw, neck and limbs. If these developed he was able to suppress them with **phenylbutazone**, but this also lessened the beneficial effect.[1] The reason is not understood. This interaction has not been confirmed by anyone else and its general importance is not known, but prescribers should be aware of this isolated case.

1. Wodak J, Gilligan BS, Veale JL, Dowty BJ. Review of 12 months' treatment with L-dopa in Parkinson's disease, with remarks on unusual side effects. *Med J Aust* (1972) 2, 1277–82.

Levodopa + Phenytoin

The therapeutic effects of levodopa can be reduced or abolished by the concurrent use of phenytoin.

Clinical evidence, mechanism, importance and management

In a study on 5 patients treated with levodopa (630–4600 mg plus 150–225 mg carbidopa daily) for Parkinson's disease, it was found that when they were additionally given **phenytoin** (100–500 mg daily) for 5–19 days the levodopa dyskinesias were relieved but the beneficial effects of the levodopa were also reduced or abolished. The patients became slow, rigidity re-emerged and some of them became unable to get out of a chair. Within 2 weeks of stopping the **phenytoin**, their parkinsonism was again well controlled by the levodopa.[1] The mechanism of this interaction is not understood. Information seems to be limited to this study, nevertheless it would seem prudent to avoid giving **phenytoin** to patients already taking levodopa. If both drugs are used it may be necessary to increase the dosage of the levodopa.

1. Mendez JS, Cotzias GC, Mena I, Papavasiliou PS. Diphenylhydantoin blocking of levodopa effects. *Arch Neurol* (1975) 32, 44.

Levodopa + Piperidine

Piperidine hydrochloride opposes both the dyskinesia associated with the use of levodopa and the beneficial effects of levodopa.

Clinical evidence, mechanism, importance and management

A study on 11 patients with Parkinson's disease and levodopa-induced dyskinesia showed that **piperidine hydrochloride** in daily doses of 700–6300 mg over periods of 10–33 days, diminished the dyskinesia, but it also opposed the effects of the levodopa so that the parkinsonian symptoms re-emerged.[1] This is probably because **piperidine** has cholinergic effects which upset the cholinergic/dopaminergic balance for which the levodopa had originally been given. This was essentially an experimental study undertaken in the hope that **piperidine** might prove to be beneficial. It would seem that there is no therapeutic value in the concurrent use of these drugs.

1. Tolosa ES, Cotzias GC, Papavasiliou PS, Lazarus CB. Antagonism by piperidine of levodopa effects in Parkinson's disease. *Neurology* (1977) 27, 875–7.

Levodopa + Pyridoxine (Vitamin B$_6$)

The effects of levodopa are reduced or abolished by the concurrent use of pyridoxine, but no adverse interaction occurs with levodopa/carbidopa or levodopa/benserazide preparations (e.g. *Sinemet, Madopar*).

Clinical evidence

(a) Levodopa + pyridoxine

A study in 25 patients being treated with levodopa showed that if they were given high doses of **pyridoxine** (750–1000 mg daily) the effects of the levodopa were completely abolished within 3–4 days, and some reduction in the effects were evident within 24 h. Daily doses of 50–100 mg also reduced or abolished the effects of levodopa, and an increase in the signs and symptoms of parkinsonism occurred in eight out of 10 patients taking only 5–10 mg **pyridoxine** daily.[1]

The antagonism of the effects of levodopa by **pyridoxine** has been described in numerous other reports.[1-8]

(b) Levodopa/carbidopa + pyridoxine

A study on 6 chronic levodopa-treated patients with Parkinson's disease found that when given 250 mg levodopa with 50 mg **pyridoxine** their mean levodopa plasma levels fell by 70% (from 356 to 109 ng/ml). With levodopa/carbidopa their mean plasma levels rose almost threefold (to 845 ng/ml) and with 50 mg **pyridoxine** as well, a further slight increase occurred (to 891 ng/ml), although the plasma-integrated area fell 22% from that obtained with levodopa/carbidopa.[8]

The absence of an interaction is confirmed in another report.[9]

Mechanism

The conversion of levodopa to dopamine within the body requires the presence of pyridoxal-5-phosphate (derived from pyridoxine) as a cofactor. When dietary amounts of pyridoxine are high, the 'wasteful' metabolism of levodopa outside the brain is increased so that less is available for entry into the CNS and its effects are reduced accordingly. Pyridoxine may also alter levodopa metabolism by Schiff-base formation. However, in the presence of dopa-decarboxylase inhibitors such as carbidopa or benserazide, this 'wasteful' metabolism of levodopa is reduced and much larger amounts are available for entry into the CNS, even if quite small doses are given. So even in the presence of large amounts of pyridoxine, the peripheral metabolism remains unaffected and the serum levels of levodopa are virtually unaltered.

Importance and management

A clinically important, well documented and well established interaction. 5 mg pyridoxine daily can reduce the effects of levodopa and should be avoided. Warn patients about proprietary pyridoxine-containing preparations. Martindale[10] lists numerous OTC preparations containing varying amounts of pyridoxine many of which could undoubtedly interact to a significant extent. Some breakfast cereals are fortified with pyridoxine and other vitamins, but the amounts are usually too small to matter (e.g. a normal serving of Kellogg's Corn Flakes or Rice Krispies (UK preparations) contains only about 0.6 mg pyridoxine, and a whole 500-g packet contains only 9 mg). There is no good clinical evidence to suggest that a low-pyridoxine diet is desirable, and indeed it may be harmful since the normal dietary requirements are about 2 mg daily.

The problem of this interaction can be totally solved by using levodopa/carbidopa or levodopa/benserazide preparations (e.g. *Sinemet* or *Madopar*) which are unaffected by pyridoxine.

1. Duvoisin RC, Yahr MD, Cote LD. Pyridoxine reversal of L-dopa effects in parkinsonism. *Trans Am Neurol Assoc* (1969) 94, 81–4.
2. Celesia GG, Barr AN. Psychosis and other psychiatric manifestations of levodopa therapy. *Arch Neurol* (1970) 23, 193–200.
3. Carter AB. Pyridoxine and parkinsonism. *BMJ* (1973) 4, 236.
4. Cotzias GC, Papavasiliou PS. Blocking the negative effects of pyridoxine on patients receiving levodopa. *JAMA* (1971) 215, 1504.

5. Leon AS, Spiegel HE, Thomas G, Abrams WB. Pyridoxine antagonism of levodopa in parkinsonism. *JAMA* (1971) 218, 1924.
6. Hildick-Smith M. Pyridoxine in parkinsonism. *Lancet* (1973) ii, 1029–30.
7. Yahr MD, Duvoisin RC. Pyridoxine and levodopa in the treatment of parkinsonism. *JAMA* (1972) 220, 861.
8. Mars H. Levodopa, carbidopa, and pyridoxine in Parkinson's disease: metabolic interactions. *Arch Neurol* (1974) 30, 444–7.
9. Papavasiliou PS, Cotzias GC, Düby SE, Steck AJ, Fehling C, Bell MA. Levodopa in parkinsonism: potentiation of central effects with a peripheral inhibitor. *N Engl J Med* (1972) 285, 8–14.
10. Sweetman SC, editor. Martindale: The complete drug reference. 33rd ed. London: Pharmaceutical Press; 2002. p.1387.

Levodopa + Rauwolfia alkaloids

The effects of levodopa are opposed by the concurrent use of rauwolfia alkaloids such as reserpine.

Clinical evidence, mechanism, importance and management

Reserpine and **other rauwolfia alkaloids** deplete the brain of monoamines, including dopamine, thereby reducing their effects.[1] This opposes the actions of administered levodopa. There are not only sound pharmacological reasons for believing this to be an interaction of clinical importance, but a reduction in the antiparkinsonian activity of levodopa by **reserpine** has been observed.[2] The **rauwolfia alkaloids** should be avoided in patients with Parkinson's disease, whether or not they are taking levodopa.

1. Bianchine JR, Sunyapridakul L. Interactions between levodopa and other drugs: significance in the treatment of Parkinson's disease. *Drugs* (1973) 6, 364.
2. Yahr MD. Personal communication (1977).

Levodopa + Spiramycin

The serum levels of levodopa are reduced by the concurrent use of spiramycin, thereby reducing its therapeutic effects.

Clinical evidence

The observation of a patient with Parkinson's disease on levodopa/carbidopa (*Sinemet*) who became less well-controlled when treated with **spiramycin**, prompted further study in seven normal subjects given 250 mg levodopa + 25 mg carbidopa. After taking 1 g **spiramycin** twice daily for 3 days, the AUC of the levodopa fell to 43% (from 253, 809 to 109, 558 ng/ml/min) while maximum serum levels fell from 2161 to 1679 ng/ml (not significant). The serum levels of the carbidopa were barely detectable (an AUC fall from 27, 706 to 1059 ng/ml/min).[1]

Mechanism

Not fully established. In some way the spiramycin markedly reduces the absorption of the carbidopa, possibly by forming a non-absorbable complex in the gut or by accelerating its transit through the gut. As a result, not enough carbidopa is absorbed to inhibit the 'wasteful' metabolism of the levodopa within the body so that the effects of the levodopa are reduced.[1]

Importance and management

Information is very limited but the interaction appears to be established and of clinical importance. If spiramycin is given, anticipate the need to increase the dosage of the levodopa/carbidopa preparation (approximately double the dose). It is not known whether other macrolide antibacterials behave in a similar way, or whether spiramycin affects levodopa/benserazide preparations. More study is needed.

1. Brion N, Kollenbach K, Marion MH, Grégoire A, Advenier C, Pays M. Effect of a macrolide (spiramycin) on the pharmacokinetics of L-dopa and carbidopa in healthy volunteers. *Clin Neuropharmacol* (1992) 15, 229–35.

Levodopa + Tacrine

A case report describes worsened parkinsonism in a patient given tacrine. The effects of levodopa were opposed.

Clinical evidence

The mild parkinsonism of an elderly woman with Alzheimer's disease worsened (severe tremor, stiffness and gait dysfunction) within two weeks of doubling her **tacrine** dosage from 10 mg to 20 mg four times daily. She improved when levodopa/carbidopa was started, but the parkinsonian symptoms (tremor) returned when **tacrine** was increased to 30 mg four times daily. The symptoms disappeared when the **tacrine** dosage was restored to 20 mg four times daily.[1]

Mechanism

Parkinsonism is due to an imbalance between two neurotransmitters, dopamine and acetylcholine, in the basal ganglia of the brain. Levodopa improves the situation by increasing the levels of dopamine, while the addition of tacrine (a centrally acting anticholinesterase) increases the amounts of acetylcholine which again upsets the balance.

Importance and management

Direct information seems to be limited to this single report, but it is consistent with the known pharmacology of both drugs and the biochemical pathology of Parkinson's disease. Be aware that if tacrine is given to any patient with parkinsonism, whether taking levodopa or any other anti-parkinson drug, the disease may possibly worsen. You may need to increase the anti-parkinson drug dosage and/or reduce the dosage of tacrine.

1. Ott BR, Lannon MC. Exacerbation of parkinsonism by tacrine. *Clin Neuropharmacol* (1992) 15, 322–5.

Levodopa + Tolcapone

Tolcapone increases the half-life and AUC of levodopa so that some reduction in the levodopa dosage may needed.

Clinical evidence, mechanism and management

Tolcapone is a reversible inhibitor of the enzyme catechol-*O*-methyltransferase (COMT) which is concerned with the metabolism of levodopa. In the presence of **tolcapone** plasma levodopa levels are increased and the levels of its inactive metabolite of levodopa, 3-*O*-methyldopa (which is implicated in the 'wearing-off' phenomenon) are reduced. **Tolcapone** can therefore be advantageously used as a useful adjunct to levodopa in the treatment of Parkinson's disease. Studies have shown that tolcapone increases the half-life and doubles the AUC of levodopa,[1-3] and the makers say that in clinical trials that the majority of patients taking 600 mg or more of levodopa (with a decarboxylase inhibitor) daily, or those with moderate/severe dyskinesias, required a reduction in levodopa dosage averaging 30%.[4] The outcome of concurrent use should therefore be monitored and the levodopa dosage reduced as required.

Tolcapone was withdrawn in countries of the European Union in November 1998 because of serious hepatic reactions.[5]

1. Dingemanse J, Jorga K, Zürcher G, Schmitt M, Sedek G, Da Prada M, Van Brummelen P. Pharmacokinetic-pharmacodynamic interaction between the COMT inhibitor tolcapone and single-dose levodopa. *Br J Clin Pharmacol* (1995) 40, 253–62.
2. Sêdek G, Jorga K, Schmitt M, Burns RS, Leese P. Effect of tolcapone on plasma levodopa concentrations after administration with levodopa/carbidopa to healthy volunteers. *Clin Neuropharmacol* (1997) 20, 531–41.
3. Sedek G, Leese P, Burns RS, Jorga K, Schmitt M. Effect of COMT inhibition on L-dopa kinetics in the presence of carbidopa. *Clin Pharmacol Ther* (1993) 53 (2), 180.
4. Tasmar (Tolcapone). Roche. US prescribing information, November 1998.
5. Committee on Safety of Medicines/Medicines Control Agency. Withdrawal of tolcapone (Tasmar). *Current Problems* (1999) 25, 2.

Levodopa + Tricyclic antidepressants

Concurrent use is usually uneventful although a small reduction in the effects of levodopa may occur. Two unexplained hypertensive crises have also occurred when both drugs were used.

Clinical evidence

(a) Reduced levodopa effects

A study in man showed that the concurrent use of **imipramine**, 100 mg daily for 3 days, reduced the absorption of a single 500-mg dose of levodopa. Peak serum concentrations of levodopa were reduced about 50% although the 24-h cumulative excretion was not significantly different from the control.[1]

(b) Hypertensive crises

A hypertensive crisis (blood pressure 210/110 mmHg) associated with agitation, tremor and generalised rigidity developed in a woman taking 6 tablets of *Sinemet* (levodopa 100 mg + 10 mg carbidopa) when she started to take 25 mg **imipramine** three times a day. It occurred again when she was later accidentally given the same dosage of **amitriptyline**.[2] A similar hypertensive reaction (a rise from 190/110 to 270/140 mmHg) occurred over 36 h in another woman taking **amitriptyline** when given half a tablet of *Sinemet* and 10 mg **metoclopramide** three times a day.[3]

Mechanisms

(a) The tricyclics have anticholinergic activity which slows gastric emptying, and this allows more time for the gastric mucosa to metabolise the levodopa 'wastefully', thereby reducing the amount available for entry into the brain. (b) The hypertensive reactions are not understood.

Importance and management

Information seems to be limited to these reports. Concurrent use is normally successful and uneventful[4-6] but it would be prudent to check that the effects of the levodopa are not undesirably reduced. Also be alert for the possibility of a hypertensive reaction which resolves if the tricyclic antidepressant is withdrawn.

1. Morgan JP, Rivera-Calimlim L, Messiha F, Sandaresan PR, Trabert N. Imipramine-mediated interference with levodopa absorption from the gastrointestinal tract in man. *Neurology* (1975) 25, 1029–34.
2. Edwards M. Adverse interaction of levodopa with tricyclic antidepressants. *Practitioner* (1982) 226, 1447 and 1449.
3. Rampton DS. Hypertensive crisis in a patient given Sinemet, metoclopramide, and amitriptyline. *BMJ* (1977) 3, 607–8.
4. Yahr MD. The treatment of Parkinsonism: current concepts. *Med Clin North Am* (1972) 56, 1377–92.
5. Calne DB, Reid JL. Antiparkinsonian drugs: pharmacological and therapeutic aspects. *Drugs* (1972) 4, 49.
6. van Wiegeren A, Wright J. Observations on patients with Parkinson's disease treated with L-dopa. I. Trial and evaluation of L-dopa therapy. *S Afr Med J* (1972) 46, 1262–6.

Levodopa + Tryptophan

Tryptophan can reduce levodopa blood levels.

Clinical evidence, mechanism, importance and management

The blood levels of dopa were markedly reduced in normal healthy subjects when 0.5 g levodopa was taken with 1.0 g **tryptophan**.[1] The reasons are not understood. The clinical importance of this was not assessed. Products containing **tryptophan** for the treatment of depression were withdrawn in the USA, UK and many other countries because of a possible association with the development of an eosinophilia-myalgia syndrome. However, since this syndrome appeared to have been associated with tryptophan from one manufacturer, tryptophan preparations were reintroduced to the UK in 1994 for restricted use.[2]

1. Weitbrecht W-U, Weigel K. Der einfluss von L-tryptophan auf die L-dopa resorption. *Dtsch Med Wochenschr* (1976) 101, 20–2.
2. Sweetman SC, editor. Martindale: The complete drug reference. 33rd ed. London: Pharmaceutical Press; 2002. p.311.

Lisuride + Erythromycin or Food

Neither erythromycin nor food interact to a clinically relevant extent with lisuride hydrogen maleate.

Clinical evidence, mechanism, importance and management

Twelve normal subjects were given 0.2 mg lisuride hydrogen maleate orally or 0.05 mg intravenously over half-an-hour after taking 1 mg **erythromycin** twice daily for 4 days. Another 30 normal subjects were given 0.2 mg lisuride hydrogen maleate orally while fasting or with **food**. It was found that neither **erythromycin** nor **food** significantly modified either the pharmacokinetics or the pharmacodynamics of the lisuride.[1] There would therefore appear to be no reason for avoiding concurrent use.

1. Gandon JM, Le Coz F, Kühne G, Hümpel M, Allain H. PK/PD interaction studies of lisuride with erythromycin and food in healthy volunteers. *Clin Pharmacol Ther* (1995) 57, 191.

Pramipexole + Cimetidine or Probenecid

Cimetidine and probenecid reduce the clearance of pramipexole from the body.

Clinical evidence, mechanism, importance and management

A study in 12 normal subjects found that multiple doses of **cimetidine** reduced the clearance of single 0.25-mg doses of pramipexole by 10.3% and increased its half-life by 29%. Multiple doses of **probenecid** reduced the pramipexole clearance by 32% in males and 35% in females.[1] The clinical significance of these interactions is uncertain.

1. Wright CE, Lasher Sisson TL, Ichhpurani AK, Peters GR. Influence of probenecid (PR) and cimetidine (C) on pramipexole (PX) pharmacokinetics. *Clin Pharmacol Ther* (1996) 59, 183.

Ropinirole + Miscellaneous drugs

Ropinirole appears not to interact adversely with amantadine, digoxin, levodopa, selegiline or trihexyphenidyl (benzhexol), but oestrogen may reduce its clearance. On theoretical grounds it is suggested that cimetidine, ciprofloxacin and fluvoxamine may increase its effects, and dopamine antagonists such as metoclopramide and sulpiride may reduce its effects.

Clinical evidence, mechanism, importance and management

Trials with ropinirole carried out by the makers found no pharmacokinetic interactions between ropinirole and **levodopa** under steady-state conditions (using clinically relevant doses) which might call for large dosage adjustments of either drug, but it is suggested that the dose of levodopa may be reduced gradually by around 20% in total.[1,2] **Amantadine, trihexyphenidyl (benzhexol)** and **selegiline** were found not to have relevant effects on ropinirole,[2] and ropinirole was also found not to affect the steady-state levels of **digoxin** in parkinsonian patients, and concurrent use was well tolerated.[1-4] During clinical trials no drugs or groups of drugs (the makers quote the **benzodiazepines**) had a clinically relevant effect on the clearance of oral ropinirole except **oestrogen** used in hormonal replacement therapy (**HRT**) which reduced the ropinirole clearance by one third. It is therefore suggested that a reduction in the ropinirole dosage may be needed if **HRT** is started, and an increase if it is withdrawn.[1,2]

In vitro studies show that the cytochrome P450 isoenzyme CYP1A2 is largely responsible for the metabolism of ropinirole, with a minor role being played by CYP3A. The potential therefore exists for the interaction with other drugs which either induce or inhibit CYP1A2. Given that in practice the doses of ropinirole are low and that *in vitro* evidence shows that it does not affect the activity of CYP1A2, it is thought that other drugs are more likely to affect ropinirole than vice versa.[2] The makers therefore suggest that concurrently used drugs such as **cimetidine**, **ciprofloxacin** and **fluvoxamine** may possibly increase the effects of ropinirole, calling for a reduction in its dosage if used concurrently.[1,2] Time alone will tell whether these largely theoretical predicted interactions are of practical importance or not, but good monitoring is advisable.

Ropinirole stimulates dopamine receptors (particularly D_2) in the nigral striatal system in the brain. The makers therefore reasonably suggest that neuroleptics and other drugs which act as central dopamine receptor antagonists (they cite **sulpiride** and **metoclopramide**) should be avoided because they may reduce the effectiveness of ropinirole.[1] The practical importance of this also awaits confirmation.

1. Requip (ropinirole). SmithKline Beecham. ABPI Compendium of Datasheets and Summaries of Product Characteristics 1998–9, p 1348.
2. SmithKline Beecham, Personal communication, September 1996.
3. Beerahee A, Taylor AC, Citerone D, Davy M, Fitzpatrick K, Lopez-Gil A, Stocchi F. Steady-state pharmacokinetics of digoxin during repeat oral administration of ropinirole in parkinsonian patients. *Br J Clin Pharmacol* (1996) 42, 668P–669P.
4. Taylor A, Beerahee A, Citerone D, Davy M, Fitzpatrick K, Lopez-Gil A, Stocchi F. The effect of steady-state ropinirole on plasma concentrations of digoxin in patients with Parkinson's disease. *Br J Clin Pharmacol* (1999) 47, 219–222.

Tolcapone + Miscellaneous drugs

No serious adverse interactions have been documented with tolcapone, but the makers contraindicate non-selective MAOIs and a combination of MAO-A and MAO-B inhibitors. They also issue a caution (on theoretical grounds) about the concurrent use of apomorphine, desipramine, dobutamine, epinephrine (adrenaline), isoprenaline (isoprenonol), maprotiline, alpha-methyldopa, venlafaxine and warfarin.

Clinical evidence, mechanism, importance and management

There appear to be no reports of any serious adverse interactions between tolcapone and other drugs, but the makers[1,2] issue a number of cautionary warnings, largely based on the pharmacological and metabolic profile of tolcapone.

The makers contraindicate the use of non-selective MAOIs (e.g. **phenelzine**, **tranylcypromine**) or with a combination of an MAO-A inhibitor (e.g. **moclobemide**) and an MAO-B inhibitor (**selegiline**), but **selegiline** alone is compatible with tolcapone provided not more than 10 mg daily is used. Whether **moclobemide** and tolcapone are compatible is not known, but the makers advise caution.

Tolcapone does not affect the pharmacokinetics of **carbidopa**, but it increases the serum levels of **benserazide** when 50 mg but not 25-mg doses are used. The clinical significance of this is uncertain but the makers advise good monitoring. Tolcapone inhibits the enzyme catechol-*O*-methyl transferase (COMT) which is concerned with the metabolism of drugs such as **apomorphine**, **epinephrine** (**adrenaline**), **dobutamine**, **isoprenaline** (**isoproterenol**) and **alpha-methyldopa**, for which reason the makers warn about the theoretical possibility of increased serum levels and related adverse effects of these drugs, but this has not been specifically studied although no adverse interactions were seen in studies with **ephedrine**. Studies with tolcapone combined with **levodopa/carbidopa** and **desipramine** demonstrated no serious interactions (although the frequency of adverse events increased slightly), however the makers suggest that caution should be exercised with any drugs which are potent norepinephrine (noradrenaline) uptake inhibitors such as **desipramine**, **maprotiline** and **venlafaxine**.

No pharmacokinetic interaction occurs with **tolbutamide** and tolcapone despite *in vitro* evidence that it inhibits cytochrome P450 isoenzyme CYP2C9, and no interaction seems likely **warfarin**, even so good monitoring is advised.

Tolcapone was withdrawn in countries of the European Union in November 1998 because of serious hepatic reactions.[3]

1. Tasmar (Tolcapone). Roche (UK). ABPI Compendium of Datasheets and Summaries of Product Characteristics 1998–9, p 1163.
2. Tasmar (Tolcapone). Roche. US prescribing information, November 1998.
3. Committee on Safety of Medicines/Medicines Control Agency. Withdrawal of tolcapone (Tasmar). *Current Problems* (1999) 25, 2.

10

Beta-blocker drug interactions

The adreno-receptors of the sympathetic nervous system are of two main types, namely alpha and beta. The beta-adreno-ceptor blocking drugs (better known as the beta-blockers) block the beta-receptors and this property is therapeutically exploited to reduce, for example, the normal sympathetic stimulation of the heart. The activity of the heart in response to stress and exercise is reduced, its consumption of oxygen is diminished, and in this way the angina of effort can be treated. Beta-blockers given orally can also be used in the treatment of cardiac arrhythmias, hypertension, myocardial infarction, and heart failure, and in the form of eye-drops for glaucoma and ocular hypertension.

Some of the beta-blockers are sufficiently selective to show that all beta-receptors are not identical but can be further sub-divided into two groups, beta-1 and beta-2. The former are found in the heart and the latter in the bronchi. Since one of the unwanted side-effects of generalised beta-blockade can be the loss of the normal norepinephrine-stimulated bronchodi-lation (leading to bronchospasm), cardioselective beta-1 blocking drugs (e.g. atenolol, metoprolol) were developed, which have less effect on beta-2 receptors. However, it should be emphasised that the selectivity is not absolute because bronchospasm can still occur with these drugs, particularly at high doses. Table 10.1 lists the cardioselective beta-blockers, and Table 10.2 the non-selective beta-blockers. Some beta-blockers also have alpha-1 blocking activity, which causes vasodilatation, and these are listed in Table 10.3. Some beta-blockers such as celiprolol and nebivolol also have vasodila-tor activity, but cause this by mechanisms other than blocking alpha-1 receptors. Other beta-blockers also possess intrinsic sympathomimetic activity in that they can activate beta-re-ceptors and are therefore partial agonists; these are listed in Table 10.4. Sotalol has additional class III antiarrhythmic ac-tivity (see introduction to chapter 4).

This chapter is generally concerned with those drugs that af-fect the activity of the beta-blockers. Where the beta-blockers are the affecting drug, the interaction is dealt with elsewhere. See the Index for a full listing.

Table 10.1 Cardioselective beta-blockers (beta-1 receptor selectivity)

Generic names	Proprietary names
Acebutolol	ACB, Acecor, Diasectral, Espesil, Monitan, Prent, Rhotral, Sectral
Atenolol	Ablock, Alinor, Alonet, Amolin, Ancoren, Angipress, Anselol, Antipressan, Aponorm, Apo-Atenol, Arcablock, Ate, Ate Lich, Atebeta, Atecor, Atehexal, Atenblock, Atendol, Atenet, Ateni, Atenil, Atenix, Ateno, Atenobene, Atenoblok, Atenodan, Atenogamma, Atenogen, Atenol, Atenolan, Atenomel, Atenor, Atenotyrol, Ateno-basan, Atermin, Aterol, Atesifar, Betasyn, Betatop, Blocotenol, Blokium, Blotex, B-Vasc, Cardaxen, Corotenol, Cuxanorm, Duratenol, Evitocor, Falitonsin, Hexa-Blok, Hypernol, Jenatenol, Juvental, Lo-Ten, Myopax, Neatenol, Neotenol, Nif-Ten, Normalol, Normaten, Normiten, Noten, Novo-Atenol, Nu-Atenol, Oraday, Plenacor, Prenolol, Primatenol, Seles Beta, Selinol, Tenat, Tenlol, Teno, Tenoblock, Tenolin, Tenolol, Tenomax, Tenoprin, Tenormin, Tenormine, Tensig, Tensotin, Ten-Bloka, Tessifol, Tonoprotect, Totamol, Trantalol, Uniloc, Vascoten, Velorin, Xaten
Betaxolol	Beofta, Bertocil, Betoptic, Betoptic-S, Betoptima, Betoquin, Davixolol, Kerlon, Kerlone, Oxodal
Bevantolol	
Bisoprolol	Bilol, Bipranix, Bisobloc, Bisocor, Bisomerck, Bisopine, Bisopral, Bisotyrol, Biso-Puren, Cardensiel, Cardicor, Cardiocor, Concor, Cordalin, Darbalan, Detensiel, Emconcor, Emcor, Euradal, Fondril, Godal, Isoten, Monocor, Nanalan, Orloc, Soprol, Zebeta
Celiprolol	Cardem, Celectol, Celipro, Celol, Cordiax, Dilanorm, Selectol
Cycloprolol (Cicloprolol)	
Esmolol	Brevibloc
Metoprolol	Arbralene, Azumetop, Beloc, Betaloc, Betazok, Bioprol, Cardeloc, Cardoxone, Denex, Dura-Zok, Jeprolol, Lanoc, Lopresor, Lopressor, Melol, Meprolol, Mepronet, Metblock, Meto, Metobeta, Metoblock, Metocor, Metodura, Metohexal, Metolol, MetoMed, Metomerck, Metop, Metopal, Metopresol, Metopress, Metoprogamma, Metoprolin, Metotyrol, Metozoc, Meto-Tablinen, Minax, Neobloc, Novo-Metoprol, Nu-Metop, Prelis, Proken M, Prolaken, Promiced, Prontol, Ritmolol, Selectadril, Selokeen, Seloken, Selopral, Selozok, Selo-Zok, Sermetrol, Sigaprolol, Slow-Lopresor, Spesicor, Toprol XL, Topromel
Nebivolol	Lobivon, Nebilet, Nebilet , Nebilox
Practolol	
Talinolol	Cordanum

Table 10.2 Non-selective beta-blockers (block beta-1 and beta-2 receptors)

Generic names	Proprietary names
Alprenolol	Aptin
Befunolol	Bentos, Betaclar, Glauconex
Bopindolol	Sandonorm
Bucindolol	
Bufetolol	
Bufuralol	
Bunitrolol	
Bupranolol	Betadrenol
Butofilolol	
Carazolol	Conduction
Carteolol	Arteolol, Arteoptic, Carteol, Cartrol, Elebloc, Endak, Mikelan, Ocupress, Teoptic
Dilevalol	
Indenolol	Securpres
Levobunolol	Ak-Beta, Betagan, Ophtho-Bunolol, Vistagan
Levomoprolol	
Mepindolol	Betagon, Corindolan
Metipranolol	Betamann, Betanol, Beta-Ophtiole, OptiPranolol, Turoptin
Nadolol	Apo-Nadol, Corgard, Solgol
Nifenalol	
Oxprenolol	Captol, Corbeton, Tevacor, Trasicor
Penbutolol	Betapressin, Levatol
Pindolol	Apo-Pindol, Barbloc, Betapindol, Durapindol, Glauco-Stulln, Hexapindol, Novo-Pindol, Nu-Pindol, Pinden, Pindocor, Pindol, Pindoptan, Pinloc, Pinsken, Viskeen, Visken, Viskene, Vypen
Propranolol	Acifol, Adrexan, Angilol, Antarol, Atensin, Avlocardyl, Bedranol, Berkolol, Betadur CR, Betalevedim, Betalol, Betapress, Betaprol, Beta-Prograne, Beta-Tablinen, Cardenol, Cardiblok, Cardinol, Cardispare, Corpendol, Deralin, Dociton, Efektolol, Elbrol, Emforal, Half Beta-Prograne, Hemipralon, Inderal, Inderalici, Indobloc, Inpanol, Lopranol LA, Nolol, Normpress, Obsidan, Palon, Perlol, Pralol, Pranolol, Prodorol, Prolol, Pronosil, Propa, Propabloc, Propal, Propalem, Prophylux, Propra, Proprahexal, Propral, Propranur, Propra-ratiopharm, Pur-Bloka, Ranoprin, Rebaten, Servanolol, Sumial, Syntonol, Syprol, Tenadren, Tiperal
Sotalol	Betades, Betapace, Beta-Cardone, Cardionorm, Cardol, CorSotalol, Darob, Dutacor, Favorex, Gilucor, Rentibloc, Rylosol, Rytmobeta, Sota, Sota Lich, Sotab, Sotabet, Sotabeta, Sotacor, Sotagamma, Sotahexal, Sotalex, Sotalin, Sotamed, Sotamol, Sotanorm, Sotaper, Sotapor, Sotaryt, Sotastad, Sotatyrol, Sota-Gry, Sota-Puren, Sota-saar, Tachytalol, Ventricor
Tertatolol	Artex, Artexal, Prenalex
Timolol	Apotil, Apo-Timol, Apo-Timop, Aquanil, Arutimol, Betim, Betimol, Blocadren, Blocanol, Chibro-Timoptol, Cusimolol, Digaol, Dispatim, Droptimol, Gaoptol, Glaucol, Glaucosan, Glauco-Oph, Glautimol, Glau-opt, Horex, Hypermol, Novo-Timol, Nyogel, Nyolol, Octil, Oftamolol, Oftan, Oftimolo, Ophtilan, Ophtim, Optimol, Shemol, Tenopt, Tiloptic, Timabak, Timacar, Timacor, Timax, Timisol , Timodrop, TimoEDO, Timoftal, Timoftol, Timoglau, Timohexal, Timolen, Timomann, Timoptic, Timoptol, Timosan, Timosil, Timosine, Timozzard, Timo-COMOD, Timo-Stulln, Tim-Ak, Tim-Ophtal, Tiof, Unitimoftol, V-Optic

Table 10.3 Drugs with both alpha and beta-blocking activity

Generic names	Proprietary names
Carvedilol	Cardilol, Cardiol, Carvipress, Coreg, Coropres, Dilatrend, Dilbloc, Dimitone, Divelol, Eucardic, Hybridil, Kredex, Querto
Labetalol	Albetol, Amipress, Hybloc, Ipolab, Labrocol, Normodyne, Presolol, Trandate
Medraxolol	

Table 10.4 Drug with beta-1-agonist and beta-blocking activity

Generic names	Proprietary names
Xamoterol	

Beta-blockers + Alcohol

The effects of atenolol and metoprolol do not appear to be changed by the concurrent use of alcohol. Some preliminary evidence suggests that the effects of alcohol and atenolol/chlortalidone or propranolol are additive on the performance of some psychomotor tests, but the importance of this is uncertain. There is some evidence that alcohol modestly reduces the haemodynamic effects of propranolol. Some of the effects of sotalol may also be changed by alcohol.

Clinical evidence, mechanism, importance and management

No clinically significant changes in blood pressure, pulse rate or the pharmacokinetics of single doses of 100 mg of **atenolol** or **metoprolol** occurred in 8 healthy subjects 6 h after drinking the equivalent of 200 ml absolute **alcohol**.[1] The performance of a number of psychomotor tests by 12 normal subjects was found to be impaired by **alcohol** (0.6 g/kg) and by one tablet of *Tenoretic* (100 mg **atenolol** + 25 mg **chlortalidone**). When taken together there was some evidence of additive effects but the practical importance of this is not clear.[2]

Propranolol 40 mg six-hourly had no effect on the alcohol-induced impairment of performance on a number of psychomotor tests in 12 healthy subjects given 50 ml/70 kg body-weight of **alcohol**, except that propranolol antagonised the effect of alcohol in one test (pursuit meter).[3] However, in another study, propranolol enhanced the effects of alcohol on some tests (inebriation and divided attention).[4]

A study in 6 healthy subjects found that **alcohol** (sufficient to maintain blood levels of 800 mg/l) raised the mean AUC of a single 80 mg oral dose of **propranolol** by 17.4% in 5 of them and decreased it by 37% in the sixth subject, but this was considered unlikely to be clinically important. No changes in heart rate or blood pressure were seen.[5] In contrast, a double-blind study in 14 healthy subjects found that **alcohol** (equivalent to 32 to 72 ml absolute alcohol) increased the clearance of a single dose of **propranolol** 80 mg and diminished its ability to lower blood pressure. **Propranolol** was not able to abolish the alcohol-induced rise in heart rate.[6] Similarly, another study found that alcohol decreased the rate of absorption and increased the rate of elimination of **propranolol**, but the clinical significance of this small alteration was not assessed.[7]

A further study in 6 healthy subjects found that although the blood pressure lowering effects of **sotalol** 160 mg were increased by alcohol, **sotalol** did not cancel out the alcohol-induced rise in heart rate.[6]

It would seem prudent to be alert for changes in response to beta-blockers that may be due to alcohol. The authors of one of the studies advise patients on **propranolol** to take an extra dose (a quarter to a third of their usual daily dose) if they develop angina or tachycardia after consuming alcohol.[6] See also, 'Antihypertensives + Alcohol', p.383.

1. Kirch W, Spahn H, Hutt HJ, Ohnhaus EE, Mutschler E. Interaction between alcohol and metoprolol or atenolol in social drinking. *Drugs* (1983) 25 (Suppl 2), 152.

2. Gerrard L, Wheeldon NM, McDevitt DG. Psychomotor effects of combined atenolol/chlortalidone administration: interaction with alcohol. *Br J Clin Pharmacol* (1994) 37, 517P–518P.

3. Lindenschmidt R, Brown D, Cerimele B, Walle T, Forney RB. Combined effects of propranolol and ethanol on human psychomotor performance. *Toxicol Appl Pharmacol* (1983) 67, 117–21.

4. Noble EP, Parker E, Alkana R, Cohen H, Birch H. Propranolol-ethanol interaction in man. *Fedn Proc* (1973) 32, 724.

5. Dorian P, Sellers EM, Carruthers G, Hamilton C, Fan T. Propranolol-ethanol pharmacokinetic interaction. *Clin Pharmacol Ther* (1982) 31, 219.

6. Sotaniemi EA, Anttila M, Rautio A, Stengård J, Saukko P, Järvensivu P. Propranolol and sotalol metabolism after a drinking party. *Clin Pharmacol Ther* (1981) 29, 705–10.

7. Grabowski BS, Cady WJ, Young WW, Emery JF. Effects of acute alcohol administration on propranolol absorption. *Int J Clin Pharmacol Ther Toxicol* (1980) 18, 317–19.

Beta-blockers + Allopurinol

Allopurinol 300 mg daily for 6 days did not affect the steady-state pharmacokinetics of atenolol 100 mg daily in 6 healthy subjects.[1]

1. Schäfer-Korting M, Kirch W, Axthelm T, Köhler H, Mutschler E. Atenolol interaction with aspirin, allopurinol, and ampicillin. *Clin Pharmacol Ther* (1983) 33, 283–8.

Beta-blockers + Ampicillin

Plasma atenolol levels are halved by 1-g doses of ampicillin. The clinical importance of this is uncertain, but probably small. No important interaction occurs with ampicillin 250 mg six hourly.

Clinical evidence

A single 1-g dose of **ampicillin** reduced the AUC of a single 100-mg dose of **atenolol** by 40%, and decreased its bioavailability from 60 to 36% in 6 healthy subjects. Similarly, when 100 mg **atenolol** was given with 1 g **ampicillin** once daily for 6 days, the mean steady-state plasma **atenolol** level was reduced by 52% (from 199 to 95 nanograms/ml), and the AUC was reduced by 52%. The blood pressure lowering effect of **atenolol** at rest was not affected, but after exercise a small rise in systolic pressure occurred (up to 17 mmHg) whereas diastolic pressure was unchanged. The effects of **atenolol** on reducing heart rate during exercise were diminished (from 24% to 11% at 12 h).[1]

Another study showed that when single doses of 50 mg **atenolol** and 1 g **ampicillin** were given concurrently by mouth, the AUC of **atenolol** was reduced by 51.5%, whereas when the **ampicillin** was given as four 250-mg doses over 24 h, the AUC was only reduced by 18.2%.[2]

Mechanism

Uncertain. Ampicillin apparently affects the absorption of the atenolol.

Importance and management

Information is limited, but the interaction appears to be established. The clinical importance awaits full evaluation but the modest effects on blood pressure and heart rate[1] suggest that it is of limited importance. Information about other beta-blockers and penicillins is lacking.

1. Schäfer-Korting M, Kirch W, Axthelm T, Köhler H, Mutschler E. Atenolol interaction with aspirin, allopurinol, and ampicillin. *Clin Pharmacol Ther* (1983) 33, 283–8.
2. McLean AJ, Tonkin A, McCarthy P, Harrison P. Dose-dependence of atenolol-ampicillin interaction. *Br J Clin Pharmacol* (1984) 18, 969–71.

Beta-blockers + Antacids or Antidiarrhoeals

Although some antacids and antidiarrhoeals may cause a modest reduction in the absorption of atenolol, propranolol, sotalol and other beta-blockers, and possibly a slight increase in the absorption of metoprolol, the clinical importance of these interactions is probably minimal.

Clinical evidence

(a) Atenolol + Aluminium, Calcium, or Magnesium containing antacids

Aluminium hydroxide 5.6 g given to 6 healthy subjects caused an insignificant fall (20%) in plasma **atenolol** levels after a single 100-mg dose, and had no effect on the reduction in exercise heart rate. When administered concurrently for 6 days, **aluminium hydroxide** had no significant effect on **atenolol** pharmacokinetics.[1] Conversely, a single dose of **calcium** 500 mg caused a 51% reduction in peak plasma level, a 32% reduction in AUC, and an increase in elimination half life from 6.2 to 11 h of atenolol after a single 100-mg dose in 6 healthy subjects. The effect of **atenolol** on heart rate was decreased by 12%. However, after 6 days' concurrent administration these changes were no longer significant, except for a 21% reduction in peak plasma **atenolol** levels. In a further 6 hypertensive subjects, neither 500 mg **calcium** daily nor 5.6 g **aluminium hydroxide** daily had any influence on the blood pressure lowering effect of **atenolol** 100 mg daily for 4 weeks.[1]

Another study showed that 30 ml *Novalucol forte* (an **aluminium and magnesium-containing antacid**) reduced the peak plasma level and AUC of a single 100-mg dose of **atenolol** by 37 and 33%, respectively, in 6 healthy subjects.[2]

(b) Indenolol + Simeco (Aluminium/Magnesium hydroxide/Simethicone) or Kaopectate (Kaolin-Pectin)

A study in *rats* showed that when given **indenolol** with either *Simeco* or *Kaopectate*, the 6 h AUCs were reduced 15 and 30% respectively.[3]

(c) Metoprolol + Aluminium/Magnesium containing antacid

In 6 healthy subjects, 30 ml *Novalucol forte* (an **aluminium and magnesium-containing antacid**) increased the peak plasma level and AUC of a single 100-mg dose of **metoprolol** by 25 and 11%, respectively.[2]

(d) Propranolol + Aluminium hydroxide or adsorbent antidiarrhoeals

Aluminium hydroxide gel 30 ml affected neither the plasma concentrations nor the reduction in exercise heart rate after a single 40-mg dose of **propranolol** in 6 healthy subjects.[4] In contrast, a study in 5 healthy subjects found that 30 ml **aluminium hydroxide gel** given with a single 80-mg dose of **propranolol** reduced the plasma **propranolol** levels and the AUC by almost 60%.[5] *In vitro* and *animal* data suggest that **bismuth subsalicylate, kaolin-pectin** and **magnesium trisilicate** can also reduce the absorption of **propranolol**.[6,7]

(e) Sotalol + Aluminium, Calcium, or Magnesium containing antacids

A study in 6 healthy subjects found that when 20 ml *Maalox* (**aluminium/magnesium hydroxide**) was given at the same time as 160 mg **sotalol**, the maximum plasma level of the **sotalol** was reduced by 26% and its AUC was reduced by 21%. Changes in heart rates reflected these pharmacokinetic changes.[8] When the **Maalox** was given 2 h after the **sotalol** no interaction occurred.[8]

Mechanism

Uncertain. The reduction in absorption could possibly be related to a delay in gastric emptying caused by the antacid, delayed dissolution due to an increase in gastric pH, or to some complexation between the two drugs in the gut which reduces absorption. However, one *in vitro* study indicated that sotalol was only subject to minor absorption or complexation interactions.[8]

Importance and management

The documentation is limited, in some instances somewhat contradictory, and largely confined to single dose or *animal* studies which may not be clinically relevant. Some changes in absorption may possibly occur but nobody seems to have shown that there is a significant effect on the therapeutic effectiveness of the beta-blockers. The one study using atenolol in patients found that the pharmacokinetic changes seen with single doses of aluminium or calcium containing antacids were not clinically significant.[1] However, be alert for any changes during concurrent use. Separating the dosages by 2 h was shown to avoid the interaction in one study,[8] and would seem a simple way of avoiding any problems.

1. Kirch W, Schäfer-Korting M, Axthelm T, Köhler H, Mutschler E. Interaction of atenolol with furosemide and calcium and aluminium salts. *Clin Pharmacol Ther* (1981) 30, 429–35.
2. Regårdh CG, Lundborg P, Persson BA. The effect of antacid, metoclopramide and propantheline on the bioavailability of metoprolol and atenolol. *Biopharm Drug Dispos* (1981) 2, 79–87.
3. Tariq M, Babhair SA. Effect of antacid and antidiarrhoeal drugs on the bioavailability of indenolol. *IRCS Med Sci* (1984) 12, 87–8.
4. Hong CY, Hu SC, Lin SJ, Chiang BN. Lack of influence of aluminium hydroxide on the bioavailability and beta-adrenoceptor blocking activity of propranolol. *Int J Clin Pharmacol Ther Toxicol* (1985) 23, 244–46.
5. Dobbs JH, Skoutakis VA, Acchardio SR, Dobbs BR. Effects of aluminium hydroxide on the absorption of propranolol. *Curr Ther Res* (1977) 21, 887–92.
6. Moustafa MA, Gouda MW, Tariq M. Decreased bioavailability of propranolol due to interactions with adsorbent antacids and antidiarrhoeal mixtures. *Int J Pharmaceutics* (1986) 30, 225–8.
7. McElnay JC, D'Arcy PF, Leonard JK. The effect of activated dimethicone, other antacid constituents, and kaolin on the absorption of propranolol. *Experentia* (1982) 38, 605–7.
8. Läer S, Neumann J, Scholz H. Interaction between sotalol and an antacid preparation. *Br J Clin Pharmacol* (1997) 43, 269–72.

Beta-blockers + Anticholinesterases

A small number of reports describe marked bradycardia and hypotension during the recovery period from anaesthesia and neuromuscular blockade in patients on beta-blockers when given anticholinesterase drugs, but normally no adverse reaction seems to occur. (See also 'Anaesthetics, general + Beta-blockers', p.745). Myasthenic symptoms and myasthenia gravis have occurred with beta-blockers, and so beta-blockers could oppose the efficacy of anticholinesterases in treating myasthenia gravis.

Clinical evidence

(a) Bradycardia

A patient on **nadolol** 40 mg daily, recovering from surgery during which succinylcholine had been used for tracheal intubation and pancuronium for general muscular relaxation, developed prolonged bradycardia (32 to 36 bpm) and hypotension (systolic pressure 60 to 70 torr) when **neostigmine** and atropine were given to reverse the neuromuscular blockade. Isoproterenol and phenylephrine infusions were required to maintain a systolic blood pressure of 90 torr, and were gradually reduced over 3 days. **Propranolol** was substituted for **nadolol**, and two-and-a-half months later she underwent general anaesthesia again (this time without a neuromuscular blocker/**neostigmine**) and she recovered uneventfully.[1] Another patient on **propranolol** 20 mg twice daily, recovering from surgery during which alcuronium had been used, received glycopyrronium and **neostigmine** without a change in heart rate. However, one hour later he developed severe bradycardia (a fall from 65 to 40 bpm) and hypotension (systolic pressure 70 mmHg) when given intravenous **physostigmine** 2 mg over 5 min for extreme drowsiness attributed to the premedication. This responded to glycopyrronium.[2] Prolonged bradycardia and hypotension, requiring isoprenaline then adrenaline (epinephrine) administration, were seen in an elderly woman on **atenolol** 50 mg daily and nitrates when given **neostigmine** and atropine for the reversal of muscle relaxation at the end of general anaesthesia.[3] Another report similarly describes bradycardia in a patient on **propranolol** when intravenous **neostigmine** was used to reverse pancuronium-induced blockade. This responded to atropine.[4] These reports contrast with a study in anaesthetised *dogs* given intravenous **propranolol** then a rapid intravenous injection of **neostigmine** or **pyridostigmine**, which failed to show any further decrease in heart rate.[5]

Another study in 8 hypertensive patients taking long-term beta-blockers (**atenolol** or **propranolol**) showed no significant changes in heart rate and no serious adverse reactions when they were given low-dose oral **pyridostigmine** (30 mg three times daily) for 2 days.[6]

(b) Antagonised effects of anticholinesterases

Three patients developed myasthenic symptoms when treated with **beta-blockers** (two on **propranolol** and, one on **oxprenolol** and the other on practolol). Two of them were effectively treated with **pyridostigmine**.[7]

Mechanism

It would appear that the heart-slowing effects of the beta-blockers and the acetylcholine-like effects of these anticholinesterase drugs can be additive. These were inadequately controlled by the use of atropine in some of the instances cited. The reason for the myasthenic symptoms is not understood.

Importance and management

(a). The information available indicates that marked adverse reactions after surgery are uncommon, but concurrent use should be well monitored to ensure that the occasional problem is dealt with promptly. Be alert when using any intravenous anticholinesterase in a patient on beta-blockers.

(b). Limited information suggests beta-blockers could oppose the efficacy of anticholinesterases in the treatment of myasthenia gravis. Strictly speaking this is a drug-disease rather than a drug-drug interaction.

1. Seidl DC, Martin DE. Prolonged bradycardia after neostigmine administration in a patient taking nadolol. *Anesth Analg* (1984) 63, 365–7.
2. Baraka A, Dajani A. Severe bradycardia following physostigmine in the presence of beta-adrenergic blockade. *Middle Eastern J Anesth* (1984) 7, 291–3.
3. Eldor J, Hoffman B, Davidson JT. Prolonged bradycardia and hypotension after neostigmine administration in a patient receiving atenolol. *Anaesthesia* (1987) 42, 1294–7.
4. Sprague DH. Severe bradycardia after neostigmine in a patient taking propranolol to control paroxysmal atrial tachycardia. *Anesthesiology* (1975) 42, 208–10.
5. Wagner DL, Moorthy SS, Stoelting RK. Administration of anticholinesterase drugs in the presence of beta-adrenergic blockade. *Anesth Analg* (1982) 61, 153–4.
6. Arad M, Roth A, Zelinger J, Zivner Z, Rabinowitz B, Atsmon J. Safety of pyridostigmine in hypertensive patients receiving beta blockers. *Am J Cardiol* (1992) 69, 518–22.
7. Herishanu Y, Rosenberg P. Beta-blockers and myasthenia gravis. *Ann Intern Med* (1975) 83, 834–5.

Beta-blockers + Barbiturates

The plasma levels and the effects of those beta-blockers that are mainly removed from the body by liver metabolism (e.g. alprenolol, metoprolol, timolol) are reduced by the concurrent use of barbiturates. Alprenolol concentrations are halved, but the others are possibly not affected as much. Beta-blockers that are mainly lost unchanged in the urine (e.g. atenolol, sotalol, nadolol) would not be expected to be affected by the barbiturates.

Clinical evidence

Pentobarbital 100 mg daily for 10 days at bedtime reduced the plasma **alprenolol** levels of 6 hypertensive patients taking 400 mg twice daily by 59%. On day 11, mean pulse rates at rest had risen from 70 to 74 bpm and blood pressures had risen from 134/89 to 145/97 mmHg. The changes were seen within 4 to 5 days of starting the barbiturate, and fell once again within 8 to 9 days of stopping.[1] These results confirm previous studies by the same research group using the same **pentobarbital** dosage in healthy subjects.[2,3] In one of these, **pentobarbital** was found to cause a 38% reduction in plasma **alprenolol** levels 90 min after a single 200-mg dose of **alprenolol**, and a 43% reduction in AUC, with no change in elimination half-life. There was also a 20% reduction in the effects of the beta-blocker on heart rate during exercise.[3] In the other study, the AUC of oral **alprenolol** was reduced by about 80%, but that of intravenous **alprenolol** was unaffected.[2]

Another study has shown that 100 mg **pentobarbital** for 10 days reduced the AUC of **metoprolol** 100 mg by 32% (range 2 to 46%) in 8 healthy subjects.[4] **Phenobarbital** 100 mg daily for 7 days reduced the AUC of **timolol** by 24% in 12 healthy subjects, which was not statistically significant.[5]

Mechanism

Barbiturates are potent liver enzyme inducing agents which can increase the metabolism and clearance of other drugs from the body. Beta-blockers that are removed from the body principally by liver metabolism (e.g. alprenolol, metoprolol, timolol) can therefore possibly be cleared more quickly in the presence of a barbiturate.

Importance and management

The alprenolol/pentobarbital interaction is well documented and likely to be of modest clinical importance when the beta-blocker is being used to treat hypertension, and possibly angina. Monitor the effects of alprenolol and increase the dose as necessary. Other barbiturates would be expected to do the same.

A reduced response is possible with any of the beta-blockers that are extensively metabolised (e.g. alprenolol, propranolol, metoprolol, timolol), but the effects on the AUCs of metoprolol and timolol appear to be less than with alprenolol (32%, 24% and 80% respectively). Detailed information about the clinical importance of this interaction with propranolol and other beta-blockers is lacking, but is likely to be minor. Any possible interaction can almost certainly be avoided by using one of the beta-blockers that are primarily lost unchanged in the urine (e.g. atenolol, nadolol).

1. Seideman P, Borg K-O, Haglund K, von Bahr C. Decreased plasma concentrations and clinical effects of alprenolol during combined treatment with pentobarbitone in hypertension. *Br J Clin Pharmacol* (1987) 23, 267–71.
2. Alvan G, Piafsky K, Lind M, von Bahr C. Effect of pentobarbital on the disposition of alprenolol. *Clin Pharmacol Ther* (1977) 22, 316–21.
3. Collste P, Seideman P, Borg K-O, Haglund K, von Bahr C. Influence of pentobarbital on effects and plasma levels of alprenolol and 4-hydroxy-alprenolol. *Clin Pharmacol Ther* (1979) 25, 423–7.
4. Haglund K, Seideman P, Collste P, Borg K-O, von Bahr C. Influence of pentobarbital on metoprolol plasma levels. *Clin Pharmacol Ther* (1979) 26, 326–9.
5. Mäntylä R, Männistö P, Nykänen S, Koponen A, Lamminsivu U. Pharmacokinetic interactions of timolol with vasodilating drugs, food and phenobarbitone in healthy human volunteers. *Eur J Clin Pharmacol* (1983) 24, 227–30.

Beta-blockers + Calcium channel blockers; Dihydropyridines

Concurrent use of beta-blockers and the dihydropyridine calcium channel blockers felodipine, isradipine, lacidipine, nicardipine, nimodipine and nisoldipine normally appears to be useful and safe. However, severe hypotension and heart failure have occurred rarely with nifedipine and nisoldipine. Changes in the pharmacokinetics of the beta-blockers and calcium channel blockers may also occur, but these changes do not appear to be clinically important.

Clinical evidence

(a) Felodipine

A double-blind crossover study in 8 healthy subjects showed that, over a 5-day period, **metoprolol** (100 mg twice daily) did not affect the pharmacokinetics of **felodipine** (10 mg twice daily). On the other hand, the bioavailability of **metoprolol** was increased by 31% and its peak plasma levels by 38%.[1] Another study in 10 healthy subjects given 10 mg **felodipine** with either 100 mg **metoprolol**, 5 mg **pindolol**, 80 mg **propranolol** or 10 mg **timolol** found no changes in heart rate, PR interval or blood pressure that might be considered to be harmful to patients with hypertension or angina. However, 7 of the 10 reported some increase in adverse reactions.[2]

(b) Isradipine

A preliminary report of a study in 24 healthy subjects found that the concurrent use of **propranolol** 40 mg twice daily and **isradipine** 5 mg twice daily caused some modest changes in the pharmacokinetics of both drugs (peak **propranolol** plasma levels increased by 17%, peak isradipine plasma levels reduced by 18%), but the AUCs were not significantly altered.[3] However, an earlier preliminary report by the same research group in 17 subjects found an increase in the **propranolol** AUC (28%), a reduction in the **isradipine** AUC (22%) and a 59% increase in the peak **propranolol** levels.[4]

(c) Lacidipine

Single-dose studies in 24 healthy subjects found that 160 mg **propranolol** reduced the peak plasma levels and AUC of lacidipine (4 mg) by 38 and 42% respectively, while the peak plasma levels and AUC of the **propranolol** were increased by 35 and 26% respectively. There was a modest additive reduction (4 to 6 mmHg) in blood pressure, and the combination reduced heart rate, but not to an extent greater than propranolol alone. No significant adverse effects were seen.[5] However, a further preliminary report of a study by the same authors, in which 12 hypertensive patients were given **propranolol** 160 mg twice daily and **lacidipine** 4 mg daily for 2 weeks, found a non-significant 30% *increase* in systemic availability of lacidipine, and no change in propranolol pharmacokinetics. In addition, no clinically significant alterations in ECG recordings, blood pressure, or pulse rate were seen.[6]

(d) Lercanidipine

The maker notes that when **lercanidipine** was administered concurrently with **metoprolol**, the bioavailability of **lercanidipine** was reduced by 50% and that of **metoprolol** was not changed. They suggest that lercanidipine dose adjustment may be needed.[7]

(e) Nicardipine

Nicardipine 30 mg did not affect the pharmacokinetics or pharmacodynamics of **atenolol** 100 mg in a single-dose study in healthy subjects.[8] In another study, 14 healthy subjects were given 50 mg **nicardipine** 12-hourly and 100 mg **metoprolol** 12-hourly, alone or together, for 5½ days. **Metoprolol** plasma levels were raised 28% by the **nicardipine** in the 7 who were extensive metabolisers, but had no significant effect in the poor metabolisers. The extent of the beta-blockade was unchanged in all of them.[9] Preliminary analysis of another study in healthy subjects found that the pharmacokinetics of both **propranolol** 80 mg twice daily and **nicardipine** 30 mg three times daily were unaffected by 6 days concurrent use.[10] However, this contrasts with two single-dose studies which found that 30 mg **nicardipine** increased the AUC and peak plasma levels of a single 80-mg dose of propranolol by 47% and 80%, respectively,[11] and of 80 mg of a sustained-release formulation to a lesser extent (17% and 22%, respectively).[12] A related single-dose study found that in elderly healthy subjects 30 mg **nicardipine** increased the maximum plasma levels and AUC of 40 mg **propranolol** by 99.6 and 80.8% respectively. **Nicardipine** caused a further decrease in blood pressure, and attenuated the reduction in heart rate seen with **propranolol** alone.[13]

(f) Nifedipine

Nifedipine 10 mg three times daily did not alter the pharmacokinetics of **atenolol** 100 mg once daily,[14,15] **metoprolol** 100 mg twice daily[14,15] or **propranolol** 80 mg twice daily.[14] However, using the same dosages, another study found an increase in **propranolol** peak plasma concentration and AUC of 56% and 23%, respectively, with **nifedipine**.[16] There was no effect on **betaxolol**,[16] and in a single-dose study, there was no pharmacokinetic interaction between **nifedipine** and **atenolol**.[17] Regardless of the pharmacokinetic changes, none of these studies in healthy subjects demonstrated any adverse haemodynamic effects from the combination of **nifedipine** and these beta-blockers.[14,16,17] Similarly, in studies in patients with normal left ventricular function there was no evidence of adverse haemodynamic effects when **nifedipine** (single-dose sublingual[18,19] or intravenously,[20] or daily dose orally[20]) was given with **atenolol**,[20] **celiprolol**[19] or **propranolol**.[18,21] However there are a few earlier isolated case reports of hypotension and heart failure with the combination:

Two patients with angina being treated with beta-blockers (**alprenolol, propranolol**) developed heart failure when additionally given 10 mg **nifedipine** three times daily. The signs of heart failure disappeared when the **nifedipine** was withdrawn.[22] One out of 15 patients with hypertension and exertional angina progressively developed hypotension (90/60 mmHg) when given 10 mg **nifedipine** twice daily in addition to treatment with **atenolol** 50 mg daily and a diuretic for 1 month.[23] Severe and prolonged hypotension (initially not recordable then 60 mmHg systolic) developed in a patient with angina treated with **propranolol** 160 mg four times daily 18 days after nifedipine 10 mg three times daily was substituted for isosorbide, and this may have been a factor which led to fatal myocardial infarction.[24] Cardiac failure is also described in another patient with angina on **atenolol** and various other drugs when additionally given **nifedipine** 20 mg three times daily.[25]

(g) Nimodipine

In a preliminary report of a study in 12 healthy subjects, nimodipine 30 mg three times daily for 4 days had no significant effect on the changes in heart rate, blood pressure or cardiac output seen with either 40 mg **propranolol** or 25 mg **atenolol** three times daily, or on the pharmacokinetics of the beta-blockers.[26]

(h) Nisoldipine

When given as a single 20-mg dose, **nisoldipine** increased the steady-state AUC of **propranolol** 160 mg daily by 35%, and the peak plasma concentrations by 55%. After combined treatment for 7 days, the AUC of **propranolol** was increased 60% and the peak plasma concentration by 55%. The combination enhanced blood pressure reduction to a small extent, but **nisoldipine** did not significantly reduce the effect of **propranolol** on heart rate.[27] Similarly, another study found that a single 20-mg dose of **nisoldipine** increased the AUC and peak plasma concentrations of a single 40-mg dose of **propranolol** by 43% and 68% respectively, and that the AUC and peak plasma concentrations of **nisoldipine** increased 30% and 57%. In this study, nisoldipine was reported to enhance beta-blockade.[28] However, the same research group later showed that the steady-state pharmacokinetics of **propranolol** 80 mg twice daily and **nisoldipine** 10 mg twice daily were not affected by combined treatment for 7 days. Nisoldipine attenuated the decrease in forearm blood flow seen with propranolol.[29] The maker of nisoldipine notes that severe hypotension can occur when nisoldipine is administered at the same time as beta-blockers, and that, in isolated cases, signs of heart failure can also occur.[30]

Mechanisms

Not understood. Where pharmacokinetic changes are seen, a possible reason is that the metabolism of the beta-blockers is changed by changes in blood flow through the liver. The pharmacodynamic changes with nifedipine may be explained by the fact that nifedipine depresses the contractility of the heart muscle. This is counteracted by a sympathetic reflex increase in heart rate due to nifedipine-induced peripheral vasodilation, so that the ventricular output stays the same or is even improved. The presence of a beta-blocker may oppose this to some extent by slowing the heart rate, which allows the negative inotropic effects of nifedipine to go unchecked.

Importance and management

The concurrent use of beta-blockers and the dihydropyridine calcium channel blockers is common, and normally valuable. However, isolated cases of severe hypotension and heart failure have been seen in a few patients on beta-blockers given nifedipine or nisoldipine. It has been suggested that those likely to be most at risk are patients with impaired left ventricular function[31] (which is a caution for the use of nifedipine anyway) and/or those taking beta-blockers in high dosage. Bear this in mind. Changes in the pharmacokinetics of the beta-blockers and calcium channel blockers may also occur, but these changes do not appear to be clinically important. It may also be worth noting that the cases with nifedipine all occurred with 'short-acting' formulations, which are now considered unsuitable for long-term management of angina or hypertension since they are associated with larger variations in blood pressure and heart rate.

1. Smith SR, Wilkins MR, Jack DB, Kendall MJ, Laugher S. Pharmacokinetic interactions between felodipine and metoprolol. *Eur J Clin Pharmacol* (1987) 31, 575–8.
2. Carruthers SG, Bailey DG. Tolerance and cardiovascular effects of single dose felodipine/β-blocker combinations in healthy subjects. *J Cardiovasc Pharmacol* (1987) 10 (Suppl 1), S169–S176.
3. Schran HF, Shepherd AM, Choc MM, Gonasun LM, Brodie CL. The effect of concomitant administration of isradipine and propranolol on their steady-state bioavailability. *Pharmacologist* (1989) 31, 153.
4. Shepherd AMM, Brodie CL, Carrillo DW, Kwan CM. Pharmacokinetic interaction between isradipine and propranolol. *Clin Pharmacol Ther* (1988) 43,194.
5. Hall ST, Harding SM, Hassani H, Keene ON, Pellegatti M. The pharmacokinetic and pharmacodynamic interaction between lacidipine and propranolol in healthy volunteers. *J Cardiovasc Pharmacol* (1991) 18, (Suppl 11), S13–S17.
6. Hall ST, Saul P, Keene ON, Hassani H. Pharmacodynamic and pharmacokinetic interaction between lacidipine and propranolol. *Pharm Res* (1992) 9 (10 Suppl), S88.
7. Zanidip (Lercanidipine). Napp Pharmaceuticals Ltd. Summary of product characteristics, March 2001.

8. Vercruysse I, Schoors DF, Musch G, Massart DL, Dupont AG. Nicardipine does not influence the pharmacokinetics and pharmacodynamics of atenolol. *Br J Clin Pharmacol* (1990) 30, 499–500.
9. Laurent-Kenesi M-A, Funck-Brentano C, Poirier J-M, Decolin D, Jaillon P. Influence of CYP2D6-dependent metabolism on the steady-state pharmacokinetics and pharmacodynamics of metoprolol and nicardipine, alone and in combination. *Br J Clin Pharmacol* (1993) 36, 531–8.
10. Macdonald FC, Dow RJ, Wilson RAG, Yee KF, Finlayson J. A study to determine potential interactions between nicardipine and propranolol in healthy volunteers. *Br J Clin Pharmacol* (1987), 23, 626P.
11. Schoors DF, Vercruysse I, Musch G, Massart DL, Dupont AG. Influence of nicardipine on the pharmacokinetics and pharmacodynamics of propranolol in healthy volunteers. *Br J Clin Pharmacol* (1990) 29, 497–501.
12. Vercruysse I, Schoors DF, Massart DL, Dupont AG. Influence of nicardipine on the pharmacokinetics of sustained release propranolol in healthy volunteers. *Br J Clin Pharmacol* (1992) 34, 445P.
13. Hartmann C, Vercruysse I, Metz T, Massart DL, Dupont AG. Influence of nicardipine on the pharmacokinetics of propranolol in the elderly. *Br J Clin Pharmacol* (1995) 39, 540P.
14. Gangji D, Juvent M, Niset G, Wathieu M, Degreve M, Bellens R, Poortmans J, Degre S, Fitzsimons TJ, Herchuelz A. Study of the influence of nifedipine on the pharmacokinetics and pharmacodynamics of propranolol, metoprolol and atenolol. *Br J Clin Pharmacol* (1984) 17, 29S–35S.
15. Kendall MJ, Jack DB, Laugher SJ, Lobo J, Smith RS. Lack of a pharmacokinetic interaction between nifedipine and the β-adrenoceptor blockers metoprolol and atenolol. *Br J Clin Pharmacol* (1984) 18, 331–5.
16. Vinceneux Ph, Canal M, Domart Y, Roux A, Cascio B, Orofiamma B, Larribaud J, Flouvat B, Carbon C. Pharmacokinetic and pharmacodynamic interactions between nifedipine and propranolol or betaxolol. *Int J Clin Pharmacol Ther Toxicol* (1986) 24, 153–8.
17. Rosenkranz B, Ledermann H, Frölich JC. Interaction between nifedipine and atenolol: pharmacokinetics and pharmacodynamics in normotensive volunteers. *J Cardiovasc Pharmacol* (1986) 8, 943–9.
18. Elkayam U, Roth A, Weber L, Kulick D, Kawanishi D, McKay C, Rahimtoola SH. Effects of nifedipine on hemodynamics and cardiac function in patients with normal left ventricular ejection fraction already treated with propranolol. *Am J Cardiol* (1986) 58, 536–40.
19. Silke B, Verma SP, Guy S. Hemodynamic interactions of a new beta blocker, celiprolol, with nifedipine in angina pectoris. *Cardiovasc Drug Ther* (1991) 5, 681–8.
20. Rowland E, Razis P, Sugrue D, Krikler DM. Acute and chronic haemodynamic and electrophysiological effects of nifedipine in patients receiving atenolol. *Br Heart J* (1983) 50, 383–9.
21. Vetrovec GW, Parker VE. Nifedipine, beta blocker interaction: effect on left ventricular function. *Clin Res* (1984) 32, 833A.
22. Anastassiades CJ. Nifedipine and beta-blocker drugs. *BMJ* (1980) 281, 1251–2.
23. Opie LH, White DA. Adverse interaction between nifedipine and β-blockade. *BMJ* (1980) 281, 1462.
24. Staffurth JS, Emery P. Adverse interaction between nifedipine and beta-blockade. *BMJ* (1981) 282, 225.
25. Robson RH, Vishwanath MC. Nifedipine and beta-blockade as a cause of cardiac failure. *BMJ* (1982) 284, 104.
26. Horstmann R, Weber H, Wingender W, Rämsch K-D, Kuhlmann J. Does nimodipine interact with beta adrenergic blocking agents? *Eur J Clin Pharmacol* (1989) 36, A258.
27. Elliott HL, Meredith PA, McNally C, Reid JL. The interactions between nisoldipine and two β-adrenoceptor antagonists—atenolol and propranolol. *Br J Clin Pharmacol* (1991) 32, 379–85.
28. Levine MAH, Ogilvie RI, Leenen FHH. Pharmacokinetic and pharmacodynamic interactions between nisoldipine and propranolol. *Clin Pharmacol Ther* (1988) 43, 39–48.
29. Shaw-Stiffel TA, Walker SE, Ogilvie RI, Leenen FH. Pharmacokinetic and pharmacodynamic interactions during multiple-dose administration of nisoldipine and propranolol. *Clin Pharmacol Ther* (1994) 55, 661–9.
30. Syscor MR (Nisoldipine). Pharmax Ltd. Summary of product characteristics, August 1998.
31. Brooks N, Cattell M, Pigeon J, Balcon R. Unpredictable response to nifedipine in severe cardiac failure. *BMJ* (1980) 281, 1324.

Beta-blockers + Calcium channel blockers; Diltiazem

The cardiac depressant effects of diltiazem and beta-blockers are additive, and although concurrent use can be beneficial, close monitoring is recommended. A number of patients, (usually those with pre-existing ventricular failure or conduction abnormalities) have developed serious and potentially life-threatening bradycardia. Diltiazem increases the serum levels of propranolol and metoprolol, but not those of atenolol, but these changes are probably not clinically important.

Clinical evidence

Ten patients were admitted to an intensive coronary care unit during one year with severe bradycardia (heart rates of 24 to 44 bpm) while receiving **diltiazem** (90 to 360 mg daily) and beta-blockers (**propranolol** 30 to 120 mg daily, **atenolol** 50 to 100 mg daily, or **pindolol** 90 mg daily). All were relatively elderly and presented with lethargy, dizziness, syncope, chest pain, and (in one case) pulmonary oedema. The ECG abnormalities were localised in the sinus node, the primary rhythm disorders being junctional escape rhythm, sinus

bradycardia and sinus pause. These resolved within 24 h of withdrawing the drugs, although a temporary pacemaker was needed in 4 patients.[1]

Symptomatic and severe bradycardia of this kind has been described in case reports in 14 other patients taking **diltiazem** and **atenolol**,[2] **metoprolol**,[2,3] **pindolol**,[4] **propranolol**,[2,3,5,6] or **sotalol**.[4] Similarly severe sinus bradycardia occurred in 8 of 59 patients in three early clinical studies of the combination of **diltiazem** and **propranolol**.[7-9] One patient developed congestive heart failure on the combination.[9] Four other similar clinical trials did not report any adverse effects.[10-13] In healthy subjects, **diltiazem** increased the AUC of **propranolol** and **metoprolol** by 48 and 33% respectively, and the maximal serum concentrations by 45 and 71%, but **atenolol** was not significantly affected.[14] Another study found a 24 to 27% reduction in **propranolol** clearance.[15]

Mechanism

The heart slowing effects of the beta-blockers can be additive with the delay in conduction through the atrioventricular node caused by the diltiazem.[4] This advantageously increases the antianginal effects in most patients, but in a few these effects may exacerbate existing cardiac abnormalities. Diltiazem apparently also inhibits the metabolism of propranolol and metoprolol, but not atenolol.[14]

Importance and management

Concurrent use is unquestionably valuable and uneventful in many patients, but severe adverse effects can develop. This is well established. A not dissimilar adverse interaction can occur with verapamil (see 'Beta-blockers + Calcium channel blockers; Verapamil', p.437). On the basis of 6 reports, the incidence of symptomatic bradyarrhythmia was estimated to be about 10 to 15%.[1] It can occur with different beta-blockers, even with very low doses, and any time from within a few hours of starting treatment up to 2 years.[1] The main risk factors seem to be ventricular dysfunction, or sinoatrial or AV nodal conduction abnormalities.[1] Note that these are usually contraindications to the use of diltiazem. Patients with normal ventricular function and no evidence of conduction abnormalities are usually not at risk. Concurrent use should be well monitored for evidence of adverse effects. Changes in the pharmacokinetics of the beta-blockers may also occur, but these changes are probably not clinically important.

1. Sagie A, Strasberg B, Kusnieck J, Sclarovsky S. Symptomatic bradycardia induced by the combination of oral diltiazem and beta blockers. *Clin Cardiol* (1991) 14, 314–16.
2. Yust I, Hoffman M, Aronson RJ. Life-threatening bradycardic reactions due to beta blocker-diltiazem interactions. *Isr J Med Sci* (1992) 28, 292–4.
3. Lan Cheong Wah LSH, Robinet G, Guiavarc'h M, Garo B, Boles JM. États de choc au cours de l'association diltiazem-β-bloquant. *Rev Med Interne* (1992) 13, 80.
4. Hassell AB, Creamer JE. Profound bradycardia after the addition of diltiazem to a beta-blocker. *BMJ* (1989) 298, 675.
5. Hossack KF. Conduction abnormalities due to diltiazem. *N Engl J Med* (1982) 307, 953–4.
6. Ishikawa T, Imamura T, Koiwaya Y, Tanaka K. Atrioventricular dissociation and sinus arrest induced by oral diltiazem. *N Engl J Med* (1983) 309, 1124–5.
7. O'Hara MJ, Khurmi NS, Bowles MJ, Raftery BB. Diltiazem and propranolol combination for the treatment of chronic stable angina pectoris. *Clin Cardiol* (1987) 10, 115–23.
8. Hung J, Lamb IH, Connolly SJ, Jutzy KR, Goris ML, Schroeder JS. The effect of diltiazem and propranolol, alone and in combination, on exercise performance and left ventricular function in patients with stable effort angina: a double-blind, randomized, and placebo-controlled study. *Circulation* (1983) 68, 560–7.
9. Strauss WE, Parisi AF. Superiority of combined diltiazem and propranolol therapy for angina pectoris. *Circulation* (1985) 71, 951–7.
10. Tilmant PY, Lablanche JM, Thieuleux FA, Dupuis BA, Bertrand ME. Detrimental effect of propranolol in patients with coronary arterial spasm countered by combination with diltiazem. *Am J Cardiol* (1983) 52, 230–33.
11. Rocha P, Baron B, Delestrain A, Pathe M, Cazor J-L, Kahn J-C. Hemodynamic effects of intravenous diltiazem in patients treated chronically with propranol. *Am Heart J* (1986) 111, 62–8.
12. Humen DP, O'Brien P, Purves P, Johnson D, Kostuk WJ. Effort angina with adequate beta-receptor blockade: comparison with diltiazem alone and in combination. *J Am Coll Cardiol* (1986) 7, 329–35.
13. Kenny J, Daly K, Bergman G, Kerkez S, Jewitt DE. Beneficial effects of diltiazem combined with beta blockade in angina pectoris. *Eur Heart J* (1985) 6, 418–23.
14. Tateishi T, Nakashima H, Shitou T, Kumagai Y, Ohashi K, Hosaka S, Ebihara A. Effect of diltiazem on the pharmacokinetics of propranolol, metoprolol and atenolol. *Eur J Clin Pharmacol* (1989) 36, 67–70.
15. Hunt BA, Bottorff MB, Herring VL, Self TH, Lalonde RL. Effects of calcium channel blockers on the pharmacokinetics of propranolol stereoisomers. *Clin Pharmacol Ther* (1990) 47, 584–91.

Beta-blockers + Calcium channel blockers; Verapamil

The cardiac depressant effects of verapamil and beta-blockers are additive, and although concurrent use can be beneficial, serious cardiodepression (bradycardia, asystole, sinus arrest) sometimes occurs. It has been suggested that the combination should only be given to those who can initially be closely supervised. An adverse interaction can occur even with beta-blockers given as eye drops (e.g. timolol).

Clinical evidence

(a) Adverse interactions

(i) Intravenous administration. Ventricular asystole developed when intravenous **verapamil** was given after the unsuccessful use of intravenous **practolol** to treat supraventricular tachycardia in a 70-year-old man and a 6-month-old baby.[1] In a later study, the combination of intravenous **verapamil** and intravenous **practolol** produced a marked reduction in cardiac contractility, which was more evident when **practolol** was given first.[2]

(ii) Oral administration. In one series, 40 out of 50 patients on 100 mg **atenolol** and 360 mg **verapamil** daily experienced a reduction in anginal episodes over a mean period of 10 months while taking both drugs. However, 16 needed a reduced dosage or withdrawal of one or both drugs. Three had bradyarrhythmias (drugs withdrawn) and 7 experienced dyspnoea (4 withdrawals and 3 dosage reductions) presumed to be secondary to left ventricular failure. Other complications were tiredness (2 patients), postural hypotension (1 patient) and dizziness (1 patient), all of which were dealt with by reducing the dosage.[3] In another study in 15 patients with angina given **atenolol** and **verapamil**, 4 experienced profound lethargy, one had left ventricular failure and 4 had bradyarrhythmias.[4]

Other case reports and studies describe heart failure,[5] dyspnoea,[5,6] sinus arrest,[7,8] heart block,[7,9,10] hypotension,[5,8,11-13] and bradycardia[4,5,8,9,11-15] in patients on **verapamil** and **alprenolol**,[7] **atenolol**,[7,8,10] **metoprolol**,[5,9,12] **propranolol**[6,11,13-15] or **pindolol**.[5] In two further cases, bradycardia occurred in patients using **timolol** in the form of eye drops.[16,17] A number of reports noted that patients had reasonable left ventricular function.[5,8,10,16]

(b) Pharmacokinetic interactions

Concurrent administration of **verapamil** and **metoprolol**, raised the **metoprolol** AUC in 10 patients by 33% and the peak plasma levels by 41%.[12] The minimum pulse rate and systolic blood pressure (1 to 3 hours post-dose) were also lower than with **metoprolol** alone. The pharmacokinetics of **atenolol** were not altered by **verapamil** in a study on a single patient,[18] nor in a study in 15 patients (unpublished data).[4] Although the mean values were not significantly increased in another study in 10 patients, individual patients showed **atenolol** AUC increases of up to 112%.[19] In healthy subjects, **verapamil** reduced the clearance of **propranolol** by 26 to 32% and increased its AUC by 46 to 58%.[20] Similarly, in 5 patients **verapamil** increased the peak plasma levels of **propranolol** by 94%, and its AUC by 66%.[15] **Propranolol** did not affect the pharmacokinetics of **verapamil**.[15] In a single-dose study, *R*-**verapamil** reduced the AUC of **talinolol** by 24% in 9 healthy subjects.[21]

Mechanism

Both beta-blockers and verapamil have negative inotropic (cardiac depressant) effects on the heart, which can be additive. Given together they can cause marked bradycardia and may even depress the contraction of the ventricle completely. Verapamil can also raise the serum levels of beta-blockers that are extensively metabolised in the liver (e.g. metoprolol, propranolol), possibly by inhibiting their metabolism.[22] It is thought that verapamil affects talinolol bioavailability by modulating intestinal P-glycoprotein.[21,23]

Importance and management

Well-documented and well-established interactions. Although concurrent use can be uneventful and successful, the reports cited here amply demonstrate that it may not always be safe, the difficulty being to identify the patients most at risk. The British National Formulary (BNF) says that oral concurrent use should only be contemplated if myocardial function is well preserved. There is a note saying that verapamil should not be injected in patients recently given beta-blockers because of the risk of hypotension and asystole. The BNF also notes that, although 30 min has been suggested as a sufficient interval before giving a beta-blocker when verapamil injection has been given first, the safety of this has not been established.[24]

It has been advised that the initiation of treatment should be restricted to hospital practice where the dose of each drug can be carefully titrated and the patient closely supervised, particularly during the first few days when adverse effects are most likely to develop.[3,4,15] Some have suggested that beta-blockers that are extensively metabolised (e.g. metoprolol, propranolol) may possibly carry some additional risk because verapamil raises their serum levels.[18] However, others contend that, since the interaction occurs with atenolol, the pharmacodynamic effects are more important than any pharmacokinetic changes.[4,8,15] Note that beta-blocker AUC changes of this size, or even more, with other enzyme inhibiting drugs have proved not to be clinically important.

1. Boothby CB, Garrard CS, Pickering D. Verapamil in cardiac arrhythmias. *BMJ* (1972) 2, 349.
2. Seabra-Gomes R, Rickards A, Sutton R. Hemodynamic effects of verapamil and practolol in man. *Eur J Cardiol* (1976) 4, 79–85.
3. McGourty JC, Silas JH. β-blockers and verapamil: a cautionary tale. *BMJ* (1984) 289, 1624.
4. Findlay IN, McInnes GT, Dargie HJ. β-blockers and verapamil: a cautionary tale. *BMJ* (1984) 289, 1074.
5. Wayne VS, Harper RW, Laufer E, Federman J, Anderson ST, Pitt A. Adverse interaction between beta-adrenergic blocking drugs and verapamil-report of three cases. *Aust N Z J Med* (1982) 12, 285–9.
6. Balasubramian V, Bowles M, Davies AB, Raferty EB. Combined treatment with verapamil and propranolol in chronic stable angina. *Br Heart J* (1981) 45, 349–50.
7. McQueen EG. New Zealand Committee on Adverse Reactions: 14th Annual Report 1979. *N Z Med J* (1980) 91, 226–9.
8. Misra M, Thakur R, Bhandari K. Sinus arrest caused by atenolol-verapamil combination. *Clin Cardiol* (1987) 10, 365–7.
9. Eisenberg JNH, Oakley GDG. Probable adverse interaction between oral metoprolol and verapamil. *Postgrad Med J* (1984) 60, 705–6.
10. Hutchison SJ, Lorimer AR, Lakhdar A, McAlpine SG. β-blockers and verapamil: a cautionary tale. *BMJ* (1984) 289, 659–60.
11. Ljungström A, Åberg H. Interaktion mellan betareceptorblockerare och verapamil. *Lakartidningen* (1973) 70, 3548.
12. Keech AC, Harper RW, Harrison PM, Pitt A, McLean AJ. Pharmacokinetic interaction between oral metoprolol and verapamil for angina pectoris. *Am J Cardiol* (1986) 58, 551–2.
13. Zatuchni J. Bradycardia and hypotension after propranolol HCl and verapamil. *Heart Lung* (1985) 14, 94–5.
14. Rumboldt Z, Baković Z, Bagatin J. Opasna kardiodepresivna interakcija izmedu verapamila i propranolola. *Lijecniki Vjesnki* (1979) 101, 430–2.
15. McCourty JC, Silas JH, Tucker GT, Lennard MS. The effect of combined therapy on the pharmacokinetics and pharmacodynamics of verapamil and propranolol in patients with angina pectoris. *Br J Clin Pharmacol* (1988) 25, 349–57.
16. Sinclair NI, Benzie JL. Timolol eye drops and verapamil — a dangerous combination. *Med J Aust* (1983) 1, 548.
17. Pringle SD, MacEwen CJ. Severe bradycardia due to interaction of timolol eye drops and verapamil. *BMJ* (1987) 294, 155–6.
18. McLean AJ, Knight R, Harrison PM, Harper RW. Clearance-based oral drug interaction between verapamil and metoprolol and comparison with atenolol. *Am J Cardiol* (1985) 55, 1628–9.
19. Keech AC, Harper RW, Harrison PM, Pitt A, McLean AJ. Extent and pharmacokinetic mechanisms of oral atenolol-verapamil interaction in man. *Eur J Clin Pharmacol* (1988) 35, 363–6.
20. Hunt BA, Bottorff MB, Herring VL, Self TH, Lalonde RL. Effects of calcium channel blockers on the pharmacokinetics of propranolol stereoisomers. *Clin Pharmacol Ther* (1990) 47, 584–91.
21. Schwarz U,Krappweis J, Berndt A, Gramatté T. Unexpected verapamil on oral bioavailability of the β-blocker talinolol in humans. *Naunyn Schmiedebergs Arch Pharmacol* (1998) 357, (4 Suppl), R167.
22. Kim M, Shen DD, Eddy AC, Nelson WL. Inhibition of the enantioselective oxidative metabolism of metoprolol by verapamil in human liver microsomes. *Drug Metab Dispos* (1993) 21, 309–17.
23. Gramatté T, Oertel R. Intestinal secretion of intravenous talinolol is inhibited by luminal *R*-verapamil. *Clin Pharmacol Ther* (1999) 66, 239–45.
24. British National Formulary. 43rd ed. London: The British Medical Association and The Pharmaceutical Press; 2002. p. 107.

Beta-blockers + Ciprofloxacin

Ciprofloxacin reduces the loss of metoprolol from the body, but this is probably clinically unimportant.

Clinical evidence, mechanism, importance and management

Preliminary evidence suggests pretreatment with five 12-hourly 500-mg doses of **ciprofloxacin** increased the AUC of (+)-**metoprolol** in 7 healthy subjects given a single dose of **metoprolol** 100 mg by 54% and reduced its clearance by 38.5%. The AUC of (−)-**metoprolol** was increased by 29% and its clearance reduced by 12%.[1] The reason would appear to be that **ciprofloxacin** inhibits the activity of the cytochrome P450 isoenzymes concerned with the metabolism and clearance from the body of metoprolol, although this is in doubt as they are metabolised, predominantly, by different isoenzymes. Beta-blocker AUC changes of this size, or even more, with other enzyme inhibiting drugs have proved not to be clinically important, and it seems probable that this will be the case with ciprofloxacin, but this needs confirmation. There appears to be no information about interactions between other beta-blockers and other quinolone antibacterials.

1. Waite NM, Rutledge DR, Warbasse LH, Edwards DJ. Disposition of the (+) and (−) isomers of metoprolol following ciprofloxacin treatment. *Pharmacotherapy* (1990) 10, 236.

Beta-blockers + Colestyramine or Colestipol

Although both colestyramine and colestipol can reduce the absorption of propranolol to some extent, this does not seem to reduce its effects.

Clinical evidence

(a) Colestyramine

When single 120-mg doses of **propranolol** and 8-g doses of **colestyramine** were taken together by 6 healthy subjects, peak propranolol plasma levels were reduced by almost 25% and the AUC was reduced 13%. An additional dose of **colestyramine** 12 h before the **propranolol** reduced the AUC by 43%. However, no changes in blood pressure or pulse rate were seen.[1] Preliminary results of another study found no significant changes in blood levels of **propranolol** in 5 patients with type II hyperlipidaemia on **propranolol** 40 mg four times daily after being given a single (unstated) dose of **colestyramine**.[2]

(b) Colestipol

When single 120-mg doses of **propranolol** and 10-g doses of **colestipol** were taken together by 6 healthy subjects, the peak plasma **propranolol** levels were raised by 30%. However, they were decreased by 36% if an additional 10 g dose of **colestipol** was taken 12 h before the **propranolol**, and the AUC was reduced by about 30%. No changes in blood pressure or pulse rates were seen.[1]

Mechanism

Uncertain. It seems probable that both the colestyramine and colestipol can bind to the propranolol in the gut, thereby reducing its absorption.

Importance and management

Information is limited. Even though both colestyramine and colestipol can apparently reduce the absorption of single-dose propranolol, no changes in its effects were reported[1] suggesting that the interaction is of minimal clinical importance. There is no obvious rea-

son for avoiding concurrent use. There seems to be no information about other beta-blockers.

1. Hibbard DM, Peters JR, Hunninghake DB. Effects of cholestyramine and colestipol on the plasma concentrations of propranolol. *Br J Clin Pharmacol* (1984) 18, 337–42.
2. Schwartz DE, Schaeffer E, Brewer HB, Franciosa JA. Bioavailability of propranolol following administration of cholestyramine. *Clin Pharmacol Ther* (1982) 31, 268.

Beta-blockers + Dextromoramide

An isolated report describes two patients who developed marked bradycardia and severe hypotension when given propranolol and dextromoramide following the induction of anaesthesia.

Clinical evidence, mechanism, importance and management

Two women about to undergo partial thyroidectomy were given 30 mg **propranolol** and **dextromoramide** (either 1.25 or 4 mg) by injection during the pre-operative period following the induction of anaesthesia with a barbiturate. Each developed marked bradycardia and severe hypotension, which responded rapidly to the intravenous injection of atropine.[1] The reasons for this response are not understood.

1. Cabanne F, Wilkening M, Caillard B, Foissac JC, Aupecle P. Interférences médicamenteuses induites par l'association propranolol-dextromoramide. *Anesth Analg Reanim* (1973) 30, 369–75.

Beta-blockers + Dextropropoxyphene (Propoxyphene)

A single-dose study has shown that the bioavailability of metoprolol is markedly increased by the concurrent use of dextropropoxyphene. The bioavailability of propranolol is also increased, but to a lesser extent. There seem to be no reports of adverse reactions when both drugs have been used.

Clinical evidence, mechanism, importance and management

Preliminary results of a study suggest that after taking **dextropropoxyphene** for a day (dose not stated) the bioavailability of a single 100-mg oral dose of **metoprolol** was increased almost 260% and the total body clearance was reduced 18% in healthy subjects. The bioavailability of a single 40-mg oral dose of **propranolol** was increased by about 70%.[1] The probable reason is that the **dextropropoxyphene** inhibits the metabolism of these beta-blockers by the liver so that they are cleared from the body more slowly.

Be alert for evidence of an increased response to **metoprolol** or **propranolol** if **dextropropoxyphene** is added, but so far there seems to be no evidence that concurrent use causes problems. No interaction would be expected with those beta-blockers which, unlike **metoprolol** and **propranolol**, are largely excreted unchanged in the urine (e.g. **nadolol, sotalol, atenolol**).

1. Lundborg P, Regård CG. The effect of propoxyphene pretreatment on the disposition of metoprolol and propranolol. *Clin Pharmacol Ther* (1981) 29, 263–4.

Beta-blockers + Diphenhydramine

Diphenhydramine inhibits the metabolism of metoprolol, but this is probably not clinically important.

Clinical evidence

A single dose of **metoprolol** 100 mg was administered to 16 healthy subjects on day 3 of a 5-day course of **diphenhydramine** 50 mg three times daily in a placebo-controlled study. **Diphenhydramine** decreased the clearance of **metoprolol** by 46% and increased its AUC by 61% in the 10 subjects who were extensive metabolisers, but had no significant effect in the 6 poor metabolisers. However, the **metoprolol** AUC in the extensive metabolisers on **diphenhydramine** was still only about one-third of that in the poor metabolisers on placebo. The effect of **metoprolol** on heart rate and systolic blood pressure during exercise was also increased by **diphenhydramine** in extensive metabolisers. However, again, it was not as great as the effect of **metoprolol** alone in poor metabolisers.[1]

Mechanism

Diphenhydramine inhibits cytochrome P450 isoenzyme CYP2D6, which is responsible, in part, for the metabolism of metoprolol and some other beta-blockers (e.g. propranolol, timolol). CYP2D6 shows polymorphism, with some individuals lacking CYP2D6 activity (poor metabolisers), in whom diphenhydramine would have no effect.

Importance and management

Information appears to be limited to this study. Increases in plasma metoprolol levels of this size are unlikely to be clinically relevant. Indeed, despite the widespread use of 'extensively-metabolised' beta-blockers and diphenhydramine, no problems seem to have been reported.

1. Hamelin BA, Bouayad A, Méthot J, Jobin J, Desgagnés P, Poirier P, Allaire J, Dumesnil J, Turgeon J. Significant interaction between the nonprescription antihistamine diphenhydramine and the CYP2D6 substrate metoprolol in healthy men with high or low CYP2D6 activity. *Clin Pharmacol Ther* (2000) 67, 466–77.

Beta-blockers + Ergot derivatives

The concurrent use of beta-blockers and ergot derivatives for the management of migraine is not uncommon, but three cases of severe peripheral vasoconstriction and one of hypertension have been described. There is also an isolated case of migraine exacerbated by propranolol alone.

Clinical evidence

A man with recurrent migraine headaches, reasonably well-controlled over a 6-year period with 2 daily suppositories of *Cafergot* (containing **ergotamine tartrate**) developed progressively painful and purple feet a short while after additionally starting to take 30 mg **propranolol** daily. When he eventually resumed taking the *Cafergot* alone there was no further evidence of peripheral vasoconstriction.[1]

A similar situation occurred in a woman taking **oxprenolol** and **ergotamine tartrate** (dosages unknown) for some considerable time, as well as a number of other drugs. Arteriography showed severe spasm in a number of arteries, which responded eventually to an intra-arterial infusion of glyceryl trinitrate and heparin.[2] Severe pain in the legs and feet occurred in another man after taking 3 mg **methysergide** and 120 mg **propranolol** daily for 2 weeks. This failed to respond to various therapies, and in 6 days it was necessary to amputate both his legs below the knee because of gangrene.[2] A woman on **propranolol** for migraine prophylaxis became hypertensive (BP 180/120 mmHg) with a crushing substernal pain immediately after being given oxygen, 5 mg prochlorperazine and 0.75 mg intravenous **dihydroergotamine** for treating an acute migraine headache. She recovered uneventfully. She was later found to be hyperthyroidic.[3]

Paradoxical exacerbation of migraine in a patient given **propranolol** 60 mg daily for angina has also been described. When taking **propranolol**, the headaches also became refractory to **ergotamine**. The migraine attacks ceased when the **propranolol** was withdrawn.[4]

These reports contrast with another stating that concurrent use of **propranolol** and **ergotamine** in 50 patients was both effective and uneventful.[5]

Mechanism

Uncertain. One suggestion is that additive vasoconstriction occurs.[1,2] Ergot derivatives cause vasoconstriction, and the beta-blockers do the same by blocking the normal (beta-2-stimulated) sympathetic vasodilatation. The beta-blockers also reduce blood flow by reducing cardiac output.

Importance and management

Concurrent use is usually safe and effective, and there are only five reports of adverse interactions. It was suggested that at least one of these could have been due to the ergotamine alone (a case of ergotism).[5] However it would clearly be prudent to be extra alert for any signs of an adverse response, particularly those suggestive of reduced peripheral circulation (coldness, numbness or tingling of the hands and feet).

1. Baumrucker JF. Drug interaction — propranolol and cafergot. *N Engl J Med* (1973) 288, 916–17.
2. Venter CP, Joubert PH, Buys AC. Severe peripheral ischaemia during concomitant use of beta blockers and ergot alkaloids. *BMJ* (1984) 289, 288–9.
3. Gandy W. Dihydroergotamine interaction with propranolol. *Ann Emerg Med* (1990) 19, 221.
4. Blank NK, Rieder MJ. Paradoxical response to propranolol in migraine. *Lancet* (1973) ii, 1336.
5. Diamond S. Propranolol and ergotamine tartrate (cont.). *N Engl J Med* (1973) 289, 159.

Beta-blockers + Erythromycin

Serum levels of talinolol and possibly nadolol are increased by concurrent use of erythromycin, but the clinical importance of this is uncertain.

Clinical evidence, mechanism, importance and management

A single-dose study in 8 healthy subjects found that the AUC and serum levels of **talinolol** 50 mg were increased by 51% and 26%, respectively, by **erythromycin** 2 g. It was suggested that the increased bioavailability of **talinolol** was due to increased intestinal absorption caused by erythromycin inhibition of P-glycoprotein.[1] Another study, in which 7 healthy subjects were given a single dose of nadolol 80 mg after 2 days of **erythromycin** 500 mg plus **neomycin** 500 mg 6-hourly, suggested an increase in the rate of beta-blocker absorption (reduced time to maximum plasma level, but no effect on AUC). A decrease in the elimination half-life was also seen.[2] More study is needed to determine the clinical significance of these findings, and to establish whether or not other beta-blockers are affected. **Sotalol** prolongs the QT interval and should generally not be given with other drugs that do the same, such as intravenous **erythromycin**, because of the increased risk of torsade de pointes arrhythmia (see also 'Drugs that prolong the QT interval + Other drugs that prolong the QT interval', p.103).

1. Schwarz UI, Gramatté T, Krappweis J, Oertel R, Kirch W. P-glycoprotein inhibitor erythromycin increases oral bioavailability of talinolol in humans. *Int J Clin Pharmacol Ther* (2000) 38, 161–7.
2. du Souich P, Caillé G, Larochelle P. Enhancement of nadolol elimination by activated charcoal and antibiotics. *Clin Pharmacol Ther* (1983) 33, 585–90.

Beta-blockers + Flecainide

Combined use may have additive cardiac depressive effects. An isolated case of bradycardia and fatal AV block has been reported.

Clinical evidence, mechanism, importance and management

A study on cardiac function and drug clearance in 10 healthy subjects found that when **propranolol** 80 mg three times daily was given with **flecainide** 200 mg twice daily for 4 days the AUCs of both drugs were increased by 20 to 30%, and they had some additive negative inotropic effects on the heart.[1] There is a report of a patient on **flecainide** 100 mg twice daily who developed bradycardia and fatal atrioventricular conduction block 3 hours after the second of 2 doses of **sotalol** 40 mg.[2] Careful monitoring has therefore been recommended if beta-blockers are added to therapy with other antiarrhythmic agents. Serious cardiac depression has been seen following the concurrent use of flecainide and other drugs with negative inotropic effects (e.g. verapamil). See the Index.

1. Holtzman JL, Kvam DC, Berry DA, Mottonen L, Borrell G, Harrison LI, Conard GJ. The pharmacodynamic and pharmacokinetic interaction of flecainide acetate with propranolol: effects on cardiac function and drug clearance. *Eur J Clin Pharmacol* (1987) 33, 97–9.
2. Warren R, Vohra J, Hunt D, Hamer A. Serious interactions of sotalol with amiodarone and flecainide. *Med J Aust* (1990) 152, 277.

Beta-blockers + Fluoxetine

Fluoxetine can increase serum pindolol and carvedilol levels, but the clinical effects of this are minimal. Two isolated reports describe lethargy and bradycardia in two men on metoprolol or propranolol shortly after starting to take fluoxetine. Sotalol was found not to interact with fluoxetine in one of them.

Clinical evidence

Metoprolol 100 mg daily improved the angina of a man who had undergone a coronary artery bypass 4 years earlier. A month later he was given 20 mg **fluoxetine** daily for depression. Within 2 days he complained of profound lethargy, and his resting heart rate was found to have fallen from 64 to 36 bpm. The **fluoxetine** was withdrawn, whereupon his heart rate returned to 64 bpm within 5 days. The **metoprolol** was replaced by 80 mg **sotalol** twice daily and **fluoxetine** reintroduced without problems.[1]

Another patient on **propranolol** 40 mg twice daily developed bradycardia (30 bpm), heart block and syncope 2 weeks after starting 20 mg **fluoxetine** daily. This patient possibly also had some pre-existing conduction disease contributing to the effect.[2]

When 9 healthy subjects were given 5 mg **pindolol** six-hourly with 20 mg **fluoxetine** daily for 3 days and then 60 mg daily for another 7 days, the pindolol AUC rose by 75.2% and its clearance fell by 45.3% compared with a single dose of **pindolol** 5 mg. Only mild to moderate alterations in pulse rate and blood pressure accompanied these changes.[3]

A double-blind crossover study in 10 patients with heart failure, maintained on carvedilol 25 to 50 mg twice daily, found that the addition of fluoxetine 20 mg daily for 28 days increased the AUC of $R(+)$-carvedilol by 77%, and decreased the clearance of both enantiomers by 44 to 56%. However, these pharmacokinetic changes were of little clinical significance, since there were no changes in blood pressure, heart rate, and heart rate variability.[4]

Mechanism

Fluoxetine inhibits the cytochrome P450 isoenzyme CYP2D6 thus inhibiting the metabolism of some beta-blockers (e.g. propranolol, metoprolol, carvedilol) so that they accumulate, the result being that their effects, such as bradycardia, may be increased.[1] Beta-blockers that are not extensively metabolised, such as sotalol, would not be expected to be affected. Bradycardia has been rarely reported with fluoxetine alone.

Pindolol may augment the antidepressant effect of fluoxetine by its antagonistic effects at 5-HT$_{1A}$ receptors.[5]

Importance and management

Direct information seems to be limited to these reports. The general importance of these interactions is uncertain but other SSRIs such as fluvoxamine can cause a very marked rise in serum propranolol levels apparently without causing problems (see 'Fluvoxamine + Miscella-

neous drugs', p.828). If problems arise the interaction can apparently be avoided by giving a water-soluble beta-blocker (such atenolol), which is not extensively metabolised. Fluoxetine may be given to patients with heart failure stabilised on carvedilol.[4] Remember that fluoxetine and particularly its metabolite have long half-lives so that this interaction may possibly still occur some days after the fluoxetine has been stopped.

1. Walley T, Pirmohamed M, Proudlove C, Maxwell D. Interaction of metoprolol and fluoxetine. *Lancet* (1993) 341, 967–8.
2. Drake WM, Gordon GD. Heart block in a patient on propranolol and fluoxetine. *Lancet* (1994) 343, 425–6.
3. Goldberg MJ, Bergstrom RF, Cerimele BJ, Thomasson HR, Hatcher BL, Simcox EA. Fluoxetine effects on pindolol pharmacokinetics. *Clin Pharmacol Ther* (1997) 61, 178.
4. Graff DW, Williamson KM, Pieper JA, Carson SW, Adams KF, Cascio WE, Patterson JH. Effect of fluoxetine on carvedilol pharmacokinetics, CYP2D6 activity, and autonomic balance in heart failure patients. *J Clin Pharmacol* (2001) 41, 97–106.
5. Dawson LA, Nguyen HQ, Smith DI, Schechter LE. Effects of chronic fluoxetine treatment in the presence and absence of (+/-)pindolol: a microdialysis study. *Br J Pharmacol* (2000) 130, 797–804.

Beta-blockers + Food

Food can increase, decrease or not affect the bioavailability of beta-blockers, but none of the changes has been shown to be of clinical importance.

Clinical evidence, mechanism, importance and management

Food increased the AUC of **propranolol** by 50 to 80%,[1-3] **metoprolol** by about 40%[1] and of **labetalol** by about 40%[4] probably by changing the extent of their metabolism during their first pass through the liver.[2-4] Food did not affect the extent of absorption of a sustained-release formulation of **propranolol**.[2] Food had very little effect on the absorption of **oxprenolol**[5,6] or **pindolol**,[7] whereas the AUC of **atenolol** was reduced by about 20%.[8] A later study suggested atenolol (and possibly other hydrophilic beta-blockers) become tightly associated with bile acid micelles, preventing their absorption.[9] None of these changes has been shown to be of clinical importance, nor is it clear whether it matters if patients take these drugs in a regular pattern in relation to meals. Beta-blocker serum concentrations vary widely between patients (a 20-fold difference in propranolol AUC has been noted between individuals),[1] and individualising the dose is therefore the major issue.

1. Melander A, Danielson K, Scherstén B, Wåhlin E. Enhancement of the bioavailability of propranolol and metoprolol by food. *Clin Pharmacol Ther* (1977) 22, 108–12.
2. Liedholm H, Melander A. Concomitant food intake can increase the bioavailability of propranolol by transient inhibition of its presystemic primary conjugation. *Clin Pharmacol Ther* (1986) 40, 29–36.
3. McLean AJ, Isbister C, Bobik A, Dudley F. Reduction of first-pass hepatic clearance of propranolol by food. *Clin Pharmacol Ther* (1981) 30, 31–4.
4. Daneshmend TK, Roberts CJC. The influence of food on the oral and intravenous pharmacokinetics of a high clearance drug: a study with labetalol. *Br J Clin Pharmacol* (1982) 14, 73–8.
5. Dawes CP, Kendall MJ, Welling PG. Bioavailability of conventional and slow-release oxprenolol in fasted and nonfasted individuals. *Br J Clin Pharmacol* (1979) 7, 299–302.
6. John VA, Smith SE. Influence of food intake on plasma oxprenolol concentrations following oral administration of conventional and Oros preparations. *Br J Clin Pharmacol* (1985) 19, 191S–195S.
7. Kiger JL, Lavene D, Guillaume MF, Guerret M, Longchampt J. The effect of food and clopamide on the absorption of pindolol in man. *Int J Clin Pharmacol Biopharm* (1976) 13, 228–32.
8. Melander A, Stenberg P, Liedholm H, Scherstén B, Wåhlin-Boll E. Food-induced reduction in bioavailability of atenolol. *Eur J Clin Pharmacol* (1979) 16, 327–30.
9. Barnwell SG, Laudanski T, Dwyer M, Story MJ, Guard P, Cole S, Attwood D. Reduced bioavailability of atenolol in man: the role of bile acids. *Int J Pharmaceutics* (1993) 89, 245–50.

Beta-blockers + Haloperidol

An isolated case report describes severe hypotension and cardiopulmonary arrest in a woman on three occasions shortly after being given haloperidol and propranolol.

Clinical evidence, importance and management

A middle-aged woman with schizophrenia and hypertension experienced 3 episodes of severe hypotension within 30 to 120 min of being given **propranolol** (40 to 80 mg) and **haloperidol** (10 mg).[1] On two of the occasions cardiopulmonary arrest took place. She fainted each time, became cyanotic, had no palpable pulses and showed severe hypotension, but rapidly responded to cardiopulmonary resuscitation. She suffered no adverse consequences. The reasons for this reaction are not understood, but one suggestion[1] is that this patient was unduly sensitive to the additive relaxant effect of both drugs on peripheral blood vessels.

This seems to be the only case of this interaction on record. Bearing in mind the widespread use of **propranolol**, other beta-blockers and **haloperidol**, this interaction is obviously rare. There would seem to be little reason for avoiding concurrent use.

1. Alexander HE, McCarty K, Giffen MB. Hypotension and cardiopulmonary arrest associated with concurrent haloperidol and propranolol therapy. *JAMA* (1984) 252, 87–8.

Beta-blockers + H$_2$-blockers; Cimetidine

The blood levels of some extensively metabolised beta-blockers (e.g. metoprolol, propranolol) can be doubled by the concurrent use of cimetidine, but normally this appears to be clinically unimportant. No important interaction normally seems to occur with other beta-blockers. An isolated report describes profound bradycardia (heart rate 36 bpm) in a patient given atenolol and cimetidine. Marked hypotension occurred in two patients on labetalol and cimetidine, and an irregular heart beat in yet another taking metoprolol and cimetidine.

Clinical evidence

(A) Beta-blockers showing raised levels

(a) Labetalol

The AUC of a single oral dose of **labetalol** 200 mg was increased by 66%, and the bioavailability by 56%, in 6 healthy subjects after 4 days treatment with **cimetidine** 400 mg four times daily.[1,2] One subject developed postural hypotension (70/40 mmHg), felt lightheaded and almost fainted on standing.[2] Conversely, the AUC of intravenous **labetalol** was unaffected by **cimetidine**.[2]

(b) Metoprolol

A study in 6 healthy subjects given 100 mg **metoprolol** twice daily for a week found that the concurrent use of 1 g **cimetidine** daily in divided doses increased the peak plasma levels by 70% and the AUC by 61%, but this did not increase the effect of **metoprolol** on the heart rate during exercise.[3,4] Three other studies confirmed that **cimetidine** increased **metoprolol** serum levels after single or multiple doses, and that this did not increase the effect of **metoprolol** on the heart rate during exercise.[5-8] However, two other studies found **cimetidine** did not affect serum levels of a single 100 mg **metoprolol** dose.[9,10] An isolated case describes one patient who complained of a "very irregular heart beat" while taking both drugs, which was much less marked when he took the two drugs separated as much time as possible.[11]

(c) Nebivolol

Cimetidine 400 mg twice daily increased the AUC of a single dose of **nebivolol** 5 mg by 48% and the peak plasma levels by 23%, but did not alter the effect of **nebivolol** on blood pressure or heart rate.[12]

(d) Pindolol

Cimetidine 1000 mg daily in divided doses increased the AUC of **pindolol** 10 mg twice daily by 30%, and the peak plasma levels by 33%, although these changes were not statistically significant.[13] In another study, **cimetidine** 400 mg twice daily increased the AUC of the **pindolol** enantiomers by 41 and 38%, and decreased the renal clearance by 39 and 30%.[14]

(e) Propranolol

Twelve healthy subjects were given 1.2 g **cimetidine** daily for a week, and from day 3 onwards they were also given **propranolol** 80 mg twelve-hourly. The mean steady-state blood levels of **propranolol** were raised by 47%, the AUC by 47% and the half-life was prolonged by 17%, but **cimetidine** did not alter the effect of **propranolol** on heart rate.[15]

A number of other single-dose and steady-state studies confirmed that **cimetidine** caused rises of 35 to 100%) in blood levels and AUC of **propranolol** whether given orally,[3,4,16-21] but that this did not increase the effect of the beta-blocker on heart rate at rest or during exercise,[3,17-20] or blood pressure.[17,19,20] In contrast, one study did show a further reduction in heart rate when **cimetidine** was given with **propranolol**.[22] A letter describes one patient given 1 g **cimetidine** daily for 6 weeks who showed an approximately threefold increase in serum **propranolol** level (AUC increased 340%) when given a single 80-mg dose.[23]

(B) Beta-blockers not affected

A brief mention of a patient taking **a beta-blocker** for angina who developed profound sinus bradycardia (36 bpm) and hypotension when additionally treated with **cimetidine** was made in a report.[23] The beta-blocker was not specified, but it was identified as **atenolol** elsewhere in a letter.[24] However, three well-controlled studies in healthy subjects and patients have shown that **cimetidine** did not significantly alter blood levels of **atenolol**, nor did it alter the affect of **atenolol** on heart rate.[3,4,9,10]

Similarly, blood levels and the pharmacokinetics of **betaxolol**,[21] carvedilol,[25] **nadolol**,[19] and **penbutolol**[13,26] were unaffected by cimetidine, and the effects of the beta-blockers on heart rate and blood pressure were not changed.[13,19,26]

A double-blind study in 12 healthy subjects found that **cimetidine** 400 mg twice daily for 3 days did not modify the effect of a single instillation of 0.25 mg **timolol** into each eye (0.05 ml of 0.5% eye drops) on heart rate or intraocular pressure to a statistically significant or clinically relevant extent.[27]

Mechanism

The blood levels of beta-blockers extensively metabolised in the liver by cytochrome P450 isoenzyme CYP2D6 (e.g. propranolol, metoprolol and nebivolol) are increased because cimetidine reduces their metabolism by inhibiting the activity of the liver enzymes. It is unclear why cimetidine affects labetalol, a beta-blocker that is extensively metabolised, but not by CYP2D6.[2] Other extensively metabolised beta-blockers *not* affected by cimetidine include betaxolol, carvedilol, and penbutolol. Pindolol is partly excreted by an active renal tubular secretion mechanism, and cimetidine increases pindolol blood levels by inhibiting this mechanism.[14] Those beta-blockers that are largely excreted unchanged in the urine (e.g. atenolol, nadolol) are not affected by cimetidine.[10,19]

Importance and management

Well studied and established interactions but, despite the considerable rises in blood levels that can occur with some beta-blockers, the effects normally appear to be clinically unimportant. Concurrent use is common, but only one isolated case of profound bradycardia involving atenolol appears to have been reported (see case cited above). Marked hypotension also seems to be rare. Combined use need not be avoided, however it has been suggested that patients with impaired liver function who are given beta-blockers that are extensively metabolised in the liver (e.g. metoprolol, propranolol) might possibly develop grossly elevated blood levels which could cause adverse effects. This needs confirmation.

1. Daneshmend TK, Roberts CJC. Cimetidine and bioavailability of labetalol. *Lancet* (1981), i, 565.
2. Daneshmend TK, Roberts CJC. The effects of enzyme induction and enzyme inhibition on labetalol pharmacokinetics. *Br J Clin Pharmacol* (1984) 18, 393–400.
3. Kirch W, Spahn H, Köhler H, Mutschler E. Accumulation and adverse effects of metoprolol and propranolol after concurrent administration of cimetidine. *Arch Toxicol* (1983) (Suppl 6), 379–83.
4. Kirch W, Spahn H, Köhler H, Mutschler E. Interaction of metoprolol, propranolol and atenolol with cimetidine. *Clin Sci* (1982) 63, 451S–453S.
5. Kendall MJ, Laugher SJ, Wilkins MR. Ranitidine, cimetidine and metoprolol: a pharmacokinetic interaction study. *Gastroenterology* (1986) 90, 1490.
6. Kirch W, Rämsch K, Janisch HD, Ohnhaus EE. The influence of two histamine H_2-receptor antagonists, cimetidine and ranitidine, on plasma levels and clinical effect of nifedipine and metoprolol. *Arch Toxicol* (1984) (Suppl 7), 256–9.
7. Chellingsworth MC, Laugher S, Akhlaghi S, Jack DB, Kendall MJ. The effects of ranitidine and cimetidine on the pharmacokinetics and pharmacodynamics of metoprolol. *Aliment Pharmacol Ther* (1988) 2, 521–7.
8. Toon S, Davidson EM, Garstang FM, Batra H, Bowes RJ, Rowland M. The racemic metoprolol H_2-antagonist interaction. *Clin Pharmacol Ther* (1988) 43, 283–9.
9. Houtzagers JJR, Streurman O, Regårdh CG. The effect of pretreatment with cimetidine on the bioavailability and disposition of atenolol and metoprolol. *Br J Clin Pharmacol* (1982) 14, 67–72.
10. Ellis ME, Hussain M, Webb AK, Barker NP, Fitzsimons TJ. The effect of cimetidine on the relative cardioselectivity of atenolol and metoprolol in asthmatic patients. *Br J Clin Pharmacol* (1984) 17, 59S–64S.
11. Anon. Adverse Drug Reactions Advisory Committee. Seven case studies. *Med J Aust* (1982) 2, 190–1.
12. Kamali F, Howes A, Thomas SHL, Ford GA, Snoeck E. A pharmacokinetic and pharmacodynamic interaction study between nebivolol and the H_2-receptor antagonists cimetidine and ranitidine. *Br J Clin Pharmacol* (1997) 43, 201–4.
13. Spahn H, Kirch W, Mutschler E. The interaction of cimetidine with metoprolol, atenolol, propranolol, pindolol and penbutolol. *Br J Clin Pharmacol* (1983) 15, 500–1.
14. Somogyi AA, Bochner F, Sallustio BC. Stereoselective inhibition of pindolol renal clearance by cimetidine in humans. *Clin Pharmacol Ther* (1992) 51, 379–87.
15. Donn KH, Powell JR, Rogers JF, Eshelman FN. The influence of H2-receptor antagonists on steady-state concentrations of propranolol and 4-hydroxypropranolol. *J Clin Pharmacol* (1984) 24, 500–8.
16. Kirch W, Köhler H, Spahn H, Mutschler E. Interaction of cimetidine with metoprolol, propranolol or atenolol. *Lancet* (1981) ii, 531–2.
17. Reimann IW, Klotz U, Frölich JC. Effects of cimetidine and ranitidine on steady-state propranolol kinetics and dynamics. *Clin Pharmacol Ther* (1982) 32, 749–57.
18. Reimann IW, Klotz U, Siems B, Frölich JC. Cimetidine increases steady-state plasma levels of propranolol. *Br J Clin Pharmacol* (1981) 12, 785–90.
19. Duchin KL, Stern MA, Willard DA, McKinstry DN. Comparison of kinetic interactions of nadolol and propranolol with cimetidine. *Am Heart J* (1984) 108, 1084–6.
20. Markiewicz A, Hartleb M, Lelek A, Boldys H, Nowak A. The effect of treatment with cimetidine and ranitidine on bioavailability of, and circulatory response to, propranolol. *Zbl Pharm* (1984) 123, 516–18.
21. Rey E, Jammet P, d'Athis P, de Lauture D, Christoforov B, Weber S, Olive G. Effect of cimetidine on the pharmacokinetics of the new beta-blocker betaxolol. *Arzneimittelforschung* (1987) 37, 953–6.
22. Feely J, Wilkinson GR, Wood AJJ. Reduction in liver blood flow and propranolol metabolism by cimetidine. *N Engl J Med* (1981) 304, 692–5.
23. Donovan MA, Heagerty AM, Patel L, Castleden M, Pohl JEF. Cimetidine and bioavailability of propranolol. *Lancet* (1981) i, 164.
24. Rowley-Jones D, Flind AC. Drug interactions with cimetidine. *Pharm J* (1981) 283, 659.
25. Data on file, database on carvedilol, SmithKline Beecham, quoted by Ruffolo RR, Boyle DA, Venuti RP, Lukas MA. Carvedilol (Kredex®): a novel multiple action cardiovascular agent. *Drugs Today* (1991) 27, 465–92.
26. Spahn H, Kirch W, Hajdu P, Mutschler E, Ohnhaus EE. Penbutolol pharmacokinetics: the influence of concomitant administration of cimetidine. *Eur J Clin Pharmacol* (1986) 29, 555–60.
27. Ishii Y, Nakamura K, Tsutsumi K, Kotegawa T, Nakano S, Natasuka K. Drug interaction between cimetidine and timolol ophthalmic solution: effect on heart rate and intraocular pressure in healthy Japanese volunteers. *J Clin Pharmacol* (2000) 40, 193–9.

Beta-blockers + H_2-blockers; Famotidine

Famotidine does not interact with beta-blockers.

Clinical evidence, mechanism, importance and management

A survey of 15 patients taking beta-blockers (acebutolol, atenolol, betaxolol, nadolol, pindolol, propranolol or sotalol) for 6 to 8 weeks found no evidence of changes in their response (increased antihypertensive effects or enhanced bradycardia) while concurrently taking 40 mg famotidine daily.[1] No interaction would be expected, and no special precautions would seem necessary if famotidine is taken with these or any other beta-blocker.

1. Chichmanian RM, Mignot G, Spreux A, Jean-Girard C, Hofliger P. Tolérance de la famotidine. Étude due réseau médecins sentinelles en pharmacovigilance. *Therapie* (1992) 47, 239–43.

Beta-blockers + H_2-blockers; Nizatidine

The heart-slowing effects of atenolol are increased by nizatidine.

Clinical evidence, mechanism, importance and management

After taking 100 mg atenolol daily for 7 days the mean resting heart rate of 12 healthy subjects fell by 10.6 bpm (from 63.7 to 53.1 bpm) 3h after dosing. A further fall of 6 bpm occurred when they were additionally given 300 mg **nizatidine** daily for 7 days. **Nizatidine** alone caused a fall in heart rate of about 8 bpm.[1] Thus the effects of nizatidine and atenolol on heart rate appear to be additive. It seems likely that **nizatidine** would have the same effects in the presence of other beta-blockers. The clinical significance of these effects is uncertain, but it might be important in elderly patients.[1] More study is needed.

1. Halabi A, Kirch W. Negative chronotropic effects of nizatidine. *Gut* (1991) 32, 630–4.

Beta-blockers + H_2-blockers; Ranitidine

Ranitidine does not alter the steady-state plasma levels of atenolol, nebivolol, propranolol or tertatolol and their therapeutic effects remain unchanged. Some studies have shown moderate rises in metoprolol levels, but these are not clinically important.

Clinical evidence

The plasma levels of **metoprolol** 100 mg twice daily were unaffected by 300 mg **ranitidine** daily for 7 days in 12 healthy subjects.[1,2] Two other studies have confirmed that **ranitidine** did not significantly affect the plasma levels of **metoprolol**.[3-6] However, these studies found increases of up to 38% in **metoprolol** AUC after single intravenous or oral doses,[3-6] and another study found that ranitidine increased the AUC and plasma concentrations of **metoprolol** 100 mg twice daily, by 55 and 34%, respectively.[7-9] All of these studies found that **ranitidine** did not alter the effect of metoprolol on heart rate during exercise.[2,3,6,7]

Ranitidine 300 mg daily for 6 days did not affect the steady-state plasma levels of **propranolol** 160 mg daily nor did it alter the effect of **propranolol** on heart rate or blood pressure in 5 healthy subjects.[10] Similarly no changes in plasma **propranolol** levels were seen in other multiple-dose[11] or single-dose studies.[12-15]

Similarly, in other studies, **ranitidine** 150 mg twice daily did not significantly alter the pharmacokinetic or pharmacodynamic effects of single 5-mg doses of **nebivolol**[16] single 5-mg doses of **tertatolol**,[17] or **atenolol** 100 mg daily for 7 days.[7,9]

Mechanism

The rises in metoprolol serum levels caused by ranitidine in the two single-dose metoprolol studies are not understood, nor is it clear why one of four studies found an increase after multiple doses.

Importance and management

The possible effects of ranitidine on the plasma levels and effects of propranolol and metoprolol have been well studied. Although some studies have shown moderate rises in metoprolol levels, particularly after single-doses, these are unlikely to be clinically important. Less is known about atenolol, nebivolol and tertatolol, although no clinically relevant interactions have been seen. There is nothing to suggest that the concurrent use of ranitidine and any beta-blocker should be avoided, nor that there is any need to take particular precautions.

1. Toon S, Batra HK, Garstang FM, Rowland M. Comparative effects of ranitidine and cimetidine on metoprolol in man. *Br J Pharmacol* (1987). Abstract presented to the British Pharmacological Society meeting, September 1986.

2. Toon S, Davidson EM, Garstang FM, Batra H, Bowers RJ, Rowland M. The racemic metoprolol H₂-antagonist interaction. *Clin Pharmacol Ther* (1988) 43, 283–9.
3. Kelly JG, Salem SAM, Kinney CD, Shanks RG, McDevitt DG. Effects of ranitidine on the disposition of metoprolol. *Br J Clin Pharmacol* (1985) 19, 219–24.
4. Kelly JG, Shanks RG, McDevitt DG. Influence of ranitidine on plasma metoprolol concentrations. *BMJ* (1983) 287, 1218–19.
5. Kendall MJ, Laugher SJ, Wilkins MR. Ranitidine, cimetidine and metoprolol–a pharmacokinetic interaction study. *Gastroenterology* (1986) 90, 1490.
6. Chellingsworth MC, Laugher S, Akhlaghi S, Jack DB, Kendall MJ. The effects of ranitidine and cimetidine on the pharmacokinetics and pharmacodynamics of metoprolol. *Aliment Pharmacol Ther* (1988) 2, 521–7.
7. Spahn H, Mutschler E, Kirch W, Ohnhaus EE, Janisch HD. Influence of ranitidine on plasma metoprolol and atenolol concentrations. *BMJ* (1983) 286, 1546–7.
8. Kirch W, Rämsch K, Janisch HD, Ohnhaus EE. The influence of two histamine H₂-receptor antagonists, cimetidine and ranitidine, on the plasma levels and clinical effect of nifedipine and metoprolol. *Arch Toxicol* (1984) 7 (Suppl), 256–9.
9. Mutschler E, Spahn H, Kirch W. The interaction between H₂-receptor antagonists and beta-adrenoceptor blockers. *Br J Clin Pharmacol* (1984) 17, 51S–57S.
10. Reimann IW, Klotz U, Frölich JC. Effects of cimetidine and ranitidine on steady-state propranolol kinetics and dynamics. *Clin Pharmacol Ther* (1982) 32, 749–57.
11. Donn KH, Powell JR, Rogers JF, Eshelman FN. The influence of H₂-receptor antagonists on steady-state concentrations of propranolol and 4-hydroxypropranolol. *J Clin Pharmacol* (1984) 24, 500–8.
12. Markiewicz A, Hartleb M, Lelek H, Boldys H, Nowak A. The effect of treatment with cimetidine and ranitidine on bioavailability of, and circulatory response to, propranolol. *Zbl Pharm* (1984) 123, 516–18.
13. Heagerty AM, Castleden CM, Patel L. Failure of ranitidine to interact with propranolol. *BMJ* (1982) 284, 1304.
14. Heagerty AM, Donovan MA, Casteleden CM, Pohl JEF, Patel L. The influence of histamine (H₂) antagonists on propranolol pharmacokinetics. *Int J Clin Pharmacol Res* (1982) 2, 203–5.
15. Patel L, Weerasuriya K. Effect of cimetidine and ranitidine on propranolol clearance. *Br J Clin Pharmacol* (1983) 15, 152P.
16. Kamali F, Howes A, Thomas SHL, Ford GA, Snoeck E. A pharmacokinetic and pharmacodynamic interaction study between nebivolol and the H₂-receptor antagonists cimetidine and ranitidine. *Br J Clin Pharmacol* (1997) 43, 201–4.
17. Kirch W, Milferstädt S, Halabi A, Rocher I, Efthymiopoulos C, Jung L. Interaction of tertatolol with rifampicin and ranitidine pharmacokinetics and antihypertensive activity. *Cardiovasc Drug Ther* (1990) 4, 487–92.

Beta-blockers + Hydralazine

Concurrent use is not uncommon in the treatment of hypertension. Plasma levels of propranolol and other extensively metabolised beta-blockers (metoprolol, oxprenolol) are increased but no adverse effects seem to have been reported.

Clinical evidence

(a) Effect of hydralazine on beta-blockers

Single 25- and 50-mg doses of **hydralazine** increased the AUC of single 40-mg doses of **propranolol** in 5 healthy subjects by 60% and 110%, and raised the peak plasma concentrations by 144 and 240% respectively.[1]

Other studies confirm that **hydralazine** increased the AUC of **propranolol** by 62 to 77%,[2] of sustained-release **oxprenolol** by 41%,[3] and of **metoprolol** by 30%[4] and 38%,[5] but not of **acebutolol** or **nadolol**.[4]

(b) Effect of beta-blockers on hydralazine

Oxprenolol was found not to have a significant effect on the pharmacokinetics of **hydralazine**.[3]

Mechanism

Uncertain. Hydralazine appears to increase the bioavailability only of those beta-blockers that undergo high hepatic extraction (e.g. propranolol, metoprolol) and not those that are largely excreted unchanged in the urine (e.g. atenolol, nadolol). It has been suggested that hydralazine may alter hepatic blood flow or inhibit hepatic enzymes.[1,4,5]

Importance and management

Moderately well documented and established interactions, but the increased beta-blocker serum levels appear to cause no adverse clinical effect. Concurrent use is usually valuable in the treatment of hypertension. No particular precautions seem to be necessary, but the outcome should be monitored.

1. Schneck DW, Vary JE. Mechanism by which hydralazine increases propranolol bioavailability. *Clin Pharmacol Ther* (1984) 35, 447–53.

2. McLean AJ, Skews H, Bobik A, Dudley FJ. Interaction between oral propranolol and hydralazine. *Clin Pharmacol Ther* (1980) 27, 726–32.
3. Hawksworth GM, Dart AM, Chiang K, Parry K, Petrie JC. Effect of oxprenolol on the pharmacokinetics and pharmacodynamics of hydralazine. *Drugs* (1983) 25 (Suppl 2), 136–40.
4. Jack DB, Kendall MJ, Dean S, Laugher SJ, Zaman R, Tenneson ME. The effect of hydralazine on the pharmacokinetics of three different beta adrenoceptor antagonists: metoprolol, nadolol, and acebutolol. *Biopharm Drug Dispos* (1982) 3, 47–54.
5. Lindeberg S, Holm B, Lundborg P, Regårdh CG, Sandström B. The effect of hydralazine on steady-state plasma concentrations of metoprolol in pregnant hypertensive women. *Eur J Clin Pharmacol* (1988) 35, 131–5.

Beta-blockers + Hydroxychloroquine

Hydroxychloroquine may increase the blood levels of metoprolol, but this is probably not clinically important.

Clinical evidence, mechanism, importance and management

Hydroxychloroquine 400 mg daily for 8 days increased the AUC and peak plasma levels of a single dose of **metoprolol** 100 mg in 7 healthy subjects who were extensive metabolisers by 65% and 72% respectively.[1] **Hydroxychloroquine** may inhibit the metabolism of **metoprolol** by cytochrome P450 isoenzyme CYP2D6. The clinical significance of this interaction is unknown, but beta-blocker AUC changes of this size, or even more, with other enzyme inhibiting drugs have proved not to be clinically important. Other beta-blockers that are extensively metabolised (e.g. propranolol) may behave similarly. More study is needed.

1. Somer M, Kallio J, Pesonen U, Pyykkö K, Huupponen R, Scheinin M. Influence of hydroxychloroquine on the bioavailability of oral metoprolol. *Br J Clin Pharmacol* (2000) 49, 549–54.

Beta-blockers + Misoprostol

Misoprostol does not interact significantly with propranolol.

Clinical evidence, mechanism, importance and management

Misoprostol 400 micrograms twice daily raised the AUC of **propranolol** 80 mg twice daily by about 20 to 40% in 12 healthy subjects, and this remained raised 7 days after **misoprostol** was discontinued.[1] However, as these findings were unexpected, the authors conducted a randomised, crossover, placebo-controlled study and ensured **propranolol** was at steady state before assessing the effect of **misoprostol**. No significant effects on the pharmacokinetics of **propranolol** were found.[2] No special precautions would seem necessary during concurrent use.

1. Bennett PN, Fenn GC, Notarianni LJ. Potential drug interactions with misoprostol: effects on the pharmacokinetics of antipyrine and propranolol. *Postgrad Med J* (1988) 64 (Suppl 1), 21–4.
2. Bennett PN, Fenn GC, Notarianni LJ, Lee CE. Misoprostol does not alter the pharmacokinetics of propranolol. *Postgrad Med J* (1991) 67, 455–7.

Beta-blockers + Morphine

Morphine may moderately raise the serum levels of esmolol, but this is unlikely to be clinically important. The fatal doses of morphine and propranolol are markedly reduced in *animals* when given together, but the clinical relevance of this in man is uncertain.

Clinical evidence, mechanism, importance and management

After being given an injection of 3 mg **morphine sulphate** the steady-state levels of **esmolol** (an infusion of 300 micrograms/kg/min over 4 h) in 10 healthy men were generally higher, but were only statistically significantly higher (by 46%) in 2 of the subjects, and were considered to be of no clinical importance. The pharmacokinetics of morphine were unchanged.[1] Studies in *animals* have shown that the median fatal dose of **propranolol** was reduced two to sevenfold in *mice* by **morphine**[2] and the median lethal dose of **morphine** was reduced fifteen to sixteenfold in *rats*[3] by **propranolol**. The same interaction has also been seen in *dogs*.[3] There do not appear to be any published reports of synergistic toxicity of morphine and propranolol, so the clinical relevance of this is uncertain.

1. Lowenthal DT, Porter RS, Saris SD, Bies CM, Slegowski MB, Staudacher A. Clinical pharmacology, pharmacodynamics and interactions with esmolol. *Am J Cardiol* (1985) 56, 14–18F.
2. Murmann W, Almirante L, Saccani-Guelfi M. Effects of hexobarbitone, ether, morphine, and urethane upon the acute toxicity of propranolol and D-(-)-INPEA. *J Pharm Pharmacol* (1966) 18, 692–4.
3. Davis WM, Hatoum NS. Possible toxic interaction of propranolol and narcotic analgesics. *Drug Intell Clin Pharm* (1981) 15, 290–1.

Beta-blockers + NSAIDs

Indometacin (indomethacin) reduces the antihypertensive effects of the beta-blockers. Piroxicam usually interacts similarly, while normally diclofenac, imidazole salicylate, naproxen, oxaprozin, sulindac and tenoxicam do not. Isolated cases have been reported with naproxen and ibuprofen. The situation with aspirin is a little uncertain. Indometacin has also been reported to cause a marked hypertensive response in two women with pre-eclampsia.

Clinical evidence

(a) Beta-blockers + Aspirin and other salicylates

A study in 11 patients taking a number of antihypertensives (which included a few on **propranolol** and **pindolol**) showed that **aspirin** 650 mg three times for 7 days daily did not affect the control of their blood pressure.[1] In contrast, another study found that 5 g of **aspirin** over 24h prevented the antihypertensive effects of a single 1 mg intravenous dose of **pindolol**, and a single 1 to 1.5 g dose of **aspirin** reduced the antihypertensive effect of a single 5 mg intravenous dose of **propranolol**.[2] **Aspirin** was reported not to affect the control of hypertension by **metipranolol**.[3] Another study in 6 healthy subjects showed that **aspirin** did not affect the kinetics of **atenolol**.[4]

Sodium salicylate was found to affect neither the pharmacokinetics of **alprenolol** nor its effects on heart rate and blood pressure during exercise in a single-dose study in healthy subjects.[5] **Imidazole salicylate** did not affect the blood pressure control of patients treated with **atenolol**.[6]

(b) Beta-blockers + Diclofenac

A study in 16 patients taking **atenolol**, **metoprolol**, **propranolol** or **pindolol** and or a diuretic found that 50 mg **diclofenac** three times daily had no effect on the control of blood pressure.[7]

(c) Beta-blockers + Ibuprofen

The antihypertensive effect of **pindolol** was antagonised by the concurrent use of **ibuprofen** in one patient.[8] However, **ibuprofen** had no effect on the control of blood pressure in patients on **propranolol** in one randomised controlled study.[9]

(d) Beta-blockers + Indometacin (Indomethacin)

The diastolic blood pressures of 7 hypertensive patients treated with **pindolol** (15 mg daily) or **propranolol** (80 to 160 mg daily) rose from 82 to 96 mmHg when they were also given **indometacin** 100 mg daily over a 10-day period. Changes in systolic pressures were not statistically significant.[10]

In another study, 50 mg **indometacin** twice daily raised the systolic/diastolic blood pressures of patients on **propranolol** (60 to 320 mg daily) by 14/5 mmHg when lying and 16/9 mmHg when standing.[11] This interaction has also been seen in other studies in patients on **metipranolol**,[3] **propranolol**,[1,12] **oxprenolol**,[13,14] **atenolol**[6,15,16] and **labetalol**.[17] Two women with pre-eclampsia treated with **pro-**

pranolol and **pindolol** became markedly hypertensive (rises from 135/85 to 240/140 mmHg, and from 130/70 to 230/130 mmHg, respectively) within 4 to 5 days of being given **indometacin** to inhibit premature contractions.[18]

(e) Beta-blockers + Naproxen

A study in hypertensive patients treated with **timolol** and hydrochlorothiazide/amiloride showed that **naproxen** 250 mg twice daily caused a significant 4 mmHg rise in diastolic blood pressure, but did not significantly increase systolic blood pressure.[19] In another study, 500 mg **naproxen** twice daily caused an average 4 mmHg rise in systolic blood pressure in patients on **atenolol,** but did not significantly increase diastolic blood pressure.[20] In contrast, another study found that **naproxen** caused no changes in hypertension controlled with **propranolol**.[21] A case report describes one patient on **propranolol** who showed a marked rise in blood pressure when given **naproxen**.[22]

(f) Beta-blockers + Oxaprozin

A study in 32 hypertensive arthritic patients found that 1200 mg **oxaprozin** daily for 4 weeks did not affect the antihypertensive effects of **metoprolol** (100 mg twice daily), although at 2 weeks there was a significant increase in systolic blood pressure.[23]

(g) Beta-blockers + Piroxicam

A double-blind study found that about one-quarter of the patients given 20 mg **piroxicam** daily and **propranolol** 80 to 160 mg daily developed diastolic pressure rises of 10 mmHg or more when lying or standing.[24] Increases in both systolic and diastolic pressures (8.1/5.2 mmHg lying and 8.5/8.9 mmHg standing) were seen in another study in 3 patients.[25] In contrast, patients taking **propranolol** and **piroxicam** for 4 weeks (doses not stated) showed systolic/diastolic blood pressure rises of 5.8/2.4 mmHg when lying and 3.5/0.5 mmHg when standing, but these were said not to be statistically significant.[26] Blood pressure showed a trend towards higher levels in another study in 20 patients given **timolol** and 20 mg **piroxicam** daily.[19]

(h) Beta-blockers + Sulindac

Sulindac 200 mg twice daily had little or no effect on the control of hypertension in patients taking hydrochlorothiazide/amiloride with **atenolol**, **metoprolol**, **propranolol** or **pindolol**.[7] In another study, diastolic blood pressure was slightly and significantly *lower* when **sulindac** was given with **timolol**.[19] No statistically significant rises in blood pressure occurred in other studies in patients on **propranolol**[21,24,25] or **atenolol**[16,20] given **sulindac** 200 mg twice daily. Another study claimed that patients given **propranolol** and **sulindac** for 4 weeks (doses not stated) showed systolic/diastolic blood pressure rises of 4.8/10.3 mmHg and 2.4/7.1 mmHg when standing or lying, but these were said not to be statistically significant.[26] In contrast, a crossover study in 26 hypertensive patients on **labetalol** found that **sulindac** 200 mg twice daily for 7 days raised the mean systolic blood pressure by 6 mmHg when sitting, and by 9 to 14 mmHg when standing, which was considered potentially clinically significant. Diastolic pressures were not affected.[17]

(i) Beta-blockers + Tenoxicam

The control of hypertension in 16 patients on **atenolol** was found not to be affected by the concurrent use of 40 mg **tenoxicam** daily.[27]

Mechanism

Indometacin alone can raise blood pressure (13 hypertensive patients given 150 mg indometacin daily for three days showed a mean systolic blood pressure rise from 118 to 131 mmHg).[28] One suggested reason is that it inhibits the synthesis and release into the circulation of two prostaglandins (PGA and PGE) from the kidney medulla which have a potent dilating effect on peripheral arterioles throughout the body. In their absence the blood pressure rises. Thus the hypotensive actions of the beta-blockers are opposed by the hypertensive actions of indometacin. This mechanism has been questioned and it is possible that other physiological and pharmacological mechanisms have a part to play.[29,30] It seems likely that NSAIDs that behave like indometacin interact by similar mechanisms.

Importance and management

Some of the beta-blocker/NSAID interactions have been well studied and are of clinical importance but others are not. The concurrent use of beta-blockers and indometacin need not be avoided (except in patients with eclampsia or pre-eclampsia) but anticipate the need to increase the dosage of the beta-blocker. Alternatively, exchange the indometacin for a non-interacting NSAID. Piroxicam may interact like indometacin while normally diclofenac, imidazole salicylate, naproxen, oxaprozin, sulindac and tenoxicam only interact minimally or not at all. The situation with aspirin is unresolved. Because the occasional patient may show a marked interaction even with NSAIDs that normally do not interact (e.g. naproxen, ibuprofen), it would be prudent to monitor the effects when any NSAID is given. Direct information about other NSAIDs seems not to be available. Many of the antihypertensive agents appear to be affected by this interaction so that exchanging one for another may not avoid the problem.

1. Mills EH, Whitworth JA, Andrews J, Kincaid-Smith P. Non-steroidal anti-inflammatory drugs and blood pressure. *Aust NZ J Med* (1982) 12, 478–82.
2. Sziegoleit W, Rausch J, Polák G, György M, Dekov E, Békés M. Influence of acetylsalicylic acid on acute circulatory effects of the beta-blocking agents pindolol and propranolol in humans. *Int J Clin Pharmacol Ther Toxicol* (1982) 20, 423–30.
3. Macek K, Jurin I. Effects of indomethacine and aspirin on the antihypertensive action of metipranolol — a clinical study. *Eur J Pharmacol* (1990) 183, 839–40.
4. Schäfer-Korting M, Kirch W, Axthelm T, Köhler H, Mutschler E. Atenolol interaction with aspirin, allopurinol, and ampicillin. *Clin Pharmacol Ther* (1983) 33, 283–8.
5. Johnsson G, Regårdh CG, Sölvell L. Lack of biological interaction of alprenolol and salicylate in man. *Eur J Clin Pharmacol* (1973) 6, 9–14.
6. Abdel-Haq B, Magagna A, Favilla S, Salvetti A. The interference of indomethacin and of imidazole salicylate on blood pressure control of essential hypertensive patients treated with atenolol. *Int J Clin Pharmacol Ther Toxicol* (1987) 25, 598–600.
7. Stokes GS, Brooks PM, Johnston HJ, Monaghan JC, Okoro EO, Kelly D. The effects of sulindac and diclofenac in essential hypertension controlled by treatment with a beta blocker and/or diuretic. *Clin Exp Hyper Theory Prac* (1991) A13, 1169–78.
8. Reid ALA. Antihypertensive effect of thiazides. *Med J Aust* (1981) 2, 109–10.
9. Davies JG, Rawlins DC, Busson M. Effect of ibuprofen on blood pressure control by propranolol and bendrofluazide. *J Int Med Res* (1988) 16, 173–81.
10. Durão V, Prata MM, Gonçalves LMP. Modification of antihypertensive effects of β-adrenoceptor blocking agents by inhibition of endogenous prostaglandin synthesis. *Lancet* (1977) ii, 1005–7.
11. Watkins J, Abbott EC, Hensby CN, Webster J, Dollery CT. Attenuation of hypotensive effects of propranolol and thiazide diuretics by indomethacin. *BMJ* (1980) 281, 702–5.
12. Lopez-Ovejero JA, Weber MA, Drayer JIM, Sealey JE, Laragh JH. Effects of indomethacin alone and during diuretic or beta-adrenoceptor blockade therapy on blood pressure and the renin system in essential hypertension. *Clin Sci Mol Med* (1978) 55, 203S–205S.
13. Salvetti A, Arzilli F, Pedrinelli R, Beggi P, Motolese M. Interaction between oxprenolol and indomethacin on blood pressure in essential hypertensive patients. *Eur J Clin Pharmacol* (1982) 22, 197–201.
14. Sörgel F, Hemmerlein M, Lang E. Wirkung von Pirprofen und Indometacin auf die Effekte von Oxprenolol und Furosemid. *Arzneimittelforschung* (1984) 34, 1330–2.
15. Ylitalo P, Pitkäjärvi T, Pyykönen M-L, Nurmi A-K, Seppälä E, Vapaatalo H. Inhibition of prostaglandin synthesis by indomethacin interacts with the antihypertensive effect of atenolol. *Clin Pharmacol Ther* (1985) 38, 443–9.
16. Salvetti A, Pedrinelli R, Alberici A, Magagna A and Abdel-Haq B. The influence of indomethacin and sulindac on some pharmacological actions of atenolol in hypertensive patients. *Br J Clin Pharmacol* (1984) 17, 108S–111S.
17. Abate MA, Neeley JL, Layne RD, D'Alessandri R. Interaction of indomethacin and sulindac with labetalol. *Br J Clin Pharmacol* (1991) 31, 363–6.
18. Schoenfeld A, Freedman S, Hod M, Ovadia Y. Antagonism of antihypertensive drug therapy in pregnancy by indomethacin? *Am J Obstet Gynecol* (1989) 161, 1204–5.
19. Wong DG, Spence JD, Lamki L, Freeman D, McDonald JWD. Effect of non-steroidal anti-inflammatory drugs on control of hypertension by beta-blockers and diuretics. *Lancet* (1986) i, 997–1001.
20. Abate MA, Layne RD, Neeley JL, D'Alessandri R. Effect of naproxen and sulindac on blood pressure response to atenolol. *DICP Ann Pharmacother* (1990) 24, 810–3.
21. Schuna AA, Vejraska BD, Hiatt JG, Kochar M, Day R, Goodfriend TL. Lack of interaction between sulindac or naproxen and propranolol in hypertensive patients. *J Clin Pharmacol* (1989) 29, 524–8.
22. Anon. Adverse Drug Reactions Advisory Committee. Seven case studies. *Med J Aust* (1982) 2, 190–1.
23. Halabi A, Linde M, Zeidler H, König J, Kirch W. Double-blind study on the interaction of oxaprozin with metoprolol in hypertensives. *Cardiovasc Drug Ther* (1989) 3, 441–3.
24. Ebel DL, Rhymer AR, Stahl E. Effect of sulindac, piroxicam and placebo on the hypotensive effect of propranolol in patients with mild to moderate essential hypertension. *Adv Therapy* (1985) 2, 131–42.
25. Pugliese F, Simonetti BM, Cinotti GA, Ciabattoni G, Catella F, Vastano S, Ghidini Ottonelli A, Pierucci A. Differential interaction of piroxicam and sulindac with the anti-hypertensive effect of propranolol. *Eur J Clin Invest* (1984) 14, 54.
26. Alvarez CR, Baez MA, Weidler DJ. Effect of sulindac and piroxicam administration on the antihypertensive effect of propranolol. *J Clin Pharmacol* (1986) 26, 544.
27. Hartmann D, Stief G, Lingenfelder M, Güzelhan C, Horsch AK. Study on the possible interaction between tenoxicam and atenolol in hypertensive patients. *Arzneimittelforschung* (1995) 45, 494–8.
28. Barrientos A, Alcazar V, Ruilope L, Jarillo D, Rodicio JL. Indomethacin and beta-blockers in hypertension. *Lancet* (1978) i, 277.
29. Frölich JC, Whorten AR, Walker L, Smigel M, Oates JA, France R, Hollifield JW, Data JL, Gerber JG, Nies AS, Williams W, Robertson GL. Renal prostaglandins: regional differences in synthesis and role in renin release and ADH action. *7th Int Congr Nephrol*, Montreal (1978). 107–114.
30. Walker LA, Frölich JC. Renal prostaglandins and leukotrienes. *Rev Physiol Biochem Pharmacol* (1987) 107, 1–72.

Beta-blockers + Omeprazole or Lansoprazole

Omeprazole does not interact with metoprolol or propranolol, and lansoprazole does not interact with propranolol.

Clinical evidence, mechanism, importance and management

Omeprazole 20 mg daily for 8 days in 8 healthy subjects had no effect on the steady-state plasma levels of propranolol (80 mg twice daily), nor on its clinical effects (resting and exercised heart rates, blood pressure).[1] Another study found that 40 mg omeprazole daily for 8 days had no effect on the steady-state plasma levels of metoprolol (100 mg daily).[2] A double-blind crossover study in 18 healthy subjects found that lansoprazole 60 mg daily for 7 days did not significantly affect the pharmacokinetics of a single 80 mg dose of propranolol.[3] No special precautions would seem necessary.

1. Henry D, Brent P, Whyte I, Mihaly G, Devenish-Meares S. Propranolol steady-state pharmacokinetics are unaltered by omeprazole. *Eur J Clin Pharmacol* (1987) 33, 369–73.
2. Andersson T, Lundborg P, Regårdh CG. Lack of effect of omeprazole treatment on steady-state plasma levels of metoprolol. *Eur J Clin Pharmacol* (1991) 40, 61–5.
3. Karol MD, Locke CS, Cavanaugh JH. Lack of interaction between lansoprazole and propranolol, a pharmacokinetic and safety assessment. *J Clin Pharmacol* (2000) 40, 301–8.

Beta-blockers + Oral contraceptives

The blood levels of metoprolol are increased in women taking oral contraceptives, but the clinical importance is probably very small. Propranolol is minimally affected.

Clinical evidence, mechanism, importance and management

The peak plasma levels and the AUC of a single 100-mg dose of metoprolol were increased by 36 and 70% respectively in 12 women on low-dose combined oral contraceptives when compared with a similar group not taking the pill, with no effect on the elimination half-life.[1] In another study, the total clearance of a single 80-mg dose of propranolol was increased (although not significantly) in 7 women given 50 micrograms ethinylestradiol daily, and an even smaller increase was seen while taking an ethinylestradiol/norethisterone contraceptive.[2] The reason for the changes appears to be that ethinylestradiol alters the metabolism of the beta-blockers. In the case of propranolol its conjugation and oxidation are increased by the ethinylestradiol.[2]

The changes seen with propranolol are almost certainly too small to matter, but with metoprolol the changes are somewhat larger. Even so, changes of this size caused by interactions of other drugs with beta-blockers are not usually clinically relevant. No special precautions therefore seem necessary if either of these beta-blockers is given to women taking combined oral contraceptives containing ethinylestradiol, or ethinylestradiol alone. Be aware, however, that some of the indications for beta-blockers preclude the use of combined oral contraceptives.

1. Kendall MJ, Quarterman CP, Jack DB, Beeley L. Metoprolol pharmacokinetics and the oral contraceptive pill. *Br J Clin Pharmacol* (1982) 14, 120–2.
2. Fagan TC, Walle T, Walle UK, Topmiller MJ. Ethinyl estradiol alters propranolol metabolism pathway-specifically. *Clin Pharmacol Ther* (1993) 53, 241.

Beta-blockers + Phenothiazines

The concurrent use of chlorpromazine and propranolol, or thioridazine and pindolol, can result in a marked rise in the plasma levels of both drugs. Propranolol also markedly increases plasma thioridazine levels. There are isolated reports of possible adverse interactions.

Clinical evidence

(a) Plasma beta-blocker levels

The mean steady-state **propranolol** levels (80 mg eight-hourly) of 4 normal subjects and one hypertensive patient were raised 70% (from 41.5 to 70.2 ng/ml) when additionally given 50 mg **chlorpromazine** 8-hourly.[1] The increase was considerable in some subjects but barely detectable in others. A sixth subject on **propranolol** promptly fainted after the first dose of **chlorpromazine** when getting out of bed. He was found to have a pulse rate of 35 to 40 bpm and a blood pressure of 70/0 mmHg. He rapidly recovered, achieving a pulse rate of 85 and blood pressure of 120/70 when given 3 mg atropine. However, it is unclear whether the adverse effect was due to **chlorpromazine** alone, or to an interaction with **propranolol**.[1]

A brief mention of an episode of minor hypotension with **chlorpromazine** that appeared to have been exacerbated by **sotalol** has been noted in a diabetic girl.[2] Serum **pindolol** levels were 2.5 times higher in 7 patients treated with **thioridazine** than in 17 patients treated with haloperidol, phenytoin, and/or phenobarbital.[3]

(b) Plasma phenothiazine levels

Propranolol (mean daily dose 8.1 mg/kg) increased the serum **chlorpromazine** levels of 7 schizophrenics by about 100 to 500%, and raised the plasma levels of the active metabolites of chlorpromazine by about 50 to 100%.[4] The same or similar work by the same authors is described elsewhere.[5] One of the patients was withdrawn from the study because he suffered a cardiovascular collapse while taking both drugs.[5] It has been suggested that the value of **propranolol** in the treatment of schizophrenia probably results from the rise in serum **chlorpromazine** levels.[5]

A schizophrenic patient taking **chlorpromazine** and **thiothixene** experienced delirium, grand mal seizures and skin photosensitivity, attributed to a rise in serum levels of the antipsychotic drugs after additionally being given **propranolol** in increasing doses up to a total of 1200 mg daily.[6]

Two patients stabilised on **thioridazine** 600 or 800 mg daily showed three and fivefold rises in plasma levels, respectively when concurrently treated over 26 to 40 days with **propranolol** given in increasing doses up to a total of 800 mg daily. No **thioridazine** toxicity was seen although plasma levels had risen into the toxic range.[7] Similarly, in another study **thioridazine** levels rose by about 55 to 370% in 5 patients taking **propranolol** in doses of 320 to 520 mg daily.[8] **Pindolol** 40 mg daily also increased serum **thioridazine** levels by about 50% in 8 patients.[3]

Mechanism

Pharmacokinetic evidence[1] and *animal* studies[9] suggest that propranolol and chlorpromazine mutually inhibit the liver metabolism of the other drug so that both accumulate within the body. The mechanism of the propranolol/thioridazine interaction is probably similar. Both beta-blockers and phenothiazines can cause hypotension, and these effects could be additive.

Importance and management

The propranolol/chlorpromazine interaction appears to be established although information is limited. Concurrent use should be well monitored and the dosages reduced if necessary. The same precautions apply with propranolol and thioridazine.[7] There seems to be no information about any other beta-blocker/phenothiazine interactions, but if the mechanism of interaction suggested above is true, it seems possible that other beta-blockers that are mainly cleared from the body by liver metabolism (e.g. alprenolol, metoprolol) might interact similarly with chlorpromazine, whereas those mainly cleared unchanged in the urine (e.g. atenolol, nadolol) are less likely to do so. See also 'Drugs that prolong the QT interval + Other drugs that prolong the QT interval', p.103.

1. Vestal RE, Kornhauser DM, Hollifield JW, Shand DG. Inhibition of propranolol metabolism by chlorpromazine. *Clin Pharmacol Ther* (1979) 25, 19–24.

2. Baker L, Barcai A, Kaye R, Haque N. Beta adrenergic blockade and juvenile diabetes: acute studies and long-term therapeutic trial. *J Pediatr* (1969) 75, 19–29.

3. Greendyke RM, Gulya A. Effect of pindolol administration on serum levels of thioridazine, haloperidol, phenytoin, and phenobarbital. *J Clin Psychiatry* (1988) 49, 105–7.

4. Peet M, Middlemiss DN, Yates RA. Pharmacokinetic interaction between propranolol and chlorpromazine in schizophrenic patients. *Lancet* (1980) ii, 978.

5. Peet M, Middlemiss DN, Yates RA. Propranolol in schizophrenia II. Clinical and biochemical aspects of combining propranolol with chlorpromazine. *Br J Psychiatry* (1981) 138, 112–17.

6. Miller FA, Rampling D. Adverse effects of combined propranolol and chlorpromazine therapy. *Am J Psychiatry* (1982) 139, 1198–9.

7. Silver JM, Yudofsky SC, Kogan M, Katz BL. Elevation of thioridazine plasma levels by propranolol. *Am J Psychiatry* (1986) 143, 1290–2.

8. Greendyke RM, Kanter DR. Plasma propranolol levels and their effect on plasma thioridazine and haloperidol concentrations. *J Clin Psychopharmacol* (1987) 7, 178–82.

9. Shand DG, Oates JA. Metabolism of propranolol by rat liver microsomes and its inhibition by phenothiazine and tricyclic antidepressant drugs. *Biochem Pharmacol* (1971) 20, 1720–3.

Beta-blockers + Propafenone

Plasma metoprolol and propranolol levels can be markedly raised (two to fivefold) by the concurrent use of propafenone. Toxicity may develop.

Clinical evidence

Four patients with ventricular arrhythmias given **metoprolol** 150 to 200 mg daily showed a two to fivefold rise in steady-state **metoprolol** serum levels when given 150 mg **propafenone** three times daily. In 4 other patients treated with **metoprolol** 50 mg three times daily and **propafenone** 150 mg three times daily, it was found that stopping **metoprolol** did not affect **propafenone** plasma levels. One of them developed distressing nightmares, and another had acute left ventricular failure with pulmonary oedema and haemoptysis, which disappeared when the **metoprolol** dosage was reduced or stopped. Single-dose studies in healthy subjects found a twofold decrease in the clearance of **metoprolol** and a further 20% reduction in exercise-induced tachycardia at 90 min when propafenone was given.[1]

A patient developed neurotoxicity (including vivid nightmares, fatigue, headache) when given 100 mg **metoprolol** daily in divided doses, which worsened while it was being withdrawn and replaced by 300 mg **propafenone** daily. The symptoms disappeared when both drugs were withdrawn.[2]

Propafenone 225 mg every 8 hours more than doubled the steady-state **propranolol** levels of 12 healthy subjects given **propranolol** 50 mg 8 hourly. The beta-blocking effects were only modestly increased. The **propafenone** pharmacokinetics remained unchanged.[3]

Mechanism

It is suggested that the propafenone reduces the metabolism of the metoprolol and propranolol by the liver, thereby reducing their clearance and raising serum levels.[1,3]

Importance and management

Information is limited but the interaction would seem to be established. Concurrent use need not be avoided but anticipate the need to reduce the dosage of metoprolol and propranolol. Monitor closely because some patients may experience adverse effects. If the suggested mechanism of interaction is correct it is possible that other beta-blockers which undergo liver metabolism will interact similarly but not those largely excreted unchanged in the urine (e.g. atenolol, nadolol). This needs confirmation.

1. Wagner F, Kalusche D, Trenk D, Jähnchen E, Roskamm H. Drug interaction between propafenone and metoprolol. *Br J Clin Pharmacol* (1987) 24, 213–20.

2. Ahmad S. Metoprolol-induced delirium perpetuated by propafenone. *Am Fam Physician* (1991) 44, 1142–3.

3. Kowey PR, Kirsten EB, Fu C-HJ, Mason WD. Interaction between propranolol and propafenone in healthy volunteers. *J Clin Pharmacol* (1989) 29, 512–17.

Beta-blockers + Quinidine

An isolated report describes a patient on quinidine who developed marked bradycardia (36 bpm) when using timolol eye drops. Another describes orthostatic hypotension with quinidine and propranolol. Both sotalol and quinidine can prolong the QT interval, which may therefore increase the risk of torsade de pointes arrhythmia if they are used together. Quinidine can raise plasma metoprolol, propranolol, and timolol levels, but the clinical relevance of this is uncertain.

Clinical evidence

(a) Metoprolol

A metabolic study found that a single 50-mg dose **quinidine** caused marked inhibition of the metabolism of a single 100-mg dose of **metoprolol** in 5 healthy subjects who were extensive metabolisers, making them effectively into poor metabolisers. The plasma levels of **metoprolol** were approximately tripled. **Quinidine** had no effect on **metoprolol** pharmacokinetics in 5 poor metabolisers.[1] Similar findings were reported in another study when 50 mg **quinidine** daily was given with **metoprolol** 100 mg twice daily for 7 days. However, the effect on heart-rate reduction was small given the increase in serum **metoprolol** concentrations.[2]

(b) Propranolol

A single-dose pharmacokinetic study showed that concurrent use of **quinidine** 200 mg and **propranolol** 20 mg doubled the AUC and the peak plasma levels of **propranolol**. Maximum heart rates during exercise were suppressed by a further 45%.[3] A similar study by the same research group found that **propranolol** AUCs were approximately tripled.[4] A further study found that **quinidine** doubled the AUC of **propranolol** and halved its clearance resulting in increased beta-blockade.[5] After a single dose of **quinidine** 200 mg, peak plasma **quinidine** levels were over 50% higher and its clearance almost 40% lower in 7 patients taking **propranolol** (40 to 400 mg daily) when compared with 8 control patients, but the **quinidine** elimination half-life did not differ.[6] However, this was not confirmed in two other studies.[7,8]

A man on **propranolol** 40 mg four times daily developed orthostatic hypotension with symptoms of dizziness and faintness on standing when additionally treated with **quinidine** 200 mg four times daily. This resolved when **quinidine** was withdrawn.[9]

(c) Sotalol

Although one study reports the safe concurrent use of **sotalol** and **quinidine**,[10] both **sotalol** and **quinidine** can prolong the QT interval, which may increase the risk of torsade de pointes arrhythmia if they are used together.

(d) Timolol

An elderly man taking 500 mg **quinidine sulfate** three times daily for atrial premature beats was hospitalised with dizziness 12 weeks after starting to use 0.5% **timolol** eye drops for open-angle glaucoma. He was found to have a sinus bradycardia of 36 bpm. The symptoms abated when the drugs were withdrawn and normal sinus rhythm returned after 24 h. The same symptoms developed within 30 h of re-starting concurrent use, but disappeared when the **quinidine** was withdrawn.[11] In a later study in healthy subjects, a single oral dose of **quinidine** 50 mg was given 30 min before 2 drops of 0.5% **timolol** ophthalmic solution were administered into each nostril. In 13 extensive metabolisers, **quinidine** caused a further decrease in heart rate and increase in plasma **timolol** concentrations compared with **timolol** alone. Administration of **quinidine** with **timolol** in these extensive metabolisers gave results similar to **timolol** alone in 5 poor metabolisers.[12]

Mechanism

Quinidine appears to increase metoprolol, propranolol and timolol plasma levels by inhibiting the cytochrome P450 isoenzyme CYP2D6, thereby reducing their clearance.[1,5,12] As CYP2D6 shows polymorphism, these interactions would be most apparent in patients with high CYP2D6 activity (extensive metabolisers), making them effectively into poor metabolisers.

Importance and management

The pharmacokinetic interaction would seem to be established, but of uncertain clinical importance. Only one isolated case of possible excessive beta-blockade has been reported (with quinidine and timolol eye drops). Concurrent use need not be avoided (and may be beneficial in the treatment of atrial fibrillation). The general consensus is that the combination of two drugs that prolong the QT interval such as quinidine and sotalol should usually be avoided, or only used with great caution. See also 'Drugs that prolong the QT interval + Other drugs that prolong the QT interval', p.103.

1. Leemann T, Dayer P, Meyer UA. Single-dose quinidine treatment inhibits metoprolol oxidation in extensive metabolizers. Eur J Clin Pharmacol (1986) 29, 739–41.
2. Schlanz KD, Yingling KW, Verme CN, Lalonde RL, Harrison DC, Bottorff MB. Loss of stereoselective metoprolol metabolism following quinidine inhibition of P450IID6. Pharmacotherapy (1991) 11, 272.
3. Sakurai T, Kawai C, Yasuhara M, Okumura K, Hori R. Increased plasma concentration of propranolol by a pharmacokinetic interaction with quinidine. Jpn Circ J (1983) 47, 872–3.
4. Yasuhara M, Yatsuzuka A, Yamada K, Okumura K, Hori R, Sakurai T, Kawai C. Alteration of propranolol pharmacokinetics and pharmacodynamics by quinidine in man. J Pharmacobio-Dyn (1990) 13, 681–7.
5. Zhou H-H, Anthony LB, Roden DM, Wood AJJ. Quinidine reduces clearance of (+)-propranolol more than (−)-propranolol through marked reduction in 4-hydroxylation. Clin Pharmacol Ther (1990) 47, 686–93.
6. Kessler KM, Humphries WC, Black M, Spann JF. Quinidine pharmacokinetics in patients with cirrhosis or receiving propranolol. Am Heart J (1978) 96, 627–35.
7. Kates RE, Blanford MF. Disposition kinetics of oral quinidine when administered concurrently with propranolol. J Clin Pharmacol (1979) 19, 378–83
8. Fenster P, Perrier D, Mayersohn M, Marcus FI. Kinetic evaluation of the propranolol-quinidine combination. Clin Pharmacol Ther (1980) 27, 450–3.
9. Loon NR, Wilcox CS, Folger W. Orthostatic hypotension due to quinidine and propranolol. Am J Med (1986) 81, 1101–4.
10. Dorian P, Newman D, Berman N, Hardy J, Mitchell J. Sotalol and type IA drugs in combination prevent recurrence of sustained ventricular tachycardia. J Am Coll Cardiol (1993) 22, 106–13.
11. Dinai Y, Sharir M, Naveh N, Halkin H. Bradycardia induced by interaction between quinidine and ophthalmic timolol. Ann Intern Med (1985) 103, 890–1.
12. Edeki TI, He H, Wood AJJ. Pharmacogenetic explanation for excessive β-blockade following timolol eye drops. JAMA (1995) 274, 1611–13.

Beta-blockers + Rifampicin (Rifampin)

Rifampicin increases the loss of bisoprolol, carvedilol, metoprolol, propranolol, tertatolol and talinolol from the body, and reduces their serum levels. The extent to which this reduces the effects of these beta-blockers is uncertain, but it is probably small.

Clinical evidence

Rifampicin 600 mg daily for 3 weeks increased the oral clearance of **propranolol** in 6 healthy subjects almost threefold. Increasing the **rifampicin** dosage to 900 or 1200 mg daily did not further increase the clearance. Four weeks after withdrawing the **rifampicin** the blood levels of **propranolol** had returned to normal.[1] In a similar study the oral clearance of **propranolol** was increased approximately fourfold by 600 mg **rifampicin** daily for 3 weeks in both poor and extensive metabolisers of propranolol.[2]

The AUC of **bisoprolol** 10 mg daily was reduced by 34% in healthy subjects given 600 mg **rifampicin** daily.[3] **Rifampicin** 600 mg daily for 12 days caused a 60% decrease in the maximum serum levels and the AUC of **carvedilol**.[4] **Rifampicin** 600 mg daily for 15 days reduced the AUC of **metoprolol** after single 100-mg doses) by 33% in 10 healthy subjects.[5] **Rifampicin** 600 mg daily for a week increased the clearance of **tertatolol** almost threefold and reduced the half-life from 9 to 3.4 h. A slight reduction in the effects of **tertatolol** on blood pressure was seen and heart rates were raised from 68 to 74 bpm.[6] **Rifampicin** 600 mg daily decreased the AUC of a single dose of **talinolol** 30 mg intravenously or 100 mg by mouth by 21 and 35%, respectively, in 8 healthy subjects.[7]

Mechanism

Rifampicin is a potent liver enzyme inducing agent which increases the metabolism and loss of extensively metabolised beta-blockers such as propranolol and metoprolol from the body. However, rifampicin may interact by mechanisms other than enzyme induction. Rifampicin administration also increases duodenal P-glycoprotein expression, so increased clearance of talinolol (which is not metabolised) may be due to induction of P-glycoprotein excretion of talinolol by rifampicin.[7]

Importance and management

These interactions are established. Their clinical importance is uncertain but probably small,[6] nevertheless concurrent use should be monitored. Increase the dosage of the beta-blocker if there is any evidence that the therapeutic response is inadequate. Beta-blockers that undergo extensive liver metabolism would be expected to be affected by the enzyme-inducing effects of rifampicin (e.g. propranolol, metoprolol, alprenolol). Those beta-blockers mainly lost unchanged in the urine (atenolol, nadolol) would not be expected to be affected, but it appears that a reaction can occur with non-metabolised drugs such as talinolol that are substrates for P-glycoprotein.

1. Herman RJ, Nakamura K, Wilkinson GR, Wood AJJ. Induction of propranolol metabolism by rifampicin. *Br J Clin Pharmacol* (1983) 16, 565–9.
2. Shaheen O, Biollaz J, Koshakji RP, Wilkinson GR, Wood AJJ. Influence of debrisoquin phenotype on the inducibility of propranolol metabolism. *Clin Pharmacol Ther* (1989) 45, 439–43.
3. Kirch W, Rose I, Klingmann I, Pabst J, Ohnhaus EE. Interaction of bisoprolol with cimetidine and rifampicin. *Eur J Clin Pharmacol* (1986) 31, 59–62.
4. Data on file, database on carvedilol, SmithKline Beecham, quoted by Ruffolo RR, Boyle DA, Venuti RP, Lukas MA. Carvedilol (Kredex®): a novel multiple action cardiovascular agent. *Drugs Today* (1991) 27, 465–92.
5. Bennett PN, John VA, Whitmarsh VB. Effect of rifampicin on metoprolol and antipyrine kinetics. *Br J Clin Pharmacol* (1982) 13, 387–91.
6. Kirch W, Milferstädt S, Halabi A, Rocher I, Efthymiopoulos C, Jung L. Interaction of tertatolol with rifampicin and ranitidine pharmacokinetics and antihypertensive activity. *Cardiovasc Drug Ther* (1990) 4, 487–92.
7. Westphal K, Weinbrenner A, Zschiesche M, Franke G, Knoke M, Oertel R, Fritz P, von Richter O, Warzok R, Hachenberg T, Kauffmann H-M, Schrenk D, Terhaag B, Kroemer HK, Siegmund W. Induction of P-glycoprotein by rifampin increases intestinal secretion of talinolol in human beings: a new type of drug/drug interaction. *Clin Pharmacol Ther* (2000) 68, 345–55.

Beta-blockers + Sulfasalazine

Sulfasalazine markedly reduces the absorption of talinolol.

Clinical evidence

The AUC of 50 mg **talinolol** in 8 healthy subjects was reduced to 9% (from 958 to 84 nanograms/ml/h) when simultaneously given with 4 g **sulfasalazine**. The maximum serum levels were also markedly reduced, from 112 to 23 nanograms/ml in 3 subjects, and to undetectable levels in the other 5 subjects.[1]

Mechanism

Not known. It is suggested that the talinolol is adsorbed onto the sulfasalazine, thereby preventing its absorption.[1]

Importance and management

Information is limited to this study, but it would appear to be an established and probably clinically important interaction. The efficacy of the talinolol would be expected to be markedly reduced, but nobody seems to have checked on this yet. If the mechanism suggested by the authors is true, their advice to separate the dosages by 2 to 3 h should minimise this interaction.[1] More study is needed to confirm how effective this is, and whether other beta-blockers behave similarly.

1. Terhaag B, Palm U, Sahre H, Richter K, Oertel R. Interaction of talinolol and sulfasalazine in the human gastrointestinal tract. *Eur J Clin Pharmacol* (1992) 42, 461–2.

Beta-blockers + Sulfinpyrazone

The antihypertensive effects of oxprenolol can be reduced or abolished by the concurrent use of sulfinpyrazone.

Clinical evidence

Ten hypertensive patients were given 80 mg **oxprenolol** twice daily for 15 days, which reduced their mean supine blood pressure from 161/101 to 149/96 mmHg, and their heart rate from 72 to 66 bpm. When additionally given 400 mg **sulfinpyrazone** twice daily for 15 days, their mean blood pressure climbed again to approximately its former level. The reduction in mean heart rate remained unaffected. **Sulfinpyrazone** halved the reduction in cardiac workload (systolic blood pressure × heart rate) seen with **oxprenolol** alone.[1]

Mechanism

Not understood. One idea is that the sulfinpyrazone inhibits the production of prostaglandins by the kidney which have vasodilatory (antihypertensive) activity. This would oppose the actions of the oxprenolol.

Importance and management

Information seems to be limited. If sulfinpyrazone is given to patients taking oxprenolol for hypertension, the effects should be monitored. It seems likely that this interaction could be accommodated by raising the dosage of the oxprenolol. The effects of this interaction on cardiac workload appear to be less important, but it would still be prudent to monitor concurrent use if oxprenolol is used for angina.

1. Ferrara LA, Mancini M, Marotta T, Pasanisi F, Fasano ML. Interference by sulphinpyrazone with the antihypertensive effects of oxprenolol. *Eur J Clin Pharmacol* (1986) 29, 717–19.

Beta-blockers + Sympathomimetics (directly-acting)

(A) Effects on blood pressure and heart rate: The hypertensive effects of epinephrine (adrenaline) can be markedly increased in patients taking non-selective beta-blockers such as propranolol. A severe and potentially life-threatening hypertensive reaction and/or marked bradycardia can develop. Cardioselective beta-blockers such as metoprolol interact minimally. An isolated report describes a fatal hypertensive reaction with propranolol and phenylephrine, but concurrent use normally seems to be uneventful.
(B) Effects on bronchi: Non-selective beta-blockers (e.g. propranolol) should not be used in asthmatic subjects because they may cause serious bronchoconstriction. Even cardioselective blockers can sometimes cause problems. No adverse interaction normally occurs during the concurrent use of beta-agonist bronchodilators (e.g. isoprenaline, salbutamol) and cardioselective beta-blockers (e.g. metoprolol).
(C) Anaphylaxis: Some evidence suggests anaphylactic shock in patients on beta-blockers may be resistant to treatment with epinephrine (adrenaline).

(A) Effects on blood pressure and heart rate

Clinical evidence

(a) Propranolol or Metoprolol + Epinephrine (Adrenaline) or Levonordefrin

An early study in 10 healthy subjects demonstrated that intravenous **epinephrine** 5 micrograms/min alone increased heart rates and caused minimal changes in blood pressure. However, after pretreatment with 10 mg **propranolol** intravenously, the same dose of **epinephrine** caused a fall in heart rate of 12 bpm and an increase in arterial pressure of 20/10 mmHg.[1] One case report describes 6 patients on 20 to 80 mg **propranolol** daily and undergoing plastic surgery who experienced marked hypertensive reactions (blood pressures in the range 190/110 to 260/150 mmHg) and bradycardia when their eyelids and/or faces were infiltrated with 8 to 40 ml of local anaesthetic solutions of lidocaine (lignocaine) containing 1:100 000 or 1:200 000 (10 or 5 microgram/ml) **epinephrine**. Cardiac arrest occurred in one patient.[2]

Similar marked increases in blood pressure, associated with marked bradycardia, sometimes severe, have been described in other studies and case reports involving **propranolol**.[3-10] In contrast, only a small blood pressure rise was seen in a comparative study with **metoprolol**.[4] This was confirmed in another study in which patients given identical infusions of **epinephrine** developed a hypertensive-bradycardial reaction while taking **propranolol** but not while taking **metoprolol**.[6] A transient hypertensive reaction has also been seen in a patient on **propranolol** when given injections of 2% mepivacaine with 1:20 000 **corbadrine** (**levonordefrin**) for dental anaesthesia.[11]

After pretreatment with a single 5-mg dose of **pindolol**, only small reductions in blood pressure (4 mmHg) and heart rate (about 5 bpm) were seen with the intra-oral injection of 3.6 ml of 2% lidocaine (lignocaine) containing 1:80 000 **epinephrine** (45 micrograms epinephrine) in healthy subjects.[12]

(b) Propranolol or Metoprolol + Phenylephrine

A woman on 40 mg **propranolol** four times daily for hypertension was given one drop of a 10% **phenylephrine hydrochloride** solution in each eye during an ophthalmic examination. About 45 min later she complained of a sudden and sharp bi-temporal pain and shortly afterwards became unconscious. She later died of an intracerebral haemorrhage due to the rupture of a berry aneurysm. She had had a similar dose of **phenylephrine** on a previous occasion in the absence of **propranolol** without any problems.[13] However, no change in blood pressure was seen in a study in both normotensive subjects and patients taking **metoprolol** who were administered 0.5 to 4-mg doses of **phenylephrine** intranasally every hour for a total of 7.5 to 15 mg (4 to 30 times the usual dose).[14] Similarly, in a placebo-controlled study in 12 hypertensive patients, neither **propranolol** nor **metoprolol** significantly altered the dose of intravenous **phenylephrine** required to cause a 25 mmHg increase in systolic blood pressure.[15]

Mechanism

Epinephrine (adrenaline) stimulates alpha- and beta-receptors of the cardiovascular system, the former results in vasoconstriction (mainly alpha-1) and the latter in both vasodilatation (mainly beta-2) and stimulation of the heart (mainly beta-1). The net result is usually a modest increase in heart rate and a small rise in blood pressure. If however the beta-receptors are blocked by a non-selective beta-blocker such as propranolol, the unopposed alpha vasoconstriction causes a marked rise in blood pressure, followed by reflex bradycardia. Cardioselective beta-blockers, which are more selective for beta-1 receptors, do not prevent the vasodilator action of adrenaline at beta-2 receptors to the same extent, and therefore the effect of any interaction is relatively small. Consequently, epinephrine has been used to assess the degree of beta-blockade after propranolol.[16] Phenylephrine is largely an alpha-stimulator, therefore beta-blockers should have a minimal effect on its action.

Importance and management

The propranolol/epinephrine (adrenaline) interaction is established. It may be serious and potentially life-threatening, depending on the dosage of epinephrine used. Marked and serious blood pressure rises and severe bradycardia have occurred in patients given 300 micrograms epinephrine (0.3 ml of 1:1000) subcutaneously[7-9] or 40 to 400 micrograms by infiltration of the skin and eyelids during plastic surgery.[2] **Epinephrine** 15 micrograms given intravenously can cause an almost 40% fall in heart rate.[10] Patients on non-selective beta-blockers such as propranolol (see Table 10.2) should only be administered epinephrine in very reduced dosages because of the marked bradycardia and hypertension that can occur. A less marked effect is likely with the cardioselective beta-blockers such as metoprolol (see

Table 10.1).[4] Local anaesthetics used in dental surgery usually contain very low concentrations of epinephrine (e.g. 5 to 20 micrograms/ml, i.e. 1 in 200 000 to 1 in 50 000) and only small volumes are usually given, so that an undesirable interaction is unlikely.

No interaction between phenylephrine and the beta-blockers would be expected. Apart from the single unexplained case cited above,[13] the literature appears to be silent. Concurrent use normally appears to be clinically unimportant,[14,15] particularly bearing in mind the widespread use of beta-blockers and the ready availability of phenylephrine in the form of OTC cough-and-cold remedies and nasal decongestants.

Acute hypertensive episodes have been controlled with chlorpromazine or phentolamine (both of which are alpha-blockers). Hydralazine and nifedipine have also been used.[2,8]

(B) Effects on bronchi

Clinical evidence

(a) Cardioselective beta-blockers + Beta-agonist bronchodilators

The cardioselective beta-blockers would not be expected to affect the beta-receptors in the bronchi, but an increasing number of reports indicate that bronchospasm can sometimes occur following their use by asthmatics and others with obstructive airways diseases, particularly if high doses are used (see also 'Antiasthmatic drugs + Beta-blockers', p.862).

No adverse interaction normally occurs between beta-agonist sympathomimetic bronchodilators and cardioselective beta-blockers. This has been demonstrated in studies with **celiprolol**,[17] **metoprolol**[18,19] or **practolol**[18] with **isoprenaline** (**isoproterenol**) infusion or inhalation; **celiprolol** with **terbutaline** infusion or inhalation;[20] or **atenolol** and **celiprolol** with **salbutamol** (**albuterol**) inhalation.[17,21,22] In contrast, another study found that the increase in forced expiratory volume (FEV) with **terbutaline** inhalation and infusion was reduced by about 0.3 litres by **atenolol** and **metoprolol**, and the authors considered this would be clinically relevant in severe asthma.[23]

(b) Non-selective beta-blockers + Beta-agonist bronchodilators

Non-selective beta-blockers (e.g. **propranolol** and **oxprenolol**) are contraindicated in asthmatic subjects because they can cause bronchospasm, reduce lung ventilation and may possibly precipitate a severe asthmatic attack in some subjects. Fatalities have occurred.[24] They also oppose the effects of bronchodilators such as **isoprenaline**,[17-19] **salbutamol** (**albuterol**),[17,21] and **terbutaline**.[20] Even eye drops containing the non-selective beta-blockers **timolol**[25,26] and **metipranolol**[27] have been reported to precipitate acute bronchospasm.

Mechanism

Non-selective beta-blockers, intended for their actions on the heart, also block the beta-2 receptors in the bronchi so that the normal bronchodilation, which is under the control of the sympathetic nervous system, is reduced or abolished. As a result the bronchoconstriction of asthma can be made worse. Cardioselective beta-blockers on the other hand, preferentially block beta-1 receptors in the heart, with less effect on the beta-2 receptors, so that beta-2 stimulating bronchodilators such as isoprenaline, salbutamol and terbutaline continue to have their bronchodilator effects.

Importance and management

A well established drug–disease interaction. Avoid non-selective beta-blockers in asthmatics and those with chronic obstructive pulmonary disease (i.e. those already likely to be taking beta-agonist bronchodilators), whether given orally or in eye-drops because serious and life-threatening bronchospasm may occur. The cardioselective beta-blockers are generally safer but not entirely free from risk in some patients, particularly in high dosage. Celiprolol (a selective blocker) appears to be exceptional in causing mild bronchodilatation in asthmatics and not bronchoconstriction, but some caution is still necessary.[22] The cardioselective and non-selective beta-blockers are listed in Tables 10.1 and 10.2, while the beta-agonist bronchodilators are listed in Table 22.2.

(C) Anaphylaxis: resistance to treatment

Clinical evidence, mechanism, importance and management

A patient on **propranolol** who suffered an anaphylactic reaction after receiving an allergy injection for desensitisation failed to respond to **epinephrine** (adrenaline) and required intubation.[28] Resistance to epinephrine treatment for anaphylaxis occurred in another patient using **timolol** eye drops.[29] A beta-agonist bronchodilator (e.g. isoprenaline, salbutamol) may be effective in patients on beta-blockers with anaphylaxis resistant to adrenaline.[30] It has also been proposed that the incidence and severity of anaphylactic reactions may be increased in those on beta-blockers,[30,31] one idea being that the adrenoceptors concerned with suppressing the release of the mediators of anaphylaxis may be blocked by either beta$_1$- or beta$_2$- antagonists.[30] However er one study failed to find any evidence to support an increased incidence of systemic reactions in patients taking beta-blockers receiving allergen immunotherapy.[32] The use of **epinephrine** to treat allergic reactions, including presumed anaphylaxis, in patients on **propranolol** has also resulted in severe hypertension, sometimes with bradycardia,[7-9] as described under (A) above.

1. Harris WS, Schoenfeld CD, Brooks RH, Weissler AM. Effect of beta adrenergic blockade on the hemodynamic responses to epinephrine in man. *Am J Cardiol* (1966) 17, 484–92.
2. Foster CA, Aston SJ. Propranolol-epinephrine interaction: a potential disaster. *Plast Reconstr Surg* (1983) 72, 74–8.
3. Kram J, Bourne HR, Melmon KL, Maibach H. Propranolol. *Ann Intern Med* (1974) 80, 282–3.
4. van Herwaarden CLA, Binkhorst RA, Fennis JFM, van'T Laar A. Effects of adrenaline during treatment with propranolol and metoprolol. *BMJ* (1977) 2, 1029.
5. Berchtold P, Bessman AN. Propranolol. *Ann Intern Med* (1974) 80, 119.
6. Houben H, Thien T, Laor VA. Effect of low-dose epinephrine infusion on hemodynamics after selective and non-selective beta-blockade in hypertension. *Clin Pharmacol Ther* (1982) 31, 685.
7. Hansbrough JF, Near A. Propranolol-epinephrine antagonism with hypertension and stroke. *Ann Intern Med* (1980) 92, 717.
8. Whelan TV. Propranolol, epinephrine and accelerated hypertension during hemodialysis. *Ann Intern Med* (1987) 106, 327.
9. Gandy W. Severe epinephrine-propranolol interaction. *Ann Emerg Med* (1989) 18, 98–9.
10. Mackie K, Lam A. Epinephrine-containing test dose during beta-blockade. *J Clin Monit* (1991) 7, 213–6.
11. Mito RS, Yagiela JA. Hypertensive response to levonordefrin in a patient receiving propranolol: report of a case. *J Am Dent Assoc* (1988) 116, 55–7.
12. Sugimura M, Hirota Y, Shibutani T, Niwa H, Hori T, Kim Y, Matsuura H. An echocardiographic study of interactions between pindolol and epinephrine contained in a local anesthetic solution. *Anesth Prog* (1995) 42, 29–35.
13. Cass E, Kadar D, Stein HA. Hazards of phenylephrine topical medication in persons taking propranolol. *Can Med Assoc J* (1979) 120, 1261–2.
14. Myers MG, Iazzetta JJ. Intranasally administered phenylephrine and blood pressure. *Can Med Assoc J* (1982) 127, 365–8.
15. Myers MG. Beta adrenoceptor antagonism and pressor response to phenylephrine. *Clin Pharmacol Ther* (1984) 36, 57–63.
16. Varma DR, Sharma KK, Arora RC. Response to adrenaline and propranolol in hyperthyroidism. *Lancet* (1976), i, 260.
17. Doshan HD, Rosenthal RR, Brown R, Slutsky A, Applin WJ, Caruso FS. Celiprolol, atenolol and propranolol: a comparison of pulmonary effects in asthmatic patients. *J Cardiovasc Pharmacol* (1986) 8 (Suppl 4), S105–S108.
18. Thiringer G, Svedmyr N. Interaction of orally administered metoprolol, practolol and propranolol with isoprenaline in asthmatics. *Eur J Clin Pharmacol* (1976) 10, 163–70.
19. Johnsson G, Svedmyr N, Thiringer G. Effects of intravenous propranolol and metoprolol and their interaction with isoprenaline on pulmonary function, heart rate and blood pressure in asthmatics. *Eur J Clin Pharmacol* (1975) 8, 175–80.
20. Matthys H, Doshan HD, Rühle K-H, Applin WJ, Braig H, Pohl M. Bronchosparing properties of celiprolol, a new β$_1$, α$_2$ blocker, in propranolol-sensitive asthmatic patients. *J Cardiovasc Pharmacol* (1986) 8 (Suppl 4), S40–S42.
21. Fogari R, Zoppi A, Tettamanti F, Poletti L, Rizzardi G, Fiocchi G. Comparative effects of celiprolol, propranolol, oxprenolol, and atenolol on respiratory function in hypertensive patients with chronic obstructive lung disease. *Cardiovasc Drugs Ther* (1990) 4, 1145–50.
22. Pujet JC, Dubreuil C, Fleury B, Provendier O, Abella ML. Effects of celiprolol, a cardioselective beta-blocker, on respiratory function in asthmatic patients. *Eur Respir J* (1992) 5, 196–200.
23. Löfdahl C-G, Svedmyr N. Cardioselectivity of atenolol and metoprolol. A study in asthmatic patients. *Eur J Respir Dis* (1981) 62, 396–404.
24. Anon. Beta-blocker caused death of asthmatic. *Pharm J* (1991) 247, 185.
25. Charan NB, Lakshminarayan S. Pulmonary effects of topical timolol. *Arch Intern Med* (1980) 140, 843–4.
26. Jones FL, Ekberg NL. Exacerbation of obstructive airway disease by timolol. *JAMA* (1980) 244, 2730.
27. Vinti H, Chichmanian RM, Fournier JP, Pesce A, Taillan B, Fuzibet JG, Cassuto JP, Dujardin P. Accidents systémiques des bêta-bloquants en collyres. A propos de six observations. *Rev Med Interne* (1989) 10, 41–4.
28. Newman BR, Schultz LK. Epinephrine-resistant anaphylaxis in a patient taking propranolol hydrochloride. *Ann Allergy* (1981) 47, 35–7.
29. Moneret-Vautrin DA, Kanny G, Faller JP, Levan D, Kohler C. Choc anaphylactique grave avec arrêt cardiaque au café et à la gomme arabique, potentialisé par un collyre bêta-bloquant. *Rev Med Interne* (1993) 14, 107–11.
30. Toogood JH. Beta-blocker therapy and the risk of anaphylaxis. *Can Med Assoc J* (1987) 136, 929–33.
31. Berkelman RL, Finton RJ, Elsea WR. Beta-adrenergic antagonists and fatal anaphylactic reactions to oral penicillin. *Ann Intern Med* (1986) 104, 134.
32. Hepner MJ, Ownby DR, Anderson JA, Rowe MS, Sears-Ewald D, Brown EB. Risk of systemic reactions in patients taking beta-blocker drugs receiving allergen immunotherapy injections. *J Allergy Clin Immunol* (1990) 86, 407–11.

Beta-blockers + Sympathomimetics (indirectly-acting)

A small but probably clinically unimportant rise in blood pressure may occur in patients on beta-blockers who take phenylpropanolamine. A marked rise has been seen in one patient on oxprenolol and methyldopa.

Clinical evidence, mechanism, importance and management

A study in 7 hypertensive patients controlled with beta-blockers (5 on **atenolol**, and the other 2 on **metoprolol** or **propranolol**) found that single 25-mg doses of rapid-release **phenylpropanolamine** (*Super Odrinex*) increased mean peak systolic/diastolic blood pressures by about 8/5 mmHg over a 6-h period.[1] Another study found that *Dimetapp Extentabs* (75 mg **phenylpropanolamine** + 12 mg **brompheniramine**) given to 5 hypertensive patients on un-named **beta-blockers** caused systolic/diastolic blood pressure rises of 1.7/0.9 mmHg over a 4-h period, which were not statistically or clinically significant.[2] These rises in blood pressure are small and relatively short-lived, and probably of little clinical importance, but they may possibly mislead the interpretation of blood pressure measurements. However a marked rise in blood pressure was seen in one patient on **methyldopa** and **oxprenolol** when given **phenylpropanolamine**, see 'Methyldopa + Sympathomimetics', p.403.

1. O'Connell MB, Gross CR. The effect of single-dose phenylpropanolamine on blood pressure in patients with hypertension controlled by β blockers. *Pharmacotherapy* (1990) 10, 85–91.
2. Petrulis AS, Imperiale TF, Speroff T. The acute effect of phenylpropanolamine and brompheniramine on blood pressure in controlled hypertension. *J Gen Intern Med* (1991) 6, 503–6.

Beta-blockers + Tasosartan

Atenolol and tasosartan have additive blood-pressure lowering effects, and no important pharmacokinetic interaction.

Clinical evidence, mechanism, importance and management

A study in 17 patients with essential hypertension found that co-administration of **atenolol** 50 mg daily and **tasosartan** 50 mg daily for 14 days reduced the peak plasma levels and the AUC of **tasosartan** by 24% and 16% respectively, but the pharmacokinetics of its active metabolite **enoltasosartan** were not affected. The peak plasma levels and AUC of **atenolol** were decreased by 22% and 18% respectively. The reduction in diastolic pressure was greater with **tasosartan** plus **atenolol** than after either treatment alone. The pharmacokinetic interaction was not considered of primary clinical importance, and the drug combination was not associated with any particular adverse events.[1] Thus, there do not appear to be any special precautions necessary for combined use. There does not appear to be any information on other beta-blockers and **tasosartan**. A single-dose study in healthy subjects suggests there is no interaction between **valsartan** and **atenolol** (see 'Valsartan + Miscellaneous drugs', p.410).

1. Andrawis NS, Battle MM, Klamerus KJ, Burghart PH, Neefe L, Weinryb I, Mayer P, Abernethy DR. A pharmacokinetic and pharmacodynamic study of the potential drug interaction between tasosartan and atenolol in patients with stage 1 and 2 essential hypertension. *J Clin Pharmacol* (2000) 40, 231–41.

Beta-blockers + Thallium scans

Beta-blockers may reduce the sensitivity of stress thallium scans used for the diagnosis of coronary heart disease.

Clinical evidence, mechanism, importance and management

A retrospective comparison of patients given **201-thallous chloride** during exercise for the diagnosis of coronary heart disease showed that there was a marked reduction in the sensitivity to stress thallium scans in those on beta-blockers when compared with other patients not taking beta-blockers. This is because beta-blockers limit the exercise-induced rise in heart rate. The suggestion was made that consideration should be given to discontinuing beta-blockers before evaluating these patients.[1] Strictly speaking this is not an interaction in the usual sense of the word. See also 'Dipyridamole + Beta-blockers', p.884.

1. Henkin RE, Chang W, Provus R. The effect of beta-blockers on thallium scans. *J Nucl Med* (1982) 23, P63.

Beta-blockers + Tobacco smoking and/or Coffee and Tea

Beta-blockers reduce heart rate and blood pressure. These therapeutically useful effects are exploited in the treatment of angina and hypertension, but are reduced to some extent if patients smoke. Some increase in the dosage of the beta-blocker may be necessary. Drinking tea or coffee may have the same but smaller effect.

Clinical evidence

(a) Beta-blockers + Tobacco smoking

A double-blind study in 10 smokers with angina pectoris, taking daily doses of either 240 mg **propranolol**, 100 mg **atenolol** or a placebo, found that **smoking** reduced their plasma **propranolol** levels by 25% when compared with a non-smoking phase. Plasma **atenolol** levels were not significantly altered. Both of the beta-blockers reduced heart rate at rest and during exercise, but the reductions were less when subjects smoked (rises of 8 to 14%).[1]

Other studies found that serum **propranolol** levels in smokers were about half those in non-smokers.[2,3] Smoking caused an increase in blood pressure and heart rate in patients with angina and these effects were evident to a reduced extent during propranolol treatment. In addition smoking abolished the beneficial effects of **propranolol** on ST segment depression.[4]

(b) Beta-blockers + Caffeine

Two 150-ml cups of **coffee** (made from 24 g coffee) increased the blood pressures of 12 healthy subjects while taking 240 mg **propranolol**, 300 mg **metoprolol** or a placebo. Mean systolic/diastolic blood pressure rises were 7%/22% with **propranolol**, 7%/19% with **metoprolol** and 4%/16% mmHg with placebo. The beta-blockers and placebo were given in divided doses over 15 hours before the test.[5]

(c) Beta-blockers + Tobacco smoking + Caffeine

Eight patients with mild hypertension taking daily doses of **propranolol** 80 mg twice daily, **oxprenolol** 80 mg twice daily or **atenolol** 100 mg daily over a 6-week period had their blood pressure monitored after smoking 2 tipped cigarettes and drinking coffee (200 mg caffeine). Their mean systolic/diastolic blood pressure rises over the following 2 h were 8.5/8 mmHg with **propranolol**, 12.1/9.1 mmHg with **oxprenolol** and 5.2/4.4 mmHg with **atenolol**.[6]

Mechanism

Smoking tobacco increases heart rate, blood pressure and the severity of myocardial ischaemia (oxygen starvation of the heart muscle), probably as a direct effect of the nicotine and due to the reduced oxygen-carrying capacity of the blood.[1,4] These actions oppose and may even totally abolish the beneficial actions of the beta-blockers. In addition, smoking stimulates the liver enzymes concerned with the metabolism of some beta-blockers (e.g. propranolol, metoprolol) so that their serum levels are reduced.

Caffeine causes the release of catecholamines into the blood, such as adrenaline, which could account for the increases in heart rate and blood pressure that are seen.[6] The blood pressure rise may be exaggerated in the presence of non-cardioselective beta-blockers, which block vasodilatation leaving the alpha (vasoconstrictor) effects of epinephrine unopposed. This too opposes the actions of the beta-blockers.

Importance and management

Established interactions. Smoking tobacco and (to a very much lesser extent) drinking tea or coffee oppose the effects of the beta-blockers in the treatment of angina or hypertension. Patients should be encouraged to stop smoking because, quite apart from its other toxic effects, it aggravates myocardial ischaemia, increases heart rate and can impair blood pressure control. If patients continue to smoke, it may be necessary to raise the dosages of the beta-blockers. The effects of the caffeine in tea, coffee, *Coca-Cola*, etc. are quite small and there seems to be no strong reason to forbid them, but the excessive consumption of large amounts may not be a good idea, particularly in those who also smoke.

1. Fox K, Deanfield J, Krikler S, Ribeiro P, Wright C. The interaction of cigarette smoking and β-adrenoceptor blockade. *Br J Clin Pharmacol* (1984) 17, 92S–93S.
2. Vestal RE, Wood AJJ, Branch RA, Shand DG, Wilkinson GR. Effects of age and cigarette smoking on propranolol disposition. *Clin Pharmacol Ther* (1979) 26, 8–15.
3. Gardner SK, Cady WJ, Ong YS. Effect of smoking on the elimination of propranolol hydrochloride. *Int J Clin Pharmacol Ther Toxicol* (1980) 18, 421–4.
4. Fox K, Jonathan A, Williams H, Selwyn A. Interaction between cigarettes and propranolol in treatment of angina pectoris. *BMJ* (1980) 281, 191–3.
5. Smits P, Hoffmann H, Thien T, Houben H, van't Laar A. Hemodynamic and humoral effects of coffee after β1-selective and nonselective β-blockade. *Clin Pharmacol Ther* (1983) 34, 153–8.
6. Freestone S and Ramsey LE. Effect of β-blockade on the pressor response to coffee plus smoking in patients with mild hypertension. *Drugs* (1983) 25 (Suppl 2), 141–5.

Beta-blockers + Vitamin C (Ascorbic acid)

Vitamin C reduces the bioavailability of propranolol but the extent is too small to matter.

Clinical evidence, mechanism, importance and management

A study in 5 healthy subjects given a single 80-mg dose of **propranolol** found that when concurrently given a single 2-g dose of **vitamin C** the maximum plasma levels of the **propranolol** were reduced by 28%, the AUC was reduced by 37% and its recovery in the urine was reduced by 66%. The fall in heart rate was also slightly less. The reason for this interaction appears to be that the **vitamin C** reduces both the absorption and the metabolic conjugation of the **propranolol**.[1] However, none of the changes seen would appear to be of clinical relevance.

1. Gonzalez JP, Valdivieso A, Calvo R, Rodríguez-Sasiaín JM, Jimenez R, Aguirre C, du Souich P. Influence of vitamin C on the absorption and first pass metabolism of propranolol. *Eur J Clin Pharmacol* (1995) 48, 295–7.

Beta-blockers + X-ray contrast media

Severe hypotension has been seen in two patients taking beta-blockers when given sodium meglumine amidotrizoate (diatrizoate) as a contrast agent.

Clinical evidence

Two patients, one taking **nadolol** and the other **propranolol**, developed severe hypotensive reactions when given **sodium meglumine**

amidotrizoate (diatrizoate) as a contrast agent for X-ray urography. Both patients developed slowly progressive erythema on the face and arms followed by tachycardia and a weak pulse. Each was successfully treated with subcutaneous epinephrine (adrenaline) and hydrocortisone.[1] See also, Anaphylaxis: resistant to treatment under 'Beta-blockers + Sympathomimetics (directly-acting)', p.448.

Mechanism

Iodinated contrast media are associated with hypersensitivity reactions due to the release of histamine. It is suggested that beta-blockers compromise the ability of the body to cope with the effects of histamine release.[1]

Importance and management

Limited documentation. Withdrawal of the beta-blocker 2 to 3 days before use of contrast media has been suggested.[1] When anaphylactic reactions do occur in patients on beta-blockers, it may be preferable to use a beta-agonist bronchodilator such as isoprenaline rather than epinephrine (adrenaline).[1]

1. Hamilton G. Severe adverse reactions to urography in patients taking beta-adrenergic blocking agents. *Can Med Assoc J* (1985) 133, 122.

Sotalol + Potassium-depleting diuretics, and other potassium-depleting drugs

The use of potassium-depleting diuretics can precipitate the development of potentially life-threatening torsade de pointes arrhythmia in patients taking sotalol unless potassium levels are maintained. This would also be expected with other potassium-depleting drugs such as corticosteroids, some laxatives, and intravenous amphotericin.

Clinical evidence

A 4-year study in cardiac clinics in South Africa identified 13 patients who developed syncope and a prolonged QT interval while taking sotalol (80 to 480 mg daily). Eleven of them were being treated for hypertension, one for ventricular asystoles, and one for both. Polymorphous ventricular tachycardia was seen in 12 of the patients, and criteria typical of torsade de pointes were seen in 10 of these 12. In 6 of them, this occurred within 72 hours of starting sotalol, and for the remaining 6, at varying intervals from 10 days to 3 years. Twelve patients were taking a combined preparation (Sotazide) containing sotalol 160 mg and hydrochlorothiazide 25 mg. Definite hypokalaemia (defined by the study as serum K^+ <3.5 mmol/l) was detected in 8 of the 13 patients. Four of the patients were also taking other drugs known to prolong the QT interval, namely disopyramide and tricyclic antidepressants. The problems resolved in all of the cases within 12 h when the sotalol was stopped and potassium supplements given when indicated.[1]

Mechanism

Potassium-depleting drugs may cause hypokalaemia, which increases the potential for torsade de pointes arrhythmia with sotalol.

Importance and management

This interaction is established, clinically important and potentially life threatening. Prolongation of the QT interval and the development of torsade de pointes in patients on sotalol, particularly with high doses, is a recognised adverse effect, but it can occur even with small doses of sotalol if potassium depletion is allowed to develop. It is clearly very important therefore to ensure that potassium levels are

maintained if potassium-depleting drugs are given with sotalol. A list of potassium-depleting diuretics is given in Table 14.2. Other drugs that may cause potassium depletion include corticosteroids, some laxatives, and intravenous amphotericin.

1. McKibbin JK, Pocock WA, Barlow JB, Scott Millar RN, Obel IWP. Sotalol, hypokalaemia, syncope, and torsade de pointes. *Br Heart J* (1984) 51, 157–62.

Sotalol + Terfenadine

Episodes of torsade de pointes arrhythmia developed in a woman on sotalol when terfenadine was added.

Clinical evidence, mechanism, importance and management

A 71-year-old woman with a history of atrial fibrillation was successfully treated with 80 mg **sotalol** twice daily. Eight days after additionally starting to take 60 mg **terfenadine** twice daily she developed repeated self-limiting episodes of torsade de pointes arrhythmia. On one occasion she required resuscitation. Both drugs were stopped and no further episodes of arrhythmia occurred 72 h after temporary pacing was discontinued.[1] It seems likely that what happened resulted from the additive effects of both drugs on the QT interval. Both can prolong the QT interval, which can lead to the development of torsade de pointes. This case confirms a previous mention of the possibility of this interaction.[2]

Although this seems to be the first report of this interaction, it is consistent with the known pharmacology of both drugs. Torsade de pointes is potentially life threatening so the concurrent use of these two drugs should be avoided. See also 'Drugs that prolong the QT interval + Other drugs that prolong the QT interval', p.103.

1. Feroze H, Suri R, Silverman DI. Torsades de pointes from terfenadine and sotalol given in combination. *Pacing Clin Electrophysiol* (1996) 19, 1519-21.
2. Woosley RL, Chen Y, Freiman JP, Gillis RA. Mechanism of the cardiotoxic actions of terfenadine. *JAMA* (1993) 269, 1532–6.

Xamoterol + Miscellaneous drugs

Xamoterol was contraindicated in patients with severe heart failure. Xamoterol has worsened COPD in patients (whether taking bronchodilators or not).

Clinical evidence, mechanism, importance and management

The makers said that xamoterol was contraindicated in those who require treatment with an ACE inhibitor,[1] not because of a direct interaction between the two but because the use of an ACE inhibitor is a probable indication that the patient has severe heart failure, which was a contraindication for xamoterol.

The beta antagonist activity of xamoterol carries the risk of increased airways resistance in patients with asthma or chronic obstructive airways disease[1] – just like conventional beta-blockers. The makers say that bronchospasm is rare, but worsening of obstructive airways disease has been seen.[2,3] For this reason the makers of xamoterol advised caution in patients with these conditions, and said that if these diseases were worsened by xamoterol it should be stopped and a bronchodilator such as salbutamol used.[1]

1. Corwin (Xamoterol). Zeneca Pharma. ABPI Compendium of Datasheets and Summaries of Product Characteristics 1999–2000, p 1780–1.
2. Lammers JWJ, Müller METM, Folgering TM, van Herwaarden CLA. A comparative study on the ventilatory and haemodynamic effects of xamoterol and atenolol in asthmatic patients. *Br J Clin Pharmacol* (1986) 22, 595–602.
3. Löfdahl C-G, Svedmyr N. Effect of xamoterol (ICI 118,587) in asthmatic patients. *Br J Clin Pharmacol* (1984) 18, 597–601.

11

Calcium channel blocker drug interactions

This chapter is primarily concerned with those interactions where the activity of the calcium channel blockers (sometimes called calcium antagonists) is changed by the presence of another drug. The table below lists all the calcium channel blockers whose interactions are described in this book, but not all are necessarily dealt with in this chapter because, where the calcium channel blocker is the affecting agent, the relevant monograph is usually categorised under the heading of the drug affected. The exceptions to this rule are the general synopses dealing with amlodipine, lercanidipine and prenylamine. The Index should be consulted for a full listing.

The calcium channel blockers have an increasingly wide application and are used for paroxysmal supraventricular tachycardia and angina, arrhythmias, hypertension, congestive heart failure, pulmonary disorders, gastrointestinal disorders and migraine headaches.

Table 11.1 Calcium channel blockers

Generic names	Proprietary names
Amlodipine	Amloprax, Amlor, Antacal, Astudal, Cordarex, Cordipina, Inovec, Istin, Lopiden, Monopina, Nicord, Norvas, Norvasc, Pressat, Prilpressin, Roxflan, Sinergen, Tensodin
Barnidipine	Cyress, Hypoca
Bepridil	Unicordium, Vascor
Darodipine	
Diltiazem	Adizem, Alandiem, Altiazem, Angiact, Angicontin, Angiodrox, Angiolong, Angiotrofin, Angiozem, Angipress, Angitil, Angizem, Anzem, Apo-Diltiaz, Auscard, Balcor, Bi-Tildiem, Calcicard, Cal-Antagon, Cardcal, Cardil, Cardiser, Cardium, Cardizem, Carreldon, Cartia, Carzem, Citizem, Clobendian, Coramil, Coras, Corazem, Corazet, Coridil, Corolater, Cronodine, Deltazen, Denazox, Diacor, Diatil, Dilaclan, Dilacor, Diladel, Dilatam, Dilcard, Dilcardia, Dilcor, Dilem, Dilfar, Diliter, Dilizem, Dilmin, Diloc, Dilpral, Dilrene, Dilsal, Dilta, Diltabeta, Diltahexal, Diltam, Diltan, Diltaretard, Diltec, Dilti, Diltia, Diltiacor, Diltiagamma, Diltiastad, Diltiem, Diltikard, Diltiuc, Diltiwas, Diltizem, Dilzatyrol, Dilzem, Dilzene, Dilzicardin, Dil-Sanorania, Dinisor, Ditizem, Doclis, Duplide, Entrydil, Escozem, Etizem, Etyzem, Gewazem, Herbesser, Horizem, Incoril, Lacerol, Levodex, Longazem, Masdil, Mdiltiwas, Medozem, Metazem, Mono-Tildiem, Myonil, Novo-Diltiazem, Nu-Diltiaz, Optil, Progor, Retalzem, Slozem, Surazem, Tiadil, Tiakem, Tiamate, Tiazac, Tilazem, Tildiem, Tilker, Trumsal, Uni Masdil, UnoCardil, Vasocardol, Viazem, Zemtard, Zildem, Zilden
Felodipine	Agon, Feloday, Felodur, Fensel, Flodil, Hydac, Modip, Munobal, Penedil, Perfudal, Plendil, Preslow, Prevex, Renedil, Splendil
Gallopamil	Algocor, Gallobeta, Procorum
Isradipine	Clivoten, Dilatol, Dynacirc, Esradin, Icaz, Lomir, Prescal, Vascal
Lacidipine	Aponil, Caldine, Lacimen, Lacipil, Lacirex, Ladip, Midotens, Motens, Tens, Viapres
Lercanidipine	Cardiovasc, Lercadip, Lercan, Lerdip, Lerzam, Vasodip, Zanedip, Zanidip
Manidipine	Calslot, Iperten, Madiplot, Manivasc, Vascoman
Nicardipine	Antagonil, Bionicard, Cardene, Cardepine, Cardibloc, Cardioten, Cardip, Cenpine, Cordipina, Dagan, Flusemide, Karden, Lecibral, Lincil, Lisanirc, Loxen, Lucenfal, Nerdipina, Nerdipine, Neucor, Nicant, Nicapress, Nicardal, Nicardium, Nicarpin, Nimicor, Niven, Perdipina, Perdipine, Ranvil, Rydene, Vasodin, Vasonase, Vasonorm, Vatrasin
Nifedipine	Adalat, Adalate, Adapine, Adcor, Adipine, Aldipin, Angiopine, Apo-Nifed, Aprical, Atenses, Bionif, Buconif, Calanif, Calcigard, Calcilat, Cardalin, Cardifen, Cardilat, Cardilate MR, Cardiopina, Cardipin, Chronadalate, Cisday, Citilat, Coracten, Coral, Cordicant, Cordilan, Cordilat, Corinfar, Coroday, Corogal, Corotrend, Dari, Dignokonstant, Dilaflux, Dilcor, Duranifin, Ecodipine, Fedip, Fenamon, Fenidina, Fortipine, Fusepina, Hexadilat, Hypolar Retard, Jedipin, Loncord, Majolat, Megalat, Nadipinia, Nelapine, Nifal, Nifangin, Nifdemin, Nife, Nife uno, Nifebene, Nifecard, Nifeclair, Nifecodan, Nifecor, Nifed, Nifedalat, Nifedate, Nifedical, Nifedicor, Nifedicron, Nifedin, Nifedipat, Nifedipat uno, Nifedipres, Nifedipress, Nifedi-Denk, Nifehexal, Nifelat, Nifelease, Nifesal, Nifezzard, Nife-basan, Nifical, Nificard, Nifidine, Nifopress, Nif-Ten, Nipin, Nivaten, Novo-Nifedin, Nu-Nifed, Nycopin, Nyefax, Osmo-Adalat, Ospocard, Oxcord, Pertensal, Pidilat, Pinifed, Pressolat, Procardia, Servidipine, Slofedipine, Systepin, Tensipine, Vascard, Vasdalat, Vasofed, Zenusin
Nimodipine	Admon, Brainal, Brainox, Calnit, Eugerial, Kenesil, Kenzolol, Modina, Modus, Nimotop, Nimovas, Noodipina, Norton, Oxigen, Periplum, Remontal, Sobrepina, Trinalion
Nisoldipine	Baymycard, Cornel, Sular, Syscor, Zadipina
Nitrendipine	Balminil, Bayotensin, Baypresol, Baypress, Caltren, Deiten, Ditrenil, Farnitran, Gericin, Hiperdipina, Hipertenol, Miniten, Nidrel, Niprina, Nitregamma, Nitren Lich, Nitrencord, Nitrendepat, Nitrendimerck, Nitrensal, Nitrepress, Nitre-Puren, Sub Tensin, Tensogradal, Trendinol, Vastensium
Prenylamine	
Tiapamil	
Verapamil	Akilen, Angimon, Anpec, Apoacor, Apo-Verap, Arpamyl LP, Azupamil, Bonceur, Calan, Calcicard, Cardioprotect, Caveril, Chronovera, Civicor, Cordilox, Corpamil, Covera, Cronovera, Dilacor, Dilacoran, Dilacoron, Durasoptin, Falicard, Flamon, Geangin, Hexasoptin, Ikacor, Ikapress, Isopamil, Isoptin, Isoptine, Jenapamil, Lodixal, Manidon, Norvil, Novo-Veramil, Nu-Verap, Quasar, Ravamil, Redupres, Securon, Univer, Vasomil, Vasopten, Vera, Verabeta, Veracaps, Veracor, Veracoron, Veraday, Veragamma, Verahexal, Verakard, Veraloc, Veramex, Veramil, Veranorm, Verapabene, Verapam, Verapin, Verapress, Verasal, Verastad, Veratensin, Veratyrol, Vera-Lich, Verelan, Verisop, Vermin, Vermine, Veroptinstada, Verpamil, Vertab, Zolvera

Amlodipine + Miscellaneous drugs

Amlodipine does not appear to interact adversely with any of the drugs cited below, and in some instances advantageous interactions may occur.

Clinical evidence, mechanism, importance and management

The makers of amlodipine say that amlodipine has been safely administered with **ACE inhibitors** (see also 'ACE inhibitors + Calcium channel blockers', p.373), **beta-blockers** and **thiazide diuretics**, and that no dosage adjustment of the amlodipine is needed. They also say that **antibacterials**, **long-acting nitrates**, **sublingual glyceryl trinitrate**, **NSAIDs** and **oral hypoglycaemic agents** have also been safely given with amlodipine.[1] None of the individual drugs studied is specifically named.

1. Istin (Amlodipine). Pfizer Ltd. Summary of product characteristics, March 2000.

Calcium channel blockers + Azole antifungals

Itraconazole can markedly raise the serum levels of felodipine which increases its side-effects, in particular ankle and leg swelling. Preliminary evidence suggests that isradipine and nifedipine can interact similarly, and that fluconazole can also interact with nifedipine.

Clinical evidence

When 9 normal subjects were given 200 mg **itraconazole** or a placebo daily for 4 days to which was then added a single 5-mg dose of **felodipine**, it was found that the **felodipine** AUC was increased sixfold and the maximum serum levels increased eightfold. The effects of the **felodipine** on blood pressure and heart rate were also increased.[1]

A woman of 54 taking 10 mg **felodipine** daily for hypertension for a year, without problems, developed ankle and leg swelling during the first week of additional treatment with 100 mg **itraconazole** daily for tinea pedis. The oedema disappeared within 2 to 4 days of stopping the **itraconazole**.[2] Virtually the same occurred in another woman taking both drugs. Later tests on her showed that the $AUC_{0-6\,h}$ of a single 5-mg dose of **felodipine** was increased at least fourfold (possibly up to tenfold) while taking **itraconazole** and ankle swelling was also noted.[2]

Ankle swelling was noted in one patient on **isradipine** when given **itraconazole**,[2] and another report describes massive pitting oedema of the legs and ankles of a patient taking **nifedipine** when given **itraconazole**.[3] Another patient similarly showed ankle oedema and markedly raised serum **nifedipine** levels (trough levels raised almost fivefold) when given **itraconazole**.[4] A patient with malignant phaeochromocytoma whose persistent hypertension was controlled with **nifedipine** showed a rise in blood pressure when his concurrent treatment with **fluconazole** (200 mg daily) was stopped. The pressure fell again when the **fluconazole** was restarted. A later study found that his maximum **nifedipine** serum levels and $AUC_{0-5\,h}$ were raised about threefold while taking the **fluconazole**.[5]

Mechanism

Ankle swelling due to precapillary vasodilatation is a not uncommon side-effect of the dihydropyridine calcium channel blockers, made worse when the plasma concentrations are high. Calcium channel blockers are metabolised in the gut wall and liver by the cytochrome P450 CYP3A subfamily of isoenzymes, which are inhibited by itraconazole, so that in the presence of this antifungal a normal oral dose becomes in effect an overdose with its attendant side-effects. Fluconazole possibly behaves in the same way.

Importance and management

Information is limited but the felodipine/itraconazole interaction would appear to be established and clinically important. It also seems that isradipine and nifedipine can interact similarly and it is possible that other calcium channel blockers may behave in the same way. If you add itraconazole to established treatment with any calcium channel blocker you should be alert for the need to lower the dosage. Information about the nifedipine/fluconazole interaction seems to be limited to the single report cited, but be alert for this interaction in any patient given both drugs.

1. Jalava K-M, Olkkola KT, Neuvonen PJ. Itraconazole greatly increases plasma concentrations and effects of felodipine. *Clin Pharmacol Ther* (1997) 61, 410–5.
2. Neuvonen PJ, Suhonen R. Itraconazole interacts with felodipine. *J Am Acad Dermatol* (1995) 33, 134–5.
3. Rosen T. Debilitating edema associated with itraconazole therapy. *Arch Dermatol* (1994) 130, 260–1.
4. Tailor SAN, Gupta AK, Walker SE, Shear NH. Peripheral edema due to nifedipine-itraconazole interaction: a case report. *Arch Dermatol* (1996) 132, 350–2.
5. Czyborra P, Kremens B, Brendel E, Bald M, Michel MC. Fluconazole enhances blood pressure-lowering effects of nifedipine in a patient with malignant phaeochromocytoma. *Naunyn Schmiedebergs Arch Pharmacol* (1998) 357 (Suppl 4), R165.

Calcium channel blockers + Bupivacaine

On theoretical grounds the potentially serious cardiac depressant effects of intravenous bupivacaine may be enhanced in patients taking calcium channel blockers.

Clinical evidence, mechanism, importance and management

A number of factors (e.g. hypoxia, hyperkalaemia, acidosis, pregnancy and age)[1] can enhance the myocardial depression of intravenous **bupivacaine**, and studies in *dogs* have now confirmed the suspicion that calcium channel blockers such as **nifedipine**[1] and **verapamil**[2] can do the same. Elderly patients with impaired cardiovascular function on calcium channel blockers would therefore appear to be at considerable risk if **bupivacaine** is accidentally given intravenously during regional anaesthesia, but so far there appear to be no clinical reports of this adverse interaction.

1. Howie MB, Mortimer W, Candler EM, McSweeney TD, Frolicher DA. Does nifedipine enhance the cardiovascular depressive effects of bupivacaine? *Reg Anesth* (1989) 14, 19–25.
2. Liu P, Feldman HS, Covino BM, Giasi R, Covion, BG. Acute cardiovascular toxicity of intravenous amide local anesthetics in anesthetized ventilated dogs. *Anesth Analg* (1982) 61, 317–22.

Calcium channel blockers + Calcium channel blockers

Blood levels of both nifedipine and diltiazem are increased by concurrent use and blood pressure is reduced accordingly. This is claimed to be an advantageous interaction.

Clinical evidence

Pretreatment of 6 normal subjects with 30 mg or 90 mg of **diltiazem** three times daily for 3 days was found to increase the AUC of single 20-mg doses of **nifedipine** two and threefold respectively.[1,2] With the **placebo** the AUC was 637 ng.h.ml^{-1}, with 30 mg **diltiazem** 1365 ng.h.ml^{-1} and with 90 mg **diltiazem** 2005 ng.h.ml^{-1}. Similar and related results are reported elsewhere.[3] In another study it was found that 10 mg **nifedipine** three times daily for 3 days increased the maximum serum levels of **diltiazem** (after a single 60-mg dose) by 54% and increased its AUC by 49%.[4] An isolated report attributes complete or partial intestinal occlusion in a patient on **diltiazem** when **nifedipine** was added on three occasions.[2]

Mechanism

A reduction in the metabolism of both the nifedipine and diltiazem in the liver seems to be the explanation.[1,5] Additive relaxant effects on smooth muscle is suggested for the case of intestinal occlusion.[6]

Importance and management

Established interactions but of uncertain clinical importance. The authors of these reports suggest that the effects of concurrent use are usually beneficial rather than adverse, and that the dosage of the nifedipine can be reduced. Fewer side effects and better compliance are predicted.[2]

1. Tateishi T, Ohashi K, Toyosaki N, Hosoda S, Sugimoto K, Kumagai Y, Kotegawa T, Ebihara A, Toyo-oka T. The effect of diltiazem on plasma nifedipine concentration in human volunteers. *Jpn Circ J* (1987) 51, 921.
2. Tateishi T, Ohashi K, Sudo T, Sakamoto K, Toyosaki N, Hosoda S, Toyo-oka T, Kumagai Y, Sugimoto K, Fujimura A, Ebihara A. Dose dependent effect of diltiazem on the pharmacokinetics of nifedipine. *J Clin Pharmacol* (1989) 29, 994–7.
3. Ohashi K, Tateishi T, Sudo T, Sakamoto K, Toyosaki N, Hosoda S, Toyo-oka T, Sugimoto K, Kumagai Y, Ebihara A. Effects of diltiazem on the pharmacokinetics of nifedipine. *J Cardiovasc Pharmacol* (1990) 15, 96–101.
4. Tateishi T, Tateishi T, Sudo T, Sakamoto K, Toyosaki N, Hosoda S, Fujimura A, Ebihara A. The effect of nifedipine on the pharmacokinetics and dynamics of diltiazem: the preliminary study in normal volunteers. *J Clin Pharmacol* (1993) 33, 738–40.
5. Ohashi K, Sudo T, Sakamoto K, Tateishi T, Fujimura A, Kumagai Y, Ebihara A. The influence of pretreatment periods with diltiazem on nifedipine kinetics. *J Clin Pharmacol* (1993) 33, 222–5.
6. Lamaison D, Abrieu V, Fialip J, Dumas R, Andronikoff M, Lavarenne J. Occlusion intestinale aiguë et antagonistes calciques. *Therapie* (1989) 44, 201–2.

Calcium channel blockers + Calcium salts

The concurrent use of verapamil and intravenous calcium salts can be therapeutically useful, but an isolated report describes antagonism of the antiarrhythmic effects of verapamil due to the use of calcium adipate and calciferol.

Clinical evidence, mechanism, importance and management

Verapamil alone is effective in treating atrial fibrillation and supraventricular arrhythmias, and if preceded by an intravenous infusion of **calcium gluconate** or **chloride**, its hypotensive and possible negative inotropic effects are reduced or prevented without compromising its antiarrhythmic effects.[1-5] Concurrent use is therefore normally valuable, but an isolated report describes an adverse response:

An elderly woman, successfully treated for over a year with **verapamil**, re-developed atrial fibrillation within a week of starting to take 1.2 g **calcium adipate** and 3000 IU **calciferol (vitamin D)** daily for diffuse osteoporosis. Her serum **calcium** levels had risen from 2.45 to 2.7 mmol/l. Normal sinus rhythm was restored by giving 500 ml saline and repeated doses of 20 mg furosemide (frusemide) and 5 mg **verapamil** by injection.[6] **Verapamil** acts by inhibiting the passage of **calcium** ions into cardiac muscle cells and it would appear that in this case the increased concentration of calcium ions outside the cells opposed the effects of the **verapamil**.

The general importance of this isolated case is uncertain, but it would clearly be prudent to monitor concurrent use for any signs of reduced **verapamil** effects.

1. Roguin N, Shapir Y, Blazer S, Zeltzer M, Berant M. The use of calcium gluconate prior to verapamil in infants with paroxysmal supraventricular tachycardia. *Clin Cardiol* (1984) 7, 613–16.
2. Salerno DM, Anderson B, Sharkey PJ, Iber C. Intravenous verapamil for treatment of multifocal atrial tachycardia with and without calcium pretreatment. *Ann Intern Med* (1987) 107, 623–8.
3. Haft JI, Habbab MA. Treatment of atrial arrhythmias: effectiveness of verapamil when preceded by calcium infusion. *Arch Intern Med* (1986) 146, 1085–9.
4. Schoen MD, Parker RB, Hoon TJ, Hariman RJ, Bauman JL, Beckman KJ. Evaluation of the pharmacokinetics and electrocardiographic effects of intravenous verapamil with intravenous calcium chloride pretreatment in normal subjects. *Am J Cardiol* (1991) 67, 300–4.
5. Weiss AT, Lewis BS, Halon DA, Hasin Y, Gotsman MS. The use of calcium with verapamil in the management of supraventricular tachyarrhythmias. *Int J Cardiol* (1983) 4, 275–84.
6. Bar-Or D, Yoel G. Calcium and calciferol antagonise effect of verapamil in atrial fibrillation. *BMJ* (1981) 282, 1585.

Calcium channel blockers + Ceftriaxone and Clindamycin

An isolated report describes the development of complete heart block in a man on long-term verapamil, attributed to the administration of intravenous ceftriaxone and clindamycin. The validity of this 'interaction' has been questioned.

Clinical evidence, mechanism, importance and management

A man of 59 who had been on 240 mg **SR verapamil** twice daily for 2 years and 300 mg phenytoin daily for several years, developed complete heart block an hour after being given 1 g intravenous **ceftriaxone** and 900 mg **clindamycin** for bilateral pneumonia. He needed cardiopulmonary resuscitation and the insertion of a temporary pacemaker, but spontaneously recovered normal sinus rhythm after 16 h. He made a full recovery. The reasons for this serious reaction are not known, but the authors of the report postulate that these two antibacterials precipitated acute **verapamil** toxicity, possibly by displacing it from its plasma protein binding sites. Although both antibacterials are highly protein-bound (+ 93%),[1] they are acidic and do not bind to the same sites as the basic **verapamil**, so that this mechanism of interaction seems very unlikely. This seems to be the first and only report of this reaction, and the suggestion by the authors that it was due to a drug interaction has been seriously questioned.[2] There seems to be no evidence that either of these antibacterials normally interact with **verapamil** if given orally.

1. Kishore K, Raina A, Misra V, Jonas E. Acute verapamil toxicity in a patient with chronic toxicity: possible interaction with ceftriaxone and clindamycin. *Ann Pharmacother* (1993) 27, 877–80.
2. Hansten PD, Horn JR. Comment: pitfalls in reporting drug interactions. *Ann Pharmacother* (1993) 27, 1545–6.

Calcium channel blockers + Cisapride

Cisapride increases the rate of absorption of nifedipine from a sustained release preparation.

Clinical evidence, mechanism, importance and management

A study in 20 patients (average age 66), and with mild to moderate hypertension found that 2.5 mg **cisapride** caused some increase in the effects of 20 mg sustained-release **nifedipine**. The mean reduction in blood pressure due to the **nifedipine** at 1 h was unchanged by the presence of the **cisapride**, but at 3 h the **nifedipine** effects were approximately doubled. These changes reflected an increase in the serum levels of the **nifedipine** (more than doubled at 3 h), probably caused by an increase in gastrointestinal motility which increases absorption.[1] What is not clear is whether this interaction has clinical importance, but the authors of this study suggest that it might result in increased **nifedipine** side-effects such as headache and dizziness. More study is needed to assess clinical relevance of this interaction.

1. Satoh C, Sakai T, Kashiwagi H, Hongo K, Aizawa O, Watanabe M, Mochizuki S, Okamura T. Influence of cisapride on the pharmacokinetics and antihypertensive effect of sustained-release nifedipine. *Int Med* (1996) 35, 941–5.

Calcium channel blockers + Clonidine or Spironolactone

Two hypertensive patients taking verapamil developed complete heart block when clonidine was added. No adverse in-

teraction appears to occur between nifedipine and clonidine, or spironolactone and felodipine.

Clinical evidence

The refractory hypertension (240/140 mmHg) of a 54-year-old woman with hyperaldosteronism partially responded with a fall to 180/100 mmHg after 10 days' treatment with 480 mg **verapamil** and 100 mg **spironolactone** daily. To this was then added 0.15 mg **clonidine** twice daily. After the second dose she became confused and her blood pressure was found to have fallen 90/70 mmHg, with a heart rate of 50 bpm. She had developed complete AV block. This resolved when all therapy was stopped. Another woman, aged 65, with persistent hypertension failed to respond well to 240 mg **verapamil** daily (blood pressure 165/100 mmHg) to which 0.15 mg **clonidine** twice daily was then added. The next day a routine ECG showed that she had a nodal rhythm of 80 bpm which developed into complete AV block. Her blood pressure had fallen to 130/80 mmHg.[1]

250 micrograms **clonidine** daily for a week increased the hypotensive effects of 20 mg **nifedipine** twice daily by about 5 mmHg (mean blood pressure) in 12 patients.[2] 50 mg **spironolactone** was found not to affect the pharmacokinetics or **felodipine** or its clinical effects.[3]

Mechanism

The verapamil/clonidine interaction is not fully understood. Verapamil very occasionally causes AV node disturbances, but both of these patients had normal sinus rhythm before the clonidine was added. Clonidine alone has been associated with AV node dysfunction in hypertensive patients. It would seem therefore that these effects were additive in these two patients.[1]

Importance and management

Information about the verapamil/clonidine interaction seems to be limited to this report.[1] Its authors say that a review of the literature from 1966 to 1992 revealed no reports of any adverse interactions between these drugs, nonetheless they suggest that it would now be prudent to administer these two drugs together with caution and good monitoring in any patient, even in those without sinus or AV node dysfunction. There seems to be no good reason for avoiding nifedipine with clonidine or spironolactone with felodipine.

1. Jaffe R, Livshits T, Bursztyn M. Adverse interaction between clonidine and verapamil. *Ann Pharmacother* (1994) 28, 881–3.
2. Salvetti A, Pedrinelli R, Magagna A, Stornello M, Scapellato L. Calcium antagonists: interactions in hypertension. *Am J Nephrol* (1986) 6 (Suppl 1), 95–9.
3. Janzon K, Edgar B. Lundborg P, Regardh CG. The influence of cimetidine and spironolactone on the pharmacokinetics and haemodynamic effects of felodipine in healthy subjects. *Acta Pharmacol Toxicol* (1986) 59 (Suppl 4), 98.

Calcium channel blockers + Co-trimoxazole

Co-trimoxazole normally appears not to interact with nifedipine, but adverse effects (leg cramps, facial flushing) have been reported in one patient.

Clinical evidence, mechanism, importance and management

The observation of a patient on **nifedipine** who developed leg cramps and facial flushing (evidence of raised serum **nifedipine** levels) when treated with **co-trimoxazole**, prompted further study of this possible interaction in 9 normal subjects. After taking 960 mg **co-trimoxazole** twice daily for 3 days the pharmacokinetics of single 20-mg doses of **nifedipine** and blood pressures in these subjects were found to be unchanged.[1] No special precautions would therefore normally seem to be necessary but monitor the outcome of concurrent use.

1. Edwards C, Monkman S, Cholerton S, Rawlins MD, Idle JR, Ferner RE. Lack of effect of co-trimoxazole on the pharmacokinetics and pharmacodynamics of nifedipine. *Br J Clin Pharmacol* (1990) 30, 889–91.

Calcium channel blockers + Dantrolene

An isolated report describes acute hyperkalaemia and cardiovascular collapse when dantrolene was given in the presence of verapamil, but not nifedipine.

Clinical evidence, mechanism, importance and management

A 90-year-old man with coronary artery disease taking 80 mg **verapamil** three times daily, with a history of malignant hyperthermia and undergoing surgery, showed marked myocardial depression and hyperkalaemia (7.1 mmol/l) within 2 h of being given **dantrolene** intravenously.[1] Six months later similar preoperative and intraoperative procedures were undertaken uneventfully when the **verapamil** was replaced by **nifedipine**. Hyperkalaemia and cardiovascular collapse have been seen in *pigs* and *dogs* given **dantrolene** and **verapamil** or **diltiazem**, but not with **nifedipine**.[2-6]

These observations would seem to link with a report of 3 patients taking **verapamil** who developed hypotension and sinus bradycardia, all of whom were noted to be hyperkalaemic. In two cases their severe left ventricular dysfunction reversed when they were given **intravenous calcium**.[6] Studies in *dogs* confirmed that hyperkalaemia reduced myocardial contractility in the presence of **verapamil**, and this was reversed by **calcium**.[6]

The overall picture is that hyperkalaemia can apparently increase the myocardial depression caused by **verapamil**, and it seems possible that drugs other than **dantrolene** which can raise blood potassium levels may be among the factors which may predispose patients to severe left ventricular dysfunction. More study is needed.

1. Rubin AS, Zablocki AD. Hyperkalaemia, verapamil, and dantrolene. *Anesthesiology* (1987) 66, 246–9.
2. Lynch C, Durbin CG, Fisher NA, Veselis RA, Althaus JS. Effects of dantrolene and verapamil on atrioventricular conduction and cardiovascular performance in dogs. *Anesth Analg* (1986) 65, 252–8.
3. San Juan AC, Port JD, Wong KC. Hyperkalaemia after dantrolene administration in dogs. *Anesth Analg* (1986) 65, S131.
4. Saltzman LS, Kates RA, Corke BC, Norfleet EA, Heath KR. Hyperkalaemia and cardiovascular collapse after verapamil and dantrolene administration in swine. *Anesth Analg* (1984) 63, 473–8.
5. Saltzman LS, Kates RA, Norfleet EA, Corke BC, Heath KR. Hemodynamic interactions of diltiazem-dantrolene and nifedipine and nifedipine-dantrolene. *Anesthesiology* (1984) 61, A11.
6. Jolly SR, Keaton N, Movahed A, Rose GC, Reeves WC. Effect of hyperkalaemia on experimental myocardial depression by verapamil. *Am Heart J* (1991) 121, 517–23.

Calcium channel blockers + Diclofenac or Naproxen

Diclofenac reduces serum verapamil levels, but naproxen appears not to interact.

Clinical evidence, mechanism, importance and management

A study in 25 hypertensive subjects taking 240 mg **slow-release verapamil** daily found that the concurrent use of 75 mg **diclofenac** twice daily reduced the AUC by 26% (from 3207 to 2389 ng/ml h), whereas 375 mg **naproxen** twice daily had no effect.[1] The reasons are not understood. Whether this interaction with **diclofenac** has a clinically important effect on treatment with **verapamil** appears not to have been assessed, but be alert for any signs of a reduced response to **verapamil**.

1. Peterson C, Basch C, Cohen A. Differential effects of naproxen and diclofenac on verapamil pharmacokinetics. *Clin Pharmacol Ther* (1990) 49, 129.

Calcium channel blockers + Erythromycin

Erythromycin markedly increases the bioavailability of felodipine. An isolated report describes increased felodipine effects and toxicity in a patient when given erythromycin.

Clinical evidence

Twelve normal subjects were given 10 mg **felodipine** before and after taking 250 mg **erythromycin** four times daily for a day.[1] The **felodipine** AUC was increased almost threefold by the **erythromycin**, the maximum serum levels were more than doubled and the half-life prolonged from 6.9 to 11.1 h.

A hypertensive woman on 10 mg **felodipine** daily developed tachycardia, flushing and massive ankle oedema within 2 to 3 days of starting to take 250 mg **erythromycin** twice daily. Her blood pressure had fallen from 120/90 to 110/70 mmHg. She fully recovered within a few days stopping the **erythromycin**.[2]

Mechanism

Ankle swelling due to precapillary vasodilatation is a not uncommon side-effect of the calcium channel blockers, made worse when the plasma concentrations are high. Calcium channel blockers are metabolised in the gut wall and liver by the cytochrome P450 CYP3A subfamily of isoenzymes, which are possibly inhibited by erythromycin, so that in its presence a normal oral dose becomes in effect an overdose with its attendant side-effects.[1,2]

Importance and management

Information seems to be limited to these two reports but the interaction would appear to be established and clinically important. Anticipate the need to reduce the felodipine dosage if erythromycin is added. There seem to be no reports of interactions between any of the other calcium channel blockers and macrolide antibacterials.

1. Bailey DG, Bend JR, Arnold MO, Tran LT, Spence JD. Erythromycin-felodipine interaction: magnitude, mechanism, and comparison with grapefruit juice. *Clin Pharmacol Ther* (1996) 60, 25–33.
2. Liedholm H, Nordin G. Erythromycin–felodipine interaction. *DICP Ann Pharmacother* (1991) 25, 1007–8.

Calcium channel blockers + Fluoxetine

Two patients on verapamil and two on nifedipine developed increased side-effects (oedema, headaches, nausea, flushing, orthostatic hypotension) due to the concurrent use of fluoxetine.

Clinical evidence

(a) Nifedipine

A patient on 60 mg **nifedipine** daily developed nausea and flushing following the addition of 20 mg **fluoxetine** every other day. The adverse effects gradually disappeared over the next 2 to 3 weeks when the **fluoxetine** dosage was halved.[1] An 80-year-old woman on **nifedipine** developed tachycardia, hypotension and profound weakness 18 days after starting 20 mg **fluoxetine** daily. On admission to hospital she was unable to stand, her upright blood pressure was 90/50 mmHg and her heart rate was 120 bpm. She fully recovered within a week of stopping the **fluoxetine**.[2]

(b) Verapamil

A woman on 240 mg **verapamil** daily developed oedema of the feet and ankles and neck vein distention within 6 weeks of starting 20 mg **fluoxetine** daily. The oedema resolved within 2 to 3 weeks of reducing the **verapamil** dosage to 120 mg daily. Another patient taking 240 mg **verapamil** daily for the prophylaxis of migraine developed morning headaches (believed by the patient not to be migraine) with-

in a week of increasing his **fluoxetine** dosage from 20 to 40 mg daily. The headaches stopped when the **verapamil** dosage was reduced and then stopped.[1]

Mechanism

What happened appeared to be the exaggeration of the side-effects of these calcium channel blockers, possibly due to inhibition of cytochrome P450 isoenzyme CYP3A4 by the fluoxetine which resulted in a marked reduction in the metabolism and clearance of the calcium channel blockers, thereby increasing their effects and side-effects.

Importance and management

Although information appears to be limited to these reports, it would seem reasonable to monitor the concurrent use of nifedipine or verapamil with fluoxetine, being alert for the need to reduce the drug dosages. More study is needed. Information about other calcium channel blockers with fluoxetine appears to be lacking.

1. Sternbach H. Fluoxetine-associated potentiation of calcium-channel blockers. *J Clin Psychopharmacol* (1991) 11, 390–1.
2. Azaz-Livshits T, Danenberg HD. Tachycardia, orthostatic hypotension and profound weakness during concomitant use of fluoxetine and nifedipine. *Eur J Clin Pharmacol* (1997) 52 (Suppl), A128.

Calcium channel blockers + Food and drinks

Food appears not to have an important effect on the absorption of bepridil, nifedipine or verapamil in a sustained-release formulation. Grapefruit juice very markedly increases the bioavailabilities of felodipine, nicardipine, nifedipine, nimodipine, nisoldipine and nitrendipine, and of amlodipine to a small extent, but these interactions appear to be of limited clinical importance. Diltiazem is not affected.

Clinical evidence

(a) Food

The absorption of two 200-mg capsules of **bepridil** in 15 normal subjects was delayed by **food** (peak serum times prolonged from 2.6 to 3.8 h) but the amount absorbed was unchanged.[1] It seems likely that steady-state levels will be unaffected by **food**. Some single dose studies suggested that **food** might delay the absorption of **nifedipine** and reduce its peak levels,[2-4] but a multiple dose study found that **food** does not have an important effect on the steady-state levels.[5] No significant effects on the absorption of **verapamil** from a multiparticulate sustained release preparation were seen when given with **food**.[6]

(b) Fruit juices

A normal-sized glass of **grapefruit juice** (200–250 ml) can increase the bioavailability of **felodipine** two to threefold in normal subjects and patients with hypertension.[7-14] Its effects are proportionately increased. One study found that diastolic pressures were reduced 20% and heart rates increased 22% when blood **felodipine** levels were at their highest.[7] Side effects such as headaches, facial flushing and lightheadedness were also increased.[7] The interaction develops after taking the first glass of **grapefruit juice** and persists for about 24 h.[13,15] The bioavailabilities of **amlodipine**,[16] **nicardipine**,[17] **nifedipine**,[7,18-21] **nimodipine**,[22,23] **nisoldipine**[24] and **nitrendipine**[25] have also been found to be increased, even approximately doubled in some instances, but without apparently normally causing adverse haemodynamic effects. The bioavailability of **diltiazem** is unaltered.[26]

Mechanism

Uncertain. One suggestion is that the increases in bioavailability are due to the flavonoid (naringin)[7,11,24] or the sesquiterpenoid[27] components (but not quercetin[18]) of the fruit juice which inhibit the activity of cytochrome P450 isoenzymes CYP3A3/4 in the intestinal wall and liver so that the metabolism of these calcium channel blockers is reduced, thereby reducing their loss from the body and increasing their effects and side-effects.

Importance and management

Established interactions but in most cases of limited clinical importance. The makers of *Plendil* (felodipine)[28] say that it should not be taken together with grapefruit juice, but generally speaking the concurrent use of the calcium channel blockers need not be avoided. However it would be worth checking the diet of any patient who complains of increased side-effects with any of the calcium channel blockers which are known to interact with grapefruit juice. Any problems can be solved either by reducing the dosage of the calcium channel blocker, swapping it for another (diltiazem does not interact), or by stopping the grapefruit juice.

1. Easterling DE, Stellar SM, Nayak RK, Desiraju RK. The effect of food on the bioavailability of bepridil. *J Clin Pharmacol* (1984) 24, 416–17.
2. Ochs HR, Rämsch K-D, Verburg-Ochs B, Greenblatt DJ, Gerloff J. Nifedipine: kinetics and dynamics after single oral doses. *Klin Wochenschr* (1984) 62, 427–9.
3. Reitberg DP, Love SJ, Quercia GT, Zinny MA. Effect of food on nifedipine pharmacokinetics. *Clin Pharmacol Ther* (1987) 42, 72–5.
4. Challenor VF, Waller DG, Gruchy BS, Renwick AG, George CF. Food and nifedipine pharmacokinetics. *Br J Clin Pharmacol* (1987) 23, 248–9.
5. Rimoy GH, Idle JR, Bhaskar NK, Rubin PC. The influence of food on the pharmacokinetics of 'biphasic' nifedipine at steady state in normal subjects. *Br J Clin Pharmacol* (1989) 28, 612–15.
6. Devane JG, Kelly JG. Effect of food on the bioavailability of a multiparticulate sustained-release verapamil formulation. *Adv Therapy* (1991) 8, 48–53.
7. Bailey DG, Spence JD, Munoz C, Arnold JMO. Interaction of citrus juices with felodipine and nifedipine. *Lancet* (1991) 337, 268–9.
8. Edgar B, Bailey DG, Bergstrand R, Johnsson G, Lurje L. Formulation dependent interaction between felodipine and grapefruit juice. *Clin Pharmacol Ther* (1990) 47, 181.
9. Bailey DG, Spence JD, Edgar B, Bayliff CD, Arnold JMO. Ethanol enhances the hemodynamic effects of felodipine. *Clin Invest Med* (1989) 12, 357–62.
10. Edgar B, Bailey D, Bergstrand R, Johnsson G, Regårdh CG. Acute effects of drinking grapefruit juice on the pharmacokinetics and dynamics on felodipine – and its potential clinical relevance. *Eur J Clin Pharmacol* (1992) 42, 313–17.
11. Bailey DG, Arnold MO, Munoz C, Spence JD. Grapefruit juice–felodipine interaction: mechanism, predictability, and effect of naringin. *Clin Pharmacol Ther* (1993) 53, 637–42.
12. Bailey DG, Bend JR, Arnold MO, Tran LT, Spence JD. Erythromycin-felodipine interaction: magnitude, mechanism, and comparison with grapefruit juice. *Clin Pharmacol Ther* (1996) 60, 25–33.
13. Lundahl JUE, Regardh CG, Edgar B, Johnsson G. The interaction of grapefruit juice maximal after the first glass. *Eur J Clin Pharmacol* (1998) 54, 75–81.
14. Lundahl J, Regårdh CG, Edgar B, Johnsson G. Effects of grapefruit juice ingestion – pharmacokinetics and haemodynamics of intravenously and orally administered felodipine in healthy men. *Eur J Clin Pharmacol* (1997) 52, 139–45.
15. Lundahl J, Regårdh CG, Edgar B, Johnsson G. Relationship between time of intake of grapefruit juice and its effect on pharmacokinetics and pharmacodynamics of felodipine in healthy subjects. *Eur J Clin Pharmacol* (1995) 49, 61–7.
16. Josefsson M, Zackrisson A-L, Ahlner J. Effect of grapefruit juice on the pharmacokinetics of amlodipine in healthy volunteers. *Eur J Clin Pharmacol* (1996) 51, 189–93.
17. Uno T, Ohkubo T, Sugarawa K, Higashlyama A, Motomura S. Effect of grapefruit juice on the disposition of nicardipine after administration of intravenous and oral doses. *Clin Pharmacol Ther* (1987) 61, 209.
18. Rashid J, McKinstry C, Renwick AG, Dirnhuber M, Waller DG, George CF. Quercetin, an *in vitro* inhibitor of CYP3A, does not contribute to the interaction between nifedipine and grapefruit juice. *Br J Clin Pharmacol* (1993) 36, 460–3.
19. Sigusch H, Hippius M, Henschel L, Kaufmann A, Hoffmann A. Influence of grapefruit juice on the pharmacokinetics of a slow release nifedipine formulation. *Pharmazie* (1994) 49, 522–4.
20. Rashid TJ, Martin U, Clarke H, Waller DG, Renwick AG, George CF. Factors affecting the absolute bioavailability of nifedipine. *Br J Clin Pharmacol* (1995) 40, 51–8.
21. Pisarík P. Blood pressure lowering effect of adding grapefruit juice to nifedipine and terazosin in a patient with severe renovascular hypertension. *Arch Fam Med* (1996) 5, 413–6.
22. Fuhr U, Maier A, Blume H, Mück W, Unger S, Staib AH. Grapefruit juice increases oral nimodipine bioavailability. *Eur J Clin Pharmacol* (1994) 47, A100.
23. Fuhr U, Maier-Brüggemann A, Blume H, Mück W, Unger S, Kuhlmann J, Huschka C, Zaigler M, Rietbrock S, Staib AH. Grapefruit juice increases oral nimodipine bioavailability. *Int J Clin Pharmacol Ther* (1998) 36, 126–32.
24. Bailey DG, Arnold JMO, Strong HA, Munoz C, Spence JD. Effect of grapefruit juice and naringin on nisoldipine pharmacokinetics. *Clin Pharmacol Ther* (1993) 54, 589–94.
25. Soons PA, Vogels BAPM, Roosemalen MCM, Schoemaker HC, Uchida E, Edgar B, Lundahl J, Cohen AF, Breimer DD. Grapefruit juice and cimetidine inhibit stereoselective metabolism of nitrendipine in humans. *Clin Pharmacol Ther* (1991) 50, 394–403.
26. Sigusch H, Henschel L, Kraul H, Merkel U, Hoffman A. Lack of effect of grapefruit juice on diltiazem bioavailability in normal subjects. *Pharmazie* (1994) 49, 675–9.
27. Chayen R, Rosenthal T. Interaction of citrus juices with felodipine and nifedipine. *Lancet* (1991) 337, 854.
28. Plendil (Felodipine). AstraZeneca. Summary of product characteristics, June 2002.

Calcium channel blockers + H₂-blockers

The serum levels of diltiazem and nifedipine are increased by cimetidine and it may possibly be necessary to reduce the dosages. Serum felodipine, lacidipine, nimodipine, nisoldipine and nitrendipine levels are also increased but this seems to be clinically unimportant. Amlodipine and cimetidine do not interact. It is uncertain whether cimetidine interacts significantly with verapamil. Ranitidine appears to interact only minimally with calcium channel blockers but famotidine may possibly reduce heart activity undesirably.

Clinical evidence

(a) Amlodipine

A crossover study in 12 normal subjects found that 400 mg **cimetidine** twice daily for 14 days had no effect on the pharmacokinetics of 10 mg **amlodipine**.[1]

(b) Diltiazem

1200 mg **cimetidine** daily for a week increased the AUC of a single 60 mg oral dose of **diltiazem in** 6 normal subjects by 50% (from 14637 to 22435 ng min/ml) and peak serum levels by 57% (from 46.4 to 73.1 ng/ml). 300 mg **ranitidine** daily for a week increased the AUC by 15% (statistically insignificant).[2] Serum **diltiazem** increases of 40% and AUC increases of 25 to 50% were seen in another study using **cimetidine**.[3]

(c) Felodipine

1 g **cimetidine** daily increased the AUC of 10 mg **felodipine** in 12 subjects by 56%, and raised the peak serum level by 54%. There was a short lasting effect on their heart rates but the clinical effects were minimal.[4]

(d) Lacidipine

A study using single doses of 4 mg **lacidipine** found that a single 800-mg dose of **cimetidine** increased the maximum serum level of **lacidipine** by 59% and increased the AUC by 74%. Pulse rates and blood pressures were unaffected.[5]

(e) Nicardipine

No adverse interaction was seen in 24 patients given **nicardipine** with **famotidine** for 6–8 weeks.[6] No changes in the pharmacokinetics or pharmacodynamics of **nicardipine** were seen in 12 normal subjects given 300 mg intravenous **cimetidine** 6-hourly for 48 h.[7]

(f) Nifedipine

1 g **cimetidine** daily for a week increased the AUC of a single 40 mg oral dose of **nifedipine** by about 60% and increased maximum serum levels by about 80% (from 46.1 to 87.7 ng/ml). 300 mg **ranitidine** daily for a week caused a non-significant rise of about 25% in maximum **nifedipine** serum levels and AUC. Seven hypertensive patients showed a fall in mean blood pressure from 127 to 109 mmHg after taking 40 mg **nifedipine** daily for 4 weeks, and a further fall to 95 mmHg after additionally taking 1 g **cimetidine** daily for two weeks. When they took 300 mg **ranitidine** instead, there was a non-significant fall to 103 mmHg.[8-10]

Other studies clearly confirm that **cimetidine** causes a very significant rise in serum **nifedipine** levels and an increase in its effects, whereas **ranitidine** interacts only minimally.[11-16] A study found no pharmacokinetic interaction between **nifedipine** and **famotidine**, but the famotidine reversed the effects of **nifedipine** on systolic time intervals and significantly reduced the stroke volume and cardiac output.[17-19] No adverse interaction was seen in 24 patients given **nifedipine** with **famotidine** for 6–8 weeks.[6]

(g) Nimodipine

Seven days' treatment with 1 g **cimetidine** daily increased the bioavailability of 30 mg **nimodipine** three times daily in 8 subjects by 75%, but the haemodynamic effects were unchanged. **Ranitidine** did not interact.[20]

(h) Nisoldipine

A study in 8 normal subjects showed that after taking 1200 mg **cimetidine** for a day the bioavailability of a single 10 mg dose of **nisoldipine** was increased by about 50%, but the haemodynamic effects of the **nisoldipine** were unaltered.[21]

(i) Nitrendipine

200 mg **cimetidine** was found to increase the bioavailability of **nitrendipine** by 154% but the haemodynamic effects were unchanged.[22] Another study showed that **ranitidine** increased the AUC of a single oral dose of **nitrendipine** by about 50% and decreased its clearance, but no changes in the haemodynamic measurements (systolic time intervals, impedance cardiography).[23] Two further studies, including one by the same authors confirmed that a pharmacokinetic interaction (AUC + 89%) occurs but it appears to be clinically unimportant.[24,25]

(j) Verapamil

A study in 8 normal subjects showed that after taking 300 mg **cimetidine** six-hourly for eight days no changes occurred in the pharmacokinetics of a single 10-mg intravenous dose of **verapamil**, but the bioavailability of a 120-mg oral dose increased from 26 to 49%. A small insignificant change in clearance occurred but no change in AUC. The changes in the PR interval caused by the **verapamil** were unaltered in the presence of **cimetidine**.[26]

Another study found that 1200 mg **cimetidine** daily for 5 days reduced the clearance of **verapamil** by 21% and increased its elimination half-life by 50%.[27] 800 mg **cimetidine** daily for a week increased its bioavailability from 35 to 42% and its clearance fell from 45.9 to 33.2 ml/min/kg in another study.[28] Yet another found a small increase in the bioavailability of both enantiomers of **verapamil**.[29] In contrast, other studies found that the pharmacokinetics of verapamil were unaffected by **cimetidine**.[27,30,31]

Mechanism

It is believed that cimetidine increases nifedipine levels by inhibiting its oxidative metabolism by the liver. Like ranitidine it may also increase the bioavailability of nifedipine by lowering gastric acidity.[12] The mechanisms of the other interactions are probably similar.

Importance and management

The diltiazem/cimetidine and nifedipine/cimetidine interactions are established. Concurrent use need not be avoided but the increase in the calcium channel blocker effects should be taken into account. It has been suggested that the dosage of diltiazem should be reduced by 30 to 35%[32] and of nifedipine by 40%.[32,33] The evidence available suggests that although cimetidine increases the serum levels of felodipine, lacidipine, nimodipine, nisoldipine and nitrendipine, the haemodynamic changes are unimportant. This needs confirmation. Amlodipine and cimetidine do not interact. The verapamil/cimetidine interaction is not well established, but monitor the effects until more is known.

Ranitidine does not interact significantly with diltiazem, nimodipine or nifedipine and is possibly a non-interacting alternative for cimetidine with other calcium channel blockers.

Famotidine does not have a pharmacokinetic interaction with nifedipine, but its negative inotropic effects may possibly be undesirable in the elderly or those with heart failure,[17-19] and therefore some care may be needed.

1. Quoted as unpublished data, Pfizer Central Research by Abernethy DR. Amlodipine: pharmacokinetic profile of a low-clearance calcium antagonist. *J Cardiovasc Pharmacol* (1991) 17 (Suppl 1), S4–S7.
2. Winship LC, McKenney JM, Wright JT, Wood JH and Goodman RP. The effect of ranitidine and cimetidine on single-dose diltiazem pharmacokinetics. *Pharmacotherapy* (1985) 5, 16–19.
3. Mazhar M, Popat KD, Sanders C. Effect of cimetidine on diltiazem blood levels. *Clin Res* (1984) 32, 741A.
4. Janzon K, Edgar B, Lundborg P, Regårdh CG. The influence of cimetidine and spironolactone on the pharmacokinetics and haemodynamic effects of felodipine in healthy subjects. *Acta Pharmacol Toxicol* (1986) 59 (Suppl 4), 98.
5. Dewland PM. A study to assess the effect of food and a single 800 mg oral dose of cimetidine on the pharmacokinetics of a single 4 mg oral dose of calcium-channel inhibitor, GR43659X (lacidipine). Boehringer Ingelheim report GMH/88/030.
6. Chichmanian RM, Mignot G, Spreux A, Jean-Girard C, Hofliger P. Tolérance de la famotidine. Étude due réseau médecins sentinelles en pharmacovigilance. *Therapie* (1992) 47, 239–43.
7. Lai C-M, McEntegart CM, Maher KE, Bell VA. Turlapaty P, Quon CY. The effects of iv cimetidine on the pharmacokinetics (PK) and pharmacodynamics (PD) of iv nicardipine in man. *Pharm Res* (1994) 11 (Suppl 10), S386.
8. Kirch W, Janisch HD, Heidemann H, Rämsch K, Ohnhaus EE. Einfluss von Cimetidin und Rantidin auf Pharmakokinetik und antihypertensiven Effekt von Nifedipin. *Dtsch Med Wochenschr* (1983) 108, 1757–61.
9. Kirch W, Rämsch K, Janisch HD, Ohnhaus EE. The influence of two histamine H₂-receptor antagonists, cimetidine and ranitidine, on the plasma levels and clinical effect of nifedipine and metoprolol. *Arch Toxicol* (1984) (Suppl 7), 256–9.
10. Kirch W, Hoensch H, Ohnhaus EE, Janisch HD. Ranitidin-Nifedipin-Interaktion. *Dtsch Med Wochenschr* (1984) 109, 1223.
11. Smith SR, Kendall MJ, Lobo J, Beerahee A, Jack DB, Wilkins MR. Ranitidine and cimetidine: drug interactions with single dose and steady-state nifedipine administration. *Br J Clin Pharmacol* (1987) 23, 311–15.
12. Adams LJ, Antonow DR, McClain CJ, McAllister R. Effect of ranitidine on bioavailability of nifedipine. *Gastroenterology* (1986) 90, 1320.
13. Kirch W, Ohnhaus EE, Hoensch H, Janisch HD. Ranitidine increases bioavailability of nifedipine. *Clin Pharmacol Ther* (1985) 37, 204.
14. Schwartz JB, Upton RA, Lin ET, Williams RL, Benet LZ. Effect of cimetidine or ranitidine administration on nifedipine pharmacokinetics and pharmacodynamics. *Clin Pharmacol Ther* (1988) 43, 673–80.
15. Renwick AG, Le Vie J, Challenor VF, Waller DG, Gruchy B, George CF. Factors affecting the pharmacokinetics of nifedipine. *Eur J Clin Pharmacol* (1987) 32, 351–5.
16. Khan A, Langley SJ, Mullins FPG, Dixon JS, Toon S. The pharmacokinetics and pharmacodynamics of nifedipine at steady state during concomitant administration of cimetidine or high dose ranitidine. *Br J Clin Pharmacol* (1991) 32, 519–22.
17. Halabi A, Ohnhaus EE, Kirch W. Influence of famotidine on non-invasive haemodynamic parameters and nifedipine plasma levels. *Eur J Clin Invest* (1988) 18, A23.
18. Kirch W, Halabi A, Linde M, Ohnhaus EE. Negativ-inotrope Wirkung von Famotidin. *Schweiz Med Wochenschr* (1988) 118, 1912–14.
19. Kirch W, Halabi A. Linde M, Santos SR, Ohnhaus EE. Negative effects of famotidine on cardiac performance assessed by noninvasive hemodynamic measurements. *Gastroenterology* (1989) 96, 1388–92.
20. Mück W, Wingender W, Seiberling M, Woelke E, Rämsch K-D, Kuhlmann J. Influence of the H2-receptor antagonists cimetidine and ranitidine on the pharmacokinetics of nimodipine in healthy volunteers. *Eur J Clin Pharmacol* (1992) 42, 325–8.
21. Van Harten J, van Brummelen P, Lodewijks MThM, Danhof M, Breimer DD. Pharmacokinetics and hemodynamic effects of nisoldipine and its interaction with cimetidine. *Clin Pharmacol Ther* (1988) 43, 332–41.
22. Soons PA, Vogels BAPM, Roosemalen MCM, Schoemaker HC, Uchida E, Edgar B, Lundahl J, Cohen AF, Breimer DD. Grapefruit juice and cimetidine inhibit stereoselective metabolism of nitrendipine in humans. *Clin Pharmacol Ther* (1991) 50, 394–403.
23. Kirch W, Nahoui R, Ohnhaus EE. Ranitidine/nitrendipine interaction. *Clin Pharmacol Ther* (1988) 43, 149.
24. Halabi A, Nahoui R, Kirch W. Influence of ranitidine on kinetics of nitrendipine and on noninvasive hemodynamic parameters. *Ther Drug Monit* (1990) 12, 303–4.
25. Santos SR, Storpirtis S, Moreira-Filho L, Donzella H, Kirch W. Ranitidine increases the bioavailability of nitrendipine in patients with arterial hypertension. *Braz J Med Biol Res* (1992) 25, 337–47.
26. Smith MS, Benyunes MC, Bjornsson TD, Shand DG, Pritchett ELC. Influence of cimetidine on verapamil kinetics and dynamics. *Clin Pharmacol Ther* (1984) 36, 551–4.
27. Loi C-M, Rollins DE, Dukes GE, Peat MA. Effect of cimetidine on verapamil disposition. *Clin Pharmacol Ther* (1985) 37, 654–7.
28. Mikus G, Stuber H. Influence of cimetidine treatment on the physiological disposition of verapamil. *Naunyn Schmiedebergs Arch Pharmacol* (1987) 335 (Suppl), R106.
29. Mikus G, Kroemer HK, Klotz U, Eichelbaum M. Stereochemical considerations of the cimetidine-verapamil interaction. *Clin Pharmacol Ther* (1988) 43, 134.
30. Abernethy DR, Schwartz JB, Todd EL. Lack of interaction between verapamil and cimetidine. *Clin Pharmacol Ther* (1985) 38, 342–9.
31. Wing LMH, Miners JO, Lillywhite KJ. Verapamil disposition—effects of sulphinpyrazone and cimetidine. *Br J Clin Pharmacol* (1985) 19, 385–91.
32. Piepho RW, Culbertson VL, Rhodes RS. Drug interactions with the calcium-entry blockers. *Circulation* (1987) 75 (Suppl V), V181–V194.
33. Piepho RW. Individualization of calcium-entry blocker dosage for systemic hypertension. *Am J Cardiol* (1985) 56, 105H–111H.

Calcium channel blockers + Macrolide antibacterials

An isolated report describes the development of marked bradycardia in an elderly woman attributed to an interaction between verapamil and clarithromycin on one occasion, and to erythromycin on another. The presence of propranolol may also have had some part to play.

Clinical evidence, mechanism, importance and management

An isolated report[1] describes a 77-year-old woman with hypertension who developed marked bradycardia (37 to 50 bpm), interpreted as a sign of either **verapamil** or **propranolol** toxicity, within 4 days of starting a course of **clarithromycin** (500 mg twice daily). The problem was solved by temporarily reducing the dose of the **verapamil** to a quarter and the **propranolol** to a half until the **clarithromycin** course was over. Essentially the same thing happened 2 years later while taking the same drugs when **erythromycin** (333 mg three times daily) was added.

The suggested mechanism of these interactions is that both macrolides inhibit the cytochrome P450 isoenzyme CYP3A4 that is responsible for the metabolism of verapamil, as a result of which the verapamil serum levels may have risen, thereby causing bradycardia. It is unlikely that the macrolides affected the metabolism of the propranolol because it is metabolised by cytochrome P450 isoenzyme CYP2D6. However the serum levels of propranolol may also have risen to some extent because the raised verapamil levels may have reduced its clearance, thus giving the propranolol a small additive part to play in the bradycardia.

This seems to be the only report of a calcium channel blocker/macrolide interaction despite the wide-spread use of both groups of drugs for a number of years, so that this interaction would appear to be of little general importance.

1. Steenbergen JA, Stauffer VL. Potential macrolide interaction with verapamil. *Ann Pharmacother* (1998) 32, 387–8.

Calcium channel blockers + Magnesium salts

Two pregnant women developed muscular weakness and then paralysis when treated concurrently with nifedipine and intravenous magnesium sulphate.

Clinical evidence

A pregnant woman at 32 weeks' gestation was effectively treated for premature uterine contractions with **nifedipine**, 60 mg orally over 3 h, and later 20 mg over 8 h. When contractions began again 12 h later she was given 500 mg **magnesium sulphate** intravenously. She developed jerky movements of the extremities, complained of difficulty in swallowing, paradoxical respirations and an inability to lift her head from the pillow. The **magnesium** was stopped and the muscle weakness disappeared over the next 25 min.[1]

A woman at 28 weeks' gestation with mild pre-eclampsia was started on an infusion of 2 g/h **magnesium sulphate**. Her plasma **magnesium** levels were found to be 2.75 mmol/l. No untoward reactions developed when she took the first dose of a course of 20 mg **nifedipine**, but 30 min after taking the second dose (by implication 3 to 4 h later) she complained of flushing and sweating and had difficulty in lifting her head and limbs. Shortly afterwards almost complete muscular paralysis developed. The **magnesium sulphate** was stopped and a dramatic improvement followed within 15 min of an intravenous injection of 1 g **calcium gluconate**.[2]

Mechanism

The probable reason is that both compounds, working in concert, can seriously reduce the amount of calcium ions needed for normal muscular contraction. Nifedipine (a calcium channel blocker) inhibits the inflow of extracellular calcium across cell membranes. Magnesium probably acts in the same way, and also reduces intracellular calcium by activating adenyl cyclase and increasing cAMP. In addition magnesium stimulates calcium-dependent ATPase which promotes calcium uptake by the sarcoplasmic reticulum. The result is muscular paralysis which is reversed by giving large amounts of calcium. Magnesium sulphate is known to have neuromuscular blocking activity which can be additive with the activity of conventional neuromuscular blockers and aminoglycoside antibacterials (see Index).

Importance and management

Direct information seems to be limited to these two reports, but the interaction appears to be established. The authors of both of these reports advise the avoidance of magnesium sulphate and nifedipine. The same interaction would be expected to occur with other calcium channel blockers but reports are lacking.

1. Snyder SW, Cardwell MS. Neuromuscular blockade with magnesium sulfate and nifedipine. *Am J Obstet Gynecol* (1989) 161, 35–6.
2. Ben-Ami M, Giladi Y, Shalev E. The combination of magnesium sulphate and nifedipine: a cause of neuromuscular blockade. *Br J Obstet Gynaecol* (1993) 101, 262–3.

Calcium channel blockers + Mizolastine

No pharmacokinetic or pharmacodynamic interaction appears to occur between diltiazem and mizolastine.

Clinical evidence, mechanism, importance and management

A double-blind crossover study in 12 normal subjects on 60 mg **diltiazem** three times daily found that the concurrent use of 10 mg **mizolastine** daily had no effect on ECGs or blood pressures. No significant increases in adverse effects were seen and the pharmacokinetics of the **diltiazem** remained unchanged.[1] There would seem to be no reason for avoiding concurrent use. Information about other calcium channel blockers appears not to be available.

1. Miget N, Herrmann WM, Bergougnan L, Dubruc C, Weber F, Rosenzweig P. Lack of interaction between mizolastine and diltiazem in healthy volunteers. *Methods Find Exp Clin Pharmacol* (1996) 18 (Suppl B), 204.

Calcium channel blockers + NSAIDs

Two reports describe abnormal bruising and prolonged bleeding times in three patients on verapamil while taking aspirin. Diclofenac reduces verapamil serum levels and raises those of isradipine but these changes are probably unimportant. Ibuprofen causes a small reduction in the antihypertensive effects of amlodipine. Indometacin (indomethacin) appears not to reduce the hypotensive effects of felodipine, nicardipine, nimodipine or verapamil but it possibly interacts with nifedipine. Diclofenac and sulindac appear not interact with nifedipine, nor ibuprofen and naproxen with verapamil or nicardipine.

Clinical evidence, mechanism, importance and management

(a) Aspirin

Abnormal bruising and prolonged bleeding times occurred in a woman on 240 mg **verapamil** daily while taking two 325 mg **aspirin** tablets several times a week for headaches. The bruising ceased when the **verapamil** was stopped. Her normal bleeding time of 1 min rose to 4.5 min while taking **verapamil**, and to 9.0 min with **verapamil** and **aspirin**. A healthy volunteer taking the same dose of **verapamil** and **aspirin** observed the appearance of new petechiae when also taking **aspirin**. Her bleeding time rose from a normal 4.5 min to more than 15 min with **verapamil** and **aspirin**.[1] A man of 85 taking 325 mg **enteric coated aspirin** daily developed wide-spread and serious ecchymoses of his arms and legs and a retroperitoneal bleed about three weeks after starting to take 240 mg **verapamil** daily.[2] The probable reason is that the **verapamil** (and other calcium channel blockers) can inhibit platelet aggregation because they interfere with the movement of calcium ions through cell membranes. These appear to be additive with those of other antiplatelet drugs. However, concurrent use of these drugs need not normally be avoided unless the outcome is clearly adverse.

(b) Diclofenac, Sulindac

Twenty-five hypertensive subjects on 240 mg slow-release **verapamil** daily showed a 26% reduction in the AUC while taking 75 mg **diclofenac** twice daily.[3] The AUC of **isradipine** (5 mg twice daily for a week) in 18 normal subjects was unaffected by a single 50-mg dose of **diclofenac** but the maximum serum levels were raised about 20%.[4] Blood aggregation was unaffected and the pharmacokinetics of the **diclofenac** were unchanged. A study in 6 elderly women with hypertension found that 100 mg **sulindac** or 25 mg **diclofenac** three times daily had no effect on the control of their blood pressure with **nifedipine**.[5] These studies suggest that no interaction of clinical relevance occurs between these calcium channel blockers and NSAIDs.

(c) Ibuprofen

Fifty-three hypertensive patients showed no changes in their blood pressure control with **verapamil** (240–480 mg daily) when also given 400 mg **ibuprofen** three times daily for three weeks.[6] A later extended study by the same group reported the same findings.[7] No special precautions seem necessary. However, another study in patients with mild or moderate essential hypertension controlled with **amlodipine** found that 400 mg **ibuprofen** three times daily for 3 days increased blood pressures by 7.8/3.9 mmHg.[8]

(d) Indometacin (Indomethacin)

100 mg **indometacin** daily for a week did not significantly affect the hypotensive effects of **nifedipine** in 21 patients with mild to moderate essential hypertension given 20 mg twice daily.[9] Four other studies, two in normal subjects[10,11] and two in patients with essential hypertension also found that **indometacin** did not alter the blood pressure lowering effects of **felodipine**,[10,12] **nicardipine**[11] or **verapamil**.[13] The haemodynamic effects of **nimodipine** (30 mg three times daily) were not affected to a clinically relevant extent by 25 mg **indometacin** twice daily in 24 normal subjects, although the AUC of **nimodipine** and its maximum serum levels were slightly increased.[14] In contrast, in another study 100 mg **indometacin** daily was found to raise the mean arterial pressure of five out of eight hypertensive patients on 15–40 mg **nifedipine** daily by 17–20 mmHg.[15] As the outcome of concurrent use is therefore not completely certain, monitor the effects if **indometacin** is started in a patient already taking a calcium channel blocker, and either raise its dosage or if necessary use another NSAID.

(e) Naproxen

375 mg **naproxen** twice daily had no effect on the pharmacokinetics of **verapamil** in 25 hypertensive subjects.[3] 55 hypertensive patients showed no changes in their blood pressure control with **verapamil** (240–480 mg daily) when given 200 mg **naproxen** twice daily for three weeks.[6] A later extended study by the same group reported the same findings.[7] 100 patients on **nicardipine** showed no clinically relevant changes in the control of their blood pressure when given 375 mg **naproxen** twice daily.[16] No special precautions seem necessary.

1. Ring ME, Martin GV, Fenster PE. Clinically significant antiplatelet effects of calcium-channel blockers. *J Clin Pharmacol* (1986) 26, 719–20.
2. Verzino E, Kaplan B, Ashley JV, Burdette M. Verapamil–aspirin interaction. *Ann Pharmacother* (1994) 28, 536–7.
3. Peterson C, Basch C, Cohen A. Differential effects of naproxen and diclofenac on verapamil pharmacokinetics. *Clin Pharmacol Ther* (1990) 49, 129.
4. Sommers De K, Kovarik JM, Meyer EC, van Wyk M, Snyman JR, Blom M, Ott S, Grass P, Kutz K. Effects of diclofenac on isradipine pharmacokinetics and platelet aggregation in volunteers. *Eur J Clin Pharmacol* (1993) 44, 391–3.
5. Takeuchi K, Abe K, Yasujima M, Sato M, Tanno M, Sato K, Yoshinaga K. No adverse effect of non-steroidal anti-inflammatory drugs, sulindac and diclofenac sodium, on blood pressure control with a calcium antagonist, nifedipine, in elderly hypertensive patients. *Tohoku J Exp Med* (1991) 165, 201–8.
6. Weir MR, Houston MC, Grey JM. Effects of NSAIDs on blood pressure controlled by verapamil. *J Am Soc Nephrol* (1993) 4, 542.
7. Houston MC, Weir M, Gray J, Ginsberg D, Szeto C, Kaihlenen PM, Sugimoto D, Runde M, Lefkowitz M. The effects of nonsteroidal anti-inflammatory drugs on blood pressures of patients with hypertension controlled by verapamil. *Arch Intern Med* (1995) 155, 1049–54.
8. Minuz P, Pancera P, Ribul M, Priante F, Degan M, Campedelli A, Arosio E, Lechi A. Amlodipine and haemodynamic effects of cyclo-oxygenase inhibition. *Br J Clin Pharmacol* (1995) 39, 45–50.
9. Slavetti A, Pedrinelli R, Magagna A, Stornello M, Scapellato L. Calcium antagonists: interactions in hypertension. *Am J Nephrol* (1986) 6 (Suppl 1), 95–99.
10. Hardy BG, Bartle WR, Myers M, Bailey DG, Edgar B. Effect of indomethacin on the pharmacokinetics and pharmacodynamics of felodipine. *Br J Clin Pharmacol* (1988) 26, 557–62.
11. Debbas NMG, Raoof NT, Al Qassab HK, Jackson SHD, Turner P. Does indomethacin antagonise the effects of nicardipine? *Acta Pharmacol Toxicol* (1986) 59 (Suppl V), 181.
12. Morgan T, Anderson A. Interaction of indomethacin with felodipine and enalapril. *J Hypertens* (1993) 11 (Suppl 5), S338–S339.
13. Perreault MM, Foster RT, Lebel M, Du Souich P, Larochelle P, Cusson JR. Pharmacodynamic effects of indomethacin in essential hypertensive patients treated with verapamil. *Clin Invest Med* (1993) 16 (Suppl 4), B17.
14. Mück W, Heine PR, Schmage N, Niklaus H, Horkulak J, Breuel H-P. Steady-state pharmacokinetics of nimodipine during chronic administration of indometacin in elderly healthy volunteers. *Arzneimittelforschung* (1995) 45, 460–2.
15. Thatte UM, Shah SJ, Salvi SS, Suraokar S, Temulkar P, Anklesaria P, Kshirsager NA. Acute drug interaction between indomethacin and nifedipine in hypertensive patients. *J Assoc Physicians India* (1988) 36, 695–8.
16. Klassen DK, Jane LH, Young DY, Peterson CA. Assessment of blood pressure during naproxen therapy in hypertensive patients treated with nicardipine. *Am J Hypertens* (1995) 8, 146–53.

Calcium channel blockers + Omeprazole

The loss from the body of both nifedipine and omeprazole is modestly reduced by concurrent use, but these changes seem unlikely to be of clinical importance.

Clinical evidence, mechanism, importance and management

After taking 20 mg **omeprazole** daily for 7 days the clearance of **nifedipine** in 10 normal subjects was reduced 21% (from 75 to 59.4 l/h). The same subjects showed a 14% reduction (from 28.8 to 24.9 l/h) in the clearance of a 40-mg intravenous dose of **omeprazole** after 5 days' treatment with 10 mg **nifedipine** three times daily.[1] In a related study the same group of workers found that 20 mg **omeprazole** increased the AUC of **nifedipine** by 26%, but no changes in blood pressures or heart rates were seen.[2] None of these changes is large and they seem not to be of clinical importance.

1. Danhof M, Soons PA, van den Berg G, Van Brummelen P, Jansen JBMJ. Interactions between nifedipine and omeprazole. *Eur J Clin Pharmacol* (1989) 36 (Suppl), A258.
2. Soons PA, van den Berg G, Danhof M, van Brummelen P, Jansen JBMJ, Lamers CBHW, Breimer DD. Influence of single- and multiple-dose omeprazole treatment on nifedipine pharmacokinetics and effects in healthy subjects. *Eur J Clin Pharmacol* (1992) 42, 319–24.

Calcium channel blockers + Rifampicin (Rifampin)

The serum levels of barnidipine, diltiazem, manidipine, nifedipine, verapamil and possibly nisoldipine are markedly reduced by rifampicin. They may become therapeutically ineffective unless their dosages are raised.

Clinical evidence

(a) Barnidipine, Manidipine

Elderly patients with hypertension well controlled on **barnidipine** or **manidipine** showed blood pressure rises when **rifampicin** was added. Increased dosages or additional antihypertensives were needed to control the blood pressures, and reduced doses when the **rifampicin** was withdrawn.[1]

(b) Diltiazem

A study in 6 extensive and 6 poor metabolisers found that the peak serum level following a single 120-mg oral dose of **diltiazem** alone was 186 ng/ml, but after taking 600 mg **rifampicin** daily for eight days maximum serum **diltiazem** levels were only 5 to 8 ng/ml.[2]

(c) Nifedipine

A hypertensive woman well controlled on **nifedipine** (40 mg twice daily) showed a blood pressure rise from 140–160/80–90 mmHg to 200/110 mmHg within 2 weeks of starting to take antitubercular treatment which included 450 mg **rifampicin** daily. When the **rifampicin** was stopped and then restarted, the blood pressure fell and then rose again. The peak **nifedipine** serum levels and the AUC fell to about 40% while taking the **rifampicin**.[3] Another patient showed reduced **nifedipine** levels (peak levels and AUCs roughly halved) and an increase in anginal attacks when given **rifampicin**,[4] and yet another showed a loss of blood pressure control when given **rifampicin**.[5]

Six normal subjects were given 20 micrograms/kg body weight **nifedipine** intravenously and 20 mg **nifedipine** orally before and after taking 600 mg **rifampicin** daily for 7 days. The pharmacokinetics of the intravenous **nifedipine** were not significantly changed by the **rifampicin**, but the oral clearance increased from 1.5 to 20.9 L/min and the bioavailability fell from 41.2 to 5.3%.[6] A pharmacokinetic study in 6 normal subjects found that 8 h after taking a single 1200-mg dose of **rifampicin** the bioavailability of a single 10-mg oral dose of **nifedipine** was reduced to 36%, its half-life was more than halved and its clearance increased threefold.[7]

(d) Nisoldipine

There is some extremely limited evidence that **nisoldipine** and **enalapril** are ineffective in reducing blood pressure while taking **rifampicin**.[1,3]

(e) Verapamil

The observation of a patient whose hypertension was not reduced by **verapamil** while on antitubercular drugs, prompted a study in 4 other patients.[8] No **verapamil** could be detected in the plasma of three of them similarly treated for tuberculosis (**rifampicin** 450–600 mg daily, isoniazid 5 mg/kg daily, ethambutol 15 mg/kg daily) after receiving a single 40 mg dose of **verapamil**. A maximum of 20 ng/ml was found in the fourth patient. Six other subjects not taking antitubercular drugs had a maximum **verapamil** serum concentration of 35 ng/ml after being given a single 40-mg dose.[8] Similar results are reported in another study.[9]

Supraventricular tachycardia was inadequately controlled in a patient taking 600 mg **rifampicin** and 300 mg isoniazid, despite the administration of 480 mg **verapamil** every 6 h.[10] Substitution of the **rifampicin** by ethambutol resulted in a fourfold rise in serum **verapamil** levels.[10] A later study in 6 normal subjects showed that after taking **rifampicin** for 2 weeks the oral bioavailability of **verapamil** was reduced from 26 to 2%, and the effects of **verapamil** on the ECG were abolished.[11] Yet another study in elderly patients similarly found a very marked increase in the clearance of 120 mg **verapamil** twice daily due to 600 mg **rifampicin** daily. The effects of **verapamil** on AV conduction were almost abolished.[12,13]

Mechanism

The evidence suggests that the rifampicin (known to be a potent enzyme inducing agent) increases the metabolism of these calcium channel blockers by the gastrointestinal wall,[6,12,14] thereby increasing their clearance from the body.

Importance and management

Established interactions of clinical importance. The documentation for nifedipine and verapamil is good, for diltiazem it is limited and for barnidipine, manidipine and nisoldipine it is very limited indeed. Monitor the effects closely if rifampicin is given with any of these calcium channel blockers, being alert for the need to make a marked increase in the dosage of the calcium channel blocker. Ethambutol is a non-interacting alternative antitubercular. There seems to be no information about other calcium channel blockers but good monitoring would seem a prudent precaution, being alert for the need to raise their dosages.

1. Yoshimoto H, Takahashi M, Saima S. Influence of rifampicin on antihypertensive effects of dihydropiridine calcium-channel blockers in four elderly patients. *Nippon Ronen Igakkai Zasshi* (1996) 33, 692–6.
2. Drda KD, Bastian TL, Self TH, Lawson J, Lanman RC, Burlew BS, Lalonde RL. Effects of debrisoquine hydroxylation phenotype and enzyme induction with rifampin on diltiazem pharmacokinetics and pharmacodynamics. *Pharmacotherapy* (1991) 11, 278.
3. Tada Y, Tsuda Y, Otsuka T, Nagasawa K, Kimura H, Kusaba T, Sakata T. Case report: nifedipine-rifampicin interaction attenuates the effect on blood pressure in a patient with essential hypertension. *Am J Med Sci* (1992) 303, 25–7.
4. Tsuchihashi K, Fukami K, Kishimoto H, Sumiyoshi T, Haze K, Saito M, Hiramori K. A case of variant angina exacerbated by administration of rifampicin. *Heart Vessels* (1987) 3, 214–17.
5. Takasugi T. A case of hypertension suggesting nifedipine and rifampicin drug interaction. *Igaku To Yakugaku* (1989) 22, 132–5.
6. Holtbecker N, Fromm MF, Kroemer HK, Ohnhaus EE, Heidemann H. The nifedipine-rifampin interaction: Evidence for induction of gut wall metabolism. *Drug Metab Dispos* (1996) 24, 1121–3.
7. Ndanusa BU, Mustapha A, Abdu-Aguye I. The effect of single dose of rifampicin on the pharmacokinetics of oral nifedipine. *J Pharm Biomed Anal* (1997) 15, 1571–5.
8. Rahn KH, Mooy K, Böhm R, vd Vet, A. Reduction of bioavailability of verapamil by rifampin. *N Engl J Med* (1985) 312, 920–1.
9. Mooy J, Böhm R, van Baak M, van Kemenade J, vd Vet A, Rahn KH. The influence of antituberculosis drugs on the plasma level of verapamil. *Eur J Clin Pharmacol* (1987) 32, 107–9.
10. Barbarash RA. Verapamil-rifampin interaction. *Drug Intell Clin Pharm* (1985) 19, 559–60.
11. Barbarash RA, Bauman JL, Fischer JH, Kondos G, Batenhorst RL. Near total reduction in verapamil bioavailability by rifampin: electrocardiographic correlates. *J Am Coll Cardiol* (1988) 11, 205A.
12. Fromm MF, Dilger K, Busse D, Klotz U, Eichelbaum M. Rifampicin induced gastrointestinal and hepatic metabolism of verapamil in the elderly. *Naunyn Schmiedebergs Arch Pharmacol* (1996) 353 (Suppl 4), R145.
13. Fromm MF, Dilger K, Busse K, Kroemer HK, Eichelbaum M, Klotz U. Gut wall metabolism of verapamil in older people: effects of rifampicin-mediated enzyme induction. *Br J Clin Pharmacol* (1998) 45, 247–55.
14. Fromm MF, Busse D, Kroemer HK, Eichelbaum M. Differential induction of prehepatic and hepatic metabolism of verapamil by rifampin. *Hepatology* (1996) 24, 796–801.

Calcium channel blockers + Sulfinpyrazone (Sulphinpyrazone)

The clearance of verapamil is markedly increased by sulfinpyrazone (sulphinpyrazone).

Clinical evidence, mechanism, importance and management

A study in 8 normal subjects showed that after taking 800 mg **sulfinpyrazone (sulphinpyrazone)** daily for a week, the clearance of a single oral dose of **verapamil** was increased about threefold (from 4.27 to 13.77 l/h/kg), possibly due to an increase in its liver metabolism.[1] The clinical importance of this is uncertain, but be alert for reduced **verapamil** effects. It seems probable that the dosage may need to be increased.

1. Wing LMH, Miners JO, Lillywhite KJ. Verapamil disposition—effects of sulphinpyrazone and cimetidine. *Br J Clin Pharmacol* (1985) 19, 385–91.

Calcium channel blockers + Vancomycin

An isolated case report suggests that the hypotensive effects of the rapid infusion of vancomycin may occur more readily in those who are already vasodilated with nifedipine.

Clinical evidence, mechanism, importance and management

A man with severe systemic sclerosis was hospitalised for Raynaud's phenomenon and dental extraction. After being started on 40 mg **nifedipine** daily, he was given intravenous **vancomycin** (1 g in 200 ml 5% dextrose) over 30 min. After 20 min he experienced a severe headache and was found to have a marked macular erythema on the upper trunk, head, neck and arms. His blood pressure fell to 100/60 mmHg and his pulse rate was 90. He recovered spontaneously.[1] The suggested reason is that the vasodilatory effects of the **nifedipine** were additive with those of the **vancomycin** (known to cause hypotension and erythema if infused quickly). The authors of this report suggest that vasodilators should be discontinued several days before giving **vancomycin**, and the blood pressure should be well monitored during infusion.

1. Daly BM, Sharkey I. Nifedipine and vancomycin-associated red man syndrome. *Drug Intell Clin Pharm* (1986) 20, 986.

Calcium channel blockers + X-ray contrast media

The hypotensive effects of an intravenous bolus of ionic X-ray contrast medium can be increased by the presence of calcium channel blockers (diltiazem, nifedipine, verapamil, etc.). No interaction or only a small interaction appears to occur with non-ionic contrast media. A case report describes serious

ventricular tachycardia in a patient on prenylamine when given sodium iotalamate (iothalamate).

Clinical evidence, mechanism, importance and management

(a) Hypotensive effects increased or unchanged

It is well recognised that ionic X-ray contrast media used for ventriculography reduce the systemic blood pressure due to peripheral vasodilation. They also have a direct depressant effect on the heart muscle. A comparative study of the haemodynamic response of 65 patients showed that the hypotensive effect of a bolus dose of an ionic agent (0.5 ml/kg **meglumine amidotrizoate (diatrizoate)** and **sodium amidotrizoate (diatrizoate)** with edetate sodium or disodium) was increased by the concurrent use of **nifedipine** or **diltiazem**: it occurred earlier (3.1 s instead of 12.9 s), was more profound (a fall in systolic pressure of 48.4 instead of 36.9 mmHg) and more prolonged (62 s instead of 36 s).[1] A similar interaction was seen in *dogs* given **verapamil**.[2] No interaction or only a minimal interaction was seen in the patients and *dogs* when non-ionic contrast media (**iopamidol** or **iohexol**) were used instead.[1,2] Concurrent use should be undertaken with care.

(b) Ventricular arrhythmia precipitated

An elderly man who had been taking 60 mg **prenylamine** and 10 mg **nifedipine** three times a day for two years experienced cardiorespiratory arrest a few seconds after a bolus intravenous injection of 80 ml **sodium iotalamate (iothalamate)** 70% (*Conray 420*), and a further arrest 90 seconds later. On the second occasion the rhythm was identified as ventricular tachycardia, converted to sinus rhythm by a 100 Joule DC shock.[3] The reason is thought to be the additive effects of the **prenylamine** and **sodium iotalamate** both of which can prolong the QT$_c$ (corrected QT interval of the heart) which predisposes the development of serious ventricular arrhythmias. Concurrent use should be avoided or undertaken with great care. The manufacturers of **sodium iotalamate** also advise the avoidance of hypokalaemia and of drugs such as **procainamide** and **quinidine** which also tend to prolong the QT$_c$ interval.

1. Morris DL, Wisneski JA, Gertz EW, Wexman M, Axelrod R, Langberg JJ. Potentiation by nifedipine and diltiazem of the hypotensive response after contrast angiography. *J Am Coll Cardiol* (1985) 6, 785–91.
2. Higgins CB, Kuber M, Slutsky RA. Interaction between verapamil and contrast media in coronary arteriography: comparison of standard ionic and new nonionic media. *Circulation* (1983) 68, 628–35.
3. Duncan JS, Ramsay LE. Ventricular tachycardia precipitated by sodium iothalamate (Conray 420) injection during prenylamine treatment: a predictable adverse drug interaction. *Postgrad Med J* (1985) 61, 415–17.

Lercanidipine + Miscellaneous drugs

The use of lercanidipine is contraindicated with ciclosporin and grapefruit juice. Lercanidipine raises the serum levels of digoxin and so increased monitoring is recommended. Metoprolol increases lercanidipine bioavailability and dose adjustments may be needed if it is used with beta-blockers. Midazolam also increases lercanidipine bioavailability, but the clinical significance of this is unclear. Ketoconazole greatly increases lercanidipine levels and so the makers predict it will also interact with amiodarone, astemizole, carbamazepine, class III antiarrhythmics, erythromycin, itraconazole, phenytoin, quinidine, rifampicin (rifampin), ritonavir, terfenadine, and troleandomycin. No interactions have been seen with lercanidipine and ACE inhibitors, cimetidine, diuretics, fluoxetine, simvastatin or warfarin.

Clinical evidence, mechanism, importance and management

(a) Antihypertensives

Lercanidipine is said to be safe with **ACE inhibitors** and **diuretics**.[1] **Metoprolol** has been shown to reduce the bioavailability of lerca-

nidipine by 50%, probably due to alterations in hepatic blood flow. The makers therefore say that concurrent use of lercanidipine and **beta-blockers** is safe, but dosage adjustments may be required.[1]

(b) Ciclosporin

The makers contraindicate the concurrent use of **ciclosporin** and lercanidipine as the plasma levels of lercanidipine were raised threefold by **ciclosporin**, and the **ciclosporin** AUC was raised by 21% by lercanidipine.[1]

(c) Cimetidine

No pharmacokinetic interaction occurs with 800 mg **cimetidine** daily,[2] but "... at higher doses caution is required since the bioavailability and the hypotensive effect of lercanidipine may be increased."[1] Whether any such increased hypotensive effects would be problematical or useful would appear to be depend on the circumstances.

(d) Digoxin

The maximum serum levels of **digoxin** rose by 33% in healthy subjects also given lercanidipine. If both drugs are used close monitoring of **digoxin** levels is advised.[1]

(e) Drugs affecting cytochrome P450 isoenzyme CYP3A4

The cytochrome P450 isoenzyme CYP3A4 is largely responsible for the metabolism of lercanidipine for which reason the makers suggest other substrates of CYP3A4 such as **terfenadine**, **astemizole**, **class III antiarrhythmics** such as **amiodarone**, and **quinidine**. **Ketoconazole** has been shown to increase the AUC of lercanidipine 15-fold. Therefore the makers suggest avoiding concurrent use with potent inhibitors of CYP3A4 such as **ketoconazole**, **itraconazole**, **ritonavir**, **erythromycin** and **troleandomycin**.[1] Similarly, they suggest caution with potent inducers of CYP3A4 such as **carbamazepine**, **phenytoin** and **rifampicin (rifampin)**.

(f) Midazolam

Midazolam appears to increase the absorption of lercanidipine by 40%. The clinical relevance of this interaction is as yet unclear.[1]

(g) Grapefruit juice

The makers point out that **grapefruit juice** can raise the serum levels of dihydropyridine calcium channel blockers, although this is normally of little clinical relevance with most other calcium channel blockers. Nevertheless grapefruit juice is a makers' contraindication.[1]

(h) Miscellaneous drugs

Studies of the concurrent use of **fluoxetine**, **simvastatin** or **warfarin** with lercanidipine have shown no clinically significant interaction. No special precautions would therefore seem necessary on concurrent use.

1. Zanidip (Lercanidipine). Napp Pharmaceuticals Limited. Summary of Product Characteristics, March 2001.
2. Barchielli M, Dolfini E, Farina P, Leoni B, Targa G, Vinaccia V, Tajana A. Clinical pharmacokinetics of lercanidipine. *J Cardiovasc Pharmacol* (1997) 29 (Suppl 2), S1–15.

Prenylamine + Miscellaneous drugs

The concurrent use of prenylamine and other drugs with negative inotropic effects such as beta-blockers and quinidine, procainamide, amiodarone or lidocaine (lignocaine) should be avoided because of the risk of the development of torsade de pointes.

Clinical evidence, mechanism, importance and management

The makers of **prenylamine** say that **prenylamine** should not be given with negative inotropic drugs such as **beta-blockers**, **quinidine**, **procainamide**, **amiodarone** or **lidocaine (lignocaine)** because there is the risk of the development of torsade de pointes associated with a prolongation of the QT interval. Other risk factors are **hypokalaemia**[1] and conduction disorders.[1] The recommendation is based on reports of atypical ventricular tachycardia (AVT or torsade de pointes) occurring in patients taking **prenylamine** and **propranolol**,[2,3] **sotalol**[4] and other **beta-blockers** or quinidine-like compounds such as **lidocaine**.[5,6] The extent of the risk seems not to have been measured but there is evidence that some of these drugs (**propranolol, acebutolol, atenolol, oxprenolol, sotalol**) have been used concurrently without problems although the QT interval was observed to be prolonged.[7] See also 'Drugs that prolong the QT interval + Other drugs that prolong the QT interval', p.103.

1. Warembourg H, Pauchant M, Ducloux G, Delbecque M, Vermeersch M, Tonnel-Levy M. Les torsades de pointe: a propos de 30 observations. *Lille Med* (1974) 19, 1–11.

2. Evans TR, Krikler DM. Drug-aggravated sinoatrial block. *Proc R Soc Med* (1975) 68, 808–9.

3. Puritz R, Henderson MA, Baker SN, Chamberlain DA. Ventricular arrhythmias caused by prenylamine. *BMJ* (1977) 2, 608–9.

4. Kontopoulos A, Filindris A, Manoudis F, Metaxas P. Sotalol-induced torsades de pointes. *Postgrad Med J* (1981) 57, 321–3.

5. Grenadier E, Alpan G, Keidar S, Palant A. Atrio-ventricular block after administration of lignocaine in patients treated with prenylamine. *Postgrad Med J* (1982) 58, 175–7.

6. Cantle J (Hoechst UK Ltd). Personal communication (1981).

7. Oakley D, Jennings K, Puritz R, Krikler D, Chamberlain D. The effect of prenylamine on the QT interval of the resting electrocardiogram in patients with angina pectoris. *Postgrad Med J* (1980) 56, 753–6.

12

Oral contraceptives and related sex hormone drug interactions

The oral contraceptives are of two main types: (i) the combined oestrogen-progestogen fixed-dose preparations, and the combined sequential preparations with the doses of each steroid varied throughout the cycle; (ii) the progestogen-only preparations or 'mini-pills'.

The oestrogens commonly used are ethinylestradiol (ethinyloestradiol) in doses of 20–50 micrograms, or mestranol in doses of 50–100 micrograms. The progestogens are either those derived from 19-norethisterone (e.g. norethynodrel, ethynodiol acetate, norgestrel, norethisterone, lynestranol (lynoestrenol)) or more uncommonly from 17 alpha-hydroxyprogesterone (e.g. megestrol) in doses ranging from about 0.25–5.0 mg. There are now very many different oral contraceptive preparations available throughout the world but most seem to be variants on these two broad themes.

The **combined and sequential preparations** are taken for 20–21 days, followed by a period of seven days during which withdrawal bleeding occurs. Some of them include six or seven tablets of lactose to be taken at this time so that the daily habit of taking a tablet is not broken. These contraceptives act in several ways: the oestrogenic component suppresses ovulation while the progestogen acts to change the endometrial structure so that even if conception were to occur, implantation would be unlikely. In addition the cervical mucus becomes unusually viscous which inhibits the free movement of the sperm.

The **progestogen-only** or '**mini-pills**' are taken continuously. They do not inhibit ovulation but probably act by increasing the viscosity of the cervical mucus so that movement of the sperm is retarded. They may also cause changes in the endometrium which inhibit successful implantation. **Contraceptive implants** are capsules which are placed under the skin and which slowly release the progestogen over a period of time, up to five years. Their actions are essentially the same as the mini-pills.

Almost all of the interactions described here in this chapter and elsewhere in this book involve the combined oral contraceptives. There is very little direct information about the interactions with the progestogen-only contraceptives or contraceptive implants so that it is unwise uncritically to assume that interactions known to occur with the former type of contraceptive also occur with the latter two types. However, it seems probable that an increased risk of failure with the progestogen-only contraceptives and contraceptive implants is likely with drugs which cause enzyme induction (e.g. phenytoin, phenobarbital (phenobarbitone), primidone, carbamazepine, rifampicin and possibly griseofulvin) which results in an increased clearance of the progestogen, with an accompanying loss of efficacy. However, much more study is needed to define the situation more clearly.

It is also not known whether interacting drugs are likely to affect the so-called **postcoital contraceptives** such as *Schering's PC4* (four tablets of 50 micrograms ethinyloestradiol + 250 micrograms levonorgestrel) although some practitioners have suggested that women taking enzyme inducers (e.g. many anticonvulsants, rifampicin) should be given a double dosage to accommodate the increased rate of metabolism by the liver. Whether this is in fact necessary or desirable is not yet known.

The preparations used for **Hormone replacement therapy (HRT)** are similar to the oral contraceptives in that they contain oestrogens alone or combined with progestogens. There are only a few reports of interactions with HRT preparations, but generally speaking they are expected to behave very much like the combined oral contraceptives.

Dianette contains cyproterone acetate and ethinylestradiol and is intended for use in women with androgen-dependent skin conditions, but it also acts as an oral contraceptive and is therefore predicted to interact like conventional oestrogen-containing oral contraceptives.

Cyproterone/Ethinylestradiol (Ethinyloestradiol) + Miscellaneous drugs

Cyproterone/Ethinylestradiol (ethinyloestrodiol) (Dianette) is expected to interact like the combined oral contraceptives with anticonvulsants and antibacterials so that the risk of contraceptive failure is increased. It also appears to interact with minocycline to increase facial pigmentation.

Clinical evidence, mechanism, importance and management

Dianette contains the anti-androgen **cyproterone acetate** (2 mg) and **ethinylestradiol (ethinyloestradiol)** (35 micrograms) and is primarily intended for the treatment of acne and moderately severe hirsutism in women, but it also acts as an oral contraceptive. It is therefore expected to interact with **antibacterials**, **antifungals** and **anticonvulsant enzyme inducers** just like the conventional combined oral contraceptives[1] so that the precautions described in this chapter for the oral contraceptives should be followed – although in fact there appear so far to be no confirmatory reports of any adverse interactions involving *Dianette*.[2] In addition *Dianette* may also possibly interact with **minocycline** to accentuate facial pigmentation (see 'Minocycline + Ethinylestradiol', p.175) which the makers say can be exacerbated by sunlight. The makers also point out that **combined oral contraceptives** must not be taken with *Dianette*.[1]

1. Dianette (cyproterone/ethinylestradiol), Schering Health Care. Summary of product characteristics, May 2000.
2. Schering Health Care. Personal Communication, June 1997.

Ethinylestradiol (Ethinyloestradiol) + Grapefruit juice

The bioavailability of ethinylestradiol (ethinyloestradiol) is increased by grapefruit juice, but this is unlikely to be clinically important.

Clinical evidence, mechanism, importance and management

A comparative study in a group of healthy young women found that the AUC and the maximum serum concentrations following a single 50-micrograms dose of ethinylestradiol (ethinyloestradiol) were raised 28% and 37% respectively when taken with 200 ml of **grapefruit juice**, compared with those when taken with 200 ml of **herb tea**. The subjects continued to take these drinks at 3 hour intervals for 12 h after taking the ethinylestradiol. It is thought that this increase in bioavailability is possibly due to the presence of **naringenin**, a plant flavonoid in the **grapefruit juice**, which inhibits some of the metabolism of the ethinylestradiol (mediated by cytochrome P450 enzymes) in the gut wall and liver.[1]

Grapefruit juice is commonly taken at breakfast time when drugs (the pill for instance) are also commonly taken, but it seems unlikely that this interaction is of practical importance because the increased bioavailability is still less than the extent of known variability between individuals.

1. Balogh A, Weber A, Klinger G. Can grapefruit juice influence the bioavailability of ethinyloestradiol? *Eur J Clin Pharmacol* (1994) 47, A93.

Gestrinone + Miscellaneous drugs

The makers say that gestrinone should not be used with oral contraceptives and that rifampicin and antiepileptic drugs may reduce its effects. An isolated report describes bleeding in a woman on warfarin given gestrinone.

Clinical evidence, mechanism, importance and management

Although gestrinone can inhibit ovulation, it is not sufficiently reliable to be used as a contraceptive. The makers strongly emphasise the importance of using a barrier method instead of **oral contraception** while on gestrinone because they say that not only are the effects of gestrinone possibly modified by **oral contraceptives**, but its use in pregnancy is totally contraindicated.[1]

The makers also suggest that **rifampicin** and **anticonvulsants** (not named, but by implication **phenytoin**, **phenobarbital (phenobarbitone)**, **primidone** and **carbamazepine**) can accelerate the metabolism of gestrinone thereby reducing its effects,[1] but so far there appear to be no reports that this actually occurs.[2] An isolated report briefly describes an increased INR with vaginal bleeding and multiple bruising in a woman on **warfarin** and gestrinone.[3] Good monitoring is advisable if any of these drugs is given concurrently, with dosage adjustments where it becomes clearly necessary.

1. Dimetriose (gestrinone). Florizel Ltd. Datasheet, May 1997.
2. Roberts G (Roussel Labs). Personal Communication 1992.
3. Beeley L, Cunningham H, Carmichael A, Brennan A. Bulletin of the West Midlands Centre for Adverse Drug Reporting (1992) 35, 13.

Intrauterine Contraceptive Devices (IUDs) + Anti-inflammatory agents

There is some evidence that the very occasional failure of an IUD to prevent pregnancy may have been due to the concurrent use of a steroidal or non-steroidal anti-inflammatory agent.

Clinical evidence, mechanism, importance and management

Two women out of a total of about 1000 fitted with *Multiload 250* (an IUD) became pregnant. One had taken **aspirin**, and the other **mefenamic acid** during the month when conception occurred. Another woman using a *Lippes C* conceived during the month when she took *Veganin* (**aspirin**, **codeine**, **paracetamol**).[1] Four women have been described who, despite being fitted with IUDs, became pregnant. Two were taking **corticosteroids** regularly and the other two often took **aspirin** for migraine.[2,3] A case-control study of 717 women who became pregnant while using IUDs suggested that **NSAIDs**, particularly **aspirin**, might have been responsible for the failures.[3] Unwanted pregnancies have also been reported elsewhere in women with IUDs treated with **corticosteroids**.[4,5]

The evidence for this possible interaction is very slim and inconclusive, but the suggestion that drugs which affect prostaglandins might possibly affect the actions of the IUDs bears further investigation.

1. Dossetor J. Personal communication (1983).
2. Buhler M, Papiernik E. Successive pregnancies in women fitted with intrauterine devices who take anti-inflammatory drugs. *Lancet* (1983) 1, 483.
3. Papiernik R, Rozenbaum H, Amblard P, Dephot N, de Mouzon J. Intra-uterine device failure: relation with drug use. *Eur J Obstet Gynecol Reprod Biol* (1989) 32, 205–12.
4. Inkeles DM, Hansen RI. Unexpected pregnancy in a woman using an intrauterine device and receiving steroid therapy. *Ann Ophthalmol* (1982) 14, 975.
5. Zerner J, Miller AB, Festino MJ. Failure of an intrauterine device concurrent with administration of corticosteroids. *Fertil Steril* (1976) 27, 1467–8.

Medroxyprogesterone or Megestrol + Aminoglutethimide

Aminoglutethimide markedly reduces the serum levels of medroxyprogesterone and megestrol. The dosage may need to be doubled to accommodate this interaction.

Clinical evidence

(a) Medroxyprogesterone

The concurrent use of **aminoglutethimide** (500–1000 mg daily) halved the plasma levels of the **medroxyprogesterone** (1500 mg daily) in 6 postmenopausal women with breast cancer.[1]

Another study in 6 postmenopausal women found that 1000 mg **aminoglutethimide** daily reduced **medroxyprogesterone** levels by 63% (from 70 to 26 ng/ml).[2] In another study on 6 women with advanced breast cancer, it was found that as the dosage of **aminoglutethimide** was gradually reduced and finally withdrawn, so the serum levels of **medroxyprogesterone** steadily climbed, although the dose remained constant.[3]

(b) Megestrol

1000 mg **aminoglutethimide** daily reduced serum **megestrol** levels in 6 postmenopausal women by 78% (from 177 to 38 ng/ml).[2]

Mechanism

The most likely reason is that the aminoglutethimide acts as an enzyme inducing agent, increasing the metabolism of the progestogens, thereby increasing their loss from the body.

Importance and management

Both interactions appear to be established and of clinical importance. A 50% reduction in the serum levels of medroxyprogesterone and megestrol should be expected during concurrent use. The authors of one report[3] say that to achieve adequate serum medroxyprogesterone acetate levels (>100 ng/ml) a daily dose of 800 mg is necessary in the presence of 125 or 250 mg aminoglutethimide twice daily. This is double the usual recommended dose of 400 mg daily.

1. Van Deijk WA, Blijham GH, Mellink WAM, Meulenberg PMM. Influence of aminoglutethimide on plasma levels of medroxyprogesterone acetate: its correlation with serum cortisol. *Cancer Treat Rep* (1985) 69, 85–90.
2. Lundgren S, Lønning PE, Aakvaag A, Kvinnsland S. Influence of aminoglutethimide on the metabolism of medroxyprogesterone acetate and megestrol acetate in postmenopausal patients with advanced breast cancer. *Cancer Chemother Pharmacol* (1990) 27, 101–5.
3. Halpenny O, Bye A, Cranny A, Feely J, Daly PA. Influence of aminoglutethimide on plasma levels of medroxyprogesterone acetate. *Med Oncol Tumor Pharmacother* (1990) 7, 241–7.

Medroxyprogesterone acetate or Megestrol + Miscellaneous drugs

High dose medroxyprogesterone acetate and megestrol do not appear to interact to a clinically relevant extent with digitoxin and antipyrine, but the half-life of warfarin is prolonged.

Clinical evidence, mechanism, importance and management

The influence of two progestogens on the pharmacokinetics of three drugs were tested on 14 patients with advanced breast cancer (13 women, one man). Single 1 g doses of **antipyrine (phenazone)** were given to 9 patients before and after five weeks' treatment with oral **medroxyprogesterone acetate** (500 mg twice daily) or **megestrol** (160 mg daily). Single 0.3 mg/kg doses of **warfarin** were similarly given to 4 patients, and the steady-state levels of **digitoxin** over three days were measured in three patients similarly treated with these progestogens over five weeks. Only small and clinically irrele-

vant effects were seen when using **antipyrine** or **digitoxin**, but the half-life of **warfarin** was increased by 71%[1] so that it might be prudent to monitor prothrombin times in patients on **warfarin** given high doses of these progestogens, being alert for any increased **warfarin** effects.

1. Lundgren S, Kvinnsland S, Utaaker E, Bakke O, Ueland PM. Effect of oral high-dose progestins on the disposition of antipyrine, digitoxin, and warfarin in advanced breast cancer. *Cancer Chemother Pharmacol* (1986) 18, 270–5.

Oestrogens (Estrogens) or Oral contraceptives + Phenothiazines

Oestrogens can increase the serum levels of butaperazine. A single report describes a very marked rise in serum chlorpromazine levels in a woman on an oral contraceptive.

Clinical evidence, mechanism, importance and management

When a severe dystonic reaction to a single dose of **prochlorperazine** was seen in a pregnant woman (presumed to be due to increased serum **butaperazine** levels resulting from the high oestrogen levels), a further study was undertaken in four postmenopausal schizophrenic women. While taking 1.25 mg **conjugated oestrogens** (*Premarin*) daily, their serum **butaperazine** levels after two 40-mg doses daily were increased by 48% (from 231 to 343 ng/ml) and the AUC was increased by 92%.[1] Another woman showed an 18-fold rise in serum **chlorpromazine** levels while taking an **oral contraceptive**.[2] The reasons are not understood but increased absorption or reduced liver metabolism are suggested.[1] The general clinical importance of these findings is not known. There seem to be no other reports of adverse reactions but it would be prudent to monitor concurrent use. There seems to be no information about other **phenothiazines** or the effects of the **oestrogens** contained in **oral contraceptives**.

1. El-Yousef MK, Manier DH. Estrogen effects on phenothiazine derivative blood levels. *JAMA* (1974) 228, 827–8.
2. Chetty M, Miller R, Moodley SV. Smoking and body weight influence the clearance of chlorpromazine. *Eur J Clin Pharmacol* (1994) 46, 523–6.

Oral contraceptives + Alcohol

The detrimental effects of alcohol may be reduced to some extent in women on oral contraceptives, but blood alcohol levels are possibly unaltered. Alcohol markedly increases the levels of circulating estradiol (oestradiol) in women using hormone replacement therapy.

Clinical evidence mechanism, importance and management

(a) Effect of contraceptives on alcohol

A controlled study in 54 women showed that those on oral contraceptives (30, 35 or 50 micrograms **oestrogen**) tolerated the effects of **alcohol** better than those not taking oral contraceptives (as measured by a reaction-time test and a bead-threading test), but their blood-alcohol levels and its rate of clearance were unchanged.[1] Two other studies suggest that blood **alcohol** levels may be reduced in those taking oral contraceptives.[2,3] The authors of the report cited[1] say that they do not recommend women on oral contraceptives to drink more than usual. No special precautions would seem to be necessary.

(b) Effect of alcohol on oestrogen/progestogens

Twelve healthy postmenopausal women on hormone replacement therapy (**estradiol (oestradiol)**) 1 mg and **medroxyprogesterone acetate** 10 mg daily) were given alcoholic drinks (0.7 g/kg bodyweight) to achieve mean peak alcohol serum levels of 21 mmol/l after about 1 h. It was found that their circulating **estradiol** levels rose threefold and were significantly above the baseline for 5 h. No significant increases in circulating estrone levels were seen.[4] The reasons for these changes are not understood, nor is it known whether they are important or not. More study is needed. No special precautions appear to be necessary at this time.

1. Hobbes J, Boutagy J, Shenfield GM. Interactions between ethanol and oral contraceptive steroids. *Clin Pharmacol Ther* (1985) 38, 371–80.
2. Jones MK, Jones BM. Ethanol metabolism in women taking oral contraceptives. *Alcohol Clin Exp Res* (1984) 8, 24–8.
3. Zeiner AR, Kegg PS. Effects of sex steroids on ethanol pharmacokinetics and autonomic reactivity. *Prog Biochem Pharmacol* (1981) 18, 130–42.
4. Ginsburg ES, Mello NK, Mendelson JH, Barbieri RL, Teoh SK, Rothman M, Gao X, Sholar JW. Effects of alcohol ingestion on estrogens in postmenopausal women. *JAMA* (1996) 276, 1747–51.

Oral contraceptives + Antacids

Despite *in vitro* evidence that magnesium trisilicate might possibly reduce the effects and the reliability of the oral contraceptives, other evidence from human studies suggests that concurrent use is safe.

Clinical evidence, mechanism, importance and management

Although *in vitro* studies[1] have clearly shown that 0.5 and 1.0% suspensions of magnesium trisilicate in water adsorb 50–90% of ethisterone, mestranol and norethisterone, a single-dose study[2] in 12 women given a single pill (30 micrograms ethinylestradiol (ethinyloestradiol) and either norethisterone acetate 1 mg or levonorgestrel 150 micrograms) with a single tablet containing magnesium trisilicate (0.5 g) and aluminium hydroxide (0.25 g), showed that the bioavailability of the contraceptive remained unchanged. This is in line with common experience. Nor does there appear to be an important interaction with any other antacid or adsorbent. No special precautions seem to be necessary.

1. Khalil SAH, Iwuagwu M. The in vitro uptake of some oral contraceptive steroids by magnesium trisilicate. *J Pharm Pharmacol* (1976) 28 (Suppl), 47P.
2. Joshi JV, Sankolli GM, Shah RS, Joshi UM. Antacid does not reduce the bioavailability of oral contraceptive steroids in women. *Int J Clin Pharmacol Ther Toxicol* (1986) 24, 192–5.

Oral contraceptives + Antiasthmatics

No recorded interactions, but asthma is included by some manufacturers of oral contraceptives among their 'special precautions' because the asthmatic condition may be worsened. Sometimes it may be improved.

Clinical evidence, mechanism, importance and management

There have been instances in which women have developed allergic conditions such as rhinitis, atopic eczema, urticaria or asthma while taking oral contraceptives.[1-3] In contrast there are other instances where pre-existing asthma and other allergic conditions have improved.[2] For this reason it has been claimed[1] that " . . . it is always worth while giving an oral contraceptive a trial for patients with any of these complaints [eczema, asthma, vasomotor rhinitis, migraine] as there is an even chance that she will be improved; if the condition is aggravated, it will return to its previous state as soon as the medication is stopped."

1. Mears E. Oral contraceptives. *Lancet* (1964) i, 981.
2. Falliers CJ. Oral contraceptives and allergy. *Lancet* (1974) ii, 515.
3. Horan JD, Lederman JJ. Possible asthmogenic effect of oral contraceptives. *Can Med Assoc J* (1968) 99, 130.

Oral contraceptives + Antibacterials and Anti-infectives

Failure of combined oral contraceptives to prevent pregnancy has been attributed to the concurrent use of a tetracycline (doxycycline, lymecycline, oxytetracycline, minocycline, tetracycline) in over 30 cases. One or two cases of failure have been reported with each of the following: chloramphenicol, cefalexin (cephalexin), cefalexin (cephalexin) with clindamycin, dapsone, erythromycin, isoniazid, spiramycin, sulfametoxypyridazine (sulphamethoxypyridazine), sulphonamides, trimethoprim and metronidazole. The risk of contraceptive failure due to these antibacterials appears to be very low indeed.

Clinical evidence

(a) Chloramphenicol, cefalexin (cephalexin)/clindamycin, dapsone, erythromycin, isoniazid, para-aminosalicylic acid, spiramycin, streptomycin, sulphonamides and trimethoprim

Two women on combined oral contraceptives are briefly reported to have shown break-through bleeding and to have become pregnant. One was taking chloramphenicol and the other sulfametoxypyridazine (sulphamethoxypyridazine).[14,15] One or two cases of failure have been attributed to concurrent treatment with each of the following: chloramphenicol, cefalexin, cefalexin/clindamycin, dapsone, erythromycin, isoniazid, spiramycin, sulfafurazole (sulphafurazole, sulfisoxazole), sulphonamides, and trimethoprim.[3,4,8,9,16] Break-through bleeding due to erythromycin, clindamycin and chloramphenicol has also been described.[13] The CSM also has on record five cases implicating co-trimoxazole in contraceptive failure (see 'Oral contraceptives + Co-trimoxazole or Trimethoprim', p.473). No evidence of ovulation or of changes in serum contraceptive steroid levels was seen in a study of 8 women treated with triple antitubercular therapy (para-aminosalicylic acid, isoniazid, streptomycin).[17]

Intravenous ^{14}C-N-methyl erythromycin was given to 6 postmenopausal women before and after two months' treatment with progesterone (5 mg). The pharmacokinetics of the erythromycin were not significantly changed.[18]

(b) Metronidazole

Three out of 25 women on combined oral contraceptives ovulated while taking metronidazole, but no cases of pregnancy were reported.[19] Pregnancy occurred in another woman on metronidazole, but she was also taking doxycycline.[5] Another study found no evidence that metronidazole affected the reliability of the combined oral contraceptives,[20] yet the CSM has 3 cases of pregnancy on their records attributed to an interaction with metronidazole.[4] Another occurs in a further report.[8]

(c) Tetracyclines

A woman on *Microgynon 30* (ethinylestradiol (ethinyloestradiol) + levonorgestrel) became pregnant, the evidence indicating that she had conceived while taking a course of tetracycline (500 mg six-hourly for three days and then 250 mg six-hourly for two days) or in the week following. There was no evidence of either nausea or vomiting which might have been an alternative explanation for the contraceptive failure.[1] A case of break-through bleeding and another pregnancy attributed to the concurrent use of tetracycline are also described in this report.[1,2]

The Committee on Safety of Medicines (CSM) in the UK has reports of 12 cases of combined oral contraceptive failure with tetracyclines (tetracycline, oxytetracycline).[3,4] Another survey describes six failures due to doxycycline, lymecycline or minocycline,[5] and a further three cases involving tetracycline are described elsewhere.[6,7] Three others describe four failures with tetracycline.[8-10] Further reports describe other failures attributed to oxytetracycline or minocycline,[7,11,12] and intermenstrual bleeding due to doxycycline or oxytetracycline.[13] See also 'Minocycline + Ethinylestradiol', p.175

for reports of facial pigmentation due to **minocycline** and **ethinylestradiol**.

These cases need to be set in the broader context of a study in three dermatological practices, over the period 1990–5, of 356 patients who had had oral contraceptives and antibacterials (said to be **cephalosporins, penicillins, tetracyclines**). In statistical terms the failure rate (3 pregnancies occurred in women on **minocycline** and two on a **cephalosporin**) was indistinguishable from the general oral contraceptive failure rate seen in 263 control patients.[7]

Mechanism

Not understood. Suppression of intestinal bacteria which results in a fall in contraceptive serum levels is one suggested explanation (see 'Mechanism' in the monograph dealing with 'Oral contraceptives + Penicillins', p.477), but two studies failed to find evidence that this actually occurs.[21,22]

Importance and management

The oral contraceptive/antibacterial–antiinfective interactions summarised here cannot be said to be adequately established and the whole issue remains very controversial. Bearing in mind the extremely wide use of both drugs, the incidence of contraceptive failure is clearly very low indeed. Much of the evidence is anecdotal with insufficient controls (if any), and in statistical terms one study indicated that the incidence of contraceptive failure due to this interaction could not be distinguished from the general and recognised failure rate of oral contraceptives,[7] although another suggested that the risk is increased sixfold.[11] Even so most women do not appear to be at risk.

On the other hand, the personal and ethical consequences of an unwanted pregnancy can be very serious, and for this reason the generally accepted current wisdom is that for maximal protection a second form of contraception (a barrier method) should be used routinely while taking a short course of an antibacterial like these and for at least 7 days afterwards. The Family Planning Association (FPA) in the UK recommends that, when using a penicillin, if the seven days run beyond the end of a packet, the new packet should be started without a break, omitting any of the inactive tablets. The same precautions would seem to be appropriate for these other antibacterials too. The FPA also say that those on long-term antibacterials (for example for acne) need only take extra precautions for the first two weeks because, after that, the gut flora becomes resistant to the antibacterial, but this was not seemingly borne out in the case of four women on oral contraceptives and minocycline[7,13] and in another on tetracycline[10] who became pregnant, although whether these failures were in fact due to interactions will never be known.

It is believed that the broad-spectrum antibacterials do not affect the reliability of the **progestogen-only contraceptives**,[23] and no interaction would be expected with **contraceptive implants**.

1. Bacon JF, Shenfield GM. Pregnancy attributable to interaction between tetracycline and oral contraceptives. *BMJ* (1980) 1, 293.
2. Lequeux A. Grossesse sous contraceptif oral après prise de tétracycline. *Louvain Med* (1980) 99, 413–4.
3. Back DJ, Breckenridge AM, Crawford FE, MacIver M, Orme ML'E, Rowe PH. Interindividual variation and drug interactions with hormonal steroid contraceptives. *Drugs* (1981) 21, 46–61.
4. Back DJ, Grimmer FM, Orme ML'E, Proudlove C, Mann RD, Breckenridge AM. Evaluation of Committee on Safety of Medicines yellow card reports on oral contraceptive-drug interactions with anticonvulsants and antibiotics. *Br J Clin Pharmacol* (1988) 25, 527–32.
5. Sparrow MJ. Pill method failures. *N Z Med J* (1987) 100, 102–5.
6. Sparrow MJ. Pregnancies in reliable pill takers. *N Z Med J* (1989) 102, 575–7.
7. Helms SE, Bredle DL, Zajic J, Jarjoura D, Brodell RT, Krishnarao I. Oral contraceptive failure rates and oral antibiotics. *J Am Acad Dermatol* (1997) 36, 705–10.
8. Kovacs GT, Riddoch G, Duncombe P, Welberry L, Chick P, Weisberg E, Leavesley GM, Baker HWG. Inadvertent pregnancies in oral contraceptive users. *Med J Aust* (1989) 150, 549–51.
9. DeSano EA, Hurley SC. Possible interactions of antihistamines and antibiotics with oral contraceptive effectiveness. *Fertil Steril* (1982) 37, 853–4.
10. London BM, Lookingbill DP. Frequency of pregnancy in acne patients taking oral antibiotics and oral contraceptives. *Arch Dermatol* (1994) 130, 392–3.
11. Hughes BR, Cunliffe WJ. Interactions between the oral contraceptive pill and antibiotics. *Br J Dermatol* (1990) 122, 717–18.
12. De Groot AC, Eshuis H, Stricker BHC. Ineffectiviteit van orale anticonceptie tijdens gebruik van minocycline. *Ned Tijdschr Geneeskd* (1990) 134, 1227–9.
13. Hetényi G. Possible interactions between antibiotics and oral contraceptives. *Ther Hung* (1989) 37, 86–9.
14. Von Hempel E, Böhm W, Carol W, Klinger G. Medikamentöse enzyminduktion und hormonal kontrazeption. *Zentralbl Gynakol* (1973) 95, 1451–7.
15. Hempel E. Personal communication (1975).
16. Pedretti E, Brunenghi GM, Morali GC. Interazione tra antibiotici e contraccettivi orali: la spiramicina. *Quad Clin Obstet Ginecol* (1991) 46, 153–4.
17. Joshi JV, Joshi UM, Sankolli GM, Gupta K, Rao AP, Hazari K, Sheth UK, Saxena BN. A study of interaction of a low-dose combination oral contraceptive with anti-tubercular drugs. *Contraception* (1980) 21, 617–29.
18. Tsunoda SM, Harris RZ, Mroczkowski PJ, Hebert MF, Benet LZ. Oral progesterone therapy does not affect the pharmacokinetics of prednisolone and erythromycin in postmenopausal women. *Clin Pharmacol Ther* (1995) 57, 182.
19. Joshi JV, Gupta KC, Joshi UM, Krishna U, Saxena BN. Interactions of oral contraceptives with other drugs and nutrition. *Contracept Delivery Syst* (1982) 3, 60.
20. Viswanathan MK, Govindarajulu P. Metronidazole therapy on the efficacy of oral contraceptive steroid pills. *J Reprod Biol Comp Endocrinol* (1985) 5, 69–72.
21. Murphy AA, Zacur HA, Charache P, Burkman RT. The effect of tetracycline on levels of oral contraceptives. *Am J Obstet Gynecol* (1991) 164, 28–33.
22. Neely JL, Abate M, Swinker M, D'Angio R. The effect of doxycycline on serum levels of ethinyl estradiol, norethindrone, and endogenous progesterone. *Obstet Gynecol* (1991) 77, 416–20.
23. McCann MF, Potter LS. Progestin-only contraception: a comprehensive review. *Contraception* (1994) 50, S1–S198.

Oral and implant contraceptives, and HRT preparations + Anticonvulsants

Oral contraceptives are unreliable during treatment with barbiturates, carbamazepine, oxcarbazepine, phenobarbital (phenobarbitone), phenytoin or primidone. Intermediate break-through bleeding and spotting can take place and pregnancies have occurred. The failure of contraceptive implants has also been reported, and, on theoretical grounds, the effectiveness of HRT preparations may be reduced. Seizure control may sometimes be disturbed. Gabapentin, lamotrigine, sodium valproate, tiagabine and vigabatrin appear not to interact.

Clinical evidence

(a) Contraceptive failure

An epileptic woman on 200 mg **phenytoin** and 50 mg **sulthiame** daily (with ferrous gluconate and folic acid) became pregnant despite the regular use of an oral contraceptive containing 0.05 mg **ethinylestradiol (ethinyloestradiol)** and 3 mg **norethisterone acetate**.[1]

Since this first report[1] in 1972, at least 29 pregnancies have been reported in the literature in epileptic women taking a range of oral contraceptives and anticonvulsants which have included either a **barbiturate** (such as **phenobarbital**), **phenytoin** or **primidone**.[2-13] **Carbamazepine** has also been clearly implicated[10,11,14-17] and possibly **ethosuximide**.[15] In addition the Committee on Safety of Medicines in the UK has received another 43 reports[15,18] in women taking antiepileptic drugs making a total of more than 70 cases in the 1968 to 1992 period. A further 5 cases over a 2-year period were reported from one major US hospital centre.[19] The precise numbers reported world-wide are difficult to confirm because some of the cases may have been reported more than once, even so the total number of unwanted pregnancies due to this interaction is very large. It is also reported that **subdermal contraceptive implants** containing **levonorgestrel** (*Norplant*) failed to prevent pregnancy in 3 women taking **phenytoin**.[20,21] and in one woman taking **phenobarbital**.[13] There is good clinical evidence (steroid levels reduced about 50% and an increased incidence of break-through bleeding) that **oxcarbazepine** may interact similarly but so far no cases of pregnancy have been reported.[22-24] In addition to these interactions, a report describes a menopausal woman on replacement treatment with **conjugated oestrogens** (*Premarin*), 1.25 mg daily, which became inadequate when she began to take 300 mg **phenytoin** daily.[25]

(b) Disturbance of seizure control

Epilepsy is included by most oral contraceptive manufacturers among the 'special precautions' to be observed because seizure control may sometimes be made worse, but it also may remain unaltered or even improve. For example, an epileptic woman under treatment with **phenytoin** and **phenobarbital (phenobarbitone)** became much worse while taking *Lyndiol* but improved when *Gynovlar* and later *Ovulen* were substituted.[26] Another report[27] describes 20 epileptics on a variety of anticonvulsants whose condition was unaltered by

Norinyl-1. A woman on **phenytoin** and **phenobarbital** was completely fit-free until she discontinued the oral contraceptive (unnamed) she had been taking.[28]

Mechanism

The likeliest explanation for the unreliability and failure of oral contraceptives is that the interacting anticonvulsants act as potent liver enzyme inducing agents which increase the metabolism and clearance of the contraceptive steroids from the body, thereby reducing their effects, and in some instances allowing ovulation to occur. A study using single doses of *Eugynon 50* in epileptic patients found that phenytoin (200–300 mg daily) or carbamazepine (300–600 mg daily) almost halved the AUC of the ethinylestradiol and levonorgestrel components.[29,30] Changes in seizure control have been attributed to changes in fluid retention which can influence seizure frequency.[26,27]

Importance and management

These are clinically important and well documented interactions. Partial or complete failure of combined oral contraceptives in the presence of **carbamazepine**, **phenobarbital (phenobarbitone)**, **phenytoin** and **primidone** is well established. It also seems likely with **oxcarbazepine**,[24] but it is uncertain with whether **ethosuximide** and **felbamate** interact (see Index). The incidence is unknown. It may be that the incidence of total failure is quite small (a failure-rate of 3.1 per 100 woman years has been reported[31]). On the other hand the incidence of spotting and break-through bleeding is high.[32-34] One study reported it in seven out of eleven patients on phenobarbital, one out of two on phenytoin, and four out of six on carbamazepine.[32] Another reported a 60% incidence in adolescents taking unnamed anticonvulsants.[33]

Several practical solutions have been proposed to increase the contraceptive reliability and reduce the unpleasant break-through bleeding:

(a) Raise the dosage of ethinylestradiol (ethinyloestradiol) (or its equivalent) from 30 to 50 micrograms by selecting a different contraceptive preparation.[14,18,32] If break-through bleeding still occurs, give two doses of 30 micrograms, or 30 micrograms plus 50 micrograms.[18,35] Reliable contraception in most patients is said to be achievable with 80–100 micrograms ethinylestradiol daily.[29,30,32,36,37] There should be no increase in side effects with these larger doses because the enzyme-inducing effects of the antiepileptics reduce the blood levels of the steroids. Ideally the blood progesterone levels should be measured on day 21 of the cycle to confirm that these increased doses are preventing ovulation.[36]

(b) Use a non-interacting anticonvulsant: **gabapentin**,[38,39] **lamotrigine**,[40] **sodium valproate**,[32,41] **tiagabine**[42] and **vigabatrin**[43] appear not to interact with the oral contraceptives.

(c) Use a barrier contraceptive method routinely while taking any of the interacting anticonvulsants. If anticonvulsants are used short-term, the Family Planning Association in the UK recommend that additional precautions should be used for at least seven days after stopping the anticonvulsants, and if the seven days run beyond the end of a packet, the new packet should be started without a break, omitting any of the inactive tablets. Allow 4–8 weeks for the liver metabolism to recover following withdrawal of long-term anticonvulsants. It is also important to be on the alert for changes in seizure control if the interacting anticonvulsants are used.

Almost all of the evidence cited here originates from studies on **combined oral contraceptives**, but the enzyme-inducing anticonvulsants (barbiturates, carbamazepine, oxcarbazepine, phenobarbital, phenytoin, primidone) can increase the metabolism of progestogens thereby reducing their efficacy, so that there is also a risk of contraceptive failure with **contraceptive implants**[13,20,21] and **progestogen-only contraceptives**.[20,21] The UK makers of *Norplant* (**levonorgestrel**) advised using additional contraceptive measures during short term use of enzyme inducers and for 7 days afterwards. Additional precautions should be taken for 4 weeks following their withdrawal if the enzyme inducers are used for more than 4 weeks (to allow liver enzymes to recover).[44] For *Depo-Provera* (**medroxyprogesterone**

acetate) one recommendation is that the time interval between injections should be reduced from 12 to 10 weeks[45] although the makers say in their datasheet that no dosage adjustment is needed.[46]

Because the preparations used for **Hormone Replacement Therapy (HRT)** contain oestrogens (estrogens) the makers quite reasonably suggest that an increased dosage of the HRT preparation may possibly be needed in patients taking anticonvulsants which are enzyme inducers (e.g. barbiturates, carbamazepine, phenobarbital, phenytoin, primidone). Concurrent use should therefore be well monitored for evidence of a reduced response but so far there seem to be no reports confirming the importance of this possible interaction.

1. Kenyon IE. Unplanned pregnancy in an epileptic. *BMJ* (1972) 1, 686–7.
2. Von Hempel E, Böhm W, Carol W, Klinger G. Medikamentöse enzyminduktion und hormonale kontrazeption. *Zentralbl Gynakol* (1973) 95, 1451–7.
3. Janz D, Schmidt D. Anti-epileptic drugs and failure of oral contraceptives. *Lancet* (1974) i, 1113.
4. Janz D, Schmidt D. Anti-epileptic drugs and the safety of oral contraceptives. Paper delivered to the German Section of the International League against Epilepsy. Berlin, 1st September 1974.
5. Belaisch J, Driguez P, Janaud A. Influence de certains médicaments sur l'action des pilules contraceptives. *Nouv Presse Med* (1976) 5, 1645–6.
6. Gagnaire JC, Tcherdchian J, Revol A, Rochet Y. Grossesses sous contraceptifs oraux chez les patientes recevant des barbituriques. *Nouv Presse Med* (1975) 4, 3008.
7. Back DJ, Orme ML'E. Drug interactions with oral contraceptive steroids. *Prescribers' J* (1977) 17, 137–42.
8. Coulam CB, Annegers JF. Do anticonvulsants reduce the efficacy of oral contraceptives? *Epilepsia* (1979) 20, 519–26.
9. Fanøe E. P-pillesvigt – antagelig på grund af interaktion med fenemal. *Ugeskr Laeger* (1977) 139, 1485.
10. Sparrow MJ. Pill method failures. *N Z Med J* (1987) 100, 102–5.
11. Kovacs GT, Riddoch G, Duncombe P, Welberry L, Chick P, Weisberg E, Leavesley GM, Baker HWG. Inadvertent pregnancies in oral contraceptive users. *Med J Aust* (1989) 150, 549–51.
12. van der Graaf WT, van Loon AJ, Postmus PE, Sleijfer DT. Twee patiënten met hersenmetastasen die zwanger werden tijdens fenytoïnegebruik. *Ned Tijdschr Geneeskd* (1992) 136, 2236–8.
13. Shane-McWhorter L, Cerveny JD, MacFarlane LL, Osborn C. Enhanced metabolism of levonorgestrel during phenobarbital treatment and resultant pregnancy. *Pharmacotherapy* (1998) 18, 1360–4.
14. Hempel E, Klinger W. Drug stimulated biotransformation of hormonal steroid contraceptives. Clinical implications. *Drugs* (1976) 12, 442–8.
15. Back DJ, Grimmer FM, Orme ML'E, Proudlove C, Mann RD, Breckenridge AM. Evaluation of Committee on Safety of Medicines yellow card reports on oral contraceptive-drug interactions with anticonvulsants and antibiotics. *Br J Clin Pharmacol* (1988) 25, 527–32.
16. Beeley L, Magee P, Hickey FM. Bulletin of the West Midlands Centre for Adverse Drug Reaction Reporting (1989) 28, 21.
17. Rapport DJ, Calabrese JR. Interactions between carbamazepine and birth control pills. *Psychosomatics* (1989) 30, 462–4.
18. Anon. Drug interaction with oral contraceptive steroids. *BMJ* (1980) 3, 93–4.
19. Krauss GL, Brandt J, Campbell M, Plate C, Summerfield M. Antiepileptic medication and oral contraceptive interactions: a national survey of neurologists and obstetricians. *Neurology* (1996) 46, 1534–9.
20. Odlind V, Olsson S-E. Enhanced metabolism of levonorgestrel during phenytoin treatment in a woman with Norplant® implants. *Contraception* (1986) 33, 257–61.
21. Haukkamaa M. Contraception by Norplant® subdermal capsules is not reliable in epileptic patients on anticonvulsant treatment. *Contraception* (1986) 33, 559–65.
22. Klosterskov Jensen P, Saano V, Haring P, Svenstrup B, Menge GP. Possible interaction between oxcarbazepine and an oral contraceptive. *Epilepsia* (1992) 33, 1149–52.
23. Sonnen AEH. Oxcarbazepine and oral contraceptives. *Acta Neurol Scand* (1990) 82 (Suppl 133), 37.
24. Fattore C, Cipolla G, Gatti G, Limido GL, Sturm Y, Bernasconi C, Perucca E. Induction of ethinylestradiol and levonorgestrel metabolism by oxcarbazepine in healthy women. *Epilepsia* (1999) 40, 783–7.
25. Notelovitz M, Tjapkes J, Ware M. Interaction between estrogen and Dilantin in a menopausal woman. *N Engl J Med* (1981) 304, 788–9.
26. McArthur J. Notes and comments. Oral contraceptives and epilepsy. *BMJ* (1967) 3, 162.
27. Espir M, Walker ME, Lawson JP. Epilepsy and oral contraception. *BMJ* (1969) 1, 294–5.
28. Copeman H. Oral contraceptives. *Med J Aust* (1963) 2, 969.
29. Orme M, Back DJ, Chadwick DJ, Crawford P, Martin C, Tjia J. The interaction of phenytoin and carbamazepine with oral contraceptive steroids. *Eur J Pharmacol* (1990) 183, 1029–30.
30. Crawford P, Chadwick DJ, Martin C, Tjia J, Back DJ, Orme M. The interaction of phenytoin and carbamazepine with combined oral contraceptive steroids. *Br J Clin Pharmacol* (1990) 30, 892–6.
31. Kay CR. Progestogen and arterial disease—evidence from the Royal College of General Practitioners' study. *Am J Obstet Gynecol* (1982) 142, 762–5.
32. Sonnen AEH. Sodium valproate and the pill. In 'Advances in Epileptology', XIIIth Epilepsy Int Symp. Akimoto H, Kazamatsuri H, Seino M, Ward A (Eds). Raven Press, NY (1982) 429–32.
33. Diamond MP, Thompson JM. Oral contraceptive use in epileptic adolescents. *J Adolesc Health Care* (1981) 2, 82.
34. Diamond MP, Greene JW, Thompson JM, VanHooydonk JE, Wentz AC. Interaction of anticonvulsants and oral contraceptives in epileptic adolescents. *Contraception* (1985) 31, 623–32.
35. Back DJ, Bates M, Bowden A, Breckenridge AM, Hall MJ, Jones H, MacIver M, Orme M, Perucca E, Richens A, Rowe PH, Smith E. The interaction of phenobarbital and other anticonvulsants with oral contraceptive steroid therapy. *Contraception* (1980) 22, 495–503.
36. O'Brien MD, Gilmour-White S. Epilepsy and pregnancy. *BMJ* (1993) 307, 492–5.
37. Orme M, Back DJ. Oral contraceptive steroids—pharmacological issues of interest to the prescribing physician. *Adv Contracept* (1991) 7, 325–31.
38. Eldon MA, Underwood BA, Randinitis EJ, Posvar EL, Sedman AJ. Lack of effect of gabapentin on the pharmacokinetics of a norethindrone acetate/ethinyl estradiol-containing oral contraceptive. *Neurology* (1993) 43 (Suppl 2), A307–A308.

39. Eldon MA, Underwood BA, Randinitis EJ, Sedman AJ. Gabapentin does not interact with a contraceptive regimen of norethindrone acetate and ethinyl estradiol. *Neurology* (1998) 50, 1146–8.
40. Holdich T, Whiteman P, Orme M, Back D, Ward S. Effect of lamotrigine on the pharmacology of the combined oral contraceptive pill. *Epilepsia* (1991) 32 (Suppl 1), 96.
41. Crawford P, Chadwick D, Cleland P, Tjia J, Cowie A, Back DJ, Orme ML'E. Sodium valproate and oral contraceptive steroids. *Br J Clin Pharmacol* (1985) 20, 288P–289P.
42. Mengel HB, Houston A, Back DJ. An evaluation of the interaction between tiagabine and oral contraceptives in female volunteers. *J Pharm Med* (1994) 4, 141–50.
43. Bartoli A, Gatti G, Cipolla G, Barzaghi N, Veliz G, Fattore C, Mumford J, Perucca E. A double-blind, placebo-controlled study on the effect of vigabatrin on in vivo parameters of hepatic microsomal enzyme induction and on the kinetics of steroid oral contraceptives in healthy female volunteers. *Epilepsia* (1997) 38, 702–7.
44. Norplant (levonorgestrel) Hoechst Marion Roussel Ltd. ABPI Compendium of Data Sheets and Summaries of Product Characterstics 1999–2000, p. 573–4.
45. Anon. Long-acting progestogen-only contraception. *Drug Ther Bull* (1996) 34, 93–6.
46. Depo-Provera (medroxyprogesterone acetate). Pharmacia. Summary of product characteristics, August 2001.

Oral contraceptives + Antihypertensives

The hypertension caused by the oral contraceptives is frequently resistant to antihypertensive therapy with guanethidine or methyldopa.

Clinical evidence, mechanism, importance and management

Virtually all women who take **oestrogen**-containing oral contraceptives show some rise in blood pressure. One study[1] on 83 women showed that the average rise in systolic/diastolic pressures was 9.2/5.0 mmHg, and that it was about twice as likely to occur as in those not on the pill. There are many reports confirming this response but, despite extensive work, the reason for it is not understood although much of the work has centred around the increases seen in the activity of the renin-angiotensin system. Once the contraceptive is withdrawn, the blood pressure usually returns to its former levels.[2]

Attempts to control gross rises in pressure using **guanethidine** or **methyldopa** have been unsatisfactory[3-5] and one report[3] states that "... concurrent medication with **guanethidine** and **oral contraceptives** made satisfactory control of hypertension difficult or impossible." It seems therefore that hypertension associated with, or exacerbated by, the use of **oral contraceptives** may not respond to drugs whose major actions are at adrenergic neurones.

1. Weir RJ, Briggs E, Mack A, Naismith L, Taylor L, Wilson E. Blood pressure in women taking oral contraceptives. *BMJ* (1974) 1, 533–5.
2. Anon. Hypertension and oral contraceptives. *BMJ* (1978) 1, 1570–1.
3. Clezy TM. Oral contraceptives and hypertension: the effect of guanethidine. *Med J Aust* (1970) 1, 638–40.
4. Wallace MR. Oral contraceptives and severe hypertension. *Aust N Z J Med* (1971) 1, 49–52.
5. Woods JW. Oral contraceptives and hypertension. *Lancet* (1967) iii, 653–4.

Oral contraceptives + Antimalarials

Chloroquine and primaquine do not reduce the serum levels of the combined oral contraceptives nor do they seem to affect their reliability. Chloroquine and quinine serum levels remain unchanged during concurrent use and their efficacy appears to be unaltered. Oral contraceptives appear not to affect the treatment of falciparum malaria with mefloquine.

Clinical evidence, mechanism, importance and management

(a) Effect of chloroquine and primaquine on oral contraceptives

A pharmacokinetic study[1] in two groups of women (12 and 7) on low-dose oral contraceptives (**ethinylestradiol (ethinyloestradiol) + norethisterone**) showed that the prophylactic use of **chloroquine phosphate**, 500 mg once a week for four weeks, caused a small increase in blood levels of the **oestrogen** (AUC + 15%), but there was nothing to suggest that the normal effects of the contraceptives were changed in any way. **Chloroquine** blood levels remained unaltered. Another study[2] in 6 women given a single dose of *Microgynon* (ethi-

nylestradiol + levonorgestrel) confirmed that neither **chloroquine** (300 mg) nor **primaquine** (45 mg) had a significant effect on the pharmacokinetics of either the **oestrogen** or the **progestogen**. Further confirmation of the absence of an interaction comes from studies[3] in *rhesus monkeys* infected with malaria in which it was shown that the efficacy of **chloroquine** was not altered by the use of either *Norinyl* or *Ovral-28*.

(b) Effect of oral contraceptives on mefloquine

A study in 12 Thai women with falciparum malaria found that their response (parasite and fever clearance) to treatment with **mefloquine** was not affected by the concurrent use of oral contraceptives. However the half-life and residence time of **mefloquine** were found to be shorter than in 6 normal healthy Thai women taking oral contraceptives.[4] There would seem to be no reason for avoiding concurrent use.

(c) Effect of oral contraceptives on quinine

A controlled study in Thai women showed that the pharmacokinetics of single 600-mg doses of **quinine** in 7 women taking oral contraceptives were not significantly different from those in 7 other women not taking contraceptives. The contraceptives were *Microgynon 30*, *Eugynon*, *Eugynon ED*, *Noriday* and *Triquilar*. There seem to be no reports that **quinine** affects the reliability of the oral contraceptives and there would seem to be no reason for avoiding concurrent use.[5]

1. Gupta KC, Joshi JV, Desai NK, Sankolli GM, Chowdhary VN, Joshi UM, Chitalange S, Satoskar RS. Kinetics of chloroquine and contraceptive steroids in oral contraceptive users during concurrent chloroquine prophylaxis. *Indian J Med Res* (1984) 80, 658–62.
2. Back DJ, Breckenridge AM, Grimmer SFM, Orme ML'E, Purba HS. Pharmacokinetics of oral contraceptive steroids following the administration of the antimalarial drugs primaquine and chloroquine. *Contraception* (1984) 30, 289–95.
3. Dutta GP, Puri SK, Kamboj KK, Srivastava SK, Kamboj VP. Interactions between oral contraceptives and malaria infections in rhesus monkeys. *Bull WHO* (1984) 62, 931–9.
4. Karbwang J, Looareesuwan S, Back DJ, Migasana S, Bunnag D, Breckenridge AM. Effect of oral contraceptive steroids on the clinical cause of malaria infection and on the pharmacokinetics of mefloquine in Thai women. *Bull WHO* (1988) 66, 763–7.
5. Wanwimolruk S, Kaewvichit S, Tanthayaphinant O, Suwannarach C, Oranratnachai A. Lack of effect of oral contraceptive use on the pharmacokinetics of quinine. *Br J Clin Pharmacol* (1991) 31, 179–81.

Oral contraceptives + Antischistosomal drugs

Early schistosomiasis and the use of praziquantel or metrifonate (metriphonate) do not appear to have any effect on the oral contraceptives.

Clinical evidence, mechanism, importance and management

Women with advanced schistosomal infections which affect the liver are not given oral contraceptives because their impaired liver function can affect the metabolism of drugs, but there seems to be no reason for withholding these contraceptives from those with only urinary or intestinal infections.[1,2] A study in 25 women with early active schistosomiasis (*S. haematobium* or *S. mansoni*) showed that neither the disease itself nor the concurrent use of antischistosomal drugs (a single 40 mg/kg dose of **praziquantel**, or **metrifonate (metriphonate)** in three doses of 10 mg/kg at fortnightly intervals) had any effect on their serum oral contraceptive steroid levels when given *Ovral* (50 micrograms **ethinylestradiol (ethinyloestradiol)** + 500 micrograms **levonorgestrel**).[3]

1. Shaaban MM, Hammad WA, Fathalla MF, Ghaneimah SA, El-Sharkawy MM, Salim TH, Liao WC, Smith SC. Effects of oral contraception on liver function tests and serum proteins in women with active schistosomiasis. *Contraception* (1982) 26, 75–82.
2. El-Raghy I, Back DJ, Osman F, Nafeh MA, Orme ML'E. The pharmacokinetics of antipyrine in patients with graded severity of schistosomiasis. *Br J Clin Pharmacol* (1985) 20, 313–6.
3. El-Raghy I, Back DJ, Osman F, Orme ML'E, Fathalla M. Contraceptive steroid concentrations in woman with early active schistosomiasis: lack of effect of antischistosomal drugs. *Contraception* (1986) 33, 373–7.

Oral contraceptives + Cimetidine or Ranitidine

Cimetidine, but not ranitidine, raises endogenous serum estradiol (oestradiol) levels but whether it raises serum contraceptive steroid levels is uncertain.

Clinical evidence, mechanism, importance and management

800 mg **cimetidine** twice daily for two weeks was found to increase the serum estradiol (oestradiol) (endogenous) levels of 9 men by about 20%, due apparently to the well-recognised inhibitory effects of **cimetidine** on the metabolism of estradiol (2-hydroxylation) by the liver. 400 mg twice daily for a week had the same effect in another 6 men,[1] but **ranitidine**, 150 mg twice daily, was found not to raise serum estradiol levels. These raised levels are a possible explanation of the signs and symptoms of oestrogen excess (gynaecomastia, sexual dysfunction) which sometimes occurs in men after taking **cimetidine** for some time. Whether **cimetidine** has the same effect on administered estradiol or other oestrogens (in oral contraceptives for instance) is uncertain but the possibility of increased effects should be borne in mind during concurrent use. There is no evidence that this is a clinically important interaction.

1. Galbraith RA, Michnovicz JJ. Effects of cimetidine on the oxidative metabolism of estradiol. *N Engl J Med* (1989) 321, 269–74.

Oral contraceptives + Clarithromycin, Dirithromycin, Roxithromycin

Clarithromycin, dirithromycin and roxithromycin appear unlikely to cause oral contraceptive failure.

Clinical evidence and mechanism

(a) Clarithromycin

Ten women on combined oral contraceptives (*Microgynon*, *Ovranette*, *Marvelon*) showed a very slight (but not statistically significant) rise in serum **ethinylestradiol (ethinyloestradiol)** levels while also taking 250 mg **clarithromycin** twice daily for seven days. No changes in **levonorgestrel** levels occurred in those taking *Microgynon* or *Ovranette*, but levels of the **active metabolite of desogestrel** were increased in those on *Marvelon*. Progesterone levels remained suppressed and FSH and LH levels were reduced. There was no evidence that **clarithromycin** reduced the effectiveness of these oral contraceptives, and some evidence (reduced levels of FSH and LH) that it actually increases their efficacy.[1]

(b) Dirithromycin

Twenty women taking *Ortho Novum 7/7/7–28* were given 500 mg **dirithromycin** daily for 14 days starting on day 21 of the cycle. A small but statistically significant decrease of 7.6% occurred in the mean **ethinylestradiol (ethinyloestradiol)** $AUC_{0–24}$, but no woman was seen to ovulate. The evidence for this was based, firstly on ultrasound studies (no cyst greater than 10 mm was seen), and secondly on the fact that no significant rises in hormone levels occurred (**ethinylestradiol** concentration of more than 50 pg/ml, a **progesterone** concentration of more than 3 ng/ml). The oral contraceptive used was a triphasic preparation containing 35 micrograms **ethinylestradiol** with 0.5, 0.75 and 1.0 mg **norethisterone** in each tablet.[2]

(c) Roxithromycin

While taking 150 mg **roxithromycin** twice daily, the anti-ovulatory effects of a low dose triphasic oral contraceptive remained unchanged during one cycle in 21 normal women. As a contrast, during another cycle while taking 300 mg **rifampicin** daily instead (known to reduce the effects of the oral contraceptives), 11 of the 21 women ovulated

(52%). Ovulation was detected by measuring serum **progesterone** levels on day 21 (a value of above 10 nmol/l being considered indicative), and confirmed by sonography of the ovaries on day 13.[3,4]

Importance and management

Information seems to be limited to these studies, on the basis of which the authors concluded that these antibacterials are unlikely to cause oral contraceptive failure in the great majority of women. However, it should be pointed out that even though contraceptive failure with other antibacterials (e.g. ampicillin) has similarly not been demonstrated in clinical studies, yet failure has nevertheless occurred in a very few individuals. See 'Oral contraceptives + Antibacterials and Anti-infectives', p.469, and 'Oral contraceptives + Penicillins', p.477.

1. Back DJ, Tjia J, Martin C, Millar E, Salmon P, Orme M. The interaction between clarithromycin and combined oral-contraceptive steroids. *J Pharm Med* (1991) 2, 81–7.
2. Wermeling DP, Chandler MHH, Sides GD, Collins D, Muse KN. Dirithromycin increases ethinyl estradiol clearance without allowing ovulation. *Obstet Gynecol* (1995) 86, 78–84.
3. Meyer BH, Müller FO, Wessels P. Lack of interaction between roxithromycin and an oral contraceptive. *Eur J Pharmacol* (1990) 183, 1031–2.
4. Meyer B, Müller F, Wessels P, Maree J. A model to detect interactions between roxithromycin and oral contraceptives. *Clin Pharmacol Ther* (1990) 47, 671–4.

Oral contraceptives + Co-trimoxazole or Trimethoprim

A human study has shown that co-trimoxazole (sulfamethoxazole (sulphamethoxazole) + trimethoprim) would be expected to increase the effectiveness of the oral contraceptives, yet there are 15 cases on record of contraceptive failure attributed to the concurrent use of co-trimoxazole.

Clinical evidence

A study in 9 women taking a triphasic contraceptive (*Trinordiol*) containing **ethinylestradiol (ethinyloestradiol)** and **levonorgestrel** showed that while taking two tablets of **co-trimoxazole** twice daily (80 mg **trimethoprim** + 400 mg **sulfamethoxazole** in each tablet) their blood levels of **ethinylestradiol** rose by 30–50% (from 29.3 to 38.2 ng/ml at 12 h and from 18.9 to 27.8 ng/ml at 24 h). **Levonorgestrel** levels remained unaltered.[1]

In contrast, the Committee on Safety of Medicines in the UK has on its records 5 cases of oral contraceptive failure attributed to the use of **co-trimoxazole**,[2,3] and another is reported elsewhere.[4] Three other surveys describe a total of 9 other cases of contraceptive failure while taking **co-trimoxazole** or **trimethoprim**.[5-7]

Mechanism

The rise in ethinylestradiol levels[1] is probably due to inhibition by the sulfamethoxazole of the liver enzymes concerned with the metabolism and clearance of the oestrogen from the body. It is not clear why co-trimoxazole should sometimes paradoxically seem to be the cause of contraceptive failure.

Importance and management

The picture is confusing and contradictory. The authors of the study cited[1] say that ". . . the effects of contraceptive steroid preparations are enhanced rather than reduced by co-trimoxazole; and it is unlikely that clinical problems will arise in women taking long-term oral contraceptive steroids who are given short courses of co-trimoxazole." This study appears to have been carefully carried out and well controlled, whereas the CSM and other reports are simply uncontrolled individual case reports. However some risk, however small, seems to exist and the precautions suggested for 'Oral contraceptives + Penicillins', p.477 would seem to be appropriate.

1. Grimmer SFM, Allen WL, Back DJ, Breckenridge AM, Orme M, Tjia T. The effect of cotrimoxazole on oral contraceptive steroids in women. *Contraception* (1983) 28, 53–9.

2. Back DJ, Breckenridge AM, Crawford FE, MacIver M, Orme ML'E, Rowe PH. Interindividual variation and drug interactions with hormonal steroid contraceptives. *Drugs* (1981) 21, 46–61.

3. Back DJ, Grimmer FM, Orme ML'E, Proudlove C, Mann RD, Breckenridge AM. Evaluation of Committee on Safety of Medicines yellow card reports on oral contraceptive-drug interactions with anticonvulsants and antibiotics. *Br J Clin Pharmacol* (1988) 25, 527–32.

4. Beeley L, Magee P, Hickey FM. Bulletin West Midlands Centre for Adverse Drug Reaction Reporting (1989) 28, 32.

5. Sparrow MJ. Pill method failures. *N Z Med J* (1987) 100, 102–5.

6. Kovacs GT, Riddoch G, Duncombe P, Welberry L, Chick P, Weisberg E, Leavesley GM, Baker HWG. Inadvertent pregnancies in oral contraceptive users. *Med J Aust* (1989) 150, 549–51.

7. Sparrow MJ. Pregnancies in reliable pill takers. *N Z Med J* (1989) 102, 575–7.

Oral and other hormonal contraceptives + Danazol

The makers say that women of child-bearing age taking danazol should use an effective non-hormonal method of contraception. There is a theoretical risk that the effects of both danazol and hormonal contraceptives might be altered or reduced.

Clinical evidence, mechanism, importance and management

Danazol can inhibit ovulation, apparently by depressing the LH surge which precedes and triggers ovulation, but in daily doses of 200 mg or more its side-effects are too unacceptable for it to be used routinely as an oral contraceptive, and at lower doses it is too unreliable.[1-3] Despite this ability of danazol to prevent conception, the makers advise the use of reliable non-hormonal contraceptive methods while taking danazol,[4] and by inference the avoidance of hormonal contraceptives. They say that there is a theoretical risk that danazol and the oral contraceptives might possibly compete for the same oestrogen, progestogen and androgen receptors, thereby altering the effects of both drugs.[5] The same reasoning would seem to apply to other hormonal preparations (such as depot preparations of etonorgestrel, medroxyprogesterone, norethisterone) but as yet there seem to be no reports of problems with the concurrent use of danazol and either oral or depot contraceptives.

1. Greenblatt RB, Oettinger M, Borenstein R, Bohler CS-S. Influence of danazol (100 mg) on conception and contraception. *J Reprod Med* (1974) 13, 201–3.

2. Colle ML, Greenblatt RB. Contraceptive properties of danazol. *J Reprod Med* (1976) 17, 98–102.

3. Lauerson NH, Wilson KH. The effect of danazol in the treatment of chronic cystic mastitis. *Obstet Gynecol* (1976) 48, 93–8.

4. Danol (danazol), Sanofi Synthelabo. Summary of product characteristics, March 2002.

5. Sterling-Winthrop, Personal communication 1990.

Oral contraceptives + Enprostil

Enprostil appears not to interact with oral contraceptives.

Clinical evidence, mechanism, importance and management

A double-blind crossover study on 22 normal women taking *Norinyl 1 + 35* (norethisterone 1 mg + ethinylestradiol (ethinyloestradiol) 0.035 mg) showed that the concurrent use of 35 micrograms enprostil for 7 days had no significant effect on the pharmacokinetics of either of the contraceptive steroids. The bioavailability of the oral contraceptives remained unaltered.[1]

1. Winters L, Wilberg C. Enprostil, a synthetic prostaglandin E₂ analogue does not affect oral contraceptive bioavailability. *Curr Ther Res* (1988) 44, 46–50.

Oral contraceptives + Felbamate

Felbamate increases the clearance of gestodene from a combined oral contraceptive, but whether this is clinically important or not is uncertain.

Clinical evidence, mechanism, importance and management

In a randomised, double-blind placebo-controlled trial 31 normal healthy women were given a low dose combined oral contraceptive (ethinylestradiol (ethinyloestradiol) 30 micrograms + gestodene 75 micrograms) for three months or more. During months 1 and 2 they were also given either felbamate (up to 2400 mg daily) or a placebo from day 15 of month 1 to day 14 of month 2. None of them showed any evidence of ovulation during the entire three months, but the $AUC_{0-24\,h}$ of the gestodene was reduced by 42% by the felbamate. The reasons are not understood. The pharmacokinetics of the ethinylestradiol were unaltered.[1] What this change means in terms of the reliability of the oral contraceptive is not known, but some reduction in its efficacy might be expected. More study is needed to find out whether this interaction is clinically important or not.

1. Saano V, Glue P, Banfield CR, Reidenberg P, Colucci RD, Meehan JW, Haring P, Radwanski E, Nomeir A, Lin C-C, Jensen PK, Affrime MB. Effects of felbamate on the pharmacokinetics of a low-dose combination oral contraceptive. *Clin Pharmacol Ther* (1995) 58, 523–31.

Oral contraceptives + Fluconazole

Five pregnancies and six cases of intermenstrual bleeding have been described in women using oral contraceptives attributed to the use of fluconazole, but other evidence suggests that no interaction would be expected or even that serum ethinylestradiol levels are raised.

Clinical evidence

(a) Contraceptive failure

Two pregnancies have been reported, despite the use of oral contraceptives, attributed to an interaction with single 150-mg doses of fluconazole. Intermenstrual bleeding has also been described in six other women on oral contraceptives when given a single 150-mg dose of fluconazole. No withdrawal bleeding was reported in one other patient.[1,2] Three other cases of unintended pregnancy have been very briefly mentioned elsewhere.[3]

(b) No interaction

A study in 10 women found no evidence that a single 50-mg dose of fluconazole or 50 mg fluconazole daily for 10 days had significant effects on the pharmacokinetics of a combined oral contraceptive (30 micrograms ethinylestradiol (ethinyloestradiol) + 150 micrograms levonorgestrel).[4] Two other studies in women taking oral contraceptives found no clinically significant changes in their endocrinological profiles while taking 50 mg fluconazole daily.[5,6] During clinical trials in which single 150-mg doses of fluconazole were used by over 700 women taking oral contraceptives, no evidence of an interaction was seen.[7]

(c) Increases in contraceptive steroid levels

A study in 14 women taking *Microgynon* (ethinylestradiol + levonorgestrel) found that 200 mg fluconazole daily for 10 days raised the levels of ethinylestradiol by 40% and of levonorgestrel by 24%.[8] Yet another study using *Ortho-Novum 7/7/7* or *Triphasil* found that a single dose of 150 mg fluconazole similarly raised serum ethinylestradiol levels.[9]

Mechanism

Unlike ketoconazole, fluconazole appears to have little effect on liver enzyme activity (cytochrome P450-mediated reactions). It is not known why such apparently contradictory results have been found.

Importance and management

A controversial situation. The weight of evidence from the trials suggests that no adverse interaction would be expected, while the pregnancies and intermenstrual bleeding attributed to the use of fluconazole come from uncontrolled reports. However these cannot simply be dismissed or ignored. The risk of contraceptive failure due to fluconazole, as with a number of other anti-infective agents, is therefore probably very small (if it actually exists) but you should consider advising the additional use of a barrier method of contraception if pregnancy is to be avoided with certainty.

1. Pfizer Ltd. Summary of unpublished reports: female reproductive disorders possibly associated with Diflucan. Data on file (Ref DIFLU:diflu41.1) (1990).
2. Bulletin of West Midlands Centre for Adverse Drug Reaction Reporting. January (1990), 30.
3. Pillans PI, Sparrow MJ. Pregnancy associated with a combined oral contraceptive and itraconazole. *N Z Med J* (1993) 106, 436.
4. Pfizer Ltd. An open study to examine the effect of fluconazole on the metabolism of an oral contraceptive in healthy female volunteers. Unpublished data on file (ref 29/VG) (1990).
5. Devenport MH, Crook D, Wynn V, Lees LJ. Metabolic effects of low-dose fluconazole in healthy female users and non-users of oral contraceptives. *Br J Clin Pharmacol* (1989) 27, 851–9.
6. Lazar JD, Wilner KD. Drug interactions with fluconazole. *Rev Infect Dis* (1990) 12 (Suppl 3), S327–33.
7. Dodd GK (Pfizer Ltd). Personal communication (1990).
8. Pfizer Ltd. A two way double blind placebo-controlled, crossover study to investigate the effect of orally administered fluconazole (200 mg) on the plasma concentration profile of an oral contraceptive in healthy female volunteers. Study No. 056–210.
9. Sinofsky FE, Pasquale SA. The effect of fluconazole on circulating ethinyl estradiol levels in women taking oral contraceptives. *Am J Obstet Gynecol* (1998) 178, 300–4.

Oral contraceptives + Genaconazole

Preliminary evidence suggests that genaconazole is unlikely to affect the reliability of the combined oral contraceptives.

Clinical evidence, mechanism, importance and management

A study in 15 women found that a single 400 mg oral dose of **genaconazole** (a triazole antifungal) on day 7 of the cycle did not interfere with the inhibitory action of a **low dose combined oral contraceptive**, as judged from the serum progesterone values.[1] This antifungal seems unlikely to affect the reliability of the oral contraceptives in most women, however it must be pointed out that other antifungals and antibacterials which have failed to show evidence of an interaction during clinical trials, have nevertheless been implicated (though rarely) in oral contraceptive failures. More study is needed.

1. Lunell N-O, Pschera H, Zador G, Carlström K. Evaluation of the possible interaction of the antifungal triazole SCH 39304 with oral contraceptives in normal healthy women. *Gynecol Obstet Invest* (1991) 32, 91–7.

Oral contraceptives + Griseofulvin

The effects of the oral contraceptives may possibly be disturbed (either intermenstrual bleeding or amenorrhoea) if griseofulvin is taken concurrently. Three women on oral contraceptives became pregnant, one while taking griseofulvin and the other two while taking griseofulvin and a sulphonamide.

Clinical evidence

Fifteen out of 22 women on **combined oral contraceptive**s experienced transient intermenstrual bleeding and 5 had amenorrhoea during the first or second cycle after starting to take **griseofulvin** (0.5–1.0 g daily). Four of the 22 (2 with intermenstrual bleeding and 2 with amenorrhoea) developed their original reactions when re-challenged with **griseofulvin**. Two other women on the pill are reported to have become pregnant while taking **griseofulvin** and a **sulphonamide** (**co-trimoxazole** in one instance and an **unknown sulphonamide** in the other).[1]

Oligomenorrhoea and irregular menses have been described in a woman on a **combined oral contraceptive** when given **griseofulvin** (250–500 mg daily). When the oral contraceptive was substituted by another with 57% more oestrogen, the menstrual flow became normal again.[2] Break-through bleeding has also been seen in three other women on the pill given **griseofulvin**[3] and one case of contraceptive failure has been reported.[4] However, a database maintained by the maker Syntex, up to 1985 contained no reports of any oral contraceptive failures due to **griseofulvin**.[5]

Mechanism

Not understood. Griseofulvin may possibly stimulate the activity of the liver enzymes concerned with the metabolism of the contraceptive steroids, thereby reducing their effects. This might explain the cases of break-through bleeding, but not those involving oligomenorrhoea and amenorrhoea. Contraceptive failure attributed to co-trimoxazole has also been reported (see 'Oral contraceptives + Co-trimoxazole or Trimethoprim', p.473).

Importance and management

Information about this interaction is very limited.[1-4] The risk of total contraceptive failure is uncertain but probably very small, however it would now be prudent for prescribers to warn women on **combined oral contraceptives** who are given griseofulvin that menstrual disturbances may possibly be signs of contraceptive unreliability, and that additional contraceptive precautions should be taken. The Committee on the Safety of Medcines in the UK has pointed out the importance of ensuring adequate contraception during and for one month after taking griseofulvin because it can induce aneuploidy (abnormal segregation of chromosomes during cell division) which carries the potential risk of teratogenicity.[6] For maximal contraceptive protection a barrier method should be used routinely while taking griseofulvin and for at least 7 days afterwards. The Family Planning Association in the UK recommend that if the 7 days run beyond the end of a packet, the new packet should be started without a break, omitting any of the inactive tablets.

The situation with **progestogen-only contraceptives** is not clear, but it has been suggested that they are not the contraceptive of choice in those taking griseofulvin, not because of reduced efficacy but because of increased menstrual irregularities.[7] In the case of **contraceptive implants**, the makers of one preparation (*Norplant*) also advise the avoidance of griseofulvin. This appears to be a recommendation based on what has been seen with oral contraceptives but there seems no hard evidence that an interaction actually occurs.

1. van Dijke CPH, Weber JCP. Interaction between oral contraceptives and griseofulvin. *BMJ* (1984) 288, 1125–6.

2. McDaniel PA, Caldroney RD. Oral contraceptives and griseofulvin interaction. *Drug Intell Clin Pharm* (1986) 20, 384.

3. Beeley L, Stewart P. Bulletin of the West Midlands Centre for Adverse Drug Reaction Reporting. (1987) 25, 23.

4. Back DJ, Grimmer FM, Orme ML'E, Proudlove C, Mann RD, Breckenridge AM. Evaluation of Committee on Safety of Medicines yellow card reports on oral contraceptive-drug interactions with anticonvulsants and antibiotics. *Br J Clin Pharmacol* (1988) 25, 527–32.

5. Szoka PR, Edgren RA. Drug interactions with oral contraceptives: compilation and analysis of an adverse experience report database. *Fertil Steril* (1988) 49 (Suppl), 31–8.

6. Committee on Safety of Medicines. Griseofulvin (Fulcin, Grisovin): contraceptive precautions. *Current Problems* (1996) 22, 8.

7. McCann MF, Potter LS. Progestin-only contraception: a comprehensive review. *Contraception* (1994) 50, S1–S198.

Oral contraceptives + Itraconazole

Two isolated reports attribute contraceptive failure to the concurrent use of itraconazole. Other reports describe break-through bleeding, delayed withdrawal bleeding and amenorrhoea.

Clinical evidence

A 25-year old who had been taking *Microgynon 30* (0.03 mg ethinylestradiol (ethinyloestradiol), 0.15 mg levonorgestrel) for a year, without problems, became pregnant when she was additionally treated for three months with 200 mg itraconazole daily for a fungal infection. The patient was said to be compliant, had suffered no gastrointestinal upset, and was not taking any other drugs which might have accounted for the failure of the pill.[1]

The Netherlands Pharmacovigilance Foundation (LAREB) have on their records nine cases of menstrual changes in women taking oral contraceptives during or after taking itraconazole (100–400 mg daily for 1–4 weeks). 7 women reported delayed withdrawal bleeding (2–5 days), in 2 of them the menstrual flow was decreased and one had previously experienced an intermenstrual blood loss. The remaining two reports were of amenorrhoea during one cycle in one case and break-through bleeding in the other. The women were taking either *Marvelon*, *Mercilon* or *Microgynon*.[2] A later report from LAREB describes 12 women taking contraceptives containing ethinylestradiol/desogestrel whose withdrawal bleeding was either delayed or did not occur at all while taking itraconazole. One of these women reported a transiently positive pregnancy test after previous break-through bleedings. Three other women taking ethinylestradiol/levonorgestrel had break-through bleeding, and yet another on ethinylestradiol/cyproterone acetate became pregnant while taking itraconazole.[3] It is not entirely clear whether this second report from LAREB is an extension of the previous report or totally new information.

Mechanism

Not understood. A study in 5 normal subjects given single oral doses of 0.05 mg ethinylestradiol and 1 mg norethisterone, before and after taking 200 mg itraconazole daily for 15 days, found no changes in the pharmacokinetics of the ethinylestradiol. In fact the bioavailability of the norethisterone was increased 40% (possibly due to inhibition of first-pass metabolism).[4]

Importance and management

The picture presented by these reports is somewhat confusing and contradictory. No interaction is firmly established, although the reports of contraceptive failure and the cases of break-through bleeding indicate that itraconazole can make oral contraception less reliable in some individuals. Bearing in mind the maker's warning that adequate contraceptive precautions should be taken by women of childbearing potential until the next menstrual period following the end of therapy because of a theoretical teratogenic risk,[5] it might therefore be a prudent to use additional barrier contraception if pregnancy is to be avoided with greater certainty while taking itraconazole. More study is needed.

1. Pillans PI, Sparrow MJ. Pregnancy associated with a combined oral contraceptive and itraconazole. *N Z Med J* (1993) 106, 436.

2. Meyboom RHB, van Puijenbroek EP, Vinks MHAM, Lastdrager CJ. Disturbance of withdrawal bleeding during concomitant use of itraconazole and oral contraceptives. *N Z Med J* (1997) 110, 300.

3. van Puijenbroek EP, Feenstra J, Meyboom RHB. Verstoring van de pilcyclus tijdens het gelijktijdig gebruik van itraconazol en orale anticonceptiva. *Ned Tijdschr Geneeskd* (1998) 142, 146–9.

4. Jones AR (Janssen). Personal communication 1994.

5. Sporanox (itraconazole). Janssen-Cilag. Summary of product characteristics, August 2001.

Oral contraceptives + Ketoconazole

Ketoconazole can reduce the effectiveness of the oral contraceptives and cause intermenstrual bleeding. So far only one pregnancy has been reported.

Clinical evidence, mechanism, importance and management

Seven out of 147 women taking low dose oral contraceptives (*Ovidon*, *Rigevidon*, *Anteovin*) experienced break-through bleeding or spotting within 2–5 days of starting a five-day course of ketoconazole, 400 mg daily. No pregnancies occurred,[1] but one unintended pregnancy attributed to contraceptive failure due to ketoconazole has been very briefly mentioned elsewhere.[2] The total picture, limited though it is, suggests that a risk of contraceptive failure exists, even though it is probably very small indeed. The precautions suggested when taking antibacterials such as the penicillins (use an additional barrier contraceptive) might be a wise precaution if pregnancy is be avoided with certainty (see 'Oral contraceptives + Penicillins', p.477).

1. Kovacs L, Somos P, Hamori M. Examination of the potential interaction between ketoconazole (Nizoral) and oral contraceptives with special regard to products of low hormone content (*Rigevidon*, *Anteovin*). *Ther Hung* (1986) 34, 167.

2. Pillans PI, Sparrow MJ. Pregnancy associated with a combined oral contraceptive and itraconazole. *N Z Med J* (1993) 106, 436.

Oral contraceptives + Lansoprazole or Pantoprazole

Lansoprazole and pantoprazole appear not to interact with combined oral contraceptives.

Clinical evidence, mechanism, importance and management

(a) Lansoprazole

Twenty-four normal healthy women were given *Microgynon 21* (0.03 mg ethinylestradiol (ethinyloestradiol) + 0.15 mg levonorgestrel) for two monthly cycles in a placebo-controlled randomised study, with and without 60 mg lansoprazole daily. The levels of the oral contraceptive steroids and endogenous hormones were not significantly altered by the lansoprazole, nor were endogenous progesterone levels raised suggesting that ovulation did not occur.[1,2] Three other studies in 30, 20 and 9 women also found no evidence that lansoprazole interacts with oral contraceptives in any way which would affect their reliability.[2]

(b) Pantoprazole

No evidence of an interaction was seen in 64 women taking low-dose triphasic contraceptives while taking 40 mg pantoprazole daily for 23 days.[3] There was no evidence that either lansoprazole or pantoprazole interacted with the oral contraceptives in any way which would affect their reliability.

1. Fuchs W, Sennewald R, Klotz U. Lansoprazole does not affect the bioavailability of oral contraceptives. *Br J Clin Pharmacol* (1994) 38, 376–80.

2. Zoton lansoprazole concommitant use of OCA. Wyeth, Personal communication, February 1998.

3. Middle MV, Müller FO, Mogilnicka EM, Hundt HKL, Beneke PC, Schall R, Steinijans VW, Hartmann M, Bliesath H, Wurst W. Pantoprazole does not impair the efficacy of hormonal contraception. *Gastroenterology* (1994) 106 (4 Suppl), A139.

Oral contraceptives + Lovastatin

Lovastatin can prevent the rise in serum lipid levels in women taking oral contraceptives.

Clinical evidence, mechanism, importance and management

Thirty non-smoking women showed a 74% rise in plasma lipid levels (from 90 to 157 mg/dl) after taking a triphasic oral contraceptive (**ethinylestradiol (ethinyloestradiol) + levonorgestrel**) for 3 months, whereas another similar group additionally taking 20 mg **lovastatin** daily showed only a non-statistically significant rise (from 105 to 113 mg/dl). It was therefore concluded that **lovastatin** may reduce the risk of atherosclerotic disease in those taking oral contraceptives. The report of this study did not comment on whether the reliability of the oral contraceptive was altered.[1]

1. Colakoglu M, Kodama H, Tanak T. The effect of combined medication of triphasic oral contraceptive with an anti-lipid agent, lovastatin, on plasma lipid levels. *Jpn J Fertil Steril* (1996) 41, 317–20.

Oral contraceptives + Nelfinavir

Nelfinavir has been found to reduce the serum levels of the ethinylestradiol (ethinyloestradiol) and the norethisterone components of a combined oral contraceptive. This is predicted to increase the risk of contraceptive failure.

Clinical evidence, mechanism, importance and management

It was found in a study in women on a combined oral contraceptive (35 micrograms **17-α-ethinylestradiol (ethinyloestradiol)** plus 0.4 mg **norethisterone (norethinderone)**) that the concurrent use of 750 mg **nelfinavir** three times daily for 7 days reduced the AUC of the **ethinylestradiol** by 47% and that of the **norethisterone** by 18%,[1] the reason being that the **nelfinavir** acts as an enzyme inducer which increases the metabolism and clearance of these steroids.

Such a large reduction in the **ethinylestradiol** levels in particular would be expected to reduce the efficacy and reliability of the contraceptive, so that although so far there appear to be no cases of contraceptive failure attributed to this interaction, to avoid this risk and that of break-through bleeding the makers reasonably recommend that alternative contraceptive measures should be considered if **nelfinavir** is used by women using combined oral contraceptives of this kind.[1]

1. Viracept (nelfinavir). Roche Products Ltd. Summary of product characteristics, October 2001.

Oral contraceptives + Nitrofurantoin

A review of the literature concluded that an alleged interaction between nitrofurantoin causing oral contraceptive failure was anecdotal and unfounded.

Clinical evidence, mechanism, importance and management

In 1966 a report was published describing oral contraceptive failure in one patient who had been taking **nitrofurantoin, mandelamine** and **amobarbital (amylobarbitone)**.[1] It is not clear why suspicion fell on the **nitrofurantoin** when the **barbiturate** was the more likely candidate. This report was the start of a chain of reviews (later said to be "tenuous and ill-cited"[2]) in which **nitrofurantoin** was listed as a cause of contraceptive failure, but no further evidence was cited until 1981 when **nitrofurantoin** was again listed among 17 other antibacterials reported to the Committee on Safety of Medicines in the UK as having caused oral contraceptive failure.[3]

D'Arcy, who undertook a survey of the evidence, offers the opinion that ". . . firm evidence for a **nitrofurantoin/oral contraceptive** interaction is, therefore, slim to non-existent: mention in the literature is based on unconfirmed hearsay . . ." and he concluded that the **nitrofurantoin/oral contraceptive** interaction is unconfirmed and anecdotal.[2] No new evidence which would be likely to alter this conclusion has appeared since the review was published in 1985.

1. Luck VR. Oral contraceptives. *Med J Aust* (1966) 2, 913–4.
2. D'Arcy PM. Nitrofurantoin. *Drug Intell Clin Pharm* (1985) 19, 540–7.
3. Back DJ, Breckenridge AM, Crawford FM, MacIver M, Orme M L'E, Rowe PH. Interindividual variation and drug interactions with hormonal steroid contraceptives. *Drugs* (1981) 21, 466–61.

Oral contraceptives + Orlistat

Orlistat does not interact with combined oral contraceptives.

Clinical evidence, mechanism, importance and management

Two groups of normal women on oral contraceptives were given 120 mg **orlistat** three times daily or a placebo on days 1–23 of two menstrual cycles.[1] Using measurements of luteinising hormone on days 12–16 and progesterone levels on days 12, 16, 19–23 to check for any evidence of ovulation, it was found that **orlistat** did not have any effect on the ovulation-suppressant effects of the contraceptives. The contraceptives which were used all contained **ethinylestradiol (ethinyloestradiol)**, but the progestogens differed: 10 with **desogestrel**, 4 **levonorgestrel**, 3 **gestodene**, 2 **cyproterone acetate**, 1 **lynestrenol**. No additional contraceptive precautions would seem necessary in women on oral contraceptives if given **orlistat**.

1. Hartmann D, Güzelhan C, Zuiderwijk PBM, Odink J. Lack of interaction between orlistat and oral contraceptives. *Eur J Clin Pharmacol* (1996) 50, 421–4.

Oral contraceptives + Penicillins

Failure of combined oral contraceptives to prevent conception and pregnancy has been attributed to the concurrent use of pencillins, but the interaction (if such it is) appears to be very rare. Failure of the progestogen-only contraceptives has also been attributed to the use of penicillins.

Clinical evidence

A woman is reported to have had two unwanted pregnancies while taking *Minovlar* (**ethinylestradiol (ethinyloestradiol) + norethisterone**). She had also been treated with wide-spectrum antibacterials, particularly **ampicillin**. Another woman on *Minovlar* for 5 years with no history of break-through bleeding, lost a quantity of blood similar to a normal period loss within a day of starting to take **ampicillin**, one capsule four times a day. There was no evidence of diarrhoea or vomiting in either case.[1,2]

The Committee on Safety of Medicines (CSM) in the UK has on record 32 further cases of contraceptive failure over the 1968–84 period attributed to penicillin antibacterials: **ampicillin, ampicillin** with either **fusidic acid, tetracycline** or **flucloxacillin; amoxicillin (amoxycillin), talampicillin, phenoxymethylpenicillin** (one also with **oxytetracycline**) and '**penicillin**'.[3,4] Another survey describes contraceptive failures due to **amoxicillin** (16 cases), **flucloxacillin, phenoxymethylpenicillin, pivampicillin** (five cases) and **amoxicillin** with **phenoxymethylpenicillin** (two cases).[5] Two other reports describe a total of 26 cases with **amoxicillin** and six cases with '**penicillin**'.[6,7] Further cases attributed to **oxacillin** and *Triplopen* (**benethamine, procaine** and **benzyl penicillins**) are reported elsewhere.[8,9]

Mechanism

Not understood. The oestrogen component of the contraceptive is cycled in the entero-hepatic shunt (i.e. it is repeatedly secreted in the bile as steroid sulphate and glucuronide conjugates which are then hydrolysed by the gut bacteria before reabsorption). One idea is that if these bacteria are decimated by the use of an antibacterial, the steroid conjugates fail to undergo bacterial hydrolysis and are very poorly reabsorbed, resulting in lower-than-normal concentrations of circulating oestrogen in a very small number of women and in an inadequate suppression of ovulation.[10] However, although the penicillins reduce urinary oestriol secretion in pregnant women,[11-15] no marked changes in serum oestrogen[3,16,17] or progestogen[18] levels in women on contraceptives have been found in formal studies. The progestogens do not take part in the entero-hepatic shunt.

Importance and management

The oral contraceptive/penicillins interaction is inadequately established and controversial. Almost all of the evidence is anecdotal with insufficient controls (if any), and in statistical terms the incidence of contraceptive failure due to this interaction seems not to be distinguishable from the general and recognised failure rate of oral contraceptives.[19] The total number of failures is extremely small when viewed against the number of women worldwide using oral contraceptives (estimated at more than 50 million) so that most women are not at risk.

On the other hand, the personal and ethical consequences of an unwanted pregnancy can be very serious, and for this reason the generally accepted current wisdom is that for maximal protection a second form of contraception (a barrier method) should be used routinely while taking a short course of a penicillin, and for at least seven days afterwards.[20] The Family Planning Association in the UK recommend that if the seven days run beyond the end of a packet, the new packet should be started without a break, omitting any of the inactive tablets. They also say that those on long-term antibacterials (for example for acne) need only take extra precautions for the first two weeks because, after that, the gut flora becomes resistant to the antibacterial, but this was not seemingly borne out in the case of four women on oral contraceptives and minocycline[19,21] and one on tetracycline[22] who became pregnant, although whether these failures resulted from an interaction will never be known.

Four contraceptive failures attributed to a **progestogen-only contraceptive**/penicillin interaction occur in the CSM records, but no definite link has been shown. It is generally believed that no increased risk of failure exists if broad-spectrum antibacterials are taken with **progestogen-only contraceptives**.[23]

1. Dossetor J. Drug interactions with oral contraceptives. *BMJ* (1975) 4, 467–8.
2. Dossetor J. Personal communication (1975).
3. Back DJ, Breckenridge AM, MacIver M, Orme M, Rowe PH, Staiger Ch, Thomas E, Tjia J. The effect of ampicillin on oral contraceptive steroids in women. *Br J Clin Pharmacol* (1982) 14, 43–8.
4. Back DJ, Grimmer FM, Orme ML'E, Proudlove C, Mann RD, Breckenridge AM. Evaluation of Committee on Safety of Medicines yellow card reports on oral contraceptive-drug interactions with anticonvulsants and antibiotics. *Br J Clin Pharmacol* (1988) 25, 527–32.
5. Sparrow MJ. Pill method failures. *N Z Med J* (1987) 100, 102–5.
6. Kovacs GT, Riddoch G, Duncombe P, Welberry L, Chick P, Weisberg E, Leavesley GM, Baker HWG. Inadvertent pregnancies in oral contraceptive users. *Med J Aust* (1989) 150, 549–51.
7. Sparrow MJ. Pregnancies in reliable pill takers. *N Z Med J* (1989) 102, 575–7.
8. Silber TJ. Apparent oral contraceptive failure associated with antibiotic administration. *J Adolesc Health Care* (1983) 4, 287–9.
9. Bainton R. Interaction between antibiotic therapy and contraceptive medication. *Oral Surg Oral Med Oral Pathol* (1986) 61, 453–5.
10. Back DJ, Breckenridge AM, Crawford FE, MacIver M, Orme ML'E, Rowe PH. Interindividual variation and drug interactions with hormonal steroid contraceptives. *Drugs* (1981) 21, 46–61.
11. Willman K, Pulkkinen MO. Reduced maternal plasma and urinary estriol during ampicillin treatment. *Am J Obstet Gynecol* (1971) 109, 893–6.
12. Tikkanen MJ, Aldercreutz H, Pulkkinen MO. Effect of antibiotics on oestrogen metabolism. *BMJ* (1973) 1, 369.
13. Pulkkinen MO, Willman K. Maternal oestrogen levels during penicillin treatment. *BMJ* (1971) 4, 48.
14. Sybulski S, Maughan GB. Effect of ampicillin administration on estradiol, estriol, and cortisol levels in maternal plasma and on estriol levels in urine. *Am J Obstet Gynecol* (1976) 124, 379–81.
15. Trybuchowski H. Effect of ampicillin on the urinary output of steroidal hormones in pregnant and non-pregnant women. *Clin Chim Acta* (1973) 45, 9–18.
16. Friedman CI, Huneke AL, Kim MH, Powell J. The effect of ampicillin on oral contraceptive effectiveness. *Obstet Gynecol* (1980) 55, 33–7.
17. Philipson A. Plasma and urine levels produced by an oral dose of ampicillin 0.5 g administered to women taking oral contraceptives. *Acta Obstet Gynecol Scand* (1979) 58, 69–71.
18. Joshi JV, Hazari KT, Sankoli GM, Mandlekar A, Joshi UM, Gupta K, Krishna U, Virkar KD, Sheth UK, Saxena BN. Interaction of an oral contraceptive with metronidazole and ampicillin therapy. *J Steroid Biochem* (1978) 9, 862.
19. Helms SE, Bredle DL, Zajic J, Jarjoura D, Brodell RT, Krishnarao I. Oral contraceptive failure rates and oral antibiotics. *J Am Acad Dermatol* (1997) 36, 705–10.
20. Orme M, Back DJ. Oral contraceptive steroids – pharmacological issues of interest to the prescribing physician. *Adv Contracept* (1991) 7, 325–31.
21. Hughes BR, Cunliffe WJ. Interactions between the oral contraceptive pill and antibiotics. *Br J Dermatol* (1990) 122, 717–18.
22. London BM, Lookingbill DP. Frequency of pregnancy in acne patients taking oral antibiotics and oral contraceptives. *Arch Dermatol* (1994) 130, 392–3.
23. McCann MF, Potter LS. Progestin-only contraception: a comprehensive review. *Contraception* (1994) 50, S1–S198.

Oral contraceptives + Pethidine (Meperidine)

Oral contraceptives do not appear to interact with pethidine (meperidine).

Clinical evidence, mechanism, importance and management

One early study suggested that women on oral contraceptives excreted more unchanged **pethidine** in the urine than a control group not taking contraceptives who were found to excrete more of the demethylated metabolite.[1] However a later, well controlled, comparative study in 24 normal subjects (eight women taking 0.5 mg **norgestrel** + 0.05 mg **ethinylestradiol (ethinyloestradiol)**, and eight women and eight men not taking contraceptives) found no differences between the serum levels or excretion patterns of the three groups.[2] There would seem to be no reason for avoiding concurrent use.

1. Crawford JS, Rudofsky S. Some alterations in the pattern of drug metabolism associated with pregnancy, oral contraceptives and the newly-born. *Br J Anaesth* (1966) 38, 446.
2. Stambaugh JE, Wainer IW. Drug interactions I: meperidine and combination oral contraceptives. *J Clin Pharmacol* (1975) 15, 46–51.

Oral contraceptives + Quinolone antibacterials

Ciprofloxacin, moxifloxacin, ofloxacin and temafloxacin have been shown not to affect the reliability of the combined oral contraceptives.

Clinical evidence

(a) Ciprofloxacin

No significant changes in gonadotropin (LH, FSH) or estradiol (oestradiol) levels occurred in 10 healthy women on combined oral contraceptives (**ethinylestradiol (ethinyloestradiol) + desogestrel**, **gestodene** or **levonorgestrel**) while also taking 500 mg **ciprofloxacin** twice daily for seven days, starting on the first day of contraceptive intake. No break-through bleeding occurred.[1] Another study in 24 normal women taking *Marvelon* (30 micrograms **ethinylestradiol** + 150 micrograms **desogestrel**) found that 500 mg **ciprofloxacin** twice daily for 10 days actually increased the ovarian suppression.[2]

(b) Moxifloxacin

A placebo-controlled, randomised, two-way crossover study in 29 young healthy women taking a combined oral contraceptive (30 micrograms **ethinylestradiol** + 150 micrograms **levonorgestrel**) found that the concurrent use of 400 mg **moxifloxacin** on menstrual cycle days 1–7 had no clinically relevant effect on the pharmacokinetics of either contraceptive steroid. The hormonal parameters measured (estradiol, progesterone, LH, FSH) were also unchanged by the presence of the quinolone indicating that ovulation continued to be suppressed.[3]

(c) Ofloxacin

A placebo-controlled, randomised crossover study over six menstrual cycles in 20 women taking *Microgynon* (30 micrograms **ethinylestradiol (ethinyloestradiol)** plus 150 micrograms **levonorgestrel**) found no evidence that 200 mg **ofloxacin** twice daily for 7 days had any effect on contraception. Evidence of ovulation was looked for by ultrasonographical measurements of the number and diameter of ovarian follicles, and by measuring FSH, estradiol (oestradiol) and progesterone levels.[4,5]

(d) Temafloxacin

Temafloxacin, now withdrawn, has been shown not interact with oral contraceptives.[6]

Mechanism

None.

Importance and management

The absence of an interaction between these combined oral contraceptives and ciprofloxacin, moxifloxacin and ofloxacin appears to be established. No special extra contraceptive precautions would therefore seem to be necessary during concurrent use. Reports of cases of contraceptive failure with these or any other quinolone antibacterial seem to be lacking.

1. Maggiolo F, Puricelli G, Dottorini M, Caprioli S, Bianchi W, Suter F. The effect of ciprofloxacin on oral contraceptive steroid treatments. *Drugs Exp Clin Res* (1991) XVII, 451–4.
2. Droppert RM, Scholten PC, Zwinkels M, Hoepelman IM, Te Velde ER. Lack of influence of ciprofloxacin on the effectiveness of oral contraceptives. *Intersci Conf Antimicrob Agents Chemother* (1994) 34, 4.
3. Staß H, Sachse R, Heinig R, Zühlsdorf M, Horstmann R. Pharmacokinetics (PK) of steroid hormons in oral contraceptives (OC) are not altered by oral moxifloxacin (MOX). *J Antimicrob Agents Chemother* (1999) 44 (Suppl A), 1398–9.
4. Csemiczky G, Alvendal C, Landgren B-M. Risk for ovulation in women taking a low-dose oral contraceptive (Microgynon) when receiving antibacterial treatment with a fluoroquinolone (ofloxacin). *Adv Contracept* (1996) 12, 101–9.
5. Scholten PC, Droppert RM, Zwinkels MG, Moesker HL, Nauta JJ, Hoepelman IM. No interaction between ciprofloxacin and an oral contraceptive. *Antimicrob Agents Chemother* (1998) 42, 3266–8.
6. Back DJ, Tija J, Martin C, Millar E, Mant T, Morrison P, Orme M. The lack of interaction between temafloxacin and combined oral contraceptives. *Contraception* (1991) 43, 317–23.

Oral contraceptives + Retinoids

There seems to be no evidence that the reliability of the combined oral contraceptives is affected by acitretin or isotretinoin. Any changes in the effects of the progestogen-only contraceptives caused by acitretin seem to be clinically unimportant.

Clinical evidence, mechanism, importance and management

(a) Acitretin

Eight women on **combined oral contraceptives** (*Stediril*, *Minidiril*, *Adepal*) and one on a **progestogen-only contraceptive** (*Microval*) were given 25–40 mg **acitretin** daily for at least two cycles. No changes in progesterone levels were seen in those taking the **combined contraceptives**, but the patient taking the **progestogen-only contraceptive** (0.03 mg **levonorgestrel**) showed a significant increase in progesterone levels after 3 cycles with **acitretin**. Plasma progesterone levels rose from 2.15 ng/ml before taking the **acitretin** to 3.87–13.46 ng/ml with **acitretin**. This rise in progesterone levels was taken as evidence that a corpus luteum had developed and hence that ovulation had occurred.[1]

Direct information seems to be limited to this report,[1] however no special precautions would seem to be necessary if **acitretin** is taken by women on **either type of contraceptive** (however see the note at the end of (b)). **Acitretin** appears to have no effect on the anti-ovulatory effects of the **combined contraceptives**, and since the **progestogen-only contraceptives** are believed to act primarily by altering the cervical mucous so that it become a sperm barrier, it probably does not matter whether **acitretin** allows ovulation to occur or not while taking this type of oral contraceptive. There seems to be no evidence in the literature that either **acitretin** (the main metabolite of **etretinate**) or **etretinate** itself has ever been responsible for oral contraceptive failure.

(b) Isotretinoin

A study in nine women on a **combined oral contraceptive** showed that the plasma concentrations of **ethinylestradiol (ethinyloestradiol)** and **levonorgestrel** were not significantly changed by the use of 0.5 mg/kg **isotretinoin** for severe pustular acne.[2] The authors concluded that oral contraceptives remain reliable during concurrent use, and they say that it seems unlikely that an interaction would occur with 1.0 mg/kg which is the dose commonly recommended in the USA.

It should however be emphasised that women who have used these retinoids should avoid becoming pregnant because of the risk of teratogenicity. The current recommendation is that pregnancy should be avoided for two years after **acitretin** is stopped and a month after **isotretinoin** is stopped.

1. Berbis Ph, Bun H, Geiger JM, Rognin C, Durand A, Serradimigni A, Hartmann D, Privat Y. Acitretin (RO10-1670) and oral contraceptives: interaction study. *Arch Dermatol Res* (1988) 280, 388–9.
2. Orme M, Back DJ, Shaw MA, Allen WL, Tjia J, Cunliffe WJ, Jones DH. Isotretinoin and contraception. *Lancet* (1984) ii, 752–3.

Oral contraceptives + Rifamycins

Oral contraceptives are very unreliable during concurrent treatment with rifampicin (rifampin). Break-through bleeding and spotting commonly occur, and conception and pregnancy may not be prevented. Rifabutin also reduces the reliability of oral contraceptives, although it interacts to a lesser extent and no contraceptive failures have been reported.

Clinical evidence

(a) Rifampicin (Rifampin)

Beginning with the first report[1] in 1971, a very marked increase in the frequency of intermenstrual break-through bleeding has been described in women on **combined oral contraceptives** when given **rifampicin**.[1] 62 out of 88 women on **combined oral contraceptives** are described in another study who had menstrual cycle disorders of various kinds (spotting, bleeding, failure to menstruate) when treated with **rifampicin**. Five pregnancies in women taking both drugs are also mentioned.[2-4] Other reports have confirmed this interaction and there have been a total of at least 15 pregnancies.[5-10] One study found that 11 out of 21 women (52%) on a **triphasic oral contraceptive** ovulated while taking 300 mg **rifampicin** daily.[11,12] In another study, 2 out of 7 on low dose **combined oral contraceptives** ovulated while taking **rifampicin**.[13] Contraceptive failure in a woman given **rifampicin**, streptomycin and isoniazid has also been described.[14] A study in 12 normal subjects taking **ethinylestradiol (ethinyloestradiol)** (0.35 micrograms) + **norethisterone (norethindrone)** (1 mg) found that after taking **rifampicin** (dosage not stated) from day 7 to 21 of the cycle, the AUC of **ethinylestradiol** fell by 62.5% and of **norethisterone** 49.4%, but no ovulation occurred and plasma progesterone levels were less than 1.0 ng/ml in all subjects on day 21.[15] **Rifampicin** serum levels are reported to be unchanged by oral contraceptives.[16]

(b) Rifabutin

A study in 22 normal women on an oral contraceptive (**ethinylestradiol (ethinyloestradiol)** plus **norethindrone**) found that when concurrently treated with 300 mg **rifabutin** or rifampicin daily for 10 days the **rifabutin**/control ratio for the **ethinylestradiol** was 0.65 and of the **norethindrone** was 0.54. (compared with 0.36 and 0.41 when taking rifampicin). Spotting was 3.6% in the controls, 17% with the **rifabutin** and 23% with rifampicin.[17] A study in 12 normal subjects taking **ethinylestradiol** (0.35 micrograms) + **norethindrone** (1 mg) found that after taking **rifabutin** (dosage not stated) from day 7 to 21 of the cycle, the AUC of **ethinylestradiol** fell by 35.5% and of **norethindrone** by 13.9%. No ovulation occurred and plasma progesterone levels were less than 0.1 ng/ml in all subjects on day 21.[15] There appear to be no reports of contraceptive failure attributed to **rifabutin**.

Mechanism

600 mg rifampicin daily for only six days was found to increase the hydroxylation of ethinylestradiol (ethinyloestradiol) fourfold[18,19] and to reduce serum norethisterone levels significantly.[20] Mestranol is probably similarly affected.[21] As a result of this enzyme induction the reduced steroid levels may be insufficient to prevent the re-establishment of a normal menstrual cycle with ovulation, which would explain the break-through bleeding and pregnancies which have occurred. The trend towards low-dose oestrogen contraceptives has possibly increased its likelihood. Rifabutin similarly acts as enzyme inducing agent but in terms of reducing contraceptive steroid levels it is less potent than rifampicin (roughly half).[15]

Importance and management

The interaction between the **combined oral contraceptives** and rifampicin is well documented, well established and clinically important. Menstrual cycle disturbances of 50–70%[2,3,11] and an ovulation rate of 52%[11,12] show very clearly that women on combined oral contraceptives should use an alternative or additional form of contraception if pregnancy is to be avoided while on rifampicin, and for 4–8 weeks after its withdrawal[22] (a UK Family Planning Association recommendation).

No failures due to rifampicin have been reported with the **progestogen-only contraceptives**, but their reliability in the presence of rifampicin is doubtful because rifampicin is known to increase the metabolism of progestogens, thereby reducing their efficacy.[20,23] The same risk is likely with **contraceptive implants**. The precautions suggested for the combined oral contraceptives should therefore be followed.

Direct information about the interaction between **combined oral contraceptives** and rifabutin seems to be limited to the reports cited, but it is supported by the well recognised enzyme inducing properties of rifabutin, so that it would now clearly be prudent for women on rifabutin to take the same precautions as with rifampicin, although the risks are lower because rifabutin is a less potent enzyme inducing agent. No cases of contraceptive failure appear so far to have been attributed to the use of rifabutin, nevertheless to be on the safe side both the makers and the CSM say that patients using these contraceptives and rifabutin should be advised to use other methods of contraception.[24,25] The risk of failure with the **progestogen-only contraceptives** and **contraceptive implants** would also seem to be similar and the same precautions would seem to be appropriate.

1. Reimers D, Jezek A. Rifampicin und andere antituberkulotika bei gleichzeitiger oraler kontrazeption. *Prax Pneumol* (1971) 25, 255.
2. Reimers D, Nocke-Finck L, Breuer H. Rifampicin causes a lowering in efficacy of oral contraceptives by influencing oestrogen excretion. Reports on Rifampicin: XXII International Tuberculosis Conference, Tokyo, September 1973, 87–9.
3. Reimers D, Nocke-Finck L, Breuer H. Rifampicin, 'pill' do not go well together. *JAMA* (1974) 227, 608.
4. Nocke-Finck L *et al.* Effects of rifampicin on menstrual cycle and estrogen excretion in patients taking oral contraceptives. *JAMA* (1973) 226, 378.
5. Kropp R. Rifampicin und ovulationshemmer. *Prax Pneumol* (1974) 28, 270–2.
6. Bessot J-C, Vandevenne A, Petitjean R, Burghard G. Effets opposés de la rifampicine et de l'isoniazide sur le métabolisme des contraceptifs oraux? *Nouv Presse Med* (1977) 6, 1568.
7. Hirsch A. Pilules endormies. *Nouv Presse Med* (1973) 2, 2957.
8. Piguet B, Muglioni JF, Chaline G. Contraception orale et rifampicine. *Nouv Presse Med* (1975) 4, 115–6.
9. Skolnik JL, Stoler BS, Katz DB, Anderson WH. Rifampicin, oral contraceptives and pregnancy. *JAMA* (1976) 236, 1382.
10. Gupta KC, Ali MY. Failure of oral contraceptive with rifampicin. *Med J Zambia* (1980/81) 15, 23.
11. Meyer BH, Müller FO, Wessels P. Lack of interaction between roxithromycin and an oral contraceptive. *Eur J Pharmacol* (1990) 183, 1031–2.
12. Meyer B, Müller F, Wessels P, Maree J. A model to detect interactions between roxithromycin and oral contraceptives. *Clin Pharmacol Ther* (1990) 47, 671–4.
13. Joshi JV, Joshi UM, Sankolli GM, Gupta K, Rao AP, Hazari K, Sheth UK, Saxena BN. A study of interaction of a low-dose combination oral contraceptive with anti-tubercular drugs. *Contraception* (1980) 21, 617–29.
14. Back DJ, Breckenridge AM, Crawford FE, MacIver M, Orme ML'E and Rowe PH. Interindividual variation and drug interactions with hormonal steroid contraceptives. *Drugs* (1981) 21, 46–61.
15. Barditch-Crovo P, Trapnell CB, Ette E, Zacur H, Flexner C. A pharmacokinetic and pharmacodynamic evaluation of the effect of rifampin and rifabutin on combination oral contraceptives. *Clin Pharmacol Ther* (1998) 63, 180.
16. Gupta KC, Joshi JV, Anklesaria PS, Shah RS, Satoskar RS. Plasma rifampicin levels during oral contraception. *J Assoc Physicians India* (1988) 36, 365–6.
17. LeBel M, Masson E, Guilbert E, Narang PK, Vallée F. Drug interaction with oral contraceptive (OC): rifabutin (FAB) versus rifampicin (FAM). *Clin Pharmacol Ther* (1998) 63, 161.
18. Bolt HM, Kappus H, Bolt M. Rifampicin and oral contraception. *Lancet* (1974) i, 1280–1.
19. Bolt HM, Kappus H, Bolt M. Effect of rifampicin treatment on the metabolism of oestradiol and 17α-ethynyloestradiol by human liver microsomes. *Eur J Clin Pharmacol* (1975) 8, 301–2.
20. Back DJ, Breckenridge AM, Crawford F, MacIver M, Orme ML'E, Park BK, Rowe PH, Smith E. The effect of rifampicin on norethisterone pharmacokinetics. *Eur J Clin Pharmacol* (1974) 15, 193–7.
21. Bolt HM, Bolt WH. Pharmacokinetics of mestranol in man in relation to its oestrogenic activity. *Eur J Clin Pharmacol* (1974) 7, 295–305.
22. Orme M, Back DJ. Oral contraceptive steroids – pharmacological issues of interest to the prescribing physician. *Adv Contracept* (1991) 7, 325–31.
23. McCann MF, Potter LS. Progestin-only contraception: a comprehensive review. *Contraception* (1994) 50, S1–S198.
24. Committee on Safety of Medicines (CSM)/Medicines Control Agency (MCA). Revised indication and drug interactions of rifabutin. *Current Problems* 1997, 23, 14.
25. Mycobutin (rifabutin). Pharmacia. Summary of product characteristics, July 1997.

Oral contraceptives + Ritonavir

Ritonavir has been found to reduce the serum levels of the ethinylestradiol (ethinyloestradiol) component of a combined oral contraceptive, but so far no cases of contraceptive failure appear to have been reported.

Clinical evidence, mechanism, importance and management

A study using a fixed combination oral contraceptive (**Demulen** – 50 micrograms **ethinylestradiol**, 1 mg **ethynodiol diacetate**) in 23 healthy women subjects found that 16 days of **ritonavir** (500 mg 12-hourly) decreased the AUC of the **ethinylestradiol** component by 41% and the maximum serum levels by 32%, probably because its metabolism by liver enzymes (glucuronosyl transferases) is increased.[1,2] This would be expected to reduce the efficacy and reliability of the contraceptive. However so far there appear to be no cases of contraceptive failure attributed to this interaction, but to avoid this risk and that of break-through bleeding the makers recommend that the dosage of **ethinylestradiol** should be increased or alternative methods of contraception considered.[3] Substitute a contraceptive preparation with a higher dose of **ethinylestradiol** or use an alternative non-hormonal form of contraception during and for one cycle after the **ritonavir** is stopped.

1. Ouellet D, Hsu A, Qian J, Cavanaugh J, Leonard J, Granneman GR. Effect of ritonavir on the pharmacokinetics of ethinyl estradiol in healthy female volunteers. 11th Int Conf AIDS (1996) Vancouver, 1, 88–9.
2. Ouellet D, Hsu A, Qian J, Locke CS, Eason CJ, Cavanaugh JH, Leonard JM, Granneman GR. Effect of ritonavir on the pharmacokinetics of ethinyl oestradiol in healthy female volunteers. *Br J Clin Pharmacol* (1998) 46, 111–16.
3. Norvir (ritonavir). Abbott Laboratories Ltd, Summary of product characteristics, January 2001.

Oral contraceptives + St John's wort (*Hypericum perforatum*)

Both breakthrough bleeding and oral contraceptive failure have been seen in women taking St John's wort. Two cases of the failure of emergency hormonal contraception attributed to the use of St John's wort have also been reported.

Clinical evidence

(a) Oral contraceptive failure

The Adverse Drug Reactions Database of the Swedish Medical Products Agency (MPA) has on record 2 cases of pregnancy due to oral contraceptive failure attributed to the use of products containing **St John's wort**.[1] This follows an earlier report from the Swedish MPA of 8 cases of intermenstrual bleeding in women aged 23 to 31 taking long term oral contraceptives when **St John's wort** was added. It occurred within about a week in five of the cases, and was known to have resolved in three cases when the **St John's wort** was stopped.[2] The Committee on the Safety of Medicines (CSM) in the UK has recorded a further 7 cases of pregnancy in women taking **St John's wort** and oral contraceptives in the 2-year period from February 2000 to February 2002.[3] Another very brief report describes 3 women who had had no problems while taking oral contraceptives (**ethinyloestradiol** 0.03 mg + **desogestrel** 0.15 mg) until break-through bleeding developed in one of them a week after starting to take **St John's wort**. In the other 2 it developed after taking **St John's wort** for 2 months.[4] The CSM has received 4 yellow card reports of interactions between oral contraceptives and **St John's wort**.[5]

(b) Emergency hormonal contraceptive failure

The CSM in the UK has received reports of 2 women who became pregnant while taking **St John's wort** and emergency hormonal contraception. One of them was also taking an oral contraceptive.[3]

Mechanism

It is believed that St John's wort can increase (induce) the metabolism by cytochrome P450 of the contraceptive steroids, thereby reducing their serum levels and their effects.[2,4,6] This can lead to breakthrough bleeding and, in some cases, total contraceptive failure. This is consistent with the way St John's wort appears to lower the serum levels of some other drugs.

Importance and management

Information appears to be limited to these reports but the oral contraceptive/St John's wort interaction appears to be established. Its incidence is not known but the evidence so far suggests that breakthrough bleeding and pregnancy resulting from this interaction are uncommon. However, since it is not known who is particularly likely to be at risk, women taking oral contraceptives should either avoid St John's wort (the recommendation of the CSM in the UK) or they should use an additional form of contraception.

Only 2 cases of emergency hormonal contraceptive failure attributed to an interaction with St John's wort have so far been reported. If this is, as believed, due to enzyme induction by the St John's wort (see 'Mechanism' above), then an increase in the dosage of the emergency hormonal contraceptive should be considered.

Although the considerable popularity of St John's wort worldwide is fairly recent, it is currently the most widely antidepressant in use in Germany and as a herb has been used for very many years in Germany and Austria. Yet there seems to be no published evidence that oral contraceptive failure in those countries is more frequent there than anywhere else. This would seem to confirm either that this interaction is very uncommon, or perhaps that it has failed to be identified as a possible cause?

1. Swedish Medical Products Agency. St John's wort may influence other medication. Available at http://www3.mpa.se/ie_engindex.html (Accessed 15/08/2002).

2. Qun-Ying Yue, Bergquist C, Gerdén B. Safety of St John's wort (Hypericum perforatum). *Lancet* (2000) 355, 576-7.

3. Committee on Safety of Medicines. Personal communication, February 15th, 2002.

4. Bon S, Hartmann K, Kubn M. Johanniskraut: Ein Enzyminduktor ? *Schweiz Apothekerzeitung* (1999) 16, 535-6.

5. Committee on Safety of Medicines. Personal communication, March 2000.

6. Committee on Safety of Medicines. Message from Professor A Breckenridge (Chairman of CSM) and Fact Sheet for Health Care Professionals, 29th February 2000.

Oral contraceptives + Tiagabine

Tiagabine appears not to interact with combined oral contraceptives.

Clinical evidence, mechanism, importance and management

A study in 10 normal women taking non-sequential combined oral contraceptives (30 micrograms **ethinylestradiol** (**ethinyloestradiol**) + 150 micrograms **levonorgestrel** or **desogestrel**) found that when 2 mg **tiagabine** four times daily was given concurrently from day 24 of the first cycle to day 7 of the next cycle, there was no evidence that the suppression of ovulation by the contraceptive was altered in any way. No significant changes in the plasma concentrations of progesterone, follicle stimulating hormone, luteinising hormone, **ethinylestradiol**, **levonorgestrel** or **desogestrel** were seen between the first and second cycles, and progesterone levels remained in the non-ovulatory range (13 nmol/l).[1] There would appear to be no reason for avoiding concurrent use.

1. Mengel HB, Houston A, Back DJ. An evaluation of the interaction between tiagabine and oral contraceptives in female volunteers. *J Pharm Med* (1994) 4, 141–50.

Oral contraceptives + Tobacco smoking

The risk of thromboembolic disease in women on oral contraceptives is increased if they smoke.

Clinical evidence, mechanism, importance and management

A study in women in the 40–41 age group on oral contraceptives who **smoked** showed that they had a lower level of high-density lipoprotein in their serum than women who neither **smoked** nor took the pill.[1] The significance of this finding is that low levels are a major risk factor in the development of coronary heart disease and related thrombotic diseases. This is borne out by epidemiological studies which show that the incidence of thromboembolic diseases in women on the pill increases both with age and if the subjects **smoke**.[2,3] For example, one study found a relative risk ("rate ratio") of non-fatal myocardial infarction in women on the pill of 4.5 in non-smokers and 39 for **heavy smokers**.[4] Another study found a relative risk of subarachnoid haemorrhage in women on the pill of 6.5 for non-smokers and 22.0 for **smokers**.[5] Just another good reason why smoking should be discouraged.

1. Arntzenius AC, van Gent CM, van der Voort H, Stegerhoek C, Styblo K. Reduced high-density lipoprotein in women aged 40–41 using oral contraceptives. *Lancet* (1978) i, 1221–3.

2. Fredriksen H, Ravenholt RT. Thromboembolism, oral contraceptives, and cigarettes. *Public Health Rep* (1970) 85, 197–205.

3. Collaborative Group for the study of stroke in young women. *JAMA* (1975) 231, 718.

4. Shapiro S, Slone D, Rosenberg L, Kaufman DW. Oral-contraceptive use in relation to myocardial infarction. *Lancet* (1979) 1, 743–7.

5. Petitti DB, Wingerd J. Use of oral contraceptives, cigarette smoking, and risk of subarachnoid haemorrhage. *Lancet* (1978) 2, 234–6.

Oral contraceptives + Topiramate

The serum levels of ethinylestradiol (ethinyloestradiol) are reduced by topiramate, increasing the risk of break-through bleeding in women taking combined oral contraceptives. It is

suggested therefore that oral contraceptives with a higher dosage of oestrogen should be used. It is not thought that contraceptive failure is likely to occur.

Clinical evidence

Twelve epileptic women stabilised on sodium valproate and taking a **combined oral contraceptive (ethinylestradiol (ethinyloestradiol) 35 micrograms + norethisterone (norethindrone)** 1 mg) were additionally given three escalating doses of **topiramate** (200, 400, 800 mg daily). The serum levels of the **norethisterone** remained unchanged, but the mean serum levels of the **ethinylestradiol** fell by 18%, 21% and 30% respectively.[1]

Mechanism

Not understood. A weak induction by topiramate of enzymes in the liver is suggested which increases the metabolism of the ethinylestradiol.[2]

Importance and management

An established interaction but supported by limited evidence. The authors of this report say that ". . . this modest interaction is not likely significantly to alter contraceptive efficacy" based on measurements of progestogen levels which suggested that no ovulation occurred or was likely to occur.[1] However, they advise the use of a combined oral contraceptive containing 50 micrograms ethinylestradiol (ethinyloestradiol) to reduce the risk of break-through bleeding,[1,2] a recommendation endorsed by the makers of topiramate.[3] The makers also say that patients should be told to report any changes in their bleeding patterns.[3] There are no reports of contraceptive failure caused by topiramate and the makers say that in a clinical trial no failures occurred in 52 patients who received topiramate for a total of 13.3 patient-years.[3]

1. Doose DR, Rosenfeld WE, Schaefer P, Walker SA, Nayak RK. Evaluation of the potential pharmacokinetic interaction between topiramate and the oral contraceptive combination, norethindrone/ethinyloestradiol. *J Clin Pharmacol* (1994) 34, 1031.
2. Rosenfeld WE, Doose DR, Walker SA, Nayak RK. Effect of topiramate on the pharmacokinetics of an oral contraceptive containing norethindrone and ethinyl estradiol in patients with epilepsy. *Epilepsia* (1997) 38, 317–23.
3. Topamax (topiramate). Janssen-Cilag Ltd. Summary of product characteristics, September 2001.

Oral contraceptives + Troleandomycin (Triacetyloleandomycin)

Severe pruritus and jaundice have been observed in women taking oral contraceptives shortly after starting treatment with troleandomycin (triacetyloleandomycin).

Clinical evidence

A report describes 10 cases of cholestatic jaundice and pruritus in women taking oral contraceptives and **troleandomycin (triacetyloleandomycin)**. All had been using the contraceptive for 7–48 months and were given the antibacterial in 250 or 500 mg doses four times a day. The pruritus was intense, lasting 2–24 days, and preceded the jaundice which, in 8 of the patients, persisted for over a month.[1]

There are numerous other reports of this adverse reaction,[2-12] one of which describes 24 cases.[5,6] The adverse reactions (fatigue, anorexia, severe itching, jaundice) can begin very rapidly, sometimes even within two days, and may last up to 14 weeks.[12]

Mechanism

Uncertain. Hepatotoxicity has been associated with the use of both types of drug, but it is not common. The reaction suggests that their damaging effects on the liver may be additive or supra-additive.

Importance and management

A well established, well documented and clinically important interaction. The incidence is unknown. Concurrent use should be avoided.

1. Miguet JP, Monange C, Vuitton D, Allemand H, Hirsch JP, Carayon P, Gisselbrecht H. Ictère cholestatique survenu après administration de triacétyloléandomycine: interférence avec les contraceptifs oraux? Dix observations. *Nouv Presse Med* (1978) 7, 4304.
2. Perol R, Hincky J, Desnos M. Hèpatites cholestatiques lors de la prise de troléandomycine chez deux femmes prenant des estrogènes. *Nouv Presse Med* (1978) 7, 4302.
3. Goldfain D, Cauveinc L, Guillan J, Verudron J. Ictère cholestatique chez des femmes prenant simultanément de la triacétyloléandomycine et des contraceptifs oraux. *Nouv Presse Med* (1979) 8, 1099.
4. Rollux R, Plottin F, Mingat J, Bessard G. Ictère apres association estroprogestatif-troléandomycine. Trois observations. *Nouv Presse Med* (1979) 8, 1694.
5. Miguet J-P, Vuitton D, Pessayre D, Allemand H, Metreau J-M, Poupon R, Capron J-P, Blanc F. Jaundice from troleandomycin and oral contraceptives. *Ann Intern Med* (1980) 92, 434.
6. Miguet J-P, Vuitton D, Allemand H, Pessayre D, Monange C, Hirsch J-P, Metreau J-M, Poupon R, Capron J-P, Blanc F. Une épidémie d'ictères due a l'association troléandomycine – contraceptifs oraux. *Gastroenterol Clin Biol* (1980) 4, 420–4.
7. Haber I, Hubens H. Cholestatic jaundice after triacetyloleandomycin and oral contraceptives. *Acta Gastroenterol Belg* (1980) 43, 475–82.
8. Claudel S, Euvrard P, Bory R, Chavaillon A, Paliard P. Cholestase intra-hépatique après association triacétyloléandomycine-estroprogestatif. *Nouv Presse Med* (1979) 8, 1182.
9. Descotes J, Evreux J Cl, Foyatier N, Gaumer R, Girard D, Savoye B, Trois nouvelles observations d'ictère après estroprogestatifs et troléandomycine. *Nouv Presse Med* (1979) 8, 1182–3.
10. Dellas JA, Hugues FC, Roussel G, Marche J. Contraception orale et troléandomycine. Un nouveau cas d'ictère. *Therapie* (1982) 37, 443–6.
11. Girard D, Pillon M, Bel A, Petigny A, Savoye B. Hepatite au decours d'un traitment a la triacetyloleandomycine chez les jeunes femmes sous estro-progestatifs. *Lyon Mediterr Med Med Sud Est* (1980) 16, 2335–44.
12. Fevery J, Van Steenbergen W, Desmet V, Deruyttere M, De Groote J. Severe intrahepatic cholestasis due to the combined intake of oral contraceptives and triacetyloleandomycin. *Acta Clin Belg* (1983) 38, 242–5.

Oral contraceptives + Vigabatrin

Vigabatrin appears not to interact with combined oral contraceptives.

Clinical evidence, mechanism, importance and management

A double-blind placebo-controlled study in 13 normal women showed that while taking 3 g **vigabatrin** daily, the single dose pharmacokinetics of an oral contraceptive containing 30 micrograms **ethinylestradiol (ethinyloestradiol)** and 150 micrograms **levonorgestrel** (*Ovranet*), given on day 21, were not statistically changed, although two of the women showed a 39% and a 50% fall in the AUC of **ethinylestradiol**. The clearance and half-life of **antipyrine (phenazone)** (a marker of enzyme induction) were also found to be unchanged, indicating that **vigabatrin** does not significantly stimulate the activity of the liver enzymes (cytochrome P450 isoenzyme CYP3A) that are concerned with the metabolism of the two components of the oral contraceptive.[1]

This study would seem to confirm the lack of reports of an **oral contraceptive/vigabatrin** interaction, however the authors of the report introduce a small note of caution because it is not clear whether the reduced **ethinylestradiol** AUCs seen in two of the women resulted from an interaction or were simply normal individual variations.[1]

1. Bartoli A, Gatti G, Cipolla G, Barzaghi N, Veliz G, Fattore C, Mumford J, Perucca E. A double-blind, placebo-controlled study on the effect of vigabatrin on in vivo parameters of hepatic microsomal enzyme induction and on the kinetics of steroid oral contraceptives in healthy female volunteers. *Epilepsia* (1997) 38, 702–7.

Oral contraceptives + Vitamins

The oral contraceptives are reported to raise serum levels of retinol (vitamin A) and lower levels of ascorbic acid, cyanocobalamin, folic acid and pyridoxine. There is conflicting evi-

dence about whether ascorbic acid does or does not raise serum ethinylestradiol (ethinyloestradiol) levels. Pyridoxine may relieve depression in women on oral contraceptives.

Clinical evidence

(a) Effects of oral contraceptives on vitamins

There is evidence that oral contraceptives can cause a biochemical deficiency of several vitamins, but clinical deficiency does not necessarily manifest itself. Serum levels of **cyanocobalamin** can be lowered,[1] **folate** deficiency with anaemia can occur,[2,3] and reduced levels of **ascorbic acid**[3-5] and **pyridoxine**[6,7] have been described. Treatment of **pyridoxine** deficiency has been shown to improve the mood of depressed women on oral contraceptives.[8] Raised levels of **retinol (vitamin A)** have also been reported.[9] These changes in vitamin requirements induced by the oral contraceptives have been reviewed in detail.[10]

(b) Effects of vitamins on oral contraceptives

One study found that 1 g **ascorbic acid** substantially raised serum **ethinylestradiol (ethinyloestradiol)** levels (+48% measured at 24 h) in women taking oral contraceptives,[11] and a single case report describes a woman on **Logynon** who experienced heavy break-through bleeding within 2–3 days of stopping her self-administered 1 g daily dose of **ascorbic acid**.[11] Another report found no significant changes in **ethinylestradiol** serum levels in women taking an oral contraceptive and given 1 g **ascorbic acid**.[12] Yet another report paradoxically attributes contraceptive failure to **ascorbic acid** and **multivitamins**.[13]

Mechanism

Not established.

Importance and management

From the point of view of reliability, there seems to be little reason for avoiding the concurrent use of oral contraceptives and vitamins (although there is one isolated and unconfirmed case involving vitamin C and multivitamins[13]) In fact routine prophylactic treatment with vitamins in women on oral contraceptives has been advised by some.[14] However, this has been questioned by others[15,16] because an increased intake of some vitamins in some circumstances might be harmful, for example, in areas of the world where protein malnutrition is rife, a pyridoxine supplement might lead to an undesirable increase in amino-acid catabolism in those on a low daily intake of protein.[15] One author's comment on the indiscriminate supplementation of the diet with multivitamin preparations in women on oral contraceptives is that it can hardly be justified.[16]

1. Wertalik LF, Metz EN, LoBuglio AF, Balcerzak SP. Decreased serum B$_{12}$ levels with oral contraceptive use. *JAMA* (1972) 221, 1371.
2. Streiff RR. Folate deficiency and oral contraceptives. *JAMA* (1970) 214, 105.
3. Meguid MM, Loebl WY. Megaloblastic anaemia associated with the oral contraceptive pill. *Postgrad Med J* (1974) 60, 470.
4. Harris AB, Pillay M, Hussein S. Vitamins and oral contraceptives. *Lancet* (1975) ii, 82.
5. Briggs M, Briggs M. Vitamin C requirements and oral contraceptives. *Nature* (1972) 238, 277.
6. Bennick HJTC, Schreurs WHP. Disturbance of tryptophan metabolism and its correction during hormonal contraception. *Contraception* (1974) 9, 347–56.
7. Doberenz AR, van Miller JP, Green JR, Beaton JR. Vitamin B6 depletion in women using oral contraceptives as determined by erythrocyte glutamic-pyruvic transaminase activities. *Proc Soc Exp Biol Med* (1971) 137, 1100.
8. Adams PW, Wynn V, Seed M, Foklhard J. Vitamin B6, depression and oral contraception. *Lancet* (1974) ii, 515.
9. Wild J, Schorah CJ, Smithells RW. Vitamin A, pregnancy, and oral contraceptives. *BMJ* (1974) 1, 57–9.
10. Larsson-Cohn U. Oral contraceptives and vitamins: a review. *Am J Obstet Gynecol* (1975) 121, 84–90.
11. Morris JC, Beeley L, Ballantine N. Interaction of ethinyloestradiol with ascorbic acid in man. *BMJ* (1981) 283, 503.
12. Zamah NM, Hümpel M, Kuhnz W, Louton T, Rafferty J, Back DJ. Absence of an effect of high vitamin C dosage on the systemic availability of ethinyl oestradiol in women using a combination oral contraceptive. *Contraception* (1993) 48, 377–91.
13. DeSano EA, Hurley SC. Possible interactions of antihistamines and antibiotics with oral contraceptive effectiveness. *Fertil Steril* (1982) 37, 853–4.
14. Briggs M, Briggs M. Oral contraceptives and vitamin requirements. *Med J Aust* (1975) 1, 407.
15. Adams PW, Wynn V, Rose DP, Folkhard J, Seed M, Strong R. Effect of pyridoxine hydrochloride (vitamin B6) upon depression associated with oral contraception. *Lancet* (1973) i, 897.
16. Back DJ, Breckenridge AM, MacIver M, Orme ML'E, Purba H, Rowe PH. Interaction of ethinyloestradiol with ascorbic acid in man. *BMJ* (1981) 282, 1516.

Tibolone + Miscellaneous drugs

On theoretical grounds the makers of tibolone suggest that it may possibly increase the effects of anticoagulants and reduce the effects of hypoglycaemic agents. They also say that the effects of tibolone may be reduced by enzyme inducing anticonvulsants and rifampicin.

Clinical evidence, mechanism, importance and management

(a) Anticoagulants

A study in 60 post-menopausal women given 2.5 mg tibolone daily for 12 weeks found no adverse effects on coagulation (prothrombin time, clotting factors VII, VIII, X) or any of the other parameters measured.[1] However, the makers say[2] that "the sensitivity of patients to **anticoagulants** may be enhanced during *Livial* (tibolone) therapy because of enhanced blood fibrinolytic activity (lower fibrinogen levels, higher antithrombin III, plasminogen and fibrin plate fibrinolytic activity values)." There seem to be no studies or case reports about concurrent use, but until more is known it would seem prudent to monitor the effects if tibolone is added to established **anticoagulant** treatment.

(b) Hypoglycaemic agents

A 1994 report from NV Organon (the makers of tibolone) says that on their adverse drug event database they only have three cases of diabetes occurring during the use of **tibolone**, and three cases of aggravation of diabetes during its use.[3] This report concludes by saying that ". . . given the available data NV Organon sees little reason to postulate a causal role of *Livial* (tibolone) use in the occurrence of aggravation of maturity onset diabetes." One case of diabetes is reported elsewhere.[4] A metabolic study in 10 non-insulin dependent diabetes given 2.5 mg tibolone daily and treated with diet and oral **hypoglycaemic agents** (not named) says that this treatment remained unchanged during the two-month study, implying that no changes were needed.[5] Even so, the makers of tibolone say in their datasheet[2] that ". . . patients should be monitored with impaired carbohydrate metabolism, since *Livial* may diminish glucose tolerance and increase the need for **insulin** or other **antidiabetic drugs**." This seems to be a simple prudent precaution until the safety of tibolone in diabetics is well established.

(c) Other drugs

The makers say[2] that "enzyme inducing compounds such as **barbiturates, carbamazepine, hydantoins [e.g. phenytoin]**, and **rifampicin** may enhance the metabolism of tibolone and thus decrease its therapeutic effect." So far this seems to be only a reasonable theoretical prediction, nevertheless it would be prudent to monitor concurrent use.

1. Cortes-Prieto J. Coagulation and fibrinolysis in post-menopausal women treated with Org OD 14. *Maturitas* (1987) (Suppl 1), 67–72.
2. Livial (tibolone), Organon Laboratories Ltd. Summary of product characteristics, April 1999.
3. Atsma WJ. Is Livial diabetogenic? *Maturitas* (1994) 19, 239–40.
4. Konstantopoulos K, Adamides S. A case of diabetes following tibolone therapy. *Maturitas* (1994) 19, 77–78.
5. Cox A, Feher MD, Levy A, Mayne PD, Lant AF. Short-term metabolic effects of tibolone in post-menopausal women with non-insulin dependent diabetes mellitus. *Br J Clin Pharmacol* (1994) 37, 510–511P.

13

Cytotoxic drug interactions

The cytotoxic drugs (antineoplastics, cytostatics) are used in the treatment of malignant disease in conjunction with radiotherapy, surgery and immunosuppressants. They also find application in the treatment of rheumatoid arthritis, skin conditions such as psoriasis, and a few are used with other immunosuppressant drugs (ciclosporin, corticosteroids) to prevent transplant rejection. These other immunosuppressant drugs are dealt with in Chapter 16. Of all the drugs discussed in this book, the cytotoxic drugs are amongst the most toxic and have a low therapeutic index. This means that a quite small increase in their activity can lead to the development of serious and life-threatening toxicity. A list of the cytotoxic

agents which are featured in this chapter appears in Table 13.1. Unlike most of the other interaction monographs in this book, some of the information on the cytotoxic drugs is derived from animal experiments and *in vitro* studies so that confirmation of their clinical relevance is still needed. The reason for including this data is that the cytotoxic drugs as a group do not lend themselves readily to the kind of clinical studies which can be undertaken with many other drugs, and there would seem to be justification in this instance for including indirect evidence of this kind. The aim is not to make definite predictions, but to warn users of the interaction possibilities.

Table 13.1 Cytotoxic and other drugs used in the treatment of cancer

Generic names	Proprietary names
Aclarubicin (Aclacinomycin A)	Aclacin, Aclaplastin
Adriamycin (see Doxorubicin)	
Altretamine (Hexamethylmelamine)	Hexalen, Hexastat
9-Aminocamptothecin	
Aminoglutethimide	Cytadren, Orimeten, Orimetene, Rodazol
Anastrozole	Arimidex
Azathioprine	Azafalk, Azahexal, Azamun, Azapress, Azatrilem, Azopi, Azopine, Immunoprin, Imunen, Imuprin, Imuran, Imurek, Imurel, Thioprine, Zytrim
Bleomycin	Blanoxan, Blenoxane, Bleo, Bleolem, Bleo-cell, Bleo-S, Blio
Busulfan (Busulphan)	Busulfex, Mielucin, Misulban, Myleran
Cactinomycin (Actinomycin C)	
Carboplatin	Blastocarb, Boplatex, B-Platin, Carboplat, Carbosin, Carbosol, Ercar, Ifacap, Kemocarb, Nealorin, Novoplatinum, Paraplatin, Paraplatine, Platicarb, Platinwas, Ribocarbo
Carmofur	Mirafur
Carmustine (BCNU)	Becenun, BiCNU, Carmubris, Gliadel, Nitrourean, Nitrumon
Chlorambucil	Chloraminophene, Leukeran, Linfolysin
Chlormethine (Mustine)	Caryolysine, Mustargen, Onco-Cloramin
Chlorozotocin	
Cisplatin (CDDP)	Abiplatin, Blastolem, Cishexal, Cisplatex, Cisplatyl, Citoplatino, Citosin, Faulplatin, Kemoplat, Lederplatin, Neoplatin, Noveldexis, Placis, Platamine, Platiblastin, Platinex, Platinol, Platiran, Platistil, Platistin, Platistine, Platosin, Pronto Platamine, Unistin
Colaspase (Asparaginase)	Elspar, Erwinase, Kidrolase, Laspar, Leunase, Paronal
Cyclophosphamide	Alkyloxan, Carloxan, Ciclosmida, Cyclan, Cycloblastin, Cycloblastine, Cyclostin, Cyclo-cell, Cytophosphan, Cytoxan, Endoxan, Endoxana, Genoxal, Genuxal, Ledoxina, Neosar, Procytox, Sendoxan
Cytarabine (Cytosine arabinoside)	Alexan, Arabine, Aracytin, Aracytine, ARA-cell, Citab, Citaloxan, Cylocide, Cytosar, Cytovis, DepoCyt, Erpalfa, Ifarab, Laracit, Medsara, Novutrax, Tabine, Udicil
Dacarbazine	Dacarb, Dacarbaziba, Dacatic, Deticene, Detilem, Detimedac, DTIC, DTIC-Dome, Fauldetic, Ifadac
Dactinomycin (Actinomycin D)	Ac-De, Bioact-D, Cosmegen

Table 13.1 Cytotoxic and other drugs used in the treatment of cancer *(continued)*

Generic names	Proprietary names
Daunorubicin (Daunomycin, Rubidomycin)	Cerubidin, Cerubidine, Daunoblastin, Daunoblastina, Daunocin, DaunoXome, Rubilem
Docetaxel	Taxotere
Doxorubicin (Adriamycin)	Adriblastin, Adriblastina, Adriblastine, Adrim, Adrimedac, Caelyx, Doxil, Doxolem, Doxorubin, DOXO-cell, Farmiblastina, Fauldoxo, Ifadox, Myocet, Ribodoxo-L, Rubex
Epirubicin	Ellence, Epilem, Farmorubicin, Farmorubicina, Farmorubicine, Pharmorubicin, Rubina
Estramustine	Cellmustin, Emcyt, Estracyt, Multosin, Prostamustin
Etoposide	Celltop, Eposid, Eposido, Eposin, ETO CS, Etomedac, Etopofos, Etopophos, Etopos, Etopul, Eto-Gry, Exitop, Fytosid, Kenazol, Lastet, Nexvep, Riboposid, Toposar, Vepesid, Vepeside
Fluorouracil (5-FU)	Actino-Hermal, Adrucil, Carac, Cinkef-U, Efudex, Efudix, Fivoflu, Fluoroplex, Flurablastin, Fluracedyl, Fluroblastin, Fluroblastine, Flurox, Ifacil, O-fluor, Ribofluor, Utora
Filgrastim (G-CSF)	Gran, Granulen, Granulokine, Neupogen
Hydroxycarbamide (Hydroxyurea)	Droxia, Hydrea, Litalir, Onco-Carbide, Syrea
Idarubicin	Idamycin, Idaralem, Zavedos
Ifosfamide	Holoxan, Holoxane, Ifex, Ifolem, Ifomida, Ifos, Ifoxan, IFO-cell, Mitoxana, Tronoxal
Lenograstim (G-CSF)	Euprotin, Granocyte, Myelostim, Neutrogin
Letrozole	Femar, Femara
Lomustine (CCNU)	Belustine, CCNU, Cecenu, CeeNU, Citostal, Prava
Melphalan	Alkeran
Mercaptopurine	Ismipur, Mercaptina, Puri-Nethol
Methotrexate (Amethopterin)	Abitrexate, Emthexat, Emthexate, Farmitrexat, Fauldexato , Ifamet, Lantarel, Ledertrexate, Maxtrex, Medsatrexate, Metex, Methoblastin, Methoblastine, Metrotex, MTX, Novatrex, O-trexat, Rheumatrex, Trexall, Trexan, Trixilem, Unitrexate
Misonidazole	
Mitomycin (Mitomycin C)	Ametycine, Ifamit, Mitocin, Mitocin-C, Mitolem, Mitostat, Mito-medac, Mixandex, Mutamycin, Mutamycine
Mitotane	Lisodren, Lysodren
Paclitaxel	Anzatax, Asotax, BrisTaxol, Ifaxol, Onxol, Paclitax, Parexel, Paxel, Praxel, Taclipaxol, Taxol
Plicamycin (Mithramycin)	Mithracin, Mithracine
Procarbazine	Matulane, Natulan, Natulanar
Streptozocin (Streptozotocin)	Zanosar
Tamoxifen	Apo-Tamox, Bilem, Clonoxifen, Cryoxifeno, Ebefen, Estroxyn, Genox, Jenoxifen, Kessar, Ledertam, Neophedan, Nolgen, Nolvadex, Nourytam, Novofen, Oncotam, Oxeprax, Ralsifen-X, Soltamox, Tadex, Tamax, Tamec, Tamexin, Tamifen, Tamizam, Tamobeta, Tamofen, Tamofene, Tamokadin, Tamooex, Tamophar, Tamoplex, Tamosin, Tamox, Tamoxan, Tamoxasta, Tamoxen, Tamoxi, Tamoxigenat, Tamoximerck, Tamoxin, Tamoxistad, Taxofen, Taxus, Tecnotax, Tuosomin, Zemide, Zitazonium
Tegafur	Citofur, Ftoral, Ftoralon, Futraful, Utefos
Teniposide	VM 26, Vumon
Thiotepa	Ledertepa, Onco Tiotepa, Thioplex
Tioguanine (Thioguanine)	Lanvis
Toremifene	Fareston
Vinblastine	Blastovin, Cellblastin, Ifabla, Lemblastine, Solblastin, Velban, Velbe
Vincristine	Cellcristin, Citomid, Farmistin, Faulcris, Ifavin, Oncovin, Pericristine, Vincasar PFS, Vincrisul, Vinracine
Vindesine	Eldisin, Eldisine, Enison, Gesidine

Aclarubicin + Cytotoxic drugs

The bone marrow depressant effects of aclarubicin can be increased by previous treatment with nitrosoureas or mitomycin. Aclarubicin appears not to interact with cyclophosphamide, cytarabine, enocitabine (behenoyl cytarabine), 5-fluorouracil, 6-mercaptopurine, 6-tioguanine or vincristine.

Clinical evidence, mechanism, importance and management

Myelosuppression is among the adverse effects of aclarubicin (aclacinomycin A). The makers warn that the concurrent use of other drugs with similar myelosuppressant actions may be expected to have additive effects and dosage reductions should be considered.[1] Prior treatment with **nitrosoureas** (not specifically named) or **mitomycin** has been shown to increase the severity of the myelosuppression.[2,3]

Aclarubicin has been given in combination with **cyclophosphamide, cytarabine, enocitabine (behenoyl cytarabine), 5-fluorouracil, 6-mercaptopurine, 6-tioguanine** or **vincristine** without signs of interaction.[1]

1. Aclarubicin. Medac GmbH. Summary of product characteristics, March 1998.
2. Van Echo DA, Whitacre MY, Aisner J, Applefeld MM, Wiernik PH. Phase I trial of aclacinomycin A. *Cancer Treat Rep* (1982) 66, 1127–32.
3. Bedikian AY, Karlin D, Stroehlein J, Valdivieso M, Korinek J, Bodey G. Phase II evaluation of aclacinomycin A (ACM-A, NSC208734) in patients with metastatic colorectal cancer. *Am J Clin Oncol (CCT)* (1983) 6, 187–190.

Altretamine (Hexamethylmelamine) + Antidepressants

Severe orthostatic hypotension has been described in patients concurrently treated with altretamine and either phenelzine, amitriptyline or imipramine.

Clinical evidence, mechanism, importance and management

Four patients experienced very severe orthostatic hypotension (described by the authors as potentially life-threatening) when concurrently treated with altretamine 150 to 250 mg/m^2 and either daily **phenelzine** 60 mg, **amitriptyline** 50 mg or **imipramine** 50 to 150 mg.[1] They experienced incapacitating dizziness, severe lightheadedness and/or fainting within a few days of taking both drugs concurrently. Standing blood pressures as low as 50/30 and 60/40 mmHg were recorded. The reasons are not known. One of the patients had no problems when **imipramine** was replaced by **nortriptyline** 50 mg daily. One other patient who had also taken altretamine with antidepressants reported dizziness while another noted nonspecific discomfort. The incidence of this interaction is unknown but it is clear that the concurrent use of these drugs should be closely monitored.

1. Bruckner HW, Schleifer SJ. Orthostatic hypotension as a complication of hexamethylmelamine antidepressant interaction. *Cancer Treat Rep* (1983) 67, 516.

9-Aminocamptothecin + Anticonvulsants

Anticonvulsants can lower the serum levels of 9-aminocamptothecin.

Clinical evidence, mechanism, importance and management

A study in 59 patients with glioblastoma multiforme or recurrent high grade astrocytomas found that the steady-state plasma levels of 9-aminocamptothecin were reduced to about one third in 29 of the pa-

tients concurrently taking anticonvulsants (**carbamazepine, phenobarbital, phenytoin, sodium valproate**). The incidence of myelosuppression was increased in those not taking anticonvulsants.[1] The reason for the reduced 9-aminocamptothecin levels is not known, but it seems likely that it was due to the enzyme inducing activity of the anticonvulsants. These results suggest that higher than usual doses of 9-aminocamptothecin are possibly needed in the presence of these anticonvulsants.

1. Grossman SA, Hochberg F, Fisher J, Chen T-L, Kim L, Gregory R, Grochow LB, Piantadosi S. Increased 9-aminocamptothecin dose requirements in patients on anticonvulsants. *Cancer Chemother Pharmacol* (1998) 42, 118–26.

Aminoglutethimide + Bendroflumethiazide (Bendrofluazide)

A single case report describes the severe loss of sodium in a patient after 10 months treatment with both drugs.

Clinical evidence, mechanism, importance and management

A woman who, for several years, had been taking four tablets daily of **bendroflumethiazide (bendrofluazide)** 2.5 mg and **potassium chloride** 578 mg for hypertension and mild cardiac incompensation, was additionally treated with aminoglutethimide, 1 g daily, and hydrocortisone, 60 mg daily, for breast cancer. After 10 months treatment she was hospitalised with severe hyponatraemia due, apparently, to the combined inhibitory effects of the aminoglutethimide on aldosterone production (which normally retains sodium in the body) and the diuretic. The serum sodium levels were subsequently kept normal by the addition of fludrocortisone (100 micrograms daily).[1]

1. Bork E, Hansen M. Severe hyponatremia following simultaneous administration of aminoglutethimide and diuretics. *Cancer Treat Rep* (1986) 70, 689–90.

Anastrozole + Miscellaneous drugs

Anastrozole should not be given with oestrogens, but it does not appear to interact with tamoxifen, aspirin, cimetidine, digoxin, oral hypoglycaemics or warfarin. It also appears not have a general effect on cytochrome P450 enzymes so that it is unlikely to interact with drugs which are affected by enzyme inducers or inhibitors.

Clinical evidence, mechanism, importance and management

A reduction in the circulating levels of estradiol (oestradiol) can have a beneficial effect on the progression of hormone-dependent breast cancer. Anastrozole achieves this by specifically inhibiting aromatase, a cytochrome P450 enzyme which is concerned with the metabolic production of estrone (oestrone) from androstenedione, and of estradiol from testosterone. Estrone is subsequently converted into estradiol. It is therefore important not to give **oestrogen-containing therapies** to women on anastrozole because that would raise the levels of circulating oestrogens and oppose the effects of anastrozole.[1] A double-blind, placebo-controlled study in 34 women with breast cancer on **tamoxifen** 20 mg daily for at least 10 weeks found that concurrent use of anastrozole 1 mg daily for 28 days did not affect the pharmacokinetics of **tamoxifen**. The oestradiol suppressant effects of anastrozole were not affected by **tamoxifen**.[2] Clinical studies with **cimetidine** have shown that it does not affect the pharmacokinetics of anastrozole[3] which suggests that anastrozole is unlikely to be affected by other drugs which inhibit cytochrome P450. Other clinical studies with **antipyrine (phenazone)** and anastrozole also showed no interaction,[4] so that it is unlikely to interact with those drugs which are known to be affected by enzyme inducers and inhibitors. The makers also say that in controlled clinical trials there was no evidence of any interactions between anastrozole and **aspirin, digoxin, oral hypogly-caemic agents** (not specifically named).[1] A randomised, double-blind, placebo-controlled, two-way crossover study in 16 healthy subjects also found that anastrozole (7 mg loading dose followed by 1 mg daily for a further 10 days) had no effect on the pharmacokinetics or pharmacodynamics of **warfarin**.[5]

1. Arimidex (Anastrozole). AstraZeneca. Summary of product characteristics, October 2001.
2. Dowsett M, Tobias JS, Howell A, Blackman GM, Welch H, King N, Ponzone R, Von Euler M, Baum M. The effect of anastrozole, on the pharmacokinetics of tamoxifen in postmenopausal women with early breast cancer. *Br J Cancer* (1999) 79, 311–15.
3. Zeneca. Effect of cimetidine on anastrozole pharmacokinetics. Data on file (1995).
4. Zeneca. Effect of anastrozole treatment on antipyrine pharmacokinetics in postmenopausal female volunteers. Data on file (1995).
5. Yates RA, Wong J, Seiberling M, Merz M, Marz W, Nauck M. The effect of anastrozole on the single-dose pharmacokinetics and anticoagulant activity of warfarin in healthy volunteers. *Br J Clin Pharmacol* (2001) 51, 429–35.

Azathioprine or Mercaptopurine + Allopurinol

The effects of azathioprine and mercaptopurine are markedly increased by the concurrent use of allopurinol. The dosage of the cytotoxic drug should be reduced to a third or a quarter if toxicity is to be avoided. No interaction possibly occurs if these cytotoxic drugs are given intravenously. This needs confirmation.

Clinical evidence

(a) Azathioprine

A patient on 300 mg **allopurinol** daily for gout was additionally given 100 mg **azathioprine** daily to treat autoimmune haemolytic anaemia. Within 10 weeks his platelet count fell from 236 to 45×10^9/l, his white cell count fell from 9.4 to 0.8×10^9/l and his haemoglobin concentration fell from 115 to 53 g/l.[1]

A number of other reports similarly describe reversible bone marrow damage associated with anaemia, pancytopenia, leucocytopenia and thrombocytopenia in patients when concurrently treated with **azathioprine** and **allopurinol**.[1-10] At least 14 cases have been reported. One fatality has been described.[7]

(b) Mercaptopurine

Seven patients with chronic granulocytic leukaemia, treated with 50 mg **mercaptopurine** daily, showed a fall in granulocyte counts equivalent to four or five times the dose of **mercaptopurine** when additionally given 400 mg **allopurinol** daily.[11]

Profound pancytopenia developed in 3 children undergoing treatment with **mercaptopurine** 2.5 mg/kg daily and **allopurinol** 10 mg/kg daily, but when the **mercaptopurine** dosage was halved no untoward effects were seen.[12] A pharmacokinetic study found that **allopurinol** caused a fivefold increase the AUC and in peak plasma **mercaptopurine** concentrations when the **mercaptopurine** was given orally. The bioavailability increased from 12 to 59%.[13] This did not occur when the **mercaptopurine** was given intravenously.[13,14] Leucopenia and thrombocytopenia occurred in another patient given both drugs.[15]

Mechanism

Azathioprine is firstly metabolised in the liver to mercaptopurine and then enzymatically oxidised in the liver and intestinal wall by xanthine oxidase to an inactive compound (6–thiouric acid) which is excreted. Allopurinol inhibits this latter enzyme (inhibition of first-pass metabolism) so that the mercaptopurine accumulates, blood levels rise and its toxic effects develop (leucopenia, thrombocytopenia, etc.). In effect the patient suffers a gross overdose.

Importance and management

A well documented, well established, clinically important and potentially life-threatening interaction. The dosages of azathioprine and mercaptopurine should be reduced to about one-third or one-quarter when given orally to reduce the development of toxicity. Despite taking these precautions toxicity may still be seen[16] and very close monitoring is advisable.

On the basis of two studies[13,14] it would seem that this precaution may not be necessary if mercaptopurine is given intravenously, even so very close monitoring is advised with any route of administration.

1. Boyd IW. Allopurinol-azathioprine interaction. *J Intern Med* (1991) 229, 386.
2. Glogner P, Heni N. Panzytopenie nach kombinationsbehandlung mit allopurinol und azathioprin. *Med Welt* (1976) 27, 1545–6.
3. Brooks RJ, Dorr RT, Durie BGM. Interaction of allopurinol with 6-mercaptopurine and azathioprine. *Biomedicine* (1982) 36, 217–22.
4. Klugkist H, Lincke HO. Panzytopenie unter Behandlung mit Azathioprin durch Interaktion mit Allopurinol bei Myasthenia gravis. *Akt Neurol* (1987) 14, 165–7.
5. Zazgornik J, Kopsa H, Schmidt P, Pils P, Kuschan K, Deutsch E. Increased danger of bone marrow damage in simultaneous azathioprine-allopurinol therapy. *Int J Clin Pharmacol Ther Toxicol* (1981) 19, 96–7.
6. Raman GV, Sharman VL, Lee HA. Azathioprine and allopurinol: a potentially dangerous combination. *J Intern Med* (1990) 228, 69–71.
7. Adverse Drug Reactions Advisory Committee. Allopurinol and azathioprine. Fatal interaction. *Med J Aust* (1980) 2, 130.
8. Adverse Drug Reactions Advisory Committee. A reminder — the allopurinol azathioprine interactions. Australian Adverse Drug Reactions Bulletin. February 1985.
9. Garcia-Ortiz RE, De Los Angeles Rodriguez M. Pancytopenia associated with the interaction of allopurinol and azathioprine. *J Pharm Technol* (1991) 7, 224–6.
10. Kennedy DT, Hayney MS, Lake KD. Azathioprine and allopurinol: the price of an avoidable drug interaction. *Ann Pharmacother* (1996) 30, 951–4.
11. Rundles RW, Wyngaarden JB, Hitchings GH, Elion GB, Silberman HR. Effects of xanthine oxidase inhibitor on thiopurine metabolism, hyperuricaemia and gout. *Trans Assoc Am Phys* (1963) 76, 126–40.
12. Levine AS, Sharp HL, Mitchell J, Krivit W, Nesbit ME. Combination therapy with 6-mercaptopurine (NSC-755) and allopurinol (NSC-1390) during induction and maintenance of remission of acute leukaemia in children. *Cancer Chemother Rep* (1969) 53, 53–7.
13. Zimm S, Collins JM, O'Neill D, Chabner BA, Poplak DG. Inhibition of first-pass metabolism in cancer chemotherapy: interaction of 6-mercaptopurine and allopurinol. *Clin Pharmacol Ther* (1983) 34, 810–17.
14. Coffey JJ, White CA, Lesk AB, Rogers WI, Serpick AA. Effect of allopurinol on the pharmacokinetics of 6–mercaptopurine (NSC 755) in cancer patients. *Cancer Res* (1972) 32, 1283–9.
15. Berns A, Rubenfeld S, Rymzo WI, and Calabro JJ. Hazard of combining allopurinol and thiopurine. *N Engl J Med* (1972) 286, 730–1.
16. Cummins D, Sekar M, Halil O, Banner N. Myelosuppression associated with azathioprine-allopurinol interaction after heart and lung transplantation. *Transplantation* (1996) 61, 1661–2.

Azathioprine or Mercaptopurine + Aminosalicylates

The toxicity of these two thiopurines can be increased by mesalazine or sulfasalazine. A case report describes bone marrow suppression with mercaptopurine and olsalazine. Balsalazide may not interact to a clinically significant extent.

Clinical evidence

There is a single case report of a 13-year old boy with severe ulcerative pancolitis and cholangitis who was being treated with 60 mg of prednisone daily, 15 mg/kg of ursodeoxycholic acid daily and 25 mg/kg **mesalazine** daily. When **azathioprine** 2 mg/kg daily was added in an attempt to reduce the prednisone dosage and its side-effects, he developed marked and prolonged **azathioprine** toxicity (severe pancytopenia).[1]

A similar case report describes a patient with Crohn's disease who had two separate episodes of bone marrow suppression while receiving 50 to 75 mg **mercaptopurine** daily and 1000 to 1750 mg **olsalazine** daily. It was found necessary to reduce the **mercaptopurine** dosage on the first occasion and to withdraw both drugs on the second.[2]

Another report describes 38 patients taking **azathioprine** (mean dose 92.8 mg) and **sulfasalazine** (mean dose 2.1 g) for rheumatoid or psoriatic arthritis. Some patients did well but in general the combination was poorly tolerated and only 45% continued after 6 months. Others (34%) withdrew because of rash (3 patients), gastrointestinal upset (7), leucopenia (1), nephrotic syndrome (1) and being generally unwell (1).[3]

A further study in 34 patients with Crohn's disease on maintenance **azathioprine** or **mercaptopurine** who were given **sulfasalazine** 4 g daily, **mesalazine** 4 g daily or **balsalazide** 6.75 g daily for 8 weeks found significant increases in whole blood 6-thioguanine nucleotide concentrations. A significant reduction in white blood cell count was noted in the group of patients on **sulfasalazine** and **mesalazine** but not for those receiving **balsalazide**. One patient on **sulfasalazine** and another on **mesalazine** withdrew from the study after 6 weeks because of leucopenia.[4]

Mechanism

Azathioprine and mercaptopurine depend for their metabolism in the body on *S*-methylation by thiopurine methyltransferase (TMPT) and oxidation by xanthine oxidase. An *in vitro* study using recombinant TMPT found that both sulfasalazine and its metabolites inhibit the activity of TMPT.[5] Therefore if these drugs are used together, the clearance of azathioprine and mercaptopurine may be reduced by the sulfasalazine, resulting in an increase in their toxicity (there is only a small margin between their therapeutic and toxic levels). About 11% of patients may be at particular risk because of genetic polymorphism resulting in TMPT enzyme activity already only half of the rest of the population.[4,5] *In vitro* studies confirmed that mesalazine,[6] olsalazine and its metabolite olsalazine-*O*-sulphate[2,6] and balsalazide[6] are inhibitors of recombinant TPMT. In patients increased levels of 6-thioguanine nucleotide are probably due to inhibition of TPMT.[4] It is suggested that the reported *in vitro* concentration (IC_{50}) of balsalazide required to halve the TPMT activity is about 1000 times higher than peak plasma levels after therapeutic doses and therefore an interaction is unlikely. Mesalazine and olsalazine peak levels may also be less than the IC_{50} concentrations but the latter in high doses (10 g daily) may result in clinically important inhibition of TPMT. Peak plasma levels of sulfasalazine are close to IC_{50} concentrations.[7]

Importance and management

These reports underline the importance of taking particular care if **azathioprine** or **mercaptopurine** are used with **mesalazine**, **olsalazine**, balsalazide or **sulfasalazine**. Balsalazide was not found to cause leucopenia in one study,[4] although the possibility that it may do so is not ruled out.[4] It has been suggested that mesalazine and olsalazine are probably safe in most patients but that balsalazide, because of low therapeutic plasma levels, indicating possibly only a minor risk for TPMT inhibition, is to be preferred.[7] In contrast, it has been suggested that the interaction may benefit patients as increased whole blood 6-thioguanine nucleotide or mild leucopenia is associated with a greater chance of remission in those treated with azathioprine or mercaptopurine.[4] The clinical benefits of the cautious use of sulfasalazine with mercaptopurine are also noted.[8] Very good monitoring is required, which is likely in patients on these types of drugs anyway. More study is needed.

1. Chouraqui JP, Serre-Debeauvais F, Armari C, Savariau N. Azathioprine toxicity in a child with ulcerative colitis: interaction with mesalazine. *Gastroenterology* (1996) 110 (4 Suppl), A883.
2. Lewis LD, Benin A, Szumlanski CL, Otterness DM, Lennard L, Weinshilboum RM, Nierenberg DW. Olsalazine and 6-mercaptopurine-related bone marrow suppression: a possible drug-drug interaction. *Clin Pharmacol Ther* (1997) 62, 464–75.
3. Helliwell PS. Combination therapy with sulphasalazine and azathioprine. *Br J Rheumatol* (1996) 35, 493–4.
4. Lowry PW, Franklin CL, Weaver AL, Szumlanski CL, Mays DC, Loftus EV, Tremaine WJ, Lipsky JJ, Weinshilboum RM, Sandborn WJ. Leucopenia resulting from a drug interaction between azathioprine or 6-mercaptopurine and mesalamine, sulphasalazine, or balsalazide. *Gut* (2001) 49, 656–64.
5. Szumlanski CL, Weinshilboum RM. Sulphasalazine inhibition of thiopurine methyltransferase: possible mechanism for interaction with 6-mercaptopurine and azathioprine. *Br J Clin Pharmacol* (1995) 39, 456–9.
6. Lowry PW, Szumlanski CL, Weinshilboum RM, Sandborn WJ. Balsalazide and azathioprine or 6-mercaptopurine: evidence for a potentially serious drug interaction. *Gastroenterology* (1999) 116, 1505–6.
7. Green JRB. Balsalazide and azathioprine or 6-mercaptopurine. *Gastroenterology* (1999) 117, 1513–14.
8. Present DH. Interaction of 6-mercaptopurine and azathioprine with 5-aminosalicylic acid agents. *Gastroenterology* (2000) 119, 276–7.

Azathioprine or Mercaptopurine + Co-trimoxazole or Trimethoprim

The risk of potentially life-threatening haematological toxicity may be increased in renal transplant patients taking azathioprine if they are treated with co-trimoxazole or trimethoprim, particularly if given for extended periods. The same interaction would be expected with mercaptopurine.

Clinical evidence

The observation that haematological toxicity often seemed to occur in renal transplant patients given **azathioprine** and **co-trimoxazole**, prompted a retrospective survey of the records of 40 patients. It was found that there was no difference in the incidence of thrombocytopenia and neutropenia in those given **azathioprine** alone or with **co-trimoxazole** (160 to 320 mg **trimethoprim** + 800 to 1600 mg **sulfamethoxazole (sulphamethoxazole)** daily) for a short time (6 to 16 days), but a significant increase occurred in the incidence and duration of these cytopenias if both drugs were given together for 22 days or more.[1]

A marked fall in white cell counts in renal transplant recipients during concurrent treatment with either **co-trimoxazole** (described as frequent) or **trimethoprim** (3 cases) has been reported elsewhere.[2] In one case the fall occurred within 5 days and was treated by temporarily withdrawing the **azathioprine** and reducing the **trimethoprim** dosage from 300 to 100 mg daily.[2]

Mechanism

Not understood. It seems possible that the bone marrow depressant effects of all three drugs may be additive. In addition, impaired renal function may allow co-trimoxazole levels to become elevated, and haemodialysis may deplete folate levels which could exacerbate the anti-folate effects of the co-trimoxazole.

Importance and management

Information appears to be limited to the studies cited, but the interaction would seem to be established. The use of co-trimoxazole or trimethoprim in renal transplant patients may clearly be hazardous and potentially life-threatening. An as yet untested suggestion by the authors of the first study[1] is that folinic acid might be an effective treatment for bone marrow suppression without affecting the antimicrobial effects of the co-trimoxazole. A similar interaction would be expected with **mercaptopurine**. More study is needed.

1. Bradley PP, Warden GD, Maxwell JG, Rothstein G. Neutropenia and thrombocytopenia in renal allograft recipients treated with trimethoprim-sulfamethoxazole. *Ann Intern Med* (1980) 93, 560–2.
2. Bailey RR. Leukopenia due to a trimethoprim-azathioprine interaction. *N Z Med J* (1984) 97, 739.

Azathioprine or Mercaptopurine + Doxorubicin (Adriamycin)

The hepatotoxicity of mercaptopurine and probably azathioprine can be increased by doxorubicin.

Clinical evidence, mechanism, importance and management

Liver damage induced by treatment with **mercaptopurine** was increased in 11 patients by the concurrent use of **doxorubicin**.[1] Since **azathioprine** is converted to **mercaptopurine** within the body, it would seem probable that increased hepatotoxicity will also be seen with **azathioprine** and **doxorubicin**.

1. Minow RA, Stern MH, Casey JH, Rodriguez V, Luna MA. Clinico-pathological correlation of liver damage in patients treated with 6-mercaptopurine and adriamycin. *Cancer* (1976) 38, 1524–8.

Bexarotene + Miscellaneous drugs

The makers say that gemfibrozil raises bexarotene plasma levels and should therefore be avoided. They warn about the theoretical possibility that inhibitors of cytochrome P450 isoenzyme CYP3A4 (clarithromycin, erythromycin, itraconazole, ketoconazole, protease inhibitors, grapefruit juice) may possibly raise bexarotene levels, whereas CYP3A4 inducers (dexamethasone, phenytoin, phenobarbital, rifampicin (rifampin)) may possibly reduce them. They also suggest the possibility of reduced oral contraceptive effects, and increased hypoglycaemic effects with insulin or oral hypoglycaemic agents. No interaction seems to occur with atorvastatin or levothyroxine.

Clinical evidence, mechanism, importance and management

No formal interaction studies appear to have been carried out so that most of drug interactions cited in this monograph are suggestions by the makers, based on theoretical considerations.[1]

(a) Effects of enzyme inducers and inhibitors

Because it is known that **bexarotene** is metabolised by cytochrome P450 isoenzyme CYP3A4, the makers point out that there is a theoretical risk that compounds which can inhibit CYP3A4 might increase **bexarotene** levels and increase its toxicity. They list **clarithromycin, erythromycin, itraconazole, ketoconazole, protease inhibitors** (none specifically named) and **grapefruit juice** as possible interacting drugs because of their known inhibitory effects on CYP3A4. They also list a number of known CYP3A4 inducers, namely **dexamethasone, phenytoin, phenobarbital** and **rifampicin (rifampin)**, because they may theoretically increase the metabolism of **bexarotene** and reduce its levels.

The makers also say that because **bexarotene** can induce liver enzymes, it may theoretically increase the metabolism of the steroids in **oral contraceptives**, thereby reducing and their serum levels and their efficacy. For this reason they advise the use of additional non-hormonal contraception (e.g. a barrier method) to avoid the risk of contraceptive failure. They point out that this is particularly important because if failure were to occur, the foetus might be exposed to the teratogenic effects of **bexarotene**.[1]

(b) Other possible drug interactions

The makers report that a population analysis of patients with cutaneous T-cell lymphoma (CTCL) found that the concurrent use of **gemfibrozil** substantially increased the plasma levels of **bexarotene** for reasons unknown. They therefore say that concurrent use is not recommended. However under similar conditions, they say that **bexarotene** levels were found not to be affected by **atorvastatin** or **levothyroxine**. Changes in thyroid function caused by **bexarotene** have been successfully treated with **thyroid hormone supplements**.[1]

The makers recommend that because **bexarotene** is related to **vitamin A**, any **vitamin A supplements** should be limited to $\leq$ 15,000 IU daily to avoid potentially additive toxic effects. The makers additionally say that although no cases of hypoglycaemia have been seen, because of the known mode of action of bexarotene it should be used with caution if given with **insulin** or agents enhancing insulin secretion (e.g. **sulphonylureas**) or insulin sensitisers (e.g. **thiazolidinediones**).[1] See the list of these drugs at the beginning of Chapter 15.

1. Targretin (Bexarotene). Elan Pharma. Summary of product characteristics, March 2001.

Bicalutamide + Phenazone (Antipyrine)

The results of an interaction study between bicalutamide and phenazone (antipyrine) suggest that bicalutamide is unlikely to interact with other drugs by causing enzyme induction.

Clinical evidence, mechanism, importance and management

The pharmacokinetics and metabolism of **phenazone (antipyrine)** (largely used as an investigational marker drug) were studied in two groups of patients with prostate cancer before and after taking either 50 mg bicalutamide daily (7 patients) or 150 mg daily (11 patients) for 12 weeks. Small changes in the **phenazone** pharmacokinetics were found (half-life shorter by 16.3% with the 50 mg bicalutamide dosage, the AUC reduced by 18.6% with the 150 mg bicalutamide dosage). Nevertheless the conclusion was reached that bicalutamide does not significantly induce the liver enzymes responsible for the metabolism of **phenazone (antipyrine)** and is therefore unlikely to interact with any other drugs by causing enzyme induction.[1]

1. Kaisary A, Klarskov P, McKillop D. Absence of hepatic enzyme induction in prostate cancer patients receiving 'Casodex' (bicalutamide). *Anticancer Drugs* (1996) 7, 54–9.

Bleomycin + Cisplatin

Cisplatin can increase the pulmonary toxicity of bleomycin by reducing its renal excretion. Raynaud's phenomenon and arterial thrombosis have also been described.

Clinical evidence

Thirty patients with carcinoma of the cervix were given bleomycin following **cisplatin** intramuscularly every 12 h for 4 days. Another 15 patients with germ cell tumours were given bleomycin following **cisplatin** by continuous infusion over 72 h. Nine of the patients with normal renal function and no previous pulmonary disease developed serious pulmonary toxicity and 6 died from respiratory failure.[1] A study in 18 patients given both drugs for the treatment of disseminated testicular non-seminoma found that the **cisplatin**-induced reduction in renal function was paralleled by an increase in bleomycin-induced pulmonary toxicity. Two patients developed pneumonitis.[2] Similar findings were made in a much larger study of 54 patients by the same group.[3] A man with unrecognised acute renal failure due to **cisplatin** treatment died from pulmonary toxicity when he was given bleomycin.[4] A study in 2 patients showed that the total clearance of bleomycin was halved (from 39 to 18 ml/min/m^2) when concurrently treated with **cisplatin** in cumulative doses exceeding 300 mg/m^2 and the renal clearance in one patient fell from 30 to 8.2 ml/min/m^2. There was no evidence of severe bleomycin toxicity in these patients.[5] Renal dysfunction caused by cisplatin has also been reported in some instances to cause bleomycin toxicity.[6] Another report describes arterial thrombosis associated with pathological vascular changes in arteries in a man treated with both drugs,[7] and Raynaud's phenomenon is reported to occur in up to 41% of patients treated.[8] A man developed fatal thrombotic microangiopathy (characterised by microangiopathic haemolytic anaemia, thrombocytopenia, renal impairment) which was attributed to the use of bleomycin and **cisplatin**.[9]

Mechanism

Excretion by the kidney accounts for almost half of the total body clearance of bleomycin. Cisplatin is nephrotoxic and reduces the glomerular filtration rate so that the clearance of the bleomycin is reduced. The accumulating bleomycin apparently causes the pulmonary toxicity.

Importance and management

Pulmonary toxicity with bleomycin is an established reaction with a potentially serious, sometimes fatal, outcome. Concurrent use should be very closely monitored and renal function checked. One of the problems is that levels of creatinine may not accurately indicate the extent of renal damage, both during and after cisplatin treatment. The renal toxicity of cisplatin may also not develop gradually. Other toxic effects on the vascular system can also occur. One group of authors strongly advises that the bleomycin should be given before the cisplatin wherever possible to prevent accumulation of bleomycin in the plasma.[1]

1. Rabinowits M, Souhami L, Gil RA, Andrade CAV, Paiva HC. Increased pulmonary toxicity with bleomycin and cisplatin chemotherapy combinations. *Am J Clin Oncol* (1990) 13, 132–8.
2. van Barneveld PWC, Sleijfer D Th, van der Mark Th W, Mulder NH, Donker AJM, Meijer S, Schraffordt Koops H, Sluiter HJ, Peset R. Influence of platinum-induced renal toxicity on bleomycin-induced pulmonary toxicity in patients with disseminated testicular carcinoma. *Oncology* (1984) 41, 4–7.
3. Sleijfer S, van der Mark TW, Schraffordt Koops H, Mulder NH. Enhanced effects of bleomycin on pulmonary function disturbances in patients with decreased renal function due to cisplatin. *Eur J Cancer* (1996) 32A, 550–2.
4. Bennett WM, Pastore L, Houghton DC. Fatal pulmonary bleomycin toxicity in cisplatin-induced acute renal failure. *Cancer Treat Rep* (1980) 64, 921–4.
5. Yee GC, Crom WR, Champion JE, Brodeur GM, Evans WE. Cisplatin-induced changes in bleomycin elimination. *Cancer Treat Rep* (1983) 67, 587–9.
6. Perry DJ, Weiss RB, Taylor HG. Enhanced bleomycin toxicity during acute renal failure. *Cancer Treat Rep* (1982) 66, 592–3.
7. Garstin IWH, Cooper GG, Hood JM. Arterial thrombosis after treatment with bleomycin and cisplatin. *BMJ* (1990) 300, 1018.
8. Vogelzang NJ, Bosl GJ, Johnson K, Kennedy BJ. Raynaud's phenomenon : a common toxicity after combination chemotherapy for testicular cancer. *Ann Intern Med* (1981) 95, 288–92.
9. Fields SM, Lindley CM. Thrombotic microangiopathy associated with chemotherapy: case report and review of the literature. *DICP Ann Pharmacother* (1989) 23, 582–8.

Bleomycin + Cytotoxic regimens and drugs used in neutropenia

There is evidence that the concurrent use of other drugs, particularly G-CSF or GM-CSF, can increase the occurrence of bleomycin-induced pulmonary reactions.

Clinical evidence, mechanism, importance and management

Of a group of patients treated for non-Hodgkin's lymphomas with bleomycin (mean total dose 36 units) in conjunction with other cytotoxic drugs (**M-BACOD, methotrexate, doxorubicin, cyclophosphamide, vincristine, dexamethasone**), 18% (15 of 83) developed acute but completely reversible pulmonary reactions.[1]

Three (possibly 4) out of 5 patients given standard **ABVD** treatment (**doxorubicin, bleomycin, vinblastine, dacarbazine**) for Hodgkin's disease developed pulmonary toxicity attributed by the author of the report to the synergistic action of **G-CSF** (**granulocyte colony stimulating factor**).[2] Eight out of 40 patients with malignant non-Hodgkin's lymphoma and treated with **G-CSF** developed cytotoxic drug-induced pneumonia. Three of them died of respiratory failure. None of 35 other patients, similarly treated but without **G-CSF** developed pneumonia. The chemotherapy regimens used were **ProMACE, MACOP-B, COP-BLAM III** and **CHOP**.[3] However it should be said that the association of pulmonary toxicity with the use of bleomycin and **G-CSF** has been questioned.[4] Non-infectious interstitial pneumonitis developed in a patient given **doxorubicin, cyclophosphamide, bleomycin, vinblastine, methotrexate** and **prednisone** with **GM-CSF** (**granulocyte macrophage colony stimulating factor**).[5]

These values are high compared with the 3 to 10% incidence of pulmonary toxicity reported in those receiving bleomycin alone. These interactions are not firmly established but good pulmonary function monitoring before, during and after giving **G-CSF** is clearly important. See also 'Bleomycin + Cisplatin', p.489 and 'Cyclophosphamide + Filgrastim (G-CSF)', p.497.

1. Bauer KA, Skarin AT, Balikian JP, Garnick MB, Rosenthal DS, Canellos GP. Pulmonary complications associated with combination chemotherapy program containing bleomycin. *Am J Med* (1983) 74, 557–63.
2. Matthews JH. Pulmonary toxicity of ABVD chemotherapy and G-CSF in Hodgkin's disease: possible synergy. *Lancet* (1993) 342, 988.
3. Iki S, Yoshinaga K, Ohbayashi Y, Urabe A. Cytotoxic drug-induced pneumonia and possible augmentation by G-CSF — clinical attention. *Ann Hematol* (1993) 66, 217–8.
4. Bastion Y, Reyes F, Bosly A, Gisselbrecht C, Yver A, Gilles E, Maral J, Coiffier B. Possible toxicity with the association of G-CSF and bleomycin. *Lancet* (1994) 343, 1221–2.
5. Philippe B, Couderc LJ, Balloul-Delclaux E, Janvier M, Caubarrere I. Pulmonary toxicity of chemotherapy and GM-CSF. *Respir Med* (1994) 88, 715.

Bleomycin + Oxygen

Serious and potentially fatal pulmonary toxicity can develop in patients treated with bleomycin who are exposed to conventional oxygen concentrations during anaesthesia.

Clinical evidence

Five patients under treatment with bleomycin, exposed to **oxygen** concentrations of 39% during and immediately following anaesthesia, developed a severe respiratory distress syndrome and died. Bleomycin-induced pneumonitis and lung fibrosis were diagnosed at postmortem. Another group of 12 matched patients who underwent the same procedures but with lower **oxygen** concentrations (22 to 25%) recovered uneventfully.[1]

Another comparative study similarly demonstrated that adult respiratory distress syndrome (ARDS) in patients on bleomycin was reduced by the use of lower **oxygen** concentrations (22 to 30%).[2] Bleomycin-induced pulmonary toxicity in man apparently related to **oxygen** concentrations has been described in other reports,[3-7] and has also been demonstrated in mice,[8] rats[9] and hamsters.[10] Other reports however found no obvious increase in pulmonary complications in patients on bleomycin exposed to **oxygen** in concentrations above 30%.[11,12]

Mechanism

Not understood. One suggestion is that bleomycin-injured lung tissue is less able to scavenge free oxygen radicals which may be present and damage occurs as a result.[3]

Importance and management

An established, well-documented, serious and potentially fatal interaction. It is advised that any patient on bleomycin undergoing general anaesthesia should have their inspired oxygen concentrations limited to less than 30% and the fluid replacement should be carefully monitored to minimise the crystalloid load. This is clearly very effective because having used these precautions Dr Goldiner writes[13] that "... since ... 1978 we have operated on more than 700 bleomycin treated patients ... we have seen no postoperative pulmonary failure in this group of patients." It has also been suggested that reduced oxygen levels should be continued during the recovery period and at any time during hospitalisation.[3] If an oxygen concentration equal or greater than 30% has to be used, short term prophylactic corticosteroid administration should be considered. Intravenous corticosteroids should be given at once if bleomycin toxicity is suspected.[3]

1. Goldiner PL, Carlon CG, Cvitkovic E, Schweizer O, Howland WS. Factors influencing postoperative morbidity and mortality in patients treated with bleomycin. *BMJ* (1978) 1, 1664–7.
2. El-Baz N, Ivankovich AD, Faber LP, Logas WG. The incidence of bleomycin lung toxicity after anesthesia for pulmonary resection: a comparison between HFV and IPPV. *Anesthesiology* (1984) 61, A107.
3. Gilson AJ,' Sahn SA. Reactivation of bleomycin lung toxicity following oxygen administration. A second response to corticosteroids. *Chest* (1985) 88, 304–6.
4. Cersosimo RJ, Matthews SJ, Hong WK. Bleomycin pneumonitis potentiated by oxygen administration. *Drug Intell Clin Pharm* (1985) 19, 921–3.
5. Hulbert JC, Grossman JE, Cummings KB. Risk factors of anesthesia and surgery in bleomycin-treated patients. *J Urol* (1983) 130, 163–4.
6. Allen SC, Riddell GS, Butchart EG. Bleomycin therapy and anaesthesia. The possible hazards of oxygen administration to patients after treatment with bleomycin. *Anaesthesia* (1981) 36, 60–3.
7. Donohue JP, Rowland RG. Complications of retroperitoneal lymph node dissection. *J Urol* (1981) 125, 338–40.
8. Toledo CH, Ross WE, Hood I, Block ER. Potentiation of bleomycin toxicity by oxygen. *Cancer Treat Rep* (1982) 66, 359–62.
9. Berend N. The effect of bleomycin and oxygen on rat lung. *Pathology* (1984) 16, 136–9.
10. Rinaldo J, Goldstein RH, Snider GL. Modification of oxygen toxicity after lung injury by bleomycin in hamsters. *Am Rev Respir Dis* (1982) 126, 1030–3.
11. Douglas MJ, Coppin CML. Bleomycin and subsequent anaesthesia: a retrospective study at Vancouver General Hospital. *Can Anaesth Soc J* (1980) 27, 449–52.
12. Mandelbaum I, Williams SD, Einhorn LH. Aggressive surgical management of testicular carcinoma metastatic to lungs and mediastinum. *Ann Thorac Surg* (1980) 30, 224–9.
13. Goldiner PL. Editorial comment. *J Urol* (1983) 130, 164.

Busulfan + Azole antifungals

Itraconazole, but not fluconazole, reduces the clearance of busulfan.

Clinical evidence, mechanism, importance and management

The pharmacokinetics of busulfan in 13 bone marrow transplant patients receiving busulfan and **itraconazole** were compared with 26 controls who took no antifungal and 13 who took **fluconazole**. The busulfan clearance was decreased 20% by **itraconazole** but not by the **fluconazole**,[1] probably because the **itraconazole** inhibits the metabolism of busulfan by the liver. The expected rise in serum busulfan levels is only likely to be moderate, but until more information is available it would be prudent to monitor for any signs of increased busulfan toxicity if **itraconazole** is used, but no special precautions seem to be needed with **fluconazole**.

1. Buggia I, Zecca N, Alessandrino EP, Locatelli F, Rosti G, Bosi A, Pession A, Rotoli B, Majolino I, Dallorso A, Regazzi MB. Itraconazole can increase systemic exposure to busulfan in patients given bone marrow transplantation. *Anticancer Res* (1996) 16, 2083–8.

Busulfan + Diazepam or Phenytoin

Phenytoin increases the loss of busulfan from the body, and lowers its serum levels. Diazepam appears not to interact.

Clinical evidence

Seven patients given high dose busulfan (1 mg/kg four times daily for 4 days) before bone marrow transplantation showed an increased clearance (from 2.80 to 3.32 ml/min/kg), a lower AUC (from 6475 to 5412 nanograms.h/ml) and a shorter half-life (from 3.94 to 3.03 h) while taking **phenytoin** (2.5 to 5 mg/kg). A continuous decline in the steady-state plasma levels of busulfan was also seen in 4 out of the 7 patients, but no pharmacokinetic changes were seen in eight other patients given **diazepam**, apart from a steady decline in steady-state serum levels in just one.[1]

Mechanism

Not established, but it seems likely that the phenytoin (a well recognised enzyme inducer) increases the metabolism of the busulfan by the liver, thereby increasing its loss from the body.

Importance and management

Information seems to be limited to this study. The authors of the study suggest that anticonvulsants with fewer enzyme inducing properties than phenytoin should be used as prophylactic anticonvulsants if busulfan is used for bone marrow transplant pretreatment.

1. Hassan M, Öberg G, Björkholm M, Wallin I, Lindgren M. Influence of prophylactic anticonvulsant therapy on high-dose busulphan kinetics. *Cancer Chemother Pharmacol* (1993) 33, 181–6.

Busulfan + Ketobemidone

Ketobemidone increases plasma levels of busulfan.

Clinical evidence

A patient with acute myeloid leukaemia was started on a course of busulfan 1 mg/kg four times daily for 4 days followed by cyclophosphamide for 2 days prior to bone marrow transplantation. At the time he was also receiving **ketobemidone** 1000 mg daily for rectal fissure. Busulfan plasma levels after the first dose were elevated (AUC increased by about one-third). Later, when the dose of **ketobemidone** was reduced and morphine substituted, busulfan levels decreased.[1]

Mechanism

Not fully understood.

Importance and management

The use of ketobemidone with high-dose busulfan is not recommended without monitoring. Dose adjustments may be required to prevent busulfan toxicity. An alternative analgesic should be considered.

1. Hassan M, Svensson J-O, Nilsson C, Hentschke P, AL-Shurbaji A, Aschan J, Ljungman P, Ringdén O. Ketobemidone may alter busulfan pharmacokinetics during high-dose therapy. *Ther Drug Monit* (2000) 22, 383–5.

Busulfan + Tioguanine (Thioguanine)

There is evidence to show that concurrent use increases the risk of oesophageal varices, nodular regenerative hyperplasia of the liver and portal hypertension.

Clinical evidence, mechanism, importance and management

Five patients on continuous busulfan 2 mg and **tioguanine (thioguanine)** 80 mg five days weekly for chronic myeloid leukaemia developed oesophageal varices associated with abnormal liver function tests. Three of them had gastrointestinal haemorrhages and one died. Endoscopy revealed varices in the other two. Liver biopsy of 4 of them showed nodular regenerative hyperplasia which was the cause of portal hypertension.[1] This report also quotes a large scale Medical Research Council trial of 677 cases, about half of whom received both drugs. Among these a total of 12 cases of oesophageal varices were found (the 5 described here, plus another 7). Nine of the 12 had gastrointestinal bleeding.[1] These serious adverse reactions would therefore seem to limit the value of this drug combination.

1. Key NS, Kelly PMA, Emerson PM, Chapman RWG, Allan NC, McGee JO'D. Oesophageal varices associated with busulphan-thioguanine combination therapy for chronic myeloid leukaemia. *Lancet* (1987) 2, 1050–2.

Capecitabine + Miscellaneous drugs

Capecitabine is contraindicated with sorivudine and its analogues because of a predicted marked and life-threatening increase in its toxicity. Its maximum tolerated dose is decreased by folinic acid and interferon alpha, and its efficacy is predicted to be reduced by allopurinol. It is reported to increase the anticoagulant effects of phenprocoumon and warfarin in some patients and to raise phenytoin serum levels, but its absorption is not affected by an aluminium/magnesium hydroxide antacid. There are no clinically significant interactions between capecitabine and paclitaxel, and probably not between capecitabine and docetaxel, although more study is needed to establish this.

Clinical evidence, mechanism, importance and management

(a) Allopurinol

Capecitabine is a precursor or prodrug which is activated by several enzymatic steps to produce active cytotoxic 5-fluorouracil (5-FU) within the body. Because **allopurinol** is reported to decrease the efficacy of 5-fluorouracil, the makers of capecitabine therefore say that **allopurinol** should be avoided.[1]

(b) Antacid

A study in 12 patients on the effects of an **aluminium and magnesium hydroxide antacid** (*Maalox*, 20 ml on the pharmacokinetics of capecitabine found that it caused a small increase in the serum levels of a single dose of capecitabine 1250 mg/m² and one metabolite

(5'-DFCR) but it had no effect on the other three major metabolites (5'DFUR, 5-FU and FBAL).[1,2] There would therefore seem to be no reason for taking special precautions if capecitabine and an antacid of this type are used concurrently.

(c) Anticoagulants

The makers report that changes in coagulation parameters and/or bleeding have been seen in a few patients on anticoagulants such as **warfarin** and **phenprocoumon** within several days or months of adding capecitabine. In one case it occurred a month after the capecitabine had been stopped. The reasons for the interaction are not understood, but what has been seen is consistent with reports of increased warfarin effects seen with another 5-fluorouracil prodrug containing **uracil** and **ftorafur** (*Orzel*) and with 5-fluorouracil itself. See 'Anticoagulants + Cytotoxic (antineoplastic) agents', p.254.

On the basis of these clinical observations the makers say that prothrombin times or INR should be regularly monitored in patients taking capecitabine with these and **other coumarin oral anticoagulants**.[1] The incidence of this interaction is not known.

(d) Docetaxel or Paclitaxel

A study in patients with advanced solid tumours found that administration of capecitabine with **docetaxel**, resulted in an almost twofold decrease in the maximum plasma concentration and AUC of fluorouracil. The authors suggest that more study is needed to assess the significance of this finding. Other pharmacokinetic parameters of capecitabine were not affected by co-administered **docetaxel**. The pharmacokinetics of **docetaxel** were not significantly affected by capecitabine or its metabolites.[3]

Another study in similar patients found that neither **paclitaxel** nor capecitabine significantly altered the pharmacokinetics of each other.[4]

(e) Folinic acid

Studies in patients with refractory advanced cancer have shown that **folinic acid** 30 mg twice daily does not have a major effect on the pharmacokinetics of capecitabine.[5] However, the pharmacodynamics of capecitabine were affected as determined by the more frequent occurrence of dose-limiting gastrointestinal disorders or the hand-foot syndrome.[5] The makers say that the maximum tolerated capecitabine dose when used alone in the intermittent regimen is 3000 mg/m^2, but it is reduced to 2000 mg/m^2 if 30 mg **folinic acid** twice daily is added.[1]

(f) Hypoglycaemic agents

There appear to be no reports of adverse interactions between **hypoglycaemic agents** and capecitabine, but it is reported that the control of diabetes mellitus may be affected by capecitabine for which reason the makers advise caution.[1]

(g) Interferon alpha

The makers[1] say that the maximum tolerated capecitabine dose when used alone is 3000 mg/m^2, but when combined with **interferon alpha-2a** (3 MIU/m^2 per day) the maximum tolerated dose is 2000 mg/m^2.

(h) Phenytoin

The makers report that increased plasma **phenytoin** levels have been seen in patients given capecitabine, and their advice is to monitor plasma **phenytoin** levels regularly during concurrent use.[1]

(i) Sorivudine and its analogues

Capecitabine is a precursor or prodrug which is activated by several enzymatic steps to produce active cytotoxic 5-fluorouracil (5-FU) within the body. On the basis of the severe and fatal toxicity seen with another 5-fluorouracil prodrug (tegafur), the makers of capecitabine contraindicate the concurrent use of **sorivudine** or any of its chemically related analogues such as **brivudine**.[1] The mechanism of this interaction appears to be that a metabolite of **sorivudine** is a potent inhibitor of an enzyme which is concerned with the metabolism of 5-fluorouracil. As a result, the serum levels of the 5-fluorouracil rise and its toxic effects develop. The patients who died of the tegafur/**sorivudine** interaction developed acute toxicity (anorexia, marked bone

marrow damage, decreases in platelet and white cell counts, atrophy of the intestinal membrane) within a few days of being given both drugs. See 'Tegafur + Sorivudine', p.523.

1. Xeloda (Capecitabine). Roche Product Limited. Summary of product characteristics, March 2002.
2. Reigner B, Clive S, Cassidy J, Jodrell D, Schulz R, Goggin T, Banken L, Roos B, Utoh M, Mulligan T, Weidekamm E. Influence of the antacid Maalox on the pharmacokinetics of capecitabine in cancer patients. *Cancer Chemother Pharmacol* (1999) 43, 309–15.
3. Pronk LC, Vasey P, Sparreboom A, Reigner B, Planting AST, Gordon RJ, Osterwalder B, Verweij J. A phase I and pharmacokinetic study of the combination of capecitabine and docetaxel in patients with advanced solid tumours. *Br J Cancer* (2000) 83, 22–9.
4. Villalona-Calero MA, Weiss GR, Durris HA, Kraynak M, Rodrigues G, Drengler RL, Eckhardt SG, Reigner B, Moczygemba J, Burger HU, Griffin T, Von Hoff DD, Roinsky EK. Phase I and pharmacokinetic study of the oral fluorpyrimidine capecitabine in combination with paclitaxel in patients with advanced solid malignancies. *J Clin Oncol* (1999) 17, 1915–25.
5. Cassidy J, Dirix L, Bissett D, Reigner B, Griffin T, Allman D, Osterwalder B, Van Oosterom AT. A phase I study of capecitabine in combination with oral leucovorin in patients with intractable solid tumours. *Clin Cancer Res* (1998) 4, 2755–61.

Carmofur + Alcohol

A disulfiram-like reaction occurred in a patient on carmofur when given coeliac plexus blockade with alcohol.

Clinical evidence, mechanism, importance and management

A man with pancreatic carcinoma treated with 500 mg carmofur daily for 25 days experienced a disulfiram-like reaction (facial flushing, diaphoresis, hypotension (BP 60/30 mmHg), and tachycardia of 128 bpm) within 30 min of being given coeliac plexus **alcohol** blockade for pain relief. Blood acetaldehyde levels were found to have risen sharply, supporting the belief that the underlying mechanism is similar to the disulfiram-alcohol interaction (see 'Alcohol + Disulfiram', p.27). It is suggested that **alcohol** blockade should be avoided for 7 days after treatment with carmofur.[1]

1. Noda J, Umeda S, Mori K, Fukunaga T, Mizoi Y. Disulfiram-like reaction associated with carmofur after celiac plexus alcohol block. *Anesthesiology* (1987) 67, 809–10.

Carmustine (BCNU) + Cimetidine

The bone marrow depressant effects of carmustine can be increased by the concurrent use of cimetidine. The fall in neutrophil and thrombocyte counts may become serious.

Clinical evidence

Six out of 8 patients treated with carmustine, 80 mg/m^2 daily, for 3 days, **cimetidine**, 300 mg six-hourly, and steroids demonstrated marked leucopenia and thrombocytopenia after the first administrations. Biopsy confirmed the marked decrease in granulocytic elements. In comparison only 6 out of 40 patients treated similarly, but without **cimetidine**, showed comparable white cell and platelet depression.[1]

This increased myelotoxicity with marked falls in neutrophil counts has been described in another report.[2]

Mechanism

Cimetidine alone occasionally causes a marked fall in neutrophil numbers[3] and in some way, as yet not understood, it can augment the bone marrow depressant effects of carmustine.

Importance and management

Information appears to be limited to the reports cited, but it seems to be an established reaction. Patients given both drugs should be closely monitored for changes in neutrophil and platelet counts because the neutropenia may be life-threatening.

1. Selker RG, Moore P, LoDolce D. Bone-marrow depression with cimetidine plus carmustine. *N Engl J Med* (1978) 299, 834.

2. Volkin RL, Shadduck RK, Winkelstein A, Zeigler ZR, Selker RG. Potentiation of car-mustine-cranial irradiation-induced myelosuppression by cimetidine. *Arch Intern Med* (1982) 142, 243–5.
3. Klotz S, Kay BF. Cimetidine and agranulocytosis. *Ann Intern Med* (1978) 88, 579.

Chlorambucil + Prednisone

A single report describes seizures in a patient possibly due to co-administered chlorambucil and prednisone.

Clinical evidence, mechanism, importance and management

A patient with non-Hodgkin's lymphoma experienced a syncopal episode with generalised tonic-clonic seizures 8 days after completing an initial 5-day course of treatment with chlorambucil 12 mg daily and **prednisone** 50 mg daily. The seizures were controlled with intravenous clonazepam. Four weeks later, on the third day of a second course, she again had generalised tonic-clonic seizures, which resolved spontaneously.

Chlorambucil-induced seizures have occurred in children with the nephrotic syndrome. Cases in adults usually involve high-dose chlorambucil or are in patients with a history of seizures. The seizures in this patient may have been due to the additive effects of both drugs in reducing the seizure threshold.[1]

1. Jourdan E, Topart D, Pinzani V, Jourdan J. Chlorambucil/prednisone-induced seizures in a patient with non-Hodgkin's lymphoma. *Am J Hematol* (2001) 67, 147.

Cisplatin + Aminoglycosides

Acute and possibly life-threatening renal failure can occur in patients treated concurrently with cisplatin and aminoglycoside antibacterials such as gentamicin and tobramycin.

Clinical evidence

Four patients treated with cisplatin in dosages ranging from low to very high (eight doses of 0.5 mg/kg, one or two doses of 3 mg/kg or a single dose of 5 mg/kg) and who were subsequently given **gentamicin/cefalotin** developed acute and fatal renal failure. Autopsy revealed extensive renal tubular necrosis.[1]

Two similar cases of severe renal toxicity attributed to the concurrent use of cisplatin with **gentamicin/cefalotin** are described elsewhere.[2,3] A very marked reduction in kidney function (as measured by a fall in creatinine clearance) has been described in 3 patients on cisplatin when they were subsequently treated with **gentamicin** or **tobramycin**.[4] A comparative study on 17 patients on cisplatin and **gentamicin** confirmed that the incidence of nephrotoxicity was increased by concurrent use, but the renal insufficiency was described as usually mild and not clinically significant.[5] There is also evidence from studies in children to show that the half-life of **gentamicin** is approximately doubled by the presence of cisplatin,[6] and **aminoglycosides** increase the risk of nephrotoxicity.[7] Both cisplatin and the **aminoglycosides** can cause the excessive loss of magnesium and combined use increases this loss.[7,8]

Mechanism

Cisplatin is nephrotoxic and it would appear that its damaging effects on the kidney are additive with the nephrotoxic and possibly the ototoxic effects of the aminoglycoside antibacterials. Enhanced renal toxicity and ototoxicity have been reported in *guinea pigs* concurrently treated with cisplatin and kanamycin.[9] The magnesium-losing effects of both also seem to be additive.

Importance and management

An established and potentially serious interaction. It has been recommended that these antibacterials should only be given with caution, or probably not at all, to patients under treatment with cisplatin,[1,2] although one report describing the use of gentamicin without cefalotin claims that concurrent use can be relatively safe.[5] There is some evidence that previous treatment with cisplatin can delay the clearance of the aminoglycosides.[10] Sequential use should therefore be well monitored and the magnesium status checked.

1. Gonzalez-Vitale JC, Hayes DM, Cvitkovic E, Sternberg SS. Acute renal failure after *cis*-Dichlorodiammineplatinum (II) and gentamicin-cephalothin therapies. *Cancer Treat Rep* (1978) 62, 693–8.
2. Salem PA, Jabboury KW, Khalil MF. Severe nephrotoxicity: a probable complication of cis-dichorodiammineplatinum (II) and cephalothin-gentamicin therapy. *Oncology* (1982) 39, 31–2.
3. Leite JBF, De Campelo Gentil F, Burchenal J, Marques A, Teixeira MIC, Abrão FA. Insuficiênza renal aguda após o uso de cis-diaminodicloroplatina, gentamicina e cefalosporina. *Rev Paul Med* (1981) 97, 75–7.
4. Dentino M, Luft FC, Yum MN, Williams SD, Einhorn LH. Long term effect of cis-diamminedichloride platinum (CDDP) on renal function and structure in man. *Cancer* (1978) 41, 1274–81.
5. Haas A, Anderson L, Lad T. The influence of aminoglycosides on the nephrotoxicity of *cis*-diamminedichloroplatinum in cancer patients. *J Infect Dis* (1983) 147, 363.
6. Stewart CF, Christensen ML, Crom WR, Evans WE. The effect of cisplatin therapy on gentamicin pharmacokinetics. *Drug Intell Clin Pharm* (1984) 18, 512.
7. Pearson ADJ, Kohli M, Scott GW, Craft AW. Toxicity of high dose cisplatinum in children — the additive role of aminoglycosides. *Proc Am Ass Cancer Res* (1987) 28, 221.
8. Flombaum CD. Hypomagnesemia associated with cisplatin combination chemotherapy. *Arch Intern Med* (1984) 144, 2336–7.
9. Schweitzer VG, Hawkins JE, Lilly DJ, Litterst CJ, Abrams G, Davis JA, Christy M. Ototoxic and nephrotoxic effects of combined treatment with *cis*-diamminedichloroplatinum and kanamycin in the guinea pig. *Otolaryngol Head Neck Surg* (1984) 92, 38–49.
10. Christensen ML, Stewart CF, Crom WR. Evaluation of aminoglycoside disposition in patients previously treated with cisplatin. *Ther Drug Monit* (1989) 11, 631–6.

Cisplatin + Antihypertensive agents

A single report describes the development of kidney failure in a patient whose cisplatin-induced hypertension was treated with furosemide (frusemide), hydralazine, diazoxide and propranolol.

Clinical evidence, mechanism, importance and management

Three hours after receiving cisplatin intravenously (70 mg/m^2 body surface area) a patient experienced severe nausea and vomiting and his blood pressure rose from 150/90 to 248/140 mmHg. This was treated with **furosemide (frusemide)** 40 mg intravenously, **hydralazine** 10 mg intramuscularly, **diazoxide** 300 mg intravenously and **propranolol** 20 mg orally twice daily for 2 days. Nine days later the patient showed evidence of renal failure which resolved within 3 weeks. The patient was subsequently similarly treated on two occasions with cisplatin and again developed hypertension, but no treatment was given and there was no evidence of kidney dysfunction.[1] The reasons for the kidney failure are not known, but studies in *dogs*[2] and *rats*[3] indicate that kidney damage may possibly be related to the concentrations of cisplatin and that **furosemide** can increase cisplatin levels in the kidney.

Information seems to be limited to the reports cited and its general clinical importance is uncertain, however the authors of the clinical report[1] ". . . advise caution in treating hypertension or altering in any way renal hemodynamics in a patient receiving cisplatin."

1. Markman M, Trump DL. Nephrotoxicity with cisplatin and antihypertensive medications. *Ann Intern Med* (1982) 96, 257.
2. Cvitkovic E, Spaulding J, Bethune V, Martin J, Whitmore WF. Improvement of cis-dichlorodiammineplatinum (NSC 119875): therapeutic index in an animal model. *Cancer* (1977) 39, 1357–61.
3. Pera MF, Zook BC, Harder HC. Effects of mannitol or furosemide diuresis on the nephrotoxicity and physiological disposition of *cis*-dichlorodiammineplatinum-(II) in rats. *Cancer Res* (1979) 39, 1269–79.

Cisplatin + Etacrynic acid

Animal studies show that the damaging effects of cisplatin on the ear can be markedly increased by the concurrent use of etacrynic acid. It seems possible that this could also occur in man.

Clinical evidence, mechanism, importance and management

Both cisplatin and **etacrynic acid** given alone can be ototoxic in man. A study[1] carried out on *guinea pigs* showed that when cisplatin 7 mg/kg or **etacrynic acid** 50 mg/kg were given alone their ototoxic effects were reversible, but when given together the damaging effects on the ear were ". . . profound, and prolonged, if not permanent." Although this adverse interaction has not yet been reported in man, in the light of this study and what is already known about the ototoxicity of these two drugs in man, it seems possible that this may be a clinically important interaction. Audiometric tests should be carried out if these drugs are used concurrently.

1. Komune S, Snow JB. Potentiating effects of cisplatin and etacrynic acid in ototoxicity. *Arch Otolaryngol* (1981) 107, 594–7.

Cisplatin + Megestrol

Megestrol acetate may antagonise the antitumour activity of cisplatin.

Clinical evidence

A study in 243 patients with advanced small-cell lung cancer treated with a regimen including cisplatin with or without **megestrol acetate** found that patients who received **megestrol** had increased non-fluid body-weight and significantly less nausea and vomiting. However, the response rate to cisplatin was significantly worse (68% compared with 80%), although the 1-year survival was similar.[1]

Mechanism

An *in vitro* study found that megestrol may antagonise cisplatin cytotoxicity by upregulating cellular detoxification mechanisms.[2]

Importance and management

The authors of the second study suggest caution with the liberal use of megestrol acetate and cisplatin. Be aware that the use of megestrol may antagonise the anti-tumour activity of cisplatin. More study is needed.

1. Rowland KM, Loprinzi CL, Shaw EG, Maksymiuk AW, Kuross SA, Jung S-H, Kugler JW, Tschetter LK, Ghosh C, Schaefer PL, Owen D, Washburn JH, Webb TA, Mailliard JA, Jett JR. Randomized double-blind placebo-controlled trial of cisplatin and etoposide plus megestrol acetate/placebo in extensive-stage small-cell lung cancer: a North Central Cancer Treatment Group Study. *J Clin Oncol* (1996) 14, 135–41.
2. Pu Y-S, Cheng A-L, Chen J, Guan J-Y, Lu S-H, Lai M-K, Hsieh C-Y. Megestrol acetate antagonises cisplatin cytotoxicity. *Anticancer Drugs* (1998) 9, 733–8.

Cisplatin + Methotrexate

The risk of fatal methotrexate toxicity appears to be markedly increased by previous treatment with cisplatin.

Clinical evidence, mechanism, importance and management

Six out of 106 patients died with clinical signs of **methotrexate** toxicity 6 to 13 days after receiving 20 to 50 mg/m^2 in the absence of the usual signs of renal dysfunction and despite having previously been treated with **methotrexate** without serious toxicity. All had received prior treatment with cisplatin. Four of the patients were regarded as good-risk.[1] A study in children and adolescents suggested that the greater the cumulative dose of cisplatin received the greater the risk of **methotrexate** toxicity.[2] Another study indicated that the sequential use of cisplatin and high-dose **methotrexate** was nephrotoxic and decreased the amount of methotrexate which could be given.[3] A report on 14 patients on high dose **methotrexate**[4] indicated that prior treatment with one course of cisplatin sharply increased their serum levels of **methotrexate**, particularly if the cumulative **methotrexate** dose exceeded 400 mg/m^2.

The picture is not totally clear but it seems possible that prior treatment with cisplatin causes kidney damage which may not necessarily be detectable with the usual creatinine clearance tests. The effect is to cause a marked reduction in the clearance of the **methotrexate**. The serum **methotrexate** levels of these patients should be closely monitored so that any delay in its clearance is detected early and appropriate measures taken.[2]

1. Haim N, Kedar A, Robinson E. Methotrexate-related deaths in patients previously treated with *cis*-diamminedichloride platinum. *Cancer Chemother Pharmacol* (1984) 13, 223–5.
2. Crom WR, Pratt CB, Green AA, Champion JE, Crom DB, Stewart CF, Evans WE. The effect of prior cisplatin therapy on the pharmacokinetics of high-dose methotrexate. *J Clin Oncol* (1984) 2, 655–61.
3. Pitman SW, Mino DR, Papac R. Sequential methotrexate-leucovorin (MTX-LCV) and cis-platinum (CDDP) in head and neck cancer. *Proc American Assoc Cancer Research/ASCO* (1979) 21, 166.
4. Crom WR, Teresi ME, Meyer WH, Green AA, Evans WE. The intrapatient effect of cis-platin therapy on the pharmacokinetics of high-dose methotrexate. *Drug Intell Clin Pharm* (1985) 19, 467.

Cisplatin + Probenecid

On the basis of studies on *animals* it is uncertain whether the nephrotoxicity of cisplatin is increased or reduced by probenecid.

Clinical evidence, mechanism, importance and management

One study[1] in *rats* showed that **probenecid** could reduce cisplatin-induced nephrotoxicity, but other studies[2] found the complete opposite. The combination of cisplatin and **probenecid** was decidedly more toxic than cisplatin alone. Until this interaction has been more thoroughly studied this drug combination should be used with great care.

1. Ross DA, Gale GR. Reduction of the renal toxicity of *cis*-dichlorodiammineplatinum (II) by probenecid. *Cancer Treat Rep* (1979) 63, 781–7.
2. Daley-Yates PT, McBrien DCH. Enhancement of cisplatin nephrotoxicity by probenecid. *Cancer Treat Rep* (1984) 68, 445–6.

Cyclophosphamide + Allopurinol

There is evidence that the incidence of serious bone marrow depression caused by cyclophosphamide can be markedly increased by the concurrent use of allopurinol, but this was not confirmed in one study.

Clinical evidence

A retrospective epidemiological survey of patients in four hospitals who, over a 4-year period, had been treated with cyclophosphamide showed that the incidence of serious bone marrow depression was 57.7% in 26 patients who had also received **allopurinol**, and 18.8% in 32 patients who had not.[1]

A study in 9 patients with malignant disease and 2 healthy subjects showed that while taking 600 mg **allopurinol** daily the concentration of the cytotoxic metabolites of cyclophosphamide increased by an average of 37.5% (range −1.5 to +109%).[2] Agranulocytosis has been reported in another patient.[3] However another study,[4] designed as a follow-up to the study cited above[1] involving cytotoxic regimens which contained cyclophosphamide, failed to confirm that **allopurinol** increased the toxicity in patients with Hodgkin's or non-Hodgkin's lymphoma.

Mechanism

Not fully resolved. Cyclophosphamide itself is inactive, but it is converted in the liver into metabolites which are cytotoxic.[5] Allopurinol possibly increases the activity of the liver enzymes concerned with the production of these metabolites.[2] Another idea is that it inhibits their loss from the kidneys.[2] Since leucocyte toxicity is related to the concentration of the metabolites,[6] the increased incidence of bone marrow depression is, in part, explained.

Importance and management

This interaction is not established with any certainty. The authors of the survey[1] cited write that ". . . there seem to be good grounds for re-evaluating the routine practice of administering allopurinol [with cyclophosphamide] prophylactically." This does not forbid concurrent use, but introduces a strong note of caution. Be alert for increased cyclophosphamide toxicity.

1. Boston Collaborative Drug Surveillance Programme. Allopurinol and cytotoxic drugs. Interaction in relation to bone marrow depression. *JAMA* (1974) 227, 1036–40.
2. Witten J, Frederiksen PL, Mouridsen HT. The pharmacokinetics of cyclophosphamide in man after treatment with allopurinol. *Acta Pharmacol Toxicol* (1980) 46, 392–4.
3. Beeley L, Daly M, Steward P. *Bulletin of the W Midlands Centre for Adverse Drug Reaction Reporting* (1987) 24, 26.
4. Stolbach L, Begg C, Bennett JM, Silverstein M, Falkson G, Harris DT, Glick J. Evaluation of bone marrow toxic reaction in patients treated with allopurinol. *JAMA* (1982) 247, 334–6.
5. Bagley CM, Bostick FW, DeVita VT. Clinical pharmacology of cyclophosphamide. *Cancer Res* (1973) 33, 226–33.
6. Mouridsen HT, Witten J, Frederiksen PL, Hulsbæk I. Studies on the correlation between rate of biotransformation and haematological toxicity of cyclophosphamide. *Acta Pharmacol Toxicol* (1978) 42, 81.

Cyclophosphamide + Amiodarone

Early-onset lung toxicity occurred in a patient on amiodarone after high-dose cyclophosphamide.

Clinical evidence, mechanism, importance and management

A patient with dendritic cell carcinoma who had been treated with **amiodarone** for 18 months, and with 6 cycles of chemotherapy including cyclophosphamide over the last 12 months, was admitted to hospital with progressive shortness of breath 18 days after a single dose of cyclophosphamide 4000 mg/m². He was found to have interstitial pneumonitis and a lung biopsy indicated drug-induced lung toxicity. The patient's condition improved rapidly over the following 10 days with discontinuation of **amiodarone** and treatment with prednisolone 60 mg daily. Over the previous year he had also received vincristine, etoposide and prednisone, cisplatin, cytarabine and dexamethasone as part of his chemotherapy regimens.[1]

Mechanism

Lung toxicity may occur in about 10% of patients treated with amiodarone.[2,3] Lung toxicity due to cyclophosphamide may occur between 1 to 6 months after exposure or occur as a more insidious form after about 6 months. The early onset on symptoms in this patient, just over 2 weeks after high-dose cyclophosphamide, suggests accelerated mechanisms of lung toxicity. Both cyclophosphamide and amiodarone lung toxicity appears to be enhanced by oxygen and the combination of cyclophosphamide with amiodarone may enhance oxidative stress and therefore lung toxicity.

Importance and management

Although information seems to be limited to the single case report cited, the potential for both cyclophosphamide and amiodarone to cause lung toxicity is established. Be alert to the possibility of enhanced lung toxicity if these drugs are co-administered.

1. Bhagat R, Sporn TA, Long GD, Folz RJ. Amiodarone and cyclophosphamide: potential for enhanced lung toxicity. *Bone Marrow Transplant* (2001) 27, 1109–1111.
2. Martin WJ, Rosenow EC. Amiodarone pulmonary toxicity. Recognition and pathogenesis (Part 1). *Chest* (1988) 93, 1067–75.
3. Martin WJ, Rosenow EC. Amiodarone pulmonary toxicity. Recognition and pathogenesis (Part 2). *Chest* (1988) 93, 1242–8.

Cyclophosphamide + Azathioprine

A report describes liver damage in four patients given cyclophosphamide who had previously been treated with azathioprine.

Clinical evidence, mechanism, importance and management

Four patients (two with systemic lupus erythematosus, one with Sjogren's syndrome, and one with Wegener's granulomatosis) developed liver injury when given cyclophosphamide. All had previously been treated with **azathioprine**. Three of them showed liver cell necrosis. Liver biopsy showed cytolytic necrosis of perihepatic venous hepatocytes. Two of them had had cyclophosphamide previously without apparent liver damage.[1] The relationship between the sequential use of these drugs is not established but these cases draw attention to the possibility of this adverse effect in other patients.

1. Shaunak S, Munro JM, Weinbren K, Walport MJ, Cox TM. Cyclophosphamide-induced liver necrosis: a possible interaction with azathioprine. *Q J Med* (1988) New Series 67, 309–17.

Cyclophosphamide + Barbiturates

Despite some *animal* data, the evidence from studies in man suggests that neither the toxicity nor the therapeutic effects of cyclophosphamide are significantly affected by the concurrent use of the barbiturates.

Clinical evidence, mechanism, importance and management

There is evidence from a number of *animal* studies that the **barbiturates** and other potent liver enzyme-inducing agents can affect the activity of cyclophosphamide,[1,2] but studies undertaken in man indicate that although some changes in the pharmacokinetics of cyclophosphamide occur, neither the toxicity nor the therapeutic effects of cyclophosphamide are significantly altered.[3,4] No special precautions seem to be necessary.

1. Donelli MG, Colombo T, Garattini S. Effect of cyclophosphamide on the activity and distribution of pentobarbital in rats. *Biochem Pharmacol* (1973) 22, 2609–14.
2. Alberts DS, van Daalen Wetters T. The effect of phenobarbital on cyclophosphamide antitumour activity. *Cancer Res* (1976) 36, 2785–9.
3. Bagley CM, Bostick FW, DeVita VT. Clinical pharmacology of cyclophosphamide. *Cancer Res* (1973) 33, 226–33.
4. Jao JY, Jusko WJ, Cohen JL. Phenobarbital effects on cyclophosphamide pharmacokinetics in man. *Cancer Res* (1972) 32, 2761–4.

Cyclophosphamide + Benzodiazepines

***Animal* studies suggest that the benzodiazepines may possibly increase the toxicity of cyclophosphamide.**

Clinical evidence, mechanism, importance and management

Studies in *mice* found that 3 days' treatment with benzodiazepines (**chlordiazepoxide, diazepam, oxazepam**) increased the lethality of the cyclophosphamide (without improving its effectiveness against Ehrlich solid tumour).[1] This may be due, it is suggested, to the induction of the liver enzymes concerned with the metabolism of cyclophosphamide to its active cytotoxic products. The importance of this possible interaction in man is uncertain, but the possibility should be borne in mind during concurrent use.

1. Sasaki K-I, Furusawa S, Takayanagi G. Effects of chlordiazepoxide, diazepam and oxazepam on the antitumour activity, the lethality and the blood level of active metabolites of cyclophosphamide and cyclophosphamide oxidase activity in mice. *J Pharm Dyn* (1983) 6, 767–72.

Cyclophosphamide + Busulfan

Cyclophosphamide serum levels may be increased if given within less than 24 h of busulfan treatment.

Clinical evidence, mechanism, importance and management

Twenty-three bone marrow transplant patients were pre-treated with **busulfan** (4 mg/kg/day) for 4 days followed by cyclophosphamide (60 mg/kg/day) for 2 days. Twelve of the patients were given the cyclophosphamide 24 to 50 h after the last **busulfan** dose, and 11 patients 7 to 15 h after. Nine others pre-treated with cyclophosphamide and total body irradiation acted as the controls. In the group with the 24 to 50 h interval between drugs, the cyclophosphamide AUC was similar to the controls, but in the 7 to 15 h interval group the AUC was more than doubled compared with the controls.[1]

It seems therefore that if the cyclophosphamide is given at least 24 h after the last busulfan dose, its serum levels will not be greatly affected, whereas if the interval is short the cyclophosphamide serum levels will be markedly increased. It is therefore important to taking this timing into consideration to achieve better drug efficacy and possibly less drug toxicity.

This interaction should be taken into account when planning a regimen.

1. Hassan M, Ljungman P, Ringdén O, Hassan Z, Öberg G, Nilsson C, Békassy A, Bielenstein M, Abdel-Rehim M, Georén S, Astner L. The effect of busulphan on the pharmacokinetics of cyclophosphamide and its 4-hydroxy metabolite: time interval influence on the therapeutic efficacy and therapy-related toxicity. *Bone Marrow Transplant* (2000) 25, 915–24.

Cyclophosphamide + Chloramphenicol

Some limited evidence suggests that chloramphenicol may reduce the production of the therapeutically active metabolites of cyclophosphamide, thereby reducing its activity.

Clinical evidence, mechanism, importance and management

Cyclophosphamide itself is inactive, but after administration it is metabolised within the body to active alkylating metabolites. *Animal* studies[1] have shown that pretreatment with **chloramphenicol** reduces the activity (lethality) of cyclophosphamide because, it is believed, the antibacterial inhibits its conversion to these active metabolites. Studies[2] in four patients showed that 1 g **chloramphenicol** twice daily for 12 days prolonged the mean half-life of cyclophosphamide from 7.5 to 11.5 h and the production of the active metabolites fell. So it seems possible that a reduction in the activity of cyclophosphamide may also occur in man, but the extent to which this affects treatment with cyclophosphamide is uncertain. Concurrent use need not be avoided, but be on the watch for evidence of a reduced response. More study is needed.

1. Dixon RL. Effect of chloramphenicol on the metabolism and lethality of cyclophosphamide in rats. *Proc Soc Exp Biol Med* (1968) 127, 1151–5.
2. Faber OK, Mouridsen HT, Skovsted L. The effect of chloramphenicol and sulphaphenazole on the biotransformation of cyclophosphamide in man. *Br J Clin Pharmacol* (1975) 2, 281–5.

Cyclophosphamide + Corticosteroids

There is evidence that single doses of prednisone can reduce the activity of cyclophosphamide, but the effects of longer term treatment is uncertain, with both increases and reduction in activity reported. Synergistic increases in enzyme induction may occur with cyclophosphamide plus dexamethasone.

Clinical evidence and mechanism

Cyclophosphamide itself is inactive, but after administration it is metabolised in the body to active metabolites. Single doses of **prednisone** have been shown to inhibit the activation of cyclophosphamide in man[1] and in *animals*,[2] probably due to competition for the drug-metabolising enzymes in the liver. In a brief report

of an *in vitro* study it was noted that the combination of cyclophosphamide with **dexamethasone** resulted in a 50 to 88% greater induction of activity of cytochrome P450 isoenzyme CYP3A4 than with either drug alone, which could result in reduced cyclophosphamide efficacy.[3] Longer-term treatment on the other hand (50 mg daily for 1 to 2 weeks) has been shown in man to have the opposite effect and increases the rate of activation of the cyclophosphamide, probably due to the induction of the liver enzymes.[1] Another study in 7 patients with systemic vasculitis given **prednisone** 1 mg/kg daily and cyclophosphamide 0.6 mg/m^2 intravenously every 3 weeks for 6 cycles found that by the last cycle the AUC of cyclophosphamide had significantly increased while that of its active metabolites had significantly decreased. The significance of this interaction is not clear but it was suggested that the cyclophosphamide dose made need to be increased for subsequent cycles,[4] and reduced when concurrent corticosteroids are withdrawn.

Importance and management

The documentation is very limited and information is conflicting, but changes in the activity of the cyclophosphamide should be watched for during concurrent use. The situation with other corticosteroids is uncertain. More study is needed.

1. Faber OK, Mouridsen HT. Cyclophosphamide activation and corticosteroids. *N Engl J Med* (1974) 291, 211.
2. Sladek NE. Therapeutic efficacy of cyclophosphamide as a function of inhibition of its metabolism. *Cancer Res* (1972) 32, 1848.
3. Lindley C, McCune J, Hawke R, Gillenwater H, Petros W, LeCluyse E. Induction of cytochrome P450 3A4 activity by cyclophosphamide alone and in combination with dexamethasone. *Clin Pharmacol Ther* (1999) 65, 175.
4. Belfayol-Pisante L, Guillevin L, Tod M, Fauvelle F. Possible influence of prednisone on the pharmacokinetics of cyclophosphamide in systemic vasculitis. *Clin Drug Invest* (1999) 18, 225–31.

Cyclophosphamide + Dapsone

Some extremely limited evidence suggests that dapsone might be capable of reducing the activity of cyclophosphamide.

Clinical evidence, mechanism, importance and management

An unexplained and undetailed report has described patients with leprosy on **dapsone** and cyclophosphamide who showed inhibition of the leucopenia normally associated with cyclophosphamide treatment.[1] Whether this indicates a reduction in the effects of cyclophosphamide is uncertain, but it would seem prudent to be on the alert for signs of a depressed therapeutic response to cyclophosphamide during concurrent treatment. More study is needed.

1. Quoted by Warren RD, Bender RA. Drug interactions with antineoplastic agents. *Cancer Treat Rep* (1977) 61, 1231–41.

Cyclophosphamide + Doxorubicin (Adriamycin)

A single case report suggests that the damaging effects of cyclophosphamide and doxorubicin on the bladder may be additive.

Clinical evidence, mechanism, importance and management

A woman was treated with cyclophosphamide (100 to 150 mg daily orally) for 3 years for the treatment of breast cancer. The cyclophosphamide was withdrawn and replaced by intravenous **doxorubicin** 30 mg weekly. After 5 doses she developed severe haemorrhagic cystitis and a bladder biopsy showed that the cyclophosphamide had caused chronic subclinical bladder damage, which apparently was further aggravated by the **doxorubicin**. The authors recommend that patients given **doxorubicin** should be carefully examined for microscopic haematuria, particularly if they have previously had cyclo-phosphamide or pelvic irradiation.[1]

1. Ershler WB, Gilchrist KW, Citrin DL. Adriamycin enhancement of cyclophosphamide-induced bladder injury. *J Urol* (1980) 123, 121–2.

Cyclophosphamide + Filgrastim (G-CSF)

A child died of respiratory failure after treatment with cyclo-phosphamide and filgrastim G-CSF.

Clinical evidence, mechanism, importance and management

A 1-year-old boy with a neuroblastoma Evans stage III died of respi-ratory insufficiency following treatment with **filgrastim (G-CSF)** and normal doses of cyclophosphamide and doxorubicin. The authors of the report suggest that the pulmonary toxicity of the cyclophospha-mide (normally only seen with high cumulative doses) is potentiated by the **filgrastim**.[1] There is some evidence that the pulmonary toxic-ity of bleomycin might possibly also be increased by **filgrastim** (see 'Bleomycin + Cytotoxic regimens and drugs used in neutropenia', p.490).

1. van Woensel JBM, Knoester H, Leeuw JA, van Aalderen WMC. Acute respiratory insuf-ficiency during doxorubicin, cyclophosphamide, and G-CSF therapy. *Lancet* (1994) 344, 759–60.

Cyclophosphamide + Indometacin (Indomethacin)

A single case report describes acute water intoxication in a patient taking indometacin when given low-dose intravenous cyclophosphamide.

Clinical evidence, mechanism, importance and management

A patient with multiple myeloma and adequate renal function on 50 mg **indometacin (indomethacin)** 8-hourly, developed acute wa-ter intoxication and salt retention after being given a single bolus in-travenous injection of 500 mg cyclophosphamide (<10 mg/kg). The reasons are not understood, but it is suggested that it was due to the additive or synergistic effects of the two drugs.[1] **Indometacin** inhib-its the production of the renal vasodilatory prostaglandins (PgE$_2$, PgI$_2$) which affect the renal blood flow and also inhibit salt and water reabsorption by the kidney. The cyclophosphamide produces metab-olites which have antidiuretic effects.

The general importance of this case is uncertain, but the authors of the report suggest caution if both drugs are used.

1. Webberley M J, Murray J A. Life-threatening acute hyponatraemia induced by low dose cyclophosphamide and indomethacin. *Postgrad Med J* (1989) 65, 950–2.

Cyclophosphamide or Chlormethine (Mustine) + Morphine or Pethidine

Animal **studies indicate that the toxicity of cyclophosphamide and chlormethine (mustine) is increased by morphine or pethidine.**

Clinical evidence, mechanism, importance and management

Studies in *mice*[1] have shown that **morphine** in doses of 5 to 25 mg/kg increases sublethal doses of **cyclophosphamide** 300 mg/kg and **chlo-rmethine (mustine)** 5 mg/kg into maximally lethal doses. The effect of **pethidine (meperidine)** was less marked. This work suggests that

there may be a need to re-evaluate the concurrent use of these drugs in man.

1. Akintonwa A. Potentiation of nitrogen mustard toxicity by narcotic analgesic. *Clin Toxi-col* (1981) 18, 451–8.

Cyclophosphamide + Pentostatin

Acute and fatal cardiotoxicity developed in two patients when pentostatin was added to high-dose cyclophosphamide treat-ment.

Clinical evidence, mechanism, importance and management

A clinical trial was started to find out if **pentostatin** would increase and improve the immunosuppression of cyclophosphamide, carmus-tine and etoposide needed to ensure the success of bone marrow trans-plantation, but when acute and fatal cardiac toxicity developed in the first two patients, the trial was stopped. Both patients had been started on 800 mg/m^2 cyclophosphamide and 200 mg/m^2 etoposide, both 12-hourly for 8 doses, and 112 mg/m^2 carmustine (BCNU) daily for 4 doses. To this was added 4 mg/m^2 **pentostatin** over 4 h on day 3. On the day after chemotherapy, cyclophosphamide was begun, but with-in 8 to 24 h both patients developed confusion, hypothermia, hypo-tension, respiratory distress, pulmonary oedema, and eventually fatal ventricular fibrillation within 45 to 120 min of the first symptoms. A later study with *rats* similarly found that **pentostatin** markedly in-creased the acute toxicity of cyclophosphamide. The reasons for this cardiotoxicity are not understood. Neither of the two patients had pre-viously shown any evidence of cardiac abnormalities.[1]

This interaction is not established beyond any doubt, but the avail-able evidence certainly suggests that it probably occurs. The part (if any) played by the carmustine and etoposide is uncertain. It is clearly not safe to combine **pentostatin** with high-dose cyclophosphamide. More study is needed.

1. Gryn J, Gordon R, Bapat A, Goldman N, Goldberg J. Pentostatin increases the acute tox-icity of high dose cyclophosphamide. *Bone Marrow Transplant* (1993) 12, 217–20.

Cyclophosphamide + Ranitidine

Ranitidine appears not to increase the bone marrow toxicity of cyclophosphamide.

Clinical evidence, mechanism, importance and management

A study in 7 cancer patients found that although 300 mg oral **raniti-dine** daily significantly prolonged the half-life and increased the AUC of cyclophosphamide (600 mg/m^2 cyclophosphamide given in-travenously), it did not significantly affect the AUCs of the two major oncolytic metabolites of cyclophosphamide nor did it affect its bone marrow toxicity (leucopenia, granulocytopenia). The authors of the study conclude that **ranitidine** can safely be given with cyclophos-phamide.[1]

1. Alberts DS, Mason-Liddil N, Plezia PM, Roe DJ, Dorr RT, Struck RF, Phillips JG. Lack of ranitidine effects on cyclophosphamide bone marrow toxicity or metabolism: a place-bo-controlled clinical trial. *J Natl Cancer Inst* (1991) 83, 1739–43.

Cyclophosphamide + Sulfaphenazole

Some very limited evidence suggests that sulfaphenazole may increase or decrease the activity of cyclophosphamide, but the clinical importance of this is uncertain.

Clinical evidence, mechanism, importance and management

A study[1] in 7 patients on a 50-mg dose of cyclophosphamide given 1 g **sulfaphenazole** twice daily for 9 to 14 days showed that the half-life of the cyclophosphamide was unchanged in 3 patients, longer in 2 patients and shorter in the remaining 2 patients. The reasons are not clear. Whether this has any practical importance or not is uncertain, but it would seem prudent to be on the watch for changes in the response to cyclophosphamide if **sulfaphenazole** is given concurrently. More study is needed. Information about other sulphonamides appears to be lacking.

1. Faber OK, Mouridsen HT, Skovsted L. The effect of chloramphenicol and sulphaphenazole on the biotransformation of cyclophosphamide in man. *Br J Clin Pharmacol* (1975) 2, 281–5.

Cyclophosphamide + Thiotepa

Pretreatment with thiotepa may inhibit the metabolism of cyclophosphamide to its active metabolite and decrease both its efficacy and toxicity. Cyclophosphamide appears not to affect the metabolism of thiotepa.

Clinical evidence, mechanism, importance and management

An *in vitro* study using human microsomes found that cyclophosphamide had no effect on the metabolism of **thiotepa** to tepa by cytochrome P450 at therapeutic concentrations.[1] However, the observation that the concentration of the active metabolite of cyclophosphamide, 4-hydroxycyclophosphamide, decreased sharply after the start of **thiotepa** administration in 20 patients suggests a possible drug interaction.[2]

In a study to investigate this, 3 patients were given high-dose cyclophosphamide 1000 or 1500 mg/m^2 as a 1-h infusion, followed by carboplatin and **thiotepa** for 4 days. The order of infusion was reversed on one treatment day in each of 4 courses. Administration of **thiotepa** 1 h before cyclophosphamide resulted in decreases in the peak plasma levels and AUC of 4-hydroxycyclophosphamide of 62% and 26% respectively when compared with those when **thiotepa** was administered 1 h after cyclophosphamide. This may affect both the efficacy and toxicity of cyclophosphamide. The authors question the practice of simultaneous infusing of cyclophosphamide and **thiotepa** and suggest that the order of administration may be of critical importance.[2]

1. Van Maanen MJ, Huitema ADR, Beijnen JH. Influence of co-medicated drugs on the biotransformation of thioTEPA to TEPA and thioTEPA-mercapturate. *Anticancer Res* (2000) 20, 1711–16.
2. Huitema ADR, Kerbusch T, Tibben MM, Rodenhuis S, Beijnen JH. Reduction of cyclophosphamide bioactivation by thioTEPA: critical sequence-dependency in high-dose chemotherapy regimens. *Cancer Chemother Pharmacol* (2000) 46, 119–27.

Cytotoxics + Calcium channel blockers

Verapamil can increase the efficacy of doxorubicin both in tissue culture systems and in patients. It raises serum doxorubicin levels. The absorption of verapamil can be reduced by COPP and VAC cytotoxic drug regimens. Nifedipine possibly reduces the clearance of vincristine.

Clinical evidence, mechanism, importance and management

(a) The effect of calcium channel blockers on cytotoxics

The efficacy of **doxorubicin** can be increased by **verapamil** and **nicardipine** in doxorubicin-resistant tissue culture systems,[1] while nifedipine has only minimal activity. A study[2] in five patients with small cell lung cancer given **doxorubicin, vincristine, etoposide** and **cyclophosphamide** showed that when given **verapamil** 240 to 480 mg daily the AUC of the **doxorubicin** was doubled, peak serum

levels were raised and the clearance was reduced. No increased toxicity was seen in this study or another study,[3] but be alert for this possibility if both drugs are used. There is also some evidence that **nifedipine** can reduce the clearance of intravenous **vincristine**,[4] but whether this increases the **vincristine** toxicity is uncertain.

(b) The effect of cytotoxics on calcium channel blockers

A study in 9 patients with a variety of malignant diseases showed that treatment with **cytotoxic drugs** reduced the absorption of 160 mg **verapamil** given orally. The AUC in 8 patients was reduced by 40% (range 7 to 58%). One patient showed a 26% increase. Five patients received a modified **COPP** regimen (**cyclophosphamide, vincristine, procarbazine, prednisone**) and four received **VAC** (**vindesine, adriamycin (doxorubicin), cisplatin**).[5] It is believed that these cytotoxics damage the lining of the upper part of the small intestine which impairs the absorption of **verapamil**. Patients should be monitored for signs of a reduced response to **verapamil** during concurrent treatment.

1. Ramu A, Spanier R, Rahamimoff H, Fuks Z. Restoration of doxorubicin responsiveness in doxorubicin-resistant P388 murine leukaemia cells. *Br J Cancer* (1984) 50, 501–7.
2. Kerr DJ, Graham J, Cummings J, Morrison JG, Thompson GG, Brodie MJ, Kaye SB. The effect of verapamil on the pharmacokinetics of adriamycin. *Cancer Chemother Pharmacol* (1986) 18, 239–42.
3. Ozols RF, Rogan AM, Hamilton TC, Klecker R, Young RC. Verapamil plus adriamycin in refractory ovarian cancer: design of a clinical trial on basis of reversal of adriamycin resistance in human ovarian cancer cell lines. *Am Assoc Cancer Res* (1986) Abstract 1186.
4. Fedeli L, Colozza M, Boschetti E, Sabalich I, Aristei C, Guerciolini R, Del Favero A, Rossetti R, Tonato M, Rambotti P, Davis S. Pharmacokinetics of vincristine in cancer patients treated with nifedipine. *Cancer* (1989) 64, 1805–11.
5. Kuhlmann J, Woodcock B, Wilke J, Rietbrock N. Verapamil plasma concentrations during treatment with cytostatic drugs. *J Cardiovasc Pharmacol* (1985) 7, 1003–6.

Cytotoxics + Food

The absorption of melphalan can be reduced by food, but etoposide is unaffected. Low-dose methotrexate appears not to be significantly affected by food.

Clinical evidence, mechanism, importance and management

(a) Etoposide

The plasma **etoposide** concentrations of 11 patients with extensive small cell lung carcinoma given 100 mg oral doses were unaffected when taken with **breakfast** (milk, cornflakes, sugar, egg, sausage, bread, margarine, marmalade, coffee or tea). Also no changes were seen when the **etoposide** was taken with **cyclophosphamide** 100 mg/m^2, **methotrexate** 12.5 mg/m^2, doxorubicin 35 mg/m^2 or **procarbazine** 60 mg/m^2 all given orally.[1]

(b) Melphalan

A study in 5 patients with multiple myeloma showed that the half-life of **melphalan** 5 mg/m^2 was unaffected when taken with a standardised **breakfast**, but the AUC was reduced to an average of 43% (range 0 to 78%). In one patient no **melphalan** was detectable when given with **food**.[2]

(c) Methotrexate

The peak serum **methotrexate** levels (measured at 1.5 h) of 10 children with lymphoblastic leukaemia, following an oral dose of 15 mg/m^2 were reduced by about 40% when taken with a **milky meal** (milk, cornflakes, sugar, white bread and butter). The area under the 4 h AUC was reduced by about 25%. A smaller reduction was seen after a 'citrus meal' (orange juice, fresh orange, white bread, butter and jam).[3] However a 4 h study is too short to assess the extent of the total absorption. Another study in 16 other children given 8 to 22.7 mg/m^2 **methotrexate** found that peak levels and AUC were not significantly affected if **methotrexate** was given before a meal.[4] Yet another study in 12 healthy subjects found that a **high fat-content breakfast** delayed the absorption of **methotrexate** 7.5 mg orally by about 30 min but the extent of the absorption was unchanged.[5]

1. Harvey VJ, Slevin ML, Joel SP, Johnston A, Wrigley PFM. The effect of food and concurrent chemotherapy on the bioavailability of oral etoposide. *Br J Cancer* (1985) 52, 363–7.
2. Kotasek D, Dale BM, Morris RG, Reece PA, Sage RE. Food reduces oral melphalan absorption. *Aust N Z J Med* (1985) 15 (Suppl 1), 120.
3. Pinkerton CR, Welshman SG, Glasgow JFT, Bridges JM. Can food influence the absorption of methotrexate in children with acute lymphoblastic leukaemia? *Lancet* (1980) 2, 944–6.
4. Madanat F, Awidi A, Shaheen O, Ottman S, Al-Turk W. Effects of food and gender on the pharmacokinetics of methotrexate in children. *Res Commun Chem Pathol Pharmacol* (1987) 55, 279–82.
5. Kozloski GD, De Vito JM, Kisicki JC, Johnson JB. The effect of food on the absorption of methotrexate sodium tablets in healthy volunteers. *Arthritis Rheum* (1992) 35, 761–4.

Cytotoxics + Gentamicin

There is evidence that the use of gentamicin with daunorubicin, tioguanine (thioguanine) and cytarabine may cause hypomagnesaemia.

Clinical evidence, mechanism, importance and management

The observation of hypomagnesaemia in 2 patients given **gentamicin** (with lincomycin or mezlocillin) during induction therapy for non-lymphoblastic leukaemia prompted further study in another 9 patients. They were all treated with the same cytotoxic regimen: intravenous **daunorubicin** 50 mg/m^2 on day 1, oral **tioguanine** (**thioguanine**) 100 mg/m^2 twice daily on days 1 to 5, and intravenous **cytarabine** 100 mg/m^2 twice daily on days 1 to 5. Six out of 11 patients demonstrated hypomagnesaemia.[1] The reasons are not known but suggestions include a direct nephrotoxic action of the cytotoxic drugs, or the cytotoxics may sensitise the kidneys to the actions of **gentamicin**. Concurrent use should be well monitored.

1. Davey P, Gozzard D, Goodall M, Leyland MJ. Hypomagnesaemia: an underdiagnosed interaction between gentamicin and cytotoxic chemotherapy for acute non-lymphoblastic leukaemia. *J Antimicrob Chemother* (1985) 15, 623–8.

Cytotoxics + Lenograstim

Lenograstim can promote the growth of myeloid cell lines *in vitro*. Since rapidly dividing myeloid cells are sensitive to cytotoxic chemotherapy the manufacturers advise that lenograstim is not used from 24 h before or until 24 h after cytotoxic chemotherapy.[1]

1. Granocyte (Lenograstim). Chugai Pharma UK Limited. Summary of product characteristics, November 2001.

Cytotoxics + Ondansetron

Cisplatin and fluorouracil do not affect the pharmacokinetics of ondansetron, but ondansetron appears to increase the nephrotoxicity of zeniplatin. Ondansetron may affect the pharmacokinetics of cyclophosphamide and cisplatin but does not appear to affect carmustine pharmacokinetics.

Clinical evidence, mechanism, importance and management

No significant changes in the pharmacokinetics of **ondansetron** occurred in 20 cancer patients on **cisplatin** (20 to 40 mg/m^2) and/or **fluorouracil** (1 g/m^2) for 5 days but the clearance was lower than in healthy subjects.[1]

A study compared the pharmacokinetics of high-dose **cyclophosphamide**, **cisplatin** and **carmustine** in 23 patients given **ondansetron**, lorazepam and diphenhydramine as antiemetics and 129 patients who received prochlorperazine instead of **ondansetron**. It was found that the AUCs of **cyclophosphamide** and **cisplatin**, but not that of

carmustine, were significantly lower in the **ondansetron group**.[2] Another study in 54 patients with breast cancer who were receiving high-dose **cyclophosphamide**, **cisplatin** and **carmustine** with lorazepam and **ondansetron** with or without prochlorperazine. This was compared to 75 matched controls who had only received prochlorperazine and lorazepam. The median AUC of **cyclophosphamide** in patients given **ondansetron** was lower than in the control patients, the **cisplatin** AUC was about 10% higher and the **carmustine** AUC was unchanged by concurrent **ondansetron**.[3] A study in 10 patients who received intravenous **cyclophosphamide** 600 mg/m^2 and **epirubicin** 90 mg/m^2 and either oral **ondansetron** 16 mg or placebo found that the pharmacokinetic parameters of **cyclophosphamide** were not significantly altered by **ondansetron**. No significant differences were found in the **cyclophosphamide metabolites** either, but there was considerable variation between subjects. It was concluded that **ondansetron** can be safely co-administered with **cyclophosphamide**.[4]

A phase II trial of **zeniplatin** in 308 patients found that nephrotoxicity occurred in 22 of them (7%). Of the 308 patients, 32 had been given **ondansetron** alone or with **dexamethasone** as antiemetic treatment, and 14 of the 32 (44%) developed nephrotoxicity of varying severity. Only 8 of the other patients (3%) who had not had **ondansetron** developed nephrotoxicity.[5] The reasons for this increased nephrotoxicity are not known but these preliminary observations suggest that concurrent use should be undertaken with caution.

1. Hsyu P-H, Bozigian HP, Pritchard JF, Kernodle A, Panella J, Hansen LA, Griffin RH. Effect of chemotherapy on the pharmacokinetics of oral ondansetron. *Pharm Res* (1991) 8 (Suppl 10), S-257.
2. Cagnoni PJ, Matthes S, Day TC, Bearman SI, Shpall EJ, Jones RB. Modification of the pharmacokinetics of high-dose cyclophosphamide and cisplatin by antiemetics. *Bone Marrow Transplant* (1999) 24, 1–4.
3. Gilbert CJ, Petros WP, Vredenburgh J, Hussein A, Ross M, Rubin P, Fehdrau R, Cavanaugh C, Berry D, McKinstry C, Peters WP. Pharmacokinetic interaction between ondansetron and cyclophosphamide during high-dose chemotherapy for breast cancer. *Cancer Chemother Pharmacol* (1998) 42, 497–503.
4. Lorenz C, Eickhoff C, Baumann F, Sehouli J, Preiss R, Schunack W, Jaehde U. Does ondansetron affect the metabolism of cyclophosphamide? *Int J Clin Pharmacol Ther* (2000) 38, 143–4.
5. Aamdal S. Can ondansetron hydrochloride (Zofran®) enhance the nephrotoxic potential of other drugs? *Ann Oncol* (1992) 3, 774.

Cytotoxics + Propofol

Severe pain may occur in patients given intravenous propofol who have previously had intravenous chemotherapy.

Clinical evidence, mechanism, importance and management

The occurrence of pain both at the injection site and up the arm on induction with propofol has been noted to occur in patients previously treated with cytotoxic drugs.[1] This would seem to link with a report of a girl of 15 with acute lymphoblastic leukaemia who been treated with several injections of **cyclophosphamide**, **methotrexate** and **vincristine** during the previous 6 months, and who was cannulated in her hand and infused with *Plasmalyte B*. An injection of 60 micrograms of **fentanyl** was painful and 20 mg lidocaine (lignocaine) helped, but 20 mg (2 ml) **propofol** caused extreme pain and a further 20 mg lidocaine was given. The whole hand became blue and congested, and blood began to move backwards up the drip tubing. The venous congestion gradually subsided over the next 15 min.[2] The authors recommend that **propofol** should be avoided in patients who have recently had intravenous chemotherapeutic agents.[2]

1. Whitlock JC, Nicol ME, Pattison J. Painful injection of propofol. *Anaesthesia* (1989) 44, 618.
2. Butt AD, James MFM. Venospasm due to propofol after chemotherapy. *S Afr Med J* (1990) 77, 168.

Cytotoxics + Vaccines

The immune response of the body is suppressed by cytotoxic drugs. The effectiveness of vaccines may be poor and gener-

alised infection may occur in patients immunised with live vaccines.

Clinical evidence, mechanism, importance and management

Since the cytotoxic drugs are immunosuppressants, the response of the body to immunisation is reduced. A study[1] in 53 patients with Hodgkin's disease showed that chemotherapy reduced the antibody response 60% when measured 3 weeks after immunisation with a **pneumococcal vaccine**. The patients were treated with **chlormethine (mustine), vincristine, prednisone and procarbazine**. A few of them also had **bleomycin, vinblastine** or **cyclophosphamide**. Subtotal radiotherapy reduced the response a further 15%. The response to **influenza immunisation** in children with various malignancies was also found to be markedly suppressed by chemotherapy. The cytotoxic drugs used were **6-mercaptopurine, methotrexate, vincristine,** and **prednisone**. Some of them were also treated with **vincristine, dactinomycin (actinomycin D)** and **cyclophosphamide**.[2] Only 9 out of 17 children with leukaemia and other malignant diseases treated with **methotrexate, cyclophosphamide, mercaptopurine** and **prednisone** developed a significant response to immunisation with **inactivated measles vaccine**.[3]

Immunisation with **live vaccines** may result in a potentially life-threatening infection. For example, a woman who was under treatment with 15 mg **methotrexate** once a month for psoriasis and who was vaccinated against **smallpox**, developed a generalised vaccinial infection.[4] Studies in *animals* given **smallpox vaccine** confirmed that they were more susceptible to infection if treated with **methotrexate, mercaptopurine** or **cyclophosphamide**.[5]

Smallpox is no longer a problem, but other live vaccines such as **rubella, measles, mumps** and others continue to be used. Extreme care should therefore be exercised in immunising patients with live vaccines who are receiving cytotoxics or other immunosuppressant drugs (see also 'Corticosteroids + Vaccines (live)', p.640).

1. Siber GR, Weitzman SA, Aisenberg AC, Weinstein HJ, Schiffman G. Impaired antibody response to pneumococcal vaccine after treatment for Hodgkins disease. *N Engl J Med* (1978) 299, 442–8.
2. Gross PA, Lee H, Wolff JA, Hall CB, Minnefore AB, Lazicki ME. Influenza immunization in immunosuppressed children. *J Pediatr* (1978) 92, 30–5.
3. Stiehm ER, Ablin A, Kushner JH, Zoger S. Measles vaccination in patients on immunosuppressive drugs. *Am J Dis Child* (1966) 111, 191–4.
4. Allison J. Methotrexate and smallpox vaccination. *Lancet* (1968) ii, 1250.
5. Rosenbaum EH, Cohen RA, Glatstein HR. Vaccination of a patient receiving immunosuppressive therapy for lymphosarcoma. *JAMA* (1966) 198, 737–40.

Docetaxel + Miscellaneous drugs

Based on *in vitro* studies, it is predicted that inhibitors of the CYP3A family of cytochrome P450 enzymes such as ciclosporin, terfenadine, erythromycin, ketoconazole, midazolam, orphenadrine and troleandomycin will increase docetaxel serum levels, whereas barbiturates are predicted to reduce them.

Clinical evidence, mechanism, importance and management

The makers[1] say that no formal clinical drug interaction studies have been carried out with docetaxel, but because it is known from *in vitro* studies that the metabolism of docetaxel is mainly mediated by the cytochrome P450 isoenzyme CYP3A family,[2] they say that drugs which are inhibitors of CYP3A might possibly increase its serum levels, increasing its toxicity. Caution is advised. The drugs named are **ciclosporin, terfenadine, erythromycin, ketoconazole** and **troleandomycin**.[1,2] Other drugs which are known to inhibit *in vitro* docetaxel metabolism include **midazolam, testosterone,** and **orphenadrine**, whereas **quinidine** (which affects CYP2D6), and **hexobarbital, mephenytoin** and **tolbutamide** (which affect CYP2C) have little or no effect.[3] *In vitro* testing of **cisplatin, diphenhydramine, doxorubicin, ranitidine, verapamil, vinblastine** and **vincristine** at concentrations usually recommended have been found not to modify

docetaxel metabolism markedly.[3] Microsomes prepared from patients treated with **pentobarbital** and/or **phenobarbital** are reported to have stimulated **docetaxel** metabolism strikingly whereas those prepared from a patient taking **prednisone** did not.[3]

None of these drugs, with the exception of **pentobarbital, phenobarbital** and **prednisone**, appear to have been studied in patients, so that the clinical importance of these predicted interactions (and non-interactions) awaits formal clinical evaluation.

1. Taxotere (Docetaxel). Aventis Pharma Ltd. Summary of product characteristics, April 2002.
2. Clarke SJ, Rivory LP. Clinical pharmacokinetics of docetaxel. *Clin Pharmacokinet* (1999) 36, 99–114.
3. Royer I, Monsarrat B, Sonnier M, Wright M, Cresteil T. Metabolism of docetaxel by human cytochromes P450: Interactions with paclitaxel and other antineoplastic drugs. *Cancer Res* (1996) 56, 58–65.

Doxorubicin (Adriamycin) + Barbiturates

The effects of doxorubicin may be reduced by the concurrent use of barbiturates.

Clinical evidence, mechanism, importance and management

A comparative study in patients treated with doxorubicin showed that those concurrently taking **barbiturates** had a plasma clearance which was 50% higher than those who were not (318 compared with 202 ml/min).[1] This clinical study is in agreement with previous studies in *mice*.[2] A possible explanation is that the **barbiturate** increases the metabolism of the doxorubicin. It seems likely that the dosage of doxorubicin will need to be increased in barbiturate-treated patients to achieve maximal therapeutic effects.

1. Riggs CE, Engel S, Wesley M, Wiernik PH, Bachur NR. Doxorubicin pharmacokinetics, prochlorperazine and barbiturate effects. *Clin Pharmacol Ther* (1982) 31, 263.
2. Reich SD, Bachur NR. Alterations in adriamycin efficacy by phenobarbital. *Cancer* (1976) 36, 3803–6.

Doxorubicin (Adriamycin) + Beta-blockers

***Animal* data suggest that additive cardiotoxicity may occur with doxorubicin and propranolol. This awaits clinical confirmation.**

Clinical evidence, mechanism, importance and management

A very well recognised problem with doxorubicin is its cardiotoxicity and cardiomyopathy. Studies in *mice*[1] showed that mortality was significantly increased when doxorubicin (18 and 23 mg/kg) and **propranolol** (1 and 10 mg/kg) were given concurrently, possibly because both drugs can inhibit the activity of two cardiac CoQ_{10} enzymes (succinoxidase, NADH-oxidase) which are essential for mitochondrial respiration. There is no clinical confirmation of this interaction in man, but the authors of this *animal* study suggest that concurrent use may be contraindicated.

1. Choe JY, Combs AB, Folkers K. Potentiation of the toxicity of adriamycin by propranolol. *Res Commun Chem Pathol Pharmacol* (1978) 21, 577–80.

Doxorubicin (Adriamycin) + Ciclosporin

High-dose ciclosporin increases the serum levels and the myelotoxicity of doxorubicin. An isolated report describes severe neurotoxicity and coma in a patient previously on ciclosporin when given doxorubicin.

Clinical evidence

Eight patients with small cell lung cancer were given an initial course of doxorubicin (25 to 70 mg/m^2 over 1 h) and a subsequent **ciclosporin**-modulated doxorubicin course (**ciclosporin** 6 mg/kg bolus, then 16 mg/kg daily for 2 days) for multidrug resistant tumour modulation. All of the patients were also given cyclophosphamide and vincristine. The **ciclosporin** increased the AUC of the doxorubicin by 48%, and of doxorubicinol by 443%. The myelotoxicity was increased by concurrent use: a fall in the leucocyte count of 84% occurred with doxorubicin and of 91% with doxorubicin + **ciclosporin** respectively. The platelet counts fell by 36% and a 73% respectively. The patients showed significant weight loss and severe myalgias.[1,2]

Three preliminary Phase I studies[3-5] are consistent with this report. **Ciclosporin** was found to increase the doxorubicin AUCs by 40 to 73%, and the doxorubicinol AUCs by 250 to 285%.

A cardiac transplant patient was given **ciclosporin** (2 mg/kg daily) for 22 months. The **ciclosporin** was stopped and he was given 60 mg doxorubicin, 2 mg vincristine, 600 mg cyclophosphamide and 80 mg prednisone to treat Burkitt's lymphoma stage IVB. Eight hours later he developed disturbances of consciousness which lead to stage I coma from which he spontaneously recovered 12 h later. A week later a similar course of chemotherapy was started. 10 to 15 min later he lost consciousness and generalised tonic clonic seizures progressively developed. He died 8 days later without recovering from the coma.[6]

Mechanisms

Uncertain. One reason may be that the ciclosporin affects the P-glycoprotein of the biliary tract so that the clearance of doxorubicin in the bile is reduced. An additional reason may be that ciclosporin inhibits the metabolism of doxorubicinol so that it accumulates.[2] The increased levels of both would explain the marked increases in bone marrow toxicity. It is not clear why such severe neurotoxicity was seen in one patient.

Importance and management

An established and clinically important interaction. The authors of one of the reports say that the use of high-dose ciclosporin for multidrug resistant tumour modulation is experimental and should only be used in clinical trials.[2] Concurrent use should be very well monitored.

1. Raber SR, Rushing DA, Rodvold KA, Piscitelli SC, Plank GS, Tewksbury DA. Effects of cyclosporin (CSA) on the pharmacokinetics (PK) and pharmacodynamics (PD) of doxorubicin (DOX). *Clin Pharmacol Ther* (1994) 55, 189.
2. Rushing DA, Raber SR, Rodvold KA, Piscitelli SC, Plank GS, Tewksbury DA. The effects of cyclosporine on the pharmacokinetics of doxorubicin in patients with small cell lung cancer. *Cancer* (1994) 74, 834–41.
3. Scheulen ME, Budach W, Skorzec M, Wiefelspütz JK, Seeber S. Influence of cyclosporin A on the pharmacokinetics and pharmacodynamics of doxorubicin. *Proc Am Assoc Cancer Res* (1993) 34, 213.
4. Bartlett NL, Fisher GA, Halsey J, Ehsan MN, Lum BL, Sikic BI. A phase I trial of doxorubicin (D) with cyclosporine (CsA) as a modulator of multidrug resistance (MDR). *Proc Am Soc Clin Oncol* (1993) 12, 142.
5. Eggert J, Scheulen ME, Schütte J, Budach W, Annweiler HM, Mengelkolch B, Skorzec M, Wiefelspütz J, Sack H, Seeber S. Influence of cyclosporin A on the pharmacokinetics and pharmacodynamics of doxorubicin and epirubicin. *Ann Hematol* (1994) 64, A26.
6. Barbui T, Rambaldi A, Parenzan L, Zucchelli M, Perico N, Remuzzi G. Neurological symptoms and coma associated with doxorubicin administration during chronic cyclosporin therapy. *Lancet* (1992) 339, 1421.

Doxorubicin (Adriamycin) + Dactinomycin (Actinomycin D) + Plicamycin (Mithramycin)

A case of fatal cardiomyopathy attributed to the concurrent use of doxorubicin (adriamycin), dactinomycin (actinomycin D) and plicamycin (mithramycin) has been described. The general importance of this is uncertain, but it would seem prudent to be on the alert for changes in cardiac function in patients treated with these drugs.[1]

1. Kushner JP, Hansen VL, Hammar SP. Cardiomyopathy after widely separated courses of adriamycin exacerbated by actinomycin-D and mithramycin. *Cancer* (1975) 36, 1577–84.

Doxorubicin (Adriamycin) + Tamoxifen

Tamoxifen appears to have no significant effect on the pharmacokinetics of doxorubicin.

Clinical evidence, mechanism, importance and management

A pharmacokinetic study in patients with non-Hodgkin's lymphoma on cyclophosphamide, vincristine, prednisone and doxorubicin (37.5 to 50 mg/m^2) found that the addition of 480 mg **tamoxifen** had no significant effect on the AUC or total clearance of doxorubicin.[1,2]

1. El-Yazigi A, Berry J, Ezzat A, Wahab FA. Pharmacokinetics of doxorubicin when combined with tamoxifen in patients with non-Hodgkin's lymphoma. *J Clin Pharmacol* (1994) 34, 1022.
2. El-Yazigi A, Berry J, Ezzat A, Wahab FA. Effect of tamoxifen on the pharmacokinetics of doxorubicin in patients with non-Hodgkin's lymphoma. *Ther Drug Monit* (1997) 19, 632–6.

Epirubicin + Miscellaneous drugs

Ciclosporin and cimetidine can increase epirubicin serum levels. Docetaxel may affect the pharmacokinetics of epirubicin. D-Verapamil can alter the pharmacokinetics of epirubicin and possibly increase its bone marrow depressant effects.

Clinical evidence, mechanism, importance and management

(a) Ciclosporin

There is evidence from studies in patients that **ciclosporin** can markedly increase the AUC of epirubicin (up to about fourfold) and increase the bone marrow suppression. A probable reason is that the excretion of epirubicin in the bile is reduced.[1] This interaction increases the efficacy of epirubicin but also increases its toxicity.

(b) Cimetidine

In a study of 8 patients, 400 mg **cimetidine** twice daily increased the AUC of epirubicin by 50%. At the same time the AUCs of two metabolites of epirubicin, epirubicinol and 7-deoxydoxorubicinol aglycone, increased 41 and 357% respectively. Liver blood flow also increased by 17%.[2] The mechanism is unknown. More study is needed of this interaction but be aware of the possibility of **cimetidine** increasing the exposure to epirubicin, monitor the patient closely and adjust epirubicin dosage if needed. **Cimetidine** can be bought over the counter in some countries so that patients may unwittingly increase the toxicity of epirubicin.

(c) Docetaxel

A short report[3] notes that in 36 patients with breast cancer given intravenous epirubicin 75 mg/m^2, a transient but significant increase in epirubicin plasma levels occurred during the subsequent infusion (after an interval of 1 h) of **docetaxel** 75 mg/m^2.

(d) D-Verapamil

When used to reduce multidrug resistance in patients with advanced colorectal cancer treated with epirubicin, the **D-isomer of verapamil** appears to increase the bone marrow depressant toxicity of the epirubicin.[4] Another study found that **D-verapamil** halved the AUC and half-life of epirubicin, and increased its clearance,[5] while yet another failed to find these changes but found that the production of the metabolites of epirubicin was increased.[6] These changes should be taken into account if both drugs are used. More study is needed to evaluate the possible advantages and disadvantages of giving these drugs together.

1. Eggert J, Scheulen ME, Schütte J, Budach W, Annweiler H, Mengelkoch B, Skorzec M, Wiefelspütz J, Sack H, Seeber S. Influence of cyclosporin A on the pharmacokinetics and pharmacodynamics of doxorubicin and epirubicin. *Ann Hematol* (1994) 68, A26.

2. Murray LS, Jodrell DI, Morrison JG, Cook A, Kerr DJ, Whiting B, Kaye SB, Cassidy J. The effect of cimetidine on the pharmacokinetics of epirubicin in patients with advanced breast cancer: preliminary evidence of a potentially common drug interaction. *Clin Oncol* (1998) 10, 35–8.

3. Cattel L, Airoldi M, Brusa P, Tagini V, Recalenda V, Marchionatti S, Bumma C, Pedani F. *Eur J Cancer* (1999) 35 (Suppl 4), S328.

4. Kornek G, Despisch D, Kastner J, Schenk T, Locker G, Raderer M, Scheithauer W. A phase II study of D-verapamil (DVPM) plus doxorubicin in advanced colorectal cancer. *Ann Hematol* (1992) 56 (Suppl), 59.

5. Scheithauer W, Schenk T, Czejka M. Pharmacokinetic interaction between epirubicin and the multidrug resistance reverting agent D-verapamil. *Br J Cancer* (1993) 68, 8–9.

6. Mross K, Hamm K, Hossfeld DK. Effects of verapamil on the pharmacokinetics and metabolism of epirubicin. *Cancer Chemother Pharmacol* (1993) 31, 369–75.

Estramustine + Food or Milk

The absorption of estramustine is reduced by milk and foods containing calcium.

Clinical evidence

A randomised three-way crossover study in 6 patients with prostatic cancer showed that the absorption of single doses of the disodium salt, equivalent to 140 mg of estramustine, were reduced to 41% when taken with 200 ml **milk**, and to 67% when taken with a standardised **breakfast** (2 pieces of white bread with margarine, ham, tomato, marmalade and water). Peak serum estramustine levels were reduced to 32 and 57% respectively.[1]

Mechanism

In vitro studies suggest that estramustine combines with calcium ions in milk and food to form a poorly-soluble complex which is not as well absorbed as the parent compound.[1]

Importance and management

An established interaction although the information is limited. The authors suggest that estramustine should be taken at a set time in relation to food intake, and not with milk, calcium-containing milk products (e.g. yoghurt) or food if maximal absorption is to be achieved. If the suggested mechanism of interaction is correct, estramustine should also not be taken with **calcium-containing drugs** (e.g. some **antacids**).

1. Gunnarsson P O, Davidsson T, Andersson S-B, Backman C, Johansson S-Å. Impairment of estramustine phosphate absorption by concurrent intake of milk and food. *Eur J Clin Pharmacol* (1990) 38, 189–93.

Etoposide + Anticonvulsants

Etoposide clearance appears to be increased by phenobarbital or phenytoin.

Clinical evidence, mechanism, importance and management

A preliminary study found that the clearance of etoposide (doses of 320 to 500 mg/m^2) was increased 170% in 5 paediatric patients with cancer taking **phenobarbital** or **phenytoin** (doses not stated).[1] Another study in 29 patients found that etoposide clearance was higher in 7 patients taking anticonvulsants (**phenobarbital**, **phenytoin** or both).[2] Be alert for the possible need to give larger doses of etoposide if these anticonvulsants are used. More study is needed.

1. Rodman JH, Murry DJ, Madden T, Santana VM. Pharmacokinetics of high doses of etoposide and the influence of anticonvulsants in pediatric cancer patients. *Clin Pharmacol Ther* (1992) 51, 156.

2. Rodman JH, Murry DJ, Madden T, Santana VM. Altered etoposide pharmacokinetics and time to engraftment in pediatric patients undergoing autologous bone marrow transplantation. *J Clin Oncol* (1994) 12, 2390–7.

Etoposide + Carboplatin or Cisplatin

The clearance of etoposide may be reduced by carboplatin, and by cisplatin given acutely but not when given chronically.

Clinical evidence, mechanism, importance and management

(a) Carboplatin

In a study of 14 young patients, an escalating dosage regimen starting with 960 mg/m^2, and increasing to 1200, and 1500 mg/m^2 of etoposide was given in three divided doses on alternate days with 400 to 700 mg/m^2 **carboplatin** given on the other days, followed by autologous marrow rescue. The etoposide clearance was substantially lower in the **carboplatin** treated patients than in previous reports about children and adults. The authors point out that the dose and the timing of **carboplatin** may be important determinants for this interaction.[1]

(b) Cisplatin

A study in 17 children with neuroblastoma found that when **cisplatin** (90 mg/m^2 intravenously) was given acutely, the clearance of etoposide (780 mg/m^2) fell and the serum levels rose. But when the **cisplatin** was given chronically, it had no effect on the clearance of etoposide.[2,3]

1. Rodman JH, Murry DJ, Madden T, Santana VM. Altered etoposide pharmacokinetics and time to engraftment in pediatric patients undergoing autologous bone marrow transplantation. *J Clin Oncol* (1994) 12, 2390–7.

2. McLeod HL, Santana VM, Bowman LC, Furman WL, Relling MV. Etoposide pharmacokinetics are influenced by acute but not by chronic cisplatin exposure. *Proc Am Assoc Cancer Res* (1992) 33, 531.

3. Relling MV, McLeod HL, Bowman LC, Santana VM. Etoposide pharmacokinetics and pharmacodynamics after acute and chronic exposure to cisplatin. *Clin Pharmacol Ther* (1994) 56, 503–11.

Etoposide + Ciclosporin

High-dose ciclosporin markedly raises etoposide serum levels and increases the suppression of white blood cell production. Severe toxicity has been reported in one patient.

Clinical evidence

In a comparative study 16 patients with multidrug resistance and advanced cancer were given 20 paired courses of etoposide alone or with **ciclosporin**. It was found that **ciclosporin** serum concentrations of either more or less than 2000 nanograms/ml increased the etoposide AUC by 80% or 50% respectively, decreased the total clearance by 38% or 28%, increased its half-life by 108 or 40%, reduced the leucocyte count nadir by −64 or −37% and altered the volume of distribution at steady state by 46 and 1.4%.[1] The patients were given 150 to 200 mg/m^2 etoposide daily for 3 consecutive days as a 2-h intravenous infusion and **ciclosporin** as a 3-day continuous infusion in doses ranging from 5 to 21 mg/kg daily.[1]

The leukaemic cells in the bone marrow of a patient with acute T-lymphocyte leukaemia were totally cleared with **ciclosporin** (8.3 mg/kg orally twice daily) and etoposide (100 to 300 mg daily for 2 to 5 days), but the side-effects were severe (mental confusion, renal and hepatic toxicity). The patient died from respiratory failure.[2]

Mechanism

It is suggested that the ciclosporin decreases the metabolism of the etoposide (by inhibiting its cytochrome P450 mediated metabolism[3] and inhibiting P-glycoprotein mediated efflux from the hepatocyte) as well as inhibiting some unknown non-renal clearance mechanism.[1] The total effect is to cause the retention of etoposide in the body, thereby increasing its effects.

Importance and management

An established interaction. The authors of report cited advise an etoposide dosage reduction of 50% if used with high-dose ciclosporin in patients with normal kidney and liver function.[1] More study is needed to find out the possible effects of low-dose ciclosporin.

1. Lum BL, Kaubisch S, Yahanda AM, Adler KM, Jew L, Ehsan MN, Brophy NA, Halsey J, Gosland MP, Sikic BI. Alteration of etoposide pharmacokinetics and pharmacodynamics by cyclosporine in a phase I trial to modulate multidrug resistance. *J Clin Oncol* (1992) 10, 1635–42.
2. Kloke O, Osieka R. Interaction of cyclosporin A with antineoplastic agents. *Klin Wochenschr* (1985) 63, 1081–2.
3. Kawashiro T, Yamashita K, Zhao X-J, Koyama E, Tani M, Chiba K, Ishizaki T. A study on the metabolism of etoposide and possible interaction with antitumor or supporting agents by human liver microsomes. *J Pharmacol Exp Ther* (1998) 386, 1294–1300.

Etoposide + Miscellaneous drugs

In vitro **studies show that some inhibitors of cytochrome P450 isoenzyme CYP3A4 may possibly increase the effects and toxicity of etoposide.**

Clinical evidence, mechanism, importance and management

In vitro studies using human liver microsomes show that **ketoconazole**, **prednisolone**, **troleandomycin**, **verapamil** and **vincristine** can inhibit the metabolism (3′-demethylation) of etoposide by cytochrome P450 isoenzyme CYP3A4. The implications of this are that these drugs might increase both the efficacy and the toxicity of etoposide when used concurrently in patients.[1] There seems as yet to be no clinical confirmation that these potential interactions have clinical relevance, but good monitoring would be a prudent precaution.

1. Kawashiro T, Yamashita K, Zhao X-J, Koyama E, Tani M, Chiba K, Ishizaki T. A study on the metabolism of etoposide and possible interactions with antitumor or supporting agents by human liver microsomes. *J Pharmacol Exp Ther* (1998) 386, 1294–1300.

Etoposide + St John's wort (*Hypericum perforatum*)

In vitro **studies suggest that hypericin, a component of St John's wort may antagonise the cytotoxic effects of etoposide. It may also stimulate the hepatic metabolism of etoposide by the cytochrome P450 isoenzyme CYP3A4. Information is very limited but it seems that it would be prudent to avoid St John's wort in patients taking etoposide or related cytotoxics.**[1] **More study is needed.**

1. Peebles KA, Baker RK, Kurz EU, Schneider AJ, Kroll DJ. Catalytic inhibition of human DNA topoisomerase IIα by hypericin, a naphthodianthrone from St. John's wort (*Hypericum perforatum*). *Biochem Pharmacol* (2001) 62, 1059–70.

Exemestane + Miscellaneous drugs

Exemestane should not be given with oestrogens (such as HRT preparations) which would oppose its actions. Ketoconazole appears not to interact.

Clinical importance, mechanism, importance and management

A reduction in the circulating levels of estradiol (oestradiol) can have a beneficial (inhibitory) effect on the progression of hormone-dependent breast cancer. Exemestane achieves this by specifically inhibiting aromatase, a cytochrome P450 enzyme which is concerned with the metabolic production of estrogens from androgens within the body, so that the breast cancer cells are deprived of oestrogens, thereby limiting their growth. It is therefore important not to give **oestro-**gen-containing therapies (such as **Hormone Replacement Therapy - HRT**) to women on exemestane because such treatment would raise the levels of circulating oestrogens and oppose the actions of exemestane.

The makers say that no formal drug interaction studies have been carried out but *in vitro* evidence shows that while exemestane is metabolised by both cytochrome P450 isoenzyme CYP3A4 and aldoketoreductases, a clinical study found that **ketoconazole** (a specific inhibitor of CYP3A4) had no significant effects on the pharmacokinetics of exemestane,[1] indicating that CYP3A4 probably only catalyses a minor metabolic pathway. Exemestane appears not to inhibit any of the major cytochrome P450 isoenzymes[1] and so far reports of clinically important interactions appear to be lacking.

1. Aromasin (Exemestane). Pharmacia. Summary of product characteristics, January 2001.

Fludarabine + Miscellaneous drugs

Fludarabine with pentostatin can cause fatal pulmonary toxicity. Dipyridamole can reduce the efficacy of fludarabine.

Clinical evidence, mechanism, importance and management

When fludarabine phosphate and **pentostatin** were used in the treatment of chronic lymphoid leukaemia, 4 out of 6 patients developed pulmonary toxicity consistent with interstitial pneumonitis, and 3 of them died. Because fludarabine phosphate is an analogue of adenine, drugs which are adenosine uptake inhibitors such as **dipyridamole** will prevent the uptake of fludarabine into cells so that its efficacy will be reduced.[1,2] These drugs should therefore be avoided in patients receiving fludarabine.

1. Schering Health Care Limited. Personal communication, February 1995.
2. Fludara (Fludarabine). Schering Health Care Limited. Summary of product characteristics, July 2000.

Fluorouracil + Aminoglycosides

Neomycin can delay the gastrointestinal absorption of fluorouracil, but the clinical importance of this is uncertain.

Clinical evidence, mechanism, importance and management

Some preliminary information from a study in 12 patients under treatment for metastatic adenocarcinoma showed that treatment with oral **neomycin** 500 mg four times daily for a week delayed the absorption of fluorouracil, but the effects were generally too small to reduce the therapeutic response, except possibly in one patient.[1] It seems probable that this interaction occurs because **neomycin** can induce a malabsorption syndrome. If **neomycin**, and most probably **paromomycin** or **kanamycin** are used in patients on fluorouracil, the possibility of this interaction should be borne in mind.

1. Bruckner HW, Creasey WA. The administration of 5-fluorouracil by mouth. *Cancer* (1974) 33, 14–18.

Fluorouracil + Cimetidine

Serum fluorouracil levels are increased about 75% by the concurrent use of cimetidine for a month.

Clinical evidence

A study in 6 patients with carcinoma under treatment with fluorouracil (15 mg/kg daily for 5 days, repeated every 4 weeks) showed that treatment with 1 g **cimetidine** daily for 4 weeks increased peak plasma fluorouracil concentrations by 74% and the AUC by 72% when given orally. When given intravenously the AUC was increased by 27%. The total body clearance was reduced by 28%.[1] The pharmacokinetics of fluorouracil were unaltered by the use of **cimetidine** for only a week.

Mechanism

Uncertain. It is probably a combination of a reduction in the metabolism of the fluorouracil caused by the cimetidine (a well-known enzyme inhibitor) and a reduction in blood flow through the liver.

Importance and management

Direct information appears to be limited to this study, but the interaction would seem to be established. Concurrent treatment should be undertaken with particular care because of the risks of fluorouracil overdosage. A reduction in the dosage may be necessary.

1. Harvey VJ, Slevin ML, Dilloway MR, Clark PI, Johnston A, Lant AF. The influence of cimetidine on the pharmacokinetics of 5-fluorouracil. *Br J Clin Pharmacol* (1984) 18, 421–30.

Fluorouracil + Cisplatin

The addition of low-dose cisplatin to fluorouracil infusion markedly increases the toxicity. Cardiotoxicity may possibly be increased with higher doses of cisplatin.

Clinical evidence, mechanism, importance and management

The addition of weekly low-dose **cisplatin** (20 mg/m^2) to continuous ambulatory fluorouracil infusions (300 mg/m^2 daily) considerably increased the toxicity (nausea, vomiting, anorexia, diarrhoea, stomatitis, myelosuppression) of 18 patients with advanced cancers. More than half developed multiple toxicities, and severe toxicity occurred in two-thirds. Leucopenia occurred in 28% given both drugs whereas it is virtually nonexistent with fluorouracil alone. Toxicity requiring treatment interruption or dose reduction was seen in 55% of patients on fluorouracil alone. This rose to 94% when given both drugs.[1] In another study of 80 patients with carcinoma of the head, neck, oesophagus and stomach it was found that concurrent use increased the cardiotoxicity (chest pain, ST-T wave changes, arrhythmias) by 15%.[2] Concurrent use clearly needs careful evaluation.

1. Jeske J, Hansen RM, Libnoch JA, Anderson T. 5-Fluorouracil infusion and low-dose weekly cisplatin: an analysis of increased toxicity. *Am J Clin Oncol (CCT)* (1990) 13, 485–8.
2. Jeremic B, Jevremovic S, Djuric L, Mijatovic L. Cardiotoxicity during chemotherapy treatment with 5-flurouracil and cisplatin. *J Chemother* (1990) 2, 264–7.

Fluorouracil + Folic acid

Two patients developed severe fluorouracil toxicity while taking multivitamin preparations containing folic acid.

Clinical evidence

A woman with carcinoma of the rectum underwent surgery and a month later was treated with 500 mg/m^2 intravenous fluorouracil daily for 5 days. At the end of this chemotherapy she was admitted with anorexia, severe mouth ulceration, bloody diarrhoea and vaginal bleeding, which was interpreted as fluorouracil toxicity. Her concurrent medication included 5 mg **folic acid** (in *Multi-B forte*) along with loperamide, sulfasalazine, Vitamins B$_{12}$ and K, and HRT. When treated again a month later with fluorouracil but without the **folic acid**, her treatment was well tolerated and without toxicity. A man similarly treated with fluorouracil for colonic cancer was admitted 2 days later with severe mouth ulceration and bloody diarrhoea. He too was found to be taking a multivitamin preparation containing 500 micrograms **folic acid**. Subsequent courses of fluorouracil at the same dosage but without the **folic acid** were well tolerated.[1]

Mechanism

It would seem that folic acid increases the inhibition by fluorouracil of thymidine formation which is important for DNA synthesis, thereby increasing the fluorouracil toxicity.

Importance and management

Direct information seem to be limited to these two cases but the interaction would appear to be established. What happened is consistent with the way **folinic acid**, another source of folate, is used therapeutically to increase the potency of fluorouracil. Patients treated with fluorouracil should therefore not be given folic acid, and should be told to avoid multivitamin preparations containing folic acid to prevent the development of severe fluorouracil side-effects.

1. Mainwaring P, Grygiel JJ. Interaction of 5-fluorouracil with folates. *Aust N Z J Med* (1995) 25, 60.

Fluorouracil + Metronidazole or Misonidazole

The toxicity of fluorouracil, but not its efficacy, is increased by metronidazole. Its toxicity is also increased by misonidazole.

Clinical evidence

Twenty-seven patients with metastatic colorectal cancer were given 750 mg/m^2 **metronidazole** intravenously 1 h before 600 mg/m^2 fluorouracil intravenously 5 days per week once every 4 weeks. The fluorouracil toxicity was markedly increased: granulocytopenia occurred in 74%, anaemia in 41%, stomatitis and oral ulceration in 34%, nausea and vomiting in 48% and thrombocytopenia in 19%.[1] A pharmacokinetic study in 10 patients showed that the **metronidazole** reduced the clearance of the fluorouracil by 27% over the 5-day period and increased the AUC by 34 %. *In vitro* studies with human colon cancer cells failed to show any increased efficacy.[1]

Studies using another nitroimidazole, **misonidazole**, in patients with colorectal cancer also found an increased incidence and severity of gastrointestinal toxicity with concurrent use,[2,3] a slightly increased incidence of leucopenia[2] and a reduction in the clearance.[3]

Mechanism

Metronidazole reduces the clearance of fluorouracil, thereby increasing its toxic effects.

Importance and management

Information is limited but the fluorouracil/metronidazole interaction appears to be established. The toxicity of fluorouracil is increased without an increase in its therapeutic efficacy. The authors of the report do not recommend use of this drug combination.[1] Be aware that misonidazole can apparently behave similarly.

1. Bardakji Z, Jolivet J, Langelier Y, Besner J-G, Ayoub J. 5-Fluorouracil-metronidazole combination therapy in metastatic colorectal cancer. *Cancer Chemother Pharmacol* (1986) 18, 140–44.
2. Spooner D, Bugden RD, Peckham MJ, Wist EA. The combination of 5-fluorouracil with misonidazole in patients with advanced colorectal cancer. *Int J Radiat Oncol Biol Phys* (1982) 8, 387–9.
3. McDermott BJ, Van den Berg HW, Martin WMC, Murphy RF. Pharmacokinetic rationale for the interaction of 5-fluorouracil and misonidazole in humans. *Br J Cancer* (1983) 48, 705–10.

Fluorouracil + Miscellaneous drugs

The toxicity and effects of fluorouracil appear to be unaffected by the drugs listed below (antihistamines, phenothiazines etc.).

Clinical evidence, mechanism, importance and management

A study in 250 patients given fluorouracil for the treatment of gastrointestinal cancer found that the following drugs did not cause any significant increase in its toxicity or decrease its therapeutic effects when compared with a placebo: **chlorprothixene, cinnarizine, pipamazine, prochlorperazine, sodium pentobarbital, thiethylperazine, thiopropazate, trimethobenzamide.**[1] No special precautions would seem necessary.

1. Moertel CG, Reitemeier RJ, Hahn RG. Effect of concomitant drug treatment on toxic and therapeutic activity of 5-fluorouracil (5-FU; NSC-19893). *Cancer Chemother Rep* (1972) 56, 245–7.

Hydroxycarbamide (Hydroxyurea) + CNS depressants

Increased CNS depression may occur.

Clinical evidence, mechanism, importance and management

Hydroxycarbamide (hydroxyurea) has CNS-depressant effects and can cause drowsiness. This may be expected to be increased by other drugs which can also cause drowsiness (e.g. **alcohol, antiemetics, antihistamines, barbiturates, cough and cold remedies, phenothiazines, opioid analgesics, tranquillisers, some tricyclic antidepressants,** etc.)

Ifosfamide + Barbiturates

Encephalopathy developed in a girl on phenobarbital when given a single first dose of ifosfamide/mesna.

Clinical evidence

A 15-year-old girl who had been taking **phenobarbital** for epilepsy since infancy developed confusion and gradually became unconscious 6 h after being given a first dose of ifosfamide for metastatic rhabdomyosarcoma. She was treated with ifosfamide 3 g/m^2, mesna 3.6 g/m^2, vincristine 2 mg and dactinomycin (actinomycin D). An ECG revealed signs of severe diffuse encephalopathy. She remained unconscious for 24 h but was asymptomatic after 48 h.[1]

Mechanism

Encephalopathy due to ifosfamide has been seen in other patients[2-4] and apparently results from the alteration in the balance of dechloroethylation of ifosfamide and the clearance of chloracetaldehyde.[3,4] However, the doses used were greater than in the case cited (>3.5 g/m^2 daily) and repeated. The reason for the encephalopathy in this case is not understood but the authors of the report suggest that the enzyme induction caused by the phenobarbital might have resulted in increased activation of the single dose of ifosfamide, resulting in increased toxicity. The vincristine may also have had additive effects.[1]

Importance and management

The relationship between this encephalopathy and the use of phenobarbital is not established, but this case serves to emphasise the need for particular caution and good monitoring if concurrent use is undertaken. More study is needed.

1. Ghosn M, Carde P, Leclerq B, Flamant F, Friedman S, Droz JP, Hayat M. Ifosfamide/mesna related encephalopathy: a case report with a possible role of phenobarbital in enhancing neurotoxicity. *Bull Cancer* (1988) 75, 391–2.
2. Cantwell BMJ, Harris AL. Ifosfamide/mesna and encephalopathy. *Lancet* (1985) i, 752.

3. Goren MP, Wright RK, Pratt CB, Pell FE. Dechloroethylation of ifosfamide and neurotoxicity. *Lancet* (1986) ii, 1219–20.
4. Salloum E, Flamant F, Ghosn M, Taleb N, Akatcherian C. Irreversible encephalopathy with ifosfamide/mesna. *J Clin Oncol* (1987) 5, 1303–4.

Ifosfamide + Cisplatin

Ifosfamide toxicity is more common in those who have had prior treatment with cisplatin. Ifosfamide increases the hearing loss due to cisplatin.

Clinical evidence

A comparative study in 36 children with malignant solid tumours on a range of drugs including some known to be potentially nephrotoxic (high dose methotrexate, aminoglycosides, cyclophosphamide), indicated that previous treatment with **cisplatin** increased their susceptibility to ifosfamide toxicity (neurotoxicity, severe leucopenia or acute tubular damage).[1]

This confirms other studies in which concurrent use[2,3] with **cisplatin** appeared to increase the nephrotoxicity of ifosfamide, but not another study which suggested that no such interaction occurs.[4] A further comparative study found that when ifosfamide was added to **cisplatin**, the hearing loss caused by **cisplatin** was exacerbated.[5]

Mechanism

It is thought that concurrent or possibly prior treatment with cisplatin damages the kidney tubules so that the clearance of the ifosfamide metabolites from the body is reduced and their toxic effects are thereby increased. Damaged kidney tubules may also be less capable of converting mesna to its active kidney-protecting form. The increase in the hearing loss is not understood.

Importance and management

These interactions appear to be established. The authors of the paper cited[1] point out that the majority of patients who develop toxicity have persistently high urinary NAG concentrations, even though serum creatinine levels remain within the acceptable range for ifosfamide treatment. They suggest that evidence of subclinical tubular damage should be sought for by monitoring the excretion of urinary NAG. The authors who reported on hearing loss advise that serial audiograms are given to patients treated with both drugs.[5]

1. Goren MP, Wright RK, Pratt CB, Horowitz ME, Dodge RK, Viar MJ, Kovnar EH. Potentiation of ifosfamide neurotoxicity, hematotoxicity, and tubular nephrotoxicity by prior *cis*-diamminedichloroplatinum(II) therapy. *Cancer Res* (1987) 47, 1457–60.
2. Niederle N, Scheulen ME, Cremer M, Schütte J, Schmidt CG, Seeber S. Ifosfamide in combination chemotherapy for sarcomas and testicular carcinomas. *Cancer Treat Rev* (1983) 10, (Suppl A), 129–35.
3. Rossi R, Danzebrink S, Hillebrand D, Linnenbürger K, Ullrich K, Jürgens H. Ifosfamide-induced subclinical nephrotoxicity and its potentiation by cisplatinum. *Med Pediatr Oncol* (1994) 22, 27–32.
4. Hacke M, Schmoll H-J, Alt JM, Baumann K, Stolte H. Nephrotoxicity of *cis*-diamminedichloroplatinum with or without ifosfamide in cancer treatment. *Clin Physiol Biochem* (1983) 1, 17–26.
5. Meyer WH, Ayers D, McHaney VA, Roberson P, Pratt CB. Ifosfamide and exacerbation of cisplatin-induced hearing loss. *Lancet* (1993) 341, 754–5.

Ifosfamide + Phenytoin

The pharmacokinetics of ifosfamide and its metabolites were altered in a child when given phenytoin (possibly due to induction of cytochrome P450 isoenzyme CYP2B6 rather than CYP3A4) which resulted in remission.[1] **This would appear to be an advantageous interaction.**

1. Ducharme MP, Bernstein ML, Granvil CP, Gehrcke B, Wainer IW. Phenytoin-induced alteration in the *N*-dechloroethylation of ifosfamide stereoisomers. *Cancer Chemother Pharmacol* (1997) 40, 531–3.

Imatinib + Miscellaneous drugs

Ketoconazole raises serum imatinib levels; other cytochrome P450 isoenzyme CYP3A4 inhibitors are predicted to do the same. Phenytoin lowers serum imatinib levels; other CYP3A4 inducers are predicted to do the same. Imatinib increases serum simvastatin levels and is predicted to interact with other drugs whose metabolism is affected by CYP3A4 inhibition. Warnings have also been issued about paracetamol (acetaminophen) and warfarin, but based on *in vitro* studies 5-fluorouracil and paclitaxel and a number of other drugs are not expected to interact.

Clinical evidence, mechanism, importance and management

(a) Drugs that may raise imatinib serum levels

In an open-label, randomised, crossover study in 14 healthy subjects found that the maximum serum levels and AUC of imatinib rose by 26% and 40% respectively when given single 400-mg doses of ketoconazole with single 200-mg doses of imatinib.[1] The reason is that **ketoconazole** is a potent inhibitor of the cytochrome P450 isoenzyme CYP3A4, which is concerned with the metabolism of imatinib. As a result its metabolism and clearance are reduced and its serum levels rise accordingly. The makers therefore advise caution with **ketoconazole** and with other CYP3A4 inhibitors (examples listed are **clarithromycin**, **erythromycin** and **itraconazole**),[2] but it is not entirely clear what action should be taken because information about excessive serum levels is very limited. The makers quote the case of a patient with myeloid blast crisis who inadvertently took 1200 mg imatinib for 6 days (the normal maximum is 800 mg). He showed elevations of serum creatinine, transaminases, bilirubin, and he developed ascites. He recovered within a week of stopping the imatinib and was later restarted on 400 mg daily.[2]

(b) Drugs that may lower imatinib serum levels

A patient on chronic treatment with **phenytoin** had a 24 hr imatinib AUC which was about one-fifth of that expected. The reason is believed to be that **phenytoin** induced the activity of the cytochrome P450 isoenzyme CYP3A4 so that the metabolism of the imatinib was markedly increased, resulting in its more rapid clearance from the body. No specific studies have been carried out with imatinib and other CYP3A4 inducing drugs, but the makers list as examples **carbamazepine**, **dexamethasone**, **phenobarbital**, **rifampicin** (**rifampin**) and **St John's wort** (*Hypericum perforatum*), all of which are predicted to reduce imatinib serum levels.[2] The makers therefore reasonably recommend caution, which means being alert for the need to raise the imatinib dosage.

(c) Drugs that may have their serum levels altered by imatinib

The makers say that the mean maximum serum levels and the AUC of **simvastatin** were found to be increased 2- and 3.5-fold by imatinib due to the inhibitory effects of imatinib on the metabolism and clearance of **simvastatin** by cytochrome P450 isoenzyme CYP3A4.[2] These rises increase the risk of **simvastatin** toxicity (rhabdomyolysis), for which reason the **simvastatin** dosage should be reduced appropriately, probably about halved. The makers name two other drugs, **pimozide** and **ciclosporin** which are also predicted to show serum levels rises with potentially serious consequences because of CYP3A4 inhibition. Other named groups of drugs which may also potentially show serum levels rises are the **triazolo-benzodiazepines** (these are **triazolam**, **midazolam**), **calcium channel blockers** and **statins**.[2]

The makers say that because **warfarin** is metabolised by CYP2C9, patients needing anticoagulation should be given low molecular weight or standard **heparin** instead. This recommendation is based on an observation in one patient[1] and on *in vitro* studies that show that imatinib can inhibit CYP2C9, but only to a moderate extent.[2] There seems to be no other evidence that a clinically relevant interaction is likely occur. The makers also say that imatinib inhibits CYP2D6 and

could therefore potentially increase the serum levels of drugs that are metabolised by this isoenzyme, but no specific *in vivo* studies of this interaction have been carried out.[2]

(d) Drugs that are not expected to interact with imatinib

In vitro studies showed no interference with the metabolism of **5-fluorouracil** by imatinib due to inhibition of cytochrome P450 isoenzyme CYP2C8. Related studies showed some competitive inhibition of the metabolism of **paclitaxel**, but only at imatinib concentrations far higher than those expected in patients, and therefore the makers predict that no interaction is likely between imatinib and either of these two cytotoxic drugs. Other *in vitro* studies with CYP3A4 also suggest that **aciclovir**, **amphotericin B**, **cytarabine**, **hydroxycarbamide** (**hydroxyurea**), **norfloxacin** and **phenoxymethylpenicillin** (**penicillin V**) are unlikely to interact with imatinib.[2]

(e) Paracetamol (Acetaminophen)

During clinical trials of imatinib one patient regularly taking **paracetamol** (**acetaminophen**) for fever, died of acute liver failure after 11 days.[3] It is not known whether this was linked to the concurrent use of these two drugs but to be on the safe side the makers now say avoid or restrict the use of paracetamol.[2]

1. Novartis Pharmaceuticals UK Limited. Personal communication, December 2001.
2. Glivec (Imatinib). Novartis Pharmaceuticals UK Ltd. Summary of product characteristics, November 2001.
3. Talpaz M, Silver RT, Druker B, Paquette R, Goldman JM, Reese SF, Capdeville R. A phase II study of STI 571 in adult patients with Philadelphia chromosome positive chronic myeloid leukaemia in accelerated phase. *Blood* (2000) 96 (Suppl 1), 469a.

Letrozole + Miscellaneous drugs

Levels of letrozole may be significantly reduced by tamoxifen. Letrozole is reported not to interact with benzodiazepines, barbiturates, cimetidine, diclofenac, furosemide (frusemide), ibuprofen, omeprazole, paracetamol (acetaminophen) or warfarin.

Clinical evidence, mechanism, importance and management

Pharmacokinetic studies have found that letrozole levels are reduced by 35 to 40% by co-administration of **tamoxifen**.[1] The pharmacokinetics of a single 2.5-mg dose of letrozole in 17 healthy subjects was unchanged by 400 mg **cimetidine** 12-hourly.[2] The makers report that no clinically significant interaction occurs between letrozole and **warfarin**, and in a large clinical trial there was no evidence of clinically relevant interactions with other commonly prescribed drugs (**benzodiazepines such as diazepam**, **barbiturates**, **diclofenac**, **furosemide** (**frusemide**), **ibuprofen**, **omeprazole**, **paracetamol** (**acetaminophen**)).[3]

1. Dowsett M. Drug and hormone interactions of aromatase inhibitors. *Endocrine-related Cancer* (1999) 6, 181–5.
2. Morgan JM, Palmisano M, Spencer S, Hirschhorn W, Piraino AJ, Rackley RJ, Choi L. Pharmacokinetic effect of cimetidine on a single 2.5-mg dose of letrozole in healthy subjects. *J Clin Pharmacol* (1996) 36, 852.
3. Femara (Letrozole). Novartis Pharmaceuticals UK Ltd. Summary of product characteristics, January 2001.

Lomustine (CCNU) + Theophylline

A single case report describes thrombocytopenia and bleeding attributed to the concurrent use of lomustine and theophylline.

Clinical evidence, mechanism, importance and management

An asthmatic woman taking **theophylline** and under treatment for medulloblastoma with lomustine, prednisone and vincristine, developed severe nose bleeding and thrombocytopenia three weeks after the third cycle of chemotherapy.[1] This was attributed to the concurrent use of the lomustine and **theophylline**. The suggested explanation is that the **theophylline** inhibited the activity of phosphodiesterase within the blood platelets, thereby increasing cyclic AMP levels and disrupting normal platelet function, which seems to be supported by an experimental study.[2] What is known is far too limited to act as more than a warning of the possibility of increased thrombocytopenia and myelotoxicity during the concurrent use of **theophylline** and lomustine.

1. Zeltzer PM, Feig SA. Theophylline-induced lomustine toxicity. *Lancet* (1979) ii, 960–1.
2. DeWys WD, Bathina S. Synergistic anti-tumour effect of cyclic AMP elevation (induced by theophylline) and cytotoxic drug treatment. *Proc Am Assoc Cancer Res* (1978) 19, 104.

Melphalan + Cimetidine

Cimetidine reduces the bioavailability of melphalan.

Clinical evidence, mechanism, importance and management

A study in 8 patients with multiple myeloma or monoclonal gammopathy showed that pretreatment with 1 g **cimetidine** daily for 6 days reduced the bioavailability of a 10 mg oral dose of melphalan by 30%.[1] The melphalan half-life was reduced from 1.94 to 1.57 h. The reasons for this reaction and its clinical importance await assessment.

1. Sviland L, Robinson A, Proctor SJ, Bateman DN. Interaction of cimetidine with oral melphalan. *Cancer Chemother Pharmacol* (1987) 20, 173–5.

Melphalan + Interferon

Interferon modestly increases the loss of melphalan, but melphalan cytotoxicity is possibly increased because of the interferon-induced fever.

Clinical evidence, mechanism, importance and management

The AUC of melphalan 0.25 mg/kg in 10 myeloma patients was reduced by 13% when given 5 h after the administration of **human interferon alfa** (7×10^6 IU/m²) due to the fever caused by the **interferon**.[1] The clinical importance of this is uncertain but the authors of the report suggest that despite this small loss, the cytotoxicity of the melphalan is increased by the fever. More study is needed.

1. Ehrsson H, Eksborg S, Wallin I, Österborg A, Mellstedt H. Oral melphalan pharmacokinetics: influence of interferon-induced fever. *Clin Pharmacol Ther* (1990) 47, 86–90.

Mercaptopurine + Food

Food reduces and delays the absorption of mercaptopurine.

Clinical evidence

A study in 17 children with acute lymphoblastic leukaemia showed that the absorption of 6-mercaptopurine (5 mg/m²) was markedly reduced if given 15 min after a standard **breakfast** (250 ml of milk and 50 g biscuits) compared with the situation when fasting. The AUC was reduced by 26% (from 143 to 105 micromol min). The maximum plasma concentration was reduced 36% (from 0.98 to 0.63 micromol) and delayed from 1.2 to 2.3 h.[1] Some individuals showed more marked effects than others. One subject showed a 2.6-fold decrease in AUC and a sixfold decrease in maximum plasma levels.[1]

This study confirms the findings of another study in 2 patients.[2]

Mechanism

Not understood. Delayed gastric emptying is a suggested reason.[1]

Importance and management

The documentation is small but this interaction appears to be established and of clinical importance. Mercaptopurine should be taken while fasting to optimise its absorption.

1. Riccardi R, Balis FM, Ferrara P, Lasorella A, Poplak DG, Mastrangelo R. Influence of food intake on bioavailability of oral 6-mercaptopurine in children with acute lymphoblastic leukaemia. *Paed Haematol Oncol* (1986) 3, 319–24.
2. Burton NK, Aherne GW, Marks VA. A novel method for the quantitation of 6-mercaptopurine in human plasma using high-performance liquid chromatography with fluorescence detection. *J Chromatogr* (1984) 309, 409–14.

Mercaptopurine + Methotrexate

High-dose methotrexate can increase the bioavailability of mercaptopurine.

Clinical evidence, mechanism, importance and management

Ten children with acute lymphoblastic leukaemia in remission were treated with 25 mg/m² of mercaptopurine daily and intravenous infusions of high dose **methotrexate** (2 or 5 g/m²) once every other week. It was found that the **methotrexate** 2 or 5 g/m² increased the AUC of mercaptopurine by 69% and 93% respectively, and raised the maximum serum mercaptopurine levels by 108% and 121% respectively. Similar results were found in studies with *rats*. The reasons for this pharmacokinetic interaction are not understood. In HL-60 human leukaemic cells incubated with mercaptopurine (250 nanograms/ml) the cumulative intracellular concentration of 6-tioguanine and 6-mercaptopurine nucleotides was not significantly altered by treatment with 20 micrograms **methotrexate**.[1] The full significance of these changes is not clear.

1. Giverhaug T, Loennechen T, Aarbakke J. The interaction of 6-mercaptopurine (6-MP) and methotrexate (MTX). *Gen Pharmacol* (1999) 33, 341–6.

Methotrexate + Alcohol

There is some inconclusive evidence that the consumption of alcohol may increase the risk of methotrexate-induced hepatic cirrhosis and fibrosis.

Clinical evidence, mechanism, importance and management

It has been claimed that **alcohol** can increase the hepatotoxic effects of methotrexate.[1] Two reports indicate that this may be so, in one 3 out of 5 patients with methotrexate-induced cirrhosis were reported to have taken **alcohol** concurrently (2 patients >85 g, 1 patient 25 to 85 g ethanol/week)[2] and in the other, the subject is known to drink excessively.[3] However, the evidence is by no means conclusive and no direct causal relationship has been established. The makers of methotrexate advise the avoidance of drugs, including **alcohol**, which have hepatotoxic potential.[4]

1. Almeyda J, Barnardo D, Baker H. Drug reactions XV. Methotrexate, psoriasis and the liver. *Br J Dermatol* (1971) 85, 302–5.
2. Tobias H, Auerbach R. Hepatotoxicity of long-term methotrexate therapy for psoriasis. *Arch Intern Med* (1973) 132, 391–400.
3. Pai SH, Werthamer S, Zak FG. Severe liver damage caused by treatment of psoriasis with methotrexate. *N Y State J Med* (1973) 73, 2585–7.
4. Methotrexate. Wyeth Laboratories. Summary of product characteristics, May 2000.

Methotrexate + Amiodarone

An isolated case report tentatively attributes the development of methotrexate toxicity to additional treatment with amiodarone.

Clinical evidence, mechanism, importance and management

An elderly woman, effectively treated for 2 years with methotrexate for psoriasis, developed ulceration of the psoriatic plaques within 2 weeks of starting treatment with **amiodarone**. The reason is not understood. A modest increase in her dosage of furosemide (frusemide) is a suggested contributory factor because it might have interfered with the excretion of the methotrexate.[1]

1. Reynolds NJ, Jones SK, Crossley J, Harman RRM. Methotrexate induced skin necrosis: a drug interaction with amiodarone? *BMJ* (1989) 299, 980–1.

Methotrexate + Aminoglycosides

There is evidence that the gastrointestinal absorption of methotrexate can be reduced by paromomycin, neomycin and possibly other oral aminoglycosides, but increased by kanamycin.

Clinical evidence

A study in 10 patients with small cell bronchogenic carcinoma treated with methotrexate found that when additionally given a range of oral anti-infectives (**paromomycin**, vancomycin, polymyxin B, nystatin) the urinary recovery of methotrexate was reduced by over one-third (from 69 to 44%).[1] The **paromomycin** was believed to have been responsible. In another study the concurrent use of **neomycin** 500 mg four times a day for 3 days reduced the methotrexate AUC and the 72-hour cumulative excretion by 50%.[2] In contrast, the same report suggests that **kanamycin** can increase the absorption of methotrexate, but no details are given.

Mechanism

Paromomycin[3] and neomycin, in common with other oral aminoglycosides, can cause a malabsorption syndrome which reduces drug absorption. Kanamycin may possibly be different because it causes less malabsorption. It also reduces the activity of the gut flora, which metabolise methotrexate so that more is available for absorption.

Importance and management

The documentation of these interactions is sparse, but it would seem prudent to be on the alert for a reduction in the response to methotrexate if patients are given oral aminoglycosides such as paromomycin or neomycin. An increased response may possibly occur with kanamycin. No interaction would be expected if the aminoglycosides are given parenterally.

1. Cohen MH, Creaven PJ, Fossieck BE, Johnston AV, Williams CL. Effect of oral prophylactic broad spectrum nonabsorbable antibiotics on the gastrointestinal absorption of nutrients and methotrexate in small cell bronchogenic carcinoma patients. *Cancer* (1976) 38, 1556–9.
2. Shen DD, Azarnoff D. Clinical pharmacokinetics of methotrexate. *Clin Pharmacokinet* (1978) 3, 1–13.
3. Keusch GT, Troncale FJ, Buchanan RD. Malabsorption due to paromomycin. *Arch Intern Med* (1970) 125, 273–6.

Methotrexate + Ascorbic acid (Vitamin C)

The urinary excretion of methotrexate is not significantly changed by the concurrent ingestion of large amounts of vitamin C (1 to 3 g daily) and it may possibly relieve the nausea of chemotherapy.

Clinical evidence, mechanism, importance and management

A patient with breast cancer, treated with methotrexate and cyclophosphamide, and who was also taking propranolol, amitriptyline, perphenazine and prochlorperazine said that the nausea caused by the cytotoxic therapy was relieved by large daily doses of **vitamin C**. A study on this patient showed that the concurrent ingestion of 1 to 3 g **vitamin C** daily had little effect on the excretion of methotrexate in the urine.[1]

1. Sketris IS, Farmer PS, Fraser A. Effect of vitamin C on the excretion of methotrexate. *Cancer Treat Rep* (1984) 68, 446–7.

Methotrexate + Barbiturates

Animal studies suggest that phenobarbital may possibly enhance the alopecia caused by methotrexate.

Clinical evidence, mechanism, importance and management

A study in *rats* showed that severe alopecia could be induced by the concurrent use of methotrexate and **phenobarbital** in dosages which when given alone failed to cause any hair loss.[1] Whether this occurs in man is uncertain.

1. Basu TK, Williams DC, Raven RW. Methotrexate and alopecia. *Lancet* (1973) ii, 331.

Methotrexate + Chloroquine

Chloroquine caused a moderate reduction in the bioavailability of methotrexate.

Clinical evidence, mechanism, importance and management

Eleven patients with rheumatoid arthritis taking regular weekly low doses of 15 mg methotrexate were studied after a single dose of methotrexate alone and after methotrexate plus 250 mg **chloroquine**. The **chloroquine** reduced the maximum plasma levels of the methotrexate by 20% and its AUC by 28%. The suggested reason is that the absorption of the methotrexate from the gut is reduced in some way.[1] These reductions would be expected to reduce both the liver toxicity and the efficacy of the methotrexate, but the clinical importance of this interaction awaits assessment.

1. Seideman P, Albertioni F, Beck O, Eksborg S, Peterson C. Chloroquine reduces the bioavailability of methotrexate in patients with rheumatoid arthritis. A possible mechanism of reduced hepatotoxicity. *Arthritis Rheum* (1994) 37, 830–3.

Methotrexate + Ciprofloxacin

A report describes methotrexate toxicity in two patients during concurrent treatment with ciprofloxacin.

Clinical evidence

When 2 patients with osteosarcoma treated with high-dose methotrexate 12 g/m^2/course were treated with **ciprofloxacin** 500 mg twice daily, during and 2 days before the start of the first methotrexate course respectively, methotrexate elimination was delayed, resulting in raised serum levels, severe cutaneous toxicity and renal failure. The first patient also had hepatic injury and haematological toxicity. Following increased folinic acid rescue, methotrexate levels normalised after several days. In earlier courses without **ciprofloxacin** in the first patient and subsequent courses in the second, methotrexate elimination was normal.[1]

Mechanism

Not fully understood. Ciprofloxacin may displace methotrexate from its plasma-protein binding sites resulting in a rise in levels of unbound methotrexate. Ciprofloxacin may also cause a decrease in renal clearance of methotrexate.

Importance and management

Information appears to be limited to one report, but it would seem prudent to monitor for raised methotrexate levels if concurrent use is necessary. Whether other quinolones behave in the same way as ciprofloxacin is uncertain. More study is needed.

1. Dalle JH, Auvrignon A, Vassal G, Leverger G. Possible ciprofloxacin-methotrexate interaction: a report of 2 cases. *Intersci Conf Antimicrob Agents Chemother* (2000) 40, 477.

Methotrexate + Colestyramine

The serum methotrexate levels of two patients (methotrexate given by infusion) were markedly reduced by the concurrent use of colestyramine.

Clinical evidence

A girl of 11 with osteosarcoma who developed colitis when treated with high-dose intravenous methotrexate, was subsequently treated with 2 g **colestyramine** six hourly from 6 to 48 h after the methotrexate. Serum methotrexate concentrations at 24 h were approximately halved. A marked fall in serum methotrexate levels were seen in another patient similarly treated.[1]

Mechanism

Methotrexate (whether given orally or by infusion) takes part in the entero-hepatic cycle, that is to say it is excreted into the gut in the bile and re-absorbed further along the gut. If colestyramine is given orally, it can bind strongly to the methotrexate[1] in the gut, thereby preventing its reabsorption and, as a result, the serum levels fall.

Importance and management

The documentation seems to be limited to this study.[1] In this instance the colestyramine was deliberately used to reduce serum methotrexate levels, but in some circumstances it might represent an unwanted interaction. Since methotrexate is excreted into the gut in the bile, separating the oral dosages of the colestyramine and methotrexate may not necessarily prevent their coming into contact and interacting together. Monitor concurrent use and make any dosage adjustments as necessary.

1. Erttmann R, Landbeck G. Effect of oral cholestyramine on the elimination of high-dose methotrexate. *J Cancer Res Clin Oncol* (1985) 110, 48–50.

Methotrexate + Corticosteroids

Methotrexate may have a 'steroid-sparing' effect, but there is evidence that the toxicity of methotrexate is increased. The efficacy of methotrexate may also possibly be reduced by hydrocortisone with cefalotin.

Clinical evidence

(a) Steroid-sparing effect

Methotrexate and the **corticosteroids** have been used together successfully, for example in the treatment of psoriatic arthritis, where a 50% reduction in the corticosteroid dosage was possible,[1,2] and in steroid-dependent asthmatics where 30 to 38% reductions in **prednisone** doses were achieved.[3,4] However, one study found no evidence of a steroid-sparing effect with **prednisone**.[5]

(b) Increased methotrexate effects, toxicity

Two patients being treated for psoriasis with methotrexate (5 mg daily for 5 to 7 days) and on long-term **corticosteroid** therapy died apparently from severe bone marrow depression. One was also on chloramphenicol.[6] Another patient taking 30 mg **prednisone** daily for psoriasis and who was given 50 mg, 100 mg and 150 mg methotrexate by injection at 10-day intervals, developed severe leucopenia

and thrombocytopenia.[1] Yet another patient, debilitated from arthritis and prolonged **corticosteroid** therapy, died of generalised systemic moniliasis after two doses of methotrexate. She had no haematological abnormalities.[7] There is some evidence that low-dose **prednisolone** 15 mg daily given long term (but not short term) can reduce the clearance of methotrexate and increase its serum levels.[8] A comparative study in children with brain tumours, treated with methotrexate either with (33 patients) or without (24 patients) **dexamethasone**, found that no serious brain oedema occurred in any of the groups and there were no differences in bone marrow toxicity or mucositis, but liver enzymes were significantly higher in the **dexamethasone** group indicating liver toxicity. AST levels were 76 compared with 19 U/l, and ALT levels were 140 compared with 39 U/l.[9]

(c) Reduced methotrexate effects with cefalotin (cephalothin)/hydrocortisone

In vitro experiments with blast cells from 7 patients with acute myelogenous leukaemia indicated that the intracellular uptake of methotrexate is reduced by the presence of **cefalotin** (21 micrograms/ml) and **hydrocortisone** (20 micrograms/ml) which are normal achievable clinical serum concentrations.[10]

Mechanisms

Not understood. The 'steroid-sparing' effect is possibly the result of a reduction in the steroid metabolism due to the methotrexate.[3]

Importance and management

These interactions between methotrexate and the corticosteroids are neither well documented nor well established, but there is sufficient evidence to suggest that particular care should be exercised during concurrent use to confirm that the clinical outcome is, as intended, advantageous. Be alert for any evidence of methotrexate toxicity.

1. Black RL, O'Brien WM, Van Scott EJ, Auerbach R, Eisen AZ, Bunim JJ. Methotrexate therapy in psoriatic arthritis. *JAMA* (1964) 189, 743–7.
2. Schewach-Millet M, Ziprkowski L. Methotrexate in psoriasis. *Br J Dermatol* (1968) 80, 534–9.
3. Sockin SM, Ostro MG, Goldman MA, Bloch KJ. The effect of methotrexate on plasma prednisolone levels in steroid dependent asthmatics. *J Allergy Clin Immunol* (1992) 89, 286.
4. Sorkness CA, Joseph J, Busse WW, Bush RK. The effect of oral methotrexate discontinuation in corticosteroid-dependent adult asthma. *J Allergy Clin Immunol* (1992) 89, 286.
5. Caldwell EJ, Vogel BM, Dziodzio JT, Bagwell S. The effects of methotrexate on prednisone dosing in steroid-dependent asthma. *Am Rev Respir Dis* (1992) 145, A420.
6. Haim S, Alroy G. Methotrexate in psoriasis. *Lancet* (1967) i, 1165.
7. Roenigk HH, Fowler-Bergfeld W, Curtis GH. Methotrexate for psoriasis in weekly oral doses. *Arch Dermatol* (1969) 99, 86–93.
8. Lafforgue P, Monjanel-Mouterde S, Durand A, Catalin J, Acquaviva PC. Is there an interaction between low doses of corticosteroids and methotrexate in patients with rheumatoid arthritis? A pharmacokinetic study in 33 patients. *J Rheumatol* (1993) 20, 263–7.
9. Wolff JEA, Hauch H, Kühl J, Egeler RM, Jürgens H. Dexamethasone increases hepatotoxicity of MTX in children with brain tumours. *Anticancer Res* (1998) 18, 2895–9.
10. Bender AR, Bleyer WA, Frisby SA, Oliverio VJ. Alterations of methotrexate uptake in human leukaemia cells by other agents. *Cancer Res* (1975) 35, 1305–8.

Methotrexate + Co-trimoxazole or Trimethoprim

Eleven cases of severe bone marrow depression have been reported, two of them fatal, caused by the concurrent use of methotrexate and co-trimoxazole (sulfamethoxazole + trimethoprim) or trimethoprim. The risk of serious pancytopenia even with low-dose methotrexate appears to be increased by co-trimoxazole, probably because the effective concentrations of methotrexate are increased.

Clinical evidence

A 61-year-old patient with rheumatoid arthritis, taking 7.5 mg methotrexate once a week, developed generalised bone marrow hypoplasia over 2 months after a 10-day course of treatment with **co-trimoxazole** for a urinary tract infection. She had taken a total of 775 mg methotrexate when the hypoplasia appeared.[1] Ten other cases of severe bone marrow depression, two of them fatal, have been described in patients on methotrexate when given **co-trimoxazole** or **trimethoprim** concurrently or sequentially.[2-10]

A 10 year (1981 to 1991) regional survey in Ottawa identified **co-trimoxazole** as one of four factors associated with serious pancytopenia in patients taking low-dose methotrexate. The other factors were increases in BUN or creatinine levels, in mean corpuscular volumes and increasing age.[11] Skin ulceration and marked pancytopenia occurred in a woman on methotrexate and **naproxen** when given **trimethoprim**,[12] and life-threatening complications (no details given) are said to have occurred in 2 patients on methotrexate given **unnamed sulphonamides**.[13]

Mechanisms

Not fully understood. Both drugs can suppress the activity of dihydrofolate reductase and it seems possible that they can act additively to produce folate deficiency which could lead to some of the bone marrow changes seen. Another possible mechanism is that the co-trimoxazole causes an increase in 'free' concentrations of methotrexate from about 37 to 52% while the renal clearance is more than halved.[14] This is calculated to increase the exposure to methotrexate by 66%.[14] Another sulphonamide, sulfafurazole (sulfisoxazole),[15] has been found to cause a small reduction in the clearance of methotrexate by the kidneys. However, one study in children with acute lymphoblastic leukaemia found that the concurrent use of co-trimoxazole had no effect on the pharmacokinetics of methotrexate.[16]

Importance and management

Information seems to be limited to the reports cited but the methotrexate/co-trimoxazole and methotrexate/trimethoprim interactions are established. Concurrent use should probably be avoided, but if these drugs are given either concurrently or sequentially, the haematological picture should be very closely monitored because the outcome can be life-threatening. One of the studies cited suggested that concurrent use might cause a mean 66% increase in the exposure to methotrexate.[14]

1. Thomas MH, Gutterman LA. Methotrexate toxicity in a patient receiving trimethoprim-sulfamethoxazole. *J Rheumatol* (1986) 13, 440–1.
2. Dan M, Shapira I. Possible role of methotrexate in trimethoprim- sulfamethoxazole-induced acute megaloblastic anemia. *Isr J Med Sci* (1984) 20, 262–3.
3. Kobrinsky NL, Ramsay NKC. Acute megaloblastic anemia induced by high-dose trimethoprim-sulfamethoxazole. *Ann Intern Med* (1981) 94, 780–1.
4. Thevenet JP, Ristori JM, Cure H, Mizony MH, Bussiere JL. Pancytopénie au cours due traitement d'une polyarthrite rheumatoïde par méthotrexate après administration de triméthoprime-sulfaméthoxazole. *Presse Med* (1987) 16, 1487.
5. Groenendal H, Rampen FHJ. Methotrexate and trimethoprim-sulphamethoxazole — a potentially hazardous combination. *Clin Exp Dermatol* (1990) 15, 358–60.
6. Maricic M, Davis M, Gall EP. Megaloblastic pancytopenia in a patient receiving concurrent methotrexate and trimethoprim-sulphamethoxazole treatment. *Arthritis Rheum* (1986) 29, 133–5.
7. Jeurissen ME, Boerbooms AM, van de Putte LB. Pancytopenia and methotrexate with trimethoprim-sulfamethoxazole. *Ann Intern Med* (1989) 111, 261.
8. Liddle BJ, Marsden JR. Drug interactions with methotrexate. *Br J Dermatol* (1989) 120, 582–3.
9. Govert JA, Patton S, Fine RL. Pancytopenia from using trimethoprim and methotrexate. *Ann Intern Med* (1992) 117, 877–8.
10. Steuer A, Gumpel JM. Methotrexate and trimethoprim: a fatal interaction. *Br J Rheumatol* (1998) 37, 105–6.
11. Al-Awadhi A, Dale P, McKendry RJR. Pancytopenia associated with low dose methotrexate therapy. A regional survey. *J Rheumatol* (1993) 20, 1121–5.
12. Ng HWK, Macfarlane AW, Graham RM, Verbov JL. Near fatal drug interactions with methotrexate given for psoriasis. *BMJ* (1987) 295, 752–3.
13. Zachariae H. Methotrexate and non-steroidal anti-inflammatory drugs. *Br J Dermatol* (1992) 126, 95.
14. Ferrazzini G, Klein J, Sulh H, Chung D, Griesbrecht E, Koren G. Interaction between trimethoprim-sulfamethoxazole and methotrexate in children with leukemia. *J Pediatr* (1990) 117, 823–6.
15. Liegler DG, Henderson ES, Hahn MA, Oliverio VT. The effect of organic acids on renal clearance of methotrexate in man. *Clin Pharmacol Ther* (1969) 10, 849–57.
16. Beach BJ, Woods WG, Howell SB. Influence of co-trimoxazole on methotrexate pharmacokinetics in children with acute lymphoblastic leukemia. *Am J Pediatr Hematol Oncol* (1981) 3, 115–9.

Methotrexate + Diuretics

Some very limited evidence suggests that triamterene may possibly increase the bone marrow suppressive effects of methotrexate. It seems doubtful if thiazides interact adversely.

Clinical evidence, mechanism, importance and management

A 57 year-old woman who had been treated for several years with diclofenac 150 mg, atenolol 50 mg and **triamterene/hydrochlorothiazide** 50/25 mg, all daily for rheumatoid arthritis and hypertension, was additionally started on 5 mg methotrexate weekly. After 2 months she was admitted to hospital with pancytopenia, extensive mucosal ulceration and renal impairment. The authors point out that **triamterene** is structurally similar to folate and has anti-folate activity which may therefore have been additive with the effects of methotrexate,[1] but the **diclofenac** may also have contributed (see 'Methotrexate + NSAIDs', p.512). There are two other reports of pancytopenia in patients on methotrexate and **triamterene**, but again the patients were also taking **NSAIDs**.[2]

A study in 9 patients showed that neither **furosemide** (**frusemide**) nor **hydroflumethiazide** had any effect on the clearance of methotrexate in the urine.[3] However, a study in women with breast cancer and under treatment with methotrexate, cyclophosphamide and fluorouracil found that the concurrent use of a **thiazide diuretic** appeared to increase the myelosuppressant effects, but it is not clear which of the cytotoxics might have been affected.[4]

1. Richmond R, McRorie ER, Ogden DA, Lambert CM. Methotrexate and triamterene — a potentially fatal combination. *Ann Rheum Dis* (1997) 56, 209–10.
2. Wyeth/Lederle. Data on file, September 1998.
3. Kristensen LØ, Weismann K, Hutters L. Renal function and the rate of disappearance of methotrexate from serum. *Eur J Clin Pharmacol* (1975) 8, 439–44.
4. Orr LE. Potentiation of myelosuppression from cancer chemotherapy and thiazide diuretics. *Drug Intell Clin Pharm* (1981) 15, 967–70.

Methotrexate + Fluorouracil

Two patients on low-dose methotrexate had a toxic skin reaction when they started to use a cream containing fluorouracil. *In vitro* and *animal* data also suggest that the cytotoxic effects of methotrexate and fluorouracil may possibly be reduced by concurrent use, but this has yet to be confirmed in man.

Clinical evidence, mechanism, importance and management

(a) Methotrexate + topical fluorouracil

Two patients with rheumatoid arthritis on low-dose methotrexate (7.5 to 12.5 mg weekly) for 6 to 14 months were given 2% **fluorouracil cream** topically for actinic keratosis. Within 2 to 3 days both patients developed erythema, blister formation and necrosis. The cream was stopped and the lesions healed over the next 2 to 3 weeks.[1] It would seem that concurrent use should be avoided.

(b) Methotrexate + systemic fluorouracil

Fluorouracil and another compound, **floxuridine**, are metabolised in the body to a third compound, **floxuridine monophosphate** which is the active cytotoxic agent. This acts by inhibiting an enzyme (thymidylate synthetase) which takes part in the biosynthesis of DNA so that DNA production is reduced. In this way **fluorouracil** and **floxuridine** impair tumour growth.[2] Tests on tumour cells in culture indicate that methotrexate interferes with and reduces the activity of **floxuridine**.[3] *In vitro* studies in the L1210 cells system, Friend leukaemia system and in human bone marrow have similarly shown that in the presence of methotrexate the activity of **fluorouracil** is also suppressed.[4] The likely reason is that the methotrexate inhibits a co-factor (5,10-methylenetetrahydrofolic acid) which is required by the **floxuridine** in order to allow it to bind to thymidylate synthetase. Thus the activity of the **floxuridine** is weakened (and by implication **fluorouracil** as well) which would explain the antagonistic effects of methotrexate.[3]

One cannot uncritically extrapolate tissue culture or *animal* experiments to man, moreover there is already debate about the time-scheduling of administration[5] and whether combinations of methotrexate and **fluorouracil** are antagonistic or even additive.[6-8] However the evidence, even if it does nothing else, emphasises that these two drugs should not be given concurrently without a full awareness that they may possibly be less effective than each drug given alone.

1. Blackburn WD, Alarcón GS. Toxic response to topical fluorouracil in two rheumatoid arthritis patients receiving low dose weekly methotrexate. *Arthritis Rheum* (1990) 33, 303–4.
2. Tattersall MNH, Jackson RC, Connors TA, Harrap KR. Combination chemotherapy: the interaction of methotrexate and 5-fluorouracil. *Eur J Cancer* (1973) 9, 733–9.
3. Maugh TH. Cancer chemotherapy: an unexpected drug interaction. *Science* (1976) 194, 310.
4. Waxman S, Bruckner H. Antitumour drug interactions: additional data. *Science* (1976) 194, 672.
5. Bertino JR, Sawicki WL, Lindquist CA, Gupta VS. Schedule-dependent antitumor effects of methotrexate and 5-fluorouracil. *Cancer Res* (1977) 37, 327–8.
6. Waxman S, Rubinoff M, Greenspan E, Bruckner H. Interaction of methotrexate (MTX) and 5-fluorouracil (5-FU); effect on de novo DNA synthesis. *Proc Am Assoc Cancer Res* (1976) 17, 157.
7. Brown I, Ward HWC. Therapeutic consequences of antitumour drug interactions: methotrexate and 5-fluorouracil in the chemotherapy of C3H mice with transplanted mammary adenocarcinoma. *Cancer Lett* (1978) 5, 291–7.
8. Bertino JR. Modulation of fluorouracil by methotrexate. *J Clin Oncol* (1991) 9, 1511–12.

Methotrexate + Folic acid or Folinic acid (Leucovorin)

Folic acid or folinic acid are sometimes added to low-dose methotrexate treatment for rheumatoid arthritis or psoriasis, but it is uncertain whether or not this reduces adverse effects and efficacy. Folinic acid (leucovorin) is frequently used as an antidote to high-dose methotrexate in cancer therapy.

Clinical evidence

(a) Folic acid

Thirty-two rheumatoid arthritis patients were treated for 24 weeks with low-dose methotrexate (median dose, 7.5 mg weekly) to which was added 1 mg **folic acid** daily. The **folic acid** was found to lower the toxicity scores significantly without affecting efficacy.[1] Preliminary results of a longer study by the same group of workers on patients with rheumatoid arthritis given low-dose methotrexate found that 5 or 50 mg **folic acid** weekly did not reduce the efficacy of the methotrexate after 51 to 53 weeks, but it was not clear from this abstract whether the methotrexate toxicity was reduced or not.[2] Another study found that patients with rheumatoid arthritis treated with low-dose methotrexate and **folic acid** were more likely to continue therapy (61 out of 85 patients, 83.5%) for more than 1 year than patients who did not take **folic acid** (26 out of 49 (53.1%)). This was attributed to the effectiveness of **folic acid** in suppressing adverse effects that result in cessation of therapy.[3] An enquiry into the use of **folic acid** supplementation in psoriasis patients on methotrexate was carried out by means of a questionnaire to dermatologists. Of those who replied, 75% used **folic acid** supplementation in methotrexate-treated patients, 46% considered that **folic acid** reduced nausea and 60% did not affect the efficacy of methotrexate in the treatment of psoriasis.[4]

(b) Folinic acid

(i) Adverse effects reduced, efficacy unaffected. A 52-week comparative trial was carried out on 92 rheumatoid arthritis patients on 7.5 to 30 mg methotrexate weekly, about half of whom were given 2.5 to 5 mg **folinic acid** weekly as a single dose 24 h after the methotrexate. Those given the **folinic acid** had significantly fewer adverse effects than the placebo group, and the efficacy was unchanged.[5] Another study in 20 patients taking low-dose methotrexate and **folinic acid** noted similar results but statistical significance was not established.[6] Two more[7,8] studies also found that **folinic acid** did not interfere with methotrexate efficacy but one of them found the **folinic acid** no more effective than placebo in reducing methotrexate-induced nausea.[7]

(ii) Efficacy reduced. In a study of 27 rheumatoid arthritis patients taking low-dose methotrexate, the clinical and laboratory indices of disease activity were worsened in 13 patients after taking 15 mg/week **folinic acid** for 4 weeks but not in 14 taking a placebo. The adverse effects were no less in the **folinic acid** group than in the placebo

group.[9] The other study in 7 patients on low-dose methotrexate (7.5 to 12 mg weekly) for rheumatoid arthritis found that **calcium folinate** (45 mg weekly taken as 15 mg daily for 3 consecutive days starting 4 to 6 h after the methotrexate) was successful in alleviating the nausea due to methotrexate, but at the same time the disease worsened in all of the patients (subjective clinical assessment, Ritchie articular index, grip strength, ESR, C-reactive protein).[10]

Mechanism

Lower AUCs and plasma methotrexate levels in patients taking folic acid may be due to its increased cellular uptake.[11] Folinic acid (leucovorin) is frequently used as an antidote to high-dose methotrexate in cancer therapy because it competes for entry into cells, and repletes the pools of tetrahydrofolate within cells (the so-called leucovorin rescue).

Importance and management

The results of these studies are inconsistent. Reduced methotrexate toxicity has been seen in four low-dose methotrexate studies[1,5,6,10] but two others[7,9] found no improvement. Efficacy was unchanged in six studies[1,2,5-8] but reduced in two others.[9,10] The outcome of concurrent use is therefore somewhat uncertain, however if adverse effects become troublesome during low-dose methotrexate treatment, folate supplementation may prove to be helpful, but good monitoring is clearly needed to make sure that the methotrexate efficacy is not reduced.

Folinic acid is also used as an antidote to high-dose methotrexate to reverse its serious toxicity – the so-called leucovorin rescue.

1. Morgan SL, Baggott JE, Vaughn WH, Young PK, Austin JS, Krumdieck CL, Alarcón GS. The effect of folic acid supplementation on the toxicity of low-dose methotrexate in patients with rheumatoid arthritis. *Arthritis Rheum* (1990) 33, 9–18.
2. Morgan SL, Baggott JE, Vaughn WH, Austin JS, Veitch TA, Krumdieck CL, Koopman WJ, Alarcón GS. 5 mg or 50 mg/week folic acid (FA) supplementation does not alter the efficacy of methotrexate (MTX)-treated rheumatoid arthritis (RA) patients. *Arthritis Rheum* (1993) 36 (9 Suppl), S79.
3. van den Berg PB, Reicher A, de Jong-van den Berg LTW. Concomitant use of folic acid prolongs duration of MTX-therapy in the treatment of RA. *Pharmacoepidemiol Drug Safety* (2000) 9 (Suppl 1), S16–S17.
4. Kirby B, Lyon CC, Griffiths CEM, Chalmers RJG. The use of folic acid supplementation in psoriasis patients receiving methotrexate: a survey in the United Kingdom. *Clin Exp Dermatol* (2000) 25, 265–8.
5. Shiroky JB, Neville C, Esdaile JM, Choquette D, Zummer M, Hazeltine M, Bykerk V, Kanji M, St-Pierre A, Robidoux L. Bourque L. Low-dose methotrexate with leucovorin (folinic acid) in the management of rheumatoid arthritis. *Arthritis Rheum* (1993) 36, 795–803.
6. Buckley LM, Vacek PM, Cooper SM. Administration of folinic acid after low dose methotrexate in patients with rheumatoid arthritis. *J Rheumatol* (1990) 17, 1158–61.
7. Hanrahan PS, Russell AS. Concurrent use of folinic acid and methotrexate in rheumatoid arthritis. *J Rheumatol* (1988) 15, 1078–80.
8. Weinblatt ME, Maier AL, Coblyn JS. Low dose leucovorin does not interfere with the efficacy of methotrexate in rheumatoid arthritis: an 8 week randomized placebo controlled trial. *J Rheumatol* (1993) 20, 950–2.
9. Joyce DA, Will RK, Hoffman DM, Laing B, Blackbourn SJ. Exacerbation of rheumatoid arthritis in patients treated with methotrexate after administration of folinic acid. *Ann Rheum Dis* (1991) 50, 913–4.
10. Tishler M, Caspi D, Fishel B, Yaron M. The effects of leucovorin (folinic acid) on methotrexate therapy in rheumatoid arthritis patients. *Arthritis Rheum* (1988) 31, 906–8.
11. Bressolle F, Kinowski JM, Morel J, Pouly B, Sany J, Combe B. Folic acid alters methotrexate availability in patients with rheumatoid arthritis. *J Rheumatol* (2000) 27, 2110–14.

Methotrexate + Miscellaneous drugs

Animal studies suggested that the toxicity of methotrexate might be increased by the use of chloramphenicol, PAS, sodium salicylate, sulfametoxypyridazine, tetracycline or tolbutamide, but confirmation of this in man has only been seen with the salicylates, sulphonamides and tetracycline.

Clinical evidence, mechanism, importance and management

Some lists, reviews and books on interactions say that the drugs listed above interact with methotrexate, apparently based largely on a study in which male *mice* were treated for 5 days with each of 4 doses of methotrexate (1.53 to 12.25 mg/kg intravenously) and immediately afterwards with non-toxic intraperitoneal doses of the drugs listed.

These drugs ". . . appeared to be capable of decreasing the lethal dose and/or decreasing the median survival time of the *mice*."[1] That is to say, the toxicity of the methotrexate was increased. The reasons are not understood, but it is suggested that displacement of the methotrexate from its plasma protein binding sites could result in a rise in the levels of unbound and active methotrexate, and in the case of **sodium salicylate** to a decrease in renal clearance.

These *animal* studies were done in 1968. Since then the clinical importance of the interaction with **salicylates** has been confirmed, there are a few cases involving another sulphonamide (**sulfamethoxazole** in the form of **co-trimoxazole**) and there is an isolated case report of an interaction with **tetracycline** (see the Index for appropriate monographs), but there appears to be no direct clinical evidence of interactions between methotrexate and any of the other drugs. The results of *animal* experiments cannot be applied directly and uncritically to man and it now seems probable that some of these suggested or alleged interactions are more theoretical than real.

1. Dixon RL. The interaction between various drugs and methotrexate. *Toxicol Appl Pharmacol* (1968) 12, 308.

Methotrexate + Nitrous oxide

Methotrexate-induced stomatitis and other toxic effects may possibly be increased by the use of nitrous oxide.

Clinical evidence, mechanism, importance and management

Studies in which intravenous methotrexate, cyclophosphamide and fluorouracil were used after mastectomy suggested that the stomatitis which can develop may be caused by a toxic interaction between methotrexate and **nitrous oxide** used during anaesthesia. A possible reason is that the effects of methotrexate on tetrahydrofolate metabolism are increased by **nitrous oxide**. It was found that the incidence of stomatitis, severe leucopenia, thrombocytopenia, and of severe systemic and local infections could be reduced by giving calcium folinate (leucovorin), intravenous hydration and withdrawal of the drugs where necessary.[1]

1. Goldhirsch A, Gelber RD, Tattersall MNH, Rudenstam C-M and Cavalli F. Methotrexate/nitrous-oxide toxic interaction in perioperative chemotherapy for early breast cancer. *Lancet* (1987) ii, 151.

Methotrexate + NSAIDs

Increased methotrexate toxicity, sometimes life-threatening, has been seen in few patients concurrently treated with some NSAIDs (amidopyrine, aspirin, azapropazone, choline magnesium trisalicylate, diclofenac, flurbiprofen, ibuprofen, indometacin (indomethacin), naproxen, phenylbutazone and sodium salicylate) whereas other patients have been treated uneventfully. The pharmacokinetics of methotrexate can also be changed by some NSAIDs (aspirin, choline magnesium trisalicylate, etodolac, ibuprofen, metamizole, naproxen, sodium salicylate, tolmetin). The development of toxicity may be related to the methotrexate dosage. The risk appears to be lowest in those taking low-dose methotrexate for psoriasis or rheumatoid arthritis with normal renal function.

Clinical evidence

(a) Aspirin and other salicylates

A study in 8 patients with rheumatoid arthritis found that 975 mg **aspirin** four times daily increased the AUC of a single 10-mg bolus of methotrexate by 28%. The methotrexate clearance was reduced.[1] A further study by the same authors in 15 rheumatoid arthritis patients (possibly using some of the same patients) also given a single 10 mg bolus dose of methotrexate, either with or without 975 mg **aspirin**

four times daily, similarly found methotrexate clearance was reduced (systemic clearance about 16%, renal clearance of unbound methotrexate about 30%) by **aspirin**. Also the unbound fraction of methotrexate was higher in patients when taking **aspirin**. Despite these changes no acute toxicity was seen.[2] Another study found that **aspirin** did not affect the pharmacokinetics of methotrexate.[3]

A study in 4 patients found that the renal clearance of methotrexate was reduced by 35% when given an infusion of **sodium salicylate** (2 g initially, then 33 mg/min).[4] Two further studies found that **choline magnesium trisalicylate** reduced the clearance, compared with **paracetamol** (acetaminophen), by 24 to 41%, and increased the unbound fraction by 28%.[5,6]

Lethal pancytopenia in 2 patients given methotrexate and **aspirin** prompted a retrospective survey of the records of other patients treated with intra-arterial infusions of methotrexate 50 mg daily for 10 days for epidermoid carcinoma of the oral cavity. Six out of 7 who developed a rapid and serious pancytopenia were found to have had **aspirin** or other **salicylates**.[7] Similar results were found in studies on *mice*.[7] There are other case reports[8,9] of methotrexate toxicity in patients taking **salicylates** but whether a causal relationship exists is uncertain. It has been suggested that pneumonitis in patients on low-dose methotrexate may have resulted from the concurrent use of 4 to 5 g **aspirin** daily.[10]

See also the report about the comparative use of **aspirin** and other NSAIDs in section (s) below.

(b) Amidopyrine

Megaloblastic pancytopenia occurred in a woman with rheumatoid arthritis given methotrexate 15 mg weekly and **amidopyrine** 1 to 1.5 g daily.[11]

(c) Azapropazone

A woman given methotrexate (25 mg weekly for 4 years) for psoriasis showed acute toxicity (oral and genital ulceration, bone marrow failure) shortly after starting to take **azapropazone** (reducing from a dose of 2.4 g on the first day, 1.8 g on the second day to 1.2 g daily for a week). She was also taking 300 mg **aspirin** daily.[12,13]

(d) Bromfenac

In a short-term study, 10 patients taking methotrexate weekly were given 50 mg **bromfenac** three times daily for 6 days. No significant changes were seen in either the pharmacokinetics of **bromfenac**, or methotrexate. However, the AUC of the major metabolite of methotrexate, 7-hydroxymethotrexate, was increased by 30% and its renal clearance was reduced by 16%. Eight of the patients had mild to moderate adverse effects and one patient had to withdraw because of moderate hypertension. No patient showed clinically important abnormal laboratory test results.[14]

(e) Celecoxib

Fourteen female patients with rheumatoid arthritis on 5 to 20 mg methotrexate weekly for at least 3 months were additionally given 200 mg **celecoxib** or a placebo twice daily for a week. It was found that the maximum serum levels of the methotrexate, its AUC, renal clearance and other pharmacokinetic parameters were unchanged by the **celecoxib**.[15]

(f) Diclofenac

A study found that **diclofenac** 100 mg daily did not affect the pharmacokinetics of methotrexate,[3] however 5 patients on low-dose methotrexate (7.5 to 12.5 mg weekly) for psoriasis or rheumatoid arthritis developed serious/fatal neutropenias. These cases probably involved other drug interactions, but **diclofenac** may have been an additional factor in two of them.[16] Other cases involving **diclofenac** are in *(j)* and*(k)*.

(g) Etodolac

A pharmacokinetic study in patients with rheumatoid arthritis found that 600 mg **etodolac** daily did not affect the AUC of methotrexate, but duration of exposure was lengthened (mean residence time increased from 8.5 to 11.4 h). No clinical toxicity was seen.[17,18]

(h) Flurbiprofen

A study in 6 patients taking low-doses of methotrexate (10 to 25 mg weekly) found no important changes in methotrexate levels when given 100 mg **flurbiprofen** three times daily.[19] In another study of 10 rheumatoid arthritis patients taking 7.5 to 17.5 mg methotrexate weekly and 3 mg/kg **flurbiprofen** daily, methotrexate oral and renal clearance were similarly unaffected by **flurbiprofen**.[20]

In contrast to these pharmacokinetic studies a case report describes an elderly woman who had been taking 2.5 mg methotrexate three times a week for 3 years for rheumatoid arthritis, who developed haematemesis, neutropenia and thrombocytopenia (diagnosed as methotrexate toxicity) within 1 to 2 weeks of starting to take 100 mg **flurbiprofen** daily.[21]

(i) Ibuprofen

A study in 7 patients found that the clearance of methotrexate (7.5 to 15 mg orally) was halved by **ibuprofen** 40 mg/kg/day when compared with **paracetamol** (**acetaminophen**).[5] In a related study the clearance was reduced by 40%.[6] Another study of 6 rheumatoid arthritis patients taking 10 to 25 mg/week methotrexate found 800 mg **ibuprofen** three times daily had no effect on methotrexate pharmacokinetics.[19] Another study similarly found that **ibuprofen** did not affect the pharmacokinetics of methotrexate.[3] A patient on methotrexate who was given **ibuprofen** required leucovorin rescue because the clearance of methotrexate had fallen by two-thirds.[22] Another patient on high-dose methotrexate (7.5 g/m^2) had severe methotrexate-induced kidney toxicity and delayed excretion of methotrexate while taking 400 mg **ibuprofen** 4-hourly.[23] A report attributes *Pneumocystis carinii* pneumonitis in a 16 year-old patient on 5 to 10 mg/week methotrexate to the concurrent use of 600 mg **ibuprofen** twice daily (also 1 mg prednisolone) daily.[24]

(j) Indometacin (Indomethacin)

A child on methotrexate 7.5 mg/m^2/week for 9 months showed an AUC increase of 140% when given **indometacin** and **aspirin**.[25] Another study found that **indometacin** did not affect the pharmacokinetics of methotrexate.[3]

Two patients on sequential intermediate dose methotrexate and fluorouracil who were concurrently taking **indometacin** 75 to 100 mg daily died from acute drug toxicity which the authors of the report attributed to **indometacin**-associated renal failure.[26] Another case of acute renal failure has been described,[27] but there were no cases of toxicity in 4 other patients on methotrexate given either **paracetamol** (**acetaminophen**) or **indometacin**.[9] An elderly woman died after a single 10 mg intramuscular dose of methotrexate while taking 50 mg **indometacin** daily rectally and 100 mg **diclofenac** daily intravenously.[28]

(k) Ketoprofen

In a study of 10 rheumatoid arthritis patients taking 7.5 to 17.5 mg methotrexate weekly and 3 mg/kg **ketoprofen** daily, the methotrexate oral and renal clearance and the fraction of methotrexate unbound were unaffected by **ketoprofen**.[20] In another study 18 rheumatoid arthritis patients who were given 15 mg methotrexate intravenously weekly, **ketoprofen** had no significant effect on the methotrexate AUC, half-life or clearance, or on those of its major metabolite 7-hydroxymethotrexate.[29] A retrospective study of 118 cycles of high-dose methotrexate treatment (800 to 8300 mg/m^2; mean 3200 mg/m^2) in 36 patients showed that 4 out the 9 patients who developed severe methotrexate toxicity had also taken **ketoprofen** (150 to 200 mg daily for 2 to 15 days). Three of them died. A marked and prolonged rise in serum methotrexate levels was observed. Another patient who showed toxicity had also been given **diclofenac** 150 mg in one day.[30] The authors of this report state that **ketoprofen** should not be given at the same time as methotrexate, but it may be safe to give it 12 to 24 h after high dose methotrexate because 50% of the methotrexate is excreted by the kidneys within 6 to 12 h. This was tried in two patients without ill-effects.[30]

(l) Meloxicam

Thirteen patients with rheumatoid arthritis were given 15 mg intravenous methotrexate before and after taking **meloxicam** 15 mg daily for a week. The pharmacokinetics of the methotrexate were unaffected by the **meloxicam** and no increase in toxicity was seen.[31]

(m) Metamizole sodium (Dipyrone)

A study in a patient with osteosarcoma showed that 4 g **metamizole sodium (dipyrone)** daily more than doubled the methotrexate AUC (from 636 to 1476 micromol.h.l^{-1}) during the first cycle of high dose methotrexate treatment.[32]

(n) Naproxen

Eighteen rheumatoid arthritis patients were given 15 mg methotrexate intravenously weekly. **Naproxen** had no significant effect on the methotrexate AUC, half-life or clearance, or on those of its major metabolite 7-hydroxymethotrexate.[29] Another study in patients with rheumatoid arthritis with normal renal function found that no toxicity was caused by 500 mg **naproxen** twice daily with 15 mg methotrexate given orally or intravenously, nor was the methotrexate clearance altered.[33] Yet another study found that **naproxen** did not affect the pharmacokinetics of methotrexate.[3]

In contrast, yet another study found that the clearance was decreased by 22%[5,6] and two children on methotrexate for 1 and 2 years showed increases in the AUC of methotrexate of 22% and 71% when given **naproxen** with **aspirin** or **indometacin** respectively.[25] A further study in 9 children on methotrexate 0.22 to 1.02 mg/kg/week found that the clearance was increased in 4 children by more than 30% when **naproxen** 14.6 to 18.8 mg/kg was given daily. There was also a 30% or more change in the pharmacokinetics of naproxen in 6 patients, but as both increases and decreases in clearance occurred, the significance is uncertain.[34]

A woman died of gross methotrexate toxicity apparently exacerbated by the concurrent use of **naproxen**.[35] A report attributes pneumonitis in a patient on 7.5 to 10 mg/week methotrexate to the concurrent use of (initially 1 g then 500 mg) **naproxen** daily.[36]

(o) Paracetamol (Acetaminophen)

Paracetamol (acetaminophen) appears not to interact with methotrexate, see *(a)*, *(i)* and *(j)*.

(p) Phenylbutazone

Two patients on methotrexate for psoriasis developed methotrexate toxicity and skin ulceration shortly after starting to take **phenylbutazone** (200 to 600 mg daily). One of them died from septicaemia following bone marrow depression.[37]

(q) Piroxicam

In a study 20 rheumatoid arthritis patients taking 10 mg/week methotrexate were given 20 mg **piroxicam** daily for at least 15 days. No effect on the pharmacokinetics of either free or bound methotrexate was seen.[38,39] In another study of 10 rheumatoid arthritis patients taking 7.5 to 17.5 mg methotrexate weekly and 20 mg **piroxicam** daily, methotrexate oral and renal clearance were similarly unaffected by **piroxicam**.[20]

(r) Tolmetin

Three children on methotrexate for between 6 months and 1 year showed increases in the AUC of methotrexate of 42%, and 18%, 25% when given **tolmetin**, and in the last two cases **tolmetin** with **aspirin**.[25]

(s) NSAIDs in general

In a study of 34 rheumatoid arthritis patients taking 5 or 10 mg/m^2 methotrexate (to nearest 2.5 mg tablet) weekly, 12 patients also took **aspirin** (average 4.5 g daily) and 22 took **alternative NSAIDs**. Twenty-one of the 34 also took prednisone. Toxicity, sometimes serious (5 patients withdrawn), was common but no clinical differences between **aspirin** or **other NSAIDs** with respect to this toxicity was seen during 12 months of therapy.[40]

A study of 87 patients on long-term treatment with methotrexate (mean weekly dose 8.19 mg), most of whom were also taking **unspecified NSAIDs**, found that the majority (72%) experienced no untoward effects and in the rest they were only relatively mild.[41]

Concurrent use of methotrexate and **NSAIDs** in more than 450 patients with psoriatic arthritis or rheumatoid arthritis ". . . without clinical problems due to interactions (with **NSAIDs**) . . ." is briefly described in another report.[42]

A literature review of methotrexate/**NSAID** interactions showed a lack of alteration of low-dose methotrexate pharmacokinetic parameters with NSAIDs with the exception of co-administered methotrexate and salicylates.[43]

In a review of the records of 315 rheumatoid arthritis patients taking low-dose methotrexate 13 patients had low platelet counts. The thrombocytopenia was believed to have resulted from an interaction with a **NSAID** or in some patients a multiple drug interaction. If multiple drug interactions were not involved, the authors found that if the **NSAID** was given on a separate day, or dosages spaced according to the **NSAID** half-life, therapy could be re-introduced avoiding the problems of thrombocytopenia.[44]

Mechanisms

Methotrexate is largely cleared unchanged from the body by renal excretion. The NSAIDs as a group inhibit the synthesis of the prostaglandins (PGE_2) resulting in a fall in renal perfusion which could lead to a rise in serum methotrexate levels, accompanied by increased toxicity. In addition, salicylates competitively inhibit the tubular secretion of methotrexate, which would further reduce its clearance.[4] NSAIDs can also cause renal failure, which would allow the methotrexate to accumulate. Phenylbutazone, amidopyrine and methotrexate cause bone marrow depression which could be additive. Protein binding displacement of methotrexate or its metabolite (7-hydroxymethotrexate) have also been suggested as possible additional mechanisms.[45,46] There is also some evidence that this metabolite is cleared more slowly in the presence of NSAIDs.[47]

Importance and management

The evidence presented here clearly shows that a few patients on methotrexate have developed very serious toxicity apparently due to the concurrent use of NSAIDs (aspirin and other salicylates, amidopyrine, azapropazone, diclofenac, flurbiprofen, ibuprofen, indometacin, ketoprofen, naproxen and phenylbutazone) whereas other patients have experienced no problems at all. There is also other evidence that the pharmacokinetics of the methotrexate are changed (in particular reduced clearance) by some NSAIDs (aspirin, choline magnesium trisalicylate, etodolac, ibuprofen, metamizole, sodium salicylate, tolmetin) which might be expected to increase its toxicity. Should all of these interacting NSAIDs therefore be totally avoided?

Because methotrexate alone is so potentially toxic, the advice of the Committee on the Safety of Medicines (CSM) in the UK is that any patient given methotrexate alone should have a full blood count and kidney and liver function tests before starting treatment. These should be repeated weekly until therapy is stabilised, and thereafter every 2 to 3 months. Patients should be told to report any sign or symptom suggestive of infection, particularly sore throat (which might possibly indicate that white cell counts have fallen) or dyspnoea or cough (suggestive of pulmonary toxicity).[48] The consensus of opinion seems to be that the risks are greatest with high dose methotrexate (150 mg or more daily to treat neoplastic diseases) and in patients with impaired kidney function, but less in those given low doses (5 to 25 mg weekly) for psoriasis or rheumatoid arthritis and with normal kidney function. But the makers of methotrexate, the CSM and British National Formulary do not advise the avoidance of NSAIDs (except azapropazone and OTC aspirin and ibuprofen), even though their use is a recognised additional risk factor for toxicity. Instead their advice is that the methotrexate dosage should be well monitored, which implies that the precautions suggested above should be stepped up.

Some of the NSAIDs cited here have not been reported to interact seriously (bromfenac, celecoxib, meloxicam, paracetamol (acetaminophen), piroxicam), and information about other NSAIDs seems to be lacking, but the same general precautions indicated above should be followed with all NSAIDs just to be on the safe side. However, the concurrent use of amidopyrine or metamizole is to be discouraged because even on their own they can cause agranulocytosis.

1. Stewart CF, Fleming RA, Magneson P, Germain B, Evans WE. Effect of aspirin on the disposition of methotrexate in patients with rheumatoid arthritis. *Clin Pharmacol Ther* (1990) 47, 139.
2. Stewart CF, Fleming RA, Germain BF, Seleznick MJ, Evans WE. Aspirin alters methotrexate disposition in rheumatoid arthritis patients. *Arthritis Rheum* (1991) 34, 1514–20.
3. Iqbal MP, Baig JA, Ali AA, Niazi SK, Mehboobali N, Hussain MA. The effects of nonsteroidal anti-inflammatory drugs on the disposition of methotrexate in patients with rheumatoid arthritis. *Biopharm Drug Dispos* (1998) 19, 163–7.
4. Liegler DG, Henderson ES, Hahn MA, Oliverio VT. The effect of organic acids on renal clearance of methotrexate in man. *Clin Pharmacol Ther* (1969) 10, 849–57.
5. Tracy TS, Jones DR, Hall SD, Brater DC, Bradley JD, Krohn K. The effect of NSAIDs on methotrexate disposition in patients with rheumatoid arthritis. *Clin Pharmacol Ther* (1990) 47, 138.
6. Tracy TS, Krohn K, Jones DR, Bradley JD, Hall SD, Brater DC. The effects of salicylate, ibuprofen, and naproxen on the disposition of methotrexate in patients with rheumatoid arthritis. *Eur J Clin Pharmacol* (1992) 42, 121–5.
7. Zuik M, Mandel MA. Methotrexate-salicylate interaction: a clinical and experimental study. *Surg Forum* (1975) 26, 567–9.
8. Dubin HV, Harrell ER. Liver disease associated with methotrexate treatment of psoriatic patients. *Arch Dermatol* (1970) 102, 498–503.
9. Baker H. Intermittent high dose oral methotrexate in psoriasis. *Br J Dermatol* (1970) 82, 65–9.
10. Maier WP, Leon-Perez R, Miller SB. Pneumonitis during low-dose methotrexate therapy. *Arch Intern Med* (1986) 146, 602–3.
11. Noskov SM. Megaloblastic pancytopenia in a female patient with rheumatoid arthritis given methotrexate and amidopyrine. *Terapeuticheskiy Arkhiv* (1990) 62, 122–3.
12. Daly HM, Scott GL, Boyle J, Roberts CJC. Methotrexate toxicity precipitated by azapropazone. *Br J Dermatol* (1986) 114, 733–35.
13. Burton JL. Drug interactions with methotrexate. *Br J Dermatol* (1991) 124, 300–1.
14. Gumbhir-Shah K, Cevallos WH, Decleene SA, Korth-Bradley JM. Lack of interaction between bromfenac and methotrexate in patients with rheumatoid arthritis. *J Rheumatol* (1996) 23, 984–9.
15. Karim A, Tolbert D, Piergies A, Hunt T, Hubbard R, Harper K, Slater M, Geis GS. Celecoxib, a specific COX–2 inhibitor, lacks significant drug-drug interactions with methotrexate or warfarin. *Arthritis Rheum* (1998) 41 (9 Suppl), S315.
16. Mayall B, Poggi G, Parkin JD. Neutropenia due to low-dose methotrexate therapy for psoriasis and rheumatoid arthritis may be fatal. *Med J Aust* (1991) 155, 480–4.
17. Anaya J-M, Fabre D, Bressolle F, Alric R, Dropsy R, Sany J. Effects of etodolac on methotrexate pharmacokinetics in rheumatoid arthritis patients. *Arthritis Rheum* (1992) 35 (9 Suppl), S343.
18. Anaya J-M, Fabre D, Bressolle F, Bolgna C, Alric R, Cocciglio M, Dropsy R, Sany J. Effect of etodolac on methotrexate pharmacokinetics in patients with rheumatoid arthritis. *J Rheumatol* (1994) 21, 203–8.
19. Skeith KJ, Russell AS, Jamali F, Coates J, Friedman H. Lack of significant interaction between low dose methotrexate and ibuprofen or flurbiprofen in patients with arthritis. *J Rheumatol* (1990) 17, 1008–10.
20. Tracy TS, Worster T, Bradley JD, Greene PK, Brater DC. Methotrexate disposition following concomitant administration of ketoprofen, piroxicam and flurbiprofen in patients with rheumatoid arthritis. *Br J Clin Pharmacol* (1994) 37, 453–6.
21. Frenia ML, Long KS. Methotrexate and nonsteroidal antiinflammatory drug interactions. *Ann Pharmacother* (1992) 26, 234–7.
22. Bloom EJ, Ignoffo RJ, Reis CA, Cadman E. Delayed clearance (CL) of methotrexate (MTX) associated with antibiotics and antiinflammatory agents. *Clin Res* (1986) 34, 560A.
23. Cassano WF. Serious methotrexate toxicity caused by interaction with ibuprofen. *Am J Pediatr Hematol Oncol* (1989) 11, 481–2.
24. Carmichael AJ, Ryatt KS. *Pneumocystis carinii* pneumonia following methotrexate. *Br J Dermatol* (1990) 122, 291.
25. Dupuis LL, Koren G, Shore A, Silverman ED, Laxer RM. Methotrexate-nonsteroidal antiinflammatory drug interaction in children with arthritis. *J Rheumatol* (1990) 17, 1469–73.
26. Ellison NM, Servi RJ. Acute renal failure and death following sequential intermediate-dose methotrexate and 5-FU: a possible adverse effect due to concomitant indomethacin administration. *Cancer Treat Rep* (1985) 69, 342–3.
27. Maiche AG. Acute renal failure due to concomitant action of methotrexate and indomethacin. *Lancet* (1986) i, 1390.
28. Gabrielli A, Leoni P, Danieli G. Methotrexate and non-steroidal anti-inflammatory drugs. *BMJ* (1987) 294, 776.
29. Christophidis N, Dawson TM, Angelis P, Ryan PFJ. A double-blind, randomised, placebo controlled pharmacokinetic and clinical study of the interaction of ketoprofen and naproxen with methotrexate in rheumatoid arthritis. *Arthritis Rheum* (1994) 37 (9 Suppl), S252.
30. Thyss A, Milano G, Kubar J, Namer M, Schneider M. Clinical and pharmacokinetic evidence of a life-threatening interaction between methotrexate and ketoprofen. *Lancet* (1986) i, 256–8.
31. Hübner G, Sander D, Degner FL, Türck D, Rau R. Lack of pharmacokinetic interaction of meloxicam with methotrexate in patients with rheumatoid arthritis. *J Rheumatol* (1997) 24, 845–51.
32. Hernández de la Figuera y Gómez T, Torres NVJ, Ronchera Oms CL, Ordovás Baines JP. Interacción farmacocinética entre metotrexato a altas dosis y dipirona. *Rev Farmacol Clin Exp* (1989) 6, 77–81.
33. Stewart CF, Fleming RA, Arkin CR, Evans WE. Coadministration of naproxen and low-dose methotrexate in patients with rheumatoid arthritis. *Clin Pharmacol Ther* (1990) 47, 540–6.
34. Wallace CA, Smith AL, Sherry DD. Pilot investigation of naproxen/methotrexate interaction in patients with juvenile rheumatoid arthritis. *J Rheumatol* (1993) 20, 1764–8.
35. Singh RR, Malaviya AN, Pandey JN, Guleria JS. Fatal interaction between methotrexate and naproxen. *Lancet* (1986) i, 1390.
36. Englebrecht JA, Calhoon SL, Scherrer JJ. Methotrexate pneumonitis after low-dose therapy for rheumatoid arthritis. *Arthritis Rheum* (1983) 26, 1275–8.
37. Adams JD, Hunter GA. Drug interaction in psoriasis. *Aust J Dermatol* (1976) 17, 39–40.
38. Combe B, Edno L, Lafforgue P, Bologna C, Bernard J-C, Acquaviva P, Sany J, Bressolle F. Total and free methotrexate pharmacokinetics, with and without piroxicam, in rheumatoid arthritis patients. *Br J Rheumatol* (1995) 34, 421–8.

39. Bressolle F, Cociglio M, Bologna C, Edno L, Lafforgue P, Acquaviva P, Sany J, Combe B. Effect of piroxicam on methotrexate and 7-OH methotrexate pharmacokinetics in rheumatoid arthritis patients. *Therapie* (1995) 50 (Suppl), 410.

40. Rooney TW, Furst DE, Koehnke R, Burmeister L. Aspirin is not associated with more toxicity than other nonsteroidal antiinflammatory drugs in patients with rheumatoid arthritis treated with methotrexate. *J Rheumatol* (1993) 20, 1297–1302.

41. Wilke WS, Calabrese LH, Segal AM. Incidence of untoward reactions in patients with rheumatoid arthritis treated with methotrexate. *Arthritis Rheum* (1983) 26 (Suppl), S56.

42. Zachariae H. Methotrexate and non-steroidal anti-inflammatory drugs. *Br J Dermatol* (1992) 126, 95.

43. Carpentier N, Ratsimbazafy V, Bertin P, Vergne P, Bonnet C, Bannwarth B, Dehais J, Treves R.Interaction méthotrexate/anti-inflammatoires non stéroïdiens: importance de la dose. *J Pharm Clin* (1999) 18, 295–9.

44. Franck H, Rau R, Herborn G. Thrombocytopenia in patients with rheumatoid arthritis on long-term treatment with low dose methotrexate. *Clin Rheumatol* (1996) 15, 163–7.

45. Slørdal L, Sager G, Aarbakke J. Pharmacokinetic interactions with methotrexate: is 7-hydroxy-methotrexate the culprit? *Lancet* (1988) i, 591–2.

46. Parish RC, Johnson V. Effect of salicylate on plasma protein binding of methotrexate. *Clin Pharmacol Ther* (1996) 59, 162.

47. Furst DE, Herman RA, Koehnke R, Erickson N,. Hash L, Riggs CE, Porras A, Veng-Pedersen P. Effect of aspirin and sulindac on methotrexate clearance. *J Pharm Sci* (1990) 79, 782–6.

48. The Committee on Safety of Medicines. *Current Problems in Pharmacovigilance* (1997) 23, 12.

Methotrexate + Omeprazole

Two reports describe a reduction in the loss of methotrexate in patients treated with omeprazole. A further report suggests that elevated methotrexate levels are not due to concomitant omeprazole.

Clinical evidence

A man with stage II_EB nodular sclerosing Hodgkin's disease developed osteosarcoma and was treated with cyclophosphamide, bleomycin, dactinomycin (actinomycin D), and methotrexate, followed by leucovorin rescue. He was also taking senna, levothyroxine, **omeprazole**, baclofen, aciclovir, ferrous sulphate and docusate sodium. During the first cycle of treatment his serum methotrexate levels remained elevated for several days, and suspicion fell on the **omeprazole**, which was stopped. The patient's serum methotrexate levels then fell rapidly, and during the following three cycles the methotrexate kinetics were normal.

An 11-year-old boy with osteoblastic osteosarcoma was given high-dose methotrexate 15 g as a 4-h infusion. He was also given **omeprazole** 20 mg twice daily (for about one week prior to methotrexate), megestrol acetate and sucralfate and folinic acid rescue. Methotrexate elimination was delayed and so further folinic acid was given. When later cycles of methotrexate were given, with ranitidine instead of omeprazole, the elimination of methotrexate was normal. The elimination half-life of the initial phase after the first dose given with **omeprazole** was 65% longer when compared to that of the second dose without omeprazole.[1]

In contrast to these findings, a further case is reported in which a man with chondroblastic osteosarcoma, who had been taking **omeprazole**, was treated with high-dose methotrexate 20 g over 6 h with hydration, urinary alkalinization and, after 24 h, folinic acid rescue. Folinic acid dose was adjusted in response to elevated methotrexate levels and **omeprazole** was stopped. A second dose of methotrexate 2 weeks later, this time without **omeprazole**, resulted in similar elevated methotrexate levels. Thus the elevated methotrexate levels in this patient could not be attributed to co-administered omeprazole.[2]

Mechanism

The suggested reason for what happened is that **omeprazole** inhibits the activity of a hydrogen-ion dependent mechanism in the kidney on which methotrexate depends for its excretion, so that its loss is diminished.[3]

The situation with lansoprazole may be similar. At pH of about 5 found in the renal tubules, pantoprazole is more slowly activated than omeprazole and this may reduce the incidence of adverse effects.[1]

The reason for the elevated methotrexate levels in the third patient were not explained but do not seen to be due to concomitant omeprazole.[2]

Importance and management

Information seems to be limited to these reports and the picture they present is somewhat contradictory. Any changes in methotrexate kinetics are important in terms of the potential for increased toxicity. Further study is required to determine whether or not omeprazole affects methotrexate levels.

The authors of one report recommend that if omeprazole therapy is necessary for a patient about to receive methotrexate, then omeprazole should be discontinued 4 to 5 days before methotrexate administration. The situation with lansoprazole may be similar. Pantoprazole may be a suitable alternative but this requires confirmation. Ranitidine was found to be a suitable alternative in one case.[1]

1. Beorlegui B, Aldaz A, Ortega A, Aquerreta I, Sierrasesúmega L, Giráldez J. Potential interaction between methotrexate and omeprazole. *Ann Pharmacother* (2000) 34, 1024–7.

2. Whelan J, Hoare D, Leonard P. Omeprazole does not alter plasma methotrexate clearance. *Cancer Chemother Pharmacol* (1999) 44, 88–9.

3. Reid T, Yuen A, Catolico M, Carlson RW. Impact of omeprazole on the plasma clearance of methotrexate. *Cancer Chemother Pharmacol* (1993) 33, 82–4.

Methotrexate + Penicillins

There is evidence that the clearance of methotrexate can be reduced by some penicillins, but acute methotrexate toxicity caused by this interaction has only been seen in a relatively small number of patients.

Clinical evidence

Four patients treated with methotrexate showed a marked reduction in its clearance when concurrently treated with different penicillins: with **penicillin** a 36% reduction; with **piperacillin** 67%; with **ticarcillin** 60%; and with **dicloxacillin** plus **indometacin (indomethacin)** 93%. Prolonged leucovorin rescue was necessary. They were given the methotrexate as an intravenous bolus (15 to 60 mg/m^2) and then 15 to 60 mg by infusion over 36 h.[1] Acute methotrexate toxicity associated with increased serum levels developed in a 16-year-old when given 1 g **amoxicillin** six-hourly.[2] Increased methotrexate serum levels were seen in another patient when given 30 g **carbenicillin** daily.[3] A marked reduction in methotrexate clearance was seen in patient when concurrently treated with **mezlocillin** 330 mg/kg daily accompanied by increased gastrointestinal toxicity.[4] Prompted by the apparent development of methotrexate-induced pneumonitis in a patient given **flucloxacillin**, a comparative study was made in two groups of 10 patients with rheumatoid arthritis on 5 to 15 mg methotrexate weekly. One of the groups was also given 500 mg **flucloxacillin** four times daily. The **flucloxacillin** had no clinically significant effect on the pharmacokinetics of the methotrexate,[5] even so the authors of the report quote another possible isolated case, and yet another has been reported.[6] Five patients on low-dose methotrexate (7.5 to 12.5 mg weekly) for psoriasis or rheumatoid arthritis developed neutropenia and thrombocytopenia when treated with penicillins (**amoxicillin with or without clavulanic acid, benzylpenicillin, flucloxacillin, piperacillin**). Three died and the other 2 were extensively hospitalised.[6] A patient on 50 mg methotrexate (weekly intravenously), diethylstilbestrol (stilboestrol), prednisone and furosemide (frusemide), developed severe toxicity within a week of starting 250 mg **phenoxymethylpenicillin** every other day.[7] A multinational survey of 79 patients on low-dose methotrexate who had developed blood dyscrasias and who had been taking concurrent medication, identified 6 patients who developed evidence of methotrexate toxicity (aplastic anaemia, neutropenia, thrombocytopenia, leucopenia, pneumonitis, toxic epidermal necrolysis, elevated serum methotrexate levels) within 5 days to 8 months of starting **penicillins**.[8]

Mechanism

It is thought that weak acids such as the penicillins can possibly successfully compete with methotrexate in the kidney tubules for excretion so that the methotrexate is retained, thereby increasing its effects and its toxicity.[2]

Importance and management

Information seems to be limited to the reports cited here which would seem to indicate that serious interactions between methotrexate and penicillins are uncommon. It is not known why only a few patients have been affected and what other factors may have contributed, but the problem does not seem to be confined to patients on high dose methotrexate. There is not enough evidence totally to forbid concurrent use, but close monitoring is obviously advisable. One published recommendation is to carry out twice-weekly platelet and white cell counts for two weeks initially, with the measurement of methotrexate levels if toxicity is suspected. Folinic acid (leucovorin) rescue should be available.[6] For the general CSM guidelines on the use of methotrexate see 'Importance and management' in 'Methotrexate + NSAIDs', p.512.

1. Bloom EJ, Ignoffo RJ, Reis CA, Cadman E. Delayed clearance (CL) of methotrexate (MTX) associated with antibiotics and anti-inflammatory agents. *Clin Res* (1986) 34, 560A.
2. Ronchera CL, Hernández T, Peris JE, Torres F, Granero L, Jiménez NV, Plá JM. Pharmacokinetic interaction between high-dose methotrexate and amoxycillin. *Ther Drug Monit* (1993) 15, 375–9.
3. Gibson DL, Bleyer AW, Savitch JL. Carbenicillin potentiation of methotrexate plasma concentration during high dose methotrexate therapy. Am Soc Hosp Pharm. Mid year clinical meeting abstracts, New Orleans, Dec 6–10 (1981) p. 111.
4. Dean R, Nachman J, Lorenzana AN. Possible methotrexate-mezlocillin interaction. *Am J Pediatr Hematol Oncol* (1992) 14, 88–9.
5. Herrick AL, Grennan DM, Giriffen K, Aarons L, Gifford LA. Lack of interaction between flucloxacillin and methotrexate in patients with rheumatoid arthritis. *Br J Clin Pharmacol* (1996) 41, 223–7.
6. Mayall B, Poggi G, Parkin JD. Neutropenia due to low-dose methotrexate therapy for psoriasis and rheumatoid arthritis may be fatal. *Med J Aust* (1991) 155, 480–4.
7. Nierenberg DW, Mamelok RD. Toxic reaction to methotrexate in a patient receiving penicillin and furosemide: a possible interaction. *Arch Dermatol* (1983) 119, 449–50.
8. Wyeth/Lederle. Personal communication, July 1996.

Methotrexate + Pristinamycin

An isolated report describes severe methotrexate toxicity in a patient when treated with pristinamycin.

Clinical evidence

A boy of 13 with acute lymphoblastic leukaemia had a relapse and began a series of regimens with methotrexate in combination with other cytotoxics including dexamethasone, mercaptopurine, vincristine, cytarabine and asparaginase, tioguanine (thioguanine) and ifosfamide. During a late cycle during which he was also taking 2 g **pristinamycin** daily for a staphylococcal infection, the clearance of the methotrexate became markedly decreased (half-life prolonged from the usual 6 h to 203 h). He developed severe methotrexate toxicity (oral mucositis, anusitis, balanitis, neutropenia and thrombocytopenia) and was given leucovorin rescue and haemodialysis.[1]

Mechanism

Not understood, but on the basis of experimental evidence the authors of the report excluded the possibilities of kidney impairment or reduction by the pristinamycin of liver metabolism.[1]

Importance and management

This appears to be the first and only report of an interaction between methotrexate and a macrolide antibacterial. Its general importance is unknown but the authors strongly advise the avoidance of pristinamycin in patients treated with methotrexate, and caution with other macrolides.[1] This report is confused by the number of different drugs being taken.

1. Thyss A, Milano G, Renée N, Cassuto-Viguier E, Jambou P, Soler C. Severe interaction between methotrexate and a macrolide-like antibiotic. *J Natl Cancer Inst* (1993) 85, 582–3.

Methotrexate + Probenecid

Probenecid markedly increases serum methotrexate levels (three to fourfold). Dosage reductions are needed to avoid toxicity.

Clinical evidence

The concurrent use of **probenecid** 500 to 1000 mg and methotrexate (200 mg/m^2 intravenous bolus injection) resulted in serum methotrexate levels in 4 patients which were four times higher at 24 h than in 4 others who had not received **probenecid** (0.4 compared with 0.09 mg/l).[1]

A three to fourfold increase in serum methotrexate levels at 24 h was seen in 4 patients given **probenecid**.[2] Pretreatment with **probenecid** (five 500-mg doses 6-hourly) doubled the serum methotrexate levels of another 4 patients.[3] Severe and life-threatening pancytopenia occurred in a woman on low-dose methotrexate 7.5 mg weekly for rheumatoid arthritis when given **probenecid**. She also had renal insufficiency, hypoalbuminaemia and was using **salicylates**.[4]

Mechanism

Probenecid inhibits the renal excretion of methotrexate in both *monkeys* and *rats*[5,6] and this is probably what also happens in man. Changes in the protein binding of methotrexate may have some part to play.[7] The increased methotrexate levels increase the risk of serious bone marrow depression.

Importance and management

An established and clinically important interaction. A marked increase in both the therapeutic and toxic effects of methotrexate can occur, apparently even with low doses if other risk factors are present.[4] Anticipate the need to reduce the dosage of the methotrexate and monitor the effects well if probenecid is used concurrently. *Animal* studies suggest that despite the rise in methotrexate levels, the clinically useful cytotoxic effects of the methotrexate may actually be reduced by the presence of probenecid.[8]

1. Aherne GW, Piall E, Marks V, Mould G, White WF. Prolongation and enhancement of serum methotrexate concentrations by probenecid. *BMJ* (1978) 1, 1097–99.
2. Howell SB, Olshen RA, Rice JA. Effect of probenecid on cerebrospinal fluid methotrexate kinetics. *Clin Pharmacol Ther* (1979) 26, 641–6.
3. Lilly MB, Omura GA. Clinical pharmacology of oral intermediate-dose methotrexate with or without probenecid. *Cancer Chemother Pharmacol* (1985) 15, 220–2.
4. Basin KS, Escalante A, Beardmore TD. Severe pancytopenia in a patient taking low dose methotrexate and probenecid. *J Rheumatol* (1991) 18, 609–10.
5. Bourke RS, Chheda G, Bremer A, Watanabe O, Tower DB. Inhibition of renal tubular transport of methotrexate by probenecid. *Cancer Res* (1975) 35, 110–6.
6. Kates RE, Tozer TN, Sorby DL. Increased methotrexate toxicity due to concurrent probenecid administration. *Biochem Pharmacol* (1976) 25, 1485–8.
7. Paxton JW. Interaction of probenecid with the protein binding of methotrexate. *Pharmacology* (1984) 28, 86–9.
8. Gangji D, Ross WE, Bleyer WA, Poplack DG, Glaubiger DL. Probenecid inhibition of methotrexate cytotoxicity in mouse L1210 leukemia cells. *Cancer Treat Rep* (1984) 68, 521–5.

Methotrexate + Retinoids

Although concurrent use can be successful, the incidence of severe liver toxicity appears to be considerably increased. The serum levels of methotrexate may be increased.

Clinical evidence

A man was given a weekly infusion of methotrexate (10 mg over 48 h) for chronic discoid psoriasis. When also given 30 mg (0.05 mg/kg) **etretinate** daily his serum methotrexate levels almost doubled. Concentrations at 12 and 24 h during the infusion were 0.11 mmol/l, compared with 0.07 and 0.05 mmol/l before the **etretinate**.[1] A later study in 6 psoriatic patients found that **etretinate** increased the maximum serum levels of methotrexate by 38%.[2]

Severe toxic hepatitis occurred in other patients when both of these drugs were used.[3-5] It may take several months to develop.[5] Signs of liver toxicity were seen in 2 out of 10 patients in one clinic given both drugs,[2] but none in another 531 patients given methotrexate alone or in 110 patients given **etretinate** alone.[3]

Mechanism

Not understood. The increased incidence of toxic hepatitis may possibly be related to the increased methotrexate serum levels.

Importance and management

Although both drugs have been used together with success for psoriasis,[6-8] the risk of severe drug-induced hepatitis seems to be very considerably increased. One author says that he has decided not to use this combination in future.[3] Concurrent use should clearly be undertaken with great care.

1. Harrison PV, Peat M, James R, Orrell D. Methotrexate and retinoids in combination for psoriasis. *Lancet* (1987) ii, 512.
2. Larsen FG, Nielsen-Kudsk F, Jakobsen P, Schrøder H, Kragballe K. Interaction of etretinate with methotrexate pharmacokinetics in psoriatic patients. *J Clin Pharmacol* (1990) 30, 802–7.
3. Zachariae H. Dangers of methotrexate/etretinate combination therapy. *Lancet* (1988) i, 422.
4. Zachariae H. Methotrexate and etretinate as concurrent therapies in the treatment of psoriasis. *Arch Dermatol* (1984) 120, 155.
5. Beck H-I, Foged EK. Toxic hepatitis due to combination therapy with methotrexate and etretinate in psoriasis. *Dermatologica* (1983) 167, 94–6.
6. Vanderveen EE, Ellis CN, Campbell JP, Case PC, Voorhees JJ. Methotrexate and etretinate as concurrent therapies in severe psoriasis. *Arch Dermatol* (1982) 118, 660–2.
7. Adams JD. Concurrent methotrexate and etretinate therapy for psoriasis. *Arch Dermatol* (1983) 119, 793.
8. Rosenbaum MM, Roenigk HH. Treatment of generalized pustular psoriasis with etretinate (Ro 10-9359) and methotrexate. *J Am Acad Dermatol* (1984) 10, 357–61.

Methotrexate + Sulfasalazine

The pharmacokinetics of methotrexate are unaffected by sulfasalazine.

Clinical evidence, mechanism, importance and management

A study in 15 patients with rheumatoid arthritis found that when 2000 mg **sulfasalazine** was added to 7.5 mg methotrexate weekly, the pharmacokinetics of the methotrexate remained unchanged.[1,2] There seems to be no reason to avoid the concurrent use of **sulfasalazine** and methotrexate.

1. Haagsma C, van Riel P, Vree T, Russel F, de Rooij DJ, van de Putte L. Combination therapy in RA: pharmacokinetic analysis of the interaction of methotrexate and sulfasalazine. *Arthritis Rheum* (1993) 36 (9 Suppl), S180.
2. Haagsma CJ, Russel FGM, Vree TB, van Riel PLCM, van de Putte LBA. Combination of methotrexate and sulphasalazine in patients with rheumatoid arthritis: pharmacokinetic analysis and relationship to clinical response. *Br J Clin Pharmacol* (1996) 42, 195–200.

Methotrexate + Tacrolimus

No adverse interaction appears to occur between methotrexate and tacrolimus.

Clinical evidence, mechanism, importance and management

A study in three bone marrow transplant patients on **tacrolimus** (0.03 mg/kg/day) found that low-dose methotrexate (15 mg/m² on day 1, and 10 mg/m² on days 3, 6 and 11) did not significantly affect clinical care and no interaction of clinical significance was seen.[1] In a further study in 40 patients given methotrexate (15 mg/m² on day 1 followed by 10 mg/m² on days 3,6 and 11 after a transplant) with 0.03 mg/kg intravenous **tacrolimus** daily, similarly found no evidence of an adverse interaction.[2,3]

1. Dix S, Devine SM, Geller RB, Wingard JR. Re: severe interaction between methotrexate and a macrolide-like antibiotic. *J Natl Cancer Inst* (1995) 87, 1641–2.
2. Wingard JR, Nash RA, Ratanatharathorn V, Fay JW, Klein JL, Przepiorka D, Devine SM, Fitzsimmons WE. Lack of interaction between tacrolimus (FK506) and methotrexate (MTX) in bone marrow transplant (BMT) recipients. *Blood* (1995) 86 (10 Suppl 1), 396a.
3. Wingard JR, Nash RA, Ratanatharathorn V, Fay JW, Klein JL, Przepiorka D, Maher RM, Devine SM, Boswell G, Bekersky I, Fitzsimmons W. Lack of interaction between tacrolimus (FK506) and methotrexate in bone marrow transplant recipients. *Bone Marrow Transplant* (1997) 20, 49–51.

Methotrexate + Tetracyclines

Two case reports describe the development of methotrexate toxicity in patients when additionally given tetracycline or doxycycline.

Clinical evidence, mechanism, importance and management

A man being successfully and uneventfully treated for psoriasis with methotrexate (25 mg weekly) was additionally started on 500 mg **tetracycline** four times daily for a mycoplasmal infection. Within 5 days he developed recurrent fever, ulcerative stomatitis and diarrhoea. His white cell count fell to 1000 and his platelet count to 30,000 (units not stated), all signs of methotrexate toxicity. The problem resolved when the methotrexate was withdrawn, but the psoriasis returned.[1] A 17-year-old girl with osteosarcoma of the femur was given **doxycycline** 100 mg every 12 hours for an abscess in her left eye at the same time as her eleventh cycle of high-dose methotrexate with folinic acid rescue. Elevated plasma methotrexate levels were observed and she developed haematological and severe vomiting requiring antiemetics, continued folinic acid, a prolonged stay in hospital and postponement of her next dose of methotrexate. **Doxycycline** had not been taken during the first 10 cycles of methotrexate therapy and the pharmacokinetic changes and symptoms seen in the eleventh cycle were attributed to concurrent **doxycycline**.[2] This interaction has also been observed in *mice*.[3] Displacement of the methotrexate from its binding sites may be part of the explanation. There appears to be the only two clinical reports of this interaction on record. Concurrent use need not be avoided, but it should be well monitored.

1. Turck M. Successful psoriasis treatment then sudden 'cytotoxicity'. *Hosp Pract* (1984) 19, 175–6.
2. Tortajada-Ituren JJ, Ordovás-Baines JP, Llopis-Salvia P, Jiménez-Torres NV. High-dose methotrexate-doxycycline interaction. *Ann Pharmacother* (1999) 33, 804–8.
3. Dixon RL. The interaction between various drugs and methotrexate. *Toxicol Appl Pharmacol* (1968) 12, 308.

Methotrexate + Urinary alkalinizers

Alkalinization increases the solubility of the methotrexate in the urine but also increases its excretion.

Clinical evidence, mechanism, importance and management

Methotrexate is much more soluble in alkaline than in acid fluids, for which reason urinary alkalinizers (and ample fluids) have been given to patients on high dose methotrexate therapy to prevent the precipitation of methotrexate in the kidney tubules, which would cause damage. However, alkalinization also increases the loss of methotrexate in the urine because at high pH values more of the drug exists in the ionised form which is not readily reabsorbed by the tubules. This increased loss was clearly shown in about 70 patients in whom alkalinization of the urine (to pH >7) with **sodium bicarbonate** and hydration reduced the serum methotrexate concentrations at 48 h by 73% and at 72 h by 76%.[1] In this instance the interaction was being exploited therapeutically to avoid toxicity. This interaction has also been shown by others.[2] The possible consequences should be recognised if concurrent use is undertaken.

1. Nirenberg A, Mosende C, Mehta BM, Gisolfi AL, Rosen G. High dose methotrexate with citrovorum factor rescue: predictive value of serum methotrexate concentrations and corrective measures to avert toxicity. *Cancer Treat Rep* (1977) 61, 779–83.
2. Sand TE, Jacobsen S. Effect of urine pH and flow on renal clearance of methotrexate. *Eur J Clin Pharmacol* (1981) 19, 453–6.

Misonidazole + Cimetidine

There is evidence that cimetidine does not interact with misonidazole.

Clinical evidence, mechanism, importance and management

Cimetidine increases the half-life and AUC of misonidazole in *mice*,[1] but 1 g **cimetidine** daily given to 6 healthy human subjects for 9 days had no effect on the pharmacokinetics of misonidazole.[2] Even so it would be prudent to monitor the effects to confirm that **cimetidine** used for longer periods does not interact.

1. Begg EJ, Williams KM, Wade DN, O'Shea KF. No significant effect of cimetidine on the pharmacokinetics of misonidazole in man. *Br J Clin Pharmacol* (1983) 15, 575–6.
2. Workman P, Donaldson J, Smith NC. Effects of cimetidine, antipyrine and pregnenolone carbonitrile on misonidazole pharmacokinetics. *Cancer Treat Rep* (1983) 67, 723–5.

Misonidazole + Miscellaneous drugs

Phenytoin, phenobarbital and dexamethasone increase the clearance of misonidazole from the body. Dexamethasone appears to reduce the neurotoxicity of misonidazole without reducing its radiosensitising effects, but this does not seem to be true for phenytoin and phenobarbital. Metoclopramide does not interact with misonidazole.

Clinical evidence, mechanism, importance and management

A study in patients suggests that the use of corticosteroids confers some protection against the peripheral neuropathy which can occur with misonidazole,[1] a possible explanation being provided by another study which showed that **dexamethasone** increased the clearance of misonidazole and reduced the AUC.[2]

After taking **phenytoin** 300 mg daily for a week or **phenobarbital** 200 mg daily for a week the half-life of misonidazole was decreased by 27 and 23% respectively in healthy subjects. The clearance increased by 42 and 31%.[3] This confirms previous human studies in which **phenytoin** shortened the misonidazole half-life by 31%[4] and 30 to 40%.[5] Both **phenytoin** and **phenobarbital** were found to reduce plasma misonidazole concentrations.[1] It seems probable that this interaction results from an increase in the metabolism of the misonidazole caused by these two enzyme-inducing drugs. Whether concurrent use helps to reduce the neurotoxicity of misonidazole is uncertain although this was not apparent in two studies.[1,6] Peak plasma concentrations of misonidazole are not affected so that its radiosensitising effects may not be reduced.[3]

A study in 6 healthy subjects indicates that **metoclopramide** has no significant effect on the pharmacokinetics of misonidazole.[7]

1. Walker MD, Strike TA. Misonidazole peripheral neuropathy. Its relationship to plasma concentration and other drugs. *Cancer Clin Trials* (1980) 3, 105–9.
2. Jones DH, Bleehen NM, Workman P, Walton MI. The role of dexamethasone in the modification of misonidazole pharmacokinetics. *Br J Cancer* (1983) 48, 553–7.
3. Williams K, Begg E, Wade D, O'Shea K. Effects of phenytoin, phenobarbital and ascorbic acid on misonidazole elimination. *Clin Pharmacol Ther* (1983) 33, 314–21.
4. Workman P, Bleehen NM, Wiltshire CR. Phenytoin shortens the half-life of the hypoxic cell radiosensitizer misonidazole in man: implications for possible reduced toxicity. *Br J Cancer* (1980) 41, 302–4.
5. Moore JL, Paterson ICM, Dawes PJD K, Henk JM. Misonidazole in patients receiving radical radiotherapy: pharmacokinetic effects of phenytoin tumor response and neurotoxicity. *Int J Radiat Oncol Biol Phys* (1982) 8, 361–4.
6. Jones DH, Bleehen NM, Workman P, Smith NC. The role of microsomal enzyme inducers in the reduction of misonidazole neurotoxicity. *Br J Radiol* (1983) 56, 865–70.
7. Williams KM, Begg EJ, Wade DN, O'Shea K. No significant effect of metoclopramide on misonidazole elimination in man. *Br J Clin Pharmacol* (1983) 15, 390–2.

Mitomycin (C) + Chlorozotocin

Pneumonitis developed in a patient concurrently treated with mitomycin and chlorozotocin.

Clinical evidence, mechanism, importance and management

A woman with pancreatic cancer developed acute interstitial pneumonitis (characterised by increasing dyspnoea and a dry cough) after receiving modest doses of mitomycin and **chlorozotocin** in combination with fluorouracil and doxorubicin (FAM-chlorozotocin). Mitomycin and **chlorozotocin** rarely cause lung damage at low doses and it is concluded that when given concurrently they may act synergistically or additively to cause lung damage. The problem responded rapidly to treatment with prednisone.[1]

1. Goedert JJ, Smith FP, Tsou E, Weiss RB. Combination chemotherapy pneumonitis: a case report of possible synergistic toxicity. *Med Pediatr Oncol* (1983) 11, 116–18.

Mitomycin (C) + Doxorubicin (Adriamycin)

An increased incidence of late onset congestive heart failure has been seen in patients treated with mitomycin who had previously been given doxorubicin.

Clinical evidence, mechanism, importance and management

Fourteen out of 91 (15.3%) patients with advanced breast cancer who had previously failed to respond to **doxorubicin** developed congestive heart failure when later treated with a combination of mitomycin (20 mg/m^2 intravenously every 4 to 6 weeks) and megestrol acetate 160 mg daily. None of them had any pre-existing heart disease. This compares with only 3 out of 89 (3.5%) other patients who had received **doxorubicin** but no mitomycin. The maximum dose of **doxorubicin** was 450 mg/m^2 and all of the patients had also been given cyclophosphamide. Some of them also received other drugs during the **doxorubicin** phase of treatment. These included fluorouracil, methotrexate, tegafur and vincristine. The heart failure developed slowly (mean time of 8.5 months) compared with those in the control group (1.5 months). The reasons for this apparent synergistic cardiotoxicity are not understood. The authors of the report suggest very close monitoring in patients treated with mitomycin if they have previously received anthracycline drugs.[1]

1. Buzdar AU, Legha SS, Tashima CK, Hortobagyi GN, Yap HY, Krutchik AN, Luna MA, Blumenschein GR. Adriamycin and mitomycin C: possible synergistic cardiotoxicity. *Cancer Treat Rep* (1978) 62, 1005–8.

Mitomycin (C) + Fluorouracil

Serious and potentially life-threatening intravascular haemolysis and kidney failure may develop after long-term use of mitomycin and fluorouracil.

Clinical evidence, mechanism, importance and management

Two patients are described in one report who developed chronic haemolysis and progressive kidney failure after long-term treatment with mitomycin and **fluorouracil (5 FU)** following partial or total gastrectomy for gastric cancer. The haemolysis was exacerbated by blood transfusions. The authors of the report[1] say that these two cases are ". . . the extreme of a syndrome we are finding increasingly in our pretransfusion patients, after 6 months or more of maintenance therapy." A similar syndrome occurred in 2 other patients, one with gastric carcinoma and one without, when treated with these two drugs.[2,3] The incidence of this severe and potentially fatal syndrome is not known, but the authors of one report suggest that this regimen should be stopped at the first sign of intravascular haemolysis, persistent proteinuria and rising serum-urea levels (two consecutive values above 8 mmol/l).[1]

1. Jones BG, Fielding JW, Newman CE, Howell A, Brookes VS. Intravascular haemolysis and renal impairment after blood transfusion in two patients on long-term 5-fluorouracil and mitomycin-C. *Lancet* (1980) 1, 1275–7.

2. Krauss S, Sonoda T, Solomon A. Treatment of advanced gastrointestinal carcinoma with 5-fluorouracil and mitomycin C. *Cancer* (1979) 43, 1598–1603.
3. Lempert KD. Haemolysis and renal impairment syndrome in patients on 5-fluorouracil and mitomycin-C. *Lancet* (1980) 2, 369–70.

Mitomycin (C) + Furosemide (Frusemide)

Furosemide (frusemide) does not interact with mitomycin C.

Clinical evidence, mechanism, importance and management

A study in 5 patients with advanced solid tumours treated with mitomycin C 10 mg/m^2 showed that **furosemide (frusemide)** given as a 40 mg intravenous bolus either 120 or 200 min after the mitomycin had no effect on its pharmacokinetics.[1]

1. Verweij J, Kerpel-Fronius S, Stuurman M, de Vries J, Pinedo HM. Absence of interaction between furosemide and mitomycin C. *Cancer Chemother Pharmacol* (1987) 19, 84–6.

Mitomycin (C) + Tamoxifen

Haemolytic anaemia, thrombocytopenia and renal dysfunction, leading to potentially fatal haemolytic uraemic syndrome, can occur in patients given tamoxifen with, or shortly after, mitomycin C.

Clinical evidence, mechanism, importance and management

When a woman with metastatic breast cancer who had previously had treatment with mitomycin C/mitoxantrone/methotrexate, developed rapidly fatal acute renal failure 21 days after starting **tamoxifen**, a comparative survey was undertaken of other patients who had also had all of these drugs.[1] Nine out of 94 (9.6%) patients developed anaemia, thrombocytopenia and renal dysfunction, compared with none in another group of 45 patients not given **tamoxifen**. One of the 9 died with renal failure. The doses used were mitomycin 7 mg/m^2 intravenously every 42 days for four courses; mitoxantrone 7 mg/m^2 and methotrexate 35 mg/m^2 intravenously every 21 days for eight courses; **tamoxifen** 20 mg orally daily.

The authors of the study concluded that the development of this haemolytic uraemic syndrome was due to a combination of subclinical endothelial damage induced by the mitomycin C, and the thrombotic effect on the platelets caused by the **tamoxifen**. They advise the avoidance of **tamoxifen** with or shortly after mitomycin C unless carefully monitored.

1. Montes A, Powles TJ, O'Brien MER, Ashley SE, Luckit J, Treleaven J. A toxic interaction between mitomycin C and tamoxifen causing the haemolytic uraemic syndrome. *Eur J Cancer* (1993) 29A, 1854–7.

Mitotane + Spironolactone

An isolated report describes the abolition of the effects of mitotane in Cushing's disease by spironolactone.

Clinical evidence, mechanism, importance and management

A woman with Cushing's disease under treatment with chlorpropamide, digoxin, furosemide (frusemide) was given 50 mg **spironolactone** four times daily to control hypokalaemia. She was additionally treated for 5 months with 3 g mitotane daily to control the elevated cortisol levels but without effect.[1] When an interaction was suspected (on the basis of *animal* studies[1]) it was decided to withdraw the **spironolactone**, whereupon severe nausea and profuse diarrhoea developed within 24 to 48 h, suggesting mitotane toxicity. This subsided and then redeveloped when the mitotane was stopped and then

restarted a week later. The mechanism of this apparent interaction is not understood. It would seem that mitotane can become ineffective in the management of Cushing's syndrome in the presence of **spironolactone**. More confirmatory study is needed.

1. Wortsman J, Soler NG. Mitotane. Spironolactone antagonism in Cushing's syndrome. *JAMA* (1977) 238, 2527.

Paclitaxel + Cisplatin or Carboplatin

One study found that low-dose paclitaxel increased the peripheral neuropathy of patients previously treated with cisplatin. Two other studies failed to find this effect. The toxicity appears to be sequence-dependent with more severe myelosuppression occurring if paclitaxel is given after cisplatin. Paclitaxel may reduce the thrombocytopenia associated with carboplatin.

Clinical evidence, mechanism, importance and management

(a) Carboplatin

As a clinical trial had found that the severity of thrombocytopenia with the combination of paclitaxel and **carboplatin** was less than expected with carboplatin alone, a study in 11 patients was carried out to determine whether there was a pharmacokinetic basis for these findings. Patients were given **carboplatin** as a 30-min infusion either alone or immediately following paclitaxel 175 mg/m^2 as a 3-h infusion and it was found that the pharmacokinetics of **carboplatin** were not significantly affected.[1] Similarly, a pharmacokinetic interaction was not noted when paclitaxel and carboplatin were given in either order,[2] and in this study platelet toxicity was also reduced. A study in patients with non-small cell lung cancer found that the AUC associated with a 50% decrease in platelet count increased from 34 to 57 micrograms/ml.h when carboplatin was given alone or after paclitaxel respectively, which suggests a pharmacodynamic basis for the attenuated toxicity of the combination.[3]

(b) Cisplatin

Twenty-two women with ovarian cancer who had relapsed after treatment with cisplatin were later treated with paclitaxel (3 h infusions of 135 or 175 mg/m^2 every three weeks) for at least six courses. The paclitaxel treatment caused the onset or worsening of pre-existing neuropathic signs and symptoms in almost all of the patients. The features were those of a distal, symmetrical, sensory polyneuropathy involving firstly the legs and secondly the arms. The motor nerves and the autonomic nervous system were unaffected. The damage was interpreted as being due to axonal damage, either primary or secondary, to dorsal root ganglia neuropathy.[4] Pharmacokinetic studies suggest that sequence-dependent differences in toxicity may be due to a 25% reduction in paclitaxel clearance when **cisplatin** is given first.[5] **Cisplatin**-induced cytotoxic lesions may be lower and thus toxicity reduced when paclitaxel is given first, as *in vitro* this order of addition to blood cells is associated with lower DNA adduct formation.[6] The apparent cumulative toxicity of these two drugs was not seen in a previous studies.[7]

The authors of the report cited here[4] do not clearly and unambiguously recommend whether these two drugs should be avoided or not, but if they are given sequentially like this it would seem prudent to monitor the effects very closely. The makers recommendation for the primary treatment of ovarian carcinoma is to give the paclitaxel first ("... when the safety profile of *Taxol* is consistent with that reported for single-agent use ..."). If the paclitaxel is given after the **cisplatin**, patients show a more profound myelosuppression and an approximately 20% decrease in paclitaxel clearance.[8]

1. Obasaju CK, Johnson SW, Rogatko A, Kilpatrick D, Brennan JM, Hamilton TC, Ozols RF, O'Dwyer PJ, Gallo JM. Evaluation of carboplatin pharmacokinetics in the absence and presence of paclitaxel. *Clin Cancer Res* (1996) 2, 549–52.

2. Huizing MT, Giaccone G, van Warmerdam LJC, Rosing H, Bakker PJM, Vermorken JB, Postmus PE, van Zandwijk, Koolen MGJ, ten Bokkel Huinink, van der Vijgh WJF, Bierhorst FJ, Lai A, Dalesio O, Pinedo HM, Veenhof CHN, Beijnen JH. Pharmacokinetics of paclitaxel and carboplatin in a dose-escalating and dose-sequencing study in patients with non-small-cell lung cancer. *J Clin Oncol* (1997) 15, 317–29.

3. Kearns CM, Belani CP, Erkmen K, Zuhowski M, Hiponia D, Ergstrom C, Ramanthan R, Trenn M, Aisner J, Ergorin MJ. Reduced platelet toxicity with combination carboplatin & paclitaxel: pharmacodynamic modulation of carboplatin associated thrombocytopenia. *Proc Am Soc Clin Oncol* (1995) 14, 170.

4. Cavaletti G, Bogliun G, Marzorati L, Zincone A, Marzola M, Colombo N, Tredici G. Peripheral neurotoxicity of taxol in patients previously treated with cisplatin. *Cancer* (1995) 75, 1141–50.

5. Rowkinsky EK, Gilbert M, McGuire WP, Noe DA, Grochow LB, Forastiere AA, Ettinger DS, Lubejko BG, Clarke B, Sartorius SE, Cornblath DR, Hendricks CB, Donehower RC. Sequences of taxol and cisplatin: a phase I and pharmacologic study. *J Clin Oncol* (1991) 9, 1692–1703.

6. Ma J, Verweij J, Planting AST, Holker HJ, Loos WJ, de Boer-Dennert M, van der Berg MEL, Stoter G, Schellens JHM. Docetaxel and paclitaxel inhibit DNA-adduct formation and intracellular accumulation of cisplatin in human leucocytes. *Cancer Chemother Pharmacol* (1996) 37, 382–4.

7. McGuire WP, Rowinsky EK, Rosenhein NB, Grumbine FC, Ettinger DS, Armstrong DK, Donehower RC. Taxol: a unique antineoplastic agent with significant activity in advanced ovarian epithelial neoplasms. *Ann Intern Med* (1989) 111, 273–9.

8. Taxol (Paclitaxel). Bristol-Myers Squibb Pharmaceuticals Ltd. Summary of product characteristics, February 2001.

Paclitaxel + Ketoconazole

Ketoconazole appears not to interact adversely with paclitaxel.

Clinical evidence, mechanism, importance and management

Women with ovarian cancer were treated with 3-h infusions of 175 mg/m^2 paclitaxel once every 21 days. It was found that when single oral doses of **ketoconazole** were given 3 h after or 3 h before the paclitaxel, the serum levels of the paclitaxel and its principal metabolite (6-alpha-hydroxypaclitaxel) remained unchanged. These findings confirmed those of other *in vitro* studies. The conclusion was reached that these two drugs can therefore be given together safely without any dosage adjustments.[1,2]

1. Jamis-Dow CA, Pearl ML, Watkins PB, Blake DS, Klecker RW, Collins JM. Predicting drug interactions in vivo from experiments in vitro: human studies with paclitaxel and ketoconazole. *Am J Clin Oncol* (1997) 20, 592–99.

2. Taxol (Paclitaxel). Bristol-Myers Squibb Pharmaceuticals Ltd. Summary of product characteristics, February 2001.

Paclitaxel + Miscellaneous drugs

In vitro studies with human liver tissue suggest that no metabolic interactions are likely between paclitaxel and cimetidine, dexamethasone or diphenhydramine. *Cremophor* levels may inhibit intracellular uptake and metabolism of paclitaxel. Ciclosporin enhances plasma paclitaxel levels after oral administration. Amifostine may affect paclitaxel pharmacokinetics. Toxicity associated with combinations of paclitaxel and cyclophosphamide, doxorubicin or epirubicin is sequence-dependent. Gemcitabine appears not to interact.

Clinical evidence, mechanism, importance and management

(a) Amifostine

A study in which 8 patients received paclitaxel at doses from 135 to 200 mg/m^2 for 2 cycles, one with **amifostine** 750 mg/m^2 as a 15-min infusion 30 min beforehand and the other without, found that **amifostine** did not affect the pharmacokinetics of paclitaxel. Six of the patients were also taking epirubicin and cisplatin.[1] Similar results have been reported in another study, which also suggested that **amifostine** did not reduce paclitaxel toxicity.[2] However, an earlier study found that pre-treatment with **amifostine** reduced the AUC of paclitaxel by 29%.[3] Further study is required.

(b) Cimetidine, Dexamethasone, Diphenhydramine

On the basis of an *in vitro* study using human liver slices and human liver microsomes it has been concluded that the metabolism of paclitaxel is unlikely to be altered by **cimetidine, dexamethasone** or **diphenhydramine**, all of which are frequently given to prevent the hypersensitivity reactions associated with paclitaxel or its vehicle.[4] The makers say that paclitaxel clearance in patients is not affected by **cimetidine** premedication.[5]

(c) Ciclosporin

Intravenous paclitaxel may be associated with adverse effects because of its vehicle, *Cremophor*. Oral paclitaxel has poor oral bioavailability because of high affinity for P-glycoprotein in the gastrointestinal tract. Studies in *mice* have shown that the combination of **ciclosporin** with oral paclitaxel produced a tenfold increase in systemic exposure to paclitaxel. This was been followed by a study in 5 patients who received an oral dose (intravenous formulation) of paclitaxel 60 mg/m^2 followed by intravenous doses of 175 mg/m^2 for subsequent courses and 9 patients who also received **ciclosporin** 15 mg/kg. Oral paclitaxel alone produced below therapeutic plasma levels, but therapeutic levels above 0.1 micromol/l were achieved when co-administered with **ciclosporin** (a ninefold increase). The combination was well-tolerated, but further study is required to determine whether oral paclitaxel is as active as intravenous paclitaxel.[6]

(d) Cremophor (paclitaxel vehicle)

In vitro, **Cremophor** was found to inhibit the metabolism of paclitaxel in human liver microsomes[4] which might be expected to increase its toxicity. This concentration may be achieved clinically in patients given paclitaxel.[7] This may be worth bearing in mind if other drugs formulated with **Cremophor** are given with paclitaxel.

(e) Cyclophosphamide

A study in patients given paclitaxel as a 24-h infusion and **cyclophosphamide** as an infusion over 1 h found that neutropenia and thrombocytopenia were more severe when paclitaxel preceded **cyclophosphamide**.[8]

(f) Doxorubicin

A study in 18 women with breast cancer, given 150 to 200 mg/m^2 paclitaxel over 3 h and 60 mg/m^2 **doxorubicin** as a bolus, found that even minor modifications of the dose and length of infusion of either drug can have unpredictable effects on the efficacy and toxicity of these drugs.[9] Other studies in patients with breast cancer have found a higher frequency of mucositis and neutropenia when paclitaxel was given before **doxorubicin**.[10,11] This may be explained by pharmacokinetic studies which found **doxorubicin** clearance was reduced if paclitaxel was given first.[10] *In vitro* studies in human breast cancer cells have shown that paclitaxel added before **doxorubicin** produces a threefold increase in cytotoxicity, which may be associated with paclitaxel-induced increase in the activity of the intracellular enzymes by which **doxorubicin** exerts its cytotoxic action.[12] Studies in *mice* have found that both paclitaxel and its vehicle, Cremophor may modify the distribution and metabolism of **doxorubicin**, in particular increasing levels in the heart. This may contribute to observed cardiac toxicity during administration with paclitaxel.[13]

If these drugs are used together a firm dosage schedule should be used. When new schedules are designed this should be done carefully with very close patient monitoring.

(g) Epirubicin

A study in 21 patients with breast cancer given intravenous **epirubicin** 90 mg/m^2 followed by paclitaxel 175 mg/m^2 as a 3-h infusion found that non-haematological toxicity was similar to that observed in 18 similar patients who were given the drugs in the reverse order. However, a lower neutrophil and platelet nadir and slower neutrophil recovery was observed when paclitaxel was given first. The AUC for **epirubicin** was also higher in this group but paclitaxel pharmacokinetics were similar in both groups. The importance of administering anthracyclines such as epirubicin before paclitaxel was noted.[14]

(h) Gemcitabine

A study in 9 patients with non-small-cell lung cancer found that when given 150 to 200 mg/m^2 paclitaxel on day 1 and 1000 mg/m^2 **gemcitabine** on days 1 and 8, the **gemcitabine** serum levels and the AUC of the deaminated metabolite of **gemcitabine** were unchanged.[15]

(i) Methotrexate

An *in vitro* study on human bladder cancer cells found the cytotoxic effect of paclitaxel in combination with **methotrexate** was dependent on the treatment sequence.[16]

1. Van den Brande J, Nannan Panday VR, Hoekman K, Rosing H, Huijskes RVHP, Verheijen RHM, Beijnen JH, Vermorken JB. Pharmacologic study of paclitaxel administered with or without the cytoprotective agent amifostine, and given as a single agent or in combination with epirubicin and cisplatin in patients with advanced solid tumours. *Am J Clin Oncol* (2001) 24, 401–3.
2. Gelmon K, Eisenhauer E, Bryce C, Tolcher A, Mayer L, Tomlinson E, Zee B, Blackstein M, Tomiak E, Yau J, Batist G, Fisher B, Iglesias J. Randomized phase II study of high-dose paclitaxel with or without amifostine in patients with metastatic breast cancer. *J Clin Oncol* (1999) 17, 3038–47.
3. Schüller J, Czejka M, Pietrzak C, Springer B, Wirth M, Schernthaner G. Influence of the cytoprotective agent amifostine (AMI) on pharmacokinetics (PK) of paclitaxel (PAC) and Taxotere® (TXT). *Proc Am Soc Clin Oncol* (1997) 16, 224a.
4. Jamis-Dow CA, Klecker RW, Katki AG, Collins JM. Metabolism of taxol by humans and rat liver in vitro: a screen for drug interactions and interspecies differences. *Cancer Chemother Pharmacol* (1995) 36, 107–14.
5. Taxol (Paclitaxel). Bristol-Myers Squibb Pharmaceuticals Ltd. Summary of product characteristics, February 2001.
6. Meerum Terwogt JM, Beijnen JH, ten Bokkel Huinink WW, Rosing H, Schellens JHM. Co-administration of cyclosporin enables oral therapy with paclitaxel. *Lancet* (1998) 352, 285.
7. Rischin D, Webster LK, Millward MJ, Linahan BM, Toner GC, Woollett AM, Morton CG, Bishop JF. Cremophor pharmacokinetics in patients receiving 3-, 6-, and 24-hour infusions of paclitaxel. *J Natl Cancer Inst* (1996) 88, 1297–1301.
8. Kennedy MJ, Zahurak ML, Donehower RC, Noe DA, Sartorius S, Chen T-L, Bowling K, Rowinsky EK. Phase I and pharmacologic study of sequences of paclitaxel and cyclophosphamide supported by granulocyte colony-stimulating factor in women with previously treated metastatic breast cancer. *J Clin Oncol* (1996) 14, 783–91.
9. Gianni L, Viganò L, Locatelli A, Capri G, Giani A, Tarenzi E, Bonadonna G. Human pharmacokinetic characterization and in vitro study of the interaction between doxorubicin and paclitaxel in patients with breast cancer. *J Clin Oncol* (1997) 15, 1906–15.
10. Holmes FA, Madden T, Newman RA, Valero V, Theriault RL, Fraschini G, Walters RS, Booser DJ, Buzdar AU, Willey J, Hortobagyi GN. Sequence-dependent alteration of doxorubicin pharmacokinetics by paclitaxel in a phase I study of paclitaxel and doxorubicin in patients with metastatic breast cancer. *J Clin Oncol* (1996) 14, 2713–21.
11. Sledge GW, Robert N, Sparano JA, Cogleigh M, Goldstein LJ, Neuberg D, Rowinsky E, Baughman L, McCaskill-Stevens W. Eastern Cooperative Oncology Group studies of paclitaxel and doxorubicin in advanced breast cancer. *Semin Oncol* (1995) 22, 105–8.
12. Baker SD. Drug interactions with taxanes. *Pharmacother* (1997) 17 (Suppl), 126S–132S.
13. Colombo T, Parisi I, Zucchetti M, Sessa C, Goldhirsch A, D'Incalci M. Pharmacokinetic interactions of paclitaxel, docetaxel and their vehicles with doxorubicin. *Ann Oncol* (1999) 10, 391–5.
14. Venturini M, Lunardi G, Del Mastro L, Vannozzi MO, Tolino G, Numico G, Viale M, Pastrone I, Angiolini C, Bertelli G, Straneo M, Rosso R, Esposito M. Sequence effect of epirubicin and paclitaxel treatment on pharmacokinetics and toxicity. *J Clin Oncol* (2000) 18, 2116–25.
15. Kroep JR, Voorn DA, van Moorsel CJA, Giaccone G, Postmust PE, Rosing H, Beijnen JH, Gall H, Smit EF, Van Groeningen CJ, Pinedo HM, Peters GJ. Pharmacokinetic interactions between paclitaxel (Tax) and gemcitabine (Gem) in patients (pts) with non-small-cell lung cancer (NSCLC). *Proc Am Assoc Cancer Res* (1998) 39, 188.
16. Cos J, Bellmunt J, Soler C, Ribas A, Lluis JM, Murio JE, Margarit C. Comparative study of sequential combinations of paclitaxel and methotrexate on a human bladder cancer cell line. *Cancer Invest* (2000) 18, 429–35.

Procarbazine + Anticonvulsants

Anticonvulsant usage seems to increase the risk of procarbazine hypersensitivity reactions.

Clinical evidence, mechanism, importance and management

A study of the records of 83 patients with primary brain tumours who were treated with procarbazine between 1981 and 1996 showed that 20 of them had procarbazine hypersensitivity reactions. There was a significant dose-response association between the development of hypersensitivity reactions and the serum levels of the anticonvulsants used (**phenytoin, phenobarbital, carbamazepine, valproate**).[1]

1. Lehmann DF, Hurteau TE, Newman N, Coyle TE. Anticonvulsant usage is associated with an increased risk of procarbazine hypersensitivity reactions in patients with brain tumours. *Clin Pharmacol Ther* (1997) 62, 225–9.

Procarbazine + Chlormethine (Mustine)

A report on two patients suggests that the concurrent use of high doses of procarbazine with chlormethine (mustine) may result in neurological toxicity.

Clinical evidence, mechanism, importance and management

Two patients with acute myelogenous leukaemia admitted to hospital for marrow transplantation and who were given high doses of procarbazine (12.5 and 15 mg/kg) and **chlormethine (mustine)** (0.75 and 1.0 mg/kg) on the same day became lethargic, somnolent and disorientated for about a week. Although no interaction has been proved, the authors suggest that the **chlormethine** may have enhanced the neurotoxic effects of the procarbazine, and advise that it would be prudent to avoid high-dose administration of these drugs on the same day.[1]

1. Weiss GB, Weiden PL, Thomas ED. Central nervous system disturbances after combined administration of procarbazine and mechlorethamine. *Cancer Treat Rep* (1977) 61, 1713–14.

Procarbazine + Miscellaneous drugs

The effects of drugs which can cause CNS depression or lower blood pressure may possibly be increased by the presence of procarbazine.

Clinical evidence, mechanisms, importance and management

Procarbazine can cause CNS depression ranging from mild drowsiness to profound stupor. The incidence is variously reported as being 31%, 14% and 8%.[1-3] Additive CNS depression may therefore be expected if other **drugs possessing CNS-depressant activity** are given concurrently.

Elsewhere a patient with hypertension and Hodgkin's disease has been reported whose blood pressure returned to normal when treated with procarbazine.[4] Additive hypotensive effects may therefore be seen with the concurrent use of **antihypertensive drugs**.

An isolated report describes an acute dystonic reaction (difficulty in speaking or moving, intermittent contractions of muscles on the left side of the neck) in a patient on procarbazine when given **prochlorperazine**.[5]

1. Brunner KW, Young CW. A methylhydrazine derivative in Hodgkin's disease and other malignant neoplasms: therapeutic and toxic effects studied in 51 patients. *Ann Intern Med* (1965) 63, 69–86.
2. Stolinsky DC, Solomon J, Pugh RP, Stevens AR, Jacobs EM, Irwin LE, Wood DA, Steinfeld JL, Bateman JR. Clinical experience with procarbazine in Hodgkin's disease, reticulum cell sarcoma, and lymphosarcoma. *Cancer* (1970) 26, 984–90.
3. Samuels ML, Leary WV, Alexanian R, Howe CD, Frei E. Clinical trials with N-isopropyl-α-(2-methylhydrazino)-p-toluamide hydrochloride in malignant lymphoma and other disseminated neoplasia. *Cancer* (1967) 20, 1187–94.
4. De Vita VT, Hahn MA, Oliverio VT. Monoamine oxidase inhibition by a new carcinostatic agent, N-isopropyl-α-(2-methylhydrazino)-p-toluamide (MIH). *Proc Soc Exp Biol Med* (1965) 120, 561–5.
5. Poster DS. Procarbazine-prochlorperazine interaction: an underreported phenomenon. *J Med* (1978) 9, 519–24.

Procarbazine + Tyramine-containing foods and Sympathomimetic amines

Despite warnings, it seems doubtful if the weak MAO-inhibitory properties of procarbazine can normally cause a hypertensive reaction with tyramine or other sympathomimetic amines.

Clinical evidence, mechanism, importance and management

The makers say that procarbazine ". . . is a weak MAO inhibitor and therefore interactions with certain foodstuffs and drugs, although very rare, must be borne in mind." This is apparently based on the results of *animal* experiments which show that the monoamine oxidase inhibitory properties of procarbazine are weaker than pheniprazine.[1] There seem to be no formal reports of hypertensive reactions in patients on procarbazine who have eaten **tyramine-containing foods** (e.g. cheese) or after using **indirectly-acting sympathomimetic amines** (e.g. **phenylpropanolamine**, **amphetamines**, etc.). The only account traced is purely anecdotal and unconfirmed: ". . . I recall one patient who described vividly reactions to wine and chicken livers which had occurred while he was taking MOPP chemotherapy several years earlier. Since he had not been forewarned, the reactions had been a frightening experience."[2] A practical way to deal with this interaction problem has been suggested by a practitioner in an Oncology unit:[2] patients on procarbazine should ideally be given a list of the potentially interacting foodstuffs (see 'Monoamine oxidase inhibitors (MAOIs) + Tyramine-rich foods', p.685), with a warning about the nature of the possible reaction but also with the advice that it very rarely occurs. The **foods** may continue to be eaten, but patients should start with small quantities to ensure that they still agree with them. Those taking MOPP should also be told that any reaction is most likely to occur during the second week while on a 14-day course of treatment with procarbazine, and during the week following when not taking it.

1. De Vita VT, Hahn MA, Oliverio VT. Monoamine oxidase inhibition by a new carcinostatic agent. N-isopropyl-α-(2-methylhydrazino)-p-toluamide (MIH). *Proc Soc Exp Biol Med* (1965) 120, 561–5.

2. Maxwell MB. Reexamining the dietary restrictions with procarbazine (an MAOI). *Cancer Nursing* (1980) 3, 451–7.

Raltitrexed + Miscellaneous drugs

On theoretical grounds the manufacturers say that folinic acid and folic acid may possibly interfere with the action of raltitrexed.

Clinical evidence, mechanism, importance and management

(a) Folinic acid, Folic acid

The antimetabolite, raltitrexed, is a folate analogue and is a potent and specific inhibitor of the enzyme thymidylate synthase. Inhibition of this enzyme ultimately interferes with the synthesis of deoxyribonucleic acid (DNA) leading to cell death. The intracellular polyglutamation of raltitrexed leads to the formation within cells of even more potent inhibitors of thymidylate synthase. **Folate** (methylene tetrahydrofolate) is a co-factor required by thymidylate synthase and therefore theoretically **folinic acid** or **folic acid** may interfere with the action of raltitrexed. Clinical interaction studies have not yet been undertaken to confirm these predicted interactions.[1]

(b) Warfarin, NSAIDs

The makers say that no specific clinical interaction studies have been conducted but a review of the clinical trial database did not reveal any evidence of interactions between raltitrexed and **warfarin**, **NSAIDs** or other drugs.[1]

1. Tomudex (Raltitrexed). AstraZeneca. Summary of product characteristics, October 2001.

Streptozocin + Phenytoin

A single case report indicates that phenytoin can reduce or abolish the cytotoxic effects of streptozocin.

Clinical evidence, mechanism, importance and management

A patient with an organic hypoglycaemic syndrome, due to a metastatic apud cell carcinoma of the pancreas, and who was treated with 2 g streptozocin daily together with 400 mg **phenytoin** daily for 4 days, failed to show the expected response until the **phenytoin** was withdrawn.[1] It would seem that the **phenytoin** protected the beta-cells of the pancreas from the cytotoxic effects of the streptozocin by some mechanism as yet unknown. Although this is an isolated case report its authors recommend that concurrent use should be avoided.

1. Koranyi L, Gero L. Influence of diphenylhydantoin on the effect of streptozotocin. *BMJ* (1979) 1, 127.

Tamoxifen + Aminoglutethimide

Aminoglutethimide markedly increases the loss of tamoxifen from the body and reduces its serum levels.

Clinical evidence, mechanism, importance and management

When given 250 mg **aminoglutethimide** four times daily for 6 weeks the serum levels of tamoxifen (20 to 80 mg daily) and most of its metabolites were markedly reduced in six menopausal women with breast cancer. The clearance of the tamoxifen was increased 222% (from 189 to 608 ml/min) and the tamoxifen AUC was reduced by 73% (range 56 to 80%).[1] The probable reason is that **aminoglutethimide** is an enzyme inducing agent which increases the metabolism of the tamoxifen by the liver, thereby increasing its loss from the body. Tamoxifen appears not to affect the pharmacokinetics of **aminoglutethimide**.[1]

The authors of this report say that their findings may explain why combined use appears to be no more effective than tamoxifen on its own. They suggest that serum tamoxifen levels should be monitored and the dosage raised if necessary to compensate for this interaction. More study is needed.

1. Lien EA, Anker G, Lønning PE, Solheim E, Ueland PM. Decreased serum concentrations of tamoxifen and its metabolites induced by aminoglutethimide. *Cancer Res* (1990) 50, 5851–7.

Tamoxifen + Herbal medicines

Indirect evidence hints at the possibility that some herbal medicines which possess oestrogenic activity may oppose the actions of competitive oestrogen receptor antagonists such as tamoxifen used in the treatment of breast cancer.

Clinical evidence, mechanism, importance and management

A letter in the Medical Journal of Australia[1] draws attention to fact that some women with breast cancer on chemotherapy or hormonal replacement therapy and who develop menopausal symptoms have found relief from hot flushes by taking a Chinese herb '**dong quai**' (or '**danggui**' root) which has been identified as *Angelica sinensis*. A possible explanation is that this and some other herbs (**vitex berry** (*Agnus castur*), **hops flower** (**lupulus**), **ginseng root**, **black cohosh** (**cimicifuga**)) have significant oestrogen binding activity and physiological oestrogenic actions.[2] The concern expressed in the letter is that the oestrogenic activity of these herbs might directly stimulate breast cancer growth and oppose the actions of competitive oestrogen receptor antagonists such as **tamoxifen**.

Although this is largely speculative at the moment, the writer of the letter suggests that such **herbal medicines** are undesirable in patients with breast cancer. In addition to tamoxifen, there are now a number of other drugs used for breast cancer which in one way or another reduce the stimulation of oestrogen receptors. More study is needed.

1. Boyle FM. Adverse interaction of herbal medicine with breast cancer treatment. *Med J Aust* (1997) 167, 286.
2. Eagon CL, Elm MS, Teepe AG, Eagon PK. Medicinal botanicals: estrogenicity in rat uterus and liver. *Proc Am Assoc Cancer Res* (1997) 38, 293.

Tamoxifen + HRT (Hormone Replacement Therapy)

HRT is reported to oppose the blood lipid lowering effects of tamoxifen.

Clinical evidence, mechanism, importance and management

A large scale comparative study was undertaken over a 12 month period in groups of women taking tamoxifen alone, **HRT** alone, or tamoxifen plus transdermal **HRT** to see whether the cardiovascular risk factors (low-density lipoprotein cholesterol, high-density lipoprotein-cholesterol levels, platelet counts) were changed by concurrent use. It was found that the decrease in total and LDL-cholesterol levels due to the tamoxifen was unchanged in current HRT users but reduced by two-thirds in women on tamoxifen who then started **HRT**.[1] It would therefore seem important to check the outcome of concurrent use. More study is needed. This report only addressed the beneficial effects of tamoxifen on lipid profiles, and not its anti-oestrogenic effects.

1. Decensi A, Robertson C, Rotmensz N, Severi G, Maisonneuve P, Sacchini V, Boyle P, Costa A, Veronesi U. Effect of tamoxifen and transdermal hormone replacement therapy on cardiovascular risk factors in a prevention trial. *Br J Cancer* (1998) 78, 572–8.

Tamoxifen + Medroxyprogesterone acetate

Medroxyprogesterone affects the metabolism of tamoxifen but the clinical importance of this is uncertain.

Clinical evidence, mechanism, importance and management

The addition of 500 mg **medroxyprogesterone acetate** twice daily only slightly reduced the tamoxifen serum levels over a 6 month period in 20 women with breast cancer given 20 mg tamoxifen twice daily, but considerably reduced the levels of the desmethyl metabolite of tamoxifen, presumably because of some effect on the metabolism of the tamoxifen by the liver.[1] The clinical importance of this interaction awaits assessment.

1. Reid AD, Horobin JM, Newman EL, Preece PE. Tamoxifen metabolism is altered by simultaneous administration of medroxyprogesterone acetate in breast cancer patients. *Breast Cancer Res Treat* (1992) 22, 153–6.

Tegafur + Sorivudine

Marked and rapidly fatal toxicity has been seen in patients given tegafur (or other fluorouracil prodrugs) and sorivudine, attributed to fluorouracil toxicity. Fluorouracil is expected to interact similarly.

Clinical evidence

The Japanese Ministry of Health reported in 1993 the deaths of 15 Japanese patients with cancer and a viral disease who died several days after being given **tegafur** (or other **fluorouracil** prodrugs) and **sorivudine**. Before death most of them developed severe toxicity including severe anorexia, marked damage to the bone marrow with decreases in white cell and platelet counts, and marked atrophy of the intestinal membrane with diarrhoea and loss of blood. Eight other patients given both drugs developed symptoms of severe toxicity.[1] Some of these details are also discussed in a Japanese journal.[2]

Mechanism

The reason for the marked toxicity (based on studies in *rats*[3]) appears to be that the **sorivudine** is converted in the gut into a metabolite (BVU or (E)-5-(2-bromovinyl)uracil) which after absorption passes to the liver where it irreversibly inhibits a liver enzyme (dihydropyrimidine dehydrogenase). This enzyme is concerned with the metabolism of the **fluorouracil** (derived from the **tegafur**) so that when it is inhibited, the metabolism and clearance of the **fluorouracil** are reduced. The consequence is that serum **fluorouracil** levels rise accompanied by toxicity. In effect these patients died from **fluorouracil** overdosage.

Importance and management

Information appears to be limited to these reports but the interaction appears to be established and of clinical importance. The concurrent use of oral **tegafur** and **sorivudine** should be strictly avoided. It is not clear whether **tegafur** given by a non-oral route would be safe.

Assuming that the mechanism of interaction has been correctly identified, it would seem equally important to avoid **sorivudine** and **fluorouracil** or **any of its prodrugs**. More study is needed to confirm this precaution.

1. Pharmaceutical Affairs Bureau, Japanese Ministry of Health and Welfare: A report on investigation of side effects of sorivudine: deaths caused by interactions between sorivudine and 5-FU prodrugs (in Japanese), June 1994, cited in ref 2.
2. Watabe T, Okuda H, Ogura K. Lethal drug interactions of the new antiviral, soruvudine, with anticancer prodrugs of 5-fluorouracil. *Yakugaku Zasshi* (1997) 117, 910–21. (In Japanese).
3. Okuda H, Nishiyama T, Ogura Y, Nagayama S, Ikeda K, Yamaguchi S, Nakamura Y, Kawaguchi K, Watabe T. Lethal drug interactions of sorivudine, a new antiviral drug, with oral 5-fluorouracil prodrugs. *Drug Metab Dispos* (1997) 25, 270–3.

Teniposide + Anticonvulsants

Carbamazepine, phenytoin and phenobarbital markedly increase the clearance of teniposide. A reduction in its cytotoxic effects may occur.

Clinical evidence, mechanism, importance and management

The clearance of teniposide was increased two to threefold (from 13 to 32 ml/min/m^2) in 6 children with acute lymphocytic leukaemia while taking **phenytoin** or **phenobarbital** concurrently.[1,2] Another patient showed a twofold increase in teniposide clearance when treated with **carbamazepine**.[2] The most probable reason is that these anticonvulsants are potent liver enzyme inducing agents which increase the metabolism of teniposide by the liver, thereby increasing its loss from the body. A previous study found that the oncolytic response to teniposide was reduced in those showing an increased teniposide clearance.[1] The authors of these two reports therefore conclude that increased dosages of teniposide will be needed in the presence of these anticonvulsants to achieve a systemic exposure to the drug comparable to that in their absence. More study is needed.

1. Baker DK, Rodman JH, Pui CH, Rivera GK, Evans WE. Anticonvulsants increase clearance of teniposide. *Clin Pharmacol Ther* (1991) 49,195.
2. Baker DK, Relling MV, Pui C-H, Christensen ML, Evans WE, Rodman JH. Increased teniposide clearance with concomitant anticonvulsant therapy. *J Clin Oncol* (1992) 10, 311–5.

Topotecan + Phenytoin

A 5-year-old child with medulloblastoma received a course of topotecan, firstly with phenytoin and then without. Phenytoin increased the total topotecan clearance by 47%.[1] This suggests that an increased topotecan dosage may possibly be needed in the presence of phenytoin in other patients.

1. Zamboni WC, Gajjar AJ, Heideman RL, Beijnen JH, Rosing H, Houghton PJ, Stewart CF. Phenytoin alters the disposition of topotecan and N-desmethyl topotecan in a patient with medulloblastoma. *Clin Cancer Res* (1998) 4, 783–9.

Toremifene + Miscellaneous drugs

Carbamazepine, phenobarbital and possibly phenytoin can reduce the serum levels of toremifene. Rifampicin and other inducers of cytochrome P450 isoenzyme CYP3A4 may also reduce the efficacy of toremifene. There are no other reports of confirmed adverse interactions with toremifene, but the makers advise care with erythromycin, ketoconazole, thiazides and troleandomycin, and the avoidance of warfarin-type anticoagulants. These latter warnings are based on theoretical considerations.

Clinical evidence, mechanism, importance and management

A pharmacokinetic study of toremifene in two groups of 10 patients, one being a control group and the other taking anticonvulsants, found that the AUC of toremifene 120 mg and its half-life in the anticonvulsant group was approximately halved. The anticonvulsants used were **carbamazepine** alone (3 patients) or with **clonazepam** (3 patients), or **phenobarbital** alone (3 patients) or with **phenytoin** (1 patient). The reason for this interaction is thought to be that these anticonvulsants induce the liver enzymes (almost certainly cytochrome P450 isoenzyme CYP3A4) so that the toremifene is metabolised and cleared from the body more quickly.[1] The makers of toremifene have therefore reasonably suggested that the toremifene dosage may need to be doubled in the presence of these anticonvulsants.[2,3] A study in 9 healthy subjects found that **rifampicin** 600 mg daily reduced the AUC, peak plasma levels and half-life of toremifene 120 mg by 87%, 55% and 44% respectively. Concomitant use of **rifampicin** or other potent CYP3A4 enzyme inducers may reduce the efficacy of toremifene.[4]

In their summary of product characteristics the makers of toremifene have made a number of recommendations as follows:

The metabolism of toremifene by the liver is mediated mainly by the cytochrome P450 isoenzymes CYP3A4 and CYP3A5 so it is suggested that drugs which can inhibit these enzymes (such as **erythromycin, troleandomycin, ketoconazole**) may possibly increase its effects.[2] Hypercalcaemia is a recognised side-effect of toremifene, and it is suggested that drugs such as the **thiazides** which decrease renal calcium excretion may increase the risk of hypercalcaemia. There is also a warning about the possibility of increased bleeding if toremifene is given with **warfarin**-type anticoagulants because it is known that other related drugs (e.g. tamoxifen) have shown this interaction, however there is no direct clinical evidence that an interaction occurs.[2,3] All of these warnings are based on indirect evidence and theoretical considerations so that their clinical importance awaits confirmation.

1. Anttila M, Laakso S, Nyländen P, Sotaniemi EA. Pharmacokinetics of the novel antiestrogenic agent toremifene in subjects with altered liver and kidney function. *Clin Pharmacol Ther* (1995) 57, 628–35.
2. Fareston (Toremifene). Orion Corporation. Summary of product characteristics, October 1996.
3. Orion Pharma UK Ltd. Personal communication, August 1996.
4. Kivistö KT, Villikka K, Nyman L, Anttila M, Neuvonen PJ. Tamoxifen and toremifene concentrations in plasma are greatly decreased by rifampin. *Clin Pharmacol Ther* (1998) 64, 648–54.

Vinblastine + Bleomycin + Cisplatin

This drug combination appears to cause serious life-threatening cardiovascular toxicity.

Clinical evidence, mechanism, importance and management

Five patients (aged 23 to 58) under treatment for germ cell tumours died from acute life-threatening vascular events (myocardial infarction, rectal infarction, cerebrovascular accident) following **VBP** therapy (**vinblastine, bleomycin, cisplatin**). A survey of the literature by the authors of this paper revealed 14 other cases of both acute and long-term cardiovascular problems (myocardial infarction, coronary heart disease, cerebrovascular accident) in patients given **VBP** therapy.[1] Raynaud's phenomenon is common (37%) in those treated with **vinblastine** and **bleomycin** or **VBP** and there is evidence that blood vessels are pathologically altered.[2] This drug combination is very effective in the treatment of testicular carcinoma but its potential toxicity is clearly very serious.[1,2]

1. Samuels BL, Vogelzang NJ, Kennedy BJ. Severe vascular toxicity associated with vinblastine, bleomycin and cisplatin chemotherapy. *Cancer Chemother Pharmacol* (1987) 19, 253–6.
2. Vogelzang NJ, Bosl GJ, Johnson K, Kennedy BJ. Raynaud's phenomenon: a common toxicity after combination chemotherapy for testicular cancer. *Ann Intern Med* (1981) 95, 288–92.

Vinblastine + Erythromycin or Ciclosporin

Erythromycin increased the toxicity of vinblastine in three patients. Ciclosporin appears not to interact with vinblastine.

Clinical evidence

Three patients with renal cell carcinoma given **erythromycin** and **ciclosporin** for 72 h to reverse multidrug resistance developed severe toxicity when treated with 9 mg/m^2 vinblastine on the third day. To rule out increased **ciclosporin** toxicity, two of them were given **erythromycin** but no **ciclosporin**. They developed vinblastine toxicity (severe neutropenia, constipation, myositis, severe myalgia) typical of much higher doses of vinblastine. Only negligible toxicity developed when they were later given vinblastine alone, and it was reported that one of the patients had twice had **ciclosporin** and vinblastine previously without problems.[1,2]

Mechanism

Uncertain, but an *in vitro* study using human liver microsomes found that erythromycin inhibits the activity of cytochrome P450 isoenzyme CYP3A4 which is also concerned with the metabolism of vinblastine.[3] This would be expected to reduce the metabolism of vinblastine resulting in an increase in its toxicity.

Importance and management

Information seems to be limited to these studies, but the interaction would appear to be established. On the basis of their findings the authors of the report cited suggest that erythromycin should be avoided at the time of vinblastine infusion and for 48 h thereafter.[1,2]

1. Tobe SW, Siu LL, Jamal SA, Skorecki KL, Warner E. Vinblastine and erythromycin: an unrecognized serious drug interaction. *Clin Invest Med* (1993) 16, (4 Suppl), B93.
2. Tobe SW, Siu LL, Jamal SA, Skorecki KL, Murphy GF, Warner E. Vinblastine and erythromycin: an unrecognized serious drug interaction. *Cancer Chemother Pharmacol* (1995) 35, 188–190.
3. Zhour-Pan X-R, Sérée E, Zhou X-J, Placidi M, Maurel P, Barra Y, Rahmani R. Involvement of human liver cytochrome P450 3A in vinblastine metabolism: drug interactions. *Cancer Res* (1993) 53, 5121–6.

Vinca Alkaloids + Mitomycin

Vinblastine and vindesine can increase the pulmonary toxicity of mitomycin. Severe and life-threatening bronchospasm and two cases of fatal acute respiratory failure have been described.

Clinical evidence, mechanism, importance and management

There are now several reports describing an increase in lung disease in patients treated with **mitomycin** and vinca alkaloids. Diffuse lung damage characterised by interstitial infiltrates and pleural effusions resulting in respiratory distress and cough have been described after treatment with **vinblastine**.[1-4] The incidence is reported to be 3 to 6%.[5] Fatal acute respiratory failure due to pulmonary oedema has been reported in 2 patients with non-small cell lung cancer treated with **vinblastine** and **mitomycin**.[6] Severe and life-threatening bronchospasm has also been described when **vindesine sulphate** was given after treatment with **mitomycin**.[4] Acute dyspnoea occurred in 3 patients receiving **mitomycin** in combination with either **vindesine** (2 patients) or **vinblastine** (1 patient) within 1 to 5 h of treatment with the vinca alkaloid.[7] The potential hazards of combining these drugs should be recognised. In view of the unpredictability of the reaction, close observation of patients receiving this combination is recommended.[6]

1. Konits PH, Aisner J, Sutherland JC, Wiernik PH. Possible pulmonary toxicity secondary to vinblastine. *Cancer* (1982) 50, 2771–4.
2. Gunstream SR, Seidenfeld JJ, Sobonya RE, McMahon LJ. Mitomycin-associated lung disease. *Cancer Treat Rep* (1983) 67, 301–4.
3. Ozols RF, Hogan WM, Ostchega T, Young RC. MVP (mitomycin, vinblastine, progesterone): a second-line regimen in ovarian cancer with a high incidence of pulmonary toxicity. *Cancer Treat Rep* (1983) 67, 721–2.
4. Dyke RW. Acute bronchospasm after a vinca alkaloid in patients previously treated with mitomycin. *N Engl J Med* (1984) 310, 389.
5. Hoelzer KL, Harrison BR, Luedke SW, Luedke DW. Vinblastine-associated pulmonary toxicity in patients receiving combination therapy with mitomycin and cisplatin. *Drug Intell Clin Pharm* (1986) 20, 287–9.
6. Rao SX, Ramaswamy G, Levin M, McCravey JW. Fatal acute respiratory failure after vinblastine-mitomycin therapy in lung carcinoma. *Arch Intern Med* (1985) 145, 1905–7.
7. Kris MG, Pablo D, Gralla J, Burke MT, Prestifillippo J, Lewin D. Dyspnea following vinblastine or vindesine administration in patients receiving mitomycin plus vinca alkaloid combination therapy. *Cancer Treat Rep* (1984) 68, 1029–31.

Vincristine + Colaspase

Some very limited evidence suggests that vincristine neurotoxicity may possibly be increased by colaspase (asparaginase).[1] A definite link between the use of these drugs and this serious toxicity has not been established, but the evidence suggests that particular care should be exercised if given concurrently.

1. Hildebrand J, Kenis Y. Vincristine neurotoxicity. *N Engl J Med* (1972) 287, 517.

Vincristine + Isoniazid

Some limited evidence suggests that vincristine neurotoxicity may possibly be increased by the concurrent use of isoniazid.

Clinical evidence, mechanism, importance and management

A woman of 85 with Hodgkin's disease was given COPP/ABVD, alternating every 28 days. She started COPP (cyclophosphamide and 2 mg vincristine on day 1, procarbazine and prednisone days 1 to 14) and was additionally given 300 mg **isoniazid** daily as prophylaxis. Five days after the start of this treatment she experienced tingling in her fingers and weakness in her legs which was interpreted by the authors of this report as being vincristine toxicity brought about by the concurrent use of **isoniazid** (paraesthesia of the feet and/or hands being a recognised early manifestation of vincristine toxicity). Their reasoning was that such a small dosage of vincristine dosage on its own was unlikely to cause severe neurotoxicity of this kind, but it is not clear just why **isoniazid** should apparently interact like this. The authors suggest that the age of this patient and her diabetes (well controlled) may have contributed to this increase in vincristine neurotoxicity.[1]

This report is consistent with another much earlier report of two patients who also developed peripheral neurotoxicity when treated with vincristine after the addition of **isoniazid** and **pyridoxine**, the cumulative doses of vincristine being 11 and 11.2 mg respectively.[2,3]

These reports appear to be the only ones implicating **isoniazid** in an increase in vincristine toxicity, but they serve to emphasise the importance of very close neurological supervision in anyone given both drugs.

1. Carrión C, Espinosa E, Herrero A, García B. Possible vincristine-isoniazid interaction. *Ann Pharmacother* (1995) 29, 201.
2. Hildebrand J, Kenis Y. Vincristine neurotoxicity. *N Engl J Med* (1972) 287, 517.
3. Hildebrand J, Kenis Y. Additive toxicity of vincristine and other drugs for the peripheral nervous system. *Acta Neurol Belg* (1971) 71, 486–91.

14

Digitalis glycoside drug interactions

Plant extracts containing cardiac glycosides have been in use for thousands of years. The ancient Egyptians were familiar with squill, as were the Romans who used it as a heart tonic and diuretic. The foxglove was mentioned in the writings of Welsh physicians in the thirteenth century and features in 'An Account of the Foxglove and some of its Medical Uses', published by William Withering in 1785, in which he described its application in the treatment of 'dropsy' or the oedema which results from heart failure.

The most commonly used cardiac glycosides are those obtained from the members of the foxglove family, *Digitalis purpurea* and *Digitalis lanata*. The leaves of these two plants are the source of a number of purified glycosides (digoxin, digitoxin, gitoxin, lanatoside C and others), of gitalin (an amorphous mixture largely composed of digitoxin and digoxin), and of powdered whole leaf digitalis. Occasionally ouabain or strophanthin (also of plant origin) are used for particular situations, while for a number of years the Russians have exploited cardiac glycosides from lily of the valley. Bufalin is a cardioactive compound obtained from toads and is found in a number of Chinese medicines. All of these cardiac glycosides have similar actions, but they differ in their potency and in their rates of elimination from the body, and this determines how much is given and how often. Table 14.1 lists many of the cardiac glycosides in use.

Digitalisation

The cardiac glycosides have two main actions and two main applications. They reduce conductivity within the atrioventricular (AV) node, hence are used for treating supraventricular tachycardias (especially atrial fibrillation), and they have a positive inotropic effect (i.e. increase the force of contraction), hence are used for congestive heart failure, although to a much lesser extent these days.

Because the most commonly used glycosides are derived from digitalis, the achievement of the desired therapeutic serum concentration of any cardiac glycoside is usually referred to as 'digitalisation'. Treatment may be started with a large 'loading dose' so that the therapeutic concentrations are achieved reasonably quickly, but once these have been reached the amount is reduced to a maintenance dose which is intended to keep a nice balance between drug intake and drug loss. This has to be done carefully because there is a relatively narrow gap between therapeutic and toxic serum concentrations. Normal therapeutic levels are about one-third of those that are fatal, and serious toxic arrhythmias begin at about two-thirds of the fatal levels. If a patient is over-digitalised, signs of intoxication will occur: firstly loss of appetite, followed by nausea and vomiting. Visual disturbances may also be experienced, headache, drowsiness, occasionally diarrhoea, and bradycardia. Death can take place from cardiac arrhythmias which are associated with total AV block. Patients under treatment for cardiac arrhythmias can therefore demonstrate arrhythmias when they are both under- as well as over-digitalised, which may complicate the decision to increase or reduce the dosage.

Interactions of the cardiac glycosides

The pharmacological actions of these glycosides are very similar, but their rates and degree of absorption, metabolism and clearance are different and this determines the dosages used. For example, the half-life of digoxin is 30 to 40 hours compared with 4 to 6 days for digitoxin, and this is reflected in their maintenance doses of 62.5 to 500 micrograms daily and 100 micrograms daily or on alternate days, respectively. It is therefore most important not to extrapolate an interaction seen with one glycoside and apply it uncritically to any other. Because the therapeutic ratio of the cardiac glycosides is low, a quite small change in serum levels may lead to inadequate digitalisation or to toxicity. For this reason interactions that have a relatively modest effect on serum levels may sometimes have serious consequences.

Table 14.1 Cardiac glycosides

Generic names	Proprietary names
Acetyldigitoxin	
Acetyldigoxin	*Cardioreg, Corotal, Digostada, Digotab, Digox, Digoxin "Didier", Gladixol N, Lanatilin, Novodigal, Stillacor*
Convallaria	*Convacard, Valdig-N Burger*
Cymarin	
Deslanoside	*Cedilanide, Desacil*
Digitalin	
Digitalis leaf	
Prepared digitalis	
Digitoxin	*Coramedan, Crystodigin, Digimed, Digimerck, Digitaline, Digitrin, Ditaven, Tardigal*
Digoxin	*Digacin, Digosin, Dilanacin, Eudigox, Grexin, Hemigoxine Nativelle, Lanacordin, Lanacrist, Lanicor, Lanoxicaps, Lanoxin, Lenoxin, Mapluxin, Novodigal, Purgoxin, Toloxin*
Gitoformate	
Lanatoside C	
Meproscillarin	
Metildigoxin (Medigoxin)	*Lanirapid, Lanitop, Miopat*
Ouabain (Stophanthin-G)	*Strodival*
Proscillaridin	*Talusin*
Strophanthin-K	*Kombetin*

Digitalis glycosides + ACE inhibitors

No significant interaction has been seen between digoxin and cilazapril, enalapril, imidapril, lisinopril, perindopril, quinapril, ramipril or spirapril. Some studies have found that serum digoxin levels rise by about 20 to 25% if captopril is used, but others have found no significant changes. It has been suggested that any interaction is likely to occur only in those patients who have pre-existing renal impairment. Digitoxin and captopril appear not to interact.

Clinical evidence

(a) Digoxin + Captopril

The serum **digoxin** levels of 20 patients with severe chronic congestive heart failure rose by 21% (from 1.4 to 1.7 nmol/l) while taking **captopril** (averaging 93.7 mg daily). Serum **digoxin** levels were above the therapeutic range (2.6 nmol/l) on 3 out of 63 occasions, but no toxicity was seen. All patients had impaired renal function and were being treated with diuretics.[1,2] Another study found a 30% rise in serum **digoxin** levels in men with congestive heart failure class II when **captopril** was given.[3]

Conversely, another study in 31 patients with stable congestive heart failure, given 25 mg **captopril** three times daily, found no significant changes in serum **digoxin** levels over a 6-month period.[4] Two other studies in healthy subjects[5] and patients with congestive heart failure[6] also found no evidence of an interaction.

(b) Digoxin + Cilazapril, Enalapril, Imidapril, Lisinopril, Perindopril, Quinapril, Ramipril or Spirapril

Cilazapril 5 mg for 14 days did not alter the trough plasma **digoxin** levels in healthy subjects.[7] **Enalapril** 20 mg daily for 30 days had no significant effect on the pharmacokinetics of **digoxin** (250 micrograms daily) in 7 patients with congestive heart failure.[8] **Imidapril** 10 mg daily had no effect on the serum **digoxin** levels of 12 healthy subjects, but slight reductions in imidaprilat levels and in ACE-inhibition (about 15%) were seen, which were of uncertain clinical relevance.[9,10] **Lisinopril** 5 mg daily for 4 weeks had no significant effect on the serum **digoxin** levels of another 9 patients.[11] This confirms the findings of 2 single dose studies.[12,13] **Perindopril** 2 to 4 mg for a month had no effect on the steady-state serum **digoxin** levels of 10 patients with mild chronic heart failure.[14] **Quinapril** is also reported not to alter the steady-state levels of **digoxin** in healthy subjects[15] and patients with congestive heart failure.[16] **Ramipril** 5 mg daily for 14 days had no effect on the serum **digoxin** levels of 12 healthy subjects.[17] **Spirapril** 12 to 48 mg daily did not significantly affect the pharmacokinetics nor the steady-state serum levels of **digoxin** in 15 healthy subjects on **digoxin** 250 micrograms twice daily.[18]

(c) Digitoxin + Captopril

A study in 12 healthy subjects given 70 micrograms **digitoxin** daily for up to 58 days found no evidence that the addition of 25 mg **captopril** daily had a relevant effect on the pharmacokinetics of **digitoxin**, or its effects on the heart.[19]

Mechanism

Not fully understood. It has been suggested that an interaction is only likely to occur in those who have renal impairment. The glomerular filtration rate of these patients may be maintained by the vasoconstrictor action of angiotensin II on the postglomerular blood vessels, which would be impaired by ACE inhibition. As a result some of the loss of digoxin through the tubules is reduced.[5]

Importance and management

The overall picture is that no clinically important adverse interaction occurs between digoxin and ACE inhibitors in patients with normal renal function, and that serum digoxin monitoring is only needed in those who have a high risk of reversible ACE inhibitor induced renal failure (e.g. patients with congestive heart failure during chronic diuretic treatment, with bilateral renal artery stenosis or unilateral renal artery stenosis in a solitary kidney).[5] It seems that in these patients their digoxin levels may rise modestly (20 to 25%). The critical factor seems to be not the particular ACE inhibitor used but the existence of abnormal renal function. This needs confirmation.

No interaction apparently occurs between digitoxin and captopril in healthy subjects, but this needs confirmation in patients.

1. Cleland JGF, Dargie HJ, Hodsman GP, Robertson JIS, Ball SG. Interaction of digoxin and captopril. Br J Clin Pharmacol (1984) 17, 214P.
2. Cleland JGF, Dargie HJ, Pettigrew A, Gillen C, Robertson JIS. The effects of captopril on serum digoxin and urinary urea and digoxin clearances in patients with congestive heart failure. Am Heart J (1986) 112, 130–5.
3. Mazurek W, Haczyński J. Interakcja kaptoprilu i digoksyny. Pol Tyg Lek (1993) 48, 834–5.
4. Magelli C, Bassein L, Ribani MA, Liberatore S, Ambrosioni E, Magnani B. Lack of effect of captopril on serum digoxin in congestive heart failure. Eur J Clin Pharmacol (1989) 36, 99–100.
5. Rossi GP, Semplicini A, Bongiovi S, Mozzato MG, Paleari CD, Pessina AC. Effect of acute captopril administration on digoxin pharmacokinetics in normal subjects. Curr Ther Res (1989) 46, 439–44.
6. Miyakawa T, Shionoiri H, Takasaki I, Kobayashi K, Ishii M. The effect of captopril on pharmacokinetics of digoxin in patients with mild congestive heart failure. J Cardiovasc Pharmacol (1991) 17, 576–80.
7. Kleinbloesem CH, van Brummelen P, Francis RJ, Wiegand U-W. Clinical pharmacology of cilazapril. Drugs (1991) 41 (Suppl 1), 3–10.
8. Douste-Blazy Ph, Blanc M, Montastruc JL, Conte D, Cotonat J, Galinier F. Is there any interaction between digoxin and enalapril? Br J Clin Pharmacol (1986) 22, 752–3.
9. Thürmann PA, Harder S. Pharmacokinetic and pharmacodynamic interaction study with digoxin and the novel ACE-inhibitor imidapril. Eur J Clin Pharmacol (1996) 50, 554.
10. Harder S, Thürmann PA. Pharmacokinetic and pharmacodynamic interaction trial after repeated oral doses of imidapril and digoxin in healthy volunteers. Br J Clin Pharmacol (1997) 43, 475–80.
11. Vandenburg MJ, Kelly JG, Wiseman HT, Mannering D, Long C, Glover DR. The effect of lisinopril on digoxin pharmacokinetics in patients with congestive heart failure. Br J Clin Pharmacol (1988) 21, 656P–657P.
12. Morris FP, Tamrazian S, Marks C, Kelly J, Stephens JD, Vandenburg MJ. An acute pharmacokinetic study of the potential interaction of lisinopril and digoxin in normal volunteers. Br J Clin Pharmacol (1985) 20, 281P–282P.
13. Vandenburg MJ, Morris F, Marks C, Kelly JG, Dews IM, Stephens JD. A study of the potential pharmacokinetic interaction of lisinopril and digoxin in normal volunteers. Xenobiotica (1988) 18, 1179–84.
14. Vandenburg MJ, Stephens JD, Resplandy G, Dews IM, Robinson J, Desche P. Digoxin pharmacokinetics and perindopril in heart failure patients. J Clin Pharmacol (1993) 33, 146–9.
15. Ferry JJ, Sedman AJ, Hengy H, Vollmer KO, Dunkey A, Klotz U, Colburn WA. Concomitant multiple dose quinapril administration does not alter steady-state pharmacokinetics of digoxin. Pharm Res (1987) 4, S98.
16. Kromer EP, Elsner D, Riegger GAJ. Digoxin, converting-enzyme inhibition (quinapril) and the combination in patients with congestive heart failure functional class II and sinus rhythm. J Cardiovasc Pharmacol (1990) 16, 9–14.
17. Doering W, Maass L, Irmisch R and König E. Pharmacokinetic interaction study with ramipril and digoxin in healthy volunteers. Am J Cardiol (1987) 59, 60D–64D.
18. Johnson BF, Wilson J, Johnson J, Flemming J. Digoxin pharmacokinetics and spirapril, a new ACE inhibitor. J Clin Pharmacol (1991) 31, 527–30.
19. de Mey C, Elich D, Schroeter V, Butzer R, Belz GG. Captopril does not interact with the pharmacodynamics and pharmacokinetics of digitoxin in healthy man. Eur J Clin Pharmacol (1992) 43, 445–7.

Digitalis glycosides + Acipimox

Acipimox does not interact with digoxin.

Clinical evidence, mechanism, importance and management

Acipimox 250 mg three times daily for a week was found to have no significant effect on the plasma **digoxin** levels, clinical condition, ECGs, plasma urea or electrolyte levels of 6 elderly patients.[1,2] No special precautions during concurrent use would seem necessary.

1. Chijioke PC, Pearson RM, Johnston A, Blackett A. Effect of acipimox on plasma digoxin levels in elderly patient volunteers. Br J Clin Pharmacol (1987) 25, 102P–103P.
2. Chijioke PC, Pearson RM, Benedetti S. Lack of acipimox-digoxin interaction in patient volunteers. Hum Exp Toxicol (1992) 11, 357–9.

Digitalis glycosides + Allopurinol

Allopurinol has been shown not to affect serum digoxin levels.

Clinical evidence, mechanism, importance and management

No significant changes in the serum **digoxin** levels of 5 healthy subjects occurred over a 7-day period while taking 300 mg **allopurinol** daily.[1] No special precautions would appear to be necessary.

1. Havelund T, Abildtrup N, Birkebaek N, Breddam E, Rosager AM. Allopurinols effekt på koncentrationen af digoksin i serum. *Ugeskr Laeger* (1984) 146, 1209–11.

Digitalis glycosides + Amiloride

Amiloride has little effect on blood digoxin levels in healthy subjects, but it reduces the contractility of the heart. In patients with renal impairment it possibly raises plasma digoxin levels.

Clinical evidence, mechanism, importance and management

Amiloride (5 mg twice daily for 8 days) virtually doubled the renal clearance of **digoxin** (from 1.3 to 2.4 ml/kg/min) in 6 healthy subjects, but almost blocked the extra-renal clearance (reduced from 2.1 to 0.1 ml/kg/min). The balance of the 2 effect was to cause a small fall in total body clearance and a small rise in plasma **digoxin** levels.[1] The positive inotropic effects of **digoxin** were reduced, but whether this is clinically important is uncertain. Studies in patients with congestive heart failure are needed. Patients with poor kidney function would be expected to show a rise in **digoxin** levels but the clinical importance of this also awaits confirmation. The effects of concurrent use should be monitored.

1. Waldorff S, Hansen PB, Kjærgård H, Buch J, Egeblad H, Steiness E. Amiloride-induced changes in digoxin dynamics and kinetics: abolition of digoxin-induced inotropism with amiloride. *Clin Pharmacol Ther* (1981) 30, 172–6.

Digitalis glycosides + Aminoglutethimide

The clearance of digitoxin is markedly increased by the concurrent use of aminoglutethimide and a reduction in its effects would be expected.

Clinical evidence, mechanism, importance and management

The clearance of **digitoxin** was increased by 109% in 5 patients while receiving **aminoglutethimide** 250 mg four times a day.[1] The likely reason is that **aminoglutethimide** increases the metabolism of the **digitoxin** by the liver. This would be expected to be clinically important, but it appears not to have been assessed. Check that patients do not become under-digitalised during concurrent treatment. No interaction would be expected with **digoxin** because it is largely excreted unchanged in the urine and therefore metabolism by the liver has little part to play in its clearance.

1. Lønning PE, Kvinnsland S and Bakke OM. Effect of aminoglutethimide on antipyrine, theophylline and digitoxin disposition in breast cancer. *Clin Pharmacol Ther* (1984) 36, 796–802.

Digitalis glycosides + Aminoglycosides

Blood levels of digoxin can be reduced by the concurrent use of neomycin.

Clinical evidence

Neomycin (1 to 3 g orally) was found to depress and delay the absorption of a single 500-microgram dose of **digoxin** in healthy subjects.[1,2] The AUC was reduced by 41 to 51%. Absorption was affected even when the **neomycin** was given 3 to 6 h before the **digoxin**. In a steady state study, 2 g **neomycin** given with 250 to 500 micrograms **digoxin** daily reduced serum concentrations of **digoxin** by 8 to 49% (mean 28.2%).[1,2]

Mechanism

The probable reason is that neomycin can cause a general but reversible malabsorption syndrome, which affects the absorption of several drugs. The extent of this is probably offset in some patients, because the neomycin also depresses the destruction of the digoxin by the bacteria in the gut.[3]

Importance and management

Information is limited, but this interaction appears to be established. Patients should be monitored for reduced digoxin effects if neomycin is given and suitable dosage adjustments made if necessary. Separating the dosages of the two drugs does not prevent this interaction. Other aminoglycosides that can be administered orally such as **kanamycin** and **paromomycin** might possibly interact similarly, but this requires confirmation. There seems to be no information about other aminoglycosides.

1. Lindenbaum J, Maulitz RM, Saha JR, Shea N, Butler VP. Impairment of digoxin absorption by neomycin. *Clin Res* (1972) 20, 410.
2. Lindenbaum J, Maulitz RM, Butler VP. Inhibition of digoxin absorption by neomycin. *Gastroenterology* (1976) 71, 399–404.
3. Lindenbaum J, Tse-Eng D, Butler VP, Rund DG. Urinary excretion of reduced metabolites of digoxin. *Am J Med* (1981) 71, 67–74.

Digitalis glycosides + Aminosalicylic acid (PAS)

Blood levels of digoxin in normal subjects are reduced to a small extent by aminosalicylic acid, but the importance of this in patients is uncertain.

Clinical evidence, mechanism, importance and management

In one study, 10 normal subjects showed a 20% reduction in the bioavailability of a single 750-microgram dose of **digoxin** (using urinary excretion as a measure) after treatment with **aminosalicylic acid** (**PAS**) 2 g four times daily for 2 weeks.[1] This seems to be just another aspect of the general malabsorption caused by **aminosalicylic acid**. The importance of this interaction in patients is not known (it is probably small) but it would be prudent to monitor concurrent use.

1. Brown DD, Juhl RP, Warner SL. Decreased bioavailability of digoxin due to hypocholesterolemic interventions. *Circulation* (1978) 58, 164–72.

Digitalis glycosides + Amiodarone

Blood levels of digoxin can be approximately doubled by the concurrent use of amiodarone. Some individuals may show even greater increases. Digitalis intoxication will occur if the dosage of digoxin is not reduced appropriately. The same interaction also appears to occur with digitoxin.

Clinical evidence

(a) Digoxin

The observation[1] that patients on **digoxin** developed digoxin intoxication when given **amiodarone** prompted study of this interaction. Seven patients on constant daily doses of **digoxin** for 14 days showed a mean rise in plasma **digoxin** levels of 69% (from 1.17 to 1.98 micrograms/l) when given 200 mg **amiodarone** three times daily. Two other patients similarly treated also showed this interaction.[1]

Numerous studies in large numbers of patients have confirmed this interaction with reported increases in serum **digoxin** levels of 75%,[2] 90%,[3] 95%[4] and 104%.[5] The occasional patient may show three- to fourfold increases, whereas others may show little or no change.[3,6] Children seem particularly sensitive with two- to threefold rises, and even as much as eightfold.[7] Other reports confirm that the **digoxin** levels are markedly increased or roughly doubled, and intoxication can occur.[6,8-15] In contrast, one group of workers state that they observed no change in serum **digoxin** levels in 5 patients given **amiodarone**.[16,17] There is also some evidence that in the treatment of resistant atrial tachyarrhythmias the risk of arrhythmias may be increased by concurrent use,[18] and another study found that combined use had an unfavourable effect on survival in patients with atrial fibrillation and sinus rhythm.[19]

(b) Digitoxin

Two elderly patients (aged 77 and 78) taking 100 micrograms **digitoxin** daily were additionally given loading doses of **amiodarone** followed by maintenance doses of 200 to 400 mg daily. Within 2 months in one case, and 4 months in the other, they were hospitalised because of bradycardia, dyspnoea, nausea and malaise. One of them had total AV block (38 bpm). The serum **digitoxin** levels of both of them were found to be elevated (54 and 45 micrograms/l respectively) well above the normal therapeutic range of 9 to 30 micrograms/l. Serum **amiodarone** and desethylamiodarone levels were normal. Both patients recovered when the **digitoxin** was stopped.[20,21]

Mechanism

Not fully understood. Amiodarone reduces both the renal and non-renal excretion of digoxin,[22] and amiodarone-induced changes in thyroid function may also have some part to play in this interaction.[23] Displacement of digoxin from its binding sites has been suggested.[24,25] One study suggests that increased absorption from the gut is responsible.[26] It is thought that amiodarone can also inhibit the metabolism of digitoxin by the liver which would explain why its serum levels are increased.[20]

Importance and management

The digoxin/amiodarone interaction is well documented, well established and of considerable clinical importance. It occurs in most patients. It is clearly evident after a few days and develops over the course of 1 to 4 weeks.[4] If no account is taken of this interaction the patient may develop digitalis intoxication. Reduce the digoxin dosage by between one-third to one-half when amiodarone is added,[1,2,11,26] with further adjustment of the dosage after a week or two, and possibly a month or more, as necessary.[11] Particular care is needed in children, who may show much larger rises in digoxin levels than adults. Amiodarone is lost from the body very slowly so that the effects of this interaction will persist for several weeks after its withdrawal.[15] Also be aware that quite apart from this pharmacokinetic interaction, there is now some evidence that concurrent use may possibly worsen the prognosis in some patients.[18,19]

Far less is known about the digitoxin/amiodarone interaction but the limited evidence available suggests that all of the precautions appropriate for digoxin should be used for digitoxin as well. Note that it may possibly take months to develop. More study of this interaction is needed.

1. Moysey JO, Jaggarao NSV, Grundy EN, Chamberlain DA. Amiodarone increases plasma digoxin concentrations. *BMJ* (1981) 282, 272.
2. Fornaro G, Rossi P, Padrini R, Piovan D, Ferrari M, Fortina A, Tomassini G, Aquili C. Ricerca farmacologico-clinica sull'interazione digitale-amiodarone in pazienti cardiopatici con insufficiencza cardiaca di vario grado. *G Ital Cardiol* (1984) 14, 990–8.
3. Oetgen WJ, Sobol SM, Tri TB, Heydorn WH, Rakita L. Amiodarone-digoxin interaction. Clinical and experimental observations. *Chest* (1984) 86, 75–9.
4. Vitale P, Jacono A, Gonzales y Reyero E, Zeuli L. Effect of amiodarone on serum digoxin levels in patients with atrial fibrillation. *Clin Trials J* (1984) 21, 199–206.
5. Nademanee K, Kannan R, Hendrickson J, Ookhtens M, Kay I, Singh BN. Amiodarone-digoxin interaction: clinical significance, time course of development, potential pharmacokinetic mechanisms and therapeutic implications. *J Am Coll Cardiol* (1984) 4, 111–16.
6. Nager G, Nager F. Interaktion zwischen Amiodaron und Digoxin. *Schweiz Med Wochenschr* (1983) 113, 1727–30.
7. Koren G, Hesslein PS, MacLeod SM. Digoxin toxicity associated with amiodarone therapy in children. *J Pediatr* (1984) 104, 467–70.
8. Nademanee K, Kannan R, Hendrickson JA, Burnam M, Kay I, Singh B. Amiodarone-digoxin interaction during treatment of resistant cardiac arrhythmias. *Am J Cardiol* (1982) 49, 1026.
9. McQueen EG. New Zealand Committee on Adverse Drug Reactions. 17th Annual Report 1982. *N Z Med J* (1983) 96, 95–9.
10. McGovern B, Garan H, Kelly E, Ruskin JN. Adverse reactions during treatment with amiodarone hydrochloride. *BMJ* (1983) 287, 175–80.
11. Marcus FI, Fenster PE. Drug therapy. Digoxin interactions with other cardiac drugs. *J Cardiovasc Med* (1983) 8, 25–8.
12. Strocchi E, Malini PL, Graziani A, Ambrosioni E, Magnani B. L'interazione tra digossina ed amiodarone. *G Ital Cardiol* (1984) 14, 12–15.
13. Robinson KC, Walker S, Johnston A, Mulrow JP, McKenna WJ, Holt DW. The digoxin-amiodarone interaction. *Circulation* (1986) 74, II-225.
14. Johnston A, Walker S, Robinson KC, McKenna WJ and Holt DW. The digoxin-amiodarone interaction. *Br J Clin Pharmacol* (1987) 24, 253P.
15. Robinson K, Johnston A, Walker S, Mulrow JP, McKenna WJ, Holt DW. The digoxin-amiodarone interaction. *Cardiovasc Drugs Therapy* (1989) 3, 25–28.
16. Achilli A, Serra N. Amiodarone increases plasma digoxin concentrations. *BMJ* (1981) 282, 1630.
17. Achilli A, Giacci M, Capezzuto A, de Luca F, Guerra R, Serra N. Interazione digossina-chinidina e digossina-amiodarone. *G Ital Cardiol* (1981) 11, 918–25.
18. Bajaj BP, Baig MW, Perrins EJ. Amiodarone-induced torsades de pointes: the possible facilitatory role of digoxin. *Int J Cardiol* (1991) 33, 335–8.
19. Mortara A, Cioffi G, Opasich C, Pozzoli M, Febo O, Riccardi G, Cobelli F, Tavazzi L. Combination of amiodarone plus digoxin in chronic heart failure: an adverse effect on survival independently of the presence of sinus rhythm or atrial fibrillation. *Circulation* (1996) 94 (8 Suppl), I-21.
20. Läer S, Scholz H, Buschmann I, Thoenes M, Meinertz T. Evidence for a new drug interaction: digitoxin toxicity after amiodarone treatment. *Eur J Clin Pharmacol* (1997) 52, A7.
21. Läer S, Scholz H, Buschmann I, Thoenes M, Meinertz T. Digitoxinintoxication during concomitant use of amiodarone. *Eur J Clin Pharmacol* (1998) 54, 95–6.
22. Fenster PE, White NW, Hanson CD. Pharmacokinetic evaluation of the digoxin-amiodarone interaction. *J Am Coll Cardiol* (1985) 5, 108–12.
23. Ben-Chetrit E, Ackerman Z, Eliakim M. Case-report: Amiodarone-associated hypothyroidism — a possible cause of digoxin intoxication. *Am J Med Sci* (1985) 289, 114–16.
24. Douste-Blazy Ph, Montastruc JL, Bonnet B, Auriol P, Conte D, Bernadet P. Influence of amiodarone on plasma and urine digoxin concentrations. *Lancet* (1984) i, 905.
25. Mingardi G. Amiodarone and plasma digoxin levels. *Lancet* (1984) i, 1238.
26. Santostasi G, Fantin M, Maragno I, Gaion RM, Basadonna O, Dalla-Volta S. Effects of amiodarone on oral and intravenous digoxin kinetics in healthy subjects. *J Cardiovasc Pharmacol* (1987) 9, 385–90.

Digitalis glycosides + Amphotericin B

Amphotericin B causes potassium loss which could lead to the development of digitalis toxicity.

Clinical evidence, mechanism, importance and management

Among the well-recognised adverse effects of **amphotericin B** treatment is increased potassium loss. The hypokalaemia can be severe. Although there seem to be no reports of adverse interactions, it would be logical to expect that digitalis toxicity could develop in patients given both drugs if the potassium levels were allowed to fall unchecked. Concurrent treatment should be well monitored and any potassium deficiency made good. Amiloride has been successfully used to counteract the potassium loss caused by **amphotericin B**.[1]

1. Smith SR, Galloway MJ, Reilly JT, Davies JM. Amiloride prevents amphotericin B related hypokalaemia in neutropenic patients. *J Clin Pathol* (1988) 41, 494–7.

Digitalis glycosides + Angiotensin II antagonists

Candesartan, eprosartan, irbesartan, losartan, and valsartan appear not to interact with digoxin but telmisartan may cause a rise in serum digoxin levels.

Clinical evidence

(a) Candesartan

There was no pharmacokinetic interaction between **candesartan** cilexetil 16 mg daily and digoxin administered as a loading dose of 750 micrograms then 250 micrograms daily in 12 healthy subjects.[1]

(b) Eprosartan

A study in 12 healthy men given single 600-microgram oral doses of digoxin found that 200 mg **eprosartan** 12-hourly for 4 days had no significant effect on the digoxin pharmacokinetics.[2]

(c) Irbesartan

A study in 10 healthy subjects taking digoxin for 2 weeks showed no changes in the AUC or maximum serum levels of the digoxin during the second week while also taking 150 mg **irbesartan** daily.[3]

(d) Losartan

When 13 healthy subjects were given single 500-microgram oral or intravenous doses of digoxin before and after taking 50 mg **losartan** daily for a week, the pharmacokinetics of digoxin were found to be unaltered.[4]

(e) Telmisartan

A study in 12 healthy subjects given a 500-microgram loading dose of **digoxin** followed by 250 micrograms daily found that the maximum serum concentration, the trough serum concentration and AUC were increased by 50, 13 and 22% respectively when **telmisartan** 120 mg daily was co-administered for 7 days.[5] The median time to maximum concentration was also shortened. No clinically relevant changes in vital signs or ECGs were noted.

(f) Valsartan

There was no adverse interaction between single doses of **valsartan** 160 mg and **digoxin** 250 micrograms in 12 healthy subjects.[6]

Mechanism

It has been suggested that there might have been more rapid adsorption of digoxin with telmisartan.[5]

Importance and management

No special precautions seem to be necessary when digoxin is used with candesartan, eprosartan, irbesartan, losartan, or valsartan. Information for eprosartan, losartan, and valsartan are from single-dose studies, although the authors of the eprosartan study consider that a clinically relevant interaction with multiple doses of digoxin is unlikely.[2] More study is needed. The small increase in trough serum digoxin level with telmisartan suggests that the dose of digoxin need not automatically be reduced when telmisartan is started, but serum digoxin levels should be monitored. Serum digoxin levels should also be monitored if the telmisartan dose is changed.

1. Jonkman JH, van Lier JJ, van Heiningen PN, Lins R, Sennewald R, Hogemann A. Pharmacokinetic drug interaction studies with candesartan cilexetil. *J Hum Hypertens* (1997) 11 (Suppl 2), S31–S35.
2. Martin DE, Tompson D, Boike SC, Tenero D, Ilson B, Citerone D, Jorkasky DK. Lack of effect of eprosartan on the single dose pharmacokinetics of orally administered digoxin in healthy male volunteers. *Br J Clin Pharmacol* (1997) 43, 661–4.
3. Marino MR, Vachharajani NN. Drug interactions with irbesartan. *Clin Pharmacokinet* (2001) 40, 605–14.
4. De Smet M, Schoors DF, De Meyer G, Verbesselt R, Goldberg MR, Fitzpatrick V, Somers G. Effect of multiple doses of losartan on the pharmacokinetics of single doses of digoxin in healthy volunteers. *Br J Clin Pharmacol* (1995) 40, 571–5.
5. Stangier J, Su C-APF, Hendricks MGC, van Lier JJ, Sollie FAE, Oosterhuis B, Jonkman JHG. The effect of telmisartan on the steady-state pharmacokinetics of digoxin in healthy male volunteers. *J Clin Pharmacol* (2000) 40, 1373–9.
6. Ciba Laboratories. Data on file, Protocols 07, 36–40, 42, 43, 52.

Digitalis glycosides + Antacids

Although some studies suggest that antacids can reduce the bioavailability of digoxin and digitoxin, there is other evidence suggesting that no clinically relevant interactions occur. Separating the dosages by 1 to 2 hours is one way of making sure.

Clinical evidence

(a) Digoxin

(i) *Evidence of an interaction.* A study in 10 healthy subjects given 750 micrograms **digoxin** (*Lanoxin*) with 60 ml of either 4% **aluminium hydroxide gel**, 8% **magnesium hydroxide gel** or **magnesium trisilicate** showed that the cumulative 6-day urinary excretion expressed as a percentage of the original dose was as follows: control 40%; **aluminium hydroxide** 31%; **magnesium hydroxide** 27%; **magnesium trisilicate** 29%.[1]

Other studies describe reductions in **digoxin** absorption of 11% with **aluminium hydroxide**, 15% with **bismuth carbonate** and **light magnesium carbonate**, and 99.5% with **magnesium trisilicate**.[2]

(ii) *Evidence of no interaction.* A study in 4 patients chronically treated with 250 to 500 micrograms **digoxin** daily, showed that concurrent treatment with either 10 ml **aluminium hydroxide mixture BP** or **magnesium trisilicate mixture BP**, three times daily, did not reduce the bioavailability of the **digoxin** and none of the patients showed any reduction in the control of their symptoms.[3]

Other bioavailability studies failed to show a significant interaction between **digoxin** (in capsule but not tablet form)[4] or **beta-acetyldigoxin**[5] and **magnesium-aluminium hydroxide**.

(b) Digitoxin

(i) *Evidence of an interaction. In vitro* studies with **digitoxin** suggest that it might possibly interact like digoxin and be absorbed by various antacids[6] (see 'Evidence of an interaction' with digoxin above) but **lanatoside C** probably does not interact.[7]

(ii) *Evidence of no interaction.* A study in 10 patients with heart failure showed that their steady-state serum **digitoxin** levels were slightly, but not significantly raised (from 13.6 to 15.1 ng/ml) while taking 20 ml **aluminium-magnesium hydroxide** gel three or four times daily, separated from the **digitoxin** dosage by at least 1 to 2 h.[8]

Mechanism

Not established. One suggestion is that the digoxin can become adsorbed onto the antacids and therefore unavailable for absorption.[1,6] This is probably also true for digitoxin. However, some results are not consistent with this idea.

Importance and management

The digoxin/antacid and digitoxin/antacid interactions are only moderately well documented, and the evidence is inconsistent. No clearly clinically relevant interactions have been reported but to be on the safe side it might be prudent to be alert for any evidence of a reduced response if antacids are added to treatment with either glycoside. Separating the dosages by 1 to 2 h to minimise admixture is effective in many other drugs which interact in the gut, and it is known to work with digoxin.

1. Brown DD, Juhl RP, Lewis K, Schrott M, Bartels B. Decreased bioavailability of digoxin due to antacids and kaolin-pectin. *N Engl J Med* (1976) 295, 1034–7.
2. McElnay JC, Harron DWG, D'Arcy PF, Eagle MRG. Interaction of digoxin with antacid constituents. *BMJ* (1978) i, 1554.
3. Cooke J, Smith JA. Absence of interaction of digoxin with antacids under clinical conditions. *BMJ* (1978) 2, 1166.
4. Allen MD, Greenblatt DJ, Harmatz JS, Smith TW. Effect of magnesium-aluminum hydroxide and kaolin-pectin on the absorption of digoxin from tablets and capsules. *J Clin Pharmacol* (1981) 21, 26–30.
5. Bonelli J, Hruby K, Magometschnigg D, Hitzenberger G, Kaik G. The bioavailability of β-acetyldigoxine alone and combined with aluminium hydroxide and magnesium hydroxide (Alucol®). *Int J Clin Pharmacol* (1977) 15, 337–9.
6. Khalil SAH. The uptake of digoxin and digitoxin by some antacids. *J Pharm Pharmacol* (1974) 26, 961–7.
7. Aldous S, Thomas R. Absorption and metabolism of lanatoside C. *Clin Pharmacol Ther* (1977) 21, 647–58.
8. Kuhlmann J. Plasmaspiegel und renale Elimination von Digitoxin bei Langzeittherapie mit Aluminium-Magnesium-Hydroxid-Gel. *Dtsch Med Wochenschr* (1984) 109, 59–61.

Digitalis glycosides + Anticonvulsants

Carbamazepine does not appear to interact significantly with digoxin, and topiramate causes only a small reduction in digoxin serum levels. See also 'Digitalis glycosides + Phenytoin', p.550.

Clinical evidence, mechanism, importance and management

Bradycardia seen in 3 patients on digitalis and **carbamazepine** was tentatively attributed to their concurrent use,[1] but as yet this has not been confirmed by other observations.

Topiramate 100 mg twice daily for 9 days caused a small reduction in the serum **digoxin** levels in 12 healthy subjects.[2,3] The maximum serum levels and the AUC were reduced by 15.8% and 12% respectively, and the oral **digoxin** clearance was increased by 13%.[3] The makers suggest good monitoring of **digoxin** if **topiramate** is added or withdrawn,[3] but changes in the pharmacokinetics of **digoxin** of this magnitude seem unlikely to be clinically relevant in most patients. See also 'Digitalis glycosides + Phenytoin', p.550.

1. Killian JM, Fromm GH. Carbamazepine in the treatment of neuralgia. Use and side effects. *Arch Neurol* (1968) 19, 129–36.
2. Liao S, Palmer M. Digoxin and topiramate drug interaction study in male volunteers. *Pharm Res* (1993) 10 (10 Suppl), S405.
3. Topamax (topiramate). Janssen-Cilag Ltd. Summary of product characteristics. March 1998.

Digitalis glycosides + Aspirin

Aspirin possibly causes a moderate rise in serum digoxin levels, but no interaction of clinical relevance seems to occur.

Clinical evidence, mechanism, importance and management

Although **aspirin** can double the serum concentrations of **digoxin** in *dogs*, a study in 8 healthy subjects demonstrated no interaction, even when taking high doses (975 mg three times daily),[1] whereas another study in 9 healthy subjects found that 1.5 g **aspirin** daily for 10 days increased the serum **digoxin** levels by 31%.[2] Bearing in mind that both drugs have been in use for a very considerable number of years, the lack of reports in the literature describing problems suggests that no clinically important interaction normally occurs.

1. Fenster PE, Comess KA, Hanson CD and Finley PR. Kinetics of digoxin-aspirin combination. *Clin Pharmacol Ther* (1982) 32, 428–30.
2. Isbary J, Doering W, König E.Der Einfluß von Tiaprofensäure auf die Digoxinkonzentration im Serum (DKS) im Vergleich zu anderen Antirheumatika (AR). *Z Rheumatol* (1982) 41, 164.

Digitalis glycosides + Azapropazone

Azapropazone normally appears not to interact with digitoxin, but the occasional patient may possibly show a small rise in plasma levels. The importance of this is uncertain.

Clinical evidence, mechanism, importance and management

Azapropazone 900 mg daily did not significantly alter the AUC of a single intravenous dose of **digitoxin** 500 micrograms in 8 arthritic patients, but its mean half-life was increased about 10%. Two of the patients showed individual half-life increases of almost one-third.[1] This suggests that concurrent use is normally likely to be uneventful, but the possibility of an interaction in the occasional patient cannot be dismissed. Information about **digoxin** appears to be lacking.

1. Faust-Tinnefeldt G, Gilfrich HJ. Digitoxin-Kinetik unter antirheumatischer Therapie mit Azapropazon. *Arzneimittelforschung* (1977) 27, 2009–11.

Digitalis glycosides + Balsalazide

The makers of balsalazide suggest that there may be an interaction with digoxin, but there seem to be no reports of such an interaction.

Clinical evidence, mechanism, importance and management

Balsalazide is a prodrug of mesalazine (a compound of 4-aminobenzoylalanine linked to mesalazine) which, like another prodrug sulfasalazine, acts by releasing mesalazine. While there is certainly a recognised, but rare, interaction between digoxin and sulfasalazine,

which results in reduced digoxin plasma levels (see 'Digitalis glycosides + Sulfasalazine', p.556), no digoxin/mesalazine interaction nor digoxin/**balsalazide** interaction has been reported. Even so the makers of **balsalazide** cautiously suggest the possibility of an interaction.[1] They recommend that plasma levels of digoxin should be monitored in digitalised patients starting **balsalazide**, although there appears to be no clinical evidence that an interaction has ever taken place,[2] nor clear reasons for believing that an interaction is likely.

1. Colazide (Balsalazide). Shire Pharmaceuticals Ltd. Summary of product characteristics, May 2001.
2. Astra Pharmaceuticals. Personal communications, November and December 1997.

Digitalis glycosides + Barbiturates

Blood levels of digitoxin can be halved by the concurrent use of phenobarbital. Its effects may be expected to be reduced accordingly.

Clinical evidence

After taking 60 mg **phenobarbital** three times daily for 12 weeks, the steady-state plasma **digitoxin** levels in a group of patients (taking 100 micrograms daily) fell by 50%.[1] In associated studies the half-life of **digitoxin** decreased from 7.8 to 4.5 days during **phenobarbital** treatment.[1,2] In another study[3] the rate of conversion of **digitoxin** to **digoxin** in one patient increased from 4% to 27% while taking 96 mg **phenobarbital** daily for 13 days.

In contrast, a study in groups of 10 normal subjects given either **digitoxin** 400 micrograms, **digoxin** 1000 micrograms or **acetyldigitoxin** 800 micrograms daily failed to find changes in the serum concentrations of any of these glycosides while concurrently taking 100 mg **phenobarbital** three times daily for 7 to 9 days.[4]

Mechanism

Phenobarbital and other barbiturates are well known as potent liver enzyme inducing agents which, it would seem, can increase the metabolism and conversion of digitoxin to digoxin.[1-3] The failure of one study to demonstrate this interaction may possibly have been because the barbiturate was taken for a relatively short time.[4]

Importance and management

An established interaction, although its clinical importance is somewhat uncertain because there seem to be few reports of the effects of concurrent use, or of problems in practice. Nevertheless, patients taking both drugs should be monitored for expected under-digitalisation and the dosage of digitoxin increased if necessary. The result of this interaction is an increase in the levels of digoxin, but as its duration of action is considerably shorter than digitoxin, a much larger dose is needed to achieve the same degree of digitalisation. Thus an increased conversion of digitoxin to digoxin means a reduction in the total activity of the two glycosides. It seems likely that digoxin itself will not be affected by the barbiturates because it is largely excreted unchanged in the urine. Other barbiturates would be expected to behave like phenobarbital.

1. Solomon HM, Abrams WB. Interactions between digitoxin and other drugs in man. *Am Heart J* (1972) 83, 277–80.
2. Solomon H, Reich S, Gaut Z, Pocelinko R, Abrams W. Induction of the metabolism of digitoxin in man by phenobarbital. *Clin Res* (1971) 19, 356.
3. Jelliffe RW, Blankenhorn DH. Effect of phenobarbital on digitoxin metabolism. *Clin Res* (1966) 14, 160.
4. Káldor A, Somogyi G, Debreczeni LA, Gachályi B. Interaction of heart glycosides and phenobarbital. *Int J Clin Pharmacol* (1975) 12, 403–7.

Digitalis glycosides + Benzodiazepines

Digoxin intoxication occurred in two elderly patients when given alprazolam, and rises in serum digoxin levels have been seen in others. A reduction in the urinary clearance of digoxin

has been described during the use of diazepam, but no inter-action seems to occur with metaclazepam.

Clinical evidence

(a) Alprazolam

An elderly woman on maprotiline, isosorbide dinitrate, furosemide (frusemide) and potassium chloride demonstrated signs of digoxin intoxication during the second week after starting 1 mg alprazolam daily. Her serum digoxin levels were later found to have risen almost 300% (from 1.6 to 4.3 ng/ml) and her apparent digoxin clearance had fallen from 126.3 to 49.8 l/day.[1] A later study in 12 patients confirmed that digoxin levels can be significantly raised by alprazolam, particularly in those aged over 65. One elderly man developed clinical digoxin toxicity.[2] In contrast, a two-way crossover study in 8 healthy subjects found no changes in the clearance of digoxin while taking 1.5 mg alprazolam daily.[3]

(b) Diazepam, Metaclazepam

The observation that 3 patients showed raised digoxin levels while taking diazepam prompted a further study in 7 healthy subjects.[4] After taking 5 mg diazepam with a single 500 micrograms dose of digoxin, and another 5 mg diazepam 12 h later, all of them were said to have a "substantial reduction in urinary excretion" and 5 of them showed a "moderate increase in the digoxin half-life." No further details were given.[4] No statistically significant interaction was seen in 9 patients on digoxin (β-acetyldigoxin) when given metaclazepam.[5]

Mechanism

Uncertain. The suggestion is that diazepam may possibly alter the extent of the protein binding of digoxin within the plasma, which may have some influence on the renal tubular excretion.[4] The reason for the digoxin/alprazolam interaction is not understood.

Importance and management

The digoxin/alprazolam interaction is established and clinically important. Monitor the effects in any patient if alprazolam is added and reduce the digoxin dosage as necessary. What is known suggests that intoxication is more likely in those over 65. Both digoxin and other benzodiazepines have been used for a very considerable time but there seem to be no other reports of adverse interactions when used together. Concurrent use therefore need not be avoided but the effects should be monitored.

1. Tollefson G, Lesar T, Grothe D, Garvey M. Alprazolam-related digoxin toxicity. *Am J Psychiatry* (1984) 141, 1612–14.
2. Guven H, Tuncok Y, Guneri S, Cavdar C, Fowler J. Age-related digoxin-alprazolam interaction. *Clin Pharmacol Ther* (1993) 54, 42–4.
3. Ochs HR, Greenblatt DJ, Verburg-Ochs B. Effect of alprazolam on digoxin kinetics and creatinine clearance. *Clin Pharmacol Ther* (1985) 38, 595–8.
4. Castillo-Ferrando JR, Garcia M, Carmona J. Digoxin levels and diazepam. *Lancet* (1980) ii, 368.
5. Völker D, Müller R, Günther C, Bode R. Digoxin-Plasmaspiegel während der Behandlung mit Metaclazepam. *Arzneimittelforschung* (1988) 38, 923–5.

Digitalis glycosides + Beta-blockers

In general digoxin and beta-blockers appear not to interact, however there is always the risk of additive bradycardia. A few cases of excessive bradycardia have been reported when propranolol was used to control digitalis-induced arrhythmias. Talinolol, and possibly carvedilol, appear to increase the bioavailability of digoxin.

Clinical evidence

(a) Pharmacokinetic interactions

In healthy subjects given digoxin 500 micrograms as a single dose, talinolol 100 mg orally substantially increased the bioavailability of digoxin. The AUC from 0 to 72 hours and the maximal serum levels of digoxin were increased by 23 and 45% respectively.[1] Conversely,

when given intravenously, talinolol 30 mg had no effect on digoxin pharmacokinetics.[1]

A single-dose study in healthy subjects given 25 mg carvedilol found that maximal plasma levels of digoxin (500-microgram dose) were increased by 0.97 ng/ml (60%) and the AUC by approximately 20%, but the clinical effects were considered likely to be small.[2] In a multiple-dose study in patients with hypertension given digoxin 250 micrograms daily, the maximum serum digoxin level was raised by 32% after 2 weeks treatment with carvedilol and the AUC was raised by 14%. Again, these changes were considered unlikely to be clinically significant.[3] No significant pharmacokinetic interaction was found in other single-dose studies of carvedilol with digitoxin,[4] or carvedilol with intravenous digoxin.[2]

A single dose of intravenous esmolol did not affect the pharmacokinetics of multiple-dose digoxin, except that a small increase in digoxin AUC over 6 h was seen.[5] The pharmacokinetics of multiple-dose digoxin have been shown to be unaffected by the concurrent use of acebutolol,[6] bevantolol 200 mg daily,[7] bisoprolol 10 mg daily,[8] or sotalol 80 to 320 mg daily.[9,10]

(b) Pharmacodynamic interactions

Increased bradycardia is expected to occur with digoxin/beta-blocker combinations, but reports of this becoming a problem seem rare. One report notes marked bradycardia (35 to 50 bpm) in a 91-year-old patient on digoxin and timolol 0.25% eye drops.[11] Bradycardia persisted on withdrawal of digoxin, and improved only after discontinuation of the timolol as well. Two cases, where propranolol 10 mg orally was used to treat arrhythmias associated with digoxin toxicity, are reported.[12] The first patient (who had heart failure) became bradycardic, asystolic and then died, while the second became bradycardic (30 bpm) but recovered when given atropine. [A further fatality was reported when intravenous propranolol was used.[13]] In a placebo-controlled study of the use of sotalol in digitalised patients with chronic atrial fibrillation, 2 of 24 sotalol recipients were withdrawn due to bradycardia compared with none of 10 placebo recipients, but the combination was considered valuable.[9]

In volunteer studies, the pharmacodynamics of digoxin were unaffected by bevantolol,[7] and esmolol,[5] with no significant changes in heart rate or blood pressure occurring.

Mechanism

In most cases where the situation has had an adverse outcome the interaction seems to be due to the additive effects on the slowing of the heart. It has been suggested that pharmacokinetic interaction with talinolol is due to competition with digoxin for intestinal P-glycoprotein, although this needs confirmation.[1] It would seem possible that this mechanism also accounts for the interaction between digoxin and carvedilol.

Importance and management

Concurrent use appears, on the whole, beneficial, but the potential for additive bradycardia should be borne in mind. Use of beta-blockers in cases of digoxin toxicity should be undertaken with great care. In addition, it may be prudent to monitor digoxin levels with talinolol, and possibly also carvedilol.

1. Westphal K, Weinbrenner A, Giessmann T, Stuhr M, Gerd F, Zschiesche M, Oertel R, Terhaag B, Kroemer HK, Siegmund W. Oral bioavailability of digoxin is enhanced by talinolol: Evidence for involvement of P-glycoprotein. *Clin Pharmacol Ther* (2000) 68, 6–12.
2. De Mey C, Brendel E, Enterling D. Carvedilol increases the systemic bioavailability of oral digoxin. *Br J Clin Pharmacol* (1990) 29, 486–90.
3. Wermeling DP, Feild CJ, Smith DA, Chandler MHH, Clifton GD, Boyle DA. Effects of long-term oral carvedilol on the steady-state pharmacokinetics of oral digoxin in patients with mild to moderate hypertension. *Pharmacotherapy* (1994) 14, 600–6.
4. Harder S, Brei R, Caspary S, Merz PG. Lack of a pharmacodynamic interaction between carvedilol and digitoxin or phenprocoumon. *Eur J Clin Pharmacol* (1993) 44, 583–6.
5. Lowenthal DT, Porter RS, Achari R, Turlapaty P, Laddu AR and Matier WL. Esmolol-digoxin drug interaction. *J Clin Pharmacol* (1987) 27, 561–6.
6. Ryan JR. Clinical pharmacology of acebutolol. *Am Heart J* (1985) 109, 1131–6.
7. Quoted as data on file, Parke-Davis, by Frishman WH, Goldberg RJ, Benfield P. Bevantolol. A preliminary review of its pharmacodynamic and pharmacokinetic properties, and therapeutic efficacy in hypertension and angina pectoris. *Drugs* (1988) 35, 1–21.
8. Vechlekar DL, Cheung WK, Pearse S, Greene DS, Dukart G, Unczowsky R, Weiss AI, Silber BM, Faulkner RD. Bisoprolol does not alter the pharmacokinetics of digoxin. *Pharm Res* (1988) 5 (Suppl), S176.
9. Singh S, Saini RK, DiMarco J, Kluger J, Gold R, Chen Y. Efficacy and safety of sotalol in digitalized patients with chronic atrial fibrillation. *Am J Cardiol* (1991) 68, 1227–30.

10. Unpublished observations (Bristol-Myers Squibb) quoted by Hanyok JJ. Clinical pharmacokinetics of sotalol. *Am J Cardiol* (1993) 72, 19–26A.
11. Rynne MV. Timolol toxicity: ophthalmic medication complicating systemic disease. *J Maine Med Ass* (1980) 71, 82.
12. Watt DAL. Sensitivity to propranolol after digoxin intoxication. *BMJ* (1968) 3, 413–14.
13. Schamroth L. The immediate effects of intravenous propranolol in various cardiac arrhythmias. *Am J Cardiol* (1966) 18, 438.

Digitalis glycosides + Beta-lactam antibacterials

No interaction normally occurs with digoxin and amoxicillin, cefazolin, flucloxacillin, phenoxymethylpenicillin or ticarcillin/clavulanic acid. No pharmacokinetic interaction occurs between ampicillin and digitoxin.

Clinical evidence

Ampicillin 500 mg four times daily for 5 days had no significant effect on **digitoxin** pharmacokinetics after a single 1000-microgram dose in 6 healthy subjects.[1] No significant changes in **digoxin** serum concentrations were found in 16 elderly patients given **amoxicillin** (2 patients also took **erythromycin** and one **flucloxacillin**), and 2 who took **flucloxacillin** and **phenoxymethylpenicillin.** However, a few patients complained of some 'toxic' symptoms (nausea, vomiting, anorexia, headache, fatigue, blurred vision, confusion) which the authors of the report attributed to the underlying illness or the antibacterials rather than to an interaction.[2,3] There was no significant change in digoxin pharmacokinetics in 15 patients given **ticarcillin/clavulanic acid** 1000 mg/200 mg intramuscularly every 12 hours for one week.[4] There was no fall in the excretion of digoxin metabolites from the gut (see Mechanism) in 3 patients receiving **cefazolin**, and a fall occurred in only 1 of 10 patients receiving **penicillins** (ampicillin 6, oxacillin 3, penicillin 1).[5]

Mechanism

Up to 10% of patients on oral digoxin excrete it in substantial amounts in the faeces and urine as inactive metabolites (digoxin reduction products or DRPs). This metabolism seems to be the responsibility of the gut flora,[6] in particular *Eubacterium lentum*, which is anaerobic and Gram positive. In the presence of some antibacterials that inhibit this organism, more digoxin is available for absorption which results in a rise in serum levels (see 'Digitalis glycosides + Macrolide antibacterials', p.544). At the same time the inactive metabolites derived from the gut disappear.[7] Despite *in vitro* susceptibility of *E. lentum* to a range of antibacterials including penicillins there is little information to suggest an interaction between penicillins and digoxin.[8] As mentioned above, there is some evidence that beta-lactam antibacterials do not interact with digoxin via this mechanism in patients.[5] One explanation could be that these antibacterials do not achieve sufficient concentrations in the gastrointestinal tract to affect *E lentum*.[8]

Importance and management

The silence of the literature on adverse interactions between digoxin and beta-lactam antibacterials, and the limited evidence given above suggest interactions are unlikely. No changes in digoxin levels occur if amoxicillin, flucloxacillin, phenoxymethylpenicillin or ticarcillin/clavulanic acid are given, and ampicillin did not affect the pharmacokinetics of digitoxin.

1. Lucena MI, Moreno A, Fernandez MC, Garcia-Morillas M, Andrade R. Digitoxin elimination in healthy subjects taking ampicillin. *Int J Clin Pharmacol Res* (1987) VII, 33–7.
2. Rhodes K, Brown NS. Does digoxin interact with the penicillin antibiotics? *J Am Geriatr Soc* (1993) 41 (10 Suppl), SA22.
3. Rhodes KM, Brown SN. Do the penicillin antibiotics interact with digoxin? *Eur J Clin Pharmacol* (1994) 46, 479–80.
4. Cazzola M, Matera MG, Santangelo G, Angrisani M, Loffreda A, de Prisco F, Paizis G, Rossi F. Serum digoxin levels after concomitant ticarcillin and clavulanic acid administration. *Ther Drug Monit* (1994) 16, 46–8.
5. Dobkin JF, Saha JR, Butler VP, Lindenbaum J. Effects of antibiotic therapy on digoxin metabolism. *Clin Res* (1982) 30, 517A.
6. Lindenbaum J, Rund DG, Butler VP, Tse-Eng D, Saha JR. Inactivation of digoxin by the gut flora: reversal by antibiotic therapy. *N Engl J Med* (1981) 305, 789–94.
7. Lindenbaum J, Tse-Eng D, Butler VP, Rund DG. Urinary excretion of reduced metabolites of digoxin. *Am J Med* (1981) 71, 67–74.
8. Ten Eick AP, Reed MD. Hidden dangers of coadministration of antibiotics and digoxin in children: focus on azithromycin. *Curr Ther Res* (2000) 61, 148–60.

Digitalis glycosides + Bosentan

Bosentan does not appear to affect the pharmacokinetics of digoxin.

Clinical evidence, mechanism, importance and management

Bosentan 500 mg twice daily for a week did not significantly affect steady-state peak or trough serum digoxin levels in 18 healthy subjects given 375 micrograms daily. There was a small reduction in the AUC of **digoxin** by about 12%, although this was not considered to be clinically relevant. There were no changes in ECG recordings and vital signs.[1]

The results suggest that **bosentan** does not interact with **digoxin**, and that concurrent use need not be avoided. However, the authors note that further studies over the longer term, and in patients with renal impairment may be necessary to confirm this.

1. Weber C, Banken L, Birnboeck H, Nave S, Schulz R. The effect of bosentan on the pharmacokinetics of digoxin in healthy male subjects. *Br J Clin Pharmacol* (1999) 47, 701–6.

Digitalis glycosides + Calcium channel blockers

Concurrent use can be valuable, but tiapamil may cause an approximately 50% and bepridil a 34 to 48% rise in serum digoxin levels, which may possibly cause toxicity if the digoxin dosage is not reduced. Felodipine, gallopamil, lacidipine, nicardipine and nisoldipine cause small but normally clinically unimportant increases, while amlodipine, isradipine and nimodipine appear not to interact. The situation with nitrendipine is uncertain but it possibly causes only a small rise. The interactions of digoxin with diltiazem, nifedipine and verapamil are dealt with individually elsewhere.

Clinical evidence

(a) Digoxin + Amlodipine

Amlodipine 5 mg daily had no significant effect on the serum **digoxin** levels or its renal clearance in 21 healthy subjects given 375 micrograms daily.[1,2]

(b) Digoxin + Bepridil

Bepridil 300 mg daily for a week raised the serum **digoxin** levels of 12 healthy subjects on 375 micrograms daily by 34% (from 0.93 to 1.25 ng/ml).[3] Five of them had mild to moderate headache, nausea and dizziness for 1 to 3 days shortly after concurrent use started. The heart-slowing effects of the two drugs were found to be additive, while the negative inotropic effects of the **bepridil** and the positive inotropism of the increased serum **digoxin** levels were almost balanced.[3]

In another study in 23 subjects given 250 micrograms **digoxin** and 300 mg **bepridil** daily for 14 days, peak plasma **digoxin** levels rose by 48% (from 1.49 to 2.2 ng/ml) and the AUC rose by 21% (from 18.7 to 22.6 ng.h/ml).[4]

(c) Digoxin + Felodipine

Felodipine 10 mg twice daily for 8 weeks raised the serum **digoxin** levels in 11 patients by a clinically non-significant amount (+15%).[5] In another study, 14 similar patients were given 10 mg **felodipine** daily for a week. Plain tablets raised the steady-state **digoxin** serum levels by 11%, but extended-release tablets had no significant effect.[6] A third study found that, when taking felodipine, peak plasma **digox-**

in levels were transiently raised by about 40% one hour after intake, but that digoxin AUCs were not significantly increased.[7]

(d) Digoxin + Gallopamil

Gallopamil 50 mg three times daily for 2 weeks raised the serum **digoxin** levels of 12 healthy subjects on 375 micrograms daily by 16% (from 0.58 to 0.67 ng/ml).[8]

(e) Digoxin + Isradipine

Isradipine (given as 2.5 mg every 12 hours for 2 days, 5 mg every 12 hours for 2 days and then 5 mg three times daily for 10 days) did not interact significantly with a single 1000-microgram dose of **digoxin** given by intravenous infusion to 24 healthy subjects.[9] A similar study by the same group found that the same dosage regimen of isradipine administered concurrently with oral digoxin 250 micrograms twice daily caused a small increase in peak-serum digoxin levels but no changes in steady-state levels or AUC.[10]

(f) Digoxin + Lacidipine

No significant changes in the **digoxin** AUC or minimum serum levels were found in 12 healthy subjects taking 250 micrograms **digoxin** daily for 7 days when given a single 4 mg oral dose of **lacidipine**, but the maximum serum levels were increased by 34%. These changes were not considered to be clinically significant.[11]

(g) Digoxin + Nicardipine

The plasma **digoxin** levels of 10 patients on 130 to 250 micrograms daily, increased by 15% (said not to be statistically significant) when given 20 mg **nicardipine** three times a day for 14 days.[12] Another 20 patients with congestive heart failure also had no significant changes in steady-state serum **digoxin** levels (doses 250 to 500 micrograms daily) while taking 30 mg **nicardipine** three times daily for 5 days.[13] Yet another study in 9 patients confirmed the absence of an interaction.[14]

(h) β-Acetyldigoxin + Nimodipine

Nimodipine 30 mg twice daily caused no change in the pharmacokinetics or haemodynamic effects of β-**acetyldigoxin** in 12 healthy subjects.[15]

(i) Digoxin + Nisoldipine

Nisoldipine 20 mg daily increased plasma trough **digoxin** levels of 10 patients with heart failure by about 15%.[16,17] **Nisoldipine** 10 mg twice daily caused no changes in the pharmacokinetics or haemodynamic effects of **digoxin** in 8 healthy subjects.[15]

(j) Digoxin or β-Acetyldigoxin + Nitrendipine

A study in 8 healthy subjects, who had been taking **digoxin** 250 micrograms twice daily for 2 weeks, showed that the concurrent use of 10 mg **nitrendipine** daily caused a slight but insignificant rise in plasma **digoxin** levels. **Nitrendipine** 20 mg daily increased the **digoxin** AUC by 15% (from 9.7 to 11.2 ng.h/ml) and maximum plasma **digoxin** levels rose from 1.34 to 2.1 ng/ml. Clearance fell by 13% (from 315 to 275 ml/min). One subject dropped out of the study because of dizziness, nausea and vomiting, palpitations, insomnia and nervousness.[18-20]

Another study found that plasma **digoxin** levels were approximately doubled when **nitrendipine** was given,[21] but other studies in healthy subjects and patients found that 20 mg **nitrendipine** twice daily caused no changes in the pharmacokinetics or haemodynamic effects of **digoxin**,[15,22] or β-**acetyldigoxin**.[23]

(k) Digoxin + Tiapamil

Eight patients on **digoxin** who were given **tiapamil** (200 mg three times a day) for 14 days, showed an approximately 50% rise in mean serum **digoxin** levels. No signs of digitalis toxicity occurred.[12]

Mechanism

Where an interaction occurs it is probably due to changes in the renal excretion of the digoxin.

Importance and management

The extent of the information varies from drug to drug, but concurrent use can be therapeutically valuable. Monitor the effects of bepridil or tiapamil to ensure that digoxin levels do not rise excessively. Reduce the digoxin dosage as necessary. The other calcium channel blockers listed here (felodipine, gallopamil, lacidipine, nicardipine, nisoldipine) either cause only minimal increases, which are unlikely to be clinically important in most patients, or do not interact at all (amlodipine, isradipine, nimodipine). The situation with nitrendipine needs clarification. The interactions of digoxin with diltiazem, nifedipine and verapamil are detailed in individual monographs.

1. Schwartz JB. Amlodipine does not affect serum digoxin concentrations or renal clearance. *Clin Res* (1987) 35, 380A.
2. Schwartz JB. Effects of amlodipine on steady-state digoxin concentrations and renal digoxin clearance. *J Cardiovasc Pharmacol* (1988) 12, 1–5.
3. Belz GG, Wistuba S, Matthews JH. Digoxin and bepridil: pharmacokinetic and pharmacodynamic interactions. *Clin Pharmacol Ther* (1986) 39, 65–71.
4. Doose DR, Wallen S, Nayak RK, Minn FL. Pharmacokinetic interaction of bepridil and digoxin at steady-state. *Clin Pharmacol Ther* (1987) 41, 204.
5. Dunselman PHJM, Scaf AHJ, Kuntze CEE, Lie KI, Wesseling H. Digoxin-felodipine interaction in patients with congestive heart failure. *Eur J Clin Pharmacol* (1988) 35, 461–5.
6. Kirch W, Laskowski M, Ohnhaus EE, Åberg J. Effects of felodipine on plasma digoxin levels and haemodynamics in patients with heart failure. *J Intern Med* (1989) 225, 237–39.
7. Rehnqvist N, Billing E, Moberg L, Lundman T, Olsson G. Pharmacokinetics of felodipine and effect on digoxin plasma levels in patients with heart failure. *Drugs* (1987) 34 (Suppl 3), 33–42.
8. Belz GG, Doering W, Munkes R, Matthews J. Interaction between digoxin and calcium antagonists and antiarrhythmic drugs. *Clin Pharmacol Ther* (1983) 33, 410–17.
9. Johnson BF, Wilson J, Marwaha R, Hoch K, Johnson J. The comparative effects of verapamil and a new dihydropyridine calcium channel blocker on digoxin pharmacokinetics. *Clin Pharmacol Ther* (1987) 42, 66–71.
10. Rodin SM, Johnson BF, Wilson J, Ritchie P, Johnson J. Comparative effects of verapamil and isradipine on steady-state digoxin kinetics. *Clin Pharmacol Ther* (1988) 43, 668–72.
11. Hall ST, Harding SM, Anderson DM, Ward C, Stevens LA. The effect of single 4 mg oral dose of calcium antagonist lacidipine on the pharmacokinetics of digoxin. In: Carpi C, Zanchetti A, eds. IVth Int Symp Calcium Antagonists: Pharmacology and Clinical Research. Florence, May 1989: 161.
12. Lessem J and Bellinetto A. Interaction between digoxin and the calcium antagonists nicardipine and tiapamil. *Clin Ther* (1983) 5, 595–602.
13. Debruyne D, Commeau Ph, Grollier G, Huret B, Scanu P, Moulin M. Nicardipine does not significantly affect serum digoxin concentrations at the steady state of patients with congestive heart failure. *Int J Clin Pharmacol Res* (1989) IX, 15–19.
14. Scanu P, Commeau P, Huret B, Gérard JL, Debruyne D, Moore N, Lamy E, Dorey H, Grolier G, Potier JC. Pharmacocinétique et effets pharmacodynamiques de la digoxine dans les myocardiopathies dilatées. Influence de la nicardipine. *Arch Mal Coeur Vaiss* (1987) 80, 1773–83.
15. Ziegler R, Horstmann R, Wingender W, Kuhlmann J. Do dihydropyridines influence pharmacokinetic and hemodynamic parameters of digoxin? *J Clin Pharmacol* (1987) 27, 712.
16. Kirch W, Stenzel J, Dylewicz P, Hutt HJ, Santos SR, Ohnhaus EE. Influence of nisoldipine on haemodynamic effects and plasma levels of digoxin. *Br J Clin Pharmacol* (1986) 22, 155–9.
17. Kirch W, Stenzel J, Santos SR, Ohnhaus EE. Nisoldipine, a new calcium channel antagonist, elevates plasma levels of digoxin. *Arch Toxicol* (1987) (Suppl 11), 310–12.
18. Kirch W, Logemann C, Heidemann H, Santos SR, Ohnhaus EE. Effect of two different doses of nitrendipine on steady-state plasma digoxin levels and systolic time intervals. *Eur J Clin Pharmacol* (1986) 31, 391–5.
19. Kirch W, Logemann C, Santos SR, Ohnhaus EE. Influence of different doses of nitrendipine on digoxin plasma concentrations. *Br J Clin Pharmacol* (1986) 23, 111P–112P.
20. Kirch W, Logemann C, Santos SR, Ohnhaus EE. Nitrendipine increases digoxin plasma levels dose dependently. *J Clin Pharmacol* (1986) 26, 553.
21. Kirch W, Hutt HJ, Heidemann H, Rämsch K, Janisch HD, Ohnhaus EE. Drug interactions with nitrendipine. *J Cardiovasc Pharmacol* (1984) 6 (Suppl 7), S982–S985.
22. Debbas NMG, Johnston A, Jackson SHD, Banim SO, Camm AJ, Turner P. The effect of nitrendipine on predose digoxin serum concentration. *Br J Clin Pharmacol* (1988) 25, 151P.
23. Ziegler R, Wingender W, Boehme K, Raemsch K, Kuhlmann J. Study of pharmacokinetic and pharmacodynamic interaction between nitrendipine and digoxin. *J Cardiovasc Pharmacol* (1987) 9 (Suppl 4), S101–S106.

Digitalis glycosides + Calcium salts

The effects of digitalis can be increased by increases in blood calcium levels, and the administration of intravenous calcium may result in the development of potentially life-threatening digitalis-induced heart arrhythmias.

Clinical evidence

Two patients developed heart arrhythmias and died after being given **digitalis** intramuscularly and either **calcium chloride** or **gluconate** intravenously. No absolutely certain causative relationship was established.[1]

There is other evidence that increases or decreases in blood **calcium** levels can increase or decrease, respectively, the effects of **digitalis**. A patient with congestive heart failure and atrial fibrillation was resistant to the actions of **digoxin** in the usual therapeutic range (1.5 to 3 ng/ml) until his serum **calcium** levels were raised from 6.7 to about 8.5 mg/100 ml by the administration of **calcium and oral vitamin D**.[2] **Disodium edetate**,[3-5] which lowers ionic blood calcium levels, has been used successfully in the treatment of digitalis intoxication, although less toxic agents are generally preferred.

Mechanism

The actions of the cardiac glycosides (even now not fully understood) are closely tied up with movement of calcium ions into heart muscle cells. Increased concentrations of calcium outside these cells increase the inflow of calcium and this enhances the activity of the glycosides. This can lead to effective over-digitalisation and even potentially life-threatening arrhythmias.

Importance and management

The report cited[1] (published in 1936) seems to be the only direct clinical evidence of a serious adverse interaction, although there is plenty of less direct evidence that an interaction is possible. Intravenous calcium should be avoided in patients on cardiac glycosides. If that is not possible, it has been suggested[6] that it should be given slowly or only in small amounts in order to avoid transient serum calcium levels higher than 15 mEq/l.

1. Bower JO, Mengle HAK. The additive effects of calcium and digitalis. A warning with a report of two deaths. *JAMA* (1936) 106, 1151.
2. Chopra D, Janson P, Sawin CT. Insensitivity to digoxin associated with hypocalcaemia. *N Engl J Med* (1977) 296, 917–8.
3. Jick S and Karsh R. The effect of calcium chelation on cardiac arrhythmias and conduction disturbances. *Am J Cardiol* (1959) 43, 287.
4. Szekely P, Wynne NA. Effects of calcium chelation on digitalis-induced cardiac arrhythmias. *Br Heart J* (1963) 25, 589–94.
5. Rosenbaum JL, Mason D, Seven MJ. The effect of disodium EDTA on digitalis intoxication. *Am J Med Sci* (1960) 240, 111–18.
6. Nola GT, Pope S, Harrison DC. Assessment of the synergistic relationship between serum calcium and digitalis. *Am Heart J* (1970) 79, 499–507.

Digitalis glycosides + Carbenoxolone

Carbenoxolone can raise blood pressure, cause fluid retention and reduce serum potassium levels. It is generally regarded as contraindicated in those using digitalis glycosides for congestive heart failure.

Clinical evidence, mechanism, importance and management

The side-effects of **carbenoxolone** treatment include an increase in blood pressure (both systolic and diastolic), fluid retention and reduced serum potassium levels. The incidence of these side-effects is said in some reports to be as high as 50%. Others quote lower figures, nevertheless it is clear that they are not an uncommon occurrence. Hypertension and fluid retention occur early in **carbenoxolone** treatment, whereas the hypokalaemia develops later and may occur in the absence of the other two side-effects.[1-4] The hypokalaemia may be exacerbated if thiazide diuretics are used to control the fluid retention without the use of suitable potassium supplements. For example, severe hypokalaemia (of 1.4 mmol/l) has been described in a patient taking **carbenoxolone** and chlortalidone without potassium supplementation.[5] **Carbenoxolone** is therefore unsuitable for patients with congestive heart failure, or those taking digitalis glycosides, unless measures to avoid hypokalaemia are taken.

1. Geismar P, Mosbech J, Myren J. A double-blind study of the effect of carbenoxolone sodium in the treatment of gastric ulcer. *Scand J Gastroenterol* (1973) 8, 251–6.
2. Turpie AGG, Thomson TJ. Carbenoxolone sodium in the treatment of gastric ulcer with special reference to side-effects. *Gut* (1965) 6, 591–4.
3. Langman MJS, Knapp DR, Wakley EJ. Treatment of chronic gastric ulcer with carbenoxolone and gefarnate: a comparative trial. *BMJ* (1973) 3, 84–6.
4. Davies GJ, Rhodes J, Calcraft BJ. Complications of carbenoxolone therapy. *BMJ* (1974) 3, 400–402.
5. Descamps C, Vandenbroucke JM, Van Ypersele de Strihou C. Rhabdomyolysis and acute tubular necrosis associated with carbenoxolone and diuretic treatment. *BMJ* (1977) 1, 272.

Digitalis glycosides + Cibenzoline (Cifenline)

Cibenzoline did not affect plasma digoxin levels.

Clinical evidence, mechanism, importance and management

A study in 12 healthy subjects taking 250 to 375 micrograms **digoxin** daily showed that the concurrent use of 160 mg **cibenzoline** twice daily for 7 days had no effect on the pharmacokinetics of the **digoxin**.[1]

1. Khoo K-C, Givens SV, Parsonnet M, Massarella JW. Effect of oral cibenzoline on steady-state digoxin concentrations in healthy volunteers. *J Clin Pharmacol* (1988) 28, 29–35.

Digitalis glycosides + Cicletanine

Cicletanine appears not to affect plasma digoxin levels.

Clinical evidence, mechanism, importance and management

Single 50 mg and 100-mg doses of **cicletanine** were found to have no effect on the plasma **digoxin** levels of 6 patients stabilised on long term treatment (125 to 250 micrograms **digoxin** daily).[1] This absence of an interaction needs further confirmation with multiple dose studies.

1. Clement DL, Teirlynck O, Belpaire F. Lack of effect of cicletanine on plasma digoxin levels. *Int J Clin Pharmacol Res* (1988) 8, 9–11.

Digitalis Glycosides + Ciclosporin

Marked rises in serum digoxin levels have been seen in some patients concurrently treated with ciclosporin.

Clinical Evidence

Four out of a series of 5 patients developed digoxin toxicity when ciclosporin was added to digoxin therapy prior to cardiac transplantation. In the 2 cases described, ciclosporin 10 mg/kg/day was added to digoxin 375 micrograms daily. Fourfold rises in digoxin levels were seen within 2 to 3 days (from 1.5 to 5.7 nmol/l and from 2.6 to 10.6 nmol/l). This was accompanied by rises in serum creatinine levels (from 110 to 120 micromol/l and from 84 to 181 micromol/l respectively) that were considered insufficient to explain the rise in digoxin levels. As a consequence of these findings, the same authors conducted a study in 4 patients given both drugs. Two patients developed acute renal failure. In the remaining 2 patients, the volume of distribution of digoxin was decreased by 69 and 72%, while the clearance was reduced by 47 and 58%.[1] In a further 7 patients, digoxin pharmacokinetics were assessed prior to cardiac transplantation, then after transplantation during maintenance ciclosporin therapy.[2] Total body clearance of digoxin remained unchanged, which appeared to be at odds with the earlier results.[1] It was suggested that haemodynamic improvements brought about by successful cardiac transplantation may have counterbalanced any inhibitory effect ciclosporin had on renal clearance.[2]

Mechanism

Not fully understood. The authors of the above studies concluded that their data show that ciclosporin has no specific inhibitory effect on the renal elimination of digoxin, but that it causes a non-specific reduction in renal function after acute administration which reduces digoxin elimination.[2] Conversely, another study in *animals* suggested that ciclosporin can reduce the secretion of digoxin by the kidney tubular cells by inhibiting P-glycoprotein.[3]

Importance and management

Information seems limited to the studies cited. The effects of concurrent use should be monitored very closely, and the digoxin dosage should be adjusted as necessary.

1. Dorian P, Cardella C, Strauss M, David T, East S, Ogilvie R. Cyclosporine nephrotoxicity and cyclosporine-digoxin interaction prior to heart transplantation. *Transplant Proc* (1987) 19, 1825–7.
2. Robieux I, Dorian P, Klein J, Chung D, Zborowska-Sluis D, Ogilvie R, Koren G. The effects of cardiac transplantation and cyclosporine therapy on digoxin pharmacokinetics. *J Clin Pharmacol* (1992) 32, 338–43.
3. Okamura N, Hirai M, Tanigawara Y, Tanaka K, Yasuhura M, Ueda K, Komano T, Hori R. Digoxin-cyclosporin A interaction: modulation of the multidrug transporter P-glycoprotein in the kidney. *J Pharmacol Exp Ther* (1993) 266, 1614–9.

Digitalis glycosides + Cimetidine or Ranitidine

Small changes in serum digoxin levels, both rises and falls, have been seen in patients given cimetidine, but these do not appear to be of clinical importance. Ranitidine appears not to interact.

Clinical evidence, mechanism, importance and management

While taking 300 mg **cimetidine** every 6 or 12 hours the steady-state serum **digoxin** levels of 11 patients with congestive heart failure fell on average by 25% (from 2.0 to 1.5 ng/ml), but none of them showed any ECG changes or signs that their condition had worsened.[1] Four other patients with stable congestive heart failure showed no significant changes in the pharmacokinetics of **digoxin** (125 to 250 micrograms daily) when treated with 300 mg **cimetidine** 6 hourly.[2] Three single dose studies in a total of 19 healthy subjects, and 6 patients with duodenal ulcers[3] found that **cimetidine** (600 to 1200 mg daily) had no significant effect on the absorption[4] or the kinetics[3,5] of **digoxin**. Another study found a small increase in **digoxin** levels in healthy subjects, but only a small statistically insignificant rise (0.02 ng/ml) in the steady-state levels of 11 patients given 400 mg **cimetidine** four times daily.[6] Six patients with chronic congestive heart failure given **metildigoxin (medigoxin)** showed no changes in their serum **digoxin** levels when concurrently treated with 150 mg **ranitidine** twice daily for a week.[7]

No interaction of clinical importance with either of these H_2-blockers has been established and no special precautions would seem to be necessary.

1. Fraley DS, Britton HL, Schwinghammer TL, Kalla R. Effect of cimetidine on steady-state serum digoxin concentrations. *Clin Pharm* (1983) 2, 163–5.
2. Mouser B, Nykamp D, Murphy JE, Krissman PH. Effect of cimetidine on oral digoxin absorption. *DICP Ann Pharmacother* (1990) 24, 286–8.
3. Garty M, Perry G, Shmueli H, Ilfeld D, Boner G, Pitlik S, Rosenfeld J. Effect of cimetidine on digoxin disposition in peptic ulcer patients. *Eur J Clin Pharmacol* (1986) 30, 489–91.
4. Jordaens L, Hoegaerts J, Belpaire F. Non-interaction of cimetidine with digoxin absorption. *Acta Clin Belg* (1981) 36, 109–10.
5. Ochs HR, Gugler R, Guthoff T, Greenblatt DJ. Effect of cimetidine on digoxin kinetics and creatinine clearance. *Am Heart J* (1984) 107, 170–2.
6. Crome P, Curl B, Holt D, Volans GN, Bennett PN, Cole DS. Digoxin and cimetidine: investigation of the potential for a drug interaction. *Hum Toxicol* (1985) 4, 391–9.
7. Enomoto N, Kurasawa T, Ichikawa M, Shimuzu T, Matsuyama T, Sakai K, Shimamura K, Oda M. Lack of interaction of β-methyldigoxin with ranitidine in patients with chronic congestive heart failure. *Eur J Clin Pharmacol* (1992) 43, 205–6.

Digitalis glycosides + Colestipol

Colestipol appears not to interfere with the absorption of either digoxin or digitoxin if it is given at least 1.5 h after the

glycoside. It may help to reduce digitoxin or digoxin levels if intoxication occurs.

Clinical evidence

(a) Digitoxin and digoxin levels reduced in intoxication

Four patients intoxicated with **digitoxin** were given 10 g **colestipol** at once and 5 g every 6 to 8 h to reduce their **digitoxin** serum levels. The average **digitoxin** half-life fell to 2.75 days compared with an untreated control patient in whom the **digitoxin** half-life was 9.3 days. Another patient intoxicated with **digoxin** was similarly treated. His **digoxin** half-life was 16 h compared with 1.8 to 2 days in two other control patients.[1]

(b) Digitoxin and digoxin levels unaffected

Ten patients on long-term treatment with either **digoxin** (125 to 250 micrograms daily) or **digitoxin** (100 to 200 micrograms daily) were concurrently treated for a year with 15 g **colestipol** daily or a placebo, taken 1.5 h after the digitalis. Their serum digitalis levels were not significantly altered by the **colestipol**.[2]

A comparative study in 11 patients with plasma **digitoxin** levels above the therapeutic range (i.e. > 40 ng/ml) showed that giving 5 g **colestipol** four times daily before meals and stopping the **digitoxin** immediately did not affect the **digitoxin** half-life (6.3 days) when compared with 11 other patients not given **colestipol** (6.8 days).[3]

Mechanism

Colestipol is an ion-exchange resin which can bind to digitalis glycosides.[1] It can apparently interfere with the entero-hepatic circulation and increase the loss during intoxication.

Importance and management

This interaction is neither well established nor apparently of great clinical importance. Giving either digoxin or digitoxin followed by the colestipol at least 1.5 h later appears to avoid any possible interaction in the gut.[2] In cases of intoxication colestipol may possibly reduce serum digitalis levels because under these circumstances the excretion of digitalis in the bile increases and more becomes available for binding in the gut.[2]

1. Bazzano G, Bazzano GS. Digitalis intoxication. Treatment with a new steroid-binding resin. *JAMA* (1972) 220, 828–30.
2. Bazzano G, Bazzano GS. Effect of digitalis-binding resins on cardiac glycosides plasma levels. *Clin Res* (1972) 20, 24.
3. van Bever RJ, Duchateau AMJA, Pluym BFM, Merkus FWHM. The effect of colestipol on digitoxin plasma levels. *Arzneimittelforschung* (1976) 26, 1891–3.

Digitalis glycosides + Colestyramine

The blood levels of both digoxin and digitoxin can be reduced by the concurrent use of colestyramine, but the clinical importance of this is uncertain. Minimise the possible effects of this interaction by separating administration.

Clinical evidence

(a) Digitalis glycoside serum levels unaffected

Ten patients on long-term treatment with either **digoxin** 125 to 250 micrograms daily or **digitoxin** 100 to 200 micrograms daily were concurrently treated for a year with 12 g **colestyramine** daily or a placebo taken 1.5 h after the digitalis. Their plasma digitalis levels were not significantly altered by the **colestyramine**.[1]

The half-life of **digitoxin** is reported to have remained unchanged when **colestyramine** was used.[2]

(b) Digitalis glycoside serum levels reduced

A study carried out in 12 subjects given 750 micrograms **digoxin** showed that the cumulative 6-day recovery of the **digoxin** from the urine was reduced almost 20% (from 40.5 to 33.1%) when 4 g **colestyramine** was given concurrently.[3]

Other reports describe a fall in serum **digoxin** levels during the concurrent use of **colestyramine**[4-6] and an increase in the loss of **digoxin** and its metabolites in the faeces during concurrent long-term use.[7] A reduction by **colestyramine** of the half-life of **digitoxin** of 35 to 40% has been described.[8-10]

Mechanism

Not totally understood. Colestyramine appears to bind with digitoxin in the gut, thereby reducing its bioavailability and interfering with the enterohepatic cycle so that its half-life is shortened. Just how digoxin interacts is uncertain.[7]

Importance and management

The overall picture is far from clear. Some interaction seems possible but the extent to which it impairs the treatment of patients on these glycosides is uncertain. Be alert for any evidence of under-digitalisation if digoxin or, more particularly, digitoxin are given with colestyramine. Give the colestyramine not less than 1.5 to 2 h after the digitalis to minimise the possibility of an interaction.[1] An alternative is to use **metildigoxin (medigoxin)**, which one study suggests may be minimally affected by colestyramine.[11] Another study showed that giving digoxin as a solution in a capsule reduced the effects of this interaction.[6]

1. Bazzano G, Bazzano GS. Effects of digitalis binding resins on cardiac glycoside plasma levels. *Clin Res* (1972) 20, 24.
2. Pabst J, Leopold J, Schad W, Meub R. Bioavailability of digitoxin during chronic administration and influence of food and cholestyramine on the bioavailability after a single dose. *Naunyn Schmiedebergs Arch Pharmacol* (1979) 307, R70.
3. Brown DD, Juhl RP, Warner SL. Decreased bioavailability of digoxin produced by dietary fiber and cholestyramine. *Am J Cardiol* (1977) 39, 297.
4. Smith TW. New approaches to the management of digitalis intoxication. In 'Symposium on Digitalis' Glydendal Norsk Forlag, Oslo (1977) 39, 312.
5. Brown DD, Juhl RP, Warner SL. Decreased bioavailability of digoxin due to hypocholesterolemic interventions. *Circulation* (1978) 58, 164–72.
6. Brown DD, Schmid J, Long RA, Hull JH. A steady-state evaluation of the effects of propantheline bromide and cholestyramine on the bioavailability of digoxin when administered as tablets or capsules. *J Clin Pharmacol* (1985) 25, 360–4.
7. Hall WH, Shappell SD, Doherty JE. Effect of cholestyramine on digoxin absorption and excretion in man. *Am J Cardiol* (1977) 39, 213–16.
8. Caldwell JH, Greenberger NJ. Cholestyramine enhances digitalis excretion and protects against lethal intoxication. *Clin Invest* (1970) 49, 16a.
9. Caldwell JH, Bush CA, Greenberger NJ. Interruption of the enterohepatic circulation of digitoxin by cholestyramine. *J Clin Invest* (1971) 50, 2638–44.
10. Carruthers SG, Dujovne CA. Cholestyramine and spironolactone and their combination in digitoxin elimination. *Clin Pharmacol Ther* (1980) 27, 184–7.
11. Hahn K-J, Weber E. Effect of cholestyramine on absorption of drugs. In 'Frontiers of Internal Medicine' 12th Int Cong Int Med, Tel Aviv 1974. *Karger, Basel* (1975), 409–11.

Digitalis glycosides + Corticosteroids

Corticosteroids can cause potassium loss and sodium and water retention which increases the risk of digitalis toxicity and possible cardiac failure.

Clinical evidence, mechanism, importance and management

The corticosteroids given systemically can increase the loss of potassium, particularly those which are naturally occurring (**cortisone**, **deoxycortone**, **hydrocortisone**) whereas the synthetic derivatives (**betamethasone**, **dexamethasone**, **methylprednisolone**, **prednisolone**, **prednisone**, **triamcinolone**) have much less mineralocorticoid activity. There is therefore the possibility of potassium depletion, particularly when used long-term, which may increase the risk of digitalis toxicity. These corticosteroids also cause sodium and water retention, resulting in oedema and hypertension, which can lead on to cardiac failure in some individuals. It is therefore important to monitor the concurrent use of these drugs well. No problems of this kind would be expected with corticosteroids used topically or by inhalation because the amounts absorbed are likely to be relatively small.

Digitalis glycosides + Cytotoxics

Treatment with radiation and/or cytotoxic agents can damage the lining of the intestine so that digoxin is much less readily absorbed when given in tablet form. This can be overcome by giving the digoxin in liquid or liquid-in-capsule form, or by substituting digitoxin.

Clinical evidence

A study in 13 patients with various forms of neoplastic disease showed that radiation therapy and/or various high dose cytotoxic regimens (including **carmustine (BCNU)**, **cyclophosphamide**, **melphalan**, **cytarabine** and **methotrexate**) reduced the absorption of **digoxin** from tablets (*Lanoxin*) by almost 46%, but the reduction was not significant (15%) when the **digoxin** was given in capsule form (*Lanoxicaps*).[1]

Other studies in patients confirm that a 50% reduction in serum **digoxin** levels (using β-**acetyldigoxin**) occurred while using drug regimens of **cyclophosphamide**, **vincristine**, **procarbazine** and **prednisone (COPP)**; **cyclophosphamide**, **vincristine** and **prednisone (COP)**; **cyclophosphamide**, **vincristine**, **cytarabine** and **prednisone (COAP)**; and doxorubicin, **bleomycin** and **prednisone (ABP)**. These effects disappeared about a week after cytotoxic therapy.[2] Radiation has a smaller effect.[3] **Digitoxin** absorption is not affected.[4]

Mechanism

The reduced absorption is thought to result from damage to the intestinal epithelium caused by the cytotoxic agents.[5]

Importance and management

The interaction appears to be established. Patients on digoxin and receiving treatment with cytotoxic drugs should be monitored for signs of under-digitalisation. The problem can be overcome by replacing digoxin tablets with digoxin in liquid form or in solution inside a capsule. The effects of the interaction are short-lived so that a downward readjustment may be necessary about a week after treatment is withdrawn. An alternative is to use digitoxin which appears not to be affected.

1. Bjornsson TD, Huang AT, Roth P, Jacob DS, Christenson R. Effects of high-dose cancer chemotherapy on the absorption of digoxin in two different formulations. *Clin Pharmacol Ther* (1986) 39, 25–8.
2. Kuhlmann J, Zilly W, Wilke J. Effects of cytostatic drugs on plasma levels and renal excretion of β-acetyldigoxin. *Clin Pharmacol Ther* (1981) 30, 518–27.
3. Sokol GH, Greenblatt DJ, Lloyd BL, Georgotas A, Allen MD, Harmatz JS, Smith TW, Shader RI. Effect of abdominal radiation therapy on drug absorption in humans. *J Clin Pharmacol* (1978) 18, 388–96.
4. Kuhlmann J, Wilke J, Rietbrock N. Cytostatic drugs are without significant effect on digitoxin plasma level and renal excretion. *Clin Pharmacol Ther* (1982) 32, 646–51.
5. Jusko WB, Conti DR, Molson A, Kuritzky P, Giller J, Schultz R. Digoxin absorption from tablets and elixir: the effect of radiation-induced malabsorption. *JAMA* (1974) 230, 1554–5.

Digitalis glycosides + Danaparoid sodium

Digoxin and danaparoid sodium appear not to interact together adversely.

Clinical evidence, mechanism, importance and management

Danaparoid sodium (bolus injection of 3250 anti-Xa units) caused a small decrease in the AUC and serum levels of **digoxin** (250 micrograms daily for 8 days), and a small increase in the clearance of plasma anti-Xa activity in 6 healthy subjects,[1] nevertheless none of these changes appears to be clinically important. More confirmatory study of this is needed.

1. de Boer A, Stiekema JCJ, Danhof M, Moolenaar AJ, Breimer DD. Interaction of ORG 10172, a low molecular weight heparinoid, and digoxin in healthy volunteers. *Eur J Clin Pharmacol* (1991) 41, 245–50.

Digitalis glycosides + Danshen

Danshen appears not to interact with digoxin, but it can falsify the results of serum immunoassay methods.

Clinical evidence, mechanism, importance and management

Danshen appears not to have been reported to affect serum **digoxin** levels, but it can falsify laboratory measurements. A study found that a fluorescent polarization immunoassay method (Abbott Laboratories) for **digoxin** gave falsely high readings in the presence of **danshen**, whereas a microparticle enzyme immunoassay (Abbott Laboratories) gave falsely low readings. These false readings could be eliminated by monitoring the free (i.e. unbound) **digoxin** concentrations.[1]

1. Wahed A, Dasgupta A. Positive and negative in vitro interference of Chinese medicine dan shen in serum digoxin measurement. Elimination of interference by monitoring free digoxin concentration. *Am J Clin Pathol* (2001) 116, 403-8.

Digitalis glycosides + Dietary fibre (bran) and Laxatives

Bisacodyl reduces serum digoxin levels to a small extent. Large amounts of dietary fibre, guar gum and bulk-forming laxatives containing ispaghula or psyllium appear to have no significant effect on the absorption of digoxin from the gut.

Clinical evidence

(a) Digoxin + Bisacodyl

Bisacodyl reduced the mean serum **digoxin** levels of 11 healthy subjects by about 12%. When the **bisacodyl** was taken 2 h before the **digoxin**, serum **digoxin** levels were slightly raised, but not to a statistically significant extent.[1]

(b) Digoxin + Fibre (bran)

The serum **digoxin** levels of 12 patients taking 125 to 250 micrograms daily 15 to 30 min before breakfast were unchanged over a 10-day period while on a diet supplemented each day with 22 g **dietary fibre**. The **fibre** was given in this way to simulate the conditions that might be encountered clinically (for example to reduce the symptoms of diverticular disease).[2]
Wheat bran 7.5 g twice daily caused a small reduction (10%) in plasma **digoxin** levels of 14 geriatric patients after 2 weeks, but no significant change after 4 weeks.[3] **Bran fibre** 11 g caused a 6 to 7% reduction in the absorption and the steady-state serum levels of **digoxin** in 16 healthy subjects.[4] The cumulative urinary recovery of single oral doses of **digoxin** in healthy subjects was reduced almost 20% by 5 g and 15 g **fibre** respectively, whereas a normal amount of **fibre** (0.75 g) had no effect.[5,6]

(c) Digoxin + Guar gum

Guar gum 5 g (*Guarem*, 95% guar gum) reduced the peak serum levels of a single 500-microgram oral dose of **digoxin** by 21% and the AUC over 0 to 6 hours was reduced by 16% in 10 healthy subjects, but the amount excreted in the urine over 24 h was only minimally reduced.[7] **Guar gum** 18 g with a test meal did not affect steady-state plasma **digoxin** levels in 11 normal subjects on **digoxin** 1000 micrograms on day 1, then 750 micrograms on day 2, then 500 micrograms daily for 3 days.[8]

(d) Digoxin + Ispaghula or psyllium

An **ispaghula** formulation (*Vi-Siblin S*) was found to have no significant effect on serum **digoxin** levels of 16 geriatric patients.[3] The same lack of effect was seen in another study in 15 patients given 3.6 g **psyllium** (*Metamucil*) three times a day.[9]

Mechanism

Not established. Bisacodyl possibly increases the absorption of digoxin from the gut. Digoxin can bind to some extent to fibre within the gut.[10] However, *in vitro* studies (with bran, carrageenan, pectin, sodium pectinate, xylan and carboxymethylcellulose) have shown that most of the binding is reversible.[11]

Importance and management

Information seems to be limited to these reports. The reduction in serum digoxin levels caused by bisacodyl is small, probably of little clinical importance, and apparently preventable by giving the bisacodyl 2 h before the digoxin. Neither dietary fibre (bran), guar gum nor the two bulk-forming laxatives (*Vi-Siblin*, *Metamucil*) have a clinically important effect on serum digoxin levels. No special precautions would appear to be necessary.

1. Wang D-J, Chu K-M, Chen J-D. Drug interaction between digoxin and bisacodyl. *J Formosan Med Assoc* (1990) 89, 913, 915–9.
2. Woods MN, Ingelfinger JA. Lack of effect of bran on digoxin absorption. *Clin Pharmacol Ther* (1979) 26, 21–3.
3. Nordström M, Melander A, Robertsson E, Steen B. Influence of wheat bran and of a bulk-forming ispaghula cathartic on the bioavailability of digoxin in geriatric in-patients. *Drug-Nutrient Interactions* (1987) 5, 67–9.
4. Johnson BF, Rodin SM, Hoch K, Shekar V. The effect of dietary fiber on the bioavailability of digoxin in capsules. *J Clin Pharmacol* (1987) 27, 487–90.
5. Brown DD, Juhl RP, Warner SL. Decreased bioavailability of digoxin produced by dietary fiber and cholestyramine. *Am J Cardiol* (1977) 39, 297.
6. Brown DD, Juhl RP, Warner SL. Decreased bioavailability of digoxin due to hypocholesterolemic interventions. *Circulation* (1978) 58, 164.
7. Huupponen R, Seppälä P, Iisalo E. Effect of guar gum, a fibre preparation, on digoxin and penicillin absorption in man. *Eur J Clin Pharmacol* (1984) 26, 279–81.
8. Lembcke B, Häsler K, Kramer P, Caspary WF, Creuzfeldt W. Plasma digoxin concentrations during administration of dietary fibre (guar gum) in man. *Z Gastroenterologie* (1982) 20, 164–7.
9. Walan A, Bergdahl B, Skoog M-L. Study of digoxin bioavailability during treatment with a bulk forming laxative (*Metamucil*). *Scand J Gastroenterol* (1977) 12 (Suppl 45), 111.
10. Floyd RA, Greenberg WM, Caldwell C. In vitro interaction between digoxin and bran. Presented at the 12th Annual ASHP Midyear Clinical Meeting, Atlanta, Georgia, December 1977.
11. Hamamura J, Burros BC, Clemens RA, Smith CH. Dietary fiber and digoxin. *Fedn Proc* (1985) 44, 759.

Digitalis glycosides + Dihydroergocryptine

Dihydroergocryptine appears not to interact with digoxin.

Clinical evidence, mechanism, importance and management

In a randomised non-blinded crossover study, 12 healthy subjects were given single doses of **digoxin** 500 micrograms with or without α-**dihydroergocryptine** 20 mg. The pharmacokinetics of **digoxin** were not significantly affected by concomitant **dihydroergocryptine**. No clinically significant changes were seen in the ability of the heart to initiate and conduct impulses, or repolarise. The slight drop in blood pressure during the first 2 to 4 hours after **digoxin** was more pronounced with the combination treatment, but there was no evidence of impaired orthostatic blood pressure control.[1] No special precautions would seem necessary during concurrent use.

1. Retzow A, Althaus M, de Mey C, Mazur D, Vens-Cappell B. Study on the interacton of the dopamine agonist α-dihydroergocryptine with the pharmacokinetics of digoxin. *Arzneimittelforschung* (2000) 50, 591–6.

Digitalis glycosides + Diltiazem

Serum digoxin levels are reported in a number of studies to be unchanged by the concurrent use of diltiazem, but others

describe increases ranging from 20 to 85%. An approximately 20% rise in serum digitoxin levels has also been described.

Clinical evidence

(a) Digoxin

(i) Evidence of no interaction. Diltiazem 30 or 60 mg four times daily had no significant effect on the serum **digoxin** levels of 9 patients treated chronically for heart disease with 250 micrograms daily.[1] Two similar studies in 12 patients[2] and 8 healthy subjects,[3] on digoxin concurrently with 120 to 360 mg **diltiazem** daily confirmed the absence of an interaction. Two further studies in healthy subjects,[4,5] found 120 mg diltiazem daily did not affect the pharmacokinetics of a single intravenous dose of digoxin 1000 micrograms.

(ii) Evidence of an interaction. A study in 17 Japanese patients (some with rheumatic valvular disease) taking either **digoxin** or **metildigoxin (medigoxin)** found that 60 mg **diltiazem** three times daily for 2 weeks increased their serum **digoxin** levels measured at 24 h by 36 and 51% respectively.[6]

Other studies in Western patients[7,8] and healthy subjects[9-12] have shown rises of 20 to 85% in plasma **digoxin** levels while taking **diltiazem.** In one case report a 143% increase was seen.[13] The authors of two of these studies noted that the effect was highly individual with some subjects showing no increase and some a large increase.[8,10]

(b) Digitoxin

Five out of 10 patients on **digitoxin** showed a 6 to 31% (mean 21%) rise in plasma digitoxin levels while taking 180 mg **diltiazem** daily for 4 to 6 weeks.[14]

Mechanism

Not understood. In those individuals showing an interaction, falls in total digoxin clearance of about 25% have been described.[8,9,15]

Importance and management

A thoroughly investigated and well documented interaction but there is no clear explanation for the inconsistent results. All patients on digoxin given diltiazem should be well monitored for signs of over-digitalisation and dosage reductions should be made if necessary. Those most at risk are patients with digoxin levels near the top end of the range. Similar precautions would appear to be necessary with digitoxin, although the documentation of this interaction is very limited.

1. Elkayam U, Parikh K, Torkan B, Weber L, Cohen JL, Rahimtoola SH. Effect of diltiazem on renal clearance and serum concentration of digoxin in patients with cardiac disease. *Am J Cardiol* (1985) 55, 1393–5.
2. Schrager BR, Pina I, Frangi M, Applewhite S, Sequeira R, Chahine RA. Diltiazem, digoxin interaction? *Circulation* (1983) 68 (Suppl), III-368.
3. Boden WE, More G, Sharma S, Bough EW, Korr KS, Young PM, Shulman RS. No increase in serum digoxin concentrations with high dose diltiazem. *Am J Med* (1986) 81, 425–8.
4. Beltrami TR, May JJ, Bertino JS. Lack of effects of diltiazem on digoxin pharmacokinetics. *J Clin Pharmacol* (1985) 25, 390–392.
5. Jones WN, Kern KB, Rindone JP, Mayersohn M, Bliss M, Goldman S. Digoxin-diltiazem interaction: a pharmacokinetic evaluation. *Eur J Clin Pharmacol* (1986) 31, 351–3.
6. Oyama Y, Fujii S, Kanda K, Akino E, Kawasaki H, Nagata M, Goto K. Digoxin-diltiazem interaction. *Am J Cardiol* (1984) 53, 1480–1.
7. Andrejak M, Hary L, Andrjak M-Th, Lesbre J Ph. Diltiazem increases steady state digoxin serum levels in patients with cardiac disease. *J Clin Pharmacol* (1987) 27, 967–70.
8. Kuhlmann J. Effects of nifedipine and diltiazem on plasma levels and renal excretion of beta-acetyldigoxin. *Clin Pharmacol Ther* (1985) 37, 150–6.
9. Rameis H, Magometschnigg D, Ganzinger U. The diltiazem-digoxin interaction. *Clin Pharmacol Ther* (1984) 36, 183–9.
10. North DS, Mattern AL, Hiser WW. The influence of diltiazem hydrochloride on trough serum digoxin levels. *Drug Intell Clin Pharm* (1986) 20, 500–3.
11. Gallet M, Aupetit JF, Lopez M, Manchon J, Lestaevel M, Lefrancois JJ. Interaction diltiazem-digoxine. Évolution de la digoxinémie et des paramtres électrocardiographiques chez le sujet sain. *Arch Mal Coeur* (1986) 79, 1216–20.
12. Larman RC. A pharmacokinetic evaluation of the digoxin-diltiazem interaction. *J Pharm Sci* (1987) 76, S79.
13. King T, Mallet L. Diltiazem-digoxin interaction in an elderly woman: a case report. *J Geriatr Drug Ther* (1991) 5, 79–83.
14. Kuhlmann J. Effects of verapamil, diltiazem, and nifedipine on plasma levels and renal excretion of digitoxin. *Clin Pharmacol Ther* (1985) 38, 667–73.
15. Yoshida A, Fujita M, Kurosawa N, Nioka M, Shichinohe T, Arakawa M, Fukuda R, Owada E, Ito K. Effects of diltiazem on plasma level and urinary excretion of digoxin in healthy subjects. *Clin Pharmacol Ther* (1984) 35, 681–5.

Digitalis glycosides + Diprafenone

Diprafenone caused a rise in serum digoxin levels.

Clinical evidence

Twelve healthy subjects were given **digoxin** 500 micrograms daily alone for a week, then **digoxin** plus **diprafenone** 300 mg daily for a week, and finally **digoxin** alone for a further week. The **diprafenone** caused a 14% increase in trough serum **digoxin** levels (from 1.4 to 1.6 ng/ml), a 41% increase in peak steady-state serum levels (from 3.9 to 5.5 ng/ml) and an increase in the AUC of 17% (from 41 to 48 ng.h/ml). When the **diprafenone** was stopped the serum **digoxin** concentrations returned to their former levels.[1]

Mechanism

It is believed that the diprafenone reduces the excretion of digoxin by the kidneys.

Importance and management

Information is limited but the interaction appears to be established. The rise in serum digoxin levels (40%) and in its AUC (almost 20%) may possibly be enough to cause problems, for which reason be alert for the need to reduce the digoxin dosage in the presence of diprafenone. Monitor well. More study is needed to confirm this interaction and to establish its clinical importance.

1. Koytchev R, Alken R-G, Mayer O. Effect of diprafenone on the pharmacokinetics of digoxin. *Eur J Clin Pharmacol* (1996) 50, 97–100.

Digitalis glycosides + Disopyramide or Procainamide

Neither disopyramide nor procainamide normally cause a significant change in serum digoxin levels. A single report describes intoxication in a patient on digitoxin and disopyramide.

Clinical evidence, mechanism, importance and management

(a) Disopyramide

A number of studies have clearly shown that **disopyramide** causes only a very small increase or no increase at all in the serum concentrations of **digoxin**.[1-6] A small but insignificant reduction in systolic time intervals has been seen[7] but the weight of evidence suggests that no adverse interaction occurs if these drugs are used together. However a very brief report describes intoxication and serious arrhythmia in one patient given **digitoxin** and **disopyramide**.[8]

(b) Procainamide

A study in patients who had been taking **digoxin** for at least 7 days showed that while taking **procainamide** their serum **digoxin** levels remained unaltered.[2,9] However, it should be noted that the makers of **procainamide** say that, in digitalis intoxication, procainamide may further depress conduction, which may result in ventricular asystole or fibrillation.[10] Considerable care and good monitoring would therefore seem necessary if both drugs are used.

1. Doering W. Quinidine-digoxin interaction. *N Engl J Med* (1979) 301, 400–4.
2. Leahey EB, Reiffel JA, Giardina E-GV, Bigger JT. The effect of quinidine and other oral antiarrhythmic drugs on serum digoxin: a prospective study. *Ann Intern Med* (1980) 92, 605–8.
3. Manolas EG, Hunt D, Sloman G. Effects of quinidine and disopyramide on serum digoxin concentrations. *Aust N Z J Med* (1980) 10, 426–9.
4. Wellens HJ, Gorgels AP, Braat SJ, Bär FW, Vanagt EJ, Phaf B. Effect of oral disopyramide on serum digoxin levels. A prospective study. *Am Heart J* (1980) 100, 934–5.
5. Risler T, Burk M, Peters U, Grabensee B, Seipel L. On the interaction between digoxin and disopyramide. *Clin Pharmacol Ther* (1983) 34, 176–80.
6. García-Barreto D, Groning E, González-Gómez A, Pérez A, Hernández-Cañero A, Toruncha A. Enhancement of the antiarrhythmic action of disopyramide by digoxin. *J Cardiovasc Pharmacol* (1981) 3, 1236–42.

7. Elliott HL, Kelman AW, Sumner DJ, Bryson SM, Campbell BC, Hillis WS, Whiting B. Pharmacodynamic and pharmacokinetic evaluation of the interaction between digoxin and disopyramide. *Br J Clin Pharmacol* (1982) 14, 141P.

8. Manchon ND, Bercoff E, Lemarchand P, Chassagne P, Senant J, Bourreille J. Fréquence et gravité des interactions médicamenteuses dans une population âgée: étude prospective concernant 63 malades. *Rev Med Interne* (1989) 10, 521–5.

9. Leahey EB, Giardina EGV, Reiffel JA, Bigger JT. Serum digoxin concentrations during administration of oral antiarrhythmic drugs. *Clin Res* (1978) 26, 602A.

10. Pronestyl (Procainamide).E.R. Squibb & Sons Ltd. ABPI Datasheet Compendium 1999–2000, 1649–51.

Digitalis glycosides + Diuretics, potassium-depleting

It is generally believed, but not unequivocally established, that the potassium loss caused by potassium-depleting diuretics (see Table 14.2) increases the toxicity of the digitalis glycosides. It is common practice to give these diuretics with potassium supplements or potassium-sparing diuretics.

Clinical evidence

(a) Evidence of an interaction

A comparative study[1] of the medical records of 418 patients on digitalis over the period 1950 to 1952, and of 679 patients over the period 1964 to 1966, showed that the incidence of digitalis toxicity had more than doubled. Of the earlier group 8.6% showed toxicity (58% on diuretics, mainly of the **organomercurial type**) compared with 17.17% of the latter group (81% taking diuretics, mainly the **chlorothiazides, furosemide (frusemide), etacrynic acid, chlortalidone**). It was concluded that the increased toxicity was related to the increased usage of potassium-depleting diuretics.

A retrospective study[2] of over 400 patients on **digoxin** showed that almost one in five had some toxic reactions attributable to the use of the glycoside. Of these 16% had demonstrable hypokalaemia (serum potassium less than 3.5 mEq/l). Almost half of the patients who showed toxicity were taking potassium-depleting diuretics, notably **hydrochlorothiazide** or **furosemide**. Similar results were found in other studies[3-9] in a considerable number of patients. There are other reports not listed here. In addition there is also some evidence that **furosemide** may raise serum **digoxin** levels,[10] however two other studies found no evidence that **furosemide** affects the urinary excretion of **digoxin**.[11,12]

(b) Evidence of no interaction

A retrospective study of patients who developed digitalis toxicity showed that the likelihood of its development in those with potassium levels below 3.5 mEq/l was no greater than those with normal potassium levels.[13]

Two other studies in a total of almost 200 patients failed to detect any association between the development of digitalis toxicity and the use of diuretics or changes in potassium levels.[14,15]

Mechanism

Not fully understood. The cardiac glycosides inhibit sodium-potassium ATP-ase which is concerned with the transport of sodium and potassium ions across the membranes of the myocardial cells, and this is associated with an increase in the availability of calcium ions concerned with the contraction of the cells. Potassium loss caused by these diuretics exacerbates the potassium loss from the myocardial cells, thereby increasing the activity and the toxicity of the digitalis. Some loss of magnesium may also have a part to play. The mechanism of this interaction is still being debated.

Importance and management

A direct link between the use of these diuretics and the development of digitalis toxicity is not established beyond doubt, but current thinking favours the belief that concurrent use can result in digitalis intoxication. Because it is only a short step from effective therapy with digitalis to a state of intoxication, those given potassium-depleting diuretics should be well monitored for signs of toxicity. Ideally serum potassium and magnesium levels should be monitored. One of the problems is that serum potassium levels and body stores of potassium are not uniformly correlated. If necessary potassium supplements should be given. It may be possible to do this with foods which are high in potassium but low in sodium (citrus fruits, bananas, peaches, dates, wheat germ, potatoes). An alternative is to use a potassium-sparing diuretic such as triamterene or spironolactone.

1. Jørgenson AW, Sørensen OH. Digitalis intoxication. A comparative study on the incidence of digitalis intoxication during the periods 1950–52 and 1964–66. *Acta Med Scand* (1970) 188, 179–83.

2. Shapiro S, Slone D, Lewis GP, Jick H. The epidemiology of digoxin. A study in three Boston Hospitals. *J Chron Dis* (1969) 22, 361–71.

3. Tawakkol AA, Nutter DO, Massumi RA. A prospective study of digitalis toxicity in a large city hospital. *Med Ann D C* (1967) 36, 402.

4. Soffer A. The changing clinical picture of digitalis intoxication. *Arch Intern Med* (1961) 107, 681–8.

5. Rodensky PL, Wasserman F. Observations on digitalis intoxication. *Arch Intern Med* (1961) 108, 171-88.

6. Steiness E, Olesen KH. Cardiac arrhythmias induced by hypokalaemia and potassium loss during maintenance digoxin therapy. *Br Heart J* (1976) 38, 167–72.

7. Binnion PF. Hypokalaemia and digoxin-induced arrhythmias. *Lancet* (1975) i, 343–4.

8. Poole-Wilson PA, Hall R, Cameron IR. Hypokalaemia, digitalis and arrhythmias. *Lancet* (1975) i, 575–6.

9. Shapiro W, Taubert K. Hypokalaemia and digoxin-induced arrhythmias. *Lancet* (1975) ii, 604–5.

10. Tsutsumi E, Fujiki H, Takeda H, Fukushima H. Effect of furosemide on serum clearance and renal excretion of digoxin. *J Clin Pharmacol* (1979) 19, 200–204.

11. Malcolm AD, Leung FY, Fuchs JCA, Duarte JE. Digoxin kinetics during furosemide administration. *Clin Pharmacol Ther* (1977) 21, 567–574.

12. Brown DD, Dormois JC, Abraham GN, Lewis K, Dixon K. Effect of furosemide on the renal excretion of digoxin. *Clin Pharmacol Ther* (1976) 20, 395–400.

13. Ogilvie RI, Ruedy J. An educational program in digitalis therapy. *JAMA* (1972) 222, 50–55.

14. Smith TW, Haber E. Digoxin intoxication: the relationship of clinical presentation to serum digoxin concentration. *J Clin Invest* (1970) 49, 2377–86.

15. Beller GA, Smith TW, Abelmann WH, Haber E, Hood WB. Digitalis intoxication. A prospective clinical study with serum level correlations. *N Engl J Med* (1971) 284, 989–97.

Table 14.2 Potassium-depleting diuretics

Carbonic anhydrase inhibitors	Acetazolamide, diclofenamide (dichlorphenamide), disulfamide (disulphamide), ethoxzolamide, methazolamide
Loop diuretics	Azosemide, bumetanide, etacrynic acid (ethacrynic acid), etozolin, furosemide (frusemide), muzolimine, piretanide, torasemide
Organomercurials	Chlormerodrin, meraluride, mercaptomerin
Thiazides and related diuretics	Althiazide, ambuside, bemetizide, bendroflumethiazide (bendrofluazide), benzthiazide, benzylhydrochlorothiazide, buthiazide, chlorothiazide, chlortalidone (chlorthalidone), clopamide, clorexolone, cyclopenthiazide, cyclothiazide, epithiazide, ethiazide, fenquizone, hydrobentizide, hydrochlorothiazide, hydroflumethiazide, indapamide, mebutizide, mefruside, methylclothiazide, meticrane, metolazone, polythiazide, quinethazone, teclothiazide, trichlormethiazide, xipamide

Digitalis glycosides + Edrophonium

Excessive bradycardia and AV-block may occur in patients on digitalis glycosides given edrophonium.

Clinical evidence, mechanism, importance and management

The rapid intravenous injection of 10 mg **edrophonium** has been used in the differentiation of cardiac arrhythmias, but in one study, 4 of 10 digitalised patients given edrophonium developed atrial tachycardia with AV block. The effect was transient; recovery of baseline ECGs occurred 15 to 20 mins after administration.[1] Nevertheless, the authors recommended that edrophonium should not be given to patients with atrial flutter or tachycardia who are taking digitalis glycosides. This recommendation is reinforced by the case of an elderly woman[2] who developed bradycardia, AV block and asystole following concurrent use. She recovered after being given atropine 1 mg.

1. Reddy RCV, Gould L, Gomprecht RF. Use of edrophonium (Tensilon) in the evaluation of cardiac arrhythmias. *Am Heart J* (1971) 82, 742–9.
2. Gould L, Zahir M, Gomprecht RF. Cardiac arrest during edrophonium administration. *Am Heart J* (1971) 81, 437–8.

Digitalis glycosides + Enoximone

Enoximone does not affect the plasma levels of either digoxin or digitoxin.

Clinical evidence, mechanism, importance and management

Studies in patients on long-term treatment with digitalis glycosides (**digoxin** or **digitoxin**) showed that the concurrent use of oral **enoximone**, 100 mg three times daily for a week, had no significant effect on the plasma levels of either of these glycosides.[1,2] Cardiac function was improved. No special precautions seem necessary.

1. Glauner T, Hertrich F, Winkelmann B, Dieterich HA, Trenk D, Jähnchen E. Lack of effect of enoximone on steady-state plasma concentrations of digoxin and digitoxin. *Eur Heart J* (1988) 9 (Suppl 1), 151.
2. Trenk D, Hertrich F, Winkelmann B, Glauner T, Dieterich HA, Jähnchen E. Lack of effect of enoximone on the pharmacokinetics of digoxin in patients with congestive heart failure. *J Clin Pharmacol* (1990) 30, 235–40.

Digitalis glycosides + Fenoldopam

Fenoldopam appears to cause a small and clinically unimportant reduction in serum digoxin levels in most patients, but more marked changes may occur in a few individuals.

Clinical evidence, mechanism, importance and management

Ten patients with congestive heart failure on chronic **digoxin** treatment (doses not stated) were additionally given 100 mg **fenoldopam** three times daily for 9 days. The mean AUC and steady-state **digoxin** levels were reduced by about 20%. In two patients, the steady-state serum levels of digoxin fell by 48% (from 1.36 to 0.71 ng/ml) and 68% (from 1.93 to 0.61 ng/ml), respectively, and in a further patient, rose by 45% (from 1.03 to 1.49 ng/ml).[1] Most patients appear therefore not to show marked changes in serum **digoxin** levels, but a few individuals may possibly need some dosage adjustment. Monitor the effects of concurrent use.

1. Strocchi E, Tartagni F, Malini PL, Valtancoli G, Ambrosioni E, Pasinelli F, Riva E, Fuccella LM. Interaction study of fenoldopam-digoxin in congestive heart failure. *Eur J Clin Pharmacol* (1989) 37, 395–7.

Digitalis glycosides + Flecainide

Plasma digoxin levels are unaltered or only modestly increased by the use of flecainide, but this is not likely to be important in most patients.

Clinical evidence

While taking 100 to 200 mg **flecainide** twice daily for 7 days the plasma **digoxin** levels of 10 patients with congestive heart failure remained unaltered. The same result was seen in 4 patients over a 4-week period.[1]

In contrast, a study in 15 healthy subjects showed that while taking 200 mg **flecainide** twice daily, their plasma **digoxin** levels measured just before and 6 h after taking a daily dose of **digoxin** 250 micrograms rose by 24% and 13% respectively.[2] The changes observed in vital signs were not clinically significant. In a single-dose study the steady-state **digoxin** levels were predicted to rise about 15% while taking 200 mg **flecainide** twice daily.[3]

Mechanism

Uncertain. It is suggested that any changes may be due to alterations in the volume of distribution.[3]

Importance and management

Documentation is limited but what is known suggests that either no interaction occurs, or any changes are small and unlikely to be clinically relevant in most patients. However the authors of one of the reports[2] suggest that patients with high drug levels, atrioventricular nodal dysfunction, or both, should be monitored during concurrent treatment.

1. McQuinn RL, Kvam DC, Parrish SL, Fox TL, Miller AM, Franciosa JA. Digoxin levels in patients with congestive heart failure are not altered by flecainide. *Clin Pharmacol Ther* (1988) 43, 150.
2. Weeks CE, Conard GJ, Kvam DC, Fox JM, Chang SF, Paone RP, Lewis GP. The effect of flecainide acetate, a new antiarrhythmic, on plasma digoxin levels. *J Clin Pharmacol* (1986) 26, 27–31.
3. Tjandramaga TB, Verbesselt R, Van Hecken A, Mullie A, De Schepper PJ. Oral digoxin pharmacokinetics during multiple-dose flecainide treatment. *Arch Int Pharmacodyn Ther* (1982) 260, 302–3.

Digitalis glycosides + Guanadrel

Guanadrel did not affect the pharmacokinetics of a single dose of digoxin.

Clinical evidence, mechanism, importance and management

No change in the pharmacokinetics of a single intravenous dose of **digoxin** occurred in 13 healthy subjects after taking 10 mg **guanadrel sulphate** orally every 12 h for 3 days before and 5 days after the digoxin dose. One subject experienced a 10 min episode of asymptomatic second degree heart block (Wenckebach) 3 h after the dose of **digoxin**, the reason for which was not clear.[1] There seem to be no reports of adverse interactions between the digitalis glycosides and any of the guanethidine-like antihypertensive drugs.

1. Wright CE, Andreadis NA. Digoxin pharmacokinetics when administered concurrently with guanadrel sulfate. *Drug Intell Clin Pharm* (1986) 20, 465.

Digitalis glycosides + Hydroxychloroquine or Chloroquine

The blood levels of digoxin were found to be markedly increased (+70%) in two elderly patients while they were treated with hydroxychloroquine. A similar increase has been seen with chloroquine in *dogs*.

Clinical evidence, mechanism, importance and management

Two women of 65 and 68 who had been taking **digoxin** 250 micrograms daily for 2 to 3 years for arrhythmias were concurrently treated with **hydroxychloroquine** 250 mg twice daily for rheumatoid arthritis. When the **hydroxychloroquine** was withdrawn the plasma **digoxin** levels of both women fell by 70 to 75% (from 3 to 0.7 nmol/l and from 3.1 to 0.9 nmol/l respectively). Neither showed any evidence of intoxication during concurrent use, and one of them claimed that the regularity of her heart rhythm had been improved.[1] The reason for this apparent interaction is not understood. It would now seem prudent to check on the effects of adding or withdrawing **hydroxychloroquine** in any patient on **digoxin**. No interaction between digoxin and **chloroquine** has been described in man, but increases (+77%) in peak serum **digoxin** levels have been seen in *dogs*.[2]

1. Leden I. Digoxin-hydroxychloroquine interaction? *Acta Med Scand* (1982) 211, 411–12.
2. McElnay JC, Sidahmed AM, D'Arcy PF and McQuade RD. Chloroquine-digoxin interaction. *Int J Pharmaceutics* (1985) 26, 267–74.

Digitalis glycosides + Itraconazole

Itraconazole can cause a marked increase in serum digoxin levels. Toxicity may occur unless the digoxin dosage is suitably reduced. Itraconazole may also oppose the positive inotropic effects of digoxin.

Clinical evidence

In a double-blind placebo-controlled crossover study 10 healthy subjects taking 250 micrograms **digoxin** daily were given either 200 mg **itraconazole** or a placebo daily for 10 days, and then the two were swapped over for a further 10 days. The serum digoxin levels of those first given the **itraconazole** fell from 1.7 to 1.0 nmol/l during the placebo period, while the others showed a rise from 0.9 to 1.8 nmol/l during the **itraconazole** period. Neither group achieved steady-state serum **digoxin** levels during the 10-day period (i.e. the graph showed that serum **digoxin** levels were still steadily climbing while taking the **itraconazole**).[1]

A man of 68 on **digoxin** 250 micrograms twice daily and ibuprofen developed nausea and fatigue (interpreted later as **digoxin** toxicity) after starting 400 mg **itraconazole** daily for an infected elbow. The symptoms disappeared when both the **itraconazole** and ibuprofen were stopped, but returned when the **itraconazole** was restarted. After 7 days his heart rate had fallen from 60 to 40 bpm and his **digoxin** level had doubled (from 1.6 to 3.2 ng/ml). He was later satisfactorily restabilised on a quarter of the **digoxin** dosage (125 micrograms daily)while taking the same dose of **itraconazole**.[2] Six other patients developed **digoxin** toxicity after taking **itraconazole** for 9 to 13 days.[3-8] The serum **digoxin** levels of 2 of them had roughly doubled and another showed a sixfold increase. Two[2,3] were restabilised on a quarter of the previous **digoxin** dosage while one of the others was restabilised on 40% of the previous dosage.[4] A further study in 3 patients with congestive heart failure found ECG changes (PVC, AV block and ST depression) during concurrent administration, and digoxin dose reductions of 50% were calculated to be required.[9] Six other cases of this interaction are reported briefly.[4]

Mechanism

Not understood. Decreased digoxin urinary clearance has been suggested.[4,10] Another suggestion is that itraconazole inhibits the action of P-glycoprotein which transports digoxin out of kidney tubule cells into the urine.[11]

Importance and management

An established and clinically important interaction of uncertain incidence but probably affecting most patients. Monitor the effects if itraconazole is started, anticipating the need to reduce the digoxin

dosage. Halving the dose was suggested in one study.[9] Two of the patients cited above were restabilised on a quarter of the digoxin dosage[2,3] and another on about one-third while taking itraconazole[4] and other patients may possibly need even greater reductions More recent findings suggest that itraconazole may possess significant negative inotropic properties, and that it should be used with caution in patients at risk of heart failure.[12] This suggests that itraconazole would oppose the pharmacological effects of digoxin.

1. Jalava K-M, Partanen J, Neuvonen PJ. Digoxin-itraconazole interaction. *Therapie* (1995) 50 (Suppl), 185.
2. Rex J. Itraconazole-digoxin interaction. *Ann Intern Med* (1992) 116, 525.
3. Kauffman CA, Bagnasco FA. Digoxin toxicity associated with itraconazole therapy. *Clin Infect Dis* (1992) 15, 886–7.
4. Sachs MK, Blanchard LM, Green PJ. Interaction of itraconazole and digoxin. *Clin Infect Dis* (1993) 16, 400–3.
5. Alderman CP, Jersmann HPA. Digoxin-itraconazole interaction. *Med J Aust* (1993) 159, 838–9.
6. McClean KL, Sheehan GJ. Interaction between itraconazole and digoxin. *Clin Infect Dis* (1994) 18, 259–60.
7. Meyboom RH, de Jonge K, Veentjer H, Dekens-Konter JA, de Koning GH. Potentiering van digoxine door itraconazol. *Ned Tijdschr Geneeskd* (1994) 138, 2353–6.
8. Cone LA, Himelman RB, Hirschberg JN, Hutcheson JW. Itraconazole-related amaurosis and vomiting due to digoxin toxicity. *West J Med* (1996) 165, 322.
9. Wagasugi H, Isizuka R, Koreeda N, Yano I, Futami T, Nohara R, Sasayoma S, Inui K. Effect of itraconazole on digoxin clearance in patients with congestive heart failure. *Yakugahu Zasshi* (2000) 120, 807–11.
10. Alderman CP, Allcroft PD. Digoxin-itraconazole interaction: possible mechanisms. *Ann Pharmacother* (1997) 31, 438–40.
11. Ito S, Koren G. Comment: possible mechanism of digoxin-itraconazole interaction. *Ann Pharmacother* (1997) 31, 1091–2.
12. Committee on Safety of Medicines/Medicines Control Agency. Cardiodepressant effects of itraconazole. *Current Problems* (2001) 27, 11.

Digitalis glycosides + Kaolin-pectin

Plasma digoxin levels can be reduced by kaolin-pectin, but the reduction is small and probably of minimal clinical importance. The interaction can be avoided by taking the two drugs 2 h apart, or by giving the digoxin in liquid or capsule form.

Clinical evidence

The concurrent use of **kaolin-pectin** suspension and **digoxin** reduced the peak plasma **digoxin** levels of 7 patients by 36%, while the $AUC_{0-24\ h}$ was reduced by 15%. Conversely, when two doses of **kaolin-pectin** were taken, one 2 h before and the other 2 h after the **digoxin**, no significant changes were seen.[1]

Single dose studies have found 42% and 62% reductions in the bioavailability of **digoxin** caused by **kaolin-pectin**.[2,3] Another study showed an interaction with **digoxin** tablets but not with **digoxin** capsules.[4]

Mechanism

Not understood. The digoxin may possibly become adsorbed onto the kaolin so that less is available for absorption. Another possibility is that the kaolin reduces the motility of the gut which normally increases mixing and brings the digoxin into contact with the absorbing surface.

Importance and management

Steady-state studies reflect the every-day situation much more closely than single dose studies, and the one cited above[1] indicates that the total reduction in digoxin absorption is small (15%). This is unlikely to be of clinical importance, however the interaction can in any case be avoided by separating the dosages (in any order) by 2 h, or by giving the digoxin in capsule or liquid form.

1. Albert KS, Elliott WJ, Abbott RD, Gilbertson TJ, Data JL. Influence of kaolin-pectin suspension on steady-state plasma digoxin levels. *J Clin Pharmacol* (1981) 21, 449–55.
2. Brown DD, Juhl RP, Lewis K, Schrott M, Bartels B. Decreased bioavailability of digoxin due to antacids and kaolin-pectin. *N Engl J Med* (1976) 295, 1034–7.
3. Albert KS, Ayres JW, Disanto AR, Weidler DJ, Sakmar E, Hallmark MR, Stoll RG, DeSante KA, Wagner JG. Influence of kaolin-pectin suspension on digoxin bioavailability. *J Pharm Sci* (1978) 67, 1582–6.
4. Allen MD, Greenblatt DJ, Harmatz JS, Smith TW. Effect of magnesium aluminum hydroxide and kaolin-pectin on absorption of digoxin from tablets and capsules. *J Clin Pharmacol* (1981) 21, 26–30.

Digitalis glycosides + Ketanserin

Experimental evidence suggests that ketanserin is unlikely to affect the serum levels of either digoxin or digitoxin.

Clinical evidence, mechanism, importance and management

Ketanserin 40 mg twice daily did not cause significant changes in the pharmacokinetics of single doses of either **digoxin** 1250 micrograms or **digitoxin** 1000 micrograms in healthy subjects, and it is concluded that ketanserin is unlikely to alter serum concentrations of either glycoside during clinical use.[1]

1. Ochs HR, Verburg-Ochs B, Höller M, Greenblatt DJ. Effect of ketanserin on the kinetics of digoxin and digitoxin. *J Cardiovasc Pharmacol* (1985) 7, 205–7.

Digitalis glycosides + Levetiracetam

Levetiracetam does not appear to interact with digoxin.

Clinical evidence, mechanism, importance and management

A double-blind, crossover, placebo-controlled study in 11 healthy subjects given an initial loading dose of **digoxin** 500 micrograms followed by 250 micrograms daily found that **levetiracetam** 1 g twice daily for one week did not significantly affect the pharmacokinetics or pharmacodynamics of **digoxin**. Also the pharmacokinetics of levetiracetam were not significantly altered by **digoxin**.[1] No special precautions seem necessary.

1. Levy RH, Ragueneau-Majlessi I, Baltes E. Repeated administration of the novel antiepileptic agent levetiracetam does not alter digoxin pharmacokinetics and pharmacodynamics in healthy volunteers. *Epilepsia* (2000) 41 (Suppl 7), 227–8.

Digitalis glycosides + Lithium

No pharmacokinetic interaction occurs between digoxin and lithium but the addition of digoxin to lithium possibly has a detrimental short-term effect on the control of mania. An isolated report describes severe bradycardia in one patient given both drugs.

Clinical evidence, mechanism, importance and management

A study in 6 healthy subjects taking **lithium carbonate** sufficient to achieve mean steady-state serum levels of 0.76 mmol/l (range 0.4 to 1 mmol/l) showed that the pharmacokinetics of **digoxin** 750 micrograms given intravenously were unchanged, and that there were no significant effects on sodium pump activity or electrolyte concentrations.[1] However an experimental 7-day study in patients with manic-depressive psychoses found that there was a greater improvement in those given **lithium** plus placebo than those given **lithium** plus **digoxin**. This may be a reflection of changes in Na-K ATPase.[2] An isolated report describes tremor, confusion and severe nodal bradycardia in a patient given both drugs. The bradycardia worsened (30 bpm) even after both drugs were stopped.[3] The clinical significance of all of these findings is uncertain. More study is needed.

1. Cooper SJ, Kelly JG, Johnston GD, Copeland S, King DJ, McDevitt DG. Pharmacodynamics and pharmacokinetics of digoxin in the presence of lithium. *Br J Clin Pharmacol* (1984) 18, 21–5.
2. Chambers CA, Smith AHW, Naylor GJ. The effect of digoxin on the response to lithium therapy in mania. *Psychol Med* (1982) 12, 57–60.
3. Winters WD, Ralph DD. Digoxin-lithium drug interaction. *Clin Toxicol* (1977) 10, 487–8.

Digitalis glycosides + Macrogol 4000

Single dose studies show that macrogol 4000, a laxative polymer, reduces the serum levels of digoxin.

Clinical evidence, mechanism, importance and management

An open, randomised, two-way crossover study in 18 healthy subjects found that 20 g **macrogol 4000** daily over an 8-day period reduced the maximum serum levels of **digoxin** by 40% following a single 500-microgram dose, and reduced the AUC by 30%. Heart rates and the PR interval were unchanged. The reason for this interaction is thought to be that the absorption of the **digoxin** is reduced.[1] The importance of this interaction awaits further assessment, but reductions in **digoxin** levels of this size are likely to be clinically relevant. If **macrogol 4000** is given with **digoxin**, be alert for the need to increase the **digoxin** dosage. Study is needed to assess the effects of this interaction on steady-state **digoxin** levels.

1. Ragueneau I, Poirier J-M, Radembino N, Sao AB, Funck-Brentano C, Jaillon P. Pharmacokinetic and pharmacodynamic drug interactions between digoxin and macrogol 4000, a laxative polymer, in healthy volunteers. *Br J Clin Pharmacol* (1999) 48, 453–6.

Digitalis glycosides + Macrolide antibacterials

A few patients can unpredictably show a rapid and marked increase in serum digoxin levels (two to fourfold) if given azithromycin, clarithromycin, erythromycin or roxithromycin. The same interaction has been seen with digitoxin and azithromycin. Digitalis intoxication can occur.

Clinical evidence

(a) Digitoxin + Azithromycin

A man with congestive heart failure on **digitoxin** 70 micrograms daily for 5 days of each week, and enalapril and furosemide (frusemide), was admitted to hospital with nausea and bradycardia (26 bpm) 4 days after starting a 3-day course of **azithromycin** (dosage not started). His serum **digitoxin** levels were found to be raised from his usual baseline range of 13 to 25 nmol/l to 44 nmol/l. His renal function was normal. The serum **digitoxin** levels of another patient treated with 250 micrograms intravenously once daily showed a marked rise from his steady-state range of 15 to 20 nmol/l after being given 500 mg **azithromycin** daily for 3 days. The **digitoxin** was withdrawn one day later but even so the levels climbed to a peak of 41.9 nmol/l after a further 3 days and remained in the toxic range for yet another 3 days.[1]

(b) Digoxin + Azithromycin

A 31-month-old boy with Down's syndrome and tetralogy of Fallot (a congenital heart defect resulting in reduced blood flow to the lungs) was discharged from hospital after repair of his heart defect. He was on **digoxin** 60 micrograms twice daily, furosemide, and potassium chloride. Eight days later when readmitted with symptoms of heart failure, intermittent fever and wheezing he was started on **azithromycin** (10 mg/kg on day 1, then 50 mg/kg daily for 4 days) was given. Three days later his steady-state serum **digoxin** levels had risen from 1.79 to 2.37 ng/ml and he experienced anorexia, nausea, and second degree atrioventricular block. All the symptoms resolved when the **digoxin** was withdrawn **Digoxin** was restarted at 50 micrograms twice daily after the **azithromycin** course was completed and steady-state **digoxin** levels of 1.42 ng/ml were noted.[2]

The makers of **azithromycin** say that, as of October 2000, there were 230 cases of the concomitant use of **azithromycin** and **digoxin** on their database. Of these, 78 cases had adverse events indicating possible digoxin toxicity. However on review, 21 cases were clearly excluded. Of the remaining cases, only 13 provided **digoxin** levels, and of these high serum **digoxin** concentrations were reported in 6, but generally, insufficient data made interpretation difficult.[3] The makers concluded that the possibility that a patient may experience an increase in digoxin concentrations during concurrent **azithromycin** therapy cannot be entirely excluded.

(c) Digoxin + Clarithromycin

A woman on warfarin, heparin, carbamazepine and **digoxin** was admitted to hospital with syncope, vomiting and an irregular heart rhythm shortly after starting 1 g **clarithromycin** daily. Her serum **digoxin** levels were found to be raised. The **clarithromycin** was decreased, the carbamazepine and **digoxin** stopped, and she was treated with digoxin-specific antibody fragments *(Digibind)* and intravenous fluids. Her serum **digoxin** levels fell again and the digitalis toxicity disappeared.[4]

Another woman of 81 developed elevated serum **digoxin** levels (increased about fourfold) within four days of starting 500 mg **clarithromycin** twice daily.[5] Another similar case in a 77-year-old man is described elsewhere.[6] A threefold rise in digoxin levels with toxicity was seen in a 66-year-old AIDS patient after taking 500 mg **clarithromycin** twice daily for 17 days,[7] and a similar rise was seen in a 91-year-old man after taking 1 g **clarithromycin** daily for 9 days.[8] Elevated serum **digoxin** levels and toxicity were seen in an 87-year-old man a few days after starting **clarithromycin** 1 g daily. After restabilisation toxicity occurred again within 2 days of re-introducing the **clarithromycin**.[9] The makers of **clarithromycin** have a few other cases on their records of raised **digoxin** levels in patients following treatment with **clarithromycin**[4] and there are other reports of this interaction in the literature.[10-17]

(d) Digoxin + Erythromycin

An elderly woman with a prosthetic heart valve being treated for left ventricular dysfunction with warfarin, furosemide (frusemide), hydralazine, isosorbide dinitrate and **digoxin**, was given **erythromycin** therapy. She took only four 250-mg doses. Four days later her serum **digoxin** levels were found to have risen to 2.6 ng/ml from a normal steady-state range of 1.4 to 1.7 ng/ml, and she showed evidence of digitalis intoxication.[18]

This report is in line with a previous report describing 2 patients on 500 micrograms **digoxin** daily whose serum **digoxin** levels roughly doubled after 5 days of **erythromycin** (1 to 2 g daily).[19] A patient on **digoxin** developed signs of toxicity (nausea, vomiting, cardiac arrhythmias) within 4 days of starting to take 500 mg **erythromycin** three times daily. Her serum **digoxin** levels were elevated. This patient recalled having similar problems during a previous course of **erythromycin**.[20] Another patient given 250 mg **erythromycin** 6-hourly similarly showed elevated serum **digoxin** levels within 6 days.[21] A study in a man who was resistant to **digoxin** found that 1 g **erythromycin** daily increased AUC of digoxin by 300%.[22]

(e) Digoxin + Rokitamycin

Rokitamycin did not affect serum **digoxin** levels in a study in 10 subjects.[23]

(f) Digoxin + Roxithromycin

A woman of 76 on **digoxin** and a number of other drugs (enalapril, isosorbide mononitrate, furosemide (frusemide), diltiazem, glyceryl trinitrate, slow-release potassium, prednisolone, omeprazole, calcitriol) developed signs of digitalis intoxication (nausea, vomiting, first degree heart block) within 4 days of starting 150 mg **roxithromycin** twice daily. Her serum **digoxin** levels were found to be raised about fourfold. She was later discharged on a lower dosage of **digoxin** and all of the other drugs except **roxithromycin**.[24]

Mechanism

Up to 10% of patients on oral digoxin excrete it in substantial amounts in the faeces and urine as inactive metabolites (digoxin reduction products or DRPs). This metabolism seems to be the responsibility of the gut flora,[19] in particular *Eubacterium lentum*, which is anaerobic and Gram positive.[21,25] In the presence of antibacterials that inhibit this organism, much more digoxin becomes available for absorption, which results in a marked rise in serum levels. At the same time the inactive metabolites derived from the gut disappear.[19,26] However, it is worth noting that most classes of antibacterials do not appear to interact with digoxin despite inhibiting *E. lentum in vitro*.[25] See also 'Digitalis glycosides + Beta-lactam antibacterials', p.534. An alternative explanation for the digoxin/erythromycin and clarithromycin interactions, is that the antibacterials inhibit the intestinal[27] or renal[14] P-glycoprotein transport of digoxin. None of these suggested mechanisms may be the whole story. The same mechanism(s) probably also explain the digitoxin/azithromycin interaction.[25]

Importance and management

The digoxin/clarithromycin and digoxin/erythromycin interactions appear to be established but unpredictable. Information is limited to a relatively small number of patients, and there is only one report about digoxin/roxithromycin. Since only a small proportion of patients (up to 10%) is likely to be at risk and the 'excreter' category of any particular patient is probably not known (see Mechanism), it is important to monitor all patients well for signs of increased digoxin effects when any of these macrolide antibacterials is first given, reducing the digoxin dosage as necessary. It has been suggested that the elderly may be more susceptible because of a reduction in renal function.[8]

The azithromycin/digoxin interaction also appears to be established, but published information is limited, however same precautions suggested for clarithromycin and erythromycin would therefore seem to be appropriate. The number of spontaneous case reports submitted to the makers indicates that the potential for this interaction should be studied further.[25] In addition remember that azithromycin has a long serum half-life (60 hours) which means that it can continue to interact for several days after it has been withdrawn.

1. Thalhammer F, Hollenstein UM, Locker GJ, Janata K, Sunder-Plassmann G, Frass M, Burgmann H. Azithromycin-related toxic effects of digitoxin. *Br J Clin Pharmacol* (1998) 45, 91–2.
2. Ten Eick AP, Sallee D, Preminger T, Weiss A, Reed DM. Possible drug interaction between digoxin and azithromycin in a young child. *Clin Drug Invest* (2000) 20, 61–4.
3. Pfizer Ltd. Personal Communication, February 2001.
4. Abbott Labs, Personal communication 1995.
5. Midoneck SR, Etingin OR. Clarithromycin-related toxic effects of digoxin. *N Engl J Med* (1995) 333, 1505.
6. Taylor JW, Gammenthaler SA, Rape JM. Clarithromycin (Biaxin) induced digoxin toxicity. Presented at the American Society of Healthcare Pharmacists Midyear Clinical Meeting, Miami, December 1994.
7. Ford A, Crocker Smith L, Baltch AL, Smith RP. Clarithromycin-induced digoxin toxicity in a patient with AIDS. *Clin Infect Dis* (1995) 21, 1051–2.
8. Brown BA, Wallace RJ, Griffith DE, Warden R. Clarithromycin-associated digoxin toxicity in the elderly. *Clin Infect Dis* (1997) 24, 92–3.
9. Guillemet C, Alt M, Arpin-Bott MP, Imler M. Clarithromycine-digoxine: une interaction méconnue chez certains patients? *Presse Med* (1997) 26, 512.
10. Nordt S, Williams S, Manoguerra A, Clark R. Clarithromycin-induced digoxin poisoning. *J Toxicol Clin Toxicol* (1997) 35, 501–2.
11. Guerriero SE, Ehrenpreis E, Gallagher KL. Two cases of clarithromycin-induced digoxin toxicity. *Pharmacotherapy* (1997) 17, 1035–7.
12. Laberge P, Martineau P. Clarithromycin-induced digoxin intoxication. *Ann Pharmacother* (1997) 31, 999–1001.
13. Trivedi S, Hyman J, Lichstein E. Clarithromycin and digoxin toxicity. *Ann Intern Med* (1998) 128, 604.
14. Wakasugi H, Yano I, Ito T, Hashida T, Futami T, Nohara R, Sasayama S, Inui K-I. Effect of clarithromycin on renal excretion of digoxin: interaction with P-glycoprotein. *Clin Pharmacol Ther* (1998) 64, 123–8.
15. Nawarskas JJ, McCarthy DM, Spinler SA. Digoxin toxicity secondary to clarithromycin therapy. *Ann Pharmacother* (1997) 31, 864–6.
16. Nordt SP, Williams SR, Manoguerra AS, Clark RF. Clarithromycin induced digoxin toxicity. *J Accid Emerg Med* (1998) 15, 194–5.
17. Juurlink DN, Ito S. Comment: clarithromycin-digoxin interaction. *Ann Pharmacother* (1999) 33, 1375–6.
18. Friedman HS, Bonventre MV. Erythromycin-induced digoxin toxicity. *Chest* (1982) 82, 202.
19. Lindenbaum J, Rund DG, Butler VP, Tse-Eng D, Saha JR. Inactivation of digoxin by the gut flora: reversal by antibiotic therapy. *N Engl J Med* (1981) 305, 789–94.
20. Maxwell DL, Gilmour-White SK, Hall MR. Digoxin toxicity due to interaction of digoxin with erythromycin. *BMJ* (1989) 298, 572.
21. Morton MR, Cooper JW. Erythromycin-induced digoxin toxicity. *DICP Ann Pharmacother* (1989) 23, 668–70.
22. Nørregaard-Hansen K, Klitgaard NA, Pedersen KE. The significance of the enterohepatic circulation on the metabolism of digoxin in patients with the ability of intestinal conversion of the drug. *Acta Med Scand* (1986) 220, 89–92.
23. Ishioka T. Effect of a new macrolide antibiotic 3′′-O-propionyl-leucomycin A₅ (Rokitamycin) on serum concentrations of theophylline and digoxin in the elderly. *Acta Ther* (1987) 13, 17–23.
24. Corallo CE, Rogers IR. Roxithromycin-induced digoxin toxicity. *Med J Aust* (1996) 165, 433–4.
25. Ten Eick AP, Reed MD. Hidden dangers of coadministration of antibiotics and digoxin in children: focus on azithromycin. *Curr Ther Res* (2000) 61, 148–60.
26. Lindenbaum J, Tse-Eng D, Butler VP, Rund DG. Urinary excretion of reduced metabolites of digoxin. *Am J Med* (1981) 71, 67–74.
27. Berndt A, Gramatté T, Kirch W. Digoxin-erythromycin interaction: in vitro evidence for competition for intestinal P-glycoprotein. *Eur J Clin Pharmacol* (1996) 50, 538.

Digitalis glycosides + Methyldopa

Methyldopa does not affect serum digoxin levels, but marked bradycardia has been seen in two elderly women when given both drugs.

Clinical evidence

(a) Serum digoxin levels unchanged

Methyldopa 250 mg daily had no effect on the steady-state serum **digoxin** levels of 8 healthy subjects taking 250 micrograms daily.[1]

(b) Bradycardia

Two elderly women with hypertension and left ventricular failure developed marked bradycardia when given **digoxin** and **methyldopa** (0.75 g or 3.75 g daily) but not with **digoxin** alone. Average and minimum heart rates of 50 and 32, and 48 and 38 bpm respectively were recorded. They were subsequently discharged on **digoxin** and hydralazine with heart rates within the normal range.[2]

Mechanism

Uncertain. Both digoxin and methyldopa[3] can cause some bradycardia, but these effects seem to have been more than simply the sum of the individual drug effects on the autonomic nervous system.[2]

Importance and management

Information is limited but it would seem that concurrent use need not be avoided, but monitor the effects for any evidence of excessive heart slowing.

1. May CA, Vlasses PH, Rocci ML, Rotmensch HH, Swanson BN, Tannenbaum RP, Ferguson RK, Abrams WB. Methyldopa does not alter the disposition of digoxin. *J Clin Pharmacol* (1984) 24, 386–9.
2. Davis JC, Reiffel JA, Bigger JT. Sinus node dysfunction caused by methyldopa and digoxin. *JAMA* (1981) 245, 1241–3.
3. Lund-Johansen P. Hemodynamic changes in long term α-methyldopa therapy of essential hypertension. *Acta Med Scand* (1972) 192, 221–6.

Digitalis glycosides + Metoclopramide

The serum levels of digoxin may be reduced by about a third if metoclopramide and slowly dissolving forms of digoxin are given concurrently. No interaction is likely with digoxin in liquid form or in fast-dissolving preparations.

Clinical evidence

A study in 11 patients taking slowly dissolving **digoxin** tablets *(Orion)* found that **metoclopramide** (10 mg three times a day for 10 days) reduced the serum **digoxin** levels by 36% (from 0.72 to 0.46 ng/ml).[1] The **digoxin** concentrations rose to their former levels when the **metoclopramide** was withdrawn.

Another study in healthy subjects found **metoclopramide** 10 mg three times daily caused a 19% reduction in the AUC of **digoxin** and a 27% reduction in peak serum **digoxin** levels (**digoxin** formulation not stated).[2] Yet another study in healthy subjects clearly showed that an interaction occurred between **metoclopramide** and **digoxin** tablets *(Lanoxin)* but not **digoxin** capsules *(Lanoxicaps)*.[3]

Mechanism

It would seem[4-6] that the metoclopramide increases the motility of the gut to such an extent that full dissolution and absorption of some digoxin formulations is unfinished by the time digoxin is lost in the faeces.

Importance and management

Information is very limited, but the interaction seems to be established. It is not likely to occur with solid form, fast-dissolving digoxin

preparations (e.g. liquid-filled capsules) or digoxin in liquid form, but only those preparations which are slowly dissolving (i.e. some tablet formulations). A reduction in digoxin levels of a third could result in under-digitalisation. There seems to be no information about **digitoxin**.

1. Manninen V, Apajalahti A, Melin J, Karesoja M. Altered absorption of digoxin in patients given propantheline and metoclopramide. *Lancet* (1973) i, 398–400.
2. Kirch W, Janisch HD, Santos SR, Duhrsen U, Dylewicz P, Ohnhaus EE. Effect of cisapride and metoclopramide on digoxin bioavailability. *Eur J Drug Metab Pharmacokinet* (1986) 11, 249–50.
3. Johnson BF, Bustrack JA, Urbach DR, Hull JH, Marwaha R. Effect of metoclopramide on digoxin absorption from tablets and capsules. *Clin Pharmacol Ther* (1984) 36, 724–30.
4. Manninen V, Apajalahti A, Simonen H, Reissell P. Effect of propantheline and metoclopramide on the absorption of digoxin. *Lancet* (1973) i, 1118–9.
5. Medin S, Nyberg L. Effect of propantheline and metoclopramide on the absorption of digoxin. *Lancet* (1973) i, 1393.
6. Fraser EJ, Leach RH, Poston JW, Bold AM, Culank LS, Lipede AB. Dissolution-rates and bioavailability of digoxin tablets. *Lancet* (1973) i, 1393.

Digitalis glycosides + Mexiletine

Serum digoxin levels are not significantly altered by mexiletine.

Clinical evidence, mechanism, importance and management

The steady-state serum **digoxin** levels of 10 healthy subjects on 250 micrograms daily were slightly but not significantly altered while concurrently taking **mexiletine** 200 mg every 8 hours for 4 days (a fall from 0.32 to 0.27 ng/ml).[1,2] When the **mexiletine** was given with 30 ml of an **aluminium magnesium hydroxide** antacid the **digoxin** AUC was approximately halved (from a range of 4.1 to 15.6 down to the range 2.6 to 8.5 ng/ml.h). This is in line with other studies showing that antacids can reduce serum digoxin levels (see 'Digitalis glycosides + Antacids', p.531). The serum mexiletine levels were not significantly altered by the antacid.[2] Two other studies in 9 patients[3] and 8 patients,[4] confirmed that **mexiletine** does not significantly affect serum **digoxin** levels.

1. Affrime MB, Lowenthal DT, Saris S. Drug interaction study of oral mexiletine and digoxin. *Drug Intell Clin Pharm* (1982) 16, 469.
2. Saris SD, Lowenthal DT, Affrime MB. Steady-state digoxin concentration during oral mexiletine administration. *Curr Ther Res* (1983) 34, 662–66.
3. Leahey EB, Reiffel JA, Giardina E-GV, Bigger T. The effect of quinidine and other oral antiarrhythmic drugs on serum digoxin. *Ann Intern Med* (1980) 92, 605–8.
4. Day T, Hunt D. Interaction between mexiletine and digoxin. *Med J Aust* (1983) 2, 630.

Digitalis glycosides + Mizolastine

Mizolastine can cause a small but clinically irrelevant rise in serum digoxin levels.

Clinical evidence, mechanism, importance and management

A double-blind placebo-controlled crossover trial in 12 healthy subjects found that 10 mg **mizolastine** daily for a week caused a significant increase (+ 17%) in maximum serum **digoxin** levels (daily dose 250 micrograms). The **digoxin** AUC and half-life were unchanged and the haemodynamic parameters measured (blood pressures, ECGs) were unaltered.[1,2] No special precautions would seem necessary during concurrent use.

1. Chaufour S, Le Coz F, Dubruc C, Cimarosti I, Rosenzweig P. Lack of effect of mizolastine on the safety and pharmacokinetics of digoxin administered orally in repeated doses in healthy volunteers. *Therapie* (1995) 50 (Suppl), 467.
2. Chaufour S, Le Coz F, Denolle T, Dubruc C, Cimarosti I, Deschamps C, Ulliac N, Delhotal-Landes B, Rosenzweig P. Lack of effect of mizolastine on the safety and pharmacokinetics of digoxin administered orally in repeated doses to healthy volunteers. *Int J Clin Pharmacol Ther* (1998) 36, 286–91.

Digitalis glycosides + Moracizine (Moricizine)

Moracizine does not significantly increase serum digoxin levels in patients with normal renal function. However, some adverse conduction effects have been seen.

Clinical evidence

Thirteen patients on **digoxin** (125 to 250 micrograms daily) showed a non-significant rise in their serum **digoxin** levels of 10 to 15% when concurrently treated with **moracizine** (10 mg/kg daily in three divided doses) for 2 weeks. Nine patients concurrently treated for 1 to 6 months showed no significant changes in their serum **digoxin** levels.[1]

No changes in the pharmacokinetics of **digoxin** were seen in a single-dose study of intravenous **digoxin** and **moracizine** in 9 healthy subjects[2] nor in another study in patients on maintenance treatment with **digoxin** over a 13-day period. However, heart arrhythmias (AV junctional rhythm and heart block) were seen, which disappeared when the **moracizine** was stopped.[3]

Mechanism

Not established. There does not appear to be a pharmacokinetic interaction between moracizine and digoxin. Concurrent use can cause a significant increase in the PR interval and QRS duration, which can result in AV block.[4]

Importance and management

Although no clinically important changes in serum digoxin levels appear to occur during concurrent use, the occurrence of arrhythmias in a few patients indicates that good monitoring is advisable. It has been pointed out that the additive effects of both drugs on intranodal and intraventricular conduction may be excessive in some patients with heart disease.[4] More study is needed.

1. Kennedy HL, Sprague MK, Redd RM, Wiens RD, Blum RI, Buckingham TA. Serum digoxin concentrations during ethmozine antiarrhythmic therapy. *Am Heart J* (1986) 111, 667–72.
2. MacFarland RT, Moeller VR, Pieniaszek HJ, Whitney CC, Marcus FI. Assessment of the potential pharmacokinetic interaction between digoxin and ethmozine. *J Clin Pharmacol* (1985) 25, 138–43.
3. Antman EM, Arnold JMO, Friedman PL, White H, Bosak M, Smith TW. Drug interactions with cardiac glycosides: evaluation of a possible digoxin-ethmozine pharmacokinetic interaction. *J Cardiovasc Pharmacol* (1987) 9, 622–7.
4. Siddoway LA, Schwartz SL, Barbey JT, Woosley RL. Clinical pharmacokinetics of moricizine. *Am J Cardiol* (1990) 65, 21D–25D.

Digitalis glycosides + Nefazodone

Nefazodone causes a moderate increase in serum digoxin levels of uncertain clinical importance.

Clinical evidence

Eighteen healthy subjects were given 200 micrograms **digoxin** alone daily for 8 days, 200 mg **nefazodone** alone twice daily for 8 days, and then both drugs together for 8 days. When taken together the steady-state AUC of **digoxin** was increased by 15%, the maximum serum levels were increased by 29% and the trough serum levels by 27%. Despite these increases no clinically significant changes in ECG measurements occurred (PR, QRS and QT intervals), nor was the heart rate nor any other vital sign altered. The pharmacokinetics of the **nefazodone** were unchanged.[1]

Mechanism

Not understood.

Importance and management

This interaction appears to be established, but its clinical importance is uncertain. Because digoxin has a narrow therapeutic index, it

would seem prudent to monitor the outcome of concurrent use in patients, being alert for the need to reduce the digoxin dosage. More study is needed.

1. Dockens RC, Greene DS, Barbhaiya RH. Assessment of pharmacokinetic and pharmacodynamic drug interactions between nefazodone and digoxin in healthy male volunteers. *J Clin Pharmacol* (1996) 36, 160–7.

Digitalis glycosides + Neuromuscular blockers

Serious cardiac arrhythmias can develop in patients receiving digitalis glycosides who are given suxamethonium (succinylcholine) or pancuronium.

Clinical evidence

Eight out of 17 digitalised patients (anaesthetised with 60 to 150 mg thiamylal and then maintained with nitrous oxide and oxygen) developed serious ventricular arrhythmias following the intravenous injection of 40 to 100 mg **suxamethonium**. Four out of the 8 patients reverted to their previous rhythm when they were given 15 to 30 mg **tubocurarine**, and one patient returned to a regular nodal rhythm from ventricular tachycardia.[1]

Of the other 9 patients, 3 had immediate and definite ST-T wave changes, and the remaining 6 showed no demonstrable changes.[1] There are other reports of this interaction,[2-4] including one that describes sinus tachycardia and atrial flutter in 6 out of 18 patients on **digoxin** when given **pancuronium**.[4]

Mechanism

Not understood. One possibility is that the suxamethonium may cause the rapid removal of potassium from the myocardial cells. Another idea is that it affects catecholamine-releasing cholinergic receptors.

Importance and management

Information is limited but the interaction appears to be established. Suxamethonium should be avoided, or used with great caution, in patients taking digitalis glycosides. Similar caution would seem appropriate with pancuronium.

1. Dowdy EG, Fabian LW. Ventricular arrhythmias induced by succinylcholine in digitalized patients: A preliminary report. *Anesth Analg* (1963) 42, 501–13.
2. Pérez HR. Cardiac arrhythmia after succinylcholine. *Anesth Analg* (1970) 49, 33–8.
3. Smith RB, Petrusack J. Succinylcholine, digitalis, and hypercalcaemia: a case report. *Anesth Analg* (1972) 51, 202–5.
4. Bartolone RS, Rao TLK. Dysrhythmias following muscle relaxant administration in patients receiving digitalis. *Anesthesiology* (1983) 58, 567–9.

Digitalis glycosides + Nifedipine

Serum digoxin levels are normally unchanged or increased only to a small extent by the concurrent use of nifedipine. One unexplained and conflicting study indicated that a 45% rise could occur. Digitoxin appears not to interact.

Clinical evidence

(a) Digoxin

(i) Serum digoxin levels unchanged. Studies in 25 patients[1-3] and 28 healthy subjects[4-6] showed that serum **digoxin** levels were not significantly altered while taking 30 to 60 mg **nifedipine** daily. Similarly no significant changes in the pharmacokinetics of **digoxin** were found in 6 patients[7] or 16 healthy subjects[8,9] on 40 to 90 mg **nifedipine** daily when given a single intravenous dose of **digoxin**. No changes in the pharmacokinetics of **nifedipine** were seen.[8]

(ii) Serum digoxin levels increased. Nifedipine 30 mg increased the plasma **digoxin** levels of 12 healthy subjects taking 375 micrograms daily by 45% (from 0.505 to 0.734 ng/ml) over 14 days.[10,11]

Nifedipine 20 mg twice daily increased the steady-state serum **digoxin** levels of 9 patients by 15% (from 0.87 to 1.04 ng/ml).[12] A 15% increase was also seen in a study[13,14] in 7 healthy subjects given 15 to 60 mg **nifedipine** daily with digoxin 250 micrograms twice daily.

(b) Digitoxin

A study in 18 subjects showed that 40 to 60 mg **nifedipine** daily had no significant effect on their steady-state plasma **digitoxin** levels over a 6-week period.[15]

Mechanism

Not understood. Changes and lack of changes in both renal and non-renal excretion of digoxin have been reported.

Importance and management

The digoxin/nifedipine interaction is well documented but the findings are inconsistent. The weight of evidence appears to be that serum digoxin levels are normally unchanged or only very moderately increased by nifedipine. Concurrent use appears normally to be safe and effective[16] but it would clearly be prudent to monitor the response. One report suggests that nifedipine has some attenuating effect on the digoxin-induced inotropism.[17] Another points out that under some circumstances (renal insufficiency or pre-existing digoxin overdosage) some risk of an undesirable interaction still exists.[13] Nifedipine appears not to interact with digitoxin significantly.

1. Schwartz JB, Raizner A, Akers S. The effect of nifedipine on serum digoxin concentrations in patients. *Am Heart J* (1984) 107, 669–73.
2. Kuhlmann J, Marcin S, Frank KH. Effects of nifedipine and diltiazem on the pharmacokinetics of digoxin. *Naunyn Schmiedebergs Arch Pharmacol* (1983) 324 (Suppl), R81.
3. Kuhlmann J. Effects of nifedipine and diltiazem on plasma levels and renal excretion of beta-acetyldigoxin. *Clin Pharmacol Ther* (1985) 37, 150–6.
4. Schwartz JB, Migliore PJ. Nifedipine does not alter digoxin level or clearance. *J Am Coll Cardiol* (1984) 3, 478.
5. Schwartz JB, Migliore PJ. Effect of nifedipine on serum digoxin concentration and renal clearance. *Clin Pharmacol Ther* (1984) 36, 19–24.
6. Pedersen KE, Madsen JL, Klitgaard NA, Kjoer K, Hvidt S. Non-interaction between nifedipine and digoxin. *Dan Med Bull* (1986) 33, 109–10.
7. Garty M, Shamir E, Ilfeld D, Pitlik S, Rosenfeld JB. Non interaction of digoxin and nifedipine in cardiac patients. *J Clin Pharmacol* (1986) 26, 304–5.
8. Koren G, Zylber-Katz E, Granit L, Levy M. Pharmacokinetic studies of nifedipine and digoxin co-administration. *Int J Clin Pharmacol Ther Toxicol* (1986) 24, 39–42.
9. Pedersen KE, Dorph-Pedersen A, Hvidt S, Klitgaard NA, Kjaer K, Nielsen-Kudsk F. Effect of nifedipine on digoxin kinetics in healthy subjects. *Clin Pharmacol Ther* (1982) 32, 562–5.
10. Belz GG, Doering W, Munkes R, Matthews J. Interaction between digoxin and calcium antagonists and antiarrhythmic drugs. *Clin Pharmacol Ther* (1983) 33, 410–17.
11. Belz GG, Aust PE, Munkes R. Digoxin plasma concentrations and nifedipine. *Lancet* (1981) i, 844–5.
12. Kleinbloesem CH, van Brummelen P, Hillers J, Moolenaar AJ, Breimer DD. Interaction between digoxin and nifedipine at steady state in patients with atrial fibrillation. *Ther Drug Monit* (1985) 7, 372–6.
13. Kirch W, Hutt HJ, Dylewicz P, Gräf KJ, Ohnhaus EE. Dose-dependence of the nifedipine-digoxin interaction? *Clin Pharmacol Ther* (1986) 39, 35–9.
14. Hutt HJ, Kirch W, Dylewicz P, Ohnhaus EE. Dose-dependence of the nifedipine/digoxin interaction? *Arch Toxicol* (1986) (Suppl 9), 209–12.
15. Kuhlmann J. Effects of quinidine, verapamil and nifedipine on the pharmacokinetics and pharmacodynamics of digitoxin during steady-state conditions. *Arzneimittelforschung* (1987) 37, 545–8.
16. Cantelli I, Pavesi PC, Parchi C, Naccarella F, Bracchetti D. Acute hemodynamic effects of combined therapy with digoxin and nifedipine in patients with chronic heart failure. *Am Heart J* (1983) 106, 308–15.
17. Hansen PB, Buch J, Rasmussen OØ, Waldorff S, Steiness E. Influence of atenolol and nifedipine on digoxin-induced inotropism in humans. *Br J Clin Pharmacol* (1984) 18, 817–22.

Digitalis glycosides + NSAIDs

Diclofenac and indometacin (indomethacin) can cause potentially toxic rises in digitalis glycoside levels, while azapropazone, fenbufen and tiaprofenic acid raise levels to a lesser degree. Two studies found that ibuprofen raised serum digoxin levels whereas another found no evidence of an interaction. Isoxicam, ketoprofen, meloxicam, piroxicam, and rofecoxib do not appear to interact significantly. In contrast, phenylbutazone appears to lower plasma digitalis glycoside levels. NSAIDs can cause deterioration of renal function, which could result in digoxin toxicity.

Clinical evidence

(a) Azapropazone

Azapropazone 900 mg daily did not significantly alter the AUC of a single intravenous dose of **digitoxin** 500 micrograms in 8 arthritic patients, but its mean half-life was increased about 10%. Two of the patients showed individual half-life increases of almost a third.[1]

(b) Diclofenac

A study in 7 healthy subjects found that 100 mg **diclofenac** daily for 10 days increased the serum levels of **digoxin** by 29%.[2] Another study in 6 healthy subjects similarly found that 50 mg **diclofenac** three times daily raised the serum **digoxin** levels by about a third.[3] The concurrent use of 100 micrograms **digitoxin** had no effect on the plasma levels of **diclofenac** 50 mg twice daily in 8 subjects; **digitoxin** levels were not reported.[4]

(c) Fenbufen

Fenbufen 900 mg daily was found to cause a slight and unimportant rise in the serum levels of patients on maintenance **digoxin therapy**.[5]

(d) Ibuprofen

The serum **digoxin** levels of 12 patients were reported to have risen by about 60% after being treated with at least 1600 mg **ibuprofen** daily for a week, but after a month of concurrent treatment they had fallen to their former levels.[6] These findings however may be unreliable because half of the patients were not satisfactorily compliant. Another study found that 1200 mg **ibuprofen** daily for 10 days raised the serum **digoxin** levels of 9 healthy subjects by 25%.[2] Yet another study found that 600 mg **ibuprofen** three times daily for 10 days had no effect on steady-state serum **digoxin** levels of 8 patients.[7]

(e) Indometacin

Neonates. A study in 11 premature neonates (aged 25 to 33 weeks) given **digoxin** showed that when 4 days later or more they were given **indometacin (indomethacin)** (mean total dose of 0.32 mg/kg over 12 to 24 h) for the treatment of patent ductus arteriosus, their mean serum **digoxin** levels rose on average by 40%. The **digoxin** was stopped in 5 of them because serum concentrations were potentially toxic.[8] This confirms the observation of digitalis toxicity in 3 other premature neonates when treated similarly,[9] and of toxic serum **digoxin** concentrations in another.[10] A further report describes very high **digoxin** levels (8.2 ng/ml) without toxicity in a full-term neonate.[11]

Adults. **Indometacin** 50 mg three times daily for 10 days increased steady-state serum **digoxin** levels of 10 adult patients by about 40% (from 0.73 to 1.02 nmol/l), with a range of 0 to 100%.[7] **Indometacin** 150 mg daily for 10 days increased the serum **digoxin** levels of 9 healthy subjects by 25%.[2] This contrasts with the results of single-dose studies in 2 groups of 6 healthy adult subjects[12,13] who had **digoxin** by infusion over 4 h. Both studies suggested that no interaction occurs.

(f) Isoxicam

Isoxicam 200 mg daily did not affect the steady-state plasma levels of 12 healthy subjects taking **beta-acetyldigoxin**.[14] This confirms the findings of a previous study.[15]

(g) Ketoprofen

Ketoprofen 50 mg four times daily for 4 days had no effect on the serum **digoxin** levels of 12 patients.[16]

(h) Meloxicam

Meloxicam 15 mg daily for 8 days had no effect on the pharmacokinetics of **digoxin** (given as **beta-acetyldigoxin**) in 12 healthy subjects.[17]

(i) Phenylbutazone

On two occasions when concurrently taking 200 or 400 mg **phenylbutazone** daily, the plasma **digitoxin** levels of 6 patients taking 100 micrograms daily were approximately halved within 8 to 10 days. They returned to their former values within roughly the same period of time after **phenylbutazone** was withdrawn.[18] A similar response has been described elsewhere in one patient.[19] Six healthy subjects showed an approximately 20% fall in their serum **digoxin** levels while taking 200 mg **phenylbutazone** three times daily for 4 days.[3]

(j) Piroxicam

In 10 patients taking **digoxin** for mild cardiac failure, 10 or 20 mg **piroxicam** daily for 15 days had no effect on the steady-state **digoxin** levels, nor were consistent effects seen on the pharmacokinetics of **digoxin**.[20] **Piroxicam** 20 mg daily for 10 days was found to have no effect on serum **digoxin** levels of 6 healthy subjects.[2]

(k) Rofecoxib

Rofecoxib 75 mg once daily did not cause significant changes in the plasma pharmacokinetics or renal elimination of single doses of **digoxin** elixir 500 micrograms in 10 healthy subjects.[21]

(l) Tiaprofenic acid

Tiaprofenic acid 200 mg three times daily for 10 days caused a non-significant rise (from 0.97 to 1.12 ng/ml, i.e. about 15%) in serum **digoxin** levels of 12 healthy subjects.[22]

Mechanism

The reasons for the altered digoxin pharmacokinetics is some of the studies are not clear. However, in the studies in neonates, the elevated digoxin levels were clearly related to indometacin-induced deterioration in renal function, which reduces the clearance of digoxin by the kidney, allowing it to accumulate in the body.[8,10,11] It should be noted that all NSAIDs have the potential to cause renal impairment.

With phenylbutazone (which remember lowers digitalis levels), it is suggested that the rate of metabolism of the digitoxin by the liver is increased.[18]

Importance and management

Be aware of the potential for NSAIDs to cause renal impairment, which could reduce digoxin clearance and result in toxicity. The digoxin/diclofenac interaction is established but the clinical importance is uncertain. It would be prudent to monitor concurrent use to ensure that the digoxin serum levels remain at acceptable levels if diclofenac is added. Reduce the digoxin dosage if necessary. The digoxin/indometacin interaction also seems established, but documentation is limited. It has been suggested that the digoxin dosage should be halved if indometacin is given to premature or full-term infants and the serum digoxin levels and urinary output monitored. You should also be alert for moderate increases in serum digoxin levels in adults if indometacin is added. The importance of the interaction with azapropazone, fenbufen and tiaprofenic acid is not known. In most cases changes to doses are unlikely to be necessary, but remain aware of the potential for interaction. No special precautions would appear to be necessary with isoxicam, ketoprofen, meloxicam, piroxicam, and rofecoxib, but note that benoxaprofen has been withdrawn from general use in most countries because of its adverse effects. More study is needed in most cases, but especially with ibuprofen, where the evidence is conflicting. Monitor digoxin carefully if ibuprofen is started or stopped.

The interaction with phenylbutazone appears to be in direct contrast to that with the other NSAIDs, but documentation is limited. The dosage of digoxin and digitoxin may possibly need to be increased to avoid under-digitalisation if phenylbutazone is added to established treatment. You should monitor concurrent use well.

1. Faust-Tinnefeldt G, Gilfrich HJ. Digitoxin-Kinetik unter antirheumatischer Therapie mit Azapropazon. *Arzneimittelforschung* (1977) 27, 2009–11.
2. Isbary J, Doering W, König E. Der Einfluß von Tiaprofensäure auf die Digoxinkonzentration im Serum (DKS) im Vergleich zu anderen Antirheumatika (AR). *Z Rheum* (1982) 41, 164.
3. Rau R, Georgiopoulos E, Neumann P, Gross D. Die Beeinflussung des Digoxinblutspiegels durch Antirheumatika. *Akt Rheum* (1980) 5, 349–58.
4. Schumacher A, Faust-Tinnefeldt G, Geissler HE, Gilfrich HJ, Mutschler E. Untersuchungen potentieller Interaktionen von Diclofenac-Natrium (Voltaren) mit einem Antazidum und mit Digitoxin. *Therapiewoche* (1983) 33, 2619–25.
5. Dunky A, Eberi R. Anti-inflammatory effects of a new anti-rheumatic drug fenbufen in rheumatoid arthritis. *XIV Int Congr Rheumatology, June 26–July 1* (1977), Abstract No 379.
6. Quattrocchi FP, Robinson JD, Curry RW, Grieco ML, Schulman SG. The effect of ibuprofen on serum digoxin concentrations. *Drug Intell Clin Pharm* (1983) 17, 286–8.
7. Jørgensen HS, Christensen HR, Kampmann JP. Interaction between digoxin and indomethacin or ibuprofen. *Br J Clin Pharmacol* (1991) 31, 108–110.

8. Koren G, Zarfin Y, Perlman M, MacLeod SM. Effects of indomethacin on digoxin pharmacokinetics in preterm infants. *Pediatr Pharmacol* (1984) 4, 25–30.
9. Mayes LC, Boerth RC. Digoxin-indomethacin interaction. *Pediatr Res* (1980) 14, 469.
10. Schimmel MS, Inwood RL, Eidelman AI, Eylath U. Toxic digitalis levels associated with indomethacin therapy in a neonate. *Clin Pediatr* (1980) 19, 768–9.
11. Haig GM, Brookfield EG. Increase in serum digoxin concentrations after indomethacin therapy in a full-term neonate. *Pharmacotherapy* (1992) 12, 334–6.
12. Finch MB, Johnston GD, Kelly JG, McDevitt DG. Pharmacokinetics of digoxin alone and in the presence of indomethacin therapy. *Br J Clin Pharmacol* (1984) 17, 353–5.
13. Sziegoleit W, Weiss M, Fahr A, Förster W. Are serum levels and cardiac effects of digoxin influenced by indometacin? *Z Rheumatol* (1984) 43, 182–4.
14. Zöller B, Engel HJ, Faust-Tinnefeldt G, Gilfrich HJ, Zimmer M. Untersuchungen zur Wechselwirkung von Isoxicam und Digoxin. *Pharmazie* (1986) 41, 340–2.
15. Chlud K. Zur Frage der Interaktionen in der Rheumatherapie: Untersuchungen von Isoxicam und Glibenclamid bei Diabetien mit rheumatischen Enkrankungen. *Tempo Medical* (1983) 12A, 15–18.
16. Lewis GR, Jacobs SG, Vavra I. Effect of ketoprofen on serum digoxin concentrations. *Curr Ther Res* (1985) 38, 494–9.
17. Degner FL, Heinzel G, Narjes H, Türck D. The effect of meloxicam on the pharmacokinetics of β-acetyl-digoxin. *Br J Clin Pharmacol* (1995) 40, 486–8.
18. Wirth KE. Arzneimittelinteraktionen bei der Anwendung herzwirksamer Glykoside. *Med Welt* (1981) 32, 234–8.
19. Solomon HM, Reich S, Spirt N, Abrams WB. Interactions between digitoxin and other drugs *in vitro* and *in vivo*. *Ann N Y Acad Sci* (1971) 179, 362–9.
20. Rau R. Interaction study of piroxicam with digoxin. In 'Piroxicam: A New Non-steroidal Anti-inflammatory Agent.' Proc IXth Eur Cong Rheumatol, Wiesbaden, September 1979, pp 41–6. Academy Professional Information Services, NY.
21. Schwartz JI, De Smet M, Larson PJ, Verbesselt R, Ebel DL, Lins R, Lens S, Porras AG, Gertz BJ. Effect of rofecoxib on the pharmacokinetics of digoxin in healthy volunteers. *J Clin Pharmacol* (2001) 41, 107–112.
22. Doering W, Isbary J. Der Einfluß von Tiaprofensäure auf die Digoxin-konzentration im Serum. *Arzneimittelforschung* (1983) 33, 167–8.

Digitalis glycosides + Orlistat

Orlistat appears not to interact with digoxin.

Clinical evidence, mechanism, importance and management

Orlistat 120 mg three times daily for 6 days was found to have no effect on the pharmacokinetics of single 400 micrograms oral doses of **digoxin** in 12 healthy subjects.[1] This suggests that no special precautions will be needed in patients who are treated with both drugs concurrently.

1. Melia AT, Zhi J, Guerciolini R, Koss-Twardy S, Min BH, Smith B, Freundlich N. Orlistat does not inhibit the absorption of digoxin in healthy volunteers. *Pharm Res* (1994) 11 (10 Suppl), S-370.

Digitalis glycosides + Penicillamine

Serum digoxin levels can be reduced by the concurrent use of penicillamine.

Clinical evidence

While taking 1 g **penicillamine** daily 2 h after taking **digoxin** orally, the serum **digoxin** levels of 10 patients measured 2, 4 and 6 h later were reduced by 13, 20 and 39% respectively. In 10 other patients similarly treated but given **digoxin** intravenously, the serum **digoxin** levels measured 4 and 6 h later were reduced by 23 and 64% respectively.[1] This interaction is reported by the same authors to occur in children.[2]

Mechanism

Unknown.

Importance and management

Information seems to be limited to the reports cited. Patients on digoxin should be checked for signs of under-digitalisation if penicillamine is added. Information about digitoxin appears to be lacking.

1. Moezzi B, Fatourechi V, Khozain R, Eslami B. The effect of penicillamine on serum digoxin levels. *Jpn Heart J* (1978) 19, 366–70.
2. Moezzi B, Khozein R, Pooymehr F, Shakibi JG. Reversal of digoxin-induced changes in erythrocyte electrolyte concentrations by penicillamine in children. *Jpn Heart J* (1980) 21, 335–9.

Digitalis glycosides + Phenytoin (Diphenylhydantoin)

Phenytoin reduces serum digoxin levels and a marked fall in serum digitoxin levels has also been seen. There is a single case report of marked bradycardia. Phenytoin was formerly used for the treatment of digitalis-induced heart arrhythmias, but sudden cardiac arrest has been reported.

Clinical evidence

(a) Bradycardia and cardiac arrest

A patient with suspected digitalis-induced heart arrhythmias developed bradycardia, then became asystolic and died, following the intravenous injection of **phenytoin**.[1] Six further fatalities after the intravenous administration of phenytoin in digitalised patients are briefly mentioned in the discussion of this case.[1] Marked bradycardia (34 bpm) and complete heart block has been described in a patient with Down's syndrome taking 250 micrograms **digoxin** daily for mitral insufficiency when his **phenytoin** dose was increased from 200 mg daily to 300 mg daily.[2]

(b) Reduced serum digoxin levels

A study in 6 healthy subjects showed that after taking 200 mg **phenytoin** twice daily for a week concurrently with β-**acetyldigoxin** 400 micrograms daily, the half-life of **digoxin** was reduced by 30% (from 33.9 to 23.7 h) and the AUC by 23% (from 31.6 to 24.4 ng/ml/h). Total clearance increased by 27% (from 258.6 to 328.3 ml/min).[3]

(c) Reduced plasma digitoxin levels

The plasma **digitoxin** levels of a man were observed to fall on 3 occasions when he was concurrently treated with **phenytoin**. On the third occasion while taking 200 micrograms **digitoxin** daily, the addition of 900 mg **phenytoin** daily caused a 60% fall (from 25 to 10 ng/ml) over a 7 to 10 day period.[4]

Mechanisms

Phenytoin has a stabilising effect on the responsiveness of the myocardial cells to stimulation so that the toxic threshold of digoxin at which arrhythmias occur is raised. But the heart-slowing effects of the digitalis glycoside are not opposed and the lethal dose is unaltered, so that the cardiac arrest would appear to be the result of the excessive bradycardia. It seems possible that the fall in plasma digitoxin levels may be due to a phenytoin-induced increase in the metabolism of the digitoxin by the liver. The reduction in serum digoxin levels by phenytoin is not understood.

Importance and management

Phenytoin was formerly used for treating digitalis-induced arrhythmias, but this use now appears to be obsolete. Intravenous phenytoin should not be used in patients with a high degree of heart block or marked bradycardia because of the risk that cardiac arrest may occur. Information about the effects of phenytoin on digitalis glycoside levels seems to be confined to these single reports, but it would now be prudent to check that patients on digoxin or digitoxin who are subsequently given phenytoin do not become under-digitalised.

1. Zoneraich S, Zoneraich O, Siegel J. Sudden death following intravenous sodium diphenylhydantoin. *Am Heart J* (1976) 91, 375–7.

2. Viukari NMA, Aho K. Digoxin-phenytoin interaction. *BMJ* (1970) 2, 51.

3. Rameis H. On the interaction between phenytoin and digoxin. *Eur J Clin Pharmacol* (1985) 29, 4953.

4. Solomon HM, Reich S, Spirt N, Abrams WB. Interactions between digitoxin and other drugs *in vitro* and *in vivo*. *Ann N Y Acad Sci* (1971) 179, 362–9.

Digitalis glycosides + Pinaverium bromide

Plasma digoxin levels are not affected by the concurrent use of pinaverium bromide in patients taking either beta-acetyldigoxin or metildigoxin (medigoxin).

Clinical evidence, mechanism, importance and management

A single-blind study in 25 patients, taking either **beta-acetyldigoxin** or **metildigoxin (medigoxin)** for congestive heart failure, found that **pinaverium bromide** 50 mg three times daily for 12 days had no significant effect on their plasma **digoxin** levels.[1] No special precautions seem necessary.

1. Weitzel O, Seidel G, Engelbert S, Berksoy M, Eberhardt G, Bode R. Investigation of possible interaction between pinaverium bromide and digoxin. *Curr Med Res Opin* (1983) 8, 600–2.

Digitalis glycosides + Prazosin

A rapid and marked rise in serum digoxin levels occurred in one study when prazosin was given.

Clinical evidence, mechanism, importance and management

Prazosin 2.5 mg twice daily increased the mean steady-state plasma **digoxin** level by 43% (from 0.94 to 1.34 ng/ml) after one day, and by 60% (0.94 to 1.51 ng/ml) after 3 days in 20 patients, although the individual response varied from an increase to a decrease, to no effect. Three days after the **prazosin** was stopped (by which time it would be totally cleared from the body), the serum **digoxin** levels had fallen to their previous values.[1] The reason for this response is not understood. There do not appear to be any other reports in the literature, and the maker notes that, in clinical experience, prazosin has been administered with digoxin without any adverse drug interaction to date.[2] However, it may be prudent to monitor serum **digoxin** levels if **prazosin** is added. More study is needed.

1. Çopur S, Tokgözoğlu L, Oto A, Oram E, Uğurlu Ş. Effects of oral prazosin on total plasma digoxin levels. *Fundam Clin Pharmacol* (1988) 2, 13–17.

2. Hypovase (Prazosin) Pfizer. Summary of product characteristics, August 1998.

Digitalis glycosides + Probenecid

Probenecid has no clinically significant effects on plasma digoxin levels.

Clinical evidence, mechanism, importance and management

A study over a 16 day period in 2 healthy subjects taking 250 micrograms **digoxin** daily showed that while concurrently taking two daily doses of *ColBenemid* (**probenecid** 500 mg + **colchicine** 500 micrograms) for 3 days, their plasma **digoxin** levels were slightly but not significantly raised (from 0.67 to 0.70 ng/ml, and from 0.60 to 0.67 ng/ml respectively).[1] Another study in 6 healthy subjects found that 2 g **probenecid** daily for 8 days had no significant effect on the pharmacokinetics of **digoxin**.[2] No special precautions would seem necessary during concurrent use.

1. Jaillon P, Weissenburger J, Cheymol G, Graves P, Marcus F. Les effets du probénécide sur la concentration plasmatique à l'équilibre de digoxine. *Therapie* (1980) 35, 655–6.

2. Hedman A, Angelin B, Arvidsson A, Dahlqvist R. No effect of probenecid on the renal and biliary clearances of digoxin in man. *Br J Clin Pharmacol* (1991) 32, 63–7.

Digitalis glycosides + Propafenone

Propafenone can increase serum digoxin levels by 30 to 90% or even more. A digoxin dosage reduction may be necessary.

Clinical evidence

Propafenone (increasing over 6 days to 300 mg every 8 hours) increased the mean steady-state serum **digoxin** levels by 83% in 5 patients taking 125 to 250 micrograms digoxin daily. Three of them continued to take both drugs for 6 months and showed a 63% rise in digoxin levels. No digitalis toxicity was seen.[1] In another study, **propafenone** 600 mg daily in divided doses increased the steady-state serum **digoxin** levels of 10 patients by 90% (from 0.97 to 1.54 ng/ml), and two of them showed symptoms of intoxication (nausea, vomiting).[2,3] Similarly, 3 children showed rises in serum digoxin levels of 112 to 254% over 3 to 24 days when given 250 to 500 mg/m^2 **propafenone** daily.[4] The mean AUC of **digoxin** increased by 13.8% in 27 patients receiving **propafenone** 10 mg/kg daily in divided doses. However, there was great inter-individual variability, with 22 patients showing an increase in AUC, and 5 a decrease. One patient experienced **digoxin** poisoning with fatal ventricular fibrillation after **propafenone**.[5]

Propafenone 450 mg daily increased the mean steady-state serum **digoxin** levels of 12 healthy subjects by about 35% (from 0.58 to 0.78 ng/ml), and the cardiac effects were increased accordingly.[6] In a study in 6 subjects[7] given a single intravenous dose of 1000 micrograms of digoxin, propafenone 150 or 300 mg every 8 h increased the AUC of **digoxin** by 28% and decreased total body clearance of digoxin by 21.9%. A similar study with oral **digoxin** found a 25% increase in **digoxin** AUC in healthy subjects.[8]

Mechanism

Not understood. One suggestion is that propafenone increases the bioavailability of the digoxin.[8] Another is that the volume of distribution and non-renal clearance of digoxin are changed by the propafenone.[7] Conversely, others reported that propafenone decreased the renal clearance of digoxin.[3,6] There is certainly some evidence that propafenone and its metabolite inhibit the P-glycoprotein transporter, which is concerned with digoxin secretion by the renal tubular cells.[9]

Importance and management

A very well established interaction of clinical importance. Monitor the effects of concurrent use and reduce the digoxin dosage appropriately in order to avoid toxicity. Most patients appear to be affected[2] and dosage reductions in the range 13 to 79% were found necessary in one of the studies cited.[2,3] The data available suggest that the extent of the rise may possibly depend on the propafenone serum concentration rather than on its dose.[7,10]

1. Salerno DM, Granrud G, Sharkey P, Asinger R, Hodges M. A controlled trial of propafenone for treatment of frequent and repetitive ventricular premature complexes. *Am J Cardiol* (1984) 53, 77–83.
2. Calvo MV, Martin-Suarez A, Avila MC, Luengo CM. Interacción digoxina-propafenona. *Medicina Clínica* (1987) 89, 171–2.
3. Calvo MV, Martin-Suarez A, Luengo CM, Avila C, Cascon M, Hurlé AD-G. Interaction between digoxin and propafenone. *Ther Drug Monit* (1989) 11, 10–15.
4. Zalzstein E, Koren G, Bryson SM, Freedom RM. Interaction between digoxin and propafenone in children. *J Pediatr* (1990) 116, 310–2.
5. Palumbo E, Svetoni N, Casini M, Spargi T, Biagi G, Martelli F, Lanzetta T. Interazione digoxina-propafenone: valori e limiti del dosaggio plasmatico dis due farmaci. *G Ital Cardiol* (1986) 16, 855–62.
6. Belz GG, Doering W, Munkes R, Matthews J. Interaction between digoxin and calcium antagonists and antiarrhythmic drugs. *Clin Pharmacol Ther* (1983) 33, 410–17.
7. Nolan PE, Marcus FI, Erstad BL, Hoyer GK, Furman C, Kirsten EB. Effects of coadministration of propafenone on the pharmacokinetics of digoxin in healthy volunteer subjects. *J Clin Pharmacol* (1989) 29, 46–52.
8. Cardaioli P, Compostella L, De Domenico R, Papalia D, Zeppellini R, Libardoni M, Pulido E, Cucchini F. Influenza del propafenone sulla farmacocinetica della digossina somministrata per via orale: studio su volontari sani. *G Ital Cardiol* (1986) 16, 237–40.
9. Woodland C, Ito S, Koren G. The mechanism of the renal tubular digoxin-propafenone interaction in vitro. *Clin Invest Med* (1994) 17 (Suppl 4), B13.
10. Bigot M-C, Debruyne D, Bonnefoy L, Grollier G, Moulin M, Potier J-C. Serum digoxin levels related to plasma propafenone levels during concomitant treatment. *J Clin Pharmacol* (1991) 31, 521–6.

Digitalis glycosides + Propantheline

Serum digoxin levels may be increased by a third or more if propantheline and slow-dissolving forms of digoxin tablets are given concurrently. No clinically significant interaction is likely with digoxin given as a liquid or in soft-gelatin capsules or in the form of fast-dissolving tablets.

Clinical evidence

The serum **digoxin** levels of 9 out of 13 patients rose by 30% (from 1.02 to 1.33 ng/ml) while taking a slow-dissolving formulation of **digoxin** tablets *(Orion)* with 15 mg **propantheline** three times daily for 10 days. Serum levels stayed the same in 3 patients and fell slightly in one. An associated study in 4 healthy subjects given **digoxin** in liquid form found that serum **digoxin** levels were unaffected by **propantheline**, and were higher than those in the patients given digoxin tablets.[1]

Another study by the same workers showed that **propantheline** increased **digoxin** serum levels by 40% with a slow-dissolving tablet formulation *(Orion)*, but had no effect on serum **digoxin** levels with a fast-dissolving tablet formulation *(Lanoxin)*.[2] In a further study, **propantheline** increased AUC of **digoxin** from *Lanoxin* tablets by 24%, compared with a non-significant increase of 13% with digoxin solution in capsule form *(Lanoxicaps)*.[3]

Mechanism

Propantheline is an anticholinergic agent which reduces gut motility. This allows the slow-dissolving formulations of digoxin more time to pass into solution so that more is available for absorption.

Importance and management

An established interaction, but only of importance if slow-dissolving digoxin formulations are used. No interaction is likely with liquid or liquid-filled capsule forms of digoxin. With slow-dissolving forms of digoxin tablets it may be necessary to reduce the digoxin dosage. No interaction seems likely with **digitoxin** because it is better absorbed from the gut than digoxin, but this requires confirmation.

1. Manninen V, Apajalahti A, Melin J, Karesoja M. Altered absorption of digoxin in patients given propantheline and metoclopramide. *Lancet* (1973) i, 398–400.
2. Manninen V, Apajalahti A, Simonen H, Reissell P. Effect of propantheline and metoclopramide on absorption of digoxin. *Lancet* (1973) i, 1118–19.
3. Brown DD, Schmid J, Long RA, Hull JH. A steady-state evaluation of the effects of propantheline bromide and cholestyramine on the bioavailability of digoxin when administered as tablets or capsules. *J Clin Pharmacol* (1985) 25, 360–4.

Digitalis glycosides + Prostaglandins

Enprostil, iloprost and rioprostil do not significantly change digoxin pharmacokinetics. Epoprostenol caused a small predicted decrease in digoxin clearance in the short-term, which is of uncertain clinical importance.

Clinical evidence, mechanism, importance and management

Enprostil 35 micrograms twice daily for 6 days in 12 healthy subjects had no effect on the pharmacokinetics of **digoxin** (250 micrograms daily). No clinically significant ECG abnormalities were seen.[1,2] **Rioprostil** 600 micrograms daily in 9 healthy subjects decreased the rate, but not the extent, of **digoxin** absorption. Steady-state **digoxin** levels were not significantly changed.[3] The **digoxin** pharmacokinetics in 12 patients showed no significant changes when they were treated concurrently for 20 days with 6-h intravenous infusions of **iloprost** (2 ng/kg/min) and **digoxin** 250 micrograms orally, although the mean time to maximum serum **digoxin** was delayed by an hour.[4,5] No special precautions would seem to be necessary with any of these prostaglandins.

In 30 patients with congestive heart failure treated with **digoxin** and **epoprostenol**, there was a predicted 15% decrease in **digoxin** clearance after 3 days concurrent use, but this effect was no longer apparent by the end of 12 weeks concurrent use. The clinical relevance of this awaits evaluation but it seems unlikely to be important, however the authors of the report suggest that you should be aware of the possible short-term changes in patients with high trough-serum **digoxin** levels and those prone to **digoxin** toxicity.[6]

1. Winters L, Windle S, Cohen A, Wolbach R. Enprostil does not interact with steady state digoxin. *Gastroenterology* (1988) 94, A500.
2. Cohen A, Winters L. Enprostil leaves steady state digoxin pharmacokinetics unaltered. *Curr Ther Res* (1988) 44, 541–6.
3. Demol P, Wingender W, Weihrauch TR, Kuhlmann J. Effect of rioprostil, a synthetic prostaglandin E1 on the bioavailability of digoxin. *Gastroenterology* (1988) 92, 1368.
4. Cabane J, Penin I, Bouslama K, Benchouieb A, Giral Ph, Picard O, Wattiaux MJ, Cheymol G, Souvignet G, Imbert JC. Traitement par iloprost des ischémies critiques des membres inférieures associées a une insuffisance cardiaque. *Therapie* (1991) 46, 235–40.
5. Penin E, Cheymol G, Bouslama K, Benchouieb A, Cabane J, Souvignet G. No pharmacokinetic interaction between iloprost and digoxin. *Eur J Clin Pharmacol* (1991) 41, 505–6.
6. Carlton LD, Patterson JH, Mattson CN, Schmith VD. The effects of epoprostenol on drug disposition I. A pilot study of the pharmacokinetics of digoxin with and without epoprostenol in patients with congestive heart failure. *J Clin Pharmacol* (1996) 36, 247–56.

Digitalis glycosides + Quinidine

The serum levels of digoxin in most patients are doubled on average within five days if quinidine is added. The digoxin dosage usually needs to be halved if intoxication is to be avoided. Digitoxin levels are also increased but this occurs more slowly and the extent may be less.

Clinical evidence

(a) Digoxin + quinidine

Arising from the observation that **quinidine** appeared to increase serum **digoxin** levels, a retrospective study of patient records revealed that 25 out of 27 patients on **digoxin** had shown a significant rise (from 1.4 to 3.2 ng/ml) in serum **digoxin** levels when given **quinidine**. Of these, 16 showed typical signs of intoxication (nausea, vomiting, anorexia) which resolved in 10 when the **digoxin** dosage was reduced or withdrawn, and in 5 when the **quinidine** was withdrawn.[1]

This is one of the first reports published in 1978 (two other groups independently reported it at a similar time[2,3]) that clearly describes this interaction, although hints of its existence can be found in papers published over the previous 50 years. Since then large numbers of research reports, both retrospective and prospective and case studies have confirmed and established the incidence and magnitude of this interaction. It occurs in over 90% of patients and, on average, there is a 100% increase in serum **digoxin** levels, although there are pronounced inter-individual differences, and the increase is somewhat dependent on the quinidine dose. There are numerous reports and reviews of this interaction, only a selection of which are listed here for economy of space. Two reviews published in 1982 and 1983 contain valuable bibliographies.[4,5]

(b) Digitoxin + quinidine

The steady-state serum **digitoxin** levels of 8 healthy subjects rose by 45% (from 13.6 to 19.7 ng/ml) over 32 days while taking 750 mg **quinidine** bisulphate daily.[6] Another study over only 10 days found a 31% increase in serum **digitoxin** levels,[7] whereas yet another found a 115% increase.[8] A study in 5 healthy subjects found that **quinidine** reduced the total body clearance of **digitoxin** by 63% and the serum **digitoxin** levels were raised.[9]

Mechanisms

Quinidine reduces the renal excretion of digoxin by 40 to 50%, and it also appears to have some effects on non-renal clearance which includes an approximate 50% reduction in its excretion in the bile.[10] It displaces digoxin from tissue binding sites and significant changes in the volume of distribution occur. There is some limited evidence that changes in the rate and extent of absorption of digoxin from the gut may have a small part to play,[11] and there is also some evidence that

P-glycoprotein may be involved.[12,13] Digoxin also appears to cause a small reduction in the renal clearance of quinidine.[14] Quinidine appears to increase digitoxin serum levels by reducing the non-renal clearance.

Importance and management

The digoxin/quinidine interaction is overwhelming well-documented, well-established and of clinical importance. Since serum digoxin levels are usually roughly doubled (up to a fivefold increases have been seen[4]) and most (90%+) patients are affected, digitalis toxicity will develop unless the dosage of digoxin is reduced appropriately (approximately halved).[1,4,15,16] A suggested rule-of-thumb is that if serum digoxin levels are no greater than 0.9 ng/ml the addition of quinidine is unlikely to cause cardiotoxic digoxin levels (if serum potassium levels are normal) whereas with levels of 1.0 ng/ml or more, toxic concentrations may develop.[17] Monitor the effects and readjust the dosage as necessary. Significant effects occur within a day of taking the quinidine and reach a maximum after about 3 to 6 days (quicker or slower in some patients), but digoxin levels will only stabilise when the quinidine has reached steady-state and that depends on whether a loading dose is given. The effects are to some extent dose-related but the correlation is not good: less than 400 to 500 mg of quinidine daily has minimal effects, and increasing doses up to 1200 mg has greater effects.[15,18] About 5 days are needed after withdrawing the quinidine before serum digoxin levels fall to their former levels. It has been recommended that patients with chronic renal failure should have their digoxin dosage reduced to one-half or one-third.[19-21] An appropriate upward readjustment will be necessary if the quinidine is subsequently withdrawn.

Far less is known about the digitoxin/quinidine interaction but the same precautions should be taken. It develops much more slowly.

Alternative non-interacting antiarrhythmics include disopyramide, mexiletine, procainamide and possibly flecainide.

1. Leahey EB, Reiffel JA, Drusin RE, Heisenbuttel RH, Lovejoy WP, Bigger JT. Interaction between quinidine and digoxin. *JAMA* (1978) 240, 533–4.
2. Ejvinsson G. Effect of quinidine on plasma concentrations of digoxin. *BMJ* (1978) i, 279–80.
3. Reid PR, Meek AG. Digoxin-quinidine interaction. *Johns Hopkins Med J* (1979) 145, 227–9.
4. Bigger JT, Leahey EB. Quinidine and digoxin. An important interaction. *Drugs* (1982) 24, 229–39.
5. Fichtl B, Doering W. The quinidine-digoxin interaction in perspective. *Clin Pharmacokinet* (1983) 8, 137–54.
6. Kuhlmann J, Dohrmann M, Marcin S. Effects of quinidine on pharmacokinetics and pharmacodynamics of digitoxin achieving steady-state conditions. *Clin Pharmacol Ther* (1986) 39, 288–94.
7. Peters U, Risler T, Grabensee B, Falkenstein U, Kroukou J. Interaktion von Chinidin und Digitoxin beim Menschen. *Dtsch Med Wochenschr* (1980) 105, 438–42.
8. Kreutz G, Keller F, Gast D and Prokein E. Digitoxin-quinidine interaction achieving steady-state conditions for both drugs. *Naunyn-Schmiedebergs Arch Toxicol* (1982) 319, R82.
9. Garty M, Sood P, Rollins DE. Digitoxin elimination reduced during quinidine therapy. *Ann Intern Med* (1981) 94, 35–7.
10. Schenck-Gustafsson K, Angelin B, Hedman A, Arvidsson A, Dahlqvist R. Quinidine-induced reduction of the biliary excretion of digoxin in patients. *Circulation* (1985) 72 (Suppl), III-19.
11. Pedersen KE, Christiansen BD, Klitgaard NA, Nielsen-Kudsk F. Effect of quinidine on digoxin bioavailability. *Eur J Clin Pharmacol* (1983) 24, 41–7.
12. Fromm MF, Kim RB, Stein CM, Roden DM. Inhibition of drug transport: mechanism for the digoxin-quinidine interaction. *Clin Pharmacol Ther* (1998) 63, 205.
13. Fromm MF, Kim RB, Stein CM, Wilkinson GR, Roden DM. Inhibition of P-glycoprotein-mediated drug transport. A unifying mechanism to explain the interaction between digoxin and quinidine. *Circulation* (1999) 99, 522–7.
14. Rameis H. Quinidine-digoxin interaction: are the pharmacokinetics of both drugs altered? *Int J Clin Pharmacol Ther Toxicol* (1985) 23, 145–53.
15. Doering W. Quinidine-digoxin interaction: pharmacokinetics, underlying mechanism and clinical implications. *N Engl J Med* (1979) 301, 400–4.
16. Leahey EB, Reiffel JA, Heissenbuttel RH, Drusin RE, Lovejoy WP, Bigger JT. Enhanced cardiac effect of digoxin during quinidine treatment. *Arch Intern Med* (1979) 139, 519–21.
17. Friedman HS, Chen T-S. Use of control steady-state serum digoxin levels for predicting serum digoxin concentration after quinidine administration. *Am Heart J* (1982) 104, 72–6.
18. Fenster PE, Powell JR, Hager WD, Graves PE, Conrad K, Goldman S. Onset and dose dependence of digoxin-quinidine interaction. *Am J Cardiol* (1980) 45, 413.
19. Fichtl B, Doering W, Seidel H. The quinidine-digoxin interaction in patients with impaired renal function. *Int J Clin Pharmacol Ther Toxicol* (1983) 21, 229–33.
20. Fenster PE, Hager WD, Perrier D, Powell JR, Graves PE, Michael UF. Digoxin-quinidine interaction in patients with chronic renal failure. *Circulation* (1982) 66, 1277–80.
21. Woodcock BG and Rietbrock N. Digitalis-quinidine interactions. *Trends Pharmacol Sci* (1982) 3, 118–22.

Digitalis + Quinidine + Pentobarbital

Digitalis toxicity arising from the digoxin/quinidine interaction only manifested itself in an elderly woman treated with digoxin, quinidine, and pentobarbital when the pentobarbital was withdrawn, and the enzyme-inducing effect of pentobarbital on quinidine ceased.

Clinical evidence, mechanism, importance and management

A woman in her nineties who had been taking 100 mg **pentobarbital** at bedtime for at least a year was given **digoxin** and **quinidine** to control paroxysmal atrial fibrillation. Her serum **quinidine** levels remained below the therapeutic range and the quinidine half-life was unusually short (1.6 h compared with the normal 10 h) until the **pentobarbital** was withdrawn, whereupon both the **quinidine** and the **digoxin** levels rose, accompanied by signs of **digoxin** toxicity.[1] It seems that the **pentobarbital** (an enzyme-inducer) kept the **quinidine** levels depressed by allowing rapid liver metabolism, as a result of which the normal **digoxin-quinidine** interaction was minimal. Once the enzyme-inducing agent was withdrawn, the **quinidine** serum levels climbed and the **digoxin/quinidine** interaction which results in elevated **digoxin** levels was able to manifest itself fully (see 'Digitalis glycosides + Quinidine', p.552). An interaction involving the interplay of 3 drugs like this is fairly unusual.

1. Chapron DJ, Mumford D, Pitegoff GJ. Apparent quinidine-induced digoxin toxicity after withdrawal of pentobarbital. A case of sequential drug interactions. *Arch Intern Med* (1979) 139, 363–5.

Digitalis glycosides + Quinine

Some but not all patients may show a marked rise (more than 60%) in serum digoxin levels if given quinine.

Clinical evidence

The steady-state **digoxin** levels of 4 healthy subjects on 250 micrograms daily rose by 63% (from 0.63 to 1.03 nmol/l) after taking 300 mg **quinine** four times daily for a day. After taking the **quinine** for a further 3 days the **digoxin** levels rose another 11% (to 1.10 nmol/l). **Digoxin** renal clearance fell by 20% (from 2.32 to 1.86 ml/min/kg).[1]

Quinine sulfate 250 mg daily for 7 days increased the mean serum **digoxin** levels of 7 healthy subjects by 25% (from 0.64 to 0.80 ng/ml). When given **quinine sulfate** 250 mg three times daily there was a further 8% rise. Considerable individual differences were seen, one subject demonstrating a 92% rise.[2] In contrast, 17 patients given 750 mg **quinine** daily showed only a small and statistically insignificant rise in mean serum **digoxin** levels (from 0.80 to 0.91 ng/ml). Serum levels were virtually unaltered in 11 patients, decreased in two and markedly increased (amount not stated) in four.[3] Another study found that **quinine** reduced the total body clearance of **digoxin** by 26%.[4]

Mechanism

Not fully understood. Unlike with quinidine, a reduction in non-renal clearance is apparently largely responsible for the rise in serum digoxin levels with quinine.[2,4,5] This is possibly due to changes in digoxin metabolism or in its biliary excretion.[4,5]

Importance and management

An established interaction of clinical importance but only moderately documented compared with the digoxin/quinidine interaction. Monitor the effects of concurrent use and reduce the digoxin dosage where necessary. Some patients may show a substantial increase in serum digoxin levels whereas others will show only small or moderate rise.

There appear to be no case reports of digoxin intoxication arising from this interaction.

1. Aronson JK, Carver JG. Interaction of digoxin with quinine. *Lancet* (1981) i, 1418.
2. Pedersen KE, Madsen JL, Klitgaard NA, Kjaer K, Hvidt S. Effect of quinine on plasma digoxin concentration and renal digoxin clearance. *Acta Med Scand* (1985) 218, 229–32.
3. Doering W. Is there a clinically relevant interaction between quinine and digoxin in human beings? *Am J Cardiol* (1981) 48, 975–6.
4. Wandell M, Powell JR, Hager WD, Fenster PE, Graves PE, Conrad KA, Goldman S. Effect of quinine on digoxin kinetics. *Clin Pharmacol Ther* (1980) 28, 425–30.
5. Hedman A, Angelin B, Arvidsson A, Dahlqvist R, Nilsson B. Interactions in the renal and biliary elimination of digoxin: stereoselective difference between quinine and quinidine. *Clin Pharmacol Ther* (1990) 47, 20–6.

Digitalis glycosides + Quinolone antibacterials

Levofloxacin, gemifloxacin, moxifloxacin and sparfloxacin do not interact pharmacokinetically with digoxin, nor moxifloxacin with beta-acetyldigoxin. Gatifloxacin may cause small increases in digoxin levels, which are probably not clinically significant.

Clinical evidence, mechanism, importance and management

No changes occurred in the pharmacokinetics of **digoxin** in a study in 12 normal subjects taking 500 mg **levofloxacin** twice daily for 5 days when given a single 400-microgram dose of **digoxin**.[1] No changes occurred in the pharmacokinetics of **digoxin** in a study in 24 healthy subjects taking 300 micrograms **digoxin** daily when treated with a 400 mg loading dose of **sparfloxacin**, followed by 200 mg daily for 10 days.[2,3] No clinically relevant pharmacokinetic changes were seen in yet another study in 14 healthy elderly subjects given 320 mg **gemifloxacin** daily for 7 days while taking 250 micrograms **digoxin** daily, nor were there any clinically important changes in vital signs or ECG changes.[4,5] No clinically relevant changes in the steady-state pharmacokinetics of **digoxin** were seen in 24 healthy subjects taking 250 micrograms **digoxin** daily when additionally given 400 mg **moxifloxacin** daily for 14 days.[6] No pharmacokinetic changes were seen in another study in 12 healthy subjects given single 600-microgram doses of **beta-acetyldigoxin** and concurrently treated with 400 mg **moxifloxacin** daily for 2 days.[7] No changes in vital signs were seen in 12 healthy volunteers given **gatifloxacin** 400 mg daily for 7 days while taking **digoxin** 250 micrograms daily. Steady-state concentrations of **digoxin** and the **digoxin** AUC were increased by 12 and 19% respectively. Dosage adjustments during concomitant use were not considered necessary.[8] There would therefore seem to be no reason for avoiding the concurrent use of **digoxin** and any of these **quinolone antibacterials**.

Information about other **digitalis glycosides** and other **quinolone antibacterials** seems to be lacking, but bearing in mind their very extensive use, this silence in the literature would suggest that no problems normally arise. In about 10% of patients, some antibacterials can increase serum digoxin levels by inhibiting the metabolism of digoxin in the gut by *Eubacterium lentum* (see 'Digitalis glycosides + Macrolide antibacterials', p.544). Despite *in vitro* susceptibility of *E. lentum* to a range of antibacterials including quinolones there is currently no information to suggest this interaction occurs between quinolones and digoxin.[9]

1. Chien SC, Chow AT, Williams R. Absence of an effect of levofloxacin on digoxin pharmacokinetics. *Am Acad Pharm Sci, Annual Meeting Program Supplement,* (1995) June 5–6, New Brunswick.
2. Johnson RD, Wilson J, Talbot G, Conway S, Heald D. The effect of sparfloxacin on the steady-state pharmacokinetics of digoxin in healthy male voluteers. *Pharm Res* (1994) 11 (10 Suppl), S429.
3. Johnson RD, Dorr MB, Hunt TL, Conway S, Talbot GH. Pharmacokinetic interaction of sparfloxacin and digoxin. *Clin Ther* (1999) 21, 368–82.
4. Vousden M, Allen A, Lewis A, Rauland M, Ehren N. Lack of effect of gemifloxacin on the pharmacokinetics of steady-state digoxin in healthy elderly volunteers. *J Antimicrob Chemother* (1999) 44 (Suppl A), 138.
5. Vousden M, Allen A, Lewis A, Ehren N. Lack of pharmacokinetic interaction between gemifloxacin and digoxin in healthy elderly volunteers. *Chemotherapy* (1999) 45, 485–90.
6. Staß H, Frey R, Kubitza J-G, Möller M, Zühlsdorf M. Influence of orally administered moxifloxacin (MOX) on the steady-state pharmacokinetics (PK) of digoxin (D) in healthy male volunteers. *J Antimicrob Chemother* (1999) 44 (Suppl A), 134–5.

7. Horstmann R, Delesen H, Dietrich H, Ochmann K, Sachse R, Stass H, Zuehlsdorf M, Kuhlmann J. No drug-drug interaction between moxifloxacin and β-acetyldigoxin. *Clin Invest Med* (1998) (Suppl), S20.

8. Olsen SJ, Uderman HD, Kaul S, Kollia GD, Birkhoffer MJ, Grasela DM. Pharmacokinetics of concomitantly administered gatifloxacin and digoxin. In: Abstracts 39th Annual ICAAC, San Francisco, 1999.

9. Ten Eick AP, Reed MD. Hidden dangers of coadministration of antibiotics and digoxin in children: focus on azithromycin. *Curr Ther Res* (2000) 61, 148–60.

Digitalis glycosides + Rauwolfia Alkaloids

Concurrent use is usually uneventful, but the incidence of arrhythmias appears to be increased, particularly in those with atrial fibrillation. Excessive bradycardia and syncope have also been described.

Clinical evidence

(a) Increased cardiac arrhythmias

Three patients on **digoxin** and either **reserpine** or **whole root Rauwolfia serpentina** developed arrhythmias: atrial tachycardia with 4:1 Wenckebach irregular block; ventricular bigeminy and tachycardia; and atrial fibrillation. A large number of other patients received both drugs without problems.[1]

The incidence of premature ventricular systoles was roughly doubled in patients taking digoxin and rauwolfia compared with a similar group taking only **rauwolfia**.[2] **Reserpine** reduced the tolerated dose of **acetyl strophanthidin** in 15 patients with congestive heart failure; 8 out of 9 with atrial fibrillation showed advanced toxic rhythms during acute digitalisation compared with only one of the 9 who responded in this way without **reserpine**.[3]

(b) Excessive bradycardia and syncope

A man on **digoxin** (250 and 375 micrograms on alternate days) and **reserpine** (25 micrograms daily) developed a very slow heart rate, sinus bradycardia and carotid sinus supersensitivity. He was hospitalised because of syncope, which remitted when the **reserpine** was withdrawn.[4]

Mechanism

Not understood. A possible explanation is that because the rauwolfia alkaloids deplete the sympathetic nerve supply (i.e. accelerator) to the heart of its neurotransmitter, this would allow the parasympathetic vagal supply (i.e. heart slowing) to have full rein. Digitalis also causes heart slowing so that the total additive bradycardia becomes excessive. In this situation the rate could become so slow that ectopic foci which would normally be swamped by a faster, more normal beat, begin to fire, leading to the development of arrhythmias. Syncope could also result from the combination of bradycardia and the hypotensive effects of reserpine elsewhere in the cardiovascular system.

Importance and management

Some caution is advisable. One group of authors who, despite having described the adverse reactions cited above,[1] conclude that ". . . time has proven the safety of the combination." However they continue with the proviso that ". . . the development of arrhythmias must be anticipated and appropriate steps taken at their appearance . . ." Particular risk of arrhythmias seems to occur in patients with atrial fibrillation (8 out of 9 in the report cited[3]), and in digitalised patients given reserpine parenterally because of the sudden release of catecholamines that takes place.[4]

1. Dick HLH, McCawley EL, Fisher WA. Reserpine-digitalis toxicity. *Arch Intern Med* (1962) 109, 503–6.

2. Schreader CJ, Etzel MM. Premature ventricular contractions due to rauwolfia therapy. *JAMA* (1956) 162, 1256.

3. Lown B, Ehrlich L, Lipschultz B, Blake J. Effect of digitalis in patients receiving reserpine. *Circulation* (1961) 24, 1185–91.

4. Bigger JT, Strauss HC. Digitalis toxicity: drug interactions promoting toxicity and the management of toxicity. *Semin Drug Treat* (1972) 2, 147–77.

Digitalis glycosides + Rifampicin (Rifampin)

The serum levels of digitoxin can be halved by the concurrent use of rifampicin. There is also some evidence that digoxin serum levels may be similarly affected.

Clinical evidence

(a) Digitoxin

A comparative study in 21 tuberculous patients and 19 healthy subjects taking 100 micrograms **digitoxin** daily showed that the serum **digitoxin** levels of the patients on **rifampicin** were approximately 50% of the levels in healthy subjects not on **rifampicin** (18.4 compared with 39.1 ng/ml).[1] The half-life of **digitoxin** was reduced by the **rifampicin** from 8.2 to 4.5 days.

There are case reports confirming that **rifampicin** can markedly reduce serum **digitoxin** levels.[2,3]

(b) Digoxin

A woman, hospitalised for endocarditis, and receiving treatment with **digoxin** (250 to 375 micrograms daily), furosemide (frusemide), aspirin, isosorbide dinitrate and potassium chloride, showed a marked fall of about 80% in her serum **digoxin** level when given 600 mg **rifampicin** daily. The serum **digoxin** climbed to its former level over the 2 weeks following **rifampicin** withdrawal.[4] She had only moderate renal impairment (serum creatinine 2.5 mg/dl). Another report describes 2 patients on renal dialysis whose **digoxin** dosage needed to be doubled while taking **rifampicin**, and similarly reduced when the **rifampicin** was withdrawn.[5] This confirms an earlier report.[6]

A study in 4 healthy subjects found that the AUC and maximum serum levels of **digoxin** following a single 1000-microgram oral dose were reduced by 30 and 54% respectively after taking 600 mg **rifampicin** daily for 6 days with 10 days pretreatment.[7] A smaller reduction (about 15%) in **digoxin** AUC and maximum serum levels was also seen when a single 1000 micrograms intravenous dose of **digoxin** was given with the same **rifampicin** regimen.[7]

Mechanism

The digitoxin/rifampicin interaction is almost certainly due to the increase in digitoxin metabolism caused by rifampicin which is a potent enzyme inducing agent.[1,8] Digoxin on the other hand is largely excreted unchanged (unmetabolised) in the urine and the interaction with rifampicin appears to be largely due to an increase in P-glycoprotein mediated efflux by the intestinal cells.[7] Poor kidney function in some patients may be an additional factor.

Importance and management

The digitoxin/rifampicin interaction is established and clinically important. Under-digitalisation may occur unless the digitoxin dosage is increased appropriately (approximately doubled). Good monitoring is obviously advisable.

The situation with digoxin is less clear. The documentation is very limited (most of it goes back to the 1980s) which is perhaps surprising considering how long both drugs have been available, but this would not be the first clinically relevant interaction to have been largely overlooked. It would now be prudent to monitor the concurrent use of these drugs, being alert for the need to increase the digoxin dosage. It may be that renal impairment increases the extent of this interaction. More study is needed.

1. Peters U, Hausamen T-U, Grosse-Brockhoff F. Einfluß von Tuberkulostatika auf die Pharmakokinetik des Digitoxins. *Dtsch Med Wochenschr* (1974) 99, 2381–6.

2. Boman G, Eliasson K, Odar-cederlöf I. Acute cardiac failure during treatment with digitoxin - an interaction with rifampicin. *Br J Clin Pharmacol* (1980) 10, 89–90.

3. Poor DM, Self TH, Davis HL. Interaction of rifampin and digitoxin. *Arch Intern Med* (1983) 143, 599.

4. Bussey HI, Merritt GJ, Hill EG. The influence of rifampin on quinidine and digoxin. *Arch Intern Med* (1984) 144, 1021–3.

5. Gault H, Longerich L, Dawe M, Fine A. Digoxin-rifampin interaction. *Clin Pharmacol Ther* (1984) 35, 750–4.

6. Novi C, Bissoli F, Simonati V, Volpini T, Baroli A, Vignati G. Rifampin and digoxin: possible drug interaction in a dialysis patient. *JAMA* (1980) 244, 2521–2.

7. Greiner B, Eichelbaum M, Fritz P, Kreichgauer H-P, von Richter O, Zundler J, Kroemer HK. The role of intestinal P-glycoprotein in the interaction of digoxin and rifampin. *J Clin Invest* (1999) 104, 147–53.

8. Zilly W, Breimer DD, Richter E. Pharmacokinetic interactions with rifampicin. *Clin Pharmacokinet* (1977) 2, 61–70.

Digitalis glycosides + Selective serotonin re-uptake inhibitors (SSRIs) and related antidepressants

Neither citalopram, clovoxamine nor fluvoxamine appear to interact with digoxin, but an isolated report describes increased serum digoxin levels attributed to the use of fluoxetine.

Clinical evidence, mechanism, importance and management

A study in 11 healthy subjects showed that **citalopram** 40 mg once daily for 28 days did not have any significant effect on the pharmacokinetics of single doses of digoxin 1000 micrograms taken on day 21. No clinically significant ECG changes were observed.[1] After taking 150 mg **clovoxamine** or 100 mg **fluvoxamine** daily for 15 days, the pharmacokinetics (distribution, elimination and clearance) of a single intravenous dose of 1250 micrograms **digoxin** were unchanged in 8 healthy subjects.[2] It seems unlikely therefore that any of these drugs will affect the steady-state serum levels of **digoxin** in patients, but this needs confirmation. No special precautions would seem to be necessary.

An isolated report describes increased serum **digoxin** levels in a woman of 93 with congestive heart failure on two occasions when **fluoxetine** was added.[3] The general importance of this interaction is not known.

1. Larsen F, Priskorn M, Overø KF. Lack of citalopram effect on oral digoxin pharmacokinetics. *J Clin Pharmacol* (2001) 41, 340–6.

2. Ochs HR, Greenblatt DJ, Verburg-Ochs B, Labedski L. Chronic treatment with fluvoxamine, clovoxamine and placebo: interaction with digoxin and effects on sleep and alertness. *J Clin Pharmacol* (1989) 29, 91–95.

3. Leibovitz A, Bilchinsky T, Gil I, Habot B. Elevated serum digoxin level associated with coadministered fluoxetine. *Arch Intern Med* (1998) 158, 1152–3.

Digitalis glycosides + Sevelamer

The pharmacokinetics of single doses of digoxin are not affected by sevelamer.

Clinical evidence, mechanism, importance and management

In an open randomised crossover study a single dose of **digoxin** 1000 micrograms by mouth was given with or without **sevelamer** 2.4 g followed by a standard breakfast. Five further doses of **sevelamer** were given immediately before subsequent meals over the following 2 days. The pharmacokinetic profile of **digoxin** was not altered by the administration of **sevelamer**.[1] **Sevelamer** is a non-absorbed phosphate-binding polymer with bile-acid binding properties. Because the bile-acid binding resins colestyramine and colestipol may interact with digoxin (see 'Digitalis glycosides + Colestyramine', p.537 and Digitalis glycosides + Colestipol'), it was suggested that sevelamer could also interact, although this appears not to be the case. This finding requires confirmation in long-term studies.

1. Burke S, Amin N, Incerti C, Plone M, Watson N. Sevelamer hydrochloride (Renagel®), a nonabsorbed phosphate-binding polymer, does not interfere with digoxin or warfarin pharmacokinetics. *J Clin Pharmacol* (2001) 41, 193–8.

Digitalis glycosides + Siberian ginseng

A man on digoxin showed grossly elevated serum digoxin levels but no toxicity while concurrently taking Siberian ginseng.

Clinical evidence, mechanism, importance and management

A 74-year-old man stabilised on **digoxin** for many years (serum levels normally in the range 0.9 to 2.2 ng/ml) was found during a routine check to have levels of 5.2 ng/ml but without evidence of toxicity or bradycardia or any other ECG changes.[1] The levels remained high even when the **digoxin** was stopped. Later it turned out he was also taking **Siberian ginseng** capsules. When the **ginseng** was stopped, the **digoxin** levels fell once again, and **digoxin** therapy was resumed. Later rechallenge with the **ginseng** caused a rise in his serum **digoxin** levels. The reasons are not known. No digoxin nor digitoxin contamination was found in the capsules, and the authors of the report also rejected the idea that the eleutherosides (chemically related to **digoxin**) in ginseng might have been converted *in vivo* into **digoxin**, or that the renal elimination of **digoxin** might have been impaired, since the patient showed no signs of toxicity. One possible explanation is that the **ginseng** affected the accuracy of the **digoxin** assay so that it gave false results.

This seems to be the only report of this reaction and its general importance is uncertain, but it acts as a reminder that "green" and other herbal remedies can sometimes interact, and that this type of **ginseng** can possibly elevate serum **digoxin** levels or affect the assay of digoxin. Be aware that **Siberian ginseng** (*Eleutherococcus senticosis*) is different from **Chinese ginseng** (*Panax* species). Siberian ginseng contains eleutherosides, which are glycosides with aglycones related to the cardiac glycosides like **digoxin**, while Chinese ginseng contains ginsenosides.

1. McRae S. Elevated serum digoxin levels in a patient taking digoxin and Siberian ginseng. *Can Med Assoc J* (1996) 155, 293–5.

Digitalis glycosides + Spironolactone

The available evidence suggests that serum digoxin levels may be increased 25% by spironolactone, but because spironolactone or its metabolite, canrenone, can interfere with some digoxin assay methods, the evaluation of this interaction is difficult. The effects of digitoxin are reported to be both increased and decreased by spironolactone.

Clinical evidence

(a) Digoxin

The serum **digoxin** levels of 9 patients were increased by about 20% (from 0.8 to 1 ng/ml) when given 200 mg **spironolactone** daily. One patient showed a three to fourfold rise.[1]

The clearance of **digoxin** in 4 patients and 4 healthy subjects after single 750 micrograms intravenous doses was reduced by about 25% following 5 days treatment with 200 mg **spironolactone** daily.[2] A marked fall in serum **digoxin** was reported in an elderly patient when **spironolactone** was withdrawn[3] but the accuracy of the assay method used is uncertain (see Importance and management below). One study found that no clinically important reduction in **digoxin** clearance occurred when *Aldactazide* (**spironolactone-hydrochlorothiazide**) was used.[4]

(b) Digitoxin

A study in 6 healthy subjects who had been taking 100 or 150 micrograms **digitoxin** daily for 30 days showed that the concurrent use of 300 mg **spironolactone** daily increased the **digitoxin** half-life by a third (from 141 to 192 h).[5]

Other studies however found that the **digitoxin** half-life was reduced (from 256 to 204 h).[6]

Mechanism

Not fully understood. Spironolactone inhibits the excretion of digoxin by the kidney (by 13%) but not its biliary clearance,[7] and probably causes a reduction in the volume of distribution.

Importance and management

The digoxin/spironolactone interaction appears to be established. What is known suggests a rise of about 25% in serum digoxin levels, although much greater increases can apparently occur.[1] Monitor concurrent use carefully for signs of over-digitalisation. The reports cited here appear to be reliable, but the total picture of this interaction is confused by a number of other reports (not cited) of doubtful reliability. The problem is that spironolactone or its metabolite, canrenone, can interfere with some assay methods. In one report, radioimmunoassay (RIA) and affinity-column-mediated immunoassay (AC-MIA) were particularly affected by spironolactone and its metabolites.[8] Conversely, falsely low digoxin readings with the Ax-Sym MEIA assay method lead to digoxin overdose and intoxication in one patient.[9] This means that monitoring is difficult unless the digoxin assay method is known to be reliable. The situation with digitoxin is even more confusing because the reports are contradictory and the outcome uncertain. Concurrent use should be well monitored.

1. Steiness E. Renal tubular secretion of digoxin. *Circulation* (1974) 50. 103–7.
2. Waldorff S, Andersen JD, Heebøll-Nielsen N, Nielsen OG, Moltke E, Sørensen U, Steiness E. Spironolactone-induced changes in digoxin kinetics. *Clin Pharmacol Ther* (1978) 24, 162–7.
3. Paladino JA, Davidson KH, McCall BB. Influence of spironolactone on serum digoxin concentration. *JAMA* (1984) 251, 470–1.
4. Finnegan TP, Spence JD, Cape R. Potassium-sparing diuretics: interaction with digoxin in elderly men. *J Am Geriatr Soc* (1984) 32, 129–31.
5. Carruthers SG, Dujovne CA. Cholestyramine and spironolactone and their combination in digitoxin elimination. *Clin Pharmacol Ther* (1980) 27, 184–7.
6. Wirth KE, Frölich JC, Hollifield JW, Falkner FC, Sweetman BS, Oates JA. Metabolism of digitoxin in man and its modification by spironolactone. *Eur J Clin Pharmacol* (1976) 9, 345–54.
7. Hedman A, Angelin B, Arvidsson A, Dahlqvist R. Digoxin-interactions in man: spironolactone reduces renal but not biliary digoxin clearance. *Eur J Clin Pharmacol* (1992) 42, 481–5.
8. Pleasants RA, Williams DM, Porter RS, Gadsden RH. Reassessment of cross-reactivity of spironolactone metabolites with four digoxin immunoassays. *Ther Drug Monit* (1989) 11, 200–4.
9. Steimer W, Müller C, Eber B, Emmanuildis K. Intoxication due to negative canrenone interference in digoxin drug monitoring. *Lancet* (1999) 354, 1176–7.

Digitalis glycosides + St. John's wort (*Hypericum perforatum*)

There is good evidence that St John's wort can reduce the blood levels of digoxin by between about one-third to one-quarter.

Clinical evidence

Thirteen healthy subjects were given **digoxin** 250 micrograms daily for 5 days until steady-state had been achieved, and then **St John's wort** extract (LI160, Lichtwer Pharma) was added for a further 10 days. When compared with another group of 12 subjects taking a placebo, the test group showed a 26.3% fall in maximum plasma **digoxin** levels, a 33.3% fall in trough **digoxin** levels and a 25% fall in the AUC.[1,2]

Mechanism

Uncertain, but the authors of the report suggest that the St John's wort possibly affects the activity of P-glycoprotein drug transporter which could alter the intestinal absorption and renal excretion of the digoxin.[2]

Importance and management

Information seems to be limited to this report, but the interaction would appear to be established. Reductions in serum digoxin levels of this size are likely to diminish the control of heart rhythm or heart failure. Digoxin serum levels should therefore be well monitored if St John's wort is either started or stopped and appropriate dosage adjustments made if necessary. The recommendation of the CSM in the UK is that St John's wort should not be used in patients taking digoxin.[3] More study of this interaction is needed. Information about the effects of St John's wort on **digitoxin** are lacking but some reduction in serum levels would seem likely.

1. Johne A, Brockmöller J, Bauer S, Maurer A, Langheinrich M, Roots I. Interaction of St John's wort extract with digoxin. *Eur J Clin Pharmacol* (1999) 55, A22.
2. Johne A, Brockmöller J, Bauer S, Maurer A, Langheinrich M, Roots I. Pharmacokinetic interaction of digoxin with an herbal extract from St John's wort (*Hypericum perforatum*). *Clin Pharmacol Ther* (1999) 66, 338–45.
3. Committee on the Safety of Medicines (UK). Message from Professor A Breckenridge (Chairman of CSM) and Fact Sheet for Health Care Professionals, 29th February 2000.

Digitalis glycosides + Sucralfate

Sucralfate caused only a small reduction in the absorption of digoxin in normal subjects, but an isolated report describes a marked reduction in one patient.

Clinical evidence

Sucralfate 1g four times daily for 2 days given to 12 normal subjects had no effect on most of the pharmacokinetic parameters of single 750-microgram doses of **digoxin.** However, the AUC was reduced by 19% (from 41.85 to 39.47 ng/ml.h) and the amount eliminated in the urine was reduced by 12%. Digoxin was also absorbed faster.[1] No interaction occurred when the **digoxin** was given 2 h before the **sucralfate.**[1] One elderly patient is reported to have had subtherapeutic serum **digoxin** levels while taking **sucralfate**, even though the dosages were separated by 2 h.[2]

Mechanism

Uncertain. One possibility is that the digoxin and sucralfate bind together in the gut, which reduces the digoxin absorption.

Importance and management

Information appears to be limited to the reports cited. The reduction in digoxin levels is apparently only small and therefore normally not likely to be clinically relevant, but the unexplained and isolated case suggests that clinicians should at least be aware of the possibility of an interaction.

1. Giesing DH, Lanman RC, Dimmitt DC, Runser DJ. Lack of effect of sucralfate on digoxin pharmacokinetics. *Gastroenterology* (1983) 84,1165.
2. Rey AM, Gums JG. Altered absorption of digoxin, sustained-release quinidine, and warfarin with sucralfate administration. *Ann Pharmacother* (1991) 25, 745–6.

Digitalis glycosides + Sulfasalazine

Serum digoxin levels can be reduced by the concurrent use of sulfasalazine.

Clinical evidence, mechanism, importance and management

The observation that a patient taking 8 g **sulfasalazine** daily had low serum **digoxin** levels, prompted a crossover study in 10 healthy subjects given 500 micrograms **digoxin** (as an elixir) alone and later after 6 days treatment with 2 to 6 g **sulfasalazine** daily. **Digoxin** absorption was reduced, ranging from 0 to 50% depending on the dosage of **sulfasalazine** used.[1] Serum **digoxin** levels were depressed accordingly.[1] The reasons are not understood. This seems to be the only report of this interaction, but it appears to be established. Concurrent use need not be avoided, but serum **digoxin** levels should be monitored and/or the patient checked for signs of under-digitalisation. In one patient examined, separating the dosages appeared not to prevent this interaction.

1. Juhl RP, Summers RW, Guillory JK, Blaug SM, Cheng FH and Brown DD. Effect of sulfasalazine on digoxin bioavailability. *Clin Pharmacol Ther* (1976) 20, 387–94.

Digitalis glycosides + Sympathomimetics (beta-agonists)

Salbutamol (albuterol) by mouth causes a small reduction in serum digoxin levels. Beta-agonists can cause hypokalaemia, which could lead to the development of digitalis toxicity.

Clinical evidence, mechanism, importance and management

A study in 10 healthy subjects who had taken 500 micrograms **digoxin** daily for 10 days[1] found that 3 h after taking 3 to 4 mg **salbutamol (albuterol)** orally their serum **digoxin** levels had fallen by 0.3 nmol/l and their serum potassium levels by 0.58 mmol/l. A follow-up study suggested that the **digoxin** distribution to skeletal muscle may have been increased.[2] Note that all beta-agonists can cause a fall in serum potassium, which can be potentiated by other potassium-depleting drugs (see 'Beta-agonist bronchodilators + Potassium-depleting drugs', p.774), and this could possibly affect the response of patients to **digoxin**. The clinical importance of these changes is uncertain but concurrent use should be monitored.

1. Edner M, Jogestrand T. Oral salbutamol decreases serum digoxin concentration. *Eur J Clin Pharmacol* (1990) 38, 195–7.
2. Edner M, Jogestrand T, Dahlqvist R. Effect of salbutamol on digoxin pharmacokinetics. *Eur J Clin Pharmacol* (1992) 42, 197–201.

Digitalis glycosides + Tetracycline

Tetracycline may cause a rise in serum digoxin levels in a few patients, which is of uncertain clinical importance.

Clinical evidence

A patient on 500 micrograms **digoxin** daily in tablet form was given 500 mg **tetracycline** 6-hourly for 5 days. His urinary excretion of digoxin metabolites (see Mechanism) fell sharply within 2 days, and his steady-state serum **digoxin** levels rose by 43%.[1]

A marked fall in the excretion of digoxin metabolites from the gut in one of 2 subjects after taking **tetracycline** is confirmed in another brief report.[2]

Mechanism

Up to 10% of patients on oral digoxin excrete it in substantial amounts in the faeces and urine as inactive metabolites (digoxin reduction products or DRPs). This metabolism seems to be the responsibility of the gut flora,[1] in particular *Eubacterium lentum*, which is anaerobic and Gram positive.[2,3] In the presence of some antibacterials such as tetracycline that can inhibit this organism, more digoxin is available for absorption, which results in a rise in serum levels. At the same time the inactive metabolites derived from the gut disappear.[2] See also 'Digitalis glycosides + Macrolide antibacterials', p.544.

Importance and management

The digoxin/tetracycline interaction is not well established and the evidence is very limited. Its general clinical importance is uncertain and it is only likely to occur with digoxin formulations with poor bioavailability (tablets rather than liquid preparations). Only a small proportion of patients (about 10%) is likely to be at risk, the difficulty being that it is usually not known if a particular patient falls into this 'excreter' category or not (see Mechanism). Monitor patients for signs of increased digoxin effects if given any tetracycline that reduces the activity of the gut flora, reducing the digoxin dosage as necessary.

1. Lindenbaum J, Rund DG, Butler VP, Tse-Eng D, Saha JR. Inactivation of digoxin by the gut flora: reversal by antibiotic therapy. *N Engl J Med* (1981) 305, 789–94.
2. Dobkin JF, Saha JR, Butler VP, Lindenbaum J. Effects of antibiotic therapy on digoxin metabolism. *Clin Res* (1982) 30, 517A.
3. Ten Eick AP, Reed MD. Hidden dangers of coadministration of antibiotics and digoxin in children: focus on azithromycin. *Curr Ther Res* (2000) 61, 148–60.

Digitalis glycosides + Thyroid hormones and Antithyroid drugs

Thyrotoxic patients are relatively resistant to the effects of digitalis glycosides and may need reduced doses as treatment with antithyroid drugs (carbimazole, thiamazole (methimazole)) progresses, whereas patients with hypothyroidism may need increased doses of digitalis glycosides as treatment with thyroid hormones proceeds. Carbimazole has been shown to reduce serum digoxin in healthy subjects.

Clinical evidence

(a) Carbimazole

The observation of relatively low plasma **digoxin** levels in a patient on **carbimazole** prompted a further study in 10 healthy subjects. In 9 out of the 10, steady-state peak serum **digoxin** levels were reduced by 23% (from 1.72 to 1.33 ng/ml) by a single 60-mg dose of **carbimazole**, but in the other subject the serum **digoxin** levels were increased. Other parameters measured (time to reach maximum serum levels and AUC) were unaffected. **Carbimazole** abolished the systolic blood pressure decrease seen in the first 3 h with **digoxin** alone, and it also reduced the duration of the **digoxin**-induced diastolic blood pressure fall from 12 to 6 h. The changes in heart rates, cardiac output and stroke volumes were not statistically significant, but inter-individual differences were large.[1-3]

(b) Thiamazole (Methimazole)

A study in 12 patients with hyperthyroidism found that normalisation of serum T3 and T4 by **thiamazole** treatment did not produce significant changes in the pharmacokinetics of the **digoxin**.[4]

Mechanism

One explanation for the changed response to digitalis is that there is a direct and altered response of the heart due to the raised or lowered thyroid hormone levels. Another is that changes in glomerular filtration rate associated with hypo- or hyperthyroidism result in increased or decreased serum digoxin, respectively.[5] Why carbimazole *reduced* serum digoxin in healthy subjects (normal thyroid status) is not known.

Importance and management

As thyroid status is returned to normal by the use of drugs (**antithyroid drugs** or **thyroid hormones**), the dosage of the digitalis glycosides may need to be adjusted appropriately. Hyperthyroidic patients may need to have their digitalis dosage gradually reduced as treatment proceeds (because initially they are relatively resistant to the effects of digitalis and start off needing higher doses). They are also relatively insensitive to the chronotropic effects of digitalis.[6,7] Hypothyroidic patients on the other hand may need a gradually increasing dosage (because initially they are relatively sensitive to digitalis).[5,6] In either of these situations it would be prudent to monitor serum digoxin levels and glomerular filtration rate as treatment continues. The reduction of serum digoxin by carbimazole in healthy

subjects does not fit with the need to decrease digoxin doses when antithyroid drugs are used in patients. Further study is needed.

1. Petereit G, Ramesh Rao B, Siepmann M, Kirch W. Influence of carbimazole on the steady state serum levels and haemodynamic effects of digoxin in healthy subjects. *Eur J Clin Pharmacol* (1995) 49, A159.
2. Rao BR, Petereit G, Ebert U, Siepmann M, Kirch W. Influence of carbimazole on the steady state serum levels and haemodynamic effects of digoxin in healthy subjects. *Therapie* (1995) 50 (Suppl), 406.
3. Rao R, Petereit G, Ebert U, Kirch W. Influence of carbimazole on serum levels and haemodynamic effects of digoxin. *Clin Drug Invest* (1997) 13, 350–4.
4. Gasińska T, Izbicka M, Dec R. Digoxin pharmacokinetics in hyperthyroid patients treated with methimazole. *J Endocrinol* (1997) 152 (Suppl), P285.
5. Croxson MS, Ibbertson HK. Serum digoxin in patients with thyroid disease. *BMJ* (1975) 3, 566–8.
6. Lawrence JR, Sumner DJ, Kalk WJ, Ratcliffe WA, Whiting B, Gray K, Lindsay M. Digoxin kinetics in patients with thyroid dysfunction. *Clin Pharmacol Ther* (1977) 22, 7–13.
7. Huffman DH, Klaassen CD, Hartman CR. Digoxin in hyperthyroidism. *Clin Pharmacol Ther* (1977) 22, 533–8.

Digitalis glycosides + Ticlopidine

**Ticlopidine causes a small and almost certainly clinically un-
important reduction in serum digoxin levels.**

Clinical evidence, mechanism, importance and management

Ticlopidine 250 mg twice daily for 10 days reduced the peak serum
digoxin concentrations by 11% and the AUC by 9% in 15 subjects
taking 125 to 500 micrograms digoxin daily.[1] These reductions are
small and unlikely to be of clinical importance.

1. Vargas R, Reitman M, Teitelbaum P, Ryan JR, McMahon FG, Jain AK, Ryan M, Regel G. Study of the effect of ticlopidine on digoxin blood levels. *Clin Pharmacol Ther* (1988) 43, 176.

Digitalis glycosides + Tolrestat

Tolrestat does not affect digoxin pharmacokinetics.

Clinical evidence, mechanism, importance and management

The steady-state pharmacokinetics of **digoxin** in 12 patients were not
significantly altered when they were additionally given 400 mg **tolrestat** daily for 7 days.[1] No special precautions appear to be necessary
during concurrent use.

1. Meng X, Parker V, Turner M, Burghart P, Battle M. Effect of tolrestat on pharmacokinetics (PK) of digoxin. *Clin Pharmacol Ther* (1994) 55, 167.

Digitalis glycosides + Trapidil

Trapidil does not alter serum digoxin levels.

Clinical evidence, mechanism, importance and management

Trapidil 400 mg daily for 8 days had no effect on the steady-state serum **digoxin** levels in 10 healthy subjects taking **digoxin**
375 micrograms daily. It was noted that the positive chronotropic effect of **trapidil** opposed the negative chronotropic effect of **digoxin**.[1]
No special precautions would seem necessary.

1. Sziegoleit W, Weiss M, Fahr A, Scharfe S. Trapidil does not affect serum levels and cardiotonic action of digoxin in healthy humans. *Jpn Circ J* (1987) 51, 1305–9.

Digitalis glycosides + Trazodone

**A rise in serum digoxin levels, accompanied by intoxication in
one instance, has been seen in two patients on digoxin when
treated with trazodone.**

Clinical evidence, mechanism, importance and management

An elderly woman stabilised on **digoxin** 125 micrograms daily (and
also taking quinidine, clonidine and a triamterene-hydrochlorothiazide diuretic) complained of nausea and vomiting within a fortnight
of starting to take **trazodone** (increased from 50 to 300 mg daily over
11 days). Her serum **digoxin** levels had risen more than threefold
(from 0.8 to 2.8 ng/ml). The **digoxin** was stopped and then restarted
at half the original dosage which maintained therapeutic levels.[1] The
patient had poor renal function, but this did not change significantly
during this incident. Another case has been reported.[2]

Even though direct information seems to be limited to these two reports, until more information is available it would now seem prudent
to monitor the effects of concurrent use.

1. Rauch PK, Jenike MA. Digoxin toxicity possibly precipitated by trazodone. *Psychosomatics* (1984) 25, 334–5.
2. Knapp JE. Mead Johnson Pharmaceutical Newsletter, 1983.

Digitalis glycosides + Trimethoprim or Co-trimoxazole

**Serum digoxin levels can be increased about 22% by trimeth-
oprim but some individuals may show a much greater rise.**

Clinical evidence

(a) Elderly patients

After taking **trimethoprim** 200 mg twice daily for 14 days the mean
serum **digoxin** levels in 9 elderly patients (aged 62 to 92) had risen by
an average of 22% (from 1.17 to 1.50 nmol/l). One patient showed a
75% rise. A 34% increase in mean serum creatinine was also seen.
When the **trimethoprim** was withdrawn, the serum **digoxin** levels
fell once again.[1,2]

(b) Young healthy adult subjects

Trimethoprim 200 mg twice daily for 10 days did not affect total
body clearance of **digoxin** after a single 1000 micrograms intravenous dose in 6 young healthy subjects (aged 24 to 31). Renal clearance was reduced, but this was compensated for by an increase in
extrarenal clearance.[2]

Mechanism

It is suggested that trimethoprim reduces the renal excretion of digoxin.[1,2] The paradoxical finding between the patients ((a) above) and the
healthy subjects ((b) above) may be the age difference, probably as
the elderly patients may not be able to accommodate with an increase
in extrarenal digoxin clearance.

Importance and management

Information seems to be limited to the information cited. Although
the serum digoxin rise in the elderly was modest, it would seem prudent to monitor the effects because some individuals can apparently
experience a marked rise. Reduce the digoxin dosage if necessary.
Trimethoprim is contained in **co-trimoxazole** but it is not known
whether prophylactic-dose co-trimoxazole (160 mg trimethoprim a
day, from 960 mg co-trimoxazole) will interact to a clinically significant degree. An interaction would seem likely with high-dose co-tri-

moxazole regimens and care with any co-trimoxazole regimen is needed in the elderly.

1. Kastrup J, Bartram R, Petersen P, Hansen JM. Trimetoprims indvirkning på serum-digoksin og serum-kreatinin. *Ugeskr Laeger* (1983) 145, 2286–8.
2. Petersen P, Kastrup J, Bartram R, Hansen JM. Digoxin-trimethoprim interaction. *Acta Med Scand* (1985) 217, 423–7.

Digitalis glycosides + Urapidil

Urapidil appears not to interact adversely with digoxin.

Clinical evidence, mechanism, importance and management

Urapidil 60 mg twice daily for 4 days (from days 5 to 8) had no significant effects on serum **digoxin** levels in 12 healthy subjects given 250 micrograms twice daily on day one, then 250 micrograms daily on days 2 to 8. Blood pressures and pulse rates were not significantly changed.[1] No special precautions seem necessary.

1. Solleder P, Haerlin R, Wurst W, Klingmann I, Mosberg H. Effect of urapidil on steady-state serum digoxin concentration in healthy subjects. *Eur J Clin Pharmacol* (1989) 37, 193–4.

Digitalis glycosides + Valaciclovir

Valaciclovir appears not to interact with digoxin.

Clinical evidence, mechanism, importance and management

In a randomised 4-period crossover study, 12 healthy subjects were given 1 g oral **valaciclovir** alone, two doses of 750 micrograms **digoxin** alone, 1 g **valaciclovir** after the second of two doses of 750 micrograms **digoxin** given 12 h apart, and finally 1 g **valaciclovir** three times daily for 8 days starting 12 h before the first **digoxin** dose.[1]

It was found that no clinically significant changes occurred in the pharmacokinetics of either drug and no ECG changes were seen. It was concluded that no dosage adjustments of either drug are needed if given concurrently.[1] Since **valaciclovir** is a prodrug of **aciclovir**, it also seems unlikely that an **aciclovir/digoxin** interaction will occur. Information about **digitoxin** seems to be lacking.

1. Soul-Lawton JH, Weatherley BC, Posner J, Layton G, Peck RW. Lack of interaction between valaciclovir, the L-valyl ester of aciclovir and digoxin. *Br J Clin Pharmacol* (1998) 45, 87–9.

Digitalis glycosides + Valspodar

There is a two to threefold increase in the digoxin AUC when valspodar is given. The digoxin dose should be halved, and digoxin levels closely monitored.

Clinical evidence, mechanism, importance and management

Twelve healthy subjects were given 1000 micrograms **digoxin** on day 1, followed by 125 micrograms daily for the next 10 days. On day 7 they were additionally given a single 400 mg dose of **valspodar**, followed by 200 mg twice daily for the following 4 days. The first single dose of **valspodar** increased the steady-state **digoxin** AUC by 76%, and by the end the period it had increased by 211%. This was apparently due to a fall in renal **digoxin** clearance (by 58 to 73%), probably because of reduced tubular secretion mediated by P-glycoprotein. No symptoms of digitalis toxicity were seen and there were no changes in vital signs or ECG parameters.[1]

Information seems to be limited to this study in healthy subjects but it suggests that the **digoxin** dosage should be reduced if valspodar is given concurrently. An initial 50% reduction has been suggested.

1. Kovarik JM, Rigaudy L, Guerret M, Gerbeau C, Rost K-L. Longitudinal assessment of a P-glycoprotein-mediated drug interaction of valspodar on digoxin. *Clin Pharmacol Ther* (1999) 66, 391–400.

Digitalis glycosides + Vasodilators

A reduction in serum digoxin levels can occur during the concurrent use of sodium nitroprusside or hydralazine, but the importance of this is as yet uncertain.

Clinical evidence, mechanism, importance and management

An experimental study in 8 patients with congestive heart failure showed that when they were given either **sodium nitroprusside** by infusion (7 to 425 micrograms/min) or **hydralazine** by intravenous injection (5 mg every 10 to 20 min to a total dose of 10 to 60 mg) their total renal **digoxin** clearance went up by 50% and their serum **digoxin** levels fell by 20% and 11% respectively.[1] It is not known whether these changes would be sustained during chronic concurrent treatment, or the extent to which the **digoxin** dosage might need to be increased. More study is needed to find out if this interaction is of practical importance.

1. Cogan JJ, Humphreys MH, Carlson CJ, Benowitz NL, Rapaport E. Acute vasodilator therapy increases renal clearance of digoxin in patients with congestive heart failure. *Circulation* (1981) 64, 973–6.

Digitalis glycosides + Verapamil

Serum digoxin levels are increased by about 40% by the concurrent use of 160 mg verapamil daily, and by about 70% by 240 mg verapamil or more daily. Digoxin toxicity may develop if the dosage is not reduced. Deaths have occurred. A rise of about 35% occurs with digitoxin.

Clinical evidence

(a) Digoxin

After 2 weeks treatment with 240 mg **verapamil** daily, in 3 divided doses, the mean serum **digoxin** levels of 49 patients with chronic atrial fibrillation had risen by 72%. The rise was seen in most patients, and 90% of it occurred within the first 7 days. The rise was less with a smaller dose of **verapamil** (160 mg). Some of the patients showed signs of **digoxin** toxicity.[1]

Reports in a total of 21 healthy subjects,[2,3] and 54 patients[4-6] describe mean rises in serum **digoxin** levels of 44 to 147% when 240 to 360 mg **verapamil** daily was added to digoxin. A 40% rise was seen with 160 mg **verapamil** daily.[7] Similar rises are reported elsewhere.[7-10]

An approximately 50% rise in digoxin levels was seen in chronic haemodialysis patients given 120 to 240 mg **verapamil**, in three divided doses daily.[11] Nine normal subjects showed a 53% rise in digoxin levels while taking 240 mg **verapamil** daily for a fortnight, which increased to a total of 155% when additionally given 160 mg quinidine three times daily.[2] Toxicity[12] and a fatality[13] occurred in patients whose **digoxin** levels became markedly increased by **verapamil**. Both asystole and sinus arrest have been described.[14,15] A single dose study indicated that cirrhosis magnifies the extent of this interaction.[16]

(b) Digitoxin

Eight out of 10 patients showed a mean 35% rise (range 14 to 97%) in plasma **digitoxin** levels over a 4 to 6 week period while taking 240 mg **verapamil** daily, in three divided doses. Two patients showed no changes, and no changes in the pharmacokinetics of a single dose **digitoxin** were found in 3 healthy subjects.[17,18]

Mechanism

The rise in serum digoxin levels is due to reductions in renal and especially extra-renal (biliary) clearance; a diminution in the volume of distribution also takes place.[6-8,19] and there is the suggestion that P-glycoprotein may also be involved.[20] Impaired extra-renal excretion is suggested as the reason for the rise in serum digitoxin levels.[17]

Importance and management

The digoxin/verapamil interaction is well documented and well established. It occurs in most patients.[8,21] Serum digoxin levels should be well monitored and downward dosage adjustments made to avoid digoxin toxicity (deaths have occurred[13]). An initial 33 to 50% dosage reduction has been recommended.[22,23] The interaction develops within 2 to 7 days, approaching or reaching a maximum within 14 days or so.[1,5] The magnitude of the rise in serum digoxin is dose-dependent[24] with a significant increase if the verapamil dosage is increased from 160 to 240 mg daily,[1] but with no further increase if the dose is raised any higher.[3] The mean rise with verapamil 160 mg daily is about 40%, and with 240 mg or more is about 60 to 80%, but the response is variable. Some patients may show rises of up to 150% while others show only a modest increase. One study found that although the rise in serum digoxin levels was 60% within a week, this had lessened to about 30% five weeks later.[8] Regular monitoring and dosage adjustments would seem to be necessary.

The documentation of the digitoxin/verapamil interaction is limited, but the interaction appears to be established. The incidence was 80% in the study cited.[17] Downward dosage adjustment may be necessary, particularly in some patients. Serum digitoxin levels rise less than digoxin levels and more slowly so they are easier to control. It has been suggested therefore that digitoxin is a valuable alternative to digoxin in this situation.[17] See also 'Digitalis glycosides + Calcium channel blockers', p.534 and 'Digitalis glycosides + Nifedipine', p.547.

1. Klein HO, Lang R, Weiss E, Di Segni E, Libhaber C, Guerrero J, Kaplinsky E. The influence of verapamil on serum digoxin concentration. *Circulation* (1982) 65, 998–1003.
2. Doering W. Effect of coadministration of verapamil and quinidine on serum digoxin concentration. *Eur J Clin Pharmacol* (1983) 25, 517–21.
3. Belz GG, Doering W, Munkes R, Matthews J. Interaction between digoxin and calcium antagonists and antiarrhythmic drugs. *Clin Pharmacol Ther* (1983) 33, 410–17.
4. Klein HO, Lang R, Di Segni E, Kaplinsky E. Verapamil-digoxin interaction. *N Engl J Med* (1980) 303, 160.
5. Merola P, Badin A, Paleari DC, De Petris A, Maragno I. Influenza del verapamile sui livelli plasmatici di digossina nell'uomo. *Cardiologia* (1982) 27, 683–7.
6. Hedman A, Angelin B, Arvidsson A, Beck O, Dahlqvist R, Nilsson B, Olsson M, Schenck-Gustafsson K. Digoxin-verapamil interaction: reduction of biliary but not renal digoxin clearance. *Clin Pharmacol Ther* (1991) 49, 256–62.
7. Lang R, Klein HO, Weiss E, Libhaber C, Kaplinsky E. Effect of verapamil on digoxin blood level and clearance. *Chest* (1980) 78, 525.
8. Pedersen KE, Dorph-Pedersen A, Hvidt S, Klitgaard NA, Pedersen KK. The long-term effect of verapamil on plasma digoxin concentration and renal digoxin clearance in healthy subjects. *Eur J Clin Pharmacol* (1982) 22, 123–7.
9. Klein HO, Lang R, Di Segni E, Sareli P, David D, Kaplinsky E. Oral verapamil versus digoxin in the management of chronic atrial fibrillation. *Chest* (1980) 78, 524.
10. Schwartz JB, Keefe D, Kates RE, Harrison DC. Verapamil and digoxin. Another drug-drug interaction. *Clin Res* (1981) 29, 501A.
11. Rendtorff C, Johannessen AC, Halck S, Klitgaard NA. Verapamil-digoxin interaction in chronic hemodialysis patients. *Scand J Urol Nephrol* (1990) 24, 137–9.
12. Gordon M, Goldenberg LMC. Clinical digoxin toxicity in the aged in association with co-administered verapamil. A report of two cases and a review of the literature. *J Am Geriatr Soc* (1986) 34, 659–62.
13. Zatuchni J. Verapamil-digoxin interaction. *Am Heart J* (1984) 108, 412–3.
14. Kounis NG. Asystole after verapamil and digoxin. *Br J Clin Pract* (1980) 34, 57.
15. Kounis NG, Mallioris C. Interactions with cardioactive drugs. *Br J Clin Pract* (1986) 40, 537–8.
16. Maragno I, Gianotti C, Tropeano PF, Rodighiero V, Gaion RM, Paleari C, Prandoni R, Menozzi L. Verapamil-induced changes in digoxin kinetics in cirrhosis. *Eur J Clin Pharmacol* (1987) 32, 309–11.
17. Kuhlmann J, Marcin S. Effects of verapamil on pharmacokinetics and pharmacodynamics of digitoxin in patients. *Am Heart J* (1985) 110, 1245–50.
18. Kuhlmann J. Effects of verapamil, diltiazem, and nifedipine on plasma levels and renal excretion of digitoxin. *Clin Pharmacol Ther* (1985) 38, 667–73.
19. Pedersen KE, Dorph-Pedersen A, Hvidt S, Klitgaard NA, Nielsen-Kudsk F. Digoxin-verapamil interaction. *Clin Pharmacol Ther* (1981) 30, 311–16.
20. Verschraagen M, Koks CHW, Schellens JHM, Beijnen JH. P-glycoprotein system as a determinant of drug interactions: the case of digoxin-verapamil. *Pharmacol Res* (1999) 40, 3016.
21. Belz GG, Aust PE, Munkes R. Digoxin plasma concentrations and nifedipine. *Lancet* (1981) i, 844–5.
22. Marcus FI. Pharmacokinetic interactions between digoxin and other drugs. *J Am Coll Cardiol* (1985) 5, 82A–90A.
23. Klein HO, Kaplinsky E. Verapamil and digoxin: their respective effects on atrial fibrillation and their interaction. *Am J Cardiol* (1982) 50, 894–902.
24. Schwartz JB, Keefe D, Kates RE, Kirsten E, Harrison DC. Acute and chronic pharmacodynamic interaction of verapamil and digoxin in atrial fibrillation. *Circulation* (1982) 65, 1163–70.

Digitalis glycosides + Zaleplon

Zaleplon appears not to interact with digoxin.

Clinical evidence, mechanism, importance and management

Zaleplon 10 mg daily given to 20 healthy subjects for 5 days had no significant effects on the steady-state pharmacokinetics of **digoxin** 375 micrograms daily. There were no significant differences in QTc or PR intervals.[1] There do not appear to be any special precautions necessary when zaleplon is given with digoxin. More study is needed.

1. Sanchez Garcia P, Paty I, Leister CA, Guerra P, Frías J, García Pérez LE, Darwish M. Effect of zaleplon on digoxin pharmacokinetics and pharmacodynamics. *Am J Health-Syst Pharm* (2000) 57, 2267–70.

Digitalis glycosides + Zileuton

Zileuton appears not to interact with digoxin.

Clinical evidence, mechanism, importance and management

In a double-blind placebo-controlled study 12 healthy subjects were given 600 mg **zileuton** or a placebo every 6 h for 13 days, and in addition 250 micrograms **digoxin** daily from days 1 to 11. The **zileuton** had no effect on the steady-state **digoxin** pharmacokinetics with the exception of the time to reach maximum plasma levels which was reduced from 1.43 to 0.95 h. Concurrent use was well tolerated.[1] This evidence suggests that no special precautions are needed if these two drugs are used together.

1. Awni WM, Hussein Z, Cavanaugh JH, Granneman GR, Dube LM. Assessment of the pharmacokinetic interaction between zileuton and digoxin in humans. *Clin Pharmacokinet* (1995) 29 (Suppl 2), 92–7.

15

Hyopglycaemic agent (Antidiabetic) drug interactions

The hypoglycaemic agents are used to control diabetes mellitus, a disease in which there is total or partial failure of the beta-cells within the pancreas to secrete into the circulation enough insulin, one of the hormones concerned with the handling of glucose. In some cases there is evidence to show that the disease results from the presence of factors which oppose the activity of insulin.

With insufficient insulin, the body tissues are unable to take up and utilise the glucose which is in circulation in the blood. Because of this, the glucose which is derived largely from the digestion of food and which would normally be removed and stored in tissues throughout the body, accumulates and boosts the glucose in the blood to such grossly elevated proportions that the kidney is unable to cope with such a load and glucose appears in the urine. Raised blood sugar levels (hyperglycaemia) with glucose and ketone bodies in the urine (glycosuria and ketonuria) are among the manifestations of a serious disturbance in the metabolic chemistry of the body which, if untreated, can lead on to the development of diabetic coma and death.

There are two main types of diabetes: one develops early in life and occurs when the ability of the pancreas suddenly, and often almost totally, fails to produce insulin. The first is called type I, Juvenile or insulin-dependent diabetes (IDDM). The other form of diabetes is the maturity-onset type and is most often seen in those over 40. This occurs when the pancreas gradually loses the ability to produce insulin over a period of months or years. It is often associated with being over-weight and can sometimes be satisfactorily controlled simply by losing weight and adhering to an appropriate diet. Its alternative names are type II or non-insulin dependent diabetes mellitus (NIDDM). A list of hypoglycaemic agents is given in Table 15.1.

The modes of action of the hypoglycaemic agents

Insulin

Insulin extracted from the pancreatic tissue of pigs and cattle is so similar to human insulin that it can be used as a replacement. However, human insulin, manufactured by genetically engineered micro-organisms, is more commonly used. It is given, not by mouth, but by injection in order to bypass the enzymes of the gut which would digest and destroy it like any other protein. There are now many formulations of insulin, some of them designed to delay absorption from the subcutaneous or intramuscular tissue into which the injection is made, so that repeated daily injections can be avoided, but all of them sooner or later release insulin into the circulation

where it acts to replace or top-up the insulin from the human pancreas.

Sulphonylurea oral hypoglycaemic agents and biguanides

The sulphonylurea and other sulphonamide-related compounds such as chlorpropamide and tolbutamide were the first synthetic compounds used in medicine as hypoglycaemic agents that had the advantage of being given by mouth. Among their actions they stimulate the remaining beta-cells of the pancreas to grow and secrete insulin which, with a restricted diet, controls blood sugar levels and permits normal metabolism to occur. Clearly they can only be effective in those diabetics whose pancreas still has the capacity to produce some insulin, so their use is confined to the maturity-onset, type II, non-insulin dependent diabetics.

The mode of action of the other synthetic oral hypoglycaemic agents, the biguanides such as metformin, is obscure, but they do not stimulate the pancreas like the sulphonylureas to release insulin, but appear to facilitate the uptake and utilisation of glucose by the cells in some way. Their use is restricted to maturity-onset diabetics because they are not effective unless insulin is also present.

Other oral hypoglycaemic agents

Acarbose acts against alphaglucosidases and specifically against sucrase in the gut to delay the digestion and absorption of monosaccharides from starch and sucrose. More recently introduced drug classes include the thiazolidinediones (e.g. rosiglitazone), which appears to increase the sensitivity of the receptors to insulin, and the meglitinides (e.g. repaglinide), which increases endogenous insulin secretion. Outside orthodox Western medicine, there are herbal preparations which are used to treat diabetes and which can be given by mouth. Blueberries were traditionally used by the Alpine peasants, and bitter gourd or karela (Momordica charantia) is an established part of herbal treatment in the Indian subcontinent and elsewhere. The Chinese herbals also contain remedies for diabetes. As yet it is not known how these herbal remedies act and their efficacy awaits formal clinical evaluation.

Interactions

The commonest interactions are those which result in a rise or fall in blood glucose levels, thereby disturbing the control of diabetes. These are detailed in this chapter. Other interactions where the hypoglycaemic agent is the affecting agent are described elsewhere. A full listing is to be found in the Index.

Table 15.1 Hypoglycaemic agents

Generic names	Proprietary names
Biguanides	
Buformin	Silubin
Metformin	Anglucid, Apophage, Biocos, Dabex, Dextin, Diabesin, Diabetase, Diabetex, Diabetmin, Diabex, Diaformin, Diamet, Diamin, Dianben, Diformin, Dimefor, Espa-formin, Formin, Glifage, Glucinan, Glucobon, Glucoformin, Glucohexal, Glucomet, Glucomin, Glucophage, Glufor, Gluformin, Glustress, Gluzolyte, Glycon, Glycoran, Glymax, Maformin, Mediabet, Meformed, Meglucon, Melbin, Mescorit, Met, Metbay, Metfin, Metfirex, Metfogamma, Metforal, Metforem, Metfor-500, Metfron, Metiguanide, Metomin, ME-F, Miformin, Novomet, Orabet, Oramet, Pocophage, Poli-Formin, Prophage, Risidon, Serformin, Siamformet, Siofor, Stagid, Thiabet
Phenformin	
Sulph(f)onylureas	
Acetohexamide	Dimelor, Dymelor
Carbutamide (Glybutamide)	Glucidoral
Chlorpropamide	Chlomide, Diabeedol, Diabemide, Diabiclor, Diabinese, Diabitex, Dibecon, Glycemin, Glymese, Hypomide, Insogen, Propamide
Glibenclamide (Glyburide)	Abuglib, Aglucil, Azuglucon, Bastiverit, Benclamin, Bevoren, Biostin, BNIL, Calabren, Clamide, Cytagon, Daonil, Debtan, Diabenol, DiaBeta, Diabetamide, Diabexil, Dia-BASF, Dia-Eptal, Dibelet, Diclanil, Diglexol, Di-Solvente, duraglucon N, Euglamin, Euglucan, Euglucon, Euglucon N, GBN, Gen-Glybe, Gewaglucon, Gilemal, Glemicid, Glib, Glibemid, Gliben, Glibenbeta, Glibendoc, Glibenhexal, Glibenil, Glibenval, Gliben-Azu, Gliben-Puren N, Glibesifar, Glibesyn, Glibetic, Glibic, Gliboral, Glib-ratiopharm, Glifarcal, Glikeyer, Glimel, Glimide, Glimidstada, Gli-basan, Gluben, Glucal, Glucobene, Glucolon, Gluconil, Gluconorm, Glucoremed, Glucostad, Glucoven, Glukoreduct, Glukovital, Gluzo, Glyben, Glycolande N, Glycomin, Glynase, Hexaglucon, Humedia, Lisaglucon, Malix, Maninil, Med-Glionil, Melix, Micronase, Miglucan, Nadib, Norboral, Norglicem, Normoglucon, Origlucon, Praeciglucon, Reglusan, Sugril
Glibornuride	Gluborid, Glutril
Gliclazide	Cadicon, Diabeside, Diabrezide, Diaclaron, Diaglyk, Dialoc, Diamexon, Diamicron, Glicron, Glimicron, Glucozide, Glyade, Glycemirex, Glycon, Glycron, Glyzide, Medoclazide, Nidem, Serviclazide, Sun-Glizide, Ziclin
Glimepiride	Amarel, Amaryl, Amarylle, Glimepil, Roname
Glipizide	Apamid, Diasef, Dipazide, Glibenese, Glidiab, Glipid, Glipiscand, Glucotrol, Gluco-Rite, Glupitel, Glygen, Luditec, Melizid, Melizide, Mindiab, Minidiab, Minodiab, Ozidia
Gliquidone	Glurenor, Glurenorm
Glisoxepide	Pro-Diaban
Glybuzole	
Glycopyramide	
Glyclyclamide	Diaborale
Tolazamide	Tolinase
Tolbutamide	Arcosal, Bioglusil, Dabetil, Diatol, Diaval, Flusan, Glyconon, Ifumelus, Orabet, Orinase, Orsinon, Rastinon
Sulph(f)onamide-related compounds	
Glymidine (Glycodiazine)	
Enzyme inhibitors	
Acarbose	Glicobase, Glucobay, Glucor, Glumida, Prandase, Precose
Voglibose	Basen, Voglisan
Other drugs	
Pioglitazone	Actos, Zactos
Repaglinide	Gluconorm, NovoNorm, Prandin
Rosiglitazone	Avandia, Tiltab

Acarbose + Miscellaneous drugs

Colestyramine may possibly increase the effects of acarbose whereas charcoal and digestive enzyme preparations are expected to reduce its effects. Neomycin may increase the efficacy and the gastrointestinal side effects of acarbose. Digoxin plasma levels can be markedly reduced, and isolated reports also describe markedly reduced valproate levels. Both increased and reduced INRs have been seen with warfarin, but normally warfarin and acarbose appear not to interact. Acarbose causes a moderate increase in the hypoglycaemic effects of insulin, the sulphonylureas and metformin. There is some indirect evidence that acarbose with alcohol may increase the hepatotoxicity of paracetamol (acetaminophen). *Maalox* and nifedipine appear not to interact.

Clinical evidence, mechanism, importance and management

Acarbose is competitive inhibitor of some intestinal carbohydrate-splitting enzymes (alpha-glucosidases), particularly sucrase, which slows the enzymic conversion of starch into absorbable monosaccharides. This means that the normal hyperglycaemia which follows a meal is less marked and smoother.

(a) Antacid

A placebo-controlled study found that 10 ml *Maalox 70* (**aluminium/magnesium hydroxide**) had no effect on the blood glucose and insulin-lowering effects of 100 mg acarbose in 24 normal subjects given a 75 g dose of sucrose. It was concluded that no special precautions are needed if this or similar antacids are used with acarbose.[1]

(b) Anticoagulants

In a double-blind, placebo-controlled study, 24 patients on **warfarin** with stable INRs between 1.8 and 3.6 were additionally given either a placebo for 4 weeks or 100 mg acarbose three times daily for 2 weeks and then 200 mg three times daily for a further 2 weeks. Their INRs, prothrombin times and partial prothrombin times were not altered to any significant extent by the acarbose.[2]

However, there are 3 isolated case reports of apparent **warfarin**/acarbose interactions, one of which describes an increased INR and two others describing reduced INRs. A 66-year-old man taking fosinopril, hydrochlorothiazide, diphenhydramine, insulin, glipizide and **warfarin** was additionally started on acarbose to improve the control of his diabetes. Four days before starting acarbose his INR was 3.09, but after 2 weeks (25 mg acarbose daily for week 1 and then 50 mg daily for week 2) his INR had risen to 4.85. The **warfarin** was temporarily stopped, then its dosage reduced, and finally the acarbose was withdrawn, resulting in the INR dropping back to 2.84. No bleeding was seen.[3] The maker, Bayer has on record 2 other cases of patients on **warfarin** whose INRs were reduced when acarbose was added. One of them stopped taking the acarbose, whereupon her INR returned to its previous value. The other patient needed an increased **warfarin** dosage.[2]

The picture presented by these reports and the absence of any others is that usually no interaction occurs, but in isolated cases some changes in **warfarin** requirements occur. To accommodate this situation it would be prudent to monitor the effects when acarbose is first added, although no interaction would be expected. Information about other anticoagulants appears to be lacking.

(c) Colestyramine

Colestyramine 12 g daily for 6 days given to 8 normal subjects taking 100 mg acarbose three times daily improved the reduction in postprandial insulin levels.[4] The mean serum insulin levels fell from 318 to 246 μUml^{-1}.h while taking both drugs, but showed a 'rebound' rise to 417 μUml^{-1}.h when both were stopped.[4] The clinical importance of this in diabetics is uncertain.

(d) Digestive enzyme preparations

The makers of acarbose reasonably suggest the avoidance of intestinal adsorbents (e.g. **charcoal**) or **digestive enzyme preparations** (such as **amylase**, **pancreatin**) because, theoretically these would be expected to reduce the effects of acarbose.[5]

(e) Digoxin

A woman on **digoxin**, insulin, nifedipine, isosorbide dinitrate, clorazepate and nabumetone had subtherapeutic plasma **digoxin** levels while taking acarbose, (0.48 to 0.64 nanograms/ml) even when her **digoxin** dosage was raised by adding 125 micrograms two days of the week to the daily dose of 250 micrograms. Later, in the absence of acarbose and with the original **digoxin** dosage, her plasma levels climbed to 1.9 nanograms/ml.[6] Two other patients similarly showed markedly reduced plasma **digoxin** levels while taking acarbose. When the acarbose was stopped, the plasma **digoxin** levels climbed again to therapeutic levels (0.23 to 1.6 nanograms/ml and 0.56 to 1.9 nanograms/ml).[7] A pharmacokinetic study in 7 normal subjects using either single 200-mg doses of **acarbose** or 100-mg doses taken three times daily similarly found that **digoxin** serum levels and AUC following single 0.5 mg **digoxin** doses were reduced. **Digoxin** levels were down about 30 to 40% and AUCs down 40%.[8] The reasons for this interaction are not understood but a reduction in the absorption of the **digoxin** from the gut has been suggested.[8] These reports contrast with another that found no interaction between **digoxin** and acarbose in 6 normal subjects.[9]

Just why there is an inconsistency between these reports is not understood but it would clearly be prudent to monitor **digoxin** levels if both drugs are used, being alert for any evidence of reduced levels.

(f) Insulin, oral hypoglycaemic agents

The makers say that while acarbose does not cause hypoglycaemia when given alone, it may increase the hypoglycaemic effects of **insulin** and the **sulphonylureas**, for which reason it may be necessary to reduce their dosages. Monitor the outcome when acarbose is first given. Any hypoglycaemic episodes should be treated with glucose, not sucrose, because acarbose delays the digestion and absorption of disaccharides, but not monosaccharides.[5] A study in normal subjects given acarbose and **thioctic acid** indicated that no clinically relevant pharmacokinetic interaction occurs between these drugs.[10,11]

A study in 6 normal subjects found that acarbose (50 to 100 mg three times daily) reduced the maximum serum levels of **metformin** (1 g) and AUC_{0-9h} by about 35%, but the 24 h urinary excretion was unchanged.[12]

Another study in 19 diabetic patients given 50 or 100 mg acarbose three times daily and 500 mg **metformin** twice daily, also found that acarbose lowered **metformin** levels (AUC reduced 12 to 13%, maximum plasma levels reduced 17 to 20%), even so the postprandial glucose levels at 3 h were still reduced 15% more by the drug combination than by **metformin** alone.[13] There would therefore appear to be no reason for avoiding concurrent use, and in fact some advantages.

(g) Neomycin

Neomycin alone can reduce postprandial blood glucose levels and may enhance the reduction in postprandial glucose levels associated with acarbose.[4] **Neomycin** (1g three times daily) increased the unpleasant gastrointestinal side-effects (flatulence, cramps and diarrhoea) of acarbose (200 mg three times daily) in 7 normal subjects.[14] The makers suggest that if these side-effects are severe the dosage of acarbose should be reduced.[5]

(h) Nifedipine

The makers say that in a pilot study of a possible interaction between **nifedipine** and acarbose, no significant or reproducible changes were seen in the plasma **nifedipine** profiles. There would seem to be no reason for avoiding concurrent use.[4,5]

(i) Paracetamol

Studies in *rats* have demonstrated that acarbose alone or in combination with alcohol may potentiate the hepatotoxicity of **paracetamol**.[15] However, it is not known whether this has any relevance to human patients.

Table 15.2 Hypoglycaemic agent/ACE inhibitor interactions: evidence for no interaction

Patients	ACE inhibitor	Hypoglycaemic agent	Notes
8 cases	Captopril 37.5 mg/day	Insulin	No change to daily insulin requirements. No evidence of symptomatic hypoglycaemia.[4]
38 cases	Captopril 50 to 100 mg/day or Enalapril 20 to 40 mg/day	Insulin or oral hypoglycaemics	Antidiabetic treatment unaltered. No evidence of unusual or unexplained hypoglycaemia.[3]
18 cases case control study	Enalapril 20 to 40 mg/day	Insulin	No change to daily insulin requirements. No evidence of unexplained hypoglycaemia.[3]
428 patients randomised controlled trial	Lisinopril 10 to 20 mg/day or placebo	Insulin	No difference in the number of hypoglycaemic episodes between lisinopril and placebo recipients.[10]
22 cases case control study	Captopril or Enalapril	Insulin and oral hypoglycaemics	Data from Centres Regionaux de Pharmacovigilance in France used. No increased risk of hypoglycaemia detected.[11]

(j) Valproate

An epileptic patient on **sodium valproate** for 10 years with stable plasma levels of 67 micrograms/ml showed a 40% fall in plasma levels to 40.5 micrograms/ml when acarbose was added. No other drugs were being taken. When the acarbose was stopped and then restarted, the **valproate** levels rose and then fell once again. The reason is not understood but the authors of the report suggest that the acarbose possibly reduces the absorption of **valproate**.[16] This is an isolated report and its general importance is unknown, but it would now be prudent to be alert for any evidence of reduced anticonvulsant effects if acarbose is added to **valproate** treatment.

1. Höpfner M, Durani B, Spengler M, Fölsch UR. Effect of acarbose and simultaneous antacid therapy on blood glucose. *Arzneimittelforschung* (1997) 47, 1108–1111.
2. Bayer. Personal communication, December 1997.
3. Morreale AP, Janetzky K. Probable interaction of warfarin and acarbose. *Am J Health-Syst Pharm* (1997) 54, 1551–2.
4. Bayer, Personal Communications, June-July 1993.
5. Glucobay (Acarbose). Bayer plc. Summary of product characteristics, September 2000.
6. Serrano JS, Jiménez CM, Serrano MI, Balboa B. A possible interaction of potential clinical interest between digoxin and acarbose. *Clin Pharmacol Ther* (1996) 60, 589–92.
7. Ben-Ami H, Krivoy N, Nagachandran P, Roguin A, Edoute Y. An interaction between digoxin and acarbose. *Diabetes Care* (1999) 22, 860-1.
8. Miura T, Ueno K, Tanaka K, Sugiura Y, Mizutani M, Takatsu F, Takano Y, Shibakawa M. Impairment of absorption of digoxin by acarbose. *J Clin Pharmacol* (1998) 38, 654-7.
9. Clissold SP, Edwards C. Acarbose: a preliminary review of its pharmacodynamic and pharmacokinetic properties, and therapeutic potential. *Drugs* (1988) 35, 214–43.
10. Gleiter CH, Schreeb KH, Thomas M, Elze M, Fieger-Büschges H, Potthast H, Schneider E, Blume HH, Hermann R. Lack of pharmacokinetic interaction between thioctic acid, glibenclamide and acarbose. *Naunyn Schmiedebergs Arch Pharmacol* (1998) 357 (4 Suppl), R171.
11. Gleiter CH, Schreeb KH, Freudenthaler S, Thomas M, Elze M, Fieger-Bueschges H, Potthast H, Schneider E, Schug BS, Blume HH, Hermann R. Lack of interaction between thioctic acid, glibenclamide and acarbose. *Br J Clin Pharmacol* (1999) 48, 819–25.
12. Scheen AJ, Fierra Alves de Magalhaes AC, Salvatore T, Lefebrve PJ. Reduction of the acute bioavailability of metformin by the α-glucosidase inhibitor acarbose in normal man. *Eur J Clin Invest* (1994) 24 (Suppl 3), 50–4.
13. Lettieri J, Liu MC, Sullivan JT, Heller AH. Pharmacokinetic (PK) and pharmacodynamic (PD) interaction between acarbose (A) and metformin (M) in diabetic (NIDDM) patients. *Clin Pharmacol Ther* (1998) 63, 155.
14. Lembcke B, Caspary WF, Fölsch UR, Creutzfeldt W. Influence of neomycin on postprandial metabolic changes and side effects of an α-glucosidehydrolase inhibitor (BAY g 5421). I. Effects on intestinal gas production and flatulence. In Frontiers of Hormone Research, vol 7. The Entero-Insular Axis. Satellite Symposium to Xth IDF-Meeting, September 7–8, Göttingen 1979, p 294–5.
15. Wang P-Y, Kaneko T, Wang Y, Sato A. Acarbose alone or in combination with ethanol potentiates the hepatotoxicity of carbon tetrachloride and acetaminophen in rats. *Hepatology* (1999) 29, 161–5.
16. Serrano JS, Jiménez CM, Serrano MI, Garrido H, Balboa B. May acarbose impair valproate bioavailability? *Methods Find Exp Clin Pharmacol* (1996) 18 (Suppl C), 98.

Hypoglycaemic agents + ACE inhibitors

Concurrent use normally appears to be uneventful but hypoglycaemia, marked in some instances, has occurred in a small number of diabetics taking insulin or sulphonylureas when treated with captopril, enalapril, lisinopril or perindo- pril. **This has been attributed, but not proved, to be due to an interaction. The problem was solved in some cases by reducing the dosage of the hypoglycaemic agent.**

Clinical evidence

Table 15.2 and Table 15.3 summarise the findings of studies[1-17] carried out in subjects taking both ACE inhibitors and hypoglycaemic agents.

Mechanism

Not understood. An increase in glucose utilisation and increased insulin sensitivity have been suggested.[1,7] Other possibilities (e.g. altered kidney function) are discussed in a series of letters in The Lancet.[18-23]

Importance and management

This interaction is not yet well established nor understood, and it remains the subject of considerable study and debate. However, some cases of severe hypoglycaemia have undoubtedly occurred due to the use of ACE inhibitors by diabetic patients. In practical terms this means that concurrent use need not be avoided but it would be prudent to warn all patients on insulin or oral hypoglycaemic agents who are just starting any ACE inhibitors (although only captopril, enalapril, lisinopril and perindopril have been implicated) that excessive hypoglycaemia has been seen very occasionally and unpredictably. The problem has been resolved in some patients by reducing the sulphonylurea dosage to a half or a quarter.[6,17] A false positive urine ketone test can also occur with captopril when using the alkaline-nitroprusside test (*Ketodiastix*).[24]

1. Ferriere M, Lachkar H, Richard J-L, Bringer J, Orsetti A, Mirouze J. Captopril and insulin sensitivity. *Ann Intern Med* (1985) 102, 134–5.
2. McMurray J and Fraser DM. Captopril, enalapril and blood glucose. *Lancet* (1986) i, 1035.
3. Passa P, Marre M, Leblanc H. Enalapril, captopril and blood glucose. *Lancet* (1986) i, 1447.
4. Winocour P, Waldek S, Anderson DC. Captopril and blood glucose. *Lancet* (1986) ii, 461.
5. Rett K, Wicklmayr M, Dietz GJ. Hypoglycemia in hypertensive diabetic patients treated with sulfonylureas, biguanides and captopril. *N Engl J Med* (1988) 319, 1609.
6. Arauz-Pacheco C, Ramirez LC, Rios JM, Raskin P. Hypoglycemia induced by angiotensin-converting enzyme inhibitors in patients with non-insulin-dependent diabetes receiving sulfonylurea therapy. *Am J Med* (1990) 89, 811–13.
7. Girardin E, Vial T, Pham E, Evreux J-C. Hypoglycémies induites par les sulfamides hypoglycémiants. *Ann Med Interne (Paris)* (1992) 143, 11–17.
8. Veyre B, Ginon I, Vial T, Dragol F, Daumont M. Hypoglycémies par interférence entre un inhibiteur de l'enzyme de conversion et un sulfamide hypoglycémiant. *Presse Med* (1993) 22, 738.
9. Aguirre C, Ayani I, Rodriguez-Sasiain JM. Hypoglycaemia associated with angiotensin converting enzyme inhibitors. *Therapie* (1995) 50 (Suppl), 198.
10. The EUCLID study group. Randomized placebo-controlled trial of lisinopril in normotensive patients with insulin-dependent diabetes and normoalbuminuria or microalbuminuria. *Lancet* (1997) 349, 1787–92.

Table 15.3 Hypoglycaemic agent/ACE inhibitor interactions: evidence for an interaction

Patients	ACE inhibitor	Hypoglycaemic agent	Notes
1 case	Captopril 50 mg/day	Glibenclamide (glyburide) 10.5 mg/day Metformin 1700 mg/day	Blood glucose 2.2 mmol/L 24 hours after the addition of captopril.[5]
1 case	Captopril	Glibenclamide 10.5 mg/day Metformin 1700 mg/day	Blood glucose of 2.9 mmol/L 48 hours after starting captopril. Hypoglycaemic drugs stopped.[5]
3 cases	Captopril	Glibenclamide	Hypoglycaemia reported to a Spanish regional Pharmacosurveillance centre.[9]
1 case	Captopril 12.5 mg/day	Glibenclamide 2.5 mg/day	Hypoglycaemia 7 hours after first dose, blood glucose 2.1 mmol/L, glibenclamide stopped.[6]
1 case	Captopril	Unspecified oral hypoglycaemic	Hypoglycaemia, oral hypoglycaemics withdrawn.[1]
5 cases	Captopril	Unspecified sulphonylureas	Hypoglycaemia reported to Centres Regionaux de Pharmacovigilance in France.[7]
3 cases case control study	Captopril	Unspecified oral hypoglycaemic	Risk of hypoglycaemia increased 3.1-fold.[16]
9 cases case control study	Captopril	Insulin	3.7-fold increase in the risk of hypoglycaemia.[16]
4 cases	Captopril	Insulin	Hypoglycaemia reported to a Spanish Regional Pharmacosurveillance centre.[9]
3 cases	Captopril	Insulin	Unexplained hypoglycaemia.[1]
1 case	Enalapril 5 mg/day	Glibenclamide 5 mg/day	Hypoglycaemia, blood glucose 2.3 mmol/L. Dose of glibenclamide reduced to 2.5 mg/day.[6]
2 cases	Enalapril 5 mg/day	Glibenclamide 5 mg/day	Hypoglycaemic attacks, glibenclamide reduced to 1.25 mg/day.[17]
9 healthy subjects	Enalapril 5 mg/day	Glibenclamide 3.5 mg/day	Hypoglycaemic effects of glibenclamide enhanced.[13]
4 cases	Enalapril	Glibenclamide	Hypoglycaemia reported to a Spanish Regional Pharmacosurveillance centre.[9]
1 case	Enalapril	Gliclazide 80 mg/day	Hypoglycaemia when enalapril dose increased from 5 to 10 mg/day.[8]
4 cases	Enalapril	Unspecified sulphonylureas	Hypoglycaemia reported to Centres Regionaux de Pharmacovigilance in France.[7]
1 case	Enalapril	Unspecified sulphonylurea	Recurrent hypoglycaemia, sulphonylurea withdrawn.[2]
10 cases case control study	Enalapril	Unspecified sulphonylurea Insulin	2.4-fold increase in the risk of hypoglycaemia with sulphonylureas. However, no increased risk was seen in insulin users. In addition when all ACE inhibitors were considered together, no significant increase in risk was seen.[14]
2 cases case control study	Enalapril	Unspecified oral hypoglycaemic	Non-significant 5.4-fold increase in the risk of hypoglycaemia.[16]
3 cases case control study	Enalapril	Insulin	Non-significant 1.7-fold increase in the risk of hypoglycaemia.[16]
1 case	Enalapril	Insulin	Reduced insulin requirements.[2]
11 cases	Enalapril	Insulin	Hypoglycaemia reported to a Spanish Regional Pharmacosurveillance centre.[9]
1 case	Lisinopril	Glibenclamide and metformin	Hypoglycaemia reported to a Spanish Regional Pharmacosurveillance centre.[9]
1 case	Lisinopril 10 mg/day	Gliclazide	Hypoglycaemia resolved on stopping gliclazide.[8]
1 case	Perindopril	Glibenclamide	Hypoglycaemia reported to a Spanish Regional Pharmacosurveillance centre.[9]
1 case	Ramipril 2.5 mg/day	Glibenclamide 5 mg/day Metformin 1700 mg/day	Patient also on naproxen, renal function deteriorated causing hypoglycaemia due to accumulation of oral hypoglycaemics.[15]
7 cases case control study	Unspecified ACE inhibitor	Insulin or oral hypoglycaemic agents	3.2-fold increase in the risk of hypoglycaemia leading to hospitalisation.[12]

11. Moore N, Kreft-Jais C, Haramburu F, Noblet C, Andrjak M, Ollanngier M, Bégaud B. Reports of hypoglycaemia associated with the use of ACE inhibitors and other drugs: a case/non-case study in the French pharmacovigilance system database. *Br J Clin Pharmacol* (1997) 44, 513–8.

12. Morris AD, Boyle DIR, McMahon AD, Pearce H, Evans JMM, Newton RW, Jung RT, MacDonald TM, The DARTS/MEMO collaboration. ACE inhibitor use is associated with hospitalization for severe hypoglycaemia in patients with diabetes. *Diabetes Care* (1997) 20, 1363–7.

13. Heise T, Hompesch BC, Flesch S, Rave K, Linkeschowa R, Heinemann L. Drug-interaction between enalapril and glibenclamide might lead to hypoglycaemia. *Diabetes* (1999) 48 (Suppl 1), A70–A71.

14. Thamer M, Ray NF, Taylor T. Association between antihypertensive drug use and hypoglycaemia: a case-control study of diabetic users of insulin or sulfonylureas. *Clin Ther* (1999) 21, 1387–1400.

15. Collin M, Mucklow JC. Drug interactions, renal impairment and hypoglycaemia in a patient with type II diabetes. *Br J Clin Pharmacol* (1999) 48, 134–7.

16. Herings RMC, de Boer A, Stricker BHC, Leufkens HGM, Porsius A. Hypoglycaemia associated with use of inhibitors of angiotensin converting enzyme. *Lancet* (1995) 345, 1195–8.

17. Ahmad S. Drug interaction induces hypoglycemia. *J Fam Pract* (1995) 40, 540–1.

18. van Haeften TW. ACE inhibitors and hypoglycaemia. *Lancet* (1995) 346, 125.

19. Kong N, Bates A, Ryder REJ. ACE inhibitors and hypoglycaemia. *Lancet* (1995) 346, 125.

20. Feher MD, Amiel S. ACE inhibitors and hypoglycaemia. *Lancet* (1995) 346, 125–6.

21. Davie AP. ACE inhibitors and hypoglycaemia. *Lancet* (1995) 346, 126.

22. Wildenborg IHM, Veenstra J, van der Voort PHJ, Verdegaal WP, Silberbusch J. ACE inhibitors and hypoglycaemia. *Lancet* (1995) 346, 126.

23. Herings RMC, de Boer A, Stricker BHC, Leufkens HGM, Porsius AJ. ACE inhibitors and hypoglycaemia. *Lancet* (1995) 346, 126–7.

24. Warren SE. False-positive urine ketone test with captopril. *N Engl J Med* (1980) 303, 1003–4.

Hypoglycaemic agents + Alcohol

Diabetics controlled on insulin or oral hypoglycaemic agents or diet alone need not abstain from alcohol, but they should drink only in moderation and accompanied by food. Alcohol makes the signs of hypoglycaemia less clear and delayed hypoglycaemia can occur. The CNS depressant effects of alcohol plus hypoglycaemia can make driving or the operation of dangerous machinery much more hazardous. A flushing reaction is common in patients on chlorpropamide who drink, but is rare with other sulphonylureas. Alcoholic patients may require above-average doses of tolbutamide.

Clinical evidence

(a) Hypoglycaemic agents in general + Alcohol

The blood glucose levels of diabetics may be reduced or may remain unchanged by **alcohol**. In one study, 2 out of 7 diabetics using **insulin** became severely hypoglycaemic after drinking the equivalent of about 3 measures of **spirits**.[1] In a hospital study over a 3-year period, 5 insulin-dependent diabetics were hospitalised with severe hypoglycaemia after going on the binge. Two of them died without recovery from the initial coma and the other 3 suffered permanent damage to the nervous system.[2] In another study it was found that **alcohol** was involved in about 4% of hypoglycaemic episodes requiring hospitalisation.[3] In contrast to these **alcohol**-induced hypoglycaemic episodes, it was found in 2 other studies[4,5] that pure **alcohol** and dry **wine** had little effect on blood glucose levels. An extensive study found that **alcohol** causes some deterioration in the metabolic control of elderly non-insulin dependent diabetics (increased lipolysis, raised triglyceride levels, ketogenesis).[6]

(b) Sulphonylureas + Alcohol

About one-third of those on **chlorpropamide** who drink **alcohol**, even in quite small amounts, experience a warm, tingling or flushing sensation of the face, and sometimes the neck and arms as well. It may also involve the conjunctivae. This can begin within 5 to 20 min of drinking, reaching a peak within 30 to 40 min, and may persist for 1 to 2 h. Very occasionally headache occurs, and light-headedness, palpitations, wheezing and breathlessness have also been experienced.[7,8]

This flushing (disulfiram-like) reaction has been described in numerous reports (far too many to list here) involving large numbers of patients on **chlorpropamide**. These reports have been extensively reviewed.[7,9–11] A similar reaction can occur, but only very rarely, with other sulphonylureas (**carbutamide**,[12] **gliclazide**,[13] **glipizide**,[8] **glib-**

enclamide (glyburide),[8,14] **tolbutamide**,[15,16] **tolazamide**[17]). A comparative study showed that the mean half-life of **tolbutamide** in alcoholics was reduced about one-third (from 384 to 232 min).[18] **Alcohol** is also reported to prolong but not increase the hypoglycaemic effects of **glipizide**.[19]

(c) Biguanides + Alcohol

A controlled study in 5 ketosis-resistant type II diabetics taking 50 to 100 mg **phenformin** daily showed that the equivalent of 3 oz **whiskey** markedly raised their blood lactate and lactate-pyruvate levels. Two of them attained blood-lactate levels of more than 50 mg%, and one of these patients had previously experienced nausea, weakness and malaise while taking **phenformin** and **alcohol**.[20] The ingestion of **alcohol** is described in other reports as having preceded the onset of **phenformin**-induced lactic-acidosis.[21–23] Some patients have complained that **alcohol** tastes metallic.

Mechanism

The exacerbation of hypoglycaemia by alcohol is not fully understood, however it is known that if hypoglycaemia occurs when liver glycogen stores are low, the liver turns to the formation of new glucose from amino acids (neoglucogenesis) which is released into the circulation. This neoglucogenesis is inhibited by the presence of alcohol so that the fall in blood glucose levels may not be prevented and a full-scale hypoglycaemic episode can result. The chlorpropamide-alcohol flush (CPAF) reaction, although extensively studied, is by no means fully understood. It seems to be related to the disulfiram-alcohol reaction and is accompanied by a rise in blood-acetaldehyde levels (see 'Alcohol + Disulfiram', p.27). It also appears to be genetically determined[8] and may involve both the prostaglandins and the endogenous opioids.[24] The decreased half-life of tolbutamide in alcoholics is probably due to the inducing effects of alcohol on liver microsomal enzymes.[18,25,26]

The reasons for the raised blood lactate levels seen during the concurrent use of phenformin and alcohol are not clear, but one suggestion is that it may possibly be related to the competitive demands for NAD by the reactions which convert alcohol to acetaldehyde, and lactate to pyruvate.[20]

Importance and management

The documentation of the hypoglycaemic agent/alcohol interactions is surprisingly patchy (with the exception of chlorpropamide and alcohol) but they are of recognised clinical importance. The following contains the main recommendations of Diabetes UK (formerly The British Diabetic Association) based on a review of what is currently known:[27,28]

General comments

Most diabetics need not avoid alcohol totally, but they are advised not to exceed 2 or 3 drinks daily. 'A drink' is defined as either half a pint (300 ml beer, a single measure of spirits (one-sixth of a gill or 25 ml or one small glass of sherry (50 ml or wine (125 ml. Drinks with a high carbohydrate content (sweet sherries, sweet wines and most liqueurs) should be avoided. Diabetics should not drink on an empty stomach and they should know that the warning signs of hypoglycaemia may possibly be obscured by the effects of the alcohol. Driving or handling dangerous machinery should be avoided because the CNS depressant effects of alcohol plus hypoglycaemia can be particularly hazardous. Warn them of the risks of hypoglycaemia occurring several hours after drinking. Those with peripheral neuropathy should be told that alcohol may aggravate the condition and they should not have more than one drink daily. Provided drinking is restricted as suggested and drinks containing a lot of carbohydrate are avoided, there is no need to include the drink in the dietary allowance. However diabetics on a weight-reducing diet should not exceed one drink daily and should include it in their daily calorie allowance.

Additional comments about the oral hypoglycaemic agents

The chlorpropamide-alcohol interaction (flushing reaction) is very well documented, but of minimal importance. It is a nuisance and possibly socially embarrassing but normally requires no treatment.

Patients should be warned. The incidence is said to lie between 13 and 33%[29,30] although one study claims that it may be as low as 4%.[31] Since it can be provoked by quite small amounts of alcohol (half a glass of sherry or wine) it is virtually impossible for sensitive patients to avoid it if they drink. Most manufacturers issue warnings about the possibility of this reaction with other sulphonylureas, but it is very rarely seen and can therefore almost always be avoided by exchanging chlorpropamide for another sulphonylurea. Alcoholic subjects may need above-average doses of tolbutamide.

Metformin does not carry the same risk of lactic acidosis seen with phenformin and it is suggested in the paper[27] prepared for and approved by the British Diabetic Association that one or two drinks a day are unlikely to be harmful. However, the drug should not be given to alcoholic patients because of the possibility of liver damage.

1. Walsh CH, O'Sullivan DJ. Effect of moderate alcohol intake on control of diabetes. *Diabetes* (1974) 23, 440–2.
2. Arky RA, Veverbrants E, Abramson EA. Irreversible hypoglycemia. A complication of alcohol and insulin. *JAMA* (1968) 206, 575–8.
3. Potter J, Clarke P, Gale EAM, Dave SH, Tattersall RB. Insulin-induced hypoglycaemia in an accident and emergency department: the tip of an iceberg? *BMJ* (1982) 285, 1180–2.
4. McMonagle J, Felig P. Effects of ethanol ingestion on glucose tolerance and insulin secretion in normal and diabetic subjects. *Metabolism* (1975) 24, 625–32.
5. Lolli G, Balboni C, Ballatore C, Risoldi L, Carletti D, Silvestri L, Pacifici De Tommaso G. Wine in the diets of diabetic patients. *QJ Stud Alcohol* (1963) 24, 412–6.
6. Ben G, Gnudi L, Maran A, Gigante A, Duner E, Iori E, Tiengo A, Avogaro A. Effects of chronic alcohol intake on carbohydrate and lipid metabolism in subjects with type II (non-insulin dependent) diabetes. *Am J Med* (1991) 90, 70–6.
7. Johnston C, Wiles PG, Pyke DA. Chlorpropamide-alcohol flush: the case in favour. *Diabetologia* (1984) 26, 1–5.
8. Leslie RDG, Pyke DA. Chlorpropamide-alcohol flushing: a dominantly inherited trait associated with diabetes. *BMJ* (1978) 2, 1519.
9. Hillson RM, Hockaday TDR. Chlorpropamide-alcohol flush: a critical reappraisal. *Diabetologia* (1984) 26, 6–11.
10. Waldhäusl W. To flush or not to flush? Comments on the chlorpropamide-alcohol flush. *Diabetologia* (1984) 26, 12–14.
11. Groop L, Eriksson CJP, Huupponen R, Ylikarhi R, Pelkonen R. Roles of chlorpropamide, alcohol and acetaldehyde in determining the chlorpropamide-alcohol flush. *Diabetologia* (1984) 26, 34–38.
12. Signorelli S. Tolerance for alcohol in patients on chlorpropamide. *Ann N Y Acad Sci* (1959) 74, 900–903.
13. Conget JI, Vendrell J, Esmatjes E, Halperin I. Gliclazide alcohol flush. *Diabetes Care* (1989) 12, 44.
14. Stowers JM. Alcohol and glibenclamide. *BMJ* (1971) 3, 533.
15. Doger H. Experience with the tolbutamide treatment of 500 cases of diabetes on an ambulatory basis. *Ann N Y Acad Sci* (1957) 71, 275.
16. Büttner H. Äthanolunverträglichkeit beim Menschen nach Sulfonylharnstoffen. *Dtsch Arch Klin Med* (1961) 207, 1–18.
17. McKendry JBR, Gfeller KF. Clinical experience with the oral antidiabetic compound tolazamide. *Can Med Assoc J* (1967) 96, 531–5.
18. Carulli N, Manenti F, Gallo M, Salvioli GF. Alcohol-drugs interaction in man: alcohol and tolbutamide. *Eur J Clin Invest* (1971) 1, 421–4.
19. Hartling SG, Faber OK, Wegmann M-L, Wahlin-Boll E and Melander A. Interaction of ethanol and glipizide in humans. *Diabetes Care* (1987) 10, 683–6.
20. Johnson HK, Waterhouse C. Relationship of alcohol and hyperlactatemia in diabetic subjects treated with phenformin. *Am J Med* (1968) 45, 98–104.
21. Davidson MB, Bozarth WR, Challoner DR, Goodner CJ. Phenformin hypoglycaemia and lactic acidosis. Report of an attempted suicide. *N Engl J Med* (1966) 275, 886–8.
22. Gottlieb A, Duberstein J, Geller A. Phenformin acidosis. *N Engl J Med* (1962) 267, 806.
23. Schaffalitzky de Muckadell OB, Koster A and Jensen SL. Fenformin-alkohol interaktion. *Ugeskr Laeger* (1973) 135, 925.
24. Johnston C, Wiles PG, Medbak S, Bowcock S, Cooke ED, Pyke DA and Rees LH. The role of endogenous opioids in the chlorpropamide alcohol flush. *Clin Endocrinol (Oxf)* (1984) 21, 489–97.
25. Kater RMH, Roggin G, Tobon F, Zieve P and Iber FL. Increased rate of clearance of drugs from the circulation of alcoholics. *Am J Med Sci* (1969) 258, 35.
26. Kater RMH, Tobon F and Iber FL. Increased rate of tolbutamide metabolism in alcoholic patients. *JAMA* (1969) 207, 363.
27. Connor H, Marks V. Alcohol and diabetes. A position paper prepared by the Nutrition Subcommittee of the British Diabetic Association's Medical Advisory Committee and approved by the Executive Council of the British Diabetic Association. *Hum Nutr Appl Nutr* (1985) 39A, 393–9.
28. Diabetes UK (formerly the British Diabetic Association). Care recommendation: alcohol. Available at http://www.diabetes.org.uk/info/carerec/alcohol.htm (accessed 27/07/2001).
29. Fitzgerald MG, Gaddie R, Malins JM and O'Sullivan DJ. Alcohol sensitivity in diabetics receiving chlorpropamide. *Diabetes* (1962) 11, 40.
30. Daeppen JP, Hofstetter JR, Curchod B and Saudan Y. Traitment oral du diabete par un nouvel hypoglycemiant, le P 607 ou Diabinese. *Schweiz Med Wochenschr* (1959) 89, 817.
31. De Silva NE, Tunbridge WMG and Alberti KGMM. Low incidence of chlorpropamide-alcohol flushing in diet-treated, non-insulin-dependent diabetics. *Lancet* (1981) i, 128–31.

Hypoglycaemic agents + Allopurinol

An increase in the half-life of chlorpropamide, and a decrease in the half-life of tolbutamide during treatment with allopurinol have been described, but the effect of these changes on the hypoglycaemic response of patients is uncertain. Marked hypoglycaemia and coma occurred in one patient on gliclazide and allopurinol.

Clinical evidence

(a) Chlorpropamide + Allopurinol

A brief report describes 6 patients given **chlorpropamide** and **allopurinol** concurrently. The half-life of **chlorpropamide** in one patient with gout and normal renal function exceeded 200 h (normally 36 h) after taking **allopurinol** for 10 days. In 2 others the half-life was extended to 44 and 55 h respectively. The other 3 patients were given **allopurinol** for only one or two days and the half-life of **chlorpropamide** remained unaltered.[1]

(b) Gliclazide + Allopurinol

Severe hypoglycaemia (1.6 mmol/l) and coma occurred in a patient taking **gliclazide** and **allopurinol**, possibly exacerbated by renal insufficiency.[2] Hypoglycaemia has been seen in another patient taking both drugs, but **enalapril** and **ranitidine** were also involved.[2]

(c) Tolbutamide + Allopurinol

Allopurinol (2.5 mg/kg twice daily for 15 days) reduced the half-life of intravenous **tolbutamide** in 10 normal subjects by 25% (from 360 to 267 min).[3,4]

Mechanism

Not understood. In the case of chlorpropamide it has been suggested that it possibly involves some competition for renal tubular mechanisms.[1]

Importance and management

Information is very limited. Only gliclazide has been implicated in severe hypoglycaemia and there seem to be no reports of either grossly enhanced hypoglycaemia with chlorpropamide, or reduced hypoglycaemia with tolbutamide. More study is needed to find out whether any of these interactions has general clinical importance, but in the meantime patients should possibly be given an appropriate warning if allopurinol is added. Information about other hypoglycaemic agents seems to be lacking.

1. Petitpierre B, Perrin L, Rudhardt M, Herrera A, Fabre J. Behaviour of chlorpropamide in renal insufficiency and under the effect of associated drug therapy. *Int J Clin Pharmacol* (1972) 6, 120–4.
2. Girardin E, Vial T, Pham E, Evreux J-C. Hypoglycémies induites par les sulfamides hypoglycémiants. *Ann Med Interne (Paris)* (1992) 143, 11–17.
3. Gentile S, Porcellini M, Loguercio C, Foglia F, Coltorti M. Modificazioni della depurazione plasmatica di tolbutamide e rifamicina-SV indotte dal trattamento con allopurino!o in volontari sano. *Progr Med (Napoli)* (1979) 35, 637–42.
4. Gentile S, Porcellini M, Foglia F, Loguercio C, Coltorti M. Influenza di allopurinolo sull'emivita plasmatica di tolbutamide e rifamicina-SV in soggetti sani. *Boll Soc Ital Biol Sper* (1979) 55, 345–8.

Hypoglycaemic agents + Anabolic steroids

Nandrolone (norandrostenolone), methandienone (methandrostenolone), testosterone and stanozolol can enhance the blood sugar reducing effects of insulin. The dosage of the hypoglycaemic agent may need to be lowered.

Clinical evidence

In a study in 54 diabetics under treatment with 25 mg **nandrolone (norandrostenolone) phenylpropionate** given weekly or 50 mg **nandrolone decanoate** given three-weekly by intramuscular injection, it was found necessary to reduce the **insulin** dosage by an average of 36% (reduction range 4–56 units) in about a third of the patients.[1]

Other reports similarly describe an enhanced reduction in blood sugar levels in diabetics treated with **insulin** and **nandrolone**,[2,3] **methandienone (methandrostenolone)**,[4] **testosterone propionate**[5] or **stanozolol**.[6] A reduction in blood sugar levels has also been seen in normal subjects given **testosterone propionate**.[7] No changes were seen when **ethylestrenol (ethyloestrenol)** was used.[1,2]

Mechanism

Uncertain.

Importance and management

Established interactions but the total picture is incomplete because not all of the anabolic steroids appear to have been studied and they may not necessarily behave identically. A fall in the dosage requirements of insulin (an 'insulin-sparing' effect) may be expected in many patients with the steroids cited. An average reduction of a third is reported.[1] Monitor concurrent use well being alert for the need to reduce the dosage of the hypoglycaemic agent.

1. Houtsmuller AJ. The therapeutic applications of anabolic steroids in ophthalmology: biochemical results. *Acta Endocrinol (Copenh)* (1961) 39 (Suppl 63), 154–74.
2. Dardenne U. The therapeutic applications of anabolic steroids in ophthalmology. *Acta Endocrinol (Copenh)* (1961) 39 (Suppl 63), 143–53.
3. Weissel W. Anaboles Hormon bei malignem oder kompliziertem Diabetes mellitus. *Wiel Klin Wsch* (1962) 74, 234.
4. Landon J, Wynn V, Samols E, Bilkus D. The effect of anabolic steroids on blood sugar and plasma insulin levels in man. *Metabolism* (1963) 12, 924–35.
5. Veil WH, Lippross O. 'Unspezifische' wirkungen der Männlichen keimdrücenhormone. *Klin Wochenschr* (1938) 17, 655–8.
6. Pergola F. El estanozolol, nuevo anabolico. *Prensa Med Argent* (1962) 49, 274–90.
7. Talaat M, Habib YA, Habib M. The effect of testosterone on the carbohydrate metabolism in normal subjects. *Arch Int Pharmacodyn Ther* (1957) 111, 215–26.

Hypoglycaemic agents + Angiotensin II antagonists

Eprosartan and glibenclamide (glyburide) appear not to interact.

Clinical evidence, mechanism, importance and management

Fifteen men and women with type II diabetes stabilised on 3.75 to 10 mg **glibenclamide** daily for at least 30 days showed no changes in their 24-h plasma glucose concentrations when additionally treated for a further 7 days with 200 mg **eprosartan** twice daily. Concurrent use was safe and well tolerated and it was concluded that there is no clinically relevant interaction between these two drugs.[1]

1. Martin DE, DeCherney GS, Ilson BE, Jones BA, Boike SC, Freed MI, Jorasky DK. Eprosartan, an angiotensin II receptor antagonist, does not affect the pharmacodynamics of glyburide in patients with type II diabetes mellitus. *J Clin Pharmacol* (1997) 37, 155–9.

Hypoglycaemic agents + Antacids

The rate of absorption of some of the oral hypoglycaemics is increased by some antacids, but there appear to be no reports of adverse responses in diabetic patients as a result of any of these interactions.

Clinical evidence

(a) Chlorpropamide + Magnesium hydroxide

Magnesium hydroxide 850 mg increased the rate of absorption of 250 mg **chlorpropamide** in normal subjects, but the insulin and glucose responses were unaffected.[1]

(b) Glibenclamide (glyburide) + Magnesium hydroxide and Aluminium hydroxide

A single-dose study in normal subjects found that **magnesium hydroxide** 850 mg had little effect on the rate or extent of absorption of a micronized **glibenclamide** preparation (*Semi-Euglucon*), but it caused a three-fold increase in the peak plasma concentration and the bioavailability of a non-micronised preparation (*Gilemid*).[2] *Maalox*

(**magnesium and aluminium hydroxides**) increased the AUC of a **glibenclamide** formulation (*Daonil*) by one-third, and its maximal serum level by 50%.[3]

(c) Glibenclamide (glyburide) + Sodium bicarbonate

Sodium bicarbonate 1 to 3 g very markedly increased the early bioavailability of non-micronised **glibenclamide** in normal subjects, but its activity remained unaltered.[4]

(d) Glipizide + Magnesium hydroxide, Sodium bicarbonate or Aluminium hydroxide

Sodium bicarbonate 3 g significantly increased the absorption of **glipizide** 5 mg and enhanced its effects to some extent, but the total absorption was unaltered.[5] The half-hour, one-hour and two-hour AUCs were increased six, four and twofold, and the time to reach the peak serum level fell from 2.5 to 1 h.[5] **Aluminium hydroxide** 1 g did not appear to affect the absorption of glipizide 5 mg.[5] **Magnesium hydroxide** 850 mg also considerably increased the rate of **glipizide** 5 mg absorption, the half-hour and 1 h AUCs being increased by 180 and 69%, respectively.[6]

(e) Tolbutamide + Magnesium hydroxide

Magnesium hydroxide 850 mg increased the 0 to 1 h and 0 to 2 h AUCs of a single 500-mg dose of **tolbutamide** by fivefold and two and a half-fold respectively in normal subjects. The total AUC was unaffected. The maximum insulin response was increased fourfold and occurred about an hour earlier, and the glucose responses were also greater and earlier.[1]

Mechanism

Uncertain. The small increase in gastric pH caused by these antacids possibly increases the solubility of these sulphonylureas and therefore increases their absorption.[7]

Importance and management

Although some interactions certainly occur in normal subjects, their clinical importance in diabetics is uncertain. No reports of adverse reactions appear to have been published, nevertheless check for any evidence of changes in diabetic control in patients given sulphonylureas and antacids, in particular with glipizide/sodium bicarbonate, glipizide/magnesium hydroxide and tolbutamide/magnesium hydroxide where some transient hypoglycaemia might occur. Separating the dosages as much as possible would probably minimise any effects. Giving glibenclamide half to one hour before the antacid has been suggested.[3]

1. Kivistö KT, Neuvonen PJ. Effect of magnesium hydroxide on the absorption and efficacy of tolbutamide and chlorpropamide. *Eur J Clin Pharmacol* (1992) 42, 675–80.
2. Neuvonen PJ, Kivistö KT. The effects of magnesium hydroxide on the absorption and efficacy of two glibenclamide preparations. *Br J Clin Pharmacol* (1991) 32, 215–20.
3. Zuccaro P, Pacifici R, Pichini S, Avico U, Federzoni G, Pini LA, Sternieri E. Influence of antacids on the bioavailability of glibenclamide. *Drugs Exp Clin Res* (1989) 15, 165–9.
4. Kivistö KT, Lehto P, Neuvonen PJ. The effects of different doses of sodium bicarbonate on the absorption and activity of non-micronized glibenclamide. *Int J Clin Pharmacol Ther Toxicol* (1993) 31, 236–40.
5. Kivistö KT, Neuvonen PJ. Differential effects of sodium bicarbonate and aluminium hydroxide on the absorption and activity of glipizide. *Eur J Clin Pharmacol* (1991) 40, 383–6.
6. Kivistö KT, Neuvonen PJ. Enhancement of absorption and effect of glipizide by magnesium hydroxide. *Clin Pharmacol Ther* (1991) 49, 39–43.
7. Lehto P, Laine K, Kivistö K, Neuvonen PJ. The effect of pH on the *in vitro* dissolution of sulfonylurea preparations — a mechanism for the antacid-sulfonylurea interaction? *Therapie* (1995) 50 (Suppl), 413.

Hypoglycaemic agents + Anticoagulants

Dicoumarol and tolbutamide mutually interact. This can result in increased hypoglycaemia (possibly coma) and increased anticoagulant effects (possibly bleeding). Dicoumarol can also increase the hypoglycaemic effects of chlorpropamide and this has also been seen in one patient given acenocoumarol (nicoumalone). Three isolated reports describe increased warfarin effects in two patients given glibenclamide (glyburide) and another given tolbutamide. The effects

of phenprocoumon are reduced by metformin but bleeding was seen in another patient on warfarin given phenformin. Other anticoagulants and hypoglycaemic agents seem not to interact together.

Clinical evidence

A. Effect of anticoagulants on hypoglycaemic agents

(a) Chlorpropamide + Dicoumarol or Acenocoumarol (Nicoumalone)

The observation of severe hypoglycaemia in a patient on **chlorpropamide** while taking **dicoumarol** prompted further study in 3 other patients and 2 non-diabetics. **Dicoumarol** doubled the serum **chlorpropamide** levels within 3 to 4 days and the half-life was more than doubled.[1] A woman with normal kidney function showed an increase in the half-life of **chlorpropamide** to 88 h (normally about 36 h) when treated with **acenocoumarol**.[2]

(b) Glibenclamide (Glyburide), Glibornuride or Tolbutamide + Phenprocoumon

Phenprocoumon has been found to cause a slight increase in the half-life of **glibornuride**,[3] but the pharmacokinetics of **glibenclamide**[4] and the hypoglycaemic effects of **tolbutamide** remained unchanged.

(c) Tolbutamide + Dicoumarol or Phenindione

Dicoumarol has been shown to increase the serum levels of **tolbutamide**, prolong its half-life (more than threefold), and reduce blood sugar levels in both diabetics[5] and normal subjects.[5,6] The hypoglycaemic effects are increased. This may become excessive in a few patients and coma has been described.[5,7-9] **Phenindione** does not affect the half-life of **tolbutamide**.[5]

B. Effect of hypoglycaemic agents on anticoagulants

(a) Dicoumarol + Tolbutamide

Two patients on **dicoumarol** showed marked increases in prothrombin times (a rise from 33 to 60 s) within 2 days of starting **tolbutamide** but no bleeding occurred. Increases were seen in 3 other patients who took **tolbutamide** and **dicoumarol** simultaneously.[10] Another patient on **dicoumarol** showed a similar increase in his prothrombin time and bled (haematuria, purpura) within 5 days of starting **tolbutamide**.[8] The half-life of **dicoumarol** was approximately halved in 2 out of 4 normal subjects given **tolbutamide**, but the hypoprothrombinaemic effects were unchanged.[11] A retrospective study on 15 patients treated concurrently found no evidence that the anticoagulant effects of the **dicoumarol** were altered by **tolbutamide**[12] but the form of the study may possibly have obscured evidence of an interaction. No change in overall anticoagulant control was seen in another study.[13]

(b) Phenprocoumon and Warfarin + Metformin

The observation that a woman diabetic needed more **phenprocoumon** while taking **metformin** prompted further study in 13 diabetics. It was found that those taking 1.1 to 3 g **metformin** daily were less well anticoagulated than those taking only 0.4 to 1 g, even though the **phenprocoumon** dosage of the former was slightly higher.[14] The half-life of **phenprocoumon** is reduced about one-third (from 123 to 85 h) while taking 1.7 g **metformin** daily.[14] Haematuria occurred in a patient on **warfarin** 3 months after concurrent treatment with **phenformin** was started. Her prothrombin values were normal.[15] The **phenformin** may have increased fibrinolysis to the point where it was additive with the effects of the **warfarin**.

(c) Other anticoagulants + Hypoglycaemic agents

Treatment of diabetic patients and normal subjects for a week with **glibenclamide** (glyburide), **glibornuride**, **tolbutamide** or **insulin** had no effect on the plasma levels or half-life of single doses of **phenprocoumon**.[16] A retrospective study of 24 patients given **dicoumarol** and 54 given **warfarin** suggested that **insulin** did not alter their anticoagulant effects; similarly **tolbutamide** is said not to have altered the anticoagulant effects of **warfarin** in 42 patients.[12] However what is not clear is whether this study would have revealed an interaction because the patients were already taking the hypoglycaemic agent and would have been routinely stabilised on the anticoagulant. A study in normal subjects found that only minor, clinically unimpor-

tant changes in the prothrombin times occurred in response to single 25-mg doses of **warfarin** when treated with 4 mg **glimepiride** daily.[17] Three isolated reports describe increased **warfarin** effects (serious in one instance) in 2 patients given **glibenclamide**,[18,19] and another given **tolbutamide**.[20]

Mechanisms

Dicoumarol appears to increase the effects of tolbutamide by inhibiting its metabolism by the liver.[5,6] This may also be true for chlorpropamide.[1] The increase in the anticoagulant effects of dicoumarol by tolbutamide may in part be due to a plasma protein binding interaction. In the case of phenprocoumon there seem to be several different mutually opposing processes going on which cancel each other out and produce a 'silent' interaction.[13] Metformin possibly reduces the effects of phenprocoumon by altering blood flow to the liver and interfering with the enterohepatic circulation. There is no clear explanation for most of these interactions.

Importance and management

Information is patchy and very incomplete. Dicoumarol with tolbutamide has been most thoroughly investigated and the interaction is clinically important. Increased hypoglycaemic effects may be expected if dicoumarol is given to patients taking tolbutamide and there is a risk of coma. If tolbutamide is given to those taking dicoumarol an increase in prothrombin times and possibly bleeding may occur. Avoid concurrent use unless the outcome can be well monitored and dosage adjustments made. The same precautions should be taken with dicoumarol and chlorpropamide, but information is limited to one study.[1] Some caution is appropriate with acenocoumarol (nicoumalone) and chlorpropamide, and warfarin with glibenclamide (glyburide) or tolbutamide although information seems to be limited to isolated observations.[2,14,20] A small increase in the dosage of phenprocoumon may be necessary if metformin is given. There appears to be no other information about interactions between other hypoglycaemic agents and anticoagulants but monitoring is advisable.

The 'Clinical Evidence' section lists those which seem to be free from interactions: tolbutamide + phenindione; glibornuride + phenprocoumon; glimepiride + warfarin; warfarin + tolbutamide; phenprocoumon + glibenclamide, glibornuride, tolbutamide or insulin; warfarin + tolbutamide. Warfarin and phenprocoumon seem to be safer than dicoumarol, nevertheless be alert for any evidence of changes in the anticoagulant or hypoglycaemic effects if either is given with any hypoglycaemic agent.

1. Kristensen M, Hansen JM. Accumulation of chlorpropamide caused by dicoumarol. *Acta Med Scand* (1968) 183, 83–6.
2. Petitpierre B, Perrin L, Rudhardt M, Herrera A, Fabre J. Behaviour of chlorpropamide in renal insufficiency and under the effect of associated drug therapy. *Int J Clin Pharmacol* (1972) 6, 120–4.
3. Eckhardt W, Rudolph R, Sauer H, Schubert WR, Undeutsch D. Zur pharmakologischen Interferenz von Glibornurid mit Sulfaphenazol, Phenylbutazon und phenprocoumon beim Menschen. *Arzneimittelforschung* (1972) 22, 2212–19.
4. Schulz E, Schmidt FH. Über den Einfluss von Sulphaphenazol, Phenylbutazon und Phenprocoumal auf die Elimination von Glibenclamid beim Menschen. *Verh Dtsch Ges Inn Med* (1970) 76, 435–8.
5. Kristensen M, Hansen JM. Potentiation of the tolbutamide effect by dicoumarol. *Diabetes* (1967) 16, 211–14.
6. Solomon HM, Schrogie JJ. Effect of phenyramidol and bishydroxycoumarin on the metabolism of tolbutamide in human subjects. *Metabolism* (1967) 16, 1029–33.
7. Spurny OM, Wolf JW, Devins GS. Protracted tolbutamide-induced hypoglycemia. *Arch Intern Med* (1965) 115, 53–6.
8. Schwartz JF. Tolbutamide-induced hypoglycemia in Parkinson's disease. A case report. *JAMA* (1961) 176, 106–9.
9. Fontana G, Addarii F, Peta G. Su di un caso di coma ipoglicemico in corso di terapia con tolbutamide e dicumarolici. *G Clin Med* (1968) 49, 849–58.
10. Chaplin H, Cassell M. Studies on the possible relationship of tolbutamide to dicoumarol in anticoagulant therapy. *Am J Med Sci* (1958) 235, 706–15.
11. Jähnchen E, Gilfrich HJ, Groth U, Meinertz T. Pharmacokinetic analysis of the dicoumarol-tolbutamide interaction in man. *Naunyn Schmiedebergs Arch Pharmacol* (1975) 287 (Suppl), R88.
12. Poucher RL, Vecchio TJ. Absence of tolbutamide effect on anticoagulant therapy. *JAMA* (1966) 197, 1069–70.
13. Jähnchen E, Meinertz T, Gilfrich H-J, Groth U. Pharmacokinetic analysis of the interaction between dicoumarol and tolbutamide in man. *Eur J Clin Pharmacol* (1976) 10, 349–56.
14. Ohnhaus EE, Berger W, Duckert F, Oesch F. The influence of dimethylbiguanide on phenprocoumon elimination and its mode of action. *Klin Wochenschr* (1983) 61, 851–8.
15. Hamblin TJ. Interaction between warfarin and phenformin. *Lancet* (1971) ii, 1323.
16. Heine P, Kewitz H, Wiegboldt K-A. The influence of hypoglycaemic sulphonylureas on elimination and efficacy of phenprocoumon following a single oral dose in diabetic patients. *Eur J Clin Pharmacol* (1976) 10, 31–6.

17. Schaaf LJ, Sisson TA, Dietz AJ, Viveash DM, Oliver LK, Knuth DW, Carel BJ. Influence of multiple dose glimepiride on the pharmacokinetics and pharmacodynamics of racemic warfarin in healthy volunteers. *Pharm Res* (1994) 11 (10 Suppl), S-359.
18. Beeley L, Stewart P, Hickey FM. Bulletin of the West Midlands Centre for Adverse Drug Reaction Reporting. (1988) 26, 27.
19. Jassal SV. Drug points. *BMJ* (1991) 303, 789.
20. Beeley L, Magee P, Hickey FN. Bulletin of the West Midlands Centre for Adverse Drug Reaction Reporting (1990) 30, 32.

Hypoglycaemic agents + Azapropazone

Two case reports and a study in three normal subjects show that azapropazone can increase the effects of tolbutamide and cause severe hypoglycaemia.

Clinical evidence

A woman whose diabetes was well controlled for 3 years on 500 mg **tolbutamide** twice daily, became confused and semi-comatose 4 days after starting to take 900 mg **azapropazone** daily. She complained of having felt agitated since starting the **azapropazone** so it was withdrawn on suspicion of causing hypoglycaemia. Later that evening she became semi-comatose and was found to have a plasma glucose level of 2 mmol/l.[1] A subsequent study in 3 normal subjects found that the same dosage of **azapropazone** increased the plasma half-life of **tolbutamide** 500 mg threefold (from 7.7 to 25.2 h) and reduced its clearance accordingly.[1] Acute hypoglycaemia occurred in another patient on **tolbutamide** 500 mg three times daily, 5.5 h after taking a single 600-mg dose of **azapropazone**.[2]

Mechanism

The clinical study suggests that azapropazone can inhibit the liver enzymes concerned with the metabolism of tolbutamide, thereby prolonging its stay in the body and increasing its effects.[1] The rapidity of the second case suggests that displacement from plasma protein binding may also occur.[2]

Importance and management

The cases cited and the associated clinical study appear to be all that is on record about this interaction so far, however it would be prudent to avoid concurrent use. Information about other sulphonylureas seems to be lacking but the makers of azapropazone say that their concurrent use is not recommended.

1. Andreasen PB, Simonsen K, Brocks K, Dimo B, Bouchelouche P. Hypoglycaemia induced by azapropazone-tolbutamide interaction. *Br J Clin Pharmacol* (1981) 12, 581–3.
2. Waller DG, Waller D. Hypoglycaemia due to azapropazone-tolbutamide interaction. *Br J Rheumatol* (1984) 23, 24–5.

Hypoglycaemic agents + Barbiturates

The hypoglycaemic effects of glymidine are reported not to be affected by phenobarbital (phenobarbitone). There appear to be no reports of adverse hypoglycaemic agent/barbiturate interactions.

Clinical evidence, mechanism, importance and management

A study in one subject showed that the hypoglycaemic effects of **glymidine** were unaffected by the concurrent use of **phenobarbital (phenobarbitone)**.[1] There seems to be nothing in the literature to suggest that an adverse interaction takes place between any of the hypoglycaemic agents and barbiturates. No special precautions would appear necessary.

1. Gerhards E, Kolb KH, Schulze PE. Über 2-Benzolsulfonylamino- 5(β-methoxy-äthoxy) pyrimidin (Glycodiazin). V. In vitro- und in vivo-Versuche zum Einfluß von Phenyläthyl-barbitursäure (Luminal) auf den Stoffwechsel und die blutzuckersenkende Wirkung des Glycodiazins. *Naunyn Schmiedebergs Arch Pharmakol Exp Pathol* (1966) 255, 200–220.

Hypoglycaemic agents + Benzodiazepines

No adverse interaction normally occurs between these drugs, but an isolated case of hyperglycaemia has been seen in an insulin-treated diabetic associated with the use of chlordiazepoxide. The effects of lorazepam were found to be increased in patients given beef/pork rather than human insulin.

Clinical evidence, mechanism, importance and management

A woman with maturity-onset diabetes of 27 years' duration, controlled on 45 units **isophane insulin suspension** daily, showed a mean fasting blood sugar rise from 220 to 380 mg/100 ml during a 3-week period while taking 40 mg **chlordiazepoxide** daily. Four other diabetics, 2 controlled on **diet** alone and the other 2 on **tolbutamide**, showed no changes in blood sugar levels while taking **chlordiazepoxide**.[1] No change in the half-life of **chlorpropamide** is reported to have occurred in another study when **diazepam** was used concurrently.[2] A preliminary report in 8 healthy type I diabetics given 2 mg **lorazepam** suggested that while taking **human insulin** they were more alert and less impaired than when taking **beef/pork insulin**.[3]

There seems to be nothing in the literature to suggest that a clinically important adverse interaction normally takes place between the hypoglycaemic agents and the benzodiazepines. No special precautions would appear to be necessary.

1. Zumoff B, Hellman L. Aggravation of diabetic hyperglycemia by chlordiazepoxide. *JAMA* (1977) 237, 1960–1.
2. Petitpierre B, Perrin L, Rudhardt M, Herrera A, Fabre J. Behaviour of chlorpropamide in renal insufficiency and under the effect of associated drug therapy. *Int J Clin Pharmacol* (1972) 6, 120–4.
3. Dahlan AA, Vrbancic MI, Hogan TE, Woo D, Herman RI. Greater sedative response to lorazepam in patients with insulin-dependent diabetes mellitus while on treatment with beef/pork versus human insulin. *Clin Invest Med* (1993) 16 (4 Suppl), B18.

Hypoglycaemic agents + Beta-blockers

In diabetics using insulin, the normal recovery reaction (blood sugar rise) if hypoglycaemia occurs may be impaired to some extent by propranolol, but serious and severe hypoglycaemia and hypertension have only been seen in a few patients. Other beta-blockers normally interact to a lesser extent or not at all. The hypoglycaemic effects of the sulphonylureas may possibly be reduced by the beta-blockers. Whether insulin or the sulphonylureas are given, be aware that some of the familiar warning signs of hypoglycaemia (tachycardia, tremor) may not occur, although sweating may be increased.

Clinical evidence

(a) Insulin + beta-blockers

(i) *Hypoglycaemia.* Although **propranolol** has occasionally been associated with spontaneous episodes of hypoglycaemia in non-diabetics,[1] and a number of studies in diabetic patients[2] and normal subjects[3-6] have shown that **propranolol** impairs the normal blood sugar rebound if blood sugar levels fall, there appear to be few reports of severe hypoglycaemia or coma in diabetics on **insulin** given **propranolol**. Marked hypoglycaemia and/or coma occurred in 5 diabetic patients on **insulin** due to the use of **propranolol**,[1,7,8] **pindolol**,[8] and **timolol** eye-drops.[9] Other contributory factors (fasting, haemodialysis, etc.) probably had some part to play.[8] **Metoprolol** interacts like **propranolol** but to a lesser extent,[3,5,10] whereas the other beta-blockers examined (**acebutolol**,[2,5] **alprenolol**,[11] **atenolol**,[2,12,13] **oxprenolol**,[10] **penbutolol**,[6] **pindolol**[14]) were found to interact minimally or not at all. The situation with **pindolol** is therefore not clear. **Propranolol** (a vasoconstrictor) has also been found to reduce the rate of absorption of subcutaneous **insulin** by almost 50%, but the importance of this is uncertain.[15]

(ii) Hypertension. Marked increases in blood pressure (systolic and diastolic) and bradycardia may develop if hypoglycaemia occurs in diabetics on **insulin** and beta-blockers.[16] Systolic/diastolic pressure rises of +38.8/+14.3 mmHg with **propranolol** 80 mg twice daily, +27.9/0 mmHg with **atenolol** 100 mg daily and +15.6/–9.2 mmHg with placebo were seen in one study in **insulin**-treated diabetics.[17] In another study rises of +27/+14 mmHg were seen with **alprenolol** 200 to 800 mg daily, but no rise with **metoprolol** 100 to 400 mg daily.[18] A report describes a pressure rise to 258/144 mmHg in a patient within 2 days of starting **propranolol**.[7] Another patient on **metoprolol** 50 mg twice daily experienced a rise from 190/96 to 230/112 mmHg during a hypoglycaemic episode.[16]

(b) Oral hypoglycaemic agents + beta-blockers

(i) Hyperglycaemia, hypoglycaemia or no interaction. The sulphonylurea-induced insulin-release from the pancreas can be inhibited by beta-blockers so that the hypoglycaemic effects are opposed to some extent. The effects of **glibenclamide (glyburide)**,[19] **chlorpropamide**[20] and **tolbutamide**[21] have been shown to be inhibited by **propranolol**. **Acebutolol** affects **glibenclamide** about the same as **propranolol** but has fewer unwanted haemodynamic effects[19] and has no effect on **tolbutamide**.[22] Two isolated cases of hypoglycaemia have been seen with **acebutolol**, in one patient taking **gliclazide** and the other taking **chlorpropamide**.[23] One study failed to find an interaction between **tolbutamide** and either **propranolol** or **metoprolol**,[24] and another found no interaction between **betaxolol** and **glibenclamide** or **metformin**.[25] No pharmacokinetic interaction was seen in a study in normal subjects given **glibenclamide** and **carvedilol**.[26] An isolated report describes hyperosmolar non-ketotic coma in a patient on **tolbutamide** and **propranolol**.[27] It is worth noting that the United Kingdom Prospective Diabetes Study Group (UKPDS) used **atenolol** 50 to 100 mg daily or captopril 25 to 50 mg twice daily as a first line agent in the control of raised blood pressure in diabetics on a range of hypoglycaemic agents. The number of patients experiencing hypoglycaemic attacks did not differ for the two antihypertensives, although weight gain was greater in the group treated with atenolol (3.4 kg for the **atenolol** group compared to 1.6 kg for the captopril group).[28] This would suggest that beta-blockers are generally useful in the treatment of diabetes.

Mechanism

Among other mechanisms, the normal physiological response to a fall in blood sugar levels is the mobilisation of glucose from the liver under the stimulation of epinephrine (adrenaline) from the adrenals. This sugar mobilisation is blocked by non-selective beta-blockers (such as propranolol) so that recovery from hypoglycaemia is delayed and may even proceed into a full-scale episode in a hypoglycaemia-prone diabetic. Normally the epinephrine would also increase the heart rate, but with the beta-receptors in the heart already blocked this fails to occur. A rise in blood pressure occurs because the stimulant effects of epinephrine on the beta-2 receptors (vasodilation) are blocked leaving the alpha (vasoconstriction) effects unopposed. Non-selective beta-blockers can also block beta-2 receptors in the pancreas concerned with insulin-release, so that the effects of the sulphonylureas may be blocked.

Importance and management

Extremely well-studied interactions. Concurrent use can be uneventful but there are some risks. The overall picture is as follows:

(A) *Diabetics on insulin* may have (i) a prolonged or delayed recovery response to hypoglycaemia while on beta-blockers, but very severe hypoglycaemia and/or coma is rare. (ii) If hypoglycaemia occurs it may be accompanied by a sharp rise in blood pressure. The risk is greatest with propranolol and possibly other non-selective blockers and least with the cardio-selective blockers (e.g. atenolol, metoprolol, etc.). Monitor the effects of concurrent use well, avoid the non-selec-

tive blockers, and check for any evidence that the insulin dosage needs some adjustment. Warn all patients that some of the normal premonitory signs of 'going hypo' may not appear, in particular tachycardia and tremors, whereas the hunger, irritability and nausea signs may be unaffected and sweating may even be increased.

(B) *Diabetics taking oral sulphonylureas* rarely seem to have serious hypoglycaemic episodes caused by beta-blockers, and any reductions in the hypoglycaemic effects of the sulphonylureas normally appear to be of little clinical importance. The selective beta-blockers are probably safer than the non-selective, however always monitor concurrent use to confirm that diabetic control is well maintained (increase the dosage if necessary), and warn all patients (as in (A) above) that some of the premonitory signs of hypoglycaemia may not occur.

(C) One experimental study indicated no interaction between betaxolol and metformin,[25] but direct information about other biguanides seems to be lacking.

There is also a hint from one report that the peripheral vasoconstrictive effects of non-selective beta-blockers and the poor peripheral circulation in diabetics could be additive.[7] Another good reason for avoiding this type of beta-blocker in diabetics.

1. Kotler MN, Berman L, Rubenstein AH. Hypoglycaemia precipitated by propranolol. *Lancet* (1966) 2, 1389–90.
2. Deacon SP, Karunanayake A, Barnett D. Acebutolol, atenolol, and propranolol and metabolic responses to acute hypoglycaemia in diabetics. *BMJ* (1977) 2, 1255–7.
3. Davidson NM, Corrall RJM, Shaw TRD, French EB. Observations in man of hypoglycaemia during selective and non-selective beta-blockade. *Scott Med J* (1976) 22, 69–72.
4. Abramson EA, Arky RA, Woeber KA. Effects of propranolol on the hormonal and metabolic responses to insulin-induced hypoglycaemia. *Lancet* (1966) ii, 1386–9.
5. Newman RJ. Comparison of propranolol, metoprolol, and acebutolol on insulin-induced hypoglycaemia. *BMJ* (1976) 2, 447–9.
6. Sharma SD, Vakil BJ, Samuel MR, Chadha DR. Comparison of penbutolol and propranolol during insulin-induced hypoglycaemia. *Curr Ther Res* (1979) 26, 252–9.
7. McMurtry RJ. Propranolol, hypoglycemia, and hypertensive crisis. *Ann Intern Med* (1974) 80, 669–70.
8. Samii K, Ciancioni C, Rottembourg J, Bisseliches F, Jacobs C. Severe hypoglycaemia due to beta-blocking drugs in haemodialysis patients. *Lancet* (1976) i, 545–6.
9. Angelo-Nielsen K. Timolol topically and diabetes mellitus. *JAMA* (1980) 244, 2263.
10. Viberti GC, Stimmler M, Keen H. The effect of oxprenolol and metoprolol on the hypoglycaemic response to insulin in normals and insulin-dependent diabetics. *Diabetologia* (1978) 15, 278.
11. Eisalo A, Heino A, Munter J. The effect of alprenolol in elderly patients with raised blood pressure. *Acta Med Scand* (1974) (Suppl) 554, 23–31.
12. Deacon SP, Barnett D. Comparison of atenolol and propranolol during insulin-induced hypoglycaemia. *BMJ* (1976) 2, 272–3.
13. Waal-Manning HJ. Atenolol and three nonselective β-blockers in hypertension. *Clin Pharmacol Ther* (1979) 25, 8–18.
14. Patsch W, Patsch JR, Sailer S. Untersuchung zur Wirkung von Pindolol auf Kohlehydrat- und Fettstoffwechsel bei Diabetes Mellitus. *Int J Clin Pharmacol Biopharm* (1977) 15, 394–6.
15. Veenstra J, van der Hulst JP, Wildenborg IH, Njoo SF, Verdegaal WP, Silberbusch J. Effect of antihypertensive drugs on insulin absorption. *Diabetes Care* (1991) 14, 1089–92.
16. Shepherd AMM, Lin M-S, Keeton TK. Hypoglycemia-induced hypertension in a diabetic patient on metoprolol. *Ann Intern Med* (1981) 94, 357–8.
17. Ryan JR, Lacorte W, Jain A, McMahon FG. Response of diabetics treated with atenolol or propranolol to insulin-induced hypoglycaemia. *Drugs* (1983) 25 (Suppl), 256–7.
18. Östman J, Arner P, Haglund K, Juhlin-Dannfelt A, Nowak J, Wennlund A. Effect of metoprolol and alprenolol on the metabolic, hormonal, and haemodynamic response to insulin-induced hypoglycaemia in hypertensive, insulin-dependent diabetics. *Acta Med Scand* (1982) 211, 381–5.
19. Zaman R, Kendall MJ, Biggs PI. The effect of acebutolol and propranolol on the hypoglycaemic action of glibenclamide. *Br J Clin Pharmacol* (1982) 13, 507–12.
20. Holt RJ, Gaskins JD. Hyperglycaemia associated with propranolol and chlorpropamide coadministration. *Drug Intell Clin Pharm* (1981) 15, 599–600.
21. Massara F, Strumia E, Camanni F, Molinatti GM. Depressed tolbutamide-induced insulin response in subjects treated with propranolol. *Diabetologia* (1971) 7, 287–9.
22. Ryan JR. Clinical pharmacology of acebutolol. *Am Heart J* (1985) 109, 1131–6.
23. Girardin E, Vial T, Pham E, Evreux J-C. Hypoglycémies induites par les sulfamides hypoglycémiants. *Ann Med Interne (Paris)* (1992) 143, 11–17.
24. Tötterman KJ, Groop LC. No effect of propranolol and metoprolol on the tolbutamide-stimulated insulin-secretion in hypertensive diabetic and non-diabetic patients. *Ann Clin Res* (1982) 14, 190–3.
25. Sinclair AJ, Davies IB, Warrington SJ. Betaxolol and glucose-insulin relationships: studies in normal subjects taking glibenclamide or metformin. *Br J Clin Pharmacol* (1990) 30, 699–702.
26. Harder S, Merz PG, Rietbrock N. Lack of pharmacokinetic interaction between carvedilol and digitoxin, phenprocoumon or glibenclamide. *Cardiovasc Drugs Ther* (1993) 7 (Suppl 2), 447.
27. Podolsky S, Pattavina CG. Hyperosmolar nonketotic diabetic coma: a complication of propranolol therapy. *Metabolism* (1973) 22, 685–93.
28. UK Prospective Diabetes Study Group. Efficacy of atenolol and captopril in reducing risk of macrovascular and microvascular complications in type 2 diabetes: UKPDS 39. *BMJ* (1998) 317, 713–20.

Hypoglycaemic agents + Calcium channel blockers

Calcium channel blockers are known to have effects on insulin secretion and glucose regulation but significant disturbances in the control of diabetes are uncommon. A report describes a patient whose diabetes worsened and who needed more insulin when treated with diltiazem. Another patient needed a 30% increase in insulin while taking nifedipine, and hypoglycaemia occurred in a patient taking gliclazide and nicardipine.

Clinical evidence

(a) Diltiazem

An insulin-dependent diabetic developed worsening and intractable hyperglycaemia (mean serum glucose levels above 13 mmol/l) when given 90 mg **diltiazem** 6-hourly. Her **insulin** requirements dropped when the **diltiazem** was withdrawn. When restarted on 30 mg **diltiazem** 6-hourly her blood sugar levels were still high, but she needed less **insulin** than when taking the higher **diltiazem** dosage.[1]

A study in 12 normal subjects showed that 60 mg **diltiazem** three times daily had no effect on the secretion of **insulin** or **glucagon**, or on plasma glucose levels.[2]

A study in 8 normal subjects found that single doses of **tolbutamide** 500 mg had no effect on the serum levels of co-administered single doses of **diltiazem** 60 mg. There was an approximately 10% increase in the AUC_{0-24} and C_{max} for **tolbutamide** in the presence of diltiazem. **Diltiazem** did not significantly affect the hypoglycaemic effects of tolbutamide.[3]

(b) Nifedipine, Nicardipine, Nimodipine or Nitrendipine

A study in 20 non-insulin dependent diabetics (5 on **metformin** and 15 **diet-controlled**) showed that neither **nifedipine** (10 mg eight-hourly) nor **nicardipine** (30 mg eight-hourly) for 4 weeks had any effect on glucose tolerance tests and no effect on the control of the diabetes, but significant reductions in blood pressures occurred (4 to 7 mmHg diastolic and systolic).[4] Another study in 8 non-diabetics and 8 diabetics (3 on **chlorpropamide**, one on **glipizide** and 4 on **diet alone**) showed that the use of 30 mg **nifedipine** daily for a month did not significantly alter their glucose tolerance tests.[5] No important changes occurred in 6 diabetic patients taking **glibenclamide (glyburide)** when chronically treated for 12 to 25 weeks with 20 to 60 mg **nifedipine** daily.[6] Another study in 6 diabetics showed that single 20-mg doses of **nifedipine** had no effect on the pharmacokinetics or actions of **glipizide** (5 to 20 mg daily).[7] This confirms other studies with **nifedipine**[8] and **nicardipine**.[9] **Nitrendipine** 30 mg daily over a 5-year period was reported to have had no adverse effect on the control of diabetes in 14 elderly patients using **insulin** or **oral hypoglycaemic agents**.[10] No clinically relevant interactions were found in 11 type 2 diabetics on **glibenclamide** while treated with **nimodipine**.[11]

There are however other reports of a deterioration in glucose tolerance during the use of **nifedipine** in 10 subjects with impaired glucose tolerance[12] and in 2 patients.[13] A further case report described a 30% increase in the insulin requirements of a diabetic man after **nifedipine** 60 mg daily was administered.[14] One study found that 10 mg **nifedipine** increased the rate of absorption of subcutaneous **insulin** by about 50%.[15] An isolated case of hypoglycaemia has been described in a patient on **gliclazide** when treated with **nicardipine**.[16]

(c) Verapamil

A study in 23 type II diabetics, 7 of whom were taking **glibenclamide (glyburide)**, showed that **verapamil** improved the oral glucose tolerance test but did not increase the hypoglycaemic effects of the **glibenclamide**.[17] Two studies in type II diabetics found that **verapamil** improved glucose tolerance tests,[18,19] but in one of the studies, no alterations in the hypoglycaemic effects of **glibenclamide** were found.[18] A study in normal subjects found that **verapamil** raised serum **glibenclamide** levels but plasma glucose levels were unchanged.[20]

Mechanism

The changes that occur are not fully understood. Suggestions include inhibition of insulin secretion by the calcium channel blockers and inhibition of glucagon secretion by glucose; changes in glucose uptake by liver and other cells; blood glucose rises following catecholamine release after vasodilation, and changes in glucose metabolism.

Importance and management

Very extensively studied, but many of the reports describe single-dose studies or multiple-dose studies in normal subjects (only a few are cited here) which do not give a clear picture of what may be expected in diabetic patients. Those studies which have concentrated on diabetics indicate that the control of the diabetes is not usually adversely affected by concurrent use although isolated cases with diltiazem, nicardipine and nifedipine have been reported.[1,14,16] No particular precautions normally seem to be necessary, nevertheless be alert for any signs of a worsening control of the diabetes. More study in diabetics is needed.

1. Pershadsingh HA, Grant N, McDonald JM. Association of diltiazem therapy with increased insulin resistance in a patient with type I diabetes mellitus. *JAMA* (1987) 257, 930–1.
2. Segrestaa JM, Caulin C, Dahan R, Houlbert D, Thiercelin JF, Herman P, Sauvanet JP, Laurribaud J. Effect of diltiazem on plasma glucose, insulin and glucagon during an oral glucose tolerance test in healthy volunteers. *Eur J Clin Pharmacol* (1984) 26, 481–3.
3. Dixit AA, Rao YM. Pharmacokinetic interaction between diltiazem and tolbutamide. *Drug Metabol Drug Interact* (1999) 15, 269–77.
4. Collins WCJ, Cullen MJ, Feely J. Calcium channel blocker drugs and diabetic control. *Clin Pharmacol Ther* (1987) 42, 420–3.
5. Donnelly T, Harrower ADB. Effect of nifedipine on glucose tolerance and insulin secretion in diabetic and non-diabetic patients. *Curr Med Res Opin* (1980) 6, 690–3.
6. Kanatsuna T, Nakano K, Mori H, Kano Y, Nishioka H, Kajiyama S, Kitagawa Y, Yoshida T, Kondo M, Nakamura N, Aochi O. Effects of nifedipine on insulin secretion and glucose metabolism in rats and hypertensive type 2 (non-insulin dependent) diabetics. *Arzneimittelforschung* (1985) 35, 514–17.
7. Connacher AA, El Debani AH, Stevenson IH. A study of the influence of nifedipine on the disposition and hypoglycaemic action of glipizide. *Br J Clin Pharmacol* (1986) 22, 240 P.
8. Abadie E, Passa PH. Diabetogenic effects of nifedipine. *BMJ* (1984) 289, 438.
9. Sakata S, Miura K. Effect of nicardipine in a hypertensive patient with diabetes mellitus. *Clin Ther* (1984) 6, 600–2.
10. Trost BN, Weidmann P. 5 years of antihypertensive monotherapy with the calcium antagonist nitrendipine do not alter carbohydrate homeostasis in diabetic patients. *Diabetes Res Clin Pract* (1988) 5 (Suppl 1), S511.
11. Mück W, Heine PR, Breuel H-P, Niklaus H, Horkulak J, Ahr G. The effect of multiple oral dosing of nimodipine on glibenclamide pharmacodynamics and pharmacokinetics in elderly patients with type-2 diabetes mellitus. *Int J Clin Pharmacol Ther* (1995) 33, 89–94.
12. Guigliano D, Torella R, Cacciapuoti F, Gentile S, Verza M, Varricchio M. Impairment of insulin secretion in man by nifedipine. *Eur J Clin Pharmacol* (1980) 18, 395–8.
13. Bhatnagar SK, Amin MMA, Al-Yusuf AR. Diabetogenic effects of nifedipine. *BMJ* (1984) 289, 19.
14. Heyman SN, Heyman A, Halperin I. Diabetogenic effect of nifedipine. *DICP Ann Pharmacother* (1989) 23, 236–7.
15. Veenstra J, van der Hulst JP, Wildenborg IH, Njoo SF, Verdegaal WP, Silberbusch J. Effect of antihypertensive drugs on insulin absorption. *Diabetes Care* (1991) 14, 1089–92.
16. Girardin E, Vial T, Pham E, Evreux J-C. Hypoglycémies induites par les sulfamides hypoglycémiants. *Ann Med Interne (Paris)* (1992) 143, 11–17.
17. Röjdmark S, Andersson DEH. Influence of verapamil on human glucose tolerance. *Am J Cardiol* (1986) 57, 39D–43D.
18. Röjdmark S, Andersson DEH. Influence of verapamil on glucose tolerance. *Acta Med Scand* (1984) (Suppl), 681, 37–42.
19. Andersson DEH, Röjdmark S. Improvement of glucose tolerance by verapamil in patients with non-insulin-dependent diabetes mellitus. *Acta Med Scand* (1981) 210, 27–33.
20. Semple CG, Omile C, Buchanan KD, Beastall GH, Paterson KR. Effect of oral verapamil on glibenclamide stimulated insulin secretion. *Br J Clin Pharmacol* (1986) 22, 187–90.

Hypoglycaemic agents + Chloramphenicol

The hypoglycaemic effects of tolbutamide and chlorpropamide can be increased by the concurrent use of chloramphenicol. Acute hypoglycaemia can occur.

Clinical evidence

While taking 2 g **chloramphenicol** daily, a man was additionally started on a course of 2 g **tolbutamide** daily. Three days later he had a typical hypoglycaemic collapse and was found to have serum **tolbutamide** levels three to fourfold higher than expected.[1]

Studies in diabetics have shown that **chloramphenicol** 2 g daily can increase the serum level and half-life of **tolbutamide** twofold and two to threefold respectively.[1,2] Blood sugar levels were reduced by about 25-30%.[2,3] Hypoglycaemia, acute in one case, developed in two other patients on **tolbutamide** given **chloramphenicol**.[4,5] Another study using 1 to 2 g **chloramphenicol** daily showed an average twofold increase in the half-life of **chlorpropamide**.[6]

Mechanism

Chloramphenicol inhibits the liver enzymes concerned with the metabolism of tolbutamide, and probably chlorpropamide as well, leading to their accumulation in the body. This is reflected in prolonged half-lives, reduced blood sugar levels and occasionally acute hypoglycaemia.[1-4,6]

Importance and management

The tolbutamide/chloramphenicol interaction is well-established and of clinical importance. The incidence is uncertain, but an increased hypoglycaemic response should be expected if both drugs are given. The chlorpropamide/chloramphenicol interaction is less well documented. The dosage of both sulphonylureas should be reduced appropriately. Some patients may show a particularly exaggerated response. The manufacturers of other sulphonylureas often list chloramphenicol as an interacting drug, based on its interactions with tolbutamide and chlorpropamide, but direct information of an interaction appears not to be available. No interaction would be expected with chloramphenicol eye drops because the systemic absorption is likely to be small. This needs confirmation.

1. Christensen LK, Skovsted L. Inhibition of drug metabolism by chloramphenicol. *Lancet* (1969) ii, 1397–9.
2. Brunová E, Slabochová Z, Platilová H, Pavlík F, Grafnetterová J, Dvořáček K. Interaction of tolbutamide and chloramphenicol in diabetic patients. *Int J Clin Pharmacol Biopharm* (1977) 15, 7–12.
3. Brunová E, Slabochová Z, Platilová H. Influencing the effect of Dirastan (tolbutamide). Simultaneous administration of chloramphenicol in patients with diabetes and bacterial urinary tract inflammation. *Cas Lek Cesk* (1974) 113, 72–5.
4. Ziegelasch H-J. Extreme hypoglykämie unter kombinierter behandlung mit tolbutamid, n-1-butylbiguanidhydrochlorid und chloramphenikol. *Z Gesamte Inn Med* (1972) 27, 63–6.
5. Soeldner JS, Steinke J. Hypoglycemia in tolbutamide-treated diabetes. *JAMA* (1965) 193, 398–9.
6. Petitpierre B, Perrin L, Rudhardt M, Herrera A, Fabre J. Behaviour of chlorpropamide in renal insufficiency and under the effect of associated drug therapy. *Int J Clin Pharmacol* (1972) 6, 120–4.

Hypoglycaemic agents + Chlorpromazine or other phenothiazines

Chlorpromazine can raise blood sugar levels, particularly in daily doses of 100 mg or more, and disturb the control of diabetes. It may be necessary to increase the dosage of the hypoglycaemic agent.

Clinical evidence

A long-term study was undertaken over the period 1955 to 1966 in a large number of women treated for a year or more with **chlorpromazine** in daily doses of 100 mg or more, or corresponding doses of other psychoactive phenothiazines (perphenazine, thioridazine, trifluoperazine). This showed that about 25% developed hyperglycaemia accompanied by glycosuria, compared with less than 9% in the control group who were not taking phenothiazines of any kind. Of those given **chlorpromazine** or **other phenothiazines**, about a quarter showed complete remission of the symptoms when the drug was withdrawn or the dosage reduced. Thioridazine appeared to be less diabetogenic than the other phenothiazines used.[1]

There are numerous other reports of this response to chlorpromazine.[2-11] One report covering 850 patients is out of step in suggesting that **chlorpromazine** has no effect on blood sugar levels; 22 diabetic patients in the study showed no significant changes in their blood sugar levels. Five patients developed diabetes, but this was believed to be due to factors other than chlorpromazine treatment.[12] **Chlorpromazine** in doses of less than 100 mg daily (50 to 70 mg) does not affect blood sugar levels significantly.[11]

Mechanism

It seems that chlorpromazine can inhibit the release of insulin, and possibly cause epinephrine (adrenaline) release from the adrenals, both of which could result in a rise in blood sugar levels.

Importance and management

A well-documented and long-established reaction first recognised in the early 1950s. The incidence is about 25% with daily doses of chlorpromazine of 100 mg or more. Increases in the dosage requirements of the hypoglycaemic agent should be anticipated during concurrent use. Smaller daily doses (50 to 70 mg) do not apparently cause hyperglycaemia. There seems to be little clinical evidence that other phenothiazines significantly disturb blood sugar levels in diabetics.

1. Thonnard-Neumann E. Phenothiazines and diabetes in hospitalized women. *Am J Psychiatry* (1968) 124, 978–82.
2. Hiles BW. Hyperglycaemia and glycosuria following chlorpromazine therapy. *JAMA* (1956) 162, 1651.
3. Dobkin AB, Lamoureux L, Letienne R, Gilbert RGB. Some studies with Largactil. *Can Med Assoc J* (1954) 70, 626–8.
4. Célice J, Porcher P, Plas F, Hélie J, Peltier A. Action de la chlorpromazine sur la vésicule biliare et le clon droit. *Therapie* (1955) 10, 30–38.
5. Charatan FBE, Bartlett NG. The effect of chlorpromazine ('Largactil') on glucose tolerance. *J Ment Sci* (1955) 101, 351–3.
6. Cooperberg AA, Eidlow S. Haemolytic anaemia, jaundice and diabetes mellitus following chlorpromazine therapy. *Can Med Assoc J* (1956) 75, 746–9.
7. Blair D, Brady DM. Recent advances in the treatment of schizophrenia: group training and tranquillizers. *J Ment Sci* (1958) 104, 625–64.
8. Amidsen A. Diabetes mellitus as a side effect of treatment with tricyclic neuroleptics. *Acta Psychiatr Scand* (1964) 40 (Suppl 180), 411–14.
9. Arneson GA. Phenothiazine derivatives and glucose metabolism. *J Neuropsychiatr* (1964) 5, 181–5.
10. Korenyi C, Lowenstein B. Chlorpromazine induced diabetes. *Dis Nerv Syst* (1971) 29, 827–8.
11. Erle G, Basso M, Federspil G, Sicolo N, Scandellari C. Effect of chlorpromazine on blood glucose and plasma insulin in man. *Eur J Clin Pharmacol* (1977) 11, 15–18.
12. Schwarz L, Munoz R. Blood sugar levels in patients treated with chlorpromazine. *Am J Psychiatry* (1968) 125, 253–5.

Hypoglycaemic agents + Cibenzoline (Cifenline)

Hypoglycaemia has been seen in a few patients while taking cibenzoline alone, and in one case with gliclazide. The risk factors appear to be age, renal insufficiency and high dosage.

Clinical evidence, mechanism, importance and management

For reasons which are not understood, **cibenzoline** occasionally and unpredictably causes hypoglycaemia which may be severe. Marked hypoglycaemia was first seen in an 67-year-old patient when given **cibenzoline**.[1] Another case described hypoglycaemia in an 84-year-old. Age, renal impairment and malnutrition acted ad facilitating factors.[2] Hypoglycaemia has been reported in another 20 cases, where the dose was not corrected for age and renal function. Hypoglycaemia also occurred in a patient aged 61 years with renal insufficiency taking **gliclazide**.[3] The reasons are not understood. This appears to be a drug–disease rather than a drug–drug interaction and diabetic patients do not seem to be more at risk than non-diabetics, but good monitoring is advisable if **cibenzoline** is given.

1. Hilleman DE, Mohiuddin SM, Ahmed IS, Dahl JM. Cibenzoline-induced hypoglycemia. *Drug Intell Clin Pharm* (1987) 21, 38–40.
2. Houdent C, Noblet C, Vandoren C, Levesque H, Morin C, Moore N, Courtois H, Wolf LM. Hypoglycémie induite par la cibenzoline chez le sujet âgè. *Rev Med Interne* (1991) 12, 143–5.
3. Girardin E, Vial T, Pham E, Evreux J-C. Hypoglycémies induites par les sulfamides hypoglycémiants. *Ann Med Interne (Paris)* (1992) 143, 11–17.

Hypoglycaemic agents + Cicletanine

Preliminary evidence suggests that cicletanine and tolbutamide do not interact adversely.

Clinical evidence, mechanism, importance and management

The hypoglycaemic responses of 10 normal subjects were studied following an intravenous infusion of 3 mg/kg **tolbutamide**, 3 days before taking 100 mg **cicletanine** daily, by mouth, for a week.[1] The **tolbutamide** infusion was repeated 1 h after the last dose of **cicletanine**. No clinically relevant changes were seen. The conclusion to be drawn is that **cicletanine** is unlikely to affect the control of diabetes in patients, but this needs confirmation from longer-term clinical studies.

1. Bayés MC, Barbanoj MJ, Vallès J, Torrent J, Obach R, Jané F. A drug interaction study between cicletanine and tolbutamide in healthy volunteers. *Eur J Clin Pharmacol* (1996) 50, 381–4.

Hypoglycaemic agents + Cimetidine or Ranitidine

Isolated cases of hypoglycaemia have been seen with gliclazide/cimetidine and glibenclamide (glyburide)/ranitidine, but marked changes in the control of diabetes in patients on most sulphonylureas when given either cimetidine or ranitidine seem to be unusual. A possible exception is glipizide with cimetidine. Cimetidine appears to reduce the clearance of metformin.

Clinical evidence

A. Studies in diabetic patients given sulphonylureas

(a) Gliclazide or Glibenclamide (Glyburide)

An elderly diabetic taking 160 mg **gliclazide** daily developed very low blood sugar levels (1 mmol/l) after starting treatment with 800 mg **cimetidine** daily.[1] Marked hypoglycaemia was seen in a patient on **glibenclamide** when treated with **ranitidine**,[2] and another report briefly describes hypoglycaemia in 2 patients given **cimetidine**, while taking **unnamed sulphonylureas**.[3]

(b) Glipizide

Non-insulin dependent diabetics were given 400 mg **cimetidine** 1 h before taking a dose of **glipizide** (average 5.7-mg dose) and then 3 h later they were given a standard meal with 200 mg of **cimetidine**. The expected rise in blood sugar levels after the meal was reduced by 40% and in some of the patients it fell to less than 3 mmol/l.[4,5] Two studies in non-insulin dependent diabetics found that 150 mg or 300 mg **ranitidine** had no significant effects on the pharmacokinetics or the effects of **glipizide**, except that the absorption was delayed,[6,7] whereas a later study by the same group of workers found that the expected rise in blood sugar levels after a meal was reduced by 25%.[5]

B. Studies in normal subjects given sulphonylureas

The pharmacokinetics of **tolbutamide** (250 mg daily for 4 days) were not significantly changed in 7 subjects when given 800 mg **cimetidine** daily for a further 4 days.[8] Other studies also found no interaction between **tolbutamide**[9,10] or **chlorpropamide**[11] and **cimetidine**, or between **tolbutamide** and **ranitidine**,[10] and the hypoglycaemic activities of **tolbutamide**, **chlorpropamide**, **glibenclamide (glyburide)** and **glipizide** remained unaltered by **cimetidine**.[12] In contrast, in another study the AUC of **tolbutamide** was found to be increased by 20% and the elimination half-life decreased by 17% by 1200 mg **cimetidine** daily, but plasma glucose levels were not significantly changed. **Ranitidine** 300 mg had no effect.[13] A later study found effectively the same results.[14] Yet another study reported that the hypoglycaemic effects of **glibenclamide** were reduced by **cimetidine** and **ranitidine**.[15] No relevant interactions, either pharmacokinetic or pharmacodynamic, were seen in a study of **glimepiride** with either **cimetidine** or **ranitidine**.[16]

C. Study in normal subjects given a biguanide

Cimetidine 800 mg daily was found to reduce the renal clearance of **metformin** in 7 normal subjects by 27% and increase the AUC by 50%.[17]

Mechanism

If an interaction occurs[13] it may be because the cimetidine inhibits the metabolism of the sulphonylurea by the liver, thereby increasing its effects. Cimetidine appears to inhibit the excretion of metformin by the kidneys.[17]

Importance and management

Information is limited and not easy to assess because of the differences between the sulphonylureas and between normal subjects and diabetics, but all the evidence cited here, as well as the relative paucity of adverse reports, suggests that most diabetics do not experience any marked changes in their diabetic control if given cimetidine. However, you may wish to issue a warning when cimetidine is first started that rarely and unpredictably hypoglycaemia has occurred. The dosage of metformin may need to be reduced if cimetidine is used, bearing in mind the possibility of lactic acidosis if levels become too high. Ranitidine normally appears not to interact.

1. Archambeaud-Mouveroux F, Nouaille Y, Nadalon S, Treves R, Merle L. Interaction between gliclazide and cimetidine. *Eur J Clin Pharmacol* (1987) 31, 631.
2. Lee K, Mize R, Lowenstein SR. Glyburide-induced hypoglycaemia and ranitidine. *Ann Intern Med* (1987) 107, 261–2.
3. Girardin E, Vial T, Pham E, Evreux J-C. Hypoglycémies induites par les sulfamides hypoglycémiants. *Ann Med Interne (Paris)* (1992) 143, 11–17.
4. Feely J, Peden N. Enhanced sulphonylurea-induced hypoglycaemia with cimetidine. *Br J Clin Pharmacol* (1983) 15, 607P.
5. Feeley J, Collins WCJ, Cullen M, El Debani AH, MacWalter RS, Peden NR, Stevenson IH. Potentiation of the hypoglycaemic response to glipizide in diabetic patients by histamine H₂–receptor antagonists. *Br J Clin Pharmacol* (1993) 35, 321–3.
6. MacWalter RS, El Debani AH, Feeley J, Stevenson IH. Potentiation by ranitidine of the hypoglycaemic response to glipizide in diabetic patients. *Br J Clin Pharmacol* (1985) 19, 121P–122P.
7. Stevenson IH, El Debani AH, MacWalter RS. Glipizide pharmacokinetics and effect in diabetic patients given ranitidine. *Acta Pharmacol Toxicol* (1986) 59 (Suppl 4), 97.
8. Stockley C, Keal J, Rolan P, Bochner F, Somogyi A. Lack of inhibition of tolbutamide hydroxylation by cimetidine in man. *Eur J Clin Pharmacol* (1986) 31, 235–7.
9. Dey NG, Castleden CM, Ward J, Cornhill J, McBurney A. The effect of cimetidine on tolbutamide kinetics. *Br J Clin Pharmacol* (1983) 16, 438–440.
10. Adebayo GI, Coker HAB. Lack of efficacy of cimetidine and ranitidine as inhibitors of tolbutamide metabolism. *Eur J Clin Pharmacol* (1988) 34, 653–6.
11. Shah GF, Ghandi TP, Patel PR, Patel MR, Gilbert RN, Shridhar PA. Tolbutamide and chlorpropamide kinetics in the presence of cimetidine in human volunteers. *Indian Drugs* (1985) 22, 455–8.
12. Shah GF, Ghandi TP, Patel PR, Patel MR, Gilbert RN, Shridhar PA. The effect of cimetidine on the hypoglycaemic activity of four commonly used sulphonylurea drugs. *Indian Drugs* (1985) 22, 570–2.
13. Cate EW, Rogers JF, Powell JR. Inhibition of tolbutamide elimination by cimetidine but not ranitidine. *J Clin Pharmacol* (1986) 26, 372–7.
14. Toon S, Holt BL, Mullins FGP, Khan A. Effects of cimetidine, ranitidine and omeprazole on tolbutamide pharmacokinetics. *J Pharm Pharmacol* (1995) 47, 85–88.
15. Kubacka RT, Antal EJ, Juhl RP. The paradoxical effect of cimetidine and ranitidine on glibenclamide pharmacokinetics and pharmacodynamics. *Br J Clin Pharmacol* (1987) 23, 743–51.
16. Schaaf LJ, Welshman IR, Viveash DM, Carel BJ. The effects of cimetidine and ranitidine on glimepiride pharmacokinetics and pharmacodynamics in normal subjects. *Pharm Res* (1994) 11 (10 Suppl), S–360.
17. Somogyi A, Stockley C, Keal J, Rolan P, Bochner F. Reduction of metformin renal tubular secretion by cimetidine in man. *Br J Clin Pharmacol* (1987) 23, 545–51.

Hypoglycaemic agents + Clonidine

There is evidence that clonidine may possibly suppress the signs and symptoms of hypoglycaemia in diabetic patients. An isolated report describes marked hyperglycaemia in a child on insulin when given clonidine.

Clinical evidence, mechanism, importance and management

(a) Non-diabetic patients

Studies in normal subjects and patients with hypertension found that their normal response to hypoglycemia (tachycardia, palpitations, perspiration) caused by a 0.1 unit/kg dose of **insulin** was markedly reduced when they were taking 450 to 900 micrograms **clonidine** daily.[1,2] The suggested reason is that **clonidine** depresses the output of the catecholamines (epinephrine (adrenaline), norepinephrine (noradrenaline)) which are secreted in an effort to raise blood sugar levels and which are also responsible for these signs. It seems possible that **clonidine** will similarly suppress the signs and symptoms of hypoglycaemia that can occur in diabetics, but there seem to be no reports confirming this. A study in normal subjects and non-diabetic patients also found that **clonidine** raises blood glucose levels, apparently by reducing **insulin** secretion.[3]

(b) Diabetic patients

A girl of 9, whose diabetes was controlled on 4 units of **insulin** daily, developed substantial hyperglycaemia and needed up to 56 units daily when she began to take 50 micrograms **clonidine** daily for Tourette syndrome. When the **clonidine** was stopped, she had numerous hypoglycaemic episodes, and within a few days it was possible to reduce her daily dosage of **insulin** to 6 units.[4] The general importance of this interaction is uncertain, but this isolated case seems to be the only one where an obviously adverse response occurred.

1. Hedeland H, Dymling J-F, Hökfelt B. The effect of insulin induced hypoglycaemia on plasma renin activity and urinary catecholamines before and following clonidine (Catapresan) in man. *Acta Endocrinol (Copenh)* (1972) 71, 321–30.
2. Hedeland H, Dymling J-F, Hökfelt B. Pharmacological inhibition of adrenaline secretion following insulin induced hypoglycaemia in man: the effect of Catapresan. *Acta Endocrinol (Copenh)* (1971) 67, 97–103.
3. Metz SA, Halter JB, Robertson RP. Induction of defective insulin secretion and impaired glucose tolerance by clonidine. Selective stimulation of metabolic alpha-adrenergic pathways. *Diabetes* (1978) 27, 554–62.
4. Mimouni-Bloch A, Mimouni M. Clonidine-induced hyperglycemia in a young diabetic girl. *Ann Pharmacother* (1993) 27, 980.

Hypoglycaemic agents + Colestyramine

There is evidence that the absorption of glipizide may be reduced about one-third if taken at the same time as colestyramine. Tolbutamide is reported not to interact.

Clinical evidence

Colestyramine 8 g in 150 ml water reduced the absorption of a single 5-mg dose of **glipizide** in 6 normal subjects by a mean of 29%. One subject had a 41% reduction. Peak serum levels were reduced by 33%. The $AUC_{0-10\,h}$ was used to measure absorption.[1]

A single dose study indicated that **colestyramine** 8 g administered 2 minutes before and 6 and 12 hours after a 500-mg dose of **tolbutamide** does not reduce the amount of **tolbutamide** absorbed, although the rate may be changed.[2]

Mechanism

Colestyramine is an anion-exchange resin, intended to bind to bile acids within the gut, but it can also bind with some acidic drugs thereby reducing the amount available for absorption.

Importance and management

Information about glipizide is limited to this single dose study so that the clinical importance of the interaction awaits further study, but it would now seem prudent to monitor the effects of concurrent use in patients. It has been suggested[1] that the glipizide should be taken 1 to 2 h before the colestyramine to minimise admixture in the gut, but this may only be partially effective because it is believed that glipizide undergoes some entero-hepatic circulation (i.e. after absorption it is excreted in the bile and reabsorbed). The effect of colestyramine on other sulphonylureas is uncertain, with the exception of tolbutamide which is reported not to interact.

1. Kivistö K T, Neuvonen P J. The effect of cholestyramine and activated charcoal on glipizide absorption. *Br J Clin Pharmacol* (1990) 30, 733–6.
2. Hunninghake D B, Pollack E. Effect of bile acid sequestering agents on the absorption of aspirin, tolbutamide and warfarin. *Fedn Proc* (1977) 35, 996.

Hypoglycaemic agents + Corticosteroids

The blood sugar lowering effects of the hypoglycaemic agents are opposed by the concurrent use of corticosteroids with glucocorticoid (hyperglycaemic) activity. It may be necessary to raise the dosage of the hypoglycaemic agent appropriately.

Clinical evidence, mechanism, importance and management

Systemic corticosteroids with glucocorticoid activity can raise blood sugar levels and induce diabetes,[1] though this is rarely seen with **topical corticosteroids**.[2] This can oppose the blood sugar lowering effects of the hypoglycaemic agents used in the treatment of diabetes mellitus. For example, a disturbance of the control of diabetes is very briefly described in a patient treated with **insulin** and **hydrocortisone**.[3] A study in 5 diabetics showed that a single 200-mg dose of **cortisone** modified their glucose tolerance curves while taking an unstated amount of **chlorpropamide**. The blood glucose levels of 4 of them rose (3 showed an initial fall), whereas in a previous test with **chlorpropamide** alone the blood sugar levels of 4 of them had fallen.[4] This almost certainly reflects a direct antagonism between the pharmacological effects of the two drugs, and this would seem to be confirmed by a study in normal subjects which showed that another glucocorticoid, **prednisone**, had no significant effect on the metabolism or clearance of **tolbutamide**.[5]

There are very few studies of this interaction, probably because the hyperglycaemic activity of the corticosteroids has been known for such a long time that the outcome of concurrent use is self-evident. The effects of corticosteroid treatment in diabetics (using **insulin** or **oral hypoglycaemic agents**) should be closely monitored and the dosage of the hypoglycaemic agent raised as necessary. Hypoglycaemic agents are sometimes deliberately given to non-diabetic patients taking corticosteroids to reduce blood sugar levels.

1. David DS, Cheigh JS, Braun DW, Fotino M, Stenzel KH, Rubin AL. HLA-A28 and steroid-induced diabetes in renal transplant patients. *JAMA* (1980) 243, 532–3.
2. Gomez EC, Frost P. Induction of glycosuria and hyperglycemia by topical corticosteroid therapy. *Arch Dermatol* (1976) 112, 1559–62.
3. Manchon ND, Bercoff E, Lemarchand P, Chassagne P, Senant J, Bourreille J. Fréquence et gravité des interactions médicamenteuses dan une population âgée: étude prospective concernant 639 malades. *Rev Med Interne* (1989) 10, 521–5.
4. Danowski TS, Mateer FM, Moses C. Cortisone enhancement of peripheral utilization of glucose and the effects of chlorpropamide. *Ann N Y Acad Sci* (1959) 74, 988–96.
5. Breimer DD, Zilly W, Richter E. Influence of corticosteroid on hexobarbital and tolbutamide disposition. *Clin Pharmacol Ther* (1978) 24, 208–12.

Hypoglycaemic agents + Cytotoxics

L-asparaginase sometimes induces diabetes mellitus. Changes in the hypoglycaemic agent dosage requirements seems a possibility in some diabetic patients. There is also evidence that the control of diabetes can also be severely disturbed in patients given cyclophosphamide.

Clinical evidence and mechanisms

(a) L-asparaginase

Three patients with acute lymphocytic leukaemia developed diabetes after treatment with **asparaginase** (colaspase); two of them 2 and 4 days after a single dose of **asparaginase**, and another patient 2 days after the fourth dose. Plasma insulin was undetectable. A normal insulin response returned in one patient after 23 days, whereas the other 2 showed a suboptimal response 2 weeks, and 9 months afterwards.[1] In another study, 5 out of 39 patients (3 adults, 2 children) developed hyperglycaemia and glycosuria after treatment with **asparaginase** (colaspase).[2] The reasons are not understood but suggestions include inhibition of **insulin** synthesis,[3] direct damage to the islets of Langerhans,[1] and reduced **insulin** binding.[3]

(b) Cyclophosphamide

Acute hypoglycaemia has been described in 2 diabetic patients under treatment with **insulin** and **carbutamide** who were concurrently treated with **cyclophosphamide**.[4] Three cases of diabetes, apparently induced by the use of **cyclophosphamide**, have also been reported.[5] The reasons are not understood.

Importance and management

Strictly speaking none of these reactions is probably an interaction, but they serve to underline the importance of monitoring the diabetic control of patients receiving either colaspase or cyclophosphamide.

1. Gailani S, Nussbaum A, Ohnuma T, Freeman A. Diabetes in patients treated with asparaginase. *Clin Pharmacol Ther* (1971) 12, 487–90.
2. Ohnuma T, Holland JF, Freeman A, Sinks LF. Biochemical and pharmacological studies with asparaginase in man. *Cancer Res* (1970) 30, 2297–2305.
3. Burghen G, Pui C-H, Yasuda K and Kitabchi AE. Decreased insulin binding and production: probable mechanism for hyperglycaemia due to therapy with prednisone (PRED) and l-asparaginase (ASP). *Pediatr Res* (1981) 15, 626.
4. Krüger H-U. Blutzuckersenkende Wirkung von Cyclophosphamid bei Diabetikern. *Med Klin* (1966) 61, 1462–3.
5. Pengelly CR. Diabetes mellitus and cyclophosphamide. *BMJ* (1965) i, 1312–13.

Hypoglycaemic agents + Danazol

On theoretical grounds danazol would be expected to oppose the effects of hypoglycaemic agents, but the practical clinical importance of this is uncertain.

Clinical evidence, mechanism, importance and management

Danazol can disturb glucose metabolism. A study in 14 non-diabetic subjects showed that 3 months treatment with 600 mg **danazol** daily caused a mild but definite deterioration in glucose tolerance, associated with high **insulin** levels. **Insulin resistance** was also seen in 5 subjects on **danazol** when given intravenous **tolbutamide**.[1] Another study in 9 non-diabetic women found that 600 mg **danazol** daily raised **insulin** levels in response to glucose or intravenous **tolbutamide**. This was attributed to the effects of **danazol** on the beta-cells of the pancreas.[2] However, the authors of another study in 9 non-diabetic women attributed the mild deterioration in glucose tolerance and the marked increase in the **insulin** response to the androgenic properties of the **danazol**.[3] **Danazol** can displace testosterone from sex hormone binding globulin sites.

For these reasons the makers of **danazol** advise caution if **danazol** is given to diabetic patients.[4] **Danazol** would be expected to oppose the actions of hypoglycaemic agents to some extent, but nobody seems to have checked to see whether this is clinically important or not.

1. Wynn V. Metabolic effects of danazol. *J Int Med Res* (1977) 5 (Suppl 3), 25–35.
2. Goettenberg N, Schlienger J L, Becmeur F, Dellenbach P. Traitement de l'endométriose pelvienne par le danazol. Incidence sur le métabolisme glucidique. *Nouv Presse Med* (1982) 11, 3703–6.
3. Vaughan-Williams C A, Shalet S M. Glucose tolerance and insulin resistance after danazol treatment. *J Obstet Gynaecol* (1989) 9, 229–32.
4. Danol (Danazol). Sanofi Synthelabo. Summary of product characteristics, June 2000.

Hypoglycaemic agents + Dextropropoxyphene (Propoxyphene)

Dextropropoxyphene (propoxyphene) does not appear to interact with tolbutamide. Hypoglycaemia was seen in a patient on an unnamed sulphonylurea and dextropropoxyphene/paracetamol (acetaminophen), and in another non-diabetic patient given dextropropoxyphene alone.

Clinical evidence, mechanism, importance and management

After taking 65 mg **dextropropoxyphene** (**propoxyphene**) 8-hourly for 4 days the clearance of **tolbutamide** (500 mg given intravenously) in 6 normal subjects was not affected.[1] Two isolated cases of hypoglycaemia have been reported, one in a patient taking an **unnamed sulphonylurea** and **dextropropoxyphene/paracetamol**,[2] and the other in a non-diabetic patient with renal failure and cervical carcinoma while taking **dextropropoxyphene** alone.[3] There would normally seem to be little reason for avoiding the concurrent use of hypoglycaemic agents and **dextropropoxyphene**, or for taking particular precautions.

1. Robson RA, Miners JO, Whitehead AG, Birkett DJ. Specificity of the inhibitory effect of dextropropoxyphene on oxidative drug metabolism in man: effects on theophylline and tolbutamide disposition. *Br J Clin Pharmacol* (1987) 23, 772–5.
2. Girardin E, Vial T, Pham E, Evreux J-C. Hypoglycémies induites par les sulfamides hypoglycémiants. *Ann Med Interne (Paris)* (1992) 143, 11–17.
3. Wiederholt IC, Genco M, Foley JM. Recurrent episodes of hypoglycemia induced by propoxyphene. *Neurology* (1967) 17, 703–6.

Hypoglycaemic agents + Disopyramide

Disopyramide occasionally causes hypoglycaemia which may be severe.

Clinical evidence, mechanism, importance and management

For reasons which are not understood **disopyramide** occasionally and unpredictably causes hypoglycaemia which may be severe.[1-5] Patients at particular risk are the elderly, the malnourished and diabetics. Impaired renal function and impaired cardiac function may be predisposing factors. The makers of **disopyramide** advise close monitoring of blood glucose levels and withdrawal of **disopyramide** if problems arise.[6] This is not simply a problem for diabetics, but certainly within the context of diabetes the hypoglycaemic effects of **disopyramide** may possibly cause particular difficulties. Although not strictly an interaction, the concurrent use of disopyramide and hypoglycaemic agents should be well monitored because of the potential for severe hypoglycaemia.

1. Goldberg IJ, Brown LK, Rayfield EJ. Disopyramide (Norpace)-induced hypoglycaemia. *Am J Med* (1980) 69, 463–6.
2. Quevedo SF, Krauss DS, Chazan JA, Crisafulli FS, Kahn CB. Fasting hypoglycemia secondary to disopyramide therapy. Report of two cases. *JAMA* (1981) 245, 2424.
3. Strathman I, Schubert EN, Cohen A, Nitzberg DM. Hypoglycemia in patients receiving disopyramide phosphate. *Drug Intell Clin Pharm* (1983) 17, 635–8.
4. Semel JD, Wortham E, Karl DM. Fasting hypoglycemia associated with disopyramide. *Am Heart J* (1983) 106, 1160–1.
5. Seriès C. Hypoglycémie induite ou favorisée par le disopyramide. *Rev Med Interne* (1988) 9, 528–9.
6. Rythmodan (Disopyramide). Borg Medicare. Summary of product characteristics. June 1998.

Hypoglycaemic agents + Disulfiram

Disulfiram appears not to disturb the control of diabetes mellitus. No pharmacokinetic interaction occurs with tolbutamide and there appears to be no evidence that disulfiram interacts with any other hypoglycaemic agent.

Clinical evidence, mechanism, importance and management

The makers of **disulfiram** say that caution should be exercised if it is used in diabetics,[1] but a reviewer[2] who has given disulfiram to over 20,000 alcoholics says that he has ". . . prescribed **disulfiram** for several hundred patients with diabetes mellitus over the past 20 years. Not a single case showed any adverse effects from this treatment. It appears that the theoretical implications of potential problems associated with disulfiram and diabetes are rarely, if ever, applicable to clinical practice." It would be reasonable to assume that many of these patients (probably most) were also taking **insulin** or one of the oral **hypoglycaemic agents**. There do not appear to be any reported cases in the literature of adverse interactions between **disulfiram** and any of the **hypoglycaemic agents**. Studies in 5 normal subjects have shown that **disulfiram** (first day 400 mg three times; second day 400 mg; third and fourth days 200 mg daily) had no significant effect on the half-life or clearance of **tolbutamide** 500 mg given intravenously.[3]

The conclusion to be drawn from all of this is that any reaction is very rare (if it ever occurs), and no special precautions would normally appear to be necessary.

1. Antabuse (Disulfiram). Dumex Ltd. Summary of product characteristics. August 1999.
2. McNichol RW. Disulfiram (Antabuse), a strategic weapon in the battle for sobriety. In McNichol RW, Ewing JA, Fairman MD (Eds) Disulfiram (Antabuse), a unique medical aid to sobriety. History, pharmacology, research, clinical use. Springfield, Il: Charles C Thomas (1987) 47–90.
3. Svendsen TL, Kristensen MB, Hansen JM, Skovsted L. The influence of disulfiram on the half life and metabolic clearance rate of diphenylhydantoin and tolbutamide in man. *Eur J Clin Pharmacol* (1976) 9, 439–41.

Hypoglycaemic agents + Diuretics; Etacrynic acid

Etacrynic acid can raise blood sugar levels in diabetics which opposes to some extent the effects of the hypoglycaemic agents. The clinical importance of this seems to be negligible.

Clinical evidence and mechanism

A double-blind study in 24 hypertensive patients, one-third of whom were diabetics, showed that daily treatment with 200 mg **etacrynic acid** over a 6-week period impaired their glucose tolerance and raised the blood sugar levels of the diabetics to the same extent as those diabetics and non-diabetics taking **hydrochlorothiazide** 200 mg daily.[1] In another study no change in carbohydrate metabolism was seen in 6 diabetics given 150 mg **etacrynic acid** daily for a week.[2] The reasons are not understood.

Importance and management

Information is very limited indeed. Some impairment of the glucose tolerance may possibly occur, but there seems to be a singular lack of evidence in the literature to show that normally etacrynic acid has much effect on the control of diabetes in most patients. Even so it would be prudent to monitor the effects of concurrent use with hypoglycaemic agents.

1. Russell RP, Lindeman RD, Prescott LF. Metabolic and hypotensive effects of ethacrynic acid. Comparative study with hydrochlorothiazide. *JAMA* (1968) 205, 81–5.
2. Dige-Petersen H. Ethacrynic acid and carbohydrate metabolism. *Nord Med* (1966) 75, 123–5.

Hypoglycaemic agents + Diuretics; Furosemide (Frusemide)

The control of diabetes is not usually disturbed by the concurrent use of furosemide (frusemide), although there are a few reports showing that it can sometimes raise blood sugar levels.

Clinical evidence, mechanism, importance and management

Although **furosemide (frusemide)** can elevate blood sugar levels[1] (but to a much lesser extent than the thiazide diuretics), worsen glucose tolerance[2] and occasionally cause glycosuria and even acute diabetes in individual patients,[3] the general picture is that the control of diabetes is not usually affected by the use of **furosemide**.[4] No clinically relevant changes in the control of diabetes were seen in a 3-month trial of 29 patients taking 40 mg **furosemide** daily and an average of 7 mg **glibenclamide (glyburide)** daily.[5] It has been described[6] as the "diuretic of choice for the diabetic patient." Even so, prescribers should be aware of its hyperglycaemic potentialities.

1. Hutcheon DE, Leonard G. Diuretic and antihypertensive action of frusemide. *J Clin Pharmacol* (1967) 7, 26–33.
2. Breckenridge A, Welborn TA, Dollery CT, Fraser R. Glucose tolerance in hypertensive patients on long-term diuretic therapy. *Lancet* (1967) i, 61–4.
3. Toivonen S, Mustala O. Diabetogenic action of frusemide. *BMJ* (1966) i, 920–21.
4. Bencomo L, Fyvolent J, Kahana S, Kahana L. Clinical experience with a new diuretic, furosemide. *Curr Ther Res* (1965) 7, 339–45.
5. Lehnert H, Schmitz H, Beyer J, Wilmbusse H, Piesche L. Controlled clinical trial investigating the influence of torasemide and furosemide on carbohydrate metabolism in patients with cardiac failure and concomitant type II diabetes. 4th Int Congr Diuretics, Boca Raton, Florida Oct 11–16th 1992. Eds. Puschett JB, Greenberrg A. *Int Congr Series 1023* (1993), 271–4.
6. Malins JM. Diuretics in diabetes mellitus. *Practitioner* (1968) 201, 529.

Hypoglycaemic agents + Diuretics; Metolazone

An isolated report describes severe hypoglycaemia in a patient on glibenclamide (glyburide) shortly after starting treatment with metolazone.

Clinical evidence, mechanism, importance and management

A diabetic man, stabilised on **glibenclamide (glyburide)** 10 mg daily and hospitalised for congestive heart failure, became clinically hypoglycaemic (blood glucose levels unmeasurable by *Labstix*) within 40 h of starting 5 mg **metolazone** daily. He was treated with intravenous glucose. Although both **glibenclamide** and **metolazone** were stopped, he had 4 further hypoglycaemic episodes over the next 30 h.[1] The reasons are not understood. *In vitro* studies failed to find any evidence that **metolazone** displaces **glibenclamide** from its protein binding sites which might possibly have provided some explanation for what happened.[1] The general importance of this apparent interaction is not clear, but until more is known it would seem prudent to monitor the effects of concurrent use. More study is needed.

1. George S, McBurney A, Cole A. Possible protein binding displacement interaction between glibenclamide and metolazone. *Eur J Clin Pharmacol* (1990) 38, 93–5.

Hypoglycaemic agents + Diuretics; Thiazides, Chlortalidone or related diuretics

By raising blood sugar levels, the thiazide diuretics, chlortalidone and other related diuretics can reduce the effects of the hypoglycaemic agents and impair the control of diabetes. Some, but by no means all, patients may need a modest increase in the dosage of their hypoglycaemic agent. Hyponatraemia also occurs occasionally.

Clinical evidence

(a) Reduced hypoglycaemic effects

Chlorothiazide, the first of the thiazide diuretics, was found within a year of its introduction in 1958 to have hyperglycaemic effects.[1] Since then a very large number of reports have described this same effect with other thiazides, the precipitation of diabetes in prediabetics, and the disturbance of blood sugar control in diabetics. One example from many:

A long-term study on 53 diabetics found that treatment with **chlorothiazide** (0.5 or 1 g daily) or **trichlormethiazide** (4 or 8 mg daily) caused a mean rise in blood sugar levels from 120 to 140 mg%. Only 7 patients needed a change in their treatment: 4 required more of their oral agent, 2 an increase in **insulin**, and one was transferred from **tolbutamide** to insulin. The oral agents used included **tolbutamide, chlorpropamide, acetohexamide** and **phenformin**.[2]

A rise in blood sugar levels has been observed with **bendroflume-**

thiazide (bendrofluazide),[3,4] benzthiazide,[5] hydrochlorothiazide (100 to 300 mg daily),[3] and chlortalidone (50 to 100 mg daily).[6]

More recent data suggests that the effects of thiazides on blood glucose may be dose related. In a double-blind randomised study comparing the effects of 1.25 or 5 mg of bendroflumethiazide on blood glucose, the lower dose had no effects on insulin action, whereas when the higher dose was given, there was evidence of impaired glucose tolerance.[7] A review of the literature on hydrochlorothiazide similarly reports that low doses (6.25 to 12.5 mg) lack significant effects on blood glucose levels.[8]

(b) Hyponatraemia

A hospital report describes 8 cases of low serum sodium concentrations observed over a 5-year period in patients taking chlorpropamide and *Moduretic* (hydrochlorothiazide 50 mg + amiloride 5 mg).[9]

Mechanisms

Not understood. One study suggested that the hyperglycaemia is due to some inhibition of insulin release by the pancreas.[10] Another is that the peripheral action of insulin is affected in some way.[5,11] There is also evidence that it may be related in part to potassium depletion.[12] The hyponatraemia appears to be due to the additive sodium-losing effects of the chlorpropamide, thiazide and amiloride.

Importance and management

The reduction in hypoglycaemia is extremely well-documented but of only moderate practical importance. A full list of references is not given here to save space. The report of the study cited above[2] stated that "in no patient was a dramatic deterioration of diabetic control observed." The incidence is said to lie between 10 and 30%.[2,13] Concurrent use need not be avoided but the outcome should be monitored. There is evidence that the full effects may take many months to develop in some patients.[4] Most patients respond to a modest increase in the dosage of the hypoglycaemic agent, or to a change from an oral drug to insulin. The adverse hyperglycaemic effects can also be reversed significantly by the use of potassium supplements.[12]

In addition to the thiazides already named, the interaction may be expected to occur with the other thiazides in common use (cyclopenthiazide, cyclothiazide, methyclothiazide, polythiazide) and possibly related diuretics such as clopamide, clorexolone, metolazone, quinethazone, etc. This requires confirmation. However, see also 'Hypoglycaemic agents + Diuretics; Metolazone', p.577.

Hyponatraemia seems to be uncommon but be aware that it can occur during concurrent use.

1. Wilkins RW. New drugs for the treatment of hypertension. *Ann Intern Med* (1959) 50, 1–10.
2. Kansal PC, Buse J, Buse MG. Thiazide diuretics and control of diabetes mellitus. *South Med J* (1969) 62, 1374–9.
3. Goldner MG, Zarowitz H, Akgun S. Hyperglycemia and glycosuria due to thiazide derivatives administered in diabetes mellitus. *N Engl J Med* (1960) 262, 403–5.
4. Lewis PJ, Kohner EM, Petrie A, Dollery CT. Deterioration of glucose tolerance in hypertensive patients on prolonged diuretic treatment. *Lancet* (1976) i, 564–6.
5. Runyan JW. Influence of thiazide diuretics on carbohydrate metabolism in patients with mild diabetes. *N Engl J Med* (1962) 267, 541–3.
6. Carliner NH, Schelling J-L, Russell RP, Okun R, Davis M. Thiazide- and phthalimidine-induced hyperglycemia in hypertensive patients. *JAMA* (1965) 191, 535–40.
7. Harper R, Ennis CN, Sheridan B, Atkinson AB, Johnston GD, Bell PM. Effects of low dose versus conventional dose thiazide diuretic on insulin action in essential hypertension. *BMJ* (1994) 309, 226–30.
8. Neutel JM. Metabolic manifestations of low-dose diuretics. *Am J Med* (1996) 101 (Suppl 3A), 71S–82S.
9. Zalin AM, Hutchinson CE, Jong M, Matthews K. Hyponatraemia during treatment with chlorpropamide and Moduretic (amiloride plus hydrochlorothiazide). *BMJ* (1984) 289, 659.
10. Fajans SS, Floyd JC, Knopf RF, Rull J, Guntsche EM, Conn JW. Benzothiadiazine suppression of insulin release from normal and abnormal islet tissue in man. *J Clin Invest* (1966) 45, 481–92.
11. Remenchik AP, Hoover C, Talso PJ. Insulin secretion by hypertensive patients receiving hydrochlorothiazide. *JAMA* (1970) 212, 869.
12. Rapoport MI, Hurd HF. Thiazide-induced glucose intolerance treated with potassium. *Arch Intern Med* (1964) 113, 405–8.
13. Wolff FW, Parmley WW, White K, Okun R. Drug-induced diabetes. Diabetogenic activity of long-term administration of benzothiadiazines. *JAMA* (1963) 185, 568–74.

Hypoglycaemic agents + Erythromycin or Clarithromycin

An isolated report describes severe liver damage with prolonged cholestasis in a patient on chlorpropamide after concurrent treatment with erythromycin. An isolated case of hypoglycaemia has been described in another patient on glibenclamide (glyburide) when given erythromycin. A study in healthy subjects showed that hypoglycaemia may occur if tolbutamide and clarithromycin are given concurrently

Clinical evidence, mechanism, importance and management

A man with type II diabetes was treated with phenformin for 10 years. Four months after the phenformin was replaced by chlorpropamide, he was treated with 1 g erythromycin ethylsuccinate daily for 3 weeks for a respiratory infection. Two weeks later he complained of increasing fatigue and fever. A short episode of pruriginous skin rash was followed by the appearance of dark urine, jaundice and hepatomegaly. The picture over the next two years was that of profound cholestasis, complicated by steatorrhoea and marked hyperlipidaemia with disappearance of interlobular bile ducts. He died of ischaemic cardiomyopathy.[1] The reasons for this serious reaction are not understood, but the authors point out that liver damage occurs in a very small number of patients given sulphonylureas, such as chlorpropamide, and also with erythromycin. They suggest that there may have been an interaction between the two drugs.[1] No general conclusions can be drawn from this unusual case.

An isolated case of hypoglycaemia occurred in a patient given glibenclamide (glyburide) and erythromycin,[2] but an earlier single-dose study in 12 non-insulin dependent diabetics found that erythromycin had little effect on glibenclamide pharmacokinetics or on its hypoglycaemic effects.[3] Nevertheless concurrent use should be well monitored.

A study in 9 healthy subjects found that clarithromycin 250 mg increased the rate of absorption of tolbutamide 500 mg by about 20% and its bioavailability by 26%. Hypoglycaemia, reported as uneasiness and giddiness, occurred on taking both drugs.[4]

1. Geubel AP, Nakad A, Rahier J, Dive C. Prolonged cholestasis and disappearance of interlobular bile ducts following chlorpropamide and erythromycin ethylsuccinate. Case of drug interaction] *Liver* (1988) 8, 350–3.
2. Girardin E, Vial T, Pham E, Evreux J-C. Hypoglycémies induites par les sulfamides hypoglycémiants. *Ann Med Interne (Paris)* (1992) 143, 11–17.
3. Fleishaker JC, Phillips JP. Evaluation of a potential interaction between erythromycin and glyburide in diabetic volunteers. *J Clin Pharmacol* (1991) 31, 259–62.
4. Jayasagar G, Dixit AA, Kirshan V, Rao YM. Effect of clarithromycin on the pharmacokinetics of tolbutamide. *Drug Metabol Drug Interact* (2000) 16, 207–15.

Hypoglycaemic agents + Fenfluramine

Fenfluramine has inherent hypoglycaemic activity which can add to, or in some instances replace, the effects of conventional hypoglycaemic agents.

Clinical evidence, mechanism, importance and management

A study of the substitution of fenfluramine (initially 40 mg daily, increased to 120 mg daily) for a biguanide hypoglycaemic agent showed that diabetes was equally well controlled by either drug in 4 of 6 patients.[1] The hypoglycaemic effects of fenfluramine are described elsewhere.[2,3] It seems that fenfluramine increases the uptake of glucose into skeletal muscle, thereby lowering blood glucose levels.[3,4]

This is a well established and, on the whole, an advantageous rather than an adverse reaction, but it would be prudent to check on the extent of the response if fenfluramine is added or withdrawn from the treatment being received by diabetics. However, note that fenfluramine was withdrawn in 1997 because its use was found to be associated with a high incidence of abnormal echocardiograms indicating abnormal functioning of heart valves.

1. Jackson WPU. Fenfluramine trials in a diabetic clinic. *S Afr Med J* (1971) 45 (Suppl), 29–30.
2. Turtle JR, Burgess JA. Hypoglycemic action of fenfluramine in diabetes mellitus. *Diabetes* (1973) 22, 858–67.
3. Dykes JRW. The effect of a low-calorie diet with and without fenfluramine, and fenfluramine alone on the glucose tolerance and insulin secretion of overweight non-diabetics. *Postgrad Med J* (1973) 49, 314–17.
4. Kirby MJ, Turner P. Effect of amphetamine, fenfluramine and norfenfluramine on glucose uptake into human isolated skeletal muscle. *Br J Clin Pharmacol* (1974) 1, 340P–341P.

Hypoglycaemic agents + Fenyramidol (Phenyramidol)

The hypoglycaemic effects of tolbutamide are increased by fenyramidol (phenyramidol) but the clinical importance of this is uncertain.

Clinical evidence, mechanism, importance and management

The half-life of intravenously administered **tolbutamide** was increased from 7 to 18 h and serum **tolbutamide** levels raised in 3 normal subjects after taking 1200 mg **fenyramidol (phenyramidol)** daily for 4 days because (so it is suggested) the **fenyramidol** inhibits the metabolism of the **tolbutamide** by the liver, thereby prolonging its stay in the body.[1] A reduction in the dosage of **tolbutamide** may be necessary to avoid excessive hypoglycaemia, but this requires confirmation. Information about other sulphonylureas is lacking.

1. Solomon HM, Schrogie JJ. Effect of phenyramidol and bishydroxycoumarin on the metabolism of tolbutamide in human subjects. *Metabolism* (1967) 16, 1029–33.

Hypoglycaemic agents + Fibrates

(a) The effects of the sulphonylurea hypoglycaemic agents can be enhanced by clofibrate in some patients and a reduction in the dosage of the hypoglycaemic agent may be necessary. (b) The antidiuretic effects of clofibrate in the treatment of diabetes insipidus are opposed by glibenclamide (glyburide).

Clinical evidence, mechanism, importance and management

(a) Increased hypoglycaemic effects

Over a 5-day period while taking 2 g **clofibrate** daily, the control of the diabetes was improved in 6 out of 13 maturity-onset diabetics on various **unnamed sulphonylureas**. Hypoglycaemia (blood glucose levels of 30 to 40 mg per 100 ml) was seen in 4 patients.[1] Other studies confirm that some, but not all, patients show a fall in blood glucose levels while taking **clofibrate** and the control of the diabetes can improve.[2-9] In one study[10] the half-life of chlorpropamide ranged from 40 to 62 h in 5 subjects treated with clofibrate compared with a mean of about 36 h in control subjects. Fasting blood glucose values decreased in 10, and increased in 4 of 14 diabetic patients on **insulin, acetohexamide, chlorpropamide** or **glipizide** when concurrently treated with **gemfibrozil** (800 mg daily initially, reduced later to 400 to 600 mg daily).[11] Another study found that of 20 patients, 9 required a slight increase in the dosage of insulin or oral hypoglycaemic agent, and one a decreased dosage, when treated with gemfibrozil 800 to 1600 mg daily.[12] A single report describes hypoglycaemia in a diabetic on **glibenclamide (glyburide)** when started on 1200 mg **gemfibrozil** daily.[13] The **glibenclamide** dosage was accordingly reduced from 5 to 1.25 mg daily with satisfactory diabetic control. When the **gemfibrozil** was later stopped and restarted, the dosage of the **glibenclamide** had to be increased and then again reduced.

Three elderly patients with mild renal dysfunction on **glibencla-**mide developed hypoglycaemia when given **bezafibrate**: one of them needed a 60% dosage reduction, another was given **tolbutamide** instead, and the third was able to stop both the **glibenclamide** and **buformin**.[14]

The French Centres Régionaux de Pharmacovigilance recorded 7 cases of hypoglycaemia during the period 1985 to 1990 in patients on **unnamed sulphonylureas** when given fibrates (one with **bezafibrate**, 3 with **ciprofibrate**, 3 with **fenofibrate**).[15]

(b) Reduced antidiuretic effects

Clofibrate 2 g daily reduced the volume of urine excreted by 2 patients with pituitary diabetes insipidus, but when given with **glibenclamide (glyburide)** the volume increased once again. Without treatment they excreted 5.8 and 6.5 litres of urine daily, and this reduced to only 2.4 and 1.7 litres while taking **clofibrate**, whereas with **glibenclamide** and **clofibrate** they excreted 3.6 and 3.7 litres daily, respectively.[16]

Mechanisms

(a) Not understood. Among the suggestions are the displacement of the sulphonylureas from their plasma protein binding sites,[4] alterations in their renal excretion,[10] and a decrease in insulin resistance.[3,17] Clofibrate has also been shown to have a hypoglycaemic action of its own which improves the glucose tolerance of diabetics.[9] It seems possible that any or all of these mechanisms might contribute towards the enhanced hypoglycaemia which is seen. (b) Not understood.

Importance and management

(a) The sulphonylurea/clofibrate interaction is established and well documented. The incidence is uncertain, but what is known suggests that between about one-third and one-half of patients may be affected. There would seem to be no good reason for avoiding the concurrent use of hypoglycaemic agents and fibrates, but patients should be warned that excessive hypoglycaemia occurs occasionally and unpredictably and it may be necessary to reduce the dosage of the hypoglycaemic agent.

(b) Information about reduced diuretic effects is limited. It would seem prudent to avoid the concurrent use of drugs with actions which are antagonistic.

1. Daubresse J-C, Luyckx AS, Lefebvre PJ. Potentiation of hypoglycemic effect of sulfonylureas by clofibrate. *N Engl J Med* (1976) 294, 613.
2. Jain AK, Ryan JR, McMahon FG. Potentiation of hypoglycemic effect of sulfonylureas by halofenate. *N Engl J Med* (1975) 293, 1283–6.
3. Ferrari C, Frezzati S, Testori GP, Bertazzoni A. Potentiation of hypoglycemic response to intravenous tolbutamide by clofibrate. *N Engl J Med* (1976) 294, 1184.
4. Jain AK, Ryan JR, McMahon FG. Potentiation of hypoglycemic effect of sulfonylureas by clofibrate. *N Engl J Med* (1976) 294, 613.
5. Daubresse J-C, Daigneux D, Bruwier M, Luyckx A, Lefebvre PJ. Clofibrate and diabetes control in patients treated with oral hypoglycaemic agents. *Br J Clin Pharmacol* (1979) 7, 599-603.
6. Miller RD. *Atromid* in the treatment of post-climacteric diabetes. *J Atheroscler Res* (1963) 3, 694-700.
7. Csögör SI, Bornemisza P. The effect of clofibrate (Atromid) on intravenous tolbutamide, oral and intravenous glucose tolerance tests. *Clin Trials J* (1977) 14, 15-19.
8. Herriott SC, Percy-Robb IW, Strong JA, Thomson CG. The effect of Atromid on serum cholesterol and glucose tolerance in diabetes mellitus. *J Atheroscler Res* (1963) 3, 679-88.
9. Barnett D, Craig JG, Robinson DS, Rogers MP. Effect of clofibrate on glucose tolerance in maturity-onset diabetes. *Br J Clin Pharmacol* (1977) 4, 455-8.
10. Petitpierre B, Perrin L, Rudhardt M, Herrera A, Fabre J. Behaviour of chlorpropamide in renal insufficiency and under the effect of associated drug therapy. *Int J Clin Pharmacol* (1972) 6, 120-4.
11. De Salcedo I, Gorringe JAL, Silva JL and Santos JA. Gemfibrozil in a group of diabetics. *Proc R Soc Med* (1976) 69 (Suppl 2), 64–70.
12. Konttinen A, Kuisma I, Ralli R, Pohjola S and Ojala K. The effect of gemfibrozil on serum lipids in diabetic patients. *Ann Clin Res* (1979) 11, 240–5.
13. Ahmad S. Gemfibrozil: interaction with glyburide. *South Med J* (1991) 84, 102.
14. Ohsawa K, Koike N, Takamura T, Nagai Y, Kobayashi KI. Hypoglycaemic attacks after administration of bezafibrate in three cases of non-insulin dependent diabetes mellitus. *J Japan Diabetes Soc* (1994) 37, 295–300.
15. Girardin E, Vial T, Pham E, Evreux J-C. Hypoglycémies induites par les sulfamides hypoglycémiants. *Ann Med Interne (Paris)* (1992) 143, 11–17.
16. Rado JP, Szende L, Marosi J, Juhos E, Sawinsky I and Tako J. Inhibition of the diuretic action of glibenclamide by clofibrate, carbamazepine and 1-deamino-8-D-arginine-vasopressin (DDAVP) in patients with pituitary diabetes insipidus. *Acta Diabetol Lat* (1974) 11, 179-97.
17. Ferrari C, Frezzati S, Romussi M, Bertazzoni A, Testori GP, Antonini S, Paracchi A. Effects of short-term clofibrate administration on glucose tolerance and insulin secretion in patients with chemical diabetes or hypertriglyceridemia. *Metabolism* (1977) 26, 129-39.

Hypoglycaemic agents + Fluconazole, Itraconazole or Clotrimazole

Fluconazole normally appears not to affect the diabetic control of most patients taking sulphonylureas, but an isolated report describes hypoglycaemic coma in one patient on glipizide and there is some evidence that the hypoglycaemic effects of both glipizide and glibenclamide (glyburide) may be modestly increased. Itraconazole also appears not to affect diabetic control in most patients, but there are reports of hypoglycaemia or hyperglycaemia associated with its use. Clotrimazole used intravaginally appears not to interact.

Clinical evidence

A. No interaction

A group of 29 postmenopausal diabetic women with vulvovaginal candidosis taking either **gliclazide** (17 patients) or **glibenclamide** (**glyburide**) (12 patients) were treated with either 50 mg **fluconazole** daily for 14 days (14 patients) or 100 mg intravaginal **clotrimazole** daily (15 patients) for the same period. None of the patients developed symptoms of hypoglycaemia and their glycosylated haemoglobin and fructosamine concentrations were unchanged. No pharmacokinetic data were reported.[1]

B. Evidence of interactions

(a) Chlorpropamide + Fluconazole

After taking 100 mg **fluconazole** daily for 7 days, the AUC of single 250-mg doses of **chlorpropamide** in 18 normal subjects was increased by 28% but the maximum plasma levels and blood glucose levels were unchanged. There was no evidence of hypoglycaemia.[2]

(b) Glibenclamide + Fluconazole

After taking 100 mg **fluconazole** daily for 7 days, the AUC of a single 5-mg dose of **glibenclamide** (**glyburide**) in 20 normal subjects was increased by 44% and maximum plasma levels rose by 19%. Blood glucose levels were not statistically significantly altered but the number of subjects who experienced symptoms of hypoglycaemia increased.[3]

(c) Glipizide + Fluconazole

After taking 100 mg **fluconazole** daily for seven days, the AUC of single 2.5-mg doses of **glipizide** in 13 normal subjects was increased by 49% and maximum serum levels rose by 17%. Blood glucose levels were not statistically significantly altered (although they went down) but the number of subjects who experienced symptoms suggestive of hypoglycaemia increased.[4]

A diabetic on **glipizide**, 2.5 mg three times daily, developed a hypoglycaemic coma within 4 days of starting to take 200 mg **fluconazole** daily. Her blood sugar levels had fallen to less than 1 g/l. She rapidly recovered when given glucose.[5]

(d) Hypoglycaemic agents + Itraconazole

Post-marketing surveillance over 10 years indicated that in most patients **itraconazole** given with either insulin or oral antidiabetic drugs did not affect diabetic control. However, there were 15 reports suggesting hyperglycaemia and 9 reports suggesting hypoglycaemia with itraconazole and hypoglycaemic agents.[6] In clinical trials only one of 189 diabetic patients experienced aggravated diabetes when given **itraconazole**.[6] The patient in question was also receiving ciclosporin for a renal transplant.

(e) Tolbutamide + Fluconazole

After taking a single dose of 150 mg and a further 6 doses of **fluconazole** 100 mg daily, the AUC of single 500-mg doses of **tolbutamide** in 13 normal subjects were increased by about 50%, and the peak plasma levels were raised. The half-life of the **tolbutamide** was increased about 40%. Blood glucose levels remained unaltered and none of the subjects showed any evidence of hypoglycaemia.[7,8] However, the authors caution against extrapolating this finding to diabetic patients taking tolbutamide regularly.[7,8]

Mechanism

Uncertain. When the plasma levels and effects of these hypoglycaemic agents are increased, a possible mechanism is that the fluconazole inhibits their metabolism by the liver.

Importance and management

The almost total absence of adverse reports implies that fluconazole and itraconazole do not usually markedly disturb the control of diabetes in those taking sulphonylureas. For fluconazole the increased plasma levels of glipizide and the single case of severe hypoglycaemia, as well as the hypoglycaemic symptoms shown by those on glibenclamide (glyburide) suggest that patients on these two sulphonylureas in particular should be warned to be alert for any evidence of hypoglycaemia. However there seems to be no reason for avoiding concurrent use.

Information about clotrimazole is very sparse, but it appears not to interact with gliclazide or glibenclamide (glyburide) (and probably not with any of the other oral hypoglycaemic agents), one reason almost certainly being because its absorption from the vagina is very small.

1. Rowe BR, Thorpe J, Barnett A. Safety of fluconazole in women taking oral hypoglycaemic agents. *Lancet* (1992) 339, 255–6.
2. Anon. A volunteer-blind, placebo-controlled study to assess potential interaction between fluconazole and chlorpropamide in healthy male volunteers. Protocol 238: Pfizer, data on file.
3. Anon. A volunteer-blind, placebo-controlled study to assess potential interaction between fluconazole and glibenclamide in healthy male volunteers. Protocol 236: Pfizer, data on file.
4. Anon. A volunteer-blind, placebo-controlled study to assess potential interaction between fluconazole and glipizide in healthy male volunteers. Protocol 237: Pfizer, data on file.
5. Fournier JP, Schneider S, Martinez P, Mahagne MH, Ducoeur S, Haffner M, Thiercelin D, Chichmanain RM, Bertrand F. Coma hypoglycémique chez une patiente traitée par glipizide et fluconazole: une possible interaction? *Therapie* (1992) 47, 446–7.
6. Verspeelt J, Marynissen G, Gupta AK, De Doneker P. Safety of itraconazole in diabetic patients. *Dermatology* (1999) 198, 382–4.
7. Lazar JD, Wilner KD. Drug interactions with fluconazole. *Rev Infect Dis* (1990) 12 (Suppl 3), S327–S333.
8. Anon. A double-blind placebo-controlled study to assess the potential interaction between fluconazole and tolbutamide in healthy male volunteers. Pfizer, data on file.

Hypoglycaemic agents + Guanethidine and related drugs

Guanethidine has hypoglycaemic activity which may possibly add to the effects of conventional hypoglycaemic agents. Soluble insulin may also exaggerate the hypotensive effects of debrisoquine.

Clinical evidence

(a) Hypoglycaemia increased

A diabetic needed an **insulin** dose increase from 70 to 94 units daily when **guanethidine** was withdrawn.[1] A later study in 3 maturity-onset diabetics showed that **guanethidine** in daily doses of 50 to 90 mg caused a significant improvement in their glucose tolerance.[2] Other reports also describe the hypoglycaemic effects of **guanethidine** in man.[3,4]

(b) Hypotension increased

An insulin-dependent man taking **debrisoquine** (20 mg twice daily) developed severe postural hypotension within an hour of using a short-acting **insulin** (28 units **soluble insulin**) plus 20 units **isophane insulin**. He became dizzy and was found to have a standing blood pressure of 97/72 mmHg. The postural fall in systolic pressure was 65 mmHg. He had no evidence of hypoglycaemia and no hypotension when using 48 units of **isophane insulin**.[5] **Insulin** can cause hypotension but this is only seen in those with an impaired reflex control of blood pressure.[5]

Mechanism

A suggested reason for the insulin/guanethidine interaction is that guanethidine can impair the homoeostatic mechanism concerned with raising blood sugar levels by affecting the release of catecholamines. The balance of the system thus impaired tends to be tipped in favour of a reduced blood sugar level, resulting in a reduced requirement for hypoglycaemic agent. The debrisoquine/insulin interaction is not understood.

Importance and management

Information about both of these interactions is very limited, and their general importance is uncertain. Check on the dosage requirements of the hypoglycaemic agent if guanethidine or related drugs (betanidine, guanadrel, debrisoquine, etc.) are started or stopped. Also check patients given debrisoquine and insulin, particularly if they are taking vasodilators, to ensure that excessive hypotension does not develop.

1. Gupta KK, Lillicrap CA. Guanethidine and diabetes. *BMJ* (1968) 2, 697–8.
2. Gupta KK. The anti-diabetic action of guanethidine. *Postgrad Med J* (1969) 45, 455–6.
3. Kansal PC, Buse J, Durling FC. Effect of guanethidine and reserpine on glucose tolerance. *Curr Ther Res* (1971) 13, 517–22.
4. Woeber KA, Arky R, Braverman LE. Reversal by guanethidine of abnormal oral glucose tolerance in thyrotoxicosis. *Lancet* (1966) i, 895–8.
5. Hume L. Potentiation of hypotensive effect of debrisoquine by insulin. *Diabetic Med* (1985) 2, 390–1.

Hypoglycaemic agents + Guar gum or Glucomannan

Guar gum appears not to affect the absorption of glipizide nor one formulation of glibenclamide (glyburide), but it reduces the absorption of metformin and enhances its postprandial hypoglycaemic effects. Glucomannan appears to reduce the absorption of glibenclamide.

Clinical evidence, mechanism, importance and management

(a) Guar gum

Guar gum granules (4.75 g **guar gum**) alone or taken 30 min later with breakfast did not significantly affect the absorption of a single 2.5-mg dose of **glipizide** in 10 healthy subjects.[1] **Guar gum** was found to reduce the absorption of **glibenclamide (glyburide)** in one formulation *(Semi-Euglucon)* but not another newer formulation *(Semi-Euglucon-N)*,[2,3] possibly because the latter preparation is more rapidly and completely absorbed. There seems to be nothing documented about any of the other sulphonylureas. **Guar gum** has also been found to reduce the absorption rate of **metformin** in normal subjects, but the total reduction in postprandial blood sugar levels was increased.[4] It seems doubtful if any of these interactions has much if any clinical relevance because among its indications **guar gum** is used to reduce oral hypoglycaemic dosage levels.[5]

(b) Glucomannan

Glucomannan 3.9 g markedly reduced the plasma levels of **glibenclamide (glyburide)** in 9 normal subjects after taking a single 2.5-mg dose. Four samples taken over 30 to 150 minutes showed reductions in the plasma levels of **glibenclamide** by about 50%.[6] The extent to which this affects the control of diabetes in patients appears not to have been studied, but a reduction in its blood sugar lowering effects might be expected. This awaits assessment.

1. Huupponen R, Karhuvaara S, Seppälä P. Effect of guar gum on glipizide absorption in man. *Eur J Clin Pharmacol* (1985) 28, 717–9.
2. Neugebauer G, Akpan W, Abshagen U. Interaktion von Guar mit Glibenclamid und Bezafibrat. *Beitr Infusionther Klin Ernahr* (1983) 12, 40–7.
3. Karttunen P, Södervik H, Silvasti M, Uusitupa M. The effects of guar gum on glibenclamide absorption and metabolic control of type II diabetics. *Acta Endocrinol (Copenh)* (1987) 115 (Suppl 282), 27.
4. Gin H, Orgerie MB, Aubertin J. The influence of guar gum on absorption of metformin from the gut in healthy volunteers. *Horm Metabol Res* (1989) 21, 81–3.
5. Guarem granules (guar gum) Rybar Laboratories. Summary of product characteristics. June 2000.
6. Shima K, Tanaka A, Ikegami H, Tabata M, Sawazaki N, Kumahara Y. Effect of dietary fiber, glucomannan, on absorption of sulfonylurea in man. *Horm Metabol Res* (1983) 15, 1–3.

Hypoglycaemic agents + Halofenate

Dose reductions of some hypoglycaemic agents may be necessary if they are given concurrently with halofenate (a lipid regulating agent no longer in use). The following dose reductions have been suggested: chlorpropamide 80%, tolazamide 46%, phenformin 33%.[1] The interaction may take 2 to 4 weeks to develop, although over 12 weeks has been suggested in other cases.[1,2] Tolbutamide levels have also been raised by concurrent use with halofenate, but insulin appears to be unaffected.[1]

1. Jain AK, Ryan JR and McMahon FG. Potentiation of hypoglycaemic effect of sulphonylureas by halofenate. *N Engl J Med* (1975) 293, 1283–6.
2. Kudzma DJ and Friedberg SJ. Potentiation of hypoglycaemic effect of chlorpropamide and phenformin by halofenate. *Diabetes* (1977) 26, 291.

Hypoglycaemic agents + Heparin

Two reports describe hypoglycaemia in a diabetic on glipizide and another on glibenclamide (glyburide), both attributed to concurrent treatment with heparin.

Clinical evidence, mechanism, importance and management

A diabetic, treated for 6 months with **glipizide** 5 mg daily with fair control, experienced recurring episodes of hypoglycaemia over a period of 4 days after taking a routine 5-mg dose of **glipizide** while hospitalised for the treatment of a foot ulcer. It was suggested that this might possibly have been due to an interaction with subcutaneous **heparin calcium** (5000 units every 12 h) which, it is postulated, might have displaced the **glipizide** from its protein binding sites.[1] The patient was also treated with **diamorphine**. Another very brief report describes hypoglycaemia in a patient treated with **glibenclamide (glyburide)** and **heparin**.[2] No other information seems to be available. Concurrent use should be monitored.

1. McKillop G, Fallon M, Slater SD. Possible interaction between heparin and a sulphonylurea a cause of prolonged hypoglycaemia? *BMJ* (1986) 293, 1073.
2. Beeley L, Daly M, Stewart P. Bulletin of the West Midlands Centre for Adverse Drug Reaction Reporting. (1987) 24, 24.

Hypoglycaemic agents + Isoniazid

Some reports state that isoniazid can raise blood sugar levels in diabetics, whereas one describes a fall. The outcome of concurrent use is uncertain. The dosage of the hypoglycaemic agent may possibly need to be adjusted to control the diabetes adequately.

Clinical evidence

A study in 6 diabetics taking **insulin** showed that while taking 300 to 400 mg **isoniazid** daily their fasting blood sugar levels were raised by 40% (from an average of 255 to 357 mg%), and their glucose tolerance curves rose and returned to normal levels more slowly. After 6 days treatment the average rise was only 20%. Two other patients needed an increased dosage of **insulin** while taking 200 mg **isoniazid** daily, but a reduction when the isoniazid was withdrawn.[1]

Another report describes glycosuria and the development of frank diabetes in 3 out of 50 patients given 300 mg **isoniazid** daily,[2] and hyperglycaemia has been seen in cases of **isoniazid** poisoning.[3]

In contrast, another study showed that **isoniazid** had a hypoglycaemic effect in 6 out of 8 diabetics.[4] A 500 mg dose of **isoniazid** caused an 18% (range 5 to 34%) reduction in blood sugar levels after 4 h; 3 g **tolbutamide** caused a 28% (19 to 43%) reduction, and together they caused a 35% (17 to 57%) reduction. One patient however showed a

10% increase in blood sugar levels after **isoniazid**, a 41% decrease after **tolbutamide**, and a 30% decrease after taking both. Another diabetic responded to neither drug.

Mechanism

Not understood.

Importance and management

The major documentation for these reactions dates back to the 1950s, since when the literature has been virtually (and perhaps significantly?) silent. The outcome of concurrent use is therefore somewhat uncertain. Nevertheless it would be prudent for diabetics given isoniazid to be monitored for changes in the control of the diabetes. Appropriate dosage adjustments (up or down?) of the hypoglycaemic agent should be made where necessary.

1. Luntz GRWN, Smith SG. Effect of isoniazid on carbohydrate metabolism in controls and diabetics. *BMJ* (1953) i, 296–9.
2. Dickson I. Glycosuria and diabetes mellitus following INAH therapy. *Med J Aust* (1962) i, 325–6.
3. Tovaryš A, Šiler Z. Diabetic syndrome and intoxication with INH. *Prakt Lekar* (1968) 48, 286; quoted in *Int Pharm Abstr* (1968) 5, 286.
4. Segarra FO, Sherman DS, Charif BS. Experiences with tolbutamide and chlorpropamide in tuberculous diabetic patients. *Ann N Y Acad Sci* (1959) 74, 656–61.

Hypoglycaemic agents + Karela (*Momordica charantia*)

The hypoglycaemic effects of chlorpropamide can be increased by the concurrent use of karela (*Momordica charantia*).

Clinical evidence, mechanism, importance and management

Karela (also known as bitter gourd, balsam pear, cundeamor) is the fruit of *Momordica charantia* which is indigenous to Asia and South America. It is used to flavour foods such as curries, and also used as a herbal medicine for the treatment of diabetes mellitus. It produces a significant improvement in glucose tolerance in non-insulin-dependent diabetics,[1-3] which may be due to its content of polypeptide-p, a hypoglycaemic peptide.[4]

A report of a diabetic who was poorly controlled on diet and **chlorpropamide**, but much better controlled when she also ate **karela**, provides evidence that the hypoglycaemic effects of **karela** and conventional oral hypoglycaemic agents can be additive.[5] What is not clear is whether excessive hypoglycaemia might occur in diabetics taking conventional hypoglycaemic agents if they were additionally to begin to take **karela** as a food or as a herbal medicine. **Karela** is available in the UK and elsewhere, and prescribers should therefore be aware that Asian patients may possibly be using **karela** as well as more orthodox drugs to control their diabetes.

1. Leatherdale BA, Panesar KR, Singh G, Atkins TW, Bailey CJ, Bignell AHC. Improvement in glucose tolerance due to Momordica charantia (karela). *BMJ* (1981) 282, 1823–4.
2. Welihinda J, Karunanayake EH, Sheriff MHR, Jaysinghe KSA . Effect of *Momordica charantia* on the glucose tolerance in maturity onset diabetes. *J Ethnopharmacol* (1986) 17, 277–82.
3. Akhtar MS. Trial of Momordica Charantia Linn (Karela) powder in patients with maturity-onset diabetes. *J Pakistan Med Assoc* (1982) 32, 106–7.
4. Khanna P, Jain SC, Panagariya A, Dixit VP. Hypoglycemic activity of polypeptide-p from a plant source. *J Nat Prod* (1981) 44, 648–55.
5. Aslam M, Stockley IH. Interaction between curry ingredient (karela) and drug (chlorpropamide). *Lancet* (1979) i, 607.

Hypoglycaemic agents + Ketoconazole

Ketoconazole increases the hypoglycaemic effects of tolbutamide in normal subjects.

Clinical evidence

After an overnight fast and breakfast the next morning, 7 normal subjects were given a single 500-mg dose of **tolbutamide** before and after taking 200 mg **ketoconazole** daily for a week. The **ketoconazole** increased the elimination half life of the **tolbutamide** more than threefold (from 3.7 to 12.3 h) and increased its AUC by 77% (from 309 to 546 micrograms ml^{-1} h). Blood glucose measurements showed that the **ketoconazole** increased the blood sugar lowering effects of the **tolbutamide** by about 10 to 15%, and 5 of the subjects experienced mild hypoglycaemic symptoms (weakness, sweating and a reeling sensation) at about 2 h.[1]

Mechanism

Not understood.

Importance and management

Information appears to be limited to this study in normal subjects. The reaction in diabetics is uncertain, but if ketoconazole is added to tolbutamide, patients should be warned to be alert for any evidence of increased hypoglycaemia. It may become necessary to reduce the tolbutamide dosage. There have been a few cases of marked hypoglycaemia in patients taking other sulphonylureas (glibenclamide (glyburide), gliclazide, glipizide, tolbutamide) with other azole antifungals (fluconazole, miconazole; see the Index), but there seems to be no information about other sulphonylureas and ketoconazole.

1. Krishnaiah YSR, Satyanarayana S, Visweswaram D. Interaction between tolbutamide and ketoconazole in healthy subjects. *Br J Clin Pharmacol* (1994) 37, 205–7.

Hypoglycaemic agents + Ketotifen

Concurrent use appears to be well tolerated, but a fall in the number of platelets has been seen in one study in patients on biguanides while taking ketotifen. The clinical importance of this is uncertain.

Clinical evidence, mechanism, importance and management

A study in 30 hospitalised diabetics (10 on **diet alone**, 10 on **unnamed sulphonylureas**, 10 on **unnamed biguanides**) found that the concurrent use of **ketotifen** 4 mg daily for 14 days was generally well tolerated. However, those on **biguanides** showed a significant decrease in platelet counts and three showed a marked fall on day 14 to slightly below 100×10^9/l which returned to normal after a few days.[1] This finding underlies the precaution issued by the makers of **ketotifen**,[2] that the combination ". . . should be avoided until this phenomenon has been satisfactorily explained." However, no other studies appear to have confirmed the fall in thrombocyte count so that its importance still remains uncertain.[3]

1. Doleček R. Ketotifen in the treatment of diabetics with various allergic conditions. *Pharmatherapeutica* (1981) 2, 568–74.
2. Zaditen (Ketotifen). Novartis Pharmaceuticals UK Ltd. Summary of product characteristics, November 2000.
3. Sandoz. Personal communication (1991).

Hypoglycaemic agents + Lithium

Lithium can raise blood sugar levels and in some instances has been associated with the development of diabetes mellitus, but the association is unclear and there is little or no evidence that its use normally causes significant changes in diabetic control.

Clinical evidence, mechanism, importance and management

A study in 10 psychiatric patients showed that when treated with **lithium carbonate** for 2 weeks their blood glucose levels were raised and their glucose tolerance tests impaired.[1] There are also a few case reports of hyperglycaemia, impaired glucose tolerance and diabetes mellitus in patients treated with lithium salts.[2-4]

Although there appear to be no reports of disturbed diabetic control in diabetics treated with **lithium** (any marked effect might be expected to have been reported by now), it would seem prudent to monitor the response if **lithium** is added to the treatment being received by diabetic patients.

1. Shopsin B, Stern S, Gershon S. Altered carbohydrate metabolism during treatment with lithium carbonate. *Arch Gen Psychiatry* (1972) 26, 566–71.
2. Craig J, Abu-Saleh M, Smith B, Evans I. Diabetes mellitus in patients on lithium. *Lancet* (1977) ii, 1028.
3. Johnstone BB. Diabetes mellitus in patients on lithium. *Lancet* (1977) ii, 935.
4. Martinez-Maldonado M, Terrell J. Lithium carbonate-induced nephrogenic diabetes insipidus and glucose intolerance. *Arch Intern Med* (1973) 132, 881–4.

Hypoglycaemic agents + Methysergide

A preliminary study indicates that methysergide may enhance the activity of tolbutamide.

Clinical evidence, mechanism, importance and management

Two days pretreatment with **methysergide** (2 mg six-hourly) increased the amount of **insulin** secreted in response to 1 g **tolbutamide** given intravenously to 8 maturity-onset diabetics by almost 40%.[1] Whether in practice the addition or withdrawal of **methysergide** adversely affects the control of diabetes is uncertain, but the possibility should be borne in mind.

1. Baldridge JA, Quickel KE, Feldman JM and Lebovitz HE. Potentiation of tolbutamide-mediated insulin release in adult onset diabetics by methysergide maleate. *Diabetes* (1974) 23, 21–4.

Hypoglycaemic agents + Mianserin

The control of diabetes appears to be unaffected by the use of mianserin.

Clinical evidence, mechanism, importance and management

Although there is some evidence of a change in glucose metabolism during treatment with **mianserin**,[1-3] the alteration failed to affect the control of diabetes in 10 patients under study and there appear to be no reports of adverse effects caused by concurrent use.[2]

1. Fell PJ, Quantock DC, van der Burg WJ. The human pharmacology of GB94–a new psychotropic agent. *Eur J Clin Pharmacol* (1973) 5, 166–73.
2. Peet M, Behagel H. Mianserin: a decade of scientific development. *Br J Clin Pharmacol* (1978) 5, 5S–9S.
3. Moonie L. Unpublished data quoted by Brogden RN, Heel RC, Speight TM, Avery GS. Mianserin: a review of its pharmacological properties and therapeutic efficacy in depressive illness. *Drugs* (1978) 16, 273–301.

Hypoglycaemic agents + Miconazole

Hypoglycaemia has been seen in few diabetics taking tolbutamide, glibenclamide (glyburide) or gliclazide when they were concurrently treated with miconazole.

Clinical evidence, mechanism, importance and management

A diabetic patient taking **tolbutamide** was hospitalised with severe hypoglycaemia about 10 days after starting to take **miconazole**.[1] In 1983 the French Commission Nationale de Pharmacovigilance reported 6 cases of hypoglycaemia in diabetics on sulphonylureas within 2 to 6 days of beginning treatment with **miconazole** (5 with **gliclazide** and one with **glibenclamide (glyburide)**).[1] The same organisation report a further 8 cases in the 1985 to 1990 period but individual sulphonylureas were not named.[2] Three other cases (two on **gliclazide** and one on **glibenclamide**) are reported elsewhere in patients given **miconazole** (up to 750 mg daily).[3]

Mechanism

Not understood. It is thought that the miconazole inhibits the metabolism of the sulphonylureas by the liver, causing them to accumulate and thereby increasing their effects.[2]

Importance and management

An established and clinically important interaction, of uncertain incidence but probably small. Concurrent use need not be avoided but it should be monitored and the dosage of the sulphonylurea reduced if necessary. Patients should be warned. Information about other sulphonylureas not cited is lacking but it seems possible that they may interact similarly.

1. Meurice JC, Lecomte P, Renard JP, Girard JJ. Interaction miconazole et sulfamides hypoglycémiants. *Presse Med* (1983) 12, 1670.
2. Girardin E, Vial T, Pham E, Evreux J-C. Hypoglycémies induites par les sulfamides hypoglycémiants. *Ann Med Interne (Paris)* (1992) 143, 11–17.
3. Loupi E, Descotes J, Lery N, Evreux JC. Interactions médicamenteuses et miconazole. A propos de 10 observations. *Therapie* (1982) 37, 437–41.

Hypoglycaemic agents + Miglitol

Miglitol causes a small reduction in serum glibenclamide (glyburide) levels, but blood glucose levels are reduced more than with glibenclamide alone.

Clinical evidence, mechanism, importance and management

In a randomised, double-blind, placebo controlled trial, 28 non-insulin dependent diabetes mellitus patients were given 2.5 mg **glibenclamide (glyburide)** twice daily with either 100 mg **miglitol** or a placebo three times daily for 2 days. It was found that the **miglitol** reduced the maximum plasma **glibenclamide** levels and its AUC by 16 and 19% respectively, even so the average blood glucose levels were reduced more by the drug combination than by the **glibenclamide** alone. Over 5 h there was a 15% greater reduction, and over 10 h a 9% greater reduction.[1] There would therefore appear to be advantages in combining these drugs together.

1. Sullivan JT, Lettieri JT, Heller AH. Effects of miglitol on pharmacokinetics and pharmacodynamics of glyburide. *Clin Pharmacol Ther* (1998) 63, 155.

Hypoglycaemic agents + Monoamine oxidase inhibitors (MAOIs)

The hypoglycaemic effects of insulin and the oral hypoglycaemic agents can be increased by the concurrent use of MAOIs. This may improve the control of blood sugar levels in most diabetics, but in a few it may cause undesirable hypoglycaemia. This can be controlled by reducing the dosage of the hypoglycaemic agent. Moclobemide appears not to interact.

Clinical evidence

A woman diabetic, stabilised on **insulin-zinc suspension**, exhibited hypoglycaemic attacks and postural syncope when treated with 15 to 25 mg **mebanazine** daily. She required a 30% reduction in the dosage of **insulin** (from 48 to 35 units daily) to achieve restabilisation. Her **insulin** requirements rose once again when the **mebanazine** was withdrawn.[1]

Other reports in diabetics showed that the concurrent use of **mebanazine** increased the hypoglycaemic activity of **insulin, tolbutamide** and **chlorpropamide**, and improved diabetic control.[2-5] No clinically relevant interaction was reported to occur between **glibenclamide (glyburide)** and **moclobemide**.[6] A study in normal subjects on 2.5 mg **glibenclamide** daily found that 200 mg **moclobemide** three times daily for a week had no effect on glucose or **insulin** concentrations after oral glucose tolerance tests.[7] Clinical trials in 8 diabetics taking **glibenclamide (glyburide), gliclazide, metformin** and **chlorpropamide** also found that **moclobemide** had no effect on blood glucose levels or any other evidence of an interaction.[7]

Mechanism

Not fully understood. A reduction in blood sugar levels has been demonstrated in man in the absence of conventional hypoglycaemic agents with mebanazine,[3] iproniazid,[8] isocarboxazid,[9] phenelzine,[3] and tranylcypromine[10] possibly due to some direct action of the MAOI on the pancreas which causes the release of insulin.[10] It would seem that this can be additive with the effects of the conventional hypoglycaemics.

Importance and management

An established interaction of only moderate clinical importance. It can benefit the control of diabetes in many patients, but some individuals may need a reduction in their hypoglycaemic agent dosage to avoid excessive hypoglycaemia. The effects of concurrent use should be monitored. Only a few MAOI/hypoglycaemic agent combinations appear to have been examined, but this interaction would seem possible with any of them. This requires confirmation.

1. Cooper AJ, Keddie KMG. Hypotensive collapse and hypoglycaemia after mebanazine-a monoamine oxidase inhibitor. *Lancet* (1964) i, 1133–5.
2. Wickström L, Pettersson K. Treatment of diabetics with monoamine-oxidase inhibitors. *Lancet* (1964) ii, 995–7.
3. Adnitt PI. Hypoglycemic action of monoamineoxidase inhibitors (MAOI's). *Diabetes* (1968) 17, 628–33.
4. Cooper AJ. The action of mebanazine, a mono amine oxidase inhibitor antidepressant drug in diabetes-part II. *Int J Neuropsychiatry* (1966) 2, 342–5.
5. Adnitt PI, Oleesky S, Schnieden H. The hypoglycaemic action of monoamineoxidase inhibitors (MAOI's). *Diabetologia* (1968) 4, 379.
6. Zimmer R, Gieschke R, Fischbach R, Gasic S. Interaction studies with moclobemide. *Acta Psychiatr Scand* (1990) (Suppl 360), 84–6.
7. Amrein R, Güntert TW, Dingemanse J, Lorscheid T, Stabl M, Schmid-Burgk W. Interactions of moclobemide with concomitantly administered medication: evidence from pharmacological and clinical studies. *Psychopharmacology (Berl)* (1992) 106, S24–S31.
8. Weiss J, Weiss S, Weiss B. Effects of iproniazid and similar compounds on the gastrointestinal tract. *Ann N Y Acad Sci* (1959) 80, 854–9.
9. van Praag HM, Leijnse B. The influence of some antidepressives of the hydrazine type on the glucose metabolism in depressed patients. *Clin Chim Acta* (1963) 8, 466–75.
10. Bressler R, Vargas-Cordon M, Lebovitz HE. Tranylcypromine: a potent insulin secretagogue and hypoglycemic agent. *Diabetes* (1968) 17, 617–24.

Hypoglycaemic agents + Naftidrofuryl oxalate

There is one very brief report describing severe hypoglycaemia during the concurrent use of glibenclamide (glyburide) and naftidrofuryl oxalate, possibly due to an interaction.[1] No details are given.

1. Beeley L, Magee P, Hickey FM. Bulletin of the West Midlands Centre for Adverse Drug Reaction Reporting (1990) 30, 17.

Hypoglycaemic agents + Naltrexone

The insulin requirements of a patient rose by about 30% when treated with naltrexone.

Clinical evidence, mechanism, importance and management

A patient with insulin-dependent type 1 diabetes was given **naltrexone** in an experimental study of the treatment of anorexia nervosa. During two periods of five days while given the **naltrexone** (dosage not stated), the blood glucose levels of the patient remained unchanged but the **insulin** dosage requirements rose from 52.8 and 61.4 units/day during the control periods to 71.4 and 76.0 units/day during the **naltrexone** periods (that is a rise of about 30%). The reason is not known but the authors of this report point out that this apparent interaction must have been on the actions of **insulin** rather than on its release because this patient had no endogenous **insulin**.[1]

The general clinical importance of this interaction is not known but it would be prudent to be alert for any evidence of increased **insulin** requirements if **naltrexone** is used in any patient.

1. Marrazzi MA, Jacober S, Luby ED. Naltrexone induced increase in insulin requirement. *Biol Psychiatry* (1994) 35, 736.

Hypoglycaemic agents + NSAIDs

No adverse interactions normally occur between chlorpropamide or tolbutamide and ibuprofen; glibenclamide (glyburide) and acemetacin, bromfenac, diclofenac, ibuprofen, tenoxicam or tolmetin; glipizide or tolbutamide and indoprofen; glibornuride and tenoxicam; or between tolbutamide and diflunisal, naproxen, sulindac or tenoxicam. There are isolated cases of hypoglycaemia in patients given fenclofenac with chlorpropamide and metformin, glibenclamide with diflunisal and glibenclamide and metformin with naproxen. Another describes loss of diabetic control attributed to indometacin. Indobufen increases the effects of glipizide, and piroxicam increases the effects of glibenclamide. See the Index for interactions with azapropazone, phenylbutazone, oxyphenbutazone and the salicylates.

Clinical evidence

(a) Chlorpropamide or Tolbutamide + Ibuprofen

Ibuprofen 1200 mg daily had no significant effect on the blood sugar levels of diabetic patients taking 62.5 to 375 mg **chlorpropamide** daily.[1] In other patients on **tolbutamide** it was found that **ibuprofen** lowered fasting blood sugar levels, but not below the normal lower limits.[2]

(b) Chlorpropamide with Metformin + Fenclofenac, Flurbiprofen or Indometacin

A woman whose diabetes was well controlled on 500 mg **chlorpropamide** and 1700 mg **metformin** daily, developed hypoglycaemia within 2 days of exchanging **flurbiprofen** 150 mg daily + **indometacin** 150 mg daily for 1200 mg **fenclofenac** daily. The hypoglycaemic agents were withdrawn the next day, but later in the evening she went into a hypoglycaemic coma. The reasons for this are not understood.[3] Conversely, another isolated report briefly describes hyperglycaemia with **chlorpropamide** possibly due to **indometacin**.[4]

(c) Glibenclamide + Acemetacin, Bromfenac, Diclofenac, Diflunisal, Ibuprofen, Naproxen, Piroxicam, Tenoxicam or Tolmetin

No changes in the control of diabetes was seen in 20 patients on **glibenclamide (glyburide)** when concurrently treated with 60 mg **acemetacin** three times daily.[5] The blood sugar levels of 12 **glibenclamide**-treated diabetics (10 mg daily) remained unchanged when given 50 mg **bromfenac** three times daily for 3 days, and the pharmacokinetics of **glibenclamide** were also unaltered.[6] The blood sugar levels of 12 **glibenclamide**-treated diabetics with rheumatic diseases remained unchanged when they were concurrently treated with 150 mg **diclofenac** daily for 4 days,[7] but an isolated case of hypoglycaemia has been reported with **diflunisal**.[8] A case of severe hypoglycaemia in a diabetic patient was attributed to the accumulation of **glibenclamide** and **metformin** due to deterioration in renal function resulting from co-administration of ramipril and **naproxen**.[9] A study in 16 healthy subjects showed that ibuprofen produced no significant changes in the pharmacokinetics of co-administered **glibenclamide**. **Ibuprofen** with **glibenclamide** caused a greater hypoglycaemic effect than **glibenclamide** alone, but the clinical significance of this was uncertain.[10] Normal subjects and diabetics showed an increased hypoglycaemic response to **glibenclamide** (blood sugar levels down by 13 to 15%) when additionally given 10 mg **piroxicam**.[11] **Tenoxicam** 20 mg daily was found not to affect the glycoregulation of 8 normal subjects given 2.5 mg **glibenclamide** daily.[12] No changes were seen in the blood sugar levels of 40 other diabetics on **glibenclamide** given either 1200 mg **tolmetin** or placebo daily for 5 days.[13]

(d) Glibornuride + Tenoxicam

A study in normal subjects found that **tenoxicam** 20 mg daily did not affect the pharmacokinetics of **glibornuride** nor the responses of plasma insulin and blood glucose to **glibornuride**.[14]

(e) Glipizide + Indobufen

Six normal subjects showed a rise in serum **glipizide** levels when treated with 200 mg **indobufen** as a single dose and then twice daily for a 5 day period, and blood sugar levels were lowered.[15]

(f) Glipizide or Tolbutamide + Indoprofen

No important changes in blood sugar levels occurred in 24 diabetic patients on **tolbutamide** or **glipizide** when given 600 mg **indoprofen** daily for 5 days.[16] A study showed that although **indoprofen** (200 mg on day 1, then 600 mg daily on days 3 to 8) lowered the plasma levels of a single 5-mg dose of **glipizide**, the blood sugar levels remained unaffected.[17]

(g) Tolbutamide + Diflunisal, Naproxen, Sulindac or Tenoxicam

A brief report states that no changes in blood **tolbutamide** or in fasting blood glucose levels were seen in diabetics given 375 mg **diflunisal** twice daily.[18] Twelve maturity-onset **tolbutamide**-treated diabetics demonstrated no changes in **tolbutamide** half-life, plasma levels, time-to-peak levels or AUC when given 400 mg **sulindac** daily. An unimportant reduction in fasting blood sugar levels was seen.[19] **Naproxen** (375 mg 12-hourly) had no effect on the pharmacokinetics or pharmacological effects of **tolbutamide** when given to 10 maturity onset diabetics over 3 days.[20] The pharmacokinetics of a single 500-mg dose of **tolbutamide** were unaffected in 7 healthy subjects after taking 20 mg **tenoxicam** daily for 14 days. The co-administration of the **tenoxicam** did not alter the blood glucose concentrations.[21]

Mechanism

Normally none.

Importance and management

The reports briefly quoted here indicate that no adverse or clinically relevant interaction normally occurs between the oral hypoglycaemic agents and the NSAIDs cited. The general quietness in the literature would seem to add confirmation, but some caution is needed with fenclofenac and indobufen. In contrast, adverse interactions can certainly occur between hypoglycaemic agents and azapropazone, phenylbutazone, oxyphenbutazone and salicylates, details of which are given in the appropriate monograph. See the Index.

1. Shah SJ, Bhandarkar SD, Satoskar RS. Drug interaction between chlorpropamide and non-steroidal anti-inflammatory drugs, ibuprofen and phenylbutazone. *Int J Clin Pharmacol Ther Toxicol* (1984) 22, 470–2.
2. Andersen LA. Ibuprofen and tolbutamide drug interaction study. *Br J Clin Pract* (1980) 34 (Suppl 6), 10–12.
3. Allen PA, Taylor RT. Fenclofenac and thyroid function tests. *BMJ* (1980) 281, 1642.
4. Beeley L, Beadle F, Elliott D. Bulletin of the West Midlands Centre for Adverse Drug Reaction Reporting (1985) 21, 19.
5. Haupt E, Hoppe FK, Rechziegler H, Zündorf P. Zur Frage der Interaktionen von nichtsteroidalen Antirheumatika mit oralen Antidiabetika: Acemetacin-Glibenclamid. *Z. Rheumatology* (1987) 46, 170–3.
6. Boni JP, Cevallos WH, DeCleene S, Korth-Bradley JM. The influence of bromfenac on the pharmacokinetics and pharmacodynamic responses to glyburide in diabetic subjects. *Pharmacotherapy* (1997) 17, 783–90.
7. Chlud K. Untersuchungen zur Wechselwirkung von Diclofenac und Glibenclamid. *Z Rheumatol* (1976) 35, 377–82.
8. Girardin E, Vial T, Pham E, Evreux J-C. Hypoglycémies induites par les sulfamides hypoglycémiants. *Ann Med Clin Pharmacol (Paris)* (1992) 143, 11–17.
9. Collin M, Mucklow JC. Drug interactions, renal impairment and hypoglycaemia in a patient with type II diabetes. *Br J Clin Pharmacol* (1999) 48, 134–7.
10. Kubacka RT, Antal EJ, Juhl RP, Welshman IR. Effects of aspirin and ibuprofen on the pharmacokinetics and pharmacodynamics of glyburide in healthy subjects. *Ann Pharmacother* (1996) 30, 20–26.
11. Diwan PV, Sastry MSP, Satyanarayana NV. Potentiation of hypoglycemic response of glibenclamide by piroxicam in rats and humans. *Indian J Exp Biol* (1992) 30, 317–9.
12. Hartmann D, Korn A, Komjati M, Heinz G, Haefelinger P, Defoin R, Waldhäusl WK. Lack of effect of tenoxicam on dynamic responses to concurrent oral doses of glucose and glibenclamide. *Br J Clin Pharmacol* (1990) 30, 245–52.
13. Chlud K, Kaik B. Clinical studies of the interaction between tolmetin and glibenclamide. *Int J Clin Pharmacol Biopharm* (1977) 15, 409–10.
14. Stoeckel K, Trueb V, Dubach UC, Heintz RC, Ascalone V, Forgo I, Hennes U. Lack of effect of tenoxicam on glibornuride kinetics and response. *Br J Clin Pharmacol* (1985) 19, 249–54.
15. Elvander-Ståhl E, Melander A, Wåhlin-Boll E. Indobufen interacts with the sulphonylurea, glipizide, but not with the β-adrenergic receptor antagonists, propranolol and atenolol. *Br J Clin Pharmacol* (1984) 18, 773–8.
16. Pedrazzi F, Bommartini F, Freddo J, Emanueli A. A study of the possible interaction of indoprofen with hypoglycemic sulfonylureas in diabetic patients. *Eur J Rheumatol Inflamm* (1981) 4, 26–31.
17. Melander A, Wåhlin-Boll E. Interaction of glipizide and indoprofen. *Eur J Rheumatol Inflamm* (1981) 4, 22–5.
18. McMahon FG, Ryan JR. Unpublished observations quoted in Tempero KF, Cirillo VJ, Steelman SL. Diflunisal: a review of the pharmacokinetic and pharmacodynamic properties, drug interactions, and special tolerability studies in humans. *Br J Clin Pharmacol* (1977) 4, 31S–36S.
19. Ryan JR, Jain AK, McMahon FG, Vargas R. On the question of an interaction between sulindac and tolbutamide in the control of diabetes. *Clin Pharmacol Ther* (1977) 21, 231–3.
20. Whiting B, Williams RL, Lorenzi M, Varady JC, Robins DS. Effect of naproxen on glucose metabolism and tolbutamide kinetics and dynamics in maturity onset diabetics. *Br J Clin Pharmacol* (1981) 11, 295–302.
21. Day RO, Geisslinger G, Paull P, Williams KM. The effect of tenoxicam on tolbutamide pharmacokinetics and glucose concentrations in healthy volunteers. *Int J Clin Pharmacol Ther* (1995) 33, 308–10.

Hypoglycaemic agents + Octreotide

Octreotide has a hypoglycaemic effect so that the dosage of insulin used by diabetics can be reduced, but it appears not to interact in this way with oral hypoglycaemic agents.

Clinical evidence

(a) Insulin

When 7 **insulin**-dependent diabetics (type 1) with poor metabolic control were given 50 micrograms **octreotide** subcutaneously three times daily (at 8, 15 and 23 h) or by continuous subcutaneous infusion, their blood glucose levels were approximately 50% lower than with **insulin** alone, when measured at 8, 12, 16, 20 and 8 h. The effects on blood glucose levels of the two modes of administration of **octreotide** were virtually the same.[1] Another study in 6 **insulin**-dependent diabetic patients also found that 50 micrograms **octreotide** before meals reduced their daily **insulin** requirements by about 50%,[2] and other studies confirm that **octreotide** behaves in this way.[3,4]

Eight obese type 2 diabetic patients whose diabetes had failed to be controlled with oral hypoglycaemic agents and who needed **insulin** treatment, showed no significant increases in blood glucose levels following a meal when they were also given 25 micrograms **octreotide**.[5]

(b) Oral hypoglycaemic agents

Octreotide appears not to have a clinically relevant effect on the hypoglycaemic effects of oral hypoglycaemic agents such as **glibenclamide (glyburide)**[6,7] in non-insulin dependent diabetics, although some metabolic changes can occur.

Mechanism

Not fully understood. Octreotide appears to act as a hypoglycaemic because it inhibits the actions of glucagon and growth hormone (which raise blood glucose levels), and because it also inhibits the absorption of carbohydrate from the gut.

Importance and management

The insulin/octreotide interaction is established. There seem to be no reports of marked hypoglycaemia during concurrent use, but if both drugs are used, anticipate the need to reduce the insulin dosage. The studies cited above[1,2] suggest that about a 50% reduction is possible.

The makers of octreotide say that octreotide may also reduce oral hypoglycaemic requirements in patients with diabetes mellitus, but two clinical studies in non-insulin dependent diabetics given glibenclamide (glyburide) failed to confirm that this occurs.[6,7] While it would certainly be prudent to monitor the effects of giving octreotide with any of the oral hypoglycaemic agents, what is known so far suggests that no clinically relevant interaction is likely.

1. Di Mauro M, Le Moli R, Nicoletti F, Lunetta M. Effects of octreotide on the glycemic levels in insulin-dependent diabetic patients. Comparative study between administration through multiple subcutaneous injections and continuous subcutaneous infusion. *Diabetologia* (1993) 36 (Suppl 1), A138.
2. Rios MS, Navascues I, Saban J, Ordoñez A, Sevilla F, Del Pozo E. Somatostatin analog SMS 201–995 and insulin needs in insulin-dependent diabetic patients studied by means of an artificial pancreas. *J Clin Endocrinol Metab* (1986) 63, 1071–4.
3. Candrina R, Giustina G. Effect of a new long-acting somatostatin analogue (SMS 201–995) on glycemic and hormonal profiles in insulin-treated type II diabetic patients. *J Endocrinol Invest* (1988) 11, 501–7.
4. Hadjidakis DJ, Halvatsiotis PG, Ioannou YJ, Mavrokefalos PJ, Raptis SA. The effects of the somatostatin analogue SMS 201–995 on carbohydrate homeostasis in insulin-dependent diabetics as assessed by the artificial endocrine pancreas. *Diabetes Res Clin Pract* (1988) 5, 91–8.
5. Giustina A, Girelli A, Buffoli MG, Cimino A, Legati F, Valentini U, Giustina G. Low-dose octreotide is able to cause a maximal inhibition of the glycemic responses to a mixed meal in obese type 2 diabetic patients treated with insulin. *Diabetes Res Clin Pract* (1991) 14, 47–54.
6. Davies RR, Miller M, Turner SJ, Watson M, McGill A, Ørskov H, Alberti KGMM, Johnston DG. Effects of somatostatin analogue SMS 201–995 in non-insulin-dependent diabetes. *Clin Endocrinol (Oxf)* (1989) 25, 739–47.
7. Williams G, Füessl HS, Burrin JM, Chilvers E, Bloom SR. Postprandial glycaemic effects of a long-acting somatostatin analogue (octreotide) in non-insulin dependent diabetes mellitus. *Horm Metabol Res* (1988) 20, 168–170.

Hypoglycaemic agents + Phenylbutazone or Oxyphenbutazone

The hypoglycaemic effects of acetohexamide, chlorpropamide, carbutamide, glymidine, glibenclamide (glyburide) and tolbutamide can be increased by the concurrent use of phenylbutazone. Severe hypoglycaemia has occurred in a few patients. Oxyphenbutazone may be expected to behave similarly but not mofebutazone.

Clinical evidence

A diabetic man under treatment with **tolbutamide** experienced an acute hypoglycaemic episode 4 days after beginning to take 200 mg **phenylbutazone** three times a day, although there was no change in his diet or in the dosage of **tolbutamide**. He was able to control the hypoglycaemia by eating a large bar of chocolate.[1]

There are numerous other case reports and studies of this interaction involving **phenylbutazone** with **acetohexamide**,[2] **carbutamide**,[3] **chlorpropamide**,[4-6] **glibenclamide (glyburide)**,[7] **glymidine**,[8] and **tolbutamide**[5,9-15] some of which describe acute hypoglycaemic episodes.[2,4,5,10,12] Several of these interactions have been fatal.[5,15] There is a report suggesting that the **glibornuride/phenylbutazone** interaction may not be clinically important.[16] In contrast to these reports, a single study describes a paradoxical rise in blood sugar levels in 3 African patients while receiving **tolbutamide** and **phenylbutazone**.[17] In addition to these reports there is some evidence that **tolbutamide** increases the metabolism of **phenylbutazone** by 42%,[14] but the extent to which this affects its therapeutic effects is uncertain.

Oxyphenbutazone has been shown to interact like **phenylbutazone** with **glymidine**[18,19] and **tolbutamide**,[20,21] but **mofebutazone** (900 mg daily) has been found not to cause any clinically important changes in blood sugar control in patients on **glibenclamide**.[22]

Mechanism

Not fully resolved. Some evidence shows that phenylbutazone can inhibit the renal excretion of glibenclamide (glyburide),[7] tolbutamide,[11] and the active metabolite of acetohexamide[2] so that they are retained in the body longer and their hypoglycaemic effects are increased and prolonged. It has also been shown that phenylbutazone can inhibit the metabolism of the sulphonylureas[14,20] as well as causing their displacement from protein binding sites.[23]

Importance and management

The hypoglycaemic agent/phenylbutazone interactions are well documented and potentially clinically important. Blood sugar levels may be lowered, but the number of reports of acute hypoglycaemic episodes seems to be small. Concurrent use should therefore be well monitored. A reduction in the dosage of the sulphonylurea may be necessary if excessive hypoglycaemia is to be avoided. Not all sulphonylureas have been shown to interact (glibornuride probably does not do so) but it would be prudent to assume that they all interact until the contrary is proved. Oxyphenbutazone may be expected to interact similarly (it is a metabolite of phenylbutazone) but, unexpectedly, not mofebutazone.

1. Mahfouz M, Abdel-Maguid R, El-Dakhakhny M. Potentiation of the hypoglycaemic action of tolbutamide by different drugs. *Arzneimittelforschung* (1970) 20, 120–2.
2. Field JB, Ohta M, Boyle C, Remer A. Potentiation of acetohexamide hypoglycemia by phenylbutazone. *N Engl J Med* (1967) 277, 889–94.
3. Kaindl F, Kretschy A, Puxkandl H, Wutte J. Zur steigerung des Wirkundseffektes peroraler Antidiabetika durch Pyrazolonderivate. *Wien Klin Wochenschr* (1961) 73, 79–80.
4. Dalgas M, Christiansen I, Kjerulf K. Fenylbutazoninduceret hypoglykaemitilfaelde hos klorpropamidbehandlet diabetiker. *Ugeskr Laeger* (1965) 127, 834–6.
5. Schulz E. Severe hypoglycemic reactions after tolbutamide, carbutamide and chlorpropamide. *Arch Klin Med* (1968) 214, 135–62.
6. Shah SJ, Bhandarkar SD, Satoskar RS. Drug interaction between chlorpropamide and non-steroidal anti-inflammatory drugs, ibuprofen and phenylbutazone. *Int J Clin Pharmacol Ther Toxicol* (1984) 22, 470–2.
7. Schulz E, Koch K, Schmidt FH. Ursachen der Potenzierung der hypoglykämischen Wirkung von Sulfonylharnstoff-derivaten durch Medikamente. II. Pharmakokinetik und Metabolismus von Glibenclamid (HN 419) in Gegenwart von Phenylbutazon. *Eur J Clin Pharmacol* (1971) 4, 32–7.
8. Held H, Kaminski B, von Olderhausen HF. Die beeinflussung der Elimination von Glycodiazin durch Leber-und Nierenfunktionsstorungen und durch eine Behandlung mit Phenylbutazon, Phenprocumarol und Doxycyclin. *Diabetologia* (1970) 6, 386–91.
9. Gulbrandsen R. Økt tolbutamid-effekt ved hjelp av fenylbutazon? *Tidsskr Nor Laegeforen* (1959) 79, 1127–8.
10. Tannenbaum H, Anderson LG, Soeldner JS. Phenylbutazone-tolbutamide drug interaction. *N Engl J Med* (1974) 290, 344.
11. Ober K-F. Mechanism of interaction of tolbutamide and phenylbutazone in diabetic patients. *Eur J Clin Pharmacol* (1974) 7, 291–4.
12. Dent LA, Jue SG. Tolbutamide-phenylbutazone interaction. *Drug Intell Clin Pharm* (1976) 10, 711.
13. Christensen LK, Hansen JM, Kristensen M. Sulphaphenazole-induced hypoglycaemic attacks in tolbutamide-treated diabetics. *Lancet* (1963) ii, 1298–1301.
14. Szita M, Gachályi B, Tornyossy M, Káldor A. Interaction of phenylbutazone and tolbutamide in man. *Int J Clin Pharmacol Ther Toxicol* (1990) 18, 378–80.
15. Slade IH, Iosefa RN. Fatal hypoglycemic coma from the use of tolbutamide in elderly patients: report of two cases. *J Am Geriatr Soc* (1967) 15, 948-50.
16. Eckhardt W, Rudolph R, Sauer H, Undeutsch D. Zur pharmackologischen Interferenz von Glibornurid mit Sulfaphenazol, Phenylbutazon und Phenprocoumon beim Menschen. *Arzneimittelforschung* (1972) 22, 2212–19.
17. Owusu SK, Ocran K. Paradoxical behaviour of phenylbutazone in African diabetics. *Lancet* (1972) i, 440–41.
18. Held H, Scheible G, von Olderhausen HF. Über Stoffwechsel und Interferenz von Arzneimitteln bei Gesunden und Leberkranken. *Tag Deut Ges Inn Med (Wiesbaden)* (1970) 76, 1153–7.
19. Held H, Scheible G. Interaktion von Phenylbutazon und Oxyphenbutazon mit glymidine. *Arzneimittelforschung* (1981) 31, 1036–8.
20. Pond SM, Birkett DJ, Wade DN. Mechanisms of inhibition of tolbutamide metabolism: Phenylbutazone, oxyphenbutazone, sulfafenazole. *Clin Pharmacol Ther* (1977) 22, 573–9.
21. Kristensen M, Christensen LK. Drug induced changes of the blood glucose lowering effect of oral hypoglycaemic agents. *Acta Diabetol Lat* (1969) 6 (Suppl 1), 116–36.
22. Speders S. Mofebutazon — Prufung einer moglichen Interaktion mit Glibornclamid. *Fortschr Med* (1993) 111, 366–8.
23. Hellman B. Potentiating effects of drugs on the binding of glibenclamide to pancreatic beta cells. *Metabolism* (1974) 23, 839–46.

Hypoglycaemic agents + Phenylephrine

Insulin-dependent diabetics can develop elevated blood pressures if treated with phenylephrine eye-drops.

Clinical evidence, mechanism, importance and management

A comparative study of 14 **insulin-dependent diabetics** who over a period of 2 h before ocular surgery were given **phenylephrine eye-drops** (a total of 4 doses of one or two drops of 10%), showed that they demonstrated an average blood pressure rise of 34/17 mmHg, whereas another 176 non-diabetic patients similarly treated showed no increases in blood pressure.[1] The reason for this pressor reaction is not understood but it would seem that enough **phenylephrine** is absorbed systemically to stimulate the adrenoceptors of the sympathetic system which innervates the cardiovascular system. The concentration of phenylephrine in the plasma is a balance between the amount absorbed and rate at which it is then inactivated. The inactivation in diabetics can be reduced (due to sympathetic denervation) so that their phenylephrine levels may rise higher than they would in normal subjects. The authors of this report say that they readily controlled these hypertensive reactions with halothane and by neuroleptanalgesia accompanying regional block with anaesthesia standby. Strictly speaking this is not a drug interaction, but a drug-disease reaction. The mydriatic dosage of **phenylephrine** should be reduced in **insulin**-dependent diabetics but whether this is also true for non insulin-dependent diabetics is uncertain.

1. Kim JM, Stevenson CE and Mathewson HS. Hypertensive reactions to phenylephrine eyedrops in patients with sympathetic denervation. *Am J Ophthalmol* (1978) 85, 862–8.

Hypoglycaemic agents + Probenecid

The clearance of chlorpropamide from the body is prolonged by probenecid, but the clinical importance of this is uncertain. Tolbutamide appears not to interact.

Clinical evidence, mechanism, importance and management

A study in 6 patients given single oral doses of **chlorpropamide** showed that the concurrent use of **probenecid** (1 to 2 g daily) increased the chlorpropamide half-life from about 36 to 50 h.[1] It seems that the **probenecid** reduces the renal excretion of **chlorpropamide**. Another report in normal subjects claimed that the half-life of **tolbutamide** was also prolonged by **probenecid**,[2] but this was not confirmed by a further properly controlled study.[3]

Information is very limited but it may possibly be necessary to reduce the dosage of the **chlorpropamide** in the presence of **probenecid**. Information about other sulphonylureas appears to be lacking.

1. Petitpierre B, Perrin L, Rudhardt M, Herrera A, Fabre J. Behaviour of chlorpropamide in renal insufficiency and under the effect of associated drug therapy. *Int J Clin Pharmacol* (1972) 6, 120–4.
2. Stowers JM, Mahler RF, Hunter RB. Pharmacology and mode of action of the sulphonylureas in man. *Lancet* (1958) i, 278–83.
3. Brook R, Schrogie JJ, Solomon HM. Failure of probenecid to inhibit the rate of metabolism of tolbutamide in man. *Clin Pharmacol Ther* (1968) 9, 314–17.

Hypoglycaemic agents + Quinine or Quinidine

Patients with falciparum malaria who are treated with quinine or quinidine may show very severe hypoglycaemia. The impact of this on the control of diabetes has yet to be determined. Quinine very occasionally causes hypoglycaemia in non-diabetics.

Clinical evidence, mechanism, importance and management

Patients with severe falciparum malaria who are treated with **quinine** may develop severe and life-threatening hypoglycaemia.[1,2] The reasons are not fully understood but it seems that in these patients the **quinine** causes the release of large amounts of **insulin** from the pancreas, possibly associated with an increase in the sensitivity to **insulin** as the malaria improves,[3] although other factors may also be involved. **Quinidine** has been shown to have a similar effect.[4] Whether these changes can also occur in patients with malaria and diabetes, despite their pancreatic beta cell impairment, seems not to have been studied, but any interpretation of disturbances in the control of the diabetes should take into account these possible effects of **quinine** or **quinidine**. **Chloroquine**, **amodiaquine**, **mefloquine** and **halofantrine** do not apparently stimulate the release of **insulin**.[4]

Quinine has also been responsible for hypoglycaemia in non-diabetic patients, one of whom was taking **quinine sulphate** 325 mg four times daily for leg muscle cramps.[5] Two other non-diabetic patients, one with congestive heart failure and the other with terminal cancer, similarly developed hypoglycaemia when given **quinine** for leg cramps.[6,7]

1. White NJ, Warrell DA, Chanthavanich P, Looareesuwan S, Warrell MJ, Krishna S, Williamson DH, Turner RC. Severe hypoglycemia and hyperinsulinemia in falciparum malaria. *N Engl J Med* (1983) 309, 61–6.
2. Looareesuwan S, Phillips RE, White NJ, Kietinun S, Karbwang J, Rackow C, Turner RC, Warrell DA. Quinine and severe falciparum malaria in late pregnancy. *Lancet* (1985) ii, 4–8.
3. Davis TME, Pukrittayakamee S, Supanaranond W, Looareesuwan S, Krishna S, Nagachinta B, Turner RC, White NJ. Glucose metabolism in quinine-treated patients with uncomplicated falciparum malaria. *Clin Endocrinol (Oxf)* (1990) 33, 739–49.
4. Phillips RE, Looareesuwan S, White NJ, Chanthavanich P, Karbwang J, Supanaranond W, Turner RC, Warrell DA. Hypoglycaemia and antimalarial drugs: quinidine and release of insulin. *BMJ* (1986) 292, 1319–21.
5. Limburg PJ, Katz H, Grant CS, Service FJ. Quinine-induced hypoglycemia. *Ann Intern Med* (1993) 119, 218–19.
6. Harats N, Ackerman Z, Shalit M. Quinine-related hypoglycemia. *N Engl J Med* (1984) 310, 1331.
7. Jones RG, Sue-Ling HM, Kear C, Wiles PG, Quirke P. Severe symptomatic hypoglycaemia due to quinine therapy. *J R Soc Med* (1986) 79, 426–8.

Hypoglycaemic agents + Quinolone antibacterials

Ciprofloxacin does not interact to clinically relevant extent with glibenclamide (glyburide), but there are two isolated reports of severe hypoglycaemia in elderly patients. Levofloxacin appears not to interact.

Clinical evidence, mechanism, importance and management

(a) Glibenclamide (glyburide) + Ciprofloxacin

A study in 12 non-insulin-dependent diabetics taking 10 mg **glibenclamide (glyburide)** in the morning, plus in some instances 5 mg in the evening, found that **ciprofloxacin** 1 g daily for a week caused rises in maximum serum **glibenclamide** levels of 20 to 30%, and of AUCs of 25 to 36%. However none of these changes were statistically significant, and more importantly blood glucose levels were not altered.[1]

However an elderly patient on **glibenclamide** 5 mg daily for over 2 years was found to be confused, with slurred speech and diaphoresis within a week after starting **ciprofloxacin** 250 mg twice daily, and was found to have serum **glibenclamide** level several times greater than that those normally seen.[2] She needed treatment with intravenous glucose to correct the hypoglycaemia. A further similar case in another elderly patient has been reported.[3]

(b) Glibenclamide + Levofloxacin

A study in 24 normal subjects found that **levofloxacin** had no effect on the pharmacokinetics of **glibenclamide** or on the plasma glucose levels observed with **glibenclamide** alone.[4]

Mechanism

Unknown. The authors of the report suggest that the ciprofloxacin may have inhibited the metabolism of the glibenclamide, thereby raising its serum levels. This may possibly be exaggerated in elderly patients whose liver function may be reduced.

Importance and management

The concurrent use of glibenclamide and ciprofloxacin need not be avoided, but when first started it might be prudent to warn patients to be alert for any problems. Levofloxacin and ofloxacin should be considered as possible alternatives in elderly patients because they are minimally involved in liver metabolism.[2] Information about other sulfonylurea/quinolone interactions seems to be lacking.

1. Ludwig E, Szekely E, Graber H, Csiba A. Study of interaction between oral ciprofloxacin and glibenclamide. *Eur J Clin Microbiol Infect Dis* (1991) 10 (Special issue) 378–9.
2. Roberge RJ, Kaplan R, Frank R, Fore C. Glyburide-ciprofloxacin interaction with resistant hypoglycaemia. *Ann Emerg Med* (2000) 36, 160–3.
3. Whitely MS, Worldling J, Patel S, Gibbs KB. Hypoglycaemia in a diabetic patient, associated with ciprofloxacin therapy. *Prac Diabetes* (1993) 10, 35.
4. Hoechst Marion Roussel, Personal Communication, March 1999.

Hypoglycaemic agents + Rifampicin (Rifampin)

Rifampicin reduces the serum levels of tolbutamide, glymidine, chlorpropamide (single case) and glibenclamide (glyburide). Dosage increases may be needed to control the diabetes effectively.

Clinical evidence

(a) Chlorpropamide

A single case report describes a diabetic man who needed an increase in his daily dosage of **chlorpropamide** from 250 to 400 mg daily when he was given 600 mg **rifampicin** daily. His serum **chlorpropamide** levels rose dramatically 12 months later when the **rifampicin** was withdrawn.[1]

(b) Glibenclamide (Glyburide)

A study in 29 well-controlled diabetics on **glibenclamide (glyburide)** found that when they were additionally given 450 or 600 mg **rifampicin** daily for 10 days, their blood sugar levels both fasting and after meals were raised. **Glibenclamide** dosage changes were needed in 15 out of 17 patients in whom the diabetes became uncontrolled. Their blood sugar levels normalised 6 days after stopping the **rifampicin**.[2] Another diabetic patient showed a marked rise in serum **glibenclamide** levels (trough levels from 40 to 200 nanograms/ml) when **rifampicin** was stopped, but no hypoglycaemia occurred.[3]

(c) Glymidine

The half-life of **glymidine** in man was reduced by about one-third by the concurrent use of **rifampicin** in one study.[4]

(d) Tolbutamide

After four weeks treatment with **rifampicin** the half-life of **tolbutamide** in 9 patients with tuberculosis was reduced by 43%, and the serum concentrations measured at 6 h were halved compared with other patients not taking **rifampicin**.[5] Similar results have been found in other studies in patients with cirrhosis or cholestasis,[6] in normal subjects[7] and in other patients.[8]

Mechanism

Rifampicin is a potent inducer of the liver microsomal enzymes concerned with the metabolism of tolbutamide and other drugs, which hastens their clearance from the body, thereby reducing their effects.[5-7]

Importance and management

Information is limited but the tolbutamide/rifampicin and glibenclamide (glyburide)/rifampicin interactions appear to be established. Patients taking either of these sulphonylureas may need an increase in the dosage while taking rifampicin (possibly roughly doubled, but this needs confirmation). This also seems possibly to be true for glymidine and chlorpropamide, but the documentation about these two

drugs is even more limited. Information about other hypoglycaemic agents does not seem to be available. More study is needed.

1. Self TH, Morris T. Interaction of rifampin and chlorpropamide. *Chest* (1980) 77, 800–801.
2. Surekha V, Peter JV, Jeyaseelan L, Cherian AM. Drug interaction: rifampicin and glibenclamide. *Natl Med J India* (1997) 10, 11–12.
3. Self TH, Tsiu SJ, Fowler JW. Interaction of rifampin and glyburide. *Chest* (1989) 96, 1443–4.
4. Held H, Schoene B, Laar HJ, Fleischmann R. Die Aktivität der Benzpyrenhydroxylase im Leberpunktat des Menschen in vitro und ihre Beziehung zur Eliminations-geschwindigkeit von Glycodiazin in vivo. *Verh Dtsch Ges Inn Med* (1974) 80, 501–3.
5. Syvälahti EKG, Pihlajamäki KK, Iisalo EJ. Rifampicin and drug metabolism. *Lancet* (1974) 2, 232–3.
6. Zilly W, Breimer DD, Richter E. Stimulation of drug metabolism by rifampicin in patients with cirrhosis or cholestasis measured by increased hexobarbital and tolbutamide clearance. *Eur J Clin Pharmacol* (1977) 11, 287–93.
7. Zilly W, Breimer DD, Richter E. Induction of drug metabolism in man after rifampicin treatment measured by increased hexobarbital and tolbutamide clearance. *Eur J Clin Pharmacol* (1975) 9, 219–27.
8. Syvälahti E, Pihlajamäki K, Iisalo E. Effect of tuberculostatic agents on the response of serum growth hormone and immunoreactive insulin to intravenous tolbutamide, and on the half-life of tolbutamide. *Int J Clin Pharmacol Biopharm* (1976) 13, 83–9.

Hypoglycaemic agents + Salicylates

Aspirin and other salicylates can lower blood sugar levels, but small analgesic doses do not normally have an adverse effect on patients taking hypoglycaemic agents. Some reduction in the dosage of the hypoglycaemic agent may be appropriate if large doses of salicylates are used.

Clinical evidence

(a) Insulin

Twelve juvenile diabetics treated with **insulin** showed a reduction in blood glucose levels averaging 15% (from 188 to 159 mg%) when additionally given either 1.2 g daily doses of **aspirin** (patients under 27.2 kg) or 2.4 g (patients over 27.2 kg) daily for a week. No significant changes in **insulin** requirements were necessary.[1]

Eight patients on 12 to 48 units **insulin zinc suspension** daily required no **insulin** when treated for 2 to 3 weeks with **aspirin** in doses large enough (3.5 to 7.5 g daily) to give maximum therapeutic serum salicylate levels of 35 to 45 mg/100 ml. Six other patients were able to reduce their **insulin** requirements by between about one-fifth to two-thirds.[2]

(b) Chlorpropamide

The blood glucose lowering effects of **chlorpropamide** and **sodium salicylate** were found to be additive in 5 normal subjects. A further study in 6 subjects showed that 100 mg **chlorpropamide** with 1.5 g **sodium salicylate** lowered blood sugar levels the same amount as either 200 mg **chlorpropamide** or 3 g **sodium salicylate** alone.[3]

The blood glucose levels of a patient on 500 mg **chlorpropamide** daily were lowered about two-thirds by **aspirin** in doses sufficient to give serum salicylate levels of 26 mg%.[4]

(c) Glibenclamide (Glyburide)

Sixteen normal subjects firstly took a single 5-mg dose of **glibenclamide**, then later they took 975 mg **aspirin** four times daily for 4 days, and then on the fourth day another single 5-mg dose of **glibenclamide**. It was found that the **aspirin** reduced the $AUC_{0-4\,h}$ of the **glibenclamide** by 68% and reduced its mean peak serum levels by 35%. The effects of this on glucose tolerance tests and insulin responses were difficult to interpret, but there was no clear evidence that any clinically relevant changes occurred.[5]

Mechanism

It has been known for over 100 years that aspirin and salicylates have hypoglycaemic properties and in relatively large doses can be used on their own in the treatment of diabetes.[6-10] The simplest explanation for this interaction with hypoglycaemic agents is that the blood sugar lowering effects are additive,[3] but there is some evidence that other mechanisms may come into play.[10] In addition aspirin can raise serum chlorpropamide levels so that its effects are increased, possibly by interfering with renal tubular excretion.[4]

Importance and management

The hypoglycaemic agent/salicylate interaction is established but of limited importance. Considering the extremely wide use of aspirin it might reasonably be expected that any generally serious interaction would have come to light by now. The data available, coupled with the common experience of diabetics,[11] is that excessive and unwanted hypoglycaemia is very unlikely with small to moderate analgesic doses. Some downward readjustment of the dosage of the hypoglycaemic agent may be appropriate if large doses of salicylates are used. Information about other hypoglycaemic agents and salicylates not cited here appears to be lacking, but they are expected to behave similarly.

1. Kaye R, Athreya BH, Kunzman EE, Baker L. Antipyretics in patients with juvenile diabetes mellitus. *Am J Dis Child* (1966) 112, 52–5.
2. Reid J, Lightbody TD. The insulin equivalence of salicylate. *BMJ* (1959) i, 897–900.
3. Richardson T, Foster J, Mawer GE. Enhancement by sodium salicylate of the blood glucose lowering effect of chlorpropamide - drug interaction or summation of similar effects? *Br J Clin Pharmacol* (1986) 22, 43–48.
4. Stowers JM, Constable LW, Hunter RB. A clinical and pharmacological comparison of chlorpropamide and other sulfonylureas. *Ann N Y Acad Sci* (1959) 74, 689–95.
5. Kubacka RT, Antal EJ, Juhl RP, Welshman IR. Effects of aspirin and ibuprofen on the pharmacokinetics and pharmacodynamics of glyburide in healthy subjects. *Ann Pharmacother* (1996) 30, 20–6.
6. Gilgore SG, Rupp JJ. The long-term response of diabetes mellitus to salicylate therapy. Report of a case. *JAMA* (1962) 180, 65–6.
7. Reid J, Macdougall AI, Andrews MM. Aspirin and diabetes mellitus. *BMJ* (1957) 2, 1071–4.
8. Ebstein W. Zur Therapie des Diabetes mellitus, insbesondere über die Anwendung des Salicylsauren Natron bei demselben. *Berl Klin Wschr* (1876) 13, 337–40.
9. Bartels K. Über die therapeutische Verwertung der Salizylsäure und ihres Nastronsalzes in der Inneren Medizin. *Dtsch Med Wschr* (1878) 4, 423.
10. Cattaneo AG, Caviezel F, Pozza G. Pharmacological interaction between tolbutamide and acetylsalicylic acid: study on insulin secretion in man. *Int J Clin Pharmacol Ther Toxicol* (1990) 28, 229–34.
11. Logie AW, Galloway DB, Petrie JC. Drug interactions and long-term antidiabetic therapy. *Br J Clin Pharmacol* (1976) 3, 1027–32.

Hypoglycaemic agents + Sex hormones

Some diabetics may require small increases or decreases in their dosage of hypoglycaemic agent while taking sex hormones such as oral contraceptives, but it is unusual for the control of diabetes to be seriously disturbed.

Clinical evidence

More than half of a group of 30 menopausal diabetics showed abnormal tolerance when given **norethynodrel** 5 mg + **mestranol** 0.075 mg but the changes in their requirements of **insulin** or **oral hypoglycaemic** agent were "few, scattered and slight in magnitude."[1]

In one study 34% of 179 diabetic women needed an increase in **insulin** and 7% a decrease when given a variety of **oral contraceptives,**[2] whereas in another study of 38 **insulin** dependent diabetics it was found that **progestogen-only** and **combined oral contraceptives** had little effect on the control of diabetes.[3] Another report[4] about women on *Orthonovin* (**norethisterone + mestranol**) stated that no **insulin** changes were necessary. More recent reports from studies using newer, low dose **oral contraceptives**, support the suggestion that changes in glucose metabolism are minimal.[5] Problems with glucose metabolism seem very unlikely when the dose of oestrogen is less then 50 micrograms.[6] However, there are a few scattered reports of individual diabetics who experienced a marked disturbance of their diabetic control when given an **oral contraceptive**, some of which were low dose.[7-10]

Mechanism

Not understood. Many mechanisms have been considered including changes in cortisol secretion, alterations in tissue glucose utilisation, production of excessive amounts of growth hormone, and alterations in liver function.[11]

Importance and management

Moderately well documented. Concurrent use need not be avoided, but because some patients need a small adjustment in their dosage of hypoglycaemic agent (increases or decreases) and because very occasionally serious disturbances occur, the diabetic response should be monitored. Also bear in mind that the lowest strength preparations (less than 20 micrograms oestrogen) are recommended for patients with risk factors for circulatory disease (such as diabetics) so the potential for interference with their diabetic control will be minimised if this recommendation is followed.

1. Cochran B and Pote WWH. C–19 nor-steroid effects on plasma lipid and diabetic control of postmenopausal women. *Diabetes* (1963) 12, 366.
2. Zeller WJ, Brehm H, Schoffling K and Melzer H. Vertraglichkeit von hormonalen Ovulationshemmern bei Diabetikerinnen. *Arzneimittelforschung* (1974) 24, 351.
3. Radberg T, Gustafson A, Skryten A and Karlsson K. Oral contraception in diabetic women. Diabetes control, serum and high density lipoprotein lipids during low-dose progestogen, combined oestrogen/progestogen and non-hormonal contraception. *Acta Endocrinol (Copenh)* (1981) 98, 246–51.
4. Tyler ET, Olsen HJ, Gotlib M, Levin M and Behne D. Long term usage of norethindrone with mestranol preparations in the control of human fertility. *Clin Med* (1964) 71, 997.
5. Miccoli R, Orlandi MC, Fruzzetti F, Giampietro O, Melis G, Ricci C, Bertolotto A, Fioretti P, Navalesi R, Masoni A. Metabolic effects of three new low-dose pills: a six-month experience. *Contraception* (1989) 39, 643–52.
6. Spellacy WN. Carbohydrate metabolism during treatment with estrogen, progestogen, and low-dose oral contraceptives. *Am J Obstet Gynecol* (1982) 142, 732–4.
7. Kopera H, Dukes NG and Ijzerman GL. Critical evaluation of clinical data on *Lyndiol*. *Int J Fertil* (1964) 9, 69.
8. Peterson WF, Steel MW and Coyne RY. Analysis of the effect of ovulatory suppressants on glucose tolerance. *Am J Obstet Gynecol* (1966) 95, 484.
9. Reder JA and Tulgan H. Impairment of diabetic control by norethynodrel with mestranol. *N Y State J Med* (1967) 67, 1073.
10. Rennie NJ. Hyperglycaemic episodes in a young woman after taking levonorgestrel-containing oral contraceptives. *N Z Med J* (1994) 107, 440–1.
11. Spellacy WN. A review of carbohydrate metabolism and the oral contraceptives. *Am J Obstet Gynecol* (1969) 104, 448.

Hypoglycaemic agents + Statins

No clinically relevant adverse interactions appear to occur with these pairs of drugs: chlorpropamide/lovastatin, glibenclamide (glyburide)/fluvastatin, glibenclamide/simvastatin, tolbutamide/fluvastatin or tolbutamide/simvastatin.

Clinical evidence

(a) Chlorpropamide + Lovastatin

A study in 7 non-insulin dependent diabetic patients with hypercholesterolaemia and on **chlorpropamide** 125 to 750 mg daily found that **lovastatin** (20 mg twice daily for 6 weeks) reduced low-density lipoprotein cholesterol by 28%, total cholesterol by 24% and apolipoprotein B by 24%. The **chlorpropamide** plasma levels were unchanged, and the diabetic control remained unaltered.[1]

(b) Tolbutamide or Glibenclamide + Fluvastatin or Simvastatin

Groups of 16 normal subjects on 40 mg **fluvastatin** or 20 mg **simvastatin** daily were given single oral doses of 3.5 mg **glibenclamide** (**glyburide**) on days 1, 8 and 15. The maximum plasma concentrations and the AUCs of the **glibenclamide** were increased by about 20%. The hypoglycaemic actions of the **glibenclamide** remained virtually unchanged by both **fluvastatin** and **simvastatin** in these subjects, and also when **fluvastatin** was tested in a group of 32 patients with non-insulin dependent diabetes.[2]

In the same series of tests, 16 normal subjects on 40 mg **fluvastatin** and 16 normal subjects on 20 mg **simvastatin** were given single 1 g oral doses of **tolbutamide**. The pharmacokinetics of the **tolbutamide** was affected only to a very minor extent, and the hypoglycaemic effects of the **tolbutamide** were unchanged.[2]

Mechanism

The small changes in the pharmacokinetics of glibenclamide caused by fluvastatin and simvastatin are not understood.

Importance and management

No special precautions appear to be needed by diabetic patients taking any of the pairs of drugs cited here. Information about other sulphonylurea hypoglycaemic agents and HMG-CoA reductase inhibitors (statins) seems not to be available.

1. Johnson BF, LaBelle P, Wilson J, Allan J, Zupkis RV, Ronca PD. Effects of lovastatin in diabetic patients treated with chlorpropamide. *Clin Pharmacol Ther* (1990) 48, 467–72.
2. Appel S, Rüfenacht T, Kalafsky G, Tetzloff W, Kallay Z, Hitzenberger G, Kutz K. Lack of interaction between fluvastatin and oral hypoglycemic agents in healthy subjects and in patients with non-insulin-dependent diabetes mellitus. *Am J Cardiol* (1995) 76, 29A–32A.

Hypoglycaemic agents + Sucralfate

Sucralfate appears not to interact significantly with chlorpropamide.

Clinical evidence, mechanism, importance and management

A two-way crossover study in 12 normal subjects showed that 1 g sucralfate four times a day 1 h before meals had no significant effect on the pharmacokinetics of a single 250-mg dose of **chlorpropamide**.[1] This seems unlikely to be clinically important. There seems to be no information about the effects of **sucralfate** on other hypoglycaemic agents.

1. Letendre PW, Carlson JD, Siefert RD, Dietz AJ, Dimmit D. Effect of sucralfate on the absorption and pharmacokinetics of chlorpropamide. *J Clin Pharmacol* (1986) 26, 622–5.

Hypoglycaemic agents + Sugar-containing pharmaceuticals

Some pharmaceutical preparations may contain sufficient amounts of sugar to affect the control of diabetes. Diabetics should be warned and advised of sugar-free alternatives where appropriate.

Clinical evidence, mechanism, importance and management

Pharmaceuticals, especially liquid formulations, may contain sugar in significant amounts. The extent to which the administration of preparations like these will affect the control of diabetes clearly depends upon the amounts ingested, but the problem is by no means merely theoretical. One report describes the loss of control in a woman given psyllium effervescent powder (*Metamucil* instant-mix) which contains **sugar**.[1] The range of other **sugar**-containing preparations is far too extensive to be listed here. Because of concerns over sugar-containing medicines and dental caries in children, in particular, the number of sugar-free preparations has grown considerably over recent years. in the UK the British National Formulary and MIMS provide guidance as to which preparations are sugar-free. Diabetics should be warned about sugar-containing medicines, and given guidance about the terminology used in labelling. Sweetening agents of not to diabetics include: invert sugar (dextrose and fructose), invert syrup (67% w/w invert sugar), syrup BP (66% w/w sucrose), glucose liquid (dextrose content 10 to 20%), glucose syrup (33.3% liquid glucose in syrup) and honey (70 to 80% glucose and fructose).[2]

1. Catellani J, Collins RJ. Drug labelling. *Lancet* (1978) ii, 98.
2. Greenwood J. Sugar content of liquid prescription medicines. *Pharm J* (1989) 243, 553–7.

Hypoglycaemic agents + Sulfinpyrazone

Sulfinpyrazone has no effect on the insulin requirements of diabetics, nor does it affect the control of patients taking glib-enclamide (glyburide). Increased hypoglycaemia might occur with tolbutamide, but as yet there appear to be no case reports of this interaction, nor of any adverse interactions with other hypoglycaemic agents.**

Clinical evidence

(a) Insulin

A double blind study, extending over 12 months, in 41 adult diabetics showed that the daily administration of 600 to 800 mg **sulfinpyrazone** had no clinically significant effects on their **insulin** requirements.[1]

(b) Glibenclamide

A study in 19 type II diabetics taking **glibenclamide (glyburide)** showed that 800 mg **sulfinpyrazone** daily did not affect the control of their diabetes.[2]

(c) Tolbutamide

A detailed study of the pharmacokinetics of **tolbutamide** in 6 normal subjects showed that after taking 200 mg **sulfinpyrazone** every 6 h for a week, the half-life of intravenously administered **tolbutamide** 500 mg was almost doubled (from 7.3 to 13.2 h) and the plasma clearance reduced by 40%.[3]

Mechanism

The available evidence suggests that the tolbutamide/sulfinpyrazone interaction occurs because the sulfinpyrazone inhibits the metabolism of tolbutamide by the liver.[3]

Importance and management

Information about the tolbutamide/sulfinpyrazone interaction appears to be limited to the report cited. So far there appear to be no reports of adverse interactions in patients, but what is known suggests that increased and possibly excessive hypoglycaemia could occur if the dosage of tolbutamide is not reduced. Such an interaction has been described with phenylbutazone with which sulfinpyrazone has a close structural similarity (see appropriate monograph). Patients should be warned if sulfinpyrazone is added to established treatment with tolbutamide. There seems to be nothing documented about any other clinically important hypoglycaemic agent/sulfinpyrazone interaction.

1. Pannebakker MAG, den Ottolander GJH, ten Pas JG. Insulin requirements in diabetic patients treated with sulphinpyrazone. *J Int Med Res* (1979) 7, 328–31.
2. Kritz H, Najemnik C, Irsigler K. Interaktionsstudie mit Sulfinpyrazon (Anturan) und Glibenclamid (Euglucon) bei Typ-II-Diabetikern. *Wien Med Wochenschr* (1983) 133, 237–43.
3. Miners JO, Foenander T, Wanwimolruk S, Gallus AS, Birkett DJ. The effect of sulphinpyrazone on oxidative drug metabolism in man: inhibition of tolbutamide elimination. *Eur J Clin Pharmacol* (1982) 22, 321–6.

Hypoglycaemic agents + Sulphonamides

The hypoglycaemic effects of some of the sulphonylureas are increased by some, but not all, sulphonamides. Occasionally and unpredictably acute hypoglycaemia has occurred in individual patients. There appear to be no reports of adverse insulin/sulphonamide interactions.

Clinical evidence

Table 15.4 summarises the information the hypoglycaemic agent/sulphonamide interactions.[1-20]

Mechanism

Not fully understood. The sulphonamides may inhibit the metabolism of the sulphonylureas so that they accumulate in the body. In this way their serum levels and hypoglycaemic effects are enhanced.[3,5,6,21] There is also evidence that the sulphonamides can displace the sulphonylureas from their protein binding sites.[21] Hypoglycaemia in-

Table 15.4 Hypoglycaemic agent/sulphonamide interactions

Drugs	Information documented	Refs
Chlorpropamide		
+ sulfafurazole (sulfisoxazole)	I case of acute hypoglycaemia	7
+ sulfadimidine	I case of acute hypoglycaemia	8
+ co-trimoxazole	2 cases of acute hypoglycaemia	9, 12
Glibenclamide		
+ co-trimoxazole		
	In a large review of glibenclamide-associated hypoglycaemia 11% were also taking co-trimoxazole	14
	8 cases of hypoglycaemia	18, 19
	Stated to be no pharmacokinetic interaction	14, 16
Glibornuride		
+ sulfaphenazole	Stated to be no interaction	10
Gliclazide		
+ co-trimoxazole	4 cases of acute hypoglycaemia	19
Glipizide		
+ co-trimoxazole	I case of acute hypoglycaemia	17
	I study stating no interaction	20
Insulin		
+ co-trimoxazole	No significant changes in blood glucose or insulin concentrations	13
Tolbutamide		
+ co-trimoxazole	Clearance reduced 25%, half-life increased 30%	15
+ sulfafurazole (sulfisoxazole)	3 cases of severe hypoglycaemia	1, 2
	4 reports state no interaction	4, 7, 11
+ sulfamethizole	Half-life of tolbutamide increased 60%. Metabolic clearance reduced 40%	3, 4
+ sulfaphenazole	2 cases of severe hypoglycaemia	6
	Half-life of tolbutamide increased x4–6	5, 6, 11
+ sulfadiazine	Half-life of tolbutamide increased	5
+ sulfadimethoxine	Stated to be no interaction	4, 6, 11
+ sulfametoxypyridazine	Stated to be no interaction	4, 6
+ sulfamethoxazole	Clearance reduced 14%, half-life increased 20%	15
	5 cases of no interaction	11
Un-named sulphonylurea		
+ co-trimoxazole	I case of acute hypoglycaemia	13

duced by sulphonamides, in the absence of a conventional hypogly-caemic agent,[22] and sometimes associated with renal failure,[18] has been described.

Importance and management

Information is very patchy and incomplete. Most sulphonamides seem to have caused marked problems (acute hypoglycaemia) in only a few patients and serious interactions are uncommon. Firm predictions cannot be made about what will, or what will not, interact in individual patients, nor how clinically important the reaction may prove to be, but Table 15.4 can be used as a broad guide. When you first add a sulphonamide to established treatment with a sulphonylurea, refer to the table and where an interaction has been recorded, warn the patient that increased hypoglycaemia, sometimes excessive, is a possibility, but that problems appear to be uncommon or rare. Co-trimoxazole does not appear to cause any significant changes in blood glucose or insulin concentrations in patients receiving insulin[13] and there appear to be no reports involving other sulphonamides.

1. Soeldner JS, Steinke J. Hypoglycemia in tolbutamide-treated diabetes. *JAMA* (1965) 193, 148–9.

2. Robinson DS. The application of basic principles of drug interaction to clinical practice. *J Urol* (1975) 113, 100–107.

3. Lumholtz B, Siersbaek-Nielsen K, Skovsted L, Kampmann J, Hansen JM. Sulphame-thizole-induced inhibition of diphenylhydantoin, tolbutamide, and warfarin metabolism. *Clin Pharmacol Ther* (1975) 17, 731–4.

4. Siersbaek-Nielsen K, Mølholm Hansen J, Skovsted L, Lumholtz B, Kampmann J. Sul-famethizole-induced inhibition of diphenylhydantoin and tolbutamide metabolism in man. *Clin Pharmacol Ther* (1973) 14, 148.

5. Kristensen M, Christensen LK. Drug induced changes of the blood glucose lowering effect of oral hypoglycemic agents. *Acta Diabetol Lat* (1969) 6 (Suppl 1), 116–23.

6. Christensen LK, Hansen JM, Kristensen M. Sulphaphenazole-induced hypoglycaemic attacks in tolbutamide-treated diabetics. *Lancet* (1963) ii, 1298–1301.

7. Tucker HSG, Hirsch JI. Sulfonamide-sulfonylurea interaction. *N Engl J Med* (1972) 286, 110–11.

8. Dall JLC, Conway H, McAlpine SG. Hypoglycaemia due to chlorpropamide. *Scott Med J* (1967) 12, 403–4.

9. Ek I. Långvarigt klorpropamidutlöst hypoglykemitillstand Läkemedelsinteraktion? *Lakartidningen* (1974) 71, 2597–8.

10. Eckhardt W, Rudolph R, Sauer H, Schubert WR, Undeutsch D. Zur pharmakologischen Interferenz von Glibornurid mit Sulfaphenazol, Phenylbutazon und Phenprocoumon beim Menschen. *Arzneimittelforschung* (1972) 22, 2212–19.

11. Dubach UC, Buckert A, Raaflaub J. Einfluss von Sulfonamiden auf die blutzuckersenk-ende Wirkung oraler Antidiabetica. *Schweiz Med Wochenschr* (1966) 96, 1483–6.

12. Baciewicz AM, Swafford WB. Hypoglycemia induced by the interaction of chlorpropa-mide and co-trimoxazole. *Drug Intell Clin Pharm* (1984) 18, 309–10.

13. Mihic M, Mautner LS, Feness JZ, Grant K. Effect of trimethoprim-sulfamethoxazole on blood insulin and glucose concentrations of diabetics. *Can Med Assoc J* (1975), 112, 80S–82S.

14. Sjöberg S, Wiholm BE, Gunnarsson R, Emilsson H, Thunberg E, Christenson I, Östman J. No evidence for pharmacokinetic interaction between glibenclamide and trimetho-prim-sulfamethoxazole. *Diabetes Res Clin Pract* (1985) (Suppl 1), S522.

15. Wing LMH, Miners JO. Cotrimoxazole as an inhibitor of oxidative drug metabolism: effects of trimethoprim and sulphamethoxazole separately and combined on tolbutamide disposition. *Br J Clin Pharmacol* (1985) 20, 482–5.

16. Sjöberg S, Wiholm BE, Gunnarsson R, Emilsson H, Thunberg E, Christenson I, Östman J. Lack of pharmacokinetic interaction between glibenclamide and trimethoprim-sulphamethoxazole. *Diabet Med* (1987) 4, 245–7.
17. Johnson JF, Dobmeier ME. Symptomatic hypoglycemia secondary to a glipizide-trimethoprim/sulfamethoxazole drug interaction. *DICP Ann Pharmacother* (1990) 24, 250–1.
18. Asplund K, Wiholm B-E, Lithner F. Glibenclamide-associated hypoglycaemia: a report on 57 cases. *Diabetologia* (1983) 24, 412–7.
19. Girardin E, Vial T, Pham E, Evreux J-C. Hypoglycémies induites par les sulfamides hypoglycémiants. *Ann Med Interne (Paris)* (1992) 143, 11–17.
20. Kradjan WA, Witt DM, Opheim KE, Wood FC. Lack of interaction between glipizide and co-trimoxazole. *J Clin Pharmacol* (1994) 34, 997–1002.
21. Hellman B. Potentiating effects of drugs on the binding of glibenclamide to pancreatic beta cells. *Metabolism* (1974) 23, 839–46.
22. Hekimsoy Z, Biberoglu S, Comlecki A, Tarhan O, Mermut C, Biberoglu K. Trimethoprim-sulfamethoxazole-induced hypoglycemia in a malnourished patient with severe infection. *Eur J Endocrinol* (1997) 136, 304–6.

Hypoglycaemic agents + Tetracyclines

A few scattered reports indicate that the hypoglycaemic effects of insulin and the sulphonylureas may sometimes be increased by oxytetracycline, and limited evidence suggests that this may also occur with doxycycline. Phenformin-induced lactic acidosis may be precipitated by tetracyclines.

Clinical evidence

(a) Insulin or Sulphonylureas + Tetracyclines

A poorly controlled diabetic needed a marked reduction in his **insulin** dosage (from 208 to 64 units daily) in order to control the hypoglycaemia which developed when also given 250 mg **oxytetracycline** four times a day. This reaction was also seen when the patient was given a second course of antibacterials, and in another patient.[1]

Marked hypoglycaemia occurred in an elderly patient on **tolbutamide** when given **oxytetracycline**,[2] and the hypoglycaemic effects of **oxytetracycline** have also been demonstrated in *dogs*.[2] Another study in diabetic subjects similarly showed that **oxytetracycline** can reduce blood sugar levels.[3] A very brief report describes hypoglycaemia in a patient on **insulin** when given **doxycycline**.[4] The half-life of **glymidine** in man has been shown to be prolonged from 4.6 to 7.6 h by **doxycycline**,[5] whereas a brief comment in another report suggests that **demeclocycline** and **doxycycline** may not affect **chlorpropamide**.[6]

(b) Biguanides + Tetracyclines

There are now at least 6 cases on record of lactic-acidosis in patients on **phenformin** that were apparently precipitated by the concurrent use of **tetracycline**.[7-10]

Mechanisms

Not understood.

Importance and management

Information about the interactions between the sulphonylureas or insulin and the tetracyclines is very limited indeed, and clinically important interactions appear to be very uncommon. Concurrent use need not be avoided but warn the patient that increased hypoglycaemia is a possibility if tetracyclines are added, particularly oxytetracycline and doxycycline. Reduce the dosage of the hypoglycaemic agent if necessary. Phenformin was withdrawn in some countries because it was associated with a high incidence of lactic acidosis; where available, concurrent use with tetracyclines should be avoided. However, there is nothing to suggest that there is an increased risk if tetracyclines are given with metformin.

1. Miller JB. Hypoglycaemic effect of oxytetracycline. *BMJ* (1966) 2, 1007.
2. Hiatt N, Bonorris G. Insulin response in pancreatectomized dogs treated with oxytetracycline. *Diabetes* (1970) 19, 307–10.
3. Sen S, Mukerjee AB. Hypoglycaemic action of oxytetracycline. A preliminary study. *J Indian Med Assoc* (1969) 52, 366–9.
4. New Zealand Committee on Adverse Drug Reactions. Ninth Annual Report. *N Z Dent J* (1975) 71, 28–32.
5. Held H, Kaminski B, von Olderhausen HF. Die beeinflussung der Elimination von Glycodiazin durch Leber- und Nierenfunctionssorungen und durch eine Behandlung mit Phenylbutazon, Phenprocoumarol und Doxycyclin. *Diabetologia* (1970) 6, 386.
6. Petitpierre B, Perrin L, Rudhardt M, Herrera A, Fabre J. Behaviour of chlorpropamide in renal insufficiency and under the effect of associated drug therapy. *Int J Clin Pharmacol* (1972) 6, 120–24.
7. Aro A, Korhonen T, Halinen M. Phenformin-induced lactic acidosis precipitated by tetracycline. *Lancet* (1978) 1, 673–4.
8. Tashima CK. Phenformin, tetracycline, and lactic acidosis. *BMJ* (1971) 4, 557–8.
9. Blumenthal SA, Streeten DHP. Phenformin-related lactic acidosis in a 30–year old man. *Ann Intern Med* (1976) 84, 55–6.
10. Phillips PJ, Pain RW. Phenformin, tetracycline and lactic acidosis. *Ann Intern Med* (1977) 86, 111.

Hypoglycaemic agents + Thioctic acid

Thioctic acid is reported not to interact with metformin or glibenclamide (glyburide).

Clinical evidence, mechanism, importance and management

A study in 24 normal subjects given tablets containing 200 mg **thioctic acid** and 500 mg **metformin** found that the pharmacokinetics of the **metformin** were unchanged by the presence of the **thioctic acid**, and the authors of the report say that there was also no pharmacodynamic interaction.[1] The report gives very few details. A further study in 24 normal subjects found that single doses of **thioctic acid** 600 mg with **glibenclamide (glyburide)** 3.5 mg did not result in any clinically relevant pharmacokinetic interactions.[2]

1. Schug BS, Schneider E, Elze M, Fieger-Büschges H, Larsimont V, Popescu G, Molz KH, Blume HH, Hermann R. Study of pharmacokinetic interaction of thioctic acid and metformin. *Eur J Clin Pharmacol* (1997) 52 (Suppl), A140.
2. Gleiter CH, Schreeb KH, Freudenthaler S, Thomas M, Elze M, Fieger-Büschges H, Potthast H, Schneider E, Schug BS, Blume HH, Hermann R. Lack of interaction between thioctic acid, glibenclamide and acarbose. *Br J Clin Pharmacol* (1999) 48, 81–25.

Hypoglycaemic agents + Tobacco smoking

Diabetics who smoke need more insulin than non-smokers.

Clinical evidence, mechanism, importance and management

A study carried out in over 100 **insulin-dependent diabetic smokers** showed that on average they needed 15 to 20% more **insulin** than non-smokers, and up to 30% more if they **smoked** heavily.[1,2] Possible mechanisms include decreased absorption of insulin from the subcutaneous tissue and a significant rise (40 to 120%) in the levels of the hormones which oppose the actions of **insulin**.[3] A consequence of this interaction is that diabetics who give up **smoking** may then need a downward adjustment of their insulin dosage.

1. Klemp P, Staberg B, Madsbad S, Kølendorf K. Smoking reduces insulin absorption from subcutaneous tissue. *BMJ* (1982) 284, 237.
2. Madsbad S, McNair P, Christensen MS, Christiansen C, Faber OK, Binder C, Transbøl I. Influence of smoking on insulin requirement and metabolic status in diabetes mellitus. *Diabetes Care* (1980) 3, 41–3.
3. Helve E, Yki-Järvinen H, Koivisto VA. Smoking and insulin sensitivity in type I diabetes. *Diabetes Res Clin Pract* (1985) (Suppl 1), S232.

Hypoglycaemic agents + Tolrestat

Tolrestat does not affect the control of diabetes in patients using diet, glibenclamide (glyburide) or insulin.

Clinical evidence, mechanism, importance and management

In a randomised double-blind placebo-controlled crossover study, 46 patients using either **diet** alone, **glibenclamide (glyburide)** or **insulin** were also treated with 400 mg **tolrestat** daily for 7 days. The pharmacokinetics of the **tolrestat** and the **glibenclamide (glyburide)** were not significantly changed and the control of their diabetes was unaltered. **Tolrestat** did not alter glucose or insulin levels. On the basis of these findings it was concluded that diabetic patients using diet and these drugs do not need to adjust their diabetic treatment if given **tolrestat**.[1] Information about other hypoglycaemic agents is lacking.

1. Meng X, Parker V, Burghart P, DiLea C, Mallett S, Gonen B, Chiang S. Effects of tolrestat (T) on plasma glucose (G) levels in diet-, glyburide- and insulin-controlled (D, Gly and I) diabetics. *Clin Pharmacol Ther* (1995) 57, 154.

Hypoglycaemic agents + Tricyclic and Tetracyclic antidepressants

Interactions between hypoglycaemic agents and these antidepressants appear to be rare, but four isolated cases of hypoglycaemia have been recorded in patients taking tolazamide with doxepin, chlorpropamide with nortriptyline, insulin with amitriptyline, and glibenclamide (glyburide)/phenformin with maprotiline.

Clinical evidence, mechanism, importance and management

A patient on **tolazamide** became hypoglycaemic 11 days after starting to take **doxepin** 250 mg/day; another on **chlorpropamide** (increased from 25 to 75 mg daily) developed marked hypoglycaemia 3 days after starting 125 mg **nortriptyline** daily;[1] a further patient on **insulin** developed violent and agitated behaviour (but no adrenergic symptoms) and hypoglycaemia when she started to take 25 mg **amitriptyline** at bedtime.[2] An elderly diabetic woman on **glibenclamide (glyburide)** and **phenformin** developed hypoglycaemia when given **maprotiline**.[3] The reasons are not understood. An earlier study suggested that no interaction was likely: 4 patients given 9 days' treatment with 75 mg **amitriptyline** daily showed no change in the half-life of a single 500-mg dose of **tolbutamide**.[4]

The patient on **doxepin** was eventually stabilised on a daily dose of **tolazamide** which was only 10% of that used before the **doxepin** was given.[1] The woman given nortriptyline stopped chlorpropamide,[1] and the woman given **maprotiline** was restabilised on half the dose of **glibenclamide/phenformin**.[3]

Apart from these cases the literature seems to be silent about interactions between these hypoglycaemics and the cyclic antidepressants. Bearing in mind the length of time these groups of drugs have been available, the risk of a clinically important interaction would seem to be very small, nevertheless be alert for any evidence of increased hypoglycaemia if both are given.

1. True BL, Perry PJ, Burns EA. Profound hypoglycemia with the addition of a tricyclic antidepressant to maintenance sulfonylurea therapy. *Am J Psychiatry* (1987) 144, 1220–1.
2. Sherman KE, Bornemann M. Amitriptyline and asymptomatic hypoglycemia. *Ann Intern Med* (1988) 109, 683–4.
3. Zogno MG, Tolfo L, Draghi E. Hypoglycemia caused by maprotiline in a patient taking oral antidiabetics. *Ann Pharmacother* (1994) 28, 406.
4. Pond SM, Graham GG, Birkett DJ, Wade DN. Effects of tricyclic antidepressants on drug metabolism. *Clin Pharmacol Ther* (1975) 18, 191–9.

Hypoglycaemic agents + Urinary alkalinizers and acidifiers

On theoretical grounds the response to chlorpropamide may be decreased if the urine is made alkaline, and increased if urine is acidified, Metabolic interactions with chlorpropamide are likely to be more apparent when the urine is acidic, but so far no adverse interactions appear to have been reported.

Clinical evidence, mechanism, importance and management

A study in 6 normal subjects given 250 mg oral doses of **chlorpropamide** showed that when the urine was made alkaline (pH 7.1 to 8.2) with **sodium bicarbonate**, the half-life of the **chlorpropamide** was reduced from 50 to 13 h, and the 72 h clearance was increased fourfold. In contrast, when the urine was acidified (pH 5.5 to 4.7) with **ammonium chloride**, the **chlorpropamide** half-life was increased from 50 to 69 h and the 72 h urinary clearance was decreased to one-twentieth, and non-renal (i.e. metabolic) clearance predominated.[1] Another study showed that the renal clearance of **chlorpropamide** was almost 100 times greater at pH 7 than at pH 5.[2] The reasons are that changes in urinary pH affect the ionisation of the **chlorpropamide**, and this affects the ability of the kidney to reabsorb it from the kidney filtrate (see more details of this interaction mechanism in the introductory chapter). Thus, urinary pH determines the relative contribution of renal and metabolic clearance.

There appear to be no reports of adverse interactions between **chlorpropamide** and drugs that can alter urinary pH, but prescribers should be aware of the possibilities: a reduced response if the pH is raised significantly and renal clearance predominates (e.g. with **sodium bicarbonate**, **acetazolamide**, some **antacids**); an increased response if the pH is made more acid than usual and metabolic clearance predominates (e.g. with **ammonium chloride**). Perhaps more importantly, the effects of drugs that alter the hepatic clearance of chlorpropamide are likely to be more significant when its renal clearance is low (i.e. when the urine is acid).[2]

1. Neuvonen PJ, Kärkkäinen S. Effects of charcoal, sodium bicarbonate, and ammonium chloride on chlorpropamide kinetics. *Clin Pharmacol Ther* (1983) 33, 386–93.
2. Neuvonen PJ, Kärkkäinen S and Lehtovaara R. Pharmacokinetics of chlorpropamide in epileptic patients: effects of enzyme induction and urine pH on chlorpropamide elimination. *Eur J Clin Pharmacol* (1987) 32, 297–301.

Hypoglycaemic agents + Vinpocetine

Vinpocetine does not interact with glibenclamide (glyburide).

Clinical evidence, mechanism, importance and management

A study in 18 elderly patients with type II diabetes and symptoms of dementia, under treatment with **glibenclamide**, showed that days treatment with 10 mg **vinpocetine**, three times daily, did not affect either the pharmacokinetics of the **glibenclamide** or the control of blood glucose levels.[1] There would seem to be no reason for avoiding concurrent use. There seems to be no information about the effects of **vinpocetine** on other hypoglycaemic agents.

1. Grandt R, Braun W, Schulz H-U, Lührmann B, Frercks H-J. Glibenclamide steady-state plasma levels during concomitant vinpocetine administration in type II diabetic patients. *Arzneimittelforschung* (1989) 39, 1451–4.

Metformin + Iodinated contrast media

Intravascular administration of iodinated contrast media may cause renal failure, which could result in lactic acidosis in patients taking metformin.

Clinical evidence, mechanism, importance and management

Intravascular administration of **iodinated contrast media** to patients on metformin may result in lactic acidosis. However, the problem is reported to occur only if the **contrast media** causes renal failure and metformin administration is continued. This is because metformin is mainly excreted by the kidneys and in renal failure toxic levels may accumulate.[1] A literature search identified 18 cases of lactic acidosis after the use of **contrast media** in patients on metformin.[2] Of these 18 cases, 14 or 15 were associated with pre-existing renal impairment and 2 with other contraindications to metformin (sepsis and cirrhosis). The remaining case was in an elderly woman with neurological disease.

The makers of metformin say that metformin should be stopped before, or at the time of giving the **contrast media** and not restarted until 48 h later, and then only after renal function has been re-checked and found to be normal.[3] Guidelines issued by the Royal College of Radiologists are based on this statement and they say that referring clinicians should assess renal function before the test.[4] However, some consider that metformin need not be stopped for 48 hours in those patients with normal renal function.[2]

1. Rasuli P, Hammond DI. Metformin and contrast media: where is the conflict? *Can Assoc Radiol J* (1998) 49, 161–6.
2. McCartney MM, Gilbert FJ, Murchison LE, Pearson D, McHardy K, Murray AD. Metformin and contrast media – a dangerous combination? *Clin Radiol* (1999) 54, 29–33.
3. Glucophage (Metformin hydrochloride). Lipha Pharmaceuticals Limited. Summary of product characteristics. March 2001.
4. The Royal College of Radiologists. Guidelines with regard to metformin-induced lactic acidosis and x-ray contrast medium agents. 19th March 1999.

Pioglitazone + Miscellaneous drugs

The makers contraindicate the use of pioglitazone with insulin and suggest caution with either ketoconazole or oral contraceptives. Pioglitazone does not interact adversely with digoxin, glipizide, metformin, phenprocoumon or warfarin and is not expected to interact with drugs such as ciclosporin, calcium channel blockers or statins.

Clinical evidence and mechanism

(a) Drugs which possibly interact

(i) Insulin. It has been noted that in patients on **insulin** the dose may need to be reduced by 10 to 25% if pioglitazone 15 or 30 mg daily is co-administered.[1] The combination is used in the US, however, in the UK, the use of pioglitazone with insulin is contraindicated because of reports of cardiac failure with this combination.[2]

(ii) Ketoconazole. Although there appear to be no adverse reports, because **ketoconazole** is known from *in vitro* studies to inhibit the liver metabolism of pioglitazone by 85%, the makers recommend that more frequent blood glucose measurements should be made[1] so as to ensure that the effects of pioglitazone are not undesirably increased.

(iii) Oral contraceptives. Although no pharmacokinetic studies have been done with pioglitazone and **oral contraceptives**, no interaction is expected because pioglitazone does not inhibit any of the enzymes which metabolise oral contraceptive hormones (see (b) below). The makers in the UK therefore do not suggest precautions are necessary. However because a related hypoglycaemic (troglitazone) reduces the levels of ethinyloestradiol and norethisterone by 30%, in the US the makers advise caution with pioglitazone and oral contraceptives.

(b) Drugs reported not to interact adversely

In healthy subjects co-administration of pioglitazone 45 mg daily with **glipizide** 5 mg daily or metformin 1 g daily for 7 days did not alter the steady-state pharmacokinetics of glipizide or **metformin**.[1,3] In normal subjects co-administration of pioglitazone with **digoxin** 250 micrograms daily for 7 days did not alter the steady-state pharmacokinetics of digoxin.[1,3] Co-administration of pioglitazone 45 mg daily with warfarin did not alter the steady-state pharmacokinetics of **warfarin** and there was no significant change in prothrombin time.[1,3] Similar results were noted with **phenprocoumon**.[3] *In vitro* studies have shown no inhibition of cytochrome P450 isoenzymes by pioglitazone.[1,3] Studies[2,3] in man suggest pioglitazone neither inhibits nor induces cytochrome P450 isoenzymes CYP3A4, CYP2C8/9 and CYP1A1/2. Interactions with drugs metabolised by these enzymes such as **ciclosporin, calcium channel blockers** and **statins** are therefore not expected.[1]

Importance and management

No special precautions seem necessary with any of these drugs (b) used concurrently with pioglitazone. Increased blood glucose monitoring is recommended when using pioglitazone with ketoconazole, and until further information is available, caution should be applied to any concurrent use with oral contraceptives.

1. Actos (Pioglitazone hydrochloride). Takeda Ltd, US product information, July 1999.
2. Actos (Pioglitazone hydrochloride). Takeda Ltd, Summary of product characteristics, October 2000.
3. Kortboyer JM, Eckland DJA. Pioglitazone has low potential for drug interactions. *Diabetologia* (1999) 42 (Suppl 1), A228.

Repaglinide + Miscellaneous drugs

On the basis of *in vitro* studies, the makers of repaglinide contraindicate erythromycin, fluconazole, itraconazole, ketoconazole, phenytoin and rifampicin, and they warn about possible changes in the response to repaglinide if taken with drugs that raise or lower blood sugar levels. Repaglinide does not interact adversely with cimetidine, digoxin, theophylline or warfarin. It may be used in combination with metformin but the makers say that there is an increased risk of hypoglycaemia.

Clinical evidence, mechanism, importance and management

The makers of repaglinide say that although no *in vivo* studies have been done, *in vitro* studies show that repaglinide is primarily metabolised by cytochrome P450 isoenzyme CYP3A4 and it is therefore predicted that CYP3A4 inhibitors such as **erythromycin, fluconazole, itraconazole** and **ketoconazole** will increase the plasma levels of repaglinide, whereas compounds which induce CYP3A4 such as **phenytoin** and **rifampicin** will decrease repaglinide plasma levels. Since the extent of these changes is not yet known, the makers contraindicate the concurrent use of these drugs until more information becomes available.[1]

The makers also point out that because a variety of drugs can affect glucose metabolism, the following interactions should be considered when prescribing repaglinide: increased hypoglycaemia with **ACE inhibitors, alcohol, anabolic steroids, non-selective beta-blockers, MAOIs, NSAIDs, octreotide** and **salicylates**; reduced hypoglycaemia with **corticosteroids, danazol, oral contraceptives, sympathomimetics, thiazides** and **thyroid hormones**. Only time will tell whether any of these predicted interactions is of clinical importance. In addition the makers also point out that **beta-blockers** may mask the signs and symptoms of hypoglycaemia, and **alcohol** may intensify and prolong the hypoglycaemic effects of repaglinide.[1]

An open label crossover single-dose and multiple-dose trial in 14 normal subjects found that single 400-mg doses of **cimetidine** and multiple 400-mg doses given twice daily had no effect on the pharmacokinetics of 2 mg repaglinide three times daily.[2] Another open label crossover multiple-dose trial in 14 normal subjects given 250 micrograms **digoxin** daily found that 2 mg repaglinide three times daily before meals had no effect on the pharmacokinetics of the **digoxin**.[3] Concurrent use was well tolerated in both studies.[2,3] A study has demonstrated that the only pharmacokinetic change with concurrent repaglinide and theophylline was a slight reduction in peak theophylline plasma levels.[4] The makers also report that repaglinide has no clinically relevant effect on the pharmacokinetics of **theophylline**.[1] A double-blind, placebo controlled study in 28 normal subjects found that repaglinide does not affect the anticoagulant effects of warfarin.[5] Repaglinide can be given with **metformin** with increased glycaemic control,[6] but the makers say that there is an increased risk of hypoglycaemia.[1]

1. NovoNorm (Repaglinide), Novo Nordisk Pharmaceuticals Ltd. Summary of product characteristics, January 2000.
2. Schwietert R, Wemer J, Jonkman JHG. No change in repaglinide pharmacokinetics with cimetidine coadministration. *Eur J Clin Pharmacol* (1997) 52, A140.
3. Schwietert R, Wemer J, Jonkman JH. Co-administration of repaglinide does not affect digoxin pharmacokinetics. *Eur J Clin Pharmacol* (1997) 52, A140.
4. Hatorp V, Thomsen MS. Drug interaction studies with repaglinide: repaglinide on digoxin or theophylline pharmacokinetics and cimetidine on repaglinide pharmacokinetics. *J Clin Pharmacol* (2000) 40, 184–92.
5. Rosenberg M, Strange P, Cohen A. Assessment of pharmacokinetic (PKP and pharmacodynamic (PD) interaction between warfarin and repaglinide. *Diabetes* (1999) 48 (Suppl 1), A356.
6. Moses R, Slobodniuk R, Boyages S, Colagiuri S, Kidson W, Carter J, Donnelly T, Moffitt P. Additional treatment with repaglinide provides significant improvement in glycaemic control in NIDDM patients poorly controlled on metformin. *Diabetologia* (1997) 40 (Suppl 1), A322.

Rosiglitazone + Miscellaneous drugs

The makers contraindicate rosiglitazone with insulin, while they issue only mild warnings about the concurrent use of paclitaxel, and of NSAIDs in those with limited cardiac reserve. Rosiglitazone is reported not to interact adversely with acarbose, alcohol, digoxin, food, glibenclamide (glyburide), metformin, nifedipine, oral contraceptives, ranitidine or warfarin.

Clinical evidence, mechanism, importance and management

(a) Drugs which may possibly interact adversely

(i) Insulin. A study in poorly controlled type-2 diabetic patients using **insulin** twice daily found that the addition of 2 or 4 mg rosiglitazone twice daily for 26 weeks improved the control of their blood sugar levels and they needed less insulin.[1] However it has also been found that there is a fourfold increase in the incidence of cardiac failure (2.5%) if both drugs are used and it is for this reason that the makers contraindicate rosiglitazone with **insulin**.[2]

(ii) Non-steroidal anti-inflammatory drugs (NSAIDs). The makers say that rosiglitazone can cause fluid retention which may exacerbate or precipitate heart failure, particularly in those with limited cardiac reserve. Because **NSAIDs** can also cause fluid retention the makers therefore issue a warning that concurrent use may possibly increase the risk of oedema in these patients.[2]

(iii) Paclitaxel. The makers say that although rosiglitazone is not expected to affect the pharmacokinetics of **paclitaxel**, because rosiglitazone is largely metabolised by cytochrome P450 isoenzyme CYP2C8 which also metabolises paclitaxel, there is the theoretical possibility of some interference. For this reason the makers advise caution with **paclitaxel**[2] although the likelihood of a clinically relevant interaction is probably small.

(b) Drugs reported not to interact adversely

Rosiglitazone 8 mg daily for 2 weeks was found to have no clinically relevant effect on the pharmacokinetics of **nifedipine** in 26 normal subjects.[3] Rosiglitazone 8 mg daily for the first two weeks of two cycles in 32 women taking an oral contraceptive (**ethinyloestradiol 0.35 mg + norethindrone 1 mg - *Ortho-Novum***) was found to have no effect on the pharmacokinetics of either steroid.[4] No special precautions are therefore needed if rosiglitazone is taken with either **nifedipine** or **oral contraceptives**. These drugs are all predominantly metabolised by cytochrome CYP3A4 which suggests that rosiglitazone is unlikely to interact to a clinically relevant extent with other drugs which are similarly metabolised by CYP3A4.

A study in normal healthy subjects found that 8 mg rosiglitazone once daily for 14 days had no effect on the steady-state pharmacokinetics of 375 micrograms **digoxin** daily. Concurrent use was safe and well tolerated.[5] However the makers contraindicate rosiglitazone in those with a history of cardiac failure because it may cause fluid retention which could lead to a deterioration in cardiac function.[6] If **digoxin** or any other **digitalis glycoside** is being used to treat cardiac failure, the use of rosiglitazone would therefore be contraindicated. This is not a drug-drug interaction but a disease-drug interaction. Rosiglitazone has been found to have no clinically relevant effect on the steady-state levels of **warfarin**.[6]

A study in 16 normal subjects found that 100 mg **acarbose** three times daily for a week slightly reduced the absorption of a single 8 mg oral dose of rosiglitazone (AUC reduced 12%) but this was not considered to be clinically relevant.[7] Rosiglitazone 2 mg twice daily for 7 days was found not to alter the mean steady-state 24 hour plasma glucose levels in diabetics taking 3.75 to 10 mg **glibenclamide (glyburide)** daily.[6] The steady-state pharmacokinetics of **metformin** (500 mg twice daily) and rosiglitazone (2 mg twice daily) were not affected by concurrent use for 4 days in normal subjects.[6] No special precautions are needed if any of these drugs is used concurrently. Indeed, the concurrent use of rosiglitazone with either **metformin** or the **sulphonylureas** is a licenced therapeutic indication because

blood sugar control is improved.[2]

A study found that pre-treatment with **ranitidine**, 150 mg twice daily for 4 days, had no effect on the pharmacokinetics of either single 4 mg oral or 2 mg intravenous doses of rosiglitazone.[8] These results suggest that absorption of rosiglitazone is not affected by a rise in gastric pH, and also suggests that other drugs which raise the pH might not interact, although this needs confirmatory study.

An 8-week study in type 2 diabetics taking 8 mg rosiglitazone or a placebo daily found that a moderate amount of **alcohol** (0.6 g/kg body weight) taken with a meal did not have a clinically relevant effect on plasma glucose levels and no episodes of hypoglycaemia were seen.[9] Another study found that the overall exposure to rosiglitazone was not affected by **food**.[10]

There would therefore appear to no reason for taking special precautions if rosiglitazone is used concurrently with **food** or any of these drugs.

(c) Metabolic studies with rosiglitazone

The makers report that *in vitro* studies demonstrate that rosiglitazone causes no significant inhibition of cytochrome P450 isoenzymes CYP1A2, CYP2A6, CYP2C19, CYP2D6, CYP2E1, CYP3A or CYP4A, so that the probability of interactions with drugs metabolised by these isoenzymes is very low. Rosiglitazone moderately inhibits CYP2C8 and causes only low inhibition of CYP2C9 *in vitro*.[2] The absence of clinically relevant interactions described in (b) above confirms that metabolic interactions are not likely to be a problem with rosiglitazone.

1. Raskin P, Dole JF, Rappaport EB. Rosiglitazone (RSG) improves glycemic control in poorly controlled, insulin-treated type 2 diabetes (T2D). *Diabetes* (1999) 48 (Suppl 1), A94.
2. Avandia (Rosiglitazone maleate). SmithKline Beecham Pharmaceuticals. Summary of product characteristics. March 2001.
3. Freed MI, Miller AK, Inglis AM, Thompson KA, Ladley D, Jorkasky DK. Rosiglitazone, a PPAR-gamma agonist, does not alter the pharmacokinetics of nifedipine, a cytochrome P450 3A4-substrate. *Diabetes* (1998) 47 (Suppl 1), A94.
4. Inglis AML, Miller AK, Culkin KT, Ladley D, Patterson SD, Jorkasky DK, Freed MI. Rosiglitazone, a PPARγ agonist, does not alter the pharmacokinetics of oral contraceptives (OC). *Diabetes* (1998) 48 (Suppl 1), A103.
5. Dicicco RA, Allen A, Jorkasky DK, Freed MI. Chronic administration of rosiglitazone (RSG) does not alter the pharmacokinetics of digoxin. *Diabetes* (1998) 47 (Suppl 1), A353.
6. Avandia (Rosiglitazone maleate). SmithKline Beecham Pharmaceuticals, Prescribing information, February 2001.
7. Inglis AML, Miller AK, Thompson KA, Jorkaksy DK, Freed MI. Coadministration of rosiglitazone and acarbose (A): Lack of a clinically relevant pharmacokinetic drug interaction. *Diabetes* (1998) 47 (Suppl 1), A353.
8. Freed MI, Miller A, Jorkasky DK, Dicicco RA. Rosiglitazone pharmacokinetics are not affected by coadministration of ranitidine. *Diabetes* (1998) 43 (Suppl 1), A353.
9. Culkin KT, Patterson SD, Jorkasky DK, Jorkasy DK, Freed MI. Rosiglitazone (RSG) does not increase the risk of alcohol-induced hypoglycemia in diet-treated type 2 diabetics. *Diabetes* (1999) 48 (Suppl 1), A350.
10. Freed MI, Allen A, Jorkasky DK, DiCicco RA. Systemic exposure to rosiglitazone is unaltered by food. *Eur J Clin Pharmacol* (1999) 55, 53-6.

Troglitazone + Miscellaneous drugs

Troglitazone was withdrawn worldwide because of reports of severe liver toxicity. For the sake of completeness, its interactions are summarised briefly here. Colestyramine causes a very marked reduction (over 70%) in the absorption of troglitazone[1] and is therefore contraindicated.[2] Troglitazone reduces the plasma levels of combined oral contraceptives by 30%,[3] which is thought to reduce their reliability. Mild hypoglycaemia may occur in a few patients when adding troglitazone to insulin or sulphonylureas.[2,4-7] Troglitazone absorption is enhanced by food,[8] and it may reduce the lipid lowering ability of gemfibrozil, but not statins.[9] It may also reduce plasma levels of ciclosporin (by up to 48%),[10] terfenadine (by 50-70%) and fexofenadine.[11] No interaction is reported to occur with digoxin,[2] paracetamol (acetaminophen),[12] or moderate amounts of alcohol,[13,14] and no interaction normally occurs with warfarin,[2] but an isolated case report describes increased anticoagulant effects.[15]

1. Young MA, Lettis S, Eastmond R. Concomitant administration of cholestyramine influences the absorption of troglitazone. *Br J Clin Pharmacol* (1998) 45, 37–40.

2. Romozin (Troglitazone). Glaxo Wellcome, Sankyo Pharma UK Ltd. Summary of product characteristics, July 1997.
3. Loi CM, Stern R, Koup JR, Vassos AB, Knowlton P, Sedman AJ. Effect of troglitazone on the pharmacokinetics of an oral contraceptive agent. *J Clin Pharmacol* (1999) 39, 410–17.
4. Akanuma Y, Kosaka K, Kuzuya T, Shigeta Y, Kaneko T. Long term study of a new oral hypoglycaemic agent CS–045 in patients with non-insulin dependent diabetes mellitus [in Japanese]. *Rinsho Iyaku* (1993) 9 (Suppl 3), 127–49.
5. Akanuma Y, Kosaka K, Toyoda T et al. Clinical evaluation of a new oral hypoglycaemic agent CS–045 in combination with insulin. Poster presented at 56th Annual Science Session of the American Diabetes Association (1996) June 8–11, San Francisco.
6. Kosaka K, Toyota T, Kuzuya T, Akanuma Y, Shigeta Y, Kaneko T, Shitiri M. Clinical evaluation of a new hypoglycemic agent CS–045 in combination with insulin. *Igaku Ayumi* (1996) 179, 951–79.
7. Püchler K, Sasahara K, Laeis P, Plenker A. Pharmacokinetic and pharmacodynamic profile of troglitazone in NIDDM patients with glibenclamide. Presented at 16th International Diabetes Federation Congress, 1997.
8. Young MA, Robinson CE, Devoy MAB, Minton NA. The influence of food on the pharmacokinetics of GR92132X, a thiazolidinedione, in healthy subjects. *Br J Clin Pharmacol* (1994) 37, 482P.
9. Bell DSH, Ovalle F. Troglitazone interferes with gemfibrozil's lipid-lowering action. *Diabetes Care* (1998) 21, 2028–9.
10. Loi CM, Young M, Randinitis E, Vassos A, Koup JR. Clinical pharmacokinetics of troglitazone. *Clin Pharmacokinet* (1999) 37, 91–104.
11. Loi CM, Stern R, Vassos AB, Koup JR, Sedman A. Effect of troglitazone on terfenadine pharmacokinetics. *Clin Pharmacol Ther* (1998) 63, 228.
12. Young MA, Lettis S, Eastmond R. Coadministration of acetaminophen and troglitazone: pharmacokinetics and safety. *J Clin Pharmacol* (1998) 38, 819–24.
13. Eckland DJA, Williams ZV, Foot EA. Troglitazone improves glycemia but does not increase the risk of hypoglycaemia following alcohol in diet-treated NIDDM subjects. 32nd Annual Meeting of the European Association for the Study of Diabetes, 1996.
14. Foot EA, Eastmond R. Good metabolic and safety profile of troglitazone alone and following alcohol in NIDDM subjects. *Diabetes Res Clin Pract* (1997) 38, 41–51.
15. Plowman BK, Morreale AP. Possible troglitazone-warfarin interaction. *Am J Health-Syst Pharm* (1998) 55, 1071.

Voglibose + Miscellaneous drugs

Voglibose does not interact adversely with digoxin, glibenclamide (glyburide), hydrochlorothiazide or warfarin.

Clinical evidence, mechanism, importance and management

(a) Digoxin

A randomised, two-way crossover study in 8 normal subjects taking 250 micrograms **digoxin** daily after breakfast for 8 days found that the concurrent use of 200 micrograms voglibose three times daily half an hour before meals had no effect on the pharmacokinetics of the **digoxin**.[1] There would therefore appear to be no reason for avoiding concurrent use. No special precautions are needed.

(b) Glibenclamide (Glyburide)

In a double-blind crossover trial, 12 normal male subjects were given either 5 mg voglibose or a placebo three times daily for 8 days and a single 1.75-mg dose of **glibenclamide** (**glyburide**) on the morning of day 8, taken at the same time as the first dose of the voglibose or placebo. The voglibose had no effect on the pharmacokinetics of the **glibenclamide** and it was concluded that concurrent use is safe.[2]

(c) Hydrochlorothiazide

A study in 12 normal subjects given a single 25-mg dose of **hydrochlorothiazide** before and after taking 5 mg voglibose three times daily for 11 days found that the **hydrochlorothiazide** plasma levels were slightly increased by the voglibose (AUC increased 7.5%, maximum plasma levels increased 15%) but these were considered to be clinically irrelevant. The combination was well tolerated and adverse events were unchanged.[3] No special precautions would appear to be needed if these two drugs are given concurrently.

(d) Warfarin

Twelve normal male subjects were given individually adjusted doses of **warfarin** to give values of 30 to 40% of normal (Quick's method), and then from day 11 to 15 they were also given 5 mg voglibose three times daily. It was found that the voglibose had no effect on the pharmacokinetics of the **warfarin** nor on its anticoagulant effects.[4] No special precautions would therefore appear to be needed if these two drugs are used concurrently.

1. Kusumoto M, Ueno K, Fujimura Y, Kameda T, Mashimo K, Takeda K, Tatami R, Shibakawa M. Lack of kinetic interaction between digoxin and voglibose. *Eur J Clin Pharmacol* (1999) 55, 79-80.
2. Kleist P, Ehrlich A, Suzuki Y, Timmer W, Wetzelsberger N, Lücker PW, Fuder H. Concomitant administration of the α-glucosidase inhibitor voglibose (AO-128) does not alter the pharmacokinetics of glibenclamide. *Eur J Clin Pharmacol* (1997) 53, 149–52.
3. Kleist P, Suzuki Y, Thomsen T, Möller M, Römer A, Hucke HP, Kurowski M, Eckl KM. Voglibose has no effect on the pharmacokinetics of hydrochlorothiazide. *Eur J Clin Pharmacol* (1998) 54, 273–4.
4. Fuder H, Kleist P, Birkel M, Ehrlich A, Emeklibas S, Maslak W, Stridde E, Wetzelsberger N, Wieckhorst G, Lücker PW. The α-glucosidase inhibitor voglibose (AO-128) does not change pharmacodynamics or pharmacokinetics of warfarin. *Eur J Clin Pharmacol* (1997) 53, 153–7.

16

Immunosuppressant drug interactions

The immunosuppressant drugs dealt with in this chapter are the corticosteroids, ciclosporin, OKT3, muromonab, mycophenolate, sirolimus and tacrolimus. Other drugs which are also used for immunosuppression (e.g. azathioprine and methotrexate) are to be found in Chapter 13 which deals with the cytotoxic drugs. When any of these drugs acts as the interacting agent the relevant monograph is categorised in the chapter dealing with the drug whose effects are changed. A list of the agents which are featured here appears in Table 16.1.

Table 16.1 Immunosuppressant drugs

Generic names	Proprietary names
Basiliximab	Simulect
Ciclosporin (A) (Cyclosporin)	Consupren, Gengraf, Immulem, Neoral, Neoral-Sandimmun, Sandimmun, Sandimmun Neoral, Sandimmune, Sigmasporin
Corticosteroids	
Cloprednol	Syntestan
Deflazacort	Calcort, Cortax, Deflan, Deflanil, Denacen, Dezacor, Flantadin, Lantadin, Rosilan, Zamene
Dexamethasone	Aacidexam, Adrecort, Aeroseb-Dex, Afpred-DEXA, Alin, Auxiloson, Bexine, Cortidex, Cortidexason, Cortisumman, Cryometasona, Dalalone, Decadran, Decadron, Decadronal, Decaject, Decasone, Decaspray, Decorex, Dectancyl, Dermadex, Dermazon, Desalark, Desocort, Dexa, Dexa Loscon mono, Dexabene, Dexacort, Dexacortal, Dexacortin, Dexacortisone, Dexadermil, Dexaflam, Dexaflan, Dexagalen, Dexagel, Dexagrin, Dexahexal, Dexalocal, Dexaltin, Dexamed, Dexametax, Dexameth, Dexaminor, Dexamonozon, Dexasone, Dexaval, Dexa-Allvoran, Dexa-Brachialin N, Dexa-clinit, Dexa-Effekton, Dexa-Helvacort, Dexa-P, Dexa-POS, Dexa-ratiopharm, Dexa-sine, Dexicar, Dexmethsone, Dexon, Dexsol, Dexthasol, Dexton, Dibasona, Diodex, Erladexone, Fortecortin, Hexadrol, Indarzona-N, Isopto Dex, Isopto Maxidex, Limethason, Lipotalon, Luxazone, Maxidex, Megacort, Mephamesone, Metax, Mexasone, Millicortine, Minidex, Oftan Dexa, Opnol, Oradexon, Polideltaxin, Soldesam, Solurex, Solutio Cordes Dexa N, Spersadex, Sterodex, Taprodex, Taxyl, Totocortin, Visumetazone
Fludrocortisone	Astonin, Astonin H, Florinef, Florinefe
Hydrocortisone (Cortisol)	Acticort, Actocortina, Aftasone, Ala-Cort, Alfacort, Alfacortone, Alfason, Anucort-HC, Anusol-HC, Apocort, Apocortal, Aquacort, Aquanil HC, A-Hydrocort, Bactine, Barriere-HC, Berlison, Biocort, BK HC, Buccalsone, Bucort, Carmol HC, Ceneo, Cetacort, Colifoam, Colofoam, Corlan, Cortacet, Cortaid, Cortamed, Cortate, Cortef, Cortenema, Cortic, Corticaine, Corticreme, Cortidro, Cortifoam, Cortisonal, Cortizone, Cortoderm, Cortop, Cortopin, Cortril, Cortrophin, Cort-Dome, Covocort, Cremicort-H, Cutaderm, Dermacort, Dermallerg, Dermarest Dri-Cort, Dermaspraid, Dermaspray demangeaison, Dermimade Hidrocortisona, Dermirit, Dermo Posterisan, Dermocortal, Dermol HC, Dermolate, Dermosa Hidrocortisona, Derm-Aid, Dilucort, Dioderm, DP HC, DP Hydrocortisone, EarSol-HC, Ebenol, Efcortelan, Efcortesol, Efficort, Egocort, Ekzemsalbe F, Emo-Cort, Fadol, Fenistil, Ficortril, Flebocortid, Foille Insetti, Glycocortison, Glycocortisone H, Gynecort, Hc45, Hemorrane, Hemril-HC, Hidalone, Hidroaltesona, Hidrocol, Hi-Cor, Hycor, Hycort, Hyderm, Hydracort, Hydrocort, Hydrocortistab, Hydrocortisyl, Hydrocortone, Hydrocutan, Hydroderm, Hydroderm HC, Hydrogalen, HydroSkin, Hydrosone, HydroTex, Hydro-Adreson, Hysone, Hytisone, Hytone, Idracemi, Isdinium, Kyypakkaus, Lacticare-HC, Lactisona, Lanacort, Laticort, Lenirit, Locoid, Locoid Crelo, Locoidon, Massengill Medicated, Mildison, Mitocortyl, Munitren H, Mylocort, Nositrol, Novocortal, Novo-Hydrocort, Nutracort, Orabase HCA, Oralsone, Pandel, Pandermil, Pannocort, Penecort, Picosyl, Posterine Corte, Prevex HC, Procort, Proctocort, Proctocream HC, Procutan, ratioAllerg, Recort Plus, Rectocort, Remederm HC, Retef, Sagittacortin, Sanadermil, Sanatison Mono, Sarna HC, Scalpicin Capilar, Schericur, Sigmacort, Siguent Hycor, Sintotrat, Skincalm, Solu-Cortef, Soventol Hydrocortison, Squibb-HC, Stiefcortil, Stopitch, Suniderma, Synacort, Systral Hydrocort, S-T Cort, Tegrin-HC, Texacort, Therasona, Uniderm, Velopural, Westcort, Zenoxone
Methylprednisolone	Advantan, Adventan, Asmacortone, Avancort, A-Methapred, Cryosolona, depMedalone, Depo Moderin, Depoject, Depopred, Depo-Medrate, Depo-Medrol, Depo-Medrone, Depo-Nisolone, Esametone, Firmacort, Medralone, Medrate, Medrol, Medrol Veriderm, Medrone, Metilbetasone Solubile, Metilpren, Metypred, Metypresol, Metysolon, M-Prednisol, Predmetil, Predni M, Prednilem, Radilem, Solomet, Solu-Medrol, Solu-Medrone, Solu-Moderin, Urbason, Vanderm etc
Prednisolone	Ak-Pred, Aprednislon, Capsoid, Corti-Clyss, Dacortin H, Decaprednil, Decortin H, Deltacortril, Deltastab, Delta-Cortef, Dhasolone, Diopred, Di-Adreson-F, Dontisolon D, duraprednisolon, Econopred, Estilsona, Farnerate, Farnezone, Fisopred, Frisolona, Gupisone, hefasolon, Hexacortone, Hydeltrasol, Hydrocortancyl, Inflamase, Inflanefran, Inf-Oph, Key-Pred, Key-Pred-SP, Klismacort, Kuhlprednon, Lenisolone, Lepicortinolo, Linola-H N, Linola-H-Fett N, Meticortelone, Ophtho-Tate, Opredsone, Orapred, Panafcortelone, Pediapred, Polypred, Precortalon aquosum, Precortisyl, Prectal, Pred, Predalone, Predcor, Predenema, Predfoam, Predisole, Predmix, Prednabene, Prednefrin SF, Prednersone, Prednesol, Predni, Predni H, Prednicortelone, Prednihexal, Predniocil, Prednisil, Prednisol, Prednisolut, Predni-Ophtal, Predni-POS, Predsim, Predsol, Pred-Clysma, Pred-Phosphate, Prelone, Prenilone, Rectopred, Redipred, Sintisone, Solone, Soludacortin, Solupred, Solu-Dacortin, Solu-Dacortina, Solu-Dacortine, Solu-Decortin-H, Sophipren, Spiricort, Sterofrin, Ultracorten H, Ultracortene-H, Ultracortenol, Walesolone, Xepasone
Prednisone	Artinisona, Cortancyl, Dacortin, Decortin, Deltacortene, Deltasone, Deltison, Liquid Pred, Meprosona-F, Meticorten, Nosipren, Ofisolona, Panafcort, Panasol-S, Predeltin, Predicor, Predicorten, Predni Tablinen, Prednicort, Prednidib, Prednitone, Premagnol, Pulmison, Rectodelt, Sone, Sterapred, Winpred
Muromonab-CD3 (OKT3)	Anti CD3, Ior-T3, Orthoclone OKT3
Mycophenolate mofetil	CellCept
Rituximab	Mabthera, Rituxan
Sirolimus	Rapamune
Tacrolimus (FK-506)	Prograf, Prograft, Protopic

Basiliximab + Miscellaneous drugs

Concurrent use of basiliximab with azathioprine, muromon-ab-CD3 or mycophenolate is not associated with an increase in adverse effects or infections. The dose requirements of ciclosporin or tacrolimus may be altered by co-administered basiliximab. Basiliximab is reported not to interact with analgesics, anti-infective drugs, diuretics or antihypertensive drugs.

Clinical evidence, mechanism, importance and management

(a) Azathioprine

Total body clearance of basiliximab was reduced by 22% when azathioprine was added to regimens also including ciclosporin for microemulsion and corticosteroids. However, the use of basiliximab in triple regimens with azathioprine did not increase adverse effects or infections.[1]

(b) Ciclosporin

A study in 39 paediatric renal transplant patients receiving ciclosporin found that lower doses of ciclosporin resulted in significantly higher trough levels, and some evidence of early ciclosporin toxicity within the first 10 days in 24 patients who also received basiliximab 10 or 20 mg on days 0 and 4 after transplantation. At days 28 to 50 ciclosporin levels declined and 20% higher doses were required in the basiliximab group to maintain adequate trough levels.[2] Another study in 54 paediatric liver transplant patients found that the addition of basiliximab to ciclosporin and corticosteroids did not significantly alter the overall ciclosporin dose requirements. However, 9 basiliximab-treated patients experienced acute rejection at 21 to 28 days after transplantation, and this was associated with low ciclosporin trough levels requiring increased ciclosporin dosage in 6 of the 9 patients.[3] It was considered that the effect on ciclosporin was due to an interleukin-2 receptor mediated alteration of the cytochrome P450 system.[2] This was considered to only play a minor role in the liver-transplant patients because of significantly lower target trough levels in these patients.[3] However, a further study failed to find an increase in rejection episodes between days 28 to 50 in kidney-transplant patients treated with basiliximab and ciclosporin.[4]

The authors of the first study[2] recommend that the initial dose of ciclosporin should be limited to 400 mg/m^2 in children receiving renal transplants who are also treated with basiliximab. Dose reductions were not considered necessary by other authors, but close monitoring was recommended.[3,4]

(c) Muromonab-CD3

The makers say that patients in phase 3 studies on basiliximab received muromonab-CD3 for episodes of rejection with no increase in adverse events or infections.[1]

(d) Mycophenolate

Total body clearance of basiliximab was reduced by 51% when azathioprine was added to regimens also including ciclosporin for microemulsion and corticosteroids. However, the use of basiliximab in triple regimens with mycophenolate mofetil did not increase adverse effects or infections.[1]

(e) Other drugs

The makers report that basiliximab has been used concurrently with analgesic, antibacterial, antifungal, antiviral, diuretics and antihypertensive drugs (beta-blockers, calcium channel blockers) without any increase in adverse reactions. None of the drugs was individually named.[1]

(f) Tacrolimus

A study in 12 adult renal-transplant patients found that trough tacrolimus levels on day 3 were increased by 63% in patients also treated with basiliximab and in 50% of these patients were associated with the development of acute tubular necrosis. By day 30, tacrolimus trough levels showed a downward trend in the basiliximab treated group, despite similar dose requirements to those on day 10. Tacrolimus dose requirements were lower in the basiliximab group compared to the control group throughout the 60-day study period.[5] Dose reductions were not considered necessary by the authors, but close monitoring was recommended.[5]

1. Simulect (Basiliximab). Novartis Pharmaceuticals UK Limited. Summary of product characteristics, January 2001.
2. Strehlau J, Pape L, Offner G, Bjoern N, Ehrich JHH. Interleukin-2 receptor antibody-induced alterations of ciclosporin dose requirements in paediatric transplant patients. *Lancet* (2000) 356, 1327–8.
3. Ganschow R, Grabhorn E, Burdelski M. Basiliximab in paediatric liver-transplant recipients. *Lancet* (2001) 357, 388.
4. Vester U, Kranz B, Treichel U, Hoyer PF. Basiliximab in paediatric liver-transplant recipients. *Lancet* (2001) 357, 388–9.
5. Sifontis NM, Benedetti E, Vasquez EM. A clinically significant drug interaction between basiliximab and tacrolimus in renal transplant recipients. *Pharmacotherapy* (2001) 10, 1297.

Ciclosporin + ACE inhibitors

Acute kidney failure developed in four kidney transplant patients on ciclosporin when given enalapril. Oliguria was seen in another patient when given captopril.

Clinical evidence

Two kidney transplant patients on ciclosporin developed acute renal failure 10 to 42 days after starting to take 5 to 10 mg enalapril twice daily. Recovery was complete when the enalapril was stopped in one of the patients, and when both drugs were stopped in the other. The latter had no problems when the ciclosporin was restarted. Both recovered renal function after 10 to 30 days. Neither had any previous evidence of renal artery stenosis or chronic rejection which are conditions known to predispose to renal failure during ACE inhibitor treatment. Two other patients appeared to tolerate concurrent use well.[1] Two further patients developed acute renal failure when given enalapril. Neither had renal arterial stenosis or acute rejection.[2] Transient oliguria was seen in another patient given ciclosporin and captopril.[3]

Mechanism

Not understood. One suggestion is that ciclosporin reduces the kidney blood flow and reduces perfusion through the glomerulus, which is worsened when the intra-renal angiotensin II is inhibited by the ACE inhibitor drug.[1]

Importance and management

Information is very limited indeed. The incidence of this interaction would appear to be low, nevertheless care and good monitoring are needed if captopril or enalapril and ciclosporin are used concurrently. More study is needed. Information about other ACE inhibitors is lacking but if the suggested mechanism is true, they too may possibly interact similarly.

1. Murray BM, Venuto RC, Kohli R, Cunningham EE. Enalapril-associated renal failure in renal transplants: possible role of cyclosporine. *Am J Kidney Dis* (1990) 16, 66–9.
2. Garcia TM, da Costa JA, Costa RS, Ferraz AS. Acute tubular renal necrosis in kidney transplant patients treated with enalapril. *Ren Fail* (1994) 16, 419–23.
3. Cockburn I. Cyclosporine A: a clinical evaluation of drug interactions. *Transplant Proc* (1986) 18 (Suppl 5), 50–5.

Ciclosporin + Acetazolamide

There is some limited evidence that acetazolamide can cause a marked and rapid rise in ciclosporin serum levels, possibly accompanied by kidney toxicity.

Clinical evidence, mechanism, importance and management

A study in 3 men found that 72 h after adding **acetazolamide** (dose not stated) their trough serum ciclosporin levels rose more than sixfold (from a range of 54 to 270 up to 517 to 1827 nanograms/ml).[1] Another man with a heart transplant demonstrated markedly increased serum ciclosporin levels (fivefold), marked renal impairment and neurotoxicity when given oral **acetazolamide** for raised intra-ocular pressure secondary to panuveitis.[2] The increase in ciclosporin serum levels has also been demonstrated in *animals*.[3]

Information seems to be limited to these reports but it is clear that the concurrent use of ciclosporin and acetazolamide should be closely monitored, being alert of the need to reduce the ciclosporin dosage. The interaction can apparently develop very rapidly. More study is needed.

1. Tabbara KF, Al-Faisal Z, Al-Rashed W. Interaction between acetazolamide and ciclosporine. *Arch Ophthalmol* (1998) 116, 832–3.
2. Keogh A, Esmore D, Spratt P, Savdie E, McClusky P, Chang V. Acetazolamide and cyclosporine. *Transplantation* (1988) 46, 478–9.
3. El-Sayed YM, Tabbara KF, Gouda MW. Effect of acetazolamide on the pharmacokinetics of cyclosporine in rabbits. *Int J Pharmaceutics* (1995) 121, 181–6.

Ciclosporin + Aciclovir

Aciclovir normally seems not to affect ciclosporin serum levels nor worsen kidney function, but a very small number of cases of nephrotoxicity and increased serum ciclosporin levels have been seen.

Clinical evidence

(a) No interaction

A retrospective study of 21 kidney transplant patients on ciclosporin (serum levels in the range 100 to 250 nanograms/ml) found that the concurrent use of oral **aciclovir** 800 mg four times daily for 3 months by 12 of them had no significant effect on their ciclosporin serum levels or on nephrotoxicity when compared with the 9 control subjects.[1]

No significant changes in renal function were seen in 11 patients on ciclosporin when given 750 to 1500 mg/m² daily **aciclovir** intravenously for at least 7 days to treat herpes infections.[2] No significant changes in serum creatinine or ciclosporin levels were seen during the 14 days following kidney transplant in 17 patients given 800 mg **aciclovir** daily.[3] Fifty-three kidney transplant patients were given ciclosporin and 800 to 3200 mg **aciclovir** daily for 12 weeks. The **aciclovir** was withdrawn from two because of unexplained and temporary increases in serum creatinine levels. The serum ciclosporin levels were not reported.[4] Five patients (2 adults and 3 children) on ciclosporin, prednisone and azathioprine were given 200 mg **aciclovir** tablets five times daily for 6 days for herpes zoster or chicken pox. Ciclosporin serum levels remained unchanged and renal function improved.[5]

(b) Toxicity

In contrast to the cases cited above, nephrotoxicity has been described in three patients given ciclosporin and **aciclovir**, and one died. Histological evidence suggested ciclosporin nephrotoxicity.[6] An increase in serum creatinine and **aciclovir** levels accompanied by reversible acute tubular necrosis has been noted during the concurrent use in another report.[7] Yet another describes a threefold increase in ciclosporin serum levels in a child with a heart transplant after starting **intravenous aciclovir**.[8]

Mechanism

Not understood.

Importance and management

Well documented. The evidence available indicates that ciclosporin levels and kidney function are usually unaltered by the concurrent use of aciclovir, but the handful of cases where problems have arisen

clearly indicate that kidney function should be well monitored. One group of workers recommends 250 mg/m² aciclovir given by slow infusion in well hydrated patients while carefully monitoring serum ciclosporin levels.[2]

1. Dugandzic RM, Sketris IS, Belitsky P, Schlech WF, Givner ML. Effect of coadministration of acyclovir and cyclosporine on kidney function and cyclosporine concentrations in renal transplant patients. *DICP Ann Pharmacother* (1991) 25, 316–7.
2. Johnson PC, Kumor K, Welsh MS, Woo J, Kahan BD. Effects of coadministration of cyclosporine and acyclovir on renal function of renal allograft recipients. *Transplantation* (1987) 44, 329–31.
3. Stoffel M, Squifflet JP, Pirson Y, Lamy M, Alexandre GPJ. Effectiveness of oral acyclovir prophylaxis in renal transplant recipients. *Transplant Proc* (1987) 19, 2190–3.
4. Balfour HH, Chace BA, Stapleton JT, Simmons RL, Fryd DS. A randomized, placebo-controlled trial of oral acyclovir for the prevention of cytomegalovirus disease in recipients of renal allografts. *N Engl J Med* (1989) 320, 1381–7.
5. Hayes K, Shakuntala V, Pingle A, Dhawan SK, Masri MA. Safe use of acyclovir (Zovirax) in renal transplant patients on cyclosporine A therapy: case reports. *Transplant Proc* (1992) 24, 1926.
6. Shepp DH, Dandliker PS, Meyers JD. Treatment of varicella-zoster virus infection in severely immunocompromised patients: a randomized comparison of acyclovir and vidarabine. *N Engl J Med* (1986) 314, 208–12.
7. Cockburn I. Cyclosporin A: a clinical evaluation of drug interactions. *Transplant Proc* (1986) 18 (Suppl 5), 50–5.
8. Boardman M, Yodur Purdy C. Cyclosporine and aciclovir; report of a drug interaction. Am Soc Hosp Pharmacists Midyear Clinical Meeting, Dallas, Texas. December 1988, Abstract SP-16.

Ciclosporin + Alcohol

An isolated report describes a marked increase in serum ciclosporin levels in a patient when he went on the binge, but a subsequent study found that moderate single doses of alcohol in other patients had no such effect. See also 'Ciclosporin + Food and Drinks', p.612.

Clinical evidence, mechanism, importance and management

The serum ciclosporin levels of a kidney transplant patient doubled (from 101 to 205 nanograms/ml) and remained high for about 4 days after going on a two-day **alcohol** binge. A subsequent study in 8 other patients with kidney transplants found no changes in serum ciclosporin or creatinine levels when they drank 50 ml of 100% **alcohol** in orange juice (equivalent to 4 oz of **whisky**).[1] Alcoholic patients with liver transplants and on ciclosporin have been reported to have a much higher rate of alcohol abstinence than other alcoholics,[2,3] but a subsequent study failed to find any evidence that this was due to the development of a disulfiram-like reaction or anything else which would make drinking unpleasant,[4] and there was no suggestion in the report cited above that such a reaction ever occurs.[1] The authors of this study say that they currently advise their patients to avoid heavy drinking but that an occasional drink probably does not affect ciclosporin levels.[1] See also 'Ciclosporin + Food and Drinks', p.612 for an interaction with red wine.

1. Paul MD, Parfrey PS, Smart M, Gault H. The effect of ethanol on serum cyclosporine A levels in renal transplant patients. *Am J Kidney Dis* (1987) 10, 133–5.
2. Starzl E, Van Thiel D, Tzakis AG. Orthoptic liver transplantation for alcoholic cirrhosis. *JAMA* (1988) 260, 2542.
3. Orrego H, Blendis LM, Blake J E, Kapur BM, Israel Y. Reliability of assessment of alcohol intake based on personal interviews in a liver clinic. *Lancet* (1979) 2, 1354.
4. Giles HG, Orrego H, Sandrin S, Saldivia V. The influence of cyclosporine on abstinence from alcohol in transplant patients. *Transplantation* (1990) 49, 1201–2.

Ciclosporin + Aminoglycosides

Both *animal* and human studies indicate that kidney toxicity may be increased by the concurrent use of ciclosporin and amikacin, gentamicin, tobramycin, framycetin or possibly other aminoglycosides.

Clinical evidence

A comparative study in patients given 30 mg **gentamicin** with **lincomycin** just prior to transplantation found that the concurrent use of ciclosporin increased the incidence of nephrotoxicity from 5% to

67%.[1] When **ampicillin, ceftazidime** and **lincomycin** were used instead the incidence of nephrotoxicity was 10%.[1] Three other reports describe increased nephrotoxicity associated with the concurrent use of ciclosporin and **gentamicin**,[2] **tobramycin**[3,4] or **framycetin**.[3] This interaction has also been well demonstrated in *animals*.[5,6] Another report describes damaged renal function in a patient on ciclosporin with **minocycline** and **amikacin**.[7]

In contrast, a retrospective analysis of the medical records of bone marrow transplant patients suggested that **aminoglycosides** can be safely given with a continuous infusion of ciclosporin without excessive nephrotoxicity, if carefully monitored.[8]

Mechanism

Uncertain. Since both ciclosporin and the aminoglycosides can individually be nephrotoxic it seems that their toxicities can be additive.

Importance and management

Established and clinically important interactions. The concurrent use of ciclosporin and aminoglycosides should be avoided, or only undertaken with care and very close monitoring.

1. Termeer A, Hoitsma AJ, Koene RAP. Severe nephrotoxicity caused by the combined use of gentamicin and cyclosporine in renal allograft recipients. *Transplantation* (1986) 42, 220–1.
2. Morales JM, Andres A, Prieto C, Diaz Rolòn JA, Rodicio JL. Reversible acute renal toxicity by toxic sinergic effect between gentamicin and cyclosporine. *Clin Nephrol* (1988) 29, 272.
3. Hows JM, Chipping PM, Fairhead S, Smith J, Baughan A, Gordon-Smith EC. Nephrotoxicity in bone marrow transplant recipients treated with cyclosporin A. *Br J Haematol* (1983) 54, 69–78.
4. Hows JM, Palmer S, Want S, Dearden C, Gordon-Smith EC. Serum levels of cyclosporin A and nephrotoxicity in bone marrow transplant patients. *Lancet* (1981) ii, 145–6.
5. Whiting PH, Simpson JG. The enhancement of cyclosporin A-induced nephrotoxicity by gentamicin. *Biochem Pharmacol* (1983) 32, 2025–8.
6. Ryffel B, Müller AM, Mihatsch MJ. Experimental cyclosporine nephrotoxicity: risk of concomitant chemotherapy. *Clin Nephrol* (1986) 25 (Suppl 1), S121–S125.
7. Thaler F, Gotainer B, Teodori G, Dubois C, Loirat Ph. Mediastinitis due to *Nocardia asteroides* after cardiac transplantation. *Intensive Care Med* (1992) 18, 127–8.
8. Chandrasekar PH, Cronin SM. Nephrotoxicity in bone marrow transplant recipients receiving aminoglycoside plus cyclosporine or aminoglycoside alone. *J Antimicrob Chemother* (1991) 27, 845–9.

Ciclosporin + Amiodarone

Ciclosporin serum levels can be increased by amiodarone. Reduce the ciclosporin dosage to avoid nephrotoxicity.

Clinical evidence

Eight patients with heart transplants and 3 with heart-lung transplants on ciclosporin were also given **amiodarone** for atrial flutter or fibrillation. Despite a 13 to 14% reduction in the ciclosporin dosage, their serum levels rose by 9%, serum creatinine levels rose by 38% (from 157 to 216 micromol/l), and blood urea nitrogen rose by 30%.[1] In another report by some of the same authors one patient is said to have shown a 50% decrease in the clearance of ciclosporin when given **amiodarone**.[2] Eight other patients with heart or heart-lung transplants were effectively treated with **amiodarone** for atrial flutter and/or atrial fibrillation, but they showed a 31% rise in serum ciclosporin levels (from 248 to 325 nanograms/ml) despite a 44% reduction in the ciclosporin dosage (from 6.2 to 3.5 mg/kg/day). Serum creatinine levels rose by 39%.[3] A kidney transplant patient doubled her serum ciclosporin levels when given **amiodarone**.[4] In 5 heart transplant patients amiodarone was discontinued and ciclosporin initiated, but the metabolism of ciclosporin was increased for 4 to 5 weeks (total plasma metabolites increased from 720 to 1437 nanograms/ml) and there was also an increase in the plasma concentration of amiodarone and its main metabolite, desethylamiodarone. During this period increased adverse effects, including pulmonary toxicity, were observed.[5]

Mechanism

Uncertain. A reduction[2] or an increase[5] in the metabolism of the ciclosporin by the amiodarone has been suggested. An interaction between amiodarone and phospholipids in the plasma membrane may inhibit transport processes. Blocking of protein in the intestinal mucosa and liver by both amiodarone and ciclosporin may result in decreased excretion and increased toxicity of amiodarone as well as accumulation of ciclosporin metabolites.[5]

Importance and management

An established and clinically important interaction. Concurrent use need not be avoided but close monitoring and ciclosporin dosage reductions are needed to minimise the potential nephrotoxicity. Remember to adjust the dosage again if the amiodarone is stopped, bearing in mind that it may take weeks before the amiodarone is totally cleared from the body.

1. Egami J, Mullins PA, Mamprin F, Chauhan A, Large SR, Wallwork J, Schofield PM. Increase in cyclosporine levels due to amiodarone therapy after heart and heart-lung transplantation. *J Am Coll Cardiol* (1993) 21, 141A.
2. Nicolau DP, Uber WE, Crumbley AJ, Strange C. Amiodarone-cyclosporine interaction in a heart transplant patient. *J Heart Lung Transplant* (1992) 11, 564–8.
3. Mamprin F, Mullins P, Graham T, Kendall S, Biocine B, Large S, Wallwork J, Schofield P. Amiodarone-cyclosporine interaction in cardiac transplantation. *Am Heart J* (1992) 123, 1725–6.
4. Chitwood KK, Abdul-Haqq AJ, Heim-Duthoy KL. Cyclosporine-amiodarone interaction. *Ann Pharmacother* (1993) 27, 569–71.
5. Preuner JG, Lehle K, Keyser A, Merk J, Rupprecht L, Goebels R. Development of severe adverse effects after discontinuing amiodarone therapy in human heart transplant recipients. *Transplant Proc* (1998) 30, 3943–4.

Ciclosporin + Amphotericin B

There is some good evidence that the risk of kidney toxicity is increased if ciclosporin and amphotericin B are used concurrently, however other evidence has shown that liposomal amphotericin B (*AmBisome*) does not increase kidney or liver toxicity when given to infants taking ciclosporin.

Clinical evidence

(a) Evidence of toxicity

The concurrent use of ciclosporin and **amphotericin B** increased the incidence of kidney toxicity in 47 patients with bone marrow transplants. Out of 10 patients who had received both drugs, 5 doubled and 3 tripled their serum creatinine levels within 5 days. In contrast only 8 out of 21 (38%) on ciclosporin alone and 3 out of 16 (19%) on **methotrexate** and **amphotericin B** doubled their serum creatinine within 14 to 30 and 5 days respectively.[1]

A study of the risk factors associated with **amphotericin B** identified the concurrent use of ciclosporin as posing a particularly significant risk for severe nephrotoxicity.[2] Two other studies in bone marrow transplant patients on ciclosporin found that **amphotericin B** contributed significantly to nephrotoxicity and renal failure.[3,4] It can apparently develop even after the **amphotericin** has been withdrawn.[3] Marked nephrotoxicity is described in one patient in another report.[5]

An isolated case report described severe tremors, later becoming myoclonic, attributed to the concurrent use of **liposomal amphotericin B (*AmBisome*)** and ciclosporin. Serum ciclosporin levels were unaltered and creatinine levels only rose slightly.[6] This alleged CNS neurotoxicity was challenged in a letter citing 187 transplant patients on ciclosporin and *AmBisome* none of whom developed neurotoxicity attributable to an interaction.[7]

(b) Evidence of no toxicity

A study which included 8 severely ill infants undergoing bone marrow transplantation for severe immunodeficiency, found no evidence of significant renal or liver toxicity when concurrently treated with **liposomal amphotericin B (*AmBisome*)** and ciclosporin. The average course of treatment lasted 29 days.[8] See also the last paragraph of (a) above.

Mechanism

Not understood. Simple additive kidney damaging effects is one possible explanation.

Importance and management

The increased kidney toxicity associated with ciclosporin/amphotericin appears to be established and clinically important. The authors of one report[1] say that "if amphotericin must be given, witholding ciclosporin until the serum level is less than about 150 nanograms/ml may be a means of decreasing renal toxicity without losing the immunosuppressive effect." However the report of no problems associated with use of liposomal amphotericin B in infants (b) provides a totally different perspective on the risks associated with concurrent use. More study is needed to sort out why these reports differ so much and whether the particular amphotericin formulation used is part of the explanation.

1. Kennedy MS, Deeg HJ, Siegel M, Crowley JJ, Storb R, Thomas ED. Acute renal toxicity with combined use of amphotericin B and cyclosporine after bone marrow transplantation. *Transplantation* (1983) 35, 211–15.
2. Guglielmo BJ, Maa L, Luber AD, Lam M. Risk factors for amphotericin B- induced nephrotoxicity. *Intersci Conf Antimicrob Agents Chemother* (1997) 37, 19.
3. Tutschka PJ, Beschorner WE, Hess AD, Santos GW. Cyclosporin-A to prevent graft-versus-host-disease: a pilot study in 22 patients receiving allogeneic marrow transplants. *Blood* (1983) 61, 318–25.
4. Miller KB, Schenkein DP, Comenzo R, Erban JK, Fogaren T, Hirsch CA, Berkman E, Rabson A. Adjusted-dose continuous-infusion cyclosporin A to prevent graft-versus-host disease following allogeneic bone marrow transplantation. *Ann Hematol* (1994) 68, 15–20.
5. Conti DJ, Tolkoff-Rubin NE, Baker GP, Doran M, Cosimi AB, Delmonico F, Auchincloss H, Russell PS, Rubin RH. Successful treatment of invasive fungal infection with fluconazole in organ transplant recipients. *Transplantation* (1989) 48, 692–5.
6. Ellis ME, Spence D, Ernst P, Meunier F. Is cyclosporin neurotoxicity enhanced in the presence of liposomal amphotericin B ? *J Infect* (1994) 29, 106–7.
7. Ringdén O, Andström EE, Remberger M, Svahn B-M, Tollemar J. No increase in cyclosporin neurotoxicity in transplant recipients treated with liposomal amphotericin B. *Infection* (1996) 24, 269.
8. Pasic S, Flannagan L, Cant AJ. Liposomal amphotericin (AmBisome) is safe in bone marrow transplantation for primary immunodeficiency. *Bone Marrow Transplant* (1997) 19, 1229–32.

Ciclosporin + Anticoagulants

The ciclosporin levels of a patient fell when given warfarin. When the ciclosporin dosage was raised an increase in the warfarin dosage was needed. Another patient on warfarin also showed an INR fall when given ciclosporin. A further report describes a rise in serum ciclosporin levels when an unnamed anticoagulant was given. Yet another describes increased acenocoumarol (nicoumalone) effects while receiving ciclosporin.

Clinical evidence, mechanism, importance and management

A man with erythrocyte aplasia effectively treated with ciclosporin for 18 months, relapsed within a week of starting **warfarin**. His ciclosporin levels had fallen from a range of 300 to 350 down to 170 nanograms/ml. He responded well when the ciclosporin dosage was increased from 3 to 7 mg/kg daily, but his prothrombin activity rose from 17% of control to 64% and he needed an increase in the **warfarin** dosage to achieve satisfactory anticoagulation. The patient was also taking phenobarbital.[1] Another woman patient with angioimmunoblastic T-cell lymphoma on a standard course of chemotherapy with CHOP, developed deep vein thrombosis and was therefore treated firstly with heparin and later **warfarin**. When 300 mg ciclosporin daily was added her INR decreased about 40% and she needed a **warfarin** dosage increase of 46% (progressively increased from 18.75 to 27.50 mg weekly).[2] Another patient on **acenocoumarol (nicoumalone)** showed quite the opposite effect. His anticoagulant dosage needed to be approximately halved when he was started on ciclosporin following a kidney transplant.[3] The reasons are not understood. Another report briefly says that serum ciclosporin levels rose in a patient when given a **warfarin derivative**.[4]

Information about oral anticoagulant/ciclosporin interactions seems to be limited to these four reports. They simply serve to emphasise the need to monitor concurrent use because the outcome is clearly uncertain.

1. Snyder DS. Interaction between cyclosporine and warfarin. *Ann Intern Med* (1988) 108, 311.
2. Turri D, Lannitto E, Caracciolo C, Mariani G. Oral anticoagulants and cyclosporin A. *Haematologica* (2000) 85, 893–4.
3. Campistol JM, Maragall D, Andreu J. Interaction between cyclosporin A and sintrom. *Nephron* (1989) 53, 291–2.
4. Cockburn I. Cyclosporin A: a clinical evaluation of drug interactions. *Transplant Proc* (1986) 18 (Suppl 5), 50–5.

Ciclosporin + Anticonvulsants

Serum ciclosporin levels are markedly reduced by the concurrent use of carbamazepine, phenobarbital or phenytoin. The dosage of ciclosporin may need to be increased two to fourfold to maintain adequate immunosuppression. Oxcarbazepine may cause a small decrease in ciclosporin levels. Sodium valproate appears not to affect ciclosporin levels but it may sometimes possibly damage renal grafts and cause liver damage.

Clinical evidence

(a) Carbamazepine, Sodium valproate

The ciclosporin serum levels of a kidney transplant patient fell from 346 to 64 nanograms/ml within 3 days of starting to take 200 mg **carbamazepine** three times daily. A week later serum levels were down to 37 nanograms/ml. They rose again when the **carbamazepine** was stopped but fell once more when it was restarted. The ciclosporin dosage was increased to keep the levels within the therapeutic range.[1]

The mean average steady state serum levels of ciclosporin per mg administered were less than 50% in a group of 3 children with kidney transplants taking **carbamazepine** than in 3 other matched patients not taking **carbamazepine**.[2] Four other individual patients have shown this interaction.[3-5] One needed her ciclosporin dosage to be doubled in order to maintain adequate serum levels while taking 800 mg **carbamazepine** daily.[3] When the **carbamazepine** was replaced by **sodium valproate** in three patients, the ciclosporin dosages became normal again.[3,4]

(b) Oxcarbazepine

A kidney-transplant patient on ciclosporin 270 mg daily and also taking daily valproate and gabapentin, prednisone, doxepin, allopurinol, levothyroxine sodium and pravastatin was also given **oxcarbazepine**. Fourteen days later, with the dose of **oxcarbazepine** at 750 mg daily, the ciclosporin trough level fell below 100 nanograms/ml and after a further 2 days was 87 nanograms/ml. The ciclosporin dose was increased to 290 mg daily and the **oxcarbazepine** dose reduced to 600 mg daily.

Ciclosporin levels then remained stable above 100 nanograms/ml and seizure frequency was reduced by 95%.[6]

(c) Phenobarbital

A 4-year-old child with a bone marrow transplant on 50 mg **phenobarbital** twice daily had serum ciclosporin levels of less than 60 nanograms/ml even after raising the dosage to 18 mg/kg daily. When the **phenobarbital** dosage was halved and later halved again the trough serum ciclosporin levels rose to 205 nanograms/ml.[7]

A threefold increase in ciclosporin clearance was seen in another child with a kidney transplant while on **phenobarbital** (12.6 compared with 3.8 ml/min/kg).[8] Reductions in ciclosporin levels due to **phenobarbital** have been described in other patients.[9-12]

(d) Phenytoin

The observation of 5 patients on ciclosporin who needed dosage increases while taking **phenytoin** prompted a further study in 6 healthy subjects. While taking 300 or 400 mg **phenytoin** daily their maximal serum ciclosporin levels and the AUC following a single 15 mg/kg dose were reduced by 37% (from 1325 to 831 micrograms/l) and 47% respectively.[13,14]

Other reports describe the need to make two to fourfold increases in the ciclosporin dosages in patients when concurrently treated with **phenytoin**.[15-19]

A report of severe gingival overgrowth in a kidney transplant patient was attributed to the additive adverse effects of ciclosporin and **phenytoin**.[20] Ciclosporin was replaced by tacrolimus, which may have fewer oral side effects, and almost complete reversal of gingival overgrowth was achieved within 6 months.

Mechanisms

Not fully resolved. It is thought that phenytoin,[13,15] carbamazepine[1,2] and phenobarbital[7,10] increase the metabolism of the ciclosporin by the liver (hepatic P450 oxygenase system) thereby increasing its loss from the body and lowering the serum levels accordingly. Oxcarbazepine produced only small reductions in ciclosporin levels, but the effect is probably due to weak induction of the cytochrome P450 isoenzyme CYP3A by oxcarbazepine.[6] Phenytoin also possibly reduces the absorption of the ciclosporin.[21]

Importance and management

None of these interactions is extensively documented but all appear to be established and of clinical importance. Serum ciclosporin levels should be well monitored if carbamazepine, phenobarbital or phenytoin are added and the ciclosporin dosage increased appropriately (by a factor of two or even more). Information about oxcarbazepine is very limited but small reductions in its dose together with an increase in ciclosporin dose may be adequate to control any interaction. However, more study is required before the concomitant use of ciclosporin and oxcarbazepine can be recommended.[6] The effects of the interaction may persist for a week or more after the anticonvulsant is withdrawn. Sodium valproate seems to be a non-interacting anticonvulsant,[3,12,22] however it may not always be without problems because interstitial nephritis was suspected in one patient with a renal graft[9] and fatal valproate-induced hepatotoxicity occurred in another.[23]

1. Lele P, Peterson P, Yang S, Jarell B, Burke JF. Cyclosporine and tegretol — another drug interaction. *Kidney Int* (1985) 27, 344.
2. Cooney GF, Mochon M, Kaiser B, Dunn SP, Goldsmith B. Effects of carbamazepine on cyclosporine metabolism in pediatric renal transplant recipients. *Pharmacotherapy* (1995) 15, 353–6.
3. Hillebrand G, Castro LA, van Scheidt W, Beukelmann D, Land W, Schmidt D. Valproate for epilepsy in renal transplant recipients receiving cyclosporine. *Transplantation* (1987) 43, 915–16.
4. Schofield OMV, Camp RDR, Levene GM. Cyclosporin A in psoriasis: interaction with carbamazepine. *Br J Dermatol* (1990) 122, 425–6.
5. Alvarez JS, Del Castillo JAC, Ortiz MJA. Effect of carbamazepine on ciclosporin blood level. *Nephron* (1991) 58, 235–6.
6. Rösche J, Fröscher W, Abendroth D, Liebel J. Possible oxcarbazepine interaction with cyclosporine serum levels: a single case study. *Clin Neuropharmacol* (2001) 24, 113–16.
7. Carstensen H, Jacobsen N, Dieperink H. Interaction between cyclosporin A and phenobarbitone. *Br J Clin Pharmacol* (1986) 21, 550–1.
8. Burckart GJ, Venkataramanan R, Starzl T, Ptachcinski JR, Gartner JC, Rosenthal T. Cyclosporine clearance in children following organ transplantation. *J Clin Pharmacol* (1984) 24, 412.
9. Kramer G, Dillmann U, Tettenborn B. Cyclosporine-phenobarbital interaction. *Epilepsia* (1989) 30, 701.
10. Beierle FA, Bailey L. Cyclosporine metabolism impeded/blocked by co-administration of phenobarbital. *Clin Chem* (1989) 35, 1160.
11. Wideman CA. Pharmacokinetic monitoring of cyclosporine. *Transplant Proc* (1983) 15 (Suppl 1), 3168–75.
12. Matsuura T, Akiyama T, Kurita T. Interaction between phenobarbital and cyclosporin following renal transplantation: a case report. *Hinyokika Kiyo* (1990) 36, 447–50.
13. Freeman DJ, Laupacis A, Keown PA, Stiller CR, Carruthers SG. Evaluation of cyclosporin-phenytoin interaction with observations on cyclosporin metabolites. *Br J Clin Pharmacol* (1984) 18, 887–93.
14. Freeman DJ, Laupacis A, Keown P, Stiller C, Carruthers G. The effect of agents that alter drug metabolizing enzyme activity on the pharmacokinetics of cyclosporine. *Ann R Coll Physicians Surg Can* (1984) 17, 301.
15. Keown PA, Laupacis A, Carruthers G, Stawecki M, Koegler J, McKenzie FN, Wall W, Stiller CR. Interaction between phenytoin and cyclosporine following organ transplantation. *Transplantation* (1984) 38, 304–6.
16. Grigg-Damberger MM, Costanzo-Nordin R, Kelly MA, Bahamon-Dussan JE, Silver M, Zucker MJ, Celesia GG. Phenytoin may compromise efficacy of cyclosporine immunosuppression in cardiac transplant patients. *Epilepsia* (1988) 29, 693.
17. Schmidt H, Naumann R, Jaschonek K, Einsele H, Dopfer R, Ehninger G. Drug interaction between cyclosporin and phenytoin in allogeneic bone marrow transplantation. *Bone Marrow Transplant* (1989) 4, 212–13.
18. Schweitzer EJ, Canafax DM, Gillingham KJ, Najarian JS, Matas AJ. Phenytoin administration in kidney recipients on CSA immunosuppression. *J Am Soc Nephrol* (1991) 2, 816.
19. Castelao AM. Cyclosporine A – drug interactions. In Sunshine I (Ed.) Recent developments in therapeutic drug monitoring and clinical toxicology. 2nd Int Conf Therapeutic Drug Monitoring Toxicology, Barcelona, Spain (1992) 203–9.
20. Hernandez G, Arriba L, Lucas M, de Andres A. Reduction of severe gingival overgrowth in a kidney transplant patient by replacing cyclosporin A with tacrolimus. *J Periodontol* (2000) 71, 1630–6.
21. Rowland M, Gupta SK. Cyclosporin-phenytoin interaction: re-evaluation using metabolite data. *Br J Clin Pharmacol* (1987) 24, 329–34.
22. Oguchi M, Kiuchi C, Akiyama H, Sakamaki H, Onozawa Y. Interaction between cyclosporin A and anticonvulsants. *Bone Marrow Transplant* (1992) 9, 391.
23. Fischman MA, Hull D, Bartus SA, Schweizer RT. Valproate for epilepsy in renal transplant recipients receiving cyclosporine. *Transplantation* (1989) 48, 542.

Ciclosporin + Azole antifungals

Ketoconazole can cause a very marked and rapid rise in serum ciclosporin levels (up to five to tenfold). Avoid concurrent use unless the ciclosporin dosage is markedly reduced. A less dramatic but still clinically important rise in ciclosporin serum levels of two to threefold has been seen in some patients when given fluconazole or itraconazole. A single report describes the same interaction with miconazole. Rhabdomyolysis has been reported in three lung transplant patients treated with ciclosporin and itraconazole, but co-administered statins may also have contributed to the adverse effects in two. The antifungal activity of fluconazole may be enhanced by ciclosporin.

Clinical evidence

(a) Fluconazole

Fluconazole 200 mg daily for 14 days approximately doubled the trough serum ciclosporin levels (from 23 to 45 nanograms/ml) of 8 kidney transplant patients. The AUC increased from 1900 to 3114 nanograms.h/ml but serum creatinine levels were unchanged.[1,2] Similar results were found by the same group of workers in a related studies.[3,4]

Other reports describe two to threefold rises in serum ciclosporin levels in kidney transplant patients within 6 to 11 days of starting treatment with 100 to 200 mg **fluconazole** daily.[5-9] One patient developed kidney toxicity which was solved by reducing the dosages of both drugs.[10]

In contrast, some patients have shown little or no changes in serum ciclosporin or creatinine levels when **fluconazole** was given.[11-16] This may have been because the interaction is dose-dependent.[15,17] One study found a lack of interaction in females and African-American patients, suggesting that gender and ethnicity may also be factors.[18]

An *in vitro* study suggests that the activity of **fluconazole** against *Candida albicans* may be enhanced by ciclosporin.[19]

(b) Itraconazole

An average 56% reduction (range 33 to 84%) in the ciclosporin dosages in four heart-lung, two heart and one lung transplant patient were needed when **itraconazole** (dosage not stated) was given. Serum creatinine levels rose temporarily until the ciclosporin dosage had been readjusted.[20] The need to reduce the ciclosporin dosage by 50 to 80% when **itraconazole** was used is briefly mentioned in another report.[21] Two to threefold rises were seen in 2 other patients given 200 mg **itraconazole** daily,[22,23] and in one case the raised levels persisted for more than 4 weeks after the **itraconazole** was stopped.[23] Unspecified reductions in the ciclosporin dosage are mentioned in yet another report.[24] Enhanced **itraconazole** absorption in the presence of a carbonated drink that increased stomach acidity was found to allow decreases in ciclosporin dose and increases in its dose interval.[25]

These reports contrast with another describing 14 bone marrow transplant patients taking ciclosporin. Those given 100 mg **itraconazole** twice daily showed no significant changes in ciclosporin or creatinine serum levels.[26]

Rhabdomyolysis has been reported in 3 lung transplant patients when **itraconazole** was used in combination with ciclosporin, but in two of these cases the concurrent use of simvastatin may have been a factor.[21,27]

(c) Ketoconazole

Ketoconazole 200 mg daily caused a marked and rapid rise in serum ciclosporin levels of 36 renal transplant patients. On the basis of experience with previous patients, the dosage was reduced by 70% when **ketoconazole** was started, and after a year the dosage reduction was 85% (from 420 mg to 66 mg daily). Minimal nephrotoxicity was seen.[28-30]

Other reports[31-46] describe essentially similar rises in serum ciclosporin levels during concurrent treatment with **ketoconazole**. See also 'Importance and management'. The effects of **ketoconazole** on ciclosporin were found to be slightly increased (from 80 to 85%) when diltiazem was added as well.[47] **Topical ketoconazole** (2% cream) has been found not interact with ciclosporin (1 mg/kg daily) in the treatment of contact allergic dermatitis and the ciclosporin dosage cannot be reduced.[48] Impaired glucose tolerance has been attributed to concurrent use in one patient.[49]

(d) Miconazole

A single case report describes an approximately 65% rise in ciclosporin serum levels within three days of starting 1 g of intravenous **miconazole** eight-hourly. Levels rose again during a subsequent treatment with **miconazole**.[50]

Mechanism

In vitro studies show that these azole antifungals inhibit the metabolism of ciclosporin by human liver microsomal enzymes, ketoconazole being the most potent.[51,52] As a result the loss of the ciclosporin from the body is reduced and its serum levels rise. Fluconazole and ketoconazole also appear to inhibit the metabolism of ciclosporin by the gut wall.[43,53]

Rhabdomyolysis may be caused by drugs including simvastatin which were also being taken by two of the patients. Itraconazole increases levels of ciclosporin, which interferes with hepatic clearance of simvastatin and this may increase the risk of muscle injury,[21] or ciclosporin may have a direct toxic effect on muscle cells.[27]

Importance and management

The ciclosporin/ketoconazole interaction is very well established and clinically important. Ciclosporin serum levels rise rapidly and sharply, but they can be controlled by reducing the ciclosporin dosage by up to about 70 to 80%[24,28,33,54-57] thereby preventing kidney damage (and also saving costs). A dosage reduction of 68 to 89% (a 75% saving) over a 13-month period with no adverse changes in immunosuppressive activity has been described, the total cost saving being about 65% because of the need to follow up more frequently and the cost of the ketoconazole.[28,29] Another study claimed an annual reduction in the 1991 costs from $6800 to $1862 (US) per heart transplant patient.[54] A projected 43% cost saving was claimed after another study in lung transplant patients,[44] and an 80% saving in one year (1994) in another in heart transplant patients.[45] Reviews of the pros and cons of concurrent use have been published.[30,58] Ketoconazole may possibly have a kidney-protective effect.[28,29,56]

Information about ciclosporin with fluconazole, itraconazole or miconazole is less extensive but concurrent use should be closely monitored, being alert for the need to reduce the ciclosporin dosage by up to 50% or more, although some patients may demonstrate no significant changes at all. A study in renal transplant patients suggested that variability in absorption and in the response to metabolic inhibition by ketoconazole made the ciclosporin blood level response difficult to predict and monitor.[59] There is some evidence that with fluconazole the interaction may possibly depend on its dosage,[15] gender and ethnicity.[18]

Additional caution is required where ciclosporin and azoles are used in patients taking statins, and either ciclosporin dose reduction[21] or replacement of ciclosporin with tacrolimus[27] has been recommended.

1. Carleton BC, Graves NM, Matas AJ, Hilligoss DM, Canafax DM. Managing the fluconazole and cyclosporine interaction: results of a double-blind randomized pharmacokinetic and safety study. *Pharmacotherapy* (1990) 10, 250.
2. Graves NM, Matas AJ, Hilligoss DM, Canafax DM. Fluconazole/cyclosporine interaction. *Clin Pharmacol Ther* (1990) 47, 208.
3. Canafax DM, Graves NM, Hilligoss DM, Carleton BC, Gardner MJ, Matas AJ. Interaction between cyclosporine and fluconazole in renal allograft recipients. *Transplantation* (1991) 51, 1014–8.
4. Canafax DM, Graves NM, Hilligoss DM, Carleton BC, Gardner MJ, Matas AJ. Increased cyclosporine levels as a result of simultaneous fluconazole and cyclosporine therapy in renal transplant recipients: a double-blind, randomized pharmacokinetic and safety study. *Transplant Proc* (1991) 23, 1041–2.
5. Torregrosa V, De la Torre M, Campistol JM, Oppenheimer F, Ricart MJ, Vilardell J, Andreu J. Interaction of fluconazole with ciclosporin A. *Nephron* (1992) 60, 125–6.
6. Sugar AM, Saunders C, Idelson BA, Bernard DB. Interaction of fluconazole and cyclosporine. *Ann Intern Med* (1989) 110, 844.
7. Barbara JAJ, Clarkson AR, LaBrooy J, McNeil JD, Woodroffe AJ. Candida albicans arthritis in a renal allograft recipient with an interaction between cyclosporin and fluconazole. *Nephrol Dial Transplant* (1993) 8, 263–6.
8. Tett S, Carey D, Lee H-S. Drug interactions with fluconazole. *Med J Aust* (1992) 156, 365.
9. Foradori A, Mezzano S, Videla C, Pefaur J, Elberg A. Modification of the pharmacokinetics of cyclosporine A and metabolites by the concomitant use of Neoral and diltiazem or ketoconazol in stable adult kidney transplants. *Transplant Proc* (1998) 30, 1685–7.
10. Collignon P, Hurley B, Mitchell D. Interaction of fluconazole with cyclosporin. *Lancet* (1989) i, 1262.
11. Ehninger G, Jaschonek K, Schuler U, Krüger HU. Interaction of fluconazole with cyclosporin. *Lancet* (1989) ii, 104–5.
12. Krüger HU, Schuler U, Zimmermann R, Ehninger G. Absence of significant interaction of fluconazole with cyclosporin. *J Antimicrob Chemother* (1989) 24, 781–6.
13. Conti DJ, Tolkoff-Rubin NE, Baker GP, Doran M, Cosimi AB, Delmonico F, Auchincloss H, Russell PS, Rubin RH. Successful treatment of invasive fungal infection with fluconazole in organ transplant recipients. *Transplantation* (1989) 48, 692–5.
14. Rubin RH, Debruin MF, Knirsch AK. Fluconazole therapy for patients with serious Candida infections who have failed standard therapies. *Intersci Conf Antimicrob Agents Chemother* (1989), 112.
15. López-Gil JA. Fluconazole-cyclosporine interaction: a dose-dependent effect? *Ann Pharmacother* (1993) 27, 427–30.
16. Lumbreras C, Cuervas-Mons V, Jara P, del Palacio A, Turrión VS, Barrios C, Moreno E, Noriega AR, Paya CV. Randomized trial of fluconazole versus nystatin for the prophylaxis of Candida infection following liver transplantation. *J Infect Dis* (1996) 174, 583–8.
17. Sud K, Singh B, Krishna VS, Thennarasu K, Kohli HS, Jha V, Gupta KL, Sakhuja V. Unpredictable cyclosporin-fluconazole interaction in renal transplant recipients. *Nephrol Dial Transplant* (1999) 14, 1698–1703.
18. Mathis AS, DiRenzo T, Friedman GS, Kaplan B, Adamson R. Sex and ethnicity may chiefly influence the interaction of fluconazole with calcineurin inhibitors. *Transplantation* (2001) 71, 1069–75.
19. Marchetti O, Moreillon P, Glauser MP, Bille J, Sanglard D. Potent synergism of the combination of fluconazole and cyclosporine in Candida albicans. *Antimicrob Agents Chemother* (2000) 44, 2373–81.
20. Kramer MR, Marshall SE, Denning DW, Keogh AM, Tucker RM, Galgiani JN, Lewiston NJ, Stevens DA, Theodore J. Cyclosporine and itraconazole interaction in heart and lung transplant recipients. *Ann Intern Med* (1990) 113, 327–9.
21. Malouf MA, Bicknell M, Glanville AR. Rhabdomyolysis after lung transplantation. *Aust N Z Med J* (1997) 27, 186.
22. Kwan JTC, Foxall PJD, Davidson DGC, Bending MR, Eisinger AJ. Interaction of cyclosporin and itraconazole. *Lancet* (1987) ii, 282.
23. Trenk D, Brett W, Jähnchen E, Birnbaum D. Time course of cyclosporin/itraconazole interaction. *Lancet* (1987) ii, 1335–6.
24. Faggian G, Livi U, Bortolotti U, Mazzucco A, Stellin G, Chiominto B, Viviani MA, Gallucci V. Itraconazole therapy for acute invasive pulmonary aspergillosis in heart transplantation. *Transplant Proc* (1989) 21, 2506–7.
25. Wimberley SL, Haug MT, Shermock K, Maurer J, Mehta A, Schilz R, Gordon S. Enhanced cyclosporine (CSA)-itraconazole (ICZ) interaction with cola in lung transplant recipients (LTR). *Intersci Conf Antimicrob Agents Chemother* (1999) 39, 4.
26. Novakova I, Donnelly P, de Witte T, de Pauw B, Boezeman J, Veltman G. Itraconazole and cyclosporin nephrotoxicity. *Lancet* (1987) i, 920–1.
27. Cohen E, Kramer MR, Maoz C, Ben-Dayan D, Garty M. Cyclosporin drug-interaction-induced rhabdomyolysis. A report of two cases in lung transplant recipients. *Transplantation* (2000) 70, 119–22.
28. First MR, Schroeder TJ, Weiskittel P, Myre SA, Alexander JW, Pesce AJ. Concomitant administration of cyclosporin and ketoconazole in renal transplant patients. *Lancet* (1989) ii, 1198–1201.
29. First MR, Schroeder TJ, Alexander JW, Stephens GW, Weiskittel P, Myre SA, Pesce AJ. Cyclosporine dose reduction by ketoconazole administration in renal transplant recipients. *Transplantation* (1991) 51, 365–70.
30. First MR, Schroeder TJ, Michael A, Hariharan S, Weiskittel P, Alexander JW. Cyclosporin-ketoconazole interaction. Long-term follow-up and preliminary results of a randomized trial. *Transplantation* (1993) 55, 1000–4.
31. Ferguson RM, Sutherland DER, Simmons RL, Najarian JS. Ketoconazole,cyclosporin metabolism and renal transplantation. *Lancet* (1982) ii, 882–3.
32. Morgenstern GR, Powles R, Robinson B, McElwain TJ. Cyclosporin interaction with ketoconazole and melphalan. *Lancet* (1982) ii, 1342.
33. Dieperink H, Møller J. Ketoconazole and cyclosporin. *Lancet* (1982) ii, 1217.
34. Lokiec F. Pharmacokinetic monitoring during graft-versus-host disease treatment following bone marrow transplantation. International Symposium on Cyclosporin A (Trinity Hall, Cambridge. September 16–18, 1981). Quoted in reference 3.
35. Gluckman E, Devergie A, Lokiec F, Poirier O, Baumelou A. Nephrotoxicity of cyclosporin in bone-marrow transplantation. *Lancet* (1981) ii, 144–5.
36. Shepard JH, Canafax DM, Simmons RL, Najarian JS. Cyclosporine-ketoconazole: a potentially dangerous drug-drug interaction. *Clin Pharm* (1986) 5, 468.
37. Schroeder TJ, Melvin DB, Clardy CW, Wadhwa NK, Myre SA, Reising JM, Wolf RK, Collins JA, Pesce AJ, First MR. Use of cyclosporine and ketoconazole without nephrotoxicity in two heart transplant recipients. *J Heart Transplant* (1987) 6, 84–9.
38. Butman SM, Wild J, Nolan P, Fagan T, Mackie M, Finley P, Copeland JG. Cyclosporine and concomitant ketoconazole after cardiac transplantation: intermediate term findings and potential savings. *J Am Coll Cardiol* (1989) 13, 62A.
39. Girardet RE, Melo JC, Fox MS, Whalen C, Lusk R, Masri ZH, Lansing AM. Concomitant administration of cyclosporine and ketoconazole for three and a half years in one heart transplant recipient. *Transplantation* (1989) 48, 887–90.
40. Schroeder TJ, Weiskittel P, Pesce AJ, Myre SA, Alexander JW, First MR. Cyclosporine pharmacokinetics with concomitant ketoconazole therapy. *Clin Chem* (1989) 35, 1176–7.

41. Charles BG, Ravenscroft PJ, Rigby RJ. The ketoconazole-cyclosporin interaction in an elderly renal transplant patient. *Aust N Z J Med* (1989) 19, 292–3.
42. Veraldi S, Menni S. Severe gingival hyperplasia following cyclosporin and ketoconazole therapy. *Int J Dermatol* (1988) 27, 730.
43. Gomez DY, Wacher VJ, Tomlanovich SJ, Hebert MF, Benet LZ. The effects of ketoconazole on the intestinal metabolism and bioavailability of cyclosporine. *Clin Pharmacol Ther* (1995) 58, 15–9.
44. Kriett JM, Jahansouz F, Smith CM, Hayden AM, Fox KJ, Kapelanski DP, Jamieson SW. The cyclosporine-ketoconazole interaction:safety and economic impact in lung transplantation. *J Heart Lung Transplant* (1994) 13, S43.
45. Keogh A, Spratt P, McCosker C, Macdonald P, Mundy J, Kaan A. Ketoconazole to reduce the need for cyclosporine after cardiac transplantation. *N Engl J Med* (1995) 333, 628–33.
46. McLachlan AJ, Tett SE. Effect of metabolic inhibitors on cyclosporine pharmacokinetics using a population approach. *Ther Drug Monit* (1998) 20, 390–5.
47. Hariharan S, Schroeder T, First MR. The effect of diltiazem on cyclosporin A (CYA) bioavailability in patients treated with CYA and ketoconazole. *J Am Soc Nephrol* (1992) 3, 861.
48. McLelland J, Shuster S. Topical ketoconazole does not potentiate oral cyclosporin A in allergic contact dermatitis. *Acta Derm Venereol (Stockh)* (1992) 72, 285.
49. Kiss D, Thiel G. Glucose-intolerance and prolonged renal-transplant insufficiency due to ketoconazole-cyclosporin A interaction. *Clin Nephrol* (1990) 33, 207–8.
50. Horton CM, Freeman CD, Nolan PE, Copeland JG. Cyclosporine interactions with miconazole and other azole-antimycotics: a case report and review of the literature. *J Heart Lung Transplant* (1992) 11, 1127–32.
51. Back DJ, Tjia JF. Comparative effects of the antimycotic drugs ketoconazole, fluconazole, itraconazole and terbinafine on the metabolism of cyclosporin by human liver microsomes. *Br J Clin Pharmacol* (1991) 32, 624–6.
52. Omar G, Whiting PH, Hawksworth GM, Humphrey MJ, Burke MD. Ketoconazole and fluconazole inhibition of the metabolism of cyclosporin A by human liver in vitro. *Ther Drug Monit* (1997) 19, 436–45.
53. Osowski CL, Dix SP, Lin LS, Mullins RE, Geller RB, Wingard JR. Evaluation of the drug interaction between intravenous high-dose fluconazole and cyclosporine or tacrolimus in bone marrow transplant patients. *Transplantation* (1996) 61, 1268–72.
54. Butman SM, Wild JC, Nolan PE, Fagan TC, Finley PR, Hicks MJ, Mackie MJ, Copeland JG. Prospective study of the safety and financial benefit of ketoconazole as adjunctive therapy to cyclosporine after heart transplantation. *J Heart Lung Transplant* (1991) 10, 351–8.
55. Schroeder TJ, Melvin DB, Clardy CW, Myre SA, Reising JM, Wolf RK, Collins JA, Pesce AJ, First MR. The use of cyclosporine and ketoconazole without nephrotoxicity in 2 heart transplant recipients. *J Heart Transplant* (1986) 5, 391.
56. First MR, Schroeder TJ, Michael A, Hariharan S, Weiskittel P, Alexander JW. Randomized controlled study of coadministration of cyclosporine and ketoconazole in renal transplant recipients. *Clin Pharmacol Ther* (1993) 53, 237.
57. Koselj M, Bren A, Kandus A, Kovac D. Drug interactions between cyclosporine and rifampicin, erythromycin, and azoles in kidney recipients with opportunistic infections. *Transplant Proc* (1994) 26, 2823–4.
58. Albengres E, Tillement JP. Cyclosporin and ketoconazole, drug interaction or therapeutic association? *Int J Clin Pharmacol Ther Toxicol* (1992) 30, 555–70.
59. Sorenson AL, Lovdahl M, Hewitt JM, Granger DK, Almond PS, Russlie HQ, Barber D, Matas AJ, Canafax DM. Effects of ketoconazole on cyclosporine metabolism in renal allograft recipients. *Transplant Proc* (1994) 26, 2822.

Ciclosporin + Aztreonam

Ciclosporin and aztreonam do not interact adversely.

Clinical evidence, mechanism, importance and management

A study in 20 kidney transplant patients found that when **aztreonam** was added for the treatment of various infections the ciclosporin serum levels were not significantly changed. The ciclosporin serum levels before, during and after **aztreonam** treatment were 517, 534 and 592 nanograms/ml respectively.[1] On the basis of this study there would seem to be no need to take special precautions if ciclosporin and **aztreonam** are used concurrently.

1. Alonso Hernandez A. Effects of aztreonam on cyclosporine levels in kidney transplant patients. *Transplantology: J Cell Organ Transplantation* (1993) 4, 85–6.

Ciclosporin + Benzbromarone

Benzbromarone does not interact adversely with ciclosporin.

Clinical evidence, mechanism, importance and management

Twenty-five kidney transplant patients on ciclosporin were given 100 mg **benzbromarone** daily to treat hyperuricaemia. The plasma uric acid levels decreased from 579 to 313 micromol/l and the urinary uric acid secretion rose from 2082 to 3233 micromol/24 h after 4 weeks treatment. The plasma uric acid levels normalised in 21 of the

patients who had creatinine clearances over 25 ml/min. No significant side-effects developed and the ciclosporin serum levels remained unchanged. The authors of the report emphasise the advantages of **benzbromarone** over allopurinol because of its efficacy, lack of significant side-effects and because unlike allopurinol it does not interact with azathioprine, which often accompanies ciclosporin treatment.[1]

1. Zürcher RM, Bock HA, Thiel G. Excellent uricosuric efficacy of benzbromarone in cyclosporin-A-treated renal transplant patients. A prospective study. *Nephrol Dial Transplant* (1994) 9, 548–51.

Ciclosporin + Benzodiazepines

Ciclosporin and midazolam appear not to interact.

Clinical evidence, mechanism, importance and management

On the basis of an experimental study in 9 patients it was concluded that the dosage of **midazolam** needs no adjustment in those on ciclosporin. **Midazolam** also appears to have no effect on ciclosporin.[1]

1. Li G, Treiber G, Meinshausen J, Wolf J, Werringloer J, Klotz U. Is cyclosporin A an inhibitor of drug metabolism? *Br J Clin Pharmacol* (1990) 30, 71–7.

Ciclosporin + Beta-blockers

There is evidence that carvedilol can cause a small to moderate rise in serum ciclosporin levels.

Clinical evidence, mechanism, importance and management

A study in 21 kidney transplant patients found that when **atenolol** was gradually replaced by **carvedilol** in a stepwise manner, starting with 6.25 mg **carvedilol** daily and gradually increasing it to 50 mg, the ciclosporin dosage had to be gradually reduced. At 90 days the daily ciclosporin dosage had been reduced by 20% (from 3.7 to 3 mg/kg body weight) to maintain levels within the therapeutic range but considerable inter-individual variations were seen.[1] The reason for this interaction is not understood. Information about other **beta-blockers** seems to be lacking, but be alert for this interaction if **carvedilol** is used.

1. Kaijser M, Johnsson C, Zezina L, Backman U, Dimeny E, Fellstrom B. Elevation of cyclosporin A blood levels during carvedilol treatment in renal transplant patients. *Clin Transplant* (1997) 11, 577–81.

Ciclosporin + Bile acids or Ursodeoxycholic acid (Ursodiol)

Ursodeoxycholic acid (ursodiol) unpredictably increases the absorption and raises the serum levels of ciclosporin in some but not all patients. Bile acids (cholic/dehydrocholic acids) appear not to interact with ciclosporin.

Clinical evidence

(a) Bile acids (cholic/dehydrocholic acids)

Eleven healthy subjects were given a single oral dose of ciclosporin on three occasions: while fasting, with breakfast, and with breakfast plus **bile acid** tablets (400 mg **cholic acid**, 100 mg **dehydrocholic acid**). The ciclosporin AUCs were 7283, 7453 and 9078 nanograms/ml respectively indicating that the **bile acids** increased the absorption of the ciclosporin by 22%. However, a related study in 19 transplant patients found that their 12 h trough ciclosporin serum levels were unchanged by the concurrent use of this daily dosage of **bile acids** over an 8-day period.[1]

(b) Ursodeoxycholic acid (Ursodiol)

A man who previously had had his entire ileum removed and about 1 m of the residual jejunum anastomosed to the transverse colon, had a heart transplant. When given **ursodeoxycholic acid** (1 to 2 g daily) it was found possible to reduce his ciclosporin dosage from 1.6 to 1.2 g daily, but later when the **ursodeoxycholic acid** was stopped his ciclosporin serum levels fell to subtherapeutic levels and severe acute rejection developed. When it was restarted the ciclosporin levels rose once again. The **ursodeoxycholic acid** increased the ciclosporin AUC by over 200%.[2] Another patient with chronic active hepatitis C showed an increase in his trough serum ciclosporin levels from 150 to 500 nanograms/ml when treated with **ursodeoxycholic acid**, and it was necessary to halve his daily ciclosporin dosage to keep his serum levels at 150 nanograms/ml.[3]

In contrast, a study in 7 liver transplant patients found no statistically significant changes in mean ciclosporin levels when administered single 600-mg doses of **ursodeoxycholic acid** at the same time as the ciclosporin.[4] Yet another study in 12 liver transplant patients, 6 of whom were cholestatic, found that after a single dose of **ursodeoxycholic acid** the ciclosporin was absorbed more rapidly in 8 patients but the mean 24 h AUC was not significantly changed although 7 patients showed some rise. There was no consistent improvement in the ciclosporin pharmacokinetics in the cholestatic patients.[5]

Mechanism

When an interaction occurs it is thought to do so because the ursodeoxycholic acid improves micellation of the oil-containing oral dosage ciclosporin formulation so that its absorption is increased.[2]

Importance and management

Information is limited but bile acids do not apparently interact with ciclosporin, while the ciclosporin/ursodeoxycholic acid interaction appears to be uncertain and unpredictable. It would therefore be prudent to monitor the effects of adding or stopping ursodeoxycholic acid in any patient on ciclosporin, being alert for the need to adjust the ciclosporin dosage. More study is needed.

1. Lindholm A, Henricsson S, Dahlqvist R. The effect of food and bile acid administration on the relative bioavailability of cyclosporin. *Br J Clin Pharmacol* (1990) 29, 541–8.
2. Gutzler F, Zimmermann R, Ring GH, Sauer P, Stiehl A. Ursodeoxycholic acid enhances the absorption of cyclosporine in a heart transplant patient with short bowel syndrome. *Transplant Proc* (1992) 24, 2620–1.
3. Sharobeem R, Bacq Y, Furet Y, Grezard O, Nivet H, Breteau M, Bagros P, Lebranchu Y. Cyclosporine A and ursodeoxycholic acid interaction. *Clin Transplant* (1993) 7, 223–6.
4. Maboundou CW, Paintaud G, Vanlemmens C, Magnette J, Bresson-Hadni S, Mantion G, Miguet JP, Bechtel PR. A single dose of ursodiol does not affect cyclosporine absorption in liver transplant patients. *Eur J Clin Pharmacol* (1996) 50, 335–7.
5. al-Quaiz MN, O'Grady JG, Tredger JM, Williams R. Variable effect of ursodeoxycholic acid on cyclosporin absorption after orthotopic liver transplantation. *Transpl Int* (1994) 7, 190–4.

Ciclosporin + Busulfan and Cyclophosphamide

The development of seizures in patients with bone marrow transplants on ciclosporin has been attributed to previous treatment with busulfan and cyclophosphamide.

Clinical evidence, mechanism, importance and management

Five of 182 patients receiving allogenic bone marrow transplants developed seizures within 22 to 61 days of starting ciclosporin and **methylprednisolone**. All of them had received 16 mg/kg **busulfan** and 120 mg/kg **cyclophosphamide** as preparative therapy without radiation.[1] Magnetic resonance imaging showed brain abnormalities which resolved a few days after the ciclosporin was withdrawn. The reasons are not understood, nor is the association between the use of the preparative drugs, the ciclosporin and the development of the sei-

zure clearly established. The authors of the report recommend that if seizures develop the ciclosporin should be stopped and anticonvulsants started.

1. Ghany AM, Tutschka PJ, McGhee RB, Avalos BR, Cunningham I, Kapoor N, Copelan EA. Cyclosporine-associated seizures in bone marrow transplant recipients given busulfan and cyclophosphamide preparative therapy. *Transplantation* (1991) 52, 310–15.

Ciclosporin + Calcium channel blockers

Diltiazem, nicardipine and verapamil raise serum ciclosporin levels but also appear to possess both kidney-tissue protective and increased immunosuppressive effects, which can improve the viability of transplanted kidneys. The interaction of diltiazem and verapamil with ciclosporin has been exploited to save costs. Felodipine, isradipine, lacidipine, nifedipine and nitrendipine normally appear not to raise serum ciclosporin levels, but rises and falls have been seen in a few patients on nifedipine. The situation with amlodipine is uncertain, but it may have kidney-protective properties.

Clinical evidence

(a) Amlodipine

Ten hypertensive patients with kidney transplants on ciclosporin (3 of them also on azathioprine) were concurrently treated with 5 to 10 mg **amlodipine** daily for 4 weeks. The hypertension was well controlled, the drug well tolerated, and the pharmacokinetics of the ciclosporin remained unaltered.[1] However, another study in 11 hypertensive kidney transplant patients found that **amlodipine** for 7 weeks raised the ciclosporin levels by an average of 40%.[2] **Amlodipine** is reported to reduce ciclosporin-associated nephrotoxicity in patients with psoriasis[3] and renal-transplant recipients.[4]

(b) Diltiazem

Sixty-five kidney transplant patients on ciclosporin and **diltiazem** needed less ciclosporin than 63 control patients not given **diltiazem** (7.3 compared with 9 mg/kg/day). There were considerable individual differences.[5]

Other studies clearly confirm that **diltiazem** can raise ciclosporin serum levels.[6-31] In some cases the serum ciclosporin levels were not only controlled by reducing the ciclosporin dosage by 30 to 60% but it appeared that **diltiazem** had a kidney protective role (reduced nephrotoxicity, fewer rejection episodes and haemodialyses).[11,22,32-36] See also cost-saving under 'Importance and management' below.

(c) Felodipine

Thirteen kidney transplant patients showed no significant changes in their serum ciclosporin levels when treated with 2.5 to 10 mg **felodipine** daily and serum creatinine levels were also unchanged. Mean blood pressures fell from 161/100 to 152/90 mmHg.[37] Another study found no significant changes in ciclosporin levels in patients also treatment with **felodipine**.[38] A single 10-mg dose of **felodipine** in ciclosporin-treated kidney transplant patients was found to have beneficial effects on blood pressure, renal haemodynamics, renal tubular sodium and water handling. The effects of long-term use were not studied.[39] A single dose study in 12 healthy subjects found that the maximum serum levels of ciclosporin 5 mg/kg were slightly raised (16%) by **felodipine** 10 mg, while the AUC and maximum serum level of the **felodipine** were raised 58% and 151% respectively but blood pressures were unchanged.[40] The same group of workers also briefly describe acute and short-term studies in groups of kidney transplant and dermatological patients which showed that 5 to 10 mg **felodipine** reduced blood pressure and opposed ciclosporin nephrotoxicity.[41] A study in heart transplant patients on ciclosporin found that **felodipine** attenuated the hypertrophic effects of ciclosporin on transplanted hearts.[42]

(d) Isradipine

Twelve kidney transplant patient showed no changes in ciclosporin levels over 4 weeks while taking up to 2.5 mg **isradipine** twice daily.[43] Similar findings are noted in another study.[38] Three other studies in 31 kidney transplant patients confirmed that ciclosporin serum levels are unchanged by **isradipine** but blood pressures are reduced.[44-46]

(e) Lacidipine

Ten kidney transplant patients on ciclosporin, prednisone and azathioprine were additionally given 4 mg **lacidipine** daily. A very small increase in the trough serum levels (6%) and AUC (14%) of the ciclosporin occurred. The blood pressures fell from 142/93 to 125/79 mmHg, and the urinary output rose from 1401 to 2050 ml/14 h.[47]

(f) Nicardipine

Nicardipine 20 mg three times a day in 9 patients raised their serum ciclosporin levels by 110% (from 226 to 430 nanograms/ml, range 24 to 341%). Their serum creatinine concentrations rose from 136 to 147 micromol/l.[48]

Other studies have found increases in serum ciclosporin levels, in some cases as much as two to threefold, when **nicardipine** was given.[49-55]

(g) Nifedipine

Five of 9 patients who showed an interaction with **nicardipine** (see above) showed no interaction when given **nifedipine**.[48] No changes in ciclosporin levels were seen in other studies,[35,56-60] but raised[17,20] and reduced levels[61] have been reported in others. Two studies found that **nifedipine** appeared to protect patients against the nephrotoxicity of ciclosporin,[62,63] however there is some evidence that the side effects of **nifedipine** (flushing, rash)[64] and gingival overgrowth may be increased.[65-68]

(h) Nitrendipine

Nitrendipine 20 mg daily for 3 weeks had no significant effect on serum ciclosporin levels of 16 kidney transplant patients.[69]

(i) Verapamil

Twenty-two kidney transplant patients on ciclosporin and **verapamil** had serum ciclosporin levels which were 50 to 70% higher than in 18 other patients not given **verapamil** although the dosages were the same. Serum creatinine levels were lower. Moreover only 3 of the 22 had rejection episodes within 4 weeks compared with 10 out of 18 not given **verapamil**.[70]

Other studies have demonstrated that 120 to 320 mg **verapamil** daily can increase, or double or even triple serum ciclosporin levels in individual patients with kidney or heart transplants.[24,38,58,61,71-75] Combined use does not apparently increase the severity or prevalence of gingival overgrowth caused by ciclosporin.[76]

Mechanism

The increased ciclosporin levels are largely due to inhibition by the calcium channel blockers of its metabolism by the liver. The reduced loss results in a serum level rise. Diltiazem also appears to reduce ischaemia-induced tubular necrosis.[77] Other calcium channel blockers also seem to have a kidney-protective effect. The raised felodipine levels are possibly due to competitive inhibition by ciclosporin of intestinal and liver metabolism, or changes in P-glycoprotein activity.

Importance and management

The interactions of ciclosporin with diltiazem, nicardipine and verapamil are established and relatively well documented. Concurrent use need not be avoided but ciclosporin levels should be well monitored and dosage reductions made as necessary. Even though ciclosporin serum levels are increased, these calcium channel blockers appear to have both a kidney-protective effect and to improve immunosuppression. One study[78] noted that ". . . calcium channel blockers lead to an alteration of the ciclosporin pharmacokinetics by increasing ciclosporin blood levels . . . this interference, however, is of no harm to the patient, since no change in kidney function was observed despite drastic elevation of ciclosporin levels." With diltiazem and verapamil the ciclosporin dosage can apparently be reduced by about 25 to 50% and possibly more with nicardipine. One study found that the costs of ciclosporin for heart transplant patients could be reduced by

using 30 mg diltiazem three times daily initially, increasing to 60 mg three times daily at 1 month: a 32% saving in year 1 and 43% in the ensuing years.[13] Another calculated a 28% saving per kidney transplant patient.[79] Yet others estimate an annual 1991 cost saving of $1700 (Can.) and $2000 (US) per patient using 60 to 360 mg diltiazem daily.[14,80,81] A $3545 (Can.) annual saving per patient (1995) has also been described.[82] Take care not to substitute one diltiazem product for another after the patient has been stabilised because there is evidence that their bioequivalence differences may alter the extent of the interaction.[27,83] A 15% saving in ciclosporin costs while using verapamil is described in one report.[24]

The situation with nifedipine is not totally clear (no effect or decreases or increases) but it appears to have a kidney-protective effect.[59] So too does felodipine. The situation with amlodipine is also uncertain, but isradipine, lacidipine and nitrendipine appear to be non-interacting alternatives. Many of the calcium channel blockers have a kidney-protective effect.

1. Toupance O, Lavaud S, Canivet E, Bernaud C, Hotton J-M, Chanard J. Antihypertensive effect of amlodipine and lack of interference with cyclosporine metabolism in renal transplant recipients. *Hypertension* (1994) 24, 297–300.
2. Pesavento TE, Jones PA, Julian BA, Curtis JJ. Amlodipine increases cyclosporine levels in hypertensive renal transplant patients: results of a prospective study. *J Am Soc Nephrol* (1996) 7, 831–5.
3. Raman GV, Campbell SK, Farrer A, Albano JDM, Cook J. Modifying effects of amlodipine on cyclosporin A-induced changes in renal function in patients with psoriasis. *J Hypertens* (1998) 16 (Suppl 4), S39–S41.
4. Schrama YC, Koomans HA. Interactions of cyclosporin A and amlodipine: blood cyclosporin A levels, hypertension and kidney function. *J Hypertens* (1998) 16 (Suppl 4), S33–S38.
5. Kohlhaw K, Wonigeit K, Frei U, Oldhafer K, Neumann K, Pichlmayr R. Effect of calcium channel blocker diltiazem on cyclosporine A blood levels and dose requirements. *Transplant Proc* (1988) 20 (Suppl 2), 572–4.
6. Pochet JM, Pirson Y. Cyclosporin-diltiazem interaction. *Lancet* (1986) i, 979.
7. Griño JM, Sabate I, Castelao AM, Alsina J. Influence of diltiazem on cyclosporin clearance. *Lancet* (1986) i, 1387.
8. Brockmöller J, Wagner K, Neumayer HH. Interaction of ciclosporine and diltiazem. *Naunyn Schmiedebergs Arch Pharmacol* (1988) 337 (Suppl), R126.
9. Kunzendorf U, Walz G, Neumayer H-H, Wagner K, Keller F, Offermann E. Einfluss von Diltiazem auf die Ciclosporin-Blutspiegel. *Klin Wochenschr* (1987) 65, 1101–3.
10. Sabaté I, Griñó JM, Castelao AM, Huguet J, Serón D, Blanco A. Cyclosporin-diltiazem interaction: comparison of cyclosporin levels measured with two monoclonal antibodies. *Transplant Proc* (1989) 21, 1460–1.
11. Ki Chul Choi, Young Joon Kang, Shin Kon Kim, Soo Bang Ryu. Effects of the calcium channel blocker diltiazem on the blood and serum levels of cyclosporin A. *Chonnam J Med Sci* (1994) 2, 131–6.
12. Campistol JM, Oppenheimer F, Vilardell J, Ricart MJ, Alcaraz A, Ponz E, Andreu J. Interaction between ciclosporin and diltiazem in renal transplant patients. *Nephron* (1991) 57, 241–2.
13. Valantine H, Keogh A, McIntosh N, Hunt S, Oyer P, Schroeder J. Cost containment-Coadministration of diltiazem with cyclosporine following cardiac transplant. *J Heart Transplant* (1990) 9, 68.
14. Bourge RC, Kirklin JK, Naftel DC, Figg WD, White-Williams C, Ketchum C. Diltiazem-cyclosporine interaction in cardiac transplant recipients: impact on cyclosporine dose and medication costs. *Am J Med* (1991) 90, 402–4.
15. Maddux MS, Veremis SA, Bauma WD, Pollak R. Significant drug interactions with cyclosporine. *Hosp Ther* (1987) 12, 56–70.
16. Brockmöller J, Neumayer H-H, Wagner K, Weber W, Heinemeyer G, Kewitz H, Roots I. Pharmacokinetic interaction between cyclosporin and diltiazem. *Eur J Clin Pharmacol* (1990) 38, 237–42.
17. Diaz C, Gillum DM. Interaction of diltiazem and nifedipine with cyclosporine in renal transplant recipients. *Kidney Int* (1989) 35, 513.
18. Wagner K, Albrecht S, Neumayer H-H. Prevention of posttransplant acute tubular necrosis by the calcium antagonist diltiazem: a propective randomized study. *Am J Nephrol* (1987) 7, 287–91.
19. McCauley J, Ptachcinski RJ, Shapiro R. The cyclosporine-sparing effects of diltiazem in renal transplantation. *Transplant Proc* (1989) 21, 3955–7.
20. Castelao AM. Cyclosporine A - drug interactions. In Sunshine I (Ed.) Recent developments in therapeutic drug monitoring and clinical toxicology. 2nd Int Conf Therapeutic Drug Monitoring Toxicology, Barcelona, Spain (1992) 203–9.
21. Shennib H, Auger J-L. Diltiazem improves cyclosporine dosage in cystic fibrosis lung transplant recipients. *J Heart Lung Transplant* (1994) 13, 292–6.
22. Macdonald P, Keogh A, Connell J, Harvison A, Richens D, Spratt P. Diltiazem co-administration reduces cyclosporine toxicity after heart transplantation: a prospective randomised study. *Transplant Proc* (1992) 24, 2259–62.
23. Masri MA, Shakuntala V, Shanwaz M, Zaher M, Dhawan I, Yasin I, Pingle A. Pharmacokinetics of cyclosporine in renal transplant patients on diltiazem. *Transplant Proc* (1994) 26, 1921.
24. Sketris IS, Methot ME, Nicol D, Belitsky P, Knox MG. Effect of calcium-channel blockers on cyclosporine clearance and use in renal transplant patients. *Ann Pharmacother* (1994) 28, 1227–31.
25. Bleck JS, Thiesemann C, Kliem V, Christians U, Hecker H, Repp H, Frei U, Westhoff-Bleck M, Manns M, Sewing KF. Diltiazem increases blood concentrations of cyclized cyclosporine metabolites resulting in different cyclosporine metabolite patterns in stable male and female renal allograft recipients. *Br J Clin Pharmacol* (1996) 41, 551–6.
26. Morris RG, Jones TE. Diltiazem disposition and metabolism in recipients of renal transplants. *Ther Drug Monit* (1998) 20, 365–70.
27. Jones TE, Morris RG, Mathew TH. Formulation of diltiazem affects cyclosporin-sparing activity. *Eur J Clin Pharmacol* (1997) 52, 55–8.
28. Jones TE, Morris RG, Mathew TH. Diltiazem-cyclosporin pharmacokinetic interaction — dose-response relationship. *Br J Clin Pharmacol* (1997) 44, 499–504.
29. Sharma A, Bell L, Drolet D, Drouin E, Gaul M, Girardin P, Goodyer P, Schreiber R. Cyclosporine (CSA) Neoral kinetics in children treated with diltiazem. *J Am Soc Nephrol* (1996) 7, 1923.

30. Wagner C, Sperschneider H, Korn A, Christians U. Influence of diltiazem on cyclosporine metabolites in renal graft recipients treated with Sandimmun® and Neoral®. *J Am Soc Nephrol* (1997) 8, 707A.

31. Åsberg A, Christiansen H, Hartmann A, Carlson E, Molden E, Berg KJ. Pharmacokinetic interactions between microemulsion formulated cyclosporine A and diltiazem in renal transplant recipients. *Eur J Clin Pharmacol* (1999) 55, 383–7.

32. Neumayer H-H, Wagner K. Diltiazem and economic use of cyclosporin. *Lancet* (1986) ii, 523.

33. Wagner K, Albrecht S, Neumayer H-H. Prevention of delayed graft function in cadaveric kidney transplantation by a calcium antagonist. Preliminary results of two prospective randomized trials. *Transplant Proc* (1986) 18, 510–15.

34. Wagner K, Albrecht S, Neumayer H-H. Prevention of delayed graft function by a calcium antagonist- a randomized trial in renal graft recipients on cyclosporine A. *Transplant Proc* (1986) 18, 1269–71.

35. Wagner K, Philipp Th, Heinemeyer G, Brockmüller F, Roots I, Neumayer HH. Interaction of cyclosporin and calcium antagonists. *Transplant Proc* (1989) 21, 1453–6.

36. Neumayer H-H, Kunzendorf U, Schreiber M. Protective effects of calcium antagonists in human renal transplantation. *Kidney Int* (1992) 41 (Suppl 36), S87–S93.

37. Cohen DJ, Teng S-N, Valeri A, Appel GB. Influence of oral felodipine on serum cyclosporine concentrations in renal transplant patients. *J Am Soc Nephrol* (1993) 4, 929.

38. Yildiz A, Sever MŞ, Türkmen A, Ecder T, Türk S, Akkaya V, Ark E. Interaction between cyclosporin A and verapamil, felodipine, and isradipine. *Nephron* (1999) 81, 117–18.

39. Pedersen EB, Sørensen SS, Eiskjær H, Skovbon H, Thomsen K. Interaction between cyclosporine and felodipine in renal transplant recipients. *Kidney Int* (1992) 41 (Suppl 36), S82–S86.

40. Madsen JK, Jensen JD, Jensen LW, Pedersen EB. Pharmacokinetic interaction between cyclosporine and the dihydropyridine calcium antagonist felodipine. *Eur J Clin Pharmacol* (1996) 50, 203–8.

41. Madsen JK, Kornerup HJ, Sørensen SS, Zachariae H, Pedersen EB. Ciclosporine nephrotoxicity can be counteracted by a calcium antagonist (felodipine) in acute and short-term studies. *J Am Soc Nephrol* (1995) 6, 1102.

42. Schwitter J, DeMarco T, Globits S, Sakuma H, Klinski C, Chatterjee K, Parmley WW, Higgins CB. Influence of felodipine on left ventricular hypertrophy and systolic function in orthoptic heart transplant recipients: possible interaction with cyclosporine medication. *J Heart Lung Transplant* (1999) 18, 1003–13.

43. Endresen L, Bergan S, Holdaas H, Pran T, Sinding-Larsen B, Berg KJ. Lack of effect of the calcium antagonist isradipine on cyclosporine pharmacokinetics in renal transplant patients. *Ther Drug Monit* (1991) 13, 490–5.

44. Martinez F, Pirson Y, Wallemacq P, van Ypersele de Strihou C. No clinically significant interaction between ciclosporin and isradipine. *Nephron* (1991) 59, 658–9.

45. Vernillet L, Bourbigot B, Codet JP, Le Saux L, Moal MC, Morin JF. Lack of effect of isradipine on cyclosporin pharmacokinetics. *Fundam Clin Pharmacol* (1992) 6, 367–74.

46. Ahmed K, Michael B, Burke JF. Effects of isradipine on renal hemodynamics in renal transplant patients treated with cyclosporine. *Clin Nephrol* (1997) 48, 307–10.

47. Ruggenenti P, Perico N, Mosconi L, Gaspari F, Benigni A, Amuchastegui CS, Bruzzi I, Remuzzi G. Calcium channel blockers protect transplant patients from cyclosporine-induced daily renal hypoperfusion. *Kidney Int* (1993) 43, 706–11.

48. Bourbigot B, Guiserix J, Airiau J, Bressollette L, Morin JF, Cledes J. Nicardipine increases cyclosporin blood levels. *Lancet* (1986) i, 1447.

49. Cantarovich M, Hiesse C, Lockiec F, Charpentier B, Fries D. Confirmation of the interaction between cyclosporine and the calcium channel blocker nicardipine in renal transplant patients. *Clin Nephrol* (1987) 28, 190–3.

50. Kessler M, Renoult E, Jonon B, Vigneron B, Huu TC, Netter P. Interaction ciclosporine-nicardipine et le transplanté rénal. *Therapie* (1987) 42, 273–5.

51. Deray G, Aupetit B, Martinez F, Baumelou A, Worcel A, Benhmida M, Legrand JC, Jacobs C. Cyclosporin-nicardipine interaction. *Am J Nephrol* (1989) 9, 349.

52. Kessler M, Netter P, Renoult E, Jonon B, Mur JM, Trechot P, Dousset B. Influence of nicardipine on renal function and plasma cyclosporin in renal transplant patients. *Eur J Clin Pharmacol* (1989) 36, 637–8.

53. Todd P, Garioch JJ, Rademaker M, Thomson J. Nicardipine interacts with cyclosporin. *Br J Dermatol* (1989) 121, 820.

54. Bouquet S, Chapelle G, Barrier L, Boutaud Ph, Menu P, Courtois Ph. Interactions ciclosporine-nicardipine chez un transplanté cardiaque, adaptation posologique. *J Pharm Clin* (1991) 11, 59.

55. Mabin D, Fourquet I, Richard P, Esnault S, Islam MS, Bourbigot B. Leucoencéphalopathie régressive au cours d'un surdosage en cyclosporine A. *Rev Neurol (Paris)* (1993) 149, 576–8.

56. McNally P, Mistry N, Idle J, Walls J, Feehally J. Calcium channel blockers and cyclosporine metabolism. *Transplantation* (1989) 48, 1071.

57. Rossi SJ, Hariharan S, Schroeder TJ, First MR. Cyclosporine dosing and blood levels in renal transplants receiving Procardia XL. *Clin Pharmacol Ther* (1993) 53, 238.

58. Ogborn MR, Crocker JFS, Grimm PC. Nifedipine, verapamil and cyclosporin A pharmacokinetics in children. *Pediatr Nephrol* (1993) 3, 314–16.

59. Propper DJ, Whiting PH, Power DA, Edward N, Catto GRD. The effect of nifedipine on graft function in renal allograft recipients treated with cyclosporin A. *Clin Nephrol* (1989) 32, 62–7.

60. Rossi SJ, Hariharan S, Schroeder TJ, First MR. Cyclosporine dosing and blood levels in renal transplant recipients receiving Procardia XL. *J Am Soc Nephrol* (1992) 3, 877.

61. Howard RL, Shapiro JI, Babcock S, Chan L. The effect of calcium channel blockers on the cyclosporine dose requirement in renal transplant recipients. *Ren Fail* (1990) 12, 89–92.

62. Feehally J, Walls J, Mistry N, Horsburgh T, Taylor J, Veitch PS, Bell PRF. Does nifedipine ameliorate cyclosporin A nephrotoxicity? *BMJ* (1987) 295, 310.

63. Morales JM, Andrés A, Alvarez C, Prieto C, Ortuño B, Ortuño T, Paternina ER, Hernandez Poblete G, Praga M, Ruilope LM, Rodicio JL. Calcium channel blockers and early cyclosporine nephrotoxicity after renal transplantation: a prospective randomized study. *Transplant Proc* (1990) 22, 1733–5.

64. McFadden JP, Pontin JE, Powles AV, Fry L, Idle JR. Cyclosporin decreases nifedipine metabolism. *BMJ* (1989) 299, 1224.

65. Thomason JM, Seymour RA, Rice N. The prevalence and severity of cyclosporin and nifedipine-induced gingival overgrowth. *J Clin Periodontol* (1993) 20, 37–40.

66. Jackson C, Babich S. Gingival hyperplasia: interaction between cyclosporin A and nifedipine? A case report. *N Y State Dent J* (1997) 63, 46–8.

67. Thomason JM, Ellis JS, Kelly PJ, Seymour RA. Nifedipine pharmacological variables as risk factors for gingival overgrowth in organ-transplant patients. *Clin Oral Investig* (1997) 1, 35–9.

68. Morgan JDT, Swarbrick MJ, Edwards CM, Donnelly PK. Cyclosporin, nifedipine and gingival hyperplasia: a randomized controlled study. *Transpl Int* (1994) 7 (Suppl 1), S320–S321.

69. Çopur MS, Tasdemir I, Turgan Ç, Yasavul Ü, Çaglar S. Effects of nitrendipine on blood pressure and blood cyclosporin A level in patients with posttransplant hypertension. *Nephron* (1989) 52, 227–30.

70. Dawidson I, Rooth P, Fry WR, Sandor Z, Willms C, Coorpender L, Alway C, Reisch J. Prevention of acute cyclosporine-induced renal blood flow inhibition and improved immunosuppression with verapamil. *Transplantation* (1989) 48, 575–80.

71. Lindholm A, Henricsson S. Verapamil inhibits cyclosporin metabolism. *Lancet* (1987) i, 1262–3

72. Hampton EM, Stewart CF, Herrod HG, Valenski WR. Augmentation of in- vitro immunosuppressive effects of cyclosporin by verapamil. *Clin Pharmacol Ther* (1987) 41, 169.

73. Robson RA, Fraenkel M, Barratt LJ, Birkett DJ. Cyclosporin-verapamil interaction. *Br J Clin Pharmacol* (1988) 25, 402–3.

74. Angermann CE, Spes CH, Anthuber M, Kemkes BM, Theisen K. Verapamil increases cyclosporin-A blood trough levels in cardiac recipients. *J Am Coll Cardiol* (1988) 11, 206A.

75. Sabatée I, Griño JM, Castelao AM, Ortolá J. Evaluation of cyclosporin-verapamil interaction, with observations on parent cyclosporin and metabolites. *Clin Chem* (1988) 34, 2151.

76. Cebeci I, Kantarci A, Firatli E, Çarin M, Tuncer Ö. The effect of verapamil on the prevalence and severity of cyclosporine-induced gingival overgrowth in renal allograft recipients. *J Periodontol* (1996) 67, 1201–5.

77. Oppenheimer F, Alcaraz A, Mañalich M, Ricart MJ, Vilardell J, Campistol JM, Andreu J, Talbot-Wright R, Fernandez-Cruz L. Influence of the calcium blocker diltiazem on the prevention of acute renal failure after renal transplantation. *Transplant Proc* (1992) 24, 50–1.

78. Wagner K, Henkel M, Heinemeyer G, Neumayer H-H. Interaction of calcium blockers and cyclosporine. *Transplant Proc* (1988) 20 (Suppl 2), 561–8.

79. Smith CL, Hampton EM, Pederson JA, Pennington LR, Bourne DWA. Clinical and medicoeconomic impact of the cyclosporine-diltiazem interaction in renal transplant recipients. *Pharmacotherapy* (1994) 14, 471–81.

80. Moody HR, Bickell-Feist L, Friesen I, Huizinga R, Halloran PF. Benefits of cyclosporine dose reduction using diltiazem. *Clin Invest Med* (1991) 14 (Suppl A), A142.

81. Smith CL, Hampton EM, Pederson JA, Pennington LR, Bourne DWA. Influence of diltiazem on the pharmacokinetics and dose/cost relationships of cyclosporine in renal transplant patients. *J Am Soc Nephrol* (1991) 2, 816.

82. Iqbal S, Holland D, Toffelmire EB. Diltiazem inhibition of cyclosporin metabolism provides cost effective therapy. *Clin Pharmacol Ther* (1995) 57, 219.

83. Cooke CE. Nontherapeutic cyclosporine levels. Sustained-release diltiazem products are not the same. *Transplantation* (1994) 57, 1687.

Ciclosporin + Cephalosporins

Very limited evidence suggests that ceftriaxone and ceftazidime may increase serum ciclosporin levels, nephrotoxicity may occur with ceftazidime and that cefuroxime does not interact.

Clinical evidence, mechanism, importance and management

Two kidney transplant patients showed two to fourfold rises in ciclosporin levels within 2 to 3 days of starting 1 g **ceftriaxone** twice daily. Levels fell when the antibacterial was stopped. The reason is uncertain but it was suggested that **ceftriaxone** possibly inhibits the metabolism of the ciclosporin by the liver.[1] However another very brief report about 51 kidney transplant patients said that **ceftriaxone** and **cefuroxime** had no effect on ciclosporin serum levels and also that they were not nephrotoxic. This report also stated that **ceftazidime** did not affect serum ciclosporin levels but it increased blood urea nitrogen and creatinine levels, indicating that it was nephrotoxic.[2] **Ceftazidime** has also been implicated in an increase in serum ciclosporin levels in another report.[3]

Information about these three cephalosporins is very limited indeed but it would certainly be prudent to monitor the outcome if **ceftriaxone** or **ceftazidime** and ciclosporin are given concurrently. More study is needed.

1. Alvarez JS, Del Castillo JAS, Ortiz MJA. Interaction between ciclosporin and ceftriaxone. *Nephron* (1991) 59, 681–2.

2. Xu F, Wu Z, Zou H. Effects on renal function and cyclosporine blood concentration by combination with three cephalosporins in renal transplant patients. *Zhongguo Kangshengsu Zashi* (1997) 22, 223–5.

3. Cockburn I. Cyclosporin A: a clinical evaluation of drug interactions. *Transplant Proc* (1986) 18 (Suppl 5), 50–5.

Ciclosporin + Chloramphenicol

Four patients have shown a marked rise in serum ciclosporin levels when treated with chloramphenicol.

Clinical evidence

A woman with a heart-lung transplant and with a trough ciclosporin serum level of 84 micrograms/l was started on **chloramphenicol** (dosage not stated) to treat *Xanthomonas maltophilia*. On the next day the ciclosporin levels had risen to 240 micrograms/l. The **chloramphenicol** was continued but the ciclosporin dosage was reduced from 300 to 225 mg daily. By day 8 the ciclosporin levels had fallen within the therapeutic range.[1]

A kidney transplant patient on ciclosporin was given several antibacterials for a variety of infections. **Chloramphenicol** increased trough ciclosporin levels at least sixfold and there was a rapid decrease in ciclosporin levels to the normal range over 4 days after **chloramphenicol** was withdrawal.[2]

Two kidney transplant patients showed marked increases in serum ciclosporin levels (almost doubled in one case) when given **chloramphenicol** to treat urinary tract infections.[3]

Mechanism

Uncertain. Chloramphenicol is a recognised enzyme inhibitor and it seems possible that it may reduce the metabolism of the ciclosporin by the liver.[2]

Importance and management

Information seems to be limited to these three reports so that although the interaction appears to be established its incidence is obviously uncertain. It would now be prudent to monitor ciclosporin levels if chloramphenicol is added, being alert for the need to reduce the ciclosporin dosage. It seems doubtful if there will be enough chloramphenicol absorbed from eye drops to interact with ciclosporin, but this needs confirmation.

1. Steinfort CL, McConachy KA. Cyclosporin-chloramphenicol drug interaction in a heart-lung transplant recipient. *Med J Aust* (1994) 161, 455.
2. Bui LL, Huang DD. Possible interaction between cyclosporine and chloramphenicol. *Ann Pharmacother* (1999) 33, 252–3.
3. Zawadzki J, Prokurat S, Smirska E, Jelonek A. Interaction between cyclosporine A and chloramphenicol after kidney transplantation. *Pediatr Nephrol* (1991) 5, C49.

Ciclosporin + Chloroquine

Three patients showed rapid rises in serum ciclosporin levels and evidence of kidney toxicity in two of them when they were given chloroquine. Some loss of kidney function has even been seen with low doses of ciclosporin used for rheumatoid arthritis.

Clinical evidence

A kidney transplant patient on ciclosporin, azathioprine and prednisolone showed a threefold rise in ciclosporin serum levels (from 148 to 420 nanograms/ml) accompanied by a rise in serum creatinine levels within 48 h of starting 900 mg **chloroquine** for suspected malarial fever. On days 2 and 3 the **chloroquine** dosage was reduced to 300 mg daily. The ciclosporin and creatinine returned to their former levels 7 days after the **chloroquine** was stopped.[1]

When another kidney transplant patient on ciclosporin, azathioprine and prednisolone was additionally given 100 mg **chloroquine** daily for 6 days, his ciclosporin serum levels rose from 105 to 470 nanograms/ml and his serum creatinine levels rose from 200 to 234 micromol/l, accompanied by a rise in blood pressure from 130/80 to 160/100 mmHg. These normalised when the **chloroquine** was stopped, and rose again when **chloroquine** was restarted.[2] The ciclosporin serum levels of another patient doubled while taking 100 mg **chloroquine** daily.[3]

A study in 88 patients with recent onset rheumatoid arthritis found that the addition of low dose ciclosporin (1.25 or 2.5 mg/kg daily) to low dose **chloroquine** was moderately effective, but changes in serum creatinine levels occurred. The creatinine was raised 2 micromol/l with placebo, and 10 micromol/l with the 2.5 mg/kg ciclosporin dosage, but decreased by 1 micromol/l with the 1.25 mg/kg ciclosporin dose, indicating that some loss in renal function can occur.[4]

Mechanism

Not understood.

Importance and management

Information is limited but it would now be prudent to monitor the effects of adding chloroquine in any patient on ciclosporin, being alert for any changes in renal function when using low doses and for increases in serum ciclosporin levels when using normal immunosuppressive doses. More study is needed.

1. Nampoory MRN, Nessim J, Gupta RK, Johny KV. Drug interaction of chloroquine and ciclosporin. *Nephron* (1992) 62, 108–9.
2. Finielz P, Gendoo Z, Chuet C, Guiserix J. Interaction between cyclosporin and chloroquine. *Nephron* (1993) 65, 333.
3. Guizerix J, Aizel A. Interactions ciclosporine-chloroquine. *Presse Med* (1996) 25, 1214.
4. van den Borne BEEM, Landewé RBM, Goei The HS, Rietveld JH, Zwinderman AH, Bruyn GAW, Breedveld FC, Dijkmans BAC. Combination therapy in recent onset rheumatoid arthritis: a randomized double blind trial of the addition of low dose cyclosporine to patients treated with low dose chloroquine. *J Rheumatol* (1998) 25, 1493–8.

Ciclosporin + Cisapride

Cisapride increases the serum levels of ciclosporin and also increases its bioavailability.

Clinical evidence, mechanism, importance and management

After taking 10 mg **cisapride** three times daily for 2 days, and then 10 mg just before and together with ciclosporin and a test meal, 10 renal transplant patients were found to have increased maximal serum ciclosporin levels by 24% and increased 4 and 6 h AUCs by 50% and 38% respectively. Peak serum levels also occurred earlier.[1] The reasons for these changes are not fully understood, but earlier gastric emptying may be involved. The clinical importance of these increases is uncertain, but it would be prudent to monitor concurrent use, reducing the dosages if necessary.

1. Finet L, Westeel PF, Hary G, Maurel M, Andrejak M, Dupas JL. Effects of cisapride on the intestinal absorption of cyclosporine in renal transplant recipients. *Gastroenterology* (1991) 100, A209.

Ciclosporin + Clindamycin

Two patients have shown a marked reduction in serum ciclosporin levels when treated with clindamycin.

Clinical evidence, mechanism, importance and management

A lung transplant patient receiving ciclosporin in a dose to achieve levels of 100 to 150 nanograms/ml required dose increases to achieve this level when additionally treated with **clindamycin** 600 mg three times daily. Initially the levels were almost halved by the addition of clindamycin. Ciclosporin was reduced to the original dose when the clindamycin was stopped. In a second lung transplant patient treatment with **clindamycin** 600 mg three times daily necessitated ciclosporin doses to be increased over 4 weeks from 325 mg daily to 1100 mg daily to maintain serum levels of about 200 nanograms/ml. The reasons for the interaction are not understood, but the authors suggest close monitoring of ciclosporin levels to prevent underdosing if clindamycin is co-administered.[1]

1. Thurnheer R, Laube I, Speich R. Possible interaction between clindamycin and cyclosporin. *BMJ* (1999) 319, 163.

Ciclosporin + Clonidine

A child taking ciclosporin showed a marked rise in serum ciclosporin levels when clonidine was added.

Clinical evidence, mechanism, importance and management

A 3-year-old renal transplant patient taking ciclosporin, azathioprine and prednisone was given a combination of propranolol, hydralazine, furosemide (frusemide) and nifedipine postoperatively in an attempt to control his blood pressure. Minoxidil was added, but was considered unacceptable because of adverse cosmetic effects. When it was replaced with **clonidine**, the ciclosporin levels increased approximately threefold to 927 nanograms/ml, in spite of a dose reduction. Ciclosporin levels fell to the normal range (150 to 300 nanograms/ml) on withdrawal of **clonidine** and blood pressure was controlled by the addition of an ACE inhibitor. It is possible that **clonidine** inhibited the metabolism of ciclosporin via the cytochrome P450 pathway.[1] Although this appears to be the only report of the interaction, it would seem advisable to avoid clonidine where possible, but if it is used, monitor the ciclosporin levels very closely.

1. Gilbert RD, Kahn D, Cassidy M. Interaction between clonidine and cyclosporine A. *Nephron* (1995) 71, 105.

Ciclosporin + Colchicine

A handful of cases of ciclosporin toxicity and serious muscle disorders (myopathy, rhabdomyolysis) have been seen when colchicine and ciclosporin were used concurrently.

Clinical evidence, mechanism, importance and management

A patient with a kidney transplant showed a transient (2 to 3 days) rise in serum creatinine and serum ciclosporin levels (from 100 to 200 up to 1519 nanograms/ml) the day after receiving a total of 4 mg **colchicine**.[1] Another kidney transplant patient on ciclosporin, azathioprine and prednisone developed **colchicine** neuromyopathy (possibly rhabdomyolysis), ciclosporin nephrotoxicity and liver function abnormalities when treated with **colchicine**.[2] Acute myopathy (muscle weakness, myalgia) occurred in a kidney transplant patient after taking **colchicine**.[3] Another case suggestive of rhabdomyolysis has been published,[4] and the makers of ciclosporin have another report on their records.[5] Two other cases of myopathy and muscle weakness in renal transplant patients have been attributed to the concurrent use of ciclosporin and **colchicine**.[6,7] There is also a report of **colchicine**-induced myopathy and hepatonephropathy in a heart transplant patient who was treated with concomitant ciclosporin and **colchicine**.[8]

The overall picture presented by these reports is very unclear. Is the **colchicine** toxicity made worse by ciclosporin, or ciclosporin toxicity made worse by **colchicine**, or both? A syndrome of myopathy, gastrointestinal disturbances and mild hepatic and renal dysfunction as a result of concurrent use has been suggested.[8,9] This may be due to inhibition of P-glycoprotein by ciclosporin and subsequent impairment of **colchicine** excretion in to the bile and urine resulting in elevated, toxic **colchicine** levels.[8]

And what is the incidence? Whatever the answers, if concurrent use is thought to be appropriate, it should be very carefully monitored because the outcome can be serious. Rhabdomyolysis appears to be a rare complication and the maker Sandoz advise a change of treatment if any signs and symptoms develop.[5] More study is needed.

1. Menta R, Rossi E, Guariglia A, David S, Cambi V. Reversible acute cyclosporin nephrotoxicity induced by colchicine administration. *Nephrol Dial Transplant* (1987) 2, 380–1.
2. Rieger EH, Halasz NA, Wahlstrom HE. Colchicine neuromyopathy after renal transplantation. *Transplantation* (1990) 49, 1196–8.
3. Lee BI, Shin SJ, Yoon SN, Choi YJ, Yang CW, Bang BK. Acute myopathy induced by colchicine in a cyclosporine-treated renal recipient. A case report and review of the literature. *J Korean Med Sci* (1997) 12, 160–1.
4. Noppen M, Velkeniers B, Dierckx R, Bruyland M, Vanhaelst L. Cyclosporine and myopathy. *Ann Intern Med* (1987) 107, 945–6.

5. Arellano F, Krupp P. Muscular disorders associated with cyclosporin. *Lancet* (1991), 337, 915.
6. Rumpf KW, Henning HV. Is myopathy in renal transplant patients induced by cyclosporin or colchicine? *Lancet* (1990) 335, 800–1.
7. Jagose JT, Bailey RR. Muscle weakness due to colchicine in a renal transplant recipient. *N Z Med J* (1997) 110, 343.
8. Gruberg L, Har-Zahav Y, Agranat O, Freimark D. Acute myopathy induced by colchicine in a cyclosporine treated heart transplant recipient: possible role of the multidrug resistance transporter. *Transplant Proc* (1999) 31, 2157–8.
9. Yussim A, Bar-Nathan N, Lustig S, Shaharabani E, Geier E, Shmuely D, Nakache R, Shapira Z. Gastrointestinal, hepatorenal, and neuromuscular toxicity caused by cyclosporine-colchicine interaction in renal transplantation. *Transplant Proc* (1994) 26, 2825–6.

Ciclosporin + Colestyramine

Colestyramine can interact with ciclosporin in some patients but the outcome appears to be unpredictable.

Clinical evidence, mechanism, importance and management

Four transplant patients on ciclosporin and prednisolone given **colestyramine** for a week had only a very small average change (+ 6%) in the AUC of the ciclosporin, but one patient had a 55% increase and another a 23% decrease.[1] Another study[2] in 6 kidney transplant patients given 4 g **colestyramine** daily found no significant changes. As **colestyramine** appears to interact unpredictably it would been prudent to monitor the outcome if it is added to established treatment with ciclosporin. More study is needed.

1. Keogh A, Day R, Critchley L, Duggin G, Baron D. The effect of food and cholestyramine on the absorption of cyclosporine in cardiac transplant patients. *Transplant Proc* (1988) 20, 27–30.
2. Jensen RA, Lal SM, Diaz-Arias A, James-Kracke M, Van Stone JC, Ross G. Does cholestyramine interfere with cyclosporine absorption? A prospective study in renal transplant patients. *ASAIO J* (1995) 41, M704–M706.

Ciclosporin + Corticosteroids

Concurrent use is very common. Some evidence suggests that ciclosporin serum levels are raised. Ciclosporin can reduce the loss of the corticosteroids from the body and corticosteroid overdosage may occur. Convulsions have also been described during concurrent use, and the incidence of diabetes mellitus is said to be increased following the use of ciclosporin and methylprednisolone.

Clinical evidence

(a) Corticosteroid levels increased

A pharmacokinetic study in 40 patients showed that the clearance of **prednisolone** was reduced about 30% in those receiving ciclosporin when compared with those on azathioprine (1.9 compared with 2.6 ml/min/kg).[1]

Another study by the same group of workers reported a 25% reduction in clearance of **prednisolone** in the presence of ciclosporin in patients with kidney transplants.[2] Other studies[3-5] confirm that ciclosporin reduces the clearance of **prednisolone** from the body by about a third, as a result some patients develop signs of overdosage (cushingoid symptoms such as steroid diabetes, osteonecrosis of the hip joints).[3] These studies have all been questioned in another study which found that the metabolism of **prednisolone** was not affected by ciclosporin.[6] A further study found that the pharmacokinetics of **methylprednisolone** in patients on ciclosporin and azathioprine varied widely between individual kidney transplant patients, but the mean values were similar to those found in normal subjects.[7]

(b) Ciclosporin levels

A comparative study over a year in two groups of kidney transplant patients taking ciclosporin and azathioprine, one group with and the other without **prednisone**, showed that the latter had higher trough ciclosporin levels (approximately 10 to 20%) despite using the same or lower doses of ciclosporin.[8] The serum ciclosporin levels of 22 out of 33 patients were reported to be more than doubled when given intravenous **methylprednisolone**. The ciclosporin dosage was reduced in 6 patients.[3,9] Other studies have found that high doses of **methylprednisolone** increased or more than doubled serum ciclosporin levels.[10-12] However another study found that the clearance of ciclosporin is increased by **high-dose steroids**, although trough ciclosporin levels were unchanged.[13] There is other evidence that **low-dose steroids** do not increase the immunosuppression of ciclosporin, but they can reduce the nephrotoxicity.[14]

(c) Convulsions

A report describes 4 young patients (aged 10, 12, 13 and 18) who had undergone bone marrow transplants for severe aplastic anaemia and who developed convulsions while treated with high dose **methylprednisolone** (5 to 20 mg/kg/day) and ciclosporin.[15] Convulsions also occurred in a woman of 25 when treated with ciclosporin and high dose **methylprednisolone**.[16]

(d) Hyperglycaemia and Diabetes Mellitus

A study of 314 kidney transplant patients over the period 1979 to 1987 found that the incidence of diabetes mellitus in those given ciclosporin and **methylprednisolone** was twice that of other patients treated with azathioprine and **methylprednisolone**. The diabetes developed within less than 2 months.[17]

Mechanisms

The evidence suggests that ciclosporin reduces the metabolism of the corticosteroids by the liver thereby reducing their loss from the body.[4,18]

Importance and management

None of these adverse interactions is well established, and the picture is confusing. Concurrent use is common and advantageous but be alert for any evidence of increased ciclosporin and corticosteroid effects. It is not clear whether high dose corticosteroids cause a rise in serum ciclosporin levels or not. Assay results should be interpreted with caution.[19] The authors of one report point out that this interaction could possibly lead to a misinterpretation of clinical data. In patients with kidney transplants a rise in serum creatinine levels is assumed to be due to rejection, unless proved otherwise. If a corticosteroid is then given, this could lead to increased ciclosporin levels which might be interpreted as ciclosporin nephrotoxicity.[9]

1. Langhoff E, Madsen S, Olgaard K, Ladefoged J. Clinical results and cyclosporine effect on prednisolone metabolism. *Kidney Int* (1984) 26, 642.
2. Langhoff E, Madsen S, Flachs H, Olgaard K, Ladefoged J, Hvidberg EF. Inhibition of prednisolone metabolism by cyclosporine in kidney-transplanted patients. *Transplantation* (1985) 39, 107–9.
3. Öst L, Klintmalm G, Ringdén O. Mutual interaction between prednisolone and cyclosporine in renal transplant patients. *Transplant Proc* (1985) 17, 1252–5.
4. Öst L. Effects of cyclosporin on prednisolone metabolism. *Lancet* (1984) i, 451.
5. Öst L. Impairment of prednisolone metabolism by cyclosporine treatment in renal graft recipients. *Transplantation* (1987) 44, 533–35.
6. Frey FJ, Schnetzer A, Horber FF, Frey BM. Evidence that cyclosporine does not affect the metabolism of prednisolone after renal transplantation. *Transplantation* (1987) 43, 494–8.
7. Tornatore KM, Morse GD, Jusko WJ, Walshe JJ. Methylprednisolone disposition in renal transplant recipients receiving triple-drug immunosuppression. *Transplantation* (1989) 48, 962–5.
8. Hricik DE, Moritz C, Mayes JT, Schulak JA. Association of the absence of steroid therapy with increased cyclosporine blood levels in renal transplant recipients. *Transplantation* (1990) 49, 221–3.
9. Klintmalm G, Säwe J. High dose methylprednisolone increases plasma cyclosporine levels in renal transplant recipients. *Lancet* (1984) i, 731.
10. Klintmalm G, Säwe J, Ringdéen O, von Bahr C, Magnusson A. Cyclosporine plasma levels in renal transplant patients. Association with renal toxicity and allograft rejection. *Transplantation* (1985) 39, 132–7.
11. Hall TG. Effect of methylprednisolone on cyclosporine blood levels. *Pharmacotherapy* (1990) 10, 248.
12. Rogerson ME, Marsden JT, Reid KE, Bewick M, Holt DW. Cyclosporine blood concentrations in the management of renal transplant recipients. *Transplantation* (1986) 41, 276–8.
13. Ptachcinski RJ, Venkataramanan R, Burckart GJ, Hakala TR, Rosenthal JT, Carpenter BJ, Taylor RJ. Cyclosporine–high-dose steroid interaction in renal transplant recipients: assessment by HPLC. *Transplant Proc* (1987) 19, 1728–9.
14. Nott D, Griffin PJA, Salaman JR. Low-dose steroids do not augment cyclosporine immunosuppression but do diminish cyclosporine nephrotoxicity. *Transplant Proc* (1985) 17, 1289–90.
15. Durrant S, Chipping PM, Palmer S, Gordon-Smith EC. Cyclosporin A, methylprednisolone and convulsions. *Lancet* (1982) ii, 829–30.
16. Boogaerts MA, Zachee P, Verwilghen RL. Cyclosporin, methylprednisolone and convulsions. *Lancet* (1982) ii, 1216–17.

17. Roth D, Milgrom M, Esquenazi V, Fuller L, Burke G, Miller J. Posttransplant hyperglycaemia. Increased incidence in cyclosporine-treated renal allograft recipients. *Transplantation* (1989) 47, 278–81.
18. Henricsson S, Lindholm A, Aravoglou M. Cyclosporin metabolism in human liver microsomes and its inhibition by other drugs. *Pharmacol Toxicol* (1990) 66, 49–52.
19. Ptachcinski RJ, Burckart GJ, Venkataramanan R, Rosenthal JT, Carpenter BJ, Hakala TR. Effect of high-dose steroids on cyclosporine blood concentrations using RIA and HPLC analysis. *Drug Intell Clin Pharm* (1987) 21, 20A.

Ciclosporin + Diphenyl-dimethyl-dicarboxylate

Two case reports show that diphenyl-dimethyl-dicarboxylate can cause a gradual fall in the serum levels of ciclosporin.

Clinical evidence, mechanism, importance and management

Two kidney transplant patients were successfully treated with ciclosporin and prednisolone for 30 and 36 months respectively. When they were started on 75 mg **diphenyl-dimethyl-dicarboxylate** daily for the treatment of chronic hepatitis, both of them showed a gradual fall in their trough serum ciclosporin levels. The ciclosporin levels of the first patient fell from 97.7 to 78 nanograms/ml at 4 weeks and to 49 nanograms/ml at 6 weeks. The other showed a fall from 127.5 to 70.5 nanograms/ml at 8 weeks and to 45 nanograms/ml at 16 weeks. The reasons are not understood. The ciclosporin dosages remained unchanged throughout, and despite the low serum levels which were reached, no graft rejection was seen. When the **diphenyl-dimethyl-dicarboxylate** was stopped, the ciclosporin levels gradually climbed again at about the same rate to approximately their former levels.[1] There would seem to be no clear reason for avoiding concurrent use but it would be prudent to monitor the outcome, being alert for the need to increase the ciclosporin dosage. **Diphenyl-dimethyl-dicarboxylate** is derived from *Schizandrae fructus* and is a 'hepatonic' preparation with actions which are not understood.

1. Kim YS, Kim DH, Kim DO, Lee BK, Kim KW, Park JN, Lee JC, Choi YS, Rim H. The effect of Diphenyl-dimethyl-dicarboxylate on cyclosporine-A blood level in kidney transplants with chronic hepatitis. *Korean J Intern Med* (1997) 12, 67–9.

Ciclosporin + Diuretics

Nephrotoxicity has been described in three patients on ciclosporin when given either amiloride-chlorothiazide, metolazone or mannitol. Furosemide (frusemide) can possibly protect the kidney against ciclosporin damage. Concurrent use of ciclosporin with thiazides, but not loop diuretics, may increase serum magnesium levels.

Clinical evidence, mechanism, importance and management

A 39-year-old man on ciclosporin whose second kidney transplant functioned subnormally and who required treatment of hypertension with **atenolol** and **minoxidil**, developed ankle oedema which was resistant to increasing doses of **furosemide (frusemide)** up to 750 mg daily. When **metolazone** 2.5 mg daily was added for 2 weeks his serum creatinine levels more than doubled (from 193 to 449 micromol/l). When it was stopped the creatinine levels fell again. Ciclosporin serum levels were unchanged and neither graft rejection nor hypovolaemia occurred.[1] The kidney transplant of another patient on ciclosporin almost ceased to function when **mannitol** was used, and biopsy indicated severe ciclosporin nephrotoxicity. Transplant function recovered when the **mannitol** was stopped.[2] The same reaction was demonstrated in *rats*.[2] A woman showed a rise in serum creatinine levels from 121 to 171 micromol/l three weeks after starting to take *Moduretic* (**amiloride + chlorothiazide**). Trough serum ciclosporin levels were unchanged.[3] Although *animal* studies suggested that **furosemide** might increase the nephrotoxicity of ciclosporin,[4] more recent human studies suggest that it may have a protective effect.[5]

The general importance of these adverse interactions is not clear, but good monitoring is obviously needed if these diuretics are given with ciclosporin.

Although ciclosporin and **loop diuretics** are both known to cause magnesium wasting, a review of magnesium serum levels, magnesium replacement doses and diuretic use in 50 heart transplant recipients indicated that magnesium requirements were not altered by concurrent use of ciclosporin and **loop diuretics**. Concurrent use of **thiazides** with ciclosporin resulted in increases in serum magnesium and decreases in magnesium replacement.[6]

1. Christensen P, Leski M. Nephrotoxic drug interaction between metolazone and cyclosporin. *BMJ* (1987) 294, 578.
2. Brunner FP, Hermle M, Mihatsch MJ, Thiel G. Mannitol potentiates cyclosporine nephrotoxicity. *Clin Nephrol* (1986) 25 (Suppl 1), S130–S136.
3. Deray G, Baumelou B, Le Hoang P, Aupetit B, Girard B, Baumelou A. Legrand JC, Jacobs C. Enhancement of cyclosporin nephrotoxicity by diuretic therapy. *Clin Nephrol* (1989) 32, 47.
4. Whiting PH, Cunningham C, Thomson AW, Simpson JG. Enhancement of high dose cyclosporin A toxicity by frusemide. *Biochem Pharmacol* (1984) 33, 1075–9.
5. Driscoll DF, Pinson CW, Jenkins RL, Bistrian BR. Potential protective effects of furosemide against early cyclosporine-induced renal injury in hepatic transplant recipients. *Transplant Proc* (1989) 21, 3549–50.
6. Arthur JM, Shamin S. Interaction of cyclosporine and FK506 with diuretics in transplant patients. *Kidney Int* (2000) 58, 325–30.

Ciclosporin + Fibrates

Increased serum ciclosporin levels have been reported in one patient and kidney deterioration in two others when given bezafibrate. The use of fenofibrate has also been associated with a reduced kidney function and possibly reduced serum ciclosporin levels. Two studies found no pharmacokinetic interaction with gemfibrozil while a third found gemfibrozil caused a significant reduction in ciclosporin levels.

Clinical evidence, mechanism, importance and management

(a) Bezafibrate

A kidney transplant patient showed a rise in his previously stable ciclosporin serum levels from about 150 to 200 nanograms/ml to a maximum of about 340 nanograms/ml over a 6-week period following the addition of 200 mg **bezafibrate** twice daily. The rise was accompanied by increases in blood urea nitrogen and creatinine levels. Renal biopsy showed evidence of kidney damage and rejection. The patient recovered when the **bezafibrate** was stopped.[1]

Two other transplant patients (one kidney and the other heart) showed reversible kidney deterioration when treated with **bezafibrate**. One was severe and the other showed the effect on two occasions. Neither showed any changes in ciclosporin serum levels.[2,3]

Another study over 3 months in heart transplant patients found that **bezafibrate** was associated with a rise in serum creatinine levels, although none of the patients had to be withdrawn from the study.[4]

Neither the incidence nor the reasons for these reactions are known, but because the outcome is uncertain and potentially serious, you should keep a close check on the effects of adding **bezafibrate** to ciclosporin in any patient. The makers of bezafibrate suggest close monitoring of kidney function.[5]

(b) Fenofibrate

Fenofibrate 200 mg once daily effectively reduced the blood cholesterol levels (from 7.7 to 6.5 mmol/l) of 10 heart transplant patients without significantly altering serum ciclosporin levels over a 2-week period. The only possible adverse effect was an increase in creatinine levels from 145 to 157 mmol/l, suggesting some possible nephrotoxicity. No other clinically adverse effects were seen, however the authors of this study suggested that longer follow-up studies were needed to confirm the safety of using these drugs together.[6] They followed this up by a 1-year study[7] in 43 heart transplant patients, only 14 of whom completed the study (67% withdrawal) for various reasons, including a rise in blood creatinine levels in 14 patients whose renal function improved when the **fenofibrate** was stopped. There was also some evidence of a reduction in ciclosporin levels in 5 patients who developed rejection, and 14 who had to stop the **fenofibrate** because ". . . of the failure to maintain adequate cyclosporine levels without adversely affecting kidney function."

The evidence from these reports emphasises the importance of monitoring the long-term concurrent use of these two drugs because there are clearly some potential hazards.

(c) Gemfibrozil

Forty kidney transplant patients under treatment with ciclosporin showed a reduction in their hypertriglyceridaemia when additionally treated with **gemfibrozil** but their ciclosporin serum levels remained unaltered.[8] Another study in which 12 patients were concurrently treated with both drugs similarly found that **gemfibrozil** did not affect serum ciclosporin levels.[9]

However, in contrast to these findings another study in 7 kidney transplant patients with hyperlipidaemia found that **gemfibrozil** 450 mg once or twice daily was associated with a decline in trough ciclosporin levels. Levels declined from 93 to 76 nanograms/ml after 6 weeks of treatment and after dose increases in 3 patients the level at 3 months was 88 nanograms/ml. In 8 similar patients not given **gemfibrozil**, and with the same ciclosporin dose throughout, trough levels changed from 99 nanograms/ml to 98 and 123 nanograms/ml at 6 weeks and 3 months. In 2 patients there was a significant increase in serum creatinine, and biopsy revealed chronic rejection in one and ciclosporin toxicity in the other. The trial was stopped at 6 months because a drug interaction was suspected. The mechanism is not known, but changes in distribution of lipoproteins during **gemfibrozil** treatment may cause changes in the free fraction of ciclosporin. Ciclosporin absorption may also be reduced. Close monitoring is recommended during concomitant use.[10]

1. Hirai M, Tatuso E, Sakurai M, Ichikawa M, Matsuya F, Saito Y. Elevated blood concentrations of cyclosporine and kidney failure after bezafibrate in renal graft recipient. *Ann Pharmacother* (1996) 30, 883–4.
2. Lipkin GW, Tomson CRV. Severe reversible renal failure with bezafibrate. *Lancet* (1993) 341, 371.
3. Jespersen B, Tvedegaard E. Bezafibrate induced reduction of renal function in a renal transplant recipient. *Nephrol Dial Transplant* (1995) 10, 702–3.
4. Barbir M, Hunt B, Kushwaha S, Kehely A, Prescot R, Thompson GR, Mitchell A, Yacoub M. Maxepa versus bezafibrate in hyperlipidemic cardiac transplant recipients. *Am J Cardiol* (1992) 70, 1596–601.
5. Bezalip (Bezafibrate). Roche Products Limited. Summary of product characteristics, August 2001.
6. deLorgeril M, Boissonnat P, Bizollon CA, Guidollet J, Faucon G, Guichard JP, Levy-Prades-Sauron R, Renaud S, Dureau G. Pharmacokinetics of cyclosporine in hyperlipidaemic long-term survivors of heart transplantation. Lack of interaction with the lipid-lowering agent, fenofibrate. *Eur J Clin Pharmacol* (1992) 43, 161–5.
7. Boissonnat P, Salen P, Guidollet J, Ferrara R, Dureau G, Ninet J, Renaud S, de Lorgeril M. The long-term effects of the lipid-lowering agent fenofibrate in hyperlipidemic heart transplant recipients. *Transplantation* (1994) 58, 245–7.
8. Pisanti N, Stanziale P, Imperatore P, D'Alessandro R, De Marino V, Capone D, De Marino V. Lack of effect of gemfibrozil on cyclosporine blood concentrations in kidney-transplanted patients. *Am J Nephrol* (1998) 18, 199–203.
9. Valino RN, Reiss WG, Hanes D, White M, Hoehn-Saric E, Klassen D, Bartlett S, Weir MR. Examination of the potential interaction between HMG-CoA reductase inhibitors and cyclosporine in transplant patients. *Pharmacotherapy* (1996) 16, 511.
10. Fehrman-Ekholm I, Jogestrand T, Angelin B. Decreased cyclosporine levels during gemfibrozil treatment of hyperlipidemia after kidney transplantation. *Nephron* (1996) 72, 483.

Ciclosporin + Food and Drinks

Food, milk and grapefruit juice, but not orange juice, can increase the bioavailability of ciclosporin. Lipid admixtures for parenteral nutrition appear not to affect ciclosporin pharmacokinetics. Red wine decreases ciclosporin bioavailability.

Clinical evidence

(a) Food and Milk

Patients taking ciclosporin with **milk** had a 39% higher AUC after **food** and 23% higher when fasting compared with others taking ciclosporin with **orange juice**.[1] **Food** more than doubled the AUC of ciclosporin (bioavailability increased from 20.7 to 53%) and almost tripled its maximal serum levels (from 783 to 2062 nanograms/ml).[2] When 18 patients with kidney transplants were given ciclosporin mixed with 240 ml **chocolate milk** and taken with a standard hospital **breakfast**, their peak ciclosporin levels rose by 31% (from 1120 to 1465 nanograms/ml), trough serum levels rose by 17% (from 228 to 267 nanograms/ml), and the AUC rose by 45%. Very considerable individual variations occurred.[3]

A study on 10 patients undergoing bone-marrow transplantation and given isocaloric and isonitrogenous parenteral nutrition with or without lipids found that ciclosporin pharmacokinetics are not affected by **lipid-enriched admixtures**.[4]

(b) Fruit juices

A considerable number of single and multiple dose studies in healthy subjects, transplant, and other patients with haematological diseases have shown that if oral ciclosporin is taken with 150 to 250 ml (5 to 8 ozs) of **grapefruit juice**, the trough and peak serum levels and the bioavailability of the ciclosporin may be increased. The increases reported vary very considerably. Increases in trough serum levels range from 23 to 85%,[5-13] in peak serum levels from 0 to 69%,[10,11,13-20] and in AUCs from 0 to 72%.[7-11,13-17,19,21,22]

The AUC of the microemulsion formulation of ciclosporin was increased by 38% (range 12 to 194%) by co-administered **grapefruit juice** but the maximum levels were unchanged.[23] A further study with the microemulsion formulation found both the peak levels and AUC increased by **grapefruit juice** but while increases of 39% and 60 % respectively were observed in African-American patients, smaller increases of 8% and 44% were observed in Caucasian patients.[24]

A study in 6 paediatric renal transplant patients found that administration of ciclosporin solution with **grapefruit juice** produced a significant increase (109%) in the 12-h trough level although the AUC was not significantly changed. The changes in the pharmacokinetics of ciclosporin in a microemulsion formulation co-administered **grapefruit juice** were similar those found with the solution but did not reach significance.[25]

Ciclosporin levels are unaffected by **orange juice**[8,15,19] and no changes are seen if the ciclosporin is given intravenously.[26]

(c) Red wine

A two-way crossover study in 12 healthy subjects given a single dose of ciclosporin 8 mg/kg with water or with 350 ml (12 oz) of **Californian red wine** found that **red wine** caused a 50% increase in the oral clearance of ciclosporin. The ciclosporin AUC was reduced by 30% and the maximum blood levels were reduced by 38% (from 1258 to 779 micrograms/l). There was a high degree of variability with increases in oral clearance ranging from 1.5% to 129% and Caucasians experiencing a greater degree of change than Asians.[27]

Mechanisms

In the case of grapefruit juice, it is suggested that the activity of cytochrome P450 isoenzyme CYP3A in the gut wall and liver is inhibited so that more ciclosporin is available.[14] Naringin (a flavonoid) has been suggested as the responsible component.

The mechanism by which red wine exerts its effect is not known. White wine does not appear to affect ciclosporin pharmacokinetics[28] so the interaction is not believed to be an effect of alcohol which may increase ciclosporin levels (see 'Ciclosporin + Alcohol', p.600). Antioxidants in red wine such as resveratrol may inactivate CYP3A4 and would also be expected to increase ciclosporin levels. The solubility of ciclosporin is decreased in red wine and it is possible that substances in red wine bind ciclosporin in the gastrointestinal tract and reduce its bioavailability.[27] Another study by the same authors suggested that ciclosporin absorption is possibly impaired through P-glycoprotein activation.[29]

Importance and management

The food, milk and grapefruit juice interactions are established and clinically important. Food, milk and grapefruit juice, but not orange juice, can increase the bioavailability of ciclosporin. The situation should therefore be monitored if any changes are made to the diet of patients on ciclosporin. Patients should be warned because increased ciclosporin levels are associated with increased nephrotoxicity.

Lipid admixtures in parenteral nutrition do not appear to affect

ciclosporin pharmacokinetics and it is speculated that they may protect against ciclosporin-induced nephrotoxicity. Close supervision and monitoring is required. There is insufficient evidence to allow extrapolation of the results to bone-marrow transplant recipients with risk factors such as dyslipidaemia, liver or renal failure.[4]

It has been suggested that the grapefruit juice/ciclosporin interaction could be exploited to save money. One group of authors has suggested that grapefruit juice is roughly as effective as diltiazem in raising ciclosporin serum levels, and has the advantage of being inexpensive, nutritious and lacking the systemic effects of diltiazem and ketoconazole which are already used in this way.[8] See 'Ciclosporin + Calcium channel blockers', p.606 and 'Ciclosporin + Azole antifungals', p.603. However, it has also been pointed out that it may be risky to try to exploit the ciclosporin/grapefruit juice interaction in this way because the increases appear to be so variable and difficult to control (if not impossible), the reasons being that batches of grapefruit juice vary so much and also that considerable patient variation occurs.[30-32]

Although patients may be advised to avoid alcohol after transplantation, those who do drink should exercise caution if drinking red wine while taking ciclosporin.[27]

1. Keogh A, Day R, Critchley L, Duggin G, Baron D. The effect of food and cholestyramine on the absorption of cyclosporine in cardiac transplant recipients. *Transplant Proc* (1988) 20, 27–30.
2. Gupta SK, Benet LZ. Food increases the bioavailability of cyclosporin in healthy volunteers. *Clin Pharmacol Ther* (1989) 45,148.
3. Ptachcinski RJ, Venkataramanan R, Rosenthal JT, Burckart GJ, Taylor RJ, Hakala TR. The effect of food on cyclosporine absorption. *Transplantation* (1985) 40, 174–6.
4. Santos P, Lourenço R, Camilo ME, Oliveira AG, Figueira I, Pereira ME, Ferreira B, Carmo JA, Lacerda JMF. Parenteral nutrition and cyclosporine: do lipids make a difference? A prospective randomized crossover trial. *Clin Nutr* (2001) 20, 31–6.
5. Edwards DJ, Ducharme MP, Provenzano R, Dehoorne-Smith M. Effect of grapefruit juice on blood concentrations of cyclosporine. *Clin Pharmacol Ther* (1993) 53, 237.
6. Ducharme MP, Provenzano R, Dehoorne-Smith M, Edwards DJ. Trough concentrations of cyclosporine in blood following administration with grapefruit juice. *Br J Clin Pharmacol* (1993) 36, 457–9.
7. Proppe D, Hoch O, McLean A. Cyclosporin A-grapefruit juice interaction in renal transplant patients. *Nephrol Dial Transplant* (1994) 9, 1055.
8. Yee GC, Stanley DL, Pessa LJ, Costa TD, Beltz SE, Ruiz J, Lowenthal DT. Effect of grapefruit juice on blood cyclosporine concentration. *Lancet* (1995) 345, 955–6.
9. Proppe DG, Hoch OD, McLean AJ, Visser KE. Influence of chronic ingestion of grapefruit juice on steady-state blood concentrations of cyclosporine A in renal transplant patients with stable graft function. *Br J Clin Pharmacol* (1995) 39, 337–8.
10. Min DI, Ku Y-M, Perry PJ, Martin MF, Lawrence G, Hunsiker LG. The effect of grapefruit juice on cyclosporine pharmacokinetics in renal allograft recipients. *Pharmacotherapy* (1996) 16, 516.
11. Herlitz H, Edgar B, Hedner T, Lidman K, Karlberg I. Grapefruit juice: a possible source of variability in blood concentration of cyclosporine A. *Nephrol Dial Transplant* (1993) 8, 375.
12. Christophidis N, Ryan P, Angelis P, Demos L, Mclean A. Grapefruit juice and cyclosporin A concentrations in patients with rheumatic diseases. *Arthritis Rheum* (1994) 37 (9 Suppl), S421.
13. Brunner L, Munar M, Bennett W. Effect of grapefruit juice on cyclosporine pharmacokinetics in renal transplant recipients. *Pharm Res* (1997) 14 (11 Suppl), S-180–S-181.
14. van Rooij J, Hollander AAMJ, Arbouw F, van Bree JB, Schoemaker HC, van Es LA, van der Woude FJ, Cohen AF. The effect of grapefruit juice on the pharmacokinetics of cyclosporine-A (CyA) in renal transplantation patients. *Br J Clin Pharmacol* (1994) 37, 479P.
15. Yee GC, Stanley DL, Ruiz J, Braddock RJ, Lowenthal DT. Effect of grapefruit juice on oral cyclosporine pharmacokinetics. *Pharmacotherapy* (1994) 14, 377.
16. Ku Y-M, Min DI, Flanigan MJ. The effect of grapefruit juice on microemulsion cyclosporine (Neoral) pharmacokinetics in healthy volunteers. *Pharmacotherapy* (1998) 18, 442.
17. Proppe D, Visser K, Hoch O, Bartels R, Meier H, McLean AJ. Differential influence on cyclosporin A metabolism by chronic grapefruit juice exposure. *Eur J Clin Invest* (1996) 26 (Suppl 1), A20.
18. Ioannides-Demos LL, Christophidis N, Ryan P, Angelis P, Liolios L, McLean AJ. Dosing implications of a clinical interaction between grapefruit juice and cyclosporine and metabolite concentrations in patients with autoimmune diseases. *J Rheumatol* (1997) 24, 49–54.
19. Edwards DJ, Woster PM, Warbasse LH. Effect of grapefruit juice and seville orange juice on cyclosporine disposition. *Clin Pharmacol Ther* (1998) 63, 149.
20. Hollander AAMJ, van Rooij J, Lentjes EGWM, Arbouw F, van Bree JB, Schoemaker RC, van Es LA, van der Woude FJ, Cohen AF. The effect of grapefruit juice on cyclosporine and prednisone metabolism in transplant patients. *Clin Pharmacol Ther* (1995) 57, 318–24.
21. Yee GC, Adams VR, Pessa L, Braddock RJ, Ruiz J, Lowenthal DT. Comparison of one versus two doses of grapefruit juice on oral cyclosporine pharmacokinetics. *Pharmacotherapy* (1997) 17, 1112.
22. Proppe D, Visser K, Bartels R, Hoch O, Meyer H, McLean AJ. Grapefruit juice selectively modifies cyclosporin A metabolite patterns in renal transplant patients. *Clin Pharmacol Ther* (1996) 59, 138.
23. Bistrup C, Nielsen FT, Jeppesen UE, Dieperink H. Effect of grapefruit juice on Sandimmun Neoral® absorption among stable renal allograft recipients. *Nephrol Dial Transplant* (2001) 16, 373–7.
24. Lee M, Min DI, Ku Y-M, Flanigan M. Effect of grapefruit juice on pharmacokinetics of microemulsion cyclosporine in African American subjects compared with Caucasian subjects: does ethnic difference matter? *J Clin Pharmacol* (2001) 41, 317–23.
25. Brunner LJ, Pai K-S, Munar MY, Lande MB, Olyaei AJ, Mowry JA. Effect of grapefruit juice on cyclosporin A pharmacokinetics in pediatric renal transplant patients. *Pediatr Transplant* (2000) 4, 313–21.

26. Ducharme MP, Warbasse LH, Edwards DJ. Disposition of intravenous and oral cyclosporine after administration with grapefruit juice. *Clin Pharmacol Ther* (1995) 57, 485–91.
27. Tsunoda SM, Harris RZ, Christians U, Velez RL, Freeman RB, Benet LZ, Warshaw A. Red wine decreases cyclosporine bioavailability. *Clin Pharmacol Ther* (2001) 70, 462–7.
28. Tsunoda SM, Harris RZ, Freeman RB, Warshaw A. Acute and chronic wine effects on cyclosporine disposition. *Br J Clin Pharmacol* (2000) 42.
29. Tsunoda SM, Christians U, Velez RL, Benet LZ, Harris RZ. Red wine (RW) effects on cyclosporine (CyA) metabolites. *Clin Pharmacol Ther* (2000) 67, 150.
30. Johnston A, Holt DW. Effect of grapefruit juice on blood cyclosporin concentration. *Lancet* (1995) 346, 122–3.
31. Hollander AAMJ, van der Woude FJ, Cohen AF. Effect of grapefruit juice on blood cyclosporin concentration. *Lancet* (1995) 346, 123.
32. Yee GC, Lowenthal DT. Effect of grapefruit juice on blood cyclosporin concentration. *Lancet* (1995) 346, 123–4.

Ciclosporin + Foscarnet

Acute but reversible renal failure occurred in two transplant patients when foscarnet was added to their treatment with ciclosporin.

Clinical evidence

A man with a kidney transplant taking steroids and ciclosporin developed a cytomegalovirus infection which was treated with **foscarnet** 85 mg/kg daily. Despite efforts to minimise the nephrotoxic effects of the **foscarnet** (hydration with 2500 ml isotonic saline daily and the administration of 80 mg nifedipine the day before and during treatment) the patient developed non-oliguric worsening of kidney function after 8 days. Nine days after stopping the **foscarnet**, the former kidney function was restored. Essentially the same thing happened to a liver transplant patient on steroids, azathioprine and ciclosporin who was very similarly treated. Acute renal failure occurred 5 days after **foscarnet** 180 mg/kg daily was started for a hepatitis B virus infection. Kidney function became normal 10 days after the **foscarnet** was stopped. The ciclosporin serum levels were therapeutic and not significantly altered at any time in either patient.[1]

Mechanism

Not understood. It seems that the nephrotoxic effects of the ciclosporin and foscarnet can be additive.

Importance and management

Direct information appears to be limited to this report, but it is consistent with the known potential toxicity of both drugs. Acute renal failure can clearly occur despite the preventative measures taken. The authors of this report[1] say that "it is mandatory to monitor renal function carefully when both drugs are administered simultaneously."

1. Morales JM, Muñoz MA, Fernández Zataraín G, Garcia Cantón C, García Rubiales MA, Andrés A, Aguado JM, Pinto IG. Reversible acute renal failure caused by the combined use of foscarnet and cyclosporin in organ transplanted patients. *Nephrol Dial Transplant* (1995) 10, 882–3.

Ciclosporin + Ganciclovir

A very small number of patients given ciclosporin and ganciclovir may develop an acute but reversible eye movement disorder.

Clinical evidence, mechanism, importance and management

In a USA hospital, 582 allogenic bone marrow transplants were carried out between 1988 and 1994. All the patients were given ciclosporin and about 45% also had **ganciclovir** at some time during the first 3 months after the transplant. Four patients (0.7%) developed an acute eye movement disorder (unilateral or bilateral sixth nerve palsies) within 4 to 34 days of starting **ganciclovir**. Three of the 4 patients also had bilateral ptosis. The problem cleared 24 to 48 h after

withdrawal of both drugs from 3 patients, and just ciclosporin from the other patient. Objective eye movement abnormality with diplopia only reoccurred in one patient when both drugs were restarted, but not when ciclosporin alone was given.[1]

The reason for this toxic reaction is not known but the authors of the report postulate a transient brain stem or neuromuscular dysfunction caused by both drugs.[1] It is an uncommon reaction and reversible, so that concurrent use need not be avoided but both drugs should be stopped if it happens. The report cited here seems to be the only report of this interaction.

1. Openshaw H, Slatkin NE, Smith E. Eye movement disorders in bone marrow transplant patients on cyclosporin and ganciclovir. *Bone Marrow Transplant* (1997) 19, 503–5.

Ciclosporin + *Geum chiloense*

A single report describes a marked and rapid increase in the serum ciclosporin levels of a man after taking an infusion of *Geum chiloense*.

Clinical evidence, mechanism, importance and management

A kidney transplant patient of 54 on ciclosporin (and also taking prednisone, azathioprine, diltiazem and nifedipine) showed a sudden and very marked rise in his ciclosporin levels from the usual range of 60 to 90 mg/dl up to a range of 469 to 600 mg/dl. He had been taking 2 to 3 mg/kg ciclosporin daily for 15 months since the transplant. His serum creatinine levels were found to be 1.3 mg/dl. It eventually turned out that about 2 weeks earlier he had started to drink an infusion of *Geum chiloense* (or *Geum quellyon*), a herbal remedy claimed to increase virility and to treat prostatism. When the herbal remedy was stopped, his serum ciclosporin levels rapidly returned to their normal values. The reasons for this apparent interaction are not known.[1]

This appears to be the only case on record but it serves, along with reports about other herbs, to emphasise that herbal remedies may not be safe just because they are 'natural'. In this instance the herbal remedy markedly increased the potential nephrotoxicity of the ciclosporin. Patients should be warned.

1. Duclos J, Goecke H. "Hierba del clavo" (*Geum chiloense*) interfiere niveles de ciclosporin: potencial riesgo para trasplantados. *Rev Med Chil* (2001) 129, 789–90.

Ciclosporin + H$_2$-blockers

Reports are inconsistent. Cimetidine, famotidine and ranitidine are reported both to cause or not to cause some increases in serum ciclosporin serum levels. Any increases in serum creatinine levels may possibly not be a reliable indicator of increased nephrotoxicity. Isolated cases of thrombocytopenia and hepatotoxicity have been reported with ranitidine.

Clinical evidence

(a) Cimetidine, Ranitidine

(i) Serum ciclosporin levels increased or unchanged. A study in 5 liver transplant patients found that **cimetidine** transiently raised peak ciclosporin levels but no changes in trough ciclosporin levels were seen after 4 h, and the conclusion was reached that it was safe to use **cimetidine** over at least a 4-week period.[1] Raised serum ciclosporin levels have been seen in 5 liver transplant patients[2] and in another patient when treated with **cimetidine** and metronidazole.[3] Higher serum ciclosporin levels were found in a study in heart transplant patients given **cimetidine**.[4] A study in 6 healthy subjects found a 30% rise in the ciclosporin AUC when 300 mg was given following a 3-day course of 400 mg **cimetidine** daily.[5]

In contrast, **cimetidine** was found not to alter the serum ciclosporin levels of groups of healthy subjects[6,7] or kidney transplant patients,[8] and no changes were seen in another group of kidney transplant patients when given either **cimetidine** or **ranitidine** for 7 days (but see (ii) below).[9] Five further reports say that **ranitidine** does not alter serum ciclosporin levels.[10-13]

(ii) Creatinine serum levels increased or unchanged. **Cimetidine** or **ranitidine** increased the mean serum creatinine levels in seven kidney transplant patients on ciclosporin by 41% (from 2.28 to 3.22 mg/dl). All of them showed a rise, whereas only 2 out of 5 other patients with heart transplants showed a serum creatinine level rise when given either **cimetidine** or **ranitidine**, nevertheless the mean rise was 37% (from 1.72 to 2.36 mg/dl).[8] A transient increase in creatinine serum levels at days 2 and 5 was seen in another study of 7 renal transplant patients given **cimetidine** 400 mg daily for 7 days.[9] Another study reported that **ranitidine** does not alter creatinine levels or inulin clearance.[11]

(iii) Toxicities. A report describes thrombocytopenia in a man with a kidney transplant on ciclosporin when given **ranitidine**.[14] Another patient experienced hepatotoxicity while taking ciclosporin when given **ranitidine**.[15]

(b) Famotidine

Famotidine is reported not to affect serum ciclosporin levels,[16-18] however higher serum ciclosporin levels were found in a study of heart transplant patients given **famotidine**.[4] No significant changes in the pharmacokinetics of ciclosporin was seen in a single dose study in 8 healthy subjects[7] and no changes serum creatinine or BUN levels in 7 kidney transplant patients.[18]

Mechanism

It is not clear why these reports are inconsistent, nor how the H_2-blockers might raise serum ciclosporin levels. It has also been suggested that any rise in serum creatinine levels could simply be because these H_2-blockers compete with creatinine for secretion by the kidney tubules, and therefore that any rises are not an indicator of kidney toxicity[19,20]

Importance and management

Information about the possible interactions of ciclosporin and cimetidine, famotidine or ranitidine is inconsistent but there appear to very few reports of confirmed toxicity. Moreover the reported increases in serum creatinine levels seen with the H_2-blockers may be not be a reflection of increased nephrotoxicity (see 'Mechanism'). Thus there is little to suggest that concurrent use should be avoided but good monitoring is advisable.

1. Puff MR, Carey WD. The effect of cimetidine on cyclosporine A levels in liver transplant recipients: a preliminary report. *Am J Gastroenterol* (1992) 87, 287–91.
2. Puff MR, Carey WD, Pippenger CE, Vogt DP. Cimetidine alters cyclosporine A metabolism in liver transplantation patients. *Gastroenterology* (1989) 96, A647.
3. Zylber-Katz E, Rubinger D, Berlatzky Y. Cyclosporine interactions with metronidazole and cimetidine. *Drug Intell Clin Pharm* (1988) 22, 504–5.
4. Reichenspurner H, Meiser BM, Muschiol F, Nolltert G, Überfuhr P, Markewitz A, Wagner F, Pfeiffer M, Reichart B. The influence of gastrointestinal agents on resorption and metabolism of cyclosporine after heart transplantation: experimental and clinical results. *J Heart Lung Transplant* (1993) 12, 987–92.
5. Choi J-S, Choi I, Min DI. Effect of cimetidine on pharmacokinetics of cyclosporine in healthy volunteers. *Pharmacotherapy* (1997) 17, 1120.
6. Freeman DJ, Laupacis A, Keown P, Stiller C, Carruthers G. The effect of agents that alter drug metabolizing enzyme activity on the pharmacokinetics of cyclosporine. *Ann R Coll Physicians Surg Can* (1984) 17, 301.
7. Shaefer MS, Rossi SJ, McGuire TR, Schaaf LJ, Collier DS, Stratta RJ. Evaluation of the pharmacokinetic interaction between cimetidine or famotidine and cyclosporine in healthy men. *Ann Pharmacother* (1995) 29, 1088–91.
8. Jarowenko MV, Van Buren CT, Kramer WG, Lorber MI, Flechner SM, Kahan BD. Ranitidine, cimetidine, and the cyclosporine-treated recipient. *Transplantation* (1986) 42, 311–12.
9. Barn YM, Ramos EL, Balagtas RS, Peterson JC, Karlix JL. Cimetidine or ranitidine in prophylactic doses do not affect renal function or cyclosporine levels in renal transplant patients (RTP). *J Am Soc Nephrol* (1993) 4, 925.
10. Zazgornik J, Schindler J, Gremmel F, Balcke P, Kopsa H, Derfler K, Minar E. Ranitidine does not influence the blood cyclosporin levels in renal transplant patients (RTP). *Kidney Int* (1985) 28, 401.
11. Jadoul M, Hené RJ. Ranitidine and the cyclosporine-treated recipient. *Transplantation* (1989) 48, 359.
12. Popovic J, Cameron JS. Effects of ranitidine on renal function in transplant recipients. *Nephrol Dial Transplant* (1990) 5, 980–1.
13. Tsang VT, Johnston A, Heritier F, Leaver N, Hodson ME, Yacoub M. Cyclosporin pharmacokinetics in heart-lung transplant recipients with cystic fibrosis. *Eur J Clin Pharmacol* (1994) 46, 261–5.
14. Bailey RR, Walker RJ, Swainson CP. Some new problems with cyclosporin A? *N Z Med J* (1985) 98, 915–6.
15. Hiesse C, Cantarovich M, Santelli C, Francais P, Charpentier B, Fries D, Buffet C. Ranitidine hepatotoxicity in a renal transplant patient. *Lancet* (1985) i, 1280.
16. Von Schütz A, Kemkes BM. Ciclosporinspiegel unter Gabe von Famotidin. *Fortschr Med* (1990) 23, 457–8.
17. Morel D, Bannwarth B, Vinçon G, Penouil F, Elouaer-Blanc L, Aparicio M, Potaux L. Effect of famotidine on renal transplant patients treated with cyclosporine A. *Fundam Clin Pharmacol* (1993) 7, 167–70.
18. Inoue S, Sugimoto H, Nagao T, Akiyama N. Does H_2-receptor antagonist alter the renal function of cyclosporine-treated kidney grafts? *Jpn J Surg* (1990) 20, 553–8.
19. Pachon J, Lorber MI, Bia MJ. Effects of H_2-receptor antagonists on renal function in cyclosporine-treated renal transplant patients. *Transplantation* (1989) 47, 254–9.
20. Lewis SM, McClosky WW. Potentiation of nephrotoxicity by H_2-antagonists in patients receiving cyclosporine. *Ann Pharmacother* (1997) 31, 363–5.

Ciclosporin + Hypoglycaemic agents

Some preliminary evidence suggests that glibenclamide (glyburide) and possibly glipizide can raise serum ciclosporin levels to a moderate extent.

Clinical evidence, mechanism, importance and management

A review of 6 post-transplant diabetic patients on ciclosporin showed that their steady-state plasma ciclosporin levels rose by 57% when concurrently treated with **glibenclamide (glyburide)**. The hepatic and renal functions of the patients were unchanged. The reasons for this reaction are not known, but it is suggested that **glibenclamide** possibly inhibits the metabolism of ciclosporin by cytochrome P450 isoenzyme CYP3A4 resulting in a reduction in its clearance.[1] Two other patients needed reductions of 20 to 30% in their ciclosporin dosage when they were additionally given 10 mg **glipizide** daily.[2] In contrast, a study in 11 post-transplant diabetic patients found no significant alterations in ciclosporin pharmacokinetics during glipizide treatment.[3]

Neither of these interactions is well established but it would now be prudent to monitor serum ciclosporin levels if either hypoglycaemic agent is added. Information about other sulphonylurea hypoglycaemic agents appears not to be available.

1. Islam SI, Masuda QN, Bolaji OO, Shaheen FM, Sheikh IA. Possible interaction between cyclosporine and glibenclamide in posttransplant diabetic patients. *Ther Drug Monit* (1996) 18, 624–6.
2. Chidester PD, Connito DJ. Interaction between glipizide and cyclosporine: report of two cases. *Transplant Proc* (1993) 25, 2136–7.
3. Sagedal S, Åsberg A, Hartmann A, Bergan S, Berg KJ. Glipizide treatment of post-transplant diabetes does not interfere with cyclosporine pharmacokinetics in renal allograft recipients. *Clin Transplant* (1998) 12, 553–6.

Ciclosporin + Ketoconazole + Famotidine

A patient taking ciclosporin and ketoconazole showed a marked fall in serum ciclosporin levels when famotidine was added.

Clinical evidence, mechanism, importance and management

A kidney transplant patient was treated with 200 mg **ketoconazole** daily to reduce her ciclosporin dosage in order to save money. A week after the operation 40 mg **famotidine** daily was added for gastritis, and shortly afterwards her serum ciclosporin levels fell to subtherapeutic levels (approximately halved). It was found necessary to raise her ciclosporin dosage from 100 to 175 mg daily.[1]

A likely explanation for what happened is that the **ketoconazole** inhibited the metabolism of the ciclosporin enabling a smaller dosage to be given (see 'Ciclosporin + Azole antifungals', p.603). When the **famotidine** was added, the dissolution and absorption of the **ketoconazole** in the stomach was reduced by the rise in pH (see 'Azole antifungals + Antacids, H_2-blockers or Sucralfate', p.139) so that less was available to inhibit the liver enzymes, resulting in a rise in the metabolism of the ciclosporin which lead on to the fall in the serum ciclosporin levels.

Direct information seems to be limited to this single case, but both the ciclosporin /**ketoconazole** and **ketoconazole/H₂-blocker** interactions are well documented and there is good reason to believe that this dual interaction might occur in other patients. Other H₂-blockers (**cimetidine, nizatidine, ranitidine**) behave like **famotidine**, and it would therefore be prudent to monitor the ciclosporin levels if drugs like these or others which can cause a significant rise in the pH of the stomach (e.g. antacids, proton pump inhibitors etc) are added to a combination of ciclosporin and **ketoconazole**.

1. Karlix JL, Cheng MA, Brunson ME, Ramos EL, Howard RJ, Peterson JC, Patton PR, Pfaff WW. Decreased cyclosporine concentrations with the addition of an H₂-receptor antagonist in a patient on ketoconazole. *Transplantation* (1993) 56, 1554–5.

Ciclosporin + Macrolide and related antibacterials

Ciclosporin levels can be markedly raised by clarithromycin, erythromycin, josamycin, pristinamycin and possibly midecamycin. Rokitamycin and troleandomycin are predicted to interact similarly. Roxithromycin appears to interact minimally, while no interaction is normally seen with azithromycin, dirithromycin or spiramycin, although there are isolated reports of an interaction with azithromycin.

Clinical evidence

(a) Azithromycin

Eight healthy subjects were given ciclosporin 3.75 to 7.5 mg/kg alone and then after taking clarithromycin 250 mg 12-hourly for 7 days or erythromycin 500 mg 8-hourly or **azithromycin**, 500 mg loading dose then 250 mg daily for 4 days. Marked increases in the maximum serum levels of ciclosporin occurred when clarithromycin and erythromycin were used, but with **azithromycin** no changes were seen.[1] Other studies also found no evidence of a ciclosporin/**azithromycin** interaction in 6 and 48 kidney transplant patients respectively,[2,3] but there are reports describing a marked increase in ciclosporin levels in two patients attributed to **azithromycin**.[4,5]

(b) Clarithromycin

The serum ciclosporin levels of a heart transplant patient on ciclosporin and azathioprine approximately doubled within 6 days of starting to take 500 mg **clarithromycin** twice daily. The makers of ciclosporin, also have on their records another case of increased ciclosporin serum levels after **clarithromycin** was started.[6] The trough serum ciclosporin levels of 3 kidney transplant patients doubled or tripled while taking 250 mg **clarithromycin** twice daily.[7] A kidney transplant patient showed a doubled ciclosporin AUC when given **clarithromycin**.[8] Another patient showed a seven to twelvefold rise in serum ciclosporin levels and acute renal failure within 3 weeks of starting to take 1 g **clarithromycin** daily. Associated with this report is a study on 5 healthy subjects which found that **clarithromycin** inhibited the CYP3A activity of all of them.[9] **Clarithromycin** 250 mg twice daily approximately doubled the serum ciclosporin levels of another kidney transplant patient within 3 days[10] and increased the maximum serum levels in 8 healthy subjects by about 50% in a week.[1] A mean 30% reduction in the dosage of ciclosporin was needed in 6 transplant patients while concurrently being treated with **clarithromycin**.[11] **Clarithromycin** 500 mg twice daily as part of a *Helicobacter pylori* eradication regimen caused a two to threefold increase in ciclosporin levels in 27 kidney transplant patients.[12,13]

(c) Dirithromycin

Fourteen days' treatment with 500 mg **dirithromycin** daily failed significantly to affect the pharmacokinetics of single 15-mg/kg oral doses of ciclosporin in 8 healthy subjects.[14]

(d) Erythromycin

A study in 9 patients with transplants on ciclosporin found that when treated with **erythromycin** the mean trough serum levels of the 3 patients with kidney transplants rose sevenfold (from 147 to 1125 nanograms/ml) and in the 6 patients with heart transplants four to fivefold (from 185 to 815 nanograms/ml). Acute nephrotoxicity occurred in all 9 patients, and 7 showed mild to severe liver toxicity caused by the increased ciclosporin serum levels.[15]

Markedly raised serum ciclosporin levels and/or toxicity have been described in a number of other studies and case reports with **erythromycin** given orally or intravenously in about 40 other patients[16-30] and demonstrated in healthy subjects.[1,31] Oral **erythromycin** may possibly have a greater effect than intravenous **erythromycin**.[27,32] **Erythromycin**-related ototoxicity, possibly associated with the use of ciclosporin has also been reported in liver transplant patients.[33]

(e) Josamycin

A man with a renal transplant on azathioprine, prednisone and ciclosporin 330 mg daily showed a marked rise in his serum ciclosporin levels from about 90 to 600 nanograms/ml when treated with 2 g **josamycin** daily for 5 days. He responded in the same way when later rechallenged with **josamycin**. Another patient reacted in the same way.[34] Two to fourfold rises have been seen in 9 other patients given 2 to 3 g (50 mg/kg) **josamycin** daily.[35-37] Another patient showed a 40% rise when given 500 mg **josamycin** twice daily.[38]

(f) Midecamycin/midecamycin diacetate

The steady-state serum ciclosporin levels of 10 kidney transplant patients were approximately doubled while taking 800 mg **midecamycin** twice daily.[39] A kidney transplant patient of 43 on ciclosporin, azathioprine and prednisone, began further treatment on day 27 following the transplant with 600 mg **midecamycin** diacetate (miocamycin; ponsinomycin) twice daily and co-trimoxazole three times daily for pneumonia. By day 33 the concentration/dose ratio of the ciclosporin had doubled, and ciclosporin levels had reached 700 nanograms/ml, accompanied by a rise in serum creatinine levels. When the **midecamyin** was replaced by **cefuroxime**, the concentrations of both ciclosporin and creatinine fell to their former levels within 3 days.[40] Ciclosporin levels in another kidney transplant patient on ciclosporin 120 mg twice daily increased from 95 nanograms/ml to 380 nanograms/ml 3 days after starting **midecamycin** 800 mg twice daily.[41] Blood levels of ciclosporin in another kidney transplant patient showed similar increases (from 97 to 203 nanograms/ml) after 4 days when she was also given **midecamycin** diacetate 600 mg twice daily.[42]

(g) Pristinamycin

A kidney transplant patient showed a tenfold rise in serum ciclosporin levels (from 30 to 290 nanograms/ml) after being given 2 g **pristinamycin** daily for 8 days. Blood creatinine levels rose from 75 to 120 micromol/l. Another patient given 1.25 g **pristinamycin** showed a rise in ciclosporin levels from 78 to 855 nanograms/ml after 6 days. Ciclosporin and creatinine levels fell to normal levels within 2 days of stopping both drugs.[43]

Pristinamycin 50 mg/kg daily raised the serum ciclosporin levels of 10 patients by 65% (from 560 to 925 nanograms/ml). Ciclosporin levels fell when the **pristinamycin** was stopped.[44,45] Within 5 days of starting to take 4 g **pristinamycin** daily the ciclosporin levels of another patient more than doubled. His serum creatinine levels also rose. Both fell back to baseline levels within 3 days of stopping the antibacterial.[46]

(h) Roxithromycin

Eight patients with heart transplants on ciclosporin 8 mg/kg daily, prednisolone and azathioprine for at least a month, were concurrently treated with 150 mg **roxithromycin** twice daily for 11 days. A rise in serum ciclosporin levels occurred, namely 37.5% (a rise from 176 to 242 nanograms/ml) at the time the **roxithromycin** was given, and +60% (from 294 to 469 nanograms/ml) four hours later. Ciclosporin levels fell again when the **roxithromycin** was stopped. A weak (10%) increase in serum creatinine levels occurred. There was no evidence of a deterioration in renal function.[47,48] The biological half-life of **roxithromycin** was found in one study to be approximately doubled (from 17 to 34.4 h) in patients with kidney transplants on ciclosporin.[49]

(i) Spiramycin

The ciclosporin serum levels of 6 heart transplant patients on steroids, azathioprine and ciclosporin remained unchanged when given 3 MIU of **spiramycin** twice daily for 10 days.[50] The same absence of an interaction between ciclosporin and **spiramycin** was found in other studies in patients with renal transplants.[51-54]

(j) Rokitamycin, Troleandomycin

In vitro studies (see 'Mechanism' below) suggest that these two macrolides behave like erythromycin,[55] but as yet there seems to be no direct clinical evidence of an interaction.

Mechanism

In vitro studies with human liver microsomes have shown that clarithromycin, erythromycin, josamycin, rokitamycin, roxithromycin and troleandomycin (but not spiramycin) inhibit ciclosporin metabolism in the liver which is catalysed by cytochrome P450 CYP3A.[9,55] This would be expected to result in raised ciclosporin levels. Erythromycin[27] and clarithromycin[8] also possibly increase the absorption of ciclosporin from the gut by inhibiting intestinal wall metabolism. Azithromycin is believed to be metabolised by routes independent of the cytochrome system. Administration of intravenous azithromycin in one of the patients was thought to have increased ciclosporin levels through P-glycoprotein inhibition and/or competition for biliary excretion.[5]

Importance and management

The ciclosporin/erythromycin interaction is well documented, well established and potentially serious. If concurrent use is thought appropriate, monitor the ciclosporin serum levels closely and reduce the dosage appropriately. An approximately 35% reduction has been calculated.[29] The dosage should be increased again when the erythromycin is stopped to maintain adequate immunosuppression. The effect of intravenous erythromycin is less than oral erythromycin so if its route of administration is changed, be alert for the need to change the ciclosporin dosage.[27,32]

Information about the interactions with clarithromycin, josamycin, midecamycin, and pristinamycin is much more limited but they appear to behave like erythromycin. The same precautions should be taken. There seems to be no direct clinical information about troleandomycin and rokitamycin but *in vitro* studies suggest that they may interact like erythromycin.[55] Be on the alert for this interaction if they are used.

Dirithromycin and spiramycin normally appear not to interact and roxithromycin appears only to interact very minimally, however bear in mind that the roxithromycin serum levels may be increased. Although most reports suggest azithromycin does not interact, increased monitoring is recommended, because of the isolated reports of increased ciclosporin levels.[5]

1. Bottorff MB, Marien ML, Clendening C. Macrolide antibiotics and inhibition of CYP3A isozymes: differences in cyclosporin pharmacokinetics. *Clin Pharmacol Ther* (1997) 56, 224.
2. Gómez E, Sánchez JE, Aguado S, Alvarez Grande J. Interaction between azithromycin and cyclosporin? *Nephron* (1996) 73, 724.
3. Bubic-Filipi Lj, Puretic Z, Thune S, Glavas-Boras S, Pasini J, Marekovic Z. Influence of azithromycin on cyclosporin levels in patients with a kidney transplant. *Nephrol Dial Transplant* (1998) 13, A276.
4. Ljutic D, Rumboldt Z. Possible interaction between azithromycin and cyclosporine: a case report. *Nephron* (1995) 70, 130.
5. Page RL, Ruscin JM, Fish D, LaPointe M. Possible interaction between intravenous azithromycin and oral cyclosporine. *Pharmacotherapy* (2001) 21, 1436–43.
6. Gersema LM, Porter CB, Russell EH. Suspected drug interaction between cyclosporine and clarithromycin. *J Heart Lung Transplant* (1994) 13, 343–5.
7. Ferrari SL, Goffin E, Mourad M, Wallemacq P, Squifflet J-P, Pirson Y. The interaction between clarithromycin and cyclosporine in kidney transplant recipients. *Transplantation* (1994) 58, 725–7.
8. Sketris IS, Wright MR, West ML. Possible role of intestinal P-450 enzyme system in a cyclosporine-clarithromycin interaction. *Pharmacotherapy* (1996) 16, 301–5.
9. Spicer ST, Liddle C, Chapman JR, Barclay P, Nankivell BJ, Thomas P, O'Connell PJ. The mechanism of cyclosporine toxicity induced by clarithromycin. *Br J Clin Pharmacol* (1997) 43, 194–6.
10. Treille S, Quoidbach A, Demol H, Vereerstraeten P, Abramowicz D. Kidney graft dysfunction after drug interaction between clarithromycin and cyclosporin. *Nephrol Dial Transplant* (1996) 11, 1192–3.
11. Sádaba B, López De Ocáriz A, Azanza JR, Quiroga J, Cienfuegos JA. Concurrent clarithromycin and cyclosporin A treatment. *J Antimicrob Chemother* (1998) 42, 393–5.
12. Skálová P, Marečková O, Skála I, Lácha J, Teplan V, Vítko Š, Petrásek R. Eradication of *Helicobacter pylori* with clarithromycin: danger of toxic levels of cyclosporin A. *Gut* (1998) 43 (Suppl 2), A109.
13. Skalova P, Mareckova O, Skala I, Lacha J, Teplan V, Vitko S, Petrasek R. Toxic levels of cyclosporin A after renal transplantation on clarithromycin therapy. *Nephrol Dial Transplant* (1998) 13, A256.
14. Bachmann K, Sullivan TJ, Resse JH, Miller K, Scott M, Jauregui L, Sides G. The pharmacokinetics of oral cyclosporine A are not affected by dirithromycin. *Intersci Conf Antimicrob Agents Chemother* (1994) 34, 4.
15. Jensen CWB, Flechner SM, Van Buren CT, Frazier OH, Cooley DA, Lorber MI, Kahan BD. Exacerbation of cyclosporine toxicity by concomitant administration of erythromycin. *Transplantation* (1987) 43, 263–70.
16. Kohan DE. Possible interaction between cyclosporine and erythromycin. *N Engl J Med* (1986), 314, 448.
17. Hourmant M, Le Bigot JF, Vernillet L, Sagniez G, Remi JP, Soulillou JP. Coadministration of erythromycin results in an increase of blood cyclosporine to toxic levels. *Transplant Proc* (1985) 17, 2723–7.
18. Wadhwa NK, Schroeder TJ, O'Flaherty E, Pesce AJ, Myre SA, Munda R, First MR. Interaction between erythromycin and cyclosporine in a kidney and pancreas allograft recipient. *Ther Drug Monit* (1987) 9, 123–5.
19. Murray BM, Edwards L, Morse GD, Kohli RR, Venuto RC. Clinically important interaction of cyclosporine and erythromycin. *Transplantation* (1987) 43, 602–4.
20. Griño JM, Sabate I, Castelao AM, Guardia M, Seron D, Alsina J. Erythromycin and cyclosporine. *Ann Intern Med* (1986) 105, 467–8.
21. Gonwa TA, Nghiem DD, Schulak JA, Corry RJ. Erythromycin and cyclosporine. *Transplantation* (1986) 41, 797–9.
22. Harnett JD, Parfrey PS, Paul MD, Gault MH. Erythromycin-cyclosporine interaction in renal transplant patients. *Transplantation* (1987) 43, 316–18.
23. Kessler M, Louis J, Renoult E, Vigneron B, Netter P. Interaction between cyclosporin and erythromycin in a kidney transplant patient. *Eur J Clin Pharmacol* (1986) 30, 633–4.
24. Godin JRP, Sketris IS, Belitsky P. Erythromycin-cyclosporine interaction. *Drug Intell Clin Pharm* (1986) 20, 504–5.
25. Martell R, Heinrichs D, Stiller CR, Jenner M, Keown PA, Dupre J. The effects of erythromycin in patients treated with cyclosporine. *Ann Intern Med* (1986) 104, 660–1.
26. Ptachcinski PJ, Carpenter BJ, Burckart GJ, Venkataramanan R, Rosenthal JT. Effect of erythromycin on cyclosporine levels. *N Engl J Med* (1985) 313, 1416–17.
27. Gupta SK, Bakran A, Johnson RWG, Rowland M. Erythromycin enhances the absorption of cyclosporin. *Br J Clin Pharmacol* (1988) 25, 401–2.
28. Morales JM, Andres A, Prieto C, Arenas J, Ortuño B, Praga M, Ruilope LM, Rodicio JL. Severe reversible cyclosporine-induced acute renal failure. A role for urinary PGE$_2$ deficiency? *Transplantation* (1988) 46, 163–5.
29. Vereerstraeten P, Thiry P, Kinnaert P, Toussaint C. Influence of erythromycin on cyclosporine pharmacokinetics. *Transplantation* (1987) 44, 155–6.
30. Ben-Ari J, Eisenstein B, Davidovits M, Shmueli D, Shapira Z, Stark H. Effect of erythromycin on blood cyclosporine concentrations in kidney transplant patients. *J Pediatr* (1988) 112, 992–3.
31. Freeman DJ, Martell R, Carruthers SG, Heinrichs D, Keown PA, Stiller CR. Cyclosporin-erythromycin interaction in normal subjects. *Br J Clin Pharmacol* (1987) 23, 776–8.
32. Zylber-Katz E. Multiple drug interactions with cyclosporine in a heart transplant patient. *Ann Pharmacother* (1995) 29, 127–31. Correction. *ibid*.; 790.
33. Moral A, Navasa M, Rimola A, García-Valdecasas JC, Grande L, Visa J, Rodés J. Erythromycin ototoxicity in liver transplant patients. *Transpl Int* (1994) 7, 62–4.
34. Kreft-Jais C, Billaud EM, Gaudry C, Bedrossian J. Effect of josamycin on plasma cyclosporine levels. *Eur J Clin Pharmacol* (1987) 32, 327–8.
35. Azanza JR, Catalán M, Alvarez MP, Sádaba B, Honorato J, Llorens R, Harreros J. Possible interaction between cyclosporine and josamycin: a description of three cases. *Clin Pharmacol Ther* (1992) 51, 572–5.
36. Torregrosa JV, Campistol JM, Franco A, Andreu J. Interaction of josamycin with cyclosporin A. *Nephron* (1993) 65, 476–7.
37. Azanza J, Catalán M, Alvarez P, Honorato J, Herreros J, Llorens R. Possible interaction between cyclosporine and josamycin. *J Heart Transplant* (1990) 9, 265–6.
38. Capone D, Gentile A, Stanziale P, Imperatore P, D'Alessandro R, D'Alto V, Basile V. Drug interaction between cyclosporine and josamycin in a kidney transplanted patient. *Fundam Clin Pharmacol* (1996) 10, 172.
39. Couet W, Istin B, Seniuta P, Morel D, Potaux L, Fourtillan JB. Effect of ponsinomycin on cyclosporin pharmacokinetics. *Eur J Clin Pharmacol* (1990) 39, 165–67.
40. Alfonso I, Alcalde G, Garcia-Sáiz M, de Cos MA, Mediavilla A. Interaction between cyclosporine a and midecamycin. *Eur J Clin Pharmacol* (1997) 52, 79–80.
41. Finielz P, Mondon J-M, Chuet C, Guiserix J. Drug interaction between midecamycin and cyclosporin. *Nephron* (1995) 70, 136.
42. Treille S, Quoidbach A, Demol H, Juvenois A, Dehout F, Abramowicz D. Kidney graft dysfunction after drug interaction between miocamycin and cyclosporin. *Transpl Int* (1999) 12, 157.
43. Gagnadoux MF, Loirat C, Pillion G, Bertheleme JP, Pouliquen M, Guest G, Broyer M. Néphrotoxicité due à l'interaction pristinamycine-cyclosporine chez le transplanté rénal. *Presse Med* (1987) 16, 1761.
44. Herbrecht R, Garcia J-J, Bergerat J-P, Oberling F. Effect of pristinamycin on cyclosporin levels in bone marrow transplant recipients. *Bone Marrow Transplant* (1990) 4, 457–8.
45. Herbrecht R, Liu KL, Bergerat J-P. Interactions of cyclosporine with antimicrobial agents. *Rev Infect Dis* (1990) 12, 371.
46. Garraffo R, Monnier B, Lapalus P, Duplay H. Pristinamycin increases cyclosporin blood levels. *Med Sci Res* (1987) 15, 461.
47. Billaud E M, Guillemain R, Fortineau N, Kitzis M-D, Dreyfus G, Amrein C, Kreft-Jaïs C, Husson J-M, Chrétien P. Interaction between roxithromycin and cyclosporin in heart transplant patients. *Clin Pharmacokinet* (1990) 19, 499–502.
48. Billaud E, Guillemain R, Kitzis M, Fortineau N, Dreyfus G, Amrein C, Kreft-Jaïs C, Chrétien P, Husson JM. Roxithromycin and cyclosporin; searching for an interaction. *Therapie* (1990) 45, Abstract 41.
49. Morávek J, Matoušovic K, Prát V, Šedivý J. Pharmacokinetics of roxithromycin in kidney grafted patients on cyclosporin A or azathioprine immunosuppression and in healthy volunteers. *Int J Clin Pharmacol Ther Toxicol* (1990) 28, 262–7.
50. Guillemain R, Billaud E, Dreyfus G, Amrein C, Kitzis M, Jebara VA and Kreft-Jais C. The effects of spiramycin on plasma cyclosporin A concentrations in heart transplant patients. *Eur J Clin Pharmacol* (1989) 36, 97–8.
51. Kessler M, Netter P, Zerrouki M, Renoult E, Trechot P, Dousset B, Jonon B, Mur JM. Spiramycin does not increase plasma cyclosporin concentrations in renal transplant patients. *Eur J Clin Pharmacol* (1988) 35, 331–2.

52. Vernillet L, Bertault-Peres P, Berland Y, Barradas J, Durand A, Olmer M. Lack of effect of spiramycin on cyclosporin pharmacokinetics. *Br J Clin Pharmacol* (1989) 27, 789–94.
53. Birmele B, Lebranchu Y, Beliveauu F, Rateau H, Furet Y, Nivet H, Bagros PH. Absence of interaction between cyclosporine and spiramycin. *Transplantation* (1989) 47, 927–8.
54. Kessler M, Netter P, Renoult E, Trechot P, Dousset B, Bannwarth B. Lack of effect of spiramycin on cyclosporine pharmacokinetics. *Br J Clin Pharmacol* (1990) 29, 370–1.
55. Marre R, de Sousa G, Orloff AM, Rahmani R. *In vitro* interaction between cyclosporin A and macrolide antibiotics. *Br J Clin Pharmacol* (1993) 35, 447–8.

Ciclosporin + Melphalan

Melphalan appears to increase the nephrotoxic effects of ciclosporin.

Clinical evidence, mechanism, importance and management

A comparative study showed that 13 out of 17 patients receiving bone marrow transplants given ciclosporin 12.5 mg/kg daily and **high-dose melphalan** (single injection of 140 to 250 mg/m²) developed kidney failure, compared with no cases of kidney failure in 7 other patients given **melphalan** but no ciclosporin.[1] In another study one out of 4 patients given both drugs developed nephrotoxicity.[2] The reasons are not understood. The effects on kidney function of concurrent use should be very closely monitored.

1. Morgenstern GR, Powles R, Robinson B, McElwain TJ. Cyclosporin interaction with ketoconazole and melphalan. *Lancet* (1982) ii, 1342.
2. Dale BM, Sage RE, Norman JE, Barber S, Kotasek D. Bone marrow transplantation following treatment with high-dose melphalan. *Transplant Proc* (1985) 17, 1711–13.

Ciclosporin + Metamizole sodium (Dipyrone)

The short term use of metamizole sodium (dipyrone) appears to have no effect on the steady-state serum levels of ciclosporin.

Clinical evidence, mechanism, importance and management

A placebo-controlled, double blind crossover study in 6 kidney and 2 heart transplant patients on ciclosporin found that while taking 500 mg **metamizole sodium (dipyrone)** three times daily for 4 days the pharmacokinetics of the ciclosporin (AUC trough and peak serum levels, elimination half-life) were unchanged, but the time to reach maximum serum levels was slightly prolonged (from 2.1 to 3.8 h). It is not known what the effects of longer use might be.[1,2]

1. Caraco Y, Zylber-Katz E, Levy M. The effect of dipyrone on cyclosporine A metabolism. *Eur J Clin Pharmacol* (1997) 52 (Suppl), A130.
2. Caraco Y, Zylber-Katz E, Fridlander M, Admon D, Levy M. The effect of short-term dipyrone administration on cyclosporin pharmacokinetics. *Eur J Clin Pharmacol* (1999) 55, 475–8.

Ciclosporin + Methotrexate

Previous or concurrent treatment with methotrexate may possibly increase the risk of liver and other toxicity, but effective and valuable concurrent use has also been reported. Ciclosporin causes a moderate rise in serum methotrexate levels, but methotrexate does not appear to affect the pharmacokinetics of ciclosporin.

Clinical evidence

(a) Evidence of toxicity

A limited comparative study in patients with chronic plaque psoriasis suggested that prior treatment with **methotrexate** (which can cause liver damage) possibly increases the risk of ciclosporin toxicity (higher serum ciclosporin and creatinine levels, hypertension).[1] This was confirmed by another study in 4 patients with resistant psoriasis in whom concurrent use (5 mg/kg ciclosporin daily and 2.5 mg **methotrexate** 12-hourly for three doses at weekly intervals) increased the serum levels of both drugs, and increased the side-effects (nausea, vomiting, mouth ulcers). Rises in creatinine levels and liver enzymes (AST, ALT) also occurred.[2]

(b) Evidence of concurrent use without toxicity

In contrast to the reports cited above, a pilot study described the effective use of both drugs for the control of acute graft-versus-host disease in marrow transplant patients, with the ciclosporin dosage reduced by 50% (1.5 mg/kg/day) during the first 2 weeks. The **methotrexate** dosages were 10 to 15 mg/m² on days 1, 3, 6 and 11 after grafting. Hepatotoxicity appeared to be reduced.[3] Another study in three bone marrow patients found that low dose **methotrexate** (15 mg/m² on day 1, and 10 mg/m² on days 3, 6 and 11) did not significantly affect clinical care and no interaction of clinical significance was seen.[4]

(c) Evidence of a pharmacokinetic interaction

An open-label pharmacokinetic study in 26 patients with rheumatoid arthritis taking **methotrexate** and 1.5 mg/kg ciclosporin 12-hourly for 14 days, found the AUC of the **methotrexate** increased by 26%, whereas the serum levels of its major metabolite (7-hydroxymethotrexate), which is much less active and may be associated with toxicity, were reduced by 80%.[5] Another study in patients with rheumatoid arthritis found that intramuscular **methotrexate** 10 mg each week for 6 months did not affect the pharmacokinetics of ciclosporin 3.2 mg/kg.[6]

Mechanism

Not understood.

Importance and management

The reports cited here give an inconsistent picture. On the one hand there is the strong recommendation by the authors of the second study[2] that combined use should be avoided, even in patients with severe unresponsive psoriasis, whereas it seems from the other studies[3,4] that concurrent use can be valuable, effective and apparently safe. If therefore you decide to use both drugs together, you should monitor closely for any evidence of ciclosporin toxicity and hepatotoxicity. More study is needed.

1. Powles AV, Baker BS, Fry L, Valdimarsson H. Cyclosporin toxicity. *Lancet* (1990) 335, 610.
2. Korstanje MJ, van Breda Vriesman CJP, van de Staak WJBM. Cyclosporine and methotrexate: a dangerous combination. *J Am Acad Dermatol* (1990) 23, 320–1.
3. Stockschlaeder M, Storb R, Pepe M, Longton G, McDonald G, Anasetti C, Appelbaum F, Doney K, Martin P, Sullivan K, Witherspoon R. A pilot study of low-dose cyclosporin for graft-versus-host prophylaxis in marrow transplantation. *Br J Haematol* (1991) 80, 49–54.
4. Dix S, Devine SM, Geller RB, Wingard JR. Re: severe interaction between methotrexate and a macrolide antibiotic. *J Natl Cancer Inst* (1995) 87, 1641–2.
5. Fox R, Morgan S, Smith H, Robbins B, Meligeni J, Caldwell J, Baggott J. Treatment of RA patients with methotrexate (MTX) plus cyclosporin A (CSA) leads to elevation of plasma MTX levels and decrease of 7 hydroxymethotrexate (7-OH) levels. *Arthritis Rheum* (1998) 41 (9 Suppl), S138.
6. Baraldo M, Ferraccioli G, Pea F, Gremese E, Furlanut M. Cyclosporine A pharmacokinetics in rheumatoid arthritis patients after 6 months of methotrexate therapy. *Pharm Res* (1999) 40, 483–6.

Ciclosporin + Metoclopramide

Metoclopramide increases the absorption of ciclosporin and raises its serum levels.

Clinical evidence, mechanism, importance and management

When 14 kidney transplant patients were given **metoclopramide** their peak serum ciclosporin levels were increased by 46% (from 388 to 567 nanograms/ml) and the AUC was increased by 22% (from 3370 to 4120 nanograms.h/ml).[1] The probable reason is that the **metoclopramide** hastens gastric emptying and ciclosporin is largely absorbed by the small intestine. The clinical importance of this interaction is uncertain but it has been suggested that it could be used to save money because it might be possible to give smaller doses of the expensive ciclosporin. Concurrent use should be well monitored to ensure that ciclosporin levels do not become toxic. More study is needed.

1. Wadhwa NK, Schroeder TJ, O'Flaherty E, Pesce AJ, Myre SA, First MR. The effect of oral metoclopramide on the absorption of cyclosporine. *Transplant Proc* (1987) 19, 1730–3.

Ciclosporin + Minoxidil

The concurrent use of ciclosporin and minoxidil can cause excessive hairiness.

Clinical evidence, mechanism, importance and management

Six kidney transplant patients on ciclosporin (serum levels of 100 to 200 nanograms/ml) were additionally given methyldopa, a diuretic and 15 to 40 mg **minoxidil** daily for intractable hypertension. After 4 weeks treatment all of them complained of severe and unpleasant hypertrichosis. Two months after stopping the **minoxidil** the hypertrichosis had significantly improved.[1] Both ciclosporin and **minoxidil** cause hypertrichosis and it would seem that their effects may be additive. The authors of the report point out that this is not a life-threatening problem, but it limits concurrent use in both men and women.[1]

1. Sever MS, Sonmez YE, Kocak N. Limited use of minoxidil in renal transplant recipients because of the additive side-effects of cyclosporine on hypertrichosis. *Transplantation* (1990) 50, 536.

Ciclosporin + Miscellaneous drugs

Isolated and unconfirmed interactions have been reported between ciclosporin and allopurinol, chlorambucil, disopyramide, doxycycline, fluoxetine, fluvoxamine, GoLytely, griseofulvin, imipenem/cilastatin, metronidazole, minocycline, latamoxef (moxalactam), quinupristin/dalfopristin, nefazodone, propafenone and quinine.

Clinical evidence and mechanism

The makers' Drug Monitoring Centre has on record a number of previously unpublished spontaneous and isolated reports of interactions between ciclosporin and other drugs.[1] There are also other isolated case reports of interactions involving ciclosporin which have been published elsewhere and are cited here.

The ciclosporin levels of a kidney transplant patient rose approximately threefold after taking 100 mg **allopurinol** daily for 12 days, accompanied by signs of renal toxicity.[2] Another showed a two to threefold rise when given 200 mg **allopurinol** daily.[3] However yet another report describes a reduction in the frequency of acute kidney transplant rejections in patients on ciclosporin, prednisolone and azathioprine when low dose **allopurinol** 25 mg on alternate days was added.[4] A woman with B-chronic lymphocytic leukaemia and autoimmune haemolytic anaemia controlled with ciclosporin, relapsed after being given a total of 200 mg **chlorambucil** 5 mg daily. Her serum ciclosporin levels dropped to 60 nanograms/ml from a range of 200 to 400 nanograms/ml, and they remained low despite a doubling of the ciclosporin dosage and withdrawal of the **chlorambucil**. Only after a month did the anaemia respond and the ciclosporin levels rise again.[5] A woman, with a year-old kidney transplant, treated with ciclosporin rapidly developed nephrotoxicity shortly after starting to take 100 mg **disopyramide** three times daily. She also experienced the anticholinergic side-effects of **disopyramide** (mucosal dryness, dysuria).[6] A patient showed an increase in serum creatinine levels when treated with **doxycycline**,[1] whereas fish oil (*Super EPA*) seems

to reduce the renal dysfunction due to ciclosporin in psoriasis.[7] The serum ciclosporin levels of a heart transplant patient doubled after taking 20 mg **fluoxetine** daily for 10 days. They fell when the ciclosporin dosage was reduced and needed to be increased again when the **fluoxetine** was stopped.[8] A patient showed increased ciclosporin and serum creatinine levels when treated with **fluvoxamine**, and it was possible to reduce the ciclosporin dosage by 33 to 50%.[9] In 5 transplant patients the pharmacokinetics of ciclosporin were not significantly affected by **citalopram** 10 to 20 mg daily.[10] The ciclosporin levels of a man were roughly halved when given 500 mg **griseofulvin** daily despite an approximately 70% increase in the ciclosporin dosage. When 16 weeks later the **griseofulvin** was stopped, his serum ciclosporin levels rose again.[11] A woman with a kidney transplant and on ciclosporin developed a urinary tract infection for which 500 mg **imipenem/cilastatin** intravenously 12-hourly was given. About 20 min after the second dose she became confused, disorientated, and agitated and developed motor aphasia and intense tremor. This was interpreted as being a combination of the adverse CNS effects of both drugs. The **imipenem/cilastatin** was not given again and these adverse effects subsided over the next few days. However it was noted that the ciclosporin serum levels climbed over the next 4 days from about 400 to 1000 nanograms/ml.[12] Four other transplant patients who were taking ciclosporin developed seizures when additionally treated with **imipenem/cilastatin**, and a fifth patient developed myoclonia.[13] In contrast **imipenem/cilastatin** with ciprofloxacin was effectively and successfully used in another patient taking ciclosporin.[14] Reduced serum ciclosporin levels following the use of **imipenem/cilastatin** have been seen in *rats*.[15] A kidney transplant patient showed a very marked fall in serum ciclosporin levels (from about 250 to 50 nanograms/ml) over 4 days when treated for persistent constipation with *GoLytely* lavage solution.[16] The serum ciclosporin levels of a kidney transplant patient more than doubled when **metronidazole** 2.25 g daily and **cimetidine** 800 mg daily were started. They fell about 50% when the **metronidazole** dosage was halved and the **cimetidine** stopped, and fell to their original levels when the **metronidazole** was withdrawn.[17] Another kidney transplant patient developed kidney toxicity with virtually doubled serum ciclosporin levels when treated with 1.5 g **metronidazole** daily.[18] Ciclosporin levels in yet another kidney transplant patient doubled (134 to 264 micrograms/l) accompanied by a modest elevation in serum creatinine when **metronidazole** 400 mg three times daily was also given. The levels fell again when metronidazole was stopped.[19] Increased ciclosporin levels associated with acute renal failure occurred in a patient given **minocycline** and **amikacin**.[14] Increased serum ciclosporin levels have been reported with **latamoxef** (**moxalactam**).[1] A kidney transplant patient showed a 70% rise in trough serum ciclosporin levels within 3 days of starting 25 mg **nefazodone** twice daily, attributed to **nefazodone's** inhibition of cytochrome P450 isoenzyme CYP3A4.[20] A cardiac transplant patient showed a tenfold increase in ciclosporin levels shortly after the addition of **nefazodone**.[21] The ciclosporin serum levels of another kidney transplant patient tripled 2 to 3 days after starting 300 mg intravenous **quinupristin/dalfopristin** 8-hourly so that the ciclosporin dosage had to be reduced by 33%.[22] A patient showed a marked rise in serum ciclosporin levels (from 450 to 750 nanograms/ml) within a week of starting 600 to 750 mg **propafenone** daily. It was controlled by reducing the ciclosporin dosage to 200 mg daily.[23] A man with a kidney transplant and mild cerebral falciparum malaria showed a gradual decrease in his serum ciclosporin levels (from 328 to 107 nanograms/ml) over 7 days when treated with 600 mg **quinine** 8-hourly, and a gradual rise when the **quinine** was stopped.[24]

Importance and management

All of the reports cited here need to be viewed in perspective because most of them are isolated and unconfirmed, and in some instances both drugs have been used together uneventfully on a number of occasions. However it should also be appreciated that many now well-recognised interactions first came to light because someone took the trouble to make a report, even though it involved only one patient.

The concurrent use of any of these drugs should therefore be well monitored if their use is thought to be necessary.

1. Cockburn I. Cyclosporin A: a clinical evaluation of drug interactions. *Transplant Proc* (1986) 18 (Suppl 5), 50–5.
2. Stevens SL, Goldman MH. Cyclosporine toxicity associated with allopurinol. *South Med J* (1992) 85, 1265–6.
3. Gorrie M, Beaman M, Nicholls A, Backwell P. Allopurinol interaction with cyclosporine. *BMJ* (1994) 308, 113.
4. Chocair P, Duley J, Simmonds HA, Cameron JS, Ianhez L, Arap S, Sabbaga E. Low-dose allopurinol plus azathioprine/cyclosporin/prednisolone, a novel immunosuppressive regimen. *Lancet* (1993) 342, 83–4.
5. Emilia G, Messora C. Interaction between cyclosporin and chlorambucil. *Eur J Haematol* (1993) 51, 179.
6. Nanni G, Magalini SC, Serino F, Castagneto M. Effect of disopyramide in a cyclosporine-treated patient. *Transplantation* (1988) 45, 257.
7. Stoof TJ, Korstanje MJ, Bilo HJG, Starink ThM, Hulsmans RFHJ, Donker AJM. Does fish oil protect renal function in cyclosporin-treated psoriasis patients? *J Intern Med* (1989) 226, 437–41.
8. Horton RC, Bonser RS. Interaction between cyclosporin and fluoxetine. *BMJ* (1995) 311, 422.
9. Vella JP, Sayegh MH. Interactions between cyclosporine and newer antidepressant medications. *Am J Kidney Dis* (1998) 31, 320–3.
10. Liston HL, Markowitz JS, Hunt N, DeVane CL, Boulton DW, Ashcraft E. Lack of citalopram effect on the pharmacokinetics of cyclosporine. *Psychosomatics* (2001) 42, 370–2.
11. Abu-Romeh SH, Rashed A. Ciclosporin A and griseofulvin: another drug interaction. *Nephron* (1991) 58, 237.
12. Zazgornik J, Schein W, Heimberger K, Shaheen FAM, Stockenhuber F. Potentiation of neurotoxic side effects by coadministration of imipenem to cyclosporine therapy in a kidney transplant recipient--synergism of side effects or drug interaction? *Clin Nephrol* (1986) 26, 265–6.
13. Bösmüller C, Steurer W, Königsrainer A, Willeit J, Margreiter R. Increased risk of central nervous system toxicity inpatients treated with ciclosporin and imipenem/cilastatin. *Nephron* (1991) 58, 362–4.
14. Thaler F, Gotainer B, Teodori G, Dubois C, Loirat Ph. Mediastinitis due to *Nocardia asteroides* after cardiac transplantation. *Intensive Care Med* (1992) 18, 127–8.
15. Mraz W, Sido B, Knedel M, Hammer C. Concomitant immunosuppressive and antibiotic therapy-reduction of cyclosporine A blood levels due to treatment with imipenem/cilastatin. *Transplant Proc* (1987) 19, 4017–20.
16. Santa T, Nishihara K, Horie S, Kotaki H, Yamamoto K, Shibuya F, Ito K, Sawada Y, Kawabe K, Iga T. Decreased cyclosporine absorption after treatment of GoLytely lavage solution in a kidney transplant patient. *Ann Pharmacother* (1994) 28, 963–4.
17. Zylber-Katz E, Rubinger D and Berlatzky Y. Cyclosporine interactions with metronidazole and cimetidine. *Drug Intell Clin Pharm* (1988) 22, 504–5.
18. Vincent F, Glotz D, Kreft-Jais C, Boudjeltia S, Duboust A, Bariety J. Insuffisance rénale aiguë chez un transplanté rénal traité par cyclosporine A et métronidazole. *Therapie* (1994) 49, 155.
19. Herzig K, Johnson DW. Marked elevation of blood cyclosporin and tacrolimus levels due to concurrent metronidazole therapy. *Nephrol Dial Transplant* (1999) 14, 521–3.
20. Helms-Smith KM, Curtis SL, Hatton RC. Apparent interaction between nefazodone and cyclosporine. *Ann Intern Med* (1996) 125, 424.
21. Wright DH, Lake KD, Bruhn PS, Emery RW. Nefazodone and cyclosporine drug-drug interaction. *J Heart Lung Transplant* (1999) 18, 913–15.
22. Stamatakis MK, Richards JG. Interaction between quinupristin/dalfopristin and cyclosporine. *Ann Pharmacother* (1997) 31, 576–8.
23. Spes CH, Angermann CE, Horn K, Strasser T, Mudra H, Landgraf R, Theisen K. Ciclosporin-propafenone interaction. *Klin Wochenschr* (1990) 68, 872.
24. Tan HW, Ch'ng SL. Drug interaction between cyclosporine A and quinine in a renal transplant patient with malaria. *Singapore Med J* (1991) 32, 189–90.

Ciclosporin + Morphine

An isolated report describes neuropsychosis in a patient when given intravenous ciclosporin and morphine.

Clinical evidence, mechanism, importance and management

A patient who underwent renal transplantation was given ciclosporin 6 mg/kg by intravenous infusion over 2 h once daily and intravenous methylprednisolone postoperatively. He also received patient-controlled analgesia as bolus doses of **morphine** 0.5 mg to a total dose of 13 mg on the first day and 11 mg on the second. On the third day he developed insomnia, anxiety, amnesia, aphasia and severe confusion. The **morphine** was discontinued and the symptoms subsided following 24 h treatment with propofol, diazepam and haloperidol. It was suggested that ciclosporin may have decreased the excitation threshold of neuronal cells, which potentiated the dysphoric effects of **morphine**.[1] This appears to be an isolated case and almost certainly not of general importance.

1. Lee P-C, Hung C-J, Lei H-Y, Tsai Y-C. Suspected acute post-transplant neuropsychosis due to interaction of morphine and cyclosporin after a renal transplant. *Anaesthesia* (2000) 55, 827–8.

Ciclosporin + Muromonab-CD3 (OKT3)

Muromonab-CD3 increases serum ciclosporin levels.

Clinical evidence, mechanism, importance and management

When **muromonab-CD3** (5 mg intravenous push daily for 10 days) was given to 10 kidney transplant patients to treat acute rejection, their mean trough ciclosporin levels on day 8 were still higher than before the **muromonab-CD3** was started, despite a 50% reduction in the ciclosporin dosage. When the **muromonab-CD3** was withdrawn, the ciclosporin dosage needed to be increased again.[1] The reasons are not understood. It is clearly necessary to titrate the dosage of ciclosporin downwards if **muromonab-CD3** is given to prevent an excessive rise in ciclosporin levels with the attendant risks of kidney toxicity.

1. Vrahnos D, Sanchez J, Vasquez EM, Pollak R, Maddux MS. Cyclosporine levels during OKT3 treatment of acute renal allograft rejection. *Pharmacotherapy* (1991) 11, 278.

Ciclosporin + NSAIDs or Aspirin or Paracetamol (Acetaminophen)

Some NSAIDs (diclofenac, indometacin (indomethacin), ketoprofen, mefenamic acid, naproxen, piroxicam and sulindac) sometimes reduce kidney function in individual patients, reflected in serum creatinine level rises and possibly in changes in ciclosporin levels, but concurrent use can also be uneventful. Diclofenac serum levels can be doubled. See also 'Ciclosporin + Topical NSAIDs', p.630. There is an isolated report of colitis in a child treated with ciclosporin and diclofenac or indometacin.

Clinical evidence

(a) Aspirin

No pharmacokinetic interaction was found between ciclosporin and **aspirin** 960 mg three times daily in healthy subjects.[1,2]

(b) Diclofenac

A study of 20 patients given ciclosporin and **diclofenac** found that 7 of them had a high probability of an interaction (rises in serum creatinine levels and blood pressures), and 9 possibly.[3] A kidney transplant patient on ciclosporin, prednisolone, digoxin, furosemide (frusemide) and spironolactone showed a marked rise in serum creatinine levels immediately after starting to take 25 mg **diclofenac** three times daily. A fall in serum ciclosporin levels (from 409 to 285 nanograms/ml) also occurred.[4] Increased nephrotoxicity was seen in another patient given 150 mg **diclofenac** daily.[5]

A 6-month study in 20 patients with severe rheumatoid arthritis and given 100 to 200 mg diclofenac with 3 mg/kg ciclosporin daily found that the **diclofenac** AUC was doubled and serum creatinine levels raised from 0.8 to 1 mg/dl. The overall pattern of adverse events and laboratory abnormalities were similar to those in patients with rheumatoid arthritis treated with ciclosporin and other NSAIDs. It was suggested that it would be prudent to start with low doses of **diclofenac** and to monitor well.[6] A study in 24 healthy subjects found no changes in the pharmacokinetics of ciclosporin after taking 50 mg **diclofenac** 8-hourly for 8 days, but there was some inconclusive evidence that **diclofenac** serum levels were increased.[7]

A child with rheumatoid arthritis on ciclosporin 10 mg/kg daily developed colitis when **diclofenac** was co-administered. The NSAID was stopped and her symptoms resolved whilst still on cyclosporine.[8]

(c) Indometacin (Indomethacin)

A study in rheumatoid arthritis patients on 2.5 mg/kg ciclosporin, found that creatinine clearances were reduced by 6% in those taking **indometacin** (doses not stated), but this was not considered to be clinically important.[9] An experimental study in healthy subjects found that ciclosporin 10 mg/kg twice daily for 4 days had no effect on effective renal plasma flow (ERPF) or the glomerular filtration rate (GFR), but when 50 mg **indometacin** twice daily was added the ERPF fell by 32% and the GFR by 37%.[10]

A child with rheumatoid arthritis on ciclosporin 10 mg/kg daily developed colitis when **indometacin** was co-administered. The NSAID was stopped and her symptoms resolved whilst still on ciclosporin.[8]

(d) Ketoprofen

A study in rheumatoid arthritis patients on 2.5 mg/kg ciclosporin, found that creatinine clearances were reduced by 2.3% in those taking **ketoprofen** (doses not stated), but this was not considered to be clinically important.[9] Another report describes increased serum creatinine levels in a patient with rheumatoid arthritis when treated with **ketoprofen**.[11]

(e) Mefenamic acid

The serum ciclosporin levels of a patient approximately doubled, accompanied by rise in creatinine levels from 113 to 168 micromol/l within a day of starting to take **mefenamic acid**. Levels fell to normal within a week of stopping the **mefenamic acid**.[12]

(f) Naproxen

Naproxen and sulindac increased serum creatinine levels by 24% in 11 patients on ciclosporin with rheumatoid arthritis, with a reduction in renal function, but accompanied by clinical improvement.[13]

(g) Paracetamol (Acetaminophen)

A study in rheumatoid arthritis patients on 2.5 mg/kg ciclosporin, found that creatinine clearances were reduced (3.5%) in those taking **paracetamol (acetaminophen)**, but this was not considered to be clinically important.[9]

(h) Piroxicam

Piroxicam is reported to have increased the serum creatinine levels of one patient.[11]

(i) Sulindac

A study in rheumatoid arthritis patients on 2.5 mg/kg ciclosporin, found that creatinine clearances were reduced by 2.6% in those taking **sulindac** (doses not stated), but this was not considered to be clinically important.[9]

A patient with a kidney transplant showed a rise in serum creatinine levels when **sulindac** was used. Serum ciclosporin levels fell and rose again when the **sulindac** was stopped.[4] Another report states that the ciclosporin levels of a woman with a kidney transplant more than doubled within 3 days of starting to take 150 mg **sulindac** twice daily.[14] Both **sulindac** and naproxen increased serum creatinine levels of 11 patients on ciclosporin with rheumatoid arthritis by 24% with a reduction in renal function, but accompanied by clinical improvement,[13] while another report describes increased serum creatinine levels in a patient with rheumatoid arthritis when treated with ketoprofen, but not when given **sulindac**.[11]

Mechanism

Uncertain. One idea is that intact kidney prostacyclin synthesis is needed to maintain the glomerular filtration rate and renal blood flow in patients given ciclosporin which possibly may protect the kidney from the development of ciclosporin-induced nephrotoxicity. If NSAIDs are used which inhibit prostaglandin production in the kidney, the nephrotoxic effects of the ciclosporin manifest themselves, possibly independently of changes in serum ciclosporin levels.[4] A study in *rats* showed that indometacin and ciclosporin together can cause rises in serum creatinine levels which are much greater than with either drug alone.[15]

The occurrence of colitis in a child receiving ciclosporin and either diclofenac or indometacin appeared to be independent of changes in ciclosporin levels and may be a result of additive effects of both drugs.[8]

Importance and management

Information about the NSAIDs listed here is sparse and limited, but the overall picture appears to be that concurrent use need not be avoided but kidney function should be well monitored and it has also been suggested that gastrointestinal symptoms should be carefully evaluated. More study is needed. It is clearly difficult to generalise about what will or will not happen if any particular NSAID is given but in the case of diclofenac it has been recommended that doses at the lower end of the range should be used at the start because its serum levels can be doubled by ciclosporin.

1. Kovarik JM, Mueller EA, Gaber M, Johnston A, Jähnchen E. Pharmacokinetics of cyclosporine and steady-state aspirin during coadministration. *J Clin Pharmacol* (1993) 33, 513–21.
2. Mueller EA, Kovarik JM, Gaber M, Jänchen E. Pharmacokinetic drug-drug interaction study with cyclosporine and acetylsalicylic acid in healthy volunteers. *Naunyn Schmiedebergs Arch Pharmacol* (1993) 347 (Suppl), R38.
3. Branthwaite JP, Nicholls A. Cyclosporin and diclofenac interaction in rheumatoid arthritis. *Lancet* (1991) 337, 252.
4. Harris KP, Jenkins D, Walls J. Nonsteroidal antiinflammatory drugs and cyclosporine. A potentially serious adverse interaction. *Transplantation* (1988) 46, 598–9.
5. Deray G, Le Hoang P, Aupetit B, Achour A, Rottembourg J, Baumelou A. Enhancement of cyclosporine A nephrotoxicity by diclofenac. *Clin Nephrol* (1987) 27, 213–14.
6. Kovarik JM, Kurki P, Mueller E, Guerret M, Markert E, Alten R, Zeidler H, Genth-Stolzenburg S. Diclofenac combined with cyclosporine in treatment of refractory rheumatoid arthritis: longitudinal safety assessment and evidence of a pharmacokinetic/dynamic interaction. *J Rheumatol* (1996) 23, 2033–8.
7. Mueller EA, Kovarik JM, Koelle EU, Merdjan H, Johnston A, Hitzenberger G. Pharmacokinetics of cyclosporine and multiple-dose diclofenac during coadministration. *J Clin Pharmacol* (1993) 33, 936–43.
8. Constantopoulos A. Colitis induced by interaction of cyclosporine A and non-steroidal anti-inflammatory drugs. *Pediatr Int* (1999) 41, 184–6.
9. Tugwell P, Ludwin D, Gent M, Roberts R, Bensen W, Grace E, Baker P. Interaction between cyclosporin A and nonsteroidal antiinflammatory drugs. *J Rheumatol* (1997) 24, 1122–5.
10. Sturrock NDC, Lang CC, Struthers AD. Indomethacin and cyclosporin together produce marked renal vasoconstriction in humans. *J Hypertens* (1994) 12, 919–24.
11. Ludwin D, Bennett KJ, Grace EM, Buchanan WA, Bensen W, Bombardier C, Tugwell PX. Nephrotoxicity in patients with rheumatoid arthritis treated with cyclosporine. *Transplant Proc* (1988) 20 (Suppl 4), 367–70.
12. Agar JWMacD. Cyclosporin A and mefenamic acid in a renal transplant patient. *Aust N Z J Med* (1991) 21, 784–5.
13. Altman RD, Perez GO, Sfakianakis GN. Interaction of cyclosporine A and nonsteroidal anti-inflammatory drugs on renal function in patients with rheumatoid arthritis. *Am J Med* (1992) 93, 396–402.
14. Sesin GP, O'Keefe E, Roberto P. Sulindac-induced elevation of serum cyclosporine concentration. *Clin Pharm* (1989) 8, 445–6.
15. Whiting PH, Burke MD, Thomson AW. Drug interactions with cyclosporine. Implications from animal studies. *Transplant Proc* (1986) 18 (Suppl 5), 56–70.

Ciclosporin + Octreotide

Octreotide causes a marked fall in the serum levels of ciclosporin and inadequate immunosuppression may result.

Clinical evidence

A diabetic man with kidney and pancreatic segment transplants was successfully immunosuppressed with azathioprine, methylprednisolone and ciclosporin. When he was additionally treated twice daily with 100 micrograms subcutaneous **octreotide** to reduce fluid collection around the pancreatic graft, his trough serum ciclosporin levels fell below the assay detection limit of 50 nanograms/ml. Nine other diabetics similarly treated with **octreotide** for peripancreatic fluid collection and fistulas after pancreatic transplantation also showed significant falls in their serum ciclosporin levels within 24 to 48 h, in three of them to undetectable levels.[1]

A similar interaction was seen in another patient.[2]

Mechanism

Uncertain. A suggestion is that the octreotide reduces the intestinal absorption of the ciclosporin.[1,2]

Importance and management

An established and clinically important interaction, although the documentation is limited. The authors of the report cited recommend that before giving octreotide the oral dosage of ciclosporin should be increased on average by 50% and the serum levels monitored daily.[1]

1. Landgraf R, Landgraf-Leurs MMC, Nusser J, Hillebrand G, Illner W-D, Abendroth D, Land W. Effect of somatostatin analogue (SMS 201–995) on cyclosporine levels. *Transplantation* (1987) 44, 724–5.
2. Rosenberg L, Dafoe DC, Schwartz R, Campbell DA, Turcotte JG, Tsai S-T, Vinik A. Administration of somatostatin analog (SMS 201–995) in the treatment of a fistula occurring after pancreas transplantation. *Transplantation* (1987) 43, 764–6.

Ciclosporin + Omeprazole or Pantoprazole

Omeprazole normally appears not to affect serum ciclosporin levels, but two isolated reports describe doubled serum ciclosporin levels in one patient, and more than halved serum ciclosporin levels in another. Pantoprazole does not affect serum ciclosporin levels.

Clinical evidence

(a) Omeprazole

Ten renal transplant patients showed no significant changes in ciclosporin levels when given 20 mg **omeprazole** daily for 2 weeks.[1,2] Eight kidney transplant patients similarly showed no significant changes in ciclosporin levels when given 20 mg **omeprazole** for 6 days.[3] No significant changes in ciclosporin levels were seen in another kidney transplant patient when 20 mg **omeprazole** daily was added for 8 weeks.[4]

In contrast, the serum ciclosporin levels of a liver transplant patient approximately doubled (from a range of 187 to 261 up to 510 nanograms/ml) about 2 weeks after starting to take 40 mg **omeprazole** daily. His ciclosporin levels were readjusted by reducing the dose from 130 to 80 mg twice daily. The levels then remained steady at about 171 nanograms/ml for the following 4 months.[5] Another patient with a bone marrow transplant showed just the opposite interaction. Her serum ciclosporin levels fell from 254 to about 100 nanograms/ml over 14 days while taking 40 mg **omeprazole** daily, and climbed again rapidly when the **omeprazole** was stopped.[6]

(b) Pantoprazole

Studies in renal transplant patients have shown that **pantoprazole** 40 mg once daily does not affect ciclosporin blood levels when given in the evening,[7] or when co-administered in the morning.[8]

Mechanism

Not understood.

Importance and management

Information is limited but what is known suggests that no interaction normally occurs. However the uncertainty of the outcome of giving omeprazole to patients on ciclosporin means that any patient given both drugs should be monitored to establish what happens. Adjust the ciclosporin dosage if necessary. Note that in the studies cited in which no interaction occurred the dose of omeprazole was 20 mg daily whereas the two cases of interaction involved 40 mg daily. There would seem to be no reason for avoiding concurrent use of ciclosporin and pantoprazole, but monitor the outcome.[9]

1. Blohmé I, Andersson T, Idström J-P. No interaction between omeprazole and cyclosporine. *Gastroenterology* (1991) 100, A721.
2. Blohmé I, Idström J-P, Andersson T. A study of the interaction between omeprazole and cyclosporine in renal transplant patients. *Br J Clin Pharmacol* (1993) 35, 156–60.
3. Kahn D, Manas D, Hamilton H, Pascoe MD. Pontin AR. The effect of omeprazole on cyclosporine metabolism in renal transplant recipients. *S Afr Med J* (1993) 83, 785.
4. Castellote E, Bonet J, Lauzurica R, Pastor C, Cofan F, Caralps A. Does interaction between omeprazole and cyclosporine exist? *Nephron* (1993) 65, 478.
5. Schouler L, Dumas F, Couzigou P, Janvier G, Winnock S, Saric J. Omeprazole-cyclosporin interaction. *Am J Gastroenterol* (1991) 86, 1097.
6. Arranz R, Yañez E, Franceschi JL, Fernandez-Rañada JM. More about omeprazole-cyclosporine interaction. *Am J Gastroenterol* (1993) 88, 154–5.
7. Lorf T, Ramadori G, Ringe B, Schwörer H. Pantoprazole does not affect cyclosporin A blood concentration in kidney-transplant patients. *Eur J Clin Pharmacol* (2000) 55, 733–5.
8. Lorf T, Ramadori G, Ringe B, Schwörer H. The effect of pantoprazole on tacrolimus and cyclosporin A blood concentration in transplant patients. *Eur J Clin Pharmacol* (2000) 56, 439–40.
9. Schwrer H, Lorf T, Ringe B, Ramadori G. Pantoprazole and cyclosporine or tacrolimus. *Aliment Pharmacol Ther* (2001) 15, 561–2.

Ciclosporin + Orlistat

The absorption of ciclosporin is significantly reduced by the concurrent use of orlistat. Acute graft rejection may occur.

Clinical evidence

The coadministration of orlistat was found in one heart transplant patient to reduce the trough blood levels, the peak levels and the AUC of ciclosporin by 47% (to 52 nanograms/ml), 86% and 75% respectively.[1] Another heart transplant patient taking ciclosporin (*Neoral*) suffered an acute rejection episode with trough ciclosporin levels of 38 nanograms/ml 24 days after starting to take **orlistat**. Ciclosporin trough levels increased to 90 to 110 nanograms/ml when the **orlistat** was stopped.[2] In a further patient taking ciclosporin (*Sandimmun*) 250 mg daily, **orlistat** 360 mg daily reduced the ciclosporin levels by two-thirds (from 150 to 50 nanograms/ml). In this patient transfer to *Neoral*, a microemulsion formulation, of ciclosporin 350 mg daily improved the bioavailability.[3] Details of this patient are also briefly reported elsewhere.[4] Another report describes 6 transplant recipients with subtherapeutic ciclosporin trough levels after the co-administration of orlistat.[5]

Mechanism

Orlistat inhibits pancreatic lipase and prevents the absorption of dietary fat and lipophilic molecules such as ciclosporin. Absorption of ciclosporin from the oil suspension formulation (*Sandimmun*) is more dependent on the lipid absorption stage and thus may be more affected by orlistat than the microemulsion form (*Neoral*).[3]

Importance and management

Information appears to be limited to these reports, but the interaction appears to be established. It has been suggested that the effects of the interaction may be reduced by using the microemulsion formulation of ciclosporin (*Neoral*).[3] Monitoring is required if the two drugs are used together, either in the standard or microemulsion form because there is a risk of subtherapeutic levels even with the microemulsion preparation.[2] Some authors recommend avoidance of the combination.[1]

1. Nägele H, Petersen B, Bonacker U, Rödiger W. Effect of orlistat on blood cyclosporin concentration in an obese heart transplant patient. *Eur J Clin Pharmacol* (1999) 55, 667–9.
2. Schnetzler B, Kondo-Oestreicher M, Vala D, Khatchatourian G, Faidutti B. Orlistat decreases the plasma level of cyclosporine and may be responsible for the development of acute rejection episodes. *Transplantation* (2000) 70, 1540–1.
3. Le Beller C, Bezie Y, Chabatte C, Guillemain R, Amrein C, Billaud EM. Co-administration or orlistat and cyclosporine in a heart transplant recipient. *Transplantation* (2000) 70, 1541–2.
4. Chavatte C, Le Beller C, Guillernain R, Arnrein C, Billaud EM. Cyclosporine/orlistat drug interaction in heart transplant recipient. *Fundam Clin Pharmacol* (2000) 14, 246.
5. Colman E, Fossler M. reduction in blood cyclosporine concentrations by orlistat. *N Engl J Med* (2000) 342, 1141–2.

Ciclosporin + Pancreatic enzyme extracts

Pancreatic enzyme extracts do not increase the bioavailability of ciclosporin in cystic fibrosis patients.

Clinical evidence, mechanism, importance and management

A study in heart-lung transplant patients with cystic fibrosis showed that they needed almost five times the oral dose of ciclosporin) as in other patients, confirming other studies showing a very much reduced bioavailability of oral ciclosporin in these patients. This is probably a reflection of the generally poor digestion and absorption in cystic fibrosis patients. The addition of **pancreatic enzymes** (*Creon*) was found not to improve this poor ciclosporin bioavailability. No adverse effects were reported.[1]

1. Tsang VT, Johnston A, Heritier F, Leaver N, Hodson ME, Yacoub M. Cyclosporin pharmacokinetics in heart-lung transplant recipients with cystic fibrosis. *Eur J Clin Pharmacol* (1994) 46, 261–5.

Ciclosporin + Penicillins

Ampicillin does not interact adversely with ciclosporin. Increased nephrotoxicity has been seen in lung transplant patients given nafcillin prophylactically. Two isolated case reports describe a fall in serum ciclosporin levels in one patient treated with nafcillin, and a rise in another treated with ticarcillin.

Clinical evidence

(a) Ampicillin

Seventy-one renal transplant patients on ciclosporin showed no changes in serum urea, creatinine or serum ciclosporin levels when **ampicillin** was given and later withdrawn.[1]

(b) Nafcillin

A retrospective study of 19 lung transplant patients on ciclosporin found that those given prophylactic **nafcillin** for a week against staphylococci showed a greater degree of kidney dysfunction than the others without **nafcillin**. Serum creatinine levels climbed steadily over six days until the **nafcillin** was stopped, whereas the 'no nafcillin' patients showed no changes. Three of the **nafcillin** group temporarily needed haemodialysis. Ciclosporin doses in the **nafcillin** group were higher but the serum levels in both groups were not significantly different. The incidence of viral infections was also greater in the **nafcillin** group.[2]

A kidney transplant patient on ciclosporin and prednisone experienced a marked fall in her serum ciclosporin levels on two occasions when treated with **nafcillin** (2 g six-hourly). Trough serum levels fell from 229 to 119 and then to 68 nanograms/ml after 3 and 7 days of **nafcillin**, before climbing again when the **nafcillin** was stopped. On the second occasion levels fell from 272 to 42 nanograms/ml after 9 days treatment with **nafcillin**.[3]

(c) Ticarcillin

Rises in serum ciclosporin levels from 90 to 230 nanograms/ml, and from 120 to 300 nanograms/ml occurred in a man within 5 to 10 days of starting to take 10 g **ticarcillin** daily.[4]

Mechanism

The authors of the study (b) postulate that the nafcillin may have interfered with the ciclosporin assay, resulting in an under-estimate of the actual levels, so that the nephrotoxicity was simply due to higher ciclosporin levels.[2] The fall in ciclosporin levels in the individual patient[3] is not understood, nor is the rise in levels seen in the patient on ticarcillin.[4]

Importance and management

Information seems to be limited to the studies cited. No special precautions would seem necessary with ampicillin, but an alternative to nafcillin should be used for anti-staphylococcal prophylaxis. Good monitoring would seem necessary if ticarcillin is given. More study is needed.

1. Xu F, Shi XH. Interaction between ampicillin, norfloxacin and cyclosporine in renal transplant recipients. *Chinese Journal of Antibiotics* (1992) 17, 290–2.
2. Jahansouz F, Kriett JM, Smith CM, Jamieson SW. Potentiation of cyclosporin nephrotoxicity by nafcillin in lung transplant recipients. *Transplantation* (1993) 55, 1045–8.
3. Veremis SA, Maddux MS, Pollak R, Mozes MF. Subtherapeutic cyclosporine concentrations during nafcillin therapy. *Transplantation* (1987) 43, 913–5.
4. Lambert C, Pointet P, Ducret F. Interaction cicloporine-ticarcilline chez un transplanté rénal. *Presse Med* (1989) 18, 230.

Ciclosporin + Prazosin

Preliminary studies show that prazosin causes a small reduction in the glomerular filtration rate of kidney transplant patients on ciclosporin.

Clinical evidence, mechanism, importance and management

A study in 8 patients with kidney transplants showed that after taking 1 mg **prazosin** twice daily for a week, their serum ciclosporin levels remained unchanged, whereas arterial blood pressures and renal vascular resistance were reduced. However the glomerular filtration rate (GFR) was reduced by about 10% (from 47 to 42 ml/min).[1] Previous studies in kidney transplant patients treated with azathioprine, prednisone and **prazosin** found no reduction in GFR.[2] There would seem to be no strong reasons for totally avoiding **prazosin** in patients on ciclosporin, but the authors of the report point out that the fall in GFR makes **prazosin** a less attractive antihypertensive than a calcium channel blocker.

1. Kiberd BA. Effects of prazosin therapy in renal allograft recipients receiving cyclosporine. *Transplantation* (1990) 49, 1200–1.
2. Curtis JR, Bateman FJA. Use of prazosin in management of hypertension in patients with chronic renal failure and in renal transplant recipients. *BMJ* (1975) 4, 432.

Ciclosporin + Probucol

Probucol reduces blood ciclosporin levels.

Clinical evidence

A study in 6 heart transplant patients taking 2.44 mg/kg ciclosporin 12-hourly daily showed that the concurrent use of 500 mg **probucol** 12-hourly decreased whole blood ciclosporin levels and the AUC. The clearance was increased by 60% and volume of distribution also increased. Comparative whole blood ciclosporin levels in nanograms/ml before and while taking the **probucol** were as follows: 1034 v 786 (1 h), 1272 v 933 (3 h), 958 v 728 (5 h), 599 v 413 (11 h).[1] This represents a 28% AUC decrease over 11 h.[1-3]

Another group of workers similarly found that 9 out 10 kidney transplant patients similarly showed a reduction in trough serum ciclosporin levels while being treated with **probucol**.[4]

Mechanism

Not understood.

Importance and management

Information appears to be limited to these studies, but the interaction appears to be well established. The ciclosporin dosage may need to be increased if probucol is added. Monitor the effects and adjust the dosage appropriately.

1. Corder CN, Sundararajan V, Liguori C, Cooper DKC, Muchmore J, Zuhdi N, Novitzky D, Barbi G, Larscheid P, Manion CV. Interference with steady state cyclosporine levels by probucol in heart transplant patients. *Clin Pharmacol Ther* (1990) 47, 204.
2. Sundararajan V, Cooper DKC, Muchmore J, Manion CV, Liguori C, Zuhdi N, Novitzky D, Chen P-N, Bourne DWA, Corder CN. Interaction of cyclosporine and probucol in heart transplant patients. *Transplant Proc* (1991) 23, 2028–32.
3. Chen P, Bourne DWA, Corder CN, Larscheid P. Clinical pharmacokinetic interaction of cyclosporine and probucol studied using a HPLC assay procedure. *Pharm Res* (1990) 7, S-254.
4. Gallego C, Sánchez P, Planells C, Sánchez S, Monte E, Romá E, Sánchez J, Pallardó LM. Interaction between probucol and cyclosporine in renal transplant patients. *Ann Pharmacother* (1994) 28, 940–2.

Ciclosporin + Pyrazinamide

Pyrazinamide appears normally not to interact with ciclosporin but one isolated report suggests that it may possi-

bly have added to the ciclosporin-lowering effects of ri-fampicin in one patient, and another patient developed toxic myopathy attributed to concurrent use.

Clinical evidence, mechanism, importance and management

A girl of 12 with a kidney transplant and on ciclosporin and pred-nisolone developed rejection while taking rifampicin and isoniazid, apparently due to the fall in serum ciclosporin levels caused by the ri-fampicin, but the rejection settled when the rifampicin was replaced by pyrazinamide.[1] Other patients taking ciclosporin have been treat-ed with pyrazinamide combined with ethambutol and/or streptomy-cin without any apparent interaction problems.[2] However an anecdotal report suggested that when pyrazinamide was added to ri-fampicin with isoniazid it appeared to add to the effects of the ri-fampicin causing an additional reduction in serum ciclosporin levels.[3] Another report attributed the development of toxic myopathy in a kid-ney transplant patient to the concurrent use of pyrazinamide and ciclosporin.[4]

There would therefore seem to be no reason for avoiding pyrazina-mide in patients taking ciclosporin, but good monitoring is clearly needed.

1. Coward RA, Raftery AT, Brown CB. Cyclosporin and antituberculous therapy. Lancet (1985) i, 1342–3.
2. Aguado JM, Herrero JA, Gavaldá J, Torre-Cisneros J, Blanes M, Rufí G, Moreno A, Gur-guí A, Hayek M, Lumbreras C and the Spanish Transplantation Infection Study Group, GESITRA. Clinical presentation and outcome of tuberculosis in kidney, liver, and heart transplant recipients in Spain. Transplantation (1997) 63, 1276–86.
3. Jiménez del Cerro LA, Hernández FR. Effect of pyrazinamide on ciclosporin levels. Ne-phron (1992) 62, 113.
4. Fernández-Solà J, Campistol JM, Miró Ó, Garcés N, Soy D. Grau JM. Acute toxic myop-athy due to pyrazinamide in a patient with renal transplantation and cyclosporine therapy. Nephrol Dial Transplant (1996) 11, 1850–2.

Ciclosporin + Quinolone antibacterials

Ciclosporin serum levels are normally unchanged by the use of ciprofloxacin and kidney toxicity is not normally in-creased, but increased serum levels and nephrotoxicity may occur in a small number of patients. There is also some evi-dence that the immunosuppressant effects are reduced by ciprofloxacin. Three reports describe rises in ciclosporin lev-els in patients given norfloxacin, but others state that no in-teraction occurs. Enoxacin, levofloxacin, ofloxacin and pefloxacin appear not to interact significantly.

Clinical evidence

(a) Ciprofloxacin

A single-dose study in 10 healthy subjects found that after taking 500 mg ciprofloxacin twice daily for 7 days the pharmacokinetics of oral ciclosporin 5 mg/kg were unchanged.[1] Five other studies confirm the lack of a pharmacokinetic interaction: in 10 renal transplant pa-tients taking 750 mg ciprofloxacin twice daily for 13 days;[2] in 15 kidney transplant patients on 500 mg ciprofloxacin twice daily for 7 days;[3] in 10 bone marrow transplant patients given 500 mg cipro-floxacin twice daily for 4 days;[4] in 4 heart transplant patients given 250 to 500 mg for 7 to 140 days;[5] and in another 3 heart transplant pa-tients given 800 to 1500 mg ciprofloxacin daily.[6] No changes in se-rum ciclosporin levels nor evidence of kidney toxicity occurred.

In contrast, a handful of cases of nephrotoxicity have been reported. A heart transplant patient developed acute renal failure within 4 days of being given ciprofloxacin 750 mg eight-hourly.[7] Another patient who had undergone a kidney transplant developed reversible nephro-toxicity.[8] Decreased renal function in a heart-lung transplant patient has been described in another report.[9] This patient and another also showed increased serum ciclosporin levels when given 500 mg cip-rofloxacin three times daily.[9] Acute interstitial nephritis in a cardiac transplant patient is reported in another.[10-12]

A case-control study in 42 kidney transplant patients suggested that the proportion of cases experiencing at least one episode of biopsy-

proved rejection within 1 to 3 months of receiving the transplant were significantly greater (45%) in those who had taken ciprofloxacin than in those (19%) who had not. There was also a marked increase in the incidence of rejection temporarily associated with cipro-floxacin use (29%) compared with the controls (2%).[13]

(b) Enoxacin, Ofloxacin, Levofloxacin, Pefloxacin

Enoxacin 400 mg twice daily for 5 days had little effect on either blood or plasma levels of single doses of ciclosporin in 10 healthy subjects.[14] A single dose study in 12 healthy subjects found that 500 mg levofloxacin had no effect on the pharmacokinetics of ciclosporin.[15] Thirty-nine patients with kidney transplants under treatment with ciclosporin and prednisolone showed no evidence of nephrotoxicity nor any other interaction when concurrently treated with 100 to 400 mg ofloxacin daily for periods of 3 to 500 days.[16] A study in kidney transplant patients treated with corticosteroids, aza-thioprine and ciclosporin found that the pharmacokinetics of the ciclosporin were not significantly changed by 400 mg pefloxacin twice daily for 4 days.[17]

(c) Norfloxacin

Six renal transplant patients given 400 mg norfloxacin twice daily for 3 to 23 days for urinary tract infections,[18] and four heart transplant patients given 400 mg for 7 to 140 days showed no changes in serum ciclosporin levels.[5] However two reports describe rises, one marked, in serum ciclosporin levels in a heart transplant patient and a kidney transplant patient when given norfloxacin.[19] A comparative study in 5 children (mean age of 8) found that while receiving 5 to 10 mg/kg/day of norfloxacin their daily dose of ciclosporin was 4.5 mg/kg/day compared with another control group of 6 children without norfloxacin who needed 7.4 mg/kg/day.[20]

Mechanisms

The ciclosporin/norfloxacin interaction probably occurs because the norfloxacin inhibits the cytochrome P450 isoenzyme CYP3A4 so that the metabolism of the ciclosporin is reduced.[20] The ciclosporin/cipro-floxacin interaction may possibly be due to some antagonism by cip-rofloxacin of the ciclosporin-dependent inhibition of interleukin-2 which thereby opposes its immunosuppressant action.[13]

Importance and management

Information seems to be limited to these reports. They indicate that in children and adults the dosage of ciclosporin will probably need to be reduced in the presence of norfloxacin. No pharmacokinetic interac-tion normally occurs between ciclosporin and ciprofloxacin but very occasionally and unpredictably an increase in serum ciclosporin lev-els and/or kidney toxicity occurs. There is also some evidence that the immunosuppressant effects of the ciclosporin may be reduced. Con-current use should therefore be well monitored. There seem to be no reports of problems with enoxacin, levofloxacin, ofloxacin or pe-floxacin but the outcome of concurrent use should nevertheless be monitored.

1. Tan KKC, Trull AK, Shawket S. Co-administration of ciprofloxacin and cyclosporin: lack of evidence for a pharmacokinetic interaction. Br J Clin Pharmacol (1989) 28, 185–7.
2. Lang J, Finaz de Villaine J, Garraffo R, Touraine J-L. Cyclosporine (cyclosporin A) pharmacokinetics in renal transplant patients receiving ciprofloxacin. Am J Med (1989) 87 (Suppl 5A), 82S–85S.
3. Van Buren DH, Koestner J, Adedoyin A, McCune T, MacDonell R, Johnson HK, Carroll J, Nylander W, Richie RE. Effect of ciprofloxacin on cyclosporine pharmacokinetics. Transplantation (1990) 50, 888–9.
4. Krüger HU, Schuler U, Proksch B, Göbel M, Ehninger G. Investigation of potential in-teraction of ciprofloxacin with cyclosporine in bone marrow transplant recipients. Anti-microb Agents Chemother (1990) 34, 1048–52.
5. Robinson JA, Venezio FR, Costanzo-Nordin MR, Pifarre R, O'Keefe PJ. Patients receiv-ing quinolones and cyclosporine after heart transplantation. J Heart Transplant (1990) 9, 30–1.
6. Hooper TL, Gould FK, Swinburn CR, Featherstone G, Odom NJ, Corris PA, Freeman R, McGregor CGA. Ciprofloxacin: a preferred tratment for legionella infections in patients receiving cyclosporin A. J Antimicrob Chemother (1988) 22, 952–3.
7. Avent CK, Krinsky JK, Kirklin JK, Bourge RC, Figg WD. Synergistic nephrotoxicity due to cyclosporine and ciprofloxacin. Am J Med (1988) 85, 452–3.
8. Elston RA, Taylor J. Possible interaction of ciprofloxacin with cyclosporin A. J Antimi-crob Chemother (1988) 21, 679–80.
9. Nasir M, Rotellar C, Hand M, Kulczycki L, Alijani MR, Winchester JF. Interaction be-tween ciclosporin and ciprofloxacin. Nephron (1991) 57, 245–6.
10. Rosado LJ, Siskind MS, Copeland JG. Acute interstitial nephritis in a cardiac transplant patient receiving ciprofloxacin. J Thorac Cardiovasc Surg (1994) 107, 1364.

11. Bourge RC. Invited letter concerning: acute interstitial nephritis in a cardiac transplant recipients receiving ciprofloxacin. *J Thorac Cardiovasc Surg* (1994) 107, 1364-5.
12. Rosado LJ, Siskind MS, Nolan PE, Copeland JG. Invited letter concerning: acute interstitial nephritis in a cardiac transplant recipients receiving ciprofloxacin. *J Thorac Cardiovasc Surg* (1994) 107, 1365-6.
13. Wrishko RE, Levine M, Primmett DRN, Kim S, Partovi N, Lewis S, Landsberg D, Keown PA. Investigation of a possible interaction between ciprofloxacin and cyclosporine in renal transplant patients. *Transplantation* (1997) 64, 996–999.
14. Ryerson BA, Toothaker RD, Posvar EL, Sedman AJ, Koup JR. Effect of enoxacin on cyclosporine pharmacokinetics in healthy subjects. *Intersci Conf Antimicrob Agents Chemother* (1991) 31, 198.
15. Doose DR, Walker SA, Chien SC, Williams RR, Nayak RK. Levofloxacin does not alter cyclosporine disposition. *J Clin Pharmacol* (1998) 38, 90–3.
16. Vogt P, Schorn T, Frei U. Ofloxacin in the treatment of urinary tract infection in renal transplant recipients. *Infection* (1988) 16, 175–8.
17. Lang J, Finaz de Villaine J, Guemei A, Touraine JL, Faucon C. Absence of pharmacokinetic interaction between pefloxacin and cyclosporin A in patients with renal transplants. *Rev Infect Dis* (1989) 11 (Suppl 5), S1094.
18. Jadoul M, Pirson Y, van Ypersele de Strihou C. Norfloxacin and cyclosporine-a safe combination. *Transplantation* (1989) 47, 747–8.
19. Thomson DJ, Menkis AH, McKenzie FN. Norfloxacin-cyclosporine interaction. *Transplantation* (1988) 46, 312–13.
20. McLellan RA, Drobitch RK, McLellan DH, Acott PD, Crocker JFS, Renton KW. Norfloxacin interferes with cyclosporine disposition in pediatric patients undergoing renal transplantation. *Clin Pharmacol Ther* (1995) 58, 322–7.

Ciclosporin + Retinoids

A considerable increase in serum ciclosporin levels occurred in one patient given etretinate, but most patients seem normally only to show minimal increases. Isotretinoin appears not to interact adversely, and acitretin possibly behaves like etretinate.

Clinical evidence

(a) Acitretin, Isotretinoin

Three reports say that **isotretinoin** has been successfully and uneventfully used for severe acne in patients on ciclosporin with heart transplants or aplastic anaemia.[1-3] An *in vitro* study using human liver microsomes found that concentrations of 100 micromol of **acitretin** and **isotretinoin** inhibited the total ciclosporin metabolism and total primary ciclosporin metabolite production to the same extent (32 to 45% respectively). These compare with figures of 36% and 38% for **etretinate**.[4]

(b) Etretinate

A woman with generalised pustular psoriasis showed a considerable rise in her serum ciclosporin levels (to 540 micrograms/l) when the dosage was raised from 200 to 300 mg daily and 50 mg **etretinate** daily was added. It was found possible to reduce the ciclosporin dosage gradually to 150 mg daily, accompanied by a fall in the trough serum ciclosporin levels to 168 micrograms/l without any loss in the control of the disease.[4]

There was no improvement in a patient with erythrodermic psoriasis treated with ciclosporin 5 to 10 mg/kg daily, but ciclosporin 5 mg/kg daily with **etretinate** 0.7 mg/kg daily cleared the psoriasis by 90%. Reducing the dose of either drug resulted in exacerbation of symptoms.[5] Another 5 patients with plaque-type psoriasis showed a relapse when the ciclosporin dosage was reduced in the presence of **etretinate**, but no additive therapeutic effect was seen. All of them showed elevated serum creatinine levels.[6] Only a modest ciclosporin dosage reduction was found in another study in which **etretinate** was also used.[7] No obvious advantages but no increase in side-effects were found in another study.[8] **Etretinate** possibly inhibits the metabolism of ciclosporin (see 'Mechanism'). See also the report of *in vitro* studies in (a).

Mechanism

Uncertain. A possible explanation is that the etretinate inhibits the metabolism of the ciclosporin by the liver, thereby reducing its loss from the body and raising its serum levels. One *in vitro* study using human liver microsomes failed to show that etretinate inhibits the metabolism of ciclosporin,[9] whereas another study using higher ciclosporin concentrations demonstrated an approximately 40% inhi-

bition.[4] The latter study found that acitretin and isotretinoin behave like etretinate[4] (see 'Clinical Evidence' above).

Importance and management

The overall picture seems to be that etretinate has only a modest effect, or no effect at all, on serum ciclosporin levels in most patients, even in dosages up to 1 mg/kg daily, nevertheless good monitoring is clearly important. There seems to be no marked therapeutic advantage in using both drugs together. Isotretinoin appears not to interact adversely with ciclosporin but monitoring for increased serum lipids has been advised because both drugs can cause an increase.[3] Acitretin (the major metabolite of etretinate) probably behaves like etretinate although this needs confirmation.

1. Hazen PE, Walker AE, Stewart JJ, Carney JF, Engstrom CW, Turgeon KL, Shurin S. Successful use of isotretinoin in a patient on cyclosporine: apparent lack of toxicity. *Int J Dermatol* (1993) 32, 466–7.
2. Bunker CB, Rustin MHA, Dowd PM. Isotretinoin treatment of severe acne in posttransplant patients taking cyclosporine. *J Am Acad Dermatol* (1990) 22, 693–4.
3. Abel EA. Isotretinoin treatment of severe cystic acne in a heart transplant patient receiving cyclosporine: consideration of drug interactions. *J Am Acad Dermatol* (1991) 24, 511.
4. Shah IA, Whiting PH, Omar G, Ormerod AD, Burke MD. The effects of retinoids and terbinafine on the human hepatic microsomal metabolism of cyclosporine. *Br J Dermatol* (1993) 129, 395–8.
5. Korstanje MJ, Bessems PJMJ, van de Staak WJBM. Combination therapy cyclosporin-etretinate effective in erythrodermic psoriasis. *Dermatologica* (1989) 179, 94.
6. Korstanje MJ, van de Staak WJBM. Combination-therapy cyclosporin-A-etretinate for psoriasis. *Clin Exp Dermatol* (1990) 15, 172–3.
7. Meinardi MMHM, Bos JD. Cyclosporine maintenance therapy in psoriasis. *Transplant Proc* (1988) 20 (Suppl 4), 42–9.
8. Brechtel B, Wellenreuther U, Toppe E, Czarnetzki BM. Combination of etretinate with cyclosporine in the treatment of severe recalcitrant psoriasis. *J Am Acad Dermatol* (1994) 30, 1023–4.
9. Webber IR, Back DJ. Effect of etretinate on cyclosporine metabolism *in vitro*. *Br J Dermatol* (1993) 128, 42–4.

Ciclosporin + Rifampicin (Rifampin), Rifabutin or Rifamycin sodium

Ciclosporin serum levels are markedly reduced by the concurrent use of rifampicin. Transplant rejection can rapidly develop if the ciclosporin dosage is not increased (three to fivefold). Rifabutin appears to interact minimally.

Clinical evidence

(a) Rifampicin (Rifampin)

A heart transplant patient on ciclosporin was started on 600 mg **rifampicin** daily in addition to amphotericin B for the treatment of an *Aspergillus fumigatus* infection. Within 11 days her serum ciclosporin levels had fallen from 473 to less than 31 nanograms/ml and severe acute graft rejection occurred. The dosage of ciclosporin was increased stepwise and the levels climbed to a plateau before suddenly falling again. The dosage had to be increased to more than 30 mg/kg daily to achieve serum levels in the range 100 to 300 nanograms/ml.[1]

A considerable number of other reports about individual patients confirm that a very marked fall in serum ciclosporin levels occurs (often to undetectable levels), accompanied by transplantation rejection in many instances,[2-25] if **rifampicin** is given without raising the ciclosporin dosage. Levels can rise to toxic proportions within two weeks of stopping the **rifampicin** unless the previously adjusted ciclosporin dosage is very much reduced.[2,4] Three patients needed increases in the dosage of ciclosporin when given **rifampicin** and **erythromycin**, although the latter normally reduces ciclosporin requirements.[18,26,27] Another patient whose ciclosporin levels had been raised by **clarithromycin** showed a fall when **rifampicin** was added.[28]

(b) Rifabutin

The clearance of ciclosporin in a patient with a kidney transplant approximately doubled (from 0.3 to 0.63 L/h/kg) when treated with isoniazid, ethambutol, pyridoxine and 600 mg **rifampicin (rifampin)** daily. When replaced by 150 mg **rifabutin** and 100 mg clofazimine daily the clearance fell to approximately its former levels, but after about three weeks rose to 0.36 L/h/kg.[14]

(c) Rifamycin sodium

Topical **rifamycin sodium** used to irrigate a wound has been reported to reduce the serum levels of ciclosporin in a kidney transplant patient.[29]

Mechanism

Rifampicin stimulates the metabolism of the ciclosporin by the liver (increased amounts of cytochrome P450 isoenzyme CYPA3)[30] resulting in a marked increase in its loss from the body, accompanied by a fall in its serum levels. In addition rifampicin decreases ciclosporin absorption from the gut by inducing its metabolism by the gut wall,[31] thus its immunosuppressant effects become markedly reduced. If rifampicin is given with erythromycin, the enzyme inhibitory effects of the latter are swamped by the more potent enzyme effects of the former. Rifabutin has some enzyme inducing properties but the extent is quite small compared with rifampicin, and is delayed.[32]

Importance and management

The ciclosporin/rifampicin interaction is very well documented, well established and clinically important. Transplant rejection may occur unless the ciclosporin dosage is markedly increased. The interaction develops within a few days (within a single day in one case[19]). Monitor the effects of concurrent use and increase the ciclosporin dosage appropriately. Three to fivefold dosage increases (sometimes frequency-increases from two to three times daily) have proved to be effective, with daily monitoring. There are also financial implications. It has been calculated that in the year 2000, the cost of post-transplant immunosuppression with ciclosporin, azathioprine and steroids may be increased 2.5-fold during 9 months concomitant antituberculosis treatment from.[33]

Remember also to reduce the dosage if the rifampicin is stopped. The authors of one large study concluded that it is better to avoid rifampicin in patients on ciclosporin and to use other tuberculostatics instead.[21] Even topical rifamycin sodium can apparently interact like rifampicin when introduced into a wound.[29]

Alternative drugs which normally do not interact with ciclosporin include **pyrazinamide**,[4,21,22] **isoniazid**[10,21,22] and **ethambutol**.[21,22] However, one report suggested that when **pyrazinamide** was added to **rifampicin** with **isoniazid** it added to the effects of the **rifampicin** further reducing serum ciclosporin levels.[34] There is one case report describing a patient who showed a gradual rise in serum ciclosporin levels when isoniazid and ethambutol were stopped,[12] and another which attributed a marked rise in ciclosporin levels to the use of isoniazid.[35] See also 'Ciclosporin + Pyrazinamide', p.623. **Rifabutin** appears to interact minimally. Another suggested alternative is to replace the ciclosporin with azathioprine and low-dose prednisolone for immunosuppression when using rifampicin.[11]

1. Modry DL, Stinson EB, Oyer PE, Jamieson SW, Baldwin JC, Shumway NE. Acute rejection and massive cyclosporine requirements in heart transplant recipients treated with rifampin. *Transplantation* (1985) 39, 313–14.
2. Langhoff E, Madsen S. Rapid metabolism of cyclosporin and prednisone in kidney transplant patients on tuberculostatic treatment. *Lancet* (1983) ii, 1303.
3. Cassidy MJD, Van Zyl-Smit R, Pascoe MD, Swanepoel CR, Jacobson JE. Effect of rifampicin on cyclosporin A blood levels in a renal transplant recipient. *Nephron* (1985) 41, 207–8.
4. Coward RA, Raferty AT, Brown CB. Cyclosporin and antituberculous therapy. *Lancet* (1985) i, 1342–3.
5. Howard P, Bixler TJ, Gill B. Cyclosporine-rifampin drug interaction. *Drug Intell Clin Pharm* (1985) 19, 763–4.
6. Van Buren D, Wideman CA, Ried M, Gibbons S, Van Buren CT, Jarowenko M, Flechner SM, Frazier OH, Cooley DA, Kahan BD. The antagonistic effect of rifampin upon cyclosporine bioavailability. *Transplant Proc* (1984) 16, 1642–5.
7. Allen RDM, Hunnisett AG, Morris PJ. Cyclosporin and rifampicin in renal transplantation. *Lancet* (1985) i, 980.
8. Langhoff E, Madsen S. Rapid metabolism of cyclosporin and prednisone in kidney transplant patient receiving tuberculostatic treatment. *Lancet* (1983) ii, 1031.
9. Offermann G, Keller F, Molzahn M. Low cyclosporin A blood levels and acute graft rejection in a renal transplant recipient during rifampin treatment. *Am J Nephrol* (1985) 5, 385–7.
10. Jurewicz WA, Gunson BK, Ismail T, Angrisani L, McMaster P. Cyclosporin and antituberculous therapy. *Lancet* (1985) i, 1343.
11. Daniels NJ, Dover JS, Schachter RK. Interaction between cyclosporin and rifampicin. *Lancet* (1984) ii, 639.
12. Leimenstoll G, Schlegelberger T, Fulde R, Niedermayer W. Interaktion von Ciclosporin und Ethambutol-Isoniazid. *Dtsch Med Wochenschr* (1988) 113, 514–15.
13. Prado A, Ramirez M, Aguirre EC, Martin RS, Zucchini A. Interaccion entre ciclosporina y rifampicina en un caso de transplante renal. *Medicina (B Aires)* (1987) 47, 521–4.
14. Vandevelde C, Chang A, Andrews D, Riggs W, Jewesson P. Rifampin and ansamycin interactions with cyclosporine after renal transplantation. *Pharmacotherapy* (1991) 11, 88–9.
15. Al-Sulaiman MH, Dhar JM, Al-Khader AA. Successful use of rifampicin in the treatment of tuberculosis in renal transplant patients immunosuppressed with cyclosporine. *Transplantation* (1990) 50, 597–8.
16. Sánchez DM, Rincón LC, Asensio JM, Serna AB. Interacción entre ciclosporina y rifampicina. *Rev Clin Esp* (1988) 183, 217.
17. Peschke B, Ernst W, Gossmann J, Kachel HG, Schoeppe W, Scheuermann EH. Antituberculous drugs in kidney transplant recipients treated with cyclosporine. *Transplantation* (1993) 56, 236–8.
18. Zylber-Katz E. Multiple drug interactions with cyclosporine in a heart transplant patient. *Ann Pharmacother* (1995) 29, 127–31.
19. Wandel C, Böhrer H, Böcker R. Rifampicin and cyclosporine dosing in heart transplant patients. *J Cardiothorac Vasc Anesth* (1995) 9, 621–2.
20. Capone D, Aiello C, Santoro GA, Gentile A, Stanziale P, D'Alessandro R, Imperatore P, Basile V. Drug interaction between cyclosporine and two antimicrobial agents, josamycin and rifampicin, in organ-transplanted patients. *Int J Clin Pharmacol Res* (1996) 16, 73–6.
21. Aguado JM, Herrero JA, Gavaldá J, Torre-Cisneros J, Blanes M, Rufí G, Moreno A, Gurguí A, Hayek M, Lumbreras C and the Spanish Transplantation Infection Study Group, GESITRA. Clinical presentation and outcome of tuberculosis in kidney, liver, and heart transplant recipients in Spain. *Transplantation* (1997) 63, 1276–86.
22. Muñoz P, Palomo J, Muños R, Rodríguez-Creixéms M, Pelaez T, Bouza E. Tuberculosis in heart transplant recipients. *Clin Infect Dis* (1995) 21, 398–402.
23. Freitag VL, Skifton RD, Lake KD. Effect of short-term rifampin on stable cyclosporine concentration. *Ann Pharmacother* (1993) 31, 871–2.
24. Carvalho GR, Mulinari A, Hauck P. Tuberculosis in renal transplant recipients. *J Am Soc Nephrol* (1997) 8, 709A.
25. Kim YH, Yoon YR, Kim YW, Shin JG, Cha IJ. Effects of rifampin on cyclosporine disposition in kidney recipients with tuberculosis. *Transplant Proc* (1998) 30, 3570–2.
26. Hooper TL, Gould FK, Swinburne CR, Featherstone G, Odom NJ, Corris PA, Freeman R, McGregor CGA. Ciprofloxacin: a preferred treatment for legionella infections in patients receiving cyclosporin A. *J Antimicrob Chemother* (1988) 22, 952–3.
27. Soto J, Sacristan JA, Alsar MJ. Effect of the simultaneous administration of rifampicin and erythromycin on the metabolism of cyclosporine. *Clin Transplant* (1992) 6, 312–14.
28. Plemmons RM, McAllister CK, Garces MC, Ward RL. Osteomyelitis due to *Mycobacterium haemophilum* in a cardiac transplant patient: case report and analysis of interactions among clarithromycin, rifampin and cyclosporine. *Clin Infect Dis* (1997) 24, 995–7.
29. Renoult E, Hubert J, Trechot Ph, Hestin D, Kessler M, L'Hermite J. Effect of topical rifamycin SV treatment on cyclosporin A blood levels in a renal transplant patient. *Eur J Clin Pharmacol* (1991) 40, 433–4.
30. Pichard L, Fabre JM, Domergue J, Fabre G, Saint-Aubert B, Mourad G, Maurel P. Molecular mechanism of cyclosporine A drug interactions: inducers and inhibitors of cytochrome P450 screening in primary cultures of human hepatocytes. *Transplant Proc* (1991) 23, 978–9.
31. Hebert MF, Roberts JP, Prueksaritanont T, Benet LZ. Bioavailability of cyclosporine with concomitant rifampin administration is markedly less than predicted by hepatic enzyme induction. *Clin Pharmacol Ther* (1992) 52, 453–7.
32. Perucca E, Grimaldi R, Frigo GM, Sardi A, Möning H, Ohnhaus EE. Comparative effects of rifabutin and rifampicin on hepatic microsomal enzyme activity in normal subjects. *Eur J Clin Pharmacol* (1988) 34, 595–9.
33. Naqvi SAA The challenge of posttransplant tuberculosis. *Transplant Proc* (2000) 32, 650–1.
34. Jiménez del Cerro LA, Hernández FR. Effect of pyrazinamide on cyclosporin levels. *Nephron* (1992) 62, 113.
35. Diaz Couselo FA, Porato F, Turin M, Etchegoyen FP, Diez RA. Interacciones de la ciclosporina en transplantados renales. *Medicina (B Aires)* (1992) 52, 296–302.

Ciclosporin + Sex hormones or Anabolic steroids and related drugs

Hepatotoxicity has been described in two patients when concurrently treated with ciclosporin and oral contraceptives. Rises in serum ciclosporin levels may also occur. Hepatotoxicity occurred in three others given ciclosporin and norethandrolone. Marked increases in serum ciclosporin levels have been seen in seven patients taking danazol and in two taking methyltestosterone. Some increase has been seen with norethisterone.

Clinical evidence

(a) Contraceptives (oral)

A woman treated for uveitis with ciclosporin 5 mg/kg daily showed an increase in trough serum ciclosporin levels (very roughly doubled) on two occasions when given an oral contraceptive (**levonorgestrel** 150 micrograms + **ethinylestradiol** 30 micrograms). She also experienced nausea, vomiting and hepatalgia, and showed evidence of severe hepatotoxicity (very marked increases in aspartate and alanine aminotransferases, and rises in serum bilirubin and alkaline phosphatase).[1]

Another report describes hepatotoxicity in a patient when concurrently treated with ciclosporin and an oral contraceptive (**desogestrel** 150 micrograms + **ethinylestradiol** 30 micrograms). Rises in serum ciclosporin levels were also seen.[2]

(b) Danazol

A 15-year-old girl with a kidney transplant for a year, taking ciclosporin and prednisone, showed a marked rise in serum ciclosporin levels over about 2 weeks (from a range of 250 to 325 up to 700 to 850 micromol/l) when given 200 mg **danazol** twice daily, even though the ciclosporin dosage was reduced from 350 to 250 mg daily.[3]

Similar rises in ciclosporin concentrations (from about 400 to 600 nanograms/ml, and from 150 to about 450 nanograms/ml) were seen in another patient on two occasions over about a 6-week period when given 400 mg and later 600 mg **danazol** daily.[4] A 12-year-old boy needed a reduction in his ciclosporin dosage from 10 to 2 mg/kg daily when 400 mg **danazol** twice daily was added.[5] A marked rise in serum ciclosporin levels has been described in two other patients when given 200 mg **danazol** three[6] or four[7] times daily. A patient with aplastic anaemia treated with ciclosporin was subsequently treated with **danazol** 200 mg daily for pancytopenia and endometriosis. Within 4 days the patient had epigastric pain and elevated serum ciclosporin and creatinine levels. **Danazol** was stopped and the ciclosporin dose was halved. Two weeks later abrupt severe hepatic injury occurred and the patient died of hepatic failure, although this was thought to be due to **danazol** toxicity rather than the interaction.[8]

A pharmacokinetic study in one kidney transplant patient found that 200 mg **danazol** three times daily for 16 days reduced the ciclosporin clearance by 50%, prolonged its half-life by 66% and raised its AUC by 65%.[9]

(c) Methyltestosterone

A man with a kidney transplant was given **methyltestosterone** for 9 months before an attempt was made to change his immunosuppressive treatment from azathioprine and prednisone to ciclosporin. Within a few days his serum ciclosporin levels rose to more than 2000 nanograms/ml and severe ciclosporin toxicity was seen (raised serum creatinine, bilirubin and alanine aminotransferase levels).[10] This interaction has been seen in another patient within 4 weeks of combined therapy.[11]

(d) Norethandrolone

Three out of four patients with bone marrow aplasia treated with ciclosporin and prednisone developed liver toxicity. It developed in two of them when **norethandrolone** was added. No toxicity occurred when they were given either of the drugs singly.[12] Jaundice associated with toxic hepatitis was attributed to the concurrent use of ciclosporin and **norethandrolone** in a girl of 14 during the post-transplant period.[13]

(e) Norethisterone

The 15-year-old girl on ciclosporin who had shown a marked increase in serum ciclosporin levels when given danazol (referred to above) continued to have elevated levels, but not as high, when the **danazol** was replaced by **norethisterone**, 5 mg three times daily, and the levels fell once again when the **norethisterone** was stopped.[3] No changes in ciclosporin levels were seen in another patient when treated with **norethisterone** intermittently.[7] Two women showed a mild rise in ciclosporin with no changes in creatinine levels when given 10 mg **norethisterone** daily for 10 days.[14]

Mechanism

Uncertain. It seems possible that some of these compounds inhibit the metabolism of the ciclosporin by the liver, thereby reducing its loss from the body and leading to an increase in its serum levels. The mechanism of the hepatotoxicity is not understood.

Importance and management

Information is limited, but what is known indicates that the concurrent use of any of these drugs and ciclosporin should be well monitored for any evidence of increases in serum ciclosporin levels or hepatotoxicity. Appropriate ciclosporin dosage adjustments should be made as necessary.

1. Deray G, le Hoang P, Cacoub P, Assogba U, Grippon P, Baumelou A. Oral contraceptive interaction with cyclosporin. *Lancet* (1987) i, 158–9.
2. Leimenstoll G, Jessen P, Zabel P, Niedermayer W. Arzneimittelschädigung der leber bei kombination von cyclosporin A und einem antikonzeptivum. *Dtsch Med Wochenschr* (1984) 109, 1989-90.
3. Ross WB, Roberts D, Griffin PJA and Salaman JR. Cyclosporin interaction with danazol and norethisterone. *Lancet* (1986) i, 330.
4. Schröder O, Schmitz N, Kayser W, Euler HH, Löffler H. Erhöhte ciclosporin-A-spiegel bei gleichzeitiger therapie mit danazol. *Dtsch Med Wochenschr* (1986) 111, 602–3.
5. Blatt J, Howrie D, Orlando S. Burckart G. Interaction between cyclosporine and danazol in a pediatric patient. *J Pediatr Hematol Oncol* (1996) 18, 95.
6. Borrás-Blasco J, Rosique-Robles JD, Peris-Marti J, Navarro-Ruiz J, Gonzalez-Delgado M, Conesa-Garcia V. Possible cyclosporin-danazol interaction in a patient with aplastic anaemia. *Am J Hematol* (1999) 62, 63–4.
7. Koneru B, Hartner C, Iwatsuki S, Starzl TE. Effect of danazol on cyclosporine pharmacokinetics. *Transplantation* (1988) 45, 1001.
8. Hayashi T, Takahashi T, Minami T, Akaike J, Kasahara K, Adachi M, Hinoda Y, Takahashi S, Hirayama T, Imai K. Fatal acute hepatic failure induced by danazol in a patient with endometriosis and aplastic anemia. *J Gastroenterol* (2001) 36, 783–6.
9. Passfall J, Keller F. Pharmacokinetics of danazol-cyclosporin interaction. *Nephrol Dial Transplant* (1994) 9, 1055.
10. Møller BB, Ekelund B. Toxicity of cyclosporine during treatment with androgens. *N Engl J Med* (1985) 313, 1416.
11. Goffin E, Pirson Y, Geubel A, van Ypersele de Strihou C. Cyclosporine-methyltestosterone interaction. *Nephron* (1991) 59, 174–5.
12. Sahnoun Z, Frikha M, Zeghal KM, Souissi T. Toxicité hépatique de la ciclosporine et interaction médicamenteuse avec les androgènes. *Sem Hop Paris* (1993) 69, 26–8.
13. Vinot O, Cochat P, Dubourg-Derain L, Bouvier R, Vial T, Philippe N. Jaundice associated with concomitant use of norethandrolone and cyclosporine. *Transplantation* (1993) 56, 470–1.
14. Castelao AM. Cyclosporine A — drug interactions. In Sunshine I (Ed.) Recent developments in therapeutic drug monitoring and clinical toxicology. 2nd Int Conf Therapeutic Drug Monitoring Toxicology, Barcelona, Spain (1992) 203–9.

Ciclosporin + Sodium clodronate

Clodronate appears not to alter serum ciclosporin levels.

Clinical evidence, mechanism, importance and management

Ten heart transplant patients treated with ciclosporin, azathioprine and diltiazem were additionally treated with 800 mg **clodronate** daily for a week. No statistically significant differences in their serum ciclosporin levels or AUCs occurred while taking the **clodronate**. Three of them were also taking simvastatin, two were taking ranitidine and one was taking propafenone, furosemide (frusemide) and cyclophosphamide. There would seem to be no reason for avoiding concurrent use, but the authors of the report suggest nevertheless that longer-term use of **clodronate** should be well monitored.[1] There seems to be no information about other **bisphosphonates**.

1. Baraldo M, Furlanut M, Puricelli C. No effect of clodronate on cyclosporin A blood levels in heart transplant patients simultaneously treated with diltiazem and azathioprine. *Ther Drug Monit* (1994) 16, 435.

Ciclosporin + St John's wort (Hypericum perforatum)

Marked falls in serum ciclosporin levels and transplant rejection can occur with few weeks of starting an extract of St John's wort.

Clinical evidence

A marked drop in ciclosporin blood levels was identified in one kidney transplant patient as being due to the addition of 300 mg **St John's wort** extract three times daily. When the **St John's wort** was stopped the ciclosporin levels climbed again. The authors of this report identified another 35 kidney and 10 liver transplant patients whose ciclosporin levels had dropped by an average of 49% (range 30 to 64%) after starting **St John's wort**. Two of them had rejection episodes.[1,2] Subtherapeutic ciclosporin levels in another 4 renal transplant patients and one liver transplant patient have been attributed to self-medication with **St John's wort**.[3-6] Graft rejection occurred in 3 cases.[3,6,7]

Two patients with heart transplants on ciclosporin developed acute transplant rejection 3 weeks after starting to take 300 mg **St John's wort** extract three times daily and it was found that their ciclosporin plasma levels had fallen well below the therapeutic range. When the **St John's wort** was stopped, the situation restabilised.[8] Three other similar cases have been reported.[9] Another heart transplant patient developed rejection within 4 weeks of starting to take **St John's wort**. Yet another patient with lung fibrosis needed an increased ciclosporin dosage when **St John's wort** was added.[10]

Mechanism

Uncertain, but it is thought that St John's wort increases the metabolism and loss of the ciclosporin from the body,[10] perhaps by affecting the microsomal cytochrome P450 complex.[2,4,8,11] It has also been suggested that an additional reason might be that St John's wort induces the intestinal P-glycoprotein drug transporter.[2,4,8,11]

Importance and management

An established and clinically important interaction. The incidence is not known but all patients on ciclosporin should avoid St John's wort because of the potentially severity of this interaction. Transplant rejection can develop within 3 to 4 weeks. It is possible to accommodate this interaction by increasing the ciclosporin dosage[10] (possibly about doubled) but this raises the costs of an already expensive drug. The advice of the CSM in the UK is that patients on ciclosporin should avoid or stop taking St John's wort. In the latter situation the serum ciclosporin levels should be well monitored and the dosage adjusted as necessary.[12]

1. Breidenbach Th, Hoffmann MW, Becker Th, Schlitt H, Klempnauer J. Drug interaction of St John's wort with ciclosporin. *Lancet* (2000) 355, 1912.
2. Breidenbach T, Kliem V, Burg M, Radermacher J, Hoffmann MW, Klempnauer J. Profound drop of cyclosporin A whole blood trough levels caused by St John's wort (Hypericum perforatum). *Transplantation* (2000) 69, 2229–30.
3. Barone GW, Gurley BJ, Ketel BL, Abul-Ezz SR. Herbal supplements: a potential for drug interactions in transplant recipients. *Transplantation* (2001) 71, 239–41.
4. Barone GW, Gurley BJ, Ketel BL, Lightfoot ML, Abul-Ezz SR. Comment: drug-herb interaction. *Ann Pharmacother* (2001) 35, 124–5.
5. Mai I, Kreuger H, Budde K, Johne A, Brockmoeller J, Neumayer H-H, Roots I. Hazardous pharmacokinetic interaction of Saint John's wort (Hypericum perforatum) with the immunosuppressant cyclosporin. *Int J Clin Pharmacol Ther* (2000) 38, 500–2.
6. Karliova M, Treichel U, Malagò M, Frilling A, Gerken G, Broelsch CE. Interaction of hypericum perforatum (St John's wort) with cyclosporin A metabolism in a patient after liver transplantation. *J Hepatol* (2000) 33, 853–5.
7. Barone GW, Gurley BJ, Ketel BL, Lightfoot ML, Abul-Ezz SR. Drug interaction between St John's wort and cyclosporine. *Ann Pharmacother* (2000) 34, 1013–16.
8. Ruschitzka F, Meier PJ, Turina M, Lüscher TF, Noll G. Acute heart transplant rejection due to Saint John's wort. *Lancet* (2000) 355, 548-9.
9. Ahmed SM, Banner NR, Dubrey SW. Low cyclosporin-A level due to Saint-John's-wort in heart-transplant patients. *J Heart Lung Transplant* (2001) 20, 795.
10. Bon S, Hartmann K, Kuhn M. Johanniskraut: ein enzyminducktor? *Schweizer Apotheker-erzeitung* (1999) 16, 535–6.
11. Cheng O. Comment: drug-herb interaction. *Ann Pharmacother* (2001) 35, 124.
12. Committee on the Safety of Medicines (UK). Message from Professor A Breckenridge (Chairman of CSM) and Fact Sheet for Health Care Professionals, 29th February 2000.

Ciclosporin + Sulfasalazine

An isolated report describes elevated ciclosporin levels in a kidney transplant patients when sulfasalazine was stopped.

Clinical evidence

A patient who had undergone a kidney transplant was treated with azathioprine, ciclosporin, prednisolone and **sulfasalazine** 1.5 g daily. After initial adjustments the dose of ciclosporin remained at 480 mg daily for 8 months. The dose of prednisone was reduced and treatment stopped at 8 months and azathioprine was stopped at 12 months without any requirement to adjust ciclosporin dosage. **Sulfasalazine** was stopped 13.5 months after transplantation and the mean ciclosporin level increased from 205 nanograms/ml to 360 nanograms/ml within 5 days and to 389 nanograms/ml after 10 days. Ciclosporin dosage was reduced over the following 2 months from 9.6 mg/kg to 5.6 mg/kg to maintain blood levels at about 200 nanograms/ml.[1]

Mechanism

Not understood. The time course of the interaction, noted after 5 days probably excludes decreased absorption. It is possible that the interaction is due to induction of cytochrome P450 enzymes.

Importance and management

Information appears to be limited to this isolated case report. However, the effect was significant and it would be prudent to monitor ciclosporin levels more closely if sulfasalazine treatment is added or discontinued.

1. Du Cheyron D, Debruyne D, Lobbedez T, Richer C, Ryckelynck J-P, Hurault de Ligny B. Effect of sulfasalazine on cyclosporin blood concentration. *Eur J Clin Pharmacol* (1999) 55, 227–8.

Ciclosporin + Sulfinpyrazone

Sulfinpyrazone can cause reduce ciclosporin serum levels. The dosage of ciclosporin may need to be increased to prevent transplant rejection.

Clinical evidence

A study in 120 heart transplant patients found that 200 mg **sulfinpyrazone** daily was effective in the treatment of hyperuricaemia. The mean uricaemia over a 4 to 8 month period fell by 22% (from 0.51 to 0.40 mmol/l) but unexpectedly the mean trough ciclosporin levels fell by 39% (from 183 to 121 micrograms/l) despite a small (7.7%) increase in the ciclosporin daily dosage. Two of the patients developed rejection: one after 4 months on **sulphinpyrazone** when the ciclosporin levels fell to 50 micrograms/l and the other after 7 months when the levels fell to 20 micrograms/l.[1] Another report describes a patient who needed unusually high doses of ciclosporin while taking **sulfinpyrazone**[2] while yet another report describes *increased* serum ciclosporin levels. In this latter case there is the possibility that it may have been an artefact due to interference with the assay method.[3]

Mechanism

Not understood.

Importance and management

Information appears to be limited to these reports but the interaction would seem to be established and clinically important. If sulfinpyrazone is added to established treatment with ciclosporin, be alert for the need to raise the ciclosporin dosage. The mean fall in trough ciclosporin levels seen in the major study cited was 39%.[1] This study does comment on how quickly this interaction develops but the two cases of transplant rejection occurred after 4 months and 7 months which implies that it can possibly be slow. Long term monitoring would therefore be a prudent precaution. The authors of this report say that sulfinpyrazone is an effective alternative to allopurinol and no additional side-effects occur including myelotoxicity when used with azathioprine.

1. Caforio ALP, Gambino A, Tona F, Feltrin G, Marchini F, Pompei E, Testolin L, Angelini A, Dalla Volta S, Casarotto D. Sulfinpyrazone reduces cyclosporine levels: a new drug interaction in heart transplant recipients. *J Heart Lung Transplant* (2000) 19, 1205–8.
2. Dossetor JB, Kovithavongs T, Salkie M, Preiksaitis J. Cyclosporine-associated lymphoproliferation, despite controlled cyclosporine blood concentrations, in a renal allograft recipient. *Proc Eur Dial Transplant Assoc Eur Renal Assoc* (1985) 21, 1021–6.
3. Cockburn I. Cyclosporin A: a clinical evaluation of drug interactions. *Transplant Proc* (1986) 18 (Suppl 5), 50–5.

Ciclosporin + Sulphonamides

Sulfadiazine given orally or sulfadimidine/trimethoprim given intravenously can cause a marked fall in serum ciclosporin levels. Sulfametoxydiazine can cause a minor fall. Although co-trimoxazole increases serum creatinine levels in kidney transplant patients on ciclosporin (normally interpreted as evidence of nephrotoxicity) it appears nevertheless normally to be safe and effective.

Clinical evidence

(a) Co-trimoxazole

A large-scale study in 132 kidney transplant patients on ciclosporin encompassing 33,876 patient-days found that **co-trimoxazole** was effective and well tolerated. Ciclosporin pharmacokinetics remained unchanged. A 15% rise in serum creatinine levels occurred which reversed when the **co-trimoxazole** was stopped. This rise was not interpreted as a sign of nephrotoxicity but appeared to be due to inhibition by the **co-trimoxazole** of the tubular excretion of creatinine.[1]

Other reports describe rises in creatinine levels (interpreted as evidence of nephrotoxicity)[2-5] interstitial nephritis,[6] granulocytopenia and thrombocytopenia[7,8] in a few patients during concurrent use of ciclosporin and **co-trimoxazole**. Apparent nephrotoxicity has also been seen with **trimethoprim**.[9]

(b) Sulfadiazine, Sulfametoxydiazine

Three heart transplant patients under treatment for toxoplasmosis showed falls in their ciclosporin levels when given **sulfadiazine** (4 to 6 g daily). Their dosage-to-level ciclosporin ratios rose by 58, 82 and 29% respectively. One out of two showed a minor fall when previously treated with **sulfametoxydiazine**.[10]

Other reports mention the use of **sulfadiazine** without commenting about any interaction.[11]

(c) Sulfadimidine/trimethoprim

A heart transplant patient on ciclosporin and prednisolone developed unmeasurably low serum ciclosporin levels 7 days after starting **sulfadimidine** (2 g four times daily intravenously) and **trimethoprim** (300 to 500 mg twice daily). Doubling the ciclosporin dosage had little effect and evidence of transplant rejection was seen. Within 10 days of starting to take the anti-infective agents orally instead of intravenously the serum ciclosporin levels climbed to approximately their former levels and the rejection problems disappeared.[12]

Another report by some of the same authors similarly describes a marked fall in serum ciclosporin levels in 5 heart transplant patients (one of them the same as the report already cited[12]) when given **sulfadimidine** and **trimethoprim** intravenously.[13]

Mechanisms

Uncertain. (a) Co-trimoxazole and trimethoprim can raise serum creatinine levels, possibly due to inhibition of creatinine secretion by the kidney tubules.[14] (b & c) The reduction in serum ciclosporin levels is not understood.

Importance and management

The documentation is only moderate but these appear to be established interactions. Be aware that intravenous sulfadimidine/trimethoprim and oral sulfadiazine can cause a marked reduction in serum ciclosporin levels with accompanying inadequate immunosuppression. The evidence suggests that oral sulfadimidine/trimethoprim, sulfametoxydiazine and co-trimoxazole do not interact adversely and are normally safe and effective, although toxicity can apparently occur in a small number of patients. Until more information is available it would be prudent to keep a close check on ciclosporin levels if any sulphonamide is given.

1. Maki DG, Fox BC, Kuntz J, Sollinger HW, Belzer FO. A prospective, randomized, double-blind study of trimethoprim-sulfamethoxazole for prophylaxis of infection in renal transplantation. Side effects of trimethoprim-sulfamethoxazole interaction with cyclosporine. *J Lab Clin Med* (1992) 119, 11–24.
2. Thompson JF, Chalmers DHK, Hunnisett AGW, Wood RFM, Morris PJ. Nephrotoxicity of trimethoprim and cotrimoxazole in renal allograft recipients treated with cyclosporine. *Transplantation* (1983) 36, 204–6.
3. Ringdén O, Myrenfors P, Klintmalm G, Tydén G, Öst L. Nephrotoxicity by co-trimoxazole and cyclosporin in transplanted patients. *Lancet* (1984) i, 1016–17.
4. Klintmalm G, Säwe J, Ringdén O, von Bahr C, Magnusson A. Cyclosporine plasma levels in renal transplant patients. Association with renal toxicity and allograft rejection. *Transplantation* (1985) 39, 132–7.
5. Klintmalm G, Ringdén O, Groth CG. Clinical and laboratory signs in nephrotoxicity and rejection in cyclosporine treated renal allograft recipients. *Transplant Proc* (1983) 15 (Suppl 1), 2815–20.
6. Smith EJ, Light JA, Filo RS, Yum MN. Interstitial nephritis caused by trimethoprim-sulfamethoxazole in renal transplant patients. *JAMA* (1980) 244, 360–1.
7. Bradley PP, Warden GD, Maxwell JG, Rothstein G. Neutropenia and thrombocytopenia in renal allograft recipients treated with trimethoprim-sulfamethoxazole. *Ann Intern Med* (1980) 93, 560–2.
8. Hulme B, Reeves DS. Leucopenia associated with trimethoprim-sulfamethoxazole after renal transplantation. *BMJ* (1971) 3, 610–2.
9. Nyberg G, Gäbel H, Althoff P, Björk S, Herlitz H, Brynger H. Adverse effect of trimethoprim on kidney function in renal transplant patients. *Lancet* (1984) i, 394–5.
10. Spes CH, Angermann CE, Stempfle HU, Wenke K, Theisen K. Sulfadiazine therapy for toxoplasmosis in heart transplant recipients decreases cyclosporine concentration. *Clin Invest* (1992) 70, 752–4.
11. Hakim M, Esmore D, Wallwork J, English TAH, Wreghitt T. Toxoplasmosis in cardiac transplantation. *BMJ* (1986) 292, 1108.
12. Wallwork J, McGregor CGA, Wells FC, Cory-Pearce R, English TAH. Cyclosporin and intravenous sulphadimidine and trimethoprim therapy. *Lancet* (1983) i, 336–7.
13. Jones DK, Hakim M, Wallwork J, Higenbottam TW, White DJG. Serious interaction between cyclosporin A and sulphadimidine. *BMJ* (1986) 292, 728–9.
14. Berg KJ, Gjellestad A, Norby G, Rootwelt K, Djøseland O, Fauchald P, Mehl A, Narverud J, Talseth T. Renal effects of trimethoprim in cyclosporin- and azathioprine-treated kidney-allografted patients. *Nephron* (1989) 53, 218–22.

Ciclosporin + Ticlopidine

No adverse interaction normally occurs between ciclosporin and ticlopidine, but two isolated case reports describe marked falls in serum ciclosporin levels.

Clinical evidence

(a) Evidence of an adverse interaction

The serum ciclosporin levels of a patient with nephrotic syndrome were roughly halved on two occasions when given 500 mg **ticlopidine** daily.[1] Another patient with a kidney transplant showed a similar fall on two occasions when given **ticlopidine** 250 mg daily.[2]

(b) Evidence of no adverse interaction

Twelve heart transplant patients were given 250 mg **ticlopidine** twice daily. The mean whole blood trough ciclosporin levels were noted to be halved but the mean ciclosporin dosage was not altered over a 3-month period. The neutrophil, platelet and whole blood leucocyte counts and haemoglobin levels were not significantly altered, but side-effects included one epistaxis, one haematuria (both necessitating half-dosage) and one neutropenia which resolved when the **ticlopidine** was withdrawn.[3]

A later study by the same group in 20 heart transplant patients given ticlopidine 250 mg daily found that the bioavailability of the ciclosporin was not clearly altered by **ticlopidine**, although one patient was withdrawn from the study after 3 days because of a 60% fall in ciclosporin levels, attributed to poor compliance rather than an interaction. No clinically significant adverse haematological, biochemical or ECG or echocardiography changes occurred.[4]

Mechanism

Not understood.

Importance and management

Information appears to be limited to the reports cited, but the broad picture is that the concurrent use of ciclosporin and ticlopidine is normally safe and effective, but the occasional patient may unpredictably show marked falls in serum ciclosporin levels. For this reason good monitoring is needed, particularly when ticlopidine is first added, so that any problems can be quickly identified.

1. Birmelé B, Lebranchu Y, Bagros Ph, Nivet H, Furet Y, Pengloan J. Interaction of cyclosporin and ticlopidine. *Nephrol Dial Transplant* (1991) 6, 150–1.
2. Verdejo A, de Cos MA, Zubimendi JA. Probable interaction between cyclosporin A and low dose ticlopidine. *BMJ* (2000) 320, 1037.

3. de Lorgeril M, Boissonnat P, Dureau G, Guidollet J, Renaud S. Evaluation of ticlopidine, a novel inhibitor of platelet aggregation, in heart transplant recipients. *Transplantation* (1993) 55, 1195–6.
4. Boissonnat P, de Lorgeril M, Perroux V, Salen P, Batt AM, Barthelemy JC, Brouard R, Serres E, Delaye J. A drug interaction study between ticlopidine and cyclosporin in heart transplant recipients. *Eur J Clin Pharmacol* (1997) 53, 39–45.

Ciclosporin + Topical NSAIDs

Adverse skin reactions have been seen in patients using ciclosporin for the treatment of psoriasis when they have used topical preparations containing flufenamic acid, nicotinate, salicylate; and indometacin.

Clinical evidence, mechanism, importance and management

A man whose psoriasis was well controlled with ciclosporin developed a localised Köbner reaction when he used a hyperaemic ointment containing **flufenamic acid, nicotinate** and **salicylate** on his chest following accidental contusion.[1] **Topical indometacin** caused exacerbation in 70% of patients using ciclosporin to treat psoriasis in another study, and improved 25%.[2] The reasons are not understood. Concurrent use, if thought appropriate, should be well monitored.

1. Mrowietz U. Köbner phenomenon in a psoriatic patient under cyclosporin therapy after contusion trauma and local application of hyperaemic ointment. *Dermatology* (1993) 187, 215–6.
2. Ellis CN, Fallon JD, Heezen JL, Voorheen JJ. Topical indomethacin exacerbates lesion of psoriasis. *J Invest Dermatol* (1983) 80, 362.

Ciclosporin + Trimetazidine

Trimetazidine appears not to alter the pharmacokinetics of ciclosporin nor its immunosuppressive effects.

Clinical evidence, mechanism, importance and management

To find out if the concurrent use of **trimetazidine** and ciclosporin was associated with any adverse effects, 12 kidney transplant patients on ciclosporin were additionally given 40 mg **trimetazidine** twice daily for 5 days. No changes in the pharmacokinetics of the ciclosporin were seen, and there were no alterations in interleukin-2 concentrations or soluble interleukin-2 receptors.[1] An associated study by the same group of workers using two models (the lymphoproliferative response of normal human lymphocytes to phytohaemagglutinin and a delayed *mouse* hypersensitivity model) similarly found that **trimetazidine** did not interfere with the ciclosporin's effects.[2] It was concluded on the basis of these two studies that the concurrent use of ciclosporin and **trimetazidine** need not be avoided.

1. Simon N, Brunet P, Roumenov D, Dussol B, Barre J, Duche JC, Albengres E, D'Athis Ph, Crevat A, Berland Y, Tillement JP. The effects of trimetazidine-cyclosporin A coadministration on interleukin 2 and cyclosporin A blood levels in renal transplant patients. *Therapie* (1995) 50 (Suppl), 498.
2. Albengres E, Tillement JP, d'Athis P, Salducci D, Chauvet-Monges AM, Crevat A. Lack of pharmacodynamic interaction between trimetazidine and cyclosporin A in human lymphoproliferative and mouse delayed hypersensitivity response models. *Fundam Clin Pharmacol* (1996) 10, 264–8.

Ciclosporin + Vitamin E (Tocopherol)

Ciclosporin absorption is increased by vitamin E.

Clinical evidence, mechanism, importance and management

Ten healthy subjects were given single 10 mg/kg oral doses of ciclosporin with and without 0.1 ml/kg oral **vitamin E** (d-alpha tocopheryl polyethylene glucose 1000 succinate). The AUC of the ciclosporin increased by 60%, the suggested reason being that ab-

sorption was increased due to improved solubilisation and micelle formation within the gut, or that decreased intestinal metabolism occurred.[1] The clinical importance of this interaction awaits assessment.

1. Chang T, Benet LZ, Hebert MF. The effect of water-soluble vitamin E (TPGS) on oral cyclosporine pharmacokinetics in healthy volunteers. *Clin Pharmacol Ther* (1995) 57, 163.

Corticosteroids + Aminoglutethimide

The effects of dexamethasone but not hydrocortisone can be reduced or abolished by the concurrent use of aminoglutethimide.

Clinical evidence

When given 500 to 750 mg **aminoglutethimide** daily the half-life of **dexamethasone** (1 mg daily) in 6 patients was reduced from 264 to 120 min. In another 22 patients it was found that increasing the **dexamethasone** dosage to 1.5 to 3 mg daily compensated for the increased **dexamethasone** metabolism and complete adrenal suppression was achieved over a prolonged period.[1]

A patient, dependent on **dexamethasone** due to brain oedema caused by a tumour, deteriorated rapidly with headache and lethargy when additionally treated with **aminoglutethimide**. The problem was solved by withdrawing the **aminoglutethimide** and temporarily increasing the **dexamethasone dosage**.[2]

Mechanism

Aminoglutethimide is an enzyme inducing agent and it seems probable that it interacts by increasing the metabolism and clearance of the steroids by the liver, thereby reducing their effects.[3]

Importance and management

Information is limited but the interaction appears to be established. The reduction in the serum corticosteroid levels can be enough to reduce or even abolish intended adrenal suppression[1] or to cause loss of control of a disease condition.[2] The former situation has been successfully accommodated by increasing the dosage of the corticosteroid or by increasing the dosage of both.[1] An alternative is to use **hydrocortisone**, which appears not to be affected by aminoglutethimide.[4] A standard fixed dose regimen of 1 g aminoglutethimide and 40 mg **hydrocortisone** daily has been shown to block adrenal steroid synthesis effectively.[4]

1. Santen RJ, Lipton A, Kendall J. Successful medical adrenalectomy with amino-glutethimide. Role of altered drug metabolism. *JAMA* (1974) 230, 1661–5.
2. Halpern J, Catane R, Baerwald H. A call for caution in the use of aminoglutethimide: negative interactions with dexamethasone and beta blocker treatment. *J Med* (1984) 15, 59–63.
3. Santen RJ, Brodie AMH. Suppression of oestrogen production as treatment of breast carcinoma: pharmacological and clinical studies with aromatase inhibitors. *Clin Oncol* (1982) 1, 77–130.
4. Santen RJ, Wells SA, Runić S, Gupta C, Kendall J, Rudy EB, Samojlik E. Adrenal suppression with aminoglutethimide. I. Differential effects of aminoglutethimide on glucocorticoid metabolism as a rationale for the use of hydrocortisone. *J Clin Endocrinol Metab* (1977) 45, 469–79.

Corticosteroids + Antacids

The absorption of prednisone can be reduced by large but not small doses of aluminium and magnesium hydroxide antacids. Prednisolone probably behaves similarly. Dexamethasone absorption is reduced by magnesium trisilicate. Phosphate-depletion caused by antacids can confuse the diagnostic picture.

Clinical evidence

(a) Prednisone or prednisolone

Gastrogel (**aluminium hydroxide**, **magnesium hydroxide** and **trisilicate**) 20 ml had no significant effect on serum levels, half-life or AUC of **prednisone** in 10 or 20-mg doses in 5 patients and 2 healthy subjects.[1]

Another study in 8 healthy subjects given 20-mg doses of **prednisolone** found that 30 ml **Magnesium Trisilicate Mixture BP** or *Aludrox* (**aluminium hydroxide gel**) caused small but not statistically significant changes in peak **prednisolone** levels and absorption, however one subject given **magnesium trisilicate** had considerably reduced levels.[2] **Aluminium phosphate** has also been found not to affect **prednisolone** absorption.[3,4] In contrast, another study in healthy subjects and patients given 60 ml of *Aldrox* or *Melox* (both containing **aluminium hydroxide** and **magnesium hydroxide**) found that the bioavailability of 10 mg **prednisone** was reduced on average by 30%, and even 40% in some individuals.[5]

(b) Dexamethasone

Magnesium trisilicate 5 g in 100 ml of water considerably reduced the bioavailability of single 1 mg oral doses of **dexamethasone** given to 6 healthy subjects. Using the urinary excretion of 11-hydroxycorticosteroids as a measure, the reduction was about 75%.[6]

Mechanism

The reduction in dexamethasone absorption is attributed to adsorption onto the surface of the magnesium trisilicate.[6,7]

Importance and management

Information seems to be limited to these studies. The indication is that large doses of some antacids can reduce bioavailability, but small doses do not. More study is needed to confirm this. Concurrent use should be monitored to confirm that the therapeutic response is adequate. Also be alert for evidence of a phosphate-depletion syndrome which can mimic steroid-induced side-effects and confuse the diagnostic picture.[8] This has been reported in a prednisolone-dependent asthmatic man given *Maalox* and *Mylanta*, both of which are phosphate-binding antacids.[8]

1. Tanner AR, Caffin JA, Halliday JW, Powell LW. Concurrent administration of antacids and prednisone: effect on serum levels of prednisolone. *Br J Clin Pharmacol* (1979) 7, 397–400.
2. Lee DAH, Taylor GM, Walker JG, James VHT. The effect of concurrent administration of antacids on prednisolone absorption. *Br J Clin Pharmacol* (1979) 8, 92–4.
3. Albin H, Vinçon G, Demotes-Mainard F, Begaud B, Bedjaoui A. Effects of aluminium phosphate on bioavailability of cimetidine and prednisolone. *Eur J Clin Pharmacol* (1984) 26, 271–3.
4. Albin H, Vinçon G, Pehourcq F, Lecorre C, Fleury B, Conri C. Influence d'un anti-acide sur la biodisponibilité de la prednisolone. *Therapie* (1983) 38, 61–5.
5. Uribe M, Casian C, Rojas S, Sierra JG, Go VLW, Muñoz RM, Gil S. Decreased bioavailability of prednisone due to antacids in patients with chronic active liver disease and in healthy volunteers. *Gastroenterology* (1981) 80, 661–5.
6. Naggar VF, Khalil SA, Gouda MW. Effect of concomitant administration of magnesium trisilicate on GI absorption of dexamethasone in humans. *J Pharm Sci* (1978) 67, 1029–30.
7. Prakash A, Verma RK. *In vitro* adsorption of dexamethasone and betamethasone on antacids. *Indian J Pharm Sci* (1984) Jan-Feb, 55–6.
8. Goodman M, Solomons CC, Miller PD. Distinction between the common symptoms of the phosphate-depletion syndrome and glucocorticoid-induced disease. *Am J Med* (1978) 65, 868–72.

Corticosteroids + Anti-infective agents

Because the corticosteroids can suppress the normal responses of the body to attack by micro-organisms, it is important to ensure that any anti-infective 'cover' is sufficient to prevent local or even generalised and potentially life-threatening infections.

Clinical evidence

A patient with severe cystic acne vulgaris given low dose oral **tetracycline**, 500 mg daily, and **betamethasone**, 2 mg daily, for 7 months became toxaemic and pyrexic with severe acne and cellulitis of the face due to the emergence of a Gram-negative organism not susceptible to the antibacterial.[1] A child with tinea corporis developed a permanently scarred knee when treated with a cream containing 1% **clotrimazole** and 0.05% **betamethasone dipropionate**.[2]

Mechanism

The corticosteroids reduce inflammation, impair antibody formation and, if given systemically, cause adrenal suppression. This increases the susceptibility of the body to infection. In both of the cases cited the infections were insufficiently controlled by the anti-infective agents during this immunosuppression.

Importance and management

Not, strictly speaking, drug-drug interactions, but the cases cited amply illustrate the importance of monitoring concurrent use. The author of one of the reports[1] points out that ". . . it appears that if oral corticoids or combined therapy are ever warranted, they should be very carefully policed because of the risk of turning a benign disease into one that is potentially fatal."

1. Paver K. Complications from combined oral tetracycline and oral corticoid therapy on acne vulgaris. *Med J Aust* (1970) 1, 509.
2. Reynolds RD, Boiko S, Lucky AW. Exacerbation of tinea corporis during treatment with 1% clotrimazole/0.05% betamethasone dipropionate (Lotrisone). *Am J Dis Child* (1991) 145, 1224–5.

Corticosteroids + Barbiturates

The therapeutic effects of systemically administered corticosteroids (dexamethasone, hydrocortisone, methylprednisolone, prednisone and prednisolone) are decreased by the concurrent use of phenobarbital (phenobarbitone) because their loss from the body is increased. An increase in the corticosteroid dosage may be needed. Other barbiturates probably interact similarly. Primidone interacts like the barbiturates.

Clinical evidence

(a) Asthmatic patients on prednisone, prednisolone, methylprednisolone

Three prednisone-dependent patients with bronchial asthma taking 10 to 40 mg **prednisone** daily showed a marked worsening of their symptoms within a few days of starting to take 120 mg **phenobarbital** daily. There was a deterioration in their pulmonary function tests (FEV1, degree of bronchospasm) and a rise in eosinophil counts, all of which improved when the **phenobarbital** was stopped. The **prednisone** clearance increased while taking the **phenobarbital**.[1]

Phenobarbital increased the clearance of **prednisolone** in asthmatic children by 41% and of **methylprednisolone** by 209%.[2] In contrast, the **prednisone** requirements of other children on **prednisone** were unaltered while taking a compound preparation containing 24 mg **phenobarbital** daily.[3]

(b) Kidney transplant patients on prednisone

The survival of kidney transplants in a group of 75 children being given **azathioprine** and **prednisone** as immunosuppressants was reduced in those given anticonvulsant treatment with 60 to 120 mg **phenobarbital** (**phenobarbitone**) daily. Two of the 11 epileptic children were also taking 100 mg **phenytoin** daily.[4] Another study found that **prednisolone** elimination is increased in renal transplant patients by concomitant **phenobarbital**.[5]

(c) Patients with rheumatoid arthritis on prednisolone

Nine patients with rheumatoid arthritis on 8 to 15 mg **prednisolone** daily showed strong evidence of clinical deterioration (worsening joint tenderness, pain, morning stiffness, fall in grip strength) when treated with **phenobarbital** for 2 weeks (plasma concentrations 0 to 2 mg% (0 to 86.2 micromol/l)). The **prednisolone** half-life fell by 25%.[6]

(d) Patients with congenital adrenal hyperplasia on dexamethasone

A 14-year-old girl with congenital adrenal hyperplasia on **dexamethasone** rapidly became over-treated (weight gain, signs of hypercortisolism) when the **primidone** (250 mg twice daily) she was taking was withdrawn over a month. Adequate control was only achieved when the **dexamethasone** dosage was reduced threefold.[7] A reduction in the effects of **dexamethasone** has also been described in another patient with congenital adrenal hyperplasia when treated with **primidone** for petit mal.[8]

Mechanism

Phenobarbital is a recognised potent liver enzyme inducing agent which increases the metabolism and loss from the body of administered corticosteroids, thereby reducing their effects. Pharmacokinetic studies in man have shown that phenobarbital reduces the half-lives of these corticosteroids and increases their clearances by 40 to 209%.[1,2,9] Primidone interacts in a similar way because it is metabolised in the body to phenobarbital.[7]

Importance and management

The corticosteroid/phenobarbital interaction is well documented, well established and of clinical importance. Concurrent use need not be avoided but the outcome should be monitored. Increase the corticosteroid dosage as necessary. The extent of the increase is variable. Dexamethasone,[1] hydrocortisone,[10] methylprednisolone,[2,9] prednisone[1,4] and prednisolone[2,6] are all known to be affected. Prednisone and prednisolone appear to be less affected than methylprednisolone and may be preferred.[2] Be alert for the same interaction with other corticosteroids and other barbiturates (which also are enzyme-inducing agents) although direct evidence seems to be lacking. The dexamethasone adrenal suppression test may be expected to be unreliable in those taking phenobarbital, however 50 mg hydrocortisone instead of dexamethasone can give reliable results in the presence of phenytoin[11] (another potent enzyme inducer) and might also be considered for those on barbiturates (see 'Corticosteroids + Phenytoin', p.638).

1. Brooks SM, Werk EE, Ackerman SJ, Sullivan I, Thrasher K. Adverse effects of phenobarbital on corticosteroid metabolism in patients with bronchial asthma. *N Engl J Med* (1972) 286, 1125-8.
2. Bartoszek M, Brenner AM, Szefler SJ. Prednisolone and methylprednisolone kinetics in children receiving anticonvulsant therapy. *Clin Pharmacol Ther* (1987) 42, 424-32.
3. Falliers CJ. Corticosteroids and phenobarbital in asthma. *N Engl J Med* (1972) 287, 201.
4. Wassner SJ, Pennisi AJ, Malekzadeh MH, Fine RN. The adverse effect of anticonvulsant therapy on renal allograft survival. *J Pediatr* (1976) 88, 134-7.
5. Gambertoglio J, Kapusnik J, Holford N, Nishikawa R, Hau T, Birnbaum J, Amend W. Enhancement of prednisolone elimination by anticonvulsants in renal transplant recipients. *Clin Pharmacol Ther* (1982) 31, 228.
6. Brooks PM, Buchanan WW, Grove M, Downie WW. Effects of enzyme induction on metabolism of prednisolone. Clinical and laboratory study. *Ann Rheum Dis* (1976) 35, 339-43.
7. Young MC, Hughes IA. Loss of therapeutic control in congenital adrenal hyperplasia due to interaction between dexamethasone and primidone. *Acta Paediatr Scand* (1991) 80, 120-4.
8. Hancock KW, Levell A. Primidone/dexamethasone interaction. *Lancet* (1978) ii, 97-8.
9. Stjernholm MR, Katz FH. Effects of diphenylhydantoin, phenobarbital, and diazepam on the metabolism of methylprednisolone and its sodium succinate. *J Clin Endocrinol Metab* (1975) 41, 887-9.
10. Burstein S, Klaiber EL. Phenobarbital-induced increase in 6-β-hydroxycortisol excretion: clue to its significance in human urine. *J Clin Endocrinol Metab* (1965) 25, 293-6.
11. Meikle AW, Stanchfield JB, West CD, Tyler FH. Hydrocortisone suppression test for Cushings syndrome: therapy with anticonvulsants. *Arch Intern Med* (1974) 134, 1068-71.

Corticosteroids + Beta-blockers

An isolated report describes hyperkalaemia in a man attributed to the concurrent use of timolol eye drops and prednisone.

Clinical evidence, mechanism, importance and management

A patient with radiation pneumonitis and glaucoma treated with **timolol eye drops** (one drop in the left eye 0.5% twice daily) developed severe hyperkalaemia shortly after starting 60 mg **prednisone** daily. His serum potassium levels fell when the **timolol** was stopped, and rose when it was restarted. Other possible contributory factors included a history of obstructive liver disease and the use of heparin.[1] This appears to be a rare and unusual case.

1. Swenson ER. Severe hyperkalaemia as a complication of timolol, a topically applied beta-adrenergic antagonist. *Arch Intern Med* (1986) 146, 1220-1.

Corticosteroids + Caffeine

The results of the dexamethasone suppression test can be falsified by the ingestion of caffeine.

Clinical evidence, mechanism, importance and management

A study in 22 healthy subjects and 6 depressed patients showed that when they were given a single 480-mg dose of **caffeine** at 2 pm following a single 1-mg dose of **dexamethasone** at 11 pm. Cortisol levels taken at 4 pm were 5.3 micrograms/dl, compared with only 2.3 micrograms/dl with placebo.[1] Thus the equivalent of about 4 to 5 cups of **coffee** might effectively falsify the results of the **dexamethasone** suppression test.

1. Uhde TW, Bierer LM, Post RM. Caffeine-induced escape from dexamethasone suppression. *Arch Gen Psychiatry* (1985) 42, 737-8.

Corticosteroids + Carbamazepine

The loss of dexamethasone, methylprednisolone and prednisolone from the body is increased in patients taking carbamazepine and a dosage increase will be needed. The results of the dexamethasone suppression test may be invalid.

Clinical evidence

A study in 8 patients on long-term treatment with **carbamazepine** showed that the elimination half-life of **prednisolone** was 27% shorter (1.98 compared with 2.73 h) and the clearance was 42% higher (4.2 versus 2.96 ml/min/kg) than in 9 healthy subjects.[1]

A study in asthmatic children found that **carbamazepine** increased the clearance of **prednisone** by 79% and of **methylprednisolone** by 342%.[2] A study in 8 healthy subjects found that while taking 800 mg **carbamazepine** daily the dosage of **dexamethasone** needed to suppress cortisol secretion (as part of the **dexamethasone** adrenal suppression test) was increased two to fourfold.[3] A further study found that it took 2 to 13 days for false-positive results to occur after **carbamazepine** was started, and 3 to 12 days to recover when the **carbamazepine** was stopped.[4]

Mechanism

The almost certain reason is that the carbamazepine stimulates the liver enzymes to metabolise the corticosteroids much faster.

Importance and management

Information is limited but the interaction appears to be established. Patients taking carbamazepine will need increased doses of dexamethasone, methylprednisolone or prednisolone. Prednisolone is less affected than methylprednisolone and is probably preferred. The same interaction seems likely with other corticosteroids but more study is needed to confirm this. Remember that corticosteroids should only be given to epileptics with care and good monitoring because of the risk that they will exacerbate the disease condition.

1. Olivesi A. Modified elimination of prednisolone in epileptic patients on carbamazepine monotherapy, and in women using low-dose oral contraceptives. *Biomed Pharmacother* (1986) 40, 301-8.

2. Bartoszek M, Brenner AM, Szefler SJ. Prednisolone and methylprednisolone kinetics in children receiving anticonvulsant therapy. *Clin Pharmacol Ther* (1987) 42, 424–32.
3. Köbberling J, v zur Mühlen A. The influence of diphenylhydantoin and carbamazepine on the circadian rhythm of free urinary corticoids and on the suppressibility of the basal and the 'impulsive' activity by dexamethasone. *Acta Endocrinol (Copenh)* (1973) 72, 303–18.
4. Privitera MR, Greden JF, Gardner RW, Ritchie JC, Carroll BJ. Interference by carbamazepine with the dexamethasone suppression test. *Biol Psychiatry* (1982) 17, 611–20.

Corticosteroids + Carbimazole or Thiamazole (Methimazole)

The loss of prednisolone from the body is increased by the use of carbimazole or thiamazole (methimazole). Its dosage may therefore need to be increased.

Clinical evidence

A comparative study was made of (a) 8 women taking **levothyroxine** and under treatment with 2.5 mg **thiamazole (methimazole)** or 5 mg **carbimazole** daily for Graves' ophthalmology, (b) 6 women on **levothyroxine** who had undergone subtotal thyroidectomy, and (c) 6 other healthy women. All were euthyroid. It was found that the clearance of 0.54 mg/kg intravenous **prednisolone** in those taking the **thiamazole** or **carbimazole** was much greater than in the other two groups (0.37, 0.24 and 0.20 l/h.kg respectively). After 6 h the plasma **prednisolone** levels in **thiamazole/carbimazole** groups were only about 10% of those in the normal women and none was detectable after 8 h, whereas total and unbound **prednisolone** levels were much higher and measurable over the 10 hour study period in the two control groups. In another group of previously hyperthyroidic patients, now euthyroid because of **carbimazole** treatment, the total **prednisolone** clearance was 0.40 l/h.[1]

Mechanism

Not established. It seems possible that the thiamazole and carbimazole increase the metabolism of the prednisolone by the liver microsomal enzymes, thereby increasing its loss from the body.

Importance and management

Direct information seems to be limited to this study although the authors point out that there is a clinical impression that higher doses of prednisolone are needed in patients with Graves' disease. Be alert for the need to use higher doses of prednisolone in patients taking either thiamazole (methimazole) or carbimazole.

1. Legler UF. Impairment of prednisolone disposition in patients with Graves' disease taking methimazole. *J Clin Endocrinol Metab* (1988) 66, 221–3.

Corticosteroids + Cimetidine or Ranitidine

Cimetidine does not interact with prednisolone, prednisone or dexamethasone, nor ranitidine with prednisone.

Clinical evidence, mechanism, importance and management

Prednisone is a pro-drug which must be converted to **prednisolone** within the body to become active. A double-blind crossover study in 9 healthy subjects showed that after taking either **cimetidine** 300 mg six-hourly or **ranitidine** 150 mg twice daily for 4 days the pharmacokinetics of the **prednisolone** after a single 40 mg oral dose of **prednisone** were little changed.[1] Another double-blind crossover study also showed that 1 g **cimetidine** daily only caused minor changes in plasma **prednisolone** levels following the administration of 10 mg of enteric-coated **prednisolone**.[2] Yet another study found that 7 days treatment with 600 mg **cimetidine** twice daily had no effect on the

pharmacokinetics of a single 8 mg intravenous dose of **dexamethasone sodium phosphate**.[3] Information about other corticosteroids appears to be lacking. There would therefore seem to be no reason, from the point of view of adverse interactions, for avoiding concurrent use, however corticosteroids are cautioned in patients with peptic ulceration.

1. Sirgo MA, Rocci ML, Ferguson RK, Eshelman FN Vlasses PH. Effects of cimetidine and ranitidine on the conversion of prednisone to prednisolone. *Clin Pharmacol Ther* (1985) 37, 534–8.
2. Morrison PJ, Rogers HJ, Bradbrook ID, Parsons C. Concurrent administration of cimetidine and enteric-coated prednisolone: effect on plasma levels of prednisolone. *Br J Clin Pharmacol* (1980) 10, 87–9.
3. Peden NR, Rewhorn I, Champion MC, Mussani R, Ooi TC. Cortisol and dexamethasone elimination during treatment with cimetidine. *Br J Clin Pharmacol* (1984) 18, 101–3.

Corticosteroids + Colestyramine or Colestipol

Colestyramine reduces the absorption of hydrocortisone, but not prednisolone, from the gut. An isolated report describes the same interaction with colestipol.

Clinical evidence

(a) Colestyramine

Colestyramine 4 g reduced the AUC of 50 mg oral **hydrocortisone** (cortisol) in 10 healthy subjects from 103.5 to 58.9 micromol/min/l. Peak levels were lower and were reached about 50 min later.[1] Two of the subjects were given both 4 g and 8 g **colestyramine**. Their AUCs were reduced by 47 and 97%, and by 59 and 86% respectively.[1]

In contrast, two patients on chronic **prednisolone** showed no changes in the bioavailability of an oral dose of **prednisolone** when given an 8 g dose of **colestyramine**.[2]

(b) Colestipol

A man with hypopituitarism taking 20 mg **hydrocortisone** each morning and 10 mg each evening became lethargic, ataxic, and with headaches (all signs of **hydrocortisone** insufficiency) within four days of starting to take 15 g **colestipol** three times daily for hypercholesterolaemia. He responded rapidly when given 100 mg intravenous **hydrocortisone**, and was discharged with the **colestipol** replaced by an **HMG Co-A reductase inhibitor**.[3]

Mechanism

It seems that hydrocortisone can become bound to colestyramine or colestipol in the gut, thereby reducing its absorption.[1,4]

Importance and management

Information is limited, but these interactions with hydrocortisone appear to be established (they are consistent with the interactions of both of these bile-acid resins with other drugs). Separate the administration of the drugs as much as possible to minimise admixture in the gut, although the authors of one report warn that this may not necessarily avoid this interaction because their data show that the colestyramine may remain in the gut for a considerable time.[1] Monitor the effects and increase the hydrocortisone dosage if necessary. Prednisolone appears to be a non-interacting alternative.

1. Johansson C, Adamsson U, Stierner U, Lindsten T. Interaction of cholestyramine on the uptake of hydrocortisone in the gastrointestinal tract. *Acta Med Scand* (1978) 204, 509–12.
2. Audétat V, Paumgartner G, Bircher J. Beeinträchtigt Cholestyramin die biologische Verfügbarkeit von Prednisolon? *Schweiz Med Wochenschr* (1977) 107, 527–8.
3. Nekl KE, Aron DC. Hydrocortisone-colestipol interaction. *Ann Pharmacother* (1993) 27, 980–1.
4. Ware AJ, Combes B. Influence of sodium taurocholate, cholestyramine and Mylanta on the intestinal absorption of glucocorticoids in the rat. *Gastroenterology* (1973) 64, 1150–5.

Corticosteroids + Contraceptives (oral) or Progesterone

The serum levels of prednisone, prednisolone, cloprednol, hydrocortisone, methylprednisolone and possibly other corticosteroids are increased by oral contraceptives. In theory both the therapeutic and toxic effects would be expected to be increased, but in practice it is uncertain whether these changes are important. Fluocortolone is not affected. Progesterone appears not to affect the metabolism of prednisolone.

Clinical evidence

(a) Contraceptives, oral

A comparative pharmacokinetic study in 6 women showed that while taking an **oral contraceptive**, the plasma clearance of a single dose of **prednisolone** was decreased by a factor of 6, the AUC was increased by a factor of 6, and the half-life increased 2.5-fold.[1] This is in broad agreement with the results of other studies,[2-9] in one of which[2] the plasma clearance of **prednisolone** was roughly halved and the AUC approximately doubled in 8 women taking an **oral contraceptive**.

A study in 6 women using **oral contraceptives** and 6 others who were not, found that the clearance of **methylprednisolone** was decreased to about half in the **oral contraceptive** users. The **oral contraceptive** users showed less sensitivity to the suppressive effects of **methylprednisolone** on the secretion of cortisol, more suppression of basophils, but no changes in the T-helper cell response patterns.[10,11]

A marked increase in plasma **cloprednol** levels has also been seen in women on oral contraceptives.[12] In another study in women with skin diseases, the use of oestrogens (**chlorotrianisene** or **hexestrol**) markedly increased the anti-inflammatory effects of **prednisone** or **hydrocortisone** given by mouth[13] and increased the concentration of serum corticosteroids threefold.

In contrast, a study in 7 women showed that the pharmacokinetics of **fluocortolone** were unaffected by the concurrent use of **oral contraceptives**.[14]

No difference was found in the plasma levels of **budesonide** (as an oral dose of 4.5 mg daily for 7 days) or in cortisol suppression in women taking **oral contraceptives** and those who were not.[9]

(b) Progesterone

Intravenous and oral **prednisolone** was given to 6 post-menopausal women before and after 2 months treatment with **progesterone** 5 mg. The pharmacokinetics of the **prednisolone** were not significantly changed.[15]

Mechanism

Not understood. The possibilities include a change in the metabolism of the corticosteroids, or in their binding to serum proteins.[5] The absence of an interaction with progesterone suggests that the oestrogenic component of the oral contraceptives is possibly responsible for any interaction.[15]

Importance and management

It is established that the pharmacokinetics of some corticosteroids are affected by oral contraceptives, but the clinical importance of any such changes is not known. The therapeutic and toxic effects would be expected to be increased but there appear to be no clinical reports of adverse reactions arising from concurrent use. In fact the authors of one study[10] concluded that ". . . women can . . . be dosed similarly with methylprednisolone irrespective of oral contraceptive use."

However until more is known it would be prudent to monitor the effects of using any corticosteroid and oral contraceptive together. Only prednisone, prednisolone, cloprednol, hydrocortisone and methylprednisolone have been reported to interact but other corticosteroids possibly behave similarly, the exception apparently being fluocortolone. Progesterone alone appears not to interact with prednisolone.

1. Legler UF, Benet LZ. Marked alterations in prednisolone elimination for women taking oral contraceptives. *Clin Pharmacol Ther* (1982) 31, 243.
2. Boekenoogen SJ, Szefler SJ, Jusko WJ. Prednisolone disposition and protein binding in oral contraceptive users. *J Clin Endocrinol Metab* (1983) 56, 702–9.
3. Kozower M, Veatch L, Kaplan MM. Decreased clearance of prednisolone, a factor in the development of corticosteroid side effects. *J Clin Endocrinol Metab* (1974) 38, 407–12.
4. Legler UF, Benet LZ. Marked alterations in dose-dependent prednisolone kinetics in women taking oral contraceptives. *Clin Pharmacol Ther* (1986) 39, 425–9.
5. Frey BM, Schaad HJ, Frey FJ. Pharmacokinetic interaction of contraceptive steroids with prednisone and prednisolone. *Eur J Clin Pharmacol* (1984) 26, 505–11.
6. Meffin PJ, Wing LMH, Sallustio BC, Brooks PM. Alterations in prednisolone disposition as a result of oral contraceptive use and dose. *Br J Clin Pharmacol* (1984) 17, 655–64.
7. Olivesi A. Modified elimination of prednisolone in epileptic patients on carbamazepine monotherapy, and in women using low-dose oral contraceptives. *Biomed Pharmacother* (1986) 40, 301–8.
8. Legler UF, Benet LZ. Veränderungen der Prednisolonkinetik in Frauen, die orale Kontrazeptiva einnehmen. *Hoppe Seylers Z Physiol Chem* (1983) 364, 348.
9. Seidegard J, Simonsson M, Edsbacker S. Effect of an oral contraceptive on the plasma levels of budesonide and prednisolone and the influence on plasma cortisol. *Clin Pharmacol Ther* (2000) 67, 373-81.
10. Slayter KL, Ludwig EA, Lew KH, Middleton E, Ferry JJ, Jusko WJ. Oral contraceptive effects on methylprednisolone pharmacokinetics and pharmacodynamics. *Clin Pharmacol Ther* (1995) 57, 182.
11. Slayter KL, Ludwig EA, Lew KH, Middleton E, Ferry JJ, Jusko WJ. Oral contraceptive effects on methylprednisolone pharmacokinetics and pharmacodynamics. *Clin Pharmacol Ther* (1996) 59, 312–21.
12. Legler UF. Altered cloprednol disposition in oral contraceptive users. *Clin Pharmacol Ther* (1987) 41, 237.
13. Spangler AS, Antoniades HN, Sotman SL, Inderbitizin TM. Enhancement of the anti-inflammatory action of hydrocortisone by estrogen. *J Clin Endocrinol Metab* (1969) 29, 650–5.
14. Legler UF. Lack of impairment of fluocortolone disposition in oral contraceptive users. *Eur J Clin Pharmacol* (1988) 35, 101–3.
15. Tsunoda SM, Harris RZ, Mroczkowski PJ, Hebert MF, Benet LZ. Oral progesterone therapy does not affect the pharmacokinetics of prednisolone and erythromycin in post-menopausal women. *Clin Pharmacol Ther* (1995) 57, 182.

Corticosteroids + Diuretics, potassium-depleting

Since both of these groups of drugs cause potassium loss, severe depletion may occur if used together.

Clinical evidence, mechanism, importance and management

There seem to be no formal clinical studies about the extent of the additive potassium depletion which can occur when these drugs are given together but an exaggeration of the potassium loss undoubtedly occurs (e.g. seen with **hydrocortisone** and **furosemide (frusemide)**[1]). Concurrent use should be well monitored and the potassium intake increased to balance this loss.

The greatest potassium loss occurs with the naturally occurring corticosteroids such as **cortisone** and **hydrocortisone**. **Corticotropin (ACTH)**, which is a pituitary hormone, and **tetracosactrin** (a synthetic polypeptide) stimulate corticosteroid secretion by the adrenal cortex and can thereby indirectly cause potassium loss. **Fludrocortisone** also causes potassium loss. The synthetic corticosteroids (glucocorticoids) have a much less marked potassium-losing effect and are less likely to cause problems. These include **betamethasone, dexamethasone, prednisolone, prednisone** and **triamcinolone**.

The potassium-depleting diuretics include **bumetanide, chlortalidone, furosemide, etacrynic acid, piretanide, the thiazides and related diuretics** (e.g. **bendroflumethiazide (bendrofluazide), benzthiazide, chlorothiazide, clopamide, cyclopenthiazide, hydrochlorothiazide, hydroflumethiazide, indapamide, mefruside, methyclothiazide, metolazone, polythiazide, xipamide**). Other potassium-depleting diuretics are listed in Table 14.2 (see 'Digitalis glycosides + Diuretics, potassium-depleting', p.541).

1. Manchon ND, Bercoff E, Lemarchand P, Chassagne P, Senant J, Bourreille J. Fréquence et gravité des interactions médicamenteuses dans une population âgée: étude prospective concernant 63 malades. *Rev Med Interne* (1989) 10, 521–5.

Corticosteroids + Ephedrine or Theophylline

Ephedrine increases the loss of dexamethasone from the body, but theophylline appears not to interact.

Clinical evidence, mechanism, importance and management

Nine asthmatic patients showed a 40% increase in the clearance of the **dexamethasone** when concurrently given 100 mg **ephedrine** daily for 3 weeks and a similar reduction in its half-life.[1] This would be expected to reduce the overall control of asthma, but this requires confirmation. Be alert for any evidence that the **dexamethasone** effects are reduced if both drugs are used. It is not clear whether other corticosteroids behave similarly. **Theophylline** appeared not to interact.[1]

1. Brooks SM, Sholiton LJ, Werk EE, Altenau P. The effects of ephedrine and theophylline on dexamethasone metabolism in bronchial asthma. *J Clin Pharmacol* (1977) 17, 308.

Corticosteroids + Glycyrrhizin

Glycyrrhizin can reduce the clearance of prednisolone from the body.

Clinical evidence, mechanism, importance and management

A study in 6 healthy subjects found that after taking four 50 mg oral doses of **glycyrrhizin** 8-hourly followed by a bolus injection of 0.096 mg/kg **prednisolone hemisuccinate**, the AUC of total **prednisolone** was increased by 50% and of free **prednisolone** by 55%.[1] This confirms the findings of two previous studies in which the **glycyrrhizin** was given by intravenous infusion.[2,3] The probable reason is that the **glycyrrhizin** inhibits the metabolism of the **prednisolone** by the liver so that it is cleared by the body more slowly. In one of the studies it was also found that **glycyrrhizin** increased the effects of **prednisolone** in some patients with rheumatoid arthritis and polyarteritis nodosa.[2]

The clinical importance of these observations is uncertain, but increased effects can be beneficial and in excess can be toxic. Concurrent use should be well monitored. More study is needed.

1. Chen M-F, Shimada F, Kato H, Yano S, Kanaoka M. Effect of oral administration of glycyrrhizin on the pharmacokinetics of prednisolone. *Endocrinol Jpn* (1991) 38, 167–74.
2. Chen M-F, Shimada F, Kato H, Yano S, Kanaoka M. Effect of glycyrrhizin on the pharmacokinetics of prednisolone following low dosage of prednisolone hemisuccinate. *Endocrinol Jpn* (1990) 37, 331–41.
3. Ojima M, Itoh N, Satoh K, Fukuchi S. The effects of glycyrrhizin preparations on patients with difficult in release of steroids treatment. *Minophagen Med Rev* (1987) (Suppl 17), 120–5.

Corticosteroids + Grapefruit juice

Grapefruit juice does not interact with prednisone or prednisolone.

Clinical evidence, mechanism, importance and management

A study in 12 kidney transplant patients found that when they were given either water or **grapefruit juice** every 3 h for 30 h, the **grapefruit juice** increased the levels of the ciclosporin they were taking, but had no significant effect on the AUC of **prednisone** or **prednisolone**. It was concluded that **grapefruit juice** does not affect the metabolism of **prednisone** or **prednisolone**.[1] No special precautions are therefore needed if these corticosteroids and **grapefruit juice** are

taken concurrently. Information about other corticosteroids is lacking but no interaction would be expected.

1. Hollander AA, van Rooij J, Lentjes EGWM, Arbouw F, van Bree JB, Schoemaker RC, van Es LA, van der Woude FJ, Cohen AF. The effect of grapefruit juice on cyclosporine and prednisone metabolism in transplant patients. *Clin Pharmacol Ther* (1995) 57, 318–24.

Corticosteroids + Itraconazole

There is evidence that itraconazole can increase the effects of deflazacort, dexamethasone, methylprednisolone and prednisone. Prednisolone appears to be affected to a lesser extent. Corticosteroid overdosage may occur if the dosage is not reduced.

Clinical evidence

A study in 14 healthy subjects found that after taking 400 mg **itraconazole** for one day and then 200 mg daily for the next 3 days, the AUC of a single 48-mg dose of **methylprednisolone** was increased more than two and a half fold (from 2773 to 7011 nanograms.h/ml). A parallel study found no interaction with 60 mg **prednisone**.[1]

A man with a lung transplant treated with **methylprednisolone**, ciclosporin (cyclosporin) and azathioprine was additionally given 200 mg **itraconazole** twice daily to treat a suspected *Aspergillus fumigatus* infection. Three weeks later signs of corticosteroid overdosage developed, namely myopathy (confirmed by electromyography) and diabetes mellitus. Ten days after stopping the **itraconazole** the muscle force had improved and the daily dose of insulin had decreased from 120 to 20 units.[2] Studies in healthy subjects have found that **itraconazole** decreases the clearance and increases the elimination half life and AUC of both oral and intravenously administered **methylprednisolone**. Enhanced adrenal suppression also occurred.[3,4]

Six patients with allergic bronchopulmonary aspergillosis (3 had underlying cystic fibrosis and 3 had severe asthma) were treated with 200 mg oral **itraconazole** twice daily for 1 to 6 months. Four of the patients concurrently treated with systemic **prednisone** were able to reduce the corticosteroid dosage by 44% (from 43 to 24 mg daily) without any clinical deterioration.[5]

A patient with cystic fibrosis on **deflazacort** developed Cushing's syndrome soon after starting 200 **itraconazole** twice daily which gradually disappeared when the **itraconazole** was stopped.[6]

A study in 8 healthy subjects found that after taking **itraconazole** 200 mg daily for 4 days the AUC, peak plasma level and elimination half-life of a single oral dose of **dexamethasone** 4.5 mg were increased by 3.7-, 1.7-, and 2.8-fold respectively. In another phase of the study **itraconazole** decreased systemic clearance of intravenous **dexamethasone** 5 mg by 68% and increased the AUC and elimination half-life by 3.3- and 3.2-fold respectively. The adrenal-suppressant effects of **dexamethasone** were enhanced by **itraconazole**.[7]

A study in 10 healthy subjects found that **itraconazole** 200 mg daily for 4 days increased the AUC of a single oral dose of **prednisolone** 20 mg by 24%, but this was considered to be of limited clinical significance.[8]

Mechanism

Uncertain. It seems probable that the itraconazole inhibits the metabolism (by cytochrome P450 isoenzyme CYP3A4) of these steroids by the liver so that they are cleared from the body less quickly and their effects (and side effects) are thereby increased. Prednisolone is less likely than methylprednisolone to interact with CYP3A4 inhibitors.[8]

Importance and management

Information appears to be limited to these reports which are not entirely consistent, but the interactions appear to be established. There is currently too little known to say whether all or only a few patients are affected, but it would now be prudent to monitor the outcome of adding itraconazole to any patient on deflazacort, dexamethasone, methylprednisolone or prednisone, being alert for the need to reduce the steroid dosage. Itraconazole appears not interact with prednisolone to a clinically significant extent. Information about other corticosteroids is lacking but good monitoring seems advisable.

1. Lebrun-Vignes B, Corbrion Archer V, Diquet B, Levron JC, Chosidow O, Puech AJ, Warot D. Effect of itraconazole on the pharmacokinetics of prednisolone and methylprednisolone and cortisol secretion in healthy subjects. Br J Clin Pharmacol (2001) 51, 443–50.
2. Linthoudt H, Van Raemdonck D, Lerut T, Demedts M, Verleden G. The association of itraconazole and methylprednisolone may give rise to important steroid-related side effects. J Heart Lung Transplant (1996) 15, 1165.
3. Varis T, Kaukonen K-M, Kivistö KT, Neuvonen PJ. Plasma concentrations and effects of oral methylprednisolone are considerably increased by itraconazole. Clin Pharmacol Ther (1998) 64, 363–8.
4. Varis T, Kivistö KT, Backman JT, Neuvonen PJ. Itraconazole decreases the clearance and enhances the effects of intravenously administered methylprednisolone in healthy volunteers. Pharmacol Toxicol (1999) 85, 29–32.
5. Denning DW, Van Wye JE, Lewiston NJ, Stevens DA. Adjunctive therapy of allergic bronchopulmonary aspergillosis with itraconazole. Chest (1991) 100, 813–9.
6. Sauty A. Leuenberger PH, Fitting JW. Cushing's syndrome in a patient with cystic fibrosis treated with itraconazole and deflazacort for allergic bronchopulmonary aspergillosis. Eur Respir J (1995) 8 (Suppl 19), 441S.
7. Varis T, Kivistö KT, Backman JT, Neuvonen PJ. The cytochrome P450 3A4 inhibitor itraconazole markedly increases the plasma concentrations of dexamethasone and enhances its adrenal-suppressant effect. Clin Pharmacol Ther (2000) 68, 487–94.
8. Varis T, Kivistö KT, Neuvonen PJ. The effect of itraconazole on the pharmacokinetics and pharmacodynamics of oral prednisolone. Eur J Clin Pharmacol (2000) 56, 57–60.

Corticosteroids + Ketoconazole

Ketoconazole reduces the metabolism and loss of methylprednisolone from the body. The corticosteroid dosage should be reduced. The situation with prednisone and prednisolone is uncertain. No clinically relevant interaction occurs with inhaled budesonide or fluticasone.

Clinical evidence

(a) Budesonide, Fluticasone (inhaled)

Sixteen healthy subjects were given single inhaled doses of 1000 micrograms **budesonide** or 500 micrograms **fluticasone** after taking two daily doses of 200 mg **ketoconazole**. Using cortisol excretion as a measure of how much of these corticosteroids was absorbed systemically, it was found that no interaction occurred between the **fluticasone** and the **ketoconazole**, and no clinically relevant interaction appeared to occur with **budesonide**.[1]
Another study in 8 healthy subjects found that **ketoconazole** 200 mg daily for 4 days increased the AUC of a single 3-mg oral dose of **budesonide** given with the last dose of **ketoconazole** 6.5-fold. When **budesonide** was administered 12 h before the last dose of **ketoconazole**, the AUC was increased 3.8-fold.[2]

(b) Methylprednisolone

Ketoconazole 200 mg daily for 6 days increased the mean AUC of a single intravenous dose of **methylprednisolone** 20 mg in 6 healthy subjects by 135% and decreased the clearance by 60%. The 24 h cortisol AUC was reduced by 44%.[3] These findings were confirmed by another study by the same group of workers.[4]

(c) Prednisone and prednisolone

Ketoconazole 200 mg daily for 6 to 7 days caused a 50% rise in the total and unbound **prednisolone** serum levels of 10 healthy subjects, following oral **prednisone** or intravenous **prednisolone**.[5] In contrast, two other studies failed to find any effect of 200 mg **ketoconazole** for 6 days on either the pharmacokinetics or the pharmacodynamics of **prednisolone**, as measured by the suppressive effects on serum cortisol, blood basophil and helper T lymphocyte values of **prednisolone**.[6,7]

Mechanism

Ketoconazole inhibits cytochrome P450 dependent enzymes (CYP3A4) in the intestinal wall and liver so that the metabolism of some oral corticosteroids is reduced, thereby reducing their loss from the body and increasing their effects. No important interaction is likely to occur with inhaled corticosteroids because they act directly on the lung tissue before any systemic absorption and metabolism can occur.

Importance and management

The methylprednisolone/ketoconazole interaction appears to be established and clinically important. A 50% reduction in the corticosteroid dosage is recommended in one study.[4] It has been pointed out that increased corticosteroid serum levels have an increased immunosuppressive effect which may be undesirable in those with a fungal infection needing treatment with ketoconazole.[5] The situation with prednisone and prednisolone is as yet uncertain.[8,9] More study is needed to clarify the situation. The study with inhaled budesonide and fluticasone indicates that no clinically important interaction occurs with ketoconazole, although a significant interaction may occur with oral budesonide. The extent of this latter interaction may be reduced by 50% by separating the administration of the two drugs by 12 hours.[2]

1. Falcoz C, Lawlor C, Hefting NR, Borgstein NG, Smeets FWM, Wemer J, Jonkman JHG, House F. Effects of CYP3A4 inhibition by ketoconazole on systemic activity of inhaled fluticasone propionate and budesonide. Eur Respir J (1997) 10 (Suppl 25), 175S-176S.
2. Seidegård J. Reduction of the inhibitory effect of ketoconazole on budesonide pharmacokinetics by separation of their time of administration. Clin Pharmacol Ther (2000) 68, 13–17.
3. Glynn AM, Slaughter RL, Brass C, D'Ambrosio R, Jusko WJ. Effects of ketoconazole on methylprednisolone pharmacokinetics and cortisol secretion. Clin Pharmacol Ther (1986) 39, 654–9.
4. Kandrotas RJ, Slaughter RL, Brass C, Jusko WJ. Ketoconazole effects on methylprednisolone disposition and their joint suppression of endogenous cortisol. Clin Pharmacol Ther (1987) 42, 465–70.
5. Zürcher RM, Frey BM, Frey FJ. Impact of ketoconazole on the metabolism of prednisolone. Clin Pharmacol Ther (1989) 45, 366–72.
6. Yamashita SK, Ludwig EA, Middleton E, Jusko WJ. Lack of pharmacokinetic and pharmacodynamic interactions between ketoconazole and prednisolone. Clin Pharmacol Ther (1991) 49, 558–70.
7. Ludwig EA, Slaughter RL, Savliwala M, Brass C, Jusko WJ. Steroid-specific effects of ketoconazole disposition: unaltered prednisolone elimination. Drug Intell Clin Pharm (1989) 23, 858–61.
8. Jusko WJ. Ketoconazole effects on corticosteroid disposition. Clin Pharmacol Ther (1990) 47, 418–9.
9. Zürcher RM, Frey BM, Frey FJ. Ketoconazole effects on corticosteroid disposition. Clin Pharmacol Ther (1990) 47, 419–21.

Corticosteroids + Macrolide antibacterials

Troleandomycin and, to a lesser extent, erythromycin can reduce the loss of methylprednisolone from the body, thereby increasing both its therapeutic and toxic effects. Prednisolone appears not to be affected except in those taking enzyme-inducing agents such as phenobarbital (phenobarbitone). Clarithromycin reduces the clearance of methylprednisolone but appears not to affect prednisone clearance although isolated case reports describe the development of acute mania and psychosis in 2 patients apparently due to an interaction between prednisone and clarithromycin.

Clinical evidence

(a) Methylprednisolone or Prednisone + Clarithromycin

A woman of 30 with no history of mental illness was treated for acute sinusitis with **prednisone** (20 mg daily for 2 days, followed by 40 mg for a further 2 days) and 1 g **clarithromycin** daily. After 5 days she stopped taking both drugs (for unknown reasons), but a further 5 days later she was hospitalised with acute mania (disorganised thoughts and behaviour, pressured speech, increased energy, reduced need for sleep and labile effect). She spontaneously recovered after a further 5 days and showed no evidence of psychiatric illness 4 months later.[1] A 50-year-old man receiving treatment for emphysema was additionally given **prednisone** 20 mg daily to improve dyspnoea. After about 2 weeks he was also given **clarithromycin** 500 mg twice daily for purulent bronchitis. Shortly afterwards his family noticed psychiatric symptoms characterised by paranoia, delusions and what was described as dangerous behaviour. He recovered following treatment with low-dose olanzapine, gradual reduction of **prednisone** dosage and discontinuation of **clarithromycin**. An interaction was suspected as the patient had previously received prednisone on a number of occasions without the development of psychosis.[2]

However, a study in 6 asthmatic patients found that although **clarithromycin** 500 mg twice daily for 9 days reduced the clearance of single doses of **methylprednisolone** by 65% and resulted in significantly higher plasma **methylprednisolone** levels it had no significant effect on **prednisone** pharmacokinetics.[3]

(b) Methylprednisolone + Erythromycin

A study in 9 adolescents aged 9 to 18 with asthma showed that after taking 250 mg **erythromycin** four times daily for a week, the clearance of **methylprednisolone** was decreased by 46% (range 28 to 61%) and the half-life was increased by 47% (from 2.34 to 3.45 h).[4]

(c) Methylprednisolone or prednisolone + Troleandomycin

A pharmacokinetic study in 4 children and 6 adult steroid-dependent asthmatics found that one weeks treatment with 14 mg/kg **troleandomycin** daily increased the half-life of **methylprednisolone** by 88% (from 2.46 to 4.63 h) and reduced the total body clearance by 64%. All 10 showed cushingoid symptoms (cushingoid facies and weight gain) which resolved when the **methylprednisolone** dosage was reduced, without any loss in the control of the asthma.[5] A later study by the same group of workers confirmed these findings but they also found that **prednisolone** clearance was not affected except in those who were also taking **phenobarbital** (**phenobarbitone**), which is an enzyme inducers.[6]

A number of other reports confirm that **troleandomycin** can act as a 'steroid-sparing' agent.[7-14] One of them reported a 50% reduction in steroid clearance.[9] However a case report suggests that the risk of disseminated varicella infection may possibly be increased by concurrent use.[10] Another study failed to find a clinically significant interaction between **methylprednisolone** and **troleandomycin**.[15]

Mechanism

What is known suggests that erythromycin and troleandomycin can inhibit the metabolism of methylprednisolone, thereby reducing its loss from the body and increasing its effects. The volume of distribution is also decreased.[4-6,16] Although the evidence is conflicting it is possible that clarithromycin can increase the serum levels and toxicity of prednisone by a similar mechanism.

Importance and management

Information about the erythromycin/methylprednisolone interaction is much more limited than with troleandomycin/methylprednisolone, but both appear to be established and of clinical importance. This 'steroid-sparing' effect should be taken into account during concurrent use and appropriate dosage reductions made to avoid the development of corticosteroid overdosage side-effects. The authors of one study[5] suggest that this reduction should be ". . . empirical and based primarily on clinical symptomatology." Another group found that a 68% reduction in methylprednisolone dosage was possible within 2 weeks,[12] and yet another group found that a four to fivefold reduction was possible.[13] Troleandomycin appears to have a greater effect than erythromycin.

Prednisolone seems not to interact with troleandomycin and is a non-interacting alternative except in those taking enzyme-inducing drugs (e.g. phenobarbital).

Methylprednisolone appears to interact with clarithromycin but the evidence on the prednisone/clarithromycin interaction is conflicting and its general importance is uncertain, but prescribers should be aware of this report if both drugs are used together.

The general silence in the literature suggests that these macrolide antibacterials do not normally interact with other corticosteroids but be on the alert for any changes until this is confirmed. There also seems to be no information about other macrolide antibacterials.

1. Finkenbine R, Gill HS. Case due to prednisone-clarithromycin interaction. *Can J Psychiatry* (1997) 42, 778.
2. Finkenbine RD, Frye MD. Case of psychosis due to prednisone-clarithromycin interaction. *Gen Hosp Psychiatry* (1998) 20, 325–6.
3. Fost DA, Leung DY, Martin RJ, Brown EE, Szefler SJ, Spahn JD. Inhibition of methylprednisolone elimination in the presence of clarithromycin therapy. *J Allergy Clin Immunol* (1999) 103, 1031–5.
4. LaForce CF, Szefler SJ, Miller MF, Ebling W, Brenner M. Inhibition of methylprednisolone elimination in the presence of erythromycin therapy. *J Allergy Clin Immunol* (1983) 72, 34–9.
5. Szefler SJ, Rose JQ, Ellis EF, Spector SL, Green AW, Jusko WJ. The effect of troleandomycin on methylprednisolone elimination. *J Allergy Clin Immunol* (1980) 66, 447–51.
6. Szefler SJ, Ellis EF, Brenner M, Rose JQ, Spector SL, Yurchak A, Andrews F, Jusko WJ. Steroid-specific and anticonvulsant interaction aspects of triacetyloleandomycin-steroid therapy. *J Allergy Clin Immunol* (1982) 69, 455–60.
7. Fox JL. Infectious asthma treated with triacetyloleandomycin. *Penn Med J* (1961) 64, 634–5.
8. Itkin IH, Menzel M. The use of macrolide antibiotic substances in the treatment of asthma. *J Allergy* (1970) 45, 146–62.
9. Ball BD, Hill M, Brenner M, Sanks R, Szefler SJ. Critical assessment of troleandomycin in severe steroid-requiring asthmatic children. *Ann Allergy* (1988) 60, 155.
10. Lantner R, Rockoff JB, DeMasi J, Boran-Ragotzy R, Middleton E. Fatal varicella in a corticosteroid-dependent asthmatic receiving troleandomycin. *Allergy Proc* (1990) 11, 83–7.
11. Eitches RW, Rachelefsky GS, Katz RM, Mendoza GR, Siegel SC. Methylprednisolone and troleandomycin in treatment of steroid-dependent asthmatic children. *Am J Dis Child* (1985) 139, 264–8.
12. Wald JA, Friedman BF, Farr RS. An improved protocol for the use of troleandomycin (TAO) in the treatment of steroid-requiring asthma. *J Allergy Clin Immunol* (1986) 78, 36–43.
13. Zeiger RS, Schatz M, Sperling W, Simon RA, Stevenson DD. Efficacy of troleandomycin in outpatients with severe, corticosteroid-dependent asthma. *J Allergy Clin Immunol* (1980) 66, 438–46.
14. Kamada AK, Hill MR, Brenner AM, Szefler SJ. Glucocorticoid reduction with troleandomycin in chronic, severe asthmatic children: implications for future trials and clinical application. *J Allergy Clin Immunol* (1992) 89, 285.
15. Nelson HS, Hamilos DL, Corsello PR, Levesque NV, Buchmeier AD, Bucher BL. A double-blind study of troleandomycin and methylprednisolone in asthmatic subjects who require daily corticosteroids. *Am Rev Respir Dis* (1993) 147, 398–404.
16. Szefler SJ, Brenner M, Jusko WJ, Spector SL, Flesher KA, Ellis EF. Dose- and time-related effect of troleandomycin on methylprednisolone elimination. *Clin Pharmacol Ther* (1982) 32, 166–171.

Corticosteroids + Miscellaneous drugs

The corticosteroids may adversely affect the drug treatment of hypertension, congestive heart failure, epilepsy, diabetes mellitus, glaucoma, peptic ulceration and acute infections.

Clinical evidence, mechanism, importance and management

A number of disease conditions, even under active treatment with drugs, can be worsened by the use of corticosteroids. Sometimes drug–drug interactions take place, whereas others are drug–disease interactions, but in each case the outcome of concurrent use needs considerable care and good monitoring.

Systemic corticosteroids can disturb the electrolyte balance of the body causing the retention of sodium and water, and can therefore oppose the treatment of **hypertension** or **congestive heart failure**. They can cause potassium loss, which can be additive with the potassium-losing effects of other drugs such as **carbenoxolone** and some **diuretics** (see 'Corticosteroids + Diuretics, potassium depleting', p.634). Very close monitoring is recommended for patients with active or quiescent **tuberculosis** (but see 'Corticosteroids + Rifampicin', p.639). They interact with **carbamazepine**, **phenytoin** and **primidone** (see the entries for 'Corticosteroids + Carbamazepine', p.632, 'Corticosteroids + Phenytoin', p.638 and 'Corticosteroids + Barbiturates', p.631 respectively) and **epilepsy** is one of the conditions which may be exacerbated by the use of the corticosteroids. Other disease conditions where great care is needed are **glaucoma**, **peptic ulceration** (see 'Corticosteroids + Cimetidine or Ranitidine', p.633), **diabetes mellitus** (see 'Hypoglycaemic agents + Corticosteroids', p.575) and **acute infections** (see 'Corticosteroids + Anti-infective agents', p.631).

Corticosteroids + NSAIDs

Concurrent use increases the incidence of gastro-intestinal bleeding and probably ulceration. Indometacin (indomethacin) and naproxen can have a 'steroid-sparing' effect.

Clinical evidence, mechanism, importance and management

(a) Gastrointestinal bleeding and ulceration

A retrospective study of more than 20,000 patients who had had corticosteroids found that the incidence of upper gastrointestinal bleeding was no greater than in the control group who had not had corticosteroids (95 compared with 91), however the risk of bleeding was increased if the patients were also taking **aspirin** or **other NSAIDs**.[1] This is consistent with the results of another study on patients taking **prednisone** and **indometacin** (**indomethacin**),[2] and gives support to the widely held belief that concurrent use of the NSAIDs (well-known as gastric irritants) can cause bleeding and ulceration. Concurrent use should be very well monitored. See also 'Aspirin or Salicylates + Corticosteroids or Corticotropin', p.46.

(b) Steroid-sparing effect

A study in 11 patients with stable rheumatoid disease on regular corticosteroid therapy showed that when given either 75 mg **indometacin** or 250 mg **naproxen** twice daily for two weeks the total plasma levels of a single 7.5-mg dose of **prednisolone** remained unchanged but the amount of unbound (free) **prednisolone** increased by 30 to 60%.[3] The probable reason is that these NSAIDs displace administered and endogenous corticosteroids from their plasma protein binding sites. It should therefore be possible to reduce the corticosteroid dosage while maintaining the therapeutic effects. One study found that the dosage of **paramethasone** could be reduced by almost 60% when **naproxen** was given.[4]

1. Carson JL, Strom BL, Schinnar R, Sim E, Maislin G, Morse ML. Do corticosteroids really cause upper GI bleeding? *Clin Res* (1987) 35, 340A.
2. Emmanuel JH, Montgomery RD. Gastric ulcer and anti-arthritic drugs. *Postgrad Med J* (1971) 47, 227.
3. Rae SA, Williams IA, English J, Baylis EM. Alteration of plasma prednisolone levels by indomethacin and naproxen. *Br J Clin Pharmacol* (1982) 14, 459–61.
4. Flores JJB, Rojas SV. Naproxen: corticosteroid-sparing effect in rheumatoid arthritis. *J Clin Pharmacol* (1975) 15, 373–7.

Corticosteroids + Omeprazole

Omeprazole normally appears not to interact with prednisone, but an isolated and unexplained report describes a reduction in the effects of prednisone in one patient when treated with omeprazole.

Clinical evidence, mechanism, importance and management

A placebo controlled, randomised, double-blind trial in 18 healthy subjects found that 40 mg **omeprazole** daily had no effect on the pharmacokinetics of a single 40-mg dose of **prednisone**.[1] This contrasts with an isolated and unexplained report of a patient suffering from pemphigus who was given **prednisone** 1 mg/kg daily, and a

week later was additionally started on **ranitidine** 200 mg daily for a gastric ulcer. Four weeks later when the skin lesions were well controlled, it was decided to replace the **ranitidine** with 40 mg **omeprazole** daily. Within 4 days the skin lesions began progressively to worsen, although the **prednisone** dosage remained unchanged, until after 3 weeks it was decided to stop the **omeprazole** and restart the **ranitidine** because an adverse interaction between the **prednisone** and the **omeprazole** was suspected. Within about a week, the skin condition had begun to improve.[2] The suggested explanation is that the **omeprazole** inhibited the liver enzyme (11β-hydroxylase) which normally converts **prednisone** into its active form (**prednisolone**) so that in effect the pemphigus became inadequately treated.[2]

It would seem therefore that an adverse interaction between **prednisone** and **omeprazole** is unlikely, nevertheless it would be prudent to be on the alert if these drugs are given concurrently because the isolated case cannot be dismissed entirely. More study is needed.

1. Cavanaugh JH, Karol M. Lack of pharmacokinetic interaction after administration of lansoprazole or omeprazole with prednisone. *J Clin Pharmacol* (1996) 36, 1064–71.
2. Joly P, Chosidow O, Laurent-Puig P, Delchier J-C, Roujeau J-C, Revuz J. Possible interaction prednisone-oméprazole dans la pemphigoïde bulleuse. *Gastroenterol Clin Biol* (1990) 14, 682–3.

Corticosteroids + Phenytoin

(a) The therapeutic effects of dexamethasone, methylprednisolone, prednisolone, prednisone (probably other glucocorticoids) and fludrocortisone can be markedly reduced by the concurrent use of phenytoin. (b) The results of the dexamethasone adrenal suppression test may prove to be unreliable, and (c) serum phenytoin levels may be changed by dexamethasone.

Clinical evidence

(a) Reduced corticosteroid levels

A comparative pharmacokinetic study in six neurological or neurosurgical patients taking **dexamethasone** (orally) and **phenytoin** showed that the average amount of **dexamethasone** which reached the general circulation was a quarter of that observed in nine other patients taking only **dexamethasone** (mean oral bioavailability fractions of 0.21 and 0.84 respectively).[1]

Other patients have been described who needed increased doses of **dexamethasone** while taking **phenytoin**.[2] The **fludrocortisone** dosages of two patients required marked increases (fourfold in one patient and 10 to 20 times in the other) while taking **phenytoin**.[3] Renal allograft survival is decreased in patients on **prednisone** taking **phenytoin** due (it is believed) to reduced immunosuppressant effects.[4] The results of studies[5-9] of the effects of **phenytoin** on the half-lives and clearance rates of other **corticosteroids** are shown in Table 16.2.

Table 16.2 A comparison of the effects of phenytoin on the kinetics of different glucocorticoids (after Petereit and colleagues[15])

Corticosteroid	Daily dosage of phenytoin (mg)	Half-life without phenytoin (min)	Decreased half-life with phenytoin (%)	Increased mean clearance rate with phenytoin (%)	Ref
Hydrocortisone	300–400	60–90	−15	+25	5
Methylprednisolone	300	165	−56	+130	6
Prednisone	Prednisolone is the biologically active metabolite of prednisone so that the values for prednisone and prednisolone should be similar				7
Prednisolone	300	190–240	−45	+77	5
Dexamethasone	300	250	−51	+140	8, 9

(b) Interference with the dexamethasone adrenal suppression test

A study on seven patients showed that while taking 300 to 400 mg **phenytoin** daily their plasma cortisol levels were only reduced by **dexamethasone** from 22 to 19 micrograms% compared with a reduction from 18 to 4 micrograms% in the absence of **phenytoin**.[10]

Other studies confirm that plasma cortisol and urinary 17-hydroxy-corticosteroid levels are suppressed far less than might be expected with small doses of **dexamethasone** (0.5 mg six-hourly for eight doses), but with larger doses (2.0 mg six-hourly for eight doses) suppression was normal.[11]

(c) Serum phenytoin levels increased or decreased

A post-traumatic epilepsy prophylaxis study showed that the serum **phenytoin** levels in those taking **dexamethasone** (16 to 150 mg: mean 63.6 mg) was 40% higher than those on **phenytoin** alone (17.3 compared with 12.5 micrograms/ml). The **phenytoin** was given as a loading dose of 11 mg/kg intravenously and then 13 mg/kg intramuscularly.[12]

A retrospective study of 40 patient records indicated that **dexamethasone** reduced serum **phenytoin** levels. The serum **phenytoin** levels of six patients on fixed doses of **phenytoin** were halved by the presence of **dexamethasone**.[13] Another patient needed a large dose of **phenytoin** (>10 mg/kg) while taking **dexamethasone**. He showed an almost 300% rise in serum **phenytoin** levels when **dexamethasone** was stopped.[14]

Mechanism

Phenytoin is a potent liver enzyme inducing agent which increases the metabolism of the corticosteroids so that they are cleared from the body more quickly, reducing both their therapeutic and adrenal suppressant effects.

Importance and management

(a). The fall in serum corticosteroid levels is established and of clinical importance where treatment depends upon transport by the circulation (e.g. in immunosuppression), but it seems unlikely to affect the response to steroids administered topically or by inhalation, intra-articular injection or enema.[15] The interaction can be accommodated in several ways: (i) Increase the corticosteroid dosage proportionally to the increase in clearance (see Table 16.2). With prednisolone an average increase of 100% (range 58–260% in five individuals) proved effective.[15] A fourfold increase may be necessary with dexamethasone,[1] and much greater increases have been required with fludrocortisone.[3] (ii) Exchange the corticosteroid for another which is less affected (see Table 16.2). A switch from dexamethasone to equivalent doses of methylprednisolone has been reported to be effective[16] but another report found that methylprednisolone was affected more than prednisolone.[17] In another case the exchange of 16 mg dexamethasone daily for 100 mg prednisone was successful.[18] (iii) Exchange the phenytoin for another anticonvulsant: Barbiturates, and to some extent primidone[19] and carbamazepine, are also enzyme-inducing agents, but sodium valproate is a successful non-interacting alternative.[2] However remember that corticosteroids should only be given to epileptics with care and good monitoring because of the risk that they will exacerbate the disease condition.

(b). The effects on the dexamethasone adrenal suppression test can apparently be accommodated by using larger-than-usual doses of dexamethasone (2 mg every 6 h for eight doses)[11] or by using an overnight test using 50 mg hydrocortisone.[16]

(c). The reports on the changes in serum phenytoin levels are inconsistent (rises and falls). The effects of concurrent use should be monitored.

1. Chalk JB, Ridgeway K, Brophy TRO'R, Yelland JDN, Eadie MJ. Phenytoin impairs the bioavailability of dexamethasone in neurological and neurosurgical patients. *J Neurol Neurosurg Psychiatry* (1984) 47, 1087–90.
2. McLelland J, Jack W. Phenytoin/dexamethasone interaction: a clinical problem. *Lancet* (1978) i, 1096–7.
3. Keilholz U, Guthrie GP. Case report: adverse effect of phenytoin on mineralocorticoid replacement with fludrocortisone in adrenal insufficiency. *Am J Med Sci* (1986) 291, 280–3.
4. Wassner SJ, Pennisi AJ, Malekzadeh MH, Fine RN. The adverse effect of anticonvulsant therapy on renal allograft survival. *J Pediatr* (1976) 88, 134–7.
5. Choi Y, Thrasher K, Werk EE, Sholiton LJ, Olinger C. Effect of diphenylhydantoin on cortisol kinetics in humans. *J Pharmacol Exp Ther* (1971) 176, 27–34.
6. Stjernholm MR, Katz FH. Effects of diphenylhydantoin, phenobarbital, and diazepam on the metabolism of methylprednisolone and its sodium succinate. *J Clin Endocrinol Metab* (1975) 41, 887–93.
7. Meikle AW, Weed JA, Tyler FH. Kinetics and interconversion of prednisolone and prednisone studies with new radio-immunoassays. *J Clin Endocrinol Metab* (1975) 41, 717.
8. Brooks SM, Werk EE, Ackerman SJ, Sullivan I, Thrasher K. Adverse effects of phenobarbital on corticosteroid metabolism in patients with bronchial asthmas. *N Engl J Med* (1972) 286, 1125–8.
9. Haque N, Thrasher K, Werk EE, Knowles HC, Sholiton LJ. Studies of dexamethasone metabolism in man. Effect of diphenylhydantoin. *J Clin Endocrinol Metab* (1972) 34, 44–50.
10. Werk EE, Choi Y, Sholiton L, Olinger C, Haque N. Interference in the effect of dexamethasone by diphenylhydantoin. *N Engl J Med* (1969) 281, 32–4.
11. Jubiz W, Meikle AW, Levinson RA, Mizutani S, West CD, Tyler FH. Effect of diphenylhydantoin on the metabolism of dexamethasone. *N Engl J Med* (1970) 283, 11–14.
12. Lawson LA, Blouin RA, Smith RB, Rapp RP, Young AB. Phenytoin-dexamethasone interaction: a previously unreported observation. *Surg Neurol* (1981) 16, 23–4.
13. Wong DD, Longenecker RG, Liepman M, Baker S, LaVergne M. Phenytoin-dexamethasone: a possible drug-drug interaction. *JAMA* (1985) 254, 2062–3.
14. Lackner TE. Interaction of dexamethasone with phenytoin. *Pharmacotherapy* (1991) 11, 344–7.
15. Petereit LB, Meikle AW. Effectiveness of prednisolone during phenytoin therapy. *Clin Pharmacol Ther* (1977) 22, 912–6.
16. Meikle AW, Stanchfield JB, West CD, Tyler FH. Hydrocortisone suppression test for Cushing syndrome: therapy with anticonvulsants. *Arch Intern Med* (1974) 134, 1068–74.
17. Bartoszek M, Brenner AM, Szefler SJ. Prednisolone and methylprednisolone kinetics in children receiving anticonvulsant therapy. *Clin Pharmacol Ther* (1987) 42, 424–32.
18. Boylan JJ, Owen DS, Chin JB. Phenytoin interference with dexamethasone. *JAMA* (1976) 235, 803–4.
19. Hancock KW, Levell MJ. Primidone/dexamethasone interaction. *Lancet* (1978) ii, 97–8.

Corticosteroids + Rifampicin (Rifampin)

The effects of the corticosteroids (cortisone, dexamethasone, fludrocortisone, hydrocortisone, methylprednisolone, prednisone, prednisolone) given systemically can be markedly reduced by the concurrent use of rifampicin, but aldosterone is not affected.

Clinical evidence

(a) Aldosterone

Seven patients with Addison's disease due to tuberculosis showed no changes in the pharmacokinetics of infused **aldosterone** after being treated with 600 mg **rifampicin** daily for 6 days.[1]

(b) Cortisone, Dexamethasone, Fludrocortisone, Hydrocortisone

A patient with Addison's disease stabilised on **cortisone** and **fludrocortisone** showed typical signs of corticosteroid overdosage when the **rifampicin** he was taking was replaced by ethambutol.[2] Another Addisonian patient needed an increase in her dosage of **cortisone** from 37.5 to 50 mg daily, plus 0.1 mg **fludrocortisone**, when 450 mg **rifampicin** daily was started.[3] When **rifampicin** was added to **prednisolone** or **dexamethasone** and **fludrocortisone** it caused an Addisonian crisis in two patients.[4] A metabolic study in an Addisonian patient on **hydrocortisone** found that **rifampicin** shortened its half-life and reduced its AUC.[5] **Rifampicin** also markedly increases the clearance of **dexamethasone**.[6,7]

(c) Prednisone, Prednisolone, Methylprednisolone

A child with nephrotic syndrome on **prednisolone**, accidentally given BCG vaccine, was treated with **rifampicin** and isoniazid to prevent possible dissemination of the vaccine. When the nephrotic condition failed to respond, the **prednisolone** dosage was raised from 2 to 3 mg/kg daily without any evidence of corticosteroid overdosage. Later when the **rifampicin** and isoniazid were withdrawn, remission of the nephrotic condition was achieved with the original dosage of **prednisolone**.[8] A number of other reports describe a reduction in the response to **prednisone, prednisolone** or **methylprednisolone** in patients when given **rifampicin**.[9-17] Pharmacokinetic studies in patients have shown that the AUC of **prednisolone** is reduced about 60% by **rifampicin**, and the half-life is decreased by 40 to 60%.[11,15,18]

Mechanism

Rifampicin is a potent liver enzyme inducing agent which increases the metabolism of the corticosteroids by the liver,[10,19] thereby increasing their loss from the body and reducing their effects.

Importance and management

The corticosteroid/rifampicin interactions are established, well documented and clinically important. The need to increase the dosages of cortisone, dexamethasone, fludrocortisone, hydrocortisone, methylprednisolone, prednisolone and prednisone should be expected if rifampicin is given. It has been suggested that as a first approximation the dosage of prednisolone should be increased two to threefold, and reduced proportionally if the rifampicin is withdrawn.[10,11,18,20] The dosage increases needed for other corticosteroids await assessment. In the case of prednisolone the interaction develops maximally by 14 days and disappears about 14 days after withdrawal of the rifampicin.[21] There seems to be no direct information about other glucocorticoids but be alert for them to be similarly affected. It is not clear whether any of the topically applied corticosteroids will interact with rifampicin but it seems unlikely. The systemic corticosteroids are usually considered as contraindicated, or only to be used with great care, in patients with active or quiescent tuberculosis. Aldosterone does not interact.

1. Schulte HM, Monig H, Benker G, Pagel H, Reinwein D, Ohnhaus EE. Pharmacokinetics of aldosterone in patients with Addison's disease: effect of rifampicin treatment on glucocorticoid and mineralocorticoid metabolism. *Clin Endocrinol (Oxf)* (1987) 27, 655–62.
2. Edwards OM, Courtenay-Evans RJ, Galley JM, Hunter J, Tait AD. Changes in cortisol metabolism following rifampicin therapy. *Lancet* (1974) ii, 549–51.
3. Maisey DN, Brown RC, Day JL. Rifampicin and cortisone replacement therapy. *Lancet* (1974) ii, 896–7.
4. Kyriazopoulou V, Parparousi O, Vagenakis AG. Rifampicin-induced adrenal crisis in Addisonian patients receiving corticosteroid replacement therapy. *J Clin Endocrinol Metab* (1984) 59, 1204–6.
5. Wang YH, Shi YF, Xiang HD. Effect of rifampin on the metabolism of glucocorticoids in Addison's disease. *Zhonghua Nei Ke Za Zhi* (1990) 29, 108–11,127.
6. Ediger SK, Isley WL. Rifampicin-induced adrenal insufficiency in the acquired immunodeficiency syndrome: difficulties in diagnosis and treatment. *Postgrad Med J* (1988) 64, 405–6.
7. Kawai SA. A comparative study of the accelerated metabolism of cortisol, prednisolone and dexamethasone in patients under rifampicin therapy. *Nippon Naibunpi Gakkai Zasshi* (1985) 61, 145–61.
8. Hendrickse W, McKiernan J, Pickup M, Lowe J. Rifampicin-induced non-responsiveness to corticosteroid treatment in nephrotic syndrome. *BMJ* (1979) i, 306.
9. van Marle W, Woods KL, Beeley L. Concurrent steroid and rifampicin therapy. *BMJ* (1979) i, 1020.
10. Buffington GA, Dominguez JH, Piering WF, Hebert LA, Kauffman HM, Lemann J. Interaction of rifampin and glucocorticoids. *JAMA* (1976) 236, 1958–60.
11. McAllister WAC, Thompson PJ, Al-Habet SM, Rogers HJ. Rifampicin reduces effectiveness and bioavailability of prednisolone. *BMJ* (1983) 286, 923–5.
12. Powell-Jackson PR, Gray BJ, Heaton RW, Costello JF, Williams R, English J. Adverse effect of rifampicin administration on steroid-dependent asthma. *Am Rev Respir Dis* (1983) 128, 307–10.
13. Bitaudeau Ph, Clément S, Chartier JPh, Papapietro PM, Bonnafoux A, Arnaud M, Trèves R, Desproges-Gotteron R. Interaction rifampicine-prednisolone. A propos de deux cas au cours d'une maladie de Horton. *Rev Rhum Mal Osteoartic* (1989) 56, 87–8.
14. Kawai S, Ichikawa Y. Drug interactions between glucocorticoids and other drugs. *Nippon Rinsho* (1994) 52, 773–8.
15. Carrie F, Roblot P, Bouquet S, Delon A, Roblot F, Becq-Giraudon B. Rifampin-induced nonresponsiveness of giant cell arteritis to prednisone treatment. *Arch Intern Med* (1994) 154, 1521–4.
16. Verma M, Singh T, Chhatwal J, Saini V, Pawar B. Rifampicin induced steroid unresponsiveness in nephrotic syndrome. *Indian Paediatr* (1994) 31, 1437.
17. Lin FL. Rifampin-induced deterioration in steroid-dependent asthma. *J Allergy Clin Immunol* (1996) 98, 1125.
18. Bergrem H, Refvem OK. Altered prednisolone pharmacokinetics in patients treated with rifampicin. *Acta Med Scand* (1983) 213, 339–43.
19. Sotaniemi EA, Medzihradsky F, Eliasson G. Glutaric acid as an indicator of use of enzyme-inducing drugs. *Clin Pharmacol Ther* (1974) 15, 417.
20. Löfdahl C-G, Mellstrand T, Svedmyr N, Wåhlén P. Increased metabolism of prednisolone and prednisolone after rifampicin treatment. *Am Rev Respir Dis* (1984) 129, A201.
21. Lee KH, Shin JG, Chong WS, Kim S, Lee JS, Jang IJ, Shin SG. Time course of the changes in prednisolone pharmacokinetics after co-administration or discontinuation of rifampicin. *Eur J Clin Pharmacol* (1993) 45, 287–89.

Corticosteroids + Sucralfate

Sucralfate appears not to interact with prednisone.

Clinical evidence, mechanism, importance and management

Sucralfate 1 g every 6 h had no effect on the pharmacokinetics of single 20-mg doses of **prednisone** in 12 healthy subjects, except that the peak plasma levels were delayed by about three-quarters of an hour when given at the same time, but not when the **sucralfate** was given 2 h after the **prednisone**.[1] No particular precautions are likely to be needed in patients given both drugs. Information about other corticosteroids is lacking.

1. Gambertoglio JG, Romac DR, Yong C-L, Birnbaum J, Lizak P, Amend WJ C. Lack of effect of sucralfate on prednisone bioavailability. *Am J Gastroenterol* (1987) 82, 42–5.

Corticosteroids + Vaccines (live)

Patients who are immunised with live virus vaccines while receiving immunosuppressive doses of corticosteroids may develop generalised, possibly life-threatening, infections.

Clinical evidence, mechanism, importance and management

The administration of corticosteroids can reduce the number of circulating lymphocytes and suppress the normal immune response so that concurrent immunisation with **live vaccines** can lead to generalised infection. It is suggested that **prednisone** in doses greater than 10 to 15 mg daily will suppress the immune response, whereas 40 to 60-mg doses on alternate days probably do not.[1] However a patient with lymphosarcoma and hypogammaglobulinaemia, taking 15 mg **prednisone** daily, developed a generalised vaccinial infection when she was **vaccinated**.[2] A fatal vaccinial infection developed in another patient treated with **cortisone**.[3] This type of problem can be controlled with immunoglobulin to give cover against a general infection while immunity develops, and this has been successfully used in steroid-dependent patients needing **smallpox vaccination**.[4]

Smallpox vaccination is no longer necessary but other live attenuated vaccines (**measles, mumps, rubella, poliomyelitis, BCG**) are still used and the principles relevant for **smallpox** are probably generally applicable, but no studies seem to have been done to establish what is safe.[1] These are some of the published warnings: ". . . extreme caution must be observed in administering **live virus vaccine** to any patient receiving steroid therapy . . . and . . . it seems unwise to administer **live virus vaccines** to any person receiving steroids for a systemic effect in any dosage."[1] Problems with topical or inhaled steroids in normal dosages seem unlikely because the amounts absorbed are relatively small,[1] however this needs confirmation. The British National Formulary says that **live vaccination** should be postponed for at least 3 months after stopping high-dose corticosteroids.[5]

1. Shapiro L. Questions and Answers. Live virus vaccine and corticosteroid therapy. Answered by Fauci AS, Bellanti JA, Polk IJ, Cherry JD. *JAMA* (1981) 246, 2075–6.
2. Rosenbaum EH, Cohen RA, Glatstein HR. Vaccination of a patient receiving immunosuppressive therapy for lymphosarcoma. *JAMA* (1966) 198, 737–40.
3. Olansky S, Smith JG, Hansen OCE. Fatal vaccinia associated with cortisone therapy. *JAMA* (1956) 162, 887–8.
4. Joseph MR. Vaccination of patients on steroid therapy. *Med J Aust* (1974) 2, 181.
5. British National Formulary. 43rd ed. London: The British Medical Association and The Pharmaceutical Press; 2002. p. 578.

Corticosteroids + Zileuton

No clinically relevant pharmacokinetic interactions occur between prednisone and zileuton.

Clinical evidence, mechanism, importance and management

In a randomised double-blind crossover study 16 healthy subjects were given 600 mg of **zileuton** 6-hourly for a week, and on day 6 they were also given either 40 mg **prednisone** or a placebo. The pharmacokinetics of the both drugs were slightly altered but these were considered to be clinically irrelevant. The **prednisone** half-life rose from 2.8 to 2.9 h, while the **zileuton** AUC fell by 13% and the time to achieve maximum serum levels fell by 26%. It was concluded that concurrent use carries a minimal risk of a clinically important pharmacokinetic interaction.[1] No special precautions would appear to be needed.

1. Awni WM, Cavanaugh JH, Tzeng T-B, Witt G, Granneman GR, Dube LM. Pharmacokinetic interactions between zileuton and prednisone. *Clin Pharmacokinet* (1995) 29 (Suppl 2), 105–111.

Daclizumab + Miscellaneous drugs

No adverse drug–drug interactions appear to have been reported with daclizumab.

Clinical evidence, mechanism, importance and management

The makers of daclizumab say that because it is an immunoglobulin, no metabolic drug-drug interactions (i.e. those mediated by inhibitory or inducing effects on cytochrome P450 enzymes) would be expected,[1] and none seems to have been reported. The makers say that daclizumab has been given in clinical trials with the following drugs without any adverse interactions: **aciclovir, azathioprine, antithymocyte immune globulin, ciclosporin, corticosteroids, ganciclovir, muromonab-CD3 (OKT3), mycophenolate mofetil** and **tacrolimus.**[1]

1. Zenapax (Daclizumab). Roche Products Limited. Summary of product characteristics, September 2000.

Everolimus + Ciclosporin

Ciclosporin increases the AUC of co-administered everolimus.

Clinical evidence

The possibility of a drug interaction was assessed by a crossover study in 24 healthy subjects who were given single doses of everolimus 2 mg, alone and with single doses of one of two **ciclosporin** formulations, namely (*Neoral* (microemulsion) 175 mg or *Sandimmune* (corn oil suspension) 300 mg). The concurrent administration of *Neoral* and everolimus increased the peak levels and the AUC of everolimus by 82% and 168% respectively. *Sandimmune* did not affect the peak levels of everolimus but its AUC was increased by 74%.[1]

Mechanism

Not fully understood. Both everolimus and ciclosporin are metabolised by the cytochrome P450 isoenzyme CYP3A4 and both are substrates of P-glycoprotein. Competition via one or both of these pathways in the liver or gut wall may contribute to the interaction.[1]

Importance and management

Information would seem limited to this single-dose study. However, it has been suggested if ciclosporin (either *Neoral* or *Sandimmune*) is removed from a everolimus-ciclosporin regimen, a two to threefold decrease in everolimus exposure could be expected. Monitoring is recommended.[1] More study is required.

1. Kovarik JM, Kalbag J, Figueiredo J, Rouilly M, O'Bannon LF, Rordorf C. Differential influence of two cyclosporine formulations on everolimus pharmacokinetics: a clinically relevant pharmacokinetic interaction. *J Clin Pharmacol* (2002) 42, 95–9.

Muromonab-CD3 (OKT3) + Indometacin (Indomethacin)

Indometacin may possibly increase the incidence of encephalopathy and psychosis in patients treated with muromonab-CD3.

Clinical evidence, mechanism, importance and management

A study of patient records found that 4 out of a total of 55 kidney transplant patients (7.3%) given muromonab-CD3 and **indometacin** 50 mg orally or rectally 6 to 8 hourly for 48 to 72 h developed serious encephalopathy and psychosis compared with only two out of 173 patients (1.2%) who had received muromonab-CD3 without **indometacin.**[1] The reasons are not understood. More study is needed to confirm the link between concurrent use and these serious adverse effects, but be particularly alert if both are used.

1. Chan GL, Weinstein SS, Wright CE, Bowers VD, Alveranga DY, Shires DL, Ackermann JR, LeFor WW, Kahana L. Encephalopathy associated with OKT3 administration. Possible interaction with indomethacin. *Transplantation* (1991) 52, 148–50.

Mycophenolate mofetil + Miscellaneous drugs

No clinically relevant interactions have so far been seen between mycophenolate mofetil and aciclovir, allopurinol, a combined oral contraceptive, co-trimoxazole, ganciclovir, or methotrexate but the makers suggest some caution nonetheless. Ciclosporin may reduce levels of mycophenolic acid and when ciclosporin is replaced by tacrolimus levels of mycophenolic acid are increased. Colestyramine and Maalox reduce its absorption but the clinical relevance of this is uncertain. It is recommended that azathioprine is not used concurrently. Oral iron preparations may significantly reduce the absorption of mycophenolate mofetil by chelation.

Clinical evidence, mechanism, importance and management

Mycophenolate mofetil is an ester pro-drug which is converted in the body into the active immunosuppressant mycophenolic acid (MPA). It is largely excreted in the urine as mycophenolic acid glucuronide (MPAG) which is inactive.

(a) Aciclovir

Healthy subjects were given single 800-mg oral doses of **aciclovir** or 1 g mycophenolate mofetil or both drugs together in a three period crossover study. The pharmacokinetics of both drugs were either minimally altered or unchanged by concurrent use, and it was concluded by the authors that any changes were unlikely to be clinically significant.[1] However the makers say that in renal impairment there may be competition for tubular secretion and increased concentrations of both drugs may occur.[2]

(b) Allopurinol

A study in 5 kidney transplant patients with gouty arthritis who were switched from azathioprine to 2 g mycophenolate mofetil daily (to avoid the risk of an azathioprine/allopurinol interaction) found that no adverse effects occurred when they were concurrently treated with **allopurinol** 100 to 200 mg daily. Ten weeks on average after the switch had taken place, the uricaemia had dropped 21%, mean serum creatinine levels were only slightly raised by 12% and white cell counts were unchanged.[3] No special precautions would therefore seem necessary.

(c) Antacids

When 10 ml of an **aluminium hydroxide/magnesium hydroxide** antacid (*Maalox TC*) was given four times daily to patients with rheumatoid arthritis, the AUC of a single 2 g dose of mycophenolate mofetil was reduced by 17% and the maximum serum concentration by 38%.[4] The clinical importance of this reduction has not been assessed but it would seem prudent to check that the immunosuppressant effects remain adequate in the presence of this or any other antacid.

(d) Azathioprine

The makers have recommended that mycophenolate mofetil should not be given with **azathioprine**[2] because they say that concurrent use has not been studied.

(e) Ciclosporin

The addition of mycophenolate mofetil to **ciclosporin** has been found to reduce the incidence of rejection episodes in a group of kidney transplant patients.[5] However, there are reports that trough levels of the active metabolite, mycophenolic acid, may be reduced in the presence of **ciclosporin**.[6] Another study found that mycophenolic acid levels in transplant patients treated with mycophenolate mofetil, prednisone and **ciclosporin** were significantly lower than levels in patients receiving only mycophenolate mofetil and prednisone.[7] In yet another study, 52 kidney transplant patients were treated with mycophenolate mofetil 1 g twice daily with **ciclosporin** and prednisone. Six months after transplantation 19 patients continued triple therapy, 19 discontinued **ciclosporin** and 14 discontinued prednisone. Three months later, patients in whom **ciclosporin** had been discontinued had higher trough mycophenolic acid levels compared to the other groups of patients. Discontinuing **ciclosporin** resulted in almost a doubling of mycophenolic acid trough levels.[8] Another study notes similar effects on mycophenolic acid levels,[9] and the problems of interpreting the results of studies comparing ciclosporin or tacrolimus with mycophenolate[10] are highlighted.[11,12] It was suggested that it could be interpreted that tacrolimus increases mycophenolic acid levels (see below) when the correct interpretation may be that ciclosporin decreases mycophenolic acid exposure.[11]

It has also been observed that the use of the triple therapy, steroids, and **ciclosporin** with mycophenolate mofetil rather than with azathioprine makes it possible to use a lower dose of **ciclosporin**.[13] Despite these alterations in the pharmacokinetics, the makers say that no pharmacokinetic interaction occurs with **ciclosporin**.[2]

(f) Colestyramine

Colestyramine 4 g three times daily for 4 days reduced the AUC of mycophenolic acid by 40% in a group of healthy subjects after taking a single 1.5 g oral dose of mycophenolate mofetil.[2] The clinical importance of this reduction has not been assessed but it would seem prudent to confirm that the immunosuppressant effects remain adequate in the presence of **colestyramine**.

(g) Contraceptives, oral

The makers say that no pharmacokinetic interaction was seen in a single-dose study between mycophenolate mofetil and *Orthonovum* (1 mg **norethisterone** + 35 micrograms **ethinylestradiol**) in 15 healthy women.[14] A study of the co-administration of mycophenolate mofetil 1 g twice daily and combined oral contraceptives (containing **ethinyl estradiol** 0.02 to 0.04 mg and **levonorgestrel** 0.05 to 0.15 mg, **desogestrel** 0.15 mg or **gestodene** 0.05 to 0.10 mg) in 18 non-transplant women (not on immunosuppressants) over 3 consecutive menstrual cycles showed no clinically relevant influence on the suppression of ovulation by the oral contraceptives.[2]

(h) Iron

A study in 7 healthy subjects found that a single dose of **ferrous sulfate** 1050 mg (210 elemental iron) reduced the AUC and maximum levels of mycophenolate mofetil by more than 90%. It is possible that a chelation complex is formed between mycophenolate mofetil and **iron** which reduces absorption. Concomitant administration of mycophenolate mofetil and **iron preparations** should be avoided.[15]

(i) Other miscellaneous drugs

The makers say that no pharmacokinetic interactions have been seen between mycophenolate mofetil and **co-trimoxazole** or intravenous **ganciclovir**.[2] A three way crossover study in 12 kidney transplant patients found no pharmacokinetic interaction between single 1500 mg oral doses of mycophenolate mofetil and intravenous **ganciclovir** (5 mg/kg) but renal clearance was slightly decreased.[16,17] However the makers point out that because these drugs act to inhibit nucleoside synthesis the possibility of some other pharmacodynamic interaction still cannot be excluded. Good monitoring would therefore be appropriate if any of these drugs is used.

A study in *monkeys* found that **probenecid** raised the AUC of the glucuronide metabolite of mycophenolate mofetil (MPAG) three-fold.[2] Whether this also happens in man is uncertain, as is the possible clinical importance of such an interaction, but it would seem prudent to monitor the outcome if **probenecid** is used concurrently.

A study in patients with rheumatoid arthritis found that the combination of **methotrexate** and mycophenolate mofetil was well-tolerated and there were no pharmacokinetic interactions.[18] There would appear to be no need for dose adjustments during concomitant administration in rheumatoid arthritis.

(j) Tacrolimus

A study in stable kidney transplant patients on long-term **tacrolimus** found that the addition of mycophenolate mofetil to their therapy resulted in a increase in the tacrolimus AUC, but this was not considered significant.[19] A 20% increase in tacrolimus levels is reported in a similar study in liver transplant patients.[2] The makers report that in one study in renal transplant patients receiving ciclosporin and mycophenolate mofetil, the AUC of mycophenolic acid increased by about 30% when ciclosporin was replaced by **tacrolimus**.[2] Similar results are reported elsewhere,[10,20] but this may be due to a reduction in mycophenolic acid levels by ciclosporin rather than an increase in levels due to **tacrolimus** (see (e) above). It is also possible that the increased levels are a factor of increased enterohepatic recirculation of mycophenolic acid.[2]

1. Shah J, Juan D, Bullingham R, Wong B, Wong R, Fu C. A single dose drug interaction study of mycophenolate mofetil and acyclovir in normal subjects. *J Clin Pharmacol* (1994) 34, 1029.
2. CellCept (Mycophenolate mofetil). Roche Product Limited. Summary of Product Characteristics, December 2001.
3. Jacobs F, Mamzer-Bruneel MF, Skhiri H, Thervet E, Legendre Ch, Kreis H. Safety of the mycophenolate mofetil-allopurinol combination in kidney transplant recipients with gout. *Transplantation* (1997) 64, 1087–8.
4. Syntex. Data on file (1994).
5. Sollinger HW. Mycophenolate mofetil for the prevention of acute rejection in primary care cadaveric renal allograft recipients. *Transplantation* (1995) 60, 225–32.
6. Weber SW, Keller F. Low mycophenolate predose levels with cyclosporine co-medication. *Kidney Blood Press Res* (1999) 22, 390.
7. Pou L, Brunet M, Cantarell C, Vidal E, Oppenheimer F, Monforte V, Vilardell J, Roman A, Martorell J, Capdevila L. Mycophenolic acid plasma concentrations: influence of co-medication. *Ther Drug Monit* (2001) 23, 35–8.

8. Gregoor PJ, de Sevaux RG, Hene RJ, Hesse CJ, Hilbrands LB, Vos P, van Gelder T, Hoitsma AJ, Weimar W. Effect of cyclosporine on mycophenolic acid trough levels in kidney transplant recipients. *Transplantation* (1999) 68, 1603–6.
9. Smak Gregoor PJ, Van Gelder T, Hesse CJ, van der Mast BJ, van Be NM, Weimar W. Mycophenolic acid plasma concentrations in kidney allograft recipients with or without cyclosporin: a cross-sectional study. *Nephrol Dial Transplant* (1999) 14, 706–8.
10. Hübner GI, Eismann R, Sziegoleit W. Drug interaction between mycophenolate mofetil and tacrolimus detectable within therapeutic mycophenolic acid monitoring in renal transplant patients. *Ther Drug Monit* (1999) 21, 536–9.
11. van Gelder T, Smak Gregoor PJH, Weimar W. Letter to the editor. *Ther Drug Monit* (2000) 22, 639.
12. Hübner GI, Sziegoleit W. Response to letter from van Gelder. *Ther Drug Monit* (2000) 22, 498–9.
13. Sanz Moreno C, Gomez Sanchez M, Fdez Fdez J, Botella J. Cyclosporine A (CsA) needs are reduced with substitution of azathioprine (Aza) by mycophenolate mofetil (MMF). *Nephrol Dial Transplant* (1998) 13, A260.
14. Syntex. Data on file. A single-dose pharmacokinetic drug interaction study of oral mycophenolate mofetil and an oral contraceptive in normal subjects. (Study No. MYCS2308) 1994.
15. Morii M, Ueno K, Ogawa A, Kato R, Yoshimura H, Wada K, Hashimoto H, Takeda M, Tanaka K, Nakatani T, Shibakawa M. Impairment of mycophenolate mofetil absorption by iron ion. *Clin Pharmacol Ther* (2000) 68, 613–16.
16. Wolfe EJ, Mathur VS, Tomlanovich S, Gaines K, Jung D, Wong R, Aweeka FT. Pharmacokinetic drug interaction study of mycophenolate mofetil and iv ganciclovir in renal transplant patients. *Clin Pharmacol Ther* (1995) 57, 148.
17. Wolfe EJ, Mathur V, Tomlanovich S, Jung D, Wong R, Griffy K, Aweeka FT. Pharmacokinetics of mycophenolate mofetil and intravenous ganciclovir alone and in combination in renal transplant recipients. *Pharmacotherapy* (1997) 17, 591–8.
18. Yocum D, Kremer J, Blackburn W, Caldwell J, Furst D, Nunez M, Zuzga J, Zeig S, Gutierrez M, Merrill J, Dumont E, B Leishman. Cellcept® (mycophenolate mofetil - MMF) and methotrexate (MTX) safety and pharmacokinetic (PK) interaction study in rheumatoid arthritis patients. *Arthritis Rheum* (1999) 42 (9 Suppl), S83.
19. Pirsch J, Bekersky I, Vincenti F, Boswell G, Woodle ES, Alak A, Kruelle M, Fass N, Facklam D, Mekki Q. Coadministration of tacrolimus and mycophenolate mofetil in stable kidney transplant patients: pharmacokinetics and tolerability. *J Clin Pharmacol* (2000) 40, 527–32.
20. Vidal E, Cantarell C, Capdevila L, Monforte V, Roman A, Pou L. Mycophenolate mofetil pharmacokinetics in transplant patients receiving cyclosporine or tacrolimus in combination therapy. *Pharmacol Toxicol* (2000) 87, 182–4.

Rituximab + Miscellaneous drugs

No adverse interactions have been reported with rituximab.

Clinical evidence, mechanism, importance and management

The makers report that there is virtually no data about possible interactions between rituximab and other drugs, but they say that no synergistic toxicity was seen in 40 patients when treated with rituximab combined with **CHOP** (**cyclophosphamide, doxorubicin, vincristine** and **prednisolone**).[1]

1. Mabthera (Rituximab). Roche Products Limited. Summary of product characteristics, March 2002.

Sirolimus + Miscellaneous drugs

Sirolimus serum levels are markedly raised by ketoconazole, moderately raised by diltiazem and markedly reduced by rifampicin. The makers recommend close monitoring with other inhibitors and inducers of cytochrome P450 isoenzyme CYP3A4. Ciclosporin raises sirolimus serum levels and possibly increases kidney toxicity, for which reason continued usage is not recommended. Sirolimus appears not to interact with oral contraceptives, and is reported not to interact to a clinically relevant extent with aciclovir, atorvastatin, co-trimoxazole, digoxin, fibrates, glibenclamide, methylprednisolone, nifedipine, prednisolone and statins.

Clinical evidence, mechanism, importance and management

(a) Ciclosporin

(i) Ciclosporin levels unchanged. A double-blind randomised study found that when sirolimus was added to a **ciclosporin**/corticosteroid regimen in kidney transplant patients, the steady-state **ciclosporin** levels remained unchanged and no differences were seen in blood pressures, glomerular filtration rates, creatinine values, triglyceride levels or serum enzymes (ALT, AST).[1] A 2-week pharmacokinetic study in 40 kidney transplant patients found that sirolimus (0.5 to 6.5 mg/m^2/12 h) did not affect the pharmacokinetics of **ciclosporin** (75 to 500 mg daily). The patients were also taking prednisone.[2] Two related studies in kidney transplant patients confirmed the absence of a sirolimus/**ciclosporin** interaction.[3] The makers also report that single doses of sirolimus were found not to affect the pharmacokinetics of microemulsion **ciclosporin** in healthy subjects when given 4 h apart.[4]

(ii) Sirolimus levels increased. Microemulsion **ciclosporin** given 4 h before sirolimus has been found to increase the maximum serum levels of the sirolimus 1.4-fold and to increase the AUC 1.8-fold, the reason being that **ciclosporin** inhibits the metabolism of sirolimus.[4]

The makers therefore recommend that sirolimus should be given 4 h after microemulsion **ciclosporin**.[4] However they also say that because higher serum creatinine levels and lower glomerular filtration rates have been seen with concurrent use, they do not recommend continued usage.[4] The makers say that if **ciclosporin** is withdrawn, the sirolimus dosage will need to be raised fourfold to take into account the absence of the interaction (twofold increase needed) and the need for increased immunosuppression (twofold increase needed). A target trough sirolimus level of 12 to 20 nanograms/ml (chromatographic assay) is recommended.[4]

(b) Contraceptives, oral

A single-dose clinical study found that the pharmacokinetics of an **oral contraceptive** (0.03 mg **ethinylestradiol** + 0.3 mg **norgestrel**) were unaffected by sirolimus. This suggests that the efficacy of the contraceptive is likely to be unchanged, but as the makers cautiously point out, the effects on oral contraception of using sirolimus long term are unknown.[4] But any interaction seems unlikely.

(c) Diltiazem

An open, three-period, randomised, crossover study in 18 healthy subjects found that a single 120-mg oral dose of **diltiazem** affected the pharmacokinetics of a single 10-mg oral dose of sirolimus. The maximum serum levels of the sirolimus increased by 43% and its AUC increased by 60%. The pharmacokinetics of the **diltiazem** and its metabolites were unchanged. The likely reason for this interaction is that the **diltiazem** inhibits the activity of cytochrome P450 isoenzyme CYP3A4 or P-glycoprotein in the gut so that the metabolism of the sirolimus is reduced and more is absorbed.[5]

This was a single dose study, but all the evidence suggests that this interaction will also occur with multiple doses of both drugs, for which reason the makers recommend whole blood monitoring and possible sirolimus dosage adjustment (a reduction) if **diltiazem** is used concurrently.[4] They do not say by how much but about 40% seems likely.

(d) Fibrates and Statins

There appear to be no reports of adverse reactions between the **fibrates** or **statins** and sirolimus, and the makers say that concurrent use is well tolerated, but they advise good monitoring.[4]

(e) Ketoconazole

A clinical study in 23 healthy subjects found that while taking multiple doses of **ketoconazole** (200 mg daily for 10 days), the maximum serum levels AUC following a single 5-mg dose of sirolimus were increased 4.3-fold and 10.9-fold respectively. The reason is believed to be that **ketoconazole** is a potent inhibitor of cytochrome P450 isoenzyme CYP3A4 which markedly reduces the metabolism of sirolimus, or possibly that it has some inhibitory action on P-glycoprotein, during absorption by the gut.[4,6]

The makers say that concurrent use is not recommended, but if the decision is made to use both drugs they suggest that the maintenance dose of sirolimus should initially be reduced to one-sixth, followed by trough sampling within 5 to 7 days. When the **ketoconazole** is withdrawn, the sirolimus dose should be gradually increased to the original maintenance dose.[4]

(f) Miscellaneous possible (?) interactions

The makers point out that sirolimus is extensively metabolised by cytochrome P450 isoenzyme CYP3A4 in the wall of the gut and by the multidrug efflux pump P-glycoprotein, so the possibility exists that interactions may occur with drugs which inhibit or induce their activity.[4] Enzyme inhibitors may raise sirolimus serum levels (**ketoconazole** described above (e) certainly does) and the makers list a number of others which also inhibit CYP3A4 which they think may possibly behave similarly. They list **cisapride, clotrimazole, clarithromycin, erythromycin, fluconazole, itraconazole, metoclopramide, nicardipine, troleandomycin** and **verapamil**.[4] Drugs which induce CYP3A4 have the opposite effect and are expected to lower sirolimus levels. **Rifampicin** does, (see (h) below), and the makers list a number of other enzyme inducers which they think may behave similarly: **carbamazepine, phenytoin, phenobarbital, rifabutin** and **St John's wort**.[4] These predictions are as yet unconfirmed, but it would certainly be prudent to monitor sirolimus' levels closely (a makers recommendation) if any of these drugs are used concurrently. What should be remembered is that the extent of the inhibitory or inducing effects of these drugs is not identical, so that very marked effects (like those observed with **ketoconazole** and **rifampicin**) may not occur, nevertheless the interaction may still be clinically important. **Grapefruit juice** inhibits CYP3A4 (potentially raising sirolimus' levels) so the makers recommendation is that it should be avoided.[4]

(g) Non-interacting drugs

The makers report that no clinically significant interactions have been observed with the following drugs: **aciclovir, atorvastatin, digoxin, glibenclamide, methylprednisolone, nifedipine, co-trimoxazole**.[4] **Nifedipine** has also been found not to interact.[2]

(h) Prednisolone

Only minor/moderate changes occurred in the pharmacokinetics of **prednisolone** (the active metabolite of prednisone) in a study in kidney transplant patients when ciclosporin, sirolimus and **prednisolone** were given concurrently (maximum serum levels +14%, AUC +18%).[7]

(i) Rifampicin.

A clinical study found that while taking multiple doses of **rifampicin**, the clearance of a single 10-mg oral dose of sirolimus was increased 5.5-fold, while the AUC and the maximum serum levels were reduced 82% and 71% respectively. The reason is that **rifampicin** is a potent inducer of cytochrome P450 isoenzyme CYP3A4 which markedly increases the metabolism and clearance of the sirolimus from the body.

The makers say that concurrent use is not recommended, but if the decision is made to use both drugs they suggest that the maintenance dose of sirolimus should initially be increased eightfold, followed by trough sampling within 5 to 7 days. When the **rifampicin** is withdrawn, the sirolimus dose should be gradually reduced to the original maintenance dose.[4]

1. Murgia MG, Jordan S, Kahan BD. The side effect profile of sirolimus: a phase I study in quiescent cyclosporine-prednisone-treated renal transplant patients. *Kidney Int* (1996) 49, 209-16.
2. Zimmerman JJ, Kahan BD. Pharmacokinetics of sirolimus in stable renal transplant patients after multiple oral dose administration. *J Clin Pharmacol* (1997) 37, 405–15.
3. Ferron GM, Mishina EV, Zimmerman JJ, Jusko WJ. Population pharmacokinetics of sirolimus in kidney transplant patients. *Clin Pharmacol Ther* (1997) 61, 416–28.
4. Rapamune (Sirolimus). Wyeth Laboratories. Summary of product characteristics, March 2001.
5. Böttinger Y, Säwe J, Brattström C, Tollemar J, Burke JT, Häss G, Zimmerman JJ. Pharmacokinetic interaction between single oral doses of diltiazem and sirolimus in healthy volunteers. *Clin Pharmacol Ther* (2001) 69, 32-40.
6. Floren LC, Christians U, Zimmerman JJ, Neefe L, Schorer R, Rushowrth D, Harper D, Renz J, Benet LZ. Sirolimus oral bioavailability increases ten-fold with concomitant ketoconazole. *Clin Pharmacol Ther* (1999) 65, 159.
7. Jusko WJ, Ferron GM, SM Mis, Kahan BD, Zimmerman JJ. Pharmacokinetics of prednisolone during administration of sirolimus in patients with renal transplants. *J Clin Pharmacol* (1996) 36, 1100–6.

Tacrolimus + Antacids

There is some *in vivo* and *in vitro* evidence that some antacids may possibly reduce the serum levels of tacrolimus, but the clinical importance of this awaits confirmation.

Clinical evidence, mechanism, importance and management

A very brief report in a review of the clinical pharmacokinetics of tacrolimus says, without giving details, that widely variable trough plasma tacrolimus levels have been seen in patients taking **sodium bicarbonate** close to the time when the tacrolimus was given, and coadministration of **sodium bicarbonate** results in lower blood concentrations of tacrolimus.[1] The advice is that if their administration is separated by at least 2 h, or the **sodium bicarbonate** is replaced by **sodium citrate** or **citric acid**, then stable trough serum tacrolimus levels are achieved.[1] The same 2 h separation has also been recommended[1] for **aluminium hydroxide gel** and **magnesium oxide** because *in vitro* studies have shown that they can cause a significant reduction in tacrolimus concentrations due to pH-mediated degradation.[2]

Study is needed to confirm and assess the extent and clinical importance of these interactions, but good monitoring would be appropriate if tacrolimus is given with any antacids, being alert for the need to separate the dosages as recommended.

1. Venkataramanan R, Swaminathan A, Prasad T, Jain A, Zuckerman S, Warty V, McMichael J, Lever J, Burckart G, Starzl T. Clinical pharmacokinetics of tacrolimus. *Clin Pharmacokinet* (1995) 29, 404–30.
2. Steeves M, Abdallah HY, Venkataramanan R, Burckart GT, Ptachcinski RJ, Abu-Elmagd K, Jain AK, Fung F, Todo S, Starzl TE. In-vitro interaction of a novel immunosuppressant, FK506, and antacids. *J Pharm Pharmacol* (1991) 43, 574–7.

Tacrolimus + Antidepressants

Marked increases in tacrolimus levels and toxicity were observed in two patients when also treated with nefazodone. Paroxetine and sertraline may not interact, but the situation is not clear.

Clinical evidence

A kidney transplant patient treated with tacrolimus 5 mg daily developed delirium and renal failure 4 weeks after starting to take **nefazodone** 150 mg daily. The level of the tacrolimus had risen about fivefold from a baseline level of 9.4 nanograms/ml some 3 months earlier (when he was on a dose of 6 mg daily) to a toxic level of 46.4 nanograms/ml (with a dose of 5 mg daily). His creatinine levels had doubled. The tacrolimus level fell to 29.6 nanograms/ml within 2 days of the dose being reduced to 3 mg daily. **Nefazodone** was then replaced by **paroxetine** 20 mg daily. After 3 days the tacrolimus dose was increased to 5 mg daily and satisfactory levels of 12.4 nanograms/ml were observed.[1] A renal transplant patient on prednisone, azathioprine and tacrolimus 5 mg daily for 2 years experienced headache, confusion and 'grey areas' in her vision within 1 week of starting **nefazodone** 50 mg twice daily in place of **sertraline** for depression. Her serum creatinine had risen from 1.5 to 2.2 mg/dl and a trough tacrolimus level was greater than 30 nanograms/ml. **Nefazodone** was replaced by **sertraline**, and tacrolimus was withheld for 4 days. Signs of tacrolimus-induced neurotoxicity disappeared within 36 hours and serum creatinine and tacrolimus levels returned to pretreatment levels within 2 weeks of stopping **nefazodone**.[2]

Mechanism

Both tacrolimus and nefazodone are metabolised by cytochrome P450 isoenzyme CYP3A4. Increased levels of tacrolimus may be due to inhibition of this isoenzyme by nefazodone. Paroxetine is a potent inhibitor of CYP2D6 with little effect on CYP3A4 and sertraline is primarily metabolised by CYP2C9 and CYP2D6 and so are unlikely to interact with tacrolimus.[1,2]

Importance and mechanism

Information appears to be limited but what is known indicates that coadministration of nefazodone and tacrolimus should be well monitored for evidence of increases in tacrolimus levels or signs of toxicity. In view of the narrow therapeutic index of tacrolimus, it may be advisable to avoid concurrent nefazodone. Paroxetine and sertraline may be a suitable alternative antidepressants, but the evidence is slim, so that additional monitoring may still be warranted.[1] Further study on the use of antidepressants with tacrolimus is needed.

1. Campo JV, Smith C, Perel JM. Tacrolimus toxic reaction associated with the use of nefazodone: paroxetine as an alternative agent. *Arch Gen Psychiatry* (1998) 55, 1050–1.

2. Olyaei AJ, deMattos AM, Norman DJ, Bennett WM. Interaction between tacrolimus and nefazodone in a stable renal transplant recipient. *Pharmacotherapy* (1998) 18, 1356–9.

Tacrolimus + Azole antifungals

Tacrolimus serum levels are considerably increased by oral fluconazole (but only minimally when given intravenously). The tacrolimus dosage will need to be halved to avoid the risk of nephrotoxicity. Preliminary information also suggests that precautions should be taken with clotrimazole, itraconazole and ketoconazole.

Clinical evidence

(a) Clotrimazole

The serum tacrolimus levels of a liver transplant patient on 6 mg daily rose from 3.5 to 5.6 nanograms/ml within a day of starting 10 mg **clotrimazole** four times daily, and to more than 9 nanograms/ml within 8 days. Later studies and rechallenge confirmed that the **clotrimazole** was responsible. The tacrolimus AUC was nearly doubled.[1]

(b) Fluconazole

Twenty organ transplant patients (11 livers, 6 kidneys, 2 hearts and one bone marrow) controlled with tacrolimus were additionally given 100 or 200 mg **fluconazole** daily for various fungal infections. On day 1 the median plasma trough levels of those given 100 mg **fluconazole** rose 1.4-fold, and in those on 200 mg it rose 3.1-fold. The dosage of the tacrolimus was reduced to accommodate this rise, the median dosage reduction being 56% (range 0 to 88%). The highest tacrolimus concentration was seen within 3 days. A pharmacokinetic study in one patient showed that when the **fluconazole** (100 mg daily) was stopped, the tacrolimus AUC fell from 13 to 5.4 nanograms/ml/h.[2]

Other studies in adult[3] and child patients[4] and individual case reports[5,6] have confirmed that the bioavailability of tacrolimus is increased by the concurrent use of oral **fluconazole**, increasing the risk of nephrotoxicity.[4] One study found that if the **fluconazole** is given intravenously, the steady-state levels of tacrolimus are only slightly increased (about 16%) which was considered to be clinically unimportant.[7]

A bone-marrow transplant patient on tacrolimus given **fluconazole** for oral candidiasis experienced headache and was found to have glycosuria, increased serum creatinine and Pelger-Huet anomaly of granulocytes, which disappeared after tacrolimus was discontinued. The effects were thought to be due to tacrolimus toxicity due to an interaction with **fluconazole**.[8]

(c) Itraconazole

Trough blood levels of tacrolimus in a heart-lung transplant patient increased threefold from 16 to 57 nanograms/ml and serum creatinine levels also rose after she was additionally given **itraconazole** 200 mg daily.[9] A renal transplant recipient on tacrolimus 6 mg daily was given **itraconazole** 100 mg twice daily for a urinary candida infection. Within a day, tacrolimus trough levels increased from 12.6 to 21 nanograms/ml and the tacrolimus dose was progressively reduced to 3 mg daily. Four days after **itraconazole** was discontinued tacrolimus had to be progressively increased to its initial dose.[10] The interaction has been reported in three other renal transplant recipients.[11-13]

(d) Ketoconazole

The addition of **ketoconazole** 200 mg daily to tacrolimus and prednisone in a renal transplant patient resulted in an increase in tacrolimus blood levels from 11.1 to 27.9 nanograms/ml, despite a 45% decrease in the dose of tacrolimus. Eventually the dose of tacrolimus had to be reduced by 80% to keep the levels within the therapeutic range. Tacrolimus levels decreased to 5.8 nanograms/ml within a week of discontinuing **fluconazole** and so the dose was raised.[14] A pharmacokinetic study in 6 healthy subjects found that 200 mg **ketoconazole** orally at bedtime for 12 days increased the bioavailability of single doses of 0.1 mg/kg oral tacrolimus from 14% to 30%.[15]

Mechanism

Not fully established but the evidence available suggests that fluconazole, itraconazole and ketoconazole inhibit the metabolism of the tacrolimus by the gut wall (by CYP3A4), and/or inhibit the activity of P-glycoprotein so that more is absorbed.[7,10,15] Other azoles probably do the same.

Importance and management

Information is limited but the tacrolimus/fluconazole interaction appears to be established, clinically important and can develop rapidly (within 3 days). The authors of one of the reports say that up to 200 mg oral fluconazole daily can be used safely and effectively provided the tacrolimus dosage is reduced by half.[2] If the fluconazole is given intravenously no clinically important interaction occurs.[7]

Information about the tacrolimus/clotrimazole, tacrolimus/itraconazole and the tacrolimus/ketoconazole interactions is also limited (seen also with in *rats*[16]) but on the basis these reports it would be prudent to follow the precautions suggested for fluconazole.

In vitro studies with human liver microsomes have shown that **miconazole**[17] also inhibits liver and small intestine microsomes which metabolize tacrolimus and it seems possible that it may interact just like fluconazole but this needs confirmation. No interaction would be expected if used topically.

1. Mieles L, Venkataramanan R, Yokoyama I, Warty VJ, Starzl TE. Interaction between FK506 and clotrimazole in a liver transplant recipient. *Transplantation* (1991) 52, 1086–7.

2. Mañez R, Martin M, Raman V, Silverman D, Jain A, Warty V, Gonzalez-Pinto I, Kusne S, Starzl TE. Fluconazole therapy in transplant recipients receiving FK506. *Transplantation* (1994) 57, 1521–23.

3. Toy S, Tata P, Jain A, Patsy K, Lever J, Burckart G, Warty V, Kusne S, Abu-Elmagd K, Fung J, Starzi T, Venkataramanan R. A pharmacokinetic interaction between tacrolimus and fluconazole. *Pharm Res* (1996) 13 (9 Suppl), S435.

4. Vincent I, Furlan V, Debray D, Jacquemin E, Taburet AM. Effects of antifungal agents on the pharmacokinetics and nephrotoxicity of FK506 in paediatric liver transplant recipients. *Intersci Conf Antimicrob Agents Chemother* (1995) 35, 5.

5. Assan R, Fredj G, Larger E, Feutren G, Bismuth H. FK 506/fluconazole interaction enhances FK506 nephrotoxicity. *Diabete Metab* (1994) 20, 49–52.

6. Chamorey E, Nouveau B, Viard L, Garcia-Credoz F, Durand A, Pisano P. Interaction tacrolimus-fluconazole chez un enfant transplanté coeur-poumons. A propos d'un cas clinique. *J Pharm Clin* (1998) 17, 51–3.

7. Osowski CL, Dix SP, Lin LS, Mullins RE, Geller RB, Wingard JR. Evaluation of the drug interaction between intravenous high-dose fluconazole and cyclosporine or tacrolimus in bone marrow transplant patients. *Transplantation* (1996) 61, 1268–72.

8. Gondo H, Okamura C, Osaki K, Shimoda K, Asano Y, Okamura T. Acquired Pelger-Huet anomaly in association with concomitant tacrolimus and fluconazole therapy following allogenic bone marrow transplantation. *Bone Marrow Transplant* (2000) 26, 1255–7.

9. Furlan V, Parquin F, Penaud JF, Cerrina J, Le Roy Ladurie F, Dartevelle P, Taburet AM. Interaction between tacrolimus and itraconazole in a heart-lung transplant recipient. *Transplant Proc* (1998) 30, 187–8.

10. Capone D, Gentile A, Imperatore P, Palmiero G, Basile V. Effects of itraconazole on tacrolimus blood concentrations in a renal transplant recipient. *Ann Pharmacother* (1999) 33, 1124–5.

11. Katari SR, Magnone M, Shapiro R, Jordan M, Scantlebury V, Vivas C, Gritsch A, McCauley J, Demetris AJ, Randhawa PS. Clinical features of acute reversible tacrolimus (FK506) nephrotoxicity in kidney transplant recipients. *Clin Transplant* (1997) 11, 237–42.

12. Macías MO, Salvador P, Hurtado JL, Martín I. Tacrolimus-itraconazole interaction in a kidney transplant patient. *Ann Pharmacother* (2000) 34, 536.

13. Ideura T, Muramatsu T, Higuchi M, Tachibana N, Hora K, Kiyosawa K. Tacrolimus/itraconazole interactions: a case report of ABO-incompatible living-related renal transplantation. *Nephrol Dial Transplant* (2000) 15, 1721–3.

14. Moreno M, Latorre C, Manzanares C, Morales E, Herrero JC, Dominguez-Gil B, Carreño A, Cubas A, Delgado M, Andres A, Morales JM. Clinical management of tacrolimus drug interactions in renal transplant patients. *Transplant Proc* (1999) 31, 2252–3.

15. Floren LC, Bekersky I, Benet LZ, Mekki Q, Dressler D, Lee JW, Roberts JP, Hebert MF. Tacrolimus oral bioavailability doubles with coadministration of ketoconazole. *Clin Pharmacol Ther* (1997) 62, 41–9.

16. Prasad TNV, Stiff DD, Subbotina N, Zemaitis MA, Burckart GJ, Starzl TE, Venkataramanan R. FK506 (tacrolimus) metabolism by rat liver microsomes and its inhibition by other drugs. *Res Commun Chem Pathol Pharmacol* (1994) 84, 35–46.

17. Christians U, Schmidt G, Bader A, Lampen A, Schottmann R, Linck A, Sewing K-F. Identification of drugs inhibiting the *in vitro* metabolism of tacrolimus by human liver microsomes. *Br J Clin Pharmacol* (1996) 41, 187–90.

Tacrolimus + Calcium channel blockers

Nifedipine, and possibly diltiazem, causes a moderate rise in serum tacrolimus levels and also appears to be kidney protective.

Clinical evidence

(a) Diltiazem

The trough blood levels of tacrolimus in a liver transplant patient stabilised on tacrolimus 8 mg twice daily increased from 12.9 to 55 nanograms/ml within 3 days of starting **diltiazem** (initially 5 to 10 mg/h intravenously for one day, then 30 mg orally every 8 h). The patient became delirious, confused and agitated. Both drugs were stopped, and over the next 3 days his mental state improved and his tacrolimus levels fell to 6.7 nanograms/ml. Tacrolimus was then restarted, gradually increasing to a dose of 5 mg twice daily, which produced levels of 9 to 10 nanograms/ml.[1] However, a study in 7 liver transplant patients given tacrolimus 0.1 mg/kg twice daily found that 90 mg of modified release **diltiazem** given daily did not significantly alter the absorption or metabolism of tacrolimus when compared to 7 similar patients not given **diltiazem**.[2]

(b) Nifedipine

A 1-year retrospective study of two groups of liver transplant patients found that in those (22 patients) taking **nifedipine** (30 or 60 mg daily) there was a 55% increase in the serum tacrolimus levels after 1 month. The cumulative dosage reduction of the tacrolimus by 6 months was 25.5% in the **nifedipine** group and by 12 months it was 31.4% when compared with the no-nifedipine group. The **nifedipine** group showed improved kidney function (lowered serum creatinine).[3]

Mechanism

Uncertain, but it seems likely that the nifedipine and possibly diltiazem inhibit the cytochrome P450 isoenzyme CYP3A4 and P-glycoprotein, thereby reducing the metabolism of tacrolimus leading to increased serum levels.[1,3] This is consistent with the findings of an *in vitro* study using human liver microsomes.[4]

Importance and management

In the case of nifedipine, this seems to be an established and clinically important interaction. If nifedipine is added to a tacrolimus regimen the serum levels should be well monitored and the tacrolimus dosage reduced appropriately. Currently the information about diltiazem is conflicting. Information about other calcium channel blockers appears to be lacking.

1. Hebert MF, Lam AY. Diltiazem increases tacrolimus concentrations. *Ann Pharmacother* (1999) 33, 680–2.

2. Teperman L, Turgut S, Negron C, John D, Diflo T, Morgan G, Tobias H. Diltiazem is a safe drug in transplant patients on Prograf and does not affect Prograf levels. *Hepatology* (1996) 24, 180A.

3. Seifeldin RA, Marcos-Alvarez A, Gordon FD, Lewis WD, Jenkins RL. Nifedipine interaction with tacrolimus in liver transplant recipients. *Ann Pharmacother* (1997) 31, 571–5.

4. Iwasaki K, Matsuda H, Nagase K, Shiraga T, Tokuma Y, Uchida K. Effects of twenty-three drugs on the metabolism of FK506 by human liver microsomes. *Res Commun Chem Pathol Pharmacol* (1993) 82, 209–16.

Tacrolimus + Chloramphenicol

A marked rise in serum tacrolimus levels has been reported in one patient when treated with systemic chloramphenicol. This is expected to be an interaction of general importance.

Clinical evidence, mechanism, importance and management

An adolescent patient with a kidney transplant developed toxic tacrolimus levels on the second day of starting **chloramphenicol** for the treatment of a vancomycin-resistant enterococcal infection. The tacrolimus dosage had to be reduced by 83% to achieve safe serum levels, and it was found that the dose-adjusted tacrolimus AUC was 7.5-fold greater while taking the **chloramphenicol**. Another report describes a similar interaction in a

liver transplant patient on tacrolimus 4 mg twice daily. The patient was given intravenous **chloramphenicol**, but at the unintentionally high dose of 1850 mg every 6 hours. After about 3 days the patient complained of lethargy, fatigue, headaches and tremors so both drugs were stopped. His tacrolimus trough concentration had increased from around 9 to 11 nanograms/ml to more than 60 nanograms/ml. Seven days later his tacrolimus level was 8.2 nanograms/ml and his symptoms had resolved.[1] The reason for the raised tacrolimus levels is thought to be that the **chloramphenicol** (a known and potent enzyme inhibitor) rapidly reduced the metabolism of the tacrolimus.[2]

These appear to be the only reports of this interaction, but it is consistent with the known metabolic characteristics of both drugs and therefore it is expected to be an interaction of general importance. Monitor the outcome closely if systemic **chloramphenicol** is added to the regimen of any patient, being alert for the need to reduce the tacrolimus dosage. It seems doubtful if a clinically relevant interaction will occur with topical **chloramphenicol** because the dosage and the systemic absorption is small, but this needs confirmation.

1. Taber DJ, Dupuis RE, Hollar KD, Strzalka AL, Johnson MW. Drug-drug interaction between chloramphenicol and tacrolimus in a liver transplant recipient. *Transplant Proc* (2000) 32, 660–62.

2. Schulman SL, Shaw LM, Jabs K, Leonard MB, Brayman KL. Interaction between tacrolimus and chloramphenicol in a renal transplant recipient. *Transplantation* (1998) 65, 1397–8.

Tacrolimus + Grapefruit juice

Grapefruit juice can markedly increase the serum levels of tacrolimus.

Clinical evidence, mechanism, importance and management

Eight liver transplant patients were given 12 oz (about 360 ml of **grapefruit juice** twice daily, which they drank within 45 min of taking their dose of tacrolimus. After a week it was found that their 12 h trough, 1 h and 4 h tacrolimus levels were raised 300%, 195% and 400% respectively. Two patients had headaches, one had diarrhoea and one had an increased creatinine level that reversed, but none of the 12 developed rejection or irreversible toxicity. Two of the patients remained on the **grapefruit juice** and it was possible to halve their tacrolimus dosage.[1]

The reason for the rise in tacrolimus levels is not known, but it seems likely that it is due to inhibition of the metabolism of tacrolimus by some component of **grapefruit juice**. In practical terms the authors of the report suggest that this interaction means that the dosage of tacrolimus can possibly be reduced (to save money) although there is a clear need to monitor the effects closely because of the difficulties of standardising **grapefruit juice**. More study is needed.

1. Westveer MK, Farquhar ML, George P, Mayes JT. Co-administration of grapefruit juice increases tacrolimus levels in liver transplant patients. Proceedings of the 15th Annual Meeting of the American Society of Transplant Physicians 1996. Abstract P-115.

Tacrolimus + Ibuprofen

Two liver transplant patients on tacrolimus developed acute renal failure after taking ibuprofen.

Clinical evidence, mechanism, importance and management

Two patients with liver transplants on tacrolimus developed acute but reversible renal failure, one after taking four *Motrin* (**ibuprofen**) tablets — dosage not stated — and the other after three 400-mg tablets of **ibuprofen** over 24 h. Both had stable renal function but some hepatic dysfunction before taking the **ibuprofen** which may have contributed to the problem. It is not clear why this adverse reaction developed but one suggestion is that the **ibuprofen**, like other NSAIDs, inhibits the production of vasodilatory prostaglandins on which good renal blood flow depends. The authors of the report say that if renal toxicity develops, the tacrolimus should be withdrawn and prostaglandin therapy started. They used intravenous PGE1 effectively in one patient. They also suggest that NSAIDs should not be given to patients on tacrolimus, especially if it is being used as rescue therapy for abnormal graft function.[1] There seems as yet to be nothing documented about adverse interactions with other NSAIDs but if the suggested mechanism is true, they may possibly behave like **ibuprofen**.

1. Sheiner PA, Mor E, Chodoff L, Glabman S, Emre S, Schwartz ME, Miller CM. Acute renal failure associated with the use of ibuprofen in two liver transplant recipients on FK506. *Transplantation* (1994) 57, 1132–3.

Tacrolimus + Macrolide antibacterials

Five patients have shown marked increases in serum tacrolimus levels accompanied by evidence of renal toxicity when treated with erythromycin. The same interaction has been seen in three patients given clarithromycin, possibly also with josamycin and is predicted with troleandomycin, but not azithromycin.

Clinical evidence

(a) Clarithromycin

A woman with a kidney transplant and taking tacrolimus, prednisone and azathioprine was started on **clarithromycin** (500 mg twice daily for 4 days, then 250 mg daily) to treat a severe *M. pneumoniae* infection. Despite a 64% reduction in the dosage of the tacrolimus, the trough tacrolimus concentrations rose sharply (from 2.8 to 36.1 nanograms/ml by day 6) and creatinine levels climbed from 3.5 to 5 mg.dl[-1]. The tacrolimus dosage was further reduced and then stopped, and not restarted until the **clarithromycin** treatment was over.[1] In another 2 kidney transplant patients, tacrolimus levels increased by 146% and 131% respectively following 9 doses of **clarithromycin** 250 mg. Creatinine levels increased by 91% and 30% respectively.[2]

(b) Erythromycin

A liver transplant patient on 6 mg tacrolimus twice daily for a year showed a marked rise in serum tacrolimus levels (from about 1.4 to 6.5 nanomol/l) when ampicillin/sulbactam (3 g intravenously 6-hourly) and **erythromycin** (250 mg orally 6-hourly) were given for 4 days to treat pneumonia, accompanied by signs of kidney toxicity (increased blood urea and creatinine levels). The **erythromycin** was stopped, and the next day the tacrolimus was stopped as well. Over the next week the serum levels of the tacrolimus, blood urea nitrogen and creatinine fell once again.[3]

A kidney transplant patient showed an increase in his serum tacrolimus levels from 1.3 to 8.5 nanograms/ml four days after starting 400 mg **erythromycin** four times a day. His serum creatinine levels almost doubled.[4] A man with a kidney transplant showed a sixfold rise in serum tacrolimus levels when treated with **erythromycin**.[5] Two children aged 3 and 7 also showed rises in serum tacrolimus levels which was accompanied by renal toxicity when **erythromycin** was added.[6]

(c) Josamycin

The makers of tacrolimus suggest that **josamycin** may increase serum tacrolimus levels, but no details are given.[7]

Mechanism

Tacrolimus inhibits the same P450 isoenzymes (CYP3A) in the liver that are involved with the metabolism of erythromycin and clarithromycin so that it is possible that competition could occur, leading to a reduction in the clearance of the tacrolimus. See also the final paragraph of 'Importance and management' below.

Importance and management

Direct information seems to be limited to these case reports, however it would now be prudent to monitor closely the effects of adding clarithromycin or erythromycin in any patient, being alert for the need to reduce the tacrolimus dosage to avoid nephrotoxicity. The same precautions would also be appropriate with **troleandomycin (triacetyloleandomycin)** and possibly most other macrolide antibacterials , for example josamycin, although they do not all behave identically.

It has been suggested that **azithromycin** is less likely to interact with tacrolimus because it has a 15-, not a 14-membered macrocyclic lactone ring structure like clarithromycin and erythromycin, and unlike these two macrolides does not form inactive complexes with cytochrome CYP3A isoenzymes.[8] This prediction awaits clinical confirmation.

1. Wolter K, Wagner K, Philipp T, Fritschka E. Interaction between FK 506 and clarithromycin in a renal transplant patient. *Eur J Clin Pharmacol* (1994) 47, 207–8.
2. Gómez G, Álvarez ML, Errasti P, Lavilla FJ, García N, Ballester B, García I, Purroy A. Acute tacrolimus nephrotoxicity in renal transplant patients treated with clarithromycin. *Transplant Proc* (1999) 31, 2250–1.
3. Shaeffer MS, Collier D, Sorrell MF. Interaction between FK506 and erythromycin. *Ann Pharmacother* (1994) 28, 280–1.
4. Jensen C, Jordan M, Shapiro R, Scantlebury V, Hakala T, Fung J, Staszrl T, Venkataramanan R. Interaction between tacrolimus and erythromycin. *Lancet* (1994) 344, 825.
5. Padhi ID, Long P, Basha M, Anandan JV. Interaction between tacrolimus and erythromycin. *Ther Drug Monit* (1997) 19, 120–2.
6. Furlan V, Perello L, Jacquemin E, Debray D, Taburet A-M. Interactions between FK506 and rifampicin or erythromycin in pediatric liver recipients. *Transplantation* (1995) 59, 1217–18.
7. Prograf (Tacrolimus). Fujisawa Limited. Summary of product characteristics, June 2002.
8. Paterson DL, Singh N. Interactions between tacrolimus and antimicrobial agents. *Clin Infect Dis* (1997) 25, 1430–40.

Tacrolimus + Miscellaneous drugs

The makers say that tacrolimus and ciclosporin should not be used concurrently because of the increased risk of kidney damage. The effects of methylprednisolone on tacrolimus are uncertain. Tacrolimus is metabolised by the cytochrome P450 isoenzyme CYP3A4, the induction and inhibition of which may affect the serum levels of tacrolimus. The makers issue warnings about the concurrent use of live attenuated vaccines, amphotericin and potassium-sparing diuretics.
See the index for a full listing of other tacrolimus interactions.

Clinical evidence, mechanism, importance and management

(a) Ciclosporin (Cyclosporin)

One study found that, in patients with normal bilirubin levels, the half-life of **ciclosporin (cyclosporin)** was prolonged from a range of 6–15 h to 26–74 h and the **ciclosporin** serum levels were raised by tacrolimus, measured by a fluorescent polarisation immunoassay.[1] On the other hand another study found no changes in the pharmacokinetics of **ciclosporin** as measured by HPLC in patients given tacrolimus, but creatinine levels were almost doubled (suggesting kidney damage)[2] which confirmed a previous report suggesting that severe renal dysfunction may develop.[3] The suggestion is that tacrolimus inhibits **ciclosporin** metabolism or its absorption.[1] The makers of tacrolimus say that it should not be co-administered with **ciclosporin** because of the risk of additive/synergistic nephrotoxicity, and if **ciclosporin** is being replaced by tacrolimus 12 to 24 h should elapse between stopping one and starting the other.[4]

(b) Corticosteroids

Tacrolimus appears to potentiate the actions of glucocorticoids by preventing their degradation.[5] Tacrolimus serum levels are said to have been increased on 10 occasions by **methylprednisolone**, decreased on 5 occasions, and unaltered on 2 out of a total of 17 occasions.[1]

(c) Other drugs

In vitro studies with *rat* and human liver microsomes have found that tacrolimus is extensively metabolised by the cytochrome P450 isoenzyme CYP3A4.[6,7] This means that drugs which inhibit or induce CYP3A4 may potentially increase or reduce the serum levels of tacrolimus. In addition tacrolimus also has an inhibitory effect on CYP3A4 so that other drugs may possibly be affected by the presence of tacrolimus. However, a report about a child who had shown an interaction with **erythromycin** (attributed to its inhibitory effect on CYP3A) apparently showed no clear interaction with **phenobarbital** (**phenobarbitone**),[8] which normally induces CYP3A4. However, the dose of **phenobarbital** was not stated.

The makers say that vaccination may be less effective in the presence of tacrolimus, and they advise the avoidance of **live attenuated vaccines**.[4] They also say that enhanced nephrotoxicity has been seen with **amphotericin** and warn about the possible risks of hyperkalaemia due to the additive effects on serum potassium levels of **potassium-sparing diuretics**.[4]

1. Venkataramanan R, Jain A, Cadoff E, Warty V, Iwasaki K, Nagase K, Krajack A, Imventarza O, Todo S, Fung JJ, Starzl TE. Pharmacokinetics of FK 506: preclinical and clinical studies. *Transplant Proc* (1990) 22 (Suppl 1), 52–6.
2. Jain AB, Venkataramanan R, Fung J, Burckart G, Emeigh J, Diven W, Warty V, Abu-Elmagd K, Todo S, Alessiani M, Starzl TE. Pharmacokinetics of cyclosporine and nephrotoxicity in orthoptic liver transplant patients rescued with FK 506. *Transplant Proc* (1991) 23, 2777–9.
3. McCauley J, Fung J, Jain A, Todo S, Starzl TE. The effects of FK506 on renal function after liver transplantation. *Transplant Proc* (1990) 22 (Suppl 1), 17–20.
4. Prograf (Tacrolimus). Fujisawa Limited. Summary of product characteristics, June 2002.
5. Thomson AW, Bonham CA, Zeevi A. Mode of action of tacrolimus (FK506): molecular and cellular mechanisms. *Ther Drug Monit* (1995) 17, 584–91.
6. Shah IA, Whiting PH, Omar G, Thomson AW, Burke MD. Effects of FK 506 on human microsomal cytochrome P–450–dependent drug metabolism in vitro. *Transplant Proc* (1991) 23, 2783–5.
7. Pichard L, Fabre I, Domergue J, Joyeux H, Maurel P. Effect of FK 506 on human hepatic cytochromes P–450: interaction with CyA. *Transplant Proc* (1991) 23, 2791–3.
8. Furlan V, Perello L, Jacquemin E, Debray D, Taburet A-M. Interactions between FK506 and rifampicin or erythromycin in pediatric liver recipients. *Transplantation* (1995) 59, 1217–18.

Tacrolimus + Nucleoside reverse transcriptase inhibitors and Protease inhibitors

Protease inhibitors including nelfinavir, ritonavir and saquinavir inhibit the metabolism of tacrolimus and increase its blood levels. Nucleoside reverse transcriptase inhibitors such as didanosine, stavudine and lamivudine appear not to interact with tacrolimus.

Clinical evidence, mechanism, importance and management

An HIV+ patient infected with the hepatitis C virus who received a liver transplant was treated with antiviral therapy consisting of **stavudine** 30 mg, and **lamivudine** 150 mg, both twice daily, and **nelfinavir** 500 mg three times daily. Tacrolimus 6 mg daily was started

postoperatively but high blood levels were observed and the dose was reduced over the next 3 months to a maintenance dose of 0.5 mg weekly to achieve levels of between 7 and 25.9 nanograms/ml.[1] There is another report of a similar patient. Without antiviral treatment his tacrolimus level, while taking 4 mg twice daily was 10.9 nanograms/ml. When on a combination of **nelfinavir**, **stavudine** and **didanosine**, tacrolimus 0.5 mg daily produced a tacrolimus level of 23.7 nanograms/ml. When his antivirals were changed to **saquinavir**, **ritonavir**, **stavudine** and **lamivudine**, tacrolimus 1 mg twice daily resulted in tacrolimus levels in excess of 120 nanograms/ml with severe prolonged toxicity. After stabilisation of the patient, **nelfinavir**, **stavudine** and **lamivudine** were restarted. A tacrolimus dose of 0.5 mg every 3 to 5 days produced satisfactory trough tacrolimus levels of 4 to 10 nanograms/ml.[2]

Mechanism

Stavudine, lamivudine and didanosine (all nucleoside reverse transcriptase inhibitors) are mainly excreted through the kidney and are unlikely to affect levels of tacrolimus. Nelfinavir, ritonavir and saquinavir (all protease inhibitors) bind strongly to cytochrome P450 CYP3A isoenzymes. Tacrolimus is metabolised by CYP3A and its metabolites are excreted in the bile. It therefore seems likely that the protease inhibitors reduced tacrolimus metabolism resulting in the extremely high levels seen.[2]

Importance and management

An established and clinically important interaction. It is advised that when protease inhibitors are given to patients taking tacrolimus, careful monitoring and a reduction in the dose of tacrolimus is required. Nucleoside reverse transcriptase inhibitors are unlikely to contribute to the interaction.[2]

1. Schvarcz R, Rudbeck G, Söderdahl G, Ståhle L. Interaction between nelfinavir and tacrolimus after orthoptic liver transplantation in a patient coinfected with HIV and hepatitis C virus (HCV). *Transplantation* (2000) 69, 2194–5.
2. Sheikh AM, Wolf DC, Lebovics E, Goldberg R, Horowitz HW. Concomitant human immunodeficiency virus protease inhibitor therapy markedly reduces tacrolimus metabolism and increases blood levels. *Transplantation* (1999) 68, 307–9.

Tacrolimus + Quinolone antibacterials

No adverse interactions appear to occur between tacrolimus and the quinolone antibacterials.

Clinical evidence, mechanism, importance and management

There seem to be no reports of clinically significant interactions between tacrolimus and the **quinolone antibacterials**. No changes in the metabolism of tacrolimus would be expected because **enoxacin**, the quinolone with the greatest effect on cytochrome P450 isoenzymes, has been found in *in vitro* studies to have almost no effect on tacrolimus metabolism by the cytochrome P450 isoenzyme CYP3A4.[1] Nor, despite some changes in interleukin-2 production caused by **ciprofloxacin**, does there appear to be a clinically relevant immunological interaction which would oppose the immunosuppressant activity of tacrolimus.[2]

On the basis of some quite unexpected rises and subsequent nephrotoxicity in a handful of patients treated with another immunosuppressant, ciclosporin (cyclosporin) and quinolone antibacterials (ciprofloxacin or norfloxacin), one well-informed review suggested that good monitoring would be appropriate if tacrolimus is given with any quinolone.[3]

Later evidence, from a study in 5 kidney transplant patients,[4] which showed that **levofloxacin** 500 mg twice daily for 5 days caused about a 25% increase in the $AUC_{0-12\,h}$ and a 18% increase in the trough tacrolimus level would seem to support this advice.

1. Iwasaki K, Matsuda H, Nagase K, Shiraga T, Tokuma Y, Uchida K. Effects of twenty-three drugs on the metabolism of FK506 by human liver microsomes. *Res Commun Chem Pathol Pharmacol* (1993) 82, 209–16.

2. Kelly PA, Burckart GJ, Anderson D, Shaprio R, Zeevi A. Ciprofloxacin does not block the antiproliferative effect of tacrolimus. *Transplantation* (1997) 63, 172–3.

3. Petersen DL, Singh N. Interactions between tacrolimus and antimicrobial agents. *Clin Infect Dis* (1997) 25, 1430–40.

4. Capone D, Carrano R, Gentile A, Palmiero G, Farella A, Andreucci VE, Basile V, Federico S. Pharmacokinetic interaction between tacrolimus and levofloxacin in kidney transplant recipients. *Nephrol Dial Transplant* (2001) 16, A207.

3. Kiuchi T, Tanaka K, Inomata Y, Uemoto S, Satomura K, Egawa H, Uyama S, Sano K, Okajima H, Yamaoka Y. Experience of tacrolimus-based immunosuppression in a living-related liver transplantation complicated with graft tuberculosis: interaction with rifampicin and side effects. *Transplant Proc* (1996) 28, 3171–2.

4. Chenhsu R-Y, Loong C-C, Chou M-H, Lin M-F, Yang W-C. Renal allograft dysfunction associated with rifampin-tacrolimus interaction. *Ann Pharmacother* (2000) 34, 27–31.

5. Hebert MF, Fisher RM, Marsh CL, Dressler D, Bekersky I. Effects of rifampin on tacrolimus pharmacokinetics in healthy volunteers. *J Clin Pharmacol* (1999) 39, 91–6.

Tacrolimus + Rifampicin (Rifampin) or Rifabutin

Four liver transplant patients needed markedly increased tacrolimus dosages when rifampicin was added, and a pharmacokinetic study has shown rifampicin increases the clearance and decreases the bioavailability of tacrolimus. Rifabutin is unlikely to interact to the same extent, but given the magnitude of the interaction with rifampicin, caution is still warranted.

Clinical evidence

The trough serum tacrolimus concentrations of a 10-year-old boy with a liver transplant fell from 10 nanograms/ml to unmeasurable levels within two days of starting 150 mg **rifampicin** (**rifampin**) twice daily. His tacrolimus dosage was therefore doubled from 4 to 8 mg twice daily. When the **rifampicin** was later stopped the tacrolimus dosage had to be reduced to 3 mg twice daily to keep the serum levels within the 10 nanogram/ml range.[1] An extremely marked reduction in serum tacrolimus levels occurred in another child (aged 10 months) with a liver transplant when **rifampicin** was added to treatment with tacrolimus. Tacrolimus levels fell to about a tenth of base-line levels.[2] This case has also been reported elsewhere.[3] In another case, this time in an adult, a tenfold increase in tacrolimus dosage was needed to keep levels within the target range when rifampicin was started. However, despite levels with the acceptable range a biopsy showed suspected tacrolimus nephrotoxicity, which was considered to be possibly due to the cumulative tacrolimus dose, or to high levels of tacrolimus metabolites (which were not measured).[4] A study in 6 healthy subjects supports the findings of these case reports. In the study, administration of **rifampicin** 600 mg daily significantly increased the clearance and decreased the bioavailability of both oral and intravenous tacrolimus.[5]

Mechanism

The reason is thought to be that the **rifampicin** increases the metabolism of the tacrolimus by the liver and in the small bowel (by inducing cytochrome CYP3A4 and P-glycoprotein) so that it is cleared more rapidly.

Importance and management

What occurred in these reports is consistent with the way rifampicin interacts with many other drugs and therefore this interaction would seem to be of general clinical importance. It would be prudent to be alert for the need to raise the dosage of tacrolimus if rifampicin is added in any patient.

Direct information about **rifabutin** seems to be lacking, but any interaction with tacrolimus is likely to much less marked than with rifampicin because its enzyme inhibitory effects are considerably less. Nevertheless until the situation is clear it would be prudent to monitor concurrent use, being alert for the need to raise the tacrolimus dosage.

1. Furlan V, Perello L, Jacquemin E, Debray D, Taburet A-M. Interactions between FK506 and rifampicin or erythromycin in pediatric liver recipients. *Transplantation* (1995) 59, 1217–18.

2. Kiuchi T, Inomata Y, Uemoto S, Satomura K, Egawa H, Okajima H, Yamaoka Y, Tanaka K. A hepatic graft tuberculosis transmitted from a living-related donor. *Transplantation* (1997) 63, 905–7.

Tacrolimus + Sex hormones or related drugs

An isolated report describes an increase in tacrolimus levels in a patient when given danazol. Ethinyloestradiol has also been seen to raise tacrolimus levels. Because tacrolimus has the potential to interfere with the metabolism of oral contraceptives the makers of tacrolimus suggest using other forms of contraception.

Clinical evidence, mechanism, importance and management

(a) Danazol

The serum tacrolimus levels of a kidney transplant patient on 10 mg daily rose from 0.7 to 2.7 nanograms/ml within 4 days of starting to take 400 to 1200 mg **danazol** daily. Despite a reduction in the **danazol** dosage to 600 mg and then 400 mg daily, her tacrolimus and creatinine serum levels remained high for a month until the **danazol** was withdrawn. The reason is not known but the authors suggest that **danazol** possibly inhibits the metabolism (demethylation and hydroxylation) of the tacrolimus by the liver so that it is cleared from the body more slowly.[1] The general importance of this interaction is uncertain but monitor the effects of concurrent use in any patient, reducing the tacrolimus dosage as necessary.

(b) Sex hormones

Tacrolimus appears to potentiate the actions of **progesterone** by preventing its degradation.[2] The makers of tacrolimus say that during clinical use **ethinyloestradiol** has been shown to increase tacrolimus levels, and *in vitro* data suggests that **gestodene** and **norethindrone** may do the same.[3] Because tacrolimus has the potential to interfere with the metabolism of **oral contraceptives**, the makers suggest that other contraceptive measures should be used.[3]

1. Shapiro R, Venkataramanan R, Warty VS, Scantlebury VP, Rybka W, McCauley J, Fung JJ, Starzl TE. FK 506 interaction with danazol. *Lancet* (1993) 341, 1344–5.

2. Thomson AW, Bonham CA, Zeevi A. Mode of action of tacrolimus (FK506): molecular and cellular mechanisms. *Ther Drug Monit* (1995) 17, 584–91.

3. Prograf (Tacrolimus). Fujisawa Limited. Summary of product characteristics, June 2002.

Tacrolimus + Theophylline

An isolated report suggests that theophylline may increase serum tacrolimus levels.

Clinical evidence, mechanism, importance and management

A kidney transplant patient on tacrolimus 7 mg daily was given **theophylline** 600 mg daily to treat post-transplant erythrocytosis. After 1 month the serum creatinine increased from 110 to 145 micromol/l and the tacrolimus trough blood concentration increased to 16 nanograms/ml (range 5 to 15 nanograms/ml). **Theophylline** dosage was reduced to 300 mg daily on 4 days each week and a month later the serum creatinine and trough tacrolimus levels were 175 micromol/l and 48.5 nanograms/ml respectively. **Theophylline** was discontinued and renal function and trough tacrolimus levels rapidly returned to normal. The pharmacokinetics of tacrolimus were later assessed in the same patient. **Theophylline** (125 mg on 4 days of the week) was associated with an almost fivefold increase in the tacrolimus AUC and an increase in the peak serum tacrolimus levels from 19.3 to 37.4 nanograms/ml, without significant alterations in renal function on this occasion.[1]

Mechanism

Unclear. Theophylline may increase tacrolimus levels by inhibiting its metabolism by cytochrome P450 isoenzyme CYP3A4, although CYP1A2 rather than CYP3A4 is considered the main enzyme in the metabolism of theophylline. However, an *in vitro* study found that tacrolimus exhibited a negligible effect on theophylline metabolism.[2]

Importance and management

Direct information seems to be limited to this single case report but any drug which inhibits cytochrome P450 3A isoenzymes may increase tacrolimus blood levels. The authors conclude that low dose theophylline may be given to transplant patients with erythrocytosis provided that tacrolimus levels are closely monitored.[1]

1. Boubenider S, Vincent I, Lambotte O, Roy S, Hiesse C, Taburet A-M, Charpentier B. Interaction between theophylline and tacrolimus in a renal transplant patient. *Nephrol Dial Transplant* (2000) 15, 1066–8.

2. Matsuda H, Iwasaki K, Shiraga T, Tozuka Z, Hata T, Guengerich FP. Interactions of FK506 (tacrolimus) with clinically important drugs. *Res Commun Mol Pathol Pharmacol* (1996) 91, 57–64.

17

Lithium drug interactions

Lithium carbonate in dosages of about 400–600 mg daily is used to treat depressive illnesses, the dosage being adjusted to give plasma concentrations of 0.8–1.5 mmol/l for acute mania, and 0.6–1.2 mmol/l for the prophylactic treatment of unipolar and bipolar affective illness. It is given under close supervision with regular monitoring of blood concentrations – initially at least once a week – because there is a narrow margin between therapeutic concentrations and those that are toxic. It is usual to take serum lithium samples about 10 to 12 hours after the last oral dose.

Side-effects which are not usually considered serious include nausea, weakness, fine tremor, mild polydipsia and polyuria. If serum concentrations rise into the 1.5 to 2.0 mmol/l range, mild intoxication occurs (lethargy, drowsiness, coarse hand tremor, muscular weakness, abdominal pain, nausea and vomiting, diarrhoea). Moderate but more serious toxicity occurs when serum concentrations rise into the 2.0 to 2.5 mmol/l range (confusion, dysarthria, nystagmus, blurred vision, ataxia, muscle twitches, ECG changes). If levels rise much above 2.5 mmol/l, serious and life-threatening toxicity can occur (coma, seizures, hyper-extension of the limbs, increased deep tendon reflexes, circulatory failure, and possibly death).[1]

In addition to these side-effects, lithium can induce diabetes insipidus and hypothyroidism in some patients, and is contraindicated in those with renal or cardiac insufficiency. Just how lithium exerts its beneficial effects is not known, but it may compete with sodium ions in various parts of the body and it alters the electrolyte composition of body fluids.

Most of the interactions involving lithium are discussed in this chapter but a few are found elsewhere in this book. The Index should be consulted for a full listing. Virtually all of the reports are concerned with the carbonate, but sometimes lithium is given as the acetate, aspartate, chloride, citrate, gluconate, orotate or sulphate instead. There is no reason to believe that these lithium salts will not interact just like lithium carbonate.

1. Finley PR, Warner MD, Peabody CA. Clinical relevance of drug interactions with lithium. *Clin Pharmacokinet* (1995) 29, 172–91.

Table 17.1 Lithium salts: generic and proprietary names

Generic names	Proprietary names
Lithium acetate	Quilonum, Quilonorm
Lithium carbonate	Acolitium, Camcolit, Carbolim, Carbolit, Carbolith, Carbolithium, Carbolitium, Duralith, Eskalith, Hypnorex, Lentolith, Leukominerase, Li 450, Licab, Licarb, Licarbium, Limed, Liskonum, Lithane, Litheum, Lithicarb, Lithobid, Lithonate, Lithosun, Litiocar, Lito, Lit-300, Maniprex, Neurolepsin, Neurolithium, Phanate, Plenur, Priadel, Quilonorm, Quilonum, Teralithe
Lithium chloride	
Lithium citrate	Litarex, Li-Liquid, Priadel
Lithium gluconate	Neurolithium
Lithium glutamate	
Lithium orotate	
Lithium sulphate	Lithiofor, Lithionit

Lithium carbonate + ACE inhibitors

No important interaction occurs in most individuals, but in some the serum lithium levels can rise by about one-third. At least 12 cases of lithium toxicity have been reported in patients when given captopril, enalapril or lisinopril (and possibly perindopril). Risk factors seem to be poor renal function and increased age.

Clinical evidence

(a) Lithium serum levels increased, intoxication

A retrospective study of patient records identified 20 who were stabilised on lithium and then started on an ACE inhibitor (13 given **lisinopril**, 6 **enalapril** and one **captopril**). Their serum lithium levels rose by an average of 35% and there was a 26% decrease in lithium clearance. 20% of the patients developed signs and symptoms suggestive of toxicity (increased tremor, confusion, ataxia) necessitating a dosage reduction or withdrawal. In three of the patients the development of the interaction was delayed for several weeks.[1,2]

A patient developed a serum lithium level of 2.35 mmol/l and intoxication (tremor, dysarthria, digestive problems) within 10 days of starting to take 50 mg **captopril** daily. He was restabilised on half his previous dose of lithium.[3] A reduced lithium dosage was found adequate in another patient on **enalapril**.[4] A woman developed signs of lithium intoxication (ataxia, dysarthria, tremor, confusion, etc.) within 2–3 weeks of starting to take 20 mg **enalapril** daily. After five weeks her serum lithium levels had risen from 0.88 to 3.3 mmol/l.[5] No toxicity occurred when the **enalapril** was later replaced by nifedipine.[5] Lithium toxicity following the use of **enalapril**, and associated in some cases with a decrease in renal function, has been seen in another five patients.[6-11] A reduced lithium dosage was found adequate in another patient on **enalapril**. A woman on lithium developed intoxication and a trough serum level of 3.0 mmol/l within 3 weeks of stopping clonidine and starting 20 mg **lisinopril** daily.[12] Four other reports similarly describe acute lithium toxicity in four patients when given **lisinopril**.[11,13-15] One of them was also taking verapamil and aspirin.[15] Toxicity took 3 months to develop in one patient when given **perindopril** and bendroflumethiazide (bendrofluazide) (also known to increase serum lithium levels).[16]

(b) Lithium serum levels unchanged

5 mg **enalapril** for 9 days had no effect on the mean serum lithium levels of 9 normal young male subjects taking 450 mg twice daily, but one subject showed a 31% increase.[17]

Mechanism

Not fully understood. One suggestion is that because the ACE inhibitors reduce drinking behaviour and both ACE inhibitors and lithium cause sodium to be lost in the urine, fluid depletion can occur. The normal compensatory reaction for this is constriction of the efferent renal arterioles to maintain the glomerular filtration rate, but this mechanism is blocked by the ACE inhibitor, as a result of which the excretion of lithium falls and toxicity develops.

Importance and management

The lithium carbonate/ACE inhibitor interaction is established but not of clinical importance in every patient. The picture seems to be that lithium levels can rise to some extent but only a few patients appear to experience a marked rise and toxicity. Just why one study[17] (quoted above) found no interaction is not clear, except that it was possibly too short. If any ACE inhibitor is added to established lithium treatment, monitor well and be alert for the need to reduce the lithium dosage (possibly by between one-third to one-half).[12] The development of the interaction may be delayed so that weekly monitoring of lithium levels for several weeks has been advised.[12] There are risk factors: the authors of one of the reports[12] say that ". . .use of this combination in patients with advanced age, congestive heart fail-

ure, renal insufficiency, or volume depletion is unjustified". Only captopril, enalapril, lisinopril (and possibly perindopril) have been implicated in this interaction but it seems likely that it could occur with any other ACE inhibitor.

1. Finley PR, O'Brien JG, Coleman RW. Lithium (Li) and angiotensin converting enzyme inhibitor (ACEI) drug interaction. *Clin Pharmacol Ther* (1994) 55, 181.
2. Finley PR, O'Brien JG, Coleman RW. Lithium and angiotensin-converting enzyme inhibitors: evaluation of a potential interaction. *J Clin Psychopharmacol* (1996) 16, 68–71.
3. Pulik M, Lida H. Interaction lithium-inhibiteurs de l'enzyme de conversion. *Presse Med* (1988) 17, 755.
4. Ahmad S. Sudden hypothyroidism and amiodarone-lithium combination: an interaction. *Cardiovasc Drugs Ther* (1995) 9, 827–8.
5. Douste-Blazy Ph, Rostin M, Livarek B, Tordjman E, Montastruc JL, Galinier F. Angiotensin converting enzyme inhibitors and lithium treatment. *Lancet* (1986) i, 1448.
6. Mahieu M, Houvenagel E, Leduc JJ, Choteau Ph. Lithium-inhibiteurs de l'enzyme conversion: une association á eviter? *Presse Med* (1988) 17, 281.
7. Drouet A, Bouvet O. Lithium et inhibiteurs de l'enzyme de conversion. *Encephale* (1990) 16, 51–2.
8. Navis GJ, de Jong PE, de Zeeuw D. Volume homeostasis, angiotensin converting enzyme inhibition, and lithium therapy. *Am J Med* (1989) 86, 621.
9. Simon G. Combination angiotensin converting enzyme inhibitor/lithium therapy contraindicated in renal disease. *Am J Med* (1988) 85, 893–4.
10. Rimmer JM, Santella RN. Combination angiotensin converting enzyme inhibitor/lithium therapy contraindicated in renal disease. *Am J Med* (1988) 85, 894.
11. Correa FJ, Eiser AR. Angiotensin-converting enzyme inhibitors and lithium toxicity. *Am J Med* (1992) 93, 108–9.
12. Baldwin CM, Safferman AZ. A case of lisinopril-induced lithium toxicity. *DICP Ann Pharmacother* (1990) 24, 946–7.
13. Griffin JH, Hahn SM. Lisinopril-induced lithium toxicity. *DICP Ann Pharmacother* (1991) 25, 101.
14. Conrad AJ. Quoted as Written Communication, July 1st 1988, in *Biol Therapies Psychiatry* (1988) 11, 43.
15. Chandragiri SS, Pasol E, Gallagher RM. Lithium, ACE inhibitors, NSAIDs, and verapamil. A possible fatal combination. *Psychosomatics* (1998) 39, 281–2.
16. Vipond AJ, Bakewell S, Telford R, Nicholls AJ. Lithium toxicity. *Anaesthesia* (1996) 51, 1156–8.
17. DasGupta K, Jefferson JW, Kobak KA, Greist JH. The effect of enalapril on serum lithium levels in healthy men. *J Clin Psychiatry* (1992) 53, 398–400.

Lithium carbonate + Aciclovir (Acyclovir)

An isolated case report describes lithium toxicity caused by the concurrent use of high-dose intravenous aciclovir.

Clinical evidence, mechanism, importance and management

A woman of 42 on 450 mg lithium carbonate twice daily developed signs of lithium toxicity 6 days after starting treatment with 10 mg/kg intravenous **aciclovir** for an herpes zoster infection. Her serum lithium levels had risen fourfold. The reasons are unknown but the authors of the report postulate that the **aciclovir** may have inhibited the renal excretion of the lithium.[1]

This appears to be the first and only report of this interaction, but it would now be prudent to monitor serum levels closely (every second or third day is the recommendation in this report) if high dose intravenous **aciclovir** is given to any patient. There appear so far to be no reports of this interaction with oral **aciclovir**, and none would be expected with topical **aciclovir**.

1. Sylvester RK, Leitch J, Granum C. Does acyclovir increase serum lithium levels? *Pharmacotherapy* (1996) 16, 466–8.

Lithium carbonate + Angiotensin II antagonists

Lithium intoxication has been seen in one patient given candesartan, one given losartan and one given valsartan.
No interaction has yet been reported with any of the other angiotensin II antagonists.

Clinical evidence

(a) Candesartan

A woman of 58 on long-term lithium treatment (stable levels between 0.6 and 0.7 mmol/l) for depression, and un-named calcium antagonists for hypertension, was additionally given 16 mg **candesartan** daily. Eight weeks later after a 10-day history of ataxia, increasing confusion, disorientation and agitation she was hospitalised and found to have toxic serum lithium levels (3.25 mmol/l). She recovered completely when all the drugs were stopped. She was later restabilised on her original lithium dosage with a change to urapidil for the hypertension.[1]

(b) Losartan

An elderly woman on lithium carbonate developed lithium intoxication (ataxia, dysarthria, confusion) after the addition of 50 mg **losartan** daily. Her serum lithium levels rose from the normally stable 0.63 mmol/l to 2.0 mmol/l over 5 weeks. When the **losartan** was replaced by nicardipine, her serum lithium levels were restabilised at 0.77 mmol/l within 2 weeks.[2]

(c) Valsartan

A woman with a long history of bipolar disorder was treated with lithium carbonate (serum levels consistently at 0.9 mmol/l) and a number of other drugs (L-tryptophan, lorazepam, glibenclamide, conjugated oestrogens and ciprofloxacin). Two weeks before being hospitalised for manic relapse she was additionally started on **valsartan**. While in hospital the ciprofloxacin was stopped, lorazepam was replaced by zopiclone, and quetiapine was added. On day 2 of her hospitalisation her serum lithium levels were 1.1 mmol/l and she became increasingly delirious, confused and ataxic over the next week. By day 11 her serum lithium levels had risen to 1.4 mmol/l. When an interaction was suspected, the **valsartan** was replaced by diltiazem. She later recovered and was stabilised at 0.8 mmol/l on her original lithium carbonate dosage.[3]

Mechanism

Not fully understood. It could be that as with the ACE-inhibitors, more lithium is retained by the kidney tubules following the increased loss of sodium brought about by the use of these angiotensin-II receptor antagonists, but inhibition of aldosterone secretion is less with these drugs than with ACE-inhibitors so that a clinically relevant interaction is less likely. *Animal* studies show that one ACE-inhibitor, ramipril, but not losartan decreases the excretion of lithium by the kidney, which would support this idea.[4,5]

Importance and management

Direct information about interactions between lithium carbonate and angiotensin II antagonists seems to be limited to just these three reports. The incidence of this interaction would therefore appear to be very low indeed although the possibility of such an interaction had been suggested, based on what can also happen with the related ACE I inhibitors. However, such sparse evidence is not enough to forbid the concurrent use of candesartan, losartan or valsartan with lithium carbonate, but it would now be prudent to monitor the outcome. The same precautions would also be appropriate with any other Angiotensin-II receptor antagonist (**eprosartan, irbesartan, telmisartan**), which is the advice of the makers of these drugs, even though the risk of an interaction is probably fairly low. Ideally serum lithium levels should be monitored. At the very least the patient should be warned to be vigilant for any evidence of lithium intoxication when any of these drugs is first added, and told what to do. Any rise in serum lithium levels may only be gradual so that intoxication might take as long as 3 to 7 weeks to develop fully.

1. Zwanzger P, Marcuse A, Boerner RJ, Walther A, Rupprecht. Lithium intoxication after administration of AT₁ blockers. *J Clin Psychiatry* (2001) 62, 208–9.

2. Blanche P, Raynaud E, Kerob D, Galezowski N. Lithium intoxication in an elderly patient after combined treatment with losartan. *Eur J Clin Pharmacol* (1997) 52, 501.

3. Leung M, Remick RA. Potential drug interaction between lithium and valsartan. *J Clin Psychopharmacol* (2000) 20, 392–3.

4. Barthelmebs M, Grima M, Imbs JL. Ramipril-induced decrease in renal excretion in the rat. *Br J Pharmacol* (1995) 116, 2161–5.

5. Barthelmebs M, Alt-Tebacher M, Madonna O, Grima M, Imbs JL. Absence of a losartan interaction with renal lithium excretion in the rat. *Br J Pharmacol* (1995) 116, 2166–9.

Lithium carbonate + Baclofen

Two patients with Huntington's chorea showed an aggravation of their hyperkinetic symptoms within a few days of starting concurrent treatment.

Clinical evidence, mechanism, importance and management

A patient with Huntington's chorea and under treatment with lithium and haloperidol, was additionally given **baclofen**. Another patient being treated with imipramine, clopenthixol, chlorpromazine and **baclofen** was also additionally given lithium. Within a few days both patients showed a severe aggravation of their hyperkinetic symptoms, which disappeared within 3 days of withdrawing the **baclofen**.[1] Other patients with Huntington's chorea showed no major changes in their mental state or movement disorder when given up to 90 mg **baclofen** daily,[2,3] which suggests that an interaction may have been the cause of the hyperkinesis in these 2 patients. Nevertheless on the basis of this very limited evidence it would now seem prudent to monitor the effects of concurrent use.

1. Andén N-E, Dalén P, Johansson B. Baclofen and lithium in Huntington's chorea. *Lancet* (1973) ii, 93.

2. Barbeau A. GABA and Huntington's chorea. *Lancet* (1973) ii, 1499–1500.

3. Paulson GW. Lioresal in Huntington's disease. *Dis Nerv Syst* (1976) 37, 465–7.

Lithium carbonate + Benzodiazepines

Preliminary evidence suggests that alprazolam is unlikely to cause a clinically important rise in serum lithium levels. Neurotoxicity may develop if clonazepam is added to treatment with lithium carbonate. An isolated case of serious hypothermia has been reported during concurrent treatment with lithium carbonate and diazepam.

Clinical evidence, mechanism, importance and management

(a) Alprazolam

2 mg **alprazolam** daily for 4 days increased the steady-state AUC of lithium (from 10.3 to 11.1 mmol/h) in 10 normal subjects taking 900 to 1500 mg daily, and reduced its urinary clearance (from a 93.6 to 78.2% recovery). It is suggested that this is unlikely to be clinically significant, but confirmation of this is needed.[1]

(b) Clonazepam

A retrospective study of patients' records revealed 5 out of 30 with bipolar affective disorder under treatment with lithium carbonate (900–2400 mg) who had developed a neurotoxic syndrome with ataxia, dysarthria, drowsiness and confusion when their neuroleptic treatment (chlorpromazine, perphenazine, haloperidol) was replaced with **clonazepam** (2–16 mg). The syndrome was reversible. The reasons are not known but suggestions include lithium toxicity or synergistic toxicity. Whatever the explanation, the authors of the report suggest that the lithium levels should be more frequently measured if **clonazepam** is added, and the effects well monitored.[2]

(c) Diazepam

A mentally retarded patient showed occasional hypothermic episodes (below 35C) while taking lithium and **diazepam**, but not while on either drug alone. After taking both drugs for 17 days during a test (lithium 1 g and **diazepam** 30 mg daily) the patient experienced a temperature fall from 35.4 to 32C over 2 h, and became comatose with reduced reflexes, dilated pupils, a systolic blood pressure of 40 to 60 mmHg, a pulse rate of 40 and no piloerector response.[3] The reasons are not known. This is an isolated case so that concurrent use need not be avoided, but be alert for any evidence of hypothermia.

There seems to be no evidence of this adverse interaction with any of the other benzodiazepines.

1. Evans RL, Nelson MV, Melethil S, Townsend R, Hornstra RK, Smith RB. Evaluation of the interaction of lithium and alprazolam. *J Clin Psychopharmacol* (1990) 10, 355–9.
2. Koczerginski D, Kennedy SH, Swinson RP. Clonazepam and lithium—a toxic combination in the treatment of mania? *Int Clin Psychopharmacol* (1989) 4, 195–9.
3. Naylor GJ, McHarg A. Profound hypothermia on combined lithium carbonate and diazepam treatment. *BMJ* (1977) 3, 22.

Lithium carbonate + Caffeine

The heavy consumption of caffeine-containing drinks may cause a small or moderate reduction in serum lithium levels. Levels may rise if the caffeine is withdrawn.

Clinical evidence, mechanism, importance and management

A study in 11 psychiatric patients on lithium carbonate (600 to 1200 mg daily) who were also regular **coffee** drinkers (4–8 cups daily containing 70 to 120 mg **caffeine** per cup) showed that when the **coffee** was withdrawn, their serum lithium levels rose by an average of 24%, although in fact only 8 of the 11 demonstrated any changes.[1] These findings are consistent with another report of two patients who had an aggravation of their lithium-induced tremor when they stopped taking **caffeine**. This was attributed to a rise in serum lithium levels.[2] Another study also found that a single dose of **caffeine** increased the urinary excretion of lithium in six subjects (extent was not quantified),[3] whereas yet another failed to find any changes in urinary clearance of lithium in 6 **coffee**-drinking subjects compared with a caffeine-free control period.[4] It is not clear exactly how the **caffeine** affects the excretion of lithium by the kidney tubules.

The weight of evidence cited here suggests that although there is no need for those on lithium to avoid **caffeine** (**coffee**, **tea**, '**Coke**', etc.), the withdrawal of **caffeine** from the diet should be done cautiously, particularly in those whose serum lithium levels are already high because of the risk of toxicity. It may be possible to use less lithium to achieve the same blood levels. In addition, remember that there is a **caffeine**-withdrawal syndrome (headache and fatigue being the major symptoms) that might worsen some of the major psychiatric disorders (such as affective and schizophrenic disorders).[1]

1. Mester R, Toren P, Mizrachi I, Wolmer L, Karni N, Weizman A. Caffeine withdrawal increases lithium blood levels. *Biol Psychiatry* (1995) 37, 348–50.
2. Jefferson JW. Lithium tremor and caffeine intake: two cases of drinking less and shaking more. *J Clin Psychiatry* (1988) 49, 72–3.
3. Thomsen K, Schou M. Renal lithium excretion in men. *Am J Physiol* (1968) 215, 823–7.
4. Bikin D, Conrad KA, Mayersohn M. Lack of influence of caffeine and aspirin on lithium elimination. *Clin Res* (1982) 30, 249.

Lithium + Calcitonin (Salcatonin)

A study in 4 depressed women found that calcitonin (salcatonin) caused a small reduction in serum lithium levels, the clinical importance of which is not known.

Clinical evidence

Prompted by the occasional observation of decreased serum lithium levels in outpatients receiving **calcitonin**, a study was undertaken in 4 manic depressive women stabilised on lithium for 10 years who were additionally treated with **salmon calcitonin** (**salcatonin**) (100 units subcutaneously for 3 consecutive days) for postmenopausal osteoporosis. It was found that their serum lithium levels fell by an average of 17% (with a minimum of −8% and a maximum of −30%). It was noted that the lithium levels of all of them dropped below the minimum therapeutic range (0.6–1.20 mmol/l) on at least one occasion. The clearance of lithium in the urine was tested in 2 of the patients and both showed increases (9.8% and 16.6%).[1]

Mechanism

Not known. Increased renal excretion and possibly some reduced intestinal absorption of the lithium is suggested by the authors of the report.[1]

Importance and management

Information seems to be limited to this report but the interaction would appear to be established. This study only lasted 3 days with only a small fall in serum lithium levels, but longer-term use might possibly be clinically important in a few patients. The authors of the report did not measure the effect on the treatment of depression. Lithium levels should be monitored in patients receiving calcitonin, being alert for the need to increase the lithium dosage, but it seems likely that this interaction will not be clinically important in most patients.

1. Passiu G, Bocchetta A, Martinelli V, Garau P, Del Zompo M, Mathieu A. Calcitonin decreases lithium plasma levels in man. Preliminary report. *Int J Clin Pharmacol Res* (1998) 18, 179–181.

Lithium carbonate + Calcium channel blockers

Concurrent use can be uneventful but neurotoxicity and decreases in serum lithium levels have been seen in a few patients also given verapamil. Profound bradycardia occurred in 2 patients, and choreoathetosis in another on lithium when given verapamil. An acute parkinsonian syndrome developed in another patient on lithium and thiothixene when given diltiazem. Marked psychosis developed in yet another patient on lithium when given diltiazem.

Clinical evidence

(a) Increased lithium effects, neurotoxicity, psychosis

A 42-year-old on 900 mg lithium carbonate daily developed toxicity (nausea, vomiting, muscular weakness, ataxia and tinnitus) within 9 days of starting to take 80 mg **verapamil** three times daily although her bipolar depressive disorder improved. Her serum lithium levels remained unchanged at 1.1 mmol/l. The toxicity disappeared within 48 h of stopping the **verapamil** but her disorder worsened. The same pattern was repeated when the **verapamil** was re-started and then withdrawn.[1] A 74-year-old woman on lithium experienced similar toxicity 2 weeks after starting 240 mg **verapamil** daily. Her serum lithium level remained stable at 0.9 mmol/l. She was later well controlled on half the dose of lithium with a serum level of 0.3 to 0.5 mmol/l.[2] A woman on lithium developed progressive ataxia and dysarthria despite a steady serum lithium level (0.60 mmol/l) on two occasions when given 240 mg **verapamil** daily, but recovered when the **verapamil** was replaced by **nifedipine**.[3] A woman well controlled on lithium developed marked psychosis within a week of starting to take 90 mg **diltiazem** daily.[4]

(b) Reduced lithium effects

A patient, well controlled on 900–1200 mg lithium daily for over eight years, showed a marked fall in serum lithium levels when given 320 mg **verapamil** daily. He was restabilised on approximately double the dose of lithium. Another patient showed an increased lithium clearance when given **verapamil** for three days, and a fall in serum lithium levels from 0.61 to 0.53 mmol/l.[5]

(c) Other toxic effects

A man given lithium for 2 weeks was started on 120 mg **verapamil**. Within four days he developed marked choreoathetoid movements of his neck, trunk and all four limbs. The problem resolved when the **verapamil** was stopped.[6] An acute parkinsonism syndrome developed in a man of 58 within four days of adding 30 mg **diltiazem** three times daily to his treatment with lithium and thiothixene.[7] Two elderly patients on lithium developed profound bradycardia when given 320–480 mg **verapamil** daily. Fatal myocardial infarction followed in one case.[8]

Mechanisms

Not understood.

Importance and management

The adverse reactions cited above contrast with other reports describing uneventful concurrent use.[9,10] This unpredictability emphasises the need to monitor the effects closely where it is thought appropriate to give lithium and calcium channel blockers. It has been suggested that particular caution should be exercised in the elderly and those with cardiovascular disease.[8]

1. Price WA, Giannini AJ. Neurotoxicity caused by lithium-verapamil synergism. *J Clin Pharmacol* (1986) 26, 717–19.
2. Price WA, Shalley JE. Lithium-verapamil toxicity in the elderly. *J Am Geriatr Soc* (1987) 35, 177–8.
3. Wright BA, Jarrett DB. Lithium and calcium channel blockers: possible neurotoxicity. *Biol Psychiatry* (1991) 30, 635–6.
4. Binder EF, Cayabyab L, Ritchie DJ, Birge SJ. Diltiazem-induced psychosis and a possible diltiazem-lithium interaction. *Arch Intern Med* (1991) 151, 373–4.
5. Weinrauch LA, Belok S, D'Elia JA. Decreased serum lithium during verapamil therapy. *Am Heart J* (1984) 108, 1378–80.
6. Helmuth D, Ljaljevic Z, Ramirez L, Meltzer HY. Choreoathetosis induced by verapamil and lithium treatment. *J Clin Psychopharmacol* (1989) 9, 454–5.
7. Valdiserri EV. A possible interaction between lithium and diltiazem: case report. *J Clin Psychiatry* (1985) 46, 540–1.
8. Dubovsky SL, Franks RD, Allen S. Verapamil: a new antimanic drug with potential interactions with lithium. *J Clin Psychiatry* (1987) 48, 371–2.
9. Brotman AW, Farhadi AM, Gelenberg AJ. Verapamil treatment of acute mania. *J Clin Psychiatry* (1986) 47, 136–8.
10. Gitlin MJ, Weiss J. Verapamil as maintenance treatment in bipolar illness: a case report. *J Clin Psychopharmacol* (1984) 4, 341–3.

Lithium carbonate + Carbamazepine

Although combined use is beneficial in many patients, mild to severe neurotoxicity is reported to have developed in some, and possibly sinus node dysfunction in others. An isolated case of lithium intoxication has been reported, caused by carbamazepine-induced renal failure.

Clinical evidence

A patient on 1800 mg lithium daily developed severe neurotoxicity (ataxia, truncal tremors, nystagmus, limb hyperreflexia, muscle fasciculation) within three days of starting to take 600 mg **carbamazepine** daily. Blood levels of both drugs remained within the therapeutic range. The symptoms resolved when each drug was withdrawn in turn and re-occurred within three days of restarting concurrent treatment.[1]

Five rapid-cycling manic patients developed similar neurotoxic symptoms (confusion, drowsiness, generalised weakness, lethargy, coarse tremor, hyperreflexia, cerebellar signs) when concurrently treated with lithium carbonate and **carbamazepine** (doses not stated). Plasma levels of both drugs remained within the accepted range.[2] Other reports describe adverse neurological effects during concurrent use which were also not accompanied by changes in drug serum levels.[3-7] The neurotoxicity disappeared in most patients when the drugs were stopped, but in one patient irreversible tardive dystonia was still present 7 years later.[8]

A nine-year study in a mental hospital found that four out of five patients on lithium who developed sinus node dysfunction were also on **carbamazepine**.[9] Another study in 10 patients found that **carbamazepine** was not effective in treating the polyuria and polydipsia associated with lithium treatment, and half of them dropped out of the study because of ataxia, dizziness, restlessness and confusion.[10] An isolated case report describes **carbamazepine**-induced acute renal failure which resulted in lithium intoxication.[11]

A systematic search through the Medline database over the 1966 to 1996 period for reports of neurotoxic adverse effects in patients on lithium at low therapeutic concentrations found a total of 41 cases, in 22% of which **carbamazepine** had been taken concurrently, in some instances with other drugs.[12]

In contrast, combined treatment in other patients is said to be well tolerated and beneficial,[13-15] but one report suggests that the dosages may need to be reduced to free the patient from side-effects.[16]

Mechanism

Not understood. A paper that plotted the serum levels of both drugs on a two-dimensional graph failed to find evidence of synergistic toxicity.[17] Another study found that concurrent use caused an approximately 10% rise in lithium levels and a 10% fall in carbamazepine levels.[18] The sinus node dysfunction caused by either lithium or carbamazepine is rare but it may possibly be additive.

Importance and management

The neurotoxic interaction is established, but its incidence is not known. It may be quite small. If concurrent use is undertaken, the outcome should be closely monitored. This is particularly important because neurotoxicity can develop even though the drug serum levels remain within the accepted therapeutic range. If any neurotoxicity develops the lithium treatment should be discontinued promptly.[12] The authors of one paper suggest that ". . .the risk factors appear to be a history of neurotoxicity with lithium therapies and the presence of concurrent compromised medical or neurological functioning. . .".[2]

1. Ghose K. Interaction between lithium and carbamazepine. *BMJ* (1980) 280, 1122.
2. Shukla S, Godwin CD, Long LEB, Miller MG. Lithium-carbamazepine neurotoxicity and risk factors. *Am J Psychiatry* (1984) 141, 1604–6.
3. Chaudhry RP, Waters BGH. Lithium and carbamazepine interaction: possible neurotoxicity. *J Clin Psychiatry* (1983) 44, 30–1.
4. Andrus PF. Lithium and carbamazepine. *J Clin Psychiatry* (1984) 45, 525.
5. Hassan MN, Thakar J, Weinberg AL, Grimes JD. Lithium-carbamazepine interaction: clinical and laboratory observations. *Neurology* (1987) 37 (Suppl 1), 172.
6. Marcoux AW. Carbamazepine-lithium drug interaction. *Ann Pharmacother* (1996) 30, 547.
7. Manto M-U, Jacquy J, Hildebrand J. Cerebellar ataxia in upper limbs triggered by addition of carbamazepine to lithium treatment. *Acta Neurol Belg* (1996) 96, 316–7.
8. Laird LK, Knox EP. The use of carbamazepine and lithium in controlling a case of chronic rapid cycling. *Pharmacotherapy* (1987) 7, 130–2.
9. Steckler TL. Lithium- and carbamazepine-associated sinus node dysfunction: nine-year experience in a psychiatric hospital. *J Clin Psychopharmacol* (1994) 14, 336–9.
10. Ghose K. Effect of carbamazepine in polyuria associated with lithium therapy. *Pharmakopsychiatr Neuropsychopharmakol* (1978) 11, 241–5.
11. Mayan H, Golubev N, Dganit D. Farfel Z. Lithium intoxication due to carbamazepine-induced renal failure. *Ann Pharmacother* (2001) 35, 560–2.
12. Emilien G, Malotoeaux JM. Lithium neurotoxicity at low therapeutic doses. Hypotheses for causes and mechanism of action a following a retrospective analysis of published case reports. *Acta Neurol Belg* (1996) 96, 281–93.
13. MacCallum WAG. Interaction of lithium and phenytoin. *BMJ* (1980) 280, 610–11.
14. Lipinski JF, Pope HG. Possible synergistic action between carbamazepine and lithium carbonate in the treatment of three acutely manic patients. *Am J Psychiatry* (1982) 139, 948–9.
15. Moss GR, James CR. Carbamazepine and lithium carbonate synergism in mania. *Arch Gen Psychiatry* (1983) 40, 588–9.
16. Kramlinger KG, Post RM. The addition of lithium to carbamazepine. *Arch Gen Psychiatry* (1989) 46, 794–800.
17. McGinness J, Kishimoto A, Hollister LE. Avoiding neurotoxicity with lithium-carbamazepine combinations. *Psychopharmacol Bull* (1990) 26, 181–4.
18. Rybakowski J, Lehmann W, Kanarkowski R, Matkowski K. Possible pharmacokinetic interaction of lithium and carbamazepine. *Lithium* (1991) 2, 183–4.

Lithium carbonate + Cisplatin

Isolated case reports describe a fall, a rise and no changes in serum lithium levels in patients given cisplatin.

Clinical evidence, mechanism, importance and management

A woman on 1200 mg lithium carbonate daily showed a fall in serum lithium levels from 1.0 to 0.3, and from 0.8 to 0.5 mmol/l on two occasions over periods of two days when given 100 mg/m² **cisplatin** intravenously over 2 h. Over the next 24 h she was also given one litre of normal saline over 4 h, 25 g sodium chloride and 20% mannitol over 4 h, and 5% dextrose in normal saline to prevent renal toxicity. Serum lithium levels returned to normal at the end of two days. No change in the control of the psychotic symptoms was seen.[1] It is not clear whether the fall in serum lithium levels was due to increased renal clearance caused by the **cisplatin**, the fluid-loading, or both.

Another patient showed clinically insignificant changes in her serum lithium levels when treated with **cisplatin**, but two months later her deteriorating kidney function resulted in a rise in her serum lithium levels.[2] A man showed a transient 64% increase in serum lithium levels, without perceptible clinical consequences, during the first of four courses of **cisplatin**, bleomycin, etoposide. The effect became less pronounced during the other courses.[3]

None of these interactions was of great clinical importance but the authors of the first report pointed out that some regimens of **cisplatin** involve the use of higher doses (40 mg/m^2) with a normal saline fluid load over 5 days, and under these circumstances it would be prudent to monitor the serum lithium levels carefully. Concurrent use should be monitored in all patients.

1. Pietruszka LJ, Biermann WA, Vlasses PH. Evaluation of cisplatin-lithium interaction. *Drug Intell Clin Pharm* (1985) 19, 31–2.
2. Beijnen JH, Vlasveld LT, Wanders J, ten Bokkel Huinik WW, Rodenhuis S. Effect of cis-platin-containing chemotherapy on lithium serum concentrations. *Ann Pharmacother* (1992) 26, 488–90.
3. Beijnen JH, Bais EM, ten Bokkel Huinink WW. Lithium pharmacokinetics during cispl-atin-based chemotherapy: a case report. *Cancer Chemother Pharmacol* (1994) 33, 523–6.

Lithium carbonate + Co-trimoxazole

Two reports describe lithium intoxication in three patients given co-trimoxazole, paradoxically accompanied by a fall in serum lithium levels.

Clinical evidence, mechanism, importance and management

Two patients stabilised on lithium carbonate (serum concentrations 0.75 mmol/l) showed signs of lithium intoxication (tremor, muscular weakness and fasciculation, apathy) within a few days of being given **co-trimoxazole** (dose not stated), yet their serum lithium levels were found to have fallen to 0.3–0.4 mmol/l. Within 48 h of withdrawing the **co-trimoxazole**, the signs of intoxication had gone and their serum lithium concentrations had climbed to their former levels.[1] Another report[2] very briefly states that ataxia, tremor and diarrhoea developed in a patient on lithium and timolol when given **co-trimox-azole**. The reasons are not understood. The general importance of this interaction is uncertain but if concurrent use is undertaken it would clearly be prudent to monitor the clinical response because it would appear that serum level monitoring may not always be a reliable guide.

1. Desvilles M, Sevestre P. Effet paradoxal de l'association lithium et sulfaméthoxazol-tri-methoprime. *Nouv Presse Med* (1982) 11, 3267–8.
2. Edwards IR. Medicines Adverse Reactions Committee: Eighteenth annual report, 1983. *N Z Med J* (1984) 97, 729–32.

Lithium carbonate + Diuretics (miscellaneous)

There is evidence that the excretion of lithium can be increased by triamterene and acetazolamide, but lithium intoxication occurred in one patient given acetazolamide. Chlormerodrin and amiloride are reported not to interact whereas serum lithium levels may rise if spironolactone is used. See also 'Lithium carbonate + Furosemide (Frusemide) or Bumetanide', p.657, and 'Lithium carbonate + Thiazides', p.665.

Clinical evidence, mechanism, importance and management

There is very little information about the interactions of any of these diuretics with lithium. A short-term study[1] on 6 subjects given lithium and **acetazolamide** demonstrated a 27–31% increase in the urinary excretion of lithium, and an increased clearance was found in another study.[2] A woman was successfully treated for a toxic overdose of lithium with **acetazolamide**, intravenous fluids, sodium bicarbonate, potassium chloride and mannitol,[3] but paradoxically lithium intoxication (a rise in serum levels from 0.8 to 5 mmol/l) occurred in another patient after treatment for a month with **acetazolamide**.[4]

Amiloride has been found to have no significant effect on serum lithium levels when used in the treatment of lithium-induced polyuria,[5,6] however it appears in one drug datasheet[7] and in the British National Formulary[8] as a diuretic which reduces the renal clearance of lithium, thereby increasing the risk of lithium toxicity. There appears to be no evidence to confirm this alleged interaction.

Chlormerodrin has been found not to interact.[1] The same study found that **spironolactone** had no effect on the excretion of lithium,[1] whereas in another report[9] the use of **spironolactone** was accompanied by a rise in serum lithium levels. **Triamterene**, administered to two patients taking lithium while on a salt-restricted diet, is said to have led to a strong lithium diuresis.[10]

These diuretics have been available for a very considerable time and it might have been expected that by now any serious adverse interactions with lithium would have emerged, but information is very sparse. None of the reports available gives a clear indication of the outcome of concurrent use, but some monitoring would be a prudent precaution.

1. Thomsen K, Schou M. Renal lithium excretion in man. *Am J Physiol* (1968) 215, 823–7.
2. Steele TH. Treatment of lithium intoxication with diuretics. In 'Clinical Chemistry and Chemical Toxicology of Metals.' (Ed SS Brown). Elsevier/North Holland (1977) p 289–92.
3. Horowitz LC, Fisher GU. Acute lithium toxicity. *N Engl J Med* (1969) 281, 1369.
4. Gay C, Plas J, Granger B, Olie JP, Loo H. Intoxication au lithium. Deux interaction in-édites: l'acétazolamide et l'acide niflumique. *Encephale* (1985) 11, 261–2.
5. Batlle DC, von Riotte AB, Gaviria M. Amelioration of polyuria by amiloride in patients receiving long-term lithium therapy. *N Engl J Med* (1985) 312, 408–14.
6. Kosten TR, Forrest JN. Treatment of severe lithium-induced polyuria with amiloride. *Am J Psychiatry* (1986) 143, 1563–8.
7. Midamor (Amiloride). Merck & Co. US prescribing information. August 2001.
8. British National Formulary. 43rd ed. London: The British Medical Association and The Pharmaceutical Press; 2002. p. 641. (Appendix 1) (1998) 36, 569.
9. Baer L, Platman SR, Kassir S, Fieve RR. Mechanism of renal lithium handling and their relationship to mineralocorticoids: a dissociation between sodium, lithium ions. *J Psychiatr Res* (1971) 8, 91–105.
10. Baer L, Platman S, Fieve RR. Lithium metabolism: its electrolyte actions and relationship to aldosterone. Recent Advances in the Psychobiology of the Depresssive Illnesses. Williams, Katz and Shield (eds) DHEW Publications, Washington DC (1972). p 49.

Lithium carbonate + Fluoxetine

Concurrent use can be advantageous and largely uneventful but unexplained neurotoxicities of various kinds have occurred in a small number of patients, and increases in serum lithium levels have been seen.

Clinical evidence

(a) Minor or no adverse reactions or interactions

A study in which 110 patients on lithium and **fluoxetine** were compared with another group of 110 on **fluoxetine** alone found no major differences between the two groups over a 7-week period. The incidence of 'serotonergic' reactions was the same and the combined use was well tolerated although a somewhat increased rate of minor side effects occurred.[1] Another report described the concurrent use of these two drugs in 5 patients with apparent success and without problems.[2] A study in 10 normal subjects given single oral doses of lithium before and after taking 20 mg **fluoxetine** three times daily for a week found only very minor changes in the pharmacokinetics of lithium, and no clinically relevant changes in haemodynamics, ECGs or laboratory parameters.[3]

(b) Marked adverse reactions

A woman with a bipolar affective disorder, successfully maintained for 20 years on 1200 mg lithium carbonate daily, developed stiffness of her arms and legs, dizziness, unsteadiness in walking and speech difficulties within a few days of starting additional treatment with 20 mg **fluoxetine** daily. Her serum lithium levels had risen from a range of 0.75–1.15 mmol/l to 1.70 mmol/l. They fell and the toxic symptoms disappeared when the lithium dosage was reduced and the

fluoxetine withdrawn.[4] Two other patients showed approximately 50% increases in serum lithium levels and developed mania (but no lithium toxicity) about a month after starting **fluoxetine** (20–40 mg daily). The problem resolved when the lithium dosage was reduced 25–33%.[5] Toxicity was seen in another patient when lithium was added to **fluoxetine** treatment, although the serum lithium levels remained in the therapeutic range,[6] and absence seizures occurred in another.[7] A woman on clonazepam developed severe hand tremor, ataxia and cogwheeling while taking 400 mg lithium carbonate and 40 mg **fluoxetine** daily. The problems resolved when the lithium and **fluoxetine** were withdrawn and replaced by maprotiline.[8] Opisthotonus and ataxia were seen in another patient on lithium and **fluoxetine**, and dystonia in another (also taking carbamazepine, captopril and trimipramine).[9] The development of the serotonin syndrome is also reported to have occurred in 2 patients on lithium and **fluoxetine**.[10,11] Heat stroke developed in a man on lithium and **fluoxetine**, attributed to synergistic impairment by the two drugs of his temperature regulatory system.[12]

Mechanisms

Not understood.

Importance and management

Concurrent use can be uneventful, but occasionally and unpredictably adverse reactions develop. The precise incidence is not known. If both drugs are used be alert for any evidence of neurotoxicity. The symptoms may include tremor, dysarthria, ataxia, confusion and absence seizures. Heat stroke has also been seen and the serum lithium levels may rise. It would clearly be prudent to monitor concurrent use.

1. Bauer M, Linden M, Schaaf B, Weber HJ. Adverse events and tolerability of the combination of fluoxetine/lithium compared with fluoxetine. *J Clin Psychopharmacol* (1996) 16, 130–4.
2. Pope HG, McElroy SL, Nixon RA. Possible synergism between fluoxetine and lithium in refractory depression. *Am J Psychiatry* (1988) 145, 1292–4.
3. Breuel H-P, Müller-Oerlinghausen B, Nickelsen T, Heine PR. Pharmacokinetic interactions between lithium and fluoxetine after single and repeated fluoxetine administration in young healthy volunteers. *Int J Clin Pharmacol Ther* (1995) 33, 415–9.
4. Salama AA, Shafey M. A case of severe lithium toxicity induced by combined fluoxetine and lithium carbonate. *Am J Psychiatry* (1989) 146, 278.
5. Hadley A, Cason MP. Mania resulting from lithium-fluoxetine combination. *Am J Psychiatry* (1989) 146, 1637–8.
6. Noveske FG, Hahn KR, Flynn RJ. Possible toxicity of combined fluoxetine and lithium. *Am J Psychiatry* (1989) 146, 1515.
7. Sacristan JA, Iglesias C, Arellano F, Lequerica J. Absence seizures induced by lithium: possible interaction with fluoxetine. *Am J Psychiatry* (1991) 148, 146–7.
8. Austin LS, Arana GW, Melvin JA. Toxicity resulting from lithium augmentation of antidepressant treatment in elderly patients. *J Clin Psychiatry* (1990) 51, 344–5.
9. Coulter DM, Pillans PI. Fluoxetine and extrapyramidal side effects. *Am J Psychiatry* (1995) 152, 122–5.
10. Karle J, Bjørndal F. Serotonergt syndrom - ved kombineret behandling med litium og fluoxetin. *Ugeskr Laeger* (1995) 157, 1204–5.
11. Muly EC, McDonald W, Steffens D, Book S. Serotonin syndrome produced by a combination of fluoxetine and lithium. *Am J Psychiatry* (1993) 150, 1565.
12. Albukrek D, Moran DS, Epstein Y. A depressed workman with heatstroke. *Lancet* (1996) 347, 1016.

Lithium carbonate + Furosemide (Frusemide) or Bumetanide

The concurrent use of lithium carbonate and furosemide (frusemide) can be safe and uneventful, but serious lithium intoxication has been described in a few individuals. Bumetanide can interact similarly.

Clinical evidence

Six normal subjects stabilised on 900 mg lithium carbonate daily (mean serum levels 4.3 mmol/l) were given 40 mg **furosemide (frusemide)** daily for 14 days. Five experienced some minor side-effects, probably attributable to the **furosemide**, and no significant changes in serum lithium levels, but one subject experienced such a marked increase in the toxic effects of lithium that she withdrew from the study after taking both drugs for only five days. Her serum lithium levels were found to have risen by over 60% (from 0.44 to 0.71 mmol/l).[1]

There are four other case reports of individual patients who experienced serious lithium intoxication or other adverse reactions when given lithium and **furosemide**.[2-5] One of the patients was also on a salt-restricted diet.[2] In contrast, 6 patients who had been stabilised on lithium for over 6 years showed no significant changes in their serum lithium levels over a 12-week period while taking 20–80 mg **furosemide** daily.[6] Another study in normal subjects also found no significant changes in lithium levels when 40 mg **furosemide** daily was given.[7] **Bumetanide** has also been responsible for the development of lithium toxicity in 2 patients[8,9] one of whom was on a salt-restricted diet.[9]

Mechanism

Not fully understood. If and when a rise in serum lithium levels occurs, it may be related to the salt depletion that can accompany the use of furosemide. As with the thiazides, such an interaction would not be expected to be immediate but would take a few days to develop. This may explain why one study in subjects given a single dose of lithium failed to demonstrate any effect on the urinary excretion of lithium after the administration of furosemide.[10]

Importance and management

Information seems to be limited to the reports cited. The incidence of this interaction is uncertain and its development unpredictable. It would therefore be imprudent to give furosemide (frusemide) or bumetanide to patients stabilised on lithium unless the effects can be well monitored because the occasional patient may develop serious intoxication.

1. Jefferson JW, Kalin NH. Serum lithium levels and long-term diuretic use. *JAMA* (1979) 241, 1134–6.
2. Hurtig HI, Dyson WL. Lithium toxicity enhanced by diuresis. *N Engl J Med* (1974) 290, 748–9.
3. Oh TE. Frusemide and lithium toxicity. *Anaesth Intensive Care* (1977) 5, 60–2.
4. Segura EG, Ogue MCP, Peral MF. Intoxicacion por sales de litio. Presentacion de uno caso. *Med Clin (Barc)* (1984) 83, 294–6.
5. Thornton WE, Pray BJ. Lithium intoxication: a report of two cases. *Can Psychiatr Assoc J* (1975) 20, 281–2.
6. Saffer D, Coppen A. Frusemide: a safe diuretic during lithium therapy? *J Affect Disord* (1983) 5, 289–92.
7. Crabtree BL, Mack JE, Johnson CD, Amyx BC. Comparison of the effects of hydrochlorothiazide and furosemide on lithium disposition. *Am J Psychiatry* (1991) 148, 1060–3.
8. Kerry RJ, Ludlow JM, Owen G. Diuretics are dangerous with lithium. *BMJ* (1980) 281, 371.
9. Huang LG. Lithium intoxication with coadministration of a loop-diuretic. *J Clin Psychopharmacol* (1990) 10, 228.
10. Thomsen K, Schou M. Renal lithium excretion in man. *Am J Physiol* (1968) 215, 823–7.

Lithium carbonate + Haloperidol

Although very serious adverse neurotoxic reactions have been described in some patients treated with lithium carbonate and haloperidol, there is ample evidence that concurrent use can also be uneventful and therapeutically valuable.

Clinical evidence

(a) Adverse effects during concurrent use

Four patients with acute mania who were treated with 1500–1800 mg lithium carbonate daily and high doses of **haloperidol** (up to 45 mg daily), developed encephalopathic syndromes (lethargy, fever, tremulousness, confusion, extrapyramidal and cerebellar dysfunction) accompanied by leukocytosis and elevated levels of serum enzymes, blood urea nitrogen and fasting blood sugar.[1] Two of them suffered irreversible widespread brain damage and 2 others were left with persistent dyskinesias.

A woman patient was observed with neuromuscular symptoms, impaired consciousness and hyperthermia after 12 days' treatment with 1500 mg lithium carbonate and 40 mg **haloperidol** daily. She recovered fully and uneventfully.[2] Three patients, two of them oligophrenic, who were given 1800 mg lithium carbonate with 10–20 mg **haloperidol** by injection for 10 days, 27 h and 24 h respectively, developed hypertonic-hypokinetic and extrapyramidal syndromes. All recovered.[3] Reversible delirium developed in one out of 29 patients given both drugs.[4] There are other reports of adverse reactions including severe extrapyramidal symptoms and organic brain damage in individual patients when given both drugs.[5-12] Another report claims that measurable brain damage may have occurred in seven patients.[13] A small rise in serum lithium levels occurs in the presence of **haloperidol**, but it is almost certainly of little or no clinical significance.[14]

A large-scale retrospective study of the literature over the 1966–96 period using the Medline database identified 41 cases of neurotoxic adverse side-effects in 41 patients on low therapeutic concentrations of lithium. Of these patients, 51.2% were also taking at least one antipsychotic (11 on **haloperidol**), 22% an antidepressant, 22% carbamazepine, and 17% an anxiolytic.[15]

Another retrospective study using both Medline and the FDA Spontaneous Reporting System over the 1969–94 period identified 237 cases of severe neurotoxicity involving lithium, of which 59 also involved the concurrent use of **haloperidol**.[16,17] Some of the cases identified in these two studies are also cited in a little more detail above.

(b) Advantageous concurrent use

In contrast to the reports cited above, there are others describing successful and uneventful use.[18] Cohen and Cohen who first described the adverse interaction[1] have also written that ". . . at least 50 other patients have been similarly treated without reported adverse effects". They also say that ". . . a survey of the experiences of leading experts indicate that although hundreds of patients have been treated with various regimens of combined lithium carbonate/**haloperidol**, there have been no previous observations of substantial irreversible brain damage or persistent dyskinesia". A retrospective search of Danish hospital records showed that 425 patients had been treated with both drugs and none of them had developed serious adverse reactions. There are other reports confirming that concurrent use can be useful and safe, involving 18 patients,[19] 59 patients[20] and 18 patients.[21]

Mechanism

Not understood. An unconfirmed suggestion is that the adverse effects are possibly due to the combined effects of lithium and haloperidol on basal striatal adenylate cyclase.[22] Another report claims that what occurs could be due to lithium toxicity alone.[23]

Importance and management

The advantageous effects of concurrent use are well documented, but the adverse effects are less clear. The Danish investigators[24] offer the opinion that ". . . the combination of lithium and haloperidol is therapeutically useful when administered to diagnostically appropriate patients. To discourage or prohibit its use would, in our opinion, be injudicious, but treatment must be carried out under proper clinical control." This implies very close monitoring to detect any signs of adverse reactions. One review[25] suggests that combined use seems to be safe if lithium levels are below 1.0 mmol/l. At the moment there seems to be no way of identifying the apparently small number of patients who are particularly at risk, but possible likely factors include a previous history of extrapyramidal reactions with antipsychotics and the use of large doses of haloperidol. If any adverse effects develop the drugs should be withdrawn immediately because irreversible brain damage can occur.

1. Cohen WJ, Cohen NH. Lithium carbonate, haloperidol, and irreversible brain damage. *JAMA* (1974) 230, 1283–7.

2. Thornton WE, Pray BJ. Lithium intoxication: a report of two cases. *Can Psychiatr Assoc J* (1975) 20, 281–2.

3. Marhold J, Zimanová J, Lachman M, Král J, Vojtěchovský M. To the incompatibility of haloperidol with lithium salts. *Acta Nerv Super (Praha)* (1974) 16, 199–200.

4. Wilson WH. Addition of lithium to haloperidol in non-affective antipsychotic non-responsive schizophrenia: a double blind, placebo controlled, parallel design clinical trial. *Psychopharmacology (Berl)* (1993) 111, 359–66.

5. Loudon JB, Waring H. Toxic reactions to lithium and haloperidol. *Lancet* (1976) ii, 1088.

6. Juhl RP, Tsuang MT, Perry PJ. Concomitant administration of haloperidol and lithium carbonate in acute mania. *Dis Nerv Syst* (1977) 38, 675.

7. Spring G, Frankel M. New data on lithium and haloperidol incompatibility. *Am J Psychiatry* (1981) 138, 818–21.

8. Menes C, Burra P, Hoaken PCS. Untoward effects following combined neuroleptic-lithium therapy. *Can J Psychiatry* (1980) 25, 573–6.

9. Keitner GI, Rahman S. Reversible neurotoxicity with combined lithium-haloperidol administration. *J Clin Psychopharmacol* (1984) 4, 104–5.

10. Kamlana SH, Kerry RJ, Khan IA. Lithium: some drug interactions. *Practitioner* (1980) 224, 1291–2.

11. Fetzer J, Kader G, Dahany S. Lithium encephalopathy: a clinical, psychiatric and EEG evaluation. *Am J Psychiatry* (1981) 138, 1622–3.

12. Thomas CJ. Brain damage with lithium/haloperidol. *Br J Psychiatry* (1979) 134, 552.

13. Thomas C, Tatham A, Jakubowski S. Lithium/haloperidol combinations and brain damage. *Lancet* (1982) i, 626.

14. Schaffer CB, Batra K, Garvey MJ, Mungas DM, Schaffer LC. The effect of haloperidol on serum levels of lithium in adult manic patients. *Biol Psychiatry* (1984) 19, 1495–9.

15. Emilien G, Maloteaux JM. Lithium neurotoxicity at low therapeutic doses. Hypotheses for causes and mechanism of action following a retrospective analysis of published case reports. *Acta Neurol Belg* (1996) 96, 281–93.

16. Goldman SA. Lithium and neuroleptics in combination: Is there enhancement of neurotoxicity leading to permanent sequelae? *J Clin Pharmacol* (1996) 36, 951–62.

17. Goldman SA. FDA MedWatch Report: Lithium and neuroleptics in combination: the spectrum of neurotoxicity. *Psychopharmacol Bull* (1996) 32, 299–309.

18. Garfinkel PE, Stancer HC, Persad E. A comparison of haloperidol, lithium carbonate and their combination in the treatment of mania. *J Affect Disord* (1980) 2, 279–88.

19. Baptista T. Lithium-neuroleptic combination and irreversible brain damage. *Acta Psychiatr Scand* (1986) 73, 111.

20. Goldney RD, Spence ND. Safety of the combination of lithium and neuroleptic drugs. *Am J Psychiatry* (1986) 143, 882–4.

21. Biederman J, Lerner Y, Belmaker H. Combination of lithium and haloperidol in schizoaffective disorder. A controlled study. *Arch Gen Psychiatry* (1979) 36, 327–33.

22. Geisler A, Klysner R. Combined effect of lithium and flupenthixol on striatal adenylate cyclase. *Lancet* (1977) i, 430–1.

23. von Knorring L. Possible mechanisms for the presumed interaction between lithium and neuroleptics. *Hum Psychopharmacol* (1990) 5, 287–92.

24. Baastrup PC, Hollnagel P, Sørensen R, Schou M. Adverse reactions in treatment with lithium carbonate and haloperidol. *JAMA* (1976) 236, 2645–6.

25. Batchelor DH, Lowe MR. Reported neurotoxicity with the lithium/haloperidol combination and other neuroleptics—a literature review. *Hum Psychopharmacol* (1990) 5, 275–80.

Lithium + Herbal remedies

A woman developed lithium toxicity after taking a herbal diuretic remedy.

Clinical evidence, mechanism, importance and management

A woman of 26, stabilised on 900 mg **lithium** twice daily for 5 months (with a serum level of 1.1 mmol/l) and also taking hydroxyzine, lorazepam, propranolol, risperidone and sertraline, came to an emergency clinic complaining of dizziness and grogginess after taking a non-prescription remedy (chlorphenamine, paracetamol (acetaminophen) and pseudoephedrine) for 2 days. The next day, after stopping the sinus remedy, she was still groggy but a little better, but 2 days later she returned, this time complaining of nausea, diarrhoea, unsteady gait, tremor, nystagmus and drowsiness, (all symptoms of **lithium** toxicity). At this visit she admitted that she had been taking a non-prescription **herbal diuretic** for the last 2 to 3 weeks to lose weight, and she was found to have a serum **lithium** level of 4.5 mmol/l. This un-named herbal preparation contained **corn silk**, *Equisetum hyemale*, **juniper**, **ovate buchu**, **parsley** and **uva ursi** (**bearberry**), all of which are believed to have diuretic actions. The other ingredients were bromelain, paprika, potassium and vitamin B6.[1]

The most likely explanation for what happened is that the **herbal diuretic** caused the **lithium** toxicity. It is unlikely that the sinus preparation had much (if any) part to play. It is impossible to know which herb or combination of herbs actually caused the toxicity, or how, but this case once again emphasises that herbal remedies are not risk-free just because they are natural. It also underscores the need for patients to avoid self-medication without first seeking informed advice and supervision if they are taking potentially hazardous drugs like **lithium**.

1. Pyevich D, Bogenschutz MP. Herbal diuretics and lithium toxicity. *Am J Psychiatry* (2001) 158, 1329.

Lithium carbonate + Iodides

The hypothyroidic and goitrogenic effects of lithium carbonate, potassium iodide and possibly other iodides may be additive if given concurrently.

Clinical evidence

A man with normal thyroid function showed evidence of hypothyroidism after 3 weeks' treatment with lithium carbonate (750–1500 mg daily). After 2 further weeks' treatment with **potassium iodide** as well, the hypothyroidism became even more marked, but resolved completely within a fortnight of the withdrawal of both drugs.[1]

A number of other reports describe the antithyroid effect of lithium when given on its own[1-8] as well as with **potassium iodide**.[9-11] There is also a case on record involving lithium, **isopropamide iodide** and haloperidol.[12]

Mechanism

Lithium accumulates in the thyroid gland and blocks the release of the thyroid hormones by thyroid-stimulating hormone. The mechanism is not well understood. Potassium iodide temporarily prevents the production of the thyroid hormones but, as time goes on, synthesis recommences. Thus, both lithium ions and iodide ions can depress the production or release of the hormones and thereby have additive hypothyroidic effects.

Importance and management

The incidence and clinical importance of this interaction are difficult to assess. Hypothyroidism due to lithium treatment is not infrequent (variously reported as 12 out of 33 patients,[2] two out of 56 men[6] and 20 out of 93 women[6]) but there are very few reports of hypothyroidism due to the concurrent use of these drugs. Nevertheless the outcome of concurrent use should be monitored. Only potassium iodide and isopropamide iodide have been implicated but it would seem possible with other iodides. It should be remembered that some OTC preparations contain iodine.

1. Shopsin B, Shenkman L, Blum M, Hollander CS. Iodine and lithium-induced hypothyroidism. Documentation of synergism. *Am J Med* (1973) 55, 695–9.
2. Schou M, Amidsen A, Jensen SE, Olsen T. Occurrence of goitre during lithium treatment. *BMJ* (1968) 3, 710.
3. Shopsin B, Blum M, Gershon S. Lithium-induced thyroid disturbance: case report and review. *Compr Psychiatry* (1969) 10, 215.
4. Emerson CH, Dyson WL, Utiger RD. Serum thyrotropin and thyroxine concentrations in patients receiving lithium carbonate. *J Clin Endocrinol Metab* (1973) 36, 338.
5. Candy J. Severe hypothyroidism — an early complication of lithium therapy. *BMJ* (1972) 3, 277.
6. Villeneuve A, Grantier J, Jus A, Perron D. Effect of lithium on thyroid in man. *Lancet* (1973) ii, 502.
7. Lloyde GG, Rosser RM, Crowe MJ. Effect of lithium on thyroid in man. *Lancet* (1973) ii, 619.
8. Bocchetta A, Bernardi F, Pedditizi M, Loviselli A, Velluzzi F, Martino E, Del Zompo M. Thyroid abnormalities during lithium treatment. *Acta Psychiatr Scand* (1991) 83, 193–8.
9. Jorgensen JD. Lithium-carbonate-induced myxedema. *JAMA* (1971) 220, 587.
10. Weiner JD. Lithium carbonate-induced myxedema. *JAMA* (1971) 220, 587.
11. Spaulding SW, Burrow GN, Ramey JN, Donabedian RK. Effect of increased iodide intake on thyroid function in subjects on chronic lithium therapy. *Acta Endocrinol (Copenh)* (1977) 84, 290–6.
12. Luby ED, Schwartz D, Rosenbaum H. Lithium carbonate-induced myxedema. *JAMA* (1971) 218, 1298.

Lithium carbonate + Ispaghula husk or Psyllium

There is evidence that ispaghula husk and psyllium can reduce serum lithium levels.

Clinical evidence

A woman, recently started on lithium, showed a fall in her serum lithium levels from 0.53 to 0.4 mmol/l when she started to take one teaspoonful of **ispaghula husk** in water twice daily, despite an increase in her lithium dosage. Four days after the **ispaghula** was stopped, her serum lithium levels rose to 0.76 mmol/l with no change in her lithium dosage.[1]

A study in 6 normal subjects similarly showed that the absorption of lithium (as measured by the urinary excretion) was reduced 14% by **psyllium**.[2]

Mechanism

Not understood. One idea is that the absorption of the lithium from the gut is reduced.[1,2] Another is that the preparations in question (not specifically named) might have had a high sodium content that would result in an increase in the excretion of the lithium by the kidneys.[2]

Importance and management

Information is very limited and the general importance of this interaction is uncertain, but it would now seem prudent to monitor the serum lithium levels in patients given ispaghula or psyllium preparations. Increase the lithium dosage if necessary.

1. Perlman BB. Interaction between lithium salts and ispaghula husk. *Lancet* (1990) 335, 416.
2. Toutoung M, Schulz P, Widmer J, Tissot R. Probable interaction entre le psyllium et le lithium. *Thérapie* (1990) 45, 357–60.

Lithium carbonate + Lamotrigine

Lamotrigine is reported not to interact with lithium to a clinically relevant extent.

Clinical evidence, mechanism, importance and management

In an open, randomised, two-period, crossover study, 21 normal men were given 2 g lithium gluconate anhydrous (9.8 mmol of lithium) every 12 h for 5½ days, either with or without 100 mg **lamotrigine** daily. It was found that the serum lithium levels were slightly lower while taking the **lamotrigine** (maximum serum levels –8.5%, AUC – 7.7%) but these small changes were not considered to be clinically relevant.[1] No special precautions or dosage adjustments would therefore appear to be needed if these drugs are used concurrently. The lithium salt used in this study was the gluconate, but there is no reason to expect other lithium salts to behave differently.

1. Chen C, Veronese L, Yin Y. The effects of lamotrigine on the pharmacokinetics of lithium. *Br J Clin Pharmacol* (2000) 50, 193–5.

Lithium carbonate + Mazindol

An isolated case report describes lithium intoxication attributed to the concurrent use of mazindol.

Clinical evidence

A manic depressive woman, well controlled on lithium carbonate, showed signs of lithium intoxication within 3 days of starting to take 2 mg **mazindol** daily. After 9 days of concurrent treatment she developed twitching, limb rigidity and muscle fasciculation, and was both dehydrated and stuporose. Her serum lithium levels were found to have risen from 0.4–1.3 mmol/l to 3.2 mmol/l. She recovered when the **mazindol** was withdrawn.[1] It is not known whether this was a direct interaction between the two drugs, or whether the mazindol-induced anorexia reduced the intake of sodium and water which then reduced the renal excretion of lithium. There seem to be no other reports of interactions between lithium and other anorectic drugs confirming this possibility.

This is an isolated case and its general importance is uncertain but the rapidity of its onset and the potentially serious outcome are good reasons for making sure that concurrent use is well monitored.

1. Hendy MS, Dove AF, Arblaster PG. Mazindol-induced lithium toxicity. *BMJ* (1980) 280, 684–5.

Lithium carbonate + Methyldopa

Lithium intoxication has been described in four patients and three normal subjects when concurrently treated with methyldopa.

Clinical evidence

A manic-depressive woman, stabilised on lithium carbonate, rapidly developed signs of lithium intoxication (blurred vision, hand tremors, mild diarrhoea, confusion, and slurred speech) when additionally given 1 g **methyldopa** daily, although her serum lithium levels remained within the range 0.5–0.7 mmol/l.[1] Later the author of this report demonstrated this interaction on himself.[2] He found that within 2 days of starting to take 1 g **methyldopa** daily the signs of lithium intoxication had clearly developed, although his serum levels had risen only moderately, reaching a maximum of 0.9 mmol/l after only 4–5 days.

This interaction has been described in 3 other patients[3-5] and in 3 normal subjects.[6] In 3 cases the signs of intoxication developed although the serum lithium levels were within the normal therapeutic range.

Mechanism

Not understood.

Importance and management

Information appears to be limited to the reports cited, but the interaction would seem to be established. Avoid concurrent use whenever possible, but if not the effects should be closely monitored. Serum lithium measurements may be unreliable because intoxication can occur even though the levels remain within the normally accepted therapeutic range.

1. Byrd GJ. Methyldopa and lithium carbonate: suspected interaction. *JAMA* (1975) 233, 320.
2. Byrd GJ. Lithium carbonate and methyldopa: apparent interaction in man. *Clin Toxicol* (1977) 11, 1–4.
3. Osanloo E, Deglin JH. Interaction of lithium and methyldopa. *Ann Intern Med* (1980) 92, 433–4.
4. O'Regan JB. Adverse interaction of lithium carbonate and methyldopa. *Can Med Assoc J* (1976) 115, 385–6.
5. Yassa R. Lithium-methyldopa interaction. *Can Med Assoc J* (1986) 134, 141–2.
6. Walker N, White K, Tornatore F, Boyd JL, Cohen JL. Lithium-methyldopa interactions in normal subjects. *Drug Intell Clin Pharm* (1980) 14, 638–9.

Lithium carbonate + Metronidazole

Three patients have been described whose serum lithium levels rose (to toxic concentrations in two of them) when concurrently treated with metronidazole.

Clinical evidence, mechanism, importance and management

A woman of 40 taking 1800 mg lithium carbonate, 0.15 mg levothyroxine and 60 mg propranolol daily whose serum lithium level two weeks previously was 1.3 mmol/l, developed signs of lithium intoxication (ataxia, rigidity, poor cognitive function, impaired co-ordination etc.) while completing a one-week course of **metronidazole** (500 mg twice daily). Her serum lithium levels had climbed by 46% (to 1.9 mmol/l).[1] Two other patients are described in another report whose serum lithium levels rose by 20% and 125% respectively 12–19 days after starting a one-week course of **metronidazole** (500–750 mg daily).[2] Both of these two patients showed evidence of kidney abnormalities possibly caused by the concurrent use of these drugs. One other patient at least is said to have taken both drugs together uneventfully.[3]

There seem to be no strong reasons for totally avoiding concurrent use but the outcome should be well monitored. The authors of one of the reports also recommend frequent analysis of creatinine and electrolyte levels and urine osmolality in order to detect any renal problems.[2]

1. Brinkley JR. Quoted as personal communication by Ayd JF in *Int Drug Ther Newslett* (1982) 17, 15–16.
2. Teicher MH, Altesman RI, Cole JO, Schatzberg AF. Possible nephrotoxic interaction of lithium and metronidazole. *JAMA* (1987) 257, 3365–6.
3. Strathman I (GD Searle and Co). Quoted as personal communication by Ayd JF in *Int Drug Ther Newslett* (1982) 17, 15.

Lithium carbonate + NSAIDs

A marked and rapid rise in serum lithium levels (+60%) with intoxication may develop in patients given clometacin or indometacin (indomethacin). A more moderate rise (+15–34%) occurs with diclofenac and ibuprofen, but much larger rises have been seen in a few patients. Increased serum lithium levels and/or intoxication have also been seen in small and variable numbers of patients when given flurbiprofen, ketoprofen, ketorolac, lornoxicam, mefenamic acid, meloxicam, naproxen, niflumic acid, phenylbutazone, piroxicam or tiaprofenic acid. Sulindac is reported to increase, reduce or have no effect on serum lithium levels. Aspirin, lysine acetylsalicylate, sodium salicylate and paracetamol (acetaminophen) appear not to interact.

Clinical evidence

(a) Aspirin and other salicylates

10 normal women stabilised on lithium sulphate showed a slight fall in serum lithium levels (from 0.63 to 0.61 mmol/l), and a slight rise in their renal excretion of lithium (from 22.0 to 23.3 ml/min) when given 4 g **aspirin** daily for 7 days.[1]

No interaction was seen in 7 patients on lithium when given 3.9 g **aspirin** daily,[2] and in one patient taking 325 mg daily.[3] Another report states that 2.4 g **aspirin** daily had no effect on the absorption or renal excretion of single doses of lithium carbonate given to six normal subjects,[4] and a further report[5] very briefly describes the absence of an interaction between lithium carbonate and **lysine acetylsalicylate** or **sodium salicylate**.[6]

(b) Clometacin

The observation of lithium intoxication in 3 patients on lithium when given **clometacin**, prompted further study of this interaction. Six women stabilised on lithium showed an almost 60% rise (from 0.64 to 1.01 mmol/l) in their serum lithium levels after receiving 450 mg **clometacin** daily for 5 days.[7] The clearance of lithium by the kidney was found to be reduced.

(c) Diclofenac

Five normal subjects[8,9] stabilised on lithium showed a 26% rise in serum lithium levels after taking 150 mg **diclofenac** daily for 7 to 10 days. Lithium excretion by the kidney fell by 23%.

(d) Flurbiprofen

11 healthy women with bipolar disorder taking immediate-release lithium (600–1200 mg daily) were additionally given 100 mg **flurbiprofen** daily or a placebo for 7 days. The mean maximum serum levels and the AUC of the lithium rose by about 18% while taking the **flurbiprofen**, and 4 of the women showed serum lithium level increases of more than 25% or 0.2 mmol/l. No lithium toxicity was seen.[10]

(e) Ibuprofen

The serum lithium levels of a patient rose by 25% (from 0.8 to 1.0 mmol/l) over a 7-day period while taking 2400 mg **ibuprofen** daily.[11,12] He experienced nausea and drowsiness. Two other patients in the study taking 1200–2400 mg **ibuprofen** daily did not show this interaction.

The serum lithium levels of 11 subjects rose by 15% when given 1600 mg **ibuprofen** daily.[13] 1800 mg **ibuprofen** daily for 6 days raised lithium levels in 9 patients by 34% (range 12–66%).[14] Lithium toxicity developed in one patient within 24 h,[15] and in 3 others within 3–7 days of starting **ibuprofen**.[16] The serum lithium levels of the latter patients doubled or tripled. Lithium toxicity has been seen in other patients attributable to the use of **ibuprofen**.[17,18]

(f) Indometacin (Indomethacin)

Indometacin (50 mg three times a day) increased the serum lithium levels of 5 subjects taking 300–900 mg lithium carbonate daily by 43% after 7 days. Renal clearance fell by 31%.[12]

Other studies have found rises of 59% and 61% in serum lithium levels in patients taking 150 mg **indometacin** daily,[9,19] and lithium intoxication has been seen.[11,20] A similar rise in serum lithium levels was found in another study on 10 normal subjects taking lithium sulphate rather than carbonate.[1] Paradoxically **indometacin** has also been successfully used to treat a lithium intoxicated patient who was polyuric, hypernatraemic and somnolent.[21]

(g) Ketoprofen

A manic-depressive patient stabilised on lithium carbonate showed a rise in his serum lithium levels from 0.9 to 1.32 mmol/l over a 3-week period when treated with 400 mg **ketoprofen** daily.[5]

(h) Ketorolac

A man of 80 taking haloperidol, procyclidine, clonazepam, aspirin, digoxin and lithium (serum levels between 0.5 and 0.7 mmol/l) was additionally given 100 mg indometacin (indomethacin) for 13 days for arthritis, then replaced by 30 mg **ketorolac** daily. On the next day his serum lithium levels were 0.9 mmol/l and 6 days later 1.1 mmol/l. When the lithium dosage was lowered from 450 to 300 mg daily, the lithium levels fell to 0.7 mmol/l, but eight days later the dosage was raised again to 450 mg daily and after another 6 days the serum levels had risen to 0.9 mmol/l.[3] Another man of 39, well controlled on lithium for cluster headache, developed neurotoxicity ("shaking of the hands and legs making it difficult to go up or down steps", masking of the face and dysarthria) shortly after starting to take 60 mg **ketorolac** daily for low back pain. His serum lithium levels were found to have risen from about 0.6 to 0.9 mmol/l.[22] When 5 normal subjects were given 900 mg lithium carbonate for 7 days and then additionally given 40 mg **ketorolac** daily for another 7 days, the 12 h trough serum lithium levels rose from 0.50 to 0.66 mmol/l.[23] The same or similar results are reported elsewhere with an increase in the incidence and severity of lithium side effects.[24]

(i) Lornoxicam

A study in 12 normal subjects found that 4 mg **lornoxicam** daily raised their maximum serum lithium levels by 20% (from 0.55 to 0.66 mmol/l) and the AUC by 9%. One of the subjects whose serum **lornoxicam** levels were unusually high showed a much higher rise in serum lithium levels (+60%), and a rise in AUC of +52%.[25]

(j) Mefenamic acid

Acute lithium toxicity accompanied by a sharp deterioration in kidney function was seen in a patient when concurrently treated with lithium carbonate and 500 mg **mefenamic acid** three times daily.[26] Withdrawal of the drugs and subsequent rechallenge confirmed this interaction. Another case of toxicity was seen in a patient but his renal function was impaired before both drugs were given.[27] Another extremely brief report describes this interaction in another patient.[28]

(k) Meloxicam

16 normal subjects taking lithium carbonate twice daily and with serum levels within the range 0.3–0.7 mmol/l showed a mean 21% increased in serum lithium levels when concurrently given 15 mg meloxicam daily.[29]

(l) Naproxen

Over a 6-day period while taking 760 mg **naproxen** daily the serum lithium levels of 7 patients rose by 16% (from 0.81 to 0.94 mmol/l). The range was 0–42% and 4 showed a rise of over 20%. One patient whose levels rose from 0.95 to 1.13 mmol/l developed signs of toxicity (staggering gait and tremors).[30]

However, a study in 9 normal subjects given 300 mg lithium carbonate 12-hourly for 7 days, followed by the addition of 220 mg **naproxen** 8-hourly for a further 5 days, found no evidence that **naproxen** increased the serum lithium levels over this short period.[31]

(m) Niflumic acid

An isolated report describes lithium intoxication in a woman after taking **niflumic acid** (three capsules) and 1.5 g aspirin daily for 5 days. Her serum lithium levels rose from 0.8 to 1.6 mmol/l.[32]

(n) Paracetamol (acetaminophen)

A study in 9 normal subjects given 300 mg lithium carbonate 12-hourly for 7 days, followed by the addition of 650 mg **paracetamol** (**acetaminophen**) 6-hourly for a further 5 days, found no evidence that **paracetamol** increased the serum lithium levels over this short period.[31]

(o) Phenylbutazone and oxyphenbutazone

The serum lithium levels of a manic depressive patient doubled (from 0.7 to 1.44 mmol/l), accompanied by signs of intoxication within 3 days of starting treatment with 750 mg **phenylbutazone** daily in the form of suppositories.[33] Renal clearance of the lithium was found to have halved (from 10 to 5 ml/min/1.73 m^2). The patient was also taking viloxazine, clorazepate, spironolactone, isosorbide and dipyridamole. The same authors describe another patient who showed a sharp rise in serum lithium levels when given 500 mg **oxyphenbutazone**.[5]

In contrast, a study in 6 patients with bipolar affective illness found that 6 days' treatment with 300 mg **phenylbutazone** daily caused only a minor increase (0–15.35%) in serum lithium levels.[34] However some CNS-related side effects (drowsiness, confusion, etc.) occurred.

(p) Piroxicam

A manic depressive woman, well controlled for over 9 years on lithium, experienced lithium toxicity (unsteadiness, trembling, confusion) and was admitted to hospital on three occasions after taking **piroxicam**. Her serum levels on two occasions had risen to 2.7 and 1.6 mmol/l, although in the latter instance the lithium had been withdrawn the previous day. In a subsequent study her serum lithium levels rose by one half (from 1.0 to 1.5 mmol/l) when given 20 mg **piroxicam** daily while continuing to take the same dose of lithium (250 mg three time a day).[35]

This interaction has also been described in 3 other patients.[18,36-39] Another report describes lithium intoxication in a man given 20 mg **piroxicam** daily which apparently took 4 months to develop completely.[4]

(q) Sulindac

(i) *Lithium levels reduced*. A patient stabilised on lithium showed a marked fall in serum lithium levels (from 0.65 to 0.39 mmol/l) after 2 weeks' concurrent treatment with **sulindac**, 200 mg daily. His serum lithium levels gradually climbed over the next 6 weeks to 0.71 mmol/l and restabilised without any change in the dosage of either lithium or **sulindac**. The serum lithium levels of another patient were approximately halved a week after his dosage of **sulindac** was doubled to 400 mg daily.[40] Control of depression was not entirely lost in either patient.

(ii) *Lithium levels unaffected*. Three studies found that serum lithium levels in 1, 4 and 6 patients respectively were unaffected by the use of **sulindac**.[30,41,42]

(iii) *Lithium levels increased*. Two patients showed increased serum lithium levels apparently due to the use of **sulindac**. In one of them the lithium levels rose from 0.9 to 2.0 mEq/l after 19 days treatment with 150 mg **sulindac** twice daily and toxicity was seen. The levels fell to 0.8 mEq/l within 5 days of stopping the **sulindac**. The other patient showed a rise from 0.9 to 1.7 mEq/l within a week of adding 150 mg **sulindac** twice daily. When the lithium dosage was reduced from 1800 to 1500 mg daily while continuing to take the **sulindac**, the serum lithium levels fell and were 1.2 mEq/l at 37 days and 1.0 mEq/l at 70 days. No lithium toxicity occurred.[43]

(r) Tiaprofenic acid

A 79-year-old woman on lithium (as well as fosinopril, nifedipine, oxazepam and haloperidol) showed a rise in her trough serum lithium levels from 0.36 to 0.57 mmol/l within 3 days of starting to take 200 mg **tiaprofenic acid** three times daily. The serum lithium levels had risen to 0.65 mmol/l by the next day and, despite halving the dosage, were found to be 0.69 mmol/l 5 days later. These rises were attributed to an interaction with the **tiaprofenic acid** exacerbated by the fosinopril.[44]

(s) Other NSAIDs

Sometimes it is claimed that most NSAIDs cause lithium toxicity because they can reduce the excretion of lithium by the kidney tubules, but there does not appear to be confirmatory documentation of this for any NSAID not already cited here. For example the drug datasheet for **azapropazone** says ". . . inhibition of renal lithium clearance by *Rheumox* (**azapropazone**) has not been reported but the possibility of this occurring should be borne in mind." The British National Formulary[45] says that the ". . . excretion of lithium [is] reduced by **azapropazone** . . . (possibility of toxicity)." The latter in particular suggests that an interaction is likely, but as yet direct clinical evidence seems to be lacking.

Mechanism

Not understood. One suggestion is that the interacting NSAIDs do so by inhibiting the synthesis of the renal prostaglandins (PGE_2) so that the renal blood flow is reduced, thereby reducing the renal excretion of the lithium. However this fails to explain why aspirin, which blocks renal prostaglandin synthesis by 65–70%, does not affect serum lithium levels.[1]

Importance and management

The documentation of these interactions is variable and limited, but what is known indicates that **clometacin** and **indometacin** (**indomethacin**) should be avoided unless serum lithium levels can be very well monitored and the dosage reduced appropriately. The other NSAIDs that have been reported to increase serum lithium levels and/or cause intoxication (**diclofenac**, **flurbiprofen**, **ibuprofen**, **ketoprofen**, **ketorolac**, **lornoxicam**, **mefenamic acid**, **meloxicam**, **naproxen**, **niflumic acid**, **phenylbutazone**, **oxyphenbutazone**, **piroxicam**, **tiaprofenic acid**) seem to be less risky. In some instances the serum lithium level rises are of little or no clinical relevance, but these NSAIDs should not be added to lithium unless the outcome can be well monitored and serum lithium dosages reduced as necessary. The effects of **sulindac** appear to be unpredictable (serum levels raised, lowered or unchanged) so that good monitoring is also necessary with this NSAID. **Aspirin**, **lysine acetylsalicylate**, **sodium salicylate** and **paracetamol** (**acetaminophen**) appear to be non-interacting alternatives. There seems to be nothing documented about any other NSAID so that they need not be avoided, nevertheless to be on the safe side good monitoring when first added would seem to be advisable.

1. Reimann IW, Diener U, Frölich JC. Indomethacin but not aspirin increases plasma lithium ion levels. *Arch Gen Psychiatry* (1983) 40, 283–6.
2. Ragheb MA. Aspirin does not significantly affect patients' serum lithium levels. *J Clin Psychiatry* (1987) 48, 425.
3. Langlois R, Paquette D. Increased serum lithium levels due to ketorolac therapy. *Can Med Assoc J* (1994) 150, 1455–6.
4. Bikin D, Conrad KA, Mayersohn M. Lack of influence of caffeine and aspirin on lithium elimination. *Clin Res* (1982) 30, 249A.
5. Singer L, Imbs JL, Danion JM, Singer P, Krieger-Finance F, Schmidt M, Schwartz J. Risque d'intoxication par le lithium en cas de traitement associé par les anti-inflammatoires non stéroïdiens. *Therapie* (1981) 36, 323–6.
6. Reimann IW, Golbs E, Fischer C, Frölich JC. Influence of intravenous acetylsalicylic acid and sodium salicylate on human renal function and lithium clearance. *Eur J Clin Pharmacol* (1985) 29, 435–41.
7. Edou D, Godin M, Colonna L, Petit M, Fillastre JP. Interaction médicamenteuse: clométacine-lithium. *Presse Med* (1983) 12, 1551.
8. Reimann IW, Frölich JC. Effects of diclofenac on lithium kinetics. *Clin Pharmacol Ther* (1981) 30, 348–52.
9. Reimann IW. Risks of non-steroidal antiinflammatory drug therapy in lithium treated patients. *Naunyn Schmiedebergs Arch Pharmacol* (1980) 311 (Suppl), R75.
10. Hughes MB, Small RE, Brink D, McKenzie ND. The effect of flurbiprofen on steady-state plasma lithium levels. *Pharmacotherapy* (1997) 17, 113–20.
11. Ragheb M, Ban TA, Buchanan D, Frölich JC. Interaction of indomethacin and ibuprofen with lithium in manic patients under a steady-state lithium level. *J Clin Psychiatry* (1980) 41, 397–8.

12. Leftwich RB, Walker LA, Ragheb M, Oates JA, Frolich JC. Inhibition of prostaglandin synthesis increases plasma lithium levels. *Clin Res* (1978) 26, 291A.
13. Kristoff CA, Hayes PE, Barr WH, Small RE, Townsend RJ, Ettigi PG. Effect of ibuprofen on lithium plasma and red blood cell concentrations. *Clin Pharm* (1986) 5, 51–5.
14. Ragheb M. Ibuprofen can increase serum lithium levels in lithium-treated patients. *J Clin Psychiatry* (1987) 48, 161–3.
15. Bailey CE, Stewart JT, McElroy RA. Ibuprofen-induced lithium toxicity. *South Med J* (1989) 82, 1197.
16. Ayd FJ. Ibuprofen-induced lithium intoxication. *Int Drug Ther Newslett* (1985) 20, 16.
17. Khan IH. Lithium and non-steroidal anti-inflammatory drugs. *BMJ* (1991) 302, 1537–8.
18. Kelly CB, Cooper SJ. Toxic elevation of serum lithium concentration by non-steroidal anti-inflammatory drugs. *Ulster Med J* (1991) 60, 240–2.
19. Frölich JC, Leftwich R, Ragheb M, Oates JA, Reimann I, Buchanan D. Indomethacin increases plasma lithium. *BMJ* (1979) 1, 1115.
20. Herschberg SN, Sierles FS. Indomethacin-induced lithium toxicity. *Am Fam Physician* (1983) 28, 155–7.
21. ter Wee PM, van Hoek B, Donker AJM. Indomethacin treatment in a patient with lithium-induced polyuria. *Intensive Care Med* (1985) 11, 103–4.
22. Iyer V. Ketorolac (Toradol®) induced lithium toxicity. *Headache* (1994) 34, 442–4.
23. Van Den Berg CM, Zum Brunnen TL, Cold JA, Jann MW, Farris F, Awad EA. Utilization of saliva lithium levels: detection of potential drug-drug interaction with NSAIDs. *Pharmacotherapy* (1997) 17, 1099.
24. Cold JA, ZumBrunnen TL, Simpson MA, Augustin BG, Awad E, Jann MW. Increased lithium serum and red blood cell concentrations during ketorolac coadministration. *J Clin Psychopharmacol* (1998) 18, 33–7.
25. Ravic M, Salas-Herrera I, Johnston A, Turner P, Foley K, Rosenow D. Influence of lornoxicam a new non-steroidal anti-inflammatory drug on lithium pharmacokinetics. *Hum Psychopharmacol* (1993) 8, 289–92.
26. MacDonald J, Neale TJ. Toxic interaction of lithium carbonate and mefenamic acid. *BMJ* (1988) 297, 1339.
27. Shelley RK. Lithium toxicity and mefenamic acid: a possible interaction and the role of prostaglandin inhibition. *Br J Psychiatry* (1987) 151, 847–8.
28. Honey J. Lithium-mefenamic acid interaction. Pharmabulletin (1982) 59, 20. Quoted by Ayd FJ. in *Int Drug Ther Newslett* (1982) 17, 16.
29. Türck D, Heinzel G, Luik G. Steady-state pharmacokinetics of lithium in healthy volunteers receiving concomitant meloxicam. *Br J Clin Pharmacol* (2000) 50, 197–204.
30. Ragheb M, Powell AL. Lithium interaction with sulindac and naproxen. *J Clin Psychopharmacol* (1986) 6, 150–4.
31. Levin GM, Grum C, Eisele G. Effect of over-the-counter dosages of naproxen sodium and acetaminophen on plasma lithium concentrations in normal volunteers. *J Clin Psychopharmacol* (1998) 18, 237–40.
32. Gay C, Plas J, Granger B, Olie JP, Loo H. Intoxication au lithium. Deux interaction inédites: l'acétazolamide et l'acide niflumique. *Encephale* (1985) 11, 261–2.
33. Singer L, Imbs JL, Schmidt M, Mack G, Sebban M, Danion JM. Baisse de la clearance rénale du lithium sous l'effet de la phénylbutazone. *Encephale* (1978) 4, 33–40.
34. Ragheb M. The interaction of lithium with phenylbutazone in bipolar affective patients. *J Clin Psychopharmacol* (1990) 10, 149–150.
35. Kerry RJ, Owen G, Michaelson S. Possible toxic interaction between lithium and piroxicam. *Lancet* (1983) i, 418–9.
36. Nadarajah J, Stein GS. Piroxicam induced lithium toxicity. *Ann Rheum Dis* (1985) 44, 502.
37. Walbridge DG, Bazire SR. An interaction between lithium carbonate and piroxicam presenting as lithium toxicity. *Br J Psychiatry* (1985) 147, 206–7.
38. Harrison TM, Wynne Davies D, Norris CM. Lithium carbonate and piroxicam. *Br J Psychiatry* (1986) 149, 124–5.
39. Shelley RK. Lithium and piroxicam. *Br J Psychiatry* (1986) 148, 343.
40. Furnell MM, Davies J. The effect of sulindac on lithium therapy. *Drug Intell Clin Pharm* (1985) 19, 374–6.
41. Ragheb MA, Powell AL. Failure of sulindac to increase serum lithium levels. *J Clin Psychiatry* (1986) 47, 33–4.
42. Miller LG, Bowman RC, Bakht F. Sparing effect of sulindac on lithium levels. *J Fam Pract* (1989) 28, 592–3.
43. Jones MT, Stoner SC. Increased lithium concentrations reported in patients treated with sulindac. *J Clin Psychiatry* (2000) 61, 527–8.
44. Alderman CP, Lindsay KSW. Increased serum lithium concentration secondary to treatment with tiaprofenic acid and fosinopril. *Ann Pharmacother* (1996) 30, 1411–13.
45. British National Formulary. 43rd ed. London: The British Medical Association and The Pharmaceutical Press; 2002. p. 641.

Lithium carbonate + Olanzapine

Olanzapine appears not to interact with lithium carbonate.

Clinical evidence, mechanism, importance and management

12 normal subjects took the following: (a) a single 32.4 mmol dose of lithium carbonate, (b) a single 32.4 mmol dose of lithium carbonate plus a 10-mg dose of **olanzapine**, (c) 10 mg **olanzapine** daily for 8 days plus, on the last day, 32.4 mmol lithium carbonate. No pharmacokinetic interactions were detected, and it was concluded that using these drugs together in recommended dosages is safe.[1,2]

1. Müller-Oerlinghausen B, Demolle D, Onkelinx C. Pharmacokinetic interaction between olanzapine and lithium in healthy male volunteers. *Pharmacopsychiatry* (1995) 28, 201.
2. Demolle D, Onkelinx C, Müller-Oerlinghausen B. Interaction between olanzapine and lithium in healthy male volunteers. *Therapie* (1995) 50 (Suppl), 486.

Lithium carbonate + Paroxetine

An isolated report describes the development of symptoms similar to those of the serotonin syndrome in a patient taking lithium and paroxetine, but it may have been that the paroxetine dosage was simply too high. Other evidence suggests that no interaction normally occurs.

Clinical evidence, mechanism, importance and management

A woman of 59 with a long-standing bipolar disorder taking 400 mg lithium and 30 mg **paroxetine** daily developed symptoms suggestive of the serotonin syndrome (shivering, tremor of her arms and legs, flushed face, agitation, and some impairment of mental focussing).[1] Her serum lithium and **paroxetine** levels were found to be 0.63 mmol/l and 693 ng/ml respectively (the latter being 6-fold higher than the upper levels seen in other patients). The lithium was continued but the **paroxetine** dosage was reduced to 10 mg daily, which reduced the serum levels to 390 ng/ml, whereupon she became symptom-free and her depression was relieved.

It is not clear whether this reaction was due to an interaction or not. It may simply have been that the **paroxetine** dosage was too high because the patient recovered when the dosage was reduced. This isolated report needs to be set in the broad context of other previous reports about successful and uneventful concurrent use in other patients, however to be on the safe side it would now be prudent to monitor well if both drugs are used.

1. Sobanski T, Bagli M, Laux G, Rao ML. Serotonin syndrome after lithium add-on medication to paroxetine. *Pharmacopsychiatry* (1997) 30, 106–7.

Lithium carbonate + Phenytoin

Signs of lithium intoxication have been seen in three patients concurrently treated with phenytoin. The serum lithium levels may remain the same.

Clinical evidence, mechanism, importance and management

A patient with a long history of depression and convulsions was treated with increasing doses of lithium carbonate and **phenytoin** over a period of about 12 years. Although the serum levels of both drugs remained within the therapeutic range, he eventually began to manifest signs of lithium intoxication (thirst, polyuria, polydipsia and tremor) that disappeared when the **phenytoin** was replaced by carbamazepine. The patient then claimed that he felt normal for the first time in years.[1] Another report[2] describes a man on **phenytoin** who became ataxic within three days of starting to take lithium. He had no other toxic symptoms and his serum lithium level was 2.0 mmol/l. A further report states that intoxication can develop during concurrent use even though the serum levels remain within the normally accepted therapeutic range.[3]

Information seems to be limited to these reports and none of them presents a clear picture of the role of **phenytoin** in the reactions described.[1-3] The interaction is not well established. However it would be prudent to be alert for signs of intoxication during concurrent use, particularly because intoxication can apparently develop even though serum levels are within the therapeutic range.

1. MacCallum WAG. Interaction of lithium and phenytoin. *BMJ* (1980) 280, 610–11.

2. Salem RB, Director K and Muniz CE. Ataxia as the primary symptom of lithium toxicity. *Drug Intell Clin Pharm* (1980) 14, 622–3.

3. Spiers J and Hirsch SR. Severe lithium toxicity with normal serum concentrations. *BMJ* (1978) 1, 185.

Lithium carbonate + Propranolol

An isolated report describes marked bradycardia in a patient on lithium when additionally given propranolol.

Clinical evidence, mechanism, importance and management

A man of 70 who had taken lithium successfully for 16 years was additionally started on 30 mg **propranolol** daily for tremor. Six weeks later he was hospitalised because of vomiting, dizziness, headache and a fainting episode. His pulse rate was 35–40 bpm and his serum lithium was 0.3 mmol/l. When later discharged on lithium without **propranolol** his pulse rate had risen to 64–80 bpm. The authors point out that both drugs reduce the production of the second messenger, cyclic adenosine monophosphate, which inhibits the influx of calcium ions across cell membranes. Lithium also reduces the mobilization of calcium ions from intracellular pools by the inositol triphosphate dependent calcium channels. These combined effects could account for the decreased contraction rate of the heart muscle in this patient.

The general importance of this interaction is uncertain, but the authors of the report suggest careful monitoring in elderly patients with atherosclerotic cardiovascular problems.[1] This interaction seems possible with other beta-blockers because they also cause heart-slowing.

1. Becker D. Lithium and propranolol: possible synergism? *J Clin Psychiatry* (1989) 50, 473.

Lithium carbonate + Sodium chloride or bicarbonate

The ingestion of marked amounts of sodium as the chloride or bicarbonate can prevent the establishment or maintenance of adequate serum lithium levels. Conversely, dietary salt restriction can cause a serum lithium rise to toxic concentrations if the lithium dosage is not reduced appropriately.

Clinical evidence

(a) Lithium response reduced by the ingestion of sodium

A depressive man, initially given 250 mg lithium carbonate four times a day, achieved a serum lithium level of 0.5 mmol/l by the following morning. When the dosage frequency was progressively increased to five, and later six times a day, his serum lithium levels failed to exceed 0.6 mmol/l because, unknown to his doctor, he was also taking **sodium bicarbonate**. In the words of the patient's wife: "... he's been taking **soda bic** for years for an ulcer, doctor, but since he started on that lithium he's been shovelling it in ..." When the **sodium bicarbonate** was stopped, relatively stable serum lithium levels of 0.8 mmol/l were achieved on the initial dosage of lithium carbonate.[1]

An investigation to find out why a number of in-patients failed to reach, or maintain, adequate therapeutic serum lithium levels, revealed that a clinic nurse had been giving the patients a proprietary saline drink (*Efferdex*), used for 'upset stomachs' and containing about 50% **sodium bicarbonate**, because the patients complained of nausea. The depression in the expected serum lithium levels was as much as 40% in some cases.[2]

Other studies confirm that the serum lithium levels can fall and the effectiveness of treatment can lessen if the intake of sodium is increased.[3-5]

(b) Lithium response increased by sodium restriction

The serum lithium levels of four manic depressives rose more rapidly and to a higher peak when salt was restricted than when taking a **dietary salt supplement**.[6]

Other studies and observations confirm that **salt** restriction can, if the effects are not monitored and dosage alterations made, lead to lithium intoxication.[5,7,8]

Mechanism

Not fully established. One suggestion is as follows. Lithium is eliminated from the body almost exclusively in the urine. The proximal tubule does not readily distinguish between sodium and lithium ions and reabsorbs 60–70% of the filtered load. It seems possible that during sodium depletion, the extracellular volume of the body is contracted so that both ions are maximally reabsorbed, leading to an increased retention of the lithium. Conversely, when the sodium levels are high (e.g. when a salt supplement is used), the extracellular volume is expanded and both sodium and lithium are excreted rather than reabsorbed. Beyond the proximal tubule, lithium and sodium appear to be handled differently, but in any case lithium reabsorption is relatively small so that any interference by sodium is likely to be minimal.[9,10]

Importance and management

Well established and clinically important interactions. The establishment and maintenance of adequate serum lithium levels can be jeopardised if the intake of ionic sodium is increased. Warn patients not to take OTC antacids or urinary alkalinizers without first seeking informed advice. Sodium bicarbonate comes in various guises and disguises (e.g. *Efferdex* (50%), *Eno's Fruit Salts* (56%), *Andrews Liver Salts* (22.6%), *Bismarex Antacid Powder* (65%), *BiSoDoL Powder* (58%)). Substantial amounts also occur in some urinary alkalinizing agents (e.g. *Citralka*, *Citravescent*).[11] There are many similar preparations available throughout the world. An antacid containing **aluminium** and **magnesium hydroxides** with simethicone has been found to have no effect on the bioavailability of lithium carbonate,[12] so that antacids of this type would appear to be safer alternatives.

Patients already stabilised on lithium should not begin to limit their intake of salt unless their serum lithium levels can be monitored and suitable dosage adjustments made, because their lithium levels can rise quite rapidly.

1. Arthur RK. Lithium levels and "Soda Bic". *Med J Aust* (1975) 2, 918.
2. McSwiggan C. Interaction of lithium and bicarbonate. *Med J Aust* (1978) 1, 38–9.
3. Bleiweiss H. Salt supplements with lithium. *Lancet* (1970) i, 416.
4. Demers RG, Heninger GR. Sodium intake and lithium treatment in mania. *Am J Psychiatry* (1971) 128, 100–4.
5. Baer L, Platman SR, Kassir S, Fieve RR. Mechanisms of renal lithium handling and their relationship to mineralocorticoids: a dissociation between sodium and lithium ions. *J Psychiatr Res* (1971) 8, 91–105.
6. Platman SR, Fieve RR. Lithium retention and excretion. *Arch Gen Psychiatry* (1969) 20, 285–9.
7. Hurtig HI, Dyson WL. Lithium toxicity enhanced by diuresis. *N Engl J Med* (1974) 290, 748–9.
8. Corcoran AC, Taylor RD, Page IH. Lithium poisoning from the use of salt substitutes. *JAMA* (1949) 139, 685–92.
9. Thomsen K, Schou M. Renal lithium excretion in man. *Am J Physiol* (1968) 215, 823–7.
10. Singer I, Rotenburg D. Mechanisms of lithium action. *N Engl J Med* (1973) 289, 254.
11. Beard TC, Wilkinson SJ, Vial JH. Hazards of urinary alkalizing agents. *Med J Aust* (1988) 149, 723.
12. Goode DL, Newton DW, Ueda CT, Wilson JE, Wulf BG, Kafonek D. Effect of antacid on the bioavailability of lithium carbonate. *Clin Pharm* (1984) 3, 284–7

Lithium carbonate + Sodium valproate

No clinically relevant adverse interaction occurs between lithium carbonate and sodium valproate.

Clinical evidence, mechanism, importance and management

16 normal subjects were given **sodium valproate** or a placebo twice daily for 12 days, to which was added lithium carbonate on days 6 to 10. The **sodium valproate** serum levels and AUC rose slightly, while the serum lithium levels were unaltered. Adverse events did not change significantly. It was concluded that the concurrent use of these drugs is safe.[1]

1. Granneman GR, Schenck DW, Cavanaugh JH, Witt GF. Pharmacokinetic interactions and side-effects resulting from concomitant administration of lithium and divalproex sodium. *J Clin Psychiatry* (1996) 57, 204–6.

Lithium carbonate + Spectinomycin

A single case report describes a patient who developed lithium intoxication when given spectinomycin.

Clinical evidence, mechanism, importance and management

A depressive woman[1] controlled on lithium developed intoxication (tremor, nausea, vomiting, ataxia and dysarthria) when given **spectinomycin** injections (dose not stated) for the treatment of gonorrhoea. Her serum lithium levels had climbed from a range of 0.8–1.1 mmol/l to 3.2 mmol/l. A likely explanation is that **spectinomycin**, particularly in multiple doses, decreases creatinine clearance, elevates BUN and reduces urine output, which would be expected to reduce the excretion of lithium, resulting in a rise in serum levels. Information seems to be limited to this report, but it would now seem prudent to monitor the effects of concurrent use in any patient.

1. Conroy RW. Quoted as a personal communication by Ayd FJ. Possible adverse drug-drug interaction report. *Int Drug Ther Newslett* (1978) 13, 15.

Lithium carbonate + Tetracyclines

Concurrent use is normally uneventful, but two isolated reports describe lithium intoxication in a woman attributed to the use of tetracycline, and in a man attributed to doxycycline.

Clinical evidence

(a) Doxycycline

A man on long term treatment with lithium carbonate became confused within a day of starting to take 100 mg **doxycycline** twice daily, and by the end of a week had signs of lithium toxicity (ataxia, dysarthria, worsened tremor, fatigue, etc.). His serum lithium levels had risen from the normal 0.8–1.1 mmol/l to 1.8 mmol/l. He recovered when the **doxycycline** was withdrawn.[1]

(b) Tetracycline

An isolated report describes a manic depressive woman, well stabilised on lithium for 3 years, with serum concentrations within the range 0.5–0.84 mmol/l. Within 2 days of starting to take a sustained-release form of **tetracycline** (*Tetrabid*) her serum lithium levels had risen to 1.7 mmol/l, and 2 days later they had climbed to 2.74 mmol/l. By then she showed clear signs of lithium intoxication (slight drowsiness, slurring of the speech, fine tremor and thirst).[2]

In contrast, 14 normal subjects taking 450 mg lithium carbonate twice daily showed a small reduction in serum lithium levels (from 0.51 to 0.47 mmol/l) when given 1 g **tetracycline hydrochloride** for seven days.[3] The incidence of adverse reactions remained largely unchanged except for a slight increase in CNS and gastrointestinal side-effects. Another report describes the uneventful use of lithium and **tetracyclines** in patients.[4]

Mechanism

Not understood. One suggested reason is that **tetracycline** (known to have nephrotoxic potentialities) may have adversely affected the renal clearance of lithium from the body.[2]

Importance and management

These two adverse reactions reports are isolated and unexplained. There would seem to be no reason for avoiding concurrent use of lithium carbonate and either tetracycline or doxycycline, but monitor the outcome.

1. Miller SC. Doxycycline-induced lithium toxicity. *J Clin Psychopharmacol* (1997) 17, 54–5.
2. McGennis AJ. Lithium carbonate and tetracycline interaction. *BMJ* (1978) 2, 1183.

3. Fankhauser MP, Lindon JL, Connolly B, Healey WJ. Evaluation of lithium–tetracycline interaction. *Clin Pharm* (1988) 7, 314–17.
4. Jefferson JW. Lithium and tetracycline. *Br J Dermatol* (1982) 107, 370.

Lithium carbonate + Theophylline

Serum lithium levels are moderately reduced (20–30%) by the concurrent use of theophylline and patients may relapse as a result.

Clinical evidence

The serum lithium levels of 10 normal subjects on 900 mg lithium carbonate daily fell by 20–30%, and the urinary clearance increased by 30%, when given 400–800 mg **theophylline** daily.[1,2]

A manic patient on lithium very rapidly relapsed when given **theophylline**. The lithium dosage had to be raised in a stepwise manner as the dosage of **theophylline** was increased, in order to maintain the serum lithium levels and to control the mania.[3] **Theophylline** has also been used to treat lithium intoxication.[4-6]

Mechanism

Uncertain. Theophylline has an effect on the renal clearance of lithium.

Importance and management

Information is very limited but the interaction appears to be established. Depressive and manic relapses may occur if the dosage of lithium is not raised appropriately when theophylline is given. Serum lithium levels should be monitored during concurrent use.

1. Perry PJ, Calloway RA, Cook BL, Smith RE. Theophylline precipitated alterations of lithium clearance. *Acta Psychiatr Scand* (1984) 69, 528–37.
2. Cook BL, Smith RE, Perry PJ, Calloway RA. Theophylline-lithium interaction. *J Clin Psychiatry* (1985) 46, 278–9.
3. Sierles FS, Ossowski MG. Concurrent use of theophylline and lithium in a patient with chronic obstructive lung disease and bipolar disorder. *Am J Psychiatry* (1982) 139, 117–18.
4. Thomsen K, Schou M. Renal lithium excretion in man. *Am J Physiol* (1968) 215, 823–7.
5. Jefferson JW, Greist JH. A Primer of Lithium Therapy. Williams and Wilkins Co., Baltimore (1977) p. 204.
6. Holstead SG, Perry PJ, Kathol RG, Carson RW, Krummel SJ. The effects of intravenous theophylline infusion versus intravenous sodium bicarbonate infusion on lithium clearance in normal subjects. *Psychiatry Res* (1988) 25, 203–11.

Lithium carbonate + Thiazides or Related diuretics

Thiazide and related diuretics can cause a rapid rise in serum lithium levels leading to intoxication unless the lithium dosage is reduced appropriately. This interaction has been seen with bendroflumethiazide (bendrofluazide), chlorothiazide, chlortalidone (chlorthalidone), hydrochlorothiazide and indapamide. Other thiazides and related diuretics are expected to behave similarly.

Clinical evidence

A patient showed a rise in serum lithium concentrations from 1.3 to 2.0 mmol/l each time he was administered 500 mg **chlorothiazide** daily.[1] A study in 4 normal subjects found that 500 mg **chlorothiazide** daily for a week reduced the clearance of lithium by the kidney by 26.5% and increased the serum lithium levels by 26.2%.[2] A fall in the urinary excretion of lithium due to the use of **chlorothiazide** has been described elsewhere.[3]

A study carried out on 22 patients found that long-term treatment with either **hydroflumethiazide** (25 mg daily) plus KCl (3.4 g daily) or **bendroflumethiazide (bendrofluazide)** (2.5 mg daily) led to a 24% reduction in the urinary excretion of lithium.[4] Normal subjects

on low doses of lithium (300 mg twice daily) showed a 23% rise (from 0.30 to 0.37 mmol/l) in serum lithium levels when additionally given 25 mg **hydrochlorothiazide** twice daily for 5 days.[5] Five subjects on 900 mg lithium carbonate daily showed an approximately 20% rise in serum lithium levels within 3 days of starting to take 50 mg **hydrochlorothiazide** daily.[6]

Lithium toxicity arising from the use of thiazide diuretics either alone[7] (**bendroflumethiazide**[8]) or with other diuretics has been seen with *Moduretic* (**hydrochlorothiazide + amiloride**),[9-11] *Aldactazide* (**hydrochlorothiazide + spironolactone**),[12] **chlorothiazide** with **spironolactone** and **amiloride**[13], and **hydrochlorothiazide** with **triamterene**.[14] One case that took 3 months to develop fully involved both **bendroflumethiazide** and **perindopril** (ACE inhibitors can also raise serum lithium levels).[15] It seems almost certain that in each of these cases the thiazide component was principally responsible for the interaction. **Chlortalidone (chlorthalidone)**[16] and **indapamide**[17] have also been responsible for the development of lithium toxicity.

Mechanism

Not fully understood. The interaction occurs even though the thiazides and similar diuretics exert their major actions in the distal part of the kidney tubule whereas lithium is reabsorbed in the proximal part. A possible reason is that thiazide diuresis is accompanied by sodium loss which, within a few days, is compensated by a retention of sodium, this time in the proximal part of the tubule. Since both sodium and lithium ions are treated virtually indistinguishably, the increased reabsorption of sodium would include lithium as well, hence a significant and measurable reduction in its excretion. This would seem to be a long-term rather than an immediate effect, which might explain why a short-term single-dose study in man with bendroflumethiazide failed to show any effect on lithium excretion.[18]

Importance and management

Established, well-documented and potentially serious interactions. The rise in serum lithium levels and the accompanying intoxication can develop within 3–10 days,[3,9,14,16] or occasionally very much longer.[15] Not every patient necessarily develops a clinically important interaction but it is not possible to predict who will, and who will not, be affected. None of the thiazide diuretics nor either of the related diuretics cited (chlortalidone (chlorthalidone), indapamide) should be given to patients on lithium unless the serum lithium levels can be closely monitored and appropriate downward dosage adjustments made.

Concurrent use under controlled conditions has been advocated for certain psychiatric conditions and for the control of lithium-induced nephrogenic diabetes insipidus. Himmelhoch and his colleagues[19] calculate that 500 mg chlorothiazide daily would increase the serum lithium levels by 40% so that an approximately 40% reduction in lithium dosage would be necessary. Reductions of 60–70% would be necessary if 750–1000 mg were used.[19,20]

Quinethazone, metolazone, clorexolone, clopamide and **several other diuretics** that are closely related to the thiazides have similar actions and are also expected to interact with lithium, but so far there appear to be no reports confirming that they do so.

1. Levy ST, Forrest JN, Heninger GR. Lithium-induced diabetes insipidus: manic symptoms, brain and electrolyte correlates, and chlorothiazide treatment. *Am J Psychiatry* (1973) 130, 1014–17.
2. Poust RI, Mallinger AG, Mallinger J, Himmelhoch JM, Neil JF, Hanin I. Effect of chlorothiazide on the pharmacokinetics of lithium in plasma and erythrocytes. *Psychopharmacol Comm* (1976) 2, 273–84.
3. Baer L, Platman S, Fieve RK. Lithium metabolism: its electrolyte actions and relationship to aldosterone. Recent Advances in the Psychobiology of the Depressive Illnesses. Williams, Katz and Shield (eds). DHEW Publications, Washington DC. (1972) p. 49.
4. Petersen V, Hvidt S, Thomsen K, Schou M. Effect of prolonged thiazide treatment on renal lithium excretion. *BMJ* (1974) 2, 143–5.
5. Crabtree BL, Mack JE, Johnson CD, Amyx BC. Comparison of the effects of hydrochlorothiazide and furosemide on lithium disposition. *Am J Psychiatry* (1991) 148, 1060–3.
6. Jefferson JW, Kalin NH. Serum lithium levels and long-term diuretic use. *JAMA* (1979) 241, 1134–6.
7. Kerry RJ, Ludlow JM, Owen G. Diuretics are dangerous with lithium. *BMJ* (1980) 281, 371.
8. Aronson JK, Reynolds DJM. ABC of monitoring drug therapy. Lithium. *BMJ* (1992) 305, 1273–6.
9. Macfie AC. Lithium poisoning precipitated by diuretics. *BMJ* (1975) 1, 516.

10. Konig P, Kufferle B, Lenz G. Ein fall von Lithium-toxikation bei therapeutischen Lithium dosaen infolge zusatzlicher Gabe eines Diuretikums. *Wien Klin Wochenschr* (1978) 90, 380.
11. Dorevitch A, Baruch E. Lithium toxicity induced by combined amiloride hcl-hydrochlorothiazide administration. *Am J Psychiatry* (1986) 143, 257–8.
12. Lutz EG. Lithium toxicity precipitated by diuretics. *J Med Soc New Jers* (1975) 72, 439–40.
13. Basdevant A, Beaufils M, Corvol P. Influence des diurétiques sur l'elimination rénale du lithium. *Nouv Presse Med* (1976) 5, 2085–6.
14. Mehta BR, Robinson BHB. Lithium toxicity induced by triamterene-hydrochlorothiazide. *Postgrad Med J* (1980) 56, 783–4.
15. Vipond AJ, Bakewell S, Telford R, Nicholls AJ. Lithium toxicity. *Anaesthesia* (1996) 51, 1156–8.
16. Solomon JG. Lithium toxicity precipitated by a diuretic. *Psychosomatics* (1980) 21, 425 and 429.
17. Hanna ME, Lobao CB, Stewart JT. Severe lithium toxicity associated with indapamide therapy. *J Clin Psychopharmacol* (1990) 10. 379–80.
18. Thomsen K, Schou M. Renal lithium excretion in man. *Am J Physiol* (1968) 215, 823–7.
19. Himmelhoch JM, Poust RI, Mallinger AG, Hanin I, Neil JF. Adjustment of lithium dosage during lithium-chlorothiazide therapy. *Clin Pharmacol Ther* (1977) 22, 225–7.
20. Himmelhoch JM, Forrest JF, Neil J, Detre TP. Thiazide-lithium synergy in refractory mood swings. *Am J Psychiatry* (1977) 134, 149–52.

Lithium carbonate + Topiramate

An isolated report describes elevated serum lithium levels and evidence of toxicity in a woman five weeks after starting to take high doses of topiramate.

Clinical evidence, mechanism, importance and management

A woman of 43 with bipolar disorder type II was started on 1500 mg lithium carbonate and 500 mg **topiramate** daily and showed a steady-state trough serum lithium level of 0.5 mEq/l over the following 10-day period. She raised the **topiramate** dose of her own accord to 800 mg daily in an attempt to lose weight, and 5 weeks later began to complain of severe anorexia, nausea, fatigue and impaired concentration. She had managed to lose 35 lb. When examined she was lethargic and showed tremors, nystagmus, bradycardia and memory loss. Her trough serum lithium level had risen to 1.4 mEq/l. The symptoms disappeared over 4 days when the lithium was stopped. Two months later she was stabilised once again at 0.5 mEq/l on 1200 mg lithium carbonate and 500 mg **topiramate** daily.[1]

The reasons for this reaction are not known but some of the toxicity could have been due to either drug, with the weight loss possibly disturbing the sodium excretion which could have affected the loss of lithium in the urine. More importantly, this case highlights the possible risk of elevated serum lithium levels if high doses of **topiramate** are used. Good monitoring would be a prudent precaution.

1. Pinniti NR, Zelinski G. Does topiramate elevate serum lithium levels? *J Clin Psychopharmacol* (2002) 22, 340.

Lithium carbonate + Tricyclic antidepressants

A combination of tricyclic antidepressants and lithium can be successful in some patients, but a few may develop adverse side-effects, some of them severe. Cases of serious neurotoxicity, the serotonin syndrome and the neuroleptic malignant syndrome have been reported.

Clinical evidence

Five out of 9 depressed patients (all under 65) tolerated combined lithium/tricyclic antidepressants without significant side-effects, but severe neurotoxic side-effects developed in the other 4 elderly patients despite the use of therapeutic doses. One of them developed tremor, memory difficulties, disorganised thinking and auditory hallucinations when given 900 mg lithium carbonate daily and 50 mg **nortriptyline** daily.[1] Another study in 14 elderly patients found that 7 showed complete improvement and 3 showed partial improvement over a period from 3–21 days when given lithium and tricyclic or related antidepressants. Side effects occurred in 6. In 4 of these the lithium was stopped as a result. One of them was successfully restarted at a lower dose. The other 3 accounted for 3 of the 4 non-responders. Tremor was the most frequent side-effect, and reversible neurotoxicity with a stroke-like syndrome was the most severe. The antidepressants used were **amitriptyline, doxepin, maprotiline and trazodone**.[2] Ten therapy-resistant patients with major depression failed to respond to lithium and **amitriptyline** within 2 weeks, but did so after 4. The blood levels of the **amitriptyline** were unchanged.[3] Seizures occurred in one woman on **amitriptyline** when lithium carbonate was added.[4]

A depressed man with a lacunar infarction at the bilateral basal ganglia and taking 175 mg **clomipramine**, 25 mg **levomepromazine** and 2 mg flunitrazepam daily, developed the serotonin syndrome (myoclonus, shivering, tremors, incoordination) a week after his dosage of lithium was raised from 600 to 1000 mg daily. As his serum lithium levels were then high (1.6 mmol/l) the lithium was stopped and the serotonin syndrome abated. The **clomipramine** dosage was reduced to 50 mg daily but some mild symptoms remained until the **clomipramine** was stopped. He responded well to 600 mg lithium alone daily without developing the serotonin syndrome.[5]

A man developed periods of confusion and disorientation over 2 weeks after starting lithium (300 mg twice daily) and **doxepin** (100 mg at bedtime). He was initially hospitalised for urine retention but despite the withdrawal of both drugs he developed an NMS (neuroleptic malignant syndrome)-like condition (fever, muscle rigidity, changes in consciousness, autonomic dysfunction) which was successfully treated with dantrolene.[6] Another patient also developed NMS when treated with lithium and **amitriptyline**.[7]

Mechanisms

Not understood.

Importance and management

The concurrent use of lithium and tricyclics can be valuable, but the case reports cited here clearly show the need to monitor the outcome closely so that any problems can be quickly dealt with. The incidence and causes of these serious reactions are not known. They are unpredictable.

1. Austin LS, Arana GW, Melvin JA. Toxicity resulting from lithium augmentation of antidepressant treatment in elderly patients. *J Clin Psychiatry* (1990) 51, 344–5.
2. Lafferman J, Solomon K, Ruskin P. Lithium augmentation for treatment-resistant depression in the elderly. *J Geriatr Psychiatry Neurol* (1988) 1, 49–52.
3. Jaspert A, Ebert E, Loew T, Martus P. Lithium increases the response to tricyclic antidepressant medication – no evidence of influences of pharmacokinetic interactions. *Pharmacopsychiatry* (1993) 26, 165.
4. Solomon JG. Seizures during lithium-amitriptyline therapy. *Postgrad Med* (1979) 66, 145–8.
5. Kojima H, Terao T, Yoshimura R. Serotonin syndrome during clomipramine and lithium treatment. *Am J Psychiatry* (1993) 150, 1897.
6. Rosenberg PB, Pearlman CA. NMS-like syndrome with a lithium/doxepin combination. *J Clin Psychopharmacol* (1991) 11, 75–6.
7. Fava S, Galizia AC. Neuroleptic malignant syndrome and lithium carbonate. *J Psychiatry Neurosci* (1995) 20, 305–6.

18

Monoamine oxidase inhibitor drug interactions

Drugs with monoamine oxidase inhibitory activity were first developed as antidepressants because it was noticed that patients with tuberculosis given isoniazid, and more particularly iproniazid, showed some degree of mood elevation. A further development occurred when postural hypotension was seen to be one of the side-effects of treatment with iproniazid and, as a result, pheniprazine and later pargyline were introduced as antihypertensive agents.

Among the serious and unexpected problems with the first generation monoamine oxidase inhibitors (MAOIs) were the serious and potentially life-threatening interactions which occurred with the sympathomimetics found in some proprietary cough and cold remedies, and with tyramine-rich foods and drinks.

The intended target of the antidepressant MAOIs is the MAO within the brain, but it is also found in other parts of the body, and in particularly high concentrations in the gut and liver where it acts as a protective detoxifying enzyme against tyramine and possibly other potentially hazardous amines which exist in foods which have undergone bacterial degradation. For this reason MAO was originally called tyramine oxidase. There are at least two forms of MAO: MAO-A

metabolises (deaminates) norepinephrine (noradrenaline) and serotonin (5 HT), and MAO-B metabolises phenylethylamine. Substances like tyramine and dopamine are metabolised by both forms of MAO.

The older MAOIs (see Table 18.1) are non-selective or non-specific. They inhibit both isoenzymes A and B, and are mostly irreversible and long-acting because the return of MAO activity depends upon the regeneration of new enzymes. As a result they can continue to have activity (both beneficial and adverse) for two to three weeks after they have been withdrawn. Tranylcypromine differs in being a reversible inhibitor of MAO so that the onset and disappearance of its actions are much quicker than the other older MAOIs.

Some of the newer and more recently developed MAOIs (see Table 18.1) are safer because they interact to a lesser extent than the first generation MAOIs. This is because they are relatively rapidly reversible and are largely selective. One group of these reversible inhibitors targets MAO-A because it is inhibition of this enzyme that is responsible for the antidepressant effect. These selective MAO-A inhibitors (brofaromine, moclobemide, toloxatone) have been given the acronym RIMA (Reversible Inhibitors of Monoamine oxi-

Table 18.1 Monoamine oxidase inhibitors (MAOI)

Generic names	Proprietary names
Older MAOI	
Irreversible MAO-inhibitors	
Iproniazid	*Marsilid*
Isocarboxazid	*Marplan*
Nialamide	*Niamid*
Phenelzine	*Nardelzine, Nardil*
Tranylcypromine	*Jarrosom N, Jatrosom N, Parnate*
Tranylcypromine with trifluoperazine	*Parmodalin, Parstelin, Stelapar*
Newer MAOI	
Reversible inhibitors of MAO-A (RIMA)	
Brofaromine	
Moclobemide	*Arima, Aurorix, Feraken, Manerix, Mobemide, Moclamine, Mohexal*
Toloxatone	*Humoryl, Umoril*
Reversible inhibitors of MAO-B	
Selegiline	*Amboneural, Amindan, Antiparkin, Apomex, Atapryl, Carbex, Clondepryl, Cognitiv, Deprenyl, Deprilan, Egibren, Eldepryl, Elegelin, Elepril, Julab, Jumex, Jumexal, Jumexil, Kinline, MAOtil, Movergan, Niar, Plurimen, Regepar, Sefmex, Selecim, Seledat, Selegam, Selegos, Selemerck, Selepark, Selgene, Selgimed, Seline, Tremorex, Zelapar*

dase A). They leave MAO-B largely uninhibited so that there is still a metabolic pathway available for the breakdown of amines such as tyramine which can cause a rise in blood pressure. In practical terms this means that the amount of tyramine needed to cause a hypertensive crisis is about tenfold greater than with the older MAOIs. The other MAOIs that specifically inhibit MAO-B are ineffective for the treatment of depression and are mainly used for Parkinson's disease. Table 18.1 is a list of the MAOIs used for depression, hypertension and Parkinson's disease. Some of them are currently available, some are still undergoing trials and a few have been withdrawn.

If you look at the drug data sheets issued by manufacturers, you will frequently see warnings about real and alleged interactions with MAOIs. Blackwell,[1] who has done so much work on the interactions of the MAOIs, has rightly pointed out that the MAOIs are among the drugs which ". . .have such a long history they accumulate much myth and misinformation. Lists of side effects and interactions are lengthy but often unsupported by recent or creditable research to establish either a cause and effect relationship or to identify the underlying mechanism. Worse still, the MAOIs have developed such a sinister reputation that manufacturers often issue a reflexive admonition to avoid co-administration with new drugs." This means that many of the warnings about potential interactions with the MAOIs may lack a sound scientific basis. Take note.

In addition to the interactions of the MAOIs described in this chapter, there are others dealt with elsewhere. The Index should be consulted for a full listing.

1. Blackwell B. Monoamine Oxidase Inhibitor interactions with other drugs. *J Clin Psychopharmacol* (1991) 11, 55–59.

Moclobemide + Cimetidine

Cimetidine increases the serum levels of moclobemide. Some dosage reduction may be necessary.

Clinical evidence, mechanism, importance and management

After taking 1 g **cimetidine** daily for two weeks the maximum serum levels of a single 100-mg dose of moclobemide in normal subjects was increased by 39% and the AUC by 123%.[1] The probable reason is that the **cimetidine** (a well-recognised enzyme inhibitor) reduces the first-pass metabolism of the moclobemide. It has therefore been recommended that patients already taking **cimetidine** should be started on the lowest therapeutic dosage of moclobemide. If **cimetidine** is added to treatment with moclobemide, the dosage of the latter should initially be reduced by 50% and later adjusted as necessary.[2]

There seems to be nothing to suggest that an adverse interaction occurs with any other MAOI and **cimetidine**.

1. Schoerlin M-P, Mayersohn M, Hoevels B, Eggers H, Dellenbach M, Pfefen J-P. Cimetidine alters the disposition kinetics of the monoamine oxidase-A inhibitor moclobemide. *Clin Pharmacol Ther* (1991) 49, 32–8.
2. Amrein R, Güntert TW, Dingemanse J, Lorscheid T, Stabl M, Schmid-Burgk W. Interactions of moclobemide with concomitantly administered medication: evidence from pharmacological and clinical studies. *Psychopharmacology (Berl)* (1992) 106, S24–S31.

Moclobemide + Miscellaneous drugs

No serious adverse interactions were seen in patients and subjects given moclobemide with the drugs named below and no special precautions would seem necessary.

Clinical evidence, mechanism, importance and management

There was no evidence of any adverse interaction when moclobemide (150–675 mg daily) was given for 3–52 weeks to 50 patients on **lithium**.[1] A study in 24 normal subjects found that 150 mg moclobemide three times daily for seven days had no effect on the absorption or disposition of **ibuprofen**, and the **ibuprofen**-induced blood loss was unaffected.[2] Studies in normal subjects found that 200 mg moclobemide three times daily increased the blood pressure lowering effects of **metoprolol** (systolic 10–15 mmHg, diastolic 5–10 mmHg), but no comparable effects were seen when given with **hydrochlorothiazide** or **nifedipine**. No orthostatic hypotension occurred with any of the drug combinations.[1]

A study in 14 patients with decompensated heart failure found that 100 mg moclobemide three times daily for eight days caused a non-significant 14% fall (from 0.99 to 0.85 ng/ml) in their serum **beta-acetyldigoxin** levels. No adverse effects attributable to an interaction were seen.[1] A study in 7 women taking combined **oral contraceptives** found no evidence of any significant alterations in estradiol (oestradiol), progesterone, FSH or LH levels while taking 200 mg moclobemide three times daily for one cycle. No serious adverse reactions occurred. The conclusion was reached that the efficacy of the **oral contraceptives** is likely to be maintained during concurrent use.[1] No serious adverse effects were seen in 110 patients given 150–400 mg moclobemide daily with **acepromazine, aceprometazine, alimemazine (trimeprazine), bromperidol, chlorpromazine, chlorprothixene, clopenthixol, clothiapine, clozapine, cyamemazine, flupenthixol, fluphenazine, fluspirilene, haloperidol, levomepromazine (methotrimeprazine), penfluridol, pipamperone, prothipendyl, sulpiride** or **thioridazine**. There was however some evidence that hypotension, tachycardia, sleepiness, tremor and constipation were more common.[1] No serious adverse effects were reported in extensive clinical trials of moclobemide when used in patients taking **antiparkinsonian drugs, antibacterials, anticonvulsants, hormones** and others, but none was specifically named.[1]

1. Amrein R, Güntert TW, Dingemanse J, Lorscheid T, Stabl M, Schmid-Burgk W. Interactions of moclobemide with concomitantly administered medication: evidence from pharmacological and clinical studies. *Psychopharmacology (Berl)* (1992) 106, S24–S31.
2. Güntert TW, Schmitt M, Dingemanse J, Jonkman JHG. Influence of moclobemide on ibuprofen-induced faecal blood loss. *Psychopharmacology (Berl)* (1992) 106, S40–S42.

Monoamine oxidase inhibitors (MAOIs) + Amantadine

An isolated report describes a rise in blood pressure in a patient on amantadine when given phenelzine.

Clinical evidence, mechanism, importance and management

A woman of 49 was treated for Parkinson's disease with **amantadine** (200 mg daily), haloperidol (5 mg daily) and flurazepam (30 mg at night). Within 72 h of starting to take 30 mg **phenelzine** daily for depression, her blood pressure rose from 140/90 to 160/110 mmHg and it remained high for a further 72 h after the **amantadine** and haloperidol had been withdrawn.[1] The reason for this hypertensive reaction is not understood. In contrast, another woman is reported to have been given **amantadine** (200 mg daily) and **phenelzine** (43 mg daily) successfully and uneventfully.[2] The general importance of this interaction is uncertain, but if concurrent use is undertaken the effects should be monitored.

1. Jack RA, Daniel DG. Possible interaction between phenelzine and amantadine. *Arch Gen Psychiatry* (1984) 41, 726.
2. Greenberg R, Meyers BS. Treatment of major depression and Parkinson's disease with combined phenelzine and amantadine. *Am J Psychiatry* (1985) 142, 273–4.

Monoamine oxidase inhibitors (MAOIs) + Antihistamines

Most of the alleged Antihistamine/MAOI interactions appear not to be based on good clinical evidence, and are probably more theoretical than real. The exception seems to be cyproheptadine (see 'Monoamine oxidase inhibitors (MAOIs) + Cyproheptadine', p.672).

Clinical evidence, mechanism, importance and management

A number of lists and charts and books about adverse interactions say that potentially serious interactions can occur between the MAOIs and the antihistamines. UK datasheets for various antihistamines contain a number of warnings but, with the exception of **cyproheptadine** (see 'Monoamine oxidase inhibitors (MAOIs) + Cyproheptadine', p.672 in this chapter), there do not appear to be any clinical reports confirming these interactions.

The UK drug datasheet says that **clemastine** may increase the effects of the MAOIs.[1] The anticholinergic effects of **cyproheptadine, diphenhydramine** and **chlorphenamine (chlorpheniramine)** are said to be increased by the MAOIs, and the latter should be avoided for 14 days.[2-4] **Azatadine**[5] and **promethazine**[6] are said to be contraindicated with the MAOIs and the later should be avoided for 14 days. The sedative effects of the MAOIs are reported to be increased by **pheniramine maleate**,[7] and **mequitazine** is said to be contraindicated with the MAOIs.[8] However, in correspondence with some of the makers of these antihistamines, none of them was able to quote direct clinical data in support of these statements.[9-14]

The Medicines Compendium 2002 also lists **alimemazine (trimeprazine), brompheniramine, cetirizine, fexofenadine, hydroxyzine, levocabastine, loratadine** and **mizolastine**, but no specific warning about interactions with MAOIs is given in the datasheets for any of these.

Some of the drug makers contacted have written to say that the authority for their warnings is Martindale's Extra Pharmacopoeia[11] or the British National Formulary,[12] or even that it was included at the request of the Medicines Control Agency[10] or the FDA,[14] but in the absence of direct, positive and clear clinical data it is difficult to avoid the conclusion that these alleged interactions are simply part of the clinical mythology which has come to surround the MAOIs. See also Blackwell's perceptive and illuminating comment quoted in the introduction to Chapter 18.

1. Tavegil (clemastine), Novartis. Datasheet, May 1997.
2. Periactin (cyproheptadine). Merck Sharp and Dohme Ltd. Summary of product characteristics, August 2001.
3. Nytol (diphenhydramine), Stafford-Miller Ltd. Summary of product characteristics, July 1998.
4. Piriton (chlorpheniramine maleate), Stafford-Miller Ltd. Summary of product characteristics, July 2000.
5. Optimine (azatadine), Schering-Plough Ltd. Summary of product characteristics, July 1997.
6. Avomine (promethazine), Manx Pharma. Datasheet, November, 1997.
7. Daneral SA (pheniramine maleate), Hoechst UK Ltd. ABPI Compendium of Data Sheets and Summaries of Product Characteristics Compendium 1996–7, p. 410–11.
8. Primalan (mequitazine). ABPI Compendium of Data Sheets and Summaries of Product Characteristics, 1998–9, p. 1104–5.
9. Intercare Products (Sandoz). Personal communication, May 1995.
10. Rhône-Poulenc Rorer, Personal communication, November 1995.
11. Glaxo Wellcome. Personal communication, December 1995.
12. Stafford Miller. Personal communication, November 1995.
13. Hoechst Roussel. Personal communication, November 1995.
14. Merck, Sharp and Dohme. Personal communication, January 1996.

Monoamine oxidase inhibitors (MAOIs) + Barbiturates

Although the MAOIs can enhance and prolong the activity of the barbiturates in *animals*, only a few isolated cases of adverse responses attributed to an interaction have been described in man.

Clinical evidence

Kline has stated,[1] without giving details, that on three or four occasions patients of his taking an MAOI continued, without his knowledge, to take their usual **barbiturate** hypnotic and thereby ". . . unknowingly raised their dose of **barbiturate** by five to ten times, and as a consequence barely managed to stagger through the day". Kline does not say whether he measured the serum **barbiturate** levels of these patients, or whether his conclusion is only a surmise.

A patient on **tranylcypromine** was inadvertently given 250 mg **amobarbital (amylobarbitone) sodium** intravenously for sedation. Within an hour she became ataxic, fell to the floor repeatedly hitting her head. After complaining of nausea and dizziness the patient became semicomatose and remained in that state for a further 36 h. To what extent the head trauma played a part is uncertain.[2]

Two other cases of coma attributed to concurrent use have been described.[3,4] In contrast, **mebanazine** is reported not to have enhanced the hypnotic activities of **secobarbital (quinalbarbitone)** or **butobarbital (butobarbitone)** in a number of patients, nor was there any evidence of a hangover effect.[5]

Mechanism

Not known. *Animal* studies[6-8] suggest that the MAOI have a general inhibitory action on the liver microsomal enzymes, thereby prolonging the activity of the barbiturates, but whether this occurs in man as well is uncertain.

Importance and management

The evidence for these interactions seem to be confined to a few unconfirmed anecdotal reports. There is no well-documented evidence showing that concurrent use should be avoided, although some cau-

tion is clearly appropriate. Mebanazine appears not to interact with secobarbital (quinalbarbitone) or butobarbital (butobarbitone).

1. Kline NS. Psychopharmaceuticals: effects and side-effects. *Bull WHO* (1959) 21, 397.
2. Domino EF, Sullivan TS, Luby ED. Barbiturate intoxication in a patient treated with a MAO inhibitor. *Am J Psychiatry* (1962) 118, 941–3.
3. Etherington L. Personal communication (1973).
4. MacLeod I. Fatal reaction to phenelzine. *BMJ* (1965) 1, 1554.
5. Gilmour SJG. Clinical trial of mebanazine—a new monoamine oxidase inhibitor. *Br J Psychiatry* (1965) 111, 899–902.
6. Wulfsohn NL, Politzer WM. 5-Hydroxytryptamine in anaesthesia. *Anaesthesia* (1962) 17, 64–8.
7. Lechat P, Lemergnan A. Monoamine oxidase inhibitors and potentiation of experimental sleep. *Biochem Pharmacol* (1961) 8, 8.
8. Buchel L, Levy J. Mecanisme des phenomenes de synergie due sommeil experimental. II. Etude des associations iproniazide-hypnotique, chez le rat et la souris. *Arch Sci Physiol (Paris)* (1965) 19, 161.

Monoamine oxidase inhibitors (MAOIs) + Benzodiazepines

The concurrent use of the MAOIs and the benzodiazepines is usually safe and effective, but a very small number of adverse reactions (chorea, severe headache, massive oedema, MAOI-toxicity) attributed to interactions have been described.

Clinical evidence, mechanism, importance and management

A patient with depression responded well when given 15 mg **phenelzine** and 10 mg **chlordiazepoxide** three times a day, but 4 to 5 months later developed choreiform movements of moderate severity and slight dysarthria. These symptoms subsided when the drugs were withdrawn.[1] Two patients on **chlordiazepoxide** and either **isocarboxazid** or **phenelzine** developed severe oedema which was attributed to the use of both drugs.[2,3] A patient on 60 mg **phenelzine** daily developed MAOI toxicity (excessive sweating, postural hypotension) within 10 days of increasing his daily dosage of **nitrazepam** to 15 mg. The patient was a slow acetylator.[4] A patient who had been taking 45 mg **phenelzine** daily for nine years developed a severe occipital headache after taking 0.5 mg **clonazepam**. A similar but milder headache occurred the next night when she took the same dose. No blood pressure measurements were taken.[5] The reasons for the development of all of these reactions are unknown. A meta-analysis of 897 patients at 31 centres is reported to have found that the use of **benzodiazepines** appeared to double the incidence of adverse effects (insomnia, restlessness, agitation, anxiety) in patients on **moclobemide**, but it is suggested that the patient groups may possibly have been different.[6] Another report found no clinically relevant interaction between **moclobemide** and **benzodiazepines**.[7]

The general picture portrayed by the reports in the literature is that concurrent use is usually effective and uneventful.[8-10] The adverse interaction reports cited here appear to be the exception, and it is by no means certain that all the responses were in fact due to drug interactions, however some caution is appropriate if these drugs are used together.

1. MacLeod DM. Chorea induced by tranquillisers. *Lancet* (1964) i, 388–9.
2. Goonewardene A, Toghill PJ. Gross oedema occurring during treatment for depression. *BMJ* (1977) 1, 879–80.
3. Pathak SK. Gross oedema during treatment for depression. *BMJ* (1977) 1, 1220.
4. Harris AL, McIntyre N. Interaction of phenelzine and nitrazepam in a slow acetylator. *Br J Clin Pharmacol* (1981) 12, 254–5.
5. Eppel AB. Interaction between clonazepam and phenelzine. *Can J Psychiatry* (1990) 35, 647.
6. Amrein R, Güntert TW, Dingesmanse J, Lorsheid T, Stabl M, Schmid-Burgk W. Interactions of moclobemide with concomitantly administered medication: evidence from pharmacological and clinical studies. *Psychopharmacology (Berl)* (1992) 106, S24–31.
7. Zimmer R, Gieschke R, Fischbach R, Gasic S. Interaction studies with moclobemide. *Acta Psychiatr Scand* (1990) (Suppl 360), 84–6.
8. Frommer EA. Treatment of childhood depression with antidepressant drugs. *BMJ* (1967) 1, 729–32.
9. Mans J, Sennes M. L'isocarboxazide, le RO 5–0690 et chlordiazepoxide, le RO-4-0403 derive des thixanthenes. Etude sur leur effect propres et leurs possibilites d'association. *J Med Bord* (1965) 141, 1909.
10. Suerinck A, Suerinck E. Etats depressifs en milieu sanatorial et inhibiteurs de la monoamine oxydase. (Resultats therepeutiques par l'association d'iproclozide et de chlodiazepoxide.) A propos de 146 observations. *J Med Lyon* (1966) 47, 573.

Monoamine oxidase inhibitors (MAOIs) + Buspirone

Elevated blood pressure has been reported in four patients taking buspirone and either phenelzine or tranylcypromine.

Clinical evidence, mechanism, importance and management

Four cases of significant blood pressure elevation during the concurrent use of **buspirone** and either **phenelzine** or **tranylcypromine** have been reported to the FDA's spontaneous Reporting System, and are described very briefly in Psychiatry Drug Alerts. One patient was a 75-year-old woman and the other three were men aged 30–42. The report does not say how much the pressures rose, or how quickly, and no other details are given.[1] On the basis of this rather sparse information the manufacturers say[2] that ". . . the administration of *BuSpar* [buspirone] to a patient taking a monoamine oxidase inhibitor (MAOI) may pose a hazard."

1. Anon. BuSpar Update. *Psychiatry Drug Alerts* (1987) 1, 43.

2. BuSpar Product Information, Mead Johnson Pharmaceuticals. 1990.

Monoamine oxidase inhibitors (MAOIs) + Chloral hydrate

A case of fatal hyperpyrexia and another of serious hypertension have been attributed to interactions between chloral and phenelzine.

Clinical evidence, mechanism, importance and management

A woman taking 45 mg **phenelzine** daily was found in bed deeply comatose with marked muscular rigidity, twitching down one side and a temperature of 41°C. She died without regaining consciousness. A postmortem failed to establish the cause of death, but it subsequently came to light that she had started drinking **whiskey** again (she had been treated for alcoholism), and she had access to **chloral hydrate**. She may have taken a fatal dose.[1] Another patient, also taking 45 mg **phenelzine** daily and **chloral hydrate** for sleeping, developed an excruciating headache followed by nausea, photophobia and a substantial rise in blood pressure.[2] This latter reaction is similar to the 'cheese reaction', but at the time the authors of the report were unaware of this type of reaction so that they failed to find out if any tyramine-rich foods had been eaten on the day of the attack.[2]

There is no clear evidence that either of these adverse reactions was due to an interaction between **phenelzine** and **chloral**, and no other reports to suggest that an interaction between these drugs is normally likely.

1. Howarth E. Possible synergistic effects of the new thymoleptics in connection with poisoning. *J Ment Sci* (1961) 107, 100–103.

2. Dillon H, Leopold RL. Acute cerebro-vascular symptoms produced by an antidepressant. *Am J Psychiatry* (1965) 121, 1012–14.

Monoamine oxidase inhibitors (MAOIs) + Choline theophyllinate

An isolated report describes the development of tachycardia and apprehension in a patient on phenelzine after taking a cough syrup containing choline theophyllinate (oxtriphylline).

Clinical evidence, mechanism, importance and management

A woman with agoraphobia, successfully treated with 45 mg **phenelzine** daily, developed tachycardia, palpitations and apprehension lasting about 4 h after taking a cough syrup (**Bronchodon**) containing **choline theophyllinate** and **guaifenesin** (**guaiphenesin**). The symptoms recurred when she was again given the syrup, and yet again when given **choline theophyllinate** (**Choledyl**) alone, but not when given **guaifenesin**.[1] The reasons are not understood. An adverse reaction with an MAOI has also been reported with caffeine which is another xanthine (see Index), but MAOI/xanthine interactions seem to be rare. It would seem prudent to check that patients given these drugs together are not experiencing any adverse effects, but there would appear to be no general need to avoid the xanthine bronchodilators.

1. Shader RI, Greenblatt DJ. MAOIs and drug interactions—a proposal for a clearinghouse. *J Clin Psychopharmacol* (1985) 5, A17.

Monoamine oxidase inhibitors (MAOIs) + Cocaine

An isolated report describes the delayed development of hyperpyrexia, coma, muscle tremors and rigidity in a patient on phenelzine after receiving a cocaine spray. Cocaine and selegiline appear not to interact adversely.

Clinical evidence, mechanism, importance and management

(a) Phenelzine

A man on 15 mg **phenelzine** twice daily underwent vocal chord surgery. He was anaesthetised with thiopental (thiopentone) and later nitrous oxide and 0.5% isoflurane in oxygen. Muscle paralysis was produced with suxamethonium and gallamine. During the operation his vocal chords were sprayed with 1 ml 10% **cocaine** spray. He regained consciousness 30 min after the surgery and was returned to the ward, but 30 min later he was found unconscious with generalised coarse tremors and marked muscle rigidity. Rectal temperature was 41.5°C. He was initially thought to have malignant hyperpyrexia and was treated accordingly with wet blankets, and largely recovered within 7 h. However later it seemed more likely that what occurred was probably due to an adverse interaction between the **phenelzine** and **cocaine** because he had been similarly and uneventfully treated with **cocaine** in the absence of **phenelzine** on two previous occasions. The reasons for the adverse reaction are not understood, but a delayed excitatory reaction because of increased concentrations of 5-HT is suggested.[1] This is an isolated report and its general importance is not known.

(b) Selegiline

A study to establish the safety of using **selegiline** to prevent **cocaine** relapse found that when 0, 20 and 40 mg intravenous doses of **cocaine** were given 1 h apart to 5 normal subjects taking 10 mg **selegiline** orally, the **cocaine** increased the heart rate, blood pressure, pupil diameter and subjective indices of euphoria and craving but the presence of **selegiline** did not alter the effects of the **cocaine**, except for miosis. It was concluded that concurrent use is safe and unlikely to increase the reinforcing effects of **cocaine**.[2]

1. Tordoff SG, Stubbing JF, Linter SPK. Delayed excitatory reaction following interaction of cocaine and monoamine oxidase inhibitor (phenelzine). *Br J Anaesth* (1991) 66, 516–8.

2. Haberny KA, Walsh SL, Ginn DH, Wilkins JN, Garner JE, Setoda D, Bigelow GW. Absence of acute cocaine interactions with the MAO-B inhibitor selegiline. *Drug Alcohol Depend* (1995) 39, 55–62.

Monoamine oxidase inhibitors (MAOIs) + Cyproheptadine

Isolated reports describe delayed hallucinations in a patient on phenelzine and the rapid re-emergence of depression in two other patients on brofaromine or phenelzine when given cyproheptadine.

Clinical evidence

A woman who had responded well to **brofaromine** rapidly became depressed again when **cyproheptadine** was added.[1] A man whose depression responded well to 75 mg **phenelzine** daily began to develop sexual dysfunction and anorgasmia. Within three days of adding 4 mg **cyproheptadine** to treat this dysfunction his depression returned but the anorgasmia did not improve. When the **cyproheptadine** was stopped his depression was relieved.[2] Hallucinations developed in a woman two months after **cyproheptadine** was added to her treatment with **phenelzine**.[3] The makers of **cyproheptadine** also say that MAOIs prolong and intensify the anticholinergic effects of antihistamines,[4] but there seems to be no clinical data to support this.

Mechanism

The reversal of the effects of the brofaromine were attributed by the authors of the second report[1] to the blockage of 5-HT receptors (brofaromine has both MAO-A inhibitory and 5-HT uptake inhibitory properties). Cyproheptadine has been observed to block the activity of another 5-HT uptake inhibitor (see 'Fluoxetine or Paroxetine + Cyproheptadine', p.824).

Importance and management

Information seems to be limited to these reports but it would now be prudent to be alert for any adverse responses if cyproheptadine is given with any MAOI. More study is needed.

1. Katz RJ, Rosenthal M. Adverse interaction of cyproheptadine with serotonergic antidepressants. *J Clin Psychiatry* (1994) 55, 314–5.
2. Zubieta JK, Demitrack MA. Depression after cyproheptadine: MAO treatment. *Biol Psychiatry* (1992) 31, 1177–8.
3. Kahn DA. Possible toxic interaction between cyproheptadine and phenelzine. *Am J Psychiatry* (1987) 144, 1242–3.
4. Periactin (cyproheptadine). Merck Sharp and Dohme Ltd. Summary of product characteristics, August 2001.

Monoamine oxidase inhibitors (MAOIs) + Dexfenfluramine or Fenfluramine

A confusing situation: the manufacturers advise against combined use of MAOIs and fenfluramine but it has also been claimed that concurrent use can be effective. Dexfenfluramine is also contraindicated with MAOIs, some other antidepressants and appetite suppressants.

Clinical evidence, mechanism, importance and management

The recommendation of the makers is that **fenfluramine** should not be used in patients with a history of depression and during treatment with antidepressants (especially the MAOIs) and there should be an interval of three weeks between stopping the MAOIs and starting **fenfluramine**.[1] Acute confusional states have been described when **fenfluramine** was used with **phenelzine**,[2] but it has also been claimed that in some instances **fenfluramine** has been used effectively with an MAOI.[3]

The makers similarly advise against the use of **dexfenfluramine** with or within two weeks of stopping an MAOI,[4] and three weeks between stopping **dexfenfluramine** and starting an MAOI because of the potential risk of the serotonin syndrome.[5] They also advise against the concurrent use of serotonergic agents (this would include **SSRIs** and some **tricyclic antidepressants**)[5] and other **appetite suppressants**.[4]

I have corresponded with the makers of **dexfenfluramine** and **fenfluramine** and they say that they have found no clinical evidence of serious problems with either of these drugs when taken with either SSRIs or MAOIs,[6] so that the published warnings about possible interactions would appear to be based on theoretical considerations. However note that more recently (in 1997) **dexfenfluramine** and **fenfluramine** were withdrawn because their use was found to be associated with a high incidence of abnormal echocardiograms indicating abnormal functioning of heart valves.

1. Ponderax Pacaps (fenfluramine). Servier Laboratories Ltd. ABPI Compendium of Data Sheets and Summaries of Product Characteristics 1998–9, p. 1307.
2. Brandon S. Unusual effect of fenfluramine. *BMJ* (1969) 4, 557.
3. Mason EC. Servier Laboratories Ltd. Personal communication (1976).
4. Adifax (dexfenfluramine). Servier Laboratories. ABPI Compendium of Data Sheets and Summaries of Product Characteristics 1998–9, p. 1302.
5. Dolan JA, Amchin L, Albano D. Potential hazard of serotonin syndrome associated with dexfenfluramine hydrochloride (Redux). *JAMA* (1996) 276, 1220–1.
6. Servier Laboratories Ltd. Personal communication, July 1997.

Monoamine oxidase inhibitors (MAOIs) + Dextromethorphan

Two fatal cases of hyperpyrexia and coma have occurred in patients on phenelzine who ingested dextromethorphan (in overdosage in one case). Three other serious but non-fatal reactions occurred in patients on isocarboxazid or phenelzine.

Clinical evidence

A woman on 60 mg **phenelzine** daily complained of nausea and dizziness before collapsing 30 min after drinking about 2 oz (55 ml of a cough mixture containing 100 mg **dextromethorphan**. She remained hyperpyrexic (42°C), hypotensive (systolic pressure not above 70 mmHg) and unconscious for 4 h before dying of cardiac arrest.[1] A 15-year-old girl taking 45 mg **phenelzine** daily (as well as thioridazine, procyclidine and metronidazole) took 13 capsules of *Romilar CF* (**dextromethorphan** 15 mg, **phenylephrine** 5 mg and **paracetamol** (**acetaminophen**) 120 mg in each capsule). She became comatose, hyperpyrexic (103°F), had a blood pressure of 100/60 mmHg, a pulse of 160 and later developed cardiac fibrillation which appeared to be the cause of her death.[2] Neither of these cases is easily understood, the latter being complicated by the overdosage and multiplicity of drugs present, particularly the phenylephrine.

A woman taking 30 mg **isocarboxazid** daily ingested 1 mg diazepam and 10 ml *Robitussin DM* (15 mg **dextromethorphan** + 100 mg **guaifenesin** (**guaiphenesin**)). Within 20 min she was nauseated and dizzy and within 45 min she began to have fine bilateral leg tremor and muscle spasms of the abdomen and lower back. These were followed by bilateral and persistent myoclonic jerks of legs, occasional choreoathetoid movements and marked urinary retention. These adverse effects persisted for about 19 h, gradually becoming less severe.[3] A further case has been described involving **phenelzine** and **dextromethorphan** (in *Robitussin-DM*).[4] Yet another patient on **phenelzine** also developed muscular rigidity, uncontrollable shaking, generalised hyperreflexia and sweating when given *Robitussin DM*. He responded within 2 h to 10 mg diazepam iv and oral activated charcoal.[5]

Mechanism

Uncertain. The authors of two of the reports[3-5] suggest that these effects may have been due to an increase in serotonin activity in the CNS (sometimes called the serotonin syndrome). A reaction (hyperpyrexia, dilated pupils, hyperexcitability and motor restlessness) has been seen in *rabbits* treated with dextromethorphan and nialamide, phenelzine or pargyline,[6] and there is some similarity to the MAOI/pethidine interaction.

Importance and management

Despite the very limited information available and our lack of understanding of why it happens, the severity of the reactions indicates that patients on MAOIs should avoid taking preparations containing dextromethorphan. Chlorpromazine opposes the development of this interaction in *rabbits* and has been used successfully in the clinical treatment of the MAOI/pethidine interaction. It might therefore also prove to be useful for treating this interaction. In one of the cases suxamethonium was used to cause paralysis, and lorazepam to reduced rigidity and myoclonus.[4] Diazepam and activated charcoal were used in another.[5]

1. Rivers N, Horner B. Possible lethal reaction between Nardil and dextromethorphan. *Can Med Assoc J* (1970) 103, 85.
2. Shamsie JC, Barriga C. The hazards of use of monoamine oxidase inhibitors in disturbed adolescents. *Can Med Assoc J* (1971) 104, 715.
3. Sovner R, Wolfe J. Interaction between dextromethorphan and monoamine oxidase inhibitor therapy with isocarboxazid. *N Engl J Med* (1988) 319, 1671.
4. Nierenberg DW, Semprebon M. The central nervous system serotonin syndrome. *Clin Pharmacol Ther* (1993) 53, 84–9
5. Sauter D, Macneil P, Weinstein E, Azar A. Phenelzine sulfate-dextromethorphan interaction: a case report. *Vet Hum Toxicol* (1991) 33, 365.
6. Sinclair JG. Dextromethorphan-monoamine oxidase inhibitor interaction in rabbits. *J Pharm Pharmacol* (1973) 25, 803–8.

Monoamine oxidase inhibitors (MAOIs) + Dextropropoxyphene (Propoxyphene)

An isolated report describes 'leg shakes', diaphoresis and severe hypotension in a woman on phenelzine when given dextropropoxyphene. Another isolated report describes a marked increase in the sedation when given these two drugs. An adverse reaction may possibly occur with moclobemide.

Clinical evidence, mechanism, importance and management

(a) Phenelzine

A woman well stabilised on **phenelzine** (15 mg three times daily) sodium valproate, lithium and trazodone, was given (**dextro)propoxyphene** 100 mg and paracetamol (acetaminophen) 650 mg for back pain and headache. 12 h later she was admitted to hospital "for leg shakes, discomfort and weakness . . .". She was confused and anxious, and intensely diaphoretic. Next day she became severely hypotensive (sbp 55–60 mmHg) and needed large fluid volume resuscitation in intensive care. She later recovered fully.[1] Another woman taking propranolol, an oestrogen and **phenelzine** became ". . . very sedated and groggy and had to lie down . . ." on two occasions within 2 h of taking **dextropropoxyphene**, 100 mg, and paracetamol (acetaminophen), 650 mg. She had had no problems with either paracetamol or **dextropropoxyphene**/paracetamol before starting the **phenelzine**.[2] The mechanisms of these interactions are not understood but some of the symptoms in the first case were not unlike those seen in the serotonin syndrome.

Apart from these two isolated reports, there seems to be no other clinical evidence of adverse interactions between irreversible MAOIs and **dextropropoxyphene**, nevertheless it would seem prudent to monitor the outcome well if both drugs are given.

(b) Moclobemide

There is *animal* data suggesting that the effects of **dextropropoxyphene** are increased by **moclobemide**, and there is an ambiguous reference to a patient taking both drugs who may have developed moderate agitation.[3] For these reasons it may be prudent to monitor concurrent use well, or avoid the drugs altogether.

1. Zornberg GL, Hegarty JD. Adverse interaction between propoxyphene and phenelzine. *Am J Psychiatry* (1993) 150, 1270–1.
2. Garbutt JC. Potentiation of propoxyphene by phenelzine. *Am J Psychiatry* (1987) 144, 251–2.
3. Amrein R, Güntert TW, Dingemanse J, Lorscheid T, Stabl M, Schmid-Burgk W. Interactions of moclobemide with concomitantly administered medication: evidence from pharmacological and clinical studies. *Psychopharmacology (Berl)* (1992) 106, S24–S31.

Monoamine oxidase inhibitors (MAOIs) + Erythromycin

An isolated case report describes severe hypotension and fainting in a woman on phenelzine shortly after starting to take a course of erythromycin.

Clinical evidence, mechanism, importance and management

A woman taking 15 mg **phenelzine** daily experienced three syncopal episodes four days after starting to take 250 mg **erythromycin** four times daily for pneumonia. When admitted to hospital her systolic blood pressure while lying down was only 70 mmHg, and unrecordable when she sat up. Even though she was not dehydrated, she was given 4 litres normal saline, but without any effect on her blood pressure. Within 24 h of stopping the **phenelzine** her blood pressure had returned to normal.[1] The reasons for this severe hypotensive reaction are not known, but it is suggested that the **erythromycin** may have caused rapid gastric emptying which resulted in a very rapid absorption of the **phenelzine** (described by the author as rapid dumping into the blood stream), thereby allowing its hypotensive side-effects to develop.[1] This seems to be the first and only report of this interaction, so that its general importance is uncertain.

1. Bernstein AE. Drug interaction. *Hosp Comm Psychiatry* (1990) 41, 806–7.

Monoamine Oxidase Inhibitors (MAOIs) + Fentanyl

A report describes the safe and uneventful use of fentanyl in a woman taking tranylcypromine.

Clinical evidence, mechanism, importance and management

A woman of 71 taking *Parstelin* (**tranylcypromine + trifluoperazine**) was given an intravenous test dose of 20 micrograms **fentanyl** and diazepam before surgery without problems. She was then anaesthetised with nitrous oxide, isoflurane and oxygen after intubation with etomidate and alcuronium. She had another 20-microgram intravenous dose of **fentanyl** and diazepam during the surgery, followed by an epidural bolus infusion of 50 micrograms **fentanyl** 15 min before the end of the surgery. She continued to receive a continuous epidural infusion of **fentanyl** at the rate of 50 to 70 micrograms/h for 4 days to control postoperative pain also without problems. The concurrent use of these drugs was successful and uneventful.[1] On the basis of this study its authors say[1] that ". . . epidural fentanyl is suggested to be a safe technique in patients who receive MAOIs." The literature seems to be silent about any problems with **fentanyl** and MAOIs which would seem to support the findings of this study.

1. Youssef MS, Wilkinson PA. Epidural fentanyl and monoamine oxidase inhibitors. *Anaesthesia* (1988) 43, 210–12.

Monoamine oxidase inhibitors (MAOIs) + Ginseng

Two patients have been reported who developed adverse effects when concurrently treated with phenelzine and ginseng.

Clinical evidence, mechanism, importance and management

A woman of 64 treated with **phenelzine** developed headache, insomnia and tremulousness on two occasions when **ginseng** was added.[1] Another depressed woman of 42 taking **ginseng** and **bee pollen** experienced a relief of her depression and became active and extremely optimistic when she was started on **phenelzine** (45 mg daily), but this was accompanied by insomnia, irritability, headaches and vague visual hallucinations. When the **phenelzine** was stopped and then restarted in the absence of the **ginseng** and **bee pollen**, her depression was not relieved.[2] It is seems unlikely that the **bee pollen** had any part to play in these reactions and suspicion therefore falls on the **ginseng**. It would seem that the psychoactive effects of the ginsenosides from the **ginseng** and the MAOI were additive, in some way as yet not understood. **Ginseng** has stimulant effects but its adverse effects include sleeplessness, nervousness, hypertension and euphoria. These two cases once again illustrate that OTC herbal or 'green' medicines are not necessarily problem-free if combined with orthodox drugs.

1. Shader RI, Greenblatt DJ. Phenelzine and the dream machine—ramblings and reflections. *J Clin Psychopharmacol* (1985) 5, 65.
2. Jones BD, Runikis AM. Interaction of ginseng with phenelzine. *J Clin Psychopharmacol* (1987) 7, 201–2.

Monoamine oxidase inhibitors (MAOIs) + Lithium carbonate

The concurrent use of phenelzine or tranylcypromine and lithium normally appears to be safe and effective but two cases of tardive dyskinesia following chronic use have been described.

Clinical evidence, mechanism, importance and management

Four severely depressed patients who had failed to respond to tricyclic antidepressants or to MAOIs, did so when **lithium** was added to their MAOI treatment. Each of them was treated with relatively modest doses of **phenelzine** (30–60 mg daily) and **lithium carbonate** (600–900 mg daily). No adverse reactions were reported.[1] 11 out of 12 patients did better on **lithium** and **tranylcypromine** than on **lithium** and other antidepressants,[2] and another previous study confirmed the effectiveness of concurrent treatment, apparently without toxicity.[3] However another report describes 2 patients with bipolar affective disorder who developed a buccolingual-masticatory syndrome after taking **tranylcypromine** (30–40 mg daily) and **lithium** (900–1200 mg daily) for 1.5–3 years attributed to dopamine receptor hypersensitivity.[4] There appear to be no reports suggesting that the combination of MAOIs and lithium is normally unsafe.

1. Fein S, Paz V, Rao N, LaGrassa J. The combination of lithium carbonate and an MAOI in refractory depressions. *Am J Psychiatry* (1988) 145, 249–50.
2. Price LH, Charney DS, Heninger GR. Efficacy of lithium-tranylcypromine treatment in refractory depression. *Am J Psychiatry* (1985) 142, 619–23.
3. Himmelhoch JM, Detre T, Kupfer DJ, Swartzburg M, Byck R. Treatment of previously intractable depressions with tranylcypromine and lithium. *J Nerv Ment Dis* (1972) 155, 216–20.
4. Stancer HC. Tardive dyskinesia not associated with neuroleptics. *Am J Psychiatry* (1979) 136, 727.

Monoamine oxidase inhibitors (MAOIs) + Mazindol

An isolated report describes a marked rise in blood pressure in a patient on phenelzine when given a single dose of mazindol.

Clinical evidence, mechanism, importance and management

A woman on **phenelzine** (30 mg three times a day) showed a blood pressure rise from 110/60 to 200/100 mmHg within 2 h of receiving a 10-mg test dose of **mazindol**. The blood pressure remained elevated for another hour, but had fallen again after another 3 h. The patient experienced no subjective symptoms.[1] It is uncertain whether this hypertensive reaction was the result of an interaction or simply a direct

response to the **mazindol** alone (the dose was large compared with the manufacturers recommended dosage of 2 mg daily). The general importance is uncertain, but it would seem wise to avoid **mazindol** in patients on MAOI. This is in line with the manufacturer's recommendations.

1. Oliver RM. Interaction between phenelzine and mazindol. Personal communication (1981).

Monoamine oxidase inhibitors (MAOIs) + Methyldopa

The concurrent use of pargyline and methyldopa appears to be safe, although an isolated report describes the delayed development of hallucinosis. The order of administration may be important. The concurrent use of antidepressant MAOI and methyldopa may not be desirable because methyldopa can sometimes cause depression.

Clinical evidence, mechanism, importance and management

A hypertensive woman on **pargyline**, 25 mg four times a day, developed hallucinosis about a month after starting to take 250 mg **methyldopa** daily, later increased to 500 mg.[1] However a number of other reports describe no unusual reactions or toxic effects during concurrent use.[2-5] The hypotensive response can be enhanced.[1]

The use of both drugs would therefore normally seem to be safe, but it has been suggested that the **methyldopa** should not be given after the **pargyline** so that the possibility of the sudden release by the methyldopa of the MAOI-accumulated stores of catecholamines can be avoided.[6] There seems to be nothing documented about the use of antidepressant MAOIs with **methyldopa**, but the potential depressant side-effects of **methyldopa** may make it an unsuitable drug for patients with depression.

1. Paykel ES. Hallucinosis on combined methyldopa and pargyline. *BMJ* (1966) 1, 803.
2. Maronde RF, Haywood LJ, Feinstein D, Sobel C. The monoamine oxidase inhibitor, pargyline hydrochloride, and reserpine. *JAMA* (1963) 184, 7.
3. Herting RL. Monoamine oxidase inhibitors. *Lancet* (1965) i, 1324.
4. Kinross-Wright J, Charalampous KD. Concurrent administration of dopa decarboxylase and monoamine oxidase inhibitors in man. *Clin Res* (1963) 11, 177.
5. Gillespsie L, Oates JA, Grout R, Sjoerdsma A. Clinical and chemical studies with alpha-methyldopa in patients with hypertension. *Circulation* (1962) 25, 281.
6. Natajaran S. Potential dangers of monoamine oxidase inhibitors and alpha-methyldopa. *Lancet* (1964) i, 1330.

Monoamine oxidase inhibitors (MAOIs) + Miscellaneous drugs

No adverse interactions between the MAOIs and either anticholinergics, carbamazepine or doxapram have been reported, although the possibility has been suggested. Bradycardia has been reported in two patients on nadolol or metoprolol and phenelzine. An isolated report suggests that the CNS stimulant effects of caffeine may possibly be increased by the MAOI.

Clinical evidence, mechanism, importance and management

Drug manufacturers often include warnings in their data sheets and package inserts about alleged interactions with the MAOIs, despite the absence of direct evidence in man that an interaction can actually take place (see Blackwell's comment at the end of the introduction to this chapter). It is usually suggested that 3 weeks should elapse between stopping the MAOI and starting the other drug. This prudent precaution protects both the health of patients and the legal liability of manufacturers, but it also means that patients may sometimes be denied the use of a drug that may be perfectly safe. If you speak to the makers many will freely admit that this is the case.

(a) Anticholinergics

Although some books and lists of drug interactions state that the effects of the **anticholinergic drugs** (by implication those which are adverse) used in the treatment of Parkinson's disease are increased by the MAOIs, there appears to be no documentary evidence of this in man, although a hyperthermic reaction has been reported in *animals*.[1]

(b) Beta-blockers

It has been claimed[2] that MAO inhibitors should be discontinued at least 2 weeks before starting **propranolol** therapy . . ., but studies in *animals*[3] using **mebanazine** as a representative MAOI failed to show . . . any undesirable property of **propranolol** following MAO inhibition. Bradycardia (46–53 bpm) has been described in two patients taking 40 mg **nadolol** or 150 mg **metoprolol** daily for hypertension within 8–11 days of starting 60 mg **phenelzine** daily. No noticeable ill effects were seen but the authors recommend careful monitoring particularly in the elderly who may tolerate bradycardia poorly.[4] Until the situation is quite clear it would prudent to monitor the concurrent use of any MAOI and beta-blocker.

(c) Caffeine

It has been claimed that a patient who normally drank 10 or 12 cups of **coffee** daily, without adverse effects, experienced extreme jitteriness during treatment with an MAOI which subsided when the **coffee** consumption was reduced to 2 or 3 cups a day. The same reaction was also said to have occurred in other patients on MAOI who drank **tea** or some of the **'Cola' drinks** which contain **caffeine**.[5] Another patient claimed that a single cup of **coffee** taken in the morning kept him jittery all day and up the entire night as well, a reaction which occurred on three separate occasions. Apart from this report and another[6] stating that the effects of **caffeine** in *mice* are enhanced by MAOI, the literature appears otherwise to be silent about this alleged interaction. Whether this reflects its mildness and unimportance, or its rarity, is not clear.

(d) Doxapram

Based on *animal* studies which reportedly show that the actions of **doxapram** are potentiated by pretreatment with MAOIs, the manufacturers[7] advise that concurrent use should be undertaken with great care. The adverse cardiovascular effects of **doxapram** (hypertension, tachycardia, arrhythmias) are said elsewhere[8] to be markedly increased in patients on MAOIs, and it is also stated that the pressor effects of MAOIs and doxapram may be additive[9] but no clinical data in support of these statements are cited.

1. Pedersen V, Nielsen IM. Hyperthermia in rabbits caused by interaction between M.A.O.I.s, antiparkinson drugs, and neuroleptics. *Lancet* (1975) i, 409–10.
2. Frieden J. Propranolol as an antiarrhythmic agent. *Am Heart J* (1967) 74, 283.
3. Barrett AM, Cullum VA. Lack of interaction between propranolol and mebanazine. *J Pharm Pharmacol* (1968) 20, 911.
4. Reggev A, Vollhardt BR. Bradycardia induced by an interaction between phenelzine and beta blockers. *Psychosomatics* (1989) 30, 106–8.
5. Kline NS. Psychopharmaceuticals: effects and side-effects. *Bull WHO* (1959) 21, 397.
6. Berkowitz BA, Spector S, Pool W. The interaction of caffeine, theophylline and theobromine with monoamine oxidase inhibitors. *Eur J Pharmacol* (1971) 16, 315–21.
7. ABPI Data Sheet Compendium 1985–6 p. 1226. Datapharm Publications (1986).
8. Esplin DW, Zablocka-Esplin B. Central nervous stimulants. In 'The Pharmacological Basis of Therapeutics' 4th edn p 335. Goodman LS and Gillman A (eds). Macmillan NY (1970).
9. Sweetman SC, editor. Martindale: The complete drug reference. 33rd ed. London: Pharmaceutical Press; 2002. p.1509.

Monoamine oxidase inhibitors (MAOIs) + Monoamine oxidase inhibitors

Two patients suffered strokes (one fatal) and another experienced a hypertensive reaction when phenelzine or isocarboxazid were replaced by tranylcypromine. Moclobemide and selegiline can safely be given together or sequentially but some dietary restrictions are necessary (no tyramine-rich foods and drinks). Marked orthostatic hypotension has been seen in two patients on iproniazid or *Parstelin* when given selegiline.

Clinical evidence, mechanism, importance and management

(a) Irreversible, non-selective MAOIs

A patient on 30 mg **isocarboxazid** daily was switched to 10 mg **tranylcypromine** and on the following day to 30 mg daily. Later she complained of feeling 'funny', had difficulty in talking, developed a headache, was restless, flushed, sweating, had a blood pressure of 210/110 mmHg (normal for the patient) and a pulse rate of 130 bpm. She died the following day. The cause of death was either a subarachnoid haemorrhage or some other unidentified reaction.[1] Another patient, switched from 75 mg **phenelzine** daily to 10, 20, 30 and then 20 mg **tranylcypromine** daily, suffered a subcortical cerebral haemorrhage on the fourth day which resulted in total right-sided hemiplegia.[2,3] Another patient taking 45 mg **phenelzine** daily, followed by a two-day drug free period and then 20 mg **tranylcypromine** daily, experienced a rise in blood pressure to 240/130 mmHg.[2]

The reasons for these reactions are not understood, but one idea is that the amphetamine-like properties of tranylcypromine may have had some part to play. Certainly there are cases of spontaneous rises in blood pressure and intracranial bleeding in patients given **tranylcypromine**, no other precipitating factor being known.[4] Not all patients experience adverse reactions when switched from one MAOI to another,[5] but until more is known it would seem prudent to have a drug-free wash-out interval when doing so, and to start dosing in a conservative and step-wise manner.

(b) Reversible, selective MAOIs (RIMAs)

A study in 24 subjects to assess the safety and tolerability of giving 100–400 mg **moclobemide** and 10 mg **selegiline** daily, sequentially or combined, found that the adverse effects were no greater under steady-state conditions than with either drug alone, but the sensitivity to tyramine was considerably increased. The mean **tyramine sensitivity factors** for moclobemide, selegiline alone, and **moclobemide** plus **selegiline** were 2–3, 1.4, and 8–9 respectively. One subject showed a value of 18 when given both drugs.[6,7] The reason is that when taken together the **moclobemide** inhibits MAO-A while **selegiline** inhibits MAO-B so that little or no MAO activity remains available to metabolise the tyramine.

In practical terms this means that patients taking **moclobemide** with **selegiline** should be given the same dietary restrictions about tyramine-rich foods and drinks (cheese, some wines and beers, etc.) which relate to the non-selective MAOIs such as phenelzine and tranylcypromine, although the risks are less. The tyramine sensitivity of these latter MAOIs is about 25 or more.[8] On the basis of work done on the *pig* (said to be similar to man in relation to the MAO isoenzymes in the brain[9]) it is suggested that if **selegiline** is replaced by **moclobemide**, the dietary restrictions can be relaxed after a wash-out period of about two weeks. If switching from **moclobemide** to **selegiline**, a wash-out period of 1–2 days is sufficient.[6] See 'Monoamine oxidase inhibitors (MAOIs) + Tyramine-rich drinks', p.684 and 'Monoamine oxidase inhibitors (MAOIs) + Tyramine-rich foods', p.685 for details of the foods and drinks to be avoided.

(c) Reversible MAOIs + Irreversible MAOIs

A patient taking 150 mg **iproniazid** daily developed severe orthostatic hypotension on two occasions within an hour of taking 5 mg **selegiline**. Another patient similarly developed postural hypotension on two occasions within 2 h of taking 5 mg **selegiline**. He had stopped taking *Parstelin* (**tranylcypromine** + **trifluoperazine**), two tablets daily, four weeks previously.[10] The reasons are not understood. This evidence suggests that **selegiline** should be given with caution to patients taking irreversible MAOIs, or who have recently stopped.

1. Bazire SR. Sudden death associated with switching monoamine oxidase inhibitors. *Drug Intell Clin Pharm* (1986) 20, 954–5.
2. Gelenberg AJ. Switching MAOI. *Biol Ther Psychiatr* (1984) 7, 36.
3. Gelenberg AJ. Switching MAOI. The sequel. *Biol Ther Psychiatr* (1985) 8, 41.
4. Cooper AJ, Magnus RV, Rose MJ. A hypertensive syndrome with tranylcypromine medication. *Lancet* (1964) 1, 527–9.
5. True BL, Alexander B, Carter BL. Comment: switching MAO inhibitors. *Drug Intell Clin Pharm* (1986) 20, 384.
6. Dingemanse J. An update of recent moclobemide interaction data. *Int Clin Psychopharmacol* (1993) 7, 167–80.
7. Korn A, Wagner B, Moritz E, Dingemanse J. Tyramine pressor sensitivity in healthy subjects during combined treatment with moclobemide and selegiline. *Eur J Clin Pharmacol* (1996) 49, 273–8.

8. Bieck PR, Antonin KH. Tyramine potentiation during treatment with MAO inhibitors: brofaromine and moclobemide vs irreversible inhibitors. *Psychopharmacology (Berl)* (1988) 96, S31.

9. Oreland L, Jossan SS, Hartvig P, Aquilonius SM, Lanström B. Turnover of monoamine oxidase B (MAO-B) in pig brain by positron emission tomography using[11]C-L-deprenyl. *J Neural Transm* (1990) 32, 55–9.

10. Pare CMB, Al Mousawi M, Sandler M, Glover V. Attempts to attenuate the 'cheese effect'. Combined drug therapy in depressive illness. *J Affect Disord* (1985) 9, 137–41.

Monoamine oxidase inhibitors (MAOIs) + Monosodium glutamate

Hypertension in patients on MAOIs who have eaten certain foods (soy sauce, chicken nuggets) has been attributed in anecdotal reports to an interaction with monosodium glutamate, however a controlled study found no evidence to support this idea.

Clinical evidence

Five normal subjects were given 400–1600 mg **monosodium glutamate** or a placebo while taking no other drugs, and after taking **tranylcypromine** for at least 2 weeks. Episodes of hypertension were seen in 2 subjects on **tranylcypromine** alone, but no changes in blood pressure or heart rate occurred which could be attributed to an interaction while taking **monosodium glutamate** as well. The largest dose of **monosodium glutamate** used was about twice the amount usually found in meals containing large amounts of **monosodium glutamate**.[1]

There are anecdotal reports of hypertensive reactions attributed to interactions with the **monosodium glutamate** contained in **soy sauce** and **chicken nuggets** in patients on MAOIs.[2,3]

Mechanism

None. Monosodium glutamate alone can cause a small rise in blood pressure, and MAOIs alone very occasionally cause hypertensive episodes. The reactions reported with soy sauce and chicken nuggets may possibly have been due to their high tyramine content (see 'Monoamine oxidase inhibitors (MAOIs) + Tyramine-rich foods', p.685).

Importance and management

The authors of the report cited suggest that any reaction is likely to be an idiosyncratic reaction and not due to an identifiable interaction between the MAOI and sodium glutamate.[1] No interaction is established. It should be pointed out that the number of subjects studied was very small.

1. Balon R, Pohl R, Yeragani VK, Berchou R, Gershon S. Monosodium glutamate and tranylcypromine administration in healthy subjects. *J Clin Psychiatry* (1990) 51, 303–6.

2. Pohl R, Balon R, Berchou R. Reaction to chicken nuggets in a patient taking an MAOI. *Am J Psychiatry* (1988) 145, 651.

3. McCabe B, Tsuang MT. Dietary consideration in MAO inhibitor regimens. *J Clin Psychiatry* (1982) 43, 178–81.

Monoamine oxidase inhibitors (MAOIs) + Morphine or Methadone

No adverse interaction normally occurs in patients on MAOIs given morphine, but there are two isolated and unexplained reports of patients on MAOIs who showed hypotension, marked in one case and accompanied by unconsciousness. Some very limited evidence also suggests that no interaction occurs with methadone.

Clinical evidence

(a) Morphine

(i) Adverse reactions. A patient taking 40 mg **tranylcypromine** and 20 mg **trifluoperazine** daily and undergoing a preoperative test with **morphine**, developed pin point pupils, became unconscious and unresponsive to stimuli, and showing a systolic blood pressure fall from 160 to 40 mmHg after receiving a total of 6 mg **morphine**. Within 2 min of being given 4 mg naloxone intravenously, the patient was awake and rational with a systolic blood pressure fully restored.[1] A moderate fall in blood pressure (from 140/90 to 90/60 mmHg) was seen in another patient on a MAOI given **morphine**.[2]

(ii) No adverse reactions. In contrast to the two reports cited above (i), a study in 15 patients who had been taking either **phenelzine, isocarboxazid, iproniazid** or *Parstelin* (**tranylcypromine + trifluoperazine**) for 3–8 weeks, showed no changes in blood pressure, pulse rate or state of awareness when given test doses of up to 4 mg **morphine**, or test doses of up to 40 mg **pethidine** (**meperidine**).[3] Another patient on **phenelzine** is reported to have developed no problems when treated with **morphine**.[4] Other patients on MAOIs who reacted adversely to **pethidine** (**meperidine**), did not do so when given **morphine**.[5-7] For more information about the MAOI/pethidine interaction see 'Monoamine oxidase inhibitors (MAOIs) + Pethidine (Meperidine)', p.676. Two other studies reported no adverse interaction in patients on **MAOIs** given **morphine**.[8,9]

(b) Methadone

A patient on **methadone** maintenance therapy (30 mg daily) was successfully and uneventfully treated for depression with **tranylcypromine**, initially 10 mg gradually increased to 30 mg daily.[10]

Mechanism

Not understood.

Importance and management

The serious MAOI/pethidine interaction also cast a shadow over morphine, which probably accounts for its inclusion on a number of lists and charts of drugs said to interact with the MAOIs, despite good evidence that patients on MAOIs who had reacted adversely with pethidine (meperidine) did not do so when given morphine.[5-7] The hypotensive reactions cited here[1,2] are of a different character and appear to be rare. There would therefore seem to be no good reason for avoiding morphine in patients on MAOIs, but be alert for the rare adverse response. Naloxone proved to be a rapid and effective treatment in one of the cases cited.[1] The extremely limited evidence available suggests that methadone can be given to patients on MAOIs, but a stepwise dosing would seem to be a prudent precaution.

1. Barry BJ. Adverse effects of MAO inhibitors with narcotics reversed with naloxone. *Anaesth Intensive Care* (1979) 7, 194.

2. Jenkins LC, Graves HB. Potential hazards of psychoactive drugs in association with anaesthesia. *Can Anaesth Soc J* (1965) 12, 121.

3. Evans-Prosser CDG. The use of pethidine and morphine in the presence of monoamine oxidase inhibitors. *Br J Anaesth* (1968) 40, 279–82.

4. Ure DS, Gillies MA, James KS. Safe use of remifentanil in a patient treated with the monoamine oxidase inhibitor phenelzine. *Br J Anaesth* (2000) 84, 414–6.

5. Palmer H. Potentiation of pethidine. *BMJ* (1960) 2, 944.

6. Denton PH, Borrelli VM, Edwards NV. Dangers of monoamine oxidase inhibitors. *BMJ* (1962) 2, 1752–3.

7. Shee JC. Dangerous potentiation of pethidine by iproniazid and its treatment. *BMJ* (1960) 2, 507–9.

8. El-Ganzouri A, Ivankovich AD, Braverman B, Land PC. Should MAOI be discontinued preoperatively? *Anesthesiology* (1983) 59, A384.

9. Ebrahim ZY, O'Hara J, Borden L, Tetzlaff J. Monoamine oxidase inhibitors and elective surgery. *Cleve Clin J Med* (1993) 60, 129–130.

10. Mendelson G. Narcotics and monoamine oxidase-inhibitors. *Med J Aust* (1979) 1, 400.

Monoamine oxidase inhibitors (MAOIs) + Pethidine (Meperidine)

The concurrent use of pethidine (meperidine) and MAOIs has resulted in a serious and potentially life-threatening reaction in a few patients. Excitement, muscle rigidity, hyperpy-

rexia, flushing, sweating and unconsciousness occur very rapidly. Respiratory depression and hypotension are also seen. Pethidine should not be given to patients on any MAOI (selective or non-selective) unless a lack of sensitivity has been confirmed.

Clinical evidence

Severe, rapid and potentially fatal toxic reactions, both excitatory and depressant can occur:

A woman on 100 mg **iproniazid** daily became restless and incoherent almost immediately after being given 100 mg **pethidine**. She was comatose within 20 min. After an hour she was flushed, sweating and showed Cheyne-Stokes respiration. Her pupils were dilated and unreactive. Deep reflexes could not be initiated and plantar reflexes were extensor. Her pulse rate was 82 and blood pressure 156/110 mmHg. She was rousable within 10 min of receiving an intravenous injection of 25 mg prednisolone hemisuccinate.[1]

A woman who, unknown to her doctor, was taking **tranylcypromine**, was given 100 mg **pethidine**. Within minutes she became unconscious, noisy and restless, having to be held down by three people. Her breathing was stertorous and the pulse impalpable. Generalised tonic spasm developed with ankle clonus, extensor plantar reflexes, shallow respiration and cyanosis. On admission to hospital she had a pulse rate of 160, a blood pressure of 90/60 mmHg and was sweating profusely (temperature 38°C). Her condition gradually improved and 4 h after admission she was conscious but drowsy. Recovery was complete the next day.[2]

This interaction has been seen in other patients treated with **iproniazid**,[1,3-5] **pargyline**,[6] **phenelzine**,[7-12] **tranylcypromine**[2] and **mebanazine**.[13] Fatalities have occurred. It has also been seen with **selegiline**, a selective inhibitor of type B monoamine oxidase (MAO-B).[14] There appear to be no reports of a human **moclobemide/pethidine** interaction but on the basis of *animal* studies it is currently recommended that the combination should be avoided or used with caution.[15]

Mechanism

Not understood, despite the extensive studies undertaken.[16-18] There is some evidence that the reactions may be due to an increase in levels of 5-HT within the brain, causing the serotonin syndrome.

Importance and management

A well-documented, serious and potentially fatal interaction first observed in the mid-1950s. Its incidence is unknown, but it is probably quite low. For example, one study found that 15 patients given various MAOIs and pethidine failed to demonstrate the interaction,[19] and no problems were seen in another study involving 45 patients on isocarboxazid given pethidine (25–75 mg) pre-operatively.[20] Bear in mind that most of the older MAOI are irreversible so that an interaction is possible for many days after their withdrawal, whereas the newer selective MAOIs (e.g. moclobemide) are reversible and unlikely still to interact 48 h after they have been stopped. Nevertheless it would be imprudent to give pethidine to anyone on an MAOI or shortly after it has been stopped, unless they are known not to be sensitive.

Sensitivity test

Churchill-Davidson has suggested[21] that sensitivity can be checked by giving a test dose of 5 mg pethidine, after which all the vital signs (pulse, respiration, blood pressure) are checked at 5 min intervals for 20 min, and then at 10 min intervals for the rest of the hour. If no obvious change has occurred, the whole check is repeated over the next hour with 10 mg pethidine, then with 20 mg, and after 3 h with 40 mg. It is not thought necessary to carry on further because by this stage any sensitivity should have revealed itself. A case is quoted of a patient who demonstrated sensitivity after 5 mg pethidine. The systolic blood pressure fell by 30 mmHg, the pulse rate rose by 20 bpm and drowsiness developed.[21]

Treatment

This interaction has been successfully treated with **prednisolone hemisuccinate**, 25 mg[1] or **chlorpromazine**, and also with **glyceryl trinitrate** sublingual spray.[22] It has also been suggested that since the latter was probably effective because it caused peripheral vasodilatation, **nifedipine** might work as well.[23]

1. Shee JC. Dangerous potentiation of pethidine by iproniazid, and its treatment. *BMJ* (1960) 2, 507–9.
2. Denton PH, Borrelli VM, Edwards NV. Dangers of monoamine oxidase inhibitors. *BMJ* (1962) 2, 1752–3.
3. Clement AJ, Benazon D. Reactions to other drugs in patients taking monoamine-oxidase inhibitors. *Lancet* (1962) ii, 197–8.
4. Papp C, Benaim S. Toxic effects of iproniazid in a patient with angina. *BMJ* (1958) 2, 1070.
5. Mitchell RS. Fatal toxic encephalitis occurring during iproniazid therapy in pulmonary tuberculosis. *Ann Intern Med* (1955) 42, 417–24.
6. Vigran IM. Dangerous potentiation of meperidine hydrochloride by pargyline hydrochloride. *JAMA* (1964) 187, 953–4.
7. Palmer H. Potentiation of pethidine. *BMJ* (1960) 2, 944.
8. Taylor DC. Alarming reaction to pethidine in patients on phenelzine. *Lancet* (1962) ii, 401–2.
9. Cocks DP, Passmore-Rowe A. Dangers of monoamine oxidase inhibitors. *BMJ* (1962) 2, 1545–6.
10. Reid NCRW, Jones D. Pethidine and phenelzine. *BMJ* (1962) 1, 408.
11. Meyer D, Halfin V. Toxicity secondary to meperidine in patients on monoamine oxidase inhibitors: a case report and critical review. *J Clin Psychopharmacol* (1981) 1, 319–21.
12. Asch DA, Parker RM. Sounding board. The Libby Zion case. One step forward or two steps backward? *N Engl J Med* (1988) 318, 771–5.
13. Anon. Death from drugs combination. *Pharm J* (1965) 195, 341.
14. Zornberg GL, Bodkin JA, Cohen BM. Severe adverse interaction between pethidine and selegiline. *Lancet* (1991) 337, 246.
15. Amrein R, Güntert TW, Dingemanse J, Lorscheid T, Stabl M, Schmid-Burgk W. Interactions of moclobemide with concomitantly administered medication: evidence from pharmacological and clinical studies. *Psychopharmacology (Berl)* (1992) 106, S24–31.
16. Leander JD, Batten J, Hargis GW. Pethidine interaction with clorgyline, pargyline or 5-hydroxytryptophan: lack of enhanced pethidine lethality or hyperpyrexia in mice. *J Pharm Pharmacol* (1978) 30, 396–8.
17. Rogers KJ, Thornton JA. The interaction between monoamine oxidase inhibitors and narcotic analgesics in mice. *Br J Pharmacol* (1969) 36, 470–80.
18. Gessner PK, Soble AG. A study of the tranylcypromine-meperidine interaction: effects of *p*-chlorophenylalanine and *l*-5-hydroxytryptophan. *J Pharmacol Exp Ther* (1973) 186, 276–87.
19. Prosser-Evans CDG. The use of pethidine and morphine in the presence of monoamine oxidase inhibitors. *Br J Anaesth* (1968) 40, 279–82.
20. Ebrahim ZY, O'Hara J, Borden L, Tetzlaff J. Monoamine oxidase inhibitors and elective surgery. *Cleve Clin J Med* (1993) 60, 129–130.
21. Churchill-Davidson HC. Anaesthesia and monoamine oxidase inhibitors. *BMJ* (1965) 1, 520.
22. Hogan C. Serotonin reaction and its treatment. *Aust Fam Physician* (1997) 26, 76–7.
23. Lyndon RW. Serotonin reaction and its treatment - reply. *Aust Fam Physician* (1997) 26, 77.

Monoamine oxidase inhibitors (MAOIs) + Phenothiazines

The concurrent use of the MAOIs and phenothiazines is usually safe and effective. The exception appears to be levomepromazine (methotrimeprazine) which has been implicated in two fatal reactions with pargyline and tranylcypromine.

Clinical evidence, mechanism, importance and management

The concurrent use of MAOIs and phenothiazines has been recommended,[1-3] and a fixed combination (**tranylcypromine** with **trifluoperazine**, *Parstelin*) is marketed. **Tranylcypromine** with **chlorpromazine** has been found valuable in the treatment of schizophrenia and it may possibly prevent the occurrence of extrapyramidal symptoms.[4] **Promazine** has been used safely and effectively in the treatment of overdosage with **tranylcypromine**.[5] A single report[6] describing the development of a severe occipital headache in a woman on an MAOI as a result of taking 30 ml of a child's cough linctus, attributed this reaction by inference to an inter-action with **promethazine**, but it is now known that the linctus in question contained **phenylpropanolamine** which is much more likely to have been the cause,[7] (see 'Monoamine oxidase inhibitors (MAOIs) + Sympathomimetics (indirectly-acting)', p.680). However, unexplained fatalities while taking **levomepromazine (methotrimeprazine)** with **pargyline**,[8] another with **levomepromazine** and **tranylcypromine**[9] and the third with an unnamed MAOI–phenothiazine combination have been reported.[9]

No special precautions would normally seem to be necessary during the concurrent use of most MAOIs and phenothiazines, with the exception of **levomepromazine** which, because it has been implicated in two fatalities, should probably be regarded as contraindicated.

1. Winkelman NW. Three evaluations of a monoamine oxidase inhibitor and phenothiazine combination (a methodological and clinical study). *Dis Nerv Syst* (1965) 26, 160–4.
2. Cheshrow EJ, Kaplitz SE. Anxiety and depression in the geriatric and chronically ill patient. *Clin Med* (1965) 72, 1281.
3. Janacek J, Schiele BC, Belville T, Anderson R. The effects of withdrawal of trifluoperazine on patients maintained on the combination of tranylcypromine and trifluoperazine. A double blind study. *Curr Ther Res* (1963) 5, 608.
4. Bucci L. The negative symptoms of schizophrenia and the monoamine oxidase inhibitors. *Psychopharmacology (Berl)* (1987) 91, 104–8.
5. Midwinter RE. Accidental overdose with 'Parstelin'. *BMJ* (1962) 2, 1755.
6. Mitchell L. Psychotropic drugs. *BMJ* (1968) 1, 381.
7. Mitchell L. (1977) Quoted as a personal communication in 'A Manual of Adverse Drug Interactions' 2nd Edn p 174. Griffin JP and D'Arcy PF. Wright, Bristol (1979).
8. Barsa JA, Saunders JC. A comparative study of tranylcypromine and pargyline. *Psychopharmacologia* (1964) 6, 295–8.
9. McQueen EG. New Zealand Committee on Adverse Drug Reactions: 14th Annual Report (1979). *N Z Med J* (1980) 91, 226.

Monoamine oxidase inhibitors (MAOIs) + Phenylephrine

The concurrent use of oral phenylephrine and the older MAOIs can result in a potentially life-threatening hypertensive crisis. Phenylephrine is commonly found in proprietary cough, cold and influenza preparations. The effects of parenteral phenylephrine may be approximately doubled. No important interaction occurs between brofaromine and phenylephrine in nose drops, and none seems likely with moclobemide.

Clinical evidence

(a) Phenelzine or Tranylcypromine + Phenylephrine

A study in four normal subjects, given 45 mg **phenelzine** or 30 mg **tranylcypromine** daily for 7 days, found that the blood pressure rise following **oral phenylephrine** was grossly enhanced. In three experiments with 45 mg given orally, the rise in blood pressure became potentially disastrous and had to be stopped with phentolamine. The enhancement was about 13 times in the only experiment that was not stopped, and 6–35 times in the two that were. The rise in blood pressure was accompanied by a severe headache. An approximately two-fold increase was seen following parenteral administration.[1]

Another study describes a 2–2.5 times increase in the effects of **parenteral phenylephrine**,[2] and an exaggerated pressor response is described in a case report.[3] A hypertensive crisis occurred in a woman on **phenelzine** who took *Robitussin-PE* which contains **phenylephrine**.[4]

(b) Brofaromine or Moclobemide + Phenylephrine

No clinically important interaction occurred in normal subjects taking 75 mg **brofaromine** twice daily when given 2.5 mg doses of **phenylephrine** (*Neo-Synephrine*) as nose drops.[5,6] Two studies in normal subjects found that 100–200 mg **moclobemide** three times daily for up to three weeks increased the blood pressure response to infusions of **phenylephrine** by a maximum of 1.8.[7]

Mechanism

Phenylephrine is given in large doses by mouth because a very large proportion is destroyed by the MAO in the gut and liver, and only a small amount gets into general circulation. If the MAO is inhibited, most of the oral dose escapes destruction and passes freely into circulation as an overdose. Hence the gross enhancement of the pressor effects. Phenylephrine has mainly direct sympathomimetic activity, but it may also have some minor indirect activity as well which would be expected to result in the release of some of the MAOI-accumulated norepinephrine (noradrenaline) at adrenergic nerve endings. This might account for the increased response to phenylephrine given parenterally.

Importance and management

The interaction between the older (irreversible) MAOIs and oral phenylephrine is established, serious and potentially life-threatening. Phenylephrine commonly occurs in oral OTC cough, cold and influenza preparations so that patients should be strongly warned about them. Whether the effects of nose drops and nasal sprays are also enhanced is uncertain, but it would be prudent to avoid them until they have been shown to be safe. The response to parenteral administration is also approximately doubled so that an appropriate dosage reduction is necessary. No interaction occurs between brofaromine and phenylephrine as nose drops,[5] and no clinically important interaction would seem likely between phenylephrine and moclobemide.[7,8] This needs confirmation.

Treatment

If a hypertensive reaction occurs it can be controlled with an alpha-adrenoreceptor blocker such as **phentolamine**, 5 mg, given intravenously,[4] or failing that an intramuscular injection of 50 mg **chlorpromazine**. The simplest alternative is to chew a capsule of 10 mg **nifedipine** to release its contents, and wash it down with a drink of water. Other calcium channel blockers would also be expected to be effective.

1. Boakes AJ, Laurence DR, Teoh PC, Barar FSK, Benedikter L, Prichard BNC. Interactions between sympathomimetic amines and antidepressant agents in man. *BMJ* (1973) 1, 311.
2. Elis J, Laurence DR, Mattie H, Prichard BNC. Modification by monoamine oxidase inhibitors of the effect of some sympathomimetics on blood pressure. *BMJ* (1967) 2, 75–8.
3. Jenkins LC, Graves HB. Potential hazards of psychoactive drugs in association with anaesthesia. *Can Anaesth Soc J* (1965) 12, 121.
4. Harrison WM, McGrath PJ, Stewart JW, Quitkin F. MAOIs and hypertensive crises: the role of OTC drugs. *J Clin Psychiatry* (1989) 50, 64–5.
5. Mühlbauer B, Gradin-Frimmer G, Bieck P. Safety of reversible monoamine oxidase inhibitors (MAOI): interaction of brofaromine with sympathomimetic drugs in healthy volunteers. *Naunyn Schmiedebergs Arch Pharmacol* (1990) 341 (Suppl), R113.
6. Gleiter CH, Mühlbauer B, Gradin-Frimmer G, Antonin KH, Bieck PR. Administration of sympathomimetic drugs with the selective MAO-A inhibitor brofaromine. Effect on blood pressure. *Drug Invest* (1992) 4, 149–54.
7. Amrein R, Güntert TW, Dingemanse J, Lorscheid T, Stabl M, Schmid-Burgk W. Interactions of moclobemide with concomitantly administered medication: evidence from pharmacological and clinical studies. *Psychopharmacology (Berl)* (1992) 106, S24–31.
8. Korn A, Eichler HG, Gasic S. Moclobemide, a new specific MAO-inhibitor does not interact with direct adrenergic agonists. The Second Amine Oxidase Workshop, Uppsala. August 1986. *Pharmacol Toxicol* (1987) 60 (Suppl I), 31.

Monoamine oxidase inhibitors (MAOIs) + Rauwolfia alkaloids or Tetrabenazine

The use of potentially depressive drugs such as the rauwolfia alkaloids or tetrabenazine is generally contraindicated in patients needing treatment for depression. Central excitation and possibly hypertension can occur if the rauwolfia is given to patients already taking MAOI, but is unlikely if the rauwolfia is given first.

Clinical evidence

A chronically depressed woman treated firstly with **nialamide** (100 mg three times a day) and on the third day with **reserpine** as well (0.5 mg three times a day) became hypomanic on the following day and almost immediately went into frank mania.[1]

Seven days after stopping 25 mg **nialamide** daily, a patient was started on **tetrabenazine**. 6 h later he collapsed and demonstrated epileptiform convulsions, partial unconsciousness, rapid respiration and tachycardia.[2]

Other reports state that the administration of **reserpine** or **tetrabenazine** after pretreatment with **iproniazid** can lead to a temporary (up to three days) disturbance of affect and memory, associated with autonomic excitation, delirious agitation, disorientation and illusions of experience and recognition.[3,4]

A delayed 'reserpine-reversal' was seen in three schizophrenics treated firstly with **phenelzine** for 12 weeks, then a placebo for 16 to

33 weeks, and lastly **reserpine**. Their blood pressures rose slightly and persistently and their psychomotor activity was considerably increased, lasting in two cases throughout the 12-week period of treatment.[5]

Mechanism

Rauwolfia alkaloids such as reserpine cause adrenergic neurones to become depleted of their normal stores of norepinephrine (noradrenaline). In this way they prevent or reduce the normal transmission of impulses at the adrenergic nerve endings of the sympathetic nervous system and thereby act as antihypertensive agents. Since the brain also possesses adrenergic neurones, failure of transmission in the CNS could account for the sedation and depression observed. If these compounds are given to patients already taking a MAOI, they can cause the sudden release of large amounts of accumulated norepinephrine, and in the brain of 5-HT as well, resulting in excessive stimulation of the receptors which is seen as gross central excitation and hypertension. This would account for the case reports cited and the effects seen in *animals*.[6-8] These stimulant effects are sometimes called 'reserpine-reversal' because instead of the expected sedation or depression, excitation or delayed depression is seen. It depends upon the order in which the drugs are given.

Importance and management

The administration of potentially depressive drugs is generally contraindicated in patients needing treatment for depression. However if concurrent use is considered desirable, the MAOIs should be given after, and not before, the other drug so that sedation rather than excitation will occur.[9] The documentation of this latter reaction in man is very limited.

1. Gradwell BG. Psychotic reactions and phenelzine. *BMJ* (1960) 2, 1018.
2. Davies TS. Monoamine oxidase inhibitors and rauwolfia compounds. *BMJ* (1960) 2, 739.
3. Voelkel A. Klinische Wirkung von Pharmaka mit Einfluss auf den Monoaminestoffwechsel de Gehirns. *Confin Neurol* (1958) 18, 144.
4. Voelkel A. Experiences with MAO inhibitors in psychiatry. *Ann N Y Acad Sci* (1959) 80, 680.
5. Esser AH. Clinical observations on reserpine reversal after prolonged MAO inhibition. *Psychiatr Neurol Neurochir* (1967) 70, 59–63.
6. Shore PA, Brodie BB. LSD-like effects elicited by reserpine in rabbits pretreated with isoniazid. *Proc Soc Exp Biol* (1957) 94, 433–5.
7. Chessin M, Kramer ER, Scott CC. Modification of the pharmacology of reserpine and serotonin by iproniazid. *J Pharmacol Exp Ther* (1957) 119, 453–60.
8. von Euler US, Bygdeman S and Persson N-A. Interaction of reserpine and monoamine oxidase inhibitors on adrenergic transmitter release. *Biochim Biol Sper* (1970) 9, 215–20.
9. Natarajan S. Potential danger of monoamineoxidase inhibitors and α-methyldopa. *Lancet* (1964) i, 1330.

Monoamine oxidase inhibitors (MAOIs) + Sulphonamides

An isolated report describes the development of weakness, ataxia and other adverse effects in a patient on phenelzine when additionally given sulfafurazole (sulphafurazole, sulfisoxazole).

Clinical evidence, mechanism, importance and management

A woman taking 45 mg **phenelzine** daily complained of weakness, ataxia, dizziness, tinnitus, muscle pains and paraesthesias within 7 days of starting to take 4 g of **sulfafurazole** daily. These adverse effects continued until the 10-day sulphonamide course was completed. All then disappeared.[1] The reasons are not understood, but as these adverse effects are a combination of the side-effects of both drugs, it seems possible that a mutual interaction (perhaps saturation of the acetylating mechanisms in the liver) was responsible. Concurrent use need not be avoided, but prescribers should be aware of this case.

1. Boyer WF, Lake CR. Interaction of phenelzine and sulfisoxazole. *Am J Psychiatry* (1983) 140, 264–5.

Monoamine oxidase inhibitors (MAOIs) + Sumatriptan

Moclobemide approximately doubles the bioavailability of subcutaneous sumatriptan but its adverse side-effects do not seem to be increased. However, the makers of sumatriptan and others say that the concurrent use of moclobemide and other MAOIs is contraindicated.

Clinical evidence

For eight days three groups of 14 subjects were given a placebo or 450 mg **moclobemide** daily or 10 mg **selegiline** daily, and then on day 8 all of the subjects were also given 6 mg **sumatriptan** subcutaneously. No statistically significant differences in pulse rates or in blood pressures were seen between any of the groups following the injection of the **sumatriptan**, however the **sumatriptan** AUC of the **moclobemide**-treated group was approximately doubled (+ 129%), its clearance was reduced by 56% and its half-life increased by 52%. The pharmacokinetic changes seen in the **selegiline** group were not consistent. There were no differences in the adverse events experienced by any of the three groups.[1]

A patient taking 900 mg **moclobemide** daily showed no adverse effects when given 100 mg oral **sumatriptan** on six occasions.[2]

A comprehensive search of the world's literature using MEDLINE, EmBASE, Biological Abstracts, Current Contents, Reaction, ClinAlert, International Pharmaceutical Abstracts, Health Protection Branch of Health Canada, WHO Collaborative Centre for International Drug Monitoring and reports from proprietary manufacturers, identified published reports of 31 patients taking **sumatriptan** and **MAOIs** concurrently, but no adverse events were reported.[3]

Mechanism

Studies with human liver have shown that MAO-A (the isoenzyme inhibited by moclobemide) is largely responsible for the metabolism of sumatriptan.[4] Thus, in the presence of moclobemide, the metabolism of sumatriptan is reduced and as a result it is cleared from the body more slowly. MAO-B (the isoenzyme inhibited by selegiline) has only a minor effect on the metabolism of sumatriptan.[4]

Importance and management

The moclobemide/sumatriptan interaction appears to be established. The same interaction seems likely to occur with any of the other selective MAO-A inhibitors and with the non-selective MAOIs too (see Table 18.1 at the beginning of this chapter), but not with the selective MAO-B inhibitors like selegiline. This needs confirmation. However the increased sumatriptan bioavailability appears not to be clinically important because, in the study cited, those subjects on moclobemide did not experience any more adverse effects than those taking the selegiline or placebo. Despite this the makers of sumatriptan quite clearly say that the concurrent use of sumatriptan and MAOIs is contraindicated, and within 2 weeks of stopping an MAOI.[5] This ultracautiousness would appear to be based on medico-legal considerations rather than on any firm clinical evidence that an increased risk actually exists.

No general adverse sumatriptan/MAOI interaction has yet been identified, but the current advice is that because experience with sumatriptan is still limited, concurrent use should continue be avoided until safety has been demonstrated.[3]

1. Glaxo, reports on file: A study to determine whether the pharmacokinetics, safety and tolerability of subcutaneously administered sumatriptan (6 mg) are altered by interaction with concurrent oral monoamine oxidase inhibitors. (Protocol C92–050).
2. Blier P, Bergeron R. The safety of combined use of sumatriptan with antidepressant treatments. *J Clin Psychopharmacol* (1995) 15, 106–9.
3. Garner DM, Lynd LD. Sumatriptan contraindications and the serotonin syndrome. *Ann Pharmacother* (1998) 32, 33–8.
4. Dixon CM, Park GR, Tarbit MH. Characterisation of the enzyme responsible for the metabolism of sumatriptan in human liver. *Biochem Pharmacol* (1994) 47, 1253–7.
5. Glaxo, Personal communication, May 1995.

Monoamine oxidase inhibitors (MAOIs) + Sympathomimetics (directly-acting)

The pressor effects of epinephrine (adrenaline), isoprenaline (isoproterenol), norepinephrine (noradrenaline) and methoxamine may be unchanged or only moderately increased in patients taking MAOIs. The increase may be somewhat greater in those who show a significant hypotensive response to the MAOI. An isolated case of tachycardia and apprehension has also been described in an asthmatic on phenelzine after taking salbutamol (albuterol). Hypomania was seen in another asthmatic after taking isoetharine. See also 'Monoamine oxidase inhibitors (MAOIs) + Phenylephrine', p.678.

Clinical evidence

(a) Effects in normal subjects

Two subjects given 45 mg **phenelzine** daily and another given 30 mg **tranylcypromine** daily for seven days showed no significant changes in their pressor responses to either **epinephrine (adrenaline)** or **isoprenaline (isoproterenol)**. Another subject on **tranylcypromine**, similarly treated, showed a twofold increase in the pressor response in the mid-range of **norepinephrine (noradrenaline)** concentrations infused, but not in the upper or low ranges.[1]

These results confirm those from two other studies, one with **norepinephrine** and **phenelzine**[2] and the other with **norepinephrine** and **methoxamine** in patients taking **nialamide**.[3] Yet another study in three volunteers on **tranylcypromine** found that the effects of **norepinephrine** were slightly increased, while with **epinephrine** a two to four fold increase in the effects on heart rate and diastolic pressure took place, but a less marked increase in systolic pressure. **Isoprenaline** behaved very much like **epinephrine**, but there was no enhancement of systolic pressure.[4] A patient using 1% **epinephrine** eye drops twice daily showed no increase in blood pressure or heart rate when treated with 20 mg rising to 50 mg **tranylcypromine** daily.[5] **Moclobemide** is reported not to interact with **norepinephrine**[6,7] or **isoprenaline (isoproterenol)**.[6] Tachycardia and apprehension in a man on **phenelzine** after taking **salbutamol (albuterol)** has also been described,[8] and hypomania in a man on **phenelzine** while taking **isoetharine**.[9]

(b) Effects in patients with MAOI-induced hypotension

In a study in seven hypertensive patients who showed postural hypotension after being given either **pheniprazine** or **tranylcypromine**, it was demonstrated that the doses of **norepinephrine (noradrenaline)** required to produce a 25 mmHg rise in systolic pressure were reduced to 13–38% and of **methoxamine** to 30–39%.[3] However another study found no significant change when **norepinephrine** was given to two patients treated with **pargyline**.[10]

Mechanism

These sympathomimetic amines act directly on the receptors at the nerve endings which innervate arterial blood vessels, so that the presence of the MAOI-induced accumulation of norepinephrine within these nerve endings would not be expected to alter the extent of direct stimulation. The enhancement seen in those patients whose blood pressure was lowered by the MAOI might possibly be due to an increased sensitivity of the receptors which is seen if the nerves are cut, and is also seen during temporary 'pharmacological severance'. The reactions of the two patients given beta-adrenergic agonists (salbutamol, isoetharine) are not understood.

Importance and management

The evidence is limited but the overall picture is that some slight to moderate enhancement of the effects of norepinephrine (noradrenaline) and epinephrine (adrenaline) may occur, but the authors of three of the reports cited[1,4,5] are in broad agreement that problems are unlikely to occur. One group says[5] that "it seems that the use of epine-

phrine, whether administered in eye drops or as a component of local anaesthesia in dental and other procedures, should not be contraindicated in patients receiving MAOIs." Direct evidence about methoxamine is even more limited but it seems to behave similarly. None of the studies demonstrated any marked changes in the effects of isoprenaline (isoproterenol).

The situation in patients who show a reduced blood pressure due to the use of an MAOI (this would normally seem to apply principally to pargyline) is less clear. One study found an increase in the pressor efforts of norepinephrine and methoxamine[3] in hypertensive patients on pheniprazine or tranylcypromine, whereas another[10] found no changes in the pressor effects of norepinephrine in patients on pargyline.

The cases involving salbutamol (albuterol) and isoetharine are isolated and possibly not of general importance. This needs confirmation. The interaction between phenylephrine and the MAOIs is dealt with earlier in this chapter (see 'Monoamine oxidase inhibitors (MAOIs) + Phenylephrine', p.678 in this chapter).

1. Boakes AJ, Laurence DR, Teoh PC, Barar FSK, Benedikter L, Prichard BNC. Interactions between sympathomimetic amines and antidepressant agents in man. *BMJ* (1973) 1, 311.
2. Elis J, Laurence DR, Mattie H, Prichard BNC. Modification by monoamine oxidase inhibitors of the effect of some sympathomimetics on blood pressure. *BMJ* (1967) 2, 75–8.
3. Horwitz D, Goldberg LI, Sjoerdsma A. Increased blood pressure responses to dopamine and norepinephrine produced by monoamine oxidase inhibitors in man. *J Lab Clin Med* (1960) 56, 747–53.
4. Cuthbert MF, Vere DW. Potentiation of the cardiovascular effects of some catecholamines by a monoamine oxidase inhibitor. *Br J Pharmacol* (1971) 43, 471P–472P.
5. Thompson DS, Sweet RA, Marzula K, Peredes JC. Lack of interaction of monoamine oxidase inhibitors and epinephrine in an older patient. *J Clin Psychopharmacol* (1997) 17, 322–3.
6. Zimmer R, Gieschke R, Fischbach R, Gasic S. Interaction studies with moclobemide. *Acta Psychiatr Scand* (1990) (Suppl 360), 84–6.
7. Cusson JR, Goldenberg E, Larochelle P. Effect of a novel monoamine-oxidase inhibitor, moclobemide on the sensitivity to intravenous tyramine and norepinephrine in humans. *J Clin Pharmacol* (1991) 31, 462–7.
8. Shader RI, Greenblatt DJ. MAOIs and drug interactions—a proposal for a clearinghouse. *J Clin Psychopharmacol* (1985) 5, A17.
9. Goldman LS, Tiller JA. Hypomania related to phenelzine and isoetharine interaction in one patient. *J Clin Psychiatry* (1987) 48, 170.
10. Pettinger WA, Oates JA. Supersensitivity to tyramine during monoamine oxidase inhibition in man. *Clin Pharmacol Ther* (1968) 9, 341–4.

Monoamine oxidase inhibitors (MAOIs) + Sympathomimetics (indirectly-acting)

The concurrent use of sympathomimetic amines with indirect activity (amphetamines, ephedrine, MDMA, metaraminol, phenylpropanolamine, pseudoephedrine, etc.) and the older MAOIs can result in a potentially fatal hypertensive crisis. These amines are found in many proprietary cough, cold and influenza preparations, or are used as appetite suppressants. No important interaction occurs with brofaromine and slow-release phenylpropanolamine but immediate-release preparations should be avoided. Indirectly-acting sympathomimetics should also be avoided by patients taking moclobemide.

Clinical evidence

(a) Non-selective MAOIs

Concurrent use can result in a rapid and serious rise in blood pressure accompanied by tachycardia, chest pains and severe occipital headache. Neck stiffness, flushing, sweating, nausea, vomiting, hypertonicity of the limbs and sometimes epileptiform convulsions can occur. Fatal intracranial haemorrhage, cardiac arrhythmias and cardiac arrest may result. Two examples from many:

A woman who, unknown to her doctors, was taking **pargyline**, was given **phenylpropanolamine** for nasal decongestion on the eve of surgery which promptly caused a hypertensive reaction. Her blood pressure rose rapidly from 130/80 to 220/160 mmHg and she complained of occipital headache, photophobia and nausea. She also exhibited sweating and vomited. Two intravenous injections of 5 mg phentolamine partially controlled her blood pressure.[1]

A 30-year-old depressed woman who was taking 45 mg **phenelzine** daily and 2 mg trifluoperazine at night, acquired some **dexamfeta-**

mine (dextroamphetamine) tablets from a friend and took 20 mg. Within 15 min she complained of severe headache which she described as if "her head was bursting". An hour later her blood pressure was 150/100 mmHg. Later she became comatose and died. A postmortem examination revealed a haemorrhage in the left cerebral hemisphere, disrupting the internal capsule and adjacent areas of the corpus striatum.[2]

This interaction has been reported with **amfetamine sulphate**,[3] **d-l amfetamine**,[4] **ephedrine**,[5,6] **isometheptene mucate**,[7] **metaraminol**,[8] **methylamphetamine**,[9-12] **mephentermine**,[13] **phenylpropanolamine**,[14-18] **pseudoephedrine**,[18-20] and **methylphenidate**,[13] in patients on **tranylcypromine**,[3,5,6,9,10,15] **phenelzine**,[2,4,5,9-12,14,16-18,21] **isocarboxazid**,[10] **iproniazid**,[20] **mebanazine**,[14] and **pargyline**.[8] **Nialamide** is expected to behave similarly but reports seem to be lacking. There are other reports and studies of this interaction not listed here. Extreme hyperpyrexia, apparently without hypertension, has with described with **tranylcypromine** and **amphetamines**.[22,23]

Marked hypertension, diaphoresis, altered mental status and hypertonicity (slow forceful twisting and arching movements) occurred in one patient on **phenelzine** after taking **MDMA (3,4-methylenedioxymethamphetamine)**.[24] Increased muscle tension, decorticate-like posturing and coma occurred in another.[25] Both recovered. **MDMA** has been prescribed by some psychiatrists in dosages of 75 to 125 mg and is also 'street-available' as a recreational drug in doses of 50 to 100 mg. Its alternative names include **AKA**, **ecstasy**, **XTC**, **MDM**, **Adam**, **doctor**, **M** and **M's**.

(b) Selective MAOIs

No interaction was seen in subjects on **brofaromine** (75 mg twice daily for 10 days) when given slow-release 75 mg **phenylpropanolamine** (*Acutrim Late Day*), but immediate-release **phenylpropanolamine** in gelatine capsules caused a 3.3-fold increase in pressor sensitivity.[26,27] The pressor effects of **ephedrine** (two doses of 50 mg with a 4-h interval) in subjects taking 300 mg **moclobemide** twice daily were increased by a factor of about 4.[28,29]

Mechanism

The reaction can be attributed to overstimulation of the adrenergic receptors of the cardiovascular system.[30] During treatment with non-selective MAOIs, large amounts of norepinephrine (noradrenaline) accumulate at adrenergic nerve endings not only in the brain, but also within the sympathetic nerve endings which innervate arterial blood vessels. Stimulation of these latter nerve endings by sympathomimetic amines with indirect actions causes the release of the accumulated norepinephrine and in the massive stimulation of the receptors. An exaggerated blood vessel constriction occurs andthe blood pressure rise is proportionately excessive. Intracranial haemorrhage can occur if the pressure is so high that a blood vessel ruptures.[2] The MAOI/MDMA reaction may also possibly be related to the serotonin syndrome. The selective MAOIs which inhibit only MAO-A (such as moclobemide) appear to behave like the irreversible non-selective MAOIs in this context.

Importance and management

(a) Non selective MAOIs

A very well-documented, serious, and potentially fatal interaction. Patients taking any of the older irreversible MAOIs, whether for depression or hypertension, should not normally take any sympathomimetic amine with indirect activity. These include the amphetamines (dexamfetamine (dextroamphetamine), hydroxyamphetamine, methylamphetamine), ephedrine, isometheptene mucate, MDMA (ecstasy), mephentermine, metaraminol, methylphenidate, phenylpropanolamine and pseudoephedrine. Direct evidence implicating amfepramone (diethylpropion), benzphetamine, chlorphentermine, cyclopentamine, mazindol,[31] methylephedrine, phendimetrazine, phenmetrazine and pholedrine seems not to have been documented, but on the basis of their known pharmacology their concurrent administration with the MAOIs should be avoided.

Many of these sympathomimetic amines occur in OTC cough, cold and influenza preparations, and as proprietary appetite suppressants.

Patients on MAOIs should be strongly warned not to take any of drugs concurrently. A possible exception to this prohibition is that under very well controlled conditions dexamfetamine and methylphenidate may sometimes be effectively (and apparently safely) used with MAOIs for refractory depression.[32,33]

(b) Selective MAOIs

No clinically important interaction appears to occur with brofaromine and slow-release phenylpropanolamine but immediate-release preparations should be avoided. Moclobemide can interact and the makers advise avoidance of sympathomimetics such as ephedrine, pseudoephedrine and phenylpropanolamine, and it would also be prudent to avoid moclobemide with any of the other indirectly-acting sympathomimetics cited here although the severity of the interactions with moclobemide is unlikely to be as great as that seen with the older MAOIs. However it should be said that ephedrine and phenylephrine were successfully and uneventfully used in the presence of moclobemide during anaesthesia to control hypotension.[34]

Treatment

If a hypertensive reaction occurs it can be controlled with an alpha-blocker such as phentolamine (5 mg intravenously) or phenoxybenzamine, or failing that an intramuscular injection of 50 mg chlorpromazine. 20 mg labetalol given intravenously over 5 min has also proved to be successful. An effective and simple alternative that is known to work is to chew a 10 mg capsule of nifedipine to release its contents, and wash it down with a drink of water.[35,36] Other calcium channel blockers would also be expected to be effective.

1. Jenkins LC, Graves HB. Potential hazards of psychoactive drugs in association with anaesthesia. *Can Anaesth Soc J* (1965) 12, 121.
2. Lloyd JTA, Walker DRH. Death after combined dexamphetamine and phenelzine. *BMJ* (1965) 2, 168–9.
3. Zeck P. The dangers of some antidepressant drugs. *Med J Aust* (1961) 2, 607–9.
4. Tonks CM, Livingstone D. Monoamineoxidase inhibitors. *Lancet* (1963) i, 1323–4.
5. Elis J, Laurence DR, Mattie H, Prichard BNC. Modification by monoamine oxidase inhibitors of the effects of some sympathomimetics on blood pressure. *BMJ* (1967) 2, 75–8.
6. Low-Beer GA, Tidmarsh D. Collapse after "Parstelin". *BMJ* (1963) 2, 683–4.
7. Kraft KE, Dore FH. Computerized drug interaction programs: how reliable ? *JAMA* (1996) 275, 1087.
8. Horler AR, Wynne NA. Hypertensive crisis due to pargyline and metaraminol. *BMJ* (1965) 2, 460–1.
9. MacDonald R. Tranylcypromine. *Lancet* (1963) i, 269.
10. Mason A. Fatal reaction associated with tranylcypromine and methylamphetamine. *Lancet* (1962) i, 1073.
11. Dally PJ. Fatal reaction associated with tranylcypromine and methylamphetamine. *Lancet* (1962) i, 1235.
12. Nymark M, Nielsen IM. Reactions due to the combination of monoamineoxidase inhibitors with thymoleptics, pethidine, or methylamphetamine. *Lancet* (1963) ii, 524–5.
13. Sherman M, Hauser GC, Glover BH. Toxic reactions to tranylcypromine. *Am J Psychiatry* (1964) 120, 1019–20.
14. Tonks CM, Lloyd AT. Hazards with monoamine oxidase inhibitors. *BMJ* (1965) 1, 589.
15. Cuthbert MF, Greenberg MP, Morley SW. Cough and cold remedies: a potential danger to patients on monoamine oxidase inhibitors. *BMJ* (1969) 1, 404–6.
16. Mason AMS, Buckle RM. "Cold" cures and monoamine oxidase inhibitors. *BMJ* (1969) 1, 845–6.
17. Humberstone PM. Hypertension from cold remedies. *BMJ* (1969) 1, 846.
18. Harrison WM, McGrath PJ, Stewart JW, Quitkin F. MAOIs and hypertensive crises: the role of OTC drugs. *J Clin Psychiatry* (1989) 50, 64–5.
19. Wright SP. Hazards with monoamine-oxidase inhibitors: a persistent problem. *Lancet* (1978) i, 284–5.
20. Davies R. Patient medication records. *Pharm J* (1982) 287, 652.
21. Stark DCC. Effects of giving vasopressors to patients on monoamine oxidase inhibitors. *Lancet* (1962) i, 1405.
22. Lewis E. Hyperpyrexia with antidepressant drugs. *BMJ* (1965) 1, 1671.
23. Kriskó I, Lewis E, Johnson JE. Severe hyperpyrexia due to tranylcypromine–amphetamine toxicity. *Ann Intern Med* (1969) 70, 559–64.
24. Smilkstein MJ, Smolinske SC, Rumack BH. A case of MAO inhibitor/MDMA interaction: agony after ecstasy. *Clin Toxicol* (1987) 25, 149–59.
25. Kaskey GB. Possible interaction between an MAOI and "Ecstasy". *Am J Psychiatry* (1992) 149, 411–2.
26. Mühlbauer B, Gradin-Frimmer G, Bieck P. Safety of reversible monoamine oxidase inhibitors (MAOI): interaction of brofaromine with sympathomimetic drugs in healthy volunteers. *Naunyn Schmiedebergs Arch Pharmacol* (1990) 341 (Suppl), R113.
27. Gleiter CH, Mühlbauer B, Gradin-Frimmer G, Antonin KH, Bieck PR. Administration of sympathomimetic drugs with the selective MAO-A inhibitor brofaromine. Effect on blood pressure. *Drug Invest* (1992) 4, 149–54.
28. Dingemanse J. An update of recent moclobemide interaction data. *Int Clin Psychopharmacol* (1993) 7, 167–80.
29. Dingemanse J, Guentert T, Gieschke R, Stabl M. Modification of the cardiovascular effects of ephedrine by the reversible monoamine oxidase A-inhibitor moclobemide. *J Cardiovasc Pharmacol* (1996) 28, 856–61.
30. Simpson LL. Mechanism of the adverse interaction between monoamine oxidase inhibitors and amphetamine. *J Pharmacol Exp Ther* (1978) 205, 392–9.
31. Magrath SM (Sandoz Products Ltd). Personal communication (1987).
32. Fawcett J, Kravitz HM, Zajecka JM, Schaff MR. CNS stimulant potentiation of monoamine oxidase inhibitors in treatment-refractory depression. *J Clin Psychopharmacol* (1991) 11, 127–32.

33. Feighner JP, Herbstein J, Damlouji N. Combined MAOI, TCA and direct stimulant therapy of treatment resistant depression. *J Clin Psychiatry* (1985) 46, 206–9.
34. Martyr JW, Orlikowski CEP. Epidural anaesthesia, ephedrine and phenylephrine in a patient taking moclobemide, a new monoamine oxidase inhibitor. *Anaesthesia* (1996) 51, 1150–2.
35. Clary C, Schweitzer E. Treatment of MAOI hypertensive crisis with sublingual nifedipine. *J Clin Psychiatry* (1987) 48, 249–50.
36. Fier M. Safer use of MAOIs. *Am J Psychiatry* (1991) 148, 391–2.

Monoamine oxidase inhibitors (MAOIs) + Tricyclic antidepressants

Because of the very toxic and sometimes fatal reactions (similar to or the same as the serotonin syndrome) which have very occasionally taken place in patients taking both MAOIs and tricyclic antidepressants, concurrent use came to be regarded as totally contraindicated, but informed opinion now considers that with extremely careful control it is permissible and advantageous to use both these drugs together for some refractory patients.

Clinical evidence

(a) Toxic reactions or other interactions

The toxic reactions have included (with variations) sweating, flushing, hyperpyrexia, restlessness, excitement, tremor, muscle twitching and rigidity, convulsions and coma. An illustrative example:

A woman who had been taking 20 mg **tranylcypromine** daily for about 3 weeks, stopped taking it 3 days before taking a single tablet of **imipramine**. Within a few hours she complained of an excruciating headache, and soon afterwards lost consciousness and started to convulse. The toxic reactions manifested were a temperature of 40°C, pulse rate of 120, severe extensor rigidity, carpal spasm, opisthotonos and cyanosis. She was treated with amobarbital and phenytoin, and her temperature was reduced with alcohol-ice-soaked towels. The treatment was effective and she recovered.[1]

Similar reactions have been recorded on a number of other occasions with normal therapeutic doses of **iproniazid**,[2] **isocarboxazid**,[2,3] **pargyline**,[4] or **phenelzine**[5-11] with **imipramine**; **phenelzine** with **desipramine**[12] or **clomipramine**;[13-15] **tranylcypromine**[16-19] with **clomipramine**; and **moclobemide** with **imipramine**.[20] **Moclobemide** is reported not to interact with **amitriptyline** or **desipramine**[17,21-23] but a reaction similar to the serotonin syndrome occurred in 2 patients when **clomipramine** (50 mg daily) was replaced by **moclobemide**,[24,25] and 4 patients developed the serotonin syndrome (3 of them died) after taking moderate overdoses of **moclobemide** and **clomipramine**.[26-29] However another study found that doses of up to 300 mg **moclobemide** could be given 24 h after the last dose of treatment with either **amitriptyline** or **clomipramine** without any major risks.[23] Another study found a 39% rise in serum **trimipramine** levels in 15 patients and a 25% rise in serum **maprotiline** levels of 6 other patients when concurrently treated with **moclobemide**. No serious toxic reactions were reported.[30] Only a minor and clinically unimportant change in the pharmacokinetics of **amitriptyline** occurs in patients given **toloxatone**.[31]

Some other reports are confused by overdosage with one or both drugs, or by the presence of other drugs and diseases. There have been fatalities.[12,16,32] In some instances the drugs were not taken together but were swapped without a washout period in between. There are far too many reports of these interactions to list all of them here, but they are extensively reviewed elsewhere.[33-35] Three patients with bipolar disorder developed mania when treated with **isocarboxazid** and **amitriptyline**.[36]

(b) Advantageous or uneventful concurrent use

Dr GA Gander of St Thomas's Hospital, London, has stated[37] that 98 out of 149 patients on combined therapy (**phenelzine, isocarboxazid** or **iproniazid** with **imipramine** or **amitriptyline**) over periods of 1 to 24 months improved significantly and that the side-effects were ". . . identical in nature and similar in frequency to those seen with a single antidepressant. . .". Side effects were easily controlled by ad-

justing the dosage. None of the serious side-effects previously reported, such as muscle twitching or loss of consciousness was seen. He also states that more than 1400 patients having combined antidepressants over a period of 4 years ". . . tend to confirm these findings described." Dr William Sargant from the same department has also written[38] that ". . . we have used combined antidepressant drugs for nearly 10 years now on some thousands of patients. We still wait to see any of the rare dangerous complications reported."

There are a number of other reports and reviews describing the beneficial use of MAOI/tricyclic antidepressant combinations.[34,35,39-42]

Mechanism

Not understood. One idea is that both drugs cause grossly elevated monoamine levels (5-HT, norepinephrine (noradrenaline)) in the brain which 'spill-over' into areas not concerned with mood elevation. It may be related to, or the same as the serotonin-syndrome seen with selective serotonin re-uptake inhibitors.[14,20] Some of the tricyclics (e.g. clomipramine, imipramine) are potent inhibitors of serotonin uptake. Less likely suggestions are that the MAOIs inhibit the metabolism of the tricyclic antidepressants, or that active and unusual metabolites of the tricyclic antidepressants are produced.[34]

Importance and management

An established, serious and life-threatening but apparently uncommon interaction. There is no precise information about its incidence but it is probably much lower than was originally thought. No detailed clinical work has been done to find out precisely what sets the scene for it to occur, but some general empirical guidelines have been suggested so that it can, as far as possible, be avoided when concurrent treatment is thought appropriate:[11,33-35,43]

- Treatment with both types of drug should only be undertaken by those well aware of the problems and who can undertake adequate supervision.
- Only patients refractory to all other types of treatment should be considered.
- Tranylcypromine, phenelzine, clomipramine and imipramine appear to be high on the list of drugs which have interacted adversely. Amitriptyline, trimipramine and isocarboxazid are possibly safer.
- Drugs should be given orally, not parenterally.
- It seems safer to give the tricyclic antidepressants first, or together with the MAOI, than to give the MAOI first. If the patient is already taking an MAOI, it may not be safe to start the tricyclic antidepressant until recovery from MAO-inhibition is complete.
- Small doses should be given initially, increasing the levels of each drug, one at a time, over a period of 2–3 weeks to levels generally below those used for each one individually.
- Do not exchange either the MAOI or the tricyclic antidepressant for other members of these drug groups without taking full precautions. A good washout period between the drugs is advisable. In the case of moclobemide, not less than 24 h, but with other MAOIs the usual advice is that washout should be up to 3 weeks. However one study reported switching 178 patients from tricyclics to MAOIs within 4 days or less. 63 of these patients were given the MAOI while still being tapered from the tricyclic, all without any apparent problems.[42]

Doses of 50 and 100 mg chlorpromazine given intramuscularly have been used successfully in the treatment of this adverse interaction[17,19] and one report suggests that patients should carry 300 mg chlorpromazine and take it if a sudden, throbbing, radiating occipital headache occurs, and seek medical help at once.[44] It has been suggested that dantrolene can probably be used to reduce the muscle rigidity and hyperpyrexia, and possibly methysergide which is a 5HT receptor antagonist.[26]

1. Brachfeld J, Wirtshafter A, Wolfe S. Imipramine-tranylcypromine incompatibility. Near-fatal toxic reaction. *JAMA* (1963) 186, 1172–3.
2. Ayd FJ. Toxic somatic and psychopathological reactions to antidepressant drugs. *J Neuropsychiatry* (1961) 2 (Suppl 1), S119–S120.
3. Kane FJ, Freeman D. Non-fatal reaction to imipramine-MAO inhibitor combination. *Am J Psychiatry* (1963), 120, 79–80.
4. McCurdy RL, Kane FJ. Transient brain syndrome as a non-fatal reaction to combined pargyline imipramine treatment. *Am J Psychiatry* (1964), 121, 397–8.
5. Loeb RH. Quoted in ref 10 below as written communication (1969).

6. Hills NF. Combining the antidepressant drugs. *BMJ* (1965) 1, 859.
7. Davies G. Side effects of phenelzine. *BMJ* (1960) 2, 1019.
8. Howarth E. Possible synergistic effects of the new thymoleptics in connection with poisoning. *J Ment Sci* (1961) 107, 100–103.
9. Singh H. Atropine-like poisoning due to tranquillizing agents. *Am J Psychiatry* (1960) 117, 360–1.
10. Lockett MF, Milner G. Combining the antidepressant drugs. *BMJ* (1965) 1, 921.
11. Graham PM, Potter JM, Paterson JW. Combination monoamine oxidase inhibitor/tricyclic antidepressant interaction. *Lancet* (1982) ii, 440.
12. Bowen LW. Fatal hyperpyrexia with antidepressant drugs. *BMJ* (1964) 2, 1465.
13. Beeley L, Daly M (eds). Bulletin of the W. Midlands Centre for Adverse Drug Reaction Reporting. (1986) 23, 16.
14. Nierenberg DW, Semprebon M. The central nervous system serotonin syndrome. *Clin Pharmacol Ther* (1993) 53, 84–8.
15. Stern TA, Schwartz JH, Shuster JL. Catastrophic illness associated with the combination of clomipramine, phenelzine, and chlorpromazine. *Ann Clin Psychiatry* (1992) 4, 81–5.
16. Beaumont G. Drug interactions with clomipramine (Anafranil). *J Int Med Res* (1973) 1, 480.
17. Tackley RM, Tregaskis B. Fatal disseminated intravascular coagulation following a monoamine oxidase inhibitor/tricyclic interaction. *Anaesthesia* (1987) 42, 760–3.
18. Richards GA, Fritz VU, Pincus P, Reyneke J. Unusual drug interactions between monoamine oxidase inhibitors and tricyclic antidepressants. *J Neurol Neurosurg Psychiatry* (1987) 50, 1240–1.
19. Gillman PK. Successful treatment of serotonin syndrome with chlorpromazine. *Med J Aust* (1996) 165, 345.
20. Brodribb TR, Downey M, Gilbar PJ. Efficacy and adverse effects of moclobemide. *Lancet* (1994) 343, 475–6.
21. Zimmer R, Gieschke R, Fischbach R, Gasic S. Interaction studies with moclobemide. *Acta Psychiatr Scand* (1990) (Suppl 360), 84–6.
22. Korn A, Eichler HG, Fischbach R, Gasic S. Moclobemide, a new reversible MAO inhibitor – interaction with tyramine and tricyclic antidepressants in healthy volunteers and depressive patients. *Psychopharmacology (Berl)* (1986) 88, 153–7.
23. Dingemanse J, Kneer J, Fotteler B, Groen H, Peeters PAM, Jonkman JHG. Switch in treatment from tricyclic antidepressants to moclobemide: a new generation monoamine oxidase inhibitor. *J Clin Psychopharmacol* (1995) 15, 41–8.
24. Spigset O, Mjorndal T, Lovheim O. Serotonin syndrome caused by a moclobemide-clomipramine interaction. *BMJ* (1993) 306, 248.
25. Gillman PK. Serotonin syndrome – clomipramine too soon after moclobemide? *Int Clin Psychopharmacol* (1997) 12, 339–42.
26. Neuvonen PJ, Pohjola-Sintonen S, Tacke U, Vuori E. Five fatal cases of serotonin syndrome after moclobemide-citalopram or moclobemide-clomipramine overdoses. *Lancet* (1993) 342, 1419.
27. Hernandez AF, Montero MN, Pla A, Vllaneuve E. Fatal moclobemide overdose or death caused by serotonin syndrome? *J Forensic Sci* (1995) 49, 128–30.
28. François B, Marquet P, Desachy A, Routson J, Lachatre G, Gastinne H. Serotonin syndrome due to an overdose of moclobemide and clomipramine: a potentially life-threatening association. *Intensive Care Med* (1997) 23, 122–4.
29. Ferrer-Dufol A, Perez-Aradros C, Murillo EC. Fatal serotonin syndrome caused by moclobemide-clomipramine overdose. *Clin Toxicol* (1998) 36, 31–2.
30. König F, Wolfersdorf M, Löble M, Wössner S, Hauger B. Trimipramine and maprotiline plasma levels during combined treatment with moclobemide in therapy-resistant depression. *Pharmacopsychiatry* (1997) 30, 125–7.
31. Vandel S, Bertschy G, Perault MC, Sandoz M, Bouguet S, Chakroun R, Guibert S, Vandel B. Minor and clinically non-significant interaction between toloxatone and amitriptyline. *Eur J Clin Pharmacol* (1993) 44, 97–9.
32. Wright SP. Hazards with monoamine-oxidase inhibitors: a persistent problem. *Lancet* (1978) i, 284–5.
33. Schuckit M, Robins E, Feighner J. Tricyclic antidepressants and monoamine oxidase inhibitors. Combination therapy in the treatment of depression. *Arch Gen Psychiatry* (1971) 24, 509–14.
34. Ponto LB, Perry PJ, Liskow BI, Seaba HH. Drug therapy reviews: tricyclic antidepressant and monoamine oxidase inhibitor combination therapy. *Am J Hosp Pharm* (1977) 34, 954–61.
35. Ananth J, Luchins D. A review of combined tricyclic and MAOI therapy. *Compr Psychiatry* (1977) 18, 221–30.
36. De la Fuente JR, Berlanga C, Leon-Andrade C. Mania induced by tricyclic-MAOI combination therapy in bipolar treatment-resistant disorder. Case reports. *J Clin Psychiatry* (1986) 47, 40–1.
37. Gander GA. In 'Antidepressant Drugs' Proc 1st Int Symp Milan (1966). Int Congr Ser No 122, p 336. Excerpta Medica.
38. Sargant W. Safety of combined antidepressant drugs. *BMJ* (1971) 1, 555–6.
39. Stockley IH. Tricyclic antidepressants. Part 1. Interaction with drugs affecting adrenergic neurones. In 'Drug Interactions and Their Mechanisms' p 14. (1974) Pharmaceutical Press, London. (1974) Pharmaceutical Press, London. (1974)
40. White K, Pistole T, Boyd JL. Combined monoamine oxidase inhibitor-tricyclic antidepressant treatment: a pilot study. *Am J Psychiatry* (1980) 137, 1422–5.
41. Berlanga C. Ortego-Soto HA. A 3-year follow-up of a group of treatment-resistant depressed patients with a MAOI/tricyclic combination. *J Affect Disord* (1995) 34, 187–92.
42. Kahn D, Silver JM, Opler LA. The safety of switching rapidly from tricyclic antidepressants to monoamine oxidase inhibitors. *J Clin Psychopharmacol* (1989) 9, 198–202.
43. Beaumont G. Personal communication (1978).
44. Schildkraut JJ, Klein DF. The classification and treatment of depressive disorders. In 'Manual of Psychiatric Therapeutics' p 61. Shader RI (ed). (1975). Little, Brown, Boston, Mass. (1975).

Monoamine oxidase inhibitors (MAOIs) + Tryptophan (L-tryptophan)

Although the concurrent use of monoamine oxidase inhibitors and tryptophan can be both safe and effective, a number of patients have developed both severe behavioural and neu-

rological signs of toxicity, and one patient died. Tryptophan has been withdrawn in some countries because of possible toxicity.

Clinical evidence

A man on **phenelzine** (90 mg daily) developed behavioural and neurological toxicity within 2 h of being given 6 g **tryptophan**.[1] He showed shivering and diaphoresis, his psychomotor retardation disappeared and he became jocular, fearful and moderately labile. His neurological signs included bilateral Babinski signs, hyperreflexia, rapid horizontal ocular oscillations, shivering of the jaw, trunk and limbs, mild dysmetria and ataxia. The situation resolved on withdrawal of the drugs.[1]

Other reports describe patients who showed severe[2] or milder[3-5] symptoms of toxicity, hypomania[6] or delirium[7] when given **pheniprazine, isocarboxazid, pargyline** or **phenelzine** with **tryptophan**. Symptoms included alcohol-like intoxication, drowsiness, delirium, myoclonus, muscle twitching, hyperreflexia, jaw quivering, teeth chattering, diaphoresis and ocular oscillations have been seen.[5,8-11] One patient showed toxicity with transient hyperthermia when the dose of **tryptophan** was increased.[12] Fatal malignant hyperpyrexia occurred in another patient on **phenelzine, tryptophan** and lithium.[13]

In contrast, concurrent use is reported elsewhere to be both safe and effective,[14] however see the note below.

Mechanism

Not understood. The reactions appears to be related to the 'serotonin syndrome' which can occur with 5-HT uptake inhibitors.

Importance and management

Information seems to be confined to the reports listed. Concurrent use can be effective in the treatment of depression,[14] but occasionally and unpredictably severe and even life-threatening toxicity occurs. The authors of the report detailed above[1] recommend that patients on MAOI should be started on a low dose of tryptophan (0.5 g). This should be gradually increased while monitoring the mental status of the patient for mental changes suggesting hypomania, and neurological changes including ocular oscillations and upper motor neurone signs. Products containing tryptophan for the treatment of depression were withdrawn in the USA, UK, and many other countries because of a possible association with the development of an eosinophilia-myalgia syndrome. However, since the syndrome appeared to have been associated with tryptophan from one manufacturer, tryptophan preparations were reintroduced in the UK in 1994 for restricted use.[15]

1. Thompson JN, Rubin EH. Case report of a toxic reaction from a combination of tryptophan and phenelzine. *Am J Psychiatry* (1984) 141, 281–3.
2. Mueller PD. Life-threatening interaction between phenelzine and L-tryptophan. *Vet Hum Toxicol* (1989) 31, 370.
3. Glassman AH, Platman SR. Potentiation of monoamine oxidase inhibitor by tryptophan. *J Psychiatr Res* (1969) 7, 83–8.
4. Pare CMB. Potentiation of monoamine-oxidase inhibitors by tryptophan. *Lancet* (1963) 2, 527–8.
5. Baloh RW, Dietz J, Spooner JW. Myoclonus and ocular oscillations induced by L-tryptophan. *Ann Neurol* (1982) 11, 95–7.
6. Goff DC. Two cases of hypomania following the addition of L-tryptophan to a monoamine oxidase inhibitor. *Am J Psychiatry* (1985) 142, 1487–8.
7. Alvine G, Black DW, Tsuang D. Case of delirium secondary to phenelzine/L-tryptophan combination. *J Clin Psychiatry* (1990) 51, 311.
8. Hodge JV, Oates JA, Sjoerdsma A. Reduction of the central effects of tryptophan by a decarboxylase inhibitor. *Clin Pharmacol Ther* (1964) 5, 149–55.
9. Pope HG, Jonas JM, Hudson JI, Kafka MP. Toxic reactions to the combination of monoamine oxidase inhibitors and tryptophan. *Am J Psychiatry* (1985) 142, 491–2.
10. Levy AB, Bucher P, Votolato N. Myoclonus, hyperreflexia and diaphoresis in patients on phenelzine-tryptophan combination treatment. *Can J Psychiatry* (1985) 30, 434–6.
11. Oates JA, Sjoerdsma A. Neurological effects of tryptophan in patients receiving a monoamine oxidase inhibitor. *Neurology* (1960) 10, 1076–8.
12. Price WA, Zimmer B, Kucas P. Serotonin syndrome: a case report. *J Clin Pharmacol* (1986) 26, 77–8.
13. Staufenberg EF, Tantam D. Malignant hyperpyrexia syndrome in combined treatment. *Br J Psychiatry* (1989) 154, 577–8.
14. Klein DF, Gittelman R, Quitkin F, Rifkin A. Diagnosis and drug treatment of psychiatric disorders: adults and children. Edition 2. Williams and Wilkins Co. (1980) 358.
15. Sweetman SC, editor. Martindale: The complete drug reference. 33rd ed. London: Pharmaceutical Press; 2002. p.311.

Monoamine oxidase inhibitors (MAOIs) + Tyramine-rich drinks

Patients taking the older MAOI (tranylcypromine, phenelzine, nialamide, pargyline, etc.) can suffer a serious hypertensive reaction if they drink some tyramine-rich drinks (some beers, lagers or wines), but no serious interaction is likely with the newer reversible and selective MAOIs (moclobemide, etc.). The hypotensive side-effects of the MAOIs may be exaggerated in a few patients by alcohol and they may experience dizziness and faintness after drinking relatively modest amounts.

Clinical evidence, mechanism, importance and management

(a) Hypertensive reactions

A severe and potentially life-threatening hypertensive reaction can occur in patients on MAOIs if they take alcoholic drinks containing significant amounts of tyramine. The details of this reaction, its mechanism, the names of the older MAOIs which interact and the newer reversible and selective MAOIs which are unlikely to do so (see Table 18.1) are described in the monograph 'Monoamine oxidase inhibitors (MAOIs) + Tyramine-rich foods', p.685. This monograph also explains what to do if a hypertensive crisis develops. A dose of 10–25 mg tyramine is believed to be required before a serious rise in blood pressure takes place. Table 18.2 summarises the reported[1-7] tyramine-content of some drinks. It can be used as broad general guide when advising patients, but it cannot be an absolute guide because all alcoholic drinks are the end-product of a biological fermentation process and no two batches are ever absolutely identical. For example there may be a 50-fold difference even between wines from the same grape stock.[5] There is no way of knowing for certain the tyramine-content of a particular drink without a detailed analysis.

(i) Ales, Beers and Lagers.
Some ales, beers and lagers in 'social' amounts contain enough tyramine to reach the 10–25 mg threshold dosage (see Table 18.2), for example a litre (a little under two pints) of some samples of Canadian ale or beer. A man on phenelzine developed a typical hypertensive reaction after drinking only 15 oz. (a little less than 0.5 L) of Upper Canada lager beer on tap (containing about 45 mg tyramine/l).[8] Alcohol-free beer and lager may have a tyramine-content which is equal to ordinary beer and lager.[9,10] One patient on tranylcypromine suffered an acute cerebral haemorrhage after drinking a de-alcoholised Irish beer,[5] and hypertensive reactions occurred in four other patients after drinking no more than 375 ml (⅔ pint) of alcohol-free beer or lager.[10,11] A very extensive study of 79 different brands of beer (from Canada, England, France, Holland, Ireland, Scotland, USA) found that the tyramine content of the bottled and canned beers examined was generally too low to matter (<10 mg/l), but four beers (all identified as being on tap) contained more than enough tyramine (26–112 mg/l) to cause a hypertensive reaction.[8] It was concluded in this report that the consumption of canned or bottled beer, including de-alcoholised beer, in moderation (fewer than four bottles, 1.5 L in a four-hour period) was safe, but ales, beers and lagers on tap should be avoided.[8] However the safety of all de-alcoholised beers is clearly still uncertain.

(ii) Spirits.
Gin, whiskey, vodka and other spirits do not contain significant amounts of tyramine because they are distilled and the volumes drunk are relatively small.[7] There seem to be no reports of hypertensive reactions in patients taking MAOIs after drinking spirits and none would be expected.

(iii) Wines.
In the context of adverse interactions with MAOIs, Chianti has developed a sinister reputation because 400 ml of one early sample of Italian Chianti wine (see Table 18.2) contained enough tyramine to reach the 10–25 mg threshold dosage. However, it is claimed by the Chianti producers[12] and others[13] that the newer methods which have replaced the ancient 'governo alla toscana' process

result in negligible amounts of tyramine in today's Chianti. This seems to be borne out by the results of recent analyses[3,5-7] two of which failed to find any tyramine at all in some samples.[3,7] Some of the other wines listed in Table 18.2 also contain tyramine, but patients would have to drink as much as 2 L or more before reaching what is believed to be the threshold dosage. This suggests that small or moderate amounts (1–2 glasses) are unlikely to be hazardous.

(b) Hypotensive reactions

Some degree of hypotension can occur in patients on MAOIs (therapeutically exploited in the case of pargyline) and this may be exaggerated by the vasodilation and reduced cardiac output caused by alcohol. Patients should therefore be warned of the possibility of orthostatic hypotension and syncope if they drink.[14] They should be advised not to stand up too quickly, and to remain sitting or lying if they feel faint or begin to 'black out'.

(c) Other reactions

In addition to the hypertensive and hypotensive reactions described in (a) and (b), the possibility that the alcohol-induced deterioration in psychomotor skills (i.e. those associated with safe driving) might be

Table 18.2 The tyramine content of some drinks

Drink	Tyramine content (mg/L)	Ref
Ale (Canada)	8.8	1
Beer (Canada)	6.4, 11.1, 11.2	2
Beer (UK)	1.34	5
Beer (USA)	1.8, 2.3, 4.4	1
Champagne (Canada)	0.2, 0.6	2
Chianti (Italy)		
Governo process	0.0, 1.76, 12.2, 10.36, 25.4	1–3, 5
Newer process	0.0–4.7	3, 5–7
Gin	0.0	7
Port	0.2	1
Reisling	0.6	1
Sauterne	0.4	1
Sherry (USA)	3.6	1
Sherry (Canada)	0.2	2
Sherry	2.65	7
Wine (from different regions in France)	3.70–5.17	4
Wine, red (Canada, France, Italy, Spain, USA)	3.51–8.64 (mean 5.18)	2, 4
Wine, red (unstated origin)	1.36	5
Wine, white (Germany, Italy, Portugal, Spain)	1.26–5.87 (mean 4.41)	2, 4
Wine, white (Germany, Former Yugoslavia)	1.22	5
Vodka	0.0	7
Whiskey	0.0	7

increased by the MAOIs has also been studied. **Moclobemide** appears to have only a minor and clinically unimportant effect[15,16] and **brofaromine**[17,18] and **befloxatone**[19] do not interact with **alcohol**.

1. Horwitz D, Lovenberg W, Engelman K, Sjoerdsma A. Monoamine oxidase inhibitors, tyramine and cheese. *JAMA* (1964) 188, 1108–10.
2. Sen NP. Analysis and significance of tyramine in foods. *J Food Sci* (1969) 34, 22–6.
3. Korn A, Eichler HG, Fischbach R, Gasic S. Moclobemide, a new reversible MAO inhibitor – interaction with tyramine and tricyclic antidepressants in healthy volunteers and depressive patients. *Psychopharmacology (Berl)* (1986) 88, 153–7.
4. Zee JA, Simard RE, L'Heureux L, Tremblay J. Biogenic amines in wines. *Am J Enol Vitic* (1983) 34, 6–9.
5. Hannah P, Glover V, Sandler M. Tyramine in wine and beer. *Lancet* (1988) i, 879.
6. Da Prada M, Zürcher G, Wüthrich I, Haefely WE. On tyramine, food, beverages and the reversible MAO inhibitor moclobemide. *J Neural Transm* (1988) (Suppl 26), 31.
7. Shulman KI, Walker SE, MacKenzie S, Knowles S. Dietary restriction, tyramine, and use of monoamine oxidase inhibitors. *J Clin Psychopharmacol* (1989) 9, 397–402.
8. Tailor SAN, Shulman KI, Walker SE, Moss J, Gardener D. Hypertensive episode associated with phenelzine and tap beer—a reanalysis of the role of pressor amines in beer. *J Clin Psychopharmacol* (1994) 14, 5–14.
9. Murray JA, Walker JF, Doyle JS. Tyramine in alcohol-free beer. *Lancet* (1988) i, 1167–8.
10. Thakore J, Dinan TG, Kelleher M. Alcohol-free beer and the irreversible monoamine oxidase inhibitors. *Int Clin Psychopharmacol* (1992) 7, 59–60.
11. Draper R, Sandler M, Walker PL. Clinical curio: monoamine oxidase inhibitors and non-alcoholic beer. *BMJ* (1984) 289, 308.
12. Anon. Statement from the Consorzio Vino Chianti Classico, London. Undated (circa 1984).
13. Kalish G. Chianti myth. The Wine Spectator, July 31st (1981).
14. Anon. MAOIs — a patient's tale. *Pulse* (1981) December 5th, p 69.
15. Berlin I, Cournot A, Zimmer R, Pedarriosse A-M, Manfredi R, Molinier P, Puech AJ. Evaluation and comparison of the interaction between alcohol and moclobemide or clomipramine in healthy subjects. *Psychopharmacology (Berl)* (1990) 100, 40–5.
16. Tiller JWG. Antidepressants, alcohol and psychomotor performance. *Acta Psychiatr Scand* (1990) (Suppl 360), 13–17.
17. Gilburt SJA, Sutton JA, Hindmarch I. The pharmacodynamics of brofaromine, alone and in combination with alcohol in young healthy volunteers. *Br J Clin Pharmacol* (1991) 33, 245P.
18. Kerr JS, Fairweather DB, Hindmarch I. The effects of brofaromine alone and in conjunction with alcohol on cognitive function, psychomotor performance, mood and sleep in healthy volunteers. *Hum Psychopharmacol* (1993) 8, 107–16.
19. Ramaekers JG, Muntjewerff ND, Uiterwijk MMC, Van Veggel LMA, Patal A, Durrieu G, O'Hanlon JF. A study of the pharmacodynamic interaction between befloxatone and ethanol on performance and mood in healthy volunteers. *J Psychopharmacol* (1996) 10, 288–94.

Monoamine oxidase inhibitors (MAOIs) + Tyramine-rich foods

A potentially life-threatening hypertensive crisis can develop in those on the older irreversible MAOIs (nialamide, pargyline, phenelzine, tranylcypromine, etc.) who eat tyramine-rich foods. Deaths from intracranial haemorrhage have occurred. Significant amounts of tyramine occur in cheese, yeast extracts (e.g. Marmite) and some types of salami. Caviar, pickled herrings, chicken and beef livers, soy sauce, avocados and other foods have been implicated in this interaction. Some of the newer selective MAOIs (brofaromine, moclobemide, selegiline, toloxatone) interact only minimally or not at all.

Clinical evidence

A rapid, serious, and potentially fatal rise in blood pressure can occur in patients on MAOI who ingest tyramine-rich foods or drinks. A violent occipital headache, pounding heart, neck stiffness, flushing, sweating, nausea and vomiting may be experienced. Two illustrative examples: the first being one of the earliest recorded observations by Rowe, a pharmacist, in a letter[1] after seeing the reaction in his wife who was taking *Parstelin* (**tranylcypromine** with trifluoperazine).

"After **cheese on toast**; within a few minutes face flushed, felt very ill; head and heart pounded most violently, and perspiration was running down her neck. She vomited several times, and her condition looked so severe that I dashed over the road to consult her GP. He diagnosed 'palpitations' and agreed to call if the symptoms had not subsided in an hour. In fact the severity diminished and after about 3 h she was normal, other than a severe headache – but 'not of the throbbing kind'. She described the early part of the attack 'as though her head must burst'."

A man on **pargyline** who, despite eating **Sweitzer cheese** uneventfully on a number of previous occasions, experienced severe subster-

Table 18.3 The tyramine content of some foods

Food	Tyramine content (µg/g)	Ref
Avocado	23, 0	15, 22
Banana pulp	7, 0	15, 22
Banana (whole)	65	15
Caviar (Iranian)	680	13
Cheese – see Table 18.4		
Country cured ham	not detectable	14
Farmer salami sausage	314	14
Genoa salami sausage	0–1237 (average 534)	14
Hard salami	0–392 (average 210)	14
Herring (pickled)	3030	16
Lebanon bologna	0–333 (average 224)	14
Liver-chicken	94–113	17
Liver-beef	0–274	18
Orange pulp	10	15
Pepperoni sausage	0–195 (average 39)	14
Plum, red	6	15
Sauerkraut	55	24
Soy sauce	0–663	23, 24
Smoked landjaeger sausage	396	14
Summer sausage	184	14
Tomato	4, 0	15, 22
Thuringer cervelat	0–162	14
Yeast extracts		
Barmene	157	4
Befit	419	4
Bovril	200–500	20
Bovril beef cubes	200–500	20
Bovril chicken cubes	50–200	20
Marmite (UK product)	500–3000	20, 22, 24
Oxo chicken cubes	130	21
Red Oxo cubes	250	21
Yeastrel	101	4
Yex	506	4
Yoghurt	0.2, 3–4	19, 22

nal chest pain and palpitations within 15 min of eating the **cheese**. His blood pressure rose to 200/114 mmHg. Two other patients experienced headache after eating **aged cheese**. One of them had a severe nose-bleed and was found to have a blood pressure of 240/140 mmHg.[2]

There are too many reports of this interaction to list them here individually, but they are reviewed extensively elsewhere.[1,3] Blackwell and his colleagues list[4] a total of 110 instances caused by tyramine-rich foods which came to their attention during the 1963–66 period. There have been many since. **Tranylcypromine, phenelzine, mebanazine** or **pargyline** have been implicated in this interaction with **cheese, yeast extracts, protein diet supplements, miso, pickled and soused herrings, tinned fish, chicken livers, caviar, soy sauce,** avocados, **peanuts**, **New Zealand prickly spinach**, **beef livers** and **Chianti wine**. Many patients recovered fully, but Blackwell lists 26 cases of intracranial haemorrhage and nine deaths.[1] Another review lists 38 cases of haemorrhage and 21 deaths.[5]

Mechanism

Tyramine is formed in foods such as cheese by the bacterial degradation of milk and other proteins, firstly to tyrosine and other amino acids, and the subsequent decarboxylation of the tyrosine to tyramine. This interaction is therefore not associated with fresh foods, but with those which have been allowed to 'mature' in some way (note that tyramine was first isolated from cheese in 1903 and is named after the Greek word for cheese: tyros).[6] Tyramine is an indirectly-acting sympathomimetic amine, one of its actions being to release norepinephrine (noradrenaline) from the adrenergic neurones associated with blood vessels which causes a rise in blood pressure by stimulating their constriction.

Normally any ingested tyramine is rapidly metabolised by the enzyme monoamine oxidase in the gut wall and liver before it escapes into general circulation. However, if the activity of the enzyme at these sites is inhibited (by the presence of an MAOI), any tyramine passes freely into circulation causing not just a rise in blood pressure, but a highly exaggerated rise due to the release from the adrenergic neurones of the large amounts of norepinephrine which accumulate there during inhibition of the MAO. This final step in the interaction is identical with that which occurs with any other indirectly-acting sympathomimetic amine in the presence of an MAOI (see 'Monoamine oxidase inhibitors (MAOIs) + Sympathomimetics', p.680). The violent headache seems to occur when the blood pressure reaches about 200 mmHg. There is also some evidence that other amines such as tryptamine and phenylethylamine may play a part in this interaction.

Importance and management

An extremely well-documented, well-established, serious and potentially fatal hypertensive reaction can occur between the older, irreversible, non-selective MAOIs (see Table 18.1) and tyramine-rich foods. The incidence is uncertain but estimates range from 1–20%.[7,8] Patients taking these MAOIs (**isocarboxazid**, **nialamide**, **phenelzine**, **pargyline**, **tranylcypromine**, and possibly also **iproniazid**) should not eat foods reported[4,9-24] to contain substantial amounts of tyramine (see Tables 18.3, 18.4). As little as 6 mg can raise the blood pressure[9] and 10–25 mg would be expected to cause a serious hypertensive reaction.[9] Because tyramine levels vary so much it is impossible to guess the amount present in any food or drink. An old and mature cheese may contain trivial amounts of tyramine compared with one that is innocuous looking and even mild-tasting. The tyramine-content can even differ significantly within a single cheese between the centre and the rind.[25] There is no guarantee that patients who have risked eating these hazardous foodstuffs on many occasions uneventfully may not eventually experience a full-scale hypertensive crisis if all the many variables conspire together.[2]

A total prohibition should be imposed on the following: **cheese** and **yeast extracts** such as *Marmite* (tyramine content up to 3 mg/g in the UK product), possibly *Bovril* (0.5 mg/g) and **pickled herrings** (3 mg/g) (see Table 18.3). Hypertensive reactions have been seen with **avocados**,[6] **beef livers**[18] and **chicken livers**,[17] **caviar**,[13] **pickled herrings**,[16] **soused herrings**,[26] **peanuts**,[26] **soy sauce**,[27] **miso**,[28] a powdered protein diet supplement (*Ever-so-slim*)[29] **sour cream** in coffee,[26] and **New Zealand prickly spinach** (*Tetragonia tetragonides*).[30] This is not a true spinach as found in the USA or Europe. A number of other foods should also be viewed with suspicion such as **sauerkraut**, **fermented bolognas** and **salamis**, **pepperoni** and **summer sausage** because some of them may contain significant amounts of tyramine (see Table 18.3). However the following are often viewed with unjustifiable suspicion: **yoghurt**, **fresh cream** and possibly **chocolate**. It also seems very doubtful if either **cream cheese** or **cottage cheese** represent a hazard. **Whole green bananas** contain up to 65 mg/g, but the **pulp** contains relatively small amounts. The need to plan a sensible and safe diet for those on MAOIs is clear. Some, but

Table 18.4 The tyramine content of some cheeses. This table should not be used to predict the probable tyramine content of a cheese. It is only intended to show the extent and the variation which can occur

Variety of cheese	Tyramine content (µg/g)	Ref
American processed	50	9
Argenti	188	11
Blue	49, 203, 266, 997	10, 11, 24
Boursault	10	
Brick	194	11
Brie	21, 180	9, 24
Brie type (Danish)	0	10
Cambozola blue vein	18	24
Camembert	86, 125	9, 11
Cheddar		
Australian	226	4
Canadian	120, 136, 192, 251, 535, 1000, 530	4, 10
English	0, 72, 182, 281, 332, 480, 953	4
Farmhouse	284	4
Kraft	214	4
New York State	1416	4
New Zealand	416, 580	4
Cream cheese	< 0.2, 9	9, 24
Cottage cheese	< 0.2	9
Danish Blue (Gorgonzola type)	31, 93, 256, 369, 294	10, 24
d'Oka	100, 310	11
Edam	100, 214	11
Emmental	24, 225	11, 24
Gorgonzola	56	24
Gouda	54, 95	11
Gouda type (Canadian)	20	10
Gourmandise	216	10
Gruyere	64 (mean of seven samples), 125, 514	12, 24
Kashar	44 (mean of seven samples)	12
Liederkrantz	1226, 1683	11
Limburger	204	11
Mozzarella	158, 410	10, 24
Munster	101, 110	11, 24
Mycelia	1340	11
Parmesan	15, 65	10, 24
Parmesan type (USA)	4, 5, 290	10
Provolone	38	10
Romano	197, 238	10, 11
Roquefort	27, 48, 520, 267	10, 11
Stilton	466, 1156, 2170	10, 24
Swiss	50, 434	11
Tulum	208 (mean of eight samples)	12
White (Turkish)	17.5	12

not all, patients may be partially protected from the cheese reaction if they are also taking a tricyclic antidepressant.[31]

It is usual to recommend avoidance of the prohibited foods for 2–3 weeks after withdrawal of the MAOI to allow full recovery of the enzymes. If a hypertensive reaction occurs it can be controlled with an alpha-blocker such as **phentolamine** (5 mg intravenously) or **phenoxybenzamine**, or failing that an intramuscular injection of 50 mg **chlorpromazine**. An intravenous infusion of 20 mg **labetalol** given over 5 min has also proved to be successful.[27] The simplest alternative is to chew a 10 mg **nifedipine** capsule to release its contents, and wash it down with a drink of water.[28,32-34]

The newer MAOIs are safer (in the context of interactions with tyramine-rich foods and drinks) than the old ones because they are reversible and selective. Thus **brofaromine**, **moclobemide** and **toloxatone** selectively inhibit MAO-A which leaves MAO-B still available to metabolize tyramine. This means that with **moclobemide** for example, tyramine only causes a modest rise in blood pressure if food is present,[35-38] so that the risk of a serious hypertensive reaction with **moclobemide**,[39-42] or any of the others in this group (**brofaromine**[43-45] and **toloxatone**[46,47]) is very much reduced. It has been calculated that while taking **moclobemide** up to 65 mg tyramine can be ingested before the capacity of the MAO to metabolize it becomes saturated.[48] Most patients therefore do not need to follow the special dietary restrictions required with the older irreversible MAO-Is, but to be on the safe side the makers of **moclobemide** (Roche) advise all patients to avoid large amounts of tyramine-rich foods because a few individuals may be particularly sensitive to tyramine. This warning would also seem appropriate for all of the other MAO-A inhibitors.

Selegiline specifically inhibits MAO-B, which leaves MAO-A still available to metabolise any tyramine. 10 mg **selegiline** daily interacts only minimally with tyramine[49] so that the makers (Britannia) say that no dietary restrictions are therefore necessary with this dosage. However higher doses (30 mg daily) have been shown to increase the sensitivity to tyramine two to fourfold,[50] and a patient on only 20 mg daily is reported to have had a hypertensive reaction after eating macaroni and **cheese**.[51] A tyramine-free diet with larger **selegiline** dosages has therefore been advised.[50]

1. Blackwell B, Marley E, Price J, Taylor D. Hypertensive interactions between monoamine oxidase inhibitors and foodstuffs. *Br J Psychiatry* (1967) 113, 349.
2. Hutchison JC. Toxic effects of monoamine oxidase inhibitors. *Lancet* (1964) ii, 151.
3. Stockley IH. Drug Interactions and their Mechanisms. Pharmaceutical Press, London (1974) p. 5.
4. Blackwell B, Marley E. Hypertensive interactions between MAOI and foodstuffs. In Neuropsychopharmacology. Proc 5th Int Congr Coll Int Neuro-psycho-pharmacologium. Brill H, Cole JO, Deniker P, Hippius H, Bradley PB (Eds). Int Congr Series no 129, Washington, March 1966. Excerpta Medica Foundation (1967).
5. Sadusk JF. The physician and the Food and Drug Administration. *JAMA* (1964) 190, 907.
6. Generali JA, Hogan LC, McFarlane M, Schwab S, Hartman CR. Hypertensive crisis resulting from avocados and a MAO inhibitor. *Drug Intell Clin Pharm* (1981) 15, 904–6.
7. Anon. Hypertensive reactions to monoamine oxidase inhibitors. *BMJ* (1964) i, 578.
8. Cooper AJ, Magnus RV, Rose MJ. A hypertensive syndrome with tranylcypromine medication. *Lancet* (1964) i, 527–9.
9. Horwitz D, Lovenberg W, Engelman K, Sjoerdsma A. Monoamine oxidase inhibitors, tyramine and cheese. *JAMA* (1964) 188, 1108.
10. Sen NP. Analysis and significance of tyramine in foods. *J Food Sci* (1969) 34, 127.
11. Kosikowsky FV, Dahlberg AC. The tyramine content of cheese. *J Dairy Sci* (1948) 31, 293–303.
12. Kayaalp SO, Renda N, Kaymakcalan S, Özer A. Tyramine content of some cheeses. *Toxicol Appl Pharmacol* (1970) 16, 459–60.
13. Isaac P, Mitchell B, Grahame-Smith DG. Monoamine-oxidase inhibitors and caviar. *Lancet* (1977) ii, 816.
14. Rice S, Eitenmiller RR, Koehler PE. Histamine and tyramine content of meat products. *J Milk Food Technol* (1975) 38, 256–8.
15. Udenfriend S, Lovenberg W, Sjoerdsma A. Physiologically active amines in common fruits and vegetables. *Arch Biochem* (1959) 85, 487.
16. Nuessle WF, Norman FC, Miller HE. Pickled herring and tranylcypromine reaction. *JAMA* (1965) 192, 726.
17. Heberg DL, Gordon MW, Glueck BC. Six cases of hypertensive crisis in patients on tranylcypromine after eating chicken livers. *Am J Psychiatry* (1966) 122, 933–5.
18. Boulton AA, Cookson B, Paulton R. Hypertensive crisis in a patient on MAOI antidepressants following a meal of beef liver. *Can Med Assoc J* (1970) 102, 1394–5.
19. van Slyke LL. Conditions affecting the proportions of fat and proteins in cows milk. *Am Chem J* (1908) 30, 8.
20. Clarke A. (Bovril Ltd). Personal communication (1987).
21. Oxo Ltd. Personal communication (1987).
22. Da Prada M, Zurcher G, Wuthrich I, Haefely WE. On tyramine, food, beverages and the reversible MAO inhibitor moclobemide. *J Neural Transm* (1988) (Suppl 26), 31–56.
23. Lee S, Wing YK. MAOI and monosodium glutamate interaction. *J Clin Psychiatry* (1991) 52, 43.
24. Shulman KI, Walker SE, MacKenzine S, Knowles S. Dietary restriction, tyramine, and the use of monoamine oxidase inhibitors. *J Clin Psychopharmacol* (1989) 9, 397–402.
25. Price K, Smith SE. Cheese reaction and tyramine. *Lancet* (1971) i, 130–1.
26. Kelly D, Guirguis W, Frommer E, Mitchell-Heggs N, Sargant W. Treatment of phobic states with antidepressants. A retrospective study of 246 patients. *Br J Psychiatry* (1970) 116, 387–98.
27. Abrams JH, Schulman P, White WB. Successful treatment of a monoamine oxidase inhibitor-tyramine hypertensive emergency with intravenous labetalol. *N Engl J Med* (1985) 313, 52.
28. Mesmer RE. Don't mix miso with MAOIs. *JAMA* (1987) 258, 3515.
29. Zetin M, Plon L, DeAntonio M. MAOI reaction with powdered protein dietary supplement. *J Clin Psychiatry* (1987) 48, 499.
30. Comfort A. Hypertensive reaction to New Zealand prickly spinach in a woman taking phenelzine. *Lancet* (1981) ii, 472.
31. Pare CMB, Al Mousavi M, Sandler M, Glover V. Attempts to attenuate the 'cheese effect.' Combined drug therapy in depressive illness. *J Affect Disord* (1985) 9, 137–41.
32. Clary C, Schweitzer E. Treatment of MAOI hypertensive crisis with sublingual nifedipine. *J Clin Psychiatry* (1987) 48, 249–50.
33. Fier M. Safer use of MAOIs. *J Psychiatry* (1991) 148, 391–2.
34. Van Harten J, Burggraaf K, Danhof M, Van Brummelen P, Breimer DD. Negligible sublingual absorption of nifedipine. *Lancet* (1987) 2, 1363–4.
35. Korn A, Eichler HG, Fischbach R, Gasic S. Moclobemide, a new reversible MAO inhibitor – interaction with tyramine and tricyclic antidepressants in healthy volunteers and depressive patients. *Psychopharmacology (Berl)* (1986) 88, 153–7.
36. Korn A, Da Prada M, Raffesberg W, Gasic S, Eichler HG. Tyramine absorption and pressure response after MAO-inhibition with moclobemide. The Second Amine Oxidase Workshop, Uppsala, August 1986. *Pharmacol Toxicol* (1987) 60, 30.
37. Burgess CD, Mellsop GW. Interaction between moclobemide and oral tyramine in depressed patients. *Fundam Clin Pharmacol* (1989) 3, 47–52.
38. Audebert C, Blin O, Monjanel-Mouterde S, Auquier P, Pedarriosse AM, Dingemanse J, Durand A, Cano JP. Influence of food on the tyramine pressor effect during chronic moclobemide treatment of healthy volunteers. *Eur J Clin Pharmacol* (1992) 43, 507–12.
39. Berlin I, Zimmer R, Cournot A, Payan C, Pedarriosse AM, Puech AJ. Determination and comparison of the pressor effect of tyramine during long-term moclobemide and tranylcypromine treatment in healthy volunteers. *Clin Pharmacol Ther* (1989) 46, 344–51.
40. Da Prada M, Zürcher G. Tyramine content of preserved and fermented foods or condiments of Far Eastern cuisine. *Psychopharmacology (Berl)* (1992) 106, S32–S34.
41. Simpson GM, Gratz SS. Comparison of the pressor effect of tyramine after treatment with phenelzine and moclobemide in healthy male volunteers. *Clin Pharmacol Ther* (1992) 52, 286–91.
42. Warrington SJ, Turner P, Mant TGK, Morrison P, Haywood G, Glover V, Goodwin BL, Sandler M, St John-Smith P, McClelland GR. Clinical pharmacology of moclobemide, a new reversible monoamine oxidase inhibitor. *J Psychopharmacol* (1991) 5, 82–91.
43. Bieck PR, Firkusny L, Schick C, Antonin K-H, Nilsson E, Schulz R, Schwenk M, Wollman H. Monoamine oxidase inhibition by phenelzine and brofaromine in healthy volunteers. *Clin Pharmacol Ther* (1989) 45, 260–9.
44. Bieck PR, Antonin KH. Tyramine potentiation during treatment with MAO inhibitors: brofaromine and moclobemide vs irreversible inhibitors. *J Neural Transm* (1989) (Suppl 28), 21–31.
45. Bieck PR, Antonin K-H, Schmidt E. Clinical pharmacology of reversible monoamine oxidase-A inhibitors. *Clin Neuropharmacol* (1993) 16 (Suppl 2), S33–S41.
46. Dollery CT, Brown MJ, Davies DS, Strolin Benedetti M. Pressor amines and monoamine oxidase inhibitors. In Monoamine Oxidase and Disease. Proc Conf Paris, Oct 1983. Tipton KF, Dostert P and Strolin Benedetti M. (Eds) Academic Press (1984) p. 429–41.
47. Provost J-C, Funck-Brentano C, Rovei V, D'Estanque J, Ego D, Jaillon P. Pharmacokinetic and pharmacodynamic interaction between toloxatone, a new reversible monoamine oxidase-A inhibitor, and oral tyramine in healthy subjects. *Clin Pharmacol Ther* (1992) 52, 384–9.
48. Karet FE, Dickerson JEC, Brown J, Brown MJ. Bovril and moclobemide: a novel therapeutic strategy for central autonomic failure. *Lancet* (1944) 344, 1263–5.
49. Elsworth JD, Glover V, Reynolds GP, Sandler M, Lees AJ, Phuapradit P, Shaw KM, Stern GM, Kumar P. Deprenyl administration in man: a selective monoamine oxidase B inhibitor without the 'cheese effect'. *Psychopharmacology (Berl)* (1978) 57, 33–8.
50. Prasad A, Glover V, Goodwin BL, Sandler M, Signy M, Smith SE. Enhanced pressor sensitivity to oral tyramine challenge following high dose selegiline treatment. *Psychopharmacology (Berl)* (1988) 95, 540–3.
51. McGrath PJ, Stewart JW, Quitkin FM. A possible L-deprenyl induced hypertensive reaction. *J Clin Psychopharmacol* (1989) 9, 310–11.

Selegiline + Maprotiline + Ephedrine

A single case report describes a severe hypertensive crisis in a man on selegiline and maprotiline when the dosage of ephedrine he was taking was raised.

Clinical evidence

A man with Parkinsonism, depression and chronic bronchitis was treated long-term with daily doses of 10 mg **selegiline**, 300 mg levodopa/30 mg carbidopa, 0.5 mg lisuride and 75 mg **maprotiline**, and since 1990 with 180 mg theophylline plus 32 mg **ephedrine**. A few months after the latter two drugs were started he was diagnosed as having hypertension and this was controlled with 100 mg **nicardipine** daily. Within two days of raising the dosage of the theophylline to 270 mg daily, and of the **ephedrine** to 48 mg daily, he was hospitalised with hypertensive crises (blood pressures up to 300/150 mmHg), intense vasoconstriction, confusion, abdominal pain, sweating, and tachycardia (110 bpm). His plasma norepinephrine (noradrenaline) levels were found to be dramatically increased. The problem was solved by stopping all of the drugs and treating with intravenous nicardipine. The patient recovered uneventfully.[1]

Mechanism

This 'pseudo-phaeochromocytoma' appears to have been due to a selegiline/maprotiline/ephedrine interaction. The suggested mechanism is that ephedrine caused some vasoconstriction by releasing norepinephrine (noradrenaline) from sympathetic nerve endings, and by its direct actions on the receptors. Maprotiline prevents the re-uptake of norepinephrine so that the effects of the norepinephrine were possibly increased and prolonged. Selegiline (an MAO-B inhibitor) possibly added to this by reducing the metabolism of the norepinephrine. Thus, apparently working in concert, the levels of norepinephrine rose, and its vasoconstrictor and hypertensive effects became grossly exaggerated.

Importance and management

This seems to be the first and only report of this interaction. There seem to be no reports of adverse interactions of this description with selegiline and other tricyclic antidepressants, or with other sympathomimetics, however it seems that together they may possibly have been responsible for the long term hypertension in this patient, which progressed to crisis proportions when the ephedrine dosage was raised.

The general importance of this single case is very difficult to assess, but it illustrates the potential risk with selegiline combined with maprotiline (possibly other tricyclics as well) if ephedrine is added. Until more is known it might be prudent to avoid sympathomimetics of this kind if taking this drug combination, and to advise patients to avoid OTC remedies which contain them. More study is needed.

1. Lefebvre H, Noblet C, Moore N, Wolf LM. Pseudo-phaeochromocytoma after multiple drug interactions involving the selective monoamine oxidase inhibitor selegiline. *Clin Endocrinol (Oxf)* (1995) 42, 95–99.

Selegiline + Sertraline or Paroxetine

Sertraline and paroxetine do not interact adversely with selegiline in many patients, but some patients have developed adverse reactions similar to the serotonin syndrome.

Clinical evidence, mechanism, importance and management

A retrospective study of 16 patients with Parkinson's disease on 5 to 10 mg selegiline daily (and other anti-parkinson agents such a levodopa/carbidopa, bromocriptine, amantadine, pergolide, anticholinergics) noted that the addition of 25 to 100 mg **sertraline** or 10 to 40 mg **paroxetine** daily caused no adverse effects and the patients appeared to benefit.[1] This contrasts with other reports where the addition of another SSRI (**fluoxetine**) to selegiline resulted in a variety of adverse reactions including the serotonin syndrome, hypertension, mania, ataxia and convulsions (see 'Fluoxetine + Monoamine oxidase inhibitors', p.826). The makers of selegiline say that similar problems have also occurred in other patients taking selegiline with **sertraline** or **paroxetine**, and they recommend that these drug combinations should be avoided.[2,3]

1. Toyama SC, Iacono RP. Is it safe to combine a selective serotonin reuptake inhibitor with selegiline? *Ann Pharmacother* (1994) 28, 405–6.
2. Eldepryl (selegiline), Orion Pharm UK, Datasheet, December 1996.
3. Zelapar (selegiline), Elan Pharma Ltd. Summary of product characteristics, December 1999.

Selegiline + Tricyclic antidepressants

Concurrent use can be useful and uneventful, but rarely and unpredictably the serotonin syndrome or other serious symptoms can develop. A hypertensive crisis occurred in one patient given selegiline, maprotiline and ephedrine.

Clinical evidence, mechanism, importance and management

Between 1989 and 1994 the FDA in the USA received 16 reports of adverse interactions between selegiline and **tricyclic antidepressants** some of which were attributed to the serotonin syndrome, for which reason the US labelling for selegiline suggests that concurrent use should be avoided.[1] The makers of selegiline in the UK also now issue a warning suggesting caution but not a contraindication. They very briefly describe severe CNS toxicity in one patient given selegiline and **amitriptyline** (hyperpyrexia and death), and in another given **protriptyline** (tremor, agitation, restlessness, followed by unresponsiveness and death).[2,3]

However these warnings need to be balanced by other reports indicating that these reactions are uncommon. One study based on the findings of 45 investigators treating 5,468 patients with selegiline and **antidepressants** (not specifically named but almost certainly including the **tricyclics**) found that only 11 patients (0.24%) experienced symptoms considered to represent the serotonin syndrome, and only 2 (0.04%) experienced symptoms considered to be serious.[4] Another small retrospective study[1] designed to evaluate the tolerability and efficacy of combining selegiline and **tricyclic antidepressants** (not specifically named) identified 28 patients who had had both drugs. Seventeen patients definitely and 6 possibly benefited, and the ". . . adverse effects were few, not life-threatening and may have occurred without selegiline." Another retrospective study of 25 patients given selegiline and un-named **tricyclic antidepressants** found no cases of the serotonin syndrome.[5]

There is also an isolated case report of a man on selegiline, levodopa/carbidopa, lisuride, **maprotiline**, theophylline and **ephedrine** who developed hypertensive crises (blood pressures up to 300/150 mmHg), intense vasoconstriction, confusion, abdominal pain, sweating, and tachycardia (110 bpm) within 2 days of raising the doses of theophylline and ephedrine. It is thought that this 'pseudo-phaeochromocytoma' was due to a selegiline/**maprotiline**/**ephedrine** interaction[6] (see 'Selegiline + Maprotiline + Ephedrine', p.687).

If therefore the decision is made to combine selegiline and any of the **tricyclic antidepressants**, the outcome should be well monitored but the likelihood of problems seems to be small. The serotonin syndrome is characterised by changes in mental status (confusion, agitation, altered levels of consciousness), motor function (hyperreflexia, rigidity, myoclonus) and in autonomic function (tremor, shivering, sweating).

1. Yu LJ, Zweig RM. Successful combination of selegiline and antidepressants in Parkinson's disease. *Neurology* (1996) 46 (2 Suppl), A374.
2. Eldepryl (Selegiline). Orion Pharma. Datasheet, December 1996.
3. Zelapar (selegiline), Elan Pharma Ltd. Summary of product characteristics, December 1999.
4. Richard I, Kurland R, Tanner C. Serotonin syndrome and the combined use of deprenyl and an antidepressant in Parkinson's disease. *Neurology* (1996) 46 (2 Suppl), A374.
5. Ritter JL, Alexander B. Retrospective study of selegiline-antidepressant drug interactions and a review of the literature. *Ann Clin Psychiatry* (1997) 9, 7–13.
6. Lefebvre H, Noblet C, Moore N, Wolf LM. Pseudo-phaeochromocytoma after multiple drug interactions involving the selective monoamine oxidase inhibitor selegiline. *Clin Endocrinol (Oxf)* (1995) 42, 95–99.

19

Neuroleptic, anxiolytic and hypnotic drug interactions

The anxiolytics include the benzodiazepines, hydroxyzine and other agents used to treat psychoneuroses such as anxiety and tension, and are intended to induce calm without causing drowsiness and sleep. Some of the benzodiazepines and related drugs are also used as anticonvulsants and hypnotics. Table 19.1 contains a list of the benzodiazepines that are referred to in this book.

The neuroleptics (or more broadly the antipsychotics) are represented by chlorpromazine (and other phenothiazines), butyrophenones and thioxanthenes. Their major use is in the treatment of psychoses such as schizophrenia and mania. These are listed in Table 19.2. Some of the phenothiazines are also used as antihistamines.

Most of the interactions involving antipsychotic, anxiolytic and hypnotic drugs are listed in this chapter, but there are other monographs elsewhere in this book where the interacting agent is a benzodiazepine or antipsychotic. A full listing is given in the Index.

Table 19.1 Benzodiazepines and other minor tranquillisers

Generic names	Proprietary names

Benzodiazepines

Alprazolam — Alcelam, Alnax, Alpralid, Alpratyrol, Alpraz, Alprox, Alzam, Alzolam, Anpress, Anxirid, Apox, Apo-Alpraz, Apraz, Azor, Calmax, Cassadan, Dizolam, Drimpam, Esparon, Frontal, Gerax, Kalma, Mialin, Neupax, Novo-Alprazol, Nu-Alpraz, Panix, Pazolam, Pharnax, Prazam, Ralozam, Siampraxol, Tafil, Trankimazin, Tranquinal, Unilan, Valeans, Xanagis, Xanax, Xanolam, Xanor, Xiemed, Zacetin, Zopax

Bromazepam — Akamon, Anxyrex, Brazepam, Bromalex, Bromam, Bromazanil, Bromaze, Bromazep, Bromidem, Bromoxon, Bropamil, Brozam, Brozepax, Compendium, Deptran, durazanil, Gityl, Lectopam, Lenitin, Lexatin, Lexilium, Lexomil, Lexostad, Lexotan, Lexotanil, Lucitan, neo OPT, Nervium, Neurilan, Normoc, Novazepan, Quietiline, Relaxil, Somalium, Ultramidol

Brotizolam — Bondormin, Lendorm, Lendormin, Lendormine, Lindormin, Sintonal

Chlordiazepoxide — Benpine, Epoxide, Huberplex, Kalmocaps, Klopoxid, Libritabs, Librium, Mitran, Multum, Novapam, Novo-Poxide, Omnalio, Paxium, Psicosedin, Radepur, Reliberan, Reposans, Risolid, Servium, Tensil, Tropium

Clobazam — Castilium, Frisium, Noiafren, Urbanil, Urbanol, Urbanyl

Clorazepate — Cloraxene, Diposef, Dipot, Dorken, Flulium, Gen-Xene, Medipax, Nansius, Novo-Clopate, Polizep, Sanor, Serene, Trancap, Tranclor, Trancon, Transene, Tranxal, Tranxene, Tranxilene, Tranxilium, Uni-Tranxene, Zetran

Clotiazepam — Clozan, Distensan, Rize, Rizen, Tienor, Veratran

Diazepam — Alboral, Aliseum, Aneurol, Ansilive, Ansiolin, Antenex, Anxicalm, Apozepam, Arzepam, Aspaserine B6 Tranq, Assival, AT-V, Benzopin, Betapam, Bialzepam, Calmociteno, Calmpose, Compaz, Complutine, Diaceplex, Dialar, Diapam, Diapanil, Diapine, Diaquel, Diatex, Diaz, Diazemuls, Diazep, Dienpax, Disopam, Dizan, Dizepam, Doval, Drenian, Ducene, D-Pam, Faustan, Freudal, Gewacalm, Gobanal, Hexalid, Kiatrium, Kratium, Lamra, Laxyl, Letansil, Medipam, Metamidol, Micronoan, Noan, Novazam, Ortopsique, Paceum, Pacium, Pax, Podium, Prizem, Propam, Psychopax, Relazepam , Rimapam, Sico Relax, Sipam, Somaplus, Stesolid, Tandial, Tensium, Tranquase, Tranquirit, Umbrium, Unisedil, V Day Zepam, Valaxona, Valclair, Valenium, Valiquid, Valium, Valix, Valocordin-Diazepam, Vatran, Vincosedan, Vival, Vivol, Zeprat, Zopam

Ketazolam — Anseren, Marcen, Sedotime, Solatran, Unakalm

Loprazolam — Dormonoct, Havlane, Somnovit, Sonin

Lorazepam — Ansilor, Anta, Anxira, Ativan, Calmogenol, Control, Donix, Duralozam, Equitam, Idalprem, Laubeel, Lora, Lorabenz, Loramed, Lorans, Lorapam, Lorasifar, Lorax, Lorazene, Lorazep, Lorenin, Loridem, Lorivan, Lorsedal, Lorzem, Max-Pax, Merlit, Mesmerin, Novo-Lorazem, Nu-Loraz, Ora, Orfidal, Placinoral, Punktyl, Sedazin, Sedicepan, Serenase, Sinestron, Somagerol, Tavor, Temesta, Tolid, Tranqipam, Vigiten

Medazepam — Rudotel

Oxazepam — Adumbran, Alepam, Alopam, Anxiolit, Azutranquil, Benzotran, durazepam, Limbial, Mirfudorm, Murelax, Noctazepam, Noripam, Opamox, Oxa, Oxabenz, Oxahexal, Oxaline, Oxamin, Oxapam, Oxapax, Oxascand, Oxepam, Ox-Pam, Praxiten, Purata, Serax, Serenal, Serepax, Seresta, Serpax, Sigacalm, Sobril, Tranquo, Uskan, Vaben

Oxazolam — Serebon

Other drugs

Alpidem —

Buspirone — Ansitec, Ansiten, Anxiolan, Axoren, Barpil, Bespar, Biron, Busansil, Buscalma, Busp, Buspanil, Buspar, Buspimen, Buspirex, Buspirol, Bustab, Effiplen, Itagil, Narol, Pasrin, Sorbon, Stesiron

Hydroxyzine — Abacus, AH 3 N, Antizine, Atano, Atarax, Aterax, Cerax, Drazine, Elroquil N, Hadarax, Histan, Hixizine, Hizin, Honsa, Hydroxin, Masarax, Med-Xyzarax, Navicalm, Otarex, Phymorax, Prurizin, Serecid, Taraxin, Trandrozine, Ucerax, Vistaril, Vistazine, Zinalerg

Zolpidem — Ambien, Bikalm, Cedrol, Cymerion, Dalparan, Ivadal, Lioram, Niotal, Nottem, Stella, Stilnoct, Stilnox

Zopiclone — Alchera, Datolan, espa-dorm, Imoclone, Imovane, Imozop, Limovan, Neurolil, Noctirex, Nocturno, Optidorm, Rhovane, Siaten, Somnal, Somnosan, Ximovan, Zilese, Zileze, Zimoclone, Zimovane, Zopimed, Zopinox, Zopitan, Zorclone, Zo-Tab

Zotepine — Lodopin, Nipolept, Zoleptil

Other benzodiazepines such as flunitrazepam (Absint, Darkene, Flunimerck, Fluninoc, Flunipam, Fluscand, Fluserin, Guttanotte, Hypnodorm, Hypnor, Narcozep, Rohipnol, Rohypnol, Roipnol, Ronal, Somnubene, Valsera), flurazepam (Dalmadorm, Dalmane, Dormodor, Felison, Flunox, Morfex, Remdue, Somnol, Staurodorm, Staurodorm Neu, Valdorm), lormetazepam (Aldosomnil, Ergocalm, Loramet, Loretam, Minias, Noctamid, Noctamide, Octonox, Pronoctan, Stilaze), midazolam (Dormicum, Dormire, Dormium, Dormonid, Hypnovel, Ipnovel, Midolam, Versed, Zolidan), nitrazepam (Alodorm, Apodorm, Arem, Dima, Dormalon, Dormo-Puren, Dumolid, Eatan N, Imeson, Insoma, Insomin, Mogadan, Mogadon, Nitrados, Nitrapan, Nitrazadon, Nitrazepol, Novanox, Numbon, Ormodon, Pacisyn, Paxadorm, Radedorm, Remnos, Serenade, Somnipar, Somnite, Sonebon), temazepam (Euhypnos, Euipnos, Levanxol, Nocturne, Norkotral Tema, Normison, Nortem, Planum, Pronervon T, Remestan, Restoril, Somapam, Temaze, temazep, Temtabs, Tenox) and triazolam (Apo-Triazo, Halcion, Hypam, Rilamir, Somese, Songar, Trilam, Trycam) may be used as sedatives and hypnotics, whereas clonazepam (Antelepsin, Clonapam, Clonex, Iktorivil, Kenoket, Klonopin, Kriadex, Paxam, Rivatril, Rivotril) and diazepam have application as anticonvulsants.

Table 19.2 Phenothiazine, butyrophenone, thioxanthene and related neuroleptics

Generic names	Proprietary names
Phenothiazines	
Butaperazine	
Chlorpromazine	Amplictil, Chloractil, Chlorazin, Chlorpromanyl, Chlorpromed, Clonazine, Hibernal, Klorproman, Largactil, Largatrex, Longactil, Matcine, Propaphenin, Prozin, Prozine, Taroctyl, Thorazine
Fluphenazine	Anatensol, Cenilene, Dapotum, Deca, Fludecate, Flufenan, Fluzine, Lyogen, Lyorodin, Modecate, Moditen, Moditen Depot, Omca, Pacinol, Permitil, Phenazin, Phenazine, Potensone, Prolixin, Sediten, Selecten, Sevinol, Siqualone
Levomepromazine (Methotrimeprazine)	Levium, Levocina, Levoprome, Levozin, Levozine, Methozane, Neozine, Neurocil, Novo-Meprazine, Nozinan, Sinogan
Mesoridazine	Serentil
Perphenazine	Conazine, Decentan, Fentazin, Leptopsique, Peratsin, Pernamed, Pernazine, Perphenan, Perzine, Porazine, Trilafon, Trilifan
Prochlorperazine	Antinaus, Buccastem, Compazine, Compro, Dhaperazine, Mitil, Nu-Prochlor, Proclozine, Proziere, Scripto-Metic, Stella, Stemetil, Stemzine
Promazine	Prazine, Protactyl, Prozine, Sinophenin, Sparine, Talofen
Thioridazine	Aldazine, Calmaril, Dazine, Mallorol, Meleril, Mellaril, Mellerette, Melleretten, Mellerettes, Melleril, Melzine, Orsanil, Ridazin, Ridazine, Rideril, Thiomed, Thiosia, Thiozine
Trifluoperazine	Eskazine, Flupazine, Modalina, Psyrazine, Stelazine, Terfluzine, Triflumed, Triplex
Butyrophenones	
Benperidol	Anquil, Benquil, Frenactil, Glianimon
Droperidol	Dehidrobenzperidol, Dehydrobenzperidol, Droleptan, Inapsine, Paxical, Sintodian
Haloperidol	Bioperidolo, Buteridol, Cereen, Dozic, Haldol, Halomed, Haloneural, Haloper, Haloperil, Halopol, Halo-P, Haricon, Haridol, H-Tab, Novo-Peridol, Pericate, Perida, Peridol, Peridor, Polyhadol, Senorm, Serenace, Serenase, Serenelfi, Sigaperidol, Tensidol
Thioxanthenes	
Chlorprothixene	Cloxan, Truquil, Truxal, Truxaletten
Flupenthixol	Depixol, Fluanxol
Tiothixene	Navane, Thixit
Other drugs	
Clozapine	Clopine, Clopsine, Clozaril, Elcrit, Froidir, Lanolept, Leponex, Zolapin
Loxapine	Desconex, Loxapac, Loxitane
Molindone	Moban
Olanzapine	Zyprexa
Quetiapine	Seroquel
Sulpiride	Aiglonyl, Arminol, Championyl, Depex, Desisulpid, Digton, Dobren, Dogmatil, Dolmatil, Eglonyl, Ekilid, Equilid, Espiride, Guastil, Intrasil, Lebopride, Lisopride, Meresa, Modal, Neogama, Pontiride, Psicocen, Rimastine, Sulp, Sulpiren, Sulpitil, Sulpivert, Sulpor, Sulpril, Suprium, Synedil, Tepavil

Ademetionine + Clomipramine

A severe reaction, diagnosed as the serotonin syndrome, developed in a woman on ademetionine (S-adenosylmethionine) shortly after her clomipramine dosage was raised.

Clinical evidence, mechanism, importance and management

An elderly woman with a major affective disorder was treated with 100 mg ademetionine (S-adenosylmethionine) daily, given intramuscularly, and 25 mg **clomipramine** daily for 10 days. About 2 to 3 days after the **clomipramine** dosage was raised to 75 mg daily, she became progressively agitated, anxious and confused. On admittance to hospital she was stuporous, with a pulse rate of 130, a breathing rate of 30 per minute, and she had diarrhoea, myoclonus, generalised tremors, rigidity, hyper-reflexia, shivering, profound diaphoresis and dehydration. Her temperature rose from 40.5 to 43°C. She had no infection, and the diagnosis was of serotonin syndrome. The drugs were withdrawn and she was given dantrolene 50 mg intravenously every 6 hours for 48 h. She made a complete recovery.[1] The reason for this severe adverse reaction is not understood.

Direct information is limited to this single case report, but clearly these two drugs should only be given together with great caution.

1. Iruela LM, Minguez L, Merino J, Monedero G. Toxic interaction of S-adenosylmethionine and clomipramine. *Am J Psychiatry* (1993) 150, 522.

Antipsychotics + Anticholinergics

These drugs are very often given together advantageously and uneventfully, but occasionally serious and even life-threatening interactions occur. These include heat-stroke in hot and humid conditions, severe constipation and adynamic ileus, and atropine-like psychoses. Anticholinergics used to counteract the extrapyramidal side-effects of antipsychotics (e.g. chlorpromazine, haloperidol, etc.) may also reduce or abolish their therapeutic effects. See also 'Phenothiazines + Tricyclic antidepressants', p.730, 'Phenothiazines + Biperiden or Orphenadrine', p.728 and 'Anticholinergics + Anticholinergics', p.414.

Clinical evidence

Concurrent use of antipsychotics and anticholinergics can result in a generalised, low grade, but not serious additive increase in the anticholinergic effects of these drugs (blurred vision, dry mouth, constipation, difficulty in urination). However sometimes serious intensification takes place. For the sake of clarity these have been subdivided here into (A) heat stroke, (B) constipation and adynamic ileus, (C) atropine-like psychoses and (D) antagonism of antipsychotic effects.

A. Heat stroke in hot and humid conditions

Three patients were admitted to hospital in Philadelphia for drug-induced hyperpyrexia during a hot and humid period. In each case their skin and mucous membranes were dry and the pulse fast (120 bpm). The first was taking daily doses of 500 mg **chlorpromazine**, 200 mg **chlorprothixene** and 6 mg **benzatropine**; the second was taking 600 mg **chlorpromazine**, 12 mg **trifluoperazine** and 2 mg **benzatropine** daily; and the third was on 8 mg **haloperidol** and 2 mg **benzatropine** daily. There was no evidence of infection.[1]

There are other reports of heat stroke, some of them fatal, in patients taking **chlorpromazine** with; **benzatropine**, **benzatropine/amitriptyline**, **benzatropine/fluphenazine/trihexyphenidyl** (**benzhexol**), **trifluoperazine**, and **promazine** with **benzatropine**.[2-4] The

danger of heat-stroke in patients on **atropine** or **atropine-like compounds** was recognised in the 1920s, and the warning has been repeated many times.[5,6]

Mechanism

Anticholinergic drugs inhibit the parasympathetic nervous system which innervates the sweat glands so that when the ambient temperature rises, the major body heat-losing mechanism can be partially or wholly put out of action.[7] Phenothiazines, thioxanthenes and butyrophenones may also have some anticholinergic effects, but additionally they impair to a varying extent the hypothalamic thermoregulatory mechanisms that control the body's ability to keep a constant temperature when exposed to heat or cold. Thus, when the ambient temperature rises, the body temperature also rises. The tricyclics can similarly disrupt the temperature control. Therefore in very hot and humid conditions, when the need to reduce the temperature is great, the additive effects of these drugs can make patients become ". . . little more able to control their internal responses to heat than are reptiles . . ."[4] However, unlike poikilothermic *animals*, they are unable to sustain life once the temperature reaches a certain point.

B. Constipation and adynamic ileus

Paralytic ileus with faecal impaction has been reported in 7 patients treated with **chlorpromazine** and **imipramine** or **trihexyphenidyl**; **levomepromazine**, **imipramine** and **benzatropine**; **levomepromazine** and **trihexyphenidyl**; **thioridazine** and **imipramine** or **thioridazine** with **trihexyphenidyl**; or **trifluoperazine** and **trihexyphenidyl**. Of the 7 patients, 4 were treated successfully, but 3 patients died because recognition of the condition was too late.[8]

A number of other cases have been described involving **chlorpromazine**, and **amitriptyline**,[9] or **nortriptyline**,[10] or **trifluoperazine** with **benzatropine**;[11] and **trifluoperazine** with **benzatropine** and **methylphenidate**.[12] Of these 4 cases, 2 were fatal. Severe constipation also occurred in a woman given **thioridazine**, **biperiden** and **doxepin**.[13]

Mechanism

Anticholinergic drugs reduce peristalsis, which in the extreme can result in total gut stasis. Additive effects can occur if two or more anticholinergic drugs are taken.

C. Atropine-like psychoses

In a double-blind study of this interaction, 3 patients given a **phenothiazine** and **benzatropine mesilate** for the parkinsonian side-effects, developed an intermittent toxic confusional state (marked disturbance of short-term memory, impaired attention, disorientation, anxiety, visual and auditory hallucinations) with peripheral anticholinergic signs.[14] Similar reactions occurred in 3 elderly patients given **imipramine** or **desipramine**, with **trihexyphenidyl**.[15] and in another man given **chlorpromazine**, **benzatropine** and **doxepin**.[13]

Mechanism

These toxic psychoses resemble the CNS effects of atropine or belladonna poisoning and appear to result from the additive effects of the drugs used.

D. Antagonism of the antipsychotic effects

A study in psychiatric patients given 300 to 800 mg **chlorpromazine** daily showed that when 6 to 10 mg **trihexyphenidyl** daily was added, the plasma **chlorpromazine** concentrations fell from a range of 100 to 300 nanograms/ml to less than 30 nanograms/ml. When the **trihexyphenidyl** was withdrawn the plasma **chlorpromazine** levels rose again and clinical improvement was seen.[16,17] Other studies confirm that **trihexyphenidyl**[18,19] and **orphenadrine**[20] reduce the plasma levels and effects of **chlorpromazine**. In contrast to these reports, another found that **trihexyphenidyl** increased **chlorpromazine** levels by 41% in 20 young schizophrenics, but no clinical change was seen. The levels dropped again over the first 4 weeks of treatment.[21] Some of the beneficial actions of **haloperidol** on social avoidance behaviour are lost during concurrent treatment with **benzatropine**, but cognitive integrative function is unaffected.[22,23]

Mechanism

The mechanism is not understood. *Animal* studies suggest that the site of interaction is in the gut.[17]

Importance and management of A–D

Established and well-documented interactions. While these drugs have been widely used together with apparent advantage and without problems, prescribers should be aware that (i) an unspectacular low-grade anticholinergic toxicity can easily go undetected, particularly in the elderly because the symptoms can be so similar to the general complaints of old people; and (ii) also be aware of the serious problems that can sometimes develop, particularly if high doses are used.

(A) Warn patients to minimise outdoor exposure and/or exercise in hot and humid climates, particularly if they are taking high doses of antipsychotic/anticholinergic drugs.

(B) Be alert for severe constipation and for the development of complete gut stasis, which can be fatal.

(C) Be aware that the symptoms of central anticholinergic psychosis can be confused with the basic psychotic symptoms of the patient. Withdrawal of one or more of the drugs, or a dosage reduction and/or appropriate symptomatic treatment can be used to control these interactions.

(D) Ensure that the concurrent use of anticholinergics to control the extrapyramidal side-effects of neuroleptics is necessary[24,25] and be aware that the therapeutic effects may possibly be reduced as a result.

See also 'Phenothiazines + Tricyclic antidepressants', p.730 and 'Drugs that prolong the QT interval + Other drugs that prolong the QT interval', p.103.

1. Westlake RJ, Rastegar A. Hyperpyrexia from drug combinations. *JAMA* (1973) 225, 1250.
2. Zelman S, Guillan R. Heat stroke in phenothiazine-treated patients: a report of three fatalities. *Am J Psychiatry* (1970) 126, 1787–90.
3. Sarnquist F, Larson CP. Drug-induced heat stroke. *Anesthesiology* (1973) 39, 348–50.
4. Reimer DR, Mohan J, Nagaswami S. Heat dyscontrol syndrome in patients receiving antipsychotic, antidepressant and antiparkinson drug therapy. *J Fla Med Assoc* (1974) 61, 573–4.
5. Willcox WH. The nature, prevention, and treatment of heat hyperpyrexia: the clinical aspect. *BMJ* (1920) 1, 392–7.
6. Litman RE. Heat sensitivity due to autonomic drugs. *JAMA* (1952) 149, 635–6.
7. Kollias J, Bullard RW. The influence of chlorpromazine on physical and chemical mechanisms of temperature regulation in the rat. *J Pharmacol Exp Ther* (1964) 145, 373–81.
8. Warnes H, Lehmann HE, Ban TA. Adynamic ileus during psychoactive medication: a report of three fatal and five severe cases. *Can Med Assoc J* (1967) 96, 1112–13.
9. Burkitt EA, Sutcliffe CK. Paralytic ileus after amitriptyline ("Tryptizol"). *BMJ* (1961) 2, 1648–9.
10. Milner G, Hills NF. Adynamic ileus and nortriptyline. *BMJ* (1966) 1, 841–2.
11. Giordano J, Huang A, Canter JW. Fatal paralytic ileus complicating phenothiazine therapy. *South Med J* (1975) 68, 351–3.
12. Spiro RK, Kysilewskyj RM. Iatrogenic ileus secondary to medication. *J Med Soc N J* (1973) 70, 565–7.
13. Ayd FJ. Doxepin with other drugs. *South Med J* (1973) 66, 465–71.
14. Davis JM. Psychopharmacology in the aged. Use of psychotropic drugs in geriatric patients. *J Geriatr Psychiatry* (1974) 7, 145.
15. Rogers SC. Imipramine and benzhexol. *BMJ* (1967) 1, 500.
16. Rivera-Calimlim L, Castañeda L, Lasagna L. Effect of mode of management on plasma chlorpromazine in psychiatric patients. *Clin Pharmacol Ther* (1973) 14, 978–86.
17. Rivera-Calimlim L, Castañeda L, Lasagna L. Chlorpromazine and trihexyphenidyl interaction in psychiatric patients. *Pharmacologist* (1973) 15, 212.
18. Chan TL, Sakalis G, Gershon S. Some aspects of chlorpromazine metabolism in humans. *Clin Pharmacol Ther* (1973) 14, 133.
19. Rivera-Calimlim L, Nasrallah H, Strauss J, Lasagna L. Clinical response and plasma levels: effect of dose, dosage schedules, and drug interactions on plasma chlorpromazine levels. *Am J Psychiatry* (1976) 133, 646–52.
20. Loga S, Curry S, Lader M. Interactions of orphenadrine and phenobarbitone with chlorpromazine: plasma concentrations and effects in man. *Br J Clin Pharmacol* (1975) 2, 197–208.
21. Rockland L, Cooper T, Schwartz F, Weber D, Sullivan T. Effects of trihexyphenidyl on plasma chlorpromazine in young schizophrenics. *Can J Psychiatry* (1990) 35, 604–7.
22. Singh MM, Smith JM. Reversal of some therapeutic effects of an antipsychotic agent by an antiparkinsonism drug. *J Nerv Ment Dis* (1973) 157, 50–8.
23. Singh MM, Smith JM. Reversal of some therapeutic effects of haloperidol in schizophrenia by anti-parkinson drugs. *Pharmacologist* (1971) 13, 207.
24. Prien RF. Unpublished surveys from the NIMH Collaborative Project on Drug Therapy in Chronic Schizophrenia and the VA Collaborative Project on Interim Drug Therapy in Chronic Schizophrenia. Quoted in *Int Drug Ther Newslett* (1974) 9, 29–32.
25. Klett CJ, Caffey EM. Evaluating the long-term need for antiparkinson drugs by chronic schizophrenics. *Arch Gen Psychiatry* (1972) 26, 374–9.

Antipsychotics + Bromocriptine

Concurrent use can be successful, but one report describes the re-emergence of schizophrenic symptoms in a patient when bromocriptine was added to molindone and imipramine.

Clinical evidence, mechanism, importance and management

Single low doses of **bromocriptine** have been found to improve the psychopathology of chronic schizophrenia in patients on antipsychotics[1] and a case report describes a reduction in psychopathology with the concurrent use of **bromocriptine** and **haloperidol**.[2] Another report describes a schizoaffective schizophrenic on **fluphenazine**, benztropine, phenytoin and phenobarbital whose psychiatric status was unaltered when **bromocriptine** was given to treat a pituitary adenoma, but the previously normal serum prolactin was reduced to less than detectable levels by the bromocriptine.[3] However, a woman with schizoaffective schizophrenia, stabilised on 100 mg **molindone** and 200 mg **imipramine** daily, relapsed (agitation, delusions, and auditory hallucinations) within 5 days of starting additional treatment with 7.5 mg **bromocriptine** daily for amenorrhoea-galactorrhoea.[4] Within 3 days of stopping the **bromocriptine** these symptoms vanished. The reason suggested by the authors of the report is that the **bromocriptine** (a dopamine agonist) opposed the actions of the antipsychotic medication (dopamine antagonists) thereby allowing the schizophrenia to re-emerge. If concurrent use is thought appropriate, the outcome should be well monitored.

1. Cutler NR, Jeste DV, Kaufmann CA, Karoum F, Schran HF, Wyatt RJ. Low dose bromocriptine: a study of acute effects in chronic medicated schizophrenics. *Prog Neuropsychopharmacol Biol Psychiatry* (1984) 8, 277–83.
2. Gattaz WF, Köllisch M. Bromocriptine in the treatment of neuroleptic-resistant schizophrenia. *Biol Psychiatry* (1986) 21, 519–21.
3. Kellner C, Harris P, Blumhardt C. Concurrent use of bromocriptine and fluphenazine. *J Clin Psychiatry* (1985) 46, 455.
4. Frye PE, Pariser SF, Kim MH, O'Shaughnessy RW. Bromocriptine associated with symptom exacerbation during neuroleptic treatment of schizoaffective schizophrenia. *J Clin Psychiatry* (1982) 43, 252–3.

Antipsychotics or Dopamine antagonists + Fluoxetine

The development of extrapyramidal symptoms and dystonia has been seen in a few patients taking fluoxetine alone or with haloperidol, fluphenazine, maprotiline, metoclopramide, perphenazine, pericyazine, pimozide, risperidone, sulpiride, thiothixene or trifluoperazine.

Clinical evidence, mechanism, importance and management

Occasionally patients taking **fluoxetine** alone develop extrapyramidal symptoms.[1,2]

Sometimes the extrapyramidal symptoms develop when an additional drug is added. A woman on 2 to 5 mg **haloperidol** daily for 2 years with only occasional mild extrapyramidal symptoms, started additionally to take 40 mg **fluoxetine** twice daily. After 5 days the **haloperidol** was stopped but restarted 9 days later. A further 2 days later she began to experience severe extrapyramidal symptoms (tongue stiffness, parkinsonism, akathisia) and for 3 days was virtually incapacitated. Both drugs were stopped and she recovered over a period of a week.[3] This case contrasts with another report describing 8 psychotic patients who showed a 20% rise in plasma **haloperidol** levels when 20 mg **fluoxetine** daily was added, without any overall increase in extrapyramidal side-effects, although one patient developed tremor and another developed akathisia.[4]

Another report describes a more than 100% rise in plasma **haloperidol** levels accompanied by clinical improvement in 7 patients given 20 to 40 mg **fluoxetine** in addition to fixed dose **haloperidol**.[5]

A man of 40 developed marked anticholinergic side-effects (urinary retention, dilated pupils, dry mouth, palpitations) and extrapyramidal effects (akathisia) within a week of starting **fluoxetine** 20 mg combined with **haloperidol** 1 mg daily and alprazolam. The problem resolved when the **haloperidol** was withdrawn. The **haloperidol** was not given alone, so the interaction is not conclusive, but the author considered these side effects very rare with **haloperidol** alone at the dose used.[6] A schizophrenic patient on **haloperidol** developed a psychoneuromotor syndrome (including nystagmus, ataxia, myoclonic jerks, hallucinations and restlessness) with features of the serotonin syndrome, when **fluoxetine** was added to his regimen.[7] A severe dystonic reaction (painful jaw tightness and throat 'closing up') occurred in a man on 40 mg **fluoxetine** daily when he took 2.5 mg **fluphenazine** on two consecutive nights.[8] The combination of **perphenazine** and **fluoxetine** was found to be effective in the treatment of psychotic depression in 30 patients, and the side effects (which included dry mouth, blurred vision, constipation, tremor or rigidity, orthostasis and hypotension) were thought to be easier to tolerate than an antipsychotic with a tricyclic antidepressant.[9] However, a woman developed marked extrapyramidal symptoms within 2 weeks of starting 4 mg **perphenazine** twice daily and 20 mg **fluoxetine** daily.[10] A patient taking **fluoxetine** and **pimozide** showed a worsening of the extrapyramidal symptoms, and another developed marked sinus bradycardia (35 to 44 bpm) with somnolence;[11] (this case was the subject of later discussion on the mechanism of the interaction[12,13]). Yet another showed no evidence of extrapyramidal symptoms but became stuporous when given both drugs.[14] An 18-year old developed extrapyramidal side-effects, and later persistent dyskinetic tongue movements when given **fluoxetine** and **risperidone**.[15] Parkinson-like symptoms developed in a patient taking **sulpiride** and **maprotiline** when **fluoxetine** was additionally given.[16] A woman developed severe urinary retention within 2 weeks of starting 10 mg **thiothixene** twice daily, 20 mg **fluoxetine** at bedtime and 2 mg benztropine twice daily. She was treated by replacing the benztropine with amantadine, urinary catheterization and urecholine.[10] A New Zealand study describes 4 out of 15 patients on **fluoxetine** and other drugs who developed extrapyramidal symptoms while taking **fluoxetine** and other psychotropics (**haloperidol**, **trifluoperazine**, **pericyazine**, **pimozide**).[1] Two patients developed extrapyramidal symptoms while taking **fluoxetine** and **metoclopramide**.[1,17]

The reasons for these marked adverse reactions are not understood but most of them appear to be an exaggeration of the side-effects of the other drugs caused by the **fluoxetine**, perhaps due to inhibition of their metabolism, or possibly additive with the direct effects of **fluoxetine**. Other possible mechanisms are discussed elsewhere.[12,13] Most of them are isolated reports and their general importance is uncertain, nevertheless if concurrent use is thought appropriate, it should be well monitored.

1. Coulter DM, Pillans PI. Fluoxetine and extrapyramidal side effects. *Am J Psychiatry* (1995) 152, 122–5.
2. Bouchard RH, Pourcher E, Vincent P. Fluoxetine and extrapyramidal side effects. *Am J Psychiatry* (1989) 146, 1352–3.
3. Tate JL. Extrapyramidal symptoms in a patient taking haloperidol and fluoxetine. *Am J Psychiatry* (1989) 146, 399–400.
4. Goff DC, Midha KK, Brotman AW, Waites M, Baldessarini RJ. Elevation of plasma concentrations of haloperidol after the addition of fluoxetine. *Am J Psychiatry* (1991) 148, 790–2.
5. Viala A, Aymard N, Leyris A, Caroli F. Corrélations pharmacocliniques lors de l'administration de fluoxétine chez des patients schizophrènes déprimés traités par halopéridol décanoate. *Therapie* (1996) 51, 19–25.
6. Benazzi F. Urinary retention with fluoxetine–haloperidol combination in a young patient. *Can J Psychiatry* (1996) 41, 606–7.
7. D'Souza DC, Bennett A, Abi-Dargham A, Krystal JH. Precipitation of a psychoneuromotor syndrome by fluoxetine in a haloperidol-treated schizophrenic patient. *J Clin Psychopharmacol* (1994) 14, 361–3.
8. Ketai R. Interaction between fluoxetine and neuroleptics. *Am J Psychiatry* (1993) 150, 836–7.
9. Rothchild AJ, Samson JA, Bessette MP, Carter-Campbell JT. Efficacy of fluoxetine and perphenazine in the treatment of psychotic depression. *J Clin Psychiatry* (1993) 54, 338–42.
10. Lock JD, Gwirtsman HE, Targ EF. Possible adverse drug interactions between fluoxetine and other psychotropics. *J Clin Psychopharmacol* (1990) 10, 383–4.
11. Ahmed I, Dagincourt PG, Miller LG, Shader RI. Possible interaction between fluoxetine and pimozide causing sinus bradycardia. *Can J Psychiatry* (1993) 38, 62–3.
12. Friedman EH. Re: bradycardia and somnolence after adding fluoxetine to pimozide regimen. *Can J Psychiatry* (1994) 39, 634.
13. Ahmed I. Re: bradycardia and somnolence after adding fluoxetine to pimozide regimen. *Can J Psychiatry* (1994) 39, 634.
14. Hansen-Grant S, Silk KR, Guthrie S. Fluoxetine-pimozide interaction. *Am J Psychiatry* (1993) 150, 1751–2.
15. Daniel DG, Egan M, Hyde T. Probable neuroleptic induced tardive dyskinesia in association with combined SSRI and risperidone treatment. *Schizophr Res* (1996) 18, 149.
16. Touw DJ, Gernaat HBPE, van der Woude J. Parkinsonisme na toevoeging van fluoxetine aan behandeling met neuroleptica of carbamazepine. *Ned Tijdschr Geneeskd* (1992) 136, 332–3.
17. Fallon BA, Liebowitz MR. Fluoxetine and extrapyramidal symptoms in CNS lupus. *J Clin Psychopharmacol* (1991) 11, 147–8.

Antipsychotics + Lithium carbonate

Serum levels of chlorpromazine can be reduced to non-therapeutic concentrations by the concurrent administration of lithium. Dosage increases may be needed. The development of severe extrapyramidal side-effects or severe neurotoxicity has been seen in one or more patients concurrently treated with lithium and amoxapine, chlorpromazine, chlorprothixene, clopenthixol, flupentixol, fluphenazine, levomepromazine, loxapine, mesoridazine, molindone, perphenazine, prochlorperazine, risperidone, thioridazine, tiotixene, trifluoperazine or zuclopenthixol. Sleep-walking has been described in some patients taking chlorpromazine-like drugs and lithium. See also 'Sulpiride + Lithium carbonate', p.735.

Clinical evidence

(a) Chlorpromazine + lithium carbonate

(i) Reduced serum chlorpromazine levels. In a double-blind study on psychiatric patients it was found that 400 to 800 mg daily doses of **chlorpromazine**, which normally produced serum levels of 100 to 300 nanograms/ml, only produced levels of 0 to 70 nanograms/ml during the concurrent use of **lithium carbonate**.[1]

Other studies confirm the reduction in serum **chlorpromazine** levels by normal therapeutic serum levels of **lithium carbonate**.[2,3] Peak serum **chlorpromazine** levels in healthy subjects were 40% lower and the AUC was 26% smaller when they were also given **lithium carbonate**.[2]

(ii) Toxic reactions. A paranoid schizophrenic maintained on 200 to 600 mg **chlorpromazine** daily for 5 years with no extrapyramidal symptoms developed stiffness of his face, arms and legs, and parkinsonian tremor of both hands within a day of starting to take 900 mg **lithium** daily. His serum **lithium** level after 3 days was 0.5 mmol/l. He was later maintained on daily doses of 1800 mg **lithium** (serum levels 1.17 mmol/l), 200 mg **chlorpromazine** and 2 mg benzatropine, which improved his condition, but he still complained of stiffness and had a persistent hand tremor.[4]

A number of other reports describe the emergence of severe extrapyramidal side-effects when **chlorpromazine** and **lithium** were used concurrently.[5-7] Ventricular fibrillation, thought to be caused by **chlorpromazine** toxicity, occurred in a patient taking both drugs when the **lithium** was suddenly withdrawn.[8] Severe neurotoxicity has also been seen in a handful of other patients on **lithium** and **chlorpromazine**.[9]

(b) Other antipsychotics + lithium carbonate

A large-scale retrospective study of the literature over the 1966 to 1996 period using the Medline database identified 41 cases of neurotoxic adverse side-effects in 41 patients on low therapeutic concentrations of **lithium**. Of these patients, 51.2% were also taking at least one antipsychotic drug.[9] Another retrospective study using both Medline and the FDA Spontaneous Reporting System over the 1969 to 1994 period identified 237 cases of severe neurotoxicity involving **lithium**, with 188 involving **lithium** plus antipsychotics.[10,11] The sudden emergence of extrapyramidal or other side-effects has also been described in other studies. The antipsychotics implicated in this interaction with **lithium** are amoxapine,[10,11] bromperidol,[10,11] chlorprothixene,[10,11] clopenthixol,[9] clozapine,[9-11] flupentixol,[12,13] fluphenazine,[9-11,13,14] haloperidol,[9,13] levomepromazine,[9-11] loxapine,[10,11,15,16] mesoridazine,[10,11] molindone,[10,11] perphenazine,[10,11] prochlorperazine[10,11] thioridazine,[9-11,17] tiotixene[9-11,18] trifluoperazine,[10,11] or **zuclopenthixol**.[9] Examples of some cases are cited in a little more detail below.

A study of 10 patients on **fluphenazine**, **haloperidol** or **thiothixene** found that the addition of **lithium** worsened their extrapyramidal symptoms.[19] Neurotoxicity (tremor, rigidity, ataxia, tiredness, vomiting, confusion) attributed to a **lithium/fluphenazine** interaction has been described in another patient. He previously took **haloperidol** and later took **chlorpromazine** concurrently with **lithium**, without problem.[20] Irreversible brain damage has been reported in a patient taking **fluphenazine decanoate** and **lithium**.[21] Severe neurotoxic complications (seizures, encephalopathy, delirium, abnormal EEGs) developed in 4 patients while taking high doses of **thioridazine** (400 mg daily or more) and **lithium**. Serum **lithium** levels remained below 1 mmol/l. **Lithium** and other phenothiazines had been used in 3 of them for extended periods without problems, and the fourth was subsequently successfully treated with **lithium** and **fluphenazine**.[22] The concurrent use of **lithium**, and **chlorpromazine**, **perphenazine**, or **thioridazine** has also been associated with sleep-walking episodes in 9% of a group of patients.[23] Somnolence, confusion, delirium, creatinine phosphokinase elevation and fever occurred in a man on **lithium** when given **risperidone**.[24]

Mechanisms

Not understood. One suggestion to account for the reduced serum levels of chlorpromazine, which is based on *animal* studies,[25,26] is that chlorpromazine can be metabolised in the gut. Therefore if lithium delays gastric emptying more chlorpromazine will be metabolised before it reaches the circulation. This exposes the chlorpromazine to the metabolism by the gut wall for a longer time. Just why severe neurotoxicity and other side effects sometimes develop in patients on lithium and neuroleptics is not understood. It is the subject of considerable discussion and debate.[9-11]

Importance and management

Information about the chlorpromazine/lithium interaction, which results in reduced serum chlorpromazine levels is limited, but it would seem to be established and of clinical importance. Serum chlorpromazine levels below 30 nanograms/ml have been shown to be ineffective, whereas clinical improvement is associated with levels within the 150 to 300 nanogram/ml range or more.[27] Thus a fall in levels to below 70 nanograms/ml (study cited above) would be expected to result in a reduced therapeutic response. Monitor the effects and increase the dosage if necessary.

The development of severe neurotoxic or severe extrapyramidal side-effects with combinations of neuroleptics and lithium appears to be uncommon and unexplained but be alert for any evidence of toxicity if lithium is given with any of these drugs. One recommendation is that the onset of neurological manifestations, such as excessive drowsiness or movement disorders, warrants electroencephalography without delay and withdrawal of the drugs. Much more study is needed to identify the patients at risk and to find out just why these serious reactions develop.

1. Kerzner B, Rivera-Calimlim L. Lithium and chlorpromazine (CPZ) interaction. *Clin Pharmacol Ther* (1976) 19, 109.
2. Rivera-Calimlim L, Kerzner B, Karch FE. Effect of lithium on plasma chlorpromazine levels. *Clin Pharmacol Ther* (1978) 23, 451–5.
3. Rivera-Calimlim L, Nasrallah H, Strauss J, Lasagna L. Clinical response and plasma levels: effect of dose, dosage schedules, and drug interactions on plasma chlorpromazine levels. *Am J Psychiatry* (1976) 133, 646–52.
4. Addonizio G. Rapid induction of extrapyramidal side effects with combined use of lithium and neuroleptics. *J Clin Psychopharmacol* (1985) 5, 296–8.
5. McGennis AJ. Hazards of lithium and neuroleptics in schizo-affective disorder. *Br J Psychiatry* (1983) 142, 99–100.
6. Yassa R. A case of lithium-chlorpromazine interaction. *J Clin Psychiatry* (1986) 47, 90–1.
7. Habib M, Khalil R, Le Pensec-Bertrand D, Ali-Cherif A, Bongrand MC, Crevat A. Syndrome neurologique persistant après traitement par les sels de lithium: toxicité de l'association lithium-neuroleptiques? *Rev Neurol (Paris)* (1986) 142, 1, 61–4.
8. Stevenson RN, Blanshard C, Patterson DLH. Ventricular fibrillation due to lithium withdrawal – an interaction with chlorpromazine? *Postgrad Med J* (1989) 65, 936–8.
9. Emilien G, Maloteaux JM. Lithium neurotoxicity at low therapeutic doses: hypotheses for causes and mechanism of action following a retrospective analysis of published case reports. *Acta Neurol Belg* (1996) 96, 281–93.
10. Goldman SA. Lithium and neuroleptics in combination: is there enhancement of neurotoxicity leading to permanent sequelae? *J Clin Pharmacol* (1996) 36, 951–62.
11. Goldman SA. FDA MedWatch Report: lithium and neuroleptics in combination: the spectrum of neurotoxicity. *Psychopharmacol Bull* (1996) 32, 299–309.
12. West A. Adverse effects of lithium treatment. *BMJ* (1977) 2, 642.
13. Kamlana SH, Kerry RJ, Khan IA. Lithium: some drug interactions. *Practitioner* (1980) 224, 1291–2.
14. Sachdev PS. Lithium potentiation of neuroleptic-related extrapyramidal side effects. *Am J Psychiatry* (1986) 143, 942.
15. de la Gandara J, Dominguez RA. Lithium and loxapine: a potential interaction. *J Clin Psychiatry* (1988) 49, 126.
16. Fuller MA, Sajatovic M. Neurotoxicity resulting from a combination of lithium and loxapine. *J Clin Psychiatry* (1989) 50, 187.
17. Bailine SH, Doft M. Neurotoxicity induced by combined lithium–thioridazine treatment. *Biol Psychiatry* (1986) 21, 834–7.
18. Fetzer J, Kader G, Danahy S. Lithium encephalopathy: a clinical, psychiatric, and EEG evaluation. *Am J Psychiatry* (1981) 138, 1622–3.
19. Addonizio G, Roth SD, Stokes PE, Stoll PM. Increased extrapyramidal symptoms with addition of lithium to neuroleptics. *J Nerv Ment Dis* (1988) 176, 682–5.
20. Alevizos B. Toxic reactions to lithium and neuroleptics. *Br J Psychiatry* (1979) 135, 482.
21. Singh SV. Lithium carbonate/fluphenazine decanoate producing irreversible brain damage. *Lancet* (1982) ii, 278.
22. Spring GK. Neurotoxicity with combined use of lithium and thioridazine. *J Clin Psychiatry* (1979) 40, 135–8.
23. Charney DS, Kales A, Soldatos CR, Nelson JC. Somnambulistic-like episodes secondary to combined lithium-neuroleptic treatment. *Br J Psychiatry* (1979) 135, 418–24.
24. Swanson CL, Price WA, McEvoy JP. Effects of concomitant risperidone and lithium treatment. *Am J Psychiatry* (1995) 152, 1096.
25. Sundaresan PR, Rivera-Calimlim L. Distribution of chlorpromazine in the gastrointestinal tract of the rat and its effects on absorptive function. *J Pharmacol Exp Ther* (1975) 194, 593–602.
26. Curry SH, D'Mello A, Mould GP. Destruction of chlorpromazine during absorption in the rat *in vivo* and *in vitro*. *Br J Pharmacol* (1971) 42, 403–11.
27. Rivera-Calimlim L, Castañeda L, Lasagna L. Significance of plasma levels of chlorpromazine. *Clin Pharmacol Ther* (1973) 14, 144.

Antipsychotics + Tea or Coffee

Tea and coffee can cause some drugs to precipitate out of solution, but so far there is no clinical evidence to show that this normally affects the bioavailability of the drugs nor that it has a detrimental effect on treatment.

Clinical evidence, mechanism, importance and management

A single report described 2 patients whose schizophrenia was said to have been exacerbated by an increased consumption of **tea** and **coffee**.[1] Subsequent *in vitro* studies[2-6] showed that a number of drugs (**chlorpromazine**, **diphenhydramine**, **promethazine**, **fluphenazine**, **orphenadrine**, **promazine**, **prochlorperazine**, **trifluoperazine**, **thioridazine**, **loxapine**, **haloperidol**, **droperidol**) form a precipitate with **tea** or **coffee** due to the formation of a drug-tannin complex, which it was thought might possibly lower the absorption of these drugs in the gut. Studies with *rats* also showed that **tea** abolished the cataleptic effects of **chlorpromazine**, which did not appear to be related to the presence of **caffeine**.[7] However, the drug-tannin complex gives up the drug into solution if it becomes acidified, as in the stomach.[6] Moreover, a clinical study of this interaction showed that the serum levels of **chlorpromazine**, **fluphenazine**, **trifluoperazine** and **haloperidol** in a group of 16 mentally retarded patients were unaffected by the consumption of **tea** or **coffee**.[8] Their behaviour also remained unchanged.[8] So there appears to be little or no direct evidence that this physio-chemical interaction is normally of any clinical importance.

1. Mikkelsen EJ. Caffeine and schizophrenia. *J Clin Psychiatry* (1978) 39, 732–5.
2. Kulhanek F, Linde OK, Meisenberg G. Precipitation of antipsychotic drugs in interaction with coffee or tea. *Lancet* (1979) ii, 1130.
3. Hirsch SR. Precipitation of antipsychotic drugs in interaction with tea or coffee. *Lancet* (1979) ii, 1130–1.
4. Lasswell WL, Wilkins JM, Weber SS. In vitro interaction of selected drugs with coffee, tea, and gallotannic acid. *Drug Nutr Interact* (1984) 2, 235–41.
5. Lasswell WL, Weber SS, Wilkins JM. *In vitro* interaction of neuroleptics and tricyclic antidepressants with coffee, tea, and gallotannic acid. *J Pharm Sci* (1984) 73, 1056–8.
6. Curry ML, Curry SH, Marroum PJ. Interaction of phenothiazine and related drugs and caffeinated beverages. *DICP Ann Pharmacother* (1991) 25, 437–8.
7. Cheeseman HJ, Neal MJ. Interaction of chlorpromazine with tea and coffee. *Br J Clin Pharmacol* (1981) 12, 165–9.
8. Bowen S, Taylor KM, Gibb IAM. Effect of coffee and tea on blood levels and efficacy of antipsychotic drugs. *Lancet* (1981) i, 1217–18.

Benzodiazepines + Acetazolamide

Although acetazolamide can be used to treat acute mountain sickness at very high altitudes, it may not protect climbers from the respiratory depressant effects of benzodiazepines such as triazolam.

Clinical evidence, mechanism, importance and management

Acetazolamide is sometimes used by climbers at very high altitudes as a prophylactic against acute mountain sickness. Benzodiazepines are used in this situation to treat insomnia, which is common at high altitude. Benzodiazepines are believed to depress breathing because they reduce the normal respiratory response to hypoxia. This was demonstrated by a Japanese climber in the Himalayas who took 500 mg **acetazolamide** daily and 500 micrograms **triazolam**, and then needed to be 'reminded' to hyperventilate in order to relieve his hypoxia while returning from a climb. The **acetazolamide** did not prevent and may possibly have increased the central ventilatory depression of the **triazolam**, possibly by increasing its delivery to the brain. The authors of the report advise against taking these two drugs together at high altitudes,[1] thus confirming a previous warning about the risks of taking benzodiazepines at high altitude.[2]

1. Masuyama S, Hirata K, Saito A. 'Ondine's curse': side effect of acetazolamide? *Am J Med* (1989) 86, 637.
2. Sutton JR, Powles ACP, Gray GW, Houston CS. Insomnia, sedation, and high altitude cerebral oedema. *Lancet* (1979) i, 165.

Benzodiazepines + Amiodarone

An isolated report describes the development of clonazepam toxicity attributed to the concurrent use of amiodarone.

Clinical evidence, mechanism, importance and management

A man of 78 with congestive heart failure and coronary artery disease was treated with furosemide (frusemide), potassium and calcium supplements, a multivitamin preparation, and with **amiodarone** 200 mg daily for sustained ventricular tachycardia. Two months after 500 micrograms **clonazepam** was added to treat restless leg syndrome, when he had been taking **amiodarone** for 6 months, he developed slurred speech, confusion, difficulty in walking, dry mouth and urinary incontinence. This was interpreted as **clonazepam** toxicity. The problems cleared when the **clonazepam** was stopped. The authors of the report suggest that the **amiodarone** may have inhibited the oxidative metabolism of the **clonazepam** by the liver, thereby allowing it to accumulate. They also point out that this patient may have been more sensitive because of a degree of hypothyroidism caused by the **amiodarone**. Hypothyroidism is known to decrease the metabolism of drugs which undergo oxidative metabolism by the liver.[1]

This is an isolated case and of doubtful general importance, nevertheless be alert for any evidence of increased effects in any patient on **amiodarone** who is taking benzodiazepines similarly metabolised (e.g. chlordiazepoxide, diazepam, flurazepam), particularly if the patient is elderly.

1. Witt DM, Ellsworth AJ, Leversee JH. Amiodarone–clonazepam interaction. *Ann Pharmacother* (1993) 27, 1463–4.

Benzodiazepines + Antacids

Although some moderate changes in the rates of absorption of chlordiazepoxide, clorazepate and diazepam can occur if given with antacids, no adverse interaction of clinical importance has been reported.

Clinical evidence

Water, low-dose *Maalox* (30 ml or high-dose *Maalox* (120 ml was given to 10 healthy subjects taking 7.5 mg **clorazepate** nightly for 10 days in a 3-period study. The mean steady-state serum levels of the active metabolite desmethyldiazepam were not affected by *Maalox*, although they varied widely between individuals.[1] This is in line with another report,[2] but contrasts with a single-dose study, in which the peak plasma concentration of desmethyldiazepam was delayed, and reduced by about one-third by the use of *Maalox*. The 48-hour AUC was reduced by about 10%.[3]

Chlordiazepoxide absorption (single dose) was delayed by *Maalox*, though the total amount of drug absorbed was not significantly affected.[4] Similar results have been found with **diazepam**.[5] Another study found that 40 ml **aluminium hydroxide gel BP** and 30 ml **sodium citrate** (0.3 mmol/l) marginally hastened the soporific effect of 10 mg oral **diazepam** when used as a premedication before minor surgery, whereas 30 ml **magnesium trisilicate mixture BPC** tended to delay the soporific effect.[6]

Mechanisms

The delay in the absorption of chlordiazepoxide and diazepam is attributed to the effect of the antacid on gastric emptying. Clorazepate on the other hand is a 'pro-drug', which needs acid conditions in the stomach for conversion by hydrolysis and decarboxylation to its active form. Antacids are presumed to inhibit this conversion by raising the pH of the stomach contents.[7]

Importance and management

Most of the reports describe single-dose studies, but what is known suggests that no adverse interaction of any clinical importance is likely during treatment with chlordiazepoxide, diazepam or clorazepate. No special precautions seem to be necessary. Whether the delay in absorption (particularly with clorazepate) has an undesirable effect in those who only take benzodiazepines during acute episodes of anxiety, and who need rapid relief is uncertain. Information about other benzodiazepines is lacking.

1. Shader RI, Ciraulo DA, Greenblatt DJ, Harmatz JS. Steady-state plasma desmethyldiazepam during long-term clorazepate use: effect of antacids. *Clin Pharmacol Ther* (1982) 31, 180–3.
2. Chun AHC, Carrigan PJ, Hoffman DJ, Kershner RP, Stuart JD. Effect of antacids on absorption of clorazepate. *Clin Pharmacol Ther* (1977) 22, 329–35.
3. Shader RI, Georgotas A, Greenblatt DJ, Harmatz JS, Allen MD. Impaired absorption of desmethyldiazepam from clorazepate by magnesium aluminium hydroxide. *Clin Pharmacol Ther* (1978) 24, 308–15.
4. Greenblatt DJ, Shader RI, Harmatz JS, Franke K, Koch-Weser J. Influence of magnesium and aluminium hydroxide mixture on chlordiazepoxide absorption. *Clin Pharmacol Ther* (1976) 19, 234–9.
5. Greenblatt DJ, Allen MD, MacLaughlin DS, Harmatz JS, Shader RI. Diazepam absorption: effect of antacids and food. *Clin Pharmacol Ther* (1978) 24, 600–9.
6. Nair SG, Gamble JAS, Dundee JW, Howard PJ. The influence of three antacids on the absorption and clinical action of oral diazepam. *Br J Anaesth* (1976) 48, 1175–80.
7. Abruzzo CW, Macasieb T, Weinfeld R, Rider JA, Kaplan SA. Changes in the oral absorption characteristics in man of dipotassium clorazepate at normal and elevated gastric pH. *J Pharmacokinet Biopharm* (1977) 5, 377–90.

Benzodiazepines + Anticonvulsants

The concurrent use of benzodiazepines with other non-benzodiazepine anticonvulsants is common and possibly accompanied by some changes in serum levels. Normally these are of limited clinical importance. Isolated interactions between alprazolam and carbamazepine, between chlordiazepoxide and phenobarbital, and between clobazam and phenytoin have been reported. The clearance of diazepam is increased by carbamazepine and phenytoin, but not phenobarbital. The hypnotic effects of midazolam are virtually abolished by carbamazepine and phenytoin.

Clinical evidence

(a) Alprazolam + Carbamazepine

A patient with atypical bipolar disorder and panic attacks, being treated with 7.5 mg **alprazolam** daily, showed a more than 50% reduction in serum **alprazolam** levels (from 43 to 19.3 nanograms/ml) when concurrently treated with 300 mg **carbamazepine** daily. This was accompanied by a deterioration in his clinical condition, which was controlled with haloperidol.[1]

(b) Chlordiazepoxide + Phenobarbital

A single case report describes a man given **phenobarbital** and **chlordiazepoxide** who demonstrated drowsiness, unsteadiness, slurred speech, nystagmus, poor memory and hallucinations, all of which disappeared once the **phenobarbital** was withdrawn. Substantial doses of **chlordiazepoxide** were well tolerated.[2]

(c) Clobazam + Anticonvulsants

Phenytoin and **carbamazepine** reduce the plasma levels of **clobazam** and increase the levels of **norclobazam** (the principal metabolite), but **phenobarbital** slightly reduces the levels of both.[3] A reduction in steady-state **clobazam** levels but a rise in norclobazam levels due to **carbamazepine** is described in another study in 6 healthy subjects.[4] Since **norclobazam** retains some anticonvulsant activity the effects of **carbamazepine** probably has no clinical significance, but this needs further study. A report describes elevated **phenytoin** serum levels and toxicity in 3 patients when concurrently treated with **clobazam**.[5] **Sodium valproate** was not reported to have a marked effect on **clobazam**,[3] but a study in children found that **clobazam** caused an 11% increase in the serum levels of **sodium valproate**, despite a reduction of at least 10% in **valproate** dosage.[6]

(d) Clonazepam + Anticonvulsants

Clonazepam in slowly increasing doses up to a maximum of 4 to 6 mg/day given over a 6-week period to patients on **phenobarbital** or **carbamazepine**, alone or in combination, had no effect on either **phenobarbital** or **carbamazepine** serum levels.[7] On the other hand, a study in 7 subjects given 1 mg **clonazepam** daily showed that **carbamazepine** 200 mg daily over a 3-week period reduced **clonazepam** plasma levels (from a range of 4 to 7 nanograms/ml down to 2.5 to 4 nanograms/ml) and half-life by about a third.[8] A retrospective analysis of the **carbamazepine/clonazepam** interaction in 183 patients also suggested an interaction. **Clonazepam** clearance was increased by 22% and **carbamazepine** clearance was decreased by 20.5% when the two drugs were used concurrently.[9]

(e) Diazepam + Anticonvulsants

No effect was found in the metabolism of **diazepam** in healthy subjects before and after taking 100 mg **phenobarbital** for 8 days.[10] Some modest additive CNS depression may possibly be expected, but the authors of this report make no comment about this. A comparative study found that the plasma clearance of a single 10 mg intravenous dose of **diazepam** in a group of 9 epileptics taking antiepileptic drugs was threefold greater and the half-life shorter than in 6 healthy subjects. Seven of the epileptics were taking **carbamazepine**.[11]

(f) Lorazepam + Valproate

Lorazepam 1 mg 12-hourly for 3 days had no effect on the pharmacokinetics of **valproate semisodium** (divalproex sodium) 500 mg 12-hourly in healthy subjects. However, **valproate semisodium** caused an increase in the AUC and maximum serum levels of **lorazepam**, of 20 and 8% respectively. Sedation scores were not affected by concurrent treatment, suggesting that the interaction is not clinically significant.[12]

(g) Midazolam + Anticonvulsants

The pharmacokinetics and pharmacodynamics of a single 15-mg oral dose of **midazolam** was studied in 6 epileptic patients taking either **carbamazepine**, **phenytoin** or both drugs together, and in 7 control subjects not taking either of these anticonvulsants. The AUC of **midazolam** in the epileptics was reduced to 5.7%, and the peak serum levels to 7.4% of their value in the control subjects. The pharmacodynamic effects (subjective drowsiness, body sway with eyes closed and open, as well as more formal tests) of the **midazolam** were also reduced. Most of the epileptics did not notice any effects of the **midazolam**, while the control subjects were clearly sedated for 2 to 4 h after taking the **midazolam** and also experienced amnesia.[13]

Mechanisms

Uncertain. Changes in the drug metabolism (increases and decreases) due to enzyme induction and inhibition are probably responsible.

Importance and management

The midazolam/anticonvulsant interactions appear to be of greatest clinical significance. You will need to use a much larger dose of midazolam in the presence of either carbamazepine or phenytoin. An alternative hypnotic may be needed. **Triazolam** is predicted to be affected just like midazolam.[13] None of the other benzodiazepine/anticonvulsant interactions appear to be of major clinical importance. It has been recommended that if clobazam is added to sodium valproate it would be prudent to monitor for any increases in valproate serum levels.

1. Arana GW, Epstein S, Molloy M, Greenblatt DJ. Carbamazepine-induced reduction of plasma alprazolam concentrations: a clinical case report. *J Clin Psychiatry* (1988) 49, 448–9.
2. Kane FJ, McCurdy RL. An unusual reaction to combined Librium-barbiturate therapy. *Am J Psychiatry* (1964) 120, 816.
3. Bun H, Monjanel-Mouterde S, Noel F, Durand A, Cano J-P. Effects of age and antiepileptic drugs on plasma levels and kinetics of clobazam and N-desmethylclobazam. *Pharmacol Toxicol* (1990) 67, 136–40.
4. Levy RH, Lane EA, Guyot M, Brachet-Liermain A, Cenraud B, Loiseau P. Analysis of parent drug-metabolite relationship in the presence of an inducer: application to the carbamazepine-clobazam interaction in normal man. *Drug Metab Dispos* (1983) 11, 286–92.
5. Zifkin B, Sherwin A, Andermann F. Phenytoin toxicity due to interaction with clobazam. *Neurology* (1991) 41, 313–14.
6. Theis JGW, Koren G, Daneman R, Sherwin AL, Menzano E, Cortez M, Hwang P. Interactions of clobazam with conventional antiepileptics in children. *J Child Neurol* (1997) 12, 208–13.
7. Johannessen SI, Strandjord RE, Munthe-Kaas AW. Lack of effect of clonazepam on serum levels of diphenylhydantoin, phenobarbital and carbamazepine. *Acta Neurol Scand* (1977) 55, 506–12.
8. Lai AA, Levy RH, Cutler RE. Time-course of interaction between carbamazepine and clonazepam in normal man. *Clin Pharmacol Ther* (1978) 24, 316–23.
9. Yukawa E, Nonaka T, Yukawa M, Ohdo S, Higuchi S, Kuroda T, Goto Y. Pharmacoepidemiologic investigation of a clonazepam-carbamazepine interaction by mixed effect modeling using routine clinical pharmacokinetic data in Japanese patients. *J Clin Psychopharmacol* (2001) 21, 588–93.
10. Brockmeyer N, Dylewicz P, Habicht H, Ohnhaus EE. The metabolism of diazepam following different enzyme inducing agents. *Br J Clin Pharmacol* (1985) 19, 544P.
11. Dhillon S, Richens A. Pharmacokinetics of diazepam in epileptic patients and normal volunteers following intravenous administration. *Br J Clin Pharmacol* (1981) 12, 841–4.
12. Samara EE, Granneman RG, Witt GF, Cavanaugh JH. Effect of valproate on the pharmacokinetics and pharmacodynamics of lorazepam. *J Clin Pharmacol* (1997) 37, 442–50.
13. Backman JT, Olkkola KT, Ojala M, Laaksovirta H, Neuvonen PJ. Concentrations and effects of oral midazolam are greatly reduced in patients treated with carbamazepine or phenytoin. *Epilepsia* (1996) 37, 253–7.

Benzodiazepines + Antipsychotics

Marked respiratory depression has been reported in 3 patients, one with hypotension, when treated with lorazepam and loxapine and neuroleptic malignant syndrome has been reported in another 3 patients on benzodiazepines and antipsychotics.

Clinical evidence, mechanism, importance and management

A woman with a psychiatric history (a DSM-III diagnosis of bipolar affective disorder, manic type) was admitted to hospital and given 2 mg **lorazepam** and 25 mg **loxapine**. After 2 h she was found to be lethargic with sonorous respirations, occasional episodes of apnoea and an irregular respiration as low as 4 breaths per minute. She was given oxygen and recovered spontaneously within 12 h. She had had no previous problems with **lorazepam**, and had none when it was later administered while she was taking perphenazine.[1] Two other cases have been reported of patients given **lorazepam** 1 to 2 mg intramuscularly and **loxapine** 50 mg orally, which resulted in prolonged stupor, a significantly lowered respiration rate (8 breaths per minute), and in one case hypotension. Both showed signs of recovery within

3 to 5 h. Both had taken each of these drugs before, alone, without problems.[2] Three cases of neuroleptic malignant syndrome following treatment with **diazepam** and **risperidone** or **clorazepate** and **zuclopenthixol** or **tiapride** and **clonazepam** are described. In 2 cases this followed the abrupt withdrawal of long-term benzodiazepines. All 3 patients recovered, one without any treatment.[3]

These reports are isolated and unexplained. There is no clear reason for avoiding concurrent use, but it should be well monitored.

1. Cohen S, Khan A. Respiratory distress with the use of lorazepam in mania. *J Clin Psychopharmacol* (1987) 7, 199–200.
2. Battaglia J, Thornton L, Young C. Loxapine-lorazepam-induced hypotension and stupor. *J Clin Psychopharmacol* (1989) 9, 227–8.
3. Bobolakis I. Neuroleptic malignant syndrome after antipsychotic drug administration during benzodiazepine withdrawal. *J Clin Psychopharmacol* (2000) 20, 281–3.

Benzodiazepines + Atropine or Hyoscine

Atropine and hyoscine do not affect the absorption or the sedative effects of diazepam.

Clinical evidence, mechanism, importance and management

A study in 8 healthy subjects given single 10 mg oral doses of **diazepam** showed that serum **diazepam** levels were not significantly changed by the concurrent use of 1 mg **atropine** or 1 mg **hyoscine hydrobromide**, nor were the sedative effects of the **diazepam** altered.[1]

1. Gregoretti SM, Uges DRA. Influence of oral atropine or hyoscine on the absorption of oral diazepam. *Br J Anaesth* (1982) 54, 1231–4.

Benzodiazepines + Azole antifungals

Fluconazole, itraconazole and ketoconazole very markedly increase the serum levels of midazolam and triazolam when given orally, thereby increasing their sedative and amnesic effects and prolonging the duration of hypnosis. This possibly does not occur with intravenous bolus administration. Ketoconazole has a small, probably clinically unimportant effect on the activity of chlordiazepoxide. The effects of alprazolam are increased by itraconazole and ketoconazole. No important interaction occurs between temazepam and itraconazole, or bromazepam and fluconazole.

Clinical evidence

(a) Alprazolam + Itraconazole

Alprazolam 800 micrograms was given to 10 healthy subjects before and after a 6 day course of **itraconazole** 200 mg daily. The **itraconazole** increased the AUC and the half-life of **alprazolam** nearly threefold, and psychomotor function was depressed.[1]

(b) Alprazolam + Ketoconazole

A study in healthy subjects found that 200 mg **ketoconazole** twice daily decreased the clearance of **alprazolam** 1 mg to about one-third, and prolonged its half-life fourfold, but the maximum serum levels remained unchanged.[2] This study is consistent with the results of *in vitro* work with human liver microsomal enzymes showing that **ketoconazole** inhibits the metabolism of **alprazolam** (due to inhibition of the cytochrome P450 isoenzyme CYP3A).[3,4]

(c) Bromazepam + Fluconazole

Fluconazole 100 mg daily for 4 days had no effect on the pharmacokinetics or pharmacodynamics of **bromazepam** in 12 healthy subjects.[5]

(d) Chlordiazepoxide + Ketoconazole

After taking 400 mg **ketoconazole** daily for 5 days the clearance of **chlordiazepoxide** (0.6 mg/kg) in 12 healthy subjects was decreased by 38%.[6]

(e) Midazolam + Fluconazole

A study in 12 healthy subjects found that 200 mg **fluconazole** daily for 5 days reduced the clearance of a single 7.5 mg oral dose of **midazolam** by 51%. The AUC of the **midazolam** was increased 3.5-fold. It was found that the subjects could hardly be wakened during the first hour after taking the **midazolam**.[7] Another study found that a single 150-mg dose of **fluconazole** increased the serum levels of single 10-mg doses of **midazolam** by about 30%.[8] Yet another study found that the route of administration of the **fluconazole** (i.e. whether oral or intravenous) made little or no difference to the pharmacodynamic effects of **midazolam**.[9] A fourfold increase in plasma **midazolam** levels was found in intensive care unit patients, stabilised on **midazolam** infusions, when **fluconazole** was added to treatment. The interaction was most marked in patients with renal failure.[10,11] These reports contrast with another, which found that 150 mg **fluconazole** only slightly increased the effects of single 10-mg doses of **midazolam**.[12]

(f) Midazolam + Itraconazole

When 9 healthy subjects were given 7.5 mg oral **midazolam** before and after taking 200 mg **itraconazole** daily for 4 days, the **itraconazole** was found to have increased the **midazolam** AUC about tenfold, increased the peak serum levels about threefold, and prolonged the half-life from 2.8 to 7.9 h. The subjects could hardly be wakened during the first hour after taking the **midazolam** and most of them experienced amnesia lasting several hours.[13] A later study found that 100 mg **itraconazole** daily for 4 days increased the **midazolam** AUC sixfold and the peak serum levels 2.5-fold.[14] A further study confirmed the marked effect of both **itraconazole** on oral **midazolam**, but found that the effects of bolus doses of intravenous **midazolam** were not increased to a clinically significant extent, although their results suggested that long-term high doses infusions of **midazolam** need to be titrated according to effect to avoid overdosage.[7]

(g) Midazolam + Ketoconazole

When 7 healthy women were given 7.5 mg oral **midazolam** before and after taking 400 mg **ketoconazole** daily for 4 days, the **ketoconazole** was found to have increased the **midazolam** AUC from 3.9 to 62 micrograms.ml^{-1}.min, increased the peak serum levels about fourfold, and prolonged the half-life from 2.8 to 8.7 h. The subjects could hardly be wakened during the first hour after taking the **midazolam** and most of them experienced amnesia lasting several hours.[13] Similar results were found in another study.[7]

(h) Temazepam + Itraconazole

Itraconazole 200 mg daily was given to 10 healthy subjects for 4 days. On day 4 a single 20-mg dose of **temazepam** was also given. A very small increase in the **temazepam** AUC was seen, but the psychomotor tests carried out were unchanged.[15]

(i) Triazolam + Fluconazole

Eight healthy subjects were given either 50, 100 or 200 mg **fluconazole** or a placebo daily for 4 days. On day 4 they were also given a single 250-microgram oral dose of **triazolam**. The **triazolam** AUCs were increased 1.6-, 2.1- and 4.4-fold by 50, 100 and 200 mg **fluconazole** respectively, and the maximum serum **triazolam** levels were more than doubled by the 200-mg **fluconazole** dose. The 100- and 200-mg **fluconazole** doses both produced significant changes in the psychomotor tests of **triazolam**, but the 50-mg dose did not.[16]

(j) Triazolam + Itraconazole

The AUC of a single 250-microgram dose of **triazolam** was increased from 5.9 to 160 nanograms.ml^{-1}.h after 9 healthy subjects were given 200 mg **itraconazole** daily for 4 days. Peak serum levels were increased threefold. Marked changes in psychomotor and other responses were seen. The subjects had amnesia and were still very tired and confused as long as 17 h after taking the **triazolam**.[17] Another study found that the interaction persists for several days after taking the **itraconazole**.[18]

(k) Triazolam + Ketoconazole

A study in healthy subjects (number not stated) found that when they were given 125 micrograms of **triazolam**, preceded by 200 mg **ketoconazole** taken 17 and 1 h before, the **triazolam** half-life was prolonged (from 4 to almost 18 h in one subject) and the clearance was increased ninefold. Pharmacodynamic testing found an increase in the impairment of a digit-symbol substitution test, and increased effects on EEG beta activity.[19] The AUC of a single 250-microgram dose of **triazolam** was increased from 5.9 to 132 nanograms.ml^{-1}.h after taking 400 mg **ketoconazole** daily for 4 days. Peak serum levels were increased threefold. Marked changes in psychomotor and other responses were seen. The subjects had amnesia and were still very tired and confused as long as 17 h after taking the **triazolam**.[17]

Mechanism

It would seem that these antifungals markedly reduce the metabolism of midazolam and triazolam by the liver, thereby reducing their loss from the body, raising their serum levels and increasing and prolonging their effects. *In vitro* evidence suggests that the cytochrome P450 isoenzyme CYP3A4 is involved.[20-23] Ketoconazole appears to inhibit the oxidation of chlordiazepoxide by the liver.[6]

Importance and management

The **midazolam/itraconazole**, **midazolam/ketoconazole**, **triazolam/itraconazole** and **triazolam/ketoconazole** interactions are established and clinically important. The authors of one of the reports cited[13] point out that the deepness of sleep caused by midazolam and its duration may be dangerously increased. Patients are unlikely to be able (for example) to drive 6 h after receiving midazolam. In very broad terms the dosage of midazolam would need to be reduced by about 75% or more in the presence of these antifungals to avoid excessive sedation, and even then the effects would still be expected to be prolonged. The same general precautions would seem equally applicable to all of these four drug pairs. Unless appropriate precautions are taken (very reduced dosages) these interactions can be dangerous. Patients should also be warned about the likelihood of increased sedation. The risk with **midazolam/fluconazole** and **triazolam/fluconazole** in doses of over 100 mg is possibly less than with the previous four drug pairs, but even so, the benzodiazepine dosage probably needs to be reduced, probably halved.

There is some evidence that *bolus doses of intravenous* **midazolam** given in the presence of **itraconazole** or **fluconazole** are not increased to a clinically significant degree, and normal doses can be used.[14] However where *high doses of intravenous* **midazolam** are used long term (e.g. during intensive care treatment) it has been suggested that the dosage will need to be titrated to avoid long-lasting hypnotic effects.[7] The *bolus or intravenous* administration of **midazolam** in the presence of **ketoconazole**, and the combinations of *bolus or intravenous* **triazolam** with any of these three antifungals seems likely to interact in the same way, but this needs confirmation.

The effects of **alprazolam**[2-4] are increased and prolonged by **ketoconazole** and **itraconazole**, but the extent of this is less than that which is seen with midazolam or triazolam. The **chlordiazepoxide/ketoconazole** and **temazepam/itraconazole** interactions are established but the effects are small and unlikely to be clinically important.

1. Yasui N, Kondo T, Otani K, Furukori H, Kaneko S, Ohkubo T, Nagasaki T, Sugawara K. Effect of itraconazole on the single oral dose pharmacokinetics and pharmacodynamics of alprazolam. *Psychopharmacology (Berl)* (1998) 139, 269–73.
2. Greenblatt DJ, Wright CE, von Moltke LL, Harmatz JS, Ehrenberg BL, Harrel LM, Corbett K, Counihan M, Tobias S, Shader RI. Ketoconazole inhibition of triazolam and alprazolam clearance: differential kinetic and dynamic consequences. *Clin Pharmacol Ther* (1998) 64, 237–47.
3. Greenblatt DJ, von Moltke LL, Harmatz JS, Ciraulo DA, Shader RI. Alprazolam pharmacokinetics, metabolism, and plasma levels: clinical implications. *J Clin Psychiatry* (1993) 54 10 (Suppl), 4–11.
4. von Moltke LL, Greenblatt DJ, Cotreau-Bibbo MM, Harmatz JS, Shader RI. Inhibitors of alprazolam metabolism *in vitro*: effect of serotonin-reuptake-inhibitor antidepressants, ketoconazole and quinidine. *Br J Clin Pharmacol* (1994) 38, 23–31.
5. Ohtani Y, Kotegawa T, Tsutsumi K, Morimoto T, Hirose Y, Nakano S. Effect of fluconazole on the pharmacokinetics and pharmacodynamics of oral and rectal bromazepam: an application of electroencephalography as the pharmacodynamic method. *J Clin Pharmacol* (2002) 42, 183–91.
6. Brown MW, Maldonado AL, Meredith CG, Speeg KV. Effect of ketoconazole on hepatic oxidative drug metabolism. *Clin Pharmacol Ther* (1985) 37, 290–7.
7. Olkkola KT, Ahonen J, Neuvonen PJ. The effect of the systemic antimycotics, itraconazole and fluconazole, on the pharmacokinetics and pharmacodynamics of intravenous and oral midazolam. *Anesth Analg* (1996) 82, 511–16.
8. Mattila MJ, Vainio P, Vanakoski J. Fluconazole moderately increases midazolam effects on performance. *Br J Clin Pharmacol* (1995) 39, 567P.
9. Ahonen J, Olkkola KT, Neuvonen PJ. Effect of route of administration of fluconazole on the interaction between fluconazole and midazolam. *Eur J Clin Pharmacol* (1997) 51, 415–19.
10. Olkkola KT, Ahonen J, Takala A, Neuvonen PJ. The interaction between fluconazole and midazolam in intensive care unit patients. *Anesthesiology* (1998) 89, A501.
11. Ahonen J, Olkkola KT, Takala A, Neuvonen PJ. Interaction between fluconazole and midazolam in intensive care patients. *Acta Anaesthesiol Scand* (1999) 43, 509–14.
12. Vanakoski J, Mattila MJ, Vainio P, Idänpään-Heikkilä JJ, Törnwall M. 150 mg fluconazole does not substantially increase the effects of 10 mg midazolam or the plasma midazolam concentrations in healthy subjects. *Int J Clin Pharmacol Ther* (1995) 33, 518–23.
13. Olkkola KT, Backman JT, Neuvonen PJ. Midazolam should be avoided in patients receiving systemic antimycotics ketoconazole or itraconazole. *Clin Pharmacol Ther* (1994) 55, 481–5.
14. Ahonen J, Olkkola KT, Neuvonen PJ. Effect of itraconazole and terbinafine on the pharmacokinetics and pharmacodynamics of midazolam in healthy volunteers. *Br J Clin Pharmacol* (1995) 40, 270–2.
15. Ahonen J, Olkkola KT, Neuvonen PJ. Lack of effect of antimycotic itraconazole on the pharmacokinetics or pharmacodynamics of temazepam. *Ther Drug Monit* (1996) 18, 124–7.
16. Varhe A, Olkkola KT, Neuvonen PJ. Effect of fluconazole dose on the extent of fluconazole-triazolam interaction. *Br J Clin Pharmacol* (1996) 42, 465–70.
17. Varhe A, Olkkola KT, Neuvonen PJ. Oral triazolam is potentially hazardous to patients receiving systemic antimycotics ketoconazole or itraconazole. *Clin Pharmacol Ther* (1994) 56, 601–7.
18. Neuvonen PJ, Varhe A, Olkkola KT. The effect of ingestion time interval on the interaction between itraconazole and triazolam. *Clin Pharmacol Ther* (1996) 60, 326–31.
19. Greenblatt DJ, von Moltke LL, Harmatz JS, Harrel LM, Tobias S, Shader RI, Wright CE. Interaction of triazolam and ketoconazole. *Lancet* (1995) 345, 191.
20. Gascon M-P, Dayer P. In vitro forecasting of drugs which may interfere with the biotransformation of midazolam. *Eur J Clin Pharmacol* (1991) 41, 573–8.
21. Hargreaves JA, Jezequel S, Houston JB. Effect of azole antifungals on human microsomal metabolism of diclofenac and midazolam. *Br J Clin Pharmacol* (1994) 38, 175P.
22. von Moltke LL, Greenblatt DJ, Duan SX, Harmatz JS, Shader RI. *In vitro* prediction of the terfenadine-ketoconazole pharmacokinetic interaction. *J Clin Pharmacol* (1994) 34, 1222–7.
23. Wrighton SA, Ring BJ. Inhibition of human CYP3A catalyzed 1′-hydroxy midazolam formation by ketoconazole, nifedipine, erythromycin, cimetidine, and nizatidine. *Pharm Res* (1994) 11, 921–4.

Benzodiazepines + Beta-blockers

Only small and clinically unimportant pharmacokinetic interactions occur between most benzodiazepines and beta-blockers, but there is some evidence that patients on diazepam may possibly be more accident-prone while taking metoprolol.

Clinical evidence, mechanism, importance and management

The clearance of **diazepam** is reduced by 17% by **propranolol**[1] and 18% by **metoprolol**,[2] but **propranolol** has only a small effect on the clearance of **clorazepate**,[3] and none on **alprazolam**,[1] **lorazepam**[1] or **oxazepam**.[4] **Labetalol** also does not affect **oxazepam**.[4] Another study found that the AUC of **diazepam** was increased by 25% by **metoprolol**, but no statistically significant changes were seen with **atenolol** or **propranolol**.[5] In another study the **bromazepam** AUC was increased by 35% by **metoprolol**, and **bromazepam** increased the effect of **metoprolol** on systolic blood pressures, but no important interactions occurred with **lorazepam** and **metoprolol**.[6]

All of these pharmacokinetic changes are either relatively small or appear not to be clinically important. However, studies of psychomotor performance have shown that simple reaction times with **oxazepam**, combined with either **propranolol** or **labetalol**, are increased,[4] and those taking **diazepam** and **metoprolol** have a reduced kinetic visual acuity,[5,7] which is related to driving ability.[8] Moreover, choice reaction times at 2 h were also found to be lengthened when taking **diazepam**, and **metoprolol**, **propranolol** or **atenolol**, but at 8 h they only persisted with **diazepam** and **metoprolol**.[7] Information is very limited indeed, but what is known so far suggests that patients who drive, and who are given **diazepam** and **metoprolol** in particular, should be given some warning. There seems to be no information about other benzodiazepines and beta-blockers. More study is needed.

1. Ochs HR, Greenblatt DJ, Verburg-Ochs B. Propranolol interactions with diazepam, lorazepam, and alprazolam. *Clin Pharmacol Ther* (1984) 36, 451–5.
2. Klotz U, Reimann IW. Pharmacokinetic and pharmacodynamic interaction study of diazepam and metoprolol. *Eur J Clin Pharmacol* (1984) 26, 223–6.
3. Ochs HR, Greenblatt DJ, Locniskar A, Weinbrenner J. Influence of propranolol coadministration or cigarette smoking on the kinetics of desmethyldiazepam following intravenous clorazepate. *Klin Wochenschr* (1986) 64, 1217–21.
4. Sonne J, Døssing M, Loft S, Olesen KL, Vollmer-Larsen A, Victor MA, Hamberg O, Thyssen H. Single dose pharmacokinetics and pharmacodynamics of oral oxazepam during concomitant administration of propranolol and labetalol. *Br J Clin Pharmacol* (1990) 29, 33–7.
5. Hawksworth G, Betts T, Crowe A, Knight R, Nyemitei-Addo I, Parry K, Petrie JC, Raffle A, Parsons A. Diazepam/β-adrenoceptor antagonist interactions. *Br J Clin Pharmacol* (1984) 17, 69S–76S.
6. Scott AK, Cameron GA, Hawksworth GM. Interaction of metoprolol with lorazepam and bromazepam. *Eur J Clin Pharmacol* (1991) 40, 405–9.
7. Betts TA, Crowe A, Knight R, Raffle A, Parsons A, Blake A, Hawksworth G, Petrie JC. Is there a clinically relevant interaction between diazepam and lipophilic β-blocking drugs? *Drugs* (1983) 25 (Suppl 2), 279–80.
8. Betts TA, Knight R, Crowe A, Blake A, Harvey P, Mortiboy D. Effect of β-blockers on psychomotor performance in normal volunteers. *Eur J Clin Pharmacol* (1985) 28 (Suppl), 39–49.

Benzodiazepines + Calcium channel blockers

The serum levels and effects of midazolam are markedly increased by diltiazem or verapamil. This also occurs with triazolam and diltiazem, and is predicted to occur with triazolam and verapamil. There appear to be no significant interactions between diazepam and diltiazem, felodipine or nimodipine; between midazolam and nitrendipine; between temazepam and diltiazem; or between triazolam and isradipine.

Clinical evidence

(a) Diazepam + Diltiazem

Single 5-mg doses of **diazepam** and 60 mg **diltiazem** were given to 6 subjects. The plasma levels of each drug were not significantly altered by the presence of the other drug.[1] Another study in which poor metabolisers and extensive metabolisers (cytochrome P450 isoenzyme CYP2C19) were given **diltiazem** 200 mg daily for 3 days before and 7 days after a single dose of **diazepam** 2 mg found no differences in the interaction between the phenotypes. Both groups showed an increase in the AUC and half-life of **diazepam**, but the clinical effects of this pharmacokinetic change were not assessed.[2]

(b) Diazepam + Felodipine

The pharmacokinetics of 10 mg intravenous **diazepam** were unchanged in 12 healthy subjects after taking **felodipine** 10 mg daily for 12 days, but the AUC and peak serum levels of desmethyldiazepam were raised by 14 and 16% respectively.[3]

(c) Diazepam + Nimodipine

The serum levels of **diazepam** 10 mg daily and **nimodipine** 30 mg three times daily were unaffected by concurrent use in 24 elderly, healthy subjects, and no clinically relevant changes in haemodynamics, ECG recordings, clinical chemistry or haematology occurred.[4]

(d) Midazolam + Diltiazem

After taking 60 mg **diltiazem** three times daily for 2 days, 9 healthy female subjects were given 15 mg **midazolam** orally. The AUC of the **midazolam** was increased fourfold, the maximum serum levels doubled and the half-life increased by 49%. It was almost impossible for the subjects to stay awake for an hour-and-a-half after taking the **midazolam**. They suffered several hours amnesia and there was a marked decrease in the performance of pharmacodynamic tests (digit symbol substitution, Maddox wing test).[5] Increased **midazolam** and **alfentanil** AUCs (15% and 24%) and half-lives (43% and 50%) were seen in 15 patients anaesthetised with **midazolam** and **alfentanil** when pretreated with 60 mg **diltiazem** 2 h before induction. Tracheal extubation was performed on average 2.5 h later than in another group given a placebo instead of the **diltiazem**.[6]

(e) Midazolam + Nitrendipine

A study in 9 healthy subjects found that the pharmacokinetics and pharmacodynamics of **midazolam** were unaffected by a single 20-mg dose of **nitrendipine**.[7]

(f) Midazolam + Verapamil

After taking 80 mg **verapamil** three times daily for 2 days, 9 healthy female subjects were given 15 mg **midazolam** orally. The AUC of the **midazolam** was increased threefold, the maximum serum levels were doubled and the half-life increased 41%. It was almost impossible for the subjects to stay awake for an hour-and-a-half after taking the **midazolam**. They suffered several hours amnesia and there was a marked decrease in the performance of pharmacodynamic tests (digit symbol substitution, Maddox wing test).[5]

(g) Temazepam + Diltiazem

Diltiazem 40 mg had no little or no effect on the hypnotic effects of **temazepam** in 16 healthy insomniacs.[8]

(h) Triazolam + Diltiazem

A study in 7 healthy subjects found that 60 mg **diltiazem** three times daily for 3 days increased the AUC of a single 250 microgram dose of **triazolam** 2.3-fold and almost doubled its peak serum levels. Pharmacodynamic tests showed an increase in the sedative effects of **triazolam**.[9,10] Yet another study in 10 healthy subjects found that 60 mg **diltiazem** three times daily for 2 days increased the AUC of a single 250 microgram dose of **triazolam** 3.4-fold, and approximately doubled its maximum plasma level and half-life. The pharmacodynamic changes were briefly described as profound and prolonged.[11,12] In contrast 40 mg **diltiazem** was found to have little or no effect on the hypnotic effects of **triazolam** in 16 healthy insomniacs in another study.[8]

(i) Triazolam + Isradipine

Isradipine 5 mg daily reduced the AUC of a single 250-microgram dose of **triazolam** by 20% in 9 healthy subjects, but no difference in the pharmacodynamic effects of **triazolam** were seen. Therefore this interaction does not appear to be of any clinical significance.[13]

Mechanism

The evidence suggests that the metabolism of midazolam and triazolam by cytochrome P450 isoenzyme CYP3A4 is inhibited by diltiazem and verapamil, leading to increased serum levels and increased effects.

Importance and management

The **midazolam/diltiazem**, **midazolam/verapamil** and **triazolam/diltiazem** interactions are established and clinically important. The authors of one report say that patients on either of these calcium channel blockers are probably incapable of doing skilled tasks (e.g. car driving) up to 6 hours after taking 15 mg **midazolam**, and possibly even after 8 to 10 h. They suggest that the usual dose of **midazolam** should be reduced at least 50% to avoid unnecessary deep sleep and prolonged hypnosis, and they also point out that since the half-life of the **midazolam** is prolonged, the effects will persist regardless of the dose.[5] The same seems likely to be true for **triazolam/diltiazem** and the interaction is also predicted to occur with **triazolam/verapamil**.[12] No special precautions appear to be necessary with **diazepam/diltiazem**, **diazepam/felodipine**, **diazepam/nimodipine**, **midazolam/nitrendipine**, **triazolam/isradipine** or **temazepam/diltiazem**.

1. Etoh A, Kohno K. Studies on the drug interaction of diltiazem. IV. Relationship between first pass metabolism of various drugs and the absorption enhancing effect of diltiazem. *Yakugaku Zasshi* (1983) 103, 581–8.
2. Kosuge K, Jun Y, Watanabe H, Kimura M, Nishimoto M, Ishizaki T, Ohashi K. Effects of CYP3A4 inhibition by diltiazem on pharmacokinetics and dynamics of diazepam in relation to CYP2C19 genotype status. *Drug Metab Dispos* (2001) 29, 1284–9.
3. Meyer BH, Müller FO, Hundt HKL, Luus HG, de la Rey N, Röthig H-J. The effects of felodipine on the pharmacokinetics of diazepam. *Int J Clin Pharmacol Ther Toxicol* (1992) 30, 117–21.
4. Heine PR, Weyer G, Breuel H-P, Mück W, Schmage N, Kuhlmann J. Lack of interaction between diazepam and nimodipine during chronic oral administration to healthy elderly subjects. *Br J Clin Pharmacol* (1994) 38, 39–43.

5. Backman JT, Olkkola KT, Aranko K, Himberg J-J, Neuvonen PJ. Dose of midazolam should be reduced during diltiazem and verapamil treatments. *Br J Clin Pharmacol* (1994) 37, 221–5.

6. Ahonen J, Olkkola KT, Salmenperä M, Hynynen M, Neuvonen PJ. Effect of diltiazem on midazolam and alfentanil disposition in patients undergoing coronary artery bypass grafting. *Anesthesiology* (1996) 85, 1246–52.

7. Handel J, Ziegler G, Gemeinhardt A, Stuber H, Fischer C, Klotz U. Lack of effect of nitrendipine on the pharmacokinetics and pharmacodynamics of midazolam during steady state. *Br J Clin Pharmacol* (1988) 25, 243–50.

8. Scharf MB, Sachais BA, Mayleben DW, Jennings SW. The effects of a calcium channel blocker on the effects of temazepam and triazolam. *Curr Ther Res* (1990) 48, 516–23.

9. Kosuge K, Nishimoto M, Kimura M, Umemura K, Nakashima K, Ohashi K. Effect of diltiazem on pharmacokinetics and dynamics of triazolam in healthy volunteers. *Jpn J Pharmacol* (1996) 71, 249P.

10. Kosuge K, Nishimoto M, Kimura M, Umemura K, Nakashima K, Ohashi K. Enhanced effect of triazolam with diltiazem. *Br J Clin Pharmacol* (1997) 43, 367–72.

11. Varhe A, Olkkola KT, Neuvonen PJ. Diltiazem interacts with triazolam. *Therapie* (1995) 50 (Suppl), 419.

12. Varhe A, Olkkola KT, Neuvonen PJ. Diltiazem enhances the effects of triazolam by inhibiting its metabolism. *Clin Pharmacol Ther* (1996) 59, 369–75.

13. Backman JT, Wang J-S, Wen X, Kivistö KT, Neuvonen PJ. Mibefradil but not isradipine substantially elevates the plasma concentrations of the CYP3A4 substrate triazolam. *Clin Pharmacol Ther* (1999) 66, 401–7.

Benzodiazepines + Ciprofloxacin or Gatifloxacin

Ciprofloxacin causes a marked reduction in the clearance of diazepam, but this does not appear to be clinically important in most individuals. Ciprofloxacin appears not to interact with temazepam. There is no pharmacokinetic interaction between gatifloxacin and midazolam.

Clinical evidence, mechanism, importance and management

(a) Ciprofloxacin

Ciprofloxacin 500 mg twice daily for 3 days was found to have no effect on the pharmacokinetics of **diazepam** in a study in 10 healthy subjects.[1] However, a later study found that 500 mg **ciprofloxacin** twice daily for 5 days increased the AUC of a single 5 mg intravenous dose of **diazepam** in 12 healthy subjects by 50% and reduced its clearance by 37%, possibly by inhibiting the metabolism of the **diazepam**. The **diazepam** half-life was doubled. This caused no significant changes in the performance of a number of psychometric tests.[2] Another study by the same group found that **ciprofloxacin** does not interact with **temazepam**.[3]

It seems unlikely that any marked increases in **diazepam** effects (drowsiness etc.) will occur in most patients, but it may possibly be significant in those who have reduced renal or hepatic clearance (e.g. the elderly).[2] More study is needed to find out whether this interaction is clinically important or not.

(b) Gatifloxacin

Gatifloxacin 400 mg daily for 5 days had no effect on the pharmacokinetics of **midazolam** in 14 healthy subjects. The pharmacokinetics of **gatifloxacin** were also unaffected by concurrent use.[4]

1. Wijnands WJA, Trooster JFG, Teunissen PC, Cats HA, Vree TB. Ciprofloxacin does not impair the elimination of diazepam in humans. *Drug Metab Dispos* (1990) 18, 954–7.

2. Kamali F, Thomas SHL, Edwards C. The influence of steady-state ciprofloxacin on the pharmacokinetics and pharmacodynamics of a single dose of diazepam in healthy volunteers. *Eur J Clin Pharmacol* (1993) 44, 365–7.

3. Kamali F, Nicholson E, Edwards C. Ciprofloxacin does not influence temazepam pharmacokinetics. *Br J Clin Pharmacol* (1994) 37, 118P.

4. Grasela DM, LaCreta FP, Kollia GD, Randall DM, Uderman HD. Open-label, nonrandomized study of the effects of gatifloxacin on the pharmacokinetics of midazolam in healthy male volunteers. *Pharmacotherapy* (2000) 20, 330–5.

Benzodiazepines + Colestyramine and Neomycin

The loss of lorazepam from the body is increased by colestyramine plus neomycin.

Clinical evidence, mechanism, importance and management

A study in 7 healthy subjects found that **neomycin** 1 g six hourly plus **colestyramine** 4 g four-hourly reduced the half-life of **oral lorazepam** by 26% (from 15.8 to 11.7 h) and increased the clearance of free **lorazepam** by 34% (from 8.5 to 11.39 ml/min/kg).[1] The reasons are not clear but parallel studies using **intravenous lorazepam**[1] suggested that these two drugs may interfere with the possible enterohepatic circulation of **lorazepam**.

The clinical importance of this interaction is uncertain but probably small, however be alert for any evidence of a reduced **lorazepam** effect. Increase the dose if necessary. Separating the dosages may not prevent this interaction if it is true that the enterohepatic circulation is involved. There is no evidence as yet that other benzodiazepines interact similarly.

1. Herman RJ, Duc Van Pham J, Szakacs CBN. Disposition of lorazepam in human beings: enterohepatic recirculation and first-pass effect. *Clin Pharmacol Ther* (1989) 46, 18–25.

Benzodiazepines or Meprobamate + Contraceptives, oral

Oral contraceptives can increase the effects of alprazolam, chlordiazepoxide, diazepam, nitrazepam and triazolam, and reduce the effects of oxazepam, lorazepam and temazepam, but whether in practice there is a need for dosage adjustments has not been determined. Chlordiazepoxide, diazepam, nitrazepam and meprobamate can also possibly increase the incidence of break-through bleeding.

Clinical evidence

(a) Alprazolam, Chlordiazepoxide, Clotiazepam, Diazepam, Nitrazepam or Triazolam + Oral contraceptives

A controlled study showed that the mean half-life of **chlordiazepoxide** (0.6 mg/kg, given intravenously) was virtually double (11.6 h compared to 20.6 h) and the total clearance was almost two-thirds lower in 6 women on **oral contraceptives** when compared to 6 women on no medication.[1]

Similar but less marked effects were found in other studies with **chlordiazepoxide**,[2] **diazepam**,[3,4] **alprazolam**[5] and to an even lesser extent with **triazolam**[5] and **nitrazepam**.[6] No changes were seen with **clotiazepam**[7] or **midazolam** given intramuscularly.[8]

(b) Lorazepam, Oxazepam or Temazepam + Oral contraceptives

A controlled study, comparing 7 women on the **oral contraceptive pill** with 8 women on no medication showed that the mean half-life of **lorazepam** (2 mg, given intravenously) was over 50% lower in the **oral contraceptives** group (6 h compared to 14 h) and the total clearance was over threefold greater.[1]

A smaller change was seen in other controlled studies with **lorazepam**,[5,9] and **temazepam**,[5] and in two other studies small falls in the half-life of **oxazepam** were observed.[1,9]

(c) Contraceptive effects decreased

A study in 72 patients taking **combined oral contraceptives** (*Rigevidon*, *Anteovin*) found that break-through bleeding occurred in 36.1% while taking daily doses of 10 to 20 mg **chlordiazepoxide**, 5 to 15 mg **diazepam**, 5 to 10 mg **nitrazepam** or 200 to 600 mg **meprobamate**, but no pregnancies occurred. Only three cases occurred with **diazepam** or **nitrazepam**.[10] The average values for break-through bleeding with these two oral contraceptives were 9.1% for *Rigevidon* and 3.3% for *Anteovin* in the absence of other drugs. It was possible to establish a causal relationship between the bleeding and the use of the tranquilliser or hypnotic in 77% of the cases either by stopping the drug or by exchanging it for another.[10]

Mechanisms

Oral contraceptives affect the metabolism of the benzodiazepines by the liver in different ways: oxidative metabolism is reduced (alprazolam, chlordiazepoxide, diazepam, etc.), whereas metabolism by glucuronide conjugation is increased (lorazepam, oxazepam, temazepam, etc.). Just why these tranquillisers should cause breakthrough bleeding is not understood.

Importance and management

Established interactions but of uncertain clinical importance. Long-term use of benzodiazepines that are highly oxidised (alprazolam, chlordiazepoxide, diazepam, nitrazepam, etc.) in women on the pill should be monitored to ensure that the dosage is not too high. Those taking glucuronidated benzodiazepines (lorazepam, oxazepam, temazepam, etc.) may need a dosage increase. Clotiazepam and midazolam appear not to interact. More study is needed to find out if any these interactions is of real practical importance. No firm conclusions could be drawn from the results of one study, which set out to evaluate the importance of this interaction.[11]

The increased incidence of break-through bleeding (more than one-third) due to these tranquillisers which is described in the report cited above, is an unpleasant reaction and it suggests that the contraceptive is possibly unreliable, but no outright contraceptive failures were actually reported.[10] Limited evidence from the study suggests that changing the tranquilliser or the contraceptive might be the answer.

1. Patwardhan RV, Mitchell MC, Johnson RF, Schenker S. Differential effects of oral contraceptive steroids on the metabolism of benzodiazepines. *Hepatology* (1983) 3, 248–53.
2. Roberts RK, Desmond PV, Wilkinson GR, Schenker S. Disposition of chlordiazepoxide: sex differences and effects of oral contraceptives. *Clin Pharmacol Ther* (1979) 25, 826–31.
3. Giles HG, Sellers EM, Naranjo CA, Frecker RC, Greenblatt DJ. Disposition of intravenous diazepam in young men and women. *Eur J Clin Pharmacol* (1981) 20, 207–13.
4. Abernethy DR, Greenblatt DJ, Divoll M, Arendt R, Ochs HR, Shader RI. Impairment of diazepam metabolism by low-dose estrogen-containing oral-contraceptive steroids. *N Engl J Med* (1982) 306, 791–2.
5. Stoehr GP, Kroboth PD, Juhl RP, Wender DB, Phillips P, Smith RB. Effect of oral contraceptives on triazolam, temazepam, alprazolam, and lorazepam kinetics. *Clin Pharmacol Ther* (1984) 36, 683–90.
6. Jochemsen R, Van der Graff M, Boejinga JK, Breimer DD. Influence of sex, menstrual cycle and oral contraception on the disposition of nitrazepam. *Br J Clin Pharmacol* (1982) 13, 319–24.
7. Ochs HR, Greenblatt DJ, Verburg-Ochs B, Harmatz JS, Grehl H. Disposition of clotiazepam: influence of age, sex, oral contraceptives, cimetidine, isoniazid and ethanol. *Eur J Clin Pharmacol* (1984) 26, 55–9.
8. Holazo AA, Winkler MB, Patel IH. Effects of age, gender and oral contraceptives on intramuscular midazolam pharmacokinetics. *J Clin Pharmacol* (1988) 28, 1040–5.
9. Abernethy DR, Greenblatt DJ, Ochs HR, Weyers D, Divoll M, Harmatz JS, Shader RI. Lorazepam and oxazepam kinetics in women on low-dose oral contraceptives. *Clin Pharmacol Ther* (1983) 33, 628–32.
10. Somos P. Interaction between certain psychopharmaca and low-dose oral contraceptives. *Ther Hung* (1990) 38, 37–40.
11. Kroboth PD, Smith RB, Stoehr GP, Juhl RP. Pharmacodynamic evaluation of the benzodiazepine–oral contraceptive interaction. *Clin Pharmacol Ther* (1985) 38, 525–32.

Benzodiazepines + Dextropropoxyphene (Propoxyphene)

Some evidence suggests that the combined CNS depressant effects of alprazolam and dextropropoxyphene may be greater than with other benzodiazepines because the serum levels of alprazolam may be increased.

Clinical evidence, mechanism, importance and management

A study in healthy subjects showed that while taking 65 mg **dextropropoxyphene** six-hourly the pharmacokinetics of single doses of **diazepam** and **lorazepam** were not significantly changed. In the case of **alprazolam**, the half-life was prolonged from 11.6 to 18.3 h, and its clearance fell from 1.3 to 0.8 ml/min/kg.[1] It would seem that **dextropropoxyphene** inhibits the metabolism (hydroxylation) of the **alprazolam** by the liver, thereby reducing its loss from the body, but has little or no effect on the *N*-demethylation or glucuronidation of

the other two benzodiazepines. The clinical importance of this is uncertain, but the inference to be drawn is that the CNS depressant effects of **alprazolam** will be increased, over and above the simple additive CNS depressant effects likely when other benzodiazepines and **dextropropoxyphene** are taken together. More study is needed.

1. Abernethy DR, Greenblatt DJ, Morse DS, Shader RI. Interaction of propoxyphene with diazepam, alprazolam and lorazepam. *Br J Clin Pharmacol* (1985) 19, 51–7.

Benzodiazepines + Disulfiram

An isolated report describes temazepam toxicity due to disulfiram. The serum levels of chlordiazepoxide and diazepam are increased by the use of disulfiram and some patients may possibly experience increased drowsiness. Alprazolam, oxazepam and lorazepam are either not affected or only minimally affected.

Clinical evidence

A man on 200 mg **disulfiram** daily developed confusion, drowsiness, slurred speech and an unsteady gait within a few days of starting to take 20 mg **temazepam** at night. This was interpreted as **temazepam** toxicity. The symptoms disappeared when both drugs were stopped.[1]

After taking 500 mg **disulfiram** daily for 14 to 16 days, the plasma clearances of single doses of **chlordiazepoxide** and **diazepam** were reduced by 54 and 41% respectively and the half-lives were increased by 84 and 37% respectively. The plasma levels of **chlordiazepoxide** were approximately doubled. Changes in the pharmacokinetic parameters of **oxazepam** were minimal. No differences were noted between the alcoholic subjects (without hepatic cirrhosis) and the healthy subjects.[2]

Another paper by the same workers shows that **lorazepam** behaves like **oxazepam**,[3] and the pharmacokinetics of **alprazolam** are unaffected by **disulfiram**.[4]

Mechanism

Disulfiram inhibits the initial metabolism (*N*-demethylation and oxidation) of both chlordiazepoxide and diazepam by the liver so that an alternative but slower metabolic pathway is used, which results in the accumulation of these benzodiazepines in the body. In contrast, the metabolism (glucuronidation) of oxazepam and lorazepam is minimally affected by disulfiram so that their clearance from the body remains largely unaffected.[2,3]

Importance and management

There seems to be only one report (with temazepam) about a clinically significant disulfiram/benzodiazepine interaction. The other reports only describe potential interactions which have been identified by single dose studies. These do not necessarily reliably predict what will happen in practice. However, it seems possible that some patients will experience increased drowsiness (a) possibly because of this interaction, and (b) because drowsiness is a very common side-effect of disulfiram. Reduce the dosage of the benzodiazepine if necessary. Other benzodiazepines which are metabolised similarly may possibly interact in the same way (e.g. bromazepam, clonazepam, clorazepate, prazepam, ketazolam, clobazam, flurazepam, nitrazepam, medazepam, triazolam) but this needs confirmation. Alprazolam, oxazepam and lorazepam appear to be non-interacting alternatives.

1. Hardman M, Biniwale A, Clarke CE. Temazepam toxicity precipitated by disulfiram. *Lancet* (1994) 344, 1231–2.
2. MacLeod SM, Sellers EM, Giles HG, Billings BJ, Martin PR, Greenblatt DJ, Marshman JA. Interaction of disulfiram with benzodiazepines. *Clin Pharmacol Ther* (1978) 24, 583–9.
3. Sellers EM, Giles HG, Greenblatt DJ, Naranjo CA. Differential effects on benzodiazepine disposition by disulfiram and ethanol. *Arzneimittelforschung* (1980) 30, 882–6.
4. Diquet B, Gujadhur L, Lamiable D, Warot D, Hayoun H, Choisy H. Lack of interaction between disulfiram and alprazolam in alcoholic patients. *Eur J Clin Pharmacol* (1990) 38, 157–60.

Benzodiazepines + Ethambutol

Ethambutol appears not to interact with diazepam.

Clinical evidence, mechanism, importance and management

A study in 6 patients, newly diagnosed as having tuberculosis and treated with **ethambutol** (25 mg/kg), showed that although some of the pharmacokinetic parameters of **diazepam** were different to those obtained in healthy control subjects, the changes were not significant.[1] There seems to be nothing in the literature to suggest that **ethambutol** interacts with other benzodiazepines.

1. Ochs HR, Greenblatt DJ, Roberts G-M, Dengler HJ. Diazepam interaction with antituberculosis drugs. *Clin Pharmacol Ther* (1981) 29, 671–8.

Benzodiazepines + Food

Food can delay and reduce the hypnotic effects of flunitrazepam and loprazolam.

Clinical evidence, mechanism, importance and management

A study in 2 groups of 8 subjects found that when they took single 2-mg doses of **flunitrazepam** or **loprazolam** 2 h after an **evening dinner** (spaghetti, meat, salad, an apple and wine) and 1 h before going to bed, the peak plasma levels of the 2 hypnotics were reduced by 63% and 41% respectively. The time to reach these levels were delayed by 2.5 and 3.6 h respectively, and the absorption half-lives of the drugs were considerably prolonged.[1] It seems probable therefore that in a 'real-life' situation the onset of sleep would be delayed and the effects of these benzodiazepines would be reduced by **food**.

1. Bareggi SR, Pirola R, Truci G, Leva S, Smirna S. Effect of after-dinner administration on the pharmacokinetics of oral flunitrazepam and loprazolam. *J Clin Pharmacol* (1988) 28, 371–5.

Benzodiazepines + Grapefruit juice

Grapefruit juice can increase the bioavailability of oral diazepam, midazolam and triazolam but there is evidence that this may be of little practical importance.

Clinical evidence

Eight healthy subjects were given either 5 mg of **intravenous midazolam** or 15 mg of **oral midazolam** after drinking 200 ml **grapefruit juice** 60 min and 15 min previously. The pharmacokinetics of the **intravenous midazolam** remained unchanged, but the AUC of the **oral midazolam** was increased by 52%, and its maximum plasma levels rose by 56%. These changes were also reflected in the psychometric measurements made.[1]

A single oral 250-microgram dose of **triazolam** was given to 10 healthy subjects with either 250 ml **grapefruit juice** or water. The mean AUC of the **triazolam** was increased 1.5-fold by the **grapefruit juice**. The peak serum levels were increased 1.3-fold, and the time when the serum levels peaked was prolonged from 1.5 to 2.5 h. A slight decrease in psychomotor performance occurred (more drowsiness and tiredness).[2] Another study of the interaction between **triazolam** and **grapefruit juice** found that the effects of the **grapefruit juice** were much more pronounced when multiple doses of **grapefruit juice** were given. The **triazolam** AUC and half-life was increased by about 50% and 6% when single doses of **grapefruit juice** were given, and by almost 150% and 54% by multiple doses. The effect of **grapefruit juice** on psychomotor tests was also greater after multiple dosing.[3]

A large scale placebo controlled study in a total of 120 healthy young medical students used psychomotor tests to measure the effect of benzodiazepines with and without **grapefruit juice**. Subjects were given 10 mg **midazolam** or 250 micrograms **triazolam** with 300 ml **grapefruit juice**. Only a minor increase in the benzodiazepine effects occurred with concurrent **grapefruit juice**, and these effects were of little or no practical importance.[4]

A study in 8 healthy subjects found that 250 ml **grapefruit juice** increased the AUC of a single 5 mg oral dose of **diazepam** 3.2-fold and the maximum serum levels were increased 1.5-fold.[5]

Mechanism

The evidence suggests that some components within the grapefruit juice (probably naringin amongst others) inhibit intestinal metabolism of these benzodiazepines by the cytochrome P450 isoenzyme CYP3A4, so that more is left to enter the circulation.[1]

Importance and management

Established interactions but probably of minor practical importance. These increases in bioavailability might be expected to increase the extent of the sedation and amnesia due to these benzodiazepines but in young healthy adults (with midazolam and triazolam at least) this is apparently of little importance. The clinical effects of this interaction with diazepam appear not to have been investigated. What is not clear is whether other factors such as old age or liver cirrhosis might increase the effects. Information about other benzodiazepines appears, as yet, to be lacking.

1. Kupferschmidt HHT, Ha HR, Ziegler WH, Meier PJ, Krähenbühl S. Interaction between grapefruit juice and midazolam in humans. *Clin Pharmacol Ther* (1995) 58, 20–8.
2. Hukkinen SK, Varhe A, Olkkola KT, Neuvonen PJ. Plasma concentrations of triazolam are increased by concomitant ingestion of grapefruit juice. *Clin Pharmacol Ther* (1995) 58, 127–31.
3. Lilja JJ, Kivistö KT, Backman JT, Neuvonen PJ. Effect of grapefruit juice dose on grapefruit juice–triazolam interaction: repeated consumption prolongs triazolam half-life. *Eur J Clin Pharmacol* (2000) 56, 411–15.
4. Vanakoski J, Mattila MJ, Seppälä T. Grapefruit juice does not enhance the effects of midazolam and triazolam in man. *Eur J Clin Pharmacol* (1996) 50, 501–8.
5. Özdemir M, Aktan Y, Boydağ BS, Cingi MI, Musmul A. Interaction between grapefruit juice and diazepam in humans. *Eur J Drug Metab Pharmacokinet* (1998) 23, 55–9.

Benzodiazepines + 5-HT$_3$ receptor antagonists

Lorazepam and granisetron, and temazepam and ondansetron appear not to interact.

Clinical evidence, mechanism, importance and management

Lorazepam 2.5 mg clearly affected the performance of a number of psychometric tests by 12 healthy subjects. Statistically significant increases occurred in drowsiness, feebleness, muzziness, clumsiness, lethargy, mental slowness, relaxation, dreaminess, incompetence, sadness and withdrawal. But there was very little evidence that 160 micrograms/kg **granisetron** alone had any effect on the performance of these tests except that clumsiness and inattentiveness were increased, nor was there evidence that **granisetron** added to the effects of **lorazepam** when taken concurrently.[1]

Temazepam 20 mg was given to 24 healthy subjects with a placebo or 8 mg **ondansetron** in a double-blind crossover study. The pharmacokinetics of the **temazepam** were found to be unchanged by the **ondansetron** and the psychomotor performances of the subjects (subjective and objective sedation, memory and other measurements) were not influenced by the presence of the **ondansetron**.[2]

No additional special precautions would seem to be necessary on concurrent use.

1. Leigh TJ, Link CGG, Fell GL. Effects of granisetron and lorazepam, alone and in combination, on psychometric performance. *Br J Clin Pharmacol* (1991) 31, 333–6.
2. Preston GC, Keene ON, Palmer JL. The effect of ondansetron on the pharmacokinetics and pharmacodynamics of temazepam. *Anaesthesia* (1996) 51, 827–30.

Benzodiazepines + H₂-blockers

The serum levels of **adinazolam, alprazolam, chlordiazepoxide, clobazam, clorazepate, diazepam, flurazepam, nitrazepam, triazolam (and probably halazepam and prazepam) are raised by cimetidine,** but normally this appears to be of little or no clinical importance and only the occasional patient may experience an increase in the effects (sedation). **Clotiazepam, lorazepam, lormetazepam, oxazepam and temazepam are not normally affected by cimetidine. Famotidine, nizatidine and ranitidine do not interact with most benzodiazepines, except possibly triazolam. The picture with midazolam is somewhat confused.**

Clinical evidence

(a) Benzodiazepines + Cimetidine

A combined serum level rise of 75% in **diazepam** and **desmethyldiazepam** (the active metabolite) was seen in 10 patients after taking 1200 mg **cimetidine** daily for 2 weeks, but reaction times and other motor and intellectual tests remained unaffected.[1] Other reports also describe a rise in the plasma levels and/or AUC of **diazepam** (associated with increased sedation in one report[2]) due to **cimetidine**.[3-10] Generalised incoordination has also been described in one individual.[11]

Cimetidine also causes rises in the serum levels of other benzodiazepines: **adinazolam,**[12] **alprazolam,**[13,14] **chlordiazepoxide,**[15] **clobazam,**[16] **clorazepate,**[17] **flurazepam,**[18] **nitrazepam,**[19] and **triazolam.**[13,14] Liver cirrhosis increases the effects of **cimetidine** on the loss of **chlordiazepoxide.**[20] Confusion has been reported in a man of 50 on **clorazepate** when given **cimetidine,**[21] and increased sedation has been seen in some patients on **adinazolam** and **cimetidine.**[12] Prolonged hypnosis in an elderly woman[22] and CNS toxicity (including lethargy and hallucinations)[23] in a woman of 49 have been attributed to a **triazolam/cimetidine** interaction but this remains unconfirmed.

In contrast **cimetidine** does not normally interact with clobazam,[24] clotiazepam,[25] **lorazepam,**[18] **lormetazepam,**[26] **oxazepam**[18] or **temazepam,**[27,28] although prolonged post-operative sedation was seen in one patient on **oxazepam** and **cimetidine.**[29]

There is some controversy about whether or not **midazolam** is affected by **cimetidine.** An increase in sedation,[30] an increase in midazolam levels[31] and no pharmacokinetic interaction[32,33] have been reported with the combination.

(b) Benzodiazepines + Famotidine, Nizatidine, Ranitidine or Roxatidine

Ranitidine does not interact significantly with **diazepam,**[34,35] **adinazolam**[36] or **temazepam.**[28,37] **Famotidine** does not interact with **bromazepam,**[38] **clorazepate,**[38] **chlordiazepoxide,**[38] **diazepam**[6,10,39] or **triazolam,**[38] but **ranitidine** can modestly increase the bioavailability (by about 10 to 30%) of oral **triazolam.**[40,41] **Nizatidine** does not interact significantly with **diazepam.**[35,42,43] There is some controversy about whether **midazolam** is or is not affected by **ranitidine.** Increases in sedation have been reported on a number of occasions,[30,31,37,44] but a lack of effect has also been documented.[32,33] **Roxatidine** does not interact with **diazepam** or **desmethyldiazepam.**[45]

Mechanism

Cimetidine inhibits the liver enzymes concerned with the *N*-dealkylation plus oxidation or nitro-reduction of diazepam, alprazolam, chlordiazepoxide, clorazepate, flurazepam, nitrazepam and triazolam. As a result their clearance from the body is reduced and their serum levels rise. Lorazepam, oxazepam and temazepam are metabolised by a different metabolic pathway involving glucuronidation, which is not affected by cimetidine and so they do not usually interact. Ranitidine, famotidine and nizatidine appear not to inhibit liver microsomal enzymes. There is some evidence that ranitidine increases the absorption of triazolam, and possibly other benzodiazepines due to changes in gastric pH.[41] Cimetidine may similarly affect absorption.[3]

Importance and management

The benzodiazepine/cimetidine interactions are well documented (not all the references are listed here) but normally they appear to be of little clinical importance, although a few patients may be adversely affected (increased effects, drowsiness, etc.). Reports of problems are very few indeed, particularly when viewed against the very common use of both drugs. Lorazepam, lormetazepam, oxazepam and temazepam are non-interacting alternative benzodiazepines. Ranitidine does not interact with diazepam or temazepam, and neither nizatidine, ranitidine nor famotidine would be expected to interact with other benzodiazepines which are metabolised similarly (see 'Mechanism' above) although the effects of oral triazolam are possibly very slightly increased. The situation with midazolam is unclear and so it would seem wise to be cautious when using any H₂-blocker with this drug.

1. Greenblatt DJ, Abernethy DR, Morse DS, Harmatz JS and Shader RI. Clinical importance of the interaction of diazepam and cimetidine. *Anesth Analg* (1986) 65, 176–80.
2. Klotz U, Reimann I. Delayed clearance of diazepam due to cimetidine. *N Engl J Med* (1980) 302, 1012–13.
3. McGowan WAW, Dundee JW. The effect of intravenous cimetidine on the absorption of orally administered diazepam and lorazepam. *Br J Clin Pharmacol* (1982) 14, 207–11.
4. Klotz U, Reimann I. Elevation of steady-state diazepam levels by cimetidine. *Clin Pharmacol Ther* (1981) 30, 513–17.
5. Gough PA, Curry SH, Araujo OE, Robinson JD, Dallman JJ. Influence of cimetidine on oral diazepam elimination with measurement of subsequent cognitive change. *Br J Clin Pharmacol* (1982) 14, 739–42.
6. Locniskar A, Greenblatt DJ, Harmatz JS, Zinny MA. Influence of famotidine and cimetidine on the pharmacokinetic properties of intravenous diazepam. *J Clin Pharmacol* (1985) 25, 459–60.
7. Klotz U, Antilla V-J. Drug interactions with cimetidine: pharmacokinetic studies to evaluate its mechanism. *Naunyn Schmiedebergs Arch Pharmacol* (1980) 311, R77.
8. Bressler R, Carter D, Winters L. Enprostil, in contrast to cimetidine, does not affect diazepam pharmacokinetics. *Adv Therapy* (1988) 5, 306–12.
9. Lima DR, Santos RM, Werneck E, Andrade GN. Effect of orally administered misoprostol and cimetidine on the steady state pharmacokinetics of diazepam and nordiazepam in human volunteers. *Eur J Drug Metab Pharmacokinet* (1991) 16, 161–70.
10. Locniskar A, Greenblatt DJ, Harmatz JS, Zinny MA, Shader RI. Interaction of diazepam with famotidine and cimetidine, two H₂-receptor antagonists. *J Clin Pharmacol* (1986) 26, 299–303.
11. Anon. Court warns on interaction of drugs. *Doctor* (1979) 9, 1.
12. Hulhoven R, Desager JP, Cox S, Harvengt C. Influence of repeated administration of cimetidine on the pharmacokinetics and pharmacodynamics of adinazolam in healthy subjects. *Eur J Clin Pharmacol* (1988) 35, 59–64.
13. Pourbaix S, Desager JP, Hulhoven R, Smith RB, Harvengt C. Pharmacokinetic consequences of long term coadministration of cimetidine and triazolobenzodiazepines, alprazolam and triazolam, in healthy subjects. *Int J Clin Pharmacol Ther Toxicol* (1985) 23, 447–51.
14. Abernethy DR, Greenblatt DJ, Divoll M, Moschitto LJ, Harmatz JS, Shader RI. Interaction of cimetidine with the triazolobenzodiazepines alprazolam and triazolam. *Psychopharmacology (Berl)* (1983) 80, 275–8.
15. Desmond PV, Patwardhan RV, Schenker S, Speeg KV. Cimetidine impairs elimination of chlordiazepoxide (Librium) in man. *Ann Intern Med* (1980) 93, 266–8.
16. Pullar T, Edwards D, Haigh JRM, Peaker S, Feeley MP. The effect of cimetidine on the single dose pharmacokinetics of oral clobazam and N-desmethylclobazam. *Br J Clin Pharmacol* (1987) 23, 317–21.
17. Divoll M, Abernethy DR, Greenblatt DJ. Cimetidine impairs drug oxidizing capacity in the elderly. *Clin Pharmacol Ther* (1982) 31, 218.
18. Greenblatt DJ, Abernethy DR, Koepke HH, Shader RI. Interaction of cimetidine with oxazepam, lorazepam, and flurazepam. *J Clin Pharmacol* (1984) 24, 187–93.
19. Ochs HR, Greenblatt DJ, Gugler R, Müntefering G, Locniskar A, Abernethy DR. Cimetidine impairs nitrazepam clearance. *Clin Pharmacol Ther* (1983) 34, 227–30.
20. Nelson DC, Schenker S, Hoyumpa AM, Speeg KV, Avant GR. The effects of cimetidine on chlordiazepoxide elimination in cirrhosis. *Clin Res* (1981) 29, 824A.
21. Bouden A, El Hechmi Z, Douki S. Cimetidine-benzodiazepine association confusiogene: a propos d'une observation. *Tunis Med* (1990) 68, 63–4.
22. Parker WA, MacLachlan RA. Prolonged hypnotic response to triazolam-cimetidine combination in an elderly patient. *Drug Intell Clin Pharm* (1984) 18, 980–1.
23. Britton ML, Waller ES. Central nervous system toxicity associated with concurrent use of triazolam and cimetidine. *Drug Intell Clin Pharm* (1985) 19, 666–8.
24. Grigoleit H-G, Hajdú P, Hundt HKL, Koeppen D, Malerczyk V, Meyer BH, Müller FO, Witte PU. Pharmacokinetic aspects of the interaction between clobazam and cimetidine. *Eur J Clin Pharmacol* (1983) 25, 139–42.
25. Ochs HR, Greenblatt DJ, Verburg-Ochs B, Harmatz JS, Grehl H. Disposition of clotiazepam: influence of age, sex, oral contraceptives, cimetidine, isoniazid and ethanol. *Eur J Clin Pharmacol* (1984) 26, 55–9.
26. Doenicke A, Dorow R, Täuber U. Die Pharmakokinetik von Lormetazepam nach Cimetidin. *Anaesthesist* (1991) 40, 675–9.
27. Greenblatt DJ, Abernethy DR, Divoll M, Locniskar A, Harmatz JS, Shader RI. Noninteraction of temazepam and cimetidine. *J Pharm Sci* (1984) 73, 399–401.
28. Elliott P, Dundee JW, Collier PS, McClean E. The influence of two H₂-receptor antagonists, cimetidine and ranitidine, on the systemic availability of temazepam. *Br J Anaesth* (1984) 56, 800P–801P.
29. Lam AM, Parkin JA. Cimetidine and prolonged post-operative somnolence. *Can Anaesth Soc J* (1981) 28, 450–2.
30. Sanders LD, Whitehead C, Gildersleve CD, Rosen M, Robinson JO. Interaction of H₂-receptor antagonists and benzodiazepine sedation. *Anaesthesia* (1993) 48, 286–92.
31. Fee JPH, Collier PS, Howard PJ, Dundee JW. Cimetidine and ranitidine increase midazolam bioavailability. *Clin Pharmacol Ther* (1987) 41, 80–4.
32. Greenblatt DJ, Locniskar A, Scavone JM, Blyden GT, Ochs HR, Harmatz JS, Shader RI. Absence of interaction of cimetidine and ranitidine with intravenous and oral midazolam. *Anesth Analg* (1986) 65, 176–80.
33. Ochs HR, Greenblatt DJ, Shader I. Absence of interaction of cimetidine and ranitidine with intravenous and oral midazolam. *Dig Dis Sci* (1986) 31 (Suppl), 194S.

34. Klotz U, Reimann IW, Ohnhaus EE. Effect of ranitidine on the steady state pharmacokinetics of diazepam. *Eur J Clin Pharmacol* (1983) 24, 357–60.
35. Klotz U, Gottlieb W, Keohane PP, Dammann HG. Nocturnal doses of ranitidine and nizatidine do not affect the disposition of diazepam. *J Clin Pharmacol* (1987) 27, 210–12.
36. Suttle AB, Songer SS, Dukes GE, Hak LJ, Koruda M, Fleishaker JC, Brouwer KLR. Ranitidine does not alter adinazolam pharmacokinetics or pharmacodynamics. *Clin Pharmacol Ther* (1991) 49, 178.
37. Dundee JW, Wilson CM, Robinson FP, Thompson EM, Elliott P. The effect of ranitidine on the hypnotic action of single doses of midazolam, temazepam and zopiclone. *Br J Clin Pharmacol* (1985) 19, 553P–554P.
38. Chichmanian RM, Mignot G, Spreux A, Jean-Girard C, Hofliger P. Tolérance de la famotidine. Étude du réseau médecins sentinelles en pharmacovigilance. *Therapie* (1992) 47, 239–43.
39. Klotz U, Arvela P, Rosenkranz B. Famotidine, a new H_2-receptor antagonist, does not affect hepatic elimination of diazepam or tubular secretion of procainamide. *Eur J Clin Pharmacol* (1985) 28, 671–5.
40. Vanderveen RP, Jirak JL, Peters GR, Cox SR, Bombardt PA. Effect of ranitidine on the disposition of orally and intravenously administered triazolam. *Clin Pharm* (1991) 10, 539–43.
41. O'Connor-Semmes RL, Kersey K, Lam R, Davis IM, Koch KM, Powell JR. Use of metabolite data to determine mechanism of ranitidine-triazolam interaction in the young and elderly. *Clin Pharmacol Ther* (1996) 59, 172.
42. Klotz U, Dammann HG, Gottlieb WR, Walter TA, Keohane P. Nizatidine (300 mg nocte) does not interfere with diazepam pharmacokinetics in man. *Br J Clin Pharmacol* (1987) 23, 105–6.
43. Klotz U. Lack of effect of nizatidine on drug metabolism. *Scand J Gastroenterol* (1987) 22 (Suppl 136), 18–23.
44. Elwood RJ, Hildebrand PJ, Dundee JW, Collier PS. Ranitidine influences the uptake of oral midazolam. *Br J Clin Pharmacol* (1983) 15, 743–5.
45. Labs RA. Interaction of roxatidine acetate with antacids, food and other drugs. *Drugs* (1988) 35 (Suppl 3), 82–9.

Benzodiazepines + Isoniazid

Isoniazid reduces the loss of both diazepam and triazolam from the body. Some increase in their effects would be expected. No interaction occurs with oxazepam or clotiazepam.

Clinical evidence

(a) Diazepam or triazolam

A study in 9 healthy subjects showed that after 3 days treatment with 90 mg **isoniazid** twice daily, the half-life of a single dose of **diazepam** was increased from about 34 to 45 h, and the total clearance reduced by 26%.[1] A study in 6 healthy subjects showed that after taking 90 mg **isoniazid** twice daily for 3 days, the half-life of a single dose of **triazolam** was increased from 2.5 to 3.3 h, the AUC was increased by 46% and the clearance was reduced by 43%.[2]

(b) Oxazepam or clotiazepam

A study in 9 healthy subjects showed that 90 mg **isoniazid** twice daily for 3 days had no effect on the pharmacokinetics of a single 30 mg oral dose of **oxazepam**.[2] Similarly the pharmacokinetics of **clotiazepam** were not altered in another study of the effects of **isoniazid**.[3]

Mechanism

What is known suggests that the isoniazid acts as an enzyme inhibitor, decreasing the metabolism and loss of diazepam and triazolam from the body, thereby increasing and prolonging their effects.

Importance and management

Information is limited but the interactions appear to be established. Their clinical importance is uncertain but be alert for the need to decrease the dosages of diazepam and triazolam if isoniazid is started. There seems to be no direct information about other benzodiazepines, but those undergoing high first-pass extraction and/or liver microsomal metabolism would be expected to interact similarly. Oxazepam and clotiazepam appear not to interact.

1. Ochs HR, Greenblatt DJ, Roberts G-M, Dengler HJ. Diazepam interaction with antituberculosis drugs. *Clin Pharmacol Ther* (1981) 29, 671–8.
2. Ochs HR, Greenblatt DJ, Knüchel M. Differential effect of isoniazid on triazolam oxidation and oxazepam conjugation. *Br J Clin Pharmacol* (1983) 16, 743–6.
3. Ochs HR, Greenblatt DJ, Verburg-Ochs B, Harmatz JS, Grehl H. Disposition of clotiazepam: influence of age, sex, oral contraceptives, cimetidine, isoniazid and ethanol. *Eur J Clin Pharmacol* (1984) 26, 55–9.

Benzodiazepines + Kava

A man on alprazolam became semicomatose a few days after starting to take kava.

Clinical evidence, mechanism, importance and management

A 54-year-old man taking **alprazolam**, cimetidine and terazosin was hospitalized in a lethargic and disorientated state three days after starting to take **kava** which he had bought from a local health food store. He denied having overdosed with any of these drugs. The patient became alert again after several hours.[1] The reason for what happened is not known, but the suggested explanation is that the **kava** α-**pyrones** might have had additive sedative effects with those of the **alprazolam**.[1,2] This is an isolated case and its general importance is not known.

1. Almeida JC, Grimsley EW. Coma from the health food store: interaction between kava and alprazolam. *Ann Intern Med* (1996) 125, 940–1.
2. Jussofie A, Schmiz A, Hiemke C. Kavapyrone enriched extract from *Piper methysticum* as modulator of GABA binding site in different regions of rat brain. *Psychopharmacology (Berl)* (1994) 116, 469–74.

Benzodiazepines + Macrolide antibacterials

The serum levels and effects of midazolam and triazolam are markedly increased and prolonged by the concurrent use of erythromycin. The same interaction has been seen between triazolam and clarithromycin, troleandomycin or josamycin, and between midazolam and clarithromycin. Roxithromycin has a weak effect on midazolam and triazolam, and erythromycin has a weak effect on diazepam, flunitrazepam, nitrazepam and temazepam, while azithromycin does not interact with midazolam. Erythromycin possibly increases the effects of alprazolam.

Clinical evidence

A. Alprazolam

(a) Alprazolam + Erythromycin

In vitro work using human liver microsomal enzymes has shown that **erythromycin** inhibits the metabolism of **alprazolam**.[1]

B. Diazepam

(a) Diazepam + Erythromycin

In a double-blind crossover study, 6 healthy subjects were given single 5 mg oral doses of **diazepam** after taking 500 mg **erythromycin** three times daily for a week. The **diazepam** AUC was increased by 15%, but its pharmacodynamic were unchanged.[2]

C. Flunitrazepam

(a) Flunitrazepam + Erythromycin

In a double-blind crossover study, 5 healthy subjects were given single 1 mg oral doses of **flunitrazepam** after taking 500 mg **erythromycin** three times daily for a week. The **flunitrazepam** AUC was increased by 25% but its pharmacodynamic effects were unchanged.[2]

D. Midazolam

(a) Midazolam + Azithromycin

A study in 64 healthy medical students found that 750 mg **azithromycin** had no effect on the metabolism of 10 or 15-mg doses of **midazolam**, and did not alter the performance of a number of psychomotor tests.[3] A study in 10 healthy subjects given 250 mg **azithromycin** daily found that some small changes in pharmacokinetics of 15 mg **midazolam** (a possible small delay in its onset of action), but its pharmacodynamic effects were unaltered.[4] Other studies confirm that **azithromycin** does not interact with **midazolam**.[5,6]

(b) Midazolam + Clarithromycin

Oral 4 mg and intravenous 0.05 mg/kg doses of **midazolam** were given simultaneously to 16 healthy subjects, before and after taking 500 mg **clarithromycin** twice daily for 7 days. It was found that the **clarithromycin** reduced the systemic clearance of the **midazolam** by about 64%, which resulted in a doubling of the **midazolam** induced sleeping time.[7] Similar results were found in another study.[6]

(c) Midazolam + Erythromycin

A study in 12 healthy subjects found that 500 mg **erythromycin** three times daily for 6 days almost tripled the peak serum levels of **midazolam** following a single 15-mg dose, more than doubled its half-life and increased the AUC more than fourfold. The subjects could hardly be wakened during the first hour after being given the **midazolam**, and most experienced amnesia lasting several hours.[8,9]

The serum **midazolam** levels (after 0.5 mg/kg premedication) of a boy of 8, about to undergo surgery, were approximately doubled when he was also given intravenous **erythromycin**. He developed nausea and tachycardia, and after 40 min (by which point he had received 200 mg **erythromycin**) he lost consciousness.[10] A patient in a coronary care unit given 300 mg intravenous **midazolam** over 14 h slept for about 6 days (apart from brief wakening when given fluma-zenil). The **midazolam** half-life was increased approximately ten-fold. This was attributed to an interaction due to the combined effects of 4 g **erythromycin** daily and 1.7 g **amiodarone** over 3 days.[11,12] An interaction between **midazolam** and **erythromycin** was suspected in another report, but it was obscured by the state of the patient and the use of other drugs.[13] A study in healthy subjects found that even a single 750-mg dose of **erythromycin** increased the sedative effects of a single 10-mg dose of **midazolam**.[14,15] Two other studies found that **erythromycin** increased the serum levels of **midazolam** two to threefold, and markedly worsened the performance of a number of psychomotor tests.[3,5]

(d) Midazolam + Roxithromycin

Roxithromycin 300 mg daily for 6 days increased the AUC of a single 15-mg dose of **midazolam** by about 47% in 10 healthy subjects, and lengthened the half-life from 1.7 to 2.2 h. Only minor psychomotor changes were seen.[16] A modest increase in the effects of **midazolam** were seen in another study in subjects given 300 mg **roxithromycin**, but the effects were very much weaker than those seen with erythromycin.[15]

E. Nitrazepam

(a) Nitrazepam + Erythromycin

When 10 healthy subjects were given 500 mg **erythromycin** three times daily for 4 days, the AUC of a single 5-mg dose of **nitrazepam** was increased by 25%, the peak serum levels were increased by 30% and the concentration peak time was reduced by over 50%. However, hardly any changes were seen in psychomotor tests undertaken, and it was concluded that this interaction is of little clinical significance.[17]

F. Temazepam

(a) Temazepam + Erythromycin

A double-blind randomised crossover study in 10 healthy subjects found that 500 mg **erythromycin** three times daily for 6 days had no significant effect on the pharmacokinetics of single 20 mg doses of **temazepam**, or on its psychomotor effects.[18]

G. Triazolam

(a) Triazolam + Azithromycin

A clinical study in 12 healthy subjects found that **azithromycin** did not affect the pharmacokinetics of a single 125-microgram dose of **triazolam**.[19] These results were supported by an *in vitro* study, which confirmed that **azithromycin** was a weak inhibitor of **triazolam** metabolism.[19]

(b) Triazolam + Clarithromycin

An *in vitro* study found **clarithromycin** to be a relatively potent inhibitor of **triazolam** metabolism. These results were confirmed in practice with 12 healthy subjects, who were given both drugs. The

oral clearance of **triazolam** was reduced to 22% of the level seen with placebo.[19]

(c) Triazolam + Erythromycin

A study in 16 healthy subjects found that 333 mg **erythromycin** three times daily for 3 days, reduced the clearance of a single 500-micro-gram dose of **triazolam** by about 50%, doubled the AUC, and increased the maximum serum levels by about one-third (from 2.8 to 4.1 nanograms/ml).[20] Other reports confirm the marked decrease in clearance and an increase in peak serum levels.[19,21] Drowsiness, weakness and slowness was seen in a patient taking **triazolam** when treated with **erythromycin** for a dental abscess.[22] Repeated visual hallucinations and abnormal body sensations occurred in one patient with acute pneumonia and chronic renal failure on 600 mg **erythromycin** daily after each dose of **triazolam** and **nitrazepam**. These symptoms had not occurred before the addition of **erythromycin**.[23]

(d) Triazolam + Roxithromycin

A study found that 300 mg **roxithromycin** had only a very small effect on the effects of **triazolam**.[15]

(e) Triazolam + Troleandomycin and Josamycin

Troleandomycin 2 g daily given to 7 healthy subjects for 7 days increased the peak **triazolam** levels by 107%, the AUC by 275% and the half-life from 1.81 to 6.48 h. Apparent oral clearance was reduced by 74%. Marked psychomotor impairment and amnesia was seen.[24] **Josamycin** and **troleandomycin** have been reported to interact similarly in 2 patients on **triazolam**, causing an increase in its effects.[25] An *in vitro* study has shown **troleandomycin** to be a potent inhibitor of **triazolam** metabolism.[19]

Mechanism

The most probable explanation is that these interacting macrolide antibacterials reduce the metabolism of midazolam and triazolam by the liver and/or the intestinal wall, thereby reducing their loss from the body, raising their serum levels and increasing and prolonging their effects. It seems probable that the cytochrome P450 CYP3A family of enzymes is involved.[26,27]

Importance and management

The **midazolam/erythromycin**, **triazolam/clarithromycin**, **triazolam/erythromycin** and **triazolam/troleandomycin** interactions appear to be established, and of clinical importance. The dosages of the midazolam and triazolam should be reduced 50 to 75% when these antibacterials are used if excessive effects (marked drowsiness, memory loss) are to be avoided. Remember too that the hypnotic effects are also prolonged so that patients should be warned about hangover effects next morning if they intend to drive. Much less is known about **midazolam/clarithromycin** and **triazolam/josamycin**, but the same precautions should be taken. Midazolam would also be expected to interact with both josamycin and troleandomycin but this needs confirmation.

Azithromycin does not interact with midazolam or triazolam, and the effects of roxithromycin on midazolam and triazolam, and of erythromycin on diazepam, flunitrazepam, nitrazepam and temazepam appear to be small and unimportant so that no special precautions seem to be necessary.

On the basis of *in vitro* studies it seems possible that the effects and side-effects of alprazolam will be increased by erythromycin but the extent is uncertain.

1. Greenblatt DJ, von Moltke LL, Harmatz JS, Ciraulo DA, Shader RI. Alprazolam pharmacokinetics, metabolism, and plasma levels: clinical implications. *J Clin Psychiatry* (1993) 54 10 (Suppl), 4–11.
2. Luurila H, Olkkola KT, Neuvonen PJ. An interaction between erythromycin and the benzodiazepines diazepam and flunitrazepam. *Therapie* (1995) 50 (Suppl), 484.
3. Mattila MJ, Vanakoski J, Idänpään-Heikkilä JJ. Azithromycin does not alter the effects of oral midazolam on human performance. *Eur J Clin Pharmacol* (1994) 47, 49–52.
4. Backman JT, Olkkola KT, Neuvonen PJ. Azithromycin does not increase plasma concentrations of oral midazolam. *Int J Clin Pharmacol Ther* (1995) 33, 356–9.
5. Zimmermann T, Yeates RA, Laufen H, Scharpf F, Leitold M, Wildfeuer A. Influence of the antibiotics erythromycin and azithromycin on the pharmacokinetics and pharmacodynamics of midazolam. *Arzneimittelforschung* (1996) 46, 213–17.
6. Yeates RA, Laufen H, Zimmermann T. Interaction between midazolam and clarithromycin: comparison with azithromycin. *Int J Clin Pharmacol Ther* (1996) 34, 400–5.

7. Gorski JC, Jones DR, Haehner-Daniels BD, Hamman MA, O'Mara EM, Hall SD. The contribution of intestinal and hepatic CYP3A to the interaction between midazolam and clarithromycin. *Clin Pharmacol Ther* (1998) 64, 133–43.

8. Aranko K, Olkkola KT, Hiller A, Saarnivaara L. Clinically important interaction between erythromycin and midazolam. *Br J Clin Pharmacol* (1992) 33, 217P–218P.

9. Olkkola KT, Aranko K, Luurila H, Hiller A, Saarnivaara L, Himberg J-J, Neuvonen PJ. A potentially hazardous interaction between erythromycin and midazolam. *Clin Pharmacol Ther* (1993) 53, 298–305.

10. Hiller A, Olkkola KT, Isohanni P, Saarnivaara L. Unconsciousness associated with midazolam and erythromycin. *Br J Anaesth* (1990) 65, 826–8.

11. Gascon M-P, Dayer P, Waldvogel F. Les interactions médicamenteuses du midazolam. *Schweiz Med Wochenschr* (1989) 119, 1834–6.

12. Gascon M-P, Dayer P. In vitro forecasting of drugs which may interfere with the biotransformation of midazolam. *Eur J Clin Pharmacol* (1991) 41, 573–8.

13. Byatt CM, Lewis LD, Dawling S, Cochrane GM. Accumulation of midazolam after repeated dosage in patients receiving mechanical ventilation in an intensive care unit. *BMJ* (1984) 289, 799–800.

14. Mattila MJ, Vanakoski J. Oral single doses of erythromycin enhance the effects of midazolam on human performance. *Br J Clin Pharmacol* (1993) 35, 77P–78P.

15. Mattila MJ, Idänpään-Heikkilä JJ, Törnwall M, Vanakoski J. Oral single doses of erythromycin and roxithromycin may increase the effects of midazolam on human performance. *Pharmacol Toxicol* (1993) 73, 180–5.

16. Backman JT, Aranko K, Himberg J-J, Olkkola KT. A pharmacokinetic interaction between roxithromycin and midazolam. *Eur J Clin Pharmacol* (1994) 46, 551–5.

17. Luurila H, Olkkola KT, Neuvonen PJ. Interaction between erythromycin and nitrazepam in healthy volunteers. *Pharmacol Toxicol* (1995) 76, 255–8.

18. Luurila H, Olkkola KT, Neuvonen PJ. Lack of interaction of erythromycin and temazepam. *Ther Drug Monit* (1994) 16, 548–51.

19. Greenblatt DJ, von Moltke LL, Harmatz JS, Counihan M, Graf JA, Durol ALB, Mertzanis P, Duan SX, Wright CE, Shader RI. Inhibition of triazolam clearance by macrolide antimicrobial agents: in vitro correlates and dynamic consequences. *Clin Pharmacol Ther* (1998) 64, 278–85.

20. Phillips JP, Antal EJ, Smith RB. A pharmacokinetic drug interaction between erythromycin and triazolam. *J Clin Psychopharmacol* (1986) 6, 297–9.

21. Hugues FC, Le Jeunne C, Munera Y. Conséquences en thérapeutique de l'inhibition microsomiale hépatique par les macrolides. *Sem Hop Paris* (1987) 63, 2280–3.

22. Matera MG. Erythromycin inhibition of triazolam metabolism. *Minerva Med* (1987) 78, 1194.

23. Tokinaga N, Kondo T, Kaneko S, Otani K, Mihara K, Morita S. Hallucinations after a therapeutic dose of benzodiazepine hypnotics with co-administration of erythromycin. *Psychiatry Clin Neurosci* (1996) 50, 337–9.

24. Warot D, Bergougnan L, Lamiable D, Berlin I, Bensimon G, Danjou P, Puech AJ. Troleandomycin-triazolam interaction in healthy volunteers: pharmacokinetic and psychometric evaluation. *Eur J Clin Pharmacol* (1987) 32, 389–93.

25. Carry PV, Ducluzeau R, Jourdan C, Bourrat C, Vigneou C, Descotes J. De nouvelles interactions avec les macrolides? *Lyon Med* (1982) 248, 189–90.

26. Lown KS, Thummel KE, Benedict PE, Shen DD, Turgeon DK, Berent S, Watkins PB. The erythromycin breath test predicts the clearance of midazolam. *Clin Pharmacol Ther* (1995) 57, 16–24.

27. Kanamitsu S, Ito K, Green CE, Tyson CA, Shimada N, Sugiyama Y. Prediction of in vivo interaction between triazolam and erythromycin based on in vitro studies using human liver microsomes and recombinant human CYP3A4. *Pharm Res* (2000) 17, 419–26.

Benzodiazepines + Metoclopramide

Intravenous but not oral metoclopramide increases the rate of absorption of diazepam and raises its maximum serum levels.

Clinical evidence, mechanism, importance and management

Metoclopramide given intravenously increased the peak plasma levels of **diazepam** by 38% and increased the rate of absorption (peak levels by 30 instead of 60 min),[1] but 10 mg oral **metoclopramide** did not increase the rate of absorption of oral **diazepam** 0.2 mg/kg in 6 healthy subjects.[2] The reason is not understood. The clinical importance of this interaction is not known, but it is probably small.

1. Gamble JAS, Gaston JH, Nair SG, Dundee JW. Some pharmacological factors influencing the absorption of diazepam following oral administration. *Br J Anaesth* (1976) 48, 1181–5.

2. Chapman MH, Woolner DF, Begg EJ, Atkinson HC, Sharman JR. Co-administered oral metoclopramide does not enhance the rate of absorption of oral diazepam. *Anaesth Intensive Care* (1988) 16, 202–5.

Benzodiazepines + Metronidazole

Metronidazole does not interact with alprazolam, diazepam, lorazepam or midazolam.

Clinical evidence, mechanism, importance and management

One study in healthy subjects found that 750 mg **metronidazole** (for an unstated time) had no effect on the pharmacokinetics of **lorazepam** or **alprazolam**.[1] Another study found that 400 mg **metronidazole** twice daily for 5 days also had no effect on the pharmacokinetics of a single 0.1-mg/kg intravenous dose of **diazepam**.[2] In vivo and in vitro studies have shown that **metronidazole** has no effect on the pharmacokinetics or pharmacodynamics of **midazolam**.[3] Interactions with other benzodiazepines seem unlikely. No special precautions seem necessary.

1. Blyden GT, Greenblatt DJ, Scavone JM. Metronidazole impairs clearance of phenytoin but not of alprazolam or lorazepam. *Clin Pharmacol Ther* (1986) 39, 181.

2. Jensen JC, Gugler R. Interaction between metronidazole and drugs eliminated by oxidative metabolism. *Clin Pharmacol Ther* (1985) 37, 407–10.

3. Wang J-S, Backman JT, Kivistö KT, Neuvonen PJ. Effects of metronidazole on midazolam metabolism in vitro and in vivo. *Eur J Clin Pharmacol* (2000) 56, 555–9.

Benzodiazepines + Nefazodone

Nefazodone increases the plasma levels, effects and side-effects of alprazolam, midazolam and triazolam, but not lorazepam. Dosage reductions may be needed.

Clinical evidence

(a) Alprazolam

A placebo-controlled study found that 200 mg **nefazodone** twice daily caused an almost twofold increase in the **alprazolam** plasma levels of 48 healthy subjects while they were taking **alprazolam** 1 mg twice daily for 7 days.[1,2] A complementary study showed that impairment of psychomotor performance and increased sedation occurred when **nefazodone** was given with **alprazolam**.[3]

(b) Lorazepam

A placebo-controlled study in healthy subjects given 200 mg **nefazodone** twice daily found that no changes in the pharmacokinetics of **lorazepam** 2 mg twice daily taken concurrently.[1] A complementary study showed that no impairment of psychomotor performance or increased sedation occurred when **nefazodone** was given with **lorazepam**.[3]

(c) Midazolam

A study in healthy subjects found that both the AUC and the maximum serum level of a single 10-mg dose of **midazolam** were increased about fivefold and doubled respectively, when given 400 mg **nefazodone** daily.[4]

(d) Triazolam

A study in 12 healthy subjects found that the pharmacokinetics of single 250-microgram doses of **triazolam** were changed by 200 mg **nefazodone** twice daily as follows: the maximum plasma levels, the half-life and the AUC were increased by 1.7-fold, 4.6-fold and 4-fold respectively.[1,5] A complementary study showed that impairment of psychomotor performance and increased sedation occurred when **nefazodone** was given with **triazolam**.[3]

Mechanism

Nefazodone appears to inhibit the oxidative metabolism of **alprazolam**, **midazolam** and **triazolam** by the liver (probably by cytochrome P450 isoenzyme CYP3A4) so that they accumulate in the body. **Lorazepam** is unaffected because it is primarily lost as a conjugate.[1]

Importance and management

The interactions of nefazodone with alprazolam, midazolam and triazolam are established and clinically important, but no interaction occurs with lorazepam. The practical consequences are that the effects and side-effects of alprazolam, midazolam and triazolam are expected to be increased by nefazodone, but the extent is uncertain. Be alert for any evidence of any psychomotor impairment, drowsiness etc. and reduce the benzodiazepine dosage (probably to about half) if necessary. More study is needed. As yet there seems to be no direct information about other benzodiazepines.

1. Greene DS, Dockens RC, Salazar DE, Barbhaiya RH. Coadministration of nefazodone (NEF) and benzodiazepines I: pharmacokinetic assessment. *Clin Pharmacol Ther* (1994) 55, 141.

2. Greene DS, Salazar DE, Dockens RC, Kroboth P, Barbhaiya RH. Coadministration of nefazodone and benzodiazepines: III. A pharmacokinetic interaction study with alprazolam. *J Clin Psychopharmacol* (1995) 15, 399–408.

3. Kroboth P, Folan M, Lush R, Chaikin PC, Barbhaiya RH, Salazar DE. Coadministration of nefazodone and benzodiazepines II: pharmacodynamic assessment. *Clin Pharmacol Ther* (1994) 55, 142.

4. Lam YWF, Alfaro CL, Ereshefsky L, Miller M. Effect of antidepressants (AD) and ketoconazole (K) on oral midazolam (M) pharmacokinetics (PK). *Clin Pharmacol Ther* (1998) 63, 229.

5. Barbhaiya RH, Shukla UA, Kroboth PD, Greene DS. Coadministration of nefazodone and benzodiazepines: II. A pharmacokinetic interaction study with triazolam. *J Clin Psychopharmacol* (1995) 15, 320–6.

Benzodiazepines + NSAIDs

Diazepam and indometacin (indomethacin) appear not to interact adversely except that feelings of dizziness may be increased. Diclofenac reduces both the sedative and hypnotic dosages of midazolam.

Clinical evidence, mechanism, importance and management

Diazepam 10 to 15 mg impaired the performance of a number of psychomotor tests (digit symbol substitution, letter cancellation, tracking and flicker fusion) in 119 healthy medical students. It also caused subjective drowsiness, mental slowness and clumsiness. When 50 or 100 mg **indometacin (indomethacin)** was given as well, the effects were little different from **diazepam** alone except that the feeling of dizziness (common to both drugs) was increased and caused subjective clumsiness.[1] A clinical study found that 75 mg **diclofenac** given intravenously to 10 patients reduced both the sedative and hypnotic dosages of **midazolam** given by infusion by 35%, when compared to 10 control subjects not given **diclofenac**.[2] The clinical importance of this is uncertain.

1. Nuotto E, Saarialho-Kere U. Actions and interactions of indomethacin and diazepam on performance in healthy volunteers. *Pharmacol Toxicol* (1988) 62, 293–7.

2. Carrero E, Castillo J, Bogdanovich A, Nalda MA. El diclofenac reduce las dosis sedante e hipnótica de midazolam. *Rev Esp Anestesiol Reanim* (1991) 38, 127.

Benzodiazepines + Opiates

There appear to be only minor pharmacokinetic interactions between midazolam and alfentanil and between flunitrazepam and buprenorphine. The increased sedation and unexpected deaths associated with these combinations respectively result from pharmacodynamic interactions.

Clinical evidence, mechanism, importance and management

A study of patients having abdominal hysterectomies under **alfentanil** and **midazolam** anaesthesia found that although the pharmacokinetics of **midazolam** were unchanged, postoperative sedation was more pronounced, when compared with a group of patients that did not receive **alfentanil**.[1] Another study investigating the mechanism behind several deaths reported with the combination of **buprenorphine** and **flunitrazepam** found that **buprenorphine** inhibited the cytochrome P450 isoenzyme CYP3A4 mediated metabolism of **flunitrazepam**, but only to a very minor extent, which is unlikely to be relevant in clinical practice.[2] The significance of these interactions is currently unclear and more study is needed on a wider range of agents.

1. Persson MP, Nilsson A, Hartvig P. Relation of sedation and amnesia to plasma concentrations of midazolam in surgical patients. *Clin Pharmacol Ther* (1988) 43, 324–31.

2. Kilicarslan T, Sellers EM. Lack of interaction of buprenorphine with flunitrazepam metabolism. *Am J Psychiatry* (2000) 157, 1164–6.

Benzodiazepines + Omeprazole

Gait disturbances (attributed to benzodiazepine toxicity) occurred in two patients on triazolam, lorazepam or flurazepam when given omeprazole, and another patient on diazepam became wobbly and sedated.

Clinical evidence

Two elderly patients, both smokers and taking **triazolam** and **lorazepam** or **flurazepam**, developed gait disturbances when concurrently treated with 20 mg **omeprazole** daily. They rapidly recovered when the **benzodiazepines** or the **omeprazole** were stopped.[1] A brief report describes a patient on **omeprazole** who became wobbly and sedated by small (unspecified) doses of **diazepam**,[2] and another report describes a patient who showed toxic levels of desmethyldiazepam and remained unconscious for 13 days after receiving a high dose of **clorazepate** (1500 mg over about 29 h) and **omeprazole** 80 mg daily.[3]

After taking 40 mg **omeprazole** daily for a week, the clearance of a single 0.1 mg/kg intravenous dose of **diazepam** in 8 healthy subjects was reduced by 54%.[4] Another study found a 40% reduction in the oral clearance of **diazepam** in white American subjects on 40 mg **omeprazole**, but only a 21% reduction in Chinese subjects.[5] Yet another study found a 27% decrease in **diazepam** clearance while taking 20 mg of **omeprazole** daily.[6]

Mechanism

In vitro studies with human liver microsomes have confirmed that omeprazole inhibits diazepam metabolism, almost certainly because of its action on cytochrome P450 isoenzyme CYP3A, although CYP2C9 also appears to be involved.[5,7] This would cause the diazepam to accumulate and its effects to be increased. Further *in vitro* study using suggests that omeprazole may possibly interact similarly with **midazolam**.[8] The reaction with lorazepam (and other glucuronidated benzodiazepines) may possibly not be an interaction (so it is suggested) but a side-effect of giving sedating medications to markedly anaemic patients.[2]

Importance and management

Information is limited, but what is currently known suggests that patients given omeprazole and the benzodiazepines cited should be monitored for any signs of increased benzodiazepine effects (sedation, unstable gait etc). If this occurs the benzodiazepine dosage should be reduced. More study is needed. See 'Mechanism' for the comment about midazolam. The effects of other proton pump inhibitors are not known, but a preliminary report suggests that **rabeprazole** does not interact with diazepam.[9]

1. Martí-Massó JF, López de Munain A, López de Dicastillo G. Ataxia following gastric bleeding due to omeprazole–benzodiazepine interaction. *Ann Pharmacother* (1992) 26, 429–30.

2. Shader RI. Question the experts. *J Clin Psychopharmacol* (1993) 13, 459.

3. Konrad A. Protracted episode of reduced consciousness following co-medication with omeprazole and clorazepate. *Clin Drug Invest* (2000) 19, 307–11.

4. Gugler R, Jensen JC. Omeprazole inhibits elimination of diazepam. *Lancet* (1984) i, 969.

5. Caraco Y, Tateishi T. Wood AJJ. Interethnic difference in omeprazole's inhibition of diazepam metabolism. *Clin Pharmacol Ther* (1995) 58, 62–72.

6. Andersson T, Andrén K, Cederberg C, Edvardsson G, Heggelund A, Lundborg P. Effect of omeprazole and cimetidine on plasma diazepam levels. *Eur J Clin Pharmacol* (1990) 39, 51–4.

7. Zomorodi K, Houston JB. Diazepam–omeprazole inhibition interaction: an *in vitro* investigation using human liver microsomes. *Br J Clin Pharmacol* (1996) 42, 157–62.

8. Li G, Klotz U. Inhibitory effect of omeprazole on the metabolism of midazolam in vitro. *Arzneimittelforschung* (1990) 40, 1105–7.

9. Merritt GJ, Humphries TJ, Spera AC, Hale JA, Laurent AL. Effect of rabeprazole sodium on the pharmacokinetics of diazepam in healthy male volunteers. *Pharm Res* (1997) 14 (Suppl 11), S-566.

Benzodiazepines + Paracetamol (Acetaminophen)

Paracetamol reduces the excretion of diazepam but plasma levels are little affected.

Clinical evidence, mechanism, importance and management

The 96-h urinary excretion of **diazepam** (given as a single 10-mg oral dose) and its metabolite (desmethyldiazepam) were reduced by a 500-mg dose of **paracetamol** in 4 healthy subjects. The reductions were from 44 to 12% and from 27 to 8% in the 2 female subjects, and from 11 to 4.5% in one of the male subjects. The reasons are not understood. Plasma levels of **diazepam** and its metabolite were not significantly affected.[1] There would seem to be no reason for avoiding concurrent use. There seems to be no information about other benzodiazepines.

1. Mulley BA, Potter BI, Rye RM, Takeshita K. Interactions between diazepam and paracetamol. *J Clin Pharm* (1978) 3, 25–35.

Benzodiazepines + Probenecid

Probenecid reduces the loss from the body of adinazolam, lorazepam and nitrazepam, but not temazepam. Increased therapeutic and toxic effects (sedation) may be expected.

Clinical evidence

(a) Adinazolam

In a single-dose study, **probenecid** 2 g increased the psychomotor effects of 60 mg sustained-release **adinazolam** in 16 healthy subjects. The tests used were symbol-digit substitution, digit span forwards and continuous performance tasks.[1] The peak serum levels of **adinazolam** and its active metabolite (*N*-desmethyl adinazolam) were increased by 37% and 49% respectively, and the clearances were reduced by 16% and 53% respectively. Both drugs have uricosuric actions, but when used together the effects appear not to be additive.[1]

(b) Lorazepam

Probenecid 500 mg six-hourly approximately halved the clearance of a single 2 mg intravenous dose of **lorazepam** in 9 healthy subjects. The elimination half-life was more than doubled, from 14.3 to 33 h.[2]

(c) Nitrazepam or temazepam

Probenecid 500 mg daily for 3 days reduced the clearance of **nitrazepam** by 25% in healthy subjects, but did not significantly affect **temazepam**.[3]

Mechanism

Probenecid inhibits the clearance of many drugs and their metabolites by the kidney tubules, including some of the benzodiazepines. It also inhibits the metabolism (glucuronidation) of nitrazepam and lorazepam by the liver.[2,3] The overall result is that the benzodiazepines accumulate and their effects are increased.

Importance and management

Established interactions but of uncertain clinical importance. Be alert for increases in both the therapeutic and toxic effects (sedation, antegrade amnesia) of adinazolam, lorazepam and possibly nitrazepam. Reduce the dosage as necessary. There seems to be no direct information about other benzodiazepines, but those that are metabolised like lorazepam and nitrazepam (e.g. oxazepam) are also possible candidates for this interaction. More study is needed.

1. Golden PL, Warner PE, Fleishaker JC, Jewell RC, Millikin S, Lyon J, Brouwer KLR. Effects of probenecid on the pharmacokinetics and pharmacodynamics of adinazolam in humans. *Clin Pharmacol Ther* (1994) 56, 133–41.

2. Abernethy DR, Greenblatt DJ, Ameer B, Shader RI. Probenecid impairment of acetaminophen and lorazepam clearance: direct inhibition of ether glucuronide formation. *J Pharmacol Exp Ther* (1985) 234, 345–9.
3. Brockmeyer NH, Mertins L, Klimek K, Goos M, Ohnhaus EE. Comparative effects of rifampin and/or probenecid on the pharmacokinetics of temazepam and nitrazepam. *Int J Clin Pharmacol Ther Toxicol* (1990) 28, 387–93.

Benzodiazepines + Prostaglandins

Enprostil and misoprostol appear not to interact significantly with diazepam.

Clinical evidence, mechanism, importance and management

Treatment with 35 micrograms **enprostil** twice daily for 5 days had no statistically significant effect on the pharmacokinetics of a single 10-mg oral dose of **diazepam** in 12 healthy subjects.[1] Another study in 12 subjects found that 200 micrograms **misoprostol** four times daily for 7 days had no effect on the steady-state serum levels of **diazepam** 10 mg daily or **nordiazepam**.[2]

No special precautions would seem to be necessary if either **enprostil** or **misoprostol** is given with **diazepam**.

1. Bressler R, Carter D, Winters L. Enprostil, in contrast to cimetidine, does not affect diazepam pharmacokinetics. *Adv Therapy* (1988) 5, 306–12.
2. Lima DR, Santos RM, Werneck E, Andrade GN. Effect of orally administered misoprostol and cimetidine on the steady state pharmacokinetics of diazepam and nordiazepam in human volunteers. *Eur J Drug Metab Pharmacokinet* (1991) 16, 161–70.

Benzodiazepines + Rifampicin (Rifampin)

Rifampicin causes a very marked increase in the loss from the body of diazepam, midazolam, nitrazepam and triazolam, but not temazepam. Benzodiazepines which are metabolised similarly are expected to interact in the same way.

Clinical evidence

(a) Diazepam

The mean half-life of **diazepam** was less than one-third (14 compared with 58 h) in 7 patients with tuberculosis treated with daily doses of isoniazid (0.5 to 2.2 g), **rifampicin** (450 to 600 mg) and ethambutol (25 mg/kg) when compared to healthy control subjects. The clearance was threefold greater in the tuberculosis patients.[1] **Rifampicin** 600 or 1200 mg daily for 7 days increased the clearance of **diazepam** in 21 healthy subjects approximately threefold.[2,3]

(b) Midazolam

A pharmacokinetic study in 10 healthy subjects found that after taking 600 mg **rifampicin** daily for 5 days the AUC of a single 15 mg oral dose of **midazolam** was reduced to 4% of the value without **rifampicin**, and its half-life was shortened by almost two-thirds. The psychomotor effects of the **midazolam** (as measured by the digit symbol substitution test, Maddox wing test, postural sway and drowsiness) were almost totally lost.[4]

(c) Nitrazepam

The total body clearance of **nitrazepam** in a study in healthy subjects was increased by 83% after taking 600 mg **rifampicin** daily for 7 days.[5]

(d) Temazepam

A study in which **temazepam** and **rifampicin** were given concurrently found that the pharmacokinetics of **temazepam** were unchanged.[5]

(e) Triazolam

Triazolam 500 micrograms orally was given to 10 healthy subjects before and after taking 600 mg **rifampicin** or a placebo daily for 5 days. The **rifampicin** reduced the **triazolam** AUC to 5% and decreased the maximum serum **triazolam** to 12% of the placebo group values. The elimination half-life fell from 2.8 to 1.3 h. Pharmacodynamic tests (drowsiness, sway, Maddox wing, etc.) showed that the **rifampicin** abolished the effects of **triazolam**.[6]

Mechanism

Rifampicin is a potent liver enzyme inducing agent which increases the metabolism of many drugs by the liver, thereby hastening their loss from the body. In the case of midazolam it is cytochrome P450 isoenzyme CYP3A4 in both liver and gut that is affected.[4] The enzyme inducing effects of the rifampicin seem to predominate if isoniazid (an enzyme inhibitor) is also present. Temazepam undergoes glucuronidation and is therefore unaffected by rifampicin.

Importance and management

The documentation of these interactions is limited but what has been reported is consistent with the way rifampicin interacts with many other drugs. The clinical importance of some of these benzodiazepine/rifampicin interactions has not yet been assessed or quantified precisely, but what is known suggests that you may need to increase the dosage of **diazepam** (possibly three or fourfold), and of **nitrazepam** (about twofold) if rifampicin is used concurrently. Be alert for a reduction in the effects of other similarly metabolised benzodiazepines (e.g. **chlordiazepoxide**, **flurazepam**). **Alprazolam** is predicted to interact because CYP3A is involved with its metabolism.[7] The effect of rifampicin on oral **midazolam** and **triazolam** is so very large that they become ineffective as hypnotics and an alternative should be used instead.

Those benzodiazepines which undergo glucuronidation like **temazepam** (e.g. **lorazepam**, **oxazepam**) are not expected to be affected by rifampicin.

1. Ochs HR, Greenblatt DJ, Roberts G-M, Dengler HJ. Diazepam interaction with antituberculosis drugs. *Clin Pharmacol Ther* (1981) 29, 671–8.
2. Brockmeyer N, Dylewicz P, Habicht H, Ohnhaus EE. The metabolism of diazepam following different enzyme inducing agents. *Br J Clin Pharmacol* (1985) 19, 544P.
3. Ohnhaus EE, Brockmeyer N, Dylewicz P, Habicht H. The effect of antipyrine and rifampin on the metabolism of diazepam. *Clin Pharmacol Ther* (1987) 42, 148–56.
4. Backman JT, Olkkola KT, Neuvonen PJ. Rifampin drastically reduces plasma concentrations and effects of oral midazolam. *Clin Pharmacol Ther* (1996) 59, 7–13.
5. Brockmeyer NH, Mertins L, Klimek K, Goos M, Ohnhaus EE. Comparative effects of rifampin and/or probenecid on the pharmacokinetics of temazepam and nitrazepam. *Int J Clin Pharmacol Ther Toxicol* (1990) 28, 387–93.
6. Villikka K, Kivostö KT, Backman JT, Olkkola KT, Neuvonen PJ. Triazolam is ineffective in patients taking rifampin. *Clin Pharmacol Ther* (1997) 61, 8–14.
7. Greenblatt DJ, von Moltke LL, Harmatz JS, Ciraulo DA, Shader RI. Alprazolam pharmacokinetics, metabolism, and plasma levels: clinical implications. *J Clin Psychiatry* (1993) 54, 10 (Suppl), 4–11.

Benzodiazepines + Saquinavir

A very marked increase in the sedative effects of midazolam has been seen in one patient treated with saquinavir, which confirms predictions based on *in vitro* studies. A study also demonstrated marked effects on midazolam pharmacokinetics when saquinavir was given.

Clinical evidence, mechanism, importance and management

A 32-year-old with advanced HIV disease on zidovudine, lamivudine and co-trimoxazole had no problems when 5 mg intravenous **midazolam** was used as sedative cover for investigations including bronchoscopy. He awoke spontaneously and was free from sedation 2 h later. He was readmitted for further investigations 8 weeks later, but was now additionally taking 600 mg **saquinavir** three times daily. Once again he was given 5 mg intravenous **midazolam**, but this time he did not wake spontaneously and after 30 min needed 300 micrograms intravenous flumazenil to revert the prolonged sedation. He was not free from sedation until 5 h later.[1] This very marked increase in the effects of the **midazolam** was attributed by the authors of this report to inhibition of its liver metabolism by the **saquinavir**.[1] A double-blind randomised study, in 12 healthy subjects found that 1200 mg **saquinavir** (soft-gel formulation) three times daily increased the bioavailability of oral **midazolam** from 41 to 90% and in-

creased the AUC fivefold. Psychomotor tests showed impaired skills and greater sedation with the addition of **saquinavir**.[2] However, in contrast to the case report above, despite some changes in the pharmacokinetics of intravenous **midazolam**, the drug effect was only marginally altered.[2] The case report is consistent with the way other protease inhibitors such as ritonavir behave, and it confirms the prediction of the makers of saquinavir, which are based on the known *in vitro* inhibition of cytochrome P450 isoenzyme CYP3A4 by **saquinavir** (although it is reported to be weak).[3]

This interaction would be expected to be of general importance, so be alert for the need to reduce the **midazolam** dosage (extent not yet established) in the presence of **saquinavir**. The authors of the study mentioned suggest that continuous intravenous **midazolam** doses should be reduced by 50%, but do not consider dose adjustments to single intravenous doses necessary.[2] The same precautions would be appropriate with **triazolam** as well (also a maker's precaution).

1. Merry C, Mulcahy F, Barry M, Gibbons S, Back D. Saquinavir interaction with midazolam: pharmacokinetic considerations when prescribing protease inhibitors for patients with HIV disease. *AIDS* (1997) 11, 268–9.
2. Palkama VJ, Ahonen J, Neuvonen PJ, Olkkola KT. Effect of saquinavir on the pharmacokinetics and pharmacodynamics of oral and intravenous midazolam. *Clin Pharmacol Ther* (1999) 66, 33–9.
3. Invirase (Saquinavir). Roche Products Limited. Summary of product characteristics, December 2000.

Benzodiazepines + Selective serotonin re-uptake inhibitors (SSRIs)

Fluvoxamine increases the serum levels and side-effects of alprazolam, bromazepam and diazepam, but not lorazepam or midazolam. Whether or not other benzodiazepines are affected depends on the way they are metabolised. Sertraline appears not to interact with alprazolam.

Clinical evidence

(a) Alprazolam

Fluvoxamine 50 mg for 3 days then 100 mg daily for 7 days, doubled the serum levels of **alprazolam** 1 mg four times daily given on days 7 to 10, in 60 healthy subjects. The **alprazolam** clearance was more than halved (from 3.72 to 1.67 L/h). Psychomotor performance and memory were found to be significantly worsened, even after only one day of the combination.[1,2] **Sertraline** 50 mg daily had no effect on the pharmacokinetics of **alprazolam** 1 mg daily in 12 healthy subjects, after 2 weeks of concurrent use. This lack of interaction is in line with *in vitro* predictions.[3]

(b) Bromazepam

Fluvoxamine 50 mg twice daily increased the plasma levels of **bromazepam** (single 12-mg doses) in 12 healthy subjects by 36% and increased the AUC from 3879 to 9195 nanograms.h/ml. Some increased impairment in cognitive functions was seen.[4]

(c) Diazepam

Fluvoxamine (50 mg on day one, 100 mg on day 2, then 150 mg daily thereafter) for 16 days decreased the clearance of a single 10-mg dose of **diazepam** (given on day 4) in 8 healthy subjects by two-thirds (from 0.40 to 0.14 ml/min/kg). The half-life was increased from 51 to 118 h, and the AUC was increased threefold.[5]

(d) Lorazepam

Fluvoxamine 50 mg twice daily caused a very small, non-significant, increase in the serum levels and AUC of single 4 mg doses of **lorazepam** in 12 healthy subjects.[4]

(e) Midazolam

A study in healthy subjects found that 200 mg **fluvoxamine** daily had minimal effects on the pharmacokinetics of single 10-mg doses of **midazolam**.[6]

Mechanism

The evidence suggests that fluvoxamine inhibits the metabolism of those benzodiazepines that undergo oxidation (e.g. alprazolam,[7] bromazepam, diazepam) thereby increasing and prolonging their effects, but not those which are metabolised by glucuronidation (e.g. lorazepam).

Importance and management

Evidence is limited, but what is known suggests that the dosages of alprazolam, bromazepam, diazepam and other benzodiazepines which are similarly metabolised (e.g. nitrazepam) should be reduced – probably halved – in the presence of fluvoxamine to avoid adverse side-effects (drowsiness, reduced psychomotor performance and memory). Fluvoxamine is unlikely to affect lorazepam and other benzodiazepines metabolised by glucuronidation (e.g. lormetazepam, oxazepam, temazepam) or midazolam. It seems unlikely that sertraline will affect any of the benzodiazepines and it may therefore be a useful alternative to fluvoxamine.

1. Fleishaker JC, Hulst LK. Effect of fluvoxamine on the pharmacokinetics and pharmacodynamics of alprazolam in healthy volunteers. *Pharm Res* (1992) 9 (Suppl 10), S-292.
2. Fleishaker JC, Hulst LK. A pharmacokinetic and pharmacodynamic evaluation of the combined administration of alprazolam and fluvoxamine. *Eur J Clin Pharmacol* (1994) 46, 35–9.
3. Preskorn SH, Greenblatt DJ, Harvey AT. Lack of effect of sertraline on the pharmacokinetics of alprazolam. *J Clin Psychopharmacol* (2000) 20, 585–6.
4. Van Harten J, Holland RL, Wesnes K. Influence of multiple-dose administration of fluvoxamine on the pharmacokinetics of the benzodiazepines bromazepam and lorazepam: a randomised, cross-over study. *Eur Neuropsychopharmacol* (1992) 2, 381.
5. Perucca E, Gatti G, Cipolla G, Spina E, Barel S, Soback S, Gips M, Bialer M. Inhibition of diazepam metabolism by fluvoxamine: a pharmacokinetic study in normal volunteers. *Clin Pharmacol Ther* (1994) 56, 471–6.
6. Lam YWF, Alfaro CL, Ereshefsky L, Miller M. Effect of antidepressants (AD) and ketoconazole (K) on oral midazolam (M) pharmacokinetics (PK). *Clin Pharmacol Ther* (1998) 63, 229.
7. von Moltke LL, Greenblatt DJ, Court MH, Duan SX, Harmatz JS, Shader RI. Inhibition of alprazolam and desipramine hydroxylation *in vitro* by paroxetine and fluvoxamine: comparison with other selective serotonin reuptake inhibitor antidepressants. *J Clin Psychopharmacol* (1995) 15, 125–31.

Benzodiazepines and related drugs + Theophylline or Caffeine

Theophylline reduces the serum levels of alprazolam. Caffeine, and to a lesser extent theophylline, may reduce the sedative (and possibly also the anxiolytic) effects of diazepam and clonazepam. Caffeine also opposes the effects of triazolam and zopiclone. Aminophylline can be used to antagonise the anaesthesia induced by benzodiazepines.

Clinical evidence

(a) Effect of caffeine and theophylline

Caffeine, and to a lesser extent **theophylline**, counteract the drowsiness and mental slowness induced by **diazepam** in single doses of 10 to 20 mg.[1-4] There is also evidence that **caffeine**, and **clonazepam**[5] or **triazolam**[6] have mutually opposing effects and that **caffeine** may interact similarly with **zopiclone**.[6]

(b) Effect of theophylline

A comparative study was made in two groups of patients given 500 micrograms **alprazolam** twice daily for 7 days. One group of 6 patients with chronic obstructive pulmonary disease were taking **theophylline**, while the other 7 patients, with chronic heart failure or atherosclerotic disease, were not. On day 7, those taking the **theophylline** were found to have trough serum **alprazolam** levels of 13.25 nanograms/ml, while in the other group the levels were 43.92 nanograms/ml.[7]

A patient who was unrousable and unresponsive following anaesthesia with **diazepam** (60 mg over 10 min) and N_2O/O_2 (60%/40%), rapidly returned to consciousness when given 56 mg **aminophylline** intravenously.[8] Other reports confirm this antagonism of the anaesthesia induced by **diazepam**, even by low doses of **aminophylline** (60 mg to 4.5 mg/kg intravenously).[9-11] **Flunitrazepam**,[12] lo-

razepam,[13] and **midazolam**[14] are also affected. There is some controversy about whether **theophylline** antagonises **midazolam** anaesthesia/sedation or not.[15,16]

Mechanism

Uncertain. One suggestion is that the xanthines can block adenosine receptors.[9] Another is that the xanthines induce the metabolism of the benzodiazepines by the liver so that they are cleared from the body more rapidly.[17]

Importance and management

The documentation is somewhat sparse and there is a need for more study over the range of benzodiazepine drugs, but the overall picture is that these interactions are established. The extent to which these xanthines actually reduce the anxiolytic effects of the benzodiazepines remains uncertain (it needs assessment) but be alert for reduced benzodiazepine effects if both are used. Caffeine in tea or coffee appears to reduce the sedative effects of triazolam and zopiclone. This would appear to be a disadvantage at night, but possibly useful the next morning.

1. Mattila MJ, Nuotto E. Caffeine and theophylline counteract diazepam effects in man. *Med Biol* (1983) 61, 337–43.
2. Mattila MJ, Palva E, Savolainen K. Caffeine antagonizes diazepam effects in man. *Med Biol* (1982) 60, 121–3.
3. Henauer SA, Hollister LE, Gillespie HK, Moore F. Theophylline antagonizes diazepam-induced psychomotor impairment. *Eur J Clin Pharmacol* (1983) 25, 743–7.
4. Meyer BH, Weis OF, Müller FO. Antagonism of diazepam by aminophylline in healthy volunteers. *Anesth Analg* (1984) 63, 900–2.
5. Gaillard J-M, Sovilla J-Y, Blois R. The effect of clonazepam, caffeine and the combination of the two drugs on human sleep. In Sleep '84, Ed by Koella WP, Rüther E, Schulz H. Publ by Gustav Fischer Verlag, Stuttgart, NY (1985) pp 314–15.
6. Mattila ME, Mattila MJ, Nuotto E. Caffeine moderately antagonizes the effects of triazolam and zopiclone on the psychomotor performance of healthy subjects. *Pharmacol Toxicol* (1992) 70, 286–9.
7. Tuncok Y, Akpinar O, Guven H, Akkoclu A. The effects of theophylline on serum alprazolam levels. *Int J Clin Pharmacol Ther* (1994) 32, 642–5.
8. Stirt JA. Aminophylline is a diazepam antagonist. *Anesth Analg* (1981) 60, 767–8.
9. Niemand D, Martinell S, Arvidsson S, Svedmyr N, Ekström-Jodal B. Aminophylline inhibition of diazepam sedation: is adenosine blockade of GABA-receptors the mechanism? *Lancet* (1984) i, 463–4.
10. Arvidsson SB, Ekström-Jodal B, Martinell SAG, Niemand D. Aminophylline antagonises diazepam sedation. *Lancet* (1982) 2, 1467.
11. Kleindienst G, Usinger P. Diazepam sedation is not antagonised completely by aminophylline. *Lancet* (1984) 1, 113.
12. Gürel A, Elevli M, Hamulu A. Aminophylline reversal of flunitrazepam sedation. *Anesth Analg* (1987) 66, 333–6.
13. Wangler MA, Kilpatrick DS. Aminophylline is an antagonist of lorazepam. *Anesth Analg* (1985) 64, 834–6.
14. Gallen JS. Aminophylline reversal of midazolam sedation. *Anesth Analg* (1989) 69, 268.
15. Kanto J, Aaltonen L, Himberg J-J, Hovi-Viander M. Midazolam as an intravenous induction agent in the elderly: a clinical and pharmacokinetic study. *Anesth Analg* (1986) 65, 15–20.
16. Sleigh JW. Failure of aminophylline to antagonize midazolam sedation. *Anesth Analg* (1986) 65, 540.
17. Ghoneim MM, Hinrichs JV, Chiang C-K, Loke WH. Pharmacokinetic and pharmacodynamic interactions between caffeine and diazepam. *J Clin Psychopharmacol* (1986) 6, 75–80.

Benzodiazepines + Tobacco smoking

Smokers may possibly need larger doses of some benzodiazepines than non-smokers.

Clinical evidence, mechanism, importance and management

Some studies have suggested that **smoking** does not affect the pharmacokinetics of **diazepam**,[1,2] **chlordiazepoxide**,[3] **clorazepate**,[4] **lorazepam**,[2] **midazolam**,[2] or **triazolam**,[5] but others have found that the clearance of **alprazolam**,[6] **clorazepate**,[7] **diazepam**,[8] **lorazepam**[9] and **oxazepam**[10,11] from the body is increased by **smoking**, but not all the changes are significant.[8] The Boston Collaborative Drug Surveillance Program reported a decreased frequency of drowsiness in those on **diazepam** or **chlordiazepoxide** who **smoked**,[12] which confirmed the findings of a previous study.[13] The probable reason is that some of the components of **tobacco** smoke are enzyme-inducing agents, which increase the rate at which the liver metabolises these benzodiazepines thereby reducing their effects and side-effects. The inference to be drawn is that **smokers** may possibly need larger doses than non-smokers to achieve the same therapeutic effects, and **smoking** also possibly reduces the drowsiness that the benzodiazepines can cause. However, one study suggested that caffeine intake,[13] and others suggest age, may affect the response to benzodiazepines, so the picture is not altogether clear. Whether any of these interactions has much clinical relevance awaits assessment.

1. Klotz U, Avant GR, Hoyumpa A, Schenker S, Wilkinson GR. The effects of age and liver disease on the disposition and elimination of diazepam in adult man. *J Clin Invest* (1975) 55, 347–59.
2. Ochs HR, Greenblatt DJ, Knüchel M. Kinetics of diazepam, midazolam, and lorazepam in cigarette smokers. *Chest* (1985) 87, 223–6.
3. Desmond PV, Roberts RK, Wilkinson GR, Schenker S. No effect of smoking on metabolism of chlordiazepoxide. *N Engl J Med* (1979) 300, 199–200.
4. Ochs HR, Greenblatt DJ, Locniskar A, Weinbrenner J. Influence of propranolol coadministration or cigarette smoking on the kinetics of desmethyldiazepam following intravenous clorazepate. *Klin Wochenschr* (1986) 64, 1217–21.
5. Ochs HR, Greenblatt DJ, Burstein ES. Lack of influence of cigarette smoking on triazolam pharmacokinetics. *Br J Clin Pharmacol* (1987) 23, 759–63.
6. Smith RB, Gwilt PR, Wright CE. Single- and multiple-dose pharmacokinetics of oral alprazolam in healthy smoking and nonsmoking men. *Clin Pharm* (1983) 2, 139–43.
7. Norman TR, Fulton A, Burrows GD, Maguire KP. Pharmacokinetics of N-desmethyldiazepam after a single oral dose of clorazepate: the effect of smoking. *Eur J Clin Pharmacol* (1981) 21, 229–33.
8. Greenblatt DJ, Allen MD, Harmatz JS, Shader RI. Diazepam disposition determinants. *Clin Pharmacol Ther* (1980) 27, 301–12.
9. Greenblatt DJ, Allen MD, Locniskar A, Harmatz JS, Shader RI. Lorazepam kinetics in the elderly. *Clin Pharmacol Ther* (1979) 26, 103–13.
10. Greenblatt DJ, Divoll M, Harmatz JS, Shader RI. Oxazepam kinetics: effects of age and sex. *J Pharmacol Exp Ther* (1980) 215, 86–91.
11. Ochs HR, Greenblatt DJ, Otten H. Disposition of oxazepam in relation to age, sex, and cigarette smoking. *Klin Wochenschr* (1981) 59, 899–903.
12. Boston Collaborative Drug Surveillance Program. Clinical depression of the central nervous system due to diazepam and chlordiazepoxide in relation to cigarette smoking and age. *N Engl J Med* (1973) 288, 277–80.
13. Downing RW, Rickels K. Coffee consumption, cigarette smoking and reporting of drowsiness in anxious patients treated with benzodiazepines or placebo. *Acta Psychiatr Scand* (1981) 64, 398–408.

Benzodiazepines + Vinpocetine

Vinpocetine does not appear to interact adversely with oxazepam.

Clinical evidence, mechanism, importance and management

No changes in the steady-state serum levels of **oxazepam** 10 mg three times daily were seen in 16 healthy subjects while taking 10 mg **vinpocetine** three times daily, for 7 days.[1] There would therefore seem to be no reason for taking special precautions if these two drugs are given together.

1. Storm G, Oosterhuis B, Sollie FAE, Visscher HW, Sommer W, Beitinger H, Jonkman JHG. Lack of pharmacokinetic interaction between vinpocetine and oxazepam. *Br J Clin Pharmacol* (1994) 38, 143–6.

Bromperidol + Carbamazepine

Even though carbamazepine reduces bromperidol serum levels, concurrent use is still apparently useful for the treatment of schizophrenia.

Clinical evidence, mechanism, importance and management

When 13 schizophrenic patients on 12 or 24 mg bromperidol daily were additionally given 200 mg **carbamazepine** twice daily for 4 weeks, the plasma levels of bromperidol and reduced bromperidol (a metabolite) were reduced by 37 and 23% respectively, on average at 4 weeks. Despite this fall in levels, the Clinical Global Impression scores (a measure of severity of illness) fell slightly. The postulated reason for the interaction is that the **carbamazepine** increases the metabolism of the bromperidol (possibly because of induction of cytochrome P450 isoenzyme CYP3A4) resulting in its increased loss from the body.[1] This study therefore suggests that even though a pharmacokinetic interaction occurs which lowers bromperidol serum

levels, combined use is nevertheless useful for the treatment of schizophrenic patients.

1. Otani K, Ishida M, Yasui N, Kondo T, Mihara K, Suzuki A, Furukori H, Kaneko S, Inoue Y. Interaction between carbamazepine and bromperidol. *Eur J Clin Pharmacol* (1997) 53, 219–22.

Bromperidol + Cisapride

An isolated report describes an increase in serum bromperidol levels, associated with clinical deterioration, in a patient when additionally treated with cisapride.

Clinical evidence, mechanism, importance and management

A schizophrenic patient on 18 mg bromperidol daily showed a marked deterioration (auditory hallucinations, persecutory delusions, etc.) within about 5 days of adding 7.5 mg **cisapride**. A retrospective study showed that the serum concentrations of the bromperidol and its reduced metabolite had been increased by the **cisapride** (bromperidol levels about doubled, the metabolite increased about 50%). When the **cisapride** was stopped his mental state recovered within a week.[1]

This is an isolated report and of uncertain general importance, but if both drugs are used concurrently the outcome should be monitored.

1. Ishida M, Iotani K, Yasui N, Inoue Y, Kaneko S. Possible interaction between cisapride and bromperidol. *Prog Neuropsychopharmacol Biol Psychiatry* (1997) 21, 235–8.

Buspirone + Calcium channel blockers

Diltiazem and verapamil can markedly raise the serum levels of buspirone, increasing the likelihood of increased side-effects.

Clinical evidence, mechanism, importance and management

A randomised crossover study in 9 healthy subjects found that after taking 60 mg **diltiazem** three times daily for 2 days (a total of 5 doses), the AUC of a single 10-mg dose of buspirone was increased 5.5-fold and the maximum serum levels 4.1-fold. When 80 mg **verapamil** three times daily for 2 days (a total of 5 doses) was given with a single 10-mg dose of buspirone, the buspirone AUC and maximum serum levels were increased 3.4-fold. The reason is thought to be that both calcium channel blockers inhibit the cytochrome P450 isoenzyme CYP3A4, which is concerned with the metabolism of the buspirone, thereby reducing its metabolism and loss from the body.[1]

The practical consequences of this interaction are that the effects and side-effects of buspirone are increased by **diltiazem** and **verapamil**. Concurrent use need not be avoided but be alert for the need to reduce the buspirone dosage. More study is needed. Information about other calcium channel blockers appears to be lacking.

1. Lamberg TS, Kivistö KT, Neuvonen PJ. Effects of verapamil and diltiazem on the pharmacokinetics and pharmacodynamics of buspirone. *Clin Pharmacol Ther* (1998) 63, 640–5.

Buspirone + Erythromycin or Itraconazole

The plasma levels of buspirone are markedly increased by erythromycin and itraconazole. Ketoconazole is predicted to interact similarly.

Clinical evidence

Eight healthy subjects were given 10 mg buspirone before and after taking 500 mg **erythromycin** three times daily or 100 mg **itracona-**

zole twice daily or a placebo for 4 days. It was found that the buspirone maximum plasma levels and its AUC were increased 5-fold and 6-fold respectively by the **erythromycin**, and the same parameters were increased 13-fold and 19-fold by the **itraconazole**. These increased buspirone concentrations caused a moderate impairment of psychomotor performance (digital symbol substitution, body sway, drowsiness, etc.) and an increase in side-effects.[1,2]

Mechanism

It is believed that erythromycin and itraconazole can reduce the metabolism and clearance of the buspirone by inhibiting cytochrome P450 isoenzyme CYP3A4 so that its effects are increased accordingly.

Importance and management

Direct information appears to be limited to this study but the interactions would seem to be established. The dosage of buspirone should be greatly reduced if erythromycin or itraconazole are given concurrently. More study is needed. **Ketoconazole** is predicted to interact similarly because it is a potent CYP3A4 inhibitor.[2]

1. Kivistö KT, Lamberg TS, Kantola T, Neuvonen PJ. Buspirone concentrations are greatly increased by erythromycin and itraconazole. *Eur J Clin Pharmacol* (1997) 52, A134.
2. Kivistö KT, Lamberg TS, Kantola T, Neuvonen PJ. Plasma buspirone concentrations are greatly increased by erythromycin and itraconazole. *Clin Pharmacol Ther* (1997) 62, 348–54.

Buspirone + Miscellaneous drugs

No adverse interactions appear to occur if buspirone and alprazolam, amitriptyline or triazolam are given together, and with diazepam the side-effects are similar to those seen with diazepam alone. Buspirone and cimetidine or terfenadine appear not to interact. An isolated report describes mania in an alcoholic patient on buspirone when given disulfiram.

Clinical evidence, mechanism, importance and management

(a) Benzodiazepines

The concurrent use of 1 mg **alprazolam** 8-hourly and 10 mg buspirone 8-hourly in 12 healthy subjects caused a 7% and 8% increase in the maximum serum levels and AUC of **alprazolam**. The maximum serum levels of buspirone were not altered, but the AUC of buspirone was increased by 29%. However, these changes were within the normal pharmacokinetic variability of these drugs. No unexpected side effects were seen.[1] Buspirone 15 mg 8-hourly had no effect on serum **diazepam** levels of 5 mg **diazepam** given to 12 healthy subjects daily for 10 days, but the **nordiazepam** levels were raised by about 20%. All subjects experienced some mild side-effects (headache, nausea, dizziness, and in two cases muscle twitching). These symptoms subsided after a few days.[2] There would seem to be no reason for avoiding concurrent use of benzodiazepines and buspirone.

(b) Cimetidine

Cimetidine 1 g daily for 7 days had no effect on serum buspirone levels nor on its excretion in 10 healthy subjects taking 45 mg buspirone daily. Some small pharmacokinetic changes were seen, but the performance of three psychomotor function tests remained unaltered.[3]

There would seem to be no reason for avoiding concurrent use.

(c) Disulfiram

An isolated report describes mania in an alcoholic patient on 20 mg buspirone daily, possibly due to an interaction with 400 mg **disulfiram** daily[4], but buspirone on its own has also apparently caused mania.[5,6] The reasons are not understood, but until more is known caution should be taken if both drugs are used in combination.

(d) Terfenadine

A single 10-mg dose of buspirone was given to 10 healthy subjects after 3 days of treatment with **terfenadine** 120 mg daily. There were

no significant effects on the pharmacokinetics or pharmacodynamics of buspirone.[7]

(e) Tricyclic antidepressants

Buspirone 15 mg eight-hourly added to 25 mg **amitriptyline** eight-hourly for 10 days had no significant effect on the steady-state serum levels of **amitriptyline** or **nortriptyline** in healthy subjects. No evidence of a pharmacodynamic interaction was seen.[2] There would seem to be no reason for avoiding concurrent use.

1. Buch AB, Van Harken DR, Seidehamel RJ, Barbhaiya RH. A study of pharmacokinetic interaction between buspirone and alprazolam at steady state. *J Clin Pharmacol* (1993) 33, 1104–9.
2. Gammans RE, Mayol RF, Labudde JA. Metabolism and disposition of buspirone. *Am J Med* (1986) 80 (Suppl 3B), 41–51.
3. Gammans RE, Pfeffer M, Westrick ML, Faulkner HC, Rehm KD, Goodson PJ. Lack of interaction between cimetidine and buspirone. *Pharmacotherapy* (1987) 7, 72–9.
4. McIvor RJ, Sinanan K. Buspirone-induced mania. *Br J Psychiatry* (1991) 158, 136–7.
5. Price WA, Bielefeld M. Buspirone-induced mania. *J Clin Psychopharmacol* (1989) 9, 150–1.
6. McDaniel JS, Ninan PT, Magnuson JV. Possible induction of mania by buspirone. *Am J Psychiatry* (1990) 147, 125–6.
7. Lamberg TS, Kivistö KT, Neuvonen PJ. Lack of effect of terfenadine on the pharmacokinetics of the CYP3A4 substrate buspirone. *Pharmacol Toxicol* (1999) 84, 165–9.

Buspirone + Rifampicin (Rifampin)

Rifampicin (rifampin) can cause a marked reduction in the plasma levels and effects of buspirone.

Clinical evidence

Buspirone 30 mg daily was given to 10 healthy subjects before and after taking 600 mg **rifampicin (rifampin)** daily for 5 days in a randomised, two-phase crossover study. It was found that the **rifampicin (rifampin)** reduced the total AUC of the buspirone by almost 90% and reduced the peak plasma levels by 87%. The pharmacodynamic effects of the buspirone were accordingly reduced (as measured by digit symbol substitution, critical flicker fusion, body sway and visual analogue scales for subjective drowsiness).[1]

Mechanism

Not fully established but it is almost certain that the rifampicin (rifampin) induces the activity of cytochrome P450 isoenzyme CYP3A4 in the gut wall and liver so that the metabolism and clearance of the buspirone are increased.

Importance and management

Direct information appears to be limited to this study but it is consistent with the way rifampicin (rifampin) interacts with many other drugs. This interaction would appear to be clinically important. If both drugs are used concurrently, be alert for the need to use a considerably increased buspirone dosage.

1. Lambert TS, Kivistö KT, Neuvonen PJ. Concentrations and effects of buspirone are considerably reduced by rifampicin. *Br J Clin Pharmacol* (1998) 45, 381–5.

Buspirone + Selective serotonin re-uptake inhibitors (SSRIs)

An isolated report describes the development of the serotonin syndrome with buspirone and citalopram. Buspirone with fluoxetine can be effective, but some adverse reactions have been reported. Fluvoxamine may possibly reduce the effects of buspirone.

Clinical evidence, mechanism, importance and management

(a) Citalopram

An isolated report describes the development of the serotonin syndrome and hyponatraemia, thought to be caused by a **citalopram-buspirone** interaction.[1] The general importance of this is unknown.

(b) Fluoxetine

A 35-year-old man with a long history of depression, anxiety and panic was started on 60 mg buspirone daily. His anxiety abated, but worsening depression prompted additional treatment for 3 weeks with 200 mg **trazodone** daily, which had little effect, so 20 mg **fluoxetine** daily was added. Within 48 h his usual symptoms of anxiety had returned and persisted even when the dose of buspirone was raised to 80 mg daily. Stopping the buspirone did not increase his anxiety.[2] Another patient with obsessive-compulsive disorder on **fluoxetine** experienced a marked worsening of the symptoms when 10 mg buspirone daily was added.[3] A patient had a grand mal seizure 3 weeks after buspirone 30 mg daily was added to **fluoxetine** 80 mg daily. The drugs were stopped and an EEG showed no signs of epilepsy, so the seizure was attributed to a drug interaction.[4] Other reports describe their effective concurrent use in patients with treatment-resistant depression[5] and with obsessive-compulsive disorder.[6,7]

The reasons for these adverse reactions are not understood, but there would seem to be little reason for avoiding concurrent use, however the outcome should be well monitored. More study is needed.

(c) Fluvoxamine

A double blind study in 9 healthy subjects found that after taking **fluvoxamine** daily (mean dose 127 mg, range 100 to 150 mg) for 3 weeks, the plasma levels of single 30-mg doses of buspirone were increased almost threefold, probably due to inhibition of liver enzymes. Even so, the psychological responses to the buspirone were reduced.[8] However, a study in 10 healthy subjects given a single 10-mg dose after 5 days of **fluvoxamine** 100 mg daily, found that although the pharmacokinetics of buspirone were altered (AUC increased 2.4-fold) the pharmacodynamic tests remained unchanged.[9] Concurrent use need not be avoided but it would be wise to remain alert to the possibility of reduced buspirone effects until more is known.

1. Spigset O, Adielsson G. Combined serotonin syndrome and hyponatraemia caused by a citalopram–buspirone interaction. *Int Clin Psychopharmacol* (1997) 12, 61–3.
2. Bodkin JA, Teicher MH. Fluoxetine may antagonize the anxiolytic action of buspirone. *J Clin Psychopharmacol* (1989) 9, 150.
3. Tanquary J, Masand P. Paradoxical reaction to buspirone augmentation of fluoxetine. *J Clin Psychopharmacol* (1990) 10, 377.
4. Grady TA, Pigott TA, L'Heureux F, Murphy DL. Seizure associated with fluoxetine and adjuvant buspirone therapy. *J Clin Psychopharmacol* (1992) 12, 70–1.
5. Bakish D. Fluoxetine potentiation by buspirone: three case histories. *Can J Psychiatry* (1991) 36, 749–50.
6. Markovitz PJ, Stagno SJ, Calabrese JR. Buspirone augmentation of fluoxetine in obsessive-compulsive disorder.*Am J Psychiatry* (1990) 147, 798–800.
7. Jenike MA, Baer L, Buttolph L. Buspirone augmentation of fluoxetine in patients with obsessive compulsive disorder. *J Clin Psychiatry* (1991) 52, 13–14.
8. Anderson IM, Deakin JFW, Miller HEJ. The effect of chronic fluvoxamine on hormonal and psychological responses to buspirone in normal volunteers. *Psychopharmacology (Berl)* (1996) 128, 74–82.
9. Lamberg TS, Kivistö KT, Laitila J, Mårtensson K, Neuvonen PJ. The effect of fluvoxamine on the pharmacokinetics and pharmacodynamics of buspirone. *Eur J Clin Pharmacol* (1998) 54, 761–6.

Chlorpromazine + Carbamazepine or Oxcarbazepine

The serum levels of chlorpromazine are not affected by oxcarbazepine.

Clinical evidence, mechanism, importance and management

Oxcarbazepine was substituted for **carbamazepine** in 4 difficult to treat schizophrenic patients. All patients were also taking chlorpromazine, and in 3 cases other antipsychotic medication (lithium or zuclopenthixol or clozapine). After 3 weeks of taking the **oxcarbazepine** all the patients showed rises in their **chlorpromazine**

levels, of 28, 63, 76 and 90%. In one case this rise was associated with increased extrapyramidal side effects.[1] The reason is that carbamazepine induces (increases) the metabolism of many drugs, including these antipsychotics. Chlorpromazine dosages initially had had to be increased to match this increase; but when the carbamazepine was replaced by **oxcarbazepine** (which is not an enzyme inducer), the metabolism returned to normal so that these dosages became in effect overdosages.[1] Information is limited but this report is consistent with the way carbamazepine often interacts with many drugs that oxcarbazepine does not interact with. No special precautions would therefore appear to be needed if **oxcarbazepine** is given with **chlorpromazine** unless it is used to replace carbamazepine (or some other similar enzyme inducing agent) in which case the antipsychotic dosages will probably need to be reduced.

1. Raitasuo V, Lehtovaara R, Huttunen MO. Effect of switching carbamazepine to oxcarbazepine on the plasma levels of neuroleptics: a case report. *Psychopharmacology (Berl)* (1994) 116, 115–16.

Clozapine + Anticonvulsants

Clozapine serum levels are markedly reduced (about halved) by carbamazepine and possibly phenytoin. Isolated cases of fatal pancytopenia and of neuroleptic malignant syndrome have been seen in two patients taking clozapine and carbamazepine. Sodium valproate can apparently lower serum clozapine levels, and an isolated case report suggests that lamotrigine may raise them.

Clinical evidence

(a) Carbamazepine

A study by a therapeutic drug monitoring service for clozapine found that the concentration/dose ratio of 17 patients also taking **carbamazepine** was 50% of that found in 124 other patients taking only clozapine.[1] A 47% decrease in the serum levels of clozapine were seen in another 12 patients when treated with **carbamazepine**. **Oxcarbazepine** did not interact.[2] The serum clozapine levels of 2 patients who had been on 600 or 800 mg clozapine daily and 600 or 800 mg **carbamazepine** daily for several months were approximately doubled (from 1.4 to 2.4 and from 1.5 to 3.0 micromol/l respectively) within 2 weeks of withdrawing the **carbamazepine**.[3]

A man with mania on 1200 mg **carbamazepine** daily and lithium developed muscle rigidity, mild hyperpyrexia, tachycardia, sweating and somnolence (diagnosed as neuroleptic malignant syndrome) 3 days after the lithium was stopped and 25 mg clozapine daily started. The symptoms immediately improved when the clozapine was stopped.[4] A patient on **carbamazepine**, lithium, benztropine and clonazepam developed fatal pancytopenia about 10 weeks after starting clozapine 400 mg daily.[5] A retrospective study of the records of other patients given clozapine and **carbamazepine** failed to find any positive evidence of increased granulopenia when both drugs were used.[6] However, it was later pointed out that there was actually a significant increase in granulopenia, the confusion being due to a statistical error.[7]

A case report describes 2 schizophrenic patients who were changed from **carbamazepine** to **oxcarbazepine** while concurrently taking clozapine. After 3 weeks their serum clozapine levels had risen from 1.4 to 1.7 micromol/l and from 1.5 to 2.5 micromolmol/l).[8] See also 'Chlorpromazine + Carbamazepine or Oxcarbazepine', p.714.

(b) Lamotrigine

A man of 35, who had been taking clozapine for 3 years, became dizzy and sedated about a month after starting to take **lamotrigine**. His plasma levels were found to have increased to 1020 micrograms/l. When the **lamotrigine** was stopped his levels returned to 450 micrograms/l.[9]

(c) Phenytoin

Two patients developed reduced clozapine levels (falls of 65 to 85%) and worsening psychoses when **phenytoin** was added to their treatment.[10]

(d) Sodium valproate

A controlled study in 11 psychotic patients found that when **sodium valproate** (at an average dose of 1060 mg daily) was added to clozapine, the steady-state serum clozapine levels were increased by 39% and of the desmethylated metabolite by 23%. However, correction of these levels for dose and weight reduced the total clozapine metabolite values to only 6% above those of the controls. No increase in clozapine side-effects was seen.[11] Another study found that **sodium valproate** and clozapine had no significant effect on the pharmacokinetics of the other drug.[12] In contrast, a study in 4 schizophrenics stabilised on clozapine 550 to 650 mg daily found that when **sodium valproate** 750 to 1000 mg daily was added, the serum clozapine levels began to fall, and by 3 weeks had dropped by an average of 41%. No deterioration in the patients' condition occurred.[13] A 15% decrease in clozapine levels was seen in another study, in 7 patients given clozapine and **sodium valproate**.[14] An isolated report describes sedation, confusion, slurred speech and impaired functioning on two occasions when **semisodium valproate** was added to clozapine in a 37-year-old man.[15]

Mechanisms

Not established, but it seems likely that both carbamazepine and phenytoin (recognised potent enzyme inducers) increase the metabolism of the clozapine by the liver, thereby reducing its effects. One suggestion is that carbamazepine induces the activity of cytochrome P450 isoenzyme CYP3A4 and possibly CYP1A2 as well.[1] The case of pancytopenia may possibly have been due to the additive bone marrow depressant effects of the clozapine and carbamazepine.

Importance and management

The interaction between clozapine and carbamazepine is much more firmly established than between clozapine and phenytoin, but both appear to be clinically important. Be alert for the need to increase the clozapine dosage (roughly doubled) if either is given concurrently, and to reduce the dosage if either is withdrawn. Oxcarbazepine is an alternative to carbamazepine which appears not to interact.[2,3] As yet there only appears to be one case report with lamotrigine, so the situation is unclear. There appears to be no pharmacokinetic mechanism for this interaction, so it awaits confirmation.

The situation with sodium valproate is not entirely clear. There are cases of successful concurrent use,[15] but in the light of the reports cited here it would clearly be prudent to monitor concurrent use closely. You should also be alert for any evidence of agranulocytosis with clozapine and any other drug (e.g. carbamazepine), which can depress the bone marrow function. See 'Clozapine + Miscellaneous drugs', p.718.

1. Jerling M, Lindström L, Bondesson U, Bertilsson L. Fluvoxamine inhibition and carbamazepine induction of the metabolism of clozapine: evidence from a therapeutic drug monitoring service. *Ther Drug Monit* (1994) 16, 368–74.
2. Tiihonen J, Vartiainen H, Hakola P. The carbamazepine-induced changes in plasma levels of neuroleptics. *Pharmacopsychiatry* (1995) 28, 26–8.
3. Raitasuo V, Lehtovaara R, Huttunen MO. Carbamazepine and plasma levels of clozapine. *Am J Psychiatry* (1993) 150, 169.
4. Müller T, Becker T, Fritze J. Neuroleptic malignant syndrome after clozapine plus carbamazepine. *Lancet* (1988) 2, 1500.
5. Gerson SL, Lieberman JA, Friedenberg WR, Lee D, Marx JJ, Meltzer H. Polypharmacy in fatal clozapine-associated agranulocytosis. *Lancet* (1991) 338, 262–3.
6. Junghan U, Albers M, Woggon B. Increased risk of hematological side-effects in psychiatric patients treated with clozapine and carbamazepin? *Pharmacopsychiatry* (1993) 26, 262.
7. Langbehm DR, Alexander B. Increased risk of side-effects in psychiatric patients treated with clozapine and carbamazepine: a reanalysis. *Pharmacopsychiatry* (2000) 33,196.
8. Raitasuo V, Lehtovaara R, Huttunen MO. Effect of switching carbamazepine to oxcarbazepine on the plasma levels of neuroleptics: a case report. *Psychopharmacology (Berl)* (1994) 116, 115–16.
9. Kossen M, Selten JP, Kahn RS. Elevated clozapine plasma level with lamotrigine. *Am J Psychiatry* (2001) 158, 1930.
10. Miller DD. Effect of phenytoin on plasma clozapine concentrations in two patients. *J Clin Psychiatry* (1991) 52, 23–5.
11. Centorrino F, Baldessarini RJ, Kando J, Frankenburg FR, Volpicelli SA, Puopolo PR, Flood JG. Serum concentrations of clozapine and its major metabolites: effects of cotreatment with fluoxetine or valproate. *Am J Psychiatry* (1994) 151, 123–5.

12. Facciolà G, Avenoso A, Scordo MG, Madia AG, Ventimiglia A, Perucca E, Spina E. Small effects of valproic acid on the plasma concentrations of clozapine and its major metabolites in patients with schizophrenic or affective disorders. *Ther Drug Monit* (1999) 21, 341–5.
13. Finley P, Warner D. Potential impact of valproic acid therapy on clozapine disposition. *Biol Psychiatry* (1994) 36, 487–8.
14. Longo LP, Salzman C. Valproic acid effects on serum concentrations of clozapine and norclozapine. *Am J Psychiatry* (1995) 152, 650.
15. Costello LE, Suppes T. A clinically significant interaction between clozapine and valproate. *J Clin Psychopharmacol* (1995) 15, 139–141.

Clozapine + Antiparkinsonian drugs

Clozapine appears not to interact adversely with *Sinemet* and pergolide, and may be used advantageously in some patients.

Clinical evidence, mechanism, importance and management

Ten out of 13 patients with Parkinson's disease with mild to moderate dementia developed psychoses when treated with *Sinemet* (**levodopa + carbidopa**), with or without **pergolide**. Their psychoses improved when they were additionally treated with clozapine.[1] Another study similarly found that 25 mg clozapine daily improved the control of parkinsonism with **levodopa**.[2] There would therefore seem to be advantages for some patients in giving these drugs in combination.

1. Greene P, Cote L, Fahn S. Treatment of drug-induced psychosis in Parkinson's disease with clozapine. In 'Advances In Neurology', Narabayashi H, Nagatsu T, Yanagisawa N, Mizuno Y (Eds.), Raven Press, NY (1993) 703–6.
2. Arevalo GJG, Gershanik OS. Modulatory effect of clozapine on levodopa response in Parkinson's disease: a preliminary study. *Mov Disord* (1993) 8, 349–54.

Clozapine + Azole antifungals

Itraconazole and ketoconazole do not interact with clozapine.

Clinical evidence, mechanism, importance and management

A double-blind study in 7 schizophrenic patients on clozapine found that when 200 mg **itraconazole** daily was added for a week, no changes in clozapine or desmethylclozapine serum levels were seen.[1]

A single 50-mg dose of clozapine was given to 5 schizophrenic patients before and after a 7-day course of **ketoconazole** 400 mg daily. The **ketoconazole** had no significant effect on the pharmacokinetics of the clozapine.[2]

The conclusion is that cytochrome P450 isoenzyme CYP3A4 is of only minor importance in clozapine metabolism, and that because no interaction takes place between clozapine and **itraconazole** or clozapine and **ketoconazole**, both it and other inhibitors of CYP3A4 can be used with clozapine.[1,2]

1. Raaska K, Neuvonen PJ. Serum concentrations of clozapine and *N*-desmethylclozapine are unaffected by the potent CYP3A4 inhibitor itraconazole. *Eur J Clin Pharmacol* (1998) 54, 167–70.
2. Lane H-Y, Chiu C-C, Kazmi Y, Desai H, Lam YWF, Jann MW, Chang W-H. Lack of CYP3A4 inhibition by grapefruit juice and ketoconazole upon clozapine administration in vivo. *Drug Metabol Drug Interact* (2001) 18, 263–78.

Clozapine + Benzodiazepines

A handful of reports describe severe hypotension, respiratory depression, unconsciousness and potentially fatal respiratory arrest in patients on benzodiazepines and clozapine. Dizziness and sedation are also increased.

Clinical evidence

A schizophrenic patient failed to respond to fluphenazine, **diazepam**, **clobazam** and **lormetazepam** after a trial over several weeks. The fluphenazine was stopped and clozapine started at a dose of 25 mg at noon and 100 mg at night. Toxic delirium and severe hypersalivation developed 3 h later. The patient collapsed (systolic pressure 50 mmHg, diastolic unrecordable) and stopped breathing. Resuscitation was started, but the patient remained unconscious for 30 min. After a few drug-free days he was successfully re-started on 12.5 mg clozapine, which was very slowly titrated upwards, and a low benzodiazepine dosage.[1]

Another patient on clozapine died suddenly and unexpectedly during the night, apparently due to respiratory arrest, after being given three 2-mg intravenous doses of **lorazepam** the previous day.[2]

There are at least 6 other cases of severe hypotension, respiratory depression or loss of consciousness in patients on clozapine and **flurazepam, lorazepam** or **diazepam**,[1,3-5] as well as 2 cases of marked sedation, hypersalivation and ataxia in patients on **lorazepam** and clozapine.[6] Two of these reports[1,3] are from the same group of workers and it is not clear whether they are about the same or different patients.

Mechanism

Not understood. Clozapine on its own very occasionally causes respiratory arrest and hypotension.

Importance and management

The authors of the first of these reports[1] say that the relative risk of the cardiovascular/respiratory reaction is only 2.1%. Another report[2] says that the death cited above is the only life-threatening event among 162 patients given clozapine and benzodiazepines between 1986 and 1991 so that the incidence of serious problems is clearly quite low. Even so, concurrent use should be very well monitored because of the severity of the reaction, even if it is rare.

1. Grohmann R, Rüther E, Sassim N, Schmidt LG. Adverse effects of clozapine. *Psychopharmacology (Berl)* (1989) 99, S101–S104.
2. Klimke A, Klieser E. Sudden death after intravenous application of lorazepam in a patient treated with clozapine. *Am J Psychiatry* (1994) 151, 780.
3. Sassim N, Grohmann R. Adverse drug reactions with clozapine and simultaneous application of benzodiazepines. *Pharmacopsychiatry* (1988) 21, 306–7.
4. Friedman LJ, Tabb SE, Worthington JJ, Sanchez CJ, Sved M. Clozapine – a novel antipsychotic agent. *N Engl J Med* (1991) 325, 518–9.
5. Tupala E, Niskanen L, Tiihonen J. Transient syncope and ECG changes associated with the concurrent administration of clozapine and diazepam. *J Clin Psychiatry* (1999) 60, 619–20.
6. Cobb CD, Anderson CB, Seidel DR. Possible interaction between clozapine and lorazepam. *Am J Psychiatry* (1991) 148, 1606–7.

Clozapine + Caffeine

Caffeine increases serum clozapine levels which can possibly increase the incidence of clozapine side effects.

Clinical evidence

A study[1] in 12 healthy subjects found that after taking 400 to 1000 mg **caffeine** daily, the AUC of a single 12.5 mg dose of clozapine was increased by 19% and its clearance was decreased by 14%. A previous study in 7 patients had found that clozapine levels were reduced by 47% after avoiding **caffeine** for 5 days, and increased again when **caffeine** consumption was resumed.[2]

A 66-year-old woman on 300 mg clozapine daily developed supraventricular tachycardia (180 bpm) when given 500 mg intravenous **caffeine** during an ECT session to increase the seizure length. Verapamil was needed to revert the arrhythmia. She had previously had up to 1000 mg **caffeine** during ECT sessions without problems before starting to take clozapine.[3] Another patient on clozapine for schizophrenia had an exacerbation of his psychotic symptoms which was attributed to **caffeinated coffee** (5 to 10 cups daily). The problem resolved when the patient stopped drinking **caffeine**. He had previously had no problems with **caffeine** while taking 30 mg haloperidol and 30 mg procyclidine daily.[4] A 31-year-old woman on 550 mg clozapine daily developed increased daytime sleepiness, sialorrhoea and withdrawn behaviour after taking about 1200 mg **caffeine** daily

(as drinks and tablets). Her plasma clozapine levels fell from 1500 to 630 nanograms/ml when her **caffeine** intake was stopped.[5]

Mechanism

Uncertain, but it seems likely that caffeine inhibits the metabolism of clozapine (by the cytochrome P450 isoenzyme CYP1A2) so that its serum levels and side effects increase.[1,2,6]

Importance and management

This would appear to be an established and clinically important interaction, but unlikely to be a problem if clozapine serum levels are established and well monitored, and caffeine intake remains fairly stable. Possible exceptions are if large doses are given during ECT treatment or if for some other reason the caffeine intake suddenly increases markedly.

1. Hägg S, Spigset O, Mjörndal T, Dahlqvist R. Effect of caffeine on clozapine pharmacokinetics in healthy volunteers. *Br J Clin Pharmacol* (2000) 49, 59–63.
2. Carrillo JA, Herraiz AG, Ramos SI, Benitez J. Effects of caffeine withdrawal from the diet on the metabolism of clozapine in schizophrenic patients. *J Clin Psychopharmacol* (1998) 18, 311–16.
3. Beale MD, Pritchett JT, Kellner CH. Supraventricular tachycardia in a patient receiving ECT, clozapine, and caffeine. *Convuls Ther* (1994) 10, 228–31.
4. Vainer JL, Chouinard G. Interaction between caffeine and clozapine. *J Clin Psychopharmacol* (1994) 14, 284–5.
5. Odom-White A, de Leon J. Clozapine levels and caffeine. *J Clin Psychiatry* (1996) 57, 175–6.
6. Carrillo JA, Jerling M, Bertilsson L. Comments to ""Interaction between caffeine and clozapine". *J Clin Psychopharmacol* (1995) 15, 376–7.

Clozapine + Ciprofloxacin

An isolated report describes the development of agitation in an elderly man on clozapine, tentatively attributed to elevated serum levels caused by an interaction with ciprofloxacin. A study supports this observation.

Clinical evidence, mechanism, importance and management

An elderly man with multi-infarct dementia and behavioural disturbances treated with clozapine, glibenclamide (glyburide), trazodone and melatonin, was hospitalised for agitation on the last day of a 10 day course of 500 mg **ciprofloxacin** twice daily. When the **ciprofloxacin** course was over his plasma clozapine serum levels fell from 90 nanograms/ml to undetectable concentrations (lower limit of detection being 50 nanograms/ml).[1] **Ciprofloxacin** 250 mg twice daily for 7 days was given to 7 schizophrenic patients, stabilised on clozapine. The mean serum clozapine and *N*-desmethylclozapine concentrations were increased by 29 and 31% respectively, but no additional side-effects were reported. Inter-individual variation in serum levels was high, so it seems likely that some patients may demonstrate a clinically significant interaction.[2] The likely mechanism is that **ciprofloxacin** inhibits the cytochrome P450 isoenzyme CYP1A2, resulting in an elevation of the clozapine levels. There seem as yet to be no other reports of a clozapine/quinolone antibacterial interaction.

1. Markowitz JS, Gill HS, Devane CL, Mintzer JE. Fluoroquinolone inhibition of clozapine metabolism. *Am J Psychiatry* (1997) 153, 881.
2. Raaska K, Neuvonen PJ. Ciprofloxacin increases serum clozapine and *N*-desmethylclozapine: a study in patients with schizophrenia. *Eur J Clin Pharmacol* (2000) 56, 585–9.

Clozapine + Erythromycin

A study in healthy subjects found no evidence of an interaction between clozapine and erythromycin, but three patients developed clozapine toxicity (seizures in one case, drowsiness, incoordination and incontinence in another and neutropenia in the third) when additionally treated with erythromycin.

Clinical evidence

A randomised crossover study in 12 healthy subjects found that when given a single 12.5-mg dose of clozapine while taking 500 mg **erythromycin** three times daily, the pharmacokinetics of the clozapine were unchanged.[1]

In contrast, a schizophrenic man, controlled on 800 mg clozapine daily without problems, was additionally started on 250 mg **erythromycin** four times daily for a fever and sore throat caused by pharyngitis. After a week he had a single tonic-clonic seizure and his serum clozapine levels were found to be 1300 micrograms/ml. Both drugs were stopped and the clozapine restarted 2 days later, initially at only 400 mg daily, but after several weeks at 800 mg daily. At this time his serum clozapine levels were noted to be 700 micrograms/ml.[2] Another schizophrenic on 600 mg clozapine daily became drowsy, with slurred speech, incontinence, difficulty in walking and incoordination within 2 to 3 days of starting to take 333 mg **erythromycin** three times daily. His serum clozapine level was found to be 1150 micrograms/l and he had leucocytosis. He recovered when both drugs were stopped. When later he was restarted on the same clozapine dosage, but without the **erythromycin**, his steady-state trough clozapine serum level was 385 micrograms/l.[3] Another case also describes a reduced white cell count when **erythromycin** was added to established clozapine therapy, but no clozapine levels were available.[4]

Mechanism

Uncertain. One suggestion is that the erythromycin might have inhibited the liver enzymes concerned with the metabolism of the clozapine (cytochrome P450 isoenzyme CYP2D6 and CYP3A4) leading to a reduced clearance with increased serum clozapine levels and accompanied toxicity.[2,3]

Importance and management

Information appears to be limited to this study and the three case reports, but just why they do not agree is not known, although it should be noted that the single dose study may not reflect the situation on multiple dosing. Under the circumstances it would seem prudent to monitor the outcome of adding erythromycin to clozapine treatment in any patient, being alert for any evidence of toxicity. Information about the possible effects of other macrolide antibacterials appears to be lacking. More study is needed.

1. Hägg S, Spigset O, Mjörndal T, Granberg K, Persbo-Lundqvist G, Dahlqvist R. Absence of interaction between erythromycin and a single dose of clozapine. *Eur J Clin Pharmacol* (1999) 55, 221–6.
2. Funderburg LG, Vertrees JE, True JE, Miller AL. Seizure following addition of erythromycin to clozapine treatment. *Am J Psychiatry* (1994) 151, 1840–1.
3. Cohen LG, Chesley S, Eugenio L, Flood JG, Fisch J, Goff DC. Erythromycin-induced clozapine toxic reaction. *Arch Intern Med* (1996) 156, 675–7.
4. Usiskin SI, Nicolson R, Lenane M, Rapoport JL. Retreatment with clozapine after erythromycin-induced neutropenia. *Am J Psychiatry* (2000) 157, 1021.

Clozapine + H₂-blockers

A single case report describes increased serum clozapine levels and toxicity due to cimetidine, but not ranitidine.

Clinical evidence, mechanism, importance and management

A man with chronic paranoid schizophrenia was treated with atenolol and clozapine 900 mg daily. When 400 mg **cimetidine** twice daily was added for gastritis, his serum clozapine levels rose almost 60% (from a range of 992 to 1081 nanograms/ml to 1559 to 1701 nanograms/ml) but without any problems. Within 3 days of raising the **cimetidine** dosage to 400 mg three times daily he developed evidence of clozapine toxicity (marked diaphoresis, dizziness, vomiting, weakness, orthostatic hypotension), all of which resolved over 5 days when the clozapine dosage was lowered to 200 mg daily and the cimetidine stopped. The serum clozapine levels during this period are not available. When the **cimetidine** was replaced by 300 mg **ranitidine** daily his clozapine serum levels were not affected.[1] The suggested reason for this interaction is that the **cimetidine** (a potent enzyme inhibitor) reduces the liver metabolism of the clozapine so that it accumulates, causing toxicity. **Ranitidine** does not cause enzyme inhibition.

Information appears to be limited to this report but it is consistent with the way **cimetidine** interacts with many other drugs. **Ranitidine**, or possibly other H₂-blockers such as **famotidine** or **nizatidine** which do not inhibit liver enzymes, would seem to be preferable and safer alternatives. This needs confirmation. More study is needed.

1. Szymanski S, Lieberman JA, Picou D, Masiar S, Cooper T. A case report of cimetidine-induced clozapine toxicity. *J Clin Psychiatry* (1991) 52, 21–2.

Clozapine + Lithium carbonate

A few patients given lithium carbonate and clozapine have developed toxic symptoms. These have included myoclonus, other reversible neurologic symptoms, neuroleptic malignant syndrome, seizures, delirium and psychoses.

Clinical evidence

A schizophrenic man, poorly controlled on 750 mg clozapine daily for 6 weeks, was additionally given 900 and then 1200 mg **lithium** daily. His serum **lithium** level was 0.86 mmol/l. Within a week he began to experience paroxysmal jerky movements of his upper and lower extremities lasting about half-an-hour. This myoclonus resolved when both drugs were stopped, and did not recur when clozapine was restarted alone.[1] Another patient developed neuroleptic malignant syndrome (stiffness, rigidity, tachycardia, diaphoresis, hypertension) 3 to 4 weeks after clozapine was added to his **lithium** treatment. The symptoms disappeared within 2 to 3 days of stopping the clozapine.[2] An elderly man also developed neuroleptic malignant syndrome 3 days after starting to take 25 mg clozapine daily. He was also taking carbamazepine and had stopped taking **lithium** 3 days before.[3]

Four out of 10 patients on **lithium carbonate** (mean dose of 1400 mg daily) and clozapine (maximum mean dose 900 mg daily) developed reversible neurological symptoms which included involuntary jerking of the limbs and tongue, facial spasm, tremor, confusion, generalised weakness, stumbling gait, leaning and falling to the right. One of them had delirium. Serum **lithium** levels remained unchanged, but the problems resolved when the **lithium** was stopped. Three of the four had a recurrence of the symptoms when rechallenged with the drug combination.[4] A man on clozapine and **lithium carbonate** developed an organic psychosis with delusions and visual hallucinations over a 5-day period when clozapine was tapered off and stopped, accompanied by a doubling in his serum **lithium** levels. He recovered completely when all drugs were stopped.[5] Two patients on clozapine developed seizures: one developed a tonic-clonic seizure within 4 days of adding 900 mg **lithium carbonate** to 600 mg clozapine daily, and the other a grand mal seizure within 6 days of adding 900 mg **lithium carbonate** to 900 mg clozapine daily.[6]

Mechanisms

Not understood.

Importance and management

Some patients develop a toxic reaction when given both drugs, and others do not, for reasons that are not understood. Concurrent use should therefore be extremely well monitored. One group of workers suggest that lithium levels of no more than 0.5 mmol/l may give therapeutic benefits while minimising side-effects, but they do not say why.[4]

1. Lemus CZ, Lieberman JA, Johns CA. Myoclonus during treatment with clozapine and lithium: the role of serotonin. *Hillside J Clin Psychiatry* (1989) 11, 127–30.
2. Pope HG, Cole JO, Choras PT, Fulwiler CE. Apparent neuroleptic malignant syndrome with clozapine and lithium. *J Nerv Ment Dis* (1986) 174, 493–5.
3. Müller T, Becker T, Fritze J. Neuroleptic malignant syndrome after clozapine plus carbamazepine. *Lancet* (1988) ii, 1500.

4. Blake LM, Marks RC, Luchins DJ. Reversible neurologic symptoms with clozapine and lithium. *J Clin Psychopharmacol* (1992) 12, 297–9.
5. Hellwig B, Hesslinger B, Walder J. Tapering off clozapine in a clozapine-lithium co-medication may cause an acute organic psychosis. A case report. *Pharmacopsychiatry* (1995) 28, 187.
6. Garcia G, Crismon ML, Dorson PG. Seizures in two patients after the addition of lithium to a clozapine regimen. *J Clin Psychopharmacol* (1994) 14, 426–7.

Clozapine + Miscellaneous drugs

There are isolated cases of apparent interactions between clozapine, and ampicillin, buspirone, caffeine, enalapril, haloperidol, nicotinic acid, tryptophan, nitrofurantoin, methazolamide, olanzapine, propranolol, thiamazole (methimazole), tobacco smoking or vitamin C. The makers of clozapine warn about the concurrent use of clozapine with anticholinergics, bone marrow depressants, CNS depressants, hypotensives or respiratory depressants. Also see the index for other clozapine monographs.

Clinical evidence, mechanism, importance and management

(a) Anticholinergics, hypotensives, respiratory depressants

The makers of clozapine, caution about the concurrent use of **anticholinergics, hypotensives** and **respiratory depressant drugs** because of the possibility of additive effects including hypotension and circulatory collapse.[1]

(i) Anticholinergics. Confirmation of the clinical relevance of the clozapine/**anticholinergic** drug interaction was seen in a patient who developed severe urinary retention while taking clozapine and **meclozine**.[2]

A man with a schizoaffective disorder on **nortriptyline**, perphenazine and propranolol was additionally given 150 mg clozapine daily. Some improvement was seen after 8 days, and over the next week the propranolol was gradually discontinued while the clozapine dosage was raised to 225 mg daily. The patient then began to complain of extreme fatigue and slurred speech, and by day 17 was delirious and confused. His serum **nortriptyline** levels were found to have doubled (from 93 to 185 nanograms/ml) from the time the clozapine was started. He recovered within 5 days of stopping all of the drugs, after which the clozapine was restarted.[3] The authors of the report interpreted the symptoms as an anticholinergic delirium arising from the additive anticholinergic effects of the clozapine, **nortriptyline** and **perphenazine**, made worse by the increased levels of **nortriptyline**.[3] Just why the **nortriptyline** levels rose is not clear, but one possible explanation is that the **nortriptyline** and clozapine compete for the same liver enzymes concerned with their metabolism, resulting in a reduction in the clearance of the **nortriptyline**. Tables 9.1 and 9.2 in Chapter 9 are lists of drugs which have anticholinergic activity.

(ii) Antihypertensives. A clozapine/**antihypertensive** interaction occurred in 2 patients who experienced syncope when given clozapine and **enalapril**. One was taking 5 mg **enalapril** and fainted within an hour of being given an initial 25-mg dose of clozapine. Later he was well controlled without problems on 2.5 mg **enalapril** daily and clozapine in doses starting at 12.5 mg and rising later to 800 mg daily. The other patient taking 10 mg **enalapril** daily fainted within 5 h of being given 25 mg clozapine. He needed resuscitation, but was later well controlled on clozapine in doses up to 600 mg daily.[4] The clozapine serum levels of a man of 39 rose from 490 to 966 nanograms/ml after the addition of **lisinopril** 5 mg daily. When the **lisinopril** dose was increased to 10 mg daily, the levels further rose to 1092 nanograms/ml. The dose of clozapine was reduced, and **lisinopril** replaced by **diltiazem**, after which his levels began to return to normal.[5] Coma developed in a woman 1.5 to 2 h after a single 150-mg dose of clozapine was added to an existing regimen of 40 mg **propranolol** daily. She had stopped taking fluphenazine 24 h earlier. The patient recovered and was then later slowly titrated up to 100 mg clozapine, in addition to the **propranolol** without any problems. Al-

though the authors state that a **propranolol/clozapine** interaction is a likely cause of the coma, the effects of fluphenazine cannot be wholly ruled out.[6] Table 8.1 lists the antihypertensive drugs.

(b) Bone marrow depressants

Because clozapine can cause blood dyscrasias and potentially fatal agranulocytosis, the makers say that it should not be given with other drugs that can also cause agranulocytosis. They list **carbamazepine, co-trimoxazole, chloramphenicol, cytotoxics, pyrazolone analgesics, phenylbutazone, penicillamine, sulphonamides** and **depot antipsychotics** (because they cannot be stopped if an adverse reaction occurs).[1] There are several cases that confirm the clinical significance of these predicted interactions.

A woman was treated with **thiamazole (methimazole)** for Graves' disease and at times with various different antipsychotics including haloperidol, flupenthixol, zuclopenthixol and perphenazine for schizophrenia. Because of the severe extrapyramidal reactions and failure to control the schizophrenia, clozapine (increased over 5 days to 250 mg daily) was started instead. Within 5 days her white cell count had fallen to 2200/mm³, which rose to 4000/mm³, a month after both drugs were stopped. Later, after the **thiamazole** was stopped she was successfully treated with the same dose of clozapine.[7] A patient who had been taking 500 mg clozapine daily for 8 months developed granulocytopenia within 8 days of starting 200 mg **nitrofurantoin** daily.[8] A patient on clozapine, 25 mg daily, showed no significant changes in his white blood cell count while taking 23.5 g **chloroquine** for malaria prophylaxis, over the course of a month.[9] An isolated report describes neutropenia in an 86-year old women 2 weeks after **methazolamide** for glaucoma was added to clozapine. Both drugs were stopped and her white cell count recovered. She later started clozapine without problem and so the toxic effect was attributed by inference to the combined use of two drugs both of which can both depress bone marrow function.[10]

Neutropenia developed 4 days after **co-trimoxazole** was started in a woman of 47 who had been stabilised on clozapine for 5 years. **Co-trimoxazole** was stopped and the white cell counts returned to normal over the next 2 weeks.[11]

Three patients have been described who showed a delay in recovery from clozapine-induced agranulocytosis when given **olanzapine**, and it has been suggested that **olanzapine** should therefore be avoided until the patient's haematological status has normalised.[12]

(c) CNS depressants

Clozapine causes drowsiness, particularly when first started, which would be expected to be additive with any other **CNS depressant**. The makers particularly list **alcohol, MAO inhibitors, narcotics** and **sedative antihistamines**.[1] See also 'Clozapine + Benzodiazepines', p.715.

(d) Miscellaneous drugs

(i) Ampicillin. An isolated report describes a 17-year-old recently started on clozapine (12.5 mg increased to 50 mg three times daily) who on day 15 was additionally given 500 mg **ampicillin** four times daily. On the next day the patient became easily distracted, very drowsy and salivated excessively. These adverse reactions stopped when the **ampicillin** was replaced by doxycycline.[13]

(ii) Buspirone. A man on clozapine for a year developed acute and potentially lethal gastrointestinal bleeding and marked hyperglycaemia about 5 weeks after starting **buspirone**, and a week after its dosage was raised to 20 mg daily. No gut pathology (e.g. ulceration) was detected and there were no problems after his recovery when later given clozapine alone, so the reaction was attributed to the drug combination.[14]

(iii) Caffeine. A schizophrenic patient who had abused **caffeine** for years, without side-effects, experienced acute exacerbation of the psychosis and abrupt onset of signs of arousal and stiffness when started on clozapine. These acute reactions were completely prevented when the patient was told to take the clozapine 40 min after any **caffeinated drink**.[15] Another patient on clozapine experienced drowsiness and sialorrhoea when taking **caffeine** tablets, **coffee** and chocolate. His serum clozapine levels more than halved when the **caffeine** was stopped.[16]

(iv) Grapefruit juice. **Grapefruit juice** did not affect the metabolism of clozapine in 2 studies in a total of 36 schizophrenic patients.[17,18]

(v) Haloperidol. A man of 68 on clozapine 600 mg daily and venlafaxine, lorazepam, aspirin, vitamin E and multivitamins was started on **haloperidol** 4 mg daily to control persistent paranoid delusions and hallucinations. After 27 days he was found collapsed and was lethargic, tachycardic, feverish and delirious. Because neuroleptic malignant syndrome was suspected the neuroleptics were withheld, and the patient recovered over the following 7 days. Clozapine was later restarted without a recurrence of symptoms.[19]

(vi) Nefazodone. A man of 40 who had been successfully treated with risperidone and clozapine 425 to 475 mg daily was started on **nefazodone** 200 mg increasing to 300 mg daily, for the treatment of persistent depression. After a week on the higher dose he became dizzy and hypotensive and it was noted that his clozapine level had risen from 133 to 233 nanograms/ml. This was thought to be due to an inhibitory effect of **nefazodone** on the cytochrome P450 isoenzyme CYP3A4.[20]

(vii) Nicotinic acid/Tryptophan/Vitamin C. A man with schizophrenia taking **tryptophan, lorazepam, vitamin C, benzatropine** and **nicotinic acid**, developed a severe urticarial rash covering his face, neck and trunk 3 days after starting 150 mg clozapine daily. All of the drugs except **lorazepam** were stopped, and the rash subsided. It did not recur when clozapine was restarted and gradually increased to 600 mg daily, nor when small doses of **benzatropine** and **fluphenazine** were briefly added. The authors draw the inference that **tryptophan, vitamin C** and **nicotinic acid** may have been responsible for this 'interaction'.[21]

(viii) Reboxetine. **Reboxetine** 8 mg daily was given to 7 patients stabilised on clozapine without any effect on the pharmacokinetics of clozapine or its major metabolite.[22]

(ix) Tobacco smoke. **Tobacco** smoking might be expected to lower serum clozapine levels because the smoke contains aromatic hydrocarbons which are potent enzyme inducers, but studies of this likely interaction have been equivocal. One group of workers found no differences in clozapine levels with **smoking**,[23] while another group found smokers had lower clozapine levels.[24] In addition a case report describes clozapine-induced seizures in a man when he gave up smoking, although no levels were available so the authors point out it is difficult to say that smoking cessation was the cause.[25]

1. Clozaril (Clozapine). Novartis Pharmaceuticals UK Ltd. Summary of product characteristics, May 2002.
2. Cohen MAA, Alfonso CA, Mosquera M. Development of urinary retention during treatment with clozapine and meclizine. *Am J Psychiatry* (1994) 151, 619–20.
3. Smith T, Riskin J. Effect of clozapine on plasma nortriptyline concentration. *Pharmacopsychiatry* (1994) 27, 41–2.
4. Aronowitz JS, Chakos MH, Safferman AZ, Lieberman JA. Syncope associated with the combination of clozapine and enalapril. *J Clin Psychopharmacol* (1994) 14, 429–30.
5. Abraham G, Grunberg B, Gratz S. Possible interaction of clozapine and lisinopril. *Am J Psychiatry* (2001) 158, 969.
6. Vetter PH, Proppe DG. Clozapine induced coma. *J Nerv Ment Dis* (1992) 180, 58–9.
7. Rocco PL. Concurrent treatment with clozapine and methimazole inducing granulocytopenia: a case report. *Hum Psychopharmacol* (1993) 8, 445–6.
8. Juul Povlsen U, Noring U, Fog R, Gerlach J. Tolerability and therapeutic effect of clozapine. *Acta Psychiatr Scand* (1985) 71, 176–85.
9. König P, Künz A. Compatibility of clozapine and chloroquine. *Lancet* (1991) 338, 948.
10. Burke WJ, Ranno AE. Neutropenia with clozapine and methazolamide. *J Clin Psychopharmacol* (1994) 14, 357–8.
11. Henderson DC, Borba CP. Trimethoprim-sulfamethoxazole and clozapine. *Psychiatr Serv* (2001) 52, 111–12.
12. Flynn SW, Altman S, MacEwan GW, Black LL, Greenidge LL, Honer WG. Prolongation of clozapine-induced granulocytopenia associated with olanzapine. *J Clin Psychopharmacol* (1997) 17, 494–5.
13. Csík V, Molnár J. Possible adverse interaction between clozapine and ampicillin in an adolescent with schizophrenia. *J Child Adolesc Psychopharmacol* (1994) 4, 123–8.
14. Good MI. Lethal interaction of clozapine and buspirone? *Am J Psychiatry* (1997) 154, 1472–3.
15. Vainer JL, Chouinard G. Caffeine and antipsychotics. *Clin Invest Med* (1993) 16 (Suppl 4), B20.
16. Odom-White A, de Leon J. Clozapine levels and caffeine. *J Clin Psychiatry* (1996) 57, 175–6.
17. Lane H-Y, Chiu C-C, Kazmi Y, Desai H, Lam YWF, Jan MW, Chang W-H. Lack of CYP3A4 inhibition by grapefruit juice and ketoconazole upon clozapine administration in vivo. *Drug Metabol Drug Interact* (2001) 18, 263–78.
18. Lane H-Y, Jann MW, Chang Y-C, Chiu C-C, Huang M-C, Lee S-H, Chang W-H. Repeated ingestion of grapefruit juice does not alter clozapine's steady-state plasma levels, effectiveness, and tolerability. *J Clin Psychiatry* (2001) 62, 812–17.
19. Garcia G, Ghani S, Poveda RA, Dansky BL. Neuroleptic malignant syndrome with antidepressant/antipsychotic drug combination. *Ann Pharmacother* (2001) 35, 784–5.
20. Khan AY, Preskorn SH. Increase in plasma levels of clozapine and norclozapine after administration of nefazodone. *J Clin Psychiatry* (2001) 62, 375–6.
21. Goumeniouk AD, Ancill RJ, MacEwan GW, Koczapski AB. A case of drug-drug interaction involving clozapine. *Can J Psychiatry* (1991) 36, 234–5.
22. Spina E, Avenoso A, Scordo MG, Ancione M, Madia A, Levita A. No effect of reboxetine on plasma concentrations of clozapine, risperidone, and their active metabolites. *Ther Drug Monit* (2001) 23, 675–8.
23. Hasegawa M, Gutierrez-Esteinou R, Way L, Meltzer HY. Relationship between clinical efficacy and clozapine concentrations in plasma in schizophrenia: effect of smoking. *J Clin Psychopharmacol* (1993) 13, 383–90.
24. Haring C, Meise U, Humpel C, Fleischhacker WW, Hinterhuber H. Dose-related plasma effects of clozapine: influence of smoking behaviour, sex and age. *Psychopharmacology (Berl)* (1989) 99, S38–S40.
25. McCarthy RH. Seizures following smoking cessation in a clozapine responder. *Pharmacopsychiatry* (1994) 27, 210–11.

Clozapine + Rifampicin

An isolated report describes a marked fall in the serum levels of a patient on clozapine when treated with rifampicin.

Clinical evidence, mechanism, importance and management

A schizophrenic patient on clozapine who developed tuberculosis was additionally treated with **rifampicin**, isoniazid and pyrazinamide. Within 2 to 3 weeks his trough serum clozapine levels had fallen dramatically from about 250 to 40 nanograms/ml) but rose again rapidly when the **rifampicin** was replaced by ciprofloxacin. The suggested reason is that the **rifampicin** (a potent enzyme inducing agent) increased the metabolism of the clozapine, probably by the cytochrome P450 isoenzymes CYP1A2 and CYP3A, thereby increasing the loss of the clozapine from the body.[1]

This appears to be an isolated case but it is consistent with the way **rifampicin** interacts with other drugs. Clozapine serum levels should be well monitored if **rifampicin** is added, being alert for the need to increase its dosage. An alternative (as in this case) is to use another antibacterial.

1. Joos AAB, Frank UG, Kaschka WP. Pharmacokinetic interaction of clozapine and rifampicin in a forensic patient with an atypical mycobacterial infection. *J Clin Psychopharmacol* (1998) 18, 83–5.

Clozapine + Risperidone

Concurrent use can be effective and well tolerated but two isolated reports describe a rise in serum clozapine levels when risperidone was added and another describes the development of atrial ectopics. Dystonia has been seen when clozapine was replaced by risperidone.

Clinical evidence

A man with a schizoaffective disorder on clozapine was additionally started on **risperidone**, firstly 0.5 mg twice daily, and then after a week 1 mg twice daily. Clinical improvement was seen and it was found that after 2 weeks his serum clozapine levels had risen by 74% (from 344 to 598 nanograms/ml) without any adverse effects.[1] The serum clozapine levels of another patient more than doubled when given **risperidone**. No signs of clozapine toxicity were seen, but mild oculogyric crises were reported.[2] A schizophrenic on clozapine and trihexyphenidyl who developed tachycardia (120 bpm), which was controlled with propranolol, developed atrial ectopics when **risperidone** 1.5 mg daily was added. The ectopics stopped when the **risperidone** was withdrawn and started again when it was re-introduced. Clozapine plasma levels were normal throughout the duration of **risperidone** treatment.[3] Four patients have been described who developed dystonia when transferred from clozapine to **risperidone**.[4] A single case of agranulocytosis has been seen 6 weeks after **risperidone** was added to stable clozapine treatment. The patient needed 3 doses of GCSF before the white cell count returned to normal.[5] Another case report describes neuroleptic malignant syndrome in a man of 20 within 2 days of clozapine being added to **risperidone** treatment. The drugs were stopped and he recovered over the following 10 days. He subsequently received clozapine alone without problem.[6] Contrasting with these reports is a study in 12 schizophrenic patients which found that the addition of **risperidone** to clozapine was both effective and well tolerated, although 4 patients complained of mild akathisia. Serum clozapine levels were not significantly changed.[7]

Mechanism, importance and management

The suggested reason for the raised clozapine levels is that both drugs compete for metabolism by the same enzyme system (cytochrome P450 isoenzyme CYP2D6) resulting in a reduction in the metabolism of the clozapine.[1,2] The dystonias are attributed to cholinergic rebound and ongoing dopamine blockade caused by a rapid switch of medication. The recommendation is that withdrawal should be tapered and possibly that an anticholinergic agent should be given.[4]

1. Tyson SC, Devane LC, Risch SC. Pharmacokinetic interaction between risperidone and clozapine. *Am J Psychiatry* (1995) 152, 1401–2.
2. Koreen AR, Lieberman JA, Kronig M, Cooper TB. Cross-tapering clozapine and risperidone. *Am J Psychiatry* (1995) 152, 1690.
3. Chong SA, Tan CH, Lee HS. Atrial ectopics with clozapine-risperidone combination. *J Clin Psychopharmacol* (1997) 17, 130–1.
4. Simpson GM, Meyer JM. Dystonia while changing from clozapine to risperidone. *J Clin Psychopharmacol* (1996) 16, 260–1.
5. Godleski LS, Sernyak MJ. Agranulocytosis after addition of risperidone to clozapine treatment. *Am J Psychiatry* (1996) 153, 735–6.
6. Kontaxakis VP, Havaki-Kontaxaki BJ, Stamouli SS, Christodoulou GN. Toxic interaction between risperidone and clozapine: a case report. *Prog Neuropsychopharmacol Biol Psychiatry* (2002) 26, 407–9.
7. Henderson DC, Goff DC. Risperidone as an adjunct to clozapine therapy in chronic schizophrenics. *J Clin Psychiatry* (1996) 57, 395–7.

Clozapine + Selective serotonin re-uptake inhibitors (SSRIs)

Fluoxetine, paroxetine sertraline and possibly citalopram can raise serum clozapine levels. Particularly large increases can occur with fluvoxamine. Toxicity has been seen in some patients.

Clinical evidence

(a) Citalopram

Preliminary studies in 5 patients found that their mean serum clozapine levels were unchanged by the concurrent use of **citalopram**.[1] Another study in 8 patients found similar results.[2] However, sedation hypersalivation and confusion were found in a patient who had recently had **citalopram** 40 mg daily added to his established clozapine treatment. When total clozapine serum levels were measured they were found to be 1097 nanograms/ml. The **citalopram** dose was reduced to 20 mg daily, the symptoms resolved over the following 2 weeks, and the total clozapine level dropped to 792 nanograms/ml.[3]

(b) Fluoxetine

Several studies and case reports have demonstrated increased clozapine levels of 30 to 75%, and increased norclozapine levels of 34 to 52% after **fluoxetine** was added to established clozapine treatment.[4-6] In one case the levels of clozapine and the metabolite, norclozapine, were raised over fivefold, accompanied by hypertension, when clozapine was given with **fluoxetine**. Clozapine levels became subtherapeutic 2 weeks after **fluoxetine** was withdrawn, necessitating an increase in dosage.[7]

A patient who had been taking 500 mg clozapine and 3 mg lorazepam daily, developed myoclonic jerks of his whole body 79 days after 20 mg **fluoxetine** was added. These decreased over the next two days when the **fluoxetine** and lorazepam were stopped.

In contrast, there are reports of successful use,[8] and no pharmacokinetic changes[9] when clozapine and **fluoxetine** were used together.

Fourteen schizophrenics showed increases of 30% and 33% in their serum levels of clozapine and norclozapine when an average of 39.3 mg of **fluoxetine** daily was added.[5] Another study found that the steady-state serum clozapine levels increased by 76% and those of norclozapine by 52% in 6 psychotic patients when an average of 36 mg **fluoxetine** was added. No increase in side-effects was seen.[4] Ten schizophrenics showed increases of 58%, 36% and 38% in the serum levels of clozapine, norclozapine and clozapine *N*-oxide when

concurrently treated with 20 mg **fluoxetine** daily for 8 weeks.[6] A man on 20 mg **fluoxetine** daily developed unexpectedly elevated serum clozapine levels when clozapine was started, accompanied by hypertension. When the **fluoxetine** was stopped, the clozapine and blood pressure fell to normal levels.[7]

An improvement in the control of chronic paranoid schizophrenia occurred in one patient when **fluoxetine** (60 mg daily) was added to clozapine (800 mg daily).[8] This contrasts with another study in a patient who showed no changes in his steady-state serum clozapine levels over eight weeks while taking 500 mg clozapine daily and 80 mg **fluoxetine** daily.[9] Another patient who had been taking 500 mg clozapine and 3 mg lorazepam daily, developed myoclonic jerks of his whole body 79 days after 20 mg **fluoxetine** was added. These decreased over the next two days when the **fluoxetine** and lorazepam were stopped. Serum clozapine levels were not measured.[10]

(c) Fluvoxamine

Three- to tenfold elevations in plasma clozapine levels have been seen in several studies and case reports where clozapine and **fluvoxamine** were used concurrently.[11-18] These elevations occurred as early as 20 days after combined treatment was started,[16] but were often not associated with any significant side-effects, in one case even after treatment had continued for a year.[14] Another study, which compared 12 patients on clozapine, with 11 patients on clozapine and **fluvoxamine** found that in the combined treatment group, clozapine doses were about half those used when clozapine was given alone. A trend towards decreased granulocyte levels was also seen in the clozapine/fluvoxamine group, but no when clozapine was used alone.[19] Other cases have also demonstrated worsening psychosis[20] or extrapyramidal side effects[21] (including, rigidity, tremors and akathisia) and sedation within days of giving **fluvoxamine** with clozapine.

A study in 16 patients on 2.5 to 3 mg/kg clozapine found that the addition of 50 mg **fluvoxamine** daily increased the steady-state serum levels of clozapine, *N*-desmethylclozapine and clozapine *N*-oxide by almost threefold.[22] Two schizophrenics showed marked rises in serum clozapine levels (from 255 to 267 nanograms/ml in one of them to a range of 1345 to 3151 nanograms/ml) when given 75 to 100 mg **fluvoxamine** daily.[11,18] Three out of four patients in another study were found to have a much higher clozapine concentration/dose ratio while taking **fluvoxamine**. The dose-normalised clozapine concentration of two of them rose by a factor of 5 to 10.[13] Three further patients showed three to ninefold increases in serum clozapine levels while taking 500 to 800 mg clozapine daily and 100 to 200 mg **fluvoxamine** daily. No significant side effects occurred while taking both drugs over extended periods (78,100 and 366 days).[14] Another two patients developed elevated serum clozapine levels when **fluvoxamine** was added, one of whom showed drowsiness, slurred speech, ataxia and hypotension.[16] Other reports describe this interaction,[17] including one about a woman whose serum clozapine rose 7.5-fold (to 7570 nanomol/l) after taking 100 mg **fluvoxamine** daily for 2 months. She was hospitalised with abdominal pain, dehydration and fever.[15] The serum clozapine levels of another patient rose more than twofold within a month of adding 50 mg **fluvoxamine** daily accompanied by worsening psychosis.[20]

Another patient showed extremely high serum clozapine levels, up to 4160 micrograms/l, as a result of also taking **fluvoxamine**.[23]

(d) Paroxetine

Sixteen schizophrenics showed increases of 57% and 50% in their serum levels of clozapine and norclozapine when an average of 31.2 mg of **paroxetine** daily was added. One patient on 300 mg clozapine daily developed reversible cerebral intoxication when given 40 mg **paroxetine** daily.[5] Another patient with a delusional disorder developed an anticholinergic syndrome with doubled serum clozapine levels within about 3 weeks of the addition of **paroxetine**.[24] In contrast, a study in 14 patients on 2.5 to 3 mg/kg clozapine found that the addition of 20 mg **paroxetine** daily had no effect on the serum levels of clozapine.[22]

(e) Sertraline

10 schizophrenics showed increases of 30% and 52% in their serum levels of clozapine and norclozapine when an average of 92.5 mg of **sertraline** daily was added.[5] Another patient on 600 mg clozapine

daily showed a fall in total clozapine serum levels of 40% within a month of stopping 300 mg **sertraline** daily.[25]

The serum clozapine levels of a schizophrenic patient doubled within a month of adding 50 mg **sertraline** daily and her psychosis worsened. When the **sertraline** was stopped she improved and her serum clozapine levels fell once again.[20]

Mechanism

It seems probable that the interacting SSRIs inhibit the clozapine metabolism by the liver (probably by inhibiting cytochrome P450 isoenzyme CYP2D6 or CYP1A2) thereby reducing its loss from the body. The levels of clozapine and norclozapine rise together, on the basis of which it has been suggested that the metabolic step inhibited is distal to *N*-dealkylation.[5]

Importance and management

These interactions are established. Concurrent use need not be avoided, but it would prudent to monitor closely because of the rises in serum clozapine and norclozapine levels which can occur (very considerable in the case of fluvoxamine) and in some cases in a deterioration in treatment. Adjust the clozapine dosage as necessary. The authors of one study suggest particularly close monitoring if the daily clozapine dosage exceeds 300 mg or 3.5 mg/kg.[5]

1. Taylor D, Ellison Z, Ementon Shaw L, Wickham H, Murray R. Co-administration of citalopram and clozapine: effect on plasma clozapine levels. *Int Clin Psychopharmacol* (1998) 13, 19–21.
2. Avenoso A, Facciolà G, Scordo MG, Gitto C, Ferrante GD, Madia AG, Spina E. No effect of citalopram on plasma levels of clozapine, risperidone and their active metabolites in patients with chronic schizophrenia. *Clin Drug Invest* (1998) 16, 393–8.
3. Borba CP, Henderson DC. Citalopram and clozapine: potential drug interaction. *J Clin Psychiatry* (2000) 61, 301–2.
4. Centorrino F, Baldessarini RJ, Kando J, Frankenburg FR, Volpicelli SA, Puopolo PR, Flood JG. Serum concentrations of clozapine and its major metabolites: effects of cotreatment with fluoxetine or valproate. *Am J Psychiatry* (1994) 151, 123–5.
5. Centorrino F, Baldessarini RJ, Frankenburg FR, Kando J, Volpicelli SA, Flood JG. Serum levels of clozapine and norclozapine in patients treated with selective serotonin reuptake inhibitors. *Am J Psychiatry* (1996) 153, 820–2.
6. Spina E, Avenoso A, Facciolà G, Fabrazzo M, Monteleone P, Maj M, Perucca E, Caputi AP. Effect of fluoxetine on the plasma concentrations of clozapine and its major metabolites in patients with schizophrenia. *Int Clin Psychopharmacol* (1998) 13, 141–5.
7. Sloan D, O'Boyle J. Hypertension and increased serum clozapine associated with clozapine and fluoxetine in combination. *Ir J Psych Med* (1977) 14, 149–51.
8. Cassady SL, Thaker GK. Addition of fluoxetine to clozapine. *Am J Psychiatry* (1992) 149, 1274.
9. Eggert AE, Crismon ML, Dorson PG. Lack of effect of fluoxetine on plasma clozapine concentrations. *J Clin Psychiatry* (1994) 55, 454–5.
10. Kingsbury SJ, Puckett KM. Effects of fluoxetine on serum clozapine levels. *Am J Psychiatry* (1995) 152, 473–4.
11. Hiemke C, Weigmann H, Müller H, Dahmen N, Wetzel H, Fuchs E. Elevated clozapine plasma levels after addition of fluvoxamine. *Soc Neurosci Abs* (1993) 19, 382.
12. Weigmann H, Müller H, Dahmen N, Wetzel H, Hiemke C. Interactions of fluvoxamine with the metabolism of clozapine. *Pharmacopsychiatry* (1993) 26, 209.
13. Jerling M, Lindström L, Bondesson U, Bertilsson L. Fluvoxamine inhibition and carbamazepine induction of the metabolism of clozapine: evidence from a therapeutic drug monitoring service. *Ther Drug Monit* (1994) 16, 368–74.
14. Dumortier G, Lochu A, Colen de Melo P, Ghribi O, Roche Rabreau D, Degrassat K, Desce JM. Elevated clozapine plasma concentrations after fluvoxamine initiation. *Am J Psychiatry* (1996) 153, 738–9.
15. Olesen OV, Starup G, Linnet K. Alvorlig lægemiddelinteraktion mellem clozapin – Leponex og fluvoxamin – Fevarin. *Ugeskr Laeger* (1996) 158, 6931–2.
16. Dequardo JR, Roberts M. Elevated clozapine levels after fluvoxamine initiation. *Am J Psychiatry* (1996) 153, 840–1.
17. Koponen HJ, Leinonen E, Lepola U. Fluvoxamine increases the clozapine serum levels significantly. *Eur Neuropsychopharmacol* (1996) 6, 69–71.
18. Hiemke C, Weigmann H, Härtter S, Dahmen N, Wetzel H, Müller H. Elevated levels of clozapine in serum after addition of fluvoxamine. *J Clin Psychopharmacol* (1994) 14, 279–81.
19. Hinze-Selch D, Deuschle M, Weber B, Heuser I, Pollmächer T. Effect of coadministration of clozapine and fluvoxamine versus clozapine monotherapy on blood cell counts, plasma levels of cytokines and body weight. *Psychopharmacology (Berl)* (2000) 149, 163–9.
20. Chong SA, Tan CH, Lee HS. Worsening of psychosis with clozapine and selective serotonin reuptake inhibitor combination: two case reports. *J Clin Psychopharmacol* (1997) 17, 68–9.
21. Kuo F-J, Lane H-Y, Chang W-H. Extrapyramidal symptoms after addition of fluvoxamine to clozapine. *J Clin Psychopharmacol* (1998) 18, 483–4.
22. Wetzel H, Anghelescu I, Szegedi A, Wiesner J, Weigmann H, Hörtter S, Hiemke C. Pharmacokinetic interactions of clozapine with selective serotonin reuptake inhibitors: differential effects of fluvoxamine and paroxetine in a prospective study. *J Clin Psychopharmacol* (1998) 18, 2–9.
23. Heeringa M, Beurskens R, Schouten W, Verduijn MM. Elevated plasma levels of clozapine after concomitant use of fluvoxamine. *Pharm World Sci* (1999) 21, 243–4
24. Joos AAB, König F, Frank UG, Kaschka WP, Mörike KE, Ewald R. Dose-dependent pharmacokinetic interaction of clozapine and paroxetine in an extensive metabolizer. *Pharmacopsychiatry* (1997) 30, 266–70.
25. Pinniniti NR, De Leon J. Interaction of sertraline with clozapine. *J Clin Psychopharmacol* (1997) 17, 119.

Droperidol/Hyoscine + Monoamine oxidase inhibitors (MAOIs)

An isolated and unexplained report describes hypotension in a patient given droperidol and hyoscine as premedication, shortly after the withdrawal of phenelzine and perphenazine.

Clinical evidence, mechanism, importance and management

Four days after the withdrawal of **phenelzine** and perphenazine, a patient was given operative premedication of 20 mg **droperidol** and 400 micrograms **hyoscine**, orally. About 2 h later he was observed to be pale, sweating profusely, slightly cyanosed, with a blood pressure of 75/60 mmHg and a pulse rate of 60. No excitement or changes in respiration were seen. The blood pressure gradually rose to 115/80 mmHg over the next 45 min, but did not return to his normal level of 160/100 mmHg for 36 h. The operation was successfully undertaken without any hypotensive episodes 11 days later, using the same premedication.[1] The response was attributed to the after-effects of **phenelzine** treatment, but there is no obvious explanation for this interaction (if indeed it is an interaction).

1. Penlington GN. Droperidol and monoamine-oxidase inhibitors. *BMJ* (1966) 1, 483–4.

Fluphenazine + Spiramycin

Acute dystonia occurred in a man on fluphenazine during treatment with spiramycin, which was attributed to an interaction.

Clinical evidence, mechanism, importance and management

A man with schizoaffective disorder taking lorazepam, orphenadrine, fluvoxamine and fluphenazine, developed acute and painful dystonia of the trunk, neck, right arm and leg legs about a week of his last injection of fluphenazine decanoate (12.5 mg every 2 weeks), on the fourth day of taking 6 million units of **spiramycin** daily for gingivitis. The problem resolved when he was given biperiden.[1] The reasons for this adverse reaction are not understood, nor is it entirely clear whether this was a fluphenazine/**spiramycin** interaction, although the author suggested that a causal link existed. This seems to be the only report of an alleged interaction between fluphenazine and a macrolide antibacterial and it is therefore of little or no general importance.

1. Benazzi F. Spiramycin-associated acute dystonia during neuroleptic treatment. *Can J Psychiatry* (1997) 42, 665–6.

Haloperidol + Antacids

There seem to be no clinical studies or reports confirming the anecdotal evidence of a possible reduction in the effects of haloperidol by antacids.

Clinical evidence, mechanism, importance and management

In 1982 a questioner in a letter asked whether haloperidol interacts with **antacids** because he had had a patient doing well on haloperidol who had begun to deteriorate when *Amphojel* (**aluminium hydroxide**) was added. In a written answer it was stated[1] that there are no reports of this interaction but ". . . several clinicians asked said that oral haloperidol and **antacids** should not be administered together . . . based on clinical impressions." There do not appear to be any reports or studies of this alleged interaction so that it remains purely anecdotal, however the advice given in the answer to the original question was to separate the administration by several hours to prevent admixture in the gut. Study is needed to find out whether such a precaution is really needed.

1. Goldstein BJ. Interaction of antacids with psychotropics. *Hosp Community Psychiatry* (1982) 33, 96.

Haloperidol + Anticonvulsants

Haloperidol serum levels are approximately halved by carbamazepine, phenobarbital and phenytoin. Neurotoxicity has been seen with haloperidol and carbamazepine. Valproate or valproic acid appear not to interact. Haloperidol can raise serum carbamazepine levels.

Clinical evidence

(a) Haloperidol + Carbamazepine

(i) Serum haloperidol levels reduced. A study in 9 schizophrenics on haloperidol (averaging 30 mg daily) showed an approximately 55% fall in serum haloperidol levels (a mean fall from 45.5 to 21.2 nanograms/ml) when given **carbamazepine** for 5 weeks (precise dose not stated, but said to be 5 to 6 tablets daily). They also took 10 mg trihexyphenidyl (benzhexol) and 30 mg oxazepam at night as necessary. **Carbamazepine** serum levels and the control of the disease remained unchanged.[1]
Other studies have similarly found approximately 40 to 60% falls in serum haloperidol levels while taking **carbamazepine**,[2-4] with the occasional patient having undetectable levels.[3,5] Decreases in serum haloperidol levels of unspecified amounts have also been described.[6-9] A few patients showed clinical worsening or increased side-effects.[3-5] Three patients showed two to fivefold increases in serum haloperidol levels and clinical improvement when **carbamazepine** 1200 to 1400 mg daily was stopped, but extrapyramidal side-effects developed within 1 to 30 days.[10] Three cases of neurotoxicity (drowsiness, slurred speech, confusion) during concurrent use have also been described.[6,11,12]
A case report describes 3 schizophrenic patients who were changed from **carbamazepine** to **oxcarbazepine** while concurrently taking haloperidol. After 2 weeks their serum haloperidol levels had dramatically risen (from 6 to 18 nanomol/l, from 6 to 14 nanomol/l and from 17 to 27 nanomol/l). This was accompanied by severe extrapyramidal side-effects, which necessitated dose reductions in 2 of the patients.[13] See 'Chlorpromazine + Carbamazepine or Oxcarbazepine', p.714.

(ii) Serum carbamazepine levels raised. A study in Japanese schizophrenic patients found that **carbamazepine** reduced the serum haloperidol levels by an unstated amount confirming (i) above, while at the same time the serum **carbamazepine** levels were raised by about 30% despite a smaller (75%) dosage.[7] An associated study by the same group of workers found that concurrent use increased the incidence of QTc lengthening.[14]

(b) Haloperidol + Phenobarbital and Phenytoin

A study in epileptic patients, 2 on **phenobarbital**, 3 on **phenytoin**, and 5 on both drugs, found that after 6 weeks their serum haloperidol levels while taking doses of 30 mg daily were approximately half of those in a control group who were not taking anticonvulsants (19.4 compared to 36.6 nanograms/ml). The patients' serum anticonvulsant levels remained unchanged.[15] Another patient showed a marked rise in serum haloperidol levels with clinical improvement when 300 mg **phenytoin** was stopped.[10] A retrospective study found that **phenobarbital** reduced the haloperidol concentration/dose ratio, suggesting that **phenobarbital** may affect the metabolism of haloperidol.[9]

(c) Haloperidol + Valproic acid or valproate

A study in 6 patients given 6 to 10 mg haloperidol daily showed no significant interaction with **valproic acid**.[16] No interaction was found in another study.[17]

Mechanism

Carbamazepine, phenobarbital and phenytoin are recognised enzyme inducing agents, therefore it seems highly likely that the reduced serum haloperidol levels occur because its metabolism by the liver is markedly increased by these anticonvulsants.

Importance and management

The interactions of haloperidol with carbamazepine, phenytoin and phenobarbital are moderately well documented and appear to be clinically important, but only a few patients have been reported to show clinical worsening. Although there are advantages in adding carbamazepine to haloperidol in treating manic patients or schizoaffective excited patients, and others with excited psychoses and schizophrenia,[18] be alert for the need to increase the haloperidol dosage if any of these anticonvulsants is given concurrently. The authors of one study with phenobarbital and phenytoin suggest a two to threefold increase in the haloperidol dosage.[15] Another study, in which intramuscular haloperidol was used, recommended shortening the interval between injections rather than raising the dosage, but it was no stated by how much.[19] Remember too that if the anticonvulsants are withdrawn it may be necessary to reduce the haloperidol dosage. Also be alert for the development of dystonic reactions and for a rise in serum carbamazepine levels. No special precautions appear to be necessary if sodium valproate is used concurrently.

1. Kidron R, Averbuch I, Klein E, Belmaker RH. Carbamazepine-induced reduction of blood levels of haloperidol in chronic schizophrenia. *Biol Psychiatry* (1985) 20, 219–22.
2. Jann MW, Ereshefsky L, Saklad SR, Seidel DR, Davis CM, Burch NR, Bowden CL. Effects of carbamazepine on plasma haloperidol levels. *J Clin Psychopharmacol* (1985) 5, 106–9.
3. Arana GW, Goff DC, Friedman H, Ornsteen M, Greenblatt DJ, Black B, Shader RI. Does carbamazepine-induced reduction of plasma haloperidol levels worsen psychotic symptoms? *Am J Psychiatry* (1986) 143, 650–1.
4. Kahn EM, Schulz SC, Perel JM, Alexander JE. Change in haloperidol level due to carbamazepine—a complicating factor in combined medication for schizophrenia. *J Clin Psychopharmacol* (1990) 10, 54–7.
5. Fast DK, Jones BD, Kusalic M, Erickson M. Effect of carbamazepine on neuroleptic plasma levels and efficacy. *Am J Psychiatry* (1986) 143, 117–18
6. Brayley J, Yellowlees P. An interaction between haloperidol and carbamazepine in a patient with cerebral palsy. *Aust N Z J Psychiatry* (1987) 21, 605–7.
7. Iwahashi K, Miyatake R, Suwaki H, Hosokawa K, Ichikawa Y. The drug–drug interaction effects of haloperidol on plasma carbamazepine levels. *Clin Neuropharmacol* (1995) 18, 233–6.
8. Jann MW, Chang W-H, Lane H-Y. Differences in haloperidol epidemiologic pharmacokinetic studies. *J Clin Psychopharmacol* (2001) 21, 628–30.
9. Hirokane G, Someya T, Takahashi S, Morita S, Shimoda K. Interindividual variation of plasma haloperidol concentrations and the impact of concomitant medications: the analysis of therapeutic drug monitoring data. *Ther Drug Monit* (1999) 21, 82–6.
10. Jann MW, Fidone GS, Hernandez JM, Amrung S, Davis CM. Clinical implications of increased antipsychotic plasma concentrations upon anticonvulsant cessation. *Psychiatry Res* (1989) 28, 153–9.
11. Kanter GL, Yerevanian BI, Ciccone JR. Case report of a possible interaction between neuroleptics and carbamazepine. *Am J Psychiatry* (1984) 141, 1101–2.
12. Yerevanian BI, Hodgman CH. A haloperidol-carbamazepine interaction in a patient with rapid-cycling bipolar disorder. *Am J Psychiatry* (1985) 142, 785–6.
13. Raitasuo V, Lehtovaara R, Huttunen MO. Effect of switching carbamazepine to oxcarbazepine on the plasma levels of neuroleptics. A case report. *Psychopharmacology (Berl)* (1994) 116, 115–16.
14. Iwahashi K, Nakamura K, Miyatake R, Suwaki H, Hosokawa K. Cardiac effects of haloperidol and carbamazepine treatment. *Am J Psychiatry* (1996) 153, 135.
15. Linnoila M, Viukari M, Vaisanen K, Auvinen J. Effect of anticonvulsants on plasma haloperidol and thioridazine levels. *Am J Psychiatry* (1980) 137, 819–21.
16. Ishizaki T, Chiba K, Saito M, Kobayashi K, Iizuka R. The effects of neuroleptics (haloperidol and chlorpromazine) on the pharmacokinetics of valproic acid in schizophrenic patients. *J Clin Psychopharmacol* (1984) 4, 254–61.
17. Normann C, Klose P, Hesslinger B, Langosch JM, Berger M, Walden J. Haloperidol plasma levels and psychopathology in schizophrenic patients with antiepileptic co-medication: a clinical trial. *Pharmacopsychiatry* (1997) 30, 204.
18. Klein E, Bental E, Lerer B, Belmaker RH. Carbamazepine and haloperidol v placebo and haloperidol in excited psychoses: a controlled study. *Arch Gen Psychiatry* (1984) 41, 165–70.
19. Pupeschi G, Agenet C, Levron J-C, Barges-Bertocchio M-H. Do enzyme inducers modify haloperidol decanoate rate of release? *Prog Neuropsychopharmacol Biol Psychiatry* (1994) 18, 1323–32.

Haloperidol + Antituberculars

The serum levels of haloperidol can be reduced by the concurrent use of rifampicin (rifampin), and possibly raised by isoniazid.

Clinical evidence

A study in schizophrenic patients on haloperidol, 7 of whom were also on a range of antitubercular drugs (**ethambutol**, **isoniazid**, **rifampicin**), and 18 of whom were on **isoniazid** only, showed that those on multiple drugs, which included **rifampicin** had significantly reduced haloperidol serum levels. The half-life of haloperidol in 2 patients on **rifampicin** was 4.9 h compared with 9.4 h in 3 other patients not taking **rifampicin**.[1] Three of the patients on **isoniazid** had increased serum haloperidol levels.[1]

The trough serum haloperidol levels of 15 schizophrenics fell to 37.4% after taking **rifampicin** 600 mg daily for 7 days.[2] After 28 days the serum level had dropped further to 30%. In another group of 5 patients stabilised on haloperidol and **rifampicin**, the serum haloperidol levels rose to 229% 7 days after stopping **rifampicin**, and to 329% after 28 days.[2] The clinical effects of the haloperidol were assessed as having being reduced by the **rifampicin**.[2]

Mechanism

The likeliest explanation is that the rifampicin, a recognised enzyme inducing agent, increases the metabolism and loss of the haloperidol from the body.

Importance and management

The haloperidol/rifampicin interaction would appear to be established and clinically important. Be alert for any evidence of reduced haloperidol effects if rifampicin alone is used, and possibly increased effects if isoniazid alone is used. Adjust the haloperidol dosage if necessary. More study is needed.

1. Takeda M, Nishinuma K, Yamashita S, Matsubayashi T, Tanino S, Nishimura T. Serum haloperidol levels of schizophrenics receiving treatment for tuberculosis. *Clin Neuropharmacol* (1986) 9, 386–97.
2. Kim Y-H, Cha I-J, Shim J-C, Shin J-G, Yoon Y-R, Kim Y-K, Kim J-I, Park G-H, Jang I-J, Woo J-I, Shin S-G. Effect of rifampin on the plasma concentration and the clinical effect of haloperidol concomitantly administered to schizophrenic patients. *J Clin Psychopharmacol* (1996) 16, 247–52.

Haloperidol + Buspirone

One report found no pharmacokinetic interaction, but two others found that buspirone can cause a rise in serum haloperidol levels of uncertain importance.

Clinical evidence, mechanism, importance and management

A pharmacokinetic study in 27 schizophrenic patients on 10 to 40 mg haloperidol daily found that 5 mg **buspirone** three times daily for 2 weeks, followed by 10 mg three times daily for 4 weeks, did not significantly affect the steady-state haloperidol levels.[1]

These findings contrast with those of another 6-week study, in which 6 out of 7 schizophrenics showed rises in haloperidol levels of 15 to 122% when given **buspirone**.[2] The authors also mention a single dose study in healthy subjects, which found a 30% rise in haloperidol levels when subjects were additionally given **buspirone**.[2]

It is not known why these findings differ, but since no adverse reactions have been reported, there would seem to be no reason for avoiding concurrent use. Even so it would seem prudent to monitor concurrent use for any evidence of increased and adverse haloperidol effects.

1. Huang HF, Jann MW, Wei F-C, Chang T-P, Chen J-S, Juang D-J, Lin S-K, Lam YFW, Chien C-P, Chang W-H. Lack of pharmacokinetic interaction between buspirone and haloperidol in patients with schizophrenia. *J Clin Pharmacol* (1996) 36, 963–9.
2. Goff DC, Midha KK, Brotman AW, McCormick S, Waites M, Amico ET. An open trial of buspirone added to neuroleptics in schizophrenic patients. *J Clin Psychopharmacol* (1991) 11, 193–7.

Haloperidol + Dexamfetamine (Dextroamphetamine)

Acute dystonia occurred in two healthy subjects when given haloperidol and dexamfetamine (dextroamphetamine).

Clinical evidence

Two healthy young women were given 5 mg haloperidol and 5 mg **dexamfetamine** (**dextroamphetamine**) as part of a neuropharmacological study. After 29 h one of them developed stiffness of neck and limbs, Parkinsonian facies, her tongue protruded and she had oropharyngeal spasm. After 34 h the other woman developed oculogyric crisis and acute dystonia of the neck with her back slightly arched. Both recovered rapidly after being given 10 mg intramuscular **procyclidine**.[1]

Mechanism

Not fully understood, but the authors of the study suggest that the acute dystonia was due to a potentiation of dopamine release.

Importance and management

This study was carried out under good supervision. It emphasises the importance of not giving these two drugs together in patients.

1. Capstick C, Checkley S, Gray J, Dawe S. Dystonia induced by amphetamine and haloperidol. *Br J Psychiatry* (1994) 165, 276.

Haloperidol + Fluvoxamine

Limited evidence suggests that fluvoxamine can increase the serum levels of haloperidol causing toxicity.

Clinical evidence, mechanism, importance and management

A study in 3 schizophrenic patients on benzatropine showed that the concurrent use of **fluvoxamine** caused their serum haloperidol levels to climb. When the **fluvoxamine** was stopped the levels fell once again. This was not a formal pharmacokinetic study, but (as an example), while taking 150 to 200 mg **fluvoxamine** from day 16 to day 37, the haloperidol serum levels of one patient rose from 17 to a maximum of 38 nanograms/ml. The **fluvoxamine** was then stopped and 54 days later his serum haloperidol levels had fallen to 9 nanograms/ml. This patient became lethargic and showed worsening of all of the clinical and cognitive functions assessed while taking all three drugs.[1] Another limited study also observed that **fluvoxamine** causes a rise in the serum levels of haloperidol.[2] The reasons are not understood, but it seems possible that **fluvoxamine** can inhibit the metabolism of haloperidol, which leads to increased serum levels.

Information seems to be limited to these studies and more work needs to be done on it to assess its general importance, but it would now seem prudent to be on the alert for this interaction if **fluvoxamine** and haloperidol are given together in any patient. It may be necessary to reduce the haloperidol dosage to avoid toxicity.

1. Daniel DG, Randolph C, Jaskiw G, Handel S, Williams T, Abi-Dargham A, Shoaf S, Egan M, Elkashef A, Liboff S, Linnoila M. Coadministration of fluvoxamine increases serum concentrations of haloperidol. *J Clin Psychopharmacol* (1994) 14, 340–3.
2. Vandel S, Bertschy G, Baumann P, Bouquet S, Bonin B, Francois T, Sechter D, Bizouard P. Fluvoxamine and fluoxetine: Interaction studies with amitriptyline, clomipramine and neuroleptics in phenotyped patients. *Pharmacol Res* (1995) 31, 347–53.

Haloperidol + Granisetron

Granisetron appears not to increase the adverse effects of haloperidol (drowsiness, mental slowness, etc.).

Clinical evidence, mechanism, importance and management

A study in 12 healthy subjects found that while 3 mg haloperidol alone caused some impaired psychometric performance (increased drowsiness, muzziness, lethargy, mental slowness, etc.), the addition of 160 micrograms/kg **granisetron** did not seem to make performance significantly worse.[1] If both drugs are used, no special precautions would seem necessary, over and above those needed for either drug alone.

1. Leigh TJ, Link CGG, Fell GL. Effects of granisetron and haloperidol, alone and in combination, on psychometric performance and the EEG. *Br J Clin Pharmacol* (1992) 34, 65–70.

Haloperidol + Imipenem

Marked but transient hypotension was seen in 3 patients on intravenous imipenem when given low dose intravenous haloperidol.

Clinical evidence, mechanism, importance and management

Three patients in intensive care who were being treated with intravenous **imipenem** (500 mg six-hourly for 48 h, 72 h and 7 days respectively) developed a rapid and short-lived episode of hypotension when given a 2.5-mg dose of intravenous haloperidol. For example, the blood pressure of one of the patients fell from 117/75 mmHg to 91/49 mmHg. After 30 min her blood pressure had risen to 100/57 mmHg. No treatment for hypotension was given to any of the patients and the reaction was brief and self-limiting. Two of them were also taking famotidine and erythromycin. No acute ECG changes were seen.[1]

The reason for this fall in blood pressure is not understood, but the authors attribute what happened to the concurrent use of haloperidol and **imipenem**, although they point out that intravenous haloperidol alone can cause orthostatic hypotension. One suggestion is that competitive protein binding displacement might have increased the levels of free haloperidol.[1]

The authors advice is that if haloperidol is used low doses should be given and the outcome well monitored. They say that no pressor agent was needed in these cases, but they suggest the possible use of **metaraminol, phenylephrine** or **norepinephrine (noradrenaline)** rather than **dopamine**, the vasopressor effects of which might be blocked or reversed by haloperidol.[1] This interaction seems not to have been reported to occur with oral haloperidol.

1. Franco-Bronson K, Gajwani P. Hypotension associated with intravenous haloperidol and imipenem. *J Clin Psychopharmacol* (1999) 19, 480–1.

Haloperidol + Indometacin (Indomethacin)

Profound drowsiness and confusion have been described in patients given haloperidol and indometacin.

Clinical evidence

A double-blind crossover study in 20 patients to find out the possible advantages of combining haloperidol 5 mg daily with **indometacin (indomethacin)** 25 mg three times daily was eventually abandoned because 13 patients (11 on haloperidol and 2 on placebo) failed to complete the trial. Profound drowsiness or tiredness caused 6 of the haloperidol treated patients to be withdrawn from the trial. The au-

thors of the paper said[1] that the combined treatment ". . . produced drowsiness and confusion so severe that in some cases the patient's independent existence was in jeopardy; this side-effect was far more intense than anything which might have been expected with haloperidol alone."

Mechanism

Not understood.

Importance and management

Evidence of this interaction appears to be very limited. The incidence (6 out of 20) is high. If concurrent use is thought appropriate, keep a close watch to ensure that this severe side-effect does not develop. It might be wiser to avoid concurrent use because many patients requiring this type of treatment may not be hospitalised and under the day-to-day scrutiny of the prescriber.

1. Bird HA, Le Gallez P, Wright V. Drowsiness due to haloperidol/indometacin in combination. *Lancet* (1983) i, 830–1.

Haloperidol + Quinidine

Blood levels of haloperidol can be markedly increased if quinidine is added.

Clinical evidence, mechanism, importance and management

An experimental study of the metabolism of haloperidol in 13 healthy subjects found that 1 h after taking 250 mg **quinidine bisulphate**, the maximum plasma levels and the AUC of haloperidol, following a single 5-mg dose, were approximately doubled. The reasons are not understood.[1] The clinical importance of this in patients has not been assessed, but it seems likely that the effects and side-effects of haloperidol will be increased if **quinidine** is added. Be alert for this interaction if both drugs are given. See also 'Drugs that prolong the QT interval + Other drugs that prolong the QT interval', p.103.

1. Young D, Midha KK, Fossler MJ, Hawes EM, Hubbard JW, McKay G, Korchinski ED. Effect of quinidine on the interconversion kinetics between haloperidol and reduced haloperidol in humans: implications for the involvement of cytochrome P450IID6. *Eur J Clin Pharmacol* (1993) 44, 433–8.

Haloperidol + Sertraline

Sertraline does not appear to worsen the effects of haloperidol on cognitive function.

Clinical evidence, mechanism, importance and management

A single 2-mg dose of haloperidol was given to 21 subjects on days 2 to 25 of a double-blind, randomised, placebo-controlled study. On days 9 to 25 the subjects received in addition either placebo, or **sertraline**, increased over 7 days to 200 mg daily. All subjects took psychomotor tests on days 1, 2 and 25 to assess the effect of haloperidol. Their cognitive function was impaired for 6 to 8 h after taking the haloperidol, but this effect had disappeared after 23 h. On day 25 cognitive impairment in some of the psychomotor tests was worse and occurred sooner after dosing. However, these effects were seen equally in both the **sertraline** and placebo groups, suggesting that **sertraline** does not worsen the cognitive impairment caused by haloperidol.[1] Another study found similar pharmacodynamic results, and also demonstrated that the pharmacokinetics of haloperidol are unaffected by **sertraline**.[2] No special precautions would therefore seem necessary during concurrent use.

1. Williams SA, Wesnes K, Oliver SD, Rapeport WG. Absence of effect of sertraline on time-based sensitization of cognitive impairment with haloperidol. *J Clin Psychiatry* (1996) 57 (Suppl 1), 7–11.
2. Lee MS, Kim YK, Lee SK, Suh KY. A double-blind study of adjunctive sertraline in haloperidol-stabilized patients with chronic schizophrenia. *J Clin Psychopharmacol* (1998) 18, 399–403.

Haloperidol + Tobacco smoking

Smokers may need more haloperidol than non-smokers.

Clinical evidence, mechanism, importance and management

Steady-state haloperidol levels were found to be lower in a group of 23 cigarette **smokers** than in another group of 27 **non-smokers** (16.83 compared with 28.8 nanograms/ml) and the clearance was increased (1.58 compared with 1.1 l/min).[1] Other studies have broadly confirmed these findings.[2,3] The probable reason is that some of the components of **tobacco smoke** act as liver enzyme inducers which increase the rate at which the liver metabolises and clears the haloperidol from the body. It seems possible that **smokers** may need larger doses of haloperidol than non-smokers, and the dosage of haloperidol may need to be adjusted if patients start or stop smoking.

1. Jann MW, Saklad SR, Ereshefsky L, Richards AL, Harrington CA, Davis CM. Effects of smoking on haloperidol and reduced haloperidol plasma concentrations and haloperidol clearance. *Psychopharmacology (Berl)* (1986) 90, 468–70.
2. Perry PJ, Miller DD, Arndt SV, Smith DA, Holman TL. Haloperidol dosing requirements: the contribution of smoking and nonlinear pharmacokinetics. *J Clin Psychopharmacol* (1993) 13, 46–51.
3. Pan L, Vander Stichele R, Rosseel MT, Berlo JA, De Schepper N, Belpaire FM. Effects of smoking, CYP2D6 genotype, and concomitant drug intake on the steady state plasma concentrations of haloperidol and reduced haloperidol in schizophrenic inpatients. *Ther Drug Monit* (1999) 21, 489–97.

Haloperidol + Venlafaxine

There is evidence that venlafaxine can increase the serum levels of haloperidol. This is consistent with an isolated report of a man who developed urinary retention when venlafaxine was added to a previously well tolerated regimen of haloperidol and alprazolam.

Clinical evidence, mechanism, importance and management

A study in 24 healthy subjects found that **venlafaxine** 75 mg 12-hourly, at steady-state, reduced the renal clearance of a single 2-mg dose of haloperidol by 42%, resulting in a 70% rise in the AUC and an 88% rise in the maximum serum levels.[1,2] This rise in haloperidol levels would seem to be consistent with an isolated report of a man of 75 who had encountered no problems while taking 1 mg haloperidol and 500 micrograms alprazolam daily, but who suddenly developed urinary retention when the drugs were given with 37.5 mg **venlafaxine** daily. Urinary retention resolved spontaneously when all the drugs were stopped. The suggested reason is that **venlafaxine** inhibited the cytochrome P450 isoenzyme CYP2D6 which is concerned with the metabolism of haloperidol. As a result the serum levels of the haloperidol rose, thereby increasing its anticholinergic effects.[3]

The evidence is very limited but what is known suggests that patients should be well monitored for increased haloperidol side-effects if **venlafaxine** is taken concurrently. It may be necessary to reduce the haloperidol dosage.

1. Efexor (Venlafaxine). Wyeth Laboratories. Summary of product characteristics, January 2002.
2. Wyeth, Personal communication, April 2001.
3. Benazzi F. Urinary retention with venlafaxine-haloperidol combination. *Pharmacopsychiatry* (1997) 30, 27.

Hydroxyzine + Miscellaneous drugs

Hydroxyzine can cause ECG abnormalities in high doses. It has been suggested that concurrent use with other drugs that can cause cardiac abnormalities might increase the likelihood of dysrhythmias and sudden death.

Clinical evidence, mechanism, importance and management

A study in 25 elderly psychotic patients on 300 mg hydroxyzine over a 9-week period showed that ECG changes were mild, except for alteration in T waves, which were definite in 9 patients and usually observed in leads 1,2 AVL and V_{3-6}. In each case the T-waves were lower in altitude, broadened and flattened and sometimes notched. The QT interval was usually prolonged. A repeat of the study in a few patients, one at least given 400 mg hydroxyzine, gave similar results, the most pronounced change being a marked attenuation of cardiac repolarisation. On the basis of these observations the authors suggest that other drugs that cause ECG abnormalities (they mention **antiparkinson drugs, atropine, lithium carbonate, phenothiazines, quinidine, procainamide, thioridazine, tricyclic antidepressants**), might aggravate and exaggerate these hydroxyzine-induced changes and increase the risk of sudden death.[1] More study is needed to assess the practical importance of these potential interactions. See also 'Drugs that prolong the QT interval + Other drugs that prolong the QT interval', p.103.

1. Hollister LE. Hydroxyzine hydrochloride: possible adverse cardiac interactions. *Psychopharmacol Comm* (1975) 1, 61–5.

Loxapine + Fluvoxamine

An isolated report describes amenorrhoea and galactorrhoea apparently due to the addition of fluvoxamine to loxapine.

Clinical evidence, mechanism, importance and management

A woman of 38 with a bipolar affective disorder was maintained on 150 mg loxapine, 30 mg oxazepam and 7.5 mg zopiclone daily. **Fluvoxamine** was then added, eventually up to 150 mg daily, and the loxapine dosage halved. After 6 weeks she complained of amenorrhoea, followed shortly by galactorrhoea. The galactorrhoea resolved within 3 weeks of stopping the **fluvoxamine**, and menstruation occurred a week later. Her prolactin levels were found to be 80 micrograms/l (normal 4 to 30 micrograms/l). The reasons for what happened are not known. Galactorrhoea is a known side-effect of phenothiazines (such as loxapine) and is due to an elevation of serum prolactin levels caused by the blockade of dopamine receptors in the hypothalamus, but just why **fluvoxamine** apparently increased this effect, particularly when the loxapine dosage had been halved, is not understood. The role (if any) of the other drugs is not known.[1]

This is the first and only report of an apparent interaction between these drugs, and it would not seem to be of general importance.

1. Jefferies J, Bezchlibnyk-Butler K, Remington G. Amenorrhea and galactorrhea associated with fluvoxamine in a loxapine-treated patient. *J Clin Psychopharmacol* (1992) 12, 296–7.

Loxapine + Sumatriptan

An isolated report describes a severe dystonic reaction in a woman on loxapine when given sumatriptan.

Clinical evidence, mechanism, importance and management

A woman was treated with 10 mg loxapine twice daily for psychotic target symptoms, benzatropine for the prophylaxis of extrapyramidal effects, carbamazepine for mood stabilisation and *Fiorcet* (paracetamol (acetaminophen), caffeine, butalbital) for migraine headaches. Two days after the loxapine was raised to 35 mg daily she was given a single 6 mg subcutaneous dose of **sumatriptan** for a migraine headache. Within 15 min she developed torticollis, which was treated with intramuscular benzatropine and intravenous diphenhydramine. The authors of the report suggest that what happened was possibly the additive dystonic effects of the loxapine and **sumatriptan**, despite the presence of the benzatropine. Dystonia is a not uncommon extrapyramidal reaction associated with antipsychotics, and neck stiffness and dystonia are recognised side effects of **sumatriptan**, but of low incidence.[1] This seems to be the first and only report this apparent interaction, but the authors suggest good monitoring if both drugs are used concurrently.

1. Garcia G, Kaufman MB, Colucci RD. Dystonic reaction associated with sumatriptan. *Ann Pharmacother* (1994) 28, 1199.

Molindone + Paroxetine

An isolated report describes the development of severe extrapyramidal symptoms in a patient on molindone when paroxetine was added.

Clinical evidence, mechanism, importance and management

An elderly woman on 10 mg molindone twice daily developed severe and disabling extrapyramidal symptoms (severe bradykinesia, tremor, inability to feed herself, delirium) within about 2 weeks of starting 10 mg **paroxetine** daily. These resolved when molindone was stopped, and no problems occurred when fluoxetine alone was started. The authors of the report postulate that the **paroxetine** may have raised the serum molindone levels, but no measurements were made.[1] No general conclusions can be drawn from this slim evidence, but it would now clearly be prudent to monitor the concurrent use of these drugs in any patient.

1. Malek-Ahmadi P, Allen SA. Paroxetine-molindone interaction. *J Clin Psychiatry* (1995) 56, 82–3.

Olanzapine + Miscellaneous drugs

Fluvoxamine causes a rise in serum olanzapine levels, whereas tobacco smoking and activated charcoal cause a fall. Postural hypotension and possibly drowsiness may be increased with alcohol. Olanzapine appears not to interact to a clinically relevant extent with aluminium/magnesium antacids, carbamazepine, cimetidine, diazepam, imipramine, theophylline or warfarin.

Clinical evidence, mechanism, importance and management

(a) Alcohol

The makers say that patients on olanzapine have shown an increased heart rate and accentuated postural hypotension when given a single dose of **alcohol** (amount not stated). No pharmacokinetic interaction has been seen.[1] In practical terms this means that patients should be warned of the risk of faintness and dizziness if they stand up quickly, and told what to do. The makers also say that olanzapine can cause drowsiness and they warn about driving or operating dangerous machinery.[2] It would be expected that alcohol might worsen this effect.

The patient information leaflet produced by the makers[3] actually says "Do not drink any alcohol while taking *Zyprexa* (olanzapine)".

(b) Antacids

The makers of olanzapine say that single doses of an **aluminium** and **magnesium-containing antacid** had no effect on the pharmacokinetics of olanzapine.[1,2] No special precautions would seem to be needed during concurrent use.

(c) Benzodiazepines

Single dose studies have shown that no pharmacokinetic interaction occurs between olanzapine and **diazepam**,[1] confirming other *in vitro* studies using human liver microsomes[1,2] which demonstrated no inhibition of the cytochrome P450 isoenzymes CYP3A4 or CYP2C19, which are concerned with the metabolism of **diazepam**. In patients taking both drugs it was noted that mild increases in heart rate, sedation and dry mouth were seen, but no dosage adjustments were thought to be necessary.[1] There would therefore appear to be no reason for avoiding concurrent use.

(d) Carbamazepine

Multiple-dose studies in healthy subjects have shown that **carbamazepine** increases the metabolism of olanzapine (by induction of cytochrome P450 isoenzyme CYP1A2). The clearance of olanzapine was increased 44% and its terminal elimination half-life was reduced 20%, but these changes were not considered significant enough to call for dosage adjustments of either drug.[1] Another study found that 5 patients taking olanzapine and **carbamazepine** had a concentration/dose ratio 36% lower than 22 patients taking olanzapine alone.[4] Clinical monitoring of the effect is recommended by the makers if both drugs are to be used concurrently.[2]

(e) Charcoal, activated

The makers report that **activated charcoal** reduces the bioavailability of oral olanzapine by 50 to 60%, and recommend that administration be separated by 2 hours.[2]

(f) Cimetidine

The makers say that *in vivo* interaction studies found that **cimetidine** had no effect on the pharmacokinetics of olanzapine.[1,2] No special precautions would seem to be needed during concurrent use.

(g) Haloperidol

A man of 67 with a long history of bipolar disorder was taking **haloperidol** 10 mg daily, with valproate and benzatropine. Because he had previously had parkinsonian symptoms, olanzapine was started, to be increased as the **haloperidol** was decreased. On day 6 he became extremely parkinsonian. The **haloperidol** was stopped and 2 days later the symptoms had resolved. It is thought that either the small amount of dopaminergic activity of olanzapine, combined with that of the **haloperidol** brought on these symptoms, or that olanzapine affected the metabolism of **haloperidol**, caused increased levels and therefore greater dopaminergic activity.[5] The significance of this interaction is not clear, but it would be wise to be aware of this interaction if the combination is used.

(h) Selective serotonin re-uptake inhibitors

Olanzapine 2.5 to 7.5 mg or a placebo was given to 10 male smokers daily for 3 days, and then on days 4 to 11 they were additionally given 50 to 100 mg **fluvoxamine** daily. It was noted that somnolence increased (by 19 to 115%) but the subjects accommodated to this within 4 days. During concurrent use the olanzapine maximum plasma levels and AUC rose by 84 and 119% respectively and the olanzapine clearance fell by 50%. It was concluded that this interaction was due **fluvoxamine** inhibition of cytochrome P450 isoenzyme CYP1A2, which is involved in the metabolism of olanzapine.[6] A retrospective study found that in patients taking **fluvoxamine**, and olanzapine, the concentration/dose ratio was 2.3-fold higher than those on olanzapine alone. In contrast **sertraline** had no effect on the concentration/dose ratio, suggesting it does not interact.[7] A case report suggests that the **fluvoxamine** interaction is clinically relevant. The olanzapine serum levels of a woman of 21 were 6 times the recommended upper limit while she was taking **fluvoxamine**. During this time she had developed rigidity and tremor. After a dose reduction from 20 mg of olanzapine to 5 mg the levels were still almost double the recommended level. When **paroxetine** was substituted for **fluvoxamine** and the olanzapine dose was left at 5 mg, the olanzapine levels became almost normal and no symptoms were seen.[8] The makers of olanzapine suggest lower olanzapine doses may be needed if **fluvoxamine** is used concurrently.[2]

(i) Tobacco smoking

Tobacco smoking induces cytochrome P450 isoenzyme CYP1A2 so that the clearance of olanzapine in smokers is increased and its half-life shortened. Non-smokers show a 33% lower clearance and a 21% longer half-life.[1] The consequences are that the effects of olanzapine will be reduced to some extent by **smoking**, but it is not clear whether smokers will therefore need to be given a significantly larger dosage to achieve the same therapeutic effects. The makers advise careful monitoring in case a dose increase is necessary.[2]

(j) Tricyclic antidepressants

A randomised, open-label three-way crossover study in 9 healthy men given single doses of 5 mg olanzapine and 75 mg **imipramine** found no clinically relevant pharmacokinetic or pharmacodynamic interactions between the two drugs.[9] This would seem to confirm *in vitro* studies using human liver microsomes, which demonstrated minimal inhibition of the cytochrome P450 isoenzyme CYP2D6, which is involved in the metabolism of the tricyclic antidepressants.[1,2] However, there is one case report on record of seizures, thought to be caused by the concurrent use of olanzapine and **clomipramine**. Neither agent alone had produced this reaction in the patient.[10] No special precautions would seem to be necessary if both drugs are used concurrently, but be aware that they both have the potential to lower the seizure threshold and that the effect may be additive.

(k) Warfarin

A three-way randomised crossover study was carried out in 15 healthy subjects given 10 mg olanzapine or 20 mg racemic **warfarin** or both drugs together as single doses. No significant changes were seen in the pharmacokinetics of either drug, and the adverse effects of the olanzapine and the anticoagulant effects of the **warfarin** were unchanged.[11] These results and those of other *in vitro* studies using human liver microsomes supports the conclusion that olanzapine has little inhibitory effect on cytochrome P450 isoenzyme CYP2C9.[1,2] The makers say that a clinically important interaction is unlikely between these two drugs.[2] However until more clinical experience has been gained it would seem prudent to monitor concurrent use.

(l) Effect of olanzapine on liver microsomal enzymes

The makers of olanzapine say that *in vitro* studies carried using human liver microsomes have shown that olanzapine has only an extremely small inhibitory effect on the cytochrome P450 isoenzymes CYP3A4, CYP2C9, CYP1A2, CYP2C19 and CYP2D6.[2] This means that olanzapine is not expected to inhibit the *in vivo* metabolism of other concurrently used drugs that are metabolised by any of these P450 isoenzymes, so that their serum levels are not expected to rise (however the possibility of interactions by other mechanisms cannot be discounted).

1. Zyprexa (Olanzapine). Eli Lilly. Clinical and Laboratory Experience - A Comprehensive Monograph. August 1996.
2. Zyprexa (Olanzapine). Eli Lilly and Company Limited. Summary of product characteristics, November 2001.
3. Zyprexa (Olanzapine). Lilly. Patient information sheet, November 2001.
4. Olesen OV, Linnet K. Olanzapine serum concentrations in psychiatric patients given standard doses: the influence of comedication. *Ther Drug Monit* (1999) 21, 87–90.
5. Gomberg RF. Interaction between olanzapine and haloperidol. *J Clin Psychopharmacol* (1999) 19, 272–3.
6. Mäenpää J, Wrighton S, Bergstrom R, Cerimele B, Tatum D, Hatcher B, Callaghan JT. Pharmacokinetic (PK) and pharmacodynamic (PD) interactions between fluvoxamine and olanzapine. *Clin Pharmacol Ther* (1997) 61, 225.
7. Weigmann H, Gerek S, Zeisig A, Müller M, Härtter S, Heimke C. Fluvoxamine but not sertraline inhibits the metabolism of olanzapine: evidence from a therapeutic drug monitoring service. *Ther Drug Monit* (2001) 23, 410–13.
8. de Jong J, Hoogenboom B, van Troostwijk LD, de Haan L. Interaction of olanzapine with fluvoxamine. *Psychopharmacology (Berl)* (2001) 155, 219–20.
9. Callaghan JT, Cerimele BJ, Kassahun KJ, Nyhart EH, Hoyes-Beehler PJ, Kondraske GV. Olanzapine: interaction study with imipramine. *J Clin Pharmacol* (1997) 37, 971–8.
10. Deshauer D, Albuquerque J, Alda M, Grof P. Seizures caused by possible interaction between olanzapine and clomipramine. *J Clin Psychopharmacol* (2000) 20, 283–4.
11. Maya JF, Callaghan JT, Bergstrom RF, Cerimele BJ, Kassahun K, Nyhart EH, Brater DC. Olanzapine and warfarin drug interaction. *Clin Pharmacol Ther* (1997) 61, 182.

Phenothiazines + Antacids

Antacids containing aluminium and magnesium hydroxide or magnesium trisilicate can reduce the serum levels of chlorpromazine, which would be expected to reduce the therapeutic response. *In vitro* studies suggest that this may possibly also occur with other antacids and phenothiazines.

Clinical evidence

A study in 10 patients taking 600 to 1200 mg **chlorpromazine** daily showed that when concurrently treated with 30 ml *Aludrox* (**aluminium and magnesium hydroxide gel**) their urinary excretion of **chlorpromazine** was reduced by 10 to 45%.[1]

A study was prompted by the observation of one psychotic patient, controlled on **chlorpromazine** who relapsed within 3 days of starting to take an **unnamed antacid**. When *Gelusil* (**aluminium hydroxide + magnesium trisilicate**) 30 ml was given with a liquid suspension of **chlorpromazine** to 6 patients, the serum **chlorpromazine** levels measured 2 h later were reduced by about 20% (from 168 to 132 nanograms/ml).[2,3] *In vitro* studies have also found that other phenothiazines (**trifluoperazine, fluphenazine, perphenazine, thioridazine**) are adsorbed to a considerable extent onto a number of antacids (**magnesium trisilicate, bismuth subnitrate, aluminium hydroxide-magnesium carbonate**) but no clinical studies of the possible effects of these interactions appear to have been done.[4]

Mechanism

Chlorpromazine and other phenothiazines become adsorbed onto these antacids,[2,5] which would seem to account for the reduced bioavailability.

Importance and management

Clinical information seems to be limited to the reports cited. Reductions in serum levels of up to 45% would be expected to be clinically important, but so far only one case seems to have been reported.[2,3] Separating the doses as much as possible (1 to 2 h) to avoid admixture in the gut should minimise any effects. An alternative would be to use one of the ionic antacids such as calcium carbonate-glycine or magnesium hydroxide gel, which seem to affect the gastrointestinal absorption of chlorpromazine to a lesser extent.[5] Other phenothiazines and antacids are known to interact *in vitro*,[4] but the clinical importance of these interactions awaits further study.

1. Forrest FM, Forrest IS, Serra MT. Modification of chlorpromazine metabolism by some other drugs frequently administered to psychiatric patients. *Biol Psychiatry* (1970) 2, 53–8.
2. Fann WE, Davis JM, Janowsky DS, Sekerke HJ, Schmidt DM. Chlorpromazine: effects of antacids on its gastrointestinal absorption. *J Clin Pharmacol* (1973) 13, 388–90.
3. Fann WE, Davis JM, Janowski DS, Schmidt D. The effects of antacids on the blood levels of chlorpromazine. *Clin Pharmacol Ther* (1973) 14, 135.
4. Moustafa MA, Babhair SA, Kouta HI. Decreased bioavailability of some antipsychotic phenothiazines due to interactions with adsorbent antacid and antidiarrhoeal mixtures. *Int J Pharmaceutics* (1987) 36, 185–9.
5. Pinell OC, Fenimore DC, Davis CM, Moreira O, Fann WE. Drug-drug interaction of chlorpromazine and antacid. *Clin Pharmacol Ther* (1978) 23, 125.

Phenothiazines + Antimalarials

Chloroquine, amodiaquine and *Fansidar* (sulfadoxine/pyrimethamine) can markedly increase serum chlorpromazine levels.

Clinical evidence

A total of 15 schizophrenic patients (in three groups of five) given 400 or 500 mg **chlorpromazine** daily for at least 2 weeks were additionally given single doses of either **chloroquine sulphate** 400 mg, **amodiaquine hydrochloride** 600 mg or three tablets of *Fansidar* (25 mg **pyrimethamine** + 500 mg **sulfadoxine**) an hour before **chlorpromazine**. Serum **chlorpromazine** levels 3 h later were found to be raised approximately threefold by the **chloroquine** and **amodiaquine**, and almost fourfold by the *Fansidar*. The plasma levels of one of the major metabolites of **chlorpromazine** (7-hydroxychlorpromazine) were also elevated, but not those of the other metabolite, chlorpromazine sulphoxide. The serum **chlorpromazine** levels of the patients given **chloroquine** or *Fansidar* still remained elevated to some extent 4 days later. There was subjective evidence that the patients were more heavily sedated when given the antimalarials.[1]

Mechanism

Not understood. Both chloroquine and *Fansidar* have relatively long half-lives compared with amodiaquine, which may explain the persistence of their effects.

Importance and management

Direct information about this interaction seems to be limited to this study. Its clinical importance is uncertain but it seems possible that these antimalarials could cause chlorpromazine toxicity. Monitor the effects of concurrent use closely and anticipate the need to reduce the chlorpromazine dosage. More study is needed. See also 'Drugs that prolong the QT interval + Other drugs that prolong the QT interval', p.103.

1. Makanjuola ROA, Dixon PAF, Oforah E. Effects of antimalarial agents on plasma levels of chlorpromazine and its metabolites in schizophrenic patients. *Trop Geogr Med* (1988) 40, 31–3.

Phenothiazines + Ascorbic acid

A single case report describes a fall in serum fluphenazine levels and deterioration in a patient when given ascorbic acid (vitamin C).

Clinical evidence, mechanism, importance and management

A man with a history of manic behaviour, taking 15 mg **fluphenazine** daily, showed a 25% fall (from 0.93 to 0.705 nanograms/ml) in his serum drug levels accompanied by a deterioration in behaviour over a 13-day period while taking 500 mg **ascorbic acid** twice daily.[1] The reason is not understood. There seem to be no other reports of this interaction with **fluphenazine** or any other phenothiazine so that this interaction would appear not to be of general importance.

1. Dysken MW, Cumming RJ, Channon RA, Davis JM. Drug interaction between ascorbic acid and fluphenazine. *JAMA* (1979) 241, 2008.

Phenothiazines + Attapulgite-pectin

An attapulgite-pectin antidiarrhoeal preparation caused a fall in the absorption of promazine in one subject.

Clinical evidence, mechanism, importance and management

A study in a healthy subject showed that **attapulgite-pectin** reduced the absorption of a single 50-mg dose of **promazine** by about 25%, possibly due to absorption of the phenothiazine onto the **attapulgite**.[1] The clinical importance of this interaction and whether other phenothiazines behave similarly appears not to have been studied, but prescribers should be aware of this possible interaction if preparations containing **attapulgite-pectin** are given. Separating the administration as much as possible (2 h or more) to avoid admixture in the gut has been shown with other drugs to minimise the effects of this type of interaction.

1. Sorby DL, Liu G. Effects of adsorbents on drug absorption II. Effect of an antidiarrhea mixture on promazine absorption. *J Pharm Sci* (1966) 55, 504–10.

Phenothiazines + Barbiturates

The serum levels of each drug are reduced by the presence of the other, but the clinical importance of these reductions is uncertain. Pentobarbital, promethazine and hyoscine in combination are said to increase the incidence of operative agitation.

Clinical evidence

(a) Serum phenothiazine levels reduced

A study in 12 schizophrenics on 100 mg **chlorpromazine** three times daily showed that when additionally treated with 50 mg **phenobarbital** three times daily, there was a 25 to 30% fall in serum **chlorpromazine** levels accompanied by changes in certain physiological measurements, which clearly reflected a reduced response. The conclusion was made that there was no advantage to be gained by concurrent use.[1]

In another study in 7 patients the serum levels of **thioridazine** were observed to be reduced by **phenobarbital**, but the clinical effects of this were uncertain.[2] However, another study found no changes in serum **thioridazine** levels, but the levels of its active metabolite (**mesoridazine**) were reduced.[3]

(b) Serum phenobarbital levels reduced

A study in a number of epileptic patients showed that their serum **phenobarbital** levels fell by 29% when treated with phenothiazines, which included **chlorpromazine**, **thioridazine** or **mesoridazine**, and increased once more when the phenothiazine was withdrawn.[4]

This study confirms another, in which 100 to 200 mg **thioridazine** daily was found to reduce serum **phenobarbital** levels by about 25%.[5] There is also some limited evidence that the concurrent use of **pentobarbital**, **promethazine** and **hyoscine** increases the incidence of pre-operative, operative and postoperative agitation, and it has been suggested that this triple combination should be avoided.[6]

Mechanisms

Uncertain. The barbiturates are potent liver enzyme inducing agents, and so it is presumed that they increase the metabolism of the phenothiazines by the liver.

Importance and management

These interactions appear to be established, but the documentation is limited. The importance of both interactions (a) and (b) is uncertain, but be alert for evidence of reductions in response during concurrent use, and to increased responses if one of the drugs is withdrawn. So far only chlorpromazine, thioridazine, mesoridazine and phenobarbital are implicated, but it seems possible that other phenothiazines and barbiturates will behave similarly.

1. Loga S, Curry S, Lader M. Interactions of orphenadrine and phenobarbitone with chlorpromazine: plasma concentrations and effects in man. *Br J Clin Pharmacol* (1975) 2, 197–208.
2. Ellenor GL, Musa MN, Beuthin FC. Phenobarbital-thioridazine interaction in man. *Res Commun Chem Pathol Pharmacol* (1978) 21, 185–8.
3. Linnoila M, Viukari M, Vaisanen K, Auvinen J. Effect of anticonvulsants on plasma haloperidol and thioridazine levels. *Am J Psychiatry* (1980) 137, 819–21.
4. Haidukewych D, Rodin EA. Effect of phenothiazines on serum antiepileptic drug concentrations in psychiatric patients with seizure disorder. *Ther Drug Monit* (1985) 7, 401–4.
5. Gay PE, Madsen JA. Interaction between phenobarbital and thioridazine. *Neurology* (1983) 33, 1631–2.
6. Macris SG, Levy L. Preanesthetic medication: untoward effects of certain drug combinations. *Anesthesiology* (1965) 26, 256.

Phenothiazines + Biperiden or Orphenadrine

Biperiden and orphenadrine do not affect the serum levels of perphenazine. An isolated report describes hypoglycaemia in a non-diabetic patient given chlorpromazine and orphenadrine. See also 'Antipsychotics + Anticholinergics', p.692.

Clinical evidence, mechanism, importance and management

A study in psychotic patients found that the addition of **biperiden** 2 mg three times daily or **orphenadrine** 50 mg three times daily for 3 weeks had no effect on the steady-state levels of **perphenazine** 24 to 48 mg daily.[1] An isolated report describes the development of a hypoglycaemic coma in a non-diabetic patient given **chlorpromazine** and **orphenadrine**.[2] The reasons are not understood.

1. Hansen LB, Elley J, Christensen TR, Larsen N-E, Naestoft J, Hvidberg EF. Plasma levels of perphenazine and its major metabolites during simultaneous treatment with anticholinergic drugs. *Br J Clin Pharmacol* (1979) 7, 75–80.
2. Buckle RM, Guillebaud J. Hypoglycaemic coma occurring during treatment with chlorpromazine and orphenadrine. *BMJ* (1967) 4, 599–600.

Phenothiazines + Cimetidine

One study found that chlorpromazine serum levels are reduced by cimetidine. Another suggested that they can be increased.

Clinical evidence, mechanism, importance and management

A study in 8 patients on 75 to 450 mg daily **chlorpromazine** found that 1 g **cimetidine** daily, in divided doses, for a week decreased their steady-state serum **chlorpromazine** levels by a third (from 37 to 24 micrograms/ml). A two-thirds fall was noted in one patient.[1] The reasons are not understood but a decrease in absorption from the gut has been suggested.[1] In contrast another report describes 2 schizophrenic patients on 100 mg **chlorpromazine** four times daily who became excessively sedated when given 400 mg **cimetidine** twice daily. The sedation disappeared when the **chlorpromazine** dosage was halved. When the **cimetidine** was later withdrawn it was found necessary to give the original **chlorpromazine** dosage.[2] **Chlorpromazine** serum levels were not measured. There is no simple explanation for these discordant reports, but they emphasise the need to monitor the concurrent use of **chlorpromazine** and **cimetidine**. More study is needed. There seems to be no information about other phenothiazines.

1. Howes CA, Pullar T, Sourindhrin I, Mistra PC, Capel H, Lawson DH, Tilstone WJ. Reduced steady-state plasma concentrations of chlorpromazine and indomethacin in patients receiving cimetidine. *Eur J Clin Pharmacol* (1983) 24, 99–102.
2. Byrne A, O'Shea B. Adverse interaction between cimetidine and chlorpromazine in two cases of chronic schizophrenia. *Br J Psychiatry* (1989) 155, 413–15.

Phenothiazines + Disulfiram

A single case report describes a man on perphenazine whose psychotic symptoms re-emerged when he began to take disulfiram.

Clinical evidence, mechanism, importance and management

A psychotic man controlled on 8 mg **perphenazine** twice daily by mouth developed marked psychosis soon after starting to take 200 mg **disulfiram** daily.[1] His serum **perphenazine** levels had fallen from 2 to 3 nanomol/l to less than 1 nanomol/l. Doubling the dosage of **perphenazine** had little effect, and no substantial clinical improvement or rise in serum levels occurred until the **perphenazine** was given as the **enantate** intramuscularly (50 mg weekly) when the levels rose to about 4 nanomol/l. The results of clinical biochemical tests suggested that the **disulfiram** was acting as a liver enzyme-inducing agent, so that the **perphenazine** was being metabolised and cleared from the body more rapidly. **Disulfiram** normally acts as an enzyme inhibitor. Too little is known to assess the general importance of this interaction, and there seems to be no information about an interaction with other phenothiazines.

1. Hansen LB, Larsen N-E. Metabolic interaction between perphenazine and disulfiram. *Lancet* (1982) ii, 1472.

Phenothiazines + Fluvoxamine

Preliminary evidence suggests that fluvoxamine does not interact with cyamemazine or levomepromazine.

Clinical evidence, mechanism, importance and management

A study in 29 inpatients taking various antipsychotics, including **cyamemazine** and **levomepromazine**, found that the concurrent use of 150 mg **fluvoxamine** daily had no effect on the serum levels of either of these phenothiazines, but the authors of the report also say that no firm conclusions should be drawn from this finding because the number of patients was too small.[1] More study is needed.

1. Vandel S, Bertschy G, Baumann P, Bouquet S, Bonin B, Francois T, Sechter D, Bizouard P. Fluvoxamine and fluoxetine: interaction studies with amitriptyline, clomipramine and neuroleptics in phenotyped patients. *Pharmacol Res* (1995) 31, 347–53.

Phenothiazines + Naltrexone

Extreme lethargy occurred in two patients on thioridazine when given naltrexone.

Clinical evidence, mechanism, importance and management

Two schizophrenic patients well stabilised on **thioridazine** (50 to 200 mg three times daily for at least one year) took part in a pilot project to assess the efficacy of **naltrexone** for the treatment of tardive dyskinesia. Both tolerated the first challenge dose of **naltrexone** (800 micrograms intravenously) without problems but experienced extreme lethargy and slept almost continuously after the second **naltrexone** dose (50 to 100 mg orally). The severe lethargy resolved within 12 h of stopping the **naltrexone**.[1] The reasons for this reaction are not understood. Information seems to be limited to this report but this would seem to be a drug combination to be avoided. There seems to be nothing documented about other phenothiazines.

1. Maany I, O'Brien CP, Woody G. Interaction between thioridazine and naltrexone. *Am J Psychiatry* (1987) 144, 966.

Phenothiazines + Phenylpropanolamine

A single case report describes fatal ventricular fibrillation attributed to the concurrent use of thioridazine and phenylpropanolamine.

Clinical evidence, mechanism, importance and management

A 27-year-old schizophrenic woman who was taking regular daily doses of 100 mg **thioridazine** and 5 mg **procyclidine** was found dead in bed 2 h after taking a single capsule of *Contac C* (**phenylpropanolamine** 50 mg + **chlorphenamine maleate** 4 mg). The principal cause of death was attributed to ventricular fibrillation.[1] Just why this happened is not understood but it is suggested that it may have been due to the combined effects of the **thioridazine** (known to be cardiotoxic and to cause T-wave abnormalities) and the **phenylpropanolamine** (possibly able to cause ventricular arrhythmias like epinephrine (adrenaline) with anaesthetics).

The general importance of this alleged interaction is uncertain but the authors of the report suggest that ephedrine-like agents such as **phenylpropanolamine** should not be given to patients on **thioridazine** or **mesoridazine**.

1. Chouinard G, Ghadirian AM, Jones BD. Death attributed to ventricular arrhythmia induced by thioridazine in combination with a single Contac C capsule. *Can Med Assoc J* (1978) 119, 729–31.

Phenothiazines + Suriclone or Zopiclone

The addition of either suriclone or zopiclone to chlorpromazine increases sedation and worsens the performance of skilled tasks related to driving.

Clinical evidence, mechanism, importance and management

No pharmacokinetic interactions were seen when 12 healthy subjects were given single oral doses of either 0.4 mg **suriclone** or 7.5 mg **zopiclone**, with 50 mg **chlorpromazine**. However the overall performance in a number of psychomotor tests (including digit symbol substitution and simulated driving) was definitely impaired more by the combination of the drugs than by **chlorpromazine** alone. Among the effects of **suriclone** with **chlorpromazine** were drowsiness, dreaminess and clumsiness. **Zopiclone** with **chlorpromazine** impaired memory and learning, and caused a marked impairment of the performance of the tests.[1] In practical terms this means that patients given **chlorpromazine** with either of these drugs should be warned that they will almost certainly feel drowsy and be less able to drive or handle potentially hazardous machinery safely.

1. Mattila MJ, Vanakoski J, Matilla-Evenden ME, Karonen S-L. Suriclone enhances the actions of chlorpromazine on human psychomotor performance but not on memory or plasma prolactin in healthy subjects. *Eur J Clin Pharmacol* (1994) 46, 215–20.

Phenothiazines + Tobacco or Cannabis smoking

Smokers of tobacco or cannabis may possibly need larger doses of chlorpromazine and fluphenazine than non-smokers.

Clinical evidence

A comparative study found that the frequency of drowsiness in 403 patients taking **chlorpromazine** was 16% in **non-smokers**, 11% in **light smokers**, and 3% in **heavy smokers** (more than 20 cigarettes daily).[1] Another report describes a patient on **chlorpromazine** who experienced increased sedation and dizziness, and higher serum **chlorpromazine** levels, when he gave up smoking.[2] A study in 31 patients found that the clearance of **chlorpromazine** was increased 38% by **tobacco smoking**, 50% by **cannabis smoking**, and 107% when **both** were **smoked**.[3]

In a retrospective study in 40 psychiatric inpatients it was found that the serum **fluphenazine** levels of **non-smokers** were more than double those of **smokers** (1.83 compared with 0.89 nanograms/ml) when given **fluphenazine hydrochloride** by mouth. When **fluphenazine decanoate** intramuscularly was given, the serum levels were little different (0.81 compared with 0.93 nanograms/ml). However in both cases the clearance of **fluphenazine** was considerably greater in the smokers than in the **non-smokers** (clearance 1.67- and 2.33-fold greater in the oral and intramuscular groups respectively).[4] No behavioural differences were seen.[4]

Mechanism

Not established. The probable reason is that some of the components of smoke act as enzyme-inducing agents, which increase the rate at which the liver metabolises these phenothiazines, thereby reducing their serum levels and clinical effects.

Importance and management

Established interactions but of uncertain clinical importance. Be alert for the need to use increased dosages of these phenothiazines in patients who smoke, and reduced dosages if smoking is stopped.

1. Swett C. Drowsiness due to chlorpromazine in relation to cigarette smoking: a report from the Boston Collaborative Drug Surveillance Program. *Arch Gen Psychiatry* (1974) 31, 211–13.

2. Stimmel GL, Falloon IRH. Chlorpromazine plasma levels, adverse effects, and tobacco smoking: case report. *J Clin Psychiatry* (1983) 44, 420–2.
3. Chetty M, Miller R, Moodley SV. Smoking and body weight influence the clearance of chlorpromazine. *Eur J Clin Pharmacol* (1994) 46, 523–6.
4. Ereshefsky L, Jann MW, Saklad SR, Davis CM, Richards AL, Burch NR. Effects of smoking on fluphenazine clearance in psychiatric inpatients. *Biol Psychiatry* (1985) 20, 329–32.

Phenothiazines + Trazodone

Undesirable hypotension occurred in two patients on chlorpromazine or trifluoperazine when given trazodone. Thioridazine causes a moderate rise in trazodone serum levels.

Clinical evidence, mechanism, importance and management

A depressed patient on **chlorpromazine** began to complain of dizziness and unstable gait within 2 weeks of starting to take 100 mg **trazodone** one to three times daily. His blood pressure had fallen to between 92/58 and 126/72 mmHg. Within 2 days of stopping the **trazodone** his blood pressure had restabilised.[1] Another patient on **trifluoperazine** was given 100 mg **trazodone** daily and within 2 days she complained of dizziness and was found to have a blood pressure of 86/52 mmHg. Within a day of stopping the **trazodone** her blood pressure was back to 100/65 mmHg.[1] It would seem that the hypotensive side-effects of the two drugs can be additive. Patients given phenothiazines and trazodone should be monitored for signs of excessive hypotension.

A study, undertaken to confirm the involvement of cytochrome P450 isoenzyme CYP2D6 in the metabolism of **trazodone**, found that when 11 depressed patients were given 150 to 300 mg **trazodone** at bedtime for 18 weeks, and then 40 mg **thioridazine** additionally for a week, the plasma levels of the **trazodone** rose by 36% and those of its active metabolite (*m*-chlorophenylpiperazine) by 54%.[2] No adverse reactions were described and there would seem to be no reason for avoiding concurrent use.

1. Asayesh K. Combination of trazodone and phenothiazines: a possible additive hypotensive effect. *Can J Psychiatry* (1986) 31, 857–8.
2. Yasui N, Otani K, Kaneko S, Ohkubo T, Osanai T, Ishida M, Mihara K, Kondo T, Sugawara K, Fukushima Y. Inhibition of trazodone metabolism by thioridazine in humans. *Ther Drug Monit* (1995) 17, 333–5.

Phenothiazines + Tricyclic antidepressants

Concurrent treatment is common, but the tricyclic antidepressant serum levels are increased by the presence of many phenothiazines, and the serum levels of some phenothiazines are also increased by the tricyclic antidepressants. Although fixed-dose combined preparations are available, it has been suggested that concurrent use might contribute to an increased incidence of tardive dyskinesia. A paradoxical reversal of the therapeutic effects of chlorpromazine after the addition of a tricyclic antidepressants has also been described.

Clinical evidence

(a) Effect of phenothiazines on tricyclic antidepressants

An extended study of 4 patients given 12.5 mg intramuscular **fluphenazine decanoate** weekly, with 6 mg **benzatropine mesilate** and 300 mg **imipramine** daily, showed that the mean combined plasma concentrations of **imipramine** and **desipramine** (a metabolite of **imipramine**) were 850 nanograms/ml. This appeared high when compared with 60 other patients described elsewhere who were taking 225 mg **imipramine** daily and had levels of 180 nanograms/ml.[1] A comparative study of 99 patients taking **amitriptyline** or **nortriptyline** alone, and 60 other patients additionally taking an average of 10 mg **perphenazine** daily, showed that although the tricyclic antidepressant dosage levels were the same, the plasma tricyclic antidepressant levels of the **perphenazine** group were up to 70% higher.[2]

Other studies have described increased tricyclic antidepressant levels with phenothiazines. There is currently evidence for this interaction between **imipramine**,[3-5] and **chlorpromazine**; between **amitriptyline**,[6] **imipramine**,[5,7] **desipramine**[8] or **nortriptyline**[9,10] and **perphenazine**; between **desipramine**,[11] **imipramine**[12] or **nortriptyline**,[13] and **thioridazine**; between **nortriptyline**,[13] and **levomepromazine** or **perphenazine**.[13]

However, other studies have found no interaction between **amitriptyline**[9,13,14] or **nortriptyline**[15] and **perphenazine**; between **amitriptyline**[13] and **thioridazine**; between **amitriptyline**[13] and **levomepromazine**; and between **amitriptyline**,[9] or **nortriptyline**[9] and **zuclopenthixol**. It should be noted that in the case of **amitriptyline**, although the levels were not affected, increased levels of **nortriptyline**, its metabolite, were raised.[13]

(b) Effect of tricyclic antidepressant on phenothiazines

In a controlled study on 8 schizophrenic patients taking 20 mg **butaperazine** daily, 6 of them on 150 mg **desipramine** or more daily showed a rise in serum **butaperazine** levels of between 50 and 300%. The 2 patients taking 100 mg or less of **desipramine** showed no changes.[16] Other studies have shown a rise in phenothiazine levels when tricyclic antidepressants are added. So far, interactions with **chlorpromazine** and **amitriptyline**,[17] **imipramine**[17] or **nortriptyline**[18] have been documented.

One study on 7 chronic schizophrenics also reported that the addition of full doses of **nortriptyline** (50 mg three times daily) to a course of **chlorpromazine** 100 mg three times daily resulted in profound worsening of the clinical state, with marked increases in agitation and tension, despite the fact the **chlorpromazine** levels were actually raised. The **nortriptyline** was withdrawn.[18] A temporary reversion of a disruptive behaviour pattern has been seen in other patients on **chlorpromazine** when given **amitriptyline**.[19]

Mechanism

The rise in the serum levels of both drugs is thought to be due to a mutual inhibition of the liver enzymes concerned with the metabolism of both drugs, which results in their accumulation. The evidence available is consistent with this idea.[3,4,7,16,18]

Importance and management

Established interactions, but the advantages and disadvantages of concurrent use are still the subject of debate. These two groups of drugs are widely used together in the treatment of schizophrenic patients who show depression, and for mixed anxiety and depression. A number of fixed-dose combinations have been marketed, e.g. *Triptafen*, *Etrafon*, *Triaval* (**amitriptyline and perphenazine**), *Motival*, *Motipress* (**nortriptyline and fluphenazine**), however the safety of using both drugs together has been questioned.

One of the problems of phenothiazine treatment is the development of tardive dyskinesia, and some evidence suggests that the higher the dosage, the greater the incidence.[20] The symptoms can be transiently masked by increasing the dosage,[21] thus the presence of a tricyclic antidepressant might not only be a factor causing the tardive dyskinesia to develop, but might also mask the condition (or so it has been suggested.[16,22]) One author has advised that, until more is known, combined treatment should be the exception rather than the rule.[22] It has also been recommended that the addition of full antidepressant doses of nortriptyline to average antipsychotic doses of chlorpromazine should be avoided because the therapeutic actions of the chlorpromazine may be reversed.[18] See also 'Antipsychotics + Anticholinergics', p.692.

Attention has also been drawn to excessive weight gain associated with several months use of amitriptyline with thioridazine for the treatment of chronic pain.[23] See also 'Drugs that prolong the QT interval + Other drugs that prolong the QT interval', p.103.

1. Siris SG, Cooper TB, Rifkin AE, Brenner R, Lieberman JA. Plasma imipramine concentrations in patients receiving concomitant fluphenazine decanoate. *Am J Psychiatry* (1982) 139, 104–6.

2. Linnoila M, George L, Guthrie S. Interaction between antidepressants and perphenazine in psychiatric patients. *Am J Psychiatry* (1982) 139, 1329–31.
3. Gram LF, Overø KF. Drug interaction: inhibitory effect of neuroleptics on metabolism of tricyclic antidepressants in man. *BMJ* (1972) 1, 463–5.
4. Crammer JL, Rolfe B. Interaction of imipramine and chlorpromazine in man. *Psychopharmacologia* (1972) 26 (Suppl), 81.
5. Gram LF. Lægemiddelinteraktion: hæmmende virkning af neuroleptica på tricykliske antidepressivas metabolisering. *Nord Psykiatr Tidsskr* (1971) 25, 357–60.
6. Perel JM, Stiller RL, Feldman BL, Lin FC, Narayanan S. Therapeutic drug monitoring (TDM) of the amitriptyline (AT)/perphenazine (PER) interaction in depressed patients. *Clin Chem* (1985) 31, 939–40.
7. Gram LF, Overø KF, Kirk L. Influence of neuroleptics and benzodiazepines on metabolism of tricyclic antidepressants in man. *Am J Psychiatry* (1974) 131, 863–6.
8. Nelson JC, Jatlow PI. Neuroleptic effect on desipramine steady-state plasma concentrations. *Am J Psychiatry* (1980) 137, 1232–4.
9. Linnet K. Comparison of the kinetic interactions of the neuroleptics perphenazine and zuclopenthixol with tricyclic antidepressives. *Ther Drug Monit* (1995) 17, 308–11.
10. Mulsant BH, Foglia JP, Sweet RA, Rosen J, Lo KH, Pollock BG. The effects of perphenazine on the concentration of nortriptyline and its hydroxymetabolites in older patients. *J Clin Psychopharmacol* (1997) 17, 318–21.
11. Hirschowitz J, Bennett JA, Zemlan FP, Garver DL. Thioridazine effect on desipramine plasma levels. *J Clin Psychopharmacol* (1983) 3, 376–9.
12. Maynard GL, Soni P. Thioridazine interferences with imipramine metabolism and measurement. *Ther Drug Monit* (1996) 18, 729–31.
13. Jerling M, Bertilsson L, Sjöqvist F. The use of therapeutic drug monitoring data to document kinetic drug interactions: an example with amitriptyline and nortriptyline. *Ther Drug Monit* (1994) 16, 1–12.
14. Cooper SF, Dugal R, Elie R, Albert J-M. Metabolic interaction between amitriptyline and perphenazine in psychiatric patients. *Prog Neuropsychopharmacol* (1979) 3, 369–76.
15. Kragh-Sørensen P, Borgå O, Garle M, Bolvig Hansen L, Hansen CE, Hvidberg EF, Larsen N-E, Sjöqvist F. Effect of simultaneous treatment with low doses of perphenazine on plasma and urine concentrations of nortriptyline and 10-hydroxynortriptyline. *Eur J Clin Pharmacol* (1977) 11, 479–83.
16. El-Yousef MK, Manier DH. Tricyclic antidepressants and phenothiazines. *JAMA* (1974) 229, 1419.
17. Rasheed A, Javed MA, Nazir S, Khawaja O. Interaction of chlorpromazine with tricyclic anti-depressants in schizophrenic patients. *J Pakistan Med Assoc* (1994) 44, 233–4.
18. Loga S, Curry S, Lader M. Interaction of chlorpromazine and nortriptyline in patients with schizophrenia. *Clin Pharmacokinet* (1981) 6, 454–62.
19. O'Connor JW. Personal communication, February 1983.
20. Crane GE. Persistent dyskinesia. *Br J Psychiatry* (1973), 122, 395–405.
21. Crane GE. Tardive dyskinesia in patients treated with major neuroleptics: a review of the literature. *Am J Psychiatry* (1968) 124 (Suppl), 40–8.
22. Ayd FJ. Pharmacokinetic interaction between tricyclic antidepressants and phenothiazine neuroleptics. *Int Drug Ther Newslett* (1974) 9, 31–2.
23. Pfister AK. Weight gain from combined phenothiazine and tricyclic therapy. *JAMA* (1978) 239, 1959.

Pimozide + Clarithromycin

Clarithromycin can increase the serum levels of pimozide, which is believed to increase its serious cardiotoxicity.

Clinical evidence, mechanism, importance and management

The sudden death of a patient taking pimozide and **clarithromycin** prompted a study of a possible interaction between the two drugs. Using human liver microsomes it was found that pimozide is partly metabolised by the cytochrome P450 isoenzyme CYP3A, and that 2 micromol of **clarithromycin** inhibits this enzyme by at least 80%.[1] The practical consequences of this were seen in a later study in 12 healthy subjects, which found that 500 mg **clarithromycin** twice daily for 5 days more than doubled the AUC of a single 6 mg oral dose of pimozide and raising its maximum serum levels by almost 50%. The QT$_c$ interval was prolonged from 19 to 28 ms.[2] The results were the same in both poor and extensive CYP2D6 metabolisers. The authors of this study concluded that **clarithromycin** can therefore increase the cardiotoxicity of pimozide during chronic use, irrespective of the CYP2D6 status of the patient.[2] Pimozide alone has been associated with ventricular arrhythmias, the prolongation of the QT interval, T-wave changes and with sudden and unexpected death, even in the young with no previous evidence of cardiac disease.[3] While the importance of this interaction is therefore still not fully established, on the basis of the evidence available and the potential severity of this interaction, it might now be prudent either to avoid concurrent use or to monitor very closely for any ECG changes. More study is needed.

1. Flockhart DA, Richard E, Woosely RL, Pearle PL, Drici M-D. A metabolic interaction between clarithromycin and pimozide may result in cardiac toxicity. *Clin Pharmacol Ther* (1996) 59, 189.

2. Desta Z, Kerbusch T, Flockhart DA. Effect of clarithromycin (CLM) on the pharmacokinetics (PK) and -dynamics (PD) of pimozide (PIM) in healthy poor (PM) and extensive (EM) metabolizers of CYP2D6. *Clin Pharmacol Ther* (1998) 63, 184.

3. Committee on Safety of Medicines. Cardiotoxic effects of pimozide. *Current Problems* (1990) 29.

Pimozide + Miscellaneous drugs

Pimozide should not be given with other drugs that can prolong the QT interval because of the risk of potentially fatal cardiac arrhythmias. Pimozide may also possibly interact with CNS depressants, levodopa, and anticonvulsants.

Clinical evidence, mechanism, importance and management

Between 1971 and 1995 the CSM received a total of 40 reports (16 fatal) of serious cardiac arrhythmias in patients taking pimozide. It is contraindicated in patients with a prolonged QT interval or with a history of cardiac arrhythmias. Patients on pimozide should have an annual ECG, and if the QT interval is prolonged the treatment should be reviewed and either withdrawn or the dosage reduced under close supervision. The CSM advises the avoidance of pimozide with the following drugs and groups of drugs that can also prolong the QT interval: **other antipsychotics** (including depot preparations), **tricyclic antidepressants**, and other drugs known to prolong the QT interval such as **antimalarials**, **antiarrhythmic agents**, **astemizole**, **terfenadine**, or drugs that can cause electrolyte disturbances, especially **diuretics**.[1] See also 'Drugs that prolong the QT interval + Other drugs that prolong the QT interval', p.103.

The makers of pimozide say that it can cause sedation and impair alertness, and therefore they give a warning about concurrent use of other CNS depressants such as **alcohol**, **hypnotics**, **sedatives** or **strong analgesics**, which may have additive effects. They also say that pimozide may impair the antiparkinson effects of **levodopa**. They suggest that the dosage of **anticonvulsants** may need to be increased because pimozide lowers the convulsive threshold.[2]

1. Committee on Safety of Medicines. Cardiac arrhythmias with pimozide (Orap). *Current Problems* (1995) 21, 2.

2. Orap (Pimozide). Janssen-Cilag Ltd. Summary of product characteristics, April 2001.

Pimozide + Paroxetine

An isolated report describes the development of oculogyric crises in a boy on pimozide when given paroxetine.

Clinical evidence, mechanism, importance and management

A boy of about 10 with various disorders (motor tics, enuresis, attention deficit hyperactivity disorder, Tourettes's disorder, impulsivity, albinism) was treated for a year with 2 mg pimozide twice daily, and later three times daily.[1] Within 3 days of additionally starting 10 mg **paroxetine** in the morning, he began to complain of his eyes hurting and his mother noted that about 4 h after taking the **paroxetine** his ". . . eyes looked like they were rolled back in his head . . ." but the problem had resolved by the evening. This oculogyric crisis occurred on a further occasion, and so the **paroxetine** was stopped. There was no other evidence of either extrapyramidal or hyperserotonergic reactions. The reasons are not understood. This isolated case needs to be viewed in its particular context (oculogyric crises are associated with albinism) so that it may not be of general importance, but this needs confirmation.

1. Horrigan JP, Barnhill LJ. Paroxetine–pimozide drug interaction. *J Am Acad Child Adolesc Psychiatry* (1994) 33, 1060–1.

Prochlorperazine + Metoclopramide

A single case report describes tongue swelling and respiratory obstruction in a patient after being given prochlorperazine followed by metoclopramide.

Clinical evidence, mechanism, importance and management

A woman of 19 experienced progressive swelling of the tongue, partial upper-airways obstruction and a sensation of choking over a period of 12 h following intramuscular doses of **metoclopramide** to a total of 30 mg. She had received a 12.5-mg intramuscular dose of prochlorperazine for nausea and headaches 24 h earlier. Her tongue on examination was strikingly blue, but within 15 min of receiving 2 mg benzatropine it returned to its normal size and colour. The respiratory distress also disappeared.[1] The reason for the reaction, suggested by the authors of the report, is that the dystonic side-effects of both drugs were additive.[1] One of the authors had seen this reaction previously in a patient on large doses of haloperidol. Oedema of the tongue has also been described with **metoclopramide** alone.[2] Prescribers should be aware of this adverse reaction, and know its simple antidote.

1. Alroe C, Bowen P. Metoclopramide and prochlorperazine: "the blue-tongue sign". *Med J Aust* (1989) 150, 724–5.
2. Robinson OPW. Metoclopramide—side effects and safety. *Postgrad Med J* (1973) 49 (Suppl July), 77–80.

Quetiapine + Miscellaneous drugs

The serum levels of quetiapine are reduced by phenytoin and predicted to be reduced by carbamazepine, barbiturates and rifampicin. A case report describes a woman on warfarin who developed a raised INR when quetiapine was added. Cautionary predictive warnings have been also issued by the makers about alcohol, erythromycin and ketoconazole, but no interaction occurs with cimetidine, fluoxetine, haloperidol, imipramine, lithium, lorazepam, risperidone or thioridazine.

Clinical evidence, mechanism, importance and management

(a) Alcohol

A single-blind randomised crossover study in 8 psychotic men on 250 mg quetiapine three times daily found that when concurrently given 0.8 g/kg **alcohol** in orange juice their mean breath **alcohol** concentrations were unaffected by quetiapine. Some statistically significant changes in the performance of psychomotor tests were seen, but these were considered to have little clinical relevance. Despite this the makers caution against the use of quetiapine in combination with other centrally acting drugs and **alcohol**.[1] This is probably because drowsiness is quetiapine's commonest side-effect, occurring in 17.5% of patients.[2] This drowsiness might be expected to be worsened by **alcohol**.

(b) Anticonvulsants or Rifampicin (Rifampin)

When 17 psychotic patients on 250 mg quetiapine three times daily were given additionally given 100 mg **phenytoin** three times daily for 10 days, the oral clearance of the quetiapine was increased fivefold.[3] The reason appears to be that **phenytoin** is a specific inducer of cytochrome P450 isoenzyme CYP3A4, which is also concerned with the metabolism of quetiapine so that the metabolism of the quetiapine is markedly increased (confirmed by *in vitro* studies). The makers of quetiapine suggest[2] that ". . . dosage adjustment [increases] will be necessary when quetiapine is administered with **phenytoin** or other enzyme inducers (e.g. **carbamazepine**, **barbiturates** or **rifampicin**)." The prediction that a similar interaction will occur with other **enzyme inducing anticonvulsants** and **rifampicin** is reasonable, but no direct clinical evidence is yet available, however be alert for the need to use an increased quetiapine dosage in patients treated with any of these drugs.

(c) Antidepressants (Fluoxetine, Imipramine, Lithium)

The makers report that 60 mg **fluoxetine** daily and 75 mg **imipramine** twice daily for 5 days had no significant effect on the steady-state serum levels of quetiapine 300 mg twice daily.[4] No special precautions would therefore appear to be necessary if either of these drugs and quetiapine are used concurrently.

The steady-state serum **lithium** levels of 10 patients with schizophrenic, schizoaffective or bipolar illness were studied while taking 250 mg quetiapine three times daily for 11 days, and after its withdrawal. The **lithium** AUC_{0-12h} and the minimum serum levels were raised 16% by the presence of the quetiapine, and concurrent use was well tolerated.[5] This small rise is unlikely to be clinically important and the makers reasonably suggest that these two drugs can be given concurrently.[2] No special precautions would appear to be necessary.

(d) Antihypertensives

The makers report that in controlled trials quetiapine caused postural hypotension (7.1%), dizziness (9.6%), tachycardia (7.1%) and rarely syncope, usually when treatment was first started.[2] Until there is more clinical experience it would seem prudent to warn patients of what can happen, and what to do if any of these effects occur. On theoretical grounds this might possibly be more likely to occur in patients already taking some **antihypertensive drugs**.

(e) Antipsychotics (Haloperidol, Risperidone, Thioridazine)

The makers report that 200 mg **thioridazine** twice daily reduced the steady-state quetiapine AUC, and its maximum and minimum serum levels by 40.8%, 47.8% and 32.5% respectively, the probable reason being that **thioridazine** increases the metabolism of the quetiapine.[6] This reduction is only moderate and its importance is not known, but until more information is available it would seem prudent to monitor concurrent use, being alert for the need to raise the quetiapine dosage.

The makers report that 7.5 mg **haloperidol** twice daily and 3 mg **risperidone** twice daily for 9 days have no significant effect on the pharmacokinetics of 300 mg quetiapine twice daily.[6] However, there is a case report describing considerable QT prolongation in a patient who took 2000 mg quetiapine whilst on **risperidone**. The authors consider this significant as the overdose was small, and because no QT prolongation was seen in toxicity studies of quetiapine when doses as large as 9600 mg were used,[7] although there is a single case of prolonged QTc interval associated with an overdose of 9600 mg.[8] No special precautions would therefore appear to be routinely necessary if either of these drugs and quetiapine are used concurrently.

(f) Cimetidine

The pharmacokinetics of quetiapine 150 mg three times daily in 7 psychotic men were not affected by 400 mg **cimetidine** three times daily for 4 days.[9] There would therefore appear to be no reason for avoiding concurrent use.

(g) Enzyme induction and inhibition

The makers report that 250 mg quetiapine three times daily given to 12 psychotic men had no effect on the pharmacokinetics of 1 g oral **antipyrine**. The significance of this is that **antipyrine** is used as a marker drug to test whether other drugs have the potential to induce liver cytochrome enzymes. The absence of an interaction suggests that quetiapine will have no effect on the oxidative function of the liver.[10] Other *in vitro* tests on human liver microsomal enzymes using quetiapine at levels several times higher than those found in plasma after high doses, found that it has little inhibitory effect of the activity of the cytochrome P450 isoenzymes CYP1A2, CYP2C9, CYP2C19, CYP2D6 and CYP3A4.[11] This suggests that quetiapine will have little inhibitory effect on drugs which are metabolised by these isoenzymes.

No studies appear to have been carried out on drugs which specifically have a potent inhibitory effect on CYP3A4 (by which quetiapine is primarily metabolised), but on theoretical grounds such drugs might be expected to raise serum quetiapine levels, thereby increasing its adverse effects. The makers particularly mention caution with

erythromycin and **ketoconazole**,[2] but so far there appear to be no clinical reports of problems with either of these drugs nor any other studies with enzyme inhibitors (except cimetidine above). See also section (b) above which concerns drugs which have enzyme inductive activity.

(h) Lorazepam

The pharmacokinetics and pharmacodynamic effects of single 2 mg doses of **lorazepam** were examined in 10 psychotic men while taking 250 mg quetiapine three times daily. It was found that the maximum serum **lorazepam** levels were not significantly changed, and the alterations in the performance of a number of psychometric tests were small and considered not to be clinically relevant.[12]

(i) Warfarin

A 71-year old woman on long-term treatment with **warfarin**, phenytoin and benztropine had her **warfarin** dosage slightly reduced (from 20 to 19.5 mg weekly) because her INR was moderately raised (from 1.6 to 2.6). After 8 days her treatment with olanzapine was changed to 200 mg quetiapine daily. Two weeks later her INR was found to have climbed to 9.2. The quetiapine was stopped and she was given two doses of vitamin K by injection. The only clinical symptoms seen were a small amount of bleeding from the injection site and a bruise on the hand. She was eventually later restabilised on phenytoin, olanzapine and **warfarin** (17.5 mg weekly) and with an INR of 1.6. The reasons for this apparent interaction are not known but the authors suggest that the quetiapine may have inhibited the metabolism of the **warfarin** (possibly by competitive inhibition of The cytochrome P450 isoenzymes CYP3A4 and CYP2C9), thereby increasing its effects. They also suggest that the phenytoin may have had some part to play.[13] This is only an isolated case but it suggests that the concurrent use of **warfarin** and quetiapine should be monitored.

1. Zeneca Pharma. Personal communication, October 1997.
2. Seroquel (Quetiapine). AstraZeneca. Summary of product characteristics, October 2001.
3. Wong YWJ, Yeh C, Thyrum PT. The effects of concomitant phenytoin administration on the steady-state pharmacokinetics of quetiapine. *J Clin Psychopharmacol* (2001) 21, 89–93.
4. Zeneca Pharma. Data on file (Study 63).
5. Potkin SG, Thyrum PT, Bera R, Vargo D, Carreon D, Kalali A, Maguire G, Yeh C, Ewing BJ, Wong YWJ. Pharmacokinetics and safety of lithium co-administered with 'Seroquel' (quetiapine). *Schizophr Res* (1997) 24, 199.
6. Zeneca Pharma. Data on file (Study 64).
7. Beelen AP, Yeo K-TJ, Lewis LD. Asymptomatic QTc prolongation associated with quetiapine fumarate overdose in a patient being treated with risperidone. *Hum Exp Toxicol* (2001) 20, 215–19.
8. Gajwani P, Pozuelo L, Tesar GE. QT interval prolongation associated with quetiapine (Seroquel) overdose. *Psychosomatics* (2000) 41, 63–5.
9. Wong YWJ, Ewing BJ, Thyrum PT, Yeh C. The effect of phenytoin and cimetidine on the pharmacokinetics of Seroquel. *Schizophr Res* (1997) 24, 200–1.
10. Zeneca Pharma. Data on file (Study 20).
11. Grimm SW, Stams KR, Bui K. In vitro prediction of potential metabolic drug interactions for Seroquel. *Schizophr Res* (1997) 24, 198.
12. Potkin SG. The pharmacokinetics and pharmacodynamics of lorazepam given before and during treatment with ICI 204,636 (Seroquel) in men with selected psychotic disorders. (5077IL/0027). Zeneca Pharma. Data on file (Study 27).
13. Rogers T, de Leon J, Atcher D. Possible interaction between warfarin and quetiapine. *J Clin Psychopharmacol* (1999) 19, 382–3.

Remoxipride + Miscellaneous drugs

The performance of skilled tasks such as car driving and handling other potentially dangerous machinery appear to be worsened if remoxipride is taken with alcohol,[1,2] diazepam[1,2] or possibly other benzodiazepines. Patients should be warned. Remoxipride appears not to interact with biperiden[2] or warfarin.[2] Remoxipride and imipramine do not affect the pharmacokinetics of each other.[3] Remoxipride serum levels can be raised by cimetidine, but the importance of this is uncertain.[4]

1. Mattila MJ, Mattila ME, Konno K, Saarialho-Kere U. Objective and subjective effects of remoxipride, alone and in combination with ethanol or diazepam, on performance in healthy subjects. *J Psychopharmacol* (1988) 2, 138–49.
2. Yisak W, von Bahr C, Farde L, Grind M, Mattila M, Ogenstad S. Drug interaction studies with remoxipride. *Acta Psychiatr Scand* (1990) 82 (Suppl 358), 58–62.

3. Yisak W, Lolk A, Hansen S, Nielsen O-W, Gram L, von Bahr C, Ogenstad S, Harring M. Remoxipride imipramine interaction. *Eur J Pharmacol* (1990) 183, 2292.
4. Yisak W, Gram LG, Brøsen K, Hansen J, Parivar K, Nilsson L. Remoxipride cimetidine interaction. *Pharm Res* (1992) 9 (Suppl 10), S-323.

Risperidone + Miscellaneous drugs

No pharmacokinetic interaction normally occurs between risperidone and amitriptyline, but extrapyramidal reactions have been reported in one patient. Carbamazepine can halve risperidone serum levels. Occasional episodes of idiopathic priapism in a man became much more prolonged when given risperidone, and increased to an almost daily occurrence when citalopram was added. No clinically relevant interaction appears to occur with risperidone and reboxetine or venlafaxine. There are case reports of adverse effects with risperidone and fluoxetine or sodium valproate, but they do not seem to be of general importance.

Clinical evidence, mechanism, importance and management

(a) Amitriptyline

A study in 12 schizophrenic patients found that 50 to 100 mg **amitriptyline** daily had no effect on the serum levels of risperidone 3 mg twice daily.[1] However, a 26-year old man developed extrapyramidal reactions when risperidone was added to 25 mg **amitriptyline** daily and its dosage increased from 2 to 4 mg daily.[2] On another occasion extrapyramidal side-effects developed after 2 mg risperidone was added to 25 mg **amitriptyline** and 20 mg fluoxetine daily.[2] Reasons for these reactions (both pharmacokinetic and pharmacodynamic) have been suggested.[3] The cases illustrate that there is the potential for an adverse interaction between these drugs in the occasional patient so that concurrent use should be well monitored.

(b) Carbamazepine

A man of 22 was taking risperidone 4 mg daily and **carbamazepine** 600 mg daily for schizophrenia. The risperidone dose was doubled due to lower than expected levels and **carbamazepine** tailed off. Ten days after **carbamazepine** had been discontinued it was noted that his plasma risperidone level was 49 micrograms/l, while it had only been 19 micrograms/l when he was taking **carbamazepine**.[4] There are 4 other cases of this interaction between risperidone and **carbamazepine**.[5-7] In one case, the addition of **carbamazepine** to established risperidone treatment resulted in a fall in the risperidone levels of about two-thirds, accompanied by the return of the patients psychotic symptoms.[7] In 2 other cases, a man of 20 and a man of 81 were stabilised on **carbamazepine** and risperidone. They both developed parkinsonian symptoms when **carbamazepine** was stopped. The symptoms resolved when the doses of risperidone were reduced by about two-thirds.[5]

These cases are supported by a study in 5 patients on **carbamazepine** and risperidone schizophrenia or bipolar disorders. The dose-normalised plasma level of risperidone and its active metabolite, 9-hydroxyrisperidone were 1.4 and 6.2 nanomol/l.mg with **carbamazepine**, compared to 4.4 and 17.3 nanomol/l without **carbamazepine**.[8]

This was attributed to the marked inducing effects of the **carbamazepine** (a recognised and potent enzyme inducer), but the precise isoenzyme affected is still debated.[4,9] It would now seem important to monitor the serum levels of risperidone in patients given **carbamazepine**, being alert for the need to raise the risperidone dosage, possibly by as much as two-thirds.

(c) Citalopram

A 29-year-old man with idiopathic priapism (about one 4 h erection every 1 to 2 months) which typically woke him up, began to experience much longer bouts lasting 6 to 8 h when treated with 4 mg risperidone daily. Within about 4 weeks of adding 40 mg **citalopram** daily to a slightly reduced risperidone dose (3 mg daily), he began to

have almost daily erections lasting 12 h. A later change in his dosages to 3 mg risperidone twice daily plus 20 mg citalopram daily resulted after 3 days in an episode of such persistent priapism that emergency detumescence treatment was needed. When both drugs were stopped he improved markedly and then only had occasional 4-h erections.[10] The reason for this adverse reaction is not known, but the authors say that since risperidone has been associated with male priapism and **citalopram** with clitoral priapism, their combined use would seem apparently to have acted additively in this man who already had an underlying predisposition. This is an isolated case, set in the particular context of idiopathic priapism, but it draws attention to the possibility that these and similar psychotropic drugs may possibly affect other patients in the same way, although the extent would be expected to be less and the incidence small.[10]

(d) Fluoxetine

A woman of 30 was treated with valproate, clonazepam, and risperidone 3 mg daily for schizophrenia. **Fluoxetine** 5 mg daily was added for a depressive disorder. The depression improved, but she noticed painful bilateral breast enlargement, which resolved when risperidone was stopped. Similar symptoms were noted when the risperidone was later restarted. It is suggested that **fluoxetine** inhibited the metabolism of risperidone by the cytochrome P450 isoenzyme CYP2D6, resulting in increased risperidone levels, which brought about increased prolactin levels and the gynaecomastia.[11]

(e) Reboxetine

Reboxetine 8 mg daily was given to 7 schizophrenic patients stabilised on risperidone 8 mg daily for a period of 3 weeks. **Reboxetine** had no significant effects on the pharmacokinetics of risperidone and its active metabolite 9-hydroxyrisperidone, suggesting that no additional precautions are necessary if **reboxetine** and risperidone are used together.[12]

(f) Sodium valproate

A study comparing 10 patients on **sodium valproate** and risperidone with 23 patients on risperidone alone found no significant difference between the 2 groups, suggesting **sodium valproate** and risperidone can be safely used concurrently.[8] However, a case report describes the development of generalised acute oedema in a schizophrenic patient when risperidone 8 mg was added to established **sodium valproate** treatment. The oedema was unresponsive to diuretics, but resolved when the risperidone dose was reduced to 2 mg. When the risperidone dose was later increased to 8 mg the oedema reappeared, so the risperidone was withdrawn.[13] No special precautions seem necessary on concurrent use, but it is worth bearing this case in mind when these two drugs are used together.

(g) Venlafaxine

Venlafaxine 75 mg 12-hourly given under steady-state conditions was found to increase the AUC of a single 1 mg oral dose of risperidone by about 32%, but the pharmacokinetic profile of the risperidone plus its active metabolite (9-hydroxyrisperidone) was not significantly changed, nor were any adverse events seen.[14] There would seem to be no reason for avoiding concurrent use.

1. Sommers DK, Snyman JR, van Wyk M, Blom MW, Huang ML, Levron JC. Lack of effect of amitriptyline on risperidone pharmacokinetics in schizophrenic patients. *Int Clin Psychopharmacol* (1997) 12, 141–5.
2. Brown ES. Extrapyramidal side effects with low-dose risperidone. *Can J Psychiatry* (1997) 42, 325–6.
3. Caley CF. Extrapyramidal reactions from concurrent SSRI and atypical antipsychotic use. *Can J Psychiatry* (1998) 43, 307–8.
4. de Leon J, Bork J. Risperidone and cytochrome P450 3A. *J Clin Psychiatry* (1997) 58, 450.
5. Takahashi H, Yoshida K, Higuchi H, Shimizu T. Development of parkinsonian symptoms after discontinuation of carbamazepine in patients concurrently treated with risperidone: two case reports. *Clin Neuropharmacol* (1999) 22, 358–60.
6. Alfaro CL, Nicolson R, Lenane M, Rapoport JL. Carbamazepine and/or fluvoxamine drug interaction with risperidone in a patient on multiple psychotropic medications. *Ann Pharmacother* (2000) 34, 122–3.
7. Spina E, Scordo MG, Avenoso A, Perucca E. Adverse drug interaction between risperidone and carbamazepine in a patient with chronic schizophrenia and deficient CYP2D6 activity. *J Clin Psychopharmacol* (2001) 21, 108–9.
8. Spina E, Avenoso A, Facciolà G, Salemi M, Scordo MG, Giacobello T, Madia AG, Perucca E. Plasma concentrations of risperidone and 9-hydroxyrisperidone: effect of comedication with carbamazepine or valproate. *Ther Drug Monit* (2000) 22, 481–5.
9. Lane H-Y, Chang W-H. Risperidone-carbamazepine interactions: is cytochrome P450 3A involved? *J Clin Psychiatry* (1998) 59, 430–1.
10. Freudenreich O. Exacerbation of idiopathic priapism with risperidone-citalopram combination. *J Clin Psychiatry* (2002) 63, 249–50.

11. Benazzi F. Gynecomastia with risperidone-fluoxetine combination. *Pharmacopsychiatry* (1999) 32, 41.
12. Spina E, Avenoso A, Scordo MG, Ancione M, Madia A, Levita A. No effect of reboxetine on plasma concentrations of clozapine, risperidone, and their active metabolites. *Ther Drug Monit* (2001) 23, 675–8.
13. Sanders RD, Lehrer DS. Edema associated with addition of risperidone to valproate treatment. *J Clin Psychiatry* (1998) 59, 689–90.
14. Amchin J, Zarycranski W, Taylor KP, Albano D, Klockowski PM. Effect of venlafaxine on the pharmacokinetics of risperidone. *J Clin Pharmacol* (1999) 39, 297–309.

Ritanserin + Miscellaneous drugs

Ritanserin does not interact with alcohol, cimetidine or ranitidine.

Clinical evidence, mechanism, importance and management

A study in 20 healthy subjects given 10 mg ritanserin, with and without 0.5 g/kg **alcohol**, found no pharmacokinetic nor pharmacodynamic interactions between these drugs.[1] **Cimetidine** 800 mg once daily or **ranitidine** 300 mg once daily for 11 days were found to cause small statistically significant changes in the pharmacokinetics of single 10-mg doses of ritanserin (given on day 3) in 9 healthy subjects, possibly due to changes in absorption,[2] but these were of little or no clinical relevance.

1. Estevez F, Parrillo S, Giusti M, Monti JM. Single-dose ritanserin and alcohol in healthy volunteers: a placebo-controlled trial. *Alcohol* (1995) 12, 541–5.
2. Trenk D, Seiler K-U, Buschmann M, Szathmary S, Benn H-P, Jähnchen E. Effect of concomitantly administered cimetidine or ranitidine on the pharmacokinetics of the 5-HT₂-receptor antagonist ritanserin. *J Clin Pharmacol* (1993) 33, 330–4.

Sertindole + Miscellaneous drugs

The makers of sertindole[1,2] contraindicate the concurrent use of astemizole, erythromycin,[3,4] itraconazole, ketoconazole, pimozide, quinidine, terfenadine,[5,6] thioridazine, tetracyclic and tricyclic antidepressants, and potassium-depleting diuretics because of an increased risk of cardiac arrhythmias. Carbamazepine and phenytoin reduce serum sertindole levels, and a dose increase may therefore be necessary.[1,7] Cimetidine,[1,2] fluoxetine and paroxetine[1,2,7,8] increase sertindole levels, and so dosage reductions may be necessary. No clinically relevant interactions occur with alprazolam,[9] antacids,[10,11] diltiazem,[7] food,[10] nifedipine,[7] propranolol,[2] tobacco smoking[7] or verapamil.[7] Sertindole was withdrawn in the UK in December 1998 because of its cardiotoxicity.[12]

1. Serdolect (Sertindole), Lundbeck Ltd. Summary of product characteristics, October 1996.
2. Lundbeck Ltd, Personal communications, July and August 1997.
3. Granneman GR, Wozniak P, Ereshefsky L, Silber C, Mack R. Effect of erythromycin on the pharmacokinetics of sertindole. Lundbeck Limited, Study summary M94–145.
4. Wong SL, Cao G, Mack RJ, Granneman GR. The effect of erythromycin on the CYP3A component of sertindole clearance in healthy volunteers. *J Clin Pharmacol* (1997) 37, 1056–61.
5. Granneman GR, Wozniak P, Ereshefsky L, Silber C, Mack R. Effect of sertindole on the pharmacokinetics of terfenadine. Lundbeck Limited, Study summary M94–146.
6. Wong SL, Cao G, Mack R, Granneman GR. Lack of CYP3A inhibition effects of sertindole on terfenadine in healthy volunteers. *Int J Clin Pharmacol Ther* (1998) 36, 146–51.
7. Granneman GR, Wozniak P, Ereshefsky L, Silber C, Mack R. Population pharmacokinetics of sertindole during long-term treatment of patients with schizophrenia. Poster presentation at the American College of Neuropsychopharmacology Annual Meeting, San Juan, Puerto Rico, December 1996.
8. Walker-Kinnear M, McNaughton S. Paroxetine discontinuation syndrome in association with sertindole therapy. *Br J Psychiatry* (1997) 170, 389.
9. Wong SL, Locke C, Staser J, Granneman GR. Lack of multiple dosing effect of sertindole on the pharmacokinetics of alprazolam in healthy volunteers. *Psychopharmacology (Berl)* (1998) 135, 236–41.
10. Granneman GR, Wozniak P, Ereshefsky L, Silber C, Mack R. Effect of food and antacid on the bioavailability of sertindole. Lundbeck Limited, Study summary M94–164.
11. Wong SL, Linnen P, Mack R, Granneman GR. Effects of food, antacid, and dosage form on the pharmacokinetics and relative bioavailability of sertindole in healthy volunteers. *Biopharm Drug Dispos* (1997) 18, 533–41.
12. Committee on Safety of Medicines/Medicines Control Agency. Suspension of availability of sertindole (Serdolect). *Current Problems* (1999) 25, 1.

Sulpiride + Antacids or Sucralfate

Sucralfate and an aluminium-magnesium hydroxide antacid can reduce the absorption of sulpiride.

Clinical evidence, mechanism, importance and management

A study in 6 healthy subjects showed that the bioavailability of a single 100-mg dose of sulpiride was reduced by 40% by 1 g **sucralfate** and 33% by 30 ml of *Simeco* (an antacid containing 215 mg **aluminium hydroxide**, 80 mg **magnesium hydroxide** and 25 mg **simethicone** in each 5 ml when taken together. When either the **sucralfate** or the antacid were taken 2 h previously the reduction in bioavailability was only about 25%. No change in bioavailability was seen in one subject when the **sucralfate** was given 2 h after the sulpiride.[1] The mechanisms of these interactions are not understood. Their clinical importance is not established but it would seem reasonable to give the sulpiride 2 h after and not before these other drugs to avoid these interactions.

1. Gouda MW, Hikal AH, Babhair SA, ElHofy SA, Mahrous GM. Effect of sucralfate and antacids on the bioavailability of sulpiride in humans. *Int J Pharmaceutics* (1984) 22, 257–63.

Sulpiride + Lithium carbonate

Serious extrapyramidal reactions developed in two patients within a few hours of starting to take sulpiride and lithium carbonate concurrently. See also 'Antipsychotics + Lithium', p.694.

Clinical evidence, mechanism, importance and management

A depressed woman who had been taking 2 g sulpiride daily for 4 weeks, then reduced to 800 mg twice daily, developed a serious parkinsonian syndrome with choreiform movements of her arms after taking a single 800-mg dose of **lithium carbonate** at night. Next morning her serum lithium level was 0.5 mmol/l. The adverse effects disappeared within 2 days of stopping the **lithium**. A man with a manic episode who had started to take 1200 mg **lithium** at night, and with a stable serum lithium level of 0.6 mmol/l, developed marked orofacial dyskinesia and acute akathisia within 12 h of starting to take 800 mg sulpiride twice daily.[1] The reasons for these reactions are not understood. One theory is that the **lithium** may have increased the binding of the sulpiride to the dopamine D_2 receptors in the brain, thereby causing extrapyramidal reactions to develop. Sulpiride is known to increase its binding in the presence of **lithium**.[2]

Information appears to be limited to these two cases. Its general importance is therefore uncertain, but the authors of the report advise caution when using this drug combination.

1. Dinan TG, O'Keane V. Acute extrapyramidal reactions following lithium and sulpiride co-administration: two case reports. *Hum Psychopharmacol* (1991) 6, 67–9.
2. Jenner P, David A, Kilpatrick G, Kupniak NM, Chivers JK, Marsden CD. Selective interaction of sulpiride with brain dopamine receptors. In: Schizophrenia: New Pharmacology and Clinical Developments, Schiff AA, Roth M, Freeman HL (eds). (1985) RSM, London.

Suriclone + Imipramine

Suriclone and imipramine appear not to interact adversely.

Clinical evidence, mechanism, importance and management

The combination of single doses of 0.4 mg suriclone and 75 mg **imipramine** was found to have a small but not statistically significant effect on the psychomotor performances of 12 healthy subjects over

9 h, and the pharmacokinetics of both drugs were unchanged.[1] There would seem to be little reason for avoiding concurrent use.

1. Perault MC, Chapelle G, Bouquet S, Chevalier P, Montay G, Gaillot J, Chakroun H, Guillet P, Vandel B. Pharmacokinetic and pharmacodynamic study of suriclone imipramine interaction in man. *Fundam Clin Pharmacol* (1994) 8, 251–5.

Tetrabenazine + Chlorpromazine

An isolated report describes severe Parkinson-like symptoms in a woman with Huntington's Chorea when given tetrabenazine and chlorpromazine.

Clinical evidence, mechanism, importance and management

A woman with Huntington's Chorea, successfully treated with 100 mg tetrabenazine daily for 9 years, became motionless, rigid, mute and only able to respond by blinking her eyes within a day of being given two intramuscular injections of 25 mg **chlorpromazine**. This was diagnosed as severe drug-induced parkinsonism, which rapidly responded to withdrawal of both drugs and treatment with benzatropine mesilate given intramuscularly and orally. She had previously tolerated **chlorpromazine** well.[1] The reason for this reaction is not understood. The authors of this report advise caution if tetrabenazine and other neuroleptics are given.

1. Moss JH, Stewart DE. Iatrogenic parkinsonism in Huntington's chorea. *Can J Psychiatry* (1986) 31, 865–6.

Thiothixene + Miscellaneous drugs

Carbamazepine, phenytoin, primidone and tobacco smoking increase the loss of thiothixene from the body, whereas cimetidine, doxepin, nortriptyline, propranolol and isoniazid reduce its loss.

Clinical evidence, mechanism, importance and management

A retrospective study in 42 patients found that the mean clearance of thiothixene in those taking enzyme-inducing drugs (**carbamazepine**, **phenytoin**, **primidone**) was threefold greater than in the control group (92.5 compared with 32. 8 l/min). Of the group taking enzyme inducers, 5 patients had non-detectable serum thiothixene levels and not surprisingly showed no clinical response. Another group taking enzyme inhibitors (**cimetidine**, **doxepin**, **nortriptyline**, **propranolol**, **isoniazid**) showed a clearance of only 9.51 l/min. **Tobacco smoking** (also an enzyme inducer) increased the clearance of thiothixene in those taking inhibitors and those taking no other drugs, but not in those taking inducers. Those who **smoked** were found to need on average 45% more thiothixene than the **non-smokers** on no other interacting drugs.[1] The reasons for the different clearances are that enzyme inducers stimulate the liver enzymes to clear the thiothixene from the body more quickly, whereas enzyme inhibitors have the opposite effect.

The conclusion to be drawn from this study is that the dosage of thiothixene should be adjusted to accommodate these changes in clearance: bigger doses for those who take enzyme inducers and/or who smoke; smaller doses for those taking inhibitors. More study is needed to find out the individual effects of these drugs.

1. Ereshefsky L, Saklad SR, Watanabe MD, Davis CM, Jann MW. Thiothixene pharmacokinetic interactions: a study of hepatic enzyme inducers, clearance inhibitors, and demographic variables. *J Clin Psychopharmacol* (1991) 11, 296–301.

Thiothixene + Paroxetine

No pharmacokinetic interaction occurs between thiothixene and paroxetine.

Clinical evidence, mechanism, importance and management

A study in 10 healthy subjects showed that after taking 20 mg **paroxetine** daily for 3 days the pharmacokinetics of single 20-mg doses of thiothixene were not significantly changed. It was inferred from this that the cytochrome P450 isoenzyme CYP2D6 is not a major pathway for the metabolism of **thiothixene**. It is unlikely that the thiothixene dosage will need to be changed if **paroxetine** is given, but there is a possibility that longer treatment with **paroxetine** may have some effect.[1]

1. Guthrie SK, Hariharan M, Kumar AA, Bader G, Tandon R. The effect of paroxetine on thiothixene pharmacokinetics. *J Clin Pharm Ther* (1997) 22, 221–6.

Zaleplon + Miscellaneous drugs

Rifampicin markedly increases the metabolism and clearance of zaleplon and is expected to reduce its hypnotic effects. Cimetidine increases the serum levels of zaleplon but this is not thought to be clinically relevant. The makers predict that erythromycin and ketoconazole may possibly increase zaleplon's effects whereas carbamazepine and phenobarbitone may possibly decrease them. Additive effects are predicted with CNS depressants, including alcohol. No clinically relevant interactions occur with digoxin, diphenhydramine, ibuprofen, imipramine, paroxetine, thioridazine or warfarin.

Clinical evidence, mechanism, importance and management

Zaleplon has been studied for possible adverse interactions using a spectrum of representative drugs as follows: Enzyme inhibitors (diphenhydramine, cimetidine) and inducers (rifampicin) of zaleplon metabolism; drugs active within the CNS (imipramine, paroxetine, thioridazine); a drug which might alter renal excretion (ibuprofen), and drugs with a narrow therapeutic index (digoxin, warfarin).

(a) Alcohol

The makers say that they do not recommend the concurrent use of zaleplon and **alcohol** because of the risk of increased sedation.[1]

(b) Cimetidine

A randomised single-dose 2-period crossover study in healthy subjects found that 800 mg of **cimetidine** decreased the clearance of a single 10-mg dose of zaleplon by 44%, resulting in an increase in its maximum serum levels and AUC of 85%.[2] The reason is that **cimetidine** inhibits both of the primary and secondary pathways by which zaleplon is metabolised (CYP3A4 and aldehyde oxidase), thereby allowing the zaleplon to accumulate.[3] Despite this increase, the makers only advise caution when both drugs are used,[1] and the advice of the author is that routine dosage adjustment of zaleplon is unnecessary because of its short half-life and good safety profile.[3]

(c) Digoxin

A non-randomised multidose study in a group of healthy subjects found that 10 mg zaleplon for 5 days had no effect on the serum levels of **digoxin** 375 micrograms daily taken for 14 days,[2] nor were the PR or QT intervals altered.[3] No special precautions would therefore appear to be needed during concurrent use.

(d) Diphenhydramine

A randomised single dose 3-period crossover study in healthy subjects found that 50 mg **diphenhydramine** had no significant effect on the pharmacokinetics of single 10-mg doses of zaleplon, despite the fact **diphenhydramine** is a moderate inhibitor of aldehyde oxidase, the primary metabolic pathway of zaleplon.[2] No special precautions would therefore appear to be needed during concurrent use. The general inference to be drawn is that other drugs which inhibit this pathway are also unlikely to interact significantly.

(e) Ibuprofen

A randomised, single-dose, 3-period crossover study in 17 healthy subjects showed that 600 mg **ibuprofen** had no effect on the pharmacokinetics of 10 mg zaleplon. The **ibuprofen** was used to test the possibility that it might affect the renal excretion of zaleplon.[4] There would appear to be no reason for avoiding concurrent use.

(f) Imipramine, Paroxetine, Thioridazine and CNS depressants

In a series of double-blind studies, groups of healthy subjects were given 20-mg doses of zaleplon plus **imipramine**, **paroxetine** or **thioridazine**. This zaleplon dose is twice the normal dose, and was used because 10 mg has only minimal effects on psychomotor performance, so 20 mg will increase the chance of detecting an interaction. It was found that 20 mg **paroxetine** for 9 days had no effect on the pharmacokinetics of 20 mg zaleplon, and psychomotor performance was unaffected.[2] Single doses of neither 75 mg **imipramine**[2] nor 50 mg **thioridazine**[5] had any effect on the pharmacokinetics of 20 mg zaleplon, and the psychomotor tests showed only short term additive effects lasting 1 to 2 h and 1 to 4 h respectively. These short-term CNS additive effects are small and unlikely to be clinically relevant, and so there would seem to be no reason for avoiding concurrent use.

The makers of zaleplon give a mild warning about taking into account the increased sedation which may occur with CNS depressants. They list **anaesthetics**, **antidepressants**, **antiepileptics**, **antipsychotics**, **anxiolytics**, **hypnotics**, **opioid analgesics** and **sedative antihistamines**.[1]

(g) Other enzyme inhibitors or inducers

Erythromycin 800 mg as a single dose increased the plasma levels of zaleplon by 34% because **erythromycin** is a potent inhibitors of the cytochrome P450 isoenzyme CYP3A4, which is concerned with the metabolism of zaleplon. Dosage adjustments are not necessary, but patients should be warned about the risk of increased sedation.[1] They makers of zaleplon predict that reduced zaleplon effects may possibly also occur with **carbamazepine** or **phenobarbital**[1] because they are potent inducers of CYP3A4, but these predictions await clinical confirmation.

(h) Rifampicin

A non-randomised, multidose, 2-period, crossover study in healthy subjects found that 600 mg **rifampicin** daily for 14 days increased the clearance of 10-mg doses of zaleplon 5.4-fold, decreasing its maximum serum levels and AUC by 80%. This is because **rifampicin** is a potent inducer of the cytochrome P450 isoenzyme CYP3A4, which increases the metabolism and clearance of zaleplon from the body.[2] This interaction would be expected to lead to a marked reduction in the hypnotic effects of zaleplon, but no studies appear to have been done to find out by how much the zaleplon dosage needs to be increased in the presence of **rifampicin**. The pharmacokinetic studies suggest at least two to threefold.

(i) Warfarin

In a non-randomised, single dose, 2-period, crossover study, a group of healthy subjects were given a single 25-mg dose of **warfarin** after taking 20 mg zaleplon daily for 12 days. The maximum serum levels of the **(S-) warfarin** were increased by 17%, but the AUC was unaffected, as were the AUC and maximum serum levels of **(R+) warfarin**.[2] Increases in the prothrombin time due to the **warfarin** were also not significantly changed.[3] No special precautions would therefore appear to be needed during concurrent use.

1. Sonata (Zaleplon). Lundbeck Limited. Summary of product characteristics, November 2001.
2. Darwish M. Overview of drug interaction studies with zaleplon. Poster presented at 13th Annual Meeting of Associated Professional Sleep Studies (APSS), Orlando, Florida, June 23rd, 1999.
3. Darwish M. Analysis of potential drug interactions with zaleplon. *J Am Geriatr Soc* (1999) 47, S62.
4. Garcia PS, Carcas A, Zapater P, Rosendo J, Paty I, Leister CA, Troy SM. Absence of an interaction between ibuprofen and zaleplon. *Am J Health-Syst Pharm* (2000) 57, 1137–41.
5. Hetta J, Broman J-E, Darwish M, Troy SM. Psychomotor effects of zaleplon and thioridazine coadministration. *Eur J Clin Pharmacol* (2000) 56, 211–17.

Ziprasidone + Miscellaneous drugs

The makers warn of the possible risks of giving ziprasidone with drugs that prolong the QT interval, and of the possible antagonism which may occur with levodopa and other dopamine agonists. Ziprasidone appears not interact to a clinically relevant extent with benztropine, carbamazepine, cimetidine, oral contraceptives, ketoconazole, lithium, lorazepam, *Maalox*, propranolol or tobacco smoking.

Clinical evidence, mechanism importance and management

(a) Carbamazepine

In a randomised, open, parallel-group study, healthy subjects were given 20-mg doses of ziprasidone twice daily, in the presence of either placebo (10 subjects), or **carbamazepine** 200 mg twice daily for 25 days, following a 4-day dose titration period (9 subjects). It was found that the 12 h AUC and maximum serum levels of the ziprasidone were reduced by 36% and 27% respectively in the **carbamazepine** group. It was concluded that while induction of the cytochrome P450 isoenzyme CYP3A4 by **carbamazepine** is responsible for this modest reduction in the steady-state levels of ziprasidone, the extent is not clinically relevant.[1] No special precautions would seem to be needed with this dosage of **carbamazepine**,[1] but there is the possibility that higher doses may interact to a greater extent.

(b) Contraceptives, oral

In a double-blind, placebo-controlled, two-way crossover study, 18 women taking an **oral contraceptive** (30 micrograms **ethinyloestradiol** + 150 micrograms **levonorgestrel**, *Microgynon* or *Ovranette*) for at least 3 months were also given 20 mg ziprasidone twice daily from days 8 to 15. The only change in the pharmacokinetics of the two steroids was a 30 min increase in the half-life of the **levonorgestrel**. No adverse effects occurred. It was concluded that combined use is safe and that ziprasidone does not affect the efficacy of this oral contraceptive[2,3] and is also unlikely to affect the safety of other similar contraceptives.

(c) Drugs which prolong the QT interval

Trials in healthy subjects found that ziprasidone 160 mg increased the QTc interval by about 10 ms. While only a relatively moderate increase in the QT interval actually occurs with ziprasidone, because of the possibility of additive effects with some other drugs (and the attendant risk of torsade de pointes), to be on the safe side the makers of ziprasidone contraindicate its use with other drugs which can prolong the QT interval. They list **dofetilide**, **moxifloxacin**, **quinidine**, **sotalol**, **sparfloxacin** and **thioridazine**, but point out that this list is not exhaustive.[4] A much longer list of QT-prolonging drugs is to be found in Chapter 4.

(d) Effects on cytochrome P450 isoenzymes

In vitro studies using human liver microsomal enzymes have shown that ziprasidone has little inhibitory effects on the cytochrome P450 isoenzymes CYP1A2, CYP2C9, CYP2C19, CYP2D6 and CYP3A4,[5,6] and a study in healthy subjects confirmed that *in vivo* ziprasidone does not inhibit CYP2D6 (using dextromethorphan has a model drug).[7] It is therefore unlikely that ziprasidone will interact with drugs whose metabolism is primarily carried out by these isoenzymes.

(e) Lithium

An open-label, randomised, placebo-controlled study in 12 healthy subjects taking 450 mg **lithium carbonate** twice daily for 15 days, found that 20 mg ziprasidone twice daily on days 9 to 11, followed by

40 mg twice daily on days 12 to 15 caused only a small increase in the steady-state serum **lithium levels** (14% compared with 11% in the placebo group). A 5% reduction in renal clearance was seen in the ziprasidone group and a 9% reduction was seen in the placebo group. These differences were neither statistically nor clinically significant.[8,9] No special precautions would therefore seem to be necessary if ziprasidone is given to patients taking **lithium**.

(f) Ketoconazole

In a randomised, open-label, crossover study, 14 healthy subjects were given a 40-mg dose of ziprasidone before and after taking 400 mg **ketoconazole** or a placebo daily for 6 days. It was found that the AUC and the maximum serum levels of the ziprasidone increased by 33% and 34% respectively in the presence of **ketoconazole**. It was concluded that while inhibition of the cytochrome P450 isoenzyme CYP3A4 by **ketoconazole** is responsible for this modest increase in the steady-state levels of ziprasidone, the extent is not believed to be clinically relevant.[10] No special precautions would seem to be needed. It also suggests that other inhibitors of CYP3A4 are unlikely to significantly alter the pharmacokinetics of ziprasidone.[10]

(g) Levodopa and dopamine agonists

The mechanism by which ziprasidone acts to control schizophrenia is not understood, but it is known to be an antagonist of dopamine type 2 (D_2) receptors and therefore it may possibly oppose the effects of **levodopa** and other dopamine agonists. There seem to be no clinical reports of problems during concurrent use, but good monitoring would be advisable if ziprasidone is given with any dopamine agonist.

(h) Maalox (Aluminium/magnesium hydroxide), or Cimetidine

Single oral doses of 40 mg ziprasidone were given to 10 healthy subjects either alone, with 800 mg **cimetidine** for 2 days, or with three doses of 30 ml *Maalox* (**aluminium hydroxide/magnesium hydroxide**). The only change in the pharmacokinetics of the ziprasidone was a 6% increase in the AUC with **cimetidine**. It was concluded that no special precautions are needed if either of these drugs and ziprasidone is given concurrently, and that any inhibition of cytochrome P450 isoenzyme CYP3A4 is irrelevant because alternative metabolic pathways are available. The results of the study with **cimetidine** also suggest that other non-specific inhibitors of cytochrome P450 are unlikely to alter the ziprasidone pharmacokinetics.[11]

(i) Miscellaneous drugs

The makers say that population pharmacokinetic analysis of schizophrenic patients who were enrolled in clinical trials showed that no significant pharmacokinetic interactions occurred with **benztropine**, **lorazepam** or **propranolol**.[4] The makers also point out that since ziprasidone is not metabolised by the cytochrome P450 isoenzyme CYP1A2, smoking should not affect its pharmacokinetics. This is borne out by studies in patients, which did not reveal any differences in the pharmacokinetics of ziprasidone between **tobacco smokers** and non-smokers.[4]

1. Miceli JJ, Anziano RJ, Robarge L, Hansen RA. Laurent A. The effect of carbamazepine on the steady-state pharmacokinetics of ziprasidone in healthy volunteers. *Br J Clin Pharmacol* (2000) 49 (Suppl 1), 65S–70S.
2. Muirhead GJ, Harness J, Holt PR, Oliver S, Anziano RJ. Ziprasidone and the pharmacokinetics of a combined oral contraceptive. *Br J Clin Pharmacol* (2000) 49 (Suppl 1), 49S–56S.
3. Muirhead GJ, Holt PR, Oliver S, Harness J, Anziano RJ. The effect of ziprasidone on steady-state pharmacokinetics of a combined oral contraceptive. *Eur Neuropsychopharmacol* (1996) 6 (Suppl 3), 38.
4. Geodon (Ziprasidone). Pfizer Inc, NY. Product Information, February 2001.
5. Prakash C, Kamel A, Cui D, Whalen RD, Miceli JJ, Tweedie D. Identification of the major human liver cytochrome P450 isoform(s) responsible for the formation of the primary metabolites of ziprasidone and prediction of possible drug interactions. *Br J Clin Pharmacol* (2000) 49 (Suppl 1), 35S–42S.
6. Prakash C, Kamel A, Cui D, Whalen RD, Miceli JJ, Tweedie DJ. Ziprasidone metabolism and cytochrome P450 isoforms. *Biol Psychiatry* (1997) 42, 40S.
7. Wilner KD, DeMattos SB, Anziano RJ, Apseloff G, Gerber N. Lack of CYP 2D6 inhibition by ziprasidone in healthy volunteers. *Biol Psychiatry* (1997) 42, 42S.
8. Wilner KD, Anziano RJ, Tensfeldt TG, Pelletier SM, Apseloff G, Gerber N. The effects of ziprasidone on steady-state lithium levels and renal clearance of lithium. *Eur Neuropsychopharmacol* (1996) 6 (Suppl 3), 38.
9. Apseloff G, Mullet D, Wilner KD, Anziano RJ, Tensfeldt TG, Pelletier SM, Gerber N. The effects of ziprasidone on steady-state lithium levels and renal clearance of lithium. *Br J Clin Pharmacol* (2000) 49 (Suppl 1), 61S–64S.
10. Miceli JJ, Smith M, Robarge L, Morse T, Laurent A. The effects of ketoconazole on ziprasidone pharmacokinetics – a placebo-controlled crossover study in healthy volunteers. *Br J Clin Pharmacol* (2000) 49 (Suppl 1), 71S–76S.
11. Wilner KD, Hansen RA, Folger CJ, Geoffroy P. The pharmacokinetics of ziprasidone in healthy volunteers treated with cimetidine or antacid. *Br J Clin Pharmacol* (2000) 49 (Suppl 1), 57S–60S.

Zolpidem + Miscellaneous drugs

The sedative effects of chlorpromazine and haloperidol (and probably other sedative drugs) are increased to some extent by zolpidem, and there may be some additive effects with alcohol. Heavy smoking possibly reduces its effects. Isolated cases of delirium and/or hallucinations have been described with zolpidem and bupropion (amfebutamone), desipramine, fluoxetine, paroxetine, sertraline or venlafaxine. Ketoconazole raises serum levels of zolpidem causing increased sedation. Zolpidem does not interact with digoxin, caffeine, cimetidine, fluconazole, fluoxetine, itraconazole, ranitidine or warfarin.

Clinical evidence, mechanism, importance and management

(a) Alcohol

No significant pharmacokinetic interaction occurs between **alcohol** and zolpidem, but some possible additive pharmacodynamic effects (e.g. drowsiness) may occur.[1,2] It seems likely that additive sedation will be seen with other sedative drugs.

(b) Antidepressants

A single-dose study using 20 mg zolpidem and 75 mg **imipramine** found no effect on the pharmacokinetics of either drug. However **imipramine** increased the sedative effects of zolpidem, and anterograde amnesia was seen.[3] Patients should be warned about the possibility of increased drowsiness if both drugs are given. Studies in healthy subjects on 20 mg **fluoxetine** daily found no significant effect on the pharmacokinetics or pharmacodynamics of 10-mg doses of zolpidem, although the onset of its action was slightly shortened.[4,5] Similar results have been found with **sertraline**.[6]

In contrast, an isolated report describes a healthy 16-year-old girl with depression who took 20 mg **paroxetine** for 3 days, and then on the evening of the third night a single 10-mg dose of zolpidem. Within 1 h she began to hallucinate, then became disorientated and was unable to recognise members of her family. She recovered spontaneously from the delirium within 4 h.[7] Other isolated cases of visual hallucinations lasting up to 7 h have been reported in patients on zolpidem who were concurrently taking **bupropion (amfebutamone), desipramine, fluoxetine, sertraline, venlafaxine** or other **antidepressants** and **neuroleptics**.[8] The reasons are not understood, but zolpidem has been associated, rarely, with delusions, short-duration hallucinations or impaired cognition. The concurrent use of these drugs need not be avoided, but the outcome should be monitored.

(c) Antifungals

Itraconazole 200 mg daily or a placebo was given to 10 healthy subjects for 4 days. On day 4 a single 10 mg oral dose of zolpidem was additionally given. The mean peak serum levels of the zolpidem were increased by 12.5% and the AUC was increased by 35%, but the performance of a number of psychomotor tests (digit symbol substitution, critical flicker fusion, subjective drowsiness, postural sway) remained unaltered. It was concluded that zolpidem can be given in normal doses in the presence of **itraconazole**.[9,10] Another study similarly found that **itraconazole** and **fluconazole** did not interact significantly with zolpidem, but the effects of **ketoconazole** were significant.[11] After taking 3 doses of **ketoconazole** 200 mg, at 12-hourly intervals, the AUC of zolpidem 5 mg was increased 1.7-fold and the 12 healthy subjects were more sedated, as shown by the digit symbol substitution test.[11]

(d) Antipsychotics

Single dose studies found that the pharmacokinetics of 20-mg doses of zolpidem were unaffected by 50 mg **chlorpromazine**[3,12] or 2 mg **haloperidol**.[3] The pharmacokinetics of both of these psychotropics were unaffected by zolpidem, except that in one study the elimination half-life of **chlorpromazine** was increased from about 5 to 8 h.[12] **Chlorpromazine** increased the sedative effects of zolpidem (as indicated by impaired performances of manual dexterity and Stroop's tests).[3,12] It seems likely that additive sedation will be seen with **other sedative drugs**.

(e) Benzodiazepines

A 56-year-old man who had been taking benzodiazepines for over 20 years, most recently **ketazolam** (30 mg at night) was changed to zolpidem 10 mg at night. Initially his sleep improved, but after 2 months he became nervous, irritable and began to sweat. After 3 months of taking zolpidem he became incapacitated. He forgot to take his zolpidem one weekend, and noticed that after 48 h his symptoms had disappeared. It was concluded that chronic use of benzodiazepines caused this reaction,[13] and so it would seem that care should be taken if any other chronic benzodiazepine user is changed over to zolpidem.

(f) Caffeine

No pharmacokinetic interaction occurred between zolpidem and **caffeine** (given as one cup of **coffee** containing 300 mg **caffeine**), and the hypnotic effects of the zolpidem were unchanged.[1]

(g) Digoxin

No significant pharmacokinetic interaction occurs between zolpidem and **digoxin**.[1]

(h) H_2-blockers

The pharmacokinetics of zolpidem in 6 healthy subjects were found in one study to be unaffected by either 1 g **cimetidine** or 300 mg **ranitidine**, given daily for 17 days, although there was some increase in sleep duration with **cimetidine**.[14] No special precautions seem to be needed.

(i) Tobacco smoking

It has been noted that two **heavy smokers** had a very high zolpidem clearance and did not experience any sedative effects.[3] This suggests that **smokers** may need above-average doses of zolpidem.

(j) Warfarin

The prothrombin times of 8 healthy subjects on **warfarin** were unaffected by 4 days treatment with 20 mg zolpidem.[3]

No special precautions would seem to be necessary on concurrent use. There seems to be no information about any other anticoagulants.

1. Priest RG. Ambieu (zolpidem 5 mg and 10 mg). UK product licence application. Paris: Registration Department (LERS) 1993. Quoted by Salvà P, Costa J. Clinical pharmacokinetics and pharmacodynamics of zolpidem: therapeutic implications. *Clin Pharmacokinet* (1995) 29, 142–53.
2. Wilkinson CJ. The acute effects of zolpidem, administered alone and with alcohol, on cognitive and psychomotor function. *J Clin Psychiatry* (1995) 56, 309–18.
3. Harvengt C, Hulhoven R, Desager JP, Coupez JM, Guillet P, Fuseau E, Lambert D, Warrington SJ. Drug interactions investigated with zolpidem. In 'Imidazopyridines in Sleep Disorders', Sauvanet JP, Langer SZ and Morselli PL (eds.). Raven Press, New York (1988) 165–73.
4. Piergies AA, Sweet J, Johnson M, Roth-Schechter BF, Allard S. The effect of co-administration of zolpidem with fluoxetine: pharmacokinetics and pharmacodynamics. *Int J Clin Pharmacol Ther* (1996) 34, 178–83.
5. Allard S, Sainati S, Roth-Schechter B, Macintyre J. Minimal interaction between fluoxetine and multiple-dose zolpidem in healthy women. *Drug Metab Dispos* (1998) 26, 617–22.
6. Allard S, Sainati S, Roth-Schechter BF. Coadministration of short-term zolpidem with sertraline in healthy women. *J Clin Pharmacol* (1999) 39, 184–91.
7. Katz SE. Possible paroxetine-zolpidem interaction. *Am J Psychiatry* (1995) 152, 1689.
8. Elko CJ, Burgess JL, Robertson WO. Zolpidem-associated hallucinations and serotonin reuptake inhibition: a possible interaction. *Clin Toxicol* (1998) 36, 195–203.
9. Luurila H, Kivistö KT, Neuvonen PJ. Lack of clinically significant interaction between itraconazole and zolpidem. *Eur J Clin Pharmacol* (1997) 52 (Suppl), A137.
10. Luurila H, Kivisto KT, Neuvonen PJ. Effect of itraconazole on the pharmacokinetics and pharmacodynamics of zolpidem. *Eur J Clin Pharmacol* (1998) 54, 163–6.
11. Greenblatt DJ, von Moltke LL, Harmatz JS, Mertzanis P, Graf JA, Durol ALB, Counihan M, Roth-Schechter B, Shader RI. Kinetic and dynamic interaction study of zolpidem with ketoconazole, itraconazole, and fluconazole. *Clin Pharmacol Ther* (1998) 64, 661–71.
12. Desager JP, Hulhoven R, Harvengt C, Hermann P, Guillet P, Thiercelin JF. Possible interactions between zolpidem, a new sleep inducer and chlorpromazine, a phenothiazine neuroleptic. *Psychopharmacology (Berl)* (1988) 96, 63–6.
13. Ortega L, Iruela LM, Ibañez-Rojo V, Baca E. Zolpidem after long-acting benzodiazepines: possible interaction. *J Drug Dev Clin Pract* (1996) 8, 45–6.
14. Hulhoven R, Desager JP, Harvengt C, Herman P, Guillet P, Thiercelin JF. Lack of interaction between zolpidem and H_2 antagonists, cimetidine and ranitidine. *Int J Clin Pharmacol Res* (1988) 8, 471–6.

Zopiclone + Anticonvulsants

Single-dose studies have shown that the sedative effects of zopiclone and carbamazepine are additive, however it has been predicted that when taken long-term both carbamazepine and phenytoin will reduce the effects of zopiclone.

Clinical evidence, mechanism, importance and management

A double-blind crossover trial in 12 healthy subjects given single doses of zopiclone 7.5 mg and **carbamazepine** 600 mg found only minor changes in the plasma levels of both drugs when taken together. Zopiclone levels were higher and **carbamazepine** levels slightly lower. Psychomotor tests confirmed that both drugs had sedative effects which were additive, and in a simulated driving test it was found that co-ordination was impaired and reaction times prolonged by concurrent use.[1] However nobody seems to have checked on what happens if zopiclone is given to patients on long-term **carbamazepine** treatment. The prediction is that because **carbamazepine** is a strong inducer of cytochrome P450 isoenzyme CYP3A4 (which is concerned with the metabolism of zopiclone) the effect would be to reduce the zopiclone serum levels and reduce its hypnotic effects accordingly.[2] **Phenytoin** is predicted to interact similarly.[2]

Zopiclone is a hypnotic so that the increased sedation with **carbamazepine** would seem normally to be an advantageous interaction, but the predicted reduction in its hypnotic effects in a 'real life' situation in patients taking **carbamazepine** or **phenytoin** long-term calls for good monitoring. Be alert for the need to increase the zopiclone dosage as necessary. More study of both of these potential interactions is needed.

1. Kuitunen T, Mattila MJ, Seppälä T, Aranko K, Mattila ME. Actions of zopiclone and carbamazepine, alone and in combination, on human skilled performance in laboratory and clinical tests. *Br J Clin Pharmacol* (1990) 30, 453–61.
2. Villikka K, Kivistö KT, Lamberg TS, Kantola T, Neuvonen PJ. Concentrations and effects of zopiclone are greatly reduced by rifampicin. *Br J Clin Pharmacol* (1997) 43, 471–4.

Zopiclone + Atropine or Metoclopramide

Atropine slows and metoclopramide hastens the absorption of zopiclone.

Clinical evidence, mechanism, importance and management

The absorption of single 7.5-mg doses of oral zopiclone in 12 healthy subjects was reduced by 600 micrograms of **atropine** given intravenously, and hastened by 10 mg **metoclopramide** given intravenously. This was presumably because these drugs alter gut motility. Mean plasma zopiclone levels at 1 h were 22.7, 6.5 and 44.4 nanograms/ml and at 2 h they were 49.3, 31.9 and 59.6 nanograms/ml, when zopiclone was given alone, with **atropine** or with **metoclopramide** respectively. The **metoclopramide** group was generally more sedated than the **atropine** group.[1] The clinical importance of these findings is not known.

1. Elliott P, Chestnutt WN, Elwood RJ, Dundee JW. Effect of atropine and metoclopramide on the plasma concentrations of orally administered zopiclone. *Br J Anaesth* (1983) 55, 1159P–1160P.

Zopiclone + Erythromycin

Erythromycin affects serum zopiclone levels, causing higher more rapid peak levels. Increased and more rapid hypnosis would be expected but no increased hangover effects.

Clinical evidence, mechanism, importance and management

Zopiclone 7.5 mg was given to 10 healthy subjects before and after taking 500 mg **erythromycin** three times daily for 6 days. The **erythromycin** increased the plasma concentration of the zopiclone fivefold at half-an-hour and twofold at one hour. Peak plasma levels rose by about 40% and occurred at 1 h instead of 2 h. The 1-hour and 2-hour AUCs were increased threefold and twofold respectively, while the total AUC was increased by nearly 80%.[1] The reasons for these changes are not understood but it seems probable that the erythromycin inhibits the metabolism of the zopiclone by cytochrome P450 isoenzyme CYP3A4, thereby increasing its serum levels. These pharmacokinetic changes were reflected in some small changes in a number of psychomotor tests.[1]

In practical terms this means that **erythromycin** speeds up the onset of zopiclone hypnosis and increases its extent, probably usefully. Zopiclone is said by the makers to have negligible residual (hangover) effects the next morning and the studies cited above[1] indicate that at 8 h (a normal nights sleep) the serum levels of the zopiclone were only raised about 27% by the presence of the **erythromycin.** This would not be expected to increase hangover effects to a relevant extent. This needs confirmation, but no special precautions would appear to be needed if these drugs are used concurrently.

1. Aranko K, Luurila H, Backman JT, Neuvonen PJ, Olkkola KT. The effect of erythromycin on the pharmacokinetics and pharmacodynamics of zopiclone. *Br J Clin Pharmacol* (1994) 38, 363–7.

Zopiclone + Itraconazole

Itraconazole raises zopiclone serum levels to some extent but this is not of clinical importance.

Clinical evidence, mechanism, importance and management

Itraconazole 200 mg daily or a placebo was given to 10 healthy young subjects for 4 days. On day 4 they were also given a single 7.5 mg oral dose of zopiclone. The **itraconazole** increased the maximum plasma levels of the zopiclone by 29% (from 49 to 63 nanograms/ml), increased its AUC by 73% and prolonged its half-life from 5 to 7 h. But despite these increases, there were no statistical or clinical differences between the performance of the psychomotor tests carried out during the placebo and **itraconazole** phases of the study. It was presumed that **itraconazole** inhibited zopiclone metabolism by the cytochrome P450 isoenzyme CYP3A.[1]

There would seem to be no reason for special precautions during concurrent use of these two drugs in young patients, although the effect in older patients awaits further study.

1. Jalava K-M, Olkkola KT, Neuvonen PJ. Effect of itraconazole on the pharmacokinetics and pharmacodynamics of zopiclone. *Eur J Clin Pharmacol* (1996) 51, 331–4.

Zopiclone + Nefazodone

A case report suggests that nefazodone may raise zopiclone levels resulting in increased sedation.

Clinical evidence, mechanism, importance and management

A woman of 86 taking diltiazem, irbesartan, lorazepam, and pravastatin was started on **nefazodone** 50 mg twice daily, increasing to 500 mg daily in divided doses, for the treatment of a major depressive episode. Because of associated insomnia zopiclone was added, starting at 15 mg each night, but reduced after 5 days to 7.5 mg, because of morning drowsiness. Plasma levels of S-zopiclone and R-zopiclone were 107 and 20.6 nanograms/ml at this time. After several months, **nefazodone** was replaced by venlafaxine, due to a lack of effect. The S-zopiclone and R-zopiclone levels were again measured and found to be only 16.9 and 1.45 nanograms/ml. It was concluded that **nefazodone**, but not venlafaxine inhibits the metabolism of zopiclone by the cytochrome P450 isoenzyme CYP3A4, resulting in elevated plasma levels.[1]

1. Alderman CP, Gebauer MG, Gilbert AL, Condon JT. Possible interaction of zopiclone and nefazodone. *Ann Pharmacother* (2001) 35, 1378–80.

Zopiclone + Rifampicin (Rifampin)

Rifampicin markedly reduces the serum levels of zopiclone. Its hypnotic effects are expected to be reduced accordingly.

Clinical evidence

In a two-phase study 8 healthy subjects were given 600 mg **rifampicin** or a placebo daily for 5 days, and then on day 6 a single 10 mg oral dose of zopiclone. The **rifampicin** reduced the zopiclone AUC by 82%, decreased the peak serum levels by 71% and reduced its half-life from 3.8 to 2.3 h. A significant reduction in the effects of zopiclone was also seen as measured by the performance of psychomotor tests.[1]

Mechanism

Not fully established, but it is thought that the rifampicin (a well recognised enzyme inducer) increases the metabolism and clearance of the zopiclone, probably by stimulating cytochrome P450 isoenzyme CYP3A4.

Importance and management

Information appears to be limited to this study, but is appears to be an established interaction and likely to be of clinical importance. If both drugs are given concurrently be alert for the need to use an increased zopiclone dosage (at least double) to achieve adequate hypnosis.

1. Villikka K, Kivistö KT, Lamberg TS, Kantola T, Neuvonen PJ. Concentrations and effects of zopiclone are greatly reduced by rifampicin. *Br J Clin Pharmacol* (1997) 43, 471–4.

Zopiclone + Trimipramine

The bioavailabilities of both drugs are modestly reduced by concurrent use.

Clinical evidence, mechanism, importance and management

When zopiclone and **trimipramine** were given concurrently for a week, in 10 healthy subjects, the bioavailability of zopiclone was reduced by almost 14% and the bioavailability of the **trimipramine** by almost 27%. Neither of these changes were statistically significant, and no other pharmacokinetic parameters were altered.[1] It seems unlikely that these changes will be of clinical relevance. There seems to be nothing documented about possible interactions of zopiclone with any of the other tricyclic antidepressants.

1. Caille G, Du Souich P, Spenard J, Lacasse Y, Vezina M. Pharmacokinetic and clinical parameters of zopiclone and trimipramine when administered simultaneously to volunteers. *Biopharm Drug Dispos* (1984) 5, 117–25.

Zotepine + Miscellaneous drugs

There appears to be little or no information about adverse interactions between zotepine and other drugs, but the makers warn about the concurrent use of anticholinergics, anticonvulsants, antihypertensives, antipsychotics, drugs which prolong the QTc interval and, by implication, uricosuric agents.

Clinical evidence, mechanism, importance and management

There appear to be no reports of adverse interactions with zotepine, but the makers issue a number of precautions and warnings based on what is currently known about its pharmacology.

(a) Anticholinergics

No pharmacokinetic interaction was seen when zotepine was given with **desipramine**, indicating that cytochrome P450 isoenzyme CYP2D6 is not involved in the metabolism of zotepine, but *in vitro* studies have shown that CYP1A2 and CYP3A4 are the major isoenzymes involved in its metabolism. Zotepine has anticholinergic properties and the makers warn about its use in patients with prostatic hypertrophy, retention of urine, narrow angle glaucoma and paralytic ileus. It would therefore be expected to have additive effects with **other anticholinergic drugs**.[1]

(b) Anticonvulsants, Antipsychotics

No specific interaction studies have been carried out with zotepine and **anticonvulsants**, but the makers point out that as with some other **antipsychotics**, zotepine has clear pro-convulsive effects which may be additive with other **antipsychotics** particularly if high doses of either or both drugs are used. They therefore recommend that zotepine doses above 300 mg daily or the concurrent use of high doses of other antipsychotics should be avoided. The makers also say that zotepine should not be used by patients with a personal or close family history of epilepsy unless individual benefit outweighs the risks.[1]

(c) Antihypertensives

Zotepine has alpha-adrenergic blocking properties which may cause orthostatic hypotension, especially when treatment is first started or if the dosage is increased. The makers advise caution when it is co-prescribed with hypotensive agents, including some **anaesthetic agents**, the implication being that any orthostatic hypotension may possibly be worsened. If patients feel faint and dizzy when they stand up, they should be advised to get up more slowly and if necessary a smaller dosage should be used.[1]

(d) Diazepam, Fluoxetine

In a clinical interaction study, **fluoxetine** and **diazepam** increased the plasma concentrations of zotepine and norzotepine. The makers advise caution if these drugs are given concurrently but none of these changes seem likely to be clinically important.[1]

(e) QTc prolonging drugs

The makers of zotepine advise caution when treating patients taking drugs known to prolong the QTc (or those with coronary heart disease or at risk of hypokalaemia) because zotepine also shows a dose-related QTc interval prolongation,[1] the implication being that the effects may be additive.

(f) Uricosuric agents

Zotepine acts as a uricosuric agent and because of a theoretical (though small) risk of renal stone formation the makers contraindicate its use by patients with acute gout or a history of kidney stones (and also by implication in those patients taking **uricosuric agents**). However, the makers also say that if treatment is undertaken, a good urine output should be maintained and zotepine should not be started within 3 weeks of resolving an episode of acute gout.[1]

1. Zoleptil (Zotepine). Knoll Limited. Summary of product characteristics, November 2001.

20

Neuromuscular blocker and anaesthetic drug interactions

This chapter is concerned with the interactions where the effects of neuromuscular blocking drugs and anaesthetics, both general and local, are affected by the presence of other drugs. Where these drugs are responsible for an interaction they are dealt with under the heading of the drug affected. See the Index for a full listing.

The modes of action of the two types of neuromuscular blocker are discussed in the monograph 'Neuromuscular

blockers + Anticholinesterases', p.755. Under some circumstances depolarising blockade (type I) is converted to the competitive block (type II). The different types of blocker are listed in Table 20.1.

The general and local anaesthetics mentioned in this chapter are listed in Table 20.2. Some of them are also used as antiarrhythmic agents and these are dealt with in the Chapter 4.

Table 20.1 Neuromuscular blockers

Generic names	Proprietary names
Non-depolarising blockers	
Alcuronium chloride	Alloferin, Alloferine
Atracurium besilate	Atracur, Faulcurium, Ifacur, Mycurium, Relatrac, Sitrac, Trablok, Tracrium
Fazadinium bromide	
Gallamine triethiodide	Flaxedil, Miowas G
Metocurine (Dimethyltubocurarine)	
Mivacurium	Mivacron, Novacrium
Pancuronium bromide	Bromurex, Curon-B, Pancuron, Pancurox, Panlem, Pavulon
Pipecuronium bromide	Arduan, Arpilon
Rocuronium	Esmeron, Zemuron
Tubocurarine chloride (Curare, d-Tubocurarine)	Curarine, Tubarine
Vecuronium bromide	Curlem, Norcuron
Depolarising blockers	
Carbolonium bromide (the blockade rapidly changes to non-depolarising)	
Decamethonium bromide	
Decamethonium iodide	
Suxamethonium bromide/chloride (Succinylcholine)	Anectine, Celocurin, Celocurine, Curacit, Ethicholine, Lysthenon, Midarine, Mioflex, Myoplegine, Myotenlis, Pantolax, Quelicin, Scoline, Succicuran, Succinolin, Succinyl, Sukolin, Uxicolin

Table 20.2 Anaesthetics

Generic names	Proprietary names
General anaesthetics	
Inhalation:	
Cyclopropane	
Diethyl ether (Ether)	
Enflurane	Alyrane, Efrane, Enfluthane, Enfran, Ethrane
Etomidate	Amidate, Hypnomidate, Radenarcon
Halothane	Fluothane
Isoflurane	AErrane, Forane, Forene, Forthane, Isoflurane, Isothane, Sofloran
Methoxyflurane	
Nitrous oxide	Entonox (N₂O/O₂)
Sevoflurane	Sevorane, Ultane
Trichloroethylene	
Parenteral:	
Alphaxalone/Alphadolone	
Ketamine hydrochloride	Brevinaze, Calypsol, Ketalar, Ketalin, Ketanest, Ketolar, Velonarcon
Propofol	Ansiven, Cryotol, Diprivan, Diprofol, Disoprivan, Fresofol, Ivofol, Klimofol, Pofol, Pronest, Propocam, Recofol
Thiopental sodium (Thiopentone)	Farmotal, Intraval, Nesdonal, Pentothal, Sodipental, Tiobarbital, Trapanal
Local anaesthetics	
Bupivacaine	Bicain, Bucain, Bupiforan, Bupyl, Buvacaina, Carbostesin, Dolanaest, Duracain, Kamacaine, Macaine, Marcain, Marcaina, Marcaine, Neocaina, Sensorcaine, Svedocain Sin Vasoconstr
Chloroprocaine	Ivracain, Nesacain, Nesacaine
Cocaine	
Lidocaine (Lignocaine)	Basicaina, Curadent, Dentipatch, Dilocaine, Docaine, Duo-Trach Kit, Dynexan, Ecocain, ELA-Max, Esracain, Gelicain, Laryng-O-Jet, Licain, Lident Adrenalina, Lident Andrenor, Lidesthesin, Lidocation, Lidocaton, Lidodan, Lidoject, Lidonostrum, Lidosen, Lidrian, Lignospan, Lignostab-A, Lincaina, Linisol, Llorentecaina Noradrenal, Luan, Mesocaine, Neo-Lidocaton, Neo-Sinedol, Neo-Xylestesin, Nervocaine, Nurocain, Octocaine, Odontalg, Ortodermina, Peterkaien, Pisacaina, Rapidocaine, Remicaine, Rowo-629, Sagittaproct, Sedagul, Xilo-Mynol, Xilonibsa, Xylanaest, Xylesine, Xylestesin, Xylocain, Xylocaina, Xylocaine, Xylocitin, Xyloneural, Xylonor, Xylotox
Mepivacaine	Carbocain, Carbocaina, Carbocaine, Carbocaine with Neo-Cobefrin, Isocaine, Isogaine, Meaverin, Meaverin hyperbar, Mecain, Mepicain, Mepicaton, Mepident, Mepiforan, Mepihexal, Mepinaest, Mepivastesin, Mepi-Mynol, Mepyl, Optocain, Pericaina, Polocaine, Scandicain, Scandicaine, Scandinibsa, Scandinor, Scandonest, Tevacaine
Procaine	Anestesia Loc Braun C/A, Aquilina, Atralcilina, Cibramicina, Cilicaine Syringe, Crysticillin, Farmaproina, Geroaslan H3, Gerovital H3, Hewedolor Procain, Jenacillin O, Lenident, Lophakomp-Procain N, Novanaest, Novocain, Novocillin, Procaneural, Procillin, Sodilin, Wycillin
Propoxycaine	

Anaesthetics, general + Alcohol

Those who regularly drink may need more thiopental (thiopentone) or propofol than those who do not. It is also probably unsafe to drink during the recovery period from anaesthesia because of the combined central nervous depressant effects.

Clinical evidence, mechanism, importance and management

A study in 532 healthy subjects aged 20–80 found that those who normally drank **alcohol** needed more **thiopental (thiopentone)** to achieve anaesthesia than non-drinkers. After adjusting for differences in age and weight distribution, men drinkers (40 g **alcohol** daily) needed 33% more **thiopental** for induction than non-drinkers, and women drinkers needed 40% more.[1] Another study found that 20 chronic alcoholics needed about one-third more **propofol** to induce anaesthesia than another 26 patients who only drank socially.[2]

When 12 normal subjects were given 0.7 g/kg **alcohol** 4 h after receiving 5 mg/kg of 2.5% **thiopental**, their performance of a number of psychomotor tests was found to be impaired.[3] This suggests that it is unsafe for ambulatory patients if they have been similarly anaesthetised to drive or handle dangerous machinery afterwards if they drink **alcohol** during the recovery period.

1. Dundee JW, Milligan KR. Induction dose of thiopentone: the effect of alcohol intake. *Br J Clin Pharmacol* (1989) 27, 693P–694P.
2. Fassoulaki A, Farinotti R, Servin F, Desmonts JM. Chronic alcoholism increases the induction dose of propofol in humans. *Anesth Analg* (1993) 77, 553–6.
3. Lichtor JL, Zacny JP, Coalson DW, Flemming DC, Uitvlugt A, Apfelbaum JL, Lane BS, Thisted RA. The interaction between alcohol and the residual effects of thiopental anesthesia. *Anesthesiology* (1993) 79, 28–35.

Anaesthetics, general + Alfentanil or Cocaine

Opisthotonus and/or grand mal seizures have been associated with the use of propofol with alfentanil, or possibly cocaine.

Clinical evidence, mechanism, importance and management

A patient with no history of epilepsy, undergoing septorhinoplasty for cosmetic reasons, was premedicated with papaveretum and hyoscine, intubated after **propofol** and **suxamethonium (succinylcholine)**, and anaesthetised with **nitrous oxide/oxygen** and 2% **isoflurane**. 10% **cocaine** paste was applied to the nasal mucosa. After the surgery he experienced a dystonic reaction during recovery which developed into a generalised convulsion. The authors of the report suggest that a possible interaction between the **propofol** and **cocaine** might have been responsible.[1] **Propofol** has been associated with opisthotonus and grand mal seizures in patients given **alfentanil**, in the absence of a history of epilepsy.[2,3] **Alfentanil** has also been found to reduce the amount of **propofol** needed to suppress the eyelash reflex and loss of consciousness, as well as increasing the blood pressure fall produced by **propofol**.[4]

1. Hendley BJ. Convulsions after cocaine and propofol. *Anaesthesia* (1990) 45, 788–9.
2. Laycock GJA. Opisthotonus and propofol: a possible association. *Anaesthesia* (1988) 43, 257.
3. Wittenstein U, Lyle DJR. Fits after alfentanil and propofol. *Anaesthesia* (1989) 44, 532–3.
4. Vuyk J, Griever GER, Engbers FHM, Burm AGL, Bovill JG, Vletter AA. The interaction between propofol and alfentanil during induction of anesthesia. *Anesthesiology* (1994) 81, A400.

Anaesthetics, general + Anaesthetics, general

An isolated report describes myoclonic seizures in a man anaesthetised with Alfathesin (alphaxalone-alphadolone) when additionally given enflurane.

Clinical evidence

Anaesthesia was induced uneventfully in a normal man of 23 with 2.5 ml *Alfathesin* (alphaxalone/alphadolone) given intravenously over 2 min, and then maintained with 2% **enflurane** in oxygen through a circle absorber system. After 8 min the patient began to have intermittent myoclonic activity (violent flexion of the extremities and contraction of trunk and facial muscles). The **enflurane** was stopped and anaesthesia maintained with **nitrous oxide** and **oxygen**. The myoclonic activity ceased within 3 min. After several minutes the **enflurane** was restarted and within 3 min the myoclonus began again, but it resolved when the **enflurane** was stopped.[1]

Mechanism

Uncertain. *Alfathesin* can causes seizures even in normal subjects and enflurane is also known to have caused seizures. It seems possible that these effects may be additive, and possibly exacerbated if hypocapnia also occurs.

Importance and management

Direct information seems to be confined to this single report. It has been suggested that concurrent use should be avoided, particularly in patients with known convulsive disorders.[1] *Alfathesin* has been withdrawn from general use.

1. Hudson R, Ethans CT. Alfathesin and enflurane: synergistic central nervous system excitation? *Can Anaesth Soc J* (1981) 28, 55–6.

Anaesthetics, general + Antihypertensives

Concurrent use normally need not be avoided but it should be recognised that the normal homoeostatic responses of the cardiovascular system will be impaired. Marked hypotension has been seen in patients on ACE inhibitors.

Clinical evidence, mechanism, importance and management

The antihypertensive drugs differ in the way they act, but they all interfere with the normal homoeostatic mechanisms which control blood pressure and, as a result, the reaction of the cardiovascular system during anaesthesia to fluid and blood losses, body positioning, etc. is impaired to some extent. For example, enhanced hypotension was seen in a study of the calcium channel blocker **nimodipine** during **general anaesthesia**.[1] This instability of the cardiovascular system needs to be recognised and allowed for, but it is widely accepted that normally any antihypertensive treatment should be continued.[2,3] In some cases there is a real risk in stopping, for example a hypertensive rebound can occur if **clonidine** or the **beta-blockers** are suddenly withdrawn. See also 'Clonidine + Beta-blockers', p.386 and 'Anaesthetics, general + Beta-blockers', p.745. However ACE inhibitors may possibly represent a risk.

Severe and unexpected hypotension has been seen during induction in patients on **captopril**.[4] Marked hypotension (75 mmHg systolic) occurred in a man of 42 on **enalapril** when anaesthetised with **propofol** which did not respond to surgical stimulation. He responded slowly to the infusion of 1 l of Hartmann's solution.[5] Although information is very limited, there would seem to be the need to take particular care with patients on **ACE inhibitors**. One recommendation is that intravenous infusion should be started in all patients on **ACE inhibitors** who are anaesthetised.[5]

1. Müller H, Kafurke H, Marck P, Zierski J, Hempelmann G. Interactions between nimodipine and general anaesthesia – clinical investigations in 124 patients during neurosurgical operations. *Act Neurochir* (1988) 45 (Suppl), 29–35.
2. Craig DB, Bose D. Drug interactions in anaesthesia: chronic antihypertensive therapy. *Can Anaesth Soc J* (1984) 31, 580–8.
3. Foëx P, Cutfield GR, Francis CM. Interactions of cardiovascular drugs with inhalational anaesthetics. *Anaesthesiol Intensivmed (Berlin)* (1982) 150, 109–28.
4. McConachie I, Healy TEJ. ACE inhibitors and anaesthesia. *Postgrad Med J* (1989) 65, 273–4.
5. Littler C, McConachie I, Healey TEJ. Interaction between enalapril and propofol. *Anaesth Intensive Care* (1989) 17, 514–5.

Anaesthetics, general + Aspirin or Probenecid

The induction of anaesthesia with midazolam is more rapid in patients who have been pretreated with aspirin or probenecid, while the anaesthetic dosage of thiopental (thiopentone) is reduced.

Clinical evidence

(a) Midazolam + Aspirin or Probenecid

A study in patients about to undergo surgery found that pretreatment with 1 g **aspirin** (given as intravenous **lysine acetylsalicylate**) 1 min before, or 1 g oral **probenecid** 1 h before induction, shortened the induction time with **midazolam** (0.3 mg/kg intravenously over 20 sec). Only 60% were 'asleep' within 3 min with **midazolam** alone, but 80–81% were 'asleep' within 3 min after the **aspirin** or **probenecid** pretreatment.[1]

(b) Thiopental (thiopentone) + Aspirin or Probenecid

The same study[1] cited above found that similar pretreatment with **aspirin** reduced the dosage of **thiopental** by 34% (from 5.3 to 3.5 mg/kg). The **thiopental** was given as a 2.5% solution intravenously, 2 mg/kg initially, followed by increments of 25 mg until the eyelash reflex was abolished.[1] The same study also found that 1 g oral **probenecid** 1 h before anaesthesia reduced the **thiopental** dosage by 15% (from 5.3 to 4.1 mg/kg).[1]

A further double-blind study in 86 women found that **probenecid** 3 h before surgery prolonged the duration of anaesthesia with **thiopental** (7 mg/kg). In patients premedicated with **pethidine** (1 mg/kg), **atropine** (0.0075 mg/kg) and either 0.5 g or 1.0 g **probenecid** prolonged the duration of anaesthesia by 65% and 46% respectively. Without the **pethidine**, 0.5 g **probenecid** caused a 26% prolongation. In patients without **pethidine** and given only 4 mg/kg **thiopental** but no surgical stimulus during anaesthesia, **probenecid** increased the duration of anaesthesia by 109%.[2]

Mechanisms

Not understood. Among the suggestions are that it could be because the aspirin and the probenecid increase the amount of free (and active) midazolam and thiopental in the plasma since they compete for the binding sites on the plasma albumins.[1,3]

Importance and management

Information is limited but what is known shows that the effects of both midazolam and thiopental (thiopentone) are increased by aspirin and probenecid. Be alert for the need to reduce the dosages.

1. Dundee JW, Halliday NJ, McMurray TJ. Aspirin and probenecid pretreatment influences the potency of thiopentone and the onset of action of midazolam. *Eur J Anaesthesiol* (1986) 3, 247–51.
2. Kaukinen S, Eerola M, Ylitalo P. Prolongation of thiopentone anaesthesia by probenecid. *Br J Anaesth* (1980) 52, 603–7.
3. Halliday NJ, Dundee JW, Collier PS, Howard PJ. Effects of aspirin pretreatment on the *in vitro* serum binding of midazolam. *Br J Clin Pharmacol* (1985) 19, 581P–582P.

Anaesthetics, general + Benzodiazepines

The sedative effects of propofol and midazolam given concurrently are greater than would be expected by simple addition.

Clinical evidence, mechanism, importance and management

Two studies have found that if **propofol** and **midazolam** are given together, the amount of sedation is greater than would be expected by the simple additive effects of both drugs. The ED_{50} is 45% less than the expected ED_{50} of the individual agents.[1,2] The reason is not known. A very modest increase in the levels of free **midazolam** in the plasma occurs (+20%), but it is too small to explain the considerable synergism which occurs.[3] Be alert for these increased effects if both drugs are used.

1. Short TG, Chui PT. Propofol and midazolam act synergistically in combination. *Br J Anaesth* (1991) 67, 539–45.
2. McClune S, McKay AC, Wright PMC, Patterson CC, Clarke RSJ. Synergistic interactions between midazolam and propofol. *Br J Anaesth* (1992) 69, 240–5.
3. Teh J, Short TG, Wong J, Tan P. Pharmacokinetic interactions between midazolam and propofol: an infusion study. *Br J Anaesth* (1994) 72, 62–5.

Anaesthetics, general + Beta-blockers

Anaesthesia in the presence of beta-blockers normally appears to be safer than withdrawal of the beta-blocker before anaesthesia, provided certain anaesthetics are avoided (methoxyflurane, cyclopropane, ether, trichloroethylene) and atropine is used to prevent bradycardia. See also 'Anaesthetics, general + Timolol', p.750 and 'Beta-blockers + Anticholinesterases', p.433.

Clinical evidence and mechanism

It used to be thought that **beta-blockers** should be withdrawn from patients before surgery because of the risk that their cardiac depressant effects would be additive with those of volatile anaesthetics, reducing cardiac output and lowering blood pressure, but it seems to depend on the anaesthetic used.[1] Lowenstein has drawn up a ranking order of compatibility (from the least to the most compatible) as follows: **methoxyflurane, ether, cyclopropane, trichloroethylene, enflurane, halothane, narcotics, isoflurane**.[1]

(a) Cyclopropane, Ether, Methoxyflurane, Trichloroethylene

A risk certainly seems to exist with **cyclopropane** and **ether** because their depressant effects on the heart are normally counteracted by the release of catecholamines, which would be blocked by the presence of a **beta-blocker**. There is also evidence (both clinical and *animal*) that unacceptable cardiac depression may also occur with **methoxyflurane** and **trichloroethylene** when a **beta-blocker** is present.[2,3] For these four anaesthetics it has been stated that an absolute indication for their use should exist before giving them in combination with a **beta-blocker**.[1]

(b) Enflurane, Halothane, Isoflurane, Narcotics

The situation with **enflurane** is not clear because it has been widely used with **propranolol** without apparent difficulties,[1] but a marked reduction in cardiac performance has also been described.[2,3] Normally **beta-blockers** and **halothane**, **isoflurane** or **narcotics** appear to be safe, but a rare and severe life-threatening allergic reaction has been described in one patient on **isoflurane**, **nitrous oxide** and oxygen when given 0.25 mg **propranolol** intravenously.[4]

On the positive side there appear to be considerable benefits to be gained from the continued use of **beta-blockers** during anaesthesia. Their sudden withdrawal from patients treated for angina or hypertension can result in the development of acute and life-threatening cardiovascular complications (possibly due to the increased sensitivity of the receptors) whether the patient is undergoing surgery or not. In the peri-operative period patients benefit from beta-blockade because it can minimise the effects of sympathetic overactivity of the cardiovascular system during anaesthesia and surgery (for example during endotracheal intubation, laryngoscopy, bronchoscopy and various surgical manoeuvres) which can cause heart dysrhythmias and hypertension.

Importance and management

The consensus of opinion is that beta-blockers should not be withdrawn before anaesthesia and surgery because the advantages of maintaining blockade and the risks accompanying withdrawal are considerable. But it is important to select the safest anaesthetics (isoflurane, halothane, narcotics), to avoid those which appear to be most risky (methoxyflurane, ether, chloroform, cyclopropane, trichloroethylene) and to ensure that the patient is protected against bradycardia by atropine (1–2 mg intravenously). See also 'Anaesthetics, general + Timolol', p.750 in this chapter, and 'Beta-blockers + Anticholinesterases', p.433 in Chapter 10.

1. Lowenstein E. Beta-adrenergic blockers. In 'Drug Interactions in Anesthesia.' Smith NT, Miller RD and Corbascio AN (eds). Lea and Febiger, Philadelphia (1981) p. 83–101.
2. Foëx P, Cutfield GR, Francis CM. Interactions of cardiovascular drugs with inhalational anaesthetics. *Anaesthesiol Intensivmed (Berlin)* (1982) 150, 109–28.
3. Foëx P, Francis CM, Cutfield GR. The interactions between β-blockers and anaesthetics. Experimental observations. *Acta Anaesthesiol Scand* (1982) (Suppl 76), 38–46.
4. Parker SD, Curry CS, Hirshman CA. A life-threatening reaction after propranolol administration in the operating room. *Anesth Analg* (1990) 70, 220–1.

Anaesthetics, general + Calcium channel blockers

Impaired myocardial conduction has been seen in two patients on diltiazem when anaesthetised with enflurane and prolonged anaesthesia has been seen with verapamil and etomidate, but it has been suggested that the concurrent use of anaesthetics and calcium channel blockers is normally without problems.

Clinical evidence, mechanism, importance and management

The author of a review about calcium channel blockers and anaesthetics concludes that concurrent use is normally beneficial except where there are other complicating factors. Thus he warns about possible decreases in ventricular function in patients undergoing open chest surgery given intravenous **verapamil** or **diltiazem**.[1] A report describes a patient on **diltiazem** and **atenolol** who had impaired AV and sinus node function before anaesthesia which worsened when given **enflurane**.[2] Another patient also on **diltiazem** demonstrated severe sinus bradycardia which progressed to asystole when **enflurane** was used.[2] The authors of this latter report suggest that **enflurane** and **diltiazem** can have additive depressant effects on myocardial conduction. Two cases of prolonged anaesthesia and Cheynes-Stokes respiration have been reported in patients who were undergoing cardioversion. Both received **verapamil** and were induced with **etomidate**.[3] Some caution is clearly appropriate.

1. Merin RG. Calcium channel blocking drugs and anesthetics: is the drug interaction beneficial or detrimental? *Anesthesiology* (1987) 66, 111–13.
2. Hantler CB, Wilton N, Learned DM, Hill AEG, Knight PR. Impaired myocardial conduction in patients receiving diltiazem therapy during enflurane anesthesia. *Anesthesiology* (1987) 67, 94–6.
3. Moore CA, Hamilton SF, Underhill AL, Fagraeus L. Potentiation of etomidate anesthesia by verapamil: a report of two cases. *Hosp Pharm* (1989) 24, 24–5.

Anaesthetics, general + Droperidol or Metoclopramide

Metoclopramide pre-treatment reduces the dosage requirements of propofol and thiopental. Droperidol seems to act similarly.

Clinical evidence

In a study of 60 surgical patients, half of whom were given 0.15 mg/kg **metoclopramide** 5 min before induction, it was found that the induction dose of **propofol** was reduced by 24% in the group given **metoclopramide**.[1] Similar results were seen in another 32 patients when pre-treated with **metoclopramide**. The **propofol** requirements were reduced by 24.5% with 10 mg **metoclopramide** and by 41.2% with 15 mg.[2] In a randomised, double-blind, placebo-controlled study in 96 women patients, both **metoclopramide** and **droperidol** reduced the amount of **thiopental** needed to induce anaesthesia.[3]

Mechanism

The mechanism is not yet known but it may involve dopamine receptors and GABA-mediated CNS transmission.

Importance and management

Although the evidence is limited these interactions would appear to be established. Droperidol has not been studied with propofol but can be expected to behave like metoclopramide. When patients are pretreated with either metoclopramide or droperidol, be alert for the need to use less propofol and thiopental to induce anaesthesia.

1. Page VJ, Chhipa JH. Metoclopramide reduces the induction dose of propofol. *Acta Anaesthesiol Scand* (1997) 41, 256–9.
2. Santiveri X, Castillo J, Buil JA, Escolano F, Castaño J. Efectos de la metoclopramida sobre las dosis hipnóticas de propofol. *Rev Esp Anestesiol Reanim* (1996) 43, 297–8.
3. Mehta D, Bradley EL Jr, Kissin I. Metoclopramide decreases thiopental hypnotic requirements. *Anesth Analg* (1993) 77, 784–7.

Anaesthetics, general + Epinephrine (Adrenaline), Norepinephrine (Noradrenaline) or Terbutaline

Patients anaesthetised with volatile anaesthetics (cyclopropane, ether, enflurane, halothane, isoflurane, fluroxene, methoxyflurane, sevoflurane can develop heart arrhythmias if given epinephrine (adrenaline) or norepinephrine (noradrenaline) unless the dosages are very low. Children appear to be less susceptible. Two patients developed arrhythmias when terbutaline was used with halothane. See also 'Anaesthetics, general + Phenylephrine', p.749.

Clinical evidence, mechanism, importance and management

(a) Epinephrine (Adrenaline) or Norepinephrine (Noradrenaline)

Oliver and Schaefer were the first to observe in 1895 that an adrenal extract could cause ventricular fibrillation in a *dog* anaesthetised with chloroform,[1] and it is now very well recognised that similar cardiac dysrhythmias can be caused by **epinephrine** and **norepinephrine** in man when anaesthetised with other **volatile anaesthetics**. A suggested[2] listing of these anaesthetics in order of decreasing sensitivity is as follows: **cyclopropane** > **halothane** > **enflurane** = **methoxyflurane** > **isoflurane** = **fluroxene** > **ether**. **Sevoflurane** appears to behave like **isoflurane**.[3]

The following recommendation has been made if **epinephrine** is used to reduce surgical bleeding in patients anaesthetised with **halothane/nitrous oxide/oxygen**: the dosage should not exceed 10 ml of 1:100,000 in any given 10 min period, nor 30 ml per h (i.e. about 100 micrograms or 1.5 micrograms/kg/10 min for a 70 kg person).[4] This dosage guide should also be safe for use with other volatile anaesthetics since **halothane** and **epinephrine** are more arrhythmogenic than the others.[2] Solutions containing 0.5% lidocaine (lignocaine) with 1:100,000 also appear to be safe because lidocaine may help to control the potential dysrhythmic effects. For example, a study in 15 adult patients showed that the dose of **epinephrine** needed to cause three premature ventricular contractions in half the group was 2.11 micrograms/kg in saline, but 3.69 micrograms/kg in 0.5% lidocaine (lignocaine).[5] However it should be borne in mind that the arrhythmogenic effects of **epinephrine** are increased if sympathetic activity is increased, and in hyperthyroidism and hypercapnia.[2]

Children appear to be much less susceptible than adults. A retrospective study of 28 children showed no evidence of dysrhythmia during **halothane** anaesthesia with **epinephrine** doses of up to 8.8 micrograms/kg, and a subsequent study on 83 children (three months to 17 years) found that 10 micrograms/kg doses were safe.[6]

(b) Terbutaline

Two patients developed ventricular arrhythmias while anaesthetised with **halothane** and nitrous oxide/oxygen when given 0.25–0.35 mg **terbutaline** subcutaneously for wheezing. Both developed unifocal premature ventricular contractions followed by bigeminy which responded to lidocaine (lignocaine).[7] Halothane was also replaced by enflurane in one case. See also 'Anaesthetics, general + Phenylephrine', p.749.

1. Oliver G, Schäefer EA. The physiological effects of extracts of the suprarenal capsules. *J Physiol* (1895) 18, 230–76.
2. Wong KC. Sympathomimetic drugs. In 'Drug Interactions in Anesthesia' Smith NT, Miller RD, Corbascio AN (eds). Lea and Febiger, Philadelphia (1981) p. 66.
3. Navarro R, Weiskopf RB, Moore MA, Lockhart S, Eger EI, Koblin D, Lu G, Wilson C. Humans anesthetized with sevoflurane or isoflurane have similar arrhythmic response to epinephrine. *Anesthesiology* (1994) 80, 545–9.
4. Katz RL, Matteo RS, Papper EM. The injection of epinephrine during general anesthesia with halogenated hydrocarbons and cyclopropane in man. 2. Halothane. *Anesthesiology* (1962) 23, 597–600.
5. Johnston RR, Eger EI, Wilson C. A comparative interaction of epinephrine with enflurane, isoflurane, and halothane in man. *Anesth Analg* (1976) 55, 709–12.
6. Karl HW, Swedlow DB, Lee KW, Downes JJ. Epinephrine–halothane interactions in children. *Anesthesiology* (1983) 58, 142–5.
7. Thiagarajah S, Grynsztejn M, Lear E, Azar I. Ventricular arrhythmias after terbutaline administration to patients anaesthetized with halothane. *Anesth Analg* (1986) 65, 417–8.

Anaesthetics, general + Fenfluramine

An isolated case of fatal cardiac arrest has been attributed to halothane anaesthesia in a woman taking fenfluramine. *Animal* studies confirm that combined use can cause serious heart arrhythmias and myocardial depression.

Clinical evidence, mechanism, importance and management

A 23-year-old woman, premedicated with diazepam and hyoscine, anaesthetised initially with **thiopental (thiopentone)** followed by **suxamethonium (succinylcholine)** and later **halothane** with oxygen, became pulseless, cyanosed and showed acute pulmonary oedema within 5 min of induction. She failed to respond to resuscitative measures including cardiac massage. It was later discovered that she had been taking **fenfluramine**. Later studies in *animals* showed that during the concurrent use of **halothane** and **fenfluramine**, marked ECG changes, sinus bradycardia, heart block, ventricular asystoles, paroxysmal ventricular tachycardia and fibrillation occurred.[1] The reasons are not understood. The authors of this isolated report recommend that patients on **fenfluramine** should not be anaesthetised with **halothane**,[1] but to keep this serious reaction in perspective it should be said that the evidence for it has come under heavy fire from at least one author.[2] However, note that **fenfluramine** was withdrawn in 1997 because its use was found to be associated with a high incidence of abnormal echocardiograms indicating abnormal functioning of heart valves.

1. Bennett JA, Eltringham RJ. Possible dangers of anaesthesia in patients receiving fenfluramine. *Anaesthesia* (1977) 32, 8–13.
2. Winnie AP. Fenfluramine and halothane. *Anaesthesia* (1979) 34, 79–81.

Anaesthetics, general + Monoamine oxidase inhibitors (MAOIs)

It used to be thought that MAOIs should be withdrawn well before anaesthesia, but there is now evidence that this may be unnecessary in most patients, although individual cases of both hypo- and hypertension have been seen. The MAOIs can however interact with other drugs sometimes used during surgery.

Clinical evidence and mechanism

The absence of problems during emergency general anaesthesia in 2 patients on MAOIs prompted further study in 6 others taking **un-**named **MAOIs** chronically. All 6 were premedicated with 10–15 mg diazepam 2 h before surgery, induced with **thiopental (thiopentone)**, given **suxamethonium (succinylcholine)** before intubation, and maintained with **nitrous oxide/oxygen** and either **halothane** or **isoflurane**. **Pancuronium** was used for muscle relaxation. **Morphine** was given postoperatively. One patient experienced hypotension that responded to repeated intravenous doses of 0.1 mg phenylephrine without hypertensive reactions. No other untoward events occurred either during or after the anaesthesia.[1]

No adverse reactions occurred in 27 other patients on MAOIs (**tranylcypromine, phenelzine, isocarboxazid, pargyline**) when anaesthetised.[2] No problems were seen in eight patients on **un-named MAOIs** when anaesthetised, nor in *dogs* on **tranylcypromine** given **enflurane** and **fentanyl**.[3] Two single case reports describe the safe and uneventful use of **propofol** in a patient on **phenelzine**[4] and another on **tranylcypromine**.[5] The latter was also given **alfentanil**. No problems were seen in one patient on **tranylcypromine** when given **ketamine**[6] and in another on **selegiline** when given **fentanyl, isoflurane** and **midazolam**.[7] No problems were seen in another patient on **phenelzine** when anaesthetised firstly with **sevoflurane** in oxygen, followed by **isoflurane**, oxygen, air and an infusion of **remifentanil**.[8] Unexplained hypertension has been described in a patient taking **tranylcypromine** when **etomidate** and **atracurium** were used.[9] **Moclobemide** was stopped on the morning of surgery in a patient who was anaesthetised with **propofol** and later **isoflurane** in **nitrous oxide** and oxygen. **Morphine** and **droperidol** were also used. No adverse reactions occurred.[10] **Ketorolac, propofol** and **midazolam** were used uneventfully in one patient on **phenelzine**.[11]

Importance and management

There seems to be little documentary evidence that the withdrawal of MAOI before anaesthesia is normally necessary. Scrutiny of reports[12] alleging an adverse reaction usually shows that what happened could be attributed to an interaction between other drugs used during the surgery (e.g. pethidine, sympathomimetics) rather than with the anaesthetics. The authors of the reports cited[1,2] here offer the opinion that . . general and regional anaesthesia may be provided safely without discontinuation of MAOI therapy, provided proper monitoring, adequate preparation, and prompt treatment of anticipated reactions are utilised.[1] This implies that the possible interactions between the MAOI and other drugs are fully recognised, but be alert for the rare unpredictable response.

1. El-Ganzouri A, Ivankovich AD, Braverman B, Land PC. Should MAOI be discontinued preoperatively? *Anesthesiology* (1983) 59, A384.
2. El-Ganzouri AR, Ivankovich AD, Braverman B, McCarthy R. Monoamine Oxidase Inhibitors: should they be discontinued preoperatively? *Anesth Analg* (1985) 64, 592–6.
3. Braverman B, Ivankovich AD, McCarthy R. The effects of fentanyl and vasopressors on anesthetized dogs receiving MAO inhibitors. *Anesth Analg* (1984) 63, 192.
4. Hodgson CA. Propofol and mono-amine oxidase inhibitors. *Anaesthesia* (1992) 47, 356.
5. Powell H. Use of alfentanil in a patient receiving monoamine oxidase inhibitor therapy. *Br J Anaesth* (1990) 64, 528–9.
6. Doyle DJ. Ketamine induction and monoamine oxidase inhibitors. *J Clin Anesth* (1990) 2, 324–5.
7. Norrily SH, Hantler CB, Sako EY. Monoamine oxidase inhibitors and cardiac anesthesia revisited. *South Med J* (1997) 90, 836–8.
8. Ure DS, Gillies MA, James KS. Safe use of remifentanil in a patient treated with the monoamine oxidase inhibitor phenelzine. *Br J Anaesth* (2000) 84, 414–16.
9. Sides CA. Hypertension during anaesthesia with monoamine oxidase inhibitors. *Anaesthesia* (1987) 42, 633–5.
10. McFarlane HJ. Anaesthesia and the new generation monoamine oxidase inhibitors. *Anaesthesia* (1994) 49, 597–99.
11. Fischer SP, Mantin R, Brock-Utne JG. Ketorolac and propofol anesthesia in a patient taking chronic monoamine oxidase inhibitors. *J Clin Anesth* (1996) 8, 245–7.
12. Jenkins LC, Graves HB. Potential hazards of psychoactive drugs in association with anaesthesia. *Can Anaesth Soc J* (1965) 12, 121–8.

Anaesthetics, general + Neuromuscular blockers

The inhalation anaesthetics (ether, halothane, enflurane, isoflurane, etc.) increase neuromuscular blockade to differing extents, but nitrous oxide appears not to interact. Propofol can cause serious bradycardia if given with suxamethonium (succinylcholine) without adequate anticholinergic premedi-

cation, and asystole has been seen with fentanyl, propofol and suxamethonium given sequentially. Propofol in its new formulation does not interact with vecuronium.

Clinical evidence, mechanism, importance and management

(a) Increased blockade

Neuromuscular blockade is increased by inhalation anaesthetics, the greater the dosage of the anaesthetic the greater the increase in blockade. In broad terms **ether**, **enflurane**, **isoflurane** and **methoxyflurane** have a greater effect than **halothane**, which is more potent than **fluroxene** and **cyclopropane**, whereas **nitrous oxide** appears not to interact.[1-5] The reasons are not fully understood but the following mechanisms have been suggested: the anaesthetic may have an effect via the CNS, or it may affect the muscle membrane, or possibly that some change in blood flow to the muscle occurs. These anaesthetics do not seem to affect either the release of acetylcholine at neuromuscular junctions or the acetylcholine receptors. The dosage of the neuromuscular blocker may need to be adjusted according to the anaesthetic in use. For example, the dosage of **atracurium** can be reduced by 25–30% if, instead of balanced anaesthesia (with **thiopental (thiopentone)**, **fentanyl** and **nitrous oxide/oxygen**),[1] **enflurane** is used, and by up to 50% if **isoflurane** or **desflurane** are used.[2,6,7] Another study showed that the reversal of blockade by **pancuronium** with neostigmine was prolonged (roughly doubled) when using **enflurane**.[8] The effects of **vecuronium** are also increased by **sevoflurane**.[9]

(b) Bradycardia and asystole

Serious sinus bradycardia (heart rates of 30–40 bpm) developed rapidly in two young women when anaesthetised with a slow intravenous infusion of **propofol** (2.5 mg/kg), followed by **suxamethonium (succinylcholine)** (1.5 mg/kg). This was controlled with 0.6 mg intravenous atropine. Four other patients premedicated with 0.6 mg atropine intramuscularly 45 min before induction of anaesthesia showed no bradycardia.[10] It would appear that **propofol** lacks central vagolytic activity and can exaggerate the muscarinic effects of **suxamethonium**.[10] Another report describes asystole in a woman given an anaesthetic induction sequence of **fentanyl**, **propofol** and **suxamethonium**.[11] Bradycardia and asystole has also been seen following the sequential administration of **propofol-fentanyl** in 2 patients.[12,13] All of these three drugs (**fentanyl**, **propofol**, **suxamethonium**) alone have been associated with bradycardia and their effects can apparently be additive. Bradycardia and asystole occurred in another patient given **propofol**, **fentanyl** and **atracurium**.[14] The authors of one report suggest that atropine or glycopyrrolate pretreatment should attenuate or prevent such reactions.[11]

(c) Propofol + Vecuronium: no interaction

The original formulation of **propofol** in *Cremophor* was found to increase the blockade due to **vecuronium**,[15] but the more recent formulation in soybean oil and egg phosphatide has been found in an extensive study in man not to interact with **vecuronium**.[16]

1. Ramsey FM, White PA, Stullken EH, Allen LL, Roy RC. Enflurane potentiation of neuromuscular blockade by atracurium. *Anesthesiology* (1982) 57, A255.
2. Sokoll MD, Gergis SD, Mehta M, Ali NM, Lineberry C. Safety and efficacy of atracurium (BW33A) in surgical patients receiving balanced or isoflurane anesthesia. *Anesthesiology* (1983) 58, 450–5.
3. Schuh FT. Differential increase in potency of neuromuscular blocking agents by enflurane and halothane. *Int J Clin Pharmacol Ther Toxicol* (1983) 21, 383–6.
4. Fogdall RP, Miller RD. Neuromuscular effects of enflurane alone and in combination with d-tubocurarine, pancuronium, and succinylcholine, in man. *Anesthesiology* (1975) 42, 173–8.
5. Miller RD, Way WL, Dolan WM, Stevens WC, Eger EI. Comparative neuromuscular effects of pancuronium, gallamine, and succinylcholine during Forane and halothane anesthesia in man. *Anesthesiology* (1971) 35, 509–14.
6. Lee C, Kwan WF, Chen B, Tsai SK, Gyermek L, Cheng M, Cantley E. Desflurane (I-653) potentiates atracurium in humans. *Anesthesiology* (1990) 73, A875.
7. Smiley RM, Ornstein E, Mathews D, Matteo RS. A comparison of the effects of desflurane and isoflurane on the action of atracurium in man. *Anesthesiology* (1990) 73, A882.
8. Delisle S, Bevan DR. Impaired neostigmine antagonism of pancuronium during enflurane anaesthesia in man. *Br J Anaesth* (1982) 54, 441–5.
9. Izawa H, Takeda J, Fukushima K. The interaction between sevoflurane and vecuronium and its reversibility by neostigmine in man. *Anesthesiology* (1992) 77, A960.
10. Baraka A. Severe bradycardia following propofol-suxamethonium sequence. *Br J Anaesth* (1988) 61, 482–3.
11. Egan TD, Brock-Utne JG. Asystole after anesthesia induction with a fentanyl, propofol, and succinylcholine sequence. *Anesth Analg* (1991) 73, 818–20.
12. Guise PA. Asystole following propofol and fentanyl in an anxious patient. *Anaesth Intensive Care* (1991) 19, 116–18.
13. Dorrington KL. Asystole with convulsion following a subanaesthetic dose of propofol plus fentanyl. *Anaesthesia* (1989) 44, 658–9.
14. Ricós P, Trillo L, Crespo MT, Guilera N, Puig MM. Bradicardia y asistolia asociadas a la administración simultánea de propofol y fentanilo en la inducción anestésica. *Rev Esp Anestesiol Reanim* (1994) 41, 194–5.
15. Robertson EN, Fragen RJ, Booij LHDJ, van Egmond J, Crul JF. Some effects of diisopropyl phenol (ICI 35 868) on the pharmacodynamics of atracurium and vecuronium in anaesthetized man. *Br J Anaesth* (1983) 55, 723–7.
16. McCarthy GJ, Mirakhur RK, Pandit SK. Lack of interaction between propofol and vecuronium. *Anesth Analg* (1992) 75, 536–8.

Anaesthetics, general + Nicotine and/or Vasopressin

A single report described coronary vasospasm attributed to surgery, anaesthesia, and nicotine from a transdermal patch. Another case report described marked hypotension and bradycardia in a young woman during surgery, attributed to the combined effects of vasopressin and the nicotine contained in a transdermal patch.

Clinical evidence

(a) Anaesthesia + Nicotine

A 47-year old woman recovering from surgery and general anaesthesia (**etomidate**, **fentanyl**, **midazolam**, **vecuronium**, **lidocaine (lignocaine)**, **nitrous oxide**, **isoflurane**) complained of chest pain and demonstrated ECG changes which were interpreted as coronary vasospasm. The authors of the report linked this response to the possible use of a **transdermal nicotine patch** which was removed just before the induction of the anaesthesia.[1]

(b) Anaesthesia + Nicotine + Vasopressin

A 22-year-old woman in good health was anaesthetised for surgery with N_2O, O_2 and **isoflurane**. 20 min after induction she was given an injection of 0.3 ml of 20 units of **vasopressin** in 30 ml saline (about 0.2 units of **vasopressin**) into the cervix. Within seconds she developed severe hypotension and bradycardia, and over the next half-an-hour blood pressures as low as 70/35 mmHg and heart rates as low as 38 bpm were recorded. She was treated with atropine and epinephrine (adrenaline), and eventually made a full recovery. This patient was wearing a **transdermal nicotine patch**.[2]

Mechanism

The authors of the first report postulate that the combination of the nicotine, the stress of surgery and the anaesthetic might have been responsible for the apparent coronary vasospasm.[1] The circulatory collapse described in the second report was attributed by the authors to the combined effects of the injected vasopressin and the nicotine from the transdermal patch. Both of these drugs can increase afterload and cause coronary artery vasoconstriction.[2]

Importance and management

Both of these are isolated reports and neither is therefore well established, nevertheless the recommendation of the authors of seems sensible, namely that nicotine patches should be removed the night before or 24 h before surgery, and that patients should be asked to avoid smoking before surgery to make sure that nicotine levels are minimal. More study is needed.

1. Williams EL, Tempelhoff R. Transdermal nicotine patch and general anesthesia. *Anesth Analg* (1993) 76, 907–8.
2. Groudine SB, Morley JN. Recent problems with paracervical vasopressin: a possible synergistic reaction with nicotine. *Med Hypoth* (1996) 47, 19–21.

Anaesthetics, general + Phenylephrine

Phenylephrine eye drops caused marked cyanosis and brady-cardia in a baby anaesthetised with halothane, and hypertension in a woman anaesthetised with isoflurane.

Clinical evidence, mechanism, importance and management

A 3-week-old baby anaesthetised with **halothane** and **nitrous oxide/oxygen** became cyanosed shortly after the instillation of two drops of 10% **phenylephrine** solution in one eye. The heart rate decreased from 160 to 60 bpm, S-T segment and T wave changes were seen, and blood pressure measurements were unobtainable. The baby recovered uneventfully when anaesthesia was stopped and oxygen administered. It was suggested that the **phenylephrine** caused severe peripheral vasodilatation and reflex bradycardia.[1] An adult patient aged 54 anaesthetised with **isoflurane** developed marked hypertension (a rise from 125/70 to 200/90 mmHg) shortly after having two drops of 10% **phenylephrine** in one eye which responded to nasal nitroglycerin and increasing concentrations of isoflurane.[1] The authors of this report say that during anaesthesia the use of **phenylephrine** should be discouraged, but if necessary use the lowest concentrations of **phenylephrine** (2.5%). They also point out that the following are effective mydriatics: single drop combinations of 0.5% cyclopentolate and 2.5% phenylephrine or 0.5% tropicamide and 2.5% phenylephrine.

1. Van der Spek AFL, Hantler CB. Phenylephrine eyedrops and anesthesia. *Anesthesiology* (1986) 64, 812–14.

Anaesthetics, general + Phenytoin, Phenobarbital (Phenobarbitone) or Rifampicin (Rifampin)

Phenytoin intoxication occurred in a child following halothane anaesthesia, and fatal hepatic necrosis occurred in a woman on phenytoin, phenobarbital (phenobarbitone) and phenylbutazone after being anaesthetised with fluroxene. Near fatal hepatic shock occurred in a woman given rifampicin (rifampin) after halothane anaesthesia.

Clinical evidence

A 10-year-old girl on long-term treatment with **phenytoin** (300 mg daily) was found to have phenytoin serum levels of 25 micrograms/ml before surgery. Three days after anaesthesia with **halothane** her serum **phenytoin** levels had risen to 41 micrograms/ml and she had marked signs of **phenytoin** intoxication.[1]

Another epileptic on 300 mg **phenytoin**, 120 mg **phenobarbital (phenobarbitone)** and **phenylbutazone** needed an increase in her **phenytoin** dosage to 2400 mg daily a week before surgery. She died of massive hepatic necrosis 36 h after anaesthesia with **fluroxene**.[2] A woman on **promethazine** and **phenobarbital** (60 mg three times daily) died from **halothane** associated hepatitis within six days of having **halothane** for the first time.[3] A nearly fatal shock-producing hepatic reaction occurred in a woman four days after having **halothane** anaesthesia immediately followed by a course of 600 mg **rifampicin** and 300 mg **isoniazid**.[4]

Mechanism

One suggested explanation is that, just as in *animals*, pre-treatment with phenobarbital and phenytoin increases the rate of drug metabolism and the hepatotoxicity of halogenated hydrocarbons including chloroform and carbon tetrachloride.[5,6] It seems possible that the general toxic effects of **halothane** on the liver can slow the normal rate

of **phenytoin** metabolism. The reason for the halothane-rifampicin interaction is not clear but additive hepatotoxicity might be the explanation.

Importance and management

No firm conclusions can be drawn from these isolated cases, but they serve to emphasise the potential hepatotoxicity of these anaesthetics with other drugs. The authors of the second report[2] suggest that patients with similar drug histories may constitute a high-risk group for liver damage after halogen or vinyl-radical anaesthetics.

1. Karlin JM, Kutt H. Acute diphenylhydantoin intoxication following halothane anesthesia. *J Pediatr* (1970) 76, 941–4.
2. Reynolds ES, Brown BR, Vandam LD. Massive hepatic necrosis after fluroxene anesthesia—a case of drug interaction? *N Engl J Med* (1972) 286, 530–1.
3. Patial RK, Sarin R, Patial SB. Halothane associated hepatitis and phenobarbitone. *J Ass Physician India* (1989) 37, 480.
4. Most JA, Markle GB. A nearly fatal hepatotoxic reaction to rifampin after halothane anesthesia. *Am J Surg* (1974) 127, 593–5.
5. Garner RC, McLean AEM. Increased susceptibility to carbon tetrachloride poisoning in the rat after pretreatment with oral phenobarbitone. *Biochem Pharmacol* (1969) 18, 645–50.
6. Munson ES, Malagodi MH, Shields RP, Tham MK, Fiserova-Bergerova V, Holday DA, Perry JC, Embro WJ. Fluroxene toxicity induced by phenobarbital. *Clin Pharmacol Ther* (1976) 18, 687–99.

Anaesthetics, general + Physostigmine

A study of 40 patients found that physostigmine pre-treatment (2 mg intravenously 5 min before induction) increased the propofol requirements by 20%.[1]

1. Fassoulaki A, Sarantopoulos C, Derveniotis C. Physostigmine increases the dose of propofol required to induce anaesthesia. *Can J Anaesth* (1998) 44, 1148–51.

Anaesthetics, general + Psychotropics

An isolated report describes a grand mal seizure in a man on chlorpromazine and flupenthixol when anaesthetised with enflurane.

Clinical evidence, mechanism, importance and management

An isolated report[1] describes the unexpected grand mal seizure in a schizophrenic patient without a history of epilepsy when given **enflurane** anaesthesia. He was taking 50 mg **chlorpromazine** three times daily (irregularly) and 40 mg **flupenthixol** intramuscularly every 2 weeks. The suggested reason is that the **enflurane** had a synergistic effect with the two psychotropic drugs, all of which are known to lower the seizure threshold. The general importance of this interaction is not known.

1. Vohra SB. Convulsions after enflurane in a schizophrenic patient receiving neuroleptics. *Can J Anaesth* (1994) 41, 420–2.

Anaesthetics, general + Sparteine sulphate

Patients induced with thiamylal sodium show a very marked increase in cardiac arrhythmias when given sparteine sulphate.

Clinical evidence, mechanism, importance and management

A group of 109 women undergoing dilatation and curretage were premedicated with **atropine** and **fentanyl**, induced with either 2% **thiamylal sodium** (5 mg/kg), 0.2% **etomidate** (0.3 mg/kg) or 2.5% **thiopental** (4 mg/kg), and given mask anaesthesia with **nitrous oxide** and **oxygen**. During the surgical procedure they were given a slow intravenous injection of 100 mg **sparteine sulphate**. 14 out of 45 patients given **thiamylal sodium** developed cardiac dysrhythmias, 10 had bigeminy and four had frequent VPCs, whereas only two patients given the other induction agents (**etomidate** or **thiopental**) showed any cardiac dysrhythmias. It is not understood why **sparteine** should interact with **thiamylal sodium** in this way. Although the dysrhythmias were effectively treated with xylocaine, the authors of this report suggest that the concurrent use of these drugs should be avoided.[1]

1. Cheng C-R, Chen S-Y, Wu K-H, Wei T-T. Thiamylal sodium with sparteine sulfate inducing dysrhythmia in anesthetized patients. *Anaesth Sinica* (1989) 27, 297–8.

Anaesthetics, general and/or Neuromuscular blockers + Theophylline

Cardiac arrhythmias can develop during the concurrent use of halothane and theophylline but this is possibly less likely with isoflurane. Seizures have been attributed to an interaction between ketamine and theophylline. Supraventricular tachycardia occurred in a patient on aminophylline when given pancuronium. The effects of pancuronium but not vecuronium can be opposed by aminophylline (theophylline).

Clinical evidence, mechanism, importance and management

(a) Development of arrhythmias

A number of reports describe arrhythmias apparently due to an interaction between **halothane** and **theophylline**. One describes intraoperative arrhythmias in four out of 67 adult asthmatics given **theophylline** and **halothane** (one had supraventricular tachycardia, two had bigeminy and one had multifocal premature ventricular contractions).[1] Nine out of another 45 patients developed heart rates exceeding 145 when given both drugs, whereas no tachycardia occurred in 22 other patients given only **halothane**.[1] There are other reports of individual adult and child patients who developed ventricular tachycardias[2] attributed to this interaction.[3-6] One child developed cardiac arrest.[6] The same interaction has been reported in *animals*.[7,8] Another report describes supraventricular tachycardia in a patient on **aminophylline** who was anaesthetised with **thiopental (thiopentone)** and **fentanyl**, followed by **pancuronium**. 3 min later his heart rate rose to 180 bpm and the ECG revealed that it was supraventricular in origin.[9] The authors of this report attributed this reaction to an interaction between the **pancuronium** and the **aminophylline**. The suggested reason for the interaction with halothane is that the **theophylline** causes the release of catecholamines (epinephrine (adrenaline), norepinephrine (noradrenaline)) from the adrenal medulla which are known to sensitise the myocardium.

The authors of one of the reports advise the avoidance of concurrent use[3] but another[10] says that: ". . . my own experience with the liberal use of these drugs has convinced me of the efficacy and wide margin of safety associated with their use in combination." A possibly safer anaesthetic may be **isoflurane**, which in studies with *dogs* has been shown not to cause cardiac arrhythmias in the presence of **aminophylline**.[11]

(b) Development of seizures

Tachycardia and extensor-type seizures occurred in four patients initially anaesthetised with **ketamine** and later with **halothane** or **enflurane**.[12] The authors attributed the seizures to an interaction between **ketamine** and **theophylline** (**aminophylline**) and they suggest avoidance of the combination or the use of antiseizure premedication in patients at risk.

(c) Altered neuromuscular blockade

A study in *rabbits* showed that at therapeutic concentrations the effects of **tubocurarine** were increased by **theophylline**, but this does not seem to have been observed in man.[13] Marked resistance to the effects of **pancuronium** was seen in two patients infused with **aminophylline**,[14,15] but no resistance was seen in one of them when

vecuronium was given instead.[14] Two other patients are reported to have shown a similar resistance but they had also had **hydrocortisone** which could have had a similar effect.[15,16]

1. Barton MD. Anesthetic problems with aspirin-intolerant patients. *Anesth Analg* (1975) 54, 376–80.
2. Roizen MF, Stevens WC. Multiform ventricular tachycardia due to the interaction of aminophylline and halothane. *Anesth Analg* (1978) 57, 738–43.
3. Roizen MF, Stevens WC. Multiform ventricular tachycardia due to the interaction of aminophylline and halothane. *Anesth Analg* (1978) 57, 738.
4. Naito Y, Arai T, Miyake C. Severe arrhythmias due to the combined use of halothane and aminophylline in an asthmatic patient. *Jpn J Anesthesiol* (1986) 35, 1126–9.
5. Bedger RC, Chang J-L, Larson CE, Bleyaert AL. Increased myocardial irritability with halothane and aminophylline. *Anesth Prog* (1980) 27, 34–6.
6. Richards W, Thompson J, Lewis G, Levy DS, Church JA. Cardiac arrest associated with halothane anesthesia in a patient receiving theophylline. *Ann Allergy* (1988) 61, 83–4
7. Takaori M, Loehning RW. Ventricular arrhythmias induced by aminophylline during halothane anaesthesia in dogs. *Can Anaesth Soc J* (1967) 14, 79–86.
8. Stirt JA, Berger JM, Roe SD, Ricker SM, Sullivan SF. Halothane-induced cardiac arrhythmias following administration of aminophylline in experimental animals. *Anesth Analg* (1981) 60, 517–20.
9. Belani KG, Anderson WW, Buckley JJ. Adverse drug interaction involving pancuronium and aminophylline. *Anesth Analg* (1982) 61, 473–4.
10. Zimmerman BL. Arrhythmogenicity of theophylline and halothane used in combination. *Anesth Analg* (1979) 58, 259–60.
11. Stirt JA, Berger JM, Sullivan SF. Lack of arrhythmogenicity of isoflurane following administration of aminophylline in dogs. *Anesth Analg* (1983) 62, 568–71.
12. Hirshman CA, Krieger W, Littlejohn G, Lee R, Julien R. Ketamine-aminophylline-induced decrease in seizure threshold. *Anesthesiology* (1982) 56, 464–7.
13. Fuke N, Martyn J, Kim C, Basta S. Concentration-dependent interaction of theophylline with *d*-tubocurarine. *J Appl Physiol* (1987) 62, 1970–4.
14. Daller JA, Erstad B, Rosado L, Otto C, Putnam CW. Aminophylline antagonizes the neuromuscular blockade of pancuronium but not vecuronium. *Crit Care Med* (1991) 19, 983–5.
15. Doll DC, Rosenberg H. Antagonism of neuromuscular blockage by theophylline. *Anesth Analg* (1979) 58, 139–40.
16. Azar I, Kumar D, Betcher AM. Resistance to pancuronium in an asthmatic patient treated with aminophylline and steroids. *Can Anaesth Soc J* (1982) 29, 280–2.

Anaesthetics, general + Thyroid hormones

Marked hypertension and tachycardia occurred in two patients taking levothyroxine when given ketamine.

Clinical evidence, mechanism, importance and management

Two patients on thyroid replacement treatment (**levothyroxine**) developed severe hypertension (240/140 and 210/130 mmHg respectively) and tachycardia (190 and 150 bpm) when given **ketamine**. Both were effectively treated with 1 mg intravenous **propranolol**.[1] It was not clear whether this was an interaction or simply a particularly exaggerated response to **ketamine**, but care is clearly needed if **ketamine** is given to patients in this category.

1. Kaplan JA, Cooperman LH. Alarming reactions to ketamine in patients taking thyroid medication — treatment with propranolol. *Anesthesiol* (1971) 35, 229–30.

Anaesthetics, general + Timolol

Marked bradycardia and hypotension occurred in a man using timolol eye-drops when he was anaesthetised.

Clinical evidence, mechanism, importance and management

A 75-year-old man being treated with **timolol eye drops** for glaucoma developed bradycardia and severe hypotension when anaesthetised (agent not named) which responded poorly to atropine, dextrose-saline infusion and elevation of his feet.[1] It would seem that there was sufficient systemic absorption of the **timolol** for it to join with the anaesthetic to cause marked depression of cardiac activity. The authors of this report suggest that if patients are to be anaesthetised, low concentrations of **timolol** should be used (possibly withhold the drops pre-operatively), and that . . . induction agents should be used judiciously and beta-blocking antagonists kept readily available. It is easy to overlook the fact that systemic absorption from eye-drops can be remarkably high. See also 'Anaesthetics, general + Beta-blockers', p.745.

1. Mostafa SM, Taylor M. Ocular timolol and induction agents during anaesthesia. *BMJ* (1985) 290, 1788.

Anaesthetics, general + Tricyclic and other antidepressants

Some very limited evidence suggests that amitriptyline may increase the likelihood of enflurane-induced seizure activity. Tachyarrhythmias have been seen in patients on imipramine when given halothane and pancuronium. A man taking maprotiline and lithium developed a tonic-clonic seizure when given propofol.

Clinical evidence, mechanism, importance and management

(a) Enflurane + Amitriptyline

Two patients taking **amitriptyline** have been described who showed clonic movements of the leg, arm and hand during surgery while anaesthetised with **enflurane** and **nitrous oxide**. The movements stopped when the **enflurane** was replaced by **halothane**.[1] A possible reason is that **amitriptyline** can lower the seizure threshold at which **enflurane**-induced seizure activity occurs. It is suggested that it may be advisable to avoid **enflurane** in patients needing tricyclic antidepressants, particularly in those who have a history of seizures or when hyperventilation or high concentrations of **enflurane** are likely to be used.[1]

(b) Halothane + Imipramine + Pancuronium

Two patients taking **imipramine** developed marked tachyarrhythmias when anaesthetised with **halothane** and given **pancuronium**.[2] This adverse interaction was subsequently clearly demonstrated in *dogs*.[2] The authors concluded on the basis of their studies that (i) gallamine should be avoided but tubocurarine would be an acceptable alternative to **pancuronium**; (ii) caution is appropriate if patients are taking any tricyclic antidepressant and **halothane** is used; (iii) **pancuronium** is probably safe in the presence of a tricyclic if **enflurane** is used. However this last (iii) conclusion does not agree with that reached by the authors of the report cited in (a) above.

(c) Propofol + Maprotiline and Lithium

A man with a bipolar mood disorder on 200 mg **maprotiline** four times daily and 300 mg **lithium carbonate** daily, underwent surgery during which he received **fentanyl**, **tubocurarine** and **propofol** (200 mg). Shortly after the injection of the **propofol** the patient complained of a burning sensation in his face. He then became rigid, his back and neck extended and his eyes turned upwards. After 15 sec rhythmic twitching developed in his eyes, arms and hands. This apparent seizure lasted about 1 min until succinylcholine was given and his trachea was intubated. The patient regained consciousness after several minutes and the surgery was cancelled.[3]

It is not known whether what occurred was due to an interaction between **propofol** and the antidepressants, or due to just one of the drugs because both **propofol**[4,5] and **maprotiline**[6] have been associated with seizures. However the authors of this report suggest that it would now be prudent to avoid using **propofol** in patients taking drugs which significantly lower the convulsive threshold. More study of this possible interaction is needed.

1. Sprague DH, Wolf S. Enflurane seizures in patients taking amitriptyline. *Anesth Analg* (1982) 61, 67–8.
2. Edwards RP, Miller RD, Roizen MF, Ham J, Way WL, Lake CR, Roderick L. Cardiac responses to imipramine and pancuronium during anesthesia with halothane or enflurane. *Anesthesiology* (1979) 50, 421–5.
3. Orser B, Oxorn D. Propofol, seizure and antidepressants. *Can J Anaesth* (1994) 41, 262–7.
4. Bevan JC. Propofol-related convulsions. *Can J Anaesth* (1993) 40, 805–9.
5. Committee on the Safety of Medicines. Propofol – convulsions, anaphylaxis and delayed recovery from anaesthesia. *Current Problems* (1989) 26.
6. Jabbari B, Bryan GE, Marsh EE, Gunderson CH. Incidence of seizures with tricyclic and tetracyclic antidepressants. *Arch Neurol* (1985) 42, 480–1.

Anaesthetics, local + Acetazolamide

Preliminary evidence suggests the possibility of procaine toxicity in patients given acetazolamide.

Clinical evidence, mechanism, importance and management

The mean plasma half-life of **procaine** in six normal subjects was increased by 66% (from 1.46 to 2.43 min) 2 h after being given 250 mg **acetazolamide** orally. The reason appears to be that the hydrolysis of the **procaine** is inhibited by the **acetazolamide**. The authors of the study suggest that higher than normal **procaine** levels (with toxicity) might possibly occur in patients given **acetazolamide** and (for example) large intramuscular doses of **procaine benzylpenicillin (procaine penicillin G)**,[1] but thus far there appear to be no reports of adverse responses due to this interaction.

1. Calvo R, Carlos R, Erill S. Effects of disease and acetazolamide on procaine hydrolysis by red blood cell enzymes. *Clin Pharmacol Ther* (1980) 27, 179–83.

Anaesthetics, local + Alcohol and Antirheumatics

The failure rate of spinal anaesthesia with bupivacaine is markedly increased in patients who are receiving antirheumatic drugs and who drink.

Clinical evidence, mechanism, importance and management

The observation that regional anaesthetic failures seemed to be particularly high among patients undergoing orthopaedic surgery who were suffering from rheumatic joint diseases, prompted further study of a possible interaction involving **antirheumatic drugs** and **alcohol**. It was found that the failure rate of low-dose spinal anaesthesia with **bupivacaine** (2 ml of 0.5%) increased from 5% in the control group (no alcohol or treatment) to 32–45% in those who had been taking **antirheumatic drugs** for at least six months or who drank at least 80 g **ethanol** daily, or both. The percentage of those patients who had a reduced response (i.e. an extended latency period and a reduced duration of action) also increased from 3 to 39–42%. **Indometacin (indomethacin)** was the specific antirheumatic drug studied in one group.[1] The reasons are not understood.

1. Sprotte G, Weis KH. Drug interaction with local anaesthetics. *Br J Anaesth* (1982) 54, 242P.

Anaesthetics, local + Anaesthetics, local

Mixtures of local anaesthetics are sometimes used to exploit the most useful characteristics of each drug. This normally seems to be safe although it is sometimes claimed that it increases the risk of toxicity. There is a case report of a man who developed toxicity when bupivacaine and mepivacaine were mixed together. The effectiveness of bupivacaine in epidural anaesthesia is reduced if preceded by chloroprocaine.

Clinical evidence and mechanism

(a) Evidence of no interaction

A study designed to assess the possibility of adverse interactions in man retrospectively studied the records of 10,538 patients over the 1952–72 period who had been given **tetracaine (amethocaine)** combined with **chloroprocaine**, **lidocaine (lignocaine)**, **mepivacaine**, **prilocaine**, **procaine** or **propoxycaine** for caudal, epidural, brachial plexus, or peripheral nerve block. The incidence of systemic toxic reactions was found to be no greater than when used singly and the conclusion was reached that combined use was advantageous and safe.[1] An *animal* study using combinations of **bupivacaine**, **lidocaine** and **chloroprocaine** also found no evidence that the toxicity was greater than if the anaesthetics were used singly.[2] **Lidocaine** does not affect the pharmacokinetics of **bupivacaine** in man.[3]

(b) Evidence of reduced analgesia

A study set up to examine the clinical impression that **bupivacaine** given epidurally did not relieve labour pain effectively if preceded by **chloroprocaine** confirmed that this was so. Using an initial 10 ml dose of 2% **chloroprocaine** followed by 8 ml 0.5% **bupivacaine**, the pain relief was less, the block was longer to set up, it had a shorter duration of action and had to be augmented more frequently than if only **bupivacaine** was used.[4,5]

(c) Evidence of a toxic interaction

An *animal* study showed that if **tetracaine (amethocaine)** was combined with other local anaesthetics the incidence of systemic toxicity and deaths increased.[1] There is a single case report of a patient given 2% **bupivacaine** and 0.75% **mepivacaine** who demonstrated lethargy, dysarthria and mild muscle tremor which the authors of the report correlated with a marked increase in the percentage of unbound (active) **bupivacaine**. They attributed this to its displacement by the **mepivacaine** from protein binding sites.[6]

Importance and management

Well examined interactions. The overall picture is that combined use does not normally result in increased toxicity although the isolated case report cited above illustrates that the possibility cannot be entirely discounted. Reduced effectiveness is seen if bupivacaine is preceded by chloroprocaine.

1. Moore DC, Bridenbaugh LD, Bridenbaugh PO, Thompson GE, Tucker GT. Does compounding of local anaesthetic agents increase their toxicity in humans? *Anesth Analg* (1972) 51, 579–85.
2. de Jong RH, Bonin JD. Mixtures of local anesthetics are no more toxic than the parent drugs. *Anesthesiology* (1981) 54, 177–81.
3. Freysz M, Beal JL, D'Athis P, Mounie J, Wilkening M, Escousse A. Pharmacokinetics of bupivacaine after axillary brachial plexus block. *Int J Clin Pharmacol Ther Toxicol* (1987) 25, 392–5.
4. Chen B-J, Kwan W-F. pH is not a determinant of 2-chloroprocaine-bupivacaine interaction: a clinical study. *Reg Anesth* (1990) 15 (Suppl 1), 25.
5. Hodgkinson R, Husain FJ, Bluhm C. Reduced effectiveness of bupivacaine 0.5% to relieve labor pain after prior injection of chloroprocaine 2%. *Anesthesiology* (1982) 57, A201.
6. Hartrick CT, Raj PP, Dirkes WE, Denson DD. Compounding of bupivacaine and mepivacaine for regional anaesthesia. A safe practice? *Reg Anesth* (1984) 9, 94–7.

Anaesthetics, local + Antihypertensives

Severe hypotension and bradycardia have been seen in patients on verapamil during epidural anaesthesia with bupivacaine, but not with lidocaine (lignocaine). Acute hypotension also occurred in a man on prazosin during epidural anaesthesia with bupivacaine.

Clinical evidence

(a) Anaesthetics, local + Alpha-blockers

A man on **prazosin** (5 mg three times daily for hypertension) developed marked hypotension (BP 60/40 mmHg) within 3–5 min of receiving **bupivacaine** through an L3–4 lumbar intradural catheter.[1] He was unresponsive to phenylephrine (five 100 micrograms boluses) but his blood pressure rose within 3–5 min of starting an infusion with epinephrine (adrenaline) 0.05 micrograms.kg^{-1}.min^{-1}.

(b) Anaesthetics, local + Calcium channel blockers

Four patients on long-term **verapamil** treatment developed severe hypotension (systolic pressures as low as 60 mmHg) and bradycardia (48 bpm) after epidural block with **bupivacaine** (0.5% with epinephrine (adrenaline)). This was totally resistant to atropine and ephedrine, and responded only to calcium gluconate or chloride. No such interaction was seen in a similar group of patients when epidural **lidocaine (lignocaine)** was used.[2]

Animal experiments have shown that the presence of **verapamil** increases the toxicity of **lidocaine**, and increases toxicity of **bupivacaine** even more.[3]

Mechanism

It would seem that some vasodilation can occur due to the local regional anaesthesia, particularly with bupivacaine, to which some patients are unable to respond by normal compensatory vasoconstriction because of the vasodilatory effects of the antihypertensive drugs. Other factors probably contributed to the development of this interaction in these particular patients.

Importance and management

Direct information seems to be limited to the reports cited. Their general importance is uncertain, but they serve to emphasise the importance of recognising that all antihypertensive drugs interfere in some way with the normal homoeostatic mechanisms which control blood pressure so that the normal physiological response to hypotension during epidural anaesthesia may be impaired. In this context lidocaine (lignocaine) would appear to be preferable to bupivacaine. Intravenous calcium effectively controls the hypotension and bradycardia produced by verapamil.[4] Particular care would seem to be important with any patient given epidural anaesthesia while taking any antihypertensive.

1. Lydiatt CA, Fee MP, Hill GE. Severe hypotension during epidural anesthesia in a prazosin-treated patient. *Anesth Analg* (1993) 76, 1152–3.
2. Collier C. Verapamil and epidural bupivacaine. *Anaesth Intensive Care* (1984) 13, 101–8.
3. Tallman RD, Rosenblatt RM, Weaver JM, Wang Y. Verapamil increases the toxicity of local anesthetics. *J Clin Pharmacol* (1988) 28, 317–21.
4. Coaldrake LA. Verapamil overdose. *Anaesth Intensive Care* (1984) 12, 174–5.

Anaesthetics, local + Benzodiazepines

There is conflicting evidence about whether diazepam can increase or decrease serum bupivacaine levels. Midazolam causes a modest decrease in lidocaine (lignocaine) but not mepivacaine levels. Spinal anaesthesia with tetracaine (amethocaine) can increase the sedative effects of midazolam.

Clinical evidence, mechanism, importance and management

(a) Effect of benzodiazepines on local anaesthetics

21 children aged 2–10 were given single caudal injections of 1 ml/kg of a mixture of 0.5% **lidocaine (lignocaine)** and 0.125% **bupivacaine** for regional anaesthesia. Pretreatment with 10 mg **diazepam** rectally half-an-hour before the surgery had no significant effect on the serum levels of **lidocaine**, but the AUC and maximal serum **bupivacaine** levels were increased by 70–75%.[1] A later study by the same workers similarly found that **diazepam** pretreatment in children raised serum **bupivacaine** levels.[2] These findings conflict with another in which intravenous **diazepam** in adult patients decreased the elimination half-life of epidural **bupivacaine**.[3] A later study in 20 children aged 2 to 7 receiving caudal block with 1 ml/kg of a 50:50 mixture of 1% **lidocaine** and 0.25% **bupivacaine**, found that 0.4 mg/kg **midazolam** given rectally as premedication caused a slight but not significant reduction in the AUC and serum levels of **bupivacaine**, whereas the **lidocaine** AUC was reduced by 25%.[4] In contrast, 0.4 mg **midazolam** given rectally as a premedication was found to have no significant effect on plasma **mepivacaine** levels.[5]

The clinical importance of these interactions is uncertain, but anaesthetists should be aware that increased **bupivacaine** serum levels have been observed with **diazepam**, and reduced **lidocaine** levels with **midazolam**. More study is needed.

(b) Effect of local anaesthetics on benzodiazepines

20 patients undergoing surgery were given repeated 1-mg intravenous doses of **midazolam** as induction anaesthesia every 30 s until they failed to respond to three repeated commands to squeeze the anaesthetist's hand. This was considered as the induction end-point 'titrated' dose. It was found that those who had been given spinal anaesthesia with 12 mg **tetracaine (amethocaine)** by subarachnoid injection needed only half the dose of **midazolam** (7.6 mg) needed by other patients who had had no spinal injection (14.7 mg). The reasons are not known. The authors of this report simply advise care in this situation.[6]

1. Giaufre E, Bruguerolle B, Morisson-Lacombe G, Rousset-Rouviere B. The influence of diazepam on the plasma concentrations of bupivacaine and lignocaine after caudal injection of a mixture of the local anaesthetics in children. *Br J Clin Pharmacol* (1988) 26, 116–18.
2. Bruguerolle B, Giaufre E, Morisson-Lacombe G, Rousset-Rouviere B, Arnaud C. Bupivacaine free plasma levels in children after caudal anaesthesia: influence of pretreatment with diazepam. *Fundam Clin Pharmacol* (1990) 4, 159–61.
3. Giasi RM, D'Agostino E, Covino BG. Interaction of diazepam in epidurally administered local anesthetic agents. *Reg Anesth* (1980) 5, 8–11.
4. Giaufre E, Bruguerolle B, Morisson-Lacombe G, Rousset-Rouviere B. The influence of midazolam on the plasma concentrations of bupivacaine and lignocaine after caudal injection of a mixture of the local anaesthetics in children. *Acta Anaesthesiol Scand* (1990) 34, 44–6.
5. Giaufre E, Bruguerolle B, Morisson-Lacombe G, Rousset-Rouviere B. Influence of midazolam on the plasma concentrations of mepivacaine after lumber epidural injection in children. *Eur J Clin Pharmacol* (1990) 38, 91–2.
6. Ben-David B, Vaida S, Gaitini L. The influence of high spinal anesthesia on sensitivity to midazolam sedation. *Anesth Analg* (1995) 81, 525–8.

Anaesthetics, local + Beta-blockers

Propranolol reduces the clearance of bupivacaine and there is the theoretical possibility that the toxicity of bupivacaine may be increased. The coronary vasoconstriction caused by cocaine is increased by propranolol. See also 'Beta-blockers + Sympathomimetics (directly-acting)', p.448.

Clinical evidence, mechanism, importance and management

(a) Bupivacaine + propranolol

The clearance of **bupivacaine** (30 to 50 mg intravenous over 10–15 min) was reduced by 35% (from 0.33 to 0.21 l/min) in 6 normal subjects after taking 40 mg **propranolol** six-hourly for a day. The reason is thought to be that the **propranolol** inhibits the activity of the liver microsomal enzymes, thereby reducing the metabolism of the **bupivacaine**. Changes in blood flow to the liver are unlikely to affect **bupivacaine** metabolism substantially because it is relatively poorly extracted from the blood. The clinical importance of this interaction is uncertain, but it is suggested that an increase in local anaesthetic toxicity might occur and caution should be exercised if multiple doses of bupivacaine are given.[1] Direct information about other beta-blockers is lacking, but some of them are known to reduce the metabolism of **lidocaine** (**lignocaine**). See 'Lidocaine (Lignocaine) + Beta-blockers', p.107.

(b) Cocaine + propranolol

A study in 30 patients being evaluated for chest pain found that **cocaine** (10% solution intranasally, 2 mg/kg) reduced coronary sinus flow by 14% and coronary artery diameter by 6–9%. The coronary vascular resistance increased by 21%. The addition of **propranolol** (0.4 mg/min by intracoronary infusion, total 2 mg) reduced coronary sinus flow by a further 15% and increased the coronary resistance by 17%. The probable reason is that the **cocaine** stimulates the alpha-receptors (vasoconstrictor) of the coronary blood vessels. When the beta-receptors (vasodilatory) are blocked by **propranolol**, the vasoconstriction is thereby increased. The clinical importance of these findings is uncertain but the authors of the report suggest that beta-blockers should be avoided in patients with myocardial ischaemia or infarction associated with the use of **cocaine**.[2]

Remember that local anaesthetic preparations often contain epinephrine (adrenaline) as a vasoconstrictor which may interact with beta-blockers. See 'Beta-blockers + Sympathomimetics (directly-acting)', p.448.

1. Bowdle TA, Freund PR, Slattery JT. Propranolol reduces bupivacaine clearance. *Anesthesiology* (1987) 66, 36–8.
2. Lange RA, Cigarroa RG, Flores ED, McBride W, Kim AS, Wells PJ, Bedotto JB, Danziger RS, Hillis LD. Potentiation of cocaine-induced coronary vasoconstriction by beta-adrenergic blockade. *Ann Intern Med* (1990) 112, 897–903.

Anaesthetics, local + Carbamazepine or Lithium carbonate

Lithium and carbamazepine appear to reduce the effects of cocaine when used as a drug of abuse.

Clinical evidence, mechanism, importance and management

Four patients were unable to get 'high' on **cocaine** while taking **lithium**.[1] A man who occasionally abused **cocaine** found that the acute **cocaine** experience (the euphoric 'rush') was very much less pleasurable while taking 1 g **carbamazepine** daily, and the 'high' was reduced.[2] Another report suggests that **cocaine** craving may be reduced by **carbamazepine**.[3] The reasons are not understood. The clinical importance of this interaction is uncertain.

1. Cronson AJ, Flemenbaum A. Antagonism of cocaine highs by lithium. *Am J Psychiatry* (1978) 135, 856–7.
2. Sherer MA, Kumor KM, Mapou RL. A case in which carbamazepine attenuated cocaine "rush". *Am J Psychiatry* (1990) 147, 950.
3. Halikas J, Kemp K, Kuhn K, Carlson G, Crea F. Carbamazepine for cocaine addiction? *Lancet* (1989) 1, 623–4.

Anaesthetics, local + Cimetidine or Ranitidine

Some studies suggest that both cimetidine and ranitidine can raise bupivacaine levels whereas other evidence suggests that no significant interaction occurs. Neither H_2-blocker appears to affect lidocaine (lignocaine) when used as an anaesthetic, but see also 'Lidocaine (Lignocaine) + Cimetidine or Ranitidine', p.108.

Clinical evidence

(a) Cimetidine + Bupivacaine

Pretreatment with 300 mg **cimetidine** intramuscularly 1–4 h before undergoing caesarian section with 0.5% **bupivacaine** had no effect on the pharmacokinetics of **bupivacaine** of 36 women or their foetuses, although the unbound **bupivacaine** levels rose by 22%.[1] Another similar study[2] in 36 women pretreated with 400 mg **cimetidine** the night before or just before surgery, and yet another[3] in 7 normal subjects given 400 mg **cimetidine** at 22.00 the previous evening and 06.00 the following morning confirmed these findings. However four normal male subjects who were given 400 mg **cimetidine** at 22.00 the previous evening and 8.00 am the following morning, followed by a 50 mg infusion of **bupivacaine** at 11.0 am, showed a 40% increase in the **bupivacaine** AUC.

(b) Cimetidine + Lidocaine (Lignocaine)

No changes in the pharmacokinetics of 400 mg **lidocaine** 2% epinephrine (adrenaline) 1:200,000 was seen in five women given epidural anaesthesia for caesarian section after a single 400-mg dose of **cimetidine** given about 2 h preoperatively.[4,5] Another very similar study in 11 women also found no statistically significant rises in whole blood **lidocaine** levels in the presence of **cimetidine**, 300 mg intramuscular at least an hour preoperatively.[6]

(c) Ranitidine + Bupivacaine

Pretreatment with 150 mg **ranitidine** orally 2 h before **bupivacaine** for extradural anaesthesia for caesarian section increased the serum levels of **bupivacaine** in 16 patients at 40 min by about 20%.[7] Similar results by the same group of authors are reported elsewhere.[8] Another study found that 150 mg **ranitidine** caused a 25% increase but it was not statistically significant.[9] No increased **bupivacaine** toxicity was reported in any of these reports. However two other studies[2,10] on 36 and 28 women respectively undergoing caesarian section found no measurable effect on the **bupivacaine** disposition when given 50 mg **ranitidine** intramuscular 2 h before or 150 mg by mouth the night before or on the morning of anaesthesia.[10]

(d) Ranitidine + Lidocaine (Lignocaine)

No changes in the pharmacokinetics of 400 mg **lidocaine** 2% epinephrine (adrenaline) 1:200,000 was seen in a study on seven women given epidural anaesthesia for caesarian section was seen after a single 150-mg dose of **ranitidine** given about 2 h preoperatively.[4,5] Another very similar study in 11 women also found no statistically significant rises in whole blood **lidocaine** levels in the presence of 150 mg **ranitidine** at least 2 h preoperatively.[6]

Mechanism

Not understood. A reduction in the metabolism of the bupivacaine by the liver caused by the cimetidine is one suggested explanation. Protein binding displacement is another.

Importance and management

A confusing situation. No clinically important interaction has been established but be alert for any evidence of increased bupivacaine toxicity resulting from raised total serum levels and rises in unbound levels during concurrent use. Cimetidine (but not ranitidine) can raise serum lidocaine (lignocaine) levels when used as an antiarrhythmic agent (see 'Lidocaine (Lignocaine) + Cimetidine or Ranitidine', p.108) but this was not demonstrated in the studies cited above. More study is needed.

1. Kuhnert BR, Zuspan KJ, Kuhnert PM, Syracuse CD, Brashear WT, Brown DE. Lack of influence of cimetidine on bupivacaine levels during parturition. *Anesth Analg* (1987) 66, 986–90.
2. O'Sullivan GM, Smith M, Morgan B, Brighouse D, Reynolds F. H₂ antagonists and bupivacaine clearance. *Anaesthesia* (1988) 43, 93–5.
3. Pihlajamäki KK, Lindberg RLP, Jantunen ME. Lack of effect of cimetidine on the pharmacokinetics of bupivacaine in healthy subjects. *Br J Clin Pharmacol* (1988) 26, 403–6.
4. Flynn RJ, Moore J, Collier PS, Howard PJ. Single dose oral H₂-antagonists do not affect plasma lidocaine levels in the parturient. *Acta Anaesthesiol Scand* (1989) 33, 593–6.
5. Flynn RJ, Moore J. Lack of effect of cimetidine and ranitidine on lidocaine disposition in the parturient. *Anesthesiology* (1988) 69, A656.
6. Dailey PA, Hughes SC, Rosen MA, Healey K, Cheek DBC, Shnider SM. Effect of cimetidine and ranitidine on lidocaine concentrations during epidural anesthesia for Cesarean section. *Anesthesiology* (1988) 69, 1013–17.
7. Wilson CM, Moore J, Ghaly RG, McLean E, Dundee JW. Plasma bupivacaine concentrations associated with extradural anaesthesia for Caesarian section: influence of pretreatment with ranitidine. *Br J Anaesth* (1986) 58, 1330P–1331P.
8. Flynn RJ, Moore J, Collier PS, McClean E. Does pretreatment with cimetidine and ranitidine affect the disposition of bupivacaine? *Br J Anaesth* (1989) 62, 87–91.
9. Noble DW, Smith KJ, Dundas CR. Effects of H-2 antagonists on the elimination of bupivacaine. *Br J Anaesth* (1987) 59, 735–7.
10. Brashear WT, Zuspan KJ, Lazebnik N, Kuhnert BR, Mann LI. Effect of ranitidine on bupivacaine disposition. *Anesth Analg* (1991) 72, 369–76.

Botulinum toxin + Miscellaneous drugs

The neuromuscular blocking effects of botulinum toxin can be increased by other drugs with neuromuscular blocking effects such as the aminoglycosides and muscle relaxants.

Clinical evidence, mechanism, importance and management

Botulinum toxin type A, derived from *Clostridium botulinum*, is used for the symptomatic relief of blepharospasm, hemifacial spasm, strabismus and other neuromuscular disorders. It is a protein neurotoxin with a large molecular weight which acts on cholinergic nerve endings, blocking the release of acetylcholine so that muscle which is innervated becomes paralysed. Predictably it has additive effects with drugs which also cause neuromuscular blockade.

A case report describes a 5-month-old baby boy who was admitted to hospital because of lethargy, poor feeding, constipation and muscle weakness (later identified as being due to a *Clostridium botulinum* infection). An hour after starting intravenous treatment with ampicillin and **gentamicin** (7.5 mg/kg daily in divided doses every 8 hours) for presumed sepsis, he stopped breathing and died. The reason appeared to be the additive neuromuscular blocking effects of the botulinum toxin and the **gentamicin**.[1]

Animal studies confirm that **gentamicin** and **tobramycin** increase the neuromuscular blocking effects of botulinum toxin,[1] and there is every reason to believe that any of the other drugs known to cause neuromuscular blockade (**aminoglycoside antibacterials**, conventional **neuromuscular blockers**, etc.) will behave similarly. The makers of botulin toxin say that the **aminoglycosides** and **spectinomycin** are contraindicated. They advise caution with **polymyxins**, **tetracyclines** and **lincomycin**, and a reduced starting dose with **muscle relaxants** with a long-lasting effect, or the use of an intermediate action drug such as vecuronium or atracurium.[2]

A very large number of drugs possess some neuromuscular blocking activity which can be additive with the effects of conventional muscle relaxants (described in detail in this chapter) and it seems likely that they will be additive with the effects of botulinum toxin. There seem to be no reports of any such interactions but it seems reasonable to expect that they will occur. You can identify these drugs by looking up 'Neuromuscular blockers' in the Index, or by browsing through this chapter.

1. Santos JI, Swenson P, Glasgow LA. Potentiation of *Clostridium botulinum* toxin by aminoglycoside antibacterials: clinical and laboratory observations. *Pediatrics* (1981) 68, 50–4.
2. Botox (botulinum toxin type A). Allergan. Drug Datasheet Compendium 1995–6, p 70.

Methoxyflurane + Antibacterials or Barbiturates

The nephrotoxic effects of methoxyflurane appear to be increased by the use of barbiturates, tetracyclines and possibly some aminoglycoside antibacterials.

Clinical evidence, mechanism, importance and management

Methoxyflurane has been withdrawn in many countries because it causes kidney damage. This damage can be exacerbated by the concurrent use of some drugs. Five out of 7 patients anaesthetised with **methoxyflurane** who had been given **tetracycline** before or after surgery showed rises in blood urea nitrogen and creatinine, and three died. Post-mortem examination showed pathological changes (oxalosis) in the kidneys.[1] Another study identified renal tubular necrosis associated with calcium oxalate crystals in six patients who had been anaesthetised with **methoxyflurane** and given **tetracycline** (four patients) and **penicillin** with **streptomycin** (two patients).[2] Other reports support the finding of increased nephrotoxicity with **tetracycline**.[3-5] Another study suggested that **penicillin**, **streptomycin** and **chloramphenicol** appear not to increase the renal toxicity,[1] but **gentamicin** and **kanamycin** possibly do so.[6] There is also some evidence that **barbiturates** can exacerbate the renal toxicity because they alter the metabolism of the **methoxyflurane** and increase the production of nephrotoxic metabolites.[7,8]

The risk of kidney damage with **methoxyflurane** would therefore appear to be increased by some of these drugs and they should only be used with great caution, if at all.

1. Kuzucu EY. Methoxyflurane, tetracycline, and renal failure. *JAMA* (1970) 211, 1162–4.
2. Dryden GE. Incidence of tubular degeneration with microlithiasis following methoxyflurane compared with other anesthetic agents. *Anesth Analg* (1974) 53, 383–5.
3. Albers DD, Leverett CL, Sandin JH. Renal failure following prostatovesiculectomy related to methoxyflurane anesthesia and tetracycline—complicated by Candida infection. *J Urol* (1971) 106, 348–50.
4. Proctor EA, Barton FL. Polyuric acute renal failure after methoxyflurane and tetracycline. *BMJ* (1971) 4, 661–2.
5. Stoelting RK, Gibbs PS. Effect of tetracycline therapy on renal function after methoxyflurane anesthesia. *Anesth Analg* (1973) 52, 431–5.
6. Cousins MJ, Mazze RI. Tetracycline, methoxyflurane anaesthesia and renal dysfunction. *Lancet* (1972) i, 751–2.

7. Churchill D, Yacoub JM, Siu KP, Symes A, Gault MH. Toxic nephropathy after low-dose methoxyflurane anesthesia: drug interaction with secobarbital? *Can Med Assoc J* (1976) 114, 326–33.
8. Cousins MJ, Mazze RI. Methoxyflurane nephrotoxicity: a study of dose response in man. *JAMA* (1973) 225, 1611–16.

Neuromuscular blockers and/or Anaesthetics + Aminoglycosides

The aminoglycoside antibacterials (amikacin, gentamicin, kanamycin, neomycin, streptomycin, tobramycin, etc.) possess neuromuscular blocking activity. Appropriate measures should be taken to accommodate the increased neuromuscular blockade and the prolonged and potentially fatal respiratory depression which can occur if these antibacterials are used with anaesthetics and conventional neuromuscular blocking drugs of any kind.

Clinical evidence

Two examples from many:

(a) Anaesthetic + Aminoglycosides

A 48-year-old patient anaesthetised with **cyclopropane** experienced severe respiratory depression after intraperitoneal irrigation with 500 mg 1% **neomycin** solution. This antibacterial-induced neuromuscular blockade was resistant to treatment with edrophonium but responded to neostigmine.[1]

(b) Anaesthetic + Neuromuscular blocker + Aminoglycosides

A 56-year-old patient, initially anaesthetised with **thiopental (thiopentone)** followed by **nitrous oxide**, was given 160 mg **gallamine** as a muscle relaxant. His respiration was depressed for 18 h following the intraperitoneal administration of 2 g **neomycin**.[2]

Many other reports confirm that some degree of respiratory embarrassment or paralysis can occur if aminoglycosides are given to anaesthetised patients. When a conventional blocker is also used, the blockade is deepened and recovery prolonged. If the antibacterial is given towards the end of surgery the result can be that a patient who is recovering normally from neuromuscular blockade suddenly develops serious apnoea which can lead on to prolonged and in some cases fatal respiratory depression. Pittinger[3] lists more than a 100 cases in the literature over the 1955–70 period involving **tubocurarine** with **neomycin** or **streptomycin; gallamine** with **neomycin, kanamycin** or **streptomycin;** and **suxamethonium (succinylcholine)** with **neomycin, kanamycin** or **streptomycin.** The routes of antibacterial administration were oral, intraperitoneal, oesophageal, intraluminal, retroperineal, intramuscular, intrapleural, cystic, beneath skin flaps, intradural and intravenous. Later reports involve irrigation of the anterior chamber of the eye with **framycetin;**[4] **gentamicin** given alone[5] or with **vecuronium,**[6] **tubocurarine**[7] or **pancuronium;**[8] **amikacin,**[9] **tobramycin**[10] or **ribostamycin**[11,12] with **tubocurarine** or **pancuronium;**[13] **pancuronium** with **streptomycin**[14,15] or **neomycin;**[12,16] **pipecuronium** with **netilmicin;**[17] **vecuronium** with **amikacin/polymyxin,**[18] **gentamicin** alone[19] (and with **clindamycin**)[20] or **tobramycin;**[19,21] **rocuronium** with **neomycin.**[22] **Dibekacin** causes a small increase in the effects of **tubocurarine** and **suxamethonium.**[11,12]

Aminoglycosides and neuromuscular blockers which appear not to interact are as follows: **tobramycin** with **alcuronium**[23] or **atracurium;**[19] **gentamicin** with **atracurium;**[19] **suxamethonium** with **ribostamycin.**[11]

Mechanism

The aminoglycosides appear to reduce or prevent the release of acetylcholine at neuromuscular junctions (related to an impairment of calcium influx) and they may also lower the sensitivity of the postsynaptic membrane, thereby reducing transmission. These effects would be additive with those of conventional neuromuscular blockers which act at the post-synaptic membrane.

Importance and management

Extremely well documented, very long established, clinically important and potentially serious interactions. Ten out of the 111 cases cited by Pittinger[3] were fatal, related directly or indirectly to aminoglycoside-induced respiratory depression. Concurrent use need not be avoided but be alert for increased and prolonged neuromuscular blockade with every aminoglycoside and neuromuscular blocker although the potencies of the aminoglycosides differ. The neuromuscular blocking potencies of the aminoglycosides seem to be in descending order (based on *animal* studies): gentamicin > streptomycin > amikacin > sisomicin > kanamycin = tobramycin > bekanamycin > dibekacin.[24] The postoperative recovery period should also be closely monitored because of the risk of recurarisation if the antibacterial is given during surgery. High risk patients appear to be those with renal disease and hypocalcaemia who may have elevated serum antibacterial levels, and those with pre-existing muscular weakness. Treatment of the increased blockade with anticholinesterases and calcium has met with variable success because the response seems to be inconsistent.

1. NY State Society of Anesthesiologists Clinical Anesthesia Conference: Postoperative neomycin respiratory depression. *N Y State J Med* (1960) 60, 1977.
2. LaPorte J, Mignault G, L'Allier R, Perron P. Un cas d'apnée à la néomycine. *Un Med Canada* (1959) 88, 149–52.
3. Pittinger CB, Eryasa Y, Adamson R. Antibiotic-induced paralysis. *Anesth Analg* (1970) 49, 487–501.
4. Clark R. Prolonged curarization due to intraocular soframycin. *Anaesth Intensive Care* (1975) 3, 79–80.
5. Holtzman JL. Gentamicin and neuromuscular blockade. *Ann Intern Med* (1976) 84, 55.
6. Harwood TN, Moorthy SS. Prolonged vecuronium-induced neuromuscular blockade in children. *Anesth Analg* (1989) 68, 534–6.
7. Warner WA, Sanders E. Neuromuscular blockade associated with gentamicin therapy. *JAMA* (1971) 215, 1153–4.
8. Regan AG, Perumbetti PPV. Pancuronium and gentamicin interaction in patients with renal failure. *Anesth Analg* (1980) 59, 393.
9. Singh YN, Marshall IG, Harvey AL. Some effects of the aminoglycoside antibiotic amikacin on neuromuscular and autonomic transmission. *Br J Anaesth* (1978) 50, 109–17.
10. Waterman PM, Smith RB. Tobramycin-curare interaction. *Anesth Analg* (1977) 56, 587–8.
11. Arai T, Hashimoto Y, Shima T, Matsukawa S, Iwatsuki K. Neuromuscular blocking properties of tobramycin, dibekacin and ribostamycin in man. *Jpn J Antibiot* (1977) 30, 281–4.
12. Hashimoto Y, Shima T, Matsukawa S, Iwatsuki K. Neuromuscular blocking properties of some antibiotics in man. *Tohoku J Exp Med* (1975) 117, 339–400.
13. Monsegur JC, Vidal MM, Beltrán J, Felipe MAN. Parálisis neuromuscular prolongada tra administración simultánea de amikacina y pancuronio. *Rev Esp Anestesiol Reanim* (1984) 31, 30–3.
14. Giala MM, Paradelis AG. Two cases of prolonged respiratory depression due to interaction of pancuronium with colistin and streptomycin. *J Antimicrob Chemother* (1979) 5, 234–5.
15. Torresi S, Pasotti EM. Su un caso di curarizzazione prolungata da interazione tra pancuronio e streptomicina. *Min Anestesiol* (1984) 50, 143–5.
16. Giala M, Sareyiannis C, Cortsaris N, Paradelis A, Lappas DG. Possible interaction of pancuronium and tubocurarine with oral neomycin. *Anaesthesia* (1982) 37, 776.
17. Stanley JC, Mirakhur RK, Clarke RSJ. Study of pipecuronium-antibiotic interaction. *Anesthesiology* (1990) 73, A898.
18. Kronenfeld MA, Thomas SJ, Turndorf H. Recurrence of neuromuscular blockade after reversal of vecuronium in a patient receiving polymyxin/amikacin sternal irrigation. *Anesthesiology* (1986) 65, 93–4.
19. Dupuis JY, Martin R, Tétrault J-P. Atracurium and vecuronium interaction with gentamicin and tobramycin. *Can J Anaesth* (1989) 36, 407–11.
20. Jedeikin R, Dolgunski E, Kaplan R, Hoffman S. Prolongation of neuromuscular blocking effect of vecuronium by antibiotics. *Anaesthesia* (1987) 42, 858–60.
21. Vanacker BF, Van de Walle J. The neuromuscular blocking action of vecuronium in normal patients and in patients with no renal function and interaction vecuronium-tobramycin in renal transplant patients. *Acta Anaesthesiol Belg* (1986) 37, 95–9.
22. Hasfurther DL, Bailey PL. Failure of neuromuscular blockade reversal after rocuronium in a patient who received oral neomycin. *Can J Anaesth* (1996) 43, 617–20.
23. Boliston TA, Ashman R. Tobramycin and neuromuscular blockade. *Anaesthesia* (1978) 33, 552.
24. Paradelis AG, Triantaphyllidis C, Giala MM. Neuromuscular blocking activity of aminoglycoside antibiotics. *Methods Find Exp Clin Pharmacol* (1980) 2, 45–51.

Neuromuscular blockers + Anticholinesterases

Anticholinesterases oppose the actions of non-depolarising neuromuscular blockers (e.g. tubocurarine) and can therefore be used as an antidote to restore muscular activity following their use, whereas they increase and prolong the actions of the depolarising neuromuscular blockers (e.g. suxamethonium (succinylcholine)).

Clinical evidence, mechanism, importance and management

Neuromuscular blockers are of two types: non-depolarising and depolarising:

The **non-depolarising** or competitive type of blockers (**tubocurarine** and others listed in Table 20.1 at the beginning of this chapter) compete with acetylcholine for the receptors on the endplate of the neuromuscular junction so that the acetylcholine is excluded. Thus the receptors fail to be stimulated and muscular paralysis results. Anticholinesterases (e.g. **ambenonium**, **edrophonium**, **neostigmine**, **physostigmine**, **pyridostigmine**, **tacrine**, etc.) can be used as an antidote to this kind of neuromuscular blockade because they inhibit the enzymes that destroy acetylcholine so that the concentration of acetylcholine at the neuromuscular junction builds up. In this way the competition between the molecules of the blocker and the acetylcholine for occupancy of the receptors swings in favour of the acetylcholine so that transmission is restored. These drugs are used routinely following surgery to reactivate paralysed muscles.

The **depolarising** blockers (**suxamethonium (succinylcholine)** and others listed in Table 20.1) also occupy the receptors on the endplate but they differ in that they act like acetylcholine to cause depolarisation. However, unlike acetylcholine, they are not immediately removed by cholinesterase so that the depolarisation persists and the muscle remains paralysed. The anticholinesterase drugs increase the concentration of acetylcholine at the neuromuscular junction, which enhances and prolongs this type of blockade, and therefore anticholinesterases cannot be used as an antidote for this kind of blocker.

Tacrine, like other anticholinesterases, has been used in anaesthetic practice to reverse the effects of non-depolarising blockers such as **tubocurarine**[1] and to prolong the effects of depolarising blockers such as **suxamethonium**.[1-5] For example, one study found that only one-third of the normal dosage of **suxamethonium** was needed in the presence of 15 mg **tacrine**.[6] However more recently **tacrine** has been increasingly used for its central effects in the treatment of Alzheimer's disease. You should therefore now be alert for changes in the effects of both types of neuromuscular blocking drugs in patients in whom **tacrine** is being used for the treatment of Alzheimer's. **Rivastigmine**, another cholinesterase inhibitor also used for Alzheimer's disease, will behave like **tacrine**.

The **organophosphorus pesticides** are potent anticholinesterases used in agriculture and horticulture to control insects on crops and in veterinary practice to control various ectoparasites. They are applied as sprays and dips. Anyone who is exposed to these toxic pesticides may therefore show changes in their responses to neuromuscular blockers (see 'Neuromuscular blockers + Insecticides', p.764). Widely used organophosphorus pesticides include **azamethiphos**, **bromophos**, **chlorpyrifos**, **clofenvinfos**, **coumafos**, **cythioate**, **dichlorvos**, **dimethoate**, **dimpylate**, **dioxation**, **ethion**, **famphur**, **fenitrothion**, **fenthion**, **heptenophos**, **iodofenphos**, **malathion**, **naled**, **parathion**, **phosmet**, **phoxim**, **pirimiphos-methyl**, **propetamphos**, **pyraclofos**, **temefos**.[7] A number of the **nerve gases** (such as **sarin**, **soman**, **tabun** and **VX**) are also potent anticholinesterases.

1. Hunter AR. Tetrahydroaminacrine in anaesthesia. *Br J Anaesth* (1965) 37, 505–13.
2. Oberoi GS, Yaubihi N. The use of tacrine (THA) and succinylcholine compared with alcuronium during laparoscopy. *Pap New Guinea Med J* (1990) 33, 25–8.
3. Davies-Lepie SR. Tacrine may prolong the effect of succinylcholine. *Anesthesiology* (1994) 81, 524.
4. Norman J, Morgan M. The effect of tacrine on the neuromuscular block produced by suxamethonium in man. *Br J Anaesth* (1975) 47, 1027.
5. Lindsay PA, Lumley J. Suxamethonium apnoea masked by tetrahydroaminacrine. *Anaesthesia* (1987) 33, 620–2.
6. El-Kammah BM, El-Gafi SH, El-Sherbiny AM, Kader MMA. Biochemical and clinical study for the role of tacrine as succinylcholine extender. *J Egypt med Assoc* (1975) 58, 559–67.
7. Sweetman SC, editor. Martindale: The complete drug reference. 33rd ed. London: Pharmaceutical Press; 2002. p.1427.

Neuromuscular blockers + Anticonvulsants

The effects of many neuromuscular blockers are reduced and shortened if anticonvulsants (carbamazepine, phenytoin) are given chronically, but they appear to be increased if the anti-convulsants are given acutely. **Mivacurium appears not to interact.**

Clinical evidence

(a) Carbamazepine given chronically: neuromuscular blocking effects reduced

The recovery from neuromuscular blockade with **pancuronium** in 18 patients undergoing craniotomy for tumours, seizure foci or cerebrovascular surgery was on average 65% shorter in those taking **carbamazepine**.[1] Another eight patients undergoing surgery and neuromuscular blockade with **doxacurium** and on **carbamazepine** for at least a week had a recovery time of 63 min compared with 161 min in the control group.[2,3] These findings are consistent with those of two other studies.[4,5] Yet another study in 18 patients found that the recovery time from **atracurium** (0.5 mg/kg intravenously) was 5.93 min in those on **carbamazepine** compared with 8.02 min in the control group.[6] Further studies found that **carbamazepine** shortened the recovery time from **vecuronium** blockade by 25–50%,[7,8] but had no effect on **atracurium**.[9-11] The effects of **pipecuronium** are also reduced by **carbamazepine**.[12] In another study it was found that the onset time for **pipecuronium** blockade was lengthened for patients with therapeutic plasma concentrations of **carbamazepine**, but not in those with subtherapeutic levels.[13] However, in yet another study nine patients on chronic phenytoin or **carbamazepine** showed an increased recovery time when **suxamethonium (succinylcholine)** was used.[14]

(b) Phenytoin given chronically: neuromuscular blocking effects reduced

The reductions in the time to recover from 25 to 75% of the response to ulnar nerve stimulation in patients given **phenytoin** chronically was found as follows: **metocurine** (58%), **pancuronium** (40%), **tubocurarine** (24%), **atracurium** (8%) (the last two were not statistically significant).[15] A similar reduction with **metocurine** is reported elsewhere.[16] 80% more **pancuronium** was needed by nine patients given chronic **phenytoin** than in 18 others without **phenytoin** (0.058 and 0.032 mg/kg/h).[17] Resistance to **pancuronium** and a shortening of the recovery period due to chronic **phenytoin** has also been described in other reports.[4,18-20] **Doxacurium**,[2,4] **pipecuronium**,[12] **rocuronium**[21] and **vecuronium**[22,23] are affected like pancuronium. In another study it was found that the, onset time for **pipecuronium** blockade was lengthened for patients with therapeutic plasma concentrations of **carbamazepine**, but not in those with subtherapeutic levels.[13] Three studies suggest that **atracurium** is normally minimally affected[5,22,24] but a reduced recovery time was found in one other study.[6] However, in yet another study nine patients on chronic **phenytoin** or carbamazepine also showed a increased recovery time when **suxamethonium** was used.[14]

(c) Phenytoin given acutely: neuromuscular blocking effects increased

A retrospective review of eight patients on chronic **phenytoin** treatment and three others given **phenytoin** acutely (within 8 h of surgery) showed that the average doses of **vecuronium** used from induction to extubation were 0.155 (chronic) and 0.0615 mg/kg/h (acute).[25] Similar results were found in another study.[23] Two other studies even suggest that the sensitivity of patients to **vecuronium** is increased by **phenytoin** given acutely,[26] and this was also seen in *animal* studies with **tubocurarine**.[27]

(d) Anticonvulsants given chronically: neuromuscular blocking effects unaffected

Carbamazepine appears not to affect **mivacurium**[28,29] or **rocuronium**,[30,31] although one case report describes a patient on **carbamazepine** therapy who showed resistance to **rocuronium**.[32] A study in patients taking **unspecified anticonvulsants** found no resistance to **mivacurium**,[33] but in a study of 13 patients on **unspecified anticonvulsants** a trend towards a shorter recovery from **mivacurium** was seen (not statistically significant).[34]

Mechanism

Not understood. Suggestions to account for the reduced response with chronic anticonvulsants include induction of liver enzyme activity which would increase the metabolism and clearance of the neuromuscular blocker, increases in the number of acetylcholine receptors on the muscle membrane (up-regulation), reduced acetylcholine release, and changes in plasma protein binding.[14,35] It is known that carbamazepine doubles the clearance of vecuronium.[8]

Importance and management

Established and clinically important interactions. More is known about phenytoin than carbamazepine. (a) Anticipate the need to use more (possibly up to twice as much) doxacurium, metocurine, pancuronium, pipecuronium, suxamethonium and vecuronium in patients given these anticonvulsants for more than a week,[23] and expect an accelerated recovery. Rocuronium seems to interact with phenytoin but the reports with carbamazepine are conflicting. The effects on tubocurarine and atracurium appear only to be small or moderate, whereas mivacurium appears not to interact. (b) Anticipate the need to use a smaller neuromuscular blocker dosage if the anticonvulsants are given acutely.

1. Roth S, Ebrahim ZY. Resistance to pancuronium in patients receiving carbamazepine. *Anesthesiology* (1987) 66, 691–3.
2. Ornstein E, Matteo RS, Weinstein JA, Halevy JD, Young WL, Abou-Donia MM. Accelerated recovery from doxacurium-induced neuromuscular blockade in patients receiving chronic anticonvulsant therapy. *J Clin Anesth* (1991) 3, 108–11.
3. Ornstein E, Matteo RS, Halevy JD, Young WL, Abou-Donia M. Accelerated recovery from doxacurium in carbamazepine treated patients. *Anesthesiology* (1989) 71, A785.
4. Desai P, Hewitt PB, Jones RM. Influence of anticonvulsant therapy on doxacurium and pancuronium-induced paralysis. *Anesthesiology* (1989) 71, A784.
5. Modica P, Tempelhoff R. Effect of chronic anticonvulsant therapy on recovery from atracurium. *Anesth Analg* (1989) 68, S198.
6. Tempelhoff R, Modica PA, Jellish WS, Spitznagel EL. Resistance to atracurium-induced neuromuscular blockade in patients with intractable seizure disorders treated with anticonvulsants. *Anesth Analg* (1990) 71, 665–9.
7. Alloul K, Varin F, Whalley D, Chutway F. Carbamazepine induced changes on vecuronium pharmacokinetics in anesthetized patients. *Clin Pharmacol Ther* (1994) 55, 143.
8. Alloul K, Varin F, Chutway RN, Ebrahim Z, Whalley D. Carbamazepine effect on vecuronium pharmacokinetic-pharmacodynamic modeling in anesthetized patients. *Anesthesiology* (1994) 81, A414.
9. Spacek A, Neiger FX, Spiss CK, Kress HG. Atracurium-induced neuromuscular blockade is not affected by chronic anticonvulsant therapy with carbamazepine. *Acta Anaesthesiol Scand* (1997) 41, 1308–11.
10. Ebrahim Z, Bulkley R, Roth S. Carbamazepine therapy and neuromuscular blockade with atracurium and vecuronium. *Anesth Analg* (1988) 67, S55.
11. Spacek A, Neiger FX, Katz RL, Watkins WD, Spiss CK. No effect of chronic carbamazepine therapy on atracurium-induced neuromuscular blockade. *Anesth Analg* (1995) 80 (Suppl 2), S464.
12. Jellish WS, Modica PA, Tempelhoff R. Accelerated recovery from pipecuronium in patients treated with chronic anticonvulsant therapy. *J Clin Anesth* (1993) 5, 105–8.
13. Hans P, Ledoux D, Bonhomme V, Brichant JF. Effect of plasma anticonvulsant level on pipecuronium-induced neuromuscular blockade: preliminary results. *J Neurosurg Anesth* (1995) 7, 254–8.
14. Melton AT, Antognini JF, Gronert GA. Prolonged duration of succinylcholine in patients receiving anticonvulsants: evidence for mild up-regulation of acetylcholine receptors? *Can J Anaesth* (1993) 40, 939–42.
15. Ornstein E, Matteo RS, Silverberg PA, Schwartz AE, Young WL, Diaz J. Chronic phenytoin therapy and nondepolarizing muscular blockade. *Anesthesiology* (1985) 63, A331.
16. Ornstein E, Matteo RS, Young WL, Diaz J. Resistance to metocurine-induced neuromuscular blockade in patients receiving phenytoin. *Anesthesiology* (1985) 63, 294–8.
17. Chen J, Kim YD, Dubois M, Kammerer W, Macnamara TE. The increased requirement of pancuronium in neurosurgical patients receiving Dilantin chronically. *Anesthesiology* (1983) 59, A288.
18. Callanan DL. Development of resistance to pancuronium in adult respiratory distress syndrome. *Anesth Analg* (1985) 64, 1126–8.
19. Messick JM, Maass L, Faust RJ, Cucchiara RF. Duration of pancuronium neuromuscular blockade in patients taking anticonvulsant medication. *Anesth Analg* (1982) 61, 203–4.
20. Liberman BA, Norman P, Hardy BG. Pancuronium-phenytoin interaction: a case of decreased duration of neuromuscular blockade. *Int J Clin Pharmacol Ther Toxicol* (1988) 26, 371–4.
21. Szenohradszky J, Caldwell JE, Sharma ML, Gruenka LD, Miller RD. Interaction of rocuronium (ORG 9426) and phenytoin in a patient undergoing cadaver renal transplantation: a possible pharmacokinetic mechanism? *Anesthesiology* (1994) 80, 1167–70.
22. Ornstein E, Matteo RS, Schwartz AE, Silverberg PA, Young WL, Diaz J. The effect of phenytoin on the magnitude and duration of neuromuscular block following atracurium or vecuronium. *Anesthesiology* (1987) 67, 191–6.
23. Platt PR, Thackray NM. Phenytoin-induced resistance to vecuronium. *Anaesth Intensive Care* (1993) 21, 185–91.
24. deBros F, Okutani R, Lai A, Lawrence KW, Basta S. Phenytoin does not interfere with atracurium pharmacokinetics and pharmacodynamics. *Anesthesiology* (1987) 67, A607.
25. Baumgardner JE, Bagshaw R. Acute versus chronic phenytoin therapy and neuromuscular blockade. *Anaesthesia* (1990) 45, 493–4.
26. Gray HSJ, Slater RM, Pollard BJ. The effect of acutely administered phenytoin on vecuronium-induced neuromuscular blockade. *Anaesthesia* (1989) 44, 379–81.
27. Gandhi IC, Jindal MN, Patel VK. Mechanism of neuromuscular blockade with some antiepileptic drugs. *Arzneimittelforschung* (1976) 26, 258–61.
28. Spacek A, Neiger FX, Spiss CK, Kress HG. Chronic carbamazepine therapy does not influence neuromuscular block. *Br J Anaesth* (1996) 77, 500–2.
29. Spacek A, Neiger FX, Katz RL, Watkins WD, Spiss CK. The influence of chronic anticonvulsants therapy with carbamazepine on mivacurium-induced neuromuscular blockade. *Anesthesiology* (1994) 81, A1063.
30. Spacek A, Neiger FX, Katz RL, Watkins WD, Spiss CK. Chronic carbamazepine therapy does not affect neuromuscular blockade by rocuronium. *Anesth Analg* (1995) 80 (Suppl 2), S463.
31. Spacek A, Neiger FX, Krenn C-G, Spiss CK, Kress HG. Does chronic carbamazepine therapy influence neuromuscular blockade by rocuronium? *Anesthesiology* (1997) 87, A833.
32. Baraka A, Idriss N. Resistance to rocuronium in an epileptic patient on long-term carbamazepine therapy. *Middle East J Anesthesiol* (1996) 13, 561–4.
33. Jellish WS, Thalji Z, Brundidge PK, Tempelhoff R. Recovery from mivacurium-induced neuromuscular blockade is not affected by anticonvulsant therapy. *J Neurosurg Anesth* (1996) 8, 4–8.
34. Thalji Z, Jellish WS, Murdoch J, Tempelhoff R. The effect of chronic anticonvulsant therapy on recovery from mivacurium induced paralysis. *Anesthesiology* (1993) 79 (Suppl 319), A965.
35. Kim CS, Arnold FJ, Itani MS, Martyn JAJ. Decreased sensitivity to metocurine during long-term phenytoin therapy may be attributable to protein binding and acetylcholine receptor changes. *Anesthesiology* (1992) 77, 500–6.

Neuromuscular blockers + Aprotinin

Apnoea developed in a number of patients after being given aprotinin (Trasylol) while recovering from neuromuscular blockade with suxamethonium (succinylcholine) with or without tubocurarine.

Clinical evidence

Three patients underwent surgery in which either **suxamethonium** alone or with **tubocurarine** was used. At the end of, or shortly after, the operation when spontaneous breathing had recommenced, **aprotinin** (*Trasylol*) in doses of 2500–12 000 KIU (Kallikrein inactivator units) was given. In each case respiration rapidly became inadequate and apnoea lasting periods of 7, 30 and 90 min occurred.[1]

Seven other cases have been reported elsewhere.[2]

Mechanism

Not fully understood. Aprotinin is only a very weak inhibitor of serum pseudocholinesterase (100,000 KIU caused a maximal 16% inhibition in man)[3] and on its own would have little effect on the metabolism of suxamethonium. But it might tip the balance in those whose cholinesterase was already very depressed.

Importance and management

The incidence of this interaction is uncertain but probably low. Only a few cases have been reported. It seems probable that it only affects those whose plasma pseudocholinesterase levels are already very low for other reasons. No difficulties should arise in those whose plasma cholinesterase levels are normal.

1. Chasapakis G, Dimas C. Possible interaction between muscle relaxants and the kallikrein-trypsin inactivator "Trasylol". *Br J Anaesth* (1966) 38, 838–9.
2. Marcello B, Porati N. Trasylol e blocco neuromusculare. *Minerva anest* (Torino) 33, 814.
3. Doenicke A, Gesing H, Krumey I, Schmidinger St. Influence of aprotinin (Trasylol) on the action of suxamethonium. *Br J Anaesth* (1970) 42, 948–60.

Neuromuscular blockers + Bambuterol

Bambuterol can prolong the recovery time from neuromuscular blockade with suxamethonium (succinylcholine).

Clinical evidence

A double-blind study found that the recovery times of 25 patients from neuromuscular blockade with **suxamethonium succinylcholine** were prolonged about 30% in those who had had 10 mg **bambuterol** 10–16 h before surgery, and about 50% by 20 mg.[1]

This confirms two previous studies,[2,3] one of which found that 30 mg **bambuterol** given about 10 h before surgery prolonged **suxamethonium** blockade by 100%.[2] In patients who are heterozygous for abnormal plasma cholinesterase, 20 mg **bambuterol** taken 2 h before surgery prolongs **suxamethonium** blockade 2–3 times, and in some patients a phase II block occurs.[4]

Mechanism

Bambuterol is an inactive prodrug which is slowly converted enzymatically in the body to its active form, terbutaline. The carbamate groups that are split off can selectively inhibit the plasma cholinesterase that is necessary for the metabolism of suxamethonium. As a result, the metabolism of the suxamethonium is reduced and its effects are thereby prolonged. The effect appears to be related to the dose of the bambuterol.

Importance and management

An established interaction but unlikely to be of great clinical importance in normal patients, although anaesthetists should certainly be aware of its existence. It may possibly be important where other factors reduce plasma cholinesterase activity or affect the extent of blockade in other ways (e.g. subjects heterozygous for abnormal plasma cholinesterase).

1. Staun P, Lennmarken C, Eriksson LI, Wirén J-E. The influence of 10 mg and 20 mg of bambuterol on the duration of succinylcholine-induced neuromuscular blockade. *Acta Anaesthesiol Scand* (1990) 34, 498–500.
2. Fisher DM, Caldwell JE, Sharma M, Wirén J-E. The influence of bambuterol (carbamylated terbutaline) on the duration of action of succinylcholine-induced paralysis in humans. *Anesthesiology* (1988) 69, 757–9.
3. Bang U, Viby-Mogensen J, Wirén JE, Theil Slovgaard L. The effect of bambuterol (carbamylated terbutaline) on plasma cholinesterase activity and suxamethonium-induced neuromuscular blockade in genotypically normal patients. *Acta Anaesthesiol Scand* (1990) 34, 596–9.
4. Bang U, Viby-Mogensen J, Wirén JE. The effect of bambuterol on plasma cholinesterase activity and suxamethonium-induced neuromuscular blockade in subjects heterozygous for abnormal plasma cholinesterase. *Acta Anaesthesiol Scand* (1990) 34, 600–4.

Neuromuscular blockers + Benzodiazepines

Some studies report that diazepam and other benzodiazepines increase the effects of neuromuscular blockers, but others say that they do not. Patients given both drugs should be monitored for possible changes in the depth and duration of neuromuscular blockade.

Clinical evidence

(a) Increased blockade

A comparative study of 10 patients given **gallamine** and four others given **gallamine** and **diazepam** (0.15–0.2 mg/kg) showed that the duration of activity of the blocker was prolonged by a factor of three by the **diazepam**, and the depression of the twitch response was doubled. Persistent muscle weakness and respiratory depression was seen in two other patients on **tubocurarine** after premedication with **diazepam**.[1,2]

Increased neuromuscular blockade has been described with **diazepam** and **tubocurarine**,[3,4] **suxamethonium (succinylcholine)**[5] and **gallamine**.[3] Another study found that recovery from 25 to 75% of the twitch height after **vecuronium** was prolonged 25% by **midazolam**, and 45% by **diazepam**.[6] The same study found a 20% prolongation of recovery from the effects of **atracurium** by **midazolam**, and 20–35% by **diazepam**.[6]

(b) Reduced blockade or no effect

The duration of paralysis due to **suxamethonium** was reduced in one study by 20% when **diazepam** (0.15 mg/kg) was used and the recovery time was shortened.[2]

In other studies **diazepam** was found to have no significant effect on the blockade due to **tubocurarine**,[7] **gallamine**,[7] **decamethonium**,[7] **pancuronium**,[8] **fazadinium**,[8] **alcuronium**[8] or **suxamethonium**.[8–10] **Lorazepam** and **lormetazepam** have little or no effects on **atracurium** or **vecuronium**,[6] and **midazolam** has no effect on **suxamethonium** or **pancuronium**.[11]

Mechanism

Not understood. One suggestion is that where some alteration in response is seen it may be a reflection of a central depressant action

rather than a direct effect on the myoneural junction.[7] Another study suggests instead a direct action on the muscle.[12]

Importance and management

There is no obvious explanation for these discordant observations. What is known shows that the benzodiazepines may sometimes unpredictably alter the depth and prolong the recovery period from neuromuscular blockade, but the extent may not be very great and may possibly be little different from the individual variations in the response of patients to neuromuscular blockers. Concurrent use need not be avoided but 'caution and monitoring' has been advised.

1. Feldman SA, Crawley BE. Diazepam and muscle relaxants. *BMJ* (1970) 1, 691.
2. Feldman SA, Crawley BE. Interaction of diazepam with muscle-relaxant drugs. *BMJ* (1970) 2, 336–8.
3. Vergano F, Zaccagna CA, Zuccaro G. Muscle relaxant properties of diazepam. *Minerva Anestesiol* (1969) 35, 91.
4. Stovner J, Endresen R. Intravenous anaesthesia with diazepam. *Acta Anaesthesiol Scand* (1965) (Suppl 24), 223–7.
5. Jörgensen H. Premedicinering med diazepam, Valium®. Jämförelse med placebo i en dubbel-blind-undersökning. *Nord Med* (1964) 72, 1395–9.
6. Driessen JJ, Cruhl JF, Vree TB, van Egmond J, Booij LHDJ. Benzodiazepines and neuromuscular blocking drugs in patients. *Acta Anaesthesiol Scand* (1986) 30, 642–6.
7. Dretchen K, Ghoneim MM, Long JP. The interaction of diazepam with myoneural blocking agents. *Anesthesiology* (1971) 34, 463–8.
8. Bradshaw EG, Maddison S. Effect of diazepam at the neuromuscular junction. A clinical study. *Br J Anaesth* (1979) 51, 955–60.
9. Stovner J, Endresen R. Diazepam in intravenous anaesthesia. *Lancet* (1965) ii, 1298–9.
10. Hunter AR. Diazepam (Valium) as a muscle relaxant during general anaesthesia: a pilot study. *Br J Anaesth* (1967) 39, 633–7.
11. Tassonyi E. Effects of midazolam (Ro 21-3981) on neuromuscular block. *Pharmatherapeutica* (1984) 3, 678–81.
12. Ludin HP, Dubach K. Action of diazepam on muscular contraction in man. *Z Neurol* (1971) 199, 30–8.

Neuromuscular blockers + Beta-blockers

Increases or decreases (often only modest) in the extent of neuromuscular blockade have been seen when beta-blockers were present. The bradycardia and hypotension caused by anaesthetics and beta-blockers may possibly be increased by alcuronium and atracurium.

Clinical evidence

(a) Reduced neuromuscular blockade

A study in 31 patients given 1 mg/15 kg body-weight **propranolol** intravenously over a 4-min period during surgery showed that the effects of **suxamethonium (succinylcholine)** were slightly reduced. The mean period of apnoea fell from 4.4 min (without propranolol) to 3.6 min. **Propranolol** was also observed to shorten the recovery from **tubocurarine**.[1] Other studies describe a shortened recovery period from **tubocurarine** due to **oxprenolol** or **propranolol**, but **pindolol** affected only a few subjects.[2]

(b) Increased neuromuscular blockade

Two patients with thyrotoxicosis showed prolonged neuromuscular blockade with **tubocurarine** or **suxamethonium** when given 120 mg **propranolol** daily.[3] A study with an infusion of **esmolol** (0.3–0.5 mg/kg/min) found that it reduced the cardioacceleration following intubation, and only prolonged the recovery from blockade with **suxamethonium** by three minutes.[4]

(c) Bradycardia and hypotension

Eight out of 42 patients on **unnamed beta-blockers** and given **atracurium** developed bradycardia (less than 50 bpm) and hypotension (systolic pressure less than 80 mmHg). Most of them had been premedicated with diazepam, induced with methohexital (methohexitone), and anaesthetised with droperidol, fentanyl and nitrous oxide/oxygen. A further 24 showed bradycardia and eight showed hypotension. All responded promptly to atropine (0.3–0.6 mg intravenously).[5]

Another patient using 0.5% **timolol eye drops** for glaucoma similarly developed bradycardia and hypotension when **atracurium** was used.[6] Bradycardia and hypotension have been seen in two other patients given **alcuronium** while using **timolol eye drops** for glaucoma or **atenolol** for hypertension.[7]

(d) No interaction

A study of 16 patients taking various beta-blockers (**propranolol** 5, **atenolol** 5, **metoprolol** 2, **bisoprolol** 2, **oxprenolol** 1, **celiprolol** 1) found no interaction with **rocuronium**.[8]

Mechanisms

The changes in the degree of blockade are not understood but it appears to occur at the neuromuscular junction. It has been seen in *animal* studies.[9,10] The bradycardia and hypotension (c) were probably due to the combined depressant effects on the heart of the anaesthetics, the beta-blocker and atracurium.

Importance and management

Information is fairly sparse, but these interactions appear normally to be of relatively minor importance. Be aware that changes in neuromuscular blockade (increases or decreases) can occur if beta-blockers are used, but they seem to be unpredictable, and then often only modest in extent. The combined cardiac depressant effects of beta-blockade and anaesthesia are well known (see 'Anaesthetics, general + Beta-blockers', p.745) and the possible additional effect of atracurium and alcuronium should also be recognised, but other neuromuscular blockers possibly do not have this effect (?). It is suggested in one report that it may be wise to avoid atracurium until more is known.[7] See also 'Beta-blockers + Anticholinesterases', p.433.

1. Varma YS, Sharma PL, Singh HW. Effect of propranolol hydrochloride on the neuromuscular blocking action of d-tubocurarine and succinylcholine in man. *Indian J Med Res* (1972) 60, 266–72.
2. Varma YS, Sharma PL, Singh HW. Comparative effect of propranolol, oxprenolol and pindolol on neuromuscular blocking action of d-tubocurarine in man. *Indian J Med Res* (1973) 61, 1382–6.
3. Rozen MS, Whan FM. Prolonged curarization associated with propranolol. *Med J Aust* (1972) 1, 467–8.
4. Murthy VS, Patel KD, Elangovan RG, Hwang T-F, Solochek SM, Steck JD, Laddu AR. Cardiovascular and neuromuscular effects of esmolol during induction of anesthesia. *J Clin Pharmacol* (1986) 26, 351–7.
5. Rowlands DE. Drug interaction? *Anaesthesia* (1984) 39, 1252.
6. Glynne GL. Drug interaction? *Anaesthesia* (1984) 39, 293.
7. Yate B, Mostafa SM. Drug interaction? *Anaesthesia* (1984) 39, 728–9.
8. Loan PB, Connolly FM, Mirakhur RK, Kumar N, Farling P. Neuromuscular effects of rocuronium in patients receiving beta-adrenoreceptor blocking, calcium entry blocking and anticonvulsant drugs. *Br J Anaesth* (1997) 78, 90–1.
9. Usubiaga JE. Neuromuscular effects of beta-adrenergic blockers and their interaction with skeletal muscle relaxants. *Anesthesiology* (1968) 29, 484–92.
10. Harrah MD, Walter WL, Katzung BG. The interaction of d-tubocurarine with antiarrhythmic drugs. *Anesthesiology* (1970) 33, 404–10.

Neuromuscular blockers + Bretylium

In theory there is the possibility of increased and prolonged neuromuscular blockade if bretylium is given with neuromuscular blockers.

Clinical evidence, mechanism, importance and management

Although case reports seem to be lacking, the muscular weakness seen in a few patients given **bretylium**[1] and the evidence from *animal* studies showing that the effects of **tubocurarine** can be increased and prolonged by **bretylium**, suggest that an interaction might occur in man.[2] One suggested possibility is that if the **bretylium** were to be given during surgery to control arrhythmias, its effects (which are delayed) might be additive with the residual effects of the neuromuscular blocker during the recovery period, resulting in apnoea. This needs confirmation.

1. Bowman WC. Effects of adrenergic activators and inhibitors on skeletal muscles. In 'Handbook of experimental pharmacology.' Szekeres L (ed). Springer-Verlag (1980) 47–128.
2. Welch GW, Waud BE. Effect of bretylium on neuromuscular transmission. *Anesth Analg* (1982) 61, 442–4.

Neuromuscular blockers + Calcium channel blockers

Limited evidence indicates that diltiazem, nicardipine, nifedipine and verapamil can increase the neuromuscular blocking effects of vecuronium. Verapamil may similarly affect tubocurarine, but it appears that rocuronium does not interact with calcium channel blockers. Calcium channel blockers do not increase the serum potassium rise due to suxamethonium (succinylcholine).

Clinical evidence

(a) Vecuronium or Tubocurarine + Calcium channel blockers

A study in 24 surgical patients anaesthetised with nitrous oxide and isoflurane found that infusions of **diltiazem** (5 or 10 micrograms/kg/min) decreased the **vecuronium** requirements by up to 50%.[1] Another study in 24 surgical patients showed that **diltiazem** (2 or 4 micrograms/kg/min) decreased the **vecuronium** requirements by 45%.[2] Reductions in the requirements for **vecuronium** was also noted in other surgical patients receiving **diltiazem** or **nicardipine**.[3] A study in patients given 0.1 mg/kg **vecuronium** for tracheal intubation found that 10 micrograms/kg **nicardipine** shortened the onset of blockade to the same extent as other patients given 0.15 mg/kg **vecuronium**. Recovery times were unaffected.[4] Yet another study showed that **nicardipine** reduced the requirements for **vecuronium** by 53% in patients undergoing surgery.[5] A study in 44 patients anaesthetised with isoflurane in nitrous oxide/oxygen found that 1 mg **nifedipine** intravenously prolonged the neuromuscular blockade due to **atracurium** or **vecuronium** from 29 up to 40 min, and increased the neuromuscular blockade from 75 up to 90%.[6] This contrasts with another study in which 30 predominantly elderly patients on chronic **nifedipine** treatment (mean daily dose 32 mg) showed no changes in the time of onset to maximum block nor the duration of clinical relaxation in response to **atracurium** or **vecuronium**.[7,8]

A woman of 66, receiving 5 mg **verapamil** intravenously three times a day for supraventricular tachycardia, underwent abdominal surgery during which she was initially anaesthetised with thiopental (thiopentone) and then maintained on nitrous oxide/oxygen with fentanyl. **Vecuronium** was used as the muscle relaxant. The effects of the **vecuronium** were increased and prolonged, and at the end of surgery reversal of the blockade using neostigmine was difficult and extended.[9] Another report similarly describes increased blockade in a patient given **tubocurarine** that was difficult to reverse with neostigmine but which responded well to edrophonium.[10] However the authors of this report say that many patients on **verapamil** do not show a clinically significant increased sensitivity to muscle relaxants.[10] **Verapamil** alone caused respiratory failure in a patient with poor neuromuscular transmission (Duchenne's dystrophy).[11]

An increase in the neuromuscular blocking effects of **pancuronium**, **vecuronium**, **atracurium** and **suxamethonium** (**succinylcholine**) by **verapamil** and **nifedipine** has been seen in *animals*.[11,12]

(b) Rocuronium + Calcium channel blockers

A study of 17 patients taking calcium channel blockers (**nifedipine** 12, **diltiazem** 2, **nicardipine** 2, **amlodipine** 1) found no changes in the neuromuscular blocking effects of **rocuronium**.[13]

(c) Suxamethonium + Calcium channel blockers

A comparative study in 21 patients taking calcium channel blockers chronically (**diltiazem**, **nifedipine**, **verapamil**) and 15 other patients not taking calcium channel blockers found that although **suxamethonium** caused a modest average peak rise of 0.5 mEq/l in plasma potassium levels, there were no differences between the two groups.[14] See also (a) above.

Mechanism

Not fully understood. One explanation for the increased blockade is as follows. Nerve impulses arriving at nerve endings release calcium ions, which in turn causes the release of acetylcholine. Calcium channel blockers can reduce the concentration of calcium ions within the nerve so that less acetylcholine is released and this would be additive with the effects of a neuromuscular blocker.[15]

Importance and management

Direct information so far seems to be limited to the cases and reports cited here. The discord between the reports remains unexplained. Until the situation is resolved, be alert for increased blockade in any patient given nicardipine, nifedipine, verapamil or any other calcium channel blocker. From the limited evidence available it appears rocuronium does not interact but it would be prudent to take care with this drug also until more is known.[13]

It would seem from the study[14] quoted above that patients on chronic calcium channel blocker treatment are at no greater risk of hyperkalaemia with suxamethonium than other patients.

1. Sumikawa K, Kawabata K, Aono Y, Kamibayashi T, Yoshiya I. Reduction in vecuronium infusion dose requirements by diltiazem in humans. *Anesthesiology* (1992) 77, A939.
2. Takasaki Y, Naruoka Y, Shimizu C, Ochi G, Nagaro T, Arai T. Diltiazem potentiates the neuromuscular blockade by vecuronium in humans. *Jpn J Anesthesiol* (1995) 44, 503–7.
3. Takiguchi M, Takaya T. Potentiation of neuromuscular blockade by calcium channel blokers. *Tokai Exp Clin Med* (1994) 19, 131–7.
4. Yamada T, Takino Y. Can nicardipine potentiate vecuronium induced neuromuscular blockade? *Masui* (1992) 41, 746–50.
5. Kawabata K, Sumikawa K, Kamibayashi T, Kita T, Takada K, Mashimo T, Yoshiya I. Decrease in vecuronium infusion dose requirements by nicardipine in humans. *Anesth Analg* (1994) 79, 1159–64.
6. Jelen-Esselborn S, Blobner M. Wirkungsverstärkung von nichtdepolarisierenden Muskelrelaxanzien durch Nifedipi i.v. in Inhalationsanaesthesie. *Anaesthesist* (1990) 39, 173–8.
7. Bell PF, Mirakhur RK, Elliott P. Onset and duration of clinical relaxation of atracurium and vecuronium in patients on chronic nifedipine therapy. *Eur J Anaesthesiol* (1989) 6, 343–6.
8. Mirakhur RK, Bell PF, Clarke RSJ. Chronic nifedipine therapy does not prolong the neuromuscular effects of vecuronium and atracurium. *Anesthesiology* (1988) 69, A506.
9. van Poorten JF, Dhasmana KM, Kuypers RSM, Erdmann W. Verapamil and reversal of vecuronium neuromuscular blockade. *Anesth Analg* (1984) 63, 155–7.
10. Jones RM, Cashman JN, Casson WR, Broadbent MP. Verapamil potentiation of neuromuscular blockade: failure of reversal with neostigmine but prompt reversal with edrophonium. *Anesth Analg* (1985) 64, 1021–5.
11. Durant NN, Nguyen N, Katz RL. Potentiation of neuromuscular blockade by verapamil. *Anesthesiology* (1984) 60, 298–303.
12. Bikhazi GB, Leung I, Foldes FF. Interaction of neuromuscular blocking agents with calcium blockers. *Anesthesiology* (1982) 57, A268.
13. Loan PB, Connolly FM, Mirakhur RK, Kumar N, Farling P. Neuromuscular effects of rocuronium in patients receiving beta-adrenoceptor blocking, calcium entry blocking and anticonvulsant drugs. *Br J Anaesth* (1997) 78, 90–1.
14. Rooke GA, Freund PR, Tomlin J. Calcium channel blockers do not enhance increases in plasma potassium after succinylcholine in humans. *J Clin Anesth* (1994) 6, 114–18.
15. Wali FA. Interactions of nifedipine and diltiazem with muscle relaxants and reversal of neuromuscular blockade with edrophonium and neostigmine. *J Pharmacol* (1986) 17, 244–53.

Neuromuscular blockers + Chloroquine

A report describes respiratory insufficiency during the recovery period following surgery, attributed to the use of chloroquine diorotate.

Clinical evidence, mechanism, importance and management

Studies were carried on the possible neuromuscular blocking actions of **chloroquine diorotate** in *animals* because it was noticed that when it was used to prevent peritoneal adhesions following abdominal surgery in man, it caused respiratory insufficiency during the recovery period. These studies found that it has a non-depolarising blocking action at the neuromuscular junction which are opposed by neostigmine.[1] It would seem therefore that during the recovery period the effects of the **chloroquine** can be additive with the residual effects of the conventional neuromuscular blocker used during the surgery.

Although this appears to be the only report of this interaction, it is consistent with the way **chloroquine** can unmask or aggravate

myasthenia gravis, or oppose the effects of drugs used in its treatment. Be alert for this reaction if **chloroquine** is used.

1. Jui-Yen T. Clinical and experimental studies on mechanism of neuromuscular blockade by chloroquine diorotate. *Jpn J Anesthesiol* (1971) 20, 491–503.

Neuromuscular blockers + Ciclosporin (Cyclosporin)

There is evidence that the neuromuscular blocking effects of atracurium, vecuronium and pancuronium may be increased in some patients treated with ciclosporin (cyclosporin).

Clinical evidence

(a) Atracurium

A retrospective study found 4 of 36 patients who experienced prolonged neuromuscular blockade when **atracurium** was used during anaesthesia for kidney transplantation. Some of them had had **ciclosporin (cyclosporin)**.[1] Extended recovery times are described in another report.[2]

(b) Pancuronium

A woman with a 2-year renal transplant controlled with 100 mg azathioprine, 300 mg **ciclosporin (cyclosporin)** and 10 mg prednisone and also taking nifedipine and furosemide (frusemide) for hypertension, underwent surgery during which she was initially anaesthetised with fentanyl and thiopental (thiopentone), and later nitrous oxide/oxygen and isoflurane. **Pancuronium** was used as the neuromuscular blocker. She was also infused with **ciclosporin** before and after surgery. Residual paralysis was seen after surgery and she was re-intubated 20 min later because of increased respiratory distress.[3]

(c) Vecuronium

A girl of 15 on 20 mg **ciclosporin (cyclosporin)** intravenously twice daily and with serum levels of 138 micrograms/litre was anaesthetised for an endoscopy and bone marrow aspiration using fentanyl, thiopental (thiopentone) and 100 micrograms/kg **vecuronium**. Anaesthesia was later maintained with nitrous oxide, oxygen and isoflurane. Attempts were later made to reverse the blockade with edrophonium, atropine and neostigmine but full neuromuscular function was not restored for 3 h and 20 min.[4]

A retrospective study of this interaction in other kidney transplant patients suggests that **ciclosporin** can increase the risk of prolonged neuromuscular blockade and ventilatory failure in those given **vecuronium**.[1] Extended recovery times are described in other reports.[2,5,6] Most reports involve **intravenous ciclosporin**, but prolongation of the effects of **vecuronium** has also been seen with **oral ciclosporin**.[7]

Mechanism

Uncertain. One idea is that *Cremophor* (polyoxyl 35 castor oil), a surface-active agent used as a vehicle for the ciclosporin[3] may increase the effective concentration of pancuronium at the neuromuscular junction. Both compounds have been observed in *animal* studies to increase vecuronium blockade[8] and *Cremophor* has been seen to decrease the onset time of pancuronium blockade in patients given *Cremophor*-containing anaesthetics.[9] However this is not the entire answer because the interaction has also been seen with oral ciclosporin which does not contain *Cremophor*.[7]

Importance and management

Direct information seems to be limited to the reports cited. The general importance is uncertain but be alert for an increase in the effects of atracurium, pancuronium or vecuronium in any patient receiving ciclosporin (cyclosporin). Not all patients appear to develop this interaction.[1] More study is needed.

1. Sidi A, Kaplan RF, Davis RF. Prolonged neuromuscular blockade and ventilatory failure after renal transplantation and cyclosporine. *Can J Anaesth* (1990) 37, 543–8.

2. Lepage JY, Malinowsky JM, de Dieulevault C, Cozian A, Pinaud M, Souron R. Interaction cyclosporine atracurium et vecuronium. *Ann Fr Anesth Reanim* (1989) 8 (Suppl), R135.

3. Crosby E, Robblee JA. Cyclosporine-pancuronium interaction in a patient with a renal allograft. *Can J Anaesth* (1988) 35, 300–2.

4. Wodd GG. Cyclosporine-vecuronium interaction. *Can J Anaesth* (1989) 36 (3 part 1), 358.

5. Takita K, Goda Y, Kawahigashi H, Okuyama A, Kubota M, Kemmotsu O. Pharmacodynamics of vecuronium in the kidney transplant recipient and the patient with normal renal function. *Jpn J Anesthesiol* (1993) 42, 190–4.

6. Wood GG. Cyclosporine-vecuronium interaction. *Can J Anaesth* (1989) 36, 358.

7. Ganjoo P, Tewari P. Oral cyclosporine-vecuronium interaction. *Can J Anaesth* (1994) 41, 1017.

8. Gramstad L, Lilleaasen P and Misaas B. Onset time for alcuronium and pancuronium after cremophor-containing anaesthetics. *Acta Anaesthesiol Scand* (1981) 25, 484–6.

9. Viby-Mogensen J. Interaction of other drugs with muscle relaxants. *Sem Anaesth* (1985) 4, 52.

Neuromuscular blockers + Cimetidine, Famotidine or Ranitidine

One report says that recovery from the neuromuscular blocking effects of suxamethonium (succinylcholine) is prolonged by cimetidine but this may possibly have been due to the presence of metoclopramide. Four other reports say that no interaction occurs between suxamethonium and either cimetidine, famotidine or ranitidine. Cimetidine, but not ranitidine, is reported to increase the effects of vecuronium, and neither affects atracurium. Cimetidine does not affect rocuronium.

Clinical evidence

(a) Evidence of increased neuromuscular blockade

A controlled study in 10 patients given 300 mg **cimetidine** orally at bedtime and another 300 mg 2 h before anaesthesia, showed that while the onset of action of **suxamethonium** (1.5 mg/kg intravenously) was unchanged, the time to recover 50% of the twitch height was prolonged 2–2.5 times (from 8.6 to 20.3 min). One patient took 57 min to recover.[1] His serum pseudocholinesterase levels were found to be normal. It was later reported that some patients were also taking **metoclopramide** which is known to interact in this way.[2]

Another study in 24 patients found that 400 mg **cimetidine** significantly prolonged the recovery (T1–25 period) from **vecuronium**, but few patients showed any response to 200 mg **cimetidine** or 100 mg **ranitidine**.[3] This prolongation of recovery from **vecuronium** due to **cimetidine** was confirmed in another study (time to return of T1 30 v 22.5 min).[4] A study using a *rat* phrenic nerve diaphragm preparation found that **cimetidine** increased the neuromuscular blocking effects of **tubocurarine** and **pancuronium**, but there seem to be no reports confirming this in man.[5]

(b) Evidence of unchanged neuromuscular blockade

A controlled study in 10 patients given 400 mg **cimetidine** at bedtime and 400 mg 90 min before anaesthesia found no evidence of an effect on the neuromuscular blockade caused by **suxamethonium**, nor on its duration or recovery period.[6] Another controlled study in patients given 300 mg **cimetidine** or 150 mg **ranitidine** the night before and 1–2 h before surgery found no evidence that the duration of action of **suxamethonium** or the activity of plasma cholinesterase were altered.[2] A study in 15 patients undergoing Caesarean section also found no evidence that either **cimetidine** or **ranitidine** affected the neuromuscular blocking effects of **suxamethonium**.[7] A study in 70 patients found no changes in the neuromuscular blocking effects of **suxamethonium** in those given 400 mg **cimetidine**, 80 mg **ranitidine** or 20 mg **famotidine**.[8] **Cimetidine** and **ranitidine** appear not to affect **atracurium**, nor does **ranitidine** affect **vecuronium**[4] or **cimetidine** affect **rocuronium**.[9]

Mechanism

Not understood. Studies with human plasma failed to find any evidence that cimetidine in normal serum concentrations inhibits the metabolism of suxamethonium,[2,10] however metoclopramide does. *In*

vitro studies with very high cimetidine concentrations found inhibition of pseudocholinesterase activity.[11] The cimetidine/vecuronium interaction is not understood.

Importance and management

Information seems to be limited to the reports cited. The most likely explanation for the discord between these results is that in the study reporting increased suxamethonium effects[1] some of the patients were also given metoclopramide which can inhibit plasma cholinesterase and prolong the effects of suxamethonium[2,8] (see also 'Neuromuscular blockers + Metoclopramide', p.766). However until the situation is clarified the possibility of an interaction should be taken into account during concurrent use. The same precautions also apply in the case of cimetidine/vecuronium.

1. Kambam JR, Dymond R, Krestow M. Effect of cimetidine on duration of action of succinylcholine. *Anesth Analg* (1987) 66, 191–2.

2. Woodworth GE, Sears DH, Grove TM, Ruff RH, Kosek PS, Katz RL. The effect of cimetidine and ranitidine on the duration of action of succinylcholine. *Anesth Analg* (1989) 68, 295–7.

3. Tryba M, Wruck G. Interaktionen von H₂-Antagonisten und nichtdepolarisierenden Muskelrelaxantien. *Anaesthesist* (1989) 38, 251–4.

4. McCarthy G, Mirakhur RK, Elliott P, Wright J. Effect of H₂-receptor antagonist pretreatment on vecuronium- and atracurium-induced neuromuscular blockade. *Br J Anaesth* (1991) 66, 713–15.

5. Galatulas I, Bossa R, Benvenuti C. Cimetidine increases the neuromuscular blocking activity of aminoglycoside antibiotics: antagonism by calcium. Organ-directed toxicity: Chem Indices Mec., Proc Symp (1981) 321–5. Pergamon Press, Oxford.

6. Stirt JA, Sperry RJ, DiFazio CA. Cimetidine and succinylcholine: potential interaction and effect on neuromuscular blockade in man. *Anesthesiology* (1989) 69, 607–8.

7. Bogod DG, Oh TE. The effect of H₂ antagonists on duration of action of suxamethonium in the parturient. *Anaesthesia* (1989) 44, 591–3.

8. Turner DR, Kao YJ, Bivona C. Neuromuscular block by suxamethonium following treatment with histamine type 2 antagonists or metoclopramide. *Br J Anaesth* (1989) 63, 348–50.

9. Latorre F, De Almeida MCS, Stanek A, Weiler N, Kleeman PP. Effect of cimetidine pretreatment on rocuronium-induced neuromuscular blockade. *Anaesthetist* (1996) 45, 900–2.

10. Cook DR, Stiller RL, Chakravorti S, Mannenhira T. Cimetidine does not inhibit plasma cholinesterase activity. *Anesth Analg* (1988) 67, 375–6.

11. Hansen WE, Bertl S. The inhibition of acetylcholinesterase and pseudocholinesterase by cimetidine? *Arzneimittelforschung* (1983) 33, 161–3.

Neuromuscular blockers + Clonidine

There is evidence that clonidine increases the duration of action of vecuronium.

Clinical evidence, mechanism, importance and management

In a study of 16 surgery patients, half received **clonidine** 90 min before their operation. Anaesthesia was induced by thiamylal and maintained by nitrous oxide/isoflurane/oxygen supplemented by fentanyl for all patients. Following administration of **vecuronium** the duration of neuromuscular blockade was increased by 26.4% in the **clonidine** group.[1]

The reasons are not understood. The clinical importance of this interaction would appear to be small.

1. Nakahara T, Akazawa T, Kinoshita Y, Nozaki J. The effect of clonidine on the duration of vecuronium-induced neuromuscular blockade in humans. *Jpn J Anesthesiol* (1995) 44, 1458–63.

Neuromuscular blockers + Corticosteroids

Three reports describe antagonism of the neuromuscular blocking effects of pancuronium by prednisone and hydrocortisone in patients with adrenocortical insufficiency. The dosage of vecuronium may need to be almost doubled in the presence of betamethasone.

Clinical evidence

A man undergoing surgery who was on 250 mg **prednisone** daily had good muscular relaxation in response to 8 mg **pancuronium** early in the operation, but an hour later began to show signs of inadequate relaxation and continued to do so for the next 1.25 h despite being given four additional 2-mg doses of **pancuronium**.[1]

A hypophysectomised man on **cortisone** developed profound paralysis when given **pancuronium**, which was rapidly reversed with 100 mg **hydrocortisone sodium succinate**.[2] Another patient on large doses of **hydrocortisone, prednisolone** and **aminophylline** proved to be resistant to the effects of **pancuronium**.[3]

Unexpected movements of head and arms occurred in a patient during surgery given **vecuronium**, and coughing in another. They had both been given **betamethasone** preoperatively (4 mg four times daily) to reduce raised intracranial pressure.[4] This prompted a retrospective search of the records of 50 other patients which revealed that those given **betamethasone** had needed almost double the dose of **vecuronium** (134 compared with 76 micrograms/kg/h).[4]

These reports contrast with another in which 25 patients who had no adrenocortical dysfunction or histories of corticosteroid therapy who were given **pancuronium, metocurine, tubocurarine** or **vecuronium**. They showed no changes in their neuromuscular blockade when given **dexamethasone** (0.4 mg/kg) or **hydrocortisone** (10 mg/kg) intravenously.[5]

Mechanism

Not understood. One idea, based on *animal* studies, is that adrenocortical insufficiency causes a defect in neuromuscular transmission (a decrease in the sensitivity of the end-plate) which is reversed by the corticosteroids. Another idea is the effects seen are connected in some way with the steroid nucleus of the pancuronium and vecuronium, or that the effects are mediated presynaptically.

Importance and management

The evidence for an interaction seem to be limited to these reports, involving only pancuronium and vecuronium. Careful monitoring is clearly needed if either is used in patients who have been treated with corticosteroids, being alert for the need to increase the dosage of the neuromuscular blocker. *Animal* studies suggest that **atracurium** may possibly be affected by betamethasone.[6]

1. Laflin MJ. Interaction of pancuronium and corticosteroids. *Anesthesiology* (1977) 47, 471–2.
2. Meyers EF. Partial recovery from pancuronium neuromuscular blockade following hydrocortisone administration. *Anesthesiology* (1977) 46, 148–50.
3. Azar I, Kumar D, Betcher AM. Resistance to pancuronium in an asthmatic patient treated with aminophylline and steroids. *Can Anaesth Soc J* (1982) 29, 280–2.
4. Parr SM, Galletly DC, Robinson BJ. Betamethasone-induced resistance to vecuronium: a potential problem in neurosurgery? *Anaesth Intensive Care* (1991) 19, 103–5.
5. Schwartz AE, Matteo RS, Ornstein E, Silverberg PA. Acute steroid therapy does not alter nondepolarizing muscle relaxant effects in humans. *Anesthesiology* (1986) 65, 326–7.
6. Robinson BJ, Lee E, Rees D, Purdie GL, Galletly DC. Betamethasone-induced resistance to neuromuscular blockade: a comparison of atracurium and vecuronium in vitro. *Anesth Analg* (1992) 74, 762–5.

Neuromuscular blockers + Cyclophosphamide

The effects of suxamethonium (succinylcholine) can be increased and prolonged in patients under treatment with cyclophosphamide because their serum pseudocholinesterase levels are depressed. Respiratory insufficiency and prolonged apnoea have been reported.

Clinical evidence

Respiratory insufficiency and prolonged apnoea occurred in a patient on two occasions while receiving **cyclophosphamide** and undergoing anaesthesia during which **suxamethonium** and **tubocurarine** were used. Plasma pseudocholinesterase levels were found to be low. Anaesthesia without the suxamethonium was uneventful. Seven out of 8 patients subsequently examined also showed depressed serum pseudocholinesterase levels while taking **cyclophosphamide**.[1]

Respiratory depression and low serum pseudocholinesterase levels have been described in other reports.[2-4] One report described a 35–70% reduction.[2]

Mechanism

Cyclophosphamide irreversibly inhibits the activity of pseudocholinesterase in the serum, as a result the metabolism of the suxamethonium is reduced and its actions are enhanced and prolonged.[4]

Importance and management

A well-documented and established interaction of clinical importance. Whether all patients are affected to the same extent is uncertain. The depression of the serum pseudocholinesterase levels may last several days, possibly weeks, so that ideally serum pseudocholinesterase levels should be checked before using suxamethonium. It should certainly be used with caution, and the dosage should be reduced.[2] Some have suggested that concurrent use should be avoided.[1] Suxethonium probably interacts similarly, but not other neuromuscular blockers because they are not metabolised by serum pseudocholinesterase.

1. Walker IR, Zapf PW, Mackay IR. Cyclophosphamide, cholinesterase and anaesthesia. *Aust N Z J Med* (1972) 3, 247–51.
2. Zsigmond EK, Robins G. The effect of a series of anti-cancer drugs on plasma cholinesterase activity. *Can Anaesth Soc J* (1972) 19, 75.
3. Mone JG, Mathie WE. Qualitative and quantitative effects of pseudocholinesterase activity. *Anaesthesia* (1967) 22, 55.
4. Wolff H. Die Hemmung der Serumcholinesterase durch Cyclophosphamid (Endoxan®). *Klin Wochenschr* (1965) 43, 819–21.

Neuromuscular blockers + Danazol, Tamoxifen

Two case reports describe prolonged atracurium effects attributed to tamoxifen and danazol.

Clinical evidence, mechanism, importance and management

A case report describes a 67-year-old mastectomy patient on methyldopa, hydrochlorothiazide, triamterene and long term 20 mg daily **tamoxifen** treatment who showed prolonged neuromuscular blockade to a single dose of 0.5 mg/kg **atracurium**, which the authors suggest might be due to an interaction between **atracurium** and **tamoxifen**.[1] The authors also point out an earlier report[2] of prolonged **atracurium** blockade where the patient was taking **danazol**. These interactions appear not be of general importance.

1. Naguib M, Gyasi HK. Antiestrogenic drugs and atracurium – a possible interaction? *Can Anaesth Soc J* (1986) 33, 682–3.
2. Bizzarri-Schmid MD, Desai SP. Prolonged neuromuscular blockade with atracurium. *Can Anaesth Soc J* (1986) 33, 209–12.

Neuromuscular blockers + Dantrolene

One patient showed increased vecuronium effects when given dantrolene, whereas two others showed no changes.

Clinical evidence, mechanism, importance and management

A woman of 60, given a total of 350 mg **dantrolene** by mouth during the 28 h before surgery to control malignant hyperthermia, showed increased neuromuscular blockade and a slow recovery rate when **vecuronium** was used subsequently.[1] This report contrasts with another describing two patients on long-term **dantrolene** (20–50 mg daily) who showed no changes in **vecuronium**-induced neuromuscular blockade during or after during surgery.[2] **Dantrolene** is a muscle relaxant which acts directly on the muscle by interfering with calcium uptake and release from the sarcoplasmic reticulum. It may also possibly interfere with the release of acetylcholine at the neuromuscular junction. Just why these reports differ is not known, but be alert for any increased effects if both drugs are used.

1. Driessen JJ, Wuis EW, Gielen MJM. Prolonged vecuronium neuromuscular blockade in a patient receiving orally administered dantrolene. *Anesthesiology* (1985) 62, 523–4.
2. Nakayama M, Iwasaki H, Fujita S, Narimatsu E, Namiki A. Neuromuscular effects of vecuronium in patients receiving long-term administration of dantrolene. *Masui — Jpn J Anesthesiol* (1993) 42, 1508–10.

Neuromuscular blockers + Dexpanthenol

An increase in the neuromuscular blocking effects of suxamethonium (succinylcholine) has been attributed to the concurrent use of dexpanthenol in one patient, but further studies failed to confirm this interaction.

Clinical evidence, mechanism, importance and management

A patient developed severe respiratory embarrassment following the intramuscular injection of 500 mg **dexpanthenol** during the recovery period from anaesthesia with nitrous oxide and cyclopropane, and neuromuscular blockade with **suxamethonium**.[1] However a later study on 6 patients under general anaesthesia showed that their response to **suxamethonium** was unaffected by the infusion of 500 mg **pantothenic acid**.[2]

Several manufacturers of products containing **pantothenic acid** have issued warnings about this interaction, but they seem to be solely based on the single unconfirmed report cited here[1] and there seems to be little other reason for avoiding concurrent use or for taking particular precautions. However, users should be aware of this case.

1. Stewart P. Case reports. *J Am Assoc Nurse Anesth* (1960) 28, 56–60.
2. Smith RM, Gottshall SC, Young JA. Succinylcholine-pantothenyl alcohol: a reappraisal. *Anesth Analg* (1969) 48, 205–208.

Neuromuscular blockers + Disopyramide

An isolated case report suggests that disopyramide may oppose the effects of neostigmine when used to reverse neuromuscular blockade with vecuronium.

Clinical evidence, mechanism, importance and management

A case report suggests that therapeutic serum levels of **disopyramide** (5 micrograms/ml) may oppose the normal antagonism by neostigmine of **vecuronium** neuromuscular blockade.[1] **Disopyramide** has also been shown to decrease the antagonism by **neostigmine** of the neuromuscular blockade of tubocurarine on the *rat* phrenic nerve-diaphragm preparation.[2] The general clinical importance of these observations are not known, but anaesthetists should be aware of these reports.

1. Baurain M, Barvais L, d'Hollander A, Hennart D. Impairment of the antagonism of vecuronium-induced paralysis and intra-operative disopyramide administration. *Anaesthesia* (1989) 44, 34–6.
2. Healy TEJ, O'Shea M, Massey J. Disopyramide and neuromuscular transmission. *Br J Anaesth* (1981) 53, 495–8.

Neuromuscular blockers + Ecothiopate iodide (Echothiophate)

The neuromuscular blocking effects of suxamethonium (succinylcholine) are markedly increased and prolonged in patients under treatment with ecothiopate iodide. The dosage of suxamethonium should be reduced appropriately.

Clinical evidence

In 1965 Murray McGavi[1] warned that the systemic absorption of **ecothiopate iodide** from eye drops could lower serum pseudocholinesterase levels to such an extent that ". . . within a few days of commencing therapy, levels are reached at which protracted apnoea could occur should these patients require general anaesthesia in which muscle relaxation is obtained with **suxamethonium**". Cases of apnoea due to this interaction were reported the following year[2,3] and the year after.[4] In one case a woman given 200 mg **suxamethonium** showed apnoea for 5½ hours. Other studies have confirmed that **ecothiopate** markedly reduces the levels of pseudocholinesterase and can prolong recovery.[5-7]

Mechanism

Suxamethonium is metabolised in the body by pseudocholinesterase. Ecothiopate iodide depresses the levels of this enzyme so that the metabolism of the suxamethonium is reduced and its effects are thereby enhanced and prolonged.[5] One study in 71 patients found that two drops of 0.06% ecothiopate iodide three times weekly in each eye caused a twofold reduction pseudocholinesterase activity in about one-third of the patients, and a fourfold reduction in one out of every seven.[8]

Importance and management

An established, adequately documented and clinically important interaction. The dosage of suxamethonium should be reduced appropriately because of the reduced plasma pseudocholinesterase levels caused by ecothiopate. The study cited above[8] suggests that prolonged apnoea is only likely in about 1 in 7. One report describes the successful use of approximately one-fifth of the normal dosage of suxamethonium in a patient receiving 0.125% ecothiopate iodide solution, one drop twice a day in both eyes, and with a plasma cholinesterase activity 62% below normal. Recovery from the neuromuscular blockade was rapid and uneventful.[9] Another report describes the successful and uneventful use of atracurium instead.[7]

1. McGavi DDM. Depressed levels of serum-pseudocholinesterase with ecothiopate-iodide eyedrops. *Lancet* (1965) ii, 272–3.
2. Gesztes T. Prolonged apnoea after suxamethonium injection associated with eye drops containing an anticholinesterase agent. *Br J Anaesth* (1966) 38, 408–409.
3. Pantuck EJ. Ecothiopate iodide eye drops and prolonged response to suxamethonium. *Br J Anaesth* (1966) 38, 406–407.
4. Mone JG, Mathie WE. Qualitative and quantitative effects of pseudocholinesterase activity. *Anaesthesia* (1967) 22, 55.
5. Cavallaro RJ, Krumperman LW, Kugler F. Effect of echothiophate therapy on the metabolism of succinylcholine in man. *Anesth Analg* (1974) 47, 570–4.
6. de Roetth A, Dettbarn W-D, Rosenberg P, Wilensky JG, Wong A. Effect of phospholine iodide on blood cholinesterase levels of normal and glaucoma subjects. *Am J Ophthalmol* (1965) 59, 586–92.
7. Messer GJ, Stoudemire A, Knos G, Johnson GC. Electroconvulsive therapy and the chronic use of pseudocholinesterase-inhibitor (echothiphate iodide) eye drops for glaucoma. A case report. *Gen Hosp Psychiatry* (1992) 14, 56–60.
8. Eilderton TE, Farmati O, Zsigmond EK. Reduction in plasma cholinesterase levels after prolonged administration of echothiophate iodide eyedrops. *Can Anaesth Soc J* (1968) 15, 291–6.
9. Donati F, Bevan DR. Controlled succinylcholine infusion in a patient receiving echothiophate eye drops. *Can Anaesth Soc J* (1981) 28, 488–90.

Neuromuscular blockers + Fentanyl citrate-Droperidol (*Innovar*)

Recovery from the neuromuscular blocking effects of suxamethonium (succinylcholine) is prolonged by fentanyl citrate-droperidol (*Innovar*).

Clinical evidence

The observation that patients who had had *Innovar* (**fentanyl citrate-droperidol**) before anaesthesia appeared to have a prolonged **suxamethonium (succinylcholine)** effects, seen as apnoea, prompted further study of this possible interaction.[1] Nineteen patients were given **suxamethonium** and thiopental (thiopentone) during the induction of anaesthesia. The average time from end fasciculation to return of full tetanus was approximately doubled (from 5.83 to 10.45 min) in 10 patients given *Innovar* (2 ml intravenously 10 min before anaesthesia) when compared with 9 patients not given *Innovar*.[1]

A much shorter delay in recovery was seen in a later study.[2] Another study[3] showed that the **droperidol** component of *Innovar* is probably responsible for this interaction.

Mechanism

Not fully understood. One suggestion[3] is that droperidol may act as a membrane stabiliser at neuromuscular junctions, and it may also reduce the levels of pseudocholinesterase which is responsible for the metabolism of suxamethonium.

Importance and management

An established interaction of moderate importance. Delayed recovery should be anticipated in patients on suxamethonium and other neuromuscular blockers if *Innovar* is used.

1. Wehner RJ. A case study: the prolongation of Anectine effect by Innovar. *J Am Assoc Nurse Anesth* (1979) 47, 576–9.
2. Moore GB, Ciresi S, Kallar S. The effect of Innovar versus droperidol or fentanyl on the duration of action of succinylcholine. *J Am Assoc Nurse Anesth* (1986) 54, 130–6.
3. Lewis RA. A consideration of prolonged succinylcholine paralysis with Innovar: is the cause droperidol or fentanyl? *J Am Assoc Nurse Anesth* (1982) 50, 55–9.

Neuromuscular blockers + Furosemide (Frusemide)

The effects of the neuromuscular blockers may possibly be changed by furosemide (frusemide).

Clinical evidence

(a) Increased neuromuscular blockade

Three patients receiving kidney transplants showed increased neuromuscular blockade with **tubocurarine** (seen as a pronounced decrease in twitch tension) when given **furosemide (frusemide)** (40 or 80 mg) and mannitol (12.5 g) intravenously. One of them showed the same reaction when later given only 40 mg **furosemide** but no mannitol. The residual blockade was easily antagonised with pyridostigmine (14 mg) or neostigmine (3 mg) with atropine (1.2 mg).[1]

(b) Decreased neuromuscular blockade

Ten patients given 1 mg/kg **furosemide (frusemide)** took 14.7 min to recover from 95 to 50% blockade with **pancuronium** (as measured by a twitch response) compared with 21.8 min in 10 other patients who had had no **furosemide**.[2]

Mechanism

Uncertain. *Animal* studies indicate that what happens probably depends on the dosage of furosemide: 0.1–10 micrograms/kg increased the blocking effects of tubocurarine and suxamethonium (succinylcholine) whereas 1–4 mg/kg opposed the blockade.[3] One suggestion is that low doses of furosemide inhibit protein kinase, whereas higher doses cause inhibition of phosphodiesterase.

Importance and management

The documentation is very limited. Be on the alert for changes in the response to any blocker if furosemide (frusemide) is used.

1. Miller RD, Sohn YJ, Matteo RS. Enhancement of *d*-tubocurarine neuromuscular blockade by diuretics in man. *Anesthesiology* (1976) 45, 442–5.
2. Azar I, Cottbell J, Gupta B, Turndorf H. Furosemide facilitates recovery of evoked twitch response after pancuronium. *Anesth Analg* (1980) 59, 55–7.
3. Scappaticci KA, Ham JA, Sohn YJ, Miller RD, Dretchen KL. Effects of furosemide on the neuromuscular junction. *Anesthesiology* (1982) 57, 381–8.

Neuromuscular blockers + Immunosuppressants

The neuromuscular blocking effects of tubocurarine are reduced by azathioprine and antilymphocytic globulin. The dosage may need to be increased two- to fourfold.

Clinical evidence, mechanism, importance and management

A retrospective study found that patients on immunosuppressant drugs following organ transplantation needed an increased dosage of **tubocurarine** to achieve satisfactory muscle relaxation. A control group of 74 patients needed 0–10 mg **tubocurarine**; 13 patients on **azathioprine** needed 12.5–25.0 mg; 11 patients on **antilymphocytic globulin** needed 10–20 mg and two patients on **azathioprine** and **guanethidine** needed 55–90 mg.[1] The reasons are not understood. Since **azathioprine** is converted within the body to **mercaptopurine** it is likely that it interacts similarly. Information is very sparse so it is not clear whether this interaction occurs with other neuromuscular blockers. More study is needed.

1. Vetten KB. Immunosuppressive therapy and anaesthesia. *S Afr Med J* (1973) 47, 767–70.

Neuromuscular blockers + Insecticides

Exposure to organophosphate insecticides such as malathion and dimpylate (diazinon) can markedly prolong the neuromuscular blocking effects of suxamethonium (succinylcholine).

Clinical evidence

A man admitted to hospital for an appendectomy became apnoeic during the early part of the operation when given 100 mg **suxamethonium** to facilitate tracheal intubation, and remained so throughout the 40 min surgery. Spontaneous restoration of neuromuscular activity did not return for 150 min. Later studies showed that he had an extremely low plasma cholinesterase activity (3–10%) although he had a normal phenotype. It subsequently turned out that he had been working with **malathion** for 11 weeks without any protection.[1]

Another report describes a man whose recovery from neuromuscular blockade with **suxamethonium** was very prolonged. He had attempted suicide nine days earlier with **dimpylate (diazinon)**, a household insecticide. His pseudocholinesterase was found to be 2.5 IU/l (normal values 7–19) and his dibucaine number was too low to be measured.[2]

Mechanism

Malathion and dimpylate are organophosphate insecticides which inhibit the activity of plasma cholinesterase, thereby reducing the metabolism of the suxamethonium and prolonging its effects.

Importance and management

An established and well understood interaction. Particular care should be exercised if suxamethonium is used in individuals known to have been exposed to **organophosphate pesticides** such as malathion and dimpylate (diazinon). Pesticides of this type are widely used in agricultural, horticultural and veterinary practice in **sprays** and **sheep dips** (see 'Neuromuscular blockers + Anticholinesterases', p.755). These anticholinesterases are expected to interact with other depolarising neuromuscular blockers in just the same way, but to oppose the actions of non-depolarising neuromuscular blockers.

1. Guillermo FP, Pretel CMM, Royo FT, Macias MJP, Ossorio RA, Gomez JAA, Vidal CJ. Prolonged suxamethonium-induced neuromuscular blockade associated with organophosphate poisoning. *Br J Anaesth* (1988) 61, 233–6.
2. Ware MR, Frost ML, Berger JJ, Stewart RB, DeVane CL. Electroconvulsive therapy complicated by insecticide ingestion. *J Clin Psychopharmacol* (1990) 10, 72–3.

Neuromuscular blockers + Lansoprazole

There is evidence that lansoprazole increases the duration of action of vecuronium.

Clinical evidence, mechanism, importance and management

In a study of 50 adult surgery patients, half of whom received 30 mg **lansoprazole** on the night before their operation, it was found that there were no differences between the time of onset of neuromuscular blockade by **vecuronium** in the two groups but **lansoprazole** increased the duration by about 34%.[1] This needs confirmation but be alert for this interaction in any patient treated with **lansoprazole**.

1. Ahmed SM, Panja C, Khan RM, Bano S. Lansoprazole potentiates vecuronium paralysis. *J Indian Med Assoc* (1997) 95, 422–3.

Neuromuscular blockers + Lidocaine (Lignocaine), Procaine or Procainamide

The neuromuscular blockade due to suxamethonium (succinylcholine) can be increased and prolonged by lidocaine (lignocaine), procaine and possibly procainamide.

Clinical evidence

A patient anaesthetised with fluroxene and nitrous oxide demonstrated 100% blockade with **suxamethonium** and **tubocurarine**. About 50 min later when twitch height had fully returned and tidal volume was 400 ml, she was given 50 mg **lidocaine (lignocaine)** intravenously for premature ventricular contractions. She immediately stopped breathing and the twitch disappeared. About 45 min later the tidal volume was 450 ml. Later it was found that the patient had a dibucaine number of 23%.[1]

Other studies in man have confirmed that **lidocaine** and **procaine** prolong the apnoea following the use of **suxamethonium** (0.7 mg/kg). A dose-relationship was established. The duration of apnoea was approximately doubled by 7.5 mg/kg of **lidocaine** or **procaine**, and tripled by 16.6 mg/kg, although the effects of **procaine** at higher doses were more marked.[2] Delirium occurred in one patient given **procaine** and **lidocaine** which was attributed to their combined neurological effects.[3]

Mechanism

Uncertain. Local anaesthetics appear to act on presynaptic, postsynaptic and muscle membranes. Procaine and lidocaine weakly inhibit pseudocholinesterase[4], which might prolong the activity of suxamethonium. There may additionally be competition between the suxamethonium and the procaine for hydrolysis by pseudocholinesterase which metabolises them both.[2] Therapeutic serum levels of 4 to 12 micrograms/ml **procainamide** have been found to inhibit cholinesterase activity by 15–30%.[5,6]

Importance and management

Information is limited but the suxamethonium/lidocaine (lignocaine) and lidocaine/procaine interactions appear to be established and of clinical importance. Be alert for signs of increased blockade and/or recurarization with apnoea during the recovery period from suxamethonium blockade if either drug is used. *Animal* studies indicate that low and otherwise safe doses of lidocaine with other drugs having neuromuscular blocking activity (e.g. polymyxin B, aminoglycoside antibacterials) may possibly be additive with conventional neuromuscular blockers and cause problems.[7]

An increase in the effects of suxamethonium by procainamide has been reported in *animals*,[8] increased muscle weakness in a myasthenic patient[5] and reductions in serum cholinesterase activity in normal subjects, but no marked interaction has yet been reported. Neverthe-

less be aware that some increase in the neuromuscular blocking effects is possible.

1. Miller RD. Neuromuscular blocking agents. In 'Drug Interactions in Anesthesia', Smith NT, Miller RD and Corbascio AN (eds). Lea and Febiger, Philadelphia 1981, p. 249.
2. Usubiaga JE, Wikinski JA, Morales RL, Usubiaga LEJ. Interaction of intravenously administered procaine, lidocaine and succinylcholine in anesthetized subjects. *Anesth Analg* (1967) 46, 39–45.
3. Ilyas M, Owens D, Kvasnicka G. Delirium induced by a combination of anti-arrhythmic drugs. *Lancet* (1969) 2, 1368.
4. Reina RA, Cannavá N. Interazione di alcuni anestetici locali con la succinilcolina. *Acta Anaesthesiol Ital* (1972) 23, 1–10
5. Drachman DA, Skom JH. Procainamide—a hazard in myasthenia gravis. *Arch Neurol* (1965) 13, 316–20.
6. Kambam JR, Naukam RJ, Sastry BVR. The effect of procainamide on plasma cholinesterase activity. *Can J Anaesth* (1987) 34, 579–81.
7. Brueckner J, Thomas KC, Bikhazi GB, Foldes FF. Neuromuscular drug interactions of clinical importance. *Anesth Analg* (1980) 59, 533–4.
8. Cuthbert MF. The effect of quinidine and procainamide on the neuromuscular blocking action of suxamethonium. *Br J Anaesth* (1966) 38, 775–9.

Neuromuscular blockers + Lithium carbonate

The concurrent use of neuromuscular blockers and lithium carbonate is normally safe and uneventful, but four patients on lithium have been described who experienced prolonged blockade and respiratory difficulties after receiving standard doses of pancuronium or suxamethonium (succinylcholine) or both.

Clinical evidence

A manic depressive woman on **lithium carbonate** and with a serum **lithium** concentration of 1.2 mmol/l, underwent surgery and was administered thiopental (thiopentone), **suxamethonium** (a total of 310 mg over 2 h) and 0.5 mg **pancuronium bromide**. Prolonged neuromuscular blockade with apnoea occurred.[1,2]

Three other patients on **lithium** are described elsewhere who experienced enhanced neuromuscular blockade when given **pancuronium** alone[3] or with **suxamethonium**,[4] or with **suxamethonium** alone.[5] The authors of one of these reports[4] say that "...We have seen potentiation of the neuromuscular blockade produced by **succinylcholine** in several patients ..." but give no further details. In contrast, a study in 17 patients failed to demonstrate any interaction in patients on **lithium carbonate** when given **suxamethonium**.[6] A **lithium/pancuronium** and **lithium/suxamethonium** interaction has been demonstrated in *dogs*[1,2,7] and a **lithium/tubocurarine** interaction in *cats*,[8] but no clear interaction has been demonstrated with any other neuromuscular blocker.[9,10] A case of **lithium** toxicity has been described in a woman on **lithium** and **suxamethonium**, but it is doubtful if it arose because of an interaction.[11]

Mechanism

Uncertain. One suggestion is that, when the interaction occurs, it may be due to changes in the electrolyte balance caused by the lithium which results in a reduction in the release of acetylcholine at the neuromuscular junction.[8,12]

Importance and management

Information is limited. There are only four definite reports of this interaction in man and good evidence that no adverse interaction normally occurs. Concurrent use need not be avoided but it would be prudent to be on the alert for this interaction in any patient on lithium carbonate who is given any neuromuscular blocker.

1. Hill G, Wong KC, Hodges M, Sentker C. Potentiation of succinylcholine neuromuscular blockade by lithium carbonate. *Fed Procn* (1976) 35, 729.
2. Hill GE, Wong KC, Hodges MR. Potentiation of succinylcholine neuromuscular blockade by lithium carbonate. *Anesthesiology* (1976) 44, 439–42.
3. Borden H, Clark MT, Katz H. The use of pancuronium bromide in patients receiving lithium carbonate. *Can Anaesth Soc J* (1974) 21, 79–82.
4. Rosner TM, Rosenberg M. Anesthetic problems in patients taking lithium. *J Oral Surg* (1981) 39, 282–5.
5. Rabolini V, Gatti G. Potenziamento del blocco neuro-muscolare di tipo depolarizzante da sali di litio (relazione su un caso). *Anest Rianim* (1988) 29, 157–9.

6. Martin BA, Kramer PM. Clinical significance of the interaction between lithium and a neuromuscular blocker. *Am J Psychiatry* (1982) 139, 1326–8.
7. Reimherr FW, Hodges MR, Hill GE, Wong KC. Prolongation of muscle relaxant effects by lithium carbonate. *Am J Psychiatry* (1977) 134, 205–6.
8. Basuray BN, Harris CA. Potentiation of d-tubocurarine (d-Tc) neuromuscular blockade in cats by lithium chloride. *Eur J Pharmacol* (1977) 45, 79–82.
9. Waud BE, Farrell L, Waud DR. Lithium and neuromuscular transmission. *Anesth Analg* (1982) 61, 399–402.
10. Hill GE, Wong KC, Hodges MR. Lithium carbonate and neuromuscular blocking agents. *Anesthesiology* (1977) 46, 122–6.
11. Jephcott G, Kerry RJ. Lithium: an anaesthetic risk. *Br J Anaesth* (1974) 46, 389–90.
12. Dehpour AR, Samadian T, Roushanzamir F. Interaction of aminoglycoside antibiotics and lithium at the neuromuscular junctions. *Drugs Exp Clin Res* (1992) 18, 383–7.

Neuromuscular blockers + Magnesium salts

The effects of rocuronium, suxamethonium (succinylcholine), tubocurarine, vecuronium, and possibly other neuromuscular blockers can be increased and prolonged by magnesium sulphate given parenterally.

Clinical evidence

A study in women undergoing caesarian section showed that those given **magnesium sulphate** for toxaemia needed less **suxamethonium (succinylcholine)** (4.73 compared with 7.39 mg/kg/h) than other normal patients.[1] A pregnant 40-year-old with severe pre-eclampsia and receiving **magnesium sulphate** by infusion, underwent emergency caesarian section during which she was initially anaesthetised with thiopental (thiopentone), maintained with nitrous oxide/oxygen and enflurane, and given firstly **suxamethonium** and later **vecuronium** as muscle relaxants. At the end of surgery she rapidly recovered from the anaesthesia but the neuromuscular blockade was very prolonged (an eightfold increase in duration).[2] Prolonged neuromuscular blockade has been described in two other women with pre-eclampsia given **magnesium sulphate** and either **tubocurarine** or **suxamethonium**.[3] A 71-year-old woman given **magnesium sulphate** and lidocaine (lignocaine) for emergency cardioversion showed delayed onset and prolonged neuromuscular blockade when given **suxamethonium**.[4] A study in patients found that 40 mg/kg **magnesium sulphate**, but not 20 mg/kg, decreased the onset and prolonged the recovery time from **vecuronium** blockade.[5] Evidence of enhanced **vecuronium** neuromuscular blockade by **magnesium sulphate** is described in two other reports.[6,7] A fourfold increase in the duration of neuromuscular blockade of **rocuronium** (1 mg/kg) was reported in a pregnant woman receiving **magnesium sulphate**.[8] Increased blockade by **magnesium** has been demonstrated with **decamethonium**, **tubocurarine** and **suxamethonium** in *animals*.[3,9]

Mechanism

Not fully understood. Magnesium sulphate has direct neuromuscular blocking activity by inhibiting the normal release of acetylcholine from nerve endings, reducing the sensitivity of the postsynaptic membrane and depressing the excitability of the muscle membranes. These effects are possibly simply additive (or possibly more than additive) with the effects of conventional blockers.

Importance and management

An established interaction but the documentation is limited. Be alert for an increase in the effects of any neuromuscular blocker if intravenous magnesium sulphate is used. Intravenous calcium gluconate was used to assist recovery in one case.[3] No interaction would be expected with magnesium sulphate given orally because its absorption is poor.

1. Morris R, Giesecke AH. Potentiation of muscle relaxants by magnesium sulfate therapy in toxemia of pregnancy. *South Med J* (1968) 61, 25–8.
2. Sinatra RS, Philip BK, Naulty JS, Ostheimer GW. Prolonged neuromuscular blockade with vecuronium in a patient treated with magnesium sulfate. *Anesth Analg* (1985) 64, 1220–2.
3. Ghoneim MM, Long JP. The interaction between magnesium and other neuromuscular blocking agents. *Anesthesiology* (1970) 32, 23–7.
4. Ip-Yam C, Allsop E. Abnormal response to suxamethonium in a patient receiving magnesium therapy. *Anaesthesia* (1994) 49, 355–6.
5. Okuda T, Umeda T, Takemura M, Shiokawa Y, Koga Y. Pretreatment with magnesium sulphate enhances vecuronium-induced neuromuscular block. *Jpn J Anesthesiol* (1998) 47, 704–8.

6. Baraka A, Yazigi A. Neuromuscular interaction of magnesium with succinylcholine-vecuronium sequence in the eclamptic parturient. *Anesthesiology* (1987) 67, 806–8.
7. Hino H, Kaneko I, Miyazawa A, Aoki T, Ishizuka B, Kosugi K, Amemiya A. Prolonged neuromuscular blockade with vecuronium in patient with triple pregnancy treated with magnesium sulfate. *Jpn J Anesthesiol* (1997) 46, 266–70.
8. Gaiser RR, Seem EH. Use of rocuronium in a pregnant patient with an open eye injury, receiving magnesium medication, for preterm labour. *Br J Anaesth* (1996) 77, 669–71.
9. Giesecke AH, Morris RE, Dalton MD, Stephen CR. Of magnesium, muscle relaxants, toxemic parturients, and cats. *Anesth Analg* (1968) 47, 689–95.

Neuromuscular blockers + Metoclopramide

The neuromuscular blocking effects of suxamethonium (succinylcholine) can be increased and prolonged in patients taking metoclopramide.

Clinical evidence

A controlled study in 22 patients undergoing elective surgery showed that the recovery from neuromuscular blockade (time from 95% to 25% suppression of the activity of the adductor pollicis muscle) due to **suxamethonium** was prolonged in those patients who had also been given 10 mg **metoclopramide** intravenously.[1]

In another study of this interaction in patients undergoing postpartum tubal ligation it was found that mean block times after 1 mg/kg **suxamethonium** were 8.0 min (control), 9.83 min (10 mg **metoclopramide**), and 12.45 min (20 mg **metoclopramide**).[2] Prolongation of the actions of **suxamethonium** (+25%) by **metoclopramide** is described in another report.[3]

Mechanism

Metoclopramide reduces the activity of plasma cholinesterase which is responsible for the metabolism of suxamethonium. As a result it is metabolised much more slowly and its effects are prolonged.[1,3] One study found that a metoclopramide serum concentration of 0.8 micrograms/ml inhibited plasma cholinesterase activity by 50%. A 10-mg dose of metoclopramide in a 70 kg adult produces serum concentrations of up to 0.14 micrograms/ml.[3]

Importance and management

An established but not extensively documented interaction of only moderate or minor clinical importance, however anaesthetists should be aware that some enhancement of blockade can occur (+25% has been reported). The authors of the first report cited[1] also point out that plasma cholinesterase activity is reduced in pregnancy and those taking ester-type local anaesthetics, which would be expected to be additive with the effects of metoclopramide.

1. Kao YJ, Turner DR. Prolongation of succinylcholine block by metoclopramide. *Anesthesiology* (1989) 70, 905–8.
2. Kao YJ, Tellez J, Turner DR. Dose-dependent effect of metoclopramide on cholinesterases and suxamethonium metabolism. *Br J Anaesth* (1990) 65, 220–4.
3. Kambam JR, Parris WCV, Franks JJ, Sastry BVR, Naukam R, Smith BE. The inhibitory effect of metoclopramide on plasma cholinesterase activity. *Can J Anaesth* (1988) 35, 476–8.

Neuromuscular blockers + Miscellaneous antibacterials or Antifungals

Colistin, colistimethate sodium (colistin sulphomethate sodium), polymyxins, lincomycin, some penicillins (apalcillin, azlocillin, mezlocillin, piperacillin), clindamycin and vancomycin possess some neuromuscular blocking activity. Increased and prolonged neuromuscular blockade is possible if these antibacterials are used with anaesthetics and conventional neuromuscular blocking drugs. In theory amphotericin B might also interact, but the tetracyclines probably do not. No interaction is seen with metronidazole, cefuroxime or chloramphenicol.

Clinical evidence

(a) Amphotericin B

Amphotericin B can induce hypokalaemia resulting in muscle weakness[1,2] which might be expected to enhance the effects of neuromuscular blockers, but there appear to be no reports in the literature confirming that this actually takes place.

(b) Clindamycin, Lincomycin

Enhanced blockade has been demonstrated in patients given **pancuronium** and **lincomycin** which was reversed by neostigmine.[3] Respiratory paralysis was seen in a man recovering from blockade with **tubocurarine**[4] and this interaction was confirmed in another report.[5] Other reports describe an increase in neuromuscular blockade in patients on **pancuronium, suxamethonium (succinylcholine)**[6] or **pipecuronium**[7] when treated with **clindamycin**. One patient developed very prolonged blockade after being unintentionally given an overdose of **clindamycin** (2400 mg instead of 600 mg) shortly after recovery from **suxamethonium** and **tubocurarine**.[8]

(c) Metronidazole

An increase in the neuromuscular blocking effects of **vecuronium** has been reported in *cats*,[9] but a later study in patients failed to find any evidence of an interaction[10] and another study with **rocuronium** also found no evidence of an interaction.[11] No interaction was also seen with **rocuronium** and **metronidazole/cefuroxime**.[11]

(d) Penicillins

A study in patients showed that the neuromuscular blocking effects of vecuronium were prolonged by a number of acylaminopenicillins: **apalcillin** + 26%, **azlocillin** + 55%, **mezlocillin** + 38%, and **piperacillin** + 46%.[12] Recurarization occurred in a patient following **vecuronium** blockade when given **piperacillin**.[13]

(e) Polymyxins

Pittinger in his literature review of antibiotic-neuromuscular blocker interactions found 17 cases over the 1955–70 period in which **colistin (polymyxin E)** or **colistimethate sodium (colistin sulphomethate sodium)**, with or without conventional neuromuscular blockers, were responsible for the development of increased blockade and respiratory muscle paralysis. Some of the patients had renal disease.[14] A later report describes prolonged respiratory depression in a patient on **pancuronium** and **colistin**.[15] Calcium gluconate was found to reverse the blockade.[15] A study found that 1 million IU of **colistin** also considerably prolonged the recovery time from **pipecuronium** blockade.[7] Pittinger also lists five cases of enhanced neuromuscular blockade with **polymyxin B**. An increase in the blockade due to **pancuronium** by **polymyxin B** is described in another report,[16] and prolonged and fatal apnoea occurred in another patient on **suxamethonium** when his peritoneal cavity was instilled with a solution containing 100 mg **polymyxin B** and 100,000 U bacitracin.[17]

(f) Tetracyclines, Cefuroxime, Chloramphenicol

Pittinger lists four cases of enhanced neuromuscular blockade with **rolitetracycline** or **oxytetracycline** in myasthenic patients[14] but

there seem to be no reports of interactions in normal patients given neuromuscular blocking drugs. No interaction was seen in the myasthenic patients when given **chloramphenicol** or **penicillin**,[18,19] nor in normal patients given **cefuroxime** in the presence of **pipecuronium**[20] or **rocuronium**.[11]

(g) Vancomycin

The neuromuscular blockade due to **vecuronium** was increased in a patient when given an infusion of **vancomycin** (1 g in 250 ml saline).[21] Transient apnoea and hypotension have also been described following rapid infusion of **vancomycin** during peritoneal dialysis of a patient.[22] A man recovering from neuromuscular blockade with **suxamethonium** (with some evidence of residual Phase II block) developed almost total muscle paralysis and apnoea when given an intravenous infusion of **vancomycin**. He recovered spontaneously when the **vancomycin** was stopped, but it took several hours.[23]

Mechanisms

Not fully understood but several sites of action have been suggested. See Table 20.3.

Importance and management

The interactions involving polymyxin B, colistin, colistimethate sodium (colistin sulphomethate sodium), lincomycin, clindamycin and vancomycin are established and clinically important. The incidence is uncertain. Concurrent use need not be avoided, but be alert for increased and prolonged neuromuscular blockade. The recovery period should be well monitored because of the risk of recurarization. Check the outcome of using amphotericin. No interaction would be expected with the tetracyclines, cefuroxime, chloramphenicol, metronidazole or metronidazole/cefuroxime, but some caution would seem appropriate with apalcillin, azlocillin, mezlocillin and piperacillin.

1. Holeman CW and Einstein H. The toxic effects of amphotericin B in man. *Calif Med* (1963) 99, 90.
2. Drutz DJ, Fan JH, Tai TY, Cheng JT, Hsieh WC. Hypokalemic rhabdomyolosis and myoglobinuria following amphotericin B therapy. *JAMA* (1970) 211, 824–6.
3. Booij LHDJ, Miller RD, Crul JF. Neostigmine and 4-aminopyrimidine antagonism of lincomycin-pancuronium neuromuscular blockade in man. *Anesth Analg* (1978) 57, 316–21.
4. Samuelson RJ, Giesecke AH, Kallus FT, Stanley VF. Lincomycin-curare interaction. *Anesth Analg* (1975) 54, 103–5.
5. Hashimoto Y, Iwatsuki N, Shima T, Iwatsuki K. Neuromuscular blocking properties of lincomycin and kanamycin in man. *Jpn J Anesth* (1971) 20, 407–11.
6. Avery D, Finn R. Succinylcholine-prolonged apnea associated with clindamycin and abnormal liver function tests. *Dis Nerv Syst* (1977) 38, 473–5.
7. de Gouw NE, Crul JF, Vandermeersch E, Mulier JP, van Egmond J, Van Aken H. Interaction of antibiotics on pipecuronium-induced neuromuscular blockade. *J Clin Anesth* (1993) 5, 212–5.
8. Al Ahdal O, Bevan DR. Clindamycin-induced neuromuscular blockade. *Can J Anaesth* (1995) 42, 614–7.
9. McInedwar IC, Marshall RJ. Interactions between the neuromuscular blocking drug ORG NC 45 and some anaesthetic, analgesic and antimicrobial agents. *Br J Anaesth* (1981) 53, 785–92.
10. D'Hollander A, Agoston S, Capouet V, Barvais L, Bomblet JP, Esselen M. Failure of metronidazole to alter a vecuronium neuromuscular blockade in humans. *Anesthesiology* (1985) 63, 99–102.
11. Cooper R, Maddineni VR, Mirakhur RK. Clinical study of interaction between rocuronium and some commonly used antimicrobial agents. *Eur J Anaesthesiol* (1993) 10, 331–5.
12. Tryba M. Wirkungsverstärkung nicht-depolarisierender muskelrelaxantien durch acylaminopenicilline. Untersuchungen am beispiel von vecuronium. *Anaesthesist* (1985) 34, 651–55.
13. Mackie K, Pavlin EG. Recurrent paralysis following piperacillin administration. *Anesthesiology* (1990) 72, 561–3.
14. Pittinger CB, Eryasa Y, Adamson R. Antibiotic-induced paralysis. *Anesth Analg* (1970) 49, 487–501.
15. Giala MM, Paradelis AG. Two cases of prolonged respiratory depression due to interaction of pancuronium with colistin and streptomycin. *J Antimicrob Chemother* (1979) 5, 234–5.
16. Fogdall RP, Miller RD. Prolongation of pancuronium-induced neuromuscular blockade by clindamycin. *Anesthesiology* (1974) 41, 407–8.
17. Small GA. Respiratory paralysis after a large dose of intraperitoneal polymyxin B and bacitracin. *Anesth Analg* (1964) 43, 137–9.
18. Gibbels E. Weitere beobachtungen zur nebenwirkung intravenöser reverin-gaben bei myasthenia gravis pseudoparalytica. *Dtsch Med Wschr* (1967) 92, 1153–4.
19. Wullen F, Kast G, Bruck A. Über nebenwirkungen bei tetracyclin-verabreichung an myastheniker. *Dtsch Med Wschr* (1967) 92, 667–9.
20. Stanley JC, Mirakhur RK, Clarke RSJ. Study of pipecuronium-antibiotic interaction. *Anesthesiology* (1990) 73, A898.
21. Huang KC, Heise A, Shrader AK, Tsueda K. Vancomycin enhances the neuromuscular blockade of vecuronium. *Anesth Analg* (1990) 71, 194–6.
22. Glicklich D, Figura I. Vancomycin and cardiac arrest. *Ann Intern Med* (1984) 101, 880–1.
23. Albrecht RF, Lanier WL. Potentiation of succinylcholine-induced phase II block by vancomycin. *Anesth Analg* (1993) 77, 1300–1302.

Table 20.3 Neuromuscular blockers + miscellaneous antibacterials

Antibacterial	Prejunctional	Receptor block	Channel block	Muscle
Colistin				+
Lincomycin	++	++	+	+
Polymyxin B	++	+++		+
Tetracyclines				+

After TA Torda, Curr Clin Prac Ser (1983) 11, Clin Exper Norcuron, pp 72–8.

Neuromuscular blockers + Monoamine oxidase inhibitors

Three patients showed an enhancement of the effects of suxamethonium (succinylcholine) during concurrent treatment with phenelzine.

Clinical evidence, mechanism, importance and management

Two patients, one taking **phenelzine** and the other who had ceased to do so six days previously, developed apnoea following electroconvulsive therapy (ECT) during which **suxamethonium** was used. Both responded to injections of nikethamide and positive pressure ventilation with oxygen.[1] A later study observed the same response in another patient taking **phenelzine**.[2] This would appear to be explained by the finding that **phenelzine** caused a reduction in the levels of serum pseudocholinesterase in four out of 10 patients studied. Since the metabolism of **suxamethonium** depends on this enzyme, reduced levels of the enzyme would result in a reduced rate of **suxamethonium** metabolism and in a prolongation of its effects. None of 12 other patients taking **tranylcypromine, isocarboxazid** or **mebanazine** showed reduced pseudocholinesterase levels.[2]

It would clearly be prudent to be on the alert for this interaction in patients on **phenelzine**, but on the basis of limited evidence it seems less likely to occur with the other MAOIs cited.

1. Bleaden FA, Czekanska G. New drugs for depression. *BMJ* (1960) 1, 200.
2. Bodley PO, Halwax K, Potts L. Low serum pseudocholinesterase levels complicating treatment with phenelzine. *BMJ* (1969) 3, 510–12.

Neuromuscular blockers and Anaesthetics + Morphine

A patient experienced hypertension and tachycardia when given pancuronium bromide after induction of anaesthesia with morphine and nitrous oxide/oxygen. The respiratory depressant effects of ketamine and morphine may be additive.

Clinical evidence, mechanism, importance and management

A woman about to receive a coronary by-pass graft was premedicated with **morphine** and hyoscine. **Morphine** (1 mg/kg) was then slowly infused while the patient was ventilated with 50% N_2O/O_2. With the onset of neuromuscular relaxation with **pancuronium**, her blood pressure rose sharply from 120/60 to 200/110 mmHg and her pulse rate increased from 54 to 96, persisting for several minutes but restabilising when 1% halothane was added.[1] The suggested reason is that **pancuronium** can antagonise the vagal tone (heart slowing) induced by the **morphine**, thus allowing the blood pressure and heart rate to rise. The authors of the report point out the undesirability of this in those with coronary heart disease.

Ketamine is a respiratory depressant like **morphine** but less potent, and its effects can be additive with morphine.[2]

1. Grossman E, Jacobi AM. Hemodynamic interaction between pancuronium and morphine. *Anesthesiology* (1974) 40, 299–301.
2. Bourke DL, Malit LA, Smith TC. Respiratory interactions of ketamine and morphine. *Anesthesiology* (1987) 66, 153–6.

Neuromuscular blockers + Ondansetron

Ondansetron does not affect neuromuscular blockade with atracurium.

Clinical evidence, mechanism, importance and management

A study[1] of patients undergoing elective surgery found that 8 or 16 mg **ondansetron** as an intravenous infusion had no effect on neuromuscular blockade with **atracurium**. No special precautions would therefore seem necessary. The authors suggest that no interaction is likely with other non-depolarising neuromuscular blockers, but this needs confirmation.

1. Lien CA, Gadalla F, Kudlak TT, Embree PB, Sharp GJ, Savarese JJ. The effect of ondansetron on atracurium-induced neuromuscular blockade. *J Clin Anesth* (1993) 5, 399–403.

Neuromuscular blockers + Promazine

An isolated report describes prolonged apnoea in a patient given promazine while recovering from neuromuscular blockade with suxamethonium (succinylcholine).

Clinical evidence, mechanism, importance and management

A woman, recovering from surgery during which she had received **suxamethonium**, was given 25 mg **promazine** intravenously for sedation. Within 3 min she had become cyanotic and dyspnoeic, and required assisted respiration for 4 h.[1] The reason is not understood but one suggestion is that **promazine** possibly depresses pseudocholinesterase levels which would reduce the metabolism of the **suxamethonium** and thereby prolong recovery. Some caution would seem appropriate if **promazine** is given to any patient who has had **suxamethonium**. There seems to be no information about other phenothiazines and other neuromuscular blockers.

1. Regan AG, Aldrete JA. Prolonged apnea after administration of promazine hydrochloride following succinylcholine infusion. *Anesth Analg* (1967) 46, 315–18.

Neuromuscular blockers + Quinidine

The effects of both depolarising (e.g. suxamethonium (succinylcholine)) and non-depolarising (e.g. tubocurarine) neuromuscular blockers can be increased by quinidine. Recurarization and apnoea have been seen in patients when quinidine was given during the recovery period from neuromuscular blockade.

Clinical evidence

A patient given **metocurine (dimethyltubocurarine)** during surgery regained her motor functions and was able to talk coherently during the recovery period. Within 15 min of additionally being given 200 mg **quinidine sulphate** by injection she developed muscular weakness and respiratory embarrassment. She needed intubation and assisted respiration for a period of 2½ hours. Edrophonium and neostigmine were used to aid recovery.[1]

This interaction has been described in man in reports involving **tubocurarine**[2] and **suxamethonium (succinylcholine)**.[3-5] It has also been seen in *animals*.[6-9]

Mechanism

Not fully understood, but it has been shown that quinidine can inhibit the enzyme (choline acetyltransferase) which is concerned with the synthesis of acetylcholine at nerve endings.[10] Neuromuscular transmission would be expected to be reduced if the synthesis of acetylcholine is reduced. Quinidine also inhibits the activity of plasma cholinesterase which is concerned with the metabolism of succinylcholine.[5]

Importance and management

An established interaction of clinical importance but the documentation in man is limited. The incidence is uncertain but it was seen to a greater or lesser extent in five of six patients studied.[3] It has only been reported in man with metocurine, tubocurarine and suxamethonium, but it occurs in *animals* with gallamine and decamethonium and it seems possible that it will occur in man with any depolarising or non-depolarising neuromuscular blocker. Be alert for increased neuromuscular blocking effects during and after surgery.

1. Schmidt JL, Vick NA, Sadove MS. The effect of quinidine on the action of muscle relaxants. *JAMA* (1963) 183, 669–73.
2. Way WL, Katzung BG, Larson CP. Recurarization with quinidine. *JAMA* (1967) 200, 163–4.
3. Grogono AW. Anesthesia for atrial defibrillation: effect of quinidine on muscular relaxation. *Lancet* (1963) ii, 1039–40.
4. Boere LA. Fehler und Gefahren. Recurarisation nach Chinidinsulfat. *Anaesthetist* (1964) 13, 368.
5. Kambam JR, Franks JJ, Naukam R, Sastry BVR. Effect of quinidine on plasma cholinesterase activity and succinylcholine neuromuscular blockade. *Anesthesiology* (1987) 67, 858–60.
6. Miller RD, Way WL, Katzung BG. The neuromuscular effects of quinidine. *Proc Soc Exp Biol Med* (1968) 129, 215–18.
7. Miller RD, Way WL, Katzung BG. The potentiation of neuromuscular blocking agents by quinidine. *Anesthesiology* (1967) 28, 1036–41.
8. Cuthbert MF. The effect of quinidine and procainamide on the neuromuscular blocking action of suxamethonium. *Br J Anaesth* (1966) 38, 775–9.
9. Usubiaga JE. Potentiation of muscle relaxants by quinidine. *Anesthesiology* (1968) 29, 1068.
10. Kambam JR, Day P, Jansen VE, Sastry BVR. Quinidine inhibits choline acetyltransferase activity. *Anesthesiology* (1989) 71, A819.

Neuromuscular blockers + Quinine

An isolated report describes recurarization and apnoea in a patient given intravenous quinine after recovering from neuromuscular blockade with suxamethonium (succinylcholine) and pancuronium.

Clinical evidence mechanism, importance and management

A patient with acute pancreatitis, taking 1800 mg **quinine** daily, was given penicillin and **gentamicin** before undergoing surgery during which **pancuronium** and **suxamethonium (succinylcholine)** were used uneventfully. After the surgery the neuromuscular blockade was reversed with neostigmine and atropine, and the patient awoke and was breathing well. After an hour and a half an intravenous infusion of 500 mg **quinine** in 500 ml isotonic saline (to run over 6 h) was started. Within 10 min (about 15 mg **quinine**) he became dyspnoeic, his breathing became totally ineffective and he needed re-intubation. Muscle flaccidity persisted for 3 h.[1] The reason for this reaction is not fully understood. A possible explanation is that it may have been the additive neuromuscular blocking effects of the **gentamicin** (well recognised as having neuromuscular blocking activity), the **quinine** (an optical isomer of quinidine which has blocking actions) and the residual effects of the **pancuronium** and **suxamethonium**.

There seem to be no other reports of problems in patients on neuromuscular blockers when given **quinine**, but this isolated case serves to emphasise the importance of being alert for any signs of recurarization in patients concurrently treated with one or more drugs possessing some neuromuscular blocking activity.

1. Sher MH, Mathews PA. Recurarization with quinine administration after reversal from anaesthesia. *Anaesth Intensive Care* (1983) 11, 241–3.

Neuromuscular blockers + Testosterone

An isolated report describes marked resistance to the effects of suxamethonium (succinylcholine) and vecuronium, apparently due to the long-term use of testosterone.

Clinical evidence, mechanism, importance and management

A woman trans-sexual who had been receiving 200 mg **testosterone enantate** intramuscularly twice monthly for 10 years was resistant to 100 mg **suxamethonium (succinylcholine)** and needed 0.1 mg/kg **vecuronium** for effective tracheal intubation before surgery. During the surgery it was found necessary to use a total of 22 mg **vecuronium** over a 50-min period to achieve acceptable relaxation of the abdominal muscles for hysterectomy and salpingo-oophorectomy to be carried out. The reasons are not understood.[1]

1. Reddy P, Guzman A, Robalino J, Shevde K. Resistance to muscle relaxants in a patient receiving prolonged testosterone therapy. *Anesthesiology* (1989) 70, 871–3.

Neuromuscular blockers + Thiotepa

An isolated report describes a marked increase in the neuromuscular blocking effects of pancuronium in a myasthenic patient when given thiotepa, but it normally appears not to interact with neuromuscular blocking agents.

Clinical evidence, mechanism, importance and management

A myasthenic patient rapidly developed very prolonged respiratory depression when given **thiotepa** intraperitoneally after receiving **pancuronium**.[1] **Thiotepa** has also been shown to increase the duration of **succinylcholine** neuromuscular blockade in *dogs*.[2] However, *in vitro* studies show that **thiotepa** is a poor inhibitor of pseudocholinesterase[3] and in a normal patient it was found not to decrease serum levels significantly.[4] The general silence in the literature would seem to confirm that no special precautions are normally necessary.

1. Bennett EJ, Schmidt GB, Patel KP, Grundy EM. Muscle relaxants, myasthenia, and mustards? *Anesthesiology* (1977) 46, 220–1.
2. Cremonesi E, Rodrigues I de J. Interação de agentes curarizantes com antineoplásico. *Rev Bra Anest* (1982) 32, 313–15.
3. Zsigmond EK, Robins G. The effect of a series of anti-cancer drugs on plasma cholinesterase activity. *Can Anaesth Soc J* (1972) 19, 75–8.
4. Mone JG, Mathie WE. Qualitative and quantitative effects of pseudocholinesterase activity. *Anaesthesia* (1967) 22, 55–7.

Neuromuscular blockers + Tobacco smoking

The neuromuscular blocking effects of rocuronium (0.6 mg/kg) are reported to be unaffected by smoking (more than 10 cigarettes daily)[1] but there is some evidence that smokers may need more vecuronium and less atracurium.[1]

1. Latorre F, de Almedia MC, Stanek A, Kleeman PP. Die Wechselwirkung von Rocuronium und Rauchen. Der Einfluss des rauchens auf die neuromuskulare Ubertragung nach Rocuronium. *Anaesthetist* (1997) 46, 493–5.

Neuromuscular blockers + Trimetaphan

Trimet(h)aphan can increase the effects of suxamethonium (succinylcholine) which may result in prolonged apnoea. This may possibly occur with other neuromuscular blocking drugs (seen also with alcuronium).

Clinical evidence

A man undergoing neurosurgery was given **tubocurarine** and **suxamethonium (succinylcholine)**. During the recovery period he developed apnoea lasting about 2.5 h attributed to the concurrent use of **trimetaphan** (4500 mg over a 90-min period). Later when he underwent further surgery using essentially the same anaesthetic techniques and drugs but with a very much smaller dose of **trimetaphan** (35 mg over a 10-min period) the recovery was normal.[1]

Nine out of 10 patients receiving ECT treatment and given **suxamethonium** showed an almost 90% prolongation in apnoea (from 142 to 265 s) when 10–20 mg **trimetaphan** was used instead of 1.2 mg atropine.[2] Prolonged apnoea has been seen in another patient given **suxamethonium** and **trimetaphan**.[3] On the basis of an *in vitro* study it was calculated that a typical dose of **trimetaphan** would double the duration of paralysis due to **suxamethonium**.[4] Prolonged neuromuscular blockade was also seen in a man given **alcuronium** and **trimetaphan**.[5]

Mechanism

Not fully understood. Trimetaphan can inhibit serum pseudocholinesterase to some extent[2] which would reduce the metabolism of the suxamethonium and thereby prolong its activity. Studies in *dogs*[6] and *rats*[7-9] and case reports in man[10] also indicate that trimetaphan has direct neuromuscular blocking activity. Its effects are additive with the neuromuscular blocking effects of the aminoglycosides.[9]

Importance and management

Information is limited but the interaction appears to be established. If trimetaphan and suxamethonium are used concurrently, be alert for enhanced and prolonged neuromuscular blockade. This has also been seen with alcuronium in man, and with other non-depolarising blockers such as tubocurarine in *animals*.[6-8] Respiratory arrest has been seen in man when large doses of trimetaphan were given in the absence of a neuromuscular blocker so that caution is certainly needed.[10] *Animal* studies suggested that the blockade might not be reversed by neostigmine or calcium chloride,[9] but one study in man successfully used neostigmine and calcium gluconate to reverse the effects of alcuronium and trimetaphan.[5]

1. Wilson SL, Miller RN, Wright C, Hasse D. Prolonged neuromuscular blockade associated with trimetaphan: a case report. *Anesth Analg* (1976) 55, 353–6.
2. Tewfik GI. Trimetaphan. Its effect on the pseudocholinesterase level of man. *Anaesthesia* (1957) 12, 326–9.
3. Poulton TJ, James FM, Lockridge O. Prolonged apnea following trimethaphan and succinylcholine. *Anesthesiology* (1979) 50, 54–6.
4. Sklar GS, Lanks KW. Effects of trimethaphan and sodium nitroprusside on hydrolysis of succinylcholine *in vitro*. *Anesthesiology* (1977) 47, 31–3.
5. Nakamura K, Koide M, Imanaga T, Ogasawara H, Takahashi M, Yoshikawa M. Prolonged neuromuscular blockade following trimetaphan infusion. *Anaesthesia* (1980) 35, 1202–7.
6. Randall LD, Peterson WG and Lehmann G. The ganglionic blocking action of thiophan derivatives. *J Pharmacol Exp Ther* (1949) 97, 48.
7. Pearcy WC, Wittenstein ES. The interactions of trimethaphan (Arfonad), suxamethonium and cholinesterase inhibitor in the rat. *Br J Anaesth* (1960) 32, 156–9.
8. Deacock AR and Davies TDW. The influence of certain ganglionic blocking agents on the neuromuscular transmission. *Br J Anaesth* (1958) 30, 217.
9. Paradelis AG, Crassaris LG, Karachalios DN, Triantaphyllidis CJ. Aminoglycoside antibiotics: interaction with trimethaphan at the neuromuscular junctions. *Drugs Exp Clin Res* (1987) 13, 233–6.
10. Dale RC, Schroeder ET. Respiratory paralysis during treatment of hypertension with trimethaphan camsylate. *Arch Intern Med* (1976) 136, 816–18.

Vecuronium + Miscellaneous drugs

Bradycardia has been seen in patients given vecuronium with alfentanil, fentanyl, sufentanil, thiopental (thiopentone) and etomidate.

Clinical evidence, mechanism, importance and management

Two patients, one aged 72 and the other aged 84, undergoing elective carotid endarterectomy developed extreme bradycardia following induction with **alfentanil** and vecuronium. The first was taking 20 mg **propranolol** 8-hourly and as the drugs were injected his heart rate fell from 50 to 35 bpm, and his blood pressure fell from 170/70 to 75/35 mmHg. He responded to ephedrine and phenylephrine. The other was taking **nifedipine** and **quinidine**. His heart rate fell from 89 to 43 bpm, and his blood pressure dropped from 210/80 to 140/45 mmHg. Both heart rate and blood pressures responded following skin incision.[1]

Bradycardia in the presence of vecuronium has been seen during induction with other drugs including **fentanyl**,[2,3] **sufentanil**,[4] **thiopental (thiopentone)**[3] and **etomidate**,[3] and may possibly be due to some effect on the CNS. Be alert for this effect if vecuronium is given with any of these agents.

1. Lema G, Sacco C, Urzúa J. Bradycardia following induction with alfentanil and vecuronium. *J Cardiothorac Vasc Anesth* (1992) 6, 774–5.
2. Mirakhur RK, Ferres CJ, Clarke RSJ, Bali M, Dundee W. Clinical evaluation of Org NC 45. *Br J Anaesth* (1983) 55, 119–24.
3. Inoue K, El-Banayosy A, Stolarksi L, Teichelt W. Vecuronium induced bradycardia following induction of anaesthesia with etomidate or thiopentone, with or without fentanyl. *Br J Anaesth* (1988) 60, 10–17.
4. Starr NJ, Sethna DH, Estafanous FG. Bradycardia and asystole following the rapid elimination of sufentanil with vecuronium. *Anesthesiology* (1986) 64, 521–3.

21

Sympathomimetic drug interactions

Norepinephrine (noradrenaline) is the principal neurotransmitter involved in the final link between nerve endings of the sympathetic nervous system and the adrenergic receptors of the organs or tissues innervated. The effects of stimulation of this system can be reproduced or mimicked by norepinephrine itself and by a number of other drugs which can also cause stimulation of these receptors. The drugs which can behave in this way are described as 'sympathomimetics' and act either directly on the adrenergic receptors like norepinephrine itself or indirectly by releasing stored norepinephrine from the nerve endings. Some of them do both. This is very simply illustrated in Figure 21.1.

We now know that the adrenergic receptors of the sympathetic system are not identical but can be subdivided into at least four main types, alpha-1, alpha-2, beta-1 and beta-2, and it is now possible broadly to categorise the sympathomimetics into groups according to their activity. The value of this categorisation is that individual sympathomimetic drugs can be selected for their stimulant actions on particular organs or tissues. For example, salbutamol and terbutaline are so-called beta-agonists which selectively stimulate the beta-2 receptors in bronchi causing bronchodilation. This represents a significant improvement on both isoprenaline (isoproterenol) which also stimulates beta-1 receptors in the heart, and on ephedrine which stimulates alpha receptors as well. Although the sympathomimetics are categorised together in this chapter, it is important to appreciate that they have a very wide range of actions and uses. One should not, therefore, extrapolate the interactions seen with one drug to any other without fully taking into account their differences and similarities. The Index should be consulted for a full listing of all interactions involving drugs with sympathomimetic activity.

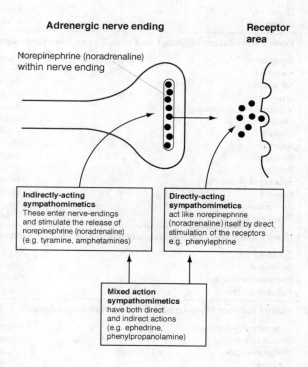

Fig. 21.1 A very simple illustration of the modes of action of indirectly-acting, directly-acting and mixed action sympathomimetics at adrenergic neurones.

Table 21.1 A categorisation of some sympathomimetic drugs

Drug	Receptors stimulated
Direct stimulators of alpha and beta receptors	
Epinephrine (Adrenaline)	Beta more marked than alpha
Mainly direct stimulators of alpha receptors	
Phenylephrine	Predominantly alpha
Methoxamine	Predominantly alpha
Metaraminol	Predominantly alpha
Norepinephrine (Noradrenaline)	Predominantly alpha
Mainly direct stimulators of beta-1 receptors	
Dopamine	Predominantly beta-1, some alpha
Dobutamine	Predominantly beta-1, some beta-2 and alpha
Direct stimulators of beta-1 and beta-2 receptors (beta-agonist bronchodilators)	
Bambuterol	Predominantly beta-2
Fenoterol	Predominantly beta-2
Formoterol	Predominantly beta-2
Isoetharine	Predominantly beta-2
Isoprenaline (Isoproterenol)	Beta-1 and beta-2
Orciprenaline	Predominantly beta-2
Pirbuterol	Predominantly beta-2
Reproterol	Predominantly beta-2
Rimiterol	Predominantly beta-2
Ritodrine	Predominantly beta-2
Salbutamol (Albuterol)	Predominantly beta-2
Salmeterol	Predominantly beta-2
Terbutaline	Predominantly beta-2
Tulobuterol	Predominantly beta-2
Direct and indirect stimulators of alpha and beta receptors	
Ephedrine	Alpha and beta
Etefedrine	Alpha and beta
Phenylpropanolamine	Alpha and beta
Pseudoephedrine	Alpha and beta
Mainly indirect stimulators of alpha and beta receptors	
Amfetamine (Amphetamine)	Alpha and beta—also central stimulant
Mephentermine	Alpha and beta—also central stimulant
Methylphenidate	Alpha and beta—also central stimulant
Tyramine	Alpha and beta

Amphetamines and Related drugs + Chlorpromazine

The appetite suppressant and other effects of amphetamines, chlorphentermine and phenmetrazine are opposed by chlorpromazine. The antipsychotic effects of chlorpromazine can be opposed by amfetamine (amphetamine).

Clinical evidence

(a) Amphetamines + Phenothiazines

20 obese schizophrenic patients being treated with phenothiazines and other drugs (including **chlorpromazine, thioridazine, imipramine and chlordiazepoxide**) failed to respond to concurrent treatment with **dexamfetamine (dextroamphetamine)** for obesity, and the expected sleep disturbance was not seen.[1] Antagonism of the effects of **amphetamines** by **chlorpromazine** has been described in other reports.[2,3]

A study in a very large number of patients taking 200–600 mg **chlorpromazine** daily indicated that the addition of 10–40 mg **amfetamine (amphetamine)** had a detrimental effect on the control of their schizophrenic symptoms.[4]

(b) Chlorphentermine or Phenmetrazine + Chlorpromazine

Chlorpromazine was found in a double-blind controlled study in patients to diminish the weight reducing effect of **phenmetrazine**.[5] The effects of both **phenmetrazine** and **chlorphentermine** on the control of obesity were found in another study to be reduced by **chlorpromazine**.[6]

Mechanism

Not understood. It is known that phenothiazines can inhibit the uptake mechanism by which the amphetamines enter neurones. If this occurs at peripheral adrenergic neurones and centrally at both adrenergic and dopaminergic neurones, some part of the antagonism of the amphetamines can be explained.

Importance and management

Established interactions. These reports amply demonstrate that it is not desirable to attempt to treat patients with chlorpromazine and amphetamines, phenmetrazine or chlorphentermine concurrently. It is not clear whether this interaction takes place with phenothiazines other than chlorpromazine, but it seems possible.

This interaction has been deliberately exploited, and with success, in the treatment of 22 children poisoned with various amphetamines (dexamfetamine (dextroamphetamine), methamphetamine, phenmetrazine).[2] They were given 1 mg/kg chlorpromazine intramuscularly initially, followed by further doses as necessary.

There seem to be no reports about interactions between other drugs related to dexamfetamine (e.g. benzphetamine, clortermine, fenproporex, phendimetrazine, phentermine, etc.) and chlorpromazine, but it would be prudent to be alert for these drugs to behave similarly.

1. Modell W, Hussar AE. Failure of dextroamphetamine sulfate to influence eating and sleeping patterns in obese schizophrenic patients: clinical and pharmacological significance. *JAMA* (1965) 193, 275–8.
2. Espelin DE, Done AK. Amphetamine poisoning: effectiveness of chlorpromazine. *N Engl J Med* (1968) 278, 1361–65.
3. Jönsson L-E. Pharmacological blockade of amphetamine effects in amphetamine-dependent subjects. *Eur J Clin Pharmacol* (1972) 4, 206–11.
4. Casey JF, Hollister LE, Klett CJ, Lasky JJ, Caffrey EM. Combined drug therapy of chronic schizophrenics. Controlled evaluation of placebo, dextro-amphetamine, imipramine, isocarboxazid and trifluoperazine added to maintenance doses of chlorpromazine. *Am J Psychiatry* (1961) 117, 997–1003.
5. Reid AA. Pharmacological antagonism between chlorpromazine and phenmetrazine in mental hospital patients. *Med J Aust* (1964) 1, 187–8.
6. Sletten IW, Ognjanov V, Menendez S, Sundland D, El-Toumi A. Weight reduction with chlorphentermine and phenmetrazine in obese psychiatric patients during chlorpromazine therapy. *Curr Ther Res* (1967) 9, 570–5.

Amphetamines + Lithium carbonate

The effects of the amphetamines can be opposed by lithium carbonate.

Clinical evidence, mechanism, importance and management

Two depressed patients spontaneously abandoned abusing amphetamines (**methamphetamine** with cannabis and **phenmetrazine**) because, while taking **lithium carbonate**, they were unable to get 'high'. Another patient complained of not feeling any effects from amphetamines taken for weight reduction until **lithium carbonate** was withdrawn.[1] A controlled study in nine depressed patients confirmed these findings.[2] The reasons for these reactions are not known, but one suggestion is that amphetamines and **lithium** have mutually opposing pharmacological actions on norepinephrine (noradrenaline) uptake at adrenergic neurones.[1] Information is very limited, but be alert for evidence of reduced amfetamine (amphetamine) effects in the presence of **lithium**.

1. Flemenbaum A. Does lithium block the effects of amphetamine? A report of three cases. *Am J Psychiatry* (1974) 131, 820–1.
2. Van Kammen DP, Murphy D. Attenuation of the euphoriant and activating effects of *d*- and *l*-amphetamine by lithium carbonate treatment. *Psychopharmacologia* (1975) 44, 215–24.

Amphetamines + Nasal decongestants

An isolated report describes the antagonism of levamphetamine in a hyperactive child by nasal decongestants containing phenylpropanolamine and chlorphenamine (chlorpheniramine).

Clinical evidence, mechanism, importance and management

Maintenance therapy with 42 mg **levamphetamine succinate** daily in a 12-year-old hyperactive boy was found to be ineffective on two occasions when he was concurrently treated with *Contac* and *Allerest* for colds. Both of these proprietary nasal decongestants contain **phenylpropanolamine** and **chlorphenamine (chlorpheniramine)**.[1] The reason is not understood. There is too little information to make any statement about the general importance of this reaction.

1. Heustis RD and Arnold LE. Possible antagonism of amphetamine by decongestant-antihistamine compounds. *J Pediatr* (1974) 85, 579.

Amphetamines + Urinary acidifiers or alkalinizers

The loss of amfetamine (amphetamine) in the urine is increased by urinary acidifiers (ammonium chloride) and reduced by urinary alkalinizers (acetazolamide, sodium bicarbonate).

Clinical evidence

A study in six normal subjects given 10–15 mg **amfetamine (amphetamine)** by mouth showed that when the urine was made alkaline (approximately pH 8) by giving **sodium bicarbonate**, only 3% of the original dose of **amfetamine** was excreted over a 16-h period compared with 54% when the urine was made acid (approximately pH 5) by taking **ammonium chloride**.[1]

Similar results have been reported elsewhere.[2] Psychoses resulting from **amfetamine** retention in patients with **alkaline urine** have been described.[3]

Mechanism

Amfetamine is a base which is excreted by the kidneys. If the urine is alkaline most of the drug exists in the un-ionised form, which is readily reabsorbed by the kidney tubules so that little is lost. In acid urine, little of the drug is in the un-ionised form so that little can be reabsorbed and much of it is lost. A more detailed and illustrated account of this interaction mechanism is given in the introductory chapter.

Importance and management

A well established and well understood interaction but reports of clinical problems arising as a result are very sparse. The interaction can be usefully exploited to clear amfetamine (amphetamine) from the body more rapidly in cases of overdosage by acidifying the urine with ammonium chloride. Conversely it can represent an undesirable interaction if therapeutic doses of amfetamine are excreted too rapidly. Care is needed to ensure that amfetamine intoxication does not develop if the urine is made alkaline with sodium bicarbonate or acetazolamide.

1. Beckett AH, Rowland M, Turner P. Influence of urinary pH on excretion of amphetamine. *Lancet* (1965) i, 303.
2. Rowland M, Beckett AH. The amphetamines: clinical and pharmacokinetic implications of recent studies of an assay procedure and urinary excretion in man. *Arzneimittelforschung* (1966) 16, 1369–73.
3. Änggård E, Jönsson L-E, Hogmark A-L, Gunne L-M. Amphetamine metabolism in amphetamine psychosis. *Clin Pharmacol Ther* (1973) 14, 870–80.

Beta-agonist bronchodilators + Potassium-depleting drugs

Beta-agonists (e.g. fenoterol, terbutaline, salbutamol (albuterol)) can cause hypokalaemia. This can be increased by other potassium-depleting drugs such as the corticosteroids, diuretics (bumetanide, etacrynic acid (ethacrynic acid), furosemide (frusemide), thiazides, etc.) and theophylline. The risk of serious heart arrhythmias in asthmatic patients may be increased.

Clinical evidence

(a) Beta-agonist bronchodilators + Corticosteroids

24 normal healthy subjects showed a fall in serum potassium levels when given either 5 mg **salbutamol (albuterol)** or 5 mg **fenoterol** by nebuliser over 30 min. These falls were increased after taking 30 mg **prednisone** daily for a week. The greatest fall (from 3.75 to 2.78 mmol/l) was found 90 min after **fenoterol** and **prednisone**. The ECG effects observed included ectopic beats and transient T wave inversion, but no significant interaction was noted for ECG disturbances in these healthy subjects.[1] However, there is evidence that the risk of mortality may be increased in corticosteroid-dependent asthmatics who take beta-agonists.[2]

(b) Beta-agonist bronchodilators + Diuretics

The serum potassium levels of 15 normal subjects were measured after inhaling 5000 micrograms **terbutaline** while taking either a placebo, or 40 mg **furosemide (frusemide)** daily, or 40 mg **furosemide** + 50 mg **triamterene** daily for four days. With **terbutaline** alone the levels fell from 3.88 to 3.35 mmol/l; after taking **furosemide** as well they fell to 3.13 mmol/l; and after **furosemide** and **triamterene** they fell to only 3.29 mmol/l. These falls were reflected in some ECG (T wave) changes.[3]

After seven days' treatment with 5 mg **bendroflumethiazide (bendrofluazide)** daily for a week the serum potassium levels of 10 normal subjects had fallen from 3.78 to 3.07 mmol/l. After taking 100–2000 micrograms inhaled **salbutamol (albuterol)** as well, the levels fell to 2.72 mmol/l. ECG changes consistent with hypokalaemia and hypomagnesaemia were also seen.[4]

Other diuretics which can cause potassium loss include **bumetanide, furosemide, etacrynic acid (ethacrynic acid)**, the **thiazides**, and many **other related diuretics**. See Table 14.2.

(c) Beta-agonist bronchodilators + Theophylline

The concurrent use of **salbutamol (albuterol)** or **terbutaline** and **theophylline** can cause a fall in serum potassium levels. There is a theoretical risk with other beta-agonists. See details under 'Theophylline + Beta-agonist bronchodilators', p.791 (refer to Index).

Mechanism

Additive potassium-losing effects.

Importance and management

Established interactions. The CSM in the UK[5] give the following advice: "Potentially serious hypokalaemia may result from beta$_2$-adrenoceptor stimulant therapy. Particular caution is required in severe asthma, as this effect may be potentiated by concomitant treatment with theophylline and its derivatives, corticosteroids, and diuretics, and hypoxia. Plasma potassium concentrations should therefore be monitored in severe asthma". Hypokalaemia may result in heart arrhythmias in patients with ischaemic heart disease and may also affect the response of patients to drugs such as the digitalis glycosides and antiarrhythmics.

1. Taylor DR, Wilkins GT, Herbison GP, Flannery EM. Interaction between corticosteroid and β-agonist drugs. Biochemical and cardiovascular effects in normal subjects. *Chest* (1992) 102, 519–24.
2. Crane J, Pearce N, Flatt A, Burgess C, Jackson R, Kwong T, Ball M, Beasley R. Prescribed fenoterol and death from asthma in New Zealand, 1981–1983: case-control study. *Lancet* (1989) i, 917–22.
3. Newnham DM, McDevitt DG, Lipworth BJ. The effects of frusemide and triamterene on the hypokalaemic and electrocardiographic responses to inhaled terbutaline. *Br J Clin Pharmacol* (1991) 32, 630–2.
4. Lipworth BJ, McDevitt DG, Struthers AD. Prior treatment with diuretic augments the hypokalemic and electrocardiographic effects of inhaled albuterol. *Am J Med* (1989) 86, 653–7.
5. Committee on Safety of Medicines. β$_2$ agonists, xanthines and hypokalaemia. *Current Problems* 28 1990.

Dobutamine or Amrinone + Calcium chloride

Calcium chloride infusion reduces the cardiotonic effects of dobutamine but not those of amrinone.

Clinical evidence, mechanism, importance and management

An experimental study of the mode of action of dobutamine in 22 patients recovering from aortocoronary bypass surgery found that an infusion of **calcium chloride** (1 mg/kg/min initially, later 0.25 mg/kg/min) reduced by 30% the increase in cardiac output produced by dobutamine (an infusion of 2.5–5.0 micrograms/kg/min). The cardiotonic actions of **amrinone** (a phosphodiesterase inhibitor) in a group of 24 similar patients were unaffected by the **calcium** infusion.[1] Just how the **calcium** alters the dobutamine effects is not known but since dobutamine is a beta-receptor agonist it is reasonable to postulate that it interferes with the signal transduction through the beta-adrenergic receptor complex. The clinical importance of these findings is uncertain.

1. Butterworth JF, Zaloga GP, Prielipp RC, Tucker WY, Royster RL. Calcium inhibits the cardiac stimulating properties of dobutamine but not of amrinone. *Chest* (1992) 101, 174–80.

Dobutamine + Cimetidine

An isolated report describes an exaggerated hypertensive response to dobutamine in a patient on cimetidine while undergoing anaesthetic induction before surgery.

Clinical evidence, mechanism, importance and management

A patient developed unexpectedly marked hypertension (210/100 mmHg) in response to the infusion of dobutamine (5 micrograms/kg/min) during induction of anaesthesia (with midazolam, fentanyl, vecuronium and oxygen) for coronary artery bypass grafting. The infusion was stopped and over the next 15 min the blood pressure fell to 90/59 mmHg. A new infusion had just the same hypertensive effect, and his blood pressure was subsequently controlled at 120/80 mmHg with only 1 micrograms/kg/min of dobutamine.[1]

The authors of the report suggest that this exaggerated response to dobutamine may have been due to the 1 g **cimetidine** which the patient was taking daily. They postulate that the **cimetidine** may possibly have inhibited the metabolism and clearance of the dobutamine by the liver, thereby increasing its effects.[1] This is an isolated case and its general importance is not known, but it would now seem prudent to reduce the dosage of dobutamine initially in patients taking **cimetidine**.

1. Baraka A, Nauphal M, Arab W. Cimetidine–dobutamine interaction? *Anaesthesia* (1992) 47, 965–66.

Dobutamine + Dipyridamole

The addition of dipyridamole to dobutamine for echocardiography can cause potentially hazardous hypotension.

Clinical evidence, mechanism, importance and management

Ten patients with a low probability of coronary artery disease underwent dobutamine echocardiography. Five were given dobutamine alone, while the other 5 had a low dose of **dipyridamole** added to the maximal dose of dobutamine to see whether the sensitivity of the test could be improved. Four of the patients given both drugs experienced severe hypotension while no hypotension was seen in the control group. The conclusion was reached that this combination of drugs can be hazardous and should not be used in patients suspected of coronary heart disease.[1]

1. Shaheen J, Rosenmann D, Tzivoni D. Severe hypotension induced by combination of dobutamine and dipyridamole. *Isr J Med Sci* (1996) 32, 1105–7.

Dobutamine + Theophylline

A man on theophylline about to undergo surgery, developed marked tachycardia when treated with dobutamine.

Clinical evidence, mechanism, importance and management

An asthmatic patient taking 150 mg **theophylline** twice daily, digoxin and spironolactone was anaesthetised for aortic valve replacement with fentanyl, midazolam and pipecuronium. Following induction, intubation and ventilation with 100% oxygen, his systolic blood pressure fell from 120 to 80 mmHg, and his heart slowed from 70 to 50 bpm. Dobutamine was then infused at 5 micrograms/kg/min, whereupon 2–3 min later his heart rate rose to 150 bpm and his systolic pressure rose to 190 mmHg. The authors of the report[1] attribute the tachycardia to a dobutamine/**theophylline** interaction resulting from a synergistic increase in cyclic AMP levels in cardiac muscle. They advise the careful titration of dobutamine in any asthmatic taking **theophylline**, particularly if a slow-release preparation is being used. More study of this apparent interaction is needed.

1. Baraka A, Darwish R, Rizkallah P. Excessive dobutamine-induced tachycardia in the asthmatic cardiac patient: possible potentiation by theophylline therapy. *J Cardiothorac Vasc Anesth* (1993) 7, 641–4.

Dopamine + Ergometrine (Ergonovine)

A single report attributes the development of gangrene in a patient to the infusion of dopamine after ergometrine.

Clinical evidence, mechanism, importance and management

Gangrene of the hands and feet has been described in one patient who was given an infusion of dopamine following the administration of **ergometrine**.[1] This would seem to have resulted from the additive peripheral vasoconstrictor effects of both drugs which reduced the circulation to such an extent that infection became unchecked. It would seem prudent to avoid concurrent use or monitor the outcome extremely closely.

1. Buchanan N, Cane RD, Miller M. Symmetrical gangrene of the extremities associated with the use of dopamine subsequent to ergometrine administration. *Intensive Care Med* (1977) 3, 55–6.

Dopamine + Phenytoin

There is some limited evidence that patients needing dopamine to support their blood pressure can become severely hypotensive if phenytoin is added to their treatment.

Clinical evidence, mechanism, importance and management

Five critically ill patients with a variety of conditions and under treatment with a number of different drugs, were given dopamine hydrochloride to maintain an adequate blood pressure. When seizures developed they were additionally given **phenytoin** at an infusion rate of 10–25 mg/min. Coincidentally their hitherto stable blood pressures fell rapidly and one patient died from cardiorespiratory arrest. A similar reaction was demonstrated in *dogs* made hypovolaemic and hypotensive by bleeding.[1] However another study in *dogs* was unable to find evidence of this serious adverse interaction,[2] and no evidence of marked hypotension occurred in a patient with cardiogenic shock on dopamine and dobutamine when a **phenytoin** infusion was added.[3]

The documentation of this adverse interaction is limited to this single report so that it is not fully established, but there is enough evidence to suggest that **phenytoin** should only be used with great caution in those requiring dopamine to maintain their blood pressure. More study is needed.

1. Bivins BA, Rapp RP, Griffin WO, Blouin R, Bustrack J. Dopamine-phenytoin interaction. A cause of hypotension in the critically ill. *Arch Surg* (1978) 113, 245–9.
2. Smith RD, Lomas TE. Modification of cardiovascular responses to intravenous phenytoin by dopamine in dogs: evidence against an adverse interaction. *Toxicol Appl Pharmacol* (1978) 45, 665–73.
3. Torres E, Garcia B, Sosa P, Alba D. No interaction between dopamine and phenytoin. *Ann Pharmacother* (1995) 29, 1300–1.

Dopamine + Tolazoline

Acute and eventually fatal hypotension occurred in a patient given dopamine and tolazoline concurrently.

Clinical evidence

A patient who had undergone surgery three days before was given dopamine to maintain his cardiac index at about 3.5 l/min/m². Pulmonary arterial pressure had been steadily rising since the surgery so that on day 4 he was given a slow bolus of **tolazoline** (2 mg/kg) to reduce the afterload of the right ventricle. Systemic arterial pressure immediately fell to 50/30 mmHg whereupon the dopamine infusion was increased, but the arterial pressure then fell even further to 38/15 mmHg. The dopamine was stopped and ephedrine, methoxamine and fresh frozen plasma were given. Two hours later his blood pressure was 70/40 mmHg. Two further attempts were made to infuse dopamine, but the arterial pressure fell to 40/15 mmHg on the first occasion, and to 38/20 mmHg on the second. The patient died of cardiac arrest.[1]

Mechanism

Not fully understood. Dopamine has both alpha (vasoconstrictor) and beta (vasodilator) activity. With the alpha effects on the systemic circulation competitively blocked by the tolazoline, its vasodilatory actions would predominate, resulting in paradoxical hypotension.

Importance and management

Information is limited but this interaction would appear to be established. The authors of this report warn that infusion of dopamine should not be considered for several hours after giving even a small dose of tolazoline. They point out that impaired renal function often accompanies severe respiratory failure which may significantly prolong the half-life of tolazoline and its effects.

1. Carlon GC. Fatal association of tolazoline and dopamine. *Chest* (1979) 76, 336.

Ephedrines + Adsorbents, Antacids, Urinary acidifiers and alkalinizers

Alkalinization of the urine by sodium bicarbonate or other urinary alkalinizers causes retention of ephedrine and pseudoephedrine in the body, leading to the possible development of toxicity (tremors, anxiety, insomnia, tachycardia). Acidification of the urine with ammonium chloride has the opposite effect because the loss is increased. Kaolin does not appear to interact significantly with pseudoephedrine but aluminium hydroxide may possibly cause a more rapid onset of activity.

Clinical evidence

(a) Ephedrine + Urinary acidifiers & alkalinizers

The excretion of **ephedrine** in the urine of three normal subjects, made acidic (about pH 5) with **ammonium chloride**, was two to fourfold higher than when the urine was made alkaline (about pH 8) with 3 g oral **sodium bicarbonate**.[1]

(b) Pseudoephedrine + Antacids or Urinary acidifiers & alkalinizers

Prompted by the observation of a patient with renal tubular acidosis and persistently alkaline urine who developed unexpected toxicity when given ordinary doses of **pseudoephedrine**, a study was made on eight adult and child subjects of the possible effects of changing the urinary pH on the loss or retention of **pseudoephedrine** by the body. When the urinary pH was made alkaline with **sodium bicarbonate**, the half-life of a single 0.5 mg/kg dose of **pseudoephedrine** increased from 1.9 to 21 h.[2]

This confirms an earlier study in which it was found that when the urinary pH of three subjects was made about 8 (using **sodium bicarbonate**), the half-lives of **pseudoephedrine** were 16, 9.2 and 15 h respectively. When the pH was made about 5 (using **ammonium chloride**), the half-lives were 4.8, 3.0 and 6.4 respectively.[3]

Another study found that 5 g **sodium bicarbonate** increased the absorption rate at 2–4 h of a single 60-mg dose of **pseudoephedrine**.[4] The same study also found that 30 ml **aluminium hydroxide gel** did not affect the total amount of **pseudoephedrine** absorbed over 24 h but the rate of absorption was briefly increased.[4]

(c) Pseudoephedrine + Kaolin

30 ml of a 30% suspension of **kaolin** was found in a study in 6 normal subjects to cause a small decrease (about 10%) in the absorption of a single 60-mg dose of **pseudoephedrine**. The rate of absorption was also decreased.[4]

Mechanism

The ephedrines are basic drugs mainly excreted unchanged in the urine. In acid urine, most of the drug is ionised in the tubular filtrate and unable to diffuse passively back into the circulation, and is therefore lost in the urine. In alkaline urine, it mostly exists in the lipid-soluble form which is retained. As a result they are lost much more slowly and accumulate. The increased rate of absorption of pseudoephedrine in the gut seen with sodium bicarbonate and aluminium hydroxide is probably also due to pH rises which favour the formation of the lipid-soluble absorbable form of pseudoephedrine. The reduced absorption with kaolin is probably due to adsorption of the pseudoephedrine onto the surface of the kaolin.

Importance and management

The ephedrines/urinary alkalinizer interaction is established but reports of adverse reactions in patients appear to be rare. Monitor the outcome of alkalinizing the urine for any evidence of toxicity due to drug retention (tremor, anxiety, insomnia, tachycardia, etc.), reducing the dosage if necessary. **Acetazolamide** makes the urine alkaline and would be expected to interact with the ephedrines in the same way as sodium bicarbonate. Acidification of the urine with ammonium chloride increases the loss of the ephedrines in the urine and could be exploited in cases of drug overdosage. Aluminium hydroxide may possibly cause a more rapid onset of pseudoephedrine activity (but this needs confirmation) whereas the effects of kaolin on absorption are small and unlikely to be clinically important.

1. Wilkinson GR, Beckett AH. Absorption, metabolism and excretion of the ephedrines in man. I. The influence of urinary pH and urine volume output. *J Pharmacol Exp Ther* (1968) 162, 139–47.
2. Brater DC, Kaojarern S, Benet LZ, Lin ET, Lockwood T, Morris RC, McSherry EJ, Melmon KL. Renal excretion of pseudoephedrine. *Clin Pharmacol Ther* (1980) 28, 690–4.
3. Kuntzman RG, Tsai I, Brand L, Mark LC. The influence of urinary pH on the plasma half-life of pseudoephedrine in man and dog and a sensitive assay for its determination in human plasma. *Clin Pharmacol Ther* (1971) 12, 62–7.
4. Lucarotti RL, Colaizzi JL, Barry H, Poust RI. Enhanced pseudoephedrine absorption by concurrent administration of aluminium hydroxide gel in humans. *J Pharm Sci* (1972) 61, 903–5.

Methylphenidate + Clonidine

Much publicised fears about the serious consequences of using methylphenidate with clonidine appear to be unfounded. There is evidence that concurrent can be both safe and effective.

Clinical evidence, mechanism, importance and management

The current summary of product characteristics for methylphenidate in the UK[1] carries the following statement. "Serious adverse events have been reported in concomitant use with clonidine, although no causality for the combination has been established. The safety of using methylphenidate in combination with clonidine or other centrally acting alpha-2 agonists has not been systematically evaluated." Similar statements are also included in the US product information.

A thumb-nail sketch of the background to this somewhat ambivalent statement is that rumours began to circulate in the US in 1995, fuelled by national radio broadcasts and newspaper reports about the deaths of 3 children who were taking methylphenidate and **clonidine**. One died from ventricular fibrillation due to cardiac abnormalities, one from cardiac arrest attributed to an overdose of fluoxetine, and the third death is unexplained. Studies of these 3 cases and one other failed to establish any link between the use of the methylphenidate/**clonidine** combination and these deaths, the final broad conclusion being that the event was largely a media-inspired scare story built on inconclusive evidence.[2,3] A small scale pilot study in 24 patients suggested that the combination is both safe and effective for the treatment of attention deficit hyperactivity disorder[4], and the makers of one formulation of methylphenidate[5] say that they are ". . . not aware of any reports describing adverse events when using *Concerta XL* (methylphenidate) in combination with **clonidine**."

1. Concerta XL (Methyphenidate). Janssen-Cilag Ltd. Summary of product characteristics, February 2002.
2. Popper CW. Editorial commentary. Combining methylphenidate and clonidine: pharmacological questions and news reports about sudden death. *J Child Adolesc Psychopharmacol* (1995) 5, 157-166.
3. Fenichel RR. Special communication. Combining methylphenidate and clonidine: the role of post-marketing surveillance. *J Child Adolesc Psychopharmacol* (1995) 5, 155-156.
4. Connor DF, Barkley RA, Davis HT. A pilot study of methylphenidate, clonidine, or the combination in ADHD comorbid with aggressive oppositional defiant or conduct disorder. *Clin Pediatr* (2000) 39, 15-25.
5. Janssen-Cilag. Personal communication, April 2002.

3,4-Methylenedioxymethamphetamine (MDMA) + Citalopram

The psychological effects of 3,4-Methylenedioxymethamphetamine (MDMA, 'Ecstasy') are markedly reduced by the concurrent use of citalopram. It seems likely that other SSRIs will also reduce or block the effects of MDMA. An isolated report describes a neurotoxic reaction in a man on citalopram when he took unknown amounts of MDMA.

Clinical evidence

(a) Reduced MDMA effects

A double-blind placebo-controlled psychometric study in 16 normal subjects found that 3,4-Methylenedioxymethamphetamine (MDMA) - 'Ecstasy' produced an emotional state with heightened mood, increased self-confidence and extroversion, moderate derealisation and an intensification of perception.[1] Most of these effects were found to be markedly reduced by pretreatment with **citalopram** (40 mg intravenous).

(b) Neurotoxic reaction

When a man on 60 mg **citalopram** daily additionally took unknown amounts of **MDMA** he became aggressive, agitated, severely grandiose, restless and performed peculiar compulsive movements (". . . in a peculiar and joyless dancelike manner."). He lacked normal movement control and said he could see little bugs. He was treated with haloperidol and chlordiazepoxide, and improved within 2 days of replacing the **citalopram** by promazine.[2] This appears to be the first and only report of this reaction.

Mechanism

The psychological effects of MDMA are believed to be due to the release of serotonin (5-HT) and dopamine within the brain, which is blocked by 5-HT uptake inhibitors such as **citalopram**. The neurotoxic reaction is not understood.

Importance and management

This MDMA/citalopram study was primarily undertaken to find out how MDMA works, but on the basis of these results and *animal* studies it seems likely that patients already taking **citalopram** may not be able to get 'high' on usual doses of 'Ecstasy'. And if the proposed mechanism of interaction is correct, the same is also likely to be true if they are taking any other SSRI (such as **fluoxetine**, **fluvoxamine**, **paroxetine**, **sertraline**). The neurotoxic reaction cited seems to be an isolated case but it illustrates some of the risks attached to using 'recreational' drugs by patients already taking other medications, particularly antidepressant and psychotropic drugs which affect the same receptors in the CNS.

1. Liechti ME, Baumann C, Gamma A, Vollenweider FX. Acute psychological effects of 3,4-methylenedioxymethamphetamine (MDMA, "Ecstasy") are attenuated by the serotonin uptake inhibitor citalopram. *Neuropsychopharmacology* (2000) 22, 513-21.
2. Lauerma H, Wuorela M, Halme M. Interaction of serotonin reuptake inhibitor and 3,4-methylenedioxymethamphetamine? *Biol Psychiatry* (1998) 43, 929.

Phenmetrazine + Amobarbital (Amylobarbitone)

The CNS side effects and the weight-reducing effects of phenmetrazine are reduced by amobarbital (amylobarbitone).

Clinical evidence, mechanism, importance and management

A comparative study in 50 overweight adults of the effects of either 75 mg phenmetrazine daily or 50 mg phenmetrazine plus 30 mg **amobarbital (amylobarbitone)** daily found that although the adverse CNS side-effects, particularly insomnia, headache and nervousness, were decreased by the presence of the barbiturate, the weight reducing effects were also decreased (by 65%).[1]

1. Hadler AJ. Phenmetrazine vs. phenmetrazine with amobarbital for weight reduction: a double-blind study. *Curr Ther Res* (1969) 11, 750-4.

Phentermine + Fluoxetine

An isolated report describes phentermine toxicity in a woman shortly after stopping fluoxetine.

Clinical evidence, mechanism, importance and management

A woman of 22 who had successfully and uneventfully taken 20 mg **fluoxetine** daily for 3 months, stopped the **fluoxetine** and then 8 days later took a single 30-mg tablet of phentermine. Within a few hours she experienced racing thoughts, stomach cramps, palpitations (pulse 84), tremors, dry eyes and diffuse hyper-reflexia. The problems had all resolved the following day after taking 1.5 mg lorazepam. The authors of this report interpreted what happened as an interaction between the phentermine and the residual inhibitory effects of the **fluoxetine** on liver cytochrome P450 enzymes, which (they postulated) lead to elevated phentermine serum levels with the resultant sympathetic hyperstimulation. It is known that **fluoxetine** and its active metabolite are only cleared from the body slowly and can persist for weeks. The authors also alternatively tentatively wondered whether some of the symptoms might have fitted the serotonin syndrome.[1]

This is an isolated case and its general importance is unknown, but the authors of the report draw attention to the possible risks of taking SSRIs and sympathomimetic drugs used for controlling diet.

1. Bostwick JM, Brown TM. A toxic reaction from combining fluoxetine and phentermine. *J Clin Psychopharmacol* (1996) 16, 189-90.

Phenylephrine + Atropine

The hypertensive and other serious adverse effects of phenylephrine absorbed from eye drops can be markedly increased by atropine.

Clinical evidence

A brief report describes seven cases of a "pseudo-phaeochromocytoma" with severe rises in blood pressure and tachycardia in young adults and children undergoing eye operations when treated with 10% phenylephrine eye drops and **atropine**. Only two of them had any pre-existing cardiovascular illness (moderate hypertension). All were under general anaesthesia with propofol, phenoperidine and vecuronium, and premedicated with intramuscular **atropine**, and some were later given more intravenous **atropine** because of the bradycardia when the oculomotor muscles were stretched. The total **atropine** doses were less than 0.01 mg/kg in adults and 0.02 mg/kg in the children. At least 0.4 ml of 10% phenylephrine was used. In three cases left ventricular failure occurred with pulmonary oedema that needed monitoring in intensive care.[1]

In a study of this interaction, six normal subjects were given a phenylephrine infusion (0.42 micrograms/kg/min) before and after being given three intravenous doses of **atropine** (0.02, 0.01, 0.01 mg/kg) at 90, 120 and 150 min. It was found that a dose of phenylephrine which raised the diastolic and systolic blood pressures by 4 mmHg before using **atropine**, raised the pressures by 17 mmHg when **atropine** was present. For safety reasons the increases in blood pressure were limited to 30 mmHg above the base line.[2]

Mechanism

Phenylephrine causes vasoconstriction which can raise the blood pressure. Normally this would be limited by a baro-reflex mediated by the vagus nerve, but if this cholinergic mechanism is blocked by atropine, the rise in blood pressure is then largely uncontrolled. Severe hypertension may occur, and other adverse cardiac events such as acute heart failure may follow.

Importance and management

A surprisingly large amount of phenylephrine can be absorbed from eye drops, and the potential adverse effects of this (severe hypertension, cardiac arrhythmias, myocardial infarction) are now well documented.[3-5] The reports cited here are good evidence that these risks are increased by the presence of atropine, and this interaction is established. It is clearly potentially serious. The authors of the report cited[1] suggest that the risks can be reduced by reducing the concentrations of phenylephrine used, swabbing to minimise the amounts which drain into the nasolachrimal duct to the nasal mucosa where rapid absorption occurs, and reducing the drop size by using a thin-walled cannula.[6] Other suggestions for reducing systemic absorption are punctal plugging, nasolachrimal duct compression, and lid closure after instillation of the eye drop.[6]

1. Daelman F, Andréjak M, Rajaonarivony D, Bryselbout E, Jezraoui P, Ossart M. Phenylephrine eyedrops, systemic atropine and cardiovascular adverse events. *Therapie* (1994) 49, 467.
2. Levine MAH, Leenen FHH. Role of vagal activity in the cardiovascular responses to phenylephrine in man. *Br J Clin Pharmacol* (1992) 33, 333–6.
3. Fraunfelder FT, Scafidi AF. Possible adverse effects from topical ocular 10% phenylephrine. *Am J Ophthalmol* (1978) 85, 447–53.
4. Van der Spek AFL, Hantler CB. Phenylephrine eyedrops and anesthesia. *Anesthesiology* (1986) 64, 812–4.
5. Lai Y-K. Adverse effect of intraoperative phenylephrine 10%: case report. *Br J Ophthalmol* (1989) 73, 468–9.
6. Craig EW, Griffiths PG. Effect on mydriasis of modifying the volume of phenylephrine in drops. *Br J Ophthalmol* (1991) 75, 222–3.

Phenylpropanolamine + Caffeine

Phenylpropanolamine can raise blood pressure and this may be further increased by caffeine. Phenylpropanolamine can also markedly raise serum caffeine levels. Combined use may result in a hypertensive crisis in a few particularly susceptible individuals and increase the risk of intracranial haemorrhage. Manic psychosis has also been seen.

Clinical evidence

After taking 75 mg phenylpropanolamine or 400 mg **caffeine** alone, or both together, the blood pressures of 16 normal subjects rose from 137/85 mmHg to 148/97 mmHg, and after 150 mg phenylpropanolamine alone they rose to 173/103 mmHg. One of the subjects had a hypertensive crisis after 150 mg phenylpropanolamine and again 2 h after 400 mg **caffeine**. This needed antihypertensive treatment.[1] The same group of workers describe a similar study in which the AUC of **caffeine** increased more than 20–fold (from 0.8 to 18.5 micrograms h/ml) when taken with 75 mg phenylpropanolamine, and the peak serum **caffeine** level increased almost fourfold (from 2.1 to 8.0 micrograms/ml).[2]

Additive effects on blood pressure are described in another report.[3] Mania with psychotic delusions occurred in a healthy woman (who

normally drank 8–10 cups of **coffee** daily) within 4 days of starting to take a phenylpropanolamine-containing decongestant. She recovered within a week of stopping both the **coffee** and the phenylpropanolamine.[4]

Mechanism

Uncertain. Simple additive hypertensive effects would seem to be part of the explanation.

Importance and management

Established interactions. These studies illustrate the potential hazards of these drugs, even in normal healthy individuals, but it has to be said that there seem to be no other reports of adverse reactions, which is perhaps surprising bearing in mind that coffee is very widely used and phenylpropanolamine is also widely available over the counter. The authors of one report[1] advise that likely users of phenylpropanolamine (those with allergies, or overweight, or postpartum women) and those particularly vulnerable (elderly or hypertensive) should be warned about taking more than the recommended doses, and of taking caffeine at the same time, because of the possible risk of intracranial haemorrhage. The effects of high levels of caffeine (insomnia, jitteriness, nervousness, agitation) are undesirable and unpleasant.

1. Lake CR, Zaloga G, Bray J, Rosenberg D, Chernow B. Transient hypertension after two phenylpropanolamine diet aids and the effects of caffeine: a placebo-controlled follow-up study. *Am J Med* (1989) 86, 427–32.
2. Lake CR, Rosenberg DB, Gallant S, Zaloga G, Chernow B. Phenylpropanolamine increases plasma caffeine levels. *Clin Pharmacol Ther* (1990) 47, 675–85.
3. Brown NJ, Ryder D, Branch RA. A pharmacodynamic interaction between caffeine and phenylpropanolamine. *Clin Pharmacol Ther* (1991) 50, 363–71.
4. Lake CR. Manic psychosis after coffee and phenylpropanolamine. *Biol Psychiatry* (1991) 30, 401–4.

Phenylpropanolamine + Indometacin (Indomethacin)

An isolated case report describes a patient on phenylpropanolamine who developed serious hypertension after taking a single dose of indometacin (indomethacin), but a controlled study in other subjects failed to find any evidence of an adverse interaction.

Clinical evidence

A woman who had been taking one *Trimolet* (85 mg D-phenylpropanolamine) daily for several months as an appetite suppressant, developed a severe bifrontal headache within 15 min of taking 25 mg **indometacin (indomethacin)**. Thirty min later her systolic blood pressure was 210 mmHg and the diastolic was unrecordable. A later study on her confirmed that neither drug on its own caused this response, but when taken together the blood pressure rose to a maximum of 200/150 mmHg within half an hour of taking the **indometacin**, and was associated with bradycardia. The blood pressure was rapidly reduced by phentolamine.[1]

In contrast, a controlled study, carried out to investigate this possible interaction, failed to find any evidence that the concurrent use of 75 mg **indometacin** twice daily and 75 mg slow release phenylpropanolamine daily in 14 healthy young women caused a rise in blood pressure.[2]

Mechanism

Not understood.

Importance and management

Direct information seems to be limited to these reports. They suggest that an adverse hypertensive response is very unlikely in most normal individuals given these doses, but it should be borne in mind that phenylpropanolamine, even on its own, can sometimes cause severe hypertension.[3-5]

1. Lee KY, Beilin LJ, Vandongen R. Severe hypertension after ingestion of an appetite suppressant (phenylpropanolamine) with indomethacin. *Lancet* (1979) i, 1110 11.
2. McKenney JM, Wright JT, Katz GM, Goodman RP. The effect of phenylpropanolamine on 24–hour blood pressure in normotensive subjects administered indomethacin. *DICP Ann Pharmacother* (1991) 25, 234–9.
3. Livingstone PH. Transient hypertension and phenylpropanolamine. *JAMA* (1966) 196, 1159.
4. Duvernoy WFC. Positive phentolamine test in hypertension induced by a nasal decongestant. *N Engl J Med* (1969) 280, 877.
5. Shapiro SR. Hypertension due to anorectic agent. *N Engl J Med* (1969) 280, 1363.

Ritodrine + Miscellaneous drugs

Supraventricular tachycardia developed in a woman on ritodrine when given glycopyrrolate (glycopyrronium). The abuse of cocaine does not appear to increase the incidence of side effects in patients given ritodrine.

Clinical evidence, mechanism, importance and management

Premature labour in a 39-year-old who was 28 weeks pregnant was arrested with an intravenous infusion of ritodrine hydrochloride. Two weeks later while on the maximum dose of ritodrine (0.3 mg.min^{-1}) her uterine contractions began again and she was scheduled for emergency caesarian section. It was noted in the operating room that she had copious oral secretions so she was given 100% oxygen by mask and 0.2 mg **glycopyrrolate (glycopyrronium)** intravenously. Shortly afterwards she developed superventricular tachycardia (a rise from 80 to 170–180 bpm) which was converted to sinus tachycardia (130 bpm) with 0.5 mg propranolol intravenously in divided doses.[1]

The reason for this reaction is not understood. Ritodrine alone has been responsible for tachyarrhythmias and one possible explanation for this interaction is that the effects of these two drugs were additive. Two other cases of tachyarrhythmia have been described in patients premedicated with **atropine** who were given ritodrine as a single intravenous bolus.[2] Information is very limited and the interaction is not well established but some caution is clearly appropriate if both drugs are used. The authors of the first report advise avoidance.

A study in patients found no evidence of an increase in adverse side-effects in pregnant patients given ritodrine for premature labour who had been abusing **cocaine**.[3]

1. Simpson JI, Giffin JP. A glycopyrrolate-ritodrine drug-drug interaction. *Can J Anaesth* (1988) 35, 187–9.
2. Sheybany S, Murphy JF, Evans D, Newcombe RG, Pearson JF. Ritodrine in the management of fetal distress. *Br J Obstet Gynaecol* (1982) 89, 723–6.
3. Darby MJ, Mazdisnian F. Does recent cocaine use increase the risk of side effects with β-adrenergic tocolysis? *Am J Obstet Gynecol* (1991) 164, 377.

Sympathomimetics (directly and indirectly-acting) + Clonidine

Experimental studies in patients show that pretreatment with clonidine can increase the blood pressure responses to ephedrine and phenylephrine, but not those of norepinephrine (noradrenaline). In the context of adverse reactions these increases appear to be of little clinical importance.

Clinical evidence, mechanism, importance and management

A study in 75 patients (38 premedicated with 5 micrograms/kg **clonidine** with 20 mg famotidine, and a control group of 39 given only famotidine and 90 min later anaesthetised with thiamylal) found that the pressor response to **phenylephrine** (2 micrograms/kg as an intravenous bolus) was augmented but not the response to **norepinephrine (noradrenaline)** (0.5 micrograms/kg). The reasons are not understood. There were no significant differences between the groups in terms of hypertension, arrhythmia or bradycardia.[1] A similar and related study by the same group of workers using enflurane and nitrous oxide for anaesthesia found that the mean maximal blood pressure increases in the **clonidine** group when given **phenylephrine** (2 micrograms/kg as an intravenous bolus) were +26% and +32% respectively for awake and anaesthetised subjects, and +13% and +18% respectively in the control group.[2] The authors of the first report[1] said that "... the degree of pressor augmentation after both agents (**phenylephrine** and **norepinephrine**) may be of little clinical importance." The findings of these studies are in line with those of other studies with patients who showed a blood pressure augmentation when given intravenous **ephedrine** 0.1 mg/kg after pretreatment with **clonidine**.[3]

1. Tanaka M, Nishikawa T. Effects of clonidine premedication on the pressor response to α-adrenergic agonists. *Br J Anaesth* (1995) 75, 593–7.
2. Inomata S, Nishikawa T, Kihara S, Akiyoshi Y. Enhancement of pressor response to intravenous phenylephrine following oral clonidine medication in awake and anaesthetized patients. *Can J Anaesth* (1995) 42, 119–25.
3. Nishikawa T, Kimura T, Taguchi N, Dohi S. Oral clonidine preanesthetic medication augments the pressor responses to intravenous ephedrine in awake or anesthetized patients. *Anesthesiology* (1991) 74, 705–10.

Sympathomimetics (directly and indirectly-acting) + Lithium carbonate

The effects of norepinephrine (noradrenaline) and phenylephrine on blood pressure are slightly reduced by lithium carbonate. Tyramine does not interact.

Clinical evidence, mechanism, importance and management

A study in 8 patients with manic depression found that after taking **lithium carbonate** for 7–10 days (serum level range 0.72–1.62 mmol/l) the dosage of **norepinephrine (noradrenaline)** had to be increased by 1.8 micrograms in 7 of the 8 to raise the blood pressure by 25 mmHg. The pressor effect of the **norepinephrine (noradrenaline)** was reduced 22% by the **lithium**.[1] Another study in 17 depressed patients with serum **lithium** levels in the range 0.8–1.2 mmol/l found that 12% more **norepinephrine (noradrenaline)** was needed to raise the blood pressure by 30 mmHg, and 31% more **phenylephrine**.[2] The reasons are not known. In both of these studies the pressor effects of **tyramine** were found to be unaffected by the presence of the **lithium**.[1,2]

These decreases in the pressor response to **norepinephrine (noradrenaline)** and to **phenylephrine** in the presence of **lithium carbonate** are both relatively small and it seems unlikely that they will present any problems in practice.

1. Fann WE, Davis JM, Jonowsky DS, Cavanaugh JH, Kaufmann JS, Griffith JD, Oates JA. Effects of lithium on adrenergic function in man. *Clin Pharmacol Ther* (1972) 13, 71–7.
2. Ghose K. Assessment of peripheral adrenergic activity and its interactions with drugs in man. *Eur J Clin Pharmacol* (1980) 17, 233–8.

Sympathomimetics (directly and indirectly-acting) + Rauwolfia alkaloids

The pressor and other effects of directly acting sympathomimetics (epinephrine (adrenaline), norepinephrine (noradrenaline), phenylephrine, etc.) are slightly increased in the presence of the rauwolfia alkaloids. The effects of indirectly acting sympathomimetics or those with mixed activity (amphetamines, mephentermine, ephedrine, phenylpropanolamine, etc.) may be reduced or abolished.

Clinical evidence

After taking 0.25–1.0 mg **reserpine** daily for two weeks the pressor responses of seven normal subjects to **norepinephrine (noradrenaline)** were slightly increased (20–40%) but their responses to **tyramine** (an indirectly acting amine) were reduced about 75%.[1] A man on **reserpine** who became hypotensive while undergoing surgery failed to respond to an intravenous injection of **ephedrine**, but did so after 30 min treatment with **norepinephrine**, presumably because the stores of **norepinephrine** at adrenergic neurones had become replenished.[2] A child who had accidentally taken **reserpine** (thought to be about 6.5 mg) also failed to respond to an intramuscular injection of **ephedrine** (16 mg).[3] The mydriatic effects of **ephedrine** in man were shown to be antagonised by pretreatment with **reserpine**,[4] but a number of patients on **reserpine** were found to have increased blood pressures (+30/+13 mmHg) during surgery if pretreated with **phenylephrine eye drops**.[5]

Experiments with *dogs* have demonstrated that **epinephrine (adrenaline)**, **norepinephrine** and **phenylephrine** – all with direct actions – remain effective vasopressors after treatment with **reserpine** and their actions are enhanced to some extent, whereas the vasopressor actions of **ephedrine**, **amfetamine (amphetamine)**, **methamphetamine**, **tyramine** and **mephentermine** – all with indirect actions – are reduced or abolished by **reserpine**.[6-8]

Mechanism

The rauwolfia alkaloids cause adrenergic neurones to lose their stores of norepinephrine, so that they can no longer stimulate adrenergic receptors and transmission ceases. Indirectly acting sympathomimetics (which depend on their ability to stimulate the release of stored noradrenaline) may therefore be expected to become ineffective, whereas the effects of directly acting sympathomimetics should remain unchanged or possibly even enhanced because of the supersensitivity of the receptors which occurs when they are deprived of stimulation by norepinephrine for any length of time. Drugs with mixed direct and indirect actions, such as ephedrine, should fall somewhere between the two, although the reports cited seem to indicate that ephedrine has predominantly indirect activity in man.[2-4]

Importance and management

These are established interactions, but the paucity of clinical information suggests that in practice these interactions do not present many problems. If a pressor drug is required, a directly acting drug such as norepinephrine (noradrenaline) or phenylephrine may be expected to be effective. Metaraminol has also been successfully used as a pressor drug in reserpine-treated patients.[9] The receptors may show some supersensitivity so that a dosage reduction may be required. Somewhat surprisingly in the light of the other evidence, one report claims that 25 mg ephedrine given orally or intramuscularly, once or twice a day, proved to be an effective treatment for reserpine-induced hypotension and bradycardia in schizophrenic patients.[10]

1. Abboud FM, Ekstein JW. Effects of small oral doses of reserpine on vascular responses to tyramine and norepinephrine in man. *Circulation* (1964) 29, 219–23.
2. Ziegler CH, Lovette JB. Operative complications after therapy with reserpine and reserpine compounds. *JAMA* (1961) 176, 916–19.
3. Phillips T. Overdose of reserpine. *BMJ* (1955) 2, 969.
4. Sneddon JM, Turner P. Ephedrine mydriasis in hypotension and the response to treatment. *Clin Pharmacol Ther* (1969) 10, 64–71.
5. Kim JM, Stevenson CE, Matthewson HS. Hypertensive reactions to phenylephrine eye-drops in patients with sympathetic denervation. *Am J Ophthalmol* (1978) 85, 862–8.
6. Stone CA, Ross CA, Wenger HC, Ludden CT, Blessing JA, Totaro JA, Porter CC. Effect of α-methyl-3,4-dihydroxyphenylalanine (methyldopa), reserpine and related agents on some vascular responses in the dog. *J Pharmacol Exp Ther* (1962) 136, 80–8.

7. Eger EI, Hamilton WK. The effect of reserpine on the action of various vasopressors. *Anesthesiology* (1959) 20, 641–5.
8. Moore JI, Moran NC. Cardiac contractile force responses to ephedrine and other sympathomimetic amines in dogs after pretreatment with reserpine. *J Pharmacol Exp Ther* (1962) 136, 89–96.
9. Smessaert AA, Hicks RG. Problems caused by rauwolfia drugs during anesthesia and surgery. *N Y State J Med* (1961) 61, 2399–2403.
10. Noce RH, Williams DB, Rapaport W. Reserpine (Serpasil) in the management of the mentally ill. *JAMA* (1955) 158, 11–15.

Terbutaline + Magnesium sulphate

Terbutaline and parenteral magnesium sulphate appear not to interact adversely.

Clinical evidence, mechanism, importance and management

Eight normal healthy adults were given two doses of 0.25 mg terbutaline subcutaneously 30 min apart, with and without 4 g **magnesium sulphate** intravenously in 250 ml saline over the same 30-min period.[1] The effects of the terbutaline were found to be moderately increased (RR interval + 0.09 s; QTc + 0.01 s; diastolic pressure + 8 mmHg; systolic pressure reduced; serum calcium + 0.13 mg/dl; glucose + 9 mg/dl) but the size of all of the changes was only small. The conclusion was reached that there appear to be no good reasons for avoiding their concurrent use, for example in the emergency treatment of asthma and other conditions.

1. Skorodin MS, Freeback PC, Yetter B, Nelson JE, Vaan de Graaff WB, Walsh JM. Magnesium sulfate potentiates several cardiovascular and metabolic actions of terbutaline. *Chest* (1994) 105, 701—5.

Tyramine-rich foods + Cimetidine

A woman on cimetidine experienced a severe headache with hypertension when she drank *Bovril* and ate some cheese.

Clinical evidence, mechanism, importance and management

A woman of 77 with hiatus hernia, on 400 mg **cimetidine** four times daily for three years, experienced a severe frontal headache and hypertension which appeared to be related to the ingestion of a cup of *Bovril* and some **English cheddar cheese**, both of which can contain substantial amounts of **tyramine**.[1] Although the authors point out the similarity between this reaction and that which is seen in patients on MAOI who eat tyramine-rich foods (see 'Monoamine oxidase inhibitors (MAOIs) + Tyramine-rich foods', p.685), there is no satisfactory explanation for what occurred. This is an isolated report and there is no reason why patients in general on **cimetidine** should avoid **tyramine-rich foods**.

1. Griffin MJJ, Morris JS. MAOI-like reaction associated with cimetidine. *Drug Intell Clin Pharm* (1987) 21, 219.

22

Theophylline and related xanthine drug interactions

The main xanthines used in medicine are theophylline and aminophylline, the latter generally being preferred when greater water solubility is needed (e.g. in the formulation of injections). Xanthines are administered in the treatment of asthma because they relax the bronchial smooth muscle. In an attempt to improve upon theophylline, various different derivatives have been made such as diprophylline and enprofylline. Table 22.1 lists these xanthines along with their proprietary names.

Caffeine is also a xanthine and it is principally used as a central nervous system stimulant, increasing wakefulness, and mental and physical activity. It is most commonly taken in the form of tea, coffee, cola drinks ('*Coke*') and cocoa. Table 22.2 lists the usual caffeine content of these drinks. Caffeine is also included in hundreds of OTC analgesic preparations with aspirin, codeine or paracetamol, but whether it enhances the analgesic effect is debatable. Caffeine is also used to assess the activity of hepatic enzyme systems (particularly cytochrome P450 isoenzyme CYP1A2) and can usefully demonstrate altered liver function, notably from drugs, as well as disease states.

Interactions

Theophylline is metabolised by hepatic cytochrome P450 enzymes, principally CYP1A2, to demethylated and hydroxylated products. Many drugs interact with theophylline by inhibition or potentiation of its metabolism. Theophylline has a narrow therapeutic range, and small increases in serum levels can result in toxicity. Moreover, symptoms of serious toxicity such as convulsions and arrhythmias can occur before minor symptoms suggestive of toxicity. Within the context of interactions, aminophylline behaves like theophylline, because it is a complex of theophylline with ethylenediamine. Caffeine also undergoes extensive hepatic metabolism, principally by CYP1A2, and interacts with many drugs, but it has a wider therapeutic range. However, other xanthines may act differently (e.g. diprophylline does not undergo hepatic metabolism), so it should not be assumed that they all share common interactions. Note though, that all xanthines can potentiate hypokalaemia caused by other drugs, and that the toxic effects of different xanthines are additive. Where xanthines affect other drugs the interactions are covered elsewhere. The Index should be consulted for a full listing.

Table 22.1 Theophylline and related xanthines

Generic names	Proprietary names
Aminophylline	Aminocont, Aminomal, Amnivent, Asmodrin, Clonofilin, Drafilyn-Z, Elixophyllin, Escophylline, Euphyllin, Euphyllina, Filotempo, Mundiphyllin, Norphyllin SR, Peterphyllin, Phyllocontin, Phyllotemp, Tefamin, Teofylamin, Truphylline
Diprophylline (Diphylline)	Austrophyllin, Dilor, Dylix, Katasma, Lufyllin, Neufil
Doxofylline	Ansimar
Enprofylline	
Theophylline	Accurbron, Aerobin, Aerodyne, Aerolate, Afonilum, afpred-THEO, Alcophyllin, Almarion, Aminomal, Apo-Theo, Aquaphyllin, Asmalix, Asmasolon, Asthma T, Austyn, Bronchoparat, Bronchophen, Bronchoretard, Bronquiasma, Chantaline, Chronophyllin, Codrinan, Contiphyllin, Cronasma, Diffumal, Dilatrane, Ditenate N, Duraphyllin, Elixifilin, Elixomin, Elixophyllin, Eufilina, Euphyllin, Euphyllina, Euphylline, Euphylong, Franol, Frivent, Glyphyllin, Histafilin, Lasma, Lepobron, Med-Phylline, Microphyllin, Novo-Theophyl, Nuelin, Perasthman N, Phenedrine, Piridasmin, Pneumogeine, Pulmeno, Pulmidur, Pulmophyllin, Pulmo-Timelets, Quibron, Respbid, Respicur, Retafyllin, Slo-Bid, Slo-Phyllin, Sodip-phylline, Solosin, Sustaire, Talofilina, Tedralan, Tefamin, Temaco, Teobid, Teolixir, Teolong, Teophyl, Teovent, Theo, Theobid Duracaps, Theochron, Theoclear, Theofol, Theolair, Theolan, Theolin, Theolong, Theophar, Theophyllard, Theoplus, Theospan-SR, Theospirex, Theostat, Theotard, Theotrim, Theovent, Theo-24, Theo-Dur, Theo-X, Tromphyllin, T-Phyl, Unicontin, Unifyl, Unilair, Unilong, Uniphyl, Uniphyllin, UniXan, Uni-Dur, Uno-Lin, Vent Retard, Xanthium, Zepholin etc.

Table 22.2 Caffeine-containing herbs and caffeine-containing drinks

Source	Caffeine-content	Caffeine-content of drink
Cocoa[3]		up to 30 mg/100 ml
Coffee beans[1]	1–2%	up to 100 mg/100 ml, decaffeinated about 3 mg/100 ml
Guarana[2*]	2.5–7.0%	
Kola (Cola)[1]	1.5–2.5%	up to 20 mg/100 ml in 'Cola' drinks
Maté[1]	0.2–2.0%	
Tea[1]	1–5%	up to 60 mg/100 ml

1. Sweetman SC, editor. Martindale: The complete drug reference. 33rd ed. London: Pharmaceutical Press; (2002) p. 1681.
2. Houghton P. Herbal products 7. Guarana. Pharm J (1995) 254, 435–6.
3. Information taken from research conducted by the US Department of Nutritional Services. Available at http://www.holymtn.com/tea/caffeine_content.htm (Accessed 27/08/02).

* Note that guarana contains guaranine (which is known to be identical to caffeine) as well as small quantities of other xanthines.

Caffeine + Antiarrhythmics

The clearance of caffeine from the body is reduced 30 to 60% by the concurrent use of mexiletine, resulting in raised serum caffeine levels. Whether this might result in caffeine toxicity is uncertain. Lidocaine (lignocaine), flecainide and tocainide appear not to interact with caffeine.

Clinical evidence

(a) Mexiletine

Seven patients with cardiac arrhythmias had a 48% reduction in caffeine clearance when given long-term treatment with 600 mg **mexiletine** daily.[1] The clearance of a single 366-mg dose of caffeine was reduced by 57% (from 126 to 54 ml/min), and the elimination half-life rose from 246 to 419 minutes, in 5 normal subjects given a single 200-mg dose of **mexiletine**.[1] Conversely, the clearance of mexiletine was not affected by caffeine. In a similar study by the same authors, the caffeine clearance was reduced by 30% (from 77 to 54 ml/min) in 7 normal subjects given 200 mg **mexiletine**.[2] In 5 patients with cardiac arrhythmias given 600 mg mexiletine daily, caffeine clearance, was reduced by 48% (from 71 to 37 ml/min). Fasting caffeine levels were almost sixfold higher during the **mexiletine** treatment period (1.99 compared with 0.35 micrograms/ml).[2] In a third study in 14 healthy volunteers, caffeine 100 mg four times daily for 2 days before and 2 days after mexiletine did not cause significant changes in plasma mexiletine levels after a single dose of **mexiletine** 200 mg.[3] Although not specifically monitored, caffeine levels tended to be increased by the mexiletine.

(b) Flecainide, Lidocaine (lignocaine), Tocainide

Single doses of 200 mg **lidocaine**, 100 mg **flecainide** and 500 mg **tocainide** had no effect on caffeine clearance in 7 healthy volunteers given a single dose of 366 mg caffeine.[2]

Mechanism

Not understood. It is likely that, as with theophylline (see 'Theophylline + Mexiletine or Tocainide', p.805), mexiletine inhibits the hepatic metabolism of caffeine.

Importance and management

The caffeine/mexiletine interaction appears to be established, but its clinical importance is uncertain. Some of the side-effects of mexiletine treatment might be partially due to caffeine-retention (from drinking tea, coffee, 'Coke', etc.).[1] In excess caffeine can cause jitteriness, tremor and insomnia. It has also been suggested that the caffeine test for liver function might be impaired by mexiletine.[1] Be alert for these possible changes.

1. Joeres R, Klinker H, Heusler H, Epping J, Richter E. Influence of mexiletine on caffeine elimination. *Pharmacol Ther* (1987) 33, 163–9.
2. Joeres R, Richter E. Mexiletine and caffeine elimination. *N Engl J Med* (1987) 317, 117.
3. Labbé L, Abolfathi Z, Robitaille NM, St-Maurice F, Gilbert M, Turegon J. Stereoselective disposition of the antiarrhythmic agent mexiletine during the concomitant administration of caffeine. *Ther Drug Monit* (1999) 21, 191–9.

Caffeine + Anticonvulsants

Phenytoin can increase the loss of caffeine from the body, and possibly invalidate the caffeine liver function test. Whether carbamazepine increases caffeine metabolism is unclear. Valproate appears not to have any effect.

Clinical evidence

The clearance of caffeine was about twofold higher, and its half-life was about 50% shorter, in patients with epilepsy taking **phenytoin** than in healthy volunteers on no medications. In the same study, there were no significant differences in caffeine pharmacokinetics between healthy volunteers and patients receiving **carbamazepine** or **sodium valproate**.[1] Conversely, **carbamazepine** was considered to have induced the metabolism of caffeine in 5 children with epilepsy, as assessed by the caffeine breath test.[2] In another study, there was a reduction in **carbamazepine** AUC when coadministered with caffeine in healthy subjects, but caffeine had no effect on the pharmacokinetics of **sodium valproate**.[3]

Mechanism

Phenytoin acts as an enzyme inducer, thereby increasing the metabolism and loss of caffeine from the body. Carbamazepine possibly has the same effect.

Importance and management

Phenytoin may possibly invalidate the caffeine liver function test, but normally no special precautions are needed if both drugs are taken. The interaction between carbamazepine and caffeine requires further study.

1. Wietholtz H, Zysset T, Kreiten K, Kohl D, Büchsel R, Matern S. Effect of phenytoin, carbamazepine, and valproic acid on caffeine metabolism. *Eur J Clin Pharmacol* (1989) 36, 401–6.
2. Parker AC, Pritchard P, Preston T, Choonara I. Induction of CYP1A2 activity by carbamazepine in children using the caffeine breath test. *Br J Clin Pharmacol* (1998) 45, 176–8.
3. Vaz J, Kulkarni C, David J, Joseph T. Influence of caffeine on pharmacokinetic profile of sodium valproate and carbamazepine in normal healthy volunteers. *Indian J Exp Biol* (1998) 36, 112–14.

Caffeine + Antifungals

Fluconazole and terbinafine cause a modest rise in serum caffeine levels. Ketoconazole appears to have less effect.

Clinical evidence, mechanism, importance and management

A study in 6 young subjects (average age 24) and 5 elderly subjects (average age 69) found that 400 or 200 mg **fluconazole** respectively daily for 10 days reduced the clearance of the caffeine from the plasma by 25% (32% in the young and 17% in the old).[1] In a single-dose study in 8 healthy subjects, **terbinafine** 500 mg and **ketoconazole** 400 mg decreased caffeine clearance by 21% and 10% respectively, and increased the half-life by 31% and 16%, respectively.[2]

It seems unlikely that the moderately increased serum caffeine levels that result will have a clinically important effect, but this needs confirmation.

1. Nix DE, Zelenitsky SA, Symonds WT, Spivey JM, Norman A. The effect of fluconazole on the pharmacokinetics of caffeine in young and elderly subjects. *Clin Pharmacol Ther* (1992) 51, 183.
2. Wahlländer A, Paumgartner G. Effect of ketoconazole and terbinafine on the pharmacokinetics of caffeine in healthy volunteers. *Eur J Clin Pharmacol* (1989) 37, 279–83.

Caffeine + Calcium channel blockers

A small and relatively unimportant increase in the effects of caffeine may occur in patients given verapamil.

Clinical evidence, mechanism, importance and management

Verapamil 80 mg three times daily for 2 days decreased the total clearance of a single 200-mg dose of caffeine by 25%, and increased its half-life by 25% (from 4.6 to 5.8 h) in 6 healthy subjects.[1] These changes are small, and unlikely to be of much importance in most patients. In excess, caffeine (including that from tea, coffee and 'Coke') can cause jitteriness and insomnia.

1. Nawoot S, Wong D, Mays DC, Gerber N. Inhibition of caffeine elimination by verapamil. *Clin Pharmacol Ther* (1988) 43, 148.

Caffeine + Cimetidine

The effects of caffeine may be increased to some extent by cimetidine.

Clinical evidence, mechanism, importance and management

Cimetidine 1000 mg daily for 6 days increased the half-life of a single dose of 300 mg caffeine in 5 subjects by about 70% and reduced caffeine clearance.[1] In another study, **cimetidine** 1200 mg daily for 4 days increased the caffeine half-life by 45% in 6 smokers and by 96% in 6 non-smokers. The caffeine clearance was reduced 31% in the smokers and by 42% in the non-smokers.[2] A further study confirmed that the caffeine half-life was increased (59%) and the clearance decreased (40%) by **cimetidine**.[3] The probable reason is that **cimetidine** inhibits the metabolism of the caffeine by the liver, resulting in its accumulation in the body. Conversely, in a further study in children, cimetidine was not found to affect caffeine metabolism as assessed by the caffeine breath test.[4]

Any increased caffeine effects are normally unlikely to be of much importance in most people, but they might have a small part to play in exaggerating the undesirable effects of caffeine from drinks (e.g. tea, coffee, 'Coke') and analgesics.

1. Broughton LJ, Rogers HJ. Decreased systemic clearance of caffeine due to cimetidine. *Br J Clin Pharmacol* (1981) 12, 155–9.
2. May DC, Jarboe CH, VanBakel AB, Williams WM. Effects of cimetidine on caffeine disposition in smokers and nonsmokers. *Clin Pharmacol Ther* (1982) 31, 656–61.
3. Beach CA, Gerber N, Ross J, Bianchine JR. Inhibition of elimination of caffeine by cimetidine in man. *Clin Res* (1982) 30, 248A.
4. Parker AC, Pritchard P, Preston T, Dalzell AM, Choonara I. Lack of inhibitory effect of cimetidine on caffeine metabolism in children using the caffeine breath test. *Br J Clin Pharmacol* (1997) 43, 467–70.

Caffeine + Contraceptives, oral or HRT (hormone replacement therapy)

The effects of caffeine may be increased and prolonged to some extent in women taking combined oral contraceptives or HRT.

Clinical evidence

(a) Contraceptives, oral

In 9 women who had been taking low-dose **combined oral contraceptives** for at least 3 months, the clearance of a single 162-mg dose of caffeine base was reduced, the half-life prolonged (5.4 compared with 7.9 h), and the serum levels raised when compared with 9 other women not taking an oral contraceptive.[1] This finding was confirmed in 3 other studies,[2-4] which found that caffeine elimination was prolonged from means of 4 and 6 h before the use of **combined oral contraceptives** to about 9 h by the end of the first cycle, and to about 11 h by the end of the third cycle.[3,4] A further study found that there was little difference between the effects of two **oral contraceptives**, one containing 30 micrograms **ethinylestradiol** + 75 micrograms **gestodene**, and the other containing 30 micrograms **ethinylestradiol** + 125 micrograms **levonorgestrel**. Both increased the half-life of caffeine by a little over 50%, but the maximum serum levels were unchanged.[5]

(b) HRT (hormone replacement therapy)

In one study, 12 healthy postmenopausal women were given a single 200-mg dose of caffeine after 8 weeks of **estradiol** therapy (*Estrace*), titrated to give estradiol plasma concentrations of 50 to 150 pg/ml. The metabolism of caffeine was reduced by 29% overall. If the data for 2 subjects who were found to have taken extra caffeine during the study period are excluded, the caffeine metabolism showed an even greater average reduction of 38%.[6]

Mechanism

Uncertain, but the probable mechanism is that estrogens inhibit the metabolism of caffeine by cytochrome P450 isoenzyme CYP1A2 resulting in its accumulation in the body.

Importance and management

An established interaction that is probably of limited clinical importance. Women on the pill or HRT who take caffeine-containing analgesics or drink caffeine-containing drinks (tea, coffee, 'Coke', etc.) may find the effects of caffeine increased and prolonged. In excess caffeine can cause jitteriness and insomnia.

1. Abernethy DR, Todd EL. Impairment of caffeine clearance by chronic use of low-dose oestrogen-containing oral contraceptives. *Eur J Clin Pharmacol* (1985) 28, 425–8.
2. Patwardhan RV, Desmond PV, Johnson RF, Schenker S. Impaired elimination of caffeine by oral contraceptive steroids. *J Lab Clin Med* (1980) 95, 603–8.
3. Meyer FP, Canzler E, Giers H, Walther H. Langzeituntersuchung zum Einfluß von Non-Ovlon auf die Pharmakokinetik von Coffein im intraindividuellen Vergleich. *Zentrabl Gynakol* (1988) 110, 1449–54.
4. Rietveld EC, Broekman MMM, Houben JJG, Eskes TKAB, van Rossum JM. Rapid onset of an increase in caffeine residence time in young women due to oral contraceptive steroids. *Eur J Clin Pharmacol* (1984) 26, 371–3.
5. Balogh A, Klinger G, Henschel L, Börner A, Vollanth R, Kuhnz W. Influence of ethinylestradiol-containing combination oral contraceptives with gestodene or levonorgestrel on caffeine elimination. *Eur J Clin Pharmacol* (1995) 48, 161–6.
6. Pollock BG, Wylie M, Stack JA, Sorisio DA, Thompson DS, Kirshner MA, Folan MM, Condifer KA. Inhibition of caffeine metabolism by estrogen replacement therapy in postmenopausal women. *J Clin Pharmacol* (1999) 39, 936–40.

Caffeine + Disulfiram

Disulfiram reduces the loss of caffeine from the body which might complicate the withdrawal from alcohol, particularly in a few individuals.

Clinical evidence, mechanism, importance and management

A study in healthy subjects and recovering alcoholics found that **disulfiram** treatment (250 or 500 mg daily) reduced the clearance of caffeine by about 30%, but a few of the alcoholics had a more than 50% reduction.[1] As a result the levels of caffeine in the body increased. Raised levels of caffeine can cause irritability, insomnia and anxiety, similar to the symptoms of alcohol withdrawal. As coffee consumption is often particularly high among recovering alcoholics, there is the risk that they may turn to alcohol to calm themselves down. To avoid this possible complication it might be wise for recovering alcoholics not to drink too much tea or coffee. Decaffeinated coffee and tea are widely available.

1. Beach CA, Mays DC, Guiler RC, Jacober CH, Gerber N. Inhibition of elimination of caffeine by disulfiram in normal subjects and recovering alcoholics. *Clin Pharmacol Ther* (1986) 39, 265–70.

Caffeine + Fluvoxamine

The clearance of caffeine is considerably reduced by fluvoxamine. An increase in the stimulant and side-effects of caffeine would be expected.

Clinical evidence

In a randomised crossover study, 8 normal healthy subjects were given a single dose of 200 mg caffeine orally alone and then on day 8 after taking **fluvoxamine** 50 mg daily for 4 days and then 100 mg daily for a further 8 days. It was found that **fluvoxamine** reduced the total clearance of caffeine by about 80% (from 107 to 21 ml/min) and increased its half-life from 5 to 31 h. Specifically, the clearance of caffeine by $N3$-, $N1$- and $N7$-demethylation was decreased.[1]

Mechanism

Fluvoxamine is a potent inhibitor of the cytochrome P450 isoenzyme CYP1A2, which is the principal enzyme concerned with the metabolism of caffeine. As a result the caffeine is cleared from the body much more slowly and accumulates.

Importance and management

The interaction would seem to be established, even though few studies exist (see also 'Theophylline + Selective serotonin re-uptake inhibitors (SSRIs)', p.813). There are no reports of caffeine toxicity arising from this interaction, but an increase in the stimulant and side-effects of caffeine (headache, jitteriness, restlessness, insomnia) is possible if patients continue to drink normal amounts of caffeine-containing drinks (tea, coffee, '*Coke*', etc.) or caffeine-containing medications. They should be warned to reduce their caffeine intake if problems develop. It has been suggested that some of the side-effects of fluvoxamine (i.e. nervousness, restlessness and insomnia) could in fact be caused by caffeine toxicity. However, a preliminary study suggested a limited effect of caffeine intake on the frequency of adverse effects of fluvoxamine.[2] More study is needed.

1. Jeppesen U, Loft S, Poulsen HE, Brøsen K. A fluvoxamine-caffeine interaction study. *Pharmacogenetics* (1996) 6, 213–222.
2. Spigset O. Are adverse drug reactions attributed to fluvoxamine caused by concomitant intake of caffeine? *Eur J Clin Pharmacol* (1998) 54, 665–6.

Caffeine + Grapefruit juice

Grapefruit juice does not interact to a clinically relevant extent with caffeine.

Clinical evidence, mechanism, importance and management

Grapefruit juice at a dose of 1.2 L decreased the clearance of caffeine from coffee by 23% and prolonged its half-life by 31% in 12 healthy subjects, but these changes were not considered clinically relevant.[1] A crossover study in 6 normal subjects given 3.3 mg/kg caffeine found that multiple doses of **grapefruit juice** (equivalent to 6 glasses) caused a non-significant increase in the AUC of caffeine. No changes in ambulatory systolic BP, diastolic BP or heart rates were seen.[2]

1. Fuhr U, Klittich K, Staib AH. Inhibitory effect of grapefruit juice and the active component, naringenin on CYP1A2 dependent metabolism of caffeine in man. *Br J Clin Pharmacol* (1993) 35, 431–6. [Title corrected by erratum]
2. Maish WA, Hampton EM, Whitsett TL, Shepard JD, Lovallo WR. Influence of grapefruit juice on caffeine pharmacokinetics and pharmacodynamics. *Pharmacotherapy* (1996) 16, 1046–52.

Caffeine + Idrocilamide

Idrocilamide given orally causes the marked retention in the body of caffeine, which can lead to caffeine toxicity.

Clinical evidence, mechanism, importance and management

The possibility that caffeine ingestion might have had some part to play in the development of psychiatric disorders seen in patients on **idrocilamide**, prompted a pharmacokinetic study in 4 healthy subjects. While taking 400 mg **idrocilamide** three times a day orally, the half-life of caffeine from a cup of coffee (150–200 mg caffeine) was prolonged by a factor of 9 (from about 7 to 59 h). The overall clearance of caffeine was decreased about 90%.[1,2] Idrocilamide causes very marked inhibition of the metabolism and clearance of caffeine from the body, leading to its accumulation.

Evidence is limited but the interaction appears to be established. Patients on oral idrocilamide should avoid caffeine, including caffeine-containing drinks (tea, coffee, '*Coke*', etc.), or only take very small

amounts, otherwise caffeine toxicity may develop. Decaffeinated teas and coffee are widely available. Non-prescription medicines may contain caffeine, so these should also be used with care.

1. Brazier JL, Descotes J, Lery N, Ollagnier M, Evreux J-C. Inhibition by idrocilamide of the disposition of caffeine. *Eur J Clin Pharmacol* (1980) 17, 37–43.
2. Evreux JC, Bayere JJ, Descotes J, Lery N, Ollagnier M, Brazier JL. Les accidents neuro-psychiques de l'idrocilamide: conséquence d'une inhibition due métabolisme de la caféine? *Lyon Med* (1979) 241, 89–91.

Caffeine + Methoxsalen

Methoxsalen markedly reduces the loss of caffeine from the body. Increased caffeine effects and possibly toxicity may occur.

Clinical evidence, mechanism, importance and management

A single 1.2 mg/kg oral dose of **methoxsalen** given to 5 subjects with psoriasis 1 h before a single 200 mg oral dose of caffeine reduced the caffeine clearance by 69% (from 110 to 34 ml/min). The elimination half-life of caffeine over the period from 2 to 16 h after taking the **methoxsalen** increased tenfold (from 5.6 to 57 h).[1] The reason is believed to be that the **methoxsalen** acts as a potent inhibitor of the metabolism of the caffeine by the liver, thereby markedly reducing its loss from the body. The practical consequences of this interaction are as yet uncertain, but it seems possible that the toxic effects of caffeine will be increased. In excess, caffeine (including that from tea, coffee and '*Coke*') can cause jitteriness, headache and insomnia. More study is needed.

1. Mays DC, Camisa C, Cheney P, Pacula CM, Nawoot S, Gerber N. Methoxsalen is a potent inhibitor of the metabolism of caffeine in humans. *Clin Pharmacol Ther* (1987) 42, 621–6.

Caffeine + Quinolone antibacterials

Enoxacin can increase the blood levels of caffeine. The effects of caffeine derived from drinks such as tea, coffee or '*Coke*', would be expected to be increased. Pipemidic acid interacts to a lesser extent, and ciprofloxacin, norfloxacin and pefloxacin interact less still. Fleroxacin, lomefloxacin, ofloxacin, rufloxacin, and trovafloxacin appear not to interact.

Clinical evidence

The effects of various quinolones on the pharmacokinetics of caffeine[1-12] are summarised in Table 22.3.

Mechanism

It would seem that the metabolism (*N*-demethylation) of caffeine is markedly reduced by some quinolones (notably pipemidic acid and enoxacin) so that it accumulates in the body, thereby enhancing its effects. Other quinolones have a much smaller effect or none at all. There appears to be a competitive interaction between the quinolones and the cytochrome P450 isoenzyme CYP1A2.[13]

Importance and management

Established interactions. Based on the results of two studies, on a scale of 100 to 0, the relative potencies of these quinolones as inhibitors of caffeine elimination have been determined as follows: enoxacin (100), pipemidic acid (29), ciprofloxacin (11), norfloxacin (9) and ofloxacin (0).[14] From further studies, clinafloxacin appears to be similar to enoxacin, pefloxacin interacts to norfloxacin (to which it is metabolised), and fleroxacin, lomefloxacin, rufloxacin, and trovafloxacin appear to behave like ofloxacin. Patients taking enoxacin, and possibly clinafloxacin, might be expected to experience an increase in the effects of caffeine (such as headache, jitteriness, rest-

Table 22.3 Effect of quinolones on caffeine pharmacokinetics in healthy subjects

Quinolone[a]	Daily caffeine intake[b]	Change in AUC	Change in clearance	Ref
Ciprofloxacin				
100 mg twice daily	220 to 230 mg	+17%		3
250 mg twice daily	220 to 230 mg	+57%	−33%	1, 3, 4
500 mg twice daily	230 mg	+58%		3
500 mg twice daily	100 mg three times daily	+127%	−49%	8
750 mg (3 × 12-hourly doses)	100 mg	+59%	−45%	7
Clinafloxacin				
400 mg twice daily	200 mg		−84%	10
Enoxacin				
100 mg twice daily	230 mg	+138%		3
200 mg twice daily	230 mg	+176%		3
400 mg twice daily	220 to 230 mg	+346%	−78%	1, 3, 4
400 mg twice daily	200 mg daily	+370%	−79%	6
400 mg twice daily	183 mg daily		−83%	12
Fleroxacin				
400 mg daily	100 mg three times daily	+18%	No change	8
Lomefloxacin				
400 mg daily	200 mg daily	No change	No change	5
Norfloxacin				
200 mg twice daily	230 mg	+16%		3
800 mg twice daily	350 mg	+52%	−35%	2
Ofloxacin				
200 mg twice daily	220 to 230 mg	No change	No change	1, 3, 4
Pefloxacin				
400 mg twice daily	183 mg daily		−47%	12
Pipedimic acid				
400 mg twice daily	230 mg	+179%		3
800 mg twice daily	350 mg	+119%	−63%	2
Rufloxacin				
400 mg (single dose)	200 mg	−18%	No change	11
Trovafloxacin				
200 mg daily	183 mg daily	+17%		9

[a] Unless otherwise stated quinolones were given for 3 to 5 days.
[b] Unless otherwise stated caffeine was given as a single dose.

lessness, insomnia) if, for example, they continue to drink normal amounts of caffeine-containing drinks (tea, coffee, 'Coke', etc.). They should be warned to cut out or reduce their intake of caffeine if this occurs. The authors of one report[1] suggest that patients with hepatic disorders, cardiac arrhythmias or latent epilepsy should avoid caffeine if they take enoxacin for a week or more. The effects of pipemidic acid are less, and those of ciprofloxacin, norfloxacin and pefloxacin are probably of little or no clinical importance. Fleroxacin, lomefloxacin, ofloxacin, rufloxacin, and trovafloxacin are non-interacting alternatives.

1. Staib AH, Stille W, Dietlein G, Shah PM, Harder S, Mieke S, Beer C. Interaction between quinolones and caffeine. *Drugs* (1987) 34 (Suppl 1), 170–4.

2. Carbó M, Segura J, De la Torre R, Badenas JM, Camí J. Effect of quinolones on caffeine disposition. *Clin Pharmacol Ther* (1989) 45, 234–40.

3. Harder S, Staib AH, Beer C, Papenburg A, Stille W, Shah PM. 4-Quinolones inhibit biotransformation of caffeine. *Eur J Clin Pharmacol* (1988) 35, 651–6.

4. Stille W, Harder S, Mieke S, Beer C, Shah PM, Frech K, Staib AH. Decrease of caffeine elimination in man during co-administration of 4-quinolones. *J Antimicrob Chemother* (1987) 20, 729–34.

5. Healy DP, Schoenle JR, Stotka J, Polk RE. Lack of interaction between lomefloxacin and caffeine in normal volunteers. *Antimicrob Agents Chemother* (1991) 35, 660–4.

6. Peloquin CA, Nix DE, Sedman AJ, Wilton JH, Toothaker RD, Harrison NJ, Schentag JJ. Pharmacokinetics and clinical effects of caffeine alone and in combination with oral enoxacin. *Rev Infect Dis* (1989) II (Suppl 5), S1095.

7. Healy DP, Polk RE, Kanawati L, Rock DT, Mooney ML. Interaction between oral ciprofloxacin and caffeine in normal volunteers. *Antimicrob Agents Chemother* (1989) 33, 474–8.

8. Nicolau DP, Nightingale CH, Tessier PR, Fu Q, Xuan D-w, Esguerra EM, Quintiliani R. The effect of fleroxacin and ciprofloxacin on the pharmacokinetics of multiple dose caffeine. *Drugs* (1995) 49 (Suppl 2), 357–9.

9. LeBel M, Teng R, Dogolo LC, Willavize S, Friedman HL, Vincent J. The influence of steady-state trovafloxacin on the steady-state pharmacokinetics of caffeine in healthy subjects. *Pharm Res* (1996) 13 (Suppl 9), S434.

10. Randinitis EJ, Koup JR, Rausch G, Vassos AB. Effect of (CLX) administration on the single-dose pharmacokinetics of theophylline and caffeine. *Intersci Conf Antimicrob Agents Chemother* (1998) 38, 6.
11. Cesana M, Broccali G, Imbimbo BP, Crema A. Effect of single doses of rufloxacin on the disposition of theophylline and caffeine after single administration. *Int J Clin Pharmacol Ther Toxicol* (1991) 29, 133–8.
12. Kinzig-Schippers M, Fuhr U, Zaigler M, Dammeyer J, Rüsing G, Labedzki A, Bulitta J, Sörgel F. Interaction of pefloxacin and enoxacin with the human cytochrome P450 enzyme CYP1A2. *Clin Pharmacol Ther* (1999) 65, 262–74.
13. Fuhr U, Wolff T, Harder S, Schymanski P, Staib AH. Quinolone inhibition of cytochrome P450-dependent caffeine metabolism in human liver microsomes. *Drug Metab Dispos* (1990) 18, 1005–10.
14. Barnett G, Segura J, de la Torre R, Carbó M. Pharmacokinetic determination of relative potency of quinolone inhibition of caffeine disposition. *Eur J Clin Pharmacol* (1990) 39, 63–9.

Caffeine + Venlafaxine

Venlafaxine does not affect the pharmacokinetics of caffeine.

Clinical evidence, mechanism, importance and management

Venlafaxine (37.5 mg twice daily for 3 days then 75 mg twice daily for 4 days) did not affect the AUC or clearance of daily (equivalent to about 3 cups of coffee) in 15 healthy subjects. A slight but significant decrease in the half-life was noted (6.1 to 5.5 h).[1] On the basis of this study, no special precautions are needed if both drugs are taken together.

1. Amchin J, Zarycranski W, Taylor KP, Albano D, Klockowski PM. Effect of venlafaxine on CYP1A2-dependent pharmacokinetics and metabolism of caffeine. *J Clin Pharmacol* (1999) 39, 252–9.

Doxofylline + Miscellaneous drugs

There is some limited evidence that erythromycin may increase the effects of doxofylline, but the clinical importance of this is uncertain. Digoxin lowers serum doxofylline levels at steady-state after an initial rise, but the bronchodilator effects do not appear to be significantly affected. Allopurinol and lithium carbonate appear to have no significant effects.

Clinical evidence, mechanism, importance and management

(a) Allopurinol, Erythromycin, Lithium carbonate

Normal subjects were given 400 mg doxofylline three times daily either alone or with **allopurinol** (100 mg once daily) or **erythromycin** (400 mg three times daily) or **lithium carbonate** (300 mg three times daily). None of the pharmacokinetic parameters measured, including the maximum serum levels, were significantly altered by any of these drugs except that the doxofylline AUCs were raised as follows: **allopurinol** (39%), **erythromycin** (70%) and **lithium carbonate** (34%). Only the erythromycin result was significant.[1]

The clinical significance of these changes is uncertain, and their mechanism is not understood. Until the situation is much clearer it would be prudent to check the outcome of adding erythromycin to established treatment with doxofylline, being alert for evidence of increased effects.

(b) Digoxin

A comparative study in 9 patients, 5 given **digoxin** (500 micrograms daily) and 4 without, found that the **digoxin** increased the serum levels of doxofylline (800 mg daily) on the first day of treatment, 3 hours after administration, by about 50%. At steady-state (30 days) the serum levels were reduced by about 30%. Nevertheless, the bronchodilating effects of the doxofylline were little different between the 2 groups. It was concluded that concurrent use is normally safe and effective, but the initial doxofylline dose should be chosen to avoid too high a serum level on the first day, and pulmonary function should be well monitored.[2]

1. Harning R, Sekora D, O'Connell K, Wilson J. A crossover study of the effect of erythromycin, lithium carbonate, and allopurinol on doxofylline pharmacokinetics. *Clin Pharmacol Ther* (1994) 55, 158.
2. Provvedi D, Rubegni M, Biffignandi P. Pharmacokinetic interaction between doxofylline and digitalis in elderly patients with chronic obstructive bronchitis. *Acta Ther* (1990) 16, 239–46.

Theophylline + Aciclovir

Preliminary evidence suggests that aciclovir can increase the serum levels of theophylline causing toxicity.

Clinical evidence

Prompted by a case of increased theophylline side-effects in a patient given **aciclovir**, a study was carried out in 5 healthy subjects who were given single 320-mg doses of theophylline (aminophylline 400 mg) before and with the sixth dose of **aciclovir** 800 mg five times daily for 2 days. The AUC of the theophylline was increased by 45% (from 189.9 to 274.9 micrograms.h/ml) and the total body clearance was reduced by 30%, when aciclovir was added.[1]

Mechanism

Uncertain, but the evidence suggests that aciclovir inhibits the oxidative metabolism of theophylline so that it accumulates.[1]

Importance and management

Evidence appears to be limited to this report, but the interaction seems to be established. Be alert for the need to reduce the dosage of theophylline if aciclovir is added to established treatment. More study is needed.

1. Maeda Y, Konishi T, Omoda K, Takeda Y, Fukuhara S, Fukuzawa M, Ohune T, Tsuya T, Tsukiai S. Inhibition of theophylline metabolism by aciclovir. *Biol Pharm Bull* (1996) 19, 1591–5.

Theophylline + Allopurinol

Some evidence from clinical studies and a single case report indicates that the effects of theophylline may be increased by the concurrent use of allopurinol.

Clinical evidence

A patient on 450 mg theophylline daily showed a 38% increase in peak serum levels after taking **allopurinol** for 3 days.[1] In 12 healthy subjects, **allopurinol** 300 mg twice daily for 14 days increased the half-life of theophylline after a single 5 mg/kg oral dose by 25%, and increased the AUC by 27%.[2] Similar increases were seen after a second dose of theophylline given 28 days after starting the **allopurinol**.[2] Two other studies of 300 mg **allopurinol** daily for 7 days failed to show any effect on the pharmacokinetics of theophylline after a single 5 mg/kg intravenous dose of aminophylline.[3,4] Similarly, steady-state theophylline concentrations were not affected by **allopurinol** 100 mg three times daily in 4 subjects receiving 125 or 250 mg theophylline three times daily. However, there was an alteration in the proportion of different urinary theophylline metabolites: methyluric acid decreased and methylxanthine increased.[4]

Mechanism

Uncertain. Allopurinol, a xanthine oxidase inhibitor, can block the conversion of methylxanthine to methyluric acid, but this had no effect on theophylline plasma levels in two studies, One suggestion is that allopurinol also inhibits oxidative metabolism of theophylline by the liver.[1]

Importance and management

Evidence appears to be limited to a single case report and the studies on normal healthy subjects. The interaction does not appear to be of more than moderate importance. Nevertheless, it would seem prudent to check for any signs of theophylline overdosage during concurrent use, particularly in patients whose disease condition may result in a reduction in the metabolism of the theophylline, or where high doses of allopurinol are used.

1. Barry M, Feeley J. Allopurinol influences aminophenazone elimination. *Clin Pharmacokinet* (1990) 19, 167–9.
2. Manfredi RL, Vesell ES. Inhibition of theophylline metabolism by long-term allopurinol administration. *Clin Pharmacol Ther* (1981) 29, 224–9.
3. Vozeh S, Powell JR, Cupit GC, Riegelman S, Sheiner LB. Influence of allopurinol on theophylline disposition in adults. *Clin Pharmacol Ther* (1980) 27, 194–7.
4. Grygiel JJ, Wing LMH, Farkas J, Birkett DJ. Effects of allopurinol on theophylline metabolism and clearance. *Clin Pharmacol Ther* (1979) 26, 660–7.

Theophylline + Alosetron

Alosetron and theophylline do not interact adversely.

Clinical evidence, mechanism, importance and management

Ten healthy women subjects were given 1 mg **alosetron** or a placebo twice daily for 16 days, to which 200 mg oral theophylline twice daily was added from day 8 to day 16. No clinically relevant changes in the pharmacokinetics of the theophylline were seen, and concurrent use was well tolerated. The effect of theophylline on **alosetron** pharmacokinetics was not measured but the authors of the report say that no metabolic interaction seems likely.[1] No special precautions would therefore appear to be needed if these drugs are used together.

1. Koch KM, Ricci BM, Hedayetullah NS, Jewel D, Kersey KE. Effect of alosetron on theophylline pharmacokinetics. *Br J Clin Pharmacol* (2001) 52, 596–600.

Theophylline + Aminoglutethimide

The loss of theophylline from the body is increased by the concurrent use of aminoglutethimide, so that a moderate reduction in its serum levels and therapeutic effects seems probable.

Clinical evidence, mechanism, importance and management

Aminoglutethimide (250 mg four times a day) increased the theophylline clearance in 3 patients taking a sustained release preparation (200 mg twice daily) by 18 to 43%.[1] Theophylline clearance was assessed before starting aminoglutethimide as well as over weeks 2 to 12 of combined therapy.

It seems probable that the aminoglutethimide, a known enzyme-inducing agent, increases the metabolism of theophylline by the liver, thereby increasing its loss from the body. The clinical importance is uncertain, but the effects of theophylline would be expected to be reduced to some extent by the addition of aminoglutethimide. Monitor the effects and increase the theophylline dosage if necessary.

1. Lønning PE, Kvinnsland S, Bakke OM. Effect of aminoglutethimide on antipyrine, theophylline and digitoxin disposition in breast cancer. *Clin Pharmacol Ther* (1984) 36, 796–802.

Theophylline + Amiodarone

An isolated case report describes raised theophylline levels and toxicity in an old man when amiodarone was added.

Clinical evidence, mechanism, importance and management

An 86-year-old man on furosemide (frusemide), digoxin, domperidone and theophylline developed signs of theophylline toxicity when **amiodarone** (600 mg daily) was added. After 9 days concurrent use his serum theophylline levels had doubled (from 93 to 194 micromol/l). The toxicity disappeared when the theophylline was stopped.[1] The reason for this adverse reaction is not understood but a reduction in the metabolism of the theophylline by the liver is suggested.[1] There was no evidence of liver dysfunction. This is an isolated case and its general importance is uncertain, but it would now seem prudent to monitor serum theophylline levels if **amiodarone** is given to any patient. More study is needed.

1. Soto J, Sacristán JA, Arellano F, Hazas J. Possible theophylline-amiodarone interaction. *DICP Ann Pharmacother* (1990) 24, 1115.

Theophylline + Ampicillin (± Sulbactam) or Amoxicillin

Neither ampicillin (± sulbactam) nor amoxicillin interacts adversely with theophylline.

Clinical evidence, mechanism, importance and management

A retrospective study in asthmatic children aged 3 months to 6 years found that the mean half-life of **theophylline** did not differ between those treated concurrently with **ampicillin** and those not.[1] Twelve adult patients with chronic obstructive pulmonary disease showed no changes in the pharmacokinetics of **theophylline** 8.5 mg/kg daily when given **ampicillin** 1 g plus **sulbactam** 500 mg 12-hourly for 7 days.[2]

A study in 9 healthy adult subjects showed that the concurrent use of **amoxicillin** 750 mg daily for 9 days did not affect the pharmacokinetics of **theophylline** given at a dosage of 540 mg twice daily.[3,4]

No special precautions would seem to be necessary during concurrent use of these antibacterials and theophylline. However, note that acute infections *per se* can alter theophylline pharmacokinetics.

1. Kadlec GJ, Ha LT, Jarboe CH, Richards D, Karibo JM. Effect of ampicillin on theophylline half-life in infants and young children. *South Med J* (1978) 71, 1584.
2. Cazzola M, Santangelo G, Guidetti E, Mattina R, Caputi M, Girbino G. Influence of sulbactam plus ampicillin on theophylline clearance. *Int J Clin Pharmacol Res* (1991) 11, 11–15.
3. Jonkman JHG, van der Boon WJV, Schoenmaker R, Holtkamp A, Hempenius J. Lack of effect of amoxicillin on theophylline pharmacokinetics. *Br J Clin Pharmacol* (1985) 19, 99–101.
4. Jonkman JHG, van der Boon WJV, Schoenmaker R, Holtkamp AH, Hempenius J. Clinical pharmacokinetics of amoxycillin and theophylline during cotreatment with both medicaments. *Chemotherapy* (1985) 31, 329–35.

Theophylline + Antacids

The extent of absorption of theophylline from the gut does not appear to be significantly affected by the concurrent use of aluminium or magnesium hydroxide antacids such as Maalox, Mylanta or Amphojel.

Clinical evidence, mechanism, importance and management

In a study in 12 healthy subjects, there was no difference in steady-state maximum serum concentrations not AUC for theophylline given as *Nuelin-Depot* or *Theodur* when an antacid (*Novalucid* – **magnesium** and **aluminium hydroxides** and **magnesium carbonate**) was given concurrently. However, the antacid caused a faster absorption of theophylline from *Nuelin-Depot*, which resulted in greater fluctuations in the serum levels. It was considered that the side effects of theophylline might be increased in those patients with serum levels at the top of the range.[1] Similar results have been found in single-dose studies using aminophylline[2] and *Theodur*[3] with **aluminium-magnesium hydroxide** antacids, and in multiple dose studies in patients using *Armophylline*,[4] *Aminophyllin*[5] or *Theodur*[5] with **aluminium-magnesium hydroxide** antacids. Care should be taken extrapolating this information to other sustained release preparations of theophylline, but generally speaking no special precautions seem to be necessary during the concurrent use of theophylline and antacids.

1. Myhre KI, Walstad RA. The influence of antacid on the absorption of two different sustained-release formulations of theophylline. *Br J Clin Pharmacol* (1983) 15, 683–7.
2. Arnold LA, Spurbeck GH, Shelver WH, Henderson WM. Effect of an antacid on gastrointestinal absorption of theophylline. *Am J Hosp Pharm* (1979) 36, 1059–62.
3. Darzentas LJ, Stewart RB, Curry SH, Yost RL. Effect of antacid on bioavailability of a sustained-release theophylline preparation. *Drug Intell Clin Pharm* (1983) 17, 555–7.
4. Muir JF, Peiffer G, Richard MO, Benhamou D, Adrejak M, Hary L, Moore N. Lack of effect of magnesium-aluminium hydroxide on the absorption of theophylline given as a pH-dependent sustained release preparation. *Eur J Clin Pharmacol* (1993) 44, 85–8.
5. Reed RC, Schwartz HJ. Lack of influence of an intensive antacid regimen on theophylline bioavailability. *J Pharmacokinetic Biopharm* (1984) 12, 315–331.

Theophylline + Anthelmintics (benzimidazole type)

Theophylline serum levels can be markedly increased by the concurrent use of tiabendazole. Toxicity may develop if the theophylline dosage is not reduced appropriately. A 50% reduction has been suggested. Neither albendazole nor mebendazole appear to interact with theophylline.

Clinical evidence

(a) Albendazole

A study in 6 healthy subjects found that the pharmacokinetics of a single dose of theophylline were unaffected by a single 400-mg dose of **albendazole**.[1]

(b) Mebendazole

A study in 6 healthy subjects found that the pharmacokinetics of a single dose of theophylline were unaffected by 100 mg **mebendazole** twice daily for 3 days.[1] The absence of a significant interaction was reported in another similar study using the same **mebendazole** dosage.[2]

(c) Tiabendazole

An elderly man on prednisone, furosemide (frusemide), terbutaline and orciprenaline had his oral theophylline switched to an infusion (45 mg/h), giving a stable serum level of 21 micrograms/ml after 48 hours. When he was also given 4 g **tiabendazole** daily for 5 days for persistence of a *Strongyloides stercoralis* infestation he developed theophylline toxicity (severe nausea) and his serum levels were found to have more than doubled (46 micrograms/ml). Three months previously, he had been treated with 3 g **tiabendazole** daily for 3 days without any symptoms of toxicity (no theophylline levels were measured).[3] Another patient developed elevated serum theophylline levels (from 15 to 22 micrograms/ml) when given 1.8 g **tiabendazole** twice daily for 3 days, despite a dosage reduction of one-third, made in anticipation of the interaction. Theophylline levels were still elevated 2 days after the **tiabendazole** was stopped, and the theophylline dose was further reduced. Levels returned to normal after 5 days, and the theophylline dose was increased again.[4]

A retrospective study of patients given both drugs found that 9 out of 40 (23%) had developed elevated serum theophylline levels and 5 of the 9 experienced significant toxicity, with 3 requiring hospitalisation. The other 31 patients did not have theophylline levels taken.[5] A further report describes a patient who had an increase in theophylline levels (from 18 to 26 micrograms/ml) within 2 days of starting **tiabendazole** 1.5 g twice daily.[2] The authors of this report then conducted a study in 6 healthy subjects who received a single dose of aminophylline before and while taking 1.5 g **tiabendazole** twice daily for 3 days. Three of the subjects had to discontinue the study because of severe nausea, vomiting or dizziness. In the remaining three, **tiabendazole** markedly affected the pharmacokinetics of aminophylline; the half-life increased (from 6.7 to 18.6 h), the clearance fell

(from 0.067 to 0.023 l/h/kg) and the elimination rate constant also decreased (from 0.11 to 0.039 h^{-1}).[2]

Mechanism

Uncertain. It is suggested that tiabendazole inhibits the metabolism of theophylline by the liver thereby prolonging its stay in the body and raising its serum levels. The nausea and vomiting may have been due to the side-effects of both the theophylline and the tiabendazole.

Importance and management

The tiabendazole/theophylline interaction is established and of clinical importance. Monitor the effects of concurrent use and reduce the theophylline dosage accordingly. A 50% theophylline dosage reduction has been suggested,[4] or, where practical, stopping theophylline for 2 to 3 days while giving the tiabendazole.[5] Where albendazole or mebendazole are suitable alternative anthelmintics, these may be preferred since no special precautions would seem to be needed if either of these is given to patients taking theophylline.

1. Adebayo GI, Mabadeje AFB. Theophylline disposition — effects of cimetidine, mebendazole and albendazole. *Aliment Pharmacol Ther* (1988) 2, 341–6.
2. Schneider D, Gannon R, Sweeney K, Shore E. Theophylline and antiparasitic drug interactions. A case report and a study of the influence of thiabendazole and mebendazole on theophylline pharmacokinetics in adults. *Chest* (1990) 97, 84–7.
3. Sugar AM, Kearns PJ, Haulk AA, Rushing JL. Possible thiabendazole-induced theophylline toxicity. *Am Rev Respir Dis* (1980) 122, 501–3.
4. Lew G, Murray WE, Lane JR, Haeger E. Theophylline—thiabendazole drug interaction. *Clin Pharm* (1989) 8, 225–7.
5. German T, Berger R. Interaction of theophylline and thiabendazole in patients with chronic obstructive lung disease. *Am Rev Respir Dis* (1992) 145, A807.

Theophylline + Antihistamines and other anti-allergic drugs

Azelastine, ketotifen, mequitazine, mizolastine, pemirolast potassium, repirinast, and terfenadine appear not to interact adversely with theophylline.

Clinical evidence, mechanism, importance and management

Azelastine 2 mg twice daily had no significant effect on the clearance of theophylline 300 mg twice daily in 10 subjects with bronchial asthma (mean decrease of 7.6%). One patient showed a 20.8% increase and another 25.3% decrease.[1]

Two studies, one in healthy adults[2] and one in asthmatic children,[3] showed that **ketotifen** did not affect the pharmacokinetics of a single dose of theophylline. It was suggested that concurrent administration might actually decrease the CNS side-effects of each drug.[2]

The pharmacokinetics of theophylline at steady state were not significantly different in 7 asthmatic patients when given 6 mg **mequitazine** daily for 3 weeks.[4]

Mizolastine 10 mg daily had virtually no effect on the steady-state pharmacokinetics of theophylline in 17 healthy subjects except for a 13% increase in mean trough level and an 8% increase in the AUC. These changes were not considered clinically relevant.[5]

Pemirolast potassium 10 mg daily for 4 days was found to have no significant effect on the steady-state serum levels or clearance of theophylline in 7 healthy subjects.[6]

Repirinast 300 mg daily had no effect on the pharmacokinetics of theophylline in 10 asthmatics given a single dose of aminophylline.[7] Another study in 7 asthmatics found that **repirinast** (dosage not clearly stated) for 3 weeks had no effect on the pharmacokinetics of theophylline given in a dosage of 400 to 800 mg in two divided doses.[8]

The pharmacokinetics of theophylline after a single dose of 250 mg were unchanged by 120 mg **terfenadine** twice daily for 16 days in 10 healthy subjects.[9] Similarly, there was no change in the steady-state pharmacokinetics of theophylline administered at a dosage of 4 mg/kg daily when administered concurrently with terfenadine

60 mg twice daily.[10] No special precautions seem to be necessary if any of these drugs is given with theophylline.

1. Asamoto H, Kokura M, Kawakami A, Sasaki Y, Fujii H, Sawano T, Iso S, Ooishi T, Horiuchi Y, Ohara N, Kitamura Y, Morishita H. Effect of azelastine on theophylline clearance in asthma patients. *Jpn J Allergol* (1988) 37, 1033–7.
2. Matejcek M, Irwin P, Neff G, Abt K, Wehrli W. Determination of the central effects of the asthma prophylactic ketotifen, the bronchodilator theophylline, and both in combination: an application of quantitative electroencephalography to the study of drug interactions. *Int J Clin Pharmacol Ther Toxicol* (1985) 23, 258–66.
3. Garty M, Scolnik D, Danziger Y, Volovitz B, Ilfeld DN, Varsano I. Non-interaction of ketotifen and theophylline in children with asthma - an acute study. *Eur J Clin Pharmacol* (1987) 32, 187–9.
4. Hasegawa T, Takagi K, Kuzuya T, Nadai M, Apichartpichean R, Muraoka I. Effect of mequitazine on the pharmacokinetics of theophylline in asthmatic patients. *Eur J Clin Pharmacol* (1990) 38, 255–8.
5. Pinquier JL, Salva P, Deschamps C, Ascalone V, Costa J. Effect of mizolastine, a new non sedative H1 antagonist on the pharmacokinetics of theophylline. *Therapie* (1995) 50 (Suppl), 148.
6. Hasegawa T, Takagi K, Nadai M, Ogura Y, Nabeshima T. Kinetic interaction between theophylline and a newly developed anti-allergic drug, pemirolast potassium. *Eur J Clin Pharmacol* (1994) 46, 55–8.
7. Nagata M, Tabe K, Houya I, Kiuchi H, Sakamoto Y, Yamamoto K, Dohi Y. The influence of repirinast, an anti-allergic drug, on theophylline pharmacokinetics in patients with bronchial asthma. *Jpn J Thoracic Dis* (1991) 29, 413–9.
8. Takagi K, Kuzuya T, Horiuchi T, Nadai M, Apichartpichean R, Ogura Y, Hasegawa T. Lack of effect of repirinast on the pharmacokinetics of theophylline in asthmatic patients. *Eur J Clin Pharmacol* (1989) 37, 301–3.
9. Brion N, Naline E, Beaumont D, Pays M, Advenier C. Lack of effect of terfenadine on theophylline pharmacokinetics and metabolism in normal subjects. *Br J Clin Pharmacol* (1989) 27, 391–5.
10. Luskin SS, Fitzsimmons WE, MacLeod CM, Luskin AT. Pharmacokinetic evaluation of the terfenadine-theophylline interaction. *J Allergy Clin Immunol* (1989) 83, 406–11.

Theophylline + Barbiturates

Theophylline serum levels can be reduced by the concurrent use of phenobarbital or pentobarbital. A single report describes a similar interaction with secobarbital (quinalbarbitone) and it would be expected to occur with other barbiturates.

Clinical evidence

(a) Pentobarbital

A single case report describes a man who had a 95% rise in the clearance of theophylline when treated with high-dose intravenous **pentobarbital**.[1] In healthy subjects, 100 mg **pentobarbital** daily for 10 days increased the clearance of theophylline by a mean of 40% and reduced the AUC by 26%, although there were marked intersubject differences.[2]

(b) Phenobarbital

After taking **phenobarbital** (2 mg/kg daily to a maximum of 60 mg) for 19 days the mean steady-state serum theophylline levels in 7 asthmatic children aged 6 to 12 years were reduced by 30%, and the clearance was increased 35% (range 12 to 71%).[3] In contrast, two earlier studies (one by the same group of authors) found no significant change in the pharmacokinetics of theophylline in asthmatic children given **phenobarbital** 2 mg/kg daily, or 16 or 32 mg three times daily.[4,5]

A mean increase in theophylline clearance of 34% was seen in normal adult subjects given **phenobarbital** for 4 weeks,[6] and, in another study, a non-significant increase of 17% was seen in the clearance of theophylline in those given phenobarbital for 2 weeks.[7] The effects of **phenobarbital** can be additive with the effects of phenytoin and smoking; one patient required theophylline doses of 4 g daily to maintain therapeutic serum levels and to control her asthma.[8]

One retrospective study found that the dose of theophylline for neonatal apnoea was higher in premature infants also being treated with **phenobarbital**,[9] but a later prospective study failed to confirm this.[10] A study in one set of newborn twins given intravenous aminophylline found that the serum theophylline levels of the twin given **phenobarbital** were about half those of the other twin not given **phenobarbital** (14 versus 40 hours).[11]

(c) Secobarbital (Quinalbarbitone)

A 337% increase in the clearance of theophylline occurred over a 4-week period in a child treated with periodic doses of **secobarbital** and regular doses of **phenobarbital**.[12]

Mechanism

Barbiturates are potent liver enzyme inducing agents which possibly increase the metabolism of theophylline by the liver, thereby hastening its removal from the body. This has been shown in *animal* studies, although *N*-demethylation (the main metabolic route for theophylline) was not affected.[13]

Importance and management

A moderately well documented, established and clinically important interaction. Patients treated with phenobarbital or pentobarbital may need above-average doses of theophylline to achieve and maintain adequate serum levels. Concurrent use should be monitored and appropriate dosage increases made. All of the barbiturates can cause enzyme induction and may, to a greater or lesser extent, be expected to behave similarly. This is illustrated by the single report involving secobarbital (quinalbarbitone), however direct information about other barbiturates seems to be lacking.

1. Gibson GA, Blouin RA, Bauer LA, Rapp RP, Tibbs PA. Influence of high-dose pentobarbital on theophylline pharmacokinetics: A case report. *Ther Drug Monit* (1985) 7, 181–4.
2. Dahlqvist R, Steiner E, Koike Y, von Bahr C, Lind M, Billing B. Induction of theophylline metabolism by pentobarbital. *Ther Drug Monit* (1989) 11, 408–10.
3. Saccar CL, Danish M, Ragni MC, Rocci ML, Greene J, Yaffe SJ, Mansmann HC. The effect of phenobarbital on theophylline disposition in children with asthma. *J Allergy Clin Immunol* (1985) 75, 716–9.
4. Goldstein EO, Eney RD, Mellits ED, Solomon H, Johnson G. Effect of phenobarbital on theophylline metabolism in asthmatic children. *Ann Allergy* (1977) 39, 69.
5. Green J, Danish M, Ragni M, Lecks H, Yaffe S. The effect of phenobarbital upon theophylline elimination kinetics in asthmatic children. *Ann Allergy* (1977) 39, 69.
6. Landay RA, Gonzalez MA, Taylor JC. Effect of phenobarbital on theophylline disposition. *J Allergy Clin Immunol* (1978) 62, 27–9.
7. Piafsky KM, Sitar DS, Ogilvie RI. Effect of phenobarbital on the disposition of intravenous theophylline. *Clin Pharmacol Ther* (1977) 22, 336–9.
8. Nicholson JP, Basile SA, Cury JD. Massive theophylline dosing in a heavy smoker receiving both phenytoin and phenobarbital. *Ann Pharmacother* (1992) 26, 334–6.
9. Yazdani M, Kissling GE, Tran TH, Gottschalk SK, Schuth CR. Phenobarbital increases the theophylline requirement of premature infants being treated for apnea. *Am J Dis Child* (1987) 141, 97–9.
10. Kandrotas RJ, Cranfield TL, Gal P, Ransom J, Weaver RL. Effect of phenobarbital administration on theophylline clearance in premature neonates. *Ther Drug Monit* (1990) 12, 139–43.
11. Delgado E, Carrasco JM, García B, Pérez E, García Lacalle C, Bermejo T, De Juana P. Interacción teofilina-fenobarbital en un neonato. *Farm Clin* (1996) 13, 142–5.
12. Paladino JA, Blumer NA, Maddox RR. Effect of secobarbital on theophylline clearance. *Ther Drug Monit* (1983) 5, 135–9.
13. Williams JF, Szentivanyi A. Implications of hepatic drug-metabolizing activity in the therapy of bronchial asthma. *J Allergy Clin Immunol* (1975) 55, 125.

Theophylline + BCG vaccine

There is evidence that BCG vaccine can increase the half-life of theophylline, but the clinical importance of this is uncertain.

Clinical evidence, mechanism, importance and management

Two weeks after receiving **BCG** vaccination (0.1 ml *Tubersol*, equivalent to five TU of **tuberculin PPD**), the clearance of single doses of 128 mg theophylline (as choline theophyllinate) in 12 normal subjects was reduced by 21% and the theophylline half-life was prolonged by 14% (range: –10% to 47%).[1] It seems possible therefore that the occasional patient may develop some signs of theophylline toxicity if their serum levels are already towards the top end of the therapeutic range but most patients are unlikely to be affected. More study is needed to determine the clinical importance of this interaction.

1. Gray JD, Renton KW, Hung OR. Depression of theophylline elimination following BCG vaccination. *Br J Clin Pharmacol* (1983) 16, 735–7.

Theophylline + Beta-agonist bronchodilators

The concurrent use of xanthines such as theophylline and beta-agonist bronchodilators is a useful option in the management of asthma and chronic obstructive pulmonary disease, but potentiation of some adverse reactions can occur, the most serious being hypokalaemia and increased heart rate particularly with high-dose theophylline. Monitoring of serum potassium is recommended in patients with severe asthma receiving concomitant therapy. Some patients may show a significant fall in serum theophylline levels if given oral or intravenous salbutamol (albuterol) or intravenous isoprenaline (isoproterenol).

Clinical evidence

(a) Formoterol

In a single-dose study, 8 healthy subjects were given oral doses of 375 mg theophylline and 144 micrograms formoterol. Combined use caused no significant pharmacokinetic interaction, but a significantly greater drop in the potassium level was seen when compared with either drug given alone.[1]

(b) Isoprenaline (Isoproterenol)

The infusion of isoprenaline increased the clearance of theophylline (given as intravenous aminophylline) by a mean of 19% in 6 children with status asthmaticus and respiratory failure. Two of them had increases of greater than 30%.[2] Another study in 12 patients with severe status asthmaticus found that an isoprenaline infusion (mean maximum rate 0.77 micrograms/kg.min) caused a mean fall in serum theophylline levels of almost 6 micrograms/ml.[3] The levels rose again when the isoprenaline was stopped.[3] A critically ill patient on intravenous aminophylline and phenytoin and nebulised terbutaline showed a marked increase in theophylline clearance (354%) when an isoprenaline infusion and intravenous methylprednisolone were added to the regimen.[4]

(c) Orciprenaline (Metaproterenol)

Orciprenaline given orally (20 mg eight-hourly) or by inhalation (1.95 mg six-hourly) for 3 days had no effect on the pharmacokinetics of theophylline after a single intravenous dose of aminophylline in 6 healthy subjects.[5] This confirms a previous finding in asthmatic children in whom it was shown that oral orciprenaline did not alter steady-state serum theophylline levels.[6]

(d) Salbutamol (Albuterol)

Pretreatment with oral theophylline for 9 days significantly increased the hypokalaemia and tachycardia caused by an infusion of salbutamol (4 micrograms/kg loading dose then 8 micrograms/kg for an hour) in normal subjects.[7] A potentially dangerous additive increase in heart rate (about 35 to 40%) was seen in one study in 9 patients with COPD given infusions of aminophylline and salbutamol.[8] Similarly, heart rate was significantly higher in 15 asthmatic children given concurrent single doses of oral theophylline and salbutamol when compared with a control group given oral theophylline alone (109 versus 91 bpm).[9] However, another study found that neither the occurrence nor the severity of arrhythmias seemed to be changed when oral theophylline was added to inhaled salbutamol therapy in 18 patients with COPD and heart disease.[10] Respiratory arrest possibly related to hypokalaemia occurred in a girl of 10 given theophylline and salbutamol.[11]

Reduced theophylline levels (clearance increased by a mean of 14%, and in 3 cases by greater than 30%), were seen when salbutamol was given orally to 10 healthy volunteers, but no changes in clearance were seen when salbutamol was given by inhalation.[12] A 25% reduction in serum theophylline levels in 10 patients while taking 16 mg oral salbutamol was reported in another study.[13] A child of 19 months given intravenous theophylline needed a threefold increase in theophylline dosage when an infusion of salbutamol was added because of an increase in the theophylline clearance.[14] Peak flow readings were decreased in 15 children (aged 5 to 13 years) giv-

en single doses of oral salbutamol and theophylline, and there was a non-significant decrease in theophylline levels.[9] These reports contrast with another study in 8 healthy subjects, which found no change in the steady-state pharmacokinetics of oral theophylline when given with oral salbutamol.[15]

(e) Terbutaline

Pretreatment with oral theophylline for at least 4 days significantly increased the fall in serum potassium levels and rises in blood glucose, pulse rates and systolic blood pressures caused by an infusion of terbutaline in 7 healthy subjects.[16] A study in children given slow-release formulations of both theophylline and terbutaline found no increases in reported side-effects and simple additive effects on the control of their asthma.[17]

Oral terbutaline decreased serum theophylline levels by about 10% in 6 asthmatics, but the control of asthma was improved.[18] Another study in asthmatic children, found that terbutaline (0.075 mg/kg three times daily) taken as an elixir, reduced steady-state serum levels of theophylline by 22%, but the symptoms of cough and wheeze improved.[19] Yet another study found no changes in the pharmacokinetics of aminophylline in asthmatic children when given terbutaline.[20]

Mechanism

Beta$_2$-agonists can cause hypokalaemia, particularly after parenteral and nebulised administration. Xanthines such as theophylline can also cause hypokalaemia, and this is a common feature of theophylline toxicity. The potassium lowering effects of beta$_2$-agonists and xanthines are additive. Why some beta-agonists lower serum theophylline levels is not known.

Importance and management

Concurrent use is beneficial, but the reports outlined above illustrate some of the disadvantages and adverse effects that have been identified. In particular, the use of intravenous beta-agonists in acutely ill patients on theophylline has been suggested to be hazardous because of the risk of profound hypokalaemia and cardiac arrhythmias.[7,16] Monitoring of serum potassium in these situations was suggested.[16] Moreover, the CSM in the UK has issued[21] the following advice: "Potentially serious hypokalaemia may result from beta$_2$-agonist therapy. Particular caution is required in severe asthma, as this effect may be potentiated by concomitant treatment with theophylline and its derivatives, corticosteroids, and diuretics, and by hypoxia. Plasma potassium concentrations should therefore be monitored in severe asthma."

1. van den Berg BTJ, Derks MGM, Koolen MGJ, Braat MCP, Butter JJ, van Boxtel CJ. Pharmacokinetic/pharmacodynamic modelling of the eosinopenic and hypokalemic effects of formoterol and theophylline combination in healthy men. *Pulm Pharmacol Ther* (1999) 12, 185–92.
2. Hemstreet MP, Miles MV, Rutland RO. Effect of intravenous isoproterenol on theophylline kinetics. *J Allergy Clin Immunol* (1982) 69, 360–4.
3. O'Rourke PP, Crone RK. Effect of isoproterenol on measured theophylline levels. *Crit Care Med* (1984) 12, 373–5.
4. Griffith JA, Kozloski GD. Isoproterenol-theophylline interaction: possible potentiation by other drugs. *Clin Pharm* (1990) 9, 54–7.
5. Conrad KA, Woodworth JR. Orciprenaline does not alter theophylline elimination. *Br J Clin Pharmacol* (1981) 12, 756–7.
6. Rachelefsky GS, Katz RM, Mickey MR, Siegel SC. Metaproterenol and theophylline in asthmatic children. *Ann Allergy* (1980) 45, 207–12.
7. Whyte KF, Reid C, Addis GJ, Whitesmith R, Reid JL. Salbutamol induced hypokalaemia: the effect of theophylline alone and in combination with adrenaline. *Br J Clin Pharmacol* (1988) 25, 571–8.
8. Georgopoulos D, Wong D, Anthonisen NR. Interactive effects of systemically administered salbutamol and aminophylline in patients with chronic obstructive pulmonary disease. *Am Rev Respir Dis* (1988) 138, 1499–1503.
9. Dawson KP, Fergusson DM. Effects of oral theophylline and oral salbutamol in the treatment of asthma. *Arch Dis Child* (1982) 57, 674–6.
10. Poukkula A, Korhonen UR, Huikuri H, Linnaluoto M. Theophylline and salbutamol in combination in patients with obstructive pulmonary disease and concurrent heart disease: effect on cardiac arrhythmias. *J Int Med* (1989) 226, 229–34.
11. Epelbaum S, Benhamou PH, Pautard JC, Devoldere C, Kremp O, Piussan C. Arrêt respiratoire chez une enfant asthmatique traitée par bêta-2-mimétiques et théophylline. Rôle possible de l'hypokaliémie dans les décès subits des asthmatiques. *Ann Pediatr (Paris)* (1989) 36, 473–5.
12. Amitai Y, Glustein J, Godfrey S. Enhancement of theophylline clearance by oral albuterol. *Chest* (1992) 102, 786–9.
13. Terra Filho M, Santos SRCJ, Cukier A, Verrastro C, Carvalho-Pinto RM, Fiss E, Vargas FS. Efeitos dos agonistas beta-2-adrenérgicos por via oral, sobre os níveis séricos de teofilina. *Revista Do Hospital Das Clinicas; Faculdade De Medicina Da Universidade De Sao Paulo* (1991) 46, 170–2.
14. Amirav I, Amitai Y, Avital A, Godfrey S. Enhancement of theophylline clearance by intravenous albuterol. *Chest* (1988) 94, 444–5.

15. McCann JP, McElnay JC, Nicholls DP, Scott MG, Stanford CF. Oral salbutamol does not affect theophylline kinetics. *Br J Pharmacol* (1986) 89 (Proc Suppl), 715P.
16. Smith SR, Kendall MJ. Potentiation of the adverse effects of intravenous terbutaline by oral theophylline. *Br J Clin Pharmacol* (1986) 21, 451–3.
17. Chow OKW, Fung KP. Slow-release terbutaline and theophylline for the long-term therapy of children with asthma: A latin square and factorial study of drug effects and interactions. *Pediatrics* (1989) 84, 119–25.
18. Garty MS, Keslin LS, Ilfeld DN, Mazar A, Spitzer S, Rosenfeld JB. Increased theophylline clearance by terbutaline in asthmatic adults. *Clin Pharmacol Ther* (1988) 43, 150.
19. Danziger Y, Garty M, Volwitz B, Ilfeld D, Versano I, Rosenfeld JB. Reduction of serum theophylline levels by terbutaline in children with asthma. *Clin Pharmacol Ther* (1985) 37, 469–71.
20. Wang Y, Yin A, Yu Z. Effects of bricanyl on the pharmacokinetics of aminophylline in asthmatic patients [In Chinese]. *Zhongguo Yiyuan Yaoxue Zazhi* (1992) 12, 389–90.
21. Committee on Safety of Medicines/Medicines Control Agency. β$_2$-Agonists, xanthines and hypokalaemia. *Current Problems* (1990) 28.

Theophylline + Beta-blockers

Propranolol reduces the clearance of theophylline. More importantly, non-selective beta-blockers such as nadolol and propranolol should not be given to asthmatic patients because they can cause bronchospasm. The concurrent use of theophylline and cardioselective beta-blockers such as atenolol, bisoprolol or metoprolol is not totally contraindicated, but some caution is still appropriate. These agents do not seem to affect the pharmacokinetics of theophylline. See also 'Antiasthmatic drugs + Beta-blockers', p.862.

Clinical evidence

(a) Pharmacokinetics

A study in 8 healthy subjects (6 of whom smoked 10–30 cigarettes daily) found that the clearance of a single dose of theophylline (as intravenous aminophylline) was reduced 37% by **propranolol** (40 mg six-hourly). **Metoprolol** (50 mg six-hourly), did not alter the clearance in the group as a whole, but the smokers showed an 11% reduction in clearance.[1] Another study found that the steady-state plasma clearance of theophylline in 7 normal subjects was reduced by 30% by 40 mg **propranolol** eight-hourly, and by 52% by 240 mg eight-hourly.[2] However, a further study found no significant pharmacokinetic interaction between theophylline and **propranolol**.[3] Three other studies found that 50 to 150 mg **atenolol**,[4,5] 10 mg **bisoprolol**,[6] both cardioselective beta-blockers, and 80 mg **nadolol**,[4] a non-selective beta-blocker, did not affect the pharmacokinetics of theophylline.

(b) Pharmacodynamics

Beta-blockers, particularly those that are non-selective, can cause bronchoconstriction, which opposes the bronchodilatory effects of theophylline.

In a study in 8 healthy volunteers, both **propranolol** 40 mg six-hourly and **metoprolol** 50 mg six-hourly prevented the mild inotropic effect seen with theophylline alone.[7]

Propranolol infusion reduced hypokalaemia and tachycardia after theophylline overdose.[8,9] **Esmolol** has been used similarly.[10]

Mechanism

Propranolol affects the clearance of theophylline by inhibiting its metabolism (demethylation and hydroxylation).[2,11]

Importance and management

The risk of severe, possibly even fatal bronchospasm when beta-blockers are used in asthmatics would seem to be far more important than any pharmacokinetic interaction between theophylline and beta-blockers. See the warning in 'Antiasthmatic drugs + Beta-blockers', p.862. Therefore, the non-selective beta-blockers such as propranolol (see the list at the beginning of Chapter 10) are contraindicated in patients with asthma or chronic obstructive pulmonary disease (COPD). Bronchospasm can occur after any route of administration of beta-blockers, even when given as eye drops. Cardioselective beta-blockers have less effect on the airways, but can still cause bronchoconstriction.

Beta-blockers can also block the inotropic effects of theophylline, which may be important in some patients with COPD.[7]

1. Conrad KA, Nyman DW. Effects of metoprolol and propranolol on theophylline elimination. *Clin Pharmacol Ther* (1980) 28, 463–7.
2. Miners JO, Wing LMH, Lillywhite KJ, Robson RA. Selectivity and dose-dependency of the inhibitory effect of propranolol on theophylline metabolism in man. *Br J Clin Pharmacol* (1985) 20, 219–23.
3. Minton NA, Turner T, Henry JA. Pharmacodynamic and pharmacokinetic interactions between theophylline and propranolol during dynamic exercise. *Br J Clin Pharmacol* (1995) 40, 521P.
4. Corsi CM, Nafziger AN, Pieper JA, Bertino JS. Lack of effect of atenolol and nadolol on the metabolism of theophylline. *Br J Clin Pharmacol* (1990) 29, 265–8.
5. Cerasa LA, Bertino JS, Ludwig EA, Savliwala M, Middleton E, Slaughter RL. Lack of effect of atenolol on the pharmacokinetics of theophylline. *Br J Clin Pharmacol* (1988) 26, 800–802.
6. Warrington SJ, Johnston A, Lewis Y, Murphy M. Bisoprolol: Studies of potential interactions with theophylline and warfarin in healthy volunteers. *J Cardiovasc Pharmacol* (1990) 16 (Suppl 5), S164–S168.
7. Conrad KA, Prosnitz EH. Cardiovascular effects of theophylline. Partial attenuation by beta-blockade. *Eur J Clin Pharmacol* (1981) 21, 109–114.
8. Kearney TE, Manoguerra AS, Curtis GP, Ziegler MG. Theophylline toxicity and the beta-adrenergic system. *Ann Intern Med* (1985) 102, 766–9.
9. Amin DN, Henry JA. Propranolol administration in theophylline overdose. *Lancet* (1985) i, 520–1.
10. Seneff M, Scott J, Freidman B, Smith M. Acute theophylline toxicity and the use of esmolol to reverse cardiovascular instability. *Ann Emerg Med* (1990) 19, 671–3.
11. Greenblatt DJ, Franke K, Huffman DH. Impairment of antipyrine clearance in humans by propranolol. *Circulation* (1978) 57, 1161–4.

Theophylline + Caffeine

Consumption of caffeine-containing beverages can raise serum theophylline levels, but the clinical relevance of this is unclear.

Clinical evidence, mechanism, importance and management

Caffeine can decrease the clearance of **theophylline** by 18–29%, prolong its half-life by up to 44% and increase its average serum levels by as much as 23%.[1-3] In addition, caffeine plasma levels were increased about twofold when theophylline was given.[2] In these studies, **caffeine** was administered in the form of tablets[1,2] or as instant **coffee** (2 to 7 cups).[3] In one study, 2 of the subjects who did not normally drink **coffee** experienced headaches and nausea.[2]

The probable mechanism of the interaction is that the 2 drugs compete for the same metabolic pathway so that they accumulate. In addition, when **caffeine** levels are high, a small percentage of it is converted to **theophylline**. There would, however, seem to be no good reason for those on **theophylline** normally to avoid **caffeine** (in coffee, tea, '*Coke*', medications, etc.), but if otherwise unexplained adverse effects occur it might be worth checking if **caffeine** is responsible. In addition, caffeine intake could have an impact on the interaction of theophylline with other drugs.

1. Loi CM, Jue SG, Bush ED, Crowley JJ, Vestal RE. Effect of caffeine dose on theophylline metabolism. *Clin Res* (1987) 35, 377A.
2. Jonkman JHG, Sollie FAE, Sauter R, Steinijans VW. The influence of caffeine on the steady-state pharmacokinetics of theophylline. *Clin Pharmacol Ther* (1991) 49, 248–55.
3. Sato J, Nakata H, Owada E, Kikuta T, Umetsu M, Ito K. Influence of usual intake of dietary caffeine on single-dose kinetics of theophylline in healthy human subjects. *Eur J Clin Pharmacol* (1993) 44, 295–8.

Theophylline + Calcium channel blockers

Concurrent use normally seems to have no adverse effect on the control of asthma, despite the small or modest changes (increases or decreases) in serum theophylline levels reported with diltiazem, felodipine, nifedipine and verapamil. However, there are isolated case reports of unexplained theophylline toxicity in two patients given nifedipine and two patients given verapamil. Israddipine appears not to interact.

Clinical evidence

(a) Diltiazem

Diltiazem 90 mg twice daily for 10 days reduced the clearance of theophylline (given as a single dose of aminophylline 6 mg/kg) by 21% in 9 healthy subjects, and increased its half-life from 6.1 to 7.5 h.[1] A 12% fall in theophylline clearance (given as a single oral dose of 5 mg/kg) was found in another study in healthy subjects given **diltiazem** 90 mg three times daily.[2] **Diltiazem** 60 mg three times daily for 5 days given to 8 patients with asthma or chronic obstructive pulmonary disease (COPD), reduced the steady-state theophylline clearance by 22% (from 87.3 to 68.3 ml/min) and increased its half-life by 24% (from 5.7 to 7.5 h).[3]

Conversely, other studies found no significant changes in peak steady-state theophylline levels in 18 patients with asthma given **diltiazem** 240 to 480 mg daily for 7 days,[4] or in 7 healthy subjects given diltiazem 120 mg twice daily for 7 days.[5] Similarly, there was no significant change in the theophylline half-life or clearance (after a single intravenous dose of aminophylline 250 mg) in healthy subjects given diltiazem 120 mg three times daily for 6 days.[6]

(b) Felodipine

Felodipine 5 mg eight-hourly for 4 days reduced the plasma AUC of theophylline in 10 normal subjects by 18.3%, but had no effect on metabolic or renal clearance.[7]

(c) Isradipine

A three-way crossover study in 11 healthy subjects found that 2.5 or 5 mg **isradipine** 12-hourly for 6 days had no significant effect on the pharmacokinetics of a single dose of theophylline (5 mg/kg orally).[8]

(d) Nifedipine

In one study, slow-release **nifedipine** 20 mg twice daily reduced the mean steady-state serum theophylline levels of 8 asthmatics by 30% (from 9.7 to 6.8 micrograms/ml). Levels fell by 50, 56 and 64% in three of the patients, but no changes in the control of the asthma were seen as measured by peak flow determinations and symptom scores.[9] However, many other studies have found no changes, or only small or modest changes, in the pharmacokinetics of theophylline in normal subjects[5,10-12] or asthmatic patients when given **nifedipine**.[4,13,14] The control of the asthma was unchanged by nifedipine.[13,14] Yet another study found that combined use improved pulmonary function and blood pressure control.[15]

In contrast, there are 2 case reports of patients who developed theophylline toxicity (theophylline levels raised to 30 and 41 micrograms/ml), apparently due to the addition of **nifedipine**.[16,17] In one case, the toxicity occurred on reinstitution of combined therapy, and resolved when the theophylline dosage was reduced by 60%.[17] During a Swan Ganz catheter study of patient response to **nifedipine** for pulmonary hypertension, 2 patients developed serious **nifedipine** side-effects, which responded dramatically to intravenous aminophylline.[18]

(e) Verapamil

In one study, **verapamil** 80 mg six-hourly for 2 days had no effect on the pharmacokinetics of theophylline (200 mg aminophylline six-hourly) given to 5 asthmatics, and no effect on their spirometric measurements (FVC, FEV$_1$, FEF$_{25-75}$).[19] Similarly, another study found **verapamil** 80 mg eight-hourly had no effect on steady-state serum theophylline levels in healthy subjects.[20] In contrast, numerous other studies in healthy subjects have found modest reductions in theophylline clearance ranging between 8% and 23% with **verapamil** 40 to 120 mg six to eight-hourly.[2,6,10,21-23] One study showed that the extent of reduction in clearance depended on the **verapamil** dosage.[23] An isolated report describes a woman on digoxin and theophylline who developed signs of toxicity (tachycardia, nausea, vomiting) after starting to take **verapamil** 80 mg, increased to 120 mg, eight-hourly. Her theophylline serum levels doubled over a 6-day period. Theophylline was later successfully reintroduced at one-third of the original dosage.[24] Another isolated report describes a patient who needed 50% less theophylline while taking 120 mg **verapamil** daily.[25]

Mechanism

It is believed that diltiazem and verapamil can decrease the metabolism of theophylline by the liver to a small extent, possibly by inhibiting cytochrome P450 isoenzyme CYP1A2.[26] Similarly, nifedipine may alter hepatic theophylline metabolism,[10] or it may increase the volume of distribution of theophylline.[11,12] Felodipine possibly reduces theophylline absorption.[7]

Importance and management

Adequately documented. The results are not entirely consistent but the overall picture is that the concurrent use of theophylline and these calcium channel blockers is normally safe. Despite the small or modest decreases in the clearance or absorption of theophylline seen with diltiazem, felodipine and verapamil, and the quite large reductions in serum levels seen in one study with nifedipine, no adverse changes in the control of the asthma were seen in any of the studies. However, very occasionally and unpredictably theophylline levels have risen enough to cause toxicity in patients given nifedipine (2 case reports) or verapamil (2 case reports), so that it would be prudent to monitor the effects.

1. Nafziger AN, May JJ, Bertino JS. Inhibition of theophylline elimination by diltiazem therapy. *J Clin Pharmacol* (1987) 27, 862–5.
2. Sirmans SM, Pieper JA, Lalonde RL, Smith DG, Self TH. Effect of calcium channel blockers on theophylline disposition. *Clin Pharmacol Ther* (1988) 44, 29–34.
3. Soto J, Sacristan JA, Alsar MJ. Diltiazem treatment impairs theophylline elimination in patients with bronchospastic airway disease. *Ther Drug Monit* (1994) 16, 49–52.
4. Christopher MA, Harman E, Hendeles L. Clinical relevance of the interaction of theophylline with diltiazem or nifedipine. *Chest* (1989) 95, 309–13.
5. Smith SR, Haffner CA, Kendall MJ. The influence of nifedipine and diltiazem on serum theophylline concentration-time profiles. *J Clin Pharm Ther* (1989) 14, 403–8.
6. Abernethy DR, Egan JM, Dickinson TH, Carrum G. Substrate-selective inhibition by verapamil and diltiazem: differential disposition of antipyrine and theophylline in humans. *J Pharmacol Exp Ther* (1988) 244, 994–9.
7. Bratel T, Billing B, Dahlqvist R. Felodipine reduces the absorption of theophylline in man. *Eur J Clin Pharmacol* (1989) 36, 481–5.
8. Perreault MM, Kazierad DJ, Wilton JH, Izzo JL. The effect of isradipine on theophylline pharmacokinetics in healthy volunteers. *Pharmacotherapy* (1993) 13, 149–53.
9. Smith SR, Wiggins J, Stableforth DE, Skinner C, Kendall MJ. Effect of nifedipine on serum theophylline concentrations and asthma control. *Thorax* (1987) 42, 794–6.
10. Robson RA, Miners JO, Birkett DJ. Selective inhibitory effects of nifedipine and verapamil on oxidative metabolism: effects on theophylline. *Br J Clin Pharmacol* (1988) 25, 397–400.
11. Jackson SHD, Shah K, Debbas NMG, Johnston A, Peverel-Cooper CA, Turner P. The interaction between i.v. theophylline and chronic oral dosing with slow release nifedipine in volunteers. *Br J Clin Pharmacol* (1986) 21, 389–92.
12. Adebayo GI, Mabadeje AFB. Effect of nifedipine on antipyrine and theophylline disposition. *Biopharm Drug Dispos* (1990) 11, 157–64.
13. Garty M, Cohen E, Mazar A, Ilfeld DN, Spitzer S, Rosenfeld JB. Effect of nifedipine and theophylline in asthma. *Clin Pharmacol Ther* (1986) 40, 195–8.
14. Yilmaz E, Canberk A, Eroğlu L. Nifedipine alters serum theophylline levels in asthmatic patients with hypertension. *Fundam Clin Pharmacol* (1991) 5, 341–5.
15. Spedini C, Lombardi C. Long-term treatment with oral nifedipine plus theophylline in the management of chronic bronchial asthma. *Eur J Clin Pharmacol* (1986) 31, 105–6.
16. Parrillo SJ, Venditto M. Elevated theophylline blood levels from institution of nifedipine therapy. *Ann Emerg Med* (1984) 13, 216–17.
17. Harrod CS. Theophylline toxicity and nifedipine. *Ann Intern Med* (1987) 106, 480.
18. Kalra L, Bone MF, Ariaraj SJP. Nifedipine-aminophylline interaction. *J Clin Pharmacol* (1988) 28, 1056–7.
19. Gotz VP, Russell WL. Effect of verapamil on theophylline disposition. *Chest* (1987) 92, 75S.
20. Rindone JP, Zuniga R, Sock JA. The influence of verapamil on theophylline serum concentrations. *Drug Metabol Drug Interact* (1989) 7, 143–7.
21. Nielsen-Kudsk JE, Buhl JS, Johannessen AC. Verapamil-induced inhibition of theophylline elimination in healthy humans. *Pharmacol Toxicol* (1990) 66, 101–3.
22. Gin AS, Stringer KA, Welage LS, Wilton JH, Matthews GE. The effect of verapamil on the pharmacokinetic disposition of theophylline in cigarette smokers. *J Clin Pharmacol* (1989) 29, 728–32.
23. Stringer KA, Mallet J, Clarke M, Lindenfeld JA. The effect of three different oral doses of verapamil on the disposition of theophylline. *Eur J Clin Pharmacol* (1992) 43, 35–8.
24. Burnakis TG, Seldon M, Czaplicki AD. Increased serum theophylline concentrations secondary to oral verapamil. *Clin Pharm* (1983) 2, 458–61.
25. Bangura L, Malesker MA, Dewan NA. Theophylline and verapamil: Clinically significant drug interaction. *J Pharm Technol* (1997) 13, 241–3.
26. Fuhr U, Woodcock BG, Siewert M. Verapamil and drug metabolism by the cytochrome P450 isoform CYP1A2. *Eur J Clin Pharmacol* (1992) 42, 463–4.

Theophylline + Carbamazepine

Two case reports describe a marked fall in serum theophylline levels during the concurrent use of carbamazepine. Another single case report and a pharmacokinetic study describe a fall in serum carbamazepine levels when theophylline was given.

Clinical evidence

(a) Theophylline serum levels reduced

Asthma in an 11-year-old girl was well controlled for 2 months with theophylline until the **phenobarbital** she was taking was replaced by **carbamazepine**. The asthma worsened, theophylline serum levels became subtherapeutic and the half-life of the theophylline halved (from 5.25 to 2.75 h). Asthmatic control was restored, and the half-life returned to pre-treatment levels 3 weeks after the **carbamazepine** was replaced by **ethotoin**.[1] The clearance of theophylline in an adult patient was doubled while taking **carbamazepine** (600 mg daily).[2]

(b) Carbamazepine serum levels reduced

A girl of 10 showed a fall in serum **carbamazepine** levels (trough concentrations roughly halved) when given theophylline for 2 days, and she experienced a grand mal seizure. Her serum theophylline levels were also unusually high (142 micromol/l, equivalent to 26 micrograms/ml) for the dosage taken (5 mg/kg six-hourly), so it may be that the convulsions were as much due to this as to the fall in **carbamazepine** levels.[3]

A single-dose pharmacokinetic study in normal subjects found that the **carbamazepine** AUC was reduced by 31% by oral aminophylline, and the maximum serum level was reduced by 45%.[4]

Mechanism

Not established, but it seems probable that each drug increases the liver metabolism and clearance of the other drug, resulting in a reduction in their effects.[1,3] It is also possible that aminophylline interferes with the absorption of carbamazepine.[4]

Importance and management

Information seems to be limited to the reports cited so that the general importance is uncertain. Concurrent use need not be avoided, but it would be prudent to check that the serum concentrations of each drug (and their effects) are not reduced to subtherapeutic levels.

1. Rosenberry KR, Defusco CJ, Mansmann HC, McGeady SJ. Reduced theophylline half-life induced by carbamazepine therapy. *J Pediatr* (1983) 102, 472–4.
2. Reed RC, Schwartz HJ. Phenytoin-theophylline-quinidine interaction. *N Engl J Med* (1983) 308, 724–5.
3. Mitchell EA, Dower JC, Green RJ. Interaction between carbamazepine and theophylline. *N Z Med J* (1986) 99, 69–70.
4. Kulkarni C, Vaz J, David J, Joseph T. Aminophylline alters pharmacokinetics of carbamazepine but not that of sodium valproate — a single dose pharmacokinetic study in human volunteers. *Ind J Physiol Pharmacol* (1995) 39, 122–6.

Theophylline + Cephalosporins

Ceftibuten and cefalexin appear not to interact with theophylline. Cefaclor has been implicated in two cases of theophylline toxicity in children, but studies in adult subjects found no pharmacokinetic interaction.

Clinical evidence, mechanism, importance and management

Ceftibuten 200 mg twice daily for 7 days was found to have no significant effect on the pharmacokinetics of single intravenous doses of theophylline given to 12 normal subjects.[1] A study in 9 healthy adults given single doses of aminophylline (5 mg/kg iv) found that **cefalexin** 500 mg, then 250 mg six-hourly for 48 h, had no significant effect on the kinetics of theophylline.[2] A case report,[3] and a brief summary in the introduction of a study,[4] have suggested that **cefaclor** might have been responsible for the development of theophylline toxicity in 2 children. However, a single-dose[4,5] and a steady-state[6] study in adult subjects found that 750 mg **cefaclor** daily for 8 and 9 days respectively had no effect on the pharmacokinetics of theophylline. No special precautions, apart from those normally taken with theophylline, seem to be necessary with any of these antibacterials. Note that acute infections *per se* can alter theophylline pharmacokinetics.

1. Bachmann K, Schwartz J, Jauregui L, Martin M, Nunlee M. Failure of ceftibuten to alter single dose theophylline clearance. *J Clin Pharmacol* (1990) 30, 444–8.
2. Pfeifer HJ, Greenblatt DJ, Friedman P. Effects of three antibiotics on theophylline kinetics. *Clin Pharmacol Ther* (1979) 26, 36–40.
3. Hammond D, Abate MA. Theophylline toxicity, acute illness, and cefaclor administration. *DICP Ann Pharmacother* (1989) 23, 339–40.
4. Jauregui L, Bachmann K, Forney R, Bischoff M, Schwartz J. The impact of cefaclor on the pharmacokinetics of theophylline. Recent Adv Chemother.*Proc Int Congr Chemother 14th Antimicrob Section 1* (1985) 694–5.
5. Bachmann K, Schwartz J, Forney RB, Jauregui L. Impact of cefaclor on the pharmacokinetics of theophylline. *Ther Drug Monit* (1986) 8, 151–4.
6. Jonkman JHG, van der Boon WJV, Schoenmaker R, Holtkamp A, Hempenius J. Clinical pharmacokinetics of theophylline during co-treatment with cefaclor. *Int J Clin Pharmacol Ther Toxicol* (1986) 24, 88–92.

Theophylline + Contraceptives, oral

Serum theophylline clearance is reduced to some extent in women taking combined oral contraceptives, but no toxicity has been reported.

Clinical evidence

The total plasma clearance of a single oral dose of aminophylline (4 mg/kg) in 8 women on **combined oral contraceptives** *(Ovral)* was about 30% lower than in 8 other women not on oral contraceptives (35.1 compared with 53.1 ml/h/kg).[1] The theophylline half-life was also prolonged by about 30% (from 7.34 to 9.79 h). Similar results were found in other studies.[2,3] In contrast, no significant differences were seen in the theophylline pharmacokinetics in 10 adolescent women (15–18 years) on low-dose **combined oral contraceptives**, when compared with age matched controls.[4] However, when theophylline clearance was measured before and after 3 to 4 months use of **combined oral contraceptives** in the same women, these authors found a 33% reduction.[5] In a retrospective analysis of factors affecting theophylline clearance, the use of oral contraceptives was associated with a reduced theophylline clearance in women who smoked.[6]

Mechanism

Uncertain, but it seems possible that the oestrogenic component may inhibit the metabolism of the theophylline by the liver microsomal enzymes, thereby reducing its clearance.

Importance and management

An established interaction, but there seem to be no reports of theophylline toxicity resulting from concurrent use. Women on combined oral contraceptives may need less theophylline than those not taking oral contraceptives. There is a small risk that patients with serum theophylline levels at the top end of the range may show some toxicity when oral contraceptives are added. It has been proposed that the effects may be more apparent with long-term, high-dose contraceptive use.[1,4]

1. Tornatore KM, Kanarkowski R, McCarthy TL, Gardner MJ, Yurchak AM, Jusko WJ. Effect of chronic oral contraceptive steroids on theophylline disposition. *Eur J Clin Pharmacol* (1982) 23, 129–34.
2. Roberts RK, Grice J, McGuffie C, Heilbronn L. Oral contraceptive steroids impair the elimination of theophylline. *J Lab Clin Med* (1983) 101, 821–5.
3. Gardner MJ, Tornatore KM, Jusko WJ, Kanarkowski R. Effects of tobacco smoking and oral contraceptive use on theophylline disposition. *Br J Clin Pharmacol* (1983) 16, 271–80.
4. Koren G, Chin TF, Correia J, Tesoro A, MacLeod S. Theophylline pharmacokinetics in adolescent females following coadministration of oral contraceptives. *Clin Invest Med* (1985) 8, 222–6.
5. Long DR, Roberts EA, Brill-Edwards M, Quaggin S, Correia J, Koren G, MacLeod SM. The effect of the oral contraceptive Ortho 7/7/7® on theophylline (T) clearance in non-smoking women aged 18–22. *Clin Invest Med* (1987) 10 (4 Suppl B), B59.
6. Jusko WJ, Gardner MJ, Mangione A, Schentag JJ, Koup JR, Vance JW. Factors affecting theophylline clearances: age, tobacco, marijuana, cirrhosis, congestive heart failure, obesity, oral contraceptives, benzodiazepines, barbiturates, and ethanol. *J Pharm Sci* (1979) 68, 1358–66.

Theophylline + Corticosteroids

Theophylline and corticosteroids have established roles in the management of asthma and their concurrent use is not uncommon. There are isolated reports of increases in serum

theophylline levels (sometimes associated with toxicity) during concurrent use of oral or parenteral corticosteroids, but others showing no changes. The general clinical importance of these findings is uncertain.

Clinical evidence

(a) Increased serum theophylline levels

Three patients in status asthmaticus with relatively stable serum concentrations of theophylline were given an intravenous 500 mg bolus of **hydrocortisone** followed 6 h later by three 2-hourly doses of 200 mg. In each case the serum theophylline levels climbed from about 20 to between 30 and 50 micrograms/ml. At least 2 of the patients complained of nausea and headache.[1] Another study in 10 children (aged 2 to 6) with status asthmaticus showed that intramuscular **methylprednisolone** tended to increase the half-life of theophylline.[2] A further study also reported a prolonged theophylline half-life (from 5 to 6.2 h) and a reduced clearance (by about one-third) when intravenous aminophylline was administered to 16 children taking corticosteroids (route and type not specified) compared with 10 who were not.[3]

(b) Reduced serum theophylline levels

An increase in the clearance of a single dose of intravenous aminophylline was seen in one of 3 normal subjects when pretreated with oral **methylprednisolone**.[4] There was no significant change in clearance in the other 2 subjects.

(c) Theophylline levels unchanged

Seven normal subjects had no significant change in steady-state theophylline clearance when given intravenous **methylprednisolone** (1.6 mg/kg) and **hydrocortisone** (33 mg/kg) in a crossover study, although there was a trend towards increased clearance.[5] Another study in 6 normal subjects showed that a single oral dose of **prednisone** (20 mg) had no significant effect on the pharmacokinetics of a single oral dose of aminophylline (200 mg).[6] Nine patients with chronic airflow obstruction showed no changes in the pharmacokinetics of a single intravenous dose of aminophylline (5.6 mg/kg) when treated with 20 mg **prednisolone** daily for three weeks.[7] Intravenous bolus doses of 500 or 1000 mg **hydrocortisone** did not affect theophylline levels in patients taking 400 mg choline theophyllinate 12-hourly for 8 days.[8] The theophylline elimination half-life was no different in premature infants who had been exposed to **betamethasone** *in utero* than in those who had not, although the exposed neonates had a wider range of theophylline metabolites indicating greater hepatic metabolism.[9,10]

Mechanism

Not understood.

Importance and management

The few reported interactions of theophylline with oral or parenteral corticosteroids are poorly documented and their clinical importance is difficult to assess because both increases, small decreases and no changes in the serum levels of theophylline have been reported. It is also questionable whether the results of studies in normal healthy subjects can validly be extrapolated to patients with status asthmaticus. There do not appear to be any data on the effect of *inhaled* corticosteroids on clearance of theophylline, and this is the combination most frequently used in asthma therapy. Both theophylline and corticosteroids can cause hypokalaemia, and the possibility that this may be potentiated by the combination should be considered.

1. Buchanan N, Hurwitz S, Butler P. Asthma—a possible interaction between hydrocortisone and theophylline. *S Afr Med J* (1979) 56, 1147–8.
2. De La Morena E, Borges MT, Garcia Rebollar C, Escorihuela R. Efecto de la metil-prednisolona sobre los niveles séricos de teofilina. *Rev Clin Esp* (1982) 167, 297–300.
3. Elvey SM, Saccar CL, Rocci ML, Mansmann HC, Martynec DM, Kester MB. The effect of corticosteroids on theophylline metabolism in asthmatic children. *Ann Allergy* (1986) 56, 520.
4. Squire EN, Nelson HS. Corticosteroids and theophylline clearance. *NER Allergy Proc* (1987) 8, 113–15.
5. Leavengood DC, Bunker-Soler AL, Nelson HS. The effect of corticosteroids on theophylline metabolism. *Ann Allergy* (1983) 50, 249–51.
6. Anderson JL, Ayres JW, Hall CA. Potential pharmacokinetic interaction between theophylline and prednisone. *Clin Pharm* (1984) 3, 187–9.
7. Fergusson RJ, Scott CM, Rafferty P, Gaddie J. Effect of prednisolone on theophylline pharmacokinetics in patients with chronic airflow obstruction. *Thorax* (1987) 42, 195–8.
8. Tatsis G, Orphanidou D, Douratsos D, Mellissinos C, Pantelakis D, Pipini E, Jordanoglou J. The effect of steroids on theophylline absorption. *J Int Med Res* (1991) 19, 326–9.
9. Jager-Roman E, Doyle PE, Thomas D, Baird-Lambert J, Cvejic M, Buchanan N. Increased theophylline metabolism in premature infants after prenatal betamethasone administration. *Dev Pharmacol Ther* (1982) 5, 127–35.
10. Baird-Lambert J, Doyle PE, Thomas D, Jager-Roman E, Cvejic M, Buchanan N. Theophylline metabolism in preterm neonates during the first weeks of life. *Dev Pharmacol Ther* (1984) 7, 239–44.

Theophylline + Co-trimoxazole

Co-trimoxazole does not interact with theophylline.

Clinical evidence, mechanism, importance and management

Eight days treatment with **co-trimoxazole** (960 mg twice daily) had no effect on the pharmacokinetics of a single intravenous dose of aminophylline (341 mg) in 6 normal subjects.[1] Another study found that **co-trimoxazole** (960 mg twice daily) for 5 days had no effect on the pharmacokinetics of a single oral dose of theophylline (267 mg) in 8 healthy subjects.[2] No special precautions would seem necessary if these drugs are given concurrently. However, note that acute infections *per se* can alter theophylline pharmacokinetics.

1. Jonkman JHG, Van Der Boon WJV, Schoenmaker R, Holtkamp AH, Hempenius J. Lack of influence of co-trimoxazole on theophylline pharmacokinetics. *J Pharm Sci* (1985) 74, 1103–4.
2. Lo KF, Nation RL, Sansom LN. Lack of effect of co-trimoxazole on the pharmacokinetics of orally administered theophylline. *Biopharm Drug Dispos* (1989) 10, 573–80.

Theophylline + Dextropropoxyphene (Propoxyphene)

Dextropropoxyphene does not interact significantly with theophylline.

Clinical evidence, mechanism, importance and management

Pre-treatment with 65 mg **dextropropoxyphene** 8-hourly for 5 days did not significantly change the total plasma clearance of theophylline (125 mg eight-hourly) at steady state in 6 normal subjects.[1] There was a small reduction in the formation of the hydroxylated metabolite of theophylline. There would seem to be no need to avoid concurrent use or to take particular precautions.

1. Robson RA, Miners JO, Whitehead AG, Birkett DJ. Specificity of the inhibitory effect of dextropropoxyphene on oxidative drug metabolism in man: effects on theophylline and tolbutamide disposition. *Br J Clin Pharmacol* (1987) 23, 772–5.

Theophylline + Disulfiram

Blood theophylline levels are increased by disulfiram. The theophylline dosage may need to be reduced to avoid toxicity.

Clinical evidence

After taking 250 mg **disulfiram** daily for a week, the clearance of theophylline (5 mg/kg infused intravenously) in 20 recovering alcoholics was decreased by a mean of about 21% (range 14.6 to 29.6%). Those taking 500 mg **disulfiram** daily showed a mean decrease of 32.5% (range 21.6 to 49.6%).[1,2] Smoking appeared to have no important effects on the extent of this interaction.

Mechanism

Disulfiram inhibits the liver enzymes concerned with the both the hydroxylation and demethylation of theophylline, thereby reducing its clearance from the body.

Importance and management

Information appears to be limited to this study but it would seem to be an established and clinically important interaction. Monitor the serum levels of theophylline and its effects if disulfiram is added, anticipating the need to reduce the theophylline dosage by up to 50%, bearing in mind that the extent of this interaction depends upon the dosage of disulfiram used.

1. Loi C-M, Day JD, Jue SG, Costello P, Vestal RE. The effect of disulfiram on theophylline disposition. *Clin Pharmacol Ther* (1987) 41, 165.
2. Loi C-M, Day JD, Jue SG, Bush ED, Costello P, Dewey LV, Vestal RE. Dose-dependent inhibition of theophylline metabolism by disulfiram in recovering alcoholics. *Clin Pharmacol Ther* (1989) 45, 476–86.

Theophylline + Ephedrine

There are some data suggesting an increased frequency of adverse effects when ephedrine is used with theophylline.

Clinical evidence, mechanism, importance and management

A double-blind randomised study in 23 children aged 4 to 14 found that when ephedrine was combined with theophylline (25 mg/130 mg), the number of adverse reactions increased significantly when compared with each drug taken separately, and moreover the combination was no more effective than theophylline alone. The combination was associated with insomnia (14 patients), nervousness (13 patients) and gastrointestinal complaints (18 patients) including vomiting (12 patients). The serum theophylline levels were unchanged by ephedrine.[1] A previous study in 12 asthmatic children by the same authors produced essentially similar results.[2] However a later study suggested that 25 mg ephedrine 8-hourly added to theophylline did produce improvements (as measured by spirometry) and no adverse effects were seen, however it was calculated that the theophylline dosage used was about half that used in the previous study.[3]

In the treatment of asthma, **ephedrine** has been largely superseded by more selective sympathomimetics, which have fewer adverse effects. **Ephedrine** is still an ingredient of a number of cough and cold remedies, when it may be combined with theophylline (e.g. *Franol*).

1. Weinberger M, Bronsky E, Bensch GW, Bock GN, Yecies JJ. Interaction of ephedrine and theophylline. *Clin Pharmacol Ther* (1975) 17, 585–92.
2. Weinberger MM, Bronsky EA. Evaluation of oral bronchodilator therapy in asthmatic children. *J Pediatr* (1974) 84, 421–7.
3. Tinkelman DG, Avner SE. Ephedrine therapy in asthmatic children. Clinical tolerance and absence of side effects. *JAMA* (1977) 237, 553–7.

Theophylline + Erythromycin

Theophylline serum levels can be increased by the concurrent use of erythromycin. Toxicity may develop in those patients whose serum levels are at the higher end of the range unless the dosage is reduced. The onset may be delayed for several days, and not all patients demonstrate this interaction. Erythromycin levels may possibly fall to subtherapeutic concentrations. For the effect of other macrolides, see 'Theophylline + Macrolide antibacterials', p.803.

Clinical evidence

(a) Theophylline serum levels increased

The peak serum theophylline levels of 12 patients with COPD given aminophylline (4 mg/kg orally 6-hourly) were raised 28% when concurrently treated with **erythromycin stearate** (500 mg 6-hourly) for 2 days. The clearance was reduced by 22%. Only one patient developed clinical signs of toxicity, although the authors suggest this may because the patients started with low theophylline levels (11 micrograms/ml) and they may not have been studied for long enough to detect the full effect of the **erythromycin**.[1] Several single-dose studies in healthy or asthmatic adults have demonstrated this interaction[2-6] and multiple dose studies have also shown altered theophylline pharmacokinetics.[7,8] A multiple-dose study in asthmatic children showed a 40% rise in theophylline levels.[9] There was often wide inter-subject variability, and not all patients demonstrated the interaction.[1,4,6-9] In addition to the studies, there are several case reports where **erythromycin** was thought to have caused previously therapeutic theophylline concentrations to rise to toxic levels. In 3 cases the level rose twofold, with accompanying symptoms of toxicity,[10-12] and in one case the patient developed a fatal cardia arrhythmia.[13]

Conversely, several studies in both healthy adults,[14-17] and adults with COPD[5,18] did not demonstrate any clinically significant interaction, although two studies did find reduced clearance of theophylline in some subjects.[14,18]

(b) Erythromycin serum levels reduced

The peak serum **erythromycin** levels of 6 healthy subjects taking 500 mg 8-hourly were almost halved and the AUC from 0 to 8 h was reduced by 38% when they were given a single 250-mg dose of theophylline intravenously.[6] Another pharmacokinetic study found that serum **erythromycin** levels fell by more than 30% when intravenous theophylline was given concurrently with oral erythromycin.[8] Earlier studies using intravenous erythromycin found no significant pharmacokinetic changes. The renal clearance was increased, but this did not affect the overall clearance.[17,19]

Mechanism

(a). Not fully understood. It seems most likely that erythromycin inhibits the metabolism of theophylline by the liver resulting in a reduction in its clearance from the body and a rise in its serum levels.

(b). It seems most likely that theophylline can affect the absorption of oral erythromycin.[17]

Importance and management

(a). The effects of erythromycin on theophylline are established (but still debated) and well documented. Not all the reports are referenced here. It does not seem to matter which erythromycin salt is used. Monitor concurrent use and anticipate the need to reduce the theophylline dosage to avoid toxicity. Not all patients will show this interaction but remember it may take several days (most commonly 2 to 7 days) to manifest itself. Limited evidence suggests that levels may return to normal 2 to 7 days after stopping erythromycin.[10-12] There are many factors, such as smoking[3,18] which affect theophylline kinetics and which may play a role in altering the significance of the interaction in different patients. Those particularly at risk are patients with already high serum theophylline levels and/or taking high dosages (20 mg/kg body weight or more) or more. Where concurrent treatment cannot be avoided, a 25% reduction in theophylline dose has been recommended for patients with levels in the 15–20 micrograms/ml range,[1,2,20] but little dosage adjustment is probably needed for those at the lower end of the range, (below 15 micrograms/ml) unless toxic symptoms appear.[1,4] In practice erythromycin can probably be safely started with theophylline, with levels monitored after 48 hours and appropriate dosage adjustments then made.

(b). The fall in erythromycin levels caused by theophylline is not well documented, but what is known suggests that it may be clinically important. Be alert for any evidence of an inadequate response to the erythromycin and increase the dosage or change the antibacterials if possible. More study is needed. Intravenous erythromycin appears not to be affected. More study is needed.

1. Reisz G, Pingleton SK, Melethil S, Ryan PB. The effect of erythromycin on theophylline pharmacokinetics in chronic bronchitis. *Am Rev Respir Dis* (1983) 127, 581–4.

2. Prince RA, Wing DS, Weinberger MM, Hendeles LS, Riegleman S. Effect of erythromycin on theophylline kinetics. *J Allergy Clin Immunol* (1981) 68, 427–31.
3. May DC, Jarboe CH, Ellenberg DT, Roe EJ, Karibo J. The effects of erythromycin on theophylline elimination in normal males. *J Clin Pharmacol* (1982) 22, 125–30.
4. Zarowitz BJM, Szefler SJ, Lasezkay GM. Effect of erythromycin base on theophylline kinetics. *Clin Pharmacol Ther* (1981) 29, 601–5.
5. Richer C, Mathieu M, Bah H, Thuillez C, Duroux P, Giudicelli J-F. Theophylline kinetics and ventilatory flow in bronchial asthma and chronic airflow obstruction: Influence of erythromycin. *Clin Pharmacol Ther* (1982) 31, 579–86.
6. Iliopoulou A, Aldhous ME, Johnston A, Turner P. Pharmacokinetic interaction between theophylline and erythromycin. *Br J Clin Pharmacol* (1982) 14, 495–9.
7. Branigan TA, Robbins RA, Cady WJ, Nickols JG, Ueda CT. The effects of erythromycin on the absorption and disposition kinetics of theophylline. *Eur J Clin Pharmacol* (1981) 21, 115–20.
8. Paulsen O, Höglund P, Nilsson L-G, Bengtsson H-I. The interaction of erythromycin with theophylline. *Eur J Clin Pharmacol* (1987) 32, 493–8.
9. LaForce CF, Miller MF, Chai H. Effect of erythromycin on theophylline clearance in asthmatic children. *J Pediatr* (1981) 99, 153–6.
10. Cummins LH, Kozak PP, Gillman SA. Erythromycin's effect on theophylline blood level. *Pediatrics* (1977) 59, 144–5.
11. Cummins LH, Kozak PP, Gillman SA. Theophylline determinations. *Ann Allergy* (1976) 37, 450–51.
12. Green JA, Clementi WA. Decrease in theophylline clearance after the administration of erythromycin to a patient with obstructive lung disease. *Drug Intell Clin Pharm* (1983) 17, 370–2.
13. Andrews PA. Interactions with ciprofloxacin and erythromycin leading to aminophylline toxicity. *Nephrol Dial Transplant* (1998) 13, 1006–8.
14. Pfeifer HJ, Greenblatt DJ, Friedman P. Effects of three antibiotics on theophylline kinetics. *Clin Pharmacol Ther* (1979) 26, 36–40.
15. Kelly SJ, Pingleton SK, Ryan PB, Melethil S. The lack of influence of erythromycin on plasma theophylline levels. *Chest* (1980) 78, 523.
16. Maddux MS, Leeds NH, Organek HW, Hasegawa GR, Bauman JL. The effect of erythromycin on theophylline pharmacokinetics at steady state. *Chest* (1982) 81, 563–5.
17. Pasic J, Jackson SHD, Johnston A, Peverel-Cooper CA, Turner P, Downey K, Chaput de Saintonge DM. The interaction between chronic oral slow-release theophylline and single-dose intravenous erythromycin. *Xenobiotica* (1987) 17, 493–7.
18. Stults BM, Felice-Johnson J, Higbee MD, Hardigan K. Effect of erythromycin stearate on serum theophylline concentration in patients with chronic obstructive lung disease. *South Med J* (1983) 76, 714–18.
19. Hildebrandt R, Möller H, Gundert-Remy U. Influence of theophylline on the renal clearance of erythromycin. *Int J Clin Pharmacol Ther Toxicol* (1987) 25, 601–4.
20. Aronson JK, Hardman M, Reynolds DJM. ABC of monitoring drug therapy. Theophylline. *BMJ* (1992) 305, 1355–8.

Theophylline + Food

The effect of food on theophylline bioavailability is unclear. In general it appears that fat or fibre in food has no effect, while high-protein and high-carbohydrate diets decrease and increase the theophylline half-life respectively. Significant changes in theophylline bioavailability have been seen with both enteral feeds and total parenteral nutrition.

Clinical evidence

(a) Theophylline and food

The bioavailability of theophylline from sustained release preparations has been shown to be reduced,[1] increased,[1,2] or unaffected[3-5] when given immediately after **breakfast**. Dose dumping, leading to signs of theophylline toxicity, was seen in 3 children with asthma who were given a dose of *Uniphyllin* immediately after **breakfast**.[5] The **fat** content[6,7] or **fibre** content[8] of meals does not seem to significantly affect theophylline absorption. **High-protein** meals appear to decrease theophylline half-life,[9,10] whereas **high-carbohydrate** meals seem to increase it.[10] There was no difference in theophylline metabolism in one study when patients were changed from a **high-carbohydrate/low-protein** diet to a **high-protein/low-carbohydrate** diet.[11] One study found that changing from a **high-protein** to a **high-carbohydrate** meal had an effect on the metabolism of theophylline similar to that of cimetidine, and that the effects of the meal change and cimetidine were additive.[12] The effects of **spicy food** have been studied, but the clinical significance of the changes are uncertain.[13]

(b) Theophylline and enteral feeds

A patient with chronic obstructive pulmonary disease showed a 53% reduction in his serum theophylline levels accompanied by bronchospasm when he was fed continuously through a nasogastric tube with *Osmolite*. The interaction occurred with both theophylline tablets (*Theo-Dur*) and liquid theophylline, but not when the theophylline was given intravenously as aminophylline. It was also found that the

interaction could be avoided by interrupting feeding 1 h either side of the oral liquid theophylline dose.[14] Conversely, hourly administration of 100 ml *Osmolite* did not affect the extent of absorption of theophylline from a slow-release preparation (*Slo-bid Gyrocaps*) in healthy subjects, although the rate of absorption was slowed.[15] Similarly, hourly administration of 100 ml *Ensure* for 10 h did not affect the rate or extent of absorption of theophylline from *Theo-24* tablets in healthy subjects.[16]

(c) Theophylline and parenteral nutrition

An isolated report describes an elderly woman treated with aminophylline by intravenous infusion who showed a marked fall in her serum theophylline levels (from 16.3 to 6.3 mg/l) when the amino acid concentration of her **parenteral nutrition** regimen was increased from 4.25 to 7%.[17] A study in 7 patients with malnutrition (marasmus-kwashiorkor) found only a small, probably clinically irrelevant increase in the elimination of a single intravenous dose of theophylline when they were **fed intravenously**.[18]

Mechanism

Not fully understood. As with any sustained-release formulation, the presence of food in the gut may alter the rate or extent of drug absorption by altering gastrointestinal transit time. It has been suggested that high-protein diets stimulate liver enzymes thereby increasing the metabolism of the theophylline and hastening its loss from the body. High carbohydrate diets have the opposite effect. Cytochrome P450 isoenzyme CYP1A2 (the principal enzyme involved in the metabolism of theophylline) is known to be induced by chemicals contained in cruciferous vegetables or formed by the action of high temperatures or smoke on meat.[19] This suggestion is supported by a study in which charcoal-grilled (broiled) beef decreased theophylline half-life by 22% on average.[20]

Importance and management

The theophylline-food interactions have been thoroughly studied but there seems to be no consistent pattern in the way the absorption of different theophylline preparations is affected. Be alert for any evidence of an inadequate response that can be related to food intake. Avoid switching between different preparations, and monitor the effects if this occurs/is necessary. Consult the product literature for any specific information on food and encourage patients to take their theophylline consistently in relation to meals where this is considered necessary. Advise patients not make major changes in their diet without consultation. Monitor the effects of both enteral and parenteral nutrition, since theophylline dosage adjustments may be required.

1. Karim A, Burns T, Wearley L, Streicher J, Palmer M. Food-induced changes in theophylline absorption from controlled-release formulations. Part I. Substantial increased and decreased absorption with Uniphyl tablets and Theo-Dur Sprinkle. *Clin Pharmacol Ther* (1985) 38, 77–83.
2. Vaughan L, Milavetz G, Hill M, Weinberger M, Hendeles L. Food-induced dose-dumping of Theo-24, a 'once-daily' slow-release theophylline product. *Drug Intell Clin Pharm* (1984) 18, 510.
3. Johansson Ö, Lindberg T, Melander A, Wåhlin-Boll E. Different effects of different nutrients on theophylline absorption in man. *Drug-Nutr Interactions* (1985) 3, 205–11.
4. Sips AP, Edelbroek PM, Kulstad S, de Wolff FA, Dijkman JH. Food does not effect bioavailability of theophylline from Theolin Retard. *Eur J Clin Pharmacol* (1984) 26, 405–7.
5. Steffensen G, Pedersen S. Food induced changes in theophylline absorption from a once-a-day theophylline product. *Br J Clin Pharmacol* (1986) 22, 571–7.
6. Thebault JJ, Aiache JM, Mazoyer F, Cardot JM. The influence of food on the bioavailability of a slow release theophylline preparation. *Clin Pharmacokinet* (1987) 13, 267–72.
7. Lefebvre RA, Belpaire FM, Bogaert MG. Influence of food on steady state serum concentrations of theophylline from two controlled-release preparations. *Int J Clin Pharmacol Ther Toxicol* (1988) 26, 375–9.
8. Fassihi AR, Dowse R, Robertson SSD. Effect of dietary cellulose on the absorption and bioavailability of theophylline. *Int J Pharmaceutics* (1989) 50, 79–82.
9. Kappas A, Anderson KE, Conney AH, Alvares AP. Influence of dietary protein and carbohydrate on antipyrine and theophylline metabolism in man. *Clin Pharmacol Ther* (1976) 20, 643–53.
10. Feldman CH, Hutchinson VE, Pippenger CE, Blumenfeld TA, Feldman BR, Davis WJ. Effect of dietary protein and carbohydrate on theophylline metabolism in children. *Pediatrics* (1980) 66, 956–62.
11. Thompson PJ, Skypala I, Dawson S, McAllister WAC, Turner Warwick M. The effect of diet upon serum concentrations of theophylline. *Br J Clin Pharmacol* (1983) 16, 267–70.

12. Anderson KE, McCleery RB, Vesell ES, Vickers FF, Kappas A. Diet and cimetidine induce comparable changes in theophylline metabolism in normal subjects. *Hepatology* (1991) 13, 941–6.

13. Bouraoui A, Toumi A, Bouchahcha S, Boukef K, Brazier JL. Influence de l'alimentation épicée et piquante sur l'absorption de la théophylline. *Therapie* (1986) 41, 467–71.

14. Gal P, Layson R. Interference with oral theophylline absorption by continuous nasogastric feedings. *Ther Drug Monit* (1986) 8, 421–3.

15. Bhargava VO, Schaaf LJ, Berlinger WG, Jungnickel PW. Effect of an enteral nutrient formula on sustained-release theophylline absorption. *Ther Drug Monit* (1989) 11, 515–19.

16. Plezia PM, Thornley SM, Kramer TH, Armstrong EP. The influence of enteral feedings on sustained-release theophylline absorption. *Pharmacotherapy* (1990) 10, 356–61.

17. Ziegenbein RC. Theophylline clearance increase from increased amino acid in a CPN regimen. *Drug Intell Clin Pharm* (1987) 21, 220–1.

18. Cuddy PG, Bealer JF, Lyman EL, Pemberton LB. Theophylline disposition following parenteral feeding of malnourished patients. *Ann Pharmacother* (1993) 27, 846–51.

19. Kelman MI, Overvik E, Poellinger L, Gustafsson JA. Induction of cytochrome P4501A isoenzymes by heterocyclic amines and other food-derived compounds. *Princess Takamatsu Symp* (1995) 23, 163–71.

20. Kappas A, Alvares AP, Anderson KE, Pantuck EJ, Pantuck CB, Chang R, Conney AH. Effect of charcoal-broiled beef on antipyrine and theophylline metabolism. *Clin Pharmacol Ther* (1979) 23, 445–50.

Theophylline + Furosemide (Frusemide)

The outcome of concurrent use is uncertain. Furosemide (frusemide) is reported to increase, decrease or to have no effect on serum theophylline levels.

Clinical evidence

The mean peak serum theophylline level of 8 asthmatics given 300 mg of a sustained-release formulation of theophylline, was reduced by 41% (from 12.14 to 7.16 micrograms/ml) by a single oral dose of 25 mg **furosemide (frusemide)**.[1] Conversely, 10 patients with asthma, chronic bronchitis or emphysema receiving a continuous maintenance infusion of aminophylline showed a 21% rise in their serum theophylline levels (from 13.7 to 16.6 micrograms/ml) 4 hours after being given a 40-mg dose of **furosemide** (intravenously over 2 min).[2] A study in 12 normal subjects failed to find any change in steady-state serum theophylline levels when two 20-mg doses of **furosemide** were given orally 4 hours apart.[3]

Four premature neonates, 2 given theophylline and **furosemide** orally and the other 2 intravenously, showed a fall in steady-state serum theophylline levels from 8 micrograms/ml down to 2 to 3 micrograms/ml when the **furosemide** was given within 30 min of the theophylline.[4]

Mechanism

Not understood, although in theory furosemide may cause increased renal excretion of theophylline, which could explain the reduced levels.

Importance and management

Information is limited and the outcome of concurrent use is inconsistent and uncertain. If both drugs are used be aware for the potential for changes in serum theophylline levels. Consider measuring levels, and make appropriate dosage adjustments as necessary. Both theophylline and diuretics can cause hypokalaemia, and the possibility that this may be potentiated by the combination should be considered.

1. Carpentiere G, Marino S, Castello F. Furosemide and theophylline. *Ann Intern Med* (1985) 103, 957.

2. Conlon PF, Grambau GR, Johnson CE, Weg JG. Effect of intravenous furosemide on serum theophylline concentration. *Am J Hosp Pharm* (1981) 38, 1345–7.

3. Jänicke U-A, Gundert-Remy U. Failure to detect a clinically significant interaction between theophylline and furosemide. *Naunyn Schmiedebergs Arch Pharmacol* (1986) 332 (Suppl), R100.

4. Toback JW, Gilman ME. Theophylline-furosemide inactivation? *Pediatrics* (1983) 71, 140–1.

Theophylline + Grapefruit juice

Grapefruit juice does not interact significantly with theophylline.

Clinical evidence, mechanism, importance and management

In one study, 12 healthy subjects were given a single 200 mg oral dose of theophylline diluted in either 100 ml of **grapefruit juice** or water, followed by 900 ml more juice or water over the next 16 h. The pharmacokinetics of the theophylline were found to be unchanged by the **grapefruit juice**.[1] The authors of the first study had previously shown that grapefruit juice had a small effect on the pharmacokinetics of caffeine (see 'Caffeine + Grapefruit juice', p.785), and that one of the constituents of grapefruit juice (naringenin) inhibited cytochrome P450 isoenzyme CYP1A2 *in vitro* (the principal enzyme in theophylline metabolism). However, most clinically relevant grapefruit juice/drug interactions are considered to be mediated via inhibition of intestinal CYP3A4 (for example, see 'Calcium channel blockers + Food and drinks', p.458). There would seem to be no reason why patients on theophylline should avoid **grapefruit juice**.

1. Fuhr U, Maier A, Keller A, Steinijans VW, Sauter R, Staib AH. Lacking effect of grapefruit juice on theophylline pharmacokinetics. *Int J Clin Pharmacol Ther* (1995) 33, 311–14.

Theophylline + Griseofulvin

Griseofulvin appears not to interact to a clinically relevant extent with theophylline.

Clinical evidence, mechanism, importance and management

A study was initiated because it was suspected that **griseofulvin** might possibly interact with theophylline. It was found that 500 mg **griseofulvin** daily for 8 days in 12 healthy subjects reduced the half-life of theophylline (a decrease from 6.6 to 5.7 h), increased its total clearance (from 80 to 84 ml/min, not significant) and also increased the clearance of 2 of its metabolites, but these changes were far too small to have any clinical relevance.[1] There would appear to be no reason for avoiding concurrent use.

1. Rasmussen BB, Jeppesen U, Gaist D, Brøsen K. Griseofulvin and fluvoxamine interactions with the metabolism of theophylline. *Ther Drug Monit* (1997) 19, 56–62.

Theophylline + H$_2$-blockers

Cimetidine raises theophylline serum levels and toxicity may develop if appropriate reductions (between one-third and one-half) are not made to the theophylline dosage. However, the extent of the interaction is unlikely to be clinically relevant in most patients with low-dose (non-prescription) cimetidine. Famotidine, nizatidine, ranitidine and roxatidine appear not to interact.

Clinical evidence

(a) Cimetidine

A number of case reports describe significantly increased theophylline levels, many to toxic levels, in patients (adults and children) treated with **cimetidine**.[1-6] A few cases describe serious effects such as seizures.[3,4]

Many pharmacokinetic studies in healthy subjects[7-15] and patients[16-20] have also clearly demonstrated that **cimetidine** (800 to 1200 mg daily in divided doses by mouth for 4 to 10 days) prolonged the theophylline half-life by about 30 to 65% and reduced the clearance by about 20 to 40%. Steady-state serum theophylline levels were raised about one-third.[16,17,20] The effect of **cimetidine** was maximal in 3 days in the one study assessing this.[16] The extent of the interaction did not differ between **cimetidine** 1200 mg and 2400 mg daily, in 1 study.[10] Two further studies found **cimetidine** 800 mg daily had less effect than 1200 mg daily.[12,21] A study investigating low-dose **cimetidine** (200 mg twice daily; non-prescription dosage) found only a 12% decrease in theophylline clearance.[22]

Two studies found that the effect of **cimetidine** did not differ between young and elderly subjects,[12,23] whereas another found it was more pronounced in the elderly.[21] The effects of **cimetidine** did not differ between smokers and non-smokers in one study,[24] but were more pronounced in smokers in another.[25] In another study the effects of **cimetidine** were not affected by gender.[21] Three studies found that the inhibitory effects of **cimetidine** and **ciprofloxacin** were additive.[23,26,27]

Three studies found that intravenous **cimetidine** also inhibited the clearance of theophylline.[28-30] In one of these, oral and intravenous **cimetidine** reduced theophylline clearance to the same extent, but when clearance was corrected for the lower bioavailability of the oral **cimetidine**, oral **cimetidine** resulted in a greater inhibition than intravenous **cimetidine**.[28] Another found no difference between the effects of **cimetidine** administered as a continuous infusion (50 mg/h) compared with an intermittent infusion (300 mg every 6 hours).[29] However, a fourth study[31] found no clinically important interaction between intravenous aminophylline and an intravenous **cimetidine** infusion, but aminophylline was administered only 12 hours after starting the **cimetidine**, which may be insufficient for **cimetidine** to have had an effect.

(b) Famotidine

Famotidine 40 mg twice daily for 5 days had no effect on the pharmacokinetics of theophylline in 10 healthy subjects.[14] In another study, 16 patients with bronchial asthma or chronic obstructive pulmonary disease (COPD) showed no changes in the clearance of theophylline while taking 20 mg **famotidine** twice daily for 3 days or more.[32] Two further studies also found no interaction between theophylline and **famotidine** 20 or 40 mg twice daily for 4 or 9 days in COPD patients.[19,33,34] In a post-marketing surveillance study it was noted that 4 asthmatics on theophylline had been treated with **famotidine** 40 mg daily for 4 to 8 weeks without any problems.[35] In contrast, in a patient with COPD and liver impairment, serum theophylline levels and the AUC after an intravenous dose were raised (+78%) and the clearance halved after taking **famotidine** 40 mg daily for 8 days.[36] A later study by the same authors in 7 patients with COPD, similarly treated but with normal liver function, found that the theophylline AUC was increased 56% and the clearance reduced by 35% by **famotidine**.[37]

(c) Nizatidine

A study in 17 COPD patients found that **nizatidine** 150 mg twice daily for a month had no effect on the steady-state pharmacokinetics of theophylline.[20] However there were 6 reports of apparent interactions in the FDA Spontaneous Adverse Drug Reaction Database up to the end of August 1989. Four patients on theophylline developed elevated serum theophylline levels, with symptoms of toxicity in at least one case, when given **nizatidine**. The problems resolved when either both drugs, or just **nizatidine** were stopped.[38]

(d) Ranitidine

Many studies in healthy subjects[10,11,15,39-41] and patients[17,20,42-45] have failed to find that **ranitidine** affects the pharmacokinetics of theophylline, even in daily doses far in excess of those used clinically (up to 4200 mg daily).[39] However, there are 7 reports describing a total of 10 patients, who developed theophylline toxicity when given **ranitidine**.[46-52] The validity of a number of these reports has been questioned,[53-56] with the authors subsequently modifying some.[57,58]

(e) Roxatidine

Roxatidine acetate hydrochloride 150 mg daily did not affect the clearance of theophylline.[59] Similarly, roxatidine 150 mg twice daily did not significantly change the pharmacokinetics of a single 250 mg intravenous dose of aminophylline in 9 healthy subjects.[60]

Mechanism

Cimetidine is an enzyme inhibitor, which depresses the metabolism (predominantly N-demethylation)[61] of theophylline by the liver, thereby prolonging its stay in the body and raising its serum levels. Famotidine, nizatidine and ranitidine do not have enzyme-inhibiting effects so that it is not clear why they sometimes appear to behave like cimetidine.

Importance and management

The theophylline/cimetidine interaction is very well documented (not all the references being listed here), very well established and clinically important. Theophylline serum levels normally rise by about one-third, but much greater increases have been seen in individual patients. Reduce the theophylline dosage to avoid toxicity (initial reductions of 30–50% have been suggested[4]) and monitor the effects. Alternatively, use one of the other H$_2$-blockers. The effect of low-dose (OTC, nonprescription) cimetidine is unlikely to be clinically relevant unless theophylline levels are at the higher end of the therapeutic range. The situation with famotidine, nizatidine and ranitidine is not totally clear. They would not be expected to interact because they are not enzyme inhibitors like cimetidine, but very occasionally and unpredictably they appear to do so, nevertheless current opinion is that normally no special precautions are needed.[54] Roxatidine appears not to interact.

1. Weinberger MM, Smith G, Milavetz G, Hendeles L. Decreased theophylline clearance due to cimetidine. *N Engl J Med* (1981) 304, 672.
2. Campbell MA, Plachetka JR, Jackson JE, Moon JF, Finley PR. Cimetidine decreases theophylline clearance. *Ann Intern Med* (1981) 95, 68–9.
3. Lofgren RP, Gilbertson RA. Cimetidine and theophylline. *Ann Intern Med* (1982) 96, 378.
4. Bauman JH, Kimelblatt BJ, Carracio TR, Silverman HM, Simon GI, Beck GJ. Cimetidine-theophylline interaction. Report of four patients. *Ann Allergy* (1982) 48, 100–102.
5. Fenje PC, Isles AF, Baltodano A, MacLeod SM, Soldin S. Interaction of cimetidine and theophylline in two infants. *Can Med Assoc J* (1982) 126, 1178.
6. Uzzan D, Uzzan B, Bernard N, Caubarrere I. Interaction médicamenteuse de la cimétidine et de la théophylline. *Nouv Presse Med* (1982) 11, 1950.
7. Jackson JE, Powell JR, Wandell M, Bentley J, Dorr R. Cimetidine decreases theophylline clearance. *Am Rev Respir Dis* (1981) 123, 615–17.
8. Roberts RK, Grice J, Wood L, Petroff V, McGuffie C. Cimetidine impairs the elimination of theophylline and antipyrine. *Gastroenterology* (1981) 81, 19–21.
9. Reitberg DP, Bernhard H, Schentag JJ. Alteration of theophylline clearance and half-life by cimetidine in normal volunteers. *Ann Intern Med* (1981) 95, 582–5.
10. Powell JR, Rogers JF, Wargin WA, Cross RE, Eshelman FN. Inhibition of theophylline clearance by cimetidine but not ranitidine. *Arch Intern Med* (1984) 144, 484–6.
11. Ferrari M, Angelini GP, Barozzi E, Olivieri M, Penna S, Accardi R. A comparative study of ranitidine and cimetidine effects on theophylline metabolism. *Giornale Ital Malattie del Torace* (1984) 38, 31–4.
12. Cohen IA, Johnson CE, Berardi RR, Hyneck ML, Achem SR. Cimetidine-theophylline interaction: effects of age and cimetidine dose. *Ther Drug Monit* (1985) 7, 426–34.
13. Mulkey PM, Murphy JE, Shleifer NH. Steady-state theophylline pharmacokinetics during and after short-term cimetidine administration. *Clin Pharm* (1983) 2, 439–41.
14. Lin JH, Chremos AN, Chiou R, Yeh KC, Williams R. Comparative effect of famotidine and cimetidine on the pharmacokinetics of theophylline in normal volunteers. . *Br J Clin Pharmacol* (1987) 24, 669–72.
15. Adebayo GI. Effects of equimolar doses of cimetidine and ranitidine on theophylline elimination. *Biopharm Drug Dispos* (1989) 10, 77–85.
16. Vestal RE, Thummel KE, Musser B, Mercer GD. Cimetidine inhibits theophylline clearance in patients with chronic obstructive pulmonary disease: A study using stable isotope methodology during multiple oral dose administration. *Br J Clin Pharmacol* (1983) 15, 411–16.
17. Boehning W. Effect of cimetidine and ranitidine on plasma theophylline in patients with chronic obstructive airways disease treated with theophylline and corticosteroids. *Eur J Clin Pharmacol* (1990) 38, 43–5.
18. Roberts RK, Grice J, McGuffie C. Cimetidine-theophylline interaction in patients with chronic obstructive airways disease. *Med J Aust* (1984) 140, 279–80.
19. Bachmann K, Sullivan TJ, Reese JH, Jauregui L, Miller K, Scott M, Yeh KC, Stepanavage M, King JD, Schwartz J. Controlled study of the putative interaction between famotidine and cimetidine in patients with chronic obstructive pulmonary disease. *J Clin Pharmacol* (1995) 35, 529–35.
20. Bachmann K, Sullivan TJ, Mauro LS, Martin M, Jauregui L, Levine L. Comparative investigation of the influence of nizatidine, ranitidine, and cimetidine on the steady-state pharmacokinetics of theophylline in COPD patients. *J Clin Pharmacol* (1992) 32, 476–82.
21. Seaman JJ, Randolph WC, Peace KE, Frank WO, Dickson B, Putterman K, Young MD. Effects of two cimetidine dosage regimens on serum theophylline levels. *Postgrad Med Custom Comm* (1985) 78, 47–53.
22. Nix DE, Di Cicco RA, Miller AK, Boyle DA, Boike SC, Zariffa N, Jorkasky DK, Schentag JJ. The effect of low-dose cimetidine (200 mg twice daily) on the pharmacokinetics of theophylline. *J Clin Pharmacol* (1999) 39, 855–65.
23. Loi C-M, Parker BM, Cusack BJ, Vestal RE. Aging and drug interactions.III. Individual and combined effects of cimetidine and ciprofloxacin on theophylline metabolism in healthy male and female nonsmokers. *J Pharmacol Exp Ther* (1997) 280, 627–37.

24. Cusack BJ, Dawson GW, Mercer GD, Vestal RE. Cigarette smoking and theophylline metabolism: effects of cimetidine. *Clin Pharmacol Ther* (1985) 37, 330–6.
25. Grygiel JJ, Miners JO, Drew R, Birkett DJ. Differential effects of cimetidine on theophylline metabolic pathways. *Eur J Clin Pharmacol* (1984) 26, 335–40.
26. Davis RL, Quenzer RW, Kelly HW, Powell JR. Effect of the addition of ciprofloxacin on theophylline pharmacokinetics in subjects inhibited by cimetidine. *Ann Pharmacother* (1992) 26, 11–13.
27. C-M Loi, Parker BM, Cusack BJ, Vestal RE. Individual and combined effects of cimetidine and ciprofloxacin on theophylline metabolism in male nonsmokers. *Br J Clin Pharmacol* (1993) 36, 195–200.
28. Cremer KF, Secor J, Speeg KV. Effect of route of administration on the cimetidine-theophylline drug interaction. *J Clin Pharmacol* (1989) 29, 451–6.
29. Gutfeld MB, Welage LS, Walawander CA, Wilton JH, Harrison NJ. The influence of intravenous cimetidine dosing regimens on the disposition of theophylline. *J Clin Pharmacol* (1989) 29, 665–9.
30. Krstenansky PM, Javaheri S, Thomas JP, Thomas RL. Effect of continuous cimetidine infusion on steady-state theophylline concentration. *Clin Pharm* (1989) 8, 206–9.
31. Gaska JA, Tietze KJ, Rocci ML, Vlasses PH. Theophylline pharmacokinetics: effect of continuous versus intermittent cimetidine IV infusion. *J Clin Pharmacol* (1991) 31, 668–72.
32. Asamoto H, Kokura M, Kawakami A, Sawano T, Sasaki Y, Kohara N, Kitamura Y, Oishi T, Morishita H. Effect of famotidine on theophylline clearance in asthma and COPD patients. *Jpn J Allergol* (1987) 36, 1012–17.
33. Verdiani P, DiCarlo S, Baronti A. Famotidine effects on theophylline pharmacokinetics in subjects affected by COPD. Comparison with cimetidine and placebo. *Chest* (1988) 94, 807–10.
34. Bachmann KA, Sullivan TJ, Reese JH, Jauregui L, Miller K, Scott M, Yeh KC, Stepanavage M, Kingd JD, Schwartz J. Absence of interaction between famotidine and theophylline in COPD patients. *J Clin Pharmacol* (1994) 34, 1012.
35. Chichmanian RM, Mignot G, Spreux A, Jean-Girard C, Hofliger P. Tolérance de la famotidine. Étude due réseau médecins sentinelles en pharmacovigilance. *Therapie* (1992) 47, 239–43.
36. Dal Negro R, Turco P, Pomari C, Trevisan F. Famotidina e teofillina: interferenza farmacocinetica cimetidino-simile? *G Ital Malattie del Torace* (1988) 42, 185–6.
37. Dal Negro R, Pomari C, Turco P. Famotidine and theophylline pharmacokinetics. An unexpected cimetidine-like interaction in patients with chronic obstructive pulmonary disease. *Clin Pharmacokinet* (1993) 24, 255–8.
38. Shinn AF. Unrecognized drug interactions with famotidine and nizatidine. *Arch Intern Med* (1991) 151, 810–14.
39. Kelly HW, Powell JR, Donohue JF. Ranitidine at very large doses does not inhibit theophylline elimination. *Clin Pharmacol Ther* (1986) 39, 577–81.
40. McEwen J, McMurdo MET, Moreland TA. The effects of once-daily dosing with ranitidine and cimetidine on theophylline pharmacokinetics. *Eur J Drug Metab Pharmacokinet* (1988) 13, 201–5.
41. Kehoe WA, Sands CD, Feng Long L, Hui Lan H, Harralson AF. The effect of ranitidine on theophylline metabolism in healthy ethnic Koreans. *Pharmacotherapy* (1994) 14, 373.
42. Seggev JS, Barzilay M, Schey G. No evidence for interaction between ranitidine and theophylline. *Arch Intern Med* (1987) 147, 179–80.
43. Zarogoulidis K, Economidis D, Paparoglou A, Pneumaticos I, Sevastou P, Tsopouridis A, Papaioanou A. Effect of ranitidine on theophylline plasma levels in patients with COPD. *Eur Resp J* (1988) 1 (Suppl 2), 195S.
44. Pérez-Blanco FJ, Huertas González JM, Morata Garcia de la Puerta IJ, Saucedo Sánchez R. Interacción de ranitidina con teofilina. *Rev Clin Esp* (1995) 195, 359–60.
45. Cukier A, Vargas FS, Santos SRCJ, Donzella H, Terra-Filho M, Teixeira LR, Light RW. Theophylline-ranitidine interaction in elderly COPD patients. *Brazil J Med Biol Res* (1995) 28, 875–9.
46. Fernandes E, Melewicz FM. Ranitidine and theophylline. *Ann Intern Med* (1984) 100, 459.
47. Gardner ME, Sikorski GW. Ranitidine and theophylline. *Ann Intern Med* (1985) 102, 559.
48. Roy AK, Cuda MP, Levine RA. Induction of theophylline toxicity and inhibition of clearance rates by ranitidine. *Am J Med* (1988) 85, 525–7.
49. Dietemann-Molard A, Popin E, Oswald-Mammosser M, Colas des Francs V, Pauli G. Intoxication à la théophylline par interaction avec la ranitidine à dose élévée. *Presse Med* (1988) 17, 280.
50. Skinner MH, Lenert L, Blaschke TF. Theophylline toxicity subsequent to ranitidine administration: a possible drug-drug interaction. *Am J Med* (1989) 86, 129–32.
51. Hegman GW, Gilbert RP. Ranitidine-theophylline interaction — fact or fiction? *DICP Ann Pharmacother* (1991) 25, 21–5.
52. Murialdo G, Piovano PL, Costelli P, Fonzi S, Barberis A, Ghia M. Seizures during concomitant treatment with theophylline and ranitidine: a case report. *Ann Ital Med Int* (1990) 5, 413–17.
53. Muir JG, Powell JR, Baumann JH. Induction of theophylline toxicity and inhibition of clearance rates by ranitidine. *Am J Med* (1989) 86, 513–14.
54. Kelly HW. Comment: ranitidine does not inhibit theophylline metabolism. *Ann Pharmacother* (1991) 25, 1139.
55. Williams DM, Figg WD, Pleasants RA. Comment: ranitidine does not inhibit theophylline metabolism. *Ann Pharmacother* (1991) 25, 1140.
56. Dobbs JH, Smith RN. Ranitidine and theophylline. *Ann Intern Med* (1984) 100, 769.
57. Roy AK. Induction of theophylline toxicity and inhibition of clearance rates by ranitidine. *Am J Med* (1989) 86, 513.
58. Hegman GW. Comment: ranitidine does not inhibit theophylline metabolism. *Ann Pharmacother* (1991) 25, 1140–41.
59. Labs RA. Interaction of roxatidine acetate with antacids, food and other drugs. *Drugs* (1988) 35 (Suppl 3), 82–9.
60. Yoshimura N, Takeuchi H, Ogata H, Ishioka T, Aoi R. Effects of roxatidine acetate hydrochloride and cimetidine on the pharmacokinetics of theophylline in healthy subjects. *Int J Clin Pharmacol Ther Toxicol* (1989) 27, 308–12.
61. Naline E, Sanceaume M, Pays M, Advenier C. Application of theophylline metabolite assays to the exploration of liver microsome oxidative function in man. *Fundam Clin Pharmacol* (1988) 2, 341–51.

Theophylline + HIV-protease inhibitors

Ritonavir can reduce the serum levels of theophylline. Indinavir appears not to interact.

Clinical evidence, mechanism, importance and management

(a) Indinavir

A study in 12 healthy subjects given a single oral 250-mg dose of theophylline before and after 5 days treatment with **indinavir** (800 mg three times a day) found an 18% increase in AUC for theophylline, which was considered clinically insignificant.[1] Further research is needed to confirm the safety in clinical practice, but it would seem unlikely that special precautions are necessary during concurrent use.

(b) Ritonavir

In one study, 27 subjects on theophylline (3 mg/kg 8-hourly) were given either **ritonavir** (300 mg increased to 500 mg twice daily) or a placebo over 10 days. **Ritonavir** reduced the maximum and minimum steady-state theophylline levels by 32% and 57%, respectively. The interaction achieved its maximal effects after 6 days' **ritonavir** use.[2] Information is very limited but the interaction appears to be established. Be alert for the need to increase the theophylline dosage if **ritonavir** and theophylline are used concurrently. More study is needed.

1. Mistry GC, Laurent A, Sterrett AT, Deutsch PJ. Effect of indinavir on the single-dose pharmacokinetics of theophylline in healthy subjects. *J Clin Pharmacol* (1999) 39, 636–42.
2. Hsu A, Granneman GR, Witt G, Cavanaugh JH, Leonard J. Assessment of multiple doses of ritonavir on the pharmacokinetics of theophylline. *11th Int Conf AIDS, Vancouver* (1996) 1, 89.

Theophylline + Idrocilamide

Idrocilamide given orally can increase serum theophylline levels. A reduction in the theophylline dosage may be needed to avoid toxicity.

Clinical evidence, mechanism, importance and management

Idrocilamide (600 mg daily by mouth for 3 days then 1200 mg for 4 days) increased the half-life of a single dose of theophylline 2.5-fold (from 8.5 to 21.6 h) in 6 normal subjects and reduced the clearance by 67%.[1] This is due to a reduction in the liver metabolism caused by the **idrocilamide** (see also 'Caffeine + Idrocilamide', p.785). Information is very limited but it indicates that concurrent use should be closely monitored. The need to reduce the theophylline dosage with oral idrocilamide should be anticipated.

1. Lacroix C, Nouveau J, Hubscher Ph, Tardif D, Ray M and Goulle JP. Influence de l'idrocilamide sur le métabolisme de la théophylline. *Rev Pneumol Clin* (1986) 42, 164–6.

Theophylline + Imipenem

Seizures developed in three patients on theophylline when given imipenem.

Clinical evidence, mechanism, importance and management

Two patients on theophylline developed seizures within 11 to 56 h of starting treatment with **imipenem** (500 mg 6 to 8 hourly intravenously), and a third patient after 6 days.[1] The reasons are not know. Theophylline serum levels appeared to be unchanged.[1] In an analysis of data from 1,754 patients who had received imipenem in dose-ranging studies, 3% had seizures, and **imipenem** was judged to be associated with 1 in 3 of these cases. However, concurrent theophylline/aminophylline therapy was not found to be a significant risk factor for the development of seizures with imipenem.[2] The general importance of these observations is uncertain but you should be aware of the cases mentioned.

1. Semel JD, Allen N. Seizures in patients simultaneously receiving theophylline and imipenem or ciprofloxacin or metronidazole. *South Med J* (1991) 84, 465–8.
2. Calandra G, Lydick E, Carrigan J, Weiss L, Guess H. Factors predisposing to seizures in seriously ill infected patients receiving antibiotics: experience with imipenem/cilastatin. *Am J Med* (1988) 84, 911–18.

Theophylline + Influenza vaccines

Normally none of the influenza vaccines (whole-virion, split-virion and surface antigen) interact with theophylline, but there are 3 reports describing rises in serum theophylline levels in a few patients attributed to the use of an influenza vaccine, accompanied by toxicity in some instances.

Clinical evidence

(a) Evidence of no interaction

Mean steady-state serum theophylline levels did not change in 12 patients with asthma given a **trivalent split-virion influenza vaccine** (*Fluzone*), although 1 patient had an increase (see (b), below). Levels were measured before vaccination and 1, 3, 7 and 14 days after vaccination.[1] Similarly, no evidence of a rise in theophylline levels was found in a number of other studies in healthy subjects, or adults and children on maintenance theophylline therapy, given various **trivalent split-virion vaccines** including *Fluzone*,[2] *Fluogen*,[3-5] *Influvac*,[6] and various **unnamed trivalent split-virion vaccines**.[7-10] In addition, no change in theophylline pharmacokinetics was found after use of a **whole-virion vaccine**.[11] No evidence of serious theophylline toxicity was seen in 119 elderly people on maintenance theophylline given an **unspecified influenza vaccine**.[12]

(b) Evidence of an interaction

Three patients who had been taking 200 mg oxtriphylline (equivalent to 128 mg theophylline) orally 6-hourly for at least 7 days showed a rise in their serum theophylline levels of 219, 89 and 85% respectively within 12 to 24 h of receiving 0.5 ml **trivalent split-virion influenza vaccine** (*Fluogen*-Parke Davis). Two of them showed signs of theophylline toxicity and in some cases effects persisted for up to 72 hours. A subsequent study in 4 normal subjects showed that the same dose of vaccine more than doubled the half-life of theophylline (from 3.3 to 7.3 h) and halved its clearance (from 52 to 25 mg/kg/h).[13]

A girl showed a rise in theophylline levels from 20 to 34 micrograms/ml (with no sign of toxicity) within 5 hours of being given a **trivalent split-virion vaccine**.[14] In a study where 11 of 12 patients had no increase in theophylline levels after vaccination with *Fluzone*, one woman showed a rise in levels (from 10 to 24.5 micrograms/ml) accompanied by headaches and palpitations.[1] Theophylline clearance was reduced 1 day after influenza vaccination (**trivalent influenza vaccine**, *Fluogen*-Parke Davis) in 8 healthy subjects, but only by 25%, which was of borderline significance. Theophylline metabolism had returned to pre-vaccination levels after 7 days.[15]

Mechanism

Uncertain. If an interaction occurs, it has been suggested it is probably due to inhibition of the liver enzymes concerned with the metabolism of theophylline, possibly secondary to interferon production, resulting in theophylline accumulation in the body.[13,15] One suggestion is that vaccine contaminants, which are potent interferon-inducing agents, may be responsible (rather than the vaccine itself), so that an interaction would seem to be less likely with modern highly-purified subunit vaccines.[16] In 1 study showing an interaction between influenza vaccine and theophylline, an increase in serum interferon levels was detected,[15] whereas, in 2 of the studies showing no interaction, no interferon production was detected.[5,11] Influenza infection

per se can result in decreased theophylline clearance and theophylline toxicity.[17]

Importance and management

A very thoroughly investigated interaction, the weight of evidence being that no adverse interaction normally occurs with any type of influenza vaccine in children, adults or the elderly. Even so, bearing in mind the occasional and unexplained reports of an interaction[1,13,14] it would seem prudent to monitor the effects of concurrent use, although problems are very unlikely to arise now that purer vaccines are available (see 'Mechanism').

1. Fischer RG, Booth BH, Mitchell DQ, Kibbe AH. Influence of trivalent influenza vaccine on serum theophylline levels. *Can Med Assoc J* (1982) 126, 1312–13.
2. Goldstein RS, Cheung OT, Seguin R, Lobley G, Johnson AC. Decreased elimination of theophylline after influenza vaccination. *Can Med Assoc J* (1982) 126, 470.
3. San Joaquin VH, Reyes S, Marks MI. Influenza vaccination in asthmatic children on maintenance theophylline therapy. *Clin Pediatr* (1982) 21, 724–6.
4. Bukowskyj M, Munt PW, Wigle R, Nakatsu K. Theophylline clearance. Lack of effect of influenza vaccination and ascorbic acid. *Am Rev Respir Dis* (1984) 129, 672–5.
5. Grabowski N, May JJ, Pratt DS, Richtsmeier WJ, Bertino JS, Sorge KF. The effect of split virus influenza vaccination on theophylline pharmacokinetics. *Am Rev Respir Dis* (1985) 131, 934–8.
6. Winstanley PA, Tjia J, Back DJ, Hobson D, Breckenridge AM. Lack of effect of highly purified subunit influenza vaccination on theophylline metabolism. *Br J Clin Pharmacol* (1985) 20, 47–53.
7. Stults BM, Hashisaki PA. Influenza vaccination and theophylline pharmacokinetics in patients with chronic obstructive lung disease. *West J Med* (1983) 139, 651–4.
8. Gomolin IH, Chapron DJ, Luhan PA. Lack of effect of influenza vaccine on theophylline levels and warfarin anticoagulation in the elderly. *J Am Geriatr Soc* (1985) 33, 269–72.
9. Feldman CH, Rabinowitz A, Levison M, Klein R, Feldman BR, Davis WJ. Effects of influenza vaccine on theophylline metabolism in children with asthma. *Am Rev Respir Dis* (1985) 131 (4 Suppl), A9.
10. Brett KA, Levy J, Pariente R, Gobert P, Falquet JCV. Influenza vaccine and theophylline metabolism. Is there an interaction? *Acta Ther* (1989) 15, 49–58.
11. Hannan SE, May JJ, Pratt DS, Richtsmeier WJ, Bertino JS. The effect of whole virus influenza vaccination on theophylline pharmacokinetics. *Am Rev Respir Dis* (1988) 137, 903–6.
12. Patriarca PA, Kendal AP, Stricof RL, Weber JA, Meissner MK, Dateno B. Influenza vaccination and warfarin or theophylline toxicity in nursing-home residents. *N Engl J Med* (1983) 308, 1601–2.
13. Renton KW, Gray JD, Hall RI. Decreased elimination of theophylline after influenza vaccination. *Can Med Assoc J* (1980) 123, 288–90.
14. Walker S, Schreiber L, Middelkamp JN. Serum theophylline levels after influenza vaccination. *Can Med Assoc J* (1981) 125, 243–4.
15. Meredith CG, Christian CD, Johnson RF, Troxell R, Davis GL, Schenker S. Effects of influenza virus vaccine on hepatic drug metabolism. *Clin Pharmacol Ther* (1985) 37, 396–401.
16. Winstanley PA, Back DJ, Breckenridge AM. Inhibition of theophylline metabolism by interferon. *Lancet* (1987) ii, 1340.
17. Kraemer MJ, Furukawa CT, Koup JR, Shapiro GG, Pierson WE, Bierman CW. Altered theophylline clearance during an influenza B outbreak. *Pediatrics* (1982) 69, 476–80.

Theophylline + Interferon

The clearance of theophylline from the body is reduced by interferon alfa. One study found that it was halved. This suggests that theophylline toxicity might occur if the dosage is not reduced appropriately.

Clinical evidence

A study in 5 patients with stable chronic active hepatitis B and 4 healthy subjects showed that 20 h after being given a single 9 or 18 million unit intramuscular injection of **interferon** (**recombinant human alfa A**, Hoffman La Roche), the theophylline clearance of in 8 of them was approximately halved (range 33 to 81%). The mean theophylline elimination half-life was increased from 6.3 to 10.7 h (1.5 to sixfold increases). One healthy subject showed no change. In the healthy subjects, 4 weeks after the study the theophylline clearances were noted to have returned to their former values.[1]

Another study in 11 healthy subjects given interferon alfa (*Roferon-A*; Hoffman La Roche) 3 million units daily for 3 days, found that the terminal half-life and AUC of the theophylline were only increased by 10 to 15%, with a similar decrease in clearance.[2] Interferon alfa 3 million units administered 3 times a week for 2 weeks decreased the clearance of a single oral dose of theophylline 150 mg by 33% in 7 patients with cancer.[3]

Mechanism

Interferon alfa inhibits the liver enzymes[4] concerned with the metabolism of some drugs, including theophylline, so that it is cleared from the body more slowly and accumulates.

Importance and management

Direct information appears to be limited to these reports, only one of which found clear evidence of a clinically important interaction. So far there appear to be no reports of toxicity but it would seem prudent to monitor concurrent use closely, reducing the theophylline dosage if necessary. Patients with enhanced metabolism (e.g. smokers) are predicted to be most at risk.[1]

1. Williams SJ, Baird-Lambert JA, Farrell GC. Inhibition of theophylline metabolism by interferon. Lancet (1987) ii, 939–41.
2. Jonkman JHG, Nicholson KG, Farrow PR, Eckert M, Grasmeijer G, Oosterhuis B, De Noorde OE, Guentert TW. Effects of α-interferon on theophylline pharmacokinetics and metabolism. Br J Clin Pharmacol (1989) 27, 795–802.
3. Israel BC, Blouin RA, McIntyre W, Shedlofsky SI. Effects of interferon-α monotherapy on hepatic drug metabolism in cancer patients. Br J Clin Pharmacol (1993) 36, 229–35.
4. Williams SJ, Farrell GC. Inhibition of antipyrine metabolism by interferon. Br J Clin Pharmacol (1986) 22, 610–12.

Theophylline + Ipriflavone

An isolated report describes increased theophylline levels in a patient given ipriflavone.

Clinical evidence, mechanism, importance and management

The theophylline serum levels of a patient with chronic obstructive pulmonary disease, taking 600 mg theophylline daily, rose from 9.5 to 17.3 micrograms/ml after additionally taking 600 mg **ipriflavone** daily for about four weeks. No toxicity occurred. The serum theophylline levels fell to about the initial level when the **ipriflavone** was stopped, and rose again when it was restarted.[1] *In vitro* studies with human liver microsomes suggest that **ipriflavone** can inhibit cytochrome P450 isoenzyme CYP1A2 and the demethylation of theophylline,[2,3] which would reduce the loss of theophylline from the body.

Although so far only one case of this interaction has been reported, the *in vitro* studies suggest that it would be prudent to monitor the theophylline levels of any patient given **ipriflavone**, making any dosage reductions as necessary.

1. Takahashi J, Kawakatsu K, Wakayama T, Sawaoka H. Elevation of serum theophylline levels by ipriflavone in a patient with chronic obstructive pulmonary disease. Eur J Clin Pharmacol (1992) 43, 207–8.
2. Monostory K, Vereczkey L. The effect of ipriflavone and its main metabolites on theophylline biotransformation. Eur J Drug Metab Pharmacokinet (1996) 21, 61–6.
3. Monostory K, Vereczkey L, Lévai F, Szatmári I. Ipriflavone as an inhibitor of human cytochrome P450 enzymes. Br J Pharmacol (1998) 123, 605–10.

Theophylline + Isoniazid

Two short-term studies found that theophylline serum levels were slightly increased by the concurrent use of isoniazid. An isolated report describes theophylline toxicity in a patient one month after starting to take theophylline with isoniazid. However, another short-term study found that isoniazid slightly increased rather than decreased theophylline clearance.

Clinical evidence

Theophylline toxicity has been described in one patient receiving concurrent treatment with **isoniazid** 5 mg/kg daily and theophylline, and this subsequently recurred on re-challenge.[1]

In 7 healthy subjects, high-dose **isoniazid** (10 mg/kg daily) for 10 days increased the AUC from 0 to 6 hours of theophylline by only 8% (from 274 to 296 micromol/h/l). The theophylline was given as an intravenous infusion and the serum levels after 6 h were 22% higher (58 micromol/l compared with 48.5 micromol/l). Five subjects also showed an increase in **isoniazid** half-life and AUC, but these were not statistically significant.[2] Another study found that 400 mg **isoniazid** daily for 2 weeks reduced the mean clearance of theophylline in 13 healthy subjects by 21%.[3]

However, another study in 4 normal subjects given 300 mg **isoniazid** daily for 6 days, found that the clearance of theophylline given orally was increased by 16%, but no consistent changes were seen in any of the other pharmacokinetic parameters measured.[4]

Mechanism

Unknown. It has been suggested that isoniazid inhibits the metabolism of theophylline by the liver, thereby reducing its loss from the body and increasing its serum levels. However, see 'Importance and management', below.

Importance and management

The reason for these inconsistent results is not understood, nor is this interaction well established. It has been suggested that it may take 3 to 4 weeks for any significant increase in theophylline levels to occur.[1] However, if enzyme inhibition was the cause, the effects would be expected more rapidly than this. All of the studies cited covered a period of only 6 to 14 days, whereas the case report describes the effects over a period up to 55 days.[1] The outcome of concurrent use is uncertain but it would clearly be prudent to be alert for any evidence of increased theophylline levels and toxicity if isoniazid is given.

1. Torrent J, Izquierdo I, Cabezas R, Jané F. Theophylline-isoniazid interaction. DICP Ann Pharmacother (1989) 23, 143–5.
2. Höglund P, Nilsson L-G, Paulsen O. Interaction between isoniazid and theophylline. Eur J Respir Dis (1987) 70, 110–16.
3. Samigun, Mulyono, Santoso B. Lowering of theophylline clearance by isoniazid in slow and rapid acetylators. Br J Clin Pharmacol (1990) 29, 570–3.
4. Thompson JR, Burckart GJ, Self TH, Brown RE, Straughn AB. Isoniazid-induced alterations in theophylline pharmacokinetics. Curr Ther Res (1982) 32, 921–5.

Theophylline + Ketoconazole or Fluconazole

Serum theophylline levels are normally affected only minimally or not at all by either fluconazole or ketoconazole. An isolated report describes a rise in serum theophylline levels due to fluconazole, and another describes falls in theophylline levels in three patients on ketoconazole.

Clinical evidence

(a) Fluconazole

A crossover study in 5 healthy subjects found that 100 mg **fluconazole** 12-hourly for 3 days, with the final dose on day 4, caused only a non-significant 16% decrease in the clearance of a single oral dose of theophylline 300 mg.[1] Another study in 10 healthy subjects found that 100 mg **fluconazole** daily for a week had no significant effect on theophylline serum levels (theophylline dosage 150 mg twice daily).[2] Nine healthy subjects had a 13.4% reduction in the clearance of theophylline (single oral dose of 6 mg/kg) after taking **fluconazole** 400 mg daily for 10 days.[3] However an isolated and brief report says that one of 2 patients given theophylline and **fluconazole** showed a rise in serum theophylline levels (degree not specified).[4]

(b) Ketoconazole

No significant changes in the pharmacokinetics of a single intravenous dose of theophylline 3 mg/kg (given as aminophylline) were seen in 12 healthy subjects after taking a single dose of 400 mg **ketoconazole,** or in 4 subjects after taking ketoconazole 400 mg daily for 5 days.[5] Similar results were found in another study in 10 healthy subjects who took **ketoconazole** 200 mg daily for 7 days.[6] **Ketoconazole** 400 mg daily for 6 days increased the theophylline half-life after a single oral dose of 250 mg by 21.7% in 6 healthy subjects, but had no effect on its clearance.[7] However, a case report describes a man whose serum theophylline levels fell sharply from about 16.5 to

9 mg/l (normal range 10 to 20 mg/l) over the 2 h immediately after taking 200 mg **ketoconazole**. A less striking fall was seen in 2 other patients.[8]

Mechanism

These antifungals appear to have minimal effects on cytochrome P450 isoenzyme CYP1A, which is concerned with the oxidative metabolism of theophylline.[1,7] It is not clear why a few individuals show some changes in theophylline levels.

Importance and management

Information seems to be limited to these reports. Neither fluconazole nor ketoconazole normally appears to interact to a relevant extent in most patients. However it seems that very occasionally some changes occur so that it would be prudent to monitor the effects if either is added to established treatment with theophylline.

1. Konishi H, Morita K, Yamaji A. Effect of fluconazole on theophylline disposition in humans. *Eur J Clin Pharmacol* (1994) 46, 309–12.
2. Feil RA, Rindone JP, Morrill GB, Habib MP. Effect of low-dose fluconazole on theophylline serum concentrations in healthy volunteers. *J Pharm Technol* (1995) 11, 267–9.
3. Foisy MM, Nix D, Middleton E, Kotas T, Symonds WT. The effects of single dose fluconazole (SD FLU) versus multiple dose fluconazole (MD FLU) on the pharmacokinetics (PK) of theophylline (THL) in young healthy volunteers. *Intersci Conf Antimicrob Agents Chemother* (1995) 39, 7.
4. Tett S, Carey D, Lee H-S. Drug interactions with fluconazole. *Med J Aust* (1992) 156, 365.
5. Brown MW, Maldonado AL, Meredith CG, Speeg KV. Effect of ketoconazole on hepatic oxidative drug metabolism. *Clin Pharmacol Ther* (1985) 37, 290–7.
6. Heusner JJ, Dukes GE, Rollins DE, Tolman KG, Galinsky RE. Effect of chronically administered ketoconazole on the elimination of theophylline in man. *Drug Intell Clin Pharm* (1987) 21, 514–17.
7. Naline E, Sanceaume M, Pays M, Advenier C. Application of theophylline metabolite assays to the exploration of liver microsome oxidative function in man. *Fundam Clin Pharmacol* (1988) 2, 341–51.
8. Murphy E, Hannon D, Callaghan B. Ketoconazole—theophylline interaction. *Ir Med J* (1987) 80, 123–4.

Theophylline + Leukotriene receptor antagonists

Montelukast in clinical doses does not appear to interact with theophylline. A single case report describes a rapid rise in theophylline levels after the addition of zafirlukast. Zafirlukast levels are reduced by theophylline, but this does not appear to be clinically important.

Clinical evidence

(a) Montelukast

The pharmacokinetics of a single intravenous dose of theophylline were not significantly changed in a group of 16 healthy subjects after taking 10 mg **montelukast** daily for 10 days, but when given doses of 200 and 600 mg montelukast daily, the AUC of theophylline was reduced by 43 and 66% respectively. These doses are 20 and 60-fold higher than the usual 10 mg daily dose.[1]

(b) Zafirlukast

When **zafirlukast** was given with theophylline, the mean serum levels of zafirlukast were reduced by 30%, but the serum theophylline levels remained unchanged.[2] In contrast, an isolated report describes a 15-year-old asthmatic taking sustained release theophylline 300 mg twice daily (as well as inhaled fluticasone, salbutamol (albuterol) and salmeterol and oral prednisolone) who became nauseous shortly after zafirlukast (dose not stated) was added to her treatment. An increase in her theophylline level from 11 to 24 mg/l was noted. The theophylline was stopped, and later attempts to reintroduce theophylline at lower doses resulted in the same dramatic increases in serum theophylline levels.[3]

Mechanism

Not understood.

Importance and management

Information about theophylline/montelukast seems to be limited. The studies indicate that when using normal clinical doses of montelukast no special precautions or dosage alterations are needed. Similarly, no adverse interaction would normally seem to occur with zafirlukast and theophylline, but the isolated (and unexplained) case suggests that concurrent use should be borne in mind when using the combination until more clinical experience has been gained.

1. Malmstrom K, Schwartz J, Reiss TF, Sullivan TJ, Reese JH, Jauregui L, Miller K, Scott M, Shingo S, Peszek I, Larson P, Ebel D, Hunt TL, Huhn RD, Bachmann K. Effect of montelukast on single-dose theophylline pharmacokinetics. *Am J Ther* (1998) 5, 189–95.
2. Accolate (Zafirlukast). AstraZeneca. Summary of product characteristics, October 2001.
3. Katial RK, Stelzle RC, Bonner MW, Marino M, Cantilena LR, Smith LJ. A drug interaction between zafirlukast and theophylline. *Arch Intern Med* (1998) 158, 1713–5.

Theophylline + Loperamide

Loperamide delays the absorption of theophylline from a sustained-release preparation.

Clinical evidence, mechanism, importance and management

A study[1] of the effects of altering the transit time of drugs through the small intestine found that when 12 healthy subjects were given high-dose **loperamide** (8 mg six-hourly for a total of eight doses), the rate, but not extent, of absorption of a single 600-mg dose of sustained-release theophylline (*Theo-24*) was decreased. The maximum serum theophylline levels were reduced from 4.6 to 3.2 micrograms/ml, and this peak level occurred at 20 instead of 11 h. One suggested reason is that **loperamide** inhibits the movement of the gut causing a relatively stagnant pool within the gut where mixing and agitation are reduced, thereby decreasing the dissolution rate of the *Theo-24* pellets. More study is needed to establish the clinical significance of the interaction in patients on long-term theophylline therapy.

1. Bryson JC, Dukes GE, Kirby MG, Heizer WD, Powell JR. Effect of altering small bowel transit time on sustained release theophylline absorption. *J Clin Pharmacol* (1989) 29, 733–8.

Theophylline + Macrolide antibacterials

Troleandomycin (triacetyloleandomycin) can increase serum theophylline levels, causing toxicity if the dosage is not reduced. Azithromycin, clarithromycin, dirithromycin, josamycin, midecamycin, rokitamycin and spiramycin normally only cause modest changes in theophylline levels or do not interact at all. There are unexplained and isolated case reports of theophylline toxicity with josamycin and with clarithromycin. Roxithromycin had no relevant interaction in 3 studies, but was reported to significantly increase serum theophylline levels in another. See also 'Theophylline + Erythromycin', p.796.

Clinical evidence

(a) Azithromycin

In an analysis of the safety data from clinical trials of **azithromycin**, there was no evidence that the plasma levels of theophylline were affected in patients treated concurrently with the two drugs.[1] Similarly, no adverse effects were reported in another clinical study of patients on **azithromycin** and theophylline.[2] **Azithromycin** 250 mg twice daily did not affect the clearance or serum levels of theophylline in patients with asthma.[3] However, a 68-year-old man experienced a marked but transient fall in serum theophylline level when **azithromycin** was withdrawn, and this was confirmed on rechallenge.[4] The same authors conducted a study in 4 healthy subjects given **azithromycin** (500 mg on day 1 then 250 mg daily for 4 days) and sustained-release theophylline (200 mg twice daily). Theophylline levels were slightly elevated during **azithromycin** therapy, and a transient drop occurred 5 days after **azithromycin** withdrawal.[5]

(b) Clarithromycin

Clarithromycin 250 mg twice daily for 7 days had no effect on the steady-state serum theophylline levels of 10 elderly patients with COPD.[6] Similarly, two other studies found that **clarithromycin** had little or no effect on theophylline pharmacokinetics.[3,7] Another study in healthy subjects given **clarithromycin** 500 mg twice daily for 4 days found a 17% rise in the AUC and an 18% rise in the maximum plasma levels of theophylline, but this was considered clinically unimportant.[8] A similar number of patients required an adjustment in theophylline dosage when treated with **clarithromycin** in two clinical trials in patients with acute bacterial exacerbation of chronic bronchitis.[9,10] However, there are isolated reports of possible theophylline toxicity, including a case of rhabdomyolysis with renal failure requiring haemodialysis.[11,12]

(c) Dirithromycin

In one study, 13 healthy subjects showed a fall in steady-state theophylline trough serum level of 18%, and a fall in peak serum level of 26% while taking 500 mg **dirithromycin** daily for 10 days, although this was not considered clinically relevant.[13] No significant changes in the theophylline pharmacokinetics were seen in 14 patients with COPD when given 500 mg **dirithromycin** daily for 10 days.[14] This is supported by a similar single-dose study in 12 healthy subjects.[15]

(d) Josamycin

No clinically significant changes in the serum theophylline levels were seen in 5 studies in patients (adults and children)[16-18] or healthy subjects[19] given **josamycin** concurrently, but a modest rise was described in one study in children.[20] Another study reported a fall of 23% in theophylline levels in 5 patients with particularly severe respiratory impairment, but no significant effect in 5 other patients with less severe disease.[21] However, an isolated report describes theophylline toxicity in a man of 80 when given **josamycin**.[22]

(e) Midecamycin/Midecamycin diacetate

In one study, 18 asthmatic children showed a slight decrease in serum theophylline levels when given **midecamycin** (40 mg/kg/day) for 10 days for a bronchopulmonary infection, but no changes were seen in 5 healthy adult subjects.[23]

Similarly, no significant changes in serum theophylline levels were seen in 20 patients on slow-release theophylline (*Theo-dur*), 300 mg twice daily, or 4 mg/kg intravenous theophylline three times daily, when concurrently treated with 1200 mg **midecamycin diacetate** (miocamycin; ponsinomycin) daily for 10 days.[24] A number of other studies confirm the absence of a clinically important interaction between theophylline and **midecamycin diacetate** in children and adults.[25-28]

(f) Rokitamycin

Two studies in 12 adults with COPD and 11 elderly patients on theophylline showed no significant changes in serum theophylline levels when given 600 to 800 mg **rokitamycin** daily for a week.[29,30]

(g) Roxithromycin

One study in 12 healthy subjects and another in 16 COPD patients showed only minor increases in steady-state theophylline levels when given 150 mg **roxithromycin** twice daily, which were not considered clinically relevant.[31,32] Yet another study in five healthy subjects similarly showed that **roxithromycin** (300 mg twice daily) did not affect the pharmacokinetics of theophylline.[33] However, another study reported a significant increase in serum theophylline levels in 14 patients with asthma after being given 150 mg **roxithromycin** twice daily, but since the amount was not stated it is difficult to assess the clinical relevance of this finding.[3]

(h) Spiramycin

A study in 15 asthmatic patients on theophylline showed that the concurrent use of 1 g **spiramycin** twice daily for at least 5 days had no significant effect on their steady-state serum theophylline levels.[34]

(i) Troleandomycin (Triacetyloleandomycin)

A series of 8 patients with severe chronic asthma showed an average 50% reduction in their theophylline clearance when treated with 250 mg **troleandomycin** four times daily. One of them had a theophylline-induced seizure after 10 days, with a serum theophylline level of 43 micrograms/ml (normal range 10 to 20 micrograms/ml). The theophylline half-life in this patient had increased from 4.6 to 11.3 h.[35] Other studies in healthy subjects[23,36] and patients[18] have also found reductions in theophylline clearance and marked rises in serum theophylline levels and half-life due to **troleandomycin**, even at low doses.[37]

Mechanism

It is believed that troleandomycin forms inactive cytochrome P-450-metabolite complexes within the liver, the effect of which is to reduce the metabolism (*N*-demethylation and 8-hydroxylation)[36] of theophylline, thereby reducing its loss from the body. Josamycin, midecamycin, clarithromycin, and roxithromycin are thought to rarely form complexes, and azithromycin, dirithromycin, rokitamycin and spiramycin are thought to not inactivate cytochrome P450.[38]

Importance and management

The theophylline/troleandomycin (triacetyloleandomycin) interaction is established and well documented. If troleandomycin is added, reduce the theophylline dosage by 25 to 50% initially, monitor the effects closely and titrate the dosage as necessary.[37,39] The situation with roxithromycin is uncertain since only 1 of 4 studies suggested an interaction, but it would be prudent to be alert for the need to reduce the theophylline dosage. Alternative macrolides which usually interact only moderately, or not at all are azithromycin, clarithromycin, dirithromycin, josamycin, midecamycin, rokitamycin and spiramycin. However, even with these it would still be prudent to monitor the outcome because a few patients, especially those with theophylline levels at the high end of the range, may need some small theophylline dosage adjustments. In the case of azithromycin, care should be taken in adjusting the dose based on theophylline levels taken after about 5 days of concurrent use, as they may only be a reflection of a transient drop. In addition, acute infection *per se* may alter theophylline pharmacokinetics.

1. Hopkins S. Clinical toleration and safety of azithromycin. *Am J Med* (1991) 91 (Suppl 3A) 40S–45S.
2. Davies BI, Maesen FPV, Gubbelman R. Azithromycin (CP-62,993) in acute exacerbations of chronic bronchitis: an open, clinical, microbiological and pharmacokinetic study. *J Antimicrob Chemother* (1989) 23, 743–51.
3. Rhee YK, Lee HB, Lee YC. Effects of erythromycin and new macrolides on the serum theophylline level and clearance. *Allergy* (1998) 53 (Suppl 43), 142.
4. Pollak PT, Slayter KL. Reduced serum theophylline concentrations after discontinuation of azithromycin: evidence for an usual interaction. *Pharmacotherapy* (1997) 17, 827–9.
5. Pollack PT, MacNeil DM. Azithromycin-theophylline inhibition-induction interaction. *Clin Pharmacol Ther* (1999) 65, 144.
6. Gaffuri-Riva V, Crippa F, Guffanti EE. Theophylline interaction with new quinolones and macrolides in COPD patients. *Am Rev Respir Dis* (1991) 143, A498.
7. Gillum JG, Israel DS, Scott RB, Climo MW, Polk RE. Effect of combination therapy with ciprofloxacin and clarithromycin on theophylline pharmacokinetics in healthy volunteers. *Antimicrob Agents Chemother* (1996) 40, 1715–16.
8. Ruff F, Chu S-Y, Sonders RC, Sennello LT. Effect of multiple doses of clarithromycin (C) on the pharmacokinetics (Pks) of theophylline (T). *Intersci Conf Antimicrob Agents Chemother* (1990) 30, 213.
9. Bachand RT. Comparative study of clarithromycin and ampicillin in the treatment of patients with acute bacterial exacerbations of chronic bronchitis. *J Antimicrob Chemother* (1991) 27 (Suppl A), 91–100.
10. Aldons PM. A comparison of clarithromycin with ampicillin in the treatment of outpatients with acute bacterial exacerbation of chronic bronchitis. *J Antimicrob Chemother* (1991) 27 (Suppl A), 101–8.
11. Abbott Labs. Personal communication, February 1995.
12. Shimada N, Omuro H, Saka S, Ebihara I, Koide H. A case of acute renal failure with rhabdomyolysis caused by the interaction of theophylline and clarithromycin. *Nippon Jinzo Gakki Shi* (1999) 41, 460–3.
13. Bachmann K, Nunlee M, Martin M, Sullivan T, Jauregui L, DeSante K, Sides GD. Changes in the steady-state pharmacokinetics of theophylline during treatment with dirithromycin. *J Clin Pharmacol* (1990) 30, 1001–5.
14. Bachmann K, Jauregui L, Sides G, Sullivan TJ. Steady-state pharmacokinetics of theophylline in COPD patients treated with dirithromycin. *J Clin Pharmacol* (1993) 33, 861–5.
15. McConnell SA, Nafziger AN, Amsden GW. Lack of effect of dirithromycin on theophylline pharmacokinetics in healthy volunteers. *J Antimicrob Chemother* (1999) 43, 733–6.
16. Ruff F, Prosper M, Puget JC. Théophylline et antibiotiques. Absence d'interaction avec la josamycine. *Therapie* (1984) 39, 1–6.

17. Jiménez Baos R, Casado de Frías E, Cadórniga R, Moreno M. Estudio de posibles inter-accinones entre josamicina y teofilina en niños. *Rev Farmacol Clin Exp* (1985) 2, 345–8.
18. Brazier JL, Kofman J, Faucon G, Perrin-Fayolle M, Lepape A, Lanoue R. Retard d'élim-ination de la théophylline dû á la troléandomycine. Absence d'effet de la josamycine. *Therapie* (1980) 35, 545–9.
19. Selles JP, Panis G, Jaber H, Bres J, Armando P. Influence of josamycine on theophylline kinetics. *Proceedings of the 13th International Congress on Chemotherapy, Vienna* (1983) Aug 28–Sept 2, 15–20.
20. Vallarino G, Merlini M, Vallarino R. Josamicina e teofillinici nella patologia respiratoria pediatrica. *G Ital Chemioter* (1982) 29 (Suppl 1), 129–33.
21. Bartolucci L, Gradoli C, Vincenzi V, Iapadre M, Valori C. Macrolide antibiotics and se-rum theophylline levels in relation to the severity of the respiratory impairment: a com-parison between the effects of erythromycin and josamycin. *Chemioterapia* (1984) 3, 286–90.
22. Barbare JC, Martin F, Biour M. Surdosage en théophylline at anomalies des tests hépa-tiques associés à la prise de josamycine. *Therapie* (1990) 45, 357–58.
23. Lavarenne J, Paire M, Talon O. Influence d'un nouveau macrolide, la midécamycine, sur les taux sanguins de théophylline. *Therapie* (1981) 36, 451–6.
24. Rimoldi R, Bandera M, Fioretti M, Giorcelli R. Miocamycin and theophylline blood lev-els. *Chemioterapia* (1986) 5, 213–16.
25. Principi N, Onorato J, Giuliani MG, Vigano A. Effect of miocamycin on theophylline ki-netics in children. *Eur J Clin Pharmacol* (1987) 31, 701–4.
26. Couet W, Ingrand I, Reigner B, Girault J, Bizouard J, Fourtillan JB. Lack of effect of ponsinomycin on the plasma pharmacokinetics of theophylline. *Eur J Clin Pharmacol* (1989) 37, 101–4.
27. Dal Negro R, Turco P, Pomari C, de Conti F. Miocamycin doesn't affect theophylline serum levels in COPD patients. *Int J Clin Pharmacol Ther Toxicol* (1988) 26, 27–9.
28. Principi N, Onorato J, Giuliani M, Viganó A. Effect of miocamycin on theophylline ki-netics in asthmatic children. *Chemioterapia* (1987) 6 (Suppl 2), 339–40.
29. Ishioka T. Effect of a new macrolide antibiotic, 3'-O-propionyl-leucomycin A5 (Rokita-mycin), on serum concentrations of theophylline and digoxin in the elderly. *Acta Ther* (1987) 13, 17–23.
30. Cazzola M, Matera MG, Paternò E, Scaglione F, Santangelo G, Rossi F. Impact of roki-tamycin, a new 16-membered macrolide, on serum theophylline. *J Chemother* (1991) 3, 240–4.
31. Saint-Salvi B, Tremblay D, Surjus A, Lefebvre MA. A study of the interaction of roxi-thromycin with theophylline and carbamazepine. *J Antimicrob Chemother* (1987) 20 (Suppl B), 121–9.
32. Bandera M, Fioretti M, Rimoldi R, Lazzarini A, Anelli M. Roxithromycin and controlled release theophylline, an interaction study. *Chemioterapia* (1988) 7, 313–16.
33. Hashiguchi K, Niki Y, Soejima R. Roxithromycin does not raise serum theophylline lev-els. *Chest* (1992) 102, 653–4.
34. Debruyne D, Jehan A, Bigot M-C, Lechevalier B, Prevost J-N, Moulin M. Spiramycin has no effect on serum theophylline in asthmatic patients. *Eur J Clin Pharmacol* (1986) 30, 505–7.
35. Weinberger M, Hudgel D, Spector S, Chidsey C. Inhibition of theophylline clearance by troleandomycin. *J Allergy Clin Immunol* (1977) 59, 228–31.
36. Naline E, Sanceaume M, Pays M, Advenier C. Application of theophylline metabolite as-says to the exploration of liver microsome oxidative function in man. *Fundam Clin Phar-macol* (1988) 2, 341–51.
37. Kamada AK, Hill MR, Brenner AM, Szefler SJ. Effect of low-dose troleandomycin on theophylline clearance: implications for therapeutic drug monitoring. *Pharmacotherapy* (1992) 12, 98–102.
38. Periti P, Mazzei T, Mini E, Novelli A. Pharmacokinetic drug interactions of macrolides. *Clin Pharmacokinet* (1992) 23, 106–31. Correction. *ibid.* (1993) 24, 70.
39. Eitches RW, Rachelefsky GS, Katz RM, Mendoza GR, Siegel SC. Methylprednisolone and troleandomycin in treatment of steroid-dependent asthmatic children. *Am J Dis Child* (1985) 139, 264–8.

Theophylline + Methotrexate

Methotrexate causes a modest reduction in the loss of theo-phylline from the body.

Clinical evidence

The apparent clearance of theophylline was reduced by 19% (from 48 to 38.9 ml/h/kg) in 8 severe steroid-dependent asthmatics after 6 weeks treatment with 15 mg intramuscular **methotrexate** weekly. Three patients complained of nausea and the theophylline dosage was reduced in one of them.[1]

Mechanism

Not known.

Importance and management

Information seems to be limited to this study and its clinical impor-tance is uncertain, but it would be prudent to monitor concurrent use.

1. Glynn-Barnhart AM, Erzurum SC, Leff JA, Martin RJ, Cochran JE, Cott GR, Szefler SJ. Effect of low-dose methotrexate on the disposition of glucocorticoids and theophylline. *J Allergy Clin Immunol* (1991) 88, 180–6.

Theophylline + Metoclopramide

Metoclopramide appears not to interact with slow-release theophylline.

Clinical evidence, mechanism, importance and management

A single dose of 10 mg **metoclopramide,** taken 20 min before two 300 mg tablets of slow-release theophylline (*Theo-Dur*), caused a small (14.5%) but not statistically significant fall in the bioavailabil-ity of the theophylline in 8 healthy subjects. However, adverse side-effects (nausea, headache, tremors, CNS stimulation) were seen more often in those taking **metoclopramide** than in those taking placebo, possibly because metoclopramide caused an earlier rise in theophyl-line levels, and because the effects of the 2 drugs may be additive.[1] A later study found that 15 mg **metoclopramide** 6-hourly had no effect on the rate or extent of absorption of 600 mg of another sustained-re-lease theophylline preparation, *Theo-24*, in 12 healthy subjects.[2] There would seem to be no reason for avoiding concurrent use.

1. Steeves RA, Robinson JD, McKenzie MW, Justus PG. Effects of metoclopramide on the pharmacokinetics of a slow-release theophylline product. *Clin Pharm* (1982) 1, 356–60.
2. Bryson JC, Dukes GE, Kirby MG, Heizer WD, Powell JR. Effect of altering small bowel transit time on sustained release theophylline absorption. *J Clin Pharmacol* (1989) 29, 733–8.

Theophylline + Metronidazole

No interaction of clinical importance normally takes place if metronidazole is given to patients taking theophylline, but an isolated report describes seizures in one patient also taking ciprofloxacin.

Clinical evidence, mechanism, importance and management

While taking **metronidazole** (250 mg three times a day) for tricho-moniasis, there were no significant changes in the pharmacokinetics of a single intravenous dose of theophylline in 5 women.[1] Another study in 10 normal subjects confirmed this finding.[2] An acutely ill elderly woman on theophylline had a generalised seizure while being treated with **metronidazole** and ciprofloxacin, although her theo-phylline level was within the therapeutic range (10 to 20 micrograms/ml).[3] Both ciprofloxacin and, more rarely, metronida-zole are associated with seizures.[3] Although the evidence is limited, no special precautions would seem to be necessary during concurrent use. However, note that acute infections *per se* can alter theophylline pharmacokinetics.

1. Reitberg DP, Klarnet JP, Carlson JK, Schentag JJ. Effect of metronidazole on theophyl-line pharmacokinetics. *Clin Pharm* (1983) 2, 441–4.
2. Adebayo GI, Mabadeje AFB. Lack of inhibitory effect of metronidazole on theophylline disposition in healthy subjects. *Br J Clin Pharmacol* (1987) 24, 110–13.
3. Semel JD, Allen N. Seizures in patients simultaneously receiving theophylline and imi-penem or ciprofloxacin or metronidazole. *South Med J* (1991) 84, 465–8.

Theophylline + Mexiletine or Tocainide

Serum theophylline levels are increased by mexiletine. The theophylline dosage will need to be reduced (approximately halved) to avoid toxicity. Tocainide has only a small and probably clinically unimportant effect on theophylline.

Clinical evidence

(a) Mexiletine

A man developed theophylline toxicity within a few days of starting 200 mg **mexiletine** three times daily. His serum theophylline concen-tration had risen from 15.3 to 25 micrograms/ml, but fell to

14.2 micrograms/ml with the disappearance of the symptoms of toxicity when the theophylline dosage was reduced by two-thirds.[1]

Other case reports describe 1.5 to threefold increases in theophylline serum levels (accompanied by clear signs of toxicity in some instances) in a total of nine patients when additionally given **mexiletine**.[2-6] Theophylline dose reductions of 50% were required in 3 cases,[2,6] although 2 cases with initial theophylline levels below the therapeutic range required no dose reductions.[3] One patient also showed arrhythmia aggravation even at therapeutic theophylline serum levels, and mexiletine was discontinued.[4]

In 15 healthy subjects, 200 mg **mexiletine** three times a day for 5 days reduced the clearance of a single intravenous dose of theophylline (5 mg/kg) by 46% in the women and 40% in the men. The theophylline half-life was prolonged by 96% in the women (from 7.4 to 14.5 h) and 71% in the men (from 8.7 to 14.9 h).[7] Two further studies in healthy subjects given theophylline concurrently with **mexiletine** for 5 days found a reduction in steady-state theophylline clearance of 44 and 43%, and an increase in the AUC of 58 and 65%, respectively.[8,9]

(b) Tocainide

After taking 400 mg **tocainide** eight-hourly for 5 days, the pharmacokinetics of a single 5 mg/kg intravenous dose of theophylline was measured in 8 subjects. The clearance was decreased about 10% (from 37.5 to 33.7 ml/h/kg) and the half-life slightly prolonged (from 9.7 to 10.4 h), but these changes were not thought to be large enough to warrant altering theophylline doses.[10]

Mechanism

Mexiletine inhibits the metabolism (demethylation) of theophylline by the liver, thereby reducing its loss from the body and increasing its effects.[7,9,11] It is possible that the interaction is due to competitive inhibition of the cytochrome P450 isoenzyme CYP1A2.[12] Studies in *rats* have shown that tocainide has a substantially smaller effect on cytochrome P450 isoenzyme CYP1A1 than mexiletine.[13]

Importance and management

The theophylline/mexiletine interaction is established and of clinical importance. Monitor concurrent use and reduce the theophylline dosage as necessary (to approximately half initially[7]) to prevent the development of theophylline toxicity. It seems doubtful if the theophylline/tocainide interaction is clinically important but this needs confirmation.

1. Katz A, Buskila D, Sukenik S. Oral mexiletine-theophylline interaction. *Int J Cardiol* (1987) 17, 227–8.
2. Stanley R, Comer T, Taylor JL, Saliba D. Mexiletine-theophylline interaction. *Am J Med* (1989) 86, 733–4.
3. Ueno K, Miyai K, Seki T, Kawaguchi Y. Interaction between theophylline and mexiletine. *DICP Ann Pharmacother* (1990) 24, 471–2.
4. Kessler KM, Interian A, Cox M, Topaz O, De Marchena EJ, Myerburg RJ. Proarrhythmia related to a kinetic and dynamic interaction of mexiletine and theophylline. *Am Heart J* (1989) 117, 964–6.
5. Kendall JD, Chrymko MM, Cooper BE. Theophylline-mexiletine interaction: a case report. *Pharmacotherapy* (1992) 12, 416–18.
6. Inafuku M, Suzuki T, Ohtsu F, Hariya Y, Nagasawa K, Yoshioka Y, Nakahara Y, Hayakawa H. The effect of mexiletine on theophylline pharmacokinetics in patients with bronchial asthma. *J Cardiol* (1992) 22, 227–33.
7. Loi C-M, Wei X, Vestal RE. Inhibition of theophylline metabolism by mexiletine in young male and female nonsmokers. *Clin Pharmacol Ther* (1991) 49, 571–80.
8. Stoysich AM, Mohiuddin SM, Destache CJ, Nipper HC, Hilleman DE. Influence of mexiletine on the pharmacokinetics of theophylline in healthy volunteers. *J Clin Pharmacol* (1991) 31, 354–7.
9. Hurwitz A, Vacek JL, Botteron GW, Sztern MI, Hughes EM, Jayaraj A. Mexiletine effects on theophylline disposition. *Clin Pharmacol Ther* (1991) 50, 299–307.
10. Loi C-M, Wei X, Parker BM, Korrapati MR, Vestal RE. The effect of tocainide on theophylline metabolism. *Br J Clin Pharmacol* (1993) 35, 437–40.
11. Ueno K, Miyai K, Kato M, Kawaguchi Y, Suzuki T. Mechanism of interaction between theophylline and mexiletine. *DICP Ann Pharmacother* (1991) 25, 727–30.
12. Nakajima M, Kobayashi K, Shimada N, Tokudome S, Yamamoto T, Kuroiwa Y. Involvement of CYP1A2 in mexiletine metabolism. *Br J Clin Pharmacol* (1998) 46, 55–62.
13. Wei X, Loi C-M, Jarvi EJ, Vestal RE. Relative potency of mexiletine, lidocaine, and tocainide as inhibitors of rat liver CYP1A1 activity. *Drug Metab Dispos* (1995) 23, 1335–8.

Theophylline + Moracizine

Moracizine increases the loss of theophylline from the body. An increase in the theophylline dosage may possibly be necessary during concurrent use.

Clinical evidence

Single oral doses of aminophylline and of a sustained-release theophylline preparation (*TheoDur*) were given to 12 healthy subjects. After additionally taking **moracizine** 250 mg three times daily for 2 weeks, the AUC of theophylline fell by 32 and 36%, theophylline clearance increased by 44 and 66%, and the elimination half-life decreased by 33 and 20% respectively.[1]

Mechanism

Uncertain. Moracizine is an enzyme-inducer and appears to increase the metabolism of theophylline.

Importance and management

Information seems to be limited to this study. The clinical importance of this interaction has not been assessed, but monitor the effects of concurrent use and be alert for the need to increase the theophylline dose and possibly its frequency. More study is needed.

1. Pieniaszek HJ, Davidson AF, Benedek IH. Effect of moricizine on the pharmacokinetics of single-dose theophylline in healthy subjects. *Ther Drug Monit* (1993) 15, 199–203.

Theophylline + Non-prescription theophylline products

Patients on theophylline should not take other medications containing theophylline (some of which are non-prescription products) unless the total dosage of theophylline can be adjusted appropriately.

Clinical evidence, mechanism, importance and management

A patient on theophylline developed elevated serum theophylline levels (35.7 micrograms/ml) when additionally given *Quinamm* for leg cramps (old formulation containing quinine 260 mg and aminophylline 195 mg). This case report highlights the need to avoid the inadvertent intake of additional doses of theophylline if toxicity is to be avoided. The newer formulation of *Quinamm* does not contain theophylline.[1] Note that OTC preparations containing theophylline are available in many countries. For example, some cough and cold preprations in the UK contain theophylline (e.g. *Do-Do Chesteze, Franol*). Patients should be warned.

1. Shane R. Potential toxicity of theophylline in combination with *Quinamm*. *Am J Hosp Pharm* (1982) 39, 40.

Theophylline + NSAIDs

Aspirin and piroxicam appear not to interact with theophylline.

Clinical evidence, mechanism, importance and management

Piroxicam 20 mg daily for 7 days had no effect on the pharmacokinetics of theophylline (given as a single intravenous dose of aminophylline 6 mg/kg) in 6 healthy subjects.[1] **Enteric-coated aspirin** 650 mg daily for 4 weeks had no effect on the steady-state serum levels of theophylline in 8 elderly patients with COPD (aged 60 to 81).[2]

Apart from checking that the patient is not sensitive to **aspirin** or any other NSAID, there would seem to be no reason for avoiding **aspirin** or **piroxicam** in patients taking theophylline.

1. Maponga C, Barlow JC, Schentag JJ. Lack of effect of piroxicam on theophylline clearance in healthy volunteers. *DICP Ann Pharmacother* (1990) 24, 123–6.
2. Daigneault EA, Hamdy RC, Ferslew KE, Rice PJ, Singh J, Harvill LM, Kalbfleisch JH. Investigation of the influence of acetylsalicylic acid on the steady state of long-term therapy with theophylline in elderly male patients with normal renal function. *J Clin Pharmacol* (1994) 34, 86–90.

Theophylline + Olanzapine

There appears to be no significant interaction between theophylline and olanzapine.

Clinical evidence, mechanism, importance and management

A study in 18 healthy subjects given **olanzapine** (5 mg on day one, 7.5 mg on day 2 and then 10 mg for 7 days) showed no significant changes in the pharmacokinetics of a single intravenous dose of aminophylline 350 mg. The pharmacokinetics of **olanzapine** also appeared to be unchanged by concurrent use. No special precautions would appear to be necessary when these two drugs are used concurrently. The authors also conclude[1] that **olanzapine** would not be expected to affect the pharmacokinetics of other drugs that are (like theophylline) substrates for the cytochrome P450 isoenzyme CYP1A2.

1. Macias WL, Bergstrom RF, Cerimele BJ, Kassahun K, Tatum DE, Callaghan JT. Lack of effect of olanzapine on the pharmacokinetics of a single aminophylline dose in healthy men. *Pharmacotherapy* (1998) 18, 1237–48.

Theophylline + Ozagrel

Ozagrel appears not to interact with theophylline.

Clinical evidence, mechanism, importance and management

Serum theophylline levels in 4 patients with asthma did not change significantly after finishing 24 weeks treatment with **ozagrel** 200 mg twice daily. Similarly, in another 8 patients with bronchial asthma, there were no significant differences in the pharmacokinetics of a single infusion of aminophylline administered before and after 7 days treatment with the same dose of **ozagrel**.[1] No special precautions would seem to be needed during concurrent use.

1. Kawakatsu K, Kino T, Yasuba H, Kawaguchi H, Tsubata R, Satake N, Oshima S. Effect of ozagrel (OKY-046), a thromboxane synthetase inhibitor, on theophylline pharmacokinetics in asthmatic patients. *Int J Clin Pharmacol Ther Toxicol* (1990) 28, 158–63.

Theophylline + Pentoxifylline (Oxpentifylline)

Pentoxifylline (oxpentifylline) can raise serum theophylline serum levels.

Clinical evidence, mechanism, importance and management

The mean trough steady-state theophylline serum levels of 9 healthy subjects given sustained-release theophylline *(TheoDur)* 200 or 300 mg twice daily for 7 days were 30% higher (range −12.8 to 94.8%) while taking 400 mg **pentoxifylline** three times daily. The subjects complained of insomnia, nausea, diarrhoea and tachycardia more frequently while taking both drugs, but this did not reach statistical significance.[1] The mechanism of this interaction is not understood, although pentoxifylline is also a xanthine derivative. Patients

should be well monitored while taking both drugs. More study is needed to clarify this highly variable interaction.

1. Ellison MJ, Horner RD, Willis SE, Cummings DM. Influence of pentoxifylline on steady-state theophylline serum concentrations from sustained-release formulations. *Pharmacotherapy* (1990) 10, 383–6.

Theophylline + Phenylpropanolamine

There is evidence that phenylpropanolamine can reduce the clearance of theophylline from the body. Increases in serum theophylline levels and toxicity may occur.

Clinical evidence, mechanism, importance and management

A single oral dose of 150 mg **phenylpropanolamine** decreased the clearance of theophylline (given as a single intravenous dose of aminophylline 4 mg/kg 1 hour after the **phenylpropanolamine**) in 8 healthy subjects by 50% (a reduction from 0.88 to 0.44 micrograms/ml/h).[1] Such a large reduction would be expected to cause a marked rise in serum theophylline levels, but so far no studies of this potentially clinically important interaction seem to have been carried out in patients. Be alert for evidence of toxicity if both drugs are used. More study is needed.

1. Wilson HA, Chin R, Adair NE, Zaloga GP. Phenylpropanolamine significantly reduces the clearance of theophylline. *Am Rev Respir Dis* (1991) 143, A629.

Theophylline + Pinacidil

Pinacidil appears not to interact with theophylline.

Clinical evidence, mechanism, importance and management

After taking **pinacidil** 12.5 mg twice daily for a week, and then 25 mg twice daily for a further week, the pharmacokinetics of a single intravenous 5 mg/kg dose of theophylline were not significantly changed in 6 healthy subjects.[1] This suggests that concurrent use in patients is likely to be safe, but further confirmation is needed.

1. Nielsen-Kudsk JE, Nielsen CB, Mellemkjær S, Siggaard C. Lack of effect of pinacidil on theophylline pharmacokinetics and metabolism in man. *Pharmacol Toxicol* (1990) 67, 156–8.

Theophylline + Pirenzepine

Pirenzepine does not appear to interact with theophylline.

Clinical evidence, mechanism, importance and management

Pirenzepine 50 mg twice daily for 5 days had no effect on the pharmacokinetics of theophylline (given as aminophylline 6.5 mg/kg, intravenously) in 5 healthy subjects.[1] This would suggest that concurrent use need not be avoided.

1. Sertl K, Rameis H, Meryn S. Pirenzepin does not alter the pharmacokinetics of theophylline. *Int J Clin Pharmacol Ther Toxicol* (1987) 25, 15–17.

Theophylline + Pneumococcal vaccine

Pneumococcal vaccination appears not to affect theophylline.

Clinical evidence, mechanism, importance and management

The pharmacokinetics of theophylline (250 mg given orally three times daily for 10 days) were unaltered in 6 healthy subjects the day after receiving 0.5 ml of a **pneumococcal vaccine**, and a week later.[1,2] These findings need confirmation in patients, but what is known suggests that no special precautions are needed during concurrent use.

1. Cupit GC, Self TH, Pieper JA, Bekemeyer WB. Effect of pneumococcal vaccine (PV) on theophylline (T) disposition. *Clin Pharmacol Ther* (1987) 41, 199.
2. Cupit GC, Self TH, Bekemeyer WB. The effect of pneumococcal vaccine on the disposition of theophylline. *Eur J Clin Pharmacol* (1988) 34, 505–7.

Theophylline or Diprophylline + Probenecid

Serum levels of theophylline are unaffected by the concurrent use of probenecid, but serum diprophylline levels can be raised.

Clinical evidence

(a) Diprophylline

A study in 12 healthy subjects showed that the half-life of a single oral dose of **diprophylline** 20 mg/kg was doubled (from 2.6 to 4.9 hours) and the clearance approximately halved by the concurrent use of 1 g **probenecid**, resulting in raised serum **diprophylline** levels.[1]

(b) Theophylline

A study in 7 healthy subjects showed that 1 g **probenecid** given 30 min before an oral dose of **aminophylline** (5.6 mg/kg) had no significant effect on the pharmacokinetics of **theophylline**.[2]

Mechanism

Diprophylline is largely excreted unchanged by the kidneys, and probenecid inhibits its renal tubular secretion.[3] **Theophylline** is largely cleared from the body by hepatic metabolism, and would therefore not be expected to be affected by probenecid.

Importance and management

Based on the findings of this single-dose study, it would seem to be prudent to monitor serum **diprophylline** levels if **probenecid** is started or stopped.

1. May DC, Jarboe CH. Effect of probenecid on dyphylline elimination. *Clin Pharmacol Ther* (1983) 33, 822–5.
2. Chen TWD, Patton TF. Effect of probenecid on the pharmacokinetics of aminophylline. *Drug Intell Clin Pharm* (1983) 17, 465–6.
3. Nadai M, Apichartpichean R, Hasegawa T, Nabeshima T. Pharmacokinetics and the effect of probenecid on the renal excretion mechanism of diprophylline. *J Pharm Sci* (1992) 81, 1024–7.

Theophylline + Propafenone

Two isolated reports describe theophylline toxicity and raised serum levels in two patients when given propafenone.

Clinical evidence

The theophylline serum levels of a 71-year-old man taking 300 mg twice daily rose from 10.2–12.8 micrograms/ml to 19 micrograms/ml with signs of theophylline toxicity when given 150 mg **propafenone** three times daily, and fell to 10.8 micrograms/ml the day after it was withdrawn. When the **propafenone** was later restarted, the theophylline levels rose again within a week to 17.7 micrograms/ml, but fell when the theophylline dosage was reduced to 200 mg twice daily.[1]

In another report, a man of 63 showed a marked reduction in the clearance of theophylline, with a rise in theophylline level from 10.8 mg/l to a maximum of 20.3 mg/l over 7 days after starting **propafenone** 150 mg, increased up to 300 mg, 8-hourly.[2] Theophylline was discontinued.

Mechanism

Uncertain. It has been suggested that propafenone may reduce the metabolism of theophylline by the liver, thereby reducing its loss from the body.

Importance and management

Information is limited to these 2 reports, but it would seem prudent to monitor the effect of adding propafenone to established treatment with theophylline in any patient. Be alert for increased serum levels and signs of toxicity. Controlled studies are needed to further investigate this potential interaction.

1. Lee BL, Dohrmann ML. Theophylline toxicity after propafenone treatment: evidence for drug interaction. *Clin Pharmacol Ther* (1992) 51, 353–5.
2. Spinler SA, Gammaitoni A, Charland SL, Hurwitz J. Propafenone-theophylline interaction. *Pharmacotherapy* (1993) 13, 68–71.

Theophylline + Proton pump inhibitors

Omeprazole and lansoprazole may cause a small increase in theophylline clearance, which is unlikely to be clinically relevant. Pantoprazole and rabeprazole do not appear to interact with theophylline.

Clinical evidence

(a) Lansoprazole

Lansoprazole 60 mg daily for 9 days caused only a very slight reduction in the steady state theophylline serum levels of 14 healthy subjects.[1] Other studies have also shown little or no change in theophylline pharmacokinetics on concurrent use.[2-5]

(b) Omeprazole

The changes in the half-life and clearance of theophylline caused by **omeprazole** were found to be small and clinically unimportant in three studies.[6,7] No changes in the steady-state pharmacokinetics of theophylline were found in other studies.[5,8] However one study found that **omeprazole** increased the clearance of theophylline in poor metabolisers by 11%.[9]

(c) Pantoprazole

A crossover study in 8 healthy subjects showed that once-daily intravenous injections of 30 mg **pantoprazole** had no clinically important effect on the pharmacokinetics of theophylline given by infusion. No clinically relevant changes in blood pressure, heart rate, ECG and routine clinical laboratory parameters were seen.[10] Other studies have also found no significant change in theophylline pharmacokinetics on concurrent use with **pantoprazole**.[4,5]

(d) Rabeprazole

A single 250 mg oral dose of theophylline was given to 25 patients before and after taking 20 mg **rabeprazole** or a placebo daily for 7 days. No significant changes in the pharmacokinetics of theophylline were seen.[11,12]

Mechanism, importance and management

Lansoprazole possibly induces cytochrome P450 isoenzyme CYP1A2 to a small extent, but this is unlikely to be significant unless an individual is particularly sensitive to this effect.[1] Other proton pump inhibitors are likely to interact similarly, and so no special precautions would seem necessary on concurrent use.

1. Granneman GR, Karol MD, Locke CS, Cavanaugh JH. Pharmacokinetic interaction between lansoprazole and theophylline. *Ther Drug Monit* (1995) 17, 460–4.
2. Kokufu T, Ihara N, Sugioka N, Koyama H, Ohta T, Mori S, Nakajima K. Effects of lansoprazole on pharmacokinetics and metabolism of theophylline. *Eur J Clin Pharmacol* (1995) 48, 391–5.

3. Ko J-W, Jang I-J, Shin S-G, Flockhart DA. Effect of lansoprazole on theophylline clearance in extensive and poor metabolizers of cytochrome P450 2C19. *Clin Pharmacol Ther* (1998) 63, 217.

4. Pan WJ, Goldwater DR, Zhang Y, Pilmer BL, Hunt RH. Lack of a pharmacokinetic interaction between lansoprazole or pantoprazole and theophylline. *Aliment Pharmacol Ther* (2000) 14, 345–52.

5. Dilger K, Zheng Z, Klotz U. Lack of drug interaction between omeprazole, lansoprazole, pantoprazole and theophylline. *Br J Clin Pharmacol* (1999) 48, 438–44.

6. Oosterhuis B, Jonkman JHG, Andersson T, Zuiderwijk PBM. No influence of single intravenous doses of omeprazole on theophylline elimination kinetics. *J Clin Pharmacol* (1992) 32, 470–5.

7. Sommers De K, van Wyk M, Snyman JR, Moncrieff J. The effects of omeprazole-induced hypochlorhydria on absorption of theophylline from a sustained-release formulation. *Eur J Clin Pharmacol* (1992) 43, 141–3.

8. Taburet AM, Geneve J, Bocquentin M, Simoneau G, Caulin C, Singlas E. Theophylline steady state pharmacokinetics is not altered by omeprazole. *Eur J Clin Pharmacol* (1992) 42, 343–5.

9. Cavuto NJ, Sukhova N, Hewett J, Balian JD, Woosley RL, Flockhart MD. Effect of omeprazole on theophylline clearance in poor metabolizers of omeprazole. *Clin Pharmacol Ther* (1995) 57, 215.

10. Schulz H-U, Hartmann M, Steinijans VW, Huber R, Lührmann B, Bliessath H, Wurst W. Lack of influence of pantoprazole on the disposition kinetics of theophylline in man. *Int J Clin Pharmacol Ther Toxicol* (1991) 29, 369–75.

11. Humphries TJ, Nardi RV, Spera AC, Lazar JD, Laurent AL, Spanyers SA. Coadministration of rabeprazole sodium (E3810) does not effect the pharmacokinetics of anhydrous theophylline or warfarin. *Gastroenterology* (1996) 110 (Suppl), A138.

12. Humphries TJ, Nardi RV, Lazar JD, Spanyers SA. Drug-drug interaction evaluation of rabeprazole sodium: a clean/expected slate? *Gut* (1996) 39 (Suppl 3), A47.

Theophylline + Pyrantel

A single case report describes increased serum theophylline levels in a child when given pyrantel embonate (pyrantel pamoate).

Clinical evidence

A boy of eight with status asthmaticus was treated firstly with intravenous aminophylline and then switched to sustained-release oral theophylline on day 3. His serum theophylline level was 15 micrograms/ml on day 3. On day 4 he was additionally given a single 160-mg dose of **pyrantel embonate** (for *Ascaris lumbricoides* infection) at the same time as his second oral theophylline dose. About 2.5 h later his serum theophylline level was 24 micrograms/ml, and a further 1.5 h later it had risen to 30 micrograms/ml. No further theophylline was given and no theophylline toxicity occurred. The patient was discharged later in the day without theophylline.[1]

Mechanism

Not understood. One suggestion is that the pyrantel inhibited the liver enzymes concerned with the metabolism of the theophylline, thereby reducing its loss from the body. However this is unlikely as the interaction occurred so rapidly. Another suggestion was that pyrantel may have increased drug release from the sustained-release theophylline preparation.

Importance and management

Information is limited to this single case report. No general conclusions can be based on such slim evidence, but concurrent use should be well monitored because, in this case, the serum theophylline concentration increase was very rapid. More study is needed.

1. Hecht L, Murray WE, Rubenstein S. Theophylline-pyrantel pamoate interaction. *DICP Ann Pharmacother* (1989) 23, 258.

Theophylline + Pyridoxal

No adverse interaction occurs if pyridoxal (a vitamin B$_6$ substance) and theophylline are taken concurrently. Some reduction in theophylline-induced hand tremor may occur.

Clinical evidence, mechanism, importance and management

In a crossover study, 15 young healthy adults were given theophylline (*Theo-Dur*) for 4 weeks (with the dose adjusted to give plasma levels of 10 mg/l) combined with daily doses of either a placebo or a **vitamin B$_6$ supplement** containing 15 mg **pyridoxal hydrochloride**. A variety of psychomotor and electrophysiological tests and self-report questionnaires failed to distinguish between the effects of the placebo or the **vitamin B$_6$ supplement** except that the hand tremor induced by the theophylline tended to be reduced.[1] There would seem to be no reason for avoiding concurrent use and it may have some advantage.

1. Bartel PR, Ubbink JB, Delport R, Lotz BP, Becker PJ. Vitamin B-6 supplementation and theophylline-related effects in humans. *Am J Clin Nutr* (1994) 60, 93–9.

Theophylline + Quinolone antibacterials

Theophylline serum levels can be markedly increased in most patients by enoxacin, and the theophylline dosage should be reduced. Pipemidic acid, clinafloxacin and grepafloxacin may interact similarly. Theophylline levels can also be markedly increased in some patients by the concurrent use of ciprofloxacin, and possibly pefloxacin. The theophylline dosage may need to be approximately halved if toxicity is to be avoided. No theophylline dosage adjustment will probably be needed in most patients given norfloxacin, ofloxacin or prulifloxacin because they normally cause a much smaller rise in theophylline levels. However, serious toxicity has been seen in few patients given norfloxacin. Fleroxacin, flumequine, gatifloxacin, gemifloxacin, levofloxacin, lomefloxacin, nalidixic acid, rufloxacin, sparfloxacin and trovafloxacin appear not to interact.

Clinical evidence

A. Pharmacokinetic studies

For comparison, the affects of the quinolone antibacterials on the pharmacokinetics of theophylline are listed[1-47] in Table 22.4.

B. Case reports

(a) Ciprofloxacin

There are numerous case reports describing this interaction, which commonly show large increases in serum theophylline levels (32 to 478% or 1.3 to 5.6-fold increases), often associated with toxicity.[48-58] From 1987 to 1988, the CSM in the UK had received 8 reports of clinically important toxic interactions between these two drugs, with one fatal case.[48] By 1991, the US FDA had 39 reports of the interaction, with three deaths.[56] Another elderly woman on theophylline developed toxic serum levels and died shortly after starting to take **ciprofloxacin**.[54] Seizures, associated with toxic levels of theophylline, were described in a number of the case reports.[52,56-58] Seizures have also occurred with the concurrent use of **ciprofloxacin** and theophylline when theophylline levels were within the therapeutic range (10 to 20 micrograms/ml).[56,59,60] **Ciprofloxacin** and toxic levels of theophylline are both known to cause seizures independently. It was suggested that, in the case of seizures, there may be a pharmacodynamic interaction between theophylline and fluoroquinolones as well as a pharmacokinetic interaction.[56] In each case, seizures began within 1 to 7 days of starting the combination and were reported as being either partial or grand mal. The addition of clarithromycin does not appear to increase the effects of ciprofloxacin on theophylline.[38]

(b) Clinafloxacin

A 78-year-old man with steroid dependent COPD and with apparently stable serum theophylline levels showed a marked increase in level (approximately doubled) after receiving 200 mg **clinafloxacin** intravenously 12-hourly for 5 days. Two theophylline dosages were withheld, and then the dosage was reduced from 300 mg 8-hourly to

Table 22.4 Effect of quinolones on theophylline pharmacokinetics in order of magnitude of the potential interaction

Quinolone (daily dose)	Increase in theophylline level	Increase in AUC	Decrease in clearance	Ref
Enoxacin 600 to 1200 mg	72 to 243%	84 to 248%	42 to 74%	2, 4, 6, 9, 11, 13, 17, 30
Pipemidic acid 800 to 1500 mg	71%	76 to 79%	49%	6, 22
Clinafloxacin 400 to 800 mg			46 to 69%	44
Grepafloxacin 200 to 600 mg	28 to 82%	93 to 113%	33 to 54%	31, 43
Ciprofloxacin 600 to 1500 mg	17 to 50%	22 to 52%	18 to 31%	1, 4, 6, 18, 26, 27, 37, 38
Pefloxacin 400 to 800 mg	17 to 20%	19 to 53%	29%	4, 6
Norfloxacin 600 to 800 mg	up to 22%	up to 17%	up to 15%	5–8, 17, 25, 27
Prulifloxacin 600 mg		16%	15%	46
Ofloxacin 400 to 600 mg	up to 10%	up to 10%	up to 12%	3, 4, 6, 8, 12, 17, 29
Trovafloxacin 200 to 300 mg		up to 8%		40, 41
Fleroxacin 400 mg	No significant change	up to 8%	up to 6%	16, 20, 21, 28
Flumequine 1200 mg	No significant change	No significant change	No significant change	36
Gatifloxacin 400 mg	No significant change	No significant change		47
Gemifloxacin 320 mg	No significant change	No significant change		45
Levofloxacin 300 to 1000 mg	No significant change	No significant change	No significant change	14, 31, 39
Lomefloxacin 400 to 800 mg	No significant change	No significant change	No significant change	10, 15, 19, 22, 26, 32
Nalidixic acid 1000 to 2000 mg		No significant change	No significant change	4, 27
Rufloxacin 200 to 400 mg	No significant change	No significant change	No significant change	23, 42
Sparfloxacin 200 to 400 mg	No significant change	No significant change	No significant change	24, 33–35

200 mg 8-hourly. Within another 5 days his serum theophylline levels had fallen to his previous steady-state level once again.[61]

(c) Enoxacin

Some patients in early studies of **enoxacin** experienced adverse effects (serious nausea and vomiting, tachycardia, seizures)[62,63] and this was found to be associated with unexpectedly high plasma theophylline levels.[2,62]

(d) Norfloxacin

No clinically significant changes in theophylline levels occurred in a patient given **norfloxacin** who subsequently showed marked changes when given **ciprofloxacin**.[50] These studies contrast with the US FDA records of 3 patients (up to 1989)[64] and 9 patients (up to 1991)[56] who experienced marked increases in theophylline levels ranging from 64 to 171% (mean 103%). Three developed seizures and one died.[56]

(e) Pefloxacin

An isolated report describes convulsions in a patient attributed to the concurrent use of theophylline and **pefloxacin**.[65]

Mechanism

The interacting quinolone antibacterials appear to inhibit the metabolism (N-demethylation) of theophylline to different extents (some hardly at all), so that it is cleared from the body more slowly and its serum levels rise. Inhibition of cytochrome P450 isoenzyme CYP1A2 is probable. The chemical structures of the different qui-

nolones have been examined in an attempt to predict the likelihood of an interaction with CYP1A2 and theophylline.[66,67] There is some evidence that combined use may amplify the epileptogenic activity of the quinolones.[56,68]

Importance and management

The theophylline/enoxacin and theophylline/ciprofloxacin interactions are well documented, well established and of clinical importance. The effect of enoxacin is marked and occurs in most patients, whereas the incidence with ciprofloxacin is uncertain and problems do not develop in a proportion of patients. Nevertheless, be alert for this interaction in all patients if ciprofloxacin is started. The risk seems greatest in the elderly[69] and those with theophylline levels already towards the top end of the therapeutic range. Toxicity may develop rapidly (within 2 to 3 days) unless the dosage of theophylline is reduced. With enoxacin, an initial reduction in theophylline dose is required, in the order of 50%,[2,4,11,70] although reductions of 75% may possibly be necessary for those with high theophylline clearances.[70] Further alterations in theophylline dose should be based on careful monitoring of theophylline levels. New steady-state serum theophylline levels are achieved within about 2 to 3 days of starting and stopping enoxacin.[13,70] With ciprofloxacin, some recommend an initial reduction in theophylline dose, in the order of 30 to 50%.[26,27,56] However, since a proportion of patients will not require a dose reduction, others suggest that the dose should be modified based on the theophylline level on day 2 of ciprofloxacin therapy.[1,4,18,37,58] Direct information about clinafloxacin, grepafloxacin and pipemidic acid is more limited, but they also appear to cause a considerable rise in serum theophylline levels, similar to enoxacin (see Table 22.4).

Keep a check on the effects if norfloxacin or ofloxacin or pefloxacin are used because theophylline serum levels may possibly rise to a small extent (10 to 22%), but these antibacterials normally appear to be much safer. However, be aware that norfloxacin has caused a much larger rise on occasions.[56,64] Fleroxacin, flumequine, gatifloxacin, gemifloxacin, levofloxacin, lomefloxacin, nalidixic acid, rufloxacin, sparfloxacin and trovafloxacin appear not to interact significantly, and no special precautions seem necessary with these drugs. However, note that acute infection can alter theophylline pharmacokinetics.

The makers of some quinolones include a warning in their product literature about the risk of combining theophylline with quinolones because of their potential additive effects on reducing the seizure threshold. Convulsions have been reported with theophylline plus ciprofloxacin, norfloxacin and pefloxacin. With some of these cases it is difficult to know whether what happened was due to increased theophylline levels, to patient pre-disposition, to potential additive effects on the seizure threshold, or to all three factors combined. However, the literature suggests that seizures attributed to concurrent use are relatively rare, so that the general warning about the risks with all quinolones may possibly be an overstatement.

1. Nix DE, DeVito JM, Whitbread MA, Schentag JJ. Effect of multiple dose oral ciprofloxacin on the pharmacokinetics of theophylline and indocyanine green. *J Antimicrob Chemother* (1987) 19, 263–9.
2. Wijnands WJA, Vree TB, van Herwaarden CLA. Enoxacin decreases the clearance of theophylline in man. *Br J Clin Pharmacol* (1985) 20, 583–8.
3. Gregoire SL, Grasela TH, Freer JP, Tack KJ, Schentag JJ. Inhibition of theophylline clearance by coadministered ofloxacin without alteration of theophylline effects. *Antimicrob Agents Chemother* (1987) 31, 375–8.
4. Wijnands WJA, Vree TB, van Herwaarden CLA. The influence of quinolone derivatives on theophylline clearance. *Br J Clin Pharmacol* (1986) 22, 677–83.
5. Bowles SK, Popovski Z, Rybak MJ, Beckman HB, Edwards DJ. Effect of norfloxacin on theophylline pharmacokinetics at steady state. *Antimicrob Agents Chemother* (1988) 32, 510–12.
6. Niki Y, Soejima R, Kawane H, Sumi M, Umeki S. New synthetic quinolone antibacterial agents and serum concentration of theophylline. *Chest* (1987) 92, 663–9.
7. Sano M, Yamamoto I, Ueda J, Yoshikawa E, Yamashina H, Goto M. Comparative pharmacokinetics of theophylline following two fluoroquinolones co-administration. *Eur J Clin Pharmacol* (1987) 32, 431–2.
8. Tierney MG, Ho G, Dales RE. Effect of norfloxacin on theophylline pharmacokinetics. *Clin Pharmacol Ther* (1988) 43, 156.
9. Beckmann J, Elsäßer W, Gundert-Remy U, Hertrampf R. Enoxacin - a potent inhibitor of theophylline metabolism. *Eur J Clin Pharmacol* (1987) 33, 227–30.
10. Nix DE, Norman A, Schentag JJ. Effect of lomefloxacin on theophylline pharmacokinetics. *Antimicrob Agents Chemother* (1989) 33, 1006–8.
11. Takagi K, Hasegawa T, Yamaki K, Suzuki R, Watanabe T, Satake T. Interaction between theophylline and enoxacin. *Int J Clin Pharmacol Ther Toxicol* (1988) 26, 288–92.
12. Al-Turk WA, Shaheen OM, Othman S, Khalaf RM, Awidi AS. Effect of ofloxacin on the pharmacokinetics of a single intravenous theophylline dose. *Ther Drug Monit* (1988) 10, 160–3.
13. Rogge MC, Solomon WR, Sedman AJ, Welling PG, Koup JR, Wagner JG. The theophylline-enoxacin interaction: II. Changes in the disposition of theophylline and its metabolites during intermittent administration of enoxacin. *Clin Pharmacol Ther* (1989) 46, 420–8.
14. Okimoto N, Niki Y, Soejima R. Effect of levofloxacin on serum concentration of theophylline. *Chemotherapy* (1992) 40, 68–74.
15. Wijnands GJA, Cornel JH, Martea M, Vree TB. The effect of multiple-dose oral lomefloxacin on theophylline metabolism in man. *Chest* (1990) 98, 1440–4.
16. Niki Y, Tasaka Y, Kishimoto T, Nakajima M, Tsukiyama K, Nakagawa Y, Umeki S, Hino J, Okimoto N, Yagi S, Kawane H, Soejima R. Effect of fleroxacin on serum concentration of theophylline. *Chemotherapy* (1990) 38, 364–71.
17. Sano M, Kawakatsu K, Ohkita C, Yamamoto I, Takeyama M, Yamashina H, Goto M. Effects of enoxacin, ofloxacin and norfloxacin on theophylline disposition in humans. *Eur J Clin Pharmacol* (1988) 35, 161–5.
18. Schwartz J, Jauregui L, Lettieri J, Bachmann K. Impact of ciprofloxacin on theophylline clearance and steady-state concentrations in serum. *Antimicrob Agents Chemother* (1988) 32, 75–7.
19. LeBel M, Vallée F, St-Laurent M. Influence of lomefloxacin on the pharmacokinetics of theophylline. *Antimicrob Agents Chemother* (1990) 34, 1254–6.
20. Seelmann R, Mahr G, Gottschalk B, Stephan U, Sörgel F. Influence of fleroxacin on the pharmacokinetics of theophylline. *Rev Infect Dis* (1989) 11 (Suppl 5), S1100.
21. Soejima R, Niki Y, Sumi M. Effect of fleroxacin on serum concentrations of theophylline. *Rev Infect Dis* (1989) 11 (Suppl 5), S1099.
22. Staib AH, Harder S, Fuhr U, Wack C. Interaction of quinolones with the theophylline metabolism in man: investigations with lomefloxacin and pipemidic acid. *Int J Clin Pharmacol Ther Toxicol* (1989) 27, 289–93.
23. Cesana M, Broccali G, Imbimbo BP, Crema A. Effect of single doses of rufloxacin on the disposition of theophylline and caffeine after single administration. *Int J Clin Pharmacol Ther Toxicol* (1991) 29, 133–8.
24. Takagi K, Yamaki K, Nadai M, Kuzuya T, Hasegawa T. Effect of a new quinolone, sparfloxacin, on the pharmacokinetics of theophylline in asthmatic patients. *Antimicrob Agents Chemother* (1991) 35, 1137–41.
25. Davis RL, Kelly HW, Quenzer RW, Standefer J, Steinberg B, Gallegos J. Effect of norfloxacin on theophylline metabolism. *Antimicrob Agents Chemother* (1989) 33, 212–4.
26. Robson RA, Begg EJ, Atkinson HC, Saunders DA, Frampton CM. Comparative effects of ciprofloxacin and lomefloxacin on the oxidative metabolism of theophylline. *Br J Clin Pharmacol* (1990) 29, 491–3.
27. Prince RA, Casabar E, Adair CG, Wexler DB, Lettieri J, Kasik JE. Effect of quinolone antimicrobials on theophylline pharmacokinetics. *J Clin Pharmacol* (1989) 29, 650–4.
28. Parent M, St-Laurent M, LeBel M. Safety of fleroxacin coadministered with theophylline to young and elderly volunteers. *Antimicrob Agents Chemother* (1990) 34, 1249–53.
29. Fourtillan JB, Granier J, Saint-Salvi B, Salmon J, Surjus A, Tremblay D, Vincent du Laurier M, Beck S. Pharmacokinetics of ofloxacin and theophylline alone and in combination. *Infection* (1986) 14 (Suppl 1), S67–S69.
30. Sörgel F, Mahr G, Granneman GR, Stephan U, Nickel P, Muth P. Effects of 2 quinolone antibacterials, temafloxacin and enoxacin, on theophylline pharmacokinetics. *Clin Pharmacokinet* (1992) 22 (Suppl 1), 65–74.
31. Niki Y, Hashiguchi K, Okimoto N, Soejima R. Quinolone antimicrobial agents and theophylline. *Chest* (1992) 101, 881.
32. Kuzuya T, Takagi K, Apichartpichean R, Muraoka I, Nadai M, Hasegawa T. Kinetic interaction between theophylline and a newly developed quinolone, NY-198. *J Pharmacobiodyn* (1989) 12, 405–9.
33. Okimoto N, Niki Y, Sumi M, Nakagawa Y, Soejima R. Effect of sparfloxacin on plasma concentration of theophylline. *Chemotherapy (Tokyo)* (1991) 39 (Suppl 4), 158–60.
34. Mahr G, Seelmann R, Gottschalk B, Stephan U, Sörgel F. No effect of sparfloxacin (SP-FX) on the metabolism of theophylline (THE) in man. *Intersci Conf Antimicrob Agents Chemother* (1990) 30, 296.
35. Yamaki K, Miyatake H, Taki F, Suzuki R, Takagi K, Satake T. Studies on sparfloxacin (SPFX) against respiratory tract infections and its effect on theophylline pharmacokinetics. *Chemotherapy* (1991) 39 (Suppl 4), 280–5.
36. Lacarelle B, Blin O, Auderbert C, Auquier P, Karsenty H, Horriere F, Durand A. The quinolone, flumequine, has no effect on theophylline pharmacokinetics. *Eur J Clin Pharmacol* (1994) 46, 477–8.
37. Batty KT, Davis TME, Ilett KF, Dusci LJ, Langton SR. The effect of ciprofloxacin on theophylline pharmacokinetics in healthy subjects. *Br J Clin Pharmacol* (1995) 39, 305–11.
38. Gillum JG, Israel DS, Scott RB, Climo MW, Polk RE. Effect of combination therapy with ciprofloxacin and clarithromycin on theophylline pharmacokinetics in healthy volunteers. *Antimicrob Agents Chemother* (1996) 40, 1715–16.
39. Gisclon LG, Curtin CR, Fowler CL, Williams RR, Hafkin B, Natarajan J. Absence of a pharmacokinetic interaction between intravenous theophylline and orally administered levofloxacin. *J Clin Pharmacol* (1997) 37, 744–50.
40. Dickens GR, Wermeling D, Vincent J. Phase I pilot study of the effects of trovafloxacin (CP-99,219) on the pharmacokinetics of theophylline in healthy men. *J Clin Pharmacol* (1997) 37, 248–52.
41. Vincent J, Teng R, Dogolo LC, Willavize SA, Friedman HL. Effect of trovafloxacin, a new fluoroquinolone antibiotic, on the steady-state pharmacokinetics of theophylline in healthy volunteers. *J Antimicrob Chemother* (1997) 39 (Suppl B), 81–6.
42. Kinzig-Schippers M, Fuhr U, Cesana M, Müller C, Staib AH, Rietbrock S. Sörgel F. Absence of effect of rufloxacin on theophylline pharmacokinetics in steady state. *Antimicrob Agents Chemother* (1998) 42, 2359–64.
43. Efthymiopoulos C, Bramer SL, Maroli A, Blum B. Theophylline and warfarin interaction studies with grepafloxacin. *Clin Pharmacokinet* (1997) 33 (Suppl 1), 39–46.
44. Randinitis EJ, Alvey CW, Koup JR, Rausch G, Abel R, Bron NJ, Hounslow NJ, Vassos AB, Sedman AJ. Drug interactions with clinafloxacin. *Antimicrob Agents Chemother* (2001) 45, 2543–52.
45. Davy M, Allen A, Bird N, Rost KL, Fuder H. Lack of effect of gemifloxacin on the steady-state pharmacokinetics of theophylline in healthy volunteers. *Chemotherapy* (1999) 45, 478–84.
46. Fattore C, Cipolla G, Gatti G, Bartoli A, Orticelli G, Picollo R, Millerioux L, Ciotolli GB, Perucca E. Pharmacokinetic interactions between theophylline and prulifloxacin in healthy volunteers. *Clin Drug Invest* (1998) 16, 387–92.
47. Stahlberg HJ, Göhler K, Guillaume M, Mignot A. Effects of gatifloxacin (GTX) on the pharmacokinetics of theophylline in healthy young volunteers. *J Antimicrob Chemother* (1999) 44 (Suppl A), 136.
48. Bem JL, Mann RD. Danger of interaction between ciprofloxacin and theophylline. *BMJ* (1988) 296, 1131.
49. Thomson AH, Thomson GD, Hepburn M, Whiting B. A clinically significant interaction between ciprofloxacin and theophylline. *Eur J Clin Pharmacol* (1987) 33, 435–6.
50. Richardson JP. Theophylline toxicity associated with the administration of ciprofloxacin in a nursing home patient. *J Am Geriatr Soc* (1990) 38, 236–8.
51. Duraski RM. Ciprofloxacin-induced theophylline toxicity. *South Med J* (1988) 81,1206.
52. Holden R. Probable fatal interaction between ciprofloxacin and theophylline. *BMJ* (1988) 297, 1339.
53. Rybak MJ, Bowles SK, Chandraseker PH, Edwards DJ. Increased theophylline concentrations secondary to ciprofloxacin. *Drug Intell Clin Pharm* (1987) 21, 879–81.
54. Paidipaty B, Erickson S. Ciprofloxacin-theophylline drug interaction. *Crit Care Med* (1990) 18, 685–6.
55. Spivey JM, Laughlin PH, Goss TF, Nix DE. Theophylline toxicity secondary to ciprofloxacin administration. *Ann Emerg Med* (1991) 20, 1131–4.
56. Grasela TH, Dreis MW. An evaluation of the quinolone-theophylline interaction using the Food and Drug Administration spontaneous reporting system. *Arch Intern Med* (1992) 152, 617–621.
57. Schlienger RG, Wyser C, Ritz R, Haefeli WE. Der klinisch-pharmakologische fall (4). Epileptischer Anfall als unerwünschte Arzneimittelwirkung bei Theophyllinintoxikation. *Schweiz Rundsch Med Prax* (1996) 85, 1407–12.
58. Andrews PA. Interactions with ciprofloxacin and erythromycin leading to aminophylline toxicity. *Nephrol Dial Transplant* (1998) 13, 1006–8.
59. Semel JD, Allen N. Seizures in patients simultaneously receiving theophylline and imipenem or ciprofloxacin or metronidazole. *South Med J* (1991) 84, 465–8.
60. Bader MB. Role of ciprofloxacin in fatal seizures. *Chest* (1992) 101, 883–4.
61. Matuschka PR, Vissing RS. Clinafloxacin-theophylline drug interaction. *Ann Pharmacother* (1995) 29, 378–80.
62. Wijnands WJA, van Herwaarden CLA, Vree TB. Enoxacin raises plasma theophylline concentrations. *Lancet* (1984) ii, 108–9.
63. Davies BI, Maesen FPV, Teengs JP. Serum and sputum concentrations of enoxacin after single oral dosing in a clinical and bacteriological study. *J Antimicrob Chemother* (1984) 14 (Suppl C), 83–9.
64. Green L, Clark J. Fluoroquinolones and theophylline toxicity: norfloxacin. *JAMA* (1989) 262, 2383.
65. Conri C, Lartigue MC, Abs L, Mestre MC, Vincent MP, Haramburu F, Constans J. Convulsions chez une malade traitée par péfloxacine et théophylline. *Therapie* (1990) 45, 358.
66. Fuhr U, Strobl G, Manaut F, Anders EM, Sorgel F, Lopez-de-Brinas E, Chu DT, Pernet AG, Mahr G, Sanz F. Quinolone antibacterial agents: relationship between structure and in vitro inhibition of the human cytochrome P450 isoform CYP1A2. *Mol Pharmacol* (1993) 43, 191–9.
67. Mizuki Y, Fujiwara I, Yamaguchi T. Pharmacokinetic interactions related to the chemical structures of fluoroquinolones. *J Antimicrob Chemother* (1996) 37 (Suppl A), 41–55.
68. Segev S, Rehavi M, Rubinstein E. Quinolones, theophylline, and diclofenac interactions with the γ-aminobutyric acid receptor. *Antimicrob Agents Chemother* (1988) 32, 1624–6.

69. Raoof S, Wollschlager C, Khan FA. Ciprofloxacin increases serum levels of theophylline. *Am J Med* (1987) 82 (Suppl 4A), 115–18.
70. Koup JR, Toothaker RD, Posvar E, Sedman AJ, Colburn WA. Theophylline dosage adjustment during enoxacin coadministration. *Antimicrob Agents Chemother* (1990) 34, 803–7.

Theophylline + Repaglinide

Repaglinide 2 mg three times a day for 4 days did not affect the steady-state pharmacokinetics of theophylline in 14 healthy subjects, except that the peak plasma concentration was slightly reduced.[1] No special precautions would appear to be necessary during concurrent use.

1. Hartop V, Thomsen MS. Drug interaction studies with repaglinide: repaglinide on digoxin or theophylline pharmacokinetics and cimetidine on repaglinide pharmacokinetics. *J Clin Pharmacol* (2000) 40, 184–92.

Theophylline + Ribavirin (Tribavirin)

Ribavirin (tribavirin) does not interact with theophylline.

Clinical evidence, mechanism, importance and management

Ribavirin (tribavirin) 200 mg six-hourly by mouth had no effect on the plasma theophylline levels of 13 healthy adult subjects given immediate or sustained-release aminophylline. Similarly, 10 mg/kg **ribavirin** daily did not affect the plasma theophylline levels in 6 children with influenza and asthma treated with theophylline.[1] No special precautions seem necessary.

1. Fraschini F, Scaglione F, Maierna G, Cogo R, Furcolo F, Gattei R, Borghi C, Palazzini E. Ribavirin influence on theophylline plasma levels in adult and children. *Int J Clin Pharmacol Ther Toxicol* (1988) 26, 30–2.

Theophylline + Rifamycins

Rifampicin (rifampin) lowers the serum levels of theophylline. An increase in the theophylline dosage may be needed (possibly up to twofold). Rifabutin appears to have little effect.

Clinical evidence

(a) Rifabutin

After taking 300 mg **rifabutin** daily for 12 days the AUC of a single dose of theophylline (5 mg/kg) was reduced by 6% (from 136 to 128 micrograms.h/ml) in 11 healthy subjects, which was not significant. Theophylline half-life and clearance were not affected.[1]

(b) Rifampicin (rifampin)

After taking 600 mg **rifampicin** daily for a week, the AUC following 450 mg of a sustained-release aminophylline preparation in 7 healthy subjects was reduced by 18%. A parallel study in another 8 healthy subjects given the same dosage of **rifampicin** showed that the metabolic clearance of intravenous aminophylline (5 mg/kg) was increased by 45%.[2]

Similarly, other studies in healthy subjects given 300 to 600 mg **rifampicin** daily for 6 to 14 days showed 25 to 82% rises in theophylline clearance, and 19 to 31% decreases in half-life.[1,3-8] A 61% fall in the 5-hour postdose serum theophylline levels occurred in a 15-month-old boy when given a 4-day course of **rifampicin** 20 mg/kg daily as meningitis prophylaxis.[9] A single report describes unexpectedly *high* serum theophylline levels when theophylline therapy was started in an alcoholic patient with hepatic impairment treated with **rifampicin** and **isoniazid**.[10]

Mechanism

Rifampicin is a potent liver enzyme inducing agent which increases the metabolism of the theophylline, thereby speeding up its clearance from the body resulting in reduced serum levels.[4] High theophylline levels in the isolated case may have been due to liver impairment brought about by the combined use of rifampicin and isoniazid or alcoholism.[10] Rifabutin is a much less potent liver enzyme-inducing agent than rifampicin and consequently has less of an effect on theophylline metabolism.

Importance and management

The theophylline/rifampicin interaction is established. Serum theophylline levels and its therapeutic effects are likely to be reduced during concurrent treatment, and this can be detected within 36 h.[9] The wide range of increases in clearance that have been reported (25–82%) and the large inter-subject variation make it difficult to predict the increase in theophylline dosage required, but in some instances a twofold increase may be needed.[4] Also, be alert for the need to decrease the theophylline dosage to avoid toxicity when rifampicin therapy is completed.

The effects of rifabutin are considerably less than rifampicin, with the one available study showing no significant interaction. On the basis of this, no special precautions appear to be necessary, but it may be prudent to monitor concurrent use.

1. Gillum JG, Sesler JM, Bruzzese VL, Israel DS, Polk RE. Induction of theophylline clearance by rifampin and rifabutin in healthy male volunteers. *Antimicrob Agents Chemother* (1996) 40, 1866–9.
2. Powell-Jackson PR, Jamieson AP, Gray BJ, Moxham J, Williams R. Effect of rifampicin administration on theophylline pharmacokinetics in humans. *Am Rev Respir Dis* (1985) 131, 939–40.
3. Straughn AB, Henderson RP, Lieberman PL, Self TH. Effect of rifampin on theophylline disposition. *Ther Drug Monit* (1984) 6, 153–6.
4. Robson RA, Miners JO, Wing LMH, Birkett DJ. Theophylline-rifampicin interaction: non-selective induction of theophylline metabolic pathways. *Br J Clin Pharmacol* (1984) 18, 445–8.
5. Löfdahl CG, Mellstrand T, Svedmyr N. Increased metabolism of theophylline by rifampicin. *Respiration* (1984) 46 (Suppl 1), 104.
6. Hauser AR, Lee C, Teague RB, Mullins C. The effect of rifampin on theophylline disposition. *Clin Pharmacol Ther* (1983) 33, 254.
7. Boyce EG, Dukes GE, Rollins DE, Sudds TW. The effect of rifampin on theophylline kinetics. *J Clin Pharmacol* (1986) 26, 696–9.
8. Rao S, Singh SK, Narang RK, Rajagopalan PT. Effect of rifampicin on theophylline pharmacokinetics in human beings. *J Assoc Physicians India* (1994) 42, 881–2.
9. Brocks DR, Lee KC, Weppler CP, Tam YK. Theophylline-rifampin interaction in a pediatric patient. *Clin Pharm* (1986) 5, 602–4.
10. Dal Negro R, Turco P, Trevisan F, De Conti F. Rifampicin-isoniazid and delayed elimination of theophylline: a case report. *Int J Clin Pharmacol Res* (1988) 8, 275–7.

Theophylline + Ropinirole

Theophylline and ropinirole do not interact.

Clinical evidence, mechanism, importance and management

In one study, 12 patients with parkinsonism were given **ropinirole**, increased from 0.5 mg to 2 mg three times daily over 28 days, then continued for a further 19 days. The pharmacokinetics of a single intravenous dose of aminophylline given before the **ropinirole** treatment was started, were compared with another single intravenous dose given on day 27. The pharmacokinetics of **ropinirole** were then compared before, during, and after, administration of oral controlled-release theophylline twice daily for 13 days (dose titrated to achieve plasma levels in the range 8 to 15 micrograms/ml). It was found that the pharmacokinetics of neither drug was altered, and concurrent use was well tolerated.[1] There would therefore appear to be no reason to take special precautions if both drugs are used concurrently, and no need to adjust the dosage of either drug. On the basis that both ropinirole and theophylline are metabolised by cytochrome P450 isoenzyme CYP1A2, the makers of **ropinirole** originally thought that an interaction might occur.

1. Thalamas C, Taylor A, Brefel-Courbon C, Eagle S, Fitzpatrick K, Rascol O. Lack of pharmacokinetic interaction between ropinirole and theophylline in patients with Parkinson's disease. *Eur J Clin Pharmacol* (1999) 55, 299–303.

Theophylline + Selective serotonin re-uptake inhibitors (SSRIs)

Theophylline serum levels can be markedly and rapidly increased by the concurrent use of fluvoxamine. Toxicity will develop if the theophylline dosage is not suitably reduced (to about a half). Some preliminary clinical evidence suggests that fluoxetine may not interact. *In vitro* evidence suggests that citalopram, paroxetine and sertraline are also unlikely to interact.

Clinical evidence

(a) Fluoxetine

A single dose of 40 mg **fluoxetine** was found to have no effect on the pharmacokinetics of theophylline when administered 8 hours before a 30 min infusion of 6 mg/kg aminophylline in 8 normal subjects.[1]

(b) Fluvoxamine

The effect of fluvoxamine on theophylline pharmacokinetics has been characterised in 2 studies in healthy subjects. In the first study, after taking **fluvoxamine** 50 mg daily for 3 days then 100 mg daily for 13 days, the AUC of a single oral dose of aminophylline 442 mg was increased almost threefold (from 115 to 308 micrograms ml^{-1}), the clearance was reduced by 62% (from 54 to 20 ml min^{-1}) and the half-life was prolonged from 7.4 to 32.1 hours.[2] In the second study, the clearance of theophylline given as a single oral dose of aminophylline 300 mg was reduced to about one-third (from 80 ml/min to 24 ml/min) and the half-life increased from 6.6 to 22 hours after taking 50 to 100 mg **fluvoxamine** daily for 7 days.[3]

A number of case reports have described fluvoxamine-induced theophylline toxicity. Agitation and tachycardia (120 bpm) developed in a man of 83 about a week after starting to take 100 mg **fluvoxamine** daily. His serum theophylline levels were found to have risen from a range of about 10–15 mg/l to 40 mg/l.[4] A man of 70 similarly developed theophylline toxicity (177 micromol/l) when **fluvoxamine** was added. Subsequently the theophylline concentrations were found to parallel a number of changes in the **fluvoxamine** dosage.[5] The clearance of theophylline in a man of 84 was approximately halved while taking **fluvoxamine**.[6] A boy of 11 complained of headaches, tiredness and vomiting within a week of starting to take **fluvoxamine**. His serum theophylline levels were found to have doubled (from 14.2 to 27.4 mg/l).[7] A woman of 78 developed evidence of theophylline toxicity (nausea) within 2 days of starting to take 50 mg **fluvoxamine** daily, and by day 6, when the fluvoxamine was stopped, her serum theophylline levels had increased about threefold.[8] She experienced a seizure and became comatose, and had supraventricular tachycardia (200 bpm) requiring intravenous digoxin and verapamil. She recovered uneventfully.

Mechanism

In vitro studies with human liver microsomes have shown that fluvoxamine inhibits cytochrome P450 isoenzyme CYP1A2, which is the principal enzyme responsible for the metabolism of theophylline.[9,10] *In vivo* this would have the effect of raising serum theophylline levels, resulting in the development of toxicity. The other SSRIs **citalopram, fluoxetine, paroxetine** and **sertraline** only weakly inhibited this enzyme *in vitro*, and consequently would not be expected to interact.[9,10]

Importance and management

The theophylline/fluvoxamine interaction is established and clinically important. The CSM says that concurrent use should usually be avoided, but that if this is not possible, reduce the theophylline dosage to a half when fluvoxamine is added.[11] Monitor well. There is good *in vitro* evidence to suggest that fluvoxamine is the only SSRI which is likely to interact (because it is the only one which affects

CYP1A2). This would seem to be borne out by the general silence in the literature about problems with any of the other SSRIs.

1. Mauro VF, Mauro LS, Klions HA. Effect of single dose fluoxetine on aminophylline pharmacokinetics. *Pharmacotherapy* (1994) 14, 367.
2. Donaldson KM, Wright DM, Mathlener IS, Harry JD. The effect of fluvoxamine at steady state on the pharmacokinetics of theophylline after a single dose in healthy male volunteers. *Br J Clin Pharmacol* (1994) 37, 492P.
3. Rasmussen BB, Jeppesen U, Gaist D, Brøsen K. Griseofulvin and fluvoxamine interactions with the metabolism of theophylline. *Ther Drug Monit* (1997) 19, 56–62.
4. Diot P, Jonville AP, Gerard F, Bonnelle M, Autret E, Breteau M, Lemarie E, Lavandier M. Possible interaction entre théophylline et fluvoxamine. *Therapie* (1991) 46, 170–71.
5. Thomson AH, McGovern EM, Bennie P, Caldwell G, Smith M. Interaction between fluvoxamine and theophylline. *Pharm J* (1992) 249, 137. Correction. *ibid.* (1992) 249, 214.
6. Puranik A, Fitzpatrick R, Ananthanarayanan TS. Monitor serum theophylline. *Care of the Elderly* (1993) 5, 237.
7. Sperber AD. Toxic interaction between fluvoxamine and sustained released theophylline in an 11-year-old boy. *Drug Safety* (1991) 6, 460–2.
8. van den Brekel AM, Harrington L. Toxic effects of theophylline caused by fluvoxamine. *Can Med Assoc J* (1994) 151, 1289–90.
9. Brøsen K, Skjelbo E, Rasmussen BB, Poulsen HE, Loft S. Fluvoxamine is a potent inhibitor of cytochrome P4501A2. *Biochem Pharmacol* (1993) 45, 1211–14.
10. Rasmussen BB, Mäenpää J, Pelkonen O, Loft S, Poulsen HE, Lykkesfeldt J, Brøsen K. Selective serotonin reuptake inhibitors and theophylline metabolism in human liver microsomes: potent inhibition by fluvoxamine. *Br J Clin Pharmacol* (1995) 39, 151–9.
11. Committee on Safety of Medicines/Medicines Control Agency. Fluvoxamine increases plasma theophylline levels. *Current Problems in Pharmacovigilance* (1994) 20, 12.

Theophylline + St John's wort (Hypericum perforatum)

A patient needed a marked increase in the dosage of theophylline while taking St John's wort.

Clinical evidence

A woman, who had previously been stabilised for several months on 300 mg theophylline twice daily, was found to need a markedly increased theophylline dosage of 800 mg twice daily to achieve serum levels of 9.2 micrograms/ml. It turned out that 2 months previously she had additionally started to take 300 mg of a **St John's wort** (0.3% hypericin) supplement each day. When she stopped taking the **St John's wort**, her serum theophylline levels doubled within a week to 19.6 micrograms/ml and her theophylline dosage was consequently adjusted downwards. This patient was also taking a whole spectrum of other drugs (amitriptyline, furosemide, ibuprofen, inhaled triamcinolone, morphine, potassium, prednisone, salbutamol (albuterol), valproic acid, zolpidem and zafirlukast) and was also a smoker. No changes in the use of these drugs or altered compliance were identified that might have offered an alternative explanation for the changed theophylline requirements.[1]

Mechanism

Uncertain, but the authors of the report briefly describe *in vitro* data that suggest one component of St John's wort (hypericin) can act as an inducer of cytochrome P450 isoenzyme CYP1A2, which would increase the metabolism and clearance of theophylline.[1]

Importance and management

Direct information about this apparent theophylline/St John's wort interaction appears to be limited to this report so that its general importance is uncertain. However, it would be prudent to monitor the effects and serum levels of theophylline if St John's wort is started or stopped. Patients should be warned. The CSM in the UK recommend that patients on theophylline should not take St John's wort. In those patients already taking the combination, the St John's wort should be stopped and the theophylline dosage monitored and adjusted if necessary.[2,3] More study is needed.

1. Nebel A, Schneider BJ, Baker RK, Kroll DJ. Potential metabolic interaction between St John's wort and theophylline. *Ann Pharmacother* (1999) 33, 502.
2. Committee on Safety of Medicines (UK). Message from Professor A Breckenridge (Chairman of CSM) and Fact Sheet for Health Care Professionals, 29th February 2000.
3. Committee on Safety of Medicines/Medicines Control Agency. Reminder: St John's wort (*Hypericum perforatum*) interactions. *Current Problems* (2000) 26, 6–7.

Theophylline + Succimer (DMSA)

A single case report describes a fall in serum theophylline levels of about one-third in a man treated with succimer.

Clinical evidence, mechanism, importance and management

A 65-year old man with chronic obstructive airways disease and chronic lead intoxication was given a 19-day course of lead chelation with **succimer (DMSA)**. His theophylline concentration was found to be reduced by about one-third on day 6 (from about 11 to 7 micrograms/ml) and remained at this level until about 9 days after the course of succimer was completed, when it had returned to pre-treatment levels. His clinical status did not alter despite these changes, possibly because he was also taking prednisone.[1] The reason for these alterations is not understood.

The general importance of this interaction is not known, but it would now be prudent to monitor the situation closely if **succimer** is added to established treatment with theophylline.

1. Harcherload R. Pharmacokinetic interaction between dimercaptosuccinic acid (DMSA) and theophylline (THEO). *Vet Hum Toxicol* (1994) 36, 376.

Theophylline + Sucralfate

Two studies found minor changes in theophylline pharmacokinetics, but another suggests that the absorption of sustained-release theophylline is significantly reduced by sucralfate.

Clinical evidence, mechanism, importance and management

While taking 1 g **sucralfate** four times daily, no clinically important changes occurred in the absorption of a single 5 mg/kg dose of an oral non-sustained release theophylline preparation (*Slo-Phyllin*) given at the same time as the sucralfate dose in 8 healthy subjects. A slight 5% decrease in the AUC was detected.[1] Another study found that 1 g **sucralfate** four times daily reduced the AUC of a single dose of a sustained-release preparation (*Theodur*) by 9% (timing of the theophylline dose in relation to the sucralfate dose not noted).[2] In contrast, another group of workers found that when 1 g **sucralfate** was given 30 min before a 350 mg sustained-release theophylline preparation (*PEG capsules*), the theophylline AUC was reduced by 40%.[3] The reasons are not understood.

Many patients are given sustained-release preparations, but neither of these studies clearly shows what is likely to happen in clinical practice, so be alert for any evidence of a reduced response to theophylline. Usually, separating the administration of sucralfate from other drugs by 2 hours is considered sufficient to avoid reduced absorption.[4] However, the study showing decreased theophylline absorption did not examine the effect of separating the doses. Further study is needed.

1. Cantral KA, Schaaf LJ, Jungnickel PW, Monsour HP. Effect of sucralfate on theophylline absorption in healthy volunteers. *Clin Pharm* (1988) 7, 58–61.
2. Kisor DF, Livengood B, Vieira-Fattahi S, Sterchele JA. Effect of sucralfate administration on the absorption of sustained released theophylline. *Pharmacotherapy* (1990) 10, 253.
3. Fleischmann R, Bozler G, Boekstegers P. Bioverfügbarkeit von Theophylline unter Ulkustherapeutika. *Verh Dtsch Ges Inn Med* (1984) 90, 1876–9.
4. Antepsin (Sucralfate). Chugai Pharma UK Limited. Summary of product characteristics, May 1995.

Theophylline + Sulfinpyrazone

Sulfinpyrazone can cause a small reduction in serum theophylline levels.

Clinical evidence, mechanism, importance and management

Sulfinpyrazone 200 mg 6-hourly increased the total clearance of theophylline (125 mg 8-hourly for four days) in 6 healthy subjects by 22% (range 8.5 to 42%).[1] This appeared to be the sum of an increase in the metabolism of the theophylline by the liver and a decrease in its renal clearance.

Information seems to be limited to this study. The fall in serum theophylline levels is unlikely to be clinically relevant in most patients, but it may possibly affect a few. Concurrent use should be monitored.

1. Birkett DJ, Miners JO, Attwood J. Evidence for a dual action of sulphinpyrazone on drug metabolism in man: theophylline-sulphinpyrazone interaction. *Br J Clin Pharmacol* (1983) 15, 567–9.

Theophylline + Teicoplanin

Clinical studies in 20 patients with chronic obstructive pulmonary disease found that the concurrent administration of 200 mg teicoplanin twice daily and 240 mg aminophylline twice daily (both given as intravenous infusions) had no significant effect on the steady-state pharmacokinetics of either drug.[1] No special precautions would seem necessary during concurrent use.

1. Angrisani M, Cazzola M, Loffreda A, Losasso C, Lucarelli C, Rossi F. Clinical pharmacokinetics of teicoplanin and aminophylline during cotreatment with both medicaments. *Int J Clin Pharmacol Res* (1992) 12, 165–71.

Theophylline + Terbinafine

Preliminary evidence indicates that terbinafine can increase the serum levels of theophylline to some extent, but the clinical importance of this is still uncertain.

Clinical evidence, mechanism, importance and management

An open-label, randomised crossover study in 12 healthy subjects given single oral doses of 5 mg/kg theophylline before and after taking 250 mg **terbinafine** daily for 3 days found that the theophylline pharmacokinetics were statistically significantly changed (AUC +16%, half-life +23%, clearance −14%). It was suggested[1] that this is due to the inhibitory effect of **terbinafine** on the activity of cytochrome P450 isoenzyme CYP1A2. The changes seen were only relatively small, but the study periods only lasted 3 days so that the effects of longer concurrent use are uncertain. Until more is known it would seem prudent to monitor the effects of adding **terbinafine** to theophylline treatment, being alert for any evidence of increased side-effects and possible toxicity. More study is needed.

1. Trépanier EF, Nafziger AN, Amsden GW. Effect of terbinafine on theophylline pharmacokinetics in healthy volunteers. *Antimicrob Agents Chemother* (1998) 42, 695–7.

Theophylline + Tetracyclines

Serum theophylline levels have been increased in two patients given minocycline or tetracycline. Some controlled studies have shown both increases and decreases in theophylline clearance with doxycycline and tetracycline, with no significant changes overall.

Clinical evidence

(a) Doxycycline

A study in 10 asthmatic subjects given **doxycycline** (100 mg twice daily on day 1 and then 100 mg daily for 4 days) showed that the mean serum theophylline level was not significantly altered, although there was large inter-individual variations with 4 of them showing rises of more than 20% (24 to 31%) and 2 having decreases of more than 20% (22 and 33%).[1] However, fluctuations of this size are not unusual with theophylline. Another study in 8 healthy subjects given doxycycline 100 mg for 7 days concurrently with theophylline 350 mg twice daily failed to find any significant changes in theophylline pharmacokinetics.[2]

(b) Minocycline

The serum theophylline levels of a woman of 70 with normal liver function increased from 9.8 to 15.5 micrograms/ml after being given 100 mg **minocycline** twice daily by infusion for 6 days. No signs of toxicity occurred. The serum concentration was 10.9 micrograms/ml 14 days after the **minocycline** was stopped.[3]

(c) Tetracycline

After taking **tetracycline hydrochloride** (250 mg four times daily) for 8 days a patient with COPD showed evidence of theophylline toxicity, and after 10 days her serum theophylline levels had risen from about 12–13 mg/l to 30.8 mg/l. Both drugs were stopped, and after 24 hours her theophylline level was 12.4 mg/l. A later rechallenge in this patient confirmed that the **tetracycline** was responsible.[4]

In an earlier study in 8 healthy subjects the same dose of **tetracycline** for 7 days did not affect the mean pharmacokinetics of theophylline after a single intravenous dose, although there was large inter-individual variation. Four subjects had a decrease in clearance of over 15%, and in one of these subjects it was 32%, and conversely, one subject had an increase in clearance of 21%.[5] Other studies in subjects and patients given **tetracycline** for shorter periods have also failed to demonstrate important interactions. A trial in 9 healthy adults given single doses of aminophylline (5 mg/kg iv) showed that the concurrent use of **tetracycline** 250 mg six-hourly for 48 h had no significant effect on the kinetics of theophylline.[6] Five non-smoking patients with COPD or asthma showed an average 14% rise in serum theophylline levels after 5 days treatment with 250 mg **tetracycline** four times a day and an 11% decrease in clearance. However, when a sixth patient was included (a smoker) the results were no longer statistically significant.[7]

Mechanism

Not understood. Inhibition of theophylline metabolism and clearance by the tetracyclines has been suggested.[4]

Importance and management

Information seems to be limited. There are two isolated cases of increased theophylline levels with minocycline and tetracycline, but controlled studies have not shown any significant changes in overall theophylline pharmacokinetics. It has been suggested that a clinically important interaction may possibly only occur in a few patients.[1,4] Consequently, it may be prudent to monitor the effects of concurrent use. Further study is needed. There seems to be no evidence of adverse interactions with any of the other tetracyclines not cited here. However, note that acute infections *per se* can alter theophylline pharmacokinetics.

1. Seggev JS, Shefi M, Schey G, Farfel Z. Serum theophylline concentrations are not affected by coadministration of doxycycline. *Ann Allergy* (1986) 56, 156–7.
2. Jonkman JHG, van der Boon WJV, Schoenmaker R, Holtkamp A, Hempenius J. No influence of doxycycline on theophylline pharmacokinetics. *Ther Drug Monit* (1985) 7, 92–4.
3. Kawai M, Honda A, Yoshida H, Goto M, Shimokata T. Possible theophylline-minocycline interaction. *Ann Pharmacother* (1992) 26, 1300–1.
4. McCormack JP, Reid SE, Lawson LM. Theophylline toxicity induced by tetracycline. *Clin Pharm* (1990) 9, 546–9.
5. Mathis JW, Prince RA, Weinberger MM, McElnay JC. Effect of tetracycline hydrochloride on theophylline kinetics. *Clin Pharm* (1982) 1, 446–8.
6. Pfeifer HJ, Greenblatt DJ, Friedman P. Effects of three antibiotics on theophylline kinetics. *Clin Pharmacol Ther* (1979) 26, 36–40.
7. Gotz VP, Ryerson GG. Evaluation of tetracycline on theophylline disposition in patients with chronic obstructive airways disease. *Drug Intell Clin Pharm* (1986) 20, 694–7.

Theophylline + Thyroid and Antithyroid compounds

Thyroid dysfunction may modestly affect theophylline requirements. There are two isolated cases of theophylline toxicity during treatment for correction of thyroid dysfunction. Monitor theophylline levels and anticipate the need to alter the dose when thyroid or antithyroid therapy is initiated until thyroid status is stabilised.

Clinical evidence

The theophylline elimination rate constant after a single intravenous dose was found to be greater in hyperthyroidic patients ($0.155 \, h^{-1}$) than in euthyroidic ($0.107 \, h^{-1}$) or hypothyroidic patients ($0.060 \, h^{-1}$); some other pharmacokinetic parameters were also changed.[1] The authors concluded that thyroid dysfunction may modestly alter theophylline requirements. It is therefore also likely that drug-induced changes in the thyroid status may alter the amount of theophylline needed to maintain therapeutic levels.

(a) Theophylline + Antithyroid compounds

The serum theophylline level of an asthmatic patient was found to have doubled (from 15.2 to 30.9 micrograms/ml), accompanied by toxicity, 3 months after treatment for hyperthyroidism with **radioactive iodine** (^{131}I). At this point the patient was hypothyroidic, and after treatment with levothyroxine was started his serum theophylline returned to about the level prior to radioactive iodine treatment (13.9 micrograms/ml).[2] Five hyperthyroidic patients showed a 20% reduction in theophylline clearance and a rise in theophylline half-life from 4.6 to 5.9 h when treated with **carbimazole** 45 mg and **propranolol** 60 mg daily. In this study, a single intravenous dose of aminophylline was administered before the treatment of thyrotoxicosis and after the euthyroid state had been achieved.[3]

(b) Theophylline + Thyroid hormones

One week after starting 1 g theophylline daily, a patient who was hypothyroidic (serum levothyroxine 1.4 micrograms/100 ml, normal range 4 to 11 micrograms/100 ml developed severe theophylline toxicity (serum levels 34.7 micrograms/ml) manifested by ventricular fibrillation (from which he was successfully resuscitated) and repeated seizures over 24 hours. After 2 months treatment with **thyroid hormones**, which increased his serum levothyroxine levels to 4.3 micrograms/100 ml, his serum theophylline level was 13.2 micrograms/ml 10 days after reinstitution of the same theophylline dosage (1 g daily).[4]

Mechanism

The thyroid status may affect the rate at which theophylline is metabolised. In hyperthyroidism it is increased, whereas in hypothyroidism it is decreased.

Importance and management

It is established that changes in thyroid status may affect how the body handles theophylline. Monitor the effects and anticipate the possible need to begin to reduce the theophylline dosage if treatment for hyperthyroidism is started (e.g. with **radioactive iodine, carbimazole, thiamazole (methimazole), propylthiouracil**, etc.). Similarly anticipate the possible need to increase the theophylline dosage if treatment is started for hypothyroidism (e.g. with **levothyroxine**). Stabilisation of the thyroid status may take weeks or even months to achieve so that if monitoring of the theophylline dosage is considered necessary, it will need to extend over the whole of this period.

1. Pokrajac M, Simić D, Varagić VM. Pharmacokinetics of theophylline in hyperthyroid and hypothyroid patients with chronic obstructive pulmonary disease. *Eur J Clin Pharmacol* (1987) 33, 483–6.
2. Johnson CE, Cohen IA. Theophylline toxicity after iodine 131 treatment for hyperthyroidism. *Clin Pharm* (1988) 7, 620–2.

3. Vozeh S, Otten M, Staub J-J, Follath F. Influence of thyroid function on theophylline kinetics. *Clin Pharmacol Ther* (1984) 36, 634–40.
4. Aderka D, Shavit G, Garfinkel D, Santo M, Gitter S, Pinkhas J. Life-threatening theophylline intoxication in a hypothyroidic patient. *Respiration* (1983) 44, 77–80.

Theophylline + Ticlopidine or Clopidogrel

Ticlopidine reduces the loss of theophylline from the body and is expected to raise its serum levels. Clopidogrel, an analogue of ticlopidine, appears not to interact.

Clinical evidence, mechanism, importance and management

(a) Clopidogrel

Clopidogrel 75 mg daily for 10 days did not alter the steady-state pharmacokinetics of theophylline given to 12 healthy subjects.[1] No problems are therefore anticipated with the concurrent use of these two drugs.

(b) Ticlopidine

Ticlopidine 250 mg twice daily for 10 days in 10 healthy subjects reduced the clearance of a single 5 mg/kg oral dose of theophylline by 37% (from 0.682 to 0.431 ml/kg/min) and increased the half-life by 44% (from 514 to 731 min).[2] The reason is not known but it seems possible that **ticlopidine** inhibits the metabolism of theophylline by the liver. Information is limited, but it would now seem prudent to monitor the effects of concurrent use. It may be necessary to reduce the dosage of theophylline, particularly when serum levels are already at the top end of the range.

1. Caplain H, Thebault J-J, Neccari J. Clopidogrel does not affect the pharmacokinetics of theophylline. *Semin Thromb Hemost* (1999) 24, 65–8.
2. Colli A, Buccino G, Cocciolo M, Parravicini R, Elli GM, Scaltrini G. Ticlopidine-theophylline interaction. *Clin Pharmacol Ther* (1987) 41, 358–62.

Theophylline + Tobacco or Cannabis smoking

Tobacco or cannabis smokers, and non-smokers heavily exposed to smoke, may need more theophylline than other non-smokers to achieve the same therapeutic benefits because the theophylline is cleared from the body more quickly. This may also occur in those who chew tobacco or take snuff but not if they chew nicotine gum.

Clinical evidence

A study found that the mean half-life of a single oral dose of theophylline in a group of **tobacco smokers** (20 to 40 cigarettes a day) was 4.3 h compared with 7 h in a group of non-smokers, and that theophylline clearance was higher (mean 126% higher) and more variable in the smokers.[1] Almost identical results were found in an earlier study,[2] and a number of later studies confirm these findings.[3-7] The ability of smoking to increase theophylline clearance occurs irrespective of age,[4] gender,[3,6] and in the presence of congestive heart failure or liver dysfunction.[7]

A similar high clearance for theophylline has been seen in a patient who **chewed tobacco** (1.11 compared with the more usual 0.59 ml/kg/min).[8] The theophylline half-life in **passive smokers** (non-smokers regularly exposed to tobacco smoke in the air they breathe, for 4 h a day in this study) is reported to be shorter than in non-smokers (6.93 compared with 8.69 h).[9]

One study found that **tobacco** or **cannabis** smoking similarly caused higher total clearances of theophylline than non-smokers (about 74 compared with 52 ml/kg/h), and that clearance was even higher (93 ml/kg/h) in those who smoked both.[5] A later analysis by the same authors of factors affecting theophylline clearance found that smoking 2 joints or more of **cannabis** weekly was associated

with a higher total clearance of theophylline than non-use (82.9 vs 56.1 ml/kg/h).[10]

In one study, 3 of 4 patients who stopped smoking for 3 months (confirmed by serum thiocyanate levels) had a longer theophylline half-life, but only 2 had a slight decrease in theophylline clearance.[1] In another study, ex-smokers who had quit heavy smoking 2 years previously had values for theophylline clearance and half-life that were intermediate between non-smokers and current heavy smokers.[3] Conversely, in another study, 7 hospitalised smokers who abstained from smoking for 7 days had a 35.8% increase in theophylline half-life and a 37.6% decrease in clearance (although clearance after abstinence was still higher than values usually found in non-smokers).[11]

Mechanism

Tobacco and cannabis smoke contain polycyclic hydrocarbons, which act as liver enzyme inducing agents, and this results in a more rapid clearance of theophylline from the body. Both the N-demethylation and 8-hydroxylation of theophylline is induced.[12]

Importance and management

Established interaction of moderate clinical importance. Heavy smokers (20–40 cigarettes daily) may need double the theophylline dosage of non-smokers,[1] and increased doses are likely for those who chew tobacco or take snuff,[8] but not for those who chew nicotine gum.[11,13] In patients who stop smoking, a reduction in theophylline dosage of up to 25 to 33% may be needed after a week,[11] but full normalisation of hepatic function appears to take many months.[1,3] Less is known about the effects of smoking cannabis, but be alert for the need to increase the theophylline dosage in regular users.

Investigators of the possible interactions of theophylline with other drugs should take into account the theophylline/tobacco[6,9] and theophylline/cannabis interactions in both smokers and passive smokers when selecting their subjects.

1. Hunt SN, Jusko WJ, Yurchak AM. Effect of smoking on theophylline disposition. *Clin Pharmacol Ther* (1976) 19, 546–51.
2. Jenne J, Nagasawa H, McHugh R, MacDonald F, Wyse E. Decreased theophylline half-life in cigarette smokers. *Life Sci* (1975) 17, 195–8.
3. Powell JR, Thiercelin J-F, Vozeh S, Sansom L, Riegelman S. The influence of cigarette smoking and sex on theophylline disposition. *Am Rev Respir Dis* (1977) 116, 17–23.
4. Cusack B, Kelly JG, Lavan J, Noel J, O'Malley K. Theophylline kinetics in relation to age: the importance of smoking. *Br J Clin Pharmacol* (1980) 10, 109–14.
5. Jusko WJ, Schentag JJ, Clark JH, Gardner M, Yurchak AM. Enhanced biotransformation of theophylline in marihuana and tobacco smokers. *Clin Pharmacol Ther* (1978) 24, 406–10.
6. Jennings TS, Nafziger AN, Davidson L, Bertino JS. Gender differences in hepatic induction and inhibition of theophylline pharmacokinetics and metabolism. *J Lab Clin Med* (1993) 122, 208–16.
7. Harralson AF, Kehoe WA, Chen J-D. The effect of smoking on theophylline disposition in patients with hepatic disease and congestive heart failure. *J Clin Pharmacol* (1996) 36, 862.
8. Rockwood R, Henann N. Smokeless tobacco and theophylline clearance. *Drug Intell Clin Pharm* (1986) 20, 624–5.
9. Matsunga SK, Plezia PM, Karol MD, Katz MD, Camilli AE, Benowitz NL. Effects of passive smoking on theophylline clearance. *Clin Pharmacol Ther* (1989) 46, 399–407.
10. Jusko WJ, Gardner MJ, Mangione A, Schentag JJ, Koup JR, Vance JW. Factors affecting theophylline clearances: age, tobacco, marijuana, cirrhosis, congestive heart failure, obesity, oral contraceptives, benzodiazepines, barbiturates, and ethanol. *J Pharm Sci* (1979) 68, 1358–66.
11. Lee BL, Benowitz NL, Jacob P. Cigarette abstinence, nicotine gum, and theophylline disposition. *Ann Intern Med* (1987) 106, 553–5.
12. Grygiel J, Birkett DJ. Cigarette smoking and theophylline clearance and metabolism. *Clin Pharmacol Ther* (1981) 30, 491–6.
13. Benowitz NL, Lee BL, Jacob P. Nicotine gum and theophylline metabolism. *Biomed Pharmacother* (1989) 43, 1–3.

Theophylline + Vidarabine

A single case report describes a woman who showed a rise in serum theophylline levels when concurrently treated with vidarabine.

Clinical evidence, mechanism, importance and management

A woman under treatment with several drugs (ampicillin, gentamicin, clindamycin, digoxin and aminophylline for congestive heart failure, chronic pulmonary disease and suspected sepsis) developed elevated serum theophylline levels (an increase from 14 mg/l to 24 mg/l) four days after starting to take **vidarabine** (400 mg daily) for herpes zoster.[1] The suggested reason is that the **vidarabine** inhibited the metabolism of the theophylline. Whether this is an interaction is uncertain, but it would now seem prudent to be on the alert for a rise in serum theophylline levels if **vidarabine** is given concurrently.

1. Gannon R, Sullman S, Levy RM, Grober J. Possible interaction between vidarabine and theophylline. *Ann Intern Med* (1984) 101, 148–9.

Theophylline + Viloxazine

Viloxazine increases serum theophylline levels and toxicity may occur unless the theophylline dosage is reduced.

Clinical evidence

A study in 8 healthy subjects given a single 200-mg dose of theophylline confirmed that pretreatment with 100 mg **viloxazine** three times daily for 3 days increased the 24-h AUC of the theophylline by 47%, increasing its maximal serum concentration and reducing its clearance.[1] An elderly woman hospitalised for respiratory failure and treated with a variety of drugs including theophylline, developed acute theophylline toxicity (a grand mal seizure) 2 days after starting to take 200 mg **viloxazine** daily. Her serum theophylline levels had increased threefold (from about 10 to 28 mg/l) and fell again when the **viloxazine** was withdrawn.[2] Nausea and vomiting, associated with raised serum theophylline levels, occurred in another patient when treated with **viloxazine**. Theophylline was stopped, and then reintroduced at one quarter of the original dose. The theophylline level then fell to subtherapeutic levels when the **viloxazine** was stopped.[3] A further case report in an elderly man describes a marked rise in serum theophylline levels to toxic concentrations (55.3 micrograms/ml) when **viloxazine**, 100 mg increased to 300 mg daily, was started.[4]

Mechanism

The suggestion is that the viloxazine competitively antagonises the metabolism of the theophylline by the liver, thereby reducing its loss from the body and resulting in an increase in its serum levels.

Importance and management

Information seems to be limited to these reports but it would appear to be a clinically important interaction. Theophylline serum levels should be well monitored if viloxazine is added, anticipating the need to reduce the dosage.

1. Perault MC, Griesemann E, Bouquet S, Lavoisy J, Vandel B. A study of the interaction of viloxazine with theophylline. *Ther Drug Monit* (1989) 11, 520–2.

2. Laaban JP, Dupeyron JP, Lafay M, Sofeir M, Rochemaure J, Fabiani P. Theophylline intoxication following viloxazine induced decrease in clearance. *Eur J Clin Pharmacol* (1986) 30, 351–3.

3. Thomson AH, Addis GJ, McGovern EM, McDonald NJ. Theophylline toxicity following coadministration of viloxazine. *Ther Drug Monit* (1988) 10, 359–60.

4. Vial T, Bertholon P, Lafond P, Pionchon C, Grangeon C, Bruel M, Antoine JC, Ollagnier M, Evreux JC. Surdosage en théophylline secondaire à un traitement par viloxazine. *Rev Med Interne* (1994) 15, 696–8.

Theophylline + Zileuton

Theophylline serum levels are raised by zileuton. The theophylline dosage should be approximately halved to avoid toxicity.

Clinical evidence

In a double-blind crossover study, 13 healthy subjects were given 200 mg theophylline four times daily for 5 days and either 800 mg **zileuton** twice daily or a placebo. The **zileuton** caused a 73% rise in the mean steady-state peak serum levels of the theophylline (from 12 to 21 mg/l), a 92% increase in the AUC (from 57 to 109 mg.h/l), and halved the apparent plasma clearance (from 3.74 to 1.91 L/h). During the use of **zileuton** the incidence of adverse effects increased (e.g. headache, gastrointestinal effects, etc.), which was attributed to theophylline toxicity, and this caused 3 of the original 16 subjects to withdraw from the study.[1]

Mechanism

Not fully established but it seems highly likely that the zileuton inhibits the metabolism of the theophylline by the liver cytochrome P450 enzymes (probably the isoenzymes CYP1A2 and CYP3A) so that its serum levels rise.

Importance and management

Information is limited but the interaction appears to be established and of clinical importance. Concurrent use need not be avoided but the dosage of theophylline should be reduced to avoid toxicity. The report[1] quoted above suggests that the typical asthma patient will need the theophylline dosage to be halved initially, followed by good monitoring. This is based on the results of a trial of over 1000 patients given 600 mg zileuton four times daily without apparent problems when their initial theophylline dosage was halved.[2]

1. Granneman GR, Braeckman RA, Locke CS, Cavanaugh JH, Dubé LM, Awni WM. Effect of zileuton on theophylline pharmacokinetics. *Clin Pharmacokinet* (1995) 29 (Suppl 2), 77–83.

2. Quoted in ref 1 as data on file, Abbott Labs.

23

Tricyclic, selective serotonin re-uptake inhibitor and related antidepressant drug interactions

The development of the tricyclic antidepressants arose out of work carried out on phenothiazine compounds related to chlorpromazine. The earlier ones possessed two benzene rings joined by a third ring of carbon atoms, with sometimes a nitrogen, and had antidepressant activity (hence their name), however some of the later ones have one, two or even four rings. Table 23.1 lists the common tricyclic antidepressants, the related selective serotonin re-uptake inhibitors (SSRIs) and a number of other compounds that are also used for depression.

Antidepressant activity

The tricyclic antidepressants inhibit the activity of the 'uptake' mechanism by which some chemical transmitters (5-HT or serotonin, norepinephrine (noradrenaline)) re-enter nerve endings in the CNS. In this way they raise the concentrations of the chemical transmitter in the receptor area. If depression represents some inadequacy in transmission between the nerves in the brain, increasing amounts of transmitter may go

some way towards reversing this inadequacy by improving transmission.

Other properties of the tricyclic antidepressants

The tricyclics also have anticholinergic (atropine-like) activity and can cause dry mouth, blurred vision, constipation, urine retention and an increase in ocular tension. Postural hypotension occurs sometimes and there are also cardiotoxic effects. Among the central side effects are sedation, the precipitation of seizures in certain individuals, and extrapyramidal reactions.

Selective serotonin re-uptake inhibitor antidepressants (SSRIs)

These antidepressants (citalopram, femoxetine, fluoxetine, fluvoxamine, paroxetine, sertraline) act on neurones in a similar way to the tricyclics but they selectively inhibit the re-uptake of serotonin (5-hydroxytryptamine or 5HT) and have fewer anticholinergic effects and are also less sedative and cardiotoxic.

Table 23.1 Cyclic and other antidepressants

Generic names	Proprietary names
Tricyclic compounds	
Amitriptyline	Adepril, ADT, Amilit-IFI, Amineurin, Amitrip, Amytril, Anapsique, Deprelio, Domical, Elatrol, Elavil, Endep, Klotriptyl, Laroxyl, Lentizol, Novoprotect, Polytanol, Protanol, Redomex, Saroten, Sarotex, Syneudon, Trepiline, Tripta, Triptizol, Triptyl, Triptyline, Tryptal, Tryptanol, Tryptine, Tryptizol
Amoxapine	Asendin, Asendis, Defanyl, Demolox
Butriptyline	Evadene
Clomipramine	Anafranil, Clofranil, Clopress, Equinorm, Hydiphen, Maronil, Novo-Clopamine, Placil
Desipramine	Deprexan, Norpramin, Nortimil, Pertofran, Petylyl
Dibenzepin	Noveril, Victoril
Dimetacrine	
Dosulepin (Dothiepin)	Dopin, Dopress, Dothep, Jardin, Prepadine, Prothiaden, Protiaden, Protiadene, Thaden, Xerenal
Doxepin	Anten, Aponal, Deptran, Desidoxepin, Doneurin, Doxal, Gilex, Mareen, Quitaxon, Sinequan, Sinquan, Sinquane, Xepin, Zonalon
Imipramine	Antidep, Celamine, Ethipramine, Imipra, Melipramine, Primonil, Pryleugan, Sermonil, Talpramin, Tofranil, Topramine
Lofepramine	Deftan, Deprimil, Emdalen, Feprapax, Gamanil, Gamonil, Lomont, Timelit, Tymelyt
Melitracen	Dixeran
Nortriptyline	Allegron, Aventyl, Martimil, Norfenazin, Noritren, Norline, Norpress, Norterol, Nortrilen, Nortyline, Ortrip, Pamelor, Paxtibi, Sensaval
Protriptyline	Concordin, Triptil, Vivactil
Trimipramine	Apo-Trimip, Herphonal, Novo-Tripramine, Rhotrimine, Stangyl, Surmontil, Tripress, Tydamine
Tetracyclic compounds	
Maprotiline	Aneural, Deprilept, Ludiomil, Maludil, Maprolu, Melodil, Mirpan, Psymion
Mianserin	Athymil, Bolvidon, Bonserin, Hopacem, Lantanon, Lerivon, Lumin, Mealin, Miabene, Mianeurin, Miaxan, Prisma, Servin, Tolimed, Tolmin, Tolvin, Tolvon
Bicyclic compounds	
Viloxazine	Vicilan, Vivalan, Vivarint
Selective serotonin re-uptake inhibitors (SSRIs)	
Citalopram	Akarin, Apertia, Celexa, Cipram, Cipramil, Elopram, Prisdal, Sepram, Seropram, Talohexal
Femoxetine	
Fluoxetine	Adofen, Afeksin, Affectine, Affex, Astrin, Atd, Auroken, Auscap, Axtin, Daforin, Deprax, Depress, Deprexin, Deproxin, Diesan, Digassim, Eufor, Felicium, Flocet, Florexal, Fluctin, Fluctine, Flumed, Fluneurin, Fluocim, Fluohexal, Fluox, Fluoxac, Fluoxemerck, Fluoxeren, Fluoxibene, Fluoxifar, Fluoxine, Fluoxistad, Fluoxityrol, Fluox-basan, Fluox-Puren, Flusol, Flutin, Flutine, Flux, Fluxantin, Fluxene, Fluxet, Fluxetil, Fluxetin, Fluxil, FluxoMed, Fluzac, Fondur, Fontex, Fonzac, Gerozac, Lorien, Lovan, Magrilan, Motivone, Mutan, Nodepe, Nortec, Norzac, Nuzak, Nycoflox, Oxetine, Oxsac, Plinzene, Positivum, Prizma, Prodep, Provatine, Prozac, Prozamel, Prozatan, Psipax, Psiquial, Reneuron, Salipax , Sanzur, Sarafem, Seromex, Seronil, Seroscand, Siqual, Tuneluz, Verotina, Zactin
Fluvoxamine	Desifluvoxamin, Dumirox, Dumyrox, Faverin, Favoxil, Felixsan, Fevarin, Floxyfral, Flox-ex, Fluvosol, Fluvoxadura, Luvox, Maveral
Paroxetine	Aropax, Casbol, Cebrilin, Deroxat, Frosinor, Motivan, Paxetil, Paxil, Pondera, Sereupin, Seroxat, Tagonis
Sertraline	Altruline, Aremis, Besitran, Gladem, Lustral, Novativ, Sealdin, Serad, Sercerin, Serlain, Tatig, Tolrest, Tresleen, Zoloft
Other compounds	
Iprindole	
Mirtazapine	Avanza, Norset, Remergil, Remeron, Rexer, Zispin
Nefazodone	Dutonin, Menfazona, Nefadar, Reseril, Rulivan, Serzone, Serzonil
Reboxetine	Davedax, Edronax, Norebox, Prolif
Trazodone	Azona, Deprax, Depyrel, Desirel, Desyrel, Donaren, Molipaxin, Thombran, Trazodil, Trazolan, Trazone, Trazorel, Triticum, Trittico
Venlafaxine	Dobupal, Efectin, Efexor, Effexor, Trevilor, Vandral
Nomifensine	(withdrawn 1986)
Zimeldine	(withdrawn 1983)

Bupropion (Amfebutamone) + Guanfacine

A grand mal seizure in a child which was attributed to a bupropion/guanfacine interaction was later identified as being more probably due to an bupropion overdose.

Clinical evidence, mechanism, importance and management

A girl of 10 being treated for attention deficit/hyperactivity disorder was prescribed increasing doses of bupropion (amfebutamone) up to 100 mg three times daily to which was subsequently added **guanfacine** 0.5 mg twice daily. 10 days later she had a grand mal seizure attributed by the author of a report to an interaction between the two drugs.[1,2] This was challenged in subsequent correspondence.[3] However two years later the author of the original report wrote to say that he had now discovered that the girl had in fact taken 5 tablets of 100 mg of bupropion and 5 tablets of 1 mg **guanfacine** before the seizure took place so that what happened was much more likely to have been due to an overdose of the bupropion than to an interaction with guanfacine.[4] Bupropion is associated with seizures at high doses. There is insufficient evidence to suggest that the concurrent use of these two drugs should be avoided.

1. Tilton P. Bupropion and guanfacine. *J Am Acad Child Adolesc Psychiatry* (1998) 37, 682–3.
2. Tilton P. Seizure associated with bupropion and guanfacine. *J Am Acad Child Adolesc Psychiatry* (1999) 38, 3.
3. Namerow LB. Seizure associated with bupropion and guanfacine. *J Am Acad Child Adolesc Psychiatry* (1999) 38, 3.
4. Tilton P. Seizure after guanfacine plus bupropion: correction. *J Am Acad Child Adolesc Psychiatry* (2000) 39, 1341.

Bupropion (Amfebutamone) + Miscellaneous drugs

The makers contraindicate bupropion with MAOIs despite evidence that serious problems are unlikely. Bupropion is contraindicated in patients with a history of seizures but those taking carbamazepine or valproate for other reasons may show marked changes in the plasma levels of bupropion and its metabolites. There are isolated reports psychosis, mania and seizures associated with the use of bupropion and fluoxetine. The makers also issue warnings about the concurrent use of drugs which can lower the convulsive threshold, levodopa, ritonavir, drugs metabolized by the cytochrome P450 isoenzymes CYP2D6 and CYP2B6, the possible of use of nicotine and following tobacco withdrawal. Cimetidine does not interact.

Clinical evidence, mechanism, importance and management

Bupropion used either as an antidepressant or as an to aid to giving up smoking seems to have few well established, clinically relevant or serious general adverse interactions, but the makers have issued a considerable number of warnings, mostly based on theoretical considerations. It seems likely that many of these warnings may be modified or prove to be unnecessary as more clinical experience is gained.

(a) Anticonvulsants

Although the incidence of seizures with bupropion is reported to be low (0.1 to 0.4%) the makers recommend that it should not be used in patients with a history of seizures and with extreme caution or not at all in those with conditions associated with an increased risk of seizures.[1,2] This means that patients taking anticonvulsants for convulsive disorders should not use bupropion, but anticonvulsant drugs have other uses and may therefore sometimes be used concurrently.

(i) *Carbamazepine, Phenobarbital, Phenytoin.* The makers warn about the outcome of using enzyme-inducing anticonvulsants such as **carbamazepine, phenytoin** and **phenobarbital**, which are expected to increase the metabolism of bupropion.[1] One study found that **carbamazepine** at steady-state decreased the maximum plasma levels and AUC of bupropion and two of its metabolites (threohydrobupropion and erythrohydrobupropion) in the region of 81 to 96%. These two metabolites have only 10 to 50% of the potency of the parent compound, whereas the AUC of another metabolite, hydroxybupropion (which has the same potency as the parent compound) was increased 50% and its AUC by 71%.[3] Two patients with bipolar illness have also been described who were initially given 450 mg bupropion daily, later increased up to 600 mg daily. They had undetectable bupropion plasma levels while taking **carbamazepine** but their plasma levels of hydroxybupropion were markedly increased.[4] What the sum of all these changes is likely to mean is uncertain, but good monitoring for any evidence of reduced efficacy and/or increased toxicity (due to the raised hydroxybupropion) is clearly needed. The same good monitoring would also be appropriate with **phenytoin** and **phenobarbital** but clinical studies appear to be lacking and the outcome equally uncertain.

(ii) *Sodium valproate, Lamotrigine.* A study found that the AUC of hydroxybupropion, an active metabolite of bupropion, almost doubled when bupropion was given with **valproate** at steady-state, but the pharmacokinetics of the parent compound and the two other metabolites were unaffected.[1,3] An increase in **valproate** levels of almost 30% was seen in another report in one patient.[4] The reasons for these changes are not known, nor is it clear what the clinical outcome of concurrent use is likely to be, but good monitoring for evidence of changed efficacy and possibly increased side-effects would seem appropriate.

The makers also say that bupropion has been found not to influence the pharmacokinetics of **lamotrigine** or its glucuronide metabolite.[1]

(b) Cimetidine

A randomised, open-label, two period crossover study in 24 normal subjects found no evidence of any clinically relevant interaction between single 300-mg doses of bupropion (sustained release preparation) and 800 mg **cimetidine**.[5] No special precautions would seem to be necessary.

(c) Drugs and circumstances which can lower the convulsive threshold

Because there is a small though finite risk of seizures (up to 0.4%) in those given bupropion at doses up to 450 mg daily,[2] the makers issue a special warning (not a contraindication) about the concurrent use of other drugs that can also lower the convulsive threshold. They name three general groups of drugs (**antipsychotics**, **antidepressants**, **systemic steroids**) and **theophylline**. The concern is that they might additively further lower the convulsive threshold. There are also warnings about clinical circumstances where an increased seizure risk associated with concurrent drug use is possible, such as diabetes treated with **hypoglycaemics** or **insulin**, withdrawal from **alcohol** or **benzodiazepines**, and the use of stimulants and anorectics.[1,3] These warnings appear to be based solely on theoretical considerations and not on any direct clinical reports, so that the real risks are unknown.

(d) Fluoxetine

The day after stopping 60 mg **fluoxetine** daily, a man aged 41 was started on 75 mg and later 100 mg bupropion three times daily. After 10 days he became "edgy and anxious" and after 12 days he developed myoclonus. After 14 days he became severely agitated and psychotic with delirium and hallucinations. His behaviour returned to normal 6 days after the bupropion was stopped.[6] It was suggested that the residual **fluoxetine** may have inhibited the metabolism of the bupropion, leading to toxic levels.[6] Another patient maintained on lithium carbonate for bipolar disorder developed anxiety, panic and eventually mania a little over a week after stopping **fluoxetine** and starting bupropion.[7] Yet another patient developed a grand mal seizure after being given **fluoxetine** and 300 mg bupropion daily.[8]

Information is very limited but these reports suggest that if concurrent or sequential use is thought appropriate, the outcome should be well monitored. More study is needed.

(e) Levodopa

The makers say that the concurrent use of bupropion and **levodopa** should be undertaken with caution because limited clinical data suggests a higher incidence of undesirable effects (nausea, vomiting, excitement, restlessness, postural tremor) in patients given both drugs. Good monitoring is therefore appropriate.[1,2]

(f) Miscellaneous drugs metabolised by cytochrome P450 isoenzyme CYP2D6 and those which affect cytochrome P450 isoenzyme CYP2B6

A pharmacokinetic study in normal healthy subjects known to be extensive metabolisers of CYP2D6 found that bupropion doubled the maximum plasma levels of **desipramine** and increased its AUC fivefold.[1] Another study in a 64-year old woman on **imipramine** (150 to 200 mg daily) found that when 225 mg bupropion daily was added, there was a fourfold rise in the plasma levels of **imipramine** and **desipramine** but no problems were reported. A comparison of the estimated clearances were: **imipramine** alone (1.7 ml/min), **desipramine** (1.7 ml/min); **imipramine** + bupropion (0.73 ml/min), **desipramine** + bupropion (0.31 ml/min).[9] The explanation would seem to be that bupropion inhibits CYP2D6, which is involved with the metabolism of these tricyclics, so that they are cleared from the body more slowly in the presence of bupropion. *In vitro* studies[1] have shown that both bupropion and its metabolite are inhibitors of CYP2D6.

Formal interaction studies with other drugs metabolized by CYP2D6 have not been carried out by the makers but they predict that a number of drugs may be similarly affected which might in theory result in a rise in their plasma levels. In addition to **desipramine** they list SSRIs (**fluoxetine, paroxetine, sertraline**), antipsychotics (**haloperidol, risperidone, thioridazine**), beta-blockers (**metoprolol**) and Type 1C antiarrhythmics (**flecainide, propafenone**). The recommendation is that if any of these drugs is added to treatment with bupropion, doses at the lower end of the range should be used. If bupropion is added to existing treatment, decreased dosages should be considered,[1,2] but there appear to be no reports of problems with the concurrent use of any of these drugs.

The makers also advise caution if bupropion is administered with drugs such as **orphenadrine, cyclophosphamide** and **ifosfamide**. The reason is that bupropion is metabolised to its major metabolite hydroxybupropion by CYP2B6 and these drugs affect this isoenzyme. The concern here is that the activity of some or all of these drugs might be altered in some way.

It should be emphasised that all of the predictions, recommendations and precautions quoted here are largely based on *in vitro* studies, not on clinical studies, and thus far there appear to be no reports of problems arising from the concurrent use of these drugs with bupropion.

(g) Monoamine oxidase inhibitors (MAOIs)

In an uncontrolled trial, 10 patients were treated for major affective disorder (8 unipolar, 2 bipolar) with bupropion (daily doses of 225 to 450 mg) and various **MAOIs** (**isocarboxazid** (1 patient), **phenelzine** (5), **tranylcypromine** (2), **selegiline** (2)). Four were transferred from the **MAOI** to bupropion without any washout period, and the other 6 were given both drugs concurrently; 7 of the 10 showed improvement. No untoward cardiovascular events occurred except for one patient on bupropion and **selegiline** who experienced orthostatic hypotension. Notable weight loss occurred in two others when transferred from the **MAOI** to bupropion.[10,11]

Despite this clear (though very limited) clinical evidence of apparent safety,[11] the makers of bupropion are apparently nervous about a possible interaction with **MAOIs** because of the toxicity seen in studies in *rats* when **phenelzine** and bupropion were given concurrently.[11] Thus at the moment the makers contraindicate bupropion with **MAOIs** and they say that at least 14 days should elapse between stopping irreversible **MAOIs** and starting bupropion.[1,2] This precaution would therefore apply particularly to the older **MAOIs** (**phenelzine, tranylcypromine, isocarboxazid** etc). For reversible (and selective) **MAOIs**, the maker's advice is that the period depends on the plasma elimination of the particular drug.[1] For **moclobemide**, which is reversible and selective for MAO-A and which has a half-life of 5 to 6 h, the period could therefore be reduced to 2 to 3 days because by

then virtually full MAO activity should have been restored. For **selegiline**, which is selective for MAO-B and has a half-life of only 1.5 h, the period could be shorter.

(h) Nicotine

Nicotine administered as transdermal patches is reported not to affect the pharmacokinetics of bupropion or its metabolites.[1] The makers say that limited data suggest that giving up smoking is more easily achieved if bupropion is taken while using a **nicotine** transdermal system, but they recommend that blood pressure measurements should be taken weekly to check for any evidence of a blood pressure increase.[1] The same warning would also seem to be applicable to the use of **nicotine** in any other form (oral or nasal).

(i) Pseudoephedrine

A man of 21 presented in a hospital emergency department with severe chest pain, radiating pain into both arms and between the shoulder blades, diaphoresis and shortness of breath. Initially this was diagnosed as acute myocardial infarction, but a later angiogram showed normal coronary arteries and it was concluded that these symptoms were due to acute myocardial ischaemia (transient Prinzmetal's variant angina) apparently brought on by the combined use of **pseudoephedrine** (9 tablets of 30 mg) over the previous 3 days, **bupropion** for smoking cessation and **nicotine** (he smoked 25 cigarettes daily). The authors of the report postulate that all these drugs acted on the alpha receptors of the coronary arteries to cause vasospasm and acute ischaemia. He had been taking both drugs and erythromycin for 3 days, and had taken **pseudoephedrine** on numerous previous occasions without problems. He recovered fully.[12]

This is an isolated case from which no general conclusions can be drawn, but some warning might be appropriate for middle-aged or elderly patients who might already be at risk of coronary ischaemia.

(j) Ritonavir

The makers of **ritonavir** contraindicate the concurrent use of bupropion[13] on theoretical grounds. They predict that the metabolism of bupropion by cytochrome P450 isoenzyme CYP2D6 might possibly be inhibited, leading to increased levels and toxicity. But the makers of bupropion do not mention the possibility of an interaction with **ritonavir** in their product literature.[1,2] There seem to be no reports of an adverse interaction.

(k) Tobacco withdrawal

Patients who give up smoking may find that the dosages of some of their medications are more than they actually need. The reason is that tobacco smoke contains compounds that induce (stimulate) the metabolism and loss from the body of certain drugs. Thus when smoking stops, the inducer is removed, the metabolism slows down and less of the drug is needed. The components of tobacco smoke are not potent enzyme inducers so that tobacco withdrawal does not usually have a marked effect, but the makers of bupropion draw attention to the following drugs which may possibly be affected by tobacco withdrawal: **clomipramine, clozapine, flecainide, imipramine, olanzapine, pentazocine, theophylline** and **tacrine**.[1] If you look in the Index under 'Tobacco smoking' you will find a more extensive list of drugs affected by tobacco smoking. Check on patients' responses to these drugs after tobacco withdrawal and make any necessary downward dosage adjustments.

1. Zyban (Bupropion). Glaxo Wellcome. Summary of product characteristics, April 2000.
2. Wellbutrin SR (Bupropion). Glaxo Wellcome, Product Information, May 2000.
3. Ketter TA, Jenkins JB, Schroeder DH, Pazzaglia PJ, Marangell LB, George MS, Callahan AM, Hinton ML, Chao J, Post RM. Carbamazepine but not valproate induced bupropion metabolism. *J Clin Psychopharmacol* (1995) 15, 327–33.
4. Popli AP, Tanquary J, Lamparella V, Masand PS. Bupropion and anticonvulsant drug interactions. *Ann Clin Psychiatry* (1995) 7, 99–101.
5. Corrigan B, Hsyu PH, Kustra R, Duncan B, Dunn J, Griffin R. A randomized, crossover study to evaluate the pharmacokinetic effect of cimetidine on *Wellbutrin* (bupropion HCl) sustained release in healthy subjects. *Pharm Res* (1997) 14 (11 Suppl), S-560.
6. van Putten T, Shaffer I. Delirium associated with bupropion. *J Clin Psychopharmacol* (1990) 10, 234.
7. Zubieta JK, Demitrack MA. Possible bupropion precipitation of mania and a mixed affective state. *J Clin Psychopharmacol* (1991) 11, 327–8.
8. Ciraulo DA, Shader RI. Fluoxetine drug-drug interactions.II. *J Clin Psychopharmacol* (1990) 10, 213–17.
9. Shad MU, Preskorn SH. A possible bupropion and imipramine interaction. *J Clin Psychopharmacol* (1997) 17, 118–19.
10. Abuzzahab Sr, FS. Combination therapy: monoamino oxidase inhibitors and bupropion HCl. *Neuropsychopharmacology* (1994) 10, (3S Pt 2), 74S.
11. Data on file, Glaxo Wellcome. Personal Communication, July 2000.

12. Pederson KJ, Kuntz DH, Garbe GJ. Acute myocardial ischemia associated with ingestion of bupropion and pseudoephedrine in a 21-year-old man. *Can J Cardiol* (2001) 17, 599–601.

13. Norvir (Ritonavir). Abbott Laboratories Ltd. Summary of product characteristics, July 1998.

Citalopram + Miscellaneous drugs

The potentially fatal serotonin syndrome can occur with moclobemide and citalopram in overdose, but it is not yet clear whether this drug combination is safe in therapeutic doses. There is preliminary evidence that citalopram may possibly increase the effects of imipramine, but not those of amitriptyline, clomipramine or maprotiline. Tricyclics and cimetidine may increase the serum levels of citalopram. Carbamazepine but not oxcarbazepine reduces serum citalopram levels. There is evidence that citalopram does not interact adversely with some benzodiazepines, chlorpromazine, fluvoxamine, haloperidol, levomepromazine, lithium, perphenazine, selegiline, thioridazine, warfarin or zuclopenthixol.

Clinical evidence, mechanism, importance and management

(a) Carbamazepine, Oxcarbazepine

Two patients with epilepsy, major depression and panic disorder showed increased citalopram levels. One showed an improved antidepressant response, but the other patient experienced tremor and increased anxiety when their treatment with **carbamazepine** was replaced by **oxcarbazepine**.[1] The most likely explanation is that **carbamazepine** (a potent liver enzyme inducing agent) reduces the serum levels of many drugs – including apparently citalopram – by increasing their clearance from the body, whereas **oxcarbazepine** does not act in this way. So if **carbamazepine** is replaced by **oxcarbazepine**, the liver metabolism returns to normal and the serum levels of the drug affected – citalopram in this case – rise. Check the serum levels and the response to citalopram if **carbamazepine** is added or withdrawn, but no interaction would be expected with **oxcarbazepine**.

(b) Cimetidine and other H₂-blockers

Twelve normal subjects were given 40 mg citalopram daily for 21 days and then for the next 8 days they were additionally given 400 mg **cimetidine** twice daily. The **cimetidine** caused a 29% decrease in the oral clearance of the citalopram, a 39% rise in its maximum serum levels and a 43% increase in its AUC. Some changes in the renal clearance of the citalopram metabolites were also seen. The apparent reason for all of these changes is that **cimetidine** inhibits the activity of cytochrome P450 isoenzymes CYP2C19 and CYP2D6 so that the metabolism of the citalopram is reduced, and as a result its serum concentrations rise.[2]

The authors of this study say that while **cimetidine** certainly causes an increase in the serum levels of citalopram, the extent is only moderate and because the drug is well tolerated and there are very considerable pharmacokinetic variations between individual subjects, they consider that there is no need to reduce the citalopram dosage.[2] There is no direct information about other H₂-blockers, but none of them (**famotidine**, **ranitidine**, etc.) normally acts as an enzyme inhibitor so that no interaction with citalopram would be expected.

(c) Fluvoxamine

A study in 7 depressed patients who had failed to respond to 3 weeks' treatment with 40 mg citalopram daily found that the addition of 50 to 100 mg **fluvoxamine** daily for another 3 weeks improved the control of the depression. Plasma *S*-and *R*-citalopram levels rose (two to threefold). No patient developed the serotonin syndrome, and no changes in vital signs or ECGs were seen.[3] More study of combined use is needed.

(d) Lithium carbonate or sulphate

No changes were seen in one study when lithium 30 mmol/day (as **lithium sulphate**) was added to citalopram.[4] Another study in 24 patients found that the concurrent use of 60 mg citalopram and 800 mg **lithium carbonate** daily was effective and did not cause problems,[5] even so the makers of citalopram suggest that concurrent use should be undertaken with caution, as they are aware of reports of enhanced serotonergic effects when lithium and SSRIs are used together.[6]

(e) Moclobemide, Selegiline and other MAOIs

Three patients developed the serotonin syndrome (tremor, convulsions, hyperthermia, unconsciousness) and died 3 to 16 h after taking overdoses of **moclobemide** and citalopram.[7] It is not clear whether the same would happen if this drug combination were to be taken in normal therapeutic doses, but additional indirect evidence suggests it may not be safe.

Moclobemide (a selective MAO-A inhibitor) can interact adversely with some of the SSRIs but not with others. It can interact with imipramine and clomipramine, both of which are potent inhibitors of serotonin uptake, causing the potentially fatal serotonin syndrome (see 'Monoamine oxidase inhibitors (MAOIs) + Tricyclic antidepressants', p.682), but is reported not to interact with fluvoxamine (see 'Fluvoxamine + Antidepressants', p.827). The makers of citalopram therefore cautiously recommend that citalopram should not be given with MAOIs or for 14 days afterwards, nor should MAOIs be added until citalopram has been stopped for 7 days.[6,8]

However, a double-blind randomised study found no important interaction between citalopram and **selegiline** (a selective MAO-B inhibitor): in normal subjects given 20 mg citalopram or a placebo daily for 10 days, there was no evidence of changes in vital signs or in the frequency of adverse events after the addition of **selegiline** daily for 4 days, but the bioavailability of the **selegiline** was slightly reduced (by about 30%). The authors of this report concluded that no clinically relevant interaction occurs between **selegiline** and citalopram.[9,10]

(f) Neuroleptics

A study in 90 schizophrenic patients found that over a 12-week period the serum levels of **chlorpromazine**, **haloperidol**, **levomepromazine**, **perphenazine**, **thioridazine** or **zuclopenthixol** were not significantly altered by the concurrent use of 40 mg citalopram daily.[11] A study in three groups of 8 normal subjects taking 40 mg citalopram daily for 10 days found that a single 50 mg oral dose of **levomepromazine** increased the initial steady-state levels of the primary metabolite of citalopram (desmethylcitalopram) by 10 to 20%.[4] These studies suggest that no special precautions are needed if these drugs are given with citalopram.

(g) Tricyclic antidepressants

In the study cited above,[4] citalopram caused an approximately 50% increase in the AUC of **desipramine** (the primary metabolite of imipramine) after a single 100 mg oral dose of **imipramine**, and a reduction in the levels of the subsequently formed metabolite of **desipramine**. In contrast, 5 patients on **amitriptyline**, **clomipramine** or **maprotiline** showed no changes in their plasma tricyclic antidepressant levels when 20 to 60 mg citalopram daily was added.[12] These preliminary observations were on only a small number of patients and require confirmation, but it would appear that, unlike other SSRIs, citalopram does not cause a marked increase in the plasma levels of some tricyclic antidepressants.

In another general study, in which 18 patients were given citalopram and tricyclic antidepressants, serum levels of citalopram were doubled in those receiving the tricyclic clomipramine; pooled results for all the tricyclics showed a 44% rise in serum citalopram levels.[13] An increase of this size might be important with some other drugs, but it is doubtful if it is of clinical importance with citalopram. See the observations made above (b) with cimetidine, which causes a similar increase.

(h) Warfarin

A study in 12 normal subjects given a single 25 mg oral dose of **warfarin** either alone or on day 15 of a 21-day course of 40 mg citalopram daily found that the pharmacokinetics of both *(R)*- and *(S)*- **warfarin** remained unchanged in the presence of the citalopram, but the maximum prothrombin time was increased by 1.6 s. This was considered to be clinically irrelevant.[14] No special precautions would appear to be needed if both drugs are used.

(i) Miscellaneous drugs

The makers of citalopram say that no pharmacodynamic interactions have been noted in clinical studies in which citalopram was given with **benzodiazepines**, **neuroleptics**, **analgesics**, **alcohol**, **antihistamines**, **antihypertensives**, **beta-blockers** and other cardiovascular drugs, but none of the individual drugs is named.[6] A general study in psychiatric patients found that **benzodiazepines** caused a modest increase (+23%) in serum citalopram levels[13] which is almost certainly too small to be clinically relevant. A study in 18 normal subjects found no pharmacokinetic interaction between **triazolam** and citalopram, and it was suggested that **triazolam** and other substrates of cytochrome P450 isoenzyme CYP3A4 can be coadministered safely with citalopram.[15]

1. Leinonen E, Lepola U, Koponen H. Substituting carbamazepine with oxcarbazepine increases citalopram levels. A report on two cases. *Pharmacopsychiatry* (1996) 29, 156–8.
2. Priskorn M, Larsen F, Segonzac A, Moulin M. Pharmacokinetic interaction study of citalopram and cimetidine in healthy subjects. *Eur J Clin Pharmacol* (1997) 52, 241–2.
3. Bondolfi G, Chautems C, Rochat B, Bertschy G, Baumann P. Non-response to citalopram in depressive patients: pharmacokinetic and clinical consequences of a fluvoxamine augmentation. *Psychopharmacol* (1996) 128, 421–5.
4. Gram LF, Hansen MG, Sindrup SH, Brøsen K, Poulsen JH, Aaes-Jørgensen T, Overø KF. Citalopram: interaction studies with levomepromazine, imipramine and lithium. *Ther Drug Monit* (1993) 15, 18–24.
5. Baumann P, Souche A, Montaldi S, Baettig D, Lambert S, Uehlinger C, Kasas A, Amey M, Jonzier-Perey M. A double-blind, placebo-controlled study of citalopram with and without lithium in the treatment of therapy-resistant depressive patients: a clinical, pharmacokinetic, and pharmacogenetic investigation. *J Clin Psychopharmacol* (1996) 16, 307–14.
6. Cipramil (Citalopram). Lundbeck Ltd. Summary of product characteristics, June 1998.
7. Neuvonen PJ, Pohjola-Sintonen S, Tacke U, Vuori E. Five fatal cases of serotonin syndrome after moclobemide-citalopram or moclobemide-clomipramine overdoses. *Lancet* (1993) 342, 1419.
8. Lundbeck Ltd, Personal communication, February 1996.
9. Laine K, Anttila M, Heinonen E, Helminen A, Huupponen R, Koulu M, Mäki-Ikola O, Reinikainen KJ, Scheinin M. Lack of adverse interactions between selegiline and citalopram. *Eur J Clin Pharmacol* (1997) 52 (Suppl), A135.
10. Laine K, Anttila M, Heinonen E, Helminen A, Huupponen R, Mäki-Ikola O, Reinikainen K, Scheinin M. Lack of adverse interactions between concomitantly administered selegiline and citalopram. *Clin Neuropharmacol* (1997) 20, 419–33.
11. Syvälahti EKG, Taiminen T, Saarijärvi S, Lehto H, Niemi H, Ahola V, Dahl M-L, Salokangas RKR. Citalopram causes no significant alterations in plasma neuroleptic levels in schizophrenic patients. *J Int Med Res* (1997) 25, 24–32.
12. Baettig D, Bondolfi G, Montaldi S, Amey M, Baumann P. Tricyclic antidepressant plasma levels after augmentation with citalopram: a case study. *Eur J Clin Pharmacol* (1993) 44, 403–5.
13. Leinonen E, Lepola U, Koponen H, Kinnunen I. The effect of age and concomitant treatment with other psychoactive drugs on serum concentrations of citalopram measured with a nonenantioselective method. *Ther Drug Monit* (1996) 18, 111–17.
14. Priskorn M, Sidhu JS, Larsen F, Davis JD, Khan AZ, Rolan PE. Investigation of multiple dose citalopram on the pharmacokinetics and pharmacodynamics of racemic warfarin. *Br J Clin Pharmacol* (1997) 44, 199–202.
15. Nolting A, Abramowitz W. Lack of interaction between citalopram and the CYP3A4 substrate triazolam. *Pharmacotherapy* (2000) 20, 750–5.

Femoxetine + Cimetidine

Femoxetine plasma levels are increased by cimetidine but no adverse effects seem to develop.

Clinical evidence, mechanism, importance and management

Cimetidine 1 g daily for 7 days raised the steady-state plasma trough levels of femoxetine in 6 normal subjects taking 600 mg daily by 140% (from 10 to 24 ng/ml). The AUC was increased but not significantly, and no increase in adverse effects was seen.[1] The probable reason for this interaction is that the **cimetidine** inhibits the oxidative metabolism of the femoxetine by the liver, reducing its loss from the body and thereby raising the plasma levels. The authors of the paper recommend that the initial femoxetine dosage should be reduced from 600 to 400 mg daily. More study is needed to confirm this interaction.

1. Schmidt J, Sørensen AS, Gjerris A, Rafaelsen OJ, Mengel H. Femoxetine and cimetidine: interaction in healthy volunteers. *Eur J Clin Pharmacol* (1986) 31, 299–302.

Fluoxetine + Benzodiazepines

Some preliminary evidence suggests that alprazolam and diazepam plasma levels (but not those of clonazepam, estazolam, midazolam or triazolam) may be raised by fluoxetine, and that combined use may impair the performance of some psychomotor tests.

Clinical evidence, mechanism, importance and management

The concurrent use of fluoxetine (60 mg) has been found to reduce **alprazolam** clearance (1 mg four times daily) by about 21%, to increase its plasma levels by about 30% accompanied by increased psychomotor impairment.[1] The reason appears to be that the **alprazolam** metabolism is reduced.[2]

Fluoxetine 30 mg, given daily for 1 or 8 days, had no effect on the pharmacokinetics of 10 mg **diazepam**.[3] A later study by the same group, using fluoxetine 60 mg, suggested that the **diazepam** half-life and AUC were increased, possibly because the fluoxetine decreased the metabolism of **diazepam**. However, they concluded that this was not of any clinical significance.[4] Another study found that fluoxetine 60 mg alone did not affect psychomotor performance but fluoxetine 60 mg plus **diazepam** 5 mg significantly impaired the Divided Attention tracking test and Vigilance test more than with **diazepam** 5 mg alone.[5] The pharmacokinetics of **clonazepam**,[6] **estazolam**,[7] **midazolam**[8] and **triazolam**[9] were not significantly affected by fluoxetine.

The practical importance of all of these findings is uncertain, but the possibility should be borne in mind that combined use of fluoxetine and the interacting drugs (**diazepam**, **alprazolam**) can possibly make patients more drowsy and adversely affect driving and other skills. Patients should be warned. More study is needed.

1. Lasher TA, Fleishaker JC, Steenwyk RC, Antal EJ. Pharmacokinetic pharmacodynamic evaluation of the combined administration of alprazolam and fluoxetine. *Psychopharmacology* (1991) 104, 323–7.
2. von Moltke LL, Greenblatt DJ, Cotreau-Bibbo MM, Harmatz JS, Shader RI. Inhibitors of alprazolam metabolism *in vitro*: effect of serotonin-reuptake-inhibitor antidepressants, ketoconazole and quinidine. *Br J Clin Pharmacol* (1994) 38, 23–31.
3. Lemberger L, Bergstrom RF, Wolen RL, Farid NA, Enas GG, Aronoff GR. Fluoxetine: clinical pharmacology and physiologic disposition. *J Clin Psychiatry* (1985) 46, 3 (Sec 2), 14–19.
4. Lemberger L, Rowe H, Bosomworth JC, Tenbarge JB, Bergstrom RF. The effect of fluoxetine on the pharmacokinetics and psychomotor responses of diazepam. *Clin Pharmacol Ther* (1988) 43, 412–19.
5. Moskowitz H, Burns M. The effects on performance of two antidepressants, alone and in combination with diazepam. *Prog Neuropsychopharmacol Biol Psychiatry* (1988) 12, 783–92.
6. Greenblatt DJ, Preskorn SH, Cotreau MM, Horst WD, Harmatz JS. Fluoxetine impairs clearance of alprazolam but not of clonazepam. *Clin Pharmacol Ther* (1992) 52, 479–86.
7. Cavanaugh J, Schneck D, Eason C, Hansen M, Gustavson L. Lack of effect of fluoxetine on the pharmacokinetics (PK) and pharmacodynamics (PD) of estazolam. *Clin Pharmacol Ther* (1994) 55, 141.
8. Lam YWF, Alfaro CL, Ereshefsky L, Miller M. Effect of antidepressants and ketoconazole on oral midazolam pharmacokinetics. *Clin Pharmacol Ther* (1998) 63, 229.
9. Wright CE, Lasher-Sisson TA, Steenwyk RC, Swanson CN. A pharmacokinetic evaluation of the combined administration of triazolam and fluoxetine. *Pharmacotherapy* (1992) 12, 103–6.

Fluoxetine + Cannabis

An isolated report describes mania in a patient on fluoxetine after smoking cannabis.

Clinical evidence, mechanism, importance and management

A woman aged 21 years with a 9-year history of bulimia and depression was treated with 20 mg fluoxetine daily. A month later, about two days after smoking two 'joints' of **cannabis** (**marijuana**), she experienced a persistent sense of well-being, increased energy, hypersexuality and pressured speech. These symptoms progressed into grandiose delusions for which she was hospitalised. Her mania and excitement were controlled with lorazepam and perphenazine, and she largely recovered after about 8 days. The reasons for this reaction are not understood but the authors of the report point out that one of the active components of **cannabis**, Δ^9-**tetrahydrocannabinol** (**dronabinol**), is, like fluoxetine, a potent inhibitor of serotonin uptake. Thus a synergistic effect on central serotonergic neurones might have occurred.[1] This seems to be the first and only report of an apparent adverse interaction between **cannabis** and fluoxetine, but it emphasises the risks of concurrent use.

1. Stoll AL, Cole JO, Lukas SE. A case of mania as a result of fluoxetine-marijuana interaction. *J Clin Psychiatry* (1991) 52, 280–1.

Fluoxetine or Paroxetine + Cyproheptadine

Three reports say that cyproheptadine can oppose the antidepressant effects of fluoxetine, and another describes the same effect on paroxetine.

Clinical evidence

(a) Fluoxetine

Three depressed men complained of anorgasmia when treated with **fluoxetine**. When this was treated with **cyproheptadine** their depressive symptoms returned, decreasing again when **cyproheptadine** was stopped.[1] Two women also complained of anorgasmia within 1 to 3 months of starting treatment with 40 to 60 mg **fluoxetine** daily for bulimia nervosa. When **cyproheptadine** was added to treat this sexual dysfunction, the urge to binge on food returned in both of them and one experienced increased depression. These symptoms resolved 4 to 7 days after stopping **cyproheptadine** treatment.[2] A woman successfully treated with 40 mg **fluoxetine** daily showed a re-emergence of her depressive symptoms on two occasions within 36 h of starting to take **cyproheptadine**.[3] In a further case, a woman who responded well to fluoxetine 20 mg daily for depression had a recurrence of her depression after she began to take **cyproheptadine** for migraine. Increasing the dose of fluoxetine to 40 mg daily controlled the depressive symptoms while **cyproheptadine** was continued for migraine.[4] In contrast, no exacerbation of depression was seen in a previous study in which both **cyproheptadine** and fluoxetine were used in 2 patients.[5]

(b) Paroxetine

The depression of a woman, which had responded well to 20 mg **paroxetine** daily, re-emerged and worsened, accompanied by confusion and psychotic symptoms, within 2 days of starting to take 2 mg **cyproheptadine** twice daily for the treatment of anorgasmia.[6] Psychotic symptoms resolved 2 days after stopping **cyproheptadine**.

Mechanism

Although the mechanism is not fully understood, cyproheptadine is a serotonin antagonist. It has therefore been suggested that cyproheptadine blocks or opposes the serotoninergic effects of these SSRIs.[1-3,6]

Importance and management

Direct information about this interaction appears to be limited to these studies although cyproheptadine has also been found to oppose the antidepressant effects of MAOIs (see 'Monoamine oxidase inhibitors (MAOIs) + Cyproheptadine', p.672). One of the studies suggests that not every patient is affected.[5] If concurrent use is thought appropriate, the outcome should be very well monitored for evidence of a reduced antidepressant response.

1. Feder R. Reversal of antidepressant activity of fluoxetine by cyproheptadine in three patients. *J Clin Psychiatry* (1991) 52, 163–4.
2. Goldbloom DS, Kennedy SH. Adverse interaction of fluoxetine and cyproheptadine in two patients with bulimia nervosa. *J Clin Psychiatry* (1991) 52, 261–2.
3. Katz RJ, Rosenthal M. Adverse interaction of cyproheptadine with serotonergic antidepressants. *J Clin Psychiatry* (1994) 55, 314–15.
4. Boon F. Cyproheptadine and SSRIs. *J Am Acad Child Adolesc Psychiatry* (1999) 38, 112.
5. McCormick S, Olin J, Brotman AW. Reversal of fluoxetine-induced anorgasmia by cyproheptadine in two patients. *J Clin Psychiatry* (1990) 51, 383–4.
6. Christensen RC. Adverse interaction of paroxetine and cyproheptadine. *J Clin Psychiatry* (1995) 56, 433–4.

Fluoxetine + Itraconazole

Anorexia developed in a patient on fluoxetine when itraconazole was started, and it disappeared when the itraconazole was stopped.

Clinical evidence, mechanism, importance and management

A man taking 20 mg fluoxetine daily, diazepam and several anti-asthmatic drugs (salbutamol (albuterol), salmeterol, budesonide, theophylline) was started on 200 mg **itraconazole** daily for allergic bronchopulmonary aspergillosis. Within 1 to 2 days he developed anorexia without nausea. He stopped the **itraconazole** after a week, and the anorexia resolved 1 to 2 days later. The author of the report attributed the anorexia to increased levels of norfluoxetine (the metabolite of fluoxetine) brought about by inhibition of its metabolism by the **itraconazole**, although the norfluoxetine levels were not measured.[1] Anorexia is a recognised adverse effect of fluoxetine.

This report and the conclusions reached are uncertain, but they draw attention to the possibility of a fluoxetine/**itraconazole** interaction. Monitor well if both drugs are used. More study is needed.

1. Black PN. Probable interaction between fluoxetine and itraconazole. *Ann Pharmacother* (1995) 29, 1048–9.

Fluoxetine + Macrolide antibacterials

An isolated case report describes what appeared to be acute fluoxetine intoxication in a man brought about by the addition of clarithromycin. See also 'Sertraline + Erythromycin', p.836.

Clinical evidence

A 53-year-old-man on long-term fluoxetine (80 mg) and nitrazepam (10 mg) at bedtime for depression and insomnia, was additionally started on 250 mg **clarithromycin** twice daily for a respiratory infection. Within a day he started to become increasingly confused and after 3 days was admitted to hospital with a diagnosis of psychosis and delirium. When no organic cause for the delirium could be found all his medications were stopped and **erythromycin** was started. His mental state returned to normal after 36 h. Once the antibacterial course had finished, the fluoxetine and nitrazepam were restarted and no further problems occurred.[1]

Mechanism

The authors of this report attribute what was seen to intoxication by fluoxetine, brought about by inhibition of its metabolism by the clarithromycin possibly mediated by cytochrome P450.[1]

Importance and management

This seems to be the first and only case of this interaction so that its general importance is uncertain, probably minor, but it would now be prudent to monitor the effects if clarithromycin is added to fluoxetine treatment. See also 'Sertraline + Erythromycin', p.836.

1. Pollak PT, Sketris IS, MacKenzie SL, Hewlett TJ. Delirium probably induced by clarithromycin in a patient receiving fluoxetine. *Ann Pharmacother* (1995) 29, 486–8.

Fluoxetine + Miscellaneous drugs

Fluoxetine normally appears not to interact with chlorothiazide, dextromethorphan or hypoglycaemic agents but isolated adverse interactions have been seen with amfetamine (amphetamine) (toxicity, psychosis), chloral (prolonged

drowsiness), dextromethorphan (hallucinations), insulin (hypoglycaemia), phenylpropanolamine (dizziness, weight loss and hyperactivity) and propofol (spontaneous movements). There is *in vitro* evidence that the effects of flecainide, mexiletine, propafenone, thioridazine, tomoxetine, and zuclopenthixol may possibly be increased by fluoxetine, and also evidence that fluoxetine's effects are increased by aminoglutethimide. See also 'Antipsychotics or Dopamine antagonists + Fluoxetine', p.693.

Clinical evidence, mechanism, importance and management

(a) Aminoglutethimide

A patient with severe obsessive-compulsive disorder resistant to clomipramine combined with SSRIs, improved when given 40 mg fluoxetine daily and 250 mg **aminoglutethimide** four times daily. Over a four-and-a-half year period whenever attempts were made to reduce the dosage of either drug, the patient started to relapse.[1] Thus at least one patient has taken both drugs together without problems, and the evidence suggests that the **aminoglutethimide** has a potentiating effect on the fluoxetine. However, more study is needed to confirm the efficacy and safety of this drug combination in other patients.

(b) Chloral hydrate

Marked drowsiness occurred for a whole day in a patient taking 20 mg fluoxetine daily after being given 500 mg **chloral hydrate** the night before. She later tolerated 1 g **chloral hydrate** in the absence of fluoxetine without adverse effects. The reason for this adverse response is not known, but the author suggests the possibility of protein binding displacement, reduced **chloral** metabolism;[2] alternatively it may have been due to the additive sedative effects of both drugs. The general importance of this interaction is unknown but concurrent use should monitored.

(c) Chlorothiazide

Fluoxetine is reported not to affect the pharmacokinetics of **chlorothiazide**.[3] No special precautions would seem necessary.

(d) Dextromethorphan

A woman who had been on 20 mg fluoxetine daily for 17 days took two teaspoonfuls of a cough syrup containing **dextromethorphan**, and two more the next morning with the next capsule of fluoxetine. Within 2 h vivid hallucinations developed (bright colours, distortions of shapes and sizes) which lasted 6 to 8 h. The patient said they were similar to her past experience with LSD 12 years earlier.[4] The reasons for this reaction are uncertain. This seems to be the first and only report of this interaction. No mention was made of adverse effects in the report of an extensive metabolic study[5] in which depressed patients on fluoxetine were given single 30-mg doses of **dextromethorphan**, nevertheless concurrent use should be well monitored. In this latter study the **dextromethorphan** was being used as an indicator or marker of changes in enzyme activity, and it was confirmed that fluoxetine inhibits the activity of cytochrome P450 isoenzyme CYP2D6, an enzyme involved in the O-demethylation of **dextromethorphan**.[5]

(e) Flecainide, Mexiletine, Propafenone, Thioridazine, Tomoxetine, Zuclopenthixol

Studies in patients and *in vitro* investigations using human liver microsomes have shown that fluoxetine and its metabolite, norfluoxetine have a strong inhibitory effect on the activity of cytochrome P450 isoenzyme CYP2D6 in the liver.[5,6] The practical consequences of this are that the effects of other drugs whose liver metabolism depends on this particular isoenzyme are likely to be increased and prolonged. A clear example of this is the increase in the effects of the tricyclic antidepressants when fluoxetine is given concurrently (see 'Tricyclic and related antidepressants + Fluoxetine', p.845). There is also a single case of markedly increased extrapyramidal side effects in a patient given **perphenazine** and fluoxetine (see 'Antipsychotics or Dopamine antagonists + Fluoxetine', p.693). Other drugs, the effects

of which are largely or partly metabolised by CYP2D6, include **flecainide**, **mexiletine**, **propafenone**, **thioridazine**, and **zuclopenthixol**. So far there appear to be no clinical cases of interactions between any of these drugs and fluoxetine, but it might now be prudent to be alert for increased and prolonged effects if fluoxetine is added.

(f) Hypoglycaemic agents

Although one study found that single or multiple doses of fluoxetine over 8 days did not affect the pharmacokinetics or the hypoglycaemic effects of 1 g **tolbutamide**,[3] the makers of fluoxetine say that hypoglycaemia has been seen in diabetic patients when fluoxetine was started, and hyperglycaemia when it was stopped.[7] An **insulin**-dependent diabetic experienced signs of hypoglycaemia (nausea, tremor, sweating, anxiety, lightheadedness) after starting to take 20 mg fluoxetine nightly. These disappeared when the fluoxetine was stopped and reappeared when it was restarted, however blood sugar levels were found to be normal (9 to 11 mmol/l).[8] The reasons are not understood. Concurrent use need not be avoided but the diabetic control should be monitored if fluoxetine is added.

(g) Propofol

Two women in their mid-twenties who had been on 20 mg fluoxetine daily for 4 to 6 months had pronounced involuntary upper limb movements lasting 20 to 30 s immediately after anaesthetic induction with 180 mg **propofol** (2.0 to 2.5 mg/kg). The movements ceased spontaneously and the rest of the anaesthesia and surgery were uneventful. Neither had any history of epilepsy or movement disorders. It is not clear whether this was a **propofol**/fluoxetine interaction or just a rare (but previously reported) reaction to **propofol**.[9]

(h) Sympathomimetics

A 16-year-old girl with an eating disorder and taking 20 mg fluoxetine once daily developed vague medical complaints of dizziness, 'hyper' feelings, diarrhoea, palpitations and a reported weight loss of 14 lbs within two weeks. The author of the report suggested that these might have been the result of an interaction with **phenylpropanolamine** (1 to 2 capsules of *Dexatrim* once daily) which the patient was surreptitiously taking, associated with a restricted food and fluid intake.[10] A man who had taken a small, unspecified, but previously tolerated dose of **amfetamine (amphetamine)** developed signs of **amfetamine** overdosage (restlessness, agitation, hyperventilation, etc.) while taking 60 mg fluoxetine daily. Another man developed first rank symptoms of schizophrenia after taking two unspecified doses of **amfetamine** while taking 20 mg fluoxetine daily.[11] The postulated reason for this fluoxetine/**amfetamine** interaction is that fluoxetine inhibits cytochrome P450 isoenzyme CYP2D6 which would be expected to result in increased **amfetamine** levels.[12] The general importance of these apparent interactions is uncertain.

1. Chouinard G, Bélanger M-C, Beauclair L, Sultan S, Murphy BEP. Potentiation of fluoxetine by aminoglutethimide, an adrenal steroid suppressant, in obsessive-compulsive disorder resistant to SSRIs: a case report. *Prog Neuropsychopharmacol Biol Psychiatry* (1996) 20, 1067–79.
2. Devarajan S. Interaction of fluoxetine and chloral hydrate. *Can J Psychiatry* (1992) 37, 590–1.
3. Lemberger L, Bergstrom RF, Wolen RL, Farid NA, Enas GG, Aronoff GR. Fluoxetine: clinical pharmacology and physiologic disposition. *J Clin Psychiatry* (1985) 46, 14–19.
4. Achamallah NS. Visual hallucinations after combining fluoxetine and dextromethorphan. *Am J Psychiatry* (1992) 149, 1406.
5. Otton SV, Wu D, Joffe RT, Cheung SW, Sellers EM. Inhibition by fluoxetine of cytochrome P450 2D6 activity. *Clin Pharmacol Ther* (1993) 53, 401–9.
6. Brøsen K, Skjelbo E. Fluoxetine and norfluoxetine are potent inhibitors of P450IID6 — the source of the sparteine/debrisoquine oxidation polymorphism. *Br J Clin Pharmacol* (1991) 32, 136–7.
7. Prozac (Fluoxetine). Eli Lilly and Company Ltd. Summary of product characteristics, July 2000.
8. Lear J, Burden AC. Fluoxetine side-effects mimicking hypoglycaemia. *Lancet* (1992) 339, 1296.
9. Armstrong TSH, Martin PD. Propofol, fluoxetine and spontaneous movement. *Anaesthesia* (1997) 52, 809–10.
10. Walters AM. Sympathomimetic-fluoxetine interaction. *J Am Acad Child Adolesc Psychiatry* (1992) 31, 565–6.
11. Barrett J, Meehan O, Fahy T. SSRI and sympathomimetic interaction. *Br J Psychiatry* (1996) 168, 253.
12. Glue P. SSRI and sympathomimetic interaction. *Br J Psychiatry* (1996) 168, 653.

Fluoxetine + Monoamine oxidase inhibitors (MAOIs)

Serious and potentially life-threatening reactions (the serotonin syndrome) can develop if fluoxetine and non-selective, irreversible MAOIs are given concurrently, or even sequentially if insufficient time is left in between. Phenelzine, tranylcypromine and selegiline have all been implicated, and there are two, possibly three, case reports involving moclobemide. Befloxatone appears not to interact.

Clinical evidence

(a) Phenelzine, Tranylcypromine

A very high incidence (25 to 50%) of adverse effects occurred in 12 patients taking fluoxetine (10 to 100 mg daily) with either **phenelzine** (30 to 60 mg daily) or **tranylcypromine** (10 to 140 mg daily), and in 6 other patients started on either of these MAOIs 10 days or more after stopping the fluoxetine. There were mental changes such as hypomania, racing thoughts, agitation, restlessness and confusion. The physical symptoms included myoclonus, hypertension, tremor, teeth chattering and diarrhoea.[1]

Uncontrollable shivering, teeth chattering, double vision, nausea, confusion, and anxiety developed in a woman given **tranylcypromine** after stopping fluoxetine. The problem resolved within a day of stopping the **tranylcypromine**, and did not recur when fluoxetine was tried again 6 weeks later.[2] Another patient developed feverishness, shivering, tremor and rigidity on the second day of replacing fluoxetine, 60 mg daily, by *Parstelin* (**tranylcypromine** + trifluoperazine).[3] Confusion, agitation and diaphoresis occurred in yet another patient when fluoxetine was stopped and **tranylcypromine** started.[4] Fever, chills, flushes, confusion, abdominal cramping, diarrhoea and other signs of the serotonin syndrome developed in a woman taking 20 mg **tranylcypromine** daily 6 weeks after stopping fluoxetine. Her blood levels of norfluoxetine were still very high (84 ng/ml).[5] The makers of fluoxetine have on record 3 unpublished reports of fatal toxic reactions attributed to the use of **tranylcypromine** after fluoxetine was stopped.[2] Another fatality occurred in a woman on **tranylcypromine**, fluoxetine, tryptophan and thioridazine.[6] A detailed review of cases reported to the makers described 8 acute cases, 7 of them fatal, in patients given fluoxetine with either **tranylcypromine** or **phenelzine**.[7] The serotonin syndrome that developed in a woman when given **tranylcypromine** 24 days after fluoxetine was stopped, lead on to rhabdomyolysis, respiratory compromise and acidosis, culminating in disseminated intravascular coagulation and myoglobinuric renal failure.[8]

(b) Moclobemide, Befloxatone

A placebo-controlled trial in 18 healthy subjects found that the concurrent use of 20 mg fluoxetine and 100 to 600 mg **moclobemide** daily for 9 days gave no evidence of an adverse interaction.[9] Another study in 18 healthy subjects given the same dosages similarly found no evidence of the serotonin syndrome.[10]

A post-marketing analysis found that at least 30 patients switched from fluoxetine to **moclobemide** within a week had experienced no ill-effects.[9,11] In an open study, 31 severely ill patients were given **moclobemide** (35 to 800 mg daily) with SSRIs, including fluoxetine (1 to 40 mg daily), initially using doses of both drugs that were lower than usual starting doses and slowly titrating them upwards. The combination was found to be safe and effective in most patients and there was no evidence of the serotonin syndrome.[12]

An open 6-week study in 50 patients with major depression on fluoxetine (or paroxetine) 20 mg daily to which was added up to 600 mg **moclobemide** daily, indicated that the combination was possibly effective. However, one patient developed symptoms suggesting the toxic serotonin syndrome. Other adverse effects occurred in other patients, the clearest one being insomnia, with dizziness, nausea and headache also occurring frequently. The high rate of adverse events suggests that there may be a clinically significant interaction.[13] Another report describes one woman who developed shivering, trem-

or, coldness, somnolence, restlessness, profound weakness, confusion, loss of appetite and incoordination the day after stopping 20 mg fluoxetine daily and starting 150 mg **moclobemide**. The same thing happened after restarting and stopping the fluoxetine, and then within a few hours of restarting the **moclobemide**.[14] There is a further report of an elderly woman who became agitated and confused, and also presented with a tremor within 3 days of her treatment with fluoxetine being replaced by **moclobemide** without a washout period.[15]

A double-blind study in 41 normal subjects found that when they were given 40 mg fluoxetine daily for 7 days, then 20 mg for 9 days, immediately followed by **befloxatone** (2.5, 5, 10 or 20 mg daily) for 5 days, no unusual adverse reactions occurred and no changes in body temperature, haemodynamics or ECGs were seen.[16]

(c) Selegiline

A woman with Parkinson's disease on **selegiline**, bromocriptine and levodopa-carbidopa was additionally started on 20 mg fluoxetine. Several days later she developed episodes of shivering and sweating in the mid-afternoon which lasted several hours. Her hands became blue, cold and mottled and her blood pressure was elevated (200/120 mmHg). These episodes disappeared when both fluoxetine and **selegiline** were stopped, and did not reappear when the fluoxetine was restarted.[17]

Another similar patient became hyperactive and apparently manic about a month after starting to take **selegiline** and fluoxetine.[17] The makers of fluoxetine are said to know of other cases of interaction.[18] Ataxia, which developed in a woman with Parkinson's disease on multiple therapy, appeared to be related to the concurrent use of fluoxetine and **selegiline**. No other toxic symptoms developed.[19] Another patient on levodopa, carbidopa, bromocriptine, **selegiline** and domperidone developed a probable tonic-clonic seizure and a pseudophaeochromocytoma syndrome (headache, flushes, palpitations, blood pressure 250/130 mmHg) when additionally given 20 mg fluoxetine daily.[20] A possible serotonin syndrome in one patient is described elsewhere.[21] These reports contrast with a series of 23 patients with parkinsonism, who received both **selegiline** and fluoxetine without the development of any serious side-effects.[22]

Mechanism

Not fully understood. The symptoms seen appear to be consistent with the serotonin-syndrome which is typified by CNS irritability, increased muscle tone, shivering, altered consciousness and myoclonus. Toxicity of this kind has been seen in patients on fluoxetine within a few days of starting additional treatment with Tryptophan, which is a precursor of serotonin (see 'Fluoxetine + Tryptophan', p.827). A not dissimilar reaction has been seen with phenelzine and tryptophan (see 'Monoamine oxidase inhibitors (MAOIs) + Tryptophan', p.683).

Importance and management

The interactions of the **older, non-selective, irreversible MAOIs** (phenelzine, tranylcypromine, etc.) and fluoxetine are established but of uncertain incidence. Because of the serious nature of the reactions, the concurrent use of these MAOIs with fluoxetine should be avoided, and sequential use should only be undertaken with great care. The makers of fluoxetine recommend that (a) five weeks should elapse between stopping the fluoxetine and starting the MAOI because the effects of fluoxetine are very persistent, and (b) two weeks between stopping an MAOI and starting fluoxetine.[23] Clonazepam has been successfully used to alleviate myoclonus, and 10 mg nifedipine to correct hypertension.[1] Other treatment has included the use of diazepam, midazolam, pancuronium, phenytoin and cooling.[3] Despite these warnings, one brief report describes the successful and apparently uneventful concurrent use of fluoxetine and **isocarboxazid** in two patients. What is not entirely clear is whether these two do not interact, or whether it was possible to combine them because very low doses were used initially, with a gradual incremental dosage increase.[24,25]

Moclobemide a selective reversible inhibitor of MAO-A, can be given safely with fluoxetine in most patients but the need to manage concurrent use with considerable care has been emphasised.[13,26] A report originating from the makers of moclobemide says that "... after discontinuation of fluoxetine therapy, moclobemide treatment can be started immediately." However, the two (possibly three) cases of serotonin syndrome cited[13-15] suggest that this combination may not be as safe as was originally thought. Good monitoring is clearly needed.

The situation with **selegiline** and fluoxetine is by no means clear cut because they have been used together apparently safely and uneventfully in some patients,[22] and only a few of the cases cited above[17,21] seems to fit the serotonin syndrome. Even so, as the serotonin syndrome is a possibility,[26] it might be prudent to avoid concurrent use unless the outcome can be closely monitored.

1. Feighner JP, Boyer WF, Tyler DL, Neborsky RJ. Adverse consequences of fluoxetine-MAOI combination therapy. *J Clin Psychiatry* (1990) 51, 222–5.
2. Sternbach H. Danger of MAOI therapy after fluoxetine withdrawal. *Lancet* (1988) ii, 850–1.
3. Ooi, TK. The serotonin syndrome. *Anaesthesia* (1991) 46, 507–8.
4. Spiller HA, Morse S, Muir C. Fluoxetine ingestion: A one year retrospective study. *Vet Hum Toxicol* (1990) 32, 153–5.
5. Coplan JD, Gorman JM. Detectable levels of fluoxetine metabolites after discontinuation: an unexpected serotonin syndrome. *Am J Psychiatry* (1993) 150, 837.
6. Kline SS, Mauro LS, Scala-Barnett DM, Zick D. Serotonin syndrome versus neuroleptic malignant syndrome as a cause of death. *Clin Pharm* (1989) 8, 510–14.
7. Beasley CM, Masica DN, Heiligenstein JH, Wheadon DE, Zerbe RL. Possible monoamine oxidase inhibitor — serotonin uptake inhibitor interaction: fluoxetine clinical data and preclinical findings. *J Clin Psychopharmacol* (1993) 13, 312–20.
8. Miller F, Friedman R, Tanenbaum J, Griffin A. Disseminated intravascular coagulation and acute myoglobinuric renal failure: a consequence of the serotoninergic syndrome. *J Clin Psychopharmacol* (1991) 11, 277–9.
9. Dingemanse J. An update of recent moclobemide interaction data. *Int Clin Psychopharmacol* (1993) 7, 167–80.
10. Dingemanse J, Wallnöfer A, Gieschke R, Guentert T, Amrein R. Pharmacokinetic and pharmacodynamic interactions between fluoxetine and moclobemide in the investigation of development of the "serotonin syndrome". *Clin Pharmacol Ther* (1998) 63, 403–13.
11. Dingemanse J, Guentert TW, Moritz E, Eckernas S-A. Pharmacodynamic and pharmacokinetic interactions between fluoxetine and moclobemide. *Clin Pharmacol Ther* (1993) 53, 178.
12. Bakish D, Hooper CL, West DL, Miller C, Blanchard A, Bashir F. Moclobemide and specific serotonin re-uptake inhibitor combination treatment of resistant anxiety and depressive disorders. *Hum Psychopharmacol* (1995) 10, 105–109.
13. Hawley CJ, Quick SJ, Ratnam S, Pattinson HA, McPhee S. Safety and tolerability of combined treatment with moclobemide and SSRIs: a systematic study of 50 patients. *Int Clin Psychopharmacol* (1996) 11, 187–91.
14. Benazzi F. Serotonin syndrome with moclobemide-fluoxetine combination. *Pharmacopsychiatry* (1996) 29, 162.
15. Chan BSH, Graudins A, Whyte IM, Dawson AH, Braitberg G, Duggin GG. Serotonin syndrome resulting from drug interactions. *Med J Aust* (1998) 169, 523–5.
16. Pinquier JL, Caplain H, Durrieu G, Zieleniuk I, Rosenzweig P. Safety and pharmacodynamic study of befloxatone after fluoxetine withdrawal. *Clin Pharmacol Ther* (1998) 63, 187.
17. Suchowersky O, deVries JD. Interaction of fluoxetine and selegiline. *Can J Psychiatry* (1990) 35, 571–2.
18. Doyle MJ (Dista Products). Personal communication (1988).
19. Jermain DM, Hughes PL, Follender AB. Potential fluoxetine-selegiline interaction. *Ann Pharmacother* (1992) 26, 1300.
20. Montastruc JL, Chamontin B, Senard JM, Tran MA, Rascol O, Llau ME, Rascol A. Pseudophaeochromocytoma in parkinsonian patient treated with fluoxetine plus selegiline. *Lancet* (1993) 341, 555.
21. Ritter JL, Alexander B. Retrospective study of selegiline-antidepressant drug interactions and a review of the literature. *Ann Clin Psychiatry* (1997) 9, 7–13.
22. Waters CH. Fluoxetine and selegiline — lack of significant interaction. *Can J Neurol Sci* (1994) 21, 259–61.
23. Prozac (Fluoxetine). Eli Lilly and Company Ltd. Summary of product characteristics, July 2000.
24. Peterson GN. Strategies for fluoxetine-MAOI combination therapy. *J Clin Psychiatry* (1991) 52, 87.
25. Boyer WF, Feighner JP. Reply. *J Clin Psychiatry* (1991) 52, 87,–8.
26. Mitchell PB. Drug interactions of clinical significance with selective serotonin reuptake inhibitors. *Drug Safety* (1997) 17, 390–406.

Fluoxetine + Pentazocine

A man on fluoxetine experienced an adverse excitatory reaction when given a single dose of pentazocine.

Clinical evidence, mechanism, importance and management

A man who had been taking 20 mg fluoxetine daily for 10 days, later increased to 40 mg daily, was given a single 100 mg oral dose of **pentazocine** (*Talwin Nx* containing 50 mg **pentazocine** and 0.5 mg **naloxone**) for a severe headache. Within 30 min he complained of lightheadedness, anxiety, nausea and paraesthesias of the hands. He was diaphoretic, flushed, and ataxic and showed a mild tremor of his arms. His blood pressure was 178/114 mmHg, pulse 62 bpm and respiration 16. He was given 50 mg diphenhydramine intramuscularly

and recovered over the following 4 h. The reasons for this reaction are not understood, but the authors of the report suggest that it may have been due to increased serotonergic activity in the CNS.[1]

The general importance of this possible interaction is uncertain, but the authors of the report advise caution if the use of both drugs is being considered.

1. Hansen TE, Dieter K, Keepers GA. Interaction of fluoxetine and pentazocine. *Am J Psychiatry* (1990) 147, 949–50.

Fluoxetine + Tryptophan

Central and peripheral toxicity developed in five patients on fluoxetine when given tryptophan.

Clinical evidence, mechanism, importance and management

Concurrent use of tryptophan with low doses of fluoxetine (20 mg daily) is said to be tolerated.[1] A more recent placebo-controlled double-blind study involving 30 patients found that fluoxetine 20 mg daily with tryptophan 2 g daily was a safe treatment for depression,[2] but problems have been seen when higher doses of both drugs have been given together. Five patients on fluoxetine (50 to 100 mg daily) for at least three months developed a number of reactions including central toxicity (agitation, restlessness, aggressivity, worsening of obsessive-compulsive disorders) and peripheral toxicity (abdominal cramps, nausea, diarrhoea) within a few days of starting 1 to 4 g **tryptophan** daily. These symptoms disappeared when the **tryptophan** was stopped. Some of the patients had taken **tryptophan** before without problems.

The reason for this reaction is not understood but the authors point out that the symptoms resemble the 'serotonin syndrome' seen in *animals* when serotonin levels are increased, and warn against the concurrent use of **tryptophan** with fluoxetine or other serotonin reuptake inhibitors.[3] Products containing **tryptophan** for the treatment of depression were withdrawn in the USA, UK, and many other countries because of a possible association with the development of an eosinophilia-myalgia syndrome. However, since the syndrome appeared to have been associated with tryptophan from one manufacturer, tryptophan preparations were reintroduced in the UK in 1994 for restricted use.[4]

1. Ciraulo DA, Shader RI. Fluoxetine drug-drug interactions II. *J Clin Psychopharmacol* (1990) 10, 213–17.
2. Levitan RD, Shen J-H, Jindal R, Driver HS, Kennedy SH, Shapiro SM. Preliminary randomized double-blind placebo-controlled trial of tryptophan combined with fluoxetine to treat major depressive disorder: antidepressant and hypnotic effects. *J Psychiatry Neurosci* (2000) 25, 337–46.
3. Steiner W, Fontaine R. Toxic reaction following the combined administration of fluoxetine and L-tryptophan: five case reports. *Biol Psychiatry* (1986) 21, 1067–71.
4. Sweetman SC, editor. Martindale: The complete drug reference. 33rd ed. London: Pharmaceutical Press; 2002. p.311.

Fluvoxamine + Antidepressants

On theoretical grounds an adverse reaction seems possible between fluvoxamine and the irreversible non-selective MAOIs or tryptophan, but moclobemide appears not to interact. Adverse reactions have been reported between fluvoxamine and lithium, but uneventful and beneficial use has also been described.

Clinical evidence, mechanism, importance and management

(a) Lithium

The CSM in the UK said that 19 reports had been received of adverse reactions when fluvoxamine was given with **lithium** (5 reports of convulsions and one of hyperpyrexia).[1] A patient on fluvoxamine became somnolent within a day of starting additional treatment with

lithium and could not stay awake. The [serum] **lithium** level 20 h after the last dose was 0.2 mmol/l. She recovered when both drugs were stopped and she was discharged on lithium alone.[2] A woman on long-term **lithium** treatment was also started on 50 mg fluvoxamine daily, increased to 200 mg daily over 10 days. She gradually developed tremor, difficulties in making fine hand movements, impaired motor co-ordination and hyperreflexia. This was interpreted as a mild form of the serotonin syndrome.[3]

In contrast to these reports, a study in 6 patients found that 750 to 1400 mg **lithium** and 100 to 150 mg fluvoxamine daily (for between 3 and 23 weeks) was safe and effective, and no adverse interaction of any kind occurred.[4] Another study in 6 depressed patients found that **lithium** did not affect the pharmacokinetics of fluvoxamine (100 mg daily) and combined use was more effective than fluvoxamine alone.[5] It would seem therefore that concurrent use can be valuable, but there is a clear need to monitor the outcome so that any problems can be quickly identified.

(b) Monoamine oxidase inhibitors (MAOIs)

The CSM in the UK has warned of possible adverse reactions if fluvoxamine is given with antidepressants such as the **MAOIs**.[1] This seems to be an extrapolation from the serious serotonin syndrome reaction seen with fluoxetine (another serotonin re-uptake inhibitor) and the MAOIs, but as yet there seems to be no direct evidence of a similar interaction involving fluvoxamine and an **MAOI**.

When 13 of 22 normal subjects on 100 mg fluvoxamine for 9 days were additionally given increasing doses (50 to 400 mg daily) of **moclobemide** for 4 days from day 7, no serious adverse reactions occurred. Any adverse events were mild to moderate (some increase in headaches, fatigue, dizziness, all of which may occur with both drugs alone) and there was no evidence of the serious serotonin syndrome.[6,7] An open study in 6 depressed patients given **moclobemide** (225 to 800 mg daily) and fluvoxamine (50 to 200 mg daily) found a marked improvement. Insomnia was the commonest side-effect (treated with trazodone) but none of the patients showed any evidence of the serotonin syndrome.[8] Another comparative 6-week study in 18 patients on both **moclobemide** (600 mg daily) and fluvoxamine (300 mg daily), and another 18 on fluvoxamine alone, found that the combination was more effective and was also safe and well tolerated. Side-effects were minimal.[9] In one study 31 severely ill patients were given **moclobemide** (35 to 800 mg daily) with SSRIs, which included fluvoxamine (5 to 300 mg daily), initially using doses of both drugs which were lower than usual starting doses and gradually titrating them slowly upwards. The combination was found to be safe and effective in most patients and there was no evidence of the serotonin syndrome.[10] However, it needs to be emphasised that **moclobemide** is a reversible and selective inhibitor of MAO-A so that it would certainly be very unwise to assume from its apparent safety with fluvoxamine that the same is true for irreversible non-selective MAOIs.

(c) Tryptophan

A warning by the CSM in the UK about the risks of giving fluvoxamine with **tryptophan** also appears to be an extrapolation from the serious reaction (the serotonin-syndrome) which has been seen with fluoxetine, another serotonin re-uptake inhibitor (see 'Fluoxetine + Tryptophan', p.827).[1] Products containing **tryptophan** for the treatment of depression were withdrawn in the USA, UK and many other countries because of a possible association with the development of an eosinophilia-myalgia syndrome. However, since this syndrome appeared to have been associated with tryptophan from one manufacturer, tryptophan preparations were reintroduced to the UK in 1994 for restricted use.[11]

1. Committee on the Safety of Medicines. Current Problems, May 1989, 26, 3. Correction. Ibid., December 1989, 27, 3.
2. Evans M, Marwick P. Fluvoxamine and lithium: an unusual interaction. *Br J Psychiatry* (1990) 156, 286.
3. Öhman R, Spigset O. Serotonin syndrome induced by fluvoxamine-lithium interaction. *Pharmacopsychiatry* (1993) 26, 263–4.
4. Hendrickx B, Floris M. A controlled pilot study of the combination of fluvoxamine and lithium. *Curr Ther Res* (1991) 49, 106–10.
5. Miljković BR, Pokrajac M, Timotijević I, Varagić V. The influence of lithium on fluvoxamine therapeutic efficacy and pharmacokinetics in depressed patients on combined fluvoxamine-lithium therapy. *Int Clin Psychopharmacol* (1997) 12, 207–12.
6. Dingemanse J. An update of recent moclobemide interaction data. *Int Clin Psychopharmacol* (1993) 7, 167–80.
7. Wallnöfer A, Guentert TW, Eckernäs SA, Dingemanse J. Moclobemide and fluvoxamine co-administration: a prospective study in healthy volunteers to investigate the potential development of the 'serotonin syndrome'. *Hum Psychopharmacol* (1995) 10, 25–31.
8. Joffe RT, Bakish D. Combined SSRI-moclobemide treatment of psychiatric illness. *J Clin Psychiatry* (1994) 55, 24–5.
9. Ebert D, Albert R, May A, Stosiek I, Kaschka W. Combined SSRI-RIMA treatment in refractory depression. Safety data and efficacy. *Psychopharmacology* (1995) 119, 342–4.
10. Bakish D, Hooper CL, West DL, Miller C, Blanchard A, Bashir F. Moclobemide and specific serotonin re-uptake inhibitor combination treatment of resistant anxiety and depressive disorders. *Hum Psychopharmacol* (1995) 10, 105–9.
11. Sweetman SC, editor. Martindale: The complete drug reference. 33rd ed. London: Pharmaceutical Press; 2002. p.311.

Fluvoxamine + Miscellaneous drugs

Warfarin plasma levels can be increased by fluvoxamine and raised INRs and bleeding have been seen in a few cases. An increased INR has also been reported in a patient on fluindione. Preliminary evidence suggests that smokers may possibly need a moderate increase in the dose of fluvoxamine. There is an isolated report of extrapyramidal disorders occurring with concurrent fluvoxamine and metoclopramide. Fluvoxamine has been reported to inhibit the clearance of tolbutamide. No clinically important interactions appear to occur if fluvoxamine is used with propranolol, atenolol, chloral hydrate or benzodiazepines.

Clinical evidence, mechanism, importance and management

(a) Anticoagulants

The concurrent use of fluvoxamine can increase plasma **warfarin** levels by up to 65% and a few cases of bleeding have been described.[1] A world-wide literature search up to 1995 by the makers of fluvoxamine identified only 11 reported drug–drug interactions between **warfarin** and fluvoxamine, all with clinical symptoms which included prolonged prothrombin times.[2] A woman aged 80 on **warfarin**, digoxin and colchicine developed an elevated INR within a week of starting to take fluvoxamine. Both the **warfarin** and fluvoxamine were stopped but her INR rose again when the **warfarin** was restarted and only stabilised 2 weeks after the fluvoxamine was withdrawn.[3] Another isolated report describes a woman anticoagulated for 4 years on **fluindione** whose INR rose to 7.13 (from a normal value of about 2.5) within 13 days of starting to take 100 mg fluvoxamine daily.[4] The reasons for this are not understood.

The general picture therefore appears to be that very occasionally and unpredictably a **warfarin**/fluvoxamine interaction occurs. It can also apparently occur with **fluindione**. Concurrent use need not be avoided but the response should be monitored when fluvoxamine is first added, being alert for the need to decrease the anticoagulant dosage. Information about other anticoagulants seems to be lacking but it would be prudent to follow the same precautions with all of them.

(b) Beta-blockers

Fluvoxamine 100 mg daily raised the plasma levels of **propranolol** (160 mg daily) fivefold in normal subjects, but the heart-slowing effects were only slightly increased (3 bpm). The diastolic pressure following exercise was slightly reduced but the general hypotensive effects remained unaltered.[1] The probable reason is that the fluvoxamine inhibits the activity of the cytochrome P450 isoenzyme concerned with the metabolism of **propranolol**.[5] No changes in plasma levels of **atenolol** were seen but the heart-slowing effects were slightly increased and the hypotensive effects slightly decreased.[1] There would seem to be little reason to avoid the concurrent use of fluvoxamine and these beta-blockers. Information about other beta-blockers appears to be lacking.

(c) Chloral hydrate, benzodiazepines

Fluvoxamine has been found not to interact adversely with **chloral hydrate** or **benzodiazepines**.[1]

(d) Metoclopramide

A 14-year-old-boy receiving fluvoxamine 50 mg daily for anorexia was, after day 7, given concomitant treatment with **metoclopramide** 10 mg daily. On the third day he developed acute movement disorders including acute dystonia, jaw rigidity, horizontal nystagmus, uncontrolled tongue movements and dysarthria. A pharmacokinetic interaction was considered unlikely. Both drugs can cause extrapyramidal reactions by blocking dopamine D_2 receptors in the basal ganglia (**metoclopramide**) or by inhibition of dopamine neurotransmission (fluvoxamine).[6] This is an isolated report, but it highlights the fact that care should be taken if two drugs with the potential to cause the same adverse effect are used together.

(e) Tobacco smoking

A comparative study in 12 **smokers** and 12 non-smokers given single 50 mg oral doses of fluvoxamine found that **smoking** reduced the fluvoxamine AUC and the maximum serum concentrations by 30.5% and 32% respectively.[7,8] What this all means in practice is still uncertain, but there may possibly be the need to raise the dosage of fluvoxamine moderately to accommodate this interaction. More study is needed to assess the clinical importance of this interaction.

(f) Tolbutamide

A study in 14 normal subjects given fluvoxamine 75 or 150 mg daily for 5 days, with a single dose of **tolbutamide** 500 mg on the third day, showed that the clearance of **tolbutamide** and its metabolites (4-hydroxytolbutamide and carboxytolbutamide) were significantly decreased. The probable reason is that fluvoxamine inhibits the cytochrome P450 isoenzyme CYP2C9. The authors suggest careful monitoring if fluvoxamine is added to a regimen that includes drugs metabolised by CYP2C9.[9]

1. Duphar files, quoted by Benfield P and Ward A. Fluvoxamine, a review of its pharmacodynamic and pharmacokinetic properties and therapeutic efficacy in depressive illness. *Drugs* (1986) 32, 313–34.
2. Wagner W, Vause EW. Fluvoxamine. A review of global drug-drug interaction data. *Clin Pharmacokinet* (1995) 29 (Suppl 1), 26–32.
3. Yap KB, Low ST. Interaction of fluvoxamine with warfarin in an elderly woman. *Singapore Med J* (1999) 40, 480–2.
4. Nezelof S, Vandel P, Bonin B. Fluvoxamine interaction with fluindione: a case report. *Therapie* (1997) 52, 608–9.
5. Brøsen K, Skjelbo E, Rasmussen BB, Poulsen HE, Loft S. Fluvoxamine is a potent inhibitor of cytochrome P4501A2. *Biochem Pharmacol* (1993) 45, 1211–14.
6. Palop V, Jimenez MJ, Catalán C, Martínez-Mir I. Acute dystonia with fluvoxamine-metoclopramide. *Ann Pharmacother* (1999) 33, 382.
7. Spigset O, Carleborg L, Hedenmalm K, Dahlqvist R. Effect of cigarette smoking on fluvoxamine pharmacokinetics in humans. *Clin Pharmacol Ther* (1995) 58, 399–403.
8. Spigset O, Carleborg L, Granberg K, Hedenmalm K, Dahlqvist R. Cigarette smoking induces the metabolism of fluvoxamine in man. *Therapie* (1995) 50 (Suppl), 46.
9. Madsen H, Enggaard TP, Hansen LL, Klitgaard NA, Brøsen K. Fluvoxamine inhibits the CYP2C9 catalysed biotransformation of tolbutamide. *Clin Pharmacol Ther* (2001) 69, 41–7.

Maprotiline + Beta-blockers

Maprotiline toxicity attributed to the concurrent use of propranolol has been described in three patients.

Clinical evidence

A patient experienced **maprotiline** toxicity (dizziness, hypotension, dry mouth, blurred vision, etc.) after taking 120 mg **propranolol** daily for two weeks. His trough [serum] **maprotiline** levels had risen by 40%. The [serum] levels fell and the side-effects disappeared when the **propranolol** was withdrawn.[1] A man on 120 mg **propranolol** daily began to experience visual hallucinations and psychomotor agitation within a few days of starting to take 200 mg **maprotiline** daily.[2] Another man on haloperidol, benztropine, triamterene, hydrochlorothiazide and **propranolol** became disorientated, agitated and uncooperative with visual hallucinations and incoherent speech within a week of starting to take 150 mg **maprotiline** daily. These symptoms disappeared when all the drugs were withdrawn. Reintroduction of the antihypertensive drugs with haloperidol and desipramine proved effective and uneventful.[3]

Mechanism

Not understood. A suggested reason is that the propranolol reduces the blood flow to the liver so that the metabolism of the maprotiline is reduced, leading to its accumulation in the body.

Importance and management

Information seems to be limited to the cases cited. The general importance of this interaction is uncertain, but if concurrent use it thought appropriate the outcome should be well monitored. The authors of one of the reports[2] say that simultaneous use is inadvisable. Another tetracyclic antidepressant, mianserin, appears not to interact with propranolol. See Index.

1. Tollefson G, Lesar T. Effect of propranolol on maprotiline clearance. *Am J Psychiatry* (1984) 141, 148–9.
2. Saiz-Ruiz J, Moral L. Delirium induced by association of propranolol and maprotiline. *J Clin Psychopharmacol* (1988) 8, 77–8.
3. Malek-Ahmadi P, Tran T. Propranolol and maprotiline toxic interaction. *Neurobehav Toxicol Teratol* (1985) 7, 203.

Maprotiline + Oral contraceptives or Tobacco smoking

Neither tobacco smoking nor the oral contraceptives affect maprotiline.

Clinical evidence, mechanism, importance and management

A study in women showed that, over a 28-day period, the use of **oral contraceptives** did not significantly affect the steady-state blood levels of **maprotiline** (75 mg nightly), nor was its therapeutic effectiveness changed.[1] **Smoking** also has no effect on **maprotiline** serum levels nor on its effectiveness.[1,2]

1. Luscombe DK. Interaction studies: the influence of age, cigarette smoking and the oral contraceptive on blood concentrations of maprotiline. In 'Depressive Illness — Far Horizons?' McIntyre JNM (ed), Cambridge Med Publ, Northampton 1982, p 61–2.
2. Holman RM. Maprotiline and cigarette smoking: an interaction study: clinical findings. In 'Depressive Illness — Far Horizons?' McIntyre JNM (ed), Cambridge Med Publ, Northampton 1982, p 66–7.

Maprotiline, Mianserin or Trazodone + Sympathomimetics (directly and indirectly-acting)

No adverse interaction would be expected in patients on maprotiline, mianserin or trazodone who are treated with sympathomimetic amines, however a single report describes toxicity in a woman on trazodone when she took pseudoephedrine.

Clinical evidence, mechanism, importance and management

The pressor (increased blood pressure) responses to **tyramine** and **norepinephrine** (**noradrenaline**) in depressed patients remained virtually unchanged after 14 days' treatment with 60 mg **mianserin** daily.[1-4] In 5 normal subjects on **maprotiline** the pressor response to **tyramine** was reduced threefold while the **norepinephrine** response remained unchanged.[5]

Other studies on normal subjects given 50 mg **trazodone** three times a day found that the pressor response to **tyramine** remained unchanged whereas the response to **norepinephrine** was reduced.[6] However an isolated report describes a woman who had been taking 250 mg **trazodone** daily for two years who took two doses of an OTC medicine containing **pseudoephedrine**. Within 6 h she experienced dread, anxiety, panic, confusion, depersonalisation and the sensation that parts of her body were separating. None of these symptoms had been experienced in the past on either preparation alone.[7] The reasons for this reaction are not understood.

The practical importance of these observations is that, unlike the tricyclic antidepressants, no special precautions normally seem necessary if patients on **maprotiline**, **mianserin** or **trazodone** are given **norepinephrine** or other directly-acting sympathomimetics. Similarly, none of the dietary precautions against eating **tyramine**-rich foods or drinks, or the administration of indirectly-acting sympathomimetics such as **phenylpropanolamine** in cough and cold remedies, need to be imposed. However, the isolated report cited indicates that the occasional patient may possibly experience unpleasant adverse effects.

1. Ghose K, Coppen A, Turner P. Autonomic actions and interactions of mianserin hydrochloride (Org GB94) and amitriptyline in patients with depressive illness. *Psychopharmacology* (1976) 49, 201–4.
2. Coppen A, Ghose K, Swade C, Wood K. Effect of mianserin hydrochloride on peripheral uptake mechanisms for noradrenaline and 5-hydroxytryptamine in man. *Br J Clin Pharmacol* (1978) 5, 13S–17S.
3. Ghose K. Studies on the interaction between mianserin and noradrenaline in patients suffering from depressive illness. *Br J Clin Pharmacol* (1977) 4, 712–14.
4. Coppen AJ, Ghose K. Clinical and pharmacological effects of treatment with a new antidepressant. *Arzneimittelforschung* (1976) 26, 1166–7.
5. Briant RH, George CF. The assessment of potential drug interactions with a new tricyclic antidepressant drug. *Br J Clin Pharmacol* (1974) 1, 113–18.
6. Larochelle P, Hamet P, Enjalbert M. Responses to tyramine and norepinephrine after imipramine and trazodone. *Clin Pharmacol Ther* (1979) 26, 24–30.
7. Weddige RL. Possible trazodone-pseudoephedrine toxicity: a case report. *Neurobehav Toxicol Teratol* (1985) 7, 204.

Mianserin + Anticonvulsants

Plasma levels of mianserin can be markedly reduced by the concurrent use of phenytoin, phenobarbital (phenobarbitone) or carbamazepine.

Clinical evidence

A comparative study[1,2] in 6 epileptics and 6 normal subjects showed that **phenytoin** with either **phenobarbital** or **carbamazepine** markedly reduced the plasma levels of single doses of **mianserin**. The mean half-life of **mianserin** was reduced by 75% (from 16.9 to 4.8 h) and the AUC by 86%. Another study in four patients found that **carbamazepine** reduced serum **mianserin** concentrations by 70%.[3]

Mechanism

It seems probable that these anticonvulsants increase the metabolism of mianserin by the liver, thereby increasing its loss from the body.

Importance and management

Information appears to be limited to these studies, but the interaction appears to be established and of clinical importance. Monitor concurrent use and increase the dosage of mianserin as necessary.

1. Nawishy S, Hathway N, Turner P. Interactions of anticonvulsant drugs with mianserin and nomifensine. *Lancet* (1981) ii, 871–2.
2. Richens A, Nawishy S, Trimble M. Antidepressant drugs, convulsions and epilepsy. *Br J Clin Pharmacol* (1983) 15, 295S–298S.
3. Leinonen E, Lillsunde P, Laukkanen V, Ylitalo P. Effects of carbamazepine on serum antidepressant concentrations in psychiatric patients. *J Clin Psychopharmacol* (1991) 11, 313–18.

Mirtazapine + Miscellaneous drugs

The sedative effects of mirtazapine may be increased by alcohol and the benzodiazepines, but pharmacokinetic interactions are unlikely. No lithium carbonate/mirtazapine interaction is reported, but the makers say that two weeks should elapse between taking an MAOI and mirtazapine.

Clinical evidence, mechanism, importance and management

Mirtazapine does not affect the absorption of **alcohol** but it adds to its CNS depressant actions[1] which underlies the maker's advice to avoid concurrent use.[2] The impairment of psychomotor performance and learning caused by **diazepam** is increased by mirtazapine and therefore the makers warn that the sedative effects of benzodiazepines in general may be potentiated[2] although the pharmacokinetics of neither mirtazapine nor **diazepam** are affected.[3] Mirtazapine seems fairly unlikely to cause pharmacokinetic interactions (i.e. by inducing or inhibiting drug metabolising enzymes) because *in vitro* data have shown that it is a very weak inhibitor of cytochromes P450 isoenzymes CYP1A2, CYP2D6 and CYP3A.[2] Twelve normal subjects were given 600 mg **lithium carbonate** or a placebo daily for 10 days and then a single 30 mg oral dose of mirtazapine on day 10. The pharmacokinetics of neither the **lithium carbonate** nor the mirtazapine were altered by concurrent use and psychomotor tests revealed no differences between those taking **lithium** and those taking the placebo.[4] No adverse mirtazapine/**MAOI** interactions have been reported[5] but to be on the safe side the makers say that the concurrent use of mirtazapine and the **MAOIs** should be avoided, and within two weeks of stopping these drugs.[2] This is a general warning which most of the makers of antidepressants issue.

1. Sitsen JMA, Zivkov M. Mirtazapine — clinical profile. *CNS Drugs* (1995) 4 (Suppl 1), 39–48.
2. Zispin (Mirtazapine). Organon Laboratories Limited. Summary of product characteristics, March 2001.
3. Mattila M, Mattila MJ, Vrijmoed-de Vries M, Kuitunen T. Actions and interactions of psychotropic drugs on human performance and mood: single doses of ORG 3770, amitriptyline and diazepam. *Pharmacol Toxicol* (1989) 65, 81–8.
4. Sitsen JMA, Voortman G, Timmer CJ. Pharmacokinetics of mirtazapine and lithium in healthy male subjects. *J Psychopharmacol* (2000) 14, 172–6.
5. Akzo Nobel, Organon Laboratories Ltd. Personal communication, January 1999.

Nefazodone + Antidepressants

An isolated report describes a woman who developed marked and acute hypotension and weakness when her treatment with desipramine, fluoxetine and venlafaxine was replaced by nefazodone. Isolated cases describe the serotonin syndrome in other patients.

Clinical evidence, mechanism, importance and management

(a) Amitriptyline

A woman who had been taking **amitriptyline** 10 mg at night and thioridazine developed the serotonin syndrome after taking half a tablet of nefazodone (dosage unspecified).[1]

(b) Desipramine, Fluoxetine, Venlafaxine

A woman with a one-year history of DSM-IV major depressive disorder and panic disorder was treated with daily doses of **desipramine** (75 mg), **fluoxetine** (20 mg), **venlafaxine** (37.5 mg), clonazepam (3 mg) and valproate (400 mg) with no side-effects except a dry mouth and sexual difficulties.[2] The first three drugs were stopped and replaced by nefazodone 100 mg twice daily started about 12 h later. Within an hour of the first dose she felt very weak and her blood pressure was found to have fallen to only 90/60 mmHg (normally 120/90). On waking the next day she had severe weakness, unsteady gait, a pale, cool and sweaty skin, and paraesthesia. During the day she took two further 100-mg doses of nefazodone and her condition persisted and worsened with continuing hypotension. The nefazodone was discontinued and by the following day the weakness had improved and disappeared over the next few days. Within a week 200 mg nefazodone daily was reintroduced without problems.

It is impossible to pin-point which of the withdrawn antidepressants interacted with the nefazodone, and why, but the suggestion is that inhibition by **fluoxetine** of the cytochrome P450 isoenzymes CYP2D6 and CYP3A3/4 resulted in elevated nefazodone levels, leading to weakness and hypotension, which was possibly exacerbated by the alpha adrenergic receptor blockade caused by the **desipramine**. No firm conclusions can be drawn from this case because of the cocktail of drugs involved, but it serves to illustrate the importance of ensuring a reasonable wash-out period when potent drugs of this kind are added or withdrawn.

(c) Paroxetine

A woman was withdrawn from nefazodone after 6 months, tapered over the last fortnight to 75 mg 12-hourly. Within a day she started **paroxetine** 20 mg daily and valproic acid, and was admitted the next day with muscle rigidity, uncoordinated muscle tremors, flailing arms and twitching legs, diaphoresis and agitation. This was identified as the serotonin syndrome. Rechallenge with **paroxetine** 7 days later was uneventful.[3]

(d) Trazodone

A woman receiving irbesartan for hypertension was also treated for depression with nefazodone at an initial dosage of 200 mg daily, followed by 400 mg daily for about 5 weeks. Four days after the dose was increased to 500 mg daily, and **trazodone** 25 to 50 mg daily also added as a hypnotic, she was admitted to hospital with a blood pressure of 240/120 mmHg. She was confused, had difficulty concentrating and had numbness on the right side of her lips, nose and right-hand fingers, flushed pruritic skin, nausea and loose stools. On examination she was restless, hyperreflexic and diaphoretic. Nefazodone and **trazodone** were discontinued. She recovered after treatment with labetalol, clonidine, amlodipine and increased irbesartan dosage. Although **trazodone** is used as a hypnotic with other serotonergic agents, it is important to be aware that this may lead to the potentially fatal serotonin syndrome.[4]

1. Chan BSH, Graudins A, Whyte IM, Dawson AH, Braitberg G, Duggin GG. Serotonin syndrome resulting from drug interactions. *Med J Aust* (1998) 169, 523–5.
2. Benazzi F. Dangerous interaction with nefazodone added to fluoxetine, desipramine, venlafaxine, valproate and clonazepam combination therapy. *J Psychopharmacol* (1997) 11, 190–1.
3. John L, Perreault MM, Tao T, Blew PG. Serotonin syndrome associated with nefazodone and paroxetine. *Ann Emerg Med* (1997) 29, 287–9.
4. Margolese HC, Chouinard G. Serotonin syndrome from addition of low-dose trazodone to nefazodone. *Am J Psychiatry* (2000) 157, 1022.

Nefazodone + Miscellaneous drugs

Nefazodone appears not to interact adversely with alcohol, cimetidine, phenytoin, propranolol, theophylline or warfarin. The makers issue warnings about possible interactions with haloperidol, lithium and MAOIs but these appear to be largely theoretical.

Clinical evidence, mechanism, importance and management

(a) Alcohol

Nefazodone 400 mg was found not to increase the sedative-hypnotic effects of **alcohol**,[1] but even so the makers of nefazodone say that it would be prudent to avoid concurrent use.[2] It is not clear just why.

(b) Cimetidine

No changes in the steady-state pharmacokinetics of either **cimetidine** or nefazodone were seen in a week long study in 18 normal subjects given 300 mg **cimetidine** four times daily and 200 mg nefazodone 12-hourly. No special precautions would seem to be necessary if both drugs are used concurrently.[3]

(c) Haloperidol

After taking 200 mg nefazodone twice daily for about 7 days to achieve steady-state pharmacokinetics, the AUC of 5 mg **haloperidol** in 12 normal subjects was found to be increased by 36% but the maximum plasma levels of **haloperidol** were unaltered. The pharmacokinetics of the nefazodone were unaltered.[4] The makers advise caution when using these two drugs together[2] but it seems fairly unlikely that the change is enough to be of clinical relevance.

(d) Lithium

The makers say that no untoward effects have been seen when nefazodone and **lithium** were used together, even so they say that caution should be exercised.[2] There appears to be no evidence that an adverse interaction occurs.

(e) Monoamine oxidase inhibitors (MAOIs)

The makers state that nefazodone should not be used in combination with an MAOI or within 2 weeks of discontinuing treatment with an MAOI. Conversely at least one week should be allowed after stopping nefazodone before starting an MAOI.[2] There appears to be no direct clinical or other evidence that an adverse interaction occurs.

(f) Phenytoin

Nefazodone 200 mg twice daily for 7 days had no effect on the pharmacokinetics of single 300-mg doses of **phenytoin** in normal subjects, and no changes in vital signs, ECGs or other physical measurements were seen. There was no evidence that a clinically significant interaction was likely.[5,6]

(g) Propranolol

A study in 18 normal subjects found that 200 mg nefazodone 12-hourly reduced the AUC of 40 mg **propranolol** 12-hourly by 14% and decreased the maximum plasma levels by 29%, but no clinically significant changes in the response to **propranolol** or relevant adverse responses were seen. The pharmacokinetics of the nefazodone were largely unchanged.[7] No special precautions would therefore seem to be necessary.

(h) Theophylline

Nefazodone 200 mg twice daily for 7 days had no effect on the pharmacokinetics or pharmacodynamics of **theophylline** (600 to 1200 mg daily) in patients with chronic obstructive airways disease, nor was there any effect on their FEV_1 values.[8,9] No special precautions would seem necessary if both drugs are used.

(i) Warfarin

In one study, 18 normal subjects stabilised on enough **warfarin** to achieve a prothrombin ratio of 1.2 to 1.5 for 14 days were then additionally given 200 mg nefazodone or placebo 12-hourly for a further 7 days. No clinically significant changes occurred in the plasma **warfarin** levels or in their prothrombin ratios.[10] No special precautions would seem necessary if both drugs are used.

1. Frewer LJ, Lader M. The effects of nefazodone, imipramine and placebo, alone and combined with alcohol, in normal subjects. *Int Clin Psychopharmacol* (1993) 8, 13–20.
2. Dutonin (Nefazodone) Bristol-Myers Squibb Pharmaceuticals Ltd. Summary of product characteristics, January 2000.
3. Barbhaiya RH, Shukla UA, Greene DS. Lack of interaction between nefazodone and cimetidine: a steady state pharmacokinetic study in humans. *Br J Clin Pharmacol* (1995) 40, 161–5.
4. Barbhaiya RH, Shukla UA, Greene DS, Breuel H-P, Midha KK. Investigation of pharmacokinetic and pharmacodynamic interactions after coadministration of nefazodone and haloperidol. *J Clin Psychopharmacol* (1996) 16, 26–34.
5. Langenbacher KM, Marino MR, Hammett JL, Nichola P, Uderman HD. Nefazodone (N) does not affect the single dose pharmacokinetics (PK) of phenytoin (P). *J Clin Pharmacol* (1996) 36, 850.
6. Marino MR, Langenbacher KM, Hammett JL, Nichola P, Uderman HD. The effect of nefazodone on the single-dose pharmacokinetics of phenytoin in healthy male subjects. *J Clin Psychopharmacol* (1997) 17, 27–33.
7. Salazar DE, Marathe PH, Fulmor IE, Lee JS, Raymond RH, Uderman HD. Pharmacokinetic and pharmacodynamic evaluation during coadministration of nefazodone and propranolol in healthy men. *J Clin Pharmacol* (1995) 35, 1109–18.
8. Dockens R, Shukla U, Roberts D, Greene R, Barbhaiya R. A placebo controlled crossover study of the effect of nefazodone on the pharmacokinetic and pharmacodynamic responses to theophylline in patients with chronic obstructive pulmonary disease. *Pharm Res* (1993) 10 (10 Suppl), S-353.
9. Dockens RC, Rapoport D, Roberts D, Greene DS, Barbhaiya RH. Lack of an effect of nefazodone on the pharmacokinetics and pharmacodynamics of theophylline during concurrent administration in patients with chronic obstructive airways disease. *Br J Clin Pharmacol* (1995) 40, 598–601.
10. Salazar DE, Dockens RC, Milbrath RL, Raymond RH, Fulmor E, Chaikin PC, Uderman HD. Pharmacokinetic and pharmacodynamic evaluation of warfarin and nefazodone coadministration in healthy subjects. *J Clin Pharmacol* (1995) 35, 730–8.

Paroxetine + Dextromethorphan

Two reports describe the development of a serotonin-like syndrome in two patients on paroxetine after taking OTC cold remedies containing dextromethorphan.

Clinical evidence

A man with multiple medical problems was admitted to hospital as an emergency, mainly because of vomiting blood. He was taking diazepam, diltiazem, glyceryl trinitrate, **paroxetine**, piroxicam, ranitidine and ticlopidine. Four days previously he had begun to take *Nyquil*, an OTC remedy for colds, containing **dextromethorphan**, pseudoephedrine, paracetamol (acetaminophen) and doxylamine. After two days he developed shortness of breath, nausea, headache and confusion, and on admittance he was also diaphoretic, tremulous, confused, and showed tachycardia and hypertension. Later he became rigid. The eventual diagnosis was that he was suffering from the serotonin syndrome, attributed to an interaction between **paroxetine** and **dextromethorphan** in the presence of vascular disease. He was treated successfully with 16 mg lorazepam intravenously over 1 h. The bleeding was thought to be from a small prepyloric ulcer.[1]

The authors of this report very briefly describe another patient on **paroxetine** who developed symptoms consistent with the serotonin syndrome within a few hours of taking an OTC cough remedy containing **dextromethorphan** and guaifenesin. She needed intensive care treatment.[2]

Mechanism

Not understood. The symptoms that developed were attributed by the authors of the report to the serotonin syndrome. Inhibition of the cytochrome P450 isoenzyme CYP2D6 has been suggested by them[2] and by others who have commented on this interaction.[3]

Importance and management

These seem to be, so far, the only reports of the serious serotonin syndrome being attributed to an interaction between a selective serotonin re-uptake inhibitor (SSRI) and dextromethorphan. One patient on another SSRI, **fluoxetine**, experienced vivid visual hallucinations after taking dextromethorphan,[4] but other patients have taken both drugs uneventfully[5] (see 'Fluoxetine + Miscellaneous drugs', p.824). The general importance of this apparent interaction is therefore very uncertain. The SSRIs are now very widely prescribed and dextromethorphan is a not uncommon ingredient of OTC remedies. More study is therefore needed to establish this apparent interaction, but in the meantime it would seem prudent for patients on paroxetine to avoid dextromethorphan-containing products because the serotonin syndrome, if it occurs, can be serious. It is not clear whether other SSRIs would interact with dextromethorphan similarly, but it has been predicted that **sertraline** and **fluvoxamine** are less likely to do so.[3] This prediction has been challenged.[2]

1. Skop BP, Finkelstein JA, Mareth TR, Magoon MR, Brown TM. The serotonin syndrome associated with paroxetine, an over-the-counter cold remedy, and vascular disease. *Am J Emerg Med* (1994) 12, 642–4.
2. Skop BP, Brown TM, Mareth TR. The serotonin syndrome associated with paroxetine. *Am J Emerg Med* (1995) 13, 606–7.
3. Harvey AT, Burke M. Comment on: The serotonin syndrome associated with paroxetine, an over-the-counter-cold remedy, and vascular disease. *Am J Emerg Med* (1995) 13, 605–6.
4. Achamallah NS. Visual hallucinations after combining fluoxetine and dextromethorphan. *Am J Psychiatry* (1992) 149, 1406.
5. Otton SV, Wu D, Joffe RT, Cheung SW, Sellers EM. Inhibition by fluoxetine of cytochrome P450 2D6 activity. *Clin Pharmacol Ther* (1993) 53, 401–9.

Paroxetine + Miscellaneous drugs

Paroxetine plasma levels may possibly be increased by cimetidine and reduced by carbamazepine, phenobarbital (phenobarbitone) or phenytoin, but the plasma levels of these anticonvulsants and sodium valproate appear to be unchanged. The dosage of alprazolam and perphenazine may need to be reduced if paroxetine is given. An increased bleeding tendency has been seen with warfarin (possibly also with acenocoumarol (nicoumalone)), but paroxetine appears not to interact to a clinically important extent with aluminium hydroxide, amobarbital (amylobarbitone), diazepam, digoxin, haloperidol, sodium valproate or food. There may possibly be a modest loss of attentiveness with oxazepam and alcohol. The antidepressant effects of paroxetine may be reversed by interferon.

Clinical evidence, mechanism, importance and management

(a) Alcohol

Studies in human subjects[1,2] found that paroxetine alone caused little impairment of a series of psychomotor tests related to car driving, and with **alcohol** the effects were unchanged except for a significant decrease in attentiveness and reaction time.[1] Another study suggested that the **alcohol**-induced sedation was antagonised by paroxetine.[3] No special precautions seem to be necessary.

(b) Aluminium hydroxide

Aludrox (**aluminium hydroxide**) 15 ml twice daily increased the absorption of a single 30-mg dose of paroxetine in normal subjects by about 12% and the maximal plasma concentration by 14%.[4] This is unlikely to be clinically important. No particular precautions would seem to be necessary.

(c) Anticoagulants

Paroxetine 30 mg daily given to subjects on 5 mg **warfarin** daily did not significantly increase their mean prothrombin times, but mild, clinically significant bleeding was seen in 5 out of 27 subjects. Two withdrew from the study because of increased prothrombin times, and another because of haematuria. The disposition of the **warfarin** and the paroxetine remained unchanged.[5] Four patients on **warfarin** whose INR was said to have increased by an average of 3 points (increases of nearly 100% in some cases) associated with the use of paroxetine and sertraline are very briefly described in one report.[6] A single case report describes severe bleeding (abdominal haematoma) in a patient on **acenocoumarol (nicoumalone)** and paroxetine when given phenytoin, but it is by no means clear whether the paroxetine had any part to play in what happened (see 'Phenytoin + Anticoagulants', p.340).[7] All of this preliminary information suggests that the response should be well monitored if paroxetine is added to established treatment with any oral anticoagulant, being alert for the need to reduce the anticoagulant dosage.

(d) Anticonvulsants

Phenobarbital 100 mg once daily for 14 days given to 10 normal subjects caused paroxetine AUC reductions of 10 to 86% in 6 subjects, but the mean values were unaltered. One subject showed a 56% increase.[8] Sixteen days' treatment with 30 mg paroxetine daily in 20 epileptics caused no changes in the plasma levels or therapeutic effects of **carbamazepine**, **phenytoin** or **sodium valproate**. Steady-state paroxetine plasma levels were lower in those taking **phenytoin** (16 nanograms/ml) than in those on **carbamazepine** (27 nanograms/ml) or **sodium valproate** (73 nanograms/ml).[9] A possible explanation is that **phenobarbital**, **phenytoin** and **carbamazepine** (well recognised enzyme inducing agents) increase the metabolism and loss of paroxetine from the body. Although there seems to be little correlation between plasma paroxetine levels and its efficacy, be alert for the need to increase its dosage if any of these anticonvulsants is given.

(e) Other Barbiturates

The sedative effects and impairment of psychomotor performance caused by 100 mg **amobarbital (amylobarbitone)** were not increased by 30 mg paroxetine.[1] An isolated report describes a spontaneous tonic-clonic seizure in a woman on paroxetine immediately after **methohexital (methohexitone)** and before electrical stimulation in the course of an ECT series. Previous ECTs under **methohexital** anaesthesia had been uneventful.[10] The general importance of this is uncertain but some caution would seem appropriate. Two cases of hepatitis in young women were considered to be caused by the concomitant use of *Atrium* (a barbiturate complex) and paroxetine, which resulted in increased hepatotoxicity of both drugs.[11]

(f) Benzodiazepines

No important changes in the pharmacokinetics of either paroxetine or **diazepam** were seen when two groups of 12 healthy subjects were given 30 mg paroxetine daily were also given 5 mg **diazepam** three times a day.[5] In another study it was found that paroxetine did not increase the impairment by **oxazepam** of a number of psychomotor tests, but the subjects said that they felt less alert and less capable while taking both drugs.[1] *In vitro* studies using human liver microsomal enzymes have shown that paroxetine inhibits the metabolism of **alprazolam** (inhibition of cytochrome P450 subfamily 3A),[12,13] so that some increased **alprazolam** effects and side-effects would be expected if both drugs are used concurrently. An isolated report describes worsening anxiety, agitation, mild abdominal cramps and diaphoresis in a woman on paroxetine, shortly after taking a tablet of **clonazepam** (dosage not stated). This toxic response was suggested as being the serotonin syndrome, although in fact many of the usual signs were absent and moreover **clonazepam** has actually been used to treat the myoclonus which occurs in the serotonin syndrome. She was effectively treated with **lorazepam**.[14]

There seem to be no strong reasons for avoiding the concurrent use of paroxetine and the benzodiazepines, but good monitoring would be a prudent precaution.

(g) Cimetidine

Cimetidine 200 mg four times daily for 8 days did not affect the mean pharmacokinetic values or bioavailability of single 30 mg doses of paroxetine in 10 normal subjects. However 2 subjects showed AUC increases of 55% and 81% respectively while on **cimetidine** and 4 others also showed some increases.[8] Another study in 11 subjects found that 300 mg **cimetidine** three times a day increased the AUC of a single 30-mg dose of paroxetine by 50%.[5] A likely reason is that **cimetidine** (a known enzyme inhibitor) reduces the metabolism of the paroxetine and its loss from the body, thereby increasing its serum levels. Monitor concurrent use and reduce the paroxetine dosage if necessary.

(h) Digoxin

No important changes in the pharmacokinetics of either paroxetine or **digoxin** were seen when two groups of 10 and 13 subjects were given 30 mg paroxetine and 0.25 mg **digoxin** daily.[5] No special precautions would seem to be needed.

(i) Food and Drink

A study in normal subjects found that paroxetine was not markedly changed by the concurrent ingestion of **food**. A 40% reduction in absorption was seen when taken with 1 litre of **milk**, but few people are likely to drink such a large amount regularly.[4]

(j) Haloperidol

The sedative effects and impairment of psychomotor performance caused by 3 mg **haloperidol** were not increased by 30 mg paroxetine.[1] No special precautions seem necessary.

(k) Interferon

A 31-year-old woman, whose mood and other depressive symptoms improved during treatment with paroxetine 50 mg daily and trazodone 50 mg at night, was later found to have essential thrombocytopenia. After unsuccessful treatment with dipyridamole, she was given **interferon alfa**, stabilised at 3 million units 3 times weekly. After 3 months her depressive symptoms returned, and worsened over a period of 6 months, in spite of increased doses of trazodone and cognitive therapy. **Interferon alfa** was discontinued and replaced by hydroxycarbamide (hydroxyurea), and then anagrelide. After a good response to a course of ECT, her depressive symptoms were controlled by paroxetine 50 mg daily and trazodone 150 mg at night.[15]

Interferon is associated with a risk of depression, but in this case is appeared to reverse the antidepressant response to paroxetine. It was suggested that this may have been due to the capacity of **interferon** to impair serotonin synthesis, by inducing enzymes that degrade the serotonin precursor tryptophan.

(l) Perphenazine

The effects of a single 0.1 mg/kg oral dose of **perphenazine** on the performance of the Digit Symbol Substitution Test and on Immediate and Delayed Recall were tested after 4, 6, 8 and 10 h later in 5 extensive metabolisers. The tests were then repeated after also taking 20 mg paroxetine daily for 10 days. The scores for these tests were worsened by the **perphenazine** when compared with a placebo and further worsened by the presence of the paroxetine. In addition to oversedation and impairment of the performance of psychomotor tests and memory, 2 of the subjects developed akathisia 10 h after taking both drugs. The AUC of the perphenazine was increased sevenfold and the maximum plasma levels sixfold.[16,17]

These results clearly demonstrated that the CNS side-effects of **perphenazine** are considerably increased by the paroxetine, almost certainly because the metabolism of the **perphenazine** by cytochrome P450 isoenzyme CYP2D6 is inhibited by the paroxetine.[16,17] This study therefore suggests that if these two drugs are given concurrently the dosage of the **perphenazine** should be reduced. More study is needed to confirm this interaction and to quantify the dosage reduction needed but the increases in AUC and maximum plasma levels suggest that very considerable reductions will be needed.

1. Cooper SM, Jackson D, Loudon JM, McClelland GR, Raptopoulos P. The psychomotor effects of paroxetine alone and in combination with haloperidol, amylobarbitone, oxazepam, or alcohol. *Acta Psychiatr Scand* (1989) 80 (Suppl 350), 53–5.
2. Hindmarch I, Harrison C. The effects of paroxetine and other antidepressants in combination with alcohol on psychomotor activity related to car driving. *Acta Psychiatr Scand* (1989) 80 (Suppl 350), 45.
3. Kerr JS, Fairweather DB, Mahendran R, Hindmarch I. The effects of paroxetine, alone and in combination with alcohol on psychomotor performance and cognitive function in the elderly. *Int Clin Psychopharmacol* (1992) 7, 101–8.
4. Greb WH, Brett MA, Buscher G, Dierdorf H-D, von Schrader HW, Wolf D, Mellows G, Zussman BD. Absorption of paroxetine under various dietary conditions and following antacid intake. *Acta Psychiatr Scand* (1989) 80 (Suppl 350), 99–101.
5. Bannister SJ, Houser VP, Hulse JD, Kisicki JC, Rasmussen JGC. Evaluation of the potential for interactions of paroxetine with diazepam, cimetidine, warfarin, and digoxin. *Acta Psychiatr Scand* (1989) 80 (Suppl 350), 102–6.
6. Askinazi C. SSRI treatment of depression with comorbid cardiac disease. *Am J Psychiatry* (1996) 153, 135–6.
7. Abad-Santos F, Carcas AJ, Capitán CF, Frias J. Case report. Retroperitoneal haematoma in a patient treated with acenocoumarol, phenytoin and paroxetine. *Clin Lab Haematol* (1995) 17, 195–7.
8. Greb WH, Buscher G, Dierdorf H-D, Köster FE, Wolf D, Mellows G. The effect of liver enzyme inhibition by cimetidine and enzyme induction by phenobarbitone on the pharmacokinetics of paroxetine. *Acta Psychiatr Scand* (1989) 80 (Suppl 350), 95–8.
9. Andersen BB, Mikkelsen M, Versterager A, Dam M, Kristensen HB, Pedersen B, Lund J, Mengel H. No influence of the antidepressant paroxetine on carbamazepine, valproate and phenytoin. *Epilepsy Res* (1991) 10, 201–4.
10. Folkerts H. Spontaneous seizure after concurrent use of methohexital anesthesia for electroconvulsive therapy and paroxetine: a case report. *J Nerv Ment Dis* (1995) 183, 115–16.
11. Cadranel J-F, Di Martino V, Cazier A, Pras V, Bachmeyer C, Olympio P, Gonzenbach A, Mofredj A, Coutarel P, Devergie B, Biour M. Atrium and paroxetine-related severe hepatitis. *J Clin Gastroenterol* (1999) 28, 52–5.
12. Greenblatt DJ, von Moltke LL, Harmatz JS, Ciraulo DA, Shader RI. Alprazolam pharmacokinetics, metabolism, and plasma levels: clinical implications. *J Clin Psychiatry* (1993) 54 (Suppl), 4–11.
13. von Moltke LL, Greenblatt DJ, Court MH, Duan SX, Harmatz JS, Shader RI. Inhibition of alprazolam and desipramine hydroxylation *in vitro* by paroxetine and fluvoxamine: Comparison with other selective serotonin reuptake inhibitor antidepressants. *J Clin Psychopharmacol* (1995) 15, 125–31.
14. Rella JG, Hoffman RS. Possible serotonin syndrome from paroxetine and clonazepam. *Clin Toxicol* (1998) 36, 257–8.
15. McAllister-Williams RH, Young AH, Menkes DB. Antidepressant response reversed by interferon. *Br J Psychiatry* (2000) 176, 93.
16. Özdemir V, Herrmann N, Walker S, Kalow W, Naranjo CA. Paroxetine potentiates CNS side effects of perphenazine. *Clin Pharmacol Ther* (1996) 59, 188.
17. Özdemir V, Naranjo CA, Herrmann N, Reed K, Sellers EM, Kalow W. Paroxetine potentiates the central nervous system side effects of perphenazine: contribution of cytochrome P4502D6 inhibition in vivo. *Clin Pharmacol Ther* (1997) 62, 334–47.

Paroxetine or Sertraline + Moclobemide

Preliminary evidence suggests that paroxetine and sertraline do not normally interact adversely with moclobemide to cause the serotonin syndrome and the combinations can be therapeutically valuable, but good monitoring is advised.

Clinical evidence, mechanism, importance and management

In one study, 31 severely ill patients were given **moclobemide** (35 to 800 mg daily) with selective serotonin re-uptake inhibitors (SSRIs), which included **paroxetine** (5 to 20 mg daily) and **sertraline** (25 to 100 mg daily), initially using lower-than-usual starting doses of both drugs and then gradually titrating them slowly upwards. The other SSRIs used were fluoxetine and fluvoxamine (see also 'Fluoxetine + Monoamine oxidase inhibitors', p.826 and 'Fluvoxamine + Antidepressants', p.827). These combinations were found to be safe and effective in most patients and there was no evidence of the serotonin syndrome.[1] An open study in 5 depressed patients given **moclobemide** (150 to 600 mg daily) and **sertraline** (25 to 200 mg daily) found improvements ranging from minimal to complete remission. Insomnia was the commonest side-effect (treated with trazodone) but none of the patients showed any evidence of the serotonin syndrome.[2] An open 6-week study in 19 patients with major depression on **paroxetine** (or fluoxetine) 20 mg daily to which was added up to 600 mg **moclobemide** daily, indicated that it was possibly effective.[3] An extension of this study with 50 patients is reported elsewhere.[4] A range of adverse effects occurred in some patients, the clearest one being insomnia, but the serotonin syndrome was not seen.[3,4] The authors of two of these reports emphasise the need to manage the concurrent use of **moclobemide** and SSRIs with care because of the potential risks, and they advise starting with low doses and monitoring well.[3,4]

1. Bakish D, Hooper CL, West DL, Miller C, Blanchard A, Bashir F. Moclobemide and specific serotonin re-uptake inhibitor combination treatment of resistant anxiety and depressive disorders. *Hum Psychopharmacol* (1995) 10, 105–9.
2. Joffe RT, Bakish D. Combined SSRI-moclobemide treatment of psychiatric illness. *J Clin Psychiatry* (1994) 55, 24–5.
3. Hawley CJ, Ratnam S, Pattinson HA, Quick SJ, Echlin D. Safety and tolerability of combined treatment with moclobemide and SSRIs: a preliminary study of 19 patients. *J Psychopharmacol* (1996) 10, 241–5.
4. Hawley CJ, Quick SJ, Ratnam S, Pattinson HA, McPhee S. Safety and tolerability of combined treatment with moclobemide and SSRIs: a systematic study of 50 patients. *Int Clin Psychopharmacol* (1996) 11, 187–91.

Reboxetine + Miscellaneous drugs

Few clinically relevant interactions have yet been identified with reboxetine. Ketoconazole may inhibit the metabolism of reboxetine and the makers advise avoidance of concurrent use with azole antifungals, macrolide antibacterials and fluvoxamine. There is a theoretical possibility that the metabolism of antiarrhythmics, antipsychotic drugs and tricyclic antidepressants could be inhibited by reboxetine, and caution is advised if they are co-prescribed. Reboxetine does not interact with alcohol although the makers advise caution, and no interaction has been seen with the MAOIs. Even so, the makers currently advise avoidance.

Clinical evidence, mechanism, importance and management

Reboxetine appears to be relatively free from adverse drug interactions. Studies with human liver microsomes using concentrations of reboxetine eight times greater than maximum plasma levels found that it has no inhibitory effects on the cytochrome P450 isoenzymes (CYP1A2, CYP2C9, CYP2D6, CYP2E1, CYP3A4) which are responsible for the metabolism of the majority of other drugs.[1] A more recent study[2] in normal subjects found that reboxetine 80 mg daily did not interact with **dextromethorphan** suggesting that there are unlikely to be clinically significant interactions with CYP2D6 substrates. However, the makers state that in high concentrations reboxetine can inhibit CYP3A4 and CYP2D6 *in vitro* and recommend that until further information is available reboxetine should be used with caution with drugs metabolised by either isoenzyme and that have a narrow therapeutic margin, such as **antiarrhythmic drugs, antipsychotics, tricyclic antidepressants**, or **ciclosporin**. The cytochrome P450 isoenzyme CYP2D6 is not thought to be involved in reboxetine metabolism. However, because of the narrow therapeutic margin of reboxetine, any inhibition of its elimination could cause adverse effects. There is little information on the potential for co-prescribed drugs to inhibit the elimination of reboxetine. The makers therefore recommend that drugs known to inhibit drug

metabolising enzymes other than CYP2D6, including **azole antifungals, macrolide antibacterials** and **fluvoxamine**, should not be given with reboxetine.[3] A study in 11 normal subjects found that **ketoconazole** 200 mg daily for 5 days decreased the clearance of single doses of reboxetine 4 mg, taken on the second day. It has been suggested that **ketoconazole**, a potent inhibitor of the cytochrome P450 isoenzyme CYP3A4, had inhibited the metabolism of reboxetine. The adverse effect profile of reboxetine was not altered, but it was concluded that caution should be used and a reduction in reboxetine dosage considered if it is given with **ketoconazole**.[4]

A mild to moderate drowsiness and an orthostatic increase in heart rate has been seen in normal subjects when reboxetine and **lorazepam** were given concurrently, but no pharmacokinetic interaction occurred.[3]

A study in 10 normal subjects found that reboxetine does not effect cognitive or psychomotor function, and there is no interaction with **alcohol**,[5,6] nevertheless the makers say that patients should be cautioned if operating machinery or driving.[3]

A study in 30 normal subjects given reboxetine 4 mg twice daily and fluoxetine 20 mg daily found no significant changes in the pharmacokinetics of either drug.[7] However, no data seem to be available about the concurrent use of reboxetine with **lithium carbonate**, or **MAOIs** and at the moment the makers currently advise the avoidance of fluvoxamine (see above) and **MAOIs** to be on the safe side.[3] They also point out the possibility of hypokalaemia if reboxetine is used with **potassium-depleting diuretics** and cautiously suggest that concurrent use of reboxetine and **ergot derivatives** might result in increased blood pressure although no clinical data are quoted.[3]

1. Dostert P, Benedetti MS, Poggesi I. Review of the pharmacokinetics and metabolism of reboxetine, a selective noradrenaline reuptake inhibitor. *Eur Neuropsychopharmacol* (1997) 7 (Suppl 1), S23–S35.
2. Avenoso A, Facciolá G, Scordo MG, Spina E. No effect of the new antidepressant reboxetine on CYP2D6 activity in healthy volunteers. *Ther Drug Monit* (1999) 21, 577–9.
3. Edronax (Reboxetine). Pharmacia & Upjohn, Summary of product characteristics, December 1997.
4. Herman BD, Fleishaker JC, Brown MT. Ketoconazole inhibits the clearance of the enantiomers of the antidepressant reboxetine in humans. *Clin Pharmacol Ther* (1999) 66, 374–9.
5. Hindmarch I, Herrman W. The effect of reboxetine on EEG, cognitive and psychomotor function in healthy volunteers. Conference on the role of reboxetine, a selective noradrenaline reuptake inhibitor (NARI) in the treatment of depression, International Conference Centre, Geneva, 23 April, 1997, Abstract book p 13–4.
6. Kerr JS, Powell J, Hindmarch I. The effects of reboxetine and amitriptyline, with and without alcohol on cognitive function and psychomotor performance. *Br J Clin Pharmacol* (1996) 42, 239–41.
7. Fleishaker JC, Herman BD, Pearson LK, Ionita A, Mucci M. Evaluation of the potential pharmacokinetic/pharmacodynamic interaction between fluoxetine and reboxetine in healthy volunteers. *Clin Drug Invest* (1999) 18, 141–50.

Selective serotonin re-uptake inhibitors (SSRIs) + Benztropine + Antipsychotics

Seven patients developed delirium when given fluoxetine, paroxetine or sertraline with benztropine in the presence of perphenazine or haloperidol. Other patients remained symptom free.

Clinical evidence, mechanism, importance and management

Five patients became confused and developed delirium when given a neuroleptic, an SSRI (4 on **fluoxetine** and one on **paroxetine**) and **benztropine**. No peripheral anticholinergic toxicity was seen. The delirium developed within 2 days in 2 cases, but took several weeks in another. The authors of the report attributed this to an interaction between the SSRIs and the **benztropine**, speculating that the SSRIs may have inhibited the metabolism of the **benztropine** thereby increasing its toxicity. Alternatively they suggest a possible additive central anticholinergic effect. They also very briefly mention 2 other patients who became delirious when given an un-named antipsychotic and either **sertraline** or **paroxetine** with **benztropine**.[1] It is noteworthy that 4 of the first group of patients were given **perphenazine** and one **haloperidol**,[1] both of which have been involved in additive anticholinergic interactions (see 'Antipsychotics + Anticholinergics', p.692). Another case of delirium associated with the use of **paroxetine** and **benztropine** has been described.[2]

In contrast, another report describes 12 patients on **fluoxetine** and **perphenazine** who also received 1 mg **benztropine** daily without showing signs of delirium.[3,4] The general clinical importance of this interaction is therefore very uncertain indeed, but it would now seem prudent to be alert for evidence of confusion and possible delirium in patients given **fluoxetine**, **paroxetine** or **sertraline** with **benztropine**, particularly if they are also taking other psychotropics that may have anticholinergic actions. The authors of the first report say that they have not seen delirium with combinations of SSRIs (not named) and other anticholinergic drugs such as **biperiden** and **diphenhydramine**.[1]

1. Roth A, Akyol S, Nelson JC. Delirium associated with the combination of a neuroleptic, an SSRI, and benztropine. *J Clin Psychiatry* (1994) 55, 492–5.
2. Armstrong SC, Schweitzer SM. Delirium associated with paroxetine and benztropine combination. *Am J Psychiatry* (1997) 154, 581–2.
3. Rothschild AJ, Samson JA, Bessette MP, Carter-Campbell JT. Efficacy of the combination of fluoxetine and perphenazine in the treatment of psychotic depression. *J Clin Psychiatry* (1993) 54, 338–42.
4. Rothschild AJ. Delirium: an SSRI-benztropine adverse effect? *J Clin Psychiatry* (1995) 56, 537.

Selective serotonin re-uptake inhibitors (SSRIs) + Tramadol

Five reports describe the development of the serotonin syndrome in patients on fluoxetine, paroxetine or sertraline when tramadol was added. Another patient developed hallucinations with tramadol and paroxetine. Other reports suggest that the SSRI/tramadol combination is therapeutically valuable and normally safe.

Clinical evidence

(a) Adverse reactions

(i) Fluoxetine. A woman who had been taking 20 mg **fluoxetine** daily for 3 years developed what was eventually diagnosed as the serotonin syndrome. A month previously she had started to take 50 mg **tramadol** four times daily, increased after a fortnight to 100 mg four times daily. Ten days before hospitalisation she had developed a tremor of the right hand and face, and in hospital she showed agitation, marked facial blepharospasm, some sweating and pyrexia, and stuttering. The symptoms began to subside 7 days after both drugs were stopped, and after 2 months she had recovered fully.[1]

(ii) Paroxetine. A man who had been taking 20 mg **paroxetine** daily for 4 months developed shivering, diaphoresis and myoclonus and became subcomatose within 12 h of taking 100 mg **tramadol**. This was diagnosed as the serotonin syndrome. The **tramadol** was stopped, the **paroxetine** dosage halved and he became conscious within a day. The other symptoms gradually disappeared over the next week.[2] Another report suggests that **tramadol** may have contributed to the development of a fatal serotonin syndrome in a patient also using moclobemide and clomipramine.[3]
A woman aged 78 taking 20 mg **paroxetine** daily developed nausea, diaphoresis and irritability 3 days after starting 50 mg **tramadol** three times a day. The next day she developed muscular weakness and confusion, and was found to have a temperature of 100.8°F and a pulse rate of 110. She recovered when the drugs were withdrawn. Similar symptoms but without an increased temperature occurred in another elderly woman on 10 mg **paroxetine** daily within 2 days of starting 50 mg **tramadol** four times daily. Both women were later able to continue on the **paroxetine** alone without problems.[4]
A tetraparetic patient with chronic pain developed nightmares and hallucinations 56 days after starting treatment with **tramadol**, **paroxetine** and dosulepin (dothiepin) which only stopped when the drugs were withdrawn.[5]

(iii) Sertraline. A 42-year-old woman was admitted to intensive care with atypical chest pain, sinus tachycardia, confusion, psychosis, sundowning, agitation, diaphoresis and tremor. Medications on admission were orciprenaline (metaproterenol), pravastatin, triamcinolone by inhalation, chlorzoxazone, nabumetone, theophylline, naphazoline ophthalmic solution, omeprazole, paracetamol (acetaminophen), terfenadine, **sertraline** and **tramadol**. She was diagnosed as having the serotonin syndrome, attributed to an increase in the dosage of **tramadol** from 150 mg daily to 300 mg daily in increments of 50 mg every 2–3 days, and an increased **sertraline** dosage (original amounts not stated but 100 mg daily when the adverse events developed). The **tramadol** had been started 3 weeks previously and she had been taking the **sertraline** for a year.[6]

(b) Advantageous reactions

6 out of 12 patients with some refractory depression and on a range of SSRI antidepressants (**fluoxetine**, **fluvoxamine**, **nefazodone**, **paroxetine**, **sertraline**) or bupropion showed a 50% or greater reduction in Hamilton Scale scores (i.e. increased control of depression) when concurrently treated with 25 mg **tramadol** three times daily for week 1, followed by 50 mg three times daily for 2 weeks. Sedation and stimulation were the most common side effects.[7] Another report[8] says ". . . we have used the **tramadol** dosing regimen [up to 50 mg 6-hourly] . . . and have achieved high patient acceptance without iatrogenic events secondary to the pharmacotherapy . . . [with] **paroxetine** at 10 mg/day to enhance pain relief, decrease depression, and increase serum levels of **tramadol**."

Mechanism

Not understood. The serotonin syndrome seems to develop unpredictably in a few patients given two or more serotoninergic drugs. See section 4.2.11 in Chapter 1 for a general discussion of the serotonin syndrome.

Importance and management

These five, possibly six cases seem to be the only reports of the serotonin syndrome or other reactions due to an SSRI/tramadol interaction, and they need to be set in the wider context of apparently uneventful and advantageous use in other patients. Even so the makers of tramadol have issued a broad warning about the possibility of an interaction of some kind with these drugs and others which enhance monoaminergic neurotransmission (see 'Tramadol + Miscellaneous drugs', p.89). There would therefore seem to be little reason for totally avoiding the concurrent use of the SSRIs and tramadol but it would clearly be prudent to monitor the outcome closely.

1. Kesavan S, Sobala GM. Serotonin syndrome with fluoxetine plus tramadol. *J R Soc Med* (1999) 92, 474–5.
2. Egberts ACG, ter Borgh J, Brodie-Meijer CCE. Serotonin syndrome attributed to tramadol addition to paroxetine therapy. *Int Clin Psychopharmacol* (1997) 12, 181–2.
3. Hernandez AF, Montero MN, Pla A, Villanueva E. Fatal moclobemide overdose or death caused by serotonin syndrome? *J Forensic Sci* (1995) 40, 128–30.
4. Lantz MS, Buchalter EN, Giambanco V. Serotonin syndrome following the administration of tramadol with paroxetine. *Int J Geriatr Psychiatry* (1998) 13, 343–5.
5. Devulder J, De Laat M, Dumoulin K, Renson A, Rolly G. Nightmares and hallucinations after long term intake of tramadol combined with antidepressants. *Acta Clin Belg* (1996) 51, 184–6.
6. Mason BJ, Blackburn KH. Possible serotonin syndrome associated with tramadol and sertraline coadministration. *Ann Pharmacother* (1997) 31, 175–7.
7. Fanelli J, Montgomery C. Use of the analgesic tramadol in antidepressant potentiation. *Psychopharmacol Bull* (1996) 32, 442.
8. Barkin RL. Alternative dosing for tramadol aids effectiveness. *Formulary* (1995) 30, 542–3.

Serotonin re-uptake inhibitors + St John's wort (Hypericum perforatum)

Four patients on sertraline and one on nefazodone developed symptoms diagnosed as the serotonin syndrome when St John's wort was taken concomitantly. Another patient on St John's wort developed severe sedation after taking a single dose of paroxetine.

Clinical evidence

(a) Lethargy and sedation

A woman who had been taking 40 mg **paroxetine** daily for 8 months stopped taking it and 10 days later started to take 600 mg **St John's wort** powder daily. No problems occurred until the next night when she took a single 20-mg dose of **paroxetine** because she thought it might help her sleep. The following day at noon she was found still to be in bed, arousable but incoherent, groggy and slow moving and almost unable to get out of bed. Two hours later she still complained of nausea, weakness and fatigue, but her vital signs and her mini mental status examinations were normal. Within 24 h she was back to normal.[1]

(b) Serotonin syndrome

Five elderly patients, 4 on **sertraline** and one on **nefazodone**, developed clinically diagnosed serotonin syndrome within 2 to 4 days of starting additional treatment with 300 mg **St John's wort** either two or three times daily. The symptoms included dizziness, nausea, vomiting, headache, anxiety, confusion, restlessness, irritability. Two of them were treated with 4 mg oral cyproheptadine either two or three times daily, and the problems of all of them resolved within a week. Four later resumed treatment with **sertraline** without problems but the other patient did not resume **nefazodone** but continued with the **St John's wort**.[2]

Mechanisms

Not understood. A very brief and undetailed report, which says that the serotonin syndrome has been seen with St John's wort alone,[3] raises the possibility that additive serotonergic effects are the explanation for what occurred in the patients described here.

Importance and management

Information appears to be limited to these reports but these interactions between paroxetine, nefazodone, sertraline and St John's wort would seem to be established. The incidence is not known but it is probably small, nevertheless because of the potential severity of the reaction it would seem prudent to avoid concurrent use. The advice of the CSM in the UK is that St John's wort should be stopped if patients are taking any SSRI (their list also includes **citalopram**, **fluoxetine**, **fluvoxamine**) because of the risk of increased serotonergic effects and an increased incidence of adverse reactions.[4]

1. Gordon JB. SSRIs and St. John's wort: possible toxicity? *Am Fam Physician* (1998) 57, 950–3.
2. Lantz MS, Buchalter E, Giambanco V. St John's wort and antidepressant drug interactions in the elderly. *J Geriatr Psychiatry Neurol* (1999) 12, 7-10.
3. Demott K. St John's wort tied to serotonin syndrome. *Clin Psychiatry News* (1998) 26, 28.
4. Committee on Safety of Medicines (UK). Message from Professor A Breckenridge (Chairman of CSM) and Fact Sheet for Health Care Professionals, 29th February 2000.

Sertraline + Cimetidine

Cimetidine causes a moderate rise in the serum levels of sertraline.

Clinical evidence

In a randomised, two-way crossover study, 12 normal subjects were given single 100 mg oral doses of sertraline after taking either 800 mg **cimetidine** or a placebo at bedtime for seven days. The **cimetidine** increased the sertraline AUC by 50%, it increased the maximum serum sertraline levels by 24%, and increased the half-life by 26%. There was a small increase in sertraline side-effects (not specified) while taking the **cimetidine**.[1]

Mechanism

Not established. The most likely reason is that the cimetidine (a known potent enzyme inhibitor) reduces the metabolism (*N*-dealkylation) of the sertraline so that it is cleared from the body more slowly, and accumulates.

Importance and management

Information seems to be limited to the study cited, but the interaction appears to be established. The increase in sertraline serum levels is only moderate, but it would be prudent to monitor the outcome for excessive side effects (dry mouth, nausea, diarrhoea, dyspepsia, tremor, ejaculatory delay, sweating) if both drugs are used. Reduce the sertraline dosage if necessary. If the suggested mechanism of interaction is true, one of the other H_2-blockers that lack enzyme inhibitory activity, such as **ranitidine** or **famotidine**, might be a non-interacting alternative for cimetidine. This needs confirmation.

1. Invicta Pharmaceuticals. Phase 1 study to assess the potential of cimetidine to alter the disposition of sertraline in normal, healthy male volunteers. Data on file (Study 050-019), 1991.

Sertraline + Erythromycin

An isolated report describes the development of what is thought to be the serotonin syndrome in a 12-year-old boy on sertraline when erythromycin was added. Also see 'Fluoxetine + Macrolide antibacterials', p.824.

Clinical evidence, mechanism, importance and management

A 12-year-old boy with severe obsessive-compulsive disorder and simple phobia, responded, without side effects, to 12.5 mg sertraline daily, titrated over 12 weeks to 37.5 mg daily. He began to feel mildly nervous within 4 days of additionally starting 400 mg **erythromycin** daily for an infection. Over the next 10 days his nervousness grew, culminating in panic, restlessness, irritability, agitation, paraesthesias, tremulousness, decreased concentration and confusion. The symptoms abated within 72 hours of stopping both drugs. The authors of this report attributed what happened to the serotonin syndrome. They postulated that the **erythromycin** (a known and potent inhibitor of cytochrome P450 isoenzyme CYP3A4) reduced the metabolism of the sertraline, thereby raising its serum levels and precipitating this toxicity.[1]

This is an isolated report and its general importance is unknown. Nor is it unequivocally established that this was the serotonin syndrome and not an idiosyncratic reaction, nevertheless this case suggests that it would now be prudent to monitor well if **erythromycin** (or possibly one of the related macrolides such as **clarithromycin**) is added to sertraline. Also see 'Fluoxetine + Macrolide antibacterials', p.824.

1. Lee DO, Lee CD. Serotonin syndrome in a child associated with erythromycin and sertraline. *Pharmacotherapy* (1999) 19, 894-6.

Sertraline + Fluoxetine

An isolated report describes an adverse reaction (hypertension, tachycardia, fever, auditory hallucinations and confusion) in a man when he started sertraline within a day of stopping fluoxetine.

Clinical evidence, mechanism, importance and management

One of 16 ostensibly normal subjects who began 50 mg sertraline daily on the day after stopping two weeks of 20 mg **fluoxetine** daily, rapidly developed hypertension, tachycardia, fever, auditory hallucinations and confusion. Most of these symptoms disappeared 48 h after stopping the sertraline, but the confusion took a week to subside.[1] The other 15 subjects showed no clinically significant adverse effects. This subject was later found to have a history of psychosis which needed treatment so that the picture is a little confused, but the rapid abatement of the symptoms when the sertraline was stopped suggests that these were due either to the sertraline alone, or to an interaction with the residual **fluoxetine**.

It is therefore not clear whether a washout period is needed between these two drugs, but a decision on this will depend on the severity of the depression in the particular patient being treated. The makers of sertraline imply caution when they say that the duration of a washout period when switching from one SSRI to another has not yet been established.[2]

1. Rosenblatt JE, Rosenblatt NC. How long a hiatus between discontinuing fluoxetine and beginning sertraline? *Curr Affect Illness* (1992) 11, 2.
2. Lustral (Sertraline). Pfizer Ltd. Summary of product characteristics, November 2000.

Sertraline + Miscellaneous drugs

An isolated report describes hypomania in a patient on sertraline when given mirtazapine and some preliminary evidence suggests the possibility of a warfarin/sertraline interaction. Sertraline appears not to interact with alcohol, alprazolam, atenolol, clonazepam, diazepam, digoxin, glibenclamide (glyburide) or tolbutamide but concurrent use should be monitored until more experience has been gained in normal clinical situations. The side-effects of lithium (tremor) are possibly increased.

Clinical evidence, mechanism, importance and management

(a) Alcohol

Sertraline (200 mg for nine days) was found not to impair cognitive or psychomotor performance, including simulated car driving, and it also appeared not to increase the effects of **alcohol**.[1] This suggests that no special precautions would seem necessary, even so the makers do not recommend concurrent use.[2]

(b) Benzodiazepines

No clinically relevant effects were found in interaction studies in which sertraline was given with **diazepam**.[1,3] Despite *in vitro* studies using human liver microsomes which showed that sertraline inhibits the metabolism of **alprazolam**[4,5] a pharmacokinetic study in 10 normal subjects found that 50 to 150 mg sertraline daily had no effect on the pharmacokinetics of **alprazolam** although some small decreases in a driving simulation score was seen.[6] The makers of sertraline say that it should not be given with benzodiazepines or other tranquillisers in patients who drive or operate machinery,[2] however a study in 13 subjects given daily doses of 1 mg **clonazepam** with 100 mg sertraline for 10 days found no evidence that the addition of sertraline to **clonazepam** made the subjects more sedated or less able to carry out simple psychometric tests.[7]

(c) Beta-blockers

No changes in the beta-blocking effects of **atenolol** were found in studies in 10 normal subjects given 100 mg sertraline with 50 mg **atenolol**.[1,8] No special precautions would seem to be necessary. There seems to be no information about other beta-blockers.

(d) Digoxin

A 17-day course of sertraline in doses of up to 200 mg daily had no significant effect on the pharmacokinetics of **digoxin** (0.25 mg daily) in 10 normal subjects, with the exception of a small decrease in the time taken to achieve maximum serum levels. Sertraline does not significantly alter steady-state plasma **digoxin** levels nor its renal clearance.[9-11] There would therefore seem to be no good reason for avoiding concurrent use and no special precautions seem necessary.

(e) Hypoglycaemic agents

After taking 200 mg sertraline daily for 22 days the clearance of a single intravenous dose of **tolbutamide** in 25 normal subjects was decreased by 16%.[12] In another study in 11 normal subjects the pharmacokinetics of single 5-mg doses of **glibenclamide** were found to be unaffected by sertraline taken in increasing doses up to 200 mg daily over 15 days. Blood glucose levels were also unchanged.[13]

There would seem to be little reason for avoiding concurrent use, but until more is known it would seem prudent to monitor the outcome.

(f) Lithium

After taking 600 mg **lithium** twice daily for 8 days, a single 100-mg dose of sertraline caused a small but statistically insignificant fall (1.4%) in steady-state serum levels in 8 normal subjects, and a statistically insignificant rise in renal **lithium** excretion (+6.9%). Seven out of the 8 also experienced side effects (mainly tremor and nausea) whereas no side effects were reported in the placebo group.[14-16] Severe priapism occurred in a patient on 500 mg **lithium carbonate** daily within 2 weeks of having the daily dosage of sertraline increased from 50 to 100 mg daily. It was not clear whether this was an interaction or simply a reaction to the increased sertraline dosage. The makers of sertraline advise caution if both drugs are used.[2]

(g) Mirtazapine

A woman with a history of depression on 250 mg sertraline daily was additionally started on 15 mg **mirtazapine** daily because of inadequately controlled depression. Within 4 days she showed hypomanic symptoms and she stopped taking the **mirtazapine**. The hypomania resolved within 3 days but her depression then recurred.[17] The reasons for this toxic reaction are not understood. This is an isolated case and its general importance is not known, but good monitoring is needed if these two drugs are given together.

(h) Warfarin

After taking sertraline in stepwise increasing doses up to 200 mg daily for 22 days, the prothrombin AUC in response to a single 0.75 mg/kg dose of **warfarin** in 6 normal subjects was increased by 7.9%. This was statistically significant, but regarded as too small to be clinically relevant.[18,19] However, another report, which gives very little detail, states that 4 patients on **warfarin** showed INR increases averaging 3 points (increases of nearly 100% in some cases) associated with the use of paroxetine and sertraline.[20] There seems to be no other reports of this possible interaction, but it would now seem prudent to check on prothrombin times if sertraline is added to treatment with **warfarin**. More study of this possible interaction is needed.

1. Warrington SJ. Clinical implications of the pharmacology of sertraline. *Int Clin Psychopharmacol* (1991) 6 (Suppl 2), 11–21.
2. Lustral (Sertraline). Pfizer Ltd. Summary of product characteristics, November 2000.
3. Gardner MJ, Baris BA, Wilner KD, Preskorn SH. Effect of sertraline on the pharmacokinetics and protein binding of diazepam in healthy volunteers. *Clin Pharmacokinet* (1997) 32 (Suppl 1), 43–9.
4. Greenblatt DJ, von Moltke LL, Harmatz JS, Ciraulo DA, Shader RI. Alprazolam pharmacokinetics, metabolism, and plasma levels: clinical implications. *J Clin Psychiatry* (1993) 54 (Suppl), 4–11.
5. von Moltke LL, Greenblatt DJ, Cotreau-Bibbo MM, Harmatz JS, Shader RI. Inhibitors of alprazolam metabolism in vitro: effect of serotonin-reuptake inhibitor antidepressants, ketoconazole and quinidine. *Br J Clin Pharmacol* (1994) 38, 23–31.
6. Hassan PC, Sproule BA, Herrmann N, Reed K, Naranjo CA. Dose-response evaluation of sertraline-alprazolam interaction in humans. *Clin Pharmacol Ther* (1998) 63, 185.
7. Kroboth PD, Bonate PL, Smith RB, Suarez E. Clonazepam (Klonopin) and sertraline (Zoloft): Absence of drug interaction in a multiple dose study. *Clin Pharmacol Ther* (1997), 61, 178.
8. Ziegler MG, Wilner KD. Sertraline does not alter the β-adrenergic blocking activity of atenolol in healthy male volunteers. *J Clin Psychiatry* (1996) 57 (Suppl 1), 12–15.
9. Invicta Pharmaceuticals. A double blind, placebo controlled, parallel group study to investigate the effects of orally administered sertraline on the plasma concentration profile and renal clearance of digoxin. Data on file. (Study 224), 1991.
10. Forster PL, Dewland PM, Muirhead D, Rapeport WG. The effects of sertraline on plasma concentrations and renal clearance of digoxin. *Biol Psychiatry* (1991) 29, 355S.
11. Rapeport WG, Coates PE, Dewland PM, Forster PL. Absence of a sertraline-mediated effect on digoxin pharmacokinetics and electrocardiographic findings. *J Clin Psychiatry* (1996) 57 (Suppl 1), 16–19.
12. Tremaine LM, Wilner KD, Preskorn SH. A study of the potential effect of sertraline on the pharmacokinetics and protein binding of tolbutamide. *Clin Pharmacokinet* (1997) 32 (Suppl 1), 31–6.
13. Invicta Pharmaceuticals. A double blind placebo controlled, multiple dose study to assess potential interaction between oral sertraline (200 mg) and glibenclamide (5 mg) in healthy male volunteers. Data on file (Study 223), 1991.
14. Invicta Pharmaceuticals. Determination of the effects of sertraline on steady state lithium levels and renal clearance of lithium in healthy volunteers. Data on file (Study 017), 1990.
15. Wilner KD, Lazar JD, Von Deutsch DA, Apseloff G, Gerber N. The effects of sertraline on steady-state lithium levels and renal clearance of lithium. *Biol Psychiatry* (1991) 29, 354S.
16. Apseloff G, Wilner KD, von Deutsch DA, Henry EB, Tremaine LM, Gerber N, Lazar JD. Sertraline does not alter steady-state concentrations or renal clearance of lithium in healthy volunteers. *J Clin Pharmacol* (1992) 32, 643–6.
17. Soutullo CA, McElroy SL, Keck PE. Hypomania associated with mirtazapine augmentation of sertraline. *J Clin Psychiatry* (1998) 59, 320.

18. Wilner KD, Lazar JD, Apseloff G, Gerber N, Yurkewick L. The effects of sertraline on the pharmacodynamics of warfarin in healthy volunteers. *Biol Psychiatry* (1991) 29, 354S–355S.

19. Apseloff G, Wilner KD, Gerber N, Tremaine LM. Effect of sertraline on protein binding of warfarin. *Clin Pharmacokinet* (1997) 32 (Suppl 1), 37–42.

20. Askinazi C. SSRI treatment of depression with comorbid cardiac disease. *Am J Psychiatry* (1996) 153, 135–6.

Sertraline + Monoamine oxidase inhibitors (MAOIs)

Four case reports describe the development of severe adverse reactions, one with a fatal outcome, attributed to the serotonin syndrome in patients given sertraline with isocarboxazid, phenelzine or tranylcypromine.

Clinical evidence

A man on **tranylcypromine** and clonazepam was additionally given 25 to 50 mg sertraline daily. Within 4 days he began to experience chills, increasing confusion, sedation, exhaustion, unsteadiness and uncoordination. Other symptoms included impotence, urinary hesitancy and constipation. These problems rapidly resolved when the sertraline was stopped and the **tranylcypromine** dosage reduced from 30 to 20 mg daily.[1]

A woman with a major depressive disorder unresponsive to lithium, thioridazine, doxepin and **phenelzine** was additionally started on 100 mg sertraline daily. Within 3 hours she became semi-comatose, with a temperature of 41°C, a heart rate of 154 bpm and symptoms of rigidity, diaphoresis and shivering. She was treated with diazepam, midazolam, ice-packs and dantrolene.[2] Another woman died from complications following the acute development of the serotonin syndrome after taking just one 100-mg dose of sertraline either with or immediately after stopping a course of **phenelzine**.[3]

A woman stopped taking **isocarboxazid** (20 to 40 mg daily) and 2 days later began to take 50 mg sertraline daily. Within 2 h she suddenly felt dizzy and began violent shaking with myoclonic jerks of her arms and legs. She had impaired gait, loss of coordination, dilated pupils poorly responsive to light, and discomfort and tightness in her back. Her temperature was normal (for her) and she was not diaphoretic. She fully recovered after 24 h, and 3 weeks later began 25 mg sertraline daily without problems.[4]

Mechanism

Not fully established. All of these 4 patients appear to have experienced the serotonin syndrome which has also been seen when other MAOIs and serotonin re-uptake inhibitors have been used together. These particular MAOIs inhibit MAO-A and MAO-B, the former being concerned with the deamination of serotonin. As a result the levels of serotonin in the CNS may rise to toxic proportions.

Importance and management

Direct information about sertraline and these three MAOIs seems to be limited to these reports so that the incidence of this adverse interaction is uncertain, but when set against the background of the severe reactions seen with other serotonin re-uptake inhibitors and MAOIs, these reactions should certainly be taken seriously. The makers say that the concurrent use of sertraline and MAOIs is contraindicated and these drugs should not be taken within two weeks of each other. However, see also 'Selegiline + Sertraline or Paroxetine', p.688.

1. Bhatara VS, Bandettini FC. Possible interaction between sertraline and tranylcypromine. *Clin Pharm* (1993) 12, 222–5.

2. Graber MA, Hoehns TB, Perry PJ. Sertraline-phenelzine interaction: a serotonin syndrome reaction. *Ann Pharmacother* (1994) 28, 732–5.

3. Keltner N. Serotonin syndrome: a case of fatal SSRI/MAOI interaction. *Perspectives in Psychiatric Care* (1994) 30, 26–31.

4. Brannan SK, Talley BJ, Bowden CL. Sertraline and isocarboxazid cause a serotonin syndrome. *J Clin Psychopharmacol* (1994) 14, 144–5.

Tianeptine + Alcohol

Alcohol reduces the absorption of tianeptine and lowered plasma levels by about 30%.

Clinical evidence, mechanism, importance and management

The absorption and peak plasma levels of tianeptine after a single 12.5-mg dose were reduced by about 30% in 12 normal subjects by concurrent **alcohol**. The subjects were given **vodka** diluted in orange juice to give blood alcohol levels between 77 and 64 mg%. The plasma levels of the major metabolite of tianeptine were unchanged.[1] No behavioural studies were done so that the clinical significance of these studies is as yet uncertain.

1. Salvadori C, Ward C, Defrance R, Hopkins R. The pharmacokinetics of the antidepressant tianeptine and its main metabolite in healthy humans — influence of alcohol co-administration. *Fundam Clin Pharmacol* (1990) 4, 115–25.

Trazodone + Haloperidol

Low dose haloperidol is reported not to interact to a clinically relevant extent with trazodone.

Clinical evidence, mechanism, importance and management

Nine depressed patients who had been taking trazodone (150 to 300 mg) at bedtime for 2 to 19 weeks were additionally given 4 mg **haloperidol** daily for a week. Plasma trazodone concentrations were not significantly changed but levels of its metabolite (*m*-chlorophenylpiperazine) were slightly raised (from 78 to 92 ng/ml). This study[1] was done to investigate the way trazodone is metabolised, but it also demonstrated that no clinically relevant pharmacokinetic interaction occurs between these two drugs at these dosages.

1. Mihara K, Otani K, Ishida M, Yasui N, Suzuki A, Ohkubo T, Osanai T, Kaneko S, Sugawara K. Increases in plasma concentration of m-chlorophenylpiperazine, but not trazodone, with low-dose haloperidol. *Ther Drug Monit* (1997) 19, 43–5.

Trazodone + Tryptophan

Concurrent use can effectively control aggression in patients with mental disorders, but a single case report describes the development of anorexia, psychosis and hypomania in one patient.

Clinical evidence, mechanism, importance and management

Trazodone with **tryptophan** can be used to treat aggressive behaviour in patients with dementia, mental retardation and other mental disorders.[1] A single report describes their effective use (100 mg and 500 mg respectively three times weekly) with clonazepam in a mildly mentally retarded patient with schizophrenia and congenital defects, but the patient stopped eating and lost 4.5 kg in three weeks and developed signs of psychosis or hypomania. Soon afterwards she became drowsy and withdrawn. When the drugs were withdrawn the aggressive behaviour restarted, but she responded again to lower doses of trazodone and **tryptophan** although the signs of psychosis reemerged.[2]

1. Wilcock GK, Stevens J, Perkins A. Trazodone/tryptophan for aggressive behaviour. *Lancet* (1987) i, 929–30.

2. Patterson BD, Srisopark MM. Severe anorexia and possible psychosis or hypomania after trazodone-tryptophan treatment of aggression. *Lancet* (1989) i, 1017.

These findings with **cimetidine** confirm those of previous studies.[9,10]

There are case reports of patients taking **imipramine** who developed severe anticholinergic side-effects (dry mouth, urine retention, blurred vision) associated with very marked rises in serum **imipramine** levels when concurrently treated with **cimetidine**.[11,12]

(e) Nortriptyline + Cimetidine

After taking 1200 mg **cimetidine** daily for 2 days, the peak plasma **nortriptyline** levels of 6 normal subjects were not significantly raised, but the AUC was increased by 20%.[9]

A case report describes a patient whose serum **nortriptyline** levels were raised about one-third while taking **cimetidine**.[13] Another patient complained of abdominal pain and distention (but no other anticholinergic side-effects) when treated with **nortriptyline** and **cimetidine**.[14]

Mechanism

Cimetidine is a potent liver enzyme inhibitor which reduces the metabolism of the tricyclic antidepressants and may also reduce the hepatic clearance of these drugs. This results in a rise in their serum levels. Ranitidine does not interact because it is not an enzyme inhibitor.

Importance and management

The interactions with cimetidine are well established, well documented and of clinical importance. The incidence is uncertain but a study with desipramine[4] showed that only 'rapid' hydroxylators demonstrate this interaction so that not all patients will be affected. Those taking amitriptyline, desipramine, doxepin, imipramine or nortriptyline who are given cimetidine should be monitored for evidence of increased toxicity (an excessive increase in mouth dryness, urine retention, blurred vision, constipation, tachycardia, postural hypotension). Other tricyclic antidepressants would be expected to be similarly affected. Ideally the antidepressant plasma levels should be monitored. Reduce the dosage of the antidepressant by 33 to 50% where necessary or replace the cimetidine with ranitidine, which, because it is not an enzyme inhibitor, does not interact with amitriptyline, doxepin or imipramine and would not be expected to interact with other tricyclic antidepressants. Other H$_2$-blockers which do not cause enzyme inhibition include **famotidine** and **nizatidine** and would therefore not be expected to interact with the tricyclic antidepressants.

1. Curry SH, DeVane CL, Wolfe MM. Cimetidine interaction with amitriptyline. *Eur J Clin Pharmacol* (1985) 29, 429–33.
2. Curry SH, DeVane CL, Wolfe MM. Lack of interaction of ranitidine with amitriptyline. *Eur J Clin Pharmacol* (1987) 32, 317–20.
3. Amsterdam JD, Brunswick DJ, Potter L, Kaplan MJ. Cimetidine-induced alterations in desipramine plasma concentrations. *Psychopharmacology* (1984) 83, 373–5.
4. Steiner E, Spina E. Differences in the inhibitory effect of cimetidine on desipramine metabolism between rapid and slow debrisoquin hydroxylators. *Clin Pharmacol Ther* (1987) 42, 278–82.
5. Abernethy DR, Todd EL. Doxepin-cimetidine interaction: increased doxepin bioavailability during cimetidine treatment. *J Clin Psychopharmacol* (1986) 6, 8–12.
6. Sutherland DL, Remillard AJ, Haight KR, Brown MA, Old L. The influence of cimetidine versus ranitidine on doxepin pharmacokinetics. *Eur J Clin Pharmacol* (1987) 32, 159–64.
7. Brown MA, Haight KR, McKay G. Cimetidine-doxepin interaction. *J Clin Psychopharmacol* (1985) 5, 245–7.
8. Wells BG, Pieper JA, Self TH, Stewart CF, Waldon SL, Bobo L, Warner C. The effect of ranitidine and cimetidine on imipramine disposition. *Eur J Clin Pharmacol* (1986) 31, 285–90.
9. Henauer SA, Hollister LE. Cimetidine interaction with imipramine and nortriptyline. *Clin Pharmacol Ther* (1984) 35, 183–7.
10. Abernethy DR, Greenblatt DJ, Shader RI. Imipramine-cimetidine interaction: impairment of clearance and enhanced absolute bioavailability. *J Pharmacol Exp Ther* (1984) 229, 702–705.
11. Shapiro PA. Cimetidine-imipramine interaction: case report and comments. *Am J Psychiatry* (1984) 141, 152.
12. Miller DD, Macklin M. Cimetidine-imipramine interaction: a case report. *Am J Psychiatry* (1983) 140, 351–2.
13. Miller DD, Macklin M. Cimetidine-imipramine interaction: case report and comments. Reply. *Am J Psychiatry* (1984) 141, 153.
14. Lerro FA. Abdominal distention syndrome in a patient receiving cimetidine-nortriptyline therapy. *J Med Soc New Jers* (1983) 80, 631–2.

Tricyclic antidepressants + Colestyramine

Colestyramine causes a moderate fall in the plasma levels of imipramine. *In vitro* evidence suggests that amitriptyline, desipramine and nortriptyline probably interact like imipramine. One patient controlled on doxepin who had an unusual gut pathology became depressed again when colestyramine was added.

Clinical evidence

Six depressed patients were treated with 75 to 150 mg **imipramine** twice daily. When 4 g **colestyramine** three times daily was added for 5 days, their plasma **imipramine** levels fell by an average of 23% (range 11 to 30%) and their plasma **desipramine** levels fell but this was less consistent and said not to be statistically significant. The effect of these reduced levels on the control of the depression was not assessed.[1]

A man whose depression was controlled with **doxepin** relapsed within a week of starting to take 6 g **colestyramine** twice daily. Within 3 weeks of increasing the dosage separation of the two drugs from 4 to 6 h his combined serum antidepressant (i.e. **doxepin** plus *n*-desmethyldoxepin) levels had risen from 39 to 81 ng/ml and his depression had improved. Reducing the **colestyramine** dosage to a single 6 g dose daily, separated from the **doxepin** by 15 h, resulted in a further rise in his serum antidepressant levels to 117 ng/ml accompanied by relief of his depression.[2]

Mechanism

It seems almost certain that these tricyclics become bound to the colestyramine (an anion-exchange resin) within the gut, thereby reducing their absorption. An *in vitro* study[3] with simulated gastric fluid (1.2 mol/l HCl) found an approximately 79 to 90% binding at pH 1 with amitriptyline, desipramine, doxepin, imipramine and nortriptyline, a 36 to 48% binding at pH 4, and a 62 to 76% binding at pH 6.5. In an earlier study,[4] binding of these tricyclics at pH 1 had ranged from 76 to 100%.

Importance and management

The imipramine/colestyramine interaction is established but of uncertain clinical importance because the fall in the plasma imipramine levels quoted above was only moderate (23%) and the effects were not measured. The single case involving doxepin[2] was unusual because the patient had an abnormal gastrointestinal tract (hemigastrectomy with pyloroplasty and chronic diarrhoea). Nevertheless it would now be prudent to be alert for any evidence of a reduced antidepressant response if colestyramine is given concurrently. A simple way of minimising the admixture of the drugs in the gut is to separate their administration. There seems to be no direct clinical information about other tricyclics but the *in vitro* studies cited in 'Mechanism', which involved amitriptyline, desipramine and nortriptyline, suggest that they also probably interact like imipramine. This needs confirmation.

1. Spina E, Avenoso A, Campo GM, Caputi AP, Perucca E. Decreased plasma concentrations of imipramine and desipramine following cholestyramine intake in depressed patients. *Ther Drug Monit* (1994) 16, 432–4.
2. Geeze DS, Wise MG, Stigelman WH. Doxepin-cholestyramine interaction. *Psychosomatics* (1988) 29, 233–6.
3. Bailey DN. Effect of pH changes and ethanol on the binding of tricyclic antidepressants to cholestyramine in simulated gastric fluid. *Ther Drug Monit* (1992) 14, 343–6.
4. Bailey DN, Coffee JJ, Anderson B, Manoguerra AS. Interactions of tricyclic antidepressants with cholestyramine in vitro. *Ther Drug Monit* (1992) 14, 339–42.

Tricyclic and related antidepressants + Co-trimoxazole

Four patients on tricyclic antidepressants and one on viloxazine relapsed when given co-trimoxazole.

Clinical evidence, mechanism, importance and management

Four patients taking tricyclic antidepressants (**imipramine, clomipramine, dibenzepin**) and one taking **viloxazine** relapsed into depression when they were concurrently treated with **co-trimoxazole (trimethoprim + sulfamethoxazole (sulphamethoxazole))** for 2 to 9 days.[1] The reasons are not known. This seems to be the first and only report of a possible interaction between these drugs so that its general importance is very uncertain, but it would now seem prudent to monitor the outcome of concurrent use.

1. Brion S, Orssaud E, Chevalier JF, Plas J, Waroquaux O. Interaction entre le cotrimoxazole et les antidépresseurs. *L'Encephale* (1987) 13, 123–6.

Tricyclic antidepressants + Dextropropoxyphene (Propoxyphene)

An elderly patient on doxepin experienced increased lethargy and daytime sedation when additionally given dextropropoxyphene. There is some evidence that dextropropoxyphene may cause moderate rises in the serum concentrations of amitriptyline and nortriptyline, possibly accompanied by increased side-effects.

Clinical evidence

An elderly man on 150 mg **doxepin** daily developed lethargy and daytime sedation when he started to take 65 mg **dextropropoxyphene** every 6 h. His plasma **doxepin** levels rose by almost 150% (from 20 to 48.5 ng/ml) and desmethyldoxepin levels were similarly increased (from 8.8 to 20.7 ng/ml).[1]

The serum **nortriptyline** levels of 10 patients were found to be 16% higher while taking **dextropropoxyphene**. The concentration/dose ratio in 12 patients was raised from 2.57 to 3.04 nmol/mg/day when compared with other patients on **nortriptyline** alone.[2] With **amitriptyline** the concentration/dose ratio was raised from 210 to 275 nmol/mg/day.[2] Fifteen patients with rheumatoid arthritis given small doses of **amitriptyline** (25 mg) and **dextropropoxyphene** (up to 65 mg three times daily) experienced some drowsiness and mental slowness. They complained of being clumsier and had more pain, but these effects were said to be mild.[3]

Mechanism

The available evidence suggests that dextropropoxyphene inhibits liver metabolism of other drugs (e.g. phenazone (antipyrine)[1]) by inhibiting the activity of the cytochrome P450 isoenzyme CYP2D6, and as a result the serum levels of the tricyclic antidepressants rise.

Importance and management

The general clinical significance of these interactions is uncertain but be alert for any evidence of increased CNS depression and increased tricyclic antidepressant side-effects if dextropropoxyphene is added. In this context it is worth noting that one report found that the incidence of hip fractures in the elderly was found to be increased by a factor of 1.6 in those taking dextropropoxyphene, and further increased to 2.6 when antidepressants, benzodiazepines or neuroleptics were added,[4] suggesting that combined use makes patients drowsier and clumsier and therefore more accident-prone. Information about other tricyclics appears to be lacking.

1. Abernethy DR, Greenblatt DJ, Steel K. Propoxyphene inhibition of doxepin and antipyrine metabolism. *Clin Pharmacol Ther* (1982) 31, 199.
2. Jerling M, Bertilsson L, Sjöqvist F. The use of therapeutic drug monitoring data to document kinetic drug interactions: an example with amitriptyline and nortriptyline. *Ther Drug Monit* (1994) 16, 1–12.
3. Saarialho-Kere U, Julkunen H, Mattila MJ, Seppälä T. Psychomotor performance of patients with rheumatoid arthritis: cross-over comparison of dextropropoxyphene, dextropropoxyphene plus amitriptyline, indomethacin and placebo. *Pharmacol Toxicol* (1988) 63, 286–92.
4. Shorr RI, Griffin MR, Daugherty JR, Ray WA. Opioid analgesics and the risk of hip fracture in the elderly: codeine and propoxyphene. *J Gerontol* (1992) 47, M111–M115.

Tricyclic antidepressants + Disulfiram

Disulfiram reduces the clearance of imipramine and desipramine from the body. The concurrent use of amitriptyline and disulfiram is reported to cause a therapeutically useful increase in the effects of disulfiram but organic brain syndrome has been seen in two patients.

Clinical evidence, mechanism, importance and management

It has been noted that **amitriptyline** increases the effects of both **disulfiram** and **citrated calcium carbimide** without any increase in side effects,[1] however there is also some evidence that an adverse interaction can occur. A study in two men showed that while taking 500 mg **disulfiram** daily, the AUC of **imipramine** 12.5 mg given intravenously after an overnight fast increased by 32.5 and 26.7% respectively, and of **desipramine** 12.5 mg given intravenously in one subject by 32.3%.[2] Peak plasma levels were also increased. The suggested reason is that the **disulfiram** inhibits the metabolism of the antidepressants by the liver. There is also a report of a man taking **disulfiram** who, when given **amitriptyline**, complained of dizziness, visual and auditory hallucinations, and who became disorientated to person, place and time. A not dissimilar reaction was seen in another patient.[3] Concurrent use should therefore be well monitored for any evidence of toxicity. More study is needed to establish the importance and extent of this interaction.

1. MacCallum WAG. Drug interactions in alcoholism treatment. *Lancet* (1969) i, 313.
2. Ciraulo DA, Barnhill J, Boxenbaum H. Pharmacokinetic interaction of disulfiram and antidepressants. *Am J Psychiatry* (1985) 142, 1373–4.
3. Maany I, Hayashida M, Pfeffer SL, Kron RE. Possible toxic interaction between disulfiram and amitriptyline. *Arch Gen Psychiatry* (1982) 39, 743–4.

Tricyclic antidepressants + Erythromycin, Josamycin or Troleandomycin

Troleandomycin increases the plasma levels of imipramine, and an isolated report suggests that josamycin may possibly increase amitriptyline serum levels. Erythromycin may interact with clomipramine, but was not found to interact with other tricyclic antidepressants.

Clinical evidence, mechanism, importance and management

(a) Amitriptyline + Josamycin

A patient taking **amitriptyline** showed a marked increase in total **amitriptyline/nortriptyline** serum levels after being treated with **josamycin**, enzyme inhibition being the suggested reason, but no toxicity was reported.[1] This is only an isolated case but be alert for any evidence of increased tricyclic side-effects and toxicity if **josamycin** is given.

(b) Desipramine, Imipramine, Doxepin, Nortriptyline, or Clomipramine + Erythromycin

Six days' treatment with 250 mg **erythromycin** four times daily was found not to affect the plasma levels of 8 patients taking tricyclic antidepressants (**desipramine, imipramine, doxepin, nortriptyline**).[2] Behavioural changes have been reported in a 15-year-old patient when **erythromycin** was added to a regimen of **clomipramine** and risperidone.[3] It has been suggested that the effects were due to increased serotonin activity related to increased **clomipramine** concentrations resulting from the inhibition of cytochrome P450 isoenzymes CYP3A3/4 by **erythromycin**.[4] Thus, the patient may have experienced a central serotonin syndrome. The authors of the original report agreed that some of the patients symptoms were compatible with the serotonin syndrome, although mental confusion and autonomic instability were absent.[5] However, caution is recommended with concurrent use of **erythromycin** (and other macrolides) with psychotropic drugs that are metabolised by cytochrome P450 isoenzymes.[3,5]

(c) Desipramine + Troleandomycin (Triacetyloleandomycin)

A study in 9 Chinese men found that when given 250 mg **troleandomycin** daily for 2 days before a single oral dose of **imipramine** 100 mg, the AUC of the **imipramine** was increased by 59% and its oral clearance was reduced by 30%. The reason is thought to be that the **troleandomycin** inhibits the activity of cytochrome P450 isoenzyme CYP3A so that the metabolism of the **imipramine** is reduced.[6] The clinical importance of this interaction is uncertain, but good monitoring is advisable.

1. Sánchez Romero A, Calzado Solaz C. Posible interacción entre josamicina y amitriptilina. *Med Clin* (1992) 98, 279.
2. Amsterdam JD, Maislin G. Effect of erythromycin on tricyclic antidepressant metabolism. *J Clin Psychopharmacol* (1991) 11, 204–6.
3. Fisman S, Reniers D, Diaz P. Erythromycin interaction with risperidone or clomipramine in an adolescent. *J Child Adolesc Psychopharmacol* (1996) 6, 133–8.
4. Oesterheld JR. Erythromycin and clomipramine: Noncompetitive inhibition of demethylation. Reply. *J Child Adolesc Psychopharmacol* (1996) 6, 211–12.
5. Fisman S, Diaz P. Erythromycin and clomipramine: Noncompetitive inhibition of demethylation. Reply. *J Child Adolesc Psychopharmacol* (1996) 6, 213.
6. Wang J-S, Wang W, Xie H-G, Huang S-L, Zhou H-H. Effect of troleandomycin on the pharmacokinetics of imipramine in Chinese: the role of CYP3A. *Br J Clin Pharmacol* (1997) 44, 195–8.

Tricyclic antidepressants + Ethchlorvynol

Transient delirium has been attributed to the concurrent use of amitriptyline and ethchlorvynol,[1] but no details were given and there appear to be no other reports confirming this alleged interaction.

1. Hussar DA. Tabular compilation of drug interactions. *Am J Pharm* (1969) 141, 109–156.

Tricyclic antidepressants + Fenfluramine

A confusing situation: some say that concurrent use is safe and effective while others say that fenfluramine can cause depression and should not be used in patients with depression.

Clinical evidence, mechanism, importance and management

Exacerbation of depression has been seen in some patients given **fenfluramine**[1] and several cases of withdrawal depression have been observed in patients on **amitriptyline** and **fenfluramine**, following episodes of severe depression.[2] The manufacturers say that **fenfluramine** should not be used in patients with a history of depression or while being treated with antidepressants.[3] On the other hand it has also been claimed that **fenfluramine** can be used safely and effectively with tricyclic antidepressants.[4,5] One report describes a rise in the plasma levels of **amitriptyline** when 60 mg **fenfluramine** was given to patients on 150 mg **amitriptyline** daily.[6]

However you should note that **fenfluramine** was withdrawn in 1997 because its use was found to be associated with a high incidence of abnormal echocardiograms indicating abnormal functioning of heart valves.

1. Gaind R. Fenfluramine (Ponderax) in the treatment of obese psychiatric out-patients. *Br J Psychiatry* (1969) 115, 963–4.
2. Harding T. Fenfluramine dependence. *BMJ* (1971) 3, 305.
3. ABPI Data Sheet Compendium, 1998–99 p 1307. Datapharm publications, London.
4. Pinder RM, Brogden RN, Sawyer PR, Speight TM, Avery GS. Fenfluramine: a review of its pharmacological properties and therapeutic efficacy in obesity. *Drugs* (1975) 10, 241–323.
5. Mason EC. Servier Laboratories Ltd. *Personal Communication* (1976).
6. Gunne L-M, Antonijevic S, Jonsson J. Effect of fenfluramine on steady state plasma levels of amitriptyline. *Postgrad Med J* (1975) 51 (Suppl 1), 117.

Tricyclic antidepressants + Fluconazole

Markedly increased serum amitriptyline levels developed in three patients and increased serum nortriptyline levels in another patient when concurrently treated with fluconazole.

Clinical evidence

(a) Amitriptyline

A man with AIDS given 200 mg fluconazole daily and 25 mg (then 50 mg) **amitriptyline** three times a day developed mental changes and visual hallucinations within 3 days. His serum **amitriptyline** levels were found to be 724 ng/ml (therapeutic levels 150 to 250 ng/ml). The confusion resolved within 4 days of stopping the **amitriptyline** when the levels had fallen to 270 ng/ml. Another man with AIDS given **amitriptyline** 50 mg daily showed a smaller rise in **amitriptyline** levels (from 185 to 349 ng/ml) over a 33-day period when given **fluconazole** (loading dose of 200 mg, followed by 100 mg daily). Yet another patient with end-stage renal disease and on peritoneal dialysis and taking 100 mg **amitriptyline** daily showed grossly elevated serum **amitriptyline** levels (1464 ng/ml) and delirium 6 days after starting **fluconazole** (1 g orally initially, then 200 to 400 mg daily).[1]

(b) Nortriptyline

An elderly woman on **nortriptyline** 75 mg daily and other drugs (ciclosporin, morphine, metoclopramide, bumetanide as well an unnamed antibacterial and antifungal) was additionally started on **fluconazole** (loading dose of 200 mg, followed by 100 mg daily). After 13 days concurrent use her trough serum **nortriptyline** levels had risen by 70% (from 149 to 252 ng/ml).[2]

Mechanism

Not understood, but it has been suggested that the fluconazole inhibits cytochrome P450 isoenzymes CYP2C9 and possibly CYP2D6 which are concerned with the metabolism of these tricyclics, and as a result their serum levels rise.[1]

Importance and management

Information about the tricyclic/fluconazole interactions seems to be limited to these two reports, which would suggest that these interactions are uncommon, bearing in mind the widespread use of these drugs. Nevertheless it would now seem prudent to be on the alert for this interaction with any tricyclic antidepressant and fluconazole. More study is needed.

1. Newberry DL, Bass SN, Mbanefo CO. A fluconazole/amitriptyline drug interaction in three male adults. *Clin Infect Dis* (1997) 24, 270–1.
2. Gannon RH, Anderson ML. Fluconazole-nortriptyline drug interaction. *Ann Pharmacother* (1992) 26, 1456–7.

Tricyclic and related antidepressants + Fluoxetine

The serum (or plasma) levels of amitriptyline, clomipramine, desipramine, imipramine and nortriptyline can be markedly increased (two to fourfold or even more) by the concurrent use of fluoxetine. Toxicity may occur unless the tricyclic antidepressant dosage is considerably reduced. This interaction can continue for many days or even weeks after fluoxetine has been withdrawn. Trazodone and fluoxetine have been used concurrently with advantage, but some patients develop increased side-effects.

Clinical evidence

(a) Amitriptyline, Clomipramine, Desipramine, Imipramine and Nortriptyline

Four patients on 300 mg **desipramine**, 150 mg **imipramine** or 100 mg **nortriptyline** daily showed two to fourfold increases in plasma tricyclic antidepressant levels within 1 to 2 weeks of starting 10 to 60 mg **fluoxetine** daily. Two of them developed typical tricyclic antidepressant anticholinergic side-effects (constipation, urinary hesitancy).[1]

A number of other reports and studies clearly confirm that marked increases occur in the serum (or plasma) levels of **amitriptyline**,[2-6] **clomipramine**,[3,7] **desipramine**,[8-18] **imipramine**[3,12-15,19,20] and **nortriptyline**,[10,11,21-23] accompanied by toxicity, if **fluoxetine** is added without reducing the dosage of the tricyclic antidepressant. Delirium and seizures have also been described[13,24] and death attributed to chronic **amitriptyline** intoxication caused by **fluoxetine**.[25] Parkinson-like symptoms developed in a patient on **amitriptyline** and **flupenthixol** when given **fluoxetine**.[26] The pharmacokinetics of **fluoxetine** appear not to be affected by **amitriptyline**.[6]

A migraine-like stroke developed in a woman 48 h after her long-standing therapy with **fluoxetine** 100 mg daily was changed, within 24 h, to **clomipramine** 200 mg daily.[27]

(b) Trazodone

A patient on **trazodone** showed a 31% increase in the antidepressant/dose ratio when given 40 mg **fluoxetine** daily. She experienced sedation and an unstable gait.[1] Five patients out of 16 stopped their medication (25 to 75 mg **trazodone** used for insomnia) because of excessive sedation the next day.[28] Three out of 8 patients had improvement in sleep and depression when given both drugs but the other 5 were either unaffected or had intolerable side effects (headaches, dizziness, daytime sedation, fatigue).[29] Another study in patients found that **fluoxetine** increases plasma **trazodone** levels.[30] However yet another report described advantageous concurrent use in 6 patients without an increase in side effects.[31] A man with traumatic brain injury showed new-onset dysarthria and speech blocking when **fluoxetine** was added to **trazodone**. His speech returned to normal when the **fluoxetine** was stopped.[32]

Mechanism

Fluoxetine reduces the metabolism (oxidation and N-demethylation) of these antidepressants by the liver, involving inhibition of cytochrome P450 isoenzyme CYP2D6, resulting in a reduction in their loss from the body.[33-35] A tenfold reduction in clearance was found in one study.[15]

Importance and management

The interactions of fluoxetine with amitriptyline, clomipramine, desipramine, imipramine and nortriptyline are established and clinically important. Monitor concurrent use (measure plasma levels), be alert for any evidence of antidepressant toxicity and reduce the dosage appropriately. Initial dosage reductions to a quarter[12] have been advised if 20 mg fluoxetine daily is added, and regular monitoring for several weeks or even months.[12] Fluoxetine's active metabolite (norfluoxetine) has a long half-life (7 to 15 days) and persists in the body so that this interaction can occur or continue for days or even weeks after the fluoxetine has been withdrawn.[36-38] Both concurrent and sequential use can therefore carry a risk. Also remember that after fluoxetine withdrawal the tricyclic dosage may eventually need to be increased when the fluoxetine effects finally disappear.[39]

Information about any other tricyclics not cited here seems to be lacking but be alert for this interaction with any of them. Monitor the outcome of using trazodone and fluoxetine together for any evidence of increased side-effects (excessive sedation).

1. Aranow RB, Hudson JI, Pope HG, Grady TA, Laage TA, Bell IR, Cole JO. Elevated antidepressant plasma levels after addition of fluoxetine. *Am J Psychiatry* (1989) 146, 911–13.
2. March JS, Moon RL, Johnston H. Fluoxetine-TCA interaction. *J Am Acad Child Adolesc Psychiatry* (1990) 29, 985–6.
3. Vandel S, Bertschy G, Bonin B, Nezelof S, François TH, Vandel B, Sechter D, Bizouard P. Tricyclic antidepressant plasma levels after fluoxetine addition. *Neuropsychobiology* (1992) 25, 202–7.
4. El-Yazigi A, Chaleby K, Gad A, Raines DA. Steady-state pharmacokinetics of fluoxetine and amitriptyline in patients treated with a combination of these drugs. *Pharm Res* (1993) 10 (10 Suppl), S-309.
5. Bertschy G, Vandel S, Perault MC. Un cas d'interaction métabolique: amitriptyline, fluoxétine, antituberculeux. *Therapie* (1994) 49, 509–12.
6. El-Yazigi A, Chaleby K, Gad A, Raines DA. Steady-state kinetics of fluoxetine and amitriptyline in patients treated with a combination of these drugs compared with those treated with amitriptyline alone. *J Clin Pharmacol* (1995) 35, 17–21.
7. Balant-Gorgia AE, Ries C, Balant LP. Metabolic interaction between fluoxetine and clomipramine: A case report. *Pharmacopsychiatry* (1996) 29, 38–41.
8. Bell IR, Cole JO. Fluoxetine induces elevation of desipramine level and exacerbation of geriatric nonpsychotic depression. *J Clin Psychopharmacol* (1988) 8, 447–8.
9. Goodnick PJ. Influence of fluoxetine on plasma levels of desipramine. *Am J Psychiatry* (1989) 146, 552.
10. Vaughan DA. Interaction of fluoxetine with tricyclic antidepressants. *Am J Psychiatry* (1988) 145, 1478.
11. von Ammon Cavanaugh S. Drug-drug interactions of fluoxetine with tricyclics. *Psychosomatics* (1990) 31, 273–6.
12. Westermeyer J. Fluoxetine-induced tricyclic toxicity: extent and duration. *J Clin Pharmacol* (1991) 31, 388–92.
13. Preskorn SH, Beber JH, Faul JC, Hirschfeld RMA. Serious adverse effects of combining fluoxetine and tricyclic antidepressants. *Am J Psychiatry* (1990) 147, 532.
14. Bergstrom RF, Lemberger L, Peyton AL. Drug interaction between fluoxetine and the tricyclic antidepressants imipramine and desipramine. *Pharm Res* (1990) 7, S-254.
15. Bergstrom RF, Peyton AL, Lemberger L. Quantification and mechanism of the fluoxetine and tricyclic antidepressant interaction. *Clin Pharmacol Ther* (1992) 51, 239–48.
16. Nelson JC, Mazure CM, Bowers MB, Jatlow PI. A preliminary, open study of the combination of fluoxetine and desipramine for rapid treatment of major depression. *Arch Gen Psychiatry* (1991) 48, 303–7.
17. Wilens TE, Biederman J, Baldessarini RJ, McDermott SP, Puopolo PR, Flood JG. Fluoxetine inhibits desipramine metabolism. *Arch Gen Psychiatry* (1992) 49, 752.
18. Preskorn SH, Alderman J, Chung M, Harrison W, Messig M, Harris S. Pharmacokinetics of desipramine coadministered with sertraline or fluoxetine. *J Clin Psychopharmacol* (1994) 14, 90–8.
19. Faynor SM, Espina V. Fluoxetine inhibition of imipramine metabolism. *Clin Chem* (1989) 35, 1180.
20. Hahn SM, Griffin JH. Comment: fluoxetine adverse effects and drug interactions. *DICP Ann Pharmacother* (1991) 25, 1273–4.
21. Kahn DG. Increased plasma nortriptyline concentration in a patient cotreated with fluoxetine. *J Clin Psychiatry* (1990) 51, 36.
22. Schraml F, Benedetti G, Hoyle K, Clayton A. Fluoxetine and nortriptyline combination therapy. *Am J Psychiatry* (1989) 146, 1636–7.
23. Downs JM, Downs AD, Rosenthal TL, Deal N, Akiskal HS. Increased plasma tricyclic antidepressant concentrations in two patients concurrently treated with fluoxetine. *J Clin Psychiatry* (1989) 50, 226–7.
24. Sternbach H. Fluoxetine-clomipramine interaction. *J Clin Psychiatry* (1995) 56, 171–2.
25. Preskorn SH, Baker B. Fatality associated with combined fluoxetine-amitriptyline therapy. *JAMA* (1997) 277, 1682.
26. Touw DJ, Gernaat HBPE, van der Woude J. Parkinsonisme na toevoeging van fluoxetine aan behandeling met neuroleptica of carbamazepine. *Ned Tijdschr Geneeskd* (1992) 136, 332–4.
27. Molaie M. Serotonin syndrome presenting with migraine like stroke. *Headache* (1997) 37, 519–21.
28. Metz A, Shader RI. Adverse interactions encountered when using trazodone to treat insomnia associated with fluoxetine. *Int Clin Psychopharmacol* (1990) 5, 191–4.
29. Nierenberg AA, Cole JO, Glass L. Possible trazodone potentiation of fluoxetine: a case series. *J Clin Psychiatry* (1992) 53, 83–5.
30. Maes M, Westenberg H, Vandoolaeghe E, Demedts P, Wauters A, Neels H, Meltzer HY. Effects of trazodone and fluoxetine in the treatment of major depression: therapeutic pharmacokinetic and pharmacodynamic interactions through formation of meta-chlorophenylpiperazine. *J Clin Psychopharmacol* (1997) 17, 358–64.
31. Swerdlow NR, Andia AM. Trazodone-fluoxetine combination for treatment of obsessive-compulsive disorder. *Am J Psychiatry* (1989) 146, 1637.
32. Patterson DE, Braverman SE, Belandres PV. Speech dysfunction due to trazodone-fluoxetine combination in traumatic brain injury. *Brain Inj* (1997) 11, 287–91.
33. Brøsen K, Skjelbo E. Fluoxetine and norfluoxetine are potent inhibitors of P450IID6 — the source of the sparteine/debrisoquine oxidation polymorphism. *Br J Clin Pharmacol* (1991) 32, 136–7.
34. Von Moltke LL, Greenblatt DJ, Cotreau-Bibbo MM, Duan SX, Harmatz JS, Shader RI. Inhibition of desipramine hydroxylation *in vitro* by serotonin-reuptake inhibitor antidepressants, and by quinidine and ketoconazole: a model system to predict drug interactions *in vivo*. *J Pharmacol Exp Ther* (1994) 268, 1278–83.
35. Brøsen K. Differences in interactions with SSRIs. *Int Clin Psychopharmacol* (1998) 13 (Suppl 5), S45–S47.
36. Downs JM, Dahmer SK. Fluoxetine and elevated plasma levels of tricyclic antidepressants. *Am J Psychiatry* (1990) 147, 1251.
37. Skowron DM, Gutierrez MA, Epstein S. Precaution with titrating nortriptyline after the use of fluoxetine. *DICP Ann Pharmacother* (1990) 24, 1008.
38. Müller N, Brockmöller J, Roots I. Extremely long plasma half-life of amitriptyline in a woman with the cytochrome P450IID6 29/29—kilobase wild-type allele — a slowly reversible interaction with fluoxetine. *Ther Drug Monit* (1991) 13, 535–6.
39. Extein IL. Recent fluoxetine treatment and complications of tricyclic therapy. *Am J Psychiatry* (1991) 148, 1601–2.

Tricyclic and related antidepressants + Fluvoxamine

Fluvoxamine can markedly raise the plasma levels of amitriptyline, clomipramine, imipramine, maprotiline and trimipramine. Toxicity may possibly occur if their dosages are not reduced. Desipramine appears to be minimally affected.

Clinical evidence

The **amitriptyline** plasma levels of 8 patients rose (range 15 to 233%) when given 100 to 300 mg **fluvoxamine** daily. Even larger rises in serum **clomipramine** levels occurred (up to eightfold) in four others given 100 to 300 mg **fluvoxamine** daily. The tricyclic dosages remained the same or were slightly lower. No toxicity was seen.[1-3]

Marked increases in tricyclic antidepressant levels (50 to 100% or more) occurred in another 5 patients on **imipramine** or **desipramine**, associated with increased side-effects in 3 of them (tremor, confusion, anticholinergic effects and one case of seizure) when given **fluvoxamine**.[4,5] However later studies by some of the same authors confirmed the interaction with **imipramine**, but suggested that **desipramine** was only slightly affected.[6,7] Increased **imipramine** serum levels were found in another study.[8] Eight patients taking **amitriptyline**, **clomipramine**, **imipramine** or **maprotiline** also demonstrated this interaction with **fluvoxamine**. **Fluvoxamine** inhibited the metabolism of the tricyclic antidepressants and **fluvoxamine** levels were seen to rise, indicating a bidirectional interaction.[9] Other studies found increased **amitriptyline**, **imipramine** and **clomipramine** serum levels in the presence of **fluvoxamine**, but despite serum **clomipramine** levels exceeding 500 ng/ml, no clinically relevant ECG changes were seen.[10,11]

Increases in the plasma levels of **amitriptyline** and **clomipramine** due to **fluvoxamine** were reported in other studies.[12,13] A depressed man who had failed to respond to **clomipramine** (150 to 225 mg daily) did so within 4 days of adding **fluvoxamine** (100 mg daily). His plasma **clomipramine** levels rose almost fourfold within a week.[14] A woman developed marked faintness and serum **clomipramine** levels raised tenfold above therapeutic levels when given **fluvoxamine**.[15] The plasma **trimipramine** levels of a man approximately doubled when given **fluvoxamine**, accompanied by worsening depression and panic attacks.[16]

Mechanism

In vivo studies and *in vitro* studies with human liver microsomes show that fluvoxamine is a non-competitive inhibitor of cytochrome P450 isoenzyme CYP1A2, which is concerned with the metabolism (*N*-demethylation) of tricyclic antidepressants. Inhibition of other enzymes involved in demethylation (CYP3A4)[13] and inhibition of hydroxylation may also occur.[9] This has the effect of raising the plasma levels of the tricyclics with possible toxicity.

Importance and management

Established interactions of clinical importance. The authors of one of the reports advise a reduction in the tricyclic antidepressant dosage based on plasma level monitoring if **fluvoxamine** is added, with an initial reduction to at least one-third to avoid toxicity,[4] although the increased levels can apparently also be advantageous.[10,11,14] There is some evidence that combined use may be valuable in the treatment of obsessive-compulsive disorder.[10,11] The effects of the interaction disappear within 1 to 2 weeks of withdrawing the **fluvoxamine**.[9] **Desipramine** appears not to interact.

1. Vandel S, Bertschy G, Allers G. Fluvoxamine tricyclic antidepressant interaction. *Therapie* (1990) 45, 21.
2. Bertschy G, Vandel S, Vandel B, Allers G, Vomat R. Fluvoxamine-tricyclic antidepressant interaction. An accidental finding. *Eur J Clin Pharmacol* (1991) 40, 119–120.
3. Bertschy G, Vandel S, Nezelof S, Bizouard P, Bechtel P. L'interaction fluvoxamine-antidépresseurs tricycliques. *Therapie* (1993) 48, 63–4.
4. Spina E, Campo GM, Avenoso A, Pollicino MA, Caputi AP. Interaction between fluvoxamine and imipramine/desipramine in four patients. *Ther Drug Monit* (1992) 14, 194–6.
5. Maskall DD, Lam RW. Increased plasma concentration of imipramine following augmentation with fluvoxamine. *Am J Psychiatry* (1993) 150, 1566.
6. Spina E, Pollicino AM, Avenso A, Campo GM, Caputi AP. Fluvoxamine-induced alterations in plasma concentrations of imipramine and desipramine in depressed patients. *Int J Clin Pharmacol Res* (1993) 13, 167–71.
7. Spina E, Pollicino AM, Avenoso A, Campo GM, Perucca E, Caputi AP. Effect of fluvoxamine on the pharmacokinetics of imipramine and desipramine in healthy patients. *Ther Drug Monit* (1993) 15, 243–6.
8. Zhen-Hua X, Song-Lin H, Hong-Hao Z. Inhibition of imipramine N-demethylation by fluvoxamine in Chinese young men. *Acta Pharmacol Sin* (1996) 17, 399–402.
9. Härtter S, Wetzel H, Hammes E, Hiemke C. Inhibition of antidepressant demethylation and hydroxylation by fluvoxamine in depressed patients. *Psychopharmacology* (1993) 110, 302–8.
10. Wetzel H, Härtter A, Szegedi A, Hammes E, Leal M, Hiemke C. Fluvoxamine co-medication to tricyclic antidepressants: metabolic interactions, clinical efficiency and side-effects. *Pharmacopsychiatry* (1993) 26, 211.
11. Szegedi A, Wetzel H, Leal M, Härtter S, Hiemke C. Combination treatment with clomipramine and fluvoxamine: drug monitoring, safety, and tolerability data. *J Clin Psychiatry* (1996) 57, 257–64.
12. Vandel S, Bertschy G, Baumann P, Bouquet S, Bonin B, Francois T, Sechter D, Bizouard P. Fluvoxamine and fluoxetine: Interaction studies with amitriptyline, clomipramine and neuroleptics in phenotyped patients. *Pharmacol Res* (1995) 31, 347–53.
13. Vandel P, Bonin B, Bertschy G, Baumann P, Bouquet S, Vandel S, Sechter D, Bizouard P. Observations of the interaction between tricyclic antidepressants and fluvoxamine in poor metabolisers of dextromethorphan and mephenytoin. *Therapie* (1997) 52, 74–6.
14. Conus P, Bondolfi G, Eap CB, Macciardi F, Baumann P. Pharmacokinetic fluvoxamine-clomipramine interaction with favorable therapeutic consequences in therapy-resistant depressive patient. *Pharmacopsychiatry* (1996) 29, 108–10.
15. Roberge C, Lecordier-Maret F, Beijean-Leymarie M, Heriault F, Starace J. Major drug interaction between fluvoxamine and clomipramine: about a case report. *J Pharm Clin* (1998) 17, 117–19.
16. Seifritz E, Holsboer-Trachsler E, Hemmeter U, Eap CB, Baumann P. Increased trimipramine plasma levels during fluvoxamine comedication. *Eur Neuropsychopharmacol* (1994) 4, 15–20.
17. Brøsen K, Skjelbo E, Rasmussen BB, Poulsen HE, Loft S. Fluvoxamine is a potent inhibitor of cytochrome P4501A2. *Biochem Pharmacol* (1993) 45, 1211–14.
18. Skjelbo E, Brøsen K. Inhibitors of imipramine metabolism by human liver microsomes. *Br J Clin Pharmacol* (1992) 34, 256–61.

Tricyclic antidepressants + Food

Some preliminary evidence suggests that very high fibre diets can reduce the serum levels of doxepin and desipramine, and thereby oppose their action.

Clinical evidence, mechanism, importance and management

Three patients showed no response to **doxepin** or **desipramine** and had reduced serum tricyclic antidepressant levels while taking very high **fibre diets** (**wheat bran**, **wheat germ**, **oat bran**, **rolled oats**, **sunflower seeds**, **coconut shreds**, **raisins**, **bran muffins**). When the diet was changed or stopped, the serum tricyclic antidepressant levels rose and the depression was relieved.[1] The reasons are not known. This interaction may possibly provide an explanation for otherwise unaccountable relapses or inadequate responses to tricyclic antidepressant treatment. Another study found that **food** (**breakfast**) had no effect on the bioavailability of **imipramine**, on its peak [serum] concentrations or the time to peak concentrations in 12 normal subjects following a 50 mg oral dose.[2]

1. Stewart DE. High-fiber diet and serum tricyclic antidepressant levels. *J Clin Psychopharmacol* (1992) 12, 438–40.
2. Abernethy DR, Divoll M, Greenblatt DJ, Shader RI. Imipramine pharmacokinetics and absolute bioavailability: effect of food. *Clin Res* (1983) 31, 626A.

Tricyclic antidepressants + Furazolidone

A report describes the development of toxic psychosis, hyperactivity, sweating and hot and cold flushes in a woman on amitriptyline when given furazolidone with diphenoxylate and atropine.

Clinical evidence, mechanism, importance and management

A depressed woman taking daily doses of 1.25 mg **conjugated oestrogen substances** and 75 mg **amitriptyline**, was additionally given 300 mg **furazolidone** and **diphenoxylate** with **atropine sulphate**. Two days later she began to experience blurred vision, profuse perspiration followed by alternate chills and hot flushes, restlessness, motor activity, persecutory delusions, auditory hallucinations and visual illusions. The symptoms cleared within a day of stopping the **furazolidone**.[1] The reasons are not understood but the authors point out that **furazolidone** has MAO-inhibitory properties and that the symptoms were similar to those seen when the tricyclic antidepressants and MAOIs interact. However the MAO-inhibitory activity of **furazolidone** normally develops over several days. Whether the concurrent use of **atropine** and **amitriptyline** (both of which have anticholinergic activity) had some part to play in the reaction is uncertain. No firm conclusions can be drawn from this slim evidence, but prescribers should be aware of this case when considering the concurrent use of tricyclic antidepressants and **furazolidone**.

1. Aderhold RM and Muniz CE. Acute psychosis with amitriptyline and furazolidone. *JAMA* (1970) 213, 2080.

Tricyclic antidepressants + Isoprenaline

Although isoprenaline (isoproterenol) and amitriptyline have been used together safely and with advantage in the treatment of asthma, an isolated case has been reported of death arising from their concurrent over-use.

Clinical evidence, mechanism, importance and management

Amitriptyline alone[1,2] and with **isoprenaline**[3] is beneficial in the treatment of asthma, and in a study of possible adverse interactions between the two, no abnormalities of heart rhythm were seen, although one out of the 4 patients studied showed potentiation of **isoprenaline**-induced tachycardia.[4] However a woman taking *Tedral* (**theophylline**, **ephedrine** and **phenobarbital**), twice daily, died as a result of aspiration of vomit in response to cardiac arrhythmias induced by the use of **amitriptyline** and **isoprenaline**.[5] It was estimated that she had taken 40 doses of **isoprenaline** 125 micrograms, daily for several days prior to her death. **Amitriptyline**, **isoprenaline**, **ephedrine** and the **fluorocarbon** inhaler propellant appear to have had additive cardiotoxic effects. This fatal interaction would seem to be due to the over-use rather than the responsible use of these drugs. However the case serves to emphasise the risk attached to the overuse of **isoprenaline** inhalers if cardiotoxic drugs such as the tricyclic antidepressants are being used concurrently.

1. Ananth J. Antiasthmatic effect of amitriptyline. *Can Med Assoc J* (1974) 110, 1131–3.
2. Meares RA, Mills JE, Horvath TB. Amitriptyline and asthma. *Med J Aust* (1971) 2, 25.
3. Mattila MJ, Muittari A. Modification by imipramine of the bronchodilator response to isoprenaline in asthmatic patients. *Ann Med Int Fenn* (1968) 57, 185–7.
4. Boakes AJ, Laurence DR, Teoh PC, Barar FSK, Benedikter LT, Prichard BNC. Interactions between sympathomimetic amines and antidepressant agents in man. *BMJ* (1973) 1, 311–5.
5. Kadar D. Amitriptyline and isoproterenol: fatal drug combination. *Can Med Assoc J* (1975) 112, 556–7.

Tricyclic antidepressants + Ketoconazole

Ketoconazole appears not to interact with desipramine, and only interacts to a small and clinically irrelevant extent with imipramine.

Clinical evidence, mechanism, importance and management

Two groups of 6 normal subjects were given either single 100 mg doses of **imipramine** or **desipramine** alone, and then again on day 10 of a 14-day course of 200 mg **ketoconazole** once daily. It was found that the **ketoconazole** caused the oral clearance of the **imipramine** to fall by 17%, its half-life to rise by 15% and the AUC of **desipramine** derived from the **imipramine** to fall by 9%. No significant changes in the pharmacokinetics of the **desipramine** were seen.[1]

These findings show that **ketoconazole** inhibits the demethylation of **imipramine** without affecting the 2-hydroxylation of **imipramine** and **desipramine**, and confirms that cytochrome P450 isoenzyme CYP3A4 has a role in the metabolism of these tricyclic antidepressants,[1] however in practical terms it would seem that any changes are small and unlikely to be of any clinical significance. No special precautions would appear necessary if **ketoconazole** is used with either of these two drugs. Information about other tricyclics seems to be lacking.

1. Spina E, Avenoso A, Campo GM, Scordo MG, Caputi AP, Perucca E. Effect of ketoconazole on the pharmacokinetics of imipramine and desipramine in healthy subjects. *Br J Clin Pharmacol* (1997) 43, 315–8.

Tricyclic antidepressants + Methadone

Methadone can double the serum levels of desipramine.

Clinical evidence

After taking 0.5 mg/kg **methadone** daily for two weeks, the mean serum **desipramine** levels of 5 men on 2.5 mg/kg daily had risen by 108%. Previous observations in patients given both drugs had shown that **desipramine** levels were higher than expected and **desipramine** side-effects developed at relatively low doses.[1]

Further evidence of an increase in plasma **desipramine** levels due to **methadone** is described in another study.[2]

Mechanism

Not understood. It is suggested that the methadone may possibly inhibit the hydroxylation of the desipramine, thereby reducing its loss from the body.[2]

Importance and management

Information seems to be limited to these two studies but the interaction would seem to be established. Monitor the effects of concurrent use and anticipate the need to reduce the desipramine dosage. There seems to be nothing reported about the effects of methadone on other tricyclic antidepressants.

1. Maany I, Dhopesh V, Arndt IO, Burke W, Woody G, O'Brien CP. Increase in desipramine serum levels associated with methadone treatment. *Am J Psychiatry* (1989) 146, 1611–13.
2. Kosten TR, Gawin FH, Morgan C, Nelson JC, Jatlow P. Desipramine and its 2-hydroxy metabolite in patients taking or not taking methadone. *Am J Psychiatry* (1990) 147, 1379–80.

Tricyclic antidepressants + Methylphenidate or Dexamfetamine (Dextroamphetamine)

Methylphenidate can cause a very marked increase in the plasma levels of imipramine resulting in clinical improvement. Toxicity appears not to have been documented but two adolescents experienced severe mood deterioration while taking both drugs. However, a review of 142 patients suggests the absence of a significant interaction. An isolated report describes a blood dyscrasia in a child given both drugs.

Clinical evidence

A study in 'several patients' demonstrated a dramatic increase in the plasma levels of **desipramine** and **imipramine** during concurrent treatment with **imipramine** and **methylphenidate**. In one patient on 150 mg **imipramine** daily it was observed that 20 mg **methylphenidate** daily increased the plasma levels of the **imipramine** from 100 to 700 micrograms/l and of **desipramine** from 200 to 850 micrograms/l over a period of 16 days.[1]

Similar effects have been described in other reports.[2,3] Study shows elevation of drug levels takes several days to occur, and several days to wear off.[3] A 9-year-old and a 15-year-old exhibited severe behavioural problems until the **imipramine** and **methylphenidate** they were taking were stopped.[4] In contrast a retrospective review in 142 children and adolescents taking either **desipramine** alone, or **desipramine** with **dexamfetamine (dextroamphetamine)** or **methylphenidate**, indicated the absence of a clinically significant interaction between **desipramine** and either stimulant. Pharmacokinetic parameters were similar in each group.[5] An isolated report describes leucopenia, anaemia, eosinophilia and thrombocytosis in a child of 10 when given **imipramine** and **methylphenidate**.[6]

Mechanisms

In vitro experiments with human liver slices indicate that methylphenidate inhibits the metabolism of imipramine, resulting in its accumulation, and this is reflected in raised blood levels.[3] The blood dyscrasia may have been due to the rare additive effects of both drugs.[6]

Importance and management

Information is limited. Some therapeutic improvement is seen because of the very marked rise in the blood levels of the antidepressant due to methylphenidate, but whether this also can lead to tricyclic antidepressant toxicity is uncertain. It does not seem to have been reported, but the possibility should be considered, although there is evidence that the pharmacokinetics of desipramine is not significantly affected by either methylphenidate or dexamfetamine. Information about other tricyclic antidepressants is lacking. It has been suggested that concurrent use in children and adolescents may be undesirable, due to case reports of adverse behavioural effects.[4]

1. Dayton PG, Perel JM, Israili ZH, Faraj BA, Rodewig K, Black N, Goldberg LI. Studies with methylphenidate: drug interactions and metabolism. In 'Clinical Pharmacology of Psychoactive Drugs', Sellers EM (ed). Alcoholism and Drug Addiction Research Foundation. *Toronto* (1975) p 183–202.
2. Cooper TB, Simpson GM. Concomitant imipramine and methylphenidate administration: a case report. *Am J Psychiatry* (1973) 130, 721.
3. Wharton RN, Perel JM, Dayton PG, Malitz S. A potential clinical use for methylphenidate with tricyclic antidepressants. *Am J Psychiatry* (1971) 127, 1619–25.
4. Grob CS, Coyle JT. Suspected adverse methylphenidate-imipramine interactions in children. *J Dev Behav Pediatrics* (1986) 7, 265–7.
5. Cohen LG, Prince J, BiedermanJ, Wilens T, Faraone SV, Whitt S, Mick E, Spencer T, Meyer MC, Polisner D, Flood JG. Absence of effect of stimulants on the pharmacokinetics of desipramine in children. *Pharmacotherapy* (1999) 19, 746–52.
6. Burke MS, Josephson A, Lightsey A. Combined methylphenidate and imipramine complication. *J Am Acad Child Adolesc Psychiatry* (1995) 34, 403–4.

Tricyclic antidepressants + Oestrogens (estrogens)/Oral contraceptives

There is evidence that oestrogens can sometimes paradoxically reduce the effects of imipramine, yet at the same time cause imipramine toxicity. The general clinical importance of this interaction has yet to be evaluated.

Clinical evidence

A study in 10 women taking 150 mg **imipramine** daily for primary depression found that those given 50 micrograms **ethinylestradiol (ethinyloestradiol)** daily for a week showed less improvement than other women given only 25 micrograms or a placebo. Four out of the 10 developed signs of **imipramine** toxicity that was dealt with by halving the **imipramine** dose.[1] Another study found that **oral contraceptives** increased the absolute bioavailability of **imipramine** by 60%.[2]

Long-standing **imipramine** toxicity was also relieved in a woman taking 100 mg daily when her dosage of **conjugated oestrogen** was reduced to a quarter.[3] In contrast, several studies which showed that serum **clomipramine** levels were raised or remained unaffected by the concurrent use of **oestrogen-containing contraceptives**, failed to confirm that tricyclic antidepressant toxicity occurs more often in those on the pill than those who are not.[4-7] Akathisia in 3 patients has been attributed to an interaction between **conjugated oestrogens** and **amitriptyline** or **clomipramine**.[8]

Mechanism

Among the possible reasons for these effects are that the oestrogens increase the bioavailability of imipramine,[2] or inhibit its metabolism.[9]

Importance and management

These interactions are inadequately established. There is no obvious reason for avoiding concurrent use, but it would seem reasonable to be alert for any evidence of toxicity and/or lack of response to tricyclic antidepressant treatment. One study suggested that the imipramine dosage should be reduced by about one-third.[2] More study is needed.

1. Prange AJ, Wilson IC, Alltop LB. Estrogen may well affect response to antidepressant. *JAMA* (1972) 219, 143–4.
2. Abernethy DR, Greenblatt DJ, Shader RI. Imipramine disposition in users of oral contraceptive steroids. *Clin Pharmacol Ther* (1984) 35, 792–7.
3. Khurana RC. Estrogen-imipramine interaction. *JAMA* (1972) 222, 702–3.
4. Beaumont G. Drug interactions with clomipramine (Anafranil). *J Int Med Res* (1973) 1, 480–84.
5. Gringras M, Beaumont G, Grieve A. Clomipramine and oral contraceptives: an interaction study — clinical findings. *J Int Med Res* (1980) 8 (Suppl 3), 76–80.
6. Luscombe DK, Jones RB. Effects of concomitantly administered drugs on plasma levels of clomipramine and desmethylclomipramine in depressive patients receiving clomipramine therapy. *Postgrad Med J* (1977) 53 (Suppl 4), 77.
7. John VA, Luscombe DK, Kemp H. Effects of age, cigarette smoking and the oral contraceptive on the pharmacokinetics of clomipramine and its desmethyl metabolite during chronic dosing. *J Int Med Res* (1980) 8 (Suppl 3), 88–95.
8. Krishnan KRR, France RD, Ellinwood EH Jr. Tricyclic-induced akathisia in patients taking conjugated estrogens. *Am J Psychiatry* (1984) 141, 696–7.
9. Somani SM, Khurana RC. Mechanism of estrogen-imipramine interaction. *JAMA* (1973) 223, 560.

Tricyclic antidepressants + Paroxetine

The serum levels of clomipramine, desipramine, imipramine and trimipramine can be markedly increased by paroxetine. The serotonin syndrome developed in a woman on paroxetine when given imipramine, and in a man who took a single paroxetine tablet shortly after stopping desipramine.

Clinical evidence

(a) Clomipramine

A 74-year-old woman, on clomipramine 75 mg daily for several years, was admitted to hospital with increasing dizziness 8 days after starting paroxetine 20 mg daily. The symptoms resolved after both drugs were discontinued. The dizziness was probably due to elevated serum levels of clomipramine and *S*-desmethylclomipramine resulting from coadministered paroxetine.[1]

(b) Desipramine

A study in 17 normal subjects who were extensive metabolisers and on 50 mg **desipramine** daily found that when additionally given 20 mg **paroxetine** daily for 10 days the maximum plasma levels of the **desipramine** rose by 358%, the trough plasma levels by 511% and the AUC by 421%. An approximately tenfold increase in the maximum serum levels and the AUC of the **paroxetine** also occurred.[2]

A 45-year-old woman on pindolol, desipramine 300 mg daily, clonazepam and olanzapine was given paroxetine, titrated up to 40 mg daily over 3 months, in an attempt to overcome inadequate antidepressant response. She developed lightheadedness, ataxia and increased confusion. Serum desipramine levels were 1810 ng/ml (therapeutic range 75–300 ng/ml). Decreasing the dose of both desipramine and paroxetine reduced the adverse effects, but serum concentrations remained high. After paroxetine was gradually withdrawn and replaced by citalopram, desipramine levels dropped into the therapeutic range. A 21-year-old man developed the serotonin syndrome when he took one tablet of paroxetine only one day after taking desipramine for 5 days. He recovered after treatment with cyproheptadine.[3]

(c) Imipramine

Paroxetine 20 mg daily increased the metabolism of **imipramine** to desipramine in 2 patients. Their serum **imipramine** levels were increased two to fourfold.[4,5] Another study found that **paroxetine** increased the half-life, AUC and maximum plasma levels of **imipramine** by about 40%, and halved its clearance.[6] Similar results were found in another study.[7] A woman on **paroxetine** 30 mg daily developed the serotonin syndrome (tachycardia, delirium, bizarre movements, myoclonus) within 2 h of taking a single dose of **imipramine** 50 mg. She recovered when treated with intravenous fluids, sedation and cyproheptadine.[8]

(d) Trimipramine

Two patients showed a marked increase (about threefold) in serum **trimipramine** and desmethyltrimipramine concentrations when concurrently treated with **paroxetine**. Both patients developed side effects (sedation and orthostatic hypotension in one patient, and dysarthria and memory impairment in the second) while taking both drugs.[9]

Mechanism

The reason is believed to be that paroxetine inhibits the cytochrome P450 isoenzyme CYP2D6 which is concerned with the metabolism of desipramine and imipramine, resulting in their accumulation.[2,6] Citalopram is considered to be a weak inhibitor of this enzyme and so is unlikely to have any significant effects.[10]

Importance and management

The paroxetine/imipramine and paroxetine/desipramine interactions appear to be established, but of uncertain importance. Since there have been reports of adverse responses in patients it would now seem prudent to be alert for the need to reduce the dosages of both desipramine and imipramine to avoid tricyclic toxicity if paroxetine is used concurrently. Replacing paroxetine with an SSRI such as citalopram, which exhibits only weak inhibition of CYP2D6, may overcome the problem, although the extents of these drug interactions requires further investigation. The paroxetine/trimipramine interaction is also established, but its incidence is uncertain. The report cited appears to be the only one documented, nevertheless you should be alert for any evidence of toxicity with this drug combination. Reduce the dosages as necessary.

1. Skjelbo EF, Brøsen K. Interaktion imellem paroxetin og clomipramin som mulig årsag til indlæggelse på medicinsk afdeling. *Ugeskr Laeger* (1998) 160, 5665–6.
2. Alderman J, Preskorn SH, Greenblatt DJ, Harrison W, Penenberg D, Allison J, Chung M. Desipramine pharmacokinetics when coadministered with paroxetine or sertraline in extensive metabolizers. *J Clin Psychopharmacol* (1997) 17, 284–91.
3. Chan BSH, Graudins A, Whyte IM, Dawson AH, Braitberg G, Duggin GG. Serotonin syndrome resulting from drug interactions. *Med J Aust* (1998) 169, 523–5.
4. Härtter S, Szegedi A, Wetzel H, Hiemke C. Differential interactions of fluvoxamine and paroxetine with the metabolism of tricyclic antidepressants. *Pharmacopsychiatry* (1993) 26, 156.
5. Härtter S, Hermes B, Szegedi A, Hiemke C. Automated determination of paroxetine and its main metabolite by column switching and on-line high-performance liquid chromatography. *Ther Drug Monit* (1994) 16, 400–6.
6. Albers LJ, Reist C, Helmeste D, Vu R, Tang SW. Paroxetine shifts imipramine metabolism. *Psychiatry Res* (1996) 59, 189–96.
7. Yoon YR, Shim JC, Shin JG, Shon JH, Kim YH, Cha IJ. Drug interaction between paroxetine and imipramine. Kor Soc Pharmacol Meeting, Seoul, S Korea, October 1997, p168.
8. Weiner AL, Tilden FF, McKay CA. Serotonin syndrome: case report and review of the literature. *Conn Med* (1997) 61, 717–21.
9. Leinonen E, Koponen HJ, Lepola U. Paroxetine increases serum trimipramine concentration. A report of two cases. *Hum Psychopharmacol* (1995) 10, 345–7.
10. Ashton AK. Lack of desipramine toxicity with citalopram. *J Clin Psychiatry* (2000) 61, 144.

Tricyclic Antidepressants + Propafenone

An isolated report describes markedly raised serum desipramine levels in a patient when concurrently treated with propafenone.

Clinical evidence, mechanism, importance and management

A man with major depression responded well to 175 mg **desipramine** daily with serum **desipramine** levels in the range 500 to 1000 nmol/l. When later he was treated for paroxysmal atrial fibrillation with digoxin (0.25 mg daily) and **propafenone** (150 mg twice daily and 300 mg at night) he developed markedly elevated serum **desipramine** levels (2092 nmol/l) and toxicity (dry mouth, sedation, shakiness) while taking 150 mg **desipramine** daily. The side effects resolved when the **desipramine** was stopped for 5 days, but when restarted at 75 mg daily his serum **desipramine** levels were still raised (1130 nmol/l).

The reason is thought to be that the **propafenone** reduced the me-

tabolism and clearance of the **desipramine** from the body.[1] The general importance of this case is uncertain, but be alert for signs of **desipramine** toxicity in any patient given **propafenone** concurrently. Reduce the **desipramine** dosage appropriately.

1. Katz MR. Raised serum levels of desipramine with the antiarrhythmic propafenone. *J Clin Psychiatry* (1991) 52, 432–3.

Tricyclic antidepressants + Quinidine

Quinidine can reduce the loss of desipramine, imipramine, nortriptyline and trimipramine from the body, thereby increasing their serum levels.

Clinical evidence

Quinidine 50 mg given 1 h before a single 50-mg dose of **nortriptyline** increased its AUC in 5 normal subjects fourfold (from 0.6 to 2.8 mg l^{-1} h), and the half-life threefold (from 14.2 to 44.7 h).[1] The clearance fell from 5.4 to 1.9 ml min^{-1}.

Another study in normal subjects found that 200 mg **quinidine** daily reduced the clearance of single doses of 100 mg **imipramine** by 30% and of 100 mg **desipramine** by 85%.[2] A further study in 2 normal subjects similarly found that 50 mg **quinidine** almost doubled the half-life of a single 75-mg dose of **trimipramine** which was reflected in some waking EEG changes (greater and longer-lasting effects on alpha and theta bands).[3]

Mechanism

Quinidine reduces the metabolism (hydroxylation) of these tricyclic antidepressants, involving inhibition of cytochrome P450 isoenzyme CYP2D6, thereby reducing their loss from the body.[4,5]

Importance and management

The clinical importance of these interactions awaits assessment, but be alert for evidence of increased tricyclic antidepressant effects and possibly the toxicity if quinidine is added. One report suggested steady-state increases of 30% with imipramine and more than 500% with desipramine in extensive metabolisers.[2] More study is needed. There seems to be no information about other tricyclics. See also 'Drugs that prolong the QT interval + Other drugs that prolong the QT interval', p.103.

1. Ayesh R, Dawling S, Widdop B, Idle JR, Smith RL. Influence of quinidine on the pharmacokinetics of nortriptyline and desipramine. *Br J Clin Pharmacol* (1988) 25, 140P–141P.
2. Brøsen K, Gram LF. Quinidine inhibits the 2-hydroxylation of imipramine and desipramine, but not the demethylation of imipramine. *Eur J Clin Pharmacol* (1989) 37, 155–60.
3. Eap CB, Laurian S, Souche A, Koeb L, Reymond P, Buclin T, Baumann P. Influence of quinidine on the pharmacokinetics of trimipramine and on its effect on the waking EEG of healthy volunteers. A pilot study on two subjects. *Neuropsychobiology* (1992) 25, 214–20.
4. Pfandl B, Mörike K, Winne D, Schareck W, Breyer-Pfaff U. Stereoselective inhibition of nortriptyline hydroxylation in man by quinidine. *Xenobiotica* (1992) 22, 721–30.
5. Von Moltke LL, Greenblatt DJ, Cotreau-Bibbo MM, Duan SX, Harmatz JS, Shader RI. Inhibition of desipramine hydroxylation *in vitro* by serotonin-reuptake-inhibitor antidepressants, and by quinidine and ketoconazole: a model system to predict drug interactions *in vivo*. *J Pharmacol Exp Ther* (1994) 268, 1278–83.

Tricyclic antidepressants + Rifampicin (Rifampin)

Two patients showed a marked reduction in serum nortriptyline or amitriptyline levels when given rifampicin.

Clinical evidence

A man with tuberculosis needed large doses of **nortriptyline** (175 mg daily) to achieve therapeutic serum concentrations while taking 300 mg isoniazid, 600 mg **rifampicin (rifampin)**, 1500 mg pyrazinamide and 25 mg pyridoxine daily. Three weeks after stopping the antitubercular drugs, the patient suddenly became drowsy and his **nortriptyline** serum levels were found to have risen from 193 to 562 nmol/l and later to 671 nmol/l. It was then found possible to maintain his **nortriptyline** serum levels in the range 150 to 500 nmol/l with only 75 mg **nortriptyline** daily.[1] A woman on **amitriptyline** and fluoxetine showed a marked fall in serum **amitriptyline** levels when treated with 600 mg **rifampicin**, 200 mg isoniazid and 1200 mg ethambutol daily. When these antitubercular drugs were stopped, her **amitriptyline** serum levels rose once again.[2]

Mechanism

It seems highly probable that the rifampicin (a well recognised and potent enzyme inducer) increased the metabolism of the nortriptyline and amitriptyline by the liver and hastened their loss from the body.

Importance and management

Information about the tricyclic antidepressant/rifampicin (rifampin) interaction seems to be limited to just these two reports which is a little surprising since both have been widely used for a considerable time. This suggests that generally this interaction may have limited clinical importance. However to be on the safe side it would be prudent to monitor the concurrent use of any of the tricyclic antidepressants and rifampicin (rifampin), being alert for reduced antidepressant effects. Increase the tricyclic dosage if necessary.

1. Bebchuk JM, Stewart DE. Drug interaction between rifampin and nortriptyline: a case report. *Int J Psychiatry Med* (1991) 21, 183–7.
2. Bertschy G, Vandel S, Perault MC. Un cas d'interaction métabolique: amitriptyline, fluoxétine, antituberculeux. *Therapie* (1994) 49, 509–12.

Tricyclic antidepressants + Sertraline

Desipramine, imipramine and nortriptyline plasma levels can be increased by 30 to 50%, or even more in some individuals, by sertraline. An isolated report describes the development of the serotonin syndrome in a patient on sertraline when amitriptyline was added.

Clinical evidence

(a) Amitriptyline

A woman who had been taking 50 mg **sertraline** daily (as well as morphine sulphate and periciazine) developed the serotonin syndrome with 3 days of starting to take 75 mg **amitriptyline** daily. She recovered when all of the psychotropic drugs were withdrawn.[1]

(b) Desipramine

Sertraline 50 mg daily increased the maximum plasma levels of **desipramine** (50 mg daily) by 31% at steady-state in 18 normal subjects and increased the AUC by 23%.[2] A later related study in 24 normal subjects by the same group of workers found that, using the same drug dosages, **sertraline** increased the **desipramine** maximum plasma levels by 44%, the minimum levels by 19% and the AUC by 37%. The maximum plasma levels and AUC of the **sertraline** were increased about twofold.[3] Another study found that 150 mg **sertraline** daily for 8 days increased the AUC of single 50-mg doses of **desipramine** in 6 subjects by 54% and the maximum plasma levels by 22%.[4] Fourteen normal subjects on **sertraline** in increasing doses up to 150 mg daily over a period of a month were then given in addition a single 100-mg dose of **desipramine**. The maximum plasma levels of the **desipramine** rose by 26% and the AUC by 72%.[5]

A depressed man on **desipramine** was additionally given 50 mg **sertraline** daily. Within a week his plasma **desipramine** levels had risen from 152 to 204 ng/ml, and after a month to 240 ng/ml, but no adverse effects were seen and the patient said he felt more energetic and motivated.[6] Another patient showed a 50% increase in **desipramine** serum levels a week after starting 50 mg **sertraline** daily, and a 250% increase after two weeks with troublesome side effects.[7]

(c) Imipramine

Sertraline 150 mg daily for 8 days increased the AUC of single doses of **imipramine** in 6 subjects by 68% and the maximum plasma levels by 39%.[4] In contrast, 7 days' treatment with 50 mg **sertraline** daily had no statistically or clinically significant effects on the pharmacokinetics of **imipramine** in 4 normal subjects. The sedation caused by the **imipramine** and other pharmacodynamic measurements taken were unaltered by concurrent use.[8,9]

(d) Nortriptyline

A study in 14 elderly patients on **nortriptyline** found that when additionally given 50 mg **sertraline** daily, the median increase in plasma **nortriptyline** levels was only 2% (with a range of –26 to 117%), but two of them showed increases of 51% and 117% respectively, changes the authors considered clinically meaningful. For those taking higher doses of **sertraline** (100 to 150 mg daily) the median increase in **nortriptyline** plasma levels was 40% (with a range of –12% to +239%).[10]

Mechanism

It is believed that sertraline inhibits the cytochrome P450 isoenzyme CYP2D6 which is concerned with the metabolism of the tricyclic antidepressants, and as a result their loss from the body is reduced and their serum levels rise.[5] Just why the serotonin syndrome developed with amitriptyline/sertraline is not understood.

Importance and management

The interactions of sertraline with desipramine, imipramine and nortriptyline are established, but the increases in the plasma concentrations are usually only moderate (about 20–50%) in most patients which may not be clinically important. It would however be prudent to be alert for any evidence of increased tricyclic antidepressant side-effects because some patients may show larger increases. The amitriptyline/sertraline interaction cited here seems to an isolated case, but there is insufficient evidence to forbid the use of this drug combination although close monitoring would be advisable.

1. Alderman CP, Lee PC. Comment: serotonin syndrome associated with combined sertraline-amitriptyline treatment. *Ann Pharmacother* (1996) 30, 1499–1500.
2. Preskorn SH, Alderman J, Chung M, Harrison W, Messig M, Harris S. Pharmacokinetics of desipramine coadministered with sertraline or fluoxetine. *J Clin Psychopharmacol* (1994) 14, 90–8.
3. Alderman J, Preskorn SH, Greenblatt DJ, Harrison W, Penenberg D, Allison J, Chung M. Desipramine pharmacokinetics when coadministered with paroxetine or sertraline in extensive metabolizers. *J Clin Psychopharmacol* (1997) 17, 284–91.
4. Kurtz DL, Bergstrom RF, Goldberg MJ, Cerimele BJ. The effect of sertraline on the pharmacokinetics of desipramine and imipramine. *Clin Pharmacol Ther* (1997) 62, 145–56.
5. Zussman BD, Davie CC, Fowles SE, Kumar R, Lang U, Wargenau M, Sourgens H. Sertraline, like other SSRIs, is a significant inhibitor of desipramine metabolism in vivo. *Br J Clin Pharmacol* (1995) 39, 550P–551P.
6. Lydiard RB, Anton RF, Cunningham T. Interactions between sertraline and tricyclic antidepressants. *Am J Psychiatry* (1993) 150, 1125–6.
7. Barros J, Asnis G. An interaction of sertraline and desipramine. *Am J Psychiatry* (1993) 150, 1751.
8. Erikson SM, Carson SW, Grimsley S, Carter JG, Kumar A, Jann MW. Effect of sertraline on steady-state serum concentrations of imipramine and its metabolites. *Pharmacotherapy* (1994) 14, 368.
9. Jann MW, Carson SW, Grimsley SR, Erikson S, Kumar A, Carter JG. Effects of sertraline upon imipramine pharmacodynamics. *Clin Pharmacol Ther* (1995) 57, 207.
10. Solai LK, Mulsant BH, Pollock BG, Sweet RA, Rosen J, Yu K, Reynolds CF. Effect of sertraline on plasma nortriptyline levels in depressed elderly. *J Clin Psychiatry* (1997) 58, 440–3.

Tricyclic antidepressants + St John's wort (*Hypericum perforatum*)

The plasma levels of amitriptyline can be reduced by St John's wort and nortriptyline seems to be similarly affected, but the clinical importance of this interaction is unknown.

Clinical evidence

12 depressed patients were given 75 mg of **amitriptyline** twice daily and 900 mg of **St John's wort extract** (Lichtwer Pharma, Berlin)

daily for at least 14 days. The $AUC_{0-12\,h}$ of the **amitriptyline** was reduced 21.7% and the AUC of **nortriptyline** by 40.6%.[1]

Mechanism

Not known, but there is evidence that St John's wort is an enzyme inducer which can increase liver metabolism, thereby reducing the plasma levels of both amitriptyline and its metabolite (nortriptyline).

Importance and management

The interaction appears to be established, but its clinical importance is uncertain. Both drugs are antidepressants, but whether the final sum of this interaction is more or less antidepressant activity is not known. It was not assessed in this study.[1] Other tricyclics probably interact similarly because they too can be affected by enzyme inducing agents (and nortriptyline clearly is). Monitor for evidence of reduced antidepressant efficacy if St John's wort is given with any tricyclic. More study is needed.

1. Roots I, Johne A, Schmider J, Brockmöller J, Maurer A, Störmer E, Donath F. Interaction of a herbal extract from St. John's wort with amitriptyline and its metabolites. *Clin Pharmacol Ther* (2000) 67, 159.

Tricyclic antidepressants + Sucralfate

Sucralfate causes a marked reduction in the absorption of amitriptyline.

Clinical evidence, mechanism, importance and management

When a single 75-mg dose of **amitriptyline** was taken by 6 normal subjects with a single 1 g dose of **sucralfate**, the AUC of the **amitriptyline** was reduced by 50% (from 680 to 320 ng h/ml).[1] Concurrent use should be monitored to confirm that the therapeutic effects of the antidepressant are not lost. An increase in the dosage may be needed. There seems to be nothing documented about other tricyclics.

1. Ryan R, Carlson J, Farris F. Effect of sucralfate on the absorption and disposition of amitriptyline in humans. *Fedn Proc* (1986) 45, 205.

Tricyclic antidepressants + Sympathomimetics (directly-acting)

Patients on tricyclic antidepressants show a grossly exaggerated response (hypertension, cardiac arrhythmias, etc.) to parenteral norepinephrine (noradrenaline), epinephrine (adrenaline) and to a lesser extent to phenylephrine. Local anaesthetics containing these vasoconstrictors do not seem to be associated with the same problems. Felypressin may be a safe alternative. Doxepin and maprotiline appear not to interact to the same extent as most tricyclic antidepressants.

Clinical evidence

The effects of intravenous infusions of **norepinephrine (noradrenaline)** were increased approximately ninefold, and of **epinephrine (adrenaline)** approximately threefold, in 6 healthy subjects who had been taking 60 mg **protriptyline** daily for 4 days.[1,2]

The pressor effects of intravenous infusions of **norepinephrine** were increased four to eightfold, of **epinephrine** two to fourfold, and to **phenylephrine** two to threefold in 4 healthy subjects who had been taking 75 mg **imipramine** daily for 5 days. There were no noticeable or consistent changes in their response to **isoprenaline (isoproterenol)**.[3]

Five patients taking **nortriptyline**, **desipramine** or **other unnamed tricyclic antidepressants** experienced adverse reactions, some of them severe (throbbing headache, chest pain) following the injection of *Xylestesin* (lidocaine (lignocaine)) with 1:25,000 **nor-epinephrine**) during dental treatment.[4] Several episodes of marked increases in blood pressure, dilated pupils, intense malaise, violent but transitory tremor and palpitations have been reported in patients taking **un-named tricyclic antidepressants** when they were given local anaesthetics containing **epinephrine** or **norepinephrine** for dental treatment.[5]

There are other reports describing this interaction of **norepinephrine** with **imipramine**,[6,7] **desipramine**,[7,8] **nortriptyline**,[9] **protriptyline**[8] and **amitriptyline**;[7,8] of **epinephrine** with **amitriptyline**,[10] and of **corbadrine** (levonordefrin) with **desipramine** (in *dogs*).[11]

Mechanism

The tricyclics and some related antidepressants block or inhibit the uptake of norepinephrine into adrenergic neurones. Thus the most important means by which norepinephrine is removed from the adreno-receptor area is inactivated and the concentration of norepinephrine outside the neurone can rise. If therefore more norepinephrine (or one of the other directly acting alpha or alpha/beta agonists) is infused into the body, the adreno-receptors of the cardiovascular system concerned with raising blood pressure become grossly stimulated by this superabundance of amines, and the normal response is accordingly exaggerated.

Importance and management

A well documented, well established and potentially serious interaction. The parenteral administration of norepinephrine (noradrenaline), epinephrine (adrenaline), phenylephrine or any other sympathomimetic amine with predominantly direct activity should be avoided in patients under treatment with tricyclic antidepressants. If these sympathomimetics must be used, the rate and amount injected must be very much reduced to accommodate the exaggerated responses that will occur. However, the situation where epinephrine or norepinephrine are used with a local anaesthetic for surface or infiltration anaesthesia, or nerve block is less clear. The cases cited are all from the 1960s or 1970s, and the preparations concerned contained concentrations of epinephrine or norepinephrine several times greater than those used currently. However, it should be noted that preparations such as *Xylocaine* + adrenaline still carry a caution about their use with tricyclic antidepressants.[11] Anecdotal evidence suggests that local anaesthetics containing sympathomimetics are, in practice, commonly used in patients receiving tricyclic antidepressants,[12] so the sparsity of reports, especially recent ones, would add weight to the argument that the interaction is only rarely significant. However, it would still seem advisable to be aware of the potential for interaction. Aspiration has been recommended to avoid inadvertent intravenous administration. **Felypressin** has been shown to be a safe alternative.[13-15] If an adverse interaction occurs it can be controlled by the use of an alpha-receptor blocking agent such as phentolamine.

Doxepin in doses of less than 150 to 200 mg daily blocks neuronal uptake much less than other tricyclic antidepressants and so is unlikely to show this interaction to the same degree, but in larger doses it will interact like other tricyclics.[16,17] **Maprotiline** (a tetracyclic antidepressant) also blocks uptake much less than most of the tricyclics and in normal therapeutic doses in a study on three subjects was shown not to increase the pressor response to norepinephrine.[18] The pressor response to norepinephrine is also not significantly increased in the presence of **iprindole**.[19] It does not seem to have been established whether the response to oral doses or nasal drops containing phenylephrine is enhanced by the presence of a tricyclic, but there seem to be no reports of problems.

1. Svedmyr N. The influence of a tricyclic antidepressive agent (protriptyline) on some of the circulatory effects of noradrenaline and adrenaline in man. *Life Sci* (1968) 7, 77–84.
2. Svedmyr N. Potentieringsrisker vid tillförsel av katekolaminer till patienter som behandlas med tricykliska antidepressiva medel. *Lakartidningen* (1968) 65 (Suppl 1), 72–6.
3. Boakes AJ, Laurence DR, Teoh PC, Barar FSK, Benedikter LT, Prichard BNC. Interactions between sympathomimetic amines and antidepressant agents in man. *BMJ* (1973) 1, 311–15.
4. Boakes AJ, Laurence DR, Lovel KW, O'Neil R, Verrill PJ. Adverse reactions to local anaesthetic/vasoconstrictor preparations. A study of the cardiovascular responses to Xylestesin and Hostacain-with-Noradrenaline. *Br Dent J* (1972) 133, 137–40.
5. Dam WH. Personal communication cited by Kristoffersen MB. Antidepressivas potensering af katekolaminvirkning. *Ugeskr Laeger* (1969) 131, 1013–14.

6. Gershon S, Holmberg G, Mattsson E, Mattsson N, Marshall A. Imipramine hydrochloride. Its effects on clinical, autonomic and psychological functions. *Arch Gen Psychiatry* (1962) 6, 96–101.
7. Fischbach R, Harrer G, Harrer H. Verstärkung der noradrenalin-wirkung durch psychopharmaka beim menschen. *Arzneimittelforschung* (1966) 16, 263–5.
8. Mitchell JR, Cavanaugh JH, Arias L, Oates JA. Guanethidine and related agents. III. Antagonism by drugs which inhibit the norepinephrine pump in man. *J Clin Invest* (1970) 49, 1596–1604.
9. Persson G, Siwers B. The risk of potentiating effect of local anaesthesia with adrenalin in patients treated with tricyclic antidepressants. *Swed Dent J* (1975) 68, 9–18.
10. Siemkowicz E. Hjertestop efter amitriptylin og adrenalin. *Ugeskr Laeger* (1975) 137, 1403–4.
11. Dreyer AC, Offermeier J. The influence of desipramine on the blood pressure elevation and heart rate stimulation of levonordefrin and felypressin alone and in the presence of local anaesthetics. *J Dent Ass SA* (1986) 41, 615–18.
12. Brown RS, Lewis VA. More on the contraindications to vasoconstrictors in dentistry. *Oral Surg Oral Med Oral Pathol* (1993) 76, 2–3.
13. Aellig WH, Laurence DR, O'Neil R, Verrill PJ. Cardiac effects of adrenaline and felypressin as vasoconstrictors in local anaesthesia for oral surgery under diazepam sedation. *Br J Anaesth* (1970) 42, 174–6.
14. Goldman V, Astrom A, Evers H. The effect of a tricyclic antidepressant on the cardiovascular effects of local anaesthetic solutions containing different vasoconstrictors. *Anaesthesia* (1971) 26, 91.
15. Perovic J, Terzic M, Todorovic L. Safety of local anaesthesia induced by prilocaine with felypressin in patients on tricyclic antidepressants. *Bull Group Int Rech Sci Stomatol Odontol* (1979) 22, 57–62.
16. Fann WE, Cavanaugh JH, Kaufmann JS, Griffith JD, Davis JM, Janowsky DS, Oates JA. Doxepin: effects on transport of biogenic amines in man. *Psychopharmacologia* (1971) 22, 111–25.
17. Oates JA, Fann WE, Cavanaugh JH. Effect of doxepin on the norepinephrine pump. *Psychosomatics* (1969) 10, 12–13.
18. Briant RH, George CF. The assessment of potential drug interactions with a new tricyclic antidepressant drug. *Br J Clin Pharmacol* (1974) 1, 113.
19. Fann WE, Davis JM, Janowsky DS, Kaufmann JS, Griffith JD, Oates JA. Effect of iprindole on amine uptake in man. *Arch Gen Psychiatry* (1972) 26, 158–62.

Tricyclic antidepressants + Sympathomimetics (indirectly-acting)

The effects of indirectly acting sympathomimetics (amphetamines, phenylpropanolamine, pseudoephedrine, tyramine, etc.) would be expected to be reduced by the tricyclic antidepressants, but so far only one case involving ephedrine and amitriptyline seems to have been reported.

Clinical evidence, mechanism, importance and management

Indirectly-acting sympathomimetic amines like **tyramine** exert their effects by causing the release of norepinephrine (noradrenaline) from adrenergic neurones rather than by a direct stimulant action on the receptors. In the presence of a tricyclic antidepressant, the uptake of these amines into adrenergic neurones is partially or totally prevented and the norepinephrine-releasing effects are therefore blocked. The reduction in the pressor response to **tyramine** due to this interaction has been used in monitoring the efficacy of treatment with the tricyclic antidepressants,[1] but **tyramine** itself is only used as a research tool, or as a model drug to test the behaviour of indirectly acting sympathomimetics. The activity of other similar sympathomimetics that are used therapeutically might therefore be expected to be blocked by the tricyclics in just the same way, but only an isolated case seems to have been reported.[2]

An elderly woman on 75 mg **amitriptyline** daily developed hypotension (70 mmHg systolic) during subarachnoid anaesthesia. Her blood pressure rose only minimally when given iv boluses of **ephedrine** (a mixed action sympathomimetic) totalling 90 mg but she responded normally when given **epinephrine (adrenaline)** (a directly-acting sympathomimetic).[2]

This single case appears to be the only report of this type of interaction occurring in a clinical situation. Bearing in mind how long and how widely both groups of drugs have been in use, the absence of any other reports would suggest that any interaction between them is rarely of practical importance, even so some drug makers include this largely theoretical interaction on their datasheets.

1. Mulgirigama LD, Pare CMB, Turner P, Wadsworth J, Witts DJ. Tyramine pressor responses and plasma levels during tricyclic antidepressant therapy. *Postgrad Med J* (1977) 53 (Suppl 4), 30–4.
2. Serle DG. Amitriptyline and ephedrine in subarachnoid anesthesia. *Anaesth Intensive Care* (1985) 13, 214.

Tricyclic antidepressants + Tamoxifen

An isolated report describes a reduction in doxepin serum levels attributed to the concurrent use of tamoxifen.

Clinical evidence, mechanism, importance and management

A 79-year-old woman with a long history of bipolar (manic-depressive) disorder, stabilised on lithium carbonate and **doxepin** 200 mg at bedtime and also taking propranolol, was additionally started on 20 mg **tamoxifen** daily after a mastectomy for breast cancer. It was noted that her total blood levels of **doxepin** and its major metabolite were reduced about 25% over the next 11 months. The control of her depression remained unchanged. The reasons for this apparent interaction are not known.[1] The makers of **tamoxifen** have another undetailed and isolated report of a possible interaction.[2]

This appears to be the first and only clear report of an interaction between a tricyclic antidepressant and **tamoxifen** so that its general importance is not known. It is probably small.

1. Jefferson JW. Tamoxifen-associated reduction in tricyclic antidepressant levels in blood. *J Clin Psychopharmacol* (1995) 15, 223–4.
2. Zeneca, Personal communication. November 1995.

Tricyclic antidepressants + Thioxanthenes

A study using C^{14}-imipramine showed that, unlike the situation between the tricyclic antidepressants and phenothiazines, flupenthixol 3 to 6 mg daily did not inhibit the metabolism of imipramine in 2 patients.[1]

1. Gram LF, Overø KF. Drug interaction: inhibitory effect of neuroleptics on metabolism of tricyclic antidepressants in man. *BMJ* (1972) 1, 463–5.

Tricyclic antidepressants + Thyroid preparations

The antidepressant response to imipramine, amitriptyline and possibly other tricyclics can be accelerated by the use of thyroid preparations. An isolated case of paroxysmal atrial tachycardia, another of thyrotoxicosis and yet another of hypothyroidism due to concurrent therapy have been described.

Clinical evidence, mechanism, importance and management

Normally an advantageous interaction. The addition of 25 micrograms **liothyronine** daily was found to increase the speed and efficacy of **imipramine** in relieving depression.[1] Similar results have been described in other studies with **desipramine**[2] and **amitriptyline**[3] but the reasons are not understood. However adverse reactions have also been seen. A patient being treated for both hypothyroidism and depression with 60 mg **thyroid** and 150 mg **imipramine** daily complained of dizziness and nausea. She was found to have developed paroxysmal atrial tachycardia.[4] A 10-year-old girl with congenital hypothyroidism, well controlled on 150 mg **desiccated thyroid** daily, developed severe thyrotoxicosis after taking 25 mg **imipramine** daily for 5 months for enuresis. The problem disappeared when the **imipramine** was withdrawn.[5] In another patient the effect of **levothyroxine** was lost and hypothyroidism developed when given **dosulepin (dothiepin)**.[6] These apparent interactions remain unexplained. There would seem to be no good reason, general speaking, for avoiding concurrent use unless problems arise.

1. Wilson IC, Prange AJ, McClane TK, Rabon AM, Lipton MA. Thyroid-hormone enhancement of imipramine in nonretarded depressions. *N Engl J Med* (1970) 282, 1063–7.
2. Extein I. Case reports of l-triiodothyronine potentiation. *Am J Psychiatry* (1982) 139, 966–7.

3. Wheatley D. Potentiation of amitriptyline by thyroid hormone. *Arch Gen Psychiatry* (1972) 26, 229–33.
4. Prange AJ. Paroxysmal auricular tachycardia apparently resulting from combined thyroid-imipramine treatment. *Am J Psychiatry* (1963) 119, 994–5.
5. Colantonio LA, Orson JM. Triiodothyronine thyrotoxicosis. Induction by desiccated thyroid and imipramine. *Am J Dis Child* (1974) 128, 396–7.
6. Beeley L, Beadle F, Lawrence R. *Bull West Mid Centre for Adverse Drug Reaction Reporting* (1984) 19, 11.

Tricyclic antidepressants + Tobacco smoking

Smoking reduces the plasma levels of amitriptyline, clomipramine, desipramine, imipramine and nortriptyline, but the concentration of the free and unbound antidepressant rises which appears to offset the effects of this interaction.

Clinical evidence

Two studies failed to find any difference between the steady-state **nortriptyline** plasma levels of **smokers** and non-smokers,[1,2] but others have found that **smoking** lowers the plasma levels of **amitriptyline**,**clomipramine**,[3] **desipramine**, **imipramine**[4] and **nortriptyline**.[5] For example a 25% reduction in plasma **nortriptyline** levels was found in one study,[5] and a 45% reduction in **imipramine + desipramine** levels in another.[4]

Mechanism

The probable reason is that some of the components of tobacco smoke are enzyme inducing agents which increase the metabolism of these antidepressants by the liver.

Importance and management

These interactions are established but it might wrongly be concluded from the figures quoted that smokers need larger doses to control their depression. Preliminary data show that the plasma concentrations of free (and pharmacologically active) nortriptyline are greater in smokers than non-smokers (10.2 compared with 7.4%), which probably offsets the fall in total plasma levels.[5] Thus the lower plasma levels in smokers may be as therapeutically effective as the higher levels in non-smokers, so that there is probably no need to raise the dosage to accommodate this interaction.

1. Norman TR, Burrows GD, Maguire KP, Rubinstein G, Scoggins BA, Davies B. Cigarette smoking and plasma nortriptyline levels. *Clin Pharmacol Ther* (1977) 21, 453–6.
2. Alexanderson B, Price Evans DA, Sjöqvist F. Steady-state plasma levels of nortriptyline in twins: influence of genetic factors and drug therapy. *BMJ* (1969) 4, 764–8.
3. John VA, Luscombe DK, Kemp H. Effects of age, cigarette smoking and the oral contraceptive on the pharmacokinetics of clomipramine and its desmethyl metabolite during chronic dosing. *J Int Med Res* (1980) 8 (Suppl 3), 88–95.
4. Perel JM, Hurwie MJ, Kanzler MB. Pharmacodynamics of imipramine in depressed patients. *Psychopharmacol Bull* (1975) 11, 16–18.
5. Perry PJ, Browne JL, Prince RA, Alexander B, Tsuang MT. Effects of smoking on nortriptyline plasma concentrations in depressed patients. *Ther Drug Monit* (1986) 8, 279–84.

Tricyclic antidepressants + Urinary acidifiers or alkalinizers

The blood levels of desipramine, nortriptyline and other tricyclic antidepressants are not significantly affected by agents which alter urinary pH.

Clinical evidence, mechanism, importance and management

Because the tricyclics are bases it might be expected that changes in the urinary pH would have an effect on their excretion, but in fact the excretion of unchanged drug is small (less than 5% with **nortriptyline** and **desipramine**) compared with the amounts metabolised by the liver.[1] Even in cases of poisoning ". . . vigorous procedures such as forced diuresis, peritoneal dialysis, or haemodialysis can therefore not be expected to markedly accelerate the elimination of these

drugs."[1] Only in the case of hepatic dysfunction is simple urinary clearance likely to take on a more important role.

1. Sjöqvist F, Berglund F, Borgå O, Hammer W, Andersson S, Thorstrand C. The pH-dependent excretion of monomethylated tricyclic antidepressants. *Clin Pharmacol Ther* (1969) 10, 826–33.

Tricyclic antidepressants + Valproate

Amitriptyline and nortriptyline serum levels can be increased by sodium valproate and valpromide. An isolated report attributes a paradoxical rise in serum desipramine levels to the withdrawal of sodium valproate.

Clinical evidence

(a) Sodium valproate or Semisodium valproate

In one study, 15 normal subjects were given a single 50-mg dose of **amitriptyline** 2 h after taking the ninth dose of 500 mg **semisodium valproate** 12-hourly. The maximum plasma levels of the **amitriptyline** and its AUC were raised by 19% and 30% respectively. The corresponding values for **nortriptyline** were 28% and 55% respectively.[1,2]

One patient developed delirium within 3 days, and another developed grossly elevated serum **nortriptyline** serum levels (393 ng/ml – about threefold higher than the normal range) and evidence of toxicity (tremulousness of hands and fingers) about two weeks after starting 500 mg **valproate** twice daily. The toxicity rapidly disappeared when both drugs were stopped. Another patient also developed elevated **nortriptyline** serum levels, attributed to the addition of **valproate**.[3] A patient on **clomipramine** 150 mg daily suffered feelings of numbness and sleep disturbances attributed to elevated serum levels of **clomipramine** and **desmethylclomipramine,** caused by the administration of **valproate** 1 to 1.4 g daily. Halving the dose of **clomipramine** restored serum concentrations to therapeutic levels.[4]

(b) Valproic acid

In contrast, a woman on thiothixene developed elevated and potentially toxic serum **desipramine** levels (a rise from 259 to 324 mg/l) at the end of a 3-month period during which **valproic acid** was gradually withdrawn and replaced by clorazepate. The authors of the report attributed this reaction to the **valproic acid** withdrawal.[5]

(c) Valpromide

The addition of 600 mg **valpromide** daily for 10 days caused a 65% rise in the serum levels of **nortriptyline** (from 61 to 100.5 ng/ml) and a 50% rise in the levels of **amitriptyline** (from 70.5 to 105.5 ng/ml) in two groups of 10 patients.[6,7]

Mechanism

Uncertain. Inhibition of the metabolism of these tricyclics by the valproate has been suggested.[3,4]

Importance and management

Information seems to be limited to these reports. It would now seem prudent to monitor the plasma levels of amitriptyline or nortriptyline if valproate is added, and to reduce the dosage of the amitriptyline if necessary. The clinical relevance of these increases is uncertain; the rises seem to be only moderate in most patients, but the gross rises seen in one patient emphasise the need to monitor concurrent use well. Information about other tricyclic antidepressants seems to be lacking.

1. Granneman GR, Carlson G, Cavanagh J, Awni WM, Wong SL. Modelling the extent of amitriptyline and nortriptyline metabolic inhibition during valproate coadministration. *Pharm Res* (1994) 11 (10 Suppl), S-434.
2. Wong SL, Cavanaugh J, Shi H, Awni WM, Granneman GR. Effects of divalproex sodium on amitriptyline and nortriptyline pharmacokinetics. *Clin Pharmacol Ther* (1996) 60, 48–53.
3. Fu C, Katzman M, Goldbloom DS. Valproate/nortriptyline interaction. *J Clin Psychopharmacol* (1994) 14, 205–6.
4. Fehr C, Gründer G, Hiemke C, Dahmen N. Increase in serum clomipramine concentrations caused by valproate. *J Clin Psychopharmacol* (2000) 20, 493–4.

5. Joseph AB, Wroblewski BA. Potentially toxic serum concentrations of desipramine after discontinuation of valproic acid. *Brain Inj* (1993) 7, 463–5.
6. Bertschy G, Vandel S, Jounet JM, Allers G. Interaction valpromide-amitriptyline. Augmentation de la biodisponibilité de l'amitriptyline et de la nortriptyline par le valpromide. *L'Encephale* (1990) 16, 43–5.
7. Vandel S, Bertschy G, Jounet JM, Allers G. Valpromide increases the plasma concentrations of amitriptyline and its metabolite nortriptyline in depressive patients. *Ther Drug Monit* (1988) 10, 386–9.

Tricyclic antidepressants + Venlafaxine

Venlafaxine can cause a marked increase in the anticholinergic side-effects of clomipramine, desipramine and nortriptyline.

Clinical evidence

A 74-year-old man on **venlafaxine** 150 mg daily and thioridazine had his treatment changed to daily doses of **venlafaxine** 75 mg, **desipramine** 50 mg, haloperidol 0.5 mg and alprazolam 0.25 mg. Within 5 days he exhibited severe anticholinergic effects (acute confusion – delirium, stupor, urinary retention and paralytic ileus). He had previously had few problems with **venlafaxine** combined with haloperidol and alprazolam.[1] A man of 75 on haloperidol, alprazolam and **venlafaxine** showed urinary retention and delirium when **desipramine** was added.[2] A woman on 20 mg of **nortriptyline** and 20 mg fluoxetine daily with only mild anticholinergic effects developed much more severe effects (dry mouth, worsened constipation, blurred vision) over 4 weeks following the replacement of the fluoxetine by 75 mg **venlafaxine daily**.[3] A man of 73 on 20 mg fluoxetine and 20 mg **nortriptyline** daily developed constipation, blurred vision and a dry mouth within a week of starting **venlafaxine**. A man of 61 on 150 mg **clomipramine** daily similarly developed anticholinergic side-effects (dry mouth, constipation, urinary retention) within a week of starting to take **venlafaxine**. These side-effects disappeared when the **venlafaxine** was stopped.[2]

A 69-year-old-man with bipolar disorder, who had been taking **venlafaxine** up to 337.5 mg daily, thioridazine 25 mg at night, and **sodium valproate** 1200 mg daily for several months with no adverse motor symptoms, experienced extrapyramidal effects 3 to 4 days after the **venlafaxine** had been gradually replaced by **nortriptyline** 50 mg daily. Symptoms persisted despite withdrawal of thioridazine, but improved on reduction of the **nortriptyline** dosage to 20 mg daily.[4] The cause of the reaction was not known, but it was suggested that there may have been an interaction between **venlafaxine** and **nortriptyline** possibly modulated by thioridazine or **sodium valproate**.

Mechanism

Not fully established but it is suggested that a possible major mechanism is that venlafaxine can inhibit the metabolism of these tricyclics by cytochrome P450 isoenzyme CYP2D6, leading to an increase in their serum levels and a marked increase in their anticholinergic side-effects.[2] Some of the patients were elderly which may have increased their sensitivity to these side-effects.

Importance and management

Information appears to be limited to these reports, three of which are by the same author. The incidence is not known but if venlafaxine and any tricyclic antidepressant are given concurrently, be alert for any evidence of increased anticholinergic side-effects. It may be necessary to withdraw one or other of the two drugs. More study is needed.

1. Benazzi F. Anticholinergic toxic syndrome with venlafaxine-desipramine combination. *Pharmacopsychiatry* (1998) 31, 36–7.
2. Benazzi F. Venlafaxine drug-drug interactions in clinical practice. *J Psychiatry Neurosci* (1998) 23, 181–2.
3. Benazzi F. Venlafaxine-fluoxetine-nortriptyline interaction. *J Psychiatry Neurosci* (1997) 22, 278–9.
4. Conforti D, Borgherini G, Fiorelli Bernardis LA, Magni G. Extrapyramidal symptoms associated with the adjunct of nortriptyline to a venlafaxine-valproic acid combination. *Int Clin Psychopharmacol* (1999) 14, 197–8.

Tricyclic antidepressants + Vinpocetine

Vinpocetine is reported not to affect plasma imipramine levels.

Clinical evidence, mechanism, importance and management

The steady-state plasma **imipramine** levels (25 mg three times daily) of 18 normal subjects were unaffected by 10 mg **vinpocetine** three times daily, taken concurrently for 10 days.[1] No special precautions would seem to be necessary. There seems to be nothing documented about any of the other tricyclic antidepressants.

1. Hitzenberger G, Schmid R, Braun W, Grandt R. Vinpocetine therapy does not change imipramine pharmacokinetics in man. *Int J Clin Pharmacol Ther Toxicol* (1990) 28, 99–104.

Venlafaxine + Fluoxetine or Paroxetine

Anticholinergic side-effects can develop in patients on fluoxetine when venlafaxine is added. The serotonin syndrome developed in one patient when fluoxetine was stopped and venlafaxine started, and in another when paroxetine was stopped and venlafaxine started.

Clinical evidence

(a) Anticholinergic side-effects

A woman on 20 mg **fluoxetine** and 1 mg clonazepam daily developed blurred vision, dry mouth, constipation, dizziness, insomnia and a hand tremor within a week of additionally starting 37.5 mg venlafaxine daily. These symptoms worsened by the second week and persisted until the venlafaxine was stopped.[1,2]

Four patients aged 21, 24, 51 and 70 on **fluoxetine** developed anticholinergic side-effects (constipation, blurred vision, urinary retention and dry mouth) within a week of adding venlafaxine, which persisted until the venlafaxine was stopped.[3] A man of 61 on 20 mg **fluoxetine** daily had extreme difficulty in urinating within 2 days of additionally starting to take 37.5 mg venlafaxine daily. The effect became intolerable after 10 days but no other obvious anticholinergic side-effects (blurred vision, constipation, dry mouth, tachycardia) were seen. This patient had some prostate enlargement and had previously had some moderate urinary problems when treated with **fluoxetine** and nortriptyline.[2,4]

(b) Serotonin syndrome

A 39-year-old woman with depression and panic attacks was treated with cimetidine, trazodone, clonazepam and **fluoxetine**. Within 24 h of abruptly stopping the latter two drugs and starting lorazepam and venlafaxine, she developed the serotonin syndrome (diaphoresis, tremors, slurred speech, myoclonus, restlessness and diarrhoea).[5]

A 21-year-old-woman whose long-term treatment with **paroxetine** was stopped a week before starting **venlafaxine** (37.5 mg daily for 5 days then 75 mg daily for 2 days) developed vomiting, dizziness, incoordination, falling anxiety and electric shock sensations in her arms and legs within 3 days of starting **venlafaxine**. She stopped **venlafaxine** after 7 days of treatment, but symptoms persisted for 5 days until treated with cyproheptadine.[6]

Mechanism

One possible explanation is that fluoxetine inhibits cytochrome P450 isoenzyme CYP2D6 which is concerned with the metabolism of venlafaxine, leading to an increase in its serum levels and in its usually minimal anticholinergic side-effects.[1-4] An alternative explanation is that these adverse effects are due to an adrenergic mechanism.[4]

Importance and management

Information about the adverse anticholinergic syndrome due to a fluoxetine/venlafaxine interaction seems to be limited to these reports, all by the same author. The incidence is not known, but if venlafaxine and fluoxetine are given concurrently, be alert for any evidence of increased anticholinergic side-effects. It may be necessary to withdraw one or other of the two drugs. You should also be aware that the development of the serotonin syndrome has been attributed to the sequential use of fluoxetine and venlafaxine in one patient, and paroxetine and venlafaxine in another.

1. Benazzi F. Severe anticholinergic side effects with venlafaxine-fluoxetine combination. *Can J Psychiatry* (1997) 42, 980–1.
2. Benazzi F. Venlafaxine-fluoxetine interaction. *J Clin Psychopharmacol* (1999) 19, 96–8.
3. Benazzi F. Venlafaxine drug-drug interactions in clinical practice. *J Psychiatry Neurosci* (1998) 23, 181–3.
4. Benazzi F. Urinary retention with venlafaxine-fluoxetine combination. *Hum Psychopharmacol* (1998) 13, 139–40.
5. Bhatara VS, Magnus RD, Paul KL, Preskorn SH. Serotonin syndrome induced by venlafaxine and fluoxetine: a case study in polypharmacy and potential pharmacodynamic and pharmacokinetic mechanisms. *Ann Pharmacother* (1998) 32, 432–26.
6. Chan BSH, Graudins A, Whyte IM, Dawson AH, Braitberg G, Duggin GG. Serotonin syndrome resulting from drug interactions. *Med J Aust* (1998) 169, 523–5.

Venlafaxine + Miscellaneous drugs

No important interactions normally appear to occur with venlafaxine and ACE inhibitors, alcohol, alprazolam, beta-blockers, cimetidine, diazepam, diuretics, hypoglycaemic agents, lithium carbonate, oral contraceptives or terfenadine, but an isolated case of the serotonin syndrome has been attributed to the concurrent use of lithium, and a handful of reports describe increased INRs and bleeding in patients on warfarin. Some caution is thought appropriate with anticonvulsants and SSRIs.

Clinical evidence, mechanism, importance and management

(a) Alcohol

Venlafaxine 50 mg 8-hourly was found to have some effect on psychomotor tests (digit symbol substitution, divided attention reaction times, POM scales) in 16 normal subjects, but these changes were small and not considered to be clinically significant, and no pharmacodynamic or pharmacokinetic interactions occurred when 0.5 g/kg alcohol was added.[1] There would seem to be no reason for avoiding concurrent use.

(b) Anticoagulants

Nobody yet seems to have studied the possible interaction of **warfarin** or **other anticoagulants** with venlafaxine but the makers have on record a handful of isolated and short case reports indicating that the effects of **warfarin** are occasionally increased by venlafaxine. These reports describe increased prothrombin times, raised INRs and bleeding (haematuria, gastrointestinal bleeding, melaena, haemarthrosis) in patients on **warfarin** who had concurrently been treated with venlafaxine.[2] Just why these adverse interactions should have occurred is not understood. The makers of venlafaxine point out that **warfarin** is possibly metabolised by the cytochrome P450 isoenzyme CYP1A and 2B subfamilies whereas venlafaxine is a weak inhibitor of isoenzyme CYP2D6.[3] From this it is not unreasonable to conclude that venlafaxine is normally unlikely to affect the metabolism of **warfarin**, but there are certainly other possible mechanisms of interaction. To be on the safe side, because an interaction can apparently occur very occasionally and unpredictably, it would be prudent to monitor prothrombin times if venlafaxine is started or stopped by patients taking any oral **anticoagulant** so that any problems can be quickly identified and dealt with. More study is needed.

(c) Anticonvulsants

No systematic studies have been done with venlafaxine and **anticonvulsants**, but during premarketing testing seizures were seen in 0.2% of patients treated. The makers suggest that venlafaxine should be used with caution in patients with a history of epilepsy, and it should be stopped if problems arise.[3,4]

(d) Antihypertensives

During the phase II and III clinical trials of venlafaxine 267 patients were also taking antihypertensive medications (**beta-blockers, diuretics, ACE-inhibitors**, etc.). Specific drugs were not named in the report.[5] There was nothing to suggest that adverse interactions of any kind occurred, but no pharmacokinetic studies were undertaken.[5] However a very small number (3%) of 2181 patients given venlafaxine showed some blood pressure rises (up to 7 mmHg diastolic) so that it is advised to check blood pressures routinely with daily doses of 200 mg or more.[4]

(e) Benzodiazepines

A double blind study in 18 normal subjects taking 50 mg venlafaxine 8-hourly found that 10 mg **diazepam** did not impair the pharmacokinetics of venlafaxine or those of its major active metabolite (*O*-desmethylvenlafaxine – ODV), nor were the pharmacokinetics of the active metabolite of diazepam (desmethyldiazepam) affected. **Diazepam** affected the performance of a battery of pharmacodynamic tests, but the additional presence of the venlafaxine had no further effect.[6,7]

A study in 16 normal subjects found that 75 mg venlafaxine twice daily reduced the AUC of a single 2 mg oral dose of **alprazolam** by 29% and reduced its half-life by 21%, but the performance of some psychometric tests were only minimally changed.[8] These two studies suggest that no special precautions are necessary during concurrent use of venlafaxine and these benzodiazepines.

(f) Cimetidine

Cimetidine 800 mg once daily for 5 days was found to reduce the oral dose clearance of venlafaxine in 18 normal subjects taking 50 mg 8-hourly by 40%, and to increase the AUC by 62%. It had no effect on the formation or elimination of its major active metabolite (ODV). A composite of plasma concentrations for venlafaxine and ODV was found to be increased by only 13%. Thus the overall pharmacological activity of the two was only slightly increased by **cimetidine**[9,10] and no special precautions would seem to be necessary. The makers of venlafaxine however suggest that the elderly and those with hepatic dysfunction may possibly show a more pronounced effect.[4]

(g) Contraceptives, oral

The makers of venlafaxine say that no systematic studies have been carried out on a possible interaction with **oral contraceptives**, but during the phase II and phase III clinical trials several women were taking **oral contraceptives**, and the inference to be drawn is that no problems arose.[3] In effect nobody yet really knows whether they interact, but they appear not to do so.

(h) Hypoglycaemic agents

During clinical trials, 18 diabetic patients took venlafaxine and **hypoglycaemic agents** (not specifically named). There was a slightly higher incidence of side-effects (nausea, somnolence, dry mouth, confusion, insomnia, impotence, decreased libido) but the makers say there was no reason to postulate that an interaction occurred.[5] Information is clearly still very limited but there is nothing to suggest that special precautions are necessary during concurrent use.

(i) Lithium carbonate

In one study 12 normal subjects were given a single 600 mg oral dose of **lithium carbonate** on day 1, followed by 50 mg venlafaxine 8-hourly from days 4 to 11, with another single 600 mg oral dose of **lithium carbonate** on day 8. The pharmacokinetic changes seen were small, the renal clearance of venlafaxine being reduced by 50% and that of its active metabolite (ODV) by 15%. Neither of these changes was considered clinically relevant. The maximum serum levels of the **lithium** were increased by 10%, and the time to reach this was reduced by about 30 min, but the other pharmacokinetic parameters of **lithium** were unchanged;[11,12] similar results had been reported earlier.[13] The general picture that emerged was that no clinically important adverse interaction normally occurs if these two drugs are used together, however an isolated report attributed the development of the serotonin syndrome to the concurrent use of venlafaxine and **lithium** in a woman described as having a sensitiveness to SSRIs.[14]

(j) Terfenadine

A study in 24 subjects given single 120 mg oral doses of **terfenadine** before and after taking 75 mg venlafaxine 12-hourly for 9 days found that the pharmacokinetic profile of the **terfenadine** was unchanged, although its acid metabolite concentrations were slightly decreased.[15] This study was undertaken to confirm that venlafaxine lacks inhibitory activity on cytochrome P450 isoenzyme CYP3A4, but at the same time it also indicates that venlafaxine does not raise the serum levels of **terfenadine,** which are associated with serious cardiotoxicity. There would therefore seem to be no reason for avoiding concurrent use.

Other *in vivo* and *in vitro* studies with venlafaxine have shown that it does not significantly, or only weakly, inhibits the activity of cytochrome P450 isoenzymes CYP2C9, CYP2D6, CYP1A2 and CYP3A3/4. This means that it is likely to be free, or largely free from clinically relevant drug–drug interactions due to changes (induction or inhibition) in drug metabolism,[16] although some studies suggest that the metabolism of venlafaxine may be inhibited by drugs which are strong inhibitors of CYP2D6, especially in patients who are extensive metabolisers of this isoenzyme.[17-19]

1. Troy SM, Turner MB, Unruh M, Parker VD, Chiang ST. Pharmacokinetic and pharmacodynamic evaluation of the potential drug interaction between venlafaxine and ethanol. *J Clin Pharmacol* (1997) 37, 1073–81.
2. Wyeth Laboratories. Personal communication, May 2000.
3. Wyeth Laboratories. Personal communication, March 1995.
4. Efexor (Venlafaxine hydrochloride) Wyeth Laboratories, Data Sheet, September 1999.
5. Wyeth Laboratories. Data on file (Study S).
6. Wyeth Laboratories. Data on file (Study 19058).
7. Troy SM, Lucki I, Peirgies AA, Parker VD, Klockowski PM, Chiang ST. Pharmacokinetic and pharmacodynamic evaluation of the potential drug interaction between venlafaxine and diazepam. *J Clin Pharmacol* (1995) 35, 410–9.
8. Amchin J, Zarycranski W, Taylor KP, Albano D, Klockowski PM. Effect of venlafaxine on the pharmacokinetics of alprazolam. *Psychopharmacol Bull* (1998) 34, 211–19.
9. Wyeth Laboratories. Data on file (Study 20276).
10. Troy SM, Rudolph R, Mayersohn M, Chiang ST. The influence of cimetidine on the disposition kinetics of the antidepressant venlafaxine. *J Clin Pharmacol* (1998) 38, 467–74.
11. Wyeth Laboratories. Data on file (Study 18840).
12. Troy SM, Parker VD, Hicks DR, Boudino FD, Chiang ST. Pharmacokinetic interaction between multiple-dose venlafaxine and single-dose lithium. *J Clin Pharmacol* (1996) 36, 175–81.
13. Parker V, Troy S, Rudolph R, Conrad K, Chiang S. The potential pharmacokinetic interaction between venlafaxine and lithium carbonate. *J Clin Pharmacol* (1991) 31, 867.
14. Mekler G, Woggon B. A case of serotonin syndrome caused by venlafaxine and lithium. *Pharmacopsychiatry* (1997) 30, 272–3.
15. Amchin J, Zarycranski W, Taylor K. Venlafaxine's lack of CYP3A4 inhibition assessed by terfenadine metabolism. *Clin Pharmacol Ther* (1997) 61, 179.
16. Ereshefsky L. Drug-drug interactions involving antidepressants: focus on venlafaxine. *J Clin Psychopharmacol* (1996) 16 (Suppl 2), 37S–50S.
17. Lessard E, Yessine MA, Hamelin BA, Turgeon J. Venlafaxine-diphenhydramine interaction in subjects with extensive or poor CYP2D6 activity. *Clin Pharmacol Ther* (1999) 65, 171.
18. Eap CB, Bertel-Laubscher R, Zullino D, Amey M, Baumann P. Marked increase of venlafaxine enantiomer concentrations as a consequence of metabolic interactions: A case report. *Pharmacopsychiatry* (2000) 33, 112–15.
19. Fogelman S, Schmider J, Greenblatt DJ, Shader RI. Inhibition of venlafaxine metabolism in vitro by index inhibitors and by SSRI antidepressants. *Clin Pharmacol Ther* (1997) 61, 181.

Venlafaxine + Monoamine oxidase inhibitors (MAOIs)

Serious and potentially life-threatening reactions (the serotonin syndrome) can develop if venlafaxine and non-selective, irreversible MAOIs (isocarboxazid, phenelzine, tranylcypromine) are given concurrently or even sequentially if insufficient time is left in between. An isolated report describes the syndrome with selegiline, but the situation with moclobemide in therapeutic doses is uncertain.

Clinical evidence

A. Irreversible non-selective MAOIs

(a) Isocarboxazid

A man with recurrent depression on 30 mg **isocarboxazid** daily was additionally given 75 mg venlafaxine. After the second dose he developed agitation, hypomania, diaphoresis, shivering and dilated pu-

pils. These symptoms subsided when the venlafaxine was stopped. He subsequently developed myoclonic jerks and diaphoresis when later given both drugs.[1]

(b) Phenelzine

A woman who had stopped taking 45 mg **phenelzine** daily 7 days previously, developed sweating, lightheadedness and dizziness within 45 min of taking a single 37.5-mg dose of venlafaxine. In the emergency department she was found to be lethargic, agitated and extremely diaphoretic. The agitation was treated with lorazepam. After she had recovered she was again started on the same regimen of venlafaxine a week later without problems.[2] A man similarly developed the serotonin syndrome when he started venlafaxine the day after he stopped taking **phenelzine**.[3] A woman developed the syndrome within less than an hour of taking **phenelzine** and venlafaxine together,[4] and 4 other patients have been described who similarly developed the reaction when **phenelzine** was replaced by venlafaxine.[5]

Twelve days after an overdose of **phenelzine** (53 tablets of 15 mg) as well as benztropine, haloperidol and lorazepam, a 31-year-old man was started on venlafaxine 75 mg every 12 hours in addition to existing treatment with olanzapine and diazepam. About an hour after the first dose, he developed leg shakiness and stiffness, diaphoresis, blurred vision, difficulty breathing, chills, nausea and palpitations. Venlafaxine and olanzapine were discontinued and the man recovered within 24 hours, after treatment with intravenous fluids, propranolol and paracetamol.[6]

(c) Tranylcypromine

A woman who had been taking **tranylcypromine** for 3 weeks developed a serious case of the serotonin syndrome within 4 hours of inadvertently taking a single tablet of venlafaxine. She recovered within 24 h when treated with ice packs, a cooling blanket, diazepam and dantrolene.[7] The serotonin syndrome developed in a man on **tranylcypromine** within 2 h of taking half a venlafaxine tablet.[8]

The makers of venlafaxine say that adverse reactions, some serious, have been seen in patients who had recently stopped taking an **MAOI** and started venlafaxine, or who had stopped venlafaxine and then started an **MAOI**. The reactions have included tremor, myoclonus, diaphoresis, nausea, vomiting, flushing, dizziness, hyperthermia with features resembling neuroleptic malignant syndrome, seizures and death.[9,10] The precise MAOIs used, their dosage, the dosage of venlafaxine, the number of patients involved and the incidence of these reactions have not been detailed.

B. Selective MAOIs

(a) Moclobemide, Selegiline

A man developed the serotonin syndrome 15 days after stopping **selegiline** 50 mg [daily] and within 30 min of starting venlafaxine 37.5 mg.[11] A 32-year-old man taking **moclobemide** 20 mg twice daily and diazepam developed the serotonin syndrome 40 minutes after taking a single dose of venlafaxine 37.5 mg.[12] Another man very rapidly developed the serotonin syndrome after taking considerable overdoses of **moclobemide** (3 g) and venlafaxine (2.625 g).[13]

Mechanism

The serotonin syndrome is thought to occur because venlafaxine can both inhibit serotonin re-uptake (its antidepressant activity is related to this activity) and because its metabolism is inhibited by MAOIs. The result is an increase in the concentrations of serotonin apparently causing overstimulation of the 5-HT$_{1A}$ receptors in the brain and spinal cord.[9]

Importance and management

An established, serious and potentially life-threatening interaction. The makers of venlafaxine recommend that it should not be used in combination with an MAOI or within 14 days of stopping treatment with the MAOI (although one patient developed the reaction 15 days after stopping selegiline[11]). Based on the half-life of venlafaxine they say that at least 7 days should elapse between stopping venlafaxine and starting an MAOI. The makers do not distinguish in this recommendation between the irreversible older MAOIs and the newer, reversible, selective MAOIs such as moclobemide. In theory the latter are probably less likely to interact, however for the time being it would be prudent to take the same precautions recommended for the non-selective MAOIs. In one of the studies was suggested that a wash-out period of several weeks is required between stopping MAOIs such as **phenelzine** and initiating a second serotonergic agent such as venlafaxine.[6]

1. Klysner R, Larsen JK, Sørensen P, Hyllested M, Pedersen BD. Toxic interaction of venlafaxine and isocarboxazide. *Lancet* (1995) 346, 1298–9.
2. Phillips SD, Ringo P. Phenelzine and venlafaxine interaction. *Am J Psychiatry* (1995) 152, 1400–1401.
3. Heisler MA, Guidry JR, Arnecke B. Serotonin syndrome induced by administration of venlafaxine and phenelzine. *Ann Pharmacother* (1996) 30, 84.
4. Weiner LA, Smythe M, Cisek J. Serotonin syndrome secondary to phenelzine-venlafaxine interaction. *Pharmacotherapy* (1998) 18, 399–403.
5. Diamond S, Pepper BJ, Diamond ML, Freitag FG, Urban GJ, Ergdemoglu AK. Serotonin syndrome induced by transitioning from phenelzine to venlafaxine: four patient reports. *Neurology* (1998) 51, 274–6.
6. Mason PJ, Morris VA, Balcezak TJ. Serotonin syndrome. Presentation of 2 cases and review of the literature. *Medicine* (2000) 79, 201–9.
7. Hodgman M, Martin T, Dean B, Krenzelok E. Severe serotonin syndrome secondary to venlafaxine and maintenance tranylcypromine therapy. *J Toxicol Clin Toxicol* (1995) 33, 554.
8. Brubacher JR, Hoffman RS, Lurin MJ. Serotonin syndrome from venlafaxine-tranylcypromine interaction. *Vet Hum Toxicol* (1996) 38, 358–61.
9. Wyeth Laboratories. Personal communication, March 1995.
10. Efexor (Venlafaxine hydrochloride) Data Sheet, Wyeth Laboratories, September 1999.
11. Gitlin MJ. Venlafaxine, monoamine oxidase inhibitors, and the serotonin syndrome. *J Clin Psychopharmacol* (1997) 17, 66–7.
12. Chan BSH, Graudins A, Whyte IM, Dawson AH, Braitberg G, Duggin GG. Serotonin syndrome resulting from drug interactions. *Med J Aust* (1998) 169, 523–5.
13. Roxanas MG, Machado JFD. Serotonin syndrome in combined moclobemide and venlafaxine ingestion. *Med J Aust* (1998) 168, 523–4.

24

Miscellaneous drug interactions

Acamprosate + Miscellaneous drugs

Acamprosate does not interact with alcohol, barbiturates, diazepam, disulfiram, imipramine, meprobamate, oxazepam or phenobarbital.

Clinical evidence, mechanism, importance and management

A 15-day phase IV study in 591 patients to assess the effects of the concurrent use of acamprosate with other drugs used during alcohol withdrawal found no evidence of interactions with **barbiturates**, **meprobamate**, **phenobarbital** or **oxazepam**.[1] Other studies found no pharmacological or clinical drug interactions with **diazepam**, **imipramine** or **disulfiram**, and the pharmacokinetics of both **alcohol** and acamprosate were unchanged by concurrent use.[2]

No special precautions would therefore appear to be needed with any of these drugs.

1. Aubin HJ, Lehert P, Beaupère B, Parot P, Barrucand D. Tolerability of the combination of acamprosate with drugs used to prevent alcohol withdrawal syndrome. *Alcoholism* (1995) 31, 25–38.
2. Durbin P, Hulot T, Chabac S. Pharmacodynamics and pharmacokinetics of acamprosate: an overview. In 'Acamprosate in relapse prevention of alcoholism.' Proceedings of the 1st Campral-Symposium ESBRA Stuttgart, September 1995.

Acipimox + Colestyramine

Acipimox does not appear to interact significantly with colestyramine.

Clinical evidence, mechanism, importance and management

A randomised crossover study in 7 healthy subjects given 150 mg of acipimox with 4 g **colestyramine**, followed by two additional 4 g doses of **colestyramine** 8 and 16 h later, showed that the pharmacokinetics of acipimox were slightly but not significantly altered by the **colestyramine**.[1] There would seem to be no good reason for avoiding concurrent use.

1. De Paolis C, Farina R, Pianezzola E, Valzelli G, Celotti F, Pontiroli AE. Lack of pharmacokinetic interaction between cholestyramine and acipimox, a new lipid lowering agent. *Br J Clin Pharmacol* (1986) 22, 496–7.

Alendronate + Miscellaneous drugs

The concurrent use of alendronate and NSAIDs should be avoided because of the increased risks of severe oesophagitis. The administration of alendronate and calcium supplements or antacids should separated by at least 30 minutes to avoid a reduction in its absorption. No other adverse interactions have been identified.

Clinical evidence, mechanism, importance and management

The makers suggest that patients should wait at least 30 minutes after taking alendronate before taking any other drug (they particularly name **calcium supplements** and **antacids**) because of the likelihood that they will interfere with the absorption of alendronate. The reason is that the bisphosphonates as a group can form complexes with a number of the divalent metallic ions (e.g. **bismuth**, **calcium**, **magnesium**).

Two of the risk factors identified with the severe oesophagitis that can occur with alendronate are pre-existing gastro-oesophageal disorders and the concurrent use of **NSAIDs** and **aspirin**.[1] A study in 26 healthy subjects found that gastric ulcers developed in 8% given alendronate alone, 12% in those given **naproxen** alone, and 38% in those given both drugs.[2] Despite the precautionary warning by the makers about this in their product literature,[3] a large-scale study in 5400 women on bisphosphonates found that 47% were also taking **NSAIDs**, 31% were taking an **H₂-blocker**, and 18% were taking all three. This suggests that prescribers are still not sufficiently aware that **NSAIDs** are best avoided by patients taking alendronate.

During clinical trials, a small number of women were given **oestrogen** while taking alendronate. No adverse reactions attributable to this concurrent use were seen.[3] The makers also say that although no interaction studies have been done, alendronate has been used in clinical studies with a wide range of other commonly prescribed drugs (not named) without any evidence of adverse interactions, and they say that none would be expected.[3]

1. Levine MAH, Grootendorst P. Alendronate co-medications may limits its use. *Clin Pharmacol Ther* (1998) 63, 197.
2. Graham DY, Malaty HM. Alendronate and naproxen are synergistic for development of gastric ulcers. *Arch Intern Med* (2001) 161, 107–110.
3. Fosamax (Alendronate). Merck Sharp & Dohme Limited. Summary of product characteristics, September 2000.

Alfacalcidol + Danazol

An isolated report describes hypercalcaemia in a woman on alfacalcidol when additionally treated with danazol.

Clinical evidence, mechanism, importance and management

A woman with idiopathic hypoparathyroidism treated with alfacalcidol developed hypercalcaemia when additionally given 400 mg **danazol** daily for endometriosis. She needed a reduction in the dosage of alfacalcidol from 4 to 0.75 micrograms daily. When the **danazol** was stopped 6 months later the alfacalcidol dosage was raised to 4 micrograms daily and she remained normocalcaemic.[1] The reasons are not understood. The general importance of this apparent interaction is unknown as it appears to be an isolated case.

1. Hepburn NC, Abdul-Aziz LAS, Whiteoak R. Danazol-induced hypercalcaemia in alphacalcidol-treated hypoparathyroidism. *Postgrad Med J* (1989) 65, 849–50.

Allopurinol + Antacids

Three haemodialysis patients showed a marked reduction in the effects of allopurinol while concurrently taking an aluminium hydroxide antacid. Separating the dosages by 3 h reduced the effects of this interaction.

Clinical evidence

Three patients on chronic haemodialysis, taking 5.7 g **aluminium hydroxide** daily and 300 mg allopurinol daily for high uric acid and phosphate levels, failed to show any fall in their hyperuricaemia until the **antacid** was given 3 h before the allopurinol, whereupon their uric acid levels fell by 40 to 65%. When one of them started once again to take both preparations together, her uric acid levels began to climb.[1]

Mechanism

Not understood.

Importance and management

Information seems to be limited to this report. Advise patients to separate the administration of these two drugs by 3 h or more to avoid admixture in the gut. Monitor the outcome. Follow the same precautions with any other antacid until more information becomes available.

1. Weissman I and Krivoy N. Interaction of aluminium hydroxide and allopurinol in patients on chronic hemodialysis. *Ann Intern Med* (1987) 107, 787.

Allopurinol + Iron

No adverse interaction occurs if iron and allopurinol are given concurrently.

Clinical evidence, mechanism, importance and management

Some early *animal* studies suggested that allopurinol might have an inhibitory effect on the metabolism of **iron**. This led the makers of allopurinol in some countries to issue a warning about their concurrent use,[1] however it now seems that no special precautions are needed.[1-3]

1. Ascione FJ. Allopurinol and iron. *JAMA* (1975) 232, 1010.
2. Emmerson BT. Effects of allopurinol on iron metabolism in man. *Ann Rheum Dis* (1966) 25, 700–703.
3. Davis PS, Deller DJ. Effect of a xanthine-oxidase inhibitor (allopurinol) on radioiron absorption in man. *Lancet* (1966) ii, 470–2.

Allopurinol + Probenecid

The theoretical possibility of an adverse interaction between allopurinol and probenecid, which could lead to uric acid precipitation in the kidneys, appears not to be realised in practice. Probenecid markedly increases the serum levels of allopurinol riboside.

Clinical evidence, mechanism, importance and management

(a) Allopurinol + Probenecid

Probenecid appears to increase the renal excretion of the active metabolite of allopurinol, oxipurinol (alloxanthine),[1] while allopurinol is thought to inhibit the metabolism of **probenecid**.[2,3] Allopurinol can increase the half-life and raise the serum plateau levels of **probenecid** by about 50 and 20% respectively.[2,3] It has been suggested that this might lead to an increase in the excretion of uric acid, which could result in the precipitation of uric acid in the kidneys. However, the clin-

ical importance of these mutual interactions seems to be minimal. No problems were reported in two studies in patients given 100 to 600 mg allopurinol and 500 to 2500 mg **probenecid** daily.[3,4]

(b) Allopurinol riboside + Probenecid

A study in 3 healthy subjects found that **probenecid** halved the clearance, increased the peak plasma levels and AUC, and extended the half-life of allopurinol riboside.[5] There is some evidence that the cure rate of American trypanosomiasis (Chagas' disease) and cutaneous leishmaniasis is better when the two drugs are used together.[5,6]

1. Elion GB, Yü T-F, Gutman AB, Hitchings GH. Renal clearance of oxipurinol, the chief metabolite of allopurinol. *Am J Med* (1968) 45, 69–77.
2. Horwitz D, Thorgeirsson SS, Mitchell JR. The influence of allopurinol and size of dose on the metabolism of phenylbutazone in patients with gout. *Eur J Clin Pharmacol* (1977) 12, 133–6.
3. Tjandramaga TB, Cucinell SA. Interaction of probenecid and allopurinol in gouty subjects. *Fedn Proc* (1971) 30, 392.
4. Yü T-F, Gutman AB. Effect of allopurinol (4-hydroxypyrazolo(3,4-d) pyrimidine) on serum and urinary uric acid in primary and secondary gout. *Am J Med* (1964) 37, 885–98.
5. Were JBO, Shapiro TA. Effects of probenecid on the pharmacokinetics of allopurinol riboside. *Antimicrob Agents Chemother* (1993) 37, 1193–6.
6. Saenz RE, Paz HM, Johnson CM, Marr JJ, Nelson DJ, Pattishall KH, Rogers MD. Treatment of American cutaneous leishmaniasis with orally administered allopurinol riboside. *J Infect Dis* (1989) 160, 153–8.

Allopurinol + Tamoxifen

A single case report describes a marked exacerbation of allopurinol hepatotoxicity in a man when given tamoxifen.

Clinical evidence, mechanism, importance and management

An elderly man who had been on 300 mg allopurinol daily for 12 years and who had mild chronic allopurinol hepatotoxicity, developed fever and marked increases in his serum levels of lactic dehydrogenase and alkaline phosphatase within a day of starting to take 10 mg **tamoxifen** twice daily.[1] This was interpreted as an exacerbation of the hepatotoxicity. He rapidly recovered when the allopurinol was stopped. The reasons for the reaction are not understood. It would now seem prudent to monitor the effects of concurrent use, but the general importance of this interaction is not known.

1. Shah KA, Levin J, Rosen N, Greenwald E, Zumoff B. Allopurinol hepatotoxicity potentiated by tamoxifen. *N Y State J Med* (1982) 82, 1745–6.

Allopurinol + Thiazides

Severe allergic reactions to allopurinol have been seen in a few patients, tentatively attributed to renal failure and the concurrent use of thiazide diuretics.

Clinical evidence, mechanism, importance and management

Most patients tolerate allopurinol very well, but life-threatening hypersensitivity reactions (rash, vasculitis, hepatitis, eosinophilia, progressive renal insufficiency, etc.) develop very occasionally with doses of 200 to 400 mg of allopurinol daily.[1] A report of 6 hypersensitivity reactions found that all of the reported cases were associated with pre-existing renal insufficiency, and in half of these, the patients were taking **thiazide diuretics**.[1] Another report describes 2 patients who developed a hypersensitivity vasculitis while taking allopurinol and **hydrochlorothiazide**.[2] Renal failure impairs the loss of oxipurinol (the major metabolite of allopurinol), but a study in healthy subjects failed to find any alteration in its clearance by **thiazides**, which might have provided a pharmacokinetic link between **thiazide** use and allopurinol toxicity.[3] A later study confirmed that in healthy subjects and patients with normal clearance of uric acid, **hydrochlorothiazide** has little effect on plasma levels and renal excretion of oxipurinol.[4] Other studies have shown that the effects of allopurinol on pyrimidine metabolism are enhanced by the use of **thiazides** (i.e.

they potentially increase hyperuricaemia, which may lead to renal damage).[5] Some caution is therefore appropriate if both drugs are used, particularly if renal function is abnormal, but more study is needed to confirm this possible interaction.

1. Hande KR, Noone RM, Stone WJ. Severe allopurinol toxicity. Description and guidelines for prevention in patients with renal insufficiency. *Am J Med* (1984) 76, 47–56.
2. Young JL, Boswell RB, Nies AS. Severe allopurinol hypersensitivity. Association with thiazides and prior renal compromise. *Arch Intern Med* (1974) 134, 553–8.
3. Hande KR. Evaluation of a thiazide-allopurinol drug interaction. *Am J Med Sci* (1986) 292, 213–16.
4. Löffler W, Landthaler R, De Vries JX, Walter-Sack I, Ittensohn A, Voss A, Zöllner N. Interaction of allopurinol and hydrochlorothiazide during prolonged oral administration of both drugs in normal subjects. I. Uric acid kinetics. *Clin Invest* (1994) 72, 1071–5.
5. Wood MH, O'Sullivan WJ, Wilson M, Tiller DJ. Potentiation of an effect of allopurinol on pyrimidine metabolism by chlorothiazide in man. *Clin Exp Pharmacol Physiol* (1974) 1, 53–8.

Almotriptan + Miscellaneous drugs

The makers of almotriptan contraindicate it with other 5-HT$_1$-agonists, lithium or ergot derivatives, despite limited evidence that the concurrent use of ergotamine may be safe. Almotriptan should not be used by patients taking nitrates, but no clinically relevant interactions occur with food, moclobemide or verapamil.

Clinical evidence, mechanism, importance and management

(a) Ergot derivatives

Ergotamine causes no differences in the rate or extent of almotriptan absorption, but a small decrease in its maximum serum levels occurs which is delayed by an hour. This is almost certainly of no clinical relevance. Nevertheless the makers contraindicate concurrent use because of a theoretical additive vasospastic risk even though no such additive effects were seen in a clinical trial in 12 healthy subjects. They also say that **ergotamine** should not be given less than 6 h after taking almotriptan, and recommend that almotriptan should not be taken less than 24 h after taking **ergotamine**.[1]

The makers similarly contraindicate other ergot derivatives (e.g. **dihydroergotamine**, **methysergide**) but make no recommendations about separating their administration.[1] The same precautions suggested for **ergotamine** would seem to be reasonable.

(b) Nitrates

The makers of almotriptan contraindicate its use in patients who have had a myocardial infarction, or have ischaemic heart disease, Prinzmetal's angina/coronary vasospasm, peripheral vascular disease or who show any evidence of ischaemic heart disease.[1] This means that any patient taking any **nitrate** (**glyceryl trinitrate**, **isosorbide mononitrate**, etc.) for angina should not use almotriptan because of the risk that it may cause vasospasm of the coronary arteries, lessen the flow of blood to the heart muscle and worsen the angina.

(c) Moclobemide

About 40% of almotriptan is lost from the body unaltered in the urine and up to 50% is lost by metabolism, mostly by deamination by monoamine oxidase (MAO-A) and to a lesser extent by cytochrome P450 isoenzymes and flavin mono-oxygenase (FMO). A multiple dose study using **moclobemide** (a reversible and selective inhibitor of MAO-A) found that the AUC of almotriptan was increased 37%, without any clinically relevant changes in maximum serum levels or half-life. No clinically significant interactions were seen[1] and it would seem therefore that concurrent use need not be avoided. There appears to be no direct clinical information about the use of **non-selective MAOIs** but it seems unlikely that a clinically relevant interaction will occur. This needs confirmation.

(d) Other 5-HT agonists or Lithium

The makers say that almotriptan is contraindicated with **other 5-HT$_{1B/1D}$-agonists**, the thinking behind it being that their effects would be expected to be additive.[1] They also say that **lithium** is contraindicated as well[1] to err on the side of caution, as patients on lithi-

um were excluded from clinical trials. There seem to be no reports of problems nor any clear theoretical reasons for this contraindication.[2]

(e) Other drugs

The makers say that no *in vivo* interaction studies have been carried out with almotriptan and other drugs, apart from those detailed in this monograph. *In vitro* studies using human liver microsomal enzymes suggest that almotriptan would not be expected to affect the metabolism of drugs metabolised by cytochrome P450 isoenzymes, or by MAO-A or MAO-B enzymes.[1]

(f) Verapamil

A study with multiple doses of **verapamil** (a cytochrome CYP3A4 substrate) found that it caused a 20% increase in the maximum serum levels and AUC of almotriptan which is not considered to be clinically relevant. No clinically significant interactions were seen.[1] There would therefore appear to be no reason for avoiding concurrent use.

1. Almogran (Almotriptan). Lundbeck Limited. Summary of product characteristics, October 2000.
2. Lundbeck Ltd. Personal communication, March 2001.

Alprostadil + Miscellaneous drugs

Intracavernous alprostadil and other drugs similarly used for erectile dysfunction should not be used concurrently.

Clinical evidence, mechanism, importance and management

There appear to be no reports of adverse interactions between intracavernous alprostadil (prostaglandin E$_1$) and other drugs, but the makers[1] say that smooth muscle relaxing drugs such as **papaverine** and other drugs used to induce erections such as **alpha-blocking drugs** (e.g. intracavernosal **moxisylyte**, **phentolamine**) should not be used concurrently because of the risks of priapism (prolonged erection).

1. Viridal (Alprostadil). Schwarz Pharma Limited. Summary of product characteristics, June 1999.

Aluminium hydroxide + Citrates or Vitamin C (ascorbic acid)

Patients with kidney failure given aluminium antacids and oral citrate can develop a potentially fatal encephalopathy due to a very marked rise in blood aluminium levels. Some drug formulations (including many non-prescription remedies) contain citrates as the effervescing or dispersing agent. There is evidence that vitamin C may interact similarly. It has also been recommended that normal subjects should not take aluminium antacids within 2 to 3 h of foods and drinks which contain citrates.

Clinical evidence

(a) Citrates

Following the death of 4 renal patients due to hyperalbuminaemia, possibly exacerbated by the concurrent use of **citrate** solutions,[1,2] a study was conducted in 34 patients and 5 healthy subjects to assess the possibility of an interaction.[2] It was found that in the 34 patients, increased serum aluminium levels were correlated with increased **citrate** intake. In the healthy subjects, aluminium levels were 11 micrograms/l at baseline. When aluminium was given the levels rose to 44 micrograms/l, and when aluminium was given concurrently with citrate, the levels rose to 98 micrograms/l. It was also found that aluminium clearance had dramatically increased in the presence of **citrate**.[2] Patients with renal failure are unlikely to be able to increase renal aluminium clearance, and so the effect of **citrate** in these patients may be even more dramatic. Another report claims to have noticed this interaction in another 8 renal patients, all of whom died.[3]

A tenfold rise in serum aluminium levels occurred in a haemodialysis patient given **effervescent co-codamol**, due to the presence of **sodium citrate** in the formulation, which is used to produce the effervescence.[4]

(b) Vitamin C (ascorbic acid)

A study in 13 healthy subjects given 900 mg aluminium hydroxide three times daily found that 2 g **vitamin C** daily increased the urinary excretion of aluminium threefold.[5] **Ascorbic acid** has been shown significantly to increase the concentration of aluminium in the liver, brain and bones of *rats* given aluminium hydroxide.[6]

Mechanism

Studies in healthy subjects clearly demonstrate that citrate markedly increases the absorption of aluminium from the gut.[2,7,8] The absorption is increased threefold, eight to tenfold and five to fiftyfold if taken with lemon juice,[9] orange juice[10,11] or citrate[2,7,8,10] respectively, but the reason is not understood. It could be that a highly soluble aluminium citrate complex is formed.[3,7]

Importance and management

The aluminium antacid/citrate interaction in patients with renal failure is established and clinically important. It is potentially fatal. Concurrent use should be strictly avoided. The authors of one report emphasise the risks associated with any of the commonly used citrates (sodium, calcium or potassium citrates, citric acid, Shohl's solution (citric acid/sodium citrate), etc.).[7] Remember too that some effervescent and dispersible tablets (including many proprietary non-prescription analgesics, indigestion and hangover remedies such as *Alka-Seltzer*) contain citric acid or citrates,[4,12] and they may also occur in soft drinks.[12] Haemodialysis patients should be strongly warned about these. The aluminium antacid/vitamin C interaction is not yet well established but the information available so far suggests that this combination should also be avoided. It is not clear whether orange juice is also unsafe but the available evidence suggests that concurrent administration probably best avoided.

The importance of the aluminium antacid/citrate interaction in non-renal subjects is by no means clear because it is still not known whether increased aluminium absorption adversely affects health. However, it has been recommended that food or drinks containing citric acid (citrus fruits and fruit juices) should not be taken at the same time as aluminium-containing medicines. Their ingestion should be separated by 2 to 3 h.[11]

1. Bakir AA, Hryhorczuk DO, Berman E, Dunea G. Acute fatal hyperaluminemic encephalopathy in undialyzed and recently dialyzed uremic patients. *Trans Am Soc Artif Intern Organs* (1986) 32, 171–6.
2. Bakir AA, Hryhorczuk DO, Ahmed S, Hessl SM, Levy PS, Spengler R, Dunea G. Hyperaluminemia in renal failure: the influence of age and citrate intake. *Clin Nephrol* (1989) 31, 40–4.
3. Kirschbaum HB, Schoolwerth AC. Acute aluminum toxicity associated with oral citrate and aluminum-containing antacids. *Am J Med Sci* (1989) 297, 9–11.
4. Main J, Hryhorczuk MK. Potentiation of aluminium absorption by effervescent analgesic tablets in a haemodialysis patient. *BMJ* (1992) 304, 1686.
5. Domingo JL, Gomez M, Llobet JM, Richart C. Effect of ascorbic acid on gastrointestinal aluminium absorption. *Lancet* (1991) 338, 1467.
6. Domingo JL, Gomez M, Llobet JM, Corbella J. Influence of some dietary constituents on aluminum absorption and retention in rats. *Kidney Int* (1991) 39, 598–601.
7. Coburn JW, Mischel MG, Goodman WG, Salusky IB. Calcium citrate markedly enhances aluminum absorption from aluminium hydroxide. *Am J Kidney Dis* (1991) 17, 708–11.
8. Walker JA, Sherman RA, Cody RP. The effect of oral bases on enteral aluminum absorption. *Arch Intern Med* (1990) 150, 2037–9.
9. Slanina P, Frech W, Ekström L-G, Lööf L, Slorach S, Cedergren A. Dietary citric acid enhances absorption of aluminum in antacids. *Clin Chem* (1986) 32, 539–41.
10. Weberg R, Berstad A. Gastrointestinal absorption of aluminium from single doses of aluminium containing antacids in man. *Eur J Clin Invest* (1986) 16, 428–32.
11. Fairweather-Tait S, Hickson K, McGaw B, Reid M. Orange juice enhances aluminium absorption from antacid preparation. *Eur J Clin Nutr* (1994) 48, 71–3.
12. Dorhout Mees EJ, Başçi A. Citric acid in calcium effervescent tablets may favour aluminium intoxication. *Nephron* (1991) 59, 322.

Anistreplase (APSAC) + Streptokinase

The effects of streptokinase or anistreplase are likely to be reduced or abolished if given some time after a prior dose of streptokinase or probably anistreplase because the persistently high levels of streptokinase antibodies reduce or prevent its activation.

Clinical evidence

A study in 25 patients who had been given **streptokinase** for the treatment of acute myocardial infarction found that 12 weeks later 24 patients had enough anti-streptokinase antibodies in circulation to neutralise an entire 1.5 million unit dose. After 4 to 8 months, 18 out of 20 still had enough antibodies to neutralise half of a 1.5 million unit dose.[1] Further study has suggested that antibody titre may remain high enough to neutralise the effects of **streptokinase** 4 years after a dose.[2] Anistreplase has been shown, in practice, to be neutralised by anti-streptokinase antibodies.[3]

Mechanism

The administration of streptokinase causes the production of anti-streptokinase antibodies. These persist in the circulation so that the clot-dissolving effects of another dose of streptokinase given many months later may be ineffective, or less effective, because it becomes bound and neutralised by these antibodies before it can activate the plasmin, which dissolves the fibrin of the clot. Many people already have a very low titre of antibodies against streptokinase even before they are given a first dose because they have become sensitised by a previous streptococcal infection, yet the incidence of allergic and anaphylactic reactions to anistreplase and streptokinase seems to be low (3% or less). At-risk patients can be identified by means of a skin test.[4]

Importance and management

An established and clinically important interaction. One author says[5] that "the real practical reason why therapy is not repeated within a year is that it simply would not work." Given that it has been suggested that the effects may be very persistent, until more is known, if a second administration is needed it would seem prudent to use a thrombolytic without antigenic effects.

1. Jalihal S, Morris GK. Antistreptokinase titres after intravenous streptokinase. *Lancet* (1990) 335, 184–5.
2. Elliott JM, Cross DB, Cederholm-Williams SA, White HD. Neutralizing antibodies to streptokinase four years after intravenous thrombolytic therapy. *Am J Cardiol* (1993) 71, 640–5.
3. Binette MJ, Agnone FA. Failure of APSAC thrombolysis. *Ann Intern Med* (1993) 119, 637.
4. Dykewicz MS, McGrath KG, Davison R, Kaplan KJ, Patterson R. Identification of patients at risk for anaphylaxis due to streptokinase. *Arch Intern Med* (1986) 146, 305–7.
5. Moriarty AJ. Anaphylaxis and streptokinase. *Hosp Update* (1987) 13, 342.

Antiasthmatic drugs + Beta-blockers

Asthmatic patients and others with a history of obstructive airways disease may experience marked, possibly life-threatening, bronchospasm if given beta-blockers. This may occur, though rarely, with beta-blockers which are classed as cardioselective, whether given orally or as eye drops.

Clinical evidence, mechanism, importance and management

The Committee on Safety of Medicines (CSM) in the UK[1] has issued the following advice: "Beta-blockers, including those considered to be cardioselective, should not be given to patients with a history of asthma/bronchospasm." An example of the danger is illustrated by an asthmatic patient who developed fatal status asthmaticus after taking just one dose of **propranolol**.[2] The CSM has had 51 reports of bronchospasm due to **propranolol**, 13 of them fatal, 5 of them in patients who had a history of asthma, bronchospasm or wheeze. The makers of **propranolol**, also highlight the dangers in their patient information leaflets.[3]

The warning applies particularly to the **non-selective beta-blockers** such as **propranolol** because asthmatics and others with chronic

Table 24.1 Non-steroidal anti-inflammatory drugs (NSAIDs) which can cause bronchoconstriction in asthmatics sensitive to aspirin (after Bianco S et al)[1]

Salicylates	Aspirin, benorylate, diflunisal, salsalate
Indole and indene-acetic acids	Indometacin (indomethacin), glucametacin, oxametacin, proglumetacin, sulindac, zomepirac
Arylacetic acids	Diclofenac, fenclofenac, fentiazac
Arylpropionic acids	Carprofen, ibuprofen, fenbufen, fenoprofen, flurbiprofen, indoprofen, ketoprofen, naproxen, tiaprofenic acid
Fenamates	Cyclofenamic acid, flufenamic acid, meclofenamic acid, mefenamic acid, niflumic acid
Pyrazolone derivatives	Aminophenazone, metamizole sodium (dipyrone), propyphenazone
Pyrazolidinediones	Azapropazone, bumadizone, feprazone, phenylbutazone, pyrazanone, oxyphenbutazone
Oxicams	Isoxicam, meloxicam, piroxicam, tenoxicam

obstructive airways disease are particularly sensitive to the effects of beta-blockade on the bronchi. However, it also extends to the so-called **selective (cardioselective) beta-blockers** because, they also can cause severe bronchospasm, particularly with high doses. The warning also applies to **beta-blockers** administered as **eye drops** since the systemic absorption can be very considerable. Strictly speaking this is not a drug–drug interaction, but a drug–disease interaction. The beta-blockers are listed as 'selective' and 'non-selective' in the introduction to Chapter 10.

The bronchoconstrictive effects of the beta-blockers can be opposed by beta-2 agonist drugs such a salbutamol, but as the makers point out, large doses may be needed and they suggest that ipratropium and intravenous aminophylline may been needed.[3] **Celiprolol** is an unusual selective beta-blocker which has been shown to cause bronchodilation rather than bronchoconstriction[4] with apparently some reduced risks for asthmatics, but this needs confirmation.

1. Committee on Safety of Medicines/Medicines Control Agency. Reminder: Beta-blockers contraindicated in asthma. *Current Problems* (1996) 22, 2.
2. Anon. Beta-blocker caused death of asthmatic. *Pharm J* (1991) 284, 185.
3. Fallowfield JM, Marlow HF. Propranolol is contraindicated in asthma. *BMJ* (1996) 313, 1486.
4. Pujet JC, Dubreuill C, Fluery B, Provendier O, Abella ML. Effects of celiprolol, a cardioselective beta-blocker, on respiratory function in asthmatic patients. *Eur Respir J* (1992) 5, 196–200.

Antiasthmatic drugs + Betel nuts (Areca)

The chewing of betel nuts may worsen the symptoms of asthma.

Clinical evidence

A study of this possible interaction was prompted by the observation of 2 Bangladeshi patients with severe asthma that appeared to have been considerably worsened by chewing **betel nuts**. One out of 4 other asthmatic patients who regularly chewed **betel nuts** developed severe bronchoconstriction (a 30% fall in the FEV_1) on two occasions when given **betel nuts** to chew, and all 4 said that prolonged **betel**

nut chewing induced coughing and wheezing. A double-blind study found that the inhalation of **arecoline** (the major constituent of the nut) caused bronchoconstriction in 6 of 7 asthmatics, and 1 of 6 healthy controls.[1]

Mechanism

Betel nut 'quids' consist of areca nut (*Areca catechu*) wrapped in betel vine leaf (*Piper betle*) and smeared with a paste of burnt (slaked) lime. It is chewed for the euphoric effects of the major constituent, arecoline, a cholinergic alkaloid, which appears to be absorbed through the mucous membrane of the mouth. Arecoline has identical properties to pilocarpine and normally has only mild systemic cholinergic properties, however asthmatic subjects seem to be particularly sensitive to the bronchoconstrictor effects of this alkaloid and possibly other substances contained in the nut.

Importance and management

Direct evidence appears to be limited to the reports cited, but the interaction seems to be established. It would appear normally not to be a serious interaction, but asthmatics should be encouraged to avoid betel nuts. This is a drug–disease interaction rather than a drug–drug interaction.

1. Taylor RFH, Al-Jarad N, John LME, Conroy DM, Barnes NC. Betel-nut chewing and asthma. *Lancet* (1992) 339, 1134–6.

Antiasthmatic drugs + NSAIDs

Aspirin and many other NSAIDs may cause bronchoconstriction in some asthmatic patients.

Clinical evidence, mechanism, importance and management

About 10% of asthmatics are sensitive to **aspirin**, and in some individuals life-threatening bronchoconstriction can occur. This is not a drug–drug interaction but an adverse response of asthmatic patients to **aspirin**, whether taking an antiasthmatic drug or not. The reasons are not understood. Those known to be sensitive to **aspirin** may also possibly react to other **NSAIDs**, in particular the **acetylated salicylates**, the **indole-** and **indene acetic acids**, and the **arylpropionic acids** (see Table 24.1). The **fenamates**, **oxicams**, **pyrazolones** and **pyrazolidinediones** are better tolerated.[1]

The nonacetylated salicylates (**sodium salicylate**, **salicylamide**, **choline magnesium trisalicylate**) are normally well tolerated.[1]

1. Bianco S, Robuschi M, Petrigni G, Scuri M, Pieroni MG, Refini RM, Vaghi A, Sestini PS. Efficacy and tolerability of nimesulide in asthmatic patients intolerant to aspirin. *Drugs* (1993) 46 (Suppl 1), 115–120.

Anticholinesterases + Antimalarials

On theoretical grounds, the neuromuscular blocking effects occasionally seen with chloroquine and quinine might be expected to worsen the symptoms of myasthenia gravis, and oppose the effects of drugs (anticholinesterases) used in its treatment.

Clinical evidence, mechanism, importance and management

Quinine and **chloroquine**[1-4] can very occasionally cause muscular weakness similar to that seen in myasthenia gravis, and rarely this neuromuscular blocking effect has been seen to be additive with the effects of conventional neuromuscular blockers (see 'Neuromuscular blockers + Quinine', p.769 and 'Neuromuscular blockers + Chloroquine', p.760). One patient developed a myasthenic syndrome within a week of starting 300 mg **chloroquine** daily, which was controllable with edrophonium, which recurred on re-challenge, and which disappeared within a few days of stopping the **chloroquine**.[2]

There seem to be no cases on record of myasthenic patients who have shown increased muscular weakness when given either of these antimalarial drugs so that the risk is still uncertain, but be alert for evidence of worsening myasthenia if either drug is used. It has been suggested that **quinine** should be avoided by myasthenics as it may aggravate their condition.[5] Strictly speaking this is a drug–disease rather than a drug–drug interaction.

1. De Bleecker J, De Reuck J, Quatacker J, Meire F. Persisting chloroquine-induced myasthenia? *Acta Clin Belg* (1991) 46, 401–6.
2. Robberecht W, Bednarik J, Bourgeois P, van Hees J, Carton H. Myasthenic syndrome caused by direct effect of chloroquine on neuromuscular junction. *Arch Neurol* (1989) 46, 464–8.
3. Sghirlanzoni A, Mantegazza R, Mora M, Pareyson D, Cornelio F. Chloroquine myopathy and myasthenia-like syndrome. *Muscle Nerve* (1988) 11, 114–19.
4. Pichon P, Soichot P, Loche D, Chapelon M. Syndrome myasthenique induit par une intoxication a la choroquine: une forme clinique inhabituelle confirmee par une atteinte oculaire. *Bull Soc Ophtalmol Fr* (1984) 84, 219–22.
5. Sweetman SC, editor. Martindale: The complete drug reference. 33rd ed. London: Pharmaceutical Press; 2002 p. 446.

Anticholinesterases + Methocarbamol

An isolated report describes a reduction in the effects of pyridostigmine in a myasthenic patient when treated with methocarbamol.

Clinical evidence, mechanism, importance and management

A woman with myasthenia gravis controlled with **pyridostigmine** developed weakness when started on 1 g **methocarbamol** four times daily and 130 mg dextropropoxyphene 6-hourly as needed, both for constant back pains. She recovered over 4 days after the **methocarbamol** was stopped and the dextropropoxyphene reduced to 65 mg 4-hourly. Rechallenge with 1 g **methocarbamol** five times daily resulted in "overwhelming weakness" 2 days later, and recovery when it was withdrawn.[1] The reasons are not understood. This seems to be the only report of this interaction but it would be prudent to monitor the effects of **methocarbamol** in any myasthenic patient, or avoid its use.

1. Podrizki A. Methocarbamol and myasthenia gravis. *JAMA* (1968) 205, 938.

Anticholinesterases + Miscellaneous drugs

Acetazolamide, ampicillin, aspirin, chlorpromazine, dipyridamole, erythromycin, imipenem/cilastatin, ketoprofen, lithium carbonate, procainamide and quinidine have all been implicated in unmasking myasthenia gravis or worsening the muscular weakness of one or more patients with the disease. Penicillamine, phenytoin and trimethadione have been associated with the development of myasthenia.

Clinical evidence, mechanism, importance and management

Acetazolamide 500 mg intravenously, was observed to worsen the muscular weakness of patients with myasthenia gravis taking anticholinesterase drugs. This was demonstrated in an electromyographic study in 7 patients given **acetazolamide** followed by **edrophonium chloride** 5 mg, and also in an isolated *animal* nerve-muscle preparation.[1] A patient well maintained on **distigmine bromide** experienced an aggravation of his myasthenic symptoms on two occasions when additionally given 75 mg **dipyridamole** three times daily.[2] **Ampicillin**,[3] **aspirin**,[4] **chlorpromazine**,[5] **erythromycin**,[6] **imipenem/cilastatin**,[7] **ketoprofen**,[4] **lithium carbonate**,[8] **procainamide**[9,10] and **quinidine**[10-13] have also been observed to increase the muscular weakness in one or more patients with myasthenia gravis, or to unmask the disease. **Phenytoin**,[14] **trimethadione**[15] and **penicillamine** alone[16-18] and possibly also the **tricyclic antidepressants**,[18] have

been associated with the development of myasthenia in a few patients. The mechanisms of these interactions are not understood.

The evidence for most of these interactions is very sparse indeed, and in most instances they are simply rare and isolated cases. It would therefore be wrong to exaggerate their importance, but it would nevertheless be prudent to be alert for any evidence of worsening myasthenia if any of the drugs listed is added to established treatment.

1. Carmignani M, Scoppetta C, Ranelletti OF, Tonali P. Adverse interaction between acetazolamide and anticholinesterase drugs at the normal and myasthenic neuromuscular junction level. *Int J Clin Pharmacol Ther Toxicol* (1984) 22, 140–4.
2. Haddad M, Zelikovski A, Reiss R. Dipyridamole counteracting distigmine in a myasthenic patient. *IRCS Med Sci* (1986) 14, 297.
3. Argov Z, Brenner T, Abramsky O. Ampicillin may aggravate clinical and experimental myasthenia gravis. *Arch Neurol* (1986) 43, 255–6.
4. McDowell IFW, McConnell JB. Cholinergic crisis in myasthenia gravis precipitated by ketoprofen. *BMJ* (1985) 291, 1094.
5. McQuillen MP, Gross M, Johns RJ. Chlorpromazine-induced weakness in myasthenia gravis. *Arch Neurol* (1963) 8, 286–90.
6. Absher JR, Bale JF. Aggravation of myasthenia gravis by erythromycin. *J Pediatr* (1991) 119, 155–6.
7. O'Riordan J, Javed M, Doherty C, Hutchinson M. Worsening of myasthenia gravis on treatment with imipenem/cilastatin. *J Neurol Neurosurg Psychiatry* (1994) 57, 383.
8. Neil JF, Himmelhoch JM, Licata SM. Emergence of myasthenia gravis during treatment with lithium carbonate. *Arch Gen Psychiatry* (1976) 33, 1090–2.
9. Drachman DA, Skom JH. Procainamide and myasthenia gravis. *Arch Neurol* (1965) 13, 316–20.
10. Kornfeld P, Horowitz SH, Genkins G, Papatestas AE. Myasthenia gravis unmasked by antiarrhythmic agents. *Mt Sinai J Med* (1976) 43, 10–14.
11. Aviado DM, Salem H. Drug action, reaction, and interaction. I. Quinidine for cardiac arrhythmias. *J Clin Pharmacol* (1975) 15, 477–85.
12. Stoffer SS, Chandler JH. Quinidine-induced exacerbation of myasthenia gravis in patient with Graves' disease. *Arch Intern Med* (1980) 140, 283–4.
13. Weisman SJ. Masked myasthenia gravis. *JAMA* (1949) 141, 917–18.
14. Brumlik J, Jacobs RS. Myasthenia gravis associated with diphenylhydantoin therapy for epilepsy. *Can J Neurol Sci* (1974) 1, 127–9.
15. Booker HE, Chun RWM, Sanguino M. Myasthenia gravis syndrome associated with trimethadione. *JAMA* (1970) 212, 2262–3.
16. Vincent A, Newsom-Davis J, Martin V. Anti-acetylcholine receptor antibodies in D-penicillamine-associated myasthenia gravis. *Lancet* (1978) i, 1254.
17. Masters CL, Dawkins RL, Zilko PJ, Simpson JA, Leedman RJ, Lindstrom J. Penicillamine-associated myasthenia gravis, antiacetylcholine receptor and antistriational antibodies. *Am J Med* (1977) 63, 689–94.
18. Ferro J, Susano R, Gómez C, de Quirós FB. Miastenia inducida por penicilamina: ¿existe interacción con los antidepresivos tricíclicos? *Rev Clin Esp* (1993) 192, 358–9.

Anticholinesterases + Propafenone

Propafenone can oppose the effects of anticholinesterases used for myasthenia gravis and has anticholinergic effects which may possibly be additive with other anticholinergic drugs.

Clinical evidence, mechanism, importance and management

Propafenone is reported to aggravate myasthenia gravis, possibly due to its anticholinergic effects on nicotinic receptors on skeletal muscle. This was seen in a patient well controlled on **pyridostigmine**. Improvement occurred when the propafenone was withdrawn. Other cases have also been described. Avoidance in patients with myasthenia gravis has been advised.[1]

1. Committee on Safety of Medicines. Respiratory and neuromuscular effects of propafenone. *Current Problems* (1990) 29, 4.

Anticholinesterases + Quinolone antibacterials

Three reports describe a worsening of the symptoms of myasthenia gravis in one patient given norfloxacin, and two given ciprofloxacin.

Clinical evidence

A woman with myasthenia gravis on 360 mg **pyridostigmine** and 20 mg prednisone daily, was started on 400 mg **norfloxacin** twice daily for a urinary tract infection. Over the next 4 h she progressively developed double vision, weakness of the neck and proximal muscles of the arms and legs, dysphagia, weakness of the chest wall muscles and shortness of breath. She complained of increasing fatigue and shortness of breath with each subsequent dose. It was necessary to double the **pyridostigmine** dosage to control the symptoms. The symptoms vanished within 2 days of stopping the **norfloxacin**. Rechallenge with 400 mg **norfloxacin** 6 months later in the absence of the prednisone produced essentially the same response.[1]

Another woman with myasthenia gravis controlled with 180 mg **pyridostigmine** 4 to 6 hourly, intravenous cyclophosphamide and prednisone, developed shortness of breath and weakness of limb and neck muscles within 8 h of starting to take 750 mg **ciprofloxacin** twice daily for a respiratory tract infection. The symptoms were initially tolerable when the **ciprofloxacin** dose was reduced to 500 mg twice daily, but over the next few days, after briefly increasing the dose back to 750 mg twice daily, it was found necessary to continue to reduce the **ciprofloxacin** dose and eventually to stop it altogether because of worsening myasthenia gravis. Improvement occurred once the **ciprofloxacin** was stopped.[2] Another report describes a man who developed myasthenic symptoms (severe dysphagia, dysarthria and ptosis) within 48 h of starting to take 250 mg **ciprofloxacin** twice daily, which was later relieved by **edrophonium** and **pyridostigmine**. He appeared to have had mild undiagnosed myasthenia for several months.[3]

Mechanism

Not understood. The inference to be drawn is that these quinolones have sufficient neuromuscular blocking activity in some myasthenic patients to oppose the actions of anticholinesterases.

Importance and management

Information seems to be limited to these three reports. Until more is known it would be prudent to monitor the effects of ciprofloxacin and norfloxacin in any patient with myasthenia gravis, although the general importance of these interactions in myasthenic patients is not known. There seems to be no information about any of the other quinolones.

1. Rauser EH, Ariano RE, Anderson BA. Exacerbation of myasthenia gravis by norfloxacin. *DICP Ann Pharmacother* (1990) 24, 207–8.
2. Moore B, Safani M, Keesey J. Possible exacerbation of myasthenia gravis by ciprofloxacin. *Lancet* (1988) 1, 882.
3. Mumford CJ, Ginsberg L. Ciprofloxacin and myasthenia gravis. *BMJ* (1990) 301, 818.

Antihistamines + Benzodiazepines

Mizolastine and lorazepam appear not to interact adversely.

Clinical evidence, mechanism, importance and management

A number of antihistamines cause sedation (see 'Alcohol + Antihistamines', p.17) and this would be expected to be increased by some of the benzodiazepines by the simple addition of their CNS depressant effects. **Mizolastine**, however, appears to lack sedative effects and does not have a detrimental effect on psychomotor performance.[1] A single oral dose of 2 mg **lorazepam** was found to impair the performance of psychomotor tests in 16 healthy subjects and caused some sedation and amnesia, but these effects were not changed while also taking 10 mg **mizolastine** daily for 8 days.[1] There would seem to be no reason for avoiding the concurrent use of these two drugs.

1. Patat A, Perault MC, Vandel B, Ulliac N, Zieleniuk I, Rosenzweig P. Lack of interaction between a new antihistamine, mizolastine, and lorazepam on psychomotor performance and memory in healthy volunteers. *Br J Clin Pharmacol* (1995) 39, 31–8.

Antihistamines + Contraceptives, oral

The effects of doxylamine and diphenhydramine appear not to be affected by the concurrent use of oral contraceptives.

Clinical evidence, mechanism, importance and management

The pharmacokinetics of 25 mg **doxylamine** in 13 subjects and the pharmacokinetics of 50 mg **diphenhydramine** in 10 subjects were not significantly altered by the use of **low dose oestrogen-containing contraceptives**.[1] One case of **oral contraceptive** failure has been attributed to the use of **unnamed antihistamines**[2] but this remains unconfirmed. No particular precautions would seem to be necessary during concurrent use.

1. Luna BG, Scavone JM, Greenblatt DJ. Doxylamine and diphenhydramine pharmacokinetics in women on low-dose estrogen oral contraceptives. *J Clin Pharmacol* (1989) 29, 257–60.
2. DeSano EA, Hurley SC. Possible interactions of antihistamines and antibiotics with oral contraceptive effectiveness. *Fertil Steril* (1982) 37, 853–4.

Antihistamines + H₂-blockers

Cimetidine does not appear to interact adversely with either cetirizine or hydroxyzine, and ranitidine is unlikely to interact with terfenadine. However, an isolated case report describes torsade de pointes in one patient on terfenadine and cimetidine.

Clinical evidence

(a) Cetirizine or Hydroxyzine + Cimetidine

Treatment with 600 mg **cimetidine** 12-hourly for 10 days had no effect on either the pharmacokinetics or pharmacodynamics of 10-mg doses of **cetirizine** in 8 patients with chronic urticaria.[1] Another 16 patients with chronic urticaria were given 25 mg **hydroxyzine** or 10 mg **cetirizine** before and after taking 600 mg **cimetidine** 12-hourly for 10 days. The **cimetidine** increased the AUC of the **hydroxyzine** by 33% and also increased its suppression of the wheal and flare response, but the pharmacokinetics of the **cetirizine** were statistically unaltered and its effects remained unchanged.[2] A previous study found that **cimetidine** raised serum **hydroxyzine** levels.[3]

(b) Terfenadine + Cimetidine or Ranitidine

Five days' treatment with 1200 mg **cimetidine** had no effect on the pharmacokinetics of single 120-mg doses of **terfenadine** in 12 healthy subjects.[4] Another study in two groups of 6 healthy subjects confirmed the lack of effect of 600 mg **cimetidine** 12-hourly or 150 mg **ranitidine** 12-hourly on the pharmacokinetics of 60 mg **terfenadine** 12-hourly. No adverse ECG changes were seen.[5] However, an isolated case report describes a woman of 63 who had 8 episodes of syncope (later identified as being due to torsade de pointes) and a convulsion 2 days after starting 60 mg **terfenadine** twice daily and 400 mg **cimetidine** twice daily. She was also taking chlorphenamine and co-proxamol (paracetamol (acetaminophen) + dextropropoxyphene (propoxyphene)).[6]

Mechanism

Cimetidine is a non-specific enzyme inhibitor, which could possibly be expected to affect the metabolism of terfenadine, which is thought to be metabolised by the cytochrome P450 isoenzyme CYP3A4. Whether other metabolic pathways are involved is not clear, but it would seem that in most cases the enzyme inhibitory effects of cimetidine do not affect terfenadine metabolism.

Importance and management

There would seem to be no good reason for avoiding the concurrent use of either cetirizine or hydroxyzine and cimetidine, nor would any of the other H₂-blockers such as famotidine, nizatidine or ranitidine be expected to interact with either of these antihistamines. The situation with terfenadine and cimetidine is not totally clear because of the isolated case report of toxicity cited here, but at the present time there is not enough evidence to advise against the use of these two drugs. Cetirizine and loratadine are non-interacting alternatives.

1. Simons KJ, Sussman GL, Simons FER. The effect of the H$_2$-antagonist cimetidine (C) on the pharmacokinetics (PK) and pharmacodynamics (PD) of the H$_1$-antagonist cetirizine (CET) in patients with chronic urticaria. *Pharm Res* (1993) 10 (10 Suppl), S-355.
2. Simons FER, Sussman GL, Simons KJ. Effect of the H$_2$-antagonist cimetidine on the pharmacokinetics and pharmacodynamics of the H$_1$-antagonists hydroxyzine and cetirizine in patients with chronic urticaria. *J Allergy Clin Immunol* (1995) 95, 685–93.
3. Salo OP, Kauppinen K, Männistö PT. Cimetidine increases the plasma concentration of hydroxyzine. *Acta Derm Venereol (Stockh)* (1986), 66, 349–50.
4. Eller MG, Okerhold RA. Effect of cimetidine on terfenadine and terfenadine metabolite pharmacokinetics. *Pharm Res* (1991) 8 (10 Suppl), S-297.
5. Honig PK, Wortham DC, Zamani K, Conner DP, Mullin JC, Cantilena LR. Effect of concomitant administration of cimetidine and ranitidine on the pharmacokinetics and electrocardiographic effects of terfenadine. *Eur J Clin Pharmacol* (1993) 45, 41–6.
6. Ng PW, Chan WK, Chan TYK. Torsade de pointes during concomitant use of terfenadine and cimetidine. *Aust N Z J Med* (1996) 26, 120–1.

Anti-ulcer preparation + Milk

Hypercalcaemia, alkalosis and renal insufficiency (milk-alkali syndrome) developed in a man while taking *Caved-S* and large amounts of milk.

Clinical evidence

A man presented with nausea, vomiting, constipation, polyuria and polydipsia, which was diagnosed as milk-alkali syndrome (hypercalcaemia, alkalosis, renal insufficiency) due to daily treatment with 6 tablets of *Caved-S* and 3.5 pints of **milk** for dyspepsia caused by a peptic ulcer.[1] This dose of *Caved-S* meant he was taking 600 mg **aluminium hydroxide**, 1200 mg **magnesium carbonate**, 600 mg **sodium bicarbonate** and 2280 mg **deglycyrrhizinised liquorice** daily.

Mechanism

The hypercalcaemia occurred because the absorbed alkali decreased the excretion of calcium by the kidneys, while the intake of calcium (in the milk) remained high. The excessive amount of calcium increased the reabsorption of bicarbonate by the kidneys (through salt and water depletion) so that the alkalosis was maintained. Hypermagnesaemia may also have had a part to play.

Importance and management

The milk-alkali syndrome is well documented but very uncommon these days because there are now other and better ways of treating peptic ulcers. This case amply illustrates that while taking this anti-ulcer preparation, well within the recommended dosage range (up to 12 tablets daily), it is still possible to develop a serious and potentially life-threatening reaction if the intake of calcium (in milk for example) is high.

1. Gibbs CJ, Lee HA. Milk-alkali syndrome due to Caved-S. *J R Soc Med* (1992) 85, 498–9.

Astemizole + Azole antifungals

Ketoconazole has been implicated in the development of life-threatening torsade de pointes arrhythmia in at least two patients taking astemizole. Itraconazole appears to interact to a much lesser extent and the evidence relating to miconazole is indirect. However, because of the severity of the interaction astemizole is contraindicated with azole antifungals.

Clinical evidence

(a) Itraconazole

Itraconazole 200 mg or a placebo were given to 12 healthy subjects twice daily for 14 days, with a single oral 10-mg dose of astemizole on day 11. The peak plasma astemizole levels were slightly but not significantly increased by the **itraconazole** but the AUC was approximately doubled and the half-life increased from 2.1 to 3.6 days. The QTc interval was unaltered.[1]

(b) Ketoconazole

A 63-year old woman developed torsade de pointes arrhythmia and was found to have a prolonged QT interval after taking astemizole and **ketoconazole**. These two drugs were withdrawn and she was successfully treated with a temporary pacemaker, magnesium sulphate and lidocaine (lignocaine). She was later discharged with a normal ECG.[2] Another patient is known to have developed torsade de pointes while taking astemizole, **erythromycin** and **ketoconazole**.[3]

(c) Miconazole

An *in vitro* study using human liver microsomal enzymes and ^{14}C-labelled compounds found that **miconazole** inhibits the metabolism of astemizole. On the basis of the values obtained it has been predicted that a clinically relevant interaction could occur *in vivo*.[4]

Mechanism

In vitro studies with human liver microsomes have shown that ketoconazole inhibits the metabolism of astemizole, which *in vivo* would result in raised serum astemizole levels.[5] High serum levels of astemizole cause a prolongation of the QT interval and may precipitate the development of torsade de pointes arrhythmia. This has been seen in young otherwise healthy individuals after astemizole overdosage.[6-8] Itraconazole and miconazole also inhibit the metabolism of astemizole but they are much less potent than ketoconazole.[4,5]

Importance and management

The astemizole/ketoconazole interaction is established and clinically important although much of the evidence for it is indirect. The risk of an astemizole/itraconazole interaction seems on the evidence currently available to be much less. The astemizole/miconazole interaction is very poorly documented and there appear to be no clinical reports of problems. Similarly there appear to be no clinical reports of problems with astemizole/fluconazole. The incidence of an azole antifungal/astemizole interaction is probably small but because of its potential severity and unpredictability, the concurrent use of these drugs is contraindicated in all patients. This is a recommendation of the makers[9] and the CSM in the UK.[10]

1. Lefebvre RA, Van Peer A, Woestenborghs R. Influence of itraconazole on the pharmacokinetics and electrocardiographic effects of astemizole. *Br J Clin Pharmacol* (1997) 43, 319–22.
2. Tsai W-C, Tsai L-M, Chen J-H. Combined use of astemizole and ketoconazole resulting in torsade de pointes. *J Formos Med Ass* (1977) 96, 144–6.
3. Gelb LN (ed). *FDA Med Bull* (1993) 23, 2.
4. Lavrijsen K, Heykants J. Interaction potential of miconazole with the metabolism of astemizole and desmethylastemizole in human liver microsomes. Data on file, Janssen Research Foundation, N 102975/1, December 1993.
5. Lavrijsen K, Van Houdt J, Meuldermans W, Janssens M, Heykants J. The interaction of ketoconazole, itraconazole and erythromycin with the in vitro metabolism of antihistamines in human liver microsomes. *Allergy* (1993) 48 (Suppl 16), 34.
6. Snook J, Boothman-Burrell D, Watkins J, Colin-Jones D. Torsade de pointes ventricular tachycardia associated with astemizole overdose. *Br J Clin Pract* (1988) 42, 257–9.
7. Craft TM. Torsade de pointes after astemizole overdose. *BMJ* (1985) 292, 660.
8. Bishop RO, Gaudry PL. Prolonged Q-T interval following astemizole overdose. *Arch Emerg Med* (1989) 6, 63–5.
9. Hismanal (Astemizole). Janssen-Cilag Ltd. Summary of product characteristics, June 1998.
10. Committee on Safety of Medicines. Ventricular arrhythmias due to terfenadine and astemizole. *Current Problems* (1992) 35, 1–2.

Astemizole + Grapefruit juice

Grapefruit juice does not interact with astemizole.

Clinical evidence, mechanism, importance and management

Astemizole 30 mg daily for 4 days, and then 10 mg daily for the next 20 days was given to 12 healthy subjects. It was found that the steady-state pharmacokinetics of the astemizole remained unaffected when the subjects drank 200 ml **grapefruit juice** at four-hourly intervals for 12 h (a total of 800 ml).[1] There would therefore appear to be no reason for avoiding **grapefruit juice** while taking astemizole, unlike the situation with terfenadine (see 'Terfenadine + Grapefruit juice', p.936).

1. Janssen-Cilag Ltd, Data on file (Study AST-BEL-7 + Amendment) 1995.

Astemizole + Macrolide antibacterials

Potentially life-threatening torsade de pointes arrhythmia has been seen in patients on astemizole and erythromycin. Troleandomycin is believed to interact similarly, but not azithromycin. There is evidence that dirithromycin interacts only minimally.

Clinical evidence

(a) Azithromycin

The makers of astemizole report that an *in vivo* study has shown that **azithromycin** had a negligible effect on the bioavailability of astemizole.[1]

(b) Dirithromycin

A 10 day course of 500 mg **dirithromycin** daily or a placebo was given to 18 healthy subjects and on day 4 they were additionally given a single 30 mg oral dose of astemizole. It was found that the pharmacokinetics of the major metabolite of astemizole (*N*-desmethylastemizole) were unchanged by the **dirithromycin**, whereas the astemizole clearance was reduced by 34%, the volume of distribution increased by 24% and the half-life extended from 25 to 45.9 h. However, no changes in the mean QTc intervals were seen.[2]

(c) Erythromycin

A woman of 87 collapsed suddenly in her kitchen 4 days after starting to take 10 mg astemizole daily and a tablet of **erythromycin** (unknown strength) twice daily. An ECG showed her to be having multiple episodes of torsade de pointes arrhythmia, the longest of 17 sec duration. Her QT_c was 720 ms and she was mildly hypokalaemic. She was given a temporary pacemaker and when eventually discharged with a normal sinus rhythm, her QT_c had fallen to 475 ms.[3] Two other patients are reported to have developed syncope and torsade de pointes arrhythmias while taking astemizole and **erythromycin**. One of them was also taking **ketoconazole**.[4]

Mechanism

Erythromycin and similar macrolides inhibit the metabolism of the astemizole by cytochrome P450 isoenzyme CYP3A4 (demonstrated in *in vitro* studies using human liver microsomes[5]) leading to its accumulation in the body. High concentrations of astemizole are known to prolong the QT_c interval which can lead to torsade de pointes arrhythmias both in overdose[6] and even in healthy teenagers at normal doses.[7]

Importance and management

Direct information about the astemizole/erythromycin interaction appears to be limited to the two reports cited, and even less is known about astemizole/clarithromycin, but this and other indirect evidence has caused the CSM[8] in the UK and the makers[1] to contraindicate the concurrent use of astemizole and macrolide antibacterials in general. This includes erythromycin, clarithromycin and **troleandomycin**, although as yet there appears to be no direct evidence implicating **troleandomycin**. However, the makers specifically except azithromycin, which does not interact,[1] and the evidence cited above indicates that dirithromycin interacts only minimally and without apparently affecting the QT_c interval. Terfenadine is not a safe alternative for astemizole because it interacts with the macrolides in the same way, but neither cetirizine (see 'Cetirizine + Erythromycin or Ketoconazole', p.872) nor loratadine (see 'Loratadine + Miscellaneous drugs', p.903) appear to do so, and are therefore safe substitutes for astemizole.

1. Hismanal (Astemizole). Janssen-Cilag Ltd. Summary of product characteristics, June 1998.

2. Bachmann K, Sullivan TJ, Reese JH, Jauregui L, Miller K, Scott M, Stotka J, Harris J. A study of the interaction between dirithromycin and astemizole in healthy adults. *Am J Ther* (1997) 4, 73–9.
3. Goss JE, Ramo BW, Blake K. Torsades de pointes associated with astemizole (Hismanal) therapy. *Arch Intern Med* (1993) 153, 2705.
4. Gelb LN (ed). *FDA Med Bull* (1993) 23, 2.
5. Lavrijsen K, Van Houdt J, Meuldermans W, Janssens M, Heykants J. The interaction of ketoconazole, itraconazole and erythromycin with the in vitro metabolism of antihistamines in human liver microsomes. *Allergy* (1993) 48 (Suppl 16), 34.
6. Snook J, Boothman-Burrell D, Watkins J, Colin-Jones D. Torsade de pointes ventricular tachycardia associated with astemizole overdose. *Br J Clin Pract* (1988) 42, 257–9.
7. Simons FER, Kesselman MS, Giddins NG, Pelech AN, Simons KJ. Astemizole-induced torsade de pointes. *Lancet* (1988) ii, 624.
8. Committee on Safety of Medicines. Ventricular arrhythmias due to terfenadine and astemizole. *Current Problems* (1992) 35, 1–2.

Astemizole + Miscellaneous drugs

The makers of astemizole contraindicate the concurrent use of SSRIs (because of possible increased astemizole serum levels) and those pro-arrhythmic drugs which might additively prolong the QT interval and thereby increase the risk of serious arrhythmias.

Clinical evidence, mechanism, importance and management

The makers of astemizole contraindicate the concurrent use of **SSRIs** because there is the risk that they will inhibit its metabolism, leading to a rise in its serum levels which could result in QT interval prolongation and the development of torsade de pointes arrhythmias. The makers say that an *in vitro* study also suggests that **nefazodone** may interact significantly.[1] These are all predicted interactions the clinical importance of which await confirmation.

The makers[1] contraindicate the ". . . concurrent use of other drugs which predispose to arrhythmias (such as **anti-arrhythmic agents, neuroleptics, tricyclic antidepressants**)" but they do not specifically name any of these drugs except for **terfenadine**. The thinking behind this warning is that some of these drugs can, like astemizole, prolong the QT interval so that their effects might possibly be additive. See 'Drugs that prolong the QT interval + Other drugs that prolong the QT interval', p.103. However, the clinical importance of all of these predicted interactions awaits confirmation.

Hypokalaemia is a contraindication for the use of astemizole,[1] and therefore care is needed with diuretics which can cause potassium depletion, such as **furosemide (frusemide)**, **bumetanide**, **etacrynic acid** and the **thiazides**.

1. Hismanal (Astemizole). Janssen-Cilag Ltd. Summary of product characteristics, June 1998.

Astemizole + Quinine

Quinine causes a marked but transient increase in plasma astemizole levels, and is therefore considered by the makers to be contraindicated to avoid the possible risk of heart arrhythmias. There are 3 reports that appear to confirm that this is a clinically important interaction.

Clinical evidence

Astemizole 30 mg daily for 4 days followed by 10 mg daily for the next 20 days, was given to 12 healthy subjects. The steady-state pharmacokinetics of the astemizole were then examined after taking 20 mg **quinine** every four hours for 12 h (a total of 80 mg **quinine**), and after a single 430-mg dose. The smaller dose of **quinine** caused only a slight increase in the maximum plasma astemizole levels and AUC, but the larger single **quinine** dose resulted in a transient threefold increase in both maximum plasma levels and AUC, especially the metabolite of astemizole, desmethylastemizole.[1]

A patient on astemizole with slight hypomagnesaemia is reported to have experienced torsade de pointes arrhythmia after taking only a single dose of **quinine sulphate**.[2]

Mechanism

Uncertain. One suggestion is that the interaction is not primarily due to inhibition of the metabolism of astemizole by the quinine, but rather to a transient quinine-induced displacement of both astemizole and its metabolite from its tissue binding sites.[1]

Importance and management

Information is very limited, but on the basis of the evidence cited above and on two case reports on file of cardiac arrhythmias possibly attributable to an astemizole/quinine interaction,[3] the makers of astemizole contraindicate the concurrent use of quinine in order to avoid the risk of cardiac arrhythmias.[4] The case report that is cited here confirms that this is a potentially clinically hazardous drug combination.[2]

The larger single dose of quinine 430 mg used in the study approached the dosage used for the treatment of malaria, whereas the smaller dose of 80 mg was equivalent to the amount contained in 2 litres of a quinine-containing soft drink.[1] There would therefore appear to be no reason for those on astemizole to avoid moderate quantities of these quinine-containing drinks. See also 'Drugs that prolong the QT interval + Other drugs that prolong the QT interval', p.103.

1. Janssen-Cilag Ltd, Data on file (Study AST-BEL-7 + Amendment) 1995.
2. Martin ES, Rogalski K, Black JN. Quinine may trigger torsades de pointes during astemizole therapy. *Pacing Clin Electrophysiol* (1997) 20, 2024–5.
3. Janssen-Cilag Ltd. Personal Communication, May 1997.
4. Hismanal (Astemizole). Janssen-Cilag Ltd. Summary of product characteristics, June 1998.

Atorvastatin + Miscellaneous drugs

Atorvastatin causes small increases in the serum levels of ethinylestradiol, norethisterone (norethindrone) and digoxin, while clarithromycin, erythromycin and grapefruit juice cause moderate increases in atorvastatin levels. Considerable increases occur with itraconazole. On theoretical grounds the makers warn of the increased risk of myopathy with niacin (nicotinic acid). No clinically relevant interactions occur with azithromycin, cimetidine, colestipol, *Maalox*, terfenadine or warfarin, nor with ACE inhibitors, beta-blockers, diuretics or hypoglycaemic agents.

Clinical evidence, mechanism, importance and management

(a) Alcohol

No adverse interactions appear to have been reported with **alcohol** and atorvastatin except that the makers say it should be used with caution in patients who drink substantial quantities of **alcohol**, the reason being that dysfunction of the liver possibly increases the risk of atorvastatin toxicity.[1]

(b) Aluminium/magnesium hydroxides (Maalox)

A study in patients given 10 mg atorvastatin daily for 15 days found that when additionally treated with 30 ml *Maalox* four times daily for a further 17 days the maximum serum levels and the AUC of the atorvastatin were reduced 34% and the absorption rate was also reduced. However the LDL-cholesterol reduction remained the same.[2] There is therefore no need to avoid the concurrent use of *Maalox*, nor does the dosage of atorvastatin need to be raised.

(c) Azole antifungals

Ten healthy subjects were given 200 mg **itraconazole** daily for 5 days, and on day 4 they were additionally given a single 40-mg dose of atorvastatin. The **itraconazole** increased the AUC of atorvastatic acid and atorvastatic lactone fourfold and threefold respective-

ly, and increased their half-lives threefold and twofold respectively. The AUC values of active and total HMG-CoA reductase inhibitors were increased 1.6 and 1.7-fold respectively.[3] The probable reason for these changes is that **itraconazole** inhibits the metabolism of atorvastatin by cytochrome P450 isoenzyme CYP3A4 so that its metabolism and clearance is reduced.

It is not known whether these increases are clinically important or not but there is evidence that the risk of myopathy is increased by increases in the serum levels of the statins in general. The makers therefore advise caution if **azole antifungals** (none specifically named) are given concurrently.[1]

(d) Cimetidine

Twelve healthy subjects were given 10 mg atorvastatin daily for 2 weeks followed by the addition of 300 mg **cimetidine** four times daily for a further 2 weeks. It was found that the **cimetidine** did not alter the atorvastatin pharmacokinetics, nor were its LDL-cholesterol reducing effects altered.[4] There would appear to be no reason for avoiding concurrent use.

(e) Colestipol

A study in which atorvastatin and **colestipol** were given concurrently found that although the serum levels of atorvastatin were reduced about 25%, the total reduction in the LDL-cholesterol levels were greater than when each drug was given alone.[1] There would therefore appear to be no reason for avoiding concurrent use, nor any need to increase the atorvastatin dosage.

(f) Contraceptives, oral

A study in 12 women taking atorvastatin and an **oral contraceptive** (*Ortho-Novum*) found that the AUC values for **norethisterone (norethindrone)** and **ethinylestradiol** were increased 28% and 19% respectively and their maximum serum levels were raised by 24% and 30% respectively.[1,5] The probable reason is that the metabolism of these steroids is reduced by inhibition of cytochrome P450 isoenzyme CYP3A4.[5] These increases are only moderate and unlikely to be clinically important but the makers say that they should be considered when selecting an oral contraceptive for women given atorvastatin.[1]

(g) Digoxin

Digoxin 250 micrograms daily was given to 24 healthy subjects for 10 days, to which was then added either 10 mg or 80 mg atorvastatin daily for a further 10 days. The mean steady-state **digoxin** levels were unaffected by 10 mg atorvastatin, but 80 mg caused a 20% rise in maximum **digoxin** levels and a 15% rise in the 24 hr AUC. The reason appears to be that atorvastatin increases the absorption of **digoxin** from the gut by inhibiting P-glycoprotein.[6] The rise is only moderate, but patients taking both drugs should be monitored, being alert for any need to reduce the **digoxin** dosage.

(h) Grapefruit juice

Twelve healthy subjects were given 200 mg double-strength **grapefruit juice** three times daily for 5 days. On day 3 they were given a single 40-mg dose of atorvastatin with the **grapefruit juice** followed by two more 200-ml doses of **grapefruit juice** at half-an-hour and one-and-a-half hour intervals. The 72-hour AUC values of the active **atorvastatin** and total HMG-CoA reductase inhibitors were increased 1.3 and 1.5-fold respectively. The probable reason is that a component of the **grapefruit juice** decreases the first-pass metabolism of the atorvastatin by the small intestine, probably by inhibiting the activity of cytochrome P450 isoenzyme CYP3A4.[7] The clinical importance of these increases is not clear but it seems doubtful if this is an important interaction when using low or moderate doses of atorvastatin.

(i) Macrolide antibacterials

Twelve healthy subjects were given a single 10-mg dose of atorvastatin on day 7 of an 11-day course of 500 mg **erythromycin** four times daily. The maximum serum atorvastatin levels were raised 38% by the **erythromycin** and the AUC was raised 33%.[5] The reason is almost certainly because the **erythromycin** inhibits cytochrome P450 isoenzyme CYP3A4 which is concerned with the metabolism of the atorvastatin.[1] **Clarithromycin** similarly increases the serum levels of atorvastatin.[1] The clinical importance of the moderate rises seen is uncertain, but the makers of atorvastatin draw attention to the risks of myopathy with increased statin levels and advise caution.[1]

Direct evidence about interactions between other macrolides and atorvastatin appears to be lacking, apart from **azithromycin** which has been shown not to interact.[1] Be alert for **troleandomycin** to behave like erythromycin whereas **dirithromycin** would not be expected to do so.

(j) Miscellaneous drugs

The makers of atorvastatin warn that the risk of myopathy is increased by the concurrent administration of **niacin (nicotinic acid)**[1] It is clearly sensible to monitor the concurrent use of these drugs, being alert for any evidence of myopathy (muscle pain, tenderness, weakness, malaise, fever, raised creatine phosphokinase (CPK) levels), particularly during the early months of treatment.[1]

The makers say that clinical studies in which atorvastatin was used with **antihypertensives** (including **ACE inhibitors**, **beta-blockers** and **diuretics**) or **hypoglycaemic agents**, no clinically significant interactions were seen.[1]

(k) Terfenadine

A group of healthy subjects was given single 120-mg doses of **terfenadine**, and then 2 weeks later another single dose of **terfenadine** on day 7 of a 9 days' course of 80 mg atorvastatin. It was found that the atorvastatin caused some small to moderate changes in the pharmacokinetics of the **terfenadine** and fexofenadine (AUC +35% and −2% respectively, maximum serum levels 8% and −16% respectively). More importantly there were no changes in the QTc interval, which indicates that atorvastatin does not increase the cardiotoxicity of the **terfenadine**.[8] There would therefore appear to be no reason for avoiding concurrent use.

(l) Warfarin

A study in 12 patients chronically treated with **warfarin** found that the addition of 80 mg atorvastatin daily for 2 weeks caused only a slight fall (about 1.7 sec) in prothrombin times for the first few days.[9] No **warfarin** dosage adjustments are likely to be needed if atorvastatin is used concurrently but the makers say that monitoring is advisable.[1]

1. Lipitor (Atorvastatin). Parke Davis. Summary of product characteristics, May 2000.
2. Yang B-B, Smithers JA, Abel RB, Stern RH, Sedman AJ, Olson SC. Effects of Maalox TC® on pharmacokinetics and pharmacodynamics of atorvastatin. *Pharm Res* (1996) 13 (9 Suppl), S437.
3. Kantola T, Kivisto KT, Neuvonen PJ. Effect of itraconazole on the pharmacokinetics of atorvastatin. *Clin Pharmacol Ther* (1998) 64, 58–65.
4. Stern RH, Gibson DM, Whitfield LR. Cimetidine does not alter atorvastatin pharmacokinetics or LDL-cholesterol reduction. *Eur J Clin Pharmacol* (1998) 53, 475–8.
5. Yang B-B, Siedlik PH, Smithers JA, Sedman AJ, Stern RH. Atorvastatin pharmacokinetic interactions with other CYP3A4 substrates: erythromycin and ethinyl estradiol. *Pharm Res* (1996) 13 (9 Suppl), S-437.
6. Boyd RA, Stern RH, Stewart RH, Wu X, Reyner EL, Zegarac EA, Randinitis EJ, Whitfield L. Atorvastatin coadministration may increase digoxin concentrations by inhibition of intestinal P-glycoprotein-mediated secretion. *J Clin Pharmacol* (2000) 40, 91–8.
7. Lilja JJ, Kivisto KT, Neuvonen PJ. Grapefruit juice increases serum concentrations of atorvastatin and has no effect on pravastatin. *Clin Pharmacol Ther* (1999) 66, 118-27.
8. Stern RH, Smithers JA, Olson SC. Atorvastatin does not produce a clinically significant effect on the pharmacokinetics of terfenadine. *J Clin Pharmacol* (1998) 38, 753–7.
9. Stern R, Abel R, Gibson GL, Besserer J. Atorvastatin does not alter the anticoagulant activity of warfarin. *J Clin Pharmacol* (1997) 37, 1062–4.

Avitriptan + Propranolol

No adverse interaction occurs if avitriptan and propranolol are used concurrently.

Clinical evidence, mechanism, importance and management

Healthy subjects were given two 150-mg doses of avitriptan and a regimen of 80 mg **propranolol** twice daily, alone and together. The pharmacokinetics of the avitriptan were unchanged by concurrent use, but the peak serum levels and the AUCs of the metabolites of avitriptan (*N*-desmethylavitriptan and methoxypyrimidinyl piperazine) were increased by about 25%. The AUC of **propranolol** was increased by 20%. A small increase in blood pressure and a small decrease in heart rate were also seen. None of these changes were considered to be clinically relevant and the conclusion was reached that avitriptan may safely be added to a steady-state regimen of **propranolol** in the treatment of migraine.[1]

1. Marathe PH, Greene DS, Kollia GD, Barghaiya RH. A pharmacokinetic interaction study of avitriptan and propranolol. *Clin Pharmacol Ther* (1998) 63, 367–8.

Azelastine + Erythromycin or Ketoconazole

No adverse interaction affecting cardiac function occurs between azelastine and erythromycin or ketoconazole.

Clinical evidence, mechanism, importance and management

(a) Erythromycin

A 3-period, open-label, crossover study in 8 healthy subjects found that when 500 mg **erythromycin** three times daily was added to 4 mg azelastine twice daily for a week, no changes in the pharmacokinetics of the azelastine were seen, suggesting that azelastine is not metabolised by cytochrome P450 isoenzyme CYP3A4. There were no adverse ECG changes when both drugs were given concurrently.[1] There would therefore appear to be no reason for avoiding concurrent use, unlike the situation with other antihistamines such as astemizole and terfenadine.

(b) Ketoconazole

In a three-period open-label study 12 healthy subjects were given azelastine 4 mg 12-hourly for 14 days, followed by a further 7 days with either 200 mg **ketoconazole** or a placebo daily. None of the treatments caused any significant ECG changes. Other *in vitro* studies indicated that no pharmacokinetic interaction is likely to occur *in vivo* between azelastine and **ketoconazole**. The authors of this study concluded that concurrent use is safe and that azelastine does not interact like astemizole or terfenadine with ketoconazole to affect cardiac function.[2] No special precautions would seem to be needed.

1. Sale M, Lyness W, Perhach J, Woosley R, Rosenberg A. Lack of effect of coadministration of erythromycin (ERY) with azelastine (AZ) on pharmacokinetic (PK) or ECG parameters. *Ann Allergy Asthma Immunol* (1996) 74, 91.
2. Morganroth J, Lyness WH, Perhach JL, Mather GG, Harr JE, Trager WF, Levy RH, Rosenberg A. Lack of effect of azelastine and ketoconazole coadministration on electrocardiographic parameters in healthy volunteers. *J Clin Pharmacol* (1997) 37, 1065–72.

Baclofen + Ibuprofen

A man developed baclofen toxicity when given ibuprofen.

Clinical evidence, mechanism, importance and management

An isolated report describes a man taking 20 mg baclofen three times a day who developed baclofen toxicity (confusion, disorientation, bradycardia, blurred vision, hypotension and hypothermia) after taking 8 doses of **ibuprofen** 600 mg three times daily. It appeared that the toxicity was caused by baclofen accumulation arising from acute renal insufficiency caused by the **ibuprofen**.[1] This is a relatively rare side-effect of **ibuprofen**. The general importance of this interaction is likely to be very small. There appears to be no information about baclofen and other NSAIDs and little reason for avoiding concurrent use.

1. Dahlin PA, George J. Baclofen toxicity associated with declining renal clearance after ibuprofen. *Drug Intell Clin Pharm* (1984) 18, 805–8.

Baclofen + Miscellaneous drugs

The makers of baclofen warn about increased sedation with CNS depressants, increased hypotension with antihyperten-

sives, and a possible increased risk of convulsions in epileptics.

Clinical evidence, mechanism, importance and management

Baclofen on its own frequently causes sedation and drowsiness, for which reason the makers warn about the possible additive effects of other **CNS depressants** and **alcohol**. Hypotension is another side-effect which is expected to be additive with **antihypertensive drugs**. The convulsive threshold is also lowered so that convulsions are possible, particularly in epileptic patients.[1] Increased care is therefore needed in those taking **anticonvulsants**.

There seem to be no direct reports describing particular problems with any of these drugs, but the warnings issued by the makers of baclofen would seem to be reasonable precautions based on the known side-effects of baclofen.

1. Lioresal (Baclofen). Cephalon UK Limited. Summary of product characteristics, July 2000.

Benzbromarone + Miscellaneous drugs

Aspirin antagonises the uricosuric effects of benzbromarone. It is not clear whether benzbromarone remains effective in the presence of pyrazinamide, but it is not affected by chlorothiazide.

Clinical evidence, mechanism, importance and management

Benzbromarone is an effective uricosuric agent, increasing the percent ratio of urate to creatinine clearance by 371% at its peak in 6 subjects with gout. When benzbromarone was given with a single 600-mg dose of **aspirin**, the peak ratio of urate to creatinine clearance with 160 mg benzbromarone was only 12%.[1] **Aspirin** in divided doses of 650 mg, up to a total of 5.2 g daily was given to 29 healthy subjects on 40 to 80 mg benzbromarone daily. The urate lowering effects of benzbromarone were most affected by aspirin 2.7 g. Alone benzbromarone reduced the urate levels by 60%, but in the presence of **aspirin** the levels were only reduced by 48%.[2]

It is not clear whether benzbromarone remains effective in patients taking **pyrazinamide**. One report claims that when 50 mg benzbromarone was given to 10 patients taking 35 mg/kg **pyrazinamide** daily for 8 to 10 days, uric acid levels were reduced by an average of 24.3% and returned to normal levels in four of them.[3] However, another report says that 160 mg benzbromarone daily had no uricosuric effect on 5 patients taking 3 g **pyrazinamide** daily,[1] and other authors also refer to this failure to reduce uric acid levels.[2]

The uricosuric effects of benzbromarone appear to be unaffected by the concurrent use of **chlorothiazide**.[4,5]

1. Sinclair DS, Fox IH. The pharmacology of hypouricemic effect of benzbromarone. *J Rheumatol* (1975) 2, 437–45.
2. Sorensen LB, Levinson DJ. Clinical evaluation of benzbromarone. *Arthritis Rheum* (1976) 19, 183–90.
3. Kropp R.Zur urikosurischen Wirkung von Benzbromaronum an Modell der pyrizinamid-bedingten Hyperurikämie. *Med Klin* (1970) 65, 1448–50.
4. Heel RC, Brogden RN, Speight TM, Avery GS. Benzbromarone: a review of its pharmacological properties and therapeutic use in gout and hyperuricaemia. *Drugs* (1977) 14, 349–66.
5. Gross A, Giraud V. Über die Wirkung von Benzbromaron auf Urikämie und Urikosurie. *Med Welt* (1972) 23, 133–6.

Betahistine + Terfenadine

A single report describes the re-emergence of the labyrinthine symptoms in a patient taking betahistine when given terfenadine.

Clinical evidence, mechanism, importance and management

An isolated and very brief report says that the effects of betahistine were opposed in a patient by the concurrent use of **terfenadine** and a multi-drug regimen (not detailed) with the return of the labyrinthine symptoms.[1] This interaction had been predicted on theoretical grounds because betahistine is an analogue of histamine which would be expected to interact like this with any antihistamine.[2] The use of antihistamines should be carefully considered in patients taking betahistine.

1. Beeley L, Cunningham H, Brennan A. Bull W Midlands Centre of Adverse Drug Reporting. (1993) 36, 28.
2. Serc (Betahistine). Solvay Healthcare Limited. Summary of product characteristics, December 1999.

Bezafibrate + Furosemide (Frusemide)

An isolated report describes acute renal failure and rhabdomyolysis in a patient attributed to treatment with 400 mg bezafibrate daily and 25 mg furosemide (frusemide) on alternate days.[1] The general importance of this is unknown.

1. Venzano C, Cordì GC, Corsi L, Dapelo M, De Micheli A, Grimaldi GP. Un caso di rabdomiolisi acuta con insufficienza renale acuta da assunzione contemporanea di furosemide e bezafibrato. *Minerva Med* (1990) 81, 909–11.

Cabergoline + Miscellaneous drugs

Dopamine antagonists (such as the phenothiazines) are expected to oppose the action of cabergoline. The makers also advise the avoidance of ergot derivatives and macrolides, which they suggest on theoretical grounds might interact. No pharmacokinetic interaction occurs between cabergoline and selegiline.

Clinical evidence, mechanism, importance and management

Cabergoline acts by directly stimulating dopamine receptors (it is a D2 agonist), which is why the makers suggest that dopamine antagonists (e.g. **phenothiazines**, **butyrophenones**, **thioxanthenes**, **metoclopramide**) should be avoided, because they would be expected to oppose the actions of cabergoline.[1] There is however no direct clinical evidence to confirm how important this is, but it is clearly a reasonable precaution to take.

Because cabergoline is an ergot derivative, the makers have looked at what happens if other **ergot derivatives** are used concurrently, but have so far found no evidence of changes in the efficacy or safety of cabergoline. Nevertheless they do not recommend their long-term concurrent use.[1] The makers also suggest, by analogy with other ergot derivatives (ergotamine, dihydroergotamine), that **macrolide antibacterials** should be avoided because of the risk that the cabergoline effects and adverse effects could be increased.[1] However, these theoretical interactions with cabergoline have yet to be shown to be of clinical importance. See also 'Ergot + Macrolide antibacterials', p.888.

No pharmacokinetic interaction was found to occur between cabergoline 1 mg daily and **selegiline** 10 mg daily in a study covering a 22 day period in 6 subjects.[2]

1. Dostinex (Cabergoline). Pharmacia. Summary of product characteristics, February 2000.
2. Dostert P, Benedetti MS, Persiani S, La Croix R, Bosc M, Fiorentini F, Deffond D, Vernay D, Dordain G. Lack of pharmacokinetic interaction between the selective dopamine agonist cabergoline and the MAO-B inhibitor selegiline. *J Neural Transm* (1995) 45 (Suppl), 247–57.

Calcium/Vitamin D + Thiazide diuretics

Hypercalcaemia and possibly metabolic alkalosis can develop in patients given high doses of vitamin D and/or large amounts of calcium if they are additionally treated with diuretics such as the thiazides, which can reduce the urinary excretion of calcium.

Clinical evidence

(a) Calcium/vitamin D + Thiazides

An elderly woman on **hydrochlorothiazide** 25 mg and **triamterene** 50 mg daily for hypertension, and 50000 units **vitamin D_2** with 1.5 g **calcium** daily for osteoporosis, became confused, disorientated and dehydrated. Her serum calcium level had risen to 13.9 mg/dl (normal range 8.2 to 10.5 mg/dl).[1]

A young woman with osteoporosis taking 3 mg **vitamin D_2** and 2 g **calcium** daily became hypercalcaemic when given **chlorothiazide**.[2] In a group of 12 patients treated for hypoparathyroidism with **vitamin D** (**dihydrotachysterol** or **ergocalciferol**), 5 patients became hypercalcaemic when treated with **bendroflumethiazide** or **methyclothiazide**.[3] A significant rise in plasma calcium levels occurred in 7 patients given **vitamin D** and a **thiazide** experimentally, and hypercalcaemia developed in 3 of them.[4]

(b) Calcium carbonate + Thiazides

A 47-year-old man was admitted to hospital complaining chiefly of dizziness and general weakness which had begun 2 months previously. He was taking 500 mg **chlorothiazide** daily for hypertension, 120 mg 'thyroid' daily for hypothyroidism and 7.5 to 10 g **calcium carbonate** daily for 'heartburn'. On examination he was found to have metabolic alkalosis with respiratory compensation, a total serum calcium concentration of 6.8 mEq/l (normal 4.3 to 5.2 mEq/l) and an abnormal ECG. He was diagnosed as having the milk-alkali syndrome. Recovery was rapid when the **thiazide** and **calcium carbonate** were withdrawn, and a sodium chloride infusion, furosemide (frusemide) and oral phosphates were given.[5]

An elderly woman with normal kidney function on **hydrochlorothiazide** 50 mg daily and 2.5 to 7.5 g **calcium carbonate** daily also developed hypercalcaemia.[6]

In both cases the **thiazide** diuretic was thought to be implicated as the levels of calcium ingestion were in the region of the normally recommended doses.

Mechanism

The thiazide diuretics (and triamterene) can cause calcium retention by reducing the urinary excretion. This, added to the increased intake of calcium, resulted in excessive calcium levels. Alkalosis (the milk-alkali syndrome associated with hypercalcaemia, alkalosis, renal insufficiency) may also occur in some individuals because the thiazide limits the excretion of bicarbonate.

Importance and management

An established interaction. The incidence is unknown but the reports cited[3,4] in (a) suggest that it can be considerable if the intake of vitamin D and calcium are high. Concurrent use need not be avoided, but the serum calcium levels should be regularly monitored to ensure that they do not become excessive. There is evidence that the hypercalcaemia may be self-limiting.[3] Patients should be warned about the ingestion of very large amounts of calcium carbonate (readily available without prescription) if they are taking thiazide diuretics.

1. Drinka PJ, Nolten WE. Hazards of treating osteoporosis and hypertension concurrently with calcium, vitamin D, and distal diuretics. *J Am Geriatr Soc* (1984) 32, 405–7.
2. Parfitt AM. Chlorothiazide-induced hypercalcaemia in juvenile osteoporosis and hyperparathyroidism. *N Engl J Med* (1969) 281, 55–9.
3. Parfitt AM. Thiazide-induced hypercalcaemia in vitamin D-treated hypoparathyroidism. *Ann Intern Med* (1972) 77, 557–63.
4. Parfitt AM. Interactions of thiazide diuretics with parathyroid hormone and vitamin D. Studies in patients with hypoparathyroidism. *J Clin Invest* (1972) 51, 1879–88.
5. Gora ML, Seth SK, Bay WH, Visconti JA. Milk-alkali syndrome associated with use of chlorothiazide and calcium carbonate. *Clin Pharm* (1989) 8, 227–9.
6. Hakim R, Tolis G, Goltzman D, Meltzer S, Friedman R. Severe hypercalcemia associated with hydrochlorothiazide and calcium carbonate therapy. *Can Med Assoc J* (1979) 121, 591–4.

Cannabis + Disulfiram

An isolated case report describes a hypomanic-like reaction in a man on disulfiram when he used cannabis.

Clinical evidence, mechanism, importance and management

A man with a 10-year history of drug abuse (alcohol, amphetamines, cocaine, cannabis) experienced a hypomanic-like reaction (euphoria, hyperactivity, insomnia, irritability) on two occasions while being treated with 250 mg **disulfiram** daily, which was attributed to the concurrent use of cannabis. The patient said that he felt as though he had been taking amfetamine.[1] The reason for this reaction is not understood. Other patients given both of these drugs did not experience this reaction.[2]

1. Lacoursiere RB, Swatek R. Adverse interaction between disulfiram and marijuana: a case report. *Am J Psychiatry* (1983) 140, 243–4.
2. Rosenberg CM, Gerrein JR, Schnell C. Cannabis in the treatment of alcoholism. *J Stud Alcohol* (1978) 39, 181.

Carbenoxolone + Antacids

There is some evidence that antacids may possibly reduce the effects of carbenoxolone.

Clinical evidence, mechanism, importance and management

The bioavailability of carbenoxolone combined with **magnesium** and **aluminium hydroxide** antacids in a liquid formulation was found to be approximately half that of carbenoxolone in granular and capsule formulations.[1] The extent to which **antacids** might reduce the ulcer-healing effects of carbenoxolone given in other formulations seems not to have been assessed, but the possibility should be borne in mind.

1. Crema F, Parini J, Visconti M, Perucca E. Effetto degli antiacidi sulla biodisponibilità del carbenoxolone. *Farmaco (Prat)* (1987) 42, 357–64.

Carbenoxolone + Antihypertensives or Diuretics

Carbenoxolone causes fluid retention and raises the blood pressure in some patients. This may be expected to oppose the effects of antihypertensive drugs. Thiazides can be used to treat the adverse side-effects of carbenoxolone. Spironolactone or amiloride oppose the ulcer-healing effects of carbenoxolone. The potassium-losing effects of the thiazides, related diuretics and carbenoxolone can be additive so that a potassium supplement may be needed to prevent hypokalaemia.

Clinical evidence, mechanism, importance and management

(a) Carbenoxolone + Antihypertensives

Carbenoxolone can raise the blood pressure. Five out of 10 patients on 300 mg carbenoxolone daily, and 2 out of 10 taking 150 mg daily, showed a rise in diastolic blood pressure of 20 mmHg or more.[1] Other reports[2-8] confirm that fluid retention and hypertension occur, the incidence of the latter being variously reported as being as low as 4%[8]

or as high as 50%,[7] and fluid retention as absent[2] or affecting 46% of patients.[7] The reason for the blood pressure rise is that carbenoxolone has mineralocorticoid-like activity. There appear to be few direct reports of adverse interactions between **antihypertensive drugs** and carbenoxolone, but patients on carbenoxolone should have regular checks on their weight and blood pressure, whether taking an **antihypertensive agent** or not. An increase in the dosage of the **antihypertensive agent** may be necessary.

(b) Carbenoxolone + Diuretics

Thiazide diuretics can be used to control the oedema and hypertension caused by carbenoxolone, but not **spironolactone**[3] (an aldosterone-antagonist) or **amiloride**[9] because they oppose its ulcer-healing effects. **Deglycyrrhizinised liquorice**, which is an analogue of carbenoxolone, has reduced mineralocorticoid activity and fewer side-effects.[7,10] If **thiazides or related drugs** are used it should be remembered the potassium-losing effects of the carbenoxolone and the diuretic will be additive, so that a potassium supplement may be needed to prevent hypokalaemia. For example, severe hypokalaemia associated with rhabdomyolysis and acute tubular necrosis occurred in a patient given carbenoxolone and **chlortalidone** without a potassium supplement.[11] Other **potassium-depleting diuretics**, which might be expected to interact similarly, are listed in Table 14.2 (see 'Digitalis glycosides + Diuretics, potassium depleting', p.541). Alternative drugs for the treatment of ulcers are the H_2-blockers, and the proton pump inhibitors.

1. Turpie AGG, Thomson TJ. Carbenoxolone sodium in the treatment of gastric ulcer with special reference to side-effects. *Gut* (1965) 6, 591.
2. Bank S, Marks IN. Maintenance carbenoxolone sodium in the prevention of gastric ulcer recurrence. In 'Carbenoxolone Sodium', Baron A and Sullivan S (eds), Butterworths, London (1970) p.103–16.
3. Doll R, Langman MJS, Shawdon HH. Treatment of gastric ulcer with carbenoxolone: antagonistic effect of spironolactone. *Gut* (1968) 9, 42–5.
4. Montgomery RD, Cookson JB. Comparative trial of carbenoxolone and a deglycyrrhizinated liquorice preparation (Cavid-S). *Clin Trials J* (1972) 9, 33–5.
5. Langman MJS, Knapp DR, Wakley EJ. Treatment of chronic gastric ulcer with carbenoxolone and gefarnate: a comparative trial. *BMJ* (1973) 3, 84–6.
6. Horwich L and Galloway R. Treatment of gastric ulcer with carbenoxolone sodium. Clinical and radiological evaluation. *BMJ* (1965) 2, 1272.
7. Fraser PM, Doll R, Langman MJS, Misiewicz JJ, Shawdon HH. Clinical trial of a new carbenoxolone analogue (BX-24), zinc sulphate, and vitamin A in the treatment of gastric ulcer. *Gut* (1972) 13, 459–63.
8. Montgomery RD. Side effects of carbenoxolone sodium: a study of ambulant therapy of gastric ulcer. *Gut* (1967) 8, 148–50.
9. Reed PI, Lewis SI, Vincent-Brown A, Holdstock DJ, Gribble RJN, Murgatroyd RE, Baron JH. The influence of amiloride on the therapeutic and metabolic effects of carbenoxolone in patients with gastric ulcer. *Scand J Gastroenterol* (1980) 15 (Suppl 65), 51–5.
10. Brogden RN, Speight TM, Avery GS. Deglycyrrhizinised liquorice: a report of its pharmacological properties and therapeutic efficacy in peptic ulcer. *Drugs* (1974) 8, 330–9.
11. Descamps C, Vandenbroucke JM, van Ypersele de Strihou C. Rhabdomyolysis and acute tubular necrosis associated with carbenoxolone and diuretic treatment. *BMJ* (1977) 1, 272.

Carbenoxolone + Miscellaneous drugs

Chlorpropamide appears to have an effect on the pharmacokinetics of carbenoxolone, causing a small reduction in serum levels. Tolbutamide, phenytoin and warfarin do not appear to have any significant effects on carbenoxolone pharmacokinetics.

Clinical evidence, mechanism, importance and management

Single doses of 500 mg **tolbutamide**, 100 mg **phenytoin**, or 10 mg **warfarin**, had no significant effect on the half-life of single 100-mg doses of carbenoxolone in 4 healthy subjects. A single 250-mg dose of **chlorpropamide** delayed the absorption of carbenoxolone in 6 patients with benign gastric ulcers taking 100 mg carbenoxolone three times daily, who showed a reduction in their carbenoxolone plasma levels. Some delay in absorption also occurred.[1] The clinical importance of this is uncertain. More study is needed.

1. Thornton PC, Papouchado M, Reed PI. Carbenoxolone interactions in man - preliminary report. *Scand J Gastroenterol* (1980) 15 (Suppl 65), 35–9.

Cerivastatin + Miscellaneous drugs

Colestyramine causes a small reduction in the serum levels of cerivastatin which can be avoided by separating their administration.[1-3] Gemfibrozil markedly raises cerivastatin levels so that this drug combination is contraindicated by the makers[3] because of a predicted increased risk of serious myopathy, but cerivastatin does not interact adversely with ciclosporin[2,4] (although it has been recommended[3] that treatment should be started at the lowest dose), cimetidine,[5] digoxin,[6,7] erythromycin,[2,8] itraconazole,[2] *Maalox*,[5] nifedipine,[9,10] omeprazole[11,12] or warfarin.[13] Cerivastatin has now been withdrawn by the makers because of severe muscle toxicity.

1. Mück W, Ritter W, Frey R, Wetzelsberger N, Lücker PW, Kuhlmann J. Influence of cholestyramine on the pharmacokinetics of cerivastatin. *Int J Clin Pharmacol Ther* (1997) 35, 250–4.
2. Mück W. Rational assessment of the interaction profile of cerivastatin supports its low propensity for drug interactions. *Drugs* (1998) 56 (Suppl 1), 15–23.
3. Lipobay (Cerivastatin). Bayer. Summary of product characteristics, September 1999.
4. Mai I, Bauer S, Fritsche J, Ochmann K, Mück W, Rohde G, Roots I, Neumayer H-H, Kuhlmann J. Single-dose pharmacokinetics of a new HMG-COA reductase inhibitor in renal transplant patients treated with cyclosporine A (CSA). *Eur J Clin Pharmacol* (1997) 52 (Suppl), A137.
5. Mück W, Ritter W, Dietrich H, Frey R, Kuhlmann J. Influence of the antacid Maalox and the H_2-antagonist cimetidine on the pharmacokinetics of cerivastatin. *Int J Clin Pharmacol Ther* (1997) 35, 261–4.
6. Lettieri J, Krol G, Mazzu A, Fiebach MZ, Heller AH. Lack of pharmacokinetic interaction between cerivastatin, a new HMG-CoA reductase inhibitor and digoxin. *Atherosclerosis* (1997) 130 (Suppl), S29.
7. Weber P, Lettieri JT, Kaiser L, Mazzu AL. Lack of mutual pharmacokinetic interaction between cerivastatin, a new HMG-CoA reductase inhibitor, and digoxin in healthy normocholesterolemic volunteers. *Clin Ther* (1999) 21, 1563-75.
8. Mück W, Ochmann K, Rhode G, Unger S, Kuhlmann J. Influence of erythromycin pre-and co-treatment on single dose pharmacokinetics of the HMG-CoA reductase inhibitor cerivastatin. *Eur J Clin Pharmacol* (1998) 53, 469–73.
9. Sachse R, Brendel E, Mück W, Rohde G, Ochmann K, Horstmann R. No drug-drug interaction between cerivastatin and nifedipine. *Naunyn Schmiedebergs Arch Pharmacol* (1998) 357 (4 Suppl), R174.
10. Sachse R, Brendel E, Mück W, Rohde G, Ochmann K, Horstmann R, Kuhlmann J. Lack of drug-drug interaction between cerivastatin and nifedipine. *Int J Clin Pharmacol Ther* (1998) 36, 409–13.
11. Mück W, Ochmann K, Rohde G, Unger S, Kuhlmann J. No drug-drug interaction between cerivastatin and omeprazole. *Naunyn Schmiedebergs Arch Pharmacol* (1998) 357 (4 Suppl), R175.
12. Sachse R, Ochmann K, Rohde G, Mück W. The effect of omeprazole pre- and cotreatment on cerivastatin absorption and metabolism in man. *Int J Clin Pharmacol Ther* (1998) 36, 517–20.
13. Schall R, Müller FO, Hundt HKL, Ritter W, Duursema L, Groenewoud G, Middle MV. No pharmacokinetic or pharmacodynamic interaction between rivastatin and warfarin. *J Clin Pharmacol* (1995) 35, 306–13.

Cetirizine + Erythromycin or Ketoconazole

Cetirizine does not interact with erythromycin or ketoconazole. No clinically important ECG changes occur if taken together.

Clinical evidence, mechanism, importance and management

Two studies in healthy subjects found that 500 mg **erythromycin** 8-hourly or 400 mg **ketoconazole** daily for 10 days had no significant effect on the pharmacokinetics of cetirizine 20 mg daily. The pharmacokinetics of neither anti-infective was changed, nor was there any evidence that the QT_c interval was significantly prolonged. Any effects on QT_c were small and inconsistent.[1] There would therefore appear to be no good reasons for avoiding cetirizine while taking either of these anti-infective agents, and in this context cetirizine would seem to be a good alternative to terfenadine and astemizole.

1. UCB Pharma. Personal communication, September 1994.

Table 24.2 Drug interactions with activated charcoal

Activated charcoal administration	Effects	Ref
Aspirin		
+ charcoal 50 g	Absorption of a 1 g dose decreased 70% by charcoal	3
+ charcoal 50 g 1 h later	Absorption of a 1 g dose decreased 10% by charcoal	3
+ charcoal 10 g	Absorption of a 975 mg dose decreased 70% by charcoal	10
Carbamazepine		
+ charcoal 50 g	Absorption of a 400 mg dose decreased 92% by charcoal	6
+ charcoal 118 g in 5 divided doses after 10 to 48 h	Half-life reduced from 32 to 17.6 h	11
Chlorpropamide		
+ charcoal 50 g	Absorption of a 250 mg dose reduced 90% by charcoal	5
Dapsone		
+ charcoal 118 g in 5 divided doses after 10 to 48 h	Half-life reduced from 32 to 17.6 h	11
Digoxin		
+ charcoal 50 g	Absorption of a 500 microgram dose decreased 98% by charcoal	3
+ charcoal 50 g 1 h later	Absorption of a 500 microgram dose decreased 40% by charcoal	3
+ charcoal 8 g	Absorption of a 500 microgram dose decreased 98% by charcoal	6
Furosemide (Frusemide)		
+ charcoal 8 g	Absorption of a 40 mg dose reduced 99% by charcoal	6
Glipizide		
+ charcoal 8 g	Absorption of a 10 mg dose reduced 81% by charcoal	4
Nizatidine		
+ charcoal 2 g 1 h later	Absorption of a 150 mg dose reduced 30% by charcoal	9
Paracetamol (Acetaminophen)		
+ charcoal 10 g	Absorption of a 2 g dose decreased 63% by charcoal	8
+ charcoal 10 g 1 h later	Absorption of a 2 g dose decreased by 23% by charcoal	8
Paroxetine		
+ charcoal 20 g 20 and 40 min later	Paroxetine became undetectable in the plasma	13
Phenobarbital (Phenobarbitone)		
+ charcoal 118 g in 5 divided doses after 10 to 48 h	Half-life reduced from 110 to 19.8 h	11
Phenylbutazone		
+ charcoal 118 g in 5 divided doses after 10 to 48 h	Half-life reduced from 51.5 to 36.7 h	11
Phenytoin (Diphenylhydantoin)		
+ charcoal 50 g	Absorption of a 500 mg dose decreased 98% by charcoal	3
+ charcoal 50 g 1 h later	Absorption of a 500 mg dose decreased 80% by charcoal	3
Rifampicin (Rifampin)		
+ charcoal 15 g	Urinary recovery reduced to 1.2%	14
+ charcoal 7.5 g	Urinary recovery reduced to 4.2%	14
Sodium valproate		
+ charcoal 50 g	Absorption of a 300 mg dose decreased 65% by charcoal	7
Theophylline		
+ charcoal 140 g in divided doses over 12 h	Half-life reduced from 6.4 to 3.3 h AUC nearly halved	12
Tolbutamide		
+ charcoal 50 g	Absorption of a 500 mg dose decreased 90% by charcoal	7

Charcoal + Miscellaneous drugs

Charcoal adsorbs drugs onto its surface and in large doses (8 to 50 g) it can markedly reduce their absorption by the gut, but smaller doses (1 to 2 g) of charcoal possibly interact minimally, or not at all.

Clinical evidence

In vitro studies have found that **carbutamide**, **chlorpropamide**, **tolazamide**, **tolbutamide**, **glibenclamide** and **glipizide** are all extensively adsorbed onto activated charcoal.[1] Activated charcoal contained in an antiemetic complementary remedy completely prevented the activity of 125 mg **mitobronitol** used to treat primary thrombocythaemia in one patient.[2] A number of other studies[3-14] have shown a variety of drugs to be affected by charcoal. See Table 24.2. In contrast, 1 g charcoal has been reported not to affect the pharmacokinetics of 500 mg **ciprofloxacin**, although repeated or higher doses may have more of an effect.[15,16]

Mechanism

Activated charcoal can adsorb gases, toxins and drugs onto its surface so that less is available for absorption through the gut wall. Separating the dosages reduces admixture in the gut.

Importance and management

Very well established interactions. Most of the reports are about the treatment of drug poisoning and overdoses where relatively large amounts of charcoal (50 g or more) are given to adsorb as much of the drug as possible. Only a few reports are concerned with smaller therapeutic doses. Activated charcoal in doses of 8 g three times a day has been used for primary hypercholesterolaemia[17] and would be expected to interact with any of the drugs cited in the table. Concurrent use should therefore be avoided or the dosages separated as much as possible. There seems to be little reported about the effects of small doses of charcoal (1 to 2 g daily) given to absorb intestinal gas or for the treatment of diarrhoea and dysentery, except that ciprofloxacin[15] is apparently not affected by 1 g charcoal, while nizatidine absorption is reduced about 30%.[9] More study is needed to define the situation more clearly and to find out the extent to which separating the dosages to prevent admixture in the gut reduces the effects of this interaction. A one hour separation was partially effective with paracetamol.[8]

1. Kannisto H, Neuvonen PJ. Adsorption of sulphonylureas onto activated charcoal *in vitro*. *J Pharm Sci* (1984) 73, 253–6.
2. Windrum P, Hull DR, Morris TCM. Herb-drug interactions. *Lancet* (2000) 355, 1019–20.
3. Neuvonen PJ, Elfving SM, Elonen E. Reduction of absorption of digoxin, phenytoin and aspirin by activated charcoal in man. *Eur J Clin Pharmacol* (1978) 13, 213–18.
4. Kivistö KT, Neuvonen PJ. The effect of cholestyramine and activated charcoal on glipizide absorption. *Br J Clin Pharmacol* (1990) 30, 733–6.
5. Neuvonen PJ, Kärkkäinen S. Effects of charcoal, sodium bicarbonate and ammonium chloride on chlorpropamide kinetics. *Clin Pharmacol Ther* (1983) 33, 386-93.
6. Neuvonen P J, Kivistö K, Hirvisalo E L. Effects of resins and activated charcoal on the adsorption of digoxin, carbamazepine and frusemide. *Br J Clin Pharmacol* (1988) 25, 229–33.
7. Neuvonen PJ, Kannisto H, Hirvisalo EL. Effect of activated charcoal on absorption of tolbutamide and valproate in man. *Eur J Clin Pharmacol* (1983) 24, 243–6.
8. Dordoni B, Willson RA, Thompson RPH, Williams R. Reduction of absorption of paracetamol by activated charcoal and cholestyramine: a possible therapeutic measure. *BMJ* (1973) 3, 86–7.
9. Knadler MP, Bergstrom RF, Callaghan JT, Obermeyer BD, Rubin A. Absorption studies of the H2-blocker nizatidine. *Clin Pharmacol Ther* (1987) 42, 514–20.
10. Juhl RP. Comparison of kaolin-pectin and activated charcoal for inhibition of aspirin absorption. *Am J Hosp Pharm* (1979) 36, 1097–8.
11. Neuvonen PJ, Elonen E, Mattila MJ. Orally given charcoal increases the rate of elimination of phenobarbital, carbamazepine, phenylbutazone, and dapsone in man. *Clin Pharmacol Ther* (1980) 27, 275–6.
12. Berlinger WG, Spector R, Goldberg MJ, Johnson GF, Quee CK, Berg MJ. Enhancement of theophylline clearance by oral activated charcoal. *Clin Pharmacol Ther* (1983) 33, 351–4.
13. Greb WH, Buscher G, Dierdorf H-D, von Schrader HW, Wolf D. Ability of charcoal to prevent absorption of paroxetine. *Acta Psychiatr Scand* (1989) 80 (Suppl 350), 156–7.
14. Orisakwe OE, Dioka CE, Okpogba AN, Orish CN, Ofoefule SI. Effect of activated charcoal on rifampicin absorption in man. *Tokai J Exp Clin Med* (1996) 21, 51–4.
15. Torre D. Influence of charcoal on ciprofloxacin activity. *Rev Infect Dis* (1988) 10, 1231.
16. Torre D, Sampietro C, Rossi S, Bianchi W, Maggiolo F. Ciprofloxacin and activated charcoal: pharmacokinetic data. *Rev Infect Dis* (1989) 11 (Suppl 5), S1015–S1016.
17. Kuusisto P, Vapaatalo H, Manninen V, Huttunen JK, Neuvonen PJ. Effect of activated charcoal on hypercholesterolaemia. *Lancet* (1986) 2, 366–7.

Chlorphenamine (Chlorpheniramine) + Ranitidine

A study in healthy subjects found that the pharmacokinetics of single 4-mg doses of racemic chlorphenamine were unaffected by 6 days treatment with 75 mg ranitidine twice daily.[1] No special precautions are needed if these drugs are used concurrently.

1. Koch KM, O'Connor-Semmes RL, Davis IM, Yin Y. Stereoselective pharmacokinetics of chlorpheniramine and the effect of ranitidine. *J Pharm Sci* (1998) 87, 1097–1100.

Chlorzoxazone + Miscellaneous drugs

The side-effects of chlorzoxazone may be increased in some patients if concurrently treated with isoniazid, in particular those who are slow acetylators of isoniazid. Disulfiram also markedly increases the plasma levels of chlorzoxazone.

Clinical evidence, mechanism, importance and management

(a) Disulfiram

A study in 6 healthy subjects to identify the activity of cytochrome P450 isoenzyme CYP2E1 found that a single 500-mg dose of **disulfiram** markedly inhibited the metabolism of a single 750-mg dose of chlorzoxazone (clearance reduced to 15%, half-life increased from 0.92 to 5.1 h, and a twofold increase in peak plasma levels).[1] No increased side-effects were seen while using these single doses, but an increase in toxicity would be expected (sedation, headache, nausea) with multiple doses. Be alert for the need to reduce the chlorzoxazone dosage if **disulfiram** is given concurrently. More study is needed.

(b) Isoniazid

Five out of 10 healthy subjects (all of them slow acetylators of isoniazid) demonstrated an increase in the side effects of 750-mg doses of chlorzoxazone (sedation, headache, nausea) after taking 300 mg **isoniazid** daily for 7 days. These symptoms disappeared within 2 days of withdrawing the **isoniazid**.[2] The reason appears to be that the **isoniazid** inhibits the activity of cytochrome P450 isoenzyme CYP2E1 so that the chlorzoxazone is metabolised by the liver and cleared from the body more slowly (a 58% reduction). Following withdrawal, the metabolism is increased.[2]

In practical terms this means that it may be necessary to reduce the chlorzoxazone dosage in some patients if concurrently treated with **isoniazid**. Only half of this group of slow acetylators developed adverse effects, and fast acetylators would not be expected to demonstrate this interaction. There is no quick and easy way to find out a patient's acetylator status. In the absence of this information you will need to monitor concurrent use carefully.

1. Kharasch ED, Thummel KE, Mhyre J, Lillibridge JH. Single-dose disulfiram inhibition of chlorzoxazone metabolism: a clinical probe for P450 2E1. *Clin Pharmacol Ther* (1993) 53, 643–50.
2. Zand R, Nelson SD, Slattery JT, Thummel KE, Kalhorn TF, Adams SP, Wright JM. Inhibition and induction of cytochrome P4502E1-catalyzed oxidation by isoniazid in humans. *Clin Pharmacol Ther* (1993) 54, 142–9.

Cilostazol + Miscellaneous drugs

Erythromycin, diltiazem and omeprazole increase the serum levels of cilostazol or its active metabolited. Other inhibitors of cytochrome P450 isoenzyme CYP3A4 (azole antifungals, grapefruit juice, macrolide antibacterials, nefazodone, SSRIs) are predicted to interact similarly. Cilostazol appears

not to interact to a clinically relevant extent with aspirin, lovastatin, quinidine, tobacco smoke or warfarin, and it is not expected to interact with clopidogrel.

Clinical evidence, mechanism, importance and management

(a) Aspirin

The makers report that although the concurrent use of cilostazol and **aspirin** for about 4 days increased the inhibition of ADP-induced platelet aggregation by 23 to 35% when compared with **aspirin** alone, there were no additive effects on arachidonic acid-induced platelet aggregation and no clinically relevant effects on prothrombin times, aPTT or bleeding times when compared with **aspirin** alone. They also report that in 8 randomised, placebo-controlled trials in 201 patients (107 patients on 75 to 81 mg **aspirin** daily for 137 days and 85 patients on 325 mg **aspirin** daily for 54 days), the incidence of bleeding was no greater than that seen with **aspirin** and placebo.[1] Another study also found no clinically significant interaction between cilostazol and aspirin.[2] This suggests that no special precautions are needed if these two drugs are used concurrently in these doses.

(b) Clopidogrel

It is not known whether there is any adverse interaction between **clopidogrel** and cilostazol, but while the FDA cautiously says that ". . . there is no experience with concomitant use . . ." the lack of any clinically relevant interactions with aspirin and clopidogrel suggests that it is likely to be safe.[3]

(c) Cytochrome P450 isoenzyme CYP3A4 inhibitors (Azole antifungals, Diltiazem, Macrolide antibacterials, SSRIs)

The makers report that 500 mg **erythromycin** 8-hourly increased the maximum serum levels and the AUC of a single 100-mg dose of cilostazol by 47% and 73% respectively, due to the inhibitory effects of the **erythromycin** on the activity of cytochrome P450 isoenzyme CYP3A4, which is concerned with the metabolism of cilostazol. Information from population pharmacokinetic analysis similarly found that **diltiazem** caused a 53% rise in serum cilostazol levels, almost certainly for the same reason. Other CYP3A4 inhibitors such as **itraconazole** and **ketoconazole** are expected to interact similarly. In view of these changes the US makers suggest halving the dose of cilastazol in the presence of CYP3A4 inhibitors such as **erythromycin**, **diltiazem** or **ketoconazole**. Other potent CYP3A4 inhibitors such as other **azole antifungals** (**fluconazole, miconazole**) and **SSRIs** (**fluvoxamine, fluoxetine, sertraline**) and **nefazodone** may also interact.[1] What is not yet clear is whether these predicted increased levels would be clinically important.

(d) Fruit juices

No studies have been done with cilostazol and **grapefruit juice**, but because it can inhibit the activity of cytochrome P450 isoenzyme CYP3A4 (see (b) above) and therefore possibly increase the activity of cilostazol, the makers say that concurrent use should be avoided.[1] It seems unlikely that a serious interaction will occur with **grapefruit juice**.

(e) Lovastatin

The makers report that when given with cilostazol at steady state, the serum levels of the **lovastatin** and its hydroxyacid metabolite following a single 80-mg dose were not significantly altered.[1] This suggests that concurrent use need not be avoided.

(f) Omeprazole

The makers report that **omeprazole** does not significantly affect the metabolism of cilostazol, but the systemic exposure to 3,4-dehydro-cilostazol (a metabolite with 4 to 7 times the activity of the parent compound) was increased 69%, probably because the **omeprazole** inhibits cytochrome P450 isoenzyme CYP2C19. For this reason the makers suggest that the dose should possibly be halved.[1]

(g) Quinidine

The concurrent use of **quinidine** with a single 100-mg dose of cilostazol did not alter the cilostazol pharmacokinetics.[1]

(h) Tobacco smoking

The makers report that population pharmacokinetic analysis suggests that **tobacco smoking** reduces the exposure to cilostazol by about 20%,[1] but this is unlikely to have much if any clinical relevance.

(i) Warfarin

A randomised, double-blind, two-way crossover study in 15 normal subjects found that 100 mg cilostazol twice daily for 7 or 13 days did not alter the pharmacokinetics of a single 25-mg dose of **warfarin** or prothrombin times, aPTT time or Ivy bleeding time.[4,5] This suggests that no interaction is likely during concurrent use, but until more experience has been gained in clinical practice it would be prudent to monitor the outcome.

1. Pletal (Cilostazol). Product information, Physicians' Desk Reference, 2002.
2. Mallikaarjun S, Bramer SL, Bortey E, Briggs A, Forbes WP. Pharmacodynamic-pharmacokinetic interaction of aspirin with cilostazol. *Clin Pharmacol Ther* (1998) 63, 231.
3. Approval of Cilostazol. FDA. Center for Drug Evaluation and Research, January 20th, 1999.
4. Millakaarjun S, Mico BA, Forbes WP, Bramer SL. A pharmacokinetic and pharmacodynamic study of the potential interaction between cilostazol and warfarin. *Pharm Res* (1997) 14 (11 Suppl), S-555.
5. Millakaarjun S, Bramer SL. Effect of cilostazol on the pharmacokinetics and pharmacodynamics of warfarin. *Clin Pharmacokinet* (1999) 37 (Suppl 2), 79-86.

Cimetidine + Rifampicin

Anti-tubercular treatment with rifampicin, isoniazid and ethambutol has been shown to increase the non-renal clearance of cimetidine by about 50%. This is probably due to enzyme induction caused by rifampicin. However, the total clearance is unchanged and so this interaction would appear to be of little clinical importance.[1]

1. Keller E, Schollmeyer P, Brandenstein U, Hoppe-Seyler G. Increased nonrenal clearance of cimetidine during antituberculous therapy. *Int J Clin Pharmacol Ther Toxicol* (1984) 22, 307–11.

Cinnarizine + Phenylpropanolamine

Phenylpropanolamine 50 mg counteracted the mild sedation caused by cinnarizine 25 or 50 mg, and improved the performance of some skills related to driving in 12 healthy subjects.[1]

1. Savolainen K, Mattila MJ, Mattila ME. Actions and interactions of cinnarizine and phenylpropanolamine on human psychomotor performance. *Curr Ther Res* (1992) 52, 160–8.

Ciprofibrate + Ibuprofen

An isolated report describes acute renal failure and rhabdomyolysis in a patient on ciprofibrate when ibuprofen was added.

Clinical evidence, mechanism, importance and management

A man of 29 with type M hyperlipidaemia who had been under treatment with 100 mg ciprofibrate daily for 6 months began to take 200 mg and then 400 mg **ibuprofen** daily for a painful heel. The pain became general, his urine turned 'muddy', he complained of having a 'stiff body', and he rapidly developed acute renal failure. His creatinine concentration was found to be 647 micromol/l and creatine kinase activity was 13740 U/l. He later fully recovered from the renal failure and rhabdomyolysis.[1]

The reasons for this reaction are not known but the authors of the report postulate that the **ibuprofen** displaced the ciprofibrate from its binding sites, thereby making a safe dose into a toxic one.[1] However, it should be said that this mechanism of interaction is rarely important on its own so it seems likely that some other factors may have contributed to what happened.

This is an isolated case so that its general importance is unknown, but it is probably very small.

1. Ramachadran S, Giles PD, Hartland A. Acute renal failure due to rhabdomyolysis in presence of concurrent ciprofibrate and ibuprofen treatment. *BMJ* (1997) 314, 1593.

Cisapride + Azole antifungals

Ketoconazole can cause a marked rise in serum cisapride levels, increasing the risk of serious and life-threatening ventricular arrhythmias including torsade de pointes. All azole antifungals are contraindicated with cisapride because of the same risk.

Clinical evidence

A report from the FDA's Medwatch program described 57 patients identified over the period September 1993 to April 1996, 34 of whom developed torsade de pointes arrhythmia and 23 of whom developed a prolonged QT interval while taking cisapride. Of these, 4 patients were reported to have died and 16 responded to resuscitation after cardiopulmonary arrest. Imidazole antifungals (**fluconazole, itraconazole, ketoconazole** or **miconazole**) or macrolide antibacterials (clarithromycin, erythromycin) were being taken by 32 out of the 57 patients (56%). The arrhythmias stopped in most patients when either or both drugs were withdrawn. Increased serum cisapride levels were seen in 9 out of 15 patients tested. Other factors may also have had some part to play in increasing the risk of arrhythmias, such as coronary disease, renal impairment, electrolyte imbalance and the concurrent use of other drugs which can prolong the QT interval.[1]

A randomised two-way crossover study in 14 healthy subjects given 4 or 5 consecutive 10-mg doses of cisapride within a 24-h period, found that the addition of 200 mg **ketoconazole** twice daily increased the AUC and the steady-state serum levels of cisapride four to eight-fold.[2]

Mechanism

In vitro studies[2] with ^{14}C-labelled human liver microsomes have shown that ketoconazole inhibits the metabolism of cisapride, probably by inhibiting the activity of cytochrome P450 isoenzyme CYP3A4. This reduces the *in vivo* clearance of the cisapride so that its serum levels rise. These raised levels appear to prolong the QT interval.[3] The same study found that to a lesser extent itraconazole and miconazole can alter cisapride metabolism.[2]

Importance and management

Information is limited but the interactions of cisapride with fluconazole, itraconazole, ketoconazole or miconazole appear to be established. The incidence is likely to be very small because market research has shown that the coprescribing of cisapride with azole antifungals is less than 0.2%.[2] Nevertheless, because of the risks the makers of cisapride now contraindicate the use of cisapride with all azole antifungals.[4]

1. Wysowski DK, Bacsanyi J. Cisapride and fatal arrhythmia. *N Engl J Med* (1996) 335, 290–1.

. 2. Janssen-Cilag Ltd. Personal communication, April 1995.

3. Ahmad SR, Wolfe SM. Cisapride and torsades de pointes. *Lancet* (1995) 345, 508.

4. Prepulsid (Cisapride) Janssen-Cilag Ltd. ABPI Compendium of Datasheets and Summaries of Product Characteristics, 1999–2000, p 655–6.

Cisapride + Diltiazem

Near syncope associated with a prolonged QT interval occurred in a woman when treated with cisapride and diltiazem.

Clinical evidence, mechanism, importance and management

A woman developed near syncope and a prolonged QT interval while taking cisapride and **diltiazem**. The QT interval returned to normal and the symptoms did not recur when the cisapride was stopped. This interaction was attributed to the inhibitory effect of the **diltiazem** on the activity of cytochrome CYP3A4, resulting in a rise in the cisapride plasma levels.[1]

This seems to be the first and only report of a cisapride/**diltiazem** interaction but what happened is consistent with the way other CYP3A4 inhibitors can interact to raise plasma cisapride levels and increase its cardiotoxicity. It would therefore now be prudent to monitor the effect of the concurrent use of these two drugs in any patient. More study is needed.

1. Thomas AR, Chan L-N, Bauman JL, Olopade CO. Prolongation of the QT interval related to cisapride-diltiazem interaction. *Pharmacotherapy* (1998) 18, 381–5.

Cisapride + Drugs that prolong the QT interval

The QT-prolonging effects of cisapride and the attendant risks of torsade de pointes arrhythmia are increased, or predicted to be increased, by the drugs listed below.

Clinical evidence, mechanism, importance and management

(a) Metabolic interactions

Some drugs can increase the QT prolonging effects of cisapride because they inhibit the activity of cytochrome P450 isoenzyme CYP3A4 which is concerned with the metabolism of cisapride, as a result of which the serum levels and the potential cardiotoxicity of the cisapride rise. The drugs which have been listed are the azole antifungals (**fluconazole, itraconazole, ketoconazole**), macrolide antibacterials (**clarithromycin, erythromycin, troleandomycin**), HIV protease inhibitors (**indinavir, ritonavir**), see the Index. Most of these drugs have been seen to interact with cisapride whereas the drugs in (b) below are only predicted to do so. **Nefazodone** is also included in the list of drugs expected to show a metabolic interaction.[1,2]

(b) Additive effects on the QT interval

The following drugs are contraindicated with cisapride because they can prolong the QT interval and it is predicted that their toxic effects may possibly be additive with those of cisapride. The drugs listed include antiarrhythmics (**amiodarone, bretylium, disopyramide, procainamide, quinidine, sotalol**), antidepressants (**amitriptyline, lithium**), antihistamines (**astemizole, terfenadine**), antimalarials (**quinine, halofantrine**), antipsychotics (**chlorpromazine, haloperidol, pimozide, thioridazine, sertindole**) and **pentamidine**.[2] The makers in the USA also list **bepridil, maprotiline, sparfloxacin** and **terodiline** as contraindicated,[3] but these are not included in the UK list.

The makers also say that cisapride should not be used in patients with uncorrected electrolyte (potassium/magnesium) disturbances (such as seen in patients taking **potassium-depleting diuretics**) or in association with the administration of **insulin** in acute settings).[1] Such diuretics would include **furosemide (frusemide), bumetanide, etacrynic acid (ethacrynic acid)**, and the **thiazides** but none of these is specifically named.

1. Prepulsid (Cisapride). Janssen-Cilag Ltd. Summary of product characteristics, August 1998.

2. Committee on Safety of Medicines/Medicines Control Agency. Cisapride (Prepulsid): Risk of arrhythmias. *Current Problems* (1998) 24, 11.
3. Janssen Pharmaceutica (US). Important Safety and Efficacy information, June 26th 1998.

Cisapride + Macrolide antibacterials

Erythromycin and clarithromycin can increase the serum levels of cisapride, resulting in a prolongation of the QT interval and increasing the risk of serious ventricular arrhythmias including torsade de pointes. The concurrent use of these macrolides and cisapride is contraindicated. Troleandomycin is predicted to interact similarly, but azithromycin probably does not.

Clinical evidence

(a) Clarithromycin

A two-period crossover study in 12 young healthy subjects given 10 mg cisapride four times daily for 10 days found that the addition of 500 mg **clarithromycin** twice daily on days 6 to 10 approximately tripled the peak and trough serum levels of the cisapride and prolonged the QTc interval by 25 to 27 ms.[1]

Two patients with chronic renal failure on cisapride developed torsade de pointes arrhythmias when treated with **clarithromycin**. The elevated serum cisapride levels of one of them fell to therapeutic levels when the **clarithromycin** was stopped.[2] A woman was involved in two motor accidents on the same day after experiencing syncopal episodes attributed to torsade de pointes arrhythmia caused by a cisapride/**clarithromycin** interaction.[3]

(b) Erythromycin

A 'Dear Doctor letter' issued in the UK by the makers of cisapride said that occasionally fatal cardiac arrhythmias, including ventricular arrhythmias and torsade de pointes associated with QT prolongation have been reported in patients taking cisapride in combination with fluconazole, **erythromycin** or clarithromycin. Most but not all of the patients were on multiple drugs and/or had other risk factors for arrhythmias.[4] The warning in this letter is based on post-marketing pharmacovigilance reports worldwide.[5]

Further evidence of the risk is contained in a report of a man with acute renal failure on dialysis who developed episodes of pulseless ventricular tachycardia (with ECG evidence of torsade de pointes) while taking 10 mg cisapride six-hourly and 1 g intravenous **erythromycin** six-hourly. The arrhythmia continued for 2 days after the **erythromycin** was stopped.[6]

However, a study in 12 healthy subjects given 10 mg cisapride four times daily found that 500 mg **erythromycin** four times daily for 5 days doubled the mean cisapride serum levels. The increase in 24 h QTc values for cisapride alone and **erythromycin** alone were 6 ms and 9 ms respectively, but there was no further increase when the drugs were taken together.[7]

Mechanism

It seems almost certain that the interacting macrolides inhibit the metabolism of the cisapride, thereby increasing its serum levels and its prolonging effects on the QT interval, which can lead to the development of cardiac arrhythmias, including torsade de pointes.

Importance and management

The cisapride/clarithromycin and cisapride/erythromycin interactions are established, clinically important and potentially life-threatening. There seem to be no reports about other macrolides, but **troleandomycin** appears to have the potential to interact and should be avoided. *In vitro* evidence indicates that **azithromycin** does not affect the metabolism of cisapride[8] and is therefore unlikely to interact with cisapride like the other macrolides. The total number of patients who have developed serious arrhythmias as a result of these interactions has not been published, but even though the figure is probably

very small, because of the potential severity of the reaction, the concurrent use of erythromycin or clarithromycin and cisapride is contraindicated in all patients.[4]

1. van Haarst AD, Van'T Klooster GEA, Van Gerven JMA, Schoemaker RC, Van Oene JC, Burggraaf J, Coene M-C, Cohen AF. The influence of cisapride and clarithromycin on QT intervals in healthy volunteers. *Clin Pharmacol Ther* (1998) 64, 542–6.
2. Sekkarie MA. Torsades de pointes in two chronic renal failure patients treated with cisapride and clarithromycin. *Am J Kidney Dis* (1997) 30, 437–9.
3. Gray VS. Syncopal episodes associated with cisapride and concurrent drugs. *Ann Pharmacother* (1998) 32, 648–51.
4. Janssen-Cilag Ltd. Dear Doctor letter, November 1995.
5. Janssen-Cilag UK Ltd. Confidential Report from Medical Information from Medical Information Department and Drug Safety Unit, December 18th 1995.
6. Jenkins IR, Gibson J. Cisapride, erythromycin and arrhythmia. *Anaesth Intensive Care* (1996) 24, 728.
7. Janssen-Cilag Ltd. Data on file, (N1251081) 1997.
8. Janssen-Cilag Ltd. Personal communication, March 1999.

Cisapride + Miscellaneous drugs

Cisapride increases the rate of absorption of diazepam and disopyramide. No clinically relevant interactions are apparent with antacids, cimetidine, digoxin, fluoxetine, morphine, paracetamol (acetaminophen), phenytoin or propranolol, but an isolated report attributes cardiotoxicity to the concurrent use of ranitidine.

Clinical evidence, mechanism, importance and management

Cisapride speeds up gastrointestinal motility. This would be expected to accelerate drug transit through the gut, to increase the absorption rate of some drugs and possibly reduce the extent of absorption. For this reason the makers of cisapride suggest that for drugs that need careful individual titration (e.g. **anticonvulsants**) it may be useful to measure their plasma concentrations.[1] However, there seems to be no direct evidence that a clinically important interaction actually occurs. In fact a study in a child of 3 found that 4 days after withdrawing cisapride, the total serum **phenytoin** levels and free **phenytoin** fraction were unchanged.[2]

Cisapride does not cause sedation but it accelerates the absorption of **diazepam** so that its sedative effects occur more quickly and may possibly be transiently increased.[3] Cisapride was found not to affect serum **propranolol** levels nor the blood pressure control of 9 mildly hypertensive patients given a sustained-release **propranolol** preparation.[4] Cisapride 20 mg was found to increase the serum levels of **morphine** (20 mg *MST Continus*, a sustained-release preparation) but the effects, as measured by pupil-constriction and sedation, were unchanged.[5] Cisapride causes no significant changes in the pharmacokinetics of **paracetamol (acetaminophen)**.[6]

Cisapride and anticholinergics have opposite effects on gastrointestinal motility (increased and decreased effects respectively). Thus one study found that cisapride 2.5 mg three times daily increased the gastric emptying, which had previously been reduced by the anticholinergic **disopyramide** (100 mg three times daily), thereby increasing the absorption and the serum levels of **disopyramide**. Its absorption rate constant was doubled and the lag time was halved. The clinical significance of this interaction is uncertain, but you should also be aware that **disopyramide** is listed by the makers as contraindicated because of the possible risk of additive cardiotoxicity (see 'Cisapride + Drugs that prolong the QT interval', p.876). In contrast, **fluoxetine** 20 mg daily, given with cisapride did not affect the QT interval in 12 healthy subjects.[7-10]

Peak serum cisapride levels are increased 45% by **cimetidine** (possibly by enzyme inhibition) whereas the bioavailability of **cimetidine** is reduced by 18% by cisapride.[11,12] Cisapride enhances the absorption rate of **ranitidine**, but reduces the AUC by 26%.[13] The 25% increase in the bioavailability of cisapride caused by **ranitidine**[14] was not confirmed in another study,[13] but a case report attributed an increase in the QT interval in a baby to the concurrent use of **ranitidine**.[9] The makers of cisapride say that the changed serum levels with these H_2-blockers is unlikely to be clinically significant.[1] Cisapride 10 mg three times a day reduced the **digoxin** AUC and the peak serum concentrations by 12 to 13% in 6 healthy subjects given a loading dose of **digoxin** followed by 250 micrograms twice daily.[8] The concurrent use of **aluminium oxide** and **magnesium hydroxide** was found in another study not to affect the absorption of cisapride.[15]

It seems doubtful if the concurrent use of cisapride with any of these drugs (with the exception of **disopyramide** and possibly **ranitidine**) is normally likely to result in a clinically relevant adverse interaction, but this needs confirmation.

Cisapride 30 mg daily for 28 days was given to 15 healthy subjects to find out if it induces or inhibits liver microsomal enzymes, using **antipyrine (phenazone)** as a marker or index drug. No changes in metabolism were found.[16]

1. Prepulsid (Cisapride). Janssen Pharmaceuticals. ABPI Compendium of Datasheets and Summaries of Product Characteristics 1998–9, p 569.
2. Roberts GW, Kowalski SR, Calabretto JP. Lack of effect of cisapride on phenytoin free fraction. *Ann Pharmacother* (1992) 26, 1016–17.
3. Bateman DN. The action of cisapride on gastric emptying and the pharmacodynamics and pharmacokinetics of oral diazepam. *Eur J Clin Pharmacol* (1986) 30, 205–8.
4. Janssen Pharmaceuticals. Effect of cisapride on the plasma concentrations of a delayed formulation of propranolol and on its clinical effects on blood pressure in mildly hypertensive patients. Data on file (Study R 51619/23-NL), 1986.
5. Rowbotham DJ, Milligan K, McHugh P. Effect of cisapride on morphine absorption after oral administration of sustained-release morphine. *Br J Anaesth* (1991) 67, 421–5.
6. Rowbotham DJ, Parnacott S, Nimmo WS. No effect of cisapride on paracetamol absorption after oral simultaneous administration. *Eur J Clin Pharmacol* (1992) 42, 235–6.
7. Kuroda T, Yoshihara Y, Nakamura H, Azumi T, Inatome T, Fukuzaki H, Takanashi H, Yogo K, Akima M. Effects of cisapride on gastrointestinal motor activity and gastric emptying of disopyramide. *J Pharmacobiodyn* (1992) 15, 395–402.
8. Kirch W, Janisch HD, Santos SR, Duhrsen U, Dylewicz P, Ohnhaus EE. Effect of cisapride and metoclopramide on digoxin bioavailability. *Eur J Drug Metab Pharmacokinet* (1986) 11, 249–50.
9. Valdes L, Champel V, Olivier C, Jonville-Bera AP, Autret E. Malaise avec allongement de l'espace QT chez un nourrisson de 39 jours traité par cisapride. *Arch Pediatr* (1997) 4, 535–7.
10. Zhao Q, Wojcik MA, Parier J-L, Pesco-Koplowitz L. Influence of coadministration of fluoxetine on cisapride pharmacokinetics and QTc intervals in healthy volunteers. *Pharmacotherapy* (2001) 21, 149–57.
11. Kirch W, Rose I, Ohnhaus EE. Cisapride and cimetidine. Both drugs alter pharmacokinetics of each other. *Clin Pharmacol Ther* (1986) 39, 202.
12. Kirch W, Janisch HD, Ohnhaus EE, van Peer A. Cisapride-cimetidine interaction: enhanced cisapride bioavailability and accelerated cimetidine absorption. *Ther Drug Monit* (1989) 11, 411–14.
13. Milligan KA, McHugh P, Rowbotham DJ. Effects of concomitant administration of cisapride and ranitidine on plasma concentrations in volunteers. *Br J Anaesth* (1989) 63, 628P.
14. Janssen Pharmaceuticals. Cisapride-ranitidine interaction. Data on file (Study R 51 619/74), 1986.
15. Janssen Pharmaceuticals. Unaltered oral absorption of cisapride on coadministration of antacids. Data on file (Study R 51 619/69), 1986.
16. Davies DS, Mills FJ, Welburn PJ. Cisapride has no effect on antipyrine clearance. *Br J Clin Pharmacol* (1988) 26, 808–9.

Clofibrate + Contraceptives, oral

Serum cholesterol and triglyceride levels can be increased by the oral contraceptives, and in at least two cases this is reported to have opposed the cholesterol-lowering effects of clofibrate. Oral contraceptives increase the loss of clofibrate from the body.

Clinical evidence, mechanism, importance and management

A woman with hypercholesterolaemia, taking clofibrate, showed a rise in her serum cholesterol levels on two occasions when concurrently using an **oral contraceptive** (*Anvolar* on one occasion, *Eugynon* on the other).[1] Another patient with type IV hyperlipoproteinaemia reacted similarly.[2] Rises in the serum levels of cholesterol and triglycerides in women taking **oral contraceptives** are well recognised.[3,4] The effect is said to be greater with increasing oestrogen content.[4] A comparative study in men, women, and women taking **oral contraceptives** found that the clearance of clofibrate was increased by 48% in those taking **oral contraceptives**, apparently due to an increase in its metabolism (glucuronidation).[5] Another study found that **oral contraceptives** increased the excretion of clofibric acid glucuronide by 25%.[6] None of these studies addressed the question of whether **oral contraceptives** are appropriate for women needing to take clofibrate, or whether concurrent use significantly reduces clofibrate efficacy, but it would seem prudent to monitor for in-

creases in blood lipid levels. More study is needed. See also 'Oral contraceptives + Lovastatin', p.477.

1. Smith RBW, Prior IAM. Oral-contraceptive opposition to hypercholesterolaemic action of clofibrate. *Lancet* (1968) i, 750–1.
2. Robertson-Rintoul J. Raised serum-lipids and oral contraceptives. *Lancet* (1972) ii, 1320–21.
3. Wynn V, Doar JWH, Mills GL, Stokes T. Fasting serum triglyceride, cholesterol, and lipoprotein levels during oral-contraceptive therapy. *Lancet* (1969) ii, 756–60.
4. Stokes T, Wynn V. Serum-lipids in women on oral contraceptives. *Lancet* (1971) ii, 677–80.
5. Miners JO, Robson RA, Birkett DJ. Gender and oral contraceptive steroids as determinants of drug glucuronidation: effects on clofibric acid elimination. *Br J Clin Pharmacol* (1984) 18, 240–3.
6. Liu H-F, Magdalou J, Nicolas A, Lafaurie C, Siest G. Oral contraceptives stimulate the excretion of clofibric acid glucuronide in women and female rats. *Gen Pharmacol* (1991) 22, 393–7.

Clofibrate + Probenecid

Plasma clofibrate levels can be approximately doubled by probenecid.

Clinical evidence, mechanism, importance and management

A pharmacokinetic study in 4 healthy subjects taking 500 mg clofibrate 12-hourly showed that 500 mg **probenecid** six-hourly for 7 days almost doubled the steady-state clofibric acid levels, from 72 to 129 mg/l, and raised the free clofibric acid levels from 2.5 to 9.1 mg/l. The suggested reason is that the **probenecid** reduces the renal and metabolic clearance of the clofibrate by inhibiting its conjugation with glucuronic acid.[1] The clinical importance of this interaction is uncertain. It appears not to have been assessed.

1. Veenendaal JR, Brooks PM, Meffin PJ. Probenecid-clofibrate interaction. *Clin Pharmacol Ther* (1981) 29, 351–8.

Clofibrate + Rifampicin (Rifampin)

Preliminary evidence shows that rifampicin can reduce the plasma levels of the active metabolite of clofibrate.

Clinical evidence, mechanism, importance and management

A reduction in the steady-state plasma levels of the active metabolite of clofibrate, chlorophenoxyisobutyric acid (CIPB), of about 35% was seen in 5 healthy subjects after taking 600 mg **rifampicin** daily for 7 days.[1] The reason appears to be that metabolism of CIPB by the liver and/or the kidneys is increased.[1] This is consistent with the well recognised and potent enzyme inducing activity of **rifampicin**. On the basis of this study it would now be prudent to monitor serum lipid levels of patients if **rifampicin** is added, increasing the clofibrate dosage if necessary. More study is needed.

1. Houin G, Tillement J-P. Clofibrate and enzymatic induction in man. *Int J Clin Pharmacol Biopharm* (1978) 16, 150–4.

Clomethiazole + Diazoxide

Clomethiazole and diazoxide given to pregnant women in labour can cause marked respiratory depression in their babies at birth or shortly afterwards.

Clinical evidence

An infusion of 0.8% clomethiazole 4 to 24 g was given to 21 pregnant women of 28 to 40 weeks gestation during labour, for eclampsia or pre-eclamptic toxaemia. **Diazoxide** 75 to 150 mg was also given intravenously to 14 of them for hypertension. All of their babies were born alive but 13 of the 21 suffered hypotonia, hypoventilation or apnoea for 24 to 36 h after birth. Three of them died of respiratory distress syndrome, one was only 28 weeks' gestation. All of the neonates affected, apart from one, came from the group of mothers who had been given **diazoxide**.[1]

Mechanism

Clomethiazole has some respiratory depressant effects and is contraindicated in patients with respiratory deficiency, but it is not clear why having passed across the placenta into the foetus its effects should apparently be so markedly increased by diazoxide.

Importance and management

Although use of this drug combination in eclampsia is historical, the interaction is included on account of its severity. The author of the report says that the respiratory depression was managed successfully with intermittent positive pressure ventilation provided that the respiratory distress syndrome was not also present.[1]

1. Johnson RA. Adverse neonatal reaction to maternal administration of intravenous chlormethiazole and diazoxide. *BMJ* (1976) 1, 943.

Clomethiazole + H₂-blockers

The sedative and hypnotic effects of clomethiazole are markedly increased by cimetidine, but not by ranitidine.

Clinical evidence

After one weeks' treatment with 1 g **cimetidine** daily (as 200 mg three times daily and 400 mg at night) the clearance of a single 1-g oral dose of clomethiazole edisilate in 8 healthy subjects was reduced by 31%, and the elimination half-life and AUC were increased by 56 and 55% respectively. Without the **cimetidine** the subjects slept for 30 to 60 min after taking clomethiazole, whereas after the **cimetidine** treatment most of them slept for at least 2 h.[1,2] Subsequent studies showed that 300 mg **ranitidine** daily does not interact significantly with clomethiazole.[3,4]

Mechanism

Cimetidine not only inhibits the liver enzymes concerned with the metabolism of the clomethiazole but it also reduces the flow of blood through the liver, both of which result in a reduction in the rate at which the clomethiazole is removed from the body. Ranitidine does not inhibit liver enzymes.

Importance and management

The clomethiazole/cimetidine interaction is established, but the documentation is limited. What occurred is consistent with the way cimetidine increases and prolongs the activity of other drugs. The authors emphasise that the risks of over-sedation and respiratory depression are likely to be greatest in the elderly and those with liver disease. Reduce the clomethiazole dosage (to about half), or replace the cimetidine with ranitidine. Other H₂-blockers that also lack enzyme inhibitory activity (e.g. famotidine, nizatidine) be expected not to interact, and no cases of interaction with these drugs have been reported to the makers of clomethiazole.[5]

1. Shaw G, Bury RW, Mashford ML, Breen KJ, Desmond PV. Cimetidine impairs the elimination of chlormethiazole. *Eur J Clin Pharmacol* (1981) 21, 83–5.
2. Desmond PV, Shaw RG, Bury RW, Mashford ML, Breen KJ. Cimetidine impairs the clearance of an orally administered high clearance drug, chlormethiazole. *Gastroenterology* (1981) 80, 1330.
3. Desmond PV, Breen KJ, Harman P, Mashford ML, Morphett B. No effect of ranitidine on the disposition or elimination of chlormethiazole or indocyanine green (ICG). *Scand J Gastroenterol* (1982) 17 (Suppl 78), 13.
4. Mashford ML, Harman PJ, Morphett BJ, Breen KJ, Desmond PV. Ranitidine does not affect chlormethiazole or indocyanine green disposition. *Clin Pharmacol Ther* (1983) 34, 23–3.
5. Astra Pharmaceuticals. Personal communication, April 1996.

Clomethiazole + Miscellaneous drugs

Clomethiazole and furosemide (frusemide) do not appear to interact adversely, nor does clomethiazole appear to interact with any of the other drugs listed below.

Clinical evidence, mechanism, importance and management

Ten female patients aged 66 to 90 were given clomethiazole edisilate syrup 500 mg each evening at 10 pm as a sedative, and 250 mg each morning with **furosemide (frusemide)** 20 to 80 mg. Other drugs being taken included **potassium chloride, ferrous sulphate, levothyroxine, lactulose, hydroxocobalamin, trihexyphenidyl (benzhexol), levodopa, digoxin, amitriptyline, folic acid, calcium with vitamin D**, and **carbidopa**. No significant changes in the serum levels or effects of clomethiazole or **furosemide** were detected, and no other significant adverse reactions were seen.[1]

1. Reid J, Judge TG. Chlormethiazole night sedation in elderly subjects receiving other medications. *Practitioner* (1980) 224, 751–3.

Clomethiazole + Propranolol

An isolated report describes marked bradycardia in an old woman on propranolol when she started to take clomethiazole.

Clinical evidence, mechanism, importance and management

An 84-year-old woman taking 40 mg **propranolol** twice daily for hypertension underwent skin grafting. Her pulse was stable (54 to 64 bpm) until the thirteenth day after the operation when she took two oral doses of clomethiazole 192 mg, 9 h apart. Her heart rate fell to 43 bpm with a PR interval of 0.24 s 3 hours after taking the second dose, and by 5 h after the dose her pulse rate was down to 36 bpm. Her pulse had risen to 70 bpm twelve hours after stopping both drugs, and had restabilised 2 days later at about 60 bpm with a PR interval of 0.20 s. At this time the **propranolol** was restarted with haloperidol.[1] The reasons for this reaction are not understood. The general importance of this interaction is not known, but it is probably small. This seems to be the only case on record.

1. Adverse Drug Reactions Advisory Committee. Chlormethiazole/propranolol interaction? *Med J Aust* (1979) 2, 553.

Clopidogrel + Miscellaneous drugs

The makers warn about possible gastrointestinal bleeding if clopidogrel is used with naproxen and other NSAIDs. They recommend caution with heparin and alteplase, and the avoidance of warfarin, although there is now some evidence of safety. No adverse interactions appear to occur with atenolol, cimetidine, digoxin, estrogen, food, *Maalox*, nifedipine, phenobarbital, phenytoin, theophylline or tolbutamide.

Clinical evidence, mechanism, importance and management

(a) Food, Antacids

Two studies, one in 12 healthy subjects (average age 23) and the other in 10 healthy subjects (average age 67), found that the bioavailability of a single 75-mg dose of clopidogrel remained unchanged when taken with **food** or two 200-mg tablets of **Maalox** taken 1 h previously.[1] No special precautions would seem to be needed.

(b) Heparin, Thrombolytics

A study in healthy subjects showed that the dosage of **heparin** did not need modification when given with clopidogrel, and the inhibitory effects of clopidogrel on platelet aggregation were unchanged.[2] They also report that in patients with recent myocardial infarction, the extent of clinical bleeding with clopidogrel/**heparin/alteplase** is similar to that seen with aspirin/**heparin/alteplase**, however, they say that the safety of other combinations has not been established and caution is required.[3]

(c) Non-interacting drugs

No clinically significant pharmacodynamic interactions were seen when clopidogrel was given with **atenolol, nifedipine** or a combination of **atenolol** and **nifedipine**,[4] and the activity of clopidogrel was not altered by the concurrent use of **cimetidine**,[3] **estrogen**[3] or **phenobarbital**.[3] Other studies have shown that clopidogrel does not alter the serum levels of **digoxin**[5] or **theophylline**.[6] Data from the CAPRIE study demonstrated that **ACE inhibitors, antidiabetic drugs** (**tolbutamide** named),[3] **anti-epileptic** therapy (**phenytoin** named),[3] **beta-blockers, calcium channel blockers, cholesterol reducing drugs, coronary/peripheral vasodilators** and **diuretics** can safely be given with clopidogrel.[7] However, *in vitro* studies with human liver microsomes had suggested that **phenytoin** and **tolbutamide** plasma levels might be raised because clopidogrel inhibits the activity of cytochrome P450 isoenzyme CYP2C9, which is concerned with **tolbutamide** metabolism.[3]

(d) NSAIDs

The makers say that **aspirin** does not modify the clopidogrel-mediated inhibition of ADP-induced platelet aggregation, but clopidogrel increases the effects of **aspirin** on collagen-induced platelet aggregation.[3] However, in practice, the concurrent use of 500 mg **aspirin** twice daily for one day was found not to increase the clopidogrel-induced prolongation of bleeding time.[3] The concurrent use of clopidogrel and **naproxen** in healthy subjects has been found to increase the occult gastrointestinal blood loss,[3] but information about the effects other **NSAIDs** is lacking. Nevertheless to be on the safe side the makers issue a broad general cautionary warning about the concurrent use of any **NSAID**. Patients should be warned about the possibility of gastrointestinal bleeding.[3]

(e) Warfarin

The makers say that the concurrent use of **warfarin** and clopidogrel is not recommended because it may increase the intensity of bleeding.[3] However, a placebo-controlled study in 20 patients who had been taking **warfarin** for at least 2 months found that found that the addition of 75 mg clopidogrel daily for 8 days had no effect on their serum **warfarin** levels or INRs. No bleeding occurred and no adverse events were reported.[8]

1. McEwen J, Strauch G, Perles P, Pritchard G, Moreland TE, Necciari J, Dickinson JP. Clopidogrel bioavailability: absence of influence of food or antacids. *Semin Thromb Hemost* (1999) 25 (Suppl 2), 47–50.
2. Caplain H, D'Honneur G, Cariou R. Prolonged heparin administration during clopidogrel treatment in healthy subjects. *Semin Thromb Hemost* (1999) 25 (Suppl 2), 61–4.
3. Plavix (Clopidogrel). Sanofi Synthelabo. Summary of product characteristics, January 2002.
4. Forbes CD, Lowe GDO, Maclaren M, Shaw BG, Dickinson JP, Keiffer G. Clopidogrel compatibility with concomitant cardiac co-medications: a study of its interactions with a beta-blocker and a calcium uptake antagonist. *Semin Thromb Hemost* (1999) 25 (Suppl 2), 55–9.
5. Peeters PAM, Crijns HJMJ, Tamminga WJ, Jonkman JHG, Dickinson JP, Necciari J. Clopidogrel, a novel antiplatelet agent, and digoxin: absence of pharmacodynamic and pharmacokinetic interaction. *Semin Thromb Hemost* (1999) 25 (Suppl 2), 51–4.
6. Caplain H, Thebault J-J, Necciari J. Clopidogrel does not affect the pharmacokinetics of theophylline. *Semin Thromb Hemost* (1999) 25 (Suppl 2), 65.
7. Morais J, on behalf of the CAPRIE investigators. Use of concomitant medications in the CAPRIE trial: clopidogrel is unlikely to be associated with clinically significant drug interactions. *Eur Heart J* (1998) 19 (Suppl) 5.
8. Lidell C, Svedberg L-E, Lindell P, Bandh S, Wallentin L. Absence of interaction between clopidogrel and warfarin in patients on long-term anticoagulation. *J Am Coll Cardiol* (2001) 37 (2 Suppl A), 314A.

CNS depressants + CNS depressants

The concurrent use of two or more drugs which depress the CNS may be expected to result in increased depression. This may have undesirable and even life-threatening consequences.

Clinical evidence, mechanism, importance and management

The primary effect of some drugs and the unwanted, secondary or side-effect of many other drugs is depression of the central nervous system causing drowsiness. If more than one CNS depressant is taken, their effects may be additive. It is not uncommon for patients, particularly the elderly, to be taking half-a-dozen drugs or more (and possibly alcohol as well). This can cause a cumulative CNS depression ranging from mild drowsiness through to a befuddled stupor, which can make the performance of the simplest everyday task more difficult or even impossible. The importance of this will depend on the context: at home and at bedtime it may even be advantageous, whereas it may considerably increase the risk of accident in the kitchen, at work, in a busy street, driving a car or handling other potentially dangerous machinery where alertness is at a premium. It has been estimated that as many as 600 traffic accident fatalities each year in the UK can be attributed to the sedative effects of psychoactive drugs alone.[1] **Alcohol** almost certainly makes things worse.

An example of the lethal effects of combining an **antihistamine**, a **benzodiazepine tranquilliser** and **alcohol** is briefly mentioned in the monograph 'Alcohol + Antihistamines', p.17. A less spectacular but socially distressing example is that of a woman accused of shop-lifting while in a confused state arising from the combined sedative effects of **Actifed**, a **Beechams Powder** and **Dolobid** (containing **triprolidine, salicylamide** and **diflunisal** respectively).[2]

Few if any well-controlled studies have been made on the cumulative or additive detrimental effects of CNS depressants (except with **alcohol**), but the following is a list of some of the groups of drugs that to a greater or lesser extent possess CNS depressant activity and which may be expected to interact in this way: **alcohol, analgesics,** some **antibacterials, anticonvulsants, antidepressants, antihistamines, antinauseants, antipsychotics, anxiolytics, cough and cold preparations, hypnotics, opioids, sedatives** and **tranquillisers**. Some of the interactions of **alcohol** with these drugs are dealt with in individual monographs. The Index should be consulted.

1. Anon. Sedative effects of drugs linked to accidents. *Pharm J* (1994) 253, 564.
2. Herxheimer A, Haffner BD. Prosecution for alleged shoplifting: successful pharmacological defence. *Lancet* (1982) i, 634.

Colchicine + Macrolide antibacterials

Two isolated case report describes acute life-threatening colchicine toxicity caused by the addition of erythromycin or clarithromycin.

Clinical evidence, mechanism, importance and management

A woman with familial Mediterranean fever and amyloidosis, under treatment with 1 mg colchicine daily, developed acute and life-threatening colchicine toxicity 16 days after starting to take 2 g **erythromycin** daily. The suggested reason is that the **erythromycin** possibly inhibited the metabolism of the colchicine by the liver, or caused more generalised hepatotoxicity. In addition this patient had both and cholestasis and renal dysfunction, which predisposed her to colchicine toxicity.[1] All of these would be expected to reduce the clearance of the colchicine from the body, resulting in its accumulation. However, the reaction is attributed, at least in part to the **erythromycin**, because in the presence of the cholestasis and renal impairment the colchicine level was 9 to 12.6 nanograms/ml, but increased to 22 nanograms/ml after the addition of **erythromycin**.[1] In a second case, a man of 67 on CAPD and colchicine 500 micrograms twice daily was admitted with symptoms of colchicine toxicity (including pancytopenia) 4 days after starting a course of **clarithromycin** 500 mg twice daily for an upper respiratory tract infection. All drugs were stopped and supportive treatment given, but he later died from multi-organ failure.[2]

Information on this interaction is limited, but it appears that macrolide antibacterials can provoke acute colchicine toxicity, at the very least in pre-disposed individuals. If any patient is given colchicine and a macrolide, be aware of the potential for toxicity, especially in patients with pre-existing renal impairment.

1. Caraco Y, Putterman C, Rahamimov R, Ben-Chetrit E. Acute colchicine intoxication - possible role of erythromycin administration. *J Rheumatol* (1992) 19, 494–6.

2. Dogukan A, Oymak FS, Taskapan H, Güven M, Tokgoz B, Utas C. Acute fatal colchicine intoxication in a patient on continuous ambulatory peritoneal dialysis (CAPD). Possible role of clarithromycin administration. *Clin Nephrol* (2001) 55, 181–2.

Colestipol + Fibrates

Over a 6-day period no adverse interaction occurred in 24 healthy subjects when given daily doses of 10 g colestipol with 500 mg clofibrate.[1] The pharmacokinetics of fenofibrate are unchanged by colestipol.[2]

1. DeSante KA, DiSante AR, Albert KS, Weber DJ, Welch RD, Vecchio TJ. The effect of colestipol hydrochloride on the bioavailability and pharmacokinetics of clofibrate. *J Clin Pharmacol* (1979) 19, 721–25.

2. Harvengt C, Desager JP. Lack of pharmacokinetic interaction of colestipol and fenofibrate in volunteers. *Eur J Clin Pharmacol* (1980) 17, 459–63.

Colestipol + Miscellaneous drugs

Colestipol is reported not to interact significantly with aspirin or methyldopa. A report suggests that the hypocholesterolaemic effects of colestipol are unaffected in insulin-treated diabetics but may be ineffective in those treated with phenformin and sulphonylureas.

Clinical evidence, mechanism, importance and management

Although colestipol can undoubtedly bind to a number of drugs in the gut, the effects on the bioavailability of most of them is usually small and clinically unimportant. The rate of absorption of **aspirin** is increased by colestipol 10 g, but the extent is unaltered and no particular precautions seem to be necessary.[1] Colestipol is also reported to have no important effect on the absorption of **methyldopa**.[2]

The concurrent use of **phenformin** and a sulphonylurea (**chlorpropamide**, **tolbutamide** or **tolazamide**) inhibited the normal hypocholesterolaemic effects of the colestipol in 12 diabetics with elevated serum cholesterol levels. No such antagonism was seen in two maturity-onset diabetics treated with **insulin**. The control of diabetes was not affected by the colestipol.[3] This suggests that colestipol may not be suitable for lowering the blood cholesterol levels of diabetics treated with these oral hypoglycaemic agents, but more study is needed to confirm these findings. **Phenformin** has been withdrawn from many countries because of severe, often fatal, lactic acidosis.

1. Hunninghake DB, Pollack E. Effect of bile acid sequestering agents on the absorption of aspirin, tolbutamide, and warfarin. *Fedn Proc* (1977) 36, 996.

2. Hunninghake DB, King S. Effect of cholestyramine and colestipol on the absorption of methyldopa and hydrochlorothiazide. *Pharmacologist* (1978) 20, 220.

3. Bandisode MS, Boshell BR. Hypocholesterolemic activity of colestipol in diabetes. *Curr Ther Res* (1975) 18, 276–84.

Colestyramine + Spironolactone

Hyperchloraemic metabolic acidosis has been seen in two patients associated with the use of colestyramine and spironolactone.

Clinical evidence, mechanism, importance and management

Two case reports describe the development of hyperchloraemic metabolic acidosis in 2 elderly patients (one with primary biliary cirrhosis the other with hepatic cirrhosis) treated with colestyramine (up to four sachets daily), who were concurrently receiving **spironolactone**.[1,2] One patient had mild renal impairment and upper respiratory tract infection.[1] This adverse reaction appears to be rare, but electrolyte monitoring during concurrent use has been advised.[1]

1. Eaves ER, Korman MG. Cholestyramine induced hyperchloremic metabolic acidosis. *Aust N Z J Med* (1984) 14, 670–2.

2. Clouston WM, Lloyd HM. Cholestyramine induced hyperchloremic metabolic acidosis. *Aust N Z J Med* (1985) 15, 271.

Cyclobenzaprine + Fluoxetine + Droperidol

A patient on cyclobenzaprine and fluoxetine developed torsade de pointes arrhythmia and ventricular fibrillation when droperidol was added.

Clinical evidence, mechanism, importance and management

A 59-year-old woman on long-term treatment with **fluoxetine** and cyclobenzaprine was additionally given **droperidol** before surgery on her Achilles tendon. Her baseline QTc was prolonged at 497 ms. During the surgery she developed torsade de pointes arrhythmia, which progressed to ventricular fibrillation. On the first postoperative day after the cyclobenzaprine had been withdrawn, her QTc had decreased towards normal (440 ms).[1]

A likely explanation is that her cyclobenzaprine serum levels were already raised by **fluoxetine** (a known inhibitor of cytochrome P450 isoenzyme CYP2D6) and as a result her QTc was already prolonged. Cyclobenzaprine is structurally like the tricyclic antidepressants and shares their adverse effects, including their dysrhythmic potentialities, so that the addition of the **droperidol**, also known to prolong the QT interval, simply further extended QTc interval and precipitated the torsade de pointes. This case not only illustrates the existence of an interaction between cyclobenzaprine and **fluoxetine**, but also the life-threatening risks of adding other drugs which can further prolong the QT interval.

1. Michalets EL, Smith LK, Van Tassel ED. Torsade de pointes resulting from the addition of droperidol to an existing cytochrome P450 drug interaction. *Ann Pharmacother* (1998) 32, 761–5.

Cyproterone acetate + Alcohol

Cyproterone acetate appears to be ineffective in alcohol excess, but there seems to be no evidence that normal social amounts of alcohol interact.

Clinical evidence, mechanism, importance and management

The makers of cyproterone acetate say that **alcohol** appears to reduce its effects, and so it is of no value in chronic alcoholics.[1] This appears to be based solely on a simple and unelaborated statement in an abstract of studies on 84 men whose hyper- or abnormal sexuality was treated with cyproterone acetate which stated[2] that "antiandrogens do not inhibit male sexual behaviour during alcohol excess."

The suggested reasons for this reaction are unknown, but it may possibly be due several factors. These include enzyme induction by the **alcohol**, which could possibly increase the metabolism and loss of the cyproterone from the body; increased sexual drive caused by **alcohol**, which might oppose the effects of cyproterone; and reduced compliance by alcoholic patients who forget to take their tablets while drinking to excess.[3] None of these possible and reasonable explanations has yet been shown to be the answer.

It seems therefore that cyproterone may not be effective in alcoholic patients, but there is nothing to suggest that the effects of cyproterone are opposed by normal moderate social amounts of **alcohol**.

1. Androcur (Cyproterone acetate). Schering Health Care Limited. Summary of product characteristics, April 2001.
2. Laschet U, Laschet L. Three years clinical results with cyproterone-acetate in the inhibiting regulation of male sexuality. *Acta Endocrinol (Copenh)* (1969) 138 (Suppl), 103.
3. Schering Health Care Limited. Personal communication, January 1997

Dantrolene + Metoclopramide

Metoclopramide increases the bioavailability of dantrolene in patients with spinal cord injury.

Clinical evidence, mechanism, importance and management

A study in 7 paraplegics and 6 quadriplegics with spinal cord injury found that a single 10-mg intravenous dose of **metoclopramide** increased the bioavailability of a single 100-mg oral dose of dantrolene by 57%. The reasons are not known, although it was suggested that absorption may have been affected. The clinical relevance of this interaction is uncertain but the authors of the study suggest that patients should be well monitored if **metoclopramide** is added or withdrawn from patients in this category who are being treated with dantrolene.[1]

1. Gilman TM, Segal JL, Brunnemann SR. Metoclopramide increases the bioavailability of dantrolene in spinal cord injury. *J Clin Pharmacol* (1996) 36, 64–71.

Desferrioxamine (Deferoxamine) + Miscellaneous drugs

High-dose vitamin C may cause cardiac disorders in some patients treated with desferrioxamine. Prochlorperazine caused unconsciousness in two patients being treated with desferrioxamine.

Clinical evidence, mechanism, importance and management

(a) Desferrioxamine + Vitamin C (ascorbic acid)

Sometimes **vitamin C** is given to increase the excretion of iron when desferrioxamine is being used. Some patients given 500 mg **vitamin C** daily whilst receiving intravenous desferrioxamine have shown a striking, but often transitory, deterioration in left ventricular function. For this reason it has been suggested that extreme caution should be used in patients with excess tissue iron.[1,2] It has been suggested that the same problem may not occur with subcutaneous desferrioxamine administration.[1] The need for the use of **vitamin C** needs to be clearly established, but under very well controlled conditions concurrent use can be undertaken.[3]

(b) Desferrioxamine + Prochlorperazine

Two patients treated with desferrioxamine lost consciousness for 48 to 72 h when given **prochlorperazine**, the presumed reason being that this drug combination removes iron from the nervous system.[4] It has also been suggested that desferrioxamine-induced damage of the retina may be more likely in the presence of phenothiazines.[5] It would seem wise to avoid the concurrent use of desferrioxamine and **prochlorperazine**, but there seems to be no direct evidence of adverse interactions with any of the other phenothiazines.

1. Henry W. Echocardiographic evaluation of the heart in thalassemia major. *Ann Intern Med* (1979) 91, 892–4.
2. Nienhuis AW. Vitamin C and iron. *N Engl J Med* (1981) 304, 170–1.
3. Cohen A, Cohen IJ, Schwartz E. Scurvy and altered iron stores in thalassemia major. *N Engl J Med* (1981) 304, 158–60.
4. Blake DR, Winyard P, Lunec J, Williams A, Good PA, Crewes SJ, Gutteridge JMC, Rowley D, Halliwell B, Cornish A, Hider RC. Cerebral and ocular toxicity induced by desferrioxamine. *Q J Med* (1985) 56, 345–55.
5. Pall H, Blake DR, Good PA, Wynyard P, Williams AC. Copper chelation and the neuro-ophthalmic toxicity of desferrioxamine. *Lancet* (1986) ii, 1279.

Desloratadine + Miscellaneous drugs

Desloratadine does not interact with alcohol, erythromycin or ketoconazole; it is not sedative and therefore will not have additive effects with CNS depressants, and it does not affect the QTc interval.

Clinical evidence, mechanism, importance and management

(a) CNS depressants, Alcohol

The makers report that desloratadine does not readily penetrate the CNS and at recommended doses does not cause drowsiness. Even 7.5 mg daily does not affect psychomotor performance.[1] This means that unlike some of the older sedative antihistamines, it will not have additive CNS depressant effects with **other CNS depressants**.

A single-dose, randomised, double-blind placebo-controlled trial in 25 healthy subjects given 7.5 mg desloratadine and enough **alcohol** to achieve blood levels averaging 100 mg/dl, found no evidence of an interaction. No increased sedation or worsening of the performance of psychomotor tests was seen.[1,2] No special precautions are therefore needed.

(b) Erythromycin, Ketoconazole and possible effects on the QTc interval

A 10-day study in 24 healthy subjects found that 500 mg **erythromycin** 8-hourly raised the AUC of desloratadine 7.5 mg daily 1.1-fold compared with a placebo, and the maximum serum levels were raised 1.2-fold. There were no statistical or clinically relevant changes in the ventricular rate, QT, PR, QRS or QTc intervals.[3] A parallel 10-day study in 24 healthy subjects found that 200 mg **ketoconazole** twice daily raised the AUC of desloratadine, 7.5 mg daily, 1.39-fold compared with a placebo, and the maximum serum levels were raised 1.45-fold. There were no statistical or clinically relevant changes in the ventricular rate, QT, PR, QRS or QTc intervals.[4] These pharmacokinetic changes are unimportant and no special precautions are needed if either of these drugs is given concurrently with desloratadine.

The enzyme responsible for the metabolism of desloratadine is not known, but this lack of interaction with **erythromycin** or **ketoconazole**, both of which are inhibitors of cytochrome P450 isoenzyme CYP3A4, suggests that this isoenzyme is not responsible. It also provides evidence that other CYP3A4 inhibitors or inducers are unlikely to interact with desloratadine.

Tests to find out if desloratadine affects the QTc interval showed that no prolongation of the QTc interval occurs (unlike with **astemizole** and **terfenadine**) even when using 45 mg daily (i.e. nine times the normal recommended dose) for 10 days.[1,3,4]

1. Neoclarityn (Desloratadine). Schering-Plough Ltd. Summary of product characteristics, July 2002.
2. Rikken G, Scharf M, Danzig M, Staudinger H. Desloratadine and alcohol coadministration: no increase in impairment of performance over that induced by alcohol alone. Poster at EAACI (European Academy of Allergy and Clinical Immunology) Conference, Lisbon, Portugal. 2–4 July 2000.
3. Glue A, Banfield C, Affrime MB, Statkevich P, Reyderman L, Pahdi D, Maxwell S, Clement R. Lack of electrocardiographic interaction between desloratadine and erythromycin. Poster at EAACI (European Academy of Allergy and Clinical Immunology) Conference, Lisbon, Portugal. 2–4 July 2000.
4. Affrime MB, Banfield C, Glue P, Keung A, Herron JM, Pahdi D, Maxwell S, Clement R. Lack of electrocardiographic effects when desloratadine and ketoconazole are coadministered. Poster at EAACI (European Academy of Allergy and Clinical Immunology) Conference, Lisbon, Portugal. 2–4 July 2000.

Dexfenfluramine or Fenfluramine + Phentermine

Fenfluramine and dexfenfluramine have been withdrawn because of the occurrence of serious and sometimes fatal valvular heart disease (aortic, mitral, tricuspid or mixed valve disease). Pulmonary hypertension has also sometimes been seen. These serious adverse effects occurred when these drugs were taken alone and when combined with phentermine as *Fen-phen* and *Dexfen-phen*, but not with phentermine alone.[1-5]

1. Committee on Safety of Medicines/Medicines Control Agency. Fenfluramine and dexfenfluramine withdrawn. *Current Problems* (1997) 23, 12.
2. Food and Drugs Administration. FDA announces withdrawal fenfluramine and dexfenfluramine (Fen-Phen). September 15th, 1997.
3. Connolly HM, Crary JL, McGoon MD, Hensrud DD, Edwards BS, Edwards WD, Schaff HV. Valvular heart disease associated with fenfluramine-phentermine. *N Engl J Med* (1997) 337, 581–8.
4. Mark EJ, Patals ED, Chang HT, Evans RJ, Kessler SC. Fatal pulmonary hypertension associated with short-term use of fenfluramine and phentermine. *N Engl J Med* (1997) 337, 602–6.
5. Graham DJ, Green L. Further cases of valvular heart disease associated with fenfluramine-phentermine. *N Engl J Med* (1997) 337, 635.

Dextromethorphan + Amiodarone

Amiodarone can increase the serum levels of dextromethorphan.

Clinical evidence

A study in 8 patients with cardiac arrhythmias (all extensive metabolisers) found that **amiodarone** (1 g daily for 10 days followed by 200 to 400 mg daily for a mean duration of 76 days) changed their excretion of dextromethorphan 40 mg and its metabolite. The amount of unchanged dextromethorphan in the urine rose by nearly 150% whereas the amount of its metabolite (dextrophan) fell by about 25%. The same study found that **amiodarone** did not affect the metabolism of **mephenytoin** or **isoniazid**.[1]

Mechanism

In vitro studies using liver microsomes have shown that amiodarone inhibits the metabolism (*O*-demethylation) of dextromethorphan by decreasing the activity of the cytochrome P450 isoenzyme CYP2D6 within the liver.[1] Thus the dextromethorphan is cleared from the body more slowly.

Importance and management

Information seems to be limited to this study. The clinical implications are (a) that amiodarone may interfere with the results of phenotyping if dextromethorphan is used to determine CYP2D6 activity, and (b) that dextromethorphan toxicity (excitation, confusion) may possibly develop in patients taking amiodarone. Be alert for any signs of toxicity if both are used. As yet too little is known about this interaction to say by how much the dextromethorphan dosage should be reduced. Remember that dextromethorphan occurs in a considerable number of proprietary cough preparations.

1. Funck-Brentano C, Jacqz-Aigrain E, Leenhardt A, Roux A, Poirier J-M, Jaillon P. Influence of amiodarone on genetically determined drug metabolism in humans. *Clin Pharmacol Ther* (1991) 50, 259–66.

Dextromethorphan + Quinidine

Quinidine markedly increases the plasma levels of dextromethorphan.

Clinical evidence

A study found that 3 out of 6 patients given 60 mg dextromethorphan twice daily had steady-state plasma levels of less than 5 nanograms/ml 12 h after the dose. The plasma dextromethorphan levels averaged only 12 nanograms/ml in the group as a whole. However, after being given 75 mg **quinidine** twice daily for a week, with only half the dose of dextromethorphan, their serum levels averaged 38 nanograms/ml.[1] Some of the patients experienced dextromethorphan toxicity (nervousness, tremors, restlessness, dizziness, shortness of breath, confusion etc.).[1]

Mechanism

Quinidine inhibits cytochrome P450 isoenzyme CYP2D6 which is involved with the metabolism of the dextromethorphan by the liver.[1] As a result, the dextromethorphan accumulates, its serum levels rise and its toxic effects manifest themselves.

Importance and management

An established and clinically important interaction but with limited documentation. If the combination is thought necessary, a low dose of dextromethorphan. Concurrent use should be well monitored for evidence of toxicity (see above).

1. Zhang Y, Britto MR, Valderhaug KL, Wedlund PJ, Smith RA. Dextromethorphan: enhancing its systemic availability by way of low-dose quinidine-mediated inhibition of cytochrome P4502D6. *Clin Pharmacol Ther* (1992) 51, 647–55.

Dihydroergotamine + Miscellaneous drugs

Three isolated cases of the serotonin syndrome have been seen in patients on paroxetine with imipramine, amitriptyline, or sertraline when given dihydroergotamine.

Clinical evidence

A woman on **imipramine**, **paroxetine** and lithium who had a 3-week continuous headache was treated with 300 micrograms of dihydroergotamine intravenously. Within 5 minutes of a subsequent 500-microgram dose she developed dysarthria, dilated pupils, diaphoresis, diffuse weakness and barely responded to commands. She was diffusely hyper-reflexive and showed occasional myoclonic jerks. She recovered after 90 min.[1]

A woman with a history of migraine headaches responded well to **amitriptyline**, metoclopramide and dihydroergotamine. Six weeks after the **amitriptyline** was replaced by **sertraline**, she was again successfully treated for acute migraine with 10 mg of intravenous metoclopramide and 1 mg of intravenous dihydroergotamine, but 2 h later she developed nausea, emesis, agitation, weakness, diaphoresis, salivation, chills and fever. All of the symptoms subsided after 24 h.[1]

A woman with a history of migraines treated prophylactically with **amitriptyline** and propranolol was admitted to hospital in status migrainosus. She was given 1 mg dihydroergotamine intravenously, 10 mg prochlorperazine intravenously and 10 mg metoclopramide intravenously. Within 20 min she became diaphoretic, tachycardic, diffusely hyper-reflexic, agitated, confused, and briefly lost consciousness twice. Diazepam 8 mg given intramuscularly calmed her agitation, and all the symptoms resolved after 6 h. A year later she was given 6 mg subcutaneous sumatriptan while taking **nortriptyline** daily with no ill effects.[1]

Mechanism

Not understood. All of these patients appeared to have developed the serotonin syndrome, which is thought to be due to hyperstimulation of 5-HT receptors in the brain. Dihydroergotamine is a 5-HT agonist while paroxetine and sertraline are both serotonin (5-HT) re-uptake inhibitors, all of which might be expected to increase 5-HT concentrations in the CNS and thereby increase receptor stimulation.

Importance and management

These appear to be isolated cases and not of general importance, nevertheless they illustrate the potential for the development of the serotonin syndrome in patients given multidrug regimens which affect 5-HT receptors. The syndrome is rare and (so it has been suggested[1]) may sometimes be an idiosyncratic reaction.

1. Mathew NT, Tietjen GE, Lucker C. Serotonin syndrome complicating migraine pharmacotherapy. *Cephalalgia* (1996) 16, 323–7.

Dimeticone + Cimetidine or Doxycycline

The bioavailabilities of cimetidine and doxycycline are not affected by dimeticone.

Clinical evidence, mechanism, importance and management

The pharmacokinetics of a 200-mg dose of **cimetidine** were not significantly changed by 2.25 g dimeticone in 11 healthy subjects.[1] Another study in 8 subjects found that 2.25 g dimeticone did not alter the bioavailability of **doxycycline**.[2]

1. Boismare F, Flipo JL, Moore N, Chanteclair G. Etude de l'effet du diméticone sur la biodisponibilité de la cimétidine. *Therapie* (1987) 42, 9–11.
2. Bistue C, Perez P, Becquart D, Vinçon G, Albin H. Effet du diméticone sur la biodisponibilité de la doxycicline. *Therapie* (1987) 42, 13–16.

Dipyridamole + Antacids, H₂-blockers or Proton pump inhibitors

The effective disintegration, dissolution and eventual absorption of dipyridamole in tablet form depends upon having a low pH in the stomach. Drugs which raise the gastric pH significantly are expected to reduce the bioavailability of dipyridamole.

Clinical evidence, mechanism, importance and management

The solubility of dipyridamole depends very much on the pH. It is very soluble at low pH values and almost insoluble at neutral pH. The following are its relative solubilities in mg/l at different pH values: >100000 (pH 1 and 2), 7000 (pH 3), 450 (pH 4), 65 (pH 5), 10 (pH 6), 5 (pH 7).[1] This indicates that dipyridamole needs a low pH in the stomach if solid formulations of the drug are to disintegrate and dissolve adequately. A consequential conclusion is that any drug which raises the stomach pH significantly would be likely to reduce the dissolution and absorption of dipyridamole. It would therefore be reasonable to expect that **antacids**, **H₂-blockers** (e.g. **cimetidine**) and **proton pump inhibitors** (e.g. **omeprazole**) which can raise the gastric pH would interact to reduce the bioavailability of dipyridamole, but nobody seems to have checked on this directly. Study is needed to find out whether this is a clinically relevant interaction or not.

1. Boehringer Ingelheim. Persantin (dipyridamole), data on file (report 1482B).

Dipyridamole + Beta-blockers

No adverse reactions normally occur in patients taking beta-blockers who undergo dipyridamole-thallium scintigraphy and echocardiography, but rarely bradycardia and asystole can occur.

Clinical evidence

A woman of 71 on 120 mg **nadolol** daily and bendroflumethiazide and with a 3-week history of chest pain was given 300 mg of oral dipyridamole as part of the diagnostic dipyridamole-echocardiography test for coronary artery disease. She was given 2.9 millicuries of thallium-201 intravenously, 45 minutes after the dipyridamole, but 3 min later while exercising she complained of chest pain and then cardiac arrest occurred. She was successfully treated with intravenous aminophylline.[1]

Adverse interactions occurred in another 2 patients on beta-blockers during diagnostic dipyridamole-echocardiography tests. One patient, on **atenolol** developed bradycardia then asystole, which was treated with aminophylline and atropine, and the other patient, on **metoprolol**, developed bradycardia, which resolved after she was given aminophylline.[2]

These reports need to be set in a broad context. A very extensive study of high-dose dipyridamole echocardiography (10,451 tests in 9,122 patients) noted particular major adverse reactions in 7 patients. Three of them developed asystole. Two of these patients were taking **unnamed beta-blockers**.[3]

Another study, over the period 1978 to 1985, of 1096 patients who had undergone intravenous dipyridamole-thallium scintigraphy found a considerable number of adverse reactions (including acute bronchospasm) but neither bradycardia nor asystole was among those listed, even though 30% of the patients were taking **propranolol**.[4] Another study in 170 patients stated that most of them were taking nitrates, **beta-blockers** and/or **calcium channel blockers** (exact numbers not stated) but neither bradycardia nor asystole were reported.[5]

Mechanism

Not established. One possible explanation is that both drugs have negative chronotropic effects on the heart.

Importance and management

The value and safety of dipyridamole perfusion scintigraphy and echocardiography have been very extensively studied in very large numbers of patients, and reports of bradycardia and asystole, attributed to a dipyridamole/beta-blocker interaction are sparse. Large numbers of patients given this test have apparently taken beta-blockers without developing these problems.[4,5] It would therefore appear to be a relatively rare interaction (if such it is), nevertheless when it occurs it is serious. See also 'Beta-blockers + Thallium scans', p.451.

1. Blumenthal MS, McCauley CS. Cardiac arrest during dipyridamole imaging. *Chest* (1988) 93, 1103–4.
2. Roach PJ, Magee MA, Freedman SB. Asystole and bradycardia during dipyridamole stress testing in patients receiving beta-blockers. *Int J Cardiol* (1993) 42, 92–4.
3. Picano E *et al* on behalf of the Echo-Persantine International Cooperative Study Group. Safety of intravenous high-dose dipyridamole echocardiography. *Am J Cardiol* (1992) 70, 252–8.
4. Ranhosky A, Kempthorne-Rawson J, and the Intravenous Dipyridamole Thallium Imaging Study Group. The safety of intravenous dipyridamole thallium myocardial perfusion imaging. *Circulation* (1990) 81, 1205–9.
5. Zhu YY, Chung WS, Botvinick EH, Dae MW, Lim AD, Ports TA, Danforth JW, Wolfe CL, Goldschlager N, Chatterjee K. Dipyridamole perfusion scintigraphy: the experience with its application in one hundred seventy patients with known or suspected unstable angina. *Am Heart J* (1991) 121, 33–43.

Dipyridamole + Caffeine

Caffeine (in tea, coffee, *Cola*, etc.) may interfere with dipyridamole-thallium-201 scintigraphy tests.

Clinical evidence, mechanism, importance and management

Caffeine 250 mg (roughly equivalent to 2 to 3 cups of **coffee**) before dipyridamole-thallium-201 scintigraphy caused a false-negative test result in a patient.[1] A further study in 8 healthy subjects confirmed that **caffeine** inhibits the haemodynamic response to the infusion of dipyridamole.[2] The authors of the report therefore say that patients should abstain from **caffeine** (**tea**, **coffee**, **chocolate**, **cocoa**, *Cola*, etc.) for at least 24 h before a test, and if during the test the haemodynamic response is low (i.e. no increase in heart rate) the presence of **caffeine** should be suspected.[2]

1. Smits P, Aengevaeren WRM, Corstens FHM, Thien T. Caffeine reduces dipyridamole-induced myocardial ischemia. *J Nucl Med* (1989) 30, 1723–6.
2. Smits P, Straatman C, Pijpers E, Thien T. Dose-dependent inhibition of the hemodynamic response to dipyridamole by caffeine. *Clin Pharmacol Ther* (1991) 50, 529–37.

Disulfiram + Monoamine oxidase inhibitors (MAOIs)

An isolated report describes delirium in a man on lithium and disulfiram when his treatment with moclobemide was replaced by tranylcypromine.

Clinical evidence, mechanism, importance and management

The treatment of a man on long-term lithium treatment and disulfiram implants, was changed from **moclobemide** (dosage not stated) to 10 mg **tranylcypromine** twice daily. Within 2 days he became acutely delirious (agitated, disoriented, incoherent, visual hallucinations) and later subcomatose, with nystagmus and a downward gaze. He was successfully treated with haloperidol and promethazine, and recovered within 24 h.[1] The reasons for this reaction are not understood.

This seems to be the only report of an adverse reaction between disulfiram and an **MAOI** so that its general importance is uncertain, but warnings about this drug combination, based on theoretical considerations, have been made previously, and **tranylcypromine** was considered to be the MAOI which presented the greatest risk.[2] MAOIs and disulfiram are generally regarded as unsafe, but just why is not clear (apart from the general and wide-spread nervousness about giving any drug with an MAOI). It seems that this particular patient had no problems while taking **moclobemide** which is a selective MAOI. If the decision is made to give disulfiram and an **MAOI**, the outcome should be very closely monitored.

1. Blansjaar BA, Egberts TCG. Delirium in a patient treated with disulfiram and tranylcypromine. *Am J Psychiatry* (1995) 152, 296.
2. Ciraulo DA. Can disulfiram (Antabuse) be safely co-administered with the monoamine oxidase (MAOI) antidepressants? *J Clin Psychopharmacol* (1989) 9, 315–16.

Donepezil + Miscellaneous drugs

Cimetidine, ketoconazole and warfarin do not appear to interact with donepezil to a clinically relevant extent.

Clinical evidence, mechanism, importance and management

Because *in vitro* studies had demonstrated that donepezil is metabolised primarily by cytochrome P450 isoenzyme CYP3A4 and to a minor extent by CYP2D6, an *in vivo* study was undertaken. Donepezil was given to 18 healthy subjects with **cimetidine**, which is an inhibitor of several cytochrome P450 isoenzymes and with **ketoconazole** which is a specific and potent inhibitor of CYP3A4. It was found that after taking **cimetidine** for a week the maximum serum levels and AUC of donepezil were increased by 13% and 10% respectively. After taking **ketoconazole** for a week the maximum serum levels and AUC of donepezil were increased 26.8% and 26.5% respectively. Donepezil had no effect on the pharmacokinetics of **cimetidine** or **ketoconazole**.[1] None of the increases in donepezil levels were considered to be clinically relevant.[1] In an open-label crossover study, 12 healthy men were given 10 mg donepezil daily for 19 days and a single 25-mg dose of **warfarin** on day 14. It was found that the pharmacokinetics of *(R)-* and *(S)*-**warfarin** and the prothrombin times were unchanged by the presence of the donepezil, and vital signs, ECG and laboratory tests were unaltered.[2] This evidence suggests that no spe-

cial precautions are needed if any of these drugs and donepezil are taken concurrently.

1. Tiseo PJ, Rogers SL, Perdomo CA, Friedhoff LT. The effect of cimetidine and ketoconazole on the pharmacokinetics of donepezil. *Clin Pharmacol Ther* (1998) 63, 234.
2. Tiseo PJ, Foley K, Friedhoff LT. The effect of multiple doses of donepezil hydrochloride on the pharmacokinetic and pharmacodynamic profile of warfarin. *Br J Clin Pharmacol* (1998) 46 (Suppl 1), 45–50.

Doxapram + Theophylline

Doxapram pharmacokinetics are unchanged in babies by theophylline, but agitation and increased muscle activity may occur in adults.

Clinical evidence, mechanism, importance and management

Theophylline does not affect the pharmacokinetics of doxapram when used to treat apnoea in premature babies. No adjustment of the dosage of doxapram is needed in the presence of **theophylline**.[1] However, the makers of doxapram say that clinical data suggests there may be an interaction between doxapram and **aminophylline** which is manifested by agitation and increased skeletal muscle activity. Care should be taken if used together.[2]

1. Jamali F, Coutts RT, Malek F, Finer NN, Peliowski A. Lack of a pharmacokinetic interaction between doxapram and theophylline in apnea of prematurity. *Dev Pharmacol Ther* (1991) 16, 78–82.
2. Dopram Infusion (Doxapram). Anpharm Limited. Product information, October 1997.

Ebastine + Miscellaneous drugs

Erythromycin causes a marked increase in the plasma levels of ebastine and of its active metabolite, accompanied by a small increase in the QTc interval. Neither cimetidine nor diazepam appear to interact with ebastine.

Clinical evidence, mechanism, importance and management

A blinded crossover study in 30 healthy subjects taking 20 mg **ebastine** daily found that the concurrent use of 2.4 g **erythromycin** daily for 10 days more than doubled the maximum ebastine plasma levels from 8.5 to 18.6 nanograms/ml and almost tripled the AUC. The maximum plasma levels of the active metabolite of ebastine, carebastine, were doubled and the AUC similarly almost tripled. Ebastine alone increased the QTc interval by 6.1 ms, **erythromycin** alone increased it by 8.9 ms, and together they increased it by 19.6 ms.[1] This increase in the QTc interval is unlikely to be clinically important unless other factors are present which also prolong the QTc interval.

Ebastine 20 mg daily was found not to impair the performance of a number of psychomotor tests in 12 healthy subjects, although body sway and flicker fusion tests were altered. When given with **diazepam** 15 mg there were no significant changes in psychomotor performance when compared to either drug alone.[2,3] **Cimetidine** 400 mg three times daily was found to have no significant effect on the conversion of single 20-mg doses of **ebastine** to carebastine in 12 healthy subjects, nor was there any evidence of any sedation or other side effects.[4] No special precautions would therefore seem to be needed if ebastine is taken with either **diazepam** or **cimetidine**.

1. Gillen M, Pentikis H, Rhodes G, Chaikin P, Morganroth J. Pharmacokinetic (PK) and pharmacodynamic (PD) interaction of ebastine (EBA) and erythromycin (ERY). *Clin Invest Med* (1998) (Suppl), S20.
2. Mattila MJ. Ebastine administered subacutely does not impair human performance or enhance diazepam effects. *Br J Clin Pharmacol* (1992) 33, 244P.
3. Mattila MJ, Aranko K, Kuitunen T. Diazepam effects on the performance of healthy subjects are not enhanced by treatment with the antihistamine ebastine. *Br J Clin Pharmacol* (1993) 35, 272–77.
4. van Rooij J, Schoemaker HC, Bruno R, Reinhoudt JF, Breimer DD, Cohen AF. Cimetidine does not influence the metabolism of the H₁-receptor antagonist ebastine to its active metabolite carebastine. *Br J Clin Pharmacol* (1993) 35, 661–3.

Eletriptan + Miscellaneous drugs

The makers of eletriptan contraindicate erythromycin and ketoconazole because they raise eletriptan levels, and they predict that other CYP3A4 inhibitors (clarithromycin, josamycin, indinavir, nelfinavir and ritonavir) will do the same. They contraindicate ergotamine, dihydroergotamine, methysergide and all 5-HT$_1$ agonists. No clinically relevant interactions occur with beta-blockers, calcium channel blockers, flunarizine, oestrogen-based HRT preparations or oral contraceptives, SSRIs or tricyclic antidepressants. MAOIs are not expected to interact. See also '5-HT$_1$ agonists (Triptans) + Selective serotonin re-uptake inhibitors (SSRIs)', p.898.

Clinical evidence, mechanism, importance and management

(a) Drugs which interact only to a clinically irrelevant extent or not at all

The makers say that in interaction studies using eletriptan with 100 mg **fluconazole**, 160 mg **propranolol** or 480 mg **verapamil**, it was found that the maximum serum levels of eletriptan were increased 1.4-, 1.1- and 2.2-fold respectively by these drugs, and the AUCs by 2-, 1.3- and 2.7-fold. However these changes were considered to be clinically unimportant. No blood pressure changes or any adverse events were seen when compared with taking eletriptan alone.[1]

In clinical trials with eletriptan taken with **beta-blockers**, **SSRIs** or **tricyclic antidepressants**, no evidence of an interaction was seen (except with **propranolol** as above). Population pharmacokinetic analysis of clinical studies suggest that these drugs as well as **calcium channel blockers** and **oestrogen-based oral contraceptives** and **HRT** are unlikely to affect the pharmacokinetics of eletriptan. **Flunarizine** appears also not to interact. The makers also say that although no formal interaction studies have been done, eletriptan is not a substrate for MAO and therefore no interaction would be expected with **MAOIs**.[1]

The makers say that there is no evidence from either *in vitro* or *in vivo* studies that eletriptan induces or inhibits cytochrome P450 isoenzymes, including CYP3A4, so that eletriptan is not expected to interact to a clinically relevant extent by altering the metabolism of other drugs.[1]

(b) Ergotamine and related drugs

The makers report that when oral **ergotamine**/caffeine was given 1h and 2 h after eletriptan, minor additive increases in blood pressure were seen. For this reason they contraindicate the concurrent use of **ergotamine** and related drugs such as **dihydroergotamine** and **methysergide**, and they recommend that at least 24 h should elapse between taking eletriptan and any of these drugs.[1]

(c) Inhibitors of cytochrome P450 isoenzyme CYP3A4

A clinical pharmacokinetic study by the makers of eletriptan found that 1000 mg **erythromycin** increased the maximum serum levels of eletriptan 2-fold, the AUC 3.6-fold and prolonged its half-life from 4.6 to 7.1 h. A parallel study using 400 mg **ketoconazole** increased the maximum serum levels of eletriptan 2.7-fold, the AUC 5.9 fold and prolonged its half-life from 4.8 to 8.3 h. The reason is that these two drugs have a potent inhibitory effect on the cytochrome P450 isoenzyme CYP3A4 which is concerned with the metabolism of eletriptan so that its metabolism and clearance are reduced, resulting in a rise in its serum levels. Because of the risk that these raised levels will result in eletriptan toxicity, the makers contraindicate the concurrent use of both of these anti-infective agents. They also contraindicate a number of other potent CYP3A4 inhibitors which are predicted to raise serum eletriptan levels similarly. These are **clarithromycin**, **josamycin** and the protease inhibitors **indinavir**, **nelfinavir** and **ritonavir**.[1]

(d) Other drugs to be avoided

The makers contraindicate the concurrent use of other 5-HT$_1$ agonists with eletriptan. This would include **naratriptan**, **rizatriptan**, **sumatriptan** and **zolmitriptan**.[1] The thinking behind this is that additive effects might lead to toxicity. They also contraindicate the use of eletriptan in patients with various disease conditions, among which are ischaemic heart disease and Prinzmetal's angina.[1]

1. Relpax (Eletriptan). Pfizer Ltd. Summary of product characteristics, June 2001.

Enoximone + Theophylline

Aminophylline reduces the beneficial cardiovascular effects of enoximone.

Clinical evidence, mechanism, importance and management

An experimental study of the mechanism of action of enoximone in 14 patients with ischaemic or idiopathic dilative cardiomyopathy found that pretreatment with **aminophylline** (7 mg/kg intravenously over 15 min) reduced the beneficial haemodynamic effects of enoximone (1 mg/kg intravenously over 15 min).[1] The reason appears to be that each drug competes for inhibition of cAMP specific phosphodiesterases in cardiac and vascular smooth muscle. The clinical importance of this awaits evaluation.

1. Morgagni GL, Bugiardini R, Borghi A, Pozzati A, Ottani F, Puddu P. Aminophylline counteracts the hemodynamic effects of enoximone. *Clin Pharmacol Ther* (1990) 47, 140.

Entacapone + Imipramine

Entacapone and imipramine appear not to interact adversely.

Clinical evidence, mechanism, importance and management

A study in 12 healthy women given 200 mg entacapone with either 75 mg **imipramine** or a placebo found no evidence that combined drug use had any relevant effect on haemodynamics or on free adrenaline or noradrenaline plasma levels.[1] There would appear to be no reason for avoiding concurrent use.

1. Illi A, Sundberg S, Ojala-Karlsson P, Scheinin M, Gordin A. Simultaneous inhibition of catecholamine-O-methylation by entacapone and neuronal uptake by imipramine: lack of interactions. *Eur J Clin Pharmacol* (1996) 51, 273–6.

Enteral tube feeding + Antacids or Sucralfate

Aluminium-containing antacids and sucralfate can interact with high-protein liquid enteral feeds within the oesophagus to produce an obstructive plug.

Clinical evidence

Three patients who were being fed with a liquid high-protein nutrient (*Fresubin liquid*) through an enteral tube developed an obstructing protein-aluminium-complex oesophageal plug when intermittently given an **aluminium/magnesium hydroxide** antacid (*Alucol-Gel*).[1]

Another report also describes blockage of a nasogastric tube in a patient treated with **aluminium hydroxide** (*Aludrox*) and *Nutrison*.[2] Other reports similarly describe the development of hard putty-like or creamy precipitations and encrustations that can block the oesophagus or stomach of patients treated with **sucralfate**, and *Ensure Plus*,[3] *Fresubin plus F*[4] or *Osmolite*.[5] Another patient developed this precipitate when treated with *Isocal* and **sucralfate** with **aluminium/magnesium hydroxide**.[6]

Mechanism

It seems that a relatively insoluble aluminium-protein complex (called a bezoar) forms between the protein in the enteral feeds and the aluminium from the antacids or sucralfate (sucralfate is about 18% aluminium). It thickens when the pH falls.[3]

Importance and management

An established and clinically important interaction that can result in the blockage of an enteral or nasogastric tube. The authors of one report say that high molecular protein solutions should not be mixed with antacids or followed by antacids, and if an antacid is needed, it should be given some time after the nutrients and the tube should be vigorously flushed beforehand.[1]

The authors of another report say that they feed for 18 hours daily and then give the sucralfate overnight.[2]

1. Valli C, Schulthess H-K, Asper R, Escher F, Häcki WH. Interaction of nutrients with antacids: a complication during enteral tube feeding. *Lancet* (1986) i, 747–8.
2. Tomlin ME, Dixon S. Aluminium and nasogastric feeds. *Pharm J* (1996) 256, 40.
3. Rowbottom SJ, Wilson J, Samuel L, Grant IS. Total oesophageal obstruction in association with combined enteral feed and sucralfate therapy. *Anaesth Intensive Care* (1993) 21, 372–4.
4. Vohra SB, Strang TI. Sucralfate therapy - a caution. *Br J Intensive Care* (1994) 4, 114.
5. Anderson W. Esophageal medication bezoar in a patient receiving enteral feedings and sucralfate. *Am J Gastroenterol* (1989) 84, 205–6.
6. Algozzine GJ, Hill G, Scoggins WG, Marr MA. Sucralfate bezoar. *N Engl J Med* (1983) 309, 1387.

Enteric coated, delayed release preparations + Antacids

It is thought that enteric-coated, delayed-release, preparations may possibly dissolve prematurely if they are taken at the same time as antacids, but positive confirmatory evidence of this seems to be lacking.

Clinical evidence, mechanism, importance and management

A number of drugs may damage the stomach wall (the NSAIDs for example) and for this reason some of them are given an enteric coating to resist gastric acid to prevent their release until they reach the more alkaline conditions within the small intestine. Other drugs are formulated as delayed release preparations to ensure that the drug is released at the optimum site for absorption. There are two British National Formulary (BNF) 'Cautionary and Advisory labels' for these preparations, one of which (No.25) says that they should be swallowed whole and not chewed to prevent mechanical damage, and the other (No.5) that advises patients not to take them at the same time of day as indigestion remedies.[1] The belief is that a rise in pH caused by the antacid might result in the premature dissolution of the preparation.

What is not clear is whether any rise in pH caused by antacids actually causes premature dissolution of these preparations. Confirmatory clinical and experimental evidence of this seems to be lacking and, moreover, **antacids** usually do not cause a marked change in the gastric pH. On the other hand the proton-pump inhibitors (**omeprazole, lansoprazole, pantoprazole, rabeprazole**) cause marked and long lasting changes in the pH which would be much more likely to affect the enteric-coating but there are no BNF warnings about using these drugs concurrently.

The BNF warnings are specifically for the enteric-coated formulations and usually do not apply to the same drugs when given in other forms (although some of these drugs may also directly interact with antacids). **Antacids** may sometimes be given intentionally with some of the non-enteric coated preparations to reduce their gastric irritant effects.

1. Appendix 10: Cautionary and advisory labels for dispensed medicines. British National Formulary (September 1998) No 36, 679.

Epoetin (recombinant human erythropoietin) + ACE inhibitors or Angiotensin II antagonists

It is not entirely clear whether captopril, enalapril, fosinopril or other ACE inhibitors affect the efficacy of epoetin or not. Epoetin may cause hypertension and thereby reduce the effects of antihypertensive drugs.

Clinical evidence

(a) Epoetin efficacy

Equal amounts of epoetin were given to haemodialysis patients either on **captopril** (20 patients), or a control group (23 patients) not taking **captopril**. The haemoglobin and haematocrit values were significantly different at 6.2 mmol/l and 29.3% in the **captopril** group and 7.1 mmol/l and 33.3% in the control group respectively.[1] Similar results were found in a small study in peritoneal dialysis patients.[2] A retrospective study of 40 dialysis patients found that the 20 patients taking an ACE inhibitor (**captopril** 12.5 to 75 mg daily, **enalapril** 2.5 to 5 mg daily or **fosinopril** 10 to 20 mg daily) showed some evidence of increased epoetin requirements after 1 year when compared with the control group. However, this was not significant until 15 months when the cumulative epoetin dosage requirements were about doubled (12092 versus 6449 units/kg).[3]

Another retrospective review of 180 haemodialysis patients, 14 of whom were taking ACE inhibitors (8 on **captopril** 35 mg daily and 6 on **enalapril** 7.85 mg daily) and epoetin over at least 32 weeks, failed to find any evidence that either the haematocrit or the dosage of epoetin were changed in any way when ACE inhibitors were added.[4] However, given the results of the other study, it is possible that this study was not continued for long enough to detect the effect. Another study in 17 patients on chronic haemodialysis found that ACE inhibitors (5 **captopril**, 12 **enalapril**) for 12 months did not increase the epoetin dose requirements or reduce the haematocrits,[5] but again this study was of shorter duration than the one that found an effect.

(b) Hypertensive effects of epoetin

One of the side-effects of epoetin is hypertension so that it is important to control any existing hypertension before epoetin is started (the makers contraindicate epoetin in uncontrolled hypertension). Blood pressure should be monitored before and during epoetin treatment, and if necessary antihypertensive drug treatment should be started or increased if the pressure rises.[6]

Mechanism

It has been argued that ACE inhibitors might possibly reduce the efficacy of epoetin in haemodialysis patients for several reasons. Firstly, because patients with chronic renal failure show haematocrit falls when given ACE inhibitors, secondly because ACE inhibitors reduce polycythaemia following renal transplantation, and thirdly because **captopril** reduces the plasma levels of endogenous erythropoietin.[1,7] A multitude of other factors have also been proposed.[8]

Importance and management

The overall picture is unclear, and it would seem that an interaction, if any truly exists, takes a long time to develop. As epoetin dosage is governed by response, no immediate intervention is necessary. The major implication of this interaction is probably cost, as ultimately higher doses of epoetin appear to be needed in patients on ACE inhibitors. More long-term study is needed. Preliminary evidence suggests that **losartan** may not interact,[9] but it is too early to draw any definite conclusions.

1. Walter J. Does captopril decrease the effect of human recombinant erythropoietin in haemodialysis patients? *Nephrol Dial Transplant* (1993) 8, 1428.
2. Mora C, Navarro JF. Negative effect of angiotensin-converting enzyme inhibitors on erythropoietin response in CAPD patients. *Am J Nephrol* (2000) 20 248.
3. Heß E, Sperschneider H, Stein G. Do ACE inhibitors influence the dose of human recombinant erythropoietin in dialysis patients? *Nephrol Dial Transplant* (1996) 11, 749–51.

4. Conlon PJ, Albers F, Butterly D, Schwab SJ. ACE inhibitors do not affect erythropoietin efficacy in haemodialysis patients. *Nephrol Dial Transplant* (1994) 9, 1358.
5. Schwenk MH, Jumani AQ, Rosenberg CR, Kulogowski JE, Charytan C, Spinowitz BS. Potential angiotensin-converting enzyme inhibitor-epoetin alfa interaction in patients receiving chronic hemodialysis. *Pharmacotherapy* (1998) 18, 627–30.
6. NeoRecormon (Epoetin beta). Roche. Summary of product characteristics, March 2001.
7. Pratt MC, Lewis-Barned NJ, Walker RJ, Bailey RR, Shand BI, Livesey J. Effect of angiotensin converting enzyme inhibitors on erythropoietin concentrations in healthy volunteers. *Br J Clin Pharmacol* (1992) 43, 363–5.
8. Macdougall IC. ACE inhibitors and erythropoietin responsiveness. *Am J Kidney Dis* (2001) 38, 649–51.
9. Kato A, Takita T, Furuhashi M, Takahashi T, Maruyama Y, Hishida A. No effect of losartan on response to erythropoietin therapy in patients undergoing hemodialysis. *Nephron* (2000) 86, 538–9.

Ergot + Glyceryl trinitrate (GTN)

The ergot alkaloids such as dihydroergotamine would be expected to oppose the anti-anginal effects of glyceryl trinitrate (nitroglycerin).

Clinical evidence, mechanism, importance and management

There seem to be no clinical reports of adverse interactions between these drugs, but since **ergot** causes vasoconstriction and can provoke angina it would therefore be expected to oppose the effects of **glyceryl trinitrate** when used as a vasodilator for the treatment of angina. Ergot derivatives are regarded as contraindicated in those with ischaemic heart disease. However, **glyceryl trinitrate** has also been shown to increase the bioavailability of **dihydroergotamine** in hypotensive subjects, which would increase its vasoconstrictor effects.[1] The clinical outcome of concurrent use is therefore uncertain. You should monitor well if the decision is taken to use both drugs.

1. Bobik A, Jennings G, Skews H, Esler M, McLean A. Low oral bioavailability of dihydroergotamine and first-pass extraction in patients with orthostatic hypotension. *Clin Pharmacol Ther* (1981) 30, 673–9.

Ergot + Macrolide antibacterials

Ergot toxicity can develop rapidly in patients on ergotamine or dihydroergotamine if they are given erythromycin or troleandomycin. A single case of toxicity has occurred with clarithromycin and also with josamycin, and toxicity is predicted to occur with midecamycin. None appears to have been described with spiramycin and none would be expected.

Clinical evidence

(a) Clarithromycin

A woman of 59 took 2 mg **ergotamine tartrate** for a typical migraine headache. After 2 h her tongue became swollen, painful and bluish in colour. She showed some hypertension (BP 200/110 mmHg) and her fingers and toes were also cold and cyanotic (blue). She had taken this dose of **ergotamine** many times previously without problems, but on this occasion she was on the fifth day of a course of 500 mg **clarithromycin** twice daily. This adverse reaction was diagnosed as ergotism. Other evidence suggests that this patient may possibly have been more than usually sensitive to vascular occlusion.[1] The authors of this report briefly quote another case, originating from the makers of clarithromycin, of a possible **dihydroergotamine/clarithromycin** interaction, although this was complicated by the concurrent use of other medications used for the treatment of AIDS.[1] A woman who had previously uneventfully taken *Cafergot* (**ergotamine tartrate** 1 mg, caffeine 100 mg) for migraine developed ergotism (leg pain, cold and cyanosed limbs and impalpable pulses) within 3 days of starting to take **clarithromycin** (dosage not stated). The authors postulated that smoking and the use of oxymetazoline (both with vasoconstrictor effects) may also have had some part to play.[2]

(b) Erythromycin

A woman who had regularly and uneventfully taken *Migral* (**ergotamine tartrate** 2 mg, cyclizine hydrochloride 50 mg, caffeine 100 mg) on a number of previous occasions, took one tablet during a course of treatment with **erythromycin** 250 mg every 6 hours. Within 2 days she developed severe ischaemic pain in her arms and legs during exercise, with a burning sensation in her feet and hands. When admitted to hospital 10 days later her extremities were cool and cyanosed. Her pulse could not be detected in the lower limbs.[3]

Eight other cases of acute ergotism are reported elsewhere[4-11] involving **ergotamine tartrate** or **dihydroergotamine** and additional treatment with **erythromycin**. The reaction has been reported to develop within a few hours,[7] but it may take several days to occur.[10] One case appeared to occur when the **erythromycin** was started 3 days after the last dose of **dihydroergotamine**.[5]

(c) Josamycin

An isolated report describes a woman of 33 who developed severe ischaemia of the legs within 3 days of starting to take 2 g **josamycin** daily and capsules containing 300 micrograms **ergotamine tartrate**. Her legs and feet were cold, white and painful, and most of her peripheral pulses were impalpable.[12]

(d) Midecamycin diacetate (miocamycin)

After taking 800 mg **midecamycin diacetate** twice daily for 8 days, peak concentrations of **dihydroergotamine** following single 9-mg doses were raised 3 to 40 fold in 12 healthy subjects.[13]

(e) Troleandomycin

A woman of 40 who had been taking **dihydroergotamine**, 90 drops daily, for 3 years without problems, developed cramp in her legs within a few hours of starting to take **troleandomycin** 250 mg four times a day. Five days later she was admitted to hospital as an emergency with severe ischaemia of her arms and legs. Her limbs were cold and all her peripheral pulses were impalpable.[14]

There are reports of several other patients who had taken normal doses of **ergotamine tartrate** or **dihydroergotamine** for months or years without problems who then developed severe ergotism within hours or days of starting to take normal doses of **troleandomycin**.[15-22] Myocardial infarction developed in one individual.[23]

Mechanism

Erythromycin and troleandomycin form metabolites in the liver, which make stable complexes with the iron of cytochrome P450 so that the normal metabolising activity of the liver enzymes (in this case the cytochrome P450 isoenzyme CYP3A4) is reduced.[24] As a result the ergot is poorly metabolised so that it accumulates in the body, thus increasing its vasoconstrictive effects resulting in ischaemia. Spiramycin, and josamycin normally do not form these complexes.[24]

Importance and management

The interactions of the ergot alkaloids with erythromycin and troleandomycin are well documented, well established and clinically important, whereas information about clarithromycin appears to be confined to a single report. There are no adverse reports about midecamycin but it is expected to interact similarly. The concurrent use of all of these macrolides and ergot alkaloids should be avoided. Some of the cases cited were effectively treated with sodium nitroprusside or naftidrofuryl oxalate, with or without heparin.[1,5,7-9,20] Spiramycin, and josamycin would not be expected to interact because they do not form cytochrome P450 complexes (see 'Mechanism'). However, there is one unexplained and unconfirmed report of an interaction with josamycin.[12]

1. Horowitz RS, Dart RC, Gomez HF. Clinical ergotism with lingual ischemia induced by a clarithromycin-ergotamine interaction. *Arch Intern Med* (1996) 156, 456–8.
2. Ausband SC, Goodman PE. An unusual case of clarithromycin associated ergotism. *J Emerg Med* (2001) 21, 411–13.
3. Francis H, Tyndall A, Webb J. Severe vascular spasm due to erythromycin-ergotamine interaction. *Clin Rheumatol* (1984) 3, 243–6.
4. Lagier G, Castot A, Riboulet G, Boesh C. Un cas d'ergotisme mineur semblant en rapport avec une potentialisation de l'ergotamine par l'éthylsuccinate d'érythromycine. *Therapie* (1979) 34, 515–21.

5. Neveux E, Lesgourgues B, Luton J-P, Guilhaume B, Bertagna, Picard J. Ergotisme aigu par association proprionate d'érythromycine-dihydroergotamine. *Nouv Presse Med* (1981) 10, 2830.
6. Collet AM, Moncharmont D, San Marco JL, Eissinger F, Pinot JJ, Laselve L. Ergotisme iatrogène: rôle de l'association tartrate d'ergotamine-propionate d'érythromycine. *Sem Hop Paris* (1982) 58, 1624–6.
7. Boucharlat J, Franco A, Carpentier P, Charignon Y, Denis B, Hommel M. Ergotisme en milieu psychiatrique par association D.H.E. propionate d'erythromicine. *Ann Med Psychol (Paris)* (1980) 138, 292–6.
8. Leroy F, Asseman P, Pruvost P, Adnet P, Lacroix D, Thery C. Dihydroergotamine-erythromycin-induced ergotism. *Ann Intern Med* (1988) 109, 249.
9. Ghali R, De Léan J, Douville Y, Noël H-P, Labbé R. Erythromycin-associated ergotamine intoxication: arteriographic and electrophysiologic analysis of a rare cause of severe ischemia of the lower extremities and associated ischemic neuropathy. *Ann Vasc Surg* (1993) 7, 291–6.
10. Bird PA, Sturgess AD. Clinical ergotism with severe bilateral upper limb ischaemia precipitated by an erythromycin-ergotamine interaction. *Aust N Z J Med* (2000) 30, 635–6.
11. Karam B, Farah E, Ashoush R, Jebara V, Ghayad E. Ergotism precipitated by erythromycin: a rare case of vasospasm. *Eur J Vasc Endovasc Surg* (2000) 19, 96–8.
12. Grolleau JY, Martin M, de la Guerrande B, Barrier J, Peltier P. Ergotisme aigu lors d'une association josamycine/tartrate d'ergotamine. *Therapie* (1981) 36, 319–21.
13. Couet W, Mathieu HP, Fourtillan JB. Effect of ponsinomycin on the pharmacokinetics of dihydroergotamine administered orally. *Fundam Clin Pharmacol* (1991) 5, 47–52.
14. Franco A, Bourlard P, Massot C, Lecoeur J, Guidicelli H, Bessard G. Ergotisme aigu par association dihyroergotamine-triacétyloléandomycine. *Nouv Presse Med* (1978) 7, 205.
15. Lesca H, Ossard D, Reynier P. Les risques de l'association tri-acétyl-oléandomycine et tartrate d'ergotamine. *Nouv Presse Med* (1976) 5, 1832–3.
16. Hayton AC. Precipitation of acute ergotism by triacetyloleandomycin. *N Z Med J* (1969) 69, 42.
17. Dupuy JC, Lardy P, Seaulau P, Kervoelen P, Paulet J. Spasmes artériels systémiques. Tartrate d'ergotamine. *Arch Mal Coeur* (1979) 72, 86–91.
18. Bigorie B, Aimez P, Soria RJ, Samama F di Maria G, Guy-Grand B, Bour H. L'association triacétyl oléandomycin-tartrate d'ergotamine est-elle dangereuse? *Nouv Presse Med* (1975) 4, 2723–5.
19. Vayssairat M, Fiessinger J-N, Becquemin M-H, Housset E. Association dihydroergotamine et triacétyloléandomycine. Rôle dans une nécrose digitale iatrogène. *Nouv Presse Med* (1978) 7, 2077.
20. Matthews NT, Havill JH. Ergotism with therapeutic doses of ergotamine tartrate. *N Z Med J* (1979) 89, 476–7.
21. Chignier E, Riou R, Descotes J, Meunier P, Courpron P, Vignon G. Ergotisme iatrogène aigu par association médicamenteuse diagnostiqué par exploration non invasive (vélocimétrie à effet Doppler). *Nouv Presse Med* (1978) 7, 2478.
22. Bacourt F, Couffinhal J-C. Ischémie des membres par association dihydroergotamine-triacétyloléandomycine. Nouvelle observation. *Nouv Presse Med* (1978) 7, 1561.
23. Baudouy PY, Mellat M, Velleteau de Moulliac M. Infarctus du myocarde provoqué par l'association tartrate d'ergotamine-troléandomycine. *Rev Med Interne* (1988) 9, 420–2.
24. Pessayre D, Larrey D, Funck-Brentano C, Benhamou JP. Drug interactions and hepatitis produced by some macrolide antibiotics. *J Antimicrob Chemother* (1985) 16 (Suppl A), 181–94.

Ergot + Methysergide

The concurrent use of ergot alkaloids and methysergide can increase the risk of severe and persistent spasm of major arteries in some patients.

Clinical evidence

A man developed right faciobrachial thermoanaesthesia, vertigo, dysphagia and hoarseness 7 days after starting combined treatment with 2 mg **methysergide** three times daily and 500 micrograms subcutaneous **ergotamine tartrate** at night. Continued use resulted in impaired pain, touch and temperature sensation over the right side of his face, shoulder and arm. Arteriography demonstrated left vertebral artery occlusion and right vertebral arterial spasm. These symptoms, apart from the faciobrachial thermoanaesthesia, resolved when the drugs were stopped.[1] Another man treated for cluster headaches with 2 mg **methysergide**, intramuscular **ergotamine tartrate** and pizotifen developed ischaemia of the right foot, with impalpable popliteal and pedal pulses. Arteriography showed that blood flow to the arteries of the leg was reduced.[1]

Another report describes prolonged myocardial ischaemia in a patient with cluster headaches when a single 2-mg dose of **ergotamine tartrate** was added to 2 mg **methysergide** three times daily. Sublingual glyceryl trinitrate relieved the pain.[2]

Mechanism

Cluster headaches are associated with abnormal dilatation of the carotid arteries, which can be constricted by both of these drugs. In the cases cited it would seem that their combined vasoconstrictor effects caused arterial spasm elsewhere in the body, resulting in serious tissue ischaemia. Parenteral ergotamine raises the risk of arterial spasm.

Importance and management

Direct information seems to be limited to these cases. Cardiovascular complications can occur with either of these drugs given alone, but these cases suggest that their concurrent use may unpredictably increase the risk in some patients. Clearly they should be used with great caution or avoided.

1. Joyce DA, Gubbay SS. Arterial complications of migraine treatment with methysergide and parenteral ergotamine. *BMJ* (1982) 285, 260–1.
2. Galer BS, Lipton RB, Solomon S, Newman LC, Spierings ELH. Myocardial ischemia related to ergot alkaloids: a case report and literature review. *Headache* (1991) 31, 446–50.

Ergot + Protease inhibitors

A patient on indinavir rapidly developed ergotism after taking normal doses of ergotamine. Five others on ritonavir also taking ergotamine showed the same interaction. Other ergot derivatives are predicted to interact similarly. Information about possible interactions between ergot and other protease inhibitors seems to be lacking.

Clinical evidence

(a) Indinavir

An HIV+ man who had been taking lamivudine, stavudine, co-trimoxazole and **indinavir** (2400 mg daily) for more than a year was additionally prescribed *Gynergene caféiné* (1 mg ergotamine tartrate + 100 mg caffeine) for migraine. He took two doses on two consecutive days and 5 days later presented in hospital with numbness and cyanosis of the toes of his left foot. The next day he complained of intermittent claudication of his left leg, and 6 days later was admitted to hospital because of worsening symptoms and night cramps. Examination showed a typical picture of ergotism with vasospasm and reduced blood flow in the popliteal, tibial and femoral arteries. He was treated with heparin and buflomedil, and recovered after 3 days.[1]

(b) Ritonavir

A man of 63 with AIDS who had taken 1 to 2 mg **ergotamine tartrate** daily for migraine headaches over the last 5 years had his treatment with zidovudine, zalcitabine and co-trimoxazole changed to zidovudine, didanosine and **ritonavir** (600 mg 12 hourly). Within 10 days he developed paraesthesias, coldness, cyanosis and skin paleness of both arms, and when admitted to hospital his axillary, brachial, radial and ulnar pulses were found to be absent. An arterial doppler test showed the absence of blood flow in both his radial and ulnar arteries and he was diagnosed as having ergotism. The ergotamine and **ritonavir** were stopped, and he recovered when treated with prostaglandin E1 and calcium nadroparin.[2]

Another man aged 31 taking 400 mg **ritonavir** twice daily (and also taking pizotifen, nelfinavir, stavudine, lamivudine, co-trimoxazole and venlafaxine) developed severe burning and numbness in both feet and paraesthesias in his hands after taking 4 tablets of 1 mg **ergotamine** and 100 mg caffeine over 10 days. He was diagnosed as having ergotism. The drugs were stopped and he was effectively treated with intravenous alprostadil and heparin.[3] At least 4 other cases of ergotism have been reported in patients on **ritonavir** after taking ergot.[4-7] The ergotism developed in two of the patients within a few hours of taking a single dose of 1 to 2 mg **ergotamine tartrate**[4,6] and in the other two within about 4 to 15 days.[5,7] One was on a combination drug (0.3 mg ergotamine tartrate, 0.2 mg belladonna extract and 20 mg phenobarbital) twice daily for gastric discomfort,[5] and the other took up to 2 mg ergotamine daily.[7]

Mechanism

Not fully established but it seems almost certain that inhibition by these protease inhibitors of the cytochrome P450 isoenzyme CYP3A4 (and possibly other isoenzymes as well) reduces the metabolism of the ergotamine, thereby increasing its serum levels and its toxicity. Ergotamine poisoning causes arterial spasm which reduces and even shuts down the flow of blood in arteries.

Importance and management

Information appears to be limited to these reports but what happened is consistent with the way other drugs which are potent liver enzyme inhibitors can interact with ergot derivatives (see 'Ergot + Macrolide antibacterials', p.888). This interaction would appear to be established and is clearly clinically important. It would now be prudent for any patient on indinavir or ritonavir to avoid the concurrent use of ergotamine or any other ergot derivative such as dihydroergotamine. Information about possible interactions between ergot derivatives and other protease inhibitors seems to be lacking, even so to be on the safe side the makers of most of the other protease inhibitors contraindicate concurrent use.

1. Rosenthal E, Sala F, Chichmanian R-M, Batt M, Cassuto J-P. Ergotism related to concurrent administration of ergotamine tartrate and indinavir. *JAMA* (1999) 281, 987.
2. Cabellero-Granada FJ, Vician P, Cordero E, Gómez-Vera MJ, de Nozal M, López-Cortés LF. Ergotism related to concurrent administration of ergotamine tartrate and ritonavir in an AIDS patient. *Antimicrob Agents Chemother* (1997), 41,1207.
3. Phan TG, Agaliotis D, White G, Britton WJ. Ischaemic peripheral neuritis secondary to ergotism associated with ritonavir therapy. *Med J Aust* (1999) 171, 502, 504.
4. Montero A, Giovannoni AG, Tvrde PL. Leg ischemia in a patient receiving ritonavir and ergotamine. *Ann Intern Med* (1999) 130, 329–30.
5. Liaudet L, Buclin T, Jaccard C, Eckert P. Severe ergotism associated with interaction between ritonavir and ergotamine. *BMJ* (1999) 318, 771.
6. Blanche P, Rigolet A, Gombert B, Ginsburg C, Salmon D, Sicard D. Ergotism related to a single dose of ergotamine tartrate in an AIDS patient treated with ritonavir. *Postgrad Med J* (1999) 75, 546–7.
7. Vila A, Mykietiuk A, Bonvehl, Temporiti E, Urueqa A, Herrera F. Clinical ergotism induced by ritonavir. *Scand J Infect Dis* (2001) 33, 788–9.

Ergot + Tetracyclines

Five patients taking ergotamine or dihydroergotamine developed ergotism when additionally treated with doxycycline or tetracycline.

Clinical evidence

A woman who had previously taken **ergotamine tartrate** successfully and uneventfully for 16 years, was treated with **doxycycline** and **dihydroergotamine** 30 drops three times a day. Five days later her hands and feet became cold and reddened, and she was diagnosed as having a mild form of ergotism.[1]

Other cases of ergotism, some of them more severe, have been described in one patient taking **ergotamine tartrate** and **doxycycline**[2] and in 3 patients taking **tetracycline** containing preparations.[2-4]

Mechanism

Unknown. One suggestion is that these antibacterials may inhibit the activity of the liver enzymes concerned with the metabolism and clearance of the ergotamine, thereby prolonging its stay in the body and enhancing its activity.[1] One of the patients had a history of alcoholism[2] and two of them were in their eighties[4] so that their liver function may have already been reduced.

Importance and management

Information is very limited indeed. The incidence and general importance of this interaction is uncertain, but it would clearly be prudent to be on the alert for any signs of ergotism in any patient given ergot derivatives and any of the tetracyclines. Impairment of liver function may possibly be a contributory factor.

1. Amblard P, Reymond JL, Franco A, Beani JC, Carpentier P, Lemonnier D, Bessard G. Ergotisme. Forme mineure par association dihydroergotamine-chlorhydrate de doxycycline, étude capillaroscopique. *Nouv Presse Med* (1978) 7, 4148–9.
2. Dupuy JC, Lardy P, Seaulau P, Kervoelen P, Paulet J. Spasmes artériels systémiques. Tartrate d'ergotamine. *Arch Mal Coeur* (1972) 86–91.
3. L'Yvonnet M, Boillot A, Jacquet AM, Barale F, Grandmottet P, Zurlinden B, Gillet JY. A propos d'un cas exceptionnel d'intoxication aigue par un dérivé de l'ergot de seigle. *Gynecologie* (1974) 25, 541–3.
4. Sibertin-Blanc M. Les dangers de l'ergotisme a propos de deux observations. *Arch Med Ouest* (1977) 9, 265–6.

Esomeprazole + Miscellaneous drugs

There appear to be no adverse drug interaction reports involving esomeprazole, but the makers suggest that it may possibly reduce the serum levels and effects of ketoconazole and itraconazole, and possibly increase those of citalopram, clomipramine and imipramine. Diazepam and phenytoin serum levels are increased but the clinical relevance of this is doubtful. No clinically relevant interaction occurs with cisapride, quinidine or warfarin.

Clinical evidence, mechanism, importance and management

(a) Cisapride

A study in healthy subjects found that 40 mg esomeprazole increased the AUC of **cisapride** by 32% and prolonged the elimination half-life by 31%, but the maximum serum levels remained unaltered. No increase in the QTc interval was seen.[1] These pharmacokinetic changes are not large enough to be clinically relevant, and any fears about QTc interval prolongation are unfounded, so there would appear to be no reason for avoiding concurrent use.

(b) Drugs metabolised by cytochrome P450 isoenzyme CYP2C19

Esomeprazole inhibits cytochrome P450 isoenzyme CYP2C19 so that the plasma levels of drugs which are metabolised by this enzyme might be expected to be increased by concurrent use. This is true for **phenytoin** which the makers say showed a 13% increase in trough plasma levels in patients given 30 mg esomeprazole, and for **diazepam** which showed a 45% decrease in clearance in those given 40 mg esomeprazole.[1] The makers suggest that monitoring would be appropriate for both of these drugs, although it seems doubtful if the plasma level rises are likely to have much if any clinical relevance. The makers also list **citalopram**, **clomipramine**, and **imipramine** as other drugs which might similarly interact with esomeprazole because they are metabolised by CYP2C19, and they issue similar warnings about possible plasma level rises and dosage reductions.[1] However, there appear to be no reports about adverse interactions with any of these drugs.

(c) Itraconazole, Ketoconazole

Esomeprazole raises the gastric pH. One study showed that after taking doses of 20 or 40 mg for 5 days the gastric pH of patients remained above 4 for a mean time of 13 and 17 h respectively.[1] Because of this the makers suggest that this might reduce the absorption of some drugs such as **itraconazole** and **ketoconazole** which depend on a low pH for optimal dissolution and absorption.[1] This was certainly found to be true for **ketoconazole** when combined with another proton pump inhibitor, omeprazole. See 'Azole antifungals + Proton pump inhibitors', p.141. Whether **itraconazole** is likely to be similarly affected is not known. One practical solution would be to use **fluconazole** instead, which is known not to be affected by omeprazole and might be expected not to interact with esomeprazole. An alternative would simply be to monitor for any inadequate response to **ketoconazole** or **itraconazole**, and to raise their dosages if necessary.

(d) Miscellaneous drugs

The makers say that esomeprazole has been shown not to have any clinically relevant effects on the pharmacokinetics of **quinidine** or **warfarin**, but a few cases of raised INRs have been seen in practice, so monitoring is recommended if treatment with esomeprazole is started or stopped.[1] However, there would therefore appear to be no reason for avoiding concurrent use.

1. Nexium (Esomeprazole), AtraZeneca. Summary of Product Characteristics, June 2002.

Ethylene dibromide + Disulfiram

The very high incidence of malignant tumours in *rats* exposed to both ethylene dibromide and disulfiram is the basis of the

However, the interaction can be avoided by separating the administration of the two drugs by at least 2 h. More study is needed.

1. Forland SC, Feng Y, Cutler RE. Apparent reduced absorption of gemfibrozil when given with colestipol. *J Clin Pharmacol* (1990) 30, 29–32.
2. Forland SC, Feng Y, Cutler RE. The effect of colestipol on the oral absorption of gemfibrozil. *J Clin Pharmacol* (1988) 28, 931.
3. East C, Bilheimer DW, Grundy SM. Combination drug therapy for familial combined hyperlipidemia. *Ann Intern Med* (1988) 109, 25–32.

Gemfibrozil + Psyllium

Psyllium causes a small, almost certainly clinically unimportant, reduction in the absorption of gemfibrozil.

Clinical evidence, mechanism, importance and management

When 600 mg gemfibrozil was taken together with or 2 h after 3 g **psyllium** in 240 ml water, the AUC in 10 healthy subjects was reduced about 10%.[1] This change in bioavailability is almost certainly too small to matter. No special precautions would seem to be necessary.

1. Forland SC and Cutler RE. The effect of psyllium on the pharmacokinetics of gemfibrozil. *Clin Res* (1990) 38, 94A.

Gemfibrozil + Rifampicin (Rifampin)

Rifampicin (rifampin) 600 mg daily for 6 days was found not to significantly affect the pharmacokinetics of 600 mg gemfibrozil in 10 healthy subjects.[1] No special precautions seem necessary.

1. Forland SC, Feng Y, Cutler RE. The effect of rifampin on the pharmacokinetics of gemfibrozil. *J Clin Pharmacol* (1988) 28, 930.

Ginkgo + Miscellaneous drugs

An isolated report describes spontaneous bleeding from the iris associated with the concurrent use of aspirin and a *Ginkgo biloba* extract. Another isolated report describes intracerebral haemorrhage associated with the concurrent use of *Ginkgo biloba* and warfarin.

Clinical evidence, mechanism, importance and management

A man of 70 developed spontaneous bleeding from the iris into the anterior chamber of his eye within a week of starting to take a *Ginkoba* tablet twice daily. He experienced recurrent episodes of blurred vision in one eye lasting about 15 minutes, during which he could see a red discoloration through his cornea. Each *Ginkoba* tablet contained 40 mg of concentrated (50:1) extract of *Ginkgo biloba*. He was also taking 325 mg **aspirin** daily which had been taking uneventfully for 3 years since having coronary bypass surgery. He stopped taking the *Ginkoba* but continued with the **aspirin**, and 3 months later had experienced no recurrence of the bleeding.[1]

The reason for this bleeding is not known, but *Ginkgo biloba* extract contains ginkgolide B which is a potent inhibitor of platelet-activating factor, which is needed for arachidonate-independent platelet aggregation, and on its own has been associated with left and bilateral subdural haematomas,[2,3] a right parietal haematoma,[4] post-laparoscopic cholecystectomy bleeding,[5] and subarachnoid haemorrhage.[6] The authors of the report suggest that the use of **aspirin**, which is also an inhibitor of platelet aggregation, may have had an additional part to play in what happened.

Another report describes an intracerebral haemorrhage in an elderly woman within 2 months of starting *Ginkgo biloba*. Her prothrombin time was found to be 16.9 and her PTT 35.5. She had been on **warfarin** uneventfully for 5 years.[7] The author of the report speculated that both drugs may have contributed towards the haemorrhage, but what happened could have been due to the *Ginkgo biloba* alone and no interaction is established.

The evidence from these reports is far too slim to forbid patients taking **warfarin** or **aspirin** to avoid *Ginkgo biloba* but they should be told to seek informed professional advice if any bleeding problems arise.

1. Rosenblatt M, Mindel J. Spontaneous hyphema associated with ingestion of *Ginkgo biloba* extract. *N Engl J Med* (1997) 336, 1108.
2. Rowin J, Lewis SL. Spontaneous bilateral subdural hematomas associated with chronic *Ginkgo biloba* ingestion. *Neurology* (1996) 46, 1775–6.
3. Gilbert GJ. *Ginkgo biloba*. *Neurology* (1997) 48, 1137.
4. Benjamin J, Muir T, Briggs K, Pentland B. A case of cerebral haemorrhage – can *Ginkgo biloba* be implicated? *Postgrad Med J* (2001) 77, 112–13.
5. Fessenden JM, Wittenborn W, Clarke L. Gingko biloba: a case report of herbal medicine and bleeding postoperatively from a laparoscopic cholecystectomy. *Am Surg* (2001) 67, 33–5.
6. Vale S. Subarachnoid haemorrhage associated with *Ginkgo biloba*. *Lancet* (1998) 352, 36.
7. Matthews MK. Association of *Ginkgo biloba* with intracerebral hemorrhage. *Neurology* (1998) 50, 1933.

Glucagon + Beta-blockers

The hyperglycaemic effects of glucagon may be reduced by propranolol.

Clinical evidence, mechanism, importance and management

The hyperglycaemic activity of glucagon was reduced to some extent in the presence of **propranolol** in 5 healthy subjects.[1] The reason is uncertain, but one suggestion is that the **propranolol** inhibits the effects of the catecholamines that are released by glucagon. A similar response would be expected in patients under treatment with **propranolol** but its clinical importance is uncertain. Whether this is also true for other beta-blockers also awaits confirmation.

1. Messerli FH, Kuchel O, Tolis G, Hamet P, Frayasse J, Genest J. Effects of β-adrenergic blockage on plasma cyclic AMP and blood sugar responses to glucagon and isoproterenol in man. *Int J Clin Pharmacol Biopharm* (1976) 14, 189–94.

Glutethimide + Tobacco smoking

The effects of glutethimide appear to be greater in smokers than in non-smokers, but this seems to be of little clinical significance.

Clinical evidence, mechanism, importance and management

A study in 7 subjects found that glutethimide worsened the performance in the tracking test (one of a battery of tests used to assess psychomotor performance) in **smokers** more than in **non-smokers**, possibly due to an increase in its absorption.[1] However there would seem to be no need for particular caution if **smokers** take glutethimide.

1. Crow JW, Lain P, Bochner F, Shoeman DW, Azarnoff DL. Glutethimide and 4-OH glutethimide: pharmacokinetics and effect on performance in man. *Clin Pharmacol Ther* (1978) 22, 458–64.

Glyceryl trinitrate (GTN, nitroglycerin) + Anticholinergics

Drugs with anticholinergic effects, such as the tricyclic antidepressants and disopyramide, depress salivation and most patients complain of having a dry mouth. In theory sublin-

gual glyceryl trinitrate will dissolve less readily under the tongue in these patients, thereby reducing its absorption and its effects, however no formal studies seem to have been done to confirm that this actually happens. Table 9.2 contains a list of drugs which are anticholinergics.

Glyceryl trinitrate (GTN, nitroglycerin) + Aspirin

Some limited evidence suggests that analgesic doses of aspirin can increase the serum levels of glyceryl trinitrate, possibly resulting in an increase in its side-effects such as hypotension and headaches. Paradoxically, long-term aspirin use appears to reduce the effects of glyceryl trinitrate used for vasodilatation in patients following coronary artery by-pass surgery.

Clinical evidence

(a) Glyceryl trinitrate effects increased

When 800 micrograms glyceryl trinitrate was given to 7 healthy subjects as a sublingual spray an hour after taking 1 g **aspirin**, the mean plasma glyceryl trinitrate levels 30 min after administration were increased by 54% (from 0.24 to 0.37 nanograms/ml). The haemodynamic effects of the glyceryl trinitrate (heart rate, reduced diastolic blood pressure, end-diastolic diameter and end-systolic diameter) were enhanced. Some changes were seen when 500 mg **aspirin** was given every 2 days (described as an anti-aggregant dose) but the effects were not statistically significant.[1]

(b) Glyceryl trinitrate effects reduced

A study in patients following coronary artery by-pass surgery found that those who had been taking 150 or 300 mg **aspirin** daily (33 patients) for at least 3 months, needed more glyceryl trinitrate (to control blood pressure) during the recovery period than those who had not taken **aspirin** (also 33 patients). To achieve the blood pressure criteria required, the **aspirin**-group needed an infusion of 8.2 micrograms/min glyceryl trinitrate. The dose remained relatively high (3.3 micrograms/min) even after 8 h, whereas the non-aspirin group only needed 5.5 micrograms/min, which was reduced to 1.9 micrograms/min after 8 h.[2]

Mechanism

Not understood. Prostaglandin-synthetase inhibitors such as aspirin can suppress the vasodilator effects of glyceryl trinitrate to some extent by blocking prostaglandin release. However, it seems that a much greater pharmacodynamic interaction also occurs, in which aspirin reduces the flow of blood through the liver so that the metabolism of the glyceryl trinitrate is reduced, thus increasing its effects.

Importance and management

A confusing and unexplained situation. It seems possible that patients taking glyceryl trinitrate may experience an exaggeration of its side-effects such as hypotension and headaches if they are taking analgesic doses of aspirin. More study is needed to find out if this is of any practical importance. Also be aware that long-term aspirin use may reduce the vasodilatory effects glyceryl trinitrate. The antiplatelet (anti-aggregant) effects of aspirin and glyceryl trinitrate appear to be additive.[3]

1. Weber S, Rey E, Pipeau C, Lutfalla G, Richard M-O, Daoud-El-Assaf H, Olive G, Degeorges M. Influence of aspirin on the hemodynamic effects of sublingual nitroglycerin. *J Cardiovasc Pharmacol* (1983) 5, 874–7.
2. Key BJ, Keen M, Wilkes MP. Reduced responsiveness to nitro-vasodilators following prolonged low dose aspirin administration in man. *Br J Clin Pharmacol* (1992) 34, 453P–454P.
3. Karlberg K-E, Ahlner J, Henriksson P, Torfgård K, Sylvén C. Effects of nitroglycerin on platelet aggregation beyond the effects of acetylsalicylic acid in healthy subjects. *Am J Cardiol* (1993) 71, 361–4.

Glyceryl trinitrate (GTN, nitroglycerin) + Nifedipine

Nifedipine 20 mg twice daily can reduce the effectiveness of glyceryl trinitrate in patients undergoing coronary artery by-pass surgery.

Clinical evidence

A comparative study of 3 groups of patients undergoing coronary by-pass graft surgery found that those given 20 mg **nifedipine** twice daily needed significantly larger doses of glyceryl trinitrate (to reduce cardiac workload, maintain graft patency and control blood pressure) than two other groups, one of them taking 10 mg **nifedipine** twice daily, and the other taking a placebo. Those taking 20 mg **nifedipine** twice daily needed an initial infusion of 9.2 mg h^{-1} whereas the other two groups needed only 6.9 and 6.3 mg h^{-1} respectively. At 8 h the infusion rates were 3.3, 1.7 and 1.6 mg h^{-1} respectively. Moreover these higher doses had little effect on the initial mean systolic blood pressure of half of the group taking 20 mg **nifedipine** twice daily, and they needed an additional infusion of nitroprusside.[1]

Mechanism

Not understood. The glyceryl trinitrate is converted to nitric oxide (NO) to elicit its vasodilator effect, and it is possible that the nifedipine affects (inhibits) the enzymic production of the NO.

Importance and management

Information is limited but the interaction appears to be established. Anticipate the need to use increased amounts of glyceryl trinitrate in patients taking 20 mg nifedipine twice daily in the situation described. Note that the smaller dose (10 mg twice daily) did not interact significantly. Whether nifedipine can reduce the effects of glyceryl trinitrate when both drugs are taken orally for the relief of angina awaits assessment.

1. Key BJ, Wilkes MP, Keen M. Reduced responsiveness to glyceryl trinitrate following antihypertensive treatment with nifedipine in man. *Br J Clin Pharmacol* (1993) 36, 499P.

H$_2$-blockers + Antacids

The absorption of cimetidine, famotidine, nizatidine and ranitidine may possibly be reduced to some extent by antacids but it seems doubtful if this significantly reduces their ulcer-healing effects. Separating the dosages by 1 to 2 h minimises any interaction. Roxatidine appears not to be affected.

Clinical evidence

(a) Cimetidine

When 12 healthy subjects were given 300 mg **cimetidine** orally four times a day, with and without 30 ml *Mylanta II* (**aluminium/magnesium hydroxide** mixture), the absorption of **cimetidine** was unaffected.[1] No interaction was found in other studies using **aluminium phosphate**[2-4] or **aluminium/magnesium hydroxide**[5] antacids.

In contrast, a number of single dose studies indicated that antacids reduce the absorption of **cimetidine**. The AUCs of 200- to 800-mg doses of cimetidine were reduced by an average of 19 to 34% by 10 to 45 ml doses of a variety of **aluminium/magnesium** containing antacids.[6-11] When the antacids were given 1 to 3 h after **cimetidine** 'marginal' or insignificant reductions occurred in the AUCs.[7,12,13]

(b) Famotidine

Mylanta II 30 ml reduced the AUC and peak serum levels of **famotidine** by about a third when taken simultaneously, but no significant interaction occurred when the antacid was taken 2 h after **famotidine**.[14] Another study found that the peak serum levels of **famotidine** were reduced by about 25% by *Mylanta II* in 17 healthy subjects.[15]

In contrast, *Mylanta Double Strength* was found to reduce the absorption of **famotidine** by 19%, a difference that was considered unimportant.[11] Two chewable tablets of *Mylanta II* were found to have no effect on the pharmacokinetics or pharmacodynamics of 10 or 20 mg **famotidine** in 18 healthy subjects.[16]

(c) Nizatidine

Mylanta Double Strength reduced the absorption of **nizatidine** by 12%, which was considered clinically insignificant.[11]

(d) Ranitidine

Mylanta II 30 ml reduced the peak **ranitidine** serum levels and the AUC after a single 150-mg dose by about one-third in 6 healthy subjects.[17] *Mylanta Double Strength* reduced the absorption of **ranitidine** by 26%, which was not thought to be clinically significant.[11] Reductions of up to 59% were found in another study.[9,10] Another study showed that **aluminium phosphate** reduced the bioavailability of **ranitidine** by 30%.[4]

(e) Roxatidine

In an open-label crossover study, 24 healthy subjects were given **roxatidine** 150 mg with 10 ml *Maalox* four times daily. The pharmacokinetics of **roxatidine** were unchanged, apart from a clinically insignificant lengthening of the half-life.[18]

Mechanism

Not fully understood. Changes in gastric pH caused by the antacid, and retarded gastric motility have been suggested as potential mechanisms.

Importance and management

A reduction in the bioavailability of cimetidine, famotidine, nizatidine and ranitidine can occur with some antacids, but none of these interactions is well established, and evidence that the ulcer-healing effects are reduced seems to be lacking. It may not prove necessary to take any special precautions, however until this is confirmed it might be prudent to follow the general recommendation that antacids should be given 1 to 2 h before or after the H$_2$-blocker if fasting, or 1 h after if the blocker is taken with food. If these precautions are followed no significant reduction in absorption should occur.[7,14,15,19] Preliminary evidence suggests that roxatidine is unaffected.

1. Shelly DW, Doering PL, Russell WL, Guild RT, Lopez LM, Perrin J. Effect of concomitant antacid administration on plasma cimetidine concentrations during repetitive dosing. *Drug Intell Clin Pharm* (1986) 20, 792–5.
2. Albin H, Vinçon G, Pehoucq F, Dangoumau J. Influence d'un antacide sur la biodisponibilité de la cimétidine. *Therapie* (1982) 37, 563–6.
3. Albin H, Vinçon G, Demotes-Mainard F, Begaud B, Bedjaoui A. Effect of aluminium phosphate on the bioavailability of cimetidine and prednisolone. *Eur J Clin Pharmacol* (1984) 26, 271–3.
4. Albin H, Vinçon G, Begaud B, Bistue C, Perez P. Effect of aluminum phosphate on the bioavailability of ranitidine. *Eur J Clin Pharmacol* (1987) 32, 97–99.
5. Burland WL, Darkin DW, Mills MW. Effect of antacids on absorption of cimetidine. *Lancet* (1976) ii, 965.
6. Bodemar G, Norlander B, Walan A. Diminished absorption of cimetidine caused by antacids. *Lancet* (1979) i, 444–5.
7. Steinberg WM, Lewis JH, Katz DM. Antacids inhibit absorption of cimetidine. *N Engl J Med* (1982) 307, 400–4.
8. Gugler R, Brand M, Somogyi A. Impaired cimetidine absorption due to antacids and metoclopramide. *Eur J Clin Pharmacol* (1981) 20, 225–8.
9. Desmond PV, Harman PJ, Gannoulis N, Kamm M, Mashford ML. The effect of antacids and food on the absorption of cimetidine and ranitidine. *Gastroenterology* (1986) 90, 1393.
10. Desmond PV, Harman PJ, Gannoulis N, Kamm M, Mashford ML. The effect of an antacid and food on the absorption of cimetidine and ranitidine. *J Pharm Pharmacol* (1990) 42, 352–4.
11. Sullivan TJ, Reese JH, Jauregui L, Miller K, Levine L, Bachmann KA. Short report: a comparative study of the interaction between antacid and H$_2$-receptor antagonists. *Aliment Pharmacol Ther* (1994) 8, 123–6.
12. Russell WL, Lopez LM, Normann SA, Doering PL, Guild RT. Effect of antacids on predicted steady-state cimetidine concentrations. *Dig Dis Sci* (1984) 29, 385–9.
13. Barzaghi N, Crema F, Mescoli G, Perucca E. Effects on cimetidine bioavailability of metoclopramide and antacids given two hours apart. *Eur J Clin Pharmacol* (1989) 37, 409–10.
14. Barzaghi N, Gatti G, Crema F, Perucca E. Impaired bioavailability of famotidine given concurrently with a potent antacid. *J Clin Pharmacol* (1989) 29, 670–2.
15. Tupy-Visich MA, Tarzian SK, Schwartz S, Lin JH, Hessey GA, Kanovsky SM, Chremos AN. Bioavailability of oral famotidine when administered with antacid or food. *J Clin Pharmacol* (1986) 26, 555.
16. Schwartz JI, Yeh KC, Bolognese J, Laskin OL, Patterson PM, Shamblen EC, Han R, Lasseter KC. Lack of effect of chewable antacid on famotidine pharmacodynamics and pharmacokinetics. *Pharmacotherapy* (1994) 14, 375.
17. Mihaly GW, Marino AT, Webster LK, Jones DB, Louis WJ, Smallwood RA. High dose of antacid (Mylanta II) reduces the bioavailability of ranitidine. *BMJ* (1982) 285, 998–9.
18. Labs RA. Interaction of roxatidine acetate with antacids, food and other drugs. *Drugs* (1988) 35 (Suppl 3), 82–9.
19. Frislid K, Berstad A. High dose of antacid reduces bioavailability of ranitidine. *BMJ* (1983) 286, 1358.

H$_2$-blockers + Sucralfate

Sucralfate normally appears not to affect the bioavailability of cimetidine, ranitidine or roxatidine, or only to reduce it moderately. There is some evidence that the healing rate may possibly be increased.

Clinical evidence, mechanism, importance and management

Most *in vitro* and human studies show that **sucralfate** does not affect the absorption of either **cimetidine**, **ranitidine**,[1-4] or **roxatidine**,[5] but two studies found 22 to 29% reductions in **ranitidine** bioavailability due to concurrent use of **sucralfate**.[6,7] There is no clear reason for avoiding concurrent use, and there is some indication that it may possibly be valuable as there is some evidence of a possible trend towards more rapid healing of duodenal ulcers if **sucralfate** and **cimetidine** are given together.[8] More confirmatory study of this is needed.

1. Mullersman G, Gotz VP, Russell WL, Derendorf H. Lack of clinically significant in vitro and in vivo interactions between ranitidine and sucralfate. *J Pharm Sci* (1986) 75, 995–8.
2. Albin H, Vincon G, Lalague MC, Couzigou P, Amouretti M. Effect of sucralfate on the bioavailability of cimetidine. *Eur J Clin Pharmacol* (1986) 30, 493–4.
3. D'Angio R, Mayersohn M, Conrad KA, Bliss M. Cimetidine absorption in humans during sucralfate coadministration. *Br J Clin Pharmacol* (1986) 21, 515–20.
4. Beck CL, Dietz AJ, Carlson JD, Letendre PW. Evaluation of potential cimetidine sucralfate interaction. *Clin Pharmacol Ther* (1987) 41, 168.
5. Seibert-Grafe M, Pidgen A. Lack of effect of multiple dose sucralfate on the pharmacokinetics of roxatidine acetate. *Eur J Clin Pharmacol* (1991) 40, 637–8.
6. Maconochie JG, Thomas M, Michael MF, Jenner WR, Tanner RJN. Ranitidine sucralfate interaction study. *Clin Pharmacol Ther* (1987) 41, 205.
7. Kimura K, Sakai H, Yoshida Y, Kasano T, Hirose M. Effects of concomitant drugs on the blood concentration of a histamine H$_2$ antagonist (the 2nd report) - concomitant or time lag administration of ranitidine and sucralfate. *Nippon Shokakibyo Gakkai Zasshi* (1986) 83, 603–7.
8. Van Deventer G, Schneidman D, Olson C, Walsh J. Comparison of sucralfate and cimetidine taken alone and in combination for treatment of active duodenal ulcer (DU). *Gastroenterology* (1984) 86, 1287.

H$_2$-blockers + Tobacco smoking

Duodenal ulcers treated with H$_2$-blockers heal less easily in smokers and are more likely to recur when treatment is over if smoking continues. Cimetidine, and to a lesser extent ranitidine, reduce the clearance of nicotine from the body, and smoking reduces the plasma levels of cimetidine and ranitidine.

Clinical evidence, mechanism, importance and management

The healing of duodenal ulcers in patients on H$_2$-blockers such as **cimetidine** and **ranitidine** is slower, and recurrence is more common in smokers than in non-smokers.[1-3] One of the possible reasons is that **smoking** reduces the plasma levels of these drugs after peak levels are achieved, although peak levels occur sooner and are higher.[4] **Cimetidine** 600 mg twice daily for a day, prior to giving **nicotine**, reduced the clearance of **nicotine** (1 microgram/kg/min given intravenously for 30 min) in 6 healthy subjects by 27 to 30%. **Ranitidine** 300 mg twice daily, for a day prior to **nicotine** reduced the clearance of **nicotine** by about 7 to 10%.[5]

Patients with ulcers should be encouraged to stop smoking, but if persuasion fails, the use of an H$_2$-blocker (**cimetidine** in particular) might possibly help them to reduce or give up smoking because it maintains **nicotine** levels with less **tobacco**.[5] There seems to be nothing documented about other H_2-blockers (**famotidine, nizatidine,** etc.) and **nicotine**.

1. Korman MG, Hansky J, Eaves ER, Schmidt GT. Cigarette smoking and the healing of duodenal ulcer. *Gastroenterology* (1982) 82, 1104.
2. Korman MG, Hetzel DJ, Hansky J, Shearman DJC, Eaves ER, Schmidt GT, Hecker R, Fitch R. Oxmetidine or cimetidine in duodenal ulcer: healing rate and effect of smoking. *Gastroenterology* (1982) 82, 1104.
3. Boyd EJS, Wilson JA, Wormsley KG. Smoking impairs therapeutic gastric inhibition. *Lancet* (1983) i, 95–7.
4. Boyd EJS, Johnston DA, Wormsley KG, Jenner WN, Salanson X. The effects of cigarette smoking on plasma concentrations of gastric antisecretory drugs. *Aliment Pharmacol Ther* (1987) 1, 57–65.
5. Bendayan R, Sullivan JT, Shaw C, Frecker RC, Sellers EM. Effect of cimetidine and ranitidine on the hepatic and renal elimination of nicotine in humans. *Eur J Clin Pharmacol* (1990) 38, 165–9.

5-HT$_1$ agonists (Triptans) + Selective serotonin re-uptake inhibitors (SSRIs)

The SSRIs normally appear not to interact with the triptans, but there are a few rare cases of dyskinesias and there is some evidence to suggest that the serotonin syndrome may occasionally develop.

Clinical evidence

(a) Almotriptan

Fluoxetine 60 mg daily was given to 14 healthy subjects for 8 days, with a single 12.5-mg dose of almotriptan on day 8. **Fluoxetine** raised the maximum plasma levels of almotriptan by about 18%, but the combination was well tolerated and caused no ECG changes, so no dose alterations were considered necessary by the authors.[1]

(b) Rizatriptan

A single 10-mg dose of rizatriptan was given to 12 healthy subjects after taking 20 mg **paroxetine** or a placebo daily for 14 days. The plasma levels of the rizatriptan and its active metabolite were not altered by the **paroxetine**, and no adverse effects were seen. Safety evaluations included blood pressure, heart rate, temperature and a visual analogue assessment of mood. There was no evidence of the serotonin syndrome.[2]

(c) Sumatriptan

A study in 11 healthy subjects found that 16 days' treatment with 20 mg **paroxetine** daily had no effect on the response to 6 mg subcutaneous sumatriptan, as measured by prolactin levels. The sumatriptan levels remained unaltered, its cardiovascular effects were unchanged and no clinically significant adverse effects occurred.[3] Other studies report that the concurrent use of sumatriptan and **SSRIs** (**fluoxetine** 20 to 60 mg daily, **fluvoxamine** 200 mg daily, **paroxetine** 20 to 50 mg daily, **ruvoxamine** 100 mg daily, **sertraline** 50 to 100 mg daily) was successful and uneventful.[4,5] No adverse effects have been noted in 148 other patients.[6]

However, post-marketing surveillance of the voluntary reports received in Canada by the makers of **fluoxetine**, identified 2 cases that showed good evidence, and another 4 cases that showed some, but not strong evidence of reactions consistent with the serotonin syndrome.[7] Other cases describe a decrease in the efficacy of sumatriptan with **fluoxetine**,[8] dyskinesias and dystonias with sumatriptan and **paroxetine**,[9] and 20 possible cases of the serotonin syndrome with sumatriptan and **SSRIs**.[6,10]

The makers of sumatriptan also say that they have rare post-marketing reports of weakness, hyper-reflexia and inco-ordination following the use of sumatriptan and **SSRIs**.[11]

(d) Zolmitriptan

A two-period crossover, double-blind study in 20 subjects given 20 mg **fluoxetine** or a placebo daily for 28 days, with the addition of 10 mg zolmitriptan on day 28, found that the pharmacokinetics of the zolmitriptan were unaffected by the **fluoxetine** and only very slight changes were seen on its active metabolite.[12]

Mechanism

Not understood. The 5-HT$_1$ agonists might possibly add to the increased levels of 5-HT at post-synaptic receptors caused by SSRIs (in theory at least), but in practice it is questionable whether this is normally clinically relevant.

Importance and management

The weight of evidence suggests that the concurrent use of the triptans and SSRIs is normally uneventful but adverse reactions do occur occasionally. The authors of some of the references above concluded that their findings do not imply that concurrent use should be avoided but that caution and close monitoring should be used.[6,7]

1. Fleishaker JC, Ryan KK, Carel BJ, Azie NE. Evaluation of the potential pharmacokinetic interaction between almotriptan and fluoxetine in healthy volunteers. *J Clin Pharmacol* (2001) 41, 217–23.
2. Goldberg MR, Lowry RC, Musson DG, Birk KL, Fisher A, DePuy ME, Shadle CR. Lack of pharmacokinetic and pharmacodynamic interaction between rizatriptan and paroxetine. *J Clin Pharmacol* (1999) 39, 192–9.
3. Wing Y-K, Clifford EM, Sheehan BD, Campling GM, Hockney RA, Cowen PJ. Paroxetine treatment and the prolactin response to sumatriptan. *Psychopharmacology (Berl)* (1996) 124, 377–9.
4. Blier P, Bergeron R. The safety of concomitant use of sumatriptan and antidepressant treatments. *J Clin Psychopharmacol* (1995) 15, 106–9.
5. Leung M. Lack of an interaction between sumatriptan and selective serotonin reuptake inhibitors. *Headache* (1995) 35, 488–9.
6. Gardner DM, Lynd LD. Sumatriptan contraindications and the serotonin syndrome. *Ann Pharmacother* (1998) 32, 33–8.
7. Joffe RT, Sokolov STH. Co-administration of fluoxetine and sumatriptan: the Canadian experience. *Acta Psychiatr Scand* (1997) 95, 551–2.
8. Szabo CP. Fluoxetine and sumatriptan: possibly a counterproductive combination. *J Clin Psychiatry* (1995) 56, 37–8.
9. Abraham JT, Brown R, Meltzer HY. Clozapine treatment of persistent paroxysmal dyskinesia associated with concomitant paroxetine and sumatriptan use. *Biol Psychiatry* (1997) 42, 144–6.
10. Mathew NT. Serotonin syndrome complicating migraine pharmacotherapy. *Cephalagia* (1996) 16, 323–7.
11. GlaxoWellcome. Personal communication, August 1997.
12. Smith DA, Cleary EW, Watkins S, Huffman CS, Polvino WJ. Zolmitriptan (311C90) does not interact with fluoxetine in healthy volunteers. *Int J Clin Pharmacol Ther* (1998) 36, 301–5.

Ifetroban + Miscellaneous drugs

No adverse interaction appears to occur between ifetroban and either heparin, *Mylanta*, ranitidine or warfarin.

Clinical evidence, mechanism, importance and management

(a) Antacids, H$_2$-blockers

A study in 18 healthy subjects to investigate the possible effects of changes in gastric pH on the pharmacokinetics of ifetroban, found that when given a single 250-mg dose of ifetroban while taking either 150 mg **ranitidine** twice daily or 30 ml *Mylanta* (**aluminium and magnesium hydroxide, simeticone**) four times daily for 5 days, no important clinical differences were seen.[1] There would appear to be no reason for avoiding concurrent use.

(b) Heparin

Heparin was administered to 37 healthy subjects to reach a stable aPTT of 1.5 times the baseline, to which 250 mg ifetroban was added, for about 5 days. The heparin was then stopped but the ifetroban continued for a further 5 days. The pharmacokinetics of the ifetroban were not changed by the **heparin** nor was the ifetroban-induced increase in the bleeding time altered by the **heparin**. Some adverse side-effects were seen but these were attributed to the use of the **heparin**.[2] On the basis of this study there would seem to be no reason for avoiding concurrent use.

(c) Warfarin

Eighteen patients with deep vein thrombosis taking **warfarin** and with INRs within the range 2 to 3, were additionally given ifetroban (dose not stated) or a placebo for 6 days. It was found that INRs were not significantly altered by the ifetroban, and no important changes in bleeding times occurred.[3] No special precautions would seem to be needed during concurrent use.

1. Beierle FA, Delaney C, Uderman H, Bourgeois ML, Jemal M, Liao WC. The effect of altered gastric acidity induced by Mylanta or ranitidine on ifetroban pharmacokinetics in healthy volunteers. *J Clin Pharmacol* (1996) 36, 854.
2. Liao W, Delaney C, Jemal M, Norton J, Uderman H, Ford N. The pharmacokinetic and pharmacodynamic (PK/PD) interaction of ifetroban, a TXA₂ receptor antagonist, and heparin. *Clin Pharmacol Ther* (1996) 59, 150.
3. Delaney C, Norton J, Briand R, Lajoie V, Beierle F, Campbell A, Whitsett T, VanNguyen P, Anderson D, Liao W. The pharmacodynamic (PD) interaction of ifetroban (IFET), a thromboxane A₂ (TXA₂) antagonist, and warfarin (W) in patients with venous thrombosis. *J Clin Pharmacol* (1996) 36, 854.

Ipratropium bromide + Salbutamol (Albuterol)

Acute angle-closure glaucoma developed rapidly in 8 patients given nebulised ipratropium and salbutamol. Increased intra-ocular pressure has been reported in others. No interaction has been seen when the drugs are given by inhaler.

Clinical evidence, mechanism, importance and management

Five patients with an acute exacerbation of chronic obstructive airways disease, given nebulised ipratropium and **salbutamol (albuterol)**, developed acute angle closure glaucoma, four of them within 1 to 36 h of starting treatment. Two of the patients had a history of angle-closure glaucoma prior to admission.[1] Three other similar cases of acute angle-closure glaucoma due to concurrent use are reported elsewhere.[2,3] An increase in intra-ocular pressure has also been reported in other patients given both drugs by nebuliser.[4]

Mechanism

The reason appears to be that the anticholinergic action of the ipratropium causes semi-dilatation of the pupil, partially blocking the flow of aqueous humour from the posterior to the anterior chamber, thereby bowing the iris anteriorly and obstructing the drainage angle. The salbutamol increases the production of aqueous humour and makes things worse. Additional factors are that higher doses of both drugs are achieved by using a nebuliser, and that some drug may escape round the edge of the mask and have a direct action on the eye.[1]

Importance and management

An established but uncommon interaction, which appears to occur mainly in patients already predisposed to angle-closure glaucoma. The authors of the first report[1] advise care in the placing of the mask to avoid the escape of droplets (the use of goggles and continuing the application of any glaucoma treatment is also effective[4]) and, if possible, the avoidance of their concurrent use by nebuliser in patients predisposed to angle-closure glaucoma. They point out that no cases of glaucoma have been reported with either drug given by inhaler.[1]

1. Shah P, Dhurjon L, Metcalfe T, Gibson JM. Acute angle closure glaucoma associated with nebulised ipratropium bromide and salbutamol. *BMJ* (1992) 304, 40–1.
2. Packe GE, Cayton RM, Mashoudi N. Nebulised ipratropium bromide and salbutamol causing closed-angle glaucoma. *Lancet* (1984) ii, 691.
3. Reuser T, Flanagan DW, Borland C, Bannerjee DK. Acute angle closure glaucoma occurring after nebulized bronchodilator treatment with ipratropium bromide and salbutamol. *J R Soc Med* (1992) 85, 499–500.
4. Kalra L, Bone M. The effect of nebulized bronchodilator therapy on intraocular pressures in patients with glaucoma. *Chest* (1988) 93, 739–41.

Iron preparations + Antacids

The absorption of iron and the expected haematological response can be reduced by the concurrent use of antacids. Separate their administration as much as possible.

Clinical evidence

(a) Aluminium and magnesium hydroxides, sodium bicarbonate and calcium carbonate

A study in 22 healthy subjects who were mildly iron-deficient (due to blood donation or menstruation) found that one teaspoonful of *Mylanta II* had little effect on the absorption at 2 h of 10 or 20 mg **ferrous sulphate**. However, 1 g **sodium bicarbonate** almost halved the absorption of **ferrous sulphate** and 500 mg **calcium carbonate** reduced it by two-thirds. **Iron** absorption from a **multivitamin-mineral** preparation was little affected by **calcium carbonate**.[1] Another study found that an antacid containing **aluminium and magnesium hydroxides** and **magnesium carbonate** reduced the absorption of **ferrous sulphate** and **ferrous fumarate** (both containing 100 mg ferrous iron) in healthy iron-replete subjects by 37% and 31% respectively.[2] Poor absorption of **iron** during treatment with **sodium bicarbonate** and **aluminium hydroxide** has been described elsewhere.[3,4] One study did not find that the absorption of **ferrous sulphate** (iron 10 mg/kg) was affected by doses of **magnesium hydroxide** (5 mg for every 1 mg of **iron**) when given 30 min apart.[5] However, it has been suggested that **iron** absorption was not measured for of a sufficient period to fully rule out a reduction in absorption.[6]

(b) Magnesium trisilicate

When oral **iron** failed to cause an expected rise in haemoglobin levels, a study was undertaken in 9 patients who were given 5 mg of isotopically labelled **ferrous sulphate**. **Magnesium trisilicate** 35 g reduced the absorption from an average of 30 to 12%, the reduction being small in some patients, but one individual showed a fall from 67 to 5%.[7]

Mechanism

Uncertain. One suggestion is that magnesium trisilicate changes ferrous sulphate into less easily absorbed salts, or increases its polymerisation.[7] Carbonates possibly cause the formation of poorly soluble iron complexes.[3] Aluminium hydroxide is believed to precipitate iron as the hydroxide and ferric ions can become intercalated into the aluminium hydroxide crystal lattice.[8]

Importance and management

Information is limited and difficult to assess because of the many variables (different dosages from very small to those mimicking overdose, a mix of subjects and patients). However, a 'blanket precaution' to achieve maximal absorption would be to separate the administration of iron preparations and antacids as much as possible to avoid admixture in the gut. This may prove not to be necessary with some preparations.

1. O'Neil-Cutting MA, Crosby WH. The effect of antacids on the absorption of simultaneously ingested iron. *JAMA* (1986) 255, 1468–70.
2. Ekenved G, Halvorsen L, Sölvell L. Influence of a liquid antacid on the absorption of different iron salts. *Scand J Haematol* (1976) 28 (Suppl), 65–77.
3. Benjamin BI, Cortell S, Conrad ME. Bicarbonate-induced iron complexes and iron absorption: one effect of pancreatic secretions. *Gastroenterology* (1967) 35, 389–96.
4. Rastogi SP, Padilla F, Boyd CM. Effect of aluminum hydroxide on iron absorption. *J Arkansas Med Soc* (1976) 73, 133–4.
5. Snyder BK, Clark RF. Effect of magnesium hydroxide administration on iron absorption after a supratherapeutic dose of ferrous sulfate in human volunteers: a randomized controlled trial. *Ann Emerg Med* (1999) 33, 400–405.
6. Wallace KL, Curry SC, LoVecchio F, Raschke RA. Effect of magnesium hydroxide on iron absorption after ferrous sulfate. *Ann Emerg Med* (1999) 34, 685–6.
7. Hall GJL, Davis AE. Inhibition of iron absorption by magnesium trisilicate. *Med J Aust* (1969) 2, 95–6.
8. Coste JF, De Bari VA, Keil LB, Needle MA. *In-vitro* interactions of oral hematinics and antacid suspensions. *Curr Ther Res* (1977) 22, 205–15.

Iron preparations or Vitamin B₁₂ + Chloramphenicol

In addition to the serious and potentially fatal bone marrow depression which can occur with chloramphenicol, it may also cause a milder, reversible bone marrow depression,

which can oppose the treatment of anaemia with iron or vitamin B_{12}.

Clinical evidence

Ten out of 22 patients on **iron-dextran** for iron-deficiency anaemia and also given **chloramphenicol**, failed to show the expected haematological response.[1] Four patients on **vitamin B_{12}** for pernicious anaemia were all similarly refractory to treatment until the **chloramphenicol** was withdrawn.[1]

Mechanism

Chloramphenicol can cause two forms of bone marrow depression. One is serious and irreversible and can result in fatal aplastic anaemia, whereas the other is probably unrelated, milder and reversible, and appears to occur at serum levels of 25 micrograms/ml or more. The reason is that chloramphenicol can inhibit protein synthesis, the first sign of which is a fall in the reticulocyte count which reflects inadequate red cell maturation. This response to chloramphenicol has been seen in *animals*,[2] healthy individuals,[3] a series of patients with liver disease,[4] and in anaemic patients[1] being treated with iron-dextran or vitamin B_{12}.

Importance and management

An established interaction of clinical importance. The authors of one study recommend that chloramphenicol dosages of 25 to 30 mg/kg are usually adequate for treating infections without running the risk of elevating serum levels to 25 micrograms/ml or more when marrow depression occurs.[5] Monitor the effects of using iron or B_{12} concurrently. A preferable alternative would be to use an alternative antibacterial. It has been claimed[6] that the optic neuritis which sometimes occurs with chloramphenicol can be reversed with large doses of vitamins B_6 and B_{12}.

1. Saidi P, Wallerstein RO, Aggeler PM. Effect of chloramphenicol on erythropoiesis. *J Lab Clin Med* (1961) 57, 247–56.
2. Rigdon RH, Crass G, Martin N. Anemia produced by chloramphenicol (chloromycetin) in the duck. *AMA Arch Pathol* (1954) 58, 85–93.
3. Jiji RM, Gangarosa EJ, de la Macorra F. Chloramphenicol and its sulfamoyl analogue. Report of reversible erythropoietic toxicity in healthy volunteers. *Arch Intern Med* (1963) 111, 116–28.
4. McCurdy PR. Chloramphenicol bone marrow toxicity. *JAMA* (1961) 176, 588–93.
5. Scott JL, Finegold SM, Belkin GA, Lawrence JS. A controlled double-blind study of the hematologic toxicity of chloramphenicol. *N Engl J Med* (1965) 272, 1137–42.
6. Cocke JC. Chloramphenicol optic neuritis. *Am J Dis Child* (1967) 114, 424–6.

Iron preparations + Colestyramine

Colestyramine binds with ferrous sulphate in the gut thereby reducing its absorption, but the clinical importance of this is uncertain.

Clinical evidence, mechanism, importance and management

Studies have shown that **colestyramine** binds with **iron** (as it does with many other drugs), and in *rats* this was found to halve the absorption from the gut of a single 100-microgram dose of **ferrous sulphate**.[1] Nobody seems to have checked on the general clinical importance of this in patients. Until more is known it would seem prudent to separate the dosages of the **iron** and **colestyramine** to avoid mixing in the gut, thereby minimising the effects of this possible interaction.

1. Thomas FB, McCullough F, Greenberger NJ. Inhibition of the intestinal absorption of inorganic and hemoglobin iron by cholestyramine. *J Lab Clin Med* (1971) 78, 70-80.

Iron preparations + Coffee or Tea

Coffee may possibly contribute towards the development of iron-deficiency anaemia in pregnant women and reduce the levels of iron in breast milk. As a result their babies may also be iron-deficient. Tea may also possibly be associated with microcytic anaemia in children.

Clinical evidence

A controlled study among pregnant low-income women in Costa Rica found that **coffee** consumption was associated with reductions in the haemoglobin levels and haematocrits of the mothers during pregnancy, and of their babies shortly after birth, despite the fact that the women were said to have been taking 60 mg of elemental **iron** (as 200 mg **ferric sulphate** [*sic*]) and 500 micrograms of **folate** daily. The babies also had a slightly lower birth weight (3189 g vs 3310 g). Almost a quarter of the mothers were considered as having iron-deficiency anaemia (haemoglobin levels of <11 g/dl) compared with none among the control group of non-coffee drinkers. Levels of **iron** in breast milk were reduced about one third. The **coffee** drinkers drank more than 450 ml of **coffee** daily, equivalent to more than 10 g **ground coffee**.[1]

A much higher incidence of microcytic anaemia has been described in **tea**-drinking infants in Israel.[2] Another report describes no change in the absorption of **iron** in daily doses of 2 to 15.8 mg/kg in 10 iron-deficient **tea**-drinking children, although the children were only given 150 ml of tea.[3]

Mechanism

Tannins are thought to form insoluble complexes with iron and thus reduce its absorption.[2,3]

Importance and management

The general importance of these findings is uncertain, but it highlights the need to keep a check on the haemoglobin levels and red cell counts of pregnant and lactating women who drink substantial amounts of coffee, and of their babies while being breast fed, even though iron supplements may be given. A similar check is needed in children who drink substantial amounts of tea. More study is needed.

1. Muñoz LM, Lönnerdal B, Keen CL, Dewey KG. Coffee consumption as a factor in iron deficiency anemia among pregnant women and their infants in Costa Rica. *Am J Clin Nutr* (1988) 48, 645–51.
2. Merhav H, Amitai Y, Palti H, Godfrey S. Tea drinking and microcytic anemia in infants. *Am J Clin Nutr* (1985) 41, 1210–13.
3. Koren G, Boichis H, Keren G. Effects of tea on the absorption of pharmacological doses of an oral iron preparation. *Isr J Med Sci* (1982) 18, 547.

Iron preparations + H$_2$-blockers

Apart from a brief and unconfirmed report alleging that cimetidine reduced the response to ferrous sulphate in 3 patients, there appears to be no other evidence that H$_2$-blockers reduce the absorption of iron to a clinically relevant extent. Iron causes only a small and clinically irrelevant reduction in the serum levels of cimetidine and famotidine.

Clinical evidence, mechanism, importance and management

(a) Effect on iron

A brief report describes 3 patients taking 1 g **cimetidine** and 600 mg **ferrous sulphate** daily whose ulcers healed after 2 months, but their anaemia and altered iron metabolism persisted. When the **cimetidine** was reduced to 400 mg daily but with the same dose of **iron**, the blood picture resolved satisfactorily within a month.[1] The author of the report attributed this response to the **cimetidine**-induced rise in gastric pH which reduced the absorption of the **iron**. However, this suggested mechanism was subsequently disputed as medicinal **iron** is already in the most absorbable form, Fe^{2+}, and so does not need an acidic environment to aid absorption.[2] A study in patients with iron deficiency, or iron deficiency anaemia found that the concurrent use of **famotidine**, **nizatidine** or **ranitidine**, did not affect their response to 2400 mg **iron succinyl-protein complex** (equivalent to 60 mg **iron** twice daily).[3] No special precautions would seem necessary.

(b) Effect on H₂-blockers

In a series of 3 experiments, healthy subjects were given a 300 mg tablet of **cimetidine** with either a 300 mg tablet of **ferrous sulphate** or 300 mg **ferrous sulphate** in solution. The reductions in the AUC and the maximum serum levels of the **cimetidine** were small (less than 16%). In the third experiment they were given 40 mg **famotidine** with a 300 mg tablet of **ferrous sulphate**. Again, the AUC and maximum serum level reductions were also very small, 10% or less. These small reductions are almost certainly due to the formation of a weak complex between the **iron** and these H₂-blockers.[4] Another study found no significant interaction between **famotidine** and **ferrous sulphate** in 6 healthy subjects.[5] An *in vitro* study with **ranitidine** found that while it also binds with **iron**, it is very weak and less than that seen with **cimetidine** or **famotidine**.[4] It was concluded that no clinically relevant interaction occurs between **ferrous sulphate** and any of these H₂-blockers.[4]

1. Esposito R. Cimetidine and iron-deficiency anaemia. *Lancet* (1977) ii, 1132.
2. Rosner F. Cimetidine and iron absorption. *Lancet* (1978) i, 95.
3. Bianchi FM, Cavassini GB, Leo P. Iron protein succynilate in the treatment of iron deficiency: Potential interaction with H₂-receptor antagonists. *Int J Clin Pharmacol Ther Toxicol* (1993) 31, 209–17.
4. Partlow ES, Campbell NRC, Chan SC, Pap KM, Granberg K, Hasinoff BB. Ferrous sulfate does not reduce serum levels of famotidine or cimetidine after concurrent ingestion. *Clin Pharmacol Ther* (1996) 59, 389–93.
5. Partlow ES, Chan SC, Pap KM, Hasinoff BB, Campbell NRC. The effect of ferrous sulfate on famotidine serum levels in healthy volunteers. *Clin Invest Med* (1994) 17 (Suppl 4), B15.

Iron preparations + Neomycin

Neomycin may alter the absorption of iron.

Clinical evidence, mechanism, importance and management

A study in 6 patients found that **neomycin** markedly reduced the absorption of **iron** (iron[59] as **ferrous citrate**) in 4 patients, but increased absorption in the other 2 patients who initially had low serum iron levels. None of the patients were anaemic.[1] The importance of this is uncertain, but monitor the outcome of concurrent use.

1. Jacobson ED, Chodos RB, Faloon WW. An experimental malabsorption syndrome induced by neomycin. *Am J Med* (1960) 28, 524–33.

Iron preparations + Pancreatic extracts

Iron absorption may possibly be reduced by pancreatic extracts.

Clinical evidence, mechanism, importance and management

A very brief study found that the absorption of **iron** in *dogs* and man was inhibited by **pancreatic extracts**, **trypsin**, **chymotrypsinogen** and **chymotrypsin**, but the extent and its importance is not clear.[1] However, be alert for any evidence of a reduced response to **iron** if pancreatic extracts are used concurrently.

1. Dietze F, Bruschke G. Inhibition of iron absorption by pancreatic extracts. *Lancet* (1970) i, 424.

Iron preparations + Vitamin E

Vitamin E impairs the response to iron in anaemic children.

Clinical evidence, mechanism, importance and management

A group of anaemic children aged 7 to 40 months was given 5 mg/kg **iron dextran** daily for 3 days. In 9 of the 26, **vitamin E** 200 units, starting 24 h before the **iron-dextran** and continued for a total of 4 days, was also given. It was noted that after 6 days those on **vitamin E** had a reticulocyte response of only 4.4% compared with 14.4% in other patients not given **vitamin E**. The **vitamin E** group also had reduced haemoglobin levels and a lower haematocrit. The reasons are not understood. Check for any evidence of a reduced haematological response in anaemic patients given **iron** and **vitamin E**. The authors of the report point out that this dosage of **vitamin E** was well above the recommended daily dietary intake.[1]

1. Melhorn DK, Gross S. Relationships between iron-dextran and vitamin E in iron deficiency anemia in children. *J Lab Clin Med* (1969) 74, 789–802.

Lanreotide + Ciclosporin

On theoretical grounds lanreotide may possibly reduce serum ciclosporin levels.

Clinical evidence, mechanism, importance and management

The makers of lanreotide say that it may possibly reduce the absorption of **ciclosporin** from the gut[1] (possibly because octreotide, another somatostatin analogue behaves in this way), but as yet there is no clinical confirmation of this interaction. Even so, it would seem prudent to monitor the outcome of concurrent use.

1. Somatuline (Lanreotide). Ipsen Ltd. Summary of product characteristics, October 2001.

Lansoprazole + Miscellaneous drugs

Lansoprazole appears not to interact to a clinically relevant extent with alcohol, diazepam, prednisone or propranolol, and seems unlikely to interact with other drugs normally affected by enzyme inducers and inhibitors. Both food and antacids can cause a moderate reduction in the bioavailability of lansoprazole which can be accommodated by separating their administration.

Clinical evidence, mechanism, importance and management

A number of drug interaction studies have been carried out with lansoprazole. A study in 30 healthy subjects given 0.6 g/kg **alcohol** before and after taking lansoprazole for 3 days found that none of the pharmacokinetic parameters for **alcohol** were significantly changed and blood **alcohol** levels were not raised by lansoprazole.[1] *Maalox* (**aluminium/magnesium hydroxides**) 30 ml reduced the AUC of 30 mg lansoprazole in a group of subjects by 13% and reduced the maximum serum level by 27%, but no changes were seen when the lansoprazole was given 1 h after the antacid.[2] **Magaldrate** also reduces the absorption of lansoprazole to some extent.[3] One study found that **food** reduces lansoprazole bioavailability by 27%.[2] Another study found a 50% reduction in lansoprazole bioavailability with food.[4] Lansoprazole 60 mg daily for 11 days had minimal effects on the pharmacokinetics of **antipyrine (phenazone)** and **indocyanine green** in a group of subjects.[5] **Antipyrine** and **indocyanine green** are used as markers of changes in drug metabolism and in liver blood flow. Lansoprazole daily for 10 days was found to have no effect on the pharmacokinetics of a single 0.1 mg/kg dose of **diazepam**.[6] The pharmacokinetics of a single 40-mg dose of **prednisone** were found to be unaffected by 30 mg lansoprazole. No changes in absorption or in the conversion of **prednisone** to **prednisolone** were seen.[7] Lansoprazole 60 mg daily for 7 days had no significant effect on the pharmacokinetics or pharmacodynamics of a single 80-mg dose of

propranolol in 15 healthy subjects.[8] All of these findings suggest that no special precautions are needed if lansoprazole is given to patients taking **diazepam**, **prednisone** or **propranolol**, and that lansoprazole is unlikely to have a clinically significant effect on other drugs which are susceptible to the actions of enzyme inducers or inhibitors. It is however recommended that lansoprazole should not be given with **food** nor at the same time as **antacids**.[2] A one hour separation is probably enough to avoid the interaction.

1. Girre C, Coutelle C, David P, Fleury B, Thomas G, Palmobo S, Dally S, Couzigou P. Lack of effect of lansoprazole on the pharmacokinetics of ethanol in male volunteers. *Gastroenterology* (1994) 106, A504.
2. Delhotal-Landes B, Cournot A, Vermerie N, Dellatolas F, Benoit M, Flouvat B. The effect of food and antacids on lansoprazole absorption and disposition. *Eur J Drug Metab Pharmacokinet* (1991), Spec No 3, 315–20.
3. Gerloff J, Barth H, Mignot A, Fuchs W, Heintze K. Does the proton pump inhibitor lansoprazole interact with antacids? *Naunyn Schmiedebergs Arch Pharmacol* (1993) 347, R31.
4. Bergstrand R, Grind M, Nyberg G, Olofsson B. Decreased oral bioavailability of lansoprazole in healthy volunteers when given with a standardised breakfast. *Clin Drug Invest* (1995) 9, 67–71.
5. Cavanaugh JH, Park YK, Awni WM, Mukherjee DX, Karol MD, Granneman GR. Effect of lansoprazole on antipyrine and ICG pharmacokinetics. *Gastroenterology* (1991) 100, A40.
6. Lefebvre RA, Flouvat B, Karolac-Tamisier S, Moerman E, Van Ganse E. Influence of lansoprazole treatment on diazepam plasma concentrations. *Clin Pharmacol Ther* (1992) 52, 458–63.
7. Cavanaugh JH, Karol MD. Lack of pharmacokinetic interaction after administration of lansoprazole or omeprazole with prednisone. *J Clin Pharmacol* (1996) 36, 1064–71.
8. Cavanaugh JH, Schneck DW, Mukherji D, Karol MD. Lack of effect of concomitant lansoprazole on single-dose propranolol pharmacokinetics and pharmacodynamics. *Gastroenterology* (1994) 106 (4 Suppl), A4.

Laxatives + Miscellaneous drugs

Sodium sulphate and castor oil used as laxatives can cause a modest but probably clinically unimportant reduction in drug absorption.

Clinical evidence, mechanism, importance and management

In an experimental study of the possible effects of laxatives on drug absorption, healthy subjects were given 10 to 20 g of oral **sodium sulphate** and 20 g of **castor oil** (doses sufficient to provoke diarrhoea). Absorption, measured by the amount of drug excreted in the urine was decreased at 4 h. The reduction was 50, 50 and 21% for **castor oil** and **isoniazid**, **sulfafurazole** (**sulfisoxazole**) and **aspirin** respectively, and 41, 33, 27% for **sodium sulphate** and **isoniazid**, **sulfafurazole** (**sulfisoxazole**) and **aspirin** respectively. However, serum levels of the drugs were relatively unchanged. The overall picture was that while these laxatives can alter the pattern of absorption, they do not seriously impair the total amount of drug absorbed.[1] More study is needed in a clinical situation.

1. Mattila MJ, Takki S, Jussila J. Effect of sodium sulphate and castor oil on drug absorption from the human intestine. *Ann Clin Res* (1974) 6, 19–24.

Levamisole + Miscellaneous drugs

There is some evidence that levamisole can increase the effects of warfarin and phenytoin, and that a disulfiram-like reaction can occur with alcohol.

Clinical evidence, mechanism, importance and management

The INR of a man of 73 on **warfarin** increased from 3 to almost 40 after being given levamisole and **fluorouracil** for 4 weeks. He again demonstrated increased **warfarin** effects when rechallenged with levamisole and **fluorouracil**.[1] A woman of 60 on **warfarin** showed an increase in her prothrombin time from a range of 13.6 to 19.7 s up to 22.6 s ten days after completing the first cycle of levamisole and **fluorouracil**. Eight days later, after completing a 3-day course of levamisole she developed gross haematuria and was found to have a prothrombin time greater than 40 s.[2] Some of the changes were probably due to the **fluorouracil** (see 'Anticoagulants + Cytotoxic (antineoplastic) agents', p.254) but the levamisole may have had some part to play because the makers refer to reports of an increase in prothrombin times with **warfarin** and levamisole in the product information.[3]

The product information for levamisole also describes an increase in the plasma levels of **phenytoin** due to **fluorouracil** with levamisole, and a disulfiram-like reaction with **alcohol**.[3] The general importance of these interactions is uncertain, but you should be aware of these reports and take appropriate precautions.

1. Scarfe MA, Israel MK. Possible drug interaction between warfarin and combination of levamisole and fluorouracil. *Ann Pharmacother* (1994) 28, 464–7.
2. Wehbe TW, Warth JA. A case of bleeding requiring hospitalization that was likely caused by an interaction between warfarin and levamisole. *Clin Pharmacol Ther* (1996) 59, 360–2.
3. Ergamisol (Levamisole). Product information. Physicians' Desk Reference (2002) 1789–91.

Levocabastine + Erythromycin or Ketoconazole

Erythromycin and ketoconazole appear not to interact with levocabastine given by nasal spray.

Clinical evidence, mechanism, importance and management

Levocabastine nasal spray 200 micrograms twice daily for 6 days, plus a single dose on day 7 was given to 38 healthy subjects. On day 7 they were also given a single oral dose of 333 mg **erythromycin** or a placebo. The **erythromycin** was found to have no effect on the steady-state serum levels of the levocabastine.[1] An essentially similar study was carried out in 37 subjects using 200 mg **ketoconazole** instead of erythromycin, with the same result.[2] These two studies suggest that no special precautions are likely if levocabastine is given with either of these drugs, although it should be pointed out that both were only given as single doses.

1. Lee P, Zhou H, Hassell AE, Mechlinski W, Wiesinger B, Gruver M, Algeo S, Hunt T, Moore LRC. Effect of erythromycin on the pharmacokinetics of steady-state intranasal levocabastine in healthy male volunteers. *J Clin Pharmacol* (1996) 36, 847.
2. Hassell AE, Zhou H, Lee P, Wiesinger B, Mechlinski W, Gruver M, Algeo S, West M, Moore LRC. Effect of ketoconazole on the pharmacokinetics of steady-state intranasal levocabastine in healthy male volunteers. *J Clin Pharmacol* (1996) 36, 847.

Levosimendan + Miscellaneous drugs

Levosimendan appears not to interact adversely with alcohol, felodipine, itraconazole or warfarin.

Clinical evidence, mechanism, importance and management

(a) Alcohol

A double-blind, randomised and crossover study in 12 healthy subjects given 0.8 g/kg **alcohol** with 1 mg levosimendan intravenously found no clinically significant pharmacokinetic or pharmacodynamic interactions.[1]

(b) Felodipine

A study of the use of levosimendan 0.5 mg four times daily and **felodipine** (dosage not stated) in 24 men with coronary heart disease found that concurrent use was well tolerated. The **felodipine** did not antagonise the positive inotropic effects of the levosimendan and had no effect on exercise capacity. Both drugs increased the heart rate during exercise, and there was a slightly additive effect of 6 to 10 bpm.[2] There would appear to be no reason for avoiding concurrent use.

(c) Itraconazole

A study in 12 healthy subjects found that pharmacokinetics of a single 2-mg dose of levosimendan were unchanged after taking 200 mg **itraconazole** daily for 5 days, and heart rates PQ, QTc and QRS intervals were unaltered. It was concluded that because **itraconazole**, which is a potent inhibitor of cytochrome P450 isoenzyme CYP3A4, does not interact significantly with levosimendan, interactions with other CYP3A4 inhibitors are unlikely.[3]

(d) Warfarin

In an open randomised crossover study 10 healthy subjects were given single 25-mg oral doses of **warfarin** before and on day 4 of a 9-day course of 0.5 mg levosimendan four times daily. No clinically relevant changes in the anticoagulant effects of the **warfarin** were seen (as measured by APTT or TT-SPA), and no interactions would therefore be expected if both drugs are used in the treatment of patients.[4]

1. Antila S, Järvinen A, Akkila J, Honkanen T, Karlsson M, Lehtonen L. Studies on psychomotoric effects and pharmacokinetic interactions of the new calcium sensitizing drug levosimendan and ethanol. *Arzneimittelforschung* (1997) 47, 816–20.
2. Lehtonen L, Antila S, Eha J, Heinpalu M, Loogna I, Mesikepp A, Planken Ü, Pöder P. No pharmacodynamic interactions between a new calcium sensitizing agent levosimendan and a calcium antagonist drug felodipine. *Eur J Clin Pharmacol* (1997) 52 (Suppl), A136.
3. Antila S, Honkanen T, Lehtonen L, Neuvonen PJ. The CYP3A4 inhibitor itraconazole does not affect the pharmacokinetics of a new calcium-sensitizing drug levosimendan. *Int J Clin Pharmacol Ther* (1998) 36, 446–9.
4. Antila S, Järvinen A, Honkanen T, Ylönen V, Lehtonen L. A new calcium sensitizing agent levosimendan has no pharmacokinetic or pharmacodynamic interactions with warfarin. *Eur J Clin Pharmacol* (1997) 52 (Suppl), A128.

Linopirdine + Antacids or H$_2$-blockers

Mylanta **and famotidine delay the absorption of linopirdine and lower its serum levels, but the total amount absorbed appears to be unchanged.**

Clinical evidence, mechanism, importance and management

A study in 24 healthy subjects found that 30 ml *Mylanta II* taken 5 min after 30 mg linopirdine, or 40 mg **famotidine** taken 1 h previously, increased the time to reach maximum plasma levels by about 75% and reduced these plasma levels by about 45%. The AUCs were unaltered.[1] The clinical importance of these changes awaits assessment.

1. Benedek IH, Connell JM, Finan WL, Fiske WD. Drug interaction study of the effect of an antacid or H$_2$-receptor antagonist on the pharmacokinetics of linopirdine. *J Clin Pharmacol* (1994) 34, 1017.

Liquorice + Miscellaneous drugs

Very large amounts of liquorice can cause pseudoaldosteronism which may adversely affect the treatment of cardiac failure and hypertension, and the control of body potassium levels.

Clinical evidence, mechanism, importance and management

The serum potassium levels of 11 out of 14 healthy subjects fell by over 0.3 mmol/l after eating 100 to 200 g liquorice daily for one to 4 weeks. Some of the subjects experienced falls as large as 1.5 mmol/l. Four subjects withdrew from the study because of hypokalaemia. Mild or uncomfortable oedema of the face, hands and ankles occurred in 6 subjects and 10 of the subjects gained weight (between 1 and 4 kg).[1] Four patients developed pseudohyperaldosteronism after taking large amounts of liquorice containing laxatives in doses of 0.5 to 8 g daily for periods of 3 months to 3 years.[2] A previously healthy patient developed fulminant congestive heart failure after eating 700 g of liquorice candy over a week.[3] The reason is that liquorice contains glycyrrhizinic acid, which has potent mineralocorticoid properties. The conclusion to be drawn is that patients under treatment for hypertension or cardiac failure, or taking drugs which lower body potassium levels, should avoid large amounts of liquorice.

1. Epstein MT, Espiner EA, Donald RA, Hughes H. Effect of eating liquorice on the renin-angiotensin aldosterone axis in normal subjects. *BMJ* (1977) 1, 488–90.
2. Scali M, Pratesi C, Zennaro MC, Zampollo V, Armanini D. Pseudohyperaldosteronism from liquorice-containing laxatives. *J Endocrinol Invest* (1990) 13, 847–8.
3. Chamberlain TJ. Licorice poisoning, pseudoaldosteronism, and heart failure. *JAMA* (1970) 213, 1343.

Loperamide + Miscellaneous drugs

An isolated report, supported by an *in vitro* **study, indicates that the effects of loperamide can be reduced by colestyramine. Co-trimoxazole and ritonavir increase the plasma levels of loperamide, but no additional side-effects are seen.**

Clinical evidence, mechanism, importance and management

(a) Colestyramine

A man who had undergone extensive surgery to the gut, with the creation of an ileostomy, needed treatment for excessive fluid loss. His fluid loss was observed to be "substantially less" (not precisely quantified) when given loperamide 2 mg six-hourly alone, than when given in combination with colestyramine 2 g every four-hourly.[1] The probable reason is that the **colestyramine** binds to the loperamide in the gut, thereby reducing its activity. An *in vitro* study using 50 ml of simulated gastric fluid showed that 64% of a 5.5-mg dose of loperamide was bound by 4 g of **colestyramine**.[1] Direct information is limited to this report but what occurred is consistent with the way **colestyramine** interacts with other drugs. It has been suggested that the two drugs should be separated as much as possible to prevent mixing in the gut, or the loperamide dosage should be increased.[1]

(b) Co-trimoxazole

Co-trimoxazole 960 mg twice daily was given to healthy subjects for 24 h before and then 48 h after taking single 4 mg doses of loperamide (12 subjects) or loperamide oxide (a prodrug of loperamide, 10 subjects). The **co-trimoxazole** increased the loperamide AUC by 89% and doubled the maximum plasma levels. The loperamide oxide AUC was raised 54% and the maximum plasma levels by 41%. It is thought that the **co-trimoxazole** inhibits the metabolism of the loperamide.[2] However, despite these rises, because loperamide has a very wide margin of safety it is thought unlikely that any dosage changes are needed.

(c) Ritonavir

In a double-blind placebo-controlled trial, 12 healthy subjects were given a single dose of **ritonavir** 600 mg, with either loperamide 16 mg or placebo. The loperamide AUC and maximum serum levels were increased threefold and by 17% respectively, but no additional side effects were seen. This was thought to be due to the effect of **ritonavir** on the cytochrome P450 isoenzyme CYP3A4.[3]

1. Ti TY, Giles HG, Sellers EM. Probable interaction of loperamide and cholestyramine. *Can Med Assoc J* (1978) 119, 607–8.
2. Kamali F, Huang ML. Increased systemic availability of loperamide after oral administration of loperamide and loperamide oxide with cotrimoxazole. *Br J Clin Pharmacol* (1996) 41, 125–8.
3. Tayrouz Y, Ganssmann B, Ding R, Klingmann A, Aderjan R, Burhenne J, Haefeli WE, Mikus G. Ritonavir increases loperamide plasma concentrations without evidence for P-glycoprotein involvement. *Clin Pharmacol Ther* (2001) 70, 405–14.

Loratadine + Miscellaneous drugs

Loratadine serum levels are considerably raised by cimetidine, clarithromycin, erythromycin and ketoconazole, but this rise seems to be clinically unimportant. No ECG changes

or heart arrhythmias appear to accompany these increased serum levels. On theoretical grounds fluconazole, fluoxetine and quinidine would not be expected to interact adversely with loratadine.

Clinical evidence

(a) Cimetidine

Loratadine 10 mg and **cimetidine** 300 mg six-hourly, were given alone and together to 24 healthy subjects, for 10 days. The AUCs of loratadine and its metabolite were increased by 203%and 106% respectively, but the safety profile of the loratadine (clinical laboratory tests, vital signs and adverse events) were unchanged. Cardiac repolarisation and all other ECG measurements were unaltered and no sedation or syncope were seen.[1]

(b) Clarithromycin

Loratadine 10 mg and 500 mg **clarithromycin** 12-hourly, were given alone and together to 24 healthy subjects, for 10 days. The AUCs of loratadine and its active metabolite were increased 76% and 49% respectively and the maximum serum levels were increased 36% and 69% respectively. The maximum QTc interval was slightly increased by 3%, but no QTc exceeded 439 ms and there was no evidence that concurrent use caused any cardiotoxicity.[2]

(c) Erythromycin

Loratadine 10 mg daily and **erythromycin** 500 mg 8-hourly, were given alone and together to 24 healthy subjects, for 10 days. The AUC of loratadine and its active metabolite was increased by about 40%, but the ECGs showed no changes in the QTc interval or any evidence of cardiotoxicity.[3] A study in 50 healthy subjects found that 40 mg loratadine daily (four times the recommended dose) for 90 days caused no changes in the ECG measurements, no episodes of dizziness or syncope, and no arrhythmias.[4]

(d) Ketoconazole

A single 20-mg dose of loratadine was given to 12 healthy subjects while they were taking either 200 mg **ketoconazole** twice daily or a placebo for 8 days. The maximum serum loratadine levels and its AUC were increased two to threefold.[5] Another study in 24 healthy subjects on 10 mg loratadine daily found that the addition of 200 mg **ketoconazole** twice daily for 10 days raised the loratadine and metabolite serum levels by 300% and 73% respectively. However, no clinically relevant changes in ECGs – in particular the QTc interval – were seen, and no syncope or sedation was reported.[6]

(e) Fluconazole, Fluoxetine, Quinidine

Fluconazole, **fluoxetine** and **quinidine** behave like cimetidine, clarithromycin, erythromycin and ketoconazole (see above) in that they also inhibit the cytochrome P450 isoenzymes CYP3A4 and CYP2D6. However, because of the safety of high-dose loratadine,[4] no clinically relevant interaction is expected, even if they cause a rise in the serum levels of loratadine.

Mechanism

Not fully established, but *in vitro* studies show that erythromycin inhibits loratadine metabolism (by cytochrome P450 isoenzymes CYP3A4 and CYP2D6)[7-9] so that the *in vivo* rise in its serum levels would seem to be explained. It seems likely that this also happens with cimetidine, clarithromycin and ketoconazole.

Importance and management

Established interactions. Although cimetidine, clarithromycin, erythromycin and ketoconazole certainly increase the serum levels of loratadine, there appears to be nothing to suggest that even a marked increase (up to fourfold) in serum loratadine levels is clinically important. None of the serious cardiotoxicity seen with some other antihistamines (astemizole, terfenadine) appears to occur. No special precautions seem to be necessary. Loratadine would therefore appear to be a safe substitute for these two interacting antihistamines if macrolide antibacterials or azole antifungals are given concurrently.

These clinically irrelevant interactions suggest that other drugs that inhibit the cytochrome P450 isoenzymes CYP3A4 and CYP2D6 may be equally safe with loratadine. The safety of these drugs with loratadine needs confirmation, but no clinically adverse interactions would be expected to occur.

1. Brannan MD, Affrime MB, Reidenberg P, Radwanski E, Lin CC. Evaluation of the pharmacokinetics and electrocardiographic pharmacokinetics of loratadine with concomitant administration of cimetidine. *Pharmacotherapy* (1994) 14, 347.
2. Carr RA, Edmonds A, Shi H, Locke CS, Gustavson LE, Craft JC, Harris SI, Palmer R. Steady-state pharmacokinetics and electrocardiographic pharmacodynamics of clarithromycin and loratadine after individual or concomitant administration. *Antimicrob Agents Chemother* (1998) 42, 1176–80.
3. Brannan MD, Reidenberg P, Radwanski E, Shneyer L, Lin C-C, Cayen MN, Affrime MB. Loratadine administered concomitantly with erythromycin: pharmacokinetic and electrocardiographic evaluations. *Clin Pharmacol Ther* (1995) 58, 269–78.
4. Affrime MB, Lorber R, Danzig M, Cuss F, Brannan MD. Three month evaluation of electrocardiographic effects of loratadine in humans. *J Allergy Clin Immunol* (1993) 91, 259.
5. Van Peer A, Crabbé R, Woestenborghs R, Heykants J, Janssens M. Ketoconazole inhibits loratadine metabolism in man. *Allergy* (1993) 48 (Suppl 16), 34.
6. Brannan MD, Reidenberg P, Radwanski E, Shneyer L, Lin C, Affrime MB. Evaluation of pharmacokinetic and electrocardiographic parameters following 10 days of concomitant administration of loratadine with ketoconazole. *J Clin Pharmacol* (1994) 34, 1016.
7. Lavrijsen K, Van Houdt J, Meuldermans W, Janssens M, Heykants J. The interaction of ketoconazole, itraconazole and erythromycin with the in vitro metabolism of antihistamines in human liver microsomes. *Allergy* (1993) 48, (Suppl 16), 34.
8. Yumibe N, Huie K, Chen KJ, Clement RP, Cayen MN. Identification of human liver cytochrome P450s involved in the microsomal metabolism of the antihistaminic drug loratadine. *J Allergy Clin Immunol* (1994) 93, 234.
9. Brannan MD, Affrime MB, Radwanski E, Cayen MN, Banfield C. Effects of various cytochrome P450 inhibitors on the metabolism of loratadine. *Clin Pharmacol Ther* (1995) 57, 193.

Lovastatin + Antihypertensives

Lovastatin normally appears not to interact adversely with ACE inhibitors, beta-blockers, potassium-sparing diuretics or thiazide diuretics. An isolated report describes severe hyperkalaemia in a diabetic when given lisinopril and lovastatin.

Clinical evidence, mechanism, importance and management

An extensive study[1] of a large group of patients with moderate hypercholesterolaemia found that the effects of lovastatin (20 to 80 mg daily for 4 years) were not altered in patients taking **selective beta-blockers** (247), or **non-selective beta-blockers** (173), **potassium-sparing diuretics** (151), or **thiazide diuretics** (97). However, a marginal enhancement of the lowering of low density lipoprotein levels was seen when lovastatin was used with **ACE inhibitors** (142). None of the drugs was individually named. A study in healthy subjects given lovastatin found that 40 mg **propranolol** twice daily caused minor reductions (of less than 18%) in the AUC of lovastatin and its metabolites.[2] These changes are small and the results seem to confirm the previous findings[1] with **beta-blockers**. No special precautions would seem to be necessary if these drugs are given concurrently

An isolated report describes a type I diabetic (on insulin) with hypertension and hyperlipidaemia who developed myositis and severe hyperkalaemia (serum potassium 8.4 mmol/l) when treated with lovastatin and **lisinopril**. The reason seemed to be a combination of the hyperkalaemic effects of the **lisinopril**, the release of intracellular potassium into the blood associated with the myositis caused by the lovastatin, and a predisposition to hyperkalaemia due to the diabetes and mild renal impairment.[3] This is an unusual case and unlikely to be of general importance.

1. Pool JL, Shear CL, Downton M, Schnaper H, Stinnett S, Dujovne C, Bradford RH, Chremos AN. Lovastatin and coadministered antihypertensive/cardiovascular agents. *Hypertension* (1992) 19, 242–8.
2. Pan HY, Triscari J, DeVault AR, Smith SA, Wang-Iverson D, Swanson BN, Willard DA. Pharmacokinetic interaction between propranolol and the HMG-CoA reductase inhibitors pravastatin and lovastatin. *Br J Clin Pharmacol* (1991) 31, 665–70.
3. Edelman S, Witztum JL. Hyperkalaemia during treatment with HMG-CoA reductase inhibitor. *N Engl J Med* (1989) 320, 1219–20.

Lovastatin + Danazol and Doxycycline

Severe rhabdomyolysis and myoglobinuria developed in a man on lovastatin about two months after danazol was added. A short course of doxycycline may have had some part to play in what happened.

Clinical evidence, mechanism, importance and management

A 72-year-old man taking atenolol, aspirin, dipyridamole and lovastatin 20 mg twice daily was admitted to hospital after complaining of myalgia over the last 12 days, and of brown urine over the last 5 days. His condition was diagnosed as severe rhabdomyolysis and myoglobinuria. About 2 months previously he had been additionally started on **danazol** 200 mg three times daily, prednisone, and one month previously a 10-day course of **doxycycline** 100 mg twice daily. The aspirin and lovastatin were stopped (**danazol** was stopped 4 days before admission and the **doxycycline** was stopped 5 days before the onset of symptoms), and all the symptoms resolved. Laboratory tests were normal within 2 weeks. The reasons for this reaction are not known, but the authors postulate that **danazol** (and the **doxycycline**) were possibly hepatotoxic, and that **danazol** may have inhibited cytochrome P450. As a result, the metabolism of the lovastatin could have been reduced, leading to the development lovastatin toxicity. It might also be that the **danazol** had a direct toxic effect on the muscles.[1]

This appears to be the first and only report of this apparent interaction. Its general importance is unknown, but it would now seem prudent to monitor the concurrent use of lovastatin and either **danazol** or **doxycycline**. The authors of the report point out that other cases of severe lovastatin toxicity have also been very slow to develop.

1. Dallaire M, Chamberland M, Rhabdomyolysis sévère chez un patient recevant lovastatine, danazol et doxycycline. *Can Med Assoc J* (1994) 150, 1991–4.

Lovastatin + Fibre or Pectin

Pectin and oat bran can reduce the blood cholesterol-lowering effects of lovastatin.

Clinical evidence, mechanism, importance and management

The serum low-density lipoprotein cholesterol levels of 3 patients on 80 mg lovastatin daily showed a marked rise from 4.48 to 6.36 mmol/l when additionally given 15 g **pectin** daily. One patient had a 59% rise.[1] Two other patients on lovastatin showed a rise from 5.03 to 6.54 mmol/l when additionally given 50 to 100 g **oat bran** daily. One patient had a 41% rise.[1] When the **pectin** and **oat bran** were stopped, the serum levels of the low-density lipoprotein cholesterol fell. It is presumed that both **pectin** and **oat bran** reduced the absorption of lovastatin from the gut.[1] Evidence is still very limited but patients should be advised not to take either of these two **fibres** at the same time as lovastatin. Separate their ingestion as much as possible. More study is needed.

1. Richter WO, Jacob BG, Schwandt P. Interaction between fibre and lovastatin. *Lancet* (1991) 338, 706.

Lovastatin + Grapefruit juice

The serum levels of lovastatin are markedly increased by grapefruit juice, increasing the risk of lovastatin toxicity.

Clinical evidence

Ten healthy subjects were given 200 ml double-strength **grapefruit juice** three times daily for 3 days, and then on day 3 they additionally took 80 mg lovastatin with 200 ml **grapefruit juice**, followed by two more 200-ml doses of **grapefruit juice** at 30 and 90 minutes. The mean peak serum levels of the lovastatin and its active metabolite, lovastatic acid, were increased 12-fold and 4-fold respectively, and the mean AUCs were increased 15-fold and 5-fold respectively.[1]

Mechanism

It seems almost certain that some component of the grapefruit juice inhibits the metabolism of the lovastatin by the intestinal wall (by CYP3A4) so that more is absorbed.

Importance and management

Information seems to be limited to this report, but it is consistent with the way grapefruit juice interacts with a number of other drugs and is of clear clinical importance. The extent of the interaction and the risks associated with elevated serum lovastatin levels (muscle damage and the possible development of rhabdomyolysis) indicate that to be on the safe side grapefruit juice should be avoided.

1. Kantola T, Kvistö KT, Neuvonen PJ. Grapefruit juice greatly increases serum concentrations of lovastatin and lovastatic acid. *Clin Pharmacol Ther* (1998) 63, 397–402.

Lovastatin or Pravastatin + Macrolide antibacterials

Erythromycin causes a very marked increase in the serum levels of lovastatin but it does not interact with pravastatin. Isolated cases of acute rhabdomyolysis have been seen with lovastatin/azithromycin, lovastatin/clarithromycin and lovastatin/erythromycin.

Clinical evidence

(a) Azithromycin

A 51-year-old man who had been taking 40 mg **lovastatin** daily for 5 years developed muscle aches and fever one day after finishing a 5-day course of 250 mg **azithromycin** daily. His creatine phosphokinase concentrations were elevated and he was diagnosed as having rhabdomyolysis. This patient was also taking colestyramine, diltiazem, doxazosin, glibenclamide (glyburide), thyroid, allopurinol, naproxen, prednisone, loratadine and inhaled beclometasone.[1]

(b) Clarithromycin

A woman of 76 who had been taking 40 mg **lovastatin** daily for 5 years developed muscle pain and weakness 2 days after completing a 10-day course of **clarithromycin** 500 mg twice daily. Later when hospitalised she was found to have elevated creatine phosphokinase concentrations and was diagnosed as having acute rhabdomyolysis. This patient was also taking famotidine, hydrochlorothiazide, triamterene, probenecid, colchicine, prednisone, aspirin, diltiazem, clonidine, insulin and inhaled salbutamol (albuterol).[1]

(c) Erythromycin

A man on **lovastatin** 20 mg three times daily, diltiazem, allopurinol and aspirin developed progressive weakness and diffuse myalgia after being treated with **erythromycin** 500 mg 6-hourly for 13 days. When admitted to hospital his creatine kinase level was high (35 200 units/l) and his urine was reddish-brown. The rhabdomyolysis was treated by stopping the lovastatin, and by giving furosemide and vigorous intravenous hydration.[2] A woman who had been on **lovastatin** for 7 years developed multiple organ toxicity (rhabdomyolysis, acute renal failure, pancreatitis, livedo reticularis and raised aminotransferase values) when **erythromycin** was added.[3] Two other cases of rhabdomyolysis attributed to a **lovastatin/erythromycin** interaction have been reported.[3]

Either **lovastatin** or **pravastatin** 40 mg daily was given to 12 healthy subjects for a week, followed by a further week with 500 mg **erythromycin** three times daily. The **erythromycin** caused the maximum serum **lovastatin** levels and the AUC to rise more than five-fold. The pharmacokinetics of the **pravastatin** remained unchanged.[4]

Mechanism

It seems possible that the erythromycin and clarithromycin inhibit cytochrome P450 isoenzyme CYP3A4 in the liver which is concerned with the metabolism of lovastatin, resulting in a reduction in its loss from the body and a consequent rise in its serum levels leading to rhabdomyolysis. Pravastatin is not affected.[4] It is not known why rhabdomyolysis developed with azithromycin or what the contribution of the other drugs might have been.

Importance and management

Information about the lovastatin/macrolide antibacterial interaction seems to be limited to the reports cited here. The lovastatin/erythromycin interaction appears to be established and of potential clinical importance. Because a marked increase in serum lovastatin levels may increase the risk of rhabdomyolysis, concurrent use should probably be avoided, or certainly very closely monitored. Temporary withdrawal of the lovastatin has also been suggested.[1] Pravastatin would appear to be an alternative, non-interacting and safer substitute.

The situation with the isolated cases involving clarithromycin and azithromycin is far from clear because of the multiplicity of other drugs being used and the disease conditions under treatment. However, clarithromycin closely parallels erythromycin in the way it interacts with many other drugs and it would therefore probably be prudent to follow the same precautions. The situation with azithromycin is also unclear, however the authors of the report cited suggest that temporary withdrawal of the lovastatin should be considered if macrolide antibacterials are needed.[1]

1. Grunden JW, Fisher KA. Lovastatin-induced rhabdomyolysis possibly associated with clarithromycin and azithromycin. *Ann Pharmacother* (1997) 31, 859–63.
2. Ayanian JZ, Fuchs CS, Stone RM. Lovastatin and rhabdomyolysis. *Ann Intern Med* (1988) 109, 682–3.
3. Wong PWK, Dillard TA, Kroenke K. Multiple organ toxicity from addition of erythromycin to long-term lovastatin therapy. *South Med J* (1998) 91, 202–5.
4. Bottorff MB, Behrens DH, Gross A, Markel M. Differences in metabolism of lovastatin and pravastatin as assessed by CYP3A inhibition with erythromycin. *Pharmacotherapy* (1997) 17, 184.

Lovastatin + Nicotinic acid (niacin)

An isolated case of rhabdomyolysis and a case of myositis have been seen in patients on lovastatin when treated with nicotinic acid (niacin).

Clinical evidence, mechanism, importance and management

Rhabdomyolysis developed in a patient on lovastatin which was attributed to the addition of **nicotinic acid** 2.5 g daily.[1] and in another also taking **ciclosporin**[2] (see also 'Statins + Ciclosporin', p.928). Myositis in another patient on lovastatin and **nicotinic acid** is also briefly reported.[1] However, no adverse effects of this kind occurred in 22 other patients concurrently treated with lovastatin, **nicotinic acid** and colestipol.[3] These adverse reports are therefore isolated and it is by no means certain that the addition of **nicotinic acid** was responsible for what happened. Myopathy does occur with lovastatin alone, although the incidence is low (0.1%).[4] However, to be on the safe side, if the decision is made to use **nicotinic acid** with lovastatin, the outcome should be very well monitored. All patients should be warned to report promptly any unexplained muscle aches, tenderness, cramps, stiffness or weakness.

1. Reaven P, Witztum JL. Lovastatin, nicotinic acid and rhabdomyolysis. *Ann Intern Med* (1988) 109, 597–8.
2. Norman DJ, Illingworth DR, Munson J, Hosenpud J. Myolysis and acute renal failure in a heart-transplant recipient receiving lovastatin. *N Engl J Med* (1988) 318, 46–7.

3. Malloy MJ, Kane JP, Kunitake ST, Tun P. Complementarity of colestipol, niacin, and lovastatin in treatment of severe familial hypercholesterolemia. *Ann Intern Med* (1987) 107, 616–23.
4. Bilheimer DW. Long term clinical tolerance of lovastatin (Mevinolin) and Simvastatin (Epistatin). An overview. *Drug Invest* (1990) 2 (Suppl 2), 58–67.

Lovastatin + Potassium-depleting diuretics

One study suggests that diuretics may reduce the lipid-lowering effects of lovastatin. Another suggests that no such interaction occurs.

Clinical evidence, mechanism, importance and management

A retrospective study of 32 patients found that the addition of the lovastatin to diuretic treatment caused an initial fall in total serum cholesterol levels for one month, followed by a rise of about 20%. The diuretics used were **furosemide (frusemide)** (16 patients), **triamterene/hydrochlorothiazide** (7), **hydrochlorothiazide** (8), **indapamide** (1). The fall and subsequent rise in serum cholesterol levels occurred in all of the patients except just the one on **indapamide**.[1] The reasons for this apparent interaction are not understood.

In contrast, another large scale study over 4 years in 8245 patients with moderate hypercholesterolaemia found that the effects of lovastatin were unaltered by the concurrent use of a range of drugs which included the **thiazides** (see 'Lovastatin + Antihypertensives', p.904).[2]

It is not clear just why the results of these two studies differ, but it would now seem prudent to monitor the effects of lovastatin in any patient concurrently treated with any of these diuretics to confirm that its cholesterol-lowering effects are maintained.

1. Aruna AS, Akula SK, Sarpong DF. Interaction between potassium-depleting diuretics and lovastatin in hypercholesterolemic ambulatory care patients. *J Pharm Technol* (1997) 13, 21–6.
2. Pool JL, Shear CL, Downton M, Schnaper H, Stinnett S, Dujovne C, Bradford RH, Chremos AN. Lovastatin and coadministered antihypertensive/cardiovascular agents. *Hypertension* (1992) 19, 242–8.

Lysergide + Selective serotonin re-uptake inhibitors (SSRIs)

Three patients with a history of lysergide (lysergic acid diethylamide, LSD) abuse experienced the new onset or worsening of the LSD flashback syndrome when given fluoxetine, paroxetine or sertraline. Grand mal convulsions occurred in one patient on LSD when given fluoxetine.

Clinical evidence

A girl of 18 with depression, panic and anxiety disorders and with a long history of illicit drug abuse experienced a 15-hour LSD flashback within 2 days of starting to take 50 mg **sertraline** daily. Another flashback lasting a day occurred when the sertraline was replaced by **paroxetine**. No further flashbacks occurred when the SSRIs were stopped. A youth of 17 with depression, also with a long history of illicit drug abuse (including LSD), began to experience LSD flashbacks 2 weeks after starting to take **paroxetine**. His father, a chronic drug abuser, had been treated with both **fluoxetine** and **paroxetine** for depression and had also reported new onset of a flashback syndrome.[1] An isolated report describes grand mal convulsions in a patient while taking **fluoxetine**, tentatively attributed to the concurrent abuse of LSD.[2]

Mechanism

Not understood. Lysergide increases serotonin in the brain, and one suggestion is that when the serotonin re-uptake is blocked in the brain, there is an increased stimulation of 5-HT$_1$ and 5-HT$_2$ receptors.[1]

Importance and management

Information is very limited indeed. The authors of the first report suggest that patients who are given SSRIs should be warned about the possibility of flashback or hallucinations if they have a known history of LSD abuse. It might be better to use other antidepressants that do not act through a 5-HT mechanism.

1. Markel H, Lee A, Holmes RD, Domino EF. Clinical and laboratory observations. LSD flashback syndrome exacerbated by selective serotonin reuptake inhibitor antidepressants in adolescents. *J Pediatr* (1994) 125, 817–9.
2. Picker W, Lerman A, Hajal F. Potential interaction of LSD and fluoxetine. *Am J Psychiatry* (1992) 149, 843–4.

MDMA (3,4-Methylenedioxymethamphetamine) + Ritonavir

A man died from a severe serotoninergic reaction after taking MDMA (Ecstasy). This was attributed to an interaction with ritonavir.

Clinical evidence, mechanism, importance and management

A man with HIV on lamivudine and zidovudine was additionally started on 600 mg **ritonavir** twice daily. About a fortnight later he went to a club and took two-and-a-half tablets of MDMA (*Ecstasy*), estimated at about 180 mg. He soon became unwell and when seen by a nurse in the club was hypertonic, tachypnoeic (45 breaths per minute), tachycardic (more than 140 bpm), cyanosed and diaphoretic. He experienced a tonic-clonic convulsion, his pulse rose to 200 bpm, he then vomited, had a cardiorespiratory arrest and died. A post mortem showed blood concentrations of 0.24 g/l alcohol and 4.56 mg/l MDMA, which was about 10 times greater than might have been expected from the MDMA dose he had taken.[1]

The mechanism this interaction is not known but a possible explanation is that **ritonavir** inhibits cytochrome P450 isoenzyme CYP2D6 which is responsible for the demethylenation of MDMA, the principle metabolic pathway, leading to a sharp rise in its serum levels. Poor liver function (due to alcoholism) may possibly have been a contributory factor.[1] An additional reason may be that MDMA may show non-linear pharmacokinetics.[2] Whatever the full explanation is, it seems that in effect this patient died from a gross overdose of MDMA. The authors say that death was consistent with a severe serotoninergic reaction.[1] Another patient who took an overdose of MDMA (18 tablets) and whose blood levels reached 4.04 mg/l showed similar life-threatening symptoms.[3]

This appears to be the only case of an MDMA/**ritonavir** interaction, but it illustrates the potential for interaction which can occur between illicit drugs and prescribed drugs. Even though this is an isolated case, what happened is consistent with the known toxic effects and pharmacology of the drugs concerned. It may be that the metabolic profile of other patients, particularly those who abuse alcohol and illicit drugs, is such that this interaction could occur again.

1. Henry JA, Hill IR. Fatal interaction between ritonavir and MDMA. *Lancet* (1998) 352, 1751–2.
2. de la Torre, R, Ortuño J, Mas M Farré M, Segura J. Fatal MDMA intoxication. *Lancet* (1999) 353, 593.
3. Roberts L, Wright H. Survival following intentional massive overdose of 'Ecstasy'. *J Accid Emerg Med* (1993) 11, 53–4.

Mequitazine + Spiramycin

An isolated report describes the development of torsade de pointes arrhythmia attributed to the use of mequitazine and spiramycin in a young woman with a congenital long QT syndrome.

Clinical evidence, mechanism, importance and management

A woman of 21 with a congenital long QT syndrome had several syncopal attacks, one at least of which was caused by torsade de pointes, attributed to the concurrent use of **mequitazine** and **spiramycin** over a 2-day period. The problem resolved when the drugs were withdrawn. The authors of this report point out that neither of these drugs is normally considered to cause torsade de pointes, but both belong to drug families which can trigger this type of arrhythmia. But when given to a patient with an already prolonged QT interval, their additive effects were apparently enough to precipitate this serious reaction.[1]

This is an isolated case and the interaction is unlikely to be of general importance, but it draws attention to the potentiality of these drugs to cause a significant prolongation of the QT interval if other factors are also present.

1. Verdun F, Mansourati J, Jobic Y, Bouquin V, Munier S, Guillo P, Pagès Y, Boschat J, Blanc J-J. Torsades de pointes sous traitement par spiramycine et méquitazine. À propos d'un cas. *Arch Mal Coeur Vaiss* (1997) 90, 103–6.

Mesalazine + Ispaghula, Lactitol or Lactulose

On theoretical grounds, delayed-release formulations designed to release mesalazine in the colon, where the pH rises, should not be given with lactulose, lactitol or other preparations which lower the pH in the colon. However ispaghula, which also lowers colonic pH, appears not to affect the bioavailability of mesalazine.

Clinical evidence, mechanism, importance and management

Asacol is a preparation of mesalazine (mesalamine) coated with an acrylic based resin (*Eudragit S*) which disintegrates above pH 7 and releases the mesalazine into the terminal ileum and colon. Since the disintegration depends upon this pH rise, the makers of *Asacol* say that the concurrent use of preparations which lower the pH in the lower part of the gut should be avoided.[1] *Salofalk* is another preparation of mesalazine with a pH-dependent enteric coating. The question is, do any of the preparations which affect colonic pH actually interact with *Asacol* and *Salofalk* in practice?

The pH in the colon can be affected by **lactulose** and **lactitol**, which are metabolised by the gut bacteria to a number of acids (acetic, butyric, propionic, lactic).[2] In healthy subjects **lactulose** (30 to 80 g/24 h) has been found to cause falls in colonic pH,[2-4] in the right colon from about 6 to 5 and in the left colon from 7.0 to 6.5. **Lactitol** (40 to 180 g/24 h) can cause similar falls in pH.[4] **Ispaghula** can also similarly lower colonic pH (from 6.5 to 5.8 in the right colon, and from 7.3 to 6.6 in the left colon).[5] However, a study in patients given mesalazine found that despite this colonic acidification by **ispaghula husk** (*Fybogel*), the release of mesalazine appeared not to be affected.[6]

Thus, although on theoretical grounds **ispaghula husk** would be expected to reduce the effects of mesalazine, no interaction of clinical importance seems to occur, and nobody as yet has shown that a clinically important interaction actually occurs with either **lactulose** or **lactitol**. More study is needed to find out whether these predicted but theoretical interactions are important or not.

1. Asacol (Mesalazine). SmithKline Beecham Pharmaceuticals. Summary of product characteristics, December 2001.
2. Patil DH, Westaby D, Mahida YR, Palmer KR, Rees R, Clark ML, Dawson AM, Silk DBA. Comparative modes of action of lactitol and lactulose in the treatment of hepatic encephalopathy. *Gut* (1987) 28, 255–9.
3. Bown RL, Gibson JA, Sladen GE, Hicks B, Dawson AM. Effects of lactulose and other laxatives on ileal and colonic pH as measured by a radiotelemetry device. *Gut* (1974) 15, 999–1004.
4. Patil DH, Westaby D, Mahida YR, Palmer KR, Rees R, Clark ML, Silk DBA. Comparison of lactulose and lactitol on ileal and colonic pH. *Gut* (1985) 26, A1125.
5. Evans DF, Crompton J, Pye G, Hardcastle JD. The role of dietary fibre on acidification of the colon in man. *Gastroenterology* (1988) 94, A118.
6. Riley SA, Tavares IA, Bishai PM, Bennett A, Mani V. Mesalazine release from coated tablets: effect of dietary fibre. *Br J Clin Pharmacol* (1991) 32, 248–50.

Mesalazine + Omeprazole

Omeprazole does not affect the release of mesalazine from a delayed-release preparation (Asacol).

Clinical evidence, mechanism, importance and management

Asacol is a preparation of mesalazine (mesalamine) coated with an acrylic based resin (*Eudragit S*) which disintegrates above pH 7 and releases the mesalazine into the terminal ileum and colon. The release is rapid at pH values of 7 and above, but it can also occur between pH 6 and 7. Since the proton-pump inhibitors can raise the pH in the stomach to 6 and above, the potential exists for the premature release of mesalazine from *Asacol*. However, a study in 6 healthy subjects given 400 mg mesalazine three times daily for 3 weeks found that when they were also given 20 mg **omeprazole** daily during the second week, and 40 mg **omeprazole** daily during the third week, the steady-state pharmacokinetics of the mesalazine remained unchanged.[1] There would therefore appear to be no reason for avoiding the concurrent use of *Asacol* and **omeprazole**, and, on the basis of this study, it seems likely that other proton-pump inhibitors will behave similarly. This needs confirmation.

1. Hussain F, Trudgill N, Riley S. Mesalazine release from a pH-dependent formulation: effect of concurrent omeprazole administration. *Gastroenterology* (1995) 108 (Suppl), A840.

Methoxsalen + Phenytoin

The serum levels of methoxsalen (8-methoxypsoralen) can be markedly reduced by the concurrent use of phenytoin, which resulted in treatment failure in one patient.

Clinical evidence, mechanism, importance and management

A patient with epilepsy failed to respond to treatment for psoriasis with PUVA (12 treatments of 30 mg methoxsalen given orally and ultraviolet A irradiation) while taking 250 mg **phenytoin** daily. Methoxsalen serum levels were normal in the absence of **phenytoin** but abnormally low while taking **phenytoin**,[1] due, it is suggested, to the enzyme inducing effects of the **phenytoin**. This interaction could lead to serious erythema and blistering if the **phenytoin** dose is reduced during therapy as photosensitivity caused by the methoxsalen may be increased. Concurrent use should be avoided or very closely monitored.

1. Staberg B, Hueg B. Interaction between 8-methoxypsoralen and phenytoin. Consequence for PUVA therapy. *Acta Derm Venereol* (1985) 65, 553–5.

Metoclopramide + Sertraline

An isolated report describes dystonia of the jaw in a patient on metoclopramide when sertraline was added.

Clinical evidence, mechanism, importance and management

A woman with gastro-oesophageal reflux, controlled with 15 mg metoclopramide four times daily, developed symptoms consistent with a mandibular dystonia (periauricular pain, jaw tightness, the sensation of her teeth clenching and grinding) on the second day of starting a course of 50 mg **sertraline** daily. A 50-mg dose of diphenhydramine resolved the problem within 30 min, but the same symptoms re-occurred the next day, 8 h after taking **sertraline**, this time relieved by 2 mg oral benzatropine mesilate. A possible explanation for this extrapyramidal side-effect is that the serotonin inhibition by the **sertraline** increased the dopamine antagonism of the metoclopramide, producing enough dopaminergic inhibition to cause the dystonia.[1] The general importance of this isolated case is not known.

1. Christensen RC, Byerly MJ. Mandibular dystonia associated with the combination of sertraline and metoclopramide. *J Clin Psychiatry* (1996) 57, 596.

Metyrapone + Cyproheptadine

Cyproheptadine may falsify the results of the metyrapone hypothalamic-hypophyseal function test.

Clinical evidence, mechanism, importance and management

Pretreatment with 4 mg **cyproheptadine** 6-hourly 2 days before and throughout a standard metyrapone test (750 mg four-hourly for 6 doses) reduced the metyrapone-induced urinary 17-hydroxycorticosteroid response in 9 healthy subjects by 32% and also reduced the serum 11-deoxycortisol response.[1] The results of metyrapone tests will therefore be unreliable in patients taking **cyproheptadine**.

1. Plonk J, Feldman JM, Keagle D. Modification of adrenal function by the anti-serotonin agent cyproheptadine. *J Clin Endocrinol Metab* (1976) 42, 291–5.

Metyrapone + Phenytoin

The results of the metyrapone test are unreliable in patients taking phenytoin. Doubling the dose of metyrapone gives results that are close to normal.

Clinical evidence, mechanism, importance and management

A study in 5 healthy subjects and 3 patients taking 300 mg **phenytoin** showed that their serum metyrapone levels 4 h after taking a regular 750-mg dose were very low indeed when compared with a control group (6.5 compared with 48.2 micrograms/100 ml. Their response to metyrapone was proportionately lower.[1] Other reports confirm that the urinary steroid response is subnormal in patients taking **phenytoin**.[2,3] The reason is that **phenytoin** is a potent liver enzyme inducing agent that increases the metabolism of the metyrapone, thereby reducing its biological activity.[1,4] As a result of this, the results of the metyrapone test for Cushing's syndrome are invalid. Doubling the dose of metyrapone from 750 mg four-hourly to two-hourly has been shown to give results similar to those in subjects not taking **phenytoin**.[1]

1. Meikle AW, Jubiz W, Matsukura S, West CD, Tyler FH. Effect of diphenylhydantoin on the metabolism of metyrapone and release of ACTH in man. *J Clin Endocrinol Metab* (1969) 29, 1553–8.
2. Krieger DT. Effect of diphenylhydantoin on pituitary-adrenal interrelations. *J Clin Endocrinol Metab* (1962) 22, 490–3.
3. Werk EE, Thrasher K, Choi Y, Sholiton LJ. Failure of metyrapone to inhibit 11-hydroxylation of 11-deoxycortisol during drug therapy. *J Clin Endocrinol Metab* (1967) 27, 1358–60.
4. Jubiz W, Levinson RA, Meikle AW, West CD, Tyler FH. Absorption and conjugation of metyrapone during diphenylhydantoin therapy: mechanism of the abnormal response to oral metyrapone. *Endocrinology* (1970) 86, 328–31.

Mifepristone + Sulprostone

An isolated report describes reversible ventricular fibrillation in a woman of 35 after being given mifepristone and sulprostone to induce an abortion. Coronary spasm may have occurred.[1]

1. Delay M, Genestal M, Carrie D, Livarek B, Boudjemaa B, Bernadet P. Arrêt cardiocirculatoire après administration de l'association mifépristone (Mifégyne) sulprostone (Nalador) pour interruption de grossesse. *Arch Mal Coeur* (1992) 85, 105–7.

Misoprostol + Alcohol

Misoprostol appears to protect the mucosal lining of the stomach from alcohol-induced damage.[1] This interaction may be clinically useful, but more study is needed.

1. Agrawal NM, Godiwala T, Arimura A, Dajani EZ. Cytoprotection by a synthetic prostaglandin against ethanol-induced gastric mucosal damage. A double-blind endoscopic study in human subjects. *Gastrointest Endosc* (1986) 32, 67–70.

Mizolastine + Miscellaneous drugs

Erythromycin, ketoconazole, and antiarrhythmics of Class I and Class III known to prolong the QT interval are contraindicated by the makers with mizolastine, and caution is advised with cimetidine, ciclosporin and nifedipine. All of these warnings are largely based on theoretical considerations and there is growing evidence that some of these precautions may not be necessary.

Clinical evidence, mechanism, importance and management

The makers say that mizolastine is contraindicated with macrolide antibacterials or systemic imidazole antifungals (only **erythromycin** and **ketoconazole** are specifically named)[1] because these drugs increase the plasma levels of mizolastine by about 50%.[2] The implication is that this will increase its prolonging effects on the QT interval, which may result in an increased risk of cardiac arrhythmias (in particular torsade de pointes).

Another study showed that when 1 g **erythromycin** twice daily was taken by 12 healthy subjects with 10 mg mizolastine daily for a week, the maximum serum levels of the mizolastine were increased by 40% and its AUC by 53%. More importantly no significant changes were seen in QT or QTc intervals when compared with the values seen before treatment.[3] A further study, showed that increasing the dosage of mizolastine fourfold (to 40 mg daily) over a week had no effect on any ECG parameters, including the QT interval in a group of healthy subjects.[4] The studies to date give little evidence to suggest this combination is a problem, and it seems likely that the warnings arise from the cardiotoxicity seen with other antihistamines. However, more study is needed before an interaction can definitely be ruled out.

In addition, the makers say that other drugs known to prolong the QT interval such as **Class I** and **Class III antiarrhythmics** are contraindicated with mizolastine. The makers also warn that care should be taken with the concurrent use of **cimetidine**, **ciclosporin** and **nifedipine** because they inhibit cytochrome CYP3A4 and might therefore raise mizolastine plasma levels.[1]

1. Mizollen (Mizolastine). Sanofi Synthelabo. Summary of product characteristics, January 2001.
2. Dubruc C, Gillet G, Chaufour S, Holt B, Jensen R, Maurel P, Thenot JP. Metabolic interaction studies of mizolastine with ketoconazole and erythromycin in rat, dog and man. *Clin Pharmacol Ther* (1998) 63, 228.
3. Chaufour S, Holt B, Jensen R, Dubruc C, Deschamp C, Rosenzweig R. Interaction study between mizolastine, a new H₁ antihistamine, and erythromycin. *Clin Pharmacol Ther* (1998) 63, 214.
4. Chaufour S, Caplain H, Lilienthal N, L'Héritier C, Deschamps C, Rosenzweig P. Mizolastine, a new H₁ antagonist, does not affect the cardiac repolarisation in healthy volunteers. *Clin Pharmacol Ther* (1998) 63, 214.

Modafinil + Miscellaneous drugs

Ciclosporin serum levels were reported to be reduced in one patient by modafinil, and clomipramine serum levels were increased in another. The makers advise an increase in the oral contraceptive dosage while taking modafinil, and vigilance if anticonvulsants, particularly phenytoin, are used. No pharmacokinetic interactions appear to occur with dexamfeta-mine (dextroamphetamine), methylphenidate or triazolam. There is also speculation, based on *in vitro* studies, about some possible interactions with other drugs.

Clinical evidence, mechanism, importance and management

(a) Anticonvulsants

Due of the enzyme inducing potential of modafinil the makers say that care should be observed with co-administration of these anticonvulsants.[1] Studies in *animals* suggest that modafinil serum levels can be reduced by **phenobarbital** (a potent enzyme inducing agent) rather than that modafinil affects anticonvulsants.[2] However, because there is some *in vitro* evidence that modafinil may possibly inhibit the metabolism of **phenytoin** by cytochromes P450 isoenzymes CYP2C9 and CYP2C19, there is some reason for monitoring concurrent use for evidence of increased **phenytoin** effects and toxicity.[3]

(b) Benzodiazepines

The makers report that single-dose studies in normal subjects given 50, 100 or 200 mg modafinil with 250 micrograms **triazolam** found no clinically important alterations in the safety of either drug.[3]

(c) Ciclosporin

A kidney transplant patient, stabilised for 9 years on 200 mg **ciclosporin** daily, developed Gélineau's syndrome and was additionally given 200 mg modafinil daily. Within a few weeks her serum **ciclosporin** levels were noted to have fallen, and it was found necessary to raise her **ciclosporin** dosage stepwise to 300 mg daily before her serum levels were back to their former values.[4] The reason is thought to be that modafinil induces cytochrome P450 isoenzyme CYP3A4 so that the metabolism and clearance of the **ciclosporin** is increased.[5] This is the first reported case of a **ciclosporin**/modafinil interaction but it highlights the need to check the **ciclosporin** levels in any patient if modafinil is started.

(d) Contraceptives, oral

The makers say that the effectiveness of oral contraceptives may be impaired due to the enzyme induction activity of modafinil. They advise using an oral contraceptive containing at least 50 micrograms of **ethinyl oestradiol**.[1] This warning is based on *in vitro* studies with human liver microsomes (not on clinical studies) which found that modafinil has some enzyme inducing activity, but the real risks of contraceptive failure are still uncertain. However, until the situation becomes clear, it would be prudent to follow the maker's advice.

(e) Dexamfetamine (Dextroamphetamine), Methylphenidate

A single dose study with 200 mg modafinil and 40 mg **methylphenidate** found that no clinically relevant changes occurred in the pharmacokinetic profile of either drug.[5,6] Another study with 200 mg modafinil and 10 mg **dexamfetamine** (**dextroamphetamine**) also found that the pharmacokinetics of neither drug appeared to be changed to a clinically relevant extent when given together.[5] These single dose studies suggest that pharmacokinetic interactions are unlikely to occur, but multiple dose studies in patients are needed to confirm the absence of clinically important interactions.

(f) Miscellaneous drugs

There is no clinical evidence of a **warfarin**/modafinil interaction but because **warfarin** can be metabolised by cytochrome P450 isoenzyme CYP2C9 (inhibited by modafinil) the US product information suggests that concurrent use should be monitored.[3] Similarly there is no clinical evidence of interactions with potent inhibitors of CYP3A4 (e.g. **itraconazole**, **ketoconazole**) which might increase the effects of modafinil, or with potent enzyme inducers (**carbamazepine**, **rifampicin**) which might reduce the effects of modafinil, but the US product information includes them under the heading of drug interactions.[3] Such interactions seem unlikely because CYP3A4 is not the only cytochrome P450 isoenzyme which is involved in the metabolism of modafinil. Nor does it seem likely that the serum levels of **theophylline** will be reduced to a clinically relevant extent by the modest enzyme inducing effects of modafinil. All of these 'interactions' are only tentative predictions based on *in vitro* evidence and confirmation in practice is awaited.

(g) Tricyclic antidepressants

A single-dose study with 50 mg **clomipramine** and 200 mg modafinil three times daily found that no pharmacokinetic changes occurred with either of the two drugs.[7] However, a single case report describes a patient on 75 mg **clomipramine** daily who showed a rise in serum **clomipramine** and desmethylclomipramine levels when 200 mg modafinil was added.[8] A postulated reason is that she was a 'poor metaboliser' and lacked cytochrome CYP2D6 so that the additional inhibition of CYP2C19 by modafinil resulted in elevated serum levels.

Information about other tricyclic antidepressants is lacking, but the makers of modafinil point out that other patients who lack CYP2D6 (about 7 to 10% of the Caucasian population) may possibly also show increased serum tricyclic antidepressants levels in the presence of modafinil.[3] Therefore monitoring would seem to be a prudent precaution.

1. Provigil (Modafinil). Cephalon. Summary of product characteristics, December 1997.
2. Moachon G, Kanmacher I, Clenet M, Matinier D. Pharmacokinetic profile of modafinil. *Drugs Today* (1996) 32 (Suppl 1), 23–33.
3. Provigil (Modafinil), Cephalon (US). Product literature, January 1999.
4. LeCacheux Ph, Charasse C, Mourtada R, Muh Ph, Boulahrouz R, Simon P. Gélineau's syndrome in a kidney-transplant patient. *Presse Med* (1997) 26, 466.
5. Provigil (Modafinil), Cephalon (USA). Product Monograph, January 1998.
6. Wong NY, Gorman S, McCormick GC, Grebow P. Single-dose pharmacokinetics of modafinil and methylphenidate given alone and in combination to healthy male volunteers. Association of Professional Sleep Societies meeting, San Francisco, June 1997, Abstract 116.
7. Wong NY, Gorman S, Simcoe D, McCormick GC, Grebow P. A double-blind placebo controlled crossover study to investigate the kinetics and acute tolerability of modafinil and clomipramine alone and in combination in healthy male volunteers. Association of Professional Sleep Societies meeting, San Francisco, June 1997, Abstract 117.
8. Grözinger M, Härtter S, Hiemke Ch, Röschke J. Does modafinil increase the blood level of tricyclic antidepressive comedication? and without lorazepam medication. *Clin Neuropharmacol* (1998) 21, 127–9.

Montelukast + Miscellaneous drugs

Montelukast in normal doses does not interact to a clinically relevant extent with corticosteroids (prednisone, prednisolone), digoxin, loratadine, oral contraceptives, phenobarbital, salbutamol (albuterol), terfenadine, or warfarin, and no important interaction seems likely with phenytoin or rifampicin (rifampin).

Clinical evidence, mechanism, importance and management

(a) Corticosteroids

A double-blind, placebo-controlled, parallel study in a large number of normal subjects (55 on montelukast and 36 on a placebo) found that the plasma profiles of 20 mg oral **prednisone** and of 250 mg intravenous **prednisolone** were unaffected by 200 mg montelukast daily for 6 weeks.[1] Other studies in patients using inhaled and/or oral **corticosteroids** have found that concurrent use is useful and well tolerated.[2,3] No special precautions appear to be needed if these drugs are used concurrently, and the makers say that montelukast can be used as add-on therapy in patients using inhaled **corticosteroids**.[4]

(b) Contraceptives, oral

The makers say that montelukast does not interact with an **ethinylestradiol** 35 micrograms + **norethisterone** 1 mg containing contraceptive.[4] No special precautions are therefore needed if both drugs are used concurrently.

(c) Digoxin

Montelukast 10 mg was given to 11 healthy subjects for 12 days, with a single 500-microgram dose of **digoxin** on day 7 in a randomised two-period crossover study. It was found that the pharmacokinetic profile of the **digoxin** was unchanged by the montelukast.[5] No special precautions are needed if both drugs are used concurrently.

(d) Miscellaneous drugs

A study in patients with moderately severe asthma found no adverse interactions when **salbutamol** (**albuterol**) and 100 mg or 250 mg montelukast were used concurrently, with or without inhaled **corticosteroids**.[6] The makers say that montelukast can be used as an add-on for the treatment of patients taking **beta-agonist drugs**.[4] No adverse interactions were seen in large numbers of patients given 10 or 20 mg montelukast and 10 mg **loratadine**, and the combination was found to be beneficial in the treatment of allergic rhinitis and conjunctivitis.[7]

(e) Phenobarbital, Phenytoin, Rifampicin (Rifampin)

Montelukast 10 mg was given to 14 healthy subjects before and after taking 100 mg **phenobarbital** daily for 14 days. It was found that the geometric mean AUC and maximum serum levels of the montelukast were reduced 38% and 20% respectively, but it was concluded that no montelukast dosage adjustment is needed.[8] The reason for these reductions is almost certainly because the **phenobarbital** induces the activity of cytochrome P450 isoenzyme CYP3A4 so that the montelukast metabolism is increased, and so the makers caution the use of montelukast and inducers of CYP3A4 such as **phenytoin**, **phenobarbital** and **rifampicin**, especially in children.[4] However, there is so far no clinical evidence that the montelukast dosage needs adjustment in the presence of any of these drugs.

(f) Terfenadine

Healthy subjects were given 60 mg **terfenadine** 12-hourly for 14 days, to which 10 mg montelukast daily was added, from day 8 to day 14. It was found that the **terfenadine** pharmacokinetics and the QTc interval were unaltered by concurrent use.[9] No special precautions are needed if both drugs are given concurrently.

(g) Warfarin

Twelve healthy subjects were given 10 mg montelukast orally for 12 days and a single 30-mg dose of **warfarin** on day 7 of a double-blind placebo-controlled and randomised study. It was found that the pharmacokinetics of the **warfarin** were virtually unchanged by the montelukast, and prothrombin times and INRs were not significantly altered.[10] No special precautions are needed if both drugs are used concurrently.

1. Noonan T, Shingo S, Kundu S, Reiss TF. A double-blind, placebo-controlled, parallel-group study in healthy male volunteers to investigate the safety and tolerability of 6 weeks of administration of MK-0476, and in subgroups, the effect of 6 weeks of administration of MK-0476 on the single dose pharmacokinetics of po and iv theophylline and corticosteroids. Merck Sharp & Dohme. Data on file.
2. Kuna P, Malstrom K, Dahlen SE, Nizankowska E, Kowalski M, Stevenson D, Bousquet J Dahlen B, Picado C, Lumry W, Holgate S, Pauwels R, Szczeklik A, Shahane A, Reiss TF. Montelukast (MK0476) a CysLT1 receptor antagonist, improves asthma control in aspirin-intolerant asthmatic patients. *Am J Respir Crit Care Med* (1997) 155, A975.
3. Knorr B, Matz J, Bernstein JA, Nguyen H, Seidenberg BC, Reiss TF, Becker A, for the Pediatric Montelukast Study Group. Montelukast for chronic asthma in 6- to 14-year-old children. A randomized, double-blind trial. *JAMA* (1998) 279, 1181–6.
4. Singulair (Montelukast). Merck Sharp & Dohme Limited. Summary of product characteristics, November 2001.
5. Depre M, Van Hecken A, Verbesselt R, Wynants K, De Lelepeire I, Freeman A, Holland S, Shahane A, Gertz B, De Schepper PJ. Effect of multiple doses of montelukast, a CysLT1 receptor agonist, on digoxin pharmacokinetics in healthy volunteers. *J Clin Pharmacol* (1999) 39, 941–4.
6. Botto A, Kundu S, Reiss T. A double-blind, placebo-controlled, 3-period, crossover study to investigate the bronchodilating ability of oral doses of MK-0476 and to investigate the interaction with inhaled albuterol in moderately severe asthmatic patients. Merck Sharp & Dohme. Data on file (Protocol 066) 1996.
7. Malstrom K, Meltzer E, Prenner B, Lu S, Weinstein S, Wolfe J, Wei LX, Reiss TF. Effects of montelukast (a leukotriene receptor antagonist), loratadine, montelukast + loratadine and placebo in seasonal allergic rhinitis and conjunctivitis. *J Allergy Clin Immunol* (1998) 101, S97.
8. Holland S, Shahane A, Rogers JD, Porras A, Grasing K, Lasseter K, Pinto M, Freeman A, Gertz B, Amin R. Metabolism of montelukast (M) is increased by multiple doses of phenobarbital (P). *Clin Pharmacol Ther* (1998) 63, 231.
9. Holland S, Gertz B, DeSmet M, Michiels N, Larson P, Freeman A, Keymeulen B. Montelukast (MON) has no effect on terfenadine (T) pharmacokinetics (PK) or QTc. *Clin Pharmacol Ther* (1998) 63, 232.
10. Van Hecken A, Depre M, Verbesselt R, Wynants K, De Lepeire I, Arnoudt J, Wong PH, Freeman A, Holland S, Gertz B, De Schepper PJ. Effect of montelukast on the pharmacokinetics and pharmacodynamics of warfarin in healthy subjects. *J Clin Pharmacol* (1999) 39, 495–500.

Naratriptan + Miscellaneous drugs

The makers of naratriptan contraindicate it with other 5-HT$_1$ agonists and they do not recommend its use with ergot derivatives, although there is some evidence for safe concurrent use. No interactions occur with alcohol, food, or tricyclic antidepressants, and none would be expected with MAOIs.

Clinical evidence, mechanism, importance and management

(a) Cardiovascular drugs

The makers report that there is no evidence of interactions with **beta-blockers** (none specifically named)[1] so that there would appear to be no problems with the concurrent use of **propranolol** used for the prophylaxis of migraine or with **other beta-blockers** for hypertension. However, naratriptan is contraindicated in patients who have had a myocardial infarction, or have ischaemic heart disease, Prinzmetal's angina/coronary vasospasm, peripheral vascular disease or who show any evidence of ischaemic heart disease and so it is not suitable for use with **beta-blockers** taken for this purpose. The situation is the same with **nitrates**.

(b) Ergot derivatives

A study by the makers in 12 normal subjects found that 1 mg intramuscular **dihydroergotamine** reduced the AUC and the maximum serum levels of a single 2.5-mg dose of naratriptan by 15% and 20% respectively but this was considered to be clinically irrelevant. Concurrent use was well tolerated and no clinically significant effects on blood pressure, heart rate or ECG were seen.[2] Another similar study using 2 mg **ergotamine** and 2.5 mg naratriptan found no clinically relevant changes in the pharmacokinetics of the naratriptan. A small rise in systolic pressure occurred (less than 5 mmHg) but no clinically significant effects on heart rate or ECG nor any other adverse effects were seen. Even so the makers say in their product literature that the use of naratriptan with **ergotamine** and its derivatives, including **methysergide**, is not recommended.[1]

(c) Non-interacting drugs

The makers report that there is no evidence of interactions with **tricyclic antidepressants**, **alcohol** or **food**. They also say that naratriptan does not inhibit monoamine oxidase so that interactions with **MAOIs** are not anticipated.[1]

(d) Sumatriptan and other 5-HT$_1$ agonists

In a study by the makers in 12 healthy subjects it was found that 2.5 mg naratriptan alone had no significant effects on blood pressure whereas a small rise in peak diastolic and systolic pressures occurred with 6 mg subcutaneous **sumatriptan** alone. When given together there was no evidence of an additive effect (i.e. no greater effect than with **sumatriptan** alone). The systemic exposure of both drugs was not increased by concurrent use, which proved to be safe and well tolerated.[3] Despite this evidence the makers say that concurrent use of naratriptan and other 5-HT$_1$ agonists is contraindicated.[1]

1. Naramig (Naratriptan). Glaxo Wellcome. Summary of product characteristics, September 2001.
2. Kempsford RD, Nicholls B, Lam R, Wintermute S. A study to investigate the potential interaction of naratriptan and dihydroergotamine. 8th International Headache Congress, Amsterdam, June 1997.
3. Williams P, Kempsford R, Fuseau E, Dow J, Smith J. Absence of a significant pharmacodynamic or pharmacokinetic interaction with naratriptan and sumatriptan co-administration. 8th International Headache Congress, Amsterdam, June 1997.

Nicorandil + Miscellaneous drugs

Nicorandil appears not to interact adversely with a wide range of drugs.

Clinical evidence, mechanism, importance and management

Studies on the safety of nicorandil in combination with other drugs have found no evidence of adverse interactions. No pharmacokinetic interactions were found with **cimetidine**, **rifampicin** or **acenocoumarol (nicoumalone)**,[1] no INR changes,[1] and no evidence of pharmacodynamic interactions was found with **furosemide (frusemide)** plus **digoxin** treatment.[2] Studies in 1152 patients using nicorandil with antianginal therapy found no evidence of increased adverse effects or withdrawals while concurrently taking **beta-blockers** (210 patients), **calcium channel blockers** (117), **long-acting nitrates** (130) (none of these drugs was individually named), **bepridil** (18), **diltiazem** (91), **verapamil** (9), **amiodarone** (23) or **molsidomine** (30). It has also been reported that **antihypertensives**, **antidiabetic** or **hypolipidaemic** agents (none of them specifically named) do not appear to interact adversely.[3] No adverse ECG effects have been seen (including QT or ST segment modifications) with nicorandil.[3] However the makers suggest that nicorandil may possibly potentiate the blood pressure lowering effects of **other vasodilators**, **tricyclic antidepressants** or **alcohol**.[4]

1. Frydman A. Pharmacokinetic profile of nicorandil in humans: an overview. *J Cardiovasc Pharmacol* (1992) 20 (Suppl 3), S34–S44.
2. Krumenacker M, Roland E. Clinical profile of nicorandil. An overview of its hemodynamic properties and therapeutic efficacy. *J Cardiovasc Pharmacol* (1992) (Suppl 3), S93–S102.
3. Witchitz S, Darmon J-Y. Nicorandil safety in the long-term treatment of coronary heart disease. *Cardiovasc Drugs Ther* (1995) 9, 237–43.
4. Ikorel (Nicorandil). Rhone-Poulenc Rorer Limited. Summary of product characteristics, June 2000.

Nicotinic acid (Niacin) + Alcohol

An isolated report describes delirium and metabolic acidosis in a patient taking nicotinic acid for hypercholesterolaemia after ingesting about 1 litre of wine, delirium had occurred on a previous similar occasion. It is suggested that the nicotinic acid may have caused liver dysfunction, which was exacerbated by the large amount of alcohol. The patient did have some elevations in liver enzymes.[1] No general conclusions can be drawn from this single case.

1. Schwab RA, Bachhuber BH. Delirium and lactic acidosis caused by ethanol and niacin coingestion. *Am J Emerg Med* (1991) 9, 363–5.

Nicotinic acid (Niacin) + Nicotine

An unpleasant flushing reaction developed in a woman taking nicotinic acid when she started to use nicotine transdermal patches.

Clinical evidence, mechanism, importance and management

A woman was treated with 250 mg nicotinic acid twice daily for 3 years without problems, as well as nifedipine, ranitidine, colestyramine and ferrous sulphate. Following laryngectomy for cancer, she restarted all of the drugs except the colestyramine and began to use **nicotine transdermal patches** 21 mg daily to try to give up smoking. She then developed unpleasant flushing episodes lasting about 30 min on several occasions shortly after taking the nicotinic acid. No further episodes developed when the nicotinic acid was stopped.[1] The reasons are not understood, but flushing is a very common side-effect of nicotinic acid, and it would seem that in this case the **nicotine patch** was responsible for its emergence. This reaction is more unpleasant than serious. Patients should be warned. A comment on this report suggests that this reaction may possibly have an immunological basis.[2]

1. Rockwell KA. Potential interaction between niacin and transdermal nicotine. *Ann Pharmacother* (1993) 27, 1283–4.
2. Sudan BJL. Comment: niacin, nicotine, and flushing. *Ann Pharmacother* (1994) 28, 1113.

Nicotinic acid (Niacin) + Salicylates

Aspirin can reduce the flushing reaction which often occurs with nicotinic acid, but it can also increase the nicotinic acid plasma levels. The importance of this latter reaction is uncertain.

Clinical evidence, mechanism, importance and management

Nicotinic acid (0.07 to 0.1 mg/kg/min as an infusion) was given to 6 healthy subjects over 6 hours. When the subjects were additionally given 1 g **aspirin** orally 2 hours after the infusion was started, the plasma nicotinic acid levels rose markedly, due to a 30 to 54% decrease in its clearance.[1] The probable reason is that the **salicylate** competes with the nicotinic acid for its metabolism by the liver (glycine conjugation) so that it clearance is reduced, resulting in a rise in its levels. The clinical importance of this is not known. However, if **aspirin** is given to reduce the annoying nicotinic acid flushing reaction,[2] check that the effects of the latter do not become excessive.

1. Ding RW, Kolbe K, Merz B, de Vries J, Weber E, Benet LZ. Pharmacokinetics of nicotinic acid-salicylic acid interaction. *Clin Pharmacol Ther* (1989) 46, 642–7.
2. Kane JP, Malloy MJ, Tun P, Phillips NR, Freedman DD, Williams ML, Rowe JS, Havel RJ. Normalization of low-density-lipoprotein levels in heterozygous familiar hypercholesterolemia with a combined drug regimen. *N Engl J Med* (1981) 304, 251–8.

Olestra + Miscellaneous drugs

Olestra does not interact with oral contraceptives or warfarin and there is evidence that it does not interact with diazepam or propranolol. It is believed that olestra is unlikely to affect the absorption of drugs taken orally.

Clinical evidence, mechanism, importance and management

While taking 18 g olestra daily for 28 days, the pharmacokinetics of the **ethinylestradiol** and **norgestrel** components of a combined oral contraceptive (*Lo/Ovral-28*) in 28 women were unchanged. Serum progesterone levels also remained unaltered.[1] This agrees with the findings of earlier single dose studies which found that olestra had no effect on the bioavailability of single doses of **ethinylestradiol**, **norethisterone (norethindrone)**, **diazepam** or **propranolol**.[2]

Another randomised, double-blind, placebo-controlled study in 40 patients found that 12 g olestra daily for 2 weeks had no significant effect on the anticoagulant effects of **warfarin**. The olestra was contained in *Pringles Original Flavor Fat Free Potato Crisps with Olean* and the patients took 1.5 servings daily.[3] Olestra, which is a sucrose polyester, is a non-absorbable, noncaloric fat replacement. It has been concluded that olestra is unlikely to reduce the absorption of oral drugs in general.[1,4]

1. Miller KW, Williams DS, Carter SB, Jones MB, Mishell DR. The effect of olestra on systemic levels of oral contraceptives. *Clin Pharmacol Ther* (1990) 48, 34–40.
2. Roberts RJ, Leff RD. Influence of absorbable and nonabsorbable lipids and lipidlike substances on drug availability. *Clin Pharmacol Ther* (1989) 45, 299–304.
3. Beckey NP, Korman LB, Parra D. Effect of the moderate consumption of olestra in patients receiving long-term warfarin therapy. *Pharmacotherapy* (1999) 19, 1075–9.
4. Goldman P. Olestra: assessing its potential to interact with drugs in the gastrointestinal tract. *Clin Pharmacol Ther* (1997) 61, 613–18.

Omeprazole + Miscellaneous drugs

An isolated report describes prolonged atracurium effects possibly due to omeprazole. A small rise in serum digoxin levels may occur. Omeprazole appears not interact to a clinically important extent with alcohol, caffeine, food, lidocaine (lignocaine), quinidine or tolbutamide, nor is omeprazole affected by the concurrent use of *Maalox* or metoclopramide. An isolated report describes confusion and catatonia in a patient when treated with disulfiram and omeprazole.

Clinical importance, mechanism, importance and management

(a) Alcohol, Caffeine, Lidocaine (Lignocaine), Maalox, Metoclopramide, Quinidine, Tolbutamide

Two studies have shown that **antacids** (such as *Maalox*) and **metoclopramide** do not affect the absorption or disposition of omeprazole.[1,2] Omeprazole is also reported not to affect either blood **alcohol** levels[3-8] or the pharmacokinetics of **lidocaine**[9] or **caffeine**.[10] Yet another study found that omeprazole does not affect the pharmacokinetics or pharmacodynamics of **quinidine**.[11]

Omeprazole has a small but almost certainly clinically irrelevant effect (+10%) on the AUC of **tolbutamide**.[12] No special precautions would seem necessary if any of these drugs is given with omeprazole.

(b) Digoxin, Food

Food delays the absorption of omeprazole, but does not affect the total amount absorbed.[13] A study using 20 mg omeprazole daily for 11 days found that only minor changes occurred in the disposition of a 1 mg oral dose of **digoxin**. On average the AUC showed a 10% increase,[14,15] a possible reason being that it increases the gastric pH. Non-selective **digoxin** assay methods may fail to detect an interaction, whereas selective HPLC assay methods and ECG studies provide evidence that the bioavailability of **digoxin** may be increased by omeprazole.[16] Until this is confirmed and quantified it would seem reasonable to monitor concurrent use although a 10% rise is almost certainly too small to matter.

(c) Disulfiram

A patient on 40 mg omeprazole daily for 7 months was additionally given 500 mg **disulfiram** daily. Six days later he gradually developed confusion, which progressed into a catatonic state with muscle rigidity and trismus after 15 days. Both drugs were withdrawn and he gradually recovered. Some months later while taking 250 mg **disulfiram** daily, he again developed confusion, disorientation and nightmares within 72 h of starting to take 40 mg omeprazole each morning. He recovered when both drugs were stopped.[17] The reason for this reaction is not understood, but the authors of the report postulate that the omeprazole may have allowed the accumulation of one of the metabolites of **disulfiram**, carbon disulphide, which could have been responsible for the toxic effects.[17]

This is the first and only report of a possible interaction between omeprazole and **disulfiram**. Other patients given both drugs are said not have shown adverse effects.[18] The general importance of this adverse interaction is therefore uncertain, but it would now seem prudent to monitor concurrent use in any patient for any evidence of this toxicity.

1. Tuynman HARE, Festern HPM, Röhss K, Meuwissen SGM. Lack of effect of antacids on plasma concentrations of omeprazole given as enteric-coated granules. *Br J Clin Pharmacol* (1987) 24, 833–5.
2. Howden CW, Reid JL. The effect of antacids and metoclopramide on omeprazole absorption and disposition. *Br J Clin Pharmacol* (1988) 25, 779–80.
3. Guram M, Holt S. Are ethanol-H₂ receptor antagonist interactions "relevant". *Gastroenterology* (1991) 100, 5 Part 2, A749.
4. Jönsson K-Å, Jones AW, Boström T. No influence of omeprazole on the pharmacokinetics of ethanol in healthy men. World Congr Gastroenterology, Sydney, August 1990. Abstracts II, PD201.
5. Roine R, DiPadova C, Frezza M, Hernández-Muñoz R, Baraona E, Lieber CS. Effects of omeprazole, cimetidine and ranitidine on blood ethanol concentrations. *Gastroenterology* (1990) 98, A114.
6. Roine R, Hernández-Muñoz R, Baraona E, Greenstein R, Lieber CS. Effect of omeprazole on gastric first-pass metabolism of ethanol. *Dig Dis Sci* (1992) 37, 891–6.

7. Jönsson K-Å, Jones AW, Boström H, Andersson T. Lack of effect of omeprazole, cimetidine, and ranitidine on the pharmacokinetics of ethanol in fasting male volunteers. *Eur J Clin Pharmacol* (1992) 42, 209–12.
8. Minocha A. Rahal PS, Brier ME, Levinson SS. Omeprazole therapy does not affect pharmacokinetics of orally administered ethanol in healthy male subjects. *J Clin Gastroenterol* (1995) 21, 107–9.
9. Noble DW, Bannister J, Lamont M, Andersson T, Scott DB. The effect of oral omeprazole on the disposition of lignocaine. *Anaesthesia* (1994) 49, 497–500.
10. Andersson T, Bergstrand R, Cederberg C, Eriksson S, Lagerström P-F, Skånberg I. Omeprazole treatment does not affect the metabolism of caffeine. *Gastroenterology* (1991) 101, 943–7.
11. Ching MS, Elliott SL, Stead CK, Murdoch RT, Devenish-Meares S, Morgan DJ, Smallwood RA. Quinidine single dose pharmacokinetics and pharmacodynamics are not affected by omeprazole. *Aliment Pharmacol Ther* (1991) 5, 523–31.
12. Oosterhuis B, Jonkman JHG, Andersson T, Zuiderwijk PBM. No influence of single intravenous doses of omeprazole on theophylline elimination kinetics. *J Clin Pharmacol* (1992) 32, 470–5.
13. Rohss K, Andren K, Heggelund A, Lagerstrom P-O, Lundborg P. Bioavailability of omeprazole given in conjuction with food. III World Conf Clin Pharmacol Ther, Stockholm July-Aug 1986. *Acta Pharmacol Toxicol* (1986) 85 (Suppl 5), Abstract 207.
14. Oosterhuis B, Jonkman JHG. Omeprazole: pharmacology, pharmacokinetics and interactions. *Digestion* (1989) 44 (Suppl 1), 9–17.
15. Oosterhuis B, Jonkman JHG, Andersson T, Zuiderwijk PBM, Jedema JN. Minor effect of multiple dose omeprazole on the pharmacokinetics of digoxin after a single oral dose. *Br J Clin Pharmacol* (1991) 32, 569–72.
16. Cohen AF, Kroon R, Schoemaker HC, Hoogkamer JFW, van Vliet-Verbeek A. Effects of gastric acidity on the bioavailability of digoxin. Evidence for a new mechanism for interactions with omeprazole. *Br J Clin Pharmacol* (1991) 31, 565P.
17. Hajela R, Cunningham G M, Kapur B M, Peachey J E, Devenyi P. Catatonic reaction to omeprazole and disulfiram in a patient with alcohol dependence. *Can Med Assoc J* (1990) 143, 1207–8.
18. Campbell L M (Astra Pharmaceuticals). Personal communication 1991.

Ondansetron + Food or Antacids

Food slightly increases the bioavailability of ondansetron but an antacid was found to have no effect.

Clinical evidence, mechanism, importance and management

When 12 normal subjects were given an 8 mg ondansetron tablet 5 min after a **meal**, its bioavailability was slightly increased (AUC + 17%) but the coadministration of a **magnesium-aluminium hydroxide** antacid had no effect.[1]

1. Bozigian HP, Pritchard JF, Gooding AW, Pakes GE. Ondansetron absorption in adults: effect of dosage form, food, and antacids. *J Pharm Sci* (1994) 83, 1011–13.

Orlistat + Miscellaneous drugs

Pravastatin serum levels are possibly moderately increased by orlistat. The makers list a number of drugs (acarbose, anorectics, biguanides) which they suggest might possibly interact adversely with orlistat. Clinical reports about these predicted interactions are lacking. It is recommended that multivitamin preparations should be taken at least 2 h after orlistat or at bedtime. The control of diabetes with oral sulphonylureas appears to be improved by orlistat. No orlistat/alcohol interaction seems to occur. See Index for further information about orlistat and other drugs.

Clinical evidence, mechanism, importance and management

(a) Alcohol

A study in healthy subjects found that orlistat for 6 days had no significant effect on the pharmacokinetics of **alcohol**.[1] There is nothing to suggest that **alcohol** should be avoided while taking orlistat, and the makers say that no interactions have been observed.[2]

(b) Hypoglycaemic agents

A placebo-controlled study in 12 healthy subjects found that 80 mg orlistat three times daily for a little over 4 days had no effect on the pharmacokinetics of single 5 mg oral doses of **glibenclamide (glyburide)** and the blood glucose lowering effects remained unchanged.[3] A later large scale 1-year clinical trial in which 139 patients took orlistat

found that 43% of the obese diabetic patients taking 120 mg orlistat three times daily were able to decrease their **sulphonylurea** dosage (**glibenclamide** or **glipizide**), and 11.7% of them were able to discontinue the **sulphonylurea**. The average dose decrease was 23% compared with 9% in the placebo group.[4] Clearly concurrent use can be advantageous. The makers say that no interactions have been seen with **biguanides**.[2]

(c) Other drugs

The makers say that in the absence of pharmacokinetic studies the concomitant administration of orlistat with **acarbose** or **anorectic drugs** is not recommended.[2] The makers also say that no interactions have been seen with **digoxin, fibrates, phenytoin, oral contraceptives, nifedipine GITS,** or **nifedipine slow release** have been observed.

(d) Pravastatin

A comparative study was undertaken in two groups of healthy subjects given **pravastatin**, either with orlistat 80 to 120 mg three times daily or without orlistat. After 10 days the orlistat group showed increased maximum serum **pravastatin** levels of 26% and an increase in the AUC of 33%, but this was not significantly different to the placebo group although it did show a tendency to be higher.[1] In contrast another study failed to find that orlistat had any effect on the pharmacokinetics of **pravastatin** and its lipid-lowering effects were unchanged.[5]

(e) Vitamins A, D, E, K and beta-carotene

Although there is good evidence that patients taking long-term orlistat have **vitamin A, D, E, K** and **beta-carotene** levels in the normal range, because orlistat may potentially impair the absorption of these fat-soluble vitamins (it blocks the ingestion of about one third of dietary fats) the makers recommend that any **multivitamin preparations** should be taken at least 2 h after the orlistat or at bedtime[2] to ensure maximum vitamin absorption. A study in healthy subjects found that about two-thirds of a supplemental dose of **beta-carotene** were absorbed in the presence of orlistat.[6]

1. Guerciolini R. Mode of action of orlistat. *Int J Obes* (1997) 21 (Suppl 3), S12–S23.
2. Xenical (Orlistat). Roche Product Limited. Summary of product characteristics, October 2001.
3. Zhi J, Melia AT, Koss-Twardy SG, Min B, Guerciolini R, Freundlich NL, Milla G, Patel IH. The influence of orlistat on the pharmacokinetics and pharmacodynamics of glyburide in healthy volunteers. *J Clin Pharmacol* (1995) 35, 521–5.
4. Hollander PA, Elbein SC, Hirsch IB, Kelley D, McGill J, Taylor T, Weiss SR, Crockett SE, Kaplan RA, Comstock J, Lucas CP, Lodewick PA, Canovatchel W, Chung J, Hauptman J. Role of orlistat in the treatment of obese patients with type 2 diabetes. A 1-year randomized double-blind study. *Diabetes Care* (1998) 21, 1288–94.
5. Oo CY, Akbari B, Lee S, Nichols G, Hellmann CR. Effect of orlistat, a novel anti-obesity agent, on the pharmacokinetics and pharmacodynamics of pravastatin in patients with mild hypercholesterolaemia. *Clin Drug Invest* (1999) 17, 217–23.
6. Zhi J, Melia AT, Koss-Twardy SG, Arora S, Patel IH. The effect of orlistat, an inhibitor of dietary fat absorption, on the pharmacokinetics of β-carotene in healthy volunteers. *J Clin Pharmacol* (1996) 36, 152–9.

Oxybutynin + Itraconazole

Itraconazole can increase the serum levels of oxybutynin, but its adverse effects are not increased and this interaction is considered to be of only minor clinical relevance.

Clinical evidence, mechanism, importance and management

A single 5-mg dose of oxybutynin was given to 10 healthy subjects after taking 200 mg **itraconazole** or a placebo daily for 4 days. The peak serum levels and the AUC of the oxybutynin were about doubled while the pharmacokinetics of the active metabolite of oxybutynin were unchanged. The sum of the oxybutynin and its metabolite concentrations were on average about 13% higher than with the placebo. No increase in adverse effects was seen. What occurred was almost certainly due to inhibition by the **itraconazole** of the metabolism (by the cytochrome P450 isoenzyme CYP3A4) of the oxybutynin in the intestinal wall and liver. The authors of this report consider that this interaction is only of minor importance and, because **itraconazole** is a known and potent enzyme inhibitor, they also predict that other CYP3A4 inhibitors which are less potent (they cite **erythromycin**, **diltiazem**, **verapamil**) are unlikely to interact with oxybutynin significantly.[1]

1. Lukkari E, Juhakoski A, Aranko K, Neuvonen PJ. Itraconazole moderately increases serum concentrations of oxybutynin but does not affect those of the active metabolite. *Eur J Clin Pharmacol* (1997) 52, 403–6.

Oxygen (hyperbaric) + Acetazolamide, Barbiturates or Opioids

It has been suggested, but not confirmed, that because increased levels of carbon dioxide in the tissues can increase the sensitivity to oxygen-induced convulsions, drugs such as acetazolamide, which are carbonic anhydrase-inhibitors, are contraindicated in those given hyperbaric oxygen, because they cause carbon dioxide to persist in the tissues. Nor should hyperbaric oxygen be given during opioid or barbiturate withdrawal because the convulsive threshold of such patients is already low.[1]

1. Gunby P. HBO can interact with preexisting patient conditions. *JAMA* (1981) 246, 1177–8.

Pantoprazole + Miscellaneous drugs

Pantoprazole appears not to interact to a clinically relevant extent with alcohol, carbamazepine, cisapride, diazepam, diclofenac, digoxin, glibenclamide (glyburide), *Maalox*, metoprolol, nifedipine, oral contraceptives, phenprocoumon, phenytoin or warfarin. Pantoprazole does not affect phenazone (antipyrine) and is therefore unlikely to interact with many drugs which are affected by enzyme inducers or inhibitors.

Clinical evidence, mechanism, importance and management

(a) Alcohol

Pantoprazole 40 mg or a placebo was given daily to 16 healthy subjects for 7 days. On day 7 they were also given 0.5 g **alcohol**/kg body weight in 200 ml orange juice 2 h after a standard breakfast. The maximum serum levels and the AUC of the **alcohol** were not significantly changed by the pantoprazole.[1] No special precautions would therefore appear to be necessary.

(b) Antacids

Pantoprazole 40 mg daily was given to 24 healthy subjects with and without 10 ml *Maalox 70*. The AUC, maximum serum levels and the half-life of the pantoprazole were unchanged by the antacid.[2] No special precautions would seem to be necessary if pantoprazole and *Maalox* are given concurrently.

(c) Anticoagulants

No change in the response to a single 25-mg oral dose of **warfarin** was seen in 26 healthy subjects while they were additionally taking 40 mg pantoprazole daily. The pharmacokinetics of *(R)*- and *(S)*-**warfarin** were unaltered and no changes in the pharmacodynamics of the **warfarin** (prothrombin time, factor VII) were seen.[3,4] No change in the responses to **phenprocoumon**, either pharmacokinetic or pharmacodynamic, was seen in 16 healthy subjects when they were additionally given 40 mg pantoprazole daily for 5 days.[5] No special precautions would seem to be necessary if pantoprazole and either **phenprocoumon** or **warfarin** are given concurrently. Information about other anticoagulants appears to be lacking.

(d) Carbamazepine

Pantoprazole 40 mg or a placebo was given daily to 20 healthy subjects for 11 days, and on day 5 they were additionally given a single 400-mg dose of **carbamazepine**. The pharmacokinetics of the **carbamazepine** and its **epoxide metabolite** were found to be unchanged by the pantoprazole.[6] No special precautions would seem to be necessary if both drugs are given concurrently.

(e) Cisapride

Single 20-mg doses of **cisapride** were given to 16 healthy subjects either alone or 1 h after the first of three 40-mg daily doses of pantoprazole. No QTc changes occurred, with or without pantoprazole, and the only pharmacokinetic changes were a 17% fall in the maximum **cisapride** concentrations and an 11% increase in clearance, possibly due to gastric hypochlorhydria caused by the pantoprazole.[7] This small interaction is almost certainly not clinically important and there would appear to be no reason for avoiding the concurrent use of these two drugs.

(f) Contraceptives, oral

A study over four menstrual cycles was completed by 64 pre-menopausal women. During cycle 1 they were given no treatment and ovulation was confirmed. In cycles 2 and 3 they were given a **low-dose triphasic oral contraceptive** (*Triphasil*), and lack of ovulation was confirmed. In cycle 4, both the **oral contraceptive** and 40 mg pantoprazole daily were given, and lack of ovulation was again checked. None of the women ovulated while taking both drugs, and so it was concluded that pantoprazole does not affect oral contraception. The study also indicates that pantoprazole does not induce cytochrome CYP3A.[8]

(g) Diazepam

Placebo or 240 mg pantoprazole (as intravenous injections) was given to 12 healthy subjects for 7 days. The half-life, clearance and AUC of 0.1 mg/kg **diazepam** given as an intravenous bolus were unchanged by the pantoprazole.[9] No special precautions would seem to be necessary if pantoprazole and **diazepam** are given concurrently.

(h) Diclofenac

Single oral doses of 40 mg pantoprazole and 100 mg **diclofenac** (enteric coated *Voltarol*) were given to 24 healthy subjects together and separately. Neither drug affected the pharmacokinetics of the other and it was concluded that the two can be given together without dosage adjustment.[10]

(i) Digoxin

β-**acetyldigoxin** 200 micrograms twice daily was given to 18 healthy subjects, with and without 40 mg pantoprazole daily, for 5 days. The pantoprazole caused a slight (10%) rise in the **digoxin** AUC and a 9% rise in the maximum **digoxin** serum levels, but both were considered to be clinically irrelevant and no changes in the **digoxin**-induced height reduction in the T-wave occurred.[11,12] This study confirmed the findings of a previous single dose study.[13] No special precautions would seem to be necessary if pantoprazole and **digoxin** are given concurrently.

(j) Glibenclamide (Glyburide)

Pantoprazole 40 mg or placebo was given to 20 healthy subjects daily for 5 days. On day 5 the subjects were additionally given 3.5 mg **glibenclamide** (**glyburide**). The pharmacokinetics of the **glibenclamide** and the pharmacodynamic profiles of glucose and insulin serum concentrations were not significantly altered, nor were the pharmacokinetics of pantoprazole affected. It was concluded that no **glibenclamide** dosage changes are needed during treatment with pantoprazole.[14,15]

(k) Metoprolol

No pharmacokinetic or pharmacodynamic interactions were seen in a randomised double-blind crossover study 18 healthy subjects given 95 mg **metoprolol** and 40 mg pantoprazole daily for 5 days. No special precautions would therefore seem necessary if both drugs are given concurrently.[16]

(l) Nifedipine

In an open, randomised, crossover study 24 healthy subjects were given 40 mg pantoprazole daily for 10 days, with 20 mg sustained-release **nifedipine** twice daily from day 6 to 10. The pharmacokinetics of the **nifedipine** were unchanged by the pantoprazole.[17] No special precautions would seem to be necessary if pantoprazole and **nifedipine** are given concurrently.

(m) Phenytoin

In a randomised crossover study 24 healthy subjects showed no changes in the pharmacokinetics (AUC, maximum serum levels, half-life) of a single 300-mg dose of **phenytoin** while taking 40 mg pantoprazole daily for 7 days.[18] No special precautions would seem to be necessary if pantoprazole and **phenytoin** are given concurrently.

(n) Phenazone (Antipyrine) and Caffeine

Single intravenous doses of pantoprazole and single 5-mg/kg oral doses of **phenazone** were given to 12 healthy subjects. In another study 12 healthy men were given 40 mg pantoprazole daily for 7 days and single 5 mg/kg oral doses of **phenazone**. No changes in the pharmacokinetics of the **phenazone** were seen in either study.[19] **Phenazone** is used as a marker or indicator of possible changes in mixed hepatic oxidase activity, so that the lack of effect of pantoprazole indicates that pantoprazole is unlikely to interact with many drugs which are affected by enzyme inducers or inhibitors. Further evidence of this is that the administration of 40 mg pantoprazole once-daily for a week was found to have no effect on the urinary excretion of 6b-hydroxycortisol and D-glucaric acid.[20] Another study using **caffeine** similarly found that pantoprazole does not induce cytochrome P450 isoenzyme CYP1A2 in man.[21]

1. Teyssen S, Singer MV, Heinze H, Pfützer R, Huber R, Harder H, Stephan S, Schneider A, Fischer R. Pantoprazole does not influence the pharmacokinetics of ethanol in healthy volunteers. *Gastroenterology* (1996) 110 (4 Suppl), A277.
2. Hartmann M, Bliesath H, Huber R, Koch H, Steinijans VW, Wurst W. Lack of influence of antacids on the pharmacokinetics of the new gastric H⁺/K⁺-ATPase inhibitor pantoprazole. *Gastroenterology* (1994) 106 (Suppl), A91.
3. Müller FO, Middle MV, Duursema L, Hundt HKL, Swart KJ, Schall R, Luus HG, Bliesath H, Steinijans VW, Wurst W. Pantoprazole does not affect the pharmacodynamics and pharmacokinetics of warfarin in healthy males. *Klin Pharmakol Akt* (1993) 4, 40.
4. Duursema L, Müller FO, Schall R, Middle MV, Hundt HKL, Groenewoud G, Steinijans VW, Bliesath H. Lack of effect of pantoprazole on the pharmacodynamics and pharmacokinetics of warfarin. *Br J Clin Pharmacol* (1995) 39, 700–3.
5. Ehrlich A, Fuder H, Hartmann M, Wieckhorst G, Timmer W, Huber R, Birkel M, Bliesath H, Steinijans VW, Wurst W, Lücker PW. Lack of pharmacokinetic and pharmacodynamic interaction between pantoprazole and phenprocoumon in man. *Eur J Clin Pharmacol* (1996) 51, 277–81.
6. Huber R, Bliesath H, Hartmann M, Koch H, Steinijans VW, Mascher H, Wurst W. Pantoprazole does not interact with the pharmacokinetics of carbamazepine. *Gastroenterology* (1996) 110 (4 Suppl), A137.
7. Ferron GM, Paul J, Fruncillo RJ, Martin PT, Yacoub L, Mayer PR. A pharmacokinetic study of the potential drug interaction between oral pantoprazole and cisapride in healthy adults. *Gastroenterology* (1998) 114, A12.
8. Middle MV, Müller FO, Schall R, Hundt HKL, Mogilnicka EM, Beneke PC. Effect of pantoprazole on ovulation suppression by a low-dose hormonal contraceptive. *Clin Drug Invest* (1995) 9, 54–6.
9. Gugler R, Hartmann M, Rudi J, Brod I, Huber R, Steinijans VW, Bliesath H, Wurst W, Klotz U. Lack of pharmacokinetic interaction of pantoprazole and diazepam in man. *Br J Clin Pharmacol* (1996) 42, 249–52.
10. Bliesath H, Huber R, Steinijans VW, Koch HJ, Wurst W, Mascher H. Lack of pharmacokinetic interaction between pantoprazole and diclofenac. *Int J Clin Pharmacol Ther* (1996) 34, 152–6.
11. Hartmann M, Huber R, Bliesath H, Steinijans VW, Koch HJ, Wurst W, Kunz K. Lack of interaction between pantoprazole and digoxin at therapeutic doses in man. In: Management of acid-related diseases: Focus on pantoprazole. Congress Abstracts, Charité, Berlin 1993, p 34-5.
12. Hartmann M, Huber R, Bliesath H, Steinijans VW, Koch HJ, Wurst W, Kunz K. Lack of interaction between pantoprazole and digoxin at therapeutic doses in man. *Int J Clin Pharmacol Ther* (1996) 34, 481–5.
13. Oosterhuis B, Jonkman JHG, Andersson T, Zuiderwijk PBM, JedeMa JN. Minor effect of multiple dose omeprazole on the pharmacokinetics of digoxin after a single oral dose. *Br J Clin Pharmacol* (1991) 32, 569–72.
14. Stötzer F, Walter-Sack I, Bliesath H, Huber R, Steinijans VW, Wurst W. No influence of pantoprazole on glibenclamide pharmacokinetics and pharmacodynamics. *Eur J Clin Pharmacol* (1996) 50, 554.
15. Walter-Sack IE, Bliesath H, Stötzer F, Huber R, Steinijans VW, Ding R, Mascher H, Wurst W. Lack of pharmacokinetic and pharmacodynamic interaction between pantoprazole and glibenclamide in humans. *Clin Drug Invest* (1998) 15, 253–60.
16. Koch HJ, Hartmann M, Bliesath H, Huber R, Steinijans VW, Mascher H, Wurst W. Pantoprazole does not interact with metoprolol pharmacokinetics and pharmacodynamics in man under steady state conditions. *Eur J Clin Pharmacol* (1996) 50, 547.
17. Bliesath H, Huber R, Hartmann M, Koch H, Steinijans VW, Wurst W. Pantoprazole does not influence the steady-state pharmacokinetics of nifedipine. *Gastroenterology* (1994) 106 (Suppl), A55.
18. Müller FO, Bliesath H, Middle MV, Hundt HKL, Hartmann M, Schall R, Steinijans VW, Huber R, Wurst W. Pantoprazole does not influence the pharmacokinetics of phenytoin in man. *Klin Pharmakol Akt* (1993) 4, 26.
19. De Mey C, Meineke I, Steinijans VW, Huber R, Hartmann M, Bliesath H, Wurst W. Pantoprazole lacks interaction with antipyrine in man, either by inhibition or induction. *Int J Clin Pharmacol Ther* (1994) 32, 98–106.
20. Reill L, Erhardt F, Fischer R, Rost KL, Roots I, Londong W. Effect of oral pantoprazole on 24-hour intragastric pH, serum gastrin profile and drug metabolizing activity in man - a placebo-controlled comparison with ranitidine. *Gut* (1993) 34 (4 Suppl), S63.
21. Steinijans VW, Huber R, Hartmann M, Zech K, Bliesath H, Wurst W, Radtke HW. Lack of pantoprazole drug interactions in man: an updated review. *Int J Clin Pharmacol Ther* (1996) 34 (Suppl 1), S31–S50.

Papaverine + Benzodiazepines

Two men given normal test doses of papaverine for the investigation of impotence had prolonged penile erections attributed to the concurrent use of diazepam.

Clinical evidence, mechanism, importance and management

Undesirably prolonged erections (duration of 5 and 6 h) occurred in 2 patients who had been given 5 or 10 mg **diazepam** intravenously for anxiety before a 60-mg papaverine injection.[1] Papaverine acts by relaxing the arterioles which supply the corpora so that the pressure rises. The increased pressure in the corpora compresses the trabecular venules so that the pressure continues to maintain the erection. **Diazepam** also relaxes smooth muscle and this it would seem can be additive with the effects of papaverine. The authors of the report say that say that caution should be exercised in the choice of papaverine dosage in patients on anxiolytics (i.e. use less) although these two cases involving **diazepam** seem to be the only ones recorded.[1]

1. Vale JA, Kirby RS, Lees W. Papaverine, benzodiazepines, and prolonged erections. *Lancet* (1991) 337, 1552.

Paraldehyde + Disulfiram

Concurrent use should be avoided because toxic reactions seem likely.

Clinical evidence, mechanism, importance and management

It is thought that paraldehyde is depolymerised in the liver to acetaldehyde, and then oxidised by acetaldehyde dehydrogenase.[1] Since **disulfiram** inhibits this enzyme, concurrent use would be expected to result in the accumulation of acetaldehyde and in a modified **disulfiram** reaction,[2] but so far there appear to be no reports of this in man. In addition, alcoholics with impaired liver function are said to be sensitive to the toxic effects of paraldehyde and may show restlessness rather than sedation. These are all good reasons for avoiding concurrent use.

1. Hitchcock P, Nelson EE. The metabolism of paraldehyde: II. *J Pharmacol Exp Ther* (1943) 79, 286–94.
2. Keplinger ML, Wells JA. Effect of Antabuse on the action of paraldehyde in mice and dogs. *Fedn Proc* (1956) 15, 445–6.

Pentoxifylline (Oxpentifylline) + Cimetidine

Cimetidine increases plasma pentoxifylline (oxpentifylline) levels to a moderate extent.

Clinical evidence, mechanism, importance and management

Cimetidine 300 mg four times daily for 7 days increased the mean steady-state plasma of pentoxifylline (taken as a 400 mg controlled-release tablet 8-hourly) in 10 healthy subjects by 27.4%.[1] The reason is not known. Side-effects such as headaches, nausea, vomiting were said to be more common and bothersome while taking the **cimetidine**,[1] however there seems to be no strong reasons for avoiding concurrent use.

1. Mauro VF, Mauro LS, Hageman JH. Alteration of pentoxifylline pharmacokinetics by cimetidine. *J Clin Pharmacol* (1988) 28, 649–54.

Pentoxifylline (Oxpentifylline) + Ciprofloxacin

Preliminary evidence suggests that ciprofloxacin increases the serum levels of pentoxifylline (oxpentifylline). Toxicity is possible.

Clinical evidence, mechanism, importance and management

Because patients taking pentoxifylline (oxpentifylline) and **ciprofloxacin** often complained of headaches, the possibility of an interaction was studied in 6 healthy subjects.[1] This showed that 500 mg **ciprofloxacin** daily for 3 days increased the peak serum levels of pentoxifylline following a single 400-mg dose, by almost 60% (from 114.5 to 179.5 nanograms/ml) and increased the AUC by 15%. The evidence suggests that the **ciprofloxacin** inhibits the metabolism of the pentoxifylline by the liver. All 6 subjects complained of a frontal headache. On the basis of these results the author of the study suggests that the dosage of pentoxifylline should be halved in those taking **ciprofloxacin**.

1. Cleary JD. Ciprofloxacin and pentoxyfylline: a clinically significant drug interaction. *Pharmacotherapy* (1992) 12, 259–60.

Perhexiline + Selective serotonin re-uptake inhibitors (SSRIs)

Three case reports describe an increase in perhexiline serum levels with toxicity due to the concurrent use of fluoxetine or paroxetine.

Clinical evidence, mechanism, importance and management

An 86-year-old woman on perhexiline was admitted to hospital because she was unable to cope at home and because of ataxia, falls, lethargy and nausea. She had started to take 20 mg **paroxetine** daily 5 weeks earlier. Her serum perhexiline levels were considerably raised, 2.02 mg/l compared with the normal range of 0.15 to 0.6 mg/l.[1] Perhexiline toxicity was also seen in two other elderly women following the use of **paroxetine** in one case, and **fluoxetine** in the other. The perhexiline serum levels fell when both drugs were stopped, but in one case the fall was very slow.[2]

The reason for the rise in perhexiline levels is not known, but it seems likely that these SSRIs can inhibit its metabolism. The general importance of these interactions is also not known, but it would now be prudent to monitor perhexiline serum levels closely if these or any other SSRIs are given concurrently, being alert for the need to reduce the perhexiline dosage. More study is needed.

1. Alderman CP. Perhexiline-paroxetine interaction. *Aust J Hosp Pharm* (1998) 28, 254–5.
2. Alderman CP, Hundertmark JD, Soetratma TW. Interaction of serotonin re-uptake inhibitors with perhexiline. *Aust N Z J Psychiatry* (1997) 31, 601–3.

Piperine + Miscellaneous drugs

Piperine can increase the bioavailability of phenytoin, propranolol, rifampicin (rifampin), theophylline and some other drugs.

Clinical evidence, mechanism, importance and management

A study in 5 healthy subjects found that piperine 20 mg, for 7 days, increased the absorption of a single 300 mg oral dose of **phenytoin** (AUC + 50%) and raised the peak serum levels.[1] In another study in 12 subjects, 20 mg piperine daily for 7 days roughly doubled the peak serum levels and the AUCs of single doses of **propranolol** and **theophylline**.[2] Piperine 50 mg was also found to increase the AUC of 450 mg **rifampicin** by 70% in 14 patients with tuberculosis.[3] Piperine 20 mg increased the bioavailability of **curcumin** (obtained from *Curcuma longa*) by 2000% in a study in man.[4] An experimental study found that *Piper longum* (containing piperine) increased the serum levels of **vasicine** (used as a test drug) by more than almost 233%, and piperine increased the serum levels of **sparteine** (another test drug) by more than 100%.[5]

Piperine is the major alkaloid of black and long peppers (*Piper nigrum* and *longum*) both of which are used in Ayurvedic formulations, the presumption being that these plant products are empirically included to increase the bioavailability of other constituents, thereby increasing their efficacy. One of the reports[1] also quotes other studies showing that the piperine increases blood levels of **sulfadiazine** and **tetracycline**. No cases of adverse interactions seem to have been reported but it seems possible that piperine might increase some drug levels to toxic concentrations.

1. Bano G, Amla V, Raina RK, Zutshi U, Chopra CL. The effect of piperine on pharmacokinetics of phenytoin in healthy volunteers. *Planta Med* (1987) 53, 568–9.
2. Bano G, Raina RK, Zutshi U, Bedi KL, Johri RK, Sharma SC. Effect of piperine on bioavailability and pharmacokinetics of propranolol and theophylline in healthy volunteers. *Eur J Clin Pharmacol* (1991) 41, 615–17.
3. Zutshi RK, Singh R, Zutshi U, Johri RK, Atal CK. Influence of piperine on rifampicin blood levels in patients of pulmonary tuberculosis. *J Assoc Physicians India* (1985) 33, 223–4.
4. Shoba G, Joy D, Joseph T, Majeed M, Rajendran R, Srinivas PSSR. Influence of piperine on the pharmacokinetics of curcumin in animals and human volunteers. *Planta Med* (1998) 64, 353–6.
5. Atal CK, Zutshi U, Rao PG. Scientific evidence on the role of Ayurvedic herbals on bioavailability of drugs. *J Ethnopharmacol* (1981) 4, 229–32.

Pirenzepine + Cimetidine, Food or Antacid

Food and *Mylanta* reduce the bioavailability of pirenzepine by about 30%. Another antacid, *Trigastril*, modestly raises the bioavailability of pirenzepine, but these changes are probably of little clinical importance. Pirenzepine and cimetidine appear to interact together, possibly advantageously.

Clinical evidence, mechanism, importance and management

The pharmacokinetics of pirenzepine and **cimetidine** are not affected by the presence of the other drug, but pirenzepine increases the **cimetidine**-induced reduction in gastric acid secretion, which is an apparently advantageous interaction.[1]

The AUC of a single 50-mg dose of pirenzepine in 20 healthy subjects was reduced by about 30% when pirenzepine was taken half-an-hour **before food, with food** or with 30 ml *Mylanta*. The **food** and **antacid** reduced the peak plasma levels by about 30% and 45% respectively, and the **food** shortened the time to achieve peak levels.[2] Another study found that the AUC of a single 50-mg dose of pirenzepine in 10 healthy subjects was increased by almost 25% by 10 ml of an **antacid** (*Trigastril*, **magnesium and aluminium hydroxides, calcium carbonate**).[3] In practical terms these modest changes in bioavailability are probably too small to matter, and in fact the makers suggest that pirenzepine should be taken half-an-hour before meals with a little fluid. The authors of this report also suggest taking it with **food** because compliance is better if associated with a convenient daily ritual.[2]

1. Jamali F, Mahachai V, Reilly PA, Thomson ABR. Lack of pharmacokinetic interaction between cimetidine and pirenzepine. *Clin Pharmacol Ther* (1985) 38, 325–30.
2. Matzek KM, MacGregor TR, Keirns JJ, Vinocur M. Effect of food and antacids on the oral absorption of pirenzepine in man. *Int J Pharmaceutics* (1986) 28, 151–5.
3. Vergin H, Herrlinger C, Gugler R. Effect of an aluminium-hydroxide containing antacid on the oral bioavailability of pirenzepine. *Arzneimittelforschung* (1989) 39, 520–3.

Polygeline + Gentamicin

The incidence of acute renal failure appears to be increased in cardiac surgical patients given polygeline (*Haemaccel*) with gentamicin.

Clinical evidence

The observation of a differing incidence of acute renal failure in patients undergoing coronary artery bypass surgery in two similar units, prompted a retrospective review of patient records. This showed that the only management differences were related to antibacterial prophylaxis and the bypass prime content.

Acute renal failure was defined as a more than 50% rise in serum creatinine on the first postoperative day in those patients whose creatinine was also greater than 120 micromol/l.

Four groups of patients were identified, and the incidence of renal failure was as follows: Group A (polygeline plus **gentamicin** and **flucloxacillin**) 31% (28 out of 91 patients); Group B (polygeline plus **cefalotin**) 12% (9 out of 72 patients); group C (crystalloid plus **gentamicin** and **flucloxacillin**) 7% (4 out of 57 patients); and group D (crystalloid plus **cefalotin**) 2% (1 out of 47 patients). Polygeline (*Haemaccel*) 1 litre, which is a urea linked gelatine colloid with a calcium concentration of 6.25 micromol/l, was used for groups A and B, with crystalloid - Hartmann's solution or Ringer's injection (calcium concentration 2 mmol/l) to make up the rest of the prime volume of 2 litres. Groups C and D received only crystalloid (no polygeline) in the prime. Albumin 100 ml was used in groups B and D.[1]

Mechanism

Not fully understood. It is thought that the relatively high calcium content of the polygeline may have potentiated the nephrotoxicity which is associated with the use of gentamicin. Hypercalcaemia has been shown in *animals* to increase aminoglycoside-induced nephrotoxicity.[2]

Importance and management

Information appears to be limited to this clinical study and *animal* studies, but the evidence available suggests that a clinically important adverse interaction occurs between these drugs. The incidence of acute renal failure in cardiac surgery patients is normally about 3 to 5%[3] which is low compared with the 31% shown by those on polygeline and gentamicin. The authors of the study advise avoidance of these two drugs. More study is needed.

1. Schneider M, Valentine S, Clarke GM, Newman MAJ, Peakcock J. Acute renal failure in cardiac surgical patients potentiated by gentamicin and calcium. *Anaesth Intensive Care* (1996) 24, 647–50.
2. Elliott WC, Patchin DS, Jones DB. Effect of parathyroid hormone activity on gentamicin nephrotoxicity. *J Lab Clin Med* (1987) 109, 48–54.
3. Hilberman M, Myers BD, Carrie BJ, Derby G, Jamison RL, Stinson EB. Acute renal failure following cardiac surgery. *J Thorac Cardiovasc Surg* (1979) 77, 880–88.

Pravastatin + Colestyramine or Colestipol

Although colestyramine and colestipol reduce serum pravastatin levels, their total lipid-lowering effects are increased by concurrent use. Separating their administration minimises this interaction. Concurrent use appears to be safe and effective.

Clinical evidence

(a) Colestyramine

Pravastatin 5, 10, or 20 mg twice daily was given to 33 patients with primary hypercholesterolaemia for 4 weeks before their morning and evening meals, to which was later added 24 g **colestyramine** daily with meals for a further 4 weeks. The **colestyramine** was taken at least an hour after the pravastatin. Despite the fact that the colesty-ramine reduced the bioavailability of the pravastatin by 18 to 49% the blood lipid level reduction caused by pravastatin was enhanced by the addition of the **colestyramine**.[1] A related study in 18 subjects found that **colestyramine** reduced the bioavailability of pravastatin by about 40% when given together, but only small and clinically insignificant pharmacokinetic changes occurred when the pravastatin was given 1 h before or 4 h after the **colestyramine**.[2]

A multicentre study involving 311 patients found that combined use of 40 mg pravastatin plus 12 g **colestyramine** daily was highly effective in the treatment of hypercholesterolaemia and without significant problems.[3]

(b) Colestipol

Colestipol reduced the bioavailability of pravastatin in 18 subjects by about 50%, but no reduction in bioavailability was seen when pravastatin was given 1 h before **colestipol**, or if the combination was given with food.[2]

Mechanism

It seems probable that these bile acid binding resins bind with pravastatin in the gut, thereby reducing its absorption.

Importance and management

Established interactions but of only relatively minor importance. Despite the reduction in the bioavailability of the pravastatin caused by the colestyramine or colestipol, the overall lipid-lowering effect is increased by concurrent use.[1,3] The effects of the interaction can be minimised by separating their administration as described above. This can be easily achieved by taking the colestyramine or colestipol with meals, and the pravastatin at bedtime.

1. Pan HY, DeVault AR, Swites BJ, Whigan D, Ivashkiv E, Willard DA, Brescia D. Pharmacokinetics and pharmacodynamics of pravastatin alone and with cholestyramine in hypercholesterolemia. *Clin Pharmacol Ther* (1990) 48, 201–7.
2. Pan HY, DeVault AR, Ivashkiv E, Whigan D, Brennan JJ, Willard DA. Pharmacokinetic interaction studies of pravastatin with bile-acid-binding resins. 8th International Symposium on Atherosclerosis, October 9-13, Rome (1988), 711.
3. Pravastatin Multicenter Study Group II. Comparative efficacy and safety of pravastatin and cholestyramine alone and combined in patients with hypercholesterolemia. *Arch Intern Med* (1993) 153, 1321–9.

Pravastatin + Mianserin

An isolated report describes rhabdomyolysis attributed to the long-term concurrent use of pravastatin and mianserin, triggered by a cold.

Clinical evidence, mechanism, importance and management

An isolated report describes a woman of 72 on **pravastatin** 20 mg and **mianserin** 10 mg daily for 2 years and who was hospitalised because of weakness in her legs which began 2 days previously, shortly after getting a cold. She could stand but not walk unaided. Laboratory data revealed evidence of increased serum enzymes, all of which suggested rhabdomyolysis. Within a week of stopping the **pravastatin** the leg weakness had disappeared and all of the laboratory readings had returned to normal. The authors of the report attributed the toxicity to the long term use of both drugs, ageing and the development of a cold.[1] But what part these factors and/or the presence of mianserin actually played in the development of this toxicity is not known. However, it does highlight the need to monitor the use of all of the statins, even pravastatin which appears normally to be relatively free of adverse interactions.

1. Takei A, Chiba S. Rhabdomyolysis associated with pravastatin treatment for major depression. *Psychiatry Clin Neurosci* (1999) 53, 539.

Pravastatin + Miscellaneous drugs

No clinically significant interactions have been seen in studies on pravastatin taken with antipyrine, aspirin, cimetidine, digoxin, grapefruit juice, itraconazole, *Maalox*, nicotinic acid, oral contraceptives or probucol. No interactions were seen in clinical trials in patients taking pravastatin and ACE inhibitors, antihypertensives, beta-blockers, calcium channel blockers, digitalis, diuretics or 'nitroglycerins'.

Clinical evidence, mechanism, importance and management

No clinically significant changes in the bioavailability of single 20-mg doses of pravastatin were seen in studies in which 20 healthy subjects took 500 mg **probucol**.[1] The concurrent use of *Maalox TC* 15 ml four times daily, given 1 h before pravastatin, reduced the bioavailability of a single 20-mg dose of pravastatin by 28%.[2] The concurrent use of **cimetidine** 300 mg four times daily, given 1 h prior to pravastatin, increased the bioavailability of a single 20-mg dose of pravastatin by 58%.[2] However, the makers say that it is unlikely that the changes caused by *Maalox* and **cimetidine** will affect the clinical efficacy of pravastatin.[2,3] Only minor and clinically irrelevant changes in the serum levels of a single 40-mg dose of pravastatin were seen in a study in 10 healthy subjects after taking 200 mg **itraconazole** daily for 4 days.[4] Other studies found that neither **aspirin** 324 mg,[5] **nicotinic acid** 1 g[5] nor **grapefruit juice**[6] significantly affected the pharmacokinetics of pravastatin.

The pharmacokinetics of a single 20-mg dose of pravastatin were found to be unaffected in 15 young women taking **oral contraceptives (ethinylestradiol + norethisterone (norethindrone), norgestrel or levonorgestrel)** when compared with similar women not taking contraceptives. No adverse effects attributable to concurrent use were seen.[7] Pravastatin 20 mg daily for 9 days had no significant effect on steady state **digoxin** serum levels of 18 healthy subjects given **digoxin** 200 micrograms daily.[8] The makers also say that during clinical trials of pravastatin no noticeable drug interactions were seen in patients taking **diuretics**, **antihypertensives**, **ACE inhibitors**, **calcium channel blockers**, **beta-blockers** or **'nitroglycerins'**.[3] A study in healthy subjects given pravastatin found that 40 mg **propranolol** twice daily reduced the AUC of total inhibitors (active plus potentially active pravastatin metabolites) by 23%, of active inhibitors (active metabolites) by 20% and of pravastatin by 16%.[9] These changes are small and would seem to confirm the lack of interaction with **beta-blockers**. No special precautions would seem to be necessary if any of these drugs is given concurrently.

Antipyrine (phenazone) is used as a model or marker drug to find out if drugs are likely to affect the metabolism of others. A study in 24 type II hypercholesterolaemic patients given 5, 10 or 20 mg pravastatin twice daily for 4 weeks found that **antipyrine** saliva samples showed no changes in either its elimination half-life or its clearance.[10] Thus pravastatin appears not to induce or inhibit liver microsomal enzymes (cytochrome P450 system) and would not be expected to interact with other drugs commonly affected in this way (e.g. **phenytoin**, **warfarin**). The lack of an interaction with **warfarin** has been confirmed (see Index).

1. Pan HY, Glaess SR, Kassalow LM, Meehan RL, Martynowicz H. A report on the bioavailability of pravastatin in the presence and absence of probucol in healthy male subjects. Data on file, ER Squibb. Protocol No. 277, 201-18 (1988).
2. Marino MR, Pan HY, Bakry D, Glaess SR, Martynowicz H. A report on the comparative pharmacokinetics of pravastatin in the presence and absence of cimetidine or antacids in healthy male subjects. Data on file, ER Squibb. Protocol No 27, 201-43 (1988).
3. Lipostat (Pravastatin).Bristol-Myers Squibb Pharmaceuticals Ltd. Summary of product characteristics, June 2001.
4. Neuvonen PJ, Kantola T, Kivostö KT. Simvastatin but not pravastatin is very susceptible to interaction with the CYP3A4 inhibitor itraconazole. *Clin Pharmacol Ther* (1998) 63, 332–41.
5. Pan HY, DeVault AR, Waclawski AP. A report on the effect of nicotinic acid alone and in the presence of aspirin on the bioavailability of SQ 31,000 in healthy male subjects. Data on file, ER Squibb. Protocol No 27, 201-6 (1987).
6. Lilja JJ, Kivistö KT, Neuvonen PJ. Grapefruit juice increases serum concentrations of atorvastatin and has no effect on pravastatin. *Clin Pharmacol Ther* (1999) 66, 118–27.
7. Pan HY, Waclawski AP, Funke PT, Whigan D. Pharmacokinetics of pravastatin in elderly versus young men and women. *Ann Pharmacother* (1993) 27, 1029–33.
8. Triscari J, Swanson BN, Willard DA, Cohen AI, Devault A, Pan HY. Steady state concentrations of pravastatin and digoxin when given in combination. *Br J Clin Pharmacol* (1993) 36, 263–5.
9. Pan HY, Triscari J, DeVault AR, Smith SA, Wang-Iverson D, Swanson BN, Willard DA. Pharmacokinetic interaction between propranolol and the HMG-CoA reductase inhibitors pravastatin and lovastatin. *Br J Clin Pharmacol* (1991) 31, 665–70.
10. Pan HY, Swanson BN, DeVault AR, Willard DA, Brescia D. Antipyrine elimination is not affected by chronic administration of pravastatin (SQ31,000), a tissue-selective HMG CoA reductase inhibitor. *Clin Res* (1988) 36, 368A.

Prostaglandins + Ciclosporin

Ciclosporin increases the serum levels of enisoprost, while ciclosporin levels are reduced. Misoprostol does not provide renal protection from ciclosporin.

Clinical evidence, mechanism, importance and management

Ciclosporin 350 mg increased the AUC of a single 400-microgram dose of **enisoprost** in 24 subjects by 93%.[1] Another study in 24 subjects found that 100 micrograms **enisoprost** or a placebo daily for 10 days reduced the AUC and maximum serum levels of a single 350-mg dose of ciclosporin by 28%.[2] The clinical importance of these interactions awaits assessment.

A multicentre trial in patients with refractory rheumatoid arthritis and treated with **ciclosporin** 5 mg/kg daily for 12 weeks found that **misoprostol** 100 micrograms four times daily for 10 days, then 200 micrograms four times daily thereafter did not show any renal protective effects. No adverse effects attributable to an interaction were seen.[3]

1. Garnett WR, Venitz J, Karim A, Neuhaus J, Moran MS, Hyndman V. Effect of cyclosporine (CSA) on the pharmacokinetics of enisoprost (E) in healthy male subjects. *Pharm Res* (1991) 8 (Suppl 10), S-65.
2. Venitz J, Garnett WR, Wang J, Karim A, Neuhaus J Moran SM, Hyndman V. Effect of enisoprost on cyclosporine pharmacokinetics in healthy male subjects. *Pharm Res* (1991) 8 (Suppl 10), S-63.
3. Weinblatt M, Germain B, Kremer J, Wall B, Weisman M, Maier A, Coblyn J. Misoprostol is not renal protective in rheumatoid arthritis patients receiving cyclosporin A; results of a randomized placebo controlled trial. *Arthritis Rheum* (1993) 36 (9 Suppl), S56.

Proton pump inhibitors + Antimicrobials

Clarithromycin almost doubles the serum levels of omeprazole, which is considered to be therapeutically useful. A small rise in the serum levels of clarithromycin also occurs. Some very limited evidence indicates that erythromycin causes a larger rise in serum omeprazole levels but paradoxically the effects of omeprazole appear to be reduced.
Glossitis, stomatitis and/or black tongue developed rapidly in a small number of patients when treated with lansoprazole and antibacterials which included amoxicillin, clarithromycin and metronidazole. The quinolones do not appear to interact significantly with omeprazole.

Clinical evidence, mechanism, importance and management

(a) Macrolides

(i) Clarithromycin. When 11 healthy subjects taking 40 mg omeprazole daily were additionally given 500 mg **clarithromycin** 8-hourly for 5 days, the maximum serum omeprazole levels rose by 30% and the 24 h AUC rose by 89%. The maximum serum **clarithromycin** levels rose by 11% (from 3.8 to 4.2 micrograms/ml) and the 8 h AUC by 15%.[1,2] None of the changes reported in the first study represent an adverse interaction, but they may help to explain why concurrent use is valuable in the eradication of *H. pylori* (a fact which the makers point out in their datasheet). **Clarithromycin** 500 mg twice daily is reported to have doubled the AUC of esomeprazole in one study, due, it is believed, to the inhibitory effect of the **clarithromycin** on the

metabolism of the esomeprazole by cytochrome P450 isoenzyme CYP3A4. Despite this increase in the AUC the makers say that dosage adjustments of the esomeprazole are not needed.[3]

(ii) Erythromycin. A study was undertaken in a patient to confirm the *in vitro* findings that **erythromycin** inhibits the metabolism of omeprazole. After taking 500 mg **erythromycin** base and 20 mg omeprazole daily for 8 weeks, it was found that the AUC of omeprazole was increased almost fourfold, and the metabolite of omeprazole was undetectable. These raised omeprazole levels might have been expected to increase its effectiveness, but in this patient the time during which the gastric pH was less than 4 decreased by 22%.[4] What is not clear is whether this reduction is clinically important, but if both drugs are used be alert for any evidence that the omeprazole is less effective.

(b) Penicillins

The hypoacidity caused by omeprazole causes a few small changes in the pharmacokinetics of **bacampicillin** and **amoxicillin**, but their bioavailabilities are not reduced[5-7] and the anti-*Helicobacter* effect of the **amoxicillin** is increased.

Six cases of glossitis, stomatitis and/or black tongue were reported to the Sicilian Regional Pharmacovigilance Centre in patients on lansoprazole when combined with antibacterials used to treat *Helicobacter pylori* infections. All 6 patients had been given daily doses of 60 mg lansoprazole for a week with 1 g **clarithromycin** and either 1 g **metronidazole** (3 patients) or 2 g **amoxicillin** (3 patients), after which the antibacterials were stopped and the lansoprazole continued at half the dose for periods of up to 3 weeks. The glossitis (1 patient), black tongue (3 patients) and stomatitis (2 patients) developed between days 2 and 19 of the courses of treatment.[8] Another 9 cases of glossitis have been reported elsewhere with lansoprazole and **amoxicillin**.[9]

Just why these drugs cause these adverse effects, and whether they are due to just one drug or to an interaction is not understood, nor is its incidence known. The incidence seems to be quite small because reports of adverse reactions seem to be fairly uncommon whereas these and related drug combinations are in increasing use for the treatment of *H. pylori* infections. However, in the light of these reports it would now be prudent to monitor the combined use of lansoprazole and these and any other antibacterials. More study is needed.

The makers say that esomeprazole has been shown not have any clinically relevant effects on the pharmacokinetics of **amoxicillin**.[3] There would therefore appear to be no reason for avoiding concurrent use.

(c) Quinolones

A single-dose study found that 20 or 80 mg omeprazole had no significant effect on the pharmacokinetics of single doses of **ofloxacin** 400 mg, **ciprofloxacin** 500 mg or **lomefloxacin** 250 or 400 mg.[10] Omeprazole 40 mg caused an 18% reduction in the AUC of a single dose of **trovafloxacin** 300 mg and a 32% reduction in the maximum serum levels, but this was considered not to be of clinical significance.[11] A double-blind, randomised, crossover study in 12 healthy subjects found that the maximum serum levels and the AUC of single 320-mg doses of **gemifloxacin** were increased 11% and 10% respectively after taking 40 mg omeprazole daily for 4 days. The confidence intervals indicated that the respective increases were unlikely to exceed 36% and 43%, and it was concluded that these two drugs could be given together without any need for dosage adjustments.[12]

1. Gustavson LE, Kaiser JF, Mukherjee DK, DeBartolo M, Schneck DW. Evaluation of the pharmacokinetic drug interactions between clarithromycin and omeprazole. *Am J Gastroenterol* (1994) 89, 1373.
2. Gustavson LE, Kaiser JF, Edmonds AL, Locke CS, DeBartolo ML, Schneck DW. Effect of omeprazole on concentrations of clarithromycin in plasma and gastric tissue at steady state. *Antimicrob Agents Chemother* (1995) 39, 2078–83.
3. Nexium (Esomeprazole). AstraZeneca. Summary of Product Characteristics, June 2002.
4. Salcedo JA, Benjamin SB, Maher KA, Sukhova N. Erythromycin inhibits the metabolism of omeprazole. *Gastroenterology* (1997) 112 (4 Suppl), A277.
5. Paulsen O, Högland P, Walder M. No effect of omeprazole-induced hypoacidity on the bioavailability of amoxycillin and bacampicillin. *Scand J Infect Dis* (1989) 21, 219–23.
6. Cardaci G, Lambert JR, Aranda-Michel J, Underwood B. Omeprazole has no effect on the gastric mucosal bioavailability of amoxicillin. *Gut* (1995) 37 (Suppl 1), A90.
7. Goddard AF, Jessa MJ, Barrett DA, Shaw PN, Idström J-P, Wason C. Wrangstadh M, Spiller RC. Effect of omeprazole on the distribution of antibiotics in gastric juice. *Gastroenterology* (1995) 108 (Suppl), A102.
8. Greco S, Mazzaglia G, Caputi AP, Pagliaro L. Glossitis, stomatitis and black tongue with lansoprazole plus clarithromycin and other antibiotics. *Ann Pharmacother* (1997) 31, 1548.
9. Hatlebakk JG, Nesje LB, Hausken T, Bang CJ, Berstad A. Lansoprazole capsules and amoxicillin oral suspension in the treatment of peptic ulcer disease. *Scand J Gastroenterol* (1995) 30, 1053–7.
10. Stuht H, Lode H, Koeppe P, Rost KL, Schaberg T. Interaction study of lomefloxacin and ciprofloxacin with omeprazole and comparative pharmacokinetics. *Antimicrob Agents Chemother* (1995) 39, 1045–9.
11. Teng R, Dogolo LC, Willavize SA, Friedman HL, Vincent J. Effect of Maalox and omeprazole on the bioavailability of trovafloxacin. *J Antimicrob Chemother* (1997) 39 (Suppl B), 93–7.
12. Allen A, Vousden M, Lewis A, Teilloi-Foo M. Effect of omeprazole on the pharmacokinetics of oral gemifloxacin in healthy volunteers. *J Antimicrob Chemother* (1999) 44 (Suppl A), 134–5.

Rabeprazole + Miscellaneous drugs

Rabeprazole causes a small to moderate rise in serum digoxin levels but it does not interact with diazepam, phenytoin or warfarin.

Clinical evidence, mechanism, importance and management

(a) Diazepam

Rabeprazole 20 mg or placebo was given to 15 patients (in 3 groups) daily for 23 days, followed by at least a 21-day washout period. On day 8 of the study they were given a single 0.1-mg/kg dose of **diazepam**. Each group contained at least two poor metabolisers and three extensive metabolisers of *(S)*-mephenytoin. No significant changes in the pharmacokinetics of the **diazepam** were seen.[1] No special precautions would therefore appear to be necessary during concurrent use.

(b) Digoxin

Sixteen patients on 375 micrograms of **digoxin** daily were concurrently treated with 20 mg rabeprazole daily or placebo for 14 days. The AUC of the **digoxin** was increased 21% and the maximum serum levels increased 28%. A statistically non-significant increase of 22% occurred in the minimum **digoxin** serum levels. The clinical importance of these increases is not known, but it has been suggested that **digoxin** levels should be monitored and dosage adjustments made as necessary if rabeprazole is given.[1]

(c) Phenytoin

Oral **phenytoin** 200 mg daily for 3 days and 250 mg intravenous phenytoin on day 4 was given to 24 patients before and after taking 20 mg rabeprazole daily for 7 days. No significant changes in the pharmacokinetics of **phenytoin** were seen.[1] No special precautions would therefore appear to be necessary during concurrent use.

(d) Warfarin

A single 0.75 mg/kg dose of **warfarin** was given to 21 patients before and after taking 20 mg rabeprazole or a placebo daily for 7 days. No significant changes in prothrombin times or in the pharmacokinetics of *(R)*- or *(S)*-warfarin were seen.[1,2] No special precautions would therefore appear to be necessary during concurrent use.

1. Humphries TJ, Nardi RV, Lazar JD, Spanyers SA. Drug-drug interaction evaluation of rabeprazole sodium: a clean/expected state? *Gut* (1996) 39 (Suppl 3), A47.
2. Humphries TJ, Nardi RV, Spera AC, Lazar JD, Laurent AL, Spanyers SA. Coadministration of rabeprazole sodium (E3810) does not affect the pharmacokinetics of anhydrous theophylline or warfarin. *Gastroenterology* (1996) 110 (Suppl), A138.

Raloxifene + Miscellaneous drugs

The absorption of raloxifene is reduced by colestyramine and their concurrent use is not recommended. A small and slow decrease in prothrombin times may occur with warfarin and possibly other anticoagulants. No clinically relevant interactions occur with ampicillin, aluminium/magnesium hydroxides, aspirin, benzodiazepines, calcium carbonate, digoxin, ibuprofen, oral antibacterials, paracetamol (acetaminophen) or antihistamines or H_2-blockers.

Clinical evidence, mechanism, importance and management

(a) Antacids

The makers of raloxifene report studies which found that an antacid containing **aluminium/magnesium hydroxides** given 1 h before and 2 h after raloxifene had no effect on its absorption. Also, no interaction was also seen with **calcium carbonate**.[1] There would therefore appear to be no reason for avoiding concurrent use.

(b) Colestyramine

The makers report[1] that the concurrent use of **colestyramine** twice daily reduced the absorption of raloxifene by about 40% due an interruption with enterohepatic cycling. It is recommended that these two drugs should not be used concurrently.[1,2]

(c) Miscellaneous drugs, clinically irrelevant interactions

Raloxifene is reported not to affect the steady-state AUC of **digoxin** over an 11-day period, while the maximum serum levels of **digoxin** were increased by only 5%. No clinically relevant changes in the plasma levels of raloxifene were seen in trials in which other drugs were used. These drugs included NSAIDs (**aspirin**, **ibuprofen**, **naproxen**, **paracetamol** (**acetaminophen**)), **oral antibacterials** (not named), **H₁- and H₂-blockers** (not named) and **benzodiazepines** (not named).[1] **Ampicillin** is reported to reduce the maximum serum levels of raloxifene but the extent of the absorption and the elimination rate are unaffected.[1] There would therefore appear to be no reason for avoiding the concurrent use of any of these drugs.

(d) Warfarin

The makers report that the concurrent use of 120 mg raloxifene and a single 20-mg dose of **warfarin** was found not to alter the pharmacokinetics of either drug.[1] However, because modest decreases in prothrombin times have been seen, which may develop over several weeks, they recommend that prothrombin times should be checked. They extend this recommendation to cover the use of other oral anticoagulants.[1,2]

1. Eli Lilly and Company Limited. Personal communication, September 1998.
2. Evista (Raloxifene). Eli Lilly and Company Limited. Summary of product characteristics, October 2001.

Retinoids + Alcohol

There is evidence that the consumption of alcohol may increase the serum levels of etretinate in patients taking acitretin. A single case report describes a marked reduction in the effects of isotretinoin following the acute intake of alcohol.

Clinical evidence, mechanism, importance and management

(a) Acitretin

A study in 10 patients with psoriasis taking **acitretin** found that concurrent intake of **alcohol** seemed to be associated with an increase in the formation of **etretinate**, which has a much longer half-life than **acitretin**. The implications of this study are not known, but it is suggested that it may have some bearing on the length of the period after **acitretin** therapy during which women are advised not to conceive.[1]

(b) Isotretinoin

A former alcoholic, who normally no longer drank, was treated for acne conglobata with some success for 3 months with 60 mg **isotretinoin** daily. When for 2 weeks he briefly started to drink again as part of his job (he was a **sherry** taster) his skin lesions reappeared and the **isotretinoin** side-effects (mucocutaneous dryness) vanished. When he stopped drinking his skin lesions became controlled again and the drug side-effects re-emerged. The following year while on another course of **isotretinoin** the same thing happened when he started and stopped drinking. The reasons are not known but one suggestion is that the **alcohol** briefly induced the liver microsomal enzymes responsible for the metabolism of **isotretinoin**, thereby reducing both

its therapeutic and side-effects.[2] The general importance of this apparent interaction is not known.

1. Larsen FG, Jakobsen P, Knudsen J, Weismann K, Kragballe K, Nielsen-Kudsk F. Conversion of acitretin to etretinate in psoriatic patients is influenced by ethanol. *J Invest Dermatol* (1993) 100, 623–7.
2. Soria C, Allegue F, Galiana J, Ledo A. Decreased isotretinoin efficacy during alcohol intake. *Dermatologica* (1991) 182, 203.

Retinoids + Food

Fatty foods increase the absorption of acitretin and etretinate.

Clinical evidence, mechanism, importance and management

The absorption of **acitretin** was increased by 90% and the peak plasma concentrations were increased by 70% when **acitretin** 50 mg was taken by 18 healthy subjects with a **standard breakfast**. The **breakfast** consisted of two poached eggs, two slices of toast, two pats of margarine and 8 oz skimmed milk.[1] Other studies have found that **high fat meals** and **milk** cause about a two to fivefold increase in the absorption of **etretinate** when compared with **high carbohydrate meals** or when **fasting**.[2,3] The reason is thought to be that because these retinoids are lipid soluble they become absorbed into the lymphatic system by becoming incorporated into the bile-acid micelles of the **fats** in the **food**. In this way losses due to first-pass liver metabolism and gut wall metabolism are minimised. The makers of acitretin recommend taking it with **food**. No special precautions appear to be necessary.

1. McNamara PJ, Jewell RC, Jensen BK, Brindley CJ. Food increases the bioavailability of acitretin. *J Clin Pharmacol* (1988) 28, 1051–5.
2. DiGiovanna JJ, Cross EG, McClean SW, Ruddel ME, Gantt G, Peck GL. Etretinate: effect of milk intake on absorption. *J Invest Dermatol* (1984) 82, 636–40.
3. Colburn WA, Gibson DM, Rodriguez LC, Buggé CJL, Blumenthal HP. Effect of meals on the kinetics of etretinate. *J Clin Pharmacol* (1985) 25, 583–9.

Retinoids + Miscellaneous drugs

The development of 'pseudotumour cerebri' (benign intracranial hypertension) has been associated with the concurrent use of isotretinoin and tetracyclines. A condition similar to vitamin A (retinol) overdosage may occur if isotretinoin and retinol are given concurrently.

Clinical evidence, mechanism, importance and management

(a) Retinoids + Tetracyclines

The concurrent use of **isotretinoin** and a **tetracycline** has resulted in the development of 'pseudotumour cerebri' (i.e. a clinical picture of cranial hypertension with headache, dizziness and dysopia). By 1983 the FDA had received reports of 10 patients with 'pseudotumour cerebri' and/or papilloedema associated with the use of **isotretinoin**. Four had retinal haemorrhages, and 5 of the 10 were also being treated with a **tetracycline**.[1] The makers also have similar reports on file of 3 patients given **isotretinoin** and either **minocycline** or **tetracycline**.[2] The same reaction has been seen in 2 patients given **etretinate** with **minocycline** or **prednisolone**.[3] It seems that the two drugs have an additive effect in increasing intracranial pressure. The makers of **isotretinoin** contraindicate its use with **tetracyclines**.[4]

(b) Retinoids + Vitamin A (Retinol)

Combined treatment may result in a condition similar to overdosage with **vitamin A**, and so concurrent use should be avoided or very closely monitored because changes in bone structure can occur, including premature fusion of the epiphyseal discs in children.[5] The makers of **isotretinoin**, say that high doses of **vitamin A** (more than

4000 to 5000 units daily, the recommended daily allowance) should be avoided.[4]

1. Anon. Adverse effects with isotretinoin. *FDA Drug Bull* (1983) 13, 21–3.
2. Shalita AR, Cunningham WJ, Leyden JJ, Pochi PE, Strauss JS. Isotretinoin treatment of acne and related disorders: an update. *J Am Acad Dermatol* (1983) 9, 629–38.
3. Viraben R, Mathieu C, Fonton B. Benign intracranial hypertension during etretinate therapy for mycosis fungoides. *J Am Acad Dermatol* (1985) 13, 515–17.
4. Roaccutane (Isotretinoin). Roche Products Limited. Summary of product characteristics, January 2002.
5. Milstone LM, McGuire J, Ablow RC. Premature epiphyseal closure in a child receiving oral 13-*cis*-retinoic acid. *J Am Acad Dermatol* (1982) 7, 663–6.

Rivastigmine + Miscellaneous drugs

Rivastigmine is expected to interact with neuromuscular blockers and to oppose the effects of anticholinergics. The makers advise the avoidance of drugs such as tacrine but say that diazepam, digoxin, fluoxetine and warfarin do not interact.

Clinical evidence, mechanism, importance and management

Rivastigmine is a cholinesterase inhibitor and is expected to interfere with the effects of **neuromuscular blockers**. See 'Neuromuscular blockers + Anticholinesterases', p.755. The makers recommend that it should not be used with other cholinomimetic drugs (**tacrine** is the obvious example) because of possible additive effects and they point out that it is expected to interfere (oppose) the activity of **anticholinergic drugs**.[1]

The makers also report that in studies in healthy subjects no pharmacokinetic interactions were seen between rivastigmine and **diazepam** or **fluoxetine**. The pharmacokinetics of **warfarin** were also unchanged by rivastigmine and no alterations in prothrombin times were seen. Similarly the pharmacokinetics of **digoxin** were unaltered and no untoward effects on cardiac conduction occurred when rivastigmine and **digoxin** were used concurrently.[1] There would therefore appear to be no reason for avoiding the concurrent use of these drugs. The makers also point out that metabolic interactions (i.e. due to enzyme induction or inhibition) are unlikely because the major cytochrome P450 isoenzymes are minimally involved in the metabolism of rivastigmine.[1]

1. Exelon (Rivastigmine). Novartis Pharmaceuticals UK Limited. Summary of Product Characteristics, October 2001.

Rizatriptan + Miscellaneous drugs

The makers of rizatriptan contraindicate the concurrent use of all MAOIs. Sumatriptan and related drugs should also not be used concurrently nor, by implication, drugs used for angina. Ergot derivatives are contraindicated except when the administration is suitably separated. Because the plasma levels of rizatriptan are almost doubled by propranolol the makers recommend a dosage reduction and a 2-h dosage separation. No adverse interaction occurs with oral contraceptives.

Clinical evidence, mechanism, importance and management

(a) Beta-blockers

The maximum plasma levels and the AUC of rizatriptan are increased 70 to 80% by the concurrent use of **propranolol** (probably because both drugs are metabolised by MAO-A) and the makers therefore recommend that the 5-mg dose of rizatriptan (rather than the more usual 10 mg) should be used in the presence of **propranolol**. They also suggest that their administration should be separated by at least 2 h. Other studies have shown that **nadolol** and **metoprolol** do not increase the plasma levels of rizatriptan, and *in vitro* studies have shown that

atenolol and **timolol** do not affect the metabolism of rizatriptan,[1] so that no reduction in the rizatriptan dosage would seem to be needed in the presence of these beta-blockers.

However it needs to be pointed out that in the case of a **beta-blocker** used for the treatment of ischaemic heart disease (see the diseases named in (d) below), the disease condition itself is a contraindication for the use of rizatriptan.

(b) Ergot derivatives

The makers of rizatriptan contraindicate the concurrent use of ergot derivatives (including **methysergide**).[1]

(c) Monoamine oxidase inhibitors (MAOIs)

In a double blind, randomised, crossover trial, 12 healthy subjects were given 150 mg **moclobemide** or a placebo three times daily for 4 days and then a single 10-mg dose of rizatriptan on day 4. The **moclobemide** increased the AUCs of rizatriptan and its active (but minor) metabolite by 2.2- and 5.3-fold respectively, and increased their maximum serum levels by 1.4- and 2.6-fold respectively. The reason appears to be that **moclobemide** is an inhibitor of MAO-A, which is concerned with the metabolism of rizatriptan. Despite these rises, the concurrent use of these drugs was well tolerated and any adverse effects were mild and similar to those seen when rizatriptan was given with the placebo.[2] The makers of rizatriptan issue a 'blanket' contraindication covering **all MAOIs** and within 2 weeks of stopping the **MAOI**, the stated reasons being that similar or greater rises in serum levels may be expected with irreversible non-selective **MAOIs**.[1]

(d) Nitrates

The makers of rizatriptan contraindicate its use in patients with established coronary heart disease, including ischaemic heart disease or Prinzmetal's angina. By implication this means that any patient taking any **nitrate (glyceryl trinitrate, isosorbide**, etc.) for angina should not use rizatriptan because of the risk that it may cause vasospasm of the coronary arteries, lessen the flow of blood to the heart muscle and worsen the angina.

(e) Oral contraceptives

A two-period, crossover, placebo controlled study in 20 healthy young women taking on an **oral contraceptive (*Ortho-Novum 1/35*, ethinylestradiol + norethindrone**) found that the concurrent use of rizatriptan (6 days on 10 mg daily and 2 days of 10 mg every 4 h for 12 h) did not effect the pharmacokinetics of either contraceptive steroid. Blood pressure, heart rate and temperature were unaffected and adverse effects were similar to those seen with the placebo.[3] There would therefore appear to be no reason for avoiding concurrent use.

(f) Sumatriptan and other 5-HT₁ receptor agonists

The makers say that **sumatriptan** and similar drugs should not be given with rizatriptan, presumably because of the risks of additive hyperstimulation of the receptors.[1] Other 5-HT₁ agonists include **naratriptan** and **zolmitriptan**.

1. Maxalt (Rizatriptan). Merck Sharpe & Dohme Limited. Summary of product characteristics, February 2002.
2. van Haarst AD, van Gerven JMA, Cohen AF, De Smet M, Sterrett A, Birk KL, Goldberg MR, Musson DG. The effects of moclobemide on the pharmacokinetics of the 5-HT₁ₓ agonist rizatriptan in healthy volunteers. *Eur J Clin Pharmacol* (1997) 52 (Suppl), A142.
3. Shadle CR, Liu G, Goldberg MR. A double-blind, placebo-controlled evaluation of the effect of oral doses of rizatriptan 10 mg on oral contraceptive pharmacokinetics in healthy female volunteers. *J Clin Pharmacol* (2000) 40, 309–15.

Sevelamer + Miscellaneous drugs

Sevelamer has been shown not to interact with digoxin, enalapril, metoprolol or warfarin and seems unlikely to interact with other drugs, but monitoring is advisable until more clinical experience has been gained.

Clinical evidence, mechanism, importance and management

Concurrent administration of single doses of sevelamer 2.418 g (equivalent to 6 capsules) and **enalapril** 20 mg did not alter the AUC of **enalapril** or its active metabolite, enalaprilat, in 28 healthy subjects.[1,2] Similarly, concurrent administration of single doses of sevelamer 2.418 g and **metoprolol** 100 mg did not alter the AUC of **metoprolol** in 31 healthy subjects.[1,2] The makers also report that other studies in healthy subjects have shown that the pharmacokinetics of single oral doses of 1000 micrograms **digoxin** and 30 mg **warfarin** were not statistically changed by the presence of 2.418 g sevelamer (equivalent to 6 capsules). In the case of **digoxin** and **warfarin** five more 2.418 g doses of the sevelamer were given over 2 days to check whether it had any effect on the enterohepatic circulation. No effect was seen.[3,4] Thus it appears that sevelamer does not bind to these drugs within the gut to reduce their absorption. The makers similarly report that in *dogs* the peak serum drug levels and AUCs of single doses of **calcitriol**, **digoxin**, **estrone**, **levothyroxine**, **propranolol**, **tetracycline**, **valproic acid**, **verapamil** and **warfarin** were not altered by sevelamer.[3] While the results of *animal* studies should never be extrapolated uncritically to the human situation, since in this instance no significant chemical or physiochemical binding apparently occurred between sevelamer and any of these drugs in the gut (and already demonstrated in the case of **digoxin** and **warfarin**), this suggests that interactions with these drugs in human gut are also unlikely.

So far the general picture is that interactions within the gut are not expected, but until more clinical experience is gained the makers suggest in the US product information[5] that "... when administering any other oral drug for which alterations in blood levels could have a clinically significant effect on safety or efficacy, the drug should be administered at least 1 hour before or 3 hours after *Renagel Capsules* (sevelamer)." This recommendation is not currently included in the UK Summary of product characteristics but if there is any evidence of reduced efficacy when other drugs are used concurrently, following this advice would seem sensible and practical.

1. Burke SK, Amin NS, Incerti C. Sevelamer hydrochloride (Renagel®), does not alter the pharmacokinetics of two commonly used antihypertensives. *Nephrol Dial Transplant* (2000) 15, A45.
2. Burke SK, Amin NS, Incerti C, Plone MA, Lee JW. Sevelamer hydrochloride (Renagel®), a phosphate-binding polymer, does not alter the pharmacokinetics of two commonly used antihypertensives in healthy volunteers. *J Clin Pharmacol* (2001) 41, 199–205.
3. Renagel (Sevelamer). Genzyme. Summary of product characteristics, January 2000.
4. Genzyme BV. Personal communication, May 2000.
5. Renagel Capsules (Sevelamer). Product profile and clinical experience. Genzyme Corporation (USA), October 1998.

Sibutramine + Miscellaneous drugs

On theoretical grounds the makers contraindicate the concurrent use of sibutramine with MAOIs and they say that is should not be given with a range of serotonergic drugs (dextromethorphan, dihydroergotamine, fentanyl, lithium, pentazocine, pethidine (meperidine), SSRIs, sumatriptan, tryptophan) because of the risk of the serious serotonin syndrome. They say that other centrally acting appetite suppressants are contraindicated and they caution about drugs that raise blood pressure or heart rate. No clinically relevant interactions have been seen between sibutramine and cimetidine, erythromycin, ketoconazole or other enzyme inhibitors or enzyme inducers. No interaction occurs with alcohol or oral contraceptives.

Clinical evidence, mechanism, importance and management

(a) Alcohol

The makers say that sibutramine did not increase the deleterious effects of **alcohol** (dose not stated) on cognitive and psychomotor function, but they point out that **alcohol** is usually not compatible with the diets used by patients who are trying to lose weight.[1]

(b) Cimetidine

When 400 mg **cimetidine** twice daily and 15 mg sibutramine once daily were given concurrently to 12 healthy subjects, there were some very small changes in the combined sibutramine metabolites (M1 and M2). Their maximum serum levels and AUC were increased 3.4 and 7.3% respectively.[2] These changes are too small to be of clinical significance, and there is no reason for avoiding the concurrent use of these two drugs.

(c) Centrally acting appetite suppressants, and drugs that raise blood pressure or heart rate

The makers say that the concurrent use of sibutramine and other **centrally acting appetite suppressants** is contraindicated. No work has been done to see what happens if sibutramine is given with **decongestants, cough, cold** and **allergy medications**, but the makers say that caution should be used if used concurrently because of the risk of raised blood pressure or heart rate. The makers in the UK and US both list **ephedrine** and **pseudoephedrine**,[1,2] while in the UK **xylometazoline**[1] is included and in the US **phenylpropanolamine**.[2]

(d) Erythromycin

Twelve uncomplicated obese patients were given 20 mg sibutramine daily for 7 days, and then together with 500 mg **erythromycin** three times daily for a further 7 days. It was found that apart from some slight and unimportant changes in the pharmacokinetics of the metabolites of sibutramine (probably caused by some inhibition of cytochrome P450 isoenzyme CYP3A4), the pharmacokinetics of sibutramine were not significantly altered by the **erythromycin**. No blood pressure changes were seen and only very small and clinically irrelevant increases in the QTc interval and heart rate occurred.[3] The extent of any interaction appears to be too small to matter, and there would seem to be no reason for avoiding the concurrent use of these two drugs, even so the makers in the UK[1] say caution should be exercised.

(e) Inducers of cytochrome P450 isoenzyme CYP3A4

The makers in the UK point out that **carbamazepine, dexamethasone, phenobarbital, phenytoin** and **rifampicin** are all inducers of CYP3A4 which is concerned with the metabolism of sibutramine.[1] These drugs might therefore possibly increase the metabolism of sibutramine resulting in a fall in its serum levels. However, this has not been studied experimentally and at the present time the existence, the extent and the possible clinical relevance of any such interaction is unknown.

(f) Inhibitors of cytochrome P450 isoenzyme CYP3A4

The makers in the UK include **clarithromycin, ciclosporin, itraconazole** and **troleandomycin**[1] as potential inhibitors of the metabolism of sibutramine (mainly due to CYP3A4 inhibition) and advise caution. But neither **erythromycin** nor **ketoconazole** which are potent CYP3A4 inhibitors interact to a clinically relevant extent with sibutramine (see (c) and (d) above), and it seems unlikely that these other inhibitors will behave very differently. The maker's warning (caution should be exercised)[1] would therefore seem to represent ultra caution.

(g) Ketoconazole

Twelve obese patients were given 20 mg sibutramine daily for 7 days, and then together with 200 mg **ketoconazole** twice daily for a further 7 days. It was found that the **ketoconazole** caused moderate increases in the serum levels of sibutramine and its two metabolites (AUC and maximum serum level increases of 58% and 36% for metabolites M1, and 20% and 19% for M2 (probably caused by some inhibition of cytochrome P450 isoenzyme CYP3A4)). Only small increases in heart rates were seen (+2.5 bpm at 4 h and +1.4 bpm at 8 h) while ECG parameters were unchanged.[4] The extent of any interaction appears to be too small to matter, and there is no reason for avoiding the concurrent use of these two drugs, even so the makers in the UK[1] say caution should be exercised.

(h) Monoamine oxidase inhibitors (MAOIs)

There are no reports of adverse reactions between sibutramine and the **MAOIs** but the makers warn that because sibutramine inhibits serotonin uptake and because the serious serotonin syndrome can occur with other drugs which inhibit serotonin uptake (such as the SSRIs) and the **MAOIs**, sibutramine is contraindicated with the **MAOIs**.

They say that 14 days should elapse between stopping either drug and starting the other.[1,2]

(i) Oral contraceptives

A crossover study in 12 women volunteers found that 15 mg sibutramine daily over 8 weeks had no clinically significant effect on the ovulation inhibitory effects of an **oral contraceptive**, and it was concluded that there is no need to use alternative contraceptive methods while taking sibutramine.[2]

(j) Serotonergic drugs

There are no reports of adverse interactions between sibutramine and any of the serotonergic drugs (the makers name **dextromethorphan**, **dihydroergotamine**, **fentanyl**, **pentazocine**, **pethidine (meperidine)**, **SSRIs, sumatriptan, tryptophan**), but because sibutramine inhibits serotonin uptake and because the serious serotonin syndrome has been seen when these drugs were taken with other serotonin re-uptake inhibitors (SSRIs), the makers say that sibutramine should not be taken with any of these serotonergic drugs.[1,2] The US makers also include **lithium** in their list.[2] The extent of the risk with these serotonergic drugs is not known but because of the potential severity of the reaction this warning would seem to be a prudent precaution.

1. Reductil (Sibutramine). Knoll Limited, UK. Summary of Product Characteristics, May 2001.
2. Meridia (Sibutramine). Product Information. Physicians' Desk Reference 2002.
3. Hinson JL, Leone MB, Leese PT, Moult JT, Carter FJ, Faulkner RD. Steady-state interaction study of sibutramine (Meridia) and erythromycin in uncomplicated obese subjects. *Pharm Res* (1996) 13 (9 Suppl), S116.
4. Hinson JL, Leone MB, Kisiki MJ, Moult JT, Trammel A and Faulkner RD. Steady-state interaction study of sibutramine (meridia) and ketoconazole in uncomplicated obese subjects. *Pharm Res* (1996) 13 (9 Suppl), S116.

Sildenafil + Dihydrocodeine

Two men using sildenafil had prolonged erections following orgasm while also taking dihydrocodeine.

Clinical evidence, mechanism, importance and management

Two men, successfully treated with 100-mg doses of sildenafil for erectile dysfunction, experienced prolonged erections after orgasm while also taking 30 to 60 mg **dihydrocodeine** 6-hourly for soft tissue injuries. One of them had erections lasting 4 and 5 hr, which resolved when the **dihydrocodeine** was stopped. The other had 2 to 3 hr erections on three occasions during the first week, but no problems over the next two weeks while continuing to take the **dihydrocodeine**.[1] The reasons are not understood.

According to the makers, 100 million tablets of sildenafil have been prescribed worldwide,[1] but priapism (prolonged erections) associated with its use is rare, and there appear to be no other reports about a sildenafil/**dihydrocodeine** interaction. Even so, it would now be prudent to warn patients about this possible (though remote) problem if **dihydrocodeine** is being used, and advise them to contact the prescriber if priapism occurs. Excessively prolonged erections can have serious consequences and may need urgent treatment.

1. Goldmeier D, Lamba H. Prolonged erections produced by dihydrocodeine and sildenafil. *BMJ* (2002) 324, 1555.

Sildenafil + Miscellaneous drugs

Erythromycin increases the serum levels of sildenafil and itraconazole and ketoconazole are predicted to behave similarly. A low starting dose of sildenafil is recommended in the presence of all these drugs. It is not entirely clear whether an increased sildenafil dosage is needed if rifampicin is used. No clinically relevant interactions occur with alcohol, aluminium/magnesium hydroxide, atorvastatin, barbiturates, cimetidine, phenytoin, SSRIs, tolbutamide, tricyclic antidepressants or warfarin.

Clinical evidence, mechanism, importance and management

A. Interacting drugs

(a) Cimetidine, erythromycin, itraconazole, ketoconazole

Erythromycin (a specific inhibitor of cytochrome P450 isoenzyme CYP3A4) 500 mg twice daily for 5 days was found to increase the AUC of single 100-mg doses of sildenafil almost threefold because it reduces the metabolism and loss of sildenafil from the body.[1] Other more potent CYP3A4 inhibitors such as **itraconazole** and **ketoconazole** are predicted to have even greater effects. Because of the expected increased efficacy and incidence of side-effects as a result of these interactions, the makers recommend that a starting dose of 25 mg sildenafil should be used if any of these drugs is being used concurrently.[2]

Cimetidine 800 mg was found to increase sildenafil concentrations (following a 50-mg dose) by 56% because **cimetidine** is a non-specific liver cytochrome P450 inhibitor.[3] No recommendation is made about **cimetidine** in the US prescribing Information[3] but the UK summary of product characteristics[2] includes it in the general warning with **erythromycin** and **ketoconazole**, although it seems doubtful if the extent of the increased effects due to **cimetidine** is likely to matter very much.

(b) Barbiturates, Phenytoin, Rifampicin

In the US prescribing information it is predicted that cytochrome P450 isoenzyme CYP3A4 inducers such as **rifampicin** (**rifampin**) will reduce the serum levels of sildenafil, so that it may therefore be necessary to use a larger dose in patients on **rifampicin**.[3] In the UK summary of product characteristics the makers say that although no specific interaction studies have been carried out, population pharmacokinetic analysis suggests that no interaction occurs with inducers of cytochrome P450 metabolism (and they specifically cite **rifampicin** and **barbiturates**).[2] They also say that no interaction was seen with **phenytoin**.[2]

B. Non-interacting drugs

(a) Alcohol, Aluminium/Magnesium hydroxide, Atorvastatin, SSRIs, Tolbutamide, Tricyclic antidepressants, Warfarin

In vivo studies have shown no significant interactions with **warfarin** 40 mg or **tolbutamide** 250 mg, probably because sildenafil is only a weak inhibitor of cytochrome P450 isoenzyme CYP2C9. Clinical trial data similarly indicate that **SSRIs** and **tricyclic antidepressants** (inhibitors of CYP2D6) do not have any effect on the pharmacokinetics of sildenafil. The bioavailability of sildenafil is not affected by single doses of an **aluminium/magnesium hydroxide** antacid, and sildenafil has been found not to increase the hypotensive effects of **alcohol** (80 mg%) in healthy subjects.[2,3]

A study in 24 healthy subjects found that the pharmacokinetics of neither sildenafil (single 100-mg dose) nor **atorvastatin** (10 mg daily for 7 days) were changed by concurrent use.[4] *In vitro* studies have shown that sildenafil is only a weak inhibitor of the cytochrome P450 isoenzymes CYP1A2, CYP2C9, CYP2C19, CYP2D6, CYP2E1 and CYP3A4, and it is predicted therefore that sildenafil is unlikely to alter the metabolism of drugs metabolised by these isoenzymes.[2,3]

1. Muirhead GJ, Faulkner S, Harness JA, Taubel J. The effects of steady-state erythromycin and azithromycin on the pharmacokinetics of sildenafil citrate in healthy volunteers. *Br J Clin Pharmacol* (2002) 53, 37S–43S.
2. Viagra (Sildenafil citrate). Pfizer Limited. Summary of product characteristics, April 2002.
3. Viagra (Sildenafil citrate). Pfizer. US Product Prescribing Information, March 1998.
4. Chung M, DiRico A, Calcagni A, Messig M, Scott R. Lack of a drug interaction between sildenafil and atorvastatin. *J Clin Pharmacol* (2000) 40, 1057.

Sildenafil + Nicorandil, Nitrates or Antihypertensive agents

The makers contraindicate the concurrent use of sildenafil and organic nitrates (glyceryl trinitrate, isosorbide mononitrate etc.) because potentially serious hypotension (dizziness, fainting) can occur and myocardial infarction may possibly

be precipitated. However, there is some preliminary and as yet unconfirmed evidence that transdermal glyceryl trinitrate may be safe. No important interactions occur with non-nitrate antihypertensive vasodilator drugs.

Clinical evidence

(a) Nicorandil

It is not yet known whether **nicorandil** interacts with sildenafil to a clinically relevant extent or not, but because part of its vasodilatory actions are (like conventional nitrates) mediated by the release of nitric oxide, to be on the safe side the makers say that the use of **nicorandil** with sildenafil is contraindicated.[1,2]

(b) Organic nitrates

Two double-blind placebo-controlled studies in groups of 15 or 16 men with angina found that the blood pressure falls seen when taking **nitrates** and a single 50-mg dose of sildenafil were approximately doubled. Those given sildenafil and on 20 mg **isosorbide dinitrate** twice daily showed a mean blood pressure fall of 44/26 mmHg compared with 22/13 mmHg with the sildenafil placebo. Those who used 500 micrograms of sublingual **glyceryl trinitrate** 1 h before the sildenafil showed a mean blood pressure fall of 36/21 mmHg compared with 26/11 mmHg with the sildenafil placebo. Individual blood pressure falls as much as 84/52 mmHg were seen.[3]

The makers[4] contraindicate the concurrent use of sildenafil and **organic nitrates** because of the potential severity of these falls in systemic blood pressure. The effect of this hypotension (so the makers suggest) could range from no symptoms to precipitating a myocardial infarction.[5]

A postmarketing report from the FDA briefly lists 69 fatalities after taking sildenafil. These were mostly middle-aged and elderly men (average age 64), 12 of whom had also taken **glyceryl trinitrate** (**nitroglycerin**) or a **nitrate** medication, but it is not clear what part (if any) the **nitrates** played in the deaths. The number of deaths needs to be set in the context of 3.6 million outpatient prescriptions for sildenafil.[6]

(c) Other antihypertensives

Pooled data suggests that patients on non-nitrate antihypertensives (**ACE inhibitors**, **alpha-blockers**, **beta-blockers**, **calcium channel blockers**, **diuretics**) showed no difference in side effect profile in patients taking sildenafil compared to placebo.[7] The makers say that this is also true for **adrenergic neurone blockers** and **angiotensin II antagonists.** They quote a study where 100 mg sildenafil was given to hypertensive patients on **amlodipine.** The mean fall in blood pressure (8/7 mmHg) was of the same magnitude as that seen when sildenafil was given alone to normal subjects.[4] The makers similarly report that **ACE inhibitors**, **calcium channel blockers** and **thiazide and related diuretics** do not to affect the pharmacokinetics of sildenafil whereas the AUC of the active metabolite of sildenafil is increased 62% by **loop** (potassium-depleting) and **potassium-sparing diuretics** and 102% by **non-selective beta-blockers.**[8] These increases would appear to be clinically irrelevant.

Mechanism

Sexual stimulation causes the endothelium of the penis to release nitric oxide (NO) which in turn activates guanylate cyclase to increase the production of cyclic guanosine monophosphate (cGMP). This relaxes the blood vessel musculature of the corpus cavernosum thus allowing it to fill with blood and causing an erection. The erection comes to an end when the guanosine monophosphate is removed by an enzyme (type 5 cGMP phosphodiesterase, or PDE5). Sildenafil inhibits this enzyme thereby increasing and prolonging the effects of the guanosine monophosphate. Because this vasodilation is usually fairly localised (sildenafil is highly selective for PDE_5) it normally only causes mild to moderate falls in blood pressure (on average about 10 mmHg) with mild headache or flushing. However, if other nitrates (e.g. glyceryl trinitrate) are taken concurrently, high levels of nitric oxide enter the circulation, the general systemic vasodilating and hypotensive effects of which can then be markedly increased.

Importance and management

The sildenafil/nitrate interaction is established, clinically important, potentially serious and even possibly fatal. Sildenafil and organic nitrates of any form should not be used concurrently. As a general rule therefore sildenafil and nitric oxide donors are contraindicated, but in a limited and preliminary study it was reported that no adverse interaction was seen when a small dose of **glyceryl trinitrate** (amount not specified) was administered in the form of a dermal patch while taking 50 mg sildenafil. No blood pressure alteration was seen and the effects of the **glyceryl trinitrate** were approximately doubled and persisted for up to 8 hours.[9] A case report also describes the deliberate and advantageous use of small doses of sildenafil with **inhaled nitric oxide** in the management of pulmonary hypertension and hypoxaemia associated with reversible right-to-left cardiac shunt.[10]

In contrast to the situation with nitric oxide donor drugs, there appears to be no reason for patients taking non-nitrate vasodilator antihypertensives (those cited in (b) above) to avoid sildenafil.[7,11]

1. Aventis Pharma, Personnal communication, February 2000.
2. Ikorel (Nicorandil). Rhone-Poulenc Rorer. Summary of product characteristics, June 2000.
3. Webb DJ, Muirhead G. Viagra (sildenafil citrate) potentiates the hypotensive effects of nitrates in men with stable angina. *J Am Coll Cardiol* (1999) 33 (2 Suppl A), p 309A. 48th Annual Science Session of the American College of Cardiology, USA.
4. Viagra (Sildenafil citrate). Pfizer Limited. Summary of product characteristics, April 2002.
5. Viagra (Sildenafil). Pfizer Inc. Dear Doctor letter, May 1998.
6. FDA (US Food and Drug Administration) postmarketing information sildenafil citrate (Viagra): Postmarketing safety of sildenafil citrate (Viagra). Reports of death in Viagra users received from marketing (late March) through July 1998. August 27th 1998.
7. Prisant LM. Safety of treatment with sildenafil citrate for erectile dysfunction in men receiving different classes of antihypertensives. *Am J Hypertens* (2000) 13, 129A–130A.
8. Viagra (Sildenafil citrate), Pfizer. US Product Prescribing Information, March 1998.
9. O'Rourke M, Jiang X-J. Sildenafil/nitrate interaction. *Circulation* (2000) 101, e90.
10. Bigatello LM, Hess D, Dennehy KC, Medoff BD, Hurford WE. Sildenafil can improve the response to inhaled nitric oxide. *Anesthesiology* (2000) 92, 1827–9.
11. Kloner RA, Siegel RL. Sildenafil and nonnitrate antihypertensive medications. *JAMA* (2000) 283, 201–2.

Sildenafil + Protease inhibitors

Indinavir, ritonavir and saquinavir cause very marked rises in serum sildenafil levels. Concurrent use need not be avoided but the sildenafil dosage should be reduced.

Clinical evidence

(a) Indinavir

A study in 6 HIV+ patients found that 25 mg sildenafil did not significantly alter the plasma levels of the **indinavir**, but the sildenafil AUC was about 4.4-fold higher than those seen in previous patients without **indinavir** taking 50 or 100 mg sildenafil.[1]

(b) Ritonavir

In an open, randomised, placebo-controlled, double-blind crossover study, 28 healthy subjects were given 100 mg sildenafil before and after taking **ritonavir** for 7 days (300, 400 and 500 mg twice daily on days 1, 2 and 3 to 7 respectively). It was found that the sildenafil AUC was increased 11-fold and the maximum serum levels 3.9-fold but the incidence and severity of sildenafil side-effects and the steady-state levels of **ritonavir** remained unchanged.[2]

(c) Saquinavir

In an open, randomised, placebo-controlled, double-blind crossover study, 28 healthy subjects were given 100 mg sildenafil before and after taking **saquinavir** 1200 mg three times daily for 7 days. It was found that the sildenafil AUC was increased 3.1-fold and the maximum serum levels 2.4-fold but the incidence and severity of sildenafil side-effects and the steady-state levels of **saquinavir** remained unchanged.[2]

Mechanism

Not understood, but it is thought that because these protease inhibitors can inhibit the activity of cytochrome P450 isoenzyme CYP3A4 which reduces the metabolism of the sildenafil, this results in an increase in its serum levels.[2]

Importance and management

Information appears to be limited to the studies cited but the interactions would seem to be established. Despite the large rises in sildenafil AUCs and sildenafil serum levels, there is no need to avoid concurrent use. However, the recommendation is that a lower starting dose (25 mg) should be considered for patients on indinavir[1] and saquinavir,[2] while those on ritonavir should not exceed a single 25-mg dose in a 48-h period.[2] Information about other protease inhibitors seems to be lacking.

1. Merry C, Barry MG, Ryan M, Tjia JF, Hennessy M, Eagling V, Mulcahy F, Back DJ. Interaction of sildenafil and indinavir when co-administered to HIV positive patients. AIDS 1999, 13, F101–F107.
2. Muirhead GJ, Wulff MB, Fielding A, Kleinermans D, Buss N. Pharmacokinetic interactions between sildenafil and saquinavir/ritonavir. Br J Clin Pharmacol (2000) 50, 99–107.

Simvastatin or Lovastatin + Azole antifungals

Itraconazole causes a very marked rise in the serum levels of simvastatin and lovastatin. Acute rhabdomyolysis occurred in three patients on simvastatin when given itraconazole. Acute rhabdomyolysis and hepatotoxicity have been reported in two patients on lovastatin and itraconazole.

Clinical evidence

(a) Lovastatin

Itraconazole 200 mg daily or a placebo was given to 12 healthy subjects for 4 days in a double-blind crossover study. On day 4 they were additionally given a single 40-mg oral dose of **lovastatin**. On average the peak plasma concentration and the 24 h AUC of the **lovastatin** were increased more than twentyfold. The peak plasma concentration of the active metabolite of **lovastatin**, lovastatin acid, was increased thirteenfold (range 10 to 23-fold) and its AUC twentyfold. The creatine kinase activity of one subject increased tenfold, but in the other 11 subjects it remained unchanged. Brief mention is also made of severe rhabdomyolysis in one patient given both drugs.[1]

A woman of 63 who had been on 80 mg **lovastatin** and 3 g nicotinic acid daily, plus timolol and aspirin for almost 10 years without problems, developed weakness and tenderness in her arms, back and legs within two weeks of starting 100 mg **itraconazole** twice daily. A few days later her urine became brown, and positive for haem. She was diagnosed as having acute rhabdomyolysis and hepatotoxicity. The **lovastatin**, nicotinic acid and **itraconazole** were stopped, and she was treated with ubiquinone. Over the next 18 days her elevated serum enzymes returned to normal, although her plasma cholesterol levels almost doubled. She was restarted on nicotinic acid 11 weeks later without problems.[2]

(b) Simvastatin

In a two-phase crossover study 10 healthy subjects were given 200 mg **itraconazole** or a placebo daily for 4 days, and then on day 4 they were given a single 40-mg dose of **simvastatin**. It was found that the peak serum levels of total simvastatin acid (simvastatin acid + simvastatin lactone) were increased 17-fold and the AUC 19-fold. The maximum serum levels of total HMG-CoA reductase inhibitors increased about threefold and the AUC fivefold.[3,4]

A 74-year-old who had been on 40 mg of **simvastatin** daily, lisinopril and aspirin for about a year without problems developed pain in his feet and then in his arms and neck within 3 weeks of starting 200 mg **itraconazole** daily. His urine turned brown, his muscles were tender, and abnormal serum creatine kinase and other enzyme levels were found. A diagnosis of rhabdomyolysis was made.[5] A 70-year-old with a kidney transplant was on, among many other drugs ciclosporin and simvastatin 40 mg daily. Despite the high dose of **simvastatin** (because of the ciclosporin) he had experienced no problems. Within 2 weeks of starting **itraconazole** 100 mg twice daily he

developed malaise and general muscle weakness with elevated creatine kinase levels, which was diagnosed as rhabdomyolysis. His serum **simvastatin** levels were found to be raised, as were those of a later volunteer subject whose **simvastatin** serum levels rose from 0.5 to 6.5 nanogram/ml within a day of starting 200 mg **itraconazole** daily.[6] A 57-year-old woman who had been on 20 mg **simvastatin** daily for 10 months without problems developed rhabdomyolysis and acute renal failure following a lung transplant when she was treated with ciclosporin and within 3 weeks of adding **itraconazole**.[7]

Mechanism

It seems likely that itraconazole inhibits cytochrome P450 isoenzyme CYP3A4 in the liver which is concerned with the metabolism of simvastatin and lovastatin. As a result they accumulate, increasing the risk of toxicity.

Importance and management

An established interaction of clinical importance. The very marked increases in statin levels considerably increases the risk of severe muscle damage. This drug combination should be avoided (the makers suggest temporary withdrawal of the statin) or it should very closely monitored with a very marked reduction in the dosage. Because of its potential seriousness any patient given this drug combination should be told to report any unexplained muscle pain, tenderness or weakness.

1. Neuvonen PJ, Jalava K-M. Itraconazole drastically increases plasma concentrations of lovastatin and lovastatin acid. Naunyn Schmiedebergs Arch Pharmacol (1996) 60 (4 Suppl), R 155.
2. Lees RS, Lees AM. Rhabdomyolysis from the coadministration of lovastatin and the antifungal agent itraconazole. N Engl J Med (1995) 333, 664-5.
3. Neuvonen PJ, Kantola T, Kivostö KT. Itraconazole greatly increases serum concentration of simvastatin acid. Eur J Clin Pharmacol (1997) 52 (Suppl), A138.
4. Neuvonen PJ, Kantola T, Kivostö KT. Simvastatin but not pravastatin is very susceptible to interaction with CYP3A4 inhibitor itraconazole. Clin Pharmacol Ther (1998) 332–41.
5. Horn M. Coadministration of itraconazole with hypolipidemic agents may induce rhabdomyolysis in healthy individuals. Arch Dermatol (1996) 132, 1254.
6. Segaert MF, De Soete C, Vandewiele I, Verbanck J. Drug-interaction-induced rhabdomyolysis. Nephrol Dial Transplant (1996) 11, 1846–7.
7. Malouf MA, Bicknell M, Glanville AR. Rhabdomyolysis after lung transplantation. Aust N Z J Med (1997) 27, 186.

Simvastatin + Miscellaneous drugs

Simvastatin causes a small but probably clinically unimportant increase in the serum levels of digoxin. It appears not to interact adversely with ACE inhibitors, beta-blockers, bile acid sequestrants, diuretics, nicotinic acid (niacin) or NSAIDs.

Clinical evidence, mechanism, importance and management

Serum **digoxin** levels can be slightly raised (0.3 nanograms/ml) by simvastatin but this appears to be of little or no clinical importance. In clinical studies no adverse interactions were seen between simvastatin and **ACE inhibitors**, **propranolol** or **beta-blockers**, **diuretics** or **NSAIDs**. No clinically relevant interactions were seen in studies with simvastatin combined with **nicotinic acid (niacin)**[1] or **ramipril**.[2]

Simvastatin is said to be effective in combination with bile-acid sequestrants (presumably **colestyramine** and **colestipol**),[3] and that it has little effect on the pharmacokinetics of **antipyrine (phenazone)** in hypercholesterolaemic patients, which suggests that simvastatin is unlikely to interact with other drugs which use the same metabolic pathway in the liver.[4]

1. Garnett WR. Interactions with hydroxymethylglutaryl-coenzyme A reductase inhibitors. Am J Health-Syst Pharm (1995) 52, 1639–45.
2. Meyer BH, Scholtz HE, Müller FO, Luus HG, de la Rey N, Seibert-Grafe M, Eckert HG, Metzger H. Lack of interaction between ramipril and simvastatin. Eur J Clin Pharmacol (1994) 47, 373–5.
3. Zocor (Simvastatin). Merck, Sharpe & Dohme. Summary of product characteristics, March 2000.
4. Walker JF. Simvastatin: the clinical profile. Am J Med (1989) 87 (Suppl 4A), 44-46S.

Simvastatin + Sildenafil

A man on simvastatin developed symptoms of rhabdomyolysis after taking a single dose of sildenafil.

Clinical evidence, mechanism, importance and management

A man of 76 who had been taking 10 mg simvastatin daily for 3 years uneventfully, presented at a clinic with a 3-day history of severe and unexplained muscle aches, particularly in the lower part of his legs and feet. The problem had started within 10 hr of taking a single 50-mg dose of **sildenafil**. When examined he showed no muscle tenderness or swelling but his creatine phosphokinase level was slightly raised (406 IU/l). There was also a mild elevation of blood-urea-nitrogen and an increase in creatinine and potassium levels. A tentative diagnosis of rhabdomyolysis was made, there being no other obvious identifiable cause for the myalgia. Both simvastatin and **sildenafil** were stopped and he made a full recovery.[1] The reasons for this possible interaction are not known.

This is an isolated case and no broad generalisations can be based on such slim evidence. Patients should be warned of the risks of rhabdomyolysis when given **statins** and based on the current evidence no further precautions currently seem necessary.

1. Gutierrez CA. Sildenafil-simvastatin interaction: possible cause of rhabdomyolysis? *Am Fam Physician* (2001) 63, 636-7.

Sodium clodronate + Aminoglycoside antibacterials

Severe hypocalcaemia occurred in two patients treated with sodium clodronate when they were given netilmicin or amikacin.

Clinical evidence

A woman of 62 with multiple myeloma was given sodium clodronate 2400 mg daily for osteolysis and bone pain. After 7 days she had grand mal seizures and her calcium was found to be 1.72 mmol/l. Despite daily calcium infusions her calcium remained low. The authors state that symptomatic hypocalcaemia with clodronate is rare, and attributed the dramatic response in this patient to a course of **netilmicin** given 5 days earlier for septicaemia[1] (see mechanism below).

A man of 69 with prostate cancer had been on sodium clodronate 2400 mg for bone pain for 13 months with a normal calcium level. After being admitted with febrile neutropenia due to a course of chemotherapy, the clodronate was withdrawn and he was given intravenous **amikacin** and ceftazidime. After 7 days he became unconscious and developed spontaneous fasciculations in his arms and legs. His calcium was found to be 1.39 mmol/l and he was diagnosed with hypocalcaemic tetany. He was given calcium infusions, and his serum calcium returned to normal over the next 12 hours.[2]

Mechanism

Not fully understood, but one suggestion is that any fall in blood calcium levels brought about by the use of clodronate is normally balanced to some extent by the excretion of parathyroid hormone which raises blood calcium levels. However, the aminoglycoside antibacterials can damage the kidneys, not only causing the loss of calcium, but of magnesium as well. Any hypomagnesaemia inhibits the activity of the parathyroids, so that the normal homoeostatic response to hypocalcaemia is reduced or even abolished.[1,2] Clodronate itself can sometimes be nephrotoxic.

Importance and management

Direct information seems to be limited to these two reports. Biochemical hypocalcaemia is believed to occur in about 10% of patients on bisphosphonates,[3] but symptomatic hypocalcaemia is said to be rare (there appear to be only four cases on record).[2] It seems therefore that the addition of the aminoglycoside in these two cases precipitated severe clinical hypocalcaemia. The authors of both reports therefore advise care if bisphosphonates are given with aminoglycosides, with close monitoring of calcium and magnesium levels. They also point out that the renal loss of calcium and magnesium can continue for weeks after the aminoglycosides are stopped, and that the bisphosphonates can also persist for weeks.[1,2] This means that the interaction is potentially possible whether the drugs are given concurrently or sequentially.

1. Pedersen-Bjergaard U, Myhre J. Severe hypoglycaemia (sic) after treatment with diphosphonate and aminoglycoside. *BMJ* (1991) 302, 295.
2. Mayordomo JI, Rivera F. Severe hypocalcaemia after treatment with oral clodronate and aminoglycoside. *Ann Oncol* (1993) 4, 432–5.
3. Jodrell DI, Iveson TJ, Smith IE. Symptomatic hypocalcaemia after treatment with high-dose aminohydroxypropylidene diphosphonate. *Lancet* (1987) i, 622.

Sodium clodronate + Miscellaneous drugs

The absorption of sodium clodronate from the gut is reduced by antacids, iron preparations, calcium supplements, milk and food containing metallic divalent ions.

Clinical evidence, mechanism, importance and management

The bisphosphonates can form complexes with a number of divalent metallic ions which can impair their absorption. For this reason sodium clodronate should be prevented from coming into contact in the gut with a range of other preparations such as **antacids** (containing **bismuth**, **calcium**, **magnesium**), **iron preparations** or **calcium supplements**. To achieve this they should be taken at least 2 h apart. It is not clear whether sodium clodronate also complexes with **aluminium** which is trivalent and found in many antacid preparations. **Food** and **milk** in particular contain calcium, and may also impair absorption, so that sodium clodronate should be separated from them by 1 to 2 h.[1] These are the makers recommendations.

The makers also say that while the concurrent use of sodium clodronate with **other bisphosphonates** is contraindicated. From clinical studies they say that there is no evidence of interactions between sodium clodronate and **steroids**, **diuretics**, **analgesics**, or **chemotherapeutic agents** (none of the drugs was specifically named). Renal impairment on concurrent use of **NSAIDs** and sodium clodronate has been reported, but a synergistic action has not been noted.[1]

1. Bonefos capsules (Sodium clodronate). Summary of product characteristics, March 1999.

Sodium polystyrene sulphonate + Antacids

The concurrent use of antacids with sodium polystyrene sulphonate can result in metabolic alkalosis.

Clinical evidence, mechanism, importance and management

A man with hyperkalaemia developed metabolic alkalosis when given 30 g sodium polystyrene sulphonate with 30 ml **magnesium hydroxide** mixture, three times daily.[1] Alkalosis has also been described in a study on a number of patients given this cation exchange resin with **Maalox** (**magnesium-aluminium hydroxides**) and **calcium carbonate**.[2] The suggested reason is that the sodium polystyrene sulphonate and **magnesium** react together within the gut to form magnesium polystyrene sulphonate and sodium chloride. As a result the normal neutralisation of the bicarbonate ions by the gastric juice and the resin within the gut fails to occur, resulting in the absorption of the bicarbonate leading to metabolic alkalosis. This interaction appears to be established. Concurrent use should be undertaken with caution and serum electrolytes should be closely monitored. Administration of the resin rectally as an enema can avoid the problem.

1. Fernandez PC, Kovnat PJ. Metabolic acidosis reversed by the combination of magnesium and a cation-exchange resin. *N Engl J Med* (1972) 286, 23–4.
2. Schroeder ET. Alkalosis resulting from combined administration of a 'nonsystemic' antacid and a cation-exchange resin. *Gastroenterology* (1969) 56, 868–74.

Sodium polystyrene sulphonate + Sorbitol

Potentially fatal colonic necrosis may occur if sodium polystyrene sulphonate is given as an enema with sorbitol.

Clinical evidence

Five patients with uraemia developed severe colonic necrosis after being given enemas containing sodium polystyrene sulphonate and **sorbitol** for the treatment of hyperkalaemia. Four of the 5 died as a result. Associated studies in *rats* (made uraemic) found that all of them died over a 2-day period after being given enemas of sodium polystyrene sulphonate with **sorbitol**, but none died after enemas without **sorbitol**. Extensive haemorrhage and transmural necrosis developed.[1]

Mechanism

Not understood.

Importance and management

Information is very limited and the interaction is not firmly established, nevertheless its seriousness indicates that sodium polystyrene sulphonate should not be given as an enema in aqueous vehicles containing sorbitol. More study is needed.

1. Lillemoe KD, Romolo JL, Hamilton SR, Pennington LR, Burdick JF, Williams GM. Intestinal necrosis due to sodium polystyrene (Kayexalate) in sorbitol enemas: clinical and experimental support for the hypothesis. *Surgery* (1987) 101, 267–72.

Sodium tiludronate + Miscellaneous drugs

The absorption of tiludronate from the gut is reduced by *Maalox* and by other antacids, iron preparations, calcium supplements, milk and calcium-rich foods containing metallic tri- and divalent ions, whereas indometacin (indomethacin) raises tiludronate bioavailability. Aspirin, diclofenac and digoxin do not interact.

Clinical evidence, mechanism, importance and management

The bisphosphonates can form complexes with a number of metallic ions which can impair their absorption from the gut. For example, when *Maalox* (**aluminium-magnesium hydroxide**) was taken by 12 healthy subjects one hour before tiludronate, the tiludronate AUC was halved and the maximum serum concentration was similarly halved, from 3.35 to 1.59 mg/l. However when the *Maalox* was taken 2 h after the tiludronate, the bioavailability was only slightly affected.[1] Other **antacid** preparations, or **calcium supplements** should similarly be prevented from coming into contact with tiludronate in the gut. **Foods**, and **milk** in particular, which are rich in calcium, may also impair absorption so that tiludronate should be separated from these drugs by 2 h. These are the makers recommendations.[2]

Studies in 12 healthy subjects found that 25 mg **diclofenac** and 600 mg **aspirin** had no significant effect on the pharmacokinetics of tiludronate. On the other hand, 50 mg **indometacin (indomethacin)** slightly increased maximum serum concentration and the AUC of the tiludronate when taken together, but not when separated by 2 h. For this reason the makers advise separating **indometacin** and tiludronate by 2 h.[1]

No significant changes in the pharmacokinetics of **digoxin** 250 micrograms daily were seen in 12 healthy subjects when additionally given tiludronate, firstly 600 mg daily for 2 days then 400 mg daily for the next 10 days.[1] No special precautions appear to be needed.

1. Sanofi Winthrop. Data on file, June 1996.
2. Skelid (Disodium tiluronate). Sanofi Synthelabo. Summary of product characteristics, January 2001.

Somatropin (human growth hormone) + Miscellaneous hormones

The glucocorticoid corticosteroids can oppose the effects of somatropin. Somatropin opposes the hypoglycaemic effects of insulin and may also reduce thyroid function.

Clinical evidence, mechanism, importance and management

Large doses of **glucocorticoid corticosteroids** can inhibit the growth stimulating effects of somatropin. Close monitoring of concurrent use is needed.[1] Somatropin raises blood sugar levels. The control of blood sugar levels in diabetic children will therefore need to be closely monitored if somatropin and **insulin** are used concurrently.[1] Somatropin can unmask hypothyroidism which can reduce the growth stimulating effects of somatropin. Monitor the thyroid function and administer **thyroid hormone** if necessary.[1]

1. Humatrope (Somatotropin). Eli Lilly and Company Limited. Summary of product characteristics, July 2001.

Statins + Calcium channel blockers

Preliminary information indicates that diltiazem causes a very marked rise in serum lovastatin levels, but pravastatin is not affected. A case report describes rhabdomyolisis in a man on diltiazem and simvastatin.

Clinical evidence

(a) Atorvastatin

The makers say that clinical studies in which atorvastatin was used with **calcium channel blockers** no clinically significant interactions were seen.[1] None of the drugs was specifically named except **amlodipine**, which is reported not to affect the pharmacokinetics of atorvastatin. However, the makers do warn that drugs that are metabolised by the cytochrome P450 isoenzyme CYP3A4 (such as diltiazem) do have the potential to interact.[1]

(b) Fluvastatin

A study in to the effects of antihypertensives on the efficacy of fluvastatin found that the concurrent use of **calcium channel blockers** was well tolerated and did not significantly affect the lipid lowering effects of fluvastatin, although there was a trend towards enhanced lowering of triglycerides.[2]

(c) Lovastatin

A study in to the effects of lovastatin and antihypertensive medication found that when **calcium channel blockers** (**diltiazem**, **nifedipine** or **verapamil**) were used in combination with lovastatin there was an additional 3 to 5% lowering in the LDL-cholesterol, which was of marginal significance.[3] Pharmacokinetic studies have shown that oral **diltiazem** increases the AUC and maximum serum levels of lovastatin about fourfold.[4,5] Lovastatin 20 mg or **isradipine** 5 mg was given to 12 healthy subjects either alone or together for 5 days. The lovastatin AUC was reduced by 40%, in males but not females, by the concurrent use of **isradipine**.[6]

(d) Pravastatin

A study in 10 subjects found that sustained-release **diltiazem** 120 mg twice daily had no effect on the pharmacokinetics of single dose pravastatin.[4]

(e) Simvastatin

A single 20-mg dose of simvastatin was given to 10 healthy subjects after they had taken sustained-release **diltiazem**, 120 mg twice daily, for 2 weeks. **Diltiazem** caused about a fivefold increase in the simvastatin AUC, a fourfold increase in the maximum serum levels and a 2.5-fold increase in the half life.[7] A similar study, in which 12 subjects were given **verapamil** 80 mg three times daily found a 4.6-fold increase in the simvastatin AUC, a 2.6-fold increase in the maximum serum levels and about a twofold increase in the half life.[8] An *in vitro* study using human liver microsomes also found that both **diltiazem** and **verapamil** moderately inhibited simvastatin metabolism.[9]

The clinical relevance of the **diltiazem** interaction was demonstrated in a man of 53, who developed rhabdomyolysis 3 months after **diltiazem** 30 mg four times daily was added to established treatment with simvastatin 40 mg daily. Both drugs were discontinued and he recovered over the following 10 days.[10]

Mechanism

Diltiazem, isradipine and verapamil inhibit the cytochrome P450 isoenzyme CYP3A4, which is involved in the metabolism of atorvastatin, simvastatin and lovastatin. Fluvastatin and pravastatin are not significantly metabolised by this isoenzyme. In one study oral diltiazem, but not intravenous diltiazem interacted, suggesting that the interaction does not occur systemically, and that intestinal CYP3A is of importance.[11]

Importance and management

The interaction with simvastatin, lovastatin and probably atorvastatin could be clinically significant, seemingly on rare occasions. It has been suggested that treatment with a statin in a patient on diltiazem (and probably verapamil and isradipine) should be started with the lowest possible dose and titrated upwards, or considerably reduced[8] if for example diltiazem is started. All patients should be warned to be alert for the signs of rhabdomyolysis. Information on other calcium channel blockers is sparse, but amlodipine does not seem to affect CYP3A4 and so is unlikely to interact by this mechanism.

1. Lipitor (Atorvastatin). Parke Davis. Summary of product characteristics, May 2000.
2. Peters TK, Jewitt-Harris J, Mehra M, Muratti EN. Safety and tolerability of fluvastatin with concomitant use of antihypertensive agents. An analysis of a clinical trial database. *Am J Hypertens* (1993) 6, 346S–352S.
3. Pool JL, Shear CL, Downton M, Schnaper H, Stinnett S, Dujovne C, Bradford RH, Chremos AN. Lovastatin and coadministered antihypertensive/cardiovascular agents. *Hypertension* (1992) 19, 242–8.
4. Agbim NE, Brater DC, Hall SD. Interaction of diltiazem with lovastatin and pravastatin. *Clin Pharmacol Ther* (1996) 61, 201.
5. Jones DR, Azie NE, Masica BA, Brater DC, Hall SD. Oral but not intravenous (IV) diltiazem impairs lovastatin clearance. *Clin Pharmacol Ther* (1999) 65, 149.
6. Zhou LX, Finley DK, Hassell AE, Holtzman JL. Pharmacokinetic interaction between isradipine and lovastatin in normal, female and male volunteers. *J Pharmacol Exp Ther* (1995) 273, 121–7.
7. Mousa O, Brater DC, Sunblad KJ, Hall SD. The interaction of diltiazem with simvastatin. *Clin Pharmacol Ther* (2000) 67, 267–74.
8. Kantola T, Kivistö KT, Neuvonen PJ. Erythromycin and verapamil considerably increase serum simvastatin and simvastatin acid concentrations. *Clin Pharmacol Ther* (1998) 64, 177–82.
9. Yeo KR, Yeo WW. Inhibitory effects of verapamil and diltiazem on simvastatin metabolism in human liver microsomes. *Br J Clin Pharmacol* (2001) 51, 461–70.
10. Kanathur N, Mathai MG, Byrd RP, Fields CL, Roy TM. Simvastatin-diltiazem drug interaction resulting in rhabdomyolisis and hepatitis. *Tenessee Med* (2001) 94, 339–41.
11. Masica AL, Azie NE, Brater C, Hall SD, Jones DR. Intravenous diltiazem and CYP3A-mediated metabolism. *Br J Clin Pharmacol* (2000) 50, 273–6.

Statins + Ciclosporin

In renal transplant patients the addition of a lovastatin or simvastatin to treatment with ciclosporin may result in muscle damage, severe rhabdomyolysis and renal failure. The interaction appears to be dose dependent. Myalgia and elevated creatine phosphokinase levels have been noted with concurrent fluvastatin and ciclosporin. Levels of pravastatin may be significantly increased during concurrent treatment with ciclosporin. Close monitoring is advised if any statin is added to therapy with ciclosporin.

Clinical evidence

(a) Atorvastatin

In a study of 10 patients on **ciclosporin** post renal-transplant, 4 showed increases in their trough **ciclosporin** levels of between 26 and 54% (necessitating a dose reduction) when **atorvastatin** 10 mg daily was added to treatment. No change was seen in the other 6 patients, and the incidence of adverse effects was no greater than in a control group of transplant patients not given **atorvastatin**.[1]

(b) Cerivastatin

No change was seen in **ciclosporin** levels in 10 patients on **ciclosporin** post renal-transplant, who were additionally given **cerivastatin** 200 micrograms daily. The incidence of adverse effects was no greater than in a control group of transplant patients not on a statin.[1] **Cerivastatin** has now been withdrawn from the market.

(c) Fluvastatin

Fluvastatin 20 mg daily was given to 16 patients on **ciclosporin** who were 21 to 103 months post renal-transplantation. No significant changes were seen in their **ciclosporin** levels, no rise was seen in creatine phosphokinase (CPK) and no additional adverse events were reported.[2,3] Similar results have been seen in other studies[4,5] one of which used **fluvastatin** 20 mg twice daily.[4] A further study reported 2 patients with mild myalgia without CPK rises, and a patient with elevated CPK without myalgia in a group of 20 renal transplant patients given **fluvastatin** 20 mg daily in addition to **ciclosporin**.[6]

(d) Lovastatin

Ciclosporin and creatine phosphokinase levels were not significantly changed in 6 renal transplant patients taking **ciclosporin** and **lovastatin** (10 mg for 8 weeks, then 20 mg for 12 weeks).[7] Similar results were found in another study.[8]

The maximum serum levels and AUC of **lovastatin** 20 mg were 40 and 47% higher respectively in a group of 21 renal transplant patients compared to values reported in patients not on **ciclosporin**.[9]

There are at least 9 documented cases of rhabdomyolysis in patients receiving **ciclosporin** and **lovastatin**,[10-14] which resulted in acute renal failure in 3 cases.[10,14] In each of these cases the patient was receiving **lovastatin** 40 to 80 mg daily. Several other studies highlight this dose-related effect. In one study, 15 patients on **ciclosporin** were additionally given **lovastatin** 20 mg without problem, but 4 of 5 other patients, who were receiving **lovastatin** 40 to 80 mg daily all developed rhabdomyolysis, which was associated with renal failure in 2 of them.[15] A further study investigated 24 patients, who were either given **lovastatin** 10 mg or **lovastatin** 20 mg in addition to **ciclosporin**. Of the 12 receiving the 20-mg dose, 7 developed either myalgia and muscle weakness or raised creatine phosphokinase levels, but only one patient from the 10-mg group did.[16]

(e) Pravastatin

Several studies have shown no rises in creatine phosphokinase levels,[17-19] no change in **ciclosporin** levels[9,18] and no increase in adverse effects[9,17,20] when **pravastatin** in doses of 10 to 40 mg daily was given concurrently with ciclosporin. However, one study demonstrated that the maximum serum levels and AUC of **pravastatin** in a group of transplant patients on **ciclosporin** were sevenfold and twentyfold greater respectively than those in a group of patients receiving **pravastatin** without **ciclosporin**.[21]

(f) Simvastatin

A group of 20 heart transplant patients were treated with both **simvastatin** 10 mg daily and **ciclosporin** over a period of 4 months.[22] No significant pharmacokinetic changes were seen and the combination was well tolerated. Similar results were found in another study over 8 months.[23]

However, a study comparing 5 renal transplant patients on **ciclosporin** and **simvastatin** 20 mg daily with 5 renal transplant patients not on **ciclosporin** found that the AUC and maximum serum levels of **simvastatin** were 2.5-fold and twofold greater respectively, in the patients on **ciclosporin**.[24] Another study found that the **ciclosporin** levels of 12 renal transplant patients dropped from 334 to 235 micrograms/l after **simvastatin** 5 to 15 mg daily was added.[25] A retrospective study of 12 patients by the same authors confirmed these results.[25] There are also two reports of rhabdomyolysis,[26,27] one fatal,[27] in patients given **ciclosporin** and **simvastatin** 20 mg daily.

Mechanism

Both statins and ciclosporin are substrates for the cytochrome P450 isoenzyme CYP3A4. The interaction seems to be largely dependent on the relative affinities of the drugs for this isoenzyme, and whether or not they are metabolised by other pathways as well (for example fluvastatin, which does not appear to interact pharmacokinetically, is also metabolised by CYP2C9, which is not affected by ciclosporin). P-glycoprotein may also play a part.[1] Any change that results in an elevation of statin levels is likely to increase the risk of myopathies.

Importance and management

The interaction of statins and ciclosporin is established and of clinical importance. For example, with lovastatin alone the incidence of myopathies is about 0.1 to 0.2%,[9] but in the presence of ciclosporin the incidence is said to be as high as 30%.[28] The drug combination has an important place in treatment post-transplantation, but if it is to be undertaken close monitoring of toxicity should take place. It is likely that any patient on ciclosporin will be monitored closely anyway, but if a statin is started be aware that dosage adjustments may be necessary. Patients should be counselled on how to recognise signs of myopathy. The interaction appears to be dose related. The makers of simvastatin suggest that if it is to be started in a patient on ciclosporin that only 10 mg is used.[29] If myopathy does occur withdrawing the statin has been shown to resolve symptoms. Reducing the dose may also be an option,[30] but don't forget there have been fatalities after patients have developed rhabdomyolysis when taking ciclosporin with a statin.

1. Renders L, Mayer-Kadner I, Koch C, Schärffe S, Burkhardt K, Veelken R, Schmieder RE, Hauser IA. Efficacy and drug interactions of the new HMG-CoA reductase inhibitors cerivastatin and atorvastatin in CsA-treated renal transplant recipients. *Nephrol Dial Transplant* (2001) 16, 141–6.
2. Li PKT, Mak TWL, Wang AYM, Lee YT, Leung CB, Lui SF, Lam CWK, Lai KN. The interaction of fluvastatin and cyclosporin A in renal-transplant patients. *Int J Clin Pharmacol Ther* (1995) 33, 246–8.
3. Li PKT, Mak TWL, Chan TH, Wang A, Lam CWK, Lai KN. Effect of fluvastatin on lipoprotein profiles in treating renal transplant recipients with dyslipoproteinemia. *Transplantation* (1995) 60, 652–6.
4. Holdaas H, Hartmann A, Stenstrøm J, Dahl KJ, Borge M, Pfister P. Effect of fluvastatin for safely lowering atherogenic lipids in renal transplant patients receiving cyclosporine. *Am J Cardiol* (1995) 76, 102A–106A.
5. Goldberg R, Roth D. Evaluation of fluvastatin in the treatment of hypercholesterolemia in renal transplant patients taking cyclosporine. *Transplantation* (1996) 62, 1559–64.
6. Goldberg RB, Roth D. A preliminary report of the safety and efficacy of fluvastatin for hypercholesterolemia in renal transplant patients receiving cyclosporine. *Am J Cardiol* (1995) 76, 107A–109A.
7. Cheung AK, DeVault GA, Gregory MC. A prospective study on treatment of hypercholesterolemia with lovastatin in renal transplant patients receiving cyclosporine. *J Am Soc Nephrol* (1993) 3, 1884–91.
8. Castelao AM, Griñó JM, Andrés E, Gilvernet S, Serón D, Castiñeiras MJ, Roca M, Galcerán JM, González MT, Alsina J. HMGCoA reductase inhibitors lovastatin and simvastatin in the treatment of hypercholesterolemia after renal transplantation. *Transplant Proc* (1993) 25, 1043–6.
9. Olbricht C, Wanner C, Eisenhauer T, Kliem V, Doll R, Boddaert M, O'Grady P, Krekler M, Mangold B, Christians U. Accumulation of lovastatin, but not pravastatin, in the blood of cyclosporine-treated kidney graft patients after multiple doses. *Clin Pharmacol Ther* (1997) 62, 311–21.
10. Alejandro DSJ, Petersen J. Myoglobinuric acute renal failure in a cardiac transplant patient taking lovastatin and cyclosporine. *J Am Soc Nephrol* (1994) 5, 153–160.
11. Corpier CL, Jones PH, Suki WN, Lederer ED, Quinones MA, Schmidt SW, Young JB. Rhabdomyolysis and renal injury with lovastatin use. Report of two cases in cardiac transplant recipients. *JAMA* (1988) 260, 239–41.
12. East C, Alivizatos PA, Grundy SM, Jones PH, Farmer JA. Rhabdomyolysis in patients receiving lovastatin after cardiac transplantation. *N Engl J Med* (1988) 318, 47–8.
13. Norman DJ, Illingworth DR, Munson J, Hosenpud J. Myolysis and acute renal failure in a heart-transplant recipient receiving lovastatin. *N Engl J Med* (1988) 318, 46–7.
14. Kobashigawa JA, Murphy F, Stevenson LW, Moriguchi JD, Kawata N, Chuck C, Wilmarth J, Leonard L, Drinkwater D, Laks H. Low dose of lovastatin safely lowers cholesterol after cardiac transplantation. *Circulation* (1989) 80 (Suppl II), II-641.
15. Ballantyne CM, Radovancevic B, Farmer JA, Frazier OH, Chandler L, Payton-Ross C, Cocanougher B, Jones PH, Young JB, Gotto AM. Hyperlipidemia after heart transplantation: report of a 6-year experience, with treatment recommendations. *J Am Coll Cardiol* (1992) 19, 1315–21.
16. Heroux AL, Thompson JA, Katz S, Hastillo AK, Katz M, Quigg RJ, Hess ML. Elimination of the lovastatin-cyclosporine adverse interaction in heart transplant patients. *Circulation* (1989) 80, II-641.
17. Yoshimura N, Oka T, Okamoto M, Ohmori Y. The effects of pravastatin on hyperlipidemia in renal transplant recipients. *Transplantation* (1992) 53, 94–9.
18. Cassem JD, Hamilton MA, Albanese E, Sabad A, Kobashigawa JA. Does pravastatin affect cyclosporine pharmacokinetics in cardiac transplant recipients. *J Invest Med* (1997) 45, 139A.
19. Muhlmeister HF, Hamilton MA, Cogert GA, Cassem JD, Sabad A, Kobashigawa JA. Long-term HMG-CoA reductase inhibition appears safe and effective after cardiac transplantation. *J Invest Med* (1997) 45, 139A.
20. Kobashigawa JA, Brownfield ED, Stevenson LW, Gleeson MP, Moriguchi JD, Kawata N, Hamilton MA, Hage AS, Minkley R, Salamandra J, Ruzevich S, Drinkwater DC, Laks H. Effects of pravastatin for hypercholesterolemia in cardiac transplant recipients. *J Am Coll Cardiol* (1993) 21, 141A.
21. Regazzi MB, Iacona I, Campana C. Raddato V, Lesi C, Perani G, Gavazzi A, Viganò M. Altered disposition of pravastatin following concomitant drug therapy with cyclosporin A in transplant recipients. *Transplant Proc* (1993) 25, 2732–4.
22. Campana C, Iacona I, Regazzi MB, Gavazzi A, Perani G, Raddato V, Montemartini C, Viganò M. Efficacy and pharmacokinetics of simvastatin in heart transplant recipients. *Ann Pharmacother* (1995) 29, 235–9.
23. Barbir M, Rose M, Kushwaha S, Akl S, Mitchell A, Yacoub M. Low-dose simvastatin for the treatment of hypercholesterolaemia in recipients of cardiac transplantation. *Int J Cardiol* (1991) 33, 241–6.
24. Arnadottir M, Eriksson L-O, Thysell H, Karkas JD. Plasma concentration profiles of simvastatin 3-hydroxy-3-methyl-glutaryl-coenzyme A reductase inhibitory activity in kidney transplant recipients with and without ciclosporin. *Nephron* (1993) 65, 410–13.
25. Akhlaghi F, McLachlan AJ, Keogh AM, Brown KF. Effect of simvastatin on cyclosporine unbound fraction and apparent blood clearance in heart transplant recipients. *Br J Clin Pharmacol* (1997) 44, 537–42.
26. Blaison G, Weber JC, Sachs D, Korganow AS, Martin T, Kretz JG, Pasquali JL. Rhabdomyolyse causée par la simvastatine chez un transplanté cardiaque sous ciclosporine. *Rev Med Interne* (1992) 13, 61–3.
27. Weise WJ, Possidente CJ. Fatal rhabdomyolysis associated with simvastatin in a renal transplant patient. *Am J Med* (2000) 108, 351–2.
28. Tobert JA. Rhabdomyolysis in patients receiving lovastatin after cardiac transplantation. *N Engl J Med* (1988) 318, 48.
29. Zocor (Simvastatin). Merck Sharp & Dohme Limited. Summary of product characteristics, March 2000.
30. Neoral (Cyclosporin). Novartis Pharmaceuticals UK Ltd. Summary of product characteristics, February 2002.

Statins + Fibrates

The risk of myopathy and/or rhabdomyolysis appears to be increased in patients given both lovastatin and gemfibrozil. Concurrent use can be effective provided stringent precautions are taken.

Severe myopathy has not been seen with pravastatin and gemfibrozil, but the safety of combined use is not yet established. Fenofibrate and pravastatin appear not to interact. An isolated case report describes the development of rhabdomyolysis in a woman treated with atorvastatin and gemfibrozil, and another report describes rhabdomyolysis in two patients when treated with simvastatin and gemfibrozil.

Clinical evidence

(a) Atorvastatin + Gemfibrozil

A 43-year-old woman with multiple medical problems was taking **gemfibrozil** (600 mg twice daily). After a recurrent attack of pancreatitis, 10 mg **atorvastatin** and 2.5 mg glibenclamide (glyburide), both twice daily were added to her treatment. Later she was also given high dose conjugated estrogens, cimetidine, fluoxetine, medroxyprogesterone, furosemide (frusemide) and trimethobenzamide suppositories. About 3 weeks after the **atorvastatin** had been added to the **gemfibrozil**, she developed brown and turbid urine (suggesting urinary myoglobin), creatine kinase levels of 4633 units/l and had myalgia. She was diagnosed as having rhabdomyolysis. Her serum creatine kinase levels rapidly fell when the **atorvastatin** and **gemfibrozil** were withdrawn.[1]

(b) Cerivastatin + Gemfibrozil

There are several cases of the combination of **cerivastatin** and **gemfibrozil** causing very severe rhabdomyolysis,[2-6] which in some cases was associated with renal failure and deaths. **Cerivastatin** has now been withdrawn from the market.

(c) Lovastatin + Bezafibrate

The pharmacokinetics of a single dose of **lovastatin** were not altered by 3 days of **bezafibrate** in 11 healthy subjects.[7]

(d) Lovastatin + Gemfibrozil

By 1990 the FDA had documented 12 case reports of severe myopathy or rhabdomyolysis associated with the concurrent use of **lovastatin** and **gemfibrozil**. The mean serum creatine kinase levels of the patients reached 15250 units/l. Four of those tested showed myoglobinuria and five had acute renal failure.[8] Details of cases of rhabdomyolysis associated with the concurrent use of these drugs,[9-13] three with renal failure,[10,11,13] have been described elsewhere. Other cases have been seen in patients taking **lovastatin** and **gemfibrozil** with ciclosporin.[14,15] In a pharmacokinetic study, 11 healthy subjects were given **gemfibrozil** 1200 mg daily for 3 days, with a single 40 mg dose of **lovastatin** on day 3. The AUC and maximum plasma level of **lovastatin acid** (a metabolite) were nearly threefold greater in the presence of **gemfibrozil**.[7]

However, in contrast, other reports[16-19] describe apparently safe and effective concurrent use in large numbers of patients under very well controlled conditions, although elevated creatine phosphokinase levels, without rhabdomyolysis, were seen in up to 8% of cases.

(e) Pravastatin + Fenofibrate

A single-dose study in 23 healthy subjects found that the concurrent use of **pravastatin** 40 mg and **fenofibrate** 201 mg had no effect on the pharmacokinetics of either drug, but a moderate increase in the formation of a non-toxic pravastatin metabolite was seen. This was not thought to be clinically important.[20]

(f) Pravastatin + Gemfibrozil

No clinically significant changes in the bioavailability of single 20-mg doses of pravastatin were seen in studies on the concurrent use of 600 mg **gemfibrozil** in 18 healthy subjects.[21] A 12-week large-scale survey found that 40 mg pravastatin daily and 600 mg **gemfibrozil** twice daily caused marked abnormalities in creatine kinase concentrations (four times the pretreatment values) in 1 of 71 patients on **pravastatin** alone, 1 of 73 patients on placebo, 2 of 72 patients on **gemfibrozil** alone, and 4 of 75 patients on combined **gemfibrozil/pravastatin** treatment. The differences between treatments were not statistically significant. Severe myopathy or rhabdomyolysis was not seen in any patient, although 14 patients had musculoskeletal pain, but in most cases this was not considered to be related to the treatment.[22]

(g) Simvastatin + Gemfibrozil

A 62-year-old with diabetes on 20 mg simvastatin and 600 mg **gemfibrozil** daily (as well as acenocoumarol (nicoumalone), glibenclamide and diclofenac) was hospitalised because of melaena, generalised myalgia, malaise and brown urine. Laboratory tests confirmed the diagnosis of rhabdomyolysis. He recovered when the **simvastatin** and **gemfibrozil** were stopped.[23] Another diabetic patient had been taking **simvastatin** and 600 mg **gemfibrozil** daily for two and a half years (and also taking felodipine, indapamide, calcium carbonate, bumetanide, psyllium, acenocoumarol (nicoumalone) and insulin). She complained of tiredness, generalised myalgia and anuria 3 months after her dosage of the **simvastatin** had been increased to 80 mg daily. Rhabdomyolysis with exaggerated renal insufficiency were diagnosed and confirmed. She recovered when the simvastatin and **gemfibrozil** were stopped.[23] A pharmacokinetic study found that the AUC of **simvastatin acid** (a **simvastatin** active metabolite) were increased nearly twofold and the peak concentration doubled, when **simvastatin** was given concurrently with **gemfibrozil**.[24]

Mechanism

Not understood. Myopathy can occur with statins and fibrates alone and their effects may therefore be additive. Limited evidence suggests a pharmacokinetic interaction concerning the cytochrome P450 isoenzyme CYP3A4 may also be involved,[24] but gemfibrozil is not generally recognised as an inhibitor of CYP3A4, so the reasons for the apparent pharmacokinetic interaction are unclear.[25]

Importance and management

The lovastatin/gemfibrozil interaction is established. The FDA discourage the concurrent use of the combination in any patient, but suggest it should be avoided in patients with compromised kidney or liver function.[8]

The other interactions are not as well established. Overall, the incidence of statin/fibrate interactions leading to myopathy has been put at 0.12%.[26] The makers of pravastatin say that the combined use of pravastatin and **fibric acid** derivatives may be useful in selected patients but because of the risks of myopathy it should generally be

avoided.[27] Other makers give similar warnings.[28] If patients are given a fibrate and a statin they should be monitored for evidence of muscle pain or tenderness (warn them to report this if it happens), and creatine kinase levels should be checked.

1. Duell PB, Connor WE, Illingworth DR. Rhabdomyolysis after taking atorvastatin with gemfibrozil. *Am J Cardiol* (1998) 81, 368–9.
2. Pogson GW, Kindred LH, Carper BG. Rhabdomyolysis and renal failure associated with *cerivastatin-gemfibrozil* combination therapy. *Am J Cardiol* (1999) 83, 1146.
3. Bermingham PR, Whitsitt TB, Smart ML, Nowak DP, Scalley RD. Rhabdomyolysis in a patient receiving the combination of cerivastatin and gemfibrozil. *Am J Health-Syst Pharm* (2000) 57, 461–4.
4. Özdemir Ö, Boran M, Gökçe V, Uzun Y, Koçak B, Korkmaz Ş. A case with severe rhabdomyolysis and renal failure associated with cerivastatin-gemfibrozil combination therapy. *Angiology* (2000) 50, 695–7.
5. Bruno-Joyce J, Dugas JM, MacCausland OE. Cerivastatin and gemfibrozil-associated rhabdomyolysis. *Ann Pharmacother* (2001) 35, 1016–19.
6. Vascónez Espinosa F, Gómez Rodríguez N, Martín Joven A, Posada García FJ. Rabdomiólisis complicada con insuficiencia renal aguda en un paciente tratado con gemfibrozilo y cerivastatina. *Rev Clin Esp* (2001) 201, 228–9.
7. Kyrklund C, Backman JT, Kivistö KT, Neuvonen M, Laitila J, Neuvonen PJ. Plasma concentrations of active lovastatin acid are markedly increased by gemfibrozil but not bezafibrate. *Clin Pharmacol Ther* (2001) 69, 340–5.
8. Pierce LR, Wysowski DK, Gross TP. Myopathy and rhabdomyolysis associated with lovastatin-gemfibrozil combination therapy. *JAMA* (1990) 264, 71–5.
9. Tobert JA. Myolysis and acute renal failure in a heart-transplant recipient receiving lovastatin. *N Engl J Med* (1988) 318, 48.
10. Marais GE, Larson KK. Rhabdomyolysis and acute renal failure induced by combination lovastatin and gemfibrozil therapy. *Ann Intern Med* (1990) 112, 228–30.
11. Manoukian AA, Bhagavan NV, Hayashi T, Nestor TA, Rios C, Scottolini AG. Rhabdomyolysis secondary to lovastatin therapy. *Clin Chem* (1990) 36, 2145–7.
12. Kogan AD, Orenstein S. Lovastatin-induced acute rhabdomyolysis. *Postgrad Med J* (1990) 66, 294–6.
13. Goldman JA, Fisherman AB, Lee JE, Johnson RJ. The role of cholesterol-lowering agents in drug-induced rhabdomyolysis and polymyositis. *Arthritis Rheum* (1989) 32, 358–9.
14. Norman DJ, Illingworth DR, Munson J, Hosenpud J. Myolysis and acute renal failure in a heart-transplant patient receiving lovastatin. *N Engl J Med* (1988) 318, 46–7.
15. East C, Alivizatos PA, Grundy SM, Jones PH, Farmer JA. Rhabdomyolysis in patients receiving lovastatin after cardiac transplantation. *N Engl J Med* (1988) 318, 47–8.
16. Illingworth DR, Bacon S. Influence of lovastatin plus gemfibrozil on plasma lipids and lipoproteins in patients with heterozygous familial hypercholesterolemia. *Circulation* (1989) 79, 590–6.
17. Glueck CJ, Oakes N, Speirs J, Tracy T, Lang J. Gemfibrozil-lovastatin therapy for primary hyperlipoproteinemias. *Am J Cardiol* (1992) 70, 1–9.
18. East C, Bilheimer DW, Grundy SM. Combination drug therapy for familial combined hyperlipidemia. *Ann Intern Med* (1988) 109, 25–32.
19. Wirebaugh SR, Shapiro ML, McIntyre TH, Whitney EJ. A retrospective review of the use of lipid-lowering agents in combination, specifically, gemfibrozil and lovastatin. *Pharmacotherapy* (1992) 12, 445–50.
20. Pan W-J, Gustavson LE, Achari R, Rieser MJ, Ye X, Gutterman C, Wallin BA. Lack of a clinically significant pharmacokinetic interaction between fenofibrate and pravastatin in healthy volunteers. *J Clin Pharmacol* (2000) 40, 316–23.
21. Pan HY, Glaess SR, Kassalow LM, Meehan RL, Martynowicz H. A report on the bioavailability of pravastatin in the presence and absence of gemfibrozil or probucol in healthy male subjects. Data on file, ER Squibb. Protocol No. 277, 201-18 (1988).
22. Wiklund O, Angelin B, Bergman M, Berglund L, Bondjers G, Carlsson A, Lindén T, Miettinen T, Ödman B, Olofsson S-O, Saarinen I, Sipilä R, Sjöström P, Kron B, Vanhanen H, Wright I. Pravastatin and gemfibrozil alone and in combination for the treatment of hypercholesterolemia. *Am J Med* (1993) 94, 13–20.
23. Van Puijenbroek EP, Du Buf-Vereijken PWG, Spooren PFMJ, Van Doormaal JJ. Possible increased risk of rhabdomyolysis during concomitant use of simvastatin and gemfibrozil. *J Intern Med* (1996) 240, 403–4.
24. Backman JT, Kyrklund C, Kivistö KT, Wang J-S, Neuvonen PJ. Plasma concentrations of active simvastatin acid are increased by gemfibrozil. *Clin Pharmacol Ther* (2001) 68, 122–9.
25. Guyton JR, Dujovne CA, Illingworth DR. Dual hepatic metabolism of *cerivastatin*—clarifications. *Am J Cardiol* (1999) 84, 497.
26. Shek A, Ferrill J. Statin-fibrate combination therapy. *Ann Pharmacother* (2001) 35, 908–17.
27. Lipostat (Pravastatin). Bristol-Myers Squibb Pharmaceuticals Ltd. Summary of product characteristics, June 2001.
28. Zocor (Simvastatin). Merck Sharpe & Dohme Limited. Summary of product characteristics, March 2000.

Statins + Nefazodone

An isolated report describes the development of myositis and rhabdomyolysis in a patient apparently due to the concurrent use of nefazodone. Another isolated report describes muscle toxicity attributed to a pravastatin/nefazodone interaction.

Clinical evidence

(a) Pravastatin + Nefazodone

A man of 74 taking atenolol, aspirin and **pravastatin** had his treatment with citalopram replaced by **nefazodone**, 50 mg twice daily. Because the possibility of an interaction was suspected, his plasma creatine kinase levels were monitored and were found at 36 h to be

877 U/l (normal 0 to 190 U/l). Lactate dehydrogenase, aspartate aminotransferase and alanine aminotransferase were all slightly elevated and this was interpreted as indicating muscle toxicity. Despite withdrawing the **nefazodone**, creatine kinase levels remained well above the normal range, though falling, and after 14 days the **pravastatin** was withdrawn as well. Later the **pravastatin** was re-introduced and then 75 mg venlafaxine twice daily was added without problems.[1]

(b) Simvastatin + Nefazodone

A man of 44 who had uneventfully taken 40 mg **simvastatin** daily for 19 weeks developed 'tea-coloured' urine a month after starting 100 mg **nefazodone** twice daily which was initially misdiagnosed as a urinary tract infection. A month later he was also complaining of severe myalgias of the thighs and calves, and was found to have muscle weakness and tenderness. Laboratory tests confirmed a new diagnosis of rhabdomyolysis and myositis. He was asymptomatic within 3 weeks of stopping both drugs, and remained problem-free 5 weeks after restarting 40 mg **simvastatin** daily.[2]

Mechanism

Uncertain. The suggestion is that nefazodone (an inhibitor of cytochrome P450 isoenzyme CYP3A4) caused a marked increase in the serum levels of the simvastatin with accompanying toxicity.[2] The same mechanism might also account for the pravastatin/nefazodone interaction.

Importance and management

Information about statin/nefazodone interactions seems to be limited to these two reports so that the risks associated with using nefazodone are uncertain, but what is known certainly suggests that concurrent use should be very well monitored.

1. Alderman CP. Possible interaction between nefazodone and pravastatin. *Ann Pharmacother* (1999) 33, 871.
2. Jacobsen RH, Wang P, Glueck CJ. Myositis and rhabdomyolysis associated with concurrent use of simvastatin and nefazodone. *JAMA* (1997) 277, 296.

St John's wort (*Hypericum perforatum*) + Miscellaneous drugs

St John's wort (*Hypericum perforatum*) is predicted to reduce the blood levels of anticonvulsants (carbamazepine, phenytoin, phenobarbital), and to increase the effects and side-effects of the triptans (naratriptan, rizatriptan, sumatriptan, zolmitriptan). All of these predicted interactions await clinical confirmation. See the Index for other interactions with St John's wort.

Clinical evidence, mechanism, importance and management

There is now good evidence that St John's wort (*Hypericum perforatum*) can interact with several drugs to reduce their serum levels, probably as a result of liver enzyme induction or induction of the drug transporter P-glycoprotein, which is concerned with intestinal absorption and renal excretion. On the basis of the interactions seen with these drugs and other evidence, the CSM in the UK predicts that the serum levels of other drugs are likely to be reduced by St John's wort.[1] These include **carbamazepine**, **phenytoin**, and **phenobarbitone**. The CSM's advice for all of these drugs is that St John's wort should be stopped. The CSM suggests that the dosage may then need to be adjusted.

St John's wort also affects the neurotransmitters in the brain and because of this it is predicted that it may also interact with triptans used for migraine (**naratriptan, rizatriptan, sumatriptan, zolmitriptan**), the expectation being that an increase in serotonergic effects and side-effects may occur. The advice of the CSM, again, is to avoid or stop St John's wort.

At the present time these are only reasonable predictions, but it would be prudent to follow the CSM's advice while clinical confirmation of these interactions is awaited or until the safety of concurrent use has been demonstrated.

1. Committee on the Safety of Medicines (UK). Message from Professor A Breckenridge (Chairman of CSM) and Fact Sheet for Health Care Professionals, 29th February 2000.

Sulfasalazine + Antibacterials

The release in the colon of the active drug (5-aminosalicylic acid) from sulfasalazine is markedly reduced by the concurrent use of ampicillin and rifampicin (rifampin), which reduce the activity of the gut bacteria. This interaction seems likely with any other oral antibacterial that similarly reduces the gut microflora, but see 'Sulfasalazine + Metronidazole', p.932.

Clinical evidence

(a) Ampicillin

The conversion and release by the bacterial microflora within the gut of the active metabolite of sulfasalazine, 5-aminosalicylic acid, was reduced by a third in 5 healthy subjects given a single 2-g dose of sulfasalazine after a 5-day course of 250 mg **ampicillin** four times daily.[1]

(b) Rifampicin (Rifampin)

A crossover trial in 11 patients with Crohn's disease on long term treatment with sulfasalazine found that while concurrently taking **rifampicin** 10 mg/kg daily and ethambutol 15 mg/kg daily their plasma levels of both 5-aminosalicylic acid and sulphapyridine fell by about 60%.[2]

Mechanism

The azo link of sulfasalazine is split by anaerobic bacteria in the colon to release sulphapyridine and 5-aminosalicylic acid, the latter being the active metabolite, which acts locally in the treatment of Crohn's disease. Antibacterials that decimate the gut flora can apparently reduce this conversion and this is reflected in lower plasma levels. Rifampicin also possibly increases the metabolism of the sulphapyridine.

Importance and management

Information is limited, but the interaction appears to be established. The extent to which these antibacterials reduce the effectiveness of sulfasalazine in the treatment of Crohn's disease or ulcerative colitis seems not to have been assessed, but watch for evidence of a reduced effect if ampicillin, rifampicin or any other oral antibacterial is given. **Neomycin**, which also affects the activity of the gut microflora, has been seen to interact similarly in *animal* studies.[3]

1. Houston JB, Day J, Walker J. Azo reduction of sulphasalazine in healthy volunteers. *Br J Clin Pharmacol* (1982) 14, 395–8.
2. Shaffer JL, Houston JB. The effect of rifampicin on sulphapyridine plasma concentrations following sulphasalazine administration. *Br J Clin Pharmacol* (1985) 19, 526–8.
3. Peppercorn MA, Goldman P. The role of intestinal bacteria in the metabolism of salicylazosulfapyridine. *J Pharmacol Exp Ther* (1972) 181, 555–62.

Sulfasalazine or Sodium Fusidate + Colestyramine

Animal studies show that colestyramine can bind with these two drugs in the gut, thereby reducing their activity, but whether this also occurs in man awaits confirmation.

Clinical evidence, mechanism, importance and management

In vitro and *in vivo* studies with *rats* have shown that **colestyramine** binds with **sodium fusidate** in the gut, thereby reducing the amount available for absorption.[1] Another study in *rats* found that **colestyramine** binds with **sulfasalazine** so that the azo-bond is protected against attack by the bacteria within the gut. As a result the active 5-aminosalicylic acid is not released and the faecal excretion of intact **sulfasalazine** increases 30-fold.[2] It seems possible that both of these interactions could also occur in man, but confirmation of this is as yet lacking. Separating the drug dosages to prevent their admixture in the gut has proved effective with other drugs that bind with **colestyramine**.

1. Johns WH, Bates TR. Drug-cholestyramine interactions. I: Physicochemical factors affecting *in vitro* binding of sodium fusidate to cholestyramine. *J Pharm Sci* (1972) 61, 730–5.
2. Pieniaszek HJ, Bates TR. Cholestyramine-induced inhibition of salicylazosulfapyridine (sulfasalazine) metabolism by rat intestinal microflora. *J Pharmacol Exp Ther* (1976) 198, 240–5.

Sulfasalazine + Cimetidine

Cimetidine does not interact with sulfasalazine.

Clinical evidence, mechanism, importance and management

A study in 14 patients with rheumatoid arthritis treated with sulfasalazine, 9 also given 400 mg **cimetidine** three times daily, found that **cimetidine** for 18 weeks did not affect the plasma or urinary levels of the sulfasalazine and there were no changes in blood cell counts or haemoglobin levels. The conclusion was reached that no clinically important interaction occurs between these two drugs.[1]

1. Pirmohamed M, Coleman MD, Galvani D, Bucknall RC, Breckenridge AM, Park BK. Lack of interaction between sulphasalazine and cimetidine in patients with rheumatoid arthritis. *Br J Rheumatol* (1993) 32, 222–6.

Sulfasalazine + Iron salts

Sulfasalazine and iron appear to bind together in the gut, but whether this reduces the therapeutic response to either compound is uncertain.

Clinical evidence, mechanism, importance and management

Ferrous iron 400 mg reduced the peak serum levels of a single 50 mg/kg dose of sulfasalazine in 5 healthy subjects by 40%. The reasons are not known, but it seems likely that the sulfasalazine chelates with the **iron** in the gut which interferes with its absorption.[1] The extent to which this suggested chelation affects the ability of the intestinal bacteria to split the sulfasalazine and release its locally active metabolite 5-aminosalicylic acid, and thereby effect a therapeutic response, seems not to have been studied. More study is needed.

1. Das KM, Eastwood MA. Effect of iron and calcium on salicylazosulphapyridine metabolism. *Scott Med J* (1973) 18, 45–50.

Sulfasalazine + Metronidazole

Metronidazole appears not to interact adversely with sulfasalazine.

Clinical evidence, mechanism, importance and management

A study in 10 patients (7 with Crohn's disease and 5 with ulcerative colitis) on long-term sulfasalazine treatment 2 to 4 g daily found no statistically significant changes in serum sulfapyridine levels occurred while they were additionally taking 400 mg **metronidazole** twice daily for 8 to 14 days.[1] There seem to be no good reasons for avoiding concurrent use.

1. Shaffer JL, Kershaw A, Houston JB. Disposition of metronidazole and its effects on sulphasalazine metabolism in patients with inflammatory bowel disease. *Br J Clin Pharmacol* (1986) 21, 431–5.

Sulfasalazine + Zileuton

Sulfasalazine and zileuton appear not to interact.

Clinical evidence, mechanism, importance and management

In randomised double-blind placebo controlled trial 14 healthy subjects were given 1 g sulfasalazine 12-hourly for 8 days, and 800 mg **zileuton** or a placebo 12-hourly on days 3 to 8. It was found that the pharmacokinetics of the sulfasalazine and its metabolites, sulphapyridine and *N*-acetyl sulphapyridine were not significantly changed. The study did not directly look at the pharmacokinetics of the **zileuton** but the parameters measured were similar to those seen in a previous study.[1] There would seem to be no reason for special precautions if both drugs are used.

1. Awni WM, Braeckman RA, Locke CS, Dubé LM, Granneman GR. The influence of multiple oral doses of zileuton on the steady-state pharmacokinetics of sulfasalazine and its metabolites, sulfapyridine and N-acetylsulfapyridine. *Clin Pharmacokinet* (1995) 29 (Suppl 2), 98–104.

Sulfinpyrazone + Flufenamic, Meclofenamic or Mefenamic acid

The uricosuric effects of sulfinpyrazone are not opposed by the concurrent use of flufenamic acid, meclofenamic acid or mefenamic acid.[1,2]

1. Latham BA, Radcliff F, Robinson RG. The effect of mefenamic acid and flufenamic acid on plasma uric acid levels. *Ann Phys Med* (1966) 8, 242–3.
2. Robinson RG, Radcliff FJ. The effect of meclofenamic acid on plasma uric acid levels. *Med J Aust* (1972) 1, 1079–80.

Sulfinpyrazone + Probenecid

Probenecid reduces the loss of sulfinpyrazone in the urine, but the uricosuria remains unaltered.

Clinical evidence, mechanism, importance and management

A study in 8 patients with gout showed that while **probenecid** was able to inhibit the renal tubular excretion of sulfinpyrazone, reducing it by about 75%, the maximal uric acid clearance was about the same as when either drug was given alone.[1] There would therefore seem to be no advantage in using these drugs together. Whether the toxic effects of sulfinpyrazone are increased seems not to have been studied.

1. Perel JM, Dayton PG, Snell MM, Yü TF, Gutman AB. Studies of interactions among drugs in man at the renal level: probenecid and sulphinpyrazone. *Clin Pharmacol Ther* (1969) 10, 834–40.

Sumatriptan + Miscellaneous drugs

Sumatriptan should not be taken by patients with ischaemic heart disease. It is not clear whether the concurrent use of the ergot alkaloids should be avoided or not, but use is contraindicated. The makers warn about the concurrent use of lithium. Sumatriptan appears not to interact with alcohol, butorphanol nasal spray, flunarizine, food or pizotifen.

Clinical evidence, mechanism, importance and management

(a) Butorphanol

No pharmacokinetic interactions were found to occur between single 1-mg doses of **butorphanol tartrate** nasal spray and a 6 mg subcutaneous dose of **sumatriptan succinate** in 24 healthy subjects, and no changes in side-effects were seen. It was concluded that concurrent use during acute migraine attacks need not be avoided.[1]

(b) Cardioactive drugs

The CSM in the UK says that sumatriptan should not be used in patients with ischaemic heart disease or Prinzmetal's angina.[2] Thus patients who are taking **nitrates** (e.g. **glyceryl trinitrate**, **isosorbide** mononitrate) or **beta-blockers** for angina should avoid sumatriptan, which may possibly cause coronary vasoconstriction. There would seem to be no reason for avoiding concurrent use when **beta-blockers** are being used for other conditions (e.g. hypertension, migraine). No pharmacokinetic interaction occurs with sumatriptan 300 mg orally and **propranolol** 80 mg twice daily for 7 days.[3]

(c) Ergot alkaloids or pizotifen

A study in 38 migraine sufferers found that 1 mg **dihydroergotamine** alone caused maximum increases in blood pressure of 13/9 mmHg, while 2 or 4 mg sumatriptan given subcutaneously caused a smaller rise in blood pressure of 7/6 mmHg. When given together the blood pressure rises were no greater than with **dihydroergotamine** alone.[4] A clinical study of sumatriptan and **dihydroergotamine** found that concurrent use was very effective and there was no evidence of adverse interactions.[5] However, another study found that sumatriptan and **ergotamine** had additive vasoconstrictive effects[6] and the makers advise the avoidance of sumatriptan with **ergotamine** because of the possible risk of additive vasospastic reactions.[7] The CSM in the UK has received 34 reports of pain or tightness in the chest caused by sumatriptan, possibly due to coronary vasoconstriction, and they too say that the concurrent use of **ergotamine** should be avoided.[2] Also, myocardial infarction has been reported in a woman of 43 after she took two 2 mg doses of **methysergide** 12 h apart, followed by sumatriptan 6 mg subcutaneously. Symptoms of the myocardial infarction began 15 minutes later.[8] However, sequential use is safe and the recommendation is that sumatriptan should not be taken sooner than 24 h after any **ergotamine**-containing preparation, and that 6 h should elapse before taking any **ergotamine** preparation after sumatriptan.[7] **Pizotifen** 500 micrograms three times daily for 8 days in 14 healthy subjects was found to have no significant effect on the pharmacokinetics of sumatriptan.[4]

(d) Lithium

A comprehensive literature search published in 1998 identified reports of only 2 patients taking sumatriptan and **lithium** concurrently who developed adverse reactions. The symptoms were suggestive of the serotonin syndrome, and were mild to moderate and self-limiting. The number of patients taking lithium and sumatriptan was not stated, so the incidence is unknown.[9] The conclusion was reached that sumatriptan can be used cautiously in patients receiving **lithium**.[9] More study is needed to clarify this situation.

(e) Miscellaneous drugs, food and drink

Studies have found that **flunarizine** 10 mg daily for 8 days had no effect on pharmacokinetics of single doses of sumatriptan, and no significant changes in blood pressure, ECG or heart rate occurred.[4,10] **Food** also does not affect the bioavailability of sumatriptan.[4] Single 0.8 g/kg doses of **alcohol** were given to 16 healthy subjects, followed half-an-hour later by 200 mg sumatriptan. No statistically significant changes in the pharmacokinetics of the sumatriptan were seen.[11] There would seem to be no reason for special precautions with **alcohol**, **flunarizine** or **food** and sumatriptan.

1. Srinivas NR, Shyu WC, Upmalis D, Lee JS, Barbhaiya RH. Lack of pharmacokinetic interaction between butorphanol tartrate nasal spray and sumatriptan succinate. *J Clin Pharmacol* (1995) 35, 432–7.
2. Committee on the Safety of Medicines. *Current Problems* (1992) 34, 2.
3. Scott AK, Walley T, Breckenridge AM, Lacey LF, Fowler PA. Lack of an interaction between propranolol and sumatriptan. *Br J Clin Pharmacol* (1991) 32, 581–4.
4. Fowler PA, Lacey LF, Thomas M, Keene ON, Tanner RJN, Baber NS. The clinical pharmacology, pharmacokinetics and metabolism of sumatriptan. *Eur Neurol* (1991) 31, 291–4.
5. Henry P, d'Allens H and the French Migraine Network Bordeaux-Lyon-Grenoble. Subcutaneous sumatriptan in the acute treatment of migraine in patients using dihydroergotamine as prophylaxis. *Headache* (1993) 33, 432–5.
6. Tfelt-Hansen P, Sperling B, Winter PDO'B. Transient additional effect of sumatriptan on ergotamine-induced constriction of peripheral arteries in man. *Clin Pharmacol Ther* (1992) 51, 149.
7. Imigran (Sumatriptan). GlaxoWellcome. Summary of product characteristics, July 2001.
8. Liston H, Bennett L, Usher B, Nappi J. The association of the combination of sumatriptan and methysergide in myocardial infarction in a premenopausal woman. *Arch Intern Med* (1999) 159, 511–13.
9. Gardner DM, Lynd LD. Sumatriptan contraindications and the serotonin syndrome. *Ann Pharmacother* (1998) 32, 33–8.
10. Van Hecken AM, Depré M, De Schepper PJ, Fowler PA, Lacey LF, Durham JM. Lack of effect of flunarizine on the pharmacokinetics and pharmacodynamics of sumatriptan in healthy volunteers. *Br J Clin Pharmacol* (1992) 34, 82–4.
11. Kempsford RD, Lacey LF, Thomas M, Fowler PA. The effect of alcohol on the pharmacokinetic profile of oral sumatriptan. *Fundam Clin Pharmacol* (1991) 5, 470.

Tacrine + Hormone replacement therapy (HRT)

There is evidence that HRT treatment can almost double the serum levels of tacrine.

Clinical evidence, mechanism, importance and management

Following the observation that **HRT** appeared to increase the response of postmenopausal Alzheimer's patients to tacrine, a study was undertaken in 10 healthy women who were given either once-daily **HRT** (2 mg **estradiol** + 0.25 mg **levonorgestrel**) or a placebo in a randomised crossover study. On day 10 of the **HRT** treatment, they were also given a single 40-mg dose of tacrine. It was found that the mean tacrine AUC was increased 60% by the **HRT**, the mean peak serum level was increased 46% and the clearance reduced by 31%. The AUC of one individual was increased threefold. The reason for these changes is thought to be that the **HRT** reduces the metabolism of the tacrine to its main metabolite (1-hydroxytacrine) by cytochrome P450 isoenzyme CYP1A2.[1]

The importance of this interaction is still uncertain, but increased tacrine levels would be expected to increase its efficacy and possibly also increase its adverse effects. Be alert therefore for the need to use a smaller tacrine dose (about half?) in patients given **HRT**. More study of this interaction is needed.

1. Laine K, Palovaara S, Tapanainen P, Manninen P. Plasma tacrine concentrations are significantly increased by concomitant hormone replacement therapy. *Clin Pharmacol Ther* (1999) 66, 602–8.

Tacrine + Ibuprofen

An isolated report describes delirium in a woman taking tacrine when ibuprofen was added.

Clinical evidence, mechanism, importance and management

A 71-year-old diabetic woman with probable Alzheimer's disease developed delirium while taking 40 mg tacrine four times daily. The symptoms included delusions, hallucinations, and fluctuating awareness. She was also bradycardic, diaphoretic and dizzy.[1] She was eventually stabilised for 8 months on 20 mg tacrine four times daily without problems, but became delirious again 2 weeks after starting to take 600 mg **ibuprofen** daily. The delirium resolved when both drugs were withdrawn. The reasons for this reaction are unknown. This is the first and only report of this apparent interaction and its general importance is probably small, but concurrent use in any patient should be monitored.

1. Hooten WM, Pearlson G. Delirium caused by tacrine and ibuprofen interaction. *Am J Psychiatry* (1996) 153, 842.

Tacrine + Miscellaneous drugs

Diazepam, quinidine, selegiline and warfarin do not appear to interact adversely with tacrine, but cimetidine, fluvoxamine and enoxacin possibly increase its effects and side-effects. Smoking reduces the serum levels of tacrine. The serum levels of theophylline are increased by tacrine. There is no pharmacokinetic interaction between digoxin and tacrine but their

heart-slowing effects may possibly be additive. The effects of tacrine are expected to be additive with those of other anticholinesterases and cholinergics, to oppose the actions of drugs with anticholinergic effects and, in its turn, to be opposed by anticholinergics. Two isolated reports describe severe parkinsonism in two patients given on haloperidol when tacrine was added.

Clinical evidence, mechanism, importance and management

(a) Cholinergics and Anticholinergics

Tacrine is an anticholinesterase drug which may therefore be expected to be additive with the actions of other **anticholinesterases** (**neostigmine**, **pyridostigmine**, etc.) and with directly acting cholinergic drugs.

Tacrine is also expected to oppose the actions of drugs with **anticholinergic** effects (see Table 9.2). This could be a disadvantage if the drug were being used for its anticholinergic effects (for example in the treatment of Parkinson's disease), but it might be useful if the anticholinergic effect is simply an unwanted side-effect. The effects of tacrine itself may also be opposed by **anticholinergics**. Those **anticholinergics** which can penetrate the brain would be expected to oppose the beneficial effects of tacrine, while those which act peripherally outside the brain could reduce the side-effects of tacrine.

All of these interactions – additive or antagonistic – would seem to be possible, but whether any of them is of real practical importance awaits confirmation. It would certainly be prudent to monitor the concurrent use of any of these potentially interacting groups of drugs.

(b) Cimetidine, Antacids

A decrease in the clearance of a single 40-mg dose of tacrine of 30% (from 23.4 to 16.3 l/min) was seen in 11 healthy subjects when given 300 mg **cimetidine** four times daily for 2 days.[1,2] The makers of tacrine also say that **cimetidine** increased the AUC and the maximum plasma level of tacrine by 64 and 54% respectively.[3] The reason is not known, but it seems probable that the **cimetidine** (a well-recognised liver enzyme inhibitor) reduces the metabolism of the tacrine by cytochrome P450 isoenzyme CYP1A2.[2] An increase in the effects of tacrine and possibly its side-effects (nausea, vomiting, diarrhoea) seems possible. One patient in the study mentioned[2] had to be withdrawn due to nausea and vomiting, but none of the other 11 subjects particularly suffered from side-effects. More study is needed to find out whether this interaction is generally clinically important. If the suggested mechanism of interaction is true, the **other H$_2$-blockers** would not be expected to interact. Tacrine also increases the secretion of gastric acid but it is not clear whether and by how much this would oppose the actions of **H$_2$-blockers** or **antacids**.

(c) Diazepam, Digoxin

Groups of 11 or 12 healthy subjects were given single doses of 2 mg **diazepam** or 500 micrograms of **digoxin** alone or while taking 20 mg tacrine 6-hourly. The pharmacokinetics of **digoxin** and **diazepam** were unchanged.[4] No special precautions would seem necessary if **diazepam** is given with tacrine, but check to see that the combined heart-slowing effects of **digoxin** and tacrine do not become excessive.

(d) Fluvoxamine

In vitro studies using human liver microsomes and human recombinant P450 isoenzymes CYP1A1 and CYP1A2 in yeast found that **fluvoxamine** inhibits CYP1A2, which is responsible for the metabolism of tacrine. It was therefore predicted that **fluvoxamine** could possibly 'dramatically' increase tacrine plasma levels in patients, possibly causing hepatotoxicity.[5] This prediction was confirmed in a study in 13 healthy subjects who showed an eightfold increase in the mean AUC of a single 40-mg dose of tacrine after taking 100 mg **fluvoxamine** for 6 days. A very large increase in the AUC of the hydroxylated metabolites of tacrine, and an eightfold fall in clearance of tacrine itself was also seen.[6] Another study in one individual found that the total clearance of tacrine was reduced about tenfold and its half-life increased tenfold by 100 mg **fluvoxamine** daily.[7]

The clinical importance of this interaction remains uncertain but an increase in gastrointestinal side-effects and possibly hepatotoxicity caused by tacrine seems likely. More study is needed.

(e) Haloperidol

An isolated report describes a man of 87 with dementia who was started on 5 mg **haloperidol** daily for symptoms of agitation and paranoia. Higher doses caused extrapyramidal symptoms. After 10 days, tacrine 10 mg four times daily was added. Within 72 h he developed severe parkinsonism, which resolved within 8 h of stopping both drugs.[8] Another isolated report describes a woman on 10 mg haloperidol daily who similarly developed a disabling parkinsonian syndrome within a week of adding tacrine 10 mg four times daily.[9] One possible reason is that the **haloperidol** blocked the dopamine receptors in striatum, thereby increasing striatal acetylcholine activity, which was further increased by the tacrine.[8] It is not clear whether other patients given other dopamine receptor blocking drugs and tacrine would similarly show this reaction.

(f) Quinidine

Quinidine 83 mg eight-hourly did not affect the clearance of a single dose of tacrine in 11 subjects.[1] Since **quinidine** inhibits cytochrome CYP2D6 in the liver, it may be concluded that this cytochrome does not have an important role to play in the metabolism of tacrine and therefore that other drugs which inhibit this enzyme are unlikely to interact with tacrine by this means. This needs confirmation.

(g) Quinolone antibacterials

In vitro studies with human and rat liver microsomes found that **enoxacin**, a specific inhibitor of the cytochrome P450 isoenzyme CYP1A2, significantly inhibited all the routes by which tacrine is metabolised.[10] A reasonable conclusion to be drawn from this is that the effects of tacrine, and its side-effects, would be increased by **enoxacin** but nobody yet seems to have studied this interaction in patients or healthy subjects. However, the same study also suggested that **enoxacin** possibly inhibits the production of the toxic metabolites of tacrine, which can damage the liver, thereby possibly reducing liver toxicity.[10]

Other quinolones vary in the extent to which they inhibit liver CYP1A2 so that any interaction would be expected to reflect this variation.

(h) Selegiline

Ten patients with Alzheimer's disease on either tacrine or physostigmine for 16 to 88 weeks showed a significant improvement when they were additionally given 5 mg **selegiline** twice daily for 4 weeks. No additional adverse effects were seen.[11] There would seem to be no good reason for avoiding concurrent use, and some apparent advantages.

(i) Theophylline

Healthy subjects were given 158 mg **theophylline** alone or while taking 20 mg tacrine 6-hourly. The clearance of the **theophylline** was reduced by 50%, probably because the tacrine inhibits its metabolism by the cytochrome P450 isoenzyme CYP1A2 in the liver.[4] Be alert for the need to reduce the **theophylline** dosage to avoid toxicity if tacrine is added. More study of this interaction is needed in patients given multiple doses of both drugs.

(j) Tobacco smoking

A comparative study in 7 **smokers** and 4 **non-smokers** found that after taking single 40-mg doses of tacrine the AUC of the tacrine in the **smokers** was about 10% of that in the **non-smokers**. The elimination half-life in the **smokers** was also reduced, to about two-thirds of that in **non-smokers**. The reason is thought to be that some of the components of **tobacco smoke** increase the activity of the cytochrome P450 isoenzyme CYP1A2 in the liver, so that the metabolism of the tacrine is markedly increased.[12] In practical terms this means that **smokers** are likely to need considerably larger doses of tacrine than **non-smokers**. More study is needed to find out how much.

(k) Warfarin

A study in 10 patients taking **warfarin** found that the addition of 20 mg tacrine four times daily for 5 days had no significant effect on prothrombin times.[13] No special precautions would therefore seem to be necessary if tacrine is given to patients on **warfarin**. Information about other anticoagulants seems to be lacking.

1. deVries TM, O'Connor-Semmes RL, Guttendorf RJ, Reece PA, Posvar EL, Sedman AJ, Koup JR, Forgue ST. Effect of cimetidine and low-dose quinidine on tacrine pharmacokinetics in humans. *Pharm Res* (1993) 10 (10 Suppl), S-337.
2. Forgue ST, Reece PA, Sedman AJ, deVries TM. Inhibition of tacrine oral clearance by cimetidine. *Clin Pharmacol Ther* (1996) 59, 444–9.
3. Cognex (Tacrine). Product Information. Physicians' Desk Reference (2002) 1351–5.
4. deVries TM, Siedlik P, Smithers JA, Brown RR, Reece PA, Posvar EL, Sedman AJ, Koup JR, Forgue ST. Effect of multiple-dose tacrine administration on single-dose pharmacokinetics of digoxin, diazepam, and theophylline. *Pharm Res* (1993) 10 (10 Suppl), S-333.
5. Becquemont L, Le Bot MA, Riche C, Beaune P. Influence of fluvoxamine on tacrine metabolism in vitro: potential implication for the hepatotoxicity in vivo. *Fundam Clin Pharmacol* (1996) 10, 156–7.
6. Becquemont L, Ragueneau I, Le Bot MA, Riche C, Funck-Brentano C, Jaillon P. Influence of the CYP1A2 inhibitor fluvoxamine on tacrine pharmacokinetics in humans. *Clin Pharmacol Ther* (1997) 61, 619–27.
7. Larsen JT, Hansen LL, Brøsen K. Tacrine-fluvoxamine interaction study in healthy volunteers. *Eur J Clin Pharmacol* (1997) 52 (Suppl), A136.
8. McSwain ML, Forman LM. Severe parkinsonian symptom development on combination treatment with tacrine and haloperidol. *J Clin Psychopharmacol* (1995) 15, 284.
9. Maany I. Adverse interaction of tacrine and haloperidol. *Am J Psychiatry* (1996) 153, 1504.
10. Madden S, Woolf TF, Pool WF, Park BK. An investigation into the formation of stable, protein-reactive and cytotoxic metabolites of tacrine *in vitro*. Studies with human and rat liver microsomes. *Biochem Pharmacol* (1993) 46, 13–20.
11. Schneider LS, Olin JT, Pawluczyk S. A double-blind crossover pilot study of *l*-deprenyl (selegiline) combined with cholinesterase inhibitor in Alzheimer's disease. *Am J Psychiatry* (1993) 150, 321–3.
12. Welty D, Pool W, Woolf T, Posvar E, Sedman A. The effect of smoking on the pharmacokinetics and metabolism of Cognex® in healthy volunteers. *Pharm Res* (1993) 10 (10 Suppl), S-334.
13. Reece PA, Garnett WR, Rock WL, Taylor JR, Underwood B, Sedman AJ, Rajagopalan R. Lack of effect of tacrine administration on the anticoagulant activity of warfarin. *J Clin Pharmacol* (1995) 35, 526–8.

Tedisamil + Beta-blockers

Atenolol does not have additive effects on the bradycardia and QT-prolonging effects of tedisamil in healthy subjects.

Clinical evidence, mechanism, importance and management

A study was carried out in 10 healthy subjects to find out whether the combination of tedisamil with a beta-blocker might induce dangerous bradycardia and prolongation of the QT interval.[1] Subjects were given 100 mg tedisamil and 50 mg **atenolol** twice daily alone or together. The falls in the heart rate at rest were not significantly different for the three treatments. When the subjects were exercised the falls in the heart rate were not significant with tedisamil, 42 bpm with **atenolol**, and 47 bpm together. Tedisamil alone and in combination with **atenolol** increased the QT interval by 12%, whereas **atenolol** alone had no effect. With both tedisamil regimens QT prolongation decreased with increasing heart rate.

Thus the combined use of these drugs is not associated with excessive bradycardia or QT prolongation greater than that seen with tedisamil alone. However, the authors of this report are at pains to point out that this study was in healthy subjects and that studies are now needed in patients with myocardial ischaemia to confirm the safety of this drug combination. It seems likely that most other beta-blockers will behave like **atenolol**, with the possible exception of **sotalol**, which is associated with QT interval prolongation.

1. Démolis J-L, Martel C, Funck-Brentano C, Sachse A, Weimann H-J, Jaillon P. Effects of tedisamil, atenolol and their combination on heart and rate-dependent QT interval in healthy volunteers. *Br J Clin Pharmacol* (1997) 44, 403–9.

Terazosin + Antihypertensives

Terazosin does not increase the effects of antihypertensive drugs nor are adverse effects increased.

Clinical evidence, mechanism, importance and management

A large multinational retrospective study of patients treated for benign prostatic hyperplasia with 5 or 10 mg terazosin daily found that it lowered the diastolic and systolic blood pressures of hypertensive patients (because it is an alpha-blocker), but in normotensive and controlled hypertensive patients no blood pressure changes or adverse effects were seen. The conclusion was reached that no special precautions are needed if terazosin is added to the drug treatment of men already taking **antihypertensive drugs**.[1]

1. Kirby RS. Terazosin in benign prostatic hyperplasia: effects on blood pressure in normotensive and hypertensive men. *Br J Urol* (1998) 82, 373–9.

Terfenadine + Azole antifungals

Five reports describe the development of terfenadine toxicity (torsade de pointes arrhythmias) in two patients concurrently taking ketoconazole and seven taking itraconazole. Potentially serious ECG changes have been demonstrated in clinical studies in other subjects. These azole antifungals as well as miconazole are contraindicated. Topical oxiconazole also appears to interact, and oral fluconazole appears not to do so in normal doses but may possibly do so with higher doses.

Clinical evidence

(a) Fluconazole

Terfenadine 60 mg 12-hourly was given to 6 healthy subjects for 6 days. None of them showed any evidence of accumulating terfenadine when additionally given 200 mg **fluconazole** daily for a week, and no significant ECG changes were seen.[1] By January 1993 no clinically significant interactions between terfenadine and **fluconazole** had been reported to the FDA.[1] However, a study in group of healthy subjects taking terfenadine 60 mg 12-hourly, demonstrated a 52% rise in the terfenadine AUC while additionally taking **high dose fluconazole** 800 mg daily for a week. An increased QT_c was also seen.[2]

(b) Itraconazole

A woman of 26 taking 60 mg terfenadine twice daily began to have fainting episodes on the third evening after starting 100 mg **itraconazole** twice daily for vaginitis. When admitted to hospital next morning her ECG showed a QT interval of 580 ms and her heart rate was 67 bpm. Several episodes of torsade de pointes were recorded, and she fainted during two of them. No arrhythmias were seen 20 h after the last **itraconazole** dose. Her QT interval returned to normal after 3 days. She was found to have 28 micrograms/l terfenadine in the first sample of serum taken (normally <5 micrograms/l) and she still had levels of 12 micrograms/l 60 h after taking the last tablet.[3,4]

A man experienced an episode of fainting and palpitations while taking 60 mg terfenadine twice daily and 200 mg **itraconazole** twice daily. His QT_c interval was found to be 538 ms. An assay showed that his serum terfenadine levels had risen to 96 micrograms/l. He later resumed **itraconazole** alone without any problems.[5] A woman on 120 mg terfenadine daily had several episodes of fainting, torsade de pointes and a long QT interval 9 days after starting to take 100 mg **itraconazole** daily. The QT interval returned to normal after both drugs were withdrawn.[6]

The FDA has on record four well-documented cases of severe cardiac complications due to this interaction.[7] Studies in healthy subjects confirm that **itraconazole** increases the AUC of terfenadine by 30%, almost doubles its half-life (from 3.4 to 6.3 h), and prolongs the QT_c interval.[7,8]

(c) Ketoconazole

A 39-year-old woman on 60 mg terfenadine twice daily developed a number of episodes of syncope and lightheadedness, preceded by palpitations, dyspnoea and diaphoresis within 2 days of starting 200 mg **ketoconazole** twice daily. ECG monitoring revealed torsade de pointes and a QT_c interval of 655 ms. Her terfenadine serum levels were 57 micrograms/l (expected levels of 10 micrograms/l or less).

Other drugs being taken were cefaclor (stopped 3 to 4 days before the problems started) and medroxyprogesterone acetate. She had taken terfenadine and cefaclor on two previous occasions in the absence of **ketoconazole** without problems.[9,10]

Another woman, aged 22, similarly developed torsade de pointes after taking 120 mg terfenadine and 200 mg **ketoconazole** daily for 5 days.[11] The FDA has on record other cases of torsade de pointes arrhythmias in patients taking both drugs.[12]

Ketoconazole 400 mg daily for a week markedly increased the serum levels of single 120-mg doses of terfenadine in 12 healthy subjects (a rise from <10 to 27 micrograms/l). The clearance of the active metabolite of terfenadine was reduced about 30% and its half-life prolonged almost threefold.[13] ECGs in patients given both drugs showed a prolongation of 10 to 20 ms of the corrected QT interval when they were compared to ECGs in patients on **ketoconazole** alone.[14] **Ketoconazole** 200 mg 12-hourly for 6 days increased the QT interval in 6 healthy subjects taking 60 mg terfenadine 12-hourly from 416 to 490 ms, and raised the plasma terfenadine levels of all of them. Terfenadine serum levels increased to 81 micrograms/l in one individual. Due to significant ECG repolarisation changes 4 subjects were withdrawn before the course of **ketoconazole** was completed.[15]

(d) Oxiconazole

A woman of 25 complained of palpitations and chest pain radiating down her left arm and was also found to be having frequent ventricular premature beats in a pattern of bigeminy. On questioning it turned out that she was taking terfenadine and using a **topical antifungal** agent containing **oxiconazole** for ringworm on her arm. Both were stopped and her symptoms disappeared the following week.[16]

Mechanism

Itraconazole and ketoconazole appear to reduce the metabolism of terfenadine by the liver by inhibition of the cytochrome P450 isoenzyme CYP3A, so that they are cleared more slowly.[17-19] The accumulating levels of terfenadine, but not its metabolites, are cardiotoxic, and can alter the repolarisation of the cardiac muscle (reflected in an increase in the QT interval) in a way as yet not fully understood. It seems to have a quinidine-like action.[20] There seems to be marked and unpredictable variability between patients. Those particularly at risk are probably are poor metabolisers of terfenadine in whom, even with normal doses, may have higher than average levels of terfenadine.

Importance and management

The terfenadine/itraconazole and terfenadine/ketoconazole interactions are established and clinically important. Terfenadine can accumulate in subjects given either of these azole antifungals, leading to the development of potentially life-threatening torsade de pointes arrhythmia in some individuals. Because of the potential severity and unpredictability of this interaction, the FDA, the CSM in the UK and the makers[21] of terfenadine now advise the avoidance of any azole antifungal (oral or topical) in all patients taking terfenadine.

The makers of terfenadine say that miconazole is contraindicated but there seems to be no direct evidence that it interacts significantly. The situation with oxiconazole used topically is uncertain. The limited evidence available[1] suggests that fluconazole is unlikely to interact in this way in doses of 200 mg daily, although there may be a risk with higher doses[2] in a few individuals.

Astemizole is not an appropriate substitute for terfenadine because it interacts with the azoles similarly, whereas **cetirizine** and **loratadine** are safer alternative antihistamines (see Index).

1. Honig PK, Wortham DC, Zamani K, Mullin JC, Conner DP, Cantilena LR. The effect of fluconazole on the steady-state pharmacokinetics and electrographic pharmacodynamics of terfenadine in humans. *Clin Pharmacol Ther* (1993) 53, 630–6.
2. Cantilena LR, Sorrels S, Wiley T, Wortham D. Fluconazole alters terfenadine pharmacokinetics and electrocardiographic pharmacodynamics. *Clin Pharmacol Ther* (1995) 57, 185.
3. Pohjola-Sintonen S, Viitasalo M, Toivonen L, Neuvonen P. Torsades de pointes after terfenadine-itraconazole interaction. *BMJ* (1993) 306, 186.
4. Pohjola-Sintonen S, Viitasalo M, Toivonen L, Neuvonen P. Itraconazole prevents terfenadine metabolism and increases risk of torsades de pointes ventricular tachycardia. *Eur J Clin Pharmacol* (1993) 45, 191–3.
5. Crane JK, Shih H-T. Syncope and cardiac arrhythmia due to an interaction between itraconazole and terfenadine. *Am J Med* (1993) 95, 445–6.
6. Romkes JH, Froger CL, Wever EFD, Westerhof PW. Wegrakingen tijdens simultaan gebruik van terfenadine en itraconazol. *Ned Tijdschr Geneeskd* (1997) 141, 950–3.
7. Honig PK, Wortham DC, Hull R, Zamani K, Smith JE, Cantilena LR. Itraconazole affects single-dose terfenadine pharmacokinetics and cardiac repolarization pharmacodynamics. *J Clin Pharmacol* (1993) 33, 1201–6.
8. Honig P, Wortham D, Hull R, Zamani K, Smith J, Cantilena L. Itraconazole affects single-dose terfenadine pharmacokinetics and cardiac repolarization pharmacodynamics. *Clin Pharmacol Ther* (1994) 55, 165.
9. Monahan BP, Ferguson CL, Killeavy ES, Lloyd BK, Troy J, Cantilena LR. Torsades de pointes occurring in association with terfenadine use. *JAMA* (1990) 264, 2788–90.
10. Cantilena LR, Ferguson CL, Monahan BP. Torsades de Pointes occurring in association with terfenadine use. *JAMA* (1991) 266, 2375–6.
11. Zimmermann M, Duruz H, Guinand O, Broccard O, Levy P, Lacatis D, Bloch A. Torsades de pointes after treatment with terfenadine and ketoconazole. *Eur Heart J* (1992) 13, 1002–3.
12. Peck CC, Temple R, Collins JM. Understanding consequences of concurrent therapies. *JAMA* (1993) 269, 1550–2.
13. Eller MG, Okerholm RA. Pharmacokinetic interaction between terfenadine and ketoconazole. *Clin Pharmacol Ther* (1991) 49, 130.
14. Mathews DR, McNutt B, Okerholm R, Flicker M, McBride G. Torsades de pointes occurring in association with terfenadine use. *JAMA* (1991) 266, 2375–6.
15. Honig PK, Wortham DC, Zamani K, Conner DP, Mullin JC, Cantilena LR. Terfenadine-ketoconazole interaction. Pharmacokinetic and electrocardiographic consequences. *JAMA* (1993) 269, 1513–18.
16. Griffith JS. Interaction between terfenadine and topical antifungal agents. *Am Fam Physician* (1995) 51, 1396–7.
17. Lavrijsen K, Van Houdt J, Meuldermans W, Janssens M, Heykants J. The interaction of ketoconazole, itraconazole and erythromycin with the in vitro metabolism of antihistamines in human liver microsomes. *Allergy* (1993) 48 (Suppl 16), 34.
18. Jurima-Romet M, Crawford K, Cyr T, Inaba T. Terfenadine metabolism in human liver. In vitro inhibition by macrolide antibiotics and azole antifungals. *Drug Metab Dispos* (1994) 22, 849–57.
19. von Moltke LL, Greenblatt DJ, Duan SX, Harmatz JS, Shader RI. *In vitro* prediction of the terfenadine-ketoconazole pharmacokinetic interaction. *J Clin Pharmacol* (1994) 34, 1222–7.
20. Woosley RL, Chen Y, Freiman JP. Mechanism of the cardiotoxic actions of terfenadine. *JAMA* (1993) 269, 1532–6.
21. Triludan (Terfenadine), Hoechst Marion Roussel Ltd, Summary of product characteristics, October 1998.

Terfenadine + Grapefruit juice

Grapefruit juice causes terfenadine to accumulate in the body, increasing the risk of serious cardiotoxicity (prolongation of the QTc interval) and the possibility of torsade de pointes arrhythmia.

Clinical evidence

Terfenadine 60 mg was given to 6 healthy subjects 12-hourly for 7 days, after which 240 ml **double-strength grapefruit juice** 12-hourly was added, for a further 7 days. Terfenadine was only detectable in the plasma while taking the **grapefruit juice**. The mean QTc interval was found to have risen from 420 to 434 ms.[1] The authors of this preliminary report have published similar and extended work under some subjects, which confirm these findings.[2,3] Another study in 4 healthy subjects by another group found that **grapefruit juice** (amount not specified) increased the maximum terfenadine plasma levels from 2.4 to 7.2 nanograms/ml and nearly doubled the $AUC_{0-24\,h}$. However, the mean QT interval was not significantly changed, but one subject showed an increase in the QTc interval of almost 50 ms.[4]

Mechanism

Not fully understood, but it seems likely that some component of the juice inhibits the metabolism of the terfenadine to its active metabolite (by cytochrome P450 isoenzyme CYP3A4) so that the parent drug accumulates.[5] Terfenadine, but not its metabolite, is a potent blocker of the delayed rectifier potassium current which probably accounts for the QTc prolongation. Increased QTc intervals are associated with the development of ventricular tachycardia and torsade de pointes cardiac arrhythmias, which are potentially life-threatening.

Importance and management

An established and potentially clinically important interaction, the toxic effects of which may possibly only affect a small subset of individuals. As yet neither the FDA nor the CSM appear to have reports of problems in patients which are attributable to this interaction.[3,6] Nevertheless because of the risk of serious cardiotoxicity (however small) it would be prudent for all patients on terfenadine to avoid grapefruit juice. The makers include grapefruit juice among their contraindications.[7] The CSM/MCA point out that there is no evidence that eating grapefruit rather than drinking the juice causes this interaction.[6]

1. Benton R, Honig P, Zamani K, Hewett RN, Cantilena LR, Woosley RL. Grapefruit juice alters terfenadine pharmacokinetics resulting in prolongation of the QTc. *Clin Pharmacol Ther* (1994) 55, 146.
2. Benton RE, Honig PK, Zamani K, Cantilena LR, Woosley RL. Grapefruit juice alters terfenadine pharmacokinetics, resulting in prolongation of repolarization on the electrocardiogram. *Clin Pharmacol Ther* (1996) 59, 383–8.
3. Honig PK, Wortham DC, Lazarev A, Cantilena LR. Grapefruit juice alters the systemic bioavailability and cardiac repolarization of terfenadine in poor metabolizers of terfenadine. *J Clin Pharmacol* (1996) 36, 345–51.
4. Clifford CP, Adams DA, Murray S, Taylor GW, Wilkins MR, Boobis AR, Davies DS. Pharmacokinetic and cardiac effects of terfenadine after inhibition of its metabolism by grapefruit juice. *Br J Clin Pharmacol* (1996) 42, 662P.
5. Anon. Grapefruit study. *Pharm J* (1997) 258, 618.
6. Committee on the Safety of Medicines. Drug interactions with grapefruit juice. *Current Problems* (1997) 23, 2.
7. Histafen (Terfenadine). Approved Prescription Services Limited. Summary of product characteristics, December 1999.

Terfenadine + Macrolide antibacterials

Erythromycin causes terfenadine to accumulate in a few individuals, which can prolong the QT_c interval in those with otherwise apparently normal cardiac function, increasing the risk of life-threatening torsade de pointes arrhythmias. Clarithromycin and troleandomycin appear to interact similarly, and probably josamycin as well, but not azithromycin nor dirithromycin. However, all macrolides are contraindicated with terfenadine.

Clinical evidence

(a) Azithromycin

No measurable plasma terfenadine was found in healthy subjects taking 60 mg terfenadine twice daily when given 250 mg **azithromycin** daily for 5 days,[1,2] nor were there any changes in the QT_c interval.[2]

(b) Clarithromycin

Clarithromycin 500 mg twice daily for 7 days increased the mean AUC of the acid metabolite of terfenadine two to threefold in 6 healthy subjects who were taking 60 mg twice daily. Four of them had detectable terfenadine in their serum (normally undetectable).[1] Almost identical results were found in another study in 14 healthy subjects, two of who had detectable plasma terfenadine levels.[3]

(c) Dirithromycin

Terfenadine 60 mg twice daily was given to 6 healthy subjects for 8 days, after which 500 mg **dirithromycin** daily was added for a further 10 days. No terfenadine was detectable (< 5 nanograms/ml) in 5 subjects throughout the study, but the remaining man had a maximum of 8.1 nanograms/ml on terfenadine alone, and 7.2 nanograms/ml when the **dirithromycin** was added. Their mean QTc was 369 ms on terfenadine alone and 367 ms on terfenadine plus **dirithromycin**. No changes in the pharmacokinetics of the acid metabolite of terfenadine were seen. These findings are consistent with the results of other related *in vitro* studies using human liver microsomes which found that **dirithromycin** had no major effect on the metabolism of terfenadine by cytochrome CYP3A4.[4,5]

(d) Erythromycin

A girl of 18 who was taking 60 mg terfenadine twice daily and 250 mg **erythromycin** 6-hourly, fainted while at school and, when later hospitalised, was seen to have repeated episodes of ventricular tachycardia and ventricular fibrillation requiring resuscitation, and later, torsade de pointes. Her QTc interval was found to be prolonged at 630 ms. The drugs were withdrawn and 9 days later, after a period on ITU she was discharged symptom free, with a normal QTc interval.[6]

Nine subjects on terfenadine 60 mg 12-hourly showed a 107% rise in the maximum serum levels of the acid metabolite of terfenadine, and a 170% rise in its AUC after additionally taking 500 mg **erythromycin** three times daily for a week. Three of the 9 subjects accumulated unmetabolised terfenadine in their serum (normally undetectable). These 3 subjects showed an increase in the QT_c interval of 33 ms on terfenadine alone, and 64 ms on the combination, whereas the other patients had no statistically significant rise in QTc interval.[7] One subject showed pronounced notching of the T wave.

Other studies have confirmed that **erythromycin** increases the AUC of terfenadine and prolongs the QT interval.[1,8] These studies contrast with another which found that 1 g **erythromycin** daily for 5 days had no effect on the serum levels of either terfenadine or its metabolite after taking a single 120-mg dose.[9] Another report documents uneventful concurrent use of **erythromycin** and terfenadine in some patients.[10]

(e) Troleandomycin

The makers of terfenadine have on record a case of a woman with a history of aortic valve disease who suffered an episode of torsade de pointes arrhythmia while taking **troleandomycin**. She had taken more than the maximum recommended dose of terfenadine.[11] Another woman taking 60 mg terfenadine three times daily developed torsade de pointes arrhythmia and a prolonged QTc interval when 500 mg **troleandomycin** three times daily was added. She recovered when both were stopped but, again developed a significantly prolonged QTc interval when both were restarted.[12]

Mechanism

Terfenadine is a prodrug, which is metabolised firstly to an active carboxylic acid metabolite, and then further oxidised to a second inactive metabolite. The interacting macrolides can apparently inhibit the second metabolic step (probably by inhibition of cytochrome P450 isoenzyme CYP3A4)[13,14] so that the acid metabolite accumulates. In a small number of susceptible individuals it may also inhibit the first step too.[1,8] Terfenadine itself, normally undetectable in the plasma, is cardiotoxic and can alter the repolarisation of the cardiac muscle (reflected in an increase in the QTc interval) in a way as yet not fully understood. It seems to have a quinidine-like action.[15] Therefore as terfenadine accumulates cardiac arrhythmias can be seen.

Importance and management

The interactions of terfenadine with erythromycin, clarithromycin and troleandomycin are established, clinically important and potentially hazardous. In fact only erythromycin and troleandomycin have actually been directly implicated, but the prolongation of the QT_c interval which occurs with clarithromycin indicates that it is similarly unsafe, and there is indirect evidence that josamycin will interact similarly. From the reports above, it does seem that only a very few individuals develop a clinically important adverse interaction with these macrolides but identifying them in advance is not as yet practical, and when they do occur, they are life-threatening.

Because of the unpredictability and potential severity of this interaction, the FDA,[10] the CSM[16] in the UK and the makers[17] of terfenadine now contraindicate macrolide antibacterials in anyone taking terfenadine, but the evidence available suggests that azithromycin and dirithromycin are safe. **Cetirizine** and **loratadine** appear to be alternative non-sedating non-interacting antihistamines (see Index). It is also known that **fexofenadine** is safe with erythromycin (see Index).

1. Honig PK, Wortham DC, Zamani K, Cantilena LR. Comparison of the effect of the macrolide antibiotics erythromycin, clarithromycin and azithromycin on terfenadine steady-state pharmacokinetics and electrocardiographic parameters. *Drug Invest* (1994) 7, 148–56.
2. Harris S, Hilligoss DM, Colangelo PM, Eller M, Okerholm R. Azithromycin and terfenadine: lack of drug interaction. *Clin Pharmacol Ther* (1995) 58, 310–15.
3. Gustavson LE, Blahunka KS, Witt GF, Harris SI, Palmer RN. Evaluation of the pharmacokinetic drug interaction between terfenadine and clarithromycin. *Pharm Res* (1993) 10 (10 Suppl), S-311.
4. Goldberg MJ, DeSante K, Cerimele B, Sides G. Effect of dirithromycin on terfenadine pharmacokinetics and QTc in healthy men. *Clin Pharmacol Ther* (1995) 57, 176.
5. Goldberg MJ, Ring B, DeSante K, Cerimele B, Hatcher B, Sides G, Wrighton S. Effect of dirithromycin on human CYP3A *in vitro* and on pharmacokinetics and pharmacodynamics of terfenadine *in vivo*. *Pharm J* (1996) 36, 1154–60.
6. Biglin KE, Faraon MS, Constance TD, Lieh-Lai M. Drug-induced torsades de pointes: a possible interaction of terfenadine and erythromycin. *Ann Pharmacother* (1994) 28, 282.
7. Honig PK, Woosley RL, Zamani K, Conner DP, Cantilena LR. Changes in the pharmacokinetics and electrocardiographic pharmacodynamics of terfenadine with concomitant administration of erythromycin. *Clin Pharmacol Ther* (1992) 52, 231–8.

8. Eller M, Russell T, Ruberg S, Okerholm R, McNutt B. Effect of erythromycin on terfenadine metabolite pharmacokinetics. *Clin Pharmacol Ther* (1993) 53, 161.
9. Mathews DR, McNutt B, Okerholm R, Flicker M, McBride G. Torsades de pointes occurring in association with terfenadine use. *JAMA* (1991) 266, 2375–6.
10. Schoenwetter WF, Kelloway JS, Lindgren D. A retrospective evaluation of potential cardiac side-effects induced by concurrent use of terfenadine and erythromycin. *J Allergy Clin Immunol* (1993) 91, 259.
11. Marion Merrell Dow. Personal Communication, August 1993.
12. Fournier P, Pacouret G, Charbonnier B. Une nouvelle cause de torsades de pointes: association terfénadine et troléandomycine. *Ann Cardiol Angeiol (Paris)* (1993) 42, 249–52.
13. Yun C-H, Okerholm RA, Guengerich FP. Oxidation of the antihistaminic drug terfenadine in human liver microsomes. Role of cytochrome P-450 3A(4) in *N*-dealkylation and C-hydroxylation. *Drug Metab Dispos* (1993) 21, 403–9.
14. Jurima-Romet M, Crawford K, Cyr T, Inaba T. Terfenadine metabolism in human liver. In vitro inhibition by macrolide antibiotics and azole antifungals. *Drug Metab Dispos* (1994) 22, 849–57.
15. Woosley RL, Chen Y, Freiman JP. Mechanism of the cardiotoxic actions of terfenadine. *JAMA* (1993) 269, 1532–6.
16. Committee on Safety of Medicines. Ventricular arrhythmias due to terfenadine and astemizole. *Current Problems* (1992) 35, 1–2 .
17. Histafen (Terfenadine). Approved Prescription Services Limited. Summary of product characteristics, December 1999.

Terfenadine + Miscellaneous drugs

Terfenadine is contraindicated with other drugs which can prolong the QT interval and those which significantly inhibit its metabolism. No pharmacokinetic interaction is likely between terfenadine and tedisamil. Zileuton causes some changes in the pharmacokinetics of terfenadine but no clinically important ECG changes occur.

Clinical evidence, mechanism, importance and management

(a) QT interval prolonging drugs

The cardiotoxicity of terfenadine is related to its ability to prolong the QT interval, which can lead to the development of potentially life-threatening arrhythmias. For this reason, the makers contraindicate the concurrent use of other drugs which prolong the QT interval and which are predicted to be additive with the effects of terfenadine. They list the following: **other antihistamines** which prolong the QT interval (this would include **astemizole**), **antiarrhythmics**, in particular those of **class I** and **III, bepridil, cisapride, halofantrine, lithium, antipsychotics, pentamidine, probucol, tricyclic antidepressants, trimethoprim** and **sparfloxacin**.[1] These lists are not exhaustive, and other drugs which prolong the QT interval are to be found in Table 4.3. The makers of terfenadine also contraindicate drugs known to induce electrolyte imbalance, which may precipitate QT interval prolongation such as **diuretics, laxatives** and the supraphysiological use of **steroid hormones** with mineralocorticoid potential (e.g. systemic **fludrocortisone**).[1]

It needs to be emphasised that while it is known that these drugs can prolong the QT interval, case reports and clinical studies demonstrating adverse reactions with most of them when combined with terfenadine are largely lacking, so that the contraindication is only a reasonable and prudent precaution. More study is needed to identify those drugs which if combined with terfenadine actually increases the QT interval to a clinically relevant extent and those which do not.

(b) Inhibitors of cytochrome P450 isoenzyme CYP3A4

Drugs which significantly inhibit cytochrome CYP3A4 can increase the serum levels of terfenadine and thereby increase its serious cardiotoxicity. Such drugs include the **azole antifungals, HIV protease inhibitors** and **macrolide antibacterials**. For this reason the concurrent use of these and other drugs is contraindicated. See the Index for the names and groups of drugs which are known to interact in this way, and the monographs where the details of the interactions are described.

(c) Tedisamil

An *in vitro* study of a possible interaction between terfenadine and **tedisamil** was carried out because terfenadine has the potential to prolong the QTc interval, and **tedisamil** can cause bradycardia and prolong the effective refractory period. Using human liver microsomes it was found that **tedisamil** (0.1 or 10 micromol) did not affect the metabolism of the terfenadine, and it was predicted that no pharmacokinetic interaction *in vivo* is likely to occur,[2] but this does not discount the possibility of some pharmacodynamic interaction. More study is needed.

(d) Zileuton

Terfenadine 60 mg 12-hourly for 7 days was given to 15 healthy subjects with either 600 mg **zileuton** 6-hourly or a placebo. The mean $AUC_{0–12\,h}$ and the maximum plasma concentrations of the terfenadine increased by 35% in the presence of **zileuton**, but the levels were still very low (less than 5 nanograms/ml). The maximum plasma concentration and AUC of the metabolite (carboxyterfenadine) were increased by about 15% while concurrently taking the **zileuton**. But much more importantly the ECG measurements showed that the addition of **zileuton** did not increase the QTc interval nor cause any other significant changes.[3,4] That is to say, despite these pharmacokinetic changes, **zileuton** appears not to increase the cardiotoxicity of terfenadine so that there would seem to be no reason for avoiding the concurrent use of these two drugs. However, the makers of terfenadine currently contraindicate **zileuton**, on the basis of a theoretical interaction.[1]

1. Histafen (Terfenadine). Approved Prescription Services Limited. Summary of product characteristics, December 1999.
2. McCully S, Cameron GA, Hawksworth GM, Bader A, Borlack JT. Investigation of the potential interaction between terfenadine and tedisamil in human liver microsomes. *Xenobiotica* (1998) 28, 219–23.
3. Awni WM, Cao G, Kasier JF, Locke CS, Machinist JM, Dube LM. The pharmacokinetic/pharmacodynamic interaction between zileuton and terfenadine. *Clin Pharmacol Ther* (1996) 59, 203.
4. Awni WM, Cavanaugh JH, Leese P, Kasier J, Cao G, Locke CS, Dube LM. The pharmacokinetic and pharmacodynamic interaction between zileuton and terfenadine. *Eur J Clin Pharmacol* (1997) 52, 49–54.

Terfenadine + Paracetamol (Acetaminophen) and Amitriptyline

An isolated report describes the development of torsade de pointes arrhythmia in an old man on very large doses of paracetamol (acetaminophen) and amitriptyline when he began to take terfenadine.

A man of 86 on 25 mg **amitriptyline** nightly, 3 mg prednisone daily and excessive amounts of **paracetamol (acetaminophen)** – up to 1 g two-hourly over a 6-month period – developed breathlessness and bradycardia shortly after starting to take 60 mg terfenadine twice daily. In hospital he became unconscious and was initially pulseless but recovered spontaneously. An ECG showed that he had AV block and a prolonged QT interval, which resulted in runs of self-limiting torsade de pointes arrhythmia.[1] The reasons for this reaction are not known, but a suggested explanation is that overdosage with **paracetamol** produced large amounts of a metabolite (*N*-acetyl-p-aminobenzoquinone imine), which could have inhibited the metabolism of the terfenadine by cytochrome P450 isoenzyme CYP3A4, resulting in terfenadine accumulation and the development of its cardiotoxic effects.[1] The **amitriptyline** may additionally have had some part to play because it can also cause torsade de pointes, although rarely.

This is an isolated case and unlikely to be of general importance. There would seem to be little reason on the basis of this report for patients on terfenadine to avoid normal therapeutic doses of **paracetamol (acetaminophen)**. There appear to be no other reports of this interaction.

1. Matsis PP, Easthorpe RN. Torsades de pointes ventricular tachycardia associated with terfenadine and paracetamol self medication. *N Z Med J* (1994) 107, 402–403.

Terfenadine + Selective serotonin re-uptake inhibitors (SSRIs) or Nefazodone

Two isolated reports provide some evidence of cardiotoxicity attributed to the concurrent use of terfenadine and fluoxetine, whereas another *in vivo* study suggests that an interaction

is unlikely. An *in vitro* study indicated that other SSRIs (desmethylsertraline, fluvoxamine, norfluoxetine, sertraline) are very unlikely to interact with terfenadine, but another suggested the remote possibility of an interaction with nefazodone. Terfenadine and paroxetine do not interact. Information about citalopram seems to be lacking.

Clinical evidence

(a) Fluoxetine

A man of 41 with no previous history of heart disease awoke one night short of breath, with a sensation of his heart missing beats and beating irregularly. He also had a few episodes of orthostasis. However a later ECG showed a normal sinus rhythm. He was taking daily doses of 120 mg terfenadine, 20 mg **fluoxetine** (started a month previously), 2400 mg ibuprofen, 400 micrograms misoprostol, *Midrin* (paracetamol (acetaminophen), dichloralphenazone, isometheptene mucate) and 300 mg ranitidine. A few days after stopping the terfenadine and 12 days after this episode, his heart function as recorded by a 24-h Holtzer monitor showed some minor abnormalities (intermittent sinus tachycardia, isolated premature beats) but nothing approaching the previous alarming episode.[1] A woman taking several drugs (topical aciclovir, beclometasone, pseudoephedrine, ibuprofen) showed a lengthened QT_c interval of 550 ms 2 weeks after starting terfenadine and **fluoxetine**, but she remained asymptomatic. Within a week of stopping the terfenadine her QT_c had returned to normal.[2]

In contrast, 12 healthy subjects who were given a single 60-mg dose of terfenadine before and after taking 60 mg **fluoxetine** daily for 8 days showed no significant changes in the pharmacokinetics of terfenadine or its acid metabolite.[3,4] Other *in vitro* studies with human liver microsomal enzymes confirmed that **fluoxetine** has only a very slight inhibitory effect on the metabolism of terfenadine, which was considered to be clinically irrelevant.[5,6]

(b) Nefazodone, Sertraline

Studies using human liver microsomes found that both **nefazodone** and **sertraline** are moderately weak inhibitors of the *N*-dealkylation and C-hydroxylation of terfenadine, but to different extents.[6] There appear to be no clinical reports of adverse interactions but **nefazodone** is currently considered to be contraindicated with terfenadine.[7] Although the CSM in the UK initially stated that terfenadine should not be used with **sertraline**, they have since reviewed the data and now consider an interaction unlikely.[8]

(c) Paroxetine

A two-period crossover study in 11 healthy subjects given 60 mg terfenadine twice daily found that the concurrent use of 20 mg **paroxetine** daily for 8 days had no effect on the AUC of terfenadine 60 mg twice daily or the QTc interval. A small, clinically unimportant reduction in the levels of carboxyterfenadine was seen. It was concluded that there is no clinically relevant interaction between terfenadine and **paroxetine**.[9,10] *In vitro* studies with human liver microsomal enzymes confirmed that **paroxetine** has only a very slight inhibitory effect on the metabolism of terfenadine, which is considered to be clinically insignificant.[5]

Mechanism

Not understood.

Importance and management

The terfenadine/fluoxetine interaction is not adequately established, but prescribers should be aware of the cases cited if both drugs are given. Terfenadine and paroxetine do not appear to interact.

An *in vitro* model study using human liver microsomal enzymes, which accurately predicted a large and potentially hazardous interaction between terfenadine and ketoconazole or itraconazole (now clinically proven) also found that six SSRIs (desmethylsertraline, fluoxetine, fluvoxamine, norfluoxetine, paroxetine, sertraline) at usual clinical doses were at least 20 times less potent than ketoconazole. This suggests that *in vivo* all of them are very unlikely to interact with terfenadine, although the authors of the study warn that if high doses

of SSRIs are used (particularly fluoxetine) some caution is appropriate.[5] Another similar *in vitro* study concluded that nefazodone inhibition of terfenadine metabolism should not cause QT interval prolongation in most individuals, although some individuals may be unusually susceptible. Thy suggest that the warning against the concomitant use of these two drugs may have contributed to the lack of reported interactions.[6] The makers of terfenadine list **citalopram** as an SSRI which might possibly increase terfenadine serum levels,[11] but direct evidence of this seems to be lacking.

1. Swims MP. Potential terfenadine-fluoxetine interaction. *Ann Pharmacother* (1993) 27, 1404–5.
2. Marchiando RJ, Cook MD, Jue SG. Probable terfenadine-fluoxetine-associated cardiac toxicity. *Ann Pharmacother* (1995) 29, 937–8.
3. Bergstrom RF, Goldberg MJ, Cerimele BJ, Hatcher BL, Simcox EA. Lack of a pharmacokinetic drug interaction between fluoxetine and terfenadine. *Pharm Res* (1996) 13 (9 Suppl), S-433.
4. Bergstrom RF, Goldberg MJ, Cerimele BJ, Hatcher BL. Assessment of the potential for a pharmacokinetic interaction between fluoxetine and terfenadine. *Clin Pharmacol Ther* (1997) 62, 643–51.
5. von Moltke LL, Greenblatt DJ, Duan SX, Harmatz JS, Wright CE, Shader RI. Inhibition of terfenadine metabolism *in vitro* by azole antifungal agents and by selective serotonin reuptake inhibitor antidepressants: relation to pharmacokinetic interactions *in vivo*. *J Clin Psychopharmacol* (1996) 16, 104–12.
6. Jurima-Romet M, Wright M, Neigh S. Terfenadine-antidepressant interactions: an *in vitro* inhibition study using human liver microsomes. *Br J Clin Pharmacol* (1998) 45, 318–21.
7. Robinson DS, Roberts DL, Smith JM, Stringfellow JC, Kaplita SB, Seminara JA, Marcus RN. The safety profile of nefazodone. *J Clin Psychiatry* (1996) 57 (Suppl 2), 31–8.
8. Committee on Safety of Medicines/Medicines Control Agency. Sertraline and terfenadine. *Current Problems* (1998) 24, 4.
9. Martin DE, Zussman B, Everitt DE, Benincosa LJ, Etheredge R, Jorkasky DK. No effect of paroxetine (P) on the cardiac safety and PK of terfenadine (T). *J Clin Pharmacol* (1996) 36, 849.
10. Martin DE, Zussman BD, Everitt DE, Benincosa LJ, Etheredge RC, Jorkasky DK. Paroxetine does not affect the cardiac safety and pharmacokinetics of terfenadine in healthy adult men. *J Clin Psychopharmacol* (1997) 17, 451–9.
11. Histafen (Terfenadine). Approved Prescription Services Limited. Summary of product characteristics, December 1999.

Thymoxamine (Moxisylyte) + Miscellaneous drugs

The makers say that intracavernosal injections of thymoxamine should not be given in combination with other drugs used for erectile dysfunction, and should be avoided by patients taking alpha- or beta-blockers. Care should also be exercised in those taking other antihypertensives such as ACE inhibitors or calcium channel blockers.

Clinical evidence, mechanism, importance and management

Thymoxamine (moxisylyte) is an alpha-1 and, to a lesser extent, an alpha-2 blocker which, if injected into the corpus cavernosum, can be used to treat erectile dysfunction. It causes relaxation of the smooth muscle fibres of the corpus cavernosum, thereby increasing the flow of blood and dilatation which results in erection of the penis. These vasodilatory effects are intended to be localised, but since some of the drug can escape into the circulation causing more general systemic effects, the makers of intracavernosal thymoxamine say that the concurrent use of other alpha-blockers (and they list **alfuzosin, doxazosin, prazosin, terazosin** and **urapidil**) and **beta-blockers** should be avoided because of the risks of additive and possibly severe orthostatic hypotension. They also suggest that if thymoxamine is to be used by patients unavoidably taking other antihypertensives (they cite **ACE inhibitors** and **calcium channel blockers**), precautions should be taken in case of potentiation of the antihypertensive effect.[1] This means, presumably, ensuring that marked hypotension (dizziness, fainting) is not a problem. The makers of intracavernosal thymoxamine also say that it should not be used in combination with other drugs used for erectile dysfunction.[1] These other drugs would include **alprostadil, papaverine, phentolamine** and **sildenafil**.

1. Érecnos (Moxisylyte hydrochloride). Fournier Pharmaceuticals. Summary of product characteristics, June 1997.

Thyroid hormones + Antacids

An isolated report describes reduced levothyroxine effects in a patient when given an aluminium-magnesium hydroxide antacid.

Clinical evidence, mechanism, importance and management

A man controlled on 150 micrograms **levothyroxine** daily for hypothyroidism developed high serum thyroid stimulating hormone levels (a rise from 1.1 up to 36 mU/l) while taking an **aluminium/magnesium hydroxide** antacid, and on two subsequent occasions when rechallenged. The reasons are not understood. He remained asymptomatic throughout.[1] The rise in the levels of thyroid stimulating hormone indicated that the dosage of the **levothyroxine** had become insufficient in the presence of the antacid. The general importance of this interaction is not known, but be alert for the need to increase the thyroid dosage in any patient on replacement treatment given this type of antacid. More study is needed.

1. Sperber AD, Liel Y. Evidence for interference with the intestinal absorption of levothyroxine sodium by aluminium hydroxide. *Arch Intern Med* (1991) 152, 183–4.

Thyroid hormones + Anticonvulsants

An isolated report describes a reduction in the effects of levothyroxine when phenytoin was given. Both carbamazepine and phenytoin can reduce serum thyroid hormone levels, but clinical hypothyroidism caused by an interaction seems to be rare.

Clinical evidence

A patient with hypothyroidism, successfully treated with 150 micrograms **levothyroxine** daily for 4 years, became hypothyroidic again when given 300 mg **phenytoin** daily. Doubling the **levothyroxine** dosage proved to be effective. Later this interaction was confirmed when stopping and restarting the **phenytoin** produced the same effect.[1]

A number of other reports describe very significant reductions in endogenous markers of thyroid function in considerable numbers of subjects and patients when treated with **phenobarbital**, **phenytoin** or **carbamazepine**,[2-6] but not **sodium valproate**.[6] However, there seem to be only two cases in which reversible hypothyroidism was seen, one with **carbamazepine** and **phenytoin**, and the other with **carbamazepine** alone.[7] There is also a report of an arrhythmia, attributed to the use of **phenytoin**, which due to protein binding increased the free **levothyroxine** in a hypothyroidic patient with rheumatic heart disease.[8] This report was later criticised by others, who suggested that the arrhythmia, if indeed there was one, was caused directly by the cardiac actions of **phenytoin**.[9,10]

Mechanism

Both phenytoin and carbamazepine can increase the metabolism of thyroid hormones, thereby reducing their serum levels. Phenytoin can also displace levothyroxine and triiodothyronine from thyroxine binding globulin.[11]

Importance and management

Despite very clear evidence that both carbamazepine and phenytoin can cause a marked reduction in serum thyroid hormone levels, the development of clinical hypothyroidism seems to be very rare and there seems to be only one case on record of an interaction between administered levothyroxine and phenytoin. There seems to be little reason for avoiding concurrent use, but the outcome should be monitored. Increase the thyroid dosage if necessary. See also 'Thyroid hormones + Barbiturates', p.940.

1. Blackshear JL, Schultz AL, Napier JS, Stuart DD. Thyroxine replacement requirements in hypothyroid patients receiving phenytoin. *Ann Intern Med* (1983) 99, 341–2.

2. Hansen JM, Skovsted L, Lauridsen UB, Kirkegaard C, Siersbæk-Nielsen K. The effect of diphenylhydantoin on thyroid function. *J Clin Endocrinol Metab* (1974) 39, 785–9.
3. Oppenheimer JH, Fisher LV, Nelson KM, Jailer JW. Depression of the serum protein-bound iodine level by diphenylhydantoin. *J Clin Endocrinol Metab* (1961) 21, 252–62.
4. Rootwelt K, Ganes T, Johannessen SI. Effect of carbamazepine, phenytoin and phenobarbitone on serum levels of thyroid hormones and thyrotropin in humans. *Scand J Clin Lab Invest* (1978) 38, 731–6.
5. Connell JMC, Rapeport WG, Gordon S, Brodie MJ. Changes in circulating thyroid hormones during short-term hepatic enzyme induction with carbamazepine. *Eur J Clin Pharmacol* (1984) 26, 453–6.
6. Larkin JG, Macphee GJA, Beastall GH, Brodie MJ. Thyroid hormone concentrations in epileptic patients. *Eur J Clin Pharmacol* (1989) 36, 213–16.
7. Aanderud S, Strandjord RE. Hypothyroidism induced by anti-epileptic therapy. *Acta Neurol Scand* (1980) 61, 330–2.
8. Fulop M, Widrow DR, Colmers RA, Epstein EJ. Possible diphenylhydantoin-induced arrhythmia in hypothyroidism. *JAMA* (1966) 196, 454–6.
9. Farzan S. Diphenylhydantoin and arrhythmia. *JAMA* (1966) 197, 133.
10. Gaspar HL. Diphenylhydantoin and arrhythmia. *JAMA* (1966) 197, 133.
11. Franklyn JA, Sheppard MC, Ramsden DB. Measurement of free thyroid hormones in patients on long-term phenytoin therapy. *Eur J Clin Pharmacol* (1984) 26, 633–4.

Thyroid hormones + Barbiturates

An isolated report describes a reduction in the response of a woman to levothyroxine when treated with a barbiturate hypnotic. See also 'Thyroid hormones + Anticonvulsants', p.940

Clinical evidence, mechanism, importance and management

An elderly woman on 300 micrograms **levothyroxine** daily for hypothyroidism complained of severe breathlessness within a week of reducing her nightly dose of *Tuinal* (**secobarbital** (**quinalbarbitone**) **sodium** 100 mg + **amobarbital sodium** 100 mg) from two capsules to one capsule. She was subsequently found to be thyrotoxic. She became symptom-free once again when the dosage of the **levothyroxine** was halved.[1] The reason is not known but **phenobarbital** is known to reduce the serum levels of endogenous thyroid hormones[2] (see 'Thyroid hormones + Anticonvulsants', p.940) and it seems possible that in this case these other two barbiturates acted in the same way, probably by enzyme induction. The general importance of this interaction is almost certainly small, but be alert for any evidence of changes in thyroid status if barbiturates are added or withdrawn from patients being treated for hypothyroidism.

1. Hoffbrand BI. Barbiturate/thyroid-hormone interaction. *Lancet* (1979) ii, 903–4.
2. Ohnhaus EE, Studer H. A link between liver microsomal enzyme activity and thyroid hormone metabolism in man. *Br J Clin Pharmacol* (1983) 15, 71–6.

Thyroid hormones + Calcium carbonate

The efficacy of levothyroxine can be reduced by the concurrent use of calcium carbonate. Separating the dosages avoids this interaction.

Clinical evidence

Twenty patients with hypothyroidism were treated with **levothyroxine** alone to which was then added 1200 mg **calcium carbonate** daily for 3 months. While taking the **calcium carbonate** their mean free thyroxine levels fell from 1.3 to 1.2 nanograms/dL and rose again to 1.4 nanograms/dL when it was stopped. The mean total thyroxine levels over the same period were 9.2, 8.6 and 9.3 micrograms/dL respectively and the mean thyroid stimulating hormone (TSH) levels were 1.6, 2.7 and 1.4 mU/l respectively.[1]

A women with thyroid cancer given **levothyroxine** 125 micrograms daily to suppress serum TSH levels showed a reduced response (fatigue, weight gain) when she took *Tums* containing **calcium carbonate** for the prevention of osteoporosis. She often took the two together. Over a 5-month period her serum TSH levels rose from 0.08 mU/l to 13.3 mU/l. Within 3 weeks of stopping the **calcium carbonate**, her serum TSH levels had fallen to 0.68 mU/l.[2] Other reports have described 4 patients who had elevations in their TSH levels while taking **calcium carbonate** concurrently with levothyroxine. All patients levels returned to normal when administration was separated by about 4 hours.[2-4]

Mechanism

In vitro studies indicate that levothyroxine is adsorbed onto the calcium carbonate when the pH is low (as in the stomach) which would reduce the amount available for absorption.[1]

Importance and management

An established interaction. The study quoted[1] shows that the mean reduction in the absorption of levothyroxine is quite small but the case histories[2,3] show that some individuals can experience a reduction in the absorption which is clearly clinically important. Since it is impossible to predict which patients are likely to be affected significantly, it would be prudent to advise all patients to separate the dosages of the two preparations by at least 4 h to avoid admixture in the gut. This interaction would be expected to occur with calcium carbonate in any form but it is not known whether other thyroid hormone preparations interact in the same way as levothyroxine.

1. Singh N, Singh PN, Hershmann JM. Effect of calcium carbonate on the absorption of levothyroxine. *JAMA* (2000) 283, 2822–25.
2. Schneyer CR. Calcium carbonate and reduction of levothyroxine efficacy. *JAMA* (1998) 279, 750.
3. Butner LE, Fulco PP, Feldman G. Calcium carbonate-induced hypothyroidism. *Ann Intern Med* (2000) 132, 595.
4. Csako G, McGriff NJ, Rotman-Pikielny P, Sarlis NJ, Pucino F. Exaggerated levothyroxine malabsorption due to calcium carbonate supplementation in gastrointestinal disorders. *Ann Pharmacother* (2001) 35, 1578–83.

Thyroid hormones + Cimetidine or Ranitidine

Cimetidine, but not ranitidine, causes a small reduction in the absorption of levothyroxine given orally.

Clinical evidence, mechanism, importance and management

When given 400 mg of **cimetidine** 90 minutes before a single capsule of **levothyroxine** containing radio-iodine (^{125}I), the absorption of **levothyroxine** in 10 women with simple goitre was reduced over the first 4 hours by 20.6% The reasons are not understood. A single 300-mg dose of **ranitidine** was found not to affect the **levothyroxine** absorption in a matched group of 10 women.[1]

The clinical importance of this interaction with **cimetidine** awaits assessment but it is probably not great, nevertheless it would be prudent to monitor the outcome if both drugs are used, being alert for the need to increase the **levothyroxine** dosage.

1. Jonderko G, Jonderko K, Marcisz CZ, Kotulska A. Effect of cimetidine and ranitidine on absorption of [^{125}I] levothyroxine administered orally. *Zhongguo Yao Li Xue Bao* (1992) 13, 391–4.

Thyroid hormones + Colestyramine

The absorption of thyroid extract, levothyroxine, and tri-iodothyronine from the gut is reduced by the concurrent use of colestyramine. Separate the dosages by 4 to 6 h to avoid the interaction.

Clinical evidence

A study was prompted when a hypothyroidic patient taking **levothyroxine** showed a fall in her basal metabolic rate, and an increase in her symptoms of hypothyroidism when she was given **colestyramine**. Two similar patients taking 60 mg **thyroid extract** or 100 micrograms **levothyroxine sodium** daily, and on 5 healthy subjects were additionally given **colestyramine** 4 g four times daily, which reduced their absorption of **levothyroxine** (^{131}I), the amount

recovered in the faeces being roughly doubled. One of the patients showed a worsening of her hypothyroidism. Separating the dosages by 4 to 5 h reduced but did not completely prevent the interaction.[1]

Another report describes a patient on **levothyroxine** whose thyroid-stimulating hormone (TSH) levels rose when given **colestyramine**, and fell again when it was stopped, indicating an impairment of **levothyroxine** absorption.[2]

Mechanism

Colestyramine binds to levothyroxine in the gut, thereby reducing its absorption. Since levothyroxine probably also undergoes enterohepatic recirculation, continued contact with the colestyramine is possible.

Importance and management

An established interaction (although the documentation is very limited) and of clinical importance. *In vitro* tests show that tri-iodothyronine interacts similarly.[1] The interaction can be minimised by separating the dosages by 4 to 6 h (but see 'Mechanism'). Even so, the outcome should be monitored so that any necessary thyroid hormone dosage adjustments can be made.

1. Northcutt RC, Stiel JN, Hollifield JW, Stant EG. The influence of cholestyramine on thyroxine absorption. *JAMA* (1969) 208, 1857–61.
2. Harmon SM, Seifert CF. Levothyroxine-cholestyramine interaction reemphasized. *Ann Intern Med* (1991) 115, 658–9.

Thyroid hormones + Ferrous sulphate

Ferrous sulphate causes a reduction in the effects of levothyroxine in patients treated for hypothyroidism.

Clinical evidence

Fourteen patients with primary hypothyroidism showed an increase in TSH levels from 1.6 to 5.4 mU/l when given 300 mg **ferrous sulphate** daily with their usual **levothyroxine** dose for 12 weeks. The symptoms of hypothyroidism in 9 of the patients worsened.[1,2] Another woman with hypothyroidism, on **levothyroxine**, showed a very marked rise in TSH levels when given **ferrous sulphate**. Her **levothyroxine** dosage was raised from 175 to 200 micrograms daily.[3]

Mechanism

The addition of iron to levothyroxine *in vitro* was found to produce a poorly soluble purple iron-levothyroxine complex suggesting that this might also occur in the gut.[1,2]

Importance and management

Information is limited to these reports but it appears to be a clinically important interaction. Monitor the effects of concurrent use and separate the dosages by 2 h or more on the assumption that reduced absorption accounts for this interaction. Monitor well. The same precautions would seem appropriate with any other iron preparation but confirmatory study is needed.

1. Campbell NRC, Wong N, Hasinoff BB, Rao B, Stalts H. Ferrous sulfate reduces thyroxine efficacy. *Clin Pharmacol Ther* (1992) 51, 165.
2. Campbell NRC, Hasinoff BB, Stalts H, Rao B, Wong NCW. Ferrous sulfate reduces thyroxine efficacy in patients with hypothyroidism. *Ann Intern Med* (1992) 117, 1010-3.
3. Schlienger JL. Accroissement des besoins en thyroxine par le sulfate de fer. *Presse Med* (1994) 23, 492.

Thyroid hormones + Lovastatin

An isolated report describes raised serum thyroid hormone levels and evidence of thyrotoxicosis in a man on levothyroxine when given lovastatin. In contrast another isolated case report describes hypothyroidism in a woman on levothyroxine when given lovastatin.

Clinical evidence, mechanism, importance and management

A 54-year-old diabetic taking 150 micrograms **levothyroxine** daily for Hashimoto's thyroiditis, and a number of other drugs (gemfibrozil, clofibrate, propranolol, diltiazem, quinidine, aspirin, dipyridamole, insulin) was started on 20 mg **lovastatin** daily. Weakness and muscle aches (with a normal creatinine phosphokinase) developed within 2 to 3 days and over a 27-day period he lost 10% of his body weight. His serum **levothyroxine** levels rose from 11.3 to 27.2 micrograms/dl. The author of the report postulated that the **lovastatin** may have displaced the thyroid hormones from their binding sites, thereby increasing their effects and causing this acute thyrotoxic state. They suggest he did not have any cardiac symptoms because of his pre-existing drug regimen.[1] In contrast, a female patient with goitrous hypothyroidism due to Hashimoto's thyroiditis, which was being treated with 125 micrograms of **levothyroxine sodium** daily, developed evidence of hypothyroidism (elevated TSH) on two occasions when additionally treated with 20 mg or 60 mg **lovastatin** daily. No clinical signs of hypothyroidism developed, apart from some increased fatigue and possibly an increased sensitivity to insulin. The authors suggest **lovastatin** may have influenced the absorption or clearance of **levothyroxine**.[2]

When the second report was published, the makers of lovastatin reported that at that time (August 1989) more than 1 million patients had taken lovastatin, and hypothyroidism had only been reported in three patients. None of the cases were confirmed by withdrawal and rechallenge.[3] It therefore seems that any interaction is a very rare event and unlikely to happen in most patients. No special precautions would seem to be necessary.

1. Lustgarten BP. Catabolic response to lovastatin therapy. *Ann Intern Med* (1988) 109, 171–2.

2. Demke DM. Drug interaction between thyroxine and lovastatin. *N Engl J Med* (1989) 321, 1341–2.

3. Gormley GJ, Tobert JA. Drug interaction between thyroxine and lovastatin. *N Engl J Med* (1989) 321, 1342.

Thyroid hormones + Rifampicin (Rifampin)

An isolated case report suggests that rifampicin might possibly reduce the effects of the thyroid hormones.

Clinical evidence, mechanism, importance and management

A woman with Turner's syndrome who had undergone a total thyroidectomy and who was being treated with 100 micrograms of **levothyroxine** daily, showed a marked fall in serum **levothyroxine** levels and free **levothyroxine** index with a dramatic rise in TSH levels when given **rifampicin**. However, no symptoms of clinical hypothyroidism developed, and the drop in serum **levothyroxine** occurred prior to starting **rifampicin**, which may reflect the clinical picture of an acute infection.[1] A possible reason for the changes is that **rifampicin** is a potent enzyme inducing agent which can markedly increase the metabolism of many drugs, thereby increasing their loss from the body and reducing their effects. **Rifampicin** given to healthy subjects also reduces endogenous serum levothyroxine levels.[2] There seem to be no reports of adverse effects in other patients given both drugs and the evidence for this interaction is by no means conclusive. Although **rifampicin** can affect thyroid hormones, it appears that healthy individuals can compensate for this. Since hypothyroid patients may not be able to compensate in the same way, bear this interaction in mind if **rifampicin** is given to a patient on **levothyroxine**.

1. Isley WL. Effect of rifampin therapy on thyroid function tests in a hypothyroid patient on replacement l-thyroxine. *Ann Intern Med* (1987) 107, 517–18.

2. Ohnhaus EE, Studer H. A link between liver microsomal enzyme activity and thyroid hormone metabolism in man. *Br J Clin Pharmacol* (1983) 15, 71–6.

Thyroid hormones + Ritonavir

A man needed to have his levothyroxine dosage doubled when given ritonavir.

Clinical evidence, mechanism, importance and management

An HIV+ man, stabilised on **levothyroxine** for autoimmune thyroiditis, developed an enlarged thyroid gland and marked lethargy about a month after his HIV treatment was changed to include stavudine, lamivudine, saquinavir and **ritonavir**. It became necessary to double his maintenance dose of levothyroxine to re-stabilise him. When the **ritonavir** and saquinavir were withdrawn and replaced by **indinavir**, the patient was able to go back to the original dose of **levothyroxine**. It is thought that this interaction occurred because **ritonavir** increases the activity of the glucuronosyl transferases, which are concerned with the metabolism (conjugation) of levothyroxine.[1]

Direct information of this apparent interaction seems to be limited to this report, but it would now be prudent to be alert for the need to a raise the dosage of **levothyroxine** if **ritonavir** is added to the drug regimen of any patient. This case report suggests that **indinavir** does not interact.

1. Tseng A, Fletcher D. Interaction between ritonavir and levothyroxine. *AIDS* (1998) 12, 2235–6.

Thyroid hormones + Sertraline

The effects of levothyroxine can be opposed in some patients by the concurrent use of sertraline.

Clinical evidence, mechanism, importance and management

Nine patients with hypothyroidism taking **sertraline** were noted to have elevated thyroid stimulating hormone (TSH) levels (indicating a decrease in the efficacy of the **levothyroxine** being taken). Two other patients with thyroid cancer whose TSH levels had been deliberately depressed developed TSH levels in the normal range while taking **sertraline**. None of the patients showed any signs of hypothyroidism at the time and all of them had been taking the same dose of **levothyroxine** for at least 6 months. TSH levels up to almost 17 µU/ml (normal range 0.3 to 5.0 µU/ml) were seen in some patients. The **levothyroxine** dosages were increased by 11 to 50% until the TSH levels were back to normal. The authors of this report say that they know of 3 patients whose TSH levels were unaltered by **sertraline**.[1]

The makers of **sertraline** say that their early-alert safety database to the end of July 1997 had identified 14 cases of hypothyroidism where a possible relation to **sertraline** could not be excluded. Seven of the patients were taking thyroxine.[2]

The mechanism of this interaction (if such it is) is not known, but these cases draw attention to the need to monitor the effects of adding **sertraline** in patients taking **thyroid hormones**, the dosage of which may need to be increased. More study is needed.

1. McCowen KC, Spark R. Elevated serum thyrotropin in thyroxine-treated patients with hypothyroidism given sertraline. *N Engl J Med* (1997) 337, 1010–11.

2. Clary CM, Harrison WM. Elevated serum thyrotropin in thyroxine-treated patients with hypothyroidism given sertraline. *N Engl J Med* (1997) 337, 1011.

Thyroid hormones + Sodium polystyrene sulphonate

A woman with hypothyroidism controlled with levothyroxine relapsed when concurrently treated with sodium polystyrene sulphonate.

Clinical evidence

A woman taking 150 micrograms **levothyroxine** daily for hypothyroidism, following total thyroidectomy later developed renal failure and began dialysis. She was also taking digoxin, clofibrate, calcium carbonate, ferrous sulphate, nicotinic acid, folic acid and magnesium sulphate. Because of persistent hyperkalaemia she took **sodium polystyrene sulphonate** 15 g daily. After 6 months, she developed lethargy, hoarse voice, facial fullness and weight gain (all signs of hypothyroidism). These symptoms resolved within 6 weeks of raising the **levothyroxine** dosage to 200 micrograms daily and separating it from the **sodium polystyrene sulphonate** by 10 h (previously taken together).[1]

Mechanism

Sodium polystyrene sulphonate is a cation-exchange resin which is used to bind potassium ions in exchange for sodium. An *in vitro* study found that when levothyroxine 200 micrograms was dispersed in 100 ml water with 15 g sodium polystyrene sulphonate, the concentration of the levothyroxine at pH 2 fell by 93% and at pH 7 by 98%.[1] This would almost certainly occur in the gut as well, thereby markedly reducing the amount of levothyroxine available for absorption.

Importance and management

Information seems to be limited to this study but the interaction would appear to be of general importance. Separate the dosages of levothyroxine and sodium polystyrene sulphonate as much as possible (10 h seems to be effective) and monitor the thyroid function to confirm that this is effective. Raise the levothyroxine dosage if necessary.

1. McLean M, Kirkwood I, Epstein M, Jones B, Hall C. Cation-exchange resin and inhibition of intestinal absorption of thyroxine. *Lancet* (1993) 341, 1286.

Thyroid hormones + Sucralfate

An isolated report describes a marked reduction in the effects of levothyroxine in a patient taking sucralfate.

Clinical evidence, mechanism, importance and management

A woman with hypothyroidism failed to respond to **levothyroxine** despite taking 4.8 micrograms/kg daily while on **sucralfate**. Her response remained inadequate (thyroid stimulating hormone (TSH) levels high, thyroxine levels low) even when the **levothyroxine** was taken 2.5 h after the **sucralfate**, but when taken 4.5 h before the **sucralfate** the thyroxine and TSH levels gradually became normal. A later *in vitro* study demonstrated that **sucralfate** binds strongly to **levothyroxine** and it is presumed that this can also occur in the gut, thereby reducing its absorption.[1] Although this seems to be the first and only report of this interaction, it would now seem prudent not to take **sucralfate** until a few hours after the **levothyroxine**. Patients should be advised accordingly and the response well monitored.

1. Havrankova J, Lahaie R. Levothyroxine binding by sucralfate. *Ann Intern Med* (1992) 117, 445–6.

Ticlopidine + Antacids or Food

Food causes a moderate increase in the absorption of ticlopidine, whereas *Maalox* causes a moderate reduction.

Clinical evidence, mechanism, importance and management

The extent of ticlopidine absorption was increased by 20% and occurred more rapidly when given after **food** to 12 healthy subjects, whereas 30 ml *Maalox* (**magnesium-aluminium hydroxides**) reduced the extent of absorption by 20%.[1] These modest changes are unlikely to be of much clinical importance. It is suggested that ticlopidine is taken with **food** to minimise gastric intolerance.[1]

1. Shah J, Fratis A, Ellis D, Murakami S, Teitelbaum P. Effect of food and antacid on absorption of orally administered ticlopidine hydrochloride. *J Clin Pharmacol* (1990) 30, 733–6.

Ticlopidine + Miscellaneous drugs

Ticlopidine decreases the clearance of phenazone (antipyrine) and increases the antiaggregant effects of aspirin and possibly other antiplatelet drugs, whereas the ticlopidine-induced increases in bleeding times are opposed by methylprednisolone. Beta-blockers, calcium channel blockers and diuretics are reported not to interact with ticlopidine. See the index for other ticlopidine interactions.

Clinical evidence, mechanism, importance and management

(a) Aspirin, other NSAIDs and Antiplatelet drugs

Aspirin combined with ticlopidine appears to inhibit platelet aggregation more than either drug alone.[1,2] The makers warn that combined use increases the risk of gastrointestinal bleeding because **aspirin** damages the gastro-duodenal lining, which can cause bleeding, and this is likely to be worsened by the platelet antiaggregant effects of the ticlopidine.[3] The same risk exists with **NSAIDs**, which can do similar damage. The makers also warn about the possible additive effects of ticlopidine with other **antiplatelet drugs** and recommend close clinical monitoring of concurrent treatment.[3]

(b) Heparins

The makers of ticlopidine say that the concurrent use of **heparins** and ticlopidine increases haemorrhagic risk, and concurrent use requires close monitoring of the APPT.[3]

(c) Phenazone (Antipyrine)

A study in healthy subjects found that 500 mg ticlopidine twice daily for 3 weeks decreased the clearance of **phenazone** (a marker of enzyme inhibition or induction). The AUC increased by 14% and the half-life increased by 27%.[4] This is consistent with the way ticlopidine appears to inhibit the metabolism of theophylline (see 'Theophylline + Ticlopidine', p.816) but so far no other drugs seem to be affected to a clinically important extent.

(d) Methylprednisolone

Intravenous **methylprednisolone** 20 mg decreases the prolongation of bleeding times caused by ticlopidine without reducing the antiplatelet effects.[1] The clinical importance of this is uncertain.

(e) Other non-interacting drugs

The makers report that in clinical studies in which ticlopidine was given with **beta-blockers**, **calcium channel blockers** and **diuretics** (none of the individual drugs was named), no clinically significant adverse interactions were reported.[3]

1. Thébault J, Blatrix C, Blanchard J, Panak E. A possible method to control prolongations of bleeding time under antiplatelet therapy with ticlopidine. *Thromb Haemost* (1982) 48, 6–8.
2. Splawinska B, Kuzniar J, Malinga K, Mazurek AP, Splawinski J. The efficacy and potency of antiplatelet activity of ticlopidine is increased by aspirin. *Int J Clin Pharmacol Ther* (1996) 34, 352–6.
3. Ticlid (Ticlopidine). Sanofi Synthelabo. Summary of product characteristics, May 2000.
4. Knudsen JB, Bastain W, Sefton CM, Allen JG, Dickinson JP. Pharmacokinetics of ticlopidine during chronic oral administration to healthy volunteers and its effects on antipyrine pharmacokinetics. *Xenobiotica* (1992) 22, 579–89.

Tirilazad mesilate + Miscellaneous drugs

Phenobarbital and phenytoin reduce the serum levels of tirilazad mesilate whereas ketoconazole increases them. Cimetidine and nimodipine appear not to interact.

Clinical evidence, mechanism, importance and management

(a) Cimetidine, Nimodipine

A study in 16 healthy subjects found that 300 mg **cimetidine** 6-hourly for 4 days had no effect on the pharmacokinetics of single 2 mg/kg doses of tirilazad mesilate given by infusion over 10 min on day 2, nor on U-89678, its metabolite.[1] There also appears to be no pharmacokinetic or pharmacodynamic interaction between tirilazad mesilate and **nimodipine**, although this was only a single-dose study.[2] No special precautions would seem necessary if either of these drugs is given with tirilazad mesilate.

(b) Ketoconazole

Tirilazad mesilate, orally (10 mg/kg) or intravenously (2 mg/kg), was given to 12 healthy subjects either alone or on day 4 of a 7-day regimen of 200 mg **ketoconazole** daily. The **ketoconazole** more than doubled the absolute bioavailability of the oral tirilazad mesilate (from 8.7 to 20.9%), apparently because its first pass liver and gut wall metabolism by cytochrome P450 isoenzyme CYP3A was inhibited.[3,4] The clinical importance of this interaction awaits assessment.

(c) Phenobarbital

The pharmacokinetics of tirilazad mesilate (1.5 mg/kg as 10 min intravenous infusions every 6 h for 29 doses) were studied in 15 healthy subjects before and after taking 100 mg **phenobarbital** daily for 8 days. The **phenobarbital** increased the clearance of the tirilazad by 25% in the male subjects and 29% in the female, and the AUC of the metabolite of tirilazad (U-89678) was reduced by 51% in the males and 69% in the females. The reason is thought to be that the **phenobarbital** acts as an enzyme inducing agent, which increases the metabolism of the tirilazad.[5,6] The clinical importance of these reductions awaits assessment, but be alert for evidence of reduced effects if both drugs are given. It is doubtful if the full enzyme-inducing effects of the **phenobarbital** would have been reached in this study after only one week, so anticipate a greater effect if it is given for a longer period.

(d) Phenytoin

After taking 200 mg **phenytoin** 8-hourly for 11 doses followed by 100 mg 8-hourly for 5 doses, the AUC (over 6 h) of tirilazad mesilate was reduced from 4.65 to 3.03 micrograms.h/ml in 12 healthy subjects. The AUC of a metabolite with possible activity (U-89678) was reduced from 1.49 to 0.2 micrograms.h/ml.[7,8] Another report by the same group of workers[9] found that **phenytoin** 8-hourly for 7 days (9 doses of 200 mg followed by 13 doses of 100 mg) reduced the clearance of tirilazad by 92% and of U-89678 by 93%. In a later study the same group of workers found that **phenytoin** increased the metabolism of tirilazad and its metabolite in men and women to similar extents.[10] The clinical importance of these reductions is still to be assessed, but you should be alert for any evidence of reduced tirilazad effects if both drugs are given.

1. Fleishaker JC, Hulst LK, Peters GR. Lack of pharmacokinetic interaction between cimetidine and tirilazad mesylate. *Pharm Res* (1994) 11, 341–4.
2. Fleishaker JC, Hulst LK, Peters GR. Lack of a pharmacokinetic/pharmacodynamic interaction between nimodipine and tirilazad mesylate in healthy volunteers. *J Clin Pharmacol* (1994) 34, 837–41.
3. Fleishaker JC, Pearson LK, Pearson PG, Wienkers LC, Peters GR. Ketoconazole (K) inhibits tirilazad mesylate (TM) metabolism and increases its oral bioavailability. *Pharm Res* (1995) 12 (9 Suppl), S-373.
4. Fleishaker JC, Pearson PG, Wienkers LC, Pearson LK, Peters GR. Biotransformation of tirilazad in humans: 2. Effect of ketoconazole on tirilazad clearance and oral bioavailability. *J Pharmacol Exp Ther* (1996) 277, 991–8.
5. Fleishaker JC, Pearson LK, Peters GR. Effect of gender on the degree of induction of tirilazad clearance by phenobarbital. *Clin Pharmacol Ther* (1995) 57, 181.
6. Fleishaker JC, Pearson LK, Peters GR. Gender does not affect the degree of induction of tirilazad clearance by phenobarbital. *Eur J Clin Pharmacol* (1996) 50, 139–45.
7. Fleishaker JC, Hulst LK, Peters GR. Interaction between phenytoin and tirilazad mesylate in man: acute induction of tirilazad metabolism? *Pharm Res* (1993) 10 (10 Suppl), S-419.
8. Fleishaker JC, Hulst LK, Peters GR. The effect of phenytoin on the pharmacokinetics of tirilazad mesylate in healthy male volunteers. *Clin Pharmacol Ther* (1994) 56, 389–97.
9. Fleishaker JC, Pearson LK, Peters GR. Induction of tirilazad clearance by phenytoin. *Biopharm Drug Dispos* (1998) 19, 91–6.
10. Fleishaker JC, Pearson LK, Peters GR. Effect of gender on the degree of induction of tirilazad clearance by phenytoin. *Clin Pharmacol Ther* (1996) 59, 168.

Tizanidine + Miscellaneous drugs

Tizanidine possibly increases the effects of antihypertensive drugs in some patients and may also increase the effects of sedative drugs and alcohol. Oral contraceptives can reduce the serum levels of tizanidine and an isolated report describes an increase in serum phenytoin levels caused by tizanidine. No interaction occurs with paracetamol (acetaminophen).

Clinical evidence, mechanism, importance and management

Tizanidine can cause a reduction in blood pressure (seen in 7 to 12% of patients)[1] for which reason the makers suggest that it may possibly increase the effects of **antihypertensive drugs**, including **diuretics**. They also say that **beta-blockers** and **digoxin** may potentiate hypotension and bradycardia[2] but there do not appear to be any reports of problems with concurrent use.

The most common side-effects of tizanidine are dry mouth and somnolence/drowsiness in up to 50% or more of patients,[1] for which reason the makers warn about the possibility of increased effects with other **sedative drugs**, and **alcohol**.[2] There is pharmacokinetic evidence that the clearance of tizanidine is reduced by about 50% in women taking **oral contraceptives**, but the clinical relevance of this is uncertain. No clinically important tizanidine/**oral contraceptive** interactions have been reported in clinical trials.[2] A trial in 20 healthy subjects found that no clinically significant interaction occurred between 325 mg **paracetamol (acetaminophen)** and 4 mg tizanidine.[1] An isolated report says that a patient showed a rise of one third (from about 75 to 100 micromol/l) in his serum **phenytoin** levels within a week of starting 6 mg tizanidine daily, and levels continued to rise despite a reduction in the **phenytoin** dosage, only returning to normal when the tizanidine was withdrawn.[3]

1. Wagstaff AJ, Bryson HM. Tizanidine. A review of its pharmacology, clinical efficacy and tolerability in the management of spasticity associated with cerebral and spinal disorders. *Drugs* (1997) 53, 435–52.
2. Zanaflex (Tizanidine hydrochloride). Elan Pharma Ltd. Summary of product characteristics, February 2001.
3. Ueno K, Miyai K, Mitsuzane K. Phenytoin-tizanidine interaction. *DICP Ann Pharmacother* (1991) 25, 1273.

Tolrestat + Aspirin

The pharmacokinetics of both drugs are changed by concurrent use, but the extent is small and unlikely to be clinically relevant.

Clinical evidence, mechanism, importance and management

Eighteen healthy subjects were given tolrestat 400 mg daily or 975 mg **aspirin** 8-hourly on study days 1 to 5, then both drugs together for days 6 to 10, and finally one or other of the drugs for days 11 to 15. The AUCs of the **aspirin** and tolrestat were raised 16% and 18% respectively, and the maximum serum levels raised 9% and lowered 2% respectively. These changes were due to reductions in the renal clearances of both drugs.[1] The clinical importance of these alterations has not been evaluated in diabetics, but all of them are quite small and unlikely to be clinically relevant. This needs confirmation.

1. Garg V, Parker V, Turner MB, Burghart P, Fruncillo R, Battle M, Chiang S. Pharmacokinetic interaction between aspirin and tolrestat in normal volunteers. *Pharm Res* (1995) 12 (9 Suppl), S-392

Tolterodine + Miscellaneous drugs

Additive anticholinergic effects may occur if tolterodine is used with other anticholinergic drugs, and the makers cur-

rently say that clarithromycin, erythromycin, itraconazole, ketoconazole and miconazole should be used with caution or avoided because of a risk of increased tolterodine effects. The makers also suggest that the effects of cisapride and metoclopramide may be reduced by tolterodine. Fluoxetine causes a small and clinically unimportant increase in the effects of tolterodine, while no interaction occurs with oral contraceptives. Tolterodine appears normally not to interact with warfarin but two cases of raised INRs have been reported.

Clinical evidence, mechanism, importance and management

(a) Anticholinergics, Cholinergic agonists and related drugs

Tolterodine and one of its 5-hydroxymethyl derivatives are cholinergic receptor antagonists with a selectivity for the urinary bladder rather than salivary glands. Even so some moderate general anticholinergic (antimuscarinic) effects can occur such as mouth dryness, dyspepsia and reduced lachrymation, and some additive anticholinergic effects and side-effects are predicted to occur if **other anticholinergic drugs** are used concurrently.[1] See 'Anticholinergics + Anticholinergics', p.414. The makers also suggest that the effects of **cisapride** and **metoclopramide** may be reduced by tolterodine.[1]

(b) Azole antifungals, Macrolide antibacterials

A study in 8 healthy subjects who were poor metabolisers (i.e. deficient in cytochrome P450 isoenzyme CYP2D6) found that after taking 200 mg **ketoconazole** daily for 4 days the clearance of a single 2-mg dose of tolterodine was reduced by 61% and its AUC was increased 2.5-fold.[2] Although tolterodine is normally metabolised to its active metabolite by CYP2D6, in low levels of this isoenzyme, CYP3A4, which is inhibited by **ketoconazole**, becomes more important. The conclusion was reached that when tolterodine is given with **ketoconazole** (or any other potent CYP3A4 inhibitor), the dosage of the tolterodine should be halved.[2] The makers of tolterodine do not recommend the use of CYP3A4 inhibitors with tolterodine because of the risk of toxicity. They name two macrolide antibacterials (**clarithromycin**, **erythromycin**) and two azole antifungals (**ketoconazole**, **itraconazole**),[1] all of which are CYP3A4 inhibitors.

(c) Fluoxetine

Thirteen psychiatric patients with symptoms of urinary incontinence were treated with 2 mg tolterodine twice daily for 3 days, followed by 20 mg **fluoxetine** daily for 3 weeks, and then for a further 3 days with tolterodine and **fluoxetine** concurrently. Nine of the 13 completed the trial, the other 4 withdrew because of the **fluoxetine**-related side-effects. The AUC of the tolterodine increased 4.8-fold with a minor decrease in its active and equipotent metabolite due, it is believed, to the enzyme inhibitory action of the **fluoxetine** on the activity of CYP2D6, which is concerned with the metabolism of the tolterodine. This change represents an approximately 25% increased in the active moiety (unbound tolterodine + metabolite).[3]

In practical terms this means that the anticholinergic (antimuscarinic) effects of the tolterodine when used for the treatment of urinary bladder overactivity are only moderately increased, and it seems unlikely that any tolterodine dosage changes are likely to be needed. The makers say that no clinically significant interaction occurs.[1]

(d) Oral contraceptives

An open-label, randomised, two-period crossover study in 24 women found that 2 mg tolterodine twice daily on days 1 to 14 for two 28-day contraceptive cycles had no effect on the pharmacokinetics of the steroids in an oral contraceptive (**ethinylestradiol** 30 micrograms + **levonorgestrel** 150 micrograms). The pharmacokinetics of the tolterodine were also not relevantly changed, and the serum levels of estradiol and progesterone indicated that suppression of ovulation continued during both periods of treatment.[4] No special precautions would seem to be needed if these drugs are used concurrently.

(e) Warfarin

The makers report that clinical studies have shown that no interactions occur between tolterodine and **warfarin**,[1] but a report describes two patients on stable doses **warfarin** who showed elevated INRs

when measured 2 weeks after tolterodine was started. Their INRs fell again when the tolterodine was stopped.[5] It would therefore now be prudent to monitor well if tolterodine is added to established **warfarin** treatment. Information about other anticoagulants appears to be lacking.

1. Detrusitol (Tolterodine). Pharmacia. Summary of product characteristics, July 2001.
2. Brynne N, Forslund C, Hallén B, Gustafsson LL, Bertilsson L. Ketoconazole inhibits the metabolism of tolterodine in subjects with deficient CYP2D6 activity. *Exp Toxic Pathol* (1998) 50, 96
3. Brynne N, Apéria B, Åberg-Wistedt A, Hallén B, Bertilsson L. Inhibition of tolterodine metabolism by fluoxetine with minor change in antimuscarinic activity. *Eur J Clin Pharmacol* (1997) 52 (Suppl), A130.
4. Olsson B, Landgren B-M. The effect of tolterodine on the pharmacokinetics and pharmacodynamics of a combination oral contraceptive containing ethinyl estradiol and levonorgestrel. *Clin Ther* (2001) 23, 1876–88.
5. Colucci VJ, Rivey MP. Tolterodine-warfarin drug interaction. *Ann Pharmacother* (1999) 33, 1173–6.

Total parenteral nutrition + Potassium-sparing diuretics

Metabolic acidosis occurred in two patients receiving total parenteral nutrition, which was attributed to the use of triamterene or amiloride.

Clinical evidence, mechanism, importance and management

Metabolic acidosis developed in two patients receiving total parenteral nutrition associated with the concurrent use of **triamterene** and **amiloride**. The cases were complicated by a number of pathological and other factors, but the suggestion is that the major reason for the acidosis was because the diuretics prevented the kidneys from responding normally to the acid load. Caution is advised during concurrent use.[1]

1. Kushner RF, Sitrin MD. Metabolic acidosis. Development in two patients receiving a potassium-sparing diuretic and total parenteral nutrition. *Arch Intern Med* (1986) 146, 343–5.

Trientine + Miscellaneous drugs

Trientine can possibly chelate with iron thereby reducing its absorption. On theoretical grounds a similar chelation interaction may occur with calcium and magnesium antacids.

Clinical evidence, mechanism, importance and management

(a) Iron preparations

Trientine is a copper chelating agent used for Wilson's disease. One of the side-effects of trientine is that it can cause iron deficiency (probably because it chelates with iron in the gut thereby reducing its absorption), and it is usual to make good this iron deficiency where necessary by giving an **iron supplement**. The makers suggest that any **iron supplement** should be given at a different time of the day from trientine to minimise their admixture in the gut.[1] A separation of at least 2 h is effective with other drugs which interact similarly and it seems likely that this will also be effective with this drug combination.

(b) Magnesium and calcium antacids

The makers say that there is no evidence that **calcium** or **magnesium antacids** alter the efficacy of trientine, but on theoretical grounds they might possibly form a chelate with the trientine in the gut.[1] It is therefore suggested that their administration should be separated. This means that if the trientine is taken on an empty stomach before meals as recommended, the antacids should be taken after meals.

1. Trientine dihydrochloride. Product summary, August 2000.

Trimetazidine + Miscellaneous drugs

Trimetazidine appears not to interact with theophylline or digoxin.

Clinical evidence, mechanism, importance and management

After taking 20 mg trimetazidine twice daily for at least 14 days the pharmacokinetics of a single 375-mg dose of **theophylline**, a single 500-microgram dose of **digoxin** and 500 mg **antipyrine** remained unchanged in 13 healthy subjects.[1] These results suggest that treatment with **theophylline** or **digoxin** is unlikely to be altered in patients concurrently treated with trimetazidine, but this needs confirmation. The non-interaction with **antipyrine** also indicates that trimetazidine is neither an inducer nor an inhibitor of drug metabolism (hydroxylation) in the liver and therefore it is unlikely to interact with many drugs that are affected by changes in liver metabolism.

1. Edeki TI, Johnston A, Campbell DB, Ings RMJ, Brownsill R, Genissel P, Turner P. An examination of the possible pharmacokinetic interaction of trimetazidine with theophylline, digoxin and antipyrine. *Br J Clin Pharmacol* (1989) 26, 657P.

Trimoprostil + Antacids

The bioavailability of trimoprostil is not affected by *Mylanta I*, *Di-Gel* or food.[1]

1. Wills RJ, Rees MMC, Rubio F, Gibson DM, Givens S, Parsonnet M, Gallo-Torres HE. Influence of antacids on the bioavailability of trimoprostil. *Eur J Clin Pharmacol* (1984) 27, 251–2.

Trinitrotoluene + Alcohol

Men exposed to trinitrotoluene in a munitions factory were found to have a greater risk of chronic liver impairment if they had a long history of drinking than if they were non-drinkers.[1]

1. Li J, Jiang QG, Zhong WD. Persistent ethanol drinking increases liver injury induced by trinitrotoluene exposure: an in-plant case-control study. *Hum Exp Toxicol* (1991) 10, 405-9.

Tripotassium dicitratobismuthate (TDB) + Miscellaneous drugs

Antacids, food and large amounts of milk can reduce the effects of tripotassium dicitratobismuthate. Omeprazole and ranitidine possibly cause an undesirable increase in the absorption of bismuth. Ciprofloxacin appears not to interact, but the effects of tetracyclines are expected to be reduced.

Clinical evidence, mechanism, importance and management

(a) Antacids, Food

TDB can bind to **antacids** and for this reason the makers suggest that **antacids** should not be taken half-an-hour before or after TDB.[1] One recommendation is that the TDB should not be taken within half-an-hour before or after **food**.[1,2]

(b) Antibacterials

TDB is expected to interact with **tetracyclines** given orally (see 'Tetracyclines + Antacids', p.223) causing a reduction in the effects of the **tetracyclines**. In two subjects it was found to have only a slight effect on the absorption of **ciprofloxacin**.[3] The clinical importance of any interaction with either quinolone or tetracycline antibacterials is not known.

(c) Omeprazole

The AUC of a single 240-mg dose of TDB was increased fourfold in 6 healthy subjects after taking 40 mg **omeprazole** daily for a week. The maximal serum levels increased from 36.7 to 86.7 micrograms/l which the authors of the study point out approaches what they describe as the "toxic range" for bismuth (100 micrograms/l). They suggest that to avoid the possibility of systemic toxicity the dosage of the TDB should be halved. However, this might then limit the activity of the TDB. In addition they also say that another preliminary study using TDB and **omeprazole** found that the eradication rates of *H. pylori* were reduced when compared with single drug treatments.[4] So all of this preliminary evidence suggests that this drug combination may not be advisable. More study is needed to confirm or deny this. A recommendation from the makers is that **omeprazole** should not be taken within 30 min before or after TDB.[1]

(d) Ranitidine

The AUC of a single 240-mg dose of TDB was increased fourfold in 12 healthy subjects treated with 300 mg **ranitidine**.[5] These figures are similar to those found in (c) above and the same reasoning about not using these drugs together would seem to be valid, but more study is needed.

1. Yamanouchi Pharma Ltd. Personal communication, November 1994.
2. De-Noltab (Tri-potassium di-citrato bismuthate). Summary of product characteristics, July 2002.
3. Brouwers JRBJ, v d Kam HJ, Sijtsma J, Koks CHW. Important drug interaction of oral ciprofloxacin with sucralfate and magnesium citrate solution. *Pharm Weekbl (Sci)* (1989) 11 (Suppl E), E13.
4. Treiber G, Walker S, Klotz U. Omeprazole-induced increase in the absorption of bismuth from tripotassium dicitrato bismuthate. *Clin Pharmacol Ther* (1994) 55, 486–91.
5. Nwokolo CU, Prewett EJ, Sawyerr AM, Hudson M, Pounder RE. The effect of histamine H_2-receptor blockade on bismuth absorption from three ulcer-healing compounds. *Gastroenterology* (1991) 101, 889–94.

Ursodeoxycholic acid + Colestilan

The absorption of ursodeoxycholic acid can be more than halved by colestilan if taken together.

Clinical evidence, mechanism, importance and management

Five healthy subjects were given 200 mg of ursodeoxycholic acid after a test meal and an overnight fast with, and then without, 1.5 g **colestilan** granules. It was found that the ursodeoxycholic acid serum levels at 30 min were reduced by the **colestilan** by more than 50% in 4 out of the 5 subjects, and the mean level was decreased from 9.2 to 3.4 micromol/l. The mechanism of this interaction would appear to be that the **colestilan** (which is an ion exchange resin) binds with the ursodeoxycholic acid in the intestine thereby reducing its absorption. The authors of this report recommend that in order to reduce the effects of this interaction, these two drugs should be given at least 2 h apart so that admixture in the gut is minimised.[1]

1. Takikawa H, Ogasawara T, Sata A, Ohashi M, Hasegawa Y, Hojo M. Effect of colestimide on intestinal absorption of ursodeoxycholic acid in men. *Int J Clin Pharmacol Ther* (2001) 39, 558–60.

Vardenafil + Miscellaneous drugs

No clinically relevant adverse interactions seem to occur between vardenafil and cimetidine, digoxin, *Maalox* or ranitidine.

Clinical evidence, mechanism, importance and management

(a) Antacids

A study in 12 healthy men found that when 20 mg vardenafil was taken with a single 10 ml dose of **Maalox** (**aluminium/magnesium hydroxides**), the pharmacokinetics of the vardenafil were slightly changed (maximum plasma levels reduced to 82%) but the mean bioavailability was unaltered.[1] There would seem to be no reason for avoiding **antacids** of this type when taking vardenafil.

(b) Digoxin

Nineteen healthy men were given 20 mg vardenafil every other day with 375 micrograms of **digoxin** daily for 14 days, and then with a **digoxin** placebo for a further 14 days. It was found that the pharmacokinetics of the **digoxin** at steady-state were unaltered by the vardenafil. The incidence of mild to moderate headache rose slightly from 7 out of 19 with the placebo to 13 out of 19 with **digoxin**.[2] There would therefore appear to be no reason to monitor **digoxin** levels while taking vardenafil concurrently.

(c) H_2-blockers

A randomised, open, three-way crossover study in 12 healthy men found that after taking 150 mg **ranitidine** twice daily for 3 days, the bioavailability of a single 20-mg dose of vardenafil, given on the fourth day, was unchanged. A similar study using 400 mg **cimetidine** twice daily found that the AUC of the vardenafil was slightly increased by 12% due, the authors of the report suggest, to its inhibitory effect on cytochrome P450 enzymes, an effect that **ranitidine** lacks.[3] There would therefore appear to be no reason for avoiding these two H_2-blockers while taking vardenafil, and it seems likely that this will be equally true for other H_2-blockers.

1. Rhode G, Wensing G, Sachse R. The pharmacokinetics of vardenafil, a new selective PDE5 inhibitor, are not affected by the antacid, Maalox 70. *Pharmacotherapy* (2001) 21, 1254.
2. Rhode G, Bauer R-J, Unger S, Ahr G, Wensing G. Vardenafil, a new selective PDE5 inhibitor, produces no interaction with digoxin. *Pharmacotherapy* (2001) 21, 1254.
3. Rhode G, Wensing G, Unger S, Sachse R. The pharmacokinetics of vardenafil, a new selective PDE5 inhibitor, is minimally affected by coadministration with cimetidine or ranitidine. *Pharmacotherapy* (2001) 21, 1254.

Vesnarinone + Miscellaneous drugs

Erythromycin increases the bioavailability of vesnarinone whereas famotidine decreases the rate but not the extent of these interactions is uncertain. The clinical relevance of these interactions is uncertain.

Clinical evidence, mechanism, importance and management

A study in 12 healthy subjects found that 500 mg **erythromycin** three times daily for a week increased the AUC of a single 60-mg dose of vesnarinone by 65% and the maximum serum levels by 11%. Systemic clearance was reduced by 36%. It was concluded from this and other *in vitro* studies that the cytochrome P450 isoenzymes CYP3A4 and CYP2E1 are involved in the metabolism of vesnarinone.[1,2] Whether this interaction with **erythromycin**, (or potentially with other inhibitors of CYP3A4) is likely to be clinically important is not yet known, but it would seem prudent to be alert for any evidence of vesnarinone toxicity if used concurrently.

A single-blind, randomised two-way crossover study was carried out in 12 healthy subjects to study the effects of changes in gastric pH on the absorption of vesnarinone. Using a pH monitor to ensure that the pH had risen from less than 2 to greater than 6, in the presence of the **famotidine** it was found that the maximum serum vesnarinone levels fell by 25% (from 3.33 to 2.5 micrograms/ml), the AUC fell by less than 2%, while the time to maximum serum levels rose from about 6 to 24 h.[3] Thus these changes in gastric pH prolong the rate but not the extent of the absorption of vesnarinone. What this is likely to mean in practical terms awaits clinical assessment. Other drugs which

raise gastric pH (e.g. other H_2-blockers, **proton pump inhibitors**) would be expected to act like famotidine.

1. Wandel C, Lang CC, Cowart DS, Girard AF, Bramer S, Flockhart DA, Wood AJ. Effect of CYP3A inhibition on vesnarinone metabolism in humans. *Clin Pharmacol Ther* (1998) 63, 506-11.
2. Wandel C, Lang CC, Cowart D, Girard A, Bramer S, Wood AJJ. CYP3A inhibition increases plasma levels of vesnarinone in humans. *Clin Pharmacol Ther* (1997) 61, 204.
3. Cowart D, Koneru B, Bramer S, Noorisa M, Kisicki J. Effect of gastric pH on the absorption and oral pharmacokinetics of the inotropic agent vesnarinone. *Clin Pharmacol Ther* (1997) 61, 157.

Vinpocetine + Antacids

Magnesium-aluminium hydroxide gel (1 sachet four times daily) had no significant effects on the serum levels of vinpocetine (20 mg three times daily) in 18 healthy subjects.[1] No special precautions seem necessary if taken together.

1. Lohmann A, Grobara P, Dingler E. Investigation of the possible influence of the absorption of vinpocetine with concomitant application of magnesium-aluminium-hydroxide gel. *Arzneimittelforschung* (1991) 41, 1164–7.

Vitamin B_{12} + Miscellaneous drugs

Although neomycin, aminosalicylic acid and the H_2-blockers can reduce the absorption of vitamin B_{12} from the gut, no interaction is likely because B_{12} is usually given by injection.

Clinical evidence, mechanism, importance and management

Neomycin causes a generalised malabsorption syndrome which has been shown to reduce the absorption of vitamin B_{12}.[1] **Colchicine** has also been shown to decrease B_{12} absorption.[1] **Aminosalicylic acid (PAS)** reduces vitamin B_{12} absorption for reasons which are not understood, but which are possibly related to a mild generalised malabsorption syndrome.[2] The H_2-blockers (such as **cimetidine**[3] and **ranitidine**[4]) can also reduce vitamin B_{12} absorption, primarily because they reduce gastric acid production. The acid is needed to release of B_{12} from dietary protein sources. There is therefore a possibility that on long-term use patients could become vitamin B_{12} deficient.

Within the context of adverse drug interactions, none of these drugs is normally likely to interact adversely because, for anaemia, vitamin B_{12} is usually given parenterally for convenience, and to avoid problems with absorption.

1. Faloon WW, Chodos RB. Vitamin B_{12} absorption studies using colchicine, neomycin and continuous 57Co B_{12} administration. *Gastroenterology* (1969) 56, 1251.
2. Palva IP, Rytkönen U, Alatulkkila M, Palva HLA. Drug-induced malabsorption of vitamin B_{12}. V. Intestinal pH and absorption of vitamin B_{12} during treatment with para-aminosalicylic acid. *Scand J Haematol* (1972) 9, 5–7.
3. Steinberg WM, King CE, Toskes PP. Malabsorption of protein-bound cobalamin but not unbound cobalamin during cimetidine administration. *Dig Dis Sci* (1980) 25, 188–92.
4. Belaiche J, Cattan D, Zittoun J, Marquet J, Yvart J. Effect of ranitidine on cobalamin absorption. *Dig Dis Sci* (1983) 28, 667–8.

Vitamin C (Ascorbic acid) + Salicylates

Aspirin reduces the absorption of ascorbic acid by about a third. Serum salicylate levels do not appear to be affected by ascorbic acid.

Clinical evidence, mechanism, importance and management

Studies in man have shown that 900 mg **aspirin** reduces the absorption of single 500-mg doses of ascorbic acid from the gut by about a third, and it reduces the urinary excretion by about a half.[1] The clinical importance of this is uncertain. It has been suggested that the normal physiological requirement of 30 to 60 mg may need to be increased to 100 to 200 mg daily in the presence of **aspirin**. More study is needed. Studies in man have shown that ascorbic acid does not significantly affect serum salicylate levels given as **choline salicylate**.[2]

1. Basu TK. Vitamin C-aspirin interactions. *Int J Vitam Nutr Res* (1982) 23 (Suppl), 83–90.
2. Hansten PD, Hayton WL. Effect of antacids and ascorbic acid on serum salicylate concentration. *J Clin Pharmacol* (1980) 24, 326–31.

Vitamin D + Phenytoin

The long-term use of phenytoin and other anticonvulsants can disturb vitamin D and calcium metabolism, which may result in osteomalacia. There are a few reports of patients taking vitamin D supplements who responded poorly to vitamin replacement while taking phenytoin. Serum phenytoin levels are not altered.

Clinical evidence

(a) Effect of phenytoin on vitamin D

A 16-year-old with grand mal epilepsy and idiopathic hypoparathyroidism failed to respond adequately to daily doses of 10 micrograms **alfacalcidol** and 6 to 12 g **calcium**, apparently due to the concurrent use of 200 mg **phenytoin** and 500 mg **primidone** daily. Replacement with 0.6 to 2.4 mg **dihydrotachysterol** daily produced a satisfactory response.[1]

Two other reports describe patients whose response to usual doses of vitamin D was poor because of concurrent anticonvulsant treatment with **phenytoin** and **primidone**.[2-4] Other reports clearly show low serum calcium levels[5,6] low serum vitamin D levels[7] osteomalacia[6] and bone structure alterations[5,7] while taking **phenytoin**.

(b) Effect of vitamin D on phenytoin

A controlled trial on 151 epileptic patients on **phenytoin** and calcium showed that the addition of 2000 units of vitamin D_2 daily over a 3-month period had no significant effect on serum **phenytoin** levels.[8]

Mechanism

The enzyme-inducing effects of phenytoin and other anticonvulsants increase the metabolism of the vitamin D, thereby reducing its effects and disturbing the calcium metabolism.[3] In addition the phenytoin may possibly reduce the absorption of the calcium from the gut.[1]

Importance and management

The disturbance of calcium metabolism by phenytoin and other anticonvulsants is very well established, but there are only a few reports describing a poor response to vitamin D. The effects of concurrent treatment should be well monitored. Those who need vitamin D supplements may probably need greater than usual doses.

1. Rubinger D, Korn-Lubetzki I, Feldman S, Popovtzer MM. Delayed response to 1 α-hydroxycholecalciferol therapy in a case of hypoparathyroidism during anticonvulsant therapy. *Isr J Med Sci* (1980) 16, 772–4.
2. Asherov J, Weinberger A, Pinkhas J. Lack of response to vitamin D therapy in a patient with hypoparathyroidism under anticonvulsant drugs. *Helv Paediatr Acta* (1977) 32, 369–73.
3. Chan JCM, Oldham SB, Holick MF, DeLuca HF. 1-α-Hydroxyvitamin D_3 in chronic renal failure. A potent analogue of the kidney hormone, 1,25-dihydroxycholecalciferol. *JAMA* (1975) 234, 47–52.
4. Maclaren N, Lifshitz F. Vitamin D-dependency rickets in institutionalized, mentally retarded children on long term anticonvulsant therapy. II. The response to 25-hydroxycholecalciferol and to vitamin D_2. *Pediatr Res* (1973) 7, 914–22.
5. Mosekilde L, Melsen F. Anticonvulsant osteomalacia determined by quantitative analyses of bone changes. Population study and possible risk factors. *Acta Med Scand* (1976) 199, 349–55.
6. Hunter J, Maxwell JD, Stewart DA, Parson V, Williams R. Altered calcium metabolism in epileptic children on anticonvulsants. *BMJ* (1971) 4, 202–4.
7. Hahn TJ, Avioli LV. Anticonvulsant osteomalacia. *Arch Intern Med* (1975) 135, 997–1000.
8. Christiansen C, Rødbro P. Effect of vitamin D_2 on serum phenytoin. A controlled therapeutical trial. *Acta Neurol Scand* (1974) 50, 661–4.

Vitamin A (Retinol) + Aminoglycoside antibacterials or Corticosteroids

Neomycin can markedly reduce the absorption of vitamin A (retinol) from the gut. It is not clear whether vitamin A improves or worsens wound healing in the presence of corticosteroids.

Clinical evidence, mechanism, importance and management

(a) Corticosteroids

A patient with systemic lupus erythematosus, taking 40 mg **prednisone** and 150 mg azathioprine daily, developed an increasingly large leg ulcer after a bump, which only healed when a topical vitamin A ointment was applied. A non-healing ulcer on a child with a kidney transplant taking 20 mg **prednisone** daily only began to heal when she started to take a vitamin A preparation containing 5000 units daily. When the vitamin A was stopped the healing continued only slowly, but dramatically increased when the vitamin A was restarted. The non-healing wounds of another 6 patients similarly improved when given vitamin A. This evidence suggests that the vitamin A raises the rate of healing to normal.[1] Conflicting results have been found in *animal* studies.[1,2]

If vitamin A is used, systemically or topically, for wounds in the presence corticosteroids, it would be prudent to confirm that wound healing is increased as intended.

(b) Neomycin

Neomycin 2 g markedly reduced the absorption of a test dose of vitamin A in 5 healthy subjects due, it is suggested, to a direct chemical interference between the **neomycin** and bile in the gut, which disrupts the absorption of fats and fat-soluble vitamins.[3] The extent to which chronic treatment with **neomycin** (or other aminoglycosides) would impair the treatment of vitamin A deficiency has not been determined.

1. Hunt TK, Ehrlich HP, Garcia JA, Dunphy JE. Effect of vitamin A on reversing the inhibitory effect of cortisone on healing of open wounds in animals and man. *Ann Surg* (1969) 170, 633–41.
2. Golan J, Mitelman S, Baruchin A, Ben-Hur N. Vitamin A and corticosteroid interaction in wound healing in rats. *Isr J Med Sci* (1980) 16, 572–5.
3. Barrowman JA, D'Mello A, Herxheimer A. A single dose of neomycin impairs absorption of vitamin A (Retinol) in man. *Eur J Clin Pharmacol* (1973) 5, 199–201.

Vitamin K + Gentamicin and Clindamycin

Seven patients in intensive care failed to respond to intravenous vitamin K for hypoprothrombinaemia while receiving gentamicin and clindamycin.

Clinical evidence, mechanism, importance and management

Some patients, particularly those in intensive care who are not eating, can quite rapidly develop acute vitamin K deficiency, which leads to prolonged prothrombin times and possibly bleeding.[1,2] This can normally be controlled by giving vitamin K parenterally. However, one report describes 7 such patients, all with normal liver function, who unexpectedly failed to respond to vitamin K. Examination of their records showed that all were receiving **gentamicin/clindamycin**.[2] Just why these two antibacterials oppose the effects of vitamin K is not understood, but it would seem prudent to avoid the use of these particular antibacterials wherever possible in patients within this category. More study is needed.

1. Ham JM. Hypoprothrombinaemia in patients undergoing prolonged intensive care. *Med J Aust* (1971) 2, 716–18.
2. Rodriguez-Erdmann F, Hoff JV, Carmody G. Interaction of antibiotics with vitamin K. *JAMA* (1981) 246, 937.

X-ray contrast media + Colestyramine

A single report describes poor radiographic visualisation of the gall bladder in a man due to an interaction between iopanoic acid and colestyramine within the gut.

Clinical evidence, mechanism, importance and management

The cholecystogram of a man on **colestyramine** with post-gastrectomy syndrome who was given oral **iopanoic acid** as an X-ray contrast medium, suggested that he had an abnormal and apparently collapsed gall bladder. A week after stopping the **colestyramine** a repeat cholecystogram gave excellent visualisation of a gall bladder of normal appearance.[1] The same effects have been observed experimentally in *dogs*.[1] The reason seems to be that the **colestyramine** binds with the **iopanoic acid** in the gut so that little is absorbed and little is available for secretion in the bile. Hence the poor visualisation of the gall bladder.

On the basis of reports about other drugs which similarly bind to **colestyramine**, it seems probable that this interaction could be avoided if the administration of the **iopanoic acid** and the **colestyramine** were to be separated as much as possible. Whether other oral acidic X-ray contrast media bind in a similar way to **colestyramine** is uncertain, but this possibility should be considered.

1. Nelson JA. Effect of cholestyramine on teleopaque oral cholecystography. *Am J Roentgenol Radium Ther Nucl Med* (1974) 122, 333–4.

X-ray contrast media + Phenothiazines

Two isolated case reports describe epileptiform reactions in two patients when metrizamide was used in the presence of chlorpromazine or dixyrazine.

Clinical evidence, mechanism, importance and management

A patient on long-term treatment with 75 mg **chlorpromazine** daily had a grand mal seizure three-and-a-half hours after being given **metrizamide** (16 ml of 170 mg iodine per ml by the lumbar route. He had another seizure 5 h later.[1] One out of 34 other patients demonstrated epileptogenic activity on an EEG when given **metrizamide** for lumbar myelography. He was taking 10 mg **dixyrazine** three times daily.[2] A clinical study of 26 patients given **levomepromazine (methotrimeprazine)** for the relief of lumbago-sciatic pain found no evidence of an increased risk of epilepsy after receiving **metrizamide**.[3] The general importance of these adverse reactions is not known.

1. Hindmarsh T, Grepe A and Widen L. Metrizamide-phenothiazine interaction. Report of a case with seizures following myelography. *Acta Radiol Diagnosis* (1975) 16, 129–34.
2. Hindmarsh T. Lumbar myelography with meglumine iocarmate and metrizamide. *Acta Radiol Diagnosis* (1975) 16, 209–22.
3. Standnes B, Oftedal S-I, Weber H. Effect of levopromazine on EEG and on clinical side effects after lumbar myelography with metrizamide. *Acta Radiol Diagnosis* (1982) 23, 111–14.

Zafirlukast + Miscellaneous drugs

Zafirlukast plasma levels are decreased by erythromycin and terfenadine whereas they are increased by aspirin, but none of these changes appears to be clinically important. Zafirlukast appears not to affect the reliability of combined oral contraceptives. Zafirlukast inhibits cytochromes CYP2C9 and CYP3A4, which may possibly affect the metabolism of a number of drugs but formal interaction studies are lacking.

Clinical evidence, mechanism, importance and management

(a) Aspirin

The concurrent use of 40 mg zafirlukast daily and 650 mg **aspirin** four times daily is reported to have resulted in a mean increase in plasma zafirlukast levels of 45%. No further details are available.[1,2] The clinical importance of this interaction awaits assessment but the makers do not suggest any alteration in the zafirlukast dosage.[3]

(b) Contraceptives, oral

A single-blind parallel group study in 39 healthy women subjects taking **oral contraceptives** (not named) found that 40 mg zafirlukast twice daily had no effect on the serum levels of **ethinylestradiol** nor on the contraceptive efficacy.[1] No further details are currently available. This study suggests that concurrent use need not be avoided but more study is needed.

(c) Erythromycin

A study in 11 asthmatic patients found that 500 mg **erythromycin** three times daily for 5 days reduced the mean plasma levels of zafirlukast by about 40%, following a single 40 mg dose.[1,2] This reduction in levels would be expected to reduce its antiasthmatic effects. No further details are available. If both drugs are given concurrently, be alert for a reduced response. The makers do not suggest any alteration in the zafirlukast dosage.[3]

(d) Miscellaneous drugs

The makers[2] say that although zafirlukast is known to inhibit the cytochrome P450 isoenzyme CYP2C9, no formal interaction studies have been done with other drugs which are metabolised by this isoenzyme. Zafirlukast is also an inhibitor of the cytochrome P450 isoenzyme CYP3A4 *in vitro*. Whether these predictions lead to clinically significant drug interactions awaits formal evaluation from clinical studies, but if zafirlukast is added to treatment with drugs which are metabolised by these isoenzymes it would be prudent to monitor for an increase in their effects.

(e) Terfenadine

A study in 16 healthy men given 320 mg zafirlukast daily found that the addition of 60 mg **terfenadine** twice daily reduced the mean maximum serum levels of the zafirlukast by 66% and reduced its AUC by 54%. **Terfenadine** serum levels remained unchanged and no ECG alterations occurred.[1] The reduction in zafirlukast serum levels would be expected to reduce its antiasthmatic effects, but this needs assessment in asthmatic patients. If both drugs are given be alert for a reduced response, but there is no need to avoid concurrent use. More study is needed.

1. Accolate (Zafirlukast). Zeneca Pharmaceuticals. Professional information brochure, April 1997.
2. Accolate (Zafirlukast). AstraZeneca. Summary of product characteristics, October 2001.
3. Zeneca Pharmaceuticals, Personal communication, July 1997.

Zinc sulphate + Calcium salts

Calcium salts reduce the absorption of zinc.

Clinical evidence, mechanism, importance and management

Elemental **calcium** (either **calcium carbonate** or **calcium citrate**) in doses of 600 mg was given to 9 healthy women with single oral doses of 20 mg zinc sulphate.[1] The AUC of zinc were reduced by 72% by the **calcium carbonate** and by 80% by the **calcium citrate**. The reason is not understood nor is the clinical importance of this interaction known, but it would seem prudent to separate zinc from the administration of any **calcium salts**. Two to three hours separation is often sufficient to achieve maximal absorption with absorption interactions. More study of this interaction is needed to confirm the extent and to determine if separation of the doses is adequate precaution.

1. Argiratos V, Samman S. The effect of calcium carbonate and calcium citrate on the absorption of zinc in healthy female subjects. *Eur J Clin Nutr* (1994) 48, 198–204.

Zolmitriptan + Miscellaneous drugs

Zolmitriptan does not interact adversely with other commonly used antimigraine preparations (dihydroergotamine,
metoclopramide, paracetamol (acetaminophen), pizotifen,
propranolol) although the makers issue a warning with ergotamine. Zolmitriptan also does not seem to interact with fluoxetine or selegiline, but when used with moclobemide a limited
daily dosage is recommended.

Clinical evidence, mechanism, importance and management

(a) Ergot derivatives

In a randomised, double-blind, placebo-controlled study, 12 healthy
subjects were given 5 mg oral **dihydroergotamine** or a placebo twice
daily for 10 days, and on day 10 they were also given 10 mg oral zolmitriptan (four times the usual dose). No significant changes in blood
pressure or ECGs were seen, nor any significant changes in the zolmitriptan pharmacokinetics. Concurrent use was well tolerated.[1] Another randomised, double-blind, placebo-controlled trial in 12
healthy subjects studied the effects of 20 mg oral zolmitriptan (eight
times the usual dose) when combined with 2 mg oral **ergotamine**
(contained in *Cafergot* tablets, 1 mg **ergotamine** + 100 mg caffeine).
Using a very detailed and thorough range of techniques, no clinically
relevant cardiovascular changes were found, even at 8 times the normal therapeutic dose of zolmitriptan, and concurrent use was generally well tolerated. No important changes in the zolmitriptan
pharmacokinetics were seen.[2]

Despite this evidence of the absence of any clinically relevant adverse interactions, the makers say that at least 6 h should elapse between taking zolmitriptan and an **ergotamine**[3] preparation, but they
also say that there is no evidence that oral **dihydroergotamine** has
any unwanted effects when used with zolmitriptan.[3]

(b) Paracetamol (Acetaminophen), Metoclopramide

In a randomised, crossover study, 15 healthy subjects were given single 10-mg doses of zolmitriptan alone or with 1 g **paracetamol** or
10 mg **metoclopramide** or with both. The **paracetamol** increased
the zolmitriptan maximum plasma levels and its AUC by 11% while
reducing its renal clearance by 9%. **Metoclopramide** had no effect.
The **paracetamol** maximum plasma levels, AUC and half-life were
reduced by 31%, 11% and 8% respectively. These small changes
were considered to be clinically irrelevant[4] and there would appear to
be no reason for avoiding concurrent use of either of these two drugs.

(c) Pizotifen

A double-blind, randomised study was carried out in 12 healthy subjects who were given 1.5 mg **pizotifen** or a placebo daily for 8 days,
and then on day 8 they were also given 10 mg oral zolmitriptan. No
clinically relevant changes in heart rates or ECGs or blood pressures
were seen as a result of concurrent use, and it was concluded that
there was no reason for avoiding the use of both drugs nor any need
to modify the dosages.[5]

(d) Propranolol

In a double-blind, randomised, crossover study, 12 healthy subjects
were given 160 mg **propranolol** or a placebo daily for 7 days, and
then on day 7 a single 10 mg oral dose of zolmitriptan. The **propranolol** increased the maximum serum levels and the AUC of the
zolmitriptan by 56% and 37% respectively, and reduced the extent of
its conversion to the active metabolite (183C91), probably due to inhibition of cytochrome P450. However the conclusion was reached
that no clinically important changes in the therapeutic effects of zolmitriptan are likely, nor are any adjustments in its dosage needed.[6]

(e) Selective MAOIs (Moclobemide, Selegiline)

In a series of 3-period, crossover and randomised studies, 12 healthy
subjects were given 10 mg oral **selegiline** daily or 150 mg oral **moclobemide** twice daily for 7 days, and then on day 7 a single oral
10-mg dose of zolmitriptan.[7] It was found that the maximum serum
levels and the AUC of the zolmitriptan were increased by 23% and
26% respectively by the **moclobemide**. A 2.5-fold increase in the
maximum plasma levels and a threefold increase in the AUC of the
active metabolite also occurred.[7] Despite these increases, because of
the good tolerability profile of zolmitriptan, no dosage reductions are
thought to be needed if given with **moclobemide**, but a maximum
intake of 7.5 mg in 24 h is the maker's recommendation.[3]

Selegiline on the other hand had no effect on the pharmacokinetics
of zolmitriptan nor its metabolites, apart from a small (7%) reduction
in its renal clearance.[7] No special precautions would therefore seem
to be necessary.

1. Veronese L, Gillotin C, Marion-Gallois R, Weatherley BC, Thebault JJ, Guillaume M, Peck RW. Lack of interaction between oral dihydroergotamine and the novel antimi-graine compound zolmitriptan in healthy volunteers. *Clin Drug Invest* (1997) 14, 217–220.
2. Dixon RM, Meire HB, Evans DH, Watt H, On N, Posner J, Rolan PE. Peripheral vascular effects and pharmacokinetics of the antimigraine compound, zolmitriptan, in combination with oral ergotamine in healthy volunteers. *Cephalalgia* (1997) 17, 639–46.
3. Zomig (Zolmitriptan). AstraZeneca. Summary of product characteristics, May 2002.
4. Seaber EJ, Ridout G, Layton G, Posner J, Peck RW. The novel anti-migraine zolmitriptan (Zomig 311C90) has no clinically significant interactions with paracetamol or metoclo-pramide. *Eur J Clin Pharmacol* (1997) 53, 229–34.
5. Seaber EJ, Gillotin C, Mohanlal R, Layton G, Posner J, Peck R. Lack of interaction be-tween pizotifen and the novel antimigraine compound zolmitriptan in healthy volunteers. *Clin Drug Invest* (1997) 14, 221–5.
6. Peck RW, Seaber EJ, Dixon R, Gillotin CG, Weatherley BC, Layton G, Posner J. The in-teraction between propranolol and the novel antimigraine agent zolmitriptan (311C90). *Br J Clin Pharmacol* (1997) 44, 595–9.
7. Rolan P. Potential drug interactions with the novel antimigraine compound zolmitriptan (Zomig™, 311C90). *Cephalalgia* (1997) 17 (Suppl 18), 21–7.

Zolpidem + Rifampicin (Rifampin)

**Rifampicin (rifampin) markedly reduces the plasma levels
and the hypnotic effects of zolpidem.**

Clinical evidence

In a randomised, placebo-controlled, crossover study, 8 healthy subjects were given 600 mg **rifampicin (rifampin)** or a placebo daily for
5 days and then on day 6 they were given a single 20 mg oral dose of
zolpidem. It was found that the **rifampicin (rifampin)** reduced the
zolpidem AUC by 73%, its maximum plasma concentration by about
60% and its half-life from 2.5 to 1.6 h. A significant reduction in the
effects of zolpidem were also seen as measured by a number of psychomotor tests (digital symbol substitution, critical flicker fusion,
subjective drowsiness, etc.).[1,2]

Mechanism

The reason is thought to be that the rifampicin (rifampin) increases
the activity of cytochrome P450 isoenzyme CYP3A4 in the liver so
that the metabolism and clearance of the zolpidem is increased.[1,2]

Importance and management

Direct information appears to be limited to this study but the interaction would seem to be established. What happens is consistent with
the way rifampicin (rifampin) interacts with other drugs. Be alert for
the need to increase the zolpidem dosage (possible doubled) if rifampicin (rifampin) is given concurrently. The authors of this report
also suggest that other drugs such as **carbamazepine** and **phenytoin**,
which similarly induce the activity of CYP3A4, will interact in the
same way. This needs confirmation.

1. Villikka K, Kivistö KT, Luurila H, Neuvonen PJ. Rifampicin reduces plasma concentra-tions and effects of zolpidem. *Eur J Clin Pharmacol* (1997) 52 (Suppl), A142.
2. Villikka K, Kivistö KT, Luurila H, Neuvonen PJ. Rifampicin reduces plasma concentra-tions and effects of zolpidem. *Clin Pharmacol Ther* (1997) 62, 629–34.

Index

All of the pairs of drugs included in the text of this book which are known to interact or not to are listed in this index. They may also be listed under the group names if two or more members of the group interact, **but you should always look up the names of both individual drugs and their groups to ensure that you have access to all the information in this book.** You can possibly get a lead on the way unlisted drugs behave if you look up those which are related or the appropriate drug group, but bear in mind that none of them are identical and any conclusions reached should only be tentative.

Whereas both recommended International Non-proprietary Names (rINNs) and United States Adopted Names (USANs) have been used in the text, entries in the index are to be found under the rINN with cross-references provided for USANs, British Approved Names (BANs), and some other widely used synonyms. Brand names have been avoided but tables of international proprietary names/generic names are included in the introductory sections of most chapters. You can find these tables by looking up the group names of the drugs in question (e.g. Anticoagulants, Anticonvulsants, etc.).

Enoximone
+ Aminophylline, 886
+ Digitoxin, 542
+ Digoxin, 542
Enprofylline
+ Adenosine, 93
+ Diazepam, 711
Enprostil
+ Contraceptives, oral, 474
+ Diazepam, 709
+ Digoxin, 551
+ Oral contraceptives, 474
Entacapone
+ Imipramine, 886
+ L-DOPA (Levodopa), 420
+ Levodopa (L-DOPA), 420
Enteral feeds (Nasogastric feeds)
+ Aluminium hydroxide, 886
+ Aminophylline, 797
+ Antacids, 886
+ Anticoagulants, 300
+ Ciprofloxacin, 210
+ Diphenylhydantoin (Phenytoin), 346
+ Hydralazine, 383
+ Magnesium hydroxide, 886
+ Ofloxacin, 210
+ Phenytoin (Diphenylhydantoin), 346
+ Quinolone antibacterials, 210
+ Ritonavir, 198
+ Sucralfate, 886
+ Theophylline, 797
+ Warfarin, 300
Enteric coated preparations (Delayed-release preparations; Modified-release preparations)
+ Antacids, 887
+ Proton pump inhibitors, 887
Enzyme induction interactions, 5
Enzyme inhibition interactions, 7
Enzyme-inducing drugs, 6
see also Hepatic drug metabolising enzyme inducers
Enzyme-inhibiting drugs, 8
see also Hepatic drug metabolising enzyme inhibitors
Ephedrine
+ Acetazolamide, 776
+ Amitriptyline, 848, 853
+ Ammonium chloride, 776
+ Clonidine, 779
+ Debrisoquin (Debrisoquine), 394
+ Debrisoquine (Debrisoquin), 394
+ Dexamethasone, 635
+ Guanethidine, 394
+ MAOIs (Monoamine oxidase inhibitors), 680
+ Maprotiline, 687
+ Methyldopa, 403
+ Moclobemide, 680
+ Monoamine oxidase inhibitors (MAOIs), 680
+ Reserpine, 779
+ Selegiline, 687
+ Sibutramine, 922
+ Sodium bicarbonate, 776
+ Theophylline, 796
+ Tolcapone, 428
+ Urinary acidifiers, 776
+ Urinary alkalinizers, 776
Epinastine
+ Alcohol (Ethanol), 17
+ Ethanol (Alcohol), 17
Epinephrine (Adrenaline)
+ Adrenergic neurone blockers, 394
+ Anaesthetics, inhalational, 746
+ Amitriptyline, 852, 853
+ Anaesthetic ether, 746
+ Beta-blockers, 448
+ Chloroform, 746
+ Cyclopropane, 746

+ Enflurane, 746
+ Ether, anaesthetic, 746
+ Guanethidine, 394
+ Halothane, 746
+ Imipramine, 852
+ Inhalational anaesthetics, 746
+ Isoflurane, 746
+ MAOIs (Monoamine oxidase inhibitors), 680
+ Methoxyflurane, 746
+ Metoprolol, 448
+ Monoamine oxidase inhibitors (MAOIs), 680
+ Nortriptyline, 852
+ Phenelzine, 680
+ Pindolol, 448
+ Propranolol, 448
+ Protriptyline, 852
+ Reserpine, 779
+ Sevoflurane, 746
+ TCAs (Tricyclic antidepressants), 852
+ Timolol, 448
+ Tolcapone, 428
+ Tranylcypromine, 680
+ Tricyclic antidepressants (TCAs), 852
Epirubicin
+ Azidothymidine (Zidovudine), 185
+ AZT (Zidovudine), 185
+ Ciclosporin (Cyclosporine), 501
+ Cimetidine, 501
+ Cyclosporine (Ciclosporin), 501
+ Docetaxel, 501
+ Ondansetron, 499
+ Paclitaxel, 520
+ Verapamil, 501
+ Zidovudine (Azidothymidine; AZT), 185
Epoetins (Erythropoietins)
+ ACE inhibitors, 887
+ Captopril, 887
+ Enalapril, 887
+ Fosinopril, 887
+ Losartan, 887
Epoprostenol
+ Digoxin, 551
+ Frusemide (Furosemide), 391
+ Furosemide (Frusemide), 391
Eprosartan
+ Amiloride, 390
+ Calcium channel blockers, 390
+ Digoxin, 530
+ Diuretics, 390
+ Diuretics, potassium-sparing, 390
+ Diuretics, thiazide, 390
+ Fenofibrate (Procetofene), 390
+ Fluconazole, 390
+ Foods, 390
+ Gemfibrozil, 390
+ Glibenclamide (Glyburide), 568
+ Glyburide (Glibenclamide), 568
+ Hydrochlorothiazide, 390
+ Hypolipidaemics (Lipid regulating drugs), 390
+ Ketoconazole, 390
+ Lipid regulating drugs (Hypolipidaemics), 390
+ Lithium carbonate, 652
+ Lovastatin, 390
+ Niacin (Nicotinic acid), 390
+ Nicotinic acid (Niacin), 390
+ Nifedipine, 390
+ Potassium compounds, 390
+ Potassium-sparing diuretics, 390
+ Pravastatin, 390
+ Procetofene (Fenofibrate), 390
+ Ranitidine, 390
+ Simvastatin, 390
+ Spironolactone, 390
+ Thiazides, 390

+ Triamterene, 390
+ Warfarin, 239
Equisetum
+ Lithium carbonate, 658
Ergocalciferol (Calciferol)
+ Bendrofluazide (Bendroflumethiazide), 871
+ Bendroflumethiazide (Bendrofluazide), 871
+ Methyclothiazide, 871
Ergoloid mesylates, *see* Co-dergocrine
Ergometrine
+ Dopamine, 775
Ergot alkaloids, *see* Ergot derivatives
Ergot derivatives (Ergot alkaloids), *see also* individual drugs
+ Almotriptan, 861
+ Azithromycin, 139
+ Beta-blockers, 439
+ Cabergoline, 870
+ Clarithromycin, 888
+ Erythromycin, 888
+ Glyceryl trinitrate (GTN; Nitroglycerin), 888
+ GTN (Glyceryl trinitrate), 888
+ HIV-protease inhibitors, 889
+ Indinavir, 889
+ Macrolides, 888
+ Midecamycin, 888
+ Naratriptan, 911
+ Nitroglycerin (Glyceryl trinitrate), 888
+ Oxymetazoline, 888
+ Reboxetine, 834
+ Ritonavir, 889
+ Rizatriptan, 921
+ Smoking, 888
+ Spiramycin, 888
+ Sumatriptan, 932
+ Tetracyclines, 890
+ Tobacco smoking, 888
+ Triacetyloleandomycin (Troleandomycin), 888
+ Troleandomycin (Triacetyloleandomycin), 888
Ergotamine
+ Almotriptan, 861
+ Beta-blockers, 439
+ Clarithromycin, 888
+ Doxycycline, 890
+ Eletriptan, 886
+ Erythromycin, 888
+ HIV-protease inhibitors, 889
+ Indinavir, 889
+ Josamycin, 888
+ Methysergide, 889
+ Naratriptan, 911
+ Oxprenolol, 439
+ Propranolol, 439
+ Ritonavir, 889
+ Sumatriptan, 932
+ Tetracycline, 890
+ Triacetyloleandomycin (Troleandomycin), 888
+ Troleandomycin (Triacetyloleandomycin), 888
+ Zolmitriptan, 950
Erythromycin
+ Acenocoumarol (Nicoumalone), 259
+ Acetazolamide, 154
+ Alcohol (Ethanol), 137, 153
+ Alfentanil, 44
+ Alprazolam, 705
+ Aluminium hydroxide, 153
+ Aminophylline, 796
+ Amprenavir, 198
+ Antacids, 153
+ Anticholinesterases, 864
+ Anticoagulants, 259
+ Anticonvulsants (Antiepileptics), 313
+ Antiepileptics (Anticonvulsants), 313